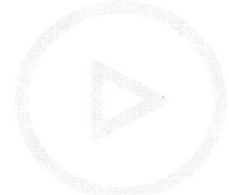

IMPORTANT:

HERE IS YOUR REGISTRATION CODE TO ACCESS
YOUR PREMIUM STUDENT ONLINE RESOURCE CENTER.

For key premium online resources you need THIS CODE to gain access. Once the code is entered, you will be able to use the Web resources for the length of your course.

Access is provided if you have purchased a new book. If the registration code is missing from this book, the registration screen on our Website will tell you how to obtain your new code.

Registering for the STUDENT ONLINE RESOURCE CENTER

TO gain access to the STUDENT ONLINE RESOURCE CENTER, simply follow the steps below:

1. USE YOUR WEB BROWSER TO GO TO: http://www.DuttonOnline.net

2. CLICK ON **FIRST TIME USER**.

3. ENTER THE REGISTRATION CODE* PRINTED ON THE RIGHT.

4. AFTER YOU HAVE ENTERED YOUR REGISTRATION CODE, CLICK **REGISTER**.

5. FOLLOW THE INSTRUCTIONS TO SET-UP YOUR PERSONAL UserID AND PASSWORD.

6. WRITE YOUR UserID AND PASSWORD DOWN FOR FUTURE REFERENCE.
KEEP IT IN A SAFE PLACE.

INSTRUCTORS! please visit: http://www.duttononline.net
click on first time user and follow the onscreen directions.

Thank you, and welcome to the STUDENT ONLINE RESOURCE CENTER!

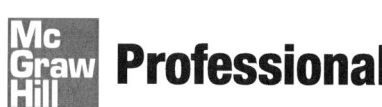 **Professional**

P/N 0-07-144521-8 PART OF 0-07-141089-9
DUTTON: ORTHOPAEDIC EXAMINATION, EVALUATION,
AND INTERVENTION

MCGRAW-HILL
STUDENT ONLINE
RESOURCE CENTER

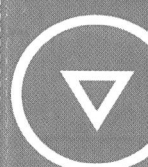

REGISTRATION CODE

Q6G3-QURM-KDV3-KBTX-3GFR

Professional

Mc Graw Hill

Orthopaedic Examination, Evaluation, and Intervention

Orthopaedic Examination, Evaluation, and Intervention

Mark Dutton, PT

Allegheny General Hospital
West Penn Allegheny Health System (WPAHS)
Pittsburgh, Pennsylvania

McGRAW-HILL
Medical Publishing Division

New York   Chicago   San Francisco   Lisbon   London   Madrid   Mexico City
Milan   New Delhi   San Juan   Seoul   Singapore   Sydney   Toronto

Orthopaedic Examination, Evaluation, & Intervention

Copyright © 2004 by The **McGraw-Hill** Companies, Inc. All rights reserved. Printed in the United States of America. Except as permitted under the United States Copyright Act of 1976, no part of this publication may be reproduced or distributed in any form or by any means, or stored in a data base or retrieval system, without the prior written permission of the publisher.

567890 DOW DOW 09876

Set ISBN: 0-07-141089-9
Book ISBN: 0-07-144520-X
Online Learning Center Resource Card ISBN: 0-07-144521-8

This book was set in Times Roman by The GTS Companies/York, PA Campus.
The editors were Michael Brown and Karen Davis.
The art coordinator was Maria Magtoto.
The production supervisor was Catherine H. Saggese.
The text designer was Marsha Cohen.
The cover designer was Mary McKeon.
The index was prepared by Deborah Tourtlotte.
RR Donnelley was printer and binder.

This book is printed on acid-free paper.

Library of Congress Cataloging-in-Publication Data

Dutton, Mark.
    Orthopaedic examination, evaluation, & intervention/Mark Dutton.
      p. cm.
    Includes bibliographical references and index.
    ISBN 0-07-141089-9 (alk. paper)
    1. Orthopaedics—Diagnosis. 2. Physical diagnosis. I. Title: Orthopaedic examination, evaluation, and intervention. II. Title.

RD734.D88 2004
616.7'075—dc21
                                                                    2003051020

Please tell the author and publisher what you think of this book by sending your comments to pt@mcgraw-hill.com. Please put the author and title of the book in the subject line.

To the Three Most Important People in My Life
My Wife Beth
My Two Daughters Leah and Lauren

I have hands,
Watch me clap.
I have feet,
Watch me stamp.
I have arms,
Watch me swing.
I have legs,
They can bend and stretch.
I have a spine,
It can twist and bend.
Oh, what a miracle I am!

Oh, what a miracle,
Oh, what a miracle,
Every little part of me.
I'm something special,
So very special, there's nobody quite like me.

Adapted from "What a Miracle" by Hap Palmer.

CONTENTS

PREFACE

The aim of this book is to fill a void in the present literature and to be of value to the student and experienced clinician alike. As a student and, later, as a practicing clinician, I found myself spending countless hours searching for the information I required and in determining what was evidence based. This search inevitably entailed poring through a multitude of texts, some of which had good illustrations, others of which provided me with materials on examination principles, and still others of which gave me insight into the many intervention approaches and techniques. However, no one book contained everything I needed, and so I began to compile my own notes and illustrations with the aim of having all of this necessary information at my fingertips, in a reader-friendly format. Over the years, this collection of notes and illustrations has grown in scope, culminating in this text. As indicated by the title, this text provides in a single volume what students and practitioners need to know about the examination, evaluation, and intervention of the orthopaedic patient.

An accurate diagnosis forms the cornerstone of any intervention. Obtaining an accurate diagnosis requires a systematic and logical approach. Such an approach should be eclectic, because no single approach works all of the time. Thus, this book attempts to incorporate the biomechanical concepts of the Norwegians and Australians; the mechanical diagnostic and classification approach of McKenzie; the selective tissue tension principles of Cyriax; the neurodynamic mobility tests of Butler; the muscle strength-length assessments of Janda, Jull, and Sahrmann; and the osteopathic approach of Mitchell.

For any intervention to be successful, accurate diagnosis must be followed by a carefully planned and specific rehabilitation program to both the affected area and its related structures. This approach must take into consideration the structure involved and the stage of healing. In this book, great emphasis is placed on the appropriate use of manual techniques and therapeutic exercise based on these considerations. Described in the intervention sections are the manual techniques of Evjenth, Maitland, Stoddard, Mitchell, and Cyriax; the stability therapy exercises of Richardson and Jull; the muscle balancing concepts of Janda and Sahrmann; and the exercise protocols of McKenzie, to name but a few. The appropriate applications of electrotherapeutic and thermal modalities are outlined throughout as adjuncts to the rehabilitative process.

It is hoped that this book will be seen as the best available textbook, guide, review, and reference for health care students and practitioners involved in the care of the orthopaedic population.

Mark Dutton

Additional materials to help students, instructors, and practitioners can be found in the Online Learning Center at www.duttononline.net. We have included video clips of techniques and patient exercises, self-testing items, resources for instructors, and other features. Comments about this book may be sent to me at pt@mcgraw-hill.com.

ACKNOWLEDGMENTS

From inception to completion, this book has taken almost a decade. Such an endeavor cannot be completed without the help of many. I would like to take this opportunity to thank the following:

▶ My parents for their continued guidance and support.

▶ The faculty of the North American Institute of Manual and Manipulative Therapy (NAIOMT)—especially, Jim Meadows, Erl Pettman, Cliff Fowler, Diane Lee, and the late Dave Lamb.

▶ The exceptional team at McGraw-Hill, for their faith and superb guidance throughout this project. Thank you especially to Julia Scardiglia who believed in this project from the start, and to other members of the initial lineup, including Janene Matragano-Oransky. Special thanks also to the crew who brought the book to its fruition: Michael Brown, Karen Davis, Jack Farrell, and Catherine Saggese.

▶ Marianne Tomnay for her help in the preparation of this manuscript.

▶ Donna Frassetto for her perceptive suggestions.

▶ Bob Davis for his creative eye and the excellent photography.

▶ Phil and Sherri Vislosky for agreeing to be the photographic models.

▶ Patrick Manning, Edward Snell, MD, and Kevin Messner for providing some of the radiographic images.

▶ The staff of Human Motion Rehabilitation, Allegheny General Hospital including Duke Rupert, Scott Rosen, Mark Orsi, Brian Lee, Ray Gronlund, Dave and Krissy Hahn, Dean Hnaras, John Karp, Brian Jones, Marie Lombardi, Melissa Saylor, Amanda Martz, Leslie Schramm, Jen Downer, Randi Marshak, Bruce Jacobs, Jan Pagonis, Craig Castor, Eric Cardwell, Vic and Missy Bauer, Pat Stauffer, Diane Ferianc, Keith Galloway, Carol Weis, Dan McCool, and Judy Hice.

▶ Tadeusz Laska, for his friendship and advice.

▶ To the countless clinicians throughout the world who continually strive to improve their knowledge and clinical skills.

▶ To the following people for their very helpful comments during the writing of this book: Tim M. Elser, MHS, PT, OCS, ATC, MTC, University of Cincinnati; Robert A. "Tony" English, PT, M.S.Ed, University of Kentucky; David Krause, PT, MBA, OCS, Mayo School of Health Sciences; Everett B. Lohman III, DPTSc, PT, OCS, Loma Linda University; Michelle Raya, PhD, PT, ATC, SCS, University of Miami; and Lisa Schwarz, MHPE, PT, ATC, Midwestern University.

INTRODUCTION

"The very first step towards success in any occupation is to become interested in it." Sir William Osler (1849–1919)

Until the beginning of the last century, knowledge about the mechanism of healing, and the methods to decrease pain and suffering, were extremely limited. Although we may scoff at many of the interventions used in the distant past, many of the interventions we use today, albeit less drastic, have yet to demonstrate much more in the way of effectiveness. That may soon change with the recent emphasis within many health care professions on evidence-based clinical practice. The demand for health care appears to have increased significantly within the past 50 years. This is thought to be the result, in part, of a change in peoples' attitudes toward suffering, which has resulted in more patients seeking help for illnesses and injuries that our forebears would have just disregarded.[1] The increased demand for health care has produced an associated increase in the demand for rehabilitation services. In response to these changes, and to alter the nature and scope of physical therapy, the American Physical Therapy Association (APTA) published the "Guide to Physical Therapist Practice."[2]

The Guide to Physical Therapist Practice

The "Guide to Physical Therapist Practice"[2] has been instrumental in moving the practice of physical therapy from the traditional biomedical model approach toward a more impairment-based, or *biopsychosocial* model.[3–7]

Biomedical Model

The biomedical model describes a patient problem in terms of a breakdown in one of the body systems. This model is based on the belief that the body is governed by certain natural laws that can be predicted and that assume a vaguely linear pattern.[8] The purpose of the examination within this model is to identify a pathologic or mechanical change that has occurred. This is achieved through the application of the differential diagnosis of disease and tissue pathology. The problem with this model is that bodies do not react along similar physiologic lines, nor is the psychosocial impact on the patient's life taken into consideration. Thus, a shift of focus was needed for the physical therapy profession so that guidelines could be outlined to identify functional impairments.[3–7]

Biopsychosocial Model

Under the biopsychosocial model, the patient presents with a problem that can encompass his or her body, psyche, or social environment. The role of the clinician is to empower the patient to deal with the problem in an individual way.[8] This model necessitates a collaborative effort between patient and clinician in the establishment of goals.

Within this model, the physical therapy diagnosis differs from the medical diagnosis because the former attempts to determine the cause, nature, and extent of the problem on the "whole" person, whereas the medical diagnosis merely identifies the pathologic entity.[9]

The "Guide to Physical Therapist Practice" is divided into two parts. Part 1 outlines patient-client management, and details the tests and measures that are used in patient management. Part 2 outlines patterns of practice for selected diagnostic categories.[2]

The preferred practice patterns (Table I-1), or categories of diagnosis, outlined in Part 2, are based on the similarities in impairments and functional limitations with which each of these categories presents. These practice patterns describe the boundaries within which physical therapists may select a number of clinical paths, and allow patients with different pathologies, but similar impairments, to be classified in the same group.

According to the "Guide," any recipient of a physical therapy examination, evaluation, diagnosis, prognosis, and intervention who has a disease, disorder, condition, impairment, functional limitation, or disability is referred to as a *patient*.[1] *Clients*, according to the "Guide" are defined as individuals who engage the services of a physical therapist and who can benefit from a physical therapist's consultation, interventions, professional advice, prevention services, or services promoting health, wellness, and fitness.[1]

The management of the patient/client is a complex process. The "Guide" lists five elements that form this process—examination, evaluation, diagnosis, prognosis, and intervention:[10]

▶ *Examination.* The examination is required prior to the initial intervention and is the cornerstone in the process leading to diagnostic classification or, as appropriate, to a referral to another practitioner. The examination includes the patient history, systems review, and tests and measures (see Chapter 8).

▶ *Evaluation.* The evaluation involves the making of clinical judgments based on the information gleaned from the

TABLE I-1   Preferred Practice Patterns[2]

Musculoskeletal Practice Pattern	Impairments
Pattern 4A	Primary prevention/risk factor reduction for skeletal demineralization
Pattern 4B	**Impaired *posture*** This pattern is often the result of a combination of other practice patterns including practice patterns C, E, F, and G, and includes impairments of motor function, muscle performance, joint mobility, localized inflammation, and range of motion. **Pathologies** associated with this pattern include vertebral pathology, neural compression syndromes, entrapment syndromes, myofascial syndromes, impingement syndromes, and referred pain. **Clinical findings** can include pain with sustained positions, limited range of motion in a noncapsular pattern of restriction, altered kinematics, positive impingement tests, neurologic findings (thoracic outlet, limb tension tests), trigger points, and palpable tenderness of specific muscles.
Pattern 4C	**Impaired *muscle performance*** This pattern is associated with a combination of other practice patterns including practice patterns D through J, and thus includes impairments of motor function, muscle performance, joint mobility, localized inflammation, and range of motion. **Pathologies** and **clinical findings** associated with this pattern include those that the pattern is associated with (practice patterns D through J).
Pattern 4D	**Impaired joint mobility, motor function, muscle performance, and range of motion associated with *connective tissue dysfunction*** Pattern D refers to an increased laxity or instability of the joint or hypomobility due to capsular restriction. **Primary impairments** in pattern D include decreased motor control and muscle performance. **Characteristic** of this pattern is the complaint of the joint "slipping" or "popping out" during activities of extreme motion. **Pathologies** associated with this pattern include osteoarthritis, rheumatoid arthropathy, adhesive capsulitis, tendinitis, capsulitis, bursitis, synovitis, and ligament pathology. **Clinical findings** associated with this pattern can include pain, altered kinematics, crepitus, and positive apprehension.
Pattern 4E	**Impaired joint mobility, motor function, muscle performance, and range of motion associated with *localized inflammation*** In addition to those conditions producing impaired range of motion, motor function, and muscle performance attributed to inflammation, practice pattern E includes conditions that cause pain and muscle guarding without the presence of structural changes. **Pathologies** include sprains and strains of the joints; internal derangements of the joint, including muscle tears; and periarticular syndromes—tendonitis, bursitis, capsulitis, and tenosynovitis. **Clinical findings** include pain with active and resisted motions, tenderness to palpation, localized edema, redness, and increased skin temperature.
Pattern 4F	**Impaired joint mobility, motor function, muscle performance, and range of motion, or reflex integrity secondary to *spinal disorders*** This pattern involves impaired motor function, muscle performance, range of motion, and joint mobility. **Pathologies** associated with this pattern include adverse neural tension and nerve root irritation. **Clinical findings** associated with this pattern can include positive limb tension tests, signs and symptoms of nerve injury, and nerve root compression

TABLE I-1 *(continued)*

Pattern 4G	**Impaired joint mobility, motor function, muscle performance, and range of motion associated with fracture.** The treatment of most fractures is beyond the scope of practice for a physical therapist.
Patterns 4H and 4I	**Impaired joint mobility, motor function, muscle performance, and range of motion associated with *joint arthroplasty, or with bony or soft tissue surgical procedures*** **Pattern H** is associated with impaired joint mobility, muscle performance, and range of motion due to joint arthroplasty. **Pattern I** involves impaired joint mobility, motor function, muscle performance, and range of motion associated with bony or soft tissue surgical procedures. **Clinical findings** and treatment following a surgical procedure will vary according to each individual and the procedure performed.
Pattern 4J	**Impaired gait, locomotion, and balance and impaired motor function, secondary to *lower extremity amputation***
Pattern 5F	**Impaired peripheral nerve integrity and muscle performance associated with *peripheral nerve injury*** This pattern involves decreased muscle strength, impaired proprioception, impaired sensory integrity, and difficulty with manipulation skills. **Pathologies** include carpal tunnel syndrome, cubital tunnel syndrome, radial tunnel syndrome, tarsal tunnel syndrome, and paroxysmal positional vertigo. **Clinical findings** can include diminished deep tendon reflexes, positive limb tension tests, and signs and symptoms of peripheral nerve compression.

examination (see Chapter 8). The clinician uses this information to establish the diagnosis, prognosis, and plan of care through the identification of factors including, but not limited to, the patient's impairments, functional limitations, disabilities, social considerations, or changes in physical health.

▶ *Diagnosis.* The diagnostic process involves assigning a diagnostic label through the classification of the patient within a specific practice pattern. This is achieved by organizing and interpreting the data from the examination. The diagnosis determines the prognosis, plan of care, and intervention strategies.

▶ *Prognosis (including the plan of care).* The prognosis is a clinical judgment made by the physical therapist based on the findings from the examination, which determines the optimal level of improvement that might be attained, and the amount of time required to reach that level.[10] The plan of care consists of statements that specify the anticipated short- and long-term goals and the expected outcomes, specific interventions to be used, and the proposed frequency and duration of the required interventions in order to attain the anticipated goals and expected outcomes.[10] Ideally, the goals should be established through a mutual agreement between patient and clinician.

▶ *Intervention.* The intervention is the purposeful and skilled interaction between the clinician and the patient to produce changes in the condition that are consistent with the diagnosis and prognosis (see Chapter 10).

It is important to remember that the "Guide" continues to be a work in progress, and there are aspects of practice that have yet to be covered within the document. Although the efforts of the APTA should be applauded for changing the emphasis from the biomedical model toward the biopsychosocial model, there appears to be room within the profession to embrace a combination of both models. This is particularly true with the advent of direct access, which has increased the importance of differential diagnosis and the detection of pathologies that require referral to a more appropriate professional.

REFERENCES

1. McKenzie R, May S. Introduction. In: McKenzie R, May S, eds. *The Human Extremities: Mechanical Diagnosis and Therapy.* Waikanae, New Zealand: Spinal Publications New Zealand Ltd; 2001:1–5.
2. Guide to physical therapist practice. *Phys Ther* 2001;81: S13–S95.
3. Dekker J, van Baar ME, Curfs EC, Kerssens JJ. Diagnosis and treatment in physical therapy: An investigation of their relationship. *Phys Ther* 1993;73:568.
4. Guccione AA. Physical therapy diagnosis and the relationship between impairment and function. *Phys Ther* 1991;71:499.

5. Sahrmann SA. Diagnosis by the physical therapist—A prerequisite for treatment: A special communication. *Phys Ther* 1988;68:1703.
6. Rose SJ. Physical therapy diagnosis: Role and function. *Phys Ther* 1989;69:535.
7. Jette AM. Diagnosis and classification by physical therapists: A special communication. *Phys Ther* 1989;69:967.
8. Coutts F. Changes in the musculoskeletal system. In: Atkinson K, Coutts F, Hassenkamp A, eds. *Physiotherapy in Orthopedics.* London: Churchill Livingstone; 1999:19–43.
9. Cocchiarella L, Andersson GBJ, eds. *Guides to the Evaluation of Permanent Impairment.* 5 ed. Chicago, Ill: American Medical Association; 2001.
10. Guide to physical therapist practice. *Phys Ther* 2001;81:S13–S95.

FUNDAMENTALS OF ORTHOPAEDICS

THE MUSCULOSKELETAL SYSTEM

CHAPTER OBJECTIVES

▶ *At the completion of this chapter, the reader will be able to:*

1. Describe the various types of biological tissue of the musculoskeletal system.

2. Describe the types of connective tissue.

3. Outline the function of collagen and elastin.

4. Describe the structural differences and similarities between fascia, tendons, and ligaments.

5. Describe the structure and function of bone.

6. Outline the different types of cartilage tissue.

7. Describe the constituents of a synovial joint.

8. Describe the cellular components of skeletal muscle.

9. Outline the sequence of events involved in a muscle contraction.

10. List the various muscle fiber types and their roles in muscle function.

OVERVIEW

A working knowledge of the musculoskeletal system forms the foundation of every orthopaedic examination, evaluation, and intervention. A basic tenet in the study of anatomy and biomechanics is that morphology relates to function, in that the function of a structure can often be determined by its design. Based on morphology and function, the tissues of the body are classified into four basic kinds: epithelial, nervous, connective, and muscle tissue.[1]

▶ *Epithelial tissue.* Epithelial tissue is found throughout the body in two forms: membranous and glandular. Membranous epithelium forms such structures as the outer layer of the skin, the inner lining of the body cavities and lumina, and the covering of visceral organs. Glandular epithelium is a specialized tissue that forms the secretory portion of glands.

▶ *Nervous tissue.* Nervous tissue, which is described in Chapter 2, helps coordinate movements via a complex motor control system of prestructured motor programs and a distributed network of reflex pathways mediated throughout the central nervous system.[2]

▶ *Connective tissue.* Connective tissue is divided into subtypes according to the matrix that binds the cells. Connective tissue provides structural and metabolic support for other tissues and organs of the body. Connective tissue includes bone, cartilage, tendons, ligaments, and blood tissue. The properties of connective tissue are described in this chapter.

▶ *Muscle tissue.* Muscle tissue is responsible for the movement of materials through the body, the movement of one part of the body with respect to another, and locomotion. There are three types of muscle tissue: smooth, cardiac, and skeletal tissue. Human skeletal and respiratory muscle tissue is described in this chapter.

Together, connective tissue and skeletal muscle tissue form the musculoskeletal system. The musculoskeletal system functions intimately with nervous tissue to produce coordinated movement and to provide adequate joint stabilization and feedback during sustained positions and purposeful movements.

Connective Tissue

Connective tissue is found throughout the body. The primary types of connective tissue cells are macrophages, which function as phagocytes to clean up debris; mast cells, which release chemicals associated with inflammation (see Chap. 5); and fibroblasts, which are the principal cells of connective tissue.[3] The connective tissue types are differentiated according to the extracellular matrix that binds the cells, as follows[1]:

1. Embryonic connective tissue
2. Connective tissue proper
   a. Loose connective tissue
   b. Dense, regular connective tissue
   c. Dense, irregular connective tissue
   d. Elastic connective tissue
   e. Reticular connective tissue
   f. Adipose connective tissue
3. Cartilage and bone tissue
   a. Hyaline cartilage
   b. Fibrocartilage
   c. Elastic cartilage
4. Blood (vascular) tissue

Connective Tissue Proper

Connective tissue proper has a loose flexible matrix, called *ground substance*. The most common cell within connective tissue proper is the fibroblast. Fibroblasts produce collagen, elastin, and reticulin fibers. Collagen and elastin are vital constituents of the musculoskeletal system.

Collagen

The collagens are a family of extracellular matrix proteins that play a dominant role in maintaining the structural integrity of various tissues and in providing tensile strength to tissues. The formation of collagen involves four steps:

1. The intracellular formation of a protocollagen chain

2. Conversion of protocollagen to procollagen (α) chains that undergo winding into a superhelix moiety

3. Secretion of procollagen from the fibroblast into the matrix followed by assembly into collagen fibrils

4. Organization of collagen fibrils into collagen fibers, which have a classic one-quarter stagger arrangement. This three-dimensional network is stabilized by both covalent and intermolecular cross-links. The collagen fibrillar network acts both as a structural framework to provide mechanical support to the tissue and as a binding surface for molecules involved in mediating either matrix-matrix or cell-matrix interactions

TABLE 1-1 Major Types of Collagen

Type	Location
I	Bone, skin, ligament, and tendon
II	Cartilage, nucleus pulposus
III	Blood vessels, gastrointestinal tract
IV	Basement membranes

Of the more than 20 types of collagen thus far identified, types I to III, V, VI, IX, XI, XII, and XIV are found mainly in connective tissue proper.[4] The major forms of collagen are outlined in Table 1-1.[5]

Elastin

Elastic fibers are composed of a protein called *elastin*. As its name suggests, elastin provides the tissues in which it is situated with elastic properties. Elastin fibers can stretch, but they normally return to their original shape when the tension is released. The elastic fibers of elastin determine the patterns of distention and recoil in most organs, including the skin and lungs, blood vessels, and connective tissue.

Elastin is synthesized as a discrete monomeric unit and secreted from several cell types, including chondroblasts, myofibroblasts, and mesothelial and smooth muscle cells.[6] Messenger RNA translation occurs on the surface of the rough endoplasmic reticulum, and with the release of a signal peptide, the protein travels through the lumen of the rough endoplasmic reticulum, where it is secreted via secretory vesicles to the plasma membrane as tropoelastin.[7] A specific elastin-binding protein apparently chaperones tropoelastin intracellularly, protecting it from proteolysis.[8] As tropoelastin is secreted from the cell, it interacts with specific glycoprotein microfibrils, which are necessary for tropoelastin alignment and the subsequent formation of elastic fibers.[9]

Elastin is synthesized to its polymeric state following the action of lysyl oxidase on epsilon amino groups of lysyl or hydroxylysyl residues.[10] Complementary DNA analysis has shown that tropoelastin is composed of a modular structure containing alternating hydrophobic domains rich in glycine, proline, valine, and highly conserved cross-linking domains rich in alanine and lysine.[11] Typically, three allysines and a small element of amino form a lysine, which spontaneously condenses to form desmosine or isodesmosine.[12] These three-dimensional cross-linking networks form helical chains that account for the remarkable elastic properties of these fibers.

Arrangement of Collagen and Elastin

Collagenous and elastic fibers are sparse and irregularly arranged in loose connective tissue but are tightly packed in dense connective tissue.[13] Fascia is an example of loose connective tissue. Tendons and ligaments are examples of dense, regular connective tissue.[14]

Fascia. Fascia is viewed as the connective tissue that provides support and protection to the joint, and acts as an interconnection between tendons, aponeuroses, ligaments, capsules, nerves, and the intrinsic components of muscle.[15,16] This type of connective tissue may be categorized as fibrous or nonfibrous, with the fibrous components consisting mainly of collagen and elastin fibers, and the nonfibrous portion consisting of amorphous ground substance, which is a viscous gel composed of long chains of carbohydrate molecules (GAG) bound to a protein and water.[17]

Tendons and Ligaments. Histologically, tendons and ligaments are similar in composition: they are densely packed connective-tissue structures that consist largely of directionally oriented, high-tensile-strength collagen.[18] Because of their function as supporting cables in an environment of high-tensile forces, ligaments and tendons must be relatively inextensible to minimize transmission loss of energy.

The collagen structural organization of tendons and ligaments is similar.[19] Both are mostly type I collagen, which is made up of two α_1 (I) and one α_2 (I) polypeptide chains in a right-handed triple helix, held together by hydrogen and covalent bonds.[20] These fibers are arranged in a quarter-stagger arrangement, which gives collagen its characteristic banding pattern and provides high strength and stability. A loose connective-tissue matrix surrounds the bundles of collagen fibrils. Bundles of collagen and elastin combine to form a matrix of connective tissue fascicles. This matrix is organized within the primary collagen bundles as well as between the bundles that surround them.[21]

Tendons

Tendons are cordlike structures that function to attach muscle to bone and to transmit the forces generated by muscles to bone in order to achieve movement or stability of the body in space.[21] The thickness of each tendon varies and is proportional to the size of the muscle from which they originate.

Within the fascicles of tendons, the collagen components are unidirectionally oriented. The fascicles are held together by loose connective tissue called *endotenon*. Endotenon contains blood vessels, lymphatics, and nerves and permits longitudinal movements of individual fascicles when tensile forces are applied to the structure. The connective tissue surrounding groups of fascicles or the entire structure is called the *epitenon*.

Gliding tendons, such as the flexor tendons of the hand, are enclosed by a tendon sheath with discrete parietal (inside surface of the sheath) and visceral (epitenon or outside layer of the tendon) synovium layers. These tendons receive vascular access only through vincula—small, loose, flexible strips of connective tissue that connect with the mesotenon and paratenon, the loose connective tissues around the sheath.[21]

Vascular tendons are surrounded by a peritendinous connective tissue paratenon, which is connected to the epitenon. If there is synovial fluid between these two layers, the paratenon is called *tenosynovium*; if not, it is termed *tenovagium*.[21]

As the tendon joins the muscle, it fans out into a much wider and thinner structure. The site where the muscle and tendon meet is called the *myotendinous junction* (MTJ). Despite its viscoelastic mechanical characteristics, the MTJ is very vulnerable to tensile failure.[22,23] Indeed, the MTJ is the location of most common muscle strains caused by tensile forces in a normal muscle-tendon unit.[21,24] In particular, a predilection for a tear near the MTJ has been reported in the biceps and triceps brachii, rotator cuff muscles, flexor pollicis longus, peroneus longus, medial head of the gastrocnemius, rectus femoris, adductor longus, iliopsoas, pectoralis major, semimembranosus, and the entire hamstring group.[25–27]

Ligaments

Skeletal ligaments are fibrous bands of dense connective tissue that connect bones across joints. Ligaments contribute to the stability of joint function by preventing excessive motion,[28] acting as guides to direct motion, and providing proprioceptive information for joint function,[29] Inman[30] feels that the ligaments are more important as checkreins than as providers of stability during movement.

The cellular organization of ligaments makes them ideal for sustaining tensile load.[31] Between the bundles are spindle-shaped fibroblasts that are responsible for creating and maintaining the matrix.[32] They are largely type I collagen (with small amounts of type III), with tendons consisting of 86 percent (dry weight) collagen and ligaments consisting of 70 percent (dry weight) collagen. Small amounts of elastin are present in ligaments, with the exception of the ligamentum flavum and the nuchal ligament of the spine. Collagen has a less unidirectional organization in ligaments than it does in tendons, but its structural framework still provides stiffness (resistance to deformation).[19]

Bone

Bone is a highly vascular form of connective tissue, composed of collagen, calcium phosphate, water, amorphous proteins, and cells. It is the most rigid of the connective tissues. Despite its rigidity, bone is a dynamic tissue that undergoes constant metabolism and remodeling. The collagen of bone is produced in the same manner as that of ligament and tendon, but by a different cell, the osteoblast.[13]

At the gross anatomical level, each bone has a distinct morphology comprising both cortical bone and cancellous bone. Cortical bone is found in the outer shell. Cancellous bone is found within the epiphyseal and metaphyseal regions of long bones as well as throughout the interior of short bones[22] (Table 1-2).

The function of bone is to provide support, enhance leverage, protect vital structures, provide attachments for both tendons and ligaments, and store minerals, particularly calcium. Bones also may serve as useful landmarks during the palpation phase of the examination. The strength of a bone is related directly to its density.

Cartilage Tissue

The development of bone is usually preceded by the formation of cartilage tissue. Cartilage tissue consists of cartilage cells called *chondrocytes*. Chondrocytes are specialized cells that are responsible for the development of cartilage and the maintenance of the extracellular matrix.[33] The extracellular matrix also contains proteoglycans, lipids, water, and dissolved electrolytes. It is the concentration of proteoglycans in solution that is responsible for the viscoelastic properties of cartilage.[34]

TABLE 1-2 General Structure of Bone[22]

Site	Comment	Conditions	Result
Epiphysis	Mainly develops under pressure Apophysis forms under traction Forms bone ends Supports articular surface	Epiphyseal dysplasias Joint surface trauma Overuse injury Damaged blood supply	Distorted joints Degenerative changes Fragmented development Avascular necrosis
Physis	Epiphyseal or growth plate Responsive to growth and sex hormones Vulnerable prior to growth spurt Mechanically weak	Physeal dysplasia Trauma Slipped epiphysis	Short stature Deformed or angulated growth or growth arrest
Metaphysis	Remodeling expanded bone end Cancellous bone heals rapidly Vulnerable to osteomyelitis Affords ligament attachment	Osteomyelitis Tumors Metaphyseal dysplasia	Sequestrum formation Altered bone shape Distorted growth
Diaphysis	Forms shaft of bone Large surface for muscle origin Significant compact cortical bone Strong in compression	Fractures Diaphyseal dysplasias Healing slower than at metaphysis	Able to remodel angulation Cannot remodel rotation Involucrum with infection Dysplasia give altered density and shape

---

Clinical Pearl

Proteoglycans are macromolecules that consist of a protein backbone to which are attached many extended polysaccharide units called *glycosaminoglycans,* of which there are two types: chondroitin sulfate and keratin sulfate.[35,36] A simple way to visualize the proteoglycan molecule is to consider a test tube brush, with the stem representing the protein core and the glycosaminoglycans representing the bristles.[37,38] Proteoglycan structure influences the mechanical properties of the tissue, including compressive stiffness, sheer stiffness, osmotic pressure, and regulation of hydration.

Chondrocytes produce aggrecan, link protein, and hyaluronan, all of which are extruded into the extracellular matrix, where they aggregate spontaneously.[36] The aggrecans form a strong, porous-permeable, fiber-reinforced composite material with collagen.

Cartilage tissue exists in three forms: hyaline, elastic, and fibrocartilage.

▶ Hyaline cartilage, commonly called *gristle*, covers the ends of long bones and, along with the synovial fluid that bathes it, provides a smoothly articulating surface. Articular cartilage plays a vital role in the function of the musculoskeletal system, permitting almost frictionless motion to occur between the articular surfaces of a diarthrodial (synovial) joint (see Chap. 4).[39] Adult articular cartilage is an avascular and noninnervated structure. Hyaline cartilage is the most abundant cartilage within the body. Most of the bones of the body form first as hyaline cartilage, and later become bone in a process called *endochondral ossification.*

▶ Elastic cartilage is a very specialized connective tissue, primarily found in locations such as the outer ear and portions of the larynx.

▶ Fibrocartilage functions as a shock absorber in both weight-bearing, and non–weight-bearing joints. Its large fiber content, reinforced with numerous collagen fibers, makes it ideal for bearing large stresses in all directions. Examples of fibrocartilage include the symphysis pubis, intervertebral disc, and menisci of the knee.

Joints

Joints are regions where bones are capped and surrounded by connective tissues that hold the bones together and determine the type and degree of movement between them.[40] Joints may be classified as *diarthrosis,* which permit free bone movement and *synarthrosis,* in which very limited or no motion occurs.

Diarthrosis. This type of joint generally unites long bones and has great mobility. Examples include but are not limited to the hip, knee and shoulder, and elbow joints. These joints are characterized by a fibroelastic joint capsule, which is filled with a lubricating substance called *synovial fluid.* Consequently these joints are often referred to as synovial joints (see later).

Synarthrosis. There are three major types of synarthroses, based on the type of tissue uniting the bone surfaces[40]:

▶ Synostosis joints, which are united by bone tissue, and which include sutures and gomphoses.

▶ Synchondrosis joints, which are joined by either hyaline or fibrocartilage. Examples include the epiphyseal plates of growing bones and the articulations between the first rib and the sternum.

▶ Syndesmosis joints, which are joined together by an interosseous membrane and include joints such as the symphysis pubis.

Synovial Joints

Synovial joints can be broadly classified according to structure into the following categories[1]:

▶ *Spheroid.* As the name suggests, a spheroid joint is a freely moving joint in which a sphere on the head of one bone fits into a rounded cavity in the other bone. Spheroid (ball and socket) joints allow motions in three planes (refer to Chap. 3). Examples of a spheroid joint surface include the heads of the femur and humerus.

▶ *Trochoid.* The trochoid joint is characterized by a pivot-like process turning within a ring, or a ring on a pivot, the ring being formed partly of bone, partly of ligament. Trochoid joints permit only rotation. Examples of a trochoid joint include the humeroradial joint and the atlanto-axial joint

▶ *Condyloid.* This type of joint is characterized by an ovoid articular surface, or condyle, which is received into an elliptical cavity in such a manner as to permit the motions of flexion, extension, adduction, abduction, and circumduction, but no axial rotation (see Chap. 3). The wrist-joint is an example of this form of articulation.

▶ *Ginglymoid.* A ginglymoid joint is a hinge joint. It is characterized by a spool-like surface and a concave surface. An example of a ginglymoid joint is the humeroulnar joint

▶ *Ellipsoid.* Ellipsoid joints are similar to spheroid joints in that they allow the same type of movement albeit to a lesser magnitude. The ellipsoid joint allows movement in two planes (flexion, extension; abduction, adduction) and is biaxial (refer to Chap. 3). Examples of this joint can be found at the radiocarpal articulation at the wrist and the metacarpophalangeal articulation in the phalanges.

▶ *Planar.* As its name suggests, a planar joint is characterized by two flat surfaces that slide over each other. Movement at this type of joint does not occur about an axis and is termed nonaxial. Examples of a planar joint include the intermetatarsal joints and some intercarpal joints.

Although the above categories give a broad description of joint structure, this classification does not sufficiently describe the articulations or the movements that occur. In reality, no joint surface is planar or resembles a true geometric form. Instead joint surfaces are either convex in all directions or concave in all directions, that is they resemble either the outer or inner surface of a piece of eggshell.[2] Because the curve of an eggshell varies from point to point, these articular surfaces are called *ovoid*. The other major type of articular surface is the *sellar* joint.[2] Sellar joints are characterized by a convex surface in one cross-sectional plane and a concave surface in the plane perpendicular

to it. Examples of a sellar joint include the interphalangeal joints, the carpometacarpal joint of the thumb, the humeroulnar joint, and the calcaneocuboid joints.

The bones that articulate in a synovial joint are capped with a smooth layer of hyaline cartilage called *articular cartilage*. Articular cartilage functions to distribute the joint forces over a large contact area, dissipating the forces associated with the load. This distribution of forces allows the articular cartilage to remain healthy and fully functional throughout decades of life.[35,39,41] Articular cartilage may be grossly subdivided into four distinct zones with differing collagen orientations[42] (Fig. 1-1), as follows:

▶ *The superficial layer (zone I).* In the superficial zone, which lies adjacent to the joint cavity, the uniform collagen fibrils are arranged parallel and tangentially to the surface in one to three layers. Zone I comprises approximately 5 to 10 percent of the matrix volume.

▶ *The middle layer (zone II).* In the middle zone, the collagen fibril orientation is less organized. Zone II comprises 40 to 45 percent of the matrix volume.

▶ *The deep or radial layer (zone III).* The deep layer comprises 40 to 45 percent of the matrix volume. It is characterized by radially aligned collagen fibers that are perpendicular to the surface of the joint, and a high proteoglycan content.

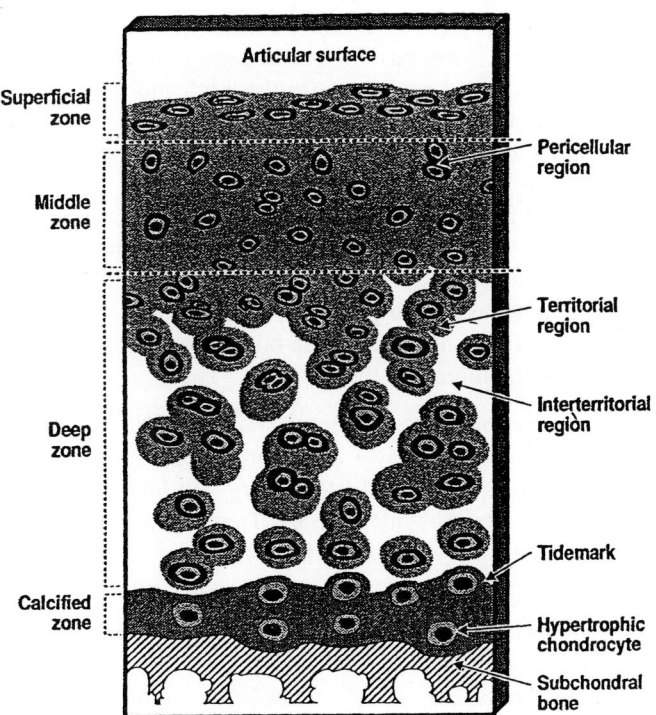

FIGURE 1-1 Regional organization of articular cartilage. (Reproduced with permission from Pool AR. Cartilage in health and disease. In: McCarty DJ, Koopman WJ, eds. *Arthritis and Allied Conditions.* 12th ed, vol 1. Philadelphia, Pa: Lea and Febiger; 1993:282.)

▶ *The tidemark.* The upper boundary of zone IV is the tidemark. The tidemark delineates the boundary between zones III and IV. The lower boundary of zone IV may mark the line of the most recent bone turnover of the calcified tissue, because it tends to migrate upward with age.[43]

▶ *The calcified zone (zone IV).* The calcified zone prevents the diffusion of nutrients from the bone tissue into the cartilage.

Synovial Fluid

Articular cartilage is subject to a great variation of loading conditions (see Chap. 4), and joint lubrication through synovial fluid is necessary to minimize frictional resistance between the weight-bearing surfaces. Fortunately, synovial joints are blessed with a very superior lubricating system, which permits a remarkably frictionless interaction at the joint surfaces. A lubricated cartilaginous interface has a coefficient of friction* of 0.002.[44] By way of comparison, ice on ice has a coefficient of friction of 0.03.[44]

The composition of synovial fluid is nearly the same as blood plasma, but with a decreased total protein content and a higher concentration of hyaluronan.[45] Indeed, synovial fluid is essentially a dialysate of plasma to which hyaluronan has been added.[46] Hyaluronan is a glycosaminoglycan that is continually synthesized and released into synovial fluid by specialized synoviocytes.[47] It is a critical constituent component of normal synovial fluid and an important contributor to joint homeostasis.[48] Hyaluronan imparts anti-inflammatory and antinociceptive properties to normal synovial fluid and contributes to joint lubrication. It also is responsible for the viscoelastic properties of synovial fluid,[45] and contributes to the lubrication of articular cartilage surfaces.[46,47] The mechanical properties of synovial fluid permit it to act as both a cushion and a lubricant to the joint.

Fluid lubrication happens by a film of synovial fluid being established, and maintained, between the two surfaces as long as movement occurs.

Numerous theories of joint lubrication exist. Two of these theories are commonly recognized: boundary lubrication[49] and fluid-film lubrication.[50]

▶ *Boundary lubrication.* Boundary lubrication is thought to occur as a single layer of hyaluronate molecules adhere to the joint surfaces and keep a very thin film of fluid between the two moving surfaces. These layers carry loads and are effective in reducing friction.[49]

▶ *Fluid-film lubrication.* As its name suggests, this type of joint lubrication is the result of a thin film of lubricant, which produces a greater bearing surface separation. The thickness, extent, and weight-bearing properties of the fluid film depend on its physical properties.[50] These physical properties include the viscosity of the joint fluid and function similarly to a biomechanical spring. The capacity of a lubricating fluid to alter its viscosity according to demand is very important. For example, with very fast velocities, a thinner, less viscous fluid film is desirable.[51]

In general, joint surface loads are sustained by fluid-film lubrication in areas of noncontact, and by boundary lubrication in areas of contact.[50] Diseases such as osteoarthritis, affect the thixotropic properties (thixotropy is the property of various gels becoming fluid when disturbed, as by shaking) of synovial fluid, resulting in reduced lubrication and subsequent wear of the articular cartilage and joint surfaces (see Chap. 4).[52,53] It is well established that damaged articular cartilage in adults has a very limited potential for healing, because it possesses neither a blood supply nor lymphatic drainage.[54]

Bursae

Closely associated with some synovial joints are flattened, saclike structures called *bursae* that are lined with a synovial membrane and filled with synovial fluid. The bursa produces small amounts of fluid, allowing for smooth and almost frictionless motion between contiguous muscles, tendons, bones, ligaments, and skin.[55–57] A tendon sheath is a modified bursa. A bursa can be a source of pain if it becomes inflamed or infected.

Skeletal Muscle Tissue

The microstructure and composition of skeletal muscle have been studied extensively. The class of tissue labeled *skeletal muscle* consists of individual muscle cells or fibers. A single muscle cell is called a *muscle fiber* or *myofiber* (Fig. 1-2). Individual muscle fibers are wrapped in a connective tissue envelope called *endomysium*. Bundles of myofibers, which form a whole muscle (fasciculus), are encased in the perimysium. The perimysium is continuous with the deep fascia. Groups of fasciculi are surrounded by a connective sheath called the epimysium. Under an electron microscope, it can be seen that each of the myofibers consists of thousands of *myofibrils*, which extend throughout its length. Myofibrils are composed of sarcomeres arranged in series.[58] The sarcomere is the contractile machinery of the muscle.

Clinical Pearl

The knowledge that muscles had contractile ability, and that nerves were composed of motor and sensory components, can be traced back to the third century BC.[59] Then, in the first century AD, Galen described the origin, insertion, and function of muscles. Galen grouped the muscles into systems and described tonic agonist and antagonist contractions of muscles[60] and their relationship to movements of the spine and to joint mechanics.[61] A major advance came in 1740 with the discovery, by von Haller (1708–1777) and Whytt (1714–1766), of the association of muscular contraction with electricity.[61]

---

* Coefficient of friction is a ratio of the force needed to make a body glide across a surface compared with the weight or force holding the two surfaces in contact.

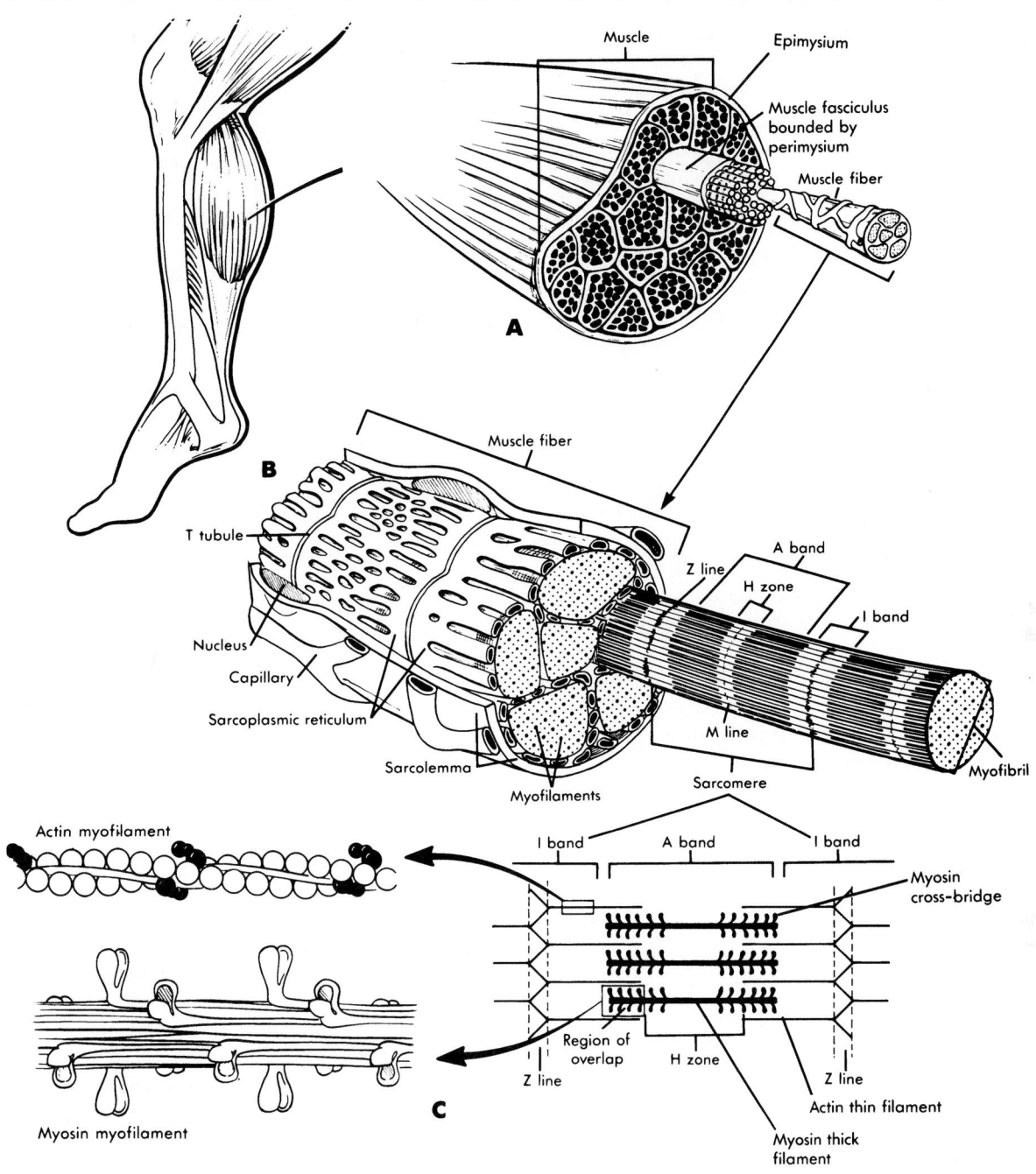

FIGURE 1-2 Components of a muscle. (Reproduced with permission from Prentice WE, Voight ML. *Techniques in Musculoskeletal Rehabilitation*, New York, NY: McGraw-Hill; 2001:31.)

Machinery of Movement

One of the most important roles of connective tissue is to mechanically transmit the forces generated by the skeletal muscle cells to provide movement. Each muscle cell contains many fibers called *myofilaments*, which run parallel to the myofibril axis (see Fig. 1-2). The myofilaments are made up of two protein filaments: actin (thin) and myosin (thick). The most distinctive feature of skeletal muscle fibers is their striated

(striped) appearance. This cross-striation is the result of an orderly arrangement within and between structures called sarcomeres and myofibrils.[62] The striations are produced by alternating dark (A) and light (I) bands that appear to span the width of the muscle fiber. The A bands are composed of myosin filaments, whereas the I bands are composed of actin filaments. The actin filaments of the I band overlap into the A band, giving the edges of the A band a darker appearance than the central region (H band), which contains only myosin.[62] At the center of each I band is a thin, dark Z line. A *sarcomere* represents the distance between each Z line.

Each muscle fiber is limited by a cell membrane called a *sarcolemma*. The protein *dystrophin* plays an essential role in the mechanical strength and stability of the sarcolemma.[63] Dystrophin is lacking in patients with Duchenne muscular dystrophy.

When a muscle contracts isotonically, the distance between the Z lines decreases, the I band and H bands disappear, but the width of the A band remains unchanged.[62] This shortening of the sarcomeres is not produced by a shortening of the actin and myosin filaments, but by a sliding of actin filaments over the myosin filaments, which pulls the Z lines together.

Structures called *cross-bridges* serve to connect the actin and myosin filaments. The myosin filaments contain two flexible, hingelike regions, which allow the cross-bridges to attach and detach from the actin filament. During contraction, the cross-bridges attach and undergo power strokes, which provide the contractile force. During relaxation, the cross-bridges detach. This attaching and detaching is asynchronous, so that some are attaching while others are detaching. Thus, at each moment, some of the cross-bridges are pulling, while others are releasing.

The regulation of cross-bridge attachment and detachment is a function of two proteins found in the actin filaments: tropomyosin and troponin. Tropomyosin attaches directly to the actin filament, whereas troponin is attached to the tropomyosin rather than directly to the actin filament. Tropomyosin and troponin function as the switch for muscle contraction and relaxation. In a relaxed state, the tropomyosin physically blocks the cross-bridges from binding to the actin. For contraction to take place, the tropomyosin must be moved.

Each muscle fiber is innervated by a somatic motor neuron. One neuron and the muscle fibers it innervates constitute a motor unit, or functional unit of the muscle. Each motor neuron branches as it enters the muscle to innervate a number of muscle fibers. The area of contact between a nerve and a muscle fiber is known as the motor end plate, or neuromuscular junction. The release of a chemical acetylcholine from the axon terminals at the neuromuscular junctions causes electrical activation of the skeletal muscle fibers (Fig. 1-3). When an action potential propagates into the transverse tubule system (narrow membranous tunnels formed from and continuous with the sarcolemma), the voltage sensors on the transverse tubule membrane signal the release of Ca^{2+} from the terminal cisternae portion of the sarcoplasmic reticulum (a series of interconnected sacs and tubes that surround each myofibril).[62] The released Ca^{2+} then diffuses into the sarcomeres and binds to troponin, displacing the tropomyosin, and allowing the actin to bind with the myosin cross-bridges. At the end of the contraction (the neural activity and action potentials cease), the sarcoplasmic reticulum actively accumulates Ca^{2+} and muscle relaxation occurs. The return of Ca^{2+} to the sarcoplasmic reticulum involves active transport, requiring the degradation of adenosine triphosphate (ATP) to adenosine diphosphate.

FIGURE 1-3   Steps in muscle contraction.

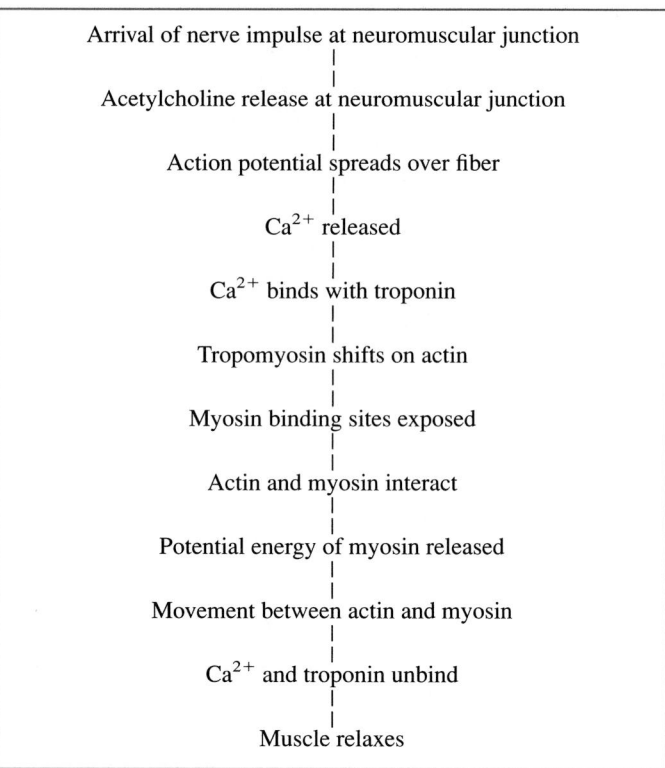

Arrival of nerve impulse at neuromuscular junction
|
Acetylcholine release at neuromuscular junction
|
Action potential spreads over fiber
|
Ca^{2+} released
|
Ca^{2+} binds with troponin
|
Tropomyosin shifts on actin
|
Myosin binding sites exposed
|
Actin and myosin interact
|
Potential energy of myosin released
|
Movement between actin and myosin
|
Ca^{2+} and troponin unbind
|
Muscle relaxes

(ADP)*.[62] Because sarcoplasmic reticulum function is closely associated with both contraction and relaxation, changes in its ability to release or sequester Ca^{2+} markedly affect both the time course and magnitude of force output by the muscle fiber.[64]

Activation of varying numbers of motor neurons results in gradations in the strength of muscle contraction. The stronger the electrical impulse, the stronger the muscle twitch. Whenever a somatic motor neuron is activated, all of the muscle fibers that it innervates are stimulated and contract with *all-or-none* twitches. Although the muscle fibers produce all-or-none contractions, muscles are capable of a wide variety of responses, ranging from activities requiring a high level of precision, to activities requiring high tension (see Chap. 3).

Clinical Pearl

The graded contractions of whole muscles occur because the number of fibers participating in the contraction varies. An increase in the force of movement is achieved by recruiting more cells into cooperative action.

---

* The most readily available energy for skeletal muscle cells is stored in the form of ATP and phosphocreatine. Through the activity of the enzyme ATPase, ATP promptly releases energy when required by the cell to perform any type of work, whether it is electrical, chemical, or mechanical.

When rapid successive impulses activate a muscle fiber already in tension, *summation* occurs and tension is progressively elevated until a maximum value for that fiber is reached.[65] A fiber repetitively activated so that its maximum tension level is maintained for a time is in *tetanus*. If the state of tetanus is sustained, fatigue causes a gradual decline in the level of tension produced.

The Energy For Movement

During physical exercise, energy turnover in skeletal muscle may increase by 400 times compared with muscle at rest, and muscle oxygen consumption may increase by more than 100 times.[66a] The energy required to power muscular activity is derived from the hydrolysis of adenosine triphosphate (ATP) to adenosine diphosphate (ADP) and inorganic phosphate (P_i). Despite the large fluctuations in energy demand just mentioned, muscle ATP remains practically constant and demonstrates a remarkable precision of the system in adjusting the rate of the ATP generating processes to the demand.[66b] There are three energy systems that contribute to the resynthesis of ATP via ADP rephosphorylation. The relative contribution of these energy systems to ATP resynthesis has been shown to depend upon the intensity and duration of exercise.[66c] These energy systems include:

▶ *Phosphagen system.* The phosphagen system is an anaerobic process—can proceed without oxygen (O_2). Within the skeletal muscle cell at the onset of muscular contraction, phosphocreatine (PCr) represents the most immediate reserve for the rephosphorylation of adenosine triphosphate (ATP). The phosphagen system provides ATP primarily for short-term, high intensity activities (i.e., sprinting) and is active at the start of all exercise regardless of intensity.[66d] One disadvantage of the phosphagen system is that because of its significant contribution to the energy yield at the onset of near maximal exercise, the concentration of PCr can be reduced to less than 40% of resting levels within 10 seconds of the start of intense exercise.[66e]

▶ *Glycolysis system.* The glycolysis system is an anaerobic process that involves the breakdown of carbohydrates—either glycogen stored in the muscle or glucose delivered in the blood—to produce ATP. Because this system relies upon a series of nine different chemical reactions, it is slower to become fully active. However, glycogenolysis has a greater capacity to provide energy than PCr, and so it supplements PCr during maximal exercise, and continues to rephosphorylate ADP during maximal exercise after PCr reserves have become essentially depleted.[66d] The process of glycolysis can go one of two ways, termed fast glycolysis and slow glycolysis, depending on the energy demands within the cell. If energy must be supplied at a high rate, fast glycolysis is used primarily. If the energy demand is not as high, slow glycolysis is activated. The main disadvantage of the fast glycolysis system is that during very high-intensity exercise, hydrogen ions dissociate from the glycogenolytic end product of lactic acid.[66b] An increase in hydrogen ion concentration is believed to inhibit glycotic reactions and directly interfere with muscle excitation-contraction and coupling, which can potentially impair contractile force during exercise.[66d]

▶ *Oxidative system.* As its name suggests, the oxidative system requires O_2 and is consequently termed the "aerobic" system. The oxidative system is the primary source of ATP at rest and during low intensity activities. It is worth noting that at no time during either rest or exercise does any single energy system provide the complete supply of energy. While being unable to produce ATP at an equivalent rate to that produced by PCr breakdown and glycogenolysis, the oxidative system is capable of sustaining low-intensity exercise for several hours.[66d] However, because of an increased complexity, the time between the onset of exercise and when this system is operating at its full potential is around 45 seconds.[66f]

Muscle Fiber Types

The basic function of a muscle is to contract. Based on their contractile properties, four different types of muscle fibers have been recognized within skeletal muscle: type I (slow-twitch red oxidative), type IIa (fast-twitch red oxidative), type IIb (fast-twitch white glycolytic), and type IIc (fast-twitch intermediate)[66] (Table 1-3). The muscle cells associated with large motor units are typically type II fibers, which are particularly suited for anaerobic metabolism and lactic acid production. These fibers contain greater concentrations of phosphagens than the type I fibers.

TABLE 1-3 Comparison of Muscle Fiber Types

Characteristics	Type I	Type IIa	Type IIb
Diameter	Small	Intermediate	Large
Capillaries	Many	Many	Few
Resistance to fatigue	High	Intermediate	Low
Glycogen content	Low	Intermediate	High
Respiration	Aerobic	Aerobic	Anaerobic
Twitch rate	Slow	Fast	Fast
Myosin ATPase content	Low	High	High

ATP, adenosine triphosphate.

TABLE 1-4 Functional Division of Muscle Groups[67]

Movement Group	Stabilization Group
Primarily type IIa	Primarily type I
Prone to develop tightness	Prone to develop weakness
Prone to develop hypertonicity	Prone to muscle inhibition
Dominate in fatigue and new movement situations	Fatigue easily
Generally cross two joints	Primarily cross one joint
EXAMPLES	EXAMPLES
Gastrocnemius/Soleus	Peronei
Tibialis posterior	Tibialis anterior
Short hip adductors	Vastus medialis and lateralis
Hamstrings	Gluteus maximus, medius, and minimus
Rectus femoris	Serratus anterior
Tensor fascia lata	Rhomboids
Erector spinae	Lower portion of trapezius
Quadratus lumborum	Short/deep cervical flexors
Pectoralis major	Upper limb extensors
Upper portion of trapezius	Rectus abdominis
Levator scapulae	
Sternocleidomastoid	
Scalenes	
Upper limb flexors	

Slow-twitch fibers are richly endowed with mitochondria and have a high capacity for oxygen uptake. They are, therefore, suitable for activities of long duration or endurance, including posture. In contrast, fast-twitch fibers are suited to quick, explosive actions, including such activities as sprinting. Fast-twitch fibers can be separated into those that have a high complement of mitochondria (type IIa), and those that are mitochondria poor (type IIb). Type IIc fibers exhibit structural features of both red and white fibers and thus have fast contraction times and good fatigue resistance.

Clinical Pearl

In fast-twitch fibers, the sarcoplasmic reticulum embraces every individual myofibril. In slow-twitch fibers, it may contain multiple myofibrils.[67]

Theory dictates that a muscle with a large percentage of the total cross-sectional area occupied by slow-twitch type I fibers should be more fatigue-resistant than one in which the fast-twitch type II fibers predominate.

Different activities place differing demands on a muscle (Table 1-4). Movement activities involve a predominance of fast-twitch fiber recruitment. Postural activities and those activities requiring stabilization entail more involvement of the slow-twitch fibers. In humans, most limb muscles contain a relatively equal distribution of each muscle fiber type, whereas the back and trunk demonstrate a predominance of slow-twitch

fibers. Although it would seem possible that physical training may cause fibers to convert from slow twitch to fast twitch or the reverse, this has not been shown to be the case.[68] However, fiber conversion from Type Ia to Type IIb, and vice versa, has been found to occur with training.[69]

The various types of muscle contraction and their relationship to impaired muscle performance are described in Chapter 6.

Clinical Pearl

For the purpose of an orthopedic examination, Cyriax subdivided musculoskeletal tissues into "contractile" and "inert" (noncontractile) tissues.[70]

- *Contractile.* As defined by Cyriax, contractile tissue is a bit of a misnomer, as the only true contractile tissue in the body is the muscle fiber. However, included under this term are the muscle belly, tendon, tenoperiosteal junction, submuscular/tendinous bursa, and bone (teno-osseous junction), because all are stressed to some degree with a muscle contraction.

- *Inert tissue.* According to Cyriax, inert tissue includes the joint capsule, ligaments, bursa, articular surfaces of the joint, synovium, dura, bone, and fascia.

The teno-osseous junction and the bursae are placed in each of the subdivisions because of their close proximity to contractile tissue, and their capacity to be compressed or stretched during movement.

Respiratory Muscles

The primary respiratory muscles of the body include the diaphragm; the internal, external, and transverse intercostals; the levator costae; and the serratus posterior inferior and superior (see Chap. 26). Although the respiratory muscles share some mechanical similarities with skeletal muscles, they are distinct from other skeletal muscles in several aspects, as follows[71,72]:

▶ Whereas skeletal muscles of the limbs overcome inertial loads, the respiratory muscles overcome primarily elastic and resistive loads.

▶ The respiratory muscles are under both voluntary and involuntary control.

▶ The respiratory muscles are similar to the heart muscles, in that they have to contract rhythmically and generate the required forces for ventilation throughout the entire life span of the individual. The respiratory muscles, however, do not contain pacemaker cells, and are under the control of mechanical and chemical stimuli, requiring neural input from higher centers to initiate and coordinate contraction.

▶ The resting length of the respiratory muscles is a relationship between the inward recoil forces of the lung and the outward recoil forces of the chest wall. Changes in the balance of recoil forces will result in changes in the resting length of the respiratory muscles. Thus, simple and everyday life occurrences such as changes in posture may alter the operational length and the contractile strength of the respiratory muscles.[73] If uncompensated, these length changes would lead to decreases in the output of the muscles and, hence, a reduction in the ability to generate volume changes.[73] The skeletal muscles of the limbs, on the other hand, are not constrained to operate at a particular resting length.

REVIEW QUESTIONS*

1. What are the three cell types associated with connective tissue?
2. What are the three types of cartilage and bone tissue?
3. Give one example of loose connective tissue
4. What is the primary type of collagen that forms tendons and ligaments?
5. What is the name of the connective tissue that surrounds groups of fascicles and/or the entire structure of a tendon?

---

* Additional questions to test your understanding of this chapter can be found in the Online Learning Center for *Orthopaedic Assessment, Evaluation, and Intervention* at www.duttononline.net. Answers for the above questions appear in the back of this book.

REFERENCES

1. Van de Graaff KM, Fox SI. Histology. In: Van de Graaff KM, Fox SI, eds. *Concepts of Human Anatomy and Physiology*. New York, NY: WCB/McGraw-Hill; 1999:130–158.

2. Williams GN, Chmielewski T, Rudolph K, Buchanan TS, Snyder-Mackler L. Dynamic knee stability: Current theory and implications for clinicians and scientists. *J Orthop Sports Phys Ther* 2001;31:546–566.

3. Prentice WE. Understanding and managing the healing process. In: Prentice WE, Voight ML, eds. *Techniques in Musculoskeletal Rehabilitation*. New York, NY: McGraw-Hill; 2001:17–41.

4. Myllyharju J, Kivirikko KI. Collagens and collagen-related diseases. *Ann Med* 2001;33:7–21.

5. Burgeson RE. New collagens new concepts. *Ann Rev Cell Biol* 1988;4:551–577.

6. Starcher BC. Lung elastin and matrix. *Chest* 2000;117(suppl 1):229S–34S.

7. Sandberg LB, Weissman N, Smith DW. The purification and partial characterization of a soluble elastin-like protein from copper-deficient porcine aorta. *Biochemistry* 1969;8: 2940–2945.

8. Hinek A, Rabinovitch M. 67-kD elastin binding protein is a protective "companion" of extracellular insoluble elastin and intracellular tropoelastin. *J Cell Biol* 1994;126:563–574.

9. Mecham RP. Elastin synthesis and fiber assembly. *Ann N Y Acad Sci* 1991;624:137–146.

10. Kagan HM, Trackman PC. Properties and function of lysyl oxidase. *Am J Respir Cell Mol Biol* 1991;5:206–210.

11. Vrhovski B, Weiss AS. Biochemistry of tropoelastin. *Eur J Biochem* 1998;259:1–18.

12. Eyre DR, Paz MA, Gallop PM. Crosslinking in collagen and elastin. *Annu Rev Biochem* 1984;53:717–748.

13. Engles M. Tissue response. In: Donatelli R, Wooden MJ, eds. *Orthopaedic Physical Therapy*. Philadelphia, Pa: Churchill Livingstone; 2001:1–24.

14. Ham AW, Cormack DH. *Histology*. 8th ed. Philadelphia, Pa: Lippincott; 1979.

15. Barnes J. *Myofascial Release: A Comprehensive Evaluatory and Treatment Approach*. Paoli, Pa: MFR Seminars; 1990.

16. Smolders JJ. Myofascial pain and dysfunction syndromes. In: Hammer WI, ed. *Functional Soft Tissue Examination and Treatment by Manual Methods—The Extremities*. Gaithersburg, Md: Aspen; 1991:215–234.

17. Ellis JJ, Johnson GS. Myofascial considerations in somatic dysfunction of the thorax. In: Flynn TW, ed. *The Thoracic Spine and Rib Cage: Musculoskeletal Evaluation and Treatment*. Boston, Mass: Butterworth-Heinemann; 1996:211–262.

18. Clancy WG Jr. Tendon trauma and overuse injuries. In: Leadbetter WB, Buckwalter JA, Gordon SL, eds. *Sports-Induced Inflammation*. Park Ridge, Ill: American Academy of Orthopaedic Surgeons; 1990:609–618.

19. Amiel D, Kleiner JB. Biochemistry of tendon and ligament. In: Nimni ME, ed. *Collagen*. Boca Raton, Fla: CRC Press; 1988:223–251.

20. Amiel D, Woo SLY, Harwood FL. The effect of immobilization on collagen turnover in connective tissue: A biochemical-biomechanical correlation. *Acta Orthop Scand* 1982;53:325–332.

21. Teitz CC, Garrett WE Jr, Miniaci A, Lee MH, Mann RA. Tendon problems in athletic individuals. *J Bone Joint Surg* 1997;79A:138–152.

22. Reid DC. *Sports Injury Assessment and Rehabilitation*. New York, NY: Churchill Livingstone; 1992.

23. Garrett W, Tidball J. Myotendinous junction: Structure, function, and failure. In: Woo SLY, Buckwalter JA, eds. *Injury and Repair of the Musculoskeletal Soft Tissues*. Rosemont, Ill: American Academy of Orthopedic Surgeons; 1988.

24. Garrett WE Jr. Muscle strain injuries: Clinical and basic aspects. *Med Sci Sports Exerc* 1990;22:436–443.

25. Garrett WE. Muscle strain injuries. *Am J Sports Med* 1996;24:S2–S8.

26. Safran MR, Seaber AV, Garrett WE. Warm-up and muscular injury prevention: An update. *Sports Med* 1989;8:239–249.

27. Huijbregts PA. Muscle injury, regeneration, and repair. *J Man Manip Ther* 2001;9:9–16.

28. Safran MR, Benedetti RS, Bartolozzi AR 3rd, Mandelbaum BR. Lateral ankle sprains: A comprehensive review: Part 1: Etiology, pathoanatomy, histopathogenesis, and diagnosis. *Med Sci Sports Exerc* 1999;31(suppl):S429–37.

29. Smith RL, Brunolli J. Shoulder kinesthesia after anterior glenohumeral dislocation. *Phys Ther* 1989;69:106–112.

30. Inman VT. Sprains of the ankle. In: Chapman MS, ed. *AAOS Instructional Course Lectures.* Rosemont, Ill: American Academy of Orthopedic Surgeons; 1975:294–308.

31. Woo SLY, et al. Anatomy, biology, and biomechanics of tendon, ligament, and meniscus. In: Simon SR, ed. *Orthopaedic Basic Science.* Rosemont, Ill: American Academy of Orthopaedic Surgeons; 1994:45–87.

32. McGaw WT. The effect of tension on collagen remodelling by fibroblasts: A stereological ultrastructural study. *Connect Tissue Res* 1986;14:229.

33. Mankin HJ, et al. Form and function of articular cartilage. In: Simon SR, ed. *Orthopaedic Basic Science.* Rosemont, Ill: American Academy of Orthopaedic Surgeons; 1994;1–44.

34. Woo SLY, Buckwalter JA. *Injury and Repair of the Musculoskeletal Tissue.* Park Ridge, Ill: American Academy of Orthopaedic Surgeons; 1988.

35. Buckwalter JA, Mankin HJ. Articular cartilage. Part I: Tissue design and chondrocyte-matrix interactions. *J Bone Joint Surg* 1997;79A:600–611.

36. Muir H. Proteoglycans as organizers of the extracellular matrix. *Biochem Soc Trans* 1983;11:613–622.

37. Junqueira LC, Carneciro J, Kelley RO. *Basic Histology.* Norwalk, Conn: Appleton and Lange; 1995.

38. Lundon K, Bolton K. Structure and function of the lumbar intervertebral disk in health, aging, and pathological conditions. *J Orthop Sports Phys Ther* 2001;31:291–306.

39. Cohen NP, Foster RJ, Mow VC. Composition and dynamics of articular cartilage: structure, function, and maintaining healthy state. *J Orthop Sports Phys Ther* 1998;28:203–215.

40. Junqueira LC, Carneciro J. Bone. In: Junqueira LC, Carneciro J, eds. *Basic Histology.* New York, NY: McGraw-Hill; 2003:141–159.

40a. Gray H: *Gray's Anatomy.* Philadelphia: Lea & Febiger, 1995.

40b. MacConnail MA, Basmajian JV: *Muscles and Movements: A Basis for Human Kinesiology.* New York: Robert Krieger, 1977.

41. Mow VC, Ratcliffe A, Poole AR. Cartilage and diarthrodial joints as paradigms for hierarchical materials and structures. *Biomaterials* 1992;13:67–97.

42. Schenk RK, Eggli PS, Hunzicker EB. Articular cartilage morphology. In: Kuettner KE, Schleyerbach R, Hascall VC, eds. *Articular Cartilage Biochemistry.* New York, NY: Raven Press; 1986:3–22.

43. Oegema TR Jr, Thompson RC Jr. Metabolism of chondrocytes derived from normal and osteoarthritic human cartilage. In: Kuettner R, Schleyerbach R, Hascall VC, eds. *Articular Cartilage Biochemistry.* New York, NY: Raven Press; 1986:257–272.

44. Chaffin D, Andersson G. *Occupational Biomechanics.* vol 53. New York: Wiley Interscience; 1985:103–107.

45. Dahl LB, Dahl IM, Engstrom-Laurent A, Granath K. Concentration and molecular weight of sodium hyaluronate in synovial fluid from patients with rheumatoid arthritis and other arthropathies. *Ann Rheum Dis* 1985;44:817–822.

46. Namba RS, Shuster S, Tucker P, Stern R. Localization of hyaluronan in pseudocapsule from total hip arthroplasty. *Clin Orthop* 1999;363:158–162.

47. Marshall KW. Intra-articular hyaluronan therapy. *Curr Opin Rheumatol* 2000;12:468–474.

48. Laurent TC, Fraser JRE. Hyaluronan. *FASEB J* 1992;6:2397–2404.

49. Swanson SA. Lubrication of synovial joints. *J Physiol* (Lond) 1972;223:22.

50. Mow VC, Flatow EL, Ateshian GA. Biomechanics. In: Buckwalter JA, Einhorn TA, Simon SR, eds. *Orthopaedic Basic Science.* Rosemont, Ill: American Academy of Orthopaedic Surgeons; 2000:142.

51. Nordin M, Frankel VH. *Basic Biomechanics of the Musculoskeletal System.* 2nd ed. Philadelphia, Pa: Lea and Febiger; 1989.

52. O'Driscoll SW. The healing and regeneration of articular cartilage. *J Bone Joint Surg* 1998;80A:1795–1812.

53. Dieppe P. The classification and diagnosis of osteoarthritis. In: Kuettner KE, Goldberg WM, eds. *Osteoarthritic Disorders.* Rosemont, Ill: American Academy of Orthopaedic Surgeons; 1995:5–12.

54. Mankin HJ. Current concepts review. The response of articular cartilage to mechanical injury. *J Bone Joint Surg* 1982;64A:460–466.

55. Ho G Jr, Tice AD, Kaplan SR. Septic bursitis in the prepatellar and olecranon bursae: An analysis of 25 cases. *Ann Intern Med* 1978;89:21–27.

56. Buckingham RB. Bursitis and tendinitis. *Compr Ther* 1981;7:52–57.

57. Reilly J, Nicholas JA. The chronically inflamed bursa. *Clin Sports Med* 1987;6:345–370.

58. Jones D, Round D. *Skeletal Muscle in Health and Disease.* Manchester, England: Manchester University Press; 1990.

59. Weinstein R, Ehni G, Wilson CB. *Lumbar Spondylosis. Diagnosis, Management and Surgical Treatment.* Chicago, Ill: Year Book Medical Publishers; 1977.

60. Bick EM. *Source Book of Orthopaedics.* 2nd ed. Baltimore, Md: Williams and Wilkins; 1948.

61. Rasch PJ, Burke RK. *Kinesiology and Applied Anatomy.* Philadelphia, Pa: Lea and Febiger; 1971.

62. Van de Graaff KM, Fox SI. Muscle tissue and muscle physiology. In: Van de Graaff KM, Fox SI, eds. *Concepts of Human Anatomy and Physiology.* New York, NY: WCB/McGraw-Hill; 1999:280–305.

63. Armstrong RB, Warren GL, Warren JA. Mechanisms of exercise-induced muscle fibre injury. *Med Sci Sports Exerc* 1990;24:436–443.

64. Williams JH, Klug GA. Calcium exchange hypothesis of skeletal muscle fatigue. A brief review. *Muscle Nerve* 1995;18:421.

65. Hall SJ. The biomechanics of human skeletal muscle. In: Hall SJ, ed. *Basic Biomechanics.* New York, NY: McGraw-Hill; 1999:146–185.

66. Brooke MH, Kaiser KK. The use and abuse of muscle histochemistry. *Ann N Y Acad Sci* 1974;228:121.

66a. Tonkonogi M, Sahlin K. Physical exercise and mitochondrial function in human skeletal muscle. *Exercise & Sport Sciences Reviews* 2002;30:129–137.

66b. Sahlin K, Tonkonogi M, Soderlund K. Energy supply and muscle fatigue in humans. *Acta Physiol Scand* 1998;162:261–266.

66c. Sahlin K, Ren JM. Relationship of contraction capacity to metabolic changes during recovery from a fatiguing contraction. *J Appl Physiol* 1989;67:648–654.

66d. McMahon S, Jenkins D. Factors affecting the rate of phosphocreatine resynthesis following intense exercise. *Sports Medicine* 2002;32:761–784.

66e. Walter G, et al. Noninvasive measurement of phosphocreatine recovery kinetics in single human muscles. *Am J Physiol* 1997; 272:C525–C534.

66f. Bangsbo J. Muscle oxygen uptake in humans at onset and during intense exercise. *Acta Physiol Scand* 2000;168:457–464.

67. Jull GA, Janda V. Muscle and motor control in low back pain. In: Twomey LT, Taylor JR, eds. *Physical Therapy of the Low Back: Clinics in Physical Therapy*. New York, NY: Churchill Livingstone; 1987:258.

68. Fitts RH, Widrick JJ. Muscle mechanics; adaptations with exercise training. *Exerc Sport Sci Rev* 1996;24:427.

69. Allemeier CA, Fry AC, Johnson P, Hikida RS, Hagerman FC, Staron RS. Effects of spring cycle training on human skeletal muscle. *J Appl Physiol* 1994;77:2385.

70. Cyriax J. *Textbook of Orthopaedic Medicine, Diagnosis of Soft Tissue Lesions*. 8th ed. London, England: Bailliere Tindall; 1982.

71. Aubier M, Farkas G, De Troyer A, Mozes R, Roussos C. Detection of diaphragmatic fatigue in man by phrenic stimulation. *J Appl Physiol* 1981;50:538–544.

72. Fenn WO. A comparison of respiratory and skeletal muscles. In: Cori CF, et al, eds. *Perspectives in Biology; Houssay Memorial Papers*. Amsterdam, Holland: Elsevier; 1963:293–300.

73. Lewit K. Relation of faulty respiration to posture, with clinical implications. *J Amer Osteopath Assoc* 1980;79:525–529.

THE NERVOUS SYSTEM

OVERVIEW

The human nervous system is an extremely complex entity that performs a multitude of functions, in much the same way as a dynamic network of interrelated computers. The nervous system can be subdivided into two anatomic divisions: the central nervous system, comprising the brain and spinal cord; and the peripheral nervous system, formed by the cranial and spinal nerves. The peripheral nervous system is further subdivided into somatic and autonomic divisions. The somatic division innervates the skin, muscles and joints, while the autonomic system innervates the glands and smooth muscle of the viscera, and the blood vessels.[1]

Basic Anatomy

The nerve cell, or neuron, which serves to store and process information, is the functional unit of the nervous system. The other cellular constituent is the neuroglial cell, or glia, which functions to provide structural and metabolic support for the neurons.[1] Glial cells outnumber the neurons 10 to 1.[2]

Although neurons come in a variety of sizes and shapes, there are four functional parts to each nerve (Fig. 2-1):

▶ *Dendrite.* Dendrites serve a receptive function and receive information from other nerve cells, or the environment.

▶ *Axon.* The axon conducts information to other nerve cells. Many axons are covered by myelin, a lipid-rich membrane. This membrane is divided into segments about 1-mm long by small gaps, called nodes of Ranvier, where the myelin is absent.[2] Myelin has a high electrical resistance and low capacitance and serves to increase the nerve conduction velocity of neural transmissions through a process called *salutatory conduction.*

▶ *Cell body.* The cell body contains the nucleus of the cell and has important integrative functions.

▶ *Axon terminal.* The axon terminal is the transmission site for action potentials, the messengers of the nerve cell.

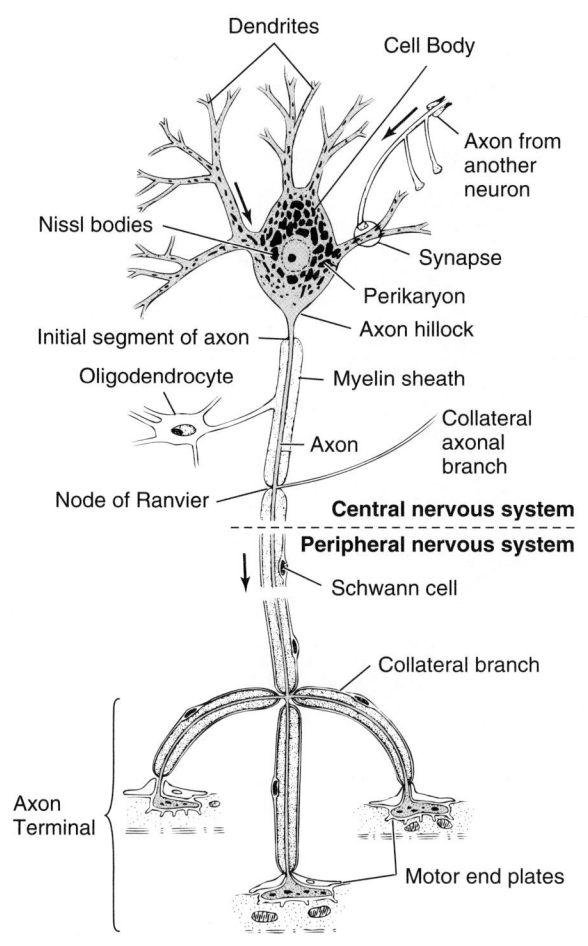

FIGURE 2-1 Schematic drawing of a neuron. (Reproduced with permission from Waxman SG. *Correlative Neuroanatomy*. 24th ed. New York, NY: McGraw-Hill; 1996.)

The communication of information from one nerve cell to another occurs at junctions called synapses, where a chemical is released in the form of a neurotransmitter.

Central Nervous System

The central nervous system consists of the brain and an elongated spinal cord. The spinal cord participates directly in the control of body movements, the processing and transmission of sensory information from the trunk and limbs, and the regulation of visceral functions.[1]

The spinal cord also provides a conduit for the two-way transmission of messages between the brain and the body. These messages travel along pathways, or tracts, which are fiber bundles of similar groups of neurons. Tracts may descend or ascend.

Clinical Pearl

Aggregates of tracts are referred to as columns, or lemnisci.

The spinal cord is normally 42 to 45 cm long in adults and is continuous with the medulla and brain stem at its upper end (Fig. 2-2).[2] The conus medullaris serves as the distal end of the cord and, in adults, the conus ends at the L1 or L2 level of the vertebral column. A series of specializations, the filum terminales and the coccygeal ligament, anchor the spinal cord and

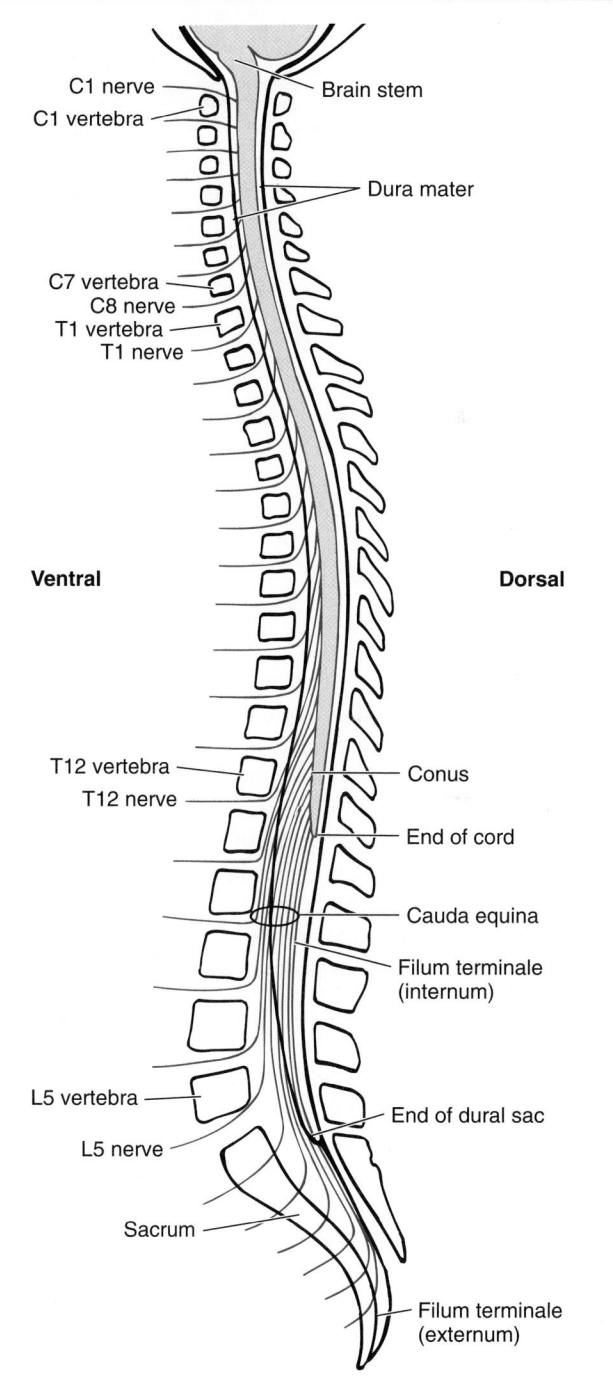

FIGURE 2-2 Schematic illustration of the spinal cord. (Reproduced with permission from Waxman SG. *Correlative Neuroanatomy*. 24th ed. New York, NY: McGraw-Hill; 1996.)

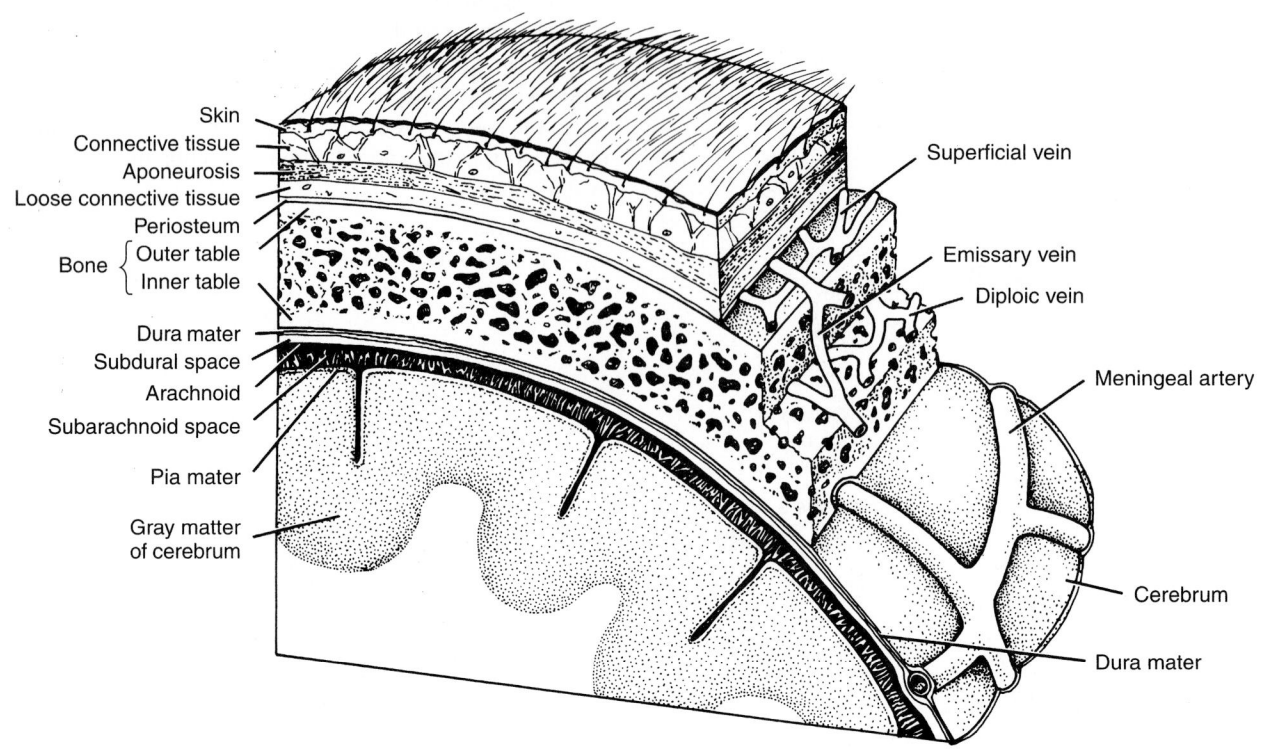

FIGURE 2-3 Schematic illustration of the relationship of the dura mater, arachnoid, and pia mater. (Reproduced with permission from Booher JM, Thibodeau GA. *Athletic Injury Assessment*. New York, NY: McGraw-Hill; 2000.)

dural sac inferiorly and ensure that tensile forces applied to the spinal cord are distributed throughout its entire length.[3]

Three membranes, or meninges, envelop the structures of the central nervous system: the dura mater, arachnoid, and pia mater (Fig. 2-3). The meninges, and related spaces, are important to both the nutrition and the protection of the spinal cord. The cerebrospinal fluid that flows through the meningeal spaces, and within the ventricles of the brain, provides a cushion for the spinal cord. The meninges also form barriers that resist the entrance of a variety of noxious organisms (see Chap. 9).

Dura Mater

The dura mater (Latin, tough mother) is the outermost and strongest of the layers and is composed of an inner meningeal layer and an outermost periosteal layer. The dura runs uninterrupted from the interior of the cranium through the foramen magnum and surrounds the spinal cord throughout its distribution from the cranium to the coccyx at the second sacral level (S2).[3] The dura also is attached to the posterior surfaces of C2 and C3.[4]

The dura forms a vertical sac (dural sac) around the spinal cord, and its short lateral projections blend with the epineurium of the spinal nerves. The dura is separated from the bones and ligaments that form the walls of the vertebral canal by an epidural space, which can become partly calcified or even ossified with age.[2]

Arachnoid

The arachnoid is a thin and delicate avascular layer, coextensive with the dura mater and the pia mater. Even though the arachnoid and pia mater are interconnected by trabeculae, there is a space between them, called the subarachnoid space, which contains the cerebrospinal fluid. The supposedly rhythmic flow of this cerebrospinal fluid is the rationale used by craniosacral therapists to explain their techniques, although there is no evidence of this finding in the literature.

Pia Mater

The pia mater is the deepest of the layers. It is intimately related and firmly attached, via connective tissue investments, to the outer surface of the spinal cord and nerve roots. The pia mater conveys the blood vessels that supply the spinal cord and has a series of lateral specializations, the denticulate (dentate) ligaments, which anchor the spinal cord to the dura mater.[3] These ligaments, which derive their name from their toothlike appearance, extend the whole length of the spinal cord.

There are no connective tissue components in the spinal nerves comparable to the epineurium and perineurium of the peripheral nerve (see later discussion); at least they are not developed to the same degree.[5] As a result, the spinal nerve roots are more sensitive to both tension and compression. The spinal nerve roots also are devoid of lymphatics and thus are predisposed to prolonged inflammation.[6]

The spinal cord has an external segmental organization. Each of the 31 pairs of spinal nerves that arise from the spinal cord has a ventral root and a dorsal root, with each root made up of 1 to 8 rootlets and consisting of bundles of nerve fibers.[2] In the dorsal root of a typical spinal nerve lies a dorsal root ganglion, a swelling that contains nerve cell bodies.[2]

Peripheral Nervous System: Somatic Nerves

The peripheral nervous system consists of the cranial nerves and the spinal nerves.

Cranial Nerves

The cranial nerves (CN) typically are described as comprising 12 pairs, which are referred to by the Roman numerals I through XII. The cranial nerve roots enter and exit the brain stem to provide sensory and motor innervation to the head and muscles of the face. CN I (olfactory) and CN II (optic) are not true nerves but rather fiber tracts of the brain. The examination of the cranial nerve system is described later in this chapter, in the section entitled "Neurologic Testing."

CN I (Olfactory)

The olfactory tract arises from the olfactory bulb on the inferior aspect of the frontal lobe, just above the cribriform plate. From here, it continues posteriorly as the olfactory tract and terminates just lateral to the optic chiasm.

The olfactory nerve is responsible for the sense of smell.

CN II (Optic)

The fibers of the optic nerve arise from the inner layer of the retina and proceed posteriorly to enter the cranial cavity via the optic foramen, to form the optic chiasm. The fibers from the nasal half of the retina decussate within the optic chiasm, whereas those from the lateral half do not.

The optic nerve is responsible for vision.

CN III (Oculomotor)

The oculomotor nerve arises in the oculomotor nucleus and leaves the brain on the medial aspect of the cerebral peduncle. It then extends from the interpeduncular fossa and runs between the posterior cerebral artery and the superior cerebellar artery before leaving the cranial cavity and entering the cavernous sinus by way of the superior orbital fissure.

The somatic portion of the oculomotor nerve supplies the levator palpebrae superioris muscle; the superior, medial, and inferior rectus muscles; and the inferior oblique muscles. These muscles are responsible for some eye movements. The visceral efferent portion of this nerve innervates two smooth intraocular muscles: the ciliary and the constrictor pupillae. These muscles are responsible for papillary constriction.

CN IV (Trochlear)

The trochlear nerve arises from the trochlear nucleus, just caudal to the oculomotor nucleus at the anterior border of the periaqueductal gray matter. The fibers cross within the midbrain and then emerge contralaterally on the posterior surface of the brain stem before entering the orbit via the superior orbital fissure to supply the superior oblique muscle.

Note: Because nerves III, IV, and VI are generally examined together, CN V is described after CN VI.

CN VI (Abducens)

The abducens nerve originates from the abducens nucleus within the inferior aspect of the pons. Its long intracranial course to the superior orbital fissure makes it vulnerable to pathology in the posterior and middle cranial fossa. The nerve innervates the lateral rectus muscle.

CN V (Trigeminal)

The trigeminal nerve is so named because of its tripartite division into the maxillary, ophthalmic, and mandibular branches. All three of these branches contain sensory cells, but the ophthalmic and maxillary are exclusively sensory, the latter supplying the soft and hard palate, maxillary sinuses, upper teeth and upper lip, and mucous membrane of the pharynx. The mandibular branch carries sensory information but also represents the motor component of the nerve, supplying the muscles of mastication, both pterygoids, the anterior belly of digastric, tensor tympani, tensor veli palatini, and mylohyoid.

The spinal nucleus and tract of the trigeminal nerve cannot be distinguished either histologically or on the basis of afferent reception from the cervical nerves. Consequently, the entire column can be viewed as a single nucleus and legitimately may be called the trigeminocervical nucleus.[7]

CN VII (Facial)

The facial nerve is made up of a sensory (intermediate) root, which conveys taste, and a motor root, the facial nerve proper, which supplies the muscles of facial expression, the platysma muscle, and the stapedius muscle of the inner ear. The intermediate root, together with the motor nerve and CN VIII, travels through the internal acoustic meatus to enter the facial canal of the temporal bone. From here, the intermediate nerve swells to form the geniculate ganglion and gives off the greater superficial petrosal nerve, which eventually innervates the lacrimal and salivary glands via the pterygopalatine ganglion and the chorda tympani nerve, respectively. The facial nerve proper exits the skull through the stylomastoid foramen.

CN VIII (Vestibulocochlear)

The vestibulocochlear nerve subserves two different senses: balance and hearing. The cochlear portion of the nerve arises from spiral ganglia and the vestibular portion arises from the vestibular ganglia in the labyrinth of the inner ear. The cochlear portion is concerned with the sense of hearing, whereas the vestibular portion is part of the system of equilibrium, the vestibular system.

The vestibular system includes the vestibular apparatus of the inner ear, the vestibular nuclei and their neural projections, and the exteroreceptors throughout the body, especially in the upper cervical spine and the eyes.[8]

FIGURE 2-4 The semicircular canals. (Reproduced with permission from Kandel ER, Schwartz JH, Jessell TM. *Principles of Neural Science.* New York, NY: McGraw-Hill; 2000.)

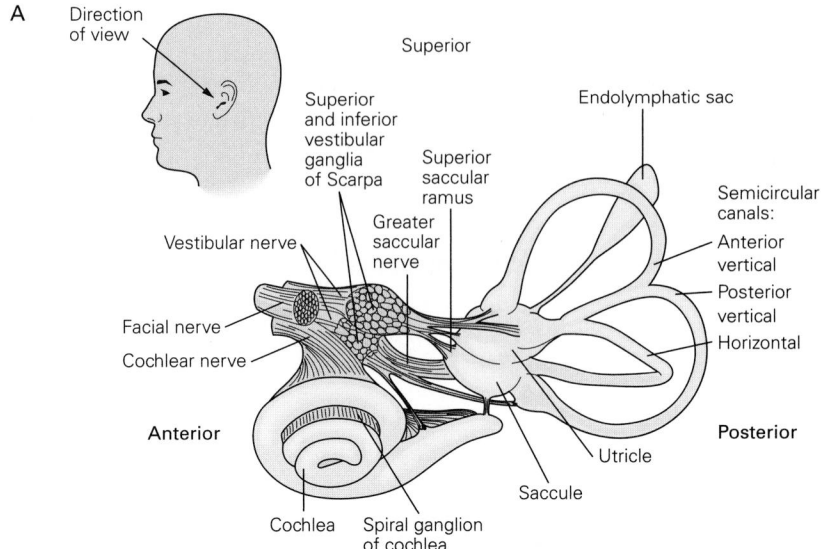

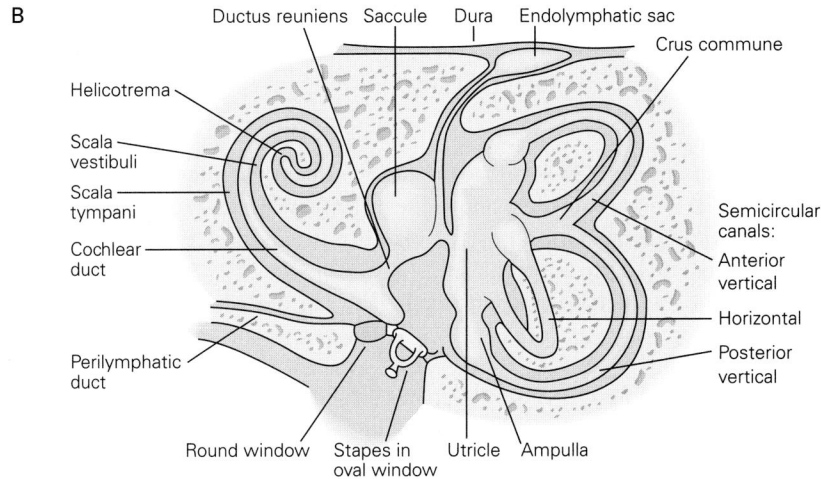

The apparatus of the inner ear consists of the static labyrinth, which comprises three semicircular canals (Fig. 2-4), each orientated at right angles to the other. The labyrinth includes specialized sensory areas that are located in the utricle and the saccule (Fig. 2-5), within which otoliths are located (Fig. 2-6).

A series of filaments line the basement membrane of the semicircular canals and project into endolymph, which deforms these filaments when head motion occurs. This deformation is registered by receptor cells, and when sudden perturbations occur, the frequency of nerve impulses along the afferent nerve supply of the cell body is altered.

Unlike the filaments of the semicircular canals, the filaments of the utricle and saccule do not project into endolymph, but instead insert into a gelatinous mass, within which is embedded the otolith. Deformation of these filaments is produced by the weight of the otolith against the cilia as the gelatinous mass is displaced during head movement.

The otoliths are responsible for providing information about gravitational forces, as well as vertical and horizontal motion: the filaments of the saccule also provide information about vertical motion. At rest, the endolymphatic fluid, or the gelatinous membrane, is stationary. When motion of the head occurs, the endolymphatic fluid, or the gelatinous membrane, initially remains stationary because of its inertia, while the canals move. This relative motion produces a dragging effect on the filaments, and either increases or decreases the discharge rate, depending on the direction of shear. At the end of the head movement, the fluid and membrane continue to move, and the cilia are now dragged in the opposite direction before coming to rest. In essence, the semicircular canal receptors transmit a positive signal when movement begins, no signal when the motion has finished, and a normal level after the sensory cell has returned to its original position. As this occurs, other sensory cells orientated in the opposite direction react in the reverse fashion.

FIGURE 2-5   The utricle. (Reproduced with permission from Kandel ER, Schwartz JH, Jessell TM. *Principles of Neural Science*. New York, NY: McGraw-Hill; 2000.)

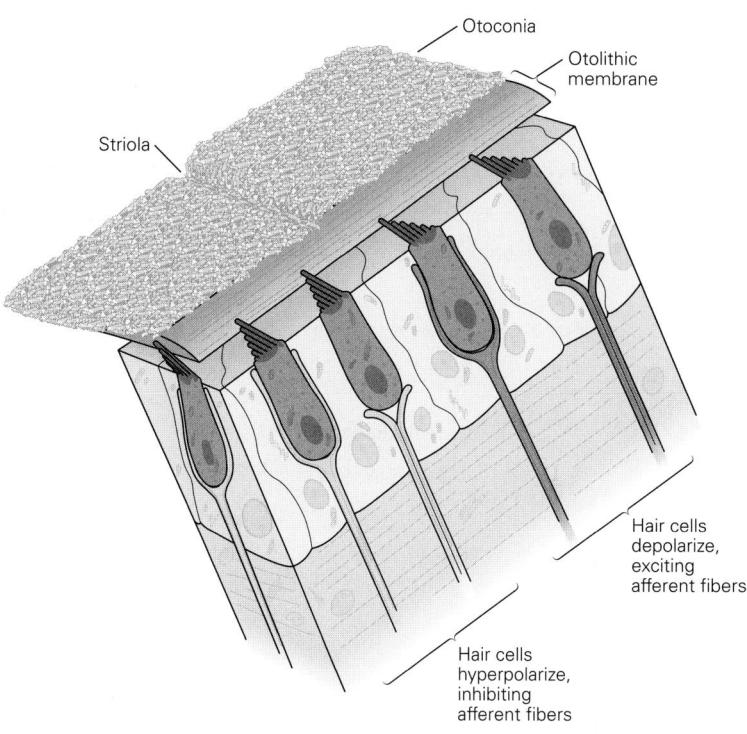

Clinical Pearl

The semicircular canal detectors are so sensitive that they can detect angular accelerations as low as 0.2 degrees per second,[9] a rate of acceleration that would turn the head through 90 degrees in 30 seconds and produce a terminal velocity of 6 degrees per second: about as fast as the movement of the second hand of a watch.[10]

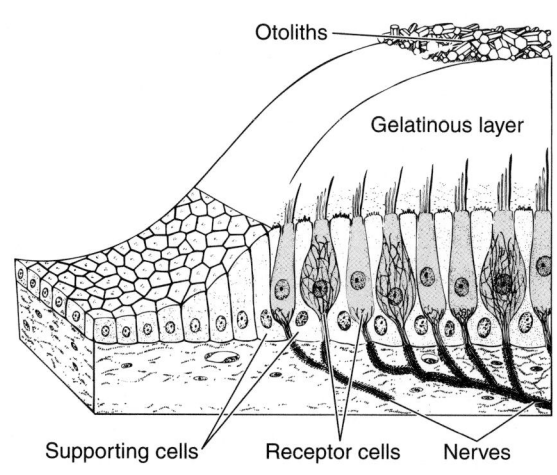

FIGURE 2-6   Macular structure. (Reproduced with permission from Waxman SG. *Correlative Neuroanatomy*. 24th ed. New York, NY: McGraw-Hill; 1996.)

CN IX (Glossopharyngeal)

The glossopharyngeal nerve contains somatic motor, visceral efferent, visceral sensory, and somatic sensory fibers. The motor fibers originate in the nucleus ambiguous, leaving the lateral medulla to join the sensory nerve, which arises from cells in the superior and petrous ganglia. The glossopharyngeal nerve exits the skull through the jugular foramen and serves a number of functions, including supplying taste fibers for the posterior third of the tongue.

CN X (Vagus)

The vagus nerve contains somatic motor, visceral efferent, visceral sensory, and somatic sensory fibers. The functions of the vagus nerve are numerous (Fig. 2-7).

CN XI (Accessory)

The accessory nerve consists of a cranial component and a spinal component. The cranial root originates in the nucleus ambiguous and is often viewed as an aberrant portion of the vagus nerve. The spinal portion of the nerve arises from the lateral parts of the anterior horns of the first five or six cervical cord segments and ascends through the foramen magnum. The spinal portion of the accessory nerve supplies the sternocleidomastoid and the trapezius muscles.

CN XII (Hypoglossal)

The hypoglossal nerve is the motor nerve of the tongue, innervating the ipsilateral side of the tongue as well as forming the descendens hypoglossi, which anastomoses with other cervical branches to form the ansa hypoglossi. The latter, in turn, innervates the infrahyoid muscles.

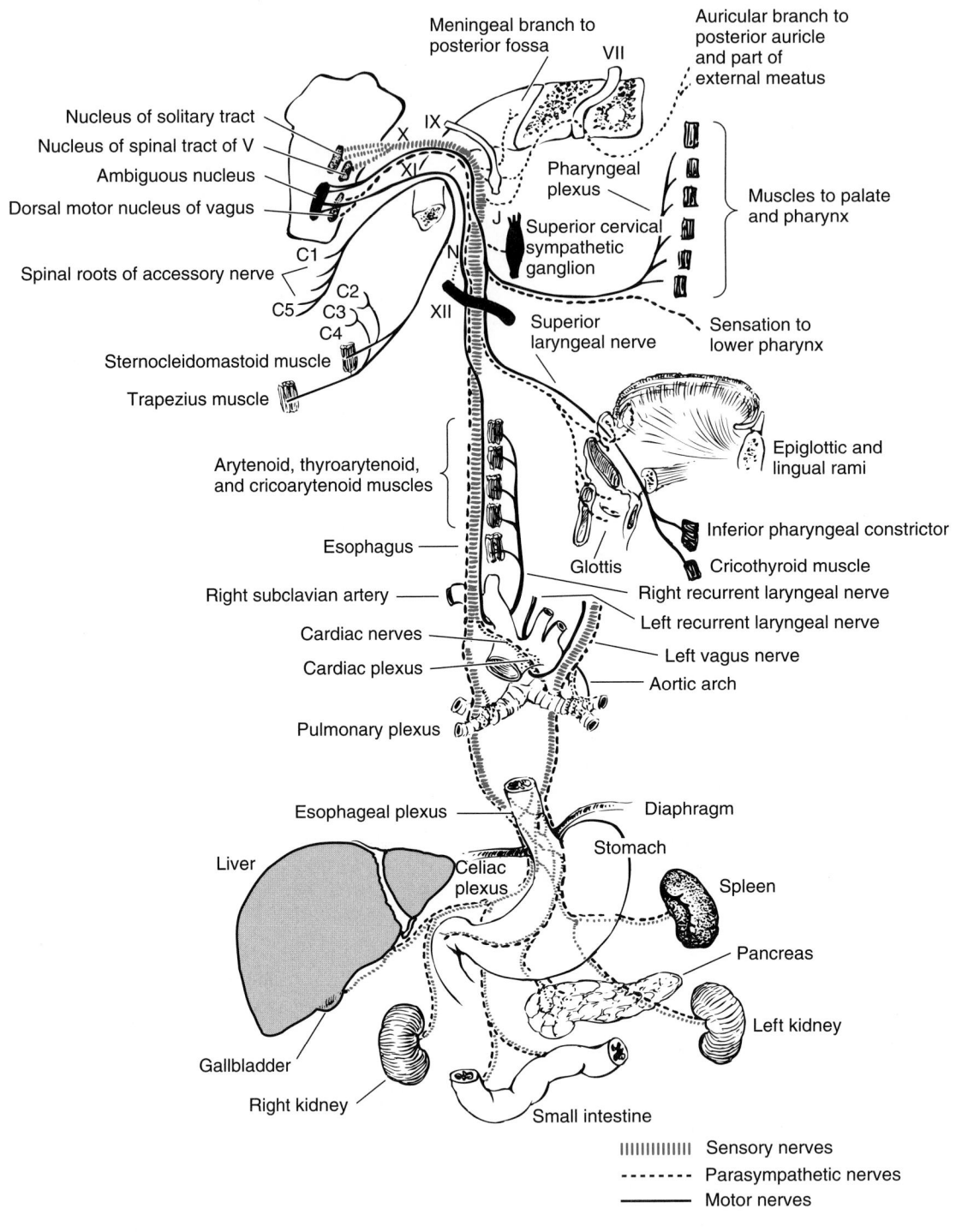

FIGURE 2-7　The vagus nerve. (Reproduced with permission from Waxman SG. *Correlative Neuroanatomy.* 24th ed. New York, NY: McGraw-Hill; 1996.)

Spinal Nerves

There are a total of 31 symmetrically arranged pairs of spinal nerves each derived from the spinal cord.[7] The spinal nerves are divided topographically into 8 cervical pairs (C1–8), 12 thoracic pairs (T1–12), 5 lumbar pairs (L1–5), 5 sacral pairs (S1–5), and a coccygeal pair (Fig. 2-8).

The dorsal and ventral roots of the spinal nerves are located within the vertebral canal. The portion of the spinal nerve that is not within the vertebral canal, and that usually occupies the intervertebral foramen, is referred to as a peripheral nerve. As the nerve roots begin to exit the vertebral canal, they must penetrate the dura mater before passing through dural sleeves

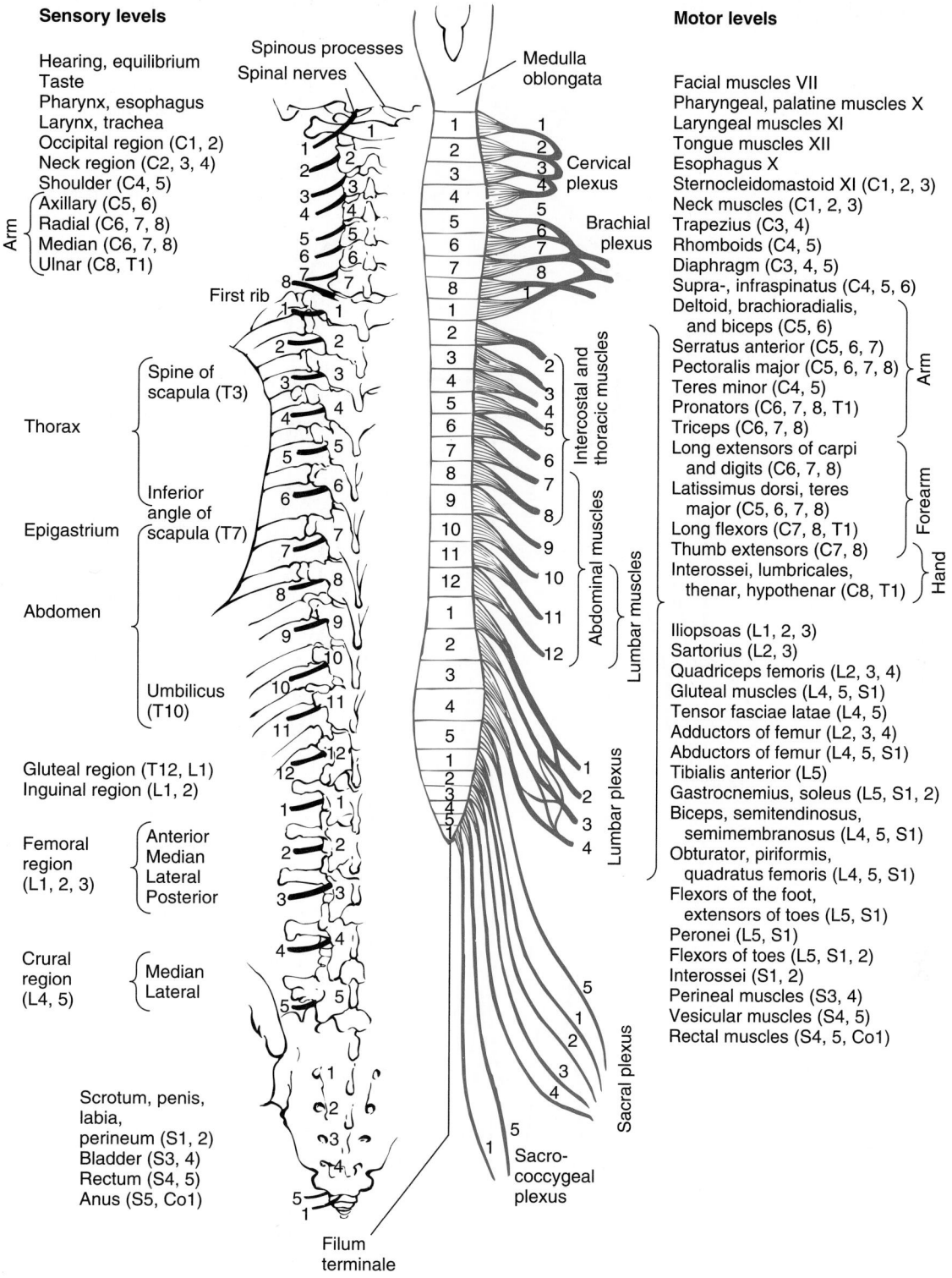

Sensory levels

Hearing, equilibrium
Taste
Pharynx, esophagus
Larynx, trachea
Occipital region (C1, 2)
Neck region (C2, 3, 4)
Shoulder (C4, 5)
Arm {
  Axillary (C5, 6)
  Radial (C6, 7, 8)
  Median (C6, 7, 8)
  Ulnar (C8, T1)
}

First rib

Spine of scapula (T3)

Thorax

Inferior angle of scapula (T7)

Epigastrium

Abdomen

Umbilicus (T10)

Gluteal region (T12, L1)
Inguinal region (L1, 2)

Femoral region (L1, 2, 3) {
  Anterior
  Median
  Lateral
  Posterior
}

Crural region (L4, 5) {
  Median
  Lateral
}

Scrotum, penis, labia, perineum (S1, 2)
Bladder (S3, 4)
Rectum (S4, 5)
Anus (S5, Co1)

Spinous processes
Spinal nerves

Medulla oblongata

Cervical plexus

Brachial plexus

Intercostal and thoracic muscles

Abdominal muscles

Lumbar muscles

Lumbar plexus

Sacral plexus

Sacro-coccygeal plexus

Filum terminale

Motor levels

Facial muscles VII
Pharyngeal, palatine muscles X
Laryngeal muscles XI
Tongue muscles XII
Esophagus X
Sternocleidomastoid XI (C1, 2, 3)
Neck muscles (C1, 2, 3)
Trapezius (C3, 4)
Rhomboids (C4, 5)
Diaphragm (C3, 4, 5)
Supra-, infraspinatus (C4, 5, 6)
Deltoid, brachioradialis, and biceps (C5, 6)   }
Serratus anterior (C5, 6, 7)   }
Pectoralis major (C5, 6, 7, 8)   } Arm
Teres minor (C4, 5)   }
Pronators (C6, 7, 8, T1)   }
Triceps (C6, 7, 8)
Long extensors of carpi and digits (C6, 7, 8)   }
Latissimus dorsi, teres major (C5, 6, 7, 8)   } Forearm
Long flexors (C7, 8, T1)   }
Thumb extensors (C7, 8)   }
Interossei, lumbricales, thenar, hypothenar (C8, T1)   } Hand

Iliopsoas (L1, 2, 3)
Sartorius (L2, 3)
Quadriceps femoris (L2, 3, 4)
Gluteal muscles (L4, 5, S1)
Tensor fasciae latae (L4, 5)
Adductors of femur (L2, 3, 4)
Abductors of femur (L4, 5, S1)
Tibialis anterior (L5)
Gastrocnemius, soleus (L5, S1, 2)
Biceps, semitendinosus, semimembranosus (L4, 5, S1)
Obturator, piriformis, quadratus femoris (L4, 5, S1)
Flexors of the foot, extensors of toes (L5, S1)
Peronei (L5, S1)
Flexors of toes (L5, S1, 2)
Interossei (S1, 2)
Perineal muscles (S3, 4)
Vesicular muscles (S4, 5)
Rectal muscles (S4, 5, Co1)

FIGURE 2-8   Motor and sensory levels of the spinal cord. (Reproduced with permission from Waxman SG. *Correlative Neuroanatomy.* 24th ed. New York, NY: McGraw-Hill; 1996.)

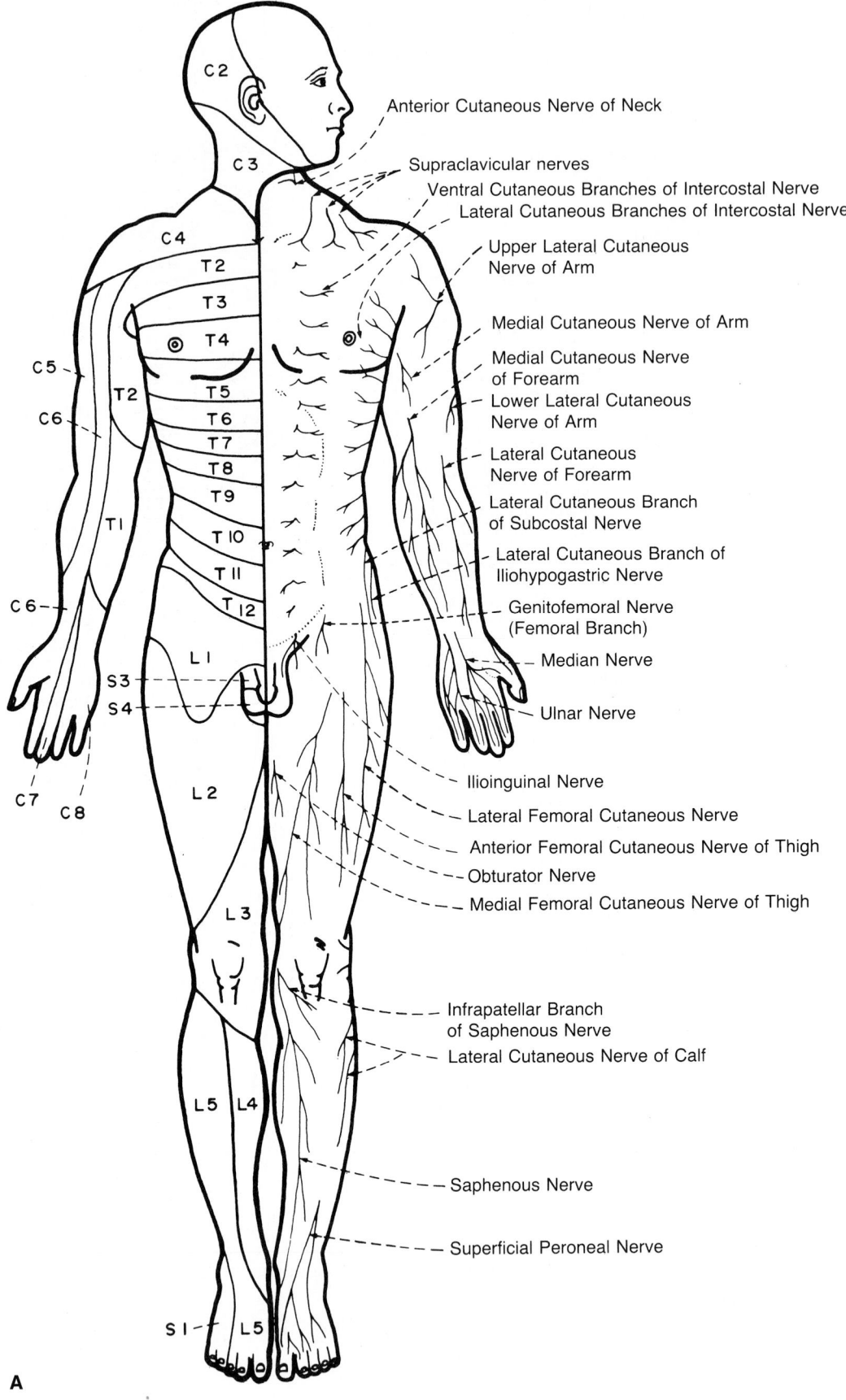

FIGURE 2-9 Segmental distribution of the body. (Reproduced with permission from Wilkins RH, Gengachary SS, eds. *Neurosurgery*. New York, NY: McGraw-Hill; 1996.)

Anterior Cutaneous Nerve of Neck

Supraclavicular nerves
Ventral Cutaneous Branches of Intercostal Nerve
Lateral Cutaneous Branches of Intercostal Nerve

Upper Lateral Cutaneous Nerve of Arm

Medial Cutaneous Nerve of Arm

Medial Cutaneous Nerve of Forearm
Lower Lateral Cutaneous Nerve of Arm

Lateral Cutaneous Nerve of Forearm

Lateral Cutaneous Branch of Subcostal Nerve

Lateral Cutaneous Branch of Iliohypogastric Nerve

Genitofemoral Nerve (Femoral Branch)

Median Nerve

Ulnar Nerve

Ilioinguinal Nerve

Lateral Femoral Cutaneous Nerve

Anterior Femoral Cutaneous Nerve of Thigh

Obturator Nerve

Medial Femoral Cutaneous Nerve of Thigh

Infrapatellar Branch of Saphenous Nerve

Lateral Cutaneous Nerve of Calf

Saphenous Nerve

Superficial Peroneal Nerve

A

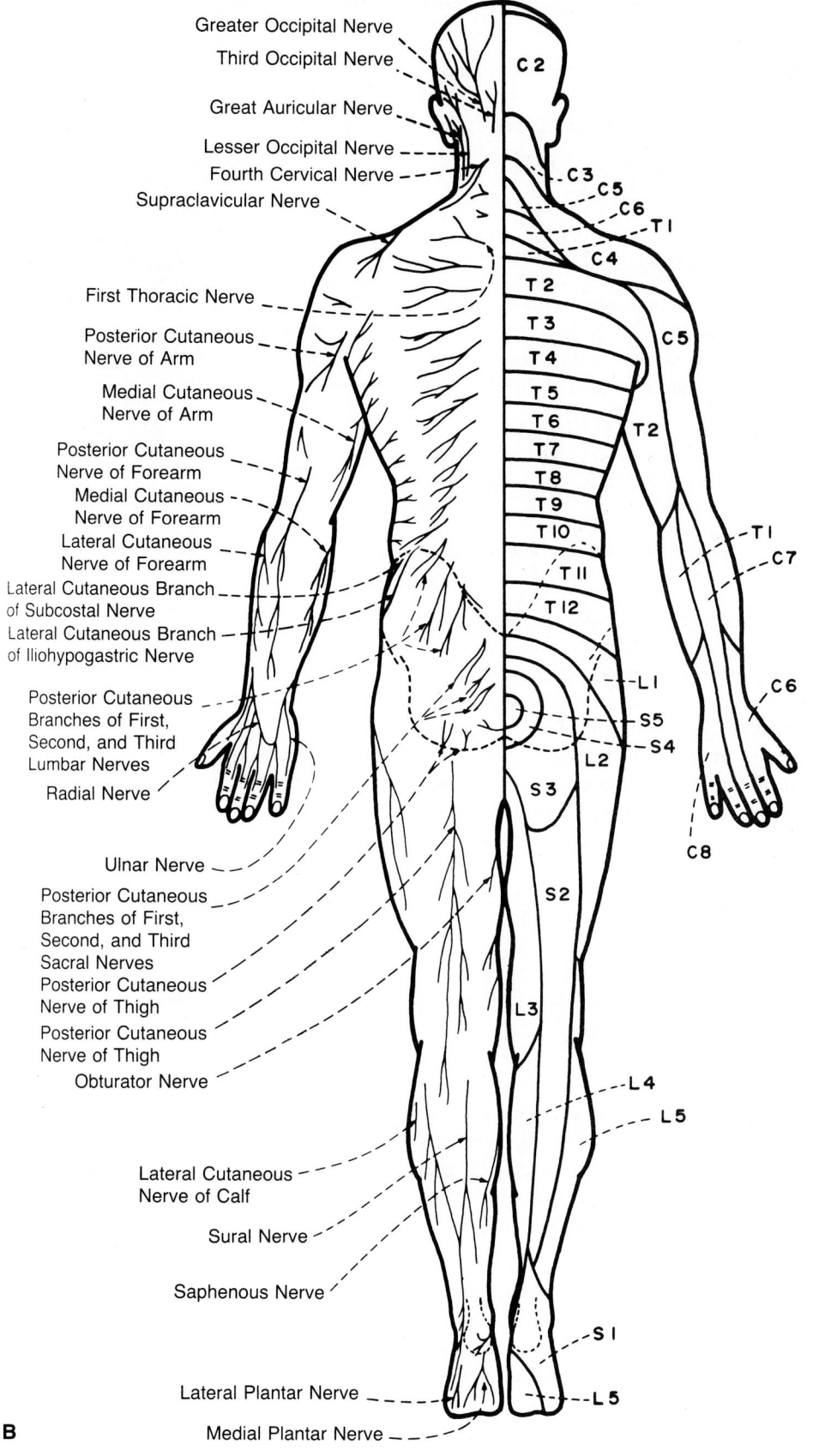

Greater Occipital Nerve

Third Occipital Nerve

Great Auricular Nerve

Lesser Occipital Nerve

Fourth Cervical Nerve

Supraclavicular Nerve

First Thoracic Nerve

Posterior Cutaneous
Nerve of Arm

Medial Cutaneous
Nerve of Arm

Posterior Cutaneous
Nerve of Forearm

Medial Cutaneous
Nerve of Forearm

Lateral Cutaneous
Nerve of Forearm

Lateral Cutaneous Branch
of Subcostal Nerve

Lateral Cutaneous Branch
of Iliohypogastric Nerve

Posterior Cutaneous
Branches of First,
Second, and Third
Lumbar Nerves

Radial Nerve

Ulnar Nerve

Posterior Cutaneous
Branches of First,
Second, and Third
Sacral Nerves

Posterior Cutaneous
Nerve of Thigh

Posterior Cutaneous
Nerve of Thigh

Obturator Nerve

Lateral Cutaneous
Nerve of Calf

Sural Nerve

Saphenous Nerve

Lateral Plantar Nerve

Medial Plantar Nerve

C 2

C 3
C 5
C 6
T 1
C 4

T 2
T 3
T 4
T 5
T 6
T 7
T 8
T 9
T 10
T 11
T 12

C 5

T 2

T 1
C 7

C 6

L 1
S 5
S 4
L 2
S 3

C 8

S 2

L 3

L 4
L 5

S 1
L 5

B

within the intervertebral foramen. The dural sleeves are continuous with the epineurium of the nerves.

Essentially, there are four branches of spinal nerves[2]:

1. **Primary dorsal.** This type usually consists of a medial sensory branch and a lateral motor branch.

2. **Primary ventral.** The primary ventral division forms the cervical, brachial, and lumbosacral plexuses.

3. **Communicating ramus.** The rami serve as a connection between the spinal nerves and the sympathetic trunk. Only the thoracic and upper lumbar nerves contain a white ramus communicans, but the gray ramus is present in all spinal nerves.

4. Meningeal or recurrent meningeal (also known as sinuvertebral). These nerves carry sensory and vasomotor innervation to the meninges.

Nerve fibers can be categorized according to function: sensory, motor, or mixed.

▶ *Sensory nerves.* The sensory nerves carry afferents from a portion of the skin. They also carry efferents to the skin structures. When a sensory nerve is compressed, the symptoms occur in the area of the nerve distribution. This area of distribution, called a dermatome, is a well-defined segmental portion of the skin (Fig. 2-9) and generally follows the segmental distribution of the underlying muscle innervation.[2] Examples of sensory nerves in the body are the lateral femoral cutaneous nerve, the saphenous nerve, and the interdigital nerves.

> ### Clinical Pearl
>
> Most individuals have no C1 dorsal root; therefore, there is no C1 dermatome. When present, the C1 dermatome covers a small area in the central part of the neck close to the occiput.[2]

▶ *Motor nerves.* The motor nerves carry efferents to muscles and return sensation from muscles and associated ligamentous structures. Any nerve that innervates a muscle also mediates the sensation from the joint upon which that muscle acts. Examples of a motor nerve include the suprascapular nerve and the dorsal scapular nerve.

▶ *Mixed nerves.* A mixed nerve is a combination of skin, sensory, and motor fibers to one trunk. Some examples of a mixed nerve are the median nerve, the ulnar nerve at the elbow as it enters the tunnel of Guyon, the peroneal nerve at the knee, and the ilioinguinal nerve.

Peripheral nerves are enclosed in three layers of tissue of differing character. From the inside outward, these are the endoneurium, perineurium, and epineurium (Fig. 2-10).[11] Nerve fibers embedded in endoneurium form a funiculus surrounded by perineurium, a thin but strong sheath of connective tissue. The nerve bundles are embedded in a loose areolar

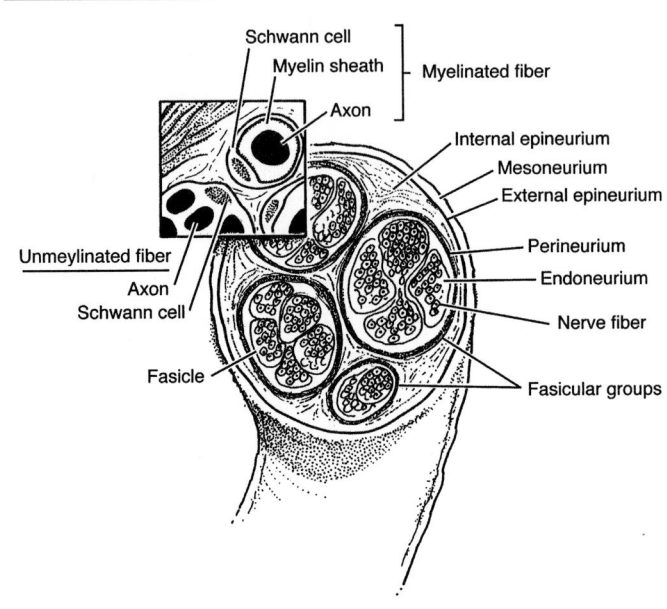

FIGURE 2-10 The epineurium, perineurium, and endoneurium. (Reproduced with permission from Dee R, Hurst LC, Gruber MA, Kottmeier SA, et al., eds. *Principles of Orthopaedic Practice.* New York, NY: McGraw-Hill; 1997.)

connective tissue framework called the epineurium (see Fig. 2-10). The epineurium that extends between the fascicles is termed the inner or interfascicular epineurium, whereas that surrounding the entire nerve trunk is called the epifascicular epineurium.[12] The connective tissue outside the epineurium is referred to as the adventitia of the nerve or epineural tissue.[12] Although the epineurium is continuous with the surrounding connective tissue, its attachment is loose, so that nerve trunks are relatively mobile except where tethered by entering vessels or exiting nerve branches.[13]

Cervical Nerves

The eight pairs of cervical nerves are derived from cord segments between the level of the foramen magnum and the middle of the seventh cervical vertebra.[14] The spinal nerves from C3 to C7, exiting from the intervertebral foramen, divide into a larger ventral ramus and a smaller dorsal ramus. The ventral ramus of the cervical spinal nerve courses on the transverse process in an anterior-lateral direction to form the cervical plexus and brachial plexus. The dorsal ramus of the spinal nerve runs posteriorly around the superior articular process, supplying the facet joint, ligaments, deep muscles, and skin of the posterior aspect of the neck.[3]

Each nerve joins with a gray communicating ramus from the sympathetic trunk and sends a small, recurrent meningeal branch back into the spinal canal to supply the dura with sensory and vasomotor innervation. It also branches into anterior and posterior primary divisions, which are mixed nerves that pass to their respective peripheral distributions. The motor branches carry a few sensory fibers that convey proprioceptive impulses from the neck muscles.

Posterior Primary Divisions. The C1 (suboccipital) nerve is the only branch of the first posterior primary divisions. It is a motor nerve, serving the muscles of the suboccipital triangle, with very few sensory fibers.[14]

Anterior Primary Divisions. The anterior primary divisions of the first four cervical nerves (C1–4) form the cervical plexus (Fig. 2-11).

Cervical Plexus (C1–4)
Sensory Branches (see Fig. 2-11).

▶ *Small occipital nerve (C2,3).* This nerve supplies the skin of the lateral occipital portion of the scalp, the upper median part of the auricle, and the area over the mastoid process.[14]

▶ *Great auricular nerve (C2,3).* This nerve supplies sensation to the ear and face over the ascending ramus of the mandible. The nerve lies on or just below the deep layer of the investing fascia of the neck. It arises from the anterior rami of the second and third cervical nerves, and emerges from behind the sternomastoid muscle, before ascending on it to cross over the parotid gland.

▶ *Cervical cutaneous nerve (cutaneous coli) (C2,3).* This nerve supplies the skin over the anterior portion of the neck.

▶ *Supraclavicular branches (C3,4).* These nerves supply the skin over the clavicle and the upper deltoid and pectoral regions, as low as the third rib.

Communicating Branches. The ansa cervicalis nerve (see Fig. 2-11) is formed by the junction of two main nerve roots derived entirely from ventral cervical rami. A loop is formed at the point of their anastomosis, and sensory fibers are carried to the dura of the posterior fossa of the skull via the recurrent meningeal branch of the hypoglossal nerve. The communication with the vagus nerve from C1 is of undetermined function.

Muscular Branches. Communication with the hypoglossal nerve from C1 to C2 carries motor fibers to the geniohyoid and thyrohyoid muscles, and to the sternohyoid and sternothyroid muscles by way of the superior root of the ansa cervicalis (see Fig. 2-11). The nerve to the thyrohyoid branches from the hypoglossal nerve, and runs obliquely across the hyoid bone to innervate the thyrohyoid. The nerve to the superior belly of the omohyoid branches from the superior root (see Fig. 2-11), and enters the muscle at a level between the thyroid notch and a horizontal plane 2-cm inferior to the notch. The nerves to the sternohyoid and sternothyroid share a common trunk, which branches from the loop (see Fig. 2-11). The nerve to the inferior belly of the omohyoid also branches from the loop (Fig. 2-11). The loop is most frequently located just deep to the site where the superior belly (or tendon) of the omohyoid muscle crosses the internal jugular vein. There is a branch to the sternocleidomastoid muscle from C2, and branches to the trapezius muscles (C3–4) via the subtrapezial plexus.

Smaller branches to the adjacent vertebral musculature supply the rectus capitis lateralis and rectus capitis anterior (C1), the longus capitis (C2,4) and longus coli (C1–4), the scalenus medius (C3,4) and scalenus anterior (C4), and the levator scapulae (C3–5).

The phrenic nerve (C3–5) passes obliquely over the scalenus anterior muscle and between the subclavian artery and vein to enter the thorax behind the sternoclavicular joint, where it descends vertically through the superior and middle mediastinum to the diaphragm (see Fig. 2-11).[14] Motor branches supply the diaphragm. Sensory branches supply the pericardium, the diaphragm, and part of the costal and mediastinal pleurae.

Phrenic nerve involvement has been described in several neuropathies, including critical illness, polyneuropathy, Guillain-Barré syndrome, brachial neuritis, and hereditary motor and sensory neuropathy type 1.[17,18] The symptoms depend largely on the degree of involvement, and whether one or both of the nerves are involved.[14]

▶ Unilateral paralysis of the diaphragm causes few or no symptoms except with heavy exertion.

▶ Bilateral paralysis of the diaphragm is characterized by dyspnea upon the slightest exertion, and difficulty with coughing and sneezing.[17,18]

▶ Phrenic neuralgia, which results from neck tumors, aortic aneurysm, and pericardial or other mediastinal infections, is characterized by pain near the free border of the ribs, beneath the clavicle, and deep in the neck.[17,18]

Brachial Plexus
The brachial plexus (Fig. 2-12) arises from the anterior primary divisions of the fifth cervical through the first thoracic nerve roots, with occasional contributions from the fourth cervical and second thoracic roots. The roots of the plexus, which consist of C5 and C6, join to form the upper trunk, C7 becomes the middle trunk, and C8 and T1 join to form the lower trunks. Each of the trunks divides into anterior and posterior divisions, which then form cords (see Fig. 2-12). The anterior divisions of the upper and middle trunk form the lateral cord, the anterior division of the lower trunk forms the medial cord, and all three posterior divisions unite to form the posterior cord. The three

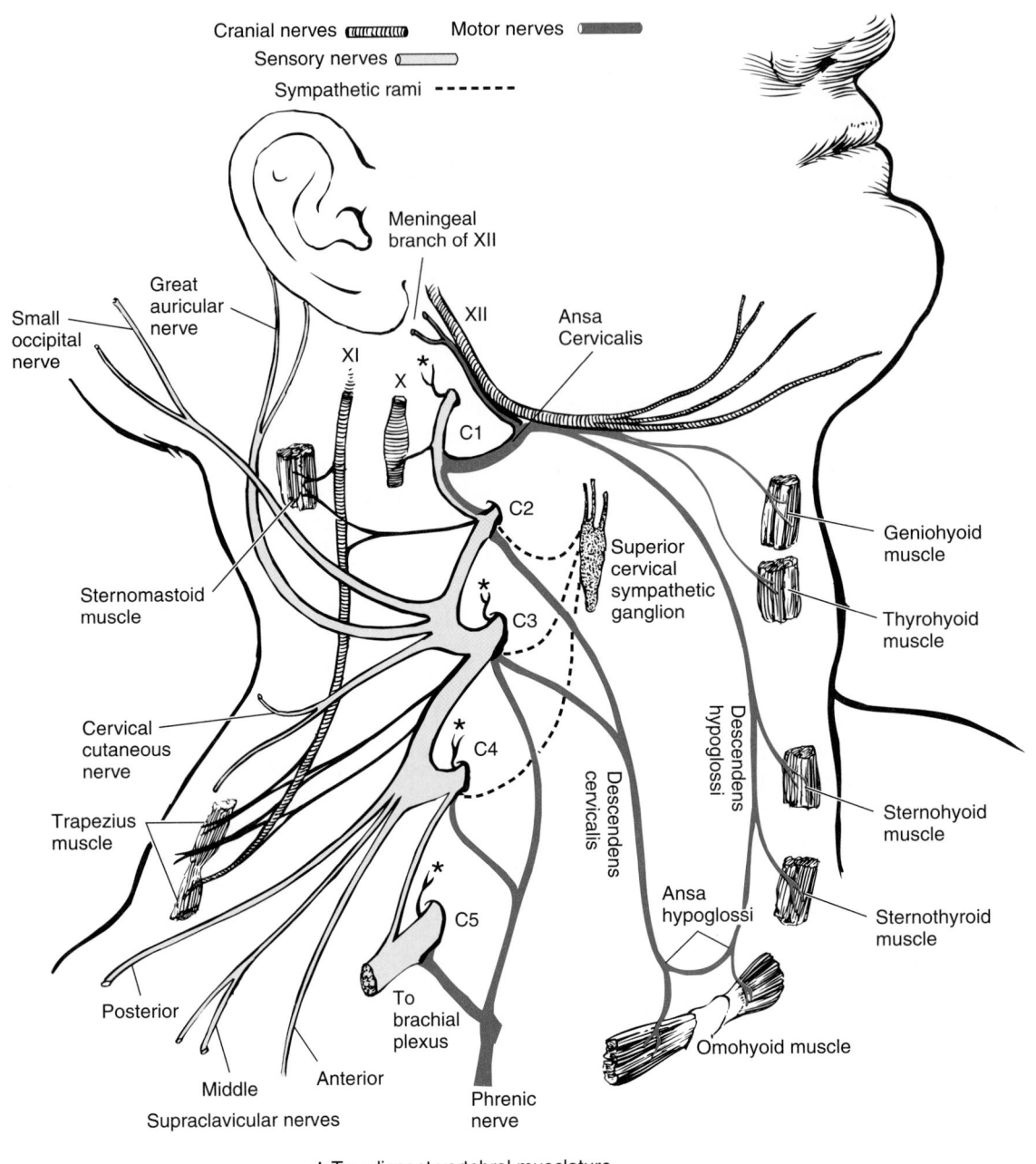

FIGURE 2-11   The cervical plexus. (Reproduced with permission from Waxman SG. *Correlative Neuroanatomy*. 24th ed. New York, NY: McGraw-Hill; 1996.)

cords, named for their relationship to the axillary artery, split to form the main branches of the plexus. These branches give rise to the peripheral nerves: musculocutaneous (lateral cord), axillary and radial (posterior cord), ulnar (medial cord), and median (medial and lateral cords).[19] Numerous smaller nerves arise from the roots, trunks, and cords of the plexus.

From the Roots

1. The origin of the dorsal scapular nerve (C5) frequently shares a common trunk with the long thoracic nerve (see

Fig. 2-12). The former passes through the scalenus medius anterior internally, and posterior, laterally, with the presence of some tendinous tissues. Leaving the long thoracic nerve, it often gives branches to the shoulder and the subaxillary region, before the branches join the long thoracic nerve again. The dorsal scapular nerve supplies the rhomboids and levator scapulae muscles.

2. The long thoracic nerve (C5–7) is purely a motor nerve that originates from the ventral rami of the fifth, sixth, and seventh cervical roots (see Fig. 2-12). It is the sole innervation to the serratus anterior muscle. The fifth and sixth cervical

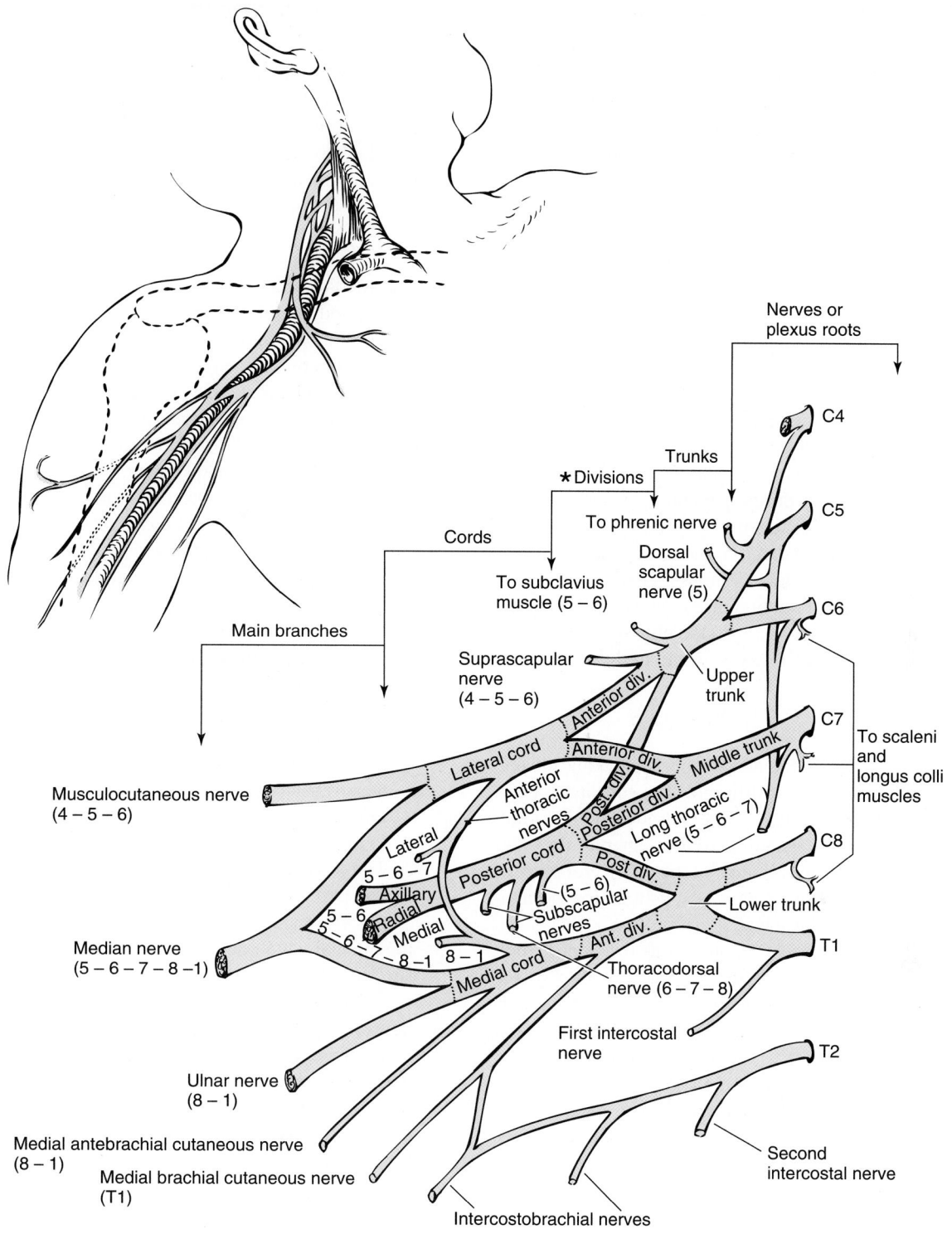

Nerves or plexus roots

C4

C5

To phrenic nerve

Dorsal scapular nerve (5)

★Divisions

Trunks

Cords

To subclavius muscle (5 – 6)

Suprascapular nerve (4 – 5 – 6)

Upper trunk

C6

Main branches

Anterior div.

Lateral cord

Anterior div.

Middle trunk

C7

To scaleni and longus colli muscles

Musculocutaneous nerve (4 – 5 – 6)

Anterior thoracic nerves

Post. div.

Posterior div.

Long thoracic nerve (5 – 6 – 7)

Lateral 5 – 6 – 7

Axillary 5 – 6

Radial

Posterior cord

Post. div.

(5 – 6) Subscapular nerves

C8

Lower trunk

Median nerve (5 – 6 – 7 – 8 –1)

5 – 6 – 7 – 8 –1

Medial 8 – 1

Ant. div.

Medial cord

Thoracodorsal nerve (6 – 7 – 8)

T1

Ulnar nerve (8 – 1)

First intercostal nerve

T2

Medial antebrachial cutaneous nerve (8 – 1)

Medial brachial cutaneous nerve (T1)

Second intercostal nerve

Intercostobrachial nerves

★ Splitting of the plexus into anterior and posterior divisions is one of the most significant features in the redistribution of nerve fibers, because it is here that fibers supplying the flexor and extensor groups of muscles of the upper extremity are separated. Similar splitting is noted in the lumbar and sacral plexuses for the supply of muscles of the lower extremity.

FIGURE 2-12   The brachial plexus. (Reproduced with permission from Waxman SG. *Correlative Neuroanatomy.* 24th ed. New York, NY: McGraw-Hill; 1996.)

roots, along with the dorsal scapular nerve, pass through the scalenus medius muscle, whereas the seventh cervical root passes anterior to it.[20] The nerve then travels beneath the brachial plexus and clavicle to pass over the first rib. From there, it descends along the lateral aspect of the chest wall, where it innervates the serratus anterior muscle. The nerve extends as far inferior as the eighth or ninth rib. Its long and relatively superficial course makes it susceptible to injury. Injury to the long thoracic nerve can occur from any of the following causes.[5,21–23]

   a. Entrapment of the fifth and sixth cervical roots as they pass through the scalenus medius muscle.

   b. Compression of the nerve during traction to the upper extremity by the undersurface of the scapula as the nerve crosses over the second rib.

   c. Compression and traction to the nerve by the inferior angle of the scapula during general anesthesia or with passive abduction of the arm.

   An injury to the long thoracic nerve may cause scapular winging; that is, the scapula assumes a position of medial translation and upward rotation of the inferior angle.[24,25]

3. A small branch from C5 passes to the phrenic nerve.

4. Smaller branches from C6 to C8 extend to the scaleni and longus coli muscles.

5. The first intercostal nerve extends from T1.

From the Trunks. A nerve extends to the subclavius muscle (C5–6) from the upper trunk, or fifth root. The subclavius muscle acts mainly on the stability of the sternoclavicular joint, with more or less intensity according to the degree of the clavicular interaction with the movements of the peripheral parts of the superior limb, and seems to act as a substitute for the ligaments of the sternoclavicular joint.[26]

   The suprascapular nerve originates from the upper trunk of the brachial plexus formed by the roots of C5 and C6 (see Fig. 2-12) at Erb's point. The nerve travels downward and laterally behind the brachial plexus and parallel to the omohyoid muscle beneath the trapezius to the superior edge of the scapula, through the suprascapular notch. The roof of the suprascapular notch is formed by the transverse scapular ligament. The notch may assume various shapes, and Rengachary and colleagues[27] describe six types of notches, depending on their configuration and enclosure. The suprascapular artery and vein initially run with the nerve and then run above the transverse suprascapular ligament over the notch. After passing through the notch, the nerve supplies the suprascapular muscle. It also provides articular branches to the glenohumeral and acromioclavicular joints and provides sensory and sympathetic fibers to two thirds of the shoulder capsule, and to the glenohumeral and acromioclavicular joints. The nerve then turns around the lateral edge of the scapular spine to innervate the infraspinatus.

   It is commonly taught that the suprascapular nerve provides the motor supply to the supraspinatus and infraspinatus muscles and sensory innervation to the shoulder joint, but that it has no cutaneous representation. However, cutaneous branches are present in the proximal one third of the arm,[28–30] and their distribution overlaps with that of the supraclavicular and axillary nerves. Pain related to suprascapular nerve entrapment may radiate to the lateral neck or posterior and lateral aspects of the shoulder capsule area.[31–35]

From the Cords

1. The medial and lateral pectoral nerves extend from the medial and lateral cords respectively (see Fig. 2-12). They supply the pectoralis major and pectoralis minor muscles. The pectoralis major muscle has dual innervation.[36] The lateral pectoral nerve (C5–7) is actually more medial in the muscle, and travels with the thoracoacromial vessels and innervates the clavicular and sternal heads. The medial pectoral nerve (C8–T1) shares a course with the lateral thoracic vessels, and provides innervation to the sternal and costal heads.[37] The main trunk of these nerves can be found near the origin of the vascular supply of the muscle.

2. The three subscapular nerves from the posterior cord consist of:

   a. The upper subscapular nerve (C5–6), which supplies the subscapularis muscle (see Fig. 2-12).

   b. The thoracodorsal nerve, or middle subscapular nerve, which arises from the posterior cord of the brachial plexus with its motor fiber contributions from C6, C7, and C8 (see Fig. 2-12). This nerve courses along the posterior-lateral chest wall, along the surface of the serratus anterior, and deep to the subscapularis, giving rise to branches that supply the latissimus dorsi.

   c. The lower subscapular nerve (C5–6) to the teres major and part of the subscapularis muscle (see Fig. 2-12).

3. Sensory branches of the medial cord (C8–T1) comprise the medial antebrachial cutaneous nerve to the medial surface of the forearm and the medial brachial cutaneous nerve to the medial surface of the arm (see Fig. 2-12). Several anatomic studies on the medial antebrachial cutaneous nerve trunk have been performed, showing variable derivation of the medial antebrachial cutaneous sensory fibers. In 1918, Kerr[38] reported that the medial antebrachial cutaneous nerve trunk branched from the medial cord in 82 percent of patients. It received contributions from the C8 and T1 segments in 97 percent of individuals, and from T1 alone in only 4 of 167 individuals. Wichman,[39] in the same year, reported 51 patients in whom the medial antebrachial cutaneous nerve trunk was derived from C8 and T1 fibers, and 38 patients in whom it was derived from T1 fibers alone.

Obstetric Brachial Plexus Lesions

The pathomorphologic spectrum of traumatic brachial plexus impairments most often includes combinations of various types of injuries: compression of spinal nerves, traction injuries of spinal roots and nerves, and avulsions of spinal roots.[195] If the rootlets are traumatically disconnected from the spinal cord, they normally exit the intradural space; in rare cases, however, they also may remain within the dural space.

Brachial plexus injuries are most commonly seen in children and usually are caused by birth injuries. Obstetric brachial plexus palsy is quite different from adult brachial plexus injury and needs a different analysis. Although the mechanisms resulting in plexus injury in both are similar (i.e., traction), in obstetric brachial plexus palsy, the traction force in energy velocity is less. Stretch (neurapraxia or axonotmesis) and incomplete rupture are more common in obstetric brachial plexus palsy than complete rupture or avulsion, which often is seen in adult brachial plexus injury. Often, there is paresis (incomplete paralysis) rather than flaccid paralysis (complete paralysis) in obstetric brachial plexus palsy. Even when there is complete rupture, the gaps are short and regeneration is still possible, whereas in adult brachial plexus injury the gaps are long and the scars are dense, which makes regeneration impossible.

Obstetrical brachial plexus palsy is classified into upper (involving C5, C6, and usually C7 roots), lower (predominantly C8 and T1), and total (C5–C8; T1) plexus palsies.[196,197] Upper brachial plexus palsy, although described first by Duchenne,[198] bears the name Erb's palsy.[199] Lower brachial plexus palsy is extremely rare in birth injuries[200] and is referred to as Klumpke's palsy.[201] Most cases of obstetric brachial plexus palsy involve Erb's palsy, and the lesion is always supraclavicular.

The infant with Erb's palsy typically shows the classic "waiter's tip" posture of the paralyzed limb.[202,203] The arm lies internally rotated at the side of the chest, the elbow is extended (paralysis of C5,6) or slightly flexed (paralysis of C5–7), the forearm is pronated, and the wrist and fingers are flexed. This posture occurs because of paralysis and atrophy of the deltoid, biceps, brachialis, and brachioradialis muscles; hence, the surgical results in patients with Erb's palsy traditionally have been expressed in terms of recovery of shoulder abduction and external rotation, elbow flexion and extension, forearm supination, and extension of the wrist, fingers, and thumb.[204]

Klumpke's paralysis is characterized by paralysis and atrophy of the small hand muscles and flexors of the wrist (so-called claw hand). Prognosis of this type is more favorable. If the sympathetic rami of T1 are involved, Horner's syndrome may be present.

Peripheral Nerves of the Upper Quadrant

Musculocutaneous Nerve (C5–6). The musculocutaneous nerve (Fig. 2-13) is the terminal branch of the lateral cord, which in turn is derived from the anterior division of the upper and middle trunks of the fifth through seventh cervical nerve roots.[40,41]

The nerve arises from the lateral cord of the brachial plexus at the level of the insertion of the pectoralis minor[41,42] and proceeds caudally and laterally, giving one or more branches to the coracobrachialis, before penetrating this muscle 3 to 8 cm below the coracoid process.[41,43] It then courses through, and supplies, the biceps brachii and brachialis muscles, before emerging between the biceps brachii and the brachioradialis muscles 2 to 5 cm above the elbow (see Fig. 2-13). At this level,

now called the lateral antebrachial cutaneous nerve, it divides into anterior and posterior divisions to innervate the anterior-lateral aspect of the forearm (Fig. 2-13).[41]

Atraumatic isolated musculocutaneous neuropathies are rare. Reported cases have been associated with positioning during general anesthesia,[44] peripheral nerve tumors,[45] and strenuous upper extremity exercise without apparent underlying disease.[46–49] Mechanisms proposed for these exercise-related cases include entrapment within the coracobrachialis,[46–48] as well as traction between a proximal fixation point at the coracobrachialis and a distal fixation point at the deep fascia at the elbow.[41]

> ### Clinical Pearl
>
> Although a musculocutaneous lesion would be expected to demonstrate weakness of elbow flexion, one would not expect to see weakness in all shoulder motions with an injury isolated to the proximal musculocutaneous nerve.

The coracobrachialis, and long and short heads of the biceps brachii, all cross the shoulder joint. They are active with shoulder flexion and abduction, and slightly active with shoulder adduction and internal rotation.[50–52] These muscles also help stabilize the shoulder joint[41] and maintain the static position of the arm.[53]

Other clinical features of musculocutaneous involvement include a loss of the biceps jerk, muscle atrophy, and loss of sensation to the anterior-lateral surface of the forearm.

Axillary Nerve (C5–6). The axillary nerve is the last nerve of the posterior cord of the brachial plexus before the latter becomes the radial nerve (see Fig. 2-13). The axillary nerve arises as one of the terminal branches of the posterior cord of the brachial plexus, with its neural origin in the fifth and sixth cervical nerve roots. The axillary nerve crosses the anterior-inferior aspect of the subscapularis muscle, where it then crosses posteriorly through the quadrilateral space and divides into two major trunks. Along its course across the subscapular muscle, the axillary nerve releases its first articular branch, which becomes separated from the main stem as it travels to the inferior-anterior glenohumeral joint capsule. The posterior trunk of the axillary nerve gives a branch to the teres minor muscle and the posterior deltoid muscle before terminating as the superior lateral brachial cutaneous nerve (see Fig. 2-13). The anterior trunk continues, giving branches to supply the middle and anterior deltoid muscle.

The axillary nerve is susceptible to injury at several sites, including the origin of the nerve from the posterior cord, the anterior-inferior aspect of the subscapularis muscle and shoulder capsule, the quadrilateral space, and within the subfascial surface of the deltoid muscle.

A deltoid paralysis causes an inability to protract or retract the arm or raise it to the horizontal position, although after some time, supplementary movements may partially take over these functions. Teres minor paralysis causes weakness of shoulder external rotation. Sensation is lost over the deltoid prominence (see Fig. 2-13).

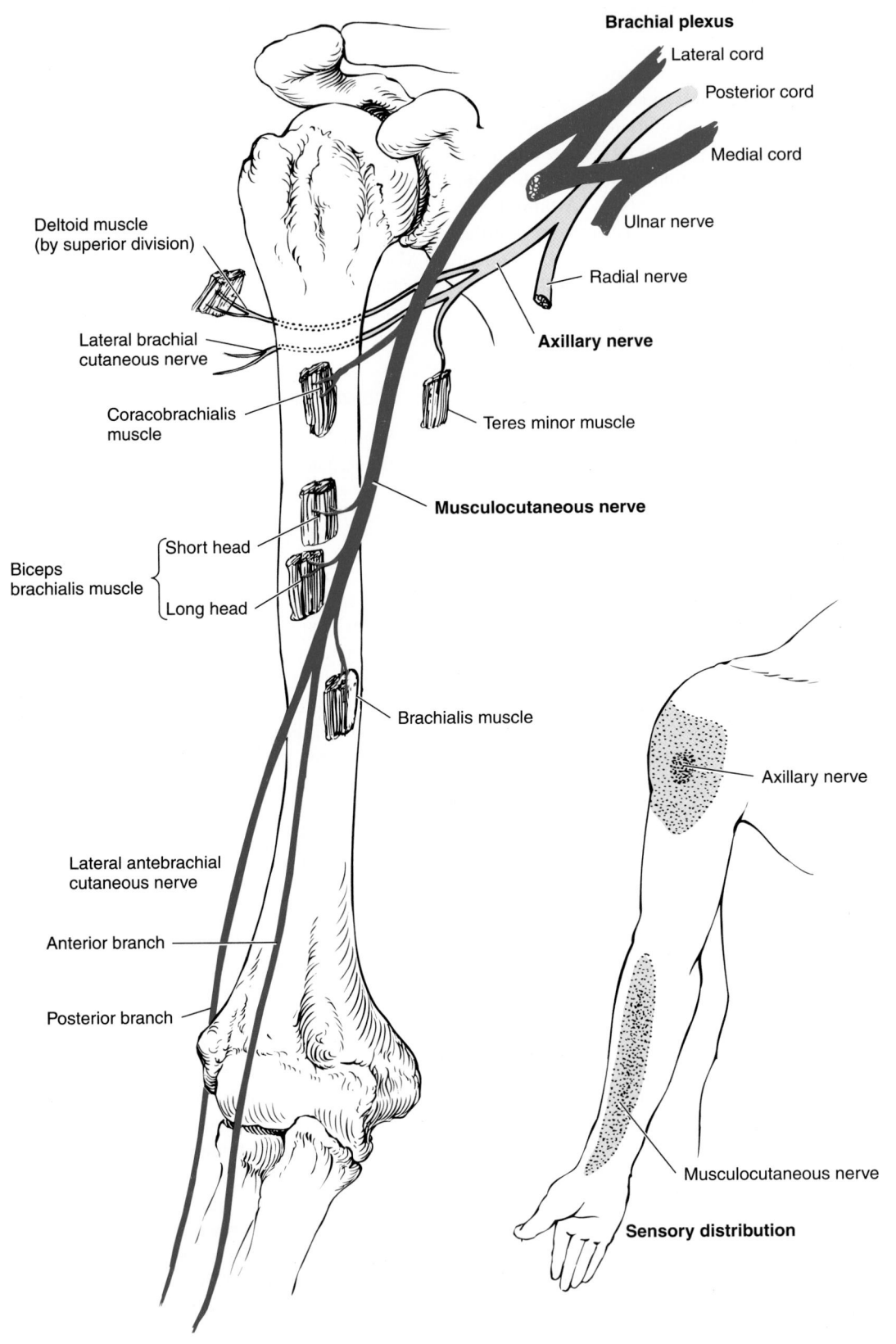

Deltoid muscle
(by superior division)

Lateral brachial
cutaneous nerve

Coracobrachialis
muscle

Biceps
brachialis muscle
{ Short head

Long head

Lateral antebrachial
cutaneous nerve

Anterior branch

Posterior branch

Brachialis muscle

Brachial plexus

Lateral cord

Posterior cord

Medial cord

Ulnar nerve

Radial nerve

Axillary nerve

Teres minor muscle

Musculocutaneous nerve

Axillary nerve

Musculocutaneous nerve

Sensory distribution

FIGURE 2-13 The musculocutaneous (C5–6) and axillary (C5–6) nerves. (Reproduced with permission from Waxman SG. *Correlative Neuroanatomy*. 24th ed. New York, NY: McGraw-Hill; 1996.)

Radial Nerve (C6–8, T1).   The radial nerve (Fig. 2-14) is the largest branch of the brachial plexus. Originating at the lower border of the pectoralis minor as the direct continuation of the posterior cord, it derives fibers from the last three cervical and first thoracic segments of the spinal cord. During its descent in the arm, the radial nerve accompanies the profunda artery behind, and around, the humerus and in the musculospiral groove. It pierces the lateral intermuscular septum and reaches the lower anterior side of the forearm, where its terminal branches arise.

> ### Clinical Pearl
> The radial nerve is frequently entrapped at its bifurcation in the region of the elbow, where the common radial nerve becomes the sensory branch and a deep or posterior interosseous branch.

The radial nerve crosses the elbow immediately anterior to the radial head, just beneath the heads of the extensor origin of the extensor carpi radialis brevis, and then divides, with the deep branch running through the body of the supinator muscle to the posterior aspect of the forearm.

The radial nerve in the arm supplies the triceps, the anconeus, and the upper portion of the extensor-supinator group of forearm muscles. In the forearm, the posterior interosseous nerve innervates all of the muscles of the six extensor compartments of the wrist, with the exception of the extensor carpi radialis brevis and extensor carpi radialis longus.

The skin areas supplied by the radial nerve include the posterior brachial cutaneous nerve, to the dorsal aspect of the arm; the posterior antebrachial cutaneous nerve, to the dorsal surface of the forearm; and the superficial radial nerve, to the dorsal aspect of the radial half of the hand (see Fig. 2-14). The isolated area of supply is a small patch of skin over the dorsum of the first interosseous space (see Fig. 2-14).

The major disability associated with radial nerve injury is a weak grip, which is weakened because of poor stabilization of the wrist and finger joints. In addition, the patient demonstrates an inability to extend the thumb, wrist, and elbow, as well as the proximal phalanges. Pronation of the forearm and adduction of the thumb also are affected, and the wrist and fingers adopt a position termed wrist drop. The triceps and other radial reflexes are absent, but the sensory loss is often slight, owing to overlapping innervation.

The site of the entrapment of the radial nerve can often be determined by the clinical findings, as follows:

▶ If the impairment occurs at a point below the triceps innervation, the strength of the triceps remains intact.

▶ If the impairment occurs at a point below the brachioradialis branch, some supination is retained.

▶ If the impairment occurs at a point in the forearm, the branches to the small muscle groups, extensors of the thumb, extensors of the index finger, extensors of the other fingers, and extensor carpi ulnaris may be affected.

▶ If the impairment occurs at a point on the dorsum of the wrist, only sensory loss on the hand is affected.

Median Nerve (C5–T1).   The trunk of the median nerve derives its fibers from the lower three (sometimes four) cervical and the first thoracic segments of the spinal cord. Although it has no branches in the upper arm, the nerve trunk descends along the course of the brachial artery, and passes onto the anterior aspect of the forearm, where it gives off muscular branches, including the anterior interosseous nerve. It then enters the hand, where it terminates with both muscular and cutaneous branches (Fig. 2-15). The sensory branches of the median nerve supply the skin of the palmar aspect of the thumb and the lateral 2½ fingers, and the distal ends of the same fingers (see Fig. 2-15).

The anterior interosseous nerve arises from the posterior aspect of the median nerve, 5 cm distal to the medial humeral epicondyle, and passes with the main trunk of the median nerve between the two heads of the pronator teres.[19] It continues along the palmar aspect of the flexor digitorum profundus and then passes between the flexor digitorum profundus and the flexor pollicis longus, running in close apposition to the interosseous membrane, to enter the pronator quadratus.[19] It provides motor innervation to the flexor pollicis longus; the medial part of flexor digitorum profundus, involving the index and sometimes the middle finger; and to the pronator quadratus. It also sends sensory fibers to the distal radioulnar, radiocarpal, intercarpal, and carpometacarpal joints.[54] Variations in the distribution of the nerve have been noted; it may supply all or none of the flexor digitorum profundus and part of the flexor digitorum superficialis.[55]

The clinical features of median nerve impairment, depending on the level of injury, include the following.[14]

1. Paralysis is noted in the flexor-pronator muscles of the forearm, all of the superficial palmar muscles except the flexor carpi ulnaris, and all of the deep palmar muscles, except the ulnar half of the flexor digitorum profundus and the thenar muscles that lie superficial to the tendon of the flexor pollices longus.
2. In the forearm, pronation is weak or lost.
3. At the wrist, there is weak flexion and radial deviation, and the hand inclines to the ulnar side.
4. In the hand, an ape-hand deformity can be present (see Fig. 2-15). This deformity is associated with:
   a. An inability to oppose or flex the thumb, or abduct it in its own plane.
   b. A weakened grip, especially in thumb and index finger, with a tendency for these digits to become hyperextended, and the thumb adducted.
   c. An inability to flex the distal phalanx of the thumb and index finger.
   d. Weakness of middle finger flexion.
   e. Atrophy of the thenar muscles.
5. There is a loss of sensation to a variable degree over the cutaneous distribution of the median nerve, most constantly over the distal phalanges of the first two fingers.
6. Pain is present in many median nerve impairments.

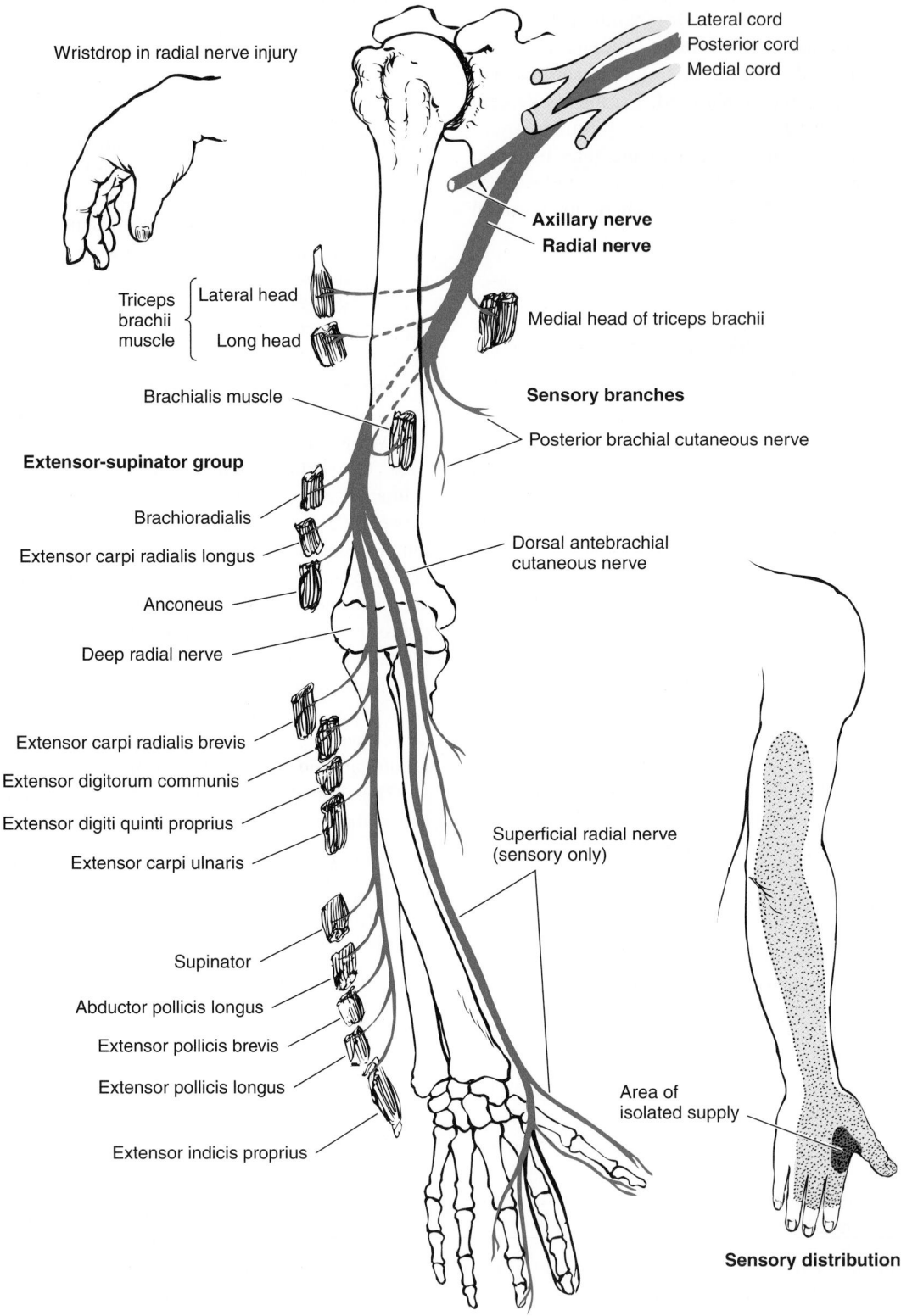

Wristdrop in radial nerve injury

Lateral cord
Posterior cord
Medial cord

Axillary nerve
Radial nerve

Triceps brachii muscle { Lateral head
Long head

Medial head of triceps brachii

Brachialis muscle

Sensory branches

Posterior brachial cutaneous nerve

Extensor-supinator group

Brachioradialis

Extensor carpi radialis longus

Dorsal antebrachial cutaneous nerve

Anconeus

Deep radial nerve

Extensor carpi radialis brevis

Extensor digitorum communis

Extensor digiti quinti proprius

Extensor carpi ulnaris

Superficial radial nerve (sensory only)

Supinator

Abductor pollicis longus

Extensor pollicis brevis

Extensor pollicis longus

Area of isolated supply

Extensor indicis proprius

Sensory distribution

FIGURE 2-14   The radial nerve (C6–8; T1). (Reproduced with permission from Waxman SG. *Correlative Neuroanatomy*. 24th ed. New York, NY: McGraw-Hill; 1996.)

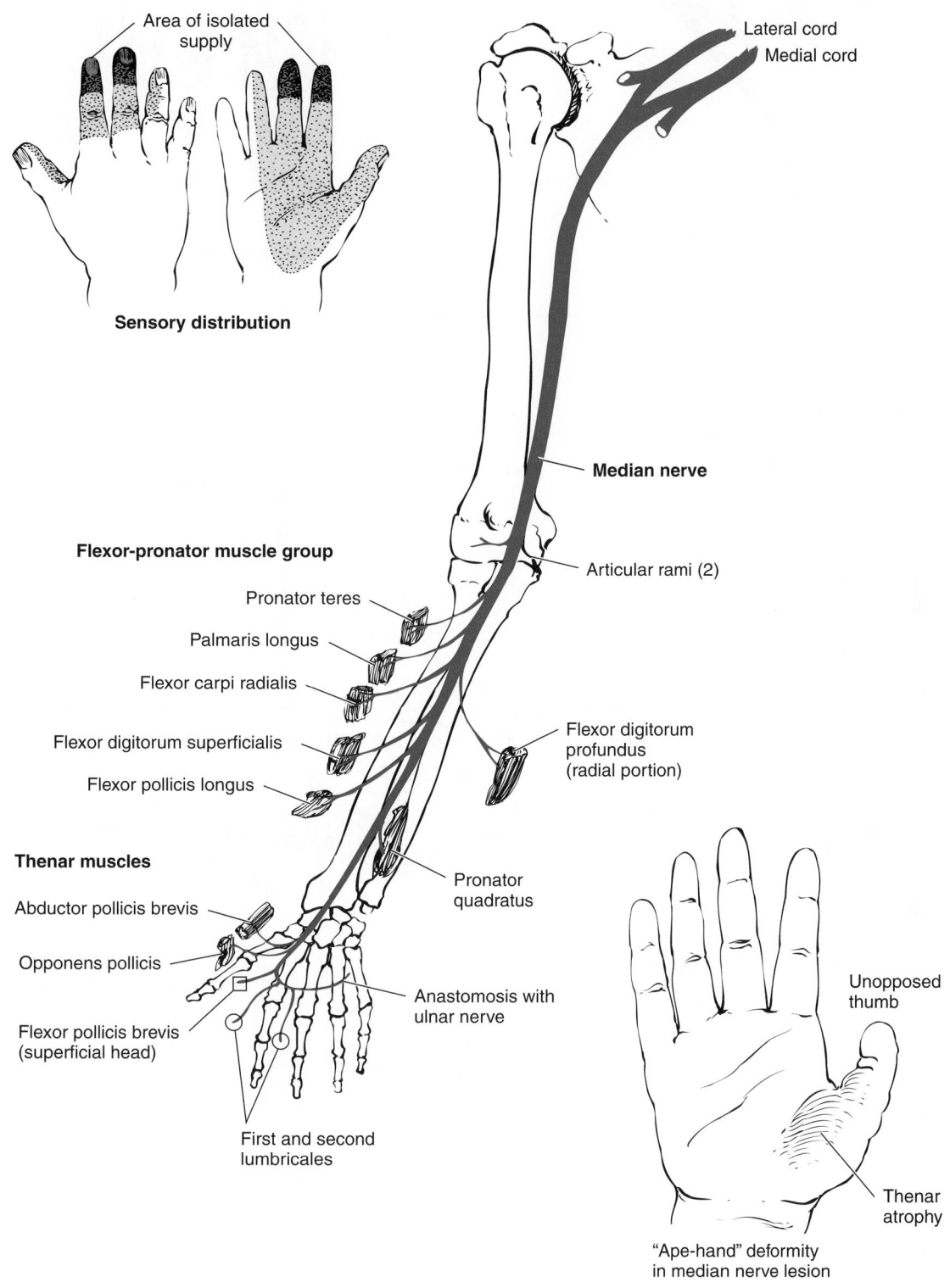

Area of isolated
supply

Sensory distribution

Lateral cord
Medial cord

Median nerve

Articular rami (2)

Flexor-pronator muscle group

Pronator teres

Palmaris longus

Flexor carpi radialis

Flexor digitorum superficialis

Flexor pollicis longus

Flexor digitorum
profundus
(radial portion)

Thenar muscles

Abductor pollicis brevis

Opponens pollicis

Flexor pollicis brevis
(superficial head)

Pronator
quadratus

Anastomosis with
ulnar nerve

First and second
lumbricales

Unopposed
thumb

Thenar
atrophy

"Ape-hand" deformity
in median nerve lesion

FIGURE 2-15 The median nerve (C6–8; T1). (Reproduced with permission from Waxman SG. *Correlative Neuroanatomy*. 24th ed. New York, NY: McGraw-Hill; 1996.)

7. Atrophy of the thenar eminence is seen early. Atrophy of the flexor-pronator groups of muscles in the forearm is seen after a few months.

8. The skin of the palm is frequently dry, cold, discolored, chapped, and at times keratotic.

Ulnar Nerve (C8, T1).   The ulnar nerve is the largest branch of the medial cord of the brachial plexus. It arises from the medial cord of the brachial plexus and contains fibers from the C8 and T1 nerve roots, although C7 may contribute some fibers (Fig. 2-16). The ulnar nerve continues along the anterior

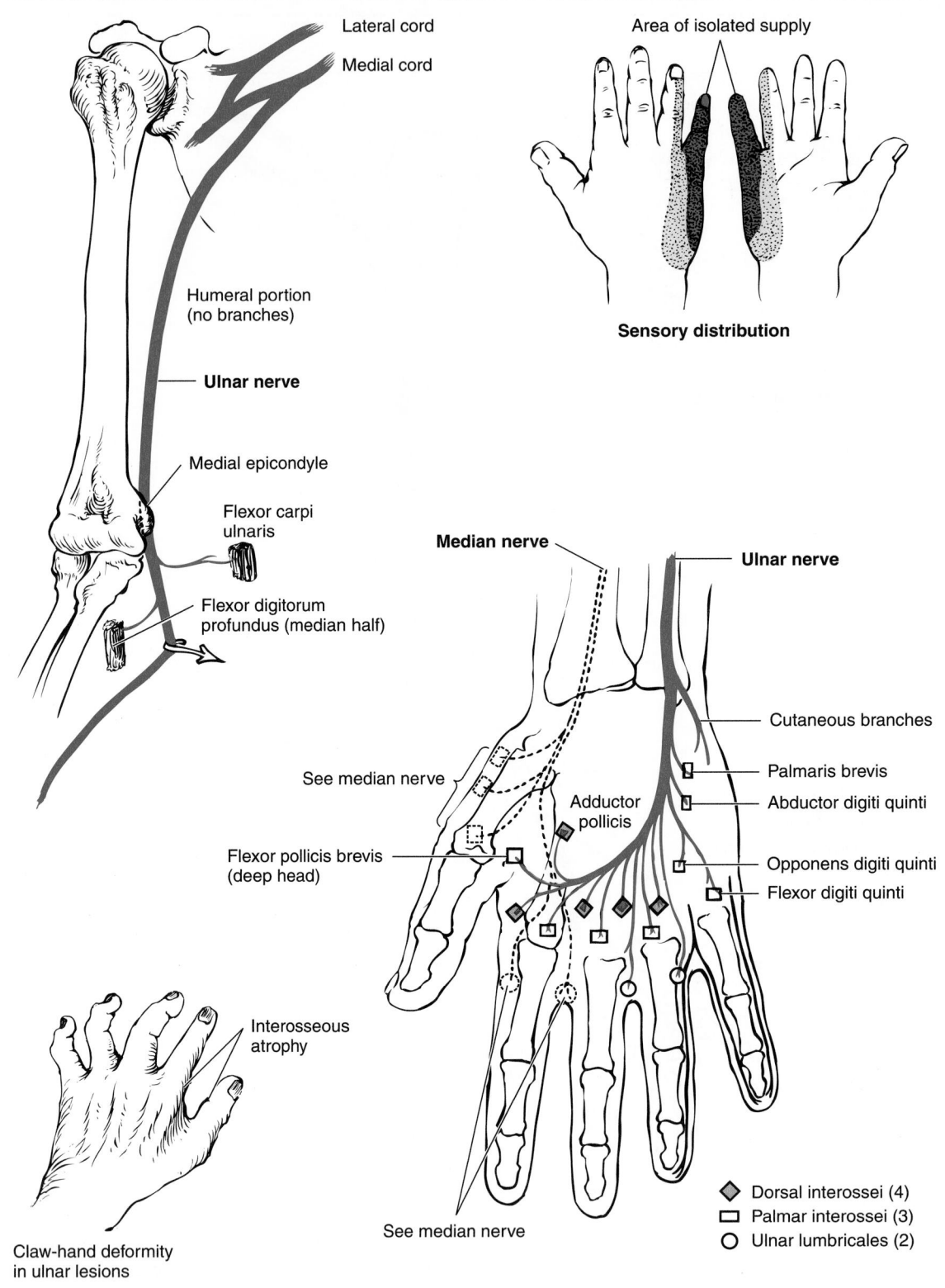

Lateral cord

Medial cord

Humeral portion
(no branches)

Ulnar nerve

Medial epicondyle

Flexor carpi
ulnaris

Flexor digitorum
profundus (median half)

Area of isolated supply

Sensory distribution

Median nerve

Ulnar nerve

See median nerve

Adductor
pollicis

Flexor pollicis brevis
(deep head)

Cutaneous branches

Palmaris brevis

Abductor digiti quinti

Opponens digiti quinti

Flexor digiti quinti

Interosseous
atrophy

See median nerve

◆ Dorsal interossei (4)
▢ Palmar interossei (3)
○ Ulnar lumbricales (2)

Claw-hand deformity
in ulnar lesions

FIGURE 2-16   The ulnar nerve (C8, T1). (Reproduced with permission from Waxman SG. *Correlative Neuroanatomy*. 24th ed. New York, NY: McGraw-Hill; 1996.)

compartment of the arm, and it passes through the medial inter-muscular septum at the level of the coracobrachialis insertion. As the ulnar nerve passes to the posterior compartment of the arm, it courses through the arcade of Struthers, which is a potential site for its compression.

At the level of the elbow, the ulnar nerve passes posterior to the medial epicondyle, where it passes through the cubital tunnel. From there, the ulnar nerve passes between the two heads of the flexor carpi ulnaris origin and traverses the deep flexor-pronator aponeurosis. This aponeurosis is superficial to the flexor digitorum profundus, but deep to the flexor carpi ulnaris and flexor digitorum superficialis muscles.[56,57]

Sunderland[58] described the intraneural topography of the ulnar nerve at various levels of the arm. At the medial epicondyle, the sensory fibers to the hand and the motor fibers to the intrinsic muscles are superficial, whereas the motor fibers to flexor carpi ulnaris and flexor digitorum profundus are deep. This may explain the common finding in "cubital tunnel syndrome" (see Chap. 15) of sensory loss and weakness of the ulnarly innervated intrinsic muscles, but relative sparing of flexor carpi ulnaris and flexor digitorum profundus strength.[59]

The ulnar nerve enters the forearm by coursing posterior to the medial humeral condyle and passing between the heads of the flexor carpi ulnaris, before resting on the flexor digitorum profundus[60] (see Fig. 2-16). It then continues distally to the wrist passing between the flexor carpi ulnaris and flexor digitorum profundus muscles, which it supplies. Proximal to the wrist, the palmar cutaneous branch of the ulnar nerve arises. This branch runs across the palmar aspect of the forearm and wrist outside of the tunnel of Guyon to supply the proximal part of the ulnar side of the palm. A few centimeters more distally to the tunnel, a dorsal cutaneous branch arises and supplies the ulnar side of the dorsum of the hand, the dorsal aspect of the fifth finger, and the ulnar half of the forefinger. The ulnar nerve supplies the flexor carpi ulnaris, the ulnar head of the flexor digitorum profundus, and all of the small muscles deep and medial to the long flexor tendon of the thumb, except the first two lumbricales (see Fig. 2-16, indicated by terminal branches in hand). Its sensory distribution includes the skin of the little finger and the medial half of the hand and the ring finger (see Fig. 2-16).

The clinical features of ulnar nerve impairment include the following.[14]

▶ Claw hand (see Fig. 2-16), resulting from unopposed action of the extensor digitorum communis in the fourth and fifth digits.

▶ An inability to extend the second and distal phalanges of any of the fingers.

▶ An inability to adduct or abduct the fingers, or to oppose all the fingertips, as in making a cone with the fingers and thumb.

▶ An inability to adduct the thumb.

▶ At the wrist, flexion is weak and ulnar deviation is lost. The ulnar reflex is absent.

▶ Atrophy of the interosseous spaces (especially the first), and of the hypothenar eminence.

▶ A loss of sensation on the ulnar side of the hand and ring finger, and most markedly over the entire little finger.

Partial lesions of the ulnar nerve may produce only motor weakness or paralysis of a few of the muscles supplied by the nerve. Lesions that occur in the distal forearm or at the wrist spare the deep flexors and the flexor carpi ulnaris.

Thoracic Nerves

Dorsal Rami. The thoracic dorsal rami (Fig. 2-17) travel posteriorly, close to the vertebral zygapophysial joints, before dividing into medial and lateral branches.

▶ The medial branches supply the short, medially placed back muscles (the iliocostalis thoracis, spinalis thoracis, semispinalis thoracis, thoracic multifidi, rotatores thoracis, and intertransversarii muscles) and the skin of the back as far as the midscapular line. The medial branches of the upper six thoracic dorsal rami pierce the rhomboids and trapezius, reaching the skin in close proximity to the vertebral spines, which they occasionally supply.

▶ The lateral branches supply smaller branches to the sacrospinalis muscles. The lateral branches increase in size the more inferior they are. They penetrate, or pass, the longissimus thoracis to the space between it and the iliocostalis cervicis, supplying both of these muscles, as well as the levatores costarum. The 12th thoracic lateral branch sends a filament medially along the iliac crest, which then passes down to the anterior gluteal skin.

As mentioned previously, the recurrent meningeal or sinuvertebral nerve is functionally also a branch of the spinal nerve. This nerve passes back into the vertebral canal through the intervertebral foramen, supplying the anterior aspect of the dura mater, outer third of the annular fibers of the intervertebral disks, vertebral body, and the epidural blood vessel walls, as well as the posterior longitudinal ligament.[61]

Ventral Rami. There are 12 pairs of thoracic ventral rami, and all but the 12th are between the ribs serving as intercostal nerves. The 12th ventral ramus, the subcostal nerve, is located below the last rib. The intercostal nerve has a lateral branch, providing sensory distribution to the skin of the lateral aspect of the trunk, and an anterior branch, supplying the intercostal muscles, parietal pleura, and the skin over the anterior aspect of the thorax and abdomen. All of the intercostal nerves mainly supply the thoracic and abdominal walls, with the upper two also supplying the upper limb. The thoracic ventral rami of T3 to T6 supply only the thoracic wall, whereas the lower five rami supply both the thoracic and abdominal walls. The subcostal nerve supplies both the abdominal wall and the gluteal skin.

Each ventral ramus is connected with an adjacent sympathetic ganglion (Fig. 2-17) by gray and white rami communicantes. The communicating rami are branches of the spinal nerves that transmit sympathetic autonomic fibers to and from the sympathetic chain of ganglia. The fibers pass from spinal nerve to chain ganglia through the white ramus, and the reverse direction through the gray. In the cervical, lower lumbar, and

FIGURE 2-17 Thoracic spinal cord, nerve roots, spinal ganglia, spinal nerves, and the paravertebral sympathetic chain ganglia. (Reproduced with permission from Harati Y. Anatomy of the spinal and peripheral autonomic nervous system. In: Low PA, ed. *Clinical Autonomic Disorders: Evaluation and Management*. Boston, Mass: Little, Brown; 1997.)

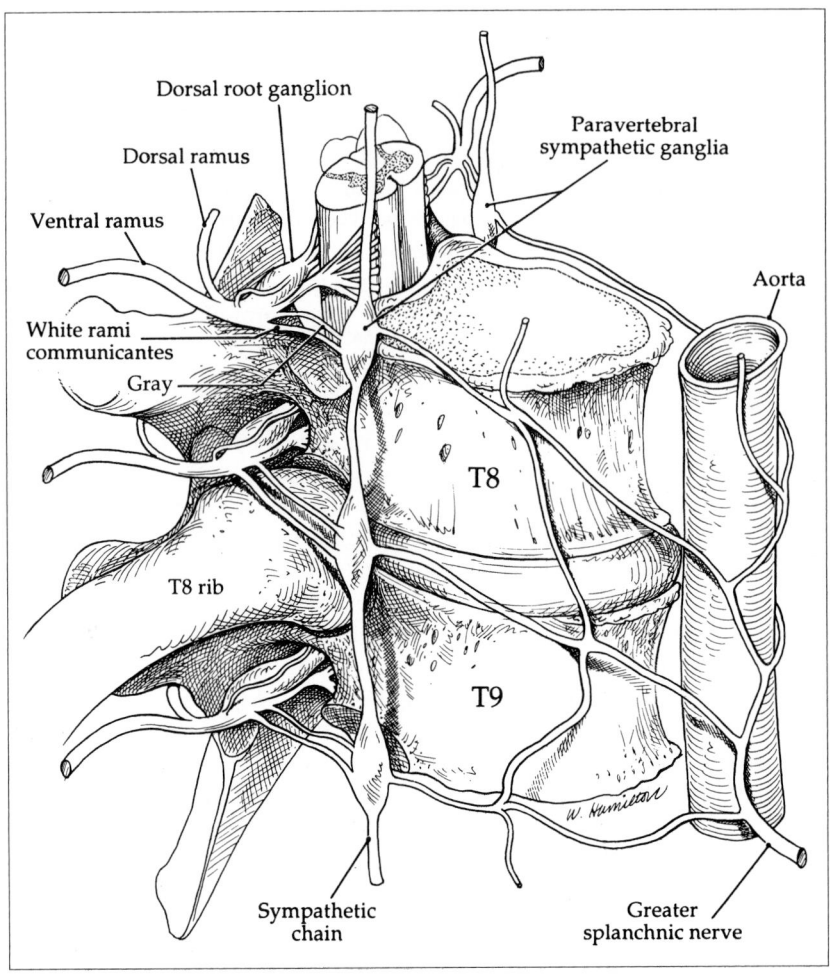

sacral levels, only gray rami are present and function to convey fibers from the chain to the spinal nerves, a mechanism that ensures that all spinal nerves contain sympathetic fibers.

From each intercostal nerve, a collateral and lateral cutaneous branch leave before the main nerve reaches the costal angle. The intercostobrachial nerve arises from the lateral collateral branch of the second intercostal nerve, pierces the intercostal muscles in the midaxillary line, and then traverses the central portion of the axilla, where a posterior axillary branch gives sensation to the posterior axillary fold. From here, the nerve passes into the upper arm along the posterior-medial border to supply the skin of this region[62] and to connect with the posterior cutaneous branch of the radial nerve.

The thoracic nerves may be involved in the same types of impairments that affect other peripheral nerves. A loss of function of one, or more of the thoracic nerves may produce partial or complete paralysis of the abdominal muscles and a loss of the abdominal reflexes in the affected quadrants. With unilateral impairments of the nerve, the umbilicus usually is drawn toward the unaffected side when the abdomen is tensed (Beevor's sign), indicating a paralysis of the lower abdominal muscles as a result of a lesion at the level of the 10th thoracic segment.

A specific syndrome called the T4 syndrome[63–65] has been shown to cause vague pain, numbness, and paresthesia in the upper extremity and generalized posterior head and neck pain (see Chap. 26).

Lumbar Plexus

The lumbar plexus (Fig. 2-18) is formed from the ventral nerve roots of the second, third, and fourth lumbar nerves (in approximately 50 percent of cases, the plexus also receives a contribution from the last thoracic nerve) as they lie between the quadratus lumborum muscle and the psoas muscle. It then travels anteriorly into the body of the psoas muscle to form the lateral femoral cutaneous, femoral, and obturator nerves.

L1, L2, and L4 divide into upper and lower branches (see Fig. 2-18). The upper branch of L1 forms the iliohypogastric and ilioinguinal nerves. The lower branch of L1 joins the upper branch of L2 to form the genitofemoral nerve (see Fig. 2-18). The lower branch of L4 joins L5 to form the lumbosacral trunk.

▶ *Iliohypogastric nerve (T12, L1) (see Fig. 2-18).* This nerve emerges from the upper lateral border of the psoas major and then passes laterally around the iliac crest between

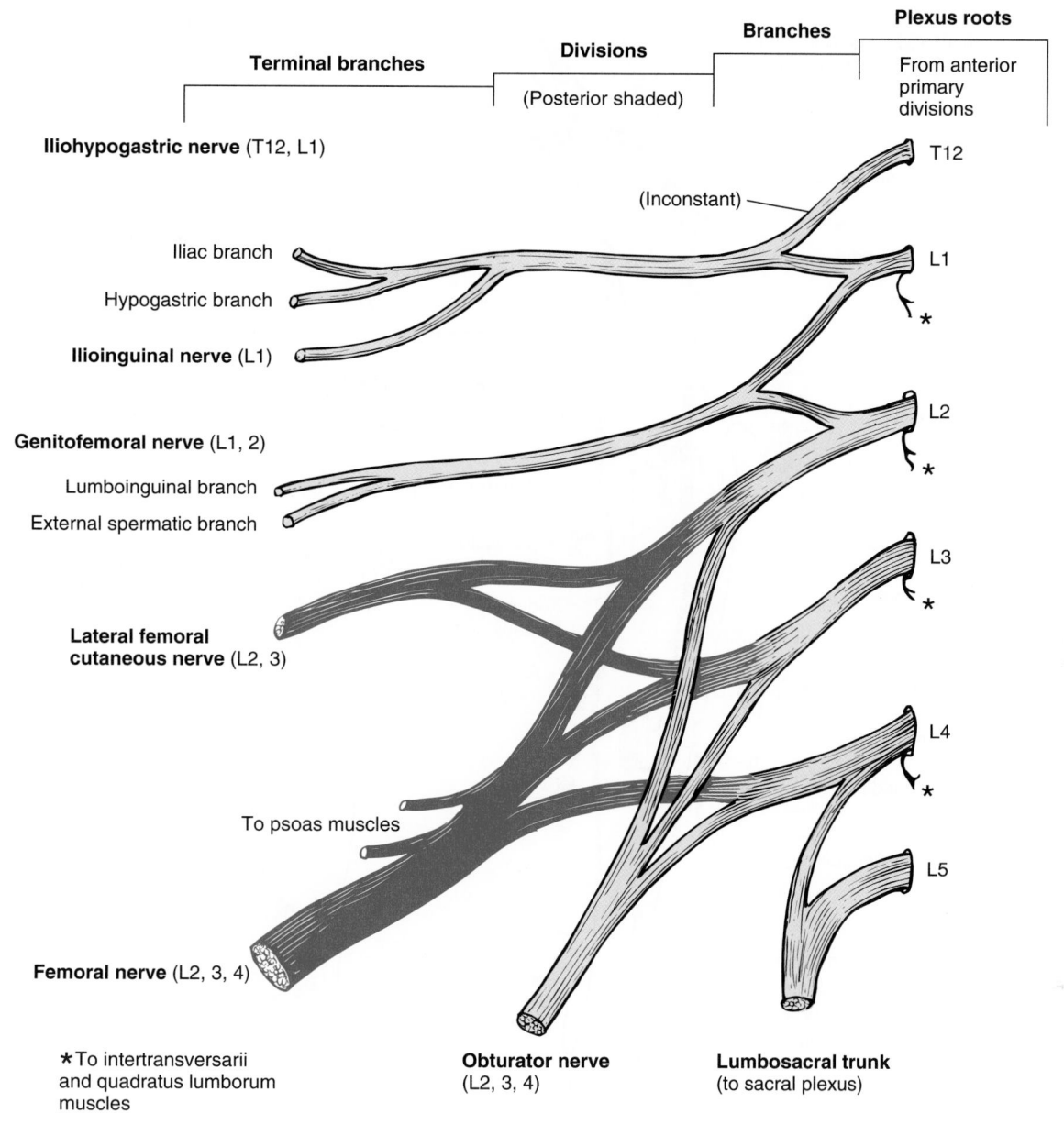

		Branches	Plexus roots
Terminal branches	Divisions		From anterior primary divisions
	(Posterior shaded)		

Iliohypogastric nerve (T12, L1) — T12

(Inconstant)

Iliac branch — L1 *

Hypogastric branch

Ilioinguinal nerve (L1)

Genitofemoral nerve (L1, 2) — L2 *

Lumboinguinal branch

External spermatic branch

Lateral femoral cutaneous nerve (L2, 3) — L3 *

— L4 *

To psoas muscles

— L5

Femoral nerve (L2, 3, 4)

★To intertransversarii and quadratus lumborum muscles

Obturator nerve (L2, 3, 4)

Lumbosacral trunk (to sacral plexus)

FIGURE 2-18   The lumbar plexus. (Reproduced with permission from Waxman SG. *Correlative Neuroanatomy.* 24th ed. New York, NY: McGraw-Hill; 1996.)

the transversus abdominis and internal oblique muscles, before dividing into lateral and anterior cutaneous branches. The lateral (iliac) branch supplies the skin of the upper lateral part of the thigh, while the anterior (hypogastric) branch descends anteriorly to supply the skin over the symphysis.

▶ *Ilioinguinal nerve (L1) (see Fig. 2-18).*   This nerve is smaller than the iliohypogastric nerve. It emerges from the lateral border of the psoas major to follow a course slightly inferior to that of the iliohypogastric, with which it may anastomose. It pierces the internal oblique, which it supplies, before emerging from the superficial inguinal ring to supply

the skin of the upper medial part of the thigh and the root of the penis and scrotum or mons pubis and labium majores. An entrapment of this nerve results in pain in the groin region, usually with radiation down to the proximal inner surface of the thigh, sometimes aggravated by increasing tension on the abdominal wall through standing erect.

▶ *Genitofemoral nerve (L1,2) (see Fig. 2-18).*   This nerve descends obliquely and anteriorly through the psoas major before emerging from the anterior surface of the psoas and dividing into genital and femoral branches. The genital branch supplies the cremasteric muscle and the skin of the scrotum or

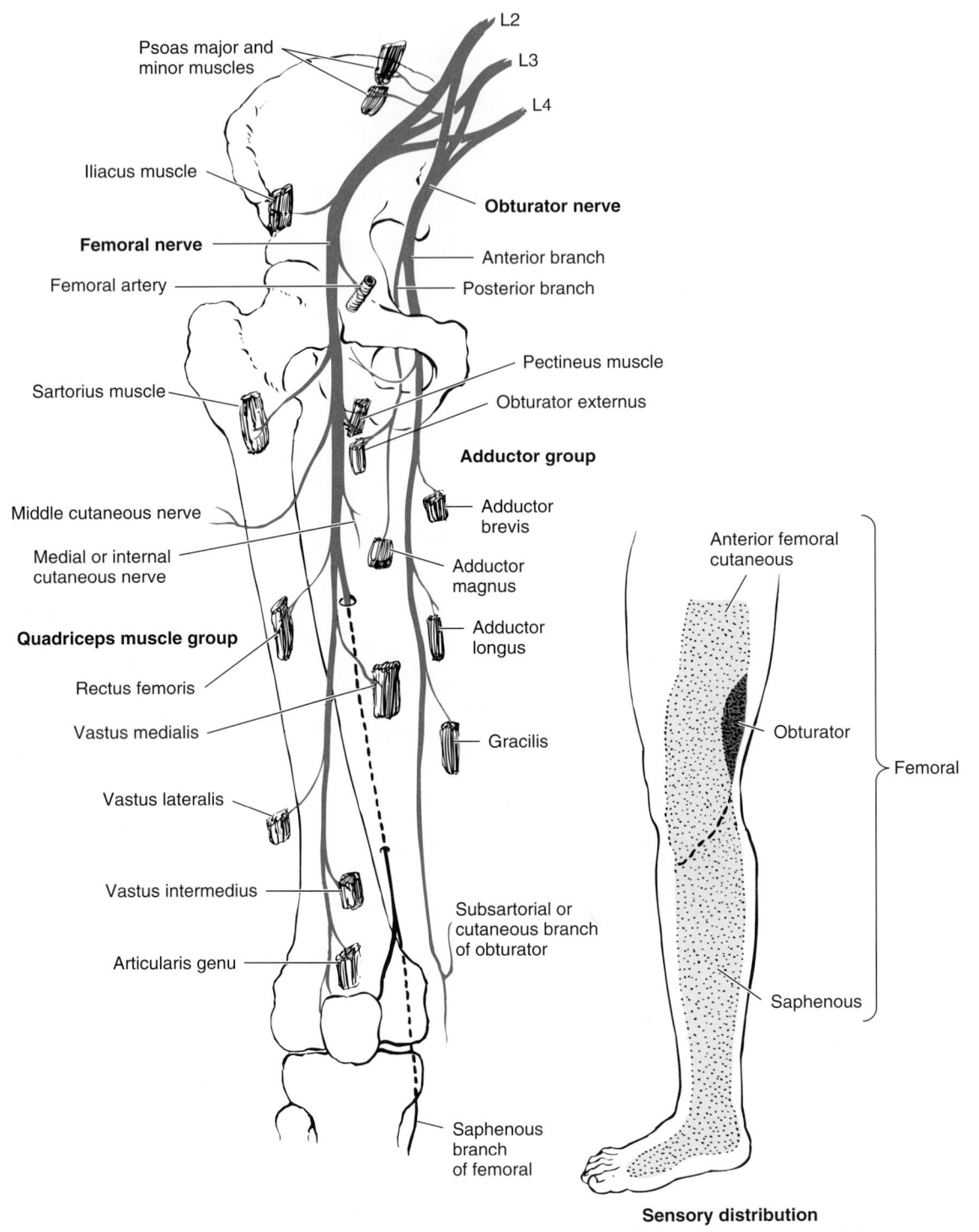

FIGURE 2-19 The femoral (L2–4) and obturator (L2–4) nerves. (Reproduced with permission from Waxman SG. *Correlative Neuroanatomy*. 24th ed. New York, NY: McGraw-Hill; 1996.)

labia, whereas the femoral branch supplies the skin of the middle upper part of the thigh and the femoral artery.

Collateral muscular branches supply the quadratus lumborum and intertransversarii from L1 and L4 and the psoas muscle from L2 and L3.

The lower branch of L2, all of L3, and the upper branch of L4 split into a small anterior and a large posterior division (see Fig. 2-18). The three anterior divisions unite to form the obturator nerve; the three posterior divisions unite to form the femoral nerve, and the lateral femoral cutaneous nerve (see Fig. 2-18).

Femoral Nerve (L2–4). The femoral nerve, the largest branch of the lumbar plexus, arises from the lateral border of the psoas just above the inguinal ligament. The nerve descends beneath this ligament to enter the femoral triangle on the lateral side of the femoral artery, where it divides into terminal branches. Above the inguinal ligament, the femoral nerve supplies the iliopsoas muscle, and in the thigh, it supplies the sartorius, pectineus, and quadriceps femoris muscles.

The sensory distribution of the femoral nerve includes the anterior and medial surfaces of the thigh via the anterior femoral cutaneous nerve, and the medial aspect of the knee, the proximal leg, and articular branches to the knee via the saphenous nerve (Fig. 2-19).

Femoral nerve palsy has been reported after acetabular fracture, cardiac catheterization, total hip arthroplasty, or anterior lumbar spinal fusion, and spontaneously in hemophilia.[66–68]

> ### Clinical Pearl
>
> An entrapment of the femoral nerve by an iliopsoas hematoma is the most likely cause of femoral nerve palsy.[69] Direct blows to the abdomen or a hyperextension moment at the hip that tears the iliacus muscle may produce an iliacus hematoma.

Obturator Nerve (L2–4). The obturator nerve (see Fig. 2-19) arises from the second, third, and fourth lumbar anterior divisions of the lumbar plexus and emerges from the medial border of the psoas, near the brim of the pelvis. It then passes behind the common iliac vessels on the lateral side of the hypogastric vessels and ureter and descends through the obturator canal in the upper part of the obturator foramen to the medial side of the thigh. While in the foramen, the obturator nerve splits into anterior and posterior branches.

▶ The anterior division of the obturator nerve gives an articular branch to the hip joint near its origin. It descends anterior to the obturator externus and adductor brevis deep to the pectineus and adductor longus and supplies muscular branches to the adductors longus and brevis, the gracilis, and, rarely, to the pectineus.[62] The anterior division divides into numerous named and unnamed branches, including the cutaneous branches to the subsartorial plexus and directly to a small area of skin on the middle internal part of the thigh, vascular branches to the femoral artery, and communicating branches to the femoral cutaneous and accessory obturator nerves.

▶ The posterior division of the obturator nerve pierces the anterior part of the obturator externus, which it supplies, and descends deep to the adductor brevis. It also supplies the adductors magnus and brevis (if it has not received supply from the anterior division) and gives an articular branch to the knee joint (see Fig. 2-19).

The obturator nerve may be involved by the same pathologic processes that affect the femoral nerve. Disability is usually minimal, although external rotation and adduction of the thigh are impaired, and crossing of the legs is difficult. The patient also may complain of severe pain, which radiates from the groin down the inner aspect of the thigh (see Fig. 2-19). The fascial development, especially with the perivascular condensations around the vessels supplying the adductor mass, constitutes a layer definite enough to create an entrapment of the anterior division of the obturator nerve.[70,71] This thickening around the vessels becomes more significant in the possible explanation of an entrapment syndrome when the intimate relationship between the nerve branches and the vessels is considered.[71]

Lateral Femoral Cutaneous Nerve. The lateral femoral cutaneous nerve (LFCN) (Fig. 2-20) is purely sensory and is derived primarily from the second and third lumbar nerve roots, with occasional contributions from the first lumbar nerve root.[72,73] Sympathetic afferent and efferent fibers also are contained within the nerve.[74] The nerve leaves the lumbar plexus and normally appears at the lateral border of the psoas, just proximal to

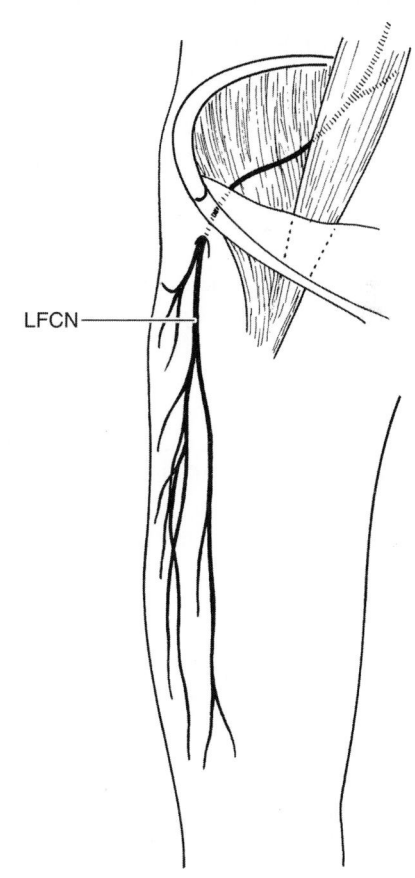

FIGURE 2-20 Lateral femoral cutaneous nerve distribution. (Reproduced with permission from Pecina M, Krmpotic-Nemanic J, Markiewitz A. *Tunnel Syndromes.* Boca Raton, Fla: CRC Press; 1991.)

the crest of the ilium. From here it courses laterally across the anterior surface of the iliacus (covered by iliac fascia) and approaches the lateral portion of the inguinal ligament posterior to the deep circumflex iliac artery. The nerve usually crosses beneath the inguinal ligament, just inferior-medial to the anterior superior iliac spine.[75] The site at which the LFCN exits the pelvis varies. Meralgia paresthetica (see Chaps. 9 and 17) has been reported with each of five known variants, as follows.[76]

▶ The split lateral attachment of the inguinal ligament. As the nerve curves medially and inferiorly around the anterior superior iliac spine, it may be subjected to repetitive trauma in this osteofibrous tunnel.[77]

▶ The nerve may pass posterior to the inguinal ligament and anterior to a sharp ridge of iliacus fascia, which can lead to a bowstring deformity of the nerve when the patient is supine.[78]

▶ Occasionally, the LFCN enters the thigh within or beneath the substance of the sartorius muscle.[79]

▶ Several cases have been reported in which the LFCN crosses over the iliac crest lateral and posterior to the anterior superior iliac spine. The nerve typically lies in a groove in the ilium and is subject to pressure from tight garments or belts.[78,79]

▶ The nerve may exit the pelvis in multiple branches with entrapment of a single branch.[80]

Alternatively, the nerve may be absent, with a branch from the femoral nerve arising below the inguinal ligament, or it may be replaced by the ilioinguinal nerve.[81]

Sacral Plexus

The lumbosacral trunk (L4, 5) descends into the pelvis, where it enters the formation of the sacral plexus.

The sacral plexus (Fig. 2-21) is formed by the ventral rami of the L4 and L5 and the S1 through S4 nerves and lies on the posterior wall of the pelvis, anterior to the piriformis and posterior to the sigmoid colon, ureter, and hypogastric vessels in front. The L4 and L5 nerves join medial to the sacral promontory, becoming the lumbosacral trunk (Fig. 2-21). The S1 through S4 nerves converge with the lumbosacral trunk in front of the piriformis muscle, forming the broad triangular band of the sacral plexus (see Fig. 2-21). The upper three nerves of the plexus divide into two sets of branches: the medial branches, which are distributed to the multifidi muscles, and the lateral branches, which become the medial cluneal nerves. The medial cluneal nerves supply the skin over the medial part of the gluteus maximus. The lower two posterior primary divisions, with the posterior division of the coccygeal nerve, supply the skin over the coccyx.

Collateral Branches of the Posterior Division

Superior Gluteal Nerve. The roots of the superior gluteal nerve (L4,5; S1) arise within the pelvis from the sacral plexus (see Fig. 2-21), and enter the buttock through the greater sciatic foramen, above the piriformis. The nerve runs laterally between gluteus medius and gluteus minimus, which it innervates before terminating in the tensor fascia lata, which it also supplies. Because the nerve passes between the gluteal muscles, it is at risk during surgery on the hip.[82]

Inferior Gluteal Nerve. The inferior gluteal nerve (L5; S1,2) passes below the piriformis muscle and through the greater sciatic foramen, and travels to the gluteus maximus muscle (see Fig. 2-21). Nerves to the piriformis consist of short smaller branches from S1 and S2.

Superior Cluneal Nerve. The medial branch of the superior cluneal nerve (see Fig. 2-21) passes superficially over the iliac crest, where it is covered by two layers of dense fibrous fascia. When the medial branch of the superior cluneal nerve passes through the fascia against the posterior iliac crest and the osteofibrous tunnel consisting of the two layers of the fascia and the superior rim of the iliac crest, the possibility of irritation or trauma to the nerve is increased, making this a potential site of nerve compression or constriction.[83]

Posterior Femoral Cutaneous Nerve. The posterior femoral cutaneous nerve constitutes a collateral branch, with roots from both anterior and posterior divisions of S1 and S2, and the anterior divisions of S2 and S3. Perineal branches pass to the skin of the upper medial aspect of the thigh and the skin of the scrotum or labium majores. Despite its close proximity to the sciatic nerve, however, injury to the posterior femoral cutaneous nerve is quite rare.

Collateral Branches of the Anterior Division. Collateral branches from the anterior divisions extend to the quadratus femoris and gemellus inferior muscles (from L4, L5, and S1) and to the obturator internus and gemellus superior muscles (from L5, S1, and S2) (see Fig. 2-21).

Sciatic Nerve. The sciatic nerve (Fig. 2-22) is the largest nerve in the body. It arises from the L4, L5, and S1 through S3 nerve roots as a continuation of the lumbosacral plexus. The nerve is composed of the independent tibial (medial) and common peroneal (lateral) divisions, which are usually united as a single nerve down to the lower portion of the thigh. The tibial division is the larger of the two divisions. Although grossly united, the funicular patterns of the tibial and common peroneal divisions are distinct, and there is no exchange of bundles between them. The common peroneal nerve is formed by the upper four posterior divisions (L4,5; S1,2) of the sacral plexus, and the tibial nerve, is formed from all five anterior divisions (L4,5; S1–3).

The sciatic nerve usually exits the pelvis through the anterior third of the greater sciatic foramen.[84] Also running through the greater sciatic foramen is the superior gluteal artery, the largest branch of the internal iliac artery, and its accompanying vein.

Numerous variations have been described for the course of the sciatic nerve, including cases in which the sciatic nerve passes through the piriformis and cases in which the tibial

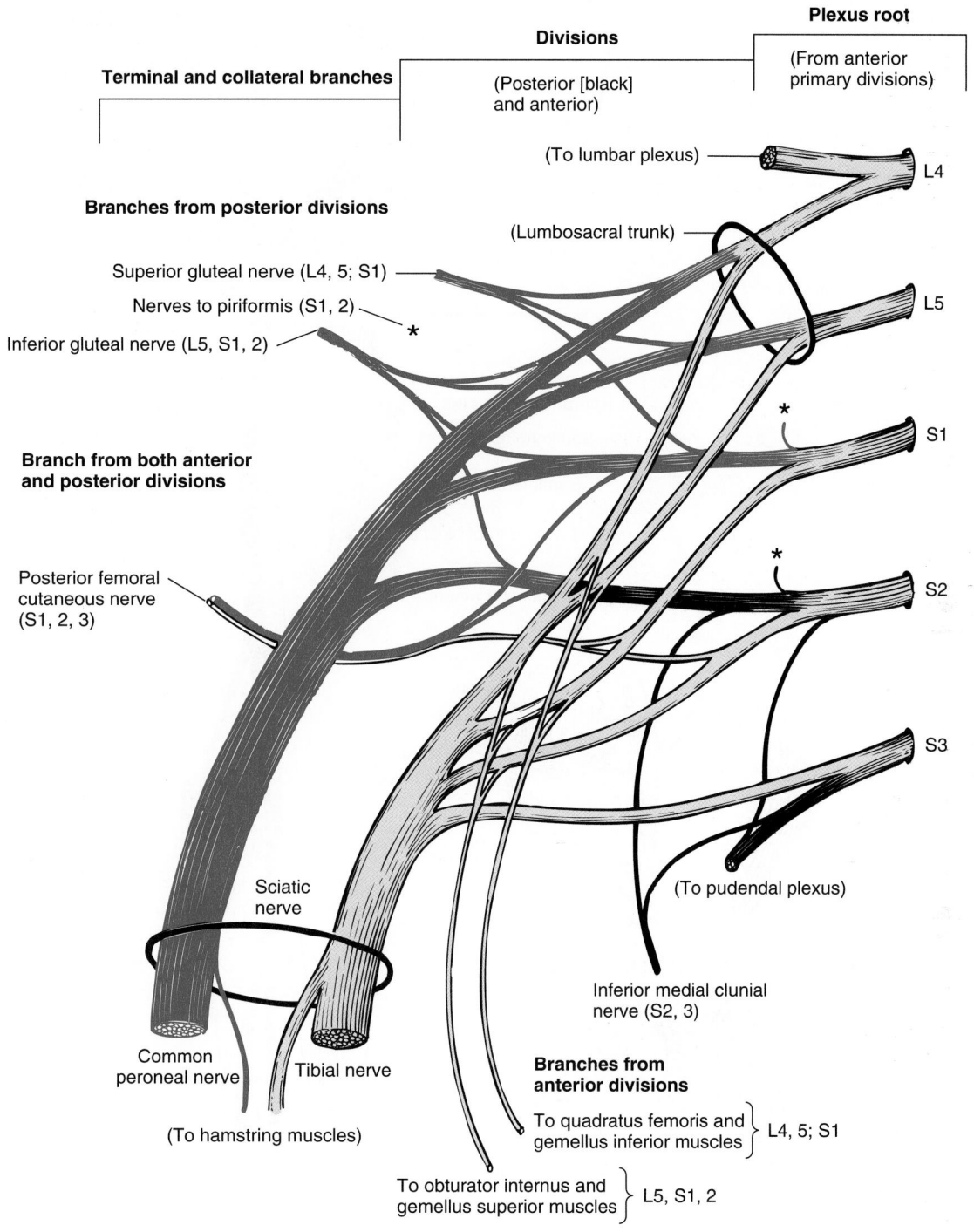

FIGURE 2-21   The sacral plexus. (Reproduced with permission from Waxman SG. *Correlative Neuroanatomy*. 24th ed. New York, NY: McGraw-Hill; 1996.)

division passes below the piriformis while the common peroneal passes above or through the muscle.[84] It seems that the tibial division always enters the gluteal region below the piriformis, and the variability is in the course of the common peroneal division. Typically, the sciatic nerve descends along the posterior surface of the thigh to the popliteal space, where it usually terminates by dividing into the tibial and common peroneal nerves (see Fig. 2-22). Innervation for the short head of the biceps comes from the common peroneal division, the only muscle innervated by this division above the knee. Rami from the tibial trunk pass to the semitendinosus and semimembranosus muscles, the long head of the biceps, and the adductor magnus muscle.

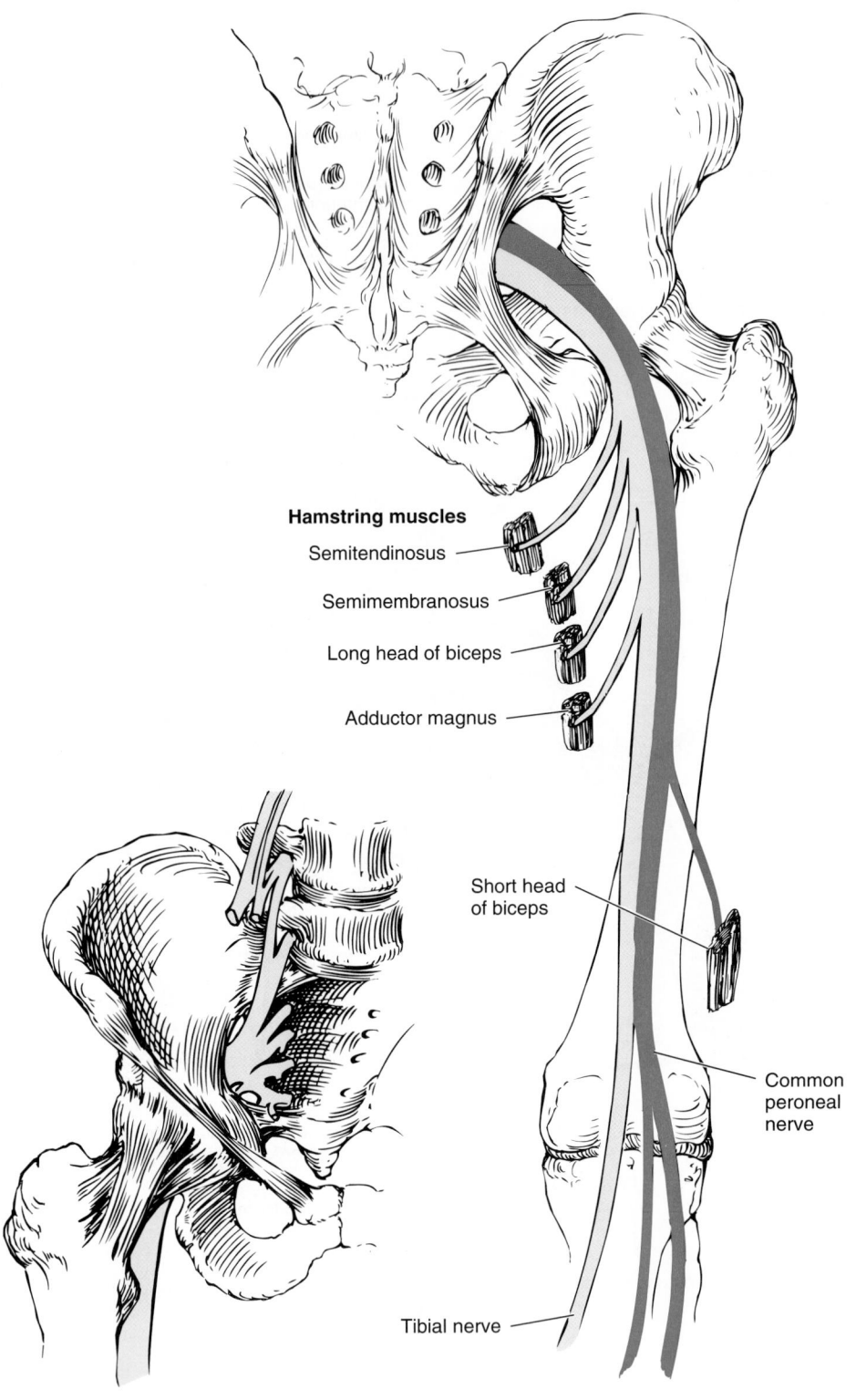

Hamstring muscles

Semitendinosus

Semimembranosus

Long head of biceps

Adductor magnus

Short head of biceps

Common peroneal nerve

Tibial nerve

FIGURE 2-22   The sciatic nerve (L4,5; S1–3). (Reproduced with permission from Waxman SG. *Correlative Neuroanatomy*. 24th ed. New York, NY: McGraw-Hill; 1996.)

In most reports of sciatic nerve injury, regardless of the cause, the common peroneal division is involved more frequently and often suffers a greater degree of damage than the tibial division, its susceptibility to injury related to several anatomic features.

Sunderland[5] performed an investigation of the cross-sectional area of the sciatic trunk, and of the tibial and common peroneal divisions, that showed differences in the relative amounts of nerve tissue (funiculi) and connective tissue within the two divisions. He found that the common peroneal division is composed of fewer and larger funiculi with less connective tissue than the tibial division. It was proposed that nerves with large and tightly packed funiculi are more vulnerable to mechanical injury than those in which the funiculi are smaller and more loosely dispersed in a greater amount of connective tissue. In the latter case, under a deforming force, the neural elements are displaced more easily and the mechanical forces can be dissipated to the intervening connective tissue.

Injury to the sciatic nerve may result indirectly from a herniated intervertebral disk (protruded nucleus pulposus), or more directly from a hip dislocation, local aneurysm, or direct external trauma of the sciatic notch, the latter of which can be confused with a compressive radiculopathy of the lumbar or sacral nerve root.[85] Following are some useful clues to help distinguish the two conditions:

1. Pain from radiculopathy should not significantly change with hip motion except in the case of a straight leg raise, whereas with a sciatic entrapment by the piriformis pain is accentuated with hip internal rotation and relieved by hip external rotation.

2. Sciatic neuropathy produces sensory changes on the sole of the foot, whereas radiculopathy generally does not, unless there is a predominant S1 involvement.

3. Compressive radiculopathy below the L4 level causes palpable atrophy of the gluteal muscles, whereas a sciatic entrapment spares these muscles.

4. The sciatic trunk is frequently tender from root compression at the foraminal level, whereas it is not normally tender in a sciatic nerve entrapment.[86]

Individual case reports of bone and soft-tissue tumors along the course of the sciatic nerve have been described as a rare cause of sciatica.[87,88]

Tibial Nerve. The tibial nerve (L4,5; S1–3) is formed by all five of the anterior divisions of the sacral plexus, thus receiving fibers from the lower two lumbar and the upper three sacral cord segments. Inferiorly, the nerve begins its own course in the upper part of the popliteal space, before descending vertically through this space, and passing between the heads of the gastrocnemius muscle, to the dorsum of the leg. The portion of the tibial trunk below the popliteal space is called the *posterior tibial nerve;* the portion within the space is called the *internal popliteal nerve* (Fig. 2-23). The tibial nerve supplies the gastrocnemius, plantaris, soleus, popliteus, tibialis posterior, flexor digitorum longus, and flexor halluces longus muscles (see Fig. 2-23).

Sural Nerve. The sural nerve (see Fig. 2-23) is a sensory branch of the tibial nerve. It is formed by the lateral sural cutaneous nerve from the common peroneal nerve and the medial calcaneal nerve from the tibial nerve. The sural nerve supplies the skin on the posterior-lateral aspect of the lower one third of the leg and the lateral side of the foot.

Terminal Branches of the Tibial Nerve. In the distal leg, the tibial nerve lies laterally to the posterior tibial vessels, and it supplies articular branches to the ankle joint and to the posterior-medial aspect of the ankle. From this point, its terminal branches include:

▶ *Medial plantar nerve* (comparable to the median nerve in the hand). This nerve supplies the flexor digitorum brevis, abductor hallucis, flexor halluces brevis, and first lumbrical muscles; and sensory branches to the medial side of the sole, the plantar surfaces of the medial 3½ toes, and the ungual phalanges of the same toes (see Fig. 2-23).

▶ *Lateral plantar nerve* (comparable to the ulnar nerve in the hand). This nerve supplies the small muscles of the foot, except those innervated by the medial plantar nerve; and sensory branches to the lateral portions of the sole, the plantar surface of the lateral 1 ½ toes, and the distal phalanges of these toes (see Fig. 2-23). The interdigital nerves are most commonly entrapped between the second and third, and the third and fourth web spaces and the intermetatarsal ligaments as a result of a forced hyperextension of the toes, eventually resulting in an interdigital neuroma.

▶ *Medial calcaneal nerve.* As it passes beneath the flexor retinaculum, the tibial nerve gives off medial calcanean branches to the skin of the heel. An irritation of this nerve may result in heel pain.

Common Peroneal Nerve. The common peroneal nerve (L4,5; S1–2) is formed by a fusion of the upper four posterior divisions of the sacral plexus, and thus derives its fibers from the lower two lumbar and the upper two sacral cord segments (see Fig. 2-24). In the thigh, it is a component of the sciatic nerve as far as the upper part of the popliteal space. The nerve gives off sensory branches in the popliteal space. These sensory branches include the superior and inferior articular branches to the knee joint, and the lateral sural cutaneous nerve (see Figs. 2-23 and 2-24).

At the apex of the popliteal fossa, the common peroneal nerve begins its independent descent along the posterior border of the biceps femoris, then crosses the dorsum of the knee joint to the upper external portion of the leg near the head of the fibula. The nerve curves around the lateral aspect of the fibula toward the anterior aspect of the bone before passing deep to the two heads of the peroneus longus muscle, where it divides into three terminal rami: the recurrent articular, superficial, and deep peroneal nerves.

▶ The recurrent articular nerve accompanies the anterior tibial recurrent artery, supplying the tibiofibular and knee joints, and a twig to the tibialis anterior muscle.

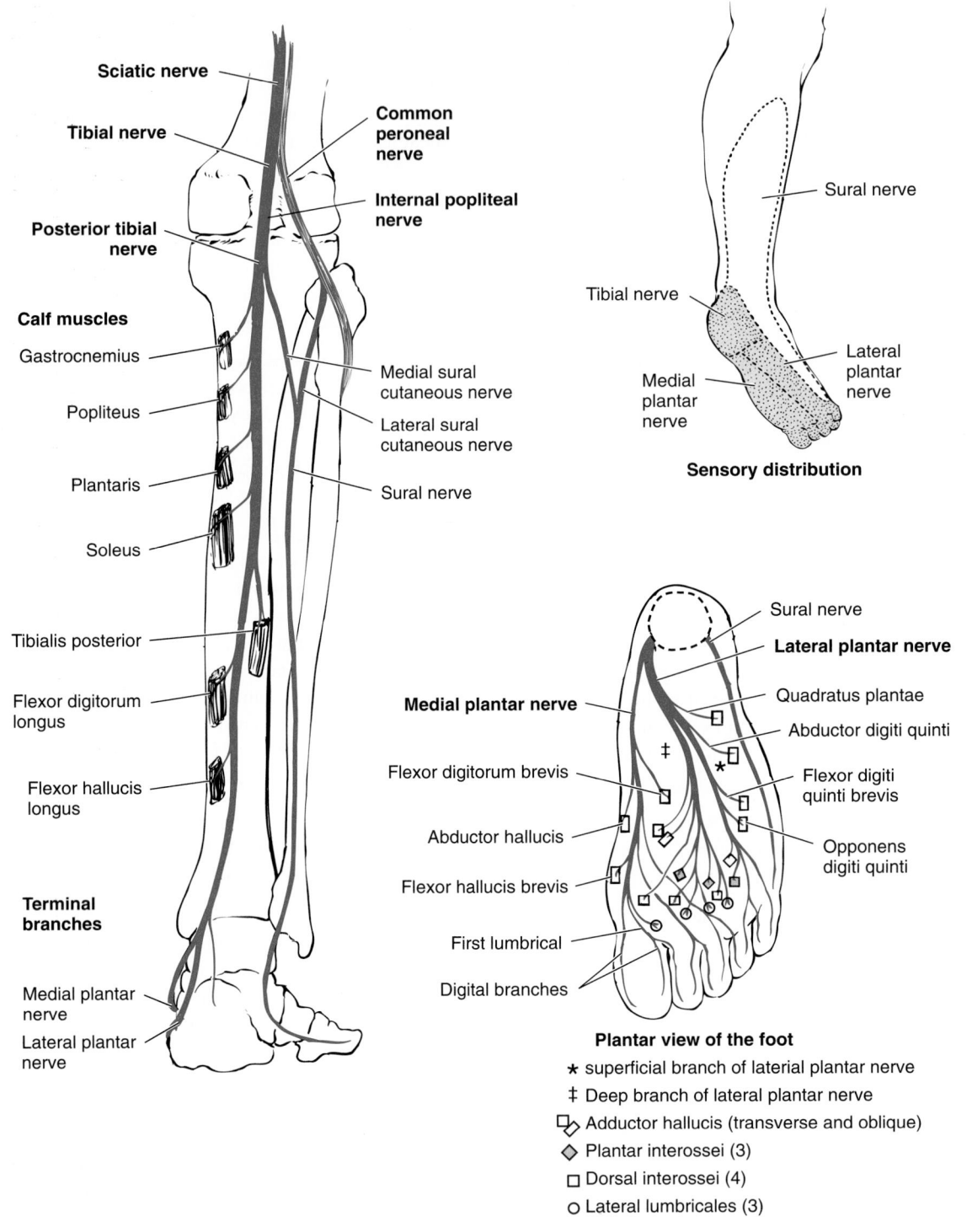

Sensory distribution

Plantar view of the foot

★ superficial branch of lateral plantar nerve
‡ Deep branch of lateral plantar nerve
⬒⬦ Adductor hallucis (transverse and oblique)
◆ Plantar interossei (3)
☐ Dorsal interossei (4)
○ Lateral lumbricales (3)

FIGURE 2-23   The tibial nerve (L4,5; S1–3). (Reproduced with permission from Waxman SG. *Correlative Neuroanatomy.* 24th ed. New York, NY: McGraw-Hill; 1996.)

▶ The superficial peroneal nerve arises deep to the peroneus longus (see Fig. 2-24). It then passes forward and downward between the peronei and the extensor digitorum longus muscles, to supply the peroneus longus and brevis muscles and provide sensory distribution to the lower front of the leg, the dorsum of the foot, part of the big toe, and adjacent sides of the second to fifth toes up to the second phalanges. When this nerve is entrapped, because it causes pain over the lateral distal aspect of the leg and ankle, it is often confused with a disk herniation involving the L5 nerve root.

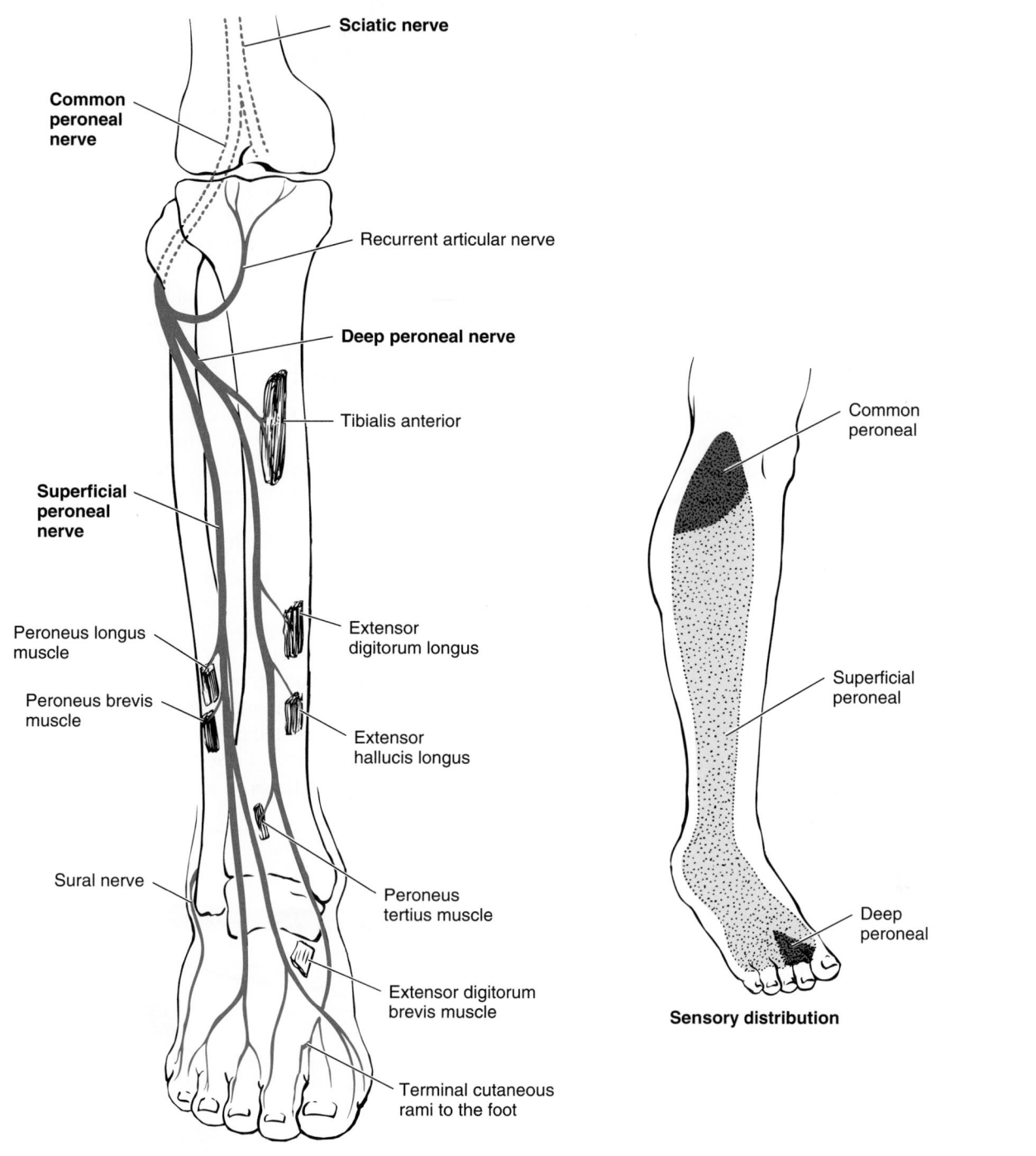

FIGURE 2-24   The common peroneal nerve (L4,5; S1,2). (Reproduced with permission from Waxman SG. *Correlative Neuroanatomy*. 24th ed. New York, NY: McGraw-Hill; 1996.)

▶ The deep peroneal nerve passes anterior and lateral to the tibialis anterior muscle, between the peroneus longus and the extensor digitorum longus muscles, and to the front of the interosseous membrane and supplies the tibialis anterior, extensor digitorum longus, extensor halluces longus, and peroneus tertius muscles (see Fig. 2-24). At the level of the ankle joint, the deep peroneal nerve passes behind the extensor halluces longus tendon and lies between it and the extensor digitorum longus tendon. The deep peroneal nerve divides into a medial and lateral branch approximately 1.5 cm above the ankle joint. These terminal branches extend to the skin of the adjacent sides of the medial two toes (medial branch), to the extensor digitorum brevis muscle (lateral branch), and the adjacent joints (see Fig. 2-24). When the deep peroneal nerve is entrapped, there is a complaint of pain in the great toe, which can be confused with a posttraumatic, sympathetic dystrophy.

> ### *Clinical Pearl*
>
> Compared with the tibial division, the common peroneal division is relatively tethered at the sciatic notch and the neck of the fibula and may, therefore, be less able to tolerate or distribute tension, such as occurs in acute stretching or with changes in limb position or length.

An insidious entrapment of the common peroneal nerve (and it is very vulnerable, especially at the fibula neck) can be confused with symptoms of a herniated disk, tendonitis of the popliteus tendon, mononeuritis, idiopathic peroneal palsy, intrinsic and extrinsic nerve tumors, and extraneural compression by a synovial cyst, ganglion cyst, soft tissue tumor, osseous mass, or a large fabella.[89] Traumatic injury of the nerve may occur secondary to a fracture, dislocation, surgical procedure, application of skeletal traction, or a tight cast.[89]

The pain from an entrapment of the common peroneal nerve is typically on the lateral surface of the knee, leg, and foot. Lateral knee pain is a common problem among patients seeking medical attention, and entrapment of the common peroneal nerve is frequently overlooked in the differential diagnostic considerations, especially in the absence of trauma or the presence of a palpable mass at the neck of the fibula.

Pudendal and Coccygeal Plexuses

The pudendal and coccygeal plexuses are the most caudal portions of the lumbosacral plexus and supply nerves to the perineal structures (Fig. 2-25).

1. The pudendal plexus supplies the coccygeus, levator ani, and sphincter ani externus muscles. The pudendal nerve is a mixed nerve, and a lesion that affects it or its ascending pathways can result in voiding and erectile dysfunctions.[90] A lesion in the afferent pathways of the pudendal nerve is often suspected clinically by suggestive patient histories, including organic neurologic disease or neurologic trauma. Lesions also are suspected when a neurologic physical examination to assess the function of signal segments S2, S3, and S4 is abnormal. The pudendal nerve divides into:
   a. The inferior hemorrhoidal nerves to the external anal sphincter and adjacent skin.
   b. The perineal nerve.
   c. The dorsal nerve of the penis.

2. The nerves of the coccygeal plexus are the small sensory anococcygeal nerves derived from the last three segments (S4,5; C). They pierce the sacrotuberous ligament and supply the skin in the region of the coccyx.

Autonomic Nervous System

The autonomic system is the division of the peripheral nervous system that is responsible for the innervation of smooth muscle, cardiac muscle, and glands of the body. It functions primarily at a subconscious level.

The autonomic nervous system has two components, sympathetic (Fig. 2-26) and parasympathetic (Fig. 2-27), each of which is differentiated by its site of origin as well as the transmitters it releases[133] (Table 2-1). In general, these two systems have antagonist effects on their end organs.

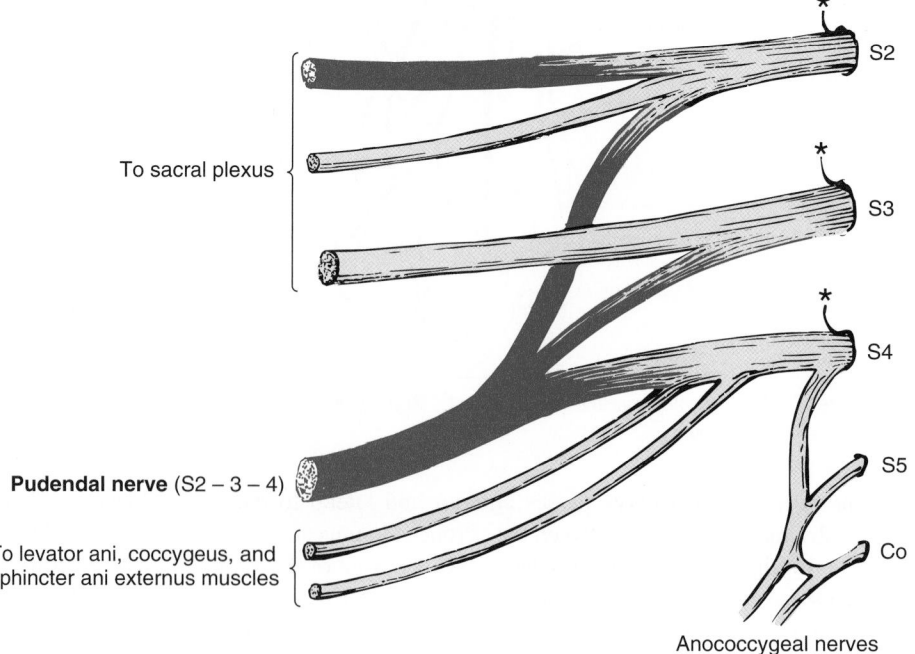

FIGURE 2-25 The pudendal and coccygeal plexuses. (Reproduced with permission from Waxman SG. *Correlative Neuroanatomy.* 24th ed. New York, NY: McGraw-Hill; 1996.)

To sacral plexus

Pudendal nerve (S2 – 3 – 4)

To levator ani, coccygeus, and sphincter ani externus muscles

S2

S3

S4

S5

Co

Anococcygeal nerves

★ Visceral branches

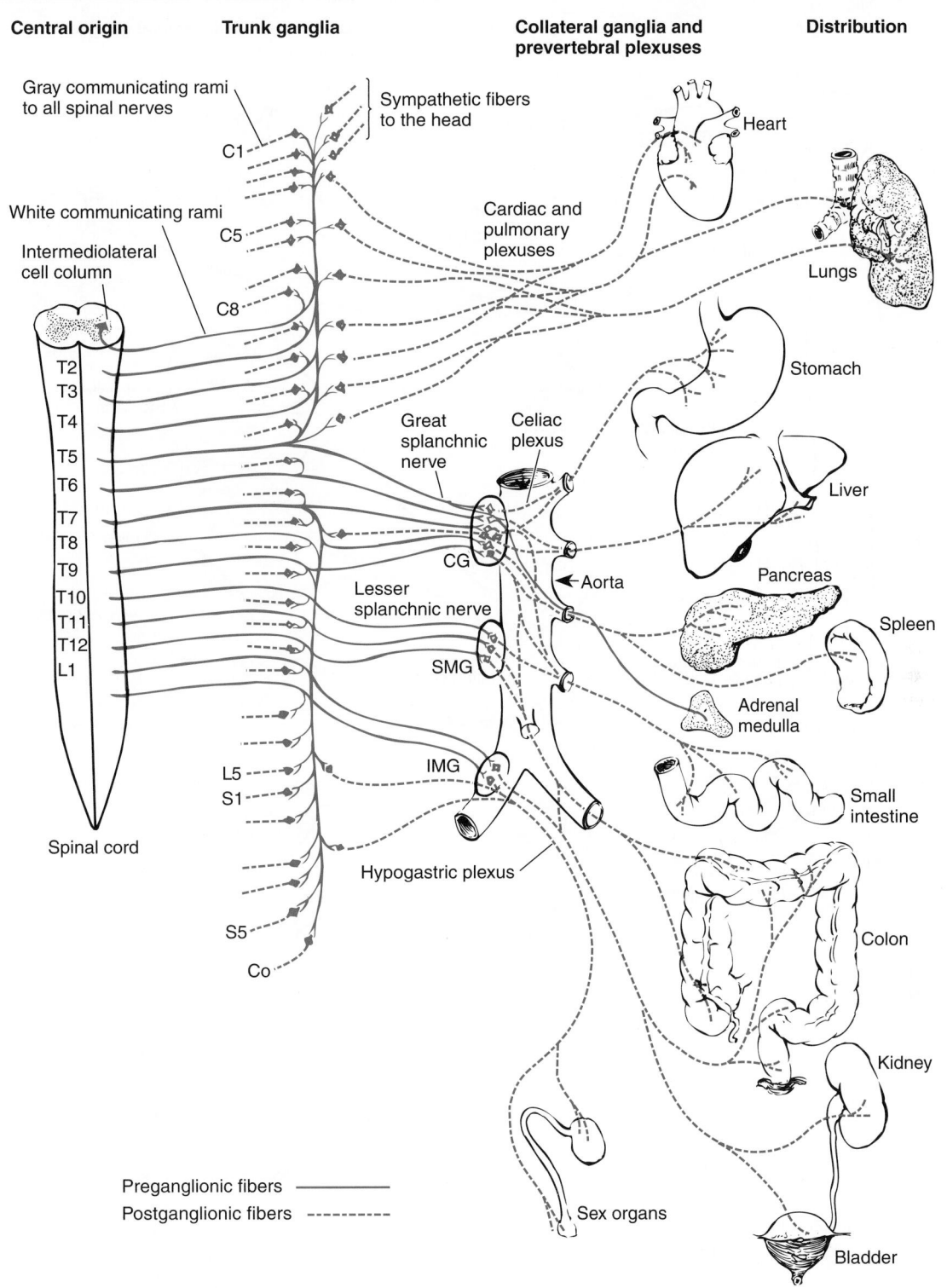

| Central origin | Trunk ganglia | Collateral ganglia and prevertebral plexuses | Distribution |

Gray communicating rami to all spinal nerves

Sympathetic fibers to the head

C1

White communicating rami

Intermediolateral cell column

C5

C8

T2
T3
T4
T5
T6
T7
T8
T9
T10
T11
T12
L1

Great splanchnic nerve

Celiac plexus

CG

Lesser splanchnic nerve

←Aorta

SMG

Spinal cord

L5
S1

IMG

S5

Co

Hypogastric plexus

Cardiac and pulmonary plexuses

Heart

Lungs

Stomach

Liver

Pancreas

Spleen

Adrenal medulla

Small intestine

Colon

Kidney

Sex organs

Bladder

Preganglionic fibers ————
Postganglionic fibers - - - - - - -

FIGURE 2-26   Sympathetic division of the autonomic nervous system (*left half*). (Reproduced with permission from Waxman SG. *Correlative Neuroanatomy*. 24th ed. New York, NY: McGraw-Hill; 1996.)

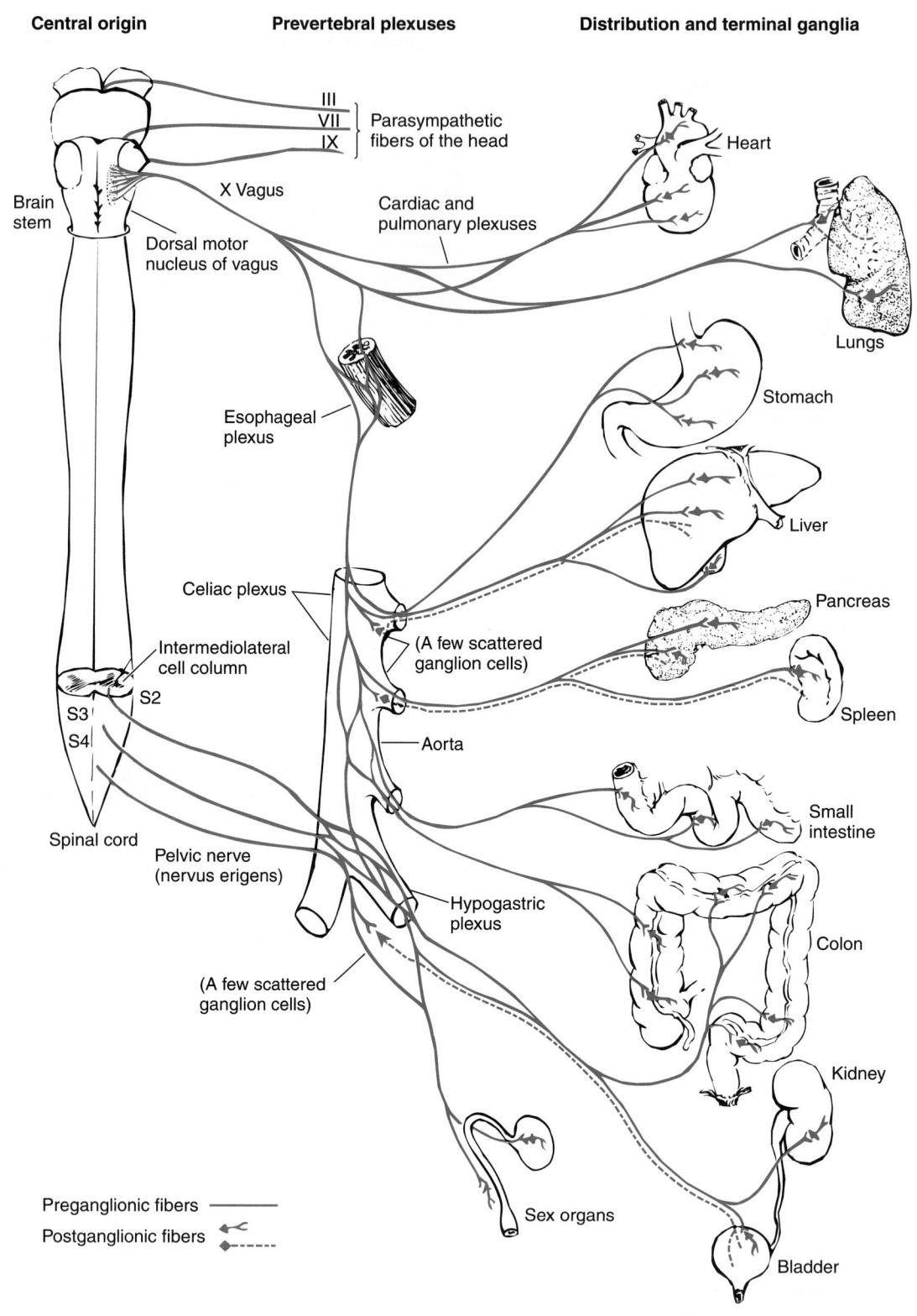

Central origin

Prevertebral plexuses

Distribution and terminal ganglia

III
VII } Parasympathetic
IX } fibers of the head

Brain stem

X Vagus

Dorsal motor nucleus of vagus

Cardiac and pulmonary plexuses

Heart

Lungs

Esophageal plexus

Stomach

Celiac plexus

Liver

(A few scattered ganglion cells)

Pancreas

Intermediolateral cell column

S2

Spleen

S3

S4

Aorta

Small intestine

Spinal cord

Pelvic nerve (nervus erigens)

Hypogastric plexus

Colon

(A few scattered ganglion cells)

Kidney

Preganglionic fibers

Postganglionic fibers

Sex organs

Bladder

FIGURE 2-27 Parasympathetic division of the autonomic nervous system (*left half*). (Reproduced with permission from Waxman SG. *Correlative Neuroanatomy*. 24th ed. New York, NY: McGraw-Hill; 1996.)

TABLE 2-1 Autonomic Nervous System Divisions[133]

	Sympathetic	Parasympathetic
General location	Thoracolumbar	Craniosacral
Specific location	Intermediolateral and medial gray matter, T1–L2	Cranial nerves III, VII, IX, X, and sacral segments S2–4
Pathway characteristics	Short preganglionic fibers	Long preganglionic fibers
	Long postganglionic fibers	Short postganglionic fibers
Principal neurotransmitter	Norepinephrine (except sweat glands)	Acetycholine

The sympathetic system can be involved in the modulation of pain, although under normal conditions, the sympathetic system has little or no effect on the activity of the peripheral afferent receptors. According to Blumberg and Janig,[134] the afferent neurons become hypersensitized as the result of direct trauma, producing allodynia, causalgia (complex regional pain syndrome type 1), and hyperalgesia.[135] Sensitized dorsal horn neurons increase their receptive fields and begin to respond to both low-threshold and high-threshold peripheral stimuli.[135,136]

A lesion to the sympathetic system also has been associated with Horner's syndrome (see later discussion) and with Raynaud's disease, a disorder of the peripheral vascular system (see Chap. 9).

Neuromuscular Control

Success in skilled performance depends on how effectively the individual detects, perceives, and uses relevant sensory information.[91] A patient cannot succeed in functional and recreational activities if his or her neuromuscular system is not prepared to meet the proprioceptive and balance demands of the specific activities.[92] The terms proprioception and balance are not synonymous.

Proprioception

Proprioception is considered a specialized variation of the sensory modality of touch, which plays an important role in coordinating muscle activity and involves the integration of sensory input concerning static joint position (joint position sensibility), joint movement (kinesthetic sensibility), velocity of movement, and force of muscular contraction from the skin, muscles, and joints.[93,94] Proprioception can be both conscious, as occurs in the accurate placement of a limb, and unconscious, as occurs in the modulation of muscle function.[94,95]

All synovial joints of the body are provided with an array of corpuscular (mechanoreceptors) and noncorpuscular (nociceptors) receptor endings imbedded in articular, muscular, and cutaneous structures with varying characteristic behaviors and distributions, depending on articular tissue (Table 2-2). These articular mechanoreceptors, which are stimulated by mechanical

forces (soft tissue elongation, relaxation, compression, and fluid tension) and which mediate proprioception, include Pacinian corpuscles, Ruffini endings, the muscle spindle, and Golgi tendon organ (GTO)-like endings.[14,97,98]

> **Clinical Pearl**
>
> The muscle spindle functions as a stretch receptor, whereas the GTO functions as a monitor for the degree of tension within a muscle and tendon (Box 2-1)

The mechanoreceptors translate mechanical deformation into electrical signals that provide information concerning joint motion and position.[94,99,105–107] Sensory information provided by the receptors travels through afferent pathways to the central nervous system, where it is integrated with information from other levels of the nervous system.[108] The central nervous system, in turn, elicits efferent motor responses (neuromuscular control) vital to mediate proprioception and influence muscle tone and function.

Freeman and Wyke categorized these mechano receptors into four different types[97,109] Types I, II, and III are articular mechanoreceptors, whereas the type IV variety is a nociceptor.[98]

▶ *Type I: small Ruffini endings.* These slow-adapting, low-threshold stretch receptors are important in signaling actual joint position or changes in joint positions. Thus, they are located in the joint capsule and in ligaments. They contribute to reflex regulation of postural tone, to coordination of muscle activity, and to a perceptional awareness of joint position. An increase in joint capsule tension by active or passive motion, posture, mobilization, or manipulation causes these receptors to discharge at a higher frequency.[98,110]

▶ *Type II: Pacinian corpuscles.* These rapidly adapting, low-threshold receptors function primarily in sensing joint motion. They are located in adipose tissue, the cruciate ligaments, the anulus fibrosus, ligaments, and the fibrous capsule. Their behavior suggests their role as a control mechanism to regulate motor unit activity of the prime movers of the joint. Type II

TABLE 2-2   Characteristics of Certain Sensory Receptors[96]

Type of Sensory Receptors	Stimulus		Receptor	
	General Term	Specific Nature	Term	Location
Mechanoreceptors	Pressure	Movement of hair in a hair follicle	Afferent nerve fiber	Base of hair follicles
		Light pressure	Meissner's corpuscle	Skin
		Deep pressure	Pacinian corpuscle	Skin
		Touch	Merkel's touch corpuscle	Skin
Nociceptors	Pain	Distention (stretch)	Free nerve endings	Wall of gastrointestinal tract, pharynx, skin
Proprioceptors	Tension	Distention	Corpuscles of Ruffini	Skin and capsules in joints and ligaments
		Length changes	Muscle spindles	Skeletal muscles
		Tension changes	Golgi tendon organs	Between muscles and tendons
Thermoreceptors	Temperature change	Cold	Krause's end bulbs	Skin
		Heat	Corpuscles of Ruffini	Skin and capsules in joints and ligaments

Box 2-1 MUSCLE SPINDLE AND GOLGI TENDON ORGAN

Muscle Spindle

Within each muscle spindle there are 2 to 12 long, slender, specialized skeletal muscle fibers called *intrafusal fibers*. The central portion of the intrafusal fiber is devoid of actin or myosin, and thus is incapable of contracting. As a result, these fibers are capable of putting tension on the spindle only. These intrafusal fibers are of two types: nuclear bag fibers and nuclear chain fibers. Nuclear bag fibers, which are primarily sensitive to changes in velocity and are innervated by type 1a phasic nerve fibers, extend beyond the capsule ends and tighten relatively slowly.[99,100] Nuclear chain fibers each contain a single row or chain of nuclei and are attached at their ends to the bag fibers.

   The muscle spindle is stimulated by a quick stretch, which reflexively produces a quick contraction of the agonistic and synergistic muscle (extrafusal) fibers. This has the effect of producing a smooth contraction and relaxation of muscle and eliminating any jerkiness during movement. The firing of the type Ia phasic nerve fibers is influenced by the rate of stretch; the faster and greater the stimulus, the greater the effect of the associated extrafusal fibers.[101,102]

Golgi Tendon Organs

Golgi tendon organs (GTOs) function to protect muscle attachments from strain or avulsion by using a postsynaptic inhibitory synapse of the muscle in which they are located.[103] The GTO receptors are arranged in series with the extrafusal muscle fibers and, therefore, become activated by stretch. The signals from the GTO may go both to local areas within the spinal cord and through the spinal cerebellar tracts to the cerebellum.[104] The local signals result in excitation of interneurons, which in turn inhibit the anterior α motor neurons of the GTO's own muscle and synergist, while facilitating the antagonists.[104] This is theorized to prevent overcontraction, or stretch, of a muscle.[103]

receptors are entirely inactive in immobile joints and become active for brief periods at the onset of movement and during rapid changes in tension. They fire during active or passive motion of a joint, or with the application of traction.

▶ *Type III: large Ruffini endings.* These slow-adapting, high-threshold receptors function to detect large amounts of tension. They only become active in the extremes of motion or when strong manual techniques are applied to the joint.

▶ *Type IV: nociceptors.* These slow-adapting, high-threshold, free nerve endings form a network of unmyelinated nerve fibers.[111,112] Type IV receptors are inactive in normal circumstances but become active with marked mechanical deformation or tension. They may also become active in response to direct mechanical or chemical irritation.

In addition to providing restraint at the extremes of joint range motion, the capsuloligamentous structures function to guide and direct normal movements.[105] However, ligaments alone are incapable of total control under situations of high load demands and require the assistance of active muscle.[113,114]

More than 50 years ago, it was proposed that extremes of motion activate the mechanoreceptors of the ligaments, initiating a spinal reflex with contraction of muscles antagonizing the movement through a ligamentomuscular reflex.[115,116] Such contraction was assumed to take place in order to prevent damage to the ligament and cartilage (a joint protective reflex).

Clinical Pearl

Proprioception can play a protective role in an acute injury through reflex muscle splinting via stimulation of the muscle spindles.[117]

These reflex actions include preparatory postural adjustments[118] and reaction movements. The former are preprogrammed neural mechanisms. The latter occur too fast for the feedback loops of the central nervous system so that they are automatic and occur subconsciously. Thus, proprioception can be viewed as the precursor of good balance and adequate function.[117]

Following an injury, alterations occur in the normal recruitment pattern and timing of muscular contractions. This is thought to result from an alteration in the ratio of muscle spindles to GTO activity, and a disruption of the proprioceptive pathway.[119–121] Any delay in response time to an unexpected load placed on the dynamic restraints can expose the static restraint structures to excessive forces, increasing the potential for injury.[91]

Fatigue also may play a part in injury, particularly if the fatigue produces a dominance of agonists or antagonists over the other.[120] Fatigue also reduces the capability of a muscle to absorb or dissipate loads. It seems plausible that some form of muscle spindle desensitization, or perhaps ligament relaxation and Golgi tendon desensitization, occurs with excessive fatigue.[122] This may then lead to a decreased efferent muscle response and reduced ability to maintain balance.

Proprioceptive deficits also can be found with aging,[123] arthrosis,[124] and joint instability.[95,117,119,125–129]

Balance

Balance is the process by which the body's center of mass is controlled with respect to the base of support, whether that base of support is stationary or moving.[129]

The visual system, which involves CN II, III, IV, and VI, assists in balance control by providing input about the position of the head or the body in space. Through the vestibulo-ocular input, signals from the muscle spindles in the extraocular muscles, the position of the eyeball is controlled so that a visual image is maintained on the fovea. The coordination of eye movements during gaze is a complex affair and is controlled by efferent signals from the trochlear, abducens, and oculomotor nuclei via the fourth, sixth, and third cranial nerves, respectively (refer to the discussion of cervico-ocular and vestibular reflexes, later in this chapter).[10] Coordination of these nuclei is achieved by gaze centers in the reticular formation, midbrain, and cortex, and by the cerebellum, which have fibers that project into the three eye muscle nuclei and control the orbital movements concerned with slow and rapid eye movements.[10]

Proprioception can be conscious or unconscious, whereas balance is typically conscious. According to Berg,[130] balance can be defined as the ability:

▶ To maintain a position.

▶ To voluntarily move.

▶ To react to a perturbation.

Position and Movement Sense

Kinesthesia refers to the sense of position and movement. Although the articular receptors quite clearly play a very active role, two other sensors, the muscle spindle and the GTO, also are important. Information about movement and position sense travels up the spinocerebellar tract (Box 2-2).

Clinical Pearl

During a concentric muscle contraction, the muscle spindle output is reduced because the muscle fibers are either shortening, or attempting to shorten, whereas during an eccentric contraction, the muscle stretch reflex generates more tension in the lengthening muscle.[101,131,132]

The Neurophysiology of Pain

Pain, at some point or other, is felt by everyone. No longer thought of as just a sensation and a symptom of many diseases, pain is considered an emotional experience that is highly individualized and extremely difficult to evaluate. Acute pain can be defined as "the normal, predicted physiological response to an adverse chemical, thermal, or mechanical stimulus . . . associated with surgery, trauma, and acute illness."[137]

Box 2-2 SPINOCEREBELLAR TRACT

The spinocerebellar tract conducts impulses related to the position and movement of muscles to the cerebellum. The cerebellum adds smoothness and precision to patterns of movement. Four tracts constitute the spinocerebellar pathway; the posterior, anterior and rostral spinocerebellar tracts, and the cuneocerebellar tract.

The posterior spinocerebellar tract conveys tactile, pressure, and proprioceptive impulses from the lower half of the body (below the level of the T6 spinal cord segment); the cuneocerebellar tract is concerned with such impulses from the body above T6. The anterior spinocerebellar tract conveys impulses from group I muscle afferents, from a wide variety of cutaneous receptors, and from fibers of descending tracts.

The axons conducting tactile, pressure, and proprioceptive impulses from muscle spindles, tendon organs, and skin in the lower half of the body are large type Ia, Ib, and type II fibers, the cell bodies of which are in the spinal ganglia of spinal nerves T6 and below.

Primary neurons below L3 send their information into the posterior columns. These processes then ascend in the columns to the L3 level. From L3 to T6, incoming impulses and those in the posterior columns project to the base of the dorsal horn called lamina VII, where there is a distinctive cell group, called *Clarke's column*. Largely limited to the thoracic cord, Clarke's column can be seen from segments L3 to C8 of the cord. The cells of Clarke's column send axons into the ipsilateral lateral funiculus where they are located posteriorly and laterally.

Clinical Pearl

Patients' attitudes, beliefs, and personalities may strongly affect their immediate experience of acute pain.

Our knowledge of the pain system has greatly improved over the past few years with discoveries that have increased our understanding of the role of nociceptors and the processing of nociceptive information. Furthermore, new findings have illuminated our knowledge about the descending pathways that modulate nociceptive activity.

Transmission of Pain

Any tissue that contains free nerve endings involved with nociception is capable of being a source of pain. The common free nerve endings have two distinct pathways into the central nervous system, which correspond to the two different types of pain represented by two distinct nerve pain pathways: fast conducting A delta and slow conducting C fibers (Table 2-3), although not all of the fibers are necessarily nociceptors. However, only three mechanisms are known by which these nociceptors can become activated: mechanical, chemical, or thermal stimuli (with a slow conduction velocity of < 2 m/s).[138] The existence of unmyelinated polymodal nociceptors, which are responsive to thermal, mechanical, and chemical stimuli, has been established in the cutaneous tissue of humans.[139] A-delta mechanothermal nociceptors and high-threshold, A-delta mechanoreceptors have also been identified. A-delta and C-fiber nociceptors have been clearly identified in fibers that innervate joints and muscles but not in viscerae, where the situation is much more complicated.[139] Thus, although certain fibers are undoubtedly nociceptors, others are activated by non-noxious stimuli but then increase their activity as the intensity of the stimulus increases.

Each of these types of fibers has different pain characteristics: A-delta fibers evoke a rapid, sharp pain reaction; C fibers cause a slow, dull pain.

Rapid Pain

The fast, or dermatomal, pain signals are transmitted in the peripheral nerves by small, myelinated A fibers. The fast pain impulse informs the subject that a threat is present and provokes an almost instantaneous and often reflexive response. This signal often is followed a second or more later by a duller pain that tells of either tissue damage or continuing stimulation.

Slow Pain

Slow, or sclerotomal, pain is transmitted in even smaller and unmyelinated C nerve fibers at much slower velocities. On entering the dorsal horn of the spinal cord, the pain signals from both visceral and somatic tissues do one of three things:

1. Synapse with interneurons that synapse directly with motor nerves and produce reflex movements.
2. Synapse with autonomic fibers from the sympathetic and parasympathetic systems and produce autonomic reflexes.
3. Synapse with interneurons that travel to the higher centers in the brain.
   a. The fast signals of the C fibers terminate in laminae I and V of the dorsal horn (see Fig. 2.29). Here they excite neurons that send long fibers to the opposite side of the cord and then upward to the brain in the lateral division of the anterior-lateral sensory pathway (lateral spinothalamic tract; Fig. 2-28 and Box 2-3).
   b. The slow signals of the C fibers terminate in laminae II and III of the dorsal horn (Fig. 2-29). Most of the information then terminates in lamina V. Here, the neuron gives off a long axon, most of which joins with

TABLE 2-3   Classification of Afferent Neurons[96]

Size	Type	Group	Subgroup	Diameter (μm)	Conduction Velocity (m/s)	Receptor	Stimulus
Large	Aα	I	Ia	12–20 (22)	70–120	Proprioceptive mechanoreceptor	Muscle velocity and length change, muscle shortening of rapid speed
	Aα	I	Ib				
	Aα	II	Muscle	6–12	36–72	Proprioceptive mechanoreceptor	Muscle length information from touch and Pacinian corpuscles
	Aβ	II	Skin			Cutaneous receptors	Touch, vibration, hair receptors
	Aδ	III	Muscle	1–5 (6)	6(12)–36 (80)	75% mechanoreceptors and thermoreceptors	Temperature change
Small	Aδ	III	Skin			25% nociceptors, mechanoreceptors, and thermoreceptors (hot and cold)	Noxious, mechanical, and temperature ($> 45°C, < 10°C$)
	C	IV	Muscle	0.3–1.0	0.4–1.0	50% mechanoreceptors and thermoreceptors	Touch and temperature
	C	IV	Skin			50% nociceptors, 20% mechanoreceptors, and 30% thermoreceptors (hot and cold)	Noxious, mechanical, and temperature ($> 45°C, < 10°C$)

the fast signal axons to cross the spinal cord and continue upward in the brain in the same spinal tract. Most of the pain fibers terminate in the reticular formation of the medulla, pons, and mesencephalon. From here, other neurons transmit the signal to the thalamus, hypothalamus (pituitary), limbic system, and the cerebral cortex.

The central pathways for processing nociceptive information begin at the level of the spinal cord (and medullary) dorsal horn. As with the periphery, the dorsal horn of the spinal cord contains many transmitters and receptors, including several peptides (substance P, calcitonin, somatostatin, neuropeptide Y, and galanin), excitatory amino acids (aspartate, glutamate), inhibitory amino acids (γ-aminobutyric acid [GABA], glycine), nitric oxide, the arachidonic acid metabolites, the endogenous opioids, adenosine, and the monoamines (serotonin, noradrenaline).[139] This list indicates that there are diverse therapeutic possibilities for the control of the transmission of nociceptive information to the brain.

Interneuronal networks in the dorsal horn are responsible not only for the transmission of nociceptive information to neurons that project to the brain, but also for the modulation of that information. The information is passed to other spinal cord neurons, including the flexor motoneurons and the nociceptive projection neurons. Other inputs result in the inhibition of projection neurons.

A small number of fast fibers pass directly to the thalamus, and then to the cerebral cortex, bypassing the brain stem. It is believed that these signals are important for recognizing and localizing pain. Of the slow signals, very few avoid the reticular system. Because most of the fast, and all of the slow, pain signals go through the reticular formation, they can have wide-ranging effects on almost the entire nervous system.

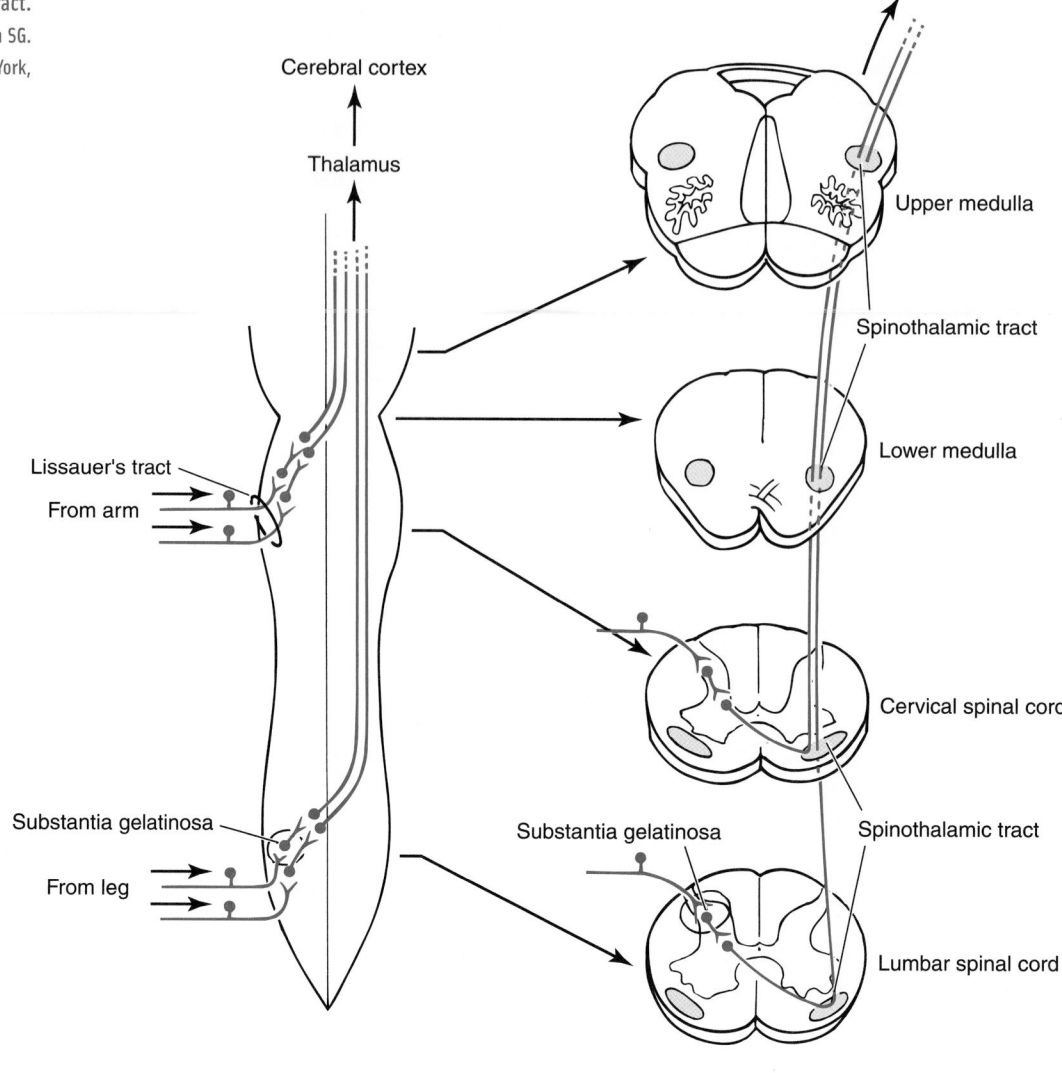

FIGURE 2-28 The spinothalamic tract. (Reproduced with permission from Waxman SG. *Correlative Neuroanatomy.* 24th ed. New York, NY: McGraw-Hill; 1996.)

Cerebral cortex

Thalamus

Upper medulla

Spinothalamic tract

Lissauer's tract

From arm

Lower medulla

Substantia gelatinosa

From leg

Substantia gelatinosa

Cervical spinal cord

Spinothalamic tract

Lumbar spinal cord

Box 2-3 SPINOTHALAMIC TRACT

The spinothalamic tract helps mediate the sensations of pain, cold, warmth, and touch from receptors throughout the body (except the face) to the brain.[112,104,140,141] Laterally projecting spinothalamic neurons are more likely to be situated in laminae I and V. Medially projecting cells are more likely to be situated in the deep dorsal horn and in the ventral horn. Most of the cells project to the contralateral thalamus, although a small fraction projects ipsilaterally.[142] Spinothalamic axons in the anterior-lateral quadrant of the spinal cord are arranged somatotopically. At cervical levels, spinothalamic axons representing the lower extremity and caudal body are placed more laterally, and those representing the upper extremity and rostral body, more anterior-medially.[143,144]

Most of the neurons respond when the skin is stimulated mechanically at a noxious intensity. However, many spinothalamic tract cells also respond, although less effectively, to innocuous mechanical stimuli, and some respond best to innocuous mechanical stimuli.[145] A large fraction of spinothalamic tract cells also respond to a noxious heating of the skin,[146] while others respond to stimulation of the receptors in muscle,[147] joints, or viscera.[111]

Spinothalamic tract cells can be inhibited effectively by repetitive electrical stimulation of peripheral nerves,[148] with the inhibition outlasting the stimulation by 20–30 minutes. Some inhibition can be evoked by stimulation of the large myelinated axons of a peripheral nerve, but the inhibition is much more powerful if small myelinated or unmyelinated afferents are included in the volleys.[149] The best inhibition is produced by stimulation of a peripheral nerve in the same limb as the excitatory receptive field, but some inhibition occurs when nerves in other limbs are stimulated. A similar inhibition results when high-intensity stimuli are applied to the skin with a clinical transcutaneous electrical nerve stimulator (TENS) unit in place of direct stimulation of a peripheral nerve.[150]

As the spinothalamic tract ascends, it migrates from a lateral position to a posterior-lateral position. In the midbrain, the tract lies adjacent to the medial lemniscus. The axons of the secondary neurons terminate in one of a number of centers in the thalamus.

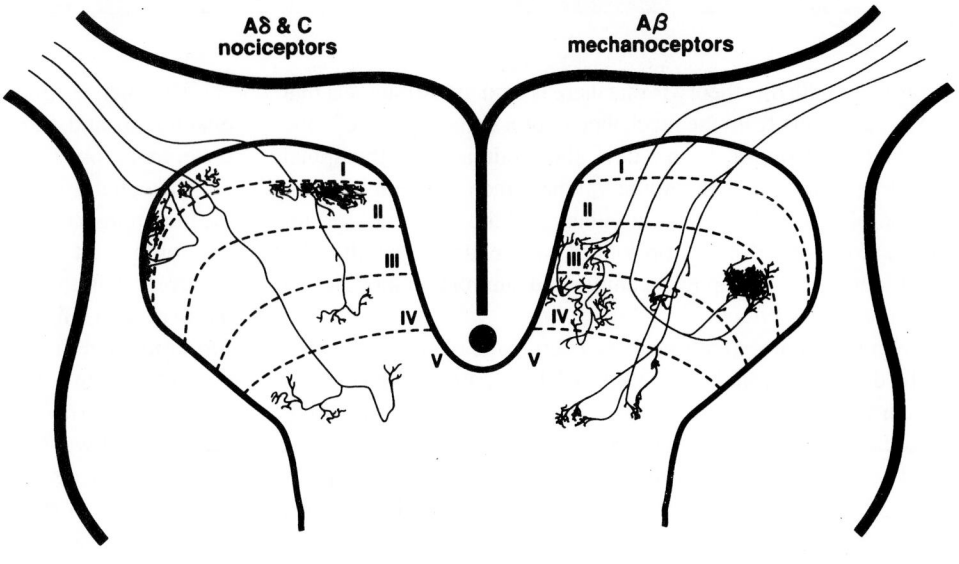

FIGURE 2-29 The termination of sensory input in the dorsal horn. (Reproduced with permission from Haldeman S, ed. *Principles and Practice of Chiropractic.* Norwalk, Conn: Appleton and Lange; 1992.)

Lamina V is the area for convergence, summation, and projection. The response of the cells in lamina V depends largely on the intensity of the stimulus. High-intensity stimulation leads to facilitation of the cell and relatively easy transmission across the cord to the other side and, from here, upward. More gentle stimulation inhibits this transmission. This inhibition is, according to theory, the result of pre- and postsynaptic effects produced by the cells of laminae II and III. Thus, the net effect at lamina V determines whether the pain signal is relayed upward. If mild mechanoreceptor input dominates, the pain signal is stopped at this point. If, however, pain input level is strong, or if the mechanoreceptor input is high, transmission of the pain signal occurs.

Control of Pain

Melzack and Wall[151] postulated that interneurons in the substantia gelatinosa act as a gate to modulate sensory input (Fig. 2-30). They proposed that the substantia gelatinosa interneuron projected to the second-order neuron of the pain-temperature pathway located in lamina V, which they called the transmission cell. It was reasoned that if the substantia gelatinosa interneuron were depolarized, it would inhibit transmission cell firing, and thus decrease further transmission of input ascending in the spinothalamic tract. The degree of modulation appeared to depend on the proportion of input from the large A fibers and the small C fibers, so that the gate could be closed by either decreasing C fiber input, or by increasing A fiber or mechanoreceptive input (see Fig. 2-30).

Melzack and Wall also believed that the gate could be modified by a descending inhibitory pathway from the brain, or brain stem,[152] suggesting that the central nervous system apparently plays a part in this modulation in a mechanism called central biasing. The gate theory was, and is, supported by practical evidence, although the experimental evidence for the theory is lacking. Researchers have identified many clinical pain states that cannot be fully explained by the gate control theory.[153]

FIGURE 2-30 Schematic representation of gate control of pain. (Reproduced with permission from Murphy DR. *Conservative Management of Cervical Spine Syndromes.* New York, NY: McGraw-Hill; 2000.)

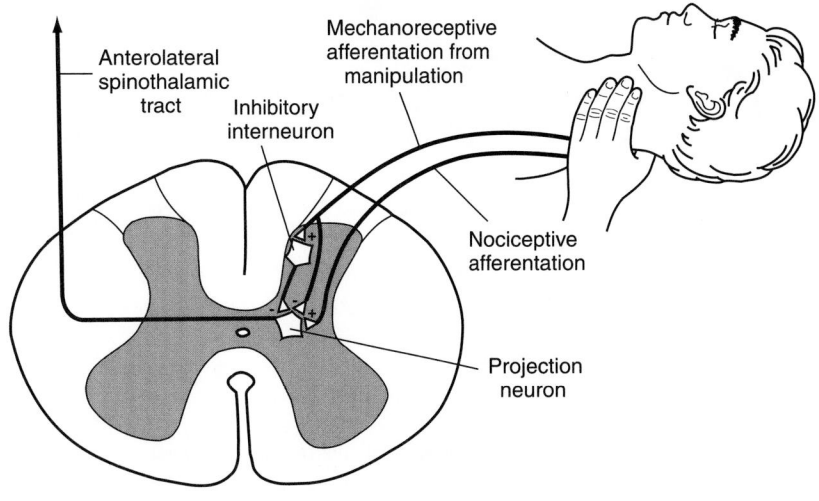

A problem with this theory is that there is evidence to suggest that the A-beta fibers from the mechanoreceptor do not synapse in the substantia gelatinosa. In this case, the modulation at the spinal cord level must occur in lamina V, where there is a simple summation of signals from the pain fibers and the mechanoreceptor fibers. However, severe or prolonged pain tends to have the segment identifying all input as painful, and summation modulation has little, if any, effect.

Numerous investigations have been made of what is known as the descending analgesia systems. These pathways have been shown to utilize several different neurotransmitters, including opioids, serotonin, and catecholamines.

The periaquaductal gray (PAG) area of the upper pons sends signals to the raphe magnus nucleus in the lower pons and upper medulla. This nucleus relays the signal down the cord to a pain inhibitory complex located in the dorsal horn of the cord (see Fig. 2-31). The PAG is believed to be involved in complex behavioral responses to stressful or life-threatening situations.

The nerve fibers derived from the gray area secrete enkephalin and serotonin, whereas the raphe magnus releases enkephalin, only.

Enkephalin is believed to produce presynaptic inhibition of the incoming pain signals to lamina I through V, thereby blocking pain signals at their entry point into the cord.[154] It is further believed that the chemical releases in the upper end of the pathway can inhibit pain signal transmission in the reticular formation and thalamus.

In the cortex, a negative feedback loop, called the corticofugal system, originates at the termination point of the various sensory pathways.[155] Excessive stimulation of this feedback loop results in a signal being transmitted down from the sensory cortex to the posterior horn of the level from which the input arose. This response prevents the spread of the signal, functioning as an automatic gain control system to prevent overloading, of the sensory system.

Neurologic Testing

The examination of the transmission capability of the nervous system is performed to detect the presence of either an upper motor neuron (UMN) lesion or a lower motor neuron (LMN) lesion.

Upper Motor Neuron Lesion

The UMN is located in the white columns of the spinal cord and the cerebral hemispheres. A UMN lesion is also known as a central palsy. Signs and symptoms associated with a UMN lesion follow.

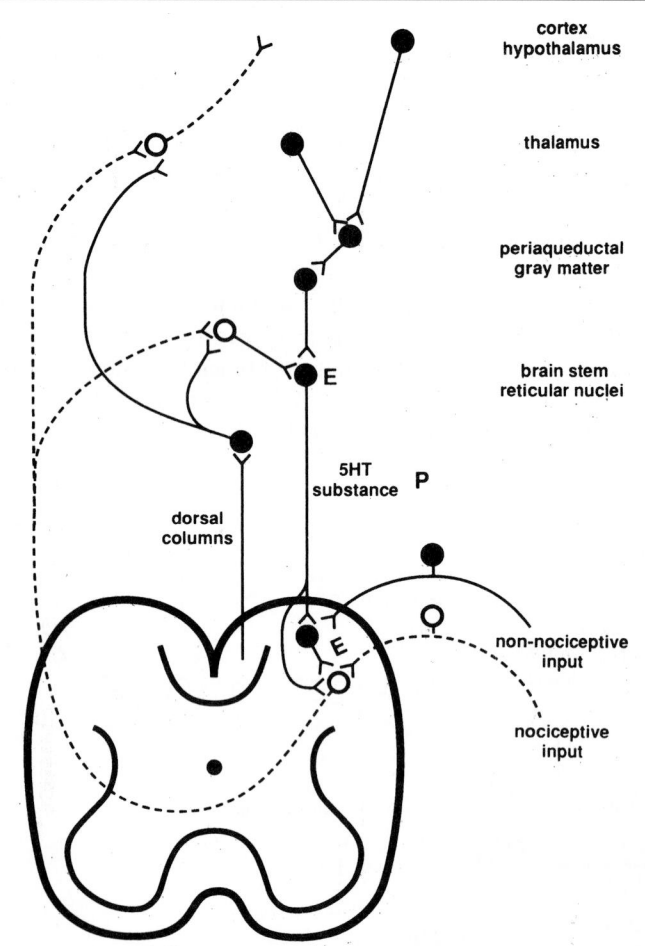

FIGURE 2-31 The primary pathways associated with the central pain control mechanism. (Reproduced with permission from Haldeman S, ed. *Principles and Practice of Chiropractic*. Norwalk, Conn: Appleton and Lange; 1992.)

> **Clinical Pearl**
>
> A UMN lesion is characterized by spastic paralysis or paresis, little or no muscle atrophy, hyperreflexive deep tendon reflexes in a nonsegmental distribution, and the presence of pathologic signs and reflexes.

Nystagmus. Nystagmus is characterized by an involuntary loss of control of the conjugate movement of the eyes (about one or more axes) involved with smooth pursuit or saccadic movement. When the eyes oscillate like a sine wave, it is called *pendular nystagmus*. If the nystagmus consists of drifts in one direction with corrective fast phases, it is called *jerk nystagmus*.

Broadly, nystagmus may be divided into one of three categories. Firstly, it may be induced physiologically (e.g., optokinetic, vestibular, and end-point). Secondly, it can be present at birth or soon after, when it is referred to as *congenital* or *infantile nystagmus*. And thirdly, it may be acquired (e.g., neurologic disease or drug toxicity).[156,157] In health, nystagmus occurs during self-rotation in order to hold images of the visual world steady on the retina and maintain clear vision. Two forms of nystagmus are induced by self-rotation: optokinetic and vestibular.[158] An optokinetic nystagmus is an involuntary, conjugate, jerk nystagmus that is seen when a person gazes into a large moving field. The vestibular form of nystagmus occurs with self-rotation.

Many forms of acquired nystagmus can be attributed to disturbances of the three mechanisms that normally ensure steady gaze: visual fixation, the vestibulo-ocular reflex, and the mechanism that makes it possible to hold the eyes at an eccentric eye position.[158] Diseases affecting the *visual system*, such as retinal disorders causing visual loss, commonly lead to nystagmus because visual fixation is no longer possible. Disease affecting the *vestibular organ* in the inner ear causes an imbalance that leads to a mixed horizontal-torsional nystagmus, usually associated with vertigo. Positional nystagmus has long been recognized as a sign of vestibular disease.[159,160] The most common form of positional nystagmus is benign paroxysmal positional nystagmus, which results from a labyrinthine lesion.[161] Disease affecting the central connections of the vestibular system, including the cerebellum, may cause several forms of nystagmus. These include down-beat, torsional, periodic alternating, and seesaw nystagmus. None of these nystagmus types are, in themselves, pathognomonic of central nervous system disease.[158]

The more serious causes of nystagmus include lesions to the brain stem or cerebellum, although the mechanisms by which the cerebellum influences eye movements are still under investigation. Nystagmus also can be a characteristic sign of vertebrobasilar compromise (see Chap. 21).

Dysphasia. Dysphasia is defined as a problem with vocabulary and results from a cerebral lesion in the speech areas of the frontal or temporal lobes. The temporal lobe receives most of its blood supply from the temporal branch of the cortical artery of the vertebrobasilar system and may become ischemic periodically, producing an inappropriate use of words.

Wallenberg's Syndrome. This is the result of a lateral medullary infarction.[162] Classically, sensory dysfunction in lateral medullary infarction is characterized by selective involvement of the spinothalamic sensory modalities with dissociated distribution (ipsilateral trigeminal and contralateral hemibody/limbs).[163] However, various patterns of sensory disturbance have been observed in lateral medullary infarction that include contralateral or bilateral trigeminal sensory impairment, restricted sensory involvement, and a concomitant deficit of lemniscal sensations.[164,165]

Ataxia. Ataxia is often most marked in the extremities. In the lower extremities, it is characterized by the so-called drunken-sailor gait pattern, with the patient veering from one side to the other and having a tendency to fall toward the side of the lesion. Ataxia of the upper extremities is characterized by a loss of accuracy in reaching for, or placing objects. Although ataxia can have a number of causes, it generally suggests central nervous system disturbance, specifically a cerebellar disorder, or a lesion of the posterior columns.[166–168]

Spasticity.[169–171] The spinal cord experiences spinal shock immediately following any trauma causing tetraplegia or paraplegia, resulting in the loss of reflexes innervated by the portion of the cord below the site of the lesion. The direct result of this spinal shock is that the muscles innervated by the traumatized portion of the cord, the portion below the lesion, as well as the bladder, become flaccid. Spinal shock, which wears off between 24 hours and 3 months after injury, can be replaced by spasticity in some, or all of these muscles.

Spasticity occurs because the reflex arc to the muscle remains anatomically intact despite the loss of cerebral innervation and control via the long tracts. During spinal shock, the arc does not function, but as the spine recovers from the shock, the reflex arc begins to function without the inhibitory or regulatory impulses from the brain, creating local spasticity and clonus.

Drop Attack. A drop attack is described as a loss of balance resulting in a fall, but with no loss of consciousness. Because it is the consequence of a loss of lower extremity control, it is never a good or benign sign. The patient, usually elderly, falls forward, with the precipitating factor being extension of the head. Recovery is usually immediate. Causes include:

▶ A vestibular system impairment.[172]

▶ Neoplastic and other impairments of the cerebellum.[173]

▶ Vertebrobasilar compromise[174] (see Chap. 21).

▶ Sudden spinal cord compression.

▶ Third ventricle cysts.

▶ Epilepsy.

▶ Type 1 Chiari malformation.[175]

Wernicke's Encephalopathy. This is an impairment, typically localized to the dorsal part of the midbrain,[176] that produces the classic triad of abnormal mental state, ophthalmoplegia, and gait ataxia.[177]

Vertical Diplopia. A history of "double vision" should alert the clinician to this condition. Patients with vertical diplopia complain of seeing two images, one atop or diagonally displaced from the other.[178]

Dysphonia. Dysphonia presents as a hoarseness of the voice. Usually, no pain is reported. Painless dysphonia is a common symptom of Wallenberg's syndrome.[164]

Hemianopia. This finding, defined as a loss in half of the visual field, is always bilateral. A visual field defect describes sensory loss restricted to the visual field and arises from damage to the primary visual pathways linking optic tract and striate cortex (see later)—Supraspinal Reflexes.

Ptosis. Ptosis is defined as a pathologic depression of the superior eyelid such that it covers part of the pupil. It results from a palsy of the levator palpebrae and Müller's muscles.

Miosis. Miosis is defined as the inability to dilate the pupil (damage to sympathetic ganglia). It is one of the symptoms of Horner's syndrome.

Horner's Syndrome. This syndrome is caused by interference to the cervicothoracic sympathetic outflow resulting from a lesion of (1) the reticular formation, (2) the descending sympathetic system, and (3) the oculomotor nerve caused by a sympathetic paralysis. The other clinical signs of Horner's syndrome are ptosis, enophthalmos, facial reddening, and anhydrosis. If Horner's syndrome is suspected, the patient should immediately be returned or referred to a physician for further examination and not treated again until the cause is found to be relatively benign.

Dysarthria. Dysarthria is defined as an undiagnosed change in articulation. Dominant or nondominant hemispheric ischemia, as well as brain stem and cerebellar impairments, may result in altered articulation.

Lower Motor Neuron Lesion

The LMN begins at the α motor neuron and includes the dorsal and ventral roots, spinal nerve, peripheral nerve, neuromuscular junction, and muscle-fiber complex.[180] The LMN consists of a cell body located in the anterior gray column and its axon, which travels to a muscle by way of the cranial or peripheral nerve. Lesions to the LMN can occur in the cell body or anywhere along the axon. An LMN lesion is also known as a peripheral palsy. These lesions can be the result of direct trauma, toxins, infections, ischemia, or compression.

> ### Clinical Pearl
>
> The characteristics of an LMN include muscle atrophy and hypotonus, diminished or absent deep tendon reflex (DTR) of the areas served by a spinal nerve root or a peripheral nerve, and absence of pathologic signs or reflexes.

The differing symptoms between a UMN lesion and an LMN lesion are the result of injuries to different parts of the nervous system. LMN impairment involves damage to a neurologic structure distal to the anterior horn cell, whereas UMN impairment involves damage to a neurologic structure proximal to the anterior horn cell; namely, the spinal cord or central nervous system.

Reflex Testing

The assessment of reflexes is extremely important in the diagnosis and localization of neurologic lesions.[2] A reflex is a subconscious, programmed unit of behavior in which a certain type of stimulus from a receptor automatically leads to the response of an effector. The response can be a simple behavior, movement, or activity. Indeed, many somatic and visceral activities are essentially reflexive. The circuitry that generates these patterns varies greatly in complexity, depending on the nature of the reflex.

A hierarchy of control mechanisms is involved with these reflexes. Reflexes can be controlled by spinal or supraspinal (brain stem) pathways.

Spinal Reflexes

The spinal reflexes are the simplest (e.g., stretch reflex, withdrawal reflex) and are entirely contained in the spinal cord. The stretch reflex (myotactic) is an example of the spinal reflex.

Myotatic Reflex. The myotatic, or deep tendon, reflex (Fig. 2-32) is one of the simplest known, depending on just two neurons and one synapse,[181] which is influenced by cortical and subcortical input, and from the stimulation of two types of receptors: the GTO and the muscle spindle. The tap of a reflex hammer on the tendon of the quadriceps femoris muscle as it crosses the knee joint causes a brief stretch of the tendon and muscle belly where the GTO and muscle spindle are stimulated.

Whenever a muscle is stretched, the intrafusal fibers are stretched with the extrafusal.[181] The sensory receptors of the spindle are excited and fire, causing a reflex contraction of the muscle that takes the stretch off the spindle (see Fig. 2-32). The subsequent impulses reach the spinal cord over the large peripheral and central processes of the sensory neurons[181] (see Fig. 2-32).

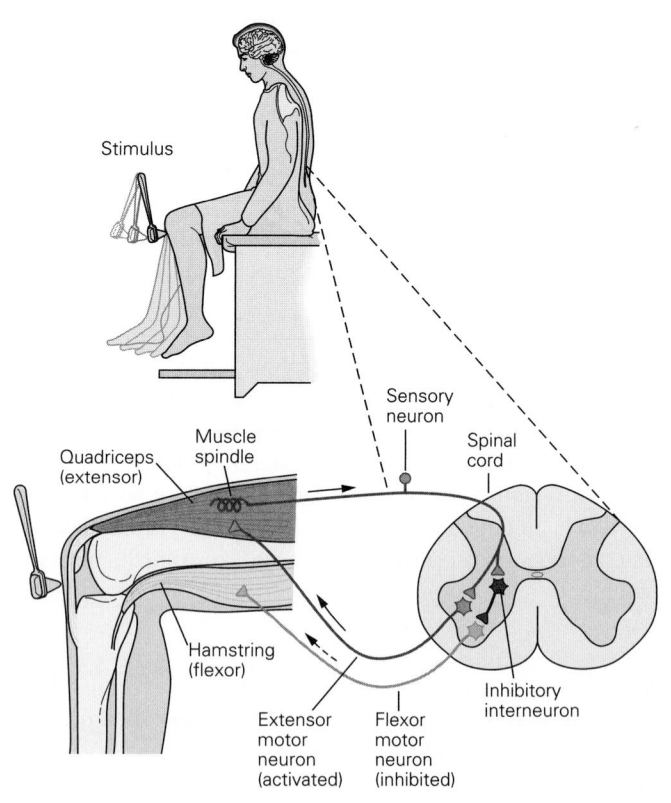

FIGURE 2-32 The myotatic reflex. (Reproduced with permission from Kandel ER, Schwartz JH, Jessell TM. *Principles of Neural Science.* New York, NY: McGraw-Hill; 2000.)

Although some impulses may head up the cord via ascending branches, most reach the synapses with the ipsilateral motor neurons of the anterior horn controlling the muscle that has been lengthened. Impulses are conducted along the axons of these motor neurons to the neuromuscular junctions, exciting the effectors (quadriceps femoris muscle), and producing a brief, weak contraction, which results in a momentary straightening of the leg (knee jerk).[181] The stretch reflex can be divided into:

1. Dynamic stretch reflex, in which the primary endings and type Ia fibers are excited by a rapid change in length (see Fig. 2-32). The speed of conduction along the type Ia fibers and the monosynaptic connection in the cord ensure that a very rapid contraction of the muscle occurs to control the sudden and potentially dangerous stretch of the muscle. The dynamic stretch reflex is over within a fraction of a second, but a secondary static reflex continues from the secondary afferent nerve fibers.

2. Static stretch reflex. As long as a stretch is applied to the muscle, both the primary and secondary endings in the nuclear chain continue to be stimulated, causing prolonged muscle contraction for as long as the excessive length of the muscle is maintained, thereby affording a mechanism for prolonged opposition to prolonged stretch.

When a load is suddenly removed from a contracting muscle, shortening of the intrafusal fibers reverses both the dynamic and static stretch reflexes, causing both sudden and prolonged inhibition of the muscle such that rebound does not occur.

Pathologic Reflexes
Refer to Table 2-4.

Babinski. In 1896, 6 years after taking his new position at the Hôpital de la Pitié, Babinski described the sign that bears his name.[182] Two years later, he presented a full account of the toe phenomenon ("phénomène des orteils") that is today regarded as a pathognomonic sign of pyramidal dysfunction.[183] Babinski later added fanning of the outer toes to the original description.[184]

In this test, the clinician applies noxious stimuli to sole of the patient's foot by running a pointed object along the plantar aspect[185] (Fig. 2-33). A positive test, demonstrated by extension of the big toe and a splaying (abduction) of the other toes, is indicative of an injury to the corticospinal tract. As Babinski observed, the pyramidal tracts are not well developed in infants, and these signs, which are abnormal past the age of 3 years, are usually present.

Oppenheim. The clinician applies noxious stimuli to the crest of the patient's tibia by running a fingernail along the crest. A positive test, demonstrated by the Babinski sign, is indicative of UMN impairment.

Clonus. The clinician passively applies a sudden dorsiflexion of the patient's ankle, and the stretch is maintained during the

TABLE 2-4 Pathologic Reflexes

Reflex	Eliciting Stimulus	Positive Response	Pathology
Babinski	Stroking of lateral aspect of side of foot	Extension of big toe and fanning of four small toes; normal reaction in newborns	Pyramidal tract lesion; organic hemiplegia
Chaddock	Stroking of lateral side of foot beneath lateral malleolus	Same response as above	Pyramidal tract lesion
Oppenheim	Stroking of anteromedial tibial surface	Same response as above	Pyramidal tract lesion
Gordon	Squeezing of calf muscles firmly	Same response as above	Pyramidal tract lesion
Brudzinski	Passive flexion of one lower limb	Similar movement occurs in opposite limb	Meningitis
Hoffmann	"Flicking" of terminal phalanx of index, middle, or ring finger	Reflex flexion of distal phalanx of thumb and of distal phalanx of index or middle finger (whichever one was not "flicked")	Increased irritability of sensory nerves in tetany; pyramidal tract lesion
Lhermitte	Neck flexion	Electric shock–like sensation that radiates down spinal column into upper or lower limbs	Abnormalities (demyelination) in posterior part of cervical spinal cord

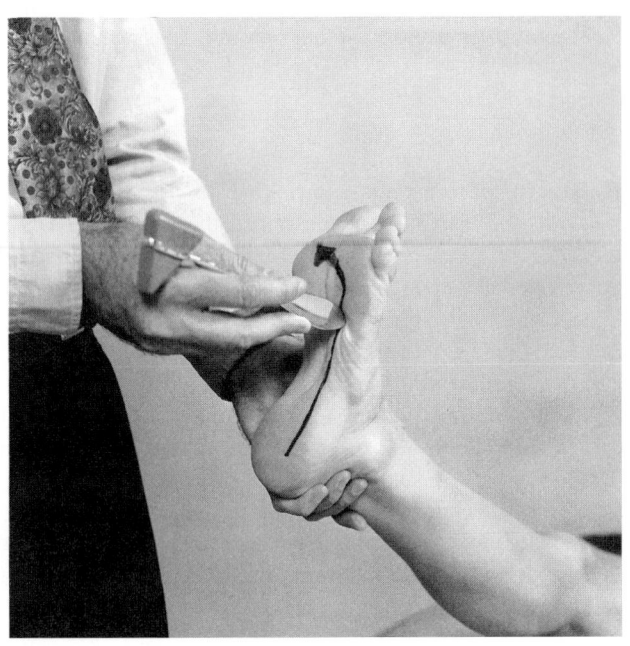

FIGURE 2-33 Babinski's reflex.

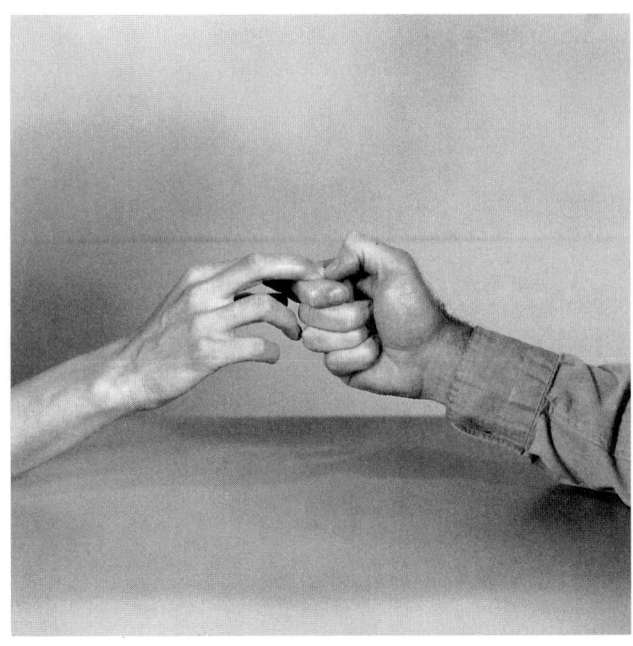

FIGURE 2-34 Hoffmann's sign.

test. The clinician notes a gradual increase in tone and then the transient occurrence of ankle clonus. In some patients, there is a more sustained clonus; in others, only a very short-lived finding. During the testing, the patient should not flex the neck as this can often increase the number of beats. A positive test, demonstrated by four or five reflex twitches of the plantar flexors (two to three twitches are considered normal), is indicative of UMN impairment.

Hoffmann. Hoffmann's sign is the upper limb equivalent of the Babinski sign. However, unlike the Babinski, some normal individuals can exhibit a present Hoffmann's sign.[186]

The clinician holds the patient's middle finger and briskly pinches the distal phalanx, thereby applying a noxious stimulus to the nail bed of the middle finger (Fig. 2-34).[186] Denno and Meadows[187] devised a dynamic version of this test, which involves the patient performing repeated flexion and extension of the head before being tested for Hoffmann's sign. A positive response for this test is the presence of Hoffmann's sign.

Supraspinal Reflexes
The supraspinal reflexes produce movement patterns that can be modulated by descending pathways and the cortex. A number of processes, which are involved in locomotor function, are oriented around these reflexes and are referred to as postural reflexes. Postural reflexes are those that help maintain postural equilibrium and stability during motion of the head, trunk, and extremities, as well as those that react in situations that have the potential to cause serious injury. The postural reflexes that constantly react and compensate for these changes require input from the somatosensory, vestibular, and visual systems.

Voluntary control of these compensatory movements would be impossible and highly inefficient, so these reactions must be reflex in nature.

The head and neck are areas of intense reflex activity. Head movements, which occur almost constantly, must be regulated to maintain normal eye-head-neck-trunk relationships, and to allow for visual fixation during head movements (Table 2-5). As noted earlier, there are three main control mechanisms for maintaining steady-gaze fixation: the vestibulo-ocular reflex; a gaze-holding system (the neural integrator), which operates whenever the eyes are required to hold an eccentric gaze position; and the cervico-ocular reflex.

For vision to be effectively integrated with balance, the subject must be capable of selecting an object for inspection and to fix the gaze on the object, regardless of head or object movement. The cervico-ocular and vestibulo-ocular reflexes work together to maintain the position and visual fixation of the eyes during movements of the head and neck. Mechanoreceptors in the cervical muscles, particularly the short-range rotators (i.e., the obliquus capitis posterior inferior, rectus capitis posterior major, splenius capitis, and sternocleidomastoid) are the primary source of afferent input in the elicitation of the cervico-ocular reflex. The vestibulo-ocular reflex is stimulated by movement of the head in space and has a strong influence on eye movement and positioning.

Visual fixation at higher speeds requires the contraction of the extraocular muscles to allow eye movements to counteract the effect of the head movements, even if the head is turning in the opposite direction. The ability to track and focus on a moving target that is moving across a visual field is termed smooth pursuit and requires a greater degree of voluntary

TABLE 2-5 Reflex Activities Involving the Cervical Spine[188]

Reflex	Eliciting Stimulus	Motor Response	Purpose
Tonic neck reflex	Neck movement that produces stretch to muscle spindles	Alteration of muscle tone in trunk and extremities	Assists with postural stability and enhances coordination
Cervicocollic reflex	Neck movement that produces stretch to muscle spindles	Eccentric contraction of the cervical muscles that oppose the initiating movement	Maintains smooth, controlled cervical movement
Cervicorespiratory reflex	Neck movement that produces stretch to muscle spindles	Alteration in respiratory rate	Assists in adjustments of respiration with changes in posture
Cervicosympathetic reflex	Neck movement that produces stretch to muscle spindles	Alteration in blood pressure	Assists in prevention of orthostatic hypotension with changes in posture
Trigeminocervical reflex	Touch stimulus to face	Head retraction	Protects against blows to face
Cervico-ocular reflex	Neck movement that produces stretch to muscle spindles	Movement of eyes in opposite direction of neck movement	Maintains gaze fixation during movements of head
Vestibulo-ocular reflex	Head movement stimulating semicircular canals	Movement of eyes in opposite direction of head movement	Maintains gaze fixation during movements of head
Smooth pursuit	Visual target moving across retinal field	Movement of eyes in direction in which target is moving	Maintains gaze fixation on moving target
Saccades	New visual target in retinal field	Movement of eyes in direction of new target	Fixates eyes on new target
Optokinetic reflex	Visual target moving across retinal field, causing perceived movement of head	Movement of eyes in opposite direction of perceived head movement	Maintains gaze fixation on moving target

control than the cervico-ocular and vestibulo-ocular reflexes can provide. The area in the brain stem where this integration of horizontal eye movements takes place is the paramedian pontine reticular formation.

The ability to read a book or to scan a page requires quick movements of the eyes called saccades. Unlike smooth pursuit, saccades can occur with a visual stimulus, by sound, verbal command, or tactile stimuli. However, like smooth pursuit, saccades are generated in the paramedian pontine reticular formation.

Visual fixation of a stationary target can be tested using the tip of a pencil. The patient is seated and is asked to look straight ahead and focus on the tip of the pencil, which is held by the clinician at arm's length from the patient. The test is repeated with the patient's eyes turned to the extremes of horizontal and vertical gaze, and the pencil tip positioned accordingly. The vestibulo-ocular reflex can be tested by asking the patient to fix vision on a distant object. The clinician holds the patient's head firmly, with the palms of the hands against the patient's cheeks, and produces a rapid but small head turn. If the reflex movement of the eyes is inappropriate (too big or too small), the abnormal eye movement will be followed by a corrective (saccadic) movement. Presence of this corrective action may indicate a lesion of the vestibular nerve.[189]

Smooth pursuit can be tested by having the patient fix his or her gaze on an object placed directly in front. The object is then moved to the right while the patient follows it with the eyes. The clinician looks for the presence of corrective saccades, which indicate that the pursuit is not holding the eye on the moving target. The object is moved back to the start position before being moved to the left while the patient again follows it with the eyes. The object can then be moved in a variety of directions, combining horizontal, vertical, and diagonal movements, to test if the patient can follow the object with the eyes without saccadic movements. Difficulty with smooth pursuit may indicate a lesion of the cerebellum, reticular formation, or cerebral cortex, or a cranial nerve lesion (oculomotor, trochlear, or abducens).[189]

Sensory Testing

The dorsal roots of the spinal nerves are represented by restricted peripheral sensory regions called dermatomes (see Fig. 2-9). The peripheral sensory nerves are represented by more distinct and circumscribed areas (see Fig. 2-9).

A degree of overlap exists with the segmental innervation of the skin,[190] and it is important to test the full area of the dermatome because the area of greater sensitivity changes. The area of sensitivity, or autogenous area, is a small region of the dermatome with no overlap and is the only area within a dermatome that is supplied exclusively by a single segmental level. Because there is so much overlap in the dermatome, spinal nerve root compression usually results in hypoesthesia rather than anesthesia within the majority of the dermatome, but anesthesia or near anesthesia in the autogenous area of the dermatome.

Paresthesia is a symptom of direct involvement of the nerve root. Paresthesia can be defined as an abnormal sensation of pins and needles, numbness, or prickling. Further irritation and destruction of the neural fibers interfere with conduction, resulting in a motor or sensory deficit, or a combination. It is, therefore, possible for a nerve root compression to cause pure motor paresis, a pure sensory deficit, or both, depending on which aspect of the nerve root is compressed. If pressure is exerted from above the nerve root, sensory impairment may result, whereas compression from below can induce motor paresis.

A full examination of the sensory system involves testing pain, temperature, pressure, vibration, position, and discriminative sensations. For patients with no apparent neurologic symptoms or signs, an abbreviated examination may be substituted.

Specific Tests[191]
Pain

▶ *Origin:*   Lateral spinothalamic tract (see Box 2-2).

▶ *Test:*   Pin-prick. This test is performed using a sharp safety pin, occasionally substituting the blunt end for the point as a stimulus. When investigating an area of cutaneous sensory loss, it is recommended that the clinician begin the pin-prick test in the area of anesthesia and work outward until the border of normal sensation is located. The clinician stimulates in the aforementioned patterns, and asks the patient "Is this sharp or dull?" or, when making comparisons using the sharp stimulus, "Does this feel the same as this?" (Note: It is important that the clinician use as light a touch as the patient can perceive and not, under any circumstances, press hard enough to draw blood.)

Temperature

▶ *Origin:*   Lateral spinothalamic tract.

▶ *Test:*   Using two test tubes, filled with hot and cold water, the clinician touches the skin and asks the patient to identify "hot" or "cold." The impulses for temperature sensation travel together with pain sensation in the lateral spinothalamic tract. The testing of skin temperature can also help the clinician to differentiate between a venous and an arterial insufficiency. With venous insufficiency, an increase in skin temperature is usually noted in the area of occlusion, and the area also appears bluish in color. Pitting edema, especially around the ankles, sacrum, and hands, also may be present. However, if pitting edema is present and the skin temperature is normal, the lymphatic system may be at fault. With arterial insufficiency, a decrease in skin temperature is usually noted in the area of occlusion, and the area appears whiter. It is also extremely painful.

Pressure

▶ *Origin:*   Spinothalamic tract.

▶ *Test:*   Firm pressure is applied to the patient's muscle belly.

Vibration

▶ *Origin:*   Dorsal column/medial lemniscal tract (Box 2-4).

▶ *Test:*   Using a relatively low-pitched tuning fork, preferably of 128 Hz, the clinician taps the fork on the heel of his or her hand and places it firmly over a bony process of the patient, such as the malleoli, patellae, epicondyles, vertebral spinous processes, and iliac crest. The patient is asked what he or she feels, and, to be certain, is asked to inform the clinician when the vibration stops. The clinician then touches the fork to stop the vibration. At this point, the patient should indicate that the vibration has stopped. If

---

Box 2-4 DORSAL MEDIAL LEMNISCUS TRACT

The dorsal medial lemniscus tract conveys impulses concerned with well-localized touch and with the sense of movement and position (kinesthesia). It is important in moment-to-moment (temporal) and point-to-point (spatial) discrimination and makes it possible for a person to put a key in a door lock without light or visualize the position of any part of his or her body without looking. Lesions to the tract from destructive tumors, hemorrhage, scar tissue, swelling, infections, and direct trauma, among others, abolish or diminish tactile sensations and movement or position sense. The cell bodies of the primary neurons in the dorsal column pathway are located in the spinal ganglion. The peripheral processes of these neurons begin at receptors in the joint capsule, muscles, and skin (tactile and pressure receptors).

vibration sense is absent, the clinician should retest, moving proximally along the extremity.

Position Sense (Proprioception)

▶ *Origin:* Dorsal column/medial lemniscal tract (see Box 2-4).

▶ *Test:* The patient is tested for ability to perceive passive movements of the extremities, especially the distal portions. Proprioception here refers to an awareness of the position of joints at rest. The clinician grasps the patient's big toe, holding it by its sides between the thumb and index finger, and then pulls it away from the other toes to avoid friction and to prevent extraneous tactile stimulation from indicating a change of position. "Down" and "up" are demonstrated to the patient as the clinician moves the patient's toe clearly upward and downward. Then, with his or her eyes closed, the patient is asked for an "up" or "down" response as the clinician moves the toe in a small arc. This movement is repeated several times on each side, avoiding simple alternation of the stimuli. If position sense is impaired, then the clinician should retest, moving proximally along the extremity. Alternatively, the patient is asked to duplicate the position with the opposite extremity.

Movement Sense (Kinesthesia)

▶ *Origin:* Dorsal column/medial lemniscal tract (see Box 2-4).

▶ *Test:* The patient is asked to indicate verbally the direction of movement while the extremity is in motion. The clinician must grip the patient's extremity over neutral borders.

Stereognosis

▶ *Origin:* Dorsal column/medial lemniscal tract (see Box 2-4).

▶ *Test:* The patient is asked to recognize, through touch alone, a variety of small objects such as comb, coins, pencils, and safety pins that are placed in his or her hand.

Graphesthesia

▶ *Origin:* Dorsal column/medial lemniscal tract (see Box 2-4).

▶ *Test:* The patient is asked to recognize letters, numbers, or designs traced on the skin. Using a blunt object, the clinician draws an image in the patient's palm, asking the patient to identify the number, letter, or design.

Two-point Discrimination

▶ *Origin:* Dorsal column/medial lemniscal tract (see Box 2-4).

▶ *Test:* A measure is taken of the smallest distance between two stimuli that can still be perceived by the patient as two distinct stimuli.

Equilibrium Reactions. The patient's ability to maintain balance in response to alterations in the body's center of gravity and base of support is tested.

Protective Reactions. The patient's ability to stabilize and support the body in response to a displacing stimulus in which the center of gravity exceeds the base of support is tested (e.g., extension of arms to protect against a fall).

Tonal Abnormality Examination[191]

Spasticity
Spasticity is defined as an increased resistance to a sudden passive stretch.

▶ *Clasped knife phenomenon.* This phenomenon is reflected by a sudden letting go by the patient when resistance is applied.

▶ *Clonus.* This is an exaggeration of the stretch reflex.

Rigidity
Rigidity is defined as an increased resistance to all motions, rendering body parts stiff and immovable.

▶ *Decorticate positioning.* Upper extremities are held in flexion and the lower extremities, in extension (Fig. 2-35).

▶ *Decerebrate positioning.* Upper and lower extremities are held in extension (see Fig. 2-35).

▶ *Cogwheel phenomenon.* This is a ratchet-like response to passive movement, characterized by an alternate giving and increased resistance to movement.

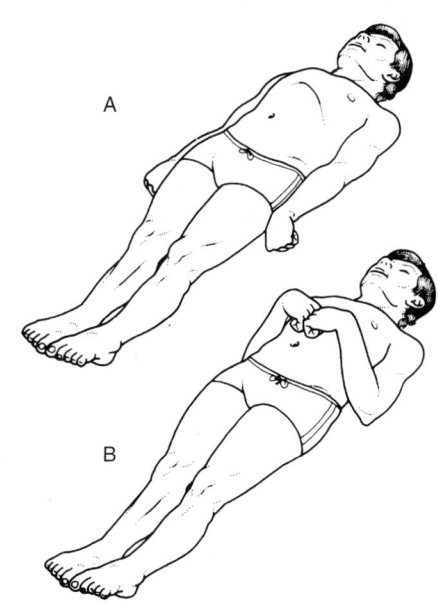

FIGURE 2-35 Posturing of the extremities. **A.** Decerebate rigidity. **B.** Decorticate rigidity. (Reproduced with permission from Booher JM, Thibodeau GA. *Athletic Injury Assessment.* New York, NY: McGraw-Hill; 2000.)

▶ *Leadpipe rigidity.* Characterized by constant rigidity, this finding is common in patients with Parkinson's disease.

Cranial Nerve Examination

With practice, the entire cranial nerve examination can be performed in approximately 5 minutes[193] (Table 2-6). The following rhyme may be used to help remember the order and tests for the cranial nerve examination[194]:

> *Smell and see*
> *And look around,*
> *Pupils large and smaller.*
> *Smile, hear!*
> *Then say ah . . .*
> *And see if you can swallow.*
> *If you're left in any doubt,*
> *Shrug and stick your tongue right out.*

CN I (Olfactory)

The sense of smell is tested by having the patient identify familiar odors (e.g., coffee, lavender, vanilla) with each nostril. The clinician should avoid irritant odors that can stimulate the trigeminal nerve.

CN II (Optic)

The optic nerve is tested by examining visual acuity and confrontation. Although the formal testing of visual acuity is presented here, in reality, it is sufficient to test this aspect of CN II at the same time that CN III, IV, and VI are being tested.

Visual Acuity. This is a test of central vision. If possible, the clinician should use a well-lit Snellen eye chart. The patient is positioned 20 feet from the chart. Patients who use corrective lenses other than reading glasses should be instructed to use them. The patient is asked to cover one eye and to read the smallest line possible. A patient who cannot read the largest letter should be positioned closer to the chart and the new distance noted. The clinician determines the smallest line of print from which the patient can identify more than half the letters. The visual acuity designated at the side of this line, together with the use of glasses, if any, is recorded.

Visual acuity is expressed as a fraction (e.g., 20/20), in which the numerator indicates the distance of the patient from the chart, the denominator the distance at which a normal eye can read the letters.

Confrontation Test. This is a rough clinical test of peripheral vision that also highlights a loss of vision in one of the visual fields. The patient and clinician sit facing each other, with their eyes level. Both the lateral and medial fields of vision are tested. The entire lateral field is tested with both eyes open, and the medial field is tested by covering one eye. When testing the medial field of vision, the clinician covers the patient's eye that is directly opposite the clinician's own (not diagonally opposite).

With arms outstretched and hands holding a small object such as a pencil, the clinician slowly brings the object into the peripheral field of vision of the patient. This is performed from eight separate directions. Each time the patient is asked to say "now" as soon as he or she sees the object. During the examination, the clinician should keep the object equidistant between his or her own eye and the patient's so that the patient's visual field can be compared to the clinician's own.

CN III (Oculomotor), CN IV (Trochlear), and CN VI (Abducens)

These three cranial nerves are tested together. The clinician:

1. Inspects the size and shape of each pupil for symmetry.

2. Tests the consensual pupillary response to light. This is tested by having the patient cover one eye, while the clinician observes the uncovered eye. The uncovered eye should undergo the same changes as the covered by first dilating, and then constricting, when the covered eye is uncovered.

3. Looks for the ability of the eyes to track movement in the six fields of gaze. The standard test is to smoothly move a target in an "H" configuration, and then in midline just above eye level toward the base of the nose (convergence).[8] The patient should be able to smoothly track a target at moderate speed, without evidence of nystagmus.

4. Looks for ptosis of the upper eyelids.

CN V (Trigeminal)

The patient is asked to clench the teeth, and the clinician palpates the temporal and masseter muscles. The three sensory branches of the trigeminal nerve are tested with pin-prick close to the midline of the face, because the skin that is more lateral is overlapped by the nerves of the face.[8] The jaw tendon reflex is assessed for the presence of hyperreflexia (Fig. 2-36).

CN VII (Facial)

The clinician inspects the face at rest and in conversation with the patient and notes any asymmetry. The patient is asked to smile. If there is asymmetry, the patient is asked to frown or wrinkle the forehead. Loss or reduced ability to smile and frown is caused by a peripheral palsy, whereas the loss of the smile, only, is caused by a supranuclear lesion.[8]

CN VIII (Vestibulocochlear)

The vestibular nerve can be tested in a number of ways, depending on the objective. Balance testing assesses the vestibulospinal reflexes. Caloric stimulation can be used to assess the vestibulo-ocular reflex. The vestibulo-ocular reflex also can be assessed by testing the ability of the eyes to follow a moving object.

The clinician assesses the function of the cochlear component of the nerve—hearing—by gently rubbing two fingers equidistant from each of the patient's ears simultaneously, or using a 256-Hz tuning fork and asking the patient to identify in which ear the noise appears to be the loudest.

There are three basic types of hearing loss.[194]

TABLE 2-6 Cranial Nerves and Methods of Testing[192]

	Nerve	Afferent (Sensory)	Efferent (Motor)	Test
I	Olfactory	Smell	—	Identify familiar odors (e.g., chocolate, coffee); test visual fields
II	Optic	Sight	—	
III	Oculomotor	—	*Voluntary motor:* levator of eyelid; superior, medial, and inferior recti; inferior oblique muscle of eyeball *Autonomic:* smooth muscle of eyeball	Upward, downward, and medical gaze; reaction to light
IV	Trochlear	—	*Voluntary motor:* superior oblique muscle of eyeball	Downward and lateral gaze
V	Trigeminal	Touch, pain: skin of face, mucous membranes of nose, sinuses, mouth, anterior tongue	*Voluntary motor:* muscles of mastication	Corneal reflex; face sensation; clench teeth, push down on chin to separate jaws
VI	Abducens	—	*Voluntary motor:* lateral rectus muscle of eyeball	Lateral gaze
VII	Facial	Taste: anterior tongue	*Voluntary motor:* facial muscles *Autonomic:* lacrimal, submandibular, and sublingual glands	Close eyes tight; smile and show teeth; whistle and puff cheeks; identify familiar tastes (e.g., sweet, sour)
VIII	Vestibulocochlear (acoustic nerve)	Hearing: ear Balance: ear	— —	Hear watch ticking Hearing tests; balance and coordination test
IX	Glossopharyngeal	Touch, pain: posterior tongue, pharynx Taste: posterior tongue	*Voluntary motor:* unimportant muscle of pharynx *Autonomic:* parotid gland	Gag reflex; ability to swallow
X	Vagus	Touch, pain; pharynx, larynx, bronchi Taste: tongue, epiglottis	*Voluntary motor:* muscles of palate, pharynx, and larynx *Autonomic:* thoracic and abdominal viscera	Gag reflex; ability to swallow; say "Ahhh"
XI	Accessory	—	*Voluntary motor:* sternocleidomastoid and trapezius muscles	Resisted shoulder shrug
XII	Hypoglossal	—	*Voluntary motor:* muscles of tongue	Tongue protrusion (if injured, tongue deviates toward injured side)

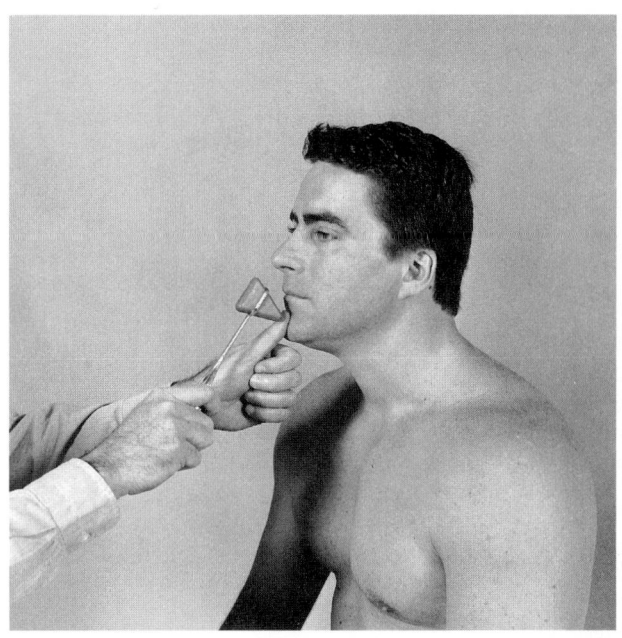

FIGURE 2-36   The jaw tendon reflex.

1. *Conductive.*   This type of hearing loss applies to any disturbance in the conduction of the sound impulse as it passes through the ear canal, tympanic membrane, middle ear, and ossicular chain to the footplate of the stapes, which is situated in the oval window. As a general rule, an individual with conductive hearing loss speaks softly, hears well on the telephone, and hears best in a noisy environment.

2. *Sensorineural.*   This type of hearing loss applies to a disturbance anywhere from the cochlea through the auditory nerve, and on to the hearing center in the cerebral cortex. As a general rule, an individual with a perceptive hearing loss usually speaks loudly, hears better in a quiet environment, and hears poorly in a crowd and on the telephone.

3. *Mixed.*   This type of hearing loss is a combination of conductive and sensorineural.

If hearing loss is present, then the clinician should test for lateralization and compare air and bone conduction.

Lateralization.   The clinician places a tuning fork over the vertex, middle of the forehead, or front teeth. The patient is asked whether the vibration is heard more in one ear (Weber's test). Normal individuals cannot lateralize the vibration to either ear. In conduction deafness (e.g., that caused by middle ear disease), the vibration is heard more in the affected ear. In sensorineural deafness, the vibration is heard more in the normal ear.

Air and Bone Conduction.   Air conduction is assessed by placing the tuning fork in front of the external auditory meatus, whereas bone conduction is assessed by placing the tuning fork on the mastoid process (Rinne's test). In a normal individual, the tuning fork is heard louder and longer by air than by bone conduction. In conduction deafness, bone conduction hearing is better. In sensorineural deafness, both air and bone conduction are reduced, although air conduction is the better of the two.

CN IX (Glossopharyngeal)

The gag reflex is used to test this nerve, but this test is reserved for severely affected patients, only.

CN X (Vagus)

The clinician listens to the patient's voice and notes any hoarseness or nasal quality. The patient is asked to open the mouth and say "Aah" while the clinician watches the movements of the soft palate and pharynx. The soft palate should rise symmetrically, the uvula should remain in the midline, and each side of the posterior pharynx should move medially.

CN XI (Spinal Accessory)

From behind the patient, the clinician notes any atrophy or fasciculation in the trapezius muscles and compares side to side. The patient is asked to shrug both shoulders upward against the clinician's hand. The strength of contraction should be noted.

The patient is asked to attempt to turn his or her head to each side against the clinician's hand. The contraction of the opposite side sternocleidomastoid, and the force of contraction should be noted.

CN XII (Hypoglossal)

The clinician inspects the tongue as it lies on the floor of the mouth, looking for fasciculation. The patient then is asked to stick out the tongue. The clinician looks for asymmetry, atrophy, or deviation from the midline. The patient is asked to move the tongue from side to side, as the clinician notes symmetry of movement.

REVIEW QUESTIONS*

1. Injury to the radial nerve in the spiral groove would result in
   A. weakness of elbow flexion
   B. inability to initiate abduction
   C. inability to control rotation during abduction
   D. inability of the rotator cuff muscles to hold the humeral head in its socket
   E. none of the above
2. A patient with a musculocutaneous nerve injury is still able to flex the elbow. The major muscle causing elbow flexion is the
   A. brachioradialis
   B. flexor carpi ulnaris
   C pronator quadratus
   D. extensor carpi ulnaris
   E. pectoralis major

*Additional questions to test your understanding of this chapter can be found in the Online Learning Center for *Orthopaedic Assessment, Evaluation, and Intervention* at www.duttononline.net.

3. Which of the following muscles is *not* innervated by the median nerve?
   A. abductor pollicis brevis
   B. flexor pollicis longus
   C. medial heads of flexor digitorum profundus
   D. superficial head of flexor pollicis brevis
   E. pronator quadratus

4. The nerve that innervates the first lumbrical muscle in the hand is the
   A. median nerve
   B. ulnar nerve
   C. radial nerve
   D. anterior interosseus nerve
   E. lateral cutaneous nerve of the hand

5. After a nerve injury, regeneration occurs proximally first and then progresses distally at a rate of about 1 mm per day. Following a radial nerve injury in the axilla, which muscle would be the last to recover?
   A. long head of the triceps
   B. anconeus
   C. extensor indicis
   D. extensor digiti minimi
   E. supinator

REFERENCES

1. Martin J. Introduction to the central nervous system. In: Martin J, ed. *Neuroanatomy: Text and Atlas*. New York, NY: McGraw-Hill; 1996:1–32.
2. Waxman SG. *Correlative Neuroanatomy*. 24th ed. New York, NY: McGraw-Hill; 1996.
3. Pratt N. Anatomy of the cervical spine. In: American Physical Therapy Association, Orthopedic Section. *Physical Therapy Home Study Course: The Cervical Spine*. La Crosse, Wis: Orthopedic Section, APTA; 1996.
4. Sunderland S. Anatomical perivertebral influences on the intervertebral foramen. In: Goldstein MN, ed. *The Research Status of Spinal Manipulative Therapy*. Bethesda, Md: HEW Publication No (NIH); 1975:76–998.
5. Sunderland S. *Nerves and Nerve Injuries*. Edinburgh, Scotland: E and S Livingstone; 1968.
6. Rydevik B, Garfin SR. Spinal nerve root compression. In: Szabo RM, ed. *Nerve Compression Syndromes: Diagnosis and Treatment*. Thorofare, NJ: Slack; 1989:247–261.
7. Bogduk N. Innervation and pain patterns of the cervical spine. In: Grant R, ed. *Physical Therapy of the Cervical and Thoracic Spine*. New York, NY: Churchill Livingstone; 1988.
8. Meadows J. *Orthopedic Differential Diagnosis in Physical Therapy*. New York, NY: McGraw-Hill; 1999.
9. Durrant JD, Freeman AR. Concepts in vestibular physiology. In: Finestone AJ, ed. *Dizziness and Vertigo*. Boston, Mass: John Wright PSG; 1982:13–43.
10. Meadows J. *A Rationale and Complete Approach to the Sub-Acute Post-MVA Cervical Patient*. Calgary, BC: Swodeam Consulting; 1995.
11. Fawcett DW. The nervous tissue. In: Fawcett DW, ed. Bloom and Fawcett: *A Textbook of Histology*. New York, NY: Chapman and Hall; 1984:336–339.
12. Millesi H, Terzis JK. Nomenclature in peripheral nerve surgery. In: Terzis JK, ed. *Microreconstruction of Nerve Injuries*. Philadelphia, Pa: WB Saunders; 1987:3–13.
13. Thomas PK, Olsson Y. Microscopic anatomy and function of the connective tissue components of peripheral nerve. In: Dyck PJ, Thomas PK, Lambert EH, Bunge R, et al, eds. *Peripheral Neuropathy*. Philadelphia, Pa: WB Saunders; 1984:97–120.
14. Chusid JG. *Correlative Neuroanatomy & Functional Neurology*. Norwalk, Conn: Appleton-Century-Crofts; 1985:144–148.
15. Daniels DL, Hyde JS, Kneeland JB, et al. The cervical nerves and foramina: Local-coil MRI imaging. *AJNR* 1986;7: 129–133.
16. Pech P, Daniels DL, Williams AL, Haughton VM. The cervical neural foramina: Correlation of microtomy and CT anatomy. *Radiology* 1985;155:143–146.
17. Carter GT, Kilmer DD, Bonekat HW, Lieberman JS, Fowler WM Jr. Evaluation of phrenic nerve and pulmonary function in hereditary motor and sensory neuropathy type 1. *Muscle Nerve* 1992;15:459–466.
18. Bolton CF. Clinical neurophysiology of the respiratory system. *Muscle Nerve* 1993;16:809–818.
19. Jenkins DB. *Hollinshead's Functional Anatomy of the Limbs and Back*. 7th ed. Philadelphia, Pa: WB Saunders; 1998.
20. Dumestre G. Long thoracic nerve palsy. *J Man Manip Ther* 1995;3:44–49.
21. Gozna ER, Harris WR. Traumatic winging of the scapula. *J Bone Joint Surg* 1979;61A:1230–1233.
22. Kauppila LI. The long thoracic nerve: Possible mechanisms of injury based on autopsy study. *J Shoulder Elbow Surg* 1993;2:244–248.
23. Kauppila LI, Vastamaki M. Iatrogenic serratus anterior paralysis: Long-term outcome in 26 patients. *Chest* 1996;109: 31–34.
24. Post M. Orthopedic management of neuromuscular disorders. In: Post M, Bigliani LU, Flatow EL, Pollock RG, et al, eds. *The Shoulder: Operative Technique*. Baltimore, Md: Williams and Wilkins; 1998:201–234.
25. Kuhn JE, Plancher KD, Hawkins RJ. Scapular winging. *J Am Acad Orthop Surg* 1995;3:319–325.
26. Reis FP, de Camargo AM, Vitti M, de Carvalho CA. Electromyographic study of the subclavius muscle. *Acta Anat* 1979;105:284–290.
27. Rengachary SS, Burr D, Lucas S, Brackett CE. Suprascapular entrapment neuropathy: A clinical, anatomical, and comparative study. Part 2: Anatomical study. *Neurosurgery* 1979;5:447–451.
28. Ajmani ML. The cutaneous branch of the human suprascapular nerve. *J Anat* 1994;185:439–442.
29. Horiguchi M. The cutaneous branch of some human suprascapular nerves. *J Anat* 1980;130:191–195.
30. Murakami T, Ohtani O, Outi H. Suprascapular nerve with cutaneous branch to the upper arm [in Japanese]. *Acta Anat Nippon* 1977;52:96.
31. Hadley MN, Sonntag VKH, Pittman HW. Suprascapular nerve entrapment: A summary of seven cases. *J Neurosurg* 1986;64:843–848.
32. Post M. Diagnosis and treatment of suprascapular nerve entrapment. *Clin Orthop* 1999;368:92–100.
33. Post M, Mayer J. Suprascapular nerve entrapment: Diagnosis and treatment. *Clin Orthop* 1987;223:126–130.
34. Vastamäki M, Goransson H. Suprascapular nerve entrapment. *Clin Orthop* 1993;297:135–143.
35. Miller T. Peripheral nerve injuries at the shoulder. *J Man Manip Ther* 1998;6:170–183.

36. Hoffman GW, Elliott LF. The anatomy of the pectoral nerves and its significance to the general and plastic surgeon. *Ann Surg* 1987;205:504.

37. Strauch B, Yu HL. *Atlas of Microvascular Surgery: Anatomy and Operative Approaches.* New York, NY: Thieme; 1993:390–391.

38. Kerr A. The brachial plexus of nerves in man, the variations in its formation and branches. *Am J Anat* 1918;23:285–376.

39. Wichman R. Die Rückenmarksnerven und ihre Segmentbezüge. In: Kerr A, ed. The brachial plexus of nerves in man, the variations in its formation and branches. *Am J Anat* 1918,23:285–376.

40. Delagi EF, Perotto A. Arm. In: Delagi EF, Perotto A, eds. *Anatomic Guide for the Electromyographer.* Springfield, Ill: Charles C Thomas, 1981:66–71.

41. Sunderland S. The musculocutaneous nerve. In: Sunderland S, ed. *Nerves and Nerve Injuries.* Edinburgh, Scotland: Churchill Livingstone, 1978:796–801.

42. de Moura WG Jr. Surgical anatomy of the musculocutaneous nerve: A photographic essay. *J Reconstr Microsurg* 1985;1: 291–297.

43. Flatow EL, Bigliani LU, April EW. An anatomic study of the musculocutaneous nerve and its relationship to the coracoid process. *Clin Orthop* 1989;244:166–171.

44. Dundore DE, DeLisa JA. Musculocutaneous nerve palsy: An isolated complication of surgery. *Arch Phys Med Rehabil* 1979;60:130–133.

45. Lusk MD, Kline DG, Garcia CA. Tumors of the brachial plexus. *Neurosurgery* 1987;21:439–453.

46. Braddom RL, Wolf C. Musculocutaneous nerve injury after heavy exercise. *Arch Phys Med Rehab* 1978;59:290–293.

47. Sander HW, Quinto CM, Elinzano H, Chokroverty S. Carpet carrier's palsy: Musculocutaneous neuropathy. *Neurology* 1997;48:1731–1732.

48. Mastaglia FL. Musculocutaneous neuropathy after strenuous physical activity. *Med J Aust* 1986;145:153–154.

49. Kim SM, Goodrich JA. Isolated proximal musculocutaneous nerve palsy. *Arch Phys Med Rehab* 1984;65:735–736.

50. Blackburn TA, McLeod WD, White B, Wofford L, et al. EMG analysis of posterior rotator cuff exercises. *Athl Training* 1990;25:40–45.

51. Blackburn TA Jr. Rehabilitation of the shoulder and elbow after arthroscopy. *Clin Sports Med* 1987;3:587–606.

52. Townsend H, Jobe FW, Pink M, Perry J. Electromyographic analysis of the glenohumeral muscles during a baseball rehabilitation program. *Am J Sports Med* 1991;3:264–272.

53. Bierman W, Yamshon LJ. Electromyography in kinesiologic evaluations. *Arch Phys Med Rehabil* 1948;29:206–211.

54. Stern PJ, Kutz JE. An unusual variant of the anterior interosseous nerve syndrome: A case report and review of the literature. *J Hand Surg* 1980;5:32–34.

55. Hope PG. Anterior interosseous nerve palsy following internal fixation of the proximal radius. *J Bone Joint Surg* 1988;70B:280–282.

56. Amadio PC, Beckenbaugh RD. Entrapment of the ulnar nerve by the deep flexor-pronator aponeurosis. *J Hand Surg Am* 1986;11A:83–87.

57. Hirasawa Y, Sawamura H, Sakakida K. Entrapment neuropathy due to bilateral epitrochlearis muscles: A case report. *J Hand Surg Am* 1979;4:181–184.

58. Sunderland S. The ulnar nerve. In: Sunderland S, ed. *Nerves and Nerve Injuries.* Edinburgh, Scotland: Churchill Livingstone;1968:816–828.

59. Apfelberg DB, Larson SJ. Dynamic anatomy of the ulnar nerve at the elbow. *Plast Reconstr Surg* 1973;51:76–81.

60. Chen FS, Rokito AS, Jobe FW. Medial elbow problems in the overhead-throwing athlete. *J Am Acad Orthop Surg* 2001;9: 99–113.

61. Mannheimer JS, Lampe GN. *Clinical Tanscutaneous Electrical Nerve Stimulation.* Philadelphia, Pa: FA Davis; 1984: 440–445.

62. Williams PL, Warwick R, Dyson M, Bannister LH, et al. *Gray's Anatomy.* 37th ed. London, England: Churchill Livingstone; 1989.

63. McGuckin N. The T 4 syndrome. In: Grieve GP, ed. *Modern Manual Therapy of the Vertebral Column.* New York, NY: Churchill Livingstone, 1986:370–376.

64. DeFranca GG, Levine LJ. The T 4 syndrome. *J Manipulative Physiol Ther* 1995;18:34–37.

65. Grieve GP. Thoracic musculoskeletal problems. In: Boyling JD, Palastanga N, eds. *Grieve's Modern Manual Therapy of the Vertebral Column.* Edinburgh, Scotland: Churchill Livingstone; 1994:401–428.

66. Warfel BS, Marini SG, Lachmann EA, Nagler W. Delayed femoral nerve palsy following femoral vessel catheterization. *Arch Phys Med Rehabil* 1993;74:1211–1215.

67. Hardy SL. Femoral nerve palsy associated with an associated posterior wall transverse acetabular fracture. *J Orthop Trauma* 1997;11:40–42.

68. Papastefanou SL, Stevens K, Mulholland RC. Femoral nerve palsy: An unusual complication of anterior lumbar interbody fusion. *Spine* 1994;19:2842–2844.

69. Fealy S, Paletta GA Jr. Femoral nerve palsy secondary to traumatic iliacus muscle hematoma: Course after nonoperative management. *J Trauma Inj Infect Crit Care* 1999;47: 1150–1152.

70. Bradshaw C, McCrory P, Bell S, Bruckner P, et al. Obturator neuropathy: A cause of chronic groin pain in athletes. *Am J Sports Med* 1997;25:402–408.

71. Harvey G, Bell S. Obturator neuropathy. An anatomic perspective. *Clin Orthop Rel Res* 1999;363:203–211.

72. Ecker AD, Woltman HW. Meralgia paresthetica: A report of one hundred and fifty cases *JAMA* 1938;110:1650–1652.

73. Keegan JJ, Holyoke EA. Meralgia paresthetica: An anatomical and surgical study. *J Neurosurg* 1962;19:341–345.

74. Reichert FL. Meralgia paresthetica; a form of causalgia relieved by interruption of the sympathetic fibers. *Surg Clin North Am* 1933;13:1443.

75. Edelson JG, Nathan H. Meralgia paresthetica. *Clin Orthop* 1977;122:255–262.

76. Ivins GK. Meralgia paresthetica, the elusive diagnosis: Clinical experience with 14 adult patients. *Ann Surg* 2000;232: 281–286.

77. Nathan H. Gangliform enlargement on the lateral cutaneous nerve of the thigh. *J Neurosurg* 1960;17:843.

78. Ghent WR. Further studies on meralgia paresthetica. *Can Med J* 1961;85:871.

79. Stookey B. Meralgia paresthetica: Etiology and surgical treatment. *JAMA* 1928;90:1705.

80. Williams PH, Trzil KP. Management of meralgia paresthetica. *J Neurosurg* 1991;74:76.

81. Sunderland S. Traumatized nerves, roots and ganglia: Musculoskeletal factors and neuropathological consequences. In: Knorr IM, Huntwork EH, eds. *The Neurobiologic Mechanisms in Manipulative Therapy.* New York, NY: Plenum Press; 1978: 137–166.

82. Kenny, P, O'Brien CP, Synnott K, Walsh MG. Damage to the superior gluteal nerve after two different approaches to the hip. *J Bone Joint Surg* 1999;81B:979–981.

83. Lu J, et al. Anatomic considerations of superior cluneal nerve at posterior iliac crest region. *Clin Orthop Rel Res* 1998;347:224–228.

84. Netter FH. Lumbar, sacral, and coccygeal plexuses (The CIBA collection of medical illustrations). In: *Nervous System*. Part I. West Caldwell, NJ: CIBA-Geigy; 1991:122–123.

85. Sogaard I. Sciatic nerve entrapment: Case report. *J Neurosurg* 1983;58:275–276.

86. Robinson DR. Pyriformis syndrome in relation to sciatic pain. *Am J Surg* 1947;73:355–358.

87. Benyahya E, Etaouil N, Janani S, et al. Sciatica as the first manifestation of leiomyosarcoma of the buttock. *Rev Rheum* 1997;64:135–137.

88. Lamki N, Hutton L, Wall WJ, Rorabeck CH. Computed tomography in pelvic liposarcoma: A case report. *J Comput Tomogr* 1984;8:249–251.

89. Resnick D. *Diagnosis of Bone and Joint Disorders*. Philadelphia, Pa: WB Saunders; 1995:2773–2777.

90. Ohsawa K, Nishida T, Kurohmaru M, Hayashi Y. Distribution pattern of pudendal nerve plexus for the phallus retractor muscles in the cock. *Okajimas Folia Anat Jpn* 1991; 67:439–441.

91. Voight ML, Cook G. Impaired neuromuscular control: Reactive neuromuscular training. In: Prentice WE, Voight ML, eds. *Techniques in Musculoskeletal Rehabilitation*. New York, NY: McGraw-Hill; 2001:93–124.

92. Voight ML, Cook G, Blackburn TA. Functional lower quarter exercises through reactive neuromuscular training. In: Bandy WD, ed. *Current Trends for the Rehabilitation of the Athlete*: Home Study Course. La Crosse, Wis: Sports Physical Therapy Section, APTA; 1997.

93. McCloskey DI. Kinesthetic sensibility. *Physiol Rev* 1978; 58:763–820.

94. Borsa PA, Lephart SM, Kocher MS, et al. Functional assessment and rehabilitation of shoulder proprioception for glenohumeral instability. *J Sport Rehabil* 1994;3:84–104.

95. Lephart SM, Warner JJP, Borsa PA, et al. Proprioception of the shoulder joint in healthy, unstable and surgically repaired shoulders. *J Shoulder Elbow Surg* 1994;3:371–380.

96. Previte JJ. *Human Physiology*. New York, NY: McGraw-Hill; 1983.

97. Freeman MAR, Wyke BD. An experimental study of articular neurology. *J Bone Joint Surg* 1967;49B:185.

98. Wyke BD. The neurology of joints: A review of general principles. *Clin Rheumat Dis* 1981;7:223–239.

99. Grigg P. Peripheral neural mechanisms in proprioception. *J Sport Rehabil* 1994;3:1–17.

100. Swash M, Fox K. Muscle spindle innervation in man. *J Anat* 1972;112:61–80.

101. Wilk KE, Voight ML, Keirns MA, Gambetta V, Andrews JR, Dillman CJ. Stretch-shortening drills for the upper extremities: theory and clinical application. *J Orthop Sports Phys Ther* 1993;17:225–239.

102. de Jarnette B. *Sacro-occipital Technique*. Nebraska City, Neb: Major Bertrand de Jarnette, DC; 1972.

103. Pollard H, Ward G. A study of two stretching techniques for improving hip flexion range of motion. *J Manipulative Physiol Ther* 1997;20:443–447.

104. Willis WD. *The Pain System*. Basel, Switzerland: Karger; 1985.

105. Grigg P, Hoffmann AH. Properties of Ruffini afferents revealed by stress analysis of isolated sections of cat knee capsule. *J Neurophysiol* 1982;47:41–54.

106. Clark R, Wyke BD. Contributions of temporomandibular articular mechanoreceptors to the control of mandibular posture: An experimental study. *J Dent Assoc S Africa* 1974;2:121–129.

107. Skaggs CD. Diagnosis and treatment of temporomandibular disorders. In: Murphy DR, ed. *Cervical Spine Syndromes*. New York, NY: McGraw-Hill; 2000:579–592.

108. Lephart SM, Pincivero DM, Giraldo JL, Fu FH. The role of proprioception in the management of and rehabilitation of athletic injuries. *Am J Sports Med* 1997;25:130–137.

109. Wyke BD. The neurology of joints. *Ann R Coll Surg Engl* 1967;41:25–50.

110. Wyke BD. Articular neurology and manipulative therapy. In: Glasgow EF, Twomey LT, Scull ER, et al. eds. *Aspects of Manipulative Therapy*. New York, NY: Churchill Livingstone; 1985:72–77.

111. Milne RJ, Foreman RD, Giesler GJ Jr, Willis WD. Convergence of cutaneous and pelvic visceral nociceptive inputs onto primate spinothalamic neurons. *Pain* 1981;11:163–183.

112. Vierck CJ, Greenspan JD, Ritz LA. Long-term changes in purposive and reflexive responses to nociceptive stimulation following anterior-lateral chordotomy. *J Neurosci* 1990; 10:2077–2095.

113. Wojtys EM, Wylie BB, Huston LJ. The effects of muscle fatigue on neuromuscular function and anterior tibial translation in healthy knees. *Am J Sports Med* 1996;24:615.

114. Abbott LC, Saunders JBDM, Bast FC, Anderson CE, et al. Injuries to the ligaments of the knee joint. *J Bone Joint Surg* 1944;26:503–521.

115. Gardner E. Reflex muscular responses to stimulation of articular nerves in cat. *Am J Physiol* 1950;161:133–141.

116. Palmer I. On injuries to ligaments of knee joint; clinical study. *Acta Chir Scand* 1938;suppl 53.

117. Lephart SM, Henry TJ. Functional rehabilitation for the upper and lower extremity. *Orthop Clin North Am* 1995;26:579–592.

118. Lee WA. Anticipatory control of postural and task muscles during rapid arm flexion. *J Mot Behav* 1980;12:185–196.

119. Barrack RL, Skinner HB, Buckley SL. Proprioception in the anterior cruciate deficient knee. *Am J Sports Med* 1989;17:1–6.

120. Skinner HB, Wyatt MP, Hodgdon JA, Conard DW, Barrack RL. Effect of fatigue on joint position sense of the knee. *J Orthop Res* 1986;4:112–118.

121. Williams GR, Chmielewski T, Rudolph KS, et al. Dynamic knee stability: Current theory and implications for clinicians and scientists. *J Orthop Sports Phys Ther* 2001;31:546–566.

122. Johnston RB 3rd, Howard ME, Cawley PW, Losse GM. Effect of lower extremity muscular fatigue on motor control performance. *Med Sci Sports Exerc* 1998;30:1703–1707.

123. Skinner HB, Barrack RL, Cook SD. Age-related decline in proprioception. *Clin Orthop* 1984;184:208–211.

124. Barrett DS, Cobb AG, Bentley G. Joint proprioception in normal, osteoarthritic and replaced knees. *J. Bone Joint Surg* 1991;73B:53–56.

125. Barrett DS. Proprioception and function after anterior cruciate ligament reconstruction. *J Bone Joint Surg* 1991;73B:833–837.

126. Beard DJ, Kyberd PJ, Fergusson CM, Dodd CA. Proprioception after rupture of the anterior cruciate ligament. An objective indication of the need for surgery? *J Bone Joint Surg* 1993; 75B:311–315.

127. Corrigan JP, Cashman WF, Brady MP. Proprioception in the cruciate deficient knee. *J Bone Joint Surg* 1992;74B: 247–250.

128. Fremerey RW, Lobenhoffer P, Zeichen J, Skutek M, Bosch U, Tscherne H. Proprioception after rehabilitation and reconstruction in knees with deficiency of the anterior cruciate ligament: a prospective, longitudinal study. *J Bone Joint Surg Br* 2000;82:801–806.

129. Voight M, Blackburn T. Proprioception and balance training and testing following injury. In: Ellenbecker TS, ed. *Knee Ligament Rehabilitation*. Philadelphia, Pa: Churchill Livingstone; 2000:361–385.

130. Berg K. Balance and its measure in the elderly: A review. *Physiother Can* 1989;41:240–246.

131. Komi PV, Buskirk E. Effects of eccentric and concentric muscle conditioning on tension and electrical activity of human muscle. *Ergonomics* 1972;15:417.

132. Komi PV. The stretch-shortening cycle and human power output. In: Jones NL, McCartney N, McComas AJ, eds. *Human Muscle Power*. Champlain, Ill: Human Kinetics; 1986:27.

133. Morgenlander JC. The autonomic nervous system. In: Gilman S, ed. *Clinical Examination of the Nervous System*. New York, NY: McGraw-Hill; 2000:213–225.

134. Blumberg H, Janig W. Clinic manifestations of reflex sympathetic dystrophy and sympathetically maintained pain. In: Wall PD, Melzack R, eds. *Textbook of Pain*. London, England: Churchill Livingstone;1994:685–698.

135. Woolf CJ. The dorsal horn: State-dependent sensory processing and the generation of pain. In: Wall PD, Melzack R, eds. *Textbook of Pain*. London, England: Churchill Livingstone; 1994: 201–220.

136. Walker SM, Cousins MJ. Complex regional pain syndromes: Including 'reflex sympathetic dystrophy' and 'causalgia'. *Anaesth Intens Care* 1997;25:113–125.

137. Federation of State Medical Boards of the United States. *Model Guidelines for the Use of Controlled Substances for the Treatment of Pain*. Euless, Tex: The Federation; 1998.

138. Bogduk N. The anatomy and physiology of nociception. In: Crosbie J, McConnell J, eds. *Key Issues in Physiotherapy*. Oxford, England: Butterworth-Heinemann; 1993:48–87.

139. Besson JM. The neurobiology of pain. *Lancet* 1999;353: 1610–1615.

140. Spiller WG, Martin E. The treatment of persistent pain of organic origin in the lower part of the body by division of the anterior-lateral column of the spinal cord. *JAMA* 1912;58:1489–1490.

141. Gowers WR. A case of unilateral gunshot injury to the spinal cord. *Trans Clin Lond* 1878;11:24–32.

142. Willis WD, Coggeshall RE. *Sensory Mechanisms of the Spinal Cord*. 2nd ed. New York, NY: Plenum Press; 1991.

143. Willis WD, Trevino DL, Coulter JD, Maunz RA. Responses of primate spinothalamic tract neurons to natural stimulation of hindlimb. *J Neurophysiol* 1974;37:358–372.

144. Hyndman OR, Van Epps C. Possibility of differential section of the spinothalamic tract. *Arch Surg* 1939;38:1036–1053.

145. Ferrington DG, Sorkin LS, Willis WD. Responses of spinothalamic tract cells in the superficial dorsal horn of the primate lumbar spinal cord. *J Physiol* 1987;388:681–703.

146. Kenshalo DR Jr, Leonard RB, Chung JM, Willis WD. Responses of primate spinothalamic neurons to graded and to repeated noxious heat stimuli. *J Neurophysiol* 1979;42:1370–1389.

147. Foreman RD, Schmidt RF, Willis WD. Effects of mechanical and chemical stimulation of fine muscle afferents upon primate spinothalamic tract cells. *J Physiol* 1979;286:215–231.

148. Chung JM, Fang ZR, Hori Y, Lee KH, Willis WD. Prolonged inhibition of primate spinothalamic tract cells by peripheral nerve stimulation. *Pain* 1984;19:259–275.

149. Chung JM, Lee KH, Hori Y, Endo K, Willis WD. Factors influencing peripheral nerve stimulation produced inhibition of primate spinothalamic tract cells. *Pain* 1984;19: 277–293.

150. Lee KH, Chung JM, Willis WD. Inhibition of primate spinothalamic tract cells by TENS. *J Neurosurg* 1985;62: 276–287.

151. Melzack R, Wall PD. On the nature of cutaneous sensory mechanisms. *Brain* 1962;85:331–356.

152. Melzack R. The gate theory revisited. In: LeRoy PL, ed. *Current Concepts in the Management of Chronic Pain*. Miami, Fla: Symposia Specialists;1977.

153. Nathan PW. The gate-control theory of pain—A critical review. *Brain* 1976;99:123–158.

154. Mayer DJ, Price DD. Central nervous system mechanisms of analgesia. *Pain* 1976;2:379–404.

155. Fields HL, Anderson SD. Evidence that raphe-spinal neurons mediate opiate and midbrain stimulation-produced analgesias. *Pain* 1978;5:333–349.

156. Dell'Osso LF, Daroff RB. Nystagmus and saccadic intrusions and oscillations. In: Glaser JS, ed. *Neuro-ophthalmology*. Baltimore, Md: Lippincott, Williams and Wilkins; 1999: 369–401.

157. Harris C. Nystagmus and eye movement disorders. In: Taylor D, ed. *Paediatric Ophthalmology*. Oxford, England: Blackwell; 1997:869–896.

158. Abadi RV. Mechanisms underlying nystagmus. *J Royal Soc Med* 2002;95:231–234.

159. Nylen CO. The otoneurological diagnosis of tumours of the brain. *Acta Otolaryngol Suppl (Stockh)* 1939;33:5–149.

160. Barany R. Diagnose von Krankheitserscheinungen im Bereiche des Otolithenapparates. *Acta Otolaryngol* 1921;2:434–437.

161. Dix MR, Hallpike CS. The pathology, symptomatology and diagnosis of certain common disorders of the vestibular system. *Ann Otol Rhinol Laryngol* 1952;61:987–1016.

162. Rigueiro-Veloso MT, Pego-Reigosa R, Branas-Fernandez F, Martinez-Vazquez F, Cortes-Laino JA. Wallenberg's syndrome: A review of 25 cases. *Rev Neurol* 1997;25:1561.

163. Norrving B, Cronqvist S. Lateral medullary infarction: Prognosis in an unselected series. *Neurology* 1991;41:244–248.

164. Chia LG, Shen WC. Wallenberg's lateral medullary syndrome with loss of pain and temperature sensation on the contralateral face: Clinical, MRI and electrophysiological studies. *J Neurol* 1993;240:462–467.

165. Kim JS, Lee JH, Suh DC, Lee MC. Spectrum of lateral medullary syndrome: Correlation between clinical findings and magnetic resonance imaging in 33 subjects. *Stroke* 1994;25:1405–1410.

166. Jenkins IH, Frackowiak RSJ. Functional studies of the human cerebellum with positron emission tomography. *Rev Neurol* 1993;149:647–653.

167. Molinari M, Leggio MG, Solida A, et al. Cerebellum and procedural learning: evidence from focal cerebellar lesions. *Brain* 1997;120:1753–1762.

168. Kim SG, Ugurbil K, Strick PL. Activation of a cerebellar output nucleus during cognitive processing. *Science* 1994;265: 949–951.

169. Pierrot-Deseilligny E, Mazieres L. Spinal mechanisms underlying spasticity. In: Delwaide PJ, Young RR, eds. *Clinical Neurophysiology in Spasticity: Contribution to Assessment and Pathophysiology*. Amsterdam, Holland: Elsevier; 1985: 63–76.

170. Hoppenfeld S. *Orthopedic Neurology—A Diagnostic Guide to Neurological Levels*. Philadelphia, Pa: JB Lippincott; 1977:97–98.

171. Ashby P, McCrea D. Neurophysiology of spinal spasticity; In: Davidoff RA, ed. *Handbook of the Spinal Cord*. New York, NY: Marcel Decker; 1987:119–143.

172. Meissner I, Weibers DO, Swanson JW, O'Fallon WM. The natural history of drop attacks. *Neurology* 1986;36: 1029–1034.

173. Zeiler K, Zeitlhofer J. Syncopal consciousness disorders and drop attacks from the neurologic viewpoint [in German]. *Wien Klin Wochenschr* 1988;100:93–99.

174. Kameyama M. Vertigo and drop attack. With special reference to cerebrovascular disorders and atherosclerosis of the vertebral-basilar system. *Geriatrics* 1965;20:892–900.

175. Bardella L, Maleci A, Di Lorenzo N. Drop attack as the only symptom of type 1 Chiari malformation. Illustration by a case [in Italian]. Riv Patol Nerv Mental 1984;105:217–222.

176. Schochet SS Jr. Intoxications and metabolic diseases of the central nervous system. In: Nelson JS, Parisi JE, Schochet SS Jr, eds. *Principles and Practice of Neuropathology*. St. Louis, Mo: Mosby; 1993:302–343.

177. Harper CG, Giles M, Finlay-Jones R. Clinical signs in the Wernicke-Korsakoff complex: A retrospective analysis of 131 cases diagnosed at necropsy. *J Neurol Neurosurg Psychiatry* 1986;49:341–345.

178. Brazis PW, Lee AG. Binocular vertical diplopia. *Mayo Clin Proc* 1998;73:55–66.

179. Giles CL, Henderson JW. Horner's syndrome: an analysis of 216 cases. *Am J Ophthalmol* 1958;46:289–296.

180. Jermyn RT. A nonsurgical approach to low back pain. *J Am Osteopath Assoc* 2001;101(suppl):S6–S11.

181. Diamond MC, Scheibel AB, Elson LM. *The Human Brain Coloring Book*. New York, NY: Harper and Row; 1985.

182. Babinski J. *Réflexes tendineux & réflexes osseux*. Paris, France: Imprimerie Typographique R. Tancrede; 1912.

183. Babinski J. Du phénomène des orteils et de sa valeur sémiologique. *Semaine Méd* 1898;18:321–322.

184. Babinski J. De l'abduction des orteils. *Rev Neurol* 1903;11:728–729.

185. Dommisse GF, Grobler L. Arteries and veins of the lumbar nerve roots and cauda equina. *Clin Orthop* 1976;115:22–29.

186. Gilman S. The physical and neurologic examination. In: Gilman S, ed. *Clinical Examination of the Nervous System*. New York, NY: McGraw-Hill; 2000:1–34.

187. Denno JJ, Meadows GR. Early diagnosis of cervical spondylotic myelopathy: A useful clinical sign. *Spine* 1991;16:1353–1355.

188. Murphy DR. *Conservative Management of Cervical Spine Syndromes*. New York, NY: McGraw-Hill; 2000.

189. Kori AA, Leigh JL. The cranial nerve examination. In: Gilman S, ed. *Clinical Examination of the Nervous System*. New York, NY: McGraw-Hill; 2000:65–111.

190. Denny-Brown D. The tract of Lissauer in relation to sensory transmission in the dorsal horn of the spinal cord of the macaque. *J Comp Neurol* 1973;151:175.

191. Meadows JTS. *Manual Therapy: Biomechanical Assessment and Treatment, Advanced Technique. Lecture and Video Supplemental Manual*. Calgary, BC: Swodeam Consulting; 1995.

192. Hollinshead WH, Jenkins DB. *Functional Anatomy of the Limbs and Back*. Philadelphia, Pa: WB Saunders; 1981.

193. Goldberg S. *The Four Minute Neurological Examination*. Miami, Fla: Medmaster; 1992.

194. Judge RD, Zuidema GD, Fitzgerald FT. Head. In: Judge RD, Zuidema GD, Fitzgerald FT, eds. *Clinical Diagnosis*. Boston, Mass: Little, Brown; 1982:123–151.

195. Beghi E, Kurland LT, Mulder DW, Nicolosi A. Brachial plexus neuropathy in the population of Rochester, Minnesota, 1970–1981. *Ann Neurol* 1985;118:320–323.

196. Terzis JK, Liberson WT, Levine R. Obstetric brachial plexus palsy. *Hand Clin* 1986;2:773.

197. Terzis JK, Liberson WT, Levine R. Our experience in obstetrical Brachial Plexus palsy. In: Terzis JK, ed. *Microreconstruction of Nerve Injuries*. Philadelphia, Pa: Saunders; 1987:513.

198. Duchenne GBA. *De l'électrisation localisée et de son application à la pathologie et à la thérapeutique par courants induits et par courants galvaniques interrompus et continus*. 3rd ed. Paris, France: Librairie JB Baillière et fils; 1872.

199. Erb W. Uber eine eigenthümliche Localisation von Lahmungen im plexus brachialis. *Naturhist Med Ver Heidelberg Verh* 1874;2:130.

200. Al-Qattan MM, Clarke HM, Curtis CG. Klumpke's birth palsy: Does it really exist? *J Hand Surg* 1995;20B:19.

201. Klumpke A. Contribution à l'étude des paralysies radiculaires du plexus brachial. *Rev Med* 1885;5:739.

202. Brown KLB. Review of obstetrical palsies: Nonoperative treatment. In: Terzis JK, ed. *Microreconstruction of Nerve Injuries*. Philadelphia, Pa: Saunders; 1987:499.

203. Brown KLB. Review of obstetrical palsies: Nonoperative treatment. *Clin Plast Surg* 1984;11:181.

204. Gilbert A, Tassin JL. Obstetrical palsy: A clinical, pathologic, and surgical review. In: Terzis JK, ed. *Microreconstruction of Nerve Injuries*. Philadelphia, Pa: Saunders; 1987:529.

CHAPTER 3

THE BIOMECHANICS OF MOVEMENT

CHAPTER OBJECTIVES

▶ **At the completion of this chapter, the reader will be able to:**

1. Give definitions for commonly used biomechanical terms.

2. Describe the different planes of the body.

3. Describe the different axes of the body and the motions that occur around them.

4. Define the terms osteokinematic motion and arthrokinematic motion.

5. Differentiate between the different types of motion that can occur at the joint surfaces.

6. Describe the basic biomechanics of joint motion in terms of their concave-convex relationships.

7. Describe the components of normal and abnormal motion.

8. Define the terms *close packed* and *open packed*.

OVERVIEW

The science of biomechanics involves the application of mechanical principles in the study of the structure and function of movement. For the physical therapist designing and supervising rehabilitation programs a working knowledge of biomechanics is essential: a fundamental skill of the physical therapist is to identify, analyze, and solve problems related to human movement. The structures involved with human movement include the muscles and tendons, which produce the movement, and the joints, around which the movements occur. Most joints in the body are capable of physiologic movement, with the synovial joints having the most motion available.

Terminology

When describing movements, it is necessary to have a starting position as the reference position. This starting position is referred to as the *anatomic reference position*. The anatomic reference position for the human body is described as the erect standing position with the feet just slightly separated and the arms hanging by the side, the elbows straight, and the palms of the hand facing forward (Fig. 3-1).

Directional Terms

Directional terms are used to describe the relationship of body parts or the location of an external object with respect to the body.[1] The following are commonly used directional terms:

▶ *Superior* or *cranial.*   Closer to the head.

▶ *Inferior* or *caudal.*   Closer to the feet.

▶ *Anterior* or *ventral.*   Toward the front of the body.

▶ *Posterior* or *dorsal.*   Toward the back of the body.

▶ *Medial.*   Toward the midline of the body.

▶ *Lateral.*   Away from the midline of the body.

▶ *Proximal.*   Closer to the trunk.

▶ *Distal.*   Away from the trunk.

▶ *Superficial.*   Toward the surface of the body.

▶ *Deep.*   Away from the surface of the body in the direction of the inside of the body.

Movements of the Body Segments

Movements of the body segments occur in three dimensions along imaginary planes and around various axes of the body.

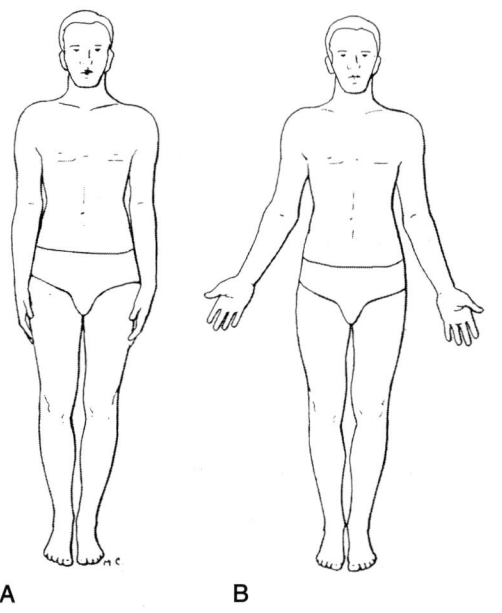

FIGURE 3-1 *A.* Fundamental standing position. *B.* The anatomic reference position of the body.

Planes of the Body

There are three traditional planes of the body corresponding to the three dimensions of space: sagittal, frontal, and transverse[1] (Fig. 3-2).

▶ *Sagittal.* The sagittal plane, also known as the *anterior-posterior or median plane,* divides the body vertically into left and right halves of equal size.

▶ *Frontal.* The frontal plane, also known as the *lateral or coronal plane,* divides the body equally into front and back halves.

▶ *Transverse.* The transverse plane, also known as the *horizontal plane,* divides the body equally into top and bottom halves.

Because each of these planes bisects the body, it follows that each plane must pass through the center of gravity.[*] If the movement described occurs in a plane that passes through the center of gravity, that movement is deemed to have occurred in a *cardinal* plane. An *arc of motion* represents the total number of degrees traced between the two extreme positions of movement in a specific plane of motion.[2] If a joint has more than one plane of motion, each type of motion is referred to as a *unit of motion.* For example, the wrist has two units of motion: flexion-extension (anterior-posterior plane), and ulnar-radial deviation (lateral plane).[2]

---

[*] The center of gravity may be defined as "the point at which the three planes of the body intersect each other."[2] The line of gravity is defined as "the vertical line at which the two vertical planes intersect each other."[2]

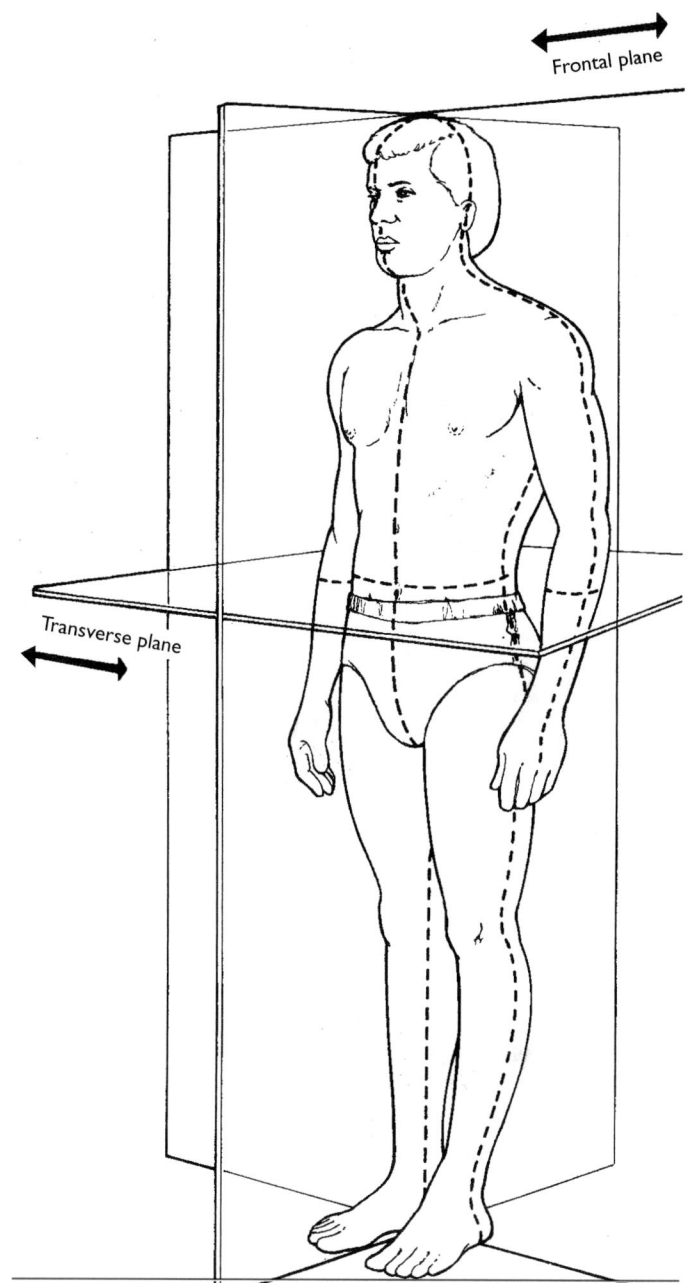

FIGURE 3-2 Planes of the body.

Few movements involved with functional activities occur in the cardinal planes. Instead, most movements occur in an infinite number of vertical and horizontal planes parallel to the cardinal planes (see discussion that follows).

Axes of the Body

Three reference axes are used to describe human motion: frontal, sagittal, and longitudinal. The axis around which the movement takes place is always perpendicular to the plane in which it occurs.

▶ *Frontal.* The frontal axis, also known as the *transverse axis,* is perpendicular to the sagittal plane.

▶ *Sagittal.* The sagittal axis is perpendicular to the frontal plane.

▶ *Longitudinal.* The longitudinal axis, also known as the *vertical axis,* is perpendicular to the transverse plane.

Most movements occur *in* planes and *around* axes that are somewhere in between the traditional planes and axes. However, nominal identification of every plane and axis of movement is impractical. The structure of the joint determines the possible axes of motion that are available. For example, a hinge joint has only a frontal-horizontal axis. Condyloid (ovoid) joints (see Chap. 1) have both a frontal-horizontal and a sagittal-horizontal axis. Ball-and-socket joints have frontal, sagittal-horizontal, and vertical axes. The planes and axes for the more common planar movements are as follows:

▶ Flexion, extension, hyperextension, dorsiflexion, and plantar flexion occur in the sagittal plane around a frontal-horizontal axis.

▶ Abduction and adduction, side flexion of the trunk, elevation and depression of the shoulder girdle, radial and ulnar deviation of the wrist, and eversion and inversion of the foot occur in the frontal plane around a sagittal-horizontal axis.

▶ Rotation of the head, neck, and trunk; internal rotation and external rotation of the arm or leg; horizontal adduction and abduction of the arm or thigh; and pronation and supination of the forearm occur in the transverse plane around the longitudinal axis.

▶ Arm circling and trunk circling are examples of *circumduction*. Circumduction involves an orderly sequence of circular movements that occur in the sagittal, frontal, and intermediate oblique planes, so that the segment as a whole incorporates a combination of flexion, extension, abduction, and adduction. Circumduction movements can occur at biaxial and triaxial joints. Examples of these joints include the tibiofemoral, radiohumeral, hip, glenohumeral, and the spinal joints.

Both the configuration of a joint and the line of pull of the muscle acting at a joint determine the motion that occurs at a joint:

▶ A muscle whose line of pull is lateral to the joint is a potential abductor.

▶ A muscle whose line of pull is medial to the joint is a potential adductor.

▶ A muscle whose line of pull is anterior to a joint has the potential to extend or flex the joint. At the knee, an anterior line of pull may cause the knee to extend, whereas at the elbow joint, an anterior line of pull may cause flexion of the elbow.

▶ A muscle whose line of pull is posterior to the joint has the potential to extend or flex a joint (refer to preceding example).

Joint Kinematics

Kinematics is the study of motion. In studying joint kinematics, two major types of motion are involved: (1) osteokinematic and (2) arthrokinematic.

Osteokinematic Motion

Osteokinematic motion occurs when any object forms the radius of an imaginary circle about a fixed point. The axis of rotation for osteokinematic motions is oriented perpendicular to the plane in which the rotation occurs.[1] The distance traveled by the motion may be a small arc or a complete circle and is measured as an angle, in degrees. All human body segment motions involve osteokinematic motions. Examples of osteokinematic motion include abduction or adduction of the arm, flexion of the hip or knee, and side bending of the trunk.

Arthrokinematic Motion

The motions occurring at the joint surfaces are termed *arthrokinematic* movements. Before discussing the various types of arthrokinematic motions, it is necessary to describe the shapes of joint surfaces.

At each synovial articulation, the articulating surface of each bone moves relative to the shape of the other articulating surface. For the sake of simplicity, the shapes of these articulating surfaces in synovial joints are described as being *ovoid* or *sellar* in shape (see Chap. 1). Under this concept, an articulating surface can be either concave (female) or convex (male) in shape (ovoid), or a combination of both shapes (sellar). An example of the former occurs at the glenohumeral joint: the humeral head would be the convex surface and the glenoid fossa would be the concave surface. An example of a joint that has a combination of both shapes is the first carpometacarpal joint (see Chap. 16).

Normal arthrokinematic motions must occur for full-range physiologic motion to take place. A restriction of arthrokinematic motion results in a decrease in osteokinematic motion. Mennell[3,4] referred to these motions as *joint-play* motions, and he introduced the concept that full, painless, active range of motion is not possible without these motions. The three types of movement that occur at the articulating surfaces include[5]:

▶ *Roll.* A roll occurs when the points of contact on each joint surface are constantly changing (Fig. 3-3). This type of movement is analogous to a tire on a car as the car rolls forward. The term *rock* is often used to describe small rolling motions.

▶ *Slide.* A slide is a pure translation. It occurs if only one point on the moving surface makes contact with varying points on the opposing surface (see Fig. 3-3). This type of movement is analogous to a car tire skidding when the brakes are applied suddenly on a wet road. This type of motion also is referred to as *translatory* or *accessory* motion. Although the roll of a joint always occurs in the same

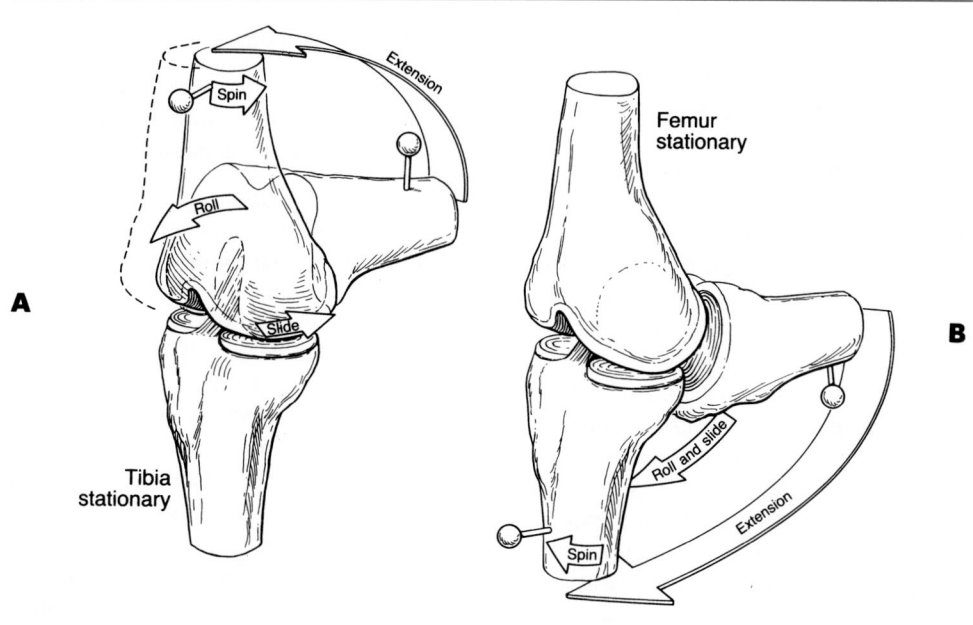

FIGURE 3-3 The kinematics of joint movements. (Reproduced with permission from Dutton M. *Manual Therapy of the Spine.* New York, NY: McGraw-Hill; 2001.)

direction as the swing of a bone, the direction of the slide is determined by the shape of the articulating surface (Fig. 3-4). This rule is often referred to as the *concave-convex rule*: If the joint surface is convex relative to the other surface, the slide occurs in the opposite direction to the osteokinematic motion (see Fig. 3-4). If, on the other hand, the joint surface is concave, the slide occurs in the same direction as the osteokinematic motion. The clinical significance of the concave-convex rule is described in Chapter 11.

▶ *Spin.* A spin is defined as any movement in which the bone moves but the mechanical axis remains stationary. A spin involves a rotation of one surface on an opposing surface around a longitudinal axis (see Fig. 3-3). This type of motion is analogous to the pirouette performed in ballet. Spin motions in the body include internal and external rotation of the glenohumeral joint when the humerus is abducted to 90 degrees; and at the radial head during forearm pronation and supination.

Most anatomic joints demonstrate composite motions involving a roll, slide, and spin.

Osteokinematic and arthrokinematic motions are directly proportional to each other, and one cannot occur completely without the other. It therefore follows that if a joint is not functioning correctly, one or both of these motions may be at fault. When examining a patient with movement impairment, it is critical that the clinician determine whether the osteokinematic

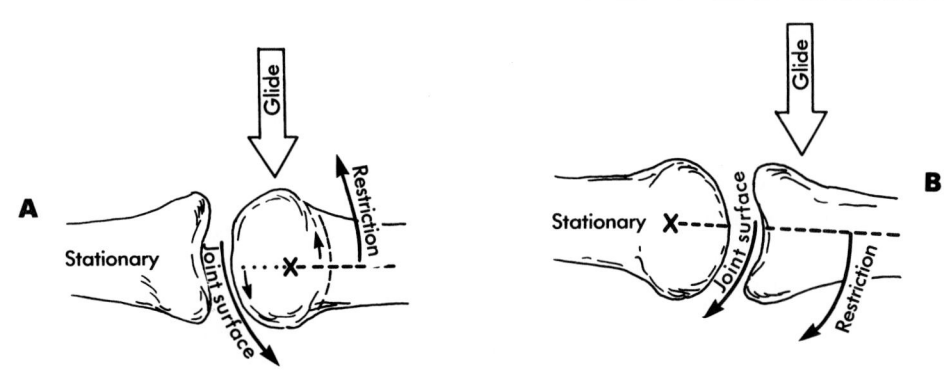

FIGURE 3-4 Gliding motions according to joint surface shapes. (Reproduced with permission from Dutton M. *Manual Therapy of the Spine.* New York, NY: McGraw-Hill; 2001.)

motion or the arthrokinematic motion is restricted so that the intervention can be made as specific as possible.

In the extremities, osteokinematic motion is controlled by the amount of flexibility of the surrounding soft tissues of the joint, where flexibility is defined as the amount of internal resistance to motion. In contrast, the arthrokinematic motion is controlled by the integrity of the joint surfaces and the supporting tissues of the joint. This characteristic can be noted clinically in a chronic rupture of the anterior cruciate ligament of the knee. Upon examination of that knee, the arthrokinematic motion (joint glide) is found to be increased, illustrated by a positive Lachman's test, but the range of motion of the knee, its osteokinematic motion, is not affected (see Chap. 18).

In the spine, the osteokinematic motion is controlled by both the flexibility of the surrounding soft tissues *and* by the integrity of the joint surfaces and the supporting tissues of the joint. This characteristic can be noted clinically when examining the cranioverertebral joint glides, where a restriction in the arthrokinematic motion (joint glide) can be caused by either a joint restriction or an adaptively shortened suboccipital muscle (see Chap. 22).

The examination of these motions and their clinical implications are described in Chapter 8.

Degrees of Freedom

The number of independent modes of motion at a joint is called the *degrees of freedom (DOF)*. If a joint can swing in one direction or can only spin, it is said to have 1 DOF.[6–9] The proximal interphalangeal joint is an example of a joint with 1 DOF. If a joint can spin and swing in one way only *or* it can swing in two completely distinct ways, but not spin, it is said to have 2 DOF.[6–9] The tibiofemoral joint, temporomandibular joint, proximal and distal radioulnar joints, subtalar joint, and talocalcaneal joint are examples of joints with 2 DOF. If the bone can spin and also swing in two distinct directions then it is said to have 3 DOF.[6–9] Ball-and-socket joints such as the shoulder and hip have 3 DOF.

Clinical Pearl

Joint motion that occurs only in one plane is designated as one degree of freedom; in two planes, two degrees of freedom; and in three planes, three degrees of freedom.

Because of the arrangement of the articulating surfaces—the surrounding ligaments and joint capsules—most motions around a joint do not occur in straight planes or along straight lines. Instead, the bones at any joint move through space in curved paths. This can best be illustrated using *Codman's paradox*.

1. Stand with your arms by your side, palms facing inward, thumbs extended. Notice that the thumb is pointing forward.

2. Flex one arm to 90 degrees at the shoulder so that the thumb is pointing up.

3. From this position, horizontally extend your arm so that the thumb remains pointing up but your arm is in a position of 90 degrees of glenohumeral abduction.

4. From this position, without rotating your arm, return the arm to your side and note that your thumb is now pointing away from your thigh.

Referring to the start position, and using the thumb as the reference, it can be seen that the arm has undergone an external rotation of 90 degrees. But where and when did the rotation take place? Undoubtedly, it occurred during the three separate, straight-plane motions or *swings* that etched a triangle in space. What you have just witnessed is an example of a conjunct rotation—a rotation that occurs as a result of joint surface shapes—and the effect of inert tissues rather than contractile tissues. Conjunct rotations can only occur in joints that can rotate internally or externally. Although not always apparent, most joints can so rotate. Consider the motions of elbow flexion and extension. While fully flexing and extending your elbow a number of times, watch the pisiform bone and forearm. If you watch carefully you should notice that the pisiform and the forearm move in a direction of supination during flexion, and pronation during extension of the elbow. The pronation and supination motions are examples of conjunct rotations.

Most habitual movements, or those movements that occur most frequently at a joint, involve a conjunct rotation. However, the conjunct rotations are not always under volitional control. In fact, the conjunct rotation is only under volitional control in joints with 3 DOF (glenohumeral and hip joints). In joints with fewer than 3 DOF (hinge joints, such as the tibiofemoral and ulnohumeral joints), the conjunct rotation occurs as part of the movement but is not under voluntary control. The implications become important when attempting to restore motion at these joints: the mobilizing techniques must take into consideration both the relative shapes of the articulating surfaces as well as the conjunct rotation that is associated with a particular motion.

Close-packed and Open-packed Positions of the Joint

Joint movements usually are accompanied by a relative compression (approximation) or distraction (separation) of the opposing joint surfaces. These relative compressions or distractions affect the level of *congruity* of the opposing surfaces. The position of maximum congruity of the opposing joint surfaces is termed the *close-packed* position of the joint. The position of least congruity is termed the *open-packed* position. Thus, movements toward the close-packed position of a joint involve an element of compression, whereas movements out of this position involve an element of distraction.

Close-packed Position

The close-packed position of a joint is the joint position that results in:

▶ Maximal tautness of the major ligaments.

▶ Maximal surface congruity.

▶ Minimal joint volume.

▶ Maximal stability of the joint.

Once the close-packed position is achieved, no further motion in that direction is possible. This is the often-cited reason why most fractures and dislocations occur when an external force is applied to a joint that is in its close-packed position. In addition, many of the traumatic injuries of the upper extremities result from falling on a shoulder, elbow or wrist, which are in their close-packed position. This type of injury, a *f*all *o*n an *o*utstretched *h*and is often referred to as a FOOSH injury. The close-packed positions for the various joints are depicted in Table 3-1.

Open-packed Position

In essence, any position of the joint, other than the close-packed position, could be considered as an open-packed position. The open-packed position, also referred to as the *loose-packed* position of a joint, is the joint position that results in:

▶ Slackening of the major ligaments of the joint.

▶ Minimal surface congruity.

▶ Minimal joint surface contact.

▶ Maximal joint volume.

▶ Minimal stability of the joint.

The open-packed position permits maximal distraction of the joint surfaces. Because the open-packed position causes the brunt of any external force to be borne by the joint capsule or surrounding ligaments, most capsular or ligamentous sprains occur when a joint is in its open-packed position. The open-packed positions for the various joints are depicted in Table 3-2.

Clinical Pearl

The open-packed position is commonly used during joint mobilization techniques (see Chap. 11).

Hypomobility, Hypermobility, and Instability

The amount of motion available at a joint is based on a number of factors, including the shape of the articulating surfaces, the health of the joint and the surrounding tissues, and the load-deformation history of the joint (see Chap. 4). A good analogy of joint motion is the door hinge and doorstop, in which the hinge represents the joint and the doorstop represents the restriction imposed by the

TABLE 3-1 Close-packed Position of the Joints

Joint	Position
Zygapophysial (spine)	Extension
Temporomandibular	Teeth clenched
Glenohumeral	Abduction and external rotation
Acromioclavicular	Arm abducted to 90 degrees
Sternoclavicular	Maximum shoulder elevation
Ulnohumeral	Extension
Radiohumeral	Elbow flexed 90 degrees; forearm supinated 5 degrees
Proximal radioulnar	5 degrees of supination
Distal radioulnar	5 degrees of supination
Radiocarpal (wrist)	Extension with radial deviation
Metacarpophalangeal	Full flexion
Carpometacarpal	Full opposition
Interphalangeal	Full extension
Hip	Full extension, internal rotation, and abduction
Tibiofemoral	Full extension and external rotation of tibia
Talocrural (ankle)	Maximum dorsiflexion
Subtalar	Supination
Midtarsal	Supination
Tarsometatarsal	Supination
Metatarsophalangeal	Full extension
Interphalangeal	Full extension

integrity of the joint and the surrounding tissues. Just as the doorstop prevents the door from swinging too far and damaging the wall, the integrity of the joint and its surrounding structures serve to prevent the joint moving past the normal range of motion.

TABLE 3-2   Open-packed (Resting) Position of the Joints

Joint	Position
Zygapophysial (spine)	Midway between flexion and extension
Temporomandibular	Mouth slightly open (freeway space)
Glenohumeral	55 degrees of abduction, 30 degrees of horizontal adduction
Acromioclavicular	Arm resting by side
Sternoclavicular	Arm resting by side
Ulnohumeral	70 degrees of flexion, 10 degrees of supination
Radiohumeral	Full extension, full supination
Proximal radioulnar	70 degrees of flexion, 35 degrees of supination
Distal radioulnar	10 degrees of supination
Radiocarpal (wrist)	Neutral with slight ulnar deviation
Carpometacarpal	Midway between abduction-adduction and flexion-extension
Metacarpophalangeal	Slight flexion
Interphalangeal	Slight flexion
Hip	30 degrees of flexion, 30 degrees of abduction, slight lateral rotation
Tibiofemoral	25 degrees of flexion
Talocrural (ankle)	10 degrees of plantar flexion, midway between maximum inversion and eversion
Subtalar	Midway between extremes of range of movement
Midtarsal	Midway between extremes of range of movement
Tarsometatarsal	Midway between extremes of range of movement
Metatarsophalangeal	Neutral
Interphalangeal	Slight flexion

If the movement of a joint is less than that considered normal, or when compared with the same joint on the opposite extremity, it may be deemed *hypomobile*. A joint that moves more than is considered normal when compared with the same joint on the opposite extremity may be deemed *hypermobile*. Hypermobility may occur as a generalized phenomenon or be localized to just one direction of movement, as follows.

▶ *Generalized hypermobility.* The more generalized form of hypermobility, as its name suggests, refers to the manifestations of multiple joint hyperlaxity, joint hypermobility, or articular hypermobility. This type of hypermobility can be seen in acrobats, gymnasts, and those individuals who are "double-jointed." In addition, generalized hypermobility occurs with genetic diseases that include joint hypermobility as an associated finding, such as Ehlers-Danlos syndrome, osteogenesis imperfecta, and Marfan's syndrome.

▶ *Localized hypermobility.* Localized hypermobility is likely to occur as a reaction to neighboring stiffness. For example, a compensatory hypermobility may occur at a joint when a neighboring joint or segment is injured. The injury to the neighboring joint results in a decrease in motion at the injured joint. This decrease in movement of the neighboring joint is often the result of the body's initial response to trauma, which is a reflexive increase in tone of muscles in an attempt to stabilize the affected area. Over time, the prolonged increased tonus may result in a decreased blood supply and an increase in the buildup of lactic acid. In addition, the nociceptors response in the muscle or the joint capsule may result in an inhibition of the segmental muscles, which, in turn, may lead to uncoordinated movements and produce myofascial trigger points.

Using the door hinge and stop analogy, it can be seen that both too much motion (resulting in damage to the wall) and too little motion (resulting in an inability to get through the door opening) can be disadvantageous. Similar consequences can be seen at a joint: a hypermobile joint may have insufficient stability to prevent damage occurring, whereas a hypomobile joint may provide insufficient motion at the joint for it to be functional. Hypermobile joints usually preserve their stability under normal conditions, remaining functional in weight bearing and within certain limits of motion.

It is essential to distinguish patients who have greater mobility in all their joints (generalized hypermobility) from those who for some other reason have one or a few joints that are more mobile than the rest (localized hypermobility). Whereas intervention is unlikely to be either warranted or of benefit with generalized hypermobility, the intervention for a localized hypermobility should address any neighboring *hypomobility*.

The term *stability*, specifically related to the joint, has been the subject of much research.[10–25] In contrast to a hypermobile joint, an unstable joint involves a disruption of the osseous and ligamentous structures of that joint and results in a loss of function. Joint stability may be viewed as a factor of joint integrity, elastic energy, passive stiffness, and muscle activation.

▶ *Joint integrity.* Joint integrity is enhanced in those ball-and-socket joints with deeper sockets or steeper sides, as opposed to those with planar sockets and shallower sides. Joint integrity is also dependent on the attributes of the supporting structures around the joint and the extent of joint disease.

▶ *Elastic energy.* Connective tissues (see Chap. 1) are elastic structures and, as such, are capable of storing elastic energy when stretched. This stored elastic energy may then be used to help return the joint to its original position when the stresses are removed.

▶ *Passive stiffness.* Individual joints have passive stiffness that increases toward the joint end range. An injury to these passive structures causing inherent loss in the passive stiffness results in joint laxity.[26]

▶ *Muscle activation.* Muscle activation increases stiffness, both within the muscle and within the joint(s) it crosses.[27] However, the synergist and antagonist muscles that cross the joint must be activated with the correct and appropriate activation in terms of magnitude or timing. A faulty motor control system may lead to inappropriate magnitudes of muscle force and stiffness, allowing a joint to buckle or undergo shear translation.[27]

Pathologic breakdown of the above factors may result in *instability.* Two types of instability are recognized: articular and ligamentous. Articular instability can lead to abnormal patterns of coupled and translational movements.[28] Ligamentous instability may lead to multiple planes of aberrant joint motion.[29]

Functional instability occurs when the severity of the instability adversely affects a patient's function. Functional instability may result in[30–33]:

▶ Long-term, nonacute pain or short-term episodic pain.

▶ Early morning stiffness.

▶ Inconsistent function and dysfunction–(e.g., full range of motion but abnormal movement, which may include angulation, hinging, or deviation).

▶ A feeling of apprehension or giving way.

REVIEW QUESTIONS*

1. Describe the anatomic reference position of the body.
2. Give the name of the plane of the body that divides the body equally into front and back halves.
3. Which plane divides the body equally into top and bottom halves?
4. Which of the body axes is perpendicular to the frontal plane?
5. List the motions that occur in the sagittal plane around a frontal-horizontal axis.

---

* Additional questions to test your understanding of this chapter can be found in the Online Learning Center for *Orthopaedic Assessment, Evaluation, and Intervention* at www.duttononline.net.

REFERENCES

1. Hall SJ. Kinematic concepts for analyzing human motion. In: Hall SJ, ed. *Basic Biomechanics.* New York, NY: McGraw-Hill; 1999:28–89.
2. Cocchierella L, Andersson GBJ, eds. *American Medical Association, Guides to the Evaluation of Permanent Impairment.* 5th ed. Chicago, Ill: American Medical Association; 2001.
3. Mennell JB. *The Science and Art of Joint Manipulation.* London, England: J and A Churchill; 1949.
4. Mennell JM. *Back Pain. Diagnosis and Treatment Using Manipulative Techniques.* Boston, Mass: Little, Brown; 1960.
5. MacConaill MA. Arthrology. In: Warwick R, Williams PL, eds. *Gray's Anatomy.* Philadelphia, Pa: WB Saunders; 1975; 484–510.
6. Lehmkuhl LD, Smith LK. *Brunnstrom's Clinical Kinesiology.* Philadelphia, Pa: FA Davis; 1983:361–390.
7. MacConnail MA, Basmajian JV. *Muscles and Movements: A Basis for Human Kinesiology.* New York, NY: Robert Krieger; 1977.
8. Rasch PJ, Burke RK. *Kinesiology and Applied Anatomy.* Philadelphia, Pa: Lea and Febiger; 1971.
9. Steindler A. *Kinesiology of the Human Body under Normal and Pathological Conditions.* Springfield, Ill: Charles C Thomas; 1955.
10. Answorth AA, Warner JJP. Shoulder instability in the athlete. *Orthop Clin North Am* 1995;26:487–504.
11. Bergmark A. Stability of the lumbar spine. *Acta Orthop Scand* 1989;60:1–54.
12. Boden BP, Pearsall AW, Garrett WE Jr, Feagin JA Jr. Patellofemoral instability: Evaluation and management. *J Am Acad Orthop Surgeons* 1997;5:47–57.
13. Callanan M, Tzannes A, Hayes K, Paxinos A, Walton J, Murrell GA. Shoulder instability. Diagnosis and management. *Aust Fam Physician* 2001;30:655–661.
14. Cass JR, Morrey BF. Ankle instability: Current concepts, diagnosis, and treatment. *Mayo Clin Proc* 1984;59:165–170.
15. Clanton TO. Instability of the subtalar joint. *Orthop Clin North Am* 1989;20:583–592.
16. Cox JS, Cooper PS. Patellofemoral instability. In: Fu FH, Harner CD, Vince KG, eds. *Knee Surgery.* Baltimore, Md: Williams and Wilkins; 1994:959–962.
17. Freeman MAR, Dean MRE, Hanham IWF. The etiology and prevention of functional instability of the foot. *J Bone Joint Surg* 1965;47B:678–685.
18. Friberg O. Lumbar instability: A dynamic approach by traction-compression radiography. *Spine* 1987;12:119–129.
19. Grieve GP. Lumbar instability. *Physiotherapy* 1982;68:2.
20. Hotchkiss RN, Weiland AJ. Valgus stability of the elbow. *J Orthop Res* 1987;5:372–377.
21. Kaigle A, Holm S, Hansson T. Experimental instability in the lumbar spine. *Spine* 1995;20:421–430.
22. Kuhlmann JN, et al. Stability of the normal wrist. In: Tubiana R, ed. *The Hand.* Philadelphia, Pa: WB Saunders; 1985:934–944.
23. Landeros O, Frost HM, Higgins CC. Post traumatic anterior ankle instability. *Clin Orthop* 1968;56:169–178.
24. Luttgens K, Hamilton N. The center of gravity and stability. In: Luttgens K, Hamilton N, eds. *Kinesiology: Scientific Basis of Human Motion.* Dubuque, Iowa: McGraw-Hill; 1997:415–442.
25. Wilke H, Wolf S, Claes LE, Arand M, Wiesend A. Stability increase of the lumbar spine with different muscle groups: A biomechanical in vitro study. *Spine* 1995;20:192–198.

26. Panjabi MM. The stabilizing system of the spine. Part 1. Function, dysfunction adaption and enhancement. *J Spinal Disord* 1992;5:383–389.

27. McGill SM, Cholewicki J. Biomechanical basis for stability: An explanation to enhance clinical utility. *J Orthop Sports Phys Ther* 2001;31:96–100.

28. Gertzbein SD, Seligman J, Holtby R, et al. Centrode patterns and segmental instability in degenerative disc disease. *Spine* 1985;10:257–261.

29. Cholewicki J, McGill S. Mechanical stability of the in vivo lumbar spine: Implications for injury and chronic low back pain. *Clin Biomech* 1996;11:1–15.

30. Terry GC, Hammon D, France P, Norwood LA. The stabilizing function of passive shoulder restraints. *Am J Sports Med* 1991;19:26–34.

31. Meadows JTS. The principles of the Canadian approach to the lumbar dysfunction patient. In: American Physical Therapy Association. *Management of Lumbar Spine Dysfunction: Independent Home Study Course*. La Cross, Wis: APTA, Orthopaedic Section; 1999.

32. Meadows J. *Orthopedic Differential Diagnosis in Physical Therapy*. New York, NY: McGraw-Hill; 1999.

33. Schneider G. Lumbar instability. In: Boyling JD, Palastanga N, eds. *Grieve's Modern Manual Therapy*. Edinburgh, Scotland: Churchill Livingstone; 1994.

THE RESPONSE OF BIOLOGICAL TISSUE TO STRESS

CHAPTER OBJECTIVES

▶ *At the completion of this chapter, the reader will be able to:*

1. Describe the various types of loading that can act on the musculoskeletal system.

2. Outline the responses of the various tissues to stress.

3. Describe the etiology and pathophysiology of various musculoskeletal injuries associated with different types of body tissue.

4. Describe the pathologic processes of articular cartilage, including osteoarthritis and rheumatoid arthritis.

5. List the detrimental effects that immobilization can have on tissues of the musculoskeletal system.

OVERVIEW

A wide range of external and internal forces are either generated or resisted by the human body during the course of daily activities. Examples of these external forces include ground reaction force, friction, gravity, and applied force through contact. Examples of internal forces include muscle contraction, joint contact, and joint shear forces.

One of the contributing factors to maintaining musculoskeletal health is the ability of the biological tissues to withstand these stresses during activity. Maintaining this health is a delicate balance, because insufficient, excessive, or repetitive stresses can prove deleterious. Whether a stress proves to be beneficial or detrimental to a tissue is very much dependent on the physiologic capacity of the tissue to accept load. This capacity is dependent on a number of factors, among them:

▶ *Age.* Increasing age reduces the capacity of the tissues to cope with stress loading.

▶ Proteoglycan and collagen content of the tissue. Both increasing age and exposure to trauma can result in unfavorable alterations in the proteoglycan and collagen content of the tissue.

▶ Ability of the tissue to undergo adaptive change. All musculoskeletal tissue has the capacity to adapt to change. This capacity to change is determined primarily by the viscoelastic property of the tissue (see later).

▶ The speed at which the adaptive change occurs. This is dependent on the type and severity of the insult to the tissue. Insults of low force and longer duration may provide the tissue an opportunity to adapt. In contrast, insults of a higher force and shorter duration are less likely to provide the tissue time to adapt (see later).

Terminology

Kinetics is the study of forces that arise as motions change. Before discussing the response of the biological tissues to stress, an understanding of the concepts and definitions used in the study of kinetics is necessary.[1,2]

▶ *Mass.* Mass is the quantity of matter composing a body. The common unit of mass is the kilogram (kg).

▶ *Inertia.* The resistance to action or to change is termed *inertia*. The body's tendency to maintain its current state, whether motionless or moving with a constant velocity, is a result of inertia. Although inertia has no units of measurement,

TABLE 4-1   Units of Force

Unit	Definition
Dyne	A force magnitude causing an acceleration of 1 cm/s^2 to a rigid body with 1 g of mass
Newton (N)	A force magnitude causing an acceleration of 1 cm/s^2 to a rigid body with 1 kg of mass
lbf	A force magnitude causing an acceleration of 1 g (32.2 ft/s^2) to a mass of 1 lb; 1 kgf = 2.2 lbf
kgf	A force magnitude causing an acceleration of 1 g (9.8 m/s^2) to a mass of 1 kg; 1 kgf = 9.8 N

the amount of inertia a body possesses is directly proportional to its mass.

▶ *Center of gravity.*   A body's center of gravity or center of mass is the point around which the weight and mass are equally balanced in all directions. From a kinetic perspective, the location of the center of mass determines the way in which the body responds to external forces.

▶ *Force.*   Force is a vector quantity, with magnitude, direction, and point of application to a body. When a force acts on an object, there are two potential effects: acceleration and deformation (see "load-deformation curve," following). The term *load* describes the type of force applied to a tissue. Body weight, friction, and air or water resistance are all forces that commonly act on the body. *Stress* is the force per unit area that develops on the cross-section of a structure in response to externally applied loads. Stress is quantified as force per unit area over which the force acts. *Strain* is the deformation that develops within a structure in response to externally applied loads. The two basic types of strain are linear strain, which causes a change in the length of a structure, and shear strain, which causes a change in the angular relationships within a structure. The various units of force are depicted in Table 4-1. A number of forces are recognized. These include compression, tension, shear, and torsion.

• *Compression.*   Compression can be viewed as a squeezing force.

• *Tension.*   Tensile force is the opposite of a compressive force and can be viewed as a pulling or stretching force.

• *Shear.*   Shear forces tend to cause one portion of an object to slide or displace with respect to another portion of the object. Whereas compressive and tensile forces act along the longitudinal axis of a structure to which they are applied, shear forces act parallel or tangent to a surface. For example, bending forward at the waist produces shear forces between the lumbar vertebral bodies and their respective intervertebral disks.

• *Torsion.*   Torsional forces occur when a structure is made to twist about its longitudinal axis, typically when one end of the structure is fixed. For example, torsional forces occur in the lower extremity if a directional change is attempted while the sole of the foot is planted firmly on the ground.

▶ *Load-deformation curve.*   The load-deformation curve, or stress-strain curve, of a structure depicts the relationship between the amount of force applied to a structure and the

structure's response in terms of deformation or acceleration (Fig. 4-1). Young's modulus is a numerical description of the relationship between the amount of stress a tissue undergoes and the deformation that results. Mathematically, Young's modulus is the slope of the load-deformation response graph for a given structure. Biological tissues are anisotropic, which means they can demonstrate differing mechanical behavior as a function of test direction. With relatively small loads, deformation occurs, but the response is elastic: when the force is removed, the structure returns to its original size and shape. If the applied force causes the deformation to exceed the structure's *yield point* or *elastic limit*, however, the response is plastic: some amount of the deformation is permanent. This permanent change results from the breaking of bonds and their subsequent inability to contribute to the recovery of the tissue. Deformations exceeding the ultimate failure point produce mechanical failure of the structure, which in the human body may be represented by the fracturing of bone or the rupturing of soft tissues. The shape and position of the load-deformation curve depends on a number of factors. These include:

• *Stiffness.*   The stiffer the structure, the steeper the slope of its stress-strain curve. Stiffness can be defined as the resistance of a structure to deformation, or the force required to produce a unit of deformation. Connective tissue that is loaded more quickly will behave more stiffly (will deform less) than the same tissue that is loaded at a slower rate.[3] In collagen fibers, the greater the density of the chemical bonds between the fibers or between the fibers and their

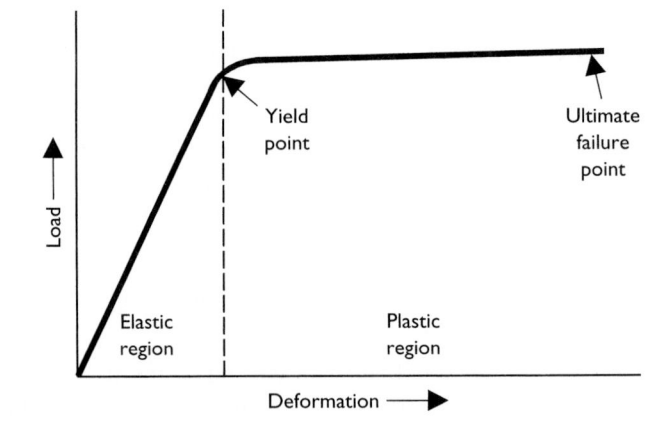

FIGURE 4-1   The stress-strain curve. (Reproduced with permission from Hall SJ. *Basic Biomechanics*. New York, NY: McGraw-Hill; 1999.)

surrounding matrix, the greater the stiffness. For example, the tendons of the digital flexors and extensors are very stiff, and their length changes very little when muscle forces are applied through them.[4] In contrast, the tendons of some muscles, particularly those involved in locomotion and ballistic performance, are more elastic.[4]

- *Viscoelasticity.* The mechanical qualities of a tissue can be separated into categories based on whether the tissue acts primarily like a solid, a fluid, or a mixture of the two. Solids are described according to their elasticity, strength, hardness, and stiffness. Bone, ligaments, tendons, and skeletal muscle are all examples of elastic solids. Biological tissues that demonstrate attributes of both solids and fluids are viscoelastic. Viscoelasticity is time-dependent behavior under load: the ability of a structure to stretch or shorten over time. The viscoelastic properties of a structure determine its response to loading. A more viscoelastic tissue causes the load-deformation curve to shift further to the right.

- *Age.* Age has effects on all aspects of the load-deformation curve. At an early age, a long failure region is observed, which is less evident at later age.

- *Exercise.* Exercise increases the stiffness and ultimate tensile strength of some structures, such as ligaments, cartilage, bone, and tendons. Conversely, immobility compromises the properties of connective tissue and skeletal muscle (see "Detrimental Effects of Immobility," later).

The various structures of the musculoskeletal system respond in a fairly predictable manner when exposed to stress. The extent of the response depends on the specific tissue involved, the type of force to which the body is subjected, the maximum force that the body tissue can tolerate without deformation, and the ability of the tissue to withstand sudden or repetitive stresses.[5] The distinction between sudden and repetitive stress is important. An acute stress (loading) occurs when a single force is large enough to cause injury on biological tissues; the causative force is termed *macrotrauma.* A repetitive stress (loading) occurs when a single force itself is insufficient to cause injury on biological tissues. However, when repeated or chronic stress over a period of time causes an injury, the injury is called a *chronic injury,* and the causative mechanism is termed *microtrauma* (see Chap. 5).

Response of Connective Tissue to Stress

Collagen fibers have a wavy, or folded, appearance at rest. When a force that lengthens the collagen fibers is initially applied to connective tissue, these folds are affected first. As the fibers unfold, the slack is taken up. This slack is called the tissue's *crimp.* The crimp of collagen is one of the major factors behind the viscoelastic properties of connective tissue and the characteristics of the load-deformation curve: the area of immediate elastic deformation on the load-deformation curve is represented by the crimp (see Fig. 4-1). Crimp is different for each type of connective tissue, and this provides each of these tissues with different viscoelastic properties.

If a load is applied to connective tissue and then removed immediately, the material recoils to its original size. If, however, the load is allowed to remain, the material continues to stretch. After a period of sustained stretch, the stretching tends to reach a steady-state value. Realignment of the collagen fibers in the direction of the stress occurs, and water and proteoglycans are displaced from between the fibers. *Creep* is the gradual rearrangement of collagen fibers, proteoglycans, and water that occurs because of a constantly applied force after the initial lengthening caused by crimp has ceased. Creep is time-dependent. Short duration stresses (less than 15 minutes) do not have sufficient time to produce this displacement; however, longer times can produce it. Once creep occurs, the tissue has difficulty returning to its initial length (see below).

Thus, stress to connective tissues can result in no change, a semipermanent change, or a permanent change to the microstructure of the collagenous tissue. The semipermanent or permanent changes may result in either *microfailure* or *macrofailure.*

Microfailure

Plastic deformation of connective tissue occurs when a tissue remains deformed and does not recover its prestress length. Once all of the possible realignment has occurred, any further loading breaks the restraining bonds, resulting in microfailure. On average, collagen fibers are able to sustain a 3 percent increase in elongation (strain) before microscopic damage occurs (see Fig. 4-1).[6] Following a brief stretch, providing the chemical bonds remain intact, the collagen and proteoglycans gradually recover their original alignment. The recovery process occurs at a slower rate and often to a lesser extent. The loss of energy that occurs between the lengthening force and the recovery activity is referred to as *hysteresis.* The more chemical bonds that are broken with applied stress, the greater is the hysteresis. If the stretch is of sufficient force and duration and a sufficient number of chemical bonds are broken, the tissue is unable to return to its original length until the bonds are re-formed. Instead, it returns to a new length and to a new level of strain resistance. Increased tissue excursion is now needed before tension develops in the structure. In essence, this has the affect of decreasing the stabilizing capabilities of the connective tissue.

Clinical Pearl

Microfailure is not always undesirable. Indeed, microfailure can be the aim of some manual stretching techniques that are intended to produce elongation of connective tissue structures. Low-level damage must occur to the connective tissue in order to produce permanent elongation.[3] Exercises also may be used to change the physical properties of both tendons and ligaments, as both have demonstrated adaptability to external loads with an increase in strength: weight ratios.[7-9] The improved strength results from an increase in the proteoglycan content and collagen cross-links.[7-9]

Macrofailure

If the stress applied is sufficient, and if enough of the bonds are broken, the tissue is no longer capable of resisting the force, and macrofailure, a complete rupture of the connective tissue occurs.

> **Clinical Pearl**
>
> Collagen does not offer much in the way of resistance to compression, but it does possess great tensile strength.[10,11] The tensile strength of collagen has been estimated at 50 to 125 N/mm^2, depending on the specimen.[12]

Articular Cartilage

Articular cartilage is a viscoelastic structure with a very high tensile strength and is resistant to compressive and shearing forces. The constitutive properties of hyaline cartilage are highly nonlinear, demonstrating an ability to undergo large deformations while still being able to return to its original shape and dimension.[2] The mechanical properties of articular cartilage change with the interstitial fluid content. The movement of this fluid helps provide nourishment to the chondrocytes, because cartilage is largely avascular. This avascularity limits the capacity of articular cartilage to repair itself (see Chap. 5).

Under stress, the interstitial fluid moves in when the tissue is dilated and out when it is compressed. The rate at which this interstitial fluid moves in or out of articular cartilage is dependent on the amplitude and, to a much smaller extent, the load application. Recovery from the deformation of the articular cartilage occurs in two phases: immediate and delayed. The early rebound of tissue height reflects the solid elastic properties of the tissue. The second part phase of the recovery occurs when the interstitial fluid begins to be slowly resorbed.

Although the cartilage matrix is filled with a normal amount of fluid, the friction forces at the joint surfaces are very low. However, the load-deformation history of a joint is important to the function and well-being of articular cartilage.[13–15] Damage to articular cartilage may result from microtrauma (degeneration), macrotrauma, or an inflammatory process.

Degeneration: Osteoarthritis

Osteoarthritis (OA), also known as degenerative joint disease, is a clinical condition of synovial joints. OA is characterized by development of fissures, cracks, and general thinning of joint cartilage; bone damage; hypertrophy of the cartilage; and synovial inflammation. The degenerative changes are most pronounced on the articular cartilage in weight-bearing areas of the large joints. In OA, the concentration and molecular weight of hyaluronan in synovial fluid is diminished as a result of dilution and fragmentation. Synovitis is minimal in the early stages of the disease but may contribute to joint damage in advanced disease.

The degenerative changes associated with OA may result in pain and stiffness of the affected joints. Two types of OA are commonly recognized: primary OA and secondary OA.

▶ Primary OA, the most common form, has no known cause, although it appears to be related to aging and heredity.[16] It most often affects the distal interphalangeal joints and less often, the proximal interphalangeal joints of the hands, hip, and knee and the metatarsophalangeal and tarsometatarsal joints of the feet. In addition, the cervical and lumbar spine may be affected.

▶ Secondary OA may occur in any joint as a result of articular injury. These injuries include fracture, repetitive joint use, obesity, or metabolic disease (osteoporosis, osteomalacia). Secondary OA may occur at any age. OA of the hip and knee represents two of the most significant causes of adult pain and physical disability.[17] It is estimated that 70 to 85 percent of people older than 55 years are afflicted with OA, and OA is listed eighth as a worldwide cause of disability.[18]

The pathogenesis of OA is multifactorial. Although specific risk factors for OA differ by anatomic joint region, age is the most consistently identified demographic risk factor for all articular sites.[16] Before the age of 50 years, men have a higher prevalence and incidence of this disease than women, but after age 50, women have a higher prevalence and incidence.[19] However, increasing age does not appear to be an absolute risk factor in the development of OA, for not every elderly person develops osteoarthritis.[21] The increase in the incidence and prevalence of OA with age is likely a consequence of several biologic changes that occur with aging, including:

▶ A decreased responsiveness of chondrocytes to growth factors that stimulate repair.

▶ An increase in the laxity of ligaments around the joints, making older joints relatively unstable and, therefore, more susceptible to injury.

▶ A failure of major shock absorbers or protectors of the joint with age, including a gradual decrease in strength, and a slowing of peripheral neurologic responses,[20] both of which protect the joint.[15]

OA is not a passive process of joint wear and tear but a metabolically active process.[22] Whether OA develops appears to depend on a variety of factors, as follows[17]:

▶ *Hormone replacement therapy.* Women receiving hormone replacement therapy have a lower prevalence of OA than women who are not receiving this therapy.

▶ *Obesity.* Studies have repeatedly confirmed the relationship of OA with body mass index. Obesity is more often associated with progressive OA of the knee than of the hip.[22–24]

▶ *Genetics and family history.* Abundant evidence supports the importance of genetic factors in some subgroups of OA.[24–26]

▶ *Activity level.* Certain forms of exercise are widely believed to increase bone density (bone mass index) in specific areas of the body. Bone mass index can be increased up to 26 percent in some locations by loading the skeleton through physical exercise.[27] Strenuous, high-intensity, and repetitive exercise, both sport and occupational, has been associated with the development of OA, although there appears to be no increased incidence of OA with moderate exercise.

▶ *Occupation.* Work-related activities that involve repetitive actions have been shown to be correlated with increased rates of osteoarthritis of the hip, knee, and other joints. Farmers, for example, have high rates of osteoarthritis of the hip,[28] and epidemiologic studies have shown that firefighters, farmers, construction workers, and miners have a higher prevalence of osteoarthritis of the knee than the general population.[29,30] In fact, workers whose jobs require knee bending, as well as lifting or regularly carrying loads of 25 lb or more, have increased radiologic evidence of osteoarthritis in the knee compared with those workers who do not.[31] This trend also has been shown to hold true for the upper extremity; for example, jackhammer operators exhibit an increased prevalence of osteoarthritis of the upper extremity when compared with the general population.[32]

▶ *Muscle loss.* A diagnosis of OA causes atrophy proximal to the involved joints because of progressive weakness and disuse.[22] The loss of supporting muscle may increase the joint load, which can lead to cartilage damage, especially in the weight-bearing joints.

▶ *Trauma.* A prior history of trauma may be an important risk factor in the development of OA in a joint damaged by ligamentous instability or meniscal tear in the knee.

The clinical findings associated with OA include:

▶ *Pain.* This is the most commonly reported complaint in OA. Early in the course of the disease, the pain may be poorly localized, asymmetric, and episodic. The pain of OA may have a nagging and aching quality. The severity and frequency of the pain increase as the disease progresses. More severe reports of pain usually are localized to the joint involved, but the pain also may be referred.[17]

▶ *Stiffness.* Early in the disease process, stiffness is experienced in the affected joints following activity resumption after a period of rest. As the disease progresses, pieces of degenerated cartilage may shed into the joint, producing loose bodies that may cause the joint to either lock or give way.[22]

▶ *Crepitus, swelling, inflammation, synovitis, and joint effusion.* All may be present. Swelling and joint effusion are seen in more advanced stages of OA. Heberden's and, less commonly, Bouchard's nodes may be present on the distal and proximal interphalangeal joints, respectively.

▶ *Tenderness.* Tenderness to palpation over the joint is common but may be mild or absent.

▶ *Impaired function.* When the knee or hip is involved, gait may be impaired. If the fingers are involved, hand function is likely to be affected.

Dramatic spontaneous restoration of the joint space in osteoarthritis is rare, although limited fibrocartilaginous repair is common. Regeneration of the joint space seems to be associated with peripheral osteophyte formation at the joint margin. An osteophyte, which consists of new cartilage and bone, likely forms in response to abnormal stresses on the joint margin, although its formation may also occur as a part of the aging process. There is experimental evidence that osteophyte formation is related to instability of joints and its growth has been described as part of the attempt of a synovial joint to adapt to injury, limiting excess movement and helping to recreate a viable joint surface.[32a]

Inflammation

Rheumatoid Arthritis.[33] Rheumatoid arthritis (RA) can be defined as a chronic, progressive, systemic, inflammatory disease of connective tissue characterized by spontaneous remissions and exacerbations (flare-ups). It is the second most common rheumatic disease after OA, but it is the most destructive to synovial joints. Unlike OA, RA involves primary tissue inflammation rather than joint degeneration. Although most individuals who develop RA do so in their early to middle adulthood, some experience a late onset RA (LORA) in their older years.

Although the exact etiology of RA is unclear, it is considered one of many autoimmune disorders. Abnormal immunoglobulin (Ig) G and IgM antibodies develop in response to IgG antigens to form circulating immune complexes. These complexes lodge in connective tissue, especially synovium, and create an inflammatory response. Inflammatory mediators, including cytokines (e.g., tumor necrosis factor), chemokines, and proteases, activate and attract neutrophils and other inflammatory cells. The synovium thickens, fluid accumulates in the joint space, and a pannus forms, eroding joint cartilage and bone. Bony ankylosis, calcifications, and loss of bone density follow.

The signs and symptoms of RA vary among individuals, depending on the rate the disease progresses. A complete musculoskeletal examination helps diagnose the disease. Clinical manifestations include both joint involvement and systemic problems; some are associated with the early stages of RA, whereas others are seen later in advanced disease.

Rheumatoid disease typically begins in the joints of the arm or hand. The individual complains of joint stiffness lasting longer than 30 minutes on awakening, pain, swelling, and heat (synovitis). Unlike with OA, the distal interphalangeal joints of the fingers usually are not involved in RA.

Complaints of fatigue, anorexia, low-grade fever, and mild weight loss are commonly associated with RA. As the disease progresses over years, systemic manifestations increase, and potentially life-threatening organ involvement begins. Cardiac problems, such as pericarditis and myocarditis, and respiratory complications, such as pleurisy, pulmonary fibrosis, and pneumonitis, are common.

As the disease worsens, joints become deformed, and secondary osteoporosis can result in fractures, especially in older adults. Hand and finger deformities are typical in the advanced stages of the disease. Palpable subcutaneous nodules, often appearing on the ulnar surface of the arm, are associated with a severe, destructive disease pattern.

Some RA patients have associated syndromes. Two such syndromes are Sjogren's and Felty's. Sjogren's syndrome is characterized by dryness of the eyes (keratoconjunctivitis), mouth (xerostomia), and other mucous membranes. Felty's syndrome is characterized by leukopenia and hepatosplenomegaly, often leading to recurrent infections. It encompasses a diverse group of pathogenic mechanisms in RA, all of which result in decreased levels of circulating neutrophils.

No single test or group of laboratory tests can confirm a diagnosis of RA, but they can support the findings from the patient's history and the physical findings. A number of immunologic tests, such as the rheumatoid factor (RF) and antinuclear antibody (ANA) titer are available to aid diagnosis. Normal values differ, depending on the precise laboratory technique used.

Juvenile Arthritis. The descriptive term *juvenile idiopathic arthritis* was adopted as an umbrella term to indicate disease of childhood onset characterized primarily by arthritis of no known etiology persisting for at least 6 weeks. Juvenile rheumatoid arthritis (JRA) is the most prevalent pediatric rheumatic diagnosis among children in the United States. Substantial evidence points to an autoimmune pathogenesis.[34]

Ligament

Skeletal ligaments consist of fibrous bands of dense connective tissue that behaves as a viscoelastic structure when exposed to stress. The cellular organization of the ligament makes it ideal for sustaining tensile load,[35] and its structural framework helps provide stiffness (resistance to deformation).[36] The stress-shielding capability of a ligament is dependent on the type and location of the ligament. The different biomechanical responses of ligaments can be explained by the anatomic and histologic variations in the substance and insertions of ligaments.[36–39] The elastic fiber content, organization of collagen fibers, and direct or indirect insertion patterns, may all contribute to these varying responses.

Point tenderness, joint effusion, and a history of trauma, are all characteristic of a ligamentous injury. Ligament injuries may be graded by severity[40] (Table 4-2).

▶ *Grade I.* Grade I sprains are painful but do not cause swelling or instability. According to O'Donoghue,[41] a grade I, or mild, sprain is characterized by tearing of only a few fibers with minimal hemorrhage. Because there is no laxity or residual instability, and full function and strength is maintained, the individual can usually return to sports in 1 to 2 weeks, with complete healing expected in 4 to 6 weeks.[42]

▶ *Grade II.* A grade II, or moderate, sprain is an incomplete tear of the ligament with mild laxity and instability, marked swelling, and pain, resulting in a slight reduction in func-

tion, possible decrease in strength, and the potential for loss of proprioception. In the case of a grade II sprain in the lower extremity, patients should be prescribed crutches until they are able to walk comfortably.[42] These individuals usually require 8 to 12 weeks to return to their sport.

▶ *Grade III.* A grade III, or severe, sprain is characterized by complete disruption of the ligament with gross instability and laxity, marked swelling, and significant pain. With grade III sprains, there is a high potential for a complete loss of full function, strength, and proprioception, particularly if the rehabilitation is deficient or inadequate. These individuals are at greater risk for chronic instability or osteochondral lesions,[43,44] which often require future surgery.

Stress tests applied perpendicular to the normal plane of joint motion can help distinguish between grade II and grade III ligament injuries. In grade III injuries, significant joint gapping occurs with the application of the stress test.[45] However, because of patient discomfort and guarding against possible pain, it is difficult to assess joint laxity by clinical examination alone. Currently, clinicians often use ancillary tests such as arthrometry or magnetic resonance imaging when diagnosing and grading soft tissue injuries.

Tendon

In general, the causes of a tendon injury center around microtrauma to tendon tissue because of repetitive mechanical load from external factors such as improper training techniques in athletes or incorrect use of equipment, and inappropriate shoe wear. In addition, patients often are found to have an anatomic predisposition resulting from inflexibility, weakness, or malposition.[46–48] Estimates of the Bureau of Labor Statistics[49] indicate that chronic tendon injuries account for 48 percent of reported occupational illnesses, whereas overuse injuries in sports account for 30 to 50 percent of all sports injuries.[50]

Mechanical overload does not seem to be the only factor to explain a tendon injury and may even be merely a permissive factor, allowing the tendon problem to become symptomatic.[51] Age and vascular supply may also be potential factors in the development of these injuries.

Tendonitis

The term *tendonitis* implies an inflammatory reaction to a tendon injury. Tendonitis usually is described as a microscopic tearing and inflammation of the tendon tissue, commonly resulting from tissue fatigue rather than direct trauma. However, histologic studies of injured tendons do not show the characteristic signs of an inflammatory response. These studies reveal few inflammatory cells, such as macrophages or polymorphonuclear leukocytes, and little formation of granulation tissue.[4] Rather, the histologic pattern is more characteristic of a degenerative condition.[4]

Tenosynovitis, Peritendonitis, and Paratenonitis

Tenosynovitis/tenovaginitis, peritendonitis, and paratenonitis indicate an inflammatory disorder of tissues surrounding the

TABLE 4-2 Ligament Injuries[40]

Grade	Signs	Implications
I (mild)	Minimal loss of structural integrity No abnormal motion Little or no swelling Localized tenderness Minimal bruising	Minimal functional loss Early return to training; some protection may be necessary
II (moderate)	Significant structural weakening Some abnormal motion Solid end feel to stress More bruising and swelling Often associated hemarthrosis and effusion	Tendency to recurrence Needs protection from risk of further injury May need modified immobilization May stretch out further with time
III (severe)	Loss of structural integrity Marked abnormal motion Significant bruising Hemarthrosis	Needs prolonged protection Surgery may be considered Often permanent functional instability

tendon such as the tendon sheath. In most cases, these conditions seem to result from a repetitive friction of the tendon and its sheath.[52]

Tendonosis

Tendonosis is a diagnosis that is used in research literature as well as clinical practice. The term *tendonosis* refers to a degenerative process (the suffix "-osis" is indicative of a degenerative process rather than a inflammatory disorder) of the tendon that is characterized by the presence of dense populations of fibroblasts, vascular hyperplasia, and disorganized collagen.[53] The disorganized collagen is termed *angiofibroblastic hyperplasia*.[54] Degenerative tendonopathy occurs in approximately one third of the population older than 35 years of age.[55]

It is commonly presumed that pain results from an inflamed structure. It is not clear why tendonosis is painful, given the absence of acute inflammatory cells, nor is it known why the collagen fails to mature. Necropsy studies have shown that these degenerative changes also may be present in asymptomatic tendons.[56] The degree of degeneration increases with age and may represent part of the normal aging process.[4] The degeneration appears to be activity related, as well.[4]

The typical clinical finding for tendonitis and tendonosis is a strong but painful response to resistance of the involved musculotendinous structure. Tenosynovitis/tenovaginitis involves an inflammation of the cellular lining membrane of fibrous sheath through which the tendons move, which can often produce pain with active motion of the involved tendon within the sheath. (See Table 4-3.)

Bone

Despite its image as a hard and inflexible structure, bone is a solid with elastic properties. The material properties of bone vary, depending on the type of bone. Test results on the ability of bone to withstand stresses are dependent on the rate and history of loading.

A lifelong pattern of bone turnover occurs. This turnover is characterized by two opposite activities: the formation of new bone by osteoblasts and the degradation (resorption) of old bone by osteoclasts. Osteoclastic cells reabsorb bony material and leave abandoned cells. Osteoblastic cells then reform bone by depositing bony material into osteoclast cell cavities. The material becomes mineralized, and bone structure is formed. The osteoblastic and osteoclastic cycle takes approximately 100 days to complete.[57] Nearly 25% of trabecular or cancellous bone, which composes vertebrae, the distal radius, and parts of the femur, is resorbed each year.[58] This resorption rate is more frequent for trabecular or cancellous bone than for cortical or compact bone, which predominately makes up long bones. This process occurs because trabecular bone has a greater surface area-to-volume ratio. Cortical bone remodeling is thought to be eightfold lower than that of trabecular bone.[58]

Bone is stiffer and stronger than other tissues at higher strain levels.[58a] The ability of bone to modify its morphology in the face of altered forces has long been recognized. However bone is not anistropic—it does not have the same capacity to absorb loads in all directions. In general, cancellous bone is less stiff than cortical bone.

Clinical Pearl

A typical load-deformation plot for cortical bone under tension reveals three distinct regions: (1) a linear region from which the elastic modulus is obtained, (2) a yield region which produces the yield strength, and (3) a post-yield region which ends in the fracture point. If the elastic strain of the cortical bone is exceeded, the yield strain of the bone is reached and a fracture occurs.

TABLE 4-3 Interventions for Tendonitis, Tendonosis, and Overuse Syndrome[40]

Grade	Symptoms	Intervention
I	Pain only after activity; does not interfere with performance; often generalized tenderness; disappears before next exercise session	Modification of activity Assessment of training pattern Possibly NSAIDs
II	Minimal pain with activity; does not interfere with intensity or distance; usually localized tenderness	Modification of activity Physical therapy; NSAIDs; consider orthotics
III	Pain interferes with activity; usually disappears between sessions; definite local tenderness	Significant modification of activity Assess training schedule Physical therapy; NSAIDs, consider orthotics Usually need to temporarily discontinue aggravating motion
IV	Pain does not disappear between activity sessions; seriously interferes with intensity of training; significant local sign of pain, tenderness, crepitus, swelling	Design alternate program May require splinting Physical therapy and NSAIDs
V	Pain interferes with sport and activities of daily living; symptoms often chronic or recurrent; signs of tissue changes and altered associated muscle function	Prolonged rest from activity NSAIDs plus other medical therapies Consider splint or cast Physical therapy May require surgery

NSAID, nonsteroidal anti-inflammatory drug.

Bone is better able to withstand compressive forces than tensile or torsional forces. The nonuniform load capacity of bone is largely attributable to the trabeculation that occurs in cancellous bone in response to Wolff's law.[58b] Wolff developed a mathematical model, now called *Wolff's law* that attempted to predict bone adaptation to stresses.[58c] Forces applied to bone, including muscle contractions and weight bearing, can alter both the internal and external configuration of bone through adaptation to these stresses. For example, when a bone is curved due to muscular pull or tension, more bone is deposited on the concave aspect than on the convex side. Frost[58d] described a process in which bone structure experiences microscopic damage from various forms of normal loading and is remodeled or repaired in a natural process of skeletal adaptation. He noted that bone loading needed to occur at a level "greater than normally experienced" to increase bone growth. When the load exceeds the bone's ability to repair, however, the structure is weakened.[58d] For example, in states of increased physical activity where the bone's adaptations do not occur fast enough, bone resorption (bone lysis) occurs faster than it is formed (osteoid synthesis). When bone resorption exceeds bone formation, a reduction in bone mass and strength occurs. This can result in stress fractures. Figure 4-2 depicts the distribution and frequency of stress fractures.

Gradual demineralization of bone (osteopenia) is a normal feature of aging. Men and women naturally begin to lose bone at around the age of 35, at a rate of 0.5% to 1% per year.[58e] Women lose bone at an accelerated rate after menopause. Major causes of generalized osteopenia are osteoporosis, osteomalacia,

hyperparathyroidism, and neoplasm. Osteopenia, however, may also result because of many other factors, such as poor nutrition, prolonged pharmacological intervention, disease, and decreased mobility.

Osteopenia may result in a compromise to bone strength, which remains undiagnosed until an osteoporotic fracture occurs.[58f] Osteopenia is best diagnosed by bone density measurement using a bone density scan.[58g] A World Health Organization panel of experts has defined *osteopenia* as bone mineral density between -1 and -2.5 standard deviations from the young adult mean.[58g] *Osteoporosis,* a more serious form of osteopenia has been defined as bone mineral density below -2.5 standard deviations from the young adult mean (see Chap. 9).[58g]

> **Clinical Pearl**
>
> Pain and tenderness and loss of function are the most common complaints associated with a fracture. These symptoms can be localized or generalized, depending on the degree of associated soft tissue injury.

Bursa

The term *bursitis,* used to describe an inflamed bursa, often is misused.[60] As a primary condition, it is thought to be present only in patients with degenerative changes, or with rheumatoid arthritis, gout, and pyogenic infections.[61,62] In contrast, secondary, or chronic, bursitis results from inflammation of the

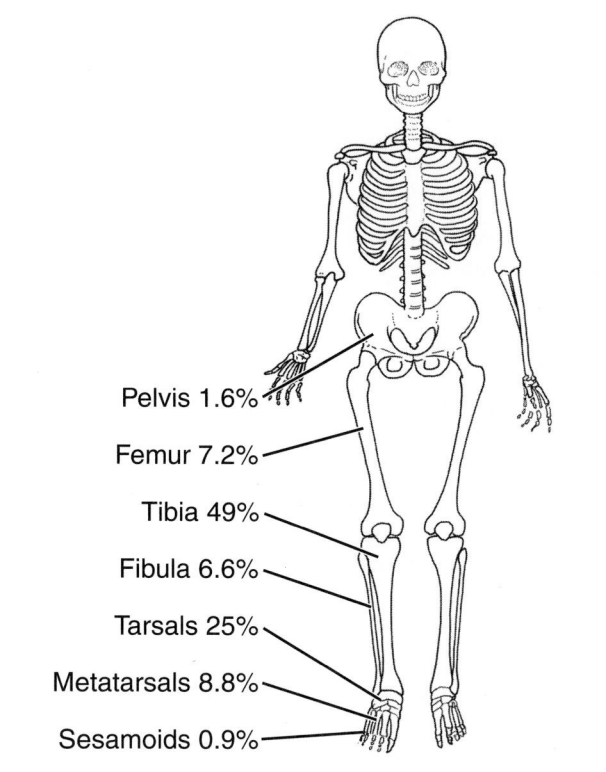

Pelvis 1.6%
Femur 7.2%
Tibia 49%
Fibula 6.6%
Tarsals 25%
Metatarsals 8.8%
Sesamoids 0.9%

FIGURE 4-2 The distribution and frequency of stress fractures. (Reproduced with permission from Simon RR, Koenigsknecht SJ. *Emergency Orthopedics: The Extremities.* 4th ed. New York, NY: McGraw-Hill; 2001.)

bursa from repeated microtrauma or direct injury.[63–66] Once traumatized, the bursa can become infected.

The wall of a chronically inflamed bursa is tough, thick, and fibrous, making its boggy structure easier to palpate. Pain is often reproduced when the nearby joint is moved, resulting in a noncapsular pattern of restriction as defined by Cyriax. In addition, at joints such as the shoulder, a painful arc may exist, and the end feel can be empty if the bursitis is acute.

Blood Vessels

Soft tissue injury may damage local blood vessels. The vascular reaction to trauma differs according to the size of the vessel involved. Larger vessels constrict under the influence of their innervation. The capillaries and small-caliber arterioles and venules rely on three mechanisms for the prevention of further blood loss: vessel and vessel wall retraction, a platelet reaction, and activation of the coagulation cascade. These smaller vessels are stimulated by vasoactive substances, including serotonin and the catecholamines that contract myofilaments in their endothelial walls. Small vessels also are subject to collapse as a result of raised extravascular pressures produced by leakage of fluid from vessels in a state of increased permeability. As the intravascular volume is reduced, increased blood viscosity helps reduce blood flow to a traumatized region.

Response of Skeletal Muscle Tissue to Stress

Muscle injury can result from excessive strain, excessive tension, contusions, lacerations, thermal stress, and myotoxic agents, such as some local anesthetics, excessive use of corticosteroids, and snake and bee venoms[67] (Table 4-4). Muscle injuries are the most common injury in sports, with an incidence varying from 10 to 55 percent of all injuries sustained in sport events.[68, 69] The majority of muscle injuries (more than 90 percent) are caused either by excessive strain of the muscle or by contusion.[70]

A distraction strain occurs in a muscle to which an excessive pulling force is applied, resulting in overstretching.[70] A contusion may occur if a muscle is injured by a heavy compressive force, such as a direct blow. At the site of the direct blow, a hematoma may develop. Two types of hematoma can be identified[71]:

1. *Intramuscular.* This type of hematoma is associated with a muscle strain or bruise. The size of the hematoma is limited by the muscle fascia. Clinical findings may include pain and loss of function.

2. *Intermuscular.* This type of hematoma develops if the muscle fascia is ruptured and the extravasated blood spreads into the interfascial and interstitial spaces. The pain is usually less severe with this type.

Muscle strains[40] may be classified according to their severity,[70] as follows:

▶ **1. *Mild (first-degree) strain.*** This type involves a tear of a few muscle fibers with minor swelling and discomfort. Grade I injuries are associated with no or minimal loss of strength and restriction of movement. Local tenderness may be present, which is increased when stress is applied to the structure. Patients with a grade I strain usually can continue normal activities as much as possible, but should be monitored for exacerbation of the existing injury.

▶ **2. *Moderate (second-degree) strain.*** This type involves greater damage to the muscle and clear loss of strength. Patients with grade II injuries have pain on activity that often prevents further participation. Moderate to severe pain is present, along with some loss of function and joint stability. Grade II strains typically require from 3 to 28 days of rehabilitation.[72]

▶ **3. *Severe (third-degree) strain.*** This type involves a tear extending across the whole muscle belly. Grade III strains are characterized by severe pain or loss of function. Whether pain increases when stress is applied to the structure is dependent on the resulting integrity of the tissue. Although grade I and II muscle strains are treated conservatively, surgical intervention is often necessary for grade III injuries.[73] Healing of grade III strains can require from 3 weeks to 3 months of rehabilitation.

The prognostic factors for muscle injury are outlined in Table 5-2.

TABLE 4-4 Classification of Muscle Injury[40]

Type	Related Factors
Exercise-induced muscle injury (delayed muscle soreness)	Increased activity Unaccustomed activity Excessive eccentric work Viral infections Secondary to muscle cell damage Onset at 24–48 hr after exercise
Strains First degree (mild): minimal structural damage; minimal hemorrhage; early resolution	Sudden overstretch Sudden contraction Decelerating limb Insufficient warm-up Lack of flexibility
Second degree (moderate): partial tear; large spectrum of injury; significant early functional loss	Increasing severity of strain associated with greater muscle fiber death, more hemorrhage, and more eventual scarring
Third degree (severe): complete tear; may require aspiration; may require surgery	Steroid use or abuse Previous muscle injury Collagen disease

Contusions
  Mild, moderate, severe
  Intramuscular versus intermuscular
	Direct blow, associated with increasing muscle trauma and tearing of fiber proportionate to severity

Avulsions Bony	Specific sites vulnerable May be complication of stress fractures Osteoporosis
Apophyseal Muscle	Skeletally immature but well-developed muscle strength Associated with steroid injection or generalized collagen disorders

Detrimental Effects of Immobilization

Continuous immobilization of connective and skeletal muscle tissues can cause some undesirable consequences. These include:

▶ *Cartilage degeneration.*[15,74–77] Immobilization of a joint causes atrophic changes in articular cartilage through a reduction in the amount of matrix proteoglycans and cartilage softening.[74] Softened articular cartilage is vulnerable to damage during weight bearing. The reduction of the matrix proteoglycans concentration has been demonstrated to be highest in the superficial zone but also occurs throughout the uncalcified cartilage, diminishing with distance from the surface of articular cartilage.[78]

▶ *Decreased mechanical and structural properties of ligaments.* One study[9] showed that after 8 weeks of immobilization, the stiffness of a ligament decreased to 69 percent of control values, and even after 1 year of rehabilitation, the ligament did not return to its prior level of strength.

> ### Clinical Pearl
>
> Following a period of immobilization, connective tissues are more vulnerable to deformation and breakdown than normal tissues subjected to similar amounts of stress.[79]

▶ *Decreased bone density.*[80–84] The interactions among systemic and local factors to maintain normal bone mass are complex. Bone mass is maintained because of a continuous coupling between bone resorption by osteoclasts and bone formation by osteoblasts, and this process is influenced by both systemic and local factors.[85] Mechanical forces acting on bone stimulate osteogenesis, and the absence of such forces inhibits osteogenesis. Marked osteopenia occurs in otherwise healthy patients in states of complete immobilization or weightlessness.[86,87] In children, bone has a high modeling rate and appears to be more sensitive to the absence of mechanical loading than bone in adults.[88]

TABLE 4-5 Structural Changes in the Various Types of Muscle Following Immobilization in a Shortened Position[90]

Structural Characteristics	Muscle Fiber Type and Changes		
	Slow Oxidative	Fast Oxidative Glycolytic	Fast Glycolytic
Number of fibers	Moderate decrease	Minimal increase	Minimal increase
Diameter of fibers	Significant decrease	Moderate decrease	Moderate decrease
Fiber fragmentation	Minimal increase	Minimal increase	Significant increase
Myofibrils	Minimal decrease and disoriented	—	Wavy
Nuclei	Degenerated and rounded	Degenerated and rounded	Degenerated and rounded
Mitochondria	Moderate decrease, degenerated,	Moderate decrease, degenerated	Minimal decrease, degenerated, swollen
Sarcoplasmic reticulum	Minimal decrease, orderly arrangement	Minimal decrease	Minimal decrease
Myofilaments	Minimal decrease, disorganized	Moderate decrease	Minimal decrease, wavy
Z band	Moderate decrease	—	Faint or absent
Vesicles	Abnormal configuration	—	—
Basement membrane	Minimal increase	—	—
Register of sarcomeres	Irregular projections, shifted with time	—	—
Fatty infiltration	Minimal increase	—	—
Collagen	Minimal increase between fibers	—	—
Macrophages	Minimal increased invasion	Minimal increased invasion	Minimal increased invasion
Satellite cells	Minimal increase	—	—
Target cells	Minimal increase	—	—

▶ *Weakness or atrophy of muscles*[89] *(Table 4-5).* Muscle atrophy is an imbalance between protein synthesis and degradation. After modest trauma, there is a decrease in whole body protein synthesis[91] rather than increased breakdown. With more severe trauma, major surgery, or multiple organ failure, both synthesis and degradation increase, the latter being more enhanced.[92,93]

Clinical Pearl

Disuse atrophy of muscle begins within 4 hours of the start of bed rest, resulting in decreases in muscle mass, muscle cell diameter, and the number of muscle fibers. However, strenuous exercise of atrophic muscle can lead to muscle damage, including sarcolemmal disruption, distortion of the contractile components of myofibrils, and cytoskeletal damage. Thus, a balance must be found.

The cause of muscle damage during exercised recovery from atrophy involves an altered ability of the muscle fibers to bear the mechanical stress of external loads (weight bearing) and movement associated with exercise. Strenuous exercise can result in primary or secondary sarcolemmal disruption, swelling or disruption of the sarcotubular system, distortion of the contractile components of myofibrils, cytoskeletal damage, and extracellular myofiber matrix abnormalities.[94] These pathologic changes are similar to those seen in healthy young adults after sprint running or resistance training.[94] It appears that the act of contracting while the muscle is in a stretched or lengthened position, known as an *eccentric contraction,* is responsible for these injuries.[95]

The clinician must remember that the restoration of full strength and range of motion may prove difficult if muscles are allowed to heal without early active motion, or in a shortened position, and that the patient may be prone to repeated strains.[96] Thus, range-of-motion exercises should be started once swelling and tenderness have subsided to the point that the exercises are not unduly painful.[96]

REVIEW QUESTIONS*

1. Give four forces that commonly act on the body.
2. What is the name given to an acute loading stress when a single force is large enough to cause injury on biological tissues?
3. When connective tissue is initially stretched what is the term used to describe the amount of slack in the tissue?
4. True/false: Collagen is well designed to resist compression.
5. What type of arthritis is also known as degenerative joint disease?

---

* Additional questions to test your understanding of this chapter can be found in the Online Learning Center for *Orthopaedic Assessment, Evaluation, and Intervention* at www.duttononline.net.

REFERENCES

1. Hall SJ. Kinetic concepts for analyzing human motion. In: Hall SJ, ed. *Basic Biomechanics.* New York, NY: McGraw-Hill; 1999:62–89.

2. Triano JJ. Interaction of spinal biomechanics and physiology. In: Haldeman S, ed. *Principles and Practice of Chiropractic*. Norwalk, Conn: Appleton and Lange; 1992:225–257.

3. Threlkeld AJ. The effects of manual therapy on connective tissue. *Phys Ther* 1992;72:893–902.

4. Teitz CC, Garrett WE Jr, Miniaci A, Lee MH, Mann RA. Tendon problems in athletic individuals. *J Bone Joint Surg* 1997;79A:138–152.

5. Zarins B. Soft tissue injury and repair: Biomechanical aspects. *Int J Sports Med* 1982;3:9–11.

6. Noyes FR, Butler DL, Paulos LE, Grood ES. Intra-articular cruciate reconstruction. I: Perspectives on graft strength, vascularization and immediate motion after replacement. *Clin Orthop* 1983;172:71–77.

7. Laros GS, Tipton CM, Cooper R. Influence of physical activity on ligament insertions in the knees of dogs. *J Bone Joint Surg* 1971;53B:275–286.

8. Nimni ME. Collagen: Structure function and metabolism in normal and fibrotic tissue. *Semin Arthritis Rheum* 1983;13: 1–86.

9. Noyes FR, Torvik PJ, Hyde WB, DeLucas JL. Biomechanics of ligament failure: II. An analysis of immobilization, exercise, and reconditioning effects in primates. *J Bone Joint Surg* 1974;56A:1406–1418.

10. Akizuki S, Mow VC, Muller F, Pita JC, Howell DS, Manicourt DH. Tensile properties of knee joint cartilage: I. Influence of ionic condition, weight bearing, and fibrillation on the tensile modulus. *J Orthop Res* 1986;4:379–392.

11. Roth V, Mow VC. The intrinsic tensile behavior of the matrix of bovine articular cartilage and its variation with age. *J Bone Joint Surg* 1980;62A:1102–1117.

12. Viidik A. On the rheology and morphology of soft collagenous tissue. *J Anat* 1969;105:184.

13. Cohen NP, Foster RJ, Mow VC. Composition and dynamics of articular cartilage: Structure, function, and maintaining healthy state. *J Orthop Sports Phys Ther* 1998;28:203–215.

14. Mankin HJ, Mow VC, Buckwalter JA, Iannotti JP, Ratcliffe A, et al. Form and function of articular cartilage. In: Simon SR, ed. *Orthopedic Basic Science*. Rosemont, Ill: American Academy of Orthopedic Surgeons; 1994:1–44.

15. O'Driscoll SW. The healing and regeneration of articular cartilage. *J Bone Joint Surg* 1998;80A:1795–1812.

16. Lawrence RC, Hochberg MC, Kelsey JL, et al. Estimates of the prevalence of selected arthritic and musculoskeletal diseases in the United States. *J Rheumatol* 1989;16:427–441.

17. Birchfield PC. Osteoarthritis overview. *Geriatr Nurs* 2001;22: 124–130; quiz 130–131.

18. Kee CK. Osteoarthritis: Manageable scourge of aging. *Rheumatology* 2000;35:199–208.

19. van Saase JLCM, van Romunde LK, Cats A, Vandenbroucke JP, Valkenburg HA. Epidemiology of osteoarthritis: Zoetermeer survey. Comparison of radiological osteoarthritis in a Dutch population with that in 10 other populations. *Ann Rheum Dis* 1989;48:271–280.

20. Sharma L, Pai YC, Holtcamp K, Rymer WZ. Is knee joint proprioception worse in the arthritic knee versus the unaffected knee in unilateral knee osteoarthritis? *Arthritis Rheum* 1997;40:1518–1525.

21. Brandt KD, Fife RS. Ageing in relation to the pathogenesis of osteoarthritis. *Clin Rheum Dis* 1986;12:117–130.

22. Townes AS. Osteoarthritis. In: Barker LR, Bruton JR, Zieve PD, eds. *Principles of Ambulatory Medicine*. Baltimore, Md: Williams and Wilkins; 1999:960–973.

23. Birchfield PC. Arthritis: Osteoarthritis and rheumatoid arthritis. In: Robinson D, Kidd P, Rogers KM, eds. *Primary Care Across the Lifespan*. St. Louis: Mosby; 2000:89–95.

24. Cardone DA, Tallia AF. Osteoarthritis. In Singleton JK, Sandowski SA, Green-Hernandez C, et al. eds. *Primary Care*. Philadelphia, Pa: Lippincott; 1999:543–548.

25. Huang J, Ushiyama T, Inoue K, Kawasaki T, Hukuda S. Vitamin D receptor gene polymorphisms and osteoarthritis of the hand, hip, and knee: a case control study in Japan. *Rheumatology* 2000;39:79–84.

26. Mustafa Z, Chapman K, Irven C, et al. Linkage analysis of candidate genes as susceptibility loci for arthritis-suggestive linkage of COL9A1 to female hip osteoarthritis. *Rheumatology* 2000;39:299–306.

27. Sharkey NA, Williams NI, Guerin JB. The role of exercise in the prevention and treatment of osteoporosis and osteoarthritis. *Rheumatology* 2000;35:209–219.

28. Croft P, Coggon D, Cruddas M, Cooper C, et al. Osteoarthritis of the hip: An occupational disease in farmers. *BMJ* 1992;304:1272.

29. Felson DT. The epidemiology of knee osteoarthritis: Results from the Framingham Osteoarthritis Study. *Sem Arthritis Rheum* 1990;20:42–50.

30. Felson DT, Hannan MT, Naimark A. Occupational physical demands, knee bending and knee osteoarthritis: Results from the Framingham study. *J Rheumatol* 1991;18:1587–1592.

31. Anderson JJ, Felson DT. Factors associated with osteoarthritis of the knee in the first National Health and Nutrition Examination Survey. *Am J Epidemiol* 1988;128:179–189.

32. Felson DT. The epidemiology of osteoarthritis: Prevalence and risk factors. In: Keuttner KE, Goldberg VM, eds. *Osteoarthritic Disorders*. Rosemont, Ill: American Academy of Orthopedic Surgeons; 1995:13–24.

32a. Bullough P, Vigorta V. *Atlas of Orthopedic Pathology*. London: Gower; 1984.

33. Ignatavicius DD. Rheumatoid arthritis and the older adult. *Geriatr Nurs* 2001;22:139–142.

34. Miller ML, Kress AM, Berry CA. Decreased physical function in juvenile rheumatoid arthritis. *Arthritis Care Res* 1999;12: 309–313.

35. Woo SLY, An KN, Arnoczky SP, et al. Anatomy, biology, and biomechanics of tendon, ligament, and meniscus. In: Simon S, ed. *Orthopedic Basic Science*. Rosemont, Ill: American Academy of Orthopedic Surgeons; 1994:45–87.

36. Amiel D, Kleiner JB. Biochemistry of tendon and ligament. In: Nimni ME, ed. *Collagen*. Boca Raton, Fla: CRC Press; 1988:223–251.

37. Francois RJ. Ligament insertions into the human lumbar vertebral body. *Acta Anat* 1975;91:467–480.

38. Attarian DE, McCrackin HJ, DeVito DP, McElhaney JH, Garrett WE Jr. Biomechanical characteristics of human ankle ligaments. *Foot Ankle* 1985;6:54–58.

39. Beynnon B, et al. The measurement of anterior cruciate ligament strain in vivo. *Int Orthop* 1992;16:1–12.

40. Reid DC. *Sports Injury Assessment and Rehabilitation*. New York, NY: Churchill Livingstone; 1992.

41. O'Donoghue DH. *Treatment of Injuries to Athletes*. Philadelphia, Pa: WB Saunders; 1976:698–746.

42. Adamson C, Cymet T. Ankle sprains: Evaluation, treatment, rehabilitation. *Md Med J* 1997;46:530–537.

43. Dias LS. Fractures of the distal tibial and fibular physes. In: Rockwood JCA, Wilkins KE, King RE, eds. *Fractures in Children*. Philadelphia, Pa: Lippincott; 1991:1314–1381.

44. Wilkerson LA. Ankle injuries in athletes. *Prim Care* 1992;19:377–392.

45. Frost HM. Does the ligament injury require surgery? *Clin Orthop* 1966;49:72.

46. Clement DB, Taunton JE, Smart GW. Achilles tendinitis and peritendinitis: Etiology and treatment. *Am J Sports Med* 1984;12:179–183.

47. James SL, Bates BT, Osternig LR. Injuries to runners. *Am J Sports Med* 1978;6:40–49.

48. Ilfeld FW. Can stroke modification relieve tennis elbow? *Clin Orthop* 1992;276:182–186.

49. Bureau of Labor Statistics. Occupational injuries and illness in the United States by industry 1988. *Bulletin* 1990:2368.

50. Renstrom P. Sports traumatology today: A review of common current sports injury problems. *Ann Chir Gynaecol* 1991;80:81–93.

51. Almekinders LC, Temple JD. Etiology, diagnosis and treatment of tendinitis: An analysis of the literature. *Med Sci Sports Exerc* 1998;30:1183–1190.

52. Backman C, Boquist L, Friden J, Lorentzon R, Toolanen G. Chronic Achilles paratenonitis with tendinosis: An experimental model in the rabbit. *J Orthop Res* 1990;8:541–547.

53. Leadbetter WB. Cell-matrix response in tendon injury. *Clin Sports Med* 1992;11:533–578.

54. Nirschl RP. Tennis elbow tendinosis: Pathoanatomy, nonsurgical and surgical management. In: Gordon SL, Blair SJ, Fine LJ, eds. *Repetitive Motion Disorders of the Upper Extremity.* Rosemont, Ill: American Academy of Orthopedic Surgeons; 1995;467–479.

55. Jozsa LG, Kannus P. Overuse injuries of tendons. In: Jozsa LG, Kannus P, eds. *Human Tendons: Anatomy, Physiology, and Pathology.* Champaign, Ill: Human Kinetics; 1997:164–253.

56. Kannus P, Jozsa L. Histopathological changes preceding spontaneous rupture of a tendon. A controlled study of 891 patients. *J Bone Joint Surg* 1991;73A:1507–1525.

57. Sinaki, M. Osteoporosis. In: Joel A, DeLisa JB, eds. *Rehabilitation Medicine: Principles and Practice.* 1993, Philadelphia, Pa: Lippincott, 1993;1018–1035.

58. Rosen CJ, Kessenich CR. The pathophysiology of osteoporosis. In: Rosen CJ, ed. *Current Clinical Practice–Osteoporosis: Diagnostic and Therapeutic Principles,* Humana Press: Totowa, NJ; 1996:47–64.

58a. Carter D, Hayes W. Bone compressive strength. *Science* 1976;194:1174–1176.

58b. Triano JJ. Interaction of spinal biomechanics and physiology. In: Haldeman S, *Principles and Practice of Chiropractic,* ed. East Norwalk, Conn. Appleton & Lange; 1992:225–257.

58c. Wolff J. *The Law of Remodeling* (Maquet P, Furlong R, trans). Berlin: Springer-Verlag. 1986 (1892).

58d. Frost, HM. Suggested fundamentals and concepts in skeletal physiology. *Calcif Tissue Int* 1993;52:1–4.

58e. Thomas J, Doherty SM. HIV infection—a risk factor for osteoporosis. *Journal of Acquired Immune Deficiency Syndromes: JAIDS* 2003;33:281–291.

58f. Eisele SA, Sammarco GJ. Fatigue fractures of the foot and ankle in the athlete. Instr Course Lect 1993;42:175–183.

58g. Kanis JA, et al. Bone measurements with DXA and ultrasound: diagnostic and prognostic use. *Osteoporosis 1996; Pro of the 1996 World Congress on Osteoporosis.* Amsterdam: Elsevier; 1996.

59. Eisele SA, Sammarco GJ. Fatigue fractures of the foot and ankle in the athlete. *Instr Course Lect* 1993;42:175–183.

60. Gordon EJ. Diagnosis and treatment of common shoulder disorders. *Med Trial Tech Q* 1981;28:25–73.

61. Neviaser TJ. The role of the biceps tendon in the impingement syndrome. *Orthop Clin North Am* 1987;18:383–386.

62. Nitz AJ. Physical therapy management of the shoulder. *Phys Ther* 1986;66:1912–1919.

63. Buckingham RB. Bursitis and tendinitis. *Compr Ther* 1981;7:52–57.

64. Reilly J, Nicholas JA. The chronically inflamed bursa. *Clin Sports Med* 1987;6:345–370.

65. Ho G Jr, Tice AD, Kaplan SR. Septic bursitis in the prepatellar and olecranon bursae: An analysis of 25 cases. *Ann Intern Med* 1978;89:21–27.

66. Frey CC, et al. The retrocalcaneal bursa: Anatomy and bursography. *Foot Ankle* 1982;13:203–207.

67. Huijbregts PA. Muscle injury, regeneration, and repair. *J Man Manipulative Ther* 2001;9:9–16.

68. Garrett WE. Muscle strain injuries. *Am J Sports Med* 1996;24:S2–S8.

69. Lehto MU, Jarvinen MJ. Muscle injuries, their healing process and treatment. *Ann Chir Gynaecol* 1991;80:102–108.

70. Jarvinen TA, Kaariainen M, Jarvinen M, Kalimo H. Muscle strain injuries. *Curr Opin Rheumatol* 2000;12:155–161.

71. Kalimo H, Rantanen J, Jarvinen M. Soft tissue injuries in sport. In: Jarvinen M, ed. *Balliere's Clinical Orthopedics.* 1997:1–24.

72. Watrous BG, Ho G Jr. Elbow pain. *Prim Care* 1988;15:725–735.

73. Glick JM. Muscle strains: Prevention and treatment. *Phys Sports Med* 1980;8:73–77.

74. Jurvelin J, Kiviranta I, Tammi M, Helminen JH. Softening of canine articular cartilage after immobilization of the knee joint. *Clin Orthop* 1986;207:246–252.

75. Behrens F, Kraft EL, Oegema TR Jr. Biochemical changes in articular cartilage after joint immobilization by casting or external fixation. *J Orthop Res* 1989;7:335–343.

76. Salter RB, Field P. The effects of continuous compression on living articular cartilage. *J Bone Joint Surg* 1960;42A:31–49.

77. Salter RB, Simmonds DF, Malcolm BW, Rumble EJ, MacMichael D, Clements ND. The biological effect of continuous passive motion on the healing of full-thickness defects in articular cartilage. *J Bone Joint Surg* 1980;62A:1232–1251.

78. Haapala J, Arokoski JP, Hyttinen MM, et al. Remobilization does not fully restore immobilization induced articular cartilage atrophy. *Clin Orthop Rel Res* 1999;362:218–229.

79. Deyo RA. Measuring functional outcomes in therapeutic trials for chronic disease. *Control Clin Trials* 1984;5:223.

80. Akeson WH, Amiel D, Woo SLY. Immobility effects on synovial joints: The pathomechanics of joint contracture. *Biorheology* 1980;17:95–110.

81. Akeson WH, Amiel D, Abel MF, Garfin SR, Woo SL. Effects of immobilization on joints. *Clin Orthop* 1987;219:28–37.

82. Akeson WH, Woo SL, Amiel D, Coutts RD, Daniel D. The connective tissue response to immobility: Biochemical changes in periarticular connective tissue of the immobilized rabbit knee. *Clin Orthop* 1973;93:356–362.

83. Bailey DA, Faulkner RA, McKay HA. Growth, physical activity, and bone mineral acquisition. In: Hollosky JO, ed. *Exercise and Sport Sciences Reviews.* Baltimore, Md: Williams and Wilkins; 1996:233–266.

84. Lane JM, Riley EH, Wirganowicz PZ. Osteoporosis: Diagnosis and treatment. *J Bone Joint Surg* 1996;78A:618–632.

85. Harris WH, Heaney RP. Skeletal renewal and metabolic bone disease. *N Engl J Med* 1969;280:193–202, 253–259, 303–311.

86. Donaldson CL, Hulley SB, Vogel JM, Hattner RS, Bayers JH, McMillan DE. Effect of prolonged bed rest on bone mineral. *Metabolism* 1970;19:1071–1084.

87. Mazess RB, Whedon GD. Immobilization and bone. *Calcif Tiss Int* 1983;35:265–267.

88. Rosen JF, Wolin DA, Finberg L. Immobilization hypercalcemia after single limb fractures in children and adolescents. *Am J Dis Child* 1978;132:560–564.

89. Gould N, Donnermeyer D, Pope M, Ashikaga T. Transcutaneous muscle stimulation as a method to retard disuse atrophy. *Clin Orthop* 1982;164:215–220.

90. Gossman MR, Sahrmann SA, Rose SJ. Review of length-associated changes in muscle. *Phys Ther* 1982;62:1799–1808.

91. Crane CW, Picou D, Smith R, Waterlow JC, et al. Protein turnover in patients before and after elective orthopedic operations. *Br J Surg* 1977;64:129–133.

92. Birkhahn RH, Long CL, Fitkin D, Geiger JW, Blakemore WS. Effects of major skeletal trauma on whole body protein turnover in man measured by L-(1,14C)-leucine. *Surgery* 1980;88: 294–300.

93. Arnold J, Campbell IT, Samuels TA, et al. Increased whole body protein breakdown predominates over increased whole body protein synthesis in multiple organ failure. *Clin Sci* 1993;84:655–661.

94. Kasper CE, Talbot LA, Gaines JM. Skeletal muscle damage and recovery. *AACN Clinical Issues* 2002;13:237–247.

95. McNeil PL, Khakee R. Disruptions of muscle fiber plasma membranes: Role in exercise-induced damage. *Am J Pathol* 1992;140:1097–1109.

96. Booher JM, Thibodeau GA. The body's response to trauma and environmental stress. In: Booher JM, Thibodeau GA, eds. *Athletic Injury Assessment.* New York, NY: McGraw-Hill; 2000:55–76.

CHAPTER 5

THE HEALING PROCESS

CHAPTER OBJECTIVES

▶ *At the completion of this chapter, the reader will be able to:*

1. Outline the various types of tissue injury.

2. Describe the etiology and pathophysiology of various musculoskeletal injuries associated with various types of body tissue.

3. Outline the pathophysiology of the healing process.

4. Identify factors that can impede the healing process.

5. Describe the stages of healing for the various musculoskeletal tissues.

OVERVIEW

The healing process is an intricate phenomenon that occurs following an injury or disease. Injuries to the musculoskeletal system can result from a wide variety of causes.[1–4] This chapter describes the physiology of healing for each of the major components of the musculoskeletal system. The reader is referred to Chapter 10 for the implications of these healing processes on the intervention of musculoskeletal injuries.

Musculoskeletal Injuries

With the exception of bone tissue, all other tissues of the body can be referred to as *soft tissue*. Injuries to the soft tissues can be classified as primary or secondary. Primary injuries can be self-inflicted, caused by another individual or entity, or caused by the environment.[5–8] Secondary injuries are essentially the inflammatory response that occurs with the primary injury.[9] Primary injuries can be subclassified into acute, chronic, or acute on chronic.

▶ *Acute.* Acute injuries occur as the result of direct trauma or a sudden overloading of the musculoskeletal tissues. These macrotraumatic injuries include fractures and dislocations, which are outside the scope of practice for a physical therapist, and subluxations, sprains, and strains, which make up the majority of conditions seen in the physical therapy clinic. In addition, the clinician may also treat contusions, which result from excessive compression to the soft tissues with resultant disruption of the muscle fibers and intramuscular bleeding.[10] Excessive tension to the soft tissues is borne by the collagen within the tissue. Although collagen fibers have the ability to elongate, if stretched sufficiently, sequential failure occurs (see Chap. 4).

▶ *Chronic.* Chronic, or overuse, injuries occur as the result of a cumulative repetitive overload, incorrect mechanics, or frictional resistance. These microtraumatic injuries include tendonitis, tenosynovitis, bursitis, and synovitis.

▶ *Acute on chronic.* This type of injury presents as a sudden rupture of a previously damaged tissue and can occur when the load applied to a tissue is too great for the level of tissue repair or remodeling.

Wound Healing

Research continues to provide us with an increasing amount of information about the biocellular events that occur as a result of tissue injury, as well as factors that interfere with the natural progression of these events. Fortunately, the majority of acute soft tissue wounds heal without complication in a predictable series of events. Chronic wounds, however, involve healing abnormalities due to some complications such as infection, compromised circulation, and neuropathy. These wounds, which can cause great physical and psychological stress to the involved patients and their families often require outside intervention. Wounds are conventionally classified as superficial (partial thickness) and deep (full thickness).[11] The healing of

TABLE 5-1   Stages of Wound Healing

Stage	General Characteristics
Coagulation and inflammation (acute)	Area is red, warm, swollen, and painful Pain is present without any motion of involved area Usually lasts 48–72 h, but can last as long as 7–10 days
Migratory and proliferative (subacute)	Pain usually occurs with activity or motion of involved area Usually lasts 10 d–6 wk
Remodeling (chronic)	Pain usually occurs after activity Usually lasts 6 wk–12 mo

superficial wounds, which involve only the epidermis or dermis, requires only the replacement of the germinating layer by re-epithelialization, whereas damage to deeper tissues, including a surgically induced wound, triggers a more complicated chain of events involving both physical and chemical activities, conveniently divided into stages or phases. The purpose of these stages is to form a scar to fill in the defect.

Stages of Wound Healing

The main stages of wound healing (Table 5-1) include coagulation and inflammation (acute), which initiates shortly after the initial injury; a migratory and proliferative process (subacute), which begins within days and includes the major processes of healing; and a remodeling process (chronic), which may last for up to a year and is responsible for scar tissue formation and development of new tissue.[5,12–16]

Whereas simplification of the complex events of healing into separate categories may facilitate understanding of the

phenomenon, in reality these events occur as an amalgamation of different reactions, both spatially and temporally.[17] Certain factors appear to determine the prognosis for healing[18] (Table 5-2). The most important factor regulating the regional time line of healing is sufficient blood flow.[16]

Coagulation and Inflammation Stage

This stage is meant to be tailored to the stimulus and to be time limited. An injury to the soft tissue triggers a process that represents the body's immediate reaction to trauma.[16,19] The reaction that occurs immediately after a wound injury includes a series of defensive events that involves the recognition of a pathogen and the mounting of a reaction against it. This reaction involves both coagulation and inflammation.

A significant component of the body's defense system is the development of tissue exudate. Following an injury to the tissues, capillary blood flow is disrupted, causing hypoxia to the area. This initial period of vasoconstriction, which lasts 5 to

TABLE 5-2   Prognostic Factors for Muscle Injury[18]

Parameter	Positive Prognostic Factors	Negative Prognostic Factors
Site	Belly tears Intermuscular contusions	Musculotendinous junction tears Intramuscular contusions
Severity	Partial tears (first degree plus mild second degree) First injury	Complete tears (severe second-degree and third-degree tears) Retear
Clinical signs	Minimal loss of range Minimal swelling Little pain	Significant loss of range Obvious tense swelling Extreme pain
Complications	Usually preserved function Compartment syndrome rare Myositis ossificans less likely Often complete resolution Early resolution expected	Loss of function Compartment syndromes with large hemorrhages Myositis ossificans more prevalent Tendency for recurrent tears Prolonged disability possible

10 minutes, causes the inflammatory phase to begin and prompts a period of vasodilation, and the extravasation of blood constituents.[16] Extravasated blood contains platelets, which secrete substances that form a clot to prevent bleeding and infection, clean dead tissue and nourish white cells. These substances include macrophages and fibroblasts.[20] Coagulation and platelet release results in the excretion of platelet-derived growth factor (PDGF),[21] platelet factor 4,[22] transforming growth factor-alpha (TGF-α),[23] and transforming growth factor-beta (TGF-β).[24] The main functions of a cell-rich tissue exudate are to provide cells capable of producing the components and biological mediators necessary for the directed reconstruction of damaged tissue while diluting microbial toxins and removing contaminants present in the wound.[17]

Inflammation is mediated by chemotactic substances, including anaphylatoxins that attract neutrophils and monocytes.

▶ *Neutrophils.* Neutrophils are white blood cells of the polymorphonuclear (PMN) leukocyte subgroup (the others being eosinophils, and basophils) that are filled with granules of toxic chemicals (phagocytes) that enable them to bind to microorganisms, internalize them, and kill them.

▶ *Monocytes.* Monocytes are white blood cells of the mononuclear leukocyte subgroup (the other being lymphocytes). The monocytes migrate into tissues and develop into macrophages, and provide immunological defences against many infectious organisms. Macrophages serve to orchestrate a "long term" response to injured cells subsequent to the acute response.[25]

The white blood cells of the inflammatory stage serve to clean the wound of foreign substances, increase vascular permeability, and promote fibroblast activity.[25] Other cell participants include local immune accessory cells, such as endothelial cells, mast cells, and tissue fibroblasts. The PMN leukocytes, through their characteristic "respiratory burst" activity, produce superoxide anion radical, which is well known to be critical for defense against bacteria and other pathogens.[26] Superoxide is rapidly converted to a membrane permeable form, hydrogen peroxide (H_2O_2), by superoxide dismutase activity or even spontaneously.[25] Release of H_2O_2 may promote formation of other oxidants that are more stable (longer half-life) including hypochlorous acid, chloramines, and aldehydes.[25] The phagocytic cells that initiate the innate immune response produce a set of proinflammatory cytokines (e.g., TNF-α, IL-1, and IL-6) in the form of a cascade that amplifies the local inflammatory response, influences the adaptive immune response, and serves to signal the CNS of an inflammatory response. The extent and severity of this inflammatory response depend on the size and the type of the injury, the tissue involved, and the vascularity of that tissue.[27–29,29a,29b]

Local vasodilation is promoted by biologically active products of the complement and kinin cascades[17]:

▶ The complement cascade involves 20 or more proteins that circulate throughout the blood in an inactive form.[17] After tissue injury, activation of the complement cascade produces a variety of proteins with activities essential to healing.

▶ The kinin cascade is responsible for the transformation of the inactive enzyme kallikrein, which is present in both blood and tissue, to its active form, bradykinin. Bradykinin also contributes to the production of tissue exudate through the promotion of vasodilation and increased vessel wall permeability.[30]

Due to the variety of vascular and other physiological responses occurring, this stage of healing is characterized by swelling, redness, heat, and impairment or loss of function. The edema is due to an increase in the permeability of the venules, plasma proteins, and leukocytes, which leak into the site of injury.[31,32] The complete removal of the wound debris marks the end of the inflammatory process.

It was traditionally thought that this stage only lasted 1 to 6 days, but more recently, it has been acknowledged that it may last for longer than 6 months.[33] This stage is characterized by pain at rest or with active motion, or when specific stress is applied to the injured structure. The pain, if severe enough, can result in muscle guarding, and a loss of function.

Two key types of inflammation are recognized: the normal acute inflammatory response and an abnormal, chronic or persistent inflammatory response. Common causes for a persistent chronic inflammatory response include infectious agents, persistent viruses, hypertrophic scarring, poor blood supply, edema, repeated direct trauma, excessive tension at the wound site, and hypersensitivity reactions.[34,35] The monocyte-predominant infiltration, angiogenesis, and fibrous change are the most characteristic morphologic features of chronic inflammation. This perpetuation of inflammation involves the binding of neutrophilic myeloperoxidase to the macrophage mannose receptor.[36]

Migratory and Proliferative Stage

The second stage of wound healing, characterized by migration and proliferation, usually occurs from the time of the initial injury and overlaps the inflammation phase. Characteristic changes include capillary growth and granulation tissue formation, fibroblast proliferation with collagen synthesis, and increased macrophage and mast cell activity. This stage is responsible for the development of wound tensile strength.

After the wound base is free of necrotic tissue, the body begins to work to close the wound. The connective tissue in healing wounds is composed primarily of collagen types I and III,[37] cells, vessels, and a matrix that contains glycoproteins and proteoglycans. Proliferation of collagen results from the actions of the fibroblasts that have been attracted to the area and stimulated to multiply by growth factors, such as PDGF, TGF-β, fibroblast growth factor (FGF), epidermal growth factor, and insulin-like growth factor-1, and tissue factors such as fibronectin.[17] This proliferation produces first fibrinogen and then fibrin, which eventually becomes organized into a honeycomb matrix and walls off the injured site.[38]

The wound matrix functions as a glue to hold the wound edges together, giving it some mechanical protection while also preventing the spread of infection. However, the wound matrix has a low tensile strength and is vulnerable to breakdown until the provisional extracellular matrix is replaced with a collagenous matrix. The collagenous matrix facilitates angiogenesis by providing time and protection to new and friable vessels. Angiogenesis occurs in response to the hypoxic state created by tissue damage as well as to factors released from cells during injury.[17]

The process of neovascularization during this phase provides a granular appearance to the wound as a result of the formation of loops of capillaries and migration of macrophages, fibroblasts, and endothelial cells into the wound matrix. Once an abundant collagen matrix has been deposited in the wound, the fibroblasts stop producing collagen, and the fibroblast-rich granulation tissue is replaced by a relatively acellular scar, marking the end of this stage.

This fibrous tissue repair process occurs gradually and lasts from 5 to 15 days, and often up to 10 weeks, depending on the type of tissue and the extent of damage. Upon progressing to this stage, the active effusion and local erythema of the inflammation stage are no longer present clinically. However, residual effusion may still be present at this time and resist resorption.[39,40]

Remodeling Stage

An optimal wound environment lessens the duration of the inflammatory and proliferative phases and protects fragile tissue from breakdown during early remodeling.

The remodeling phase of wound healing involves a conversion of the initial healing tissue to scar tissue. This lengthy phase of contraction, tissue remodeling, and increasing tensile strength in the wound lasts for up to 1 year. Fibroblasts are responsible for the synthesis, deposition, and remodeling of the extracellular matrix. Following the deposition of granulation tissue, some fibroblasts are transformed into myofibroblasts, which congregate at the wound margins and start pulling the edges inward, reducing the size of the wound. Increase in collagen types I and III and other aspects of the remodeling process are responsible for wound contraction and visible scar formation. Epithelial cells migrate from the wound edges and continue to migrate until similar cells from the opposite side are met. This contracted tissue, or scar tissue, is functionally inferior to original tissue and is a barrier to diffused oxygen and nutrients.[41] Eventually, the new epidermis becomes toughened by the production of the protein keratin. The visible scar changes color from red or purple that blanches with slight pressure to nonblanchable white as the scar matures.

Imbalances in collagen synthesis and degradation during this phase of healing may result in hypertrophic scarring or keloid formation with superficial wounds. If left untreated, the scar formed is less than 20 percent of its original size.[42] Contraction of the scar results from cross-linking of the collagen fibers and bundles, and adhesions between the immature collagen and surrounding tissues, producing hypomobility. In areas where the skin is loose and mobile, this creates minimal effect.

However, in areas such as the dorsum of the hand where there is no extra skin, wound contracture can have a significant effect on function. Consequently, controlled stresses must always be applied to new scar tissue to help prevent it from shortening.[16,29] If the healing tissues are kept immobile, the fibrous repair is weak and there are no forces influencing the collagen. Scarring that occurs parallel to the line of force of a structure is less vulnerable to reinjury than a scar that is perpendicular to those lines of force.[43]

Clinical Pearl

Despite the presence of an intact epithelium at 3 to 4 weeks after the injury, the tensile strength of the wound has been measured at approximately 25 percent of its normal value. Several months later, only 70 to 80 percent of the strength may be restored.[44] This would appear to demonstrate that the remodeling process may last many months or even years, making it extremely important to continue applying controlled stresses to the tissue long after healing appears to have occurred.[44]

Normally, the remodeling phase is characterized by a progression to pain-free function and activity. In the ideal world, the injured patient makes a smooth transition through the various stages of healing, and the sharp and burning acute pain is replaced by a duller ache, which then subsides to a point where no pain is felt. However, a persistent chronic inflammatory response involving the continued release of inflammatory products occasionally may occur. This failure during the healing phase continuum can result in chronic pathologic changes in the tissue. Characteristics of this chronic inflammation include a physiologic response that is resistant to both physical and pharmacologic intervention, resulting in a failure to remodel adequately, an imperfect repair, and a persistence of symptoms.[34,45] In addition, fibrosis can occur in synovial structures, as in extra-articular tissues, including tendons and ligaments; in bursa; or in muscle (see Chap. 10).

Examination of Wounds[46]

The examination of postsurgical wounds as part of the overall comprehensive examination is becoming more common. The outline below should provide the clinician with a guideline to perform a comprehensive wound assessment.

1. Wound history
   a. Mechanism, force, and duration of injury
   b. Time interval between injury and onset of intervention: acute versus chronic
2. Patient history
   a. Age
   b. Occupation and avocational interests
   c. Alcohol, tobacco, or caffeine use
   d. Metabolic comorbidity (diabetes mellitus, vascular disorders)
   e. Nutritional status

   f. Medications (e.g., corticosteroids, anticoagulants)
   g. Pain (location, description, frequency) and pain scale rating
   h. Presence of paresthesias or sensory loss
3. Wound examination
   a. General inspection of extremity
      (1) Edema
         (a) Description (pitting, brawny, hard, or mobile)
         (b) Measurement (circumferential or volumetric)
      (2) Color
      (3) Temperature
   b. Location of wound
   c. Wound type[47]
      (1) Tidy: clean laceration, minimal tissue damage, minimal contamination
      (2) Untidy: significant amount of tissue damage, uncertainty regarding viability of deeper structures, higher degree of contamination
      (3) Wound with tissue loss: deeper structures involved (vessels, tendons, nerve, or bone); may require soft tissue coverage, as follows:
         (a) Split-thickness (epidermis and part of dermis) or full-thickness (epidermis and entire underlying dermis) graft
         (b) Flap coverage (a flap is a portion of tissue *partly* severed from its place of origin to correct a defect in the body)
      (4) Infected wound (presently or potentially)
   d. Type of closure
      (1) Primary closure
      (2) Delayed primary closure
      (3) Secondary intention
      (4) Closure (sutures, staples, Steri-strips, graft, or flap)
      (5) Fixation (K-wire, pull-out wire, external fixator)
   e. Wound configuration
      (1) Size
      (2) Shape
      (3) Depth
   f. Integrity of tissue[48]
      (1) Viability of wound edges
      (2) Maceration: moist and white appearance of skin
      (3) Hematoma/seroma: collection of blood, serum, or both
      (4) Bleb (a blood- or serum-filled blister)
   g. Exudate
      (1) Color consistency: bloody, serous, serosanguinous, pus, purulent, dark red
      (2) Amount: slight, minimal, moderate, severe
      (3) Odor: presence or absence of foul odor
   h. Wound bed
      (1) Color and extent of granulation tissue (red wound[49])
      (2) Presence of epithelial budding (small pink islets forming within the wound)
      (3) Presence of adherent fibrinous exudates and debris (yellow wound[49])
      (4) Presence of dark, thick eschar (black wound[49])

Muscle Healing

Skeletal muscle has considerable regenerative capabilities, and the process of skeletal muscle regeneration after injury is a well-studied cascade of events.[50–52] The capacity for regeneration is based primarily on the type and extent of injury.[10,53]

The essential process of muscle regeneration is similar irrespective of the cause of injury, but the outcome and time course of regeneration vary according to the type, severity, and extent of the injury (Table 5-2).[50] Broadly speaking, there are three phases in the healing process of an injured muscle: the destruction phase, the repair phase, and the remodeling phase.[54]

Destruction Phase

The muscle fibers and their connective tissue sheaths are totally disrupted, and a gap appears between the ends of the ruptured muscle fibers when the muscle fibers retract.[52] This phase is characterized by the necrosis of muscle tissue, degeneration, and an infiltration by PMN leukocytes as hematoma and edema form at the site of injury.

Repair Phase

The repair phase usually involves the following steps:

▶ *Hematoma formation.* The gap between the ruptured ends of the fibers is at first filled by a hematoma. During the first day, the hematoma is invaded by inflammatory cells, including phagocytes, which begin disposal of the blood clot.[52]

▶ *Matrix formation.* Blood-derived fibronectin and fibrin cross-link to form a primary matrix, which acts as a scaffold and anchorage site for the invading fibroblasts.[51,52] The matrix gives the initial strength for wound tissue to withstand the forces applied to it.[55] Fibroblasts begin to synthesize proteins of the extracellular matrix.

▶ *Collagen formation.* The production of type I collagen by fibroblasts increases the tensile strength of the injured muscle. An excessive proliferation of fibroblasts can rapidly lead to an excessive formation of dense scar tissue, which creates a mechanical barrier that restricts or considerably delays complete regeneration of the muscle fibers across the gap.[52,54]

During the first week of healing the injury site is the weakest point of the muscle-tendon unit. This phase also includes regeneration of the striated muscle, production of a connective-tissue scar, and capillary ingrowth. The regeneration of the myofibers begins with the activation of satellite cells, located between the basal lamina and the plasma membrane of each individual myofiber.[56]

Satellite cells, myoblastic precursor cells, proliferate to reconstitute the injured area.[53] During muscle regeneration, it is presumed that trophic substances released by the injured muscle activate the satellite cells.[57] Unlike the multinucleated myofibers, these mononuclear cells maintain mitotic potential and respond to cellular signals by entering the cell cycle to provide the substrate for muscle regeneration and growth.[56]

The satellite cells proliferate and differentiate into multinucleated myotubes and eventually into myofibers, which mature and increase in length and diameter to span the muscle injury. Many of these myoblasts are able to fuse with existing necrosed myofibers and may prevent the muscle fibers from completely degenerating.[56]

The final stage in the regenerative process involves the integration of the neural elements and the formation of a functional neuromuscular junction.[1,58] Provided that the continuity of the muscle fiber is not disrupted and the innervation, vascular supply, and extracellular matrix are left intact, muscle will regenerate with loss of normal tissue architecture and function.[59]

Remodeling Phase

In this phase, the regenerated muscle matures and contracts with reorganization of the scar tissue. There is often incomplete restoration of the functional capacity of the injured muscle.

The pathology of skeletal muscle damage varies, depending on the initiating cause. Muscle damage can occur during the prolonged immobility of hospitalization and from external sources such as mechanical injury.[60] One of the potential consequences of muscle injury is atrophy. The amount of muscle atrophy that occurs depends on the usage prior to bed rest and the function of the muscle.[60] Antigravity muscles (such as the quadriceps) tend to have greater atrophy than antagonist muscles (such as the hamstrings). Research has shown that a single bout of exercise protects against muscle damage, with the effects lasting between 6 weeks[61] and 9 months.[62]

Muscle resistance to damage may result from an eccentric exercise-induced morphologic change in the number of sarcomeres connected in series.[63] This finding appears to support initiating a reconditioning program with gradual progression from lower intensity activities with minimal eccentric actions to protect against muscle damage.[60,64]

Ligament and Tendon Healing

The process of ligament and tendon healing is complex. Healing of ligaments and tendons generally can be broken down into four overlapping phases.

Phase I: Hemorrhagic

After disruption of the tissue, the gap is filled quickly with a blood clot. PMN leukocytes and lymphocytes appear within several hours, triggered by cytokines released within the clot. The PMN leukocytes and lymphocytes respond to autocrine and paracrine signals to expand the inflammatory response and recruit other types of cells to the wound.[58]

Phase II: Inflammatory

Macrophages arrive within 24 to 48 hours and are the predominant cell type within several days. Macrophages perform phagocytosis of necrotic tissues and also secrete multiple types of growth factors that induce neovascularization and the formation of granulation tissue. By the third day after injury, the wound contains macrophages, PMN leukocytes, lymphocytes, and multipotential mesenchymal cells, and platelets. Platelets

have been shown to release PDGF, TGF-β, and EGF. Macrophages produce basic FGF, TGF-α, TGF-β, and PDGF. These growth factors are not only chemotactic for fibroblasts and other cells, but also stimulate fibroblast proliferation and the synthesis of collagen types I, III, and V, as well as noncollagenous proteins.[65,66]

Phase III: Proliferation

The last cell type to arrive within the wound is the fibroblast. Although debate continues, it currently is thought that fibroblasts are recruited from neighboring tissue and the systemic circulation.[67] These fibroblasts have abundant rough endoplastic reticulum and begin producing collagen and other matrix proteins within 1 week of injury. By the second week after disruption, the original blood clot becomes more organized because of cellular and matrix proliferation. Capillary buds begin to form. Total collagen content is greater than in the normal ligament or tendon, but collagen concentration is lower and the matrix remains disorganized.

Phase IV: Remodeling and Maturation

Phase IV is marked by a gradual decrease in the cellularity of the healed tissue. The matrix becomes denser and longitudinally oriented. Collagen turnover, water content, and the ratio of collagen types I to III begin to approach normal levels.[68] An integrated sequence of biochemical and biomechanical signals are critical to ligament remodeling. These signals regulate the expression of structural and enzymatic proteins, including degradation enzymes such as collagenase, stromelysin, and plasminogen activator.[65] The healed tissue continues to mature for many months but will never attain normal morphologic characteristics or mechanical properties.

Ligament injuries can take as long as 3 years to heal to the point of regaining near-normal tensile strength,[69] although some tensile strength is regained by about the fifth week following injury, depending on the severity.[13,70–72] A ligament may have 50 percent of its normal tensile strength by 6 months after injury, 80 percent after 1 year, and 100 percent only after 1 to 3 years.[73–75] Forces applied to the ligament during its recovery help it to develop strength in the direction that the force is applied.[73–77]

Articular Cartilage Healing

It is well known that the capacity of articular cartilage for repair is limited. Cartilage cells, or chondrocytes, are responsible for the maintenance of the cartilage matrix. The repair response of articular cartilage varies with the depth of the injury.

Injuries of the articular cartilage that do not penetrate the subchondral bone become necrotic and do not heal. These lesions usually progress to the degeneration of the articular surface.[78] Although a short-lived tissue response may occur, it fails to provide sufficient cells and matrix to repair even small defects.[79,80]

Injuries that penetrate the subchondral bone undergo repair as a result of access to the blood supply of the bone. These repairs usually are characterized as fibrous, fibrocartilaginous, or hyaline-like cartilaginous, depending on the species, the age of the animal, and the location and size of the injury.[81] However, these reparative tissues, even those that resemble hyaline cartilage histologically, differ from normal hyaline cartilage both biochemically and biomechanically. Thus, by 6 months, fibrillation, fissuring, and extensive degenerative changes occur in the reparative tissues of approximately half of the full-thickness defects.[82,83] Similarly, the degenerated cartilage seen in osteoarthrosis does not usually undergo repair but instead progressively deteriorates.[78]

Current surgical treatment for damaged cartilage may consist of debridement or removal of loose flaps or pieces of cartilage, abrasion or burr arthroplasty at the site of the lesion, or subchondral drilling. An experimental technique undergoing active investigation is the transplantation of chondrocytes or chondrogenic cells or periosteal, perichondrial, of mesenchymal origin.[84,85]

Bone Healing

Bone healing is a complex physiologic process. The striking feature of bone healing, compared with healing in other tissues, is that repair is by the original tissue, not scar tissue. Regeneration is perhaps a better descriptor than repair. This is linked to the capacity for remodeling that intact bone possesses. Like other forms of healing, the repair of bone fracture includes the processes of inflammation, repair, and remodeling; however, the type of healing varies, depending on the method of treatment.

In classic histologic terms, fracture healing has been divided into two broad phases: primary fracture healing and secondary fracture healing.

▶ Primary healing, or primary cortical healing, involves a direct attempt by the cortex to reestablish itself once it has become interrupted. In primary cortical healing, bone on one side of the cortex must unite with bone on the other side of the cortex to reestablish mechanical continuity.

▶ Secondary healing involves responses in the periosteum and external soft tissues with the subsequent formation of a callus. The majority of fractures heal by secondary fracture healing.

Within these broader phases, the process of bone healing involves a combination of intramembranous and endochondral ossification. These two processes participate in the fracture repair sequence by at least four discrete stages of healing: the hematoma formation (inflammation or granulation) phase, the soft callus formation (proliferative) phase, the hard callus formation (maturing or modeling) phase, and the remodeling phase.[86]

▶ *Hematoma formation (inflammatory) phase.* This phase is characterized by the release of a variety of products, including fibronectin, PDGF, and TGF, by the activated platelets. These products trigger the influx of inflammatory cells.

▶ *Soft callus formation (reparative) phase.* This phase is characterized by the formation of connective tissues, including cartilage, and formation of new capillaries from preexisting vessels (angiogenesis). During the first 7 to 10 days of fracture healing, the periosteum undergoes an intramembranous bone formation response, and histologic evidence shows formation of woven bone opposed to the cortex within a few millimeters of the site of the fracture. By the middle of the second week, abundant cartilage overlies the fracture site, and this chondroid tissue initiates biochemical preparations to undergo calcification. Thus, the callus becomes a triple-layered structure consisting of an outer proliferating part, a middle cartilaginous layer, and an inner portion of new bony trabeculae (Fig. 5-1). The cartilage portion is usually replaced with bone as the healing progresses.

▶ *Hard callus formation (modeling) phase.* This phase is characterized by the production of woven bone. The calcification of fracture callus cartilage occurs by a mechanism almost identical to that which takes place in the growth plate. This calcification can occur either directly from mesenchymal tissue (intramembranous) or via an intermediate stage of cartilage (endochondral or chondroid routes). Osteoblasts can form woven bone rapidly, but the result is randomly arranged and mechanically weak. Nonetheless, bridging of a fracture by woven bone constitutes so-called clinical union. Once cartilage is calcified, it becomes a target for the ingrowth of blood vessels.

▶ *Remodeling phase.* By replacing the cartilage with bone, and converting the cancellous bone into compact bone, the callus is gradually remodeled. During this phase, the woven bone is remodeled into stronger lamellar bone by the orchestrated action of osteoclast bone resorption and osteoblast bone formation.

Radiologically or histologically, fracture gap bridging occurs by three mechanisms[86]:

1. *Intercortical bridging (primary cortical union).* This mechanism occurs when the fracture gap is reduced by normal cortical remodeling under conditions of rigid fixation. This mode of healing is the principle behind rigid internal fixation.[87]

2. *External callus bridging by new bone arising from the periosteum and the soft tissues surrounding the fracture.* Small degrees of movement at the fracture stimulate external callus formation.[88] This mode of healing is the aim in functional bracing[89] and intramedullary nailing.

3. *Intramedullary bridging by endosteal callus.*

Normal periods of immobilization following a fracture range from as short as 3 weeks for small bones to about 8 weeks for the long bones of the extremities. During the period of casting, submaximal isometrics are initiated. Once the cast is removed, it is important that controlled stresses continue to be

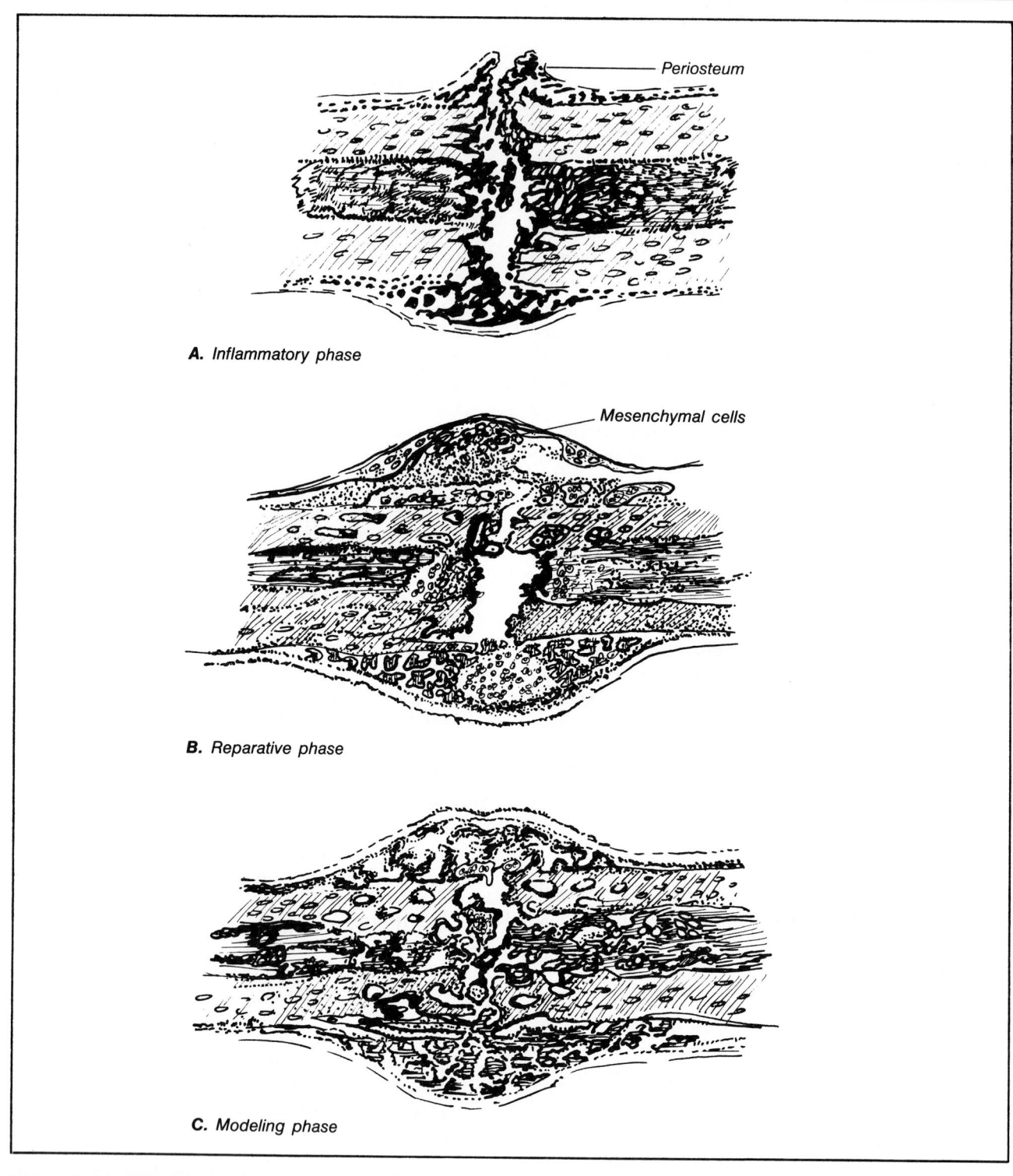

FIGURE 5-1 The various phases of fracture healing. (Reproduced with permission from Simon RR, Koenigsknecht SJ. Emergency Orthopedics, The Extremities. 4th ed. New York, NY: McGraw-Hill; 2001.)

applied to the bone, because the period of bone healing continues for up to 1 year.[90,91]

According to Wolff's law, bone remodels along lines of stress.[92] Bone is constantly being remodeled as the circumferential lamellar bone is resorbed by osteoclasts and replaced with dense osteonal bone by osteoblasts.[93]

The two key determinants of fracture healing are the blood supply and the degree of motion experienced by the fracture ends.

▶ Angiogenesis is the outgrowth of new capillaries from existing vessels. The degree of angiogenesis that occurs depends on well-vascularized tissue on either side of the gap and sufficient mechanical stability to allow new capillaries to survive. Angiogenesis leads to osteogenesis.

▶ The amount of movement that occurs between fracture ends can be stimulatory or inhibitory, depending on their magnitude. Excessive interfragmentary movement prevents the establishment of intramedullary blood vessel bridging. However, small degrees of micromotion have been shown to stimulate blood flow at the fracture site and stimulate periosteal callus.[94] A fracture that is rigidly internally fixed produces no periosteal callus and heals by a combination of endosteal callus and primary cortical union.[86] An intermedullary nail blocks endosteal healing but allows enough movement to trigger periosteal callus.[86] External fixation, particularly with fine wires in a circular fixator, is least damaging to the medullary blood supply.[86] This type of fixation may provide enough stability to allow rapid endosteal healing without external callus.[95]

REVIEW QUESTIONS*

1. Explain the difference between *primary* and *secondary* injuries.
2. Outline the differences between a *microtrauma* and a *macrotrauma*.
3. What are the three main stages of wound healing?
4. What are neutrophils?
5. What is the function of monocytes in the inflammation stage of wound healing?

---

* Additional questions to test your understanding of this chapter can be found in the Online Learning Center for *Orthopaedic Assessment, Evaluation, and Intervention* at www.duttononline.net.

REFERENCES

1. Barlow Y, Willoughby J. Pathophysiology of soft tissue repair. *Br Med Bull* 1992;48:698–711.
2. Biundo JJ Jr, Irwin RW, Umpierre E. Sports and other soft tissue injuries, tendinitis, bursitis, and occupation-related syndromes. *Curr Opin Rheumatol* 2001;13:146–149.
3. Cailliet R. *Soft Tissue Pain and Disability*. Philadelphia, Pa: FA Davis; 1980.
4. Cummings GS. Comparison of muscle to other soft tissue in limiting elbow extension. *J Orthop Sports Phys Ther* 1984;5:170.
5. Oakes BW. Acute soft tissue injuries: Nature and management. *Austr Fam Physician* 1982;10:3–16.
6. Garrick JG. The sports medicine patient. *Nurs Clin N Am* 1981;16:759–766.
7. Muckle DS. Injuries in sport. *Royal S Health J* 1982;102: 93–94.
8. Kellett J. Acute soft tissue injuries: A review of the literature. *Med Sci Sports Exerc* 1986;18:5.
9. Prentice WE. Understanding and managing the healing process. In: Prentice WE, Voight ML, eds. *Techniques in Musculoskeletal Rehabilitation*. New York, NY: McGraw-Hill; 2001:17–41.
10. Zarins B. Soft tissue injury and repair: Biomechanical aspects. *Int J Sports Med* 1982;3:9–11.
11. Clancy J, McVicar A. Wound healing: A series of homeostatic responses. *Br J Theatre Nurs* 1997;7:25–34.
12. Van der Mueulin JHC. Present state of knowledge on processes of healing in collagen structures. *Int J Sports Med* 1982;3:4–8.
13. Clayton ML, Wier GJ. Experimental investigations of ligamentous healing. *Am J Surg* 1959;98:373–378.
14. Hunt TK. Wound healing and wound infection: Theory and surgical practice. New York, NY: Appleton-Century-Crofts; 1980.
15. Mason ML, Allen HS. The rate of healing of tendons. An experimental study of tensile strength. *Ann Surg* 1941;113:424–459.
16. Singer AJ, Clark RAF. Cutaneous wound healing. *N Engl J Med* 1999;341:738–746.
17. Wong MEK, Hollinger JO, Pinero GJ. Integrated processes responsible for soft tissue healing. *Oral Surg Oral Med Oral Pathol Oral Radiol Endod* 1996;82:475–492.
18. Reid DC. *Sports Injury Assessment and Rehabilitation*. New York, NY: Churchill Livingstone; 1992.
19. Bryant MW. Wound healing. *CIBA Clin Symposia* 1977; 29:2–36.
20. Heldin CH, Westermark B. Role of platelet-derived growth factor in vivo. In: Clark RAF, ed. *The Molecular and Cellular Biology of Wound Repair*. New York, NY: Plenum Press; 1996:249–273.
21. Katz MH, Alvarez Af, Kirsner RS, Eagleston WH, Falanga V. Human wound fluid from acute wounds stimulates fibroblast and endothelial cell growth. *J Am Acad Dermatol* 1991;25:1054–1058.
22. Deuel TF, Senior RM, Ghang D, Griffin GL, Heinrikson RL, Kaiser ET. Platelet factor 4 is a chemotactic factor for neutrophils and monocytes. *Proc Natl Acad Sci U S A* 1981;74:4584–4587.
23. Schultz G, Rotatari DS, Clark W. EGF and TGF-alpha in wound healing and repair. *J Cell Biochem* 1991;45:346–352.
24. Sporn MB, Roberts AB. Transforming growth factor beta: Recent progress and new challenges. *J Cell Biol* 1992;119:1017–1021.
25. Sen CK, Khanna S, Gordillo G, et al. Oxygen, oxidants, and antioxidants in wound healing: An emerging paradigm. *Ann N Y Acad Sci* 2002;957:239–249.
26. Babior BM. Phagocytes and oxidative stress. *Am J Med* 2000;109:33–44.
27. Kellett, J., Acute soft tissue injuries: a review of the literature. *Med Sci Sports Exerc,* 1986;18:5.
28. Amadio PC. Tendon and ligament. In: Cohen IK, Diegelman RF, Lindblad WJ, eds. *Wound Healing: Biomechanical and Clinical Aspects*. Philadelphia, Pa: WB Saunders; 1992:384–395.
29. Hunt, T.K. Wound Healing and Wound Infection: Theory and Surgical Practice. New York: Appleton-Century-Crofts; 1980.
29a. Peacock EE. *Wound Repair*. 3rd ed. Philadelphia, Pa: WB Saunders; 1984.
29b. Ross R. The fibroblast and wound repair. *Biol Rev* 1968;43:51–96.
30. McAllister BS, Leeb-Lundberg JM, Javors MA, Olson MS. Bradykinin receptors and signal transduction pathways in human fibroblasts: Integral role for extracellular calcium. *Arch Biochem Biophys* 1993;304:294–301.

31. Evans RB. Clinical application of controlled stress to the healing extensor tendon: A review of 112 cases. *Phys Ther* 1989; 69:1041–1049.

32. Emwemeka CS. Inflammation, cellularity, and fibrillogenesis in regenerating tendon: Implications for tendon rehabilitation. *Phys Ther* 1989;69:816–825.

33. Merskey H, Bogduk N. Classification of chronic pain: Descriptions of chronic pain syndromes and definition of pain terms. *Report by the International Association for the Study of Pain Task Force on Taxonomy.* Seattle, Wash: IASP Press;1994.

34. Garrett WE, Lohnes J. Cellular and matrix response to mechanical injury at the myotendinous junction. In: Leadbetter WB, Buckwalter JA, Gordon SL, eds. *Sports-Induced Inflammation: Clinical and Basic Science Concepts.* Park Ridge, Ill: American Academy of Orthopedic Surgeons; 1990:215–224.

35. Di Rosa F, Barnaba V. Persisting viruses and chronic inflammation: Understanding their relation to autoimmunity. *Immunol Rev* 1998;164:17–27.

36. Lefkowitz DL, Mills K, Lefkowitz SS, Bollen A, Moguilevsky N. Neutrophil–macrophage interaction: A paradigm for chronic inflammation. *Med Hypotheses* 1995;44:68–72.

37. Thomas DW, O'Neill ID, Harding KG, Shepherd JP. Cutaneous wound healing: A current perspective. *J Oral Maxillofac Surg* 1995;53:442–447.

38. Arem A, Madden J. Effects of stress on healing wounds: Intermittent non-cyclical tension. *J Surg Res* 1971;42:528–543.

39. Safran MR, Zachazeswski JE, Benedetti RS, Bartolozzi AR 3rd, Mandelbaum R. Lateral ankle sprains: A comprehensive review part 2: Treatment and rehabilitation with an emphasis on the athlete. *Med Sci Sports Exerc* 1999;31(suppl):S438–S447.

40. Safran MR, Benedetti RS, Bartolozzi AR 3rd, Mandelbaum BR. Lateral ankle sprains: A comprehensive review: Part 1: Etiology, pathoanatomy, histopathogenesis, and diagnosis. *Med Sci Sports Exerc* 1999;31(suppl):S429–S437.

41. Chvapil M, Koopman CF. Scar formation: Physiology and pathological states. *Otolaryngol Clin North Am* 1984;17:265–272.

42. Levenson SM, Geever EF, Crowley LV, et al. The healing of rat skin wounds. *Ann Surg* 1965;161:293–308.

43. Farfan HF. The scientific basis of manipulative procedures. *Clin Rheum Dis* 1980;6:159–177.

44. Orgill D, Demling RH. Current concepts and approaches to wound healing. *Crit Care Med* 1988;16:899.

45. Stauber WT. Repair models and specific tissue responses in muscle injury. In: Leadbetter WB, Buckwalter JA, Gordon SL, eds. *Sports-Induced Inflammation: Clinical and Basic Science Concepts.* Park Ridge, Ill: American Academy of Orthopedic Surgeons; 205–213.

46. Anthony MS. Wounds. In: Clark GL, Shaw-Wilgis EF, Aiello B, et al, eds. *Hand Rehabilitation: A Practical Guide.* Philadelphia, Pa: Churchill Livingstone; 1998:1–15.

47. Noe JM. *Wound Care.* 2nd ed. Greenwich, Conn: Chesebrough-Pond; 1985.

48. Baldwin JE, Weber LJ, Simon CLS, eds. *Clinical Assessment Recommendations.* 2nd ed. Chicago, Ill: American Society of Hand Therapists; 1992.

49. Cozzell J. The new red, yellow, black color code. *Am J Nurs* 1989;10:1014.

50. Allbrook DB. Skeletal muscle regeneration. *Muscle Nerve* 1981;4:234–245.

51. Hurme T, Kalimo H. Activation of myogenic precursor cells after muscle injury. *Med Sci Sports Exerc* 1992;24:197–205.

52. Hurme T, Kalimo H, Lehto M, Jarvinen M. Healing of skeletal muscle injury: An ultrastructural and immunohistochemical study. *Med Sci Sports Exerc* 1991;23:801–810.

53. Kasemkijwattana C, Menetrey J, Bosch P, et al. Use of growth factors to improve muscle healing after strain injury. *Clin Orthop* 2000;370:272–285.

54. Kalimo H, Rantanen J, Jarvinen M. Soft tissue injuries in sport. In: Jarvinen M, ed. *Balliere's Clinical Orthopedics.* 1997:1–24.

55. Lehto M, Duance VJ, Restall D. Collagen and fibronectin in a healing skeletal muscle injury: An immunohistochemical study of the effects of physical activity on the repair of the injured gastrocnemius muscle in the rat. *J Bone Joint Surg* 1985; 67B:820–828.

56. Menetrey J, Kasemkijwattana C, Day CS, et al. Growth factors improve muscle healing in vivo. *J Bone Joint Surg* 2000; 82B:131–137.

57. Alameddine HS, Dehaupas M, Fardeau M. Regeneration of skeletal muscle fibers from autologous satellite cells multiplied in vitro: An experimental model for testing cultured cell myogenicity. *Muscle Nerve* 1989;12:544–555.

58. Frank CB, et al. Soft tissue healing. In: Fu F, Harner CD, Vince KG, eds. *Knee Surgery.* Baltimore, Md: Williams and Wilkins; 1994:189–229.

59. Injeyan HS, Fraser IH, Peek WD. Pathology of musculoskeletal soft tissues. In: Hammer WI, ed. *Functional Soft Tissue Examination and Treatment by Manual Methods.* Gaithersburg, Md: Aspen; 1991:9–23.

60. Kasper CE, Talbot LA, Gaines JM. Skeletal muscle damage and recovery. *AACN Clin Issues* 2002;13:237–247.

61. Byrnes WC, Clarkson PM, White JS, Hsieh SS, Frykman PN, Maughan RJ. Delayed onset muscle soreness following repeated bouts of downhill running. *J Appl Physiol* 1985;59:710.

62. Nosaka K, Sakamoto K, Newton M, Sacco P. How long does the protective effect on eccentric exercise-induced muscle damage last. *Med Sci Sports Exerc* 2001;33:1490–1495.

63. Lynn R, Talbot JA, Morgan DA. Differences in rat skeletal muscles after incline and decline running. *J Appl Physiol* 1998;85:98–104.

64. Nosaka K, Clarkson P. Influence of previous concentric exercise on eccentric exercise-induced muscle damage. *J Sports Sci* 1997;15:477.

65. Murphy PG, Loitz BJ, Frank CB, Hart DA. Influence of exogenous growth factors on the expression of plasminogen activators by explants of normal and healing rabbit ligaments. *Biochem Cell Biol* 1993;71:522–529.

66. Pierce GF, Mustoe TA, Lingelbach J, et al. Platelet-derived growth factor and transforming growth factor-beta enhance tissue repair activities by unique mechanisms. *J Cell Biol* 1989;109:429–440.

67. Woo SLY, Suh JK, Parsons IM, et al. Biological intervention in ligament healing effect of growth factors. *Sports Med Arthrosc Rev* 1998;6:74–82.

68. Steenfos HH. Growth factors in wound healing. *Scand J Plast Hand Surg* 1994;28:95–105.

69. Booher JM, Thibodeau GA. The body's response to trauma and environmental stress. In: Booher JM, Thibodeau GA, eds. *Athletic Injury Assessment.* New York, NY: McGraw-Hill; 2000: 55–76.

70. Frank G, Woo SLY, Amiel D, et al. Medial collateral ligament healing. A multidisciplinary assessment in rabbits. *Am J Sports Med* 1983;11:379.

71. Balduini FC, Vegso JJ, Torg JS, Torg E. Management and rehabilitation of ligamentous injuries to the ankle. *Sports Med* 1987;4:364–380.

72. Gould N, Selingson D, Gassman J. Early and late repair of lateral ligaments of the ankle. *Foot Ankle* 1980;1:84–89.

73. Vailas AC, Tipton CM, Matthes RD, Gart M. Physical activity and its influence on the repair process of medial collateral ligaments. *Connect Tissue Res* 1981;9:25–31.

74. Tipton CM, Matthes RD, Maynard JA, Carey RA. The influence of physical activity on ligaments and tendons. *Med Sci Sports Exerc* 1975;7:165–175.

75. Tipton CM, James SL, Mergner W, Tcheng TK. Influence of exercise in strength of medial collateral knee ligaments of dogs. *Am J Physiol* 1970;218:894–902.

76. Laban MM. Collagen tissue: implications of its response to stress in vitro. *Arch Phys Med Rehab* 1962;43:461.

77. McGaw WT. The effect of tension on collagen remodelling by fibroblasts: A stereological ultrastructural study. *Connect Tissue Res* 1986;14:229.

78. Wakitani S, Goto T, Pineda SJ, et al. Mesenchymal cell-based repair of large, full-thickness defects of articular cartilage. *J Bone Joint Surg* 1994;76A:579–592.

79. Fuller JA, Ghadially FN. Ultrastructural observations on surgically produced partial-thickness defects in articular cartilage. *Clin Orthop* 1972;86:193–205.

80. Ghadially FN, Thomas I, Oryschak AF, Lalaonde JM. Long-term results of superficial defects in articular cartilage: A scanning electron-microscope study. *J Pathol* 1977;121:213–217.

81. Convery FR, Akeson WH, Keown GH. The repair of large osteochondral defects. An experimental study in horses. *Clin Orthop* 1972;82:253–262.

82. Coletti JM Jr, Akeson WH, Woo SLY. A comparison of the physical behavior of normal articular cartilage and the arthroplasty surface. *J Bone Joint Surg* 1972;54A:147–160.

83. Furukawa T, Eyre DR, Koide S, Glimcher MJ. Biochemical studies on repair cartilage resurfacing experimental defects in the rabbit knee. *J Bone Joint Surg* 1980;62A:79–89.

84. Chu CR, Convery FR, Akeson WH, Meyers M, Amiel D. Articular cartilage transplantation. Clinical results in the knee. *Clin Orthop* 1999;360:159–168.

85. Perka C, Sittinger M, Schultz O, Spitzer RS, Schenzka D, Burmester GR. Tissue engineered cartilage repair using cryopreserved and noncryopreserved chondrocytes. *Clin Orthop* 2000;378:245–254.

86. Marsh DR, Li G. The biology of fracture healing: Optimising outcome. *Br Med Bull* 1999;55:856–869.

87. Muller ME. Internal fixation for fresh fractures and nonunion. *Proc R Soc Med* 1963;56:455–460.

88. McKibbin B. The biology of fracture healing in long bones. *J Bone Joint Surg* 1978;60B:150–161.

89. Sarmiento A, Mullis DL, Latta LL, Tarr RR, Alvarez R. A quantitative comparative analysis of fracture healing under the influence of compression plating vs. closed weight-bearing treatment. *Clin Orthop* 1980;149:232–239.

90. Bailey DA, Faulkner RA, McKay HA. Growth, physical activity, and bone mineral acquisition. In: Hollosky JO, ed. *Exercise and Sport Sciences Reviews*. Baltimore, Md: Williams and Wilkins; 1996:233–266.

91. Stone MH. Implications for connective tissue and bone alterations resulting from rest and exercise training. *Med Sci Sports Exerc* 1988;20:S162–S168.

92. Monteleone GP. Stress fractures in the athlete. *Orthop Clin North Am* 1995;26:423.

93. Hockenbury RT. Forefoot problems in athletes. *Med Sci Sports Exerc* 1999;31(suppl):S448–S458.

94. Wallace AL, Draper ER, Strachan RK, McCarthy ID, Hughes SP. The vascular response to fracture micromovement. *Clin Orthop* 1994;301:281–290.

95. Marsh D. Concepts of fracture union, delayed union, and nonunion. *Clin Orthop* 1998;355:S22–S230.

MANAGING IMPAIRED MUSCLE PERFORMANCE

CHAPTER OBJECTIVES

▶ *At the completion of this chapter, the reader will be able to:*

1. Outline the biomechanical properties of human skeletal muscle.

2. Define active insufficiency and passive insufficiency of a muscle.

3. Describe the various factors that may influence the amount of tension developed in muscle.

4. Differentiate among muscle strength, endurance, and power.

5. Describe strategies to increase muscle strength.

6. List the different types of resistance that can be used to strengthen muscles.

7. List the different types of muscle contractions and the advantages and disadvantages of each.

8. Outline the various types of exercise progression and the components of each.

9. Describe strategies to increase muscle endurance.

10. Describe strategies to increase muscle power.

11. Explain the basic principles behind plyometrics.

12. Describe the importance of specificity of training.

13. List and describe two types of flexibility.

14. Describe strategies to increase muscle flexibility using different stretching techniques.

15. Define delayed onset muscle soreness and explain why it occurs.

16. Define senescence sarcopenia.

17. List the changes that can occur with muscles during aging.

OVERVIEW

Muscle is the only biological tissue capable of actively generating tension. This characteristic enables human skeletal muscle to perform the important functions of maintaining upright body posture, moving body parts, and absorbing shock. The maximum tension that is generated within a fully activated muscle is not a constant, and depends on a number of factors. These factors are outlined in this chapter.

Biomechanical Properties of Skeletal Muscle

"No muscle uses its power in pushing but always in drawing to itself the parts that are joined to it."
Leonardo Da Vinci (1452–1519)

Human skeletal muscle possesses four biomechanical properties:

1. *Extensibility.* Extensibility is the ability to be stretched or to increase in length.

2. *Elasticity.* Elasticity is the ability to return to normal resting length following a stretch.

3. *Irritability.* Irritability is the ability to respond to a stimulus. With reference to skeletal muscle, this stimulus is provided electrochemically (see Chap. 1).

4. *Ability to develop tension.* The ability of skeletal muscle is referred to as a contraction. As discussed later in this chapter, a contraction may or may not result in shortening of a muscle.

Muscle Function

There are approximately 430 muscles in the body, each of which can be considered anatomically as a separate organ. About 75 pairs of muscle provide the majority of body movements and posture.[1] Muscles around a joint typically function as pairs, referred to as *agonists* and *antagonists.* An agonist muscle contracts to produce the desired movement, whereas the antagonist muscle opposes the desired movement. Antagonists resist the agonist movement by relaxing and lengthening in a gradual manner to ensure that the desired motion occurs, and that it does so in a coordinated and controlled fashion. Muscle groups that work together to produce a desired movement are called *synergists.*[2]

Most muscles span only one joint. Among the muscles that cross two or more joints are the erector spinae, biceps brachii, long head of the triceps brachii, hamstrings, rectus femoris, and several muscles crossing the wrist and hand joints, and ankle and foot joints.

Development of Muscle Tension

The effectiveness of a muscle to produce movement is dependent on a number of factors. These include the location and orientation of the muscle attachment relative to the joint, the tightness or laxity present in the musculotendinous unit, and the actions of other muscles that cross the joint.[1]

When an activated muscle develops tension, the amount of tension present is constant throughout the length of the muscle in both tendons, and at the sites of the musculotendinous attachments to bone.[1] The tensile force produced by the muscle pulls on the attached bones and creates torque at the joints crossed by the muscle. The magnitude of the tensile force is dependent on a number of factors, as discussed next.

Type of Muscle Contraction

The word *contraction*, used to describe the generation of tension within muscle fibers, conjures up an image of shortening of muscle fibers. However, a contraction can produce shortening or lengthening of the muscle, or no change in the muscle length. Thus, three types of contraction are commonly recognized: isometric, concentric, and eccentric.

▶ *Isometric contraction.* An isometric contraction occurs when tension is produced in the muscle without any appreciable change in muscle length.[3]

▶ *Concentric contraction.* A concentric contraction (Fig. 6-1) produces a shortening of the muscle. This occurs when the tension generated by the agonist muscle is sufficient to overcome an external resistance and to move the body segment of one attachment toward the segment of its other attachment.[3]

▶ *Eccentric contraction.* An eccentric contraction (Fig. 6-2) occurs when a muscle slowly lengthens as it gives in to an external force that is greater than the contractile force it is exerting.[3] In reality, the muscle does not actually lengthen, it merely returns from its shortened position to its normal resting length. Eccentric muscle contractions, which are capable of generating greater forces than either isometric or concentric contractions,[4–6] are involved in activities that require a deceleration to occur. Such activities include slowing to a stop when running, lowering an object, or sitting down. Because the load exceeds the bond between the actin and myosin filaments during an eccentric contraction, some of the myosin filaments probably are torn from the binding sites on the actin filament while the remainder are completing the contraction cycle.[7] The resulting force is substantially larger for a torn cross-bridge than for one being created during a normal cycle of muscle contraction. Consequently, the combined increase in force per cross-bridge and the number of active cross-bridges results in a maximum lengthening muscle tension that is greater than the tension that could be created during a shortening muscle action.[7]

A comparison of the three types of muscle actions in terms of force production, according to Elftman's proposal, shows that[8]:

Eccentric maximum tension
> Isometric maximum tension
> Concentric maximum tension

Four other contractions are worth mentioning.

▶ *Isotonic contraction.* An isotonic contraction is a contraction in which the tension within the muscle remains constant as the muscle shortens or lengthens.[3] This state is very difficult to produce and measure. Although the term

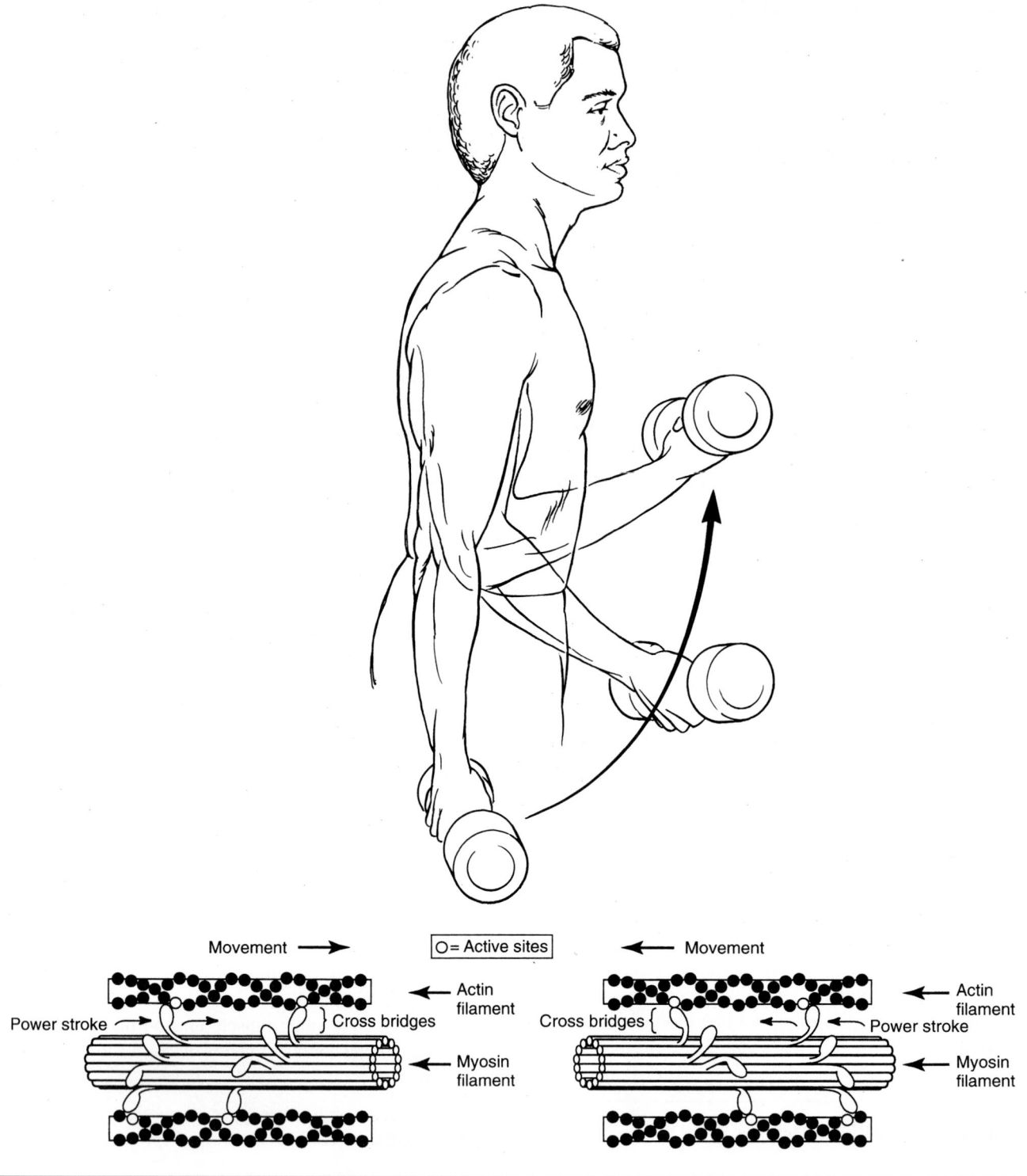

FIGURE 6-1   Contractile properties of concentric contraction. (Reproduced with permission from Zachazewski JE, Magee DJ, Quillen WS, eds. *Athletic Injuries and Rehabilitation.* Philadelphia, Pa: WB Saunders; 1996.)

isotonic is used to describe concentric and eccentric contractions alike, its use in this context is erroneous because in most exercise forms, the tension produced in muscles varies with muscle length and with the variation in external torque.[3]

▶ *Isokinetic contraction.*   An isokinetic contraction occurs when a muscle is maximally contracting at the same speed throughout the whole range of its related lever.[3] Isokinetic contractions require the use of special equipment that produces an accommodating resistance. Both high-speed/low-resistance,

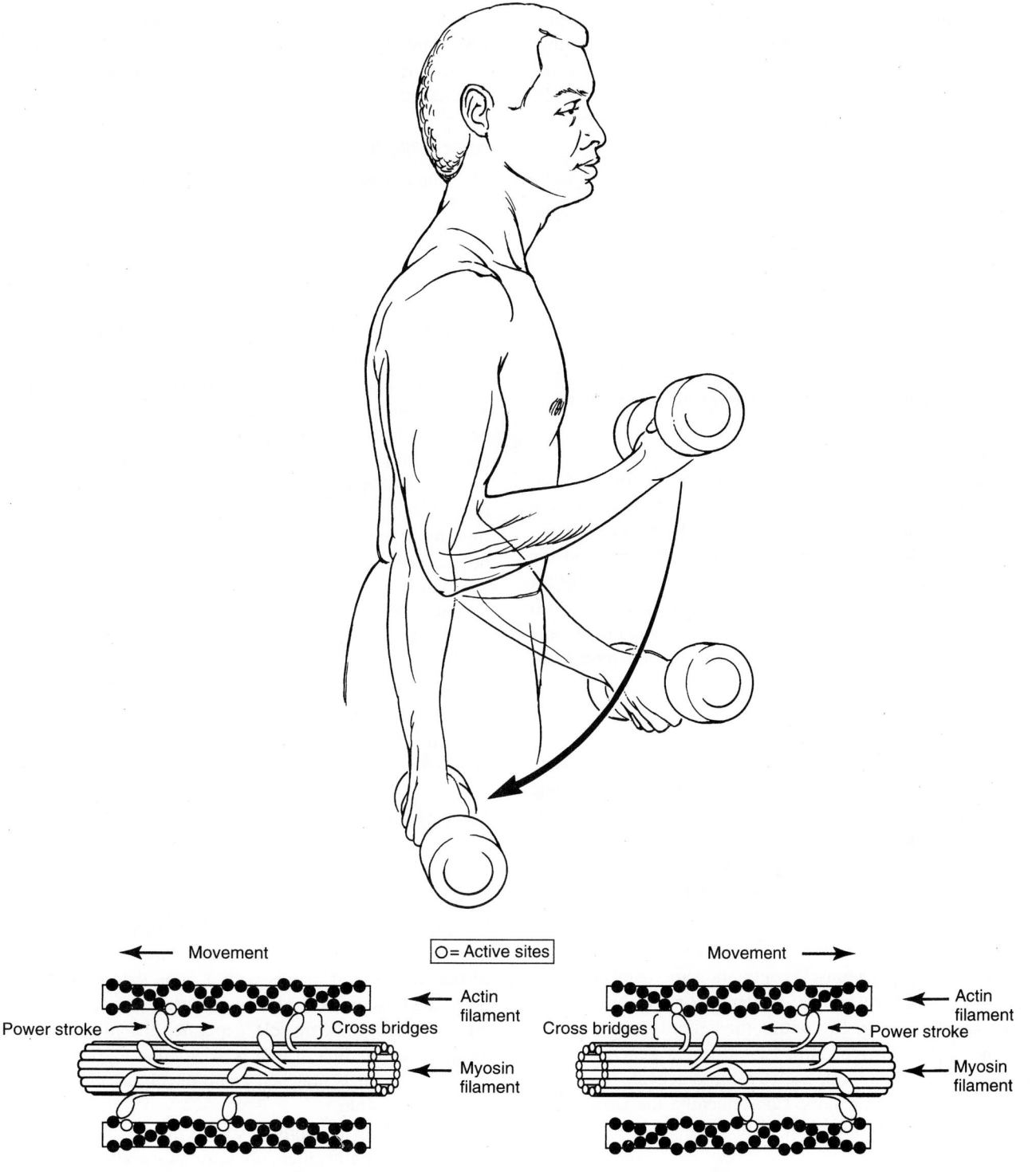

FIGURE 6-2   Contractile properties of eccentric contraction. (Reproduced with permission from Zachazewski JE, Magee DJ, Quillen WS, eds. *Athletic Injuries and Rehabilitation.* Philadelphia, Pa: WB Saunders; 1996.)

and low-speed/high-resistance regimens result in excellent strength gains.[9–12] The disadvantage of this type of exercise is its expense. In addition, there is the potential for impact loading and incorrect joint axis alignment.[13] Isokinetic exercises may also have questionable functional carryover.[14]

▶ *Econcentric contraction.*   This type of contraction combines both a controlled concentric and a simultaneous eccentric contraction of the same muscle over two separate joints.[15] Examples of an econcentric contraction include the standing hamstring curl, in which the hamstrings work concentrically to flex the knee while the hip tends to flex eccentrically, lengthening the hamstrings; and the squat. When rising from a squat, the hamstrings work concentrically as the hip extends and work eccentrically as the knee extends. Conversely, the rectus femoris work eccentrically as the hip extends and work concentrically as the knee extends.

▶ *Isolytic contraction.* An isolytic contraction is a type of eccentric isotonic contraction that makes use of a greater force than the patient can overcome. This type of contraction is used with some muscle energy techniques to stretch fibrotic tissue (see Chap. 11).

Force–Velocity Relationship

The rate of muscle shortening or lengthening substantially affects the force that a muscle can develop during contraction.

Shortening Contractions

As the speed of a muscle shortening increases, the force it is capable of producing decreases.[4,6] The slower rate of shortening is thought to produce greater forces than can be produced by increasing the number of cross-bridges formed. This relationship can be viewed as a continuum, with the optimum velocity for the muscle somewhere between the slowest and fastest rates. At very slow speeds, the force that a muscle can resist or overcome rises rapidly up to 50 percent greater than the maximum isometric contraction.[4,6]

Lengthening Contractions

When a muscle contracts while lengthening (an eccentric contraction), the force production differs from that of a shortening (concentric) contraction. Rapid lengthening contractions generate more force than do slow ones (slower lengthening contractions). During slow lengthening muscle actions, the work produced approximates that of an isometric contraction.[4,6]

Recruitment of Motor Units[1]

The force and speed of a muscle contraction are based on the requirement of an activity and are dependent on the ability of the central nervous system to control the recruitment of motor units. The motor units of slow-twitch fibers generally have lower thresholds and are relatively easier to activate than those of the fast-twitch motor units. Consequently, the slow-twitch fibers are the first to be recruited, even when the resulting limb movement is rapid.[16]

As the force requirement, speed requirement, or duration of the activity increases, motor units with higher thresholds are recruited. Type IIa units are recruited before type IIb.[17]

Electromechanical Delay

Following the stimulation of a muscle, a brief period elapses before the muscle begins to develop tension. This period is referred to as the *electromechanical delay* (EMD). The length of the EMD varies considerably among muscles. Fast-twitch fibers have shorter periods of EMD when compared with slow-twitch fibers.[18] It has been suggested that injury increases the EMD and, therefore, increases the susceptibility to injury.[19] One of the purposes of neuromuscular reeducation (see Chap. 10) is to return the EMD to a normal level.[20]

Force–Length Relationship

The number of cross-bridges that can be formed is dependent on the extent of the overlap between the actin and myosin filaments.[21] Thus, the force a muscle is capable of exerting depends on its length. For each muscle cell, there is an optimum length, or range of lengths, at which the contractile force is strongest. At the optimum length of the muscle, there is near-optimal overlap of actin and myosin, allowing for the generation of maximum tension at this length.

If the muscle is in a shortened position, the overlap of actin and myosin reduces the number of sites available for cross-bridge formation. *Active insufficiency* of a muscle occurs when the muscle is incapable of shortening to the extent required to produce full range of motion at all joints crossed simultaneously.[1,15,22,23] For example, the finger flexors cannot produce a tight fist when the wrist is fully flexed, as they can when it is in neutral position.

If the muscle is in a lengthened position compared with the optimum length, the actin filaments are pulled away from the myosin heads such that they cannot create as many cross-bridges.[7] *Passive insufficiency* of the muscle occurs when the two-joint muscle cannot stretch to the extent required for full range of motion in the opposite direction at all joints crossed.[1,15,22,23] For example, a larger range of hyperextension is possible at the wrist when the fingers are not fully extended.

Angle of Insertion

Although each muscle contains the contractile machinery to produce the forces for movement, it is the tendon that transmits these forces to the bones in order to achieve movement or stability of the body in space.[24] The interface between the muscle and tendon is called the *myotendinous junction*. The angle of insertion the tendon makes with a bone determines the line of pull. The tension generated by a muscle is a function of its angle of insertion. A muscle generates the greatest amount of torque when its line of pull is oriented at a 90-degree angle to the bone and it is attached anatomically as far from the joint center as possible.[1]

Just as there are optimal speeds of length change, and optimal muscle lengths, there are optimal insertion angles for each of the muscles. The angle of insertion of a muscle, and therefore its line of pull, can change during dynamic movements.[7]

Angle of Pennation

The *angle of pennation* is the angle created between the fiber direction and the line of pull. When the fibers of a muscle lie parallel to the long axis of the muscle, there is no angle of pennation. The number of fibers within a fixed volume of muscle increases with the angle of pennation.[7] Although maximum tension can be improved with pennation, the range of shortening of the muscle is reduced. Muscles that need to have large changes in length without the need for very high tension, such as the sartorius, do not have pennate muscle fibers.[7] In contrast, pennate muscle fibers are found in those muscles in which the emphasis is on a high capacity for tension generation rather than range of motion (e.g., gluteus maximus).

Stored Elastic Capabilities

It has been demonstrated that when a concentric contraction is preceded by a phase of active or passive stretching, elastic energy is stored in the muscle. This stored energy is then used in the following contractile phase. For example, during functional activities, the muscles operate with a strong concentric action, which is usually preceded by a *passive* eccentric loading, as part of a stretch-shortening cycle.[25] The stretch-shortening cycle includes the ability of the muscle to absorb or dissipate shock, while also preparing the stretched muscle for response.[26] Plyometric exercises, described later (in the section on "Increasing Muscle Power") are used to improve the ability of the muscles to perform these actions by enhancing their power, speed, and agility.

Gravity

With respect to gravity, muscle actions may occur:

▶ In the same direction as gravity (downward)

▶ In the opposite direction to gravity (upward)

▶ In a direction perpendicular to gravity (horizontal)

▶ In the same or opposite direction to gravity, but at an angle

The direction in which the muscle is working determines the role that gravity plays and the role that the muscle must play in order to counteract the forces of gravity. For example, if an arm muscle is working to lower a book to a table, the muscle works eccentrically against the force of gravity to control the speed of the lowering. If the muscle works to lift the book from the table, the muscle must work concentrically against the force of gravity.

Fatigue

Skeletal muscle fatigue can compromise exercise tolerance and work productivity while retarding rehabilitation of diseased or damaged muscle. It is now clear that the development of fatigue probably involves several factors that influence force production in a manner dependent on muscle fiber type and activation pattern, and that one of these factors may be the regulation of Ca^{2+} by the sarcoplasmic reticulum.[27] Characteristics of muscle fatigue include reduction in muscle force production capability and shortening velocity, reduction in the release and uptake of intracellular calcium by the sarcoplasmic reticulum, and prolonged relaxation of motor units between recruitment.[27,28]

Muscle Temperature

As body temperature elevates, the speeds of nerve and muscle functions increase, resulting in a higher value of maximum isometric tension and a higher maximum velocity of shortening possible with fewer motor units at any given load.[29] Muscle function is most efficient at 38.5° C (101° F).[30]

Clinical Pearl

Skeletal muscle blood flow increases 20-fold during muscle contractions.[31] The muscle blood flow generally increases in proportion to the metabolic demands of the tissue, a relationship reflected by positive correlations between muscle blood flow and exercise.

Improving Muscle Performance

Muscle performance can be measured using a number of parameters. These include strength, endurance, and power.

▶ *Strength* is defined as the ability of a muscle to generate force against a specific resistance, or to produce torque at a joint.

▶ *Endurance* is defined as the ability of a muscle to sustain or perform repetitive muscular contractions for an extended period.

▶ *Mechanical power* is the product of force and velocity. *Muscular power* is, therefore, the product of muscular force and the velocity of muscle shortening.

These components of muscle performance are important in functional activities. An increase in strength and endurance invariably results in the potential to allow the patient to interact with their environment in a more efficient and pain-free way, through increased movement control and capacity. Muscular power is an important contributor to activities requiring both strength and speed.

Increasing Strength

Muscular strength is derived both from the amount of tension a muscle can generate and from the moment arms of contributing muscles with respect to the joint center.

To understand the concept of moment arm, an understanding of the anatomy and movement (kinematics) of the joint of interest is necessary. Although muscles produce linear forces, motions at joints are all rotary. For example, some joints can be considered to rotate about a fixed point. A good example of such a joint is the elbow. At the elbow joint, where the humerus and ulna articulate, the resulting rotation occurs primarily about a fixed point, referred to as the center of rotation. In the case of the elbow joint, this center of rotation is relatively constant throughout the joint range of motion. However, in other joints (for example the knee) the center of rotation moves in space as the knee joint rotates because the articulating surfaces are not perfect circles. In the case of the knee, it is not appropriate to discuss a single center of rotation—rather we must speak of a center of rotation corresponding to a particular joint angle, or, using the terminology of joint kinematics, we must speak of the instant center of rotation (ICR), that is, the center of rotation at any "instant" in time or space. Thus, the moment arm is defined as the perpendicular distance from the line of force application to the axis of rotation.

Both the amount of tension a muscle can generate and the moment arms of the contributing muscles are affected by several factors (discussed earlier).

As with prescriptions for medications, a successful exercise prescription requires the correct balance between the dose (exercise) and the response (specific health or fitness adaptations).[31a] An over-prescription of resistance training exercise may result in overstress injuries, whereas underprescription will result in a failure to achieve the necessary or desired strength improvement. Depending on the specific program design, resistance training is known to enhance muscular strength, power, or endurance and can provide a potent stimulus to the neuromuscular system. Other variables such as speed, balance, coordination, jumping ability, flexibility, and other measures of motor performance have also been positively enhanced by resistance training.[31b] Resistance training, particularly when incorporated into a comprehensive fitness program, reduces the risk factors associated with coronary heart disease, non–insulin-dependent diabetes, and colon cancer; prevents osteoporosis; promotes weight loss and maintenance; improves dynamic stability and preserves functional capacity; and fosters psychological well-being.[31b]

To increase strength, the load or resistance must be gradually increased during the muscle contraction. Strengthening of a muscle occurs when the muscle is forced to work at a higher level than that to which it is accustomed. To most effectively increase muscle strength, a muscle must work with increasing effort against progressively increasing resistance.[5,32] If resistance is applied to a muscle as it contracts so that the metabolic capabilities of the muscle are progressively overloaded, adaptive changes occur within the muscle, which make it stronger over time.[6,33] These adaptive changes include[4,5,25,30,34–36]:

▶ *An increase in the size of the muscle (hypertrophy).* In normal individuals an increase in strength after a resisted exercise program is thought to initially occur as a result of neural adaptation, followed by hypertrophy of muscle fibers if the exercise program is continued for a longer period. *Mitochondria* are the main subcellular structures that determine the oxygen demand of muscle. There is consensus that there is a dilution of mitochondrial volume density through an increase in myofibrillar (i.e., contractile protein) volume density as a consequence of strength-type exercise training.[36a,36b] This increase in myofibrillar volume density, or hypertrophy that occurs with strength training is regarded as the main cause for the overall increase in the anatomical cross-sectional area (CSA) of an entire muscle group. The fiber hypertrophy is typically greater for fast- than for slow-twitch muscle fibers.[36c]

▶ *An increase in the force per unit area.* Strength training has also been shown to lead to an increase in the force per unit CSA of the muscle. This effect has been attributed either to an increase in neural drive[36d] or to an actual increase in muscle specific tension due to a denser packing of muscle filaments.[36e] A denser packing of contractile tissue along the tendon, could theoretically increase the angle of pennation of muscle fibers.[36f]

▶ *A reduction in the time to peak force.*[36g]

▶ *An increase in the rate of force development.*[36g]

Conversely, a muscle can become weak or atrophied through:

▶ Disease

▶ Neurologic compromise

▶ Immobilization (see Chap. 5)

▶ Disuse

Types of Exercise

Isometric Exercises.   Studies have demonstrated that a 6-second hold of 75 percent of maximal resistance is sufficient to increase strength when performed repetitively.[37,38] Isometric exercises have an obvious role when joint movement is restricted, either by pain or by bracing and casting. The primary role in this regard is to prevent atrophy and a decrease of ligament, bone, and muscle strength. Isometric exercises have the following disadvantages:

▶ Strength gains are not increased throughout the range (unless performed at multiple angles).

▶ They do not activate all of the muscle fibers (primary activation is of slow-twitch fibers).

▶ There are no flexibility or cardiovascular fitness benefits.

▶ Peak effort can be injurious to the tissues because of vasoconstriction and joint compression forces.

▶ There is limited functional carryover.[14]

▶ Considerable internal pressure can be generated, especially if the breath is held during contraction. This can prove injurious to patients with weakness in the abdominal wall (hernia) or cardiovascular impairment (increase in blood pressure through the Valsalva maneuver)[39] even if performed correctly.

Concentric Exercises.   Concentric contractions commonly are used in the rehabilitation process and in activities of daily living. The biceps curl and the lifting of a cup to the mouth are examples, respectively.

Eccentric Exercises.   The clinical indications for the use of eccentric exercise are numerous[40] (Table 6-1).

Functional Exercises.   Functional strength is the ability of the neuromuscular system to perform the various types of contractions involved with functional activities in an efficient manner and in a multiplanar environment.[42] Functional exercises use

TABLE 6-1 Clinical Indications for Eccentric-biased Exercise[40,41]

Mechanical, reproducible joint pain
Joint pain resistant to modality intervention
Unidirectional joint crepitus or pain arc
Deconditioned or low endurance patients
Plateaus in strength gains
Tendonitis presentations
Late-stage rehabilitation and performance training

combinations of concentric and eccentric contractions in the performance of activities that relate to a patient's needs and requirements (see later section on "Specificity of Training"). Affective rehabilitation targets specific muscles with regard to functional muscle activity patterns and overall conditioning and uses a progression of increased activity, while preventing further trauma.[43] Incremental gains in function should be seen as strength increases.

Types of Resistance

Resistance can be applied to a muscle by any external force or mass, including gravity. Cuff weights, dumbbells, and surgical tubing (elastic resistance) are economical ways of applying resistance. The use of elastic resistance in rehabilitation protocols has been discussed by several authors.[11,44–49]

According to a recent study, 96 percent of rehabilitation professionals use elastic resistance with their patients, and 85 percent of home exercise programs prescribed by rehab professionals require elastic resistance bands or tubing.[44–47,47a,48,49,49a] Elastic resistance offers a unique type of resistance that cannot be classified within the traditional subcategories of strengthening such as isometric or isotonic. The amount of variable resistance offered by elastic bands or tubing is a factor of the internal tension produced by the material. This internal tension is a factor of the elastic material's coefficient of elasticity, the surface area of the elastic material, and how much the elastic material is stretched.[49a] It is commonly believed that the resistance provided by these bands or tubing increases exponentially at the end range of motion. However, the forces produced by elastic resistance are linear until approximately 500 percent elongation, at which point the forces increase exponentially.[49a] As the elastic resistance is not stretched more than 300 percent in prescribed exercises, the exponential increase should not be attained. In addition, the torque production of elastic-resistance exercises is similar to that produced by isotonic dumbbell exercise: a bell-shaped curve.[49b]

In situations where the larger muscle groups require strengthening, a multitude of specific indoor exercise machines can be used. Examples of these machines include the Multi-hip, the Lat pull-down, the leg extension, and the leg curl machine. Although these machines are a more expensive alternative to dumbbell or elastic resistance, they do offer greater levels of resistance. Thus, these machines are often used in the more advanced stages of a rehabilitation program.

Manual resistance also can be applied. The advantages of manually applied resistance by a skilled clinician are[43] as follows:

▶ Control of the position of the extremity

▶ More effective reeducation of the muscle or extremity

▶ Critical sensory input to the patient through tactile stimulation

▶ Accurate accommodation and alterations in the resistance applied throughout the range

▶ Ability to limit the range

One of the more popular uses of manual resistance, proprioceptive neuromuscular facilitation, is detailed in Chapter 11.

Exercise Progressions

Progression is defined as "the act of moving forward or advancing toward a specific goal." In resistance training, progression entails the continued improvement in a desired variable over time until the target goal has been achieved.[49c] Optimal resistance training progressions should always be based on sound rationale and symptomatic response, and should always be individualized to meet specific training goals. A number of programs have been designed for the progression of resistance exercise programs. Some of these programs are summarized in Tables 6-2 and 6-3. Much has been written about the merits of these different training regimens. For more detail, and for scientific references about these and other programs, the reader is referred to the Fleck and Kraemer text.[49d]

The extent of the functional and health benefits from resistance training depend on factors such as initial performance and health status, along with the specification of program design variables such as frequency, duration, intensity, variation, and rest intervals.[49e]

Clinical Pearl

Three terms are commonly used with resistance training:

- *Repetitions.* The number of times a specific movement or exercise is repeated.

- *Repetition maximum (RM).* The repetition maximum is the maximum number of repetitions an individual can perform at a given weight. For example a 10-RM is the weight the patient can lift a maximum of 10 times.

- *Set.* A particular number of repetitions. Whatever exercise progression is used to achieve an increase in the total number of repetitions while maintaining a sufficient effort, the number of sets must also be increased. This increase in sets must occur in conjunction with a reduction in the number of repetitions per set by 10 to 20 percent,[52] or a reduction in the amount of resistance. Generally speaking, no more than 3–5 sets are used.

TABLE 6-2 Exercise Progressions

	Set(s) of 10	Amount of Weight	Repetitions
DeLorme program	1	50% of 10 RM	10
	2	75% of 10 RM	10
	3	100% of 10 RM	10
Oxford technique	1	100% of 10 RM	10
	2	75% of 10 RM	10
	3	50% of 10 RM	10
MacQueen technique	3 (beginning/intermediate)	100% of 10 RM	10
	4–5 (advanced)	100% of 2–3 RM	2–3
Sander program	Total of 4 sets (3 times per week)	100% of 5 RM	5
	Day 1: 4 sets	100% of 5 RM	5
	Day 2: 4 sets	100% of 3 RM	5
	Day 3: 1 set	100% of 5 RM	5
	2 sets	100% of 3 RM	5
	2 sets	100% of 2 RM	5
Knight DAPRE program	1	50% of RM	10
	2	75% of RM	6
	3	100% of RM	Maximum
	4	Adjusted working weight	Maximum

DAPRE, daily adjustable progressive resistive exercise; RM, repetition maximum.

TABLE 6-3 Adjustment Sequence for DAPRE Isotonic Program

Number of Repetitions Performed During Set	Adjusted Working Weight for Fourth Set	Next Exercise Session
0–2	−5–10 lb	−5–10 lb
3–4	0–5 lb	Same weight
5–6	Same weight	+5–10 lb
7–10	+5–10 lb	+5–15 lb
11	+10–20 lb	+10–20 lb

DAPRE, daily adjustable progressive resistive exercise.

Frequency. Optimal training frequency (the number of workouts per week) depends on several factors such as training volume, intensity, exercise selection, level of conditioning, recovery ability, and the number of muscle groups trained per workout session. Strength is most effectively enhanced by a program featuring high resistance and few repetitions. Based on studies of isokinetic and isotonic exercise,[49f,50] muscle strength recovery follows a steady, nonlinear, and predictable increase over time.[51]

Initial selection of a starting weight may require some trial and error. For any given exercise, the amount of weight selected should be sufficient to allow 6–12 RM per exercise in each of the three sets with a recovery period between sets of 60 to 90 seconds. A typical exercise prescription for high school, collegiate, and professional athletes includes three or more sets of a 6–12 RM per exercise performed 3 days/week.[53] The American College of Sports Medicine recommends 8 to 12 repetitions/set to elicit improvements in muscular strength and endurance as well as muscle hypertrophy.[49d] It is important to note that orthopaedic injury may occur in older (>65 years) and/or more frail participants when performing efforts to volitional fatigue using a high-intensity, low-to-moderate RM training regimen. Therefore, a 10 to 15 RM is generally recommended for this population.[49c] In the rehabilitation population, strengthening exercises are typically performed on a daily basis initially, with the weight and frequency governed by the individual's response to the exercise. As healing progresses, evidenced by a decrease in pain and swelling and an increase in range of motion, the exercises should be performed every other day. When expressed as a weekly percentage, the Albert 5 Percent Rule states that a 5 percent strength increase in a given week can be maintained for many weeks of resistive training providing that the patient trains three times a week at a minimum resistance load of 70 percent of maximal voluntary muscle contractile force.[51] While seemingly esoteric, the 5 percent rule can be used in determining the prognosis. For example, a patient with a 40 percent deficit in strength of the biceps can be assumed to take approximately 8 weeks to recover, barring any illness, or disease states.[51] Once sufficient strength is attained, even if the patient only performs the strength training at a minimum of once per week, their strength can be fairly well maintained over a 3-month period.[54]

Duration. Duration refers to the length of the exercise session. In most functional exercises, fatigue of the muscle being exercised is the goal. Fatigue may occur as a lack of coordination, insufficient balance, or the addition of compensatory movements. Fatigue may also be governed by the patient's level of motivation. In the rehabilitation population, fatigue should be achieved without exceeding the patient's tolerance and while protecting the injury site.

Intensity. Intensity refers to the power output (rate of performing work) or how much effort is required to perform the exercise. In clinical terms, intensity refers to the weight or resistance lifted by the patient. It is now recognized that an individual's perception of effort (relative perceived exertion or RPE) is closely related to the level of physiological effort (Table 6-4).[55,56] It is important therefore, to closely monitor the patient's response to exercise. Any discomfort or reproduction of symptoms that last more than 1–2 hours after the intervention is unacceptable.

Patient responses that can modify the intensity include increases in pain level, muscle fatigue, time taken to recover from fatigue, cardiovascular response, compensatory movements, level of motivation, and degree of comprehension.

Variation. Variation in training is a fundamental principle that supports the need for alterations in one or more program variables over time to allow for the training stimulus to remain optimal.[49c] The concept of variation has been rooted in program design universally for many years. The most commonly examined resistance training theory including planned variation is periodization. Periodization is the systematic process of planned variations in a resistance-training program over a specified training cycle.[57] Two models of periodization are recognized: classic (linear) and undulating (nonlinear)[49c]:

▶ *Classic.* This model is characterized by high initial training volume and low intensity. As training progresses, volume decreases and intensity increases in order to maximize strength, power, or both.

TABLE 6-4 Rating of Perceived Exertion[65,66]

Scale	Verbal Rating
6	
7	Very, very light
8	
9	Very light
10	
11	Fairly light
12	
13	Somewhat hard
14	
15	Hard
16	
17	Very hard
18	
19	Very, very hard
20	

▶ *Undulating.* The nonlinear program enables variation in intensity and volume within each 7- to 10-day cycle by rotating different protocols over the course of the training program. Nonlinear methods attempt to train the various components of the neuromuscular system within the same 7- to 10-day cycle. During a single workout, only one characteristic is trained in a given day (e.g., strength, power, local muscular endurance).

It has been shown that systematically varying volume and intensity is most effective for long-term progression.[49c,57,58]

Rest Intervals. Rest is an important component of any exercise progression. The rest period must be sufficient to allow for muscular recuperation and development while alleviating the potential for overtraining; however, extended periods between sessions can result in detraining.[49a] The rest period between sets is determined by the time the breathing rate, or pulse, of the patient returns to the steady state. A 48-hour rest period between concurrent training sessions is generally recommended.[49c]

When prescribing a resistance-exercise regimen, the clinician, coach, or fitness instructor should consider the individual's current health and fitness status, goals, access to appropriate equipment, and time available for training.[53] Training programs prescribed for competitive athletes, which often include exercises designed specifically to improve the development of explosive power, are generally inappropriate for children, untrained adults, elderly persons, or patients with chronic disease(s). Exercise progression in the orthopedic population, including the postsurgical population (Chaps. 28 and 29), is determined by the stage of healing and the degree of irritability of the structure, which are factors of patient response, as healing relates to signs and symptoms.

▶ If pain is present before resistance or the end-feel, the patient's symptoms are considered irritable. The intervention in the presence of irritability should not be aggressive, particularly inclusive of exercise.[59]

▶ If pain occurs after resistance, then the patient's symptoms are not considered irritable and exercise, particularly stretching, can be more aggressive.

Increasing Muscle Endurance

To increase muscle endurance, exercises are performed against light resistance for many repetitions (no fewer than 20 per set), so that the amount of energy expended is equal to the amount of energy supplied. The nature of muscular endurance encourages the body to work aerobically. This phenomenon, called *steady state*, occurs after some 5 to 6 minutes of exercise at a constant intensity level. Working at a level to which the muscle is accustomed improves the endurance of that muscle but does not increase its strength.

It is well established that endurance training results in enhanced performance and delayed onset of fatigue during endurance exercise. As mitochondria characterize muscle oxygen demand, endurance exercise training has been the intervention of choice to explore the malleability of mitochondrial structure and function.[59a] During steady state, the rate of mitochondrial ATP production is closely matched to the rate of ATP hydrolysis and demonstrates the existence of efficient cellular mechanisms to control mitochondrial ATP synthesis in a wide dynamic range.[59b] Endurance exercise training produces an increase in mitochondrial volume density in all three muscle fiber types[59c] and thus muscle aerobic power. With a higher mitochondrial density in trained muscle, the rate of substrate flux per individual mitochondrion will be less at any given rate of ATP hydrolysis.[59b] Therefore, the required activation of mitochondrial respiration by ADP to achieve a given rate of ATP formation will be less, resulting in increased ADP sensitivity of muscle oxidative phosphorylation.[59b]

Endurance exercise training also leads to a shift of skeletal muscle mitochondria toward an increased use of lipids as a substrate source both at the same absolute and at the same relative exercise intensity.[59a,59d]

Muscular endurance training is typically prescribed during the general preparation phase of training to prepare the body for the increased work demands that will be required and to program the body's neuromuscular coordination systems.

The amount of weight used during muscular endurance training can be determined by using a relative perceived exertion (RPE) scale, in which 1 is very light exertion and 10 is intense exertion. Using the example of a bench press, if an athlete plans to work at around level 3 and his maximum weight for the bench press is 220 pounds, he should reduce his workout weight by 70 percent (154 pounds) and increase the number of repetitions.

The number of repetitions used is a factor of the speed of 1 rep, and how many reps the athlete can complete in 60 seconds. For example if, under normal training conditions,

the athlete takes 3 seconds to raise the weight during a biceps curl, and 3 seconds to lower it, the muscle is under tension for 6 seconds and the athlete is working at a speed of ten repetitions per minute. By increasing the speed of the repetition to 4 seconds (the time the muscle is under tension), the athlete must achieve at least 15 reps in order to build muscular endurance.

The major drawback to muscular endurance training is the increased potential for overuse injuries. This can be offset by manipulating one or more of the training variables, such as sets, loads, tempo, rest periods between sets, number of exercises, hand position, and grip width.

Increasing Muscle Power

Muscular power is the product of muscular force and velocity of muscle shortening. Maximum power occurs at approximately one third of maximum velocity.[60] Muscular power is an important contributor to activities requiring both speed and strength. Muscles with a predominance of fast-twitch fibers generate more power at a given load than those with a high composition of slow-twitch fibers.[61] The ratio for mean peak power production by type IIb, type IIa, and type I fibers in skeletal tissue is 10:5:1.[62]

Power is increased by having a muscle work dynamically against resistance within a specified period. In the context of rehabilitation, plyometric training can be viewed as the bridge between strength and power exercises.[63]

Plyometrics

Plyometric exercises were traditionally designed to enable lower extremity muscles—primarily the thighs, quadriceps, hamstrings, and calves—to attain maximal strength using high-intensity workouts in short spurts of hops, leaps, or bounds. Although it is not possible in this text to give a detailed description of all of the physiologic principles behind plyometrics, a brief summary is presented to increase the reader's awareness of the importance of this type of exercise in the rehabilitation program.

The training system of plyometrics is credited to Yuri Verhoshanski,[64] the renowned Soviet jump coach of the late 1960s, although the actual term *plyometrics* was first introduced in the mid-1970s by an American track coach Fred Wilt.[65] The term *plyometrics*, when broken down to the roots of the words, is a little confusing. *Plyo* comes from the Greek word *pleythein*, which means to increase, and *metric*, which means to measure. The traditional definition of plyometrics was associated with rapid movement involving a prestretch of the contracting muscle, which stores elastic energy in the muscle, and activates the myotatic reflex.[66–69] The muscle's ability to use the stored elastic energy is affected by time, the magnitude of the stretch, and the velocity of the stretch.[70]

The nerve receptors involved in plyometrics are the muscle spindle, the Golgi tendon organ, and the joint capsule/ligamentous receptors (see Chap. 2).

Movement patterns in both athletics and activities of daily living involve repeated stretch-shortening cycles, in which a downward eccentric movement must be stopped and converted into an upward concentric movement in a desired direction. The degree of enhanced muscle performance is dependent on the time frame between the eccentric and concentric contractions.[69]

Acceleration and deceleration are the most important components of all task-specific activities.[51] These activities use variable speed and resistance throughout the range of contraction, stimulating neurologic receptors and increasing their excitability. These neurologic receptors play an important role in fiber recruitment and physiologic coordination. Plyometric activities serve to improve the reactivity of these receptors by involving muscle stretch-shortening exercises, which consist of three distinct phases:

1. A setting, or eccentric, phase in which the muscle is eccentrically stretched and slowly loaded. This phase begins when the athlete mentally prepares for the activity and lasts until the stretch stimulus is initiated.[70]

2. A rapid amortization (reversal) phase. This phase is the amount of time between undergoing the yielding eccentric contraction and the initiation of a concentric force.[70] If the amortization phase is slow, elastic energy is wasted as heat and the stretch reflex is not activated.[70]

3. A concentric response contraction to develop a large amount of momentum and force.

By reproducing these stretch-shortening cycles at positions of physiologic function, plyometric activities stimulate proprioceptive feedback to fine-tune muscle activity patterns. Stretch-shortening exercise trains the neuromuscular system by exposing it to increased strength loads and improving the stretch reflex[70] (see Chap. 2).

The goal of plyometric training is to decrease the amount of time required between the yielding eccentric contraction and the initiation of the overcoming concentric contraction. This improvement is particularly useful in activities that require a maximum amount of muscular force in a minimum amount of time. These parameters are difficult to imitate using traditional exercise tools but are nonetheless a very important component of the rehabilitative process in order for the patient to make a safe return to sport.

Although plyometric exercises were primarily designed for the lower extremities, the exercises can also be used for the trunk and upper extremities. Before initiating plyometric exercises, the clinician must ensure that the patient has an adequate strength and physical condition base.[70] Minimal performance criteria for safe plyometrics include the ability to perform one repetition of a parallel squat with a load of body weight on the back (for jumps over 12 inches) for the lower extremity, and a bench press with one third of body weight for the upper extremity.[63] In addition, success in the static stability tests[63] (Table 6-5) and dynamic stability tests (vertical jump for the

TABLE 6-5 Static Stability Tests for Performance of Plyometrics[63]

1. Single-leg stance: 30 sec
   Eyes open
   Eyes closed

2. Single-leg quarter squat: 30 sec
   Eyes open
   Eyes closed

3. Single-leg half squat: 30 sec
   Eyes open
   Eyes closed

lower extremities and medicine ball throw for the upper extremities) may be used as a measure of preparation.[40] Initially, the patient is instructed to perform fewer sets and repetitions. Later, the patient is permitted to do more sets, but not more repetitions.

Many different activities and devices can be used in plyometric exercises. Plyometric exercises may include diagonal and multiplanar motions with tubing (Fig. 6.3) or isokinetic machines. These exercises may be used to mimic any of the needed motions and can be performed in the standing, sitting, or supine positions.

Lower Extremity Plyometric Exercises. Lower extremity plyometric exercises involve the manipulation of the role of gravity

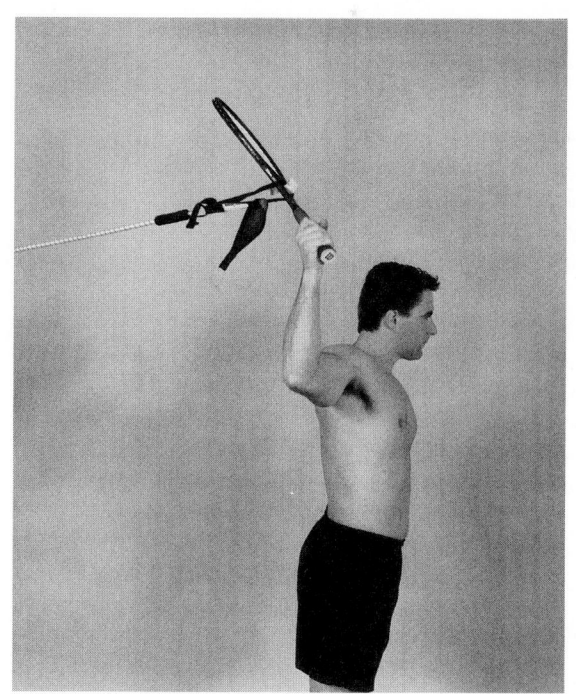

FIGURE 6-3 Plyometric exercise for tennis.

to vary the intensity of the exercise. Thus, plyometric exercises can be performed horizontally or vertically.

▶ Horizontal plyometrics are performed perpendicular to the line of gravity. These exercises are preferable for most initial clinical rehabilitation plans, because the concentric force is reduced and the eccentric phase is not facilitated.[40] Examples of these types of exercises include the sled and the leg press.

▶ Vertical plyometric exercises (against or with gravitational forces) are more advanced (Table 6-6). These exercises require a greater level of control.[40]

The footwear and landing surfaces used in plyometric drills must have shock-absorbing qualities, and the protocol should allow sufficient recovery time between sets to prevent fatigue of the muscle groups being trained.[71]

Upper Extremity Plyometric Exercises.   Plyometric exercises for the upper extremity involve relatively rapid movements in planes that approximate normal joint function. For example, at the shoulder this would include 90-degree abduction in shoulder, trunk rotation and diagonal arm motions, and rapid external and internal rotation exercises.

Plyometrics should be performed for all body segments involved in the activity. Hip rotation, knee flexion and extension, and trunk rotation are power activities that require plyometric activation.

Plyometric exercises for the upper extremity include wall push-offs (Fig. 6-4), corner push-ups, box push-offs (Fig. 6-5), and weighted ball throws (Fig. 6-6). Medicine and other weighted balls are very effective plyometric devices (Fig. 6-7). The weight of the ball creates a prestretch and an eccentric load when it is caught. This combination creates resistance and demands a powerful agonist contraction to propel it forward again. The exercises can be performed using one arm (see Fig. 6-6) or both arms at the same time (Fig. 6-8). The former emphasizes trunk rotation and the latter emphasizes trunk extension and flexion, as well as shoulder motion.

Although force-dependent motor firing patterns should be reestablished, special care must be taken to completely

TABLE 6-6   Lower Extremity Plyometric Drills[63]

WARM-UP DRILLS	ADVANCED-LEVEL DRILLS
Double-leg squats	*Single-leg box jumps*
Double-leg leg press	One-box side jumps
Double-leg squat-jumps	Two-box side jumps
Jumping jacks	Single-leg plyometric leg press (4 corners)
	Two-box side jumps with foam
ENTRY-LEVEL DRILLS–TWO LEGGED	Four-box diagonal jumps
Two-legged drills	One-box side jumps with rotation
Side-to-side (floor/line)	Two-box side jumps with rotation
Diagonal jumps (floor/4 corners)	One-box side jump with catch
Diagonal jumps (4 spots)	One-box side jump rotation with catch
Diagonal zig-zag (6 spots)	Two-box side jump with catch
Plyometric leg press	Two-box side jump rotation with catch
Plyometric leg press (4 corners)	
	ENDURANCE/AGILITY PLYOMETRICS
INTERMEDIATE-LEVEL DRILLS	Side-to-side bounding (20 ft)
Two-legged box jumps	Side jump lunges (cone)
One-box side jump	Side jump lunges (cone with foam)
Two-box side jumps	Altering rapid step-up (forward)
Two-box side jumps with foam	Lateral step-overs
Four-box diagonal jumps	High stepping (forward)
Two-box with rotation	High stepping (backward)
One/two-box with catch	Depth jump with rebound jump
One/two-box with catch (foam)	Depth jump with catch
	Jump and catch (plyoball)
Single-leg movements	
Single-leg plyometric leg press	
Single-leg side jumps (floor)	
Single-leg side-to-side jumps (floor/4 corners)	
Single-leg diagonal jumps (floor/4 corners)	

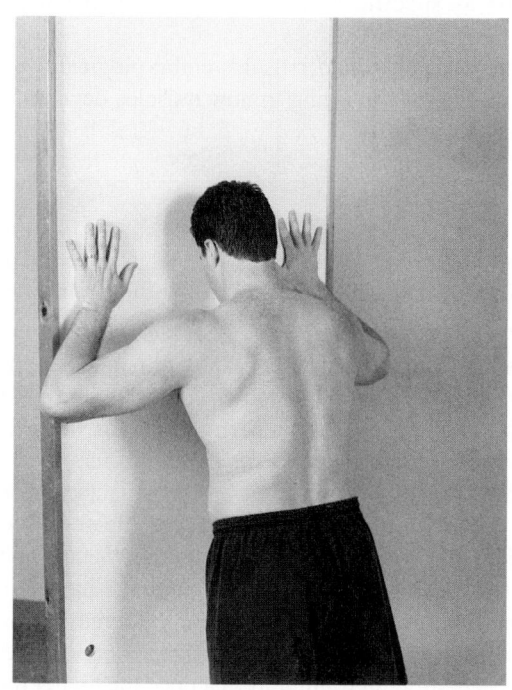

FIGURE 6-4   Wall push-off.

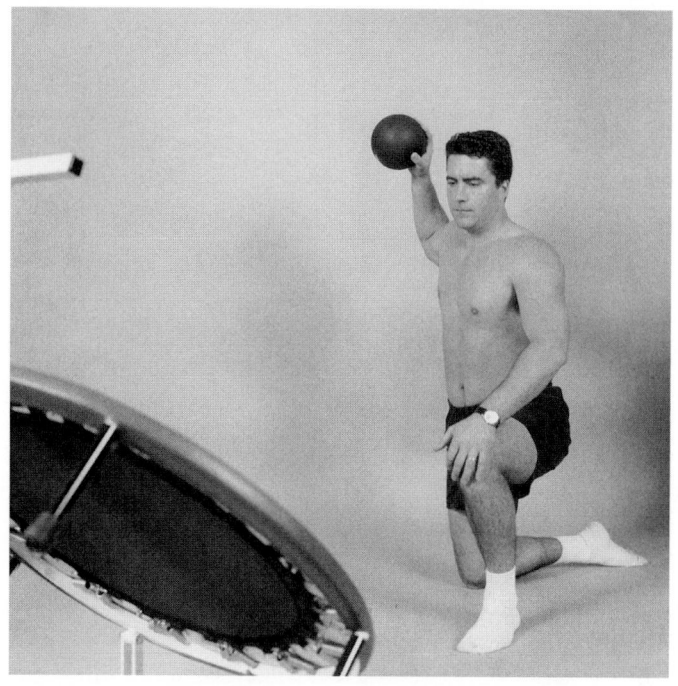

FIGURE 6-6   Weighted ball toss.

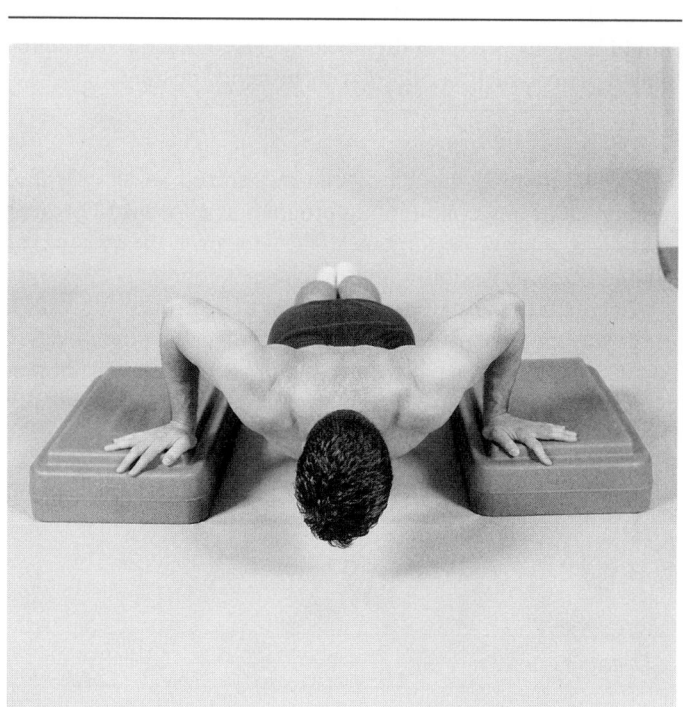

FIGURE 6-5   Box push-off.

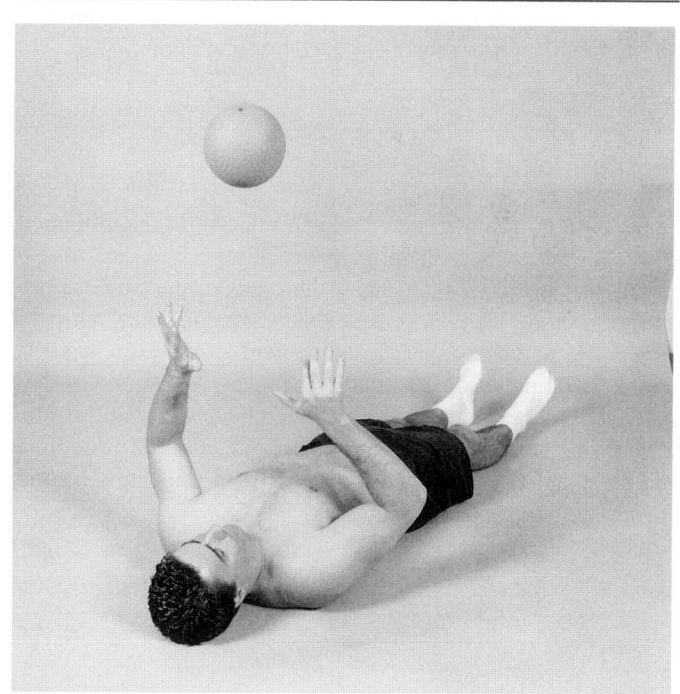

FIGURE 6-7   Medicine ball exercise.

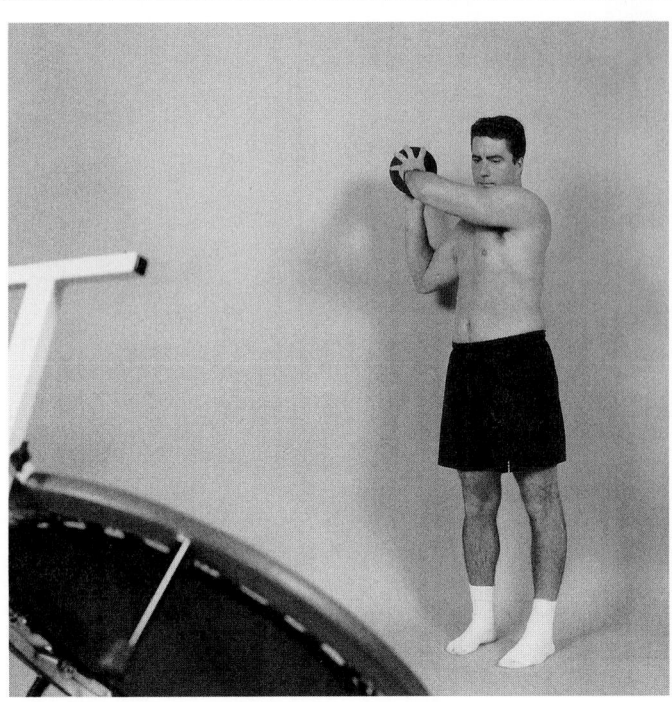

FIGURE 6-8   Double hand toss with trunk rotation.

integrate all of the components of the kinetic chain to generate and funnel the proper forces to the appropriate joint.

Specificity of Training

Specificity of training is an accepted concept in rehabilitation. This concept involves the principle of the specific adaptation to imposed demand (SAID). Thus, the focus of the exercise prescription should be to improve the strength and coordination of functional or sports-specific movements with exercises that approximate the desired activity.

The SAID principle can be applied by exercising the muscles along each extremity and within the trunk in functional patterns.[72] The exercise component of the intervention

should be as specific as the manual technique used in the clinic.

Patten[73] has classified muscles embryologically into tonic and phasic groups according to how muscles develop from the myotomes[70] (Table 6-7).

> ### Clinical Pearl
>
> In general, tonic muscles function as endurance (postural) muscles, whereas phasic muscles function as the power muscles.[74,75]

Speed-strength training applies the principles of specificity of training and is typically used with highly conditioned athletes who want to take their performance to the next level. Speed-strength training involves taking some of the basic movements of a task and increasing the resistance. For sports, such as baseball and golf, athletes can use devices, such as an oversized ball or weighted golf club, to train the arms and trunk to work against a greater resistance. Sprinters have long benefited from the use of a small parachute to increase wind resistance, or by dragging a tire fastened by a rope. The theory behind speed-strength training is that once the higher resistance is removed the athlete's speed is improved when they perform the activity under normal resistance. Wherever possible, strength testing by the clinician should assess the function of a muscle. If a power muscle is assessed, its ability to produce power should be assessed. In contrast, an endurance muscle should be tested for its ability to sustain a contraction for a prolonged period, such as occurs with sustained postures.

Increasing Flexibility

Flexibility training has long been recognized as an essential component of any conditioning program as a means to prevent injury and improve performance.[76–80] However, the question of whether muscle flexibility or stretching before activity results in a decrease in muscle injuries has yet to be proven.[9,76,81–84]

The techniques of stretching all involve the stretch reflex (see Chap. 2). A reflex is a programmed unit of behavior in which a certain type of stimulus from a receptor automatically leads to the response of an effector.

To stretch a muscle appropriately, the stretch must be applied parallel to the muscle fibers. The orientation of the

TABLE 6-7   The Various Muscle Types and Their Primary Innervation[70]

Muscle Type	Characteristics	Primary Innervation	Examples
Type I	Tonic Slow twitch Small neuron	Type 1a phasic nerve endings	Extensors External rotators Abductors
Types IIa and IIb	Phasic Fast twitch Large neuron	Anterior divisions of the nerve plexus	Flexors Adductors Two-joint muscles

fibers can be determined by palpation. Typically, in the extremities, the muscle fibers run parallel to the bone. Viscoelastic changes are not permanent, whereas plasticity changes, which are more difficult to achieve, result in a residual or permanent change in length. Frequent stretching ensures that the lengthening is maintained before the muscle has the opportunity to recoil to its shortened state.[85]

It is important for the patient to realize that the initial session of stretching may increase symptoms.[86] However, this increase in symptoms should be temporary, lasting for a couple of hours, at most.[85,87] The stretch should be performed at the point just shy of the pain, although some discomfort may be necessary to achieve results.[88] The muscle usually requires a greater stretching force initially, possibly to break up adhesions or cross-linkages, and to allow for viscoelastic and plastic changes to occur in the collagen and elastin fibers.[88]

Static Flexibility

Static flexibility is defined as the passive range or motion available to a joint or series of joints.[76,80] Increased static flexibility should not be confused with joint hypermobility, or laxity, which is a function of the joint capsule and ligaments. Decreased static flexibility indicates a loss of motion. The end-feel (see Chap. 8) encountered may help the clinician differentiate the cause among adaptive shortening of the muscle (muscle stretch), a tight joint capsule (capsular), and an arthritic joint (hard). Static flexibility can be measured by a goniometer or by a number of tests, such as the toe touch and the sit and reach, all of which have been found to be valid and reliable.[89,90]

Dynamic Flexibility

Dynamic flexibility refers to the ease of movement within the obtainable range of motion. Dynamic flexibility is measured actively. The important measurement in dynamic flexibility is *stiffness*, a mechanical term defined as the resistance of a structure to deformation.[91,92] An increase in range of motion around a joint does not necessarily equate to a decrease in the passive stiffness of a muscle.[93–95] However, strength training, immobilization, and aging have been shown to increase stiffness.[96–99] The converse of stiffness is pliability. When a soft tissue demonstrates a decrease in pliability, it has usually undergone an adaptive shortening, or an increase in tone, termed *hypertonus*.

Methods of Stretching

A variety of stretching techniques can be used to increase the extensibility of the soft tissues.

Passive Stretching. Passive stretching can be performed by the clinician or another individual partner. Because of the higher risk of injury with this type of stretching when the operator is unskilled, it should be administered only after close supervision, and with the assurance that there is excellent communication between the operator and the patient. Ideally, the passive stretch should involve a gentle, controlled, low-intensity, and prolonged elongation of the tissues.

TABLE 6-8 Progressive Velocity Flexibility Program[100]

Static stretching
↓
SSER (slow, short-end-range stretching)
↓
FSER (fast, short-end-range stretching)
↓
FFR (fast, full-range stretching)

Static Stretching. Static stretching involves the application of a steady force for a sustained period (Table 6-8). Small loads applied for long periods produce greater residual lengthening than heavy loads applied for short periods.[101] Weighted traction or pulley systems may be used for this type of stretching.

> ### Clinical Pearl
>
> Applying small loads to tendons for 20 minutes or more in an exercise session is necessary for adequate soft-tissue lengthening to occur.[101,102]

Ballistic Stretching. This technique of stretching uses bouncing movements to stretch a particular muscle. In comparisons of the ballistic and static methods, two studies[103,104] have found that both produce similar improvements in flexibility. However, this method appears to cause more residual muscle soreness or muscle strain, than those techniques that incorporate relaxation into the technique.[105–107]

Neuromuscular Facilitation. The proprioceptive neuromuscular facilitation (PNF) techniques of hold-relax, stretch-relax, and agonist contract-relax can be used to actively stretch the soft tissues (see Chap. 11). The majority of studies have shown the PNF technique to be the most effective stretching technique for increasing range of motion through muscle lengthening when compared with the static or slow-sustained, and the ballistic or bounce techniques,[79,108–111] although one study found it to be not necessarily better.[112]

Delayed Onset Muscle Soreness

Muscular soreness may result from all forms of exercise. One type of soreness that is a potential negative effect related to eccentric exercise is delayed-onset muscle soreness (DOMS).[47] This type of soreness, which occurs between 48 and 72 hours after exercise, may last up to 10 days. Prevention of this type of muscle soreness involves careful design of the eccentric program, including prepatory techniques, accurate training variables, and appropriate aftercare.[47] The intervention for DOMS includes aerobic submaximal exercise with no eccentric component (swimming, biking, or stepper machines), pain-free flexibility exercises, and high-speed (300 degrees per second) concentric-only isokinetic training.[47,113]

Muscle and Aging

With age, there is a reduction in the ability to produce and sustain muscular power. This age-related phenomenon, termed *senescence sarcopenia*, can result in a 20 to 25 percent loss of skeletal muscle mass.[114]

> ### Clinical Pearl
>
> Sarcopenia (*sarco* = muscle, *penia* = lack of) is not a disease, but rather refers specifically to the universal, involuntary decline in lean body mass that occurs with age, primarily as a result of the loss of skeletal muscle.

Sarcopenia has important consequences. The loss of lean body mass reduces function, and loss of approximately 40 percent of lean body mass is fatal.[115,116] Sarcopenia is distinct from wasting—involuntary weight loss resulting from inadequate intake, which is seen in starvation, advanced cancer, or acquired immunodeficiency syndrome.

Whereas a variety of studies have investigated the underlying mechanisms and treatments of age-related muscle loss, very few epidemiologic studies have looked at the prevalence, incidence, pathogenesis, and consequences of sarcopenia in elderly populations. It is likely that the determinants of sarcopenia are multifactorial and include genetic factors, environmental factors, and age-related changes in muscle tissue.[117]

The effects of aging on muscle morphology have been studied. Aging causes a decrease in muscle volume,[118] with type II fiber apparently being more affected by gradual atrophy.[119] Specifically, there is a disproportionate atrophy of type IIa muscle fibers with aging. These losses of muscular strength and muscle mass can have important health consequences, because they can predispose the elderly to disability, an increased risk of falls and hip fractures, and a decrease in bone mineral density.

> ### Clinical Pearl
>
> When older people maintain muscular activity, the losses in strength with age are reduced substantially. Age-related muscle fiber atrophy and weakness may be completely reversed in some individuals with resistance training.[120,121]

REVIEW QUESTIONS*

1. What are the four biomechanical properties of skeletal muscle?
2. Give three examples of a muscle that cross two or more joints.

* Additional questions to test your understanding of this chapter can be found in the Online Learning Center for *Orthopaedic Assessment, Evaluation, and Intervention* at www.duttononline.net.

3. What are the three main types of muscle contraction?
4. Define the characteristics of an isotonic contraction.
5. True/false: Rapid lengthening contractions generate more force than do slower lengthening contractions.

REFERENCES

1. Hall SJ. The biomechanics of human skeletal muscle. In: Hall SJ, ed. *Basic Biomechanics*. New York, NY: McGraw-Hill; 1999:146–185.
2. MacConnail MA, Basmajian JV. *Muscles and Movements: A Basis for Human Kinesiology*. New York, NY: Robert Krieger; 1977.
3. Luttgens K, Hamilton K. The musculoskeletal system: The musculature. In: Luttgens K, Hamilton K, eds. *Kinesiology: Scientific Basis of Human Motion*. New York: McGraw-Hill; 1997:49–75.
4. Astrand PO, Rodahl K. *The Muscle and Its Contraction: Textbook of Work Physiology*. New York, NY: McGraw-Hill; 1986.
5. Komi PV. *Strength and Power in Sport*. London, England: Blackwell; 1992.
6. McArdle W, et al. *Exercise Physiology: Energy, Nutrition, and Human Performance*. Philadelphia, Pa: Lea and Febiger; 1991.
7. Lakomy HKA. The biomechanics of human movement. In: Maughan RJ, ed. *Basic and Applied Sciences for Sports Medicine*. Woburn, Mass: Butterworth-Heinemann; 1999:124–125.
8. Elftman H. Biomechanics of muscle. *J Bone Joint Surg* 1966;48A:363.
9. Worrell TW, et al. Comparison of isokinetic strength and flexibility measures between hamstring injured and non-injured athletes. *J Orthop Sports Phys Ther* 1991;13:118–125.
10. Anderson MA, et al. The relationship among isokinetic, isotonic, and isokinetic concentric and eccentric quadriceps and hamstrings force and three components of athletic performance. *J Orthop Sports Phys Ther* 1991;14:114–120.
11. Steadman JR, Forster RS, Silfverskold JP. Rehabilitation of the knee. *Clin Sports Med* 1989;8:605–627.
12. Montgomery JB, Steadman JR. Rehabilitation of the injured knee. *Clin Sports Med* 1985;4:333–343.
13. Delsman PA, Losee GM. Isokinetic shear forces and their effect on the quadriceps active drawer. *Med Sci Sports Exerc* 1984;16:151.
14. Albert MS. Principles of exercise progression. In: Greenfield B, ed. *Rehabilitation of the Knee: A Problem Solving Approach*. Philadelphia, Pa: FA Davis; 1993.
15. Deudsinger RH. Biomechanics in clinical practice. *Phys Ther* 1984;64:1860–1868.
16. Desmedt JE, Godaux E. Fast motor units are not preferentially activated in rapid voluntary contractions in man. *Nature* 1977;267:717.
17. Gans C. Fiber architecture and muscle function. *Exerc Sport Sci Rev*; 1982;10:160.
18. Nilsson J, Tesch PA, Thorstensson A. Fatigue and EMG of repeated fast and voluntary contractions in man. *Acta Physiol Scand* 1977;101:194.
19. Sell S, Zacher J, Lack S. Disorders of proprioception of arthrotic knee joint. *Z Rheumatol* 1993;52:150–155.
20. Mattacola CG, Lloyd JW. Effects of a 6-week strength and proprioception training program on measures of dynamic balance: A single case design. *J Athl Training* 1997;32:127–135.
21. Edman KA, Reggiani C. The sarcomere length-tension relation determined in short segments of intact muscle fibres of the frog. *J Physiol* 1987;385:729–732.

22. Boeckmann RR, Ellenbecker TS. Biomechanics. In: Ellenbecker TS, ed. *Knee Ligament Rehabilitation*. Philadelphia, Pa: Churchill Livingstone; 2000:16–23.

23. Brownstein B, Noyes FR, Mangine RE, Kryger S, et al. Anatomy and biomechanics. In: Mangine RE, ed. *Physical Therapy of the Knee*. New York, NY: Churchill Livingstone; 1988:1–30.

24. Teitz CC, Garrett WE Jr, Miniaci A, Lee MH, Mann RA. Tendon problems in athletic individuals. *J Bone Joint Surg* 1997;79A: 138–152.

25. Komi PV. The stretch-shortening cycle and human power output. In: Jones NL, McCartney N, McComas AJ, eds. *Human Muscle Power*. Champlain, Ill: Human Kinetics; 1986:27.

26. Malone T, et al. Neuromuscular concepts. In: Ellenbecker TS, ed. *Knee Ligament Rehabilitation*. Philadelphia, Pa: Churchill Livingstone; 2000:399–411.

27. Williams JH, Klug GA. Calcium exchange hypothesis of skeletal muscle fatigue. A brief review. *Muscle Nerve* 1995;18:421.

28. Allen DG, Lannergren J, Westerblad H. Muscle cell function during prolonged activity: Cellular mechanisms of fatigue. *Exp Physiol* 1995;80:497.

29. Rosenbaum D, Henning EM. The influence of stretching and warm-up exercises on Achilles tendon reflex activity. *J Sports Sci* 1995;13:481.

30. Astrand PO, Rodahl K. *Physical Training: Textbook of Work Physiology*. New York, NY: McGraw-Hill; 1986.

31. Lash JM. Regulation of skeletal muscle blood flow during contractions. *Proc Soc Exp Biol Med* 1996;211:218–235.

31a. Rhea MR, Alvar BA, Burkett LN, Ball SD. A meta-analysis to determine the dose response for strength development. *Med Sci Sports Exer* 2003;35:456–464.

31b. Pollock ML, Gaesser GA, Butcher JD, et al. The recommended quantity and quality of exercise for developing and maintaining cardiorespiratory and muscular fitness, and flexibility in healthy adults: American College of Sports Medicine Position Stand. *Med Sci Sports Exerc* 1998;30:975–991.

32. Matsen FA III, Lippitt SB, Sidles JA, et al. Strength. In: Matsen FA III, et al, eds. *Practical Evaluation and Management of the Shoulder*. Philadelphia, Pa: WB Saunders; 1994:111–150.

33. Kisner C, Colby LA. *Therapeutic Exercise. Foundations and Techniques*. Philadelphia, Pa: FA Davis; 1997.

34. DeLorme T, Watkins A. *Techniques of Progressive Resistance Exercise*. New York, NY: Appleton-Century; 1951.

35. Soest A, Bobbert M. The role of muscle properties in control of explosive movements. *Biol Cybern* 1993;69:195–204.

36. Bandy W, Lovelace-Chandler V, Bandy B, et al. Adaptation of skeletal muscle to resistance training. *J Orthop Sports Phys Ther* 1990;12:248–255.

36a. Luethi JM, Howald H, Claassen H, Roesler K, Vock P, Hoppeler H. Structural changes in skeletal muscle tissue with heavy-resistance exercise. *Int J Sports Med* 1986;7:123–127.

36b. Hoppeler H, Fluck M. Plasticity of skeletal muscle mitochondria: structure and function. *Med Sci Sports Exer* 2003;35:95–104.

36c. Tesch PA, Larsson L. Muscle hypertrophy in bodybuilders. *Eur J Appl Physiol* 1982;49:301–306.

36d. Moritani T, de Vries HA. Neural factors vs. hypertrophy in the time course of muscle strength gain. *Am J Phys Med* 1979;58:115–130.

36e. Jones DA, Rutherford OM. Human muscle strength training: The effects of three different regimes and the nature of the resultant changes. *J Physiol* 1987;391:1–11.

36f. Gollinck PD, Timson BF, Moore RL, Riedy M. Muscular enlargement and number of muscle fibers in skeletal muscles of rats. *J Appl Physiol* 1981;50:936–943.

36g. Hakkinen K, Alen M, Komi PV. Changes in isometric force and relaxation time, electromyographic and muscle fibre characteristics of human skeletal muscle during strength training and de-training. *Acta Physiol Scand* 1985;125:573–585.

37. Hettinger T. *Isometrisches Muskeltraining*. Stuttgart, Germany: M Thun; 1964.

38. Mueller K. *Statische und Dynamische Muskelkraft*. Frankfurt, Germany: M Thun; 1987.

39. Green DJ, O'Driscoll G, Blanksby BA, Taylor RR. Control of skeletal blood flow during dynamic exercise: Contribution of endothelial derived nitric oxide. *Sports Med* 1996;21:119–146.

40. Albert M. Concepts of muscle training. In: Wadsworth C, ed. *Orthopaedic Physical Therapy: Topic—Strength and Conditioning Applications in Orthopaedics*. Home Study Course 98A. La Crosse, Wis: Orthopaedic Section, American Physical Therapy Association; 1998.

41. Albert MS. *Eccentric Muscle Training in Sports and Orthopedics*. 2nd ed. New York, NY: Churchill Livingstone; 1995.

42. Clark MA. *Integrated Training for the New Millenium*. Thousand Oaks, Calif: National Academy of Sports Medicine; 2001.

43. Lange GW, Hintermeister RA, Schlegel T, Dillman CJ, Steadman JR. Electromyographic and kinematic analysis of graded treadmill walking and the implications for knee rehabilitation. *J Orthop Sports Phys Ther* 1996;23:294–301.

44. Antich TJ, Brewster CE. Rehabilitation of the nonreconstructed anterior cruciate ligament-deficient knee. *Clin Sports Med* 1988;7:813–826.

45. Bynum EB, Barrack RL, Alexander AH. Open versus closed kinetic chain exercises in rehabilitation after anterior cruciate ligament reconstruction: A prospective randomized study. In: *Annual Conference of the American Academy of Orthopaedic Surgeons*. New Orleans, La: 1994.

46. Mangine RE, Noyes FR, DeMaio M. Minimal protection program: Advanced weight bearing and range of motion after ACL reconstruction—Weeks 1 to 5. *Orthopedics* 1992;15:504–515.

47. Steadman JR. Rehabilitation of acute injuries of the anterior cruciate ligament. *Clin Orthop* 1983;172:129–132.

47a. Steadman JR, Forster RS, Silfverskold JP. Rehabilitation of the knee. *Clin Sports Med*, 1989;8:605–627.

48. Steadman JR, Sterett WI. The surgical treatment of knee injuries in skiers. *Med Sci Sports Exerc* 1995;27:328–333.

49. Zappala FG, Taffel CB, Scuderi GR. Rehabilitation of patellofemoral joint disorders. *Orthop Clin North Am* 1992;23:555–565.

49a. Simoneau GG, et al. Biomechanics of elastic resistance in therapeutic exercise programs. *J Ortho Sports Phys Ther* 2001;31:16–24.

49b. Rogers ME, et al. Effects of dumbbell and elastic band training on physical function in older inner-city African-American women. *Women & Health* 2002;36:33–41.

49c. Pollock ML, Gaesser GA, Butcher JD, et al. The recommended quantity and quality of exercise for developing and maintaining cardiorespiratory and muscular fitness, and flexibility in healthy adults: American College of Sports Medicine Position Stand. *Med Sci Sports Exerc* 1998;30:975–991.

49d. Fleck SJ, Kraemer WJ. *Designing Resistance Training Programs*, 2 ed. Champaign Ill: Human Kinetics Books; 1997.

49e. Deschenes MR, Kraemer WJ. Performance and physiologic adaptations to resistance training. *Am J Phys Med Rehab* 2002;81:S3–S16.

49f. Grimby G, Thomee R. Principles of rehabilitation after injuries. In: Dirix A, Knuttgen HG, Tittel K, eds. *The Olympic Book of*

Sports Medicine, Vol 1. Oxford, England: Blackwell Scientific Publications; 1984.

50. Thomee R, Renstrom P, Grimby G, Peterson L. Slow or fast isokinetic training after surgery. *J Orthop Sports Phys Ther* 1987;8:476.

51. Albert M. Concepts of muscle training. In: Wadsworth C, ed. *Orthopaedic Physical Therapy: Topic—Strength and Conditioning Applications in Orthopaedics*. Home Study Course 98A. La Crosse, Wis: Orthopaedic Section, American Physical Therapy Association; 1998.

52. Grimsby O, Power B. Manual therapy approach to knee ligament rehabilitation. In: Ellenbecker TS, ed. *Knee Ligament Rehabilitation*. Philadelphia, Pa. Churchill Livingstone, 2000;236–251.

53. Hass CJ, Feigenbaum MS, Franklin BA. Prescription of resistance training for healthy populations. *Sports Med* 2001;31:953–964.

54. Graves JE, Pollock SH, Leggett SH, et al. Effect of reduced training frequency on muscular strength. *Sports Med* 1988; 9:316–19.

55. Borg GAV. Psychophysical basis of perceived exertion. *Med Sci Sports Exerc* 1992;14:377–381.

56. Borg GAV. Perceived exertion as an indicator of somatic stress. *Scand J Rehabil Med* 1970;2:92–98.

57. Pearson D, Faigenbaum A, Conley M, et al. The National Strength and Conditioning Association's basic guidelines for resistance training of athletes. *Strength Cond* 2000;22:14–27.

58. Kraemer WJ, Ratamess NA, Fry AC, et al. Influence of resistance training volume and periodization on physiological and performance adaptations in collegiate tennis players. *Am J Sports Med* 2000; 28:626–633.

59. Cyriax J. *Textbook of Orthopaedic Medicine, Diagnosis of Soft Tissue Lesions*, 8th ed. London: Bailliere Tindall; 1982.

59a. Hoppeler H, Fluck M. Plasticity of skeletal muscle mitochondria: structure and function. *Med Sci Sports Exerc* 2003;35:95–104.

59b. Tonkonogi M, Sahlin K. Physical exercise and mitochondrial function in human skeletal muscle. *Exerc Sport Sci Rev* 2002;30:129–137.

59c. Howald H, Hoppeler H, Claassen H, Mathieu O, Straub R: Influences of endurance training on the ultrastructural composition of the different muscle fiber types in humans. *Pflugers Arch* 1985;403:369–376.

59d. Holloszy JO, Coyle EF. Adaptations of skeletal muscle to endurance exercise and their metabolic consequences. *J Appl Physiol* 1984;56:831–838.

60. Hill AV. The heat and shortening and the dynamic constants of muscle. *Proc R Soc Lond* 1938;B126:136.

61. Tihanyi J, Apor P, Fekete GY. Force-velocity–power characteristics and fiber composition in human knee extensor muscles. *Eur J Appl Physiol* 1982;48:331.

62. Fitts RH, Widrick JJ. Muscle mechanics; adaptations with exercise training. *Exerc Sport Sci Rev* 1996;24:427.

63. Voight ML, Draovitch P, Tippett SR. Plyometrics. In: Albert MS, ed. *Eccentric Muscle Training in Sports and Orthopedics*. New York, NY: Churchill Livingstone; 1995;67–98.

64. Verhoshanski Y, Chornonson G. Jump exercises in sprint training. *Track Field Quart* 1967;9:1909.

65. Wilt F. Plyometrics—what it is and how it works. *Athletic J* 1975;55b:76.

66. Assmussen E, Bonde-Peterson F. Storage of elastic energy in skeletal muscle in man. *Acta Physiol Scand* 1974;91:385–392.

67. Bosco C, Komi PV. Potentiation of the mechanical behavior of the human skeletal muscle through prestretching. *Acta Physiol Scand* 1979;106:467–472.

68. Cavagna GA, Saibene FP, Margaria R. Effect of negative work on the amount of positive work performed by an isolated muscle. *J Appl Physiol* 1965;20:157.

69. Cavagna GA, Disman B, Margarai R. Positive work done by a previously stretched muscle. *J Appl Physiol* 1968;24:21–32.

70. Wilk KE, Voight ML, Keirns ME, Gambetta V, Andrews JR, Dillman CJ. Stretch-shortening drills for the upper extremities: Theory and clinical application. *J Orthop Sports Phys Ther* 1993;17:225–239.

71. Wathen D. Literature review: Explosive/plyometric exercises. *NSCA J* 1993;15:16–19.

72. Palmitier RA, An KN, Scott SG, Chao EY. Kinetic chain exercises in knee rehabilitation. *Sports Med* 1991;11:402–413.

73. Patten BM. *Human Embryology*. New York, NY: McGraw-Hill; 1953.

74. Janda V. *Muscle Function Testing*. London, England: Butterworths; 1983:163–167.

75. Jull GA, Janda V. Muscle and motor control in low back pain. In: Twomey LT, Taylor JR, eds. *Physical Therapy of the Low Back: Clinics in Physical Therapy*. New York, NY: Churchill Livingstone; 1987:258.

76. Gleim GW, McHugh MP. Flexibility and its effects on sports injury and performance. *Sports Med* 1997;24:289–299.

77. Payne KA, Berg K, Latin RW. Ankle injuries and ankle strength, flexibility and proprioception in college basketball players. *J Athl Training* 1997;32:221–225.

78. Saal JS. Flexibility training. In: *Physical Medicine and Rehabilitation: State of the Art Reviews*. Philadelphia, Pa: Hanley and Belfus; 1987:537–554.

79. Sady SP, Wortman MA, Blanke D. Flexibility training: Ballistic, static or proprioceptive neuromuscular facilitation? *Arch Phys Med Rehab* 1982;63:261–263.

80. American Orthopaedic Society for Sports Medicine. *Flexibility*. Chicago, Ill: AOSSM; 1988.

81. Worrell TW, Perrin DH. Hamstring muscle injury: The influence of strength, flexibility, warm-up, and fatigue. *J Orthop Sports Phys Ther* 1992;16:12–18.

82. Sutton G. Hamstrung by hamstring strains: A review of the literature. *J Orthop Sports Phys Ther* 1984;5:184–195.

83. Worrell TW. Factors associated with hamstring injuries: An approach to treatment and preventative measures. *Sports Med* 1994;17:338–345.

84. Jonhagen S, Nemeth G, Eriksson E. Hamstring injuries in sprinters: The role of concentric and eccentric hamstring strength and flexibility. *Am J Sports Med* 1994;22:262–266.

85. Kottke FJ. Therapeutic exercise to maintain mobility. In: Kottke FJ, Stillwell GK, Lehman JF, eds. *Krusen's Handbook of Physical Medicine and Rehabilitation*. Baltimore, Md: WB Saunders; 1982:389–402.

86. Travell JG, Simons DG. *Myofascial Pain and Dysfunction: The Trigger Point Manual*. Baltimore, Md: Williams and Wilkins; 1983.

87. Swezey RL. Arthrosis. In: Basmajian JV, Kirby RL, eds. *Medical Rehabilitation*. Baltimore, Md: Williams and Wilkins; 1984:216–218.

88. Joynt RL. Therapeutic exercise. In: DeLisa JA, ed. *Rehabilitation Medicine: Principles and Practice*. Philadelphia, Pa: JB Lippincott; 1988:346–371.

89. Kippers V, Parker AW. Toe-touch test: A measure of validity. *Phys Ther* 1987;67:1680–1684.

90. Jackson AW, Baker AA. The relationship of the sit and reach test to criterion measures of hamstring and back flexibility in young females. *Res Q Exerc Sport* 1986;57:183–186.

91. Litsky AS, Spector M. Biomaterials. In: Simon SR, ed. *Orthopaedic Basic Science*. Chicago, Ill: American Orthopaedic Society for Sports Medicine; 1994:447–486.

92. Johns R, Wright V. Relative importance of various tissues in joint stiffness. *J Appl Physiol* 1962;17:824–830.

93. Toft E, Espersen GT, Kalund S, Sinkjaer T, Hornemann BC. Passive tension of the ankle before and after stretching. *Am J Sports Med* 1989;17:489–494.

94. Halbertsma JPK, Goeken LNH. Stretching exercises: Effect of passive extensibility and stiffness in short hamstrings of healthy subjects. *Arch Phys Med Rehab* 1994;75:976–981.

95. Magnusson SP, Simonsen EB, Aagaard P, Sorensen H, Kjaer M. A mechanism for altered flexibility in human skeletal muscle. *J Physiol* 1996;497:291–298.

96. Klinge K, Magnusson SP, Simonsen EB, Aagaard P, Klausen K, Kjaer M. The effect of strength and flexibility on skeletal muscle EMG activity, stiffness and viscoelastic stress relaxation response. *Am J Sports Med* 1997;25:710–716.

97. Lapier TK, Burton HW, Almon RF. Alterations in intramuscular connective tissue after limb casting affect contraction-induced muscle injury. *J Appl Physiol* 1995;78:1065–1069.

98. McNair PJ, Wood GA, Marshall RN. Stiffness of the hamstring muscles and its relationship to function in ACL-deficient individuals. *Clin Biomech* 1992;7:131–137.

99. McHugh MP, Magnusson SP, Gleim GW, et al. A cross-sectional study of age-related musculoskeletal and physiological changes in soccer players. *Med Exerc Nutr Health* 1993;2:261–268.

100. Zachazewski JE. Flexibility for sports. In: Sanders B, ed. *Sports Physical Therapy*. Norwalk, Conn: Appleton and Lange; 1990:201–238.

101. Yoder E. Physical therapy management of nonsurgical hip problems in adults. In: Echternach JL, ed. *Physical Therapy of the Hip*. New York, NY: Churchill Livingstone; 1990:103–137.

102. Bohannon RW. Effect of repeated eight-minute muscle loading on the angle of straight-leg-raising. *Phys Ther* 1984;64:491.

103. DeVries HA. Evaluation of static stretching procedures for improvement of flexibility. *Res Quart* 1962;33:222–229.

104. Logan GA, Egstrom GH. Effects of slow and fast stretching on sacrofemoral angle. *J Assoc Phys Ment Rehabil* 1961;15:85–89.

105. Davies CT, White MJ. Muscle weakness following eccentric work in man. *Pflugers Arch* 1981;392:168–171.

106. Friden J, Sjostrom M, Ekblom B. A morphological study of delayed muscle soreness. *Experientia* 1981;37:506–507.

107. Hardy L. Improving active range of hip flexion. *Res Q Exerc Sport* 1985;56:111–114.

108. Markos PD. Ipsilateral and contralateral effects of proprioceptive neuromuscular facilitation techniques on hip motion and electromyographic activity. *Phys Ther* 1979;59:1366.

109. Holt LE, Travis TM, Okita T. Comparative study of three stretching techniques. *Percep Motor Skills* 1970;31:611–616.

110. Tanigawa MC. Comparison of hold-relax procedure and passive mobilization on increasing muscle length. *Phys Ther* 1972;52:725–735.

111. Prentice WE. A comparison of static stretching and PNF stretching for improving hip joint flexibility. *Athl Train* 1983;18:56–59.

112. Hartley-O'Brien SJ. Six mobilization exercises for active range of hip flexion. *Res Quart* 1980;51:625–635.

113. Hasson S, Barnes W, Hunter M, Williams J, et al. Therapeutic effect of high-speed voluntary muscle contractions on muscle soreness and muscle performance. *J Orthop Sports Phys Ther* 1989;10:499.

114. Dutta C, Hadley EC. The significance of sarcopenia in old age. *J Gerontol* Series A 1995;50A:1–4.

115. Kotler D, Tierney A, Pierson R. Magnitude of body cell mass depletion and the timing of death from wasting in AIDS. *Am J Clin Nutr* 1989;50:444–447.

116. Roubenoff R, Castaneda C. Sarcopenia—understanding the dynamics of aging muscle. *JAMA* 2001;286:1230–1231.

117. Castaneda C, Charnley J, Evans W, Crim M, et al. Elderly women accommodate to a low-protein diet with losses of body cell mass, muscle function, and immune response. *Am J Clin Nutr* 1995;62:30–39.

118. Jubrias SA, Odderson IR, Esselman PC, Conley KE. Decline in isokinetic force with age: Muscle cross-sectional area and specific force. *Pflugers Arch* 1997;434:246–253.

119. Larsson L, Sjodin B, Karlsson J. Histochemical and biochemical changes in human skeletal muscle with age in sedentary males, age 22–65 years. *Acta Physiol Scand* 1978;103:31–39.

120. Frontera WR, Meredith CN, O'Reilly KP, Evans WJ. Strength training and determinants of VO2 max in older men. *J Appl Physiol* 1990;68:329–333.

121. Roman WJ, Fleckenstein J, Stray-Gundersen J, Always SE, Peshock R, Gonyea WJ. Adaptations in the elbow flexors of elderly males following heavy resistance training. *J Appl Physiol* 1993;72:750–754.

CHAPTER 7

THE CONCEPT OF FUNCTION

CHAPTER OBJECTIVES

▶ *At the completion of this chapter, the reader will be able to:*

1. List and discuss the various components of the disablement process.

2. Differentiate among impairments, functional limitations, and disability.

3. Describe some of the models of the disablement process.

4. Discuss the variables that can influence the pathology–disability process.

5. Describe the purposes of disease specific measurement tools.

6. Demonstrate an awareness of the various methods of measuring impairment, functional limitations, and disability.

OVERVIEW

Perhaps one of the most important developments in health care in the past decade has been the increased recognition of the importance of the patient's perception of health and functional outcomes.[1] This increased recognition has shifted the focus of the physical therapy examination, evaluation, and subsequent diagnosis to the recognition of impairments, and their relationship to any functional limitation or disability.

▶ *Impairments.* Impairments, according to the "Guide to Physical Therapist Practice," represent the consequences of disease, pathologic processes, or lesions.[2]

▶ *Disability.* The term *disability* has traditionally referred to a broad category of diverse limitations in the ability to meet social or occupational demands.[3] *Handicap* was the term historically used to describe disability. Because of the negative connotations associated with the latter term, a number of organizations now prefer to use the term *disability* to encourage an emphasis on the specific activities the individual can perform, and to identify how the environment can be modified to enable the individual to perform the activities associated with various social or occupational needs.[3]

Disablement Models

A disablement model is designed to detail the functional consequences and relationships of disease, impairment, and functional limitations. Many disablement models have been proposed over the years.[4–10] Most of these models are based on Nagi's model, which depicts the relationship between the following series of linked events[7,11]: *Pathology/Pathophysiology* (the presence of disease), which may lead to *impairments* (anatomic and structural abnormalities), which may in turn lead to *functional limitations* (restrictions in basic physical and mental actions), which may then lead to *disability* (difficulty doing activities of daily life).

Disablement models can provide an idea of the mechanism, or pathway, of an association.[12] Using rheumatoid arthritis as an example of pathology, one such association includes evidence that impairment, such as an articular deformity, may lead to disability by causing functional limitations. A similar pattern of association exists between disease duration and articular signs and symptoms, which supports the idea that the association between disease duration and disability is mediated by the articular signs and symptoms.[12]

Although a degree of inevitability is implied in many of the disablement models, many factors can have an impact on the pathology–disability pathway or disablement process. Some of these factors are modifiable; some are not. Characteristics of an illness that are not amenable to modification may be termed *contextual variables*. These innate characteristics of a person include age, sex, ethnic background, and socioeconomic status. In contrast, modifiable factors are characteristics that an individual can control or adjust. The impact that the modifiable factors have on the pathology–disability pathway or disablement process can depend on both the capacities of the individual and the expectations that are imposed on the individual by those in the immediate social and occupational environment.[13] Escalante and del Rincon[12] use the term *external modifiers* to

FIGURE 7-1 The disablement process. (Reproduced with permission from Dutton M. *Manual Therapy of the Spine.* New York, NY: McGraw-Hill; 2001.)

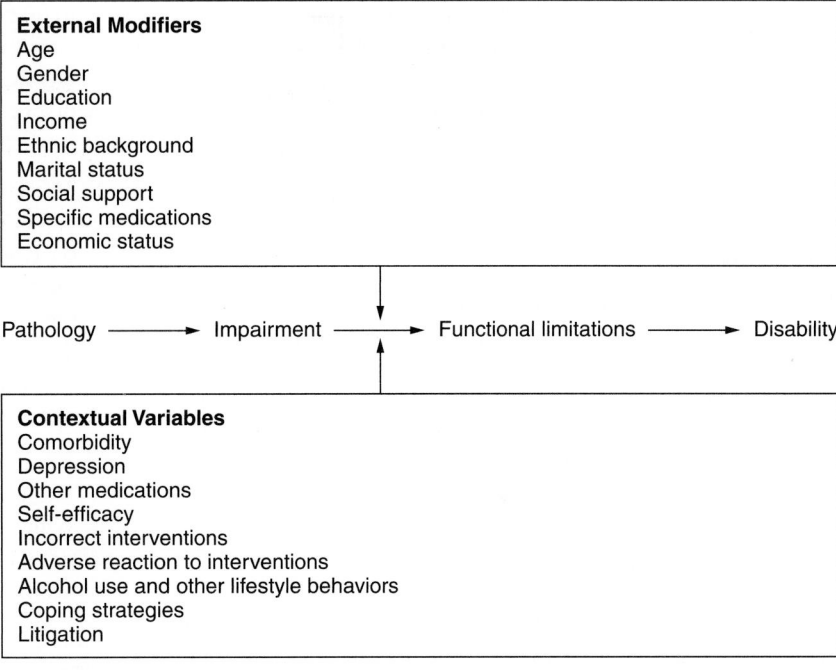

describe those secondary conditions that may influence the level of disability but are not directly related to the disease process itself (Fig. 7-1). These external modifiers can include the presence of depression or comorbidity (e.g., pressure sores, contractures, urinary tract infections). Broader definitions for these conditions include self-concept, work and social participation, health-related economic consequences for the individual or family, and other family members.[10,14]

Specific examples of modifiable patient factors include:

▶ *Level of activity.* A number of studies have made associations between physical activity levels and the onset of disability.[15–26]

▶ *Reaction to the illness.* Different cultural backgrounds are associated with different beliefs about pain, coping strategies, expressions of pain, and response to health care.[27,28] The term *sick role* has been used to define a status accorded to the individual by himself or herself and other members of society that may be variably associated with a medical condition.[13] An individual's sick role reflects not only his or her primary condition but also any additional or secondary conditions.[5,29]

▶ *Educational background.* Patient with less formal education tend to have an increased frequency of disability.[30,31]

▶ *Compensatory and coping strategies.* Some people simply do not have the emotional and social resources to deal with life, particularly in times of adversity.[32]

▶ *Pain tolerance and motivation.* Various studies[28,33] have revealed ethnic and gender differences in responses to both clinical and experimental pain. Specifically, investigators have recently indicated that African Americans report greater levels of pain than whites for such conditions as glaucoma, acquired immunodeficiency syndrome, migraine headache, jaw pain, postoperative pain, myofascial pain, angina pectoris, joint pain, nonspecific daily pain, and arthritis.[34] Interpretations of such findings remain difficult, however, because of potential group differences in disease severity and physician management.[34] There are also disparate reports about gender differences in sensitivity to pain in humans and in animals, indicating that women have a lower tolerance of pain than men.[35–37] Whether women are more willing to report pain than men are, or experience pain differently than men do, is unclear. Whatever the reasons for the differences in pain tolerance and motivation, there is perhaps reason to suppose that improved pain tolerance and motivation might be instrumental in reducing impairment and disability. The chronic pain-adaptation model of Lund and colleagues[38] describes a decreased activation of the muscles during movements in which they act as agonists and an increased activation during movements that require that they adopt the role of antagonists. These changes in muscle activation, characteristic of several types of chronic musculoskeletal pain, are described as a normal protective adaptation to avoid further pain and possible damage.[38]

▶ *Personal and health habits.* The link between disability and a health behavior, such as excessive alcohol use, is subtle because there are many potential pathways. The link between body weight and both morbidity and mortality has been examined extensively, but relatively little research has investigated the relation between body weight and disability. Among the studies that have investigated this relation, the findings are inconsistent.[39–42]

▶ *Level of social support.* The *family* is the primary unit of society and the one in which the earliest and most powerful social learning occurs.[13] The literature on the role of the family in the development and maintenance of chronic pain and disability is extensive. Dysfunctional family systems may promote, permit, and maintain chronic pain and disability.[13]

▶ *Marital status.* Considerable research shows that the spouse's reaction can modify behavior of patients with chronic pain and disability.[13]

▶ *Extent to which involved in litigation and compensation.* Few issues around disability have given rise to more controversy than the question of litigation, compensation, and secondary gain. Anecdotal clinical and legal experience shows general agreement that some claimants magnify or exaggerate their symptoms and disability to varying degree during medical examination carried out specifically for legal proceedings.[13]

Pathology and Pathophysiology

The term *pathology* is perhaps self-explanatory. It refers to any diagnosed disease, injury, disorder, or abnormal condition that is (1) characterized by a particular cluster of signs and symptoms, and (2) recognized by either the patient or clinician as abnormal.[2,3,43]

Pathology may result in a change that manifests itself as a health condition producing an alteration in, or attribute of, an individual's health status. Pathology is primarily identified at the cellular level and usually is determined by the physician's medical diagnosis.[2,3] The presence of pathology may lead to distress or interference with functional status. The severity of the pathology, and thus the impact that it has on a patient's functional status, depends on several factors. These factors include, but are not limited to:

▶ Comorbidity (the degree and location of edema, the quality of the vascular supply, the presence of infection, and the degree of atrophy)

▶ The patient's general physical health

▶ The age of the patient

▶ The patient's nutritional status

Patients generally are referred to physical therapy services with a medical diagnosis that is based on pathology (e.g., osteoarthritis of the hip). Although knowledge of pathology and pathophysiology can help the clinician predict the range, severity, and prognosis of a particular condition, a medical diagnosis does not tell the clinician how to manage the patient. A physical therapy diagnosis, on the other hand, is a diagnostic label that identifies the impact of a condition on function. When a patient is referred from a physician with a medical diagnosis, there may be four possible scenarios following the physical therapy examination.[2]

1. The clinical findings are consistent with the physician's medical diagnosis. This scenario permits the physical therapist to proceed with interventions that are justified by changes in the patient's functional status.

2. The clinical findings suggest a pathologic or pathophysiologic condition that is inconsistent with the referring physician's diagnosis and is out of the scope of the practice of physical therapy. This scenario requires the physical therapist to either return the patient to the referring physician or make a referral to another practitioner.

3. The clinical findings suggest the presence of an additional pathologic or pathophysiologic condition that was not previously identified. If the newly identified pathophysiologic condition is within the scope of physical therapy practice, the physical therapist can continue to treat the patient. If, however, the newly identified pathophysiologic condition is not within the scope of physical therapy practice, the physical therapist is required to return the patient to the referring physician or to make a referral to another practitioner (e.g., speech therapist).

4. The clinical findings fail to identify the underlying cause. With this scenario, the physical therapist continues to test the signs and symptoms while providing interventions that are justified by changes in the patient's functional status.

If a physical therapy intervention is warranted, the goal of the intervention is to restore function, with the focus of the intervention on reducing and preventing risk factors, and decreasing the impact of impairments, functional limitations, and disabilities.[2]

Impairments

The "Guide to Physical Therapist Practice" defines impairment as any loss or abnormality of anatomic, physiologic, mental, or psychological structure or function that both (1) results from underlying changes in the normal state and (2) contributes to illness.[2] Thus, impairments can be viewed as abnormalities of structure or function as indicated by signs and symptoms. Verbrugge and Jette[4] suggest that disease symptoms are essentially impairments, and thus downstream from the pathologic process of the disease.

Impairments have the potential to create pain and subtle alterations in the normal functions of the involved joint and surrounding tissues (Tables 7-1, 7-2, and 7-3). Impairments can be manifested objectively, for example, by reduced range of motion, articular deformity, abnormal gait, and the loss of strength, power, endurance, or proprioception. Impairments also can be manifested subjectively, for example, through pain (see later), tenderness, morning stiffness, or fatigue.

The definition of *impairment* refers to some form of loss. *Loss* or *loss of use* refers to a change from the normal or preexisting state. The term *normal* refers to a range representing healthy functioning, which can vary with age, gender, and other factors such as environmental conditions. For example, normal range of motion for knee flexion is deemed to be 150 degrees.[3] Although a loss of more than 70 degrees of knee flexion may prevent a patient from performing such activities as getting in and out of a bathtub, and walking up and down steps, the patient may still be able to ambulate around the house. It is important to note that physical impairment and physical functioning appear to be separate constructs that do not necessarily have a clear linear relationship.[43a,43b] Furthermore, some measures of

TABLE 7-1   Criteria for Rating Impairment Due to Lumbar Spine Injury[3]

Category I (0% impairment of the whole person)	Category II (5–8% impairment of the whole person)	Category III (10–13% impairment of the whole person)	Category IV (20–23% impairment of the whole person)	Category V (25–28% impairment of the whole person)
No significant clinical findings, no observed muscle guarding or spasm, no documentable neurologic impairment, no documented alteration in structural integrity, and no other indication of impairment related to injury or illness; no fractures	Clinical history and examination findings are compatible with a specific injury; findings may include significant muscle guarding or spasm observed at time of examination, asymmetric loss of range of motion, or nonverifiable radicular complaints, defined as complaints of radicular pain without objective findings; no alteration of structural integrity and no significant radiculopathy *or* Individual had clinically significant radiculopathy and has imaging study that demonstrates herniated disk at level and on side that would be expected based on previous radiculopathy, but no longer has radiculopathy following conservative treatment *or* Fractures: (1) < 25% compression of one vertebral body; (2) posterior element fracture without dislocation (not developmental spondylolysis) that has healed without alteration of motion segment integrity; (3) spinous or transverse process fracture with displacement without vertebral body fracture, which does not disrupt spinal canal	Significant signs of radiculopathy, such as dermatomal pain and/or in dermatomal distribution, sensory loss, loss of relevant reflex(es), loss of muscle strength or measured unilateral atrophy above or below knee compared with measurements on contralateral side at same location; impairment may be verified by electrodiagnostic findings *or* History of herniated disk at level and on side that would be expected from objective clinical findings, associated with radiculopathy, or individuals who had surgery for radiculopathy, but are now asymptomatic *or* Fractures: (1) 25–50% compression of one vertebral body; (2) posterior element fracture with displacement disrupting spinal canal: in both cases, fracture has healed without alteration of structural integrity	Loss of motion segment integrity defined from flexion and extension radiographs as at least 4.5 mm of translation of one vertebra on another or angular motion greater than 15% at L1-2, L2-3, and L3-4, greater than 20 degrees at L4-5, and greater than 25 degrees at L5-S1; may have complete or near-complete loss of motion of motion segment due to developmental fusion, or successful or unsuccessful attempt at surgical arthrodesis *or* Fractures: (1) > 50% compression of one vertebral body without residual neurologic compromise	Meets criteria categories III and IV; that is, both radiculopathy and alteration of motion segment integrity are present; significant lower extremity impairment is present as indicated by atrophy or loss of reflex(es), pain and/or sensory changes within anatomic distribution (dermatomal), or electromyographic findings as stated in lumbosacral category III and alteration of spine motion segment integrity as defined in lumbosacral category IV *or* Fractures: (1) greater than 50% compression of one vertebral body with unilateral neurologic compromise

TABLE 7-2 Criteria for Rating Impairment Due to Thoracic Spine Injury[3]

Category I (0% impairment of the whole person)	Category II (5–8% impairment of the whole person)	Category III (10–18% impairment of the whole person)	Category IV (20–23% impairment of the whole person)	Category V (25–28% impairment of the whole person)
No significant clinical findings, no observed muscle guarding, no documentable neurologic impairment, no documented changes in structural integrity, and no other indication of impairment related to injury or illness; no fractures	History and examination findings are compatible with specific injury or illness; findings may include significant muscle guarding or spasm observed at time of examination, asymmetric loss of range of motion (dysmetria), or nonverifiable radicular complaints, defined as complaints of radicular pain without objective findings; no alteration of motion segment integrity *or* Herniated disk at level and on side that would be expected from objective clinical findings, but without radicular signs following conservative treatment *or* Fractures: (1) < 25% compression of one vertebral body; (2) posterior element fracture without dislocation that has healed without alteration of motion segment integrity or radiculopathy; (3) spinous or transverse process fracture with displacement, but without vertebral body fracture	Ongoing neurologic impairment of lower extremity related to thoracolumbar injury, documented by examination of motor and sensory functions, reflexes, or findings of unilateral atrophy above or below knee related to no other condition; impairment may be verified by electrodiagnostic testing *or* Clinically significant radiculopathy verified by imaging study that demonstrates herniated disk at level and on side that would be expected from objective clinical findings; history of radiculopathy, which has improved following surgical treatment *or* Fractures: (1) 25–50% compression fracture of one vertebral body; (2) posterior element fracture with mild displacement disrupting spinal canal: in both cases, fracture has healed without alteration of structural integrity; differentiation from congenital or developmental condition should be accomplished, if possible, by examining preinjury roentgenograms, if available, or by bone scan performed after onset of condition	Alteration of motion segment integrity or bilateral or multilevel radiculopathy; alteration of motion segment integrity is defined from flexion and extension radiographs as translation of one vertebra on another of more than 2.5 mm; radiculopathy as defined in thoracic category III need not be present if there is alteration of motion segment integrity; if individual is to be placed in DRE thoracic category IV due to radiculopathy; the latter must be bilateral or involve more than one level *or* Fractures: (1) > 50% compression of one vertebral body without residual neurologic compromise	Impairment of lower extremity as defined in thoracolumbar category III and loss of structural integrity as defined in thoracic category IV *or* Fractures: (1) > 50% compression of one vertebral body with neural motor compromise but not bilateral involvement that would qualify individual for corticospinal tract evaluation

DRE, diagnosis-related estimate.

TABLE 7-3 Criteria for Rating Impairment Due to Cervical Disorders[3]

Category I (0% impairment of the whole person)	Category II (5–8% impairment of the whole person)	Category III (10–18% impairment of the whole person)	Category IV (20–23% impairment of the whole person)	Category V (25–28% impairment of the whole person)
No significant clinical findings, no muscle guarding, no documentable neurologic impairment, no significant loss of motion segment integrity, and no other indication of impairment related to injury or illness; no fractures	Clinical history and examination findings are compatible with specific injury; findings may include muscle guarding or spasm observed at time of examination by physician, asymmetric loss of range of motion, or nonverifiable radicular complaints, defined as complaints of radicular pain without objective findings; no alteration of structural integrity *or* Individual had clinically significant radiculopathy and imaging study that demonstrated herniated disk at level and on side that would be expected based on radiculopathy, but has improved following nonoperative treatment *or* Fractures: (1) < 25% compression of one vertebral body; (2) posterior element fracture without dislocation that has healed without loss of structural integrity or radiculopathy; (3) spinous or transverse process fracture with displacement	Significant signs of radiculopathy, such as pain and/or sensory loss in dermatomal distribution, loss of relevant reflex(es), loss of muscle strength or unilateral atrophy compared with unaffected side, measured at same distance above or below elbow; neurologic impairment may be verified by electrodiagnostic findings *or* Individual had clinically significant radiculopathy, verified by imaging study that demonstrates herniated disk at level and on side expected from objective clinical findings with radiculopathy or with improvement of radiculopathy following surgery *or* Fractures: (1) 25–50% compression of one vertebral body; (2) posterior element fracture with displacement disrupting spinal canal: in both cases, fracture has healed without alteration of structural integrity; radiculopathy may or may not be present; differentiation from congenital and developmental conditions may be accomplished, if possible, by examining preinjury roentgenograms or bone scan performed after onset of condition	Alteration of motion segment integrity or bilateral or multilevel radiculopathy; alteration of motion segment integrity is defined from flexion and extension radiographs as at least 3.5 mm of translation of one vertebra on another, or angular motion of more than 11 degrees greater than at each adjacent level; alternatively, individual may have loss of motion of motion segment due to developmental fusion or successful or unsuccessful attempt at surgical arthrodesis; radiculopathy as defined in cervical category III need not be present if there is alteration of motion segment integrity *or* Fractures: (1) > 50% compression of one vertebral body without residual neural neurologic compromise	Significant upper extremity impairment requiring the use of upper extremity external functional or adaptive device(s); there may be total neurologic loss at single level or severe, multilevel neurologic dysfunction *or* Fractures: structural compromise of spinal canal is present with severe upper extremity motor and sensory deficits but without lower extremity involvement

impairment are not correlated with patient function, bringing into question their meaningfulness as measurement tools.[43a]

The "Guide to Physical Therapist Practice"[2] uses preferred practice patterns to group clusters of musculoskeletal impairments that occur together:

▶ Pattern 4B refers to conditions resulting from impaired posture.

▶ Pattern 4C refers to conditions resulting from impaired muscle performance.

▶ Pattern 4D refers to conditions resulting from impaired joint mobility, motor function, muscle performance, and range of motion associated with connective tissue dysfunction.

▶ Pattern 4E refers to conditions resulting from impaired joint mobility, motor function, muscle performance, and range of motion associated with localized inflammation.

▶ Pattern 4F refers to conditions resulting from impaired joint mobility, motor function, muscle performance, range of motion, and reflex integrity associated with spinal disorders.

▶ Pattern 4G refers to conditions resulting from impaired joint mobility, motor function, muscle performance, and range of motion associated with fracture.

▶ Pattern 4H refers to conditions resulting from impaired joint mobility, motor function, muscle performance, and range of motion associated with joint arthroplasty.

▶ Pattern 4I refers to conditions resulting from impaired joint mobility, motor function, muscle performance, and range of motion associated with bony or soft tissue surgery.

▶ Pattern 4J refers to conditions resulting from impaired motor function, muscle performance, range of motion, gait, locomotion, balance, and motor function associated with amputation.

▶ Pattern 5F refers to conditions resulting from impaired peripheral nerve integrity and muscle performance associated with peripheral nerve injury.

Each of these patterns represents a diagnostic or impairment classification. Impairments resulting primarily from pain are integrated in all of the preferred practice patterns. Pain can greatly influence an individual's ability to function, depending on its location and severity. However, the perception of pain is highly individual, and different individuals may be impaired by pain to different degrees.[4] Although absolute quantification of pain is not possible, its severity may be estimated using a visual analogue scale or a numeric scale. More complex scales include the Pain Disability Index (PDI)[1,44,45] (Table 7-4) and the McGill Pain Questionnaire (MPQ)[46-48] (see Chap. 8).

The PDI is a self-report instrument that has been used to assess the degree to which chronic pain interferes with various daily activities. The PDI consists of a series of 0-to-10 scales on which an individual rates pain-related interference. The seven categories that make up the scale are family/home responsibilities, recreation, social activity, occupation, sexual behavior, self-care, and life-support activities (e.g., eating, sleeping, and breathing). An initial study[1] found the PDI to be effective in discriminating patients immediately postsurgery (high impairment) from patients several months removed from surgery (low impairment).[1] A subsequent study[45] showed the PDI to be sensitive to differences between outpatients (low impairment) and inpatients (high impairment) with chronic pain.[44]

The MPQ[46-48] contains a list of words chosen to reflect the sensory, affective, and evaluative components of the pain experience (see Chap. 8).

One of the goals of the examination process is to determine which impairments are related to the patient's functional limitations. Once these have been identified, the clinician must then determine which impairments may be remedied by physical therapy intervention.

Clinical Pearl

It is worth noting that various definitions of impairment exist outside the realm of physical therapy. For example, the American Medical Association's (AMA) *Guide to the Evaluation of Permanent Impairment*[3] rate impairment using a whole person (WP) rating scale. Within this scale, a percentage score is assigned to an individual, depending on the amount of impairment. A WP rating of 0 percent is given to an individual with impairment if the impairment has no significant organ or body system functional consequences and does not limit the performance of the common activities of daily living (ADLs) outlined in Table 7-5. A 90 to 100 percent WP impairment indicates a very severe organ or body system impairment requiring the individual to be fully dependent on others for self-care, approaching death.

Functional Limitations

A functional limitation is defined by the "Guide to Physical Therapist Practice" as a restriction of the ability to perform a fundamental physical action, task, or activity in an efficient, typically expected, or competent manner.[2] In other words, functional limitations are restrictions in performing expected basic physical and mental actions. Examples of such functional limitations include difficulty with walking and an inability to put on shoes. The vast majority of the traditional tests used in physical therapy clinics, such as range of motion and strength, are measures of impairments, not function. Measurements of functional limitations include sensorimotor performance testing during such activities as walking, climbing, bending, transferring, lifting, and carrying.[2] It is important that these measurements assess the patient's ability to perform tasks that the patient feels are important (Table 7-6).

The process of identifying meaningful, achievable functional goals should be a collaborative effort between the clinician and the patient, the patient's family, or the patient's significant other.[2] To identify functional goals, Randall and McEwen[49] recommend the following steps:

1. Determine the patient's desired outcome of the intervention.

2. Develop an understanding of the patient's self-care, work, and leisure activities and the environments in which these activities occur.

TABLE 7-4   The Pain Disability Index[1]

The rating scales below are designed to measure the degree to which several aspects of your life are presently disrupted by chronic pain. In other words, we would like to know how much your pain is preventing you from doing what you would normally do, or from doing it as well as you normally would. Respond to each category by indicating the *overall* impact of pain in your life, not just the pain at its worst.

For each of the 7 categories of life activity listed, please circle the number on the scale that describes the level of disability you typically experience. A score of 0 means no disability at all, and a score of 10 signifies that all of the activities in which you would normally be involved have been totally disrupted or prevented by your pain.

(1) FAMILY/HOME RESPONSIBILITIES

This category refers to activities related to the home or family. It includes chores or duties performed around the house (e.g., yard work) and errands or favors for other family members (e.g., driving children from school).

0   1   2   3   4   5   6   7   8   9   10

No   Total
disability   disability

(2) RECREATION

This category includes hobbies, sports, and other similar leisure-time activities.

0   1   2   3   4   5   6   7   8   9   10

No   Total
disability   disability

(3) SOCIAL ACTIVITY

This category refers to activities that involve participation with friends and acquaintances other than family members. It includes parties, theater, concerts, dining out, and other social functions.

0   1   2   3   4   5   6   7   8   9   10

No   Total
disability   disability

(4) OCCUPATION

This category refers to activities that are a part of or directly related to one's job. This includes nonpaying jobs as well, such as that of a housewife or volunteer worker.

0   1   2   3   4   5   6   7   8   9   10

No   Total
disability   disability

(5) SEXUAL BEHAVIOR

This category refers to the frequency and quality of one's sex life.

0   1   2   3   4   5   6   7   8   9   10

No   Total
disability   disability

(6) SELF-CARE

This category includes activities that involve personal maintenance and independent daily living (e.g., taking a shower, driving, getting dressed, etc.).

0   1   2   3   4   5   6   7   8   9   10

No   Total
disability   disability

(7) LIFE-SUPPORT ACTIVITY

This category refers to basic life-supporting behaviors such as eating, sleeping, and breathing.

0   1   2   3   4   5   6   7   8   9   10

No   Total
disability   disability

TABLE 7-5   Activities Commonly Measured in Activities of Daily Living (ADL) and Instrumental Activities of Daily Living (IADL) Scales[3]

Activity	Example
Self-care, personal hygiene	Urinating, defecating, brushing teeth, combing hair, bathing, dressing oneself, eating
Communication	Writing, typing, seeing, hearing, speaking
Physical activity	Standing, sitting, reclining, walking, climbing stairs
Sensory function	Hearing, seeing, tactile feeling, tasting, smelling
Nonspecialized hand activities	Grasping, lifting, tactile, discrimination
Travel	Riding, driving, flying
Sexual function	Orgasm, ejaculation, lubrication, erection
Sleep	Restful, nocturnal sleep pattern

3. Establish goals with the patient that relate to the desired outcomes (see Table 7-6).

Once the goals have been agreed upon, the clinician must write the goals so that they contain the following elements[49,51]:

▶ Who (the patient)

▶ Will do what (activities)

▶ Under what conditions (the home or work environment)

▶ How well (the amount of assistance, or number of attempts required for successful completion)

▶ By when (target date)

Thus, the functional examination creates a functional diagnosis, with functional goals. Once these functional goals are established, the clinician can grade them according to difficulty. Functional tasks can reproduce the whole task in its entirety or can break down the task to its required fundamental components and the physical demands necessary to perform each task. Regaining the smaller requirements may constitute the short-term goals, whereas completion of the whole task may become the long-term goal. For example, exercises to improve sit-to-stand transfers could be initiated by having the patient perform triceps push-ups on the chair handle, perform bilateral

TABLE 7-6   Questions to Determine Desired Outcomes[49,50]

1. If you were to concentrate your energies on one thing for yourself, what would it be?

2. What activities do you need help with that you would rather perform yourself?

3. What are your concerns about returning to work, home, school, or leisure activities?

4. What about your current situation would you like to be different in about 6 months? What would you like to be the same?

mini-squats, or exercise on the leg press, before progressing to the functional activity.

Disability

Disability may be defined as difficulty in the performance of social roles and tasks within a sociocultural and physical environment (from hygiene to hobbies, errands, to sleep), as a result of a health or physical problem.[7,8,10,52–55] Disability, which may be temporary or permanent, is the gap between what a person can do and what the person needs or wants to do. The Americans with Disabilities Act (ADA) of 1989[56] marked the first explicit national goal of achieving equal opportunity, independent living, and economic self-sufficiency for individuals with disabilities.[13] Disability is a problem that encompasses a wide range of issues, from very specific topics to the basic question of what it means to be human.

Three main models are generally used to describe disability: the moral, medical, and social models.[57] Table 7-7 compares these three models along seven dimensions: the meaning of disabilities, moral implications of disability, sample ideas, origins, goals of intervention, and benefits and negative effects of the model.[57] The moral and medical models share in common the perspective that disability resides within the individual and carries with it a degree of stigma or pathology.[57] In contrast, the social model locates the disablement in the environment and in society, which fail to appropriately accommodate and include people with disabilities.[57]

Disability is not necessarily related to any health impairment or medical condition, although a medical condition or impairment may cause or contribute to disability. For example, associations between pathology and disability have been found for several health conditions. These include diabetes,[18,21,58] cardiovascular diseases,[59,60] musculoskeletal diseases,[38,54,61] and vision-related diseases.[62]

For any given level of health or specific diagnosis, some people will be disabled and others will not. Thus, impairments and functional limitations are not related to disability in a linear fashion. It is even possible for two patients who have the same disease and similar impairments and functional limitations to have two different levels of disability. For example, degenerative joint disease of the spine that prevents heavy lifting likely has a greater impact on a construction worker than it does on a bank president.

TABLE 7-7   Comparison of the Moral, Medical, and Social Models of Disability[57]

Measure	Moral	Medical	Social
Meaning of disability	A defect caused by moral lapse or sins, failure of faith, evil; test of faith	A defect in or failure of a bodily system that is inherently abnormal and pathological	A social construct; problems reside in the environment that fails to accommodate people with disability
Moral implications	Brings shame to the person with the disability and his or her family	A medical abnormality due to genetics, bad health habits, person's behavior	Society has failed a segment of its citizens and oppresses them
Sample ideas	"God gives us only what we can bear" or "There's a reason I was chosen to have this disability"	Clinical descriptions of "patient" in medical terminology; isolation of body parts	"Nothing about us without us" or "Civil rights, not charity"
Origins	Oldest model and still most prevalent worldwide	Mid-19th century; most common model in the United States; entrenched in most rehabilitation clinics and journals	1975, following demonstrations by people with disabilities in support of the yet-unsigned Rehabilitation Act
Goals of intervention	Spiritual or divine, acceptance	"Cure" or amelioration of the disability to the greatest extent possible	Political, economic, social, and policy systems, increased access and inclusion
Benefits of model	An acceptance of being selected; a special relationship with God; a sense of greater purpose to the disability	A lessened sense of shame and stigma; faith in medical intervention; spurs medical and technologic advances	Promotes integration of the disability into their self; a sense of community and pride; depathologizing of disability
Negative effects	Shame; ostracization; need to conceal the disability or person with the disability	Paternalistic; promotes benevolence and charity; services for but not by people with disabilities	Powerlessness in the face of necessary broad social and political changes; challenges to prevailing ideas

It is now commonly agreed that a satisfactory measure of disability should include both subjective and objective measures of quality-of-life issues. *Health-related quality of life* (HRQL) represents the total effect of individual and environmental factors on an individual's function and health status.[2] The term *health-related quality of life* is often used interchangeably with the terms functional status, health status, and health outcomes. The definitions of these terms however, might range from negatively valued aspects of life, such as death, to more positively valued aspects, such as social functioning or happiness.[10,14,63–67]

Health-related quality-of-life issues may be measured by condition-specific and generic health status questionnaires. The rating of perceived difficulty in performing various activities can be considered the primary assessment of disability, whereas the rating of actual dependence on assistance is an assessment of the consequence of disability.[68]

Felce and Perry[66] have proposed a model of HRQL that integrates subjective and objective indicators, reflecting a broad range of life domains, through an individual ranking of the relative importance of each domain (Fig. 7-2). These domains are physical well-being, material well-being, social well-being, development and activity, and emotional well-being. The Felce and Perry model[66] is designed to address the concern that objective data should not be interpreted without reference to personal autonomy, preferences, and concerns. In addition Felce and Perry feel that expressions of satisfaction are themselves relative to the individual's temperament and the circumstances and experiences that have shaped their frame of reference.[66]

It is important that the clinician avoid viewing the disablement process as a unidirectional pathway with an inevitable progression toward disability. Various factors, including the patient's level of interaction with the environment and the potential effects of rehabilitation, may cause a bidirectional interaction or reversal between the components of the disablement process.[2,69] This bidirectional interaction may be referred to as the *enabling process.*[69]

FIGURE 7-2   A model of quality of life. (Reproduced with permission from Felce D, Perry J. Quality of life: Its definition and measurement. *Res Devel Disabil* 1995;16:51–74.)

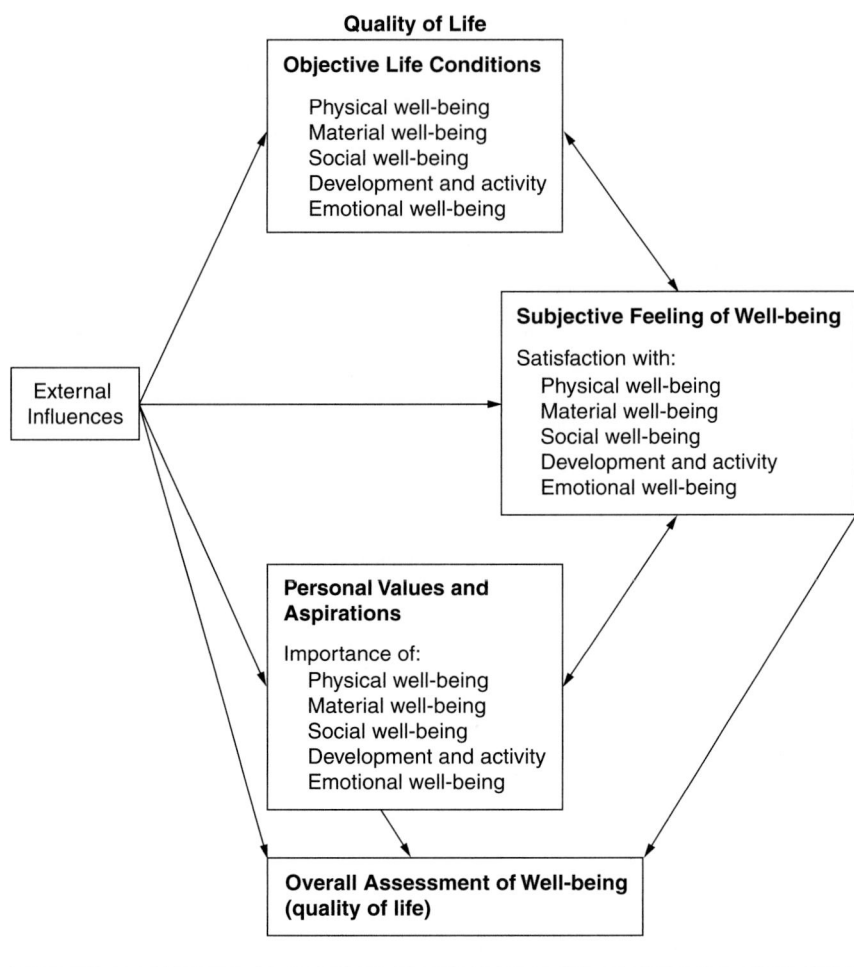

Measurement of Functional Outcomes

Outcomes measurement is a process that describes a systematic method to gauge the effectiveness and efficiency of an intervention in daily clinical practice.[70] Effectiveness in this context refers to the outcome of an intervention during the rigors of ordinary and customary care delivery.[70] The efficiency of an intervention is a factor of utilization (number of outpatient visits, length of inpatient stay) with the costs of care and outcome. The trend in using outcome measures in the decision-making process is consistent with the evidence-based approach (EBP) and represents the final step in the evaluation of clinical performance.[71,71a] The clinician should be able to evaluate and choose the appropriate outcome measure for a specific patient population since the caliber of information that an outcome measurement provides is a function of the sophistication, predictability, and accuracy of the tools or instruments used.[71b] Sensitivity and specificity are used to describe the accuracy of diagnostic tests (see Chap. 8). Measurement instruments must be able to detect change when it has occurred and to remain stable when change has not occurred.[71c] The better the sophistication, predictability, and accuracy of the measurement tool, the

less chance there is for errors in measurement that make it difficult to ascertain whether true progress has occurred. In an effort to counteract the potential for these measurement errors, the term minimal detectable change has been introduced. Minimal detectable change (MDC) is defined as the minimal amount of change that exceeds measurement error.[71c] The MDC is a statistical measure of meaningful change and is related to an instrument's reliability.[71c] Although various methods for calculating the MDC have been proposed, consensus has yet to be reached as to what is the optimal method.[71d] Unfortunately, statistically significant change using the MDC may not indicate that the change is clinically relevant. The minimally clinically important difference (MCID) is a measure of clinical relevance, and indicates the amount of change in scale points that must occur before the change may be considered meaningful.[71e] The sensitivity of the MCID is represented by the number of patients the outcome measure correctly identifies as having changed an important amount divided by all of the patients who truly changed an important amount.[71f] The specificity of the MCID is represented by the number of patients the outcome measure correctly identifies as not having changed an important amount divided by all of the patients who truly did not change an important amount.[71f] Although, it is tempting to make the assumption that the minimum level of statistical change (MDC) would be less than or equal to the MCID, the relationship between the MDC and the MCID scores has yet to be determined.[71e]

In addition to these clinical and statistical measures, the success of an intervention is based on the perspective of the stakeholder.[71c,71g] For example, to the patient, success may be considered as the relief of symptoms. To the payers of healthcare, a successful outcome is likely viewed as one that involved cost-efficient patient management.[71c] Clinicians tend to define good outcomes as the learning of long-term management strategies, relief of symptoms, and improved function.[71g]

The traditional outcome measurements have been divided into those that assess upper extremity function, those that assess lower extremity function, and those that measure the performance of basic and instrumental activities of daily living (BADLs and IADLs). Functional measurement tools for the upper extremity have involved an assessment of coordination and dexterity measurements, whereas functional measurements for the lower extremity have included the ability of the patient to perform sit-to-stand transfers, standing balance, ambulation, and stair negotiation. Some of the measurement tools that have been devised to assess the performance of BADLs and IADLs include:

▶ *Physical Performance Test (PPT).*[72] The PPT is a performance-based measure of both BADL and IADL that has been used to describe and monitor physical performance. The PPT takes about 10 minutes to administer. Scoring is based on the time taken to complete a series of usual daily tasks, such as writing a sentence, simulated eating, donning and doffing a jacket, turning 360 degrees when standing, lifting a book, picking up a penny from the floor, and walking 50 feet.

▶ *Functional Status Questionnaire (FSQ).*[73] The FSQ is a self-report measure of physical, psychological, and social role functions in patients who are ambulatory. The test takes about 15 minutes and has been found to have both construct and convergent reliability.[73]

▶ *Sickness Impact Profile (SIP).*[74] The SIP is a widely used health status measure. It measures both physical and psychosocial outcomes from the patient's perspective. The SIP is composed of 136 items that address the following areas: ambulation, mobility, body care and movement, social interaction, communication, alertness, emotional behavior, sleep and rest, eating, work, home management, and recreation and pastime activities. The SIP questionnaire has been extensively and successfully tested for its internal consistency, external validity, responsiveness to changes over time, and test-retest reliability in a wide range of clinical situations.[75]

▶ *Functional Rating Index (FRI).*[76] The FRI is an instrument specifically designed to quantitatively measure the subjective perception of function and pain of the spinal musculoskeletal system. The FRI consists of 10 items that measure both pain and function of the neck and back (Table 7-8). Of these 10 items, 8 refer to activities of daily living

TABLE 7-8 Functional Rating Index[76]

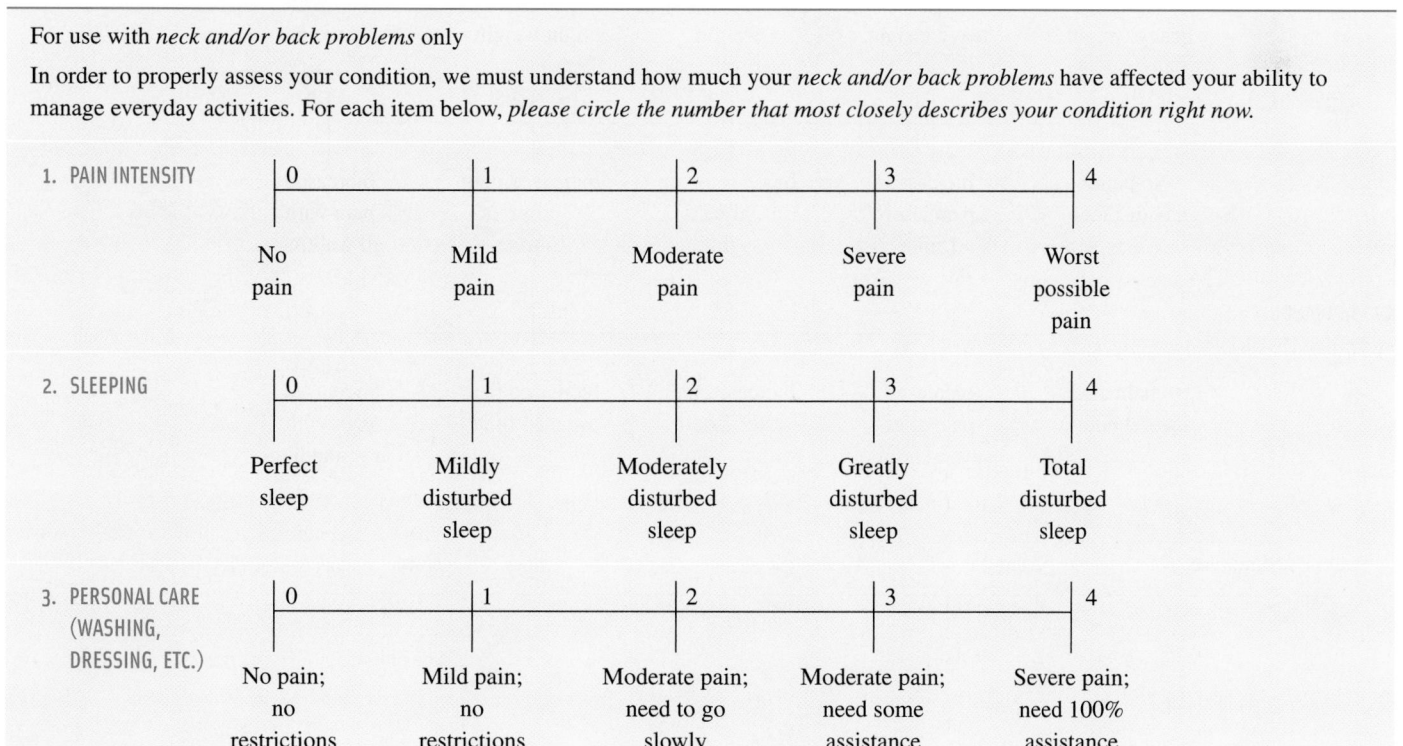

For use with *neck and/or back problems* only

In order to properly assess your condition, we must understand how much your *neck and/or back problems* have affected your ability to manage everyday activities. For each item below, *please circle the number that most closely describes your condition right now.*

1. PAIN INTENSITY	0	1	2	3	4
	No pain	Mild pain	Moderate pain	Severe pain	Worst possible pain
2. SLEEPING	0	1	2	3	4
	Perfect sleep	Mildly disturbed sleep	Moderately disturbed sleep	Greatly disturbed sleep	Total disturbed sleep
3. PERSONAL CARE (WASHING, DRESSING, ETC.)	0	1	2	3	4
	No pain; no restrictions	Mild pain; no restrictions	Moderate pain; need to go slowly	Moderate pain; need some assistance	Severe pain; need 100% assistance

TABLE 7-8   *(cont.)*

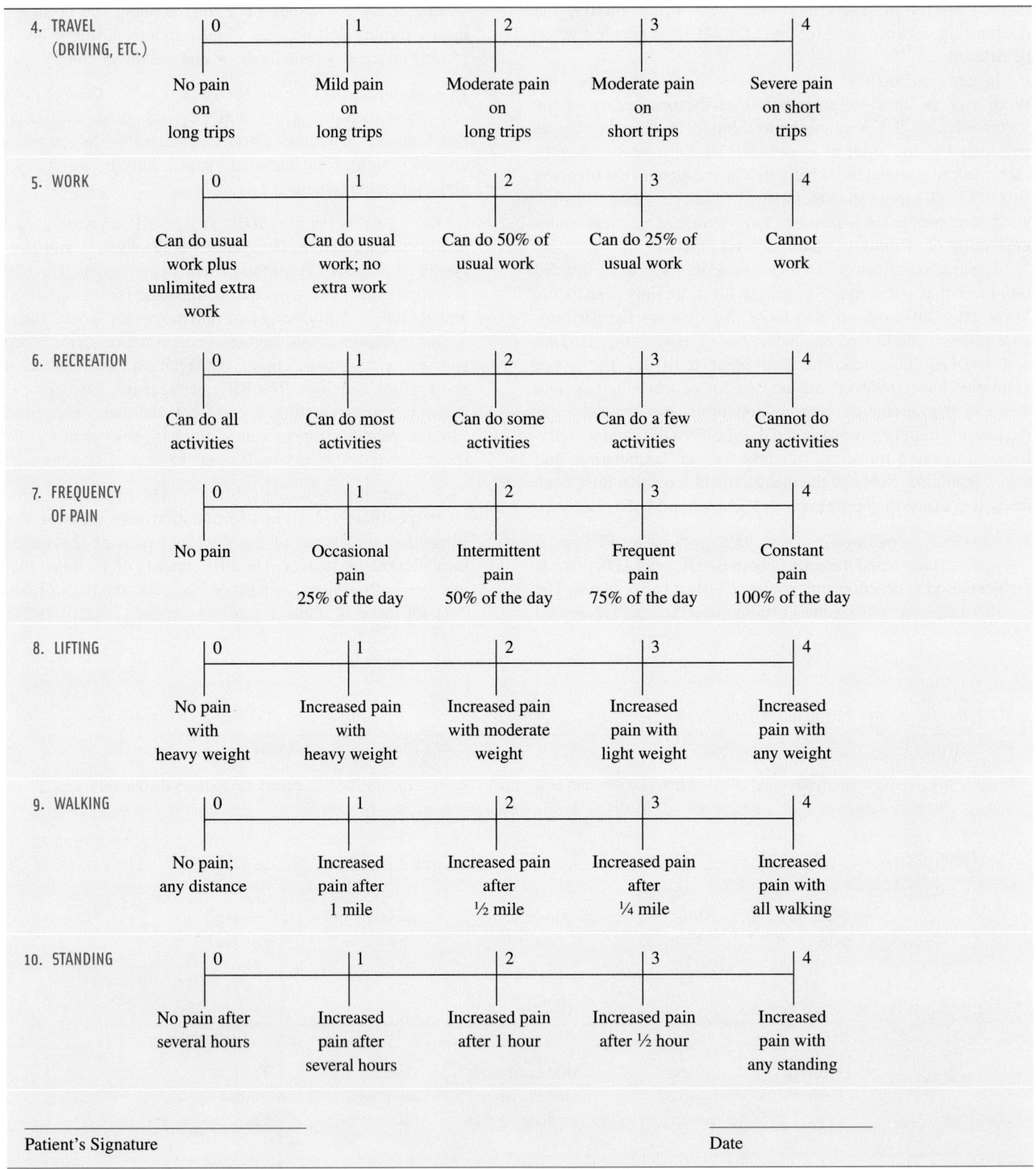

	0	1	2	3	4
4. TRAVEL (DRIVING, ETC.)	No pain on long trips	Mild pain on long trips	Moderate pain on long trips	Moderate pain on short trips	Severe pain on short trips
5. WORK	Can do usual work plus unlimited extra work	Can do usual work; no extra work	Can do 50% of usual work	Can do 25% of usual work	Cannot work
6. RECREATION	Can do all activities	Can do most activities	Can do some activities	Can do a few activities	Cannot do any activities
7. FREQUENCY OF PAIN	No pain	Occasional pain 25% of the day	Intermittent pain 50% of the day	Frequent pain 75% of the day	Constant pain 100% of the day
8. LIFTING	No pain with heavy weight	Increased pain with heavy weight	Increased pain with moderate weight	Increased pain with light weight	Increased pain with any weight
9. WALKING	No pain; any distance	Increased pain after 1 mile	Increased pain after ½ mile	Increased pain after ¼ mile	Increased pain with all walking
10. STANDING	No pain after several hours	Increased pain after several hours	Increased pain after 1 hour	Increased pain after ½ hour	Increased pain with any standing

_____   _____
Patient's Signature   Date

that might be adversely affected by a spinal condition. The remaining 2 items refer to two different attributes of pain. Using a 5-point scale for each item, the patient ranks his or her perceived ability to perform a function and/or the quantity of pain at the present time.[76] When all 10 items are completed the FRI score is calculated as follows: (total score divided by 40) times 100 percent.

▶ *Short Musculoskeletal Function Assessment (SMFA).*[77] The SMFA consists of a 46-item questionnaire (Table 7-9). The first 34 items refer to activities of daily living. The

patient ranks his or her perceived difficulty or problems with these tasks to provide a *dysfunction index.* The 12 remaining items are ranked according to how much they bother the patient and provide the clinician with a *bother index.*

▶ *36-Item Short-Form Health Survey (SF-36).*[78] The SF-36 is a general measure of health status, using a self-report with eight subscales of health. The acute version of the test takes about 7 to 10 minutes to complete, is moderately easy to score, and asks questions about physical, social, emotional role, and physical role function; mental health; energy; pain;

TABLE 7-9 Short Musculoskeletal Function Assessment (SMFA)[77]

INSTRUCTIONS

We are interested in finding out how you are managing with your injury or arthritis this week. We would like to know about any problems you may be having with your daily activities because of your injury or arthritis.

Please answer each question by putting a check in the box corresponding to the choice that best describes you.

These questions are about how much difficulty you may be having *this week* with your daily activities because of your injury or arthritis.

	Not at All Difficult	A Little Difficult	Moderately Difficult	Very Difficult	Unable to Do
1. How difficult is it for you to get in or out of a low chair?	☐	☐	☐	☐	☐
2. How difficult is it for you to open medicine bottles or jars?	☐	☐	☐	☐	☐
3. How difficult is it for you to shop for groceries or other things?	☐	☐	☐	☐	☐
4. How difficult is it for you to climb stairs?	☐	☐	☐	☐	☐
5. How difficult is it for you to make a tight fist?	☐	☐	☐	☐	☐
6. How difficult is it for you to get in or out of the bathtub or shower?	☐	☐	☐	☐	☐
7. How difficult is it for you to get comfortable to sleep?	☐	☐	☐	☐	☐
8. How difficult is it for you to bend or kneel down?	☐	☐	☐	☐	☐
9. How difficult is it for you to use buttons, snaps, hooks, or zippers?	☐	☐	☐	☐	☐
10. How difficult is it for you to cut your own fingernails?	☐	☐	☐	☐	☐
11. How difficult is it for you to dress yourself?	☐	☐	☐	☐	☐
12. How difficult is it for you to walk?	☐	☐	☐	☐	☐
13. How difficult is it for you to get moving after you have been sitting or lying down?	☐	☐	☐	☐	☐
14. How difficult is it for you to go out by yourself?	☐	☐	☐	☐	☐
15. How difficult is it for you to drive?	☐	☐	☐	☐	☐
16. How difficult is it for you to clean yourself after going to the bathroom?	☐	☐	☐	☐	☐
17. How difficult is it for you to turn knobs or levers (for example, to open doors or to roll down car windows)?	☐	☐	☐	☐	☐
18. How difficult is it for you to write or type?	☐	☐	☐	☐	☐
19. How difficult is it for you to pivot?	☐	☐	☐	☐	☐
20. How difficult is it for you to do your usual physical recreational activities, such as bicycling, jogging, or walking?	☐	☐	☐	☐	☐
21. How difficult is it for you to do your usual leisure activities, such as hobbies, crafts, gardening, card-playing, or going out with friends?	☐	☐	☐	☐	☐
22. How much difficulty are you having with sexual activity?	☐	☐	☐	☐	☐
23. How difficult is it for you to do *light* housework *or* yard work, such as dusting, washing dishes, or watering plants?	☐	☐	☐	☐	☐
24. How difficult is it for you to do *heavy* housework *or* yard work; such as washing floors, vacuuming, or mowing lawns?	☐	☐	☐	☐	☐
25. How difficult is it for you to do your usual work, such as a paid job, housework, or volunteer activities?	☐	☐	☐	☐	☐

TABLE 7-9   Short Musculoskeletal Function Assessment (SMFA)[77] *(cont.)*

The following questions ask how often you are experiencing problems *this week* because of your injury or arthritis.

	None of the Time	A Little of the Time	Some of the Time	Most of the Time	All of the Time
26. How often do you walk with a limp?	☐	☐	☐	☐	☐
27. How often do you avoid using your painful limb(s) or back?	☐	☐	☐	☐	☐
28. How often does your leg lock or give way?	☐	☐	☐	☐	☐
29. How often do you have problems with concentration?	☐	☐	☐	☐	☐
30. How often does doing too much in one day affect what you do the next day?	☐	☐	☐	☐	☐
31. How often do you act irritable toward those around you (for example, snap at people, give sharp answers, or criticize easily)?	☐	☐	☐	☐	☐
32. How often are you tired?	☐	☐	☐	☐	☐
33. How often do you feel disabled?	☐	☐	☐	☐	☐
34. How often do you feel angry or frustrated that you have this injury or arthritis?	☐	☐	☐	☐	☐

These questions are about how much you are bothered by problems you are having *this week* because of your injury or arthritis.

	Not at All Bothered	A Little Bothered	Moderately Bothered	Very Bothered	Extremely Bothered
35. How much are you bothered by problems using your hands, arms, or legs?	☐	☐	☐	☐	☐
36. How much are you bothered by problems using your back?	☐	☐	☐	☐	☐
37. How much are you bothered by problems doing work around your home?	☐	☐	☐	☐	☐
38. How much are you bothered by problems with bathing, dressing, toileting, or other personal care?	☐	☐	☐	☐	☐
39. How much are you bothered by problems with sleep and rest?	☐	☐	☐	☐	☐
40. How much are you bothered by problems with leisure or recreational activities?	☐	☐	☐	☐	☐
41. How much are you bothered by problems with your friends, family, or other important people in your life?	☐	☐	☐	☐	☐
42. How much are you bothered by problems with thinking, concentrating, or remembering?	☐	☐	☐	☐	☐
43. How much are you bothered by problems adjusting or coping with your injury or arthritis?	☐	☐	☐	☐	☐
44. How much are you bothered by problems doing your usual work?	☐	☐	☐	☐	☐
45. How much are you bothered by problems with feeling dependent on others?	☐	☐	☐	☐	☐
46. How much are you bothered by problems with stiffness and pain?	☐	☐	☐	☐	☐

and general health perception. Previous research has shown that, compared with other generic instruments, the SF-36 is a reliable and valid generic measure of the health of patients who have a musculoskeletal condition.[79] Although this test is a good tool for overall function, it is not specific to functional problems at specific joints, and it is recommended that it be used in conjunction with tests that are specific to the patient's dysfunctional joint.[79]

Although these tests measure some of the components of function, they are not multidimensional. For example, they do not always address the patient's value system or the patient's overall physical performance in his or her own environment.

The Future

Part of the problem in designing a functional measurement tool is that function is highly individual, with multiple levels of difficulty and a high degree of specificity. It is very difficult to extrapolate examination results from the clinical outcomes of pain, strength, and range of motion to specific and meaningful changes in function and quality of life. What is needed is a functional measurement tool that recognizes and classifies impairments, functional limitations, and disability using clinical measurements by qualifying and quantifying the impairments.[80] These measures can then be used as evidence of the success at returning patients to their desired level of function, in their own environment. Thus, it is critical that the outcomes chosen evaluate functional improvement as perceived by the patient. In addition, functional measures must be valid, reliable, and responsive to clinically meaningful change.[81]

Various conceptual models exist in the literature that attempt to address these issues.[4,53,63] Patrick's model of health promotion for people with disabilities is perhaps the best of these.[63] Patrick's model depicts four broad planes of outcome: total environment, opportunity, disabling process, and quality of life[63,70] (Fig. 7-3).

▶ *Total environment.* This plane includes the individual's biologic and genetic makeup, demographic characteristics (race, gender, age), lifestyle behaviors (smoking, exercise, diet, risk-taking), health and social care systems, and physical and social characteristics of the environment.

▶ *Opportunity.* This plane represents outcomes related to independent living, economic self-sufficiency, equality of rights or status, and full participation in community life. Opportunity represents the interaction between the total environment of the individual at his or her particular stage of life course, and the disabling process.

▶ *Disabling process.* This plane represents the theoretical progression from disease or injury to the restriction of activities. The disablement outcomes represented in this plane include disease or injury, impairment, functional limitation, and activity restriction or disability.

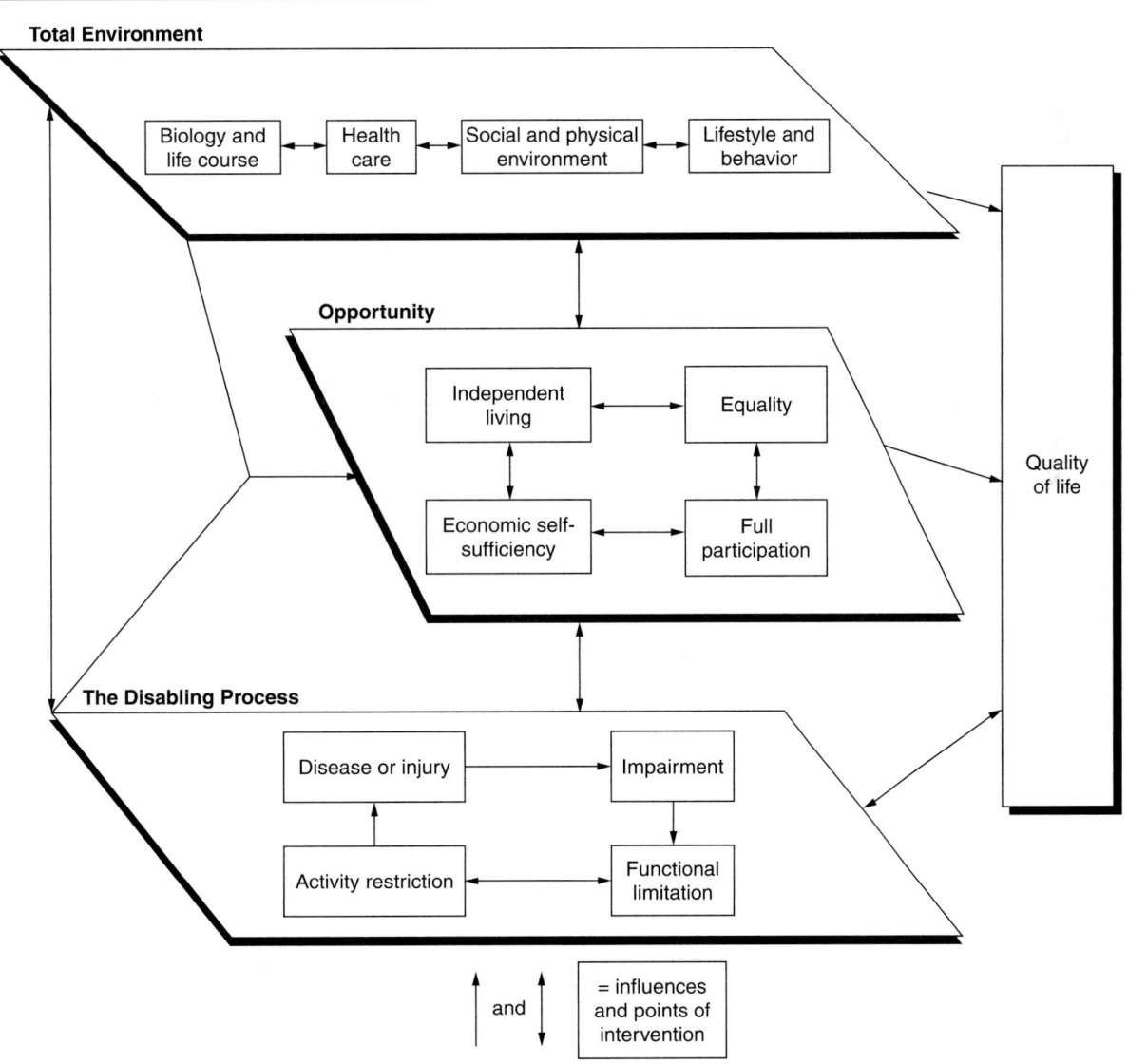

FIGURE 7-3 Patrick's model.

▶ *Quality of life.* This plane represents a distinct outcome that includes people's perceptions of their position in life in the context of their particular culture and value system and in relation to their personal goals, expectations, standards, and concerns.

According to Patrick, the elements within these planes do not constitute a linear or temporal process, in that they do not occur in an entirely unilateral direction.[63] Patrick suggests that quality-of-life outcomes are influenced by the other three planes, and that the disabling process may be halted or reversed at any of the interaction points in the model. Under such a model, the intervention includes the restoration or maintenance of functional status, the promotion of opportunity, and alterations to the patient's environment, and individual behavior.[63]

The correct selection and application of standardized outcome measurement instruments is a fundamental component of the clinical decision-making process. Resnik and Dobrzykowski[71c] recommend the following guidelines to assist the clinician in their selection:

1. Select an instrument with known reliability, validity, and demonstrated sensitivity to change.

2. Administer the instrument on intake, reassessment, and upon discharge, and know the suggested time frame for repeat administration.

3. Be familiar with the scoring procedure for the instrument.

4. Complete the scoring.

5. Document the Health Related Quality of Life (HRQL) intake, discharge, and change in scores on the patient record.

6. Understand the clinical meaning of the range of scores.

7. Be familiar with the medical detectable change (MDC) and the minimally clinically important difference (MCID) for the scale.

8. Establish a treatment goal for change of the HRQL score that is greater than the MDC or MCID for the instrument, if these are known.

9. Assess changes in HRQL scores and compare to the known MDC for the instrument to determine if true change has been made.

10. Analyze outcomes to evaluate treatment effectiveness and efficiency.

REVIEW QUESTIONS*

1. What is an *impairment* according to the *Guide to Physical Therapist Practice?*
2. Which term is preferred over *handicap* to describe limitations in the ability to meet social or occupational demands?
3. What is the term used to describe the characteristics of an illness that are not amenable to modification?
4. How does a physical therapy diagnosis differ from a medical diagnosis?
5. List three ways in which impairments may be measured objectively.

*Additional questions to test your understanding of this chapter can be found in the Online Learning Center for *Orthopaedic Assessment, Evaluation, and Intervention* at www.duttononline.net.

REFERENCES

1. Pollard CA. Preliminary validity study of Pain Disability Index. *Percep Motor Skills* 1984;59:974.
2. Guide to physical therapist practice. *Phys Ther* 2001;81:S13–S95.
3. Cocchiarella L, Andersson GBJ, eds. *American Medical Association Guides to the Evaluation of Permanent Impairment.* 5th ed. Chicago, Ill: AMA; 2001.
4. Verbrugge LM, Jette AM. The disablement process. *Soc Sci Med* 1994;38:1–14.
5. Jette AM. Physical disablement concepts for physical therapy research and practice. *Phys Ther* 1994;74:375–382.
6. Lawrence R, Jette A. Disentangling the disablement process. *J Gerontol B Psychol Sci Soc Sci* 1996;51B:S173–S182.
7. Nagi S. Disability concepts revisited: Implications for prevention. In: Pope A, Tartov A, eds. *Disability in America: Toward a National Agenda for Prevention.* Washington, DC: National Academy Press; 1991:309–327.
8. Pope A, Tartov A. *Disability in America: Toward a National Agenda for Prevention.* Washington, DC: National Academy Press; 1991.
9. Salen BO, Spangfort EV, Nygren AL, et al. The disability rating index: An instrument for the assessment of disability in clinical settings. *J Clin Epidemiol* 1994;47:1423–1434.
10. Simeonsson RJ, Leskinen M. Disability, secondary conditions and quality of life: Conceptual issues. In: Simeonsson RJ, McDevitt LN, eds. *Issues in Disability and Health: The Role of Secondary Conditions and Quality of Life.* Chapel Hill, NC: University of North Carolina Press; 1999:51–72.
11. Nagi S. Some conceptual issues in disability and rehabilitation. In: Sussman M, ed. *Sociology and Rehabilitation.* Washington, DC: American Sociological Association; 1965:100–113.
12. Escalante A, del Rincon I. How much disability in rheumatoid arthritis is explained by rheumatoid arthritis? *Arthritis Rheum* 1999;42:1712–1721.
13. Waddell G, Waddell H. A review of social influences on neck and back pain disability. In: Nachemson AL, Jonsson E, eds. *Neck and Back Pain: The Scientific Evidence of Causes, Diagnosis, and Treatment.* Philadelphia, Pa: Lippincott Williams and Wilkins; 2000:13–55.
14. Krause JS, Bell RB. Measuring quality of life and secondary conditions: Experiences with spinal cord injury. In: Simeonsson RJ, McDevitt LN, eds. *Issues in Disability and Health: The Role of Secondary Conditions and Quality of Life.* Chapel Hill, NC: University of North Carolina Press; 1999:129–143.
15. Buchner DM, Beresford SA, Larson EB, LaCroix AZ, Wagner EH. Effects of physical activity on health status in older adults. II: Intervention studies. *Annu Rev Public Health* 1992;13:469–488.
16. Caspersen CJ, Powell KE, Christenson GM. Physical activity, exercise and physical fitness. *Public Health Rep* 1985;100:125–131.
17. Gregg EW, Pereira MA, Caspersen CJ. Physical activity, falls, and fractures among older adults: A review of the epidemiologic evidence. *J Am Geriatr Soc* 2000;48:883–893.

18. Helmrich SP, Ragland DR, Leung RW, Paffenbarger RS Jr. Physical activity and reduced occurrence of non-insulin-dependent diabetes mellitus. *N Engl J Med* 1991;325:147–152.

19. Lee I, Paffenbarger RS, Hsieh C. Physical activity and risk of developing colorectal cancer among college alumni. *J Natl Cancer Inst* 1991;83:1324–1329.

20. Leon AS, Connett J, Jacobs DR Jr, Rauramaa R. Leisure-time physical activity levels and risk of coronary heart disease and death: The Multiple Risk Factor Intervention Trial (MRFIT). *JAMA* 1987;258:2388–2395.

21. Manson JE, Rimm EB, Stampfer MJ, et al. Physical activity and incidence of non-insulin-dependent diabetes mellitus in women. *Lancet* 1991;338:774–778.

22. Paffenbarger RS Jr, Wing AL, Hyde RT, Jung DL. Physical activity and incidence of hypertension in college alumni. *Am J Epidemiol* 1983;117:245–257.

23. Paffenbarger RS Jr, Hyde RT, Wing AL, Hsieh CC. Physical activity, all-cause mortality, and longevity of college alumni. *N Engl J Med* 1986;314:605–613.

24. Powell KE, Thompson PD, Caspersen CJ, Kendrick JS. Physical activity and the incidence of coronary heart disease. *Annu Rev Public Health* 1987;8:253–287.

25. Fried LP, Guralnik JM. Disability in older adults: Evidence regarding significance, etiology, and risk. *J Am Geriatr Soc* 1997;45:92–100.

26. Steultjens MP, Dekker J, Bijlsma JW. Avoidance of activity and disability in patients with osteoarthritis of the knee: The mediating role of muscle strength. *Arthritis Rheum* 2002;46:1784–1788.

27. Elton D, Stanley G. Cultural expectations and psychological factors in prolonged disability. *Adv Behav Med* 1982;2:33–42.

28. Zborowski M. Cultural components in responses to pain. *J Soc Issues* 1952;8:16–30.

29. Nordin M, Hiebert R, Pietrek M, Alexander M, Crane M, Lewis S. Association of comorbidity and outcome in episodes of nonspecific low back pain in occupational populations. *J Occup Envir Med* 2002;44:677–684.

30. Callahan LF, Pincus T. Formal education level as a significant marker of clinical status in rheumatoid arthritis. *Arthritis Rheum* 1988;31:1346–1357.

31. Nordin M. Education and return to work. In: Gunzburg R, Szpalski M, eds. Whiplash Injuries: *Current Concepts in Prevention, Diagnosis and Treatment of the Cervical Whiplash Syndrome.* Philadelphia, Pa: Lippincott-Raven; 1998:199–210.

32. Cavalieri F, Salaffi F, Ferraccioli GF. Relationship between physical impairment, psychological variables and pain in rheumatoid disability: An analysis of their relative impact. *Clin Exp Rheumatol* 1991;9:47–50.

33. Encandela J. Social science and the study of pain since Zborowski: A need for a new agenda. *Soc Sci Med* 1993;36:783–791.

34. Edwards RR, Doleys DM, Fillingim RB, Lowery D. Ethnic differences in pain tolerance: Clinical implications in a chronic pain population. *Psychosom Med* 2001;63:316–323.

35. Lautenbacher S, Rollman GB. Sex differences in responsiveness to painful and non-painful stimuli are dependent upon the stimulation method. *Pain* 1993;53:255–264.

36. Walker JS, Carmody JJ. Experimental pain in healthy human subjects: Gender differences in nociception and in response to ibuprofen. *Anesth Analg* 1998;86:1257–1262.

37. Ellermeier W, Westphal W. Gender differences in pain ratings and pupil reactions to painful pressure stimuli. *Pain* 1995;61:435–439.

38. Lund JP, Donga R, Widmer CG, Stohler CS. The pain-adaptation model: A discussion of the relationship between chronic musculoskeletal pain and motor activity. *Can J Physiol Pharmacol* 1991;69:683–694.

39. Aro S, Leino P. Overweight and musculoskeletal morbidity: A ten-year follow-up. *Int J Obesity* 1985;9:267–275.

40. Deyo RA, Bass JE. Lifestyle and low-back pain. The influence of smoking and obesity. *Spine* 1989;14:501–506.

41. Lilienfeld DE, Vladov D, Tenney JH, McLaughlin JS. Obesity and diabetes as risk factors for postoperative wound infections after cardiac surgery. *Am J Infect Control* 1988;16:3–6.

42. National Center for Health Statistics. *Prevalence of Overweight and Obesity Among Adults: United States.* Hyattsville, Md: NCHS; 2000.

43. Goodman CC, Boissonnault WG. *Pathology: Implications for the Physical Therapist.* Philadelphia, Pa: WB Saunders; 1998:791–797.

43a. Resnik L, Dobrzykowski. Guide to outcome measurement for patients with low back pain syndromes. *J Orthop Sports Phys Ther* 2003;33:307–318.

43b. Jette AM. Outcomes research: Shifting the dominant research paradigm in physical therapy. *Phys Ther* 1995; 75:965–970.

44. Tait RC, Chibnall JT, Krause S. The Pain Disability Index: Psychometric properties. *Pain* 1990;40:171–182.

45. Tait RC, Pollard CA, Margolis RB, Duckro PN, Krause SJ. The Pain Disability Index: Psychometric and validity data. *Arch Phys Med Rehab* 1987;68:438–441.

46. Burkhardt CS. The use of the McGill Pain Questionnaire in assessing arthritis pain. *Pain* 1984;19:305.

47. Melzack R. The McGill Pain Questionnaire: Major properties and scoring methods. *Pain* 1975;1:277.

48. Pearce J, Morley S. An experimental investigation of the construct validity of the McGill Pain Questionnaire. *Pain* 1989;115:115.

49. Randall KE, McEwen IR. Writing patient-centered goals. *Phys Ther* 2000;80:1197–1203.

50. Winton PJ, Bailey DB. Communicating with families: Examining practices and facilitating change. In: Simeonsson JP, Simeonsson RJ, eds. *Children with Special Needs: Family, Culture, and Society.* Orlando, Fla: Harcourt Brace Jovanovich; 1993;86–98.

51. O'Neill DL, Harris SR. Developing goals and objectives for handicapped children. *Phys Ther* 1982;62:295–298.

52. Badley EM, Wagstaff S, Wood PHN. Measures of functional ability (disability) in arthritis in relation to impairment of range of joint movement. *Ann Rheum Dis* 1984;43:563–569.

53. Dijkers MPJM, Whiteneck G, El-Jaroudi R. Measures of social outcomes in disability. *Arch Phys Med Rehabil* 2000;81(suppl):S63–S80.

54. McFarlane AC, Brooks PM. The assessment of disability and handicap in musculoskeletal disease. *J Rheumatol* 1997;24:985–989.

55. Verbrugge LM. Disability. *Rheum Dis Clin North Am* 1990;16:741–761.

56. Americans with Disabilities Act of 1989, 104 Stat 327 (1989) pp 101–336, 42 USC §12101 s2 (a) (8).

57. Olkin R. Could you hold the door for me? Including disability in diversity. *Cult Div Ethnic Minor Psychol* 2002;8:130–137.

58. Yassin AS, Beckles GL, Messonnier ML. Disability and its economic impact among adults with diabetes. *J Occup Envir Med* 2002;44:136–142.

59. Pinsky JL, Branch LG, Jette AM, et al. Framingham Disability Study: Relationship of disability to cardiovascular risk factors among persons free of diagnosed cardiovascular disease. *Am J Epidemiol* 1985;122:644–656.

60. Ettinger WH Jr, Fried LP, Harris T, Shemanski L, Schulz R, Robbins J. Self-reported causes of physical disability in older people: The cardiovascular health study. *J Am Geriatr Soc* 1994;42:1035–1044.

61. Raine S, Twomey LT. Attributes and qualities of human posture and their relationship to dysfunction or musculoskeletal pain. *Crit Rev Phys Rehabil Med* 1994;6:409–437.

62. West CG, Gildengorin G, Haegerstrom-Portnoy G, Schneck ME, Lott L, Brabyn JA. Is vision function related to physical functional ability in older adults? *J Am Geriatr Soc* 2002;50:136–145.

63. Patrick DL. Rethinking prevention for people with disabilities. Part I: A conceptual model for promoting health. *Am J Health Prom* 1997;11:257–260.

64. Barnett D. Assessment of quality of life. *Am J Cardiol* 1991;67: 41c–44c.

65. Carr A, Thompson P, Kirwan J. Quality of life measures. *Br J Rheumatol* 1996;35:275–281.

66. Felce D, Perry J. Quality of life: Its definition and measurement. *Res Dev Disabil* 1995;16:51–74.

67. Patrick DL, Deyo RA. Generic and disease-specific measures in assessing health status and quality of life. *Med Care* 1989;27(suppl):217–232.

68. Voight ML, Cook G. Impaired neuromuscular control: Reactive neuromuscular training. In: Prentice WE, Voight ML, eds. *Techniques in Musculoskeletal Rehabilitation.* New York, NY: McGraw-Hill; 2001:93–124.

69. Brandt EN Jr, Pope AM, eds. *Enabling America: Assessing the Role of Rehabilitation Science and Engineering.* Washington, DC: Institute of Medicine, National Academy Press; 1997.

70. Salive ME, Mayfield JA, Weissman NW. Patient outcomes research teams and the agency for health care policy and research. *Health Serv Res* 1990;25:697–708.

71. American Physical Therapy Association. Guide to physical therapist practice. *Phys Ther* 2001;81:S13–S95.

71a. Jette AM, Keysor JJ. Uses of evidence in disability outcomes and effectiveness research. *Milbank Q* 2002;80:325–345.

71b. Blair SJ, McCormick E, Bear-Lehman J, Fess EE, Rader E. Evaluation of impairment of the upper extremity. *Clin Orthop* 1987;221:42–58.

71c. Resnik L, Dobrzykowski E. Guide to outcome measurement for patients with low back pain syndromes. *J Orthop Sports Ther* 2003;33:307–318.

71d. Hebert R, Spiegelhalter DJ, Brayne C. Setting the minimal metrically detectable change on disability rating scales. *Arch Phys Med Rehab* 1997;78:1305–1308.

71e. Fritz JM, Irrgang JJ. A comparison of a modified Oswestry Low Back Pain Disability Questionnaire and the Quebec Back Pain Disability Scale. *Phys Ther* 2001;81:776–788.

71f. Stratford PW. Invited commentary: Guide to outcome measurement for patients with low back pain syndromes. *J Orthop Sports Phys Ther* 2003;33:317–318.

71g. Grimmer K, et al., Differences in stakeholder expectations in the outcome of physiotherapy management of acute low back pain. *Int J Qual Health Care* 1999;11:155–162.

72. Reuben DB, Siu AL. Measuring physical function in community dwelling older persons: A comparison of self administered, interviewer administered, and performance-based measures. *J Am Geriatr Soc* 1995;43:17–23.

73. Tager IB, Swanson A, Satariano WA. Reliability of physical performance and self-reported functional measures in an older population. *J Gerontol* 1998;53:M295–M300.

74. de Bruin AF, De Witte LP, Stevens F, Diederiks JP. Sickness Impact Profile: The state of the art of a generic functional status measure. *Soc Sci Med* 1992;35:1003–1014.

75. Bergner M, Bobbitt RA, Carter WB, Gilson BS. The Sickness Impact Profile: Development and final revision of a health status measure. *Med Care* 1981;19:787.

76. Feise RJ, Menke JM. Functional rating index: A new valid and reliable instrument to measure the magnitude of clinical change in spinal conditions. *Spine* 2001;26:78–86, discussion 87.

77. Swiontkowski MF, Engelberg R, Martin DP, Agel J. Short musculoskeletal function assessment questionnaire: Validity, reliability, and responsiveness. *J Bone Joint Surg* 1999;81A:1256–1258.

78. Ware JE Jr, Snow KK, Kosinski M, Gardek B, et al. *SF-36 Health Survey: Manual and Interpretation Guide.* Boston, Mass: The Health Institute; 1993.

79. Beaton DE, Richards RR. Measuring function of the shoulder. A cross-sectional comparison of five questionnaires. *J Bone Joint Surg* 1996;78A:882–890.

80. Cook G, Voight ML. Essentials of functional exercise: A four-step clinical model for therapeutic exercise prescription. In: Prentice WE, Voight ML, eds. *Techniques in Musculoskeletal Rehabilitation.* New York, NY: McGraw-Hill; 2001:387–407.

81. Davies GM, Watson DJ, Bellamy N. Comparison of the responsiveness and relative effect size of the Western Ontario and McMaster Universities Osteoarthritis Index and the Short-Form Medical Outcomes Study Survey in a randomized, clinical trial of osteoarthritis patients. *Arthritis Care Res* 1999;12:172–179.

CHAPTER 8

THE EXAMINATION AND EVALUATION

CHAPTER OBJECTIVES

▶ *At the completion of this chapter, the reader will be able to:*

1. Understand the principles of a comprehensive examination.

2. Describe the differences between the examination and the evaluation.

3. Understand the value of a complete observation of the patient and the information that can be gleaned from such an assessment.

4. Take a complete history.

5. Describe the importance of a systems review.

6. List the components of the tests and measures portion of the examination.

7. Describe the different types of imaging studies and their relative value in the examination and evaluation process.

8. Describe the different types of diagnostic models.

The Clinician's Journey

The examination process involves a complex relationship between the clinician and the patient. The aims of the examination process are to provide an efficient and effective exchange, and to develop a rapport between clinician and patient. The success of this interaction involves a myriad of skills. Successful clinicians are those who demonstrate effective communication skills, clinical reasoning, critical judgment, creative decision-making, knowledge, and competence.

The primary responsibility of a clinician is to make decisions in the best interest of the patient. These decisions are based on an evaluation of the available information gleaned from the examination. Although the approach to the examination should vary with each patient, and from condition to condition, there are several fundamental components to the examination process. The principles outlined in this chapter, and integrated throughout this text, are based on the views of a number of experts,[1-11] as well as principles I have learned, and used, over the years.

Principle 1: Utilize Your Resources

All clinicians should be life-long students of their profession and should strive toward a process of continual self-education. Part of this process involves the utilization of the expertise of more experienced clinicians. This necessitates that the early years of practice are spent in an environment in which the novice is surrounded by a staff of varying levels of clinical and life experiences, both of which can serve as valuable resources. The clinician can also improve by investing time reading relevant material, attending continuing education courses, completing home study courses, watching videos specializing in techniques, and observing exceptional clinicians. Exceptional clinicians are those who demonstrate excellent *technical* skills, combined with excellent *people* skills.

> **Clinical Pearl**
>
> From the patient's point of view, there is no substitute for interest, acceptance, and especially empathy on the part of the clinician.[12]

Finally, one must also never forget that the patient serves as perhaps the most valuable resource. Each interaction with a patient is an opportunity to increase knowledge, skill, and understanding. Integral to this relationship is patient confidentiality. Patient confidentiality must always be strictly adhered to. Except when discussing the patient's condition with other clinicians with the object of teaching or learning, the clinician should not discuss the patient's condition with anyone without the patient's permission.

Principle 2: Be an Effective Communicator

Much about becoming a clinician relates to an ability to communicate with the patient, the patient's family, and to the other members of the health-care team. The nonverbal cues are especially important, because they often are performed subconsciously. Special attention needs to be paid to one's body language, tone of voice, and attitude. The appearance of the clinician is also important if a professional image is to be projected.

Communication between clinician and patient begins when the clinician first meets the patient, and continues throughout any future sessions. Communication involves interacting with the patient using terms he or she can understand. The introduction to the patient should be handled in a professional yet empathetic tone. Listening with empathy involves understanding the ideas being communicated and the emotion behind the ideas. In essence, empathy is seeing another person's viewpoint, so that a deep and true understanding of what the person is experiencing can be obtained.

At the end of the first visit and at subsequent visits, the clinician should ask if there are any questions. Each session should have closure, which may include a handshake, if appropriate.

Examination Principles

Principle 1: Make a Complete and Accurate Functional Diagnosis

> "He who wants to know man must look upon him as a whole and not as a patched-up piece of work. If he finds a part of the human body diseased, he must look for the causes which produce disease, and not merely treat the external effects."
>
> Paracelsus (1493–1541)

The success of any rehabilitation intervention depends on the quality and accuracy of the examination and the subsequent evaluation. An *examination* refers to the gathering of data and information concerning a topic.[13] In contrast, an *evaluation* refers to the making of a value judgment based on the collected data and information.[13]

The examination must be performed with a scientific rigor that follows a predictable and strictly ordered thought process. The purpose of the examination is to obtain information that identifies and measures a change from normal. This is determined using information related by the patient in conjunction with clinical signs and findings.

Clinical Pearl

The clinician must always remember that measurements may appear to be objective, but that the interpretation of any measurement is always subjective.[14]

Patient discomfort should always be kept to a minimum. It is important that examination procedures only be performed to the point at which symptoms are provoked or begin to increase, if they are not present at rest.

The examination consists of three components of equal importance: (1) history, (2) systems review, and (3) tests and measures.[13] These components are closely related, in that they often occur concurrently. One further element, observation, occurs throughout.

> "In all experimental knowledge there are three phases: an observation made, a comparison established, and a judgment rendered."
>
> Claude Bernard (1813–1878)

Observation

Observation of the patient begins when the patient enters the clinic. As the clinician greets the patient and takes him or her to the treatment room, an initial observation is made. This early observation can provide the clinician with information that includes, but is not limited to how the patient holds the extremity, whether an antalgic gait is present, and how much discomfort appears to be present.

Much can be learned from thorough observation. Throughout the history, systems review, and tests and measures, collective observations form the basis for diagnostic deductions. Some of the observations made may be very subtle. Hoarseness of the voice could suggest laryngeal cancer, whereas a weakened, thickened, and lowered voice may indicate hypothyroidism.[15] Warm, moist hands felt during a handshake may indicate hyperthyroidism.[15] Cold, moist hands may indicate an anxious patient. Patients react differently to injury. Some patients may exaggerate the symptoms through facial expressions and gestures, whereas others remain stoic. Patients may appear calm and pleasant, defensive, angry, apprehensive, or depressed. Anxious patients, or patients in severe pain, often appear restless. Clinicians must learn to adopt their approaches to these different reactions. For example, an anxious or apprehensive patient may require more reassurance than a calm and pleasant patient.

Changes in the contours of the body shape or posture can be so specific that it often is possible to isolate the single muscle involved, the movements affected, and the related joint dysfunction from observation alone.[16] The patient's position of comfort can provide the clinician with valuable information. For example, patients with lateral recess spinal stenosis, congestive heart failure, or pulmonary disease often prefer the sitting position, whereas patients with pericarditis often sit and lean forward.[15] Patients with a posterior-lateral disk herniation often prefer to stand or lie rather than sit.

The more formal observation, which is included in each of the relevant chapters, includes but is not limited to an analysis of posture, structural alignment or deformity, and the presence of any asymmetry, scars, crepitus, color changes, swelling, and muscle atrophy.

History

The history taking specific to each joint is detailed in each of the chapters. The history usually precedes the systems review and the tests and measures components of the examination, but it also may occur concurrently. It is estimated that 80 percent of the necessary information to explain the presenting patient problem can be provided by a thorough history[17] (Table 8-1). This may be an underestimation. The clinician must record the history in a systematic fashion so that no subject areas are

TABLE 8-1 Data Generated from a Patient History

General demographics
Social history and social habits
Occupation/Employment
Growth and development
Living environment
History of current condition
Functional status and activity level
Medications
Other tests and measures
Past history of current condition
Past medical/surgical history
Family history
Health status

neglected. The method of questioning should be altered from patient to patient as the level of understanding and answering ability varies between each individual. A transfer of accurate information must occur between patient and clinician. A successful learning process requires the clinician to have patience, focus, and self-criticism.[5]

Open-ended questions or statements, such as "Tell me why you are here" are used initially to encourage the patient to provide narrative information and to decrease the opportunity for bias on the part of the clinician.[17] More specific questions are asked as the examination proceeds (Table 8-2). The specific questions help to focus the examination and deter irrelevant information. *Neutral* questions should be used whenever possible. These questions are structured in such a way so as to avoid leading the patient into giving a particular response. Leading questions, such as "Does it hurt more when you walk?" should be avoided. A more neutral question would be, "What activities make your symptoms worse?" The clinician should provide the patient with encouraging responses, such as a nod of the head, when the information is relevant, and when needed to steer the patient into supplying necessary information.

The purposes of the history are to:

▶ Develop a working relationship with the patient and establish lines of communication with the patient. Formal questioning, using a questionnaire (Table 8-3), helps to ensure that all of the important questions are asked. To help establish a rapport with the patient, the clinician should discuss the information provided on these forms with the patient at either the initial or subsequent visits.

▶ Elicit reports of potentially dangerous symptoms, or *red flags* that require an immediate medical referral[19] (Table 8-4).

▶ Determine the chief complaint, its mechanism of injury, its severity, and its impact on the patient's function.

▶ Ascertain the specific location and nature of the symptoms.

▶ Determine the irritability of the symptoms.

▶ Establish a base-line of measurements.

▶ Elicit information about the history and past history of the current condition.

▶ Gather information about the patient's past general medical and surgical history. Although this information is not always related to the presenting condition, it does afford the clinician some insight as to the impact the information may have on the patient's tolerance or response to the planned intervention.

▶ Determine the goals and expectations of the patient from the physical therapy intervention, and the functional demands of a specific vocational or avocational activity to which the patient is planning to return.

Clinical Pearl

It is important to remember that symptoms can be experienced without the presence of recognized clinical signs, and that signs can be present in the absence of symptoms. The former scenario is more common, but the latter can occur when a pathologic reflex or positive cranial nerve test is detected in the absence of any subjective complaints. In such a scenario, a positive finding could be a false positive result, or it could be prognostic.[3]

The components of the patient history described in this section are based on the "Guide to Physical Therapist Practice."[13]

General Demographics. This section includes information about the patient's age, height, weight, marital status, and primary language spoken.[13]

Certain conditions are related to age, race, and gender. For example:

▶ Among African Americans in the United States, 1 in 600 has sickle cell anemia.[21]

▶ Basal cell carcinoma and melanoma are more common among whites.

▶ Degenerative and overuse syndromes are more frequent in the over-40 age group.

▶ The onset of ankylosing spondylitis often occurs between the ages of 15 and 35 years.[22]

▶ Both osteoporosis and osteoarthritis are associated with the older population.

▶ Prostate cancer has a higher incidence in men older than 50 years.[23]

▶ The male-to-female ratio of bladder cancer is 2:1 to 4:1, and the disease is twice as common in white men as in black men in the United States.[24,25]

▶ Breast cancer is the most frequently diagnosed cancer and the second leading cause of cancer-related deaths among women in the United States.[26]

▶ Melanoma is the leading cause of cancer death in women aged 25 to 36 years.[27]

TABLE 8-2   Contents of the History[18]

HISTORY OF CURRENT CONDITION

   Did condition begin insidiously or was trauma involved?

   How long has patient had symptoms?

   Where are symptoms?

   How does patient describe symptoms? Reports about numbness and tingling suggest neurologic compromise. Reports of pain suggest chemical or mechanical irritant. Pain needs to be carefully evaluated in terms of its site, distribution, quality, onset, frequency, nocturnal occurrence, aggravating factors, and relieving factors.

PAST HISTORY OF CURRENT CONDITION

   Has patient had a similar injury in the past?

   Was it treated or did it resolve on its own? If it was treated, how was it treated and did intervention help?

   How long did most recent episode last?

PAST MEDICAL/SURGERY HISTORY

   How is patient's general health?

   Does patient have any allergies?

MEDICATIONS PATIENT IS PRESENTLY TAKING

OTHER TESTS AND MEASURES

   Has patient had any imaging tests such as x-ray, MRI, CT scan, bone scan?

   Has patient had an EMG test, or a nerve conduction velocity test, which would suggest compromise to muscle tissue and/or neurologic system?

SOCIAL HABITS (PAST AND PRESENT)

   Does patient smoke? If so, how many packs per day?

   Does patient drink alcohol? If so, how often and how much?

   Is patient active or sedentary?

SOCIAL HISTORY

   Is patient married, living with a partner, single, divorced, widowed?

   Is patient a parent or single parent?

FAMILY HISTORY

   Is there a family history of present condition?

GROWTH AND DEVELOPMENT

   Is patient right- or left-handed?

   Were there any congenital problems?

LIVING ENVIRONMENT

   What type of home does patient live in with reference to accessibility?

   Is there any support at home?

   Does patient use any extra pillows or special chairs to sleep?

OCCUPATIONAL/EMPLOYMENT/SCHOOL

   What does patient do for work?

   How long has he or she worked there?

   What does the job entail in terms of physical requirements?

   What level of education did patient achieve?

FUNCTIONAL STATUS/ACTIVITY LEVEL

   How does present condition affect patient's ability to perform activities of daily living?

   How does present condition affect patient at work?

   How does patient's condition affect sleep?

   Is patient able to drive? If so, for how long?

CT, computed tomography; EMG, electromyogram; MRI, magnetic resonance imaging.

TABLE 8-3   Sample Medical History Questionnaire

GENERAL MEDICAL HISTORY
GENERAL INFORMATION

_____ Date: _____

Last Name   First Name

The information requested may be needed if you have a medical emergency.

_____ _____ _____

Person to be notified in emergency Phone   Relationship

Are you currently working? (Y) or (N) Type of work: _____ If not, why?

GENERAL MEDICAL HISTORY:

Please check (✓) if you have been treated for:

( ) Heart problems   ( ) Lung disease/problems
( ) Fainting or dizziness   ( ) Arthritis
( ) Shortness of breath   ( ) Swollen and painful joints
( ) Calf pain with exercise   ( ) Irregular heart beat
( ) Severe headaches   ( ) Stomach pains or ulcers
( ) Recent accident   ( ) Pain with cough or sneeze
( ) Head trauma/concussion   ( ) Back or neck injuries
( ) Muscular weakness   ( ) Diabetes
( ) Cancer   ( ) Stroke(s)
( ) Joint dislocation(s)   ( ) Balance problems
( ) Broken bone   ( ) Muscular pain with activity
( ) Difficulty sleeping   ( ) Swollen ankles or legs
( ) Frequent falls   ( ) Jaw problems
( ) Unexplained weight loss   ( ) Circulatory problems
( ) Tremors   ( ) Epilepsy/seizures/convulsions
( ) High blood pressure (hypertension) ( ) Chest pain or pressure at rest
( ) Kidney disease   ( ) Allergies (latex, medication, food)
( ) Liver disease   ( ) Constant pain unrelieved by rest
( ) Weakness or fatigue   ( ) Pregnancy
( ) Hernias   ( ) Night pain (while sleeping)
( ) Blurred vision   ( ) Nervous or emotional problems
( ) Bowel/bladder problems   ( ) Any infectious disease (TB, AIDS, hepatitis)
( ) Difficulty swallowing   ( ) Tingling, numbness, or loss of feeling? If yes, where?
( ) A wound that does not heal   ( ) Constant pain or pressure during activity
( ) Unusual skin coloration

Do you use tobacco? (Y) or (N)   If yes, how much?

Are you presently taking any medications or drugs? (Y) or (N)

If yes, what are you taking them for?

1. Pain

On the line provided, mark where your "pain status" is today.

|——|

No pain   Most severe pain

2. Function. On a scale of 0 to 10 with 0 being able to perform all of your normal daily activities, and 10 being unable to perform any of your normal daily activities, give yourself a score for your _current ability_ to perform your activities of daily living. _____

Please list any major surgery or hospitalization:

Hospital: _____ Approx. Date: _____

Reasons:

Hospital: _____ Approx. Date: _____

Reasons:

Have you recently had an x-ray, MRI, or CT scan for your condition? (Y) or (N)

Facility: _____ Approx. date: _____

Findings: _____

Please mention any additional problems or symptoms you feel are important: _____

Have you been evaluated and/or treated by another physician, physical therapist, chiropractor, osteopath or health care practitioner for this condition? (Y) or (N) If yes, please circle which one.

TABLE 8-4   Red Flag Findings[20]

History	Possible Condition
Constant and severe pain, especially at night	Neoplasm, acute neuromusculoskeletal injury
Unexplained weight loss	Neoplasm
Loss of appetite	Neoplasm
Unusual fatigue	Neoplasm, thyroid dysfunction
Visual disturbances (blurriness or loss of vision)	Neoplasm
Frequent or severe headaches	Neoplasm
Arm pain lasting > 2–3 mo	Neoplasm or neurologic dysfunction
Persistent root pain	Neoplasm or neurologic dysfunction
Radicular pain with coughing	Neoplasm or neurologic dysfunction
Pain worsening after 1 mo	Neoplasm
Paralysis	Neoplasm or neurologic dysfunction
Trunk and limb paresthesia	Neoplasm or neurologic dysfunction
Bilateral nerve root signs and symptoms	Neoplasm, spinal cord compression, vertebrobasilar ischemia
Signs worse than symptoms	Neoplasm
Difficulty with balance and coordination	Spinal cord or CNS lesion
Fever or night sweats	Common findings in systemic infection and many diseases
Frequent nausea or vomiting	Common findings in many diseases, particularly of the gastrointestinal system
Dizziness	Upper cervical impairment, vertebrobasilar ischemia, craniovertebral ligament tear, inner ear dysfunction, CNS involvement, cardiovascular dysfunction
Shortness of breath	Cardiovascular and/or pulmonary dysfunction, asthma
Quadrilateral paresthesia	Spinal cord compression (cervical myelopathy), vertebrobasilar ischemia

CNS, central nervous system.

▶ Anterior knee pain caused by patellofemoral syndrome (see Chap. 18) is most common in young teenage girls and in young men in their 20s.[28]

Social History.   The clinician should procure information about the patient's social history, including support systems, family and caregiver resources, and cultural beliefs and behaviors.[13] An individual's response to pain and dysfunction is, in large part, determined by his or her cultural background, social standing, educational and economical status, and anticipation of functional compromise (see Chap. 7).[29]

Occupation, Employment, and Work Environment.   The clinician should acquire information about the patient's occupation, employment, and work environment, including current and previous community and work activities.[13] The clinician must determine the patient's work demands, the activities involved, and the activities or postures that appear to be aggravating the condition. Work-related low back injuries and repetitive motion disorders of the upper extremities are common in patients whose workplaces involve physical labor. Habitual postures may be the source of the problem in those with sedentary occupations. Patients who have sedentary occupations may also be at increased risk for overuse injuries when they are not at work, as a result of recreational pursuits (the *weekend warrior*).

Functional Status, Activity Level, and Current Level of Fitness.   The clinician must obtain information about the patient's current and prior level of function, with particular reference to the type of activities performed and the percentage of time spent performing those activities.

Growth and Development.   This section includes information about the patient's developmental background and hand or foot dominance. Developmental or congenital disorders that the clinician should note include such conditions as Legg-Calvé-Perthes disease, cerebral palsy, Down syndrome, spina bifida, scoliosis, and congenital hip dysplasia.

Living Environment.   The clinician should be aware of the living situation of the patient, including entrances and exits to the house, the number of stairs, and the location of bathrooms within the house.

History of Current Condition.   This portion of the history taking can prove the most challenging and involves the gathering of both positive and negative findings, followed by the dissemination of the information into a working hypothesis. An understanding of the patient's history of the current condition can often help determine the prognosis and guide the intervention. For example, joint locking and twinges of pain may indicate a loose body moving within the joint. Reports of a joint "giving-way" usually indicate joint instability or a reflex inhibition or weakness of muscles. If a specific intervention has been used in the past for the same condition, the clinician should ask about the effectiveness of that intervention.

The presence of any of the following findings may indicate serious pathology requiring a medical referral[30] (see Chap. 9):

► *Fevers, chills, or night sweats.* These signs and symptoms are almost always associated with a systemic disorder such as disease or infection.

► *Recent unexplained weight changes.* An unexplained weight gain could be caused by congestive heart failure, hypothyroidism, or cancer.[31] An unexplained weight loss could be the result of a gastrointestinal disorder, hyperthyroidism, cancer, or diabetes.[31]

► *Malaise, or fatigue.* These complaints, which can help to determine the general health of the patient, may be associated with a systemic disease.

► *Unexplained nausea or vomiting.* This is never a good symptom or sign.

► *Unilateral, bilateral, or quadrilateral paresthesias.* The distribution of neurologic symptoms can give the clinician clues as to the structures involved. Quadrilateral paresthesia always indicates the presence of central nervous system (CNS) involvement.

► *Shortness of breath.* Shortness of breath can indicate a myriad of conditions. These can range from anxiety and asthma to a serious cardiac or pulmonary dysfunction.

► *Bowel or bladder dysfunction.* Bowel and bladder dysfunction may indicate involvement of the cauda equina. *Cauda equina syndrome* is associated with compression of the spinal nerve roots that supply neurologic function to the bladder and bowel. A massive disk herniation may cause spinal cord or cauda equina compression. One of the early signs of cauda equina compromise is the inability to urinate while sitting down, because of the increased levels of pressure. The most common sensory deficit occurs over the buttocks, posterior-superior thighs, and perianal regions (so-called saddle anesthesia), with a sensitivity of approximately 0.75.[32] Anal sphincter tone is diminished in 60 to 80 percent of cases.[32,33] Rapid diagnosis and surgical decompression of this abnormality is essential to prevent permanent neurologic dysfunction.

► An insidious onset of severe pain with no specific mechanism of injury (see later).

► Neurologic symptoms from more than two lumbar levels, or more than one cervical level. With the exception of central protrusions or a disk lesion at L4 through L5, disk protrusions typically only affect one spinal nerve root. Multiple level involvement could suggest the presence of a tumor or other growth or it may indicate symptom magnification. The presence or absence of objective findings should help determine the cause.

► Pain at night that awakens the patient from a deep sleep, usually at the same time every night and which is unrelated to a movement. This finding may indicate the presence of a tumor.

► Painful weakness (see "Muscle Performance: Strength, Power, and Endurance," in the later discussion of tests and measures)

► A gradual increase in the intensity of the pain. This symptom typically indicates that the condition is worsening, especially if it continues with rest.

Pain receptors (nociceptors), unlike other receptors, are nonadapting in nature; that is, they will continue to fire for as long as the stimulus is present (see Chap. 2). Nociceptor stimulation can only occur in one of three ways[34]:

1. Mechanical deformation resulting in the application of sufficient mechanical forces to stress, deform, or damage a structure.

2. Excessive heat or cold.

3. The presence of chemical irritants in sufficient quantities or concentrations. Examples of chemical irritants include the chemical released as part of the inflammatory process, or the release of lactic acid in muscles producing delayed onset of muscle soreness (DOMS) (see Chap. 6).

If pain is present, the clinician's major focus should be to seek methods to control the pain. However, it is important to remember that the focus is on the cause of the pain, not on the pain itself. Pain may be constant, variable, or intermittent. Variable pain is pain that is perpetual, but that varies in intensity. Variable pain usually indicates the involvement of both a chemical, and a mechanical source. The mechanical cause of constant pain is less understood, but is thought to be the result of the deformation of collagen, which compresses or stretches the nociceptive free nerve endings, with the excessive forces being perceived as pain.[34] Thus, specific movements or positions should influence pain of a mechanical nature.

Chemical, or inflammatory, pain is more constant and is less affected by movements or positions than mechanical pain. Intermittent pain is unlikely to be caused by a chemical irritant. Usually this type of pain is caused by prolonged postures, a loose intra-articular body, or an impingement of a musculoskeletal structure.

> ### Clinical Pearl
>
> Constant pain following an injury continues until the healing process has sufficiently reduced the concentration of noxious irritants.

Unfortunately, the source of the pain is not always easy to identify, because most patients present with both mechanical and chemical pain, which is commonly manifested as pain and stiffness.

Onset. The clinician should determine the circumstances and manner in which the symptoms began, and the progression of those symptoms.[5] The mode of onset, or mechanism of injury, can be either traumatic (macrotraumatic) or atraumatic (microtraumatic), and can give clues as to the extent and nature of damage caused (see Chap. 4).

If the injury is traumatic, the clinician should determine the specific mechanism, in terms of both the direction and force, and relate the mechanism to the presenting symptoms. If the injury is recent, an inflammatory source of pain is likely. A sudden onset of pain, associated with trauma, could indicate the presence of an acute injury such as a tear, whereas immediate pain and locking is most likely to result from an intra-articular block.

If the onset is gradual or insidious, the clinician must determine if there are any predisposing factors, such as changes in the patient's daily routines or exercise programs. Symptoms of pain or limitations of movement, with no apparent reason, are usually a result of inflammation, early degeneration, repetitive activity (microtrauma), or sustained positioning and postures.[35] However, such symptoms may also be associated with something more serious, such as vascular insufficiency, a tumor, or an infection.

Intensity. One of the simplest methods to quantify the intensity of pain is to use a 10-point visual analogue scale (VAS). The VAS is a numerically continuous scale that requires the pain level be identified by making a mark on a 100-mm line or by circling the appropriate number in a 1-to-10 series[36] (Table 8-5). The patient is asked to rate his or her present pain compared with the worst pain ever experienced, with 0 representing no pain, 1 representing minimally perceived pain, and 10 representing pain that requires immediate attention.[37]

Pain Perception. It is important to remember that pain perception is highly subjective. Pain is a broad and significant symptom that can be described using many descriptors. Perhaps the simplest descriptors are acute and chronic.

Acute pain is the type of pain that usually precipitates a visit to a physician, because it has one or more of the following characteristics[38]:

▶ It is new and has not been experienced before.

▶ It is severe and disabling.

▶ It is continuous, lasting for more than several minutes, or recurs very frequently.

▶ The site of the pain may cause alarm (e.g., chest, eye).

▶ In addition to the sensory and affective components, acute pain is typically characterized by anxiety. This may produce a fight-or-flight autonomic response, which is normally used for survival needs. This autonomic reaction is also associated with an increase in systolic and diastolic blood pressure, a decrease in gut motility and salivatory flow, increased muscle tension, and papillary distention.[39,40]

Acute pain following trauma, or the insidious onset of a musculoskeletal condition, is typically chemical in nature. Although motions aggravate the pain, they cannot be used to alleviate the symptoms. In contrast, cessation of movement (absolute rest) tends to alleviate the pain, although not necessarily immediately. However, this cessation of movement should not continue beyond 2 to 5 days in order to prevent any deleterious effects (see Chap. 4).

Clinical Pearl

The aching type of pain, associated with degenerative arthritis and muscle disorders is often accentuated by activity and lessened by rest. Pain that is not alleviated by rest, and that is not associated with acute trauma, may indicate the presence of a serious disorder such as a tumor or aneurysm. This pain is often described as deep, constant, and boring, and is apt to be more noticeable and more intense at night.[41]

Chronic pain is typically more aggravating than worrying, and has the following characteristics[38]:

▶ It has been experienced before and has remitted spontaneously, or after simple measures.

▶ It is usually mild to moderate in intensity.

▶ It is usually of limited duration, although it can persist for long periods.

▶ The pain site does not cause alarm (e.g., knee, ankle).

▶ There are no alarming associated symptoms.

The symptoms of chronic pain typically behave in a mechanical fashion, in that they are provoked by activity or repeated movements and reduced with rest or a movement in the opposite direction.

Clinical Pearl

Patients with chronic pain may be more prone to depression and disrupted interpersonal relationships.[42–45]

Quality of Symptoms. The quality of the symptoms depends on the type of receptor being stimulated (see Chap. 2).

▶ Stimulation of the cutaneous A-delta nociceptors leads to pricking pain.[46]

▶ Stimulation of the cutaneous C nociceptors results in burning or dull pain.[47]

▶ Activation of the nociceptors in muscle by electrical stimulation produces aching pain.[48]

▶ Electrical stimulation of visceral nerves at low intensities results in vague sensations of fullness and nausea, but higher intensities cause a sensation of pain.[49]

Because motor and sensory axons run in the same nerves, disorders of the peripheral nerves (neuropathies) usually affect both motor and sensory functions. Peripheral neuropathies can manifest as abnormal, frequently unpleasant sensations, which are variously described by the patient as numbness, pins and needles, and tingling.[50] When these sensations occur spontaneously without an external sensory stimulus, they are called *paresthesias*[50] (Table 8-6). Patients with paresthesias typically demonstrate a reduction in the perception of cutaneous and proprioceptive sensations.

TABLE 8-5   Patient Pain Evaluation Form

Name: _____

Date: _____   Signature: _____

Please use the diagram below to indicate where you feel symptoms right now. Use the following key to indicate different types of symptoms.

KEY: Pins and Needles = 000000   Stabbing = ///////   Burning = XXXXX   Deep Ache = ZZZZZZ

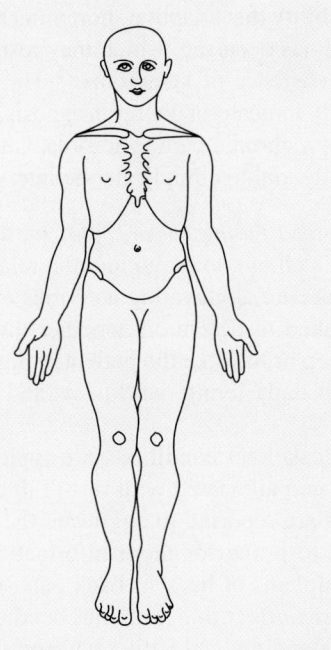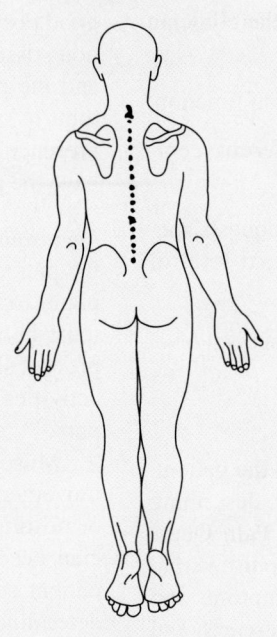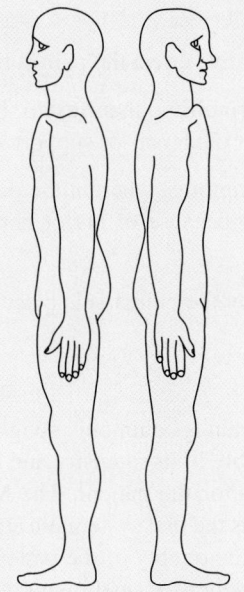

Please use the three scales below to rate your pain over the past 24 hours. Use the upper line to describe your pain level right now. Use the other scales to rate your pain at its worst and best over the past 24 hours.

RATE YOUR PAIN: 0 = NO PAIN, 10 = EXTREMELY INTENSE

1. Right now	0	1	2	3	4	5	6	7	8	9	10
2. At its worst	0	1	2	3	4	5	6	7	8	9	10
3. At its best	0	1	2	3	4	5	6	7	8	9	10

TABLE 8-6   Causes of Paresthesia

Paresthesia Location	Probable Cause
Lip (perioral)	Vertebral artery occlusion
Bilateral lower or bilateral upper extremities	Central protrusion of disk impinging on spine
All extremities simultaneously	Spinal cord compression
One half of body	Cerebral hemisphere
Segmental (in dermatomal pattern)	Disk or nerve root
Glove-and-stocking distribution	Diabetes mellitus neuropathy, lead or mercury poisoning
Half of face and opposite half of body	Brain stem impairment

Motivational-affective circuits may also mimic pain states, most notably in patients with anxiety, neurotic depression, or hysteria.[44] The mnemonic MADISON outlines the behavioral indicators that suggest motivational-affective pain.[51,52]

Multiple complaints, including complaints about unrelated body parts

Authenticity claims in an attempt to convince the clinician the symptoms exist

Denial of the negative effect the pain is having on function

Interpersonal variability, manifested by different complaints to different clinicians or support staff

Singularity of symptoms, wherein the patient requests special consideration because of his or her type and level of pain

Only you, whereby the clinician is placed at a special level of expertise

Nothing works

A description of pain is commonly sought from the patient. Because pain is variable in its intensity and quality, describing pain is often difficult for the patient. The McGill Pain Questionnaire (MPQ)[53] was the first systematic attempt to use verbal descriptors to assess the quality of the patient's symptoms and has been the most widely used instrument in pain research and practice (Table 8-7). The MPQ is a self-report inventory of 78 pain descriptors distributed across 20 subcategories (with six additional descriptors in the present pain index). The subcategories are further grouped into three broad categories, termed *sensory, affective,* and *evaluative,* respectively, in addition to a miscellaneous category. The implication is that each word reflects a particular sensory quality of pain.

The patient is asked to indicate on a body diagram the location of the pain, and to rate his or her symptoms based on the 20 categories of verbal descriptors of pain.[54] The 20 categories are ranked according to severity.[55] The patient is then asked to describe how the pain changes with time (continuous, rhythmic, brief), and how strong the pain is (mild, discomforting, distressing, horrible, excruciating).

The most commonly reported measure from the MPQ instrument, the pain-rating index total (PRIT), provides an estimate of overall pain intensity. This measure, obtained by summing all the descriptors selected from the 20 subclasses, has a possible range of 0 to 78. Separate scores for each class may be obtained by summing the values associated with the words selected from subclasses that comprise that dimension. Scores for each of these dimensions vary in range from 0 to 42 for the sensory class (PRIS), and 0 to 14 and 0 to 5 for the affective (PRIA) and evaluative classes (PRIE), respectively.

The strength of the MPQ is its ability to distinguish patients with a sensory pain experience from those who have an affective pain experience. The MPQ has been found to be sensitive to intervention effects,[43] and to have a high test-retest reliability,[53] and good construct validity.[56]

Frequency and Duration. The frequency and duration of the patient's symptoms can help the clinician to classify the injury according to its stage of healing: acute (inflammatory), subacute (migratory and proliferative), and chronic (remodeling) (Table 8-8).

In the case of a musculoskeletal injury that has been present without any formal intervention for a few months, there is a good possibility that adaptive shortening of the healing collagenous tissue has occurred, which may result in a failure to heal, and the persistence of symptoms.[35] The persistence of symptoms usually indicates a poorer prognosis, as it may indicate the presence of a chronic pain syndrome. Chronic pain syndromes have the potential to complicate the intervention process.[35]

Aggravating and Easing Factors. Of particular importance are the patient's chief complaint and the relationship of that complaint to specific aggravating activities or postures. Questions must be asked to determine whether the pain is sufficient to prevent sleep or to wake the patient at night, and the effect that activities of daily living, work, sex, and so forth, have on the pain.

Musculoskeletal conditions are typically aggravated with movement and alleviated with rest (Table 8-9). If no activities or postures are reported to aggravate the symptoms, the clinician needs to probe for more information. For example, if a patient complains of neck or back pain, the clinician needs to determine the effect that walking, bending, sleeping position, prolonged standing, and sitting have on the symptoms. Sitting or standing upright increases the lordosis and can aggravate symptoms in patients with an anterior instability, spondylolisthesis, stenosis, or a zygapophysial joint irritation. Sitting in a slouched posture typically aggravates symptoms of a lumbar disk protrusion. Nonmechanical events that provoke the symptoms could indicate a nonmusculoskeletal source for the pain[31]:

▶ *Night pain.* Pain at night that is unrelated to movement and disturbs or prevents sleep may indicate a malignancy.

▶ *Eating.* Pain that increases with eating may suggest gastrointestinal involvement.

▶ *Stress.* An increase in overall muscle tension prevents muscles from resting.

▶ *Cyclical pain.* Cyclical pain can often be related to systemic events (e.g., menstrual pain).

If aggravating movements or positions have been reported, they should be tested at the end of the tests and measures portion of the examination, to avoid any overflow of symptoms, which could confuse the clinician.

Clinical Pearl

Any relieving factors reported by the patient can often provide sufficient information to assist the clinician in the intervention plan.

TABLE 8-7 Modified McGill Pain Questionnaire

Patient's Name _____ Date _____

Directions: Many words can describe pain. Some of these words are listed below. If you are experiencing any pain, check (✓) every word that describes your pain.

A. Flickering Quivering Pulsing Throbbing Beating Pounding	H. Tingling Itchy Smarting Stinging	O. Wretched Blinding
	I. Dull Sore Hurting Aching Heavy	P. Annoying Troublesome Intense Unbearable
B. Jumping Flashing Shooting		Q. Spreading Radiating Penetrating Piercing
C. Pricking Boring Drilling Stabbing	J. Tender Taut Rasping Splitting	R. Tight Numb Drawing Squeezing Tearing
D. Sharp Cutting Lacerating	K. Tiring Exhausting	
E. Pinching Pressing Gnawing Cramping Crushing	L. Sickening Suffocating	S. Cool Cold Freezing
	M. Fearful Frightful Terrifying	T. Nagging Nauseating Agonizing Dreadful Torturing
F. Tugging Pulling Wrenching	N. Punishing Grueling Cruel Vicious Killing	
G. Hot Burning Scalding Searing		

KEY TO PAIN QUESTIONNAIRE

    Group A: Suggests vascular disorder
    Groups B–H: Suggests neurogenic disorder
    Group I: Suggests musculoskeletal disorder
    Groups J–T: Suggests emotional disorder

SCORING GUIDE: ADD UP TOTAL NUMBER OF CHECKS (✓):

Total: 4–8 = NORMAL
        8–10 = Focusing too much on pain
      10–16 = May be helped more by a clinical psychologist than by a physical therapist
      > 16 = Unlikely to respond to therapy procedures

Location. The clinician should determine the location of the symptoms, because this can indicate which areas need to be included in the physical examination. Information about how the location of the symptoms has changed since the onset can indicate whether a condition is worsening or improving. In general, as a condition worsens the pain distribution becomes more widespread and distal (peripheralized). As the condition improves, the symptoms tend to become more localized (centralized). A body chart may be used to record the location of symptoms (see Table 8-5).

TABLE 8-8   Stages of Healing

Stage	General Characteristics
Acute or inflammatory	Area is red, warm, swollen, and painful Pain is present without any motion of involved area Usually lasts for 48–72 h.
Subacute or tissue formation (neovascularization)	Pain usually occurs with activity or motion of involved area Usually lasts for 10 days to 6 wk
Chronic or remodeling	Pain usually occurs after the activity Usually lasts from 6 wk to 12 mo

TABLE 8-9   Differentiation Between Musculoskeletal and Systemic Pain[3]

Musculoskeletal Pain	Systemic Pain
Usually decreases with cessation of activity	Reduced by pressure
Generally lessens at night	Disturbs sleep
Aggravated with mechanical stress	Not aggravated by mechanical stress
Usually continuous or intermittent	Usually constant or in waves

---

> **Clinical Pearl**
>
> Symptoms that are distal and superficial are easier for the patient to specifically localize than those that are proximal and deep.

It must be remembered that the location of symptoms for many musculoskeletal conditions is quite separate from the source, especially in those peripheral joints that are more proximal, such as the shoulder and the hip. The term *referred pain* is used to describe symptoms that have their origin at a site other than where the patient feels the pain (see Chap. 9). If the extremity appears to be the source of the symptoms, the clinician should attempt to reproduce the symptoms by loading the peripheral tissues. If this proves unsuccessful, a full investigation of the spinal structures must ensue.

Behavior of Symptoms.   The presence of pain should not always be viewed negatively by the clinician. After all, its presence helps to determine the location of the injury, and its behavior aids the clinician in determining the stage of healing and the impact it has on the patient's function. For example, whether the pain is worsening, improving, or unchanging provides information on the effectiveness of an intervention. In addition, a gradual increase in the intensity of the symptoms over time may indicate to the clinician that the condition is worsening, or that the condition is nonmusculoskeletal in nature.[5,31]

Maitland[6] introduced the concept of the *degree of irritability*. An irritable structure has the following characteristics:

▶ *A progressive increase in the severity of the pain with movement or a specific posture.*   An ability to reproduce

constant pain with a specific motion or posture indicates an irritable structure.

▶ *Symptoms increased with minimal activity.*   An irritable structure is one that requires very little to increase the symptoms.

▶ *Increased latent response of symptoms.*   Symptoms that do not resolve within a few minutes following a movement or posture indicate an irritable structure.

According to McKenzie,[35] intervention for the patient whose symptoms have a low degree of irritability and are gradually resolving should focus only on education initially. However, if the improvement ceases, a mechanical intervention may then be necessary.[35]

Nature of the Symptoms.   The clinician must determine whether pain is the only symptom, or whether there are other symptoms that accompany the pain, such as dizziness, bowel and bladder changes, tingling (paresthesia), radicular pain or numbness, weakness, and increased sweating.

▶ *Dizziness.*   Although most causes of dizziness can be relatively benign, dizziness may signal a more serious problem, especially if it is associated with trauma to the neck or head, or with motions of cervical rotation and extension (e.g., vertebral artery compromise; see Chap. 21). The clinician must ascertain whether the symptoms result from vertigo, nausea, giddiness, unsteadiness, or fainting, among others. If vertigo is suspected, the patient's physician should be informed, for further investigation. However, in and of itself, vertigo is not usually a contraindication to the continuation of the examination.

▶ *Bowel or bladder dysfunction.* This finding usually indicates a compromise (compression) of the cauda equina.

▶ *Paresthesia.* The seriousness of the paresthesia depends on its distribution. Although complaints of paresthesia can be the result of a relatively benign impingement of a peripheral nerve, the reasons for its presence can vary in severity and seriousness (see Table 8-6).

▶ *Radicular pain.* This type of pain is produced by nerve root irritation and is typically described as sharp or shooting. Numbness that has a dermatomal pattern indicates spinal nerve root compression. Radiating pain refers to an increase in pain intensity and distribution. Radiating pain typically travels distally from the site of the injury.

▶ *Weakness.* Any weakness should be investigated by the clinician to determine whether it is the result of spinal nerve root compression, peripheral nerve lesion, disuse, inhibition resulting from pain or swelling, injury to the contractile or inert tissues (muscle, tendon, bursa, etc.), or a more serious pathology such as a fracture (see "Muscle Performance: Power, Strength, and Endurance, in the later discussion of tests and measures).

▶ *Increased sweating.* This finding can have a myriad of causes, ranging from increased body temperature as a result of exertion, fever, apprehension, and compromise to the autonomic system. Night sweats are of particular concern, because they often indicate the presence of a systemic problem.[57]

Issues of Symptom Magnification. Symptom magnification, an exaggerated subjective response to symptoms in the absence of adequate objective findings, is an increasingly common occurrence in the clinic. The patients who display this type of behavior are a difficult population to deal with. The causes of symptom magnification can be categorized into two main patient types:

1. Patients with a psychosomatic overlay, and those whose symptoms have a psychogenic cause.

2. Patients who are involved in litigation.

Symptom magnification is discussed in Chapter 9.

Past History of Current Condition. It is important for the clinician to determine whether the patient has had successive onsets of similar symptoms in the past, because recurrent injury tends to have a detrimental affect on the potential for recovery. If the patient's history indicates a recurrent injury, the clinician should note how often, and how easily, the injury has recurred and the success or failure of previous interventions.

Past Medical and Surgical History. The patient's past medical history can be obtained through a questionnaire (see Table 8-3). The past medical history can provide information with regard to allergies, childhood illnesses, and previous trauma. In addition,

information on any health conditions, such as cardiac problems, high blood pressure, or diabetes, should be elicited as these may impact exercise tolerance (cardiac problems, high blood pressure) and speed of healing (diabetes).

If the surgical history (see Table 8-3) is related to the current problem, the clinician should obtain as much detail about the surgery as possible from the surgical report, including any complications, precautions, or postsurgical protocols (see Chaps. 28 and 29).

Family History and General Health Status. Certain diseases, such as rheumatoid arthritis, diabetes, cardiovascular disease, and cancer, have familial tendencies.

The general health status refers to a review of the patient's health perception, physical and psychological function, as well as any specific questions related to a particular body region, or complaint.[13]

Medications. Although the dispensing of medications is out of the scope of practice for a physical therapist, questioning the patient about prescribed medication use can reveal medical conditions that the patient might not consider related to his or her present problem.[18] Medications also can have an impact on clinical findings and on the success of an intervention (see Chap. 10).[58]

▶ Pain medications, muscle relaxants, and nonsteroidal anti-inflammatory drugs (NSAIDs) can mask signs and symptoms, thereby affecting examination findings and increasing the potential for injury during the performance of prescribed exercises.[30] However, if the patient has a significant amount of pain, appropriate use of these medications may enhance treatment, allowing a more rapid progression than would otherwise be possible. However, as the patient improves, the need for this medication should lessen.

▶ Certain medications can produce changes in musculoskeletal structures. For example, prolonged use of corticosteroids may produce osteoporosis and weakening of connective tissues.[59]

▶ A patient undergoing anticoagulant therapy has a reduced clotting ability and is more susceptible to bruising or hemarthrosis. It is worth remembering that aspirin and aspirin-based products have an anticoagulant affect.

Based on the history, there may be times when the extent of the remainder of the examination may have to be limited. The decision to limit the examination is based on the presence of any subjective features that indicate the need for caution. These features include[58]:

▶ An irritable or severe disorder.

▶ Worsening symptoms.

▶ Subjective evidence of potential involvement of vital structures, such as the vertebrobasilar system (see Chap. 21), the spinal cord or CNS, or spinal nerve roots.

▶ Symptoms that do not behave in a predictable manner.

Systems Review

The systems review (Table 8-10), in addition to the scanning examination (see Tables 8-11–8-13 and later), is the part of the examination that identifies possible health problems that require consultation with, or referral to, another health care provider[13] (see Chap. 9). The systems review consists of a limited examination of[13]:

The anatomic and physiologic status of the cardiovascular, pulmonary, integumentary, musculoskeletal, and neuromuscular systems. Examples include:

▶ *Cardiovascular/pulmonary system.* Circulation is covered in the "Tests and Measures," later. Other areas of the cardiovascular/pulmonary system to assess include:

- *Pulse.* The pulse can be taken at a number of points. The most accessible is usually the radial pulse, at the distal aspect of the radius. The normal resting pulse is between 60 and 100 beats per minute. Lower rates (bradycardia) indicate athletic conditioning. Higher rates (tachycardia) may indicate an anxious patient, recent exertion, or underlying pathology. There is normally a transient increase in pulse rate with inspiration, followed by a slowing with expiration.[59a]

- *Respiratory rate.* Normal respiratory rate is between 8 and 14 per minute in adults, and slightly quicker in children. The following breathing patterns are characteristic of disease[59a]:

  - Cheyne-Stokes respiration, characterized by a periodic, regular, sequentially increasing depth of respiration, occurs with serious cardiopulmonary or cerebral disorders.

  - Biot's respiration, characterized by irregular spasmodic breathing and periods of apnea, is almost always associated with hypoventilation due to central nervous system disease.

  - Kussmaul's respiration, characterized by deep, slow breathing, indicates acidosis as the body attempts to blow off carbon dioxide.

- *Blood pressure.* The normal adult blood pressure can vary over a wide range. The normal systolic range varies from 95 to 140 mm Hg, generally increasing with age. The normal diastolic range is 60 to 90 mm Hg. The pressure should be determined in both arms. Causes of marked asymmetry (>10 Torr difference) in blood pressure of the arms are the following: errors in measurements, marked difference in arm size, thoracic outlet syndromes, embolic occlusion of an artery, dissection of an aorta, external arterial occlusion, coarctation of the aorta, and atheromatous occlusion.[59a]

▶ *Integumentary system.* Integumentary integrity is the intactness of the skin, including the ability of the skin to serve as a barrier to environmental threats (e.g., bacteria, parasites).[59b]

- *Temperature.* "Normal" body temperature of the adult is 98.4° F (37° C). However, a temperature in the range of 96.5° and 99.4° F are not at all uncommon. Fever is a temperature exceeding 100° F.[59a] The temperature is generally taken by placing the bulb of a thermometer under the patient's tongue for 1–3 minutes depending on the device. In most individuals there is a diurnal (occurring everyday) variation in body temperature of 0.5° to 2° F. The lowest ebb is reached during sleep. Menstruating women have a well-known temperature pattern that reflects the effects of ovulation, with the temperature dropping slightly before menstruation, and then dropping further 24–36 hours prior to ovulation.[59a] Coincident with ovulation, the temperature rises and remains at a somewhat higher level until just before the next menses.

- *Edema*

- *Skin changes.* These include but are not limited to rashes, blemishes, scarring, color, and pliability.

▶ *Musculoskeletal system.* The clinician observes and notes any impairments in gross symmetry, gross range of motion, or gross strength.

▶ *Neuromuscular system.* The clinician observes and notes any impairment of gait, locomotion, balance (see "Gait, Locomotion, and Balance," later), coordination, motor control, and motor learning (see "Motor Function," later). In addition, the clinician observes for peripheral and cranial

TABLE 8-10 The Systems Review

System	Focus of Assessment
Musculoskeletal	Gross range of motion, functional strength, symmetry
Neuromuscular	General movement patterns
Integumentary	Skin integrity, color, scar, temperature, patient's height, weight
Communication/Learning ability	Ability of patient to make needs known, consciousness, orientation, expected emotional and behavioral responses, patient learning preferences

nerve integrity (see Chap. 2) and notes any indication of neurological compromise such as tremors, or facial tics.

▶ *The communication ability, affect, cognition, language, and learning style of the patient.* The clinician notes whether the patient's communication level is age appropriate, whether the patient is oriented to person, place, and time, and whether the emotional and behavioral responses appear to be appropriate to his or her circumstances. It is important to verify that the patient can communicate their needs. The clinician should determine whether the patient has a good understanding about their condition, the planned intervention, and their prognosis. The clinician should also determine the learning style that best suits the patient.

Note: In the various case studies throughout this book, only the pertinent information from the history and systems review is given, with the understanding that the examiner has inquired about the other topics.

Scanning Examination. Designed by Cyriax,[60] the scanning examination is based on sound anatomic and pathologic principles. The Cyriax scanning (screening) examination traditionally follows the history and often is incorporated as part of the sys-

tems review. Although two studies[61,62] questioned the validity of some aspects of the selective tissue tension examination, no definitive conclusions were drawn from these studies. The scarcity of research to refute the work of Cyriax would suggest that its principles are sound, and that its use should be continued.

The entire scanning examination should take no more than a few minutes to complete and should be performed as part of the initial physical examination of all patients. The exception to this rule is perhaps for patients who have a definite history of trauma, or surgery, to a specific joint.

The purpose of the scanning examination is to help rule out the possibility of symptom referral from other areas, and to ensure that all possible causes of the symptoms are examined. It was Grieve[63] who coined the term *Masqueraders* to indicate conditions that may not be musculoskeletal in origin and may require skilled intervention elsewhere (Table 8-11).

The scanning examination is used when there is no history to explain the signs and symptoms, or when the signs and symptoms are unexplainable. The scanning examination is divided into two examinations: one for the lower quarter or quadrant (Table 8-12) and the other for the upper quadrant (Table 8-13). The tests that comprise the scanning examination are designed to detect neurologic weakness, the patient's ability

TABLE 8-11 Examination Findings and the Possible Conditions Causing Them[3]

Findings	Possible Condition
Dizziness	Upper cervical impairment, vertebrobasilar ischemia, craniovertebral ligament tear; may also be relatively benign
Quadrilateral paresthesia	Cord compression, vertebrobasilar ischemia
Bilateral upper limb paresthesia	Cord compression, vertebrobasilar ischemia
Hyper-reflexia	Cord compression, vertebrobasilar ischemia
Babinski or clonus sign	Cord compression, vertebrobasilar ischemia
Consistent swallow on transverse ligament stress tests	Instability, retropharyngeal hematoma, rheumatoid arthritis
Nontraumatic capsular pattern	Rheumatoid arthritis, ankylosing spondylitis, neoplasm
Arm pain lasting > 6–9 mo	Neoplasm
Persistent root pain < 30 yr	Neoplasm
Radicular pain with coughing	Neoplasm
Pain worsening after 1 mo	Neoplasm
> 1 level involved (cervical region)	Neoplasm
Paralysis	Neoplasm or neurologic disease

TABLE 8-11 (*cont.*)

Trunk and limb paresthesia	Neoplasm
Bilateral root signs and symptoms	Neoplasm
Nontraumatic strong spasm	Neoplasm
Nontraumatic strong pain in elderly patient	Neoplasm
Signs worse than symptoms	Neoplasm
Radial deviator weakness	Neoplasm
Thumb flexor weakness	Neoplasm
Hand intrinsic weakness and/or atrophy	Neoplasm, thoracic outlet syndrome, carpal tunnel syndrome
Horner's syndrome	Superior sulcus tumor, breast cancer, cervical ganglion damage, brain stem damage
Empty end-feel	Neoplasm
Severe post-traumatic capsular pattern	Fracture
Severe post-traumatic spasm	Fracture
Loss of range of motion post-trauma	Fracture
Post-traumatic painful weakness	Fracture

TABLE 8-12 Lower Quarter/Quadrant Scanning Motor Examination

Muscle Action	Muscle Tested	Root Level	Peripheral Nerve
Hip flexion	Iliopsoas	L1–2	Femoral to iliacus and lumbar plexus to psoas
Knee extension	Quadriceps	L2–4	Femoral
Hamstrings	Biceps femoris, semimembranosus, and semitendinosus	L4–S3	Sciatic
Dorsiflexion with inversion	Tibialis anterior	Primarily L4	Deep peroneal
Great toe extension	Extensor hallicus longus	Primarily L5	Deep peroneal
Ankle eversion	Peroneus longus and brevis	Primarily S1	Superficial peroneal nerve
Ankle plantarflexion	Gastrocnemius and soleus	Primarily S1	Tibial
Hip extension	Gluteus maximus	L5–S2	Inferior gluteal nerve

TABLE 8-13 Upper Quarter/Quadrant Scanning Motor Examination

Muscle Action	Muscle Tested	Root Level	Peripheral Nerve
Shoulder abduction	Deltoid	Primarily C5	Axillary
Elbow flexion	Biceps brachii	Primarily C6	Musculocutaneous
Elbow extension	Triceps brachii	Primarily C7	Radial
Wrist extension	Extensor carpi radialis longus, brevis, and extensor carpi ulnaris	Primarily C6	Radial
Wrist flexion	Flexor carpi radialis and flexor carpi ulnaris	Primarily C7	Median nerve for radialis and ulnar nerve for ulnaris
Finger flexion	Flexor digitorum superficialis, flexor digitorum profundus, and lumbricales	Primarily C8	Median nerve for superficialis, both median and ulnar nerves for profundus and lumbricales
Finger abduction	Dorsal interossei	Primarily T1	Ulnar

to perceive sensations and the inhibition of the deep tendon reflexes and other reflexes by the CNS. The components of the scanning examinations are described in Chap. 9.

The scanning examination should be carried out until the clinician is confident that there is no serious pathology present, and is routinely carried out unless there is some good reason for postponing it (e.g., recent trauma, in which case a modified differential diagnostic examination is used).[3] The tests used in the scanning examination may produce a medical diagnosis rather than a physical therapy one.[64] Those diagnoses can include:

▶ Fracture.

▶ Neurologic pathology, which either can be treated (mechanical nerve root compression from a disk protrusion, or inflammation) or is out of the scope of a physical therapist (tumor, upper motor neuron impairment, and cauda equina impairment) (Table 8-14).

▶ Tendonitis, bursitis, muscle tear.

▶ Tendon avulsion.

TABLE 8-14 Signs and Symptoms Requiring Neurologic Assessment[65]

Headaches that are sudden, severe, and diffuse
Headaches that awaken one from sleep
Headaches associated with projectile vomiting, but no nausea
Unilateral pulsating pain in synchrony with heartbeat
Headaches that worsen with activity or exertion
Headaches that begin or worsen with recumbency
Focal tenderness over the temporal artery in someone over the age of 60
Sudden, intense, sharp pain of short duration that is either spontaneous or triggered by a mild stimulus
Severe pain around sinuses or teeth
Headaches associated with other symptoms
   Cognitive impairment
   Visual disturbances (i.e., blindness, diplopia, distortions, spots, or loss of vision on one side)
   Numbness or altered sensation
Loss of strength or coordination
Loss or alteration of smell, taste, or hearing
Fever or associated systemic illness
Difficulty swallowing
Loss or impairment of voice; chronic cough

TABLE 8-15 Scan Findings and Interventions

Conditions	Findings	Protocol
Disk protrusion, prolapse, and extrusion	Severe pain All movements reduced	Gentle manual traction in progressive extension
Anterior-posterior instability	Flexion and extension reduction greater than rotation	Traction and/or traction manipulation in extension
Arthritis	Hot capsular pattern	PRICEMEM (Protection, Rest, Ice, Compression, Elevation, Medication Electrotherapeutics, Manual therapy)
Subluxation of segment	One direction restricted	Exercises in pain-free direction
Arthrosis of segment	All directions restricted	Exercises in pain-free direction

If a diagnosis is rendered from the scan, an intervention may be initiated using the guidelines outlined in Table 8-15. The scan or history, or both, also may have indicated to the clinician that the patient's condition is in the acute stage of healing. Although this is not a diagnosis in the true sense, it can be used for the purpose of the intervention plan.

Often though, the scanning examination does not generate enough signs and symptoms to formulate a working hypothesis or a diagnosis. In this case, further testing with the tests and measures is required in order to proceed.

Tests and Measures

The tests and measures (Table 8-16) component of the examination, which serves as an adjunct to the history and the systems review, involves the physical examination of the patient. The information from the history and the systems review serves as a guide for the clinician in determining which structures and systems require further investigation. The physical examination may also be modified based on the history; for example, the examination of an acutely injured patient differs greatly from that of a patient in less discomfort or distress. In addition, the examination of a child differs in some respects from that of an adult.

The tests and measures now currently used in physical therapy have been largely influenced by the work of a number of clinicians over the years, including Cyriax,[60,66–69] Maitland,[6,70] Grieve,[71] Kaltenborn,[4] Butler,[11] Sahrmann,[10] and McKenzie.[72,73]

The traditional goals of the physical examination have been to determine the structure involved, reproduce the patient's symptoms, confirm or refute the working hypothesis, and establish an objective data baseline.[5,30]

More recently, the focus of the examination has shifted to include the identification of impairments, functional limitations, disabilities, or changes in physical function and health status resulting from injury, disease, or other causes. This information is then used through the evaluation process to establish the diagnosis and the prognosis, and to determine the intervention.[13] The concept of function is described in Chapter 7.

The decision about which tests to use should be based on the best available research evidence. A good test must differentiate the target disorder from other disorders with which it might otherwise be confused.[74] Several examination approaches are available to the clinician. These include[75]:

▶ *Hypothetico-deductive clinical reasoning process.* This process is described as a method of hypothesis generation with hypothesis testing, followed by pattern recognition. Using the data from the history, examination, imaging, and laboratory results, a hypothetical diagnosis is developed through deductive reasoning. This method allows the

TABLE 8-16 Tests and Measures[13]

Aerobic capacity and endurance
Anthropometric characteristics
Arousal, attention, and cognition
Assistive and adaptive devices
Circulation (arterial, venous, lymphatic)
Cranial and peripheral nerve integrity
Environmental, home, and work (job, school, play) barriers
Ergonomics and body mechanics
Gait, locomotion, and balance
Integumentary integrity
Joint integrity and mobility
Motor function (motor control and learning)
Muscle performance (strength, power, endurance)
Neuromotor development and sensory integration
Orthotic, protective, and supportive devices
Pain
Posture
Prosthetic requirements
Range of motion (including muscle length)
Reflex integrity
Self-care and home management (ADLs, IADLs)
Sensory integrity (including proprioception and kinesthesia)
Ventilation and respiration, gas exchange
Work, community, and leisure integration or reintegration

ADLs, activities of daily living; IADLs, instrumental activities of daily living.

clinician to develop a list of potential causes (differential diagnoses) that may explain the patient's signs and symptoms. The clinician is then able to test those hypotheses and conclude the most plausible cause of the patient's symptoms by process of deduction and pattern recognition.[75a,75b,75c] Using clinical reasoning will most likely lead to the correct differential diagnosis (see Chap. 9). One of the disadvantages about using this method is that the process of hypothetico-deductive reasoning does not take into account the prevalence of a disorder.[76] As prevalence of a disorder decreases, the possibility of false positive test results increases.[76]

▶ *Anatomic method.* The anatomic method involves the application of stress to a specific structure to determine its response. This is the principle behind the Cyriax examination.[60]

▶ *Evidence-based practice (EBP).* According to Sackett and colleagues,[77] the definition of EBP is the integration of best research evidence with clinical expertise and patient values. The gathering of evidence occurs in a systematic and unbiased manner to select and interpret diagnostic tests and to assess potential interventions.[76] This method is similar to the hypothetico-deductive method, except that rules of evidence rather than signs and symptoms of pathophysiology are used. The choice of which tests to use with EBP is based on pretest probabilities, which are used to assess the diagnostic possibility of a disorder. However, these probabilities are often based on the clinician's experience, rather than on published data. Ideally, the chosen tests are based to some degree on the patient's history or presentation. The results from these tests are then combined with value judgments to arrive at the correct diagnosis. Using the EBP approach is believed to significantly increase a clinician's probability of making the correct diagnosis and selecting the best intervention.[76] This is because the clinician is only using those elements of a physical examination that have been found to be reliable and valid.[78] Unfortunately, many tests and procedures used in physical therapy practice are not, as yet, evidence based.

Before proceeding with the tests and measures, a full explanation must be provided to the patient as to what procedures are to be performed and the reasons for these. At times a complete examination cannot be performed. For example, if the joint to be examined is too acutely inflamed, the clinician may defer some of the examination to the subsequent visit. The tests and measures that relate to the neuromusculoskeletal system are listed in Table 8-17.

Pain. Pain is a disturbed sensation that causes suffering or distress.[13] The examination of pain is discussed in the history section. The mechanisms behind pain transmission are described in Chapter 2.

Range of Motion. The amount of available joint motion is based on a number of factors, including:

▶ Integrity of the joint surfaces and the amount of joint motion.

▶ Mobility and pliability of the soft tissues that surround a joint.

TABLE 8-17 Tests and Measures Related to Neuromusculoskeletal Patterns

Aerobic capacity and endurance
Anthropometric characteristics
Circulation
Cranial and peripheral nerve integrity
Environmental, home, and work barriers
Ergonomics and body mechanics
Gait, locomotion, and balance
Integumentary integrity
Joint integrity and mobility
Motor function
Muscle performance (including strength, power, and endurance)
Orthotic, protective, and supportive devices
Pain
Posture
Range of motion
Reflex integrity
Sensory integrity
Work, community, and leisure integration

▶ Degree of soft tissue approximation that occurs.

▶ Amount of scarring that is present.[79] Interstitial scarring or fibrosis can occur in and around the joint capsules, within the muscles, and within the ligaments as a result of previous trauma.

▶ Age. Joint motion tends to decrease with increasing age.

▶ Gender. In general, females have more joint motion than males.

Active Range of Motion. During the history, the patient will have indicated the general motions that aggravate or provoke the pain. The range of motion examination should determine the exact directions of motion that elicit the symptoms. The diagnosis of restricted movement in the extremities can usually be simplified by comparing both sides, provided that at least one side is uninvolved. The presence of arthritis, owing to its bilateral nature, can confuse the diagnosis, and it may be difficult to ascertain how much of the restriction is caused by myofascial dysfunction and how much by a disease of the joint lining.

In assessing motion, the clinician should first observe what an individual can do by asking him or her to move the joint through its full range of active motion. Active range of motion testing may be deferred if small and unguarded motions provoke intense pain, because this may indicate a high degree of joint irritability. The normal active range of motion for each of the joints is depicted in Table 8-18.

Active range of motion testing gives the clinician information about:

▶ Quantity of available physiologic motion.

▶ Presence of muscle substitutions.

▶ Willingness of the patient to move.

TABLE 8-18 Active Ranges of Joint Motions

Joint	Action	Degrees of Motion
Shoulder	Flexion	0–180
	Extension	0–40
	Abduction	0–180
	Internal rotation	0–80
	External rotation	0–90
Elbow	Flexion	0–150
Forearm	Pronation	0–80
	Supination	0–80
Wrist	Flexion	0–60
	Extension	0–60
	Radial deviation	0–20
	Ulnar deviation	0–30
Hip	Flexion	0–100
	Extension	0–30
	Abduction	0–40
	Adduction	0–20
	Internal rotation	0–40
	External rotation	0–50
Knee	Flexion	0–150
Ankle	Plantarflexion	0–40
	Dorsiflexion	0–20
Foot	Inversion	0–30
	Eversion	0–20

▶ Integrity of the contractile and inert tissues.

▶ Quality of motion. A painful arc during range of motion, with or without a painful limitation of movement, indicates the presence of a derangement.[80] For example, there may be an arc of pain between 60 and 120 degrees on shoulder abduction, indicating an impingement of the structures under the acromion process or coracoacromial ligament.

▶ Symptom reproduction.

▶ Pattern of motion restriction.

Full and pain-free active range of motion suggests normalcy for that movement, although it is important to remember that normal *range* of motion is not synonymous with normal motion.[81] Normal motion implies that the control of motion must also be present. This control is a factor of muscle flexibility, joint stability, and central neurophysiologic mechanisms. These factors are highly specific in the body.[82] A loss of motion at one joint may not prevent the performance of a functional task, although it may result in the task being performed in an

abnormal manner. For example, the act of walking can still be accomplished in the presence of a knee joint that has been fused into extension. Because the essential mechanisms of knee flexion in the stance period and foot clearance in the swing period are absent, the patient compensates for these losses by hiking the hip on the involved side, side bending the lumbar spine to the involved side, and through excessive motion of the foot.

Single motions in the cardinal planes are usually tested first. These tests are followed by dynamic and static testing. Dynamic testing involves repeated movements. Static testing involves sustaining a position. Sustained static positions may be used to help detect postural syndromes.[72] McKenzie[80] advocates the use of repeated movements in specific directions in the spine and the extremities. Repeated movements can give the clinician some valuable insight into the patient's condition[80]:

▶ Internal derangements tend to worsen with repeated motions.

▶ Symptoms of a postural dysfunction remain unchanged with repeated motions.

▶ Pain from a dysfunction syndrome is increased with tissue loading, but ceases at rest.

▶ Repeated motions can indicate the irritability of the condition.

▶ Repeated motions can indicate to the clinician the direction of motion to be used as part of the intervention. If pain increases during repeated motion in a particular direction, exercising in that direction is not indicated. If pain only worsens in part of the range, repeated motion exercises can be used for that part of the range that is pain-free, or that does not worsen the symptoms.

▶ Pain that is increased after the repeated motions may indicate a retriggering of the inflammatory response, and repeated motions in the opposite direction should be explored.

Combined motion testing may be used when the symptoms are not reproduced with the cardinal plane motions (flexion, extension, abduction etc.), repeated motions, or sustained positions. Compression and distraction also may be added to all of the active motion tests in an attempt to reproduce the symptoms.

Clinical Pearl

Apprehension from the patient during active range of motion that limits a movement at near or full range suggests instability, whereas apprehension in the early part of the range suggests anxiety caused by pain.

Passive Range of Motion. If the active motions do not reproduce the patient's symptoms, because the patient avoids going into the painful part of the range, or the active range of motion appears incomplete, it is important to perform gentle passive range of motion, and overpressure, at the end of the active range. The passive overpressure should be applied carefully in the presence of pain.

Passive range of motion testing gives the clinician information about the integrity of the contractile and inert tissues, and the *end-feel* (see later discussion). Passive movements are performed in the anatomic range of motion for the joint. The barrier to active motion should occur earlier in the range than the barrier to passive motion. Pain that occurs at the mid- end range of active and passive movement is suggestive of a capsular contraction or scar tissue that has not been adequately remodeled.[80]

> ### Clinical Pearl
>
> According to Cyriax, if active and passive motions are limited or painful in the same direction, the lesion is in the inert tissue, whereas if the active and passive motions are limited or painful in the opposite direction, the lesion is in the contractile tissue.[60]

The quantity and quality of movement refers to the ability to achieve end range without deviation from the intended movement plane.

Both passive and active range of motion can be measured using a goniometer, which has been shown to have a satisfactory level of intraobserver reliability.[83–85] Visual observation in experienced clinicians has been found to be equal to measurements by goniometry.[86]

The recording of range of motion varies. The measurements depicted in Tables 8-19, 8-20, and 8-21 highlight one method. The American Medical Association (AMA) recommends recording the range of motion on the basis of the neutral position of the joint being zero, with the degrees of motion increasing in the direction the joint moves from the zero starting point.[87] A plus sign (+) is used to indicate joint hyperextension and a minus sign (−) to indicate an extension lag. The method of recording chosen is not important, provided the clinician chooses a recognized method and documents it consistently with the same patient.

TABLE 8-19 Recording Range of Motion Measurements for the Spine[87]

Spinal Area	Plane	ROM-0-ROM (in degrees)*	Clinical Examples	
			Text Description	Documentation Recording (in degrees)
Cervical	Sagittal	Extension-0-Flexion (60)-0-(50)	Extends to 30 degrees, flexes to 45 degrees	S: 30-0-45
Cervical	Frontal	Left lateral bend-0-Right lateral bend (45)-0-(45)	Bends 30 degrees to left, 40 degrees to right	F: 30-0-40
Cervical		Left rotation-0-Right rotation (80)-0-(80)	Rotates left 40 degrees, right 50 degrees	R: 40-0-50
Thoracic	Sagittal	Extension-0-Flexion (5)-0-(45)	Extends to 0 degrees, flexes to 45 degrees	S: 0-0-45
Thoracic	Frontal	Left lateral bend-0-Right lateral bend (45)-0-(45)	Bends left 45 degrees, right 20 degrees	F: 45-0-20
Thoracic		Left rotation-0-Right rotation (30)-0-(30)	Rotates left 15 degrees, right 20 degrees	R: 15-0-20
Lumbar	Sagittal	Extension-0-Flexion (25)-0-(60)	Extends to 25 degrees, flexes to 40 degrees	S: 25-0-40
Lumbar	Frontal	Left lateral bend-0-Right lateral bend (25)-0-(25)	Ankylosis of the spine in 20 degrees left lateral flexion	F: 20-0
			Ankylosis in 20 degrees right lateral flexion	F: 0-20
			Restricted motion from 20–30 degrees of left lateral bending[†]	F: 30-20-0

ROM, range of motion.
* Normal ranges are in parentheses.
[†] A non-0-degree starting position is noted in the ankylosis table.

TABLE 8-20   Recording Range of Motion Measurements for the Upper Extremities[87]

Joint	Plane	Normal Active ROM ROM-0-ROM (in degrees)*	Clinical Examples	
			Text Description	Documentation Recording (in degrees)
Shoulder	Sagittal	Extension-0-Flexion (40)-0-(180)	Left extends to 40 degrees, flexes to 150 degrees	Left S: 40-0-150
			Right extends to 30 degrees, flexes to 110 degrees	Right S: 30-0-110
Shoulder	Frontal	Abduction-0-Adduction (180)-0-(30)	Left abducts to 100 degrees, adducts to 10 degrees	Left F: 100-0-10
			Right abducts to 150 degrees, adducts to 30 degrees	Right F: 150-0-30
Shoulder	Rotation	External rotation-0-Internal rotation (90)-0-(80)	Left external rotation to 90 degrees, internal rotation to 80 degrees	Left R: 90-0-80
			Right external rotation to 80 degrees, internal rotation to 40 degrees	Right R: 80-0-40
Elbow	Sagittal	Extension-0-Flexion (0)-0-(150)	Left extends to 0 degrees, flexes to 150 degrees	Left S: 0-0-150
			Right hyperextends to 0 degrees, flexes to 110 degrees	Right S: 0-0-110
Forearm	Rotation	Supination-0-Pronation (80)-0-(80)	Left supinates to 60 degrees, pronates to 80 degrees	Left R: 60-0-80
			Right supinates to 80 degrees, pronates to 80 degrees	Right R: 80-0-80
Wrist	Sigittal	Extension-0-Flexion (60)-0-(60)	Ankylosis of left wrist in 20-degree extension	Left S: 20-0
			Right extends to 20 degrees, flexes to 50 degrees	Right S: 20-0-50
Wrist	Frontal	Radial deviation-0-Ulnar deviation (20)-0-(30)	Left radial deviates to 20 degrees, ulnar deviates to 30 degrees	Left F: 20-0-30
			Right radial deviates to 10 degrees, ulnar deviates to 10 degrees	Right F: 10-0-10

ROM, range of motion.
* Normal ranges are in parentheses.

Flexibility.   The examination of flexibility is performed to determine if a particular structure, or group of structures, has sufficient extensibility to perform a desired activity. The extensibility and habitual length of connective tissue is a factor of the demands placed upon it (see Chap. 4). These demands produce changes in the viscoelastic properties and, thus, the length-tension relationship of a muscle or muscle group, resulting in an increase or decrease in the length of those structures. A decrease in the length of the soft tissue structures, or adaptive shortening, is very common in postural dysfunctions. Adaptive shortening also can be produced by:

▶ Restricted mobility.

▶ Tissue damage secondary to trauma.

▶ Prolonged immobilization.

▶ Disease.

▶ Hypertonia. Hypertonic muscles which are superficial can be identified through observation and palpation. Observation will reveal the muscle to be raised, and light palpation will provide information about tension, as the muscle will feel hard and may stand out from those around it.

TABLE 8-21 Recording Range of Motion Measurements for the Lower Extremities[87]

Joint	Plane	Normal Active ROM ROM-0-ROM (in degrees)	Clinical Examples	
			Text Description	Documentation Recording (in degrees)
Hip	Sagittal	Extension-0-Flexion (30)-0-(100)	Left extends to 30 degrees, flexes to 80 degrees	Left S: 30-0-80
			Right extends to 10 degrees, flexes to 60 degrees	Right S: 10-0-60
Hip	Frontal	Abduction-0-Adduction (40)-0-(20)	Left abducts to 30 degrees, adducts to 10 degrees	Left F: 30-0-10
			Right abducts to 20 degrees, adducts to 10 degrees	Right F: 20-0-10
Hip	Rotation	External rotation-0-Internal rotation (50)-0-(40)	Left external rotation to 30 degrees, internal rotation to 30 degrees	Left R: 30-0-30
			Right external rotation to 20 degrees, internal rotation to 15 degrees	Right R: 20-0-15
Knee	Sagittal	Extension-0-Flexion (0)-0-(150)	Left extends to 0 degrees, flexes to 150 degrees	Left S: 0-0-150
			Right hyperextends to 10 degrees, flexes to 120 degrees	Right S: 0-0-120
Ankle (Talocrural)	Sagittal	Extension-0-Flexion (20)-0-(40)	Left extends to 10 degrees, flexes to 10 degrees	Left R: 10-0-10
			Right extends to 20 degrees, flexes to 40 degrees	Right R: 20-0-40
Ankle (Subtalar)	Frontal	Extension-0-Inversion (20)-0-(30)	Left eversion 20 degrees, inversion 30 degrees	Left S: 20-0-30
			Right eversion 10 degrees, inversion 20 degrees	Right S: 10-0-20

ROM, range of motion.
* Normal ranges are in parentheses.

Flexibility can be measured objectively using standardized tests, or a goniometer. A more subjective test for flexibility includes an examination of the end-feel, which can detect a loss of motion resulting from excessive tension of the agonist muscle. Visual observation can be used. This has been found to have a variability of 30 percent in patients with low back pain and sciatica.[88]

Capsular and Non-capsular Patterns of Restriction. Cyriax[60] gave us the terms *capsular* and *noncapsular* pattern of restriction, which link impairment to pathology (Table 8-22). A capsular pattern of restriction is a limitation of pain and movement in a joint-specific ratio, which is usually present with arthritis, or following prolonged immobilization.[60] It is worth remembering that a consistent capsular pattern for a particular joint might not exist, and that these patterns are based on empirical findings and tradition, rather than research.[61,89] Significant

degeneration of the articular cartilage presents with crepitus (joint noise) on movement when compression of the joint surfaces is maintained.

A noncapsular pattern of restriction is a limitation in a joint in any pattern other than a capsular one, and may indicate the presence of either a derangement, a restriction of one part of the joint capsule, or an extra-articular lesion, that obstructs joint motion.[60]

A positive finding for hypomobility would be a reduced range in a capsular or noncapsular pattern. The hypomobility can be painful, suggesting an acute sprain of a structure, or painless, suggesting a contracture or adhesion of the tested structure.

End-feel. Cyriax[60] introduced the concept of the end-feel, which is the quality of resistance at end range. The end-feel can

TABLE 8-22   Capsular Patterns of Restriction[60]

Joint	Limitation of Motion (Passive Angular Motion)
Glenohumeral	External rotation > abduction > internal rotation (3:2:1)
Acromioclavicular	No true capsular pattern; possible loss of horizontal adduction, pain (and sometimes slight loss of end range) with each motion
Sternoclavicular	See acromioclavicular joint
Humeroulnar	Flexion > extension (±4:1)
Humeroradial	No true capsular pattern; possible equal limitation of pronation and supination
Superior radioulnar	No true capsular pattern; possible equal limitation of pronation and supination with pain at end ranges
Inferior radioulnar	No true capsular pattern; possible equal limitation of pronation and supination with pain at end ranges
Wrist (carpus)	Flexion = extension
Radiocarpal	See wrist (carpus)
Carpometacarpal	
Midcarpal	
Carpometacarpal 1	Retroposition
Carpometacarpals 2–5	Fan > fold
Metacarpophalangeal 2–5	Flexion > extension (±2:1)
Interphalangeal	Flexion > extension (±2:1)
Proximal (PIP)	
Distal (DIP)	
Hip	Internal rotation > flexion > abduction = extension > other motions
Tibiofemoral	Flexion > extension (±5:1)
Superior tibiofibular	No capsular pattern; pain at end range of translatory movements
Talocrural	Plantar flexion > dorsiflexion
Talocalcaneal (subtalar)	Varus > valgus
Midtarsal	Inversion (plantar flexion, adduction, supination)
Talonavicular calcaneocuboid	> dorsiflexion
Metatarsophalangeal 1	Extension > flexion (±2:1)
Metatarsophalangeals 2–5	Flexion ≥ extension
Interphalangeals 2–5	
Proximal	Flexion ≥ extension
Distal	Flexion ≥ extension

indicate to the clinician the cause of the motion restriction (Tables 8-23 and 8-24).

To execute the end-feel, the point at which resistance is encountered is evaluated for quality and tenderness. Additional forces are needed as the end-range of a joint is reached and the elastic limits are challenged. This space termed the *end-play zone* requires a force of overpressure to be reached so that when that force is released, the joint springs back from its elastic limits.

Although some clinicians feel that overpressure should not be applied in the presence of pain, this is erroneous. Most, if not all, of the end-feels that suggest acute or serious pathology are to be found in the painful range, including spasm and the empty end-feel.

The end-feel is very important in joints that have only very small amounts of normal range, such as those of the spine. The type of end-feel can help the clinician determine the presence of dysfunction. For example, a hard, capsular end-feel indicates a pericapsular hypomobility, whereas a jammed or pathomechanical end-feel indicates a pathomechanical hypomobility. A normal

end-feel would indicate normal range, whereas an abnormal end-feel would suggest abnormal range, either hypomobile or hypermobile. An association between an increase in pain and abnormal pathologic end-feels compared with normal end-feels has been demonstrated.[91]

The planned intervention, and its intensity, is based on the type of tissue resistance to movement demonstrated by the end-feel, and on the acuteness of the condition[60] (see Table 8-25 later). This information may indicate whether the resistance is caused by pain, muscle, capsule ligament, disturbed mechanics of the joint, or a combination.

One study that looked at the intrarater and interrater reliability of assessing end-feel, and pain and resistance sequence in subjects with painful shoulders and knees, found the end-feel to have good intrarater reliability, but unacceptable interrater reliability.[61]

Joint Integrity and Mobility.   Joint integrity and mobility testing can provide valuable information about the status and the mobility of each joint and its capsule. A normal joint has an

TABLE 8-23 Normal End-feels[64]

Type	Cause	Characteristics and Examples

Bony	Produced by bone-to-bone approximation	Abrupt and unyielding; gives impression that further forcing will break something
		Examples:
		    Normal: Elbow extension
		    Abnormal: Cervical rotation (may indicate osteophyte)

Elastic	Produced by muscle-tendon unit; may occur with adaptive shortening	Stretches with elastic recoil and exhibits constant-length phenomenon; further forcing feels as if it will snap something
		Examples:
		    Normal: Wrist flexion with finger flexion, the straight-leg raise, and ankle dorsiflexion with the knee extended
		    Abnormal: Decreased dorsiflexion of the ankle with the knee flexed

Soft tissue approximation	Produced by contact of two muscle bulks on either side of a flexing joint where joint range exceeds other restraints	Very forgiving end-feel that gives impression that further normal motion is possible if enough force could be applied
		Examples:
		    Normal: Knee flexion, elbow flexion in extremely muscular subjects
		    Abnormal: Elbow flexion with obese subject

Capsular	Produced by capsule or ligaments	Various degrees of stretch without elasticity; stretch ability is dependent on thickness of tissue
		    Strong capsular or extracapsular ligaments produce hard capsular end-feel whereas thin capsule produces softer one
		    Impression given to clinician is that if further force is applied, something will tear.
		Examples:
		    Normal: Wrist flexion (soft), elbow flexion in supination (medium), and knee extension (hard)
		    Abnormal: Inappropriate stretch ability for specific joint; if too hard, may indicate hypomobility due to arthrosis; if too soft, hypermobility

available range of active, or physiologic, motion, which is limited by a physiologic barrier as tension develops within the surrounding tissues, such as the joint capsule, ligaments, and connective tissue (Fig. 8-1). At the physiologic barrier, there is an additional amount of passive, or accessory, range of motion (see Fig. 8-1). The small motion, which is available at the joint surfaces, is referred to as *accessory* motion (see Chap. 3). This motion can only occur when resistance to active motion is applied, or when the patient's muscles are completely relaxed.[91]

Beyond the available passive range of motion, the anatomic barrier is found (see Fig. 8-1). This barrier cannot be exceeded without disruption to the integrity of the joint.

Both the physiologic (osteokinematic) and accessory (arthrokinematic) motions occur simultaneously during movement and are directly proportional to each other, with a small increment of accessory motion resulting in a larger increment of osteokinematic motion. As discussed in Chapter 3, in order for a joint to function completely, both the physiologic and accessory motions have to occur normally. It therefore follows that if a joint is not functioning completely, either the physiologic range of motion is limited compared with the expected norm, or there is no passive range of motion available between the physiologic barrier and the anatomic barrier. The assessment of the end-feel perceived by the clinician during the passive motion tests can help determine the cause of the restriction.[60] In general, the physiologic motion is controlled by the contractile tissues, whereas the accessory motion is controlled by the integrity of the joint surfaces and the noncontractile (inert) tissues. This rule may change in the case of a joint that has undergone degenerative changes, as this can result in a decrease in the physiologic motions, demonstrated by the capsular pattern of restriction. It is important that the intervention to restore the complete function of the joint be aimed at the specific cause.

TABLE 8-24 Abnormal End-feels[64]

Type	Causes	Characteristics and Examples

Springy	Produced by articular surface rebounding from intra-articular meniscus or disk; impression is that if forced further, something will collapse	Rebound sensation as if pushing off from a rubber pad
		Examples:
		  Normal: Axial compression of cervical spine
		  Abnormal: Knee flexion or extension with displaced meniscus

Boggy	Produced by viscous fluid (blood) within joint	"Squishy" sensation as joint is moved toward its end range; further forcing feels as if it will burst joint
		Examples:
		  Normal: None
		  Abnormal: Hemarthrosis at knee

Spasm	Produced by reflex and reactive muscle contraction in response to irritation of nociceptor, predominantly in articular structures and muscle; forcing it further feels as if nothing will give	Abrupt and "twangy" end to movement that is unyielding while the structure is being threatened, but disappears when threat is removed (kicks back)
		With joint inflammation, it occurs early in range, especially toward close-packed position, to prevent further stress
		With irritable joint hypermobility, it occurs at end of what should be normal range as it prevents excessive motion from further stimulating the nociceptor
		Spasm in grade II muscle tears becomes apparent as muscle is passively lengthened and is accompanied by a painful weakness of that muscle
		Note: Muscle guarding is not a true end-feel as it involves co-contraction
		Examples:
		  Normal: None
		  Abnormal: Significant traumatic arthritis, recent traumatic hypermobility, grade II muscle tears

Empty	Produced solely by pain; frequently caused by serious and severe pathologic changes that do not affect joint or muscle and so do not produce spasm; demonstration of this end-feel is, with exception of acute subdeltoid bursitis, de facto evidence of serious pathology; further forcing simply increases pain to unacceptable levels	Limitation of motion has no tissue resistance component and resistance is from patient being unable to tolerate further motion due to severe pain; it is not same feeling as voluntary guarding but rather it feels as if patient is both resisting and trying to allow movement simultaneously
		Examples:
		  Normal: None
		  Abnormal: Acute subdeltoid bursitis, sign of the buttock

Facilitation	Not truly an end-feel as facilitated hypertonicity does not restrict motion; it can, however, be perceived near end range	Light resistance as from constant light muscle contraction throughout latter half of range that does not prevent end of range being reached; resistance is unaffected by rate of movement
		Examples:
		  Normal: None
		  Abnormal: Spinal facilitation at any level

Joint pain and dysfunction do not occur in isolation.[92,93] A variety of different measurement scales have been proposed for judging the amount of accessory joint motion present between two joint surfaces, most of which are based on a comparison with a comparable contralateral joint using manually applied forces in a logical and precise manner[94] (see "Passive Accessory Mobility Tests," later). Using these techniques, joint accessory motion can be determined as being hypomobile, normal, or hypermobile.[4–6] Kaltenborn[4] introduced the concept of motion restriction of a joint based on its arthrokinematics.

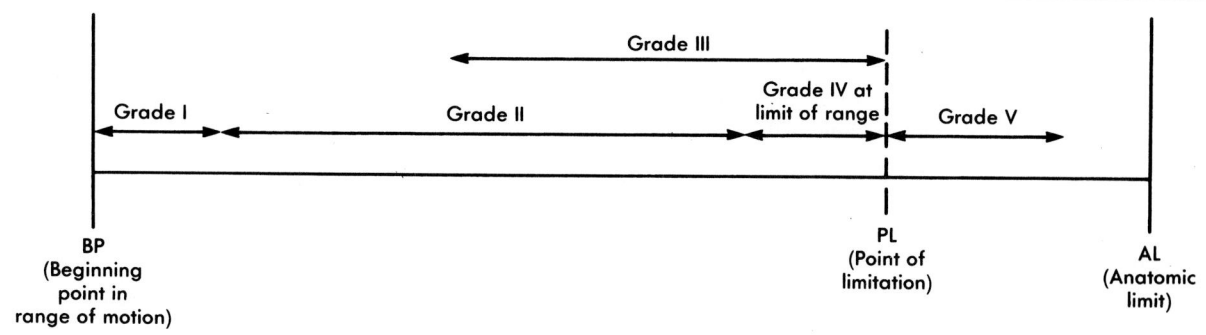

FIGURE 8-1   Available joint range of motion. (Reproduced with permission from Dutton M. *Manual Therapy of the Spine*. New York, NY: McGraw-Hill; 2002:44.)

> ### *Clinical Pearl*
>
> In general, if the concave-on-convex glide is restricted, there is a contracture of the trailing portion of the capsule, whereas if the convex-on-concave glide is restricted, there is an inability of the moving surface to glide into the contracted portion of the capsule.

Close- and Open-packed Positions of the Joint.   Two joint positions are recognized for joint mobility testing and joint mobilizations: close-packed and open-packed (see Chap. 3). The close-packed position allows the least amount of distraction of the joint surfaces and reduces the available degrees of freedom to zero (see Table 3-1). This position is avoided when the clinician is attempting to assess the accessory motion of a joint. In contrast, the open-packed, or resting, position of the joint (see Table 3-1) is used for joint mobilizations.

Active Physiologic Intervertebral Mobility Tests.   Active physiologic intervertebral mobility, or active mobility, tests were originally designed by osteopaths to assess the ability of each joint in the spine to move actively through its normal range of motion by palpating over the transverse processes of a joint during the motion. Theoretically, by palpating over the transverse processes, the clinician can indirectly assess the motions occurring at the zygapophysial joints at either side of the intervertebral disk. However, the clinician must remember that, although it is convenient to describe the various motions of the spine occurring in a certain direction, these involve the integration of movements of a multijoint complex.

The human zygapophysial joints are capable of only two major motions: gliding upward and gliding downward. If these movements occur in the same direction, flexion or extension occurs, while the movements occur in opposite directions, side-flexion occurs.

Osteopaths use the terms *opening* and *closing* to describe flexion and extension motions, respectively, at the zygapophysial joint. Under normal circumstances, an equal amount of gliding occurs at each zygapophysial joint with these motions.

▶ During flexion, both zygapophysial joints glide superiorly (open).

▶ During extension, both zygapophysial joints glide inferiorly (close).

▶ During side-flexion, one joint is gliding inferiorly (closing), while the other joint is gliding superiorly (opening). For example, during right side-flexion, the right joint is gliding inferiorly (closing), while the left joint is gliding superiorly (opening).

By combining flexion or extension movements with side-flexion, the joint can be "opened" or "closed" to its limits. Thus, flexion and right side-flexion of a segment assesses the ability of the left joint to maximally open, whereas extension and left side-flexion assesses the ability of the left joint to maximally close.

There is a point that may be considered as the center of segmental rotation, about which all segmental motion must occur. In the case of a zygapophysial joint impairment (hypermobility or hypomobility), it is presumed that this center of rotation will be altered.

If one zygapophysial joint is rendered hypomobile (i.e., the superior facet cannot move to the extreme of superior or inferior motion), then the pure motions of flexion and extension cannot occur. This results in a relative asymmetric motion of the two superior facets as the end of range of flexion or extension is approached, (i.e., a side-flexion motion will occur). However, this side-flexion motion will not be about the normal center of segmental rotation. The structure responsible for the loss of zygapophysial joint motion, whether it is a muscle, disk protrusion, or the zygapophysial joint itself, will become the new axis of vertebral motion, and a new component of rotation about a vertical axis, normally unattainable, will be introduced into the segmental motion. The degree of this rotational deviation is dependent on the distance of the impairment from the original center of rotation.

Because the zygapophysial joints in the spine are posterior to the axis of rotation, an obvious rotational change occurring between full flexion and full extension (in the position of a vertebral segment), is indicative of zygapophysial joint motion impairment.

By observing any marked and obvious rotation of a vertebral segment occurring between the positions of full flexion and full extension, one may deduce the probable pathologic impairment (see the introduction to Section IV).

Passive Physiological Intervertebral Mobility Tests. The passive physiologic intervertebral mobility (PPIVM), or passive mobility, tests use the same principles as the active physiologic intervertebral mobility tests to assess the ability of each joint in the spine to move passively through its normal range of motion while the clinician palpates over the interspinous spaces. During extension, the spinous processes should approximate, whereas during flexion, they should separate.

If pain is reproduced, it is useful to associate the pain with the onset of tissue resistance to gain an appreciation of the acuteness of the problem (Table 8-25).

According to Meadows,[95] one of three conclusions can be drawn from combining the findings from the passive mobility tests, the stability tests, and the results of the end-feel:

1. ***The joint is determined to be normal.*** If the passive mobility test of a spinal joint has a normal range and end-feel, the joint usually can be considered normal because in the spine, instability will invariably produce a hypermobility (see Chap. 9). However, in a peripheral joint, it is possible to have a normal range in the presence of articular instability. Thus, if a peripheral joint demonstrates a normal physiologic range, the stability of the joint needs to be tested before the clinician can deem the joint to be normal.

2. ***The motion is determined as being excessive (hypermobile).*** If the articular restraints are irritable, the range will be about normal but will be accompanied by a spasm end-feel, as a reflex muscle contraction prevents the motion into an abnormal, and painful, range. If non-irritable, the physiologic range will be increased and the end-feel will be softer than the expected capsular one, suggesting a complete tear of the structure under examination. If the motion is determined to be excessive, its stability needs to be assessed. Stability can be assessed using stress tests, which help determine the integrity of the inert tissues, particularly the ligaments (see "Special Tests").

3. ***The motion at the joint is determined to be reduced (hypomobile).***

If the joint motion is determined to be reduced or excessive, passive articular mobility testing is performed to determine the cause.

Passive Accessory Mobility Tests. The passive articular mobility (PAM) tests involve the clinician assessing the arthrokinematic, or accessory, motions of a joint. In the spine these tests are referred to as passive physiologic accessory intervertebral motion (PPAIVM) testing.

Accessory motions are involuntary motions (see Chap. 3). With few exceptions, muscles cannot restrict the glides of a joint, especially if the glides are tested in the open-packed position of a peripheral joint and, at the end of available range, in the spinal joints.

Thus, if the clinician assesses the accessory motion of the joint by performing a joint glide, information about the integrity of the inert structures will be given. There are two scenarios:

1. ***The joint glide is unrestricted.*** An unrestricted joint glide indicates two differing conclusions:
   a. The integrity of both the joint surface and the periarticular tissue is good. If the joint surface and periarticular structures are intact, the patient's loss of motion must be the result of a contractile tissue. The intervention for this type involves soft tissue mobilization techniques designed to change the length of a contractile tissue.
   b. The joint glide is both unrestricted and excessive. The excessive motion may indicate a pathological hypermobility or instability or it may be normal for the individual. In these cases, the end feel can provide some useful information. The intervention for this type concentrates on stabilizing techniques designed to give secondary support to the joint through muscle action.

2. ***The joint glide is restricted.*** If the joint glide is restricted, the joint surface and periarticular tissues are implicated as the cause of the patient's loss of motion, although as previously mentioned, the contractile tissues cannot definitively be ruled out. The intervention for this type of finding initially involves a specific joint mobilization to restore the glide. Once the joint glide is restored following these mobilizations, the osteokinematic motion can

TABLE 8-25 Abnormal Barriers to Motion and Recommended Manual Techniques[60]

Barrier	End-feel	Technique
Pain	Empty	None
Pain	Spasm	None
Pain	Capsular	Oscillations (I, IV)
Joint adhesions	Early capsular	Passive articular motion stretch (I–V)
Muscle adhesions	Early elastic	Passive physiologic motion stretch
Hypertonicity	Facilitation	Hold/relax
Bone	Bony	None

be assessed again. If it is still reduced, the contractile tissues are at fault. Distraction and compression can be used to help differentiate the cause of the restriction.

a. ***Distraction.*** Traction is a force imparted passively by the clinician that results in a distraction of the joint surfaces.

(1) If the distraction is limited, a contracture of connective tissue should be suspected.

(2) If the distraction increases the pain, it may indicate a tear of connective tissue and may be associated with increased range.

(3) If the distraction eases the pain, it may indicate an involvement of the joint surface.

b. ***Compression.*** Compression is the opposite force to distraction, and involves an approximation of joint surfaces.

(1) If the compression increases the pain, a loose body or internal derangement of the joint may be present.

(2) If the compression decreases the pain, it may implicate the joint capsule.

Thus, by assessing these joint motions, the clinician can determine[91]:

▶ Cause of a limitation in a joint's physiologic range of motion.[96]

▶ End-feel response of the tissues.[60]

▶ Stage of healing.[71]

▶ Integrity of the ligaments around a joint (for example, the Lachman test).

Based on the information gleaned from the joint play assessment, the clinician makes clinical decisions as to which intervention to use. If the joint play is felt to be restricted, and there is no indication of a bony end-feel or severe irritability, joint mobilization techniques are used (refer to the discussion of joint mobilization in Chap. 11). If the joint play is found to be unrestricted, the clinician may decide to employ a technique that increases the extensibility of the surrounding connective tissues, because abnormal shortness of these connective tissues, including the ligaments, joint capsule, and periarticular tissues, can restrict joint mobility.

Clinical Pearl

Caution must be used when basing clinical judgments on the results of accessory motion testing because few studies have examined the validity and reliability of accessory motion testing of the spine or extremities and little is known about the validity of these tests for most inferences.[94]

Position Testing in the Spine. The position tests are screening tests designed by osteopaths to examine the relative position of a zygapophysial joint, or joints, to the joint below. As with all screening tests, position testing is valuable in focusing the attention of the clinician to a specific area but is not appropriate for making a definitive statement concerning the movement status of the segment. However, when combined with the results of the passive movement testing, position tests help to form the working hypothesis.

Position testing of the spine is described in the Section IV introduction.

Muscle Performance: Strength, Power, and Endurance. Strength measures the power with which musculotendinous units act across a bone-joint lever-arm system to actively generate motion, or passively resist movement against gravity and variable resistance.[87]

Clinical Pearl

According to Cyriax, musculoskeletal tissues can be subdivided into contractile and inert (noncontractile) tissues.[60]

- *Contractile.* The term *contractile tissue,* as defined by Cyriax, is a bit of a misnomer, because the only true contractile tissue in the body is the muscle fiber. However, included under this term are the muscle belly, tendon, tenoperiosteal junction, submuscular/tendinous bursa, and bone (tendoosseous junction), because all are stressed to some degree with a muscle contraction.

- *Inert.* Inert tissue, according to Cyriax, includes the joint capsule, ligaments, bursa, articular surfaces of the joint, synovium, dura, bone, and fascia.

The tendoosseous junction and the bursae are placed in each of the subdivisions owing to their close proximity to contractile tissue and their capacity to be compressed or stretched during movement.

By definition, a contractile tissue is a tissue involved with a muscle contraction, and one that can be tested using an isolated muscle contraction. However, contractile tissues, such as tendons, which have no ability to contract, could be classified as inert, because although they are strongly affected by the contraction of their respective muscle bellies, they also are affected if passively stretched (Tables 8-26 and 8-27). Conversely, inert tissues, which also have no ability to contract, can be compressed, and therefore affected, during a contraction.

According to Cyriax, pain with a contraction generally indicates an injury to the muscle or a capsular structure.[60] This suspicion can be confirmed by combining the findings from the isometric test with the findings of the passive motion and the joint distraction and compression tests. In addition to examining the integrity of the contractile and inert structures, strength testing may be used to examine the integrity of the myotomes (see Chap. 9). A myotome is defined as a muscle or group of muscles served by a single nerve root. *Key muscle* is a better, more accurate term, because the muscles tested are the most representative of the supply from a particular segment. Voluntary muscle strength testing must remain somewhat subjective until a precise way of measuring muscle contraction is generally

TABLE 8-26   Differential Diagnosis of Contractile, Inert, and Neural Tissue Injury

	Contractile Tissue	Inert Tissue	Neural Tissue
Pain	Cramping, dull, ache	Dull-sharp	Burning, lancinating
Paresthesia	No	No	Yes
Duration	Intermittent	Intermittent	Intermittent-constant
Dermatomal distribution	No	No	Yes
Peripheral nerve sensory distribution	No	No	Yes (if peripheral nerve involved)
End-feel	Muscle spasm	Boggy, hard capsular	Stretch

available.[87] Cyriax reasoned that if you isolated and then applied tension to a structure, you could make a conclusion as to the integrity of that structure.[60] His work also introduced the concept of tissue reactivity. Tissue reactivity is the manner in which different stresses and movements can alter the clinical signs and symptoms. This knowledge can be used to gauge any subtle changes to the patient's condition.[97]

Pain that occurs consistently with resistance, at whatever the length of the muscle, may indicate a tear of the muscle belly.

Pain with muscle testing may indicate a muscle injury, a joint injury, or a combination of both. According to Cyriax,[60,66] strength testing can provide the clinician with the following findings:

▶ A weak and painless contraction may indicate palsy or a complete rupture of the muscle-tendon unit. The motor disorder of peripheral neuropathy is first manifested by weakness, and diminished or absent tendon reflex.[50]

TABLE 8-27   Differential Diagnosis of Muscle and Ligament Tissue Pathology

	Muscle	Ligament
Mechanism of injury	Overstretching, direct trauma	Overstretching
Contributing factors	Fatigue, muscle imbalance, inflexibility, inadequate warm-up	Fatigue, hypermobility/instability, decreased articular stability
Active movement	Pain on contraction or stretch (grade I or II), no pain on contraction (grade III), weakness on contraction (grades I–III)	Pain on stretch or distraction (grade I or II), no pain on stretch (grade III), decreased range of motion
Passive movement	Pain on stretch or compression	Pain on stretch (grade I or II), no pain on stretch (grade III), decreased range of motion
Resisted isometric movement	Pain on contraction (grades I or II), no pain on contraction (grade III), weakness on contraction (grades I–III)	No pain (Grades I–III)
Special tests	If test isolates muscles, weakness and pain on contraction (grade I or II) or weakness and no pain on contraction (grade III)	Stress tests positive
Reflexes	Normal unless grade III	Normal
Cutaneous distribution	Normal	Normal
Joint play/glide	Normal	Increased
Palpation of structure	Point tenderness, swelling (blood), spasm	Point tenderness; swelling (blood/synovial fluid)
Diagnostic imaging	Positive MRI, arthrogram, and CT scan	Positive MRI, arthrogram, and CT scan; stress radiograph shows increased ROM

CT, computed tomography; MRI, magnetic resonance imaging; ROM, range of motion. Modified from Magee DJ. *Orthopedic Physical Assessment,* 4th ed. Philadelphia: Saunders; 2002.

▶ A strong and painless contraction indicates a normal finding.

▶ A weak and painful contraction indicates serious pathology such as a significant muscle tear or tumor.

▶ A strong and painful contraction indicates a grade I contractile lesion.

Pain that does not occur during the test, but occurs upon the release of the contraction, is thought to have an articular source, produced by the joint glide that occurs following the release of tension.

> ### Clinical Pearl
>
> Pain that occurs with resistance, accompanied by pain at the opposite end of passive range, indicates muscle impairment.

The degree of certainty regarding the findings just described depends on a combination of the length of the muscle tested and the force applied (see Chap. 1). To fully test the integrity of the muscle-tendon unit, a maximum contraction must be performed in the fully lengthened position of the muscle-tendon unit. Although this position fully tests the muscle-tendon unit, there are some problems with testing in this manner:

▶ The joint and its surrounding inert tissues are in a more vulnerable position and could be the source of the pain.

▶ It is difficult to differentiate between damage to the contractile tissue of varying severity. The degree of significance with the findings in resisted testing depends on the position of the muscle and the force applied (Table 8-28). For example, pain reproduced with a minimal contraction in the rest position for the muscle is more strongly suggestive of a contractile lesion than pain reproduced with a maximal contraction in the lengthened position for the muscle.

▶ As a muscle lengthens, it reaches a point of passive insufficiency where it is not capable of generating its maximum force output (see Chap. 6).

TABLE 8-28   Strength Testing Related to Joint Position and Muscle Length

Muscle Length	Rationale
Fully lengthened	Muscle in position of passive insufficiency Tightens the inert component of the muscle Tests for muscle tears (tendoperiosteal tears) while using minimal force
Mid-range	Muscle in strongest position Tests overall power of muscle
Fully shortened	Muscle in its weakest position Used for the detection of palsies, especially if coupled with an eccentric contraction

If the same muscle is tested on the opposite side, using the same testing procedure, the concern about the length of the muscle is removed, because the focus of the test is to provide a comparison with same muscle on the opposite side, rather than to assess the absolute force output.

To assess strength, strength values have traditionally been made between similar muscle groups on opposite extremities, or antagonistic ratios. This information is then used to determine whether a patient was fully rehabilitated.

Manual muscle testing is traditionally used by the clinician to assess the strength of a muscle or muscle group. Valuable information can be gleaned from these tests, including:

▶ The amount of force the muscle is capable of producing and whether the amount of force produced varies with the joint angle.

▶ Whether any pain or weakness is produced with the contraction.

▶ The endurance of the muscle, and how much substitution occurs during the test.

Manual muscle testing is an ordinal level of measurement,[98] and has been found to have both interrater and intrarater reliability, especially when the scale is expanded to include plus or minus a half or a full grade.[99–101]

Several scales have been devised to assess muscle strength. Janda[102] uses a 0-to-5 scale with the following descriptions:

▶ *Grade 5: N (normal).*   A normal, very strong muscle with a full range of movement and able to overcome considerable resistance. This does not mean that the muscle is normal in all circumstances (e.g., when at the onset of fatigue or in a state of exhaustion).

▶ *Grade 4: G (good).*   A muscle with good strength and a full range of movement, and able to overcome moderate resistance.

▶ *Grade 3: F (fair).*   A muscle with a complete range of movement against gravity only when resistance is not applied.

▶ *Grade 2: P (poor).*   A very weak muscle with a complete range of motion only when gravity is eliminated by careful positioning of the patient.

▶ *Grade 1: T (trace).*   A muscle with evidence of slight contractility but no effective movement.

▶ *Grade 0.*   A muscle with no evidence of contractility.

Sapega[98] uses the descriptions in Table 8-29.

To be a valid test, strength testing must elicit a maximum contraction of the muscle being tested. Four strategies ensure that this occurs:

1. *Placing the muscle to be tested in a shortened position.* This puts the muscle in an ineffective physiologic position and has the effect of increasing motor neuron activity.

2. *Having the patient perform an eccentric muscle contraction by using the command "Don't let me move you."*

TABLE 8-29   Muscle Grading

Grade	Value	Movement
5	Normal (100%)	Complete range of motion against gravity with maximal resistance
4	Good (75%)	Complete range of motion against gravity with some (moderate) resistance
3+	Fair+	Complete range of motion against gravity with minimal resistance
3	Fair (50%)	Complete range of motion against gravity
3−	Fair−	Some but not complete range of motion against gravity
2+	Poor+	Initiates motion against gravity
2	Poor (25%)	Complete range of motion with gravity eliminated
2−	Poor−	Initiates motion if gravity eliminated
1	Trace	Evidence of slight contractility but no joint motion
0	Zero	No contraction palpated

Because the tension at each cross-bridge and the number of active cross-bridges is greater during an eccentric contraction, the maximum eccentric muscle tension developed is greater with an eccentric contraction than with a concentric one (see Chap. 6).

3. *Breaking the contraction.*   It is important to break the patient's muscle contraction in order to ensure that the patient is making a maximal effort and that the full power of the muscle is being tested.

4. *Holding the contraction for at least 5 seconds.*   Weakness resulting from nerve palsy has a distinct fatigability. The muscle demonstrates poor endurance, because usually it is only able to sustain a maximum muscle contraction for about 2 to 3 seconds before complete failure occurs. This strategy is based on the theories behind muscle recruitment, wherein a normal muscle, while performing a maximum contraction, uses only a portion of its motor units, keeping the remainder in reserve to help maintain the contraction. A palsied muscle with its fewer functioning motor units, has very few, if any, in reserve. If a muscle appears to be weaker than normal, further investigation is required, as follows:

   a. The test is repeated three times. Muscle weakness resulting from disuse will be consistently weak and should not become weaker with several repeated contractions.

b. Another muscle that shares the same innervation is tested. Knowledge of both spinal nerve and peripheral nerve innervation will aid the clinician in determining which muscle to select (see Chap. 2).

Substitutions by other muscle groups during testing indicates the presence of weakness. It does not, however, tell the clinician the cause of the weakness.

As always, these tests cannot be evaluated in isolation but have to be integrated into a total clinical profile before drawing any conclusion about the patient's condition.

Other grades of muscle strength are covered in several other texts.[98,102,103] If the popular methods to grade muscles are analyzed, the frailties and similarities become obvious. If the muscle strength is less than grade 3, these testing grades are perhaps useful, but it is the grades of 3 and higher that produce the most confusion. Some of the confusion arises from the descriptions of maximal, moderate, and minimal, or considerable, which removes much of the objectivity from the tests.

Although the grading of muscle strength has its role in the clinic, and the ability to isolate the various muscles is very important in determining the source of nerve palsy, specific grading does not give the clinician much information on the ability of the structure to perform functional tasks. In addition, measurements of isometric muscle force are specific to a point or small range in the joint range excursion and thus cannot be used to predict dynamic force capabilities.[104–106] More recently, the examination of strength has involved:

▶ An analysis of the ratio between the eccentric contraction and concentric contraction of a muscle at various positions and speeds.[107] This ratio is aptly named the *eccentric/concentric ratio* (E/C ratio).[108] The ratio is calculated by dividing the eccentric strength value by the concentric strength value. Various authors[109,110] have demonstrated that the upper limit of this ratio is 2.0 and that lower ratios indicate pathology[108,111] (Table 8-30).

▶ An examination of the functional strength of a muscle, or a group of muscles. Within this text, functional testing methods are outlined with special emphasis on assessing those muscles that are prone to weakness (Table 8-31).

Functional muscle function testing provides the clinician with the following information[116]:

▶ Strength of individual muscles or muscle groups that form a functional unit.

▶ Nature, range, and quality of simple movement patterns.

▶ Relationship between the strength and the flexibility of a muscle or muscle group.

Muscle function testing, therefore, should address the production and control of motion in functional activities. Although there is general agreement about the role of the trunk and pelvic musculature in normal functioning of the vertebral column, protection against pain, and recurrence of low back disorders,[72,117,118] more research is needed to determine the role of functional strength in the extremities.

TABLE 8-30   Ranges of Eccentric/Concentric Ratios for Normals[108]

Reference	Joint	Range	Velocity (degrees/s)
Kramer and MacDermid[112]	Knee	1.1–1.5	45–180
Rizzardo et al[113]	Knee	1.3–1.7	60–180
Colliander and Tesch[114]	Knee	1.2–1.6	30–150
Griffin[109]	Elbow	1.1–1.3	30–120
Hortobagyi and Katch[110]	Elbow	1.4–1.7	30–120
Dvir[115]	Shoulder (IR)	1.1–1.2	60–180
Hartsell and Spaulding[108]	Shoulder (ER)	1.2–1.7	60–180

ER, external rotation; IR, internal rotation.

Motor Function. Motor function is the ability to learn or demonstrate the skillful and efficient assumption, maintenance, modification, and control of voluntary postures and movement patterns.[13] The clinician observes for any indication of signs indicating a systemic neurologic compromise. These include abnormal movement patterns, movement synergies, or gait disturbances.

The criteria for simple motor patterns are that the movement[16,102]:

▶ Is performed exactly in the desired direction.

▶ Is smooth and of a constant speed.

▶ Follows the shortest and most efficient path.

▶ Is performed in its full range.

Most human movements involve complex movement patterns that include trunk, bilateral extremity, and unilateral extremity combinations.[119] The trunk flexes or extends with symmetric movements, rotates with reciprocal movements, and moves in combinations of flexion or extension with rotation and side-flexion in asymmetric movements. Each of the limb movements affects the trunk differently.

The criteria for complex motor patterns are as follows[16]:

▶ Synchronization between the primary movers in the distal regions with those more proximal.

▶ Smooth propagation of motion from one region of the body to another.

▶ Absence of inefficient movement patterns or muscle recruitment.

▶ Optimal relationship between the speed of motion initiated in one region and the speed of motion in other regions.

The upper extremities can work together when they are in direct or indirect contact with each other (clasping the hands together, holding an object with two hands), or separately. The lower extremities can work together off a stable base, or

TABLE 8-31   Functional Division of Muscle Groups[116]

Movement Group	Stabilization Group
Primarily type IIa	Primarily type I
Prone to develop tightness	Prone to develop weakness
Prone to develop hypertonicity	Prone to muscle inhibition
Dominate in fatigue and new movement situations	Fatigue easily
Generally cross two joints	Primarily cross one joint
Examples	*Examples*
Gastrocnemius/soleus	Peronei
Tibialis posterior	Tibialis anterior
Short hip adductors	Vastus medialis and lateralis
Hamstrings	Gluteus maximus, medius, minimus
Rectus femoris	Serratus anterior
Tensor fascia latae	Rhomboids
Erector spinae	Lower portion trapezius
Quadratus lumborum	Short and deep cervical flexors
Pectoralis major	Upper limb extensors
Upper portion of trapezius	Rectus abdominis
Levator scapulae	
Sternocleidomastoid	
Scalenes	
Upper limb flexors	

separately. In the bilateral combinations, the two limbs are separated, but both are involved in the activity. The limbs may be
moved in the same direction, termed *symmetric* (breaststroke
swimming); in opposite directions, termed *reciprocal* (swimming the crawl); toward one side of the body (pulling on a rope
above one side of the head), termed *asymmetric*; or toward opposite sides of the body (swimming side stroke), termed *cross-
diagonal* or *reciprocal asymmetric*.[119]

Primitive movement patterns are those seen with compromise to the CNS, such as the flexor withdrawal pattern.[120]

Mass movement patterns involve combined motions of the
joints within the kinetic chain, depending on the desired motion.[121] For example, a mass pattern of the lower extremity
could involve hip, knee, and ankle dorsiflexion, with the rotation and abduction-adduction component varying.

Advanced movement patterns involve such combinations as
hip extension, knee flexion, and plantar flexion, or hip flexion,
knee extension, and dorsiflexion—motions that occur with normal gait.[121]

Reflex Integrity. Reflex integrity is defined as the intactness of
the neural path involved in a reflex.[13] The neural mechanisms
associated with reflex testing are described in Chapter 2.

Deep Tendon Reflexes. Deep tendon reflex tests (see Chap. 2)
utilize the muscle spindle to determine the state of both the afferent and efferent peripheral nervous systems, and the ability
of the CNS to inhibit the reflex. A reflex is a programmed unit
of behavior in which a certain type of stimulus from a receptor
automatically leads to the response of an effector.

Any muscle that possesses a tendon is capable of producing
a deep tendon reflex. Five of these are regularly tested: the biceps (C5), brachioradialis (C6), and triceps (C7) in the upper
extremity, and the quadriceps (L4) and Achilles (S1) in the
lower extremities.

> ### Clinical Pearl
>
> The abdominal and cremaster reflexes (superficial skin reflexes)
> are decreased or absent on the side affected by a corticospinal
> tract lesion and, thus, serve as adjuncts to the muscle stretch and
> plantar reflexes[122] (Table 8-32).

The tendon is struck directly and smartly with the reflex
hammer. The biceps reflex is best tested by tapping the thumb,
which has been placed over the tendon. The limb to be tested
should be relaxed and in a flexed or semiflexed position. The
Jendrassik maneuver can be used during testing to enhance a
muscle reflex that is difficult to elicit.[123]

▶ For the upper extremity reflexes, the patient is asked to cross
the ankles and then to isometrically attempt to abduct the legs.

▶ For the lower extremity reflexes, the patient is asked to interlock the fingers and then to isometrically attempt to pull
the elbows apart (Fig. 8-2).

Deep tendon reflexes may be graded as follows:

0 Absent (areflexia)

1+ Decreased (hyporeflexia)

2+ Normal

3+ Hyperactive (brisk)

4+ Hyperactive with clonus (hyperreflexive)

Each of these categories can occur as a generalized, or local,
phenomenon. The absence of a reflex signifies an interruption
of the reflex arc. A hyperactive reflex denotes a release from
cortical inhibitory influences. Reflex asymmetry has more
pathologic significance than the absolute activity of the reflex.
For example, a bilateral patella reflex of 3+ is less significant
than a 3+ on the left and a 2+ on the right.

The causes of generalized hyporeflexia run the gamut from
neurologic disease, chromosomal metabolic conditions, and
hypothyroidism to schizophrenia and anxiety.[39]

▶ Nongeneralized hyporeflexia can result from peripheral
neuropathy, spinal nerve root compression, and cauda
equina syndrome. It is thus important to test more than one
reflex and to evaluate the information gleaned from the
examination, before reaching a conclusion as to the relevance of the findings.

▶ Hyporeflexia, if not generalized to the whole body, indicates a lower motor neuron or sensory paresis, which may
be segmental (root), multisegmental (cauda equina) or nonsegmental (peripheral nerve).

TABLE 8-32 Superficial Reflexes

Reflex	Normal Response	Pertinent Central Nervous System Segment
Upper abdominal	Umbilicus moves up and toward area being stroked	T7–9
Lower abdominal	Umbilicus moves down and toward area being stroked	T11–12
Cremasteric	Scrotum elevates	T12, L1
Plantar	Flexion of toes	S1–2
Gluteal	Skin tenses in gluteal area	L4–5, S1–3
Anal	Contraction of anal sphincter muscles	S2–4

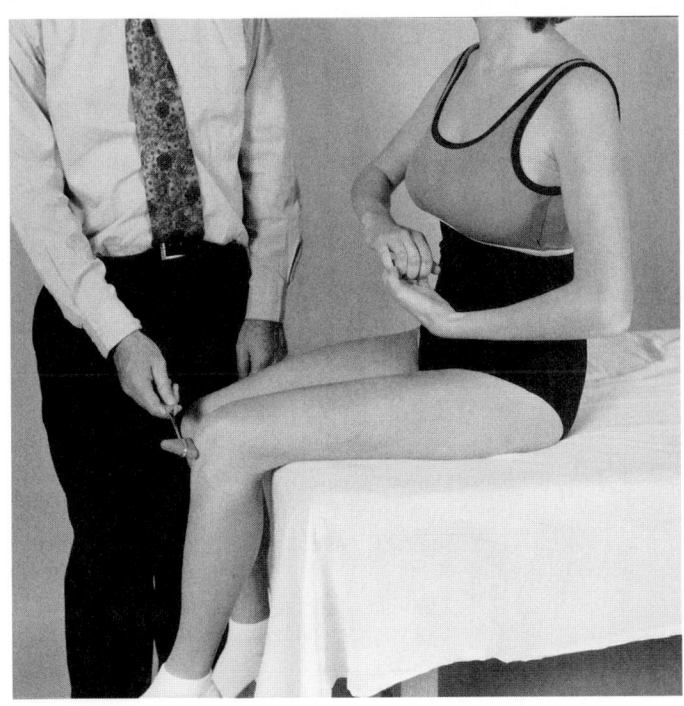

FIGURE 8-2 The Jendrassik maneuver during reflex testing.

True neurological hyperreflexia contains a clonic component and is suggestive of CNS (upper motor neuron) impairment, such as a brain stem or cerebral impairment, spinal cord compression, or a neurologic disease. The clinician also should note any additional recruitment that occurs during the reflex contraction of the target. As with hyporeflexia, the clinician should assess more than one reflex before coming to a conclusion about a hyperreflexia. The presence of an upper motor neuron impairment can be confirmed by the presence of the pathologic reflexes (see next section).

A brisk reflex is a normal finding, provided that it is not masking a hyperreflexia caused by an incorrect testing technique. Unlike hyperreflexia, a brisk reflex does not have a clonic component.

Pathologic Reflexes. There are two basic pathologic reflexes: the Babinski and its variants (Chaddock, Oppenheim, Gordon), and the Hoffman and its variants (ankle and wrist clonus). A number of primitive reflexes are normally integrated by individuals as they develop. Pathologic reflexes occur when an injury or disease process results in a loss of this normal suppression by the cerebrum on the segmental level of the brain stem or spinal cord, resulting in a release of the primitive reflex.[37] Thus, the presence of pathologic reflexes is suggestive of CNS (upper motor neuron) impairment, and requires an appropriate referral. These tests are described in Chapter 2.

Sensory Integrity. Sensory integrity is the intactness of cortical sensory processing, including proprioception, pallesthesia (the ability to sense mechanical vibration), stereognosis (the ability to perceive, recognize, and name familiar objects), and topognosis (the ability to localize exactly a cutaneous sensation).[13]

> **Clinical Pearl**
>
> The sensory distribution of each nerve is called a *dermatome* (Fig. 8-3).

A motor or sensory deficit is a symptom of direct involvement of the nerve root. It is possible for nerve root compression to cause pure motor paresis, a pure sensory deficit, or both, depending on which aspect of the nerve root is compressed[3] (see Chap. 2). Pain results if there is irritation of the neural fibers. In general, if a patient has a sensory deficit involving a peripheral nerve, he or she is able to accurately localize the area of anesthesia.[124]

Sensory testing is performed throughout the dermatomal areas (see Fig. 8-3). The segmental innervation of the skin has a high degree of overlap, especially in the thoracic spine, requiring that the clinician test the full area of the dermatome. This is done to seek out the area of sensitivity, or autogenous area, which is a small region of the dermatome with no overlap, and the only area within a dermatome that is supplied exclusively by a single segmental level.[125]

There are two components to the dermatome tests:

1. ***Light touch.*** Information about light touch, two-point discrimination, vibration, and proprioception are carried by the dorsal column–medial lemniscal tract. Light touch tests for hypoesthesia throughout the dermatome. In terms of sensation loss, light touch is the most sensitive and the first to be affected with palsy. If the light touch test is positive, the areas of reduced sensation are mapped out for the autogenous area, and then the pinprick test is performed to map out the whole of the autogenous area.[3] The use of a vibrating tuning fork has been found to be a valid and reliable test of the functional integrity of the large myelinated nerve fibers.[126]

2. ***Pinprick.*** The pinprick test examines for near-anesthesia in the autonomous, no-overlap area. Pinprick testing is the most common way of determining the sensory "level" caused by a spinal cord lesion, because information about pain, temperature, and crude touch are carried by the spinothalamic tract.[123] Pinprick sensation is difficult to test because of the natural variations in the pressure put on the pin and the sensitivity of different parts of the skin.

> **Clinical Pearl**
>
> Pain dermatomes have less overlap than light touch dermatomes.[127]

Aerobic Capacity and Endurance. Aerobic capacity endurance is the ability to perform work or participate in activity over time using the body's oxygen uptake, delivery, and energy-release mechanisms.[13] Clinical indications for the use of the tests and

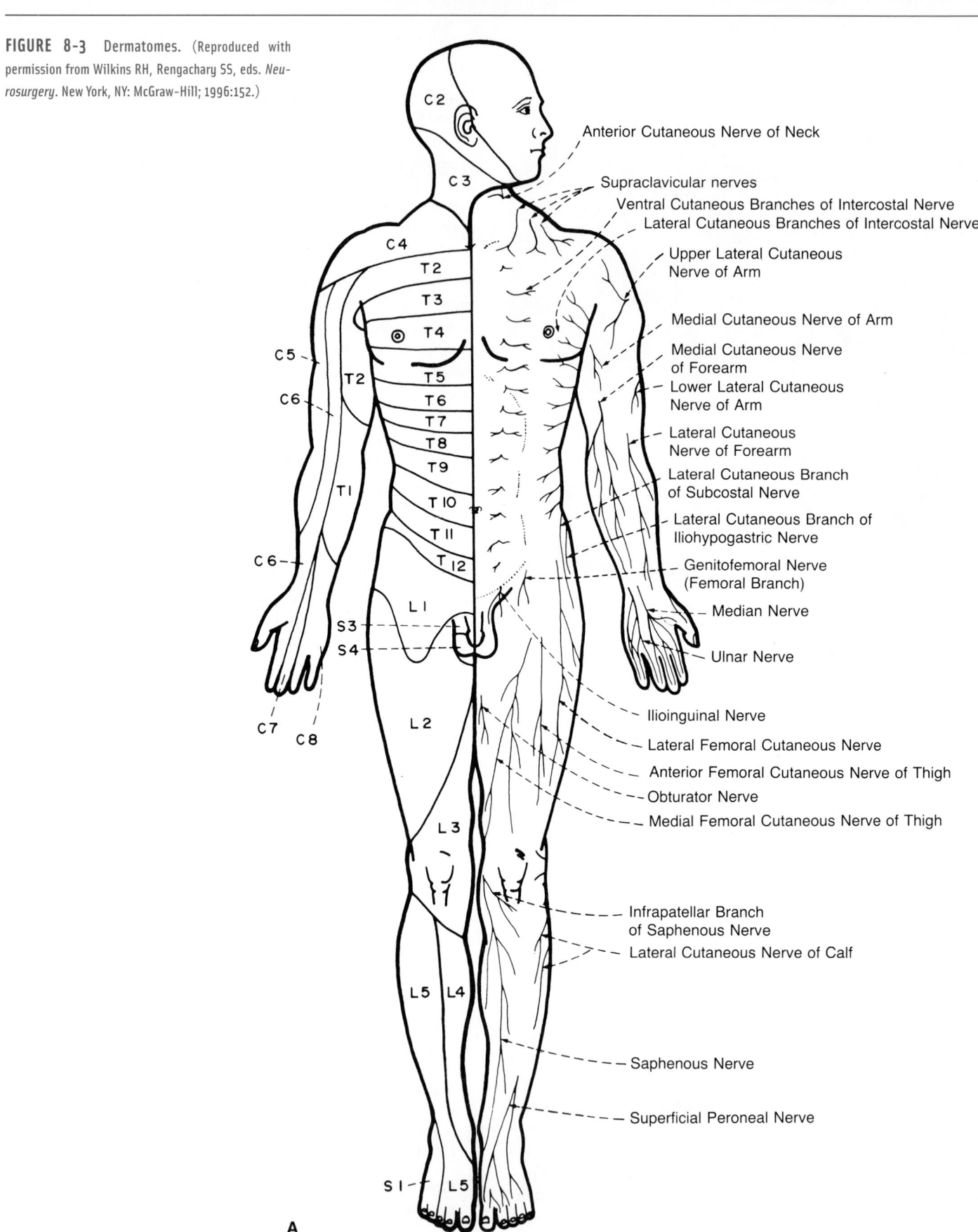

FIGURE 8-3 Dermatomes. (Reproduced with permission from Wilkins RH, Rengachary SS, eds. *Neurosurgery.* New York, NY: McGraw-Hill; 1996:152.)

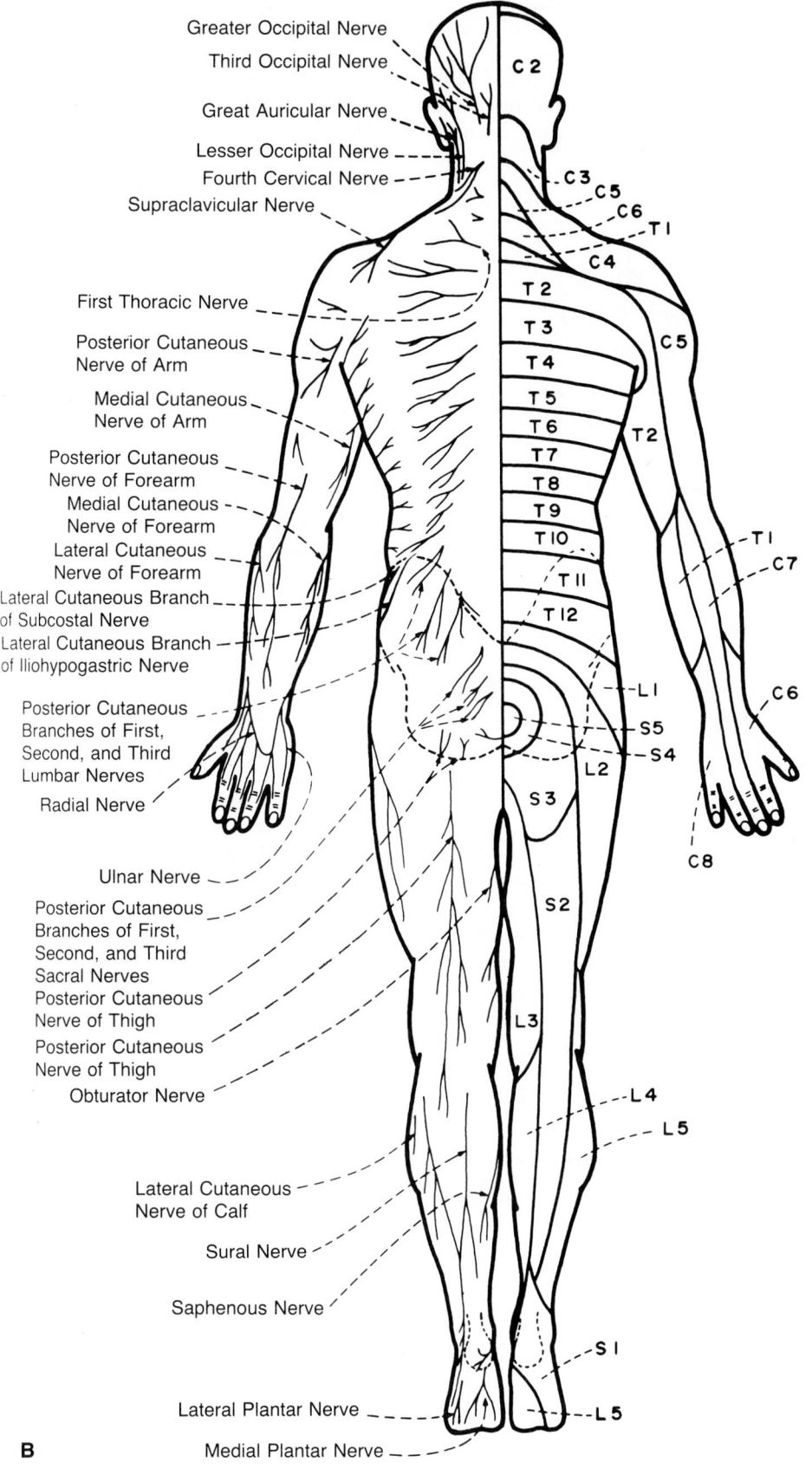

Greater Occipital Nerve

Third Occipital Nerve

Great Auricular Nerve

Lesser Occipital Nerve

Fourth Cervical Nerve

Supraclavicular Nerve

First Thoracic Nerve

Posterior Cutaneous
Nerve of Arm

Medial Cutaneous
Nerve of Arm

Posterior Cutaneous
Nerve of Forearm

Medial Cutaneous
Nerve of Forearm

Lateral Cutaneous
Nerve of Forearm

Lateral Cutaneous Branch
of Subcostal Nerve

Lateral Cutaneous Branch
of Iliohypogastric Nerve

Posterior Cutaneous
Branches of First,
Second, and Third
Lumbar Nerves

Radial Nerve

Ulnar Nerve

Posterior Cutaneous
Branches of First,
Second, and Third
Sacral Nerves

Posterior Cutaneous
Nerve of Thigh

Posterior Cutaneous
Nerve of Thigh

Obturator Nerve

Lateral Cutaneous
Nerve of Calf

Sural Nerve

Saphenous Nerve

Lateral Plantar Nerve

Medial Plantar Nerve

B

C 2
C 3
C 5
C 6
T 1
C 4
T 2
T 3
T 4
C 5
T 5
T 6
T 2
T 7
T 8
T 9
T 10
T 1
C 7
T 11
T 12
L 1
C 6
S 5
S 4
L 2
C 8
S 3
S 2
L 3
L 4
L 5
S 1
L 5

measures for this category are based on the findings of the history and systems review. These indications include, but are not limited to, pathology, pathophysiology, and impairment to the following[13]:

▶ Cardiovascular system (abnormal heart rate, rhythm, blood pressure).

▶ Endocrine/metabolic system (osteoporosis).

▶ Multiple systems (trauma, systemic disease).

▶ Neuromuscular system (generalized muscle weakness, decreased endurance).

▶ Pulmonary system (abnormal respiratory pattern, rate, rhythm).

The aerobic capacity and endurance of a patient can be measured using standardized exercise test protocols (e.g., ergometry, step tests, time or distance walk or run tests, treadmill tests), and the patient's response to such tests.[13]

Anthropometric Characteristics. Anthropometric characteristics are traits that describe body dimensions, such as height, weight, girth, and body fat composition.[13] The use of an anthropometric examination and the subsequent measurements varies. Clearly, if a noticeable amount of effusion or swelling is present, these measurements serve as an important baseline from which to judge the effectiveness of the intervention.

Swelling or edema may be localized at the site of the injury or diffused over a larger area. In general, the amount of swelling is related to the severity of the injury. However, in some cases, serious injuries produce very limited swelling, whereas in others, minor injuries cause significant swelling. These changes occur as a result of changes in the local circulation and an inability of the lymphatic system to maintain equilibrium.

A report of rapid joint swelling (within 2 to 4 hours) following a traumatic event may indicate bleeding into the joint. Swelling of a joint that is more gradual, occurring 8 to 24 hours following the trauma, is likely caused by an inflammatory process or synovial swelling.

An edematous limb indicates poor venous return. Pitting edema is characterized by an indentation of the skin after the pressure has been removed.

The more serious reasons for swelling include fracture, tumor, congestive heart failure, and deep vein thrombosis.

Circulation. Circulation is defined by the "Guide" as the movement of blood through organs and tissues to both deliver oxygen and to remove carbon dioxide and cellular byproducts.[13] Circulation also involves the passive movement of lymph through channels. The examination of the circulation includes an examination of those cardiovascular signs not tested in the aerobic capacity and endurance and anthropometric characteristics portions of the examination, including the patient's physiologic response to position change, an inspection of the nail beds, capillary refill, and monitoring of the pulses of the extremities.

In general, the dorsal pedis pulse is used in the lower extremities to assess the patency of the lower extremity vessels, whereas the radial pulse is used for the upper extremities.

Work, Environmental, and Home Barriers (Job, School, Play). Work, environmental, and home barriers are the physical impediments that keep patients from functioning optimally in their surroundings.[13] The concept of function is described in Chapter 7.

Ergonomics and Body Mechanics. Ergonomics is the relationship among the worker; the work that is done; the actions, tasks, or activities inherent in that work (job, school, play); and the environment in which the work (job, school, play) is performed.[13] Body mechanics are the interrelationships of the muscles and joints as they maintain or adjust posture in response to forces placed on or generated by the body.

It is not within the scope of this text to detail the scientific and engineering principles related to ergonomics and the numerous tests used to quantify these measures. Ergonomics as it relates to posture is discussed later, and within the related chapters.

Gait, Locomotion, and Balance. Gait analysis is an important component of the examination process (see Chap. 13) and should not be reserved only for those patients with lower extremity dysfunction. Although the act of walking is often taken for granted, normal and reciprocal gait requires a finely tuned series of reflexes.[128] The examination of gait is performed to highlight any breakdown within these reflexes, including imbalances of flexibility or strength, or compensatory motions.[129]

Gait, like posture, varies between individuals, and a gait that differs from normal is not necessarily pathologic.

The maintenance of balance involves an integration of information from the vestibular, visual, and somatosensory systems. The vestibular system, which includes the apparatus of the inner ear or cochlear system (cranial nerve VIII; see Chap. 2), is important for maintaining equilibrium, a component of balance control. Table 8-33 outlines some equilibrium coordination tests. Balance is an essential component for participation in sports and for activities of daily living.

Several sophisticated systems are available to assess balance. These include stabilometers, force platforms, and motion analysis systems. However, this equipment is costly and, thus, is impractical for most clinicians.

Balance can be measured using static testing or dynamic tests. Static balance analyzes the ability of an individual to maintain a stationary position within a base of support. Dynamic balance involves the ability of maintaining balance while in motion.

The Balance Error Scoring System (BESS) is a quantifiable clinical test for static balance.[131] The test includes three different stances: double leg support, single leg support, and tandem (one leg in front of the other). For each of the tests, the individual places his or her hands on the iliac crests. These three positions are completed twice with the eyes closed, once while on a firm surface, and once while on a piece of medium density foam, for a total of six trials.[131] Each stance test lasts 20 seconds and begins as soon as the subject closes the eyes. During the single stances,

TABLE 8-33 Equilibrium Coordination tests[130]

Stand in normal, comfortable posture
Stand with feet together (narrow base of support)
Stand with one foot directly in front of the other (toe of one foot touching heel of opposite foot)
Stand on one foot *Note:* Arm position may be altered in each of these positions (by side, overhead, etc.); also, unexpected displacement of patient can be used to increase difficulty (ensuring that patient is carefully guarded)
Stand, alternating between forward trunk flexion and return to neutral
Stand and laterally flex trunk to each side
Walk, placing heel of one foot directly in front of toe of opposite foot
Walk along a straight line drawn or taped on floor, or place feet on foot markers while walking
Walk sideways and backward
March in place
Alter speed of ambulatory activities
Stop and start abruptly while walking
Walk in a circle, alternating directions
Walk on heels or toes

TABLE 8-34 Balance Error Scoring System (BESS)

ERRORS
Hands lifted off iliac crest
Opening eyes
Step, stumble, or fall
Moving hip into more than 30 degrees of flexion or abduction
Lifting forefoot or heel
Remaining out of test position for more than 5 seconds

The BESS score is calculated by adding 1 error point for each error or any combination of errors occurring during 1 movement.

the patient is asked to maintain the uninvolved lower extremity in 20 to 30 degrees of hip flexion, and 40 to 50 degrees of knee flexion. Any loss of balance is to be corrected as soon as possible. The performance for each of the six tests is scored by adding one error point for each error committed (Table 8-34). If the subject is unable to maintain the static balance for longer than 5 seconds during the entire 20-second test, the test is considered incomplete, and the subject scores the maximum error score of 10.

Dynamic balance can be tested using functional reach tests,[132] timed agility tests such as the figure-of-eight test,[133,134] carioca or hop test,[135] BESS test for dynamic balance,[136] timed T-band kicks, and timed balance beam walking with eyes open or closed.[131]

Orthotic, Adaptive, Protective, and Assistive Devices. These devices are implements and equipment used to support or protect weak or ineffective joints or muscles and serve to enhance performance.[13] Examples of such devices include canes, crutches, walkers, reachers, and ankle foot orthoses (AFO). The uses of appropriate orthotic, adaptive, protective, and assistive devices is outlined in later chapters.

Posture. Posture describes the relative positions of different joints at any given moment.[29] Over the course of time, various definitions have been put forward to describe the attributes of good posture.[103,129,137,138] Any posture that does not satisfy these requirements has thus been considered faulty posture.

The following factors appear to influence adult posture:

▶ *Heredity.*[139]

▶ *Environment.*[139]

▶ *Disease.*

▶ *Habit.*

Each joint has a direct effect on both its neighboring joint, and on the joints further away. Individuals have characteristics about their posture, which can often define them. As with so-called good movement, *good posture* is a subjective term reflecting what the clinician believes to be correct based on ideal models. Various attempts have been made to define ideal posture.[103,129,138,140,141] Good posture may be defined as "the optimal alignment of the patient's body that allows the neuromuscular system to perform actions requiring the least amount of energy to achieve the desired effect."[129]

The postural examination gives an overall view of the patient's muscle function in both chronic and acute pain states. The examination enables the clinician to differentiate between possible provocative causes, such as structural variations, altered joint mechanics, muscle imbalances, and the residual effects of pathology.

Skeletal malalignment may be defined as either abnormal joint alignment or deformity within a bone. Abnormal, or *nonneutral* alignment, is defined as "positioning that deviates from the midrange position of function."[142] To be classified as abnormal, nonneutral alignment must produce physical functional limitations. Nonneutral alignment may produce neuromusculoskeletal pathology at adjacent or distal joints through compensatory motions or postures. Nonneutral alignment, whether maintained statically, or performed repetitively, appears to be a key precipitating factor in soft tissue and neurologic pain.[143]

This may be the result of an alteration in joint load distribution or in the force transmission of the muscles.

Nonneutral alignment can occur in the frontal (scoliosis, leg-length discrepancy) and the sagittal plane (forward head, anteriorly rotated pelvis, decrease in lumbar lordosis, knee recurvatum, shoulder protraction) and can progress to a somatic dysfunction.[144–146]

Sustained postures also can produce muscle imbalances and pain, especially if the joint is held at the end of its range.[147]

> ### *Clinical Pearl*
>
> A muscle imbalance occurs when the resting length of the agonist and the antagonist changes, with one adopting a shorter resting length than normal and the other adopting a longer resting length than normal. The inert tissues, such as the ligaments and joint capsules, react in a similar fashion, thereby altering joint play, which in turn alters arthrokinematic function and force transmission as the muscles around that joint alter their length in an attempt to minimize the stresses at that joint.[143,148,149]

It is theorized that, if a muscle lengthens as part of a compensation, muscle spindle activity increases within that muscle, producing reciprocal inhibition of that muscle's functional antagonist, and resulting in an alteration in the normal force-couple and arthrokinematic relationship, thereby effecting the efficient and ideal operation of the movement system.[10,102,150–152]

The pain from sustained positions is thought to result from ischemia of the isometrically contracting muscles, localized fatigue, or an excessive mechanical strain on the structures. Intramuscular pressure can compress the blood vessels and prevent the removal of metabolites and the supply of oxygen, either of which can cause temporary pain.[153]

Although most clinicians can appreciate that repeated movement patterns performed in a therapeutic manner may be beneficial, it must also be remembered that repeated motions performed erroneously can produce changes in muscle tension, muscle strength, length, and stiffness.[10]

It is quite normal for muscles to frequently change their lengths during movements. However, this change in resting length may become pathologic when it is sustained through incorrect habituation or as a response to pain.

> ### *Clinical Pearl*
>
> A sustained change in muscle length is postulated to influence the information sent by the proprioceptors, which can cause alterations in recruitment patterns and the dominance of one synergist over another.[10,154]

Muscles maintained in a shortened or lengthened position eventually will adapt to their new positions. These muscles initially are incapable of producing a maximal contraction in the newly acquired positions[155]; however, changes at the sarcomere level eventually allow the muscle to produce maximal

tension at this new length.[10] Although this may appear to be a satisfactory adaptation, the changes in length produce changes in tension development, as well as changes in the angle of pull.[156] For example, a passively insufficient muscle is activated earlier in a movement than a normal muscle and has a tendency to be more hypertonic, thereby producing a reflex inhibition of the antagonists.[102,116,149,157]

Jull[116] and Janda[158] developed a system that characterized muscles, based on common patterns of kinetic chain dysfunction, into two functional divisions: a movement group and a stabilization group (see Table 8-31).

More recently, Sahrmann[10] has stressed the importance of observation along both directions of the kinetic chain, and the importance of examining joints proximal to the site of the disorder, or symptomology, to determine the mechanical cause of the symptoms, rather than identifying the painful tissues. Once the mechanical source is identified, the focus of the intervention is the simultaneous retraining of the muscles, by contracting the lengthened muscle when it is in a shortened position, and stretching the shortened muscle.[10]

> ### *Clinical Pearl*
>
> Postural imbalances involve the entire body, as should any corrections. It is important to remember that prior to any intervention an appropriate examination must take place.

Common lower limb skeletal malalignments and possible correlated and compensatory motions or postures are compiled in Table 8-35.

Work (Job, School, Play), Community, and Leisure Integration and Reintegration. In short, this category refers to the process of assuming or resuming roles and functions.

Self-care and Home Management (Including ADL and IADL) This section addresses the patient's perception of his or her condition, namely issues regarding the patient's perception on their functional level and quality-of-life (see Chap. 7).

Palpation

Palpation is a fundamental skill used in a number of the tests and measures. Both Gerwin and colleagues[159] and Njoo and Van der Does[160] found that training and experience are essential in performing reliable palpation tests. Palpation, which can play a central role in the performance of several manual therapy techniques,[161] is performed to[162,163]:

▶ Check for any vasomotor changes such as an increase in skin temperature that might suggest an inflammatory process.

▶ Localize specific sites of swelling.

▶ Identify specific anatomic structures and their relationship to one another.

▶ Identify sites of point tenderness. Hyperalgic skin zones can be detected using skin drag, which consists of moving the

TABLE 8-35 Skeletal Malalignment of the Lower Quarter and Correlated and Compensatory Motions or Postures

Malalignment	Possible Correlated Motions or Postures	Possible Compensatory Motions or Postures
ANKLE AND FOOT Ankle equinus		Hypermobile first ray Subtalar or midtarsal excessive pronation Hip or knee flexion Genu recurvatum
Rearfoot varus Excessive subtalar supination (calcaneal valgus)	Tibial; tibial and femoral; or tibial, femoral, and pelvic external rotation	Excessive internal rotation along the lower quarter chain Hallux valgus Plantar flexed first ray Functional forefoot valgus Excessive or prolonged midtarsal pronation
Rearfoot valgus Excessive subtalar pronation (calcaneal valgus)	Tibial; tibial and femoral; or tibial, femoral, and pelvic internal rotation Hallux valgus	Excessive external rotation along the lower quarter chain Functional forefoot varus
Forefoot varus	Subtalar supination and related rotation along lower quarter	Plantar flexed first ray Hallux valgus Excessive midtarsal or subtalar pronation or prolonged pronation Excessive tibial; tibial and femoral; or tibial, femoral, and pelvic internal rotation, or all with contralateral lumbar spine rotation
Forefoot valgus	Hallux valgus Subtalar pronation and related rotation along lower quarter	Excessive midtarsal or subtalar supination Excessive tibial; tibial and femoral; or tibial, femoral, and pelvic external rotation, or all with ipsilateral lumbar spine rotation
Metatarsus adductus	Hallux valgus Internal tibial torsion Flat foot In-toeing	
Hallux valgus	Forefoot valgus Subtalar pronation and related rotation along the lower quarter[33]	Excessive tibial; tibial and femoral; or tibial, femoral, and pelvic external rotation, or all with ipsilateral lumbar spine rotation
KNEE AND TIBIA Genu valgus	Pes planus Excessive subtalar pronation External tibial torsion Lateral patellar subluxation Excessive hip adduction Ipsilateral hip excessive internal rotation Lumbar spine contralateral rotation	Forefoot varus Excessive subtalar supination to allow lateral heel to contact ground In-toeing to decrease lateral pelvic sway during gait Ipsilateral pelvic external rotation
Genu varus	Excessive lateral angulation of tibia in frontal plane; (tibial varum); (tibia vara) Internal tibial torsion Ipsilateral hip external rotation Excessive hip abduction	Forefoot valgus Excessive subtalar pronation to allow medial heel to contact ground Ipsilateral pelvic internal rotation

TABLE 8-35   *(cont.)*

Genu recurvatum	Ankle plantar flexion Excessive anterior pelvic tilt	Posterior pelvic tilt Flexed trunk posture Excessive thoracic kyphosis
External tibial torsion	Out-toeing Excessive subtalar supination with related rotation along lower quarter	Functional forefoot varus Excessive subtalar pronation with related rotation along lower quarter
Internal tibial torsion	In-toeing Metatarsus adductus Excessive subtalar pronation with related rotation along lower quarter	Functional forefoot valgus Excessive subtalar supination with related rotation along lower quarter
Excessive tibial retroversion (posterior slant of tibial plateaus)	Genu recurvatum	
Inadequate tibial retrotorsion (posterior deflection of proximal tibia due to hamstrings pull)	Flexed knee posture	
Inadequate tibial retroflexion (bowing of the tibia)	Altered alignment of Achilles tendon causing altered associated joint motion	
Bowleg deformity of tibia (tibia vara, tibial varum)	Internal tibial torsion	Forefoot valgus Excessive subtalar pronation
HIP AND FEMUR Excessive femoral anteversion (anteversion)	In-toeing Excessive subtalar pronation Lateral patellar subluxation	Excessive external tibial torsion Excessive knee external rotation Excessive tibial; tibial and femoral; or tibial, femoral, and pelvic external rotation; or all with ipsilateral lumbar spine rotation
Femoral retrotorsion (retroversion)	Out-toeing Excessive subtalar supination	Excessive knee internal rotation Excessive tibial; tibial and femoral; or tibial, femoral, and pelvic internal rotation; or all with contralateral lumbar spine rotation
Excessive femoral neck to shaft angle (coxa valga)	Long ipsilateral lower limb and correlated motions or postures of a long limb Posterior pelvic rotation Supinated subtalar joint and related external rotation along the lower quarter	Excessive ipsilateral subtalar pronation Excessive contralateral subtalar supination Contralateral plantar flexion Ipsilateral genu recurvatum Ipsilateral hip or knee flexion Ipsilateral forward pelvis with contralateral lumbar spine rotation
Decreased femoral neck to shaft angle (coxa vara)	Pronated subtalar joint and related internal rotation along lower quarter Short ipsilateral lower limb and correlated motions or postures along lower quarter: anterior pelvic rotation	Excessive ipsilateral subtalar supination Excessive contralateral subtalar pronation Ipsilateral plantar flexion Contralateral genu recurvatum Contralateral hip or knee flexion Ipsilateral backward pelvic rotation with ipsilateral lumbar spine rotation

From Riegger-Krugh C, Keysor JJ. Skeletal malalignments of the lower quarter: correlated and compensatory motions and postures. *J Orthop Sports Phys Ther* 1996;23(2):164–170.

pads of the fingertips over the surface of the skin and attempting to sense resistance or drag.

▶ Identify soft tissue texture changes or myofascial restriction. Normal tissue is soft and mobile and moves equally in all directions. Abnormal tissue may feel hard, sensitive, or somewhat crunchy or stringy.[164]

▶ Locate changes in muscle tone resulting from trigger points, muscle spasm, hypertonicity, or hypotonicity. However, a study by Hsieh and colleagues[165] found that among nonexpert physicians, physiatric or chiropractic, trigger point palpation is not reliable for detecting taut band and local twitch response, and only marginally reliable for referred pain after training. The most useful diagnostic test to detect these changes is to create a fold in the tissue, and to stretch it.[166] The tissue should be soft and supple, and there should be no resistance to the stretch.

▶ Determine circulatory status by checking distal pulses.

▶ Detect changes in the moisture of the skin.

The pertinent palpation areas for each of the joints are described later, within the relevant chapters.

Special Tests

Special tests for each area are dependent on the special needs and structure of each joint. Numerous tests exist for each joint. These tests are only performed if there is some indication that they would by helpful in arriving at a diagnosis. The tests help confirm or implicate a particular structure and may also provide information as to the degree of tissue damage.

In the joints of the spine, examples of special tests include directional stress tests (posterior-anterior pressures; anterior, posterior, and rotational stressing), joint quadrant testing, vascular tests, and repeated movement testing. Examples of special tests in the peripheral joints include ligament stress tests (i.e., Lachman for the anterior cruciate ligament), articular stress testing (valgus stress applied at the elbow), and glenohumeral impingement tests. The special tests for each of the joints are described in the various chapters of this book.

The interpretation of the findings from the special tests depends on the skill and experience of the clinician, as well as the degree of familiarity with the tests.

Neuromeningeal Mobility Tests

The neurodynamic mobility tests (see Chap. 12) examine for the presence of any abnormalities of the dura, both centrally and peripherally. These tests are used if a dural adhesion or irritation is suspected. The tests employ a sequential and progressive stretch to the dura until the patient's symptoms are reproduced.[11] Theoretically, if the dura is scarred, or inflamed, a lack of extensibility with stretching occurs. Because the sinuvertebral nerve innervates the dural sleeve, the pain caused by an inflamed dura is felt by the patient at multisegmental levels and is described as having an achelike quality. If the patient experiences sharp or stabbing pain during the test, a more serious underlying condition should be suspected.

Imaging Studies

Although the ordering of imaging studies is not within the scope of physical therapy practice, clinicians frequently receive imaging study reports. Thus, it is important for the clinician to know what relevance to attach to these reports, and the strengths and weaknesses of the various imaging techniques. In general, imaging tests have a high sensitivity (few false negatives), but low specificity (high false-positive rate).

Radiology. X-rays are part of the electromagnetic spectrum and have the ability to penetrate through body tissues of varying densities. The amount of beam that is absorbed is dependent on the density of the tissue. The film plate is positioned to capture the particles of the beam that are not absorbed by the tissues of the body. Tissues of greater density allow less penetration of the X-rays. Exposure to the X-ray particles causes the film to darken, whereas areas of absorption appear lighter on the film. The denser a tissue is, the lighter it appears on the film.

The following structures are listed in order of descending density: metal, bone, soft tissue, water or body fluid, fat, and air. Because air is the least dense material in the body, it absorbs the least amount of x-ray particles, resulting in the darkest portion of the film. Bone can have varying densities within the body. For example, cancellous bone is less dense than cortical bone and thus appears lighter than the cortical bone on the radiograph.

When evaluating radiographs, the clinician should use a systematic method. One such system uses the mnemonic ABCS[167]:

▶ *A: Architecture or alignment.* The normal shape of each bone should be apparent. The outline of each bone should be smooth and continuous. Breaks in continuity usually represent fractures.

▶ *B: Bone density.* The cortex of the bone should appear denser than the remainder of the bone. Subchondral bone becomes sclerosed in the presence of stress in accordance with Wolff's law[168] and increases its density.

▶ *C: Cartilage spaces.* Each joint should have a well-preserved joint space between the articulating surfaces. A decreased joint space typically indicates osteoarthritis.

▶ *S: Soft tissue evaluation.* Trauma to soft tissues produces abnormal images, resulting from effusion and distention.

Conventional Radiography. Plain-film, or conventional, radiographs are relatively inexpensive and give an excellent view of cortical bone (Figs. 8-4 through 8-11). They are thus very helpful in detecting fractures and subluxations in patients with a history of trauma.[169] For example, in patients with cervical trauma, the physician often orders lateral (Fig. 8-4), anterior-posterior, and oblique views, together with an open-mouth view. Radiographs also may be used to highlight the presence of degenerative joint disease, which is characterized by an approximation of the joint surface on the radiograph. However, radiographs do not provide an image of soft tissue

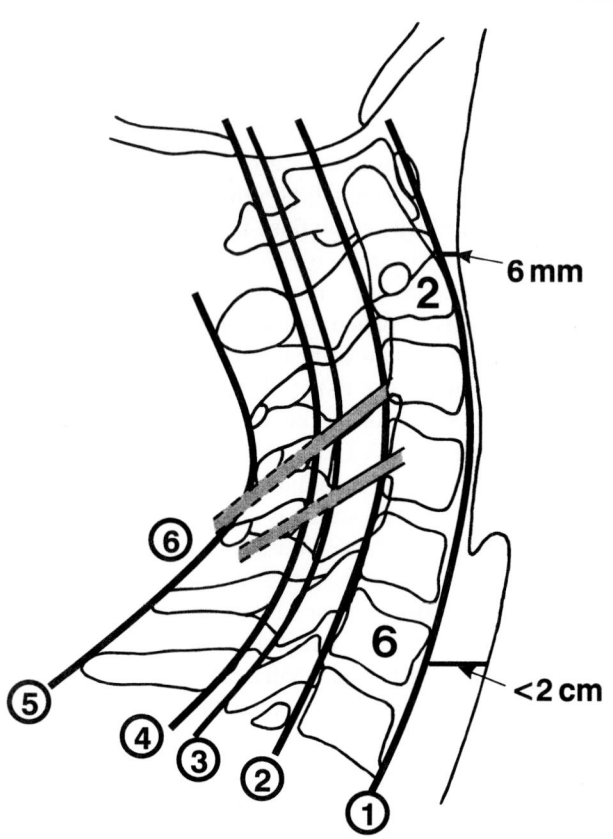

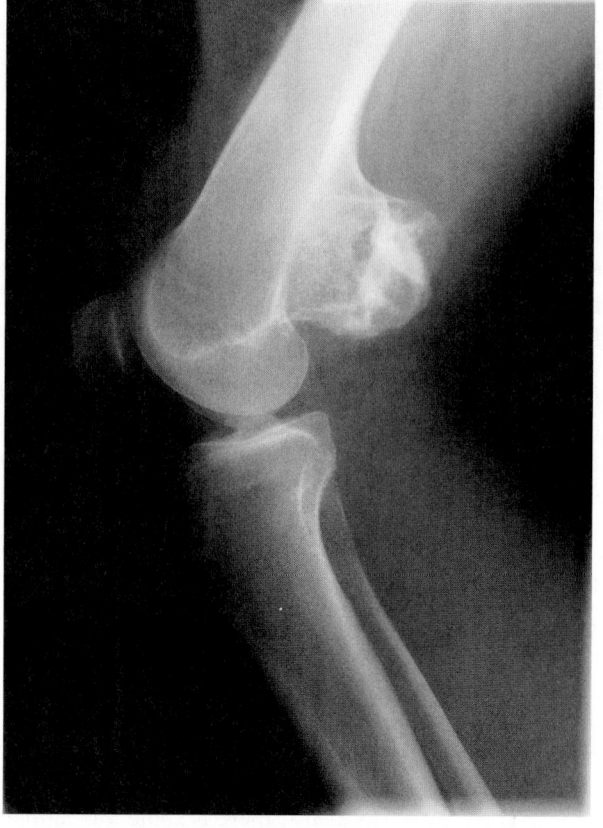

FIGURE 8-5 Radiograph showing abnormal bone growth of femur.

structures such as muscles, tendons, ligaments, and intervertebral disks.

Stress Radiograph. Flexion and extension views can be helpful in assessing spinal mobility and stability in the spine and should be ordered in the acutely injured athlete when there is a high degree of suspicion of spine injury. Greater than 2 mm of motion at any segment would suggest instability and warrant further examination.

A stress radiograph is a procedure using radiographs taken while the stress is applied to a joint. An unstable joint demonstrates widening of the joint space when the stress is applied.

Contrast-enhanced Radiography. Contrast-enhanced radiography procedures involve the use of a contrasting agent to highlight different structures. These agents may be administered orally, rectally, or by injection. Different contrast media may be used and include radiopaque organic iodides and radiotranslucent gases. Contrast-enhanced radiography procedures include:

▶ *Arthrography.* Arthrography is the study of structures within an encapsulated joint using a contrast medium, with or without air that is injected into the joint space. The contrast medium distends the joint capsule. This type of radiograph

is called an *arthrogram.* An arthrogram outlines the soft tissue structures of a joint that would otherwise not be visible with a plain-film radiograph. This procedure is commonly performed on patients with injuries involving the shoulder or the knee.

▶ *Myelography.* Myelography is the radiographic study of the spinal cord, nerve roots, dura mater, and spinal canal. The contrast medium is injected into the subarachnoid space, and a radiograph is taken. This type of radiograph is called a *myelogram.* Myelography is used frequently to diagnose intervertebral disk herniations, spinal cord compression, stenosis, nerve root injury, or tumors. The nerve root and its sleeve can be observed clearly on direct myelograms. When myelography is enhanced with computed tomography (CT) scanning, the image is called a *CT myelogram.*

▶ *Diskography.* Diskography is the radiographic study of the intervertebral disk. A radiopaque dye is injected into the disk space between two vertebrae. A radiograph is then taken. This type of radiograph is called a *diskogram.* An abnormal dye pattern between the intervertebral disks indicates a rupture of the disk.

▶ *Angiography.* Angiography is the radiographic study of the vascular system. A water-soluble radiopaque dye is injected either intra-arterially (arteriogram) or intravenously (venogram). A rapid series of radiographs is then taken to follow the course of the contrast medium as it travels through the blood vessels. Angiography is used to help detect injury to or partial blockage of blood vessels.

Computed Tomography. Computed tomography (CT), also known as computerized axial tomography (CAT) and computerized transaxial tomography (CTI), uses a fanlike beam of X-rays to provide an almost three-dimensional, or tomographic, image. The CT scan provides good visualization of the shape, symmetry, and position of structures by delineating specific areas (Fig. 8-12). This information can be helpful in the examination of acute fractures, aneurysms, infections, hematomas, cysts, and tumors.

In the cervical spine, the accuracy of CT imaging ranges from 72 to 91 percent in the diagnosis of disk herniation, but approaches 96 percent when combining CT with myelography.[170,171] The addition of contrast allows for the visualization of the subarachnoid space and examination of the spinal cord and nerve roots.

Magnetic Resonance Imaging. Magnetic resonance imaging (MRI) has been a viable imaging technique since the early 1980s. These images are the result of the interaction of body tissues with electromagnetic forces. The advantages of MRI include its excellent tissue contrast, ability to provide cross-sectional images, noninvasive nature, and complete lack of ionizing radiation. MRI provides an excellent view of anatomic and physiologic tissues (Figs. 8-13 and 8-14). It commonly is used to assess the CNS and soft tissue injuries. However, MRI studies are expensive and offer poor visualization of cortical bone.

MRI has demonstrated excellent sensitivity in the diagnosis of lumbar disk herniation. It is considered the imaging study of choice for nerve root impingement, although this is tempered by the prevalence of abnormal findings in asymptomatic subjects.[172] It can, however, detect ligament and disk disruption, which cannot be demonstrated by other imaging studies.[173,174]

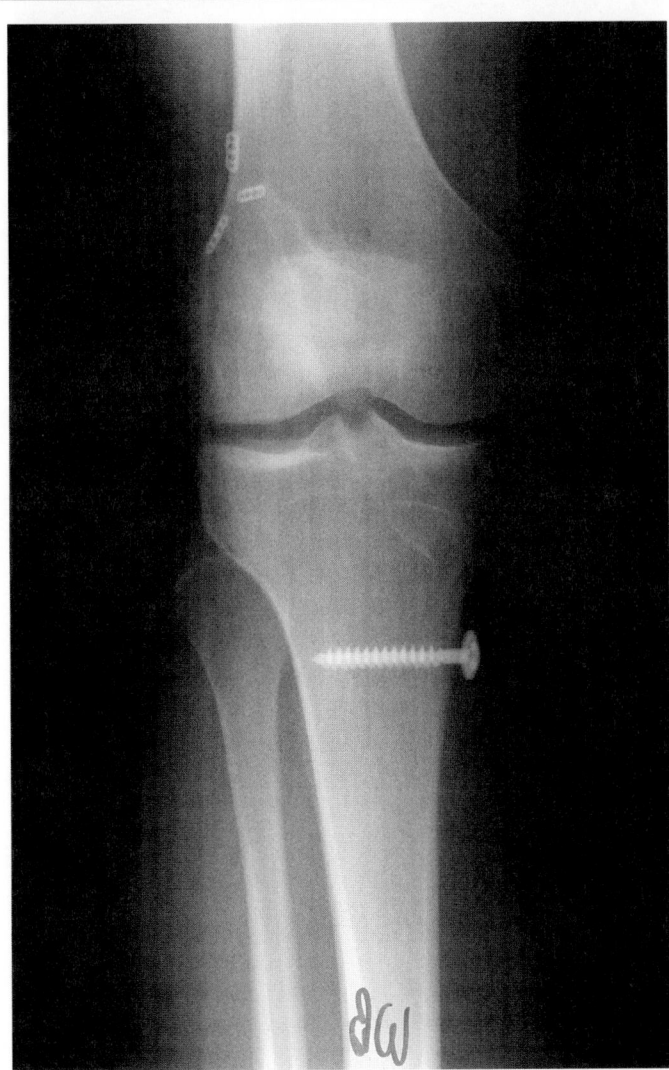

FIGURE 8-6 Radiograph of knee showing a history of three prior anterior cruciate ligament repairs.

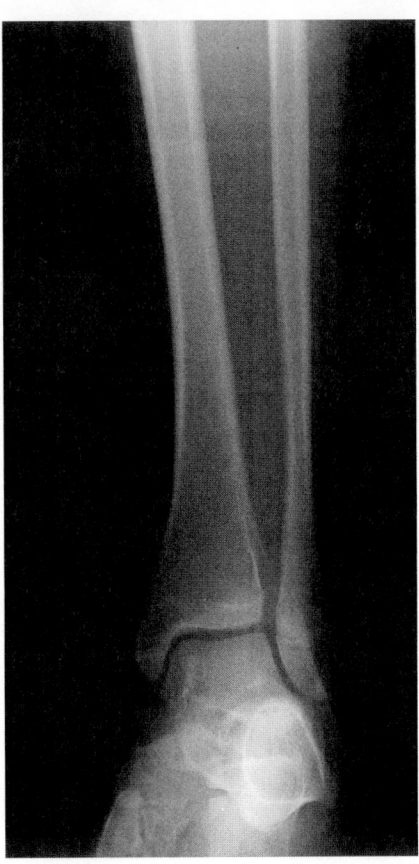

FIGURE 8-7 Radiograph showing grade I Salter-Harris fracture of fibula.

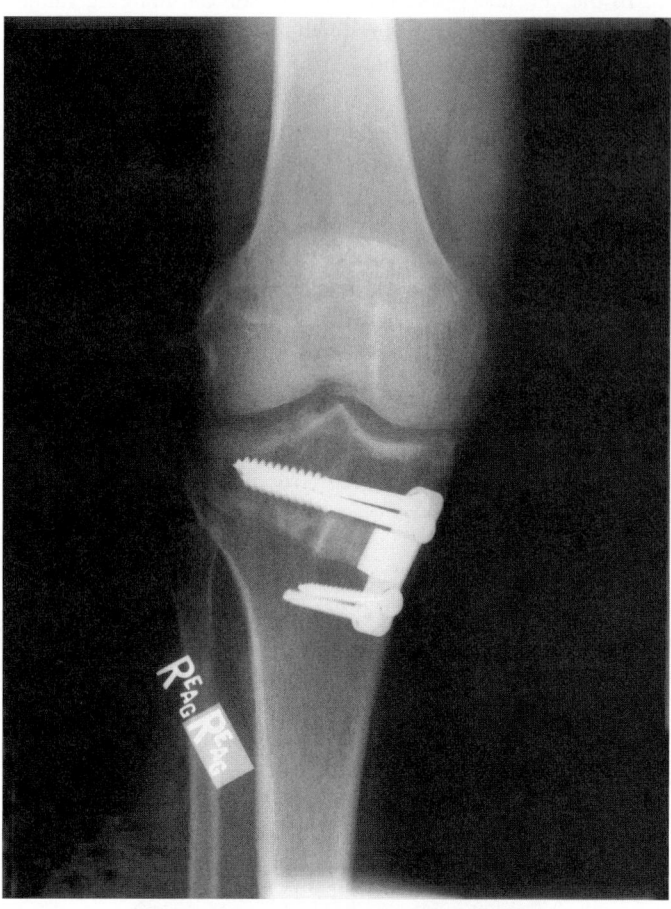

FIGURE 8-8   Radiograph of right knee following medial wedge osteotomy.

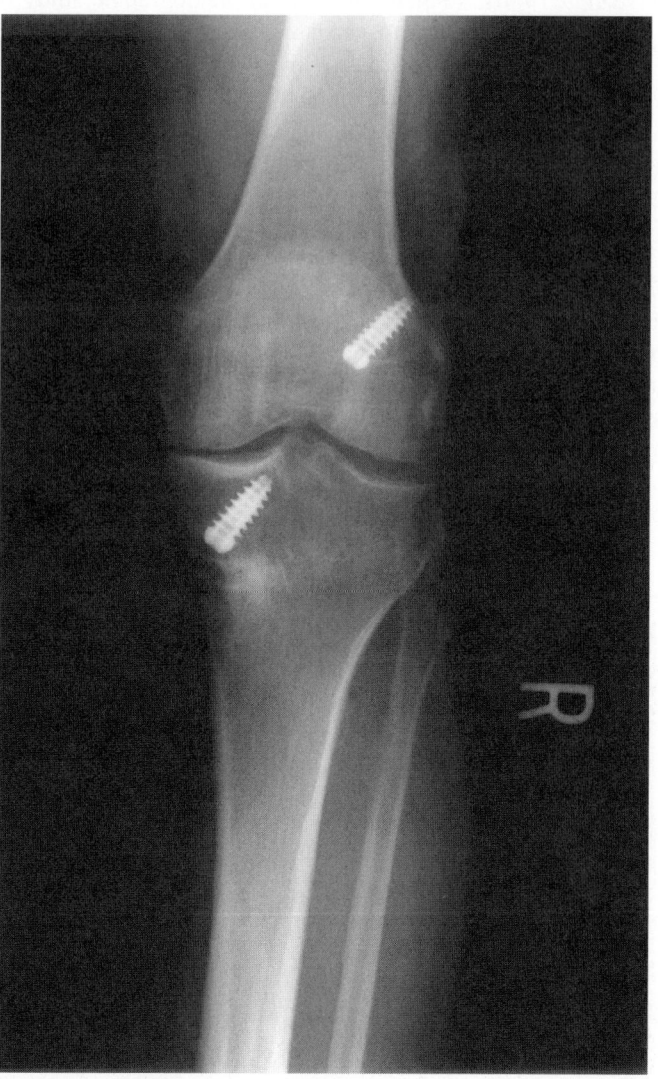

FIGURE 8-9   Radiograph following anterior cruciate ligament reconstruction (allogaft) of right knee.

Diagnostic Ultrasound.   Ultrasound is a modality based on the transmission of sound waves through tissue and the time it takes for the waves to be reflected back to the transducing probe. Ultrasound is readily available, noninvasive, and inexpensive. Different tissues transmit sound waves at different velocities and, therefore, create different images.

Although initially used primarily for abdominal imaging, ultrasound imaging is rapidly becoming appreciated for it musculoskeletal applications. Ultrasound imaging currently is used to help detect soft tissue injuries, tumors, bone infections, and arthropathy; and to evaluate bone mineral density. It also may be used to assess the degree and quality of fracture healing, and in the detection of synovitis and wood and plastic foreign bodies.

Radionucleotide Scanning.   Radionucleotide scanning studies involve the diagnostic use of radioactive material or isotopes. These materials are administered orally or intravenously. The most common radionuclide scanning test is the bone scan (Fig. 8-15). This test is used to detect particular areas of abnormal metabolic activity within a bone. The abnormality shows up as a so-called hot spot, which is darker in appear-

ance than normal tissue. An abnormality may indicate tumor, avascular necrosis, bone infection (osteomyelitis), Paget's disease, or recent fracture. Bone scans can detect sites of stress fracture in a bone before a conventional radiograph shows any abnormality, and often before they are symptomatic.

Fluoroscopy.   Fluoroscopic procedures involve the use of X-rays to demonstrate motions in joints or to guide injections. Because of the high exposure of radiation with this technique, it is used only rarely.

Evaluation

Following the history, systems review, and the tests and measures, an evaluation is made based on the information gathered.[175] According to Grieve,[72] an evaluation is the level of judgment necessary to make sense of the findings in order to identify a relationship between the symptoms reported and the signs of disturbed function. The evaluation is used to determine the diagnosis, prognosis, and plan of care. The diagnosis guides the intervention.

Prior to performing the examination, the clinician has some idea of the likelihood that the patient has the condition of interest, based on the history.[176] Once the examination is complete, the clinician should be able to add and subtract the various findings and determine the accuracy of the working hypothesis. One of the problems for the clinician is how to attach relevance to all of the information gleaned from the examination. This judgment process can be viewed as a continuum. At one end of the continuum is the novice who uses very clear-cut signposts, while at the other end there is the experienced clinician who has a vast bank of clinical experiences from which to draw.[177]

The clinician's knowledge base is, therefore, critical in the evaluation process.[178] Experienced clinicians appear to have a superior organization of knowledge, and they use a combination of hypothetico-deductive reasoning and pattern recognition to derive the correct diagnosis or working hypothesis.[178] The experienced clinician is able to recognize patterns and extrapolate information from them to develop an accurate working hypothesis.[179] According to Kahney,[180] the expert seems to do less problem-solving than the novice, because the former has already stored solutions to many of the clinical problems previously encountered.[177] However, this experience does not always bear fruit. Although the novice may jump to the wrong conclusion, the expert can fall into a similar trap of taking short cuts in the examination and making a diagnosis after just the history. In this scenario, the clinician only attends to data that supports his or her working hypothesis while ignoring (probably unconsciously) negating factors.[177]

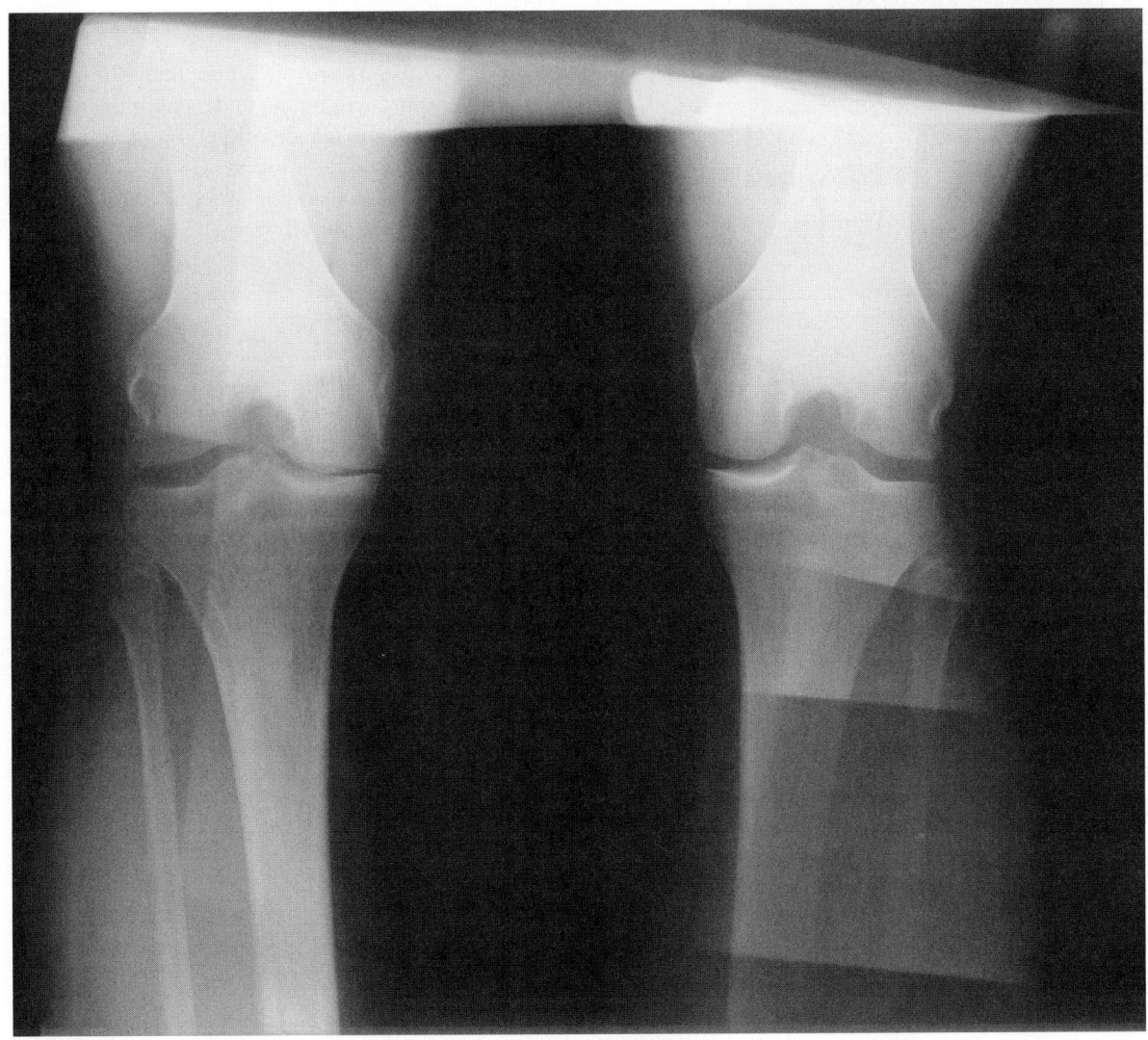

FIGURE 8-10   Radiograph showing end-stage medial compartment degeneration (varus malalignment) of right knee.

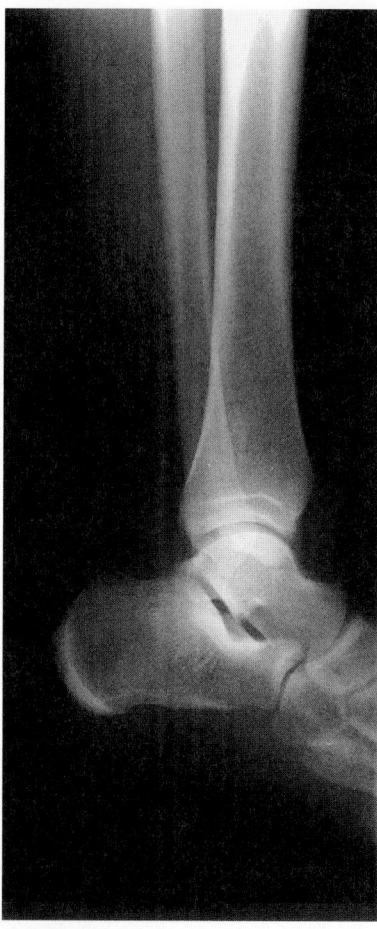

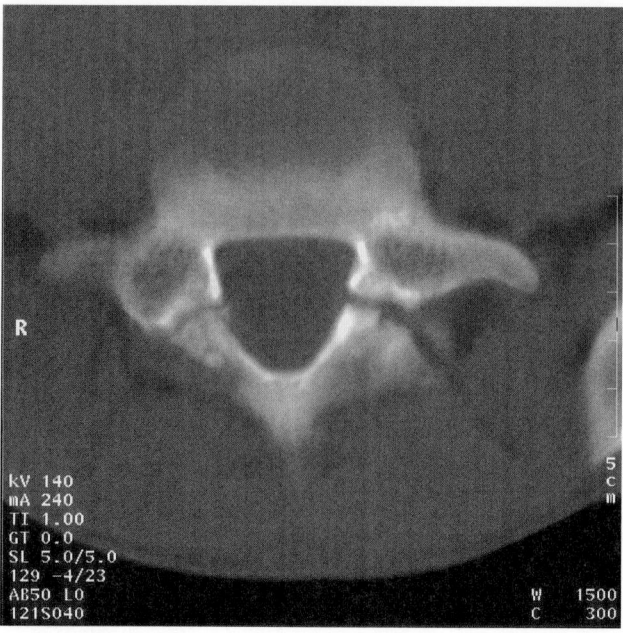

FIGURE 8-12   Computed tomographic image of lumbar spine showing bilateral spondylolysis at level of L5-S1.

Clinical Decision Making. When integrating evidence into clinical decision-making, an understanding of how to appraise the quality of the evidence offered by the clinical tests is important. One of the major problems in evaluating studies in the literature is that of deciding whether the results are definite enough to indicate an effect other than chance. Judging the

FIGURE 8-11   Radiograph showing right ankle avulsion fracture and deltoid sprain.

FIGURE 8-13   Magnetic resonance imaging (MRI) scan showing anterior cruciate ligament–deficient left knee.

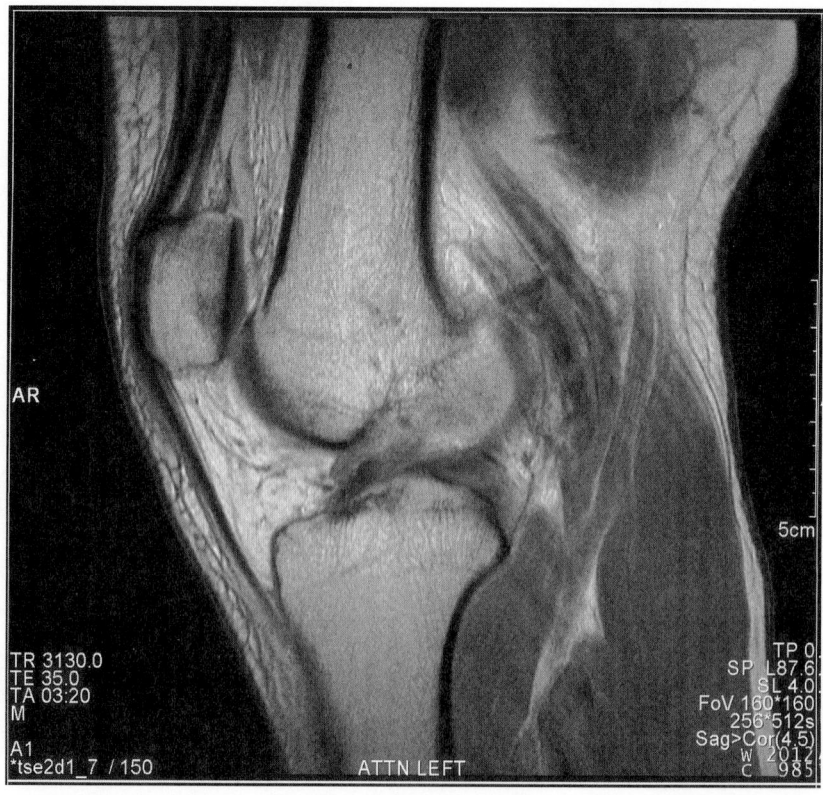

FIGURE 8-14 MRI showing the same knee as in Figure 8-13 from a different view.

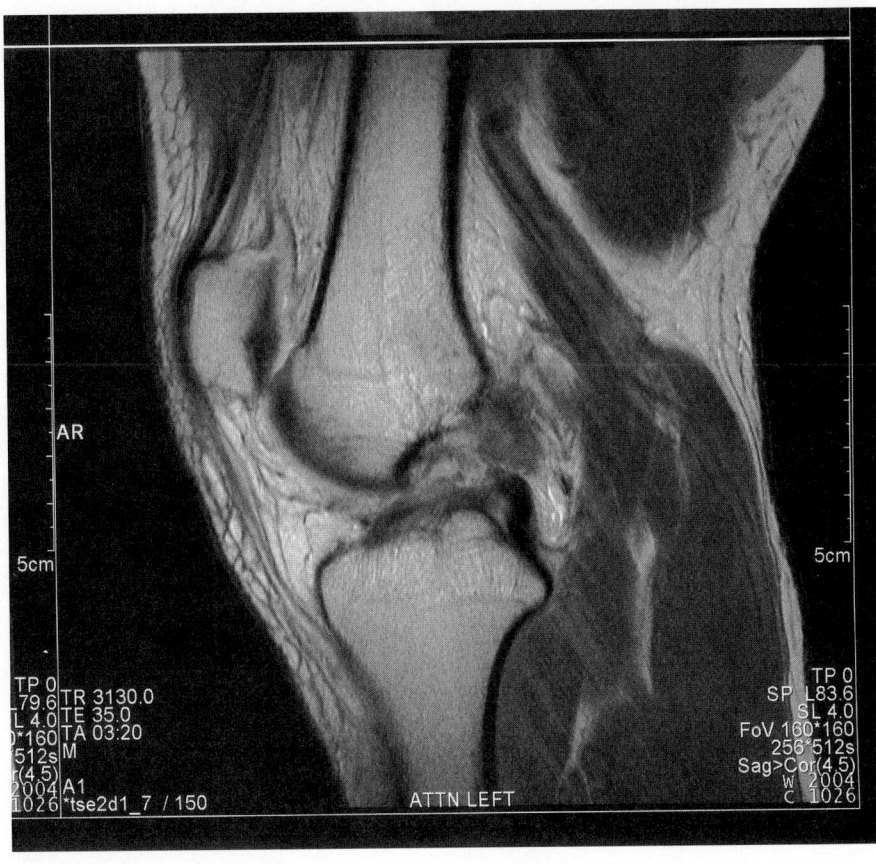

strength of the evidence becomes an important part of the decision-making process. The standard for the assessment of the efficacy and value of a test or intervention is the clinical trial; that is, a prospective study assessing the effect and value of a test or intervention against a control in human subjects.[181] Unfortunately, many of the experimental studies that deal with physical therapy topics are not clinical trials, because there is no control to judge the efficacy of the test or intervention and there are no tests or interventions from which to draw comparisons.[182] The ideal clinical trial includes a blinded, randomized design and a control group (Table 8-36). The control can be current standard practice, a placebo, or no active intervention.[181] Clinicians must constantly remind themselves that without information gathered from controlled clinical trials, they have limited scientific basis for their tests or interventions.[183]

Reliability, *validity*, and *significance* are essential to measurements and research procedure designs.

Reliability. Reliability is defined as the extent to which repeated measurements of a relatively stable phenomenon are close to each other.[184] Test-retest reliability is the consistency of repeated measurements that are separated in time when there is no change in what is being measured. Any difference between the two sets of scores represents measurement error, which can arise from a number of factors including intrarater variability, interrater reliability, or a lack of consistency of results. Reliability may be measured as repeatability between measurements performed by the same examiner (intrarater reliability), or between measurements by different examiners (interrater reliability).

Reliability is quantitatively expressed by way of an index of agreement, with the simplest index being the percentage agreement value. The percentage agreement value is defined as the ratio of the number of agreements to the total number of ratings made.[185] However, because this value does not correct for chance agreement, it can provide a misleadingly high estimate of reliability.[99,185–187]

The results of an examination are of limited value if they are not consistently repeatable.[99,188] The kappa statistic (κ) is a chance-corrected index of agreement that overcomes the problem of chance agreement when used with nominal and ordinal data[189] (Table 8-37). However, with higher scale data, it ends to underestimate reliability.[190] Theoretically, κ can be negative if agreement is worse than chance. Practically, in clinical reliability studies, κ usually varies between 0.00 and 1.00.[190] The κ statistic does not differentiate among disagreements; it assumes that all disagreements are of equal significance.[190]

The *Pearson product moment correlation coefficient* (*r*) quantitatively describes the strength and direction of the relationship between two variables. It is designed for use with

FIGURE 8-15   Bone scan showing stress fracture of right tibia.

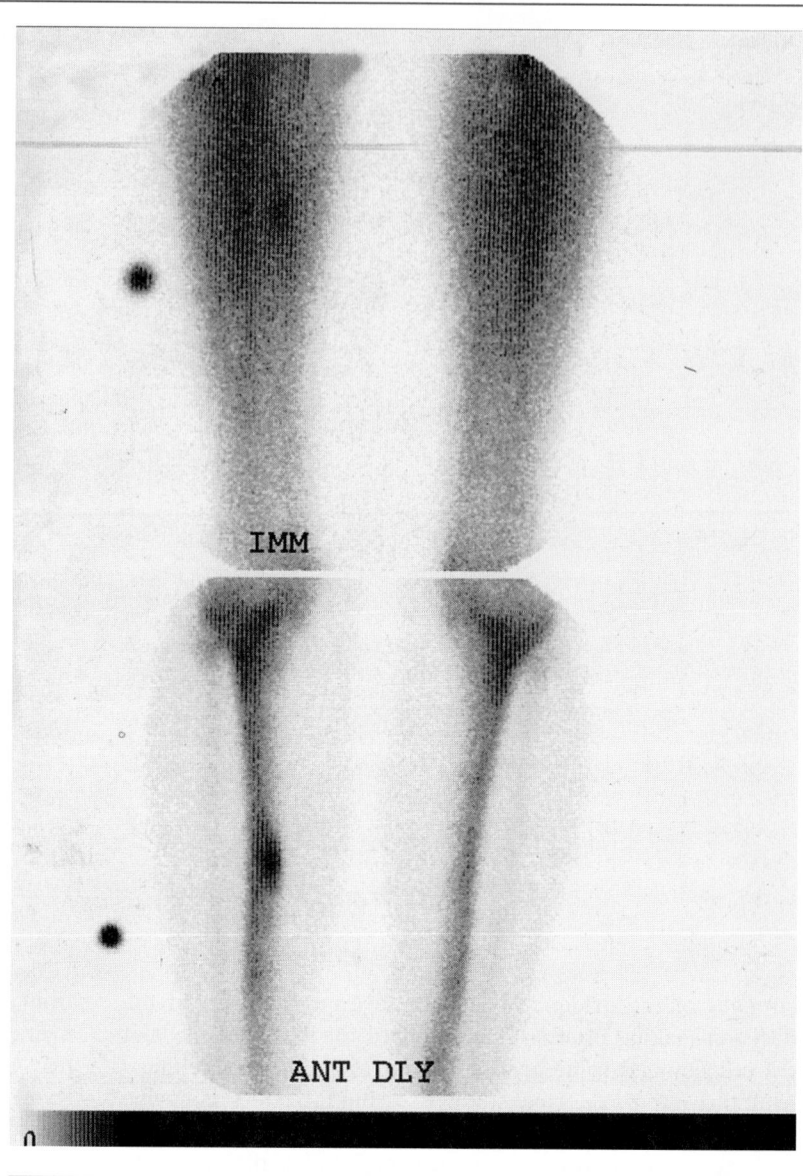

TABLE 8-36   Hierarchy of Evidence Grading

	Level of Evidence Grading = A	Level of Evidence Grading = B	Level of Evidence Grading = C	Level of Evidence Grading = D	Level of Evidence Grading = E
Type of Study	Randomized clinical trials	Cohort study	Nonrandomized trial with concurrent or historical controls Case study Study of sensitivity and specificity of a diagnostic test Population-based descriptive study	Cross-sectional study Case series Case report	Expert consensus Clinical experience

TABLE 8-37 Kappa (κ) Benchmark Values[190]

Value (%)	Description
< 40	Poor to fair agreement
40–60	Moderate agreement
60–80	Substantial agreement
> 80	Excellent agreement
100	Perfect agreement

continuous data with underlying normal distributions on an interval or ratio scale[191] (Table 8-38). Correlation coefficients are limited in their use as indices of agreement, because they are designed to assess only two ratings, or two raters,[190] and are measures of covariance rather than reflecting agreement.[191]

The *intraclass correlation coefficient* (ICC) is a reliability coefficient calculated with variance estimates obtained through an *analysis of variance* (ANOVA)[191] (Table 8-39). The advantage of the ICC over correlation coefficients is that it does not require the same number of raters per subject, and it can be used for two or more raters or ratings.[191]

Validity.   Test validity is defined as the degree to which a test measures what it purports to be measuring, and how well it correctly classifies individuals with or without a particular disease.[99,188,192] Validity is directly related to the notion of sensitivity and specificity.

▶ Sensitivity represents the proportion of a population with the target disorder that has a positive result with the diagnostic test. A test that can correctly identify every person who has the target disorder has a sensitivity of 1.0. *SnNout* is an acronym for when *Sen*sitivity of a symptom or sign is high, a *N*egative response rules *out* the target disorder. Thus, a so-called highly sensitive test helps rule out a disorder.

▶ Specificity is the proportion of the study population without the target disorder, in whom the test result is negative[193] (Table 8-40). A test that can correctly identify every person who does not have the target disorder has a specificity of 1.0. *SpPin* is an acronym for when *Sp*ecificity is extremely high, a *P*ositive test result rules *in* the target disorder. Thus, a so-called highly specific test helps rule in a disorder or condition.

TABLE 8-38 Pearson Coefficient (*r*) Benchmark Values for Health Sciences[190]

Value	Description
0.00–0.25	Little or no relationship
0.25–0.50	Fair relationship
0.50–0.75	Moderate to good relationship
> 0.75	Good to excellent relationship

TABLE 8-39 Intraclass Correlation Coefficient Benchmark Values[190]

Value	Description
< 0.75	Poor to moderate agreement
> 0.75	Good agreement
> 90	Reasonable agreement for clinical measurements

A test with a very high sensitivity, but low specificity, and vice versa, is of little value, and the acceptable levels are generally set at between 50 percent (unacceptable test) and 100 percent (perfect test), with an arbitrary cut off at about 80 percent.[193]

There are several types of validity, including construct validity, face validity, content validity, external validity, concurrent validity, and criterion-referenced validity.

▶ *Construct validity.*   Construct validity refers to the ability of a test to represent the underlying construct (the theory developed to organize and explain some aspects of existing knowledge and observations). Construct validity refers to overall validity.

▶ *Face validity.*   Face validity refers to the degree to which the questions or procedures incorporated within a test make sense to the users. The assessment of face validity is generally informal and nonquantitative.

▶ *Content validity.*   Content validity refers to the assessment by experts that the content of the measure is consistent with what is to be measured. Content validity is concerned with sample-population representativeness, i.e., the knowledge and skills covered by the test items should be representative of the larger domain of knowledge and skills. In many instances, it is difficult, if not impossible, to administer a test covering all aspects of knowledge or skills. Therefore, only several tasks are sampled from the population of knowledge

TABLE 8-40 Concept Definitions of Sensitivity, Specificity, and Predictive Values

Concept	Definition
Sensitivity	Proportion of patients with a disease who test positive
Specificity	Proportion of patients without the disease who test negative
Positive predictive value	Proportion of patients who actually have the disease who test positive
Negative predictive value	Proportion of patients who do not actually have the disease and who test negative

or skills. In these circumstances, the proportion of the score attributable to a particular component ability should be proportional to the importance of that component to total performance. In content validity, evidence is obtained by looking for agreement in judgments by judges. In short, face validity can be determined by one person, but content validity should be confirmed by a panel.

▶ *External validity.* External validity deals with the degree to which study results can be generalized to different subjects, settings, and times.[194,194a]

▶ *Criterion-referenced validity.* Criterion-referenced validity is determined by comparing the results of a test to those of a test that is accepted as a "gold standard" test (a test that is nearly 100% valid).[194b] There are three types of criterion-referenced validity: concurrent, predictive, and discriminant.

▶ *Concurrent validity.* Concurrent validity is determined by correlating a test with another test done at the same time.[194b]

▶ *Predictive validity.* Predictive validity is the extent to which test scores are associated with future behavior or performance.

▶ *Discriminant validity.* Discriminant validity is the ability of a test to distinguish between two different constructs and is evidenced by a low correlation between the results of the test and those of tests of a different construct.

Diagnostic tests are used for the purpose of discovery, confirmation, and exclusion.[195] Tests for discovery and exclusion must have high sensitivity for detection, whereas confirmation tests require high specificity[196] (see Table 8-40). The sensitivity and specificity of any physical test to discriminate relevant dysfunction must be appreciated to make meaningful decisions.[197]

Other points used in testing include the prediction value, confidence interval, and likelihood ratio:

▶ *Prediction value.* The prediction value of a positive test indicates that those members of the study population who have a positive test outcome will have the condition under investigation.[193] The diagnostic power of the negative test outcome relates to those of the study population with a negative test outcome who do not suffer from the condition under investigation.[193]

▶ *Confidence interval.* The 95 percent confidence interval expresses the limits within which the actual association of 95 percent acceptance is positioned.[74,193]

▶ *Likelihood ratio.* The likelihood ratio is the index measurement that combines sensitivity and specificity values and indicates how much a given diagnostic test result will lower or raise the pretest probability of the target disorder.[74,193]

Significance. The symbol p is used in statistics to describe the probability of something happening. A study generally will give a value of p for any conclusions they draw. The p values, or significance levels, measure the strength of the evidence against the null hypothesis. The null hypothesis is defined as the hypothesis that is statistically tested. In most scenarios, the researcher is trying to disprove the null hypothesis. For example, in an experiment designed to test the ability of stretching technique A versus stretching technique B to improve hamstring length, the null hypothesis would be that there is no difference in benefit between technique A and technique B. The researcher would hope to show that one technique is better than the other.

Accepting or rejecting the null hypothesis does not prove that the null hypothesis is true or false. The p value is a measure of the strength of the null hypothesis. The smaller the p value, the stronger is the evidence against the null hypothesis. In general, an effect that shows up in a study is regarded as being significant (i.e., not just random) if the probability of it happening by chance is less than .05 (1 chance in 20). For instance, if the conclusion of a study finds that the intervention is better than the control with $p < .00001$, that is a very strong conclusion indeed. A conclusion that involves $p < .25$, however, would be regarded by most people as too weak to rely on.

Physical Therapy Diagnosis. Patients may be referred to physical therapy with a nonspecific diagnosis, an incorrect diagnosis, or no diagnosis at all.[198] Physical therapists are responsible for thoroughly examining each patient and then either treating the patient according to established guidelines or referring the patient elsewhere.[199]

Making a physical therapy diagnosis involves a combination of hypothesis testing and pattern recognition.[175] The best indicator for the correctness of a diagnosis is the quality of the hypothesis considered, because if the appropriate diagnosis is not considered from the start, any subsequent inquiries will be misdirected.[178]

A diagnosis can only be made when all potential causes for the signs and symptoms have been ruled out. The clinician should resist the urge to categorize a condition based on a small number of findings. In such cases, knowledge of differential diagnosis is essential, so that the clinician can systematically rule out all of the potential causes for the pain (see Chap. 9).

The physical therapy diagnosis is a label ascribed to a cluster of signs and symptoms. With the implementation of the "Guide," the focus of the examination process has changed to one in which an accurate diagnosis is made within appropriate practice patterns[13] (see Table I-1, in the introduction to this section). Most of the time, these patterns do not occur in isolation. Patients often present with a mixture of signs and symptoms that indicate one or more possible problem areas. For example, patterns such as impaired posture (practice pattern B), impaired muscle performance (practice pattern C), and impairment due to localized inflammation (practice pattern E), can occur concurrently with each other.

The diagnostic process is essentially an exercise in probability revision.[176,200] Musculoskeletal impairments that have a traumatic origin and specific mechanism are often relatively easy to diagnose from the history. Impairments with an insidious onset, however, are more puzzling and, at the same time often more interesting. Once these impairments have been highlighted, a determination can be made as to the reason for those impairments, and the relationship between the impairments and the patient's functional limitations or disabilities.

The McKenzie System.   The McKenzie system[72,201] has been reported as the most commonly used classification system by physical therapists for diagnostic purposes.[202] This system uses pain behavior, and its relationship to movements and positions, to determine the appropriate plan of intervention, and allows the classification of patients into broad rather than tissue-specific categories[203] (Fig. 8-16). Each syndrome in the McKenzie classification is broad in terms of pathology, but is specific in terms of clinical behavior, and can lead to the formulation of an intervention strategy.[204,205]

The McKenzie approach uses pain behavior, and its relationship to movements and positions, to categorize the patient into three broad rather than tissue-specific categories for the vast majority of mechanical disorders of the musculoskeletal system:

1. Posture syndrome.

2. Dysfunction syndrome.

3. Derangement syndrome.

The McKenzie system is based on the information gained from the history and examination, which determine the stage of the disorder, and the patient's response to mechanical loading.[28]

▶ *Postural syndrome.*   Pain from the postural syndrome is caused by mechanical deformation or vascular deprivation of the normal soft tissues, which results from prolonged positioning or sustained postures. The syndrome is characterized by intermittent pain provoked by prolonged static loading of normal tissues. Patients who experience pain arising from end-range stress of normal tissue require postural correction and interruption of end-range stress at frequent intervals.[206]

▶ *Dysfunction syndrome.*   The pain from a dysfunction syndrome results from the mechanical deformation of abnormal tissues, such as contracted or fibrosed, adaptively shortened, or adherent tissues. This deformation can result from previous trauma, inflammation, or degeneration, which causes scarring, or adaptive shortening. Dysfunction syndrome is characterized by intermittent pain and a restriction of end-range motion. Patients with this syndrome require exercises at end range to remodel the affected structures.[206]

▶ *Derangement syndrome.*   The pain from the derangement syndrome is caused by an internal disruption and displacement of a tissue. This syndrome often is characterized by constant pain, although certain positions may alleviate the symptoms for as long as the position is maintained (see Fig. 8-16). Patients with this syndrome can be taught to perform movements to reduce the internal derangements and

maintain stability.[206] If these self-applied exercises fail to reduce the derangement, skilled intervention is required.[206]

The McKenzie system is described further in the introduction to Part IV.

Prognosis.   The prognosis is the predicted level of function that the patient will attain within a certain time frame. This prediction helps guide the intensity, duration, and frequency of the intervention, and aids in justifying the intervention. Knowledge of the severity of an injury, the age and physical status of a patient, and the healing processes of the various tissues involved, are among the factors used in determining the prognosis.

The intervention cannot speed up the healing process, but it can prevent further injury or a delay in the process.[207] As the clinician cannot be with the patient at all times, patient education and patient responsibility become extremely important in determining the prognosis.

Principle 2: Examine, Progress, and Reexamine

The selection of intervention procedures, and the intervention progression, must be guided by continuous reexamination of the patient's response to a given procedure, making the reexamination of patient dysfunction before, during, and after each intervention essential.[208]

At each visit, the clinician must reexamine the patient's status. To evaluate progress, comparisons are made between the findings from the initial examination. There are three possible scenarios following a reexamination:

1. ***The patient's function has improved.***   In this scenario, the intensity of the intervention may be incrementally increased.

2. ***The patient's function has diminished.***   In this scenario, the intensity and the focus of the intervention must be changed. Further review of the home exercise program may be needed. The patient may require further education on activity modification and the use of heat and ice at home. The working hypothesis must be reviewed. Further investigation is needed.

3. ***There is no change in the patient's function.***   Depending on the time that has elapsed since the last visit, there may be a reason for the lack of change. This finding may indicate the need for a change in the intensity of the intervention. If the patient is in the acute or subacute stage of healing (see Chap. 5), a decrease in the intensity may be warranted to allow the tissues more of an opportunity to heal. In the chronic stage, an increase in intensity may be warranted (refer to principle 2 of Chapter 10).

The developing health care system of the last decade has dramatically limited patients' access to rehabilitation services, and has increased the accountability of the health care provider.[209] This development has placed a burden on the physical therapy profession to make the necessary changes to deal effectively with health care reform, so that physical therapists

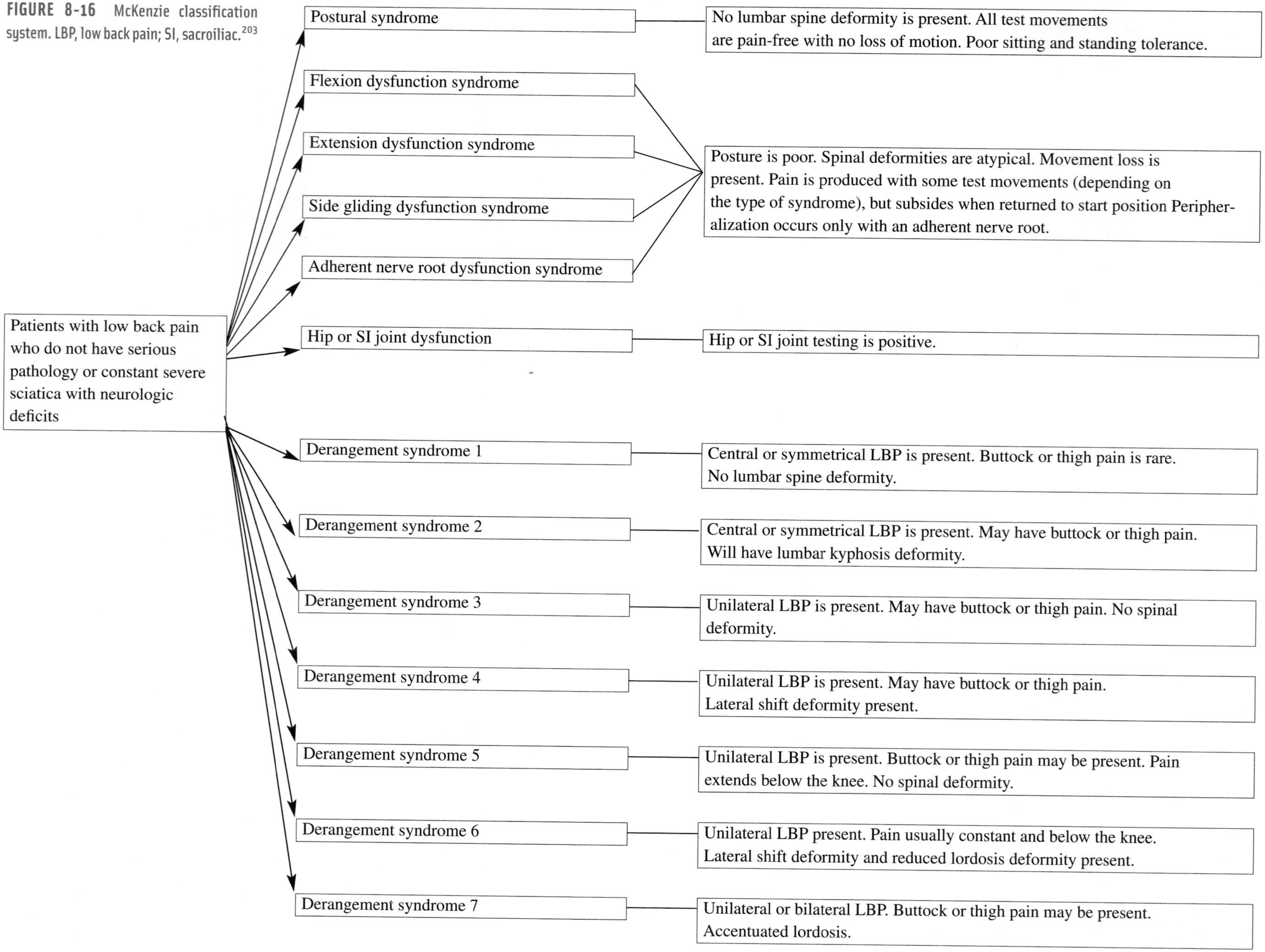

FIGURE 8-16 McKenzie classification system. LBP, low back pain; SI, sacroiliac.[203]

Patients with low back pain who do not have serious pathology or constant severe sciatica with neurologic deficits

Postural syndrome — No lumbar spine deformity is present. All test movements are pain-free with no loss of motion. Poor sitting and standing tolerance.

Flexion dysfunction syndrome
Extension dysfunction syndrome
Side gliding dysfunction syndrome
Adherent nerve root dysfunction syndrome — Posture is poor. Spinal deformities are atypical. Movement loss is present. Pain is produced with some test movements (depending on the type of syndrome), but subsides when returned to start position Peripheralization occurs only with an adherent nerve root.

Hip or SI joint dysfunction — Hip or SI joint testing is positive.

Derangement syndrome 1 — Central or symmetrical LBP is present. Buttock or thigh pain is rare. No lumbar spine deformity.

Derangement syndrome 2 — Central or symmetrical LBP is present. May have buttock or thigh pain. Will have lumbar kyphosis deformity.

Derangement syndrome 3 — Unilateral LBP is present. May have buttock or thigh pain. No spinal deformity.

Derangement syndrome 4 — Unilateral LBP is present. May have buttock or thigh pain. Lateral shift deformity present.

Derangement syndrome 5 — Unilateral LBP is present. Buttock or thigh pain may be present. Pain extends below the knee. No spinal deformity.

Derangement syndrome 6 — Unilateral LBP present. Pain usually constant and below the knee. Lateral shift deformity and reduced lordosis deformity present.

Derangement syndrome 7 — Unilateral or bilateral LBP. Buttock or thigh pain may be present. Accentuated lordosis.

become more accountable for their professional performance and more cost-effective in their provision of patient care.[209] It is important that examination and intervention techniques continue to be verified through peer-reviewed research, patient outcome databases, and an increased efficiency and effectiveness.[210,211]

REVIEW QUESTIONS*

1. Give a definition of empathy.
2. Differentiate between the terms examination and evaluation.
3. What are the three components of the examination?
4. Give three medical conditions that are capable of producing an unexplained weight gain.
5. What is cauda equina syndrome?

* Additional questions to test your understanding of this chapter can be found in the Online Learning Center for *Orthopaedic Assessment, Evaluation, and Intervention* at www.duttononline.net.

REFERENCES

1. Kibler WB. Shoulder rehabilitation: Principles and practice. *Med Sci Sports Exerc* 1998;30(suppl 1):40–50.
2. Nirschl RP, Sobel J. Arm care. In: Nirschl RP, Sobel J, eds. *A Complete Guide to Prevention and Treatment of Tennis Elbow.* Arlington, Virginia: Medical Sports; 1996.
3. Meadows J. *Orthopedic Differential Diagnosis in Physical Therapy.* New York, NY: McGraw-Hill; 1999.
4. Kaltenborn FM. *Manual Mobilization of the Extremity Joints: Basic Examination and Treatment Techniques.* 4th ed. Oslo, Norway: Olaf Norlis Bokhandel, Universitetsgaten; 1989.
5. Maitland G. *Vertebral Manipulation.* Sydney, Australia: Butterworth; 1986.
6. Maitland G. *Peripheral Manipulation.* 3rd ed. London, England: Butterworth; 1991.
7. Evjenth O, Hamberg J. *Muscle Stretching in Manual Therapy, A Clinical Manual.* Alfta, Sweden: Alfta Rehab Forlag; 1984.
8. Lee DG. Biomechanics of the thorax. In: Grant R, ed. *Physical Therapy of the Cervical and Thoracic Spine.* New York, NY: Churchill Livingstone; 1988:47–76.
9. Lee DG. *The Pelvic Girdle: An Approach to the Examination and Treatment of the Lumbo-Pelvic-Hip Region.* 2nd ed. Edinburgh, Scotland: Churchill Livingstone; 1999.
10. Sahrmann SA. *Diagnosis and Treatment of Movement Impairment Syndromes.* St Louis, Mo: Mosby; 2001.
11. Butler DS. *Mobilization of the Nervous System.* New York, NY: Churchill Livingstone; 1992.
12. Judge RD, Zuidema GD, Fitzgerald FT. Introduction. In: Judge RD, Zuidema GD, Fitzgerald FT, eds. *Clinical Diagnosis.* Boston, Mass: Little, Brown; 1982:3–8.
13. Guide to physical therapist practice. *Phys Ther* 2001;18:513–595.
14. Delitto A. Subjective measures and clinical decision making. *Phys Ther* 1989;69:580.
15. Judge RD, Zuidema GD, Fitzgerald FT. General appearance. In: Judge RD, Zuidema GD, Fitzgerald FT, eds. *Clinical Diagnosis.* Boston, Mass: Little, Brown; 1982:29–47.
16. Vasilyeva LF, Lewit K. Diagnosis of muscular dysfunction by inspection. In: Liebenson C, ed. *Rehabilitation of the Spine: A Practitioner's Manual.* Baltimore, Md: Lippincott Williams and Wilkins; 1996:113–142.
17. Goodman CC, Snyder TK. Introduction to the interviewing process. In: Goodman CC, Snyder TK, eds. *Differential Diagnosis in Physical Therapy.* Philadelphia, Pa: Saunders; 1990:7–42.
18. Clarnette RG, Miniaci A. Clinical exam of the shoulder. *Med Sci Sports Exerc* 1998;30(suppl):1–6.
19. Boissonnault WG. *Examination in Physical Therapy Practice: Screening for Medical Disease.* New York, NY: Churchill Livingstone; 1991.
20. Meadows J. *A Rationale and Complete Approach to the Sub-Acute Post-MVA Cervical Patient.* Calgary, Canada: Swodeam Consulting; 1995.
21. Steinberg MH. Management of sickle cell disease. *N Engl J Med* 1999;340:1021–1030.
22. Haslock I. Ankylosing spondylitis. *Baillieres Clin Rheumatol* 1993;7:99.
23. Potosky AL, Feuer EJ, Levin DL. Impact of screening on incidence and mortality of prostate cancer in the United States. *Epidemiol Rev* 2001;23:181–186.
24. Wingo PA, Tong T, Bolden S. Cancer statistics, 1995. *CA Cancer J Clin* 1995;45:8.
25. Parkin DM, Muir CS. Cancer incidence in five continents. Comparability and quality of data. *IARC Sci Pub* 1992;66:45.
26. Ries LAG, Elsner MP, Kosary CL. *SEER Cancer Statistics Review, 1973–1997.* Bethesda, Md: National Cancer Institute; 2000.
27. Martinez JC, Otley CC. The management of melanoma and nonmelanoma skin cancer: A review for the primary care physician. *Mayo Clin Proc* 2001;76:1253–1265.
28. McKenzie R, May S. Mechanical diagnosis. In: McKenzie R, May S, eds. *The Human Extremities: Mechanical Diagnosis and Therapy.* Waikanae, New Zealand: Spinal Publications New Zealand Ltd, 2000:79–88.
29. Judge RD, Zuidema GD, Fitzgerald FT. The medical history and physical. In: Judge RD, Zuidema GD, Fitzgerald FT, eds. *Clinical Diagnosis.* Boston, Mass: Little, Brown; 1982:9–19.
30. Stetts DM. Patient examination. In: Wadsworth C, ed. *Current Concepts of Orthopaedic Physical Therapy—Home Study Course 11.2.2.* LaCrosse, Wis: Orthopaedic Section, American Physical Therapy Association; 2001.
31. Goodman CC, Snyder TEK. *Differential Diagnosis in Physical Therapy.* Philadelphia, Pa: Saunders; 1990.
32. Kostuik JP, Harrington J, Alexander D, Rand W, Evans D. Cauda equina syndrome and lumbar disc herniation. *J Bone Joint Surg* 1986;68A:386–391.
33. O'Laoire SA, Crockard HA, Thomas DG. Prognosis for sphincter recovery after operation for cauda equina compression owing to lumbar disc prolapse. *BMJ* 1981;282:1852–1854.
34. Bogduk N. The anatomy and physiology of nociception. In: Crosbie J, McConnell J, eds. *Key Issues in Physiotherapy.* Oxford, England: Butterworth-Heinemann; 1993:48–87.
35. McKenzie R, May S. History. In: McKenzie R, May S, eds. *The Human Extremities: Mechanical Diagnosis and Therapy.* Waikanae, New Zealand: Spinal Publications New Zealand Ltd; 2000:89–103.
36. Huskisson EC. Measurement of pain. *Lancet* 1974;2:127.
37. Halle JS. Neuromusculoskeletal scan examination with selected related topics. In: Flynn TW, ed. *The Thoracic Spine and Rib*

Cage: Musculoskeletal Evaluation and Treatment. Boston, Mass: Butterworth-Heinemann; 1996:121–146.

38. Wiener SL. *Differential Diagnosis of Acute Pain by Body Region.* New York, NY: McGraw-Hill; 1993:1–4.

39. Adams RD, Victor M. *Principles of Neurology.* 5th ed. New York, NY: McGraw-Hill; 1993.

40. Chusid JG. *Correlative Neuroanatomy & Functional Neurology.* Norwalk, Conn: Appleton-Century-Crofts; 1985:144–148.

41. Judge RD, Zuidema GD, Fitzgerald FT. Musculoskeletal system. In: Judge RD, Zuidema GD, Fitzgerald FT, eds. *Clinical Diagnosis.* Boston, Mass: Little, Brown; 1982:365–403.

42. Bonica JJ. Neurophysiological and pathological aspects of acute and chronic pain. *Arch Surg* 1977;112:750–761.

43. Burkhardt CS. The use of the McGill Pain Questionnaire in assessing arthritis pain. *Pain* 1984;19:305.

44. Chaturvedi SK. Prevalence of chronic pain in psychiatric patients. *Pain* 1987;29:231–237.

45. Dunn D. Chronic regional pain syndrome, type 1: Part I. *AORN J* 2000;72:421–458.

46. Konietzny F, Perl ER, Trevino D, Light A, Hensel H. Sensory experiences in man evoked by intraneural electrical stimulation of intact cutaneous afferent fibers. *Exp Brain Res* 1981;42:219–222.

47. Ochoa J, Torebjörk E. Sensations evoked by intraneural microstimulation of C nociceptor fibres in human skin nerves. *J Physiol* 1989;415:583–599.

48. Torebjörk HE, Ochoa JL, Schady W. Referred pain from intraneural stimulation of muscle fascicles in the median nerve. *Pain* 1984;18:145–156.

49. Ness TJ, Gebhart GF. Visceral pain: A review of experimental studies. *Pain* 1990;41:167–234.

50. Rowland LP. Diseases of the motor unit. In: Kandel ER, Schwartz JH, Jessell TM, eds. *Principles of Neural Science.* New York, NY: McGraw-Hill; 2000:695–712.

51. Goldstein R. Psychological evaluation of low back pain. *Spine* 1986;1:103.

52. Norris TR. History and physical examination of the shoulder. In: Nicholas JA, Hershman EB, Posner MA, eds. *The Upper Extremity in Sports Medicine.* St. Louis, Mo: Mosby Year-Book; 1995:39–83.

53. Melzack R. The McGill Pain Questionnaire: Major properties and scoring methods. *Pain* 1975;1:277.

54. Melzack R, Torgerson WS. On the language of pain. *Anaesthesiology* 1971;34:50.

55. Liebenson C. Pain and disability questionnaires in chiropractic rehabilitation. In: Liebenson C, ed. *Rehabilitation of the Spine: A Practitioner's Manual.* Baltimore, Md: Lippincott Williams and Wilkins; 1996:57–71.

56. Pearce J, Morley S. An experimental investigation of the construct validity of the McGill Pain Questionnaire. *Pain* 1989;115:115.

57. D'Ambrosia R. *Musculoskeletal Disorders: Regional Examination and Differential Diagnosis.* 2nd ed. Philadelphia, Pa: Lippincott; 1986.

58. Magarey ME. Examination of the cervical and thoracic spine. In: Grant R, ed. *Physical Therapy of the Cervical and Thoracic Spine.* New York, NY: Churchill Livingstone; 1994:109–144.

59. Hertling D, Kessler RM. *Management of Common Musculoskeletal Disorders: Physical Therapy Principles and Methods.* 3rd ed. Philadelphia, Pa: Lippincott Williams and Wilkins; 1996.

59a. Judge RD, Zuidema GD, Fitzgerald FT. Vital signs. In: Judge RD, Zuidema GD, Fitzgerald FT, eds. *Clinical Diagnosis.* Boston, Mass: Little, Brown; 1982:49–58.

59b. American Physical Therapy Association. Guide to physical therapist practice, *Phys Ther,* 2001;81:S13–S95.

60. Cyriax J. *Textbook of Orthopaedic Medicine, Diagnosis of Soft Tissue Lesions.* 8th ed. London, England: Bailliere Tindall; 1982.

61. Hayes KW. An examination of Cyriax's passive motion tests with patients having osteoarthritis of the knee. *Phys Ther* 1994;74:697.

62. Franklin ME. Assessment of exercise induced minor lesions: The accuracy of Cyriax's diagnosis by selective tissue tension paradigm. *J Orthop Sports Phys Ther* 1996;24:122.

63. Grieve GP. The masqueraders. In: Boyling JD, Palastanga N, eds. *Grieve's Modern Manual Therapy.* Edinburgh, Scotland: Churchill Livingstone; 1994:841–856.

64. Meadows JTS. *Manual Therapy: Biomechanical Assessment and Treatment, Advanced Technique.* Lecture and video supplemental manual. Calgary, Canada: Swodeam Consulting; 1995.

65. Isaacs E, Bookout M. Screening for pathological origins of head and facial pain. In: Boissonnault WG, ed. *Examination in Physical Therapy Practice: Screening for Medical Disease.* Philadelphia, Pa: Saunders;1995:175–189.

66. Judge RD, Zuidema GD, Fitzgerald FT. Vital signs. In: Judge RD, Zuidema GD, Fitzgerald FT, eds. *Clinical Diagnosis.* Boston, Mass: Little, Brown; 1982:49–58.

67. Cyriax J. *Examination of the Shoulder. Limited Range Diagnosis of Soft Tissue Lesions.* 8th ed. Vol 1. London, England: Balliere Tindall; 1982:127–142.

68. Cyriax JH, Cyriax PJ. *Illustrated Manual of Orthopaedic Medicine.* London, England: Butterworth; 1983.

69. Cyriax J. Diagnosis of soft tissue lesions. In: *Textbook of Orthopaedic Medicine.* Baltimore, Md: Williams and Wilkins; 1980:682.

70. Maitland GD. The hypothesis of adding compression when examining and treating synovial joints. *J Orthop Sports Phys Ther* 1980;2:7.

71. Grieve GP. *Common Vertebral Joint Problems.* New York, NY: Churchill Livingstone; 1981.

72. McKenzie RA. *The Lumbar Spine: Mechanical Diagnosis and Therapy.* Waikanae, New Zealand: Spinal Publications New Zealand Ltd; 1981.

73. McKenzie R, May S. Introduction. In: McKenzie R, May S, eds. *The Human Extremities: Mechanical Diagnosis and Therapy.* Waikanae, New Zealand: Spinal Publications New Zealand Ltd; 2000:1–5.

74. Jaeschke R, Guyatt G, Sackett DL. Users guides to the medical literature. III. How to use an article about a diagnostic test. B. What are the results and will they help me in caring for my patients? *JAMA* 1994;27:703–707.

75. Cibulka MT, Aslin K. How to use evidence-based practice to distinguish between three different patients with low back pain. *J Orthop Sports Phys Ther* 2001;31:678–695.

75a. Jones M. Clinical reasoning and pain. *Man Ther* 1995; 1:118–127.

75b. Jones MA. Clinical reasoning in manual therapy. *Phys Ther;* 1992;72:875–884.

75c. Higgs J, Jones M. *Clinical Reasoning in the Health Professions,* 2nd ed. London: Butterworth-Heinemann: 2000;118–127.

76. Sackett DL, Haynes RB, Tugwell P. *Clinical Epidemiology: A Basic Science for Clinical Medicine.* Boston, Mass: Little, Brown; 1985.

77. Sackett DL, Strauss SE, Richardson WS et al. *Evidence Based Medicine: How to Practice and Teach EBM.* 2nd ed. Edinburgh, Scotland: Churchill Livingstone; 2000.

78. Fess EE. The need for reliability and validity in hand assessment instruments [editorial]. *J Hand Surg* 1986;11A:621–623.

79. Gleim GW, McHugh MP. Flexibility and its effects on sports injury and performance. *Sports Med* 1997;24:289–299.

80. McKenzie R, May S. Physical examination. In: McKenzie R, May S, eds. *The Human Extremities: Mechanical Diagnosis and Therapy*. Waikanae, New Zealand: Spinal Publications New Zealand Ltd; 2000:105–121.

81. Farfan HF. The scientific basis of manipulative procedures. *Clin Rheum Dis* 1980;6:159–177.

82. Harris ML. Flexibility. *Phys Ther* 1969;49:591–601.

83. Boone DC, Azen SP, Lin CM, Spence C, Baron C, Lee L. Reliability of goniometric measurements. *Phys Ther* 1978; 58:1355–1360.

84. Mayerson NH, Milano RA. Goniometric measurement reliability in physical medicine. *Arch Phys Med Rehab* 1984;65:92–94.

85. Riddle DL, Rothstein JM, Lamb RL. Goniometric reliability in a clinical setting: Shoulder measurements. *Phys Ther* 1987; 67:668–673.

86. Williams JG, Callaghan M. Comparison of visual estimation and goniometry in determination of a shoulder joint angle. *Physiotherapy* 1990;76:655–657.

87. Cocchiarella L, Andersson GBJ, eds. *American Medical Association. Guides to the Evaluation of Permanent Impairment*. 5th ed. Chicago, Ill: AMA; 2001.

88. Nelson MA, Allen P, Clamp SE, de Dombal FT. Reliability and reproducibility of clinical findings in low-back pain. *Spine* 1979;4:97–101.

89. Rothstein JM. Cyriax reexamined. *Phys Ther* 1994;74:1073.

90. Petersen CM, Hayes KW. Construct validity of Cyriax's selective tension examination: Association of end-feels with pain path the knee and shoulder. *J Orthop Sports Phys Ther* 2000; 30:512–527.

91. Williams PL, Warwick R, Dyson M, Bannister LH et al. *Gray's Anatomy*. 37th ed. London, England: Churchill Livingstone; 1989.

92. Stokes M, Young A. The contribution of reflex inhibition to arthrogenous muscle weakness. *Clin Sci* 1984;67:7–14.

93. Watson D, Trott P. Cervical headache: An investigation of natural head posture and upper cervical flexor muscle performance. *Cephalalgia* 1993;13:272–284.

94. Riddle DL. Measurement of accessory motion: Critical issues and related concepts. *Phys Ther* 1992;72:865–874.

95. Meadows JTS. The principles of the Canadian approach to the lumbar dysfunction patient. In: *Management of Lumbar Spine Dysfunction—Independent Home Study Course*. La Crosse, Wis: Orthopaedic Section, American Physical Therapy Association; 1999.

96. Maitland GD. Passive movement techniques for intra-articular and periarticular disorders. *Aust J Physiother* 1985;31:3–8.

97. Tovin BJ, Greenfield BH. Impairment-based diagnosis for the shoulder girdle. In: *Evaluation and Treatment of the Shoulder: An Integration of the Guide to Physical Therapist Practice*. Philadelphia, Pa: FA Davis; 2001:55–74.

98. Sapega AA. Muscle performance evaluation in orthopedic practice. *J Bone Joint Surg* 1990;72A:1562–1574.

99. Marx RG, Bombardier C, Wright JG. What do we know about the reliability and validity of physical examination tests used to examine the upper extremity? *J Hand Surg* 1999; 24A:185–193.

100. Iddings DM, Smith LK, Spencer WA. Muscle testing: Part 2. Reliability in clinical use. *Phys Ther Rev* 1961;41:249–256.

101. Silver M, McElroy A, Morrow L, Heafner BK. Further standardization of manual muscle test for clinical study: applied in chronic renal disease. *Phys Ther* 1970;50:1456–1465.

102. Janda V. *Muscle Function Testing*. London, England: Butterworth; 1983:163–167.

103. Kendall FP, McCreary EK, Provance PG. *Muscles: Testing and Function*. Baltimore, Md: Williams and Wilkins; 1993.

104. Astrand PO, Rodahl K. *Textbook of Work Physiology*. New York, NY: McGraw-Hill; 1973:411–420.

105. Astrand PO, Rodahl K. *The Muscle and Its Contraction: Textbook of Work Physiology*. New York, NY: McGraw-Hill; 1986.

106. Muller EA. Influences of training and inactivity of muscle strength. *Arch Phys Med Rehab* 1970;51:449–462.

107. Hartsell HD, Forwell L. Postoperative eccentric and concentric isokinetic strength for the shoulder rotators in the scapular and neutral planes. *J Orthop Sports Phys Ther* 1997;25:19–25.

108. Hartsell HD, Spaulding SJ. Eccentric/concentric ratios at selected velocities for the invertor and evertor muscles of the chronically unstable ankle. *Br J Sports Med* 1999;33:255–258.

109. Griffin JW. Differences in elbow flexion torque measured concentrically, eccentrically and isometrically. *Phys Ther* 1987;67:1205–1208.

110. Hortobagyi T, Katch FI. Eccentric and concentric torque-velocity relationships during arm flexion and extension. *J Appl Physiol* 1995;60:395–401.

111. Trudelle-Jackson E, Meske N, Highenboten C et al. Eccentric/concentric torque deficits in the quadriceps muscle. *J Orthop Sports Phys Ther* 1989;11:142–145.

112. Kramer JF, MacDermid J. Isokinetic measures during concentric-eccentric cycles of the knee extensors. *Aust J Physiother* 1989;35:9–14.

113. Rizzardo M, Wessel J, Bay G. Eccentric and concentric torque and power of the knee extensors of females. *Can J Sport Sci* 1988;3:166–169.

114. Colliander EB, Tesch PA. Bilateral eccentric and concentric torque of quadriceps and hamstring muscles in females and males. *Eur J Appl Physiol* 1989;59:227–232.

115. Dvir Z. *Isokinetics: Muscle Testing, Interpretation and Clinical Applications*. New York, NY: Churchill Livingstone; 1995.

116. Jull GA, Janda V. Muscle and motor control in low back pain. In: Twomey LT, Taylor JR, eds. *Physical Therapy of the Low Back: Clinics in Physical Therapy*. New York, NY: Churchill Livingstone; 1987:258.

117. Woolbright JL. Exercise protocol for patients with low back pain. *J Am Osteopath Assoc* 1983;82:919.

118. Nachemson A. Work for all. For those with low back pain as well. *Clin Orthop* 1982;179:77.

119. Knott M, Voss DE. *Proprioceptive Neuromuscular Facilitation*. 2nd ed. New York, NY: Harper and Row; 1968.

120. Brunnstrom S. *Movement Therapy in Hemiplegia*. New York, NY: Harper and Row; 1970.

121. Voss DE, Ionta MK, Myers DJ. *Proprioceptive Neuromuscular Facilitation: Patterns and Techniques*. Philadelphia, Pa: Harper and Row; 1985:1–342.

122. Gilman S. The physical and neurologic examination. In: Gilman S, ed. *Clinical Examination of the Nervous System*. New York, NY: McGraw-Hill; 2000:1–34.

123. Currier RD, Fitzgerald FT. Nervous system. In: Judge RD, Zuidema GD, Fitzgerald FT, eds. *Clinical Diagnosis*. Boston, Mass: Little, Brown; 1982:405–445.

124. Goldberg S. *The Four Minute Neurological Examination*. Miami, Fla: Medmaster; 1992.

125. Dutton M. *Manual Therapy of the Spine: An Integrated Approach*. New York, NY: McGraw-Hill; 2002.

126. Dellon AL. Clinical use of vibratory stimuli to evaluate peripheral nerve injury and compression neuropathy. *Plast Reconstr Surg* 1980;65:466–476.

127. Martin JH, Jessell TM. Anatomy of the somatic sensory system. In: Kandel ER, Schwartz JH, Jessell TM, eds. *Principles of Neural Science*. New York, NY: Elsevier; 1991:353–366.

128. Mann RA. Biomechanics of the foot. *Instr Course Lect* 1982;31:167–180.

129. Ayub E. Posture and the upper quarter. In: Donatelli RA, ed. *Physical Therapy of the Shoulder*. New York, NY: Churchill Livingstone; 1991:81–90.

130. Schmitz TJ. Sensory assessment. In: O'Sullivan SB, Schmitz TJ, eds. *Physical Rehabilitation: Assessment and Treatment*. Philadelphia, Pa: FA Davis; 1994:83–95.

131. Guskiewicz KM. Impaired postural stability: Regaining balance. In: Prentice WE, Voight ML, eds. *Techniques in Musculoskeletal Rehabilitation* New York, NY: McGraw-Hill; 2001:125–150.

132. Donahoe B, Turner D, Worrell T. The use of functional reach as a measurement of balance in healthy boys and girls aged 5–15. *Phys Ther* 1993;73:S71.

133. Fisher A, Wietlisbach S, Wilberger J. Adult performance on three tests of equilibrium. *Am J Occup Ther* 1988;42:30–35.

134. Newton R. Review of tests of standing balance abilities. *Brain Inj* 1992;3:335–343.

135. Irrgang JJ, Harner C. Recent advances in ACL rehabilitation: Clinical factors. *J Sports Rehabil* 1997;6:111–124.

136. Trulock SC. *A Comparison of Static, Dynamic and Functional Methods of Objective Balance Assessment*. Chapel Hill, NC: University of North Carolina Press; 1996.

137. Janda V. On the concept of postural muscles and posture in man. *Aust J Physiother* 1983;29:83–84.

138. Turne, M. Posture and pain. *Phys Ther* 1957;37:294.

139. Darnell MW. A proposed chronology of events for forward head posture. *J Craniomandib Prac* 1983;1:49–54.

140. Greenfield B, Catlin P, Coats PW, Green E, McDonald JJ, North C. Posture in patients with shoulder overuse injuries and healthy individuals. *J Orthop Sports Phys Ther* 1995;21:287–295.

141. Oatis CA. Role of the hip in posture and gait. In: Echternach J, ed. *Clinics in Physical Therapy: Physical Therapy of the Hip*. New York, NY: Churchill Livingstone; 1983:165–179.

142. Putz-Anderson V. *Cumulative Trauma Disorders: A Manual for Musculoskeletal Diseases of the Upper Limbs*. Bristol, Pa: Taylor and Francis; 1988.

143. Keller K, Corbett J, Nichols D. Repetitive strain injury in computer keyboard users: Pathomechanics and treatment principles in individual and group intervention. *J Hand Ther* 1998; 11:9–26.

144. Korr IM, Wright HM, Thomas PE. Effects of experimental myofascial insults on cutaneous patterns of sympathetic activity in man. *J Neural Transm* 1962;23:330–355.

145. Travell JG, Simons DG. *Myofascial Pain and Dysfunction—The Trigger Point Manual*. Baltimore, Md: Williams and Wilkins; 1983.

146. Beal MC. The short leg problem. *J Am Osteopath Assoc* 1977;76:745–751.

147. Wilder DG, Pope MH, Frymoyer JW. The biomechanics of lumbar disc herniation and the effect of overload and instability. *J Spinal Disord* 1988;1:16.

148. Kiser DM. Physiological and biomechanical factors for understanding repetitive motion injuries. *Semin Occup Med* 1987; 2:11–17.

149. Greenfield B. Upper quarter evaluation: Structural relationships and interindependence. In: Donatelli R, Wooden M, eds. *Orthopedic Physical Therapy*. New York, NY: Churchill Livingstone; 1989:43–58.

150. Janda V. Muscle strength in relation to muscle length, pain and muscle imbalance. In: Harms-Ringdahl K, ed. *Muscle Strength*. New York, NY: Churchill Livingstone; 1993:83.

151. Lewit K. *Manipulative Therapy in Rehabilitation of the Motor System*. 3rd ed. London, England: Butterworth; 1999.

152. Lewit K, Simons DG. Myofascial pain: Relief by post-isometric relaxation. *Arch Phys Med Rehabil* 1984;65:452–456.

153. Smith A. Upper limb disorders—Time to relax? *Physiotherapy* 1996;82:31–38.

154. Babyar SR. Excessive scapular motion in individuals recovering from painful and stiff shoulders: Causes and treatment strategies. *Phys Ther* 1996;76:226–247.

155. Tardieu C, Tabary JC, Tardieu G, et al. Adaptation of sarcomere numbers to the length imposed on muscle. In: Guba F, Marechal G, Takacs O, eds. *Mechanism of Muscle Adaptation to Functional Requirements*. Elmsford, NY: Pergamon; 1981:99.

156. Seidel-Cobb D, Cantu R. Myofascial treatment. In: Donatelli RA, ed. *Physical Therapy of the Shoulder*. New York, NY: Churchill Livingstone; 1997:383–401.

157. Janda V. Muscles, motor regulation and back problems. In: Korr IM, ed. *The Neurological Mechanisms in Manipulative Therapy*. New York, NY: Plenum; 1978:27.

158. Janda V. Muscles and motor control in cervicogenic disorders: Assessment and management. In: Grant R, ed. *Physical Therapy of the Cervical and Thoracic Spine*. New York, NY: Churchill Livingstone; 1994:195–216.

159. Gerwin RD, Shannon S, Hong CZ, Hubbard D, Gevirtz R. Interrater reliability in myofascial trigger point examination. *Pain* 1997;17:591–595.

160. Njoo KH, Van der Does E. The occurrence and inter-rater reliability of myofascial trigger points in the quadratus lumborum and gluteus medius: A prospective study in non-specific low back patients and controls in general practice. *Pain* 1994;58:317–321.

161. Farrell JP. Cervical passive mobilization techniques: The Australian approach. *Phys Med Rehabil* 1990;4:309–334.

162. Dyson M, Pond JB, Joseph J, Warwick R. The stimulation of tissue regeneration by means of ultrasound. *Clin Sci* 1968; 35:273–285.

163. Dyson M, Suckling J. Stimulation of tissue repair by ultrasound: A survey of the mechanisms involved. *Physiotherapy* 1978; 64:105–108.

164. Ramsey SM. Holistic manual therapy techniques. *Prim Care* 1997;24:759–785.

165. Hsieh CY, Hong CZ, Adams AH, et al. Interexaminer reliability of the palpation of trigger points in the trunk and lower limb muscles. *Arch Phys Med Rehabil* 2000;81:258–264.

166. Dvorak J, Dvorak V. General principles of palpation. In: Gilliar WG, Greenman PE, eds. *Manual Medicine: Diagnostics*. New York, NY: Thieme; 1990:71–75.

167. Swain JH. An introduction to radiology of the lumbar spine. In: Wadsworth C, ed. *Orthopedic Physical Therapy Home Study Course*. La Crosse, Wis: Orthopedic Section, American Physical Therapy Association; 1994.

168. Wolff J. *The Law of Remodeling*. Maquet P, Furlong R, trans Berlin, Germany: Springer-Verlag; 1986 (1892).

169. Schutter H. Intervertebral disc disorders. In: *Clinical Neurology*. Philadelphia, Pa: Lippincott-Raven; 1995:chap. 41.

170. Jahnke RW, Hart BL. Cervical stenosis, spondylosis, and herniated disc disease. *Radiol Clin North Am* 1991;29:777–791.

171. Modic MT, Ross JS, Masaryk TJ. Imaging of degenerative disease of the cervical spine. *Clin Orthop* 1989;239:109–120.

172. Forristall RM, Marsh HO, Pay NT. Magnetic resonance imaging and contrast CT of the lumbar spine: Comparison of diagnostic methods and correlation with surgical findings. *Spine* 1988; 13:1049–1054.

173. Harris JH, Yeakley JW. Hyperextension-dislocation of the cervical spine: Ligament injuries demonstrated by magnetic resonance imaging. *J Bone Joint Surg* 1992;74B:567.

174. Ellenberg MR, Honet JC, Treanor WJ. Cervical radiculopathy. *Arch Phys Med Rehabil* 1994;75:342–352.

175. Cwynar DA, McNerney T. A primer on physical therapy. *Prim Care* 1999;3:451–459.

176. Fritz JM, Wainner RS. Examining diagnostic tests: An evidence-based perspective. *Phys Ther* 2001;81:1546–1564.

177. Coutts F. Changes in the musculoskeletal system. In: Atkinson K, Coutts F, Hassenkamp A, eds. *Physiotherapy in Orthopedics.* London, England: Churchill Livingstone; 1999:19–43.

178. Jones MA. Clinical reasoning in manual therapy. *Phys Ther* 1992;72:875–884.

179. Brooks LR, Norman GR, Allen SW. The role of specific similarity in a medical diagnostic task. *J Exp Psychol Gen* 1991; 120:278–287.

180. Kahney H. *Problem Solving: Current Issues.* Buckingham, England: Open University Press; 1993.

181. Friedman LM, Furberg CD, DeMets DL. *Fundamentals of Clinical Trials.* Chicago, Ill: Mosby-Year Book; 1985:2, 51, 71.

182. Bloch R. Methodology in clinical back pain trials. *Spine* 1987;12:430–432.

183. Schiffman EL. The role of the randomized clinical trial in evaluating management strategies for temporomandibular disorders. In: Fricton JR, Dubner R, eds. *Orofacial Pain and Temporomandibular Disorders. Advances in Pain Research and Therapy.* Vol 21. New York, NY: Raven; 1995:415–463.

184. Wright JG, Feinstein AR. Improving the reliability of orthopaedic measurements. *J Bone Joint Surg* 1992;74B: 287–291.

185. Haas M. Statistical methodology for reliability studies. *J Manipulative Physiol Ther* 1991;14:119–132.

186. Cooperman JM, Riddle DL, Rothstein JM. Reliability and validity of judgments of the integrity of the anterior cruciate ligament of the knee using the Lachman's test. *Phys Ther* 1990;70:225–233.

187. Shields RK, Enloe LJ, Evans RE, Smith KB, Steckel SD. Reliability, validity, and responsiveness of functional tests in patients with total joint replacement. *Phys Ther* 1995;75:169.

188. Feinstein AR. *Clinimetrics.* Westford, Mass: Murray Printing; 1987.

189. Laslett M, Williams M. The reliability of selected pain provocation tests for sacroiliac joint pathology. *Spine* 1994;19: 1243–1249.

190. Portney L, Watkins MP. *Foundations of Clinical Research: Applications to Practice.* Norwalk, Conn: Appleton and Lange; 1993.

191. Huijbregts PA. Spinal motion palpation: A review of reliability studies. *J Man Manipulative Ther* 2002;10:24–39.

192. Roach KE, Brown MD, Albin RD, Delaney KG, Lipprandi HM, Rangelli D. The sensitivity and specificity of pain response to activity and position in categorizing patients with low back pain. *Phys Ther* 1997;77:730–738.

193. Van der Wurff P, Meyne W, Hagmeijer RHM. Clinical tests of the sacroiliac joint, a systematic methodological review. Part 2: Validity. *Man Ther* 2000;5:89–96.

194. Domholdt E. *Physical Therapy Research: Principles and Applications.* Philadelphia, Pa: Saunders; 1993.

194a. Huijbregts PA. Spinal motion palpation: A review of reliability studies. *J Man & Manip Ther* 2002;10:24–39.

194b. Van der Wurff P, Meyne W, Hagmeijer RHM. Clinical tests of the sacroiliac joint, a systematic methodological review, Part 2: Validity. *Man Ther* 2000;5:89–96.

195. Feinstein AR. Clinical biostatistics XXXI: On the sensitivity, specificity & discrimination of diagnostic tests. *Clin Pharmacol Ther* 1975;17:104–116.

196. Anderson MA, Foreman TL. Return to competition: Functional rehabilitation. In: Zachazewski JE, Magee DJ, Quillen WS, eds. *Athletic Injuries and Rehabilitation.* Philadelphia, Pa: Saunders; 1996:229–261.

197. Jull GA. Physiotherapy management of neck pain of mechanical origin. In: Giles LGF, Singer KP, eds. *Clinical Anatomy and Management of Cervical Spine Pain.* London, England: Butterworth-Heinemann; 1998:168–191.

198. Clawson AL, Domholdt E. Content of physician referrals to physical therapists at clinical education sites in Indiana. *Phys Ther* 1994;74:356–360.

199. Leerar PJ. Differential diagnosis of tarsal coalition versus cuboid syndrome in an adolescent athlete. *J Orthop Sports Phys Ther* 2001;31:702–707.

200. Sox HC Jr. Probability theory in the use of diagnostic tests: An introduction to critical study of the literature. *Ann Intern Med* 1986;104:60–66.

201. McKenzie RA. *The Cervical and Thoracic Spine: Mechanical Diagnosis and Therapy.* Waikanae, New Zealand: Spinal Publications New Zealand Ltd; 1990.

202. Battie MC, Cherkin DC, Dunn R, Ciol MA, Wheeler KJ. Managing low back pain: Attitudes and treatment preferences of physical therapists. *Phys Ther* 1994;74:219–226.

203. Riddle DL. Classification and low back pain; a review of the literature and critical analysis of selected systems. *Phys Ther* 1998;78:708–737.

204. Stankovic R, Johnell O. Conservative management of acute low back pain. A prospective randomized trial: McKenzie method of treatment versus patient education in "mini back school." *Spine* 1990;15:120–123.

205. Donelson R. The McKenzie approach to evaluating and treating low back pain. *Orthop Rev* 1990;19:681–686.

206. McKenzie R. Patient heal thyself. Paper presented at the American Back Society Annual Meeting; 1999; Las Vegas, Nev.

207. Evans P. The healing process at cellular level: A review. *Physiotherapy* 1980;66:256–260.

208. Yoder E. Physical therapy management of nonsurgical hip problems in adults. In: Echternach JL, ed. *Physical Therapy of the Hip.* New York, NY: Churchill Livingstone; 1990:103–137.

209. DeCarlo MS, Sell KE. The effects of the number and frequency of physical therapy treatments on selected outcomes of treatment in patients with anterior cruciate ligament reconstructions. *J Orthop Sports Phys Ther* 1997;26:332–339.

210. Coile RC. Forcasting the future—Part two. *Rehab Manage* 1994;7:59–63.

211. Nugent J. Blaze your trails through managed care. *PT Mag* 1994;2:19–20.

CHAPTER 9

DIFFERENTIAL DIAGNOSIS

CHAPTER OBJECTIVES

▶ *At the completion of this chapter, the reader will be able to:*

1. Understand the importance of differential diagnosis.

2. Recognize signs and symptoms that require medical referral.

3. List the various systemic or medical pathologies that can mimic musculoskeletal pathology.

OVERVIEW

With the advent of direct access laws in a growing number of states, many physical therapists now have the primary responsibility for being the gatekeepers of health care and for making medical referrals. This responsibility requires that the clinician have a high level of knowledge, including an understanding of the concepts of differential diagnosis. Differential diagnosis involves the ability to quickly differentiate problems of a serious nature from those that are not, using the history and physical examination. Problems of a serious nature include, but are not limited to, visceral diseases, cancer, infections, fractures, and vascular disorders. These conditions can often be highlighted with a systems review. The systems review is the part of the physical examination that helps to identify any health problem that requires consultation with, or referral to, another health care provider.[1] The systems review includes the following components[1]:

▶ For the cardiovascular/pulmonary system, the assessment of heart rate, respiratory rate, blood pressure, and edema.

▶ For the integumentary system, the assessment of skin integrity, skin color, and presence of scar formation.

▶ For the musculoskeletal system, the assessment of gross symmetry, gross range of motion, gross strength, weight, and height.

▶ For the neuromuscular system, a general assessment of gross coordinated movement (e.g., balance, locomotion, transfers, and transitions).

▶ For communication ability, affect, cognition, language, and learning style, the assessment of the ability to make needs known; consciousness, orientation (person, place, and time); expected emotional and behavioral responses; and learning preferences (e.g., learning barriers, education needs).

Referred Pain

Pain is the most common determinant for a patient to seek intervention. It is important to assume that all reports of pain by the patient are serious in nature until proven otherwise with a thorough examination.[2]

Clinical Pearl

In general, the greater the degree of pain radiation, the greater the chance that the problem is acute or that it is occurring from a proximal structure, or both.

Although pain intensity and the functional response to symptoms are subjective, patterns of pain response to stimulation of the pain generator are quite objective (e.g., antalgic gait).[3] Referred pain can be generated by[4]:

▶ Convergence of sensory input from separate parts of the body to the same dorsal horn neuron via primary sensory fibers (convergence-projection theory).[5–8]

▶ Secondary pain resulting from a myofascial trigger point.[9]

▶ Sympathetic activity elicited by a spinal reflex.[10]

▶ Pain-generating substances.[7]

Macnab[11] recommends the following classification for referred pain:

1. Viscerogenic.

2. Vasculogenic.

3. Neurogenic.

4. Psychogenic.

5. Spondylogenic.

Viscerogenic Pain

The pain in this category can be referred from any viscera in the trunk or abdomen. Visceral pain can be produced by chemical damage, ischemia, or spasm of the smooth muscles.

Viscerogenic pain may be produced when the nociceptive fibers from the viscera synapse in the spinal cord with some of the same neurons that receive pain from the skin. When the visceral nociceptors are stimulated, some are transmitted by the same neurons that conduct skin nociception and take on the same characteristics. Visceral pain has five important clinical characteristics:

1. It is not evoked from all viscera.

2. It is not always linked to visceral injury.

3. It is diffuse and poorly localized.

4. It is referred to other locations.

5. It is often accompanied by autonomic reflexes, such as nausea and vomiting.

Viscerogenic pain (Table 9-1) tends to be diffuse because of the organization of visceral nociceptive pathways in the central nervous system. This organization demonstrates an absence of a separate pathway for visceral sensory information and a low proportion of visceral afferent nerve fibers compared with those of somatic origin.

Pain arising from problems in the peritoneum, pleura, or pericardium differs from that of other visceral impairments because of the innervation of these structures. The parietal walls of these structures are supplied extensively with both fast and slow pain fibers and, thus, can produce the sharp pain of superficial impairments.

> ### Clinical Pearl
>
> A visceral source of the symptoms should always be suspected if the symptoms are not altered with movement or position changes.

In general, symptoms from a musculoskeletal condition are provoked by certain postures, movements, or activities, and relieved by others. However, this generalization must be viewed as such. Determining the mechanism often will clarify the cause of the symptoms. For example, pain that occurs following eating may have a gastric source.

Vasculogenic Pain

Vasculogenic pain tends to result from venous congestion or arterial deprivation to the musculoskeletal areas. Vasculogenic pain may mimic a wide variety of musculoskeletal, neurologic, and arthritic disorders, because this type of pain is often worsened by activity.

To help exclude a vasculogenic cause, it is important to review the cardiopulmonary, hematologic, and neurologic systems during the examination. Clinical evidence of arterial insufficiency includes lower extremity asymmetry, skin condition changes, skin temperature and color changes, and diminishing pulses.

Doppler examination is the cornerstone of the vascular examination and is based on waveform and sound. This test examines blood flow in the major arteries and veins in the arms and legs with the use of ultrasound. The ultrasound transducer produces high-frequency sound waves that echo off the blood vessels, resulting in a "swishing" noise during blood flow. A faster flow produces a higher pitch and a steeper waveform. To produce a frequency change detectable by the Doppler examination, blood velocity must be greater than 3 cm/s. However, an absent signal does not necessarily mean there is no blood flow. It may simply mean that the flow is slower than 3 cm/s. In the lower extremity, segmental pressures are usually taken from six sites:

1. High thigh.

2. Above the knee.

3. Below the knee.

4. Ankle.

5. Forefoot.

6. Digit.

A pressure gradient of less than 20 mm Hg is normal, 20 to 30 mm Hg is borderline, and greater than 30 mm Hg is considered abnormal. Pressure differences of less than 20 mm Hg between limbs are considered normal.

After the segmental pressures of the lower extremity are measured, brachial pressure on both sides is measured.

TABLE 9-1 Potential Areas of Cutaneous Referral from Various Viscera[11a]

Visceral Organ	Pain Referral
Heart (T1–5) Bronchi and Lung (T2–4)	Under sternum, base of neck, over shoulders, over pectorals, and down one or both arms (L > R)
Esophagus (T5–6)	Pharynx, lower neck, arms, midline chest from upper to lower sternum
Gastric (T6–10)	Lower thoracic to upper abdomen
Gallbladder (T7–9)	Upper abdomen, lower scapular, and thoracolumbar
Pancreas	Upper lumbar or upper abdomen
Kidneys (T10–L1)	Upper lumbar, occasionally anterior abdomen about 4–5 cm lateral to umbilicus
Urinary Bladder (T11–12)	Lower abdomen or low lumbar
Uterus	Lower abdomen or low lumbar

Comparisons are made between ankle–arm, forefoot–arm, and digit–arm ratios. Normal values are > 1 for the ankle–arm index, > 0.75 for the forefoot–arm, and > 0.65 for each digit–arm index.

Neurogenic Pain

The neurologic tissues comprise those tissues that are involved in nerve conduction (see Chap. 2). Neurogenic causes of pain may include:

▶ Tumor compressing and irritating a neural structure of the spinal cord or the meninges.

▶ Spinal nerve root irritation.

▶ Peripheral nerve entrapment.

▶ Neuritis.

The presenting signs and symptoms requiring a neurological assessment are outlined in Table 8-14.

Scanning Examination

The tests of the Cyriax[12] upper or lower quarter scanning examination (Table 9-2) can be used to:

▶ Examine the patient's neurologic status.

▶ Highlight the presence of a lesion to the central or peripheral nervous systems (see Chap. 2).

TABLE 9-2 Components of the Scan and Structures Tested

Component	Description
Active ROM	Willingness to move, ROM, integrity of contractile and inert tissues, pattern of restriction (capsular, or noncapsular), quality of motion, and symptom reproduction
Passive ROM	Integrity of inert and contractile tissues, ROM, end-feel, sensitivity
Resisted	Integrity of contractile tissues (strength, sensitivity)
Stress	Integrity of inert tissues (ligamentous-disk stability)
Dural	Dural mobility
Neurologic	Nerve conduction
Dermatome	Afferent (sensation)
Myotome	Efferent (strength, fatigability)
Reflexes	Afferent-efferent and central nervous systems

ROM, range of motion.

▶ Help determine whether the symptoms are being referred.

▶ Confirm the physician's diagnosis.

▶ Help rule out any serious pathology, such as a fracture or tumor.

▶ Assess the status of the contractile and inert tissues.

▶ Generate a working hypothesis.

The clinician must choose which scanning examination to use based on the presenting signs and symptoms. The upper quarter scanning examination (see Table 8-12) is appropriate for upper thoracic, upper extremity, and cervical problems, whereas the lower quarter scanning examination (see Table 8-13) is typically used for thoracic, lower extremity, and lumbosacral problems. The preferred sequence of the scanning examination is outlined in Table 9-3.

The thoroughness of the scanning examination is influenced by both patient tolerance and professional judgment. A general guideline is that the examination must continue until the clinician is confident that the patient's symptoms are not the result of a serious condition that demands medical attention.

The tests included in the scanning examination include strength testing, sensation testing (light touch and pinprick), deep tendon reflexes (Table 9-4), and the pathological reflexes (see Table 2-4). The various tests of the scanning examinations specific to the cervical, lumbar, and thoracic spine are described in the relevant chapters (see Chaps. 23, 25, and 26, respectively).

At the end of each of the scanning examinations, either a medical diagnosis (disk protrusion, prolapse, or extrusion; acute arthritis; specific tendonitis; muscle belly tear; spondylolisthesis; or stenosis) can be made, or the scanning examination is considered negative (see Table 9-3). A negative scanning examination does not imply that there were no findings; rather, the results of examination were insufficient to generate a diagnosis upon which an intervention could be based. In this case, further examination is required.

Psychogenic Pain

It is common to find emotional overtones in the presence of pain, particularly with low back and neck pain. These overtones are thought to result from an inhibition of the pain control mechanisms of the central nervous system from such causes as grief, the side effects of medications, or fear of reinjury. Somatosensory amplification refers to the tendency to experience somatic sensation as intense, noxious, and disturbing. Barsky and colleagues[13] introduced the concept of somatosensory amplification as an important feature of hypochondriasis. Somatosensory amplification is observed in patients whose extreme anxiety leads to an increase in their perception of pain.

The term *nonorganic* was proposed by Waddell[14] to define the abnormal illness behaviors exhibited by patients suffering from depression, emotional disturbance, or anxiety states. The presence of three of five of the following Waddell signs has been correlated significantly with disability.[15]

TABLE 9-3 Typical Sequence of Upper or Lower Quarter Scanning Examinations

1. Initial Observation: Involves everything from initial entry of patient, including gait, demeanor, standing, and sitting postures, obvious deformities and postural defects, scars, radiation burns, creases, and birthmarks
2. Patient history
3. Scanning Examination
4. Active Range of Motion
5. Passive Overpressure
6. Resistive Tests
7. Deep Tendon Reflexes
8. Sensation Testing
9. Special Tests

NEGATIVE SCAN

If, at end of scan, clinician has determined that patient's condition is appropriate for physical therapy but has not determined diagnosis to treat patient, clinician will need to perform further testing

POSITIVE SCAN (RESULTS IN A DIAGNOSIS)

1. Specific interventions (traction, manual techniques, and specific exercises) can be given if diagnosis is one that will benefit from physical therapy
2. Patient is returned to physician for more tests if signs and symptoms are cause for concern

TABLE 9-4 Common Deep Tendon Reflexes

Reflex	Site of Stimulus	Normal Response	Pertinent Central Nervous System Segment
Jaw	Mandible	Mouth closes	CNV
Biceps	Biceps tendon	Biceps contraction	C5–6
Brachioradialis	Brachioradialis tendon or just distal to musculotendinous junction	Flexion of elbow and/or pronation of forearm	C5–6
Triceps	Distal triceps tendon above olecranon process	Elbow extension	C7–8
Patella	Patellar tendon	Leg extension	L3–4
Medial hamstrings	Semimembranosus tendon	Knee flexion	L5, S1
Lateral hamstrings	Biceps femoris tendon	Knee flexion	S1–2
Tibialis posterior	Tibialis posterior tendon behind medial malleolus	Plantar flexion of foot with inversion	L4–5
Achilles	Achilles tendon	Plantar flexion of foot	S1–2

CN, cranial nerve.

▶ Superficial or nonanatomic tenderness to light touch that is widespread and refers pain to other areas.

▶ Simulation tests. These are a series of tests that should be comfortable to perform. Examples include axial loading of the spine through the patient's head with light pressure to the skull and passive hip and shoulder rotation with the patient positioned standing. Neither of these tests should produce low back pain. If pain is reported with these tests, a nonorganic origin should be suspected.

▶ Distraction test.[16] This test involves checking a positive finding elicited during the examination on the distracted patient. For example, if a patient is unable to perform a seated trunk flexion maneuver, the same patient can be observed when asked to remove his or her shoes. A difference of 40 to 45 degrees is significant for inconsistency.

▶ Regional disturbances. These signs include sensory or motor disturbances that have no neurologic basis.

▶ Overreaction. This includes disproportionate verbalization, muscle tension, tremors, and grimacing during the examination.

The Somatosensory Amplification Rating Scale (SARS; Table 9-5) is a version of Waddell's nonorganic physical signs that has been modified to allow for a more accurate appraisal of the patient with exaggerated illness behavior.[13]

Clinical Pearl

It is important to remember that the Waddell and SARS assessment tools are designed not to detect whether patients are malingering, but only to indicate whether they have symptoms of a nonorganic origin.

Litigation

Patients pursuing litigation may be subdivided into two groups:

1. Those patients with a legitimate injury and cause for litigation who genuinely want to improve.

2. Those patients who are merely motivated by the lure of the litigation settlement, and who have no intention of showing signs of improvement until their case is settled. Termed *malingerers,* these patients are a frustrating group for clinicians to deal with because, like the nonorganic patient type, they display exaggerated complaints of pain, tenderness, and suffering.

Malingering is defined as the intentional production of false symptoms or the exaggeration of symptoms that truly exist.[17] These symptoms may be physical or psychological but have in common the intention of achieving a certain goal. Any individual involved in litigation, whether the result of a motor vehicle accident, work injury, or accident has the potential for

malingering.[18] Malingering can be thought of as synonymous with faking, lying, or fraud, and it represents a frequently unrecognized and mismanaged medical diagnosis.[17] Unfortunately, due to the similarity between malingerers and nonorganic patients, this deception often causes a significant, negative response from the clinician toward malingerers and nonorganic patients alike.

It is most important that the clinician address any suspected deception in a structured and unemotional manner, and that interactions with the patient be performed in a problem-oriented, constructive, and helpful fashion.[17]

Clinical Pearl

The diagnosis of malingering should be made based on the production of actions in the attainment of a known goal, without elaboration of those actions based on the negative emotional response of the clinician.[17]

With very few exceptions, patients in significant pain look and feel miserable, move extremely slowly, and present with consistent findings during the examination. In contrast, malingerers present with severe symptoms and exaggerated responses during the examination but can often be observed to be in no apparent distress at other times. This is particularly true if the malingering patient is observed in an environment outside of the clinic.

However, it cannot be stressed enough that all patients should be given the benefit of the doubt until the clinician, with a high degree of confidence, can rule out an organic cause for the pain.

A number of clinical signs and symptoms can alert the clinician to the possibility of a patient who is malingering. These include:

▶ Subjective complaints of paresthesia with only stocking-glove anesthesia (conditions including diabetic neuropathy and the T4 syndrome must be ruled out; see Chap. 26).

▶ Inappropriate scoring on the Oswestry Low Back Disability Questionnaire (Table 9-6), Neck Disability Index (Table 9-7), and McGill Pain Questionnaire (see Table 8-7).

▶ Reflexes inconsistent with the presenting problem, or symptoms.

▶ Cogwheel motion of muscles during strength testing for weakness.

▶ The ability of the patient to complete a straight leg raise in a supine position, but difficulty performing the equivalent range in a seated position.

Whatever the reasoning or motivation behind the malingering patient, the success rate from the clinician's viewpoint will be low, and so it is well worth recognizing these individuals from the outset.

TABLE 9-5 Somatosensory Amplification Rating Scale (SARS)[13]

Examination	Percent	Score*
SENSORY EXAMINATION:		
A. No deficit or deficit well localized to dermatome		0
Deficit related to dermatome(s) but some inconsistency		1
Nondermatomal or very inconsistent deficit		2
Blatantly impossible (i.e., split down midline or entire body with positive tuning fork test)		3
B. Amount of body involved:		
Evaluate similar to burn (% of surface areas	< 15%	0
for an entire leg is 18%)	15–35%	1
	36–60%	2
	> 60%	3
MOTOR EXAMINATION:		
A. No deficit or deficit well localized to myotomes		0
Deficit related to myotome(s) but some inconsistency		1
Nonmyotomal or very inconsistent weakness, exhibits		2
cogwheeling or giving way, weakness is coachable		
Blatantly impossible, significant weakness which disappears when distracted		3
B. Amount of body involved:	< 15%	0
	15–35%	1
	36–60%	2
	> 60%	3
TENDERNESS:		
A. No tenderness or tenderness clearly localized		
to discrete, anatomically sensible structures		0
Tenderness not well localized, some inconsistency		1
Diffuse or very inconsistent tenderness, multiple anatomic		2
structures involved (skin, muscle, bone, etc.)		
Blatantly impossible, significant tenderness of multiple anatomic structures		
(skin, muscle, bone, etc.), which disappears when distracted		3
B. Amount of body involved:	< 15%	0
	15–35%	1
	36–60%	2
	> 60%	3

Examination		Score*
ADDITIONAL TESTS: DISTRACTION TESTS		
Distraction straight leg raise (SLR) rating determined by	< 20°	0
the difference in measurements between supine and seated	20–45°	1
	> 45°	2
SLR supine at less than 45 degrees		3
Standing flexion vs. long sit test		
Rating determined by two factors		
1. Difference between hip ROM, standing vs. supine	< 20°	0
	20–40°	1
	41–50°	2
	> 50°	3
2. Distance measurement from middle		
finger to toes, standing vs. supine (long sit)	< 5 cm	0
	6–10 cm	1
	11–18 cm	2
	> 18 cm	3
Total score possible:		27

ROM, range of motion.
* SARS scores of 5 or greater are indicative of inappropriate illness behavior. The higher the score, the greater the exaggerated behavior.

TABLE 9-6   Oswestry Low Back Disability Questionnaire

PLEASE READ: This questionnaire is designed to enable us to understand how much your low back pain has affected your ability to manage your everyday activities. Please answer each section by marking the **ONE BOX** that most applies to you. We realize that you feel that more than one statement may relate to your problem, but please just mark the one box that most closely describes your problem at this point in time.

Name:

Date:

Section 1—Pain Intensity
( ) The pain comes and goes and is very mild
( ) The pain is mild and does not vary much
( ) The pain comes and goes and is moderate
( ) The pain is moderate and does not vary much
( ) The pain comes and goes and is severe
( ) The pain is severe and does not vary much

Section 2—Personal Care
( ) I have no pain when I wash or dress
( ) I do not normally change my way of washing and dressing even though it causes some pain
( ) I have had to change the way I wash and dress because these activities increase my pain
( ) Because of pain I am unable to do **some** washing and dressing without help
( ) Because of pain I am unable to do **most** washing and dressing without help
( ) Because of pain I am unable to do **any** washing and dressing without help

Section 3—Lifting (*Skip if you have not attempted lifting since the onset of your back pain.*)
( ) Can lift heavy weights without increasing my pain
( ) Can lift heavy weights but it increases my pain
( ) Pain prevents me from lifting heavy weights off the floor
( ) Pain prevents me from lifting heavy weights off the floor but I can manage if they are conveniently positioned, e.g., on a table
( ) Pain prevents me from lifting heavy weights but I can manage light to medium weights if they are conveniently positioned
( ) I can only lift very light weight at the most

Section 4—Walking
( ) I have **no** pain when I walk
( ) I have **some** pain when I walk but it does not prevent me from walking normal distances
( ) Pain prevents me from walking **long** distances
( ) Pain prevents me from walking **intermediate** distances
( ) Pain prevents me from walking **short** distances
( ) Pain prevents me from walking at all

Section 5—Sitting
( ) Sitting does not cause me any pain
( ) I can sit as long as I need to provided I have my choice of chair
( ) Pain prevents me from sitting more than 1 hour
( ) Pain prevents me from sitting more than ½ hour

( ) Pain prevents me from sitting more than 10 minutes
( ) Pain prevents me from sitting at all

Section 6—Standing
( ) Standing does not cause me any pain
( ) I have some pain when I stand but it does not increase with time
( ) Pain prevents me from standing more than 1 hour
( ) Pain prevents me from standing more than ½ hour
( ) Pain prevents me from standing more than 10 minutes
( ) Pain prevents me from standing at all

Section 7—Sleeping
( ) I have no pain when I lie in bed
( ) I have some pain when I lie in bed but it does not prevent me from sleeping well
( ) Because of pain my sleep is reduced by 25%
( ) Because of pain my sleep is reduced by 50%
( ) Because of pain my sleep is reduced by 75%
( ) Pain prevents me from sleeping at all

Section 8—Sex Life (if applicable)
( ) My sex life is normal and causes no pain
( ) My sex life is normal but increases my pain
( ) My sex life is nearly normal but is very painful
( ) My sex life is severely restricted
( ) My sex life is nearly absent because of pain
( ) Pain prevents any sex life at all

Section 9—Social Life
( ) My social life is normal and causes no pain
( ) My social life is normal but increases my pain
( ) Pain has no significant effect on my social life, apart from limiting my more energetic interests (sports, etc.)
( ) Pain has restricted my social life and I do not go out often
( ) Pain has restricted social life to my home
( ) I have no social life because of pain

Section 10—Traveling
( ) I have no pain when I travel
( ) I have some pain when I travel but none of my usual forms of travel make it worse
( ) Traveling increases my pain but has not required that I seek alternative forms of travel
( ) I have had to change the way I travel because my usual form of travel increases my pain
( ) Pain has restricted all forms of travel
( ) I can only travel while lying down

TABLE 9-7   Neck Disability Index[18a]

This questionnaire has been designed to give the doctor information as to how your neck pain has affected your ability to manage in everyday life. Please answer every section and mark in each section only the **ONE BOX** that applies to you. We realize you may consider that two of the statements in any one section relate to you, but please just mark the box that most closely describes your problem.

Section 1—Pain Intensity
- ☐ I have no pain at the moment.
- ☐ The pain is very mild at the moment.
- ☐ The pain is moderate at the moment.
- ☐ The pain is fairly severe at the moment.
- ☐ The pain is the worst imaginable at the moment.

Section 2—Personal Care (Washing, Dressing, etc.)
- ☐ I can look after myself normally without causing extra pain.
- ☐ I can look after myself normally but it causes extra pain.
- ☐ It is painful to look after myself and I am slow and careful.
- ☐ I need some help but manage most of my personal care.
- ☐ I need help every day in most aspects of self care.
- ☐ I do not get dressed, I wash with difficulty and stay in bed.

Section 3—Lifting
- ☐ I can lift heavy weights without extra pain.
- ☐ I can lift heavy weights but it gives extra pain.
- ☐ Pain prevents me from lifting heavy weights off the floor, but I can manage if they are conveniently positioned, for example on a table.
- ☐ Pain prevents me from lifting heavy weights, but I can manage light to medium weights if they are conveniently positioned.
- ☐ I can lift very light weights.
- ☐ Cannot lift or carry anything at all.

Section 4—Reading
- ☐ I can read as much as I want to with no pain in my neck.
- ☐ I can read as much as I want to with slight pain in my neck.
- ☐ I can read as much as I want with moderate pain in my neck.
- ☐ I can't read as much as I want because of moderate pain in my neck.
- ☐ I can hardly read at all because of severe pain in my neck.
- ☐ I cannot read at all.

Section 5—Headaches
- ☐ I have no headaches at all.
- ☐ I have slight headaches which come infrequently.
- ☐ I have moderate headaches which come infrequently.
- ☐ I have moderate headaches which come frequently.
- ☐ I have severe headaches which come frequently.
- ☐ I have headaches almost all the time

Section 6—Concentration
- ☐ I can concentrate fully when I want to with no difficulty.
- ☐ I can concentrate fully when I want to with slight difficulty.

- ☐ I have a fair degree of difficulty in concentrating when I want to.
- ☐ I have a lot of difficulty in concentrating when I want to.
- ☐ I have a great deal of difficulty in concentrating when I want to.
- ☐ I cannot concentrate at all.

Section 7—Work
- ☐ I can do as much work as I want to.
- ☐ I can only do my usual work, but no more.
- ☐ I can do most of my usual work, but no more.
- ☐ I cannot do my usual work.
- ☐ I can hardly do any work at all.
- ☐ I can't do any work at all.

Section 8—Driving
- ☐ I can drive my car without any neck pain.
- ☐ I can drive my car as long as I want with slight pain in my neck.
- ☐ I can drive my car as long as I want because of moderate pain in my neck.
- ☐ I can't drive my car as long as I want because of moderate pain in my neck.
- ☐ I can hardly drive at all because of severe pain in my neck.
- ☐ I can't drive my car at all.

Section 9—Sleeping
- ☐ I have no trouble sleeping.
- ☐ My sleep is slightly disturbed (less than 1 hour sleepless).
- ☐ My sleep is mildly disturbed (1–2 hours sleepless).
- ☐ My sleep is moderately disturbed (2–3 hours sleepless).
- ☐ My sleep is greatly disturbed (3–5 hours sleepless).
- ☐ My sleep is completely disturbed (5–7 hours sleepless).

Section 10—Recreation
- ☐ I am able to engage in all my recreation activities with no neck pain at all.
- ☐ I am able to engage in all my recreation activities, with some pain in my neck.
- ☐ I am able to engage in most, but not all of my usual recreation activities because of pain in my neck.
- ☐ I am able to engage in a few of my usual recreation activities because of pain in my neck.
- ☐ I can hardly do any recreation activities because of pain in my neck.
- ☐ I can't do any recreation activities at all.

Spondylogenic Pain

Severe pathologic processes involving the bone, such as infections, neoplasms, and metabolic disorders, frequently produce pain. Several findings are helpful in diagnosing such pathologic processes. These findings may include:

- ▶ Severe and unrelenting pain.
- ▶ The presence of a fever.
- ▶ Bone tenderness.
- ▶ Unexplained weight loss.

Osseous Impairments

Infective Disease: Osteomyelitis. Osteomyelitis is an infectious process of the bone and its marrow. The term can refer to infections caused by pyogenic microorganisms but also can be used to describe other sources of infection, such as tuberculosis, or specific fungal infections (mycotic osteomyelitis), parasitic infections (hydatid disease), viral infections, or syphilitic infections (Charcot arthropathy).

Hematogenous spread from a primary source of infection is the most common route of infection. The pyogenic form usually results from a pelvic inflammatory disease but may be the result of spread from the skin or from pulmonary sites. Infection also can result from surgery, a penetrating wound, or poor dental hygiene.

The tuberculosis infection spreads to bone from the lungs or urinary tract. The proximal tibia is the most common site. Osteomyelitis may produce a fever or an abnormality in white blood cell count.

> ### Clinical Pearl
>
> The most common clinical finding in patients with osteomyelitis is constant pain with marked tenderness over the involved bone.

Neoplastic Disease

Benign Tumors: Osteoblastoma and Osteoid Osteoma. Osteoblastoma and osteoid osteoma are benign bone-forming tumors with similar clinical findings.

▶ Osteoblastoma is a solitary bone neoplasm. It is most common in the vertebrae of children and young adults. Short and flat bones are more commonly affected than the long bones (76.5 percent versus 23.5 percent).[19] In the vertebrae, the body is only rarely affected primarily; usually it is involved only secondarily by tumors extending from other segments of the same or of the nearest vertebra.[19]

▶ Osteoid osteoma is a benign osteoblastic tumor of unknown etiology. It occurs most often in the long bones, although the spine is the location of 10 percent of all osteoid osteomas.[20]

Painful scoliosis is a well-recognized presentation of spinal osteoid osteoma and osteoblastoma and is thought to be caused by pain-provoked muscle spasm on the side of the lesion.[19]

Malignant Tumors. Metastatic disease of the spine is the most frequent neoplastic disorder of the axial skeleton. Malignant tumors can be primary or secondary.

1. *Primary.* Primary tumors include:
    a. *Multiple myeloma.* Myeloma is a plasma cell tumor. It is the most common malignant primary bone tumor. Early in its course, it can easily be overlooked as the cause of back pain. Common presentations of myeloma include bone pain, recurrent or persistent infection, anemia, renal impairment, or a combination of these. Some patients are asymptomatic. Presenting features, which require urgent specialist referral, include:
        (1) Persistent, unexplained backache associated with loss of height and osteoporosis.
        (2) Symptoms suggestive of spinal cord or nerve root compression.
    b. *Chordoma.* Chordomas are rare tumors of notochordal origin representing approximately 5 percent of all malignant tumors of bone.[21] They typically are slow-growing, locally aggressive tumors. Chordomas usually are diagnosed in patients with pain or symptoms caused by compression of the surrounding structures. The clinical presentation initially may be mild in nature, leading to considerable delay in seeking medical attention. Vertebral chordomas involve the spinal cord and nerve roots progressively, resulting in pain, numbness, motor weakness, and, eventually, paralysis.
    c. *Osteosarcoma.* Osteosarcoma is a relatively uncommon malignancy. The peak incidence of osteosarcoma occurs in the second decade, with an additional smaller peak after age 50.[22] These tumors typically arise in the metaphyseal regions of long bones, with the rib, distal femur, proximal tibia, and proximal humerus representing the four most common sites. The metaphysis of the vertebra is also predilected.[19] Osteosarcomas frequently penetrate and destroy the cortex of the bone and extend into the surrounding soft tissues.

        The initial clinical symptom of a malignant tumor is frequently pain in the affected area, which also may be associated with localized soft tissue swelling or limitation of motion in the adjacent joint.[23]

2. *Secondary.* Metastases to the spine most commonly arise from breast and lung cancer and from lymphoma.[24,25] Lesions associated with primary tumors from the breast, prostate, kidney, and thyroid, and lesions associated with lymphoma and myeloma account for 75 percent of all spinal metastases.[24,25] When lung cancer is included, the percentage is greater than 90 percent.[26] The clinical findings for a secondary spinal tumor are similar to those of a primary tumor.

Metabolic Disease

Osteoporosis. Osteoporosis can result from insufficient bone formation, excessive bone resorption, or a combination of these two phenomena. The result is decreased bone mineral density (BMD) and a progressive loss of trabecular connectivity that is irreversible and diminishes the bone quality in terms of its mechanical resistance to deformity under loading.[27]

Osteoporosis has been classified into two broad general types: type 1 (postmenopausal) and type 2 (involutional).[28] Type 2 osteoporosis generally is seen in the older age population and has been referred to as senile osteoporosis.[28]

> ### Clinical Pearl
>
> Women are more prone to develop osteoporosis because of the contribution of the loss of estrogen to accelerated bone loss in the postmenopausal female population.

It has been estimated that 15 percent of postmenopausal Caucasian women in the United States and 35 percent of women older than 65 years have osteoporosis.[28] Further,

50 percent of women older than 50 years have osteopenia of the femoral neck, and 20 percent have osteoporosis at this site.[29] The incidence of hip fracture rises dramatically with age, to 3.4 per 100 in the 65-to-74-year-old age group, and 9.4 per 100 in those older than 85 years.[27]

Numerous risk factors have been identified as contributing to the likelihood that an individual will develop bone loss. Genetics plays a major role, and female gender, positive family history, and racial characteristics associated with Caucasian, Asian, or Hispanic background increase the risk of osteoporosis.[30] Low body weight (less than 85 percent ideal body weight, or less than 127 lb) also has been correlated with the development of osteoporosis.[28]

Modifiable risk factors associated with osteoporosis include early or iatrogenic menopause, pregnancy at an early age, smoking, sedentary lifestyle, alcoholism, low body fat, low calcium intake, high caffeine intake, prolonged bed rest, and anorexia.[28,31,32] Medications such as corticosteroids, some diuretics, and thyroid hormone preparations also can significantly increase bone loss and the risk of osteoporosis.[33,34]

In addition to risk factors for the disease, there are independent risk factors for fractures, including use of medications in elderly patients with central nervous system side effects, balance problems, poor muscle strength, visual impairment, home environmental factors such as stairs, and medical comorbidities that increase the likelihood of falls.[27,31]

The diagnosis of osteoporosis often is first established by the presence of an osteoporotic fracture. However, a physical therapist may treat a patient with an undiagnosed low BMD. These patients have a lowered fracture threshold. It is important to be able to identify this patient type so that safer choices can be made with regard to the types of intervention. At present, the only diagnostic tool available that is within the scope of practice of the physical therapist is the identification of those risk factors previously mentioned.[35]

The specific effects of physical activity on bone health have been investigated in several studies.[32,33,35–39] The conclusions drawn from these studies suggest that there is:

▶ Strong evidence that physical activity early in life contributes to higher peak bone mass.[38]

▶ Some evidence that resistance and high-impact exercise are likely the most beneficial.

▶ Some evidence that high-intensity aerobic exercise (70 to 90 percent of maximal heart rate) may reverse or attenuate BMD loss.

▶ Some evidence that high-load low-repetition routines are more effective at increasing BMD than low-load high-repetition regimens.

Exercise during the middle years of life has numerous health benefits, but there are few studies of the effects of exercise on BMD.[38] Exercise during the later years, in the presence of adequate calcium and vitamin D intake, probably has a modest effect on slowing the decline in BMD, but it is clear that exercise late in life, even beyond age 90 years, can increase muscle mass and strength twofold or more in frail persons.[38]

Randomized clinical trials of exercise have been shown to reduce the risk of falls by approximately 25 percent,[40,41] but there is no experimental evidence that exercise affects fracture rates.[38] It also is possible that regular exercisers might fall differently, thereby reducing the risk of fracture caused by falls, but this hypothesis requires testing.[38]

The availability of new, effective drug therapies in the past decade has revolutionized the intervention for osteoporosis, and it is important that clinicians at least be aware of the intervention options.

Diagnostic tools have focused on bone density. New minimally invasive procedures are finding a place among interventions for patients with osteoporotic fractures. The use of injected hydroxyapatite cements into distal radius fractures for percutaneous stabilization has shown efficacy as an intervention for patients with these fractures.[42]

> ### Clinical Pearl
>
> It should be the responsibility of health care providers to educate their young female patients about the benefits of sufficient exercise, and the recommended dietary calcium intake to build healthy bone.

What we know about prevention is that a key factor in the development of osteoporosis in later life is a deficient level of peak bone mass at physical maturity,[43] and that physical activity and calcium intake play substantial roles in the development of bone mass during these developmental years.[44]

Osteomalacia. Osteomalacia is the least common of the traditional forms of metabolic bone disease. It is characterized by impairment of bone mineralization, leading to accumulation of unmineralized matrix or osteoid in the skeleton.[45] Among the causes of osteomalacia, the most important are disorders of vitamin D availability, synthesis, or action.[46]

Clinically, osteomalacia is manifested by progressive generalized bone pain, muscle weakness, hypocalcemia, and pseudofractures. In its late stages, osteomalacia is characterized by a waddling gait.[47] Osteomalacia is believed to be rare in the United States because of the routine fortification of milk and a few other foods with vitamin D. However, patients with various gastrointestinal diseases are known to be at risk.[47]

Paget's Disease. Paget's disease (osteitis deformans) of the bone is an osteometabolic disorder. The disease is described as a focal disorder of accelerated skeletal remodeling that may affect one or more bones. This remodeling produces a slowly progressive enlargement and deformity of multiple bones.

Despite intensive studies and widespread interest, the etiology of Paget's disease remains obscure. The pathologic process consists of three phases:

▶ *Phase I:* an osteolytic phase characterized by prominent bone resorption and hypervascularization.

▶ *Phase II:* a sclerotic phase, reflecting previously increased bone formation, but currently decreased cellular activity and vascularity.

▶ *Phase III:* a mixed phase, with both active bone resorption and compensatory bone formation, resulting in a disorganized skeletal architecture. The bones become spongelike, weakened, and deformed.

Complications include pathologic fractures, delayed union, progressive skeletal deformities, chronic bone pain, neurologic compromise of the peripheral and central nervous systems with facial or ocular nerve compression and spinal stenosis, and pagetic arthritis.

Involvement of the lumbar spine may produce symptoms of clinical spinal stenosis. Involvement of the cervical and thoracic spine may predispose patients to myelopathy.

Although this disorder may be asymptomatic, when symptoms do occur, they occur insidiously. Paget's disease is managed either medically or surgically.

Spondylolisthesis. Spondylolisthesis usually occurs in the lumbar spine. During the past century, the etiology of spondylolisthesis has been discussed extensively in the literature.[48–62] Newman[57] described five groups represented by this deformity, based on etiology:

1. *Congenital spondylolisthesis.* This condition results from dysplasia of the fifth lumbar and sacral arches and zygapophysial joints.

2. *Isthmic spondylolisthesis.* This condition is caused by a defect in the pars interarticularis, which can be an acute fracture, a stress fracture, or an elongation of the pars.

3. *Degenerative spondylolisthesis.* This condition occurs as a result of disk and zygapophysial joint degeneration. Degenerative spondylolisthesis usually affects older people and occurs most commonly at L4 to L5. The slip occurs because of arthritis in the zygapophysial joint, with loss of the ligamentous support. The zygapophysial joints sustain approximately 33 percent of the static compression load on the lumbar motion segment and dynamically as much as 33 percent of the axial load, depending on spine position.[63]

4. *Traumatic spondylolisthesis.* This condition occurs with a fracture or acute dislocation of the zygapophysial joint. It is fairly rare.

5. *Pathologic spondylolisthesis.* This condition may result from a systemic disease causing a weakening of the pars, pedicle, or zygapophysial joint, or from a local condition such as a tumor.

Spondylolisthesis aquisita, a sixth etiologic category, was added to represent the slip caused by the surgical disruption of ligaments, bone, and disk.

Clinically, these patients complain of low back pain that is mechanical in nature. Mechanical pain is worsened with activity and alleviated with rest. Patients also may complain of leg pain, which can have a radicular type pattern or, more commonly, will manifest as neurogenic claudication. If neurogenic claudication is present, the patient may complain of bilateral thigh and leg tiredness, aches, and fatigue.[53] Questions regarding bicycle use versus walking can help the clinician to differentiate neurogenic from vascular claudication. Both cycling and walking increase symptoms in vascular claudication due to the increased demand for blood supply. However, patients with neurogenic claudication worsen with walking but are unaffected by cycling due to the differing positions of the lumbar spine adopted in each of these activities. Patients with neurogenic claudication are far more comfortable leaning forward or sitting, which flexes the spine, than walking.[59] The position of forward flexion increases the anteroposterior diameter of the canal, which allows a greater volume of the neural elements and improves the microcirculation.

Range of motion for flexion of the lumbar spine frequently is normal with both types of claudication. Some patients are able to touch their toes without difficulty. Strength is usually intact in the lower extremities. Sensation also is usually intact. A check of distal pulses is important to rule out any coexisting vascular insufficiency. Findings such as hairless lower extremities, coldness of the feet, or absent pulses are signs of peripheral vascular disease. Sensory defects in a stocking-glove distribution are more suggestive of diabetic neuropathy. The deep tendon reflexes generally will be normal or diminished. If hyperreflexic symptoms and other upper motor neuron signs, such as clonus or a positive Babinski test, are found, the cervical, thoracic, and lumbar spine should be investigated to rule out a lesion of the spinal cord or cauda equina.

Differential diagnosis includes coexisting osteoarthritis of the hip, myelopathy, spinal tumors, and infections.

Generalized Body Pain

When discussing the issue of differential diagnosis with generalized body pain, it is well worth mentioning two conditions: fibromyalgia, and myofascial pain syndrome. Although these conditions share several features, they are distinct entities whose physical findings and interventions differ significantly.[64]

Fibromyalgia

Primary fibromyalgia is a common, but poorly understood, complex of generalized body aches that can cause pain or paresthesias, or both, in a nonradicular pattern.[65] Fibromyalgia was first described in 1904[66] as a pathologic state.[67] However, fibromyalgia is not a disease, but rather a syndrome with a common set of characteristic symptoms, including widespread pain and the presence of a defined number of tender points.[68]

The relationship of tender points to fibromyalgia has been the focus of much research[69–72] and, according, to the criteria of the American College of Rheumatology, a positive tender point is defined as a point that becomes painful (not merely tender) when approximately 4 kg of pressure is applied.[73] A positive tender point count of 11 or more of 18 standardized sites, when present in combination with the history of widespread pain, yields a sensitivity of 88.4 percent and a specificity of 81.1 percent in the diagnosis of fibromyalgia.

Tender points are the single most powerful way to discriminate patients with fibromyalgia from controls with other painful conditions.[73] The pathology and pathophysiology of the tender point remain elusive, and it has been hypothesized that the myalgias may result from neurohumeral changes rather than local metabolic or pathophysiologic features.[74] Prevalence of fibromyalgia is about 10 to 20 times greater in women than in men, although the reason for this is unknown. Sleep is usually poor, and sleep studies show stage 4 sleep is the most interrupted; however, sleep disturbances are common in the general population and not endemic to fibromyalgia patients.[75]

A multifaceted approach involving cardiovascular fitness training, spray and stretch, strength and endurance training, massage, and electrotherapeutic and physical modalities, including microstimulation, may help to reduce some of the disease consequences.[76]

Myofascial Pain Syndrome

Myofascial pain syndrome (MPS) often manifests with symptoms suggestive of neurologic disorders, including diffuse pain and tenderness, headache, vertigo, visual disturbances, paresthesias, incoordination, and referred pain that often can be clarified by the musculoskeletal and neurologic examination.[77] MPS is characterized by the presence of myofascial trigger points (MTrPs).[67,78–81] MPS should always be considered as a diagnosis in the presence of persistent pain.[80,82–86]

An MTrP is a hyperirritable location, approximately 2 to 5 cm in diameter,[87] within a taut band of muscle fibers that is painful when compressed and that can give rise to characteristic referred pain, tenderness, and tightness[83] (Box 9-1). The patient's reaction to firm palpation of the MTrP is a distinguishing characteristic of MPS and is termed a *positive jump sign*.[84] This reaction may include withdrawal, wrinkling of the face, or a verbal response. This hyperirritability appears to be a result of sensitization of the chemonociceptors and mechanonociceptors located within the muscle.

Clinical Pearl

Some confusion exists as to the difference between trigger points and tender points. Although MTrPs can occur in the same sites as the tender points of fibromyalgia, MTrPs can cause referral of pain in a distinct and characteristic area, remote from the trigger point site, not necessarily in a dermatomal distribution[78] (Table 9-8). Referred pain is, by definition, absent in the tender points of fibromyalgia.[73,81]

Healthy muscles do not contain trigger points, are not tender to firm palpation, and do not refer pain.

MTrPs are thought to begin after a microtrauma or macrotrauma, or a sustained muscle contraction from a postural dysfunction, which can become a site of sensitized nerves with altered metabolism.[88] Stimulation of these receptors can cause[79,89]:

Box 9-1 CLASSIFICATION OF TRIGGER POINTS[79]

- *Active trigger points* are those that are symptomatic with respect to pain, and refer a pattern of pain at rest or during motion (or both) that is specific for that muscle.[87a] An active trigger point usually produces restricted range of motion and a visible or palpable local twitch response during mechanical stimulation of the myofascial trigger point (MTrP),[78–80] but failure to elicit this response does not exclude myofascial pain syndrome.[78] MTrPs are always tender and cause muscle weakness.
- *Latent trigger points*, which represent the majority of trigger points, are usually asymptomatic but may have all the other clinical characteristics of active trigger points.[87a]
- *Associated trigger points* develop in response to compensatory overload, shortened range of motion, or referred phenomena caused by trigger point activity in another muscle.[87a] There are two kinds of such trigger points[79]:
  - *Satellite trigger points* are in the zone of referral of another muscle.
  - *Secondary trigger points* are activated because the muscle was overloaded as a synergist or an antagonist of a muscle harboring a primary trigger point.[87a]

▶ *Localized ischemia.* Ischemia to the nerves and muscles results in a bombardment of the nervous system with abnormal impulses, creating hyperalgesia in the segmentally related muscles and referral zones.[85,89,90]

▶ *Edema.*

▶ *Fibrosis.*

▶ *Temperature changes.*

▶ Focal or regional autonomic dysfunction, including localized vasoconstriction, persistent hyperemia after palpation, diaphoresis, lacrimation, salivation, and pilomotor activity.

Thus, MTrPs are typically located in areas that are prone to increased mechanical strain or impaired circulation (e.g., upper trapezius, levator scapulae, infraspinatus, quadratus lumborum, and gluteus minimus). As with all chronic pain conditions, concomitant social, behavioral, and psychological disturbances often precede or follow their development.[91,92]

Whatever the etiologic factors, it would appear that the development of MTrPs may be a progressive process, with a stage of neuromuscular dysfunction of muscle hyperactivity and irritability that is sustained by numerous perpetuating factors and then followed by a stage of organic dystrophic changes in the muscle bands with MTrPs.[84]

TABLE 9-8   Muscles Most Likely to Refer Pain to a Given Area[79]

Location	Potential Muscles Involved
Chest pain	Pectoralis major
	Pectoralis minor
	Scaleni
	Sternocleidomastoid (sternal)
	Sternalis
	Iliocostalis cervicis
	Subclavius
	External abdominal oblique
Side of chest pain	Serratus anterior
	Latissimus
Abdominal pain	Rectus abdominis
	External abdominal oblique
	Transversus abdominis
	Iliocostalis thoracis
	Multifidi
	Quadratus lumborum
	Pyramidalis
Low thoracic back pain	Iliocostalis thoracis
	Multifidi
	Serratus posterior inferior
	Rectus abdominis
	Latissimus dorsi
Lumbar pain	Gluteus medius
	Multifidi
	Iliopsoas
	Longissimus thoracis
	Iliocostalis lumborum
	Iliocostalis thoracis
	Rectus abdominis
Pelvic pain	Coccygeus
	Levator ani
	Obturator internus
	Adductor magnus
	Piriformis
	Obliquus internus abdominis
Buttock pain	Gluteus medius
	Quadratus lumborum
	Gluteus maximus
	Iliocostalis lumborum
	Longissimus thoracis
	Semitendinosus
	Semimembranosus
	Piriformis
	Gluteus minimus
	Rectus abdominis

MTrPs, which can give rise to both referred pain and autonomic phenomena, are classified as either active or latent. Active MTrPs are believed to cause pain, whereas latent trigger points are said to restrict range of motion and produce weakness of the affected muscle, with the patient unaware of the tender area until the examination.[88] Latent trigger points can persist for years after a patient recovers from an injury and may become active and create acute pain in response to minor overstretching, overuse, or chilling of the muscle.[79,93]

According to Simons,[94] the diagnosis of MPS can be made if five major criteria and at least one out of three minor criteria are met. The major criteria are:

1. Localized spontaneous pain.

2. Spontaneous pain or altered sensations in the expected referred pain area for a given trigger point.

3. Presence of a taut palpable band in an accessible muscle.

4. Exquisite localized tenderness in a precise point along the taut band.

5. Some degree of reduced range of movement when measurable.

Minor criteria include:

1. Reproduction of spontaneously perceived pain and altered sensations by pressure on the trigger point.

2. Elicitation of a local twitch response of muscular fibers by "transverse" snapping palpation, or by needle insertion into the trigger point.

3. Pain relieved by muscle stretching or injection of the trigger point.

The conservative intervention for MPS is described in Chapter 11.

Pain Related to Specific Regions

Causes of Head and Facial Pain

The causes of head and facial pain include, but are not limited to, those listed in Table 9-9.

Trauma

Head pain is common following trauma to the head and neck. The traumatic episodes that do not produce profound neurologic damage are termed *concussions* (contusions). Concussion is not always associated with some degree of loss of consciousness and typically involves a sudden acceleration (or deceleration) force, which causes the brain to move suddenly within the skull. For a loss of consciousness to occur, these forces must disconnect the alerting system in the brain stem, resulting in a temporary lack of activity in the reticular formation, probably secondary to hypoxia resulting from induced ischemia.[95] It is estimated that a velocity of only 20 mph can

TABLE 9-9 Potential Causes of Head and Facial Pain

Trauma
Headache
Occipital neuralgia
Osteoarthritis
Rheumatoid arthritis and related rheumatoid arthritis variants (dermatomyositis, temporal arteritis)
Lyme disease
Fibromyalgia
Arteriovenous malformation
Intracranial infection (meningitis)
Cerebrovascular disease
Tumor
Encephalitis
Systemic infections
Multiple sclerosis
Miscellaneous

cause concussion from inertial loading (no head impact) in most healthy adults.[96]

Headache

Headaches are a common complaint. Approximately 85 to 95 percent of the adult population in the United States experience a headache during a given 1-year period,[97] although only 1.7 to 2.5 percent of patients visit the emergency department for a complaint of headache,[98] with most choosing to treat themselves with over-the-counter medications.[99,100]

Headaches, in general, can be grouped into two main divisions: benign or nonbenign (see Table 8-14), and primary or secondary. Primary headaches are the result of some underlying structural abnormality, or disease process, whereas secondary headaches are the result of an underlying pathologic process.[101] The origin of benign headaches can vary. Common causes include neurologic (trigeminal neuralgia, cervical neuralgia, atypical facial pain, post-traumatic, post–lumbar puncture), musculoskeletal (tension headache, occipital headache, cervicogenic headache), and vascular (migraine, cluster, hypertension).[102,103] Other headaches, such as chronic daily and rebound, are thought to be related to a combination of neurologic and musculoskeletal causes. Osteoarthritis, rheumatoid arthritis, and related rheumatoid arthritis variants (dermatomyositis, temporal arteritis), Lyme disease, fibromyalgia, and reflex sympathetic dystrophy also have been indicated as additional sources of head and neck pain.[103] Diseases of the sinus (maxillary sinusitis, frontal sinusitis, or malignancy), diseases of the eye (inflammation of the iris, glaucoma), and infection and inflammation of the ear apparatus also may cause headaches.[102,104] Sensitivity to tapping over the sinuses is fairly diagnostic for sinusitis, whereas diminished vision is characteristic of glaucoma.[102,104]

Migraine Headache. Migraines are equally distributed among the sexes in childhood, but two out of every three adults with migraine headaches are women.[103] According to the International Headache Society,[105] there are two types of migraine headaches: migraine without aura (common migraine), and migraine with aura. The migraine without aura type involves episodes lasting 4 to 72 hours, and symptoms are typically unilateral and with a pulsating quality of moderate or severe intensity, which is thought to result from a change in the blood vessels of the brain. This type of headache is aggravated by routine physical activity and is associated with nausea, auras, photophobia, and phonophobia.

The migraine with aura type is characterized by reversible aura symptoms, which typically develop gradually over more than 4 minutes, but last no longer than 60 minutes.[105]

It is thought that migraine headaches are a different expression of a common underlying problem.[103] As with cluster headaches, it has long been recognized that migraine headaches are exacerbated by disturbances or irregularities in sleep patterns.[101]

Cluster Headache. Cluster headaches are severe, unilateral, retro-orbital headaches. This type of headache is more common in men than women. As their name suggests, cluster headaches occur in groups or clusters, and they tend to occur at predictable times of day. Cluster headaches also may develop because of specific sleep disorders, such as sleep apnea, bruxism, or sleep deprivation.[101]

Cluster headaches are often accompanied by nasal congestion, eyelid edema, rhinorrhea, miosis, lacrimation, and ptosis (drooping eyelid) on the symptomatic side.[101] These headaches can last from 15 to 180 minutes if untreated.[105]

Unlike migraine sufferers, who feel obliged to lie down during a severe headache, individuals with cluster headaches feel better during a headache by remaining in an erect posture and moving about.[103] Cluster headaches are thought to result from vasodilation in branches of the external carotid artery, because they often are triggered by vasodilating substances, such as nitroglycerine and alcohol.[106]

Tension-type Headache. The term *tension-type headache* is designated by the International Headache Society to describe what was previously called *tension headache,* muscle contraction headache, psychomyogenic headache, stress headache, ordinary headache, and psychogenic headache.[105] The International Headache Society distinguishes between the episodic and the chronic varieties of tension-type headaches, and divides them into two groups: those associated with a disorder of the pericranial muscles, and those not associated with this type of disorder.[105]

Tension headaches, which constitute up to 70 percent of headaches and which occur more often in women than in men, are thought to result from emotional stress.[103,107] They are characterized by a bilateral, non-throbbing ache in the frontal or temporal areas, and spasm or hypertonus of the neck muscles.[106] Unlike migraine headaches, tension-type headache is typically relieved by physical activity and usually responds well to soft tissue and specific traction techniques.

Benign Exertional Headache. Benign exertional headache (BEH) has been recognized as a separate entity for more than 70 years.[108] Characteristic features of BEH include[109]:

▶ Headache that is specifically brought on by physical exercise, particularly with straining and Valsalva-type maneuvers, such as those seen in weightlifting.

▶ Bilateral and throbbing at onset and may develop migrainous features in patients susceptible to migraine.

▶ Duration of 5 minutes to 24 hours.

▶ Prevented by avoiding excessive exertion.

▶ Not associated with any systemic or intracranial disorder.

Clearly, the major differential diagnosis to be considered in this situation would be a subarachnoid hemorrhage, which needs to be excluded by the appropriate investigations.

Effort-induced Headache. Effort headaches have been reported to be the most common type of headache in athletes.[110] These headaches differ from BEH in that they are not necessarily associated with a power or straining type of exercise. The clinical features of this effort headache syndrome include[109]:

▶ An onset of mild to severe headache with aerobic-type exercise.

▶ More frequent in hot weather.

▶ Vascular-type headache (i.e., throbbing).

▶ Short duration of headache (4 to 6 hours).

▶ Provoking exercise may be maximal or submaximal.

▶ Patient may have prodromal "migrainous" symptoms.

▶ Headache tends to recur in individuals with exercise.

▶ Patient may have a past history of migraine.

▶ Norm neurological examination and investigations.

Occipital Headache. The occipital headache is felt by many clinicians to be referred pain from a cervical disorder,[111–113] especially when cervical traction temporarily decreases the headache pain.[103]

The underlying musculoskeletal mechanism for this type of headache is often structural, including cervical hypomobility or hypermobility, joint subluxation, degenerative bony changes, or poor posture. Postures, movements, or activities that put strain on the neck have been associated with headaches.[114] In one study,[115] 51 percent of patients associated their headaches with particular sustained neck flexion during reading, studying, typing, or driving a car. Sixty-five percent of headache patients reported a chronic course lasting between 2 and 20 years, and only 7 percent reported pain of less than one week's duration.[115]

The general misunderstanding is that there is no cervical sensory reference to the head area, because the C1 dorsal ramus has no sensory component, and that only the trigeminal nerve has sensory input to the vertex and frontal regions. In fact, there is considerable sensory input into the C1 root, but not from a cutaneous source (see "Occipital Neuralgia," later).[116] Experiments have confirmed a close trigeminocervical relationship.[117,118] Because the head and neck comprise one functional unit, cervical musculoskeletal disorders can refer as headache, temporomandibular, or facial pain—with or without neck pain.[119] Cervical headaches are described in more detail in Chapter 23.

Hypertension Headache. Hypertension headaches usually occur in individuals with diastolic readings above 120 mm Hg, although the intensity of these headaches does not necessarily parallel the height of the blood pressure levels.[120] Typically, the headache begins in the early morning, reaches a peak upon awakening, and then diminishes once the patient rises and begins daily activity.[102] The headache usually is described as a nonlocalized, dull, and throbbing ache that is aggravated by activities that increase blood pressure, such as bending, coughing, or exertion.[104] The distribution of the headache can vary and may extend over the entire cranium.[102]

External Compression Headache. This entity, formerly known as *swim-goggle headache,* manifests with pain in the facial and temporal areas that results from wearing excessively tight face masks or swimming goggles.[109,121] It is commonly seen in swimmers and divers. The etiology is believed to be related to continuous stimulation of cutaneous nerves by the application of pressure, although neuralgia of the supraorbital nerve also has been implicated.[109]

Idiopathic Carotidynia Headache.[122] Idiopathic carotidynia is associated with unilateral facial or orbital pain in half of the patients with this condition. The pain remains isolated in about 10 percent of patients, but usually there is an ipsilateral headache. The characteristic unilateral headache is most commonly located in the frontotemporal area, but it occasionally involves the entire hemicranium or the occipital area. The onset of headache is usually gradual, but it may be an instantaneous, excruciating, "thunderclap" headache that mimics a subarachnoid hemorrhage. The headache is most commonly described as a constant steady aching, but it may also be throbbing or steady and sharp. About one fourth of patients with a history of migraine consider the headache to resemble a migraine, but most patients consider the headache or facial pain to be unlike any other such pain. The median interval between the onset of neck pain and the appearance of other symptoms is 2 weeks, whereas other symptoms occur only 15 hours after the onset of headache.

Chronic Daily Headache. Chronic daily headaches, following trauma to the head or neck, are a common occurrence,[123] with the duration of these headaches unrelated to the severity or type of trauma.[124,125] These headaches typically consist of a group of disorders that can be subclassified into primary and secondary types.[126]

▶ The primary chronic daily headache disorders include transformed migraine, chronic tension-type headache, new daily persistent headache, and hemicrania continua. This type of headache is defined as a constant tension headache with migrainous exacerbations.[127,128]

▶ The secondary chronic daily headaches include cervical spine disorders, headache associated with vascular disorders, and nonvascular intracranial disorders.

Chronic daily headache usually evolves over time from episodic migraine, but the cause is still controversial. Individuals suffering from chronic daily headache often suffer from rebound headache as well. Rebound headache is the worsening of head pain in chronic headache sufferers. It is caused by the frequent and excessive use of nonnarcotic analgesics.[129] Several studies have demonstrated that as many as three quarters of patients with chronic daily headache suffer from drug-induced rebound headache.[130,131]

The role of trauma in chronic daily headaches, however, may be understated. Tension headaches may well initiate a headache in patients predisposed by some previous and forgotten traumatic incident.

Post-traumatic Headache. In addition to the immediate pain following a head injury, post-traumatic headache, a more prolonged and enduring headache, may develop.[132] This condition, resembling either migraine or tension-type headache, may last for weeks, months, or years. It also may be associated with post-traumatic syndrome, which includes a variety of symptoms, such as irritability, insomnia, anxiety, seizure, amnesia, depression, and reduced ability to concentrate.[132]

The more serious causes of headache associated with trauma include subdural hematoma, epidural hematoma, intracerebral hematoma, aneurysm, subarachnoid hemorrhage, or cerebral contusion.

The clinician should attempt to establish the overall health of the patient through a review of systems[106]:

▶ *Nervous system.* The physical examination of the nervous system can include sensory and motor testing of the cranial and spinal nerves, reflex testing, and an examination of gait, balance, and coordination. The need for such testing often can be determined through the presence of the signs and symptoms outlined in Table 8-14.

▶ *Cardiovascular system.* Fluctuations in blood pressure often are associated with headaches.

▶ *Endocrine system.* Headaches may be associated with hormonal changes and hormonal replacement therapy.[133]

▶ *Musculoskeletal system.* An examination must be made of the middle and upper cervical segments, and the temporomandibular joint. In addition, a thorough postural examination should be performed to assess for muscle imbalances and overall alignment. Relative flexibility and strength are assessed during upper limb movements. Finally, the clinician should examine for MTrPs and the presence of adverse neural tension (see Chap. 12).

Occipital Neuralgia

Occipital neuralgia is a rare neuralgic disorder that involves the greater occipital nerve.[134] The greater occipital nerve originates from the second cervical root (C2). Occipital neuralgia is a headache syndrome that is characterized by occipital and sub-occipital headache that may radiate to the frontal, periorbital, retro-orbital, maxillary, and mandibular regions.[135] It also may be associated with neck pain, dizziness, paresthesias, or hyperesthesia of the posterior scalp, and loss of the normal cervical lordosis. Occipital neuralgia is more common in women than men.[136] The pain usually awakens the patient from sleep in the morning but may occur at any time of day.[136] The causes of occipital neuralgia include:

▶ Scalp trauma from a direct blow.

▶ Compression neuropathy.

▶ Sustained contraction (spasm) of the posterior neck muscles,[134] especially the semispinalis capitis, obliquus capitis inferior, and trapezius muscles.[137]

▶ Hyperextension injury and resultant compression of the ganglion and root of C2.

▶ Fracture of the atlas or axis.

▶ Gout.

▶ Mastoiditis.

▶ Osteoarthritis of the craniovertebral joints.

Diagnosis usually is made using palpation over the greater occipital nerve as it passes the superior nuchal line.

The intervention for patients with occipital neuralgia involves infiltrating the nerve with a mixture of local anesthetic and corticosteroid.[137]

Glossopharyngeal Neuralgia

The cause of glossopharyngeal neuralgia is at present unknown, although most authors place the site of disturbance in the region of the posterior root[138,139] or in the spinal tract of the nerve.[140] Glossopharyngeal neuralgia is characterized by intense unilateral attacks of pain in the retrolingual area, radiating to the depth of the ear.[104] The pain typically is aggravated by movement or contact with the pharynx, especially with swallowing.

Trigeminal Neuralgia

Trigeminal neuralgia (TN), or tic douloureux, is a severe chronic pain syndrome characterized by dramatic, brief stabbing or electric shock-like pain paroxysms felt in one or more divisions of the trigeminal distribution, either spontaneously or on gentle tactile stimulation of a trigger point on the face or in the oral cavity.[140a] It is unclear whether TN is a neuropathic pain state of the central or peripheral nervous system.

Bell's Palsy

Bell's palsy is a lower motor neuron disease of the facial nerve characterized by a wide range of facial muscle movement dysfunction from mild paresis to total paralysis. Individual patients display a spectrum of symptoms: some maintain reduced movement throughout the course of the disorder while others rapidly become totally paralyzed over a 24-hour period. Bell's palsy is the most common form of facial paralysis, with an incidence of 20 to 30 per 100,000 persons.[141] The diagnosis is established by the exclusion of several localized lesions, such as temporal bone fracture, acoustic neuroma, suppuration or tumor of the middle ear, and disorders of the parotid gland.[142]

Bell's palsy induces a wide range of facial muscle movement dysfunction, from mild paresis to total paralysis. Fundamental to management issues of this disorder is the question of its etiology, once thought to be idiopathic. Two recent independent studies[143,144] strongly support the concept that the facial paralysis associated with Bell's palsy is the result of a viral inflammatory response that induces edema and ischemia of the facial nerve as it passes through its bony canal. The infectious agents associated with Bell's palsy are herpes simplex virus type 1, varicella-zoster virus, and the spirochete *Borrelia burgdorferi,* the causative organism of Lyme disease.[145]

The intervention for this condition is empiric, varying from observation alone to the use of corticosteroids, electric stimulation, surgical decompression, and antiviral agents. Transcranial magnetic stimulation of the facial nerve also has been reported to be useful.[146]

Healing is occasionally incomplete, resulting in residual nerve dysfunction, including partial palsy and motor synkinesis (involuntary movement accompanying a voluntary one) and autonomic synkinesis (involuntary lacrimation after a voluntary muscle movement). On the basis of the study of Peitersen,[146a] all patients regain some function, and 85% of all patients will regain normal or very near normal function within 6–8 weeks.

Surgical management of Bell's palsy has been controversial since its inception because of the following points: issues of patient selection criteria based on electrodiagnostic studies; site of decompression; limited number of patients who require decompression at any single center; and the inability to transfer results from study to study because of the continued use of independent facial function grading systems.[147,148]

Ramsay Hunt Syndrome

Ramsay Hunt syndrome, a herpetic inflammation of the geniculate or facial nerve ganglia, or both, manifests as a peripheral facial nerve palsy accompanied by an erythematous vesicular rash on the ear (zoster oticus) or in the mouth.[149] It is the second most common cause of atraumatic peripheral facial paralysis. Other frequent symptoms and signs can include tinnitus, hearing loss, nausea, vomiting, vertigo, and nystagmus.

Compared with Bell's palsy, patients with Ramsay Hunt syndrome often have more severe paralysis at onset and are less likely to recover completely.

The intervention for Ramsay Hunt syndrome can involve medication. Prednisone and acyclovir may improve outcome, although a prospective randomized treatment trial remains to be undertaken.[149]

Arteriovenous Malformation

This congenital malformation may manifest with an abrupt onset of head and facial pain.

Meningitis

The brain is protected from infection by the skull, pia, arachnoid, and dural meninges covering its surface, and by the blood-brain barrier. When any of these defenses are broached by a pathogen, infection of the meninges and subarachnoid space can occur, resulting in meningitis.[150]

Rigidity of the neck can occur with neuralgia, and with other irritative lesions of the meninges, such as meningitis.[151]

Since the fifth century BC, the seriousness of infectious meningitis has been recognized.[152] In the 20th century, the annual incidence of bacterial meningitis ranges from approximately 3 per 100,000 population in the United States[153] to 500 per 100,000 in the so-called meningitis belt of Africa.[154]

Predisposing factors for the development of community-acquired meningitis include preexisting diabetes mellitus, otitis media, pneumonia, sinusitis, and alcohol abuse.[155]

The clinical features of meningitis reflect the underlying pathophysiologic processes.[151] The blood-brain barrier is breached, and an inflammatory response within the cerebrospinal fluid occurs. The resultant meningeal inflammation and irritation elicit a protective reflex to prevent stretching of the inflamed and hypersensitive nerve roots, which is detectable clinically as neck stiffness (Kernig or Brudzinski sign).[156,157] The meningeal inflammation also may cause a generalized headache, cranial nerve palsies, vomiting, and nausea.[158] If the inflammatory process progresses to cerebral vasculitis or causes cerebral edema and elevated intracranial pressure, alterations in mental status, headache, vomiting, seizures, and cranial nerve palsies may ensue.[150]

Despite classic descriptions of meningeal signs, and sweeping statements about its clinical presentation, the signs and symptoms of meningitis have been inadequately studied.[151] Based on the limited studies, the following points should be remembered during the examination[151]:

▶ The absence of all three signs of the classic triad of fever, neck stiffness, and an altered mental status virtually eliminates a diagnosis of meningitis. Fever is the most sensitive of the classic triad of signs, and occurs in a majority of patients, with neck stiffness the next most sensitive sign. Alterations in mental status also have a relatively high sensitivity, indicating that normal mental status helps to exclude meningitis in low-risk patients. Changes in mental status are more common in bacterial than viral meningitis.

▶ Among the signs of meningeal irritation, Kernig and Brudzinski signs appear to have low sensitivity but high specificity.

Cerebrovascular Disease

The frequency of headache with cerebrovascular disease is dependent on the size and location of the hemorrhage. Small hemorrhages may occur without an associated headache. The headache may be the presenting symptom of cerebrovascular disease, and associated neurological changes are likely. These could include, but are not limited to, loss of the ability to sit, stand, and walk; right- or left-sided weakness; visual disturbances; aphasia; apraxia; dysphasia; seizures; and mental status changes.

Intracranial Bleeding

Depending on the rate of arterial or venous bleeding, signs of intracranial bleeding may take minutes to days. A meningeal artery or branch laceration with an associated overlying skull fracture is a frequent source of delayed epidural bleeding.[159] However, venous bleeding also is associated with delayed and chronic hematomas by nature of the low pressure and slow rate of bleeding.[159] Other causes of low-tension hemorrhages are small dural lesions or diffuse cerebral contusion sites.

A subarachnoid hemorrhage can be the cause of head, facial, orbital, or neck pain. The pain, which is usually severe, may occur in one region or over all of the areas. Neck stiffness and pain on movement are common findings and often are associated with nausea and vomiting. Other possible findings include:

▶ Upper motor neuron signs and symptoms (Babinski, clonus, hyperreflexia, ataxia, and so on).

▶ Photophobia.

▶ Motor or sensory disturbances.

▶ Syncope.

▶ Somnolence and lethargy.

▶ Seizures.

▶ Visual disturbances.

▶ Dysphasia.

Patients with intracranial bleeding usually prefer to remain still with their eyes closed. Often they become disoriented and demonstrate judgment and memory abnormalities.

Tumors

A complete discussion of each type of brain tumor is beyond the scope of this text. Tumors of the brain may be classified according to type, as follows:

▶ *Astrocytomas.* Astrocytomas are benign brain tumors. Glioblastoma multiforme, a type of astrocytoma, is the most common adult brain neoplasm.

▶ *Oligodendrogliomas.* These are benign primary brain tumors that arise from oligodendrocytes.

▶ *Meningiomas.* These tumors are slow growing and benign, and comprise about 20 percent of all intracranial tumors in adults.

▶ *Metastatic tumors.* These are tumors that originate from tissues outside of the brain. They can occur as single or multiple tumors.

The term *benign* is misleading when referring to brain tumors. Although benign may mean curable, this is not always true with brain tumors. Tumors, benign or otherwise, are space-occupying lesions that may increase to a size that compresses nearby structures or increases intracranial pressure. Patients with tumors of the brain may present acutely with the following symptoms:

▶ Abrupt onset of severe headache.

▶ Facial pain.

▶ Episodes of loss of consciousness.

▶ Changes in mental status.

▶ Nausea and vomiting.

▶ Focal neurologic signs and symptoms.

▶ Neck stiffness or pain.

Encephalitis

Encephalitis is an inflammation of the brain. The inflammation may be caused by an arthropod-borne virus, or it may occur as a sequela of influenza, measles, German measles, chickenpox, herpes simplex, or other infectious diseases. Clinical findings include:

▶ Signs of meningeal irritation (Kernig or Brudzinski sign).

▶ Changes in mental status.

▶ Signs of increased intracranial pressure, including increased restlessness, vomiting, seizures, and pupil irregularities.

▶ Behavioral changes.

Systemic Infections

Systemic infections that are capable of provoking head or facial pain include Rocky Mountain spotted fever, Lyme disease, pneumonia, and pyelonephritis.

Rocky Mountain Spotted Fever. This condition begins abruptly with a high fever and bilateral frontal or frontotemporal headache. The classic rash begins on the distal aspects of the extremities and spreads proximally. Serologic tests are required to confirm the diagnosis.

Lyme Disease.[160] Lyme disease is a bacterial infection that is transmitted to humans by ticks that usually live on mice or deer. Most infections are acquired in three distinct sections of the United States: along the northeast coast, in areas of Wisconsin and Minnesota, and, to a lesser extent, in northern California and southern Oregon. People who hike, camp, or live in or near wooded areas in these locations during summer months are most at risk for Lyme disease. Following a bite from a deer tick, a red bump may occur at the site of the bite. If the tick is infected, a larger rash may form around the bite. The classic description of the rash is an enlarging area of redness with partial central clearing. However, it may take several days before the lesion expands enough to have the classic appearance.

The most common signs and symptoms associated with the rash are nonspecific flulike symptoms, including myalgia, arthralgias, fever, joint pain and swelling, headache, fatigue, motor or sensory radiculoneuritis, mononeuritis multiplex, or neck stiffness.[161]

Cardiac symptoms can include fluctuating degrees of atrioventricular block, occasionally acute myopericarditis or mild left ventricular dysfunction, and, rarely, cardiomegaly or fatal pancarditis.[161]

The initial diagnosis usually is based on the recognition of the characteristic clinical findings. The culture of *B. burgdorferi* from specimens in Barbour-Stoenner-Kelly medium permits a definitive diagnosis.[161]

Pneumonia.   Patients with pneumonia may present with fever and severe headache.

Pyelonephritis.   Acute pyelonephritis is an inflammation of the kidney and renal pelvis. Clinical signs and symptoms of acute pyelonephritis include fever; shaking chills; thoracolumbar, interscapular, neck, and flank pain; nausea and vomiting; costovertebral angle tenderness; and, less commonly, symptoms of cystitis such as dysuria and increased frequency.[162] In addition, a bifrontal or generalized headache may accompany the neck pain and stiffness.

Multiple Sclerosis

Multiple sclerosis (MS) is a chronic demyelinating disorder with a wide range of clinical manifestations that reflects multifocal areas of central nervous system myelin destruction. In adults, the clinical presentation of MS at onset is characterized by motor system (26.5 percent), sensory system (25 percent), or optic nerve (21 percent) involvement, or a combination of all three.[163] Cerebellar and sphincteric involvement are less frequent (14.1 percent each).[163]

Patients with motor weakness may develop paralysis affecting one or more, or all, limbs. Sensory dysfunction may occur in one modality (e.g., to light touch, temperature, or deep sensation), and may manifest as hypoesthesia/anesthesia or hypersensitivity with numbness, burning sensation, paresthesia, and dysesthesia in various parts of the body.[163] Optic neuritis is associated with a decrease in visual acuity, sometimes resulting in blindness, accompanied by orbital pain when the involved eye moves. Examples of acute or paroxysmal pain include head and facial pain, painful tonic spasms, radicular pain, and dysesthesia.[164] Other manifestations include fatigue, cognitive loss, and mood disturbance.

Most patients with MS (85 percent) have a relapsing-remitting course of disease, with each relapse being associated with new neurologic symptoms or worsening of existing ones. With additional relapses, the possibility of complete recovery is reduced and permanent disability may develop.[163] In the remaining 15 percent of patients, the disease course is primary progressive, with continuous neurologic deterioration.[163]

MS usually manifests between 20 and 40 years of age, with a peak onset at around 30 years and a female-to-male ratio of 2:1. At present, MS is regarded as being modifiable, but incurable.

Miscellaneous Causes

Temporal Arteritis.   This condition is characterized by severe headache, which can begin abruptly or gradually. Associated symptoms may include jaw weakness, scalp tenderness, and visual loss.

Acute Sinusitis.   Sinusitis is an infection or inflammation of the sinuses. Sinuses are hollow air spaces located within the skull or bones of the head surrounding the nose. Each sinus has an opening into the nose for the free exchange of air and mucus, and each is joined with the nasal passages by a continuous mucous membrane lining. Anything that causes a swelling in the nose, such as an infection, an allergic reaction, or an immune reaction, may affect the sinuses. Sinusitis involves an infection or inflammation of one or more of the following:

- ▶ *Frontal sinuses* over the eyes in the brow area.

- ▶ *Maxillary sinuses* inside each cheekbone.

- ▶ *Ethmoid sinuses* just behind the bridge of the nose and between the eyes.

- ▶ *Sphenoid sinuses* behind the ethmoids in the upper region of the nose and behind the eyes.

Air trapped within a blocked sinus, along with pus or other secretions, may cause pressure on the sinus wall and subsequent pain. Similarly, when air is prevented from entering a sinus by a swollen membrane at the opening, a vacuum can be created that also causes pain. The location of the sinus pain depends on which sinus is affected. Symptoms can include:

- ▶ Headache upon awakening in the morning, and tenderness to palpation over the frontal sinuses.

- ▶ Upper jaw, cheek, and tooth pain (maxillary sinuses).

- ▶ Pain and swelling of tear ducts in the corner of the eyes and pain between the eyes and sides of the nose (ethmoid sinuses).

- ▶ Earaches, neck pain, and deep aching at the top of the head (sphenoid sinuses).

Other symptoms of sinusitis include:

- ▶ Fever.

- ▶ Weakness.

- ▶ Tiredness.

- ▶ Cough that may be more severe at night.

- ▶ Runny nose (rhinitis) or nasal congestion.

On rare occasions, acute sinusitis may result in brain infection and other serious complications.

Eclampsia.   Eclampsia is the most commonly occurring hypertensive disease in pregnancy. Worldwide, preeclampsia and eclampsia contribute to the death of a pregnant woman every

3 minutes.[165] The classic clinical presentation consists of epileptic seizures or coma manifesting during the third trimester or early puerperium in women who already have the preeclamptic symptom triad of edema, proteinuria, and hypertension.[166] The diagnosis of eclampsia requires the exclusion of other medical or neurologic disorders underlying the symptomatology. The differential diagnostic considerations include sinus or cerebral vein thrombosis, subarachnoid hemorrhage from an aneurysm, infectious or autoimmune-inflammatory disorders, and sickle cell crisis.

Cerebrospinal Fluid (CSF) Hypotension.   This condition commonly occurs following a lumbar puncture, which can produce leakage of CSF through a dural tear. A lumbar puncture is a routine procedure performed for a variety of functions: spinal anesthesia, intrathecal administration of cytotoxic and antibiotic drugs, myelography, obtaining CSF samples, and pressure measurement.[167] The leak of CSF results in CSF hypovolemia and downward shifting of the brain, causing pressure on the pain-sensitive dural sinuses that is amplified in the upright posture and relieved with recumbence.[168] The clinical manifestations of CSF hypotension are headache and backache, which usually start within hours to a week following the lumbar puncture. More serious complications may include labyrinthine and ocular cranial nerve disturbances, meningitis, subdural hematomas, and fistulas.

Temporomandibular Joint Dysfunction.   See Chapter 24.

Periodontal Disease.   Periodontal disease may be associated with a small increased risk of coronary heart disease.[169] Clinically, periodontitis starts as an acute inflammation of the apical periodontal ligament and the neighboring spongiosa, accompanied by well-known imminent symptoms such as pain, tenderness to percussion, and swelling.

Thyroiditis.   Acute bacterial thyroiditis (or pyogenic thyroiditis) is a rare, potentially life-threatening complication of bacterial infection elsewhere in the body, especially following an upper respiratory tract infection.[170] The condition occurs in all age groups, although women with preexisting thyroid disease constitute the group most likely to develop thyroid infection. In childhood, it is often linked to local anatomic defects. The ample blood supply and lymphatic drainage, high iodine content, and protective thyroid capsule contribute to the low incidence of infection.

Common pathogens include *Streptococcus pyogenes, S. pneumoniae,* and *Staphylococcus.* Less common organisms include *Salmonella, Bacteroides, Haemophilus influenzae, Streptococcus viridans,* and other streptococcal organisms.[170] Clinical signs and symptoms include fever (92 percent), anterior neck pain (100 percent), tenderness (94 percent), warmth (70 percent), erythema (82 percent), dysphagia (91 percent), dysphonia (82 percent), and pharyngitis (69 percent).[170,171]

Fracture of the Facial Bones or Skull.   The examination of the face for a fracture requires knowledge not only of normal anatomy, but also of common fracture patterns in the face. Computed tomography is currently the imaging procedure of choice for most facial fractures, because it highlights the complex anatomy and fractures of the facial bones and their related soft tissue complications extremely well. Approximately 60 to 70 percent of all facial fractures involve the orbit.[172] The exceptions to this are a local nasal bone fracture, or a zygomatic arch fracture. The most common mechanism producing facial fractures is auto accidents. Other mechanisms include fights or assaults, falls, sports, industrial accidents, and gunshot wounds. Less than 10 percent of all facial fractures occur in children, perhaps because of the increased resiliency of a child's facial skeleton.[172] The nose is the most frequently injured facial structure, and the most commonly missed facial fracture of the face is a fracture of the nasal bone. Patients with a temporal bone fracture may present with a conductive hearing loss caused by dislocations in the ossicular chain. Facial nerve paralysis also may occur secondary to either transection or edema of the facial nerve.

Trochleitis.[173]   Trochleitis is a local inflammatory process of the superior oblique tendon trochlea characterized by periocular pain. Eye movement in supraduction typically aggravates the pain. Physical examination demonstrates exquisite point tenderness over the trochlea of the superior oblique muscle. The cause often is unknown, but trochleitis can occur in rheumatoid arthritis, systemic lupus erythematosus, psoriasis, or enteropathic arthropathy. Rare causes include sinusitis, trauma, and metastasis.

Causes of Cervical Pain

The causes of cervical pain are numerous, as outlined in Table 9-10 and Figure 9-1.

TABLE 9-10   Potential Causes of Cervical Pain

Thyroid disease
Subarachnoid hemorrhage
Retropharyngeal abscess
Carotodynia
Cardiac disease
Trauma
Myofascial pain syndrome
Tumors
Temporomandibular joint dysfunction
Meningitis
Epidural hematoma
Lyme disease
Cervical disk disease or herniation
Vertebral artery disorders
Torticollis
Rheumatoid arthritis
Ankylosing spondylitis
Gout
Osteoarthritis
Occipital neuralgia

Potential Causes of Cervical, Thoracic, Lumbar, Pelvic and Lower Extremity Pain

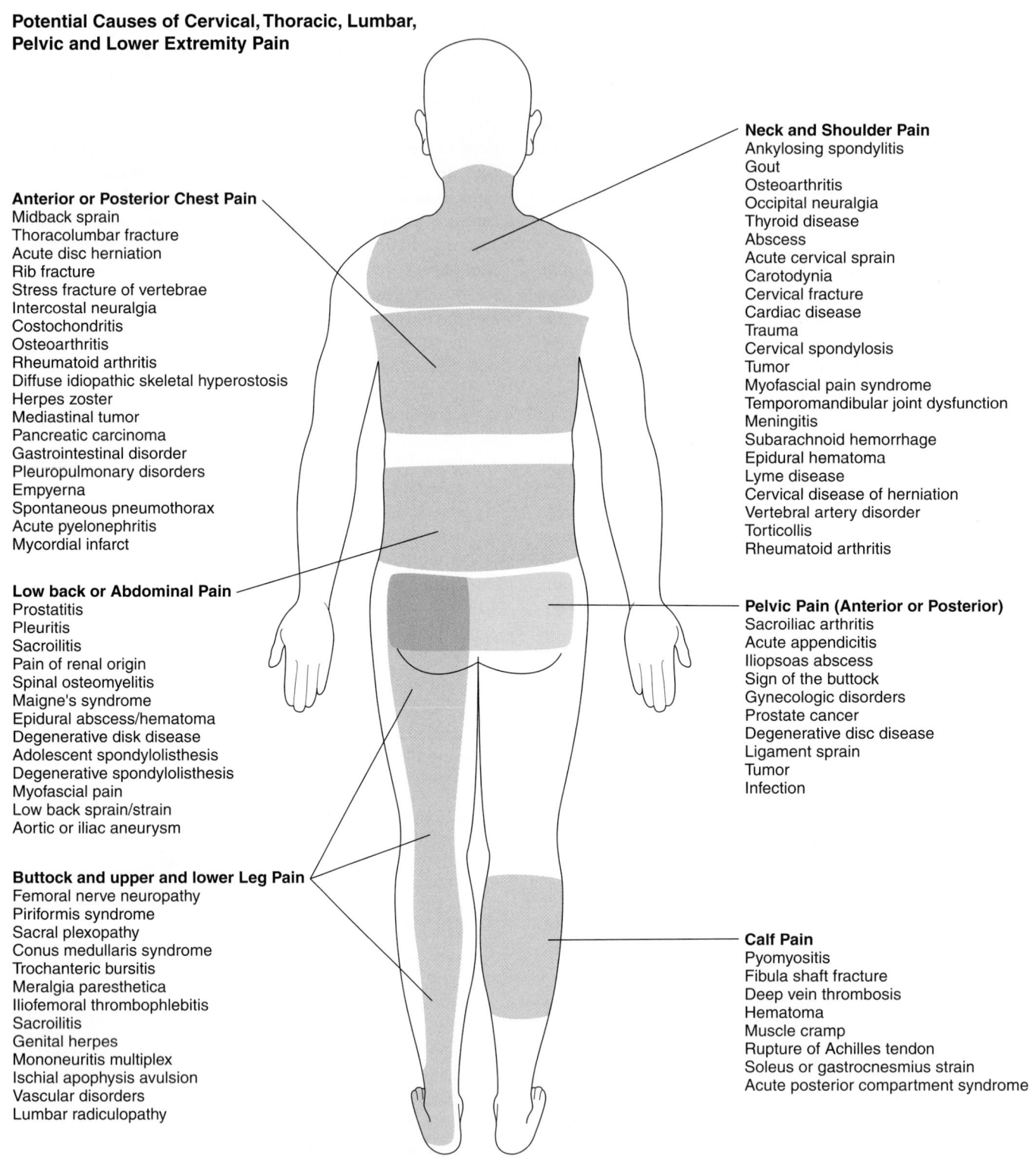

Neck and Shoulder Pain
Ankylosing spondylitis
Gout
Osteoarthritis
Occipital neuralgia
Thyroid disease
Abscess
Acute cervical sprain
Carotodynia
Cervical fracture
Cardiac disease
Trauma
Cervical spondylosis
Tumor
Myofascial pain syndrome
Temporomandibular joint dysfunction
Meningitis
Subarachnoid hemorrhage
Epidural hematoma
Lyme disease
Cervical disease of herniation
Vertebral artery disorder
Torticollis
Rheumatoid arthritis

Anterior or Posterior Chest Pain
Midback sprain
Thoracolumbar fracture
Acute disc herniation
Rib fracture
Stress fracture of vertebrae
Intercostal neuralgia
Costochondritis
Osteoarthritis
Rheumatoid arthritis
Diffuse idiopathic skeletal hyperostosis
Herpes zoster
Mediastinal tumor
Pancreatic carcinoma
Gastrointestinal disorder
Pleuropulmonary disorders
Empyerna
Spontaneous pneumothorax
Acute pyelonephritis
Mycordial infarct

Low back or Abdominal Pain
Prostatitis
Pleuritis
Sacroilitis
Pain of renal origin
Spinal osteomyelitis
Maigne's syndrome
Epidural abscess/hematoma
Degenerative disk disease
Adolescent spondylolisthesis
Degenerative spondylolisthesis
Myofascial pain
Low back sprain/strain
Aortic or iliac aneurysm

Pelvic Pain (Anterior or Posterior)
Sacroiliac arthritis
Acute appendicitis
Iliopsoas abscess
Sign of the buttock
Gynecologic disorders
Prostate cancer
Degenerative disc disease
Ligament sprain
Tumor
Infection

Buttock and upper and lower Leg Pain
Femoral nerve neuropathy
Piriformis syndrome
Sacral plexopathy
Conus medullaris syndrome
Trochanteric bursitis
Meralgia paresthetica
Iliofemoral thrombophlebitis
Sacroilitis
Genital herpes
Mononeuritis multiplex
Ischial apophysis avulsion
Vascular disorders
Lumbar radiculopathy

Calf Pain
Pyomyositis
Fibula shaft fracture
Deep vein thrombosis
Hematoma
Muscle cramp
Rupture of Achilles tendon
Soleus or gastrocnesmius strain
Acute posterior compartment syndrome

FIGURE 9-1   Potential causes of cervical, thoracic, lumbar, pelvic, and lower extremity pain.

Thyroid Disease

The thyroid gland synthesizes, stores, and secretes thyroid hormones, mainly L-thyroxine (T_4). L-triiodothyronine (T_3) is produced from T_4 by deiodination, mainly in liver, kidney, and muscle. The thyroid gland controls the metabolic rate of many organs and tissues. The thyroid gland cannot function normally unless it is exposed to thyroid-stimulating hormone (TSH), which is produced by the thyrotrophs of the anterior pituitary.[174] Underactivity (hypothyroidism) and overactivity of thyroid function (hyperthyroidism) represent the most common endocrine problems, have widespread manifestations, including cervical pain, and often require long-term treatment.

Hypothyroidism.   Most patients with hypothyroidism have disease of the thyroid gland. Occasionally, hypothyroidism develops in patients with normal thyroid glands because of inadequate stimulation by TSH. Such individuals have disorders of the anterior pituitary or hypothalamus. Thyroid hormone deficiency affects practically all body functions. The complaints and physical findings vary widely from patient to patient, depending on the severity of the deficiency. Patients may present with weakness, fatigue, arthralgias and myalgias, muscle cramps, cold intolerance, constipation, lethargy, dryness of the skin, headache, neck pain, menorrhagia, hoarseness, edema, and weight gain.[174] Most patients have varying degrees of brittle nails and hair, pallor, delayed relaxation time of the deep tendon reflexes, keratinic skin color, thickening of the tongue, mental status changes, and diastolic hypertension.[174] In some patients, severe hypothermia, edema, and even effusions into the pleura, and peritoneal and pericardial cavities may occur.[174]

Hyperthyroidism.   Hyperthyroidism denotes clinical disorders associated with increased serum concentrations of free T_4 estimate or free T_3, or both. The most common causes of hyperthyroidism are Graves' disease, nodular goiter, and thyroiditis. Excessive thyroid hormone concentrations affect many body functions. Such symptoms include[174]:

▶ Nervousness.

▶ Restlessness.

▶ Heat intolerance.

▶ Increased and inappropriate perspiration.

▶ Fatigue.

▶ Muscle cramps.

▶ Paratracheal neck pain.

▶ Increased frequency of bowel movements.

▶ Weight loss in association with unchanged or increased food ingestion.

▶ Palpitations.

The clinical signs of hyperthyroidism, which also vary widely among patients, may include exophthalmus, tachycardia, fine resting tremors, moist warm skin, heat radiation from the skin, hyperreflexia, onycholysis, an enlarged thyroid gland with or without a bruit, and diplopia.[174] Patients who are found to have relatively specific symptoms and signs (such as goiter, nodule, eye findings of Graves' disease, or tremor) should be referred to an endocrinologist for consideration of treatment.

Subarachnoid Hemorrhage
See the discussion of intracranial bleeding under "Causes of Head and Facial Pain," earlier.

Retropharyngeal Abscess
Retropharyngeal abscess (RPA) is a relatively uncommon infection of the space anterior to the prevertebral layer of the deep cervical fascia. This infection is most common in children younger than 3 or 4 years, because of the rich concentration of lymph nodes in this space.[175] The infection in children classically results from extension of oropharyngeal infections, including pharyngitis, tonsillitis, and adenitis.[176] Trauma, often caused by a fall while holding a pencil or stick in the mouth, and dental infections are the usual underlying causes of RPA in older children and adults.[176] The major causative organisms are *Streptococcus pyogenes, Staphylococcus aureus,* and oropharyngeal anaerobic bacteria.[177] The infection progresses through three stages: cellulitis, phlegmon, and abscess.

RPA can produce posterior neck and shoulder pain and stiffness. These symptoms are also associated with hyperextension of the neck, torticollis, fever, irritability, muffled voice, stertor, and other signs of upper airway obstruction.[176] The pain often is worsened with swallowing. Swelling of the lateral or posterior aspect of the neck can be present.

The differential diagnosis includes acute epiglottitis, foreign body aspiration, vertebral osteomyelitis, hematoma (particularly in boys with hemophilia), and lymphoma.[176]

Carotodynia
In addition to sinus and dental abnormalities and stress, several different neurologic conditions can cause facial pain. These include various neuralgias (trigeminal, vagoglossopharyngeal, cranial), carotodynia (a painful carotid artery), and optic neuritis. Pain characteristics and results of specific neurologic tests establish the diagnosis. Carotodynia is associated with neck pain, tenderness, and a unilateral headache.

Cardiac Disease
See the discussion of myocardial infarction under "Causes of Thoracic Pain," later.

Trauma or Whiplash
See Chapter 23.

Tumors
Tumors of the adult cervical spine may be primary, arising from the bone, or secondary (i.e., metastatic from a distant primary site.) Tumors of the cervical cord may cause neck pain. These tumors may be primary, metastatic, extramedullary, or intramedullary. Pain of insidious onset, with or without neurologic signs and symptoms (e.g., progressive leg weakness, bladder paralysis, and sensory loss), may occur.

Temporomandibular Joint Dysfunction
See Chapter 24.

Meningitis
See the discussion under "Causes of Head and Facial Pain, earlier".

Epidural Hematoma

Most cervical epidural hematomas are spontaneous, with precipitating factors that include coagulopathy, vascular malformation, neoplasm, and pregnancy.[178] Cervical epidural hematoma also can be caused by trauma, although this is uncommon. Traumatic causes of spontaneous epidural hematoma include vertebral trauma, epidural steroid injection, lumbar puncture, penetrating injuries, birth trauma, and spinal manipulation.[179] Excessive movement of the cervical spine, such as may occur with a cervical manipulation, can injure the epidural veins, either by direct trauma or by a sudden increase in venous pressure, resulting in a cervical epidural hematoma.[178,180] The clinician must be particularly mindful of the risk factors for the complications of spinal manual therapy, such as misdiagnosis, unrecognized neurologic manifestations, improper technique, presence of coagulation disorder or herniated nucleus pulposus, and manipulation of the cervical spine.[181]

Presenting signs and symptoms vary. The onset of neck pain is often the first symptom, but epidural hematoma has been diagnosed in its absence. Compression of the spinal cord also can produce sensory deficits, motor deficits, and bowel or bladder incontinence.

Lyme Disease

See the discussion of systemic infections under "Causes of Head and Facial Pain," earlier.

Cervical Disk Disease or Herniation

See Chapter 20.

Vertebral Artery Disorders

See Chapter 21.

Torticollis

As many as 80 different causes of torticollis have been documented in the literature.[182] Torticollis is not a specific diagnosis but, rather, a sign of an underlying disorder resulting in the characteristic tilting of the head to one side. Differential diagnosis of torticollis ranges from innocuous abnormalities that require no specific therapy to potentially life-threatening tumors of the central nervous system. The neuromuscular causes of torticollis may be classified as congenital or acquired. Congenital muscular torticollis is the most common type of torticollis.[183] Several causes are implicated, including fetal positioning, difficult labor and delivery, cervical muscle abnormalities, Sprengel's deformity, and Klippel-Feil syndrome.[184] In addition to torticollis, patients with Klippel-Feil syndrome have the classic clinical triad described by Klippel and Feil in 1912: short, broad necks; restricted movement; and low hairlines.[185,186] The restricted neck mobility is the result of the fusion of a variable number of cervical vertebrae, sometimes reducing their number, and cervical spina bifida.[187] Extraosseous changes, hemivertebra, vertebral body clefts, and thoracolumbar abnormalities sometimes also are seen.[188]

Acquired torticollis, which includes spasmodic torticollis, is clinically similar but has different etiologies.[189] Acquired torticollis in children may be related to trauma or infections, as in Grisel's syndrome, which occurs after head, neck, and pharyngeal infections.[190] In this syndrome, the soft tissue inflammation associated with pharyngitis, mastoiditis, or tonsillitis results in accumulation of fluid in the nearby cervical joints.[191] This edema may then lead to subluxation of the atlantoaxial joint.

Spasmodic torticollis is the involuntary hyperkinesis of neck musculature, causing turning of the head on the trunk, sometimes with additional forward flexion (anterocollis), backward extension (retrocollis), or lateral flexion (laterocollis).[189] It also is marked by abnormal head postures.[191] The sternocleidomastoid muscle is involved in 75 percent of cases and the trapezius in 50 percent.[191] Other muscles that might become involved include the rectus capitis, obliquus inferior, and splenius capitis.[192] In some cases, the spasm generalizes to the muscles of the shoulder, girdle, trunk, or limbs.[193]

Neck movements can vary from jerky to smooth[193,194] and are aggravated by standing, walking, or stressful situations, but usually do not occur with sleep.[195]

Spontaneous remissions (partial or complete) have been reported in up to 60 percent of patients in some series[194]; others note full remission in 16 percent, with sustained remission for 12 months of 6 to 12 percent.[196,197]

Various treatments for torticollis have been described. Spencer and colleagues[198] described a single-subject study using behavioral therapies that consisted of progressive relaxation, positive practice, and visual feedback. Their patient had significant improvements in all areas, which were maintained at a 2-year follow-up examination.

Agras and Marshall[199] used massed negative practice (i.e., repeating the spasmodic positioning), 200 to 400 repetitions of the movement daily, which achieved full resolution of symptoms in one of two patients. Results persisted for 22 months.

Another single-case study used positive practice (exercising against the spasmodic muscle groups) in a bed-ridden woman who had symptoms of spasmodic torticollis for 8 years. After 3 months of positive practice, she was able to ambulate unassisted; her therapeutic gains were maintained at a 1-year follow-up examination.[198]

Biofeedback also has been used successfully as an intervention for torticollis.[200]

Rheumatoid Arthritis

Involvement of the cervical spine is common in rheumatoid arthritis (RA), ankylosing spondylitis (AS), and juvenile polyarthritis.[95] Fifty percent or more of patients with RA have evidence of neck involvement, especially at the atlanto-axial joint.[95] These patients are prone to a cervical derangement, of which an anterior subluxation of C1 on C2, during head flexion, is the most common.[201] Although most patients with anterior subluxation have no neurologic complications, the more advanced and unstable lesions may result in myelopathy.[95]

Patients also can experience severe bony erosions of one or both of the lateral zygapophysial joints. This erosion can result in occipital pain with cervical rotation, and a rotational head-tilt deformity, if the lesion is unilateral.[201]

The symptoms of these spondyloarthropathies typically fall into two categories:

1. *Pain resulting from the inflammatory process.* RA of the cervical spine may cause generalized aching posterior neck, shoulder, and occipital pain. This pain is often worse with neck flexion.

2. *Derangement or deformity.* This finding results from joint damage, typically with a concomitant risk to the nearby neural structures. Radicular symptoms may be present in one or both upper extremities. With myelopathy, spastic weakness, hyperreflexia, and other upper motor neuron signs are present. Depending on the level of involvement within the cervical spine, signs and symptoms of vertebral artery compromise also may be present.

Ankylosing Spondylitis

Ankylosing spondylitis (AS) also commonly affects the C1 to C2 segment, although this is usually a late manifestation of the disease process. Following ankylosing of the sacroiliac, lumbar, and thoracic segments, the atlanto-axial joint becomes painful initially, only to be less symptomatic as the joint begins to lose motion.[95]

Neurologic injury associated with AS is usually the result of cervical fracture of the syndesmophytes and resulting pseudoarticulation.[95,202] AS is described further under "Causes of Thoracic Pain," later.

Gout

Gout is the most common form of inflammatory arthritis in men older than 40 years of age, and appears to be on the increase.[203] In the United States, the self-reported prevalence of gout almost trebled in men aged 45 to 64 years between 1969 and 1981.[204] The rising prevalence of gout is thought to stem from dietary changes, environmental factors, increasing longevity, subclinical renal impairment, and the increased use of drugs causing hyperuricemia, particularly diuretics.[205] Although the occurrence of gout in the neck is distinctly uncommon, the medications used to treat it can have serious side effects in this region. These complications include ligament laxity with resultant instability and neck pain.[206]

Osteoarthritis

Degenerative osteoarthrosis (OA) of the subaxial cervical spine is common in elderly patients[207] and is typically characterized by posterior neck, shoulder, and arm pain in a specific dermatomal pattern rather than occipitocervical pain.[208] Diffuse or focal trigger point tenderness may be present in the posterior neck on the involved side.

OA of the atlanto-axial joints may be overlooked when the patient has occipitocervical pain associated with degenerative changes in the subaxial spine.

Occipital Neuralgia

See the discussion under "Causes of Head and Facial Pain," earlier.

Causes of Thoracic Pain

Thoracic pain has a wide differential diagnosis (see Fig. 9-1). Pain may originate from structures within the thorax, such as the heart, lungs, or esophagus. However, musculoskeletal causes of chest pain must be considered. Musculoskeletal problems of the chest wall can occur in the ribs, sternum, articulations, or myofascial structures. The cause is usually evident in the case of direct trauma.

Systemic origins of musculoskeletal pain in the thoracic spine (Table 9-11) usually are accompanied by constitutional symptoms affecting the whole body, and by other associated symptoms that the patient may not relate to the back pain, and, therefore, may fail to mention to the clinician. These additional symptoms should be discovered during the subjective examination by the careful interviewer. When the patient (or the examination) indicates the presence of a fever (or night sweats), a referral to a physician is indicated.

The close proximity of the thoracic spine to the chest and respiratory organs may result in a correlation between respiratory movements and increased thoracic symptoms. When

TABLE 9-11 Systemic Causes of Thoracic Pain[209]

Systemic Origin	Location
Gallbladder disease	Midback between scapula
Acute cholecystitis	Right subscapular area
Peptic ulcer: stomach or duodenal ulcers	5th–10th thoracic vertebrae
PLEUROPULMONARY DISORDERS Basilar pneumonia	Right upper back
Empyema	Scapula
Pleurisy	Scapula
Spontaneous pneumothorax	Ipsilateral scapula
Pancreatic carcinoma	Middle thoracic or lumbar spine
Acute pyelonephritis	Costovertebral angle (posteriorly)
Esophagitis	Midback between scapula
Myocardial infarction	Midthoracic spine
Biliary colic	Right upper back; midback between scapula; right interscapular or subscapular areas

TABLE 9-12   Potential Causes of Thoracic Pain

Mediastinal tumors
Pancreatic carcinoma
Gastrointestinal disorders
Pleuropulmonary conditions
Spontaneous pneumothorax
Myocardial infarction
Herpes zoster
Acute disk herniation
Vertebral fracture
Rib fracture
Stress fracture
Intercostal neuralgia
Costochondritis
Osteoarthritis
Rheumatoid arthritis
Diffuse idiopathic skeletal hyperostosis (DISH)
Manubriosternal dislocations

screening the patient through the subjective history, the clinician should remember that symptoms of pleural, intercostal muscular, costal, and dural origin all increase on coughing or deep inspiration; thus, only pain of a cardiac origin is ruled out when symptoms increase in association with respiratory movements.

The causes of thoracic pain include those listed in Table 9-12.

Gastrointestinal Conditions

The subjective history often provides several clues to a gastrointestinal cause of chest pain.

Peptic Ulcer Disease.   Peptic ulceration of the stomach or duodenum is often accompanied by abnormalities of the gastric mucosa, and the key to determining the cause of ulcer disease often lies in histologic diagnosis of the associated *gastritis* or *gastropathy.*

The terms *ulcer disease* and *peptic ulcer* are used synonymously to refer to erosions or ulcers of the stomach and duodenum.

Ulcer disease was long assumed to be idiopathic, caused by acid hypersecretion or psychologic stress, or a combination. *Helicobacter pylori* is now well recognized as a major risk factor for the development of peptic ulcer disease.[210]

The patient usually describes a typical history of ulcers characterized by periodic symptoms, relief with antacids, and the relationship of pain to certain foods and the timing of meals. For example, the patient may have relief from pain after eating initially, but the pain then returns and increases 1 to 2 hours after eating, when the stomach is emptied. In the pediatric age group, abdominal pain is a very common reason for seeking medical advice. It is also the most common presenting symptom of peptic ulcer disease. However, peptic and other erosive or ulcerative gastritides and gastropathies of the stomach and duodenum are relatively uncommon in this age group.[211]

The pain of a peptic ulcer occasionally occurs only in the back between the eighth and tenth thoracic vertebrae. Duodenal ulcers may refer pain from the fifth thoracic vertebra, either at the midline or just to either side of the spine. This localization may accompany penetration through the viscera (organs). When questioned further, the patient may indicate that blood is present in the feces.

The differential diagnosis of ulcer disease includes esophagitis, gastritis, gastropathy, nonulcer dyspepsia, gallbladder or liver disease, pneumonia, and pancreatitis, among others.[211]

Acute Cholecystitis.   Acute cholecystitis is the result of cystic duct obstruction by gallstones or biliary sludge. In this condition, ductal obstruction is soon followed by chemical inflammation and a superimposed infection of the gallbladder. Acute cholecystitis may refer intense, sudden, paroxysmal pain to the right scapula, midback, or right shoulder. Pain intensity often increases with movement or respirations. Rebound tenderness and abdominal muscle guarding are often present. A low-grade fever also may be present. There may be reports of nausea and vomiting. Finally, mild jaundice, which is more apparent in fair-skinned patients, may be observed in those experiencing acute cholecystitis.[212] This finding is attributable to edema of the common bile duct, which causes bilirubin to diffuse across the inflamed gallbladder mucosa.[212]

Biliary Colic.   Biliary colic is a common initial presentation of gallstone disease. The pain of biliary colic is referred to the right posterior upper quadrant, with pain in the right shoulder. There may be interscapular pain with referred pain to the right side. Occasionally, the pain beneath the right costal margin may be confused with the shoulder girdle pain secondary to intracostal nerve compression. The pain is initially intermittent. Pain usually recurs, but the interval to the next attack of pain is quite variable.

Severe Esophagitis.   Gastroesophageal reflux disease is defined as symptoms or mucosal damage (esophagitis) resulting from the exposure of the distal esophagus to refluxed gastric contents. Esophageal pain has many patterns. It is often described as burning, sometimes as gripping, and it can also be pressing, boring, or stabbing. It may be associated with a foul taste, morning pain, worsening pain after a meal, and epigastric tenderness. Severe esophagitis may refer pain to the anterior chest. It tends to be felt mainly in the throat or epigastrium. On occasion, it can radiate to the neck, back, or upper arms—all of which may equally apply to cardiac pain.

Pancreatic Carcinoma

The most frequent symptom of a pancreatic carcinoma is pain. It first may be noted as a paroxysmal (sudden, recurrent, or intensifying) or steady, dull pain, radiating from the epigastrium into the back. The pain is usually slowly progressive, is worse at night, and is unrelated to digestive activities. Other signs and symptoms may include jaundice, anorexia, severe weight loss, and gastrointestinal difficulties unrelated to meals. The disease is predominantly found in men (3:1) and occurs in the sixth and seventh decades.

Mediastinal Tumors

Most spinal tumors occur in the first half of life. Although primary tumors of the thoracic spine are rare, the thoracic spine is the most common site for metastases. Tumors occur in the thoracic spine because of its length and proximity to the mediastinum. The vascularization of the vertebrae in the mid to lower thoracic spine is generally through a watershed effect rather than by direct segmental arteries, which leaves the region susceptible to a secondary metastatic invasion from lymph nodes involved with lymphoma, breast, or lung cancer.[213,214]

Tumors of T12 to L2 (typically, multiple myeloma) may compress the conus medullaris containing the S3 to S5 nerve roots. This may lead to an impairment of the urinary or anal sphincter, which is sometimes associated with saddle anesthesia.

Myocardial Infarction

Pain of myocardial origin, resulting from a sudden and complete occlusion of the coronary artery, frequently radiates over the left pectoral region, left shoulder, medial left arm, right upper extremity, epigastrium, and jaw, and can therefore mimic musculoskeletal pain. The pain typically has a crushing or gripping quality over the substernal region. Angina pectoris pain, which is a symptom that represents an imbalance between myocardial perfusion and demand, may be exertional or variant, making it difficult for the clinician to recognize. The distribution of symptoms for angina pectoris includes substernal and chest pressure, shoulder pain, and neck or jaw pain, which worsens with exertion and improves with rest. This condition constitutes a medical emergency.

Pleuropulmonary Conditions

Pneumothorax.   Pneumothorax is defined as the entry of air into the pleural space with secondary lung collapse.[215] The pleura is a thin serous layer that covers the lungs (visceral pleura). The pleural space extends from 3 cm above the midpoint of the clavicle down to the 12th rib overlying the kidney. Three types of pneumothorax may cause thoracic pain: spontaneous, iatrogenic, and traumatic.

Spontaneous pneumothorax, in contrast to iatrogenic and traumatic pneumothorax, occurs without any precipitating event. Primary spontaneous pneumothorax, seen in otherwise healthy individuals, is rarely life threatening. Secondary spontaneous pneumothorax, seen in patients with underlying lung disease, is a more serious condition and is associated with substantial mortality.

Several findings in the examination of the respiratory and cardiovascular systems may help establish the diagnosis of pneumothorax. Patients with pneumothorax present with pleuritic pain or breathlessness. The pain is localized to the side of the pneumothorax. This pain may be referred to the ipsilateral scapula or shoulder, across the chest, or over the abdomen. Pneumothorax also may be associated with hemoptysis (blood in sputum), tachycardia (increased heart rate), tachypnea (rapid respirations), and cyanosis (blue lips and skin resulting from lack of oxygen).[209] The patient may be most comfortable sitting in an upright position.

A chest radiograph is usually sufficient to confirm the diagnosis. Intervention can range from simple aspiration, tube drainage, and chemical sclerosis of the pleura, to thoracoscopy and thoracotomy.

Pleural Effusion.   Pleural effusion describes fluid (transudative or exudative) within the pleural space. Pleural effusion usually results from an underlying disease, such as heart failure, or from medical disorders leading to hypoalbuminaemia.[216] It also may be caused by infection (bacterial or mycobacterial), malignancy, collagen vascular disease, pancreatitis, or pulmonary embolism.[217]

Pleural effusions may be asymptomatic but if large, produce breathlessness or pain, or both.[216] Breath sounds are reduced on the affected side, and the percussion note is stony dull.[216]

Intervention usually involves drainage of the fluid.

Acute Disk Herniation

Disk lesions account for a high percentage of the causes of anterior and posterior thoracic pain syndromes (see Chap. 20).[218] Thoracic disk herniations do not have a characteristic clinical presentation, and the symptomatology may be confused with other diagnoses. In a review of the literature, covering 280 cases of thoracic disk herniation,[219] only 23 percent had sensory symptoms, most commonly numbness, paresthesias, or dysesthesias. A thoracic disk herniation can produce posterior, anterior, or radicular (bilateral or unilateral) pain, which can be so severe as to mimic a myocardial infarction. All movements are severely limited and extremely painful and may reproduce radicular pain.

Vertebral Fracture

A high percentage of spinal fractures involve the thoracic spine. The most common thoracic fracture is the compression fracture, which results from an axial loading of the thoracic spine, combined with flexion and side flexion. Osteoporotic fractures are most common in the mid to low thoracic spine and result from an inability of the vertebral body to sustain the compression forces involved with everyday activities.[37] Thus, most patients with this problem do not have a history of an identifiable trauma (sensitivity, 0.30).[220] Fractures that occur at the levels of T1 to T10 can have associated damage to the spinal cord, whereas fractures at T11 to T12 can manifest as mixed spinal cord, conus medullaris, or spinal nerve root injuries.[221] Traumatic fractures of the thoracic spine include compression and burst fractures.

▶ Compression fractures are relatively benign, because they involve only the anterior column (Fig. 9-2). They are thought to occur because of the relative stiffness of the thoracic spine compared with the greater mobility of the neighboring lumbar spine.[222] These fractures, which most commonly occur in the midthoracic and midlumbar spine, are typically stable, unless severe. Diagnosis is confirmed with a lateral radiograph, which demonstrates anterior wedging.

▶ Burst fractures involve both the anterior and middle columns and also may involve ligamentous or bony injury of the posterior column. Although the mechanism for this

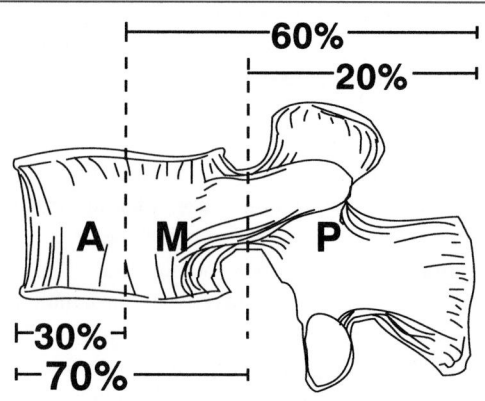

FIGURE 9-2 Compression fractures of the vertebral column. A, anterior; M, middle; P, posterior. (Reproduced with permission from Dee R, et al, eds. *Principles of Orthopaedic Practice.* New York, NY: McGraw-Hill; 1997.)

type of fracture is the same as for compression fractures, the axial loading is of a greater magnitude and typically is combined with flexion. Consequently, the anterior body undergoes a bursting effect, with retropulsion of part of the posterior vertebral body wall (middle column) into the canal, decreasing the canal size.[223]

Rib Fracture

Rib fractures are very common in the blunt trauma population, with one review demonstrating that 10 percent of patients admitted to a level 2 trauma center had evidence of rib fractures.[224] However, the true incidence of rib fractures is not known because up to 50 percent of rib fractures may be missed on a standard chest x-ray film.[225] The primary symptom of a rib fracture is pain on inspiration, resulting in hypoventilation.[221] On physical examination, there is local tenderness, crepitation, and, on occasion, a palpable defect.

Stress Fracture of the Rib

There are more reports of stress fractures of the first rib than any other single rib.[226] A contraction of the anterior scalene muscle produces bending forces at the subclavian sulcus, which is the usual site of the fracture.[227] This mechanism usually occurs in overhead activities, such as pitching, basketball, tennis or weightlifting.[228,229]

Pain occurs in the region of shoulder, anterior cervical triangle, or clavicular region.[229] The pain may radiate to the sternum or pectoral region. The onset is usually insidious, although it may start with acute pain. Pain may occur with deep breathing.[230]

Tenderness to palpation may be present medial to the superior angle of the scapula, at the base of the neck, supraclavicular triangle, or deep in the axilla.[226] Shoulder movements may be painful or restricted.

The recommended treatment of a first rib stress fracture involves immobilization of the shoulder girdle on the affected side with a sling.[226] Pain resolves within 2 to 8 weeks of immobilization.[229]

Stress fractures of the other ribs also may occur. The most common cause is a change in technique or training load. Exam-

ination may reveal local tenderness to palpation. Rib springing is usually positive for pain.

Intercostal Neuralgia

Neurogenic pain of the thorax can be the result of infection, such as varicella-zoster (shingles); mechanical compression of the nerve by a disk protrusion; an osteophyte; a neuroma; a fracture; or a condition called *postherpetic neuralgia.* Neuralgic pain, which typically has a burning quality, is unchanged by analgesics or rest.

Epidemic Myalgia

Epidemic myalgia, also known as epidemic pleurodynia or Bornholm disease, is characterized by the abrupt onset of chest or abdominal pain, usually accompanied by fever, and was first described in the late 1800s.[231] This acute viral illness is caused mainly by coxsackie B virus, but other enteroviruses may be implicated.[226] The mode of transmission is via a shared water source,[232] and there is a 3- to 5-day incubation period. Peak incidence is during the soccer and American football seasons, and outbreaks involving athletic teams have been reported.[232]

Presentation usually follows a nonspecific prodromal illness, with sudden onset of sharp lateral chest or abdominal pains.[226] The intercostal and upper abdominal wall muscles are most commonly involved, with the pleura involved rarely.[233] The pain is intermittent and exacerbated by movement, coughing, and deep inspiration.[226] It is accompanied by fever and malaise.

Diagnosis is made by isolation of the virus from the feces or on throat swab in the early stages of the disease. The condition is self-limiting and rarely requires any specific treatment.[226] Symptoms usually resolve after a few days but may recur.

Costochondritis

Costochondritis is a common but poorly understood condition that manifests as chest wall pain. It is usually characterized by pain and tenderness on the costochondral or chondrosternal joints in the absence of swelling. The second to fifth costal cartilages are the most commonly affected.[233]

Diagnosis is based on a history of chest pain with associated anterior chest wall tenderness that is localized to the costochondral junction of one or more ribs. Swelling, heat, and erythema usually are absent. The pain may be provoked by certain movements, such as adduction of the arm on the affected side with accompanying rotation of the head to the same side.[226]

Costochondritis is a mostly benign, self-limiting condition. Symptoms usually resolve within 1 year.[234]

Osteoarthritis

Osteoarthritis (OA) of the thoracic spine affects three sites: the intervertebral disk, the zygapophysial joints, and the articulations of the rib with the vertebral body and transverse process.[218]

Osteoarthritic changes in the zygapophysial joints and costovertebral joints occur most commonly at T11 and L1, which coincides with those joints whose orientation is more sagittal, and the area that sustains the peak incidence of traumatic fractures in the thoracic spine.[222,235] OA of the costovertebral and costotransverse joints is a frequent source of chronic pain, but is not typically associated with neurologic changes.[218] This condition is associated with local pain and tenderness at the site of degeneration. Rib joint pain typically is exacerbated by exaggerated respiratory movements.[236]

Spondylosis, disk degeneration, and Schmorl's nodes are most frequently encountered within the T10 to T12 vertebrae,[235] probably as a result of a reduced resistance to torsion in this area.[237]

The relationship between zygapophysial joint orientation and OA suggests that repeated torsional trauma might well have a significant role in the development of OA in zygapophysial joints that are sagittally oriented.[235]

Rheumatoid Arthritis

Thoracic pain related to rheumatoid arthritis (RA) is associated with pain and stiffness that is greatest in the morning and usually improves with movement.[218,238] Inspection usually shows a flat lumbar spine, and a gross limitation of side flexion in both directions is demonstrated.

Ankylosing Spondylitis

Ankylosing spondylitis (AS, also known as Bekhterev's or Marie-Strümpell disease) is a chronic rheumatoid disorder that affects 1 to 3 per 1000 people. Thoracic involvement in AS occurs almost universally. The patient is usually between 15 and 40 years of age. There is a 10 to 20 percent risk that offspring of patients with the disease will later develop it.[239] Although males are affected more frequently than females, mild courses of AS are more common in the latter.[240]

The disease includes involvement of the anterior longitudinal ligament and ossification of the disk, thoracic zygapophysial joint joints, costovertebral joints, and manubrio sternal joint. This multijoint involvement makes the checking of chest expansion measurements a required test in this region.

In time, AS progresses to involve the whole spine and results in spinal deformities, including flattening of the lumbar lordosis, kyphosis of the thoracic spine, and hyperextension of the cervical spine. These changes, in turn, result in flexion contractures of the hips and knees, with significant morbidity and disability.[240]

The most characteristic feature of the back pain associated with AS is pain at night.[241] Patients often awaken in the early morning (between 2 and 5 AM) with back pain and stiffness, and usually either take a shower or exercise before returning to sleep.[240] Back ache during the day is typically intermittent irrespective of exertion or rest.[240]

Calin and colleagues[242] describe five screening questions for AS:

1. Is there morning stiffness?

2. Is there improvement in discomfort with exercise?

3. Was the onset of back pain before age 40 years?

4. Did the problem begin slowly?

5. Has the pain persisted for at least 3 months?

Using at least four positive answers to define a "positive" result, the sensitivity of these questions was 0.95 and specificity, 0.85.[242]

Peripheral arthritis is uncommon in AS, but when it occurs, it is usually late in the course of the arthritis.[243] Peripheral arthritis developing early in the course of the disease is a predictor of disease progression.[244] The arthritis usually occurs in the lower extremities in an asymmetric distribution, with involvement of the "axial" joints, including shoulders and hips, more common than involvement of more distal joints.[240,245]

Inspection usually reveals a flat lumbar spine and gross limitation of side bending in both directions. Mobility loss tends to be bilateral and symmetric. There is loss of spinal elongation on flexion (Schober's test), although this can occur in patients with chronic low back pain or spinal tumors and is thus not specific for inflammatory spondylopathies.[220] The patient may relate a history of costochondritis and, upon examination, rib springing may give a hard end-feel. Basal rib expansion often is decreased. The glides of the costotransverse joints and distraction of the sternoclavicular joints are decreased, and the lumbar spine exhibits a capsular pattern.

As the disease progresses, the pain and stiffness can spread up the entire spine, pulling it into forward flexion, so that the patient adopts the typical stooped-over position. The patient gazes downward, the entire back is rounded, the hips and knees are semiflexed, and the arms cannot be raised beyond a limited amount at the shoulders.[246]

Longitudinal studies in patients with AS have revealed that deformities and disability occur within the first 10 years of disease.[244] Most of the loss of function occurs during the first 10 years and correlates significantly with the occurrence of peripheral arthritis, radiographic changes of AS in the spine, and the development of so-called bamboo spine.

An exercise program is particularly important for these patients to maintain functional spinal outcomes.[247] The goal of exercise therapy is to maintain the mobility of the spine and involved joints for as long as possible, and to prevent the spine from stiffening in an unacceptable kyphotic position. A strict regimen of daily exercises, which include positioning and spinal extension exercises, breathing exercises, and exercises for the peripheral joints, must be followed. Several times a day, patients should lie prone for 5 minutes, and they should be encouraged to sleep on a hard mattress and avoid the side lying position. Swimming is the best routine sport.

Diffuse Idiopathic Skeletal Hyperostosis

Diffuse idiopathic skeletal hyperostosis (DISH), or Forestier disease, is a metabolic disease that typically affects men older than 40 years of age and does not usually result in severe disability.[248] The disease is characterized by an ossification of the anterior longitudinal ligaments and all related, anatomically similar ligaments,[218] without marked disk disease, which results in overall stiffness of the spine, particularly in the morning, and palpable tenderness.

Manubriosternal Dislocations

Traumatic disruption of the manubriosternal joint most often occurs via one of two mechanisms.[249,250] The first and most common mechanism results from a direct compression injury to the anterior chest. The direction of applied force displaces the fragment posteriorly and downward. The second type of mechanism follows hyperflexion with compression injury to the upper thorax. The force is transmitted to the sternum through the clavicles, chin, or upper two ribs.

Causes of Lumbar Pain

Numerous systemic disorders may cause low back discomfort, as indicated in Figure 9-1 and Table 9-13.

Renal Origin

Pain of renal origin is associated with pelvic, flank, or low back pain.

Acute Pyelonephritis.   See the discussion of pyelonephritis under "Causes of Head and Facial Pain," earlier.

Renal Cortical Abscess.   Renal abscess has been described as an elusive diagnosis in patients with variable symptoms of insidious onset. This condition can cause flank pain, chills, and fever, and may be associated with a history of recent infection.

Urologic management of renal abscesses includes surgical exploration, percutaneous drainage, intravenous antibiotic therapy, or nephrectomy.[251,252]

Acute Glomerulonephritis.   This condition occasionally can manifest with bilateral flank pain, costovertebral angle tenderness, and fever. Malaise, fatigue, anorexia, and nausea frequently accompany this condition.

Ureteral Colic.   Ureteral colic causes constant severe pain in the right lower abdomen. The pain is caused by passage of a calculus (kidney stone), blood clot, or tissue fragment in the lower half of the ureter. The pain, which may be intermittent, radiates down the course of the ureter into the urethra or groin area. Accompanying signs and symptoms include nausea, vomiting, sweating, and tachycardia.

Kidney stones are associated with conditions of hypercalcemia (excess calcium in the blood) such as hyperparathyroidism, metastatic carcinoma, multiple myeloma, senile osteoporosis, specific renal tubular disease, hyperthyroidism, and

TABLE 9-13   Potential Causes of Lumbar Pain

Renal dysfunction
Epidural abscess and epidural hematoma
Sacroilitis
Metastasis
Maigne's syndrome
Aortic or iliac aneurysm
Prostatitis
Pleural dysfunction
Ankylosing spondylitis
Stiff person syndrome

Cushing's disease.[209] Other conditions associated with calculus formation are infection, urinary stasis, dehydration, and excessive ingestion or absorption of calcium.[209]

Urinary Tract Infection.   A urinary tract infection (UTI) affecting the lower urinary tract is related directly to an irritation of the bladder and urethra. The intensity of symptoms depends on the severity of the infection, and although low back pain may be the patient's chief complaint, further questioning usually elicits additional urologic symptoms, such as urinary frequency, urinary urgency, or hematuria. The diagnosis of UTI is based on symptoms and the presence of pathogens and white blood cells in urine.

Epidural Abscess

Most spinal epidural abscesses or infections are thought to result from the spread of bacteria, usually from a cutaneous or mucosal source. Infection in the spinal epidural space is an uncommon but potentially fatal condition that often constitutes a surgical emergency. The infectious agent may enter the epidural space by several routes[253]:

▶ Insertion of an epidural needle and catheter.

▶ Migration along the outside of a catheter.

▶ Local spread through soft tissue and bone.

▶ Hematogenous spread.

▶ Injection or infusion of contaminated fluid.

Early diagnosis is essential for successful treatment.[254] The diagnosis of spinal abscess can be difficult because of its rarity and the insidious presentation. The signs and symptoms may develop slowly over days to several weeks. Fever is not always present.[255] Localized back pain or radicular pain is frequently the first sign of epidural infection.[255,256] This initial finding is followed by progressive radicular and cord compression signs.[255,256] Pain is the most consistent symptom and occurs in virtually all patients at some time during their illness.[254]

Intervention depends on the cause, and ranges from antibiotic therapy to surgery.

Prostatitis

Prostatitis is an inflammation of the prostate gland. The cause of the inflammation is usually infection, which can be bacterial or nonbacterial. In acute bacterial prostatitis, patients complain of a sudden onset of fever, chills, and low back or perineal pain. Typically, dysuria, frequency, or hesitancy is present. Patients with chronic bacterial prostatitis may have no systemic symptoms; that is, they may not have fever or chills, although complaints of perineal or low back pain usually are present. Patients with nonbacterial prostatitis have a variable presentation and lack systemic symptoms. These patients have mild pain and may have voiding symptoms.

Differential diagnosis includes prostatodynia, cystitis, urethritis, and benign prostatic hypertrophy.

Pleural Dysfunction

Although usually associated with thoracic pain, pleuritic pain can produce right lower abdomen pain. The cause is usually pneumonia or pulmonary embolism. The symptoms accompanying pneumonia include fever, coughing, rales, wheezes, chills, and purulent sputum. Pulmonary embolism usually is associated with dyspnea, fever, cough, rales, and wheezes. High-risk patients for pulmonary embolism include those with recent:

▶ Trauma.

▶ Surgery.

▶ Pregnancy.

▶ Heart failure.

▶ Malignancy.

▶ Previous embolism.

▶ Prolonged travel in automobile or airplane.

▶ Prolonged immobilization.

Aortic Aneurysm

The aorta is segmentally described in three sections: ascending aorta, aortic arch, and descending aorta. The portion of the aorta above the diaphragm is designated as thoracic, and the abdominal aorta is that portion below the diaphragm. The aorta consists of three layers: adventitia (the outermost), media, and intima.

An acute aortic dissection is caused by a transverse disruption in the intima and media.[257] This disruption results in the formation of a hematoma within the media. Aortic aneurysms can be described as either fusiform (circumferential dilatation) or saccular (balloonlike).[258]

The underlying causes of aortic disease are associated with many factors, including atherosclerosis, hypertension, medial degeneration and aging, aortitis, congenital abnormalities, trauma, smoking, cellular enzyme dysfunction, and hyperlipidemia.[257]

Acute aortic dissection is characterized by the onset of intense pain, described as sharp, tearing, or stabbing. The pain occurs in the chest and spreads toward the back and into the abdomen. The pain associated with this condition is unaffected by position. Distal pulses frequently are decreased or absent. This is a potentially life-threatening condition requiring immediate transport of the patient to an emergency department. The patient is admitted to the intensive care unit for further evaluation and to temporarily manage the crisis with antihypertensive medications.[257]

Metastasis

Malignant neoplasm (primary or metastatic) is the most common systemic disease affecting the spine, although it accounts for less than 1 percent of episodes of low back pain.[220] Metastatic lesions affecting the lumbar spine occur most commonly from the ovary, breast, kidney, thyroid, lung, or prostate gland.

A previous history of cancer has such high specificity (0.98) that such patients should be considered to have cancer until proven otherwise.[220] Most patients with back pain caused by cancer report that pain is unrelieved by bed rest (sensitivity > 0.90).[220]

Ankylosing Spondylitis

See the discussion under "Causes of Thoracic Pain," earlier.

Stiff Person Syndrome (SPS)

Stiff person syndrome (SPS), also known as Moersch-Woltmann syndrome, or stiff-man syndrome (SMS) is a rare, disabling neurological disorder, which is often under-diagnosed because of a lack of awareness of its clinical manifestations. Variants of the syndrome may involve one limb only (stiff leg syndrome), a variety of additional neurological symptoms and signs such as eye movement disturbances, ataxia, or Babinski signs (progressive encephalomyelitis with rigidity and myoclonus), or be associated with malignant disease (paraneoplastic SPS).[220a]

SPS has an insidious onset, usually in the fourth or fifth decades, with a slow progression over months or years followed by long-lasting stabilization. SPS is characterized by fluctuating symmetrical muscle rigidity and back pain with superimposed painful episodic spasms of the axial and proximal limb muscles.[220b]

▶ The muscle rigidity associated with SPS can lead to contractures, and simultaneous contraction of the thoracolumbar paraspinal and abdominal wall muscles causes lumbar hyperlordosis.

▶ The episodic spasms, which are often provoked by noise, touch, emotional upset or sudden movement, may manifest as an excessive startle reaction. These spasms can be violent enough to cause excruciating pain and, in rare cases, generate forces capable of fracturing long bones. Patients with SPS may exhibit excessive fear and avoidance of circumscribed situations that are assumed by patients to be difficult to master because of an increase in stiffness, paroxysmal spasms, or sudden falls.[220c] Such situations include crossing a street, climbing downstairs without banisters, or walking unaided. Patients may be incapacitated by the phobia to the same degree as the motor symptoms themselves. It has been suggested that the presence of this particular anxiety is one of the reasons for the frequent misdiagnosis of *psychogenic movement disorder* in these patients.[220c]

The rigidity and spasms gradually impair voluntary movements and postural reflexes, resulting in slow, restricted movements and an increased risk of falls. Intellect is not affected, and motor and sensory nerve examination is also normal. However, almost all patients have an abnormal EMG pattern, which shows continuous motor unit activity in affected muscles.

The cause of SPS is unknown, but an autoimmune-mediated chronic encephalomyelitis is suggested due to its frequent association with other autoimmune disorders such as type 1 diabetes or thyroiditis. Antibodies against GAD are present in about 60% of patients with SPS. GAD is the rate-limiting enzyme in the synthesis of γ-aminobutyric acid (GABA), one of the main inhibitory central neurotransmitters. Reductions in GABA production may therefore impair transmission at central nervous system inhibitory synapses, resulting in the continuous motor unit activity seen in this disease. However, approximately 40% of patients have no evidence of autoantibodies, suggesting that the pathogenesis of this syndrome may be heterogeneous.

The mainstays of treatment for SPS are drugs that enhance GABA-mediated central inhibition (diazepam, baclofen, sodium valproate, and vigabatrin) and antispastic physical therapy. SPS should be considered in all patients with unexplained back pain, stiffness and muscle spasms as early recognition and therapeutic intervention can significantly decrease morbidity and improve quality of life. Stiffness and spasms resembling SPS may occur as dominant symptoms in a variety of recognized neurological diseases such as multiple sclerosis, brain stem or spinal cord tumors, paraneoplastic or circulatory diseases of the spinal cord.[220a]

Causes of Buttock and Upper and Lower Leg Pain

The causes for buttock and upper and lower leg pain include those listed in Figure 9-1 and Table 9-14.

Lumbar Disk Herniation
See Chapter 20.

Femoral Nerve Neuropathy
Femoral neuropathy has been described as a complication of compression resulting from [259]:

▶ Hematoma.

▶ Hemophilia.

TABLE 9-14 Potential Causes of Buttock and Upper and Lower Leg Pain

Femoral nerve neuropathy
Lumbar disk herniation
Piriformis syndrome
Intermittent claudication
Sacral plexopathy
Conus medullaris syndrome
Trochanteric bursitis
Meralgia paresthetica
Iliofemoral thrombophlebitis
Sacroiliitis
Mononeuritis multiplex
Ischial apophysis and avulsion
Gluteal compartment syndrome
Genital herpes
Vascular disorders

▶ Leukemia.

▶ Hysterectomy and pelvic surgery.

▶ Lithotomy position.

▶ Blunt trauma.

▶ Iliac artery aneurysm.

▶ Inguinal herniorrhaphy.

▶ Malignancy and radiation therapy.

▶ Epstein-Barr virus infection.

▶ Diabetes mellitus.

Typical signs of femoral neuropathy are weakness of ipsilateral hip flexion, knee extension, and paresthesias of the anteromedial thigh. Symptoms may vary with both degree and location of injury. The more distal injuries may have either sensory or motor symptoms, whereas the proximal injuries tend to have both. A decreased or absent knee jerk is usually present. The differential diagnoses of upper lumbar nerve root symptoms include spondylolisthesis, disk prolapse, or an infective cause such as diskitis or an epidural abscess.

Piriformis Syndrome
The "piriformis syndrome," an uncommon and often undiagnosed cause of buttock and leg pain, has been described as an anatomic abnormality of the piriformis muscle and the sciatic nerve which can result in irritation of the sciatic nerve by the piriformis muscle causing buttock and hamstring pain. Piriformis syndrome may also be described as a sensation in which the hamstring muscles feel "tight" or are "about to tear."[260]

Multiple etiologies have been proposed to explain the compression or irritation of the sciatic nerve that occurs with the piriformis syndrome:[261]

▶ *Hypertrophy of the piriformis muscle.*[262,263]

▶ *Trauma.*[264,265,265a] Trauma, direct or indirect, to the sacroiliac or gluteal region can lead to piriformis syndrome and is a result of hematoma formation and subsequent scarring between the sciatic nerve and the short external rotators.

▶ *Hip flexion contracture.* A flexion contracture at the hip has been associated with piriformis syndrome. This flexion contracture increases the lumbar lordosis, which increases the tension in the pelvic–femoral muscles as these muscles try to stabilize the pelvis and spine in the new position. This increased tension causes the involved muscles to hypertrophy with no corresponding increase in the size of the bony foramina, resulting in neurological signs of sciatic compression.[266]

▶ *Gender.* Females are more commonly affected by piriformis syndrome, with as much as a 6:1 female-to-male incidence.[265a,267–270]

▶ *Ischial bursitis.*

▶ *Pseudoaneurysm of the inferior gluteal artery.*[264]

▶ *Excessive exercise to the hamstring muscles.*[271]

▶ *Inflammation and spasm of the piriformis muscle.*[272] This is often in association with trauma,[262,272a] infection, and anatomical variations of the muscle.[266,273,274]

▶ *Anatomical anomalies.* In 1938, anomalies of the piriformis muscle, with a subsequent alteration in the relationship between the piriformis muscle and the sciatic nerve were implicated in sciatica.[273] Local anatomical anomalies may contribute to the likelihood that symptoms will develop. Patients with this condition report radicular pain that is much like the nerve-root pain associated with lumbar disk disease with movement of the hip.[275] These patients typically present with a history of gluteal trauma, symptoms of pain in the buttock and intolerance to sitting, tenderness to palpation of the greater sciatic notch, and pain with flexion, adduction, and internal rotation of the hip.

As early as 1937, two findings on physical examination were attributed to sciatic pain, with the piriformis as the cause[276]:

1. Positive straight leg raise (pain in the vicinity of the greater sciatic notch on extension of the knee with the hip flexed to 90 degrees, and tenderness to palpation of the greater sciatic notch).

2. Freiberg's sign (pain with passive internal rotation of the hip).

Robinson[277] has been credited with introducing the term *piriformis syndrome* and outlining its six classic findings:

1. A history of trauma to the sacroiliac and gluteal regions.

2. Pain in the region of the sacroiliac joint, greater sciatic notch, and piriformis muscle that usually causes difficulty with walking.

3. Acute exacerbation of pain caused by stooping or lifting (and moderate relief of pain by traction on the affected extremity with the patient in the supine position).

4. A palpable sausage-shaped mass, tender to palpation, over the piriformis muscle on the affected side.

5. A positive straight leg raise.

6. Gluteal atrophy, depending on the duration of the condition.

Other clinical signs have since been introduced. Pace and Nagle[277a] described a diagnostic maneuver that is now referred to as Pace's sign: pain and weakness in association with resisted abduction and external rotation of the involved thigh.

Local muscle spasm usually is palpable in the obturator internus or, less commonly, in the piriformis muscle. The neurologic examination is usually normal.[278] An examination of the hip and lower leg usually demonstrates restricted external rotation of the hip and lumbosacral muscle tightness.[278]

Conservative intervention for this condition includes gentle, pain-free static stretching of the piriformis muscle, strain–counterstrain techniques, ice massage to the gluteal region, and spray and stretch techniques.

Sacral Plexopathy

The sciatic nerve is the most frequently injured lower extremity nerve. Sciatic nerve compression has been reported secondary to piriformis entrapment, heterotopic ossification around the hip,[279] ruptured aneurysm, retroperitoneal bleeding, pelvic fracture, dislocation or fracture of the hip, tumor, misplaced intramuscular injections, myofascial bands in the distal thigh,[280] and myositis ossificans of the biceps femoris muscle.[281] Additional causes include post-traumatic or anticoagulant-induced extraneural hematomas[282] and compartment syndrome of the posterior thigh.[283] Entrapment sciatic neuropathy complicating total hip arthroplasty has been described secondary to escaped cement, subfascial hematoma, and nerve impingement during trochanteric wiring.[284]

In the usual situation, the patient complains of an immediate onset of painful paresthesia, radiating down the posterior and posterolateral thigh and calf, and into the foot. Differential diagnosis also includes an L5-to-S1 radiculopathy caused by a herniated disk, or zygapophysial joint disease with lateral recess or foramen stenosis.

Intermittent Claudication

The blood supply of the lumbar and sacral plexuses usually derives from branches of the internal iliac artery (iliolumbar artery, superior and inferior gluteal artery, lateral sacral artery), and the deep iliac circumflex artery.[285] Acute ischemic impairments of the lumbosacral plexus are caused by high-grade stenosis and occlusion of the iliac arteries, or of the distal abdominal aorta.

The most frequent cause of such acute ischemic impairments of the lumbosacral plexus is surgery of the aortic bifurcation and the pelvic arteries, or radiation therapy.[286] Finally, intra-arterial injections into the iliac arteries or gluteal arteries may result in persistent ischemic plexopathy.[287]

Reduced perfusion within the area of the internal iliac artery can result in a temporary ischemic impairment of the lumbosacral plexus. This impairment occurs only during muscular activity of the legs. In this condition, the pain is mostly localized to the pelvis and is followed by paresthesia, a diminishing of the tendon reflexes, with possible motor weakness. This special type of intermittent claudication is usually associated with stenosis of the pelvic arteries, including the internal iliac arteries.[287]

The diagnosis is confirmed by changes in the lumbar motor evoked potentials after exertion. These changes exclude the diagnosis of ischemia of the lower spinal cord or conus medullaris.

Peripheral nerves have a high tolerance to ischemia because of collateral circulation.[288] However, during leg activity, the muscles supplied by branches of the external iliac arteries, experience a steal-phenomenon that privileges the leg muscles over the pelvic organs.[287]

Although the neurologic examination of the inactive patient usually discloses no abnormality, the clinical diagnosis of this type of intermittent claudication caused by exercise-induced ischemia of the lumbosacral plexus is based mainly on two specific features[287]:

1. The symptoms appear in correlation with the degree of muscle activity. In early stages of the disease, complaints only occur during walking uphill or riding a bicycle. This allows a distinction from the intermittent claudication caused by spinal stenosis. In the latter symptoms predominantly appear during walking downhill. In addition, patients with spinal stenosis can ride a bicycle for a long distance without complaints.

2. In addition to pain, progressive sensorimotor deficits in the area of the lumbosacral plexus occur during exertion. This cannot be seen in patients with peripheral arterial occlusive disease.

Conus Medullaris Syndrome

Conus medullaris syndrome results from an injury to the spinal cord. The injury can be caused by trauma, such as bone or bullet fragments. It may also result from cyst formation, aortic surgery, and vascular disease.

The symptoms include severe low back and buttock pain, lower limb weakness, and saddle hyperesthesia or anesthesia. Bowel and bladder changes also frequently are reported.

Meralgia Paresthetica

In 1885, the German surgeon Werner Hager[289] gave the first description of an injury to the lateral femoral cutaneous nerve. This syndrome was described independently by both Bernhardt[290] and Roth[291] in 1895. Roth named the syndrome *meralgia paresthetica* from the Greek words *meros* (thigh) and *algos* (pain).

Meralgia paresthetica is a mononeuropathy of the lateral femoral cutaneous nerve (LFCN), diagnosis of which is often missed or delayed.[292] It also can occur to other nerves that traverse the hip, such as the ilioinguinal, genitofemoral, obturator, and anterior cutaneous nerves of the thigh.[293]

The LFCN is primarily a sensory nerve but also includes efferent sympathetic fibers carrying vasomotor, pilomotor, and sudomotor impulses.[294] It is quite variable and may be derived from several different combinations of lumbar nerves, including L2 and L3, L1 and L2, L2 alone, and L3 alone.[295] The LFCN may be associated with the femoral nerve as it passes through the inguinal ligament, or it may anastomose with the femoral nerve distal to the inguinal ligament.[292]

Toxic and metabolic disorders, such as diabetes mellitus, alcoholism, and lead poisoning, which have been reported to be causative in several cases, have all been described to increase susceptibility of individual peripheral nerves, including the lateral femoral cutaneous nerve, to mechanical insults.[296,297] This apparent vulnerability of the lateral femoral cutaneous nerve has been investigated by a number of authors.[298,299] The compression of the nerve may be at the level of the roots, but it also may be compressed along the retroperitoneal course.

Numerous direct and indirect causes for the disease have been suggested in the literature including[290,300–303]:

- ▶ Obesity.
- ▶ Direct trauma.
- ▶ Abdominal distention.
- ▶ Metastatic carcinoma in the iliac crest.
- ▶ Anatomic variation at the site of passage.[302]
- ▶ Retroperitoneal tumors.
- ▶ Leg-length discrepancy.
- ▶ Idiopathic causes.
- ▶ Tight clothing around the waist.
- ▶ Complications after thoraco-abdominal surgery.
- ▶ Complications after iliac bone graft harvesting.

Neuropathy of this nerve may cause pain, numbness, and dysesthesia in the anterolateral aspect of the thigh that is most marked on walking and standing, resulting in restriction of activities.[304] Sitting may relieve the symptoms in some patients but exacerbate them in others. Eventually, no position provides relief. Patients may have secondary hip, knee, and calf pain. Entrapment of the lateral cutaneous nerve of the thigh also can be the cause of chronic groin pain.[305–307] It is most common in middle-aged men and may occur as the first sign of a lumbar cord tumor.

Differential diagnosis includes back, hip, and groin pathology. Intervention is dependent on the cause.

Iliofemoral Thrombophlebitis

Thrombophlebitis of the superficial veins of the leg is usually regarded as a mild and uncomplicated disease. Although this is generally true in the case of acute thrombosis of the branches of the saphenous vein, the natural history of superficial venous thrombophlebitis (SVT) involving the main trunk may not be as benign. The relationship between SVT and deep venous thrombosis (DVT) with attendant pulmonary embolus has become the focus of more recent studies. An association with DVT has been reported with frequencies of 12 to 44 percent,[308] and there have been several reports of pulmonary embolism in thrombophlebitis.[309]

The clinical signs and symptoms of iliofemoral thrombophlebitis include generalized leg pain, bluish discoloration, and swelling. This condition also may be associated with acute lower abdominal, groin and flank pain, fever, chills, and localized tenderness.

Mononeuritis Multiplex

Mononeuritis multiplex can occur in association with a number of other medical conditions including rheumatoid arthritis, vasculitis, polyarteritis nodosa, diabetes mellitus, sarcoidosis, and amyloidosis. An ischemic mechanism is the most likely cause of mononeuritis multiplex. It is generally accepted that mononeuritis multiplex in rheumatoid arthritis results from ischemia caused by vasa nervorum vasculitis. Involvement of peripheral nerves precedes involvement of the central nervous system. The classic symptoms for mononeuritis multiplex include a sudden onset of severe aching, burning, or lancinating leg pain, paresthesias, sensory loss, and motor weakness.[310] The symptoms can involve one or more nerves in each leg, usually in an asymmetric pattern.[310]

Ischial Apophysitis and Avulsion

The ischial apophysis constitutes the insertion of the hamstrings and the adductor magnus muscles. Ischial tuberosity pain may be caused by several clinical entities, which include acute and old bony or periosteal avulsions and apophysitis. The clinical diagnostic criterion for ischial apophysitis consists of a gradual increase in functional and palpatory pain at the ischial tuberosity without any major trauma at the beginning of the symptoms. Usually there is asymmetry on plain radiographs of the ischial tuberosities in apophysitis. The radiograph demonstrates a sclerotic area, and osteoporotic patches on the lower margin of the ischial tuberosity. Patients with an avulsion usually report an acute traumatic incident. An avulsion fragment may be visible on plain radiograph immediately after injury or later. The pain is usually local, but may also radiate down the thigh. Active or resisted knee flexion increases the pain, unless the avulsion is complete. Complete avulsions can be painless.

The healing process of an avulsion may lead to heterotrophic bone formation.

Differential diagnosis includes intervertebral disk disease, piriformis syndrome, ischial bursitis, and pubic arch stress fracture.

Conservative intervention for apophysitis consists of modification of activities. Avulsions require at least 1 month of rest from training, depending on the displacement. Urgent surgical intervention is recommended in cases of a complete or nearly complete soft tissue avulsion of the hamstring muscle insertion.[311]

Gluteal Compartment Syndrome[312]

The characteristic finding for a gluteal compartment syndrome is a tense, swollen buttock following a mechanism of severe contusion, such as a fall from a height. The swelling in the buttock can result in necrosis of the gluteal muscles or sciatic neuropathy, or both. The patient should be referred immediately to an orthopedic surgeon. A fasciotomy is typically performed if the pressure within the gluteal compartment is 30 mm Hg or higher for a duration of 6 to 8 hours.[313]

Genital Herpes

Genital herpes is a chronic, viral, sexually transmitted disease for which there is no cure. It affects over 30 million people in the United States and continues to increase worldwide.[314] The majority of individuals are asymptomatic; however, some present with painful and recurrent genital lesions and systemic complications. As a chronic illness, the individual's response to the disease may produce serious psychosocial morbidity.[315] Women are more likely to have genital herpes than are men.[316]

Vascular Disorders

Gradual obstruction of the aortic bifurcation produces[209]:

▶ Bilateral buttock and leg pain.

▶ Weakness and fatigue of the lower extremities.

▶ Atrophy of the leg musculature.

▶ Absent femoral pulses.

▶ Color and temperature changes in the lower extremities.

▶ Pain that is often aggravated with lumbar extension.

▶ A pulsing sensation in the abdomen. On occasion, an abdominal aortic aneurysm can cause severe back pain. Prompt medical attention is imperative because rupture can result in death. The patients are usually men in their sixth or seventh decade, who present with a deep, boring pain in the mid-lumbar region. Other historical clues of coronary disease or intermittent claudication of the lower extremities may be present. An examination may reveal a pulsing abdominal mass. Peripheral pulses may be diminished or absent.[317]

Involvement of the femoral artery along its course, or at the femoral-popliteal junction, produces[209]:

▶ Thigh and calf pain.

▶ Absent pulses below the femoral pulse.

Obstruction of the popliteal artery or its branches produces pain in the calf, ankle, or foot.

Causes of Pelvic Pain

The causes of pelvic pain include those listed in Figure 9-1 and Table 9-15.

Sacroiliac Arthritis

Sacroiliac arthritis is characterized by pain in the posterior aspect of the sacrum, or by groin pain (uncommon), which can radiate into the posterior thigh. The pain is usually increased with walking, either at heel strike or at midstance. Frequently the pain wakes the patient when turning in bed.

Lumbar extension is the most painful motion, ipsilateral side bending and rotation less so, and flexion least of all. If pain is increased with unilateral weight bearing or hopping but is reduced if a sacroiliac belt is worn, sacroiliac joint arthritis may be present.

TABLE 9-15   Potential Causes of Pelvic Pain

Sacroiliac arthritis
Acute appendicitis
Iliopsoas abscess
Iliopsoas hematoma
Sign of the buttock
Gynecologic disorders
Prostate cancer

The sacroiliac joint stress tests described in Chapter 27 are used to help with the clinical diagnosis. Imaging studies are used to confirm the diagnosis.

Acute Appendicitis

This condition frequently begins with dull and aching pain in the right lower abdomen. The pain is intensified with walking, coughing, and trunk movements. There is usually an associated low-grade fever. Dysuria, diarrhea, constipation, or increased urinary frequency also may be reported. The patient is often able to localize the pain to McBurney's point, which is located by palpation at the mid-point between the anterior superior iliac spine and the umbilicus.

Less common signs include rectal or testicular tenderness and right lower abdominal skin hyperesthesia.

Iliopsoas Abscess

The pain associated with an iliopsoas abscess occurs in the right lower abdomen. The pain is usually mild to moderate and is increased with hip extension and palpation in the right iliac fossa. The abscess is caused by an infection of the thoracolumbar spine, such as tuberculosis, or is secondary to an intestinal disorder, such as Crohn's disease.[318]

Iliopsoas Hematoma

Hematomas are more frequently seen in the iliacus muscle than the psoas.[319] The causes of these hematomas include:

► Heparin anticoagulation or DVT prophylaxis therapy.

► Hemophilia.

► Trauma from either a direct blow to the abdomen or a hyperextension moment at the hip, such as occurs in a slip or fall.

Nontraumatic hematomas often manifest insidiously with no obvious lesion or ecchymosis. Patients initially may complain of flank pain but frequently will develop motor and sensory deficits along the femoral nerve distribution of the affected side. Flank pain refers to pain in the side of the trunk between the right or left upper abdomen and the back. A palpable lower abdominal mass may be present, depending on the size and location of the hematoma.

Iliopsoas hematomas have been successfully managed with conservative treatment. This intervention involves bed rest for 24 to 48 hours, followed by gentle hip range of motion exercises. Progressive strengthening exercises are then initiated according to patient tolerance.

Surgical intervention involves evacuation of the clot.

Sign of the Buttock

The sign of the buttock is not technically a cause of pain but is, rather, a collection of signs indicating a serious pathology present posterior to the axis of flexion and extension in the hip.[12] Among the causes of the syndrome are osteomyelitis, infectious sacroiliitis, fracture of the sacrum or pelvis, septic bursitis, ischiorectal abscess, gluteal hematoma, gluteal tumor, and rheumatic bursitis.

The sign of the buttock typically includes almost all of the following:

► Limited straight leg raising.

► Limited hip flexion.

► Limited trunk flexion.

► Noncapsular pattern of restriction at the hip.

► Painful and weak hip extension.

► Gluteal swelling.

► Empty end-feel on hip flexion.

Greenwood and colleagues[320] have suggested that a noncapsular pattern of the hip in the presence of a positive sign of the buttock indicates that the pathology is not amenable to a physical therapy intervention.

Gynecologic Disorders

Gynecologic disorders have the potential to cause midpelvic or low back discomfort.

Pelvic Inflammatory Disease. Pelvic inflammatory disease (PID) is the general term describing endometritis, salpingitis, tubo-ovarian abscess, or pelvic peritonitis. The microbial etiology of pelvic inflammatory disease is unclear but is assumed to occur by the ascending spread of microorganisms from the vagina or endocervix into the upper genital tract.[321] PID has been considered primarily a sexually transmitted disease caused in large part by the sexually transmitted pathogens *Neisseria gonorrhoeae* and *Chlamydia trachomatis*.[321] However, endogenous microorganisms that are part of the lower genital tract flora can also be recovered from the endometrium, fallopian tubes, and peritoneal fluid of women with acute PID.[321]

The characteristic presentation of PID is one of suprapubic pain. The pain is usually constant or crampy and may be associated with fever, chills, and direct abdominal tenderness.[318] The use of an intrauterine device (IUD) doubles the risk of endometritis.[318]

The onset of PID is usually within 7 days of the beginning of a menstrual cycle. There may be fever and vaginal discharge.

Tubal Pregnancy. In its early stages, this condition usually produces mild and colicky lower abdominal pain. The pain is caused by an ectopic pregnancy, in which the embryo locates itself in the fallopian tube instead of the uterus. Tubal pregnancy is usually associated with abnormal menstruation and irregular spotting or staining.

Endometriosis. Endometriosis affects up to 1 in 7 women and as many as 30 to 50 percent of all infertile women.[322] Endometriosis can be found anywhere in the pelvis, including the broad ligaments, uterosacral ligaments, and ovaries. The condition is linked to abdominal, midline, and pelvic pain. Associated signs and symptoms include pain on defecation, diarrhea, dysmenorrhea, dyspareunia (difficult or painful coitus), and dysuria.[323] The diagnosis of endometriosis can be elusive, because its most common symptoms are also symptoms of multiple disorders.[322] Although endometriosis is not considered a malignant disorder, it has characteristics in common with malignant cells. For instance, endometriosis, like cancer, can be both locally and distantly metastatic; it attaches to other tissues, invades, and damages them.[324]

Interstitial Cystitis. Interstitial cystitis is a clinical syndrome of urinary frequency or pelvic pain, or both, in a patient in whom no other pathology can be established. Interstitial cystitis has no single, definable presentation. The pain that occurs with this syndrome is not limited to pain on voiding (dysuria); it can refer to locations throughout the pelvis, including the urethra, vagina, suprapubic area, lower abdomen, lower back, medial aspect of the thigh, and inguinal area, in any combination.[325]

Prostate Cancer

Prostate cancer is the most common nonskin cancer and the second leading cause of male cancer deaths among U.S. men. Risk factors for prostate cancer include age, familial history of cancer, and ethnicity. Whether chronic or recurrent prostatic inflammation contributes to prostate cancer development has not been ascertained.

Prostate cancer often is diagnosed when a man seeks medical assistance because of urinary obstruction or sciatica. The sciatic (low back, hip, and leg) pain is caused by metastasis of the cancer to the bones of the pelvis, lumbar spine, or femur.

Prostate cancer screening or early detection has been accomplished using digital rectal examination, measurement of serum prostate-specific antigen (PSA), and its various forms, transrectal ultrasonography, and combinations of these tests.

► *Digital rectal examination.* The vast majority of prostatic carcinomas arise in the peripheral zone of the prostate, which comprises the posterior surface of the gland, including the apical, lateral, posterolateral, and anterolateral portions of the prostate. It is this part of the gland that is accessible by digital rectal examination.

► *PSA.* Measurement of PSA levels is regarded widely as the most clinically useful tool for the early diagnosis of prostate cancer. The routine use of serum PSA testing in men beginning at age 50 years also has led to a marked decrease in the age at diagnosis of prostate cancer patients.

Causes of Trochanteric, Pubic, and Thigh Pain

Potential causes of trochanteric, pubic, and thigh pain include those listed in Figure 9-3 and Table 9-16.

Dislocation and Fracture Dislocation of the Hip

A posterior dislocation of the hip usually occurs in a motor vehicle accident or fall. There is usually severe groin and lateral hip pain. The leg is shortened and held flexed, adducted, and internally rotated. Posterior dislocations are more common than anterior dislocations.

Potential Causes of Trochanteric, Pubic, and Thigh Pain

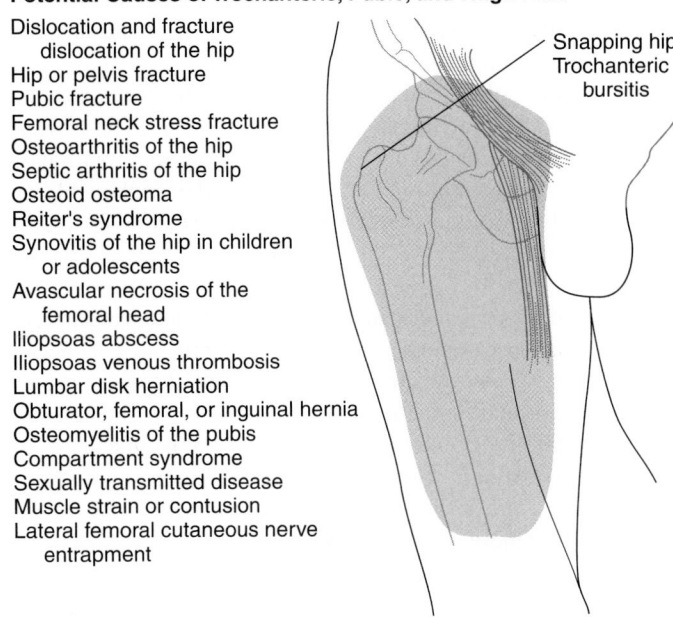

Dislocation and fracture
   dislocation of the hip
Hip or pelvis fracture
Pubic fracture
Femoral neck stress fracture
Osteoarthritis of the hip
Septic arthritis of the hip
Osteoid osteoma
Reiter's syndrome
Synovitis of the hip in children
   or adolescents
Avascular necrosis of the
   femoral head
Iliopsoas abscess
Iliopsoas venous thrombosis
Lumbar disk herniation
Obturator, femoral, or inguinal hernia
Osteomyelitis of the pubis
Compartment syndrome
Sexually transmitted disease
Muscle strain or contusion
Lateral femoral cutaneous nerve
   entrapment

Snapping hip
Trochanteric
bursitis

FIGURE 9-3   Potential causes of trochanteric, pubic, and thigh pain.

An anterior dislocation usually occurs as the result of forced abduction. Anterior dislocations cause groin pain and tenderness. In a superior anterior (pubic) dislocation, the leg is held extended and externally rotated. In an inferior anterior (obturator) dislocation, the thigh is abducted, externally rotated, and held in flexion.

The intervention for a hip dislocation is early closed reduction under spinal or general anesthesia.

Congenital dislocations of the hip are described in Chapter 17.

TABLE 9-16   Potential Causes of Trochanteric, Pubic, and Thigh Pain

Dislocation and fracture dislocation of the hip
Labral tear
Hip or pelvis fracture
Pubic stress fracture
Femoral neck stress fracture
Osteoarthritis of the hip
Septic arthritis of the hip
Reiter's syndrome
Transient synovitis of hip in children or adolescents
Avascular necrosis of femoral head
Iliopsoas abscess
Iliofemoral venous thrombosis
Obturator, femoral, or inguinal hernia
Osteomyelitis pubis
Compartment syndrome
Genital herpes

Labral Tear

Labral tears of the hip are more common than previously thought.[326] Because a labral lesion produces a decrease of pressure within the joint and causes an increase in the laxity of that joint, symptoms of a labral tear are usually mechanical: a history of trauma, buckling, twinges, and painful clicking. The labrum can be assessed using passive extension and external rotation of the hip, with the patient lying supine at the edge of the table. A positive finding with this test is apprehension or exquisite pain.

Hip Fracture

A fracture of the proximal femur (femoral neck, intertrochanteric or subtrochanteric) usually results from a fall but can occur spontaneously. The characteristic findings include severe groin, anterior thigh, and, sometimes, trochanteric pain and tenderness. Fracture of the femoral neck typically occurs in an elderly osteoporotic patient, with a female-to-male ratio of 4:1.[327] Depending on the severity and location of the fracture, there may be a shortening of the involved leg.

Pubic Stress Fracture

Pubic rami fractures are the most commonly seen pubic fractures, with the superior ramus more commonly involved than the inferior ramus. Pubic rami and pubic bone fractures account for more than 70 percent of all pelvic fractures.[328] Pubic stress fractures are associated with a gradual onset of groin pain, which is intensified with weight bearing, walking, or abduction of the thigh.

Femoral Neck Stress Fracture

See Chapter 17.

Osteitis Pubis

See Chapter 27.

Adductor Muscle Strain

See Chapter 17.

Reiter's Syndrome

Reiter's syndrome refers to the clinical triad of nongonococcal urethritis, conjunctivitis, and arthritis first described by Reiter in 1916.[329] This form of arthritis usually follows an infection of the genitourinary or gastrointestinal tract. It usually manifests at least one other extra-articular feature, with asymmetric involvement of the large weight-bearing joints.[245] The joints of the mid-foot, and the metatarsophalangeal and interphalangeal joints of the toes are most commonly affected. Onset is usually between the ages of 20 and 40 years, with males predominantly affected.[245]

The association of Reiter's syndrome with HLA-B27, occurring in 70 to 90 percent of patients, has been recognized for nearly as long as the association of HLA-B27 with ankylosing spondylitis.[330]

Transient Synovitis of the Hip in Children or Adolescents

Transient synovitis of the hip is one of the most common causes of hip pain and limp in young children. It is defined as an acute, self-limiting inflammation of the synovial lining of the hip joint. The cause of the inflammation is still a subject of great discussion. Proposed causes have included[331]:

▶ Virus.

▶ Trauma.

▶ Allergy.

The classic patient with transient synovitis of the hip is a 3- to 8-year-old boy with a history of acute unilateral hip pain associated with a limp. Anterior thigh or medial knee, pain is occasionally the predominant complaint. Because of the pain and the reactive effusion, hip motion is limited. The hip is usually held in a position of flexion and external rotation so that the hip capsule is lax as much as possible and the elevated intracapsular pressure is slightly relieved.[331]

Transient synovitis usually lasts 3 to 10 days. The intervention involves methods to alleviate the symptoms. This includes rest, avoidance of weight bearing on the involved extremity, and anti-inflammatory therapy. Traction may be considered as a temporary means of relieving pressure on the joint.

Osteoarthritis of the Hip

Osteoarthritis (OA) of the hip is one of many causes of hip and groin pain in older patients. It is important to identify patients with symptomatic OA correctly and to exclude conditions that may be mistaken for, or coexist, with it.[332,333] Periarticular pain that is not reproduced by passive motion suggests an alternate etiology such as bursitis, tendonitis, or periostitis. The distribution of painful joints also helps to distinguish OA from other types of arthritis, because metacarpophalangeal, wrist, elbow, ankle, and shoulder arthritis are unlikely locations for OA, except after trauma. Symptoms that include prolonged morning stiffness (greater than 1 hour) should raise suspicion of an inflammatory arthritis, such as rheumatoid arthritis.

The primary goals of treatment are to relieve pain, maintain joint function and mobility, and reduce joint swelling. This intervention approach involves focusing on modifying risk factors, particularly obesity, and engaging specific treatments, such as moderate exercise and pharmacotherapy.[334]

Septic Arthritis of the Hip

The clinical presentation of septic arthritis of the hip is similar to that of synovitis of the hip. However, because delayed diagnosis of septic arthritis can be life threatening, correct and early differentiation of septic arthritis and transient synovitis is important.[331] Compared with patients who have transient synovitis, those with septic arthritis usually have more severe pain and spasm. The leg is rigid and is held in the standard flexed and externally rotated position to increase capsular capacity.[331]

Avascular Necrosis of the Femoral Head

Avascular necrosis of the femoral head is also known as aseptic necrosis or osteonecrosis. According to Kenzora[335] and colleagues,[336] the term *avascular necrosis* should be reserved exclusively for post-traumatic causes, because they originate in ischemia as a result of blood flow interruption. When the etiology of the necroses has not been established clearly or is obscure, it is best to use the general term *idiopathic osteonecrosis*.

Several etiologic factors have been implicated in the development of nontraumatic avascular necrosis of the hip, but the precipitating event that is common to most, if not all, is a mechanical interruption of the circulation of the femoral head. If the affected area is sufficiently large and the collateral circulation is inadequate, avascular necrosis will develop. This may occur by direct external vascular occlusion without disruption of the vessels, as in marrow infiltrative diseases. Arterial thrombosis probably occurs in the vascular disorders, and emboli have been implicated in sickle-cell disease and caisson disease (dysbaric osteonecrosis). The systemic administration of steroids and an excessive intake of alcohol are the two factors most often associated with nontraumatic avascular necrosis.[337] Overall, etiologic factors can be clearly identified in most patients; perhaps only 10 to 20 percent of patients have truly idiopathic avascular necrosis.

The symptoms of avascular necrosis are nonspecific and usually insidious in onset. The pain, which is typically felt in the groin, proximal thigh, or buttock area, is usually exacerbated by weight bearing, but it is often present at rest. The clinical findings vary, and it is only when the femoral head becomes deformed that limitations of motion in a noncapsular pattern occur. Axial loading of the joint, as in the scour test, may reproduce the symptoms. A limp or an antalgic gait is typically a late finding, and the functional disability is proportionate to the level of pain.[337] Usually, the pain becomes more severe as fragmentation and collapse of the femoral head take place. Sometimes the pain will lessen if spontaneous improvement occurs, and small lesions may remain asymptomatic and resolve spontaneously.[337]

Clinically diagnosed avascular necrosis is progressive in 70 to 80 percent of patients who are managed nonoperatively, and this progression usually results in collapse of the femoral head.[337] Although conservative intervention is aimed at limiting the stresses through the hip joint, and utilizing a support, operative intervention generally is recommended.

Iliopsoas Abscess
See the discussion under "Causes of Pelvis Pain," earlier.

Trochanteric Bursitis
See Chapter 17.

Obturator, Femoral, or Inguinal Hernia
The clinical diagnosis of inguinal and femoral hernias is usually straightforward. A few hernias, however, present a diagnostic problem. This diagnostic difficulty is usually encountered in obese patients or in patients with reducible hernias that are not protruding at the time of physical examination. False-positive findings include lipoma of the spermatic cord and preperitoneal lipoma. A cord lipoma appears as a smooth, finger-like projection of fat parallel to the cord vessels at rest. During straining, longitudinal sliding occurs. Unlike indirect inguinal hernias, the anteroposterior diameter of the inguinal canal does not increase during the Valsalva maneuver.

Osteomyelitis Pubis
Bony infection or inflammation of the pubic area is rare. Osteomyelitis pubis is an entity characterized by pelvic pain, a wide-based gait, and bony destruction of the margins of the pubic symphysis.[338] Delay in its diagnosis is common because the presentation is similar to that of osteitis pubis and urologic, gynecologic, and abdominal lesions. Osteomyelitis pubis should be considered when a patient presents with the following signs: pain or pubic tenderness, painful hip abduction, and fever.[338]

Antibiotic treatment is essential, with the specific drug therapy depending on identification of the causative agent.

Compartment Syndrome
Compartment syndrome is a condition in which myoneural anoxia results from a prolonged increase in tissue pressure within a closed osseofascial space. This compromises local blood flow of skeletal muscle, resulting in ischemia and necrosis.

Local blood flow may be impaired by:

▶ An increase in the pressure of the compartment resulting from the application of a tight bandage or plaster cast.

▶ A decrease in arterial flow, as in peripheral vascular disease.

▶ An increase in venous pressure that can reduce the gradient for local blood flow.

False aneurysms of the profunda femoris artery are a rare but recognized complication following orthopedic procedures in the upper thigh. Such procedures include internal fixation of intertrochanteric, subtrochanteric, and intracapsular femoral neck fractures; subtrochanteric osteotomy; and intramedullary nailing of the femur.[339]

A compartment syndrome of the thigh usually manifests as a pulsating, expanding swelling of the upper thigh with an audible bruit. Potential complications include expansion and extensive soft tissue destruction and pressure to neighboring structures.[339] This can result in neuropathy or venous outflow obstruction and thrombosis. Rupture and severe hemorrhage, infection of the aneurysm, and sepsis of the nearby prosthesis, as well as fracture non-union, also have been reported.[339]

Early recognition and repair of the aneurysm is of paramount importance to avoid life- and limb-threatening complications from delayed diagnosis.[339] Any unexplained thigh swelling encountered following a surgical procedure on the proximal femur and shaft should alert the clinician to a potential injury to the profunda femoris artery.[339]

Genital Herpes
See the discussion under "Causes of Buttock and Upper and Lower Leg Pain," earlier.

Causes of Shoulder and Upper Arm Pain
The causes of shoulder and upper arm pain include those listed in Tables 9-17 and 9-18.

TABLE 9-17   Potential Causes of Shoulder Pain

Tendinous and capsular lesions
Traumatic synovitis
Subluxation
Dislocation
Spondyloarthropy
Acute arthritis
Infections
Tumor
Clay shoveler's fracture
Degenerative conditions
Metabolic conditions
Cerebrovascular disease
Multiple sclerosis
Amyotrophic lateral sclerosis
Guillain-Barré syndrome
Syringomyelia
Cervical radicular pain
Elbow dysfunction
Peripheral nerve entrapment
Brachial plexopathy
Herpes zoster
Gallbladder dysfunction
Cardiac dysfunction
Pulmonary dysfunction
Diaphragm
Spleen

Local Conditions

Tendinous and Capsular Lesions.   See Chapter 14.
Synovitis.   The shoulder joint is composed of two synovial cavities: the subacromial–subdeltoid bursa and the glenohumeral joint. In rotator cuff diseases, subacromial synovitis is responsible for the generation of shoulder pain, and its severity may correlate with the intensity of pain. During inflammation, so-called hyperalgesia occurs, which is characterized by intensified pain with a reduced threshold to somatic stimulation.

Pigmented villonodular synovitis is one of a group of benign, proliferative lesions arising from the synovium of joints, bursae, and tendon sheaths.[340] Traditionally, these lesions have been identified as benign giant cell tumor of the tendon sheath, hemorrhagic villous synovitis, and proliferative synovitis.[341] Pigmented villonodular synovitis in the knee and hand has been described frequently, but its occurrence at the shoulder is rare.

The cause of pigmented villonodular synovitis is unclear, but it may be related to inflammation or trauma. The lesions develop slowly, and patients usually present with gradual onset of pain at the affected joint.[340] A palpable, tender, soft tissue mass may be present. Pigmented villonodular synovitis is regarded as a locally aggressive but benign tumor. Early diagnosis and treatment are essential to preserve joint function and integrity. The treatment of choice is complete synovectomy or bursectomy, or arthroscopic synovectomy.[340]

Subluxation.   Shoulder subluxation can be caused by trauma, overuse, or hemiplegia. The traumatic and overuse causes of shoulder subluxation, which can often be diagnosed on the basis of history and physical examination, are described in Chapter 14. The most common complaints are of instability, restricted activities, and pain. Strength and range of motion are usually normal. The most common significant finding on physical examination is apprehension.

Shoulder pain is a common complication of hemiplegia. One of the most commonly cited causes of shoulder pain in hemiplegia is shoulder subluxation. Shoulder subluxation occurs in hemiplegia because of the paralysis of active restraints,

TABLE 9-18   Origin and Location of Shoulder Pain[209]

Right Shoulder		Left Shoulder	
Systemic Origin	Location	Systemic Origin	Location
Peptic ulcer	Lateral border of right scapula	Ruptured spleen Myocardial ischemia	Left shoulder Left pectoral/shoulder area
Myocardial ischemia	Right shoulder, down arm	Pancreas	Left shoulder
Hepatic/biliary			
Acute cholecystitis	Right shoulder; between scapulae; right subscapular area		
Liver abscess	Right shoulder		
Gallbladder	Right upper trapezius		
Liver disease (hepatitis, cirrhosis, metastatic tumors)	Right shoulder, right subscapular area		

which play a critical role in maintaining glenohumeral joint integrity. In this population, glenohumeral joint subluxation may inhibit functional recovery by limiting glenohumeral range of motion.

Unfortunately, the available options for preventing and treating shoulder subluxation are limited. Armboards and laptrays have not been shown to be effective and may lead to an overcorrection of inferior subluxation.[342] This overcorrection may predispose the involved shoulder to impingement syndromes. The use of slings remains controversial. Slings may cause lateral subluxation, contribute to the deleterious effects of joint immobilization, or promote undesirable synergistic patterns of muscle activation.[342] Intramuscular neuromuscular electrical stimulation (NMES) delivered via percutaneously placed electrodes may address the limitations of transcutaneous systems and increase the use of NMES to treat shoulder subluxation and pain.[342]

Dislocation. In contrast to the hip, in which the ball-and-socket joint is deep and well stabilized, the articular surface of the shoulder rests in the shallow glenoid cavity. Ninety-five percent of shoulder dislocations occur in the anterior direction and result in stretching and detachment of the anterior capsule and labrum.[343] Dislocation of the shoulder is a common and often disabling injury, resulting in damage to nerves, blood vessels, and the rotator cuff muscles. Most shoulder dislocations are traumatic in origin. The most common mechanisms are a fall on an outstretched hand, a blow against the anterior arm when the limb is extended and externally rotated, or, rarely, a blow to the back of the shoulder.

Traumatic shoulder dislocations are accompanied by extreme pain that worsens as the supporting musculature goes into spasm.[344] Generally, patients present with the arm somewhat abducted and externally rotated, often grasped tightly by the opposite hand to minimize movement.[344]

The examination of a patient who has recently dislocated the shoulder is often difficult because of associated pain and muscle guarding. It is important to examine for axillary nerve function (deltoid power and overlying sensation), supraspinatus power, and glenohumeral range of motion.[345] Axillary nerve palsy and avulsion of the supraspinatus are common complications of a dislocated shoulder. Associated fractures may be present. Vascular compromise is uncommon in this injury, but when it occurs, rapid surgical referral is necessary to save the limb.[344]

Spondyloarthropathy. Rheumatoid arthritis (RA) affects the joints in a characteristic and symmetric fashion. In addition to the smaller joints, RA can affect the larger joints, including the shoulders. It results in pain and stiffness, which are usually greatest in the morning.[346–348] This condition should be considered when patients have symmetric involvement of the shoulder, morning stiffness, constitutional signs, and physical signs of joint inflammation.[349] Synovial inflammation of the subacromial–subdeltoid bursae can occur, resulting in pain on abduction to 90 degrees in both shoulders.[349] Chronic inflammation or long-term corticosteroid use, or both, may also result in rotator cuff

tearing, another viable cause of pain and function loss in the patient with RA. This should be suspected when significant weakness is noted on abduction or external rotation.[349] The clinician also should look for other signs of inflammatory arthritis, which include synovial thickening of the metacarpophalangeal joints and thickening at, and loss of range of motion of, the wrists. The rheumatoid factor is often negative in older patients with RA.[349]

> ### Clinical Pearl
>
> Polymyalgia rheumatica is another cause of shoulder pain in older individuals. These patients have pain in the shoulder and hip girdle muscles, profound morning stiffness, and malaise.[349] This condition can be difficult to distinguish from RA in older people.

Rheumatoid arthritis can affect body image, self-esteem, and sexuality in the older adult. The person with RA loses control over body changes, is chronically fatigued, and eventually may lose independence in activities of daily living (ADLs). As a reaction to these losses, individuals may display the phases of the grieving process, such as anger or denial. Some people become depressed, feeling helpless and hopeless because no cure exists for the condition at this time. Chronic pain and suffering interfere with quality of life.

Because RA affects multiple body systems, lessens quality of life, and affects functional ability, the approach to managing the client with this condition must be interdisciplinary. Management typically includes drug therapy, physical or occupational therapy, and recreational therapy. Some clients also need psychologic counseling to help cope with the disease.

Rest and energy conservation are crucial for managing RA. Pacing activities, obtaining assistance, and allowing rest periods helps conserve the older adult's energy. Positioning joints in their optimal functional position helps prevent deformities. Ambulatory and adaptive devices can help individuals maintain independence in ADLs. For example, a long-handled shoehorn may help in putting on shoes. Velcro attachments on shoes often are a better option than laces. Styrofoam or paper cups may collapse or bend, whereas a hard plastic or china cup may be easier to handle. The clinician also should review principles of joint protection with the patient and family and provide adaptive equipment as needed to perform ADLs independently.

Strengthening exercises and other pain-relief measures, such as the use of ice and heat, can be prescribed. Ice application is used for hot, inflamed joints. Heat is used for painful joints that are not acutely inflamed. Showers, hot packs (not too heavy), and paraffin dips are ideal for heat application.

Acute Arthritis. Septic arthritis of the shoulder is uncommon but can occur in patients who are debilitated from generalized disease,[350] in those taking immunosuppressive medications, or in combination with an underlying shoulder disease process, such as rotator cuff tearing[351] or RA.[352,353]

Diabetic patients are at higher risk of developing monoarticular steroid-sensitive arthritis.[354] A condition of unknown etiology, it can affect the rotator cuff and the glenohumeral joint capsule.[355] As the name suggests, the condition is provoked by the patient's reaction to hydrocortisone.

Diagnosis requires joint aspiration and bacteriologic testing. Monoarticular arthritis, which usually resolves spontaneously in 2 years with medical intervention,[356] is an absolute contraindication to capsular stretching.[357]

Degenerative Conditions. Intrinsic glenohumeral arthritis is an infrequent cause of shoulder pain, but loss of glenohumeral motion often is seen in patients with periarticular syndromes (see Chap. 14).[349] Although the rotator cuff often is intact, the subscapularis muscle often is shortened, limiting external rotation.[358] X-ray findings include[358]:

▶ Flattening posterior erosion of the glenoid and an enlarged or deformed humeral head.[359,360]

▶ Inferiorly located osteophytes.

▶ Acromioclavicular arthritic changes.[359]

Infections

Osteomyelitis. The bones most commonly involved in acute hematogenous osteomyelitis, in order of frequency, are femur, tibia, humerus, fibula, radius, phalanges, calcaneus, ulna, ischium, metatarsals, and vertebral bodies.[361] Patients with sickle cell disease are at an increased risk for bacterial infections, and osteomyelitis is the second most common infection in these patients.[362]

Patients usually present with fever, malaise, irritability, pain, and localized tenderness at the site of infection. Muscle guarding also may be a feature, as well as decreased movement and pain of the affected limb and adjacent joints. These symptoms may be accompanied by edema and erythema over the involved area.

Cat-scratch Disease. Cat-scratch disease is generally a benign, self-limited infectious disease in immunocompetent patients. It is caused by *Bartonella henselae,* a small, Gram-negative, argyrophilic, non–acid-fast, pleomorphic bacillus.[363] Domestic cats, especially kittens, serve as a reservoir for *B. henselae.*[363] In general, patients present with a history of a scratch, bite, or close contact with a kitten or cat. A red-brown, nontender papule often develops at the region of the inoculation within 3 to 10 days and may persist for several weeks. Most patients develop tender regional lymphadenopathy, particularly in the axilla, and many develop fever.

Tumors. The differential diagnosis of all painful shoulders includes tumors of a wide variety. Evaluation of a shoulder tumor has several areas in common with other musculoskeletal neoplasms. Thorough evaluation of patients requires not only routine radiography, but also radionuclide imaging, computed tomographic (CT) scanning, magnetic resonance imaging (MRI),

and angiography. The typical clinical features of a bone tumor include variable pain, which is often worse at night and markedly responsive to salicylates. Surgical treatment of shoulder tumors depends on the patient's age and the type, extent, and aggressiveness of the tumor.

Vascular Conditions. Nontraumatic avascular necrosis of the humeral head may be idiopathic or associated with the systemic use of corticosteroids, dysbaric conditions, transplantation, systemic illness, alcoholism, sickle cell disease, hyperuricemia, pancreatitis, lymphoma, or Gaucher's disease.[353,364–367]

Diagnosis is through imaging, particularly MRI, which detects the pathology at its earliest stage.

Metabolic Conditions. Gout is a metabolic disease characterized by recurrent episodes of acute arthritis. High blood levels of uric acid lead to inflammation, joint swelling, and severe pain. Symptoms are caused by deposits of microcrystals in joints and periarticular tissues. Several factors have been identified as predisposing a person to gout, including lifestyle elements of obesity, high-purine diet, and habitual alcohol ingestion.

Onset is usually sudden, often during the night or early morning. The classic finding of gouty arthritis (gout) is warmth, swelling, cutaneous erythema, and severe pain of the first metatarsophalangeal joint. However, other joints also may be involved. These include the shoulder, knee, wrist, ankle, elbow bursa, heel, or fingers. Fever, chills, and malaise accompany an episode of gout. As the condition becomes chronic, the patient may report morning stiffness and joint deformity, progressive loss, and disability. Chronic gouty nephropathy may occur.

Differential diagnosis includes cellulitis, septic arthritis, rheumatoid arthritis, bursitis related to bunion, sarcoidosis, multiple myeloma, and hyperparathyroidism.

Fractures. See Chapter 14.

Referred Pain

Referred pain from the cervical region may be experienced in the shoulder or interpreted as a distal sensation.[368]

Referral sources for this region include the heart,[369] pleura, lung tissue, diaphragm,[370] lymph nodes of the neck, shoulder, chest, and breast tissue.[370]

Pain in the shoulder area can be caused by direct or referred pain from an underlying malignancy, such as a Pancoast's tumor (see later).[370] The scapula and humerus are frequently sites of metastases involving tumors of the kidney, breast, lung, and prostate.[349] These patients have persistent pain that is unaffected by movement but is associated with fatigue, weight loss, and other constitutional signs. A history of gradually progressive pain, starting as a mild ache but developing into persistent severe pain, should initiate a search for a malignancy.[349] Severe shoulder pain in a patient with an otherwise normal physical examination of the shoulder and cervical spine should increase the suspicion of a malignancy.

Intrinsic neck pathology can cause referred pain to the head, anterior and posterior chest wall, shoulder girdle, and upper limb.[368] In the case of radiculopathy, muscle function might be affected directly. Cervical spine symptoms are usually affected by head position, with neck extension causing an exacerbation and flexion producing some relief.[349]

Intracerebral and Intraspinal Conditions

Cerebrovascular Disease.   See the discussion under "Causes of Head and Facial Pain," earlier.

Subclavian Steal Syndrome.   The subclavian steal syndrome was described in 1960.[371] This initial report described a proximal subclavian artery obstruction, reversed vertebral flow with resultant siphoning of blood from the brain and cerebrovascular symptoms. The syndrome was described again in 1961[372] and given its name in an accompanying editorial.[373]

This condition results in signs and symptoms of cerebral ischemia. Ischemia is the result of subclavian artery stenosis proximal to the origin of the vertebral artery and subsequently "stealing" blood from the cerebral circulation of the circle of Willis and basilar vessel.

This condition is not within the scope of physical therapy practice. It is mentioned because many of its symptoms mimic a musculoskeletal lesion of the shoulder or upper arm. The symptoms usually are precipitated or aggravated by arm exercises.[374]

The subclavian steal syndrome can also produce vertebral artery symptoms such as a "drop attack,"[375] a sudden loss of postural tone without loss of consciousness that can occur while walking and turning the neck to look to the side or up. Other vertebral artery symptoms associated with this condition include headache, dizziness, and vertigo.[376]

More recently, a related syndrome known as the *coronary-subclavian steal* has been recognized. This syndrome has the same pathologic anatomy as a proximal left subclavian artery stenosis or occlusion. But the steal consists of the siphoning of blood from the myocardium through the left internal mammary artery graft to the subclavian artery.[377] This syndrome may be manifested by diminished pulses in the left arm, blood pressure difference of 20 mm Hg or more in the upper extremities, and the development of myocardial ischemia.[378]

Multiple Sclerosis.   Pain, either acute or chronic, occurs in more than 65 percent of patients with multiple sclerosis[379] during all stages of the disease. Chronic pain may be characterized by dysesthetic extremities, back and shoulder pain, and pain secondary to spasticity.[164] Complications of disuse, such as frozen shoulder, and osteoporosis are other painful syndromes that may develop.[164]

Amyotrophic Lateral Sclerosis.   Amyotrophic lateral sclerosis (ALS) is a neurodegenerative disorder that causes rapid loss of motor neurons in the brain and spinal cord, leading to paralysis and death. Diagnosis is based solely on clinical data and depends on the recognition of a characteristic constellation of symptoms and signs and supportive electrophysiologic findings. For clinically definitive diagnosis of ALS, upper and lower motor neuron signs in bulbar and two spinal regions or in three spinal regions are required. The lower motor neuron weakness and muscle atrophy involves both peripheral nerve and myotomal distributions.

The clinical hallmark of ALS is the coexistence of muscle atrophy, weakness, fasciculations, and cramps (caused by lower motor neuron degeneration), together with hyperactive or inappropriately brisk deep tendon reflexes, pyramidal tract signs, and increased muscle tone (the result of corticospinal tract involvement).[380] Muscle cramps are often already present before other symptoms develop. Most patients present with asymmetric, distal weakness of the arm or leg.

ALS is a progressive disease. The symptoms usually progress first in the affected extremity, then gradually spread to adjacent muscle groups and to remote ipsilateral or contralateral regions. Although disability is usually limited in the early stages, ALS progresses relentlessly. Most patients are ultimately unable to walk, care for themselves, speak, and swallow.[380] However, there is usually no clinical involvement of parts of the central nervous system other than the motor pathways.[380]

Respiratory weakness resulting from high cervical (phrenic nerve, C4) and thoracic spinal cord involvement is the most common cause of death in ALS, often in conjunction with aspiration pneumonia.[380]

Guillain-Barré Syndrome.   Guillain-Barré syndrome (GBS) is challenging to identify because of its multitude of presentations and manifestations. GBS may be defined as a postinfectious, acute, paralytic peripheral neuropathy. It can affect any age group, although there is a peak incidence in young adults. GBS appears to be an inflammatory or immune-mediated condition.

The majority of patients describe an antecedent febrile illness. Upper respiratory infections are seen in 50 percent of cases and are caused by a variety of viruses. The illness is usually an acute respiratory or gastrointestinal condition that lasts for several days and then resolves. This is followed in 1 to 2 weeks by the development of a progressive ascending weakness or paralysis, which is usually symmetric and occurs over several days or weeks. The progression of the weakness or paralysis can be gradual (1 to 3 weeks) or rapid (1 to 2 days). The patient reports difficulty or instability with walking, arising from a chair, and ascending or descending stairs. Associated signs and symptoms include cranial nerve involvement (facial weakness), paresthesias, sensory deficits, difficulty breathing, diminished stretch reflexes, autonomic dysfunction (tachycardia, vasomotor symptoms), oropharyngeal weakness, and ocular involvement.[381]

The differential diagnosis for GBS is quite large and includes the spectrum of illnesses causing acute or subacute paralysis. These include spinal cord compression (myelopathy), upper motor neuron disorders, poliomyelitis, transverse myelitis, polyneuropathy, systemic lupus erythematosus, tick paralysis, polyarteritis nodosa, myasthenia gravis, and sarcoidosis.[381]

All patients with suspected GBS should be hospitalized for vigilant monitoring because of the high risk of respiratory failure, which occurs in approximately one third of patients.[381]

Syringomyelia. Syringomyelia is a disease that produces fluid-containing cysts (syrinx) within the spinal cord, often associated with stenosis of the foramen magnum. The syrinx can occur within the spinal cord (syringomyelia) or brain stem (syringobulbia). Syringomyelia has been found in association with various disorders, including spinal column or brain stem abnormalities (scoliosis, Klippel-Feil syndrome, Chiari I malformation), intramedullary tumors, and traumatic degeneration of the spinal cord. Chiari I malformation is the most common condition in patients with syringomyelia.

Painful dysesthesias, which have been described variously as burning pain, pins-and-needles sensations, and stretching or pressure of the skin, occur in up to 40 percent of patients with syringomyelia.[382] The pain tends to arise in a dermatomal pattern and is accompanied, in most cases, by hyperesthesia.

Radiologic features that suggest syringomyelia include an increase in the width and depth of the cervical canal, bony abnormalities at the craniovertebral junction, diastematomyelia, and occipitalization of the atlas.

Extraspinal Conditions. The extraspinal causes of shoulder pain include tumor, clay shoveler's fracture, brachial plexopathy, and herpes zoster.

Tumor. Pancoast's syndrome is a constellation of characteristic symptoms and signs that includes shoulder and arm pain along the distribution of the eighth cervical nerve trunk and first and second thoracic nerve trunks, Horner's syndrome, and weakness and atrophy of the muscles of the hand, most commonly caused by local extension of an apical lung tumor at the superior thoracic inlet.[383,384] These tumors are called *superior pulmonary sulcus tumors* or *Pancoast's tumors.*

The most common initial symptom is shoulder pain caused by localization of the Pancoast tumors in the superior pulmonary sulcus. Pain can radiate up to the head and neck or down to the medial aspect of the scapula, axilla, anterior part of the chest, or ipsilateral arm, often along the distribution of the ulnar nerve.[385] This radicular causalgic pain is often difficult to treat. Sensory loss and motor deficit in the upper extremity also may occur. Weakness and atrophy of the intrinsic muscles of the hand sometimes occur, along with pain and paresthesia of the medial aspect of the arm, forearm, and fourth and fifth digits along the distribution of the ulnar nerve, caused by extension of the tumor to C8 and T1 nerve roots.[385]

The differential diagnosis of Pancoast's syndrome includes other primary thoracic neoplasms, metastatic and hematologic conditions, infectious diseases, thoracic outlet syndromes, and pulmonary amyloid nodules.[385]

Clay Shoveler's Fracture. Clay shoveler's fracture is a rare condition that was first described by McKellar,[386] based on a few cases reported found in Englishmen who spent long hours digging heavy clay. It has since been described in power lifters.[387] The condition is characterized by a traction fracture of the lower cervical or upper thoracic spine resulting from an excessive pull of the trapezius and rhomboid muscles during heavy work. The patient reports a sudden onset of sharp neck, shoulder, and arm pain and exhibits limited active bilateral elevation to around 150 degrees. Passive elevation remains unaffected. Other conditions that mimic these symptoms include a fracture of the first rib, mononeuritis of the long thoracic nerve, mononeuritis of the accessory nerve, C5 full-root palsy, and total rupture of the supraspinatus.[357]

Brachial Plexopathy.[388] Idiopathic brachial plexopathy (IBP) is a syndrome of shoulder pain and weakness. IBP has a number of pseudonyms, including neuralgic amyotrophy, Parsonage-Turner syndrome, and idiopathic brachial neuritis. The initial symptom typically seen with IBP is sudden, sharp, and throbbing pain in the shoulder girdle, followed by weakness in the scapular and proximal arm muscles. Sensory loss is usually not prominent. The pain usually subsides within 24 hours to 3 weeks, and the weakness and atrophy are recognized as the pain resolves. Weakness is maximal within 2 to 3 weeks of the onset of symptoms and often is accompanied by muscle wasting and scapular winging. Slow resolution of the weakness follows in nearly all patients, but recovery may be incomplete.

Herpes Zoster.[389] Herpes zoster is characterized by deep, boring, or stabbing thoracic and arm pain. Varicella-zoster virus infection is unique because of its two clinical manifestations: varicella (chickenpox) and herpes zoster (shingles). After an individual has chickenpox, the virus lies dormant in the dorsal root ganglia and sensory ganglia of cranial nerves. Herpes zoster occurs if the virus becomes reactivated, causing an acute, painful infection of a sensory nerve and its corresponding cutaneous area of innervation. Herpes zoster, therefore, occurs only in individuals previously infected with the chickenpox virus.

Postherpetic neuralgia is the most common complication of herpes zoster. It arises from inflammatory injury to sensory nerves, ganglia, and nerve roots and from maladaptive responses to pain signaling and the likely inability of pain receptors to return to normal after the inflammation subsides. The nerve dysfunction can result in hyperesthesia, hypoesthesia, dysesthesia, and allodynia (pain as the result of an innocuous stimuli, such as clothing touching the affected skin).

The characteristic rash begins as erythematous macules and papules that progress to vesicles within 24 hours, then to pustules (3 to 4 days), and finally to crusts (7 to 10 days). The most common distribution of herpes zoster is unilateral involvement of the thoracic dermatome, followed by the cranial, cervical, and lumbar dermatomes. Involvement of the maxillary division of the trigeminal nerve causes vesicles of the uvula and tonsillar area. Involvement of the mandibular branch produces vesicles on the floor of the mouth, buccal membranes, and the anterior part of the tongue. Herpes zoster near or involving the eyes is considered an emergency, because this potentially serious development can lead to blindness.

In general, the diagnosis of herpes zoster is based on the history and the clinical examination, which shows the characteristic painful, grouped vesicular rash in a dermatomal distribution. Acute herpes zoster infection is a self-limiting condition, and the primary treatment goals are to reduce and manage the acute pain and modify the duration of the rash and inflammation.

Causes of Elbow and Forearm Pain

The causes of elbow and forearm pain include those listed in Table 9-19.

Fracture
See Chapter 15.

Dislocation
See Chapter 15.

Osteochondritis
Osteochondritis occurs in many areas of the adolescent skeleton, and patients usually present with as an insidious onset of diffuse lateral elbow pain accompanied by a decrease in range of motion, including locking.[390] The etiology of this condition is not completely understood, but its occurrence in the elbows of adolescents probably relates to focal arterial injury and subsequent bone necrosis resulting from increased radiohumeral compression forces.[391]

Physical examination usually demonstrates a loss of full elbow extension. Resistive testing can produce crepitus, in addition to pain at the humeroradial joint.[391]

Intervention for these lesions depends on the findings from the radiographic, clinical, and, on occasion, arthroscopic examination and usually focuses on the control of pain.[391] A motion-limiting brace can be used to reduce stress.

Surgical intervention is reserved for patients who do not respond to conservative measures, or those with loose bodies or separation of the cartilage cap.[391]

Ligament Sprain
See Chapter 15.

TABLE 9-19 Potential Causes of Elbow and Forearm Pain

Fracture
Dislocation
Osteochondritis
Ligament sprain
Arthrosis
Peripheral nerve entrapment
Soft tissue injury or tendonitis (lateral epicondylitis, medial epicondylitis, triceps tendonitis, bicipital tendonitis, brachialis tendonitis, Little League elbow)
Infective arthritis
Polyarthritis
Gout
Bursitis
Vascular disorders
Referred pain

Arthrosis
Arthrosis of the elbow is often the result of a previous micro- or macrotraumatic injury to the elbow. Unless the case is severe, the patient does not complain of much pain, except perhaps with vigorous activity. However, complaints of early morning stiffness and pain at the end of the day are common. Motion testing reveals a capsular pattern, with a bony end-feel, in both flexion and extension, and crepitus is felt during both motions. There is no specific treatment for this condition. Surgery to remove loose bodies or for debridement is used in severe cases.

Peripheral Nerve Entrapment
See Chapter 15.

Soft Tissue Injury or Tendonitis
See Chapter 15.

Infective Arthritis
The source of infective arthritis is commonly tooth decay or a pelvic disease. The pain is described as a severe aching or throbbing. A history of a puncture wound of the skin also should arouse suspicion. The involved joint feels hot and appears swollen. The involved elbow is usually held stiffly in slight flexion. Associated findings include fever and joint tenderness.

Polyarthritis
The polyarthritides that can affect the elbow include acute rheumatic fever, Reiter's syndrome, and Lyme disease arthritis.

Gout
Gout at the elbow is characterized by acute pain, swelling, redness, and tenderness of the elbow joint. See the discussion under "Metabolic Conditions," earlier.

Bursitis
See Chapter 15.

Vascular Disorders
Volkmann's Ischemia (Anterior Compartment Syndrome). This condition occurs as the result of increased tissue fluid pressure within a fascial muscle compartment that reduces capillary blood perfusion below a level necessary for tissue viability.[392] In the upper extremity, acute compartment syndrome that involves the forearm is the most common type of compartment syndrome. Nerve injury resulting from the compression produces a deformed limb known as *Volkmann's ischemic contracture.*[393]

Acute compartment syndrome can be caused by constrictive casts or dressings, limb placement during surgery, blunt trauma, hematoma, burns, frostbite, snake bite, strenuous exercise, and fractures.[392] Clinical findings include[392]:

▶ A swollen and tense tender compartment.

▶ Severe pain, exacerbated with passive stretch of the forearm muscles.

▶ Sensibility deficits.

▶ Motor weakness or paralysis.

▶ No absence of radial and ulnar pulses at the wrist.

The clinical diagnosis is confirmed by measuring the intracompartmental tissue fluid pressure.

Conservative intervention involves the removal of the constricting splint, dressing, or cast. Surgical intervention, by performing a fasciotomy, is reserved for patients whose symptoms do not resolve quickly.[392]

Acute Axillary or Brachial Artery Occlusion.[394] The causes of arterial occlusion include emboli from the heart or from an atheromatous plaque or aneurysm of the innominate or subclavian-axillary arteries. Trauma to the chest, shoulder, or upper arm also may cause arterial obstruction. The five P's describe the signs and symptoms of this medical emergency:

▶ Pain.

▶ Paralysis.

▶ Paresthesias.

▶ Pallor.

▶ Pulses (absent).

The pain is usually severe and constant, involving the forearm, hand, and fingers. Paralysis and paresthesia indicate severe ischemia of the arm. Gangrene can begin to develop 6 hours after the onset of symptoms in such scenarios. The pallor occurs because of lack of blood flow and cutaneous vasoconstriction. The absence of pulses confirms occlusion.

Referred Pain

Referred pain to the elbow can have a number of causes, including coronary heart disease, polyarthritis, or an acute C8 radiculopathy.

Causes of Wrist, Hand, and Finger Pain

The causes of wrist, hand, and finger pain include, but are not limited to those listed in Table 9-20 and shown in Figure 9-4.

Fracture
See Chapter 16.

Sprains and Dislocations
See Chapter 16.

Triangular Fibrocartilage Complex (TFCC) Lesions
See Chapter 16.

Tenosynovitis
See Chapter 16.

Tendonitis
See Chapter 16.

TABLE 9-20   Potential Causes of Wrist, Hand, and Finger Pain

Fracture
Sprains and dislocations
Triangular fibrocartilage complex (TFCC) lesions
Tenosynovitis
Tendonitis
Carpal instability
Gout and pseudogout
Rheumatoid arthritis
Psoriatic arthritis
Osteoarthritis
Carpal tunnel syndrome
Infection
Kienböck's disease
Ganglia
Tumors
Peripheral nerve entrapment
Reflex sympathetic dystrophy/Complex regional pain syndrome
Vascular occlusion
Mononeuritis multiplex
Referred pain

Carpal Instability
See Chapter 16.

Gout and Pseudogout
Gouty arthritis and pseudogout are metabolic joint diseases caused by deposition of sodium urate or calcium pyrophosphate crystals in the joint, leading to arthritis (see also, earlier discussions). The wrists are the second most commonly affected joint in pseudogout, after the knees. Radiographs demonstrate crystal deposits in articular fibrocartilage of the wrist.[395] Septic arthritis of the wrist can cause destruction of joint cartilage and bony structures. Generally, the diagnosis of acute infection is not problematic, but differentiation between pure soft tissue infection and infection involving the bony structures can be complicated.[396] Furthermore, identification of a chronic infection as the cause of chronic wrist pain may be difficult.[397,398] If there is a clinical suspicion an (ultrasound-guided) needle aspiration or synovial biopsy should be taken.[396] The new generation of ultrasonography has proved to be a valuable technique, with a high success rate, for obtaining synovial fluid or membrane samples for pathologic and bacteriologic examinations.[399]

Rheumatoid Arthritis
See Chapter 16.

Psoriatic Arthritis
Psoriatic arthritis is an inflammatory arthritis associated with psoriasis. It affects men and women with equal frequency.[245] Its peak onset is in the fourth decade of life, although it may occur in children and in older adults. Psoriatic arthritis can manifest in one of a number of patterns, including distal joint disease (affecting the distal interphalangeal joints of the hands and feet),

Potential Causes of Wrist and Hand Pain

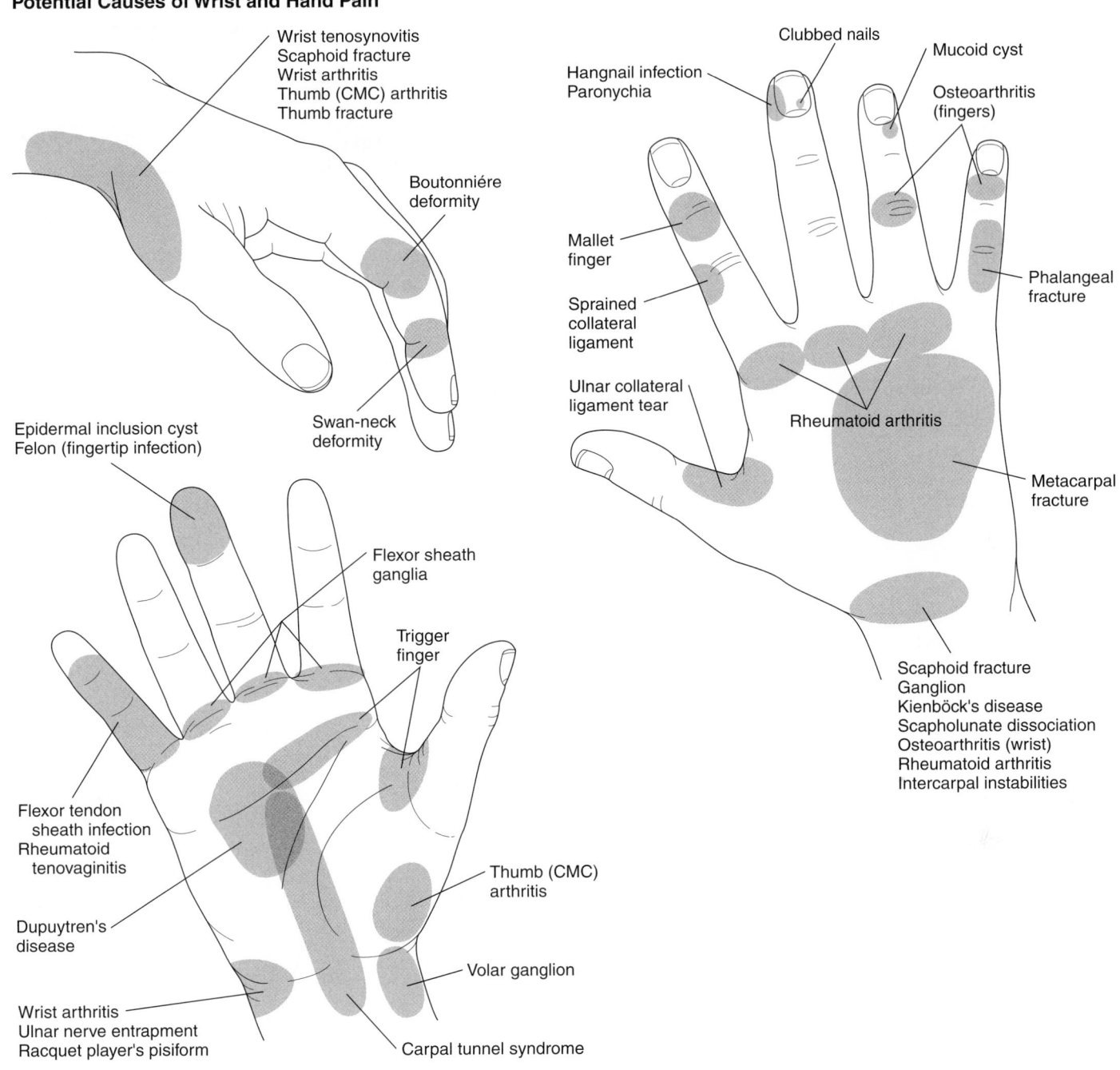

Wrist tenosynovitis
Scaphoid fracture
Wrist arthritis
Thumb (CMC) arthritis
Thumb fracture

Boutonniére deformity

Swan-neck deformity

Epidermal inclusion cyst
Felon (fingertip infection)

Flexor sheath ganglia

Trigger finger

Flexor tendon sheath infection
Rheumatoid tenovaginitis

Dupuytren's disease

Wrist arthritis
Ulnar nerve entrapment
Racquet player's pisiform

Thumb (CMC) arthritis

Volar ganglion

Carpal tunnel syndrome

Clubbed nails

Mucoid cyst

Hangnail infection
Paronychia

Osteoarthritis (fingers)

Mallet finger

Phalangeal fracture

Sprained collateral ligament

Ulnar collateral ligament tear

Rheumatoid arthritis

Metacarpal fracture

Scaphoid fracture
Ganglion
Kienböck's disease
Scapholunate dissociation
Osteoarthritis (wrist)
Rheumatoid arthritis
Intercarpal instabilities

FIGURE 9-4 Potential causes of wrist and hand pain.

asymmetric oligoarthritis, polyarthritis (which tends to be asymmetric in half the cases), and arthritis mutilans (a severe destructive form of arthritis and the spondyloarthropathy that occurs in 40 percent of patients, but most commonly in the presence of one of the peripheral patterns).[245] Patients with psoriatic arthritis have less tenderness over both affected joints and tender points than patients with rheumatoid arthritis.[400]

The spondyloarthropathy of psoriatic arthritis may be distinguished from ankylosing spondylitis (AS) by the pattern of the sacroiliitis.[401] Whereas sacroiliitis in AS tends to be symmetric, affecting both sacroiliac joints to the same degree, it tends to be asymmetric in psoriatic arthritis,[245] and patients with psoriatic arthritis do not have as severe a spondyloarthropathy as patients with AS.[239]

Another articular feature of psoriatic arthritis is the presence of dactylitis, tenosynovitis (often digital, in flexor and extensor tendons and in the Achilles tendon), and enthesitis.[401] The presence of erosive disease in the distal interphalangeal joints is typical.[401]

Nail lesions occur in more than 80 percent of the patients with psoriatic arthritis, and have been found to be the only clinical feature distinguishing patients with psoriatic arthritis from patients with uncomplicated psoriasis.[402] Other extra-articular features include iritis, urethritis, and cardiac impairments similar to those seen in AS, although less frequently.[401]

Psoriatic arthritis may result in significant joint damage and disability.

Osteoarthritis
See Chapter 16.

Carpal Tunnel Syndrome
See Chapter 16.

Infection

Wrist. The most common infection of the wrist is infectious tenosynovitis of the flexor pollices longus.

Hand. These infections include:

▶ Bursal infections.

▶ Space infections.

▶ Infected bites.

▶ Cellulitis. Cellulitis is an infection of the skin and underlying structures. With treatment, it usually follows a relatively benign course. However, in some cases, the same pathogens can cause other diseases, such as necrotizing fasciitis or toxic shock syndrome, and even death. The most common pathogens in cellulitis are *Staphylococcus aureus* and β-hemolytic streptococci. Symptoms include localized redness, swelling, and pain. Associated symptoms include fever, chills, and nausea and vomiting. Cellulitis typically is treated with systemic antibiotics, via either the oral or intravenous route.

Fingers

Paronychia and Eponychia. Paronychia is an acute inflammation of the lateral or proximal nail folds that is usually caused by infection, producing a red, tender, throbbing, and intensely painful swelling of the proximal or lateral nail folds.[403] It is the most common infection of the hand. If the infection involves the eponychium as well as the lateral fold, it is called *eponychia.*

Mild cases of paronychia typically are treated with warm soaks two to four times daily, and splinting with or without systemic antibiotics. The more severe cases require incision and drainage.[404]

Differential diagnosis includes apical abscess, felon, and subungual infection.[405] A subungual infection may result from an extension of the paronychia under the nail.[405]

Felon. A felon is an abscess of the terminal phalanx pulp (Fig. 9-5). The most common cause is a puncture wound. Initially, the condition is characterized by mild swelling, erythema, and

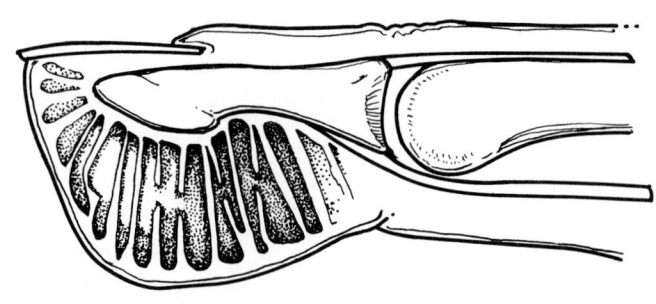

FIGURE 9-5 A felon. (Reproduced with permission from Dee R, et al, eds. *Principles of Orthopaedic Practice.* New York, NY: McGraw-Hill; 1997.)

tenderness. Over a period of a few days, the pulp becomes tense, red and exquisitely tender.[405]

Mild cases are treated with antibiotics and elevation. Most cases, however, require a combination of incision and drainage, and systemic antibiotics.

Web Space Infections. A web space abscess usually is caused by a puncture in the skin between the fingers (Fig. 9-6). It is characterized by its collar-button or dumbbell shape as the expanding abscess penetrates the palmar fascia.[405] Swelling and tenderness are noted on the palmar and dorsal aspects of the web space. The adjacent fingers adopt an abducted position. Intervention involves incision and drainage.

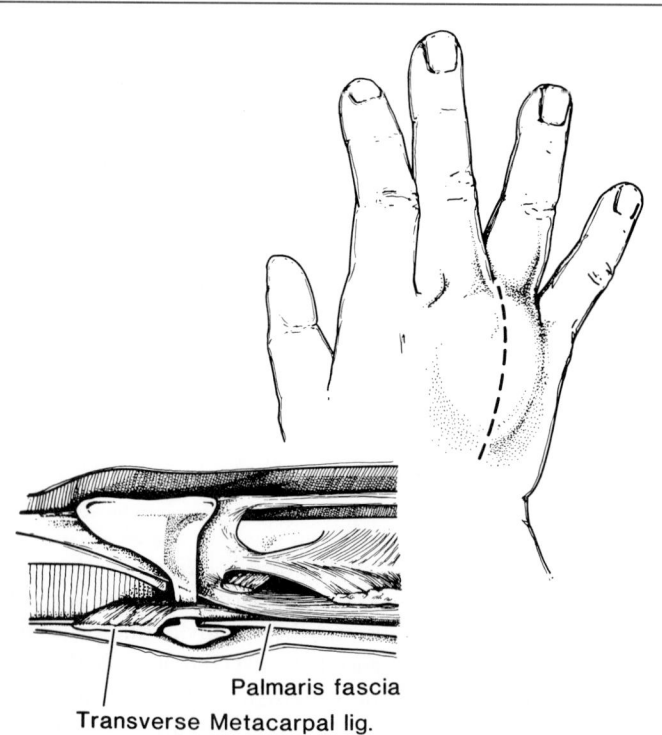

Palmaris fascia
Transverse Metacarpal lig.

FIGURE 9-6 Web space infection. (Reproduced with permission from Dee R, et al, eds. *Principles of Orthopaedic Practice.* New York, NY: McGraw-Hill; 1997.)

Herpetic Whitlow.   Herpetic whitlow is a viral infection of the fingers. It is caused by contact with the herpes simplex virus.[405] The condition usually manifests with intense throbbing and erythema of the involved finger. The condition is self-limiting and typically lasts for 2 to 3 weeks. The intervention is conservative and symptomatic.[405]

Kienböck's Disease

Kienböck's disease, or lunatomalacia, is a complication of injury to the lunate. It is defined as an aseptic or avascular necrosis of the lunate. The etiology of this disease remains elusive, although it is thought that trauma plays a large part in disrupting the blood supply to the bone.[406] The disease occurs predominantly in males, with a 2:1 prevalence,[407] and the majority of patients are 20 to 40 years of age.[408]

Subjective complaints include pain on the central-dorsal aspect of the wrist, especially during and after activities. Stiffness of the hand is another common complaint.[409] With time, the pain becomes severe and constant, with accompanying weakness of grip strength and loss of wrist motion, especially wrist extension.[409] Imaging techniques are needed to make a definitive diagnosis.

The intervention for Kienböck's disease depends on the stage of the disease. Conservative measures involve immobilization during the acute phase. Surgical options include joint leveling by radial shortening or ulnar lengthening, intercarpal fusion, arthroplasty, and vascularized bone grafts.[410]

Ganglia.   Ganglia are thin-walled cysts containing mucoid hyaluronic acid that develop spontaneously over a joint capsule or tendon sheath. They are the most common soft-tissue tumor in the hand.[411,412] Ganglia, seen primarily in 20- to 30-year-olds, also may occur in association with such systemic diseases as arthritis, or with trauma.[413,414] The exact cause of the ganglia is controversial. However, there is consensus that a one-way connection to the synovial sheath allows fluid to enter the cyst but not to flow freely back into the sheath.[411]

Common sites for ganglia are the volar or dorsal surfaces of the wrist and fingers.[415] Ganglia may not cause pain.[407] Frequently, as the ganglion begins to grow, the patient reports aching that is irritated by flexion and extension of the joint.[415]

At times, ganglia occur at other parts of the wrist, causing compression of the ulnar or median nerve.[415] When compression occurs, associated sensory symptoms in the digits or intrinsic muscle weakness may develop.[411]

Upon examination, a ganglion is smooth, round, or multi-lobulated, and tender with applied pressure. The key to distinguishing a ganglion from other soft-tissue tumors is the history of size variation. Suspicious soft-tissue masses require evaluation and further diagnostic testing or excisional biopsy.[415]

For symptom relief, immobilization of the wrist through splinting is effective. This may cause the ganglion to shrink temporarily, although it is uncommon for the immobilization to be effective in resolving the ganglion.[415] Needle aspiration can resolve the ganglion. Occasionally, surgical excision is indicated for the patient with significant pain or cosmetic irritation.

Tumors

Benign tumors account for the majority of tumors of the wrist and hand, although malignancies can occur.[416] The clinical presentation is variable and depends on the condition, location, size, and degree of soft tissue involvement, although there are a number of scenarios that warrant suspicion of a possible occult lesion[417]:

▶ A young patient complaining of bone pain that is not related to any preceding trauma.

▶ Presence of swelling, or of a mass, in the absence of trauma.

▶ Pain or swelling that persists despite intervention.

Peripheral Nerve Entrapment

Pain of a neurogenic origin can be referred to the wrist and hand. These can include C5 to T1 nerve root lesions, thoracic outlet syndrome, and brachial plexus tension syndromes. In addition, neurogenic causes can be secondary to adhesion formation, or trauma.

Proximal Nerve Entrapment.   Proximal causes of pain, paresthesias, and numbness in the lateral hand, thumb, and index and middle fingers include:

▶ C6 or C7 radiculopathy (see Chap. 20).

▶ Thoracic outlet syndrome (see Chap. 23).

▶ Pronator teres syndrome (see Chap. 15).

Proximal causes of these symptoms in the medial hand and the fourth and fifth fingers include:

▶ C8 radiculopathy.

▶ Brachial plexus compression at the thoracic outlet.

▶ Cubital tunnel syndrome (see Chap. 15).

Distal Nerve Entrapment (see Chap. 16).   Entrapment of the following nerves may occur:

▶ Median nerve (carpal tunnel syndrome).

▶ Ulnar nerve (Guyon canal entrapment).

▶ Radial nerve.

Complex Regional Pain Syndrome (Reflex Sympathetic Dystrophy)

See Chapter 16.

Vascular Occlusion

An embolus or trauma may obstruct the brachial, ulnar or radial artery. The amount of pain distal to the obstruction is dependent on the degree of collateral circulation. Prolonged restriction to the blood flow may result in gangrene.

Raynaud's Phenomenon.   Raynaud's phenomenon is a vascular disorder that can affect one or both hands and the feet. Reversible vasospasm of the extremities occurs either as an isolated symptom without underlying disorder (primary Raynaud's phenomenon) or in association with another disorder or condition (secondary Raynaud's phenomenon).

The clinical findings include digital pallor followed by cyanosis and then rubor.[418] Throbbing and tingling sensations usually accompany the rubor stage.

Raynaud's phenomenon is usually managed with simple measures, such as using warm clothes, mittens (not gloves), hand warmers, and automatic car starters.[419] The most frequently used drugs are calcium channel antagonists.

Scleroderma

Scleroderma means "hard skin." The term is used to describe two distinct diseases: localized scleroderma and systemic scleroderma. Localized scleroderma is primarily a cutaneous disease. Systemic sclerosis is a multisystem connective tissue disease. The etiology of both of these diseases is not known.

There are two main subsets of systemic sclerosis, limited scleroderma (the old CREST syndrome), and diffuse scleroderma[419]:

▶ *Limited scleroderma.* Patients generally have a long history of Raynaud's phenomenon, in some cases 10 to 15 years, and mildly puffy or swollen fingers before they present to their physicians with a digital ulcer, heartburn, or shortness of breath.

▶ *Diffuse scleroderma.* Patients have a much more acute onset of disease. They have arthralgias, carpal tunnel syndrome, swollen hands, swollen legs, and crepituslike friction rubs over tendon areas of hands, wrists, and ankles. These patients potentially have severe problems not only from skin thickening and contractures but also from other organ systems, including gastrointestinal, pulmonary, cardiovascular, and renal.

Raynaud's phenomenon is present in almost all patients with scleroderma.

Mononeuritis Multiplex

This condition is associated with a sudden onset of severe aching or sharp forearm and hand pain, paresthesias, and dysesthesias in the distribution of the median, ulnar, or radial nerves.[418] Mononeuritis multiplex can occur in association with a number of other medical conditions, including rheumatoid arthritis, vasculitis, polyarteritis nodosa, diabetes mellitus, sarcoidosis, and amyloidosis. An ischemic mechanism is the most likely cause of mononeuritis multiplex. It is generally accepted that mononeuritis multiplex in rheumatoid arthritis results from ischemia caused by vasa nervorum vasculitis.

Referred Pain: Viscerogenic

The heart, apical lung, and bronchus are all capable of referring pain to the wrist and hand.

Causes of Knee Pain

Generalized Knee Pain

Causes of generalized knee pain include:

▶ Fracture (supracondylar, patellar, proximal tibia).

▶ Acute dislocation of the knee.

▶ Acute dislocation of the patella.

▶ Intra-articular ligament injury (see Chap. 18).

▶ Monoarthritis.

▶ Polyarthritis.

▶ Reactive arthritis.

▶ Complex regional pain syndrome (Reflex Sympathetic Dystrophy)

▶ Referred pain.

Anterior Knee Pain

Anterior knee pain is a common problem in active adolescents and young adults. The causes of anterior knee pain generally fall under three categories:[420]

▶ *Focal musculoskeletal lesions.* This group consists mainly of lesions that can be clinically and radiologically defined. Such lesions include Osgood-Schlatter's disease, jumper's knee, bipartite patella, tumors, plical irritation, and ligamentous injuries. These lesions normally respond well to locally applied interventions.

▶ *Traumatic lesions.* This group includes all of the conditions with a specific mechanism of injury involving direct trauma. These conditions include osteochondritis dissicans and bone contusions.

▶ *Miscellaneous lesions.* This group includes the more obscure causes of anterior knee pain including dynamic problems, such as maltracking of the patella and the excessive lateral pressure syndrome, as well as idiopathic chondromalacia, referred pain, complex regional pain syndrome, and psychogenic pain.

Musculoskeletal Causes

Osgood Schlatter's Disease. See Chapter 18.
Bursitis. (See Chapter 18.)
Jumper's Knee. See Chapter 18.
Bipartite Patella. This condition is common in childhood. It is often bilateral and usually is regarded as a variation of normal ossification. Very rarely, in response to overuse or acute injury, the synchondrosis separating the two centers of ossification may become painful and the site of local tenderness. There are three sites at which bipartite patella is found and each has an important soft-tissue attachment[420]:

▶ Distal pole of the patella with attachment of the patellar tendon. This type may represent the end stage of Sinding-Larsen-Johansson syndrome.

▶ Lateral margin of the patella with attachment of the lateral retinaculum.

▶ Superior-lateral corner of the patella, the insertion of vastus lateralis. This is the most common site for symptoms.

Trauma-related Causes

Osteochondritis Dissecans.[420] Osteochondritis dissecans is a rare cause of anterior knee pain in the young athlete. It involves the weight-bearing portions of the medial and lateral femoral condyles. Occasionally, pain may not be the most prominent symptom, but a catching sensation with knee flexion or an extensor weakness may be the primary complaint. Sometimes the lesion is associated with maltracking. If the lesion is small, a painful arc is produced as it passes over the articular surface of the femur during movement.

MRI, CT, and bone scans often are used to characterize these lesions.

Conservative intervention with rest is appropriate for intact lesions, which usually will show no sclerosis, and in patients younger than 13 or 14 years of age, in whom healing is the rule.[420]

Surgical techniques can be used to securely attach the loose osteochondral fragments to the underlying bone.

Bone Contusion. Bone bruises are related to trauma. There is no unique mechanism of injury, but they seem to result from direct impact, axial overloading, and impingement. Bone bruises can occur in sites other than the knee. They pose a potential risk for chondrolysis and stress fracture, and mobilization and weight bearing should be increased gradually.

Miscellaneous Causes

Tumors. Neoplastic involvement of the knee is a less common cause of knee pain. Malignant primary tumors arising from the patella include hemangioendothelioma, hemangiosarcoma, lymphoma, fibrous histiocytoma, osteoblastoclastoma, and plasmacytoma.[421] Soft tissue sarcomas are the most common malignant tumor of the knee, and these include osteosarcomas, Ewing's sarcoma, rhabdomyosarcoma, and synovial sarcomas.[422,423] Metastasis to the patella is rare.[424]

Benign tumors are more prevalent at this site. In a published series of 42 patellar tumors,[425] 90 percent were benign, with the most common diagnosis being chondroblastoma. Other benign tumors of the knee may include osteochondromas, nonossifying fibromas, and osteoid osteomas. Very rarely, soft tissue tumors may occur within the fat pad; in addition, synovial lesions, such as pigmented villonodular synovitis, can cause anterior knee pain, clicking, and catching.[420]

A history of knee pain worsened by activity and relieved by rest suggests benign involvement. However, pain that is constant, unrelenting, severe, and occurs at night suggests a malignant process.[426–428] In malignant tumors of the patella, pathologic fracture is often the presenting complaint.

Plicae. See Chapter 18.
Hoffa's Syndrome. See Chapter 18.
Osteomyelitis of the Patella. Osteomyelitis of the patella usually affects children between the ages of 5 and 15 years. It is exceedingly rare in adults and in children younger than 5 years of age.[429]

The patient may present with complaints of insidious onset of pain and swelling in the knee and calf. Pain localized to the patella may be mild or severe, causing a limp and restriction of motion. Motion is less severely affected than in patients with septic arthritis. Swelling may be minimal in the more indolent cases, or marked with distention of the prepatellar bursa or the knee, which may divert attention from the patella. Cellulitis overlying the patella also may be present. Isolated pinpoint tenderness over the patella is probably the single most useful clinical sign.[429]

Differential diagnosis of the swollen knee in an individual with sepsis includes septic arthritis; osteomyelitis of the distal femur, proximal tibia, or patella; and septic bursitis.[430] With more benign symptoms and the presence of a lytic lesion of the patella, neoplasm and Brodie's abscess must be considered.[430]

Excessive Lateral Pressure Syndrome. See Chapter 18.
Maltracking of the Patella. See Chapter 18.

Iatrogenic Causes: Infrapatellar Contracture Syndrome. See Chapter 18.

Medial Knee Pain

The causes of medial knee pain include the following:

Medial Meniscus Tear. See Chapter 18.
Medial Collateral Ligament (MCL) Sprain. See Chapter 18.
MCL Bursitis. See Chapter 18.
Hoffa's Disease. See Chapter 18.
Pes Anserine Bursitis. See Chapter 18.
Semimembranosus Tendonitis. See Chapter 18.

Lateral Knee Pain

The causes of lateral knee pain include the following:

Iliotibial Band Friction Syndrome. See Chapter 18.
Popliteus Tenosynovitis.
Popliteus Tendon Rupture.
Lateral Meniscal Tear. See Chapter 18.
Lateral Collateral Ligament Sprain.
Tibiofibular Disorder. See Chapter 18.
Biceps Femoris Tendonitis. See Chapter 18.
Osteochondral Fracture of the Lateral Femoral Condyle.

Posterior Knee Pain

The causes of posterior knee pain include the following:

Gastrocnemius Muscle Strain or Rupture.
Plantaris Muscle Strain or Rupture.
Hamstring Muscle and Tendon Disorder.
Muscle Spasm or Cramp.
Posterior Cruciate Ligament or Posterior Capsule Tear. See Chapter 18.
Baker's Cyst. See Chapter 18.

Causes of Lower Leg Pain

Anterolateral Lower Leg Pain

The causes of anterolateral lower leg pain include those listed in Table 9-21.

Anterior Compartment Syndrome. Compartment syndrome is a condition of pain associated with increased tissue pressure in the involved muscular compartment. This condition is suggested by lower-leg muscular pain with running or other activity and is relieved, very rapidly, by stopping the activity. The clinical signs of compartment syndrome can be remembered using the mnemonic of the five Ps: pain, paralysis, paresthesia, pallor, and pulses. Pain, especially disproportionate pain, is often the earliest sign, but the loss of normal neurologic sensation is the most reliable sign.[431,432]

Palpation of the compartment in question may demonstrate swelling or a tense compartment.[433] Decrease or loss of two-point discrimination also can be an early finding of compartment syndrome.[431,432] Clinical findings also may include shiny, erythematous skin overlying the involved compartment (described as a "woody" feeling), and excessive swelling. Intracompartmental tissue pressure is usually lower than arterial blood pressure, making peripheral pulses and capillary refill poor indicators of blood flow within the compartment.[433]

Compartment syndrome is confirmed by elevated compartment pressures. Normal tissue pressure ranges between zero and 10 mm Hg.[433] Capillary blood flow within the compartment may be compromised at pressures greater than 20 mm Hg. Muscle and nerve fibers are at risk for ischemic necrosis at pressures greater than 30 to 40 mm Hg.

Differential diagnosis includes tibial stress fracture, anterior tibialis tendonitis, and the catch-all group of "shin splints." Acute compartment syndrome requires emergent surgical fasciotomy.

Lateral Compartment Syndrome. Lateral compartment syndrome is very rare. It is often misdiagnosed as tenosynovitis of the tibialis anterior and flexor hallucis longus, fibular stress fracture, or a lateral gastrocnemius strain. Characteristic findings include tenderness along the proximal half of the leg, with swelling and tightness over the lateral compartment. On occasion, there may be complaints of numbness over the dorsum of the foot caused by compression of the superficial peroneal nerve.[432,433]

Intervention is based on the severity of the symptoms. In mild cases, treatment involves relative rest, education, and examination for underlying etiologies.[434] These include lower extremity malalignment, muscle imbalances, training errors, inadequate footwear, and poor technique.[434]

An acute compartment syndrome, or one that does not respond to conservative intervention, requires an open fasciotomy.

Irritation of the Superficial Peroneal Nerve. Compression of a peripheral nerve causes deformation of the nerve fibers, local ischemia, edema, and increased endoneurial pressure caused by accelerated vascular permeability, resulting in the loss of nerve fiber function (see Chap. 18).

Muscle Strain. See Chapter 18.

Calf Pain

The causes of calf pain include those listed in Table 9-22.

Pyomyositis. *Pyomyositis* is a term used to denote spontaneous muscle abscess of skeletal muscle. It is predominantly a disease of tropical countries. The etiology of pyomyositis is poorly understood. Local mechanical trauma at the time of incidental bacteremia is frequently postulated as a mechanism. Underlying conditions, such as immunodeficiency, or chronic illness, such as diabetes mellitus, may predispose to pyomyositis.

The natural history of pyomyositis may be divided into three stages: invasive, purulent, and late.[435]

1. ***Invasive stage.*** This stage occurs when the organism enters the muscle. It is characterized by an insidious onset of dull, cramping pain, with or without fever and anorexia. There is localized edema, sometimes described as indurated or woody, but usually little or no tenderness. This stage lasts from 10 to 21 days.

2. ***Purulent stage.*** This stage occurs when a deep collection of pus has developed in the muscle. The muscle usually but not always is tender, and fever and chills are common. The overlying skin may be normal or show mild erythema.

3. ***Late stage.*** This stage is characterized by exquisite tenderness of the site, which is red and fluctuant. The patient has high fever and occasionally may be in septic shock.

TABLE 9-21   Potential Causes of Anterolateral Leg Pain

Anterior compartment syndrome
Lateral compartment syndrome
Irritation of the superficial peroneal nerve
Muscle strain of one or more peroneals or of anterior tibialis

TABLE 9-22   Potential Causes of Calf Pain

Pyomyositis
Fibula shaft fracture
Deep vein thrombosis
Hematoma
Rupture of Achilles tendon
Soleus muscle strain
Acute posterior compartment syndrome
Muscle cramps

The iliopsoas is one of the most common sites of pyomyositis (see the discussion of iliopsoas abscess under "Causes of Pelvic Pain," earlier).

Fibula Shaft Fracture.   Direct trauma is the most common cause of isolated fibular fractures.[436] Another cause is a forced muscle contraction of the soleus.[437] Fibular stress fractures are common in long-distance runners. Loading of the fibula occurs maximally during the initial period of stance, and forces up to three times body weight are transmitted through the leg.[438] Thus, pain with this condition is typically reported with weight bearing during the initial period of stance. There also may be tenderness over the fracture site.

Deep Venous Thrombosis.   Muscle veins drain into the deep veins of the lower extremity. Soleal muscle veins drain into the peroneal and tibial posterior veins. The veins of the gastrocnemius drain into the popliteal vein. Thrombosis usually develops as a result of venous stasis or slow-flowing blood around venous valve sinuses. Extension of the primary thrombus occurs within or between the deep and superficial veins of the leg, and the propagating clot causes venous obstruction, damage to valves, and possible venous thromboembolism (VTE). Most episodes of VTE are clinically silent. The most common cause of leg swelling is edema, but expansion of all or part of a limb may result from an increase in any tissue component (muscle, fat, blood, etc.).[439]

The clinical features of a VTE include[439]:

▶ Calf pain or tenderness, or both.

▶ Swelling with pitting edema.

▶ Swelling below the knee (distal deep vein thrombosis) or up to the groin (proximal deep vein thrombosis).

▶ Increased skin temperature.

▶ Superficial venous dilation.

▶ Cyanosis, in patients with severe obstruction.

The intervention is aimed at reducing symptoms and preventing complications. The main complications of deep vein thrombosis are pulmonary embolism, post-thrombotic syndrome, and recurrence of thrombosis.[439] Proximal thrombi are a major source of morbidity and mortality. Distal thrombi are generally smaller and more difficult to detect noninvasively, and their prognosis and clinical importance are less clear.[439]

Hematoma.   A strain of the gastrocnemius muscle may follow a trivial trauma. Complete or partial tears of the musculotendinous unit may result in a hematoma. Clinical manifestations of gastrocnemius hematoma may include local swelling, pain, and tenderness aggravated by passive dorsiflexion of the ankle joint. This condition can mimic a deep venous thrombosis. The subjective history may help with the diagnosis. A definite diagnosis is established by CT scanning examination, which will reveal a local soft tissue mass within the gastrocnemius consistent with a hematoma.

Rupture of the Achilles Tendon.   See Chapter 19.
Soleus Muscle Strain.   See Chapter 19.
Acute Posterior Compartment Syndrome.   Acute calf pain can occur as a result of a posterior compartment syndrome. Causes include a deep venous thrombosis, rupture of a Baker's cyst, and spontaneous rupture of the medial head of the gastrocnemius. The diagnosis of posterior compartment syndrome is made by measuring the pressure in the posterior compartment. The intervention usually involves a fasciotomy.

Anteromedial Lower Leg Pain

The causes of anteromedial lower leg pain include those listed in Table 9-23.

Stress Fracture of the Tibia.   Tibial stress fractures are a common cause of shin soreness and a very common cause of exertional leg pain. Simple muscle strains are probably the most common cause of acute exercise induced leg pain, whereas more subacute or chronic pain may be caused by stress fractures or chronic (exertional) compartment syndrome.

Recognition of anterior tibial stress fractures is important because these fractures are prone to nonunion and avascular necrosis. They also are at greater risk for becoming displaced than are posterior tibial stress fractures. This increased susceptibility to complication has been attributed to a predominance of tensile forces along the anterior diaphysis rather than compressive forces along the posterior diaphysis.

Bone grafting, electrical stimulation, and internal localization sometimes are needed.

Medial Tibial Stress Syndrome.   See Chapter 19.
Saphenous Neuritis.[440]   Saphenous neuritis, also known as *gonalgia paresthetica,* is a painful condition caused by either irritation or compression at the adductor canal or elsewhere along the course of the saphenous nerve. The condition also may be associated with surgical or nonsurgical trauma to the nerve, especially at the medial or anterior aspect of the knee.

Saphenous neuritis can imitate other pathology around the knee or calf, particularly a medial meniscal tear, muscle injury, or osteoarthritis. As an isolated entity, saphenous neuritis may appear in conjunction with other common problems, such as osteoarthritis and patellofemoral pain syndrome. Its clinical appearance is characterized by a dull or achy pain along the course of the saphenous nerve on the medial side of the thigh,

TABLE 9-23   Potential Causes of Anteromedial Lower Leg Pain

Stress fracture of tibia
Medial tibial stress syndrome
Saphenous neuritis
Osteomyelitis of tibia
Soleus syndrome
Shin splints
Greater saphenous vein thrombosis

Potential Causes of Foot and Ankle Pain

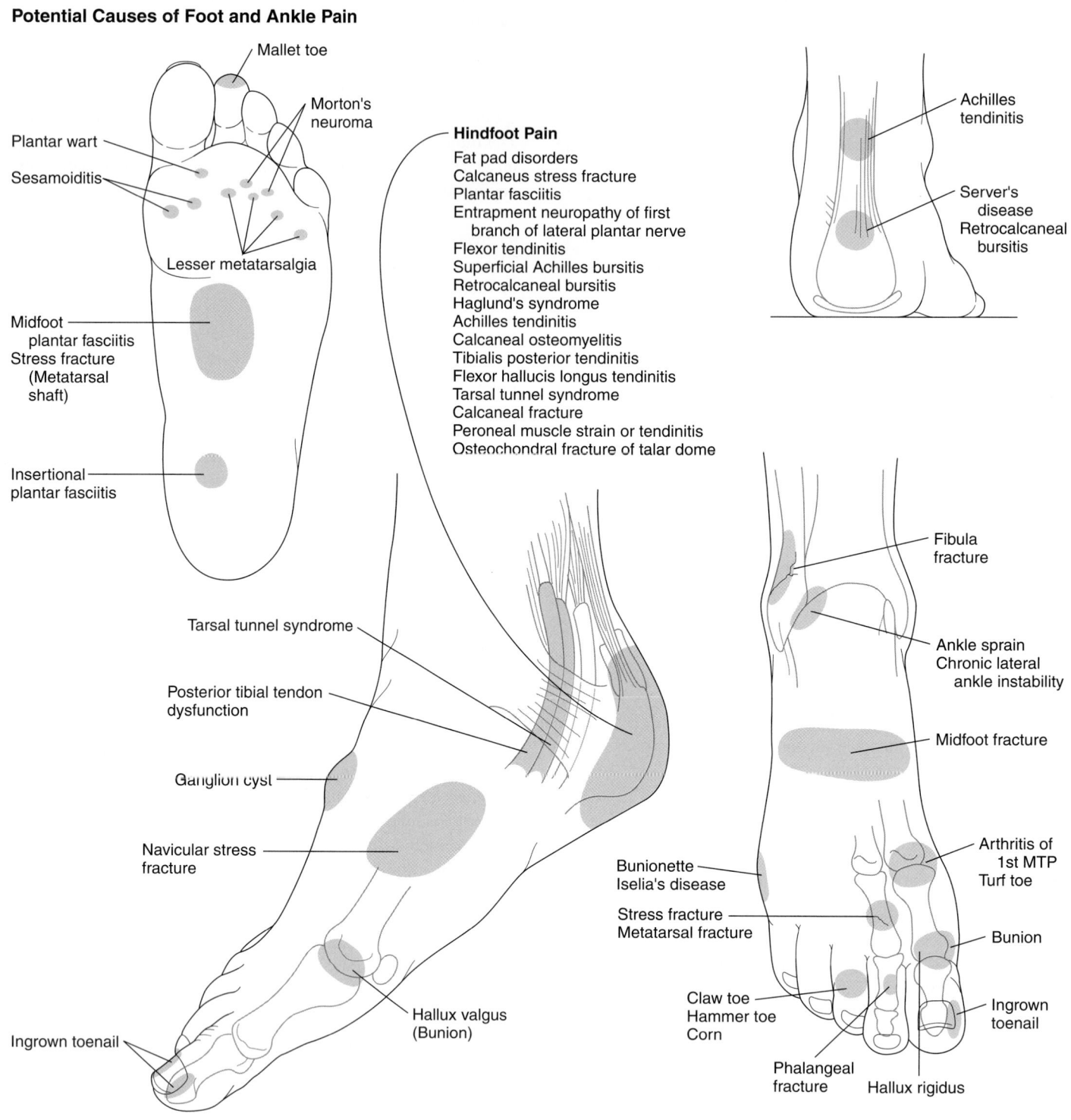

Hindfoot Pain

Fat pad disorders
Calcaneus stress fracture
Plantar fasciitis
Entrapment neuropathy of first
    branch of lateral plantar nerve
Flexor tendinitis
Superficial Achilles bursitis
Retrocalcaneal bursitis
Haglund's syndrome
Achilles tendinitis
Calcaneal osteomyelitis
Tibialis posterior tendinitis
Flexor hallucis longus tendinitis
Tarsal tunnel syndrome
Calcaneal fracture
Peroneal muscle strain or tendinitis
Osteochondral fracture of talar dome

FIGURE 9-7   Potential causes of foot and ankle pain.

knee, or calf. Hyperesthesia of the nerve is common. There is usually tenderness to light palpation along the course of the nerve, especially at the exit of the nerve from the adductor canal, near the medial joint line, or along the nerve in the proximal third of the leg. The diagnosis is confirmed by relief of

symptoms after injection of the affected area with local anesthetic.

Initial treatment can include nonsurgical symptomatic care, treatment of associated pathology, desensitization therapy, transcutaneous electrical nerve stimulation, and diagnostic or therapeutic injections of local anesthetic. In recalcitrant cases, surgical decompression and neurectomy are potential options. The key to treatment is prompt recognition; palpation of the saphenous nerve should be part of every routine examination of the knee.

Osteomyelitis of the Tibia. Osteomyelitis is a severe infection that can arise after operative treatment of bone and from acute penetrating trauma to the bone. The tibia is the most common site of post-traumatic osteomyelitis.[441] Post-traumatic tibial osteomyelitis results from trauma or nosocomial infection from the treatment of trauma that allows organisms to enter bone, proliferate in traumatized tissue, and cause subsequent bone infection.[441] The resulting infection is usually polymicrobial.

Patients with post-traumatic osteomyelitis of the tibia may present with localized bone and joint pain, erythema, swelling, and drainage around the area of trauma, surgery, or wound infection.[441] Signs of bacteremia, such as fever, chills, and night sweats, may be present in the acute phase of osteomyelitis, but not in the chronic phases.[441]

Radiographs are important for the diagnosis, staging, and evaluation of the progression of post-traumatic osteomyelitis.[441]

Causes of Ankle Pain

The causes of generalized ankle pain include those shown in Figure 9-7 and listed in Table 9-24.

Crystal-induced Arthropathies

Two types of arthritis, gout and pseudogout, are quite common in the ankle joint. Episodes of acute arthritis in this region, without an apparent cause, should arouse suspicion of a gout attack, especially in a middle-aged man.

Ligament Sprain

See Chapter 19.

Tendonitis

See Chapter 19.

TABLE 9-24   Potential Causes of Generalized Ankle Pain

Crystal-induced arthropathies
Ligament sprain
Tendonitis
Fracture
Bursitis
Os trigonum
Osteochondritis dissecans of talus
Acute monarthritis
Transient migratory osteoporosis
Polyarthritis
Lyme arthritis
Reiter's syndrome
Rheumatoid arthritis

Fracture

See Chapter 19.

Bursitis

See Chapter 19.

Os Trigonum

The term *os trigonum* refers to a failure of the lateral tubercle of the posterior process to unite with the body of the talus during ossification, producing an impingement with extreme plantar flexion.[442] The posterior aspect of the talus often exhibits a separate ossification center, appearing at 8 to 10 years of age in girls and 11 to 13 years of age in boys. Fusion usually occurs 1 year after its appearance.[443,444] When fusion does not occur, an os trigonum is formed. It has been reported to be present in approximately 10 percent of the general population and is often unilateral.[443,445–447]

The origin of this ossicle may be congenital or acquired. Congenitally, it can be a persistent separation of the secondary center of the lateral tubercle from the remainder of the posterior talus secondary to repeated microtrauma during development.[443,447] The acquired form may be secondary to an actual fracture that has not united.[443,447,448] With either form, the os trigonum is usually asymptomatic.[442] However, it can become symptomatic in young athletes who actively plantar flex the ankle, such as ballet dancers, gymnasts, ice skaters, or, on occasion, soccer players.[443,445,447,449,450]

The pain, which is typically in the posterolateral ankle, results from a mechanical impingement of the posterior talus between the posterior tibia and the calcaneus.[442] Repetitive impingement of the soft tissues in this interval also can result in hypertrophic capsulitis.[443,446,451–453] Associated posteromedial pain[443,449,452] may indicate a concurrent flexor hallucis longus tendonitis. The diagnosis is confirmed with imaging studies.

Plain radiographs should include a lateral view of the ankle, and a lateral view in plantarflexion. A bone scan may be used to determine the reactivity of the os trigonum,[443,454] but absence of uptake does not exclude impingement.[442]

Differential diagnosis includes posterior ankle impingement, Achilles tendonitis, peroneal tendonitis, and flexor hallucis longus tendonitis.[443]

Conservative intervention may include rest, anti-inflammatory medications, avoidance of plantarflexion casting and injection.[443,449] The pain, however, usually returns once the young athletes resume their sports.

Osteochondritis Dissecans

Osteochondritis dissecans (OCD) of the talus may result from an inversion stress to the ankle. This is actually a "transchondral fracture" secondary to trauma.[455] More commonly, onset of pain is insidious and some prior macrotrauma is evident.[442] Young patients may present with pain over the anterolateral or posteromedial talus. They often report recurrent ankle effusions or weakness. Plain radiographs of the ankle usually show the lesion, but sometimes a bone scan or MRI is necessary for diagnosis.[456] The Berndt-Harty[457] classification of talus OCD is as follows:

► *Type I.* Small area of compression of subchondral bone.

► *Type II.* Partially detached osteochondral fragment.

► *Type III.* Completely detached osteochondral fragment but remaining in its crater.

► *Type IV.* Displaced osteochondral fragment.

Berndt and Harty[457] reported that 43 percent of OCD lesions involve the middle third of the lateral talus, with 57 percent involving the posterior third of the medial talus.[455] One study[458] reported that lateral OCD lesions rarely heal on their own, whereas most medial lesions do.[455]

The intervention for type I and II lesions begins with casting and orthotics.[442] The intervention for type III medial lesions starts off conservatively, as well, but may require arthroscopic or open debridement. Type III lateral lesions and type IV lesions all require arthroscopic removal or pinning for the best chance of healing.[459]

Causes of Foot Pain

Generalized Foot Pain

The causes of generalized foot pain include those shown in Figure 9-7 and listed in Table 9-25.

Infection. Infection of the foot includes such diagnoses as cellulites, necrotizing fasciitis, and osteomyelitis.

Cellulitis. Cellulitis is common after foot and ankle surgery. It is important to distinguish a superficial infection from one that involves the deeper soft tissue envelope and possibly the joint or bone.

► *Superficial.* With a superficial infection, the skin is warm, tender, and erythematous, but joint motion is painless. Occasionally, lymphangitis or lymphadenopathy is present.

TABLE 9-25   Potential Causes of Generalized Foot Pain

Trauma
Infection
Rheumatoid arthritis
Gout
Pseudogout
Systemic lupus erythematosus
Sickle cell disease
Reflex sympathetic dystrophy/Complex regional pain syndrome
Peripheral vascular disease
Peripheral polyneuropathy
Systemic disorders
Nerve and root compression syndromes
Foot cramps
Cold injury
Bites
Cutaneous disorders

The area is tender to palpation. The most common causative organisms in uncompromised hosts are *Staphylococcus aureus* and β-hemolytic streptococci.

► *Deep.* Deep infections with abscess formation are a serious complication. In patients with deep infections, the skin is warm, tender, swollen, and possibly fluctuant. White blood cell count and temperature may be increased. Plain radiographs, MRI, and needle aspiration are helpful in making the diagnosis.

Necrotizing Fasciitis. Necrotizing fasciitis is characterized by rapidly progressive necrosis and edema of the subcutaneous fat and fascia that can result in septic shock, end-organ failure, and loss of limb or life. Patients who are immunocompromised, such as those with human immunodeficiency virus infections, diabetes mellitus, and alcoholism, are at increased risk for necrotizing fasciitis. Clinical signs of necrotizing fasciitis include tense edema and erythema that do not respond to antibiotics or elevation. Patients are usually febrile.

Osteomyelitis. Fever, local pain, edema, exudative drainage, and elevated leukocyte count and sedimentation rate are typical findings with osteomyelitis. Surgical treatment of patients with osteomyelitis consists of debridement of all necrotic and infected tissue and appropriate antibiotic therapy. Treatment also may include the use of antibiotic-impregnated methylmethacrylate beads, local or vascularized soft tissue flaps, autogenous bone grafts, or vascularized bone grafts once the infection is eradicated.

Rheumatoid Arthritis. Rheumatoid arthritis characteristically involves the synovial tissues of the small joints of the feet, rather than the talocrural or subtalar joint. Three times more women than men are affected. In 17 percent of cases, the disease first manifests in the foot.[460]

The early stage of the disease should be suspected in young women presenting with bilateral foot pain and a tendency to morning stiffness in the metatarsophalangeal (MTP) joints of the feet.

Gout. About 60 percent of initial attacks of gout involve the great toe (podagra), which becomes swollen and excruciatingly painful.[460]

Pseudogout. Pseudogout involves joints in addition to the MTP joint, including the talonavicular or subtalar joints.[460]

Systemic Lupus Erythematosus. Systemic lupus erythematosus (SLE) is a systemic autoimmune disease with clinical features that include glomerulonephritis, rashes, serositis, hemolytic anemia, thrombocytopenia, and central nervous system involvement.[461] This disease occurs most commonly in women of childbearing age.

The variety of neurologic presentations of SLE can include cranial neuropathies, stroke syndromes, movement disorders, spinal cord lesions, seizure disorders, dementias, cognitive disturbances, psychoses, and mood disorders. Peripheral nervous system manifestations include symmetric polyneuropathies, mononeuritis multiplex, acute inflammatory demyelinating polyneuropathies, chronic relapsing inflammatory demyelinating polyneuropathies, and autonomic failure.

SLE is considered to be the prototypical human autoimmune disease mediated by pathogenic immune complexes.

Sickle Cell Disease.[462]   Sickle cell disease is an inherited blood disorder that affects mostly African Americans. It leaves patients vulnerable to repeated crises that can cause severe pain, multisystem organ damage, and early death. Sickle cell crises typically begin during the preschool or early elementary school years. How often they recur and how long each attack lasts vary considerably.

The crisis begins when a trigger—such as an acute infection (especially viral), stress, dehydration, or extremely hot or cold temperatures—causes the red blood cells to release oxygen. People with sickle cell disease have abnormal hemoglobin, called *hemoglobin S (HbS)*, which forms long polymers upon deoxygenation. The rodlike polymers change the normally round and pliable red blood cells into stiff cells with a crescent, or sickle, shape.

Bundles of these deformed cells plug up the capillaries throughout the body, reducing blood flow. This vaso-occlusion causes localized tissue hypoxia, which in turn promotes further sickling. Tissue infarction and necrosis soon follow.

Pain is usually the main symptom. It may be localized or diffuse, constant or intermittent. About half of all patients also have fever, swelling in the joints of the hands or feet, long bone pain, tachypnea, hypertension, nausea, and vomiting. Hospitalization becomes necessary when these complications are severe. Acute chest syndrome and cerebrovascular accidents are life-threatening complications of sickle cell disease. In addition, the patient may develop an infarct in a lung, causing acute chest syndrome, characterized by a combination of chest pain, dyspnea, fever, and leukocytosis.

Complex Regional Pain Syndrome (Reflex Sympathetic Dystrophy).[463]   Complex regional pain syndrome (CRPS), formerly known as reflex sympathetic dystrophy (RSD), is a regional, post-traumatic, neuropathic pain problem that most often affects one or more limbs (see Chap. 16 for CRPS of the upper extremity).

Most patients with CRPS have an identifiable inciting or initiating injury, which may be trivial, such as a minor limb sprain, or severe, such as trauma involving a major nerve or nerves. Adults can present with CRPS after a fracture or trauma with immobilization. With children, CRPS occurs most often in athletic girls (1:6 boys to girls) with an average age of 12 years.[464]

Most of the cases of CRPS in the lower extremity, including the foot and ankle, have a history of minor trauma. The key features are pain, allodynia and hyperalgesia, abnormal vasomotor

activity, and abnormal sudomotor activity persisting beyond the period of normal healing. Allodynia is defined as a disproportionately increased pain response to a non-noxious stimulus. Hyperalgesia is defined as a disproportionately increased pain response to a mildly noxious stimulus.

Patients with CRPS often adopt a protective posture to protect the affected extremity from mechanical and thermal stimulation. They may wear a stocking to guard the involved extremity. Allodynia may be so severe that the patient will not allow the physician or therapist to examine or even touch the affected limb.

Successful treatment of CRPS depends on an aggressive and multidisciplinary approach. Because pain and limb dysfunction are the major clinical problems, physical rehabilitation and pain control are the main treatment objectives. Early referral to a pain clinic for possible sympathetic nerve blocks or neurosuppressive medications may be indicated.

Peripheral Vascular Disease.[465]   Peripheral vascular disease (PVD) is common in the western world. PVD typically begins its progression in midlife (for men at approximately 45 years of age, and for women, 55 to 60 years). Arteries generally have smooth linings, which allow blood to flow unimpaired. Arteriosclerosis is a degenerative arterial disease that refers to a so-called hardening of the arteries. In this condition, muscle and elastic tissue are replaced with fibrous tissue, and calcification may occur.

Atherosclerosis is the most common type of arteriosclerosis. It is characterized by the formation of atheromatous plaques, which are deposits of fatty material in the lining of medium and large-sized arteries. These arteries then become narrowed and rough as more fat is deposited. Blood clots form more easily because of the roughness of the vessel wall, further narrowing the artery, and thus potentially limiting blood flow. A reduction of blood supply to the organs and tissues prevents them from performing adequately. In addition, the plaques are liable to break down and form ulcers. Thromboses may then develop as a result of the roughening and ulceration of the inner coat of the arteries.

Patients suffering reduced blood supply to the lower limbs often experience effort-related cramp in the calves, thighs, and buttocks, which disappears at rest. This condition is known as *intermittent claudication.*

PVD with claudication can be confused with neurogenic claudication and spinal stenosis. The major difference is the response of the pain to rest or to the position of the spine. Unlike the pain from spinal stenosis, the pain from PVD is not relieved by trunk flexion or aggravated with sustained trunk extension (Table 9-26).

The site of claudication indicates the most likely site of the narrowing or blockage. When severe, claudication can become debilitating, can limit mobility, and sometimes is associated with a worsened quality of life and loss of functional independence. Pain may occur at more regular intervals as the disease process continues to its end stage—critical limb ischemia—until finally it occurs when the patient is at rest (rest

TABLE 9-26 Differentiating Causes of Claudication[209]

Vascular Claudication	Neurogenic Claudication	Spinal Stenosis
Pain* is usually bilateral	Pain is usually bilateral, but may be unilateral	Usually bilateral pain
Occurs in calf (foot, thigh, hip, or buttocks)	Occurs in back, buttocks, thighs, calves, feet	Occurs in back, buttocks, thighs, calves, feet
Pain consistent in all spinal positions	Pain is decreased in spinal flexion, increased in spinal extension and with walking	Pain is decreased in spinal flexion, increased in spinal extension and with walking
Pain is brought on by physical exertion (e.g., walking), relieved promptly by rest (1–5 min), and increased by walking uphill	Pain is decreased by recumbency	Pain is relieved with prolonged rest (may persist hours after resting), decreased when walking uphill
No burning or dysesthesia	Burning and dysesthesia from back to buttocks and leg(s)	Burning and numbness present in lower extremities
Decreased or absent pulses in lower extremities	Normal pulses	Normal pulses
Color and skin changes in feet; cold, numb, dry, or scaly skin; poor nail and hair growth	Good skin nutrition	Good skin nutrition
Affects ages 40–60+	Affects ages 40–60+	Peaks in the seventh decade, affects men primarily

* Pain associated with vascular claudication also may be described as an "aching," "cramping," or "tired" feeling.

pain). At this stage, rest pain is usually worse when the legs are elevated and during sleep, with the patient gaining relief by hanging the foot over the side of the bed. The development of nonhealing wounds or gangrene (tissue death) may occur at this stage.

This disease process can lead to loss of limb and life; therefore, investigation and early diagnosis are important. The patient who presents with typical, reproducible, exertional discomfort in the buttocks, thighs, or calves that disappears with rest is likely to have claudication and symptomatic PVD.

Peripheral Polyneuropathy. Polyneuropathy is a syndrome with many different causes. Clinical features in painful neuropathies include sensory loss, paresthesia, paradox hyperalgesia, paroxysms, and increased pain on repetitive stimulation.

Systemic Disorders. The systemic disorders that can cause foot pain include:

▶ Carcinoma.

▶ Leukemia.

▶ Lymphoma.

▶ Myeloma.

▶ Amyloidosis.

▶ Connective tissue diseases (polyarteritis nodosa, SLE).

▶ Renal failure.

▶ Acquired immunodeficiency syndrome (AIDS).

▶ Sarcoidosis.

▶ Cutaneous disorders.

Nerve and Root Compression Syndromes. See Chapter 19.

Forefoot Pain
The causes of forefoot pain include those shown in Fig. 9-7 and listed in Table 9-27.

Metatarsalgia. Metatarsalgia, in its broadest definition, includes discomfort around the metatarsal heads or the plantar aspects of the metatarsal heads. Metatarsalgia is discussed in Chapter 19.

Freiberg's Disease. Freiberg's disease, an avascular necrosis of the second metatarsal epiphysis, is a source of metatarsalgia.[442] The disease is an osteochondrosis of congenital, traumatic, or vascular etiology that leads to eventual collapse and deformity of

TABLE 9-27   Potential Causes of Forefoot Pain

Metatarsalgia
Freiberg's disease
Morton's neuroma
Arthritis
Fracture
Forefoot sprain
Bursitis
Idiopathic synovitis
Arterial insufficiency

a lesser metatarsal head. It is unlikely that an athletic injury is the sole cause of Freiberg's disease, although a mechanical stress to the forefoot may exacerbate a previously subclinical condition. The condition is most common in the second metatarsal head, with a predilection of 68 to 82 percent.[466,467] Less commonly, it may occur at the third, fourth, or fifth metatarsal heads.

The female-to-male ratio in Freiberg's disease is 5:1, and the typical patient is a female adolescent aged 11 to 17 years.[468] The condition may be asymptomatic early in its course and manifest in young adulthood to middle age.

Physical examination usually reveals unilateral pain over the second metatarsal head, that is worse with activity, limited range of motion, periarticular swelling, and, occasionally, a plantar callosity under the second metatarsal head.[469]

This condition is usually self-limiting and requires only conservative treatment in the form of rest from high-impact activities, an orthosis to correct pronation,[470] a range-of-motion walking boot, or a short leg cast for more severe acute pain. Patients with severe antalgia should use crutches. Hoskinson[467] reported success with conservative treatment in 11 of 28 patients, although all had restriction of joint motion.

The surgical intervention for Freiberg's disease involves debridement of the joint, removal of loose bodies, and removal of metatarsal head osteophytes, with reshaping of the head.[471] A dorsiflexion osteotomy of the metatarsal head also has been advocated to rotate the healthy plantar cartilage up into articulation with the proximal phalanx.

Morton's Neuroma.   An interdigital neuroma, or Morton's neuroma (Fig. 9-8), is a mechanical entrapment neuropathy of the interdigital nerve. The entrapment may occur as the nerve courses on the plantar side of the distal aspect of the transverse intermetatarsal ligament, where it is vulnerable to traction injury and compression during the toe-off phase of running or during repetitive positions of toe rise.[472]

The most commonly involved nerve is the third interdigital nerve, between the third and fourth metatarsal heads, followed in incidence by the second interdigital nerve and, rarely, the first and fourth interdigital nerves.[472,473]

The individual with an interdigital neuroma will complain of symptoms of forefoot burning, cramping, tingling, and numbness in the toes of the involved interspace, with occasional proximal radiation in the foot.[472]

Morton's neuroma is described further in Chapter 19.

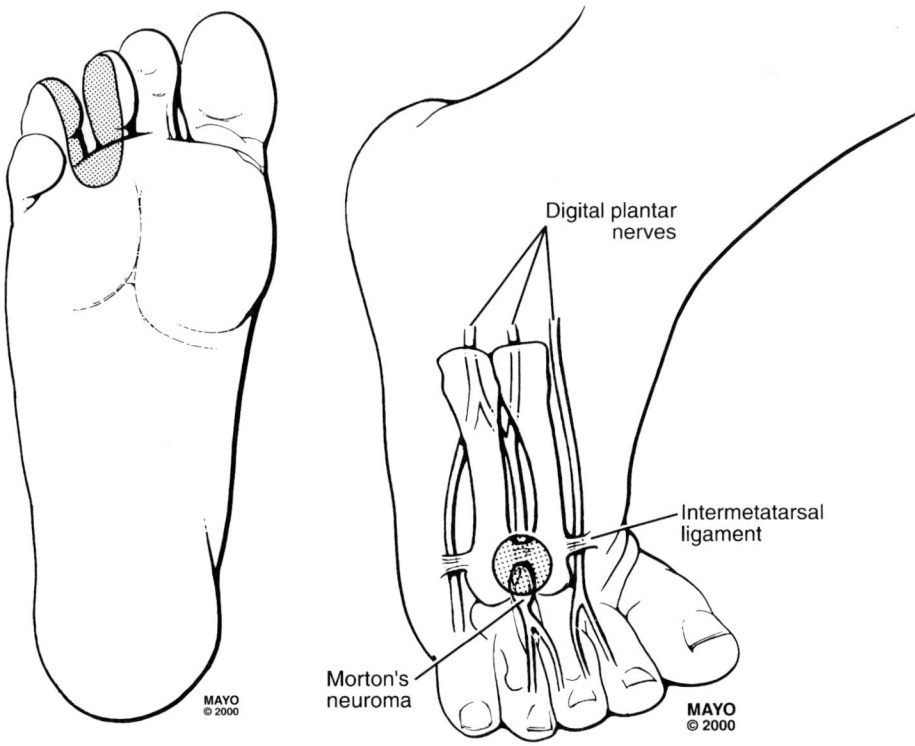

FIGURE 9-8   Morton's neuroma. (Reproduced with permission from O'Connor FG, Wilder RP, eds. *Textbook of Running Medicine.* New York, NY: McGraw-Hill; 2001.)

Digital plantar nerves

Intermetatarsal ligament

Morton's neuroma

MAYO
© 2000

Arthritis. See Chapter 19.
Fracture. See Chapter 19.
Forefoot Sprain. See Chapter 19.
Bursitis. See Chapter 19.

Medial Forefoot and Great Toe Pain

The causes of medial forefoot and great toe pain include those shown in Figure 9-7 and listed below:

Nail Lesions. See Chapter 19.
Hallux Valgus. See Chapter 19.
Hallux Rigidus. See Chapter 19.
Arthritis of the First Metatarsophalangeal Joint. See Chapter 19.

Midfoot Pain

The causes of midfoot pain include those shown in Figure 9-7 and listed below:

Longitudinal Arch Strain.
Aseptic Necrosis of the Navicular.
Tendonitis of the Flexor Hallucis Longus or Peroneal Tendonitis. See Chapter 19.
Subtalar Osteochondral Fracture. See Chapter 19.
Accessory Navicular. The accessory navicular is the most common accessory bone in the foot. It occurs on the medial plantar border of the navicular at the site of insertion of the tibialis posterior tendon.[474] The incidence in the general population has been reported to be between 4 and 14 percent,[474,475] but few patients actually become symptomatic.[442] A histologic study by Grogan and colleagues[476] suggested that tensile failure in the cartilaginous synchondrosis was the cause of pain.

In the adolescent athletic population, symptoms may arise secondary to pressure over the bony prominence, a tear in the actual synchondrosis, or tibialis posterior tendonitis.[475]

The patient usually presents with pain and a prominence over the navicular in a pronated foot. There is usually local tenderness to palpation and pain with resisted foot inversion.[474] It has been hypothesized that the tibialis posterior tendon inserts into the accessory navicular, a weaker insertion point, thereby causing a drop in the medial arch of the foot and a pes planus.[477] However, Sullivan and Miller[478] found no difference in the longitudinal arches of those with an accessory navicular and those without.[442]

Physical examination is supplemented by radiographic assessment. The anteroposterior view or a 45-degree eversion oblique view is usually diagnostic.[474]

The intervention for this condition consists of orthotics, trial of casting, range of motion exercises, and eventual removal if symptoms continue.[474–476,478–481]

Köhler's Bone Disease. Köhler's bone disease is an aseptic necrosis of unknown etiology that typically affects the tarsal navicular bone.[442] The condition usually is caused by repetitive microtrauma to the maturing epiphysis.[442] It is largely found in active boys aged 4 to 7 years.

Köhler's bone disease is typically self-limiting and should not require any type of surgery. Initial intervention involves de-

creased activity or a short leg cast for 3 to 6 weeks.[482] Orthotics may be necessary to maintain the longitudinal arch.

Stress Fracture of the Navicular. See Chapter 19.
Acquired Flatfoot. See Chapter 19.
Osteoarthritis. See Chapter 19.
Plantar Fascial Pain. See Chapter 19.
Cuboid Subluxation Syndrome. See Chapter 19.

Dorsal Foot Pain

Tendonitis of the Extensor Hallucis Longus, Extensor Digitorum Longus, or Tibialis Anterior. See Chapter 19.

Hindfoot Pain

The causes of generalized hindfoot pain include those shown in Figure 9-7 and as follows:

Generalized Hindfoot Pain
Intra-articular Calcaneal Fractures. The calcaneus is the most frequently fractured tarsal bone, with calcaneal fractures accounting for 65 percent of tarsal injuries and approximately 2 percent of all fractures.[483] Acute complications include swelling, fracture blisters, and compartment syndromes. Late complications include arthritis; malunion, including calcaneofibular abutment; and heel pad problems. Complications associated with operative treatment include wound dehiscence, infection, and iatrogenic nerve injury.

Plantar Hindfoot Pain
Fat Pad Disorders.
Calcaneus Stress Fracture. See Chapter 19.
Plantar Fasciitis. See Chapter 19.
Entrapment Neuropathy of the First Branch of the Lateral Plantar Nerve. See Chapter 19.
Flexor Tendonitis.

Posterior Hindfoot Pain
Superficial Achilles Bursitis. See Chapter 19.
Retrocalcaneal Bursitis. See Chapter 19.
Haglund's Syndrome. See Chapter 19.
Achilles Tendonitis. See Chapter 19.
Achilles Tendon Rupture. See Chapter 19.
Calcaneal Osteomyelitis. Primary hematogenous osteomyelitis of the calcaneus is uncommon and accounts for 3 to 10 percent of all acute bone infections in children.[484] The calcaneus has a so-called metaphyseal equivalent region that borders the apophysis and is susceptible to hematogenous infection, as in long bones.[485] *S. aureus* has been found to be the most common bacterial agent in hematogenous calcaneal osteomyelitis.

Clinical findings include fever, pain, and swelling around the foot and ankle. The differential diagnosis may include septic arthritis of the ankle, cellulitis, stress fracture, calcaneal apophysitis, Achilles enthesopathy, and subcutaneous abscess.

Medial Hindfoot Pain
Tibialis Posterior Tendonitis. See Chapter 19.
Flexor Hallucis Longus Tendonitis. See Chapter 19.

Tarsal Tunnel Syndrome.   Tarsal tunnel syndrome (TTS) is a compressive neuropathy of the posterior tibial nerve (Fig. 9-9), or one of its branches, which usually occurs at the level of the ankle. This relatively rare syndrome was first described by Keck[486] and Lam[487] in two separate reports in 1962.

The posterior tibial nerve often is entrapped as it courses through the tarsal tunnel, passing under the deep fascia, the flexor retinaculum, and within the abductor hallucis muscle.[488] The most common site of entrapment is at the anterior inferior aspect of the tunnel, where the nerves wind around the medial malleolus.[489]

The etiology is multifactorial and may be post-traumatic, neoplastic, inflammatory,[490] or a result of rapid weight gain,[491] fluid retention,[491] abnormal foot or ankle mechanics,[492–494] or a valgus foot deformity.[495–497]

The diagnosis is based on history and clinical examination. The typical patient reports a poorly localized burning sensation or pain and paresthesia at the medial plantar surface of the foot, with the distribution correlating with the level of entrapment of the medial or lateral plantar nerve as they join to form the posterior tibial nerve.[460] Discomfort is worse after activity and typically is accentuated during the end of a working day.[488] Some patients have cramps in the longitudinal foot arch. Resting pain is reported infrequently but can disturb sleep.[460] Plantar fasciitis has similar findings and must be ruled out.[498]

The physical examination can reveal any one, or all, of the following:

▶ Positive Tinel's sign, sometimes with pain radiating distally toward the midsole, along the posterior branch of the nerve.[499] Percussion should be performed with and without weight bearing.[500]

▶ Pain with passive dorsiflexion[490] or eversion.[499]

▶ Decreased two-point discrimination on the plantar aspect of the foot.[499]

▶ Varus or valgus deformity of the heel.[491,495,497,499]

▶ Weakness of the foot intrinsics with sustained plantar flexion of the toes.

▶ Normal results from the neurologic examination.[501]

The most effective conservative interventions for TTS are local corticosteroid injections, an orthoses for foot deformity,[497,502] strengthening of the foot intrinsics to restore the medial longitudinal arch,[494] weight loss for obese patients,[494] and a 1-inch heel lift to decrease tension on the tibial nerve.[490]

Surgical intervention, which typically occurs after a trial course of conservative measures, involves decompression of the nerve.[495,496] The overall results from early surgical decompression are beneficial in most patients.[491]

Calcaneal Fracture.   See Chapter 19.
Medial Ankle Sprain.   See Chapter 19.

Lateral Hindfoot Pain
Peroneal Muscle Strain or Tendonitis.   See Chapter 19.
Lateral Ankle Sprain.   See Chapter 19.
Osteochondral Fracture of the Talar Dome.   See Chapter 19.
Sural Nerve Entrapment.
Stress Fracture of the Lateral Malleolus.   See Chapter 19.

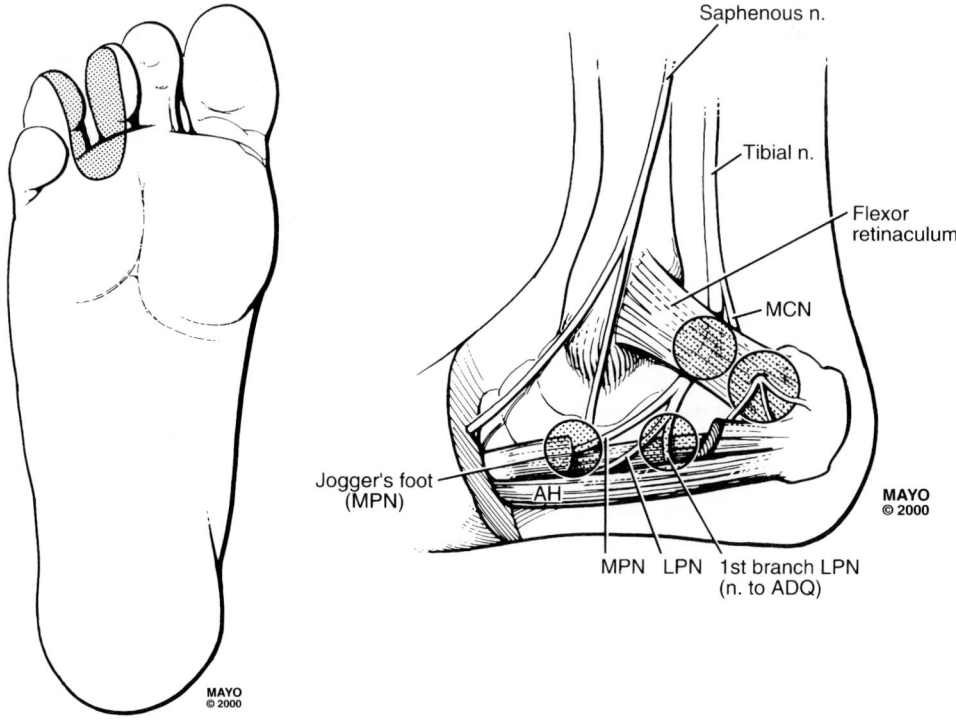

FIGURE 9-9   Tarsal tunnel syndrome. (Reproduced with permission from O'Connor FG, Wilder RP, eds. *Textbook of Running Medicine.* New York, NY: McGraw-Hill; 2001.)

Saphenous n.
Tibial n.
Flexor retinaculum
MCN
Jogger's foot (MPN)
AH
MPN   LPN   1st branch LPN (n. to ADQ)
MAYO © 2000

CASE STUDY NECK PULSING

HISTORY

A 37-year-old woman presented to the office complaining that her head "wanted to go back." Her symptoms began approximately 6 months earlier with painless "pulsing" on the left side of her neck that became worse with stressful situations and physical activity but was relieved by relaxation and sleep. She could briefly stop the pulsing by placing her hand on the right posterior aspect of the neck. Her symptoms had progressed to an extension of the neck with spasm, which caused her to lean forward to maintain eye contact with others. She also noted an occasional "eye tic," which seemed to come and go spontaneously. She denied any paresthesias, weakness, dysphasia, visual changes or hearing loss, or bowel or bladder changes. Although she had no family history of specific neurologic problems, the patient reported a maternal aunt who had "facial tics." The patient had a medical history notable for anxiety and several phobias for which she had received psychological counseling. Vascular studies had ruled out vascular disease and the presence of an aneurysm in the neck and trunk. Imaging studies had ruled out fracture or tumor.

TEST AND MEASURES

On physical examination, her neck was positioned in extension, side bent slightly to the left, and rotated to the right, and there was a palpable spasm and hypertrophy of the left cervical paravertebral musculature. She had full range of motion of the neck in all planes with intact motor strength, and there were no other motor or sensory deficits. Cranial nerve tests and reflexes were normal bilaterally, and no other tremor, tic, or dystonia was observed.

EVALUATION

A provisional diagnosis of spasmodic torticollis was made. Given the fact that this patient had no sensory, motor, or range of motion deficits, the case was discussed with her physician. The physician agreed to a trial period of physical therapy using the principles of positive practice.[198]

INTERVENTION

* *Electrotherapeutic modalities and thermal agents.* A moist heat pack was applied to the left side of the cervical spine when the patient arrived for each treatment session. Ultrasound at 3 MHz was administered to the cervical musculature on the left side of the neck for 10 minutes following the moist heat.
* *Manual therapy.* Following the ultrasound, soft tissue techniques of massage and gentle stretching were performed. The neck was gently stretched into flexion, right side bending, and left rotation.
* *Therapeutic exercises.* The patient performed repetitive active range-of-motion exercises into the combined motion of flexion, right side bending, and left rotation against the spasmodic muscle group.

* *Patient-related instruction.* Explanation was given as to the potential causes of the patient's symptoms. The patient was advised to perform the active range-of-motion exercises as many times as possible when in the upright position. Her husband was instructed on the same stretching and massage techniques. The patient also received instruction on the use of heat at home. Instructions to sleep on the left side using a medium-sized pillow were given.
* *Goals/outcomes.* Both the patient's goals from the intervention and the expected therapeutic goals from the clinician were discussed with the patient. It was concluded that the clinical sessions would occur until the patient, and her husband, felt comfortable with their ability to perform the treatment protocol independently, at which time the patient would be discharged to a home exercise program. The patient attended therapy sessions for 6 visits. At a 2-month follow-up, the patient reported a marked improvement in her symptoms, but noticed that they returned in a few days if the exercise regimen was not continued.

CASE STUDY GROIN PAIN IN A MIDDLE-AGED FEMALE

HISTORY

A 56-year-old, moderately obese woman presents with a prescription that reads "Hip OA, evaluate and treat."

Patient presented with left groin pain of an insidious onset that is worsening. The pain started approximately 3 months ago when the patient commenced a walking program to lose some weight. The symptoms improve with rest, but worsen with activity, especially with walking and stair negotiation. The series of radiographs taken at the physician's office reveal slight degenerative changes at the hip joint.

WORKING HYPOTHESIS

Given the age of the patient, the insidious onset and location of pain, the radiograph findings, and the fact that the pain improves with rest, the diagnosis from the physician could be correct. However, any insidious onset of symptoms should always alert the clinician.

Less intuitive clinicians would proceed with the following tests, with the physician diagnosis in the back of their minds, tainting their judgment.

A lower quarter scanning examination is performed with the following results:

* Slight groin discomfort with lumbar flexion.
* Slight groin discomfort at 90 degrees of left straight leg raise.
* Slight groin discomfort with the prone knee bend test if the hip is extended
* No neurologic signs present.
* No pain reproduced with active, passive, and resisted testing of the hip except with passive hip extension.
* The scour test and the FABER (flexion in abduction and external rotation) test both reproduce the groin pain.

At this point, the clinician could decide to treat the patient for osteoarthritis of the hip. However, some important points are raised from the examination findings. For example, no capsular pattern was noted at the hip. In fact, the only hip motion that was painful—extension—is not even mentioned in the capsular pattern. The only other tests that could be deemed positive were the scour test and the FABER test, both of which examine more than just the hip joint.

The focus of every examination should be to consider all potential causes for the patient's symptoms and to find ways to both provoke *and* alleviate the symptoms. It would be prudent in this case to perform an examination of the lumbar and sacroiliac joints. These tests would reveal:

- No capsular pattern of left hip.
- Groin pain also reproduced with lumbar extension.
- Slight pain with hip flexion (L1–2), but only with the hip extended.
- Bilateral tightness of the rectus femoris and hip flexors.
- Left rotation of all of the lumbar segments.

As is often the case, a more detailed examination reveals more information, but does not always make the diagnosis easier. The clinician needs to use the mental list of all the structures in the body that can refer pain to the groin and begin to rule out each one with a series of tests until only one remains. Groin pain is a common finding in patients, and the findings thus far could suggest a number of candidates.

Groin pain could suggest hip osteoarthritis:

- The age of the patient, the insidious onset and location of pain, the radiographic findings, and the fact that the pain improves with rest support this conclusion.
- A positive scour test and FABER test somewhat support this conclusion.
- The noncapsular pattern somewhat refutes this conclusion.

Groin pain could suggest pelvic impairment:

- The positive FABER test somewhat supports this conclusion.
- All of the other sacroiliac tests are negative, which refutes this conclusion.

Groin pain could suggest a lumbar or thoracic impairment:

- Pain reproduced with lumbar extension could support this conclusion.
- The positive prone knee bend somewhat supports this conclusion.
- The positive FABER test somewhat supports this conclusion.
- The pain with resisted hip flexion, with the hip in extension, could confirm this conclusion based on the anatomy of the hip flexors.

Groin pain could suggest a contractile structure:

- Pain reproduced by resisted hip flexion supports this conclusion.
- The positive scour test refutes this conclusion.
- The insidious onset could refute or support this conclusion, depending on whether it was a muscle or tendon impairment.

Groin pain could suggest a host of other pathologies.

In fact, this patient was diagnosed with an iliopectineal bursitis. It should be clear from this case study that an examination draws on all of the clinician's resources. The more experienced clinician would now begin to wonder why the left iliopsoas became adaptively shortened.

This case also highlights a problem that many clinicians face: the potential invasion of a patient's intimate areas. Although most clinicians routinely palpate the spine and the extremities if they suspect dysfunction, many are reluctant to palpate in more intimate areas. It is essential to protect the patient's dignity and modesty at all times; however, the clinician needs to examine all potential causes for the pain. A thorough explanation as to the reasons for an examination of these areas must be given to the patient. It is also a wise policy for the clinician to be accompanied by a member of staff who is of the same sex as the patient, if the examination may involve such procedures.

CASE STUDY BACK AND LEG PAIN

HISTORY

A 55-year-old man presented with complaints of an insidious onset of severe back and left leg pain. Progressively worsening symptoms of pain over the past few months were followed by left foot drop. A magnetic resonance imaging (MRI) examination was interpreted as mild lumbar spine degenerative disk disease without evidence of nerve root compromise. The patient could report no specific aggravating or relieving activities, but did report pain at night, not related to movement in bed. The patient's past medical history was significant for a renal transplantation approximately 20 years previously.

QUESTIONS

1. What aspects of the history should alert the clinician to the possibility of a serious pathology?
2. What is the significance of night pain that is unrelated to movement?
3. Does this presentation/history warrant further investigation? Why or why not?

EXAMINATION

The patient appeared to be a well-nourished and healthy-looking individual with no obvious postural deformities. Given the insidious nature of his back pain and the history suggesting a nerve root impairment, a lower quarter scanning examination was performed with the following results:

- Active lumbar range of motion, with passive overpressure and resistance, was full and pain free in all directions, although some trunk pain was elicited with end-range extension. No other positions or activities appeared to change the pain.

- Fatigable muscle weakness, graded at 4/5, was found in the L5 to S1 distribution.
- The Achilles tendon reflex on the left was diminished.

QUESTIONS

1. Did the scanning examination confirm your working hypothesis? How?
2. What is the significance of the fatigable weakness?
3. What is the significance of having pain that is not reproducible with activities or positions?

The distribution of the patient's symptoms appeared to fit that of a disk herniation at L5 to S1, but the clinician returned the patient to his physician for further testing because:

- The clinician was unable to reproduce the pain with movement.
- There was a history of night pain.
- There were no relieving or aggravating positions or activities.

The results of the physical therapy examination prompted the physician to order a second MRI examination of the lumbosacral spine, and an electromyographic study. The MRI uncovered an aneurysm extending posteromedially, and adjacent to the left lumbosacral nerve plexus. Arteriography verified the origin of the aneurysm from the left internal iliac artery. After prompt excision of the aneurysm, the patient reported significant reduction of back and limb pain in the immediate postoperative period.

EVALUATION

In addition to demonstrating how a visceral source of pain can mimic a musculoskeletal impairment, this case illustrates two other points.

1. The importance of a good history.
2. How, on occasions imaging studies can be used to determine the cause of "suspicious" clinical findings. The initial MRI showed no significant evidence for nerve root compromise in the lumbosacral spine, and yet the history indicated the possibility of nerve root irritation. However, it is not unusual for MRI results to give both false-positive or false-negative results while clinical findings are more reliable.

Although this patient's symptoms resembled a radiculopathy and strength testing did little to refute the hypothesis, there was nothing in the motion tests to confirm the diagnosis. Visceral lumbosacral radiculopathy, although uncommon, is reported to develop secondary to abdominal aortic aneurysms, retroperitoneal abscesses, neoplasms, and hemorrhages.[503,504]

CASE STUDY   RIGHT BUTTOCK PAIN

HISTORY

A 55-year-old woman presented for physical therapy with a physician diagnosis of "right lumbosacral radiculitis." The patient had a 10-month history of right buttock pain with radiation to the posterolateral right lower limb, which was associated with intermittent numbness and tingling of the distal lower limb and foot. She denied any low back pain or any radiation of pain down her left lower limb. The pain was exacerbated by walking uphill, by lying on her right side, and after exercise. It was not worse with bending or with Valsalva maneuver. Past medical history was significant for chronic low back pain, lymphoma (diagnosed at age 23 and treated successfully with local radiation to the neck and axillae), status postmeningioma resection, status post–bilateral modified radical mastectomy for carcinoma in situ, and hypothyroidism.[505] A magnetic resonance image (MRI) of the lumbosacral spine revealed multilevel degenerative disk disease from L3 and L4 through L5 to S1, with mild foraminal narrowing bilaterally. There was no evidence of focal herniation or canal stenosis.

QUESTIONS

1. What structure(s) could be the cause of these symptoms?
2. Does the history of the symptoms follow a pattern associated with a musculoskeletal disorder? If not, why not?
3. What in the patient's past medical history needs to be noted?
4. What tests or questions would you use to help rule out the potentially serious causes of these symptoms such as cauda equina compression?
5. What impairment could cause an increase in these symptoms when walking uphill and lying on the right side?
6. Why would the patient's symptoms increase after exercise?
7. What is your working hypothesis at this stage based on the various diagnoses that could manifest with leg pain and paresthesia, and what tests you would use to rule out each one?
8. Does this presentation/history warrant a scanning examination? Why or why not?

EXAMINATION

This type of history certainly warrants a scan. A lumbar scanning examination produced the following results:

- A negative straight leg raise test on the left; but a positive straight leg raise on the right side at approximately 45 degrees, which reproduced right buttock and posterior thigh pain.
- Motor and sensory examinations were otherwise intact in bilateral lower limbs.
- No spinal or paraspinal tenderness or spasm on palpation.
- Moderate spasm and tenderness of the right piriformis and gluteus medius muscles, and marked tenderness over the right sciatic notch.
- Active range of motion of the lumbar spine was full and pain-free in all directions.
- Active and passive range of motion of the patient's hips were somewhat decreased in internal and external rotation as well as abduction bilaterally.

QUESTIONS

1. Did the scanning examination confirm your working hypothesis? How?
2. What findings from the preceding list surprised you, given the history?
3. What do you do now?

The scan findings were inconclusive for a right lumbosacral radiculitis, so a further investigation was warranted. After a discussion with the patient's physician, however, a trial of physical therapy was ordered for symptomatic pain relief. The patient underwent a physical therapy program, which consisted of modalities to her right piriformis and gluteal muscles, stretching exercises, hip range-of-motion exercises, instruction in proper posture and body mechanics, and generalized conditioning exercises. Her symptoms improved somewhat initially, but then returned to the previous level, and the patient was returned to her physician.

QUESTIONS

1. What are some of the problems associated with proceeding to treat this patient?
2. How would you describe this condition to the patient?
3. Based on the findings thus far, and the rationale to provide pain relief, is there anything else you would add to the patient's intervention?
4. Given the lack of progress from the patient, how long would you wait before returning her to the physician?

EVALUATION

Because of persistent pain, an MRI of the pelvis was obtained. The MRI examination of the pelvis revealed a markedly enlarged uterus with a large pedunculated myoma that was impinging on the right sciatic foramen at the level of exit of the right sciatic nerve.

The impression at that time was right sciatic neuropathy secondary to uterine myoma. Because of her persistent complaints, the patient was referred for a subtotal abdominal hysterectomy, which was performed without complications. At follow-up, approximately 6 months postoperatively, the patient reported a very rare, mild right buttock pain without any lower limb radiation, which was a significant improvement compared with her preoperative pain.

A history of sciatica that is worse with certain positions, is not worse with Valsalva maneuver, and is not associated with low back pain, should prompt clinicians to consider a uterine fibroid as a potential cause, especially in women with a history of uterine fibroids. Likewise, failure to respond to an intervention for the more common causes of sciatica, such as herniated intervertebral disk, should initiate a return to the physician for further workup, which may include pelvic ultrasound, computed axial tomography, or MRI.

CASE STUDY INTERMITTENT LEG NUMBNESS

HISTORY

A 46-year-old man presented to the clinic with a 10-year history of sensations that he described as a mixture both of pins and needles and of cotton wool around the second and third toes of his feet. The symptoms developed suddenly while at work and had progressed to intermittent numbness of both legs from the waist down. Over the following 10 years, the patient suffered momentarily from electric-type sensations radiating down into his legs, more so on the right than the left. In addition, he noticed stiffness in his gait and reduced sensation on passing urine, and an aching sensation had developed in the buttocks. He had a history of infrequent low back pain over a number of years. The patient's physician had given him a workup for multiple sclerosis, but the results were negative.

QUESTIONS

1. What aspects of the history should alert the clinician to the possibility of a serious pathology?
2. What is the significance of the gait stiffness?
3. What is the significance of the reduced sensation on passing urine?
4. Does this presentation/history warrant a scanning examination? Why or why not?

EXAMINATION

Given the history and symptoms of this patient, a thoracic and lumbar scan was performed with the following positive findings:

- A broad-based gait pattern.
- Weakness of hip flexion on the right.
- Brisk knee and ankle jerks with clonus on the right.
- Positive Lhermitte's symptom.
- Sensory examination was normal, although it appeared that vibration sensation was absent in the left leg.
- Abdominal reflexes were absent.
- Nystagmus on lateral gaze was present.

QUESTIONS

1. Did the findings from scanning examination provide a working hypothesis?
2. List those findings from this patient that could indicate the presence of a serious pathology.
3. What is the significance of the Lhermitte's symptom?
4. What do you do now?

EVALUATION

All of the signs and symptoms of this patient indicate upper motor neuron impairment. He was referred back to his physician, where a magnetic resonance image (MRI) of the thoracic spine showed a thoracic disk prolapse at T9 to T10, with an osteo-phyte impinging the theca and just indenting the cord. A computed tomography myelogram showed a large calcified disk prolapse at T9 to T10, with calcification in the remaining disk space and considerable compression of the spinal cord from right to left.

REVIEW QUESTIONS*

1. List the five categories of referred pain as described by Macnab.
2. Give a broad definition of malingering.
3. True or false: Osteoid osteomas are malignant tumors.
4. Degenerative spondylolisthesis occurs most commonly at which spinal levels?
5. Which type of headache is associated with auras?

*Additional questions to test your understanding of this chapter can be found in the Online Learning Center for *Orthopaedic Assessment, Evaluation, and Intervention* at www.duttononline.net.

REFERENCES

1. Guide to physical therapist practice. *Phys Ther* 2001; 81:S13–S95.
2. Grieve GP. The masqueraders. In: Boyling JD, Palastanga N, eds. *Grieve's Modern Manual Therapy*. Edinburgh, Scotland: Churchill Livingstone; 1994:841–856.
3. Donelson R, et al. A prospective study of centralization in lumbar referred pain. *Spine* 1997;22:1115–1122.
4. Takahashi Y, et al., Regional correspondence between the ventral portion of the lumbar intervertebral disc and the groin mediated by a spinal reflex. A possible basis of discogenic referred pain. *Spine* 1998;23:1853–1858; discussion 1859.
5. Akeyson EW, Schramm LP. Processing of splanchnic and somatic input in thoracic spinal cord of the rat. *Am J Physiol* 1994;266:R257–R267.
6. Bryan RN, et al. Location and somatotopic organization of the cells of origin of the spinocervical tract. *Exp Brain Res* 1973;17:177–189.
7. Bonica JJ. Neurophysiological and pathological aspects of acute and chronic pain. *Arch Surg* 1977;112:750–761.
8. Dawson NJ, Schmid H, Pierau FK. Pre-spinal convergence between thoracic and visceral nerves of the rat. *Neurosci Lett* 1992;138:149–152.
9. Schmidt RF. *Fundamentals of Sensory Physiology* in Japanese. Tokyo, Japan: Kinpodo; 1980:120–125.
10. Jinkins JR, Whittemore AR, Bradley WG. The anatomic basis of vertebrogenic pain and the autonomic syndrome associated with lumbar disc extrusion. *Am J Roentgenol* 1989;152:1277–1289.
11. MacNab I. *Backache*. Baltimore, Md: Williams and Wilkins; 1978:98–100.
11a. Head H. *Studies in Neurology*. London, England: Oxford Medical Publications; 1920:653.
12. Cyriax J. *Textbook of Orthopaedic Medicine, Diagnosis of Soft Tissue Lesions*. 8th ed. London, England: Bailliere Tindall; 1982.
13. Barsky AJ, et al. The amplification of somatic symptoms. *Psychosom Med* 1988;50:510–519.
14. Waddell G, et al. Chronic low back pain, psychological distress and illness behavior. *Spine* 1984;9:209–213.
15. Werneke MW, Harris DE, Lichter RL. Clinical effectiveness of behavioral signs for screening low-back pain patients in a work oriented physical rehabilitation program. *Spine* 1993;18:2412.
16. Kenna O, Murtagh A. The physical examination of the back. *Aust Fam Physician* 1985;14:1244–1256.
17. LoPiccolo CJ, Goodkin K, Baldewicz TT. Current issues in the diagnosis and management of malingering. *Ann Med* 1999;31:166–174.
18. American Psychiatric Association. *Diagnostic and Statistical Manual of Mental Disorders*. 4th ed. Washington, DC: APA; 1994.
18a. Vernon H, Mior S. The neck disability index: A study of reliability and validity. *J Manipulative Physiol Ther* 1991;14:409–415.
19. Della Rocca C, Huvos AG. Osteoblastoma: Varied histological presentations with a benign clinical course. An analysis of 55 cases. *Am J Surg Pathol* 1996;20:841–850.
20. Azouz EM, et al. Osteoid osteoma and osteoblastoma of the spine in children: Report of 22 cases with brief literature review. *Pediatr Radiol* 1986;16:25–31.
21. Bjornsson J, et al. Chordoma of the mobile spine: A clinicopathologic analysis of 40 patients. *Cancer* 1993;71:735–740.
22. Dorfman HD, Czerniak B. Bone cancers. *Cancer* 1995;75:203–210.
23. Dahlin DC, Coventry MB. Osteogenic sarcoma: A study of six hundred cases. *J Bone Joint Surg* 1967;49A:101–110.
24. Boland PJ, Lane JM, Sundaresan N. Metastatic disease of the spine. *Clin Orthop* 1982;169:95–102.
25. Harrington KD. Metastatic disease of the spine. *J Bone Joint Surg* 1986;68A:1110–1115.
26. Bell GR. Surgical treatment of spinal tumors. *Clin Orthop Rel Res* 1997;335:54–63.
27. Rosier RN. Expanding the role of the orthopaedic surgeon in the treatment of osteoporosis. *Clin Orthop Rel Res* 2001;385:57–67.
28. Lane JM, Russell L, Khan SN. Osteoporosis. *Clin Orthop* 2000;372:139–150.
29. Praemer A, Furner S, Rice DP. Musculoskeletal conditions in the United States. In: Paremer A, Furner S, and Rice DP, eds. *Osteoporosis*. Rosemont, Ill: American Academy of Orthopaedic Surgeons; 1999:40–47.
30. Eisman JA. Genetics of osteoporosis. *Endocr Rev* 1999; 20:788–804.
31. Cummings SR, et al. Risk factors for hip fracture in white women. *N Engl J Med* 1995;332:767–773.
32. Scheiber LB, Torregrosa L. Early intervention for postmenopausal osteoporosis. *J Musculoskel Med* 1999; 16:146–157.
33. Lane JM, Riley EH, Wirganowicz PZ. Osteoporosis: Diagnosis and treatment. *J Bone Joint Surg* 1996;78A:618–632.
34. Bukata SV, Rosier RN. Diagnosis and treatment of osteoporosis. *Curr Opin Orthop* 2000;11:336–340.
35. Huijbregts PA. Osteoporosis: Diagnosis and conservative treatment. *J Man Manipulative Ther* 2001;9:143–153.
36. Block J, et al. Does exercise prevent osteoporosis? *JAMA* 1987;257:345.
37. Cummings SR, et al. Epidemiology of osteoporosis and osteoporotic fractures. *Epidemiol Rev* 1985;7:178–208.
38. NIH Consensus Development Panel on Osteoporosis Prevention and Therapy. Osteoporosis prevention, diagnosis, and therapy. *JAMA* 2001;94:785–795.

39. Snow-Harter C, Marcus R. Exercise, bone mineral density, and osteoporosis. *Exerc Sport Sci Rev* 1991;19:351–388.

40. Buchner DM, et al. Effects of physical activity on health status in older adults. II: Intervention studies. *Annu Rev Public Health* 1992;13:469–488.

41. Nelson ME, et al. Effects of high intensity strength training on multiple risk factors for osteoporotic fractures. A randomized controlled trial. *JAMA* 1994;272:1909–1914.

42. Jupiter JB, et al. Repair of five distal radius fractures with an investigational cancellous bone cement: A preliminary report. *J Orthop Trauma* 1997;11:110–116.

43. Bailey DA, Faulkner RA, McKay HA. Growth, physical activity, and bone mineral acquisition. In: Hollosky JO, ed. *Exercise and Sport Sciences Reviews*. Baltimore, Md: Williams and Wilkins; 1996:233–266.

44. Recker R, et al. Bone gain in young adult women. *JAMA* 1992;268:2403–2408.

45. Frame B, Parfitt M. Osteomalacia: Current concepts. *Ann Intern Med* 1978;89:966–982.

46. Strewler GJ. Mineral metabolism and metabolic bone disease. In: Greenspan FS, Stewler GJ, eds. *Basic and Clinical Endocrinology*. Stamford, Conn: Appleton and Lange; 1997:263–316.

47. Basha B, et al. Osteomalacia due to vitamin D depletion: A neglected consequence of intestinal malabsorption. *Am J Med* 2000;108:296–300.

48. Barash HL. Spondylolisthesis and tight hamstrings. *J Bone Joint Surg* 1970;52:1319.

49. Bradford DS, Hu SS. Spondylolysis and spondylolisthesis. In: Weinstein SL, ed. *The Pediatric Spine*. New York, NY: Raven; 1994.

50. Edelman B. Conservative treatment considered best course for spondylolisthesis. *Orthop Today* 1989;9:6–8.

51. Friberg S. Studies on spondylolisthesis. *Acta Chir Orthop* 1939;60:1.

52. Grobler LJ, et al. Etiology of spondylolisthesis: Assessment of the role played by lumbar facet joint morphology. *Spine* 1993;18:80–91.

53. Laus M, et al. Degenerative spondylolisthesis: Lumbar stenosis and instability. *Chir Organi Mov* 1992;77:39–49.

54. Love TW, Fagan AB, Fraser RD. Degenerative spondylolisthesis: Developmental or acquired? *J Bone Joint Surg* 1999; 81B:670–674.

55. Matsunaga S, et al. Natural history of degenerative spondylolisthesis: Pathogenesis and natural course of slippage. *Spine* 1990;15:1204–1210.

56. Meschan I. Spondylolisthesis: A commentary on etiology and on improved method of roentgenographic mensuration and detection of instability. *AJR Am J Roentgenol* 1945;55:230.

57. Newman PH. The etiology of spondylolisthesis. *J Bone Joint Surg* 1963;45B:39–59.

58. O'Sullivan P, Twomey L, Allison G. Evaluation of specific stabilizing exercise in the treatment of chronic low back pain with radiologic diagnosis of spondylolysis or spondylolisthesis. *Spine* 1997;22:2959–2967.

59. Postacchinia F, Perugia D. Degenerative lumbar spondylolisthesis. Part I: Etiology, pathogenesis, pathomorphology, and clinical features. *Ital J Orthop Traumatol* 1991;17:165–173.

60. Rosenberg NJ. Degenerative spondylolisthesis. *J Bone Joint Surg* 1975;57A:467–474.

61. Seitsalo S, et al. Progression of the spondylolisthesis in children and adolescents. *Spine* 1991;16:417–421.

62. Spring WE. Spondylolisthesis—a new clinical test. Proceedings of the Australian Orthopedics Association. *J Bone Joint Surg* 1973;55B:229.

63. Yang K, King A. Mechanism of facet load transmission as a hypothesis for low back pain. *Spine* 1984;9:557–565.

64. Borg-Stein J, Stein J. Trigger points and tender points: One and the same? Does injection treatment help? *Rheum Dis Clin North Am* 1996;22:305–322.

65. Freundlich B, Leventhal L. The fibromyalgia syndrome. In: Schumacher HR, Klippel JH, Koopman WJ, eds. *Primer on the Rheumatic Diseases*. Atlanta, Ga: Arthritis Foundation; 1993: 227–230.

66. Stockman R. The courses, pathology and treatment of chronic rheumatism. *Edinb Med J* 1904;15:107–116.

67. Grodin AJ, Cantu RI. Soft tissue mobilization. In: Basmajian JV, Nyberg R, eds. *Rational Manual Therapies*. Baltimore, Md: Williams and Wilkins; 1993:199–221.

68. Schneider MJ. Tender points/fibromyalgia vs. trigger points/myofascial pain syndrome: A need for clarity in terminology and differential diagnosis. *J Manipulative Physiol Ther* 1995; 18:398–406.

69. Campbell SM. Is the tender point concept valid? *Am J Med* 1986;81:33–37.

70. Campbell SM, et al. Clinical characteristics of fibrositis: I. A "Blinded" controlled study of symptoms and tender points. *Arthritis Rheum* 1983;26:817–824.

71. Cott A, et al. Interrater reliability of the tender point criterion for fibromyalgia. *J Rheumatol* 1992;19:1955–1959.

72. Croft P, Schollum J, Silman A. Population study of tender point counts and pain as evidence of fibromyalgia. *BMJ* 1994; 309:696–699.

73. Wolfe F, et al. The American College of Rheumatology 1990 criteria for the classification of fibromyalgia. *Arthritis Rheum* 1990; 33:160–172.

74. Simms RW. Muscle studies in fibromyalgia syndrome. *J Musculoskel Pain* 1994;2:117–123.

75. Farney RJ, Walker JM. Office management of common sleep/wake disorders. *Med Clin North Am* 1995;79:391–414.

76. Offenbacher M, Stucki G. Physical therapy in the treatment of fibromyalgia. *Scand J Rheumatol* 2000;29:78–85.

77. Aronoff GM. Myofascial pain syndrome and fibromyalgia: A critical assessment and alternate view. *Clin J Pain* 1998;14:74–85.

78. McClaflin RR. Myofascial pain syndrome: Primary care strategies for early intervention. *Postgrad Med* 1994;96:56–73.

79. Travell JG, Simons DG. *Myofascial Pain and Dysfunction—The Trigger Point Manual*. Baltimore, Md: Williams and Wilkins; 1983.

80. Fricton JR. Myofascial pain. *Baillieres Clin Rheumatol* 1994;8:857–880.

81. Vecchiet L, Giamberardino MA, Saggini R. Myofascial pain syndromes: Clinical and pathophysiological aspects. *Clin J Pain* 1991;7(suppl):16–22.

82. Chen SH, Wu YC, Hong CZ. Current management of myofascial pain syndrome. *Clin J Pain* 1996;6:27–46.

83. Esenyel M, Caglar N, Aldemir T. Treatment of myofascial pain. *Am J Phys Med Rehabil* 2000;79:48–52.

84. Fricton JR. Clinical care for myofascial pain. *Dent Clin North Am* 1991;35:1–29.

85. Goldman LB, Rosenberg NL. Myofascial pain syndrome and fibromyalgia. *Semin Neurol* 1991;11:274–280.

86. Krause H, Fischer AA. Diagnosis and treatment of myofascial pain. *Mt Sinai J Med* 1991;58:235–239.

87. Fricton JR. Management of masticatory myofascial pain. *Semin Orthodont* 1995;1:229–243.

87a. Smolders JJ. Myofascial pain and dysfunction syndromes. In: Hammer WI, ed. *Functional Soft Tissue Examination and Treatment by Manual Methods—The Extremities.* Gaithersburg, Md: Aspen; 1991:215–234.

88. Dreyer SJ, Boden SD. Nonoperative treatment of neck and arm pain. *Spine* 1998;23:2746–2754.

89. Keller K, Corbett J, Nichols D. Repetitive strain injury in computer keyboard users: Pathomechanics and treatment principles in individual and group intervention. *J Hand Ther* 1998;11:9–26.

90. Quinter J, Elvey R. Understanding "RSI": A review of the role of peripheral neural pain and hyperalgesia. *J Man Manipulative Ther* 1993;1:99–105.

91. Fricton JR., et al. Myofascial pain syndrome of the head and neck: A review of clinical characteristics of 164 patients. *Oral Surg Oral Med Oral Pathol* 1985;60:615–623.

92. Fricton JR. Behavioral and psychosocial factors in chronic craniofacial pain. *Anesth Progr* 1985;32:7–12.

93. Stratton SA, Bryan JM. Dysfunction, evaluation, and treatment of the cervical spine and thoracic inlet. In: Donatelli R, Wooden M, eds. *Orthopaedic Physical Therapy.* New York, NY: Churchill Livingstone; 1993:77–122.

94. Simons DG. Muscular pain syndromes. In: Fricton JR, Awad E, eds. *Advances in Pain Research and Therapy.* New York, NY: Raven; 1990:1–41.

95. Hardin J Jr. Pain and the cervical spine. *Bull Rheum Dis* 2001;50:1–4.

96. Nordhoff LS Jr. Cervical trauma following motor vehicle collisions. In: Murphy DR, ed. *Cervical Spine Syndromes.* New York, NY: McGraw-Hill; 2000:131–150.

97. Barton CW. Evaluation and treatment of headache patients in the emergency department: A survey. *Headache* 1994;34:91–94.

98. Thomas SH, Stone CK. Emergency department treatment of migraine, tension and mixed-type headache. *J Emerg Med* 1994;12:657–664.

99. Oates LN, Scholz MJ, Hoffert MJ. Polypharmacy in a headache centre population. *Headache* 1993;33:436–438.

100. Robinson RG. Pain relief for headaches: Is self-medication a problem? *Can Fam Physician* 1993;39:867–872.

101. Biondi DM. Headaches and their relationship to sleep. *Dent Clin North Am* 2001;45:685–700.

102. Esposito CJ, Crim GA, Binkley TA. Headaches: A differential diagnosis. *J Craniomand Pract* 1986;4:318–322.

103. Friedman MH, Nelson AJ Jr. Head and neck pain review: Traditional and new perspectives. *J Orthop Sports Phys Ther* 1996;24:268–278.

104. Appenzeller O. *Pathogenesis and Treatment of Headache.* New York, NY: Spectrum Publications; 1976.

105. International Headache Society Headache Classification and Diagnostic Criteria for Headache Disorders. Cranial neuralgias and facial pain. *Cephalalgia* 1988;8:19–22,71,72.

106. Nicholson GG, Gaston J. Cervical headache. *J Orthop Sports Phys Ther* 2001;31:184–193.

107. Cohen MJ, McArthur DL. Classification of migraine and tension headache from a survey of 10,000 headache diaries. *Headache* 1981;21:25–29.

108. Tinel J. La cephelee a l'effort, syndrome de distension des vienes intracraniences. *La Medicine* 1932;13:113–118.

109. McCrory P. Headaches and exercise. *Sports Med* 2000; 30:221–229.

110. Williams S, Nukada H. Sport and exercise headache. Part 2: Diagnosis and classification. *Br J Sports Med* 1994;28:96–100.

111. Fredriksen TA, Hovdal H, Sjaastad O. Cervicogenic headache: Clinical manifestation. *Cephalalgia* 1987;7:147–160.

112. Hunter CR, Mayfield FH. Role of the upper cervical roots in the production of pain in the head. *Am J Surg* 1949;48:743–751.

113. Wilson PR. Chronic neck pain and cervicogenic headache. *Clin J Pain* 1991;7:5–11.

114. Lewit K. Vertebral artery insufficiency and the cervical spine. *Br J Geriatr Pract* 1969;6:37–42.

115. Jull GA. Headaches associated with cervical spine: A clinical review. In: Boyling JD, Palastanga N, eds. *Grieve's Modern Manual Therapy.* Edinburgh, Scotland: Churchill Livingstone; 1994.

116. Kimmel DL. The cervical sympathetic rami and the vertebral plexus in the human foetus. *J Comp Neurol* 1959;112:141–161.

117. Abrahams VC, Richmond FJR, Rose PK. Absence of monosynaptic reflex in dorsal neck muscles of the cat. *Brain Res* 1975;92:130–131.

118. Kerr FWL, Olafsson RA. Trigeminal cervical volleys: Convergency on single units in the spinal gray at C1 and C2. *Arch Neurol* 1961;5:171–178.

119. Friedman MH, Weisberg J. *Temporomandibular Joint Disorders.* Chicago, Ill: Quintessence Publishing; 1985.

120. Campbell CD, et al. TMJ symptoms and referred pain patterns. *J Prosthet Dent* 1982;47:430–433.

121. Pestronk A, Pestronk S. Goggle migraine. *N Engl J Med* 1983;308:226–227.

122. Silbert PL, Mokri B, Schievink WI. Headache and neck pain in spontaneous internal carotid and vertebral artery dissections. *Neurology* 1995;45:1517–1522.

123. Appenzeller O. Post-traumatic headaches. In: Dalessio DJ, ed. *Wolff's Headache and Other Head Pain.* New York, NY: Oxford University Press; 1987:289–303.

124. Packard RC. Posttraumatic headache: Permanency and relationship to legal settlement. *Headache* 1992;32:496–500.

125. Yamaguchi M. Incidence of headache and severity of head injury. *Headache* 1992;32:427–431.

126. Silberstein SD. Tension-type headaches. *Headache* 1994;34:S2–S7.

127. Mathew NT, Subits E, Nigam M. Transformation of migraine into daily chronic headache. Analysis of factors. *Headache* 1982;22:66–68.

128. Sheftell FD. Chronic daily headache. *Neurol Clin* 1992;42:32–36.

129. Kudrow L. Paradoxical effects of frequent analgesic use. *Adv Neurol* 1982;33:335–341.

130. Warner JS, Fenichel GM. Chronic post-traumatic headache often a myth? *Neurology* 1996;46:915–916.

131. Mathew NT. Chronic refractory headache. *Neurology* 1993; 43:S26–S33.

132. Saper JR, Magee KR. *Freedom from Headaches.* New York, NY: Simon and Schuster; 1981.

133. Goodman CC, Boissonnault WG. *Pathology: Implications for the Physical Therapist.* Philadelphia, Pa: Saunders; 1998:791–797.

134. Sulfaro MA, Gobetti JP. Occipital neuralgia manifesting as orofacial pain. *Oral Surg Oral Med Oral Pathol Oral Radiol Endod* 1995;80:751–755.

135. Shankland W. Differential diagnosis of headaches. *J Craniomand Pract* 1986;4:47–51.

136. Cox C, Cocks R. Occipital neuralgia. *J Med Assoc Alabama* 1979;1:23–28.

137. Vital JM, et al. An anatomic and dynamic study of the greater occipital nerve (n. of Arnold): Applications to the treatment of Arnold's neuralgia. *Surg Radiol Anat* 1989;11:205–210.

138. Wolff HG. *Headache and Other Head Pain.* New York, NY: Oxford University Press; 1987:53–76.

139. Dandy WE. An operation for the cure of tic douloureux. Partial section of the sensory root at the pons. *Arch Surg* 1929;18:687.

140. Sjoqvist O. Surgical section of pain tracts and pathways in the spinal cord and brain stem. In: *4th Congress de Neurologique Internationale.* Paris, France: Masson; 1949.

140a. Devor M, Amir R, Rappaport ZH: Pathophysiology of trigeminal neuralgia: the ignition hypothesis. *Clin J Pain* 2002;18:4–13.

141. Hadar T, et al. Specific IgG and IgA antibodies to herpes simplex virus and varicella zoster virus in acute peripheral facial palsy patients. *J Med Virol* 1983;12:237–245.

142. Morgan M, Nathwani D. Facial palsy and infection: The unfolding story. *Clin Infec Dis* 1992;14:263–271.

143. Murakami S, et al. Bell's palsy and herpes simplex virus: Identification of viral DNA in endoneurial fluid and muscle. *Ann Intern Med* 1996;124:27–30.

144. Burgess RC, et al. Polymerase chain reaction amplification of herpes simplex viral DNA from the geniculate ganglion of a patient with Bell's palsy. *Ann Otol Rhinol Laryngol* 1994;103:775–779.

145. Nasatzky E, Katz J. Bell's palsy associated with herpes simplex gingivostomatitis. A case report. *Oral Surg Oral Med Oral Pathol Oral Radiol Endod* 1998;86:293–296.

146. Maccabee PJ, et al. Intracranial stimulation of facial nerve in humans with magnetic coil. *Electroencephalogr Clin Neurophysiol* 1988;70:350–354.

146a. Peitersen E. The natural history of Bell's palsy. *Am J Otol* 1982;4:107–111.

147. Gantz BJ, et al. Surgical management of Bell's palsy. *Laryngoscope* 1999;109:1177–1188.

148. Peitersen E. The natural history of Bell's palsy. *Am J Otol* 1982;4:107–111.

149. Sweeney CJ, Gilden DH. Ramsay Hunt syndrome. *J Neurol Neurosurg Psychiatry* 2001;71:149–154.

150. Lindsay KW, Bone I, Callander R. *Neurology and Neurosurgery Illustrated.* New York, NY: Churchill Livingstone; 1991.

151. Attia J, et al. Does this adult patient have acute meningitis? *JAMA* 1999;282:175–181.

152. Sprengell C. *The Aphorisms of Hippocrates, and the Sentences of Celsus.* 2nd ed. London, England: R Wilkin; 1735.

153. Tunkel AR, Scheld WM. Pathogenesis and pathophysiology of bacterial meningitis. *Clin Microbiol Rev* 1993;6:118–136.

154. Scheld WM. Meningococcal diseases. In: Warren KS, Mahmoud AAF, eds. *Tropical and Geographical Medicine.* New York, NY: McGraw-Hill; 1990:798–814.

155. Durand ML, et al. Acute bacterial meningitis in adults: A review of 493 episodes. *N Engl J Med* 1993;328:21–28.

156. Brody IA, Wilkins RH. The signs of Kernig and Brudzinski. *Arch Neurol* 1969;21:215–218.

157. O'Connell JEA. The clinical signs of meningeal irritation. *Brain* 1946;69:9–21.

158. Harvey AM, et al. *The Principles and Practice of Medicine.* Norwalk, Conn: Appleton and Lange; 1988.

159. Pozzati E, et al. Subacute and chronic extradural hematomas: A study of 30 cases. *J Trauma* 1980;20:795–799.

160. Summary for patients. Rashes and symptoms in early Lyme disease. *Ann Intern Med* 2002;136:124.

161. Steere AC. Lyme disease. *N Engl J Med* 2001;345:115–125.

162. Gilstrap LC III, Cunningham FG, Whalley PJ. Acute pyelonephritis in pregnancy: An anterospective study. *Obstet Gynecol* 1981;57:409–413.

163. Pinhas-Hamiel O, Sarova-Pinhas I, Achiron A. Multiple sclerosis in childhood and adolescence: Clinical features and management. *Paediatr Drugs* 2001;3:329–336.

164. Krupp LB, Rizvi SA. Symptomatic therapy for underrecognized manifestations of multiple sclerosis. *Neurology* 2002;58:S32–S39.

165. Myers JE, Baker PN. Hypertensive diseases and eclampsia. *Curr Opin Obstet Gynecol* 2002;14:119–125.

166. Thomas SV. Neurological aspects of eclampsia. *J Neurol Sci* 1998;155:37–43.

167. Carson D, Serpell M. Choosing the best needle for diagnostic lumbar puncture. *Neurology* 1996;47:33–37.

168. Raymond JR, Raymond PA. Post lumbar puncture headache: Etiology and management. *West J Med* 1988;148:551–554.

169. DeStefano F, et al. Dental disease and risk of coronary heart disease and mortality. *BMJ* 1993;306:688–691.

170. Andres JC, Nagalla R. Acute bacterial thyroiditis secondary to urosepsis. *J Am Board Fam Pract* 1995;8:128–129.

171. Filipchuk, D. Classic trigeminal neuralgia: a surgical perspective. *J. Neurosci Nur* 2003;35(2):82–86.

172. Dolan KD, Jacoby C, Smoker WR. The radiology of facial fractures. *Radiographics* 1984;4:575–663.

173. Yanguela J, et al. Trochleitis and migraine headache. *Neurology* 2002;58:802–805.

174. Surks MI, Ocampo E. Subclinical thyroid disease. *Am J Med* 1996;100:217–223.

175. Thompson JW, Cohen SR, Reddix P. Retropharyngeal abscess in children: A retrospective and historical analysis. *Laryngoscope* 1988;98:589–592.

176. Lee SS, Schwartz RH, Bahadori RS. Retropharyngeal abscess: Epiglottitis of the new millennium. *J Pediatr* 2001;138:435–437.

177. Asmar BL. Bacteriology of retropharyngeal abscess in children. *Pediatr Infect Dis J* 1990;9:595–596.

178. Segal DH, Lidov MW, Camins MB. Cervical epidural hematoma after chiropractic manipulation in a healthy young woman: case report. *Neurosurgery* 1996;39:1043–1045.

179. Pan G, et al. Traumatic epidural hematoma of the cervical spine: Diagnosis with magnetic resonance imaging. *J Neurosurg* 1988;68:798–801.

180. Tseng SH, et al. Cervical epidural hematoma after spinal manipulation therapy: Case report. *J Trauma Inj Infect Crit Care* 2002;52:585–586.

181. Powell F, Hanigan W, Olivero W. A risk/benefit analysis of spinal manipulation therapy for relief of lumbar or cervical pain. *Neurosurgery* 1993;33:73–79.

182. Kiwak KJ. Establishing an etiology for torticollis. *Postgrad Med* 1984;75:126–134.

183. Kiesewetter WB, et al. Neonatal torticollis. *JAMA* 1955;157:1281–1285.

184. Gorlin RJ, Cohen MM, Levin LS. *Syndromes of the Head and Neck.* 3rd ed. New York, NY: Oxford University Press; 1990.

185. Klippel M, Feil A. Anomalie de la colonne vertebrale par absence des vertebres cervicale. *Bull Mem Soc Anat* 1912;87:185–188.

186. Klippel M, Feil A. Un cas d'absence des vertebres cervicales avec cage thoracique remontant jusqu'a la base du crane. *Nouv Iconogr Salpetriere* 1912;25:223–224.

187. Chaumien JP, et al. Le soi-disant syndrome de Klippel-Feil et ses incidences orthopediques. *Rev Chir Orthop* 1990;76:30–38.

188. Gonzalez-Reimers E, et al. Klippel-Feil syndrome in the prehispanic population of El Hierro (Canary Islands). *Ann Rheum Dis* 2001;60:174.

189. Smith DL, DeMario MC. Spasmodic torticollis: A case report and review of therapies. *J Am Board Fam Pract* 1996;9:435–441.

190. Wilson BC, Jarvis BL, Haydon RC. Nontraumatic subluxation of the atlantoaxial joint: Grisel's syndrome. *Larynoscope* 1987;96:705–708.

191. Britton TC. Torticollis—what is straight ahead? *Lancet* 1998;351:1223–1224.

192. Colbassani HJ Jr, Wood JH. Management of spastic torticollis. *Surg Neurol* 1986;25:153–158.

193. Adams RD, Victor M. *Principles of Neurology*. 5th ed. New York, NY: McGraw-Hill; 1993.

194. Lowenstein DH, Aminoff MJ. The clinical course of spasmodic torticollis. *Neurology* 1988;38:530–532.

195. Ackerman J, Chau V, Gilbert-Barness E. Pathological case of the month. Congenital muscular torticollis. *Arch Pediatr Adol Med* 1996;150:1101–1102.

196. Rondot P, Marchand MP, Dellatolas G. Spasmodic torticollis—review of 220 patients. *Can J Neurol Sci* 1991;18:143–151.

197. Jahanshahi M, Marion MH, Marsden CD. Natural history of adult-onset idiopathic torticollis. *Arch Neurol* 1990;47:548–552.

198. Spencer J, et al. Behavior therapy for spasmodic torticollis: A case study suggesting a causal role for anxiety. *J Behav Ther Exp Psychiatry* 1991;22:305–311.

199. Agras S, Marshall C. The application of negative practice to spasmodic torticollis. *Am J Psychiatry* 1965;121:579–582.

200. Leplow B. Heterogeneity of biofeedback training effects in spasmodic torticollis. A single-case approach. *Behav Res Ther* 1990;28:359–365.

201. Halla JT, Hardin JG. The spectrum of atlantoaxial (C1-2) facet joint involvement in rheumatoid arthritis. *Arthr Rheum* 1990;22:325–329.

202. Murray G, Persellin R. Cervical fracture complicating ankylosing spondylitis. *Am J Med* 1981;70:1033–1041.

203. Roubenoff R. Gout and hyperuricaemia. *Rheum Dis Clin North Am* 1990;16:539–550.

204. Lawrence RC, et al. Estimates of the prevalence of selected arthritic and musculoskeletal diseases in the United States. *J Rheumatol* 1989;16:427–441.

205. Isomaki H, von Essen R, Ruutsalo HM. Gout, particularly diuretic-induced, is on the increase in Finland. *Scand J Rheumatol* 1977;6:213–216.

206. Patte D, et al. Over-extension lesions. *Rev Chir Orthop* 1988;74:314–318.

207. Bohlman HH. Degenerative arthritis of the lower cervical spine. In: McEvarts C, ed. *Surgery of the Musculoskeletal System*. New York, NY: Churchill Livingstone; 1990:1857–1886.

208. Emery SE, Bohlman HH. Osteoarthritis of the cervical spine. In: Moskowitz RW, et al, eds. *Osteoarthritis. Diagnosis and Medical/Surgical Management*. Philadelphia, Pa: Saunders; 1992:651–668.

209. Goodman CC, Snyder TEK. *Differential Diagnosis in Physical Therapy*. Philadelphia, Pa: Saunders; 1990.

210. Marshall BJ, et al. Attempt to fulfill Koch's postulates for pyloric campylobacter. *Med J Aust* 1985;142:436–439.

211. Hassall E. Peptic ulcer disease and current approaches to *Helicobacter pylori*. *J Pediatr* 2001;138:462–468.

212. Farrar JA. Emergency! Acute cholecystitis. *Am J Nurs* 2001;101:35–36.

213. Sim FH. Metastatic bone disease and myeloma. In: Evarts CM, ed. *Surgery of the Musculoskeletal System*. Philadelphia, Pa: Churchill Livingstone; 1983:320–393.

214. Chade HO. Metastatic tumours of the spine. In: Vinken PJ, Bruyn GW, eds. *Spinal Tumors*. Amsterdam, Holland: North Holland Publishers; 1976:415–433.

215. Light RW. Pneumothorax. In: Light RW, ed. *Pleural Diseases*. Baltimore, Md: Williams and Wilkins; 1995:242–277.

216. Peek GJ, Morcos S, Cooper G. The pleural cavity. *BMJ* 2000;320:1318–1321.

217. Jay SJ. Pleural effusions, 1: Preliminary evaluation-recognition of the transudate. *Postgrad Med* 1986;80:164–167.

218. Bland JH. Diagnosis of thoracic pain syndromes. In: Giles LGF, Singer KP, eds. *Clinical Anatomy and Management of the Thoracic Spine*. Oxford, England: Butterworth-Heinemann; 2000:145–156.

219. Acre CA, Dohrmann GJ. Thoracic disc herniation: Improved diagnosis with computed tomographic scanning and a review of the literature. *Surg Neurol* 1985;23:356–361.

220. Deyo RA, Rainville J, Kent DL. What can the history and physical examination tell us about low back pain? *JAMA* 1992;268:760–765.

220a. Meinck HM: Stiff man syndrome. *CNS Drugs* 2001;15:515–26.

220b. Bastin A, Gurmin V, Mediwake R, Gibbs J, Beynon H: Stiff man syndrome presenting with low back pain. *Ann Rheum Dis [Letter]* 2002;61:939–940.

220c. Henningsen P, Meinck HM: Specific phobia is a frequent nonmotor feature in stiff man syndrome. *J Neurol, Neurosurg & Psych* 2003;74:462–465.

221. Reid ME. Bone trauma and disease of the thoracic spine and ribs. In: Flynn TW, ed. *The Thoracic Spine and Rib Cage*. Boston, Mass: Butterworth-Heinemann; 1996:87–105.

222. Singer KP, et al. The influence of zypophysial joint orientation on spinal injuries at the thoracolumbar junction. *Surg Radiol Anat* 1989;11:233–239.

223. O'Brien MF, Lenke LG. Fractures and dislocations of the spine. In: Dee R, et al, ed. *Principles of Orthopaedic Practice*. New York, NY: McGraw-Hill; 1997:1237–1293.

224. Ziegler DW, Agarwal NN. The morbidity and mortality of rib fractures. *J Trauma* 1994;37:975–979.

225. Trunkey D. Cervicothoracic trauma. In: Blaisdell F, Trunkey D, eds. *Trauma Management*. Vol. 3. New York, NY: Thieme; 1986.

226. Gregory PL, Biswas AC, Batt ME. Musculoskeletal problems of the chest wall in athletes. *Sports Med* 2002;32:235–250.

227. Gupta A, Jamshidi M, Robin JR. Traumatic first rib fractures: Is angiography necessary? A review of 73 cases. *Cardiovasc Surg* 1997;5:48–53.

228. Jenkins SA. Spontaneous fractures of both first ribs. *J Bone Joint Surg* 1952;34B:9–13.

229. Lankenner PAJ, Micheli LJ. Stress fractures of the first rib: A case report. *J Bone Joint Surg* 1985;67A:159–160.

230. Mintz AC, et al. Stress fracture of the first rib from serratus anterior tension: An unusual mechanism of injury. *Ann Emerg Med* 1990;19:411–414.

231. Sylvest E. *Epidemic Myalgia: Bornholm Disease.* London, England: Oxford University Press; 1934.

232. Ikeda RM, et al. Pleurodynia among football players at a high school. *JAMA* 1993;270:2205–2206.

233. Fam AG, Smythe HA. Musculoskeletal chest wall pain. *Can Med Assoc J* 1985;133:379–389.

234. Disla E, et al. Costochondritis: A prospective analysis in an emergency department setting. *Arch Int Med* 1994;154:2466–2469.

235. Singer KP, Malmivaara A. Pathoanatomical characteristics of the thoracolumbar junctional region. In: Giles LGF, Singer KP, eds. *Clinical Anatomy and Management of the Thoracic Spine.* Oxford, England: Butterworth-Heinemann; 2000:100–113.

236. Lawrence DJ, Bakkum B. Chiropractic management of thoracic spine pain of mechanical origin. In: Giles LGF, Singer KP, eds. *Clinical Anatomy and Management of Thoracic Pain.* Oxford, England: Butterworth-Heinemann; 2000:244–256.

237. Markolf KL. Deformation of the thoracolumbar intervertebral joints in response to external loads. *J Bone Joint Surg* 1972;54A:511–533.

238. Heywood AWB, Meyers OL. Rheumatoid arthritis of the thoracic and lumbar spine. *J Bone Joint Surg* 1986;68B:362–368.

239. Gladman DD, et al. Differences in the expression of spondyloarthropathy: A comparison between ankylosing spondylitis and psoriatic arthritis: genetic and gender effects. *Clin Invest Med* 1993;16:1–7.

240. Haslock I. Ankylosing spondylitis. *Baillieres Clin Rheumatol* 1993;7:99.

241. Gran JT. An epidemiologic survey of the signs and symptoms of ankylosing spondylitis. *Clin Rheumatol* 1985;4:161–169.

242. Calin A, et al. Clinical history as a screening test for ankylosing spondylitis. *JAMA* 1977;237:2613–2614.

243. Cohen MD, Ginsurg WW. Late onset peripheral joint disease in ankylosing spondylitis. *Ann Rheum Dis* 1982;42:574–578.

244. Carrett S, et al. The natural disease course of ankylosing spondylitis. *Arthritis Rheum* 1993;26:186–190.

245. Gladman DD. Clinical aspects of the spondyloarthropathies. *Am J Med Sci* 1998;316:234–238.

246. Turek SL. *Orthopaedics—Principles and Their Application.* 4th ed. Vol. 2. Philadelphia, Pa: JB Lippincott; 1984.

247. Kraag G, et al. The effects of comprehensive home physiotherapy and supervision on patients with ankylosing spondylitis: An 8-month follow-up. *J Rheumatol* 1994;21:261–263.

248. Weinfeld RM, et al. The prevalence of diffuse idiopathic skeletal hyperostosis (DISH) in two large metropolitan hospital populations. *Skel Radiol* 1997;26:222–225.

249. Cameron HU. Traumatic disruption of the manubriosternal joint in the absence of rib fractures. *J Trauma* 1980;20:892.

250. Thirupathi R, Husted C. Traumatic disruption of the manubriosternal joint. *Bull Hosp Jt Dis* 1982;42:242–247.

251. Anderson KA, McAninch JW. Renal abscesses: Classification and review of 40 cases. *Urology* 1980;16:333.

252. Siegel JF, Smith A, Moldwin R. Minimally invasive treatment of renal abscess. *J Urol* 1996;155:52–55.

253. Goucke CR, Graziotti P. Extradural abscess following local anaesthetic and steroid injection for chronic back pain. *Br J Anaesth* 1990;65:427–429.

254. Mackenzie AR, et al. Spinal epidural abscess: The importance of early diagnosis and treatment. *J Neurol Neurosurg Psychiatry* 1998;65:209–212.

255. Baker AS, et al. Spinal epidural abscess. *N Engl J Med* 1975;293:463–468.

256. Obrador GT, Levenson DJ. Spinal epidural abscess in hemodialysis patients: Report of three cases and review of the literature. *Am J Kidney Dis* 1996;27:75–83.

257. Nauer KA. Acute dissection of the aorta: A review for nurses. *Crit Care Nurs Q* 2000;23:20–27.

258. Gruendemann BJ, Fernsebner B. *Comprehensive Perioperative Nursing.* Vol. 2. Boston, Mass: Jones and Bartlett; 1995.

259. Sharma KR, et al. Incidence of acute femoral neuropathy following renal transplantation. *Arch Neurol* 2002;59:541–545.

260. McCrory P: The "piriformis syndrome"—myth or reality? *Brit J Sports Med* 2001;35:209–210.

261. Beauchesne RP, Schutzer SF. Myositis ossificans of the piriformis muscle: An unusual cause of piriformis syndrome. A case report. *J Bone Joint Surg* 1997;79A:906–910.

262. Jankiewicz JJ, Hennrikus WL, Houkom JA. The appearance of the piriformis muscle syndrome in computed tomography and magnetic resonance imaging. A case report and review of the literature. *Clin Orthop* 1991;262:205–209.

263. Palliyath S, Buday J. Sciatic nerve compression: Diagnostic value of electromyography and computerized tomography. *Electromyogr Clin Neurophysiol* 1989;29:9–11.

264. Papadopoulos SM, McGillicuddy JE, Albers JW. Unusual cause of piriformis muscle syndrome. *Arch Neurol* 1990;47:1144–1146.

265. Tesio L, Bassi L, Galardi G. Transient palsy of hip abductors after a fall on the buttocks. *Arch Orthop Trauma Surg* 1990;109:164–165.

265a. Pace JB, Nagle D: Piriformis syndrome. *West J Med* 1976;124:435–439.

266. Pecina M. Contribution to the etiological explanation of the piriformis syndrome. *Acta Anat Nippon* 1979;105:181–187.

267. Boyd KT, Pierce NS, Batt ME. Common hip injuries in sport. *Sports Med* 1997;24:273–288.

268. Durrani Z, Winnie AP. Piriformis muscle syndrome: An underdiagnosed cause of sciatica. *J Pain Symptom Manage* 1991;6:374–379.

269. Solheim LF, Siewers P, Paus B. The piriformis syndrome. Sciatic nerve entrapment treated with section of the piriformis muscle. *Acta Orthop Scand* 1981;52:73–75.

270. Steiner C, et al. Piriformis syndrome: Pathogenesis, diagnosis, and treatment. *J Am Osteopath Assoc* 1987;87:318–323.

271. Julsrud ME. Piriformis syndrome. *J Am Podiatr Med Assoc* 1989;79:128–131.

272. Pfeifer T, Fitz WFK. Das Piriformis-Syndrom. *Zeitschr Orthop* 1989;127:691–694.

272a. Robinson DR. Pyriformis syndrome in relation to sciatic pain. *Am J Surg* 1947;73:355–358.

273. Beaton LE, Anson BJ. The sciatic nerve and the piriformis muscle: Their interrelation a possible cause of coccygodynia. *J Bone Joint Surg* 1938;20:686–688.

274. Hughes SS, et al. Extrapelvic compression of the sciatic nerve. An unusual cause of pain about the hip: Report of five cases. *J Bone Joint Surg* 1992;74A:1553–1559.

275. Benson ER, Schutzer SF. Posttraumatic piriformis syndrome: Diagnosis and results of operative treatment. *J Bone Joint Surg* 1999;81A:941–949.

276. Freiberg AH. Sciatic pain and its relief by operations on muscle and fascia. *Arch Surg* 1937;34:337–350.

277. Robinson DR. Pyriformis syndrome in relation to sciatic pain. *Am J Surg* 1947;73:355–358.

277a. Pace JB, Nagle D. Piriformis syndrome. *West J Med* 1976;124:435–439.

278. McCrory P. The "piriformis syndrome"—myth or reality? *Br J Sports Med* 2001;35:209–210.

279. Thakkar DH, Porter RW. Heterotopic ossification enveloping the sciatic nerve following posterior fracture-dislocation of the hip: A case report. *Injury* 1981;13:207–209.

280. Banerjee T, Hall CD. Sciatic entrapment neuropathy. *Neurosurgery* 1976;45:216–217.

281. Jones BV, Ward MW. Myositis ossificans in the biceps femoris muscles causing sciatic nerve palsy: A case report. *J Bone Joint Surg* 1980;62B:506–507.

282. Richardson RR, Hahn YS, Siqueira EB. Intraneural hematoma of the sciatic nerve: Case report. *J Neurosurg* 1978;49:298–300.

283. Zimmerman JE, et al. Posterior compartment syndrome of the thigh with a sciatic palsy. *J Neurosurg* 1977;46:369–372.

284. Johanson NA, et al. Nerve injury in total hip arthroplasty. *Clin Orthop* 1983;179:214–222.

285. Day MH. The blood supply of the lumbar and sacral plexuses in the human foetus. *J Anat* 1964;98:104–116.

286. Wohlgemuth WA, Rottach KG, Stoehr M. Radiogene Amyotrophie: Cauda equina Läsion als Strahlenspätfolge. *Nervenarzt* 1998;69:1061–1065.

287. Wohlgemuth WA, Rottach KG, Stoehr M. Intermittent claudication due to ischaemia of the lumbosacral plexus. *J Neurol Neurosurg Psychiatry* 1999;67:793–795.

288. Roberts JT. The effect of occlusive arterial diseases of the extremities on the blood supply of nerves. Experimental and clinical studies on the role of the vasa nervorum. *Am Heart J* 1948;35:369–392.

289. Hager W. Neuralgia femoris. Resection des Nerv. cutan. femoris anterior externus. *Heilung Dtsch Med Wochenschr* 1885;11:218.

290. Bernhardt M. Ueber eine wenig bekannte Form der Beschäftigungsneuralgie. *Neurolog Centralbl* 1896;15:13–17.

291. Roth VK. Meralgia paraesthetica. *Med Obozr Mosk* 1895;43:678.

292. Ivins GK. Meralgia paresthetica, the elusive diagnosis: Clinical experience with 14 adult patients. *Ann Surg* 2000;232:281–286.

293. Lambert SD. Athletic injuries to the hip. In: Ecternach J, ed. *Physical Therapy of the Hip*. New York, NY: Churchill Livingstone; 1990:143–164.

294. Reichert FL. Meralgia paresthetica; a form of causalgia relieved by interruption of the sympathetic fibers. *Surg Clin North Am* 1933;13:1443.

295. Sunderland S. *Nerves and Nerve Injuries*. Edinburgh, Scotland: E and S Livingstone; 1968.

296. Dellon AL, Mackinnon SE, Seiler WA IV. Susceptibility of the diabetic nerve to chronic compression. *Ann Plast Surg* 1988;20:117.

297. Asbury AK. Focal and multifocal neuropathies of diabetes. In: Dyck PJ, et al, eds. *Diabetic Neuropathy*. Philadelphia, Pa: Saunders; 1987:45–55.

298. Lee FC. An osteoplastic neurolysis operation for the cure of meralgia paresthetica. *Ann Surg* 1941;113:85.

299. Macnicol MF, Thompson WJ. Idiopathic meralgia paresthetica. *Clin Orthop* 1990;254:270.

300. Yamamoto T, Nagira K, Kurosaka M. Meralgia paresthetica occurring 40 years after iliac bone graft harvesting: Case report. *Neurosurgery* 2001;49:1455–1457.

301. Nathan H. Gangliform enlargement on the lateral cutaneous nerve of the thigh. *J Neurosurg* 1960;17:843.

302. Stookey B. Meralgia paresthetica: Etiology and surgical treatment. *JAMA* 1928;90:1705.

303. Lorei MP, Hershman EB. Peripheral nerve injuries in athletes: Treatment and prevention. *Sports Med* 1993;16:130–147.

304. Edelson R, Stevens P. Meralgia paresthetica in children. *J Bone Joint Surg* 1994;76A:993–999.

305. Ashby EC. Chronic obscure groin pain is commonly caused by enthesopathy: "Tennis elbow" of the groin. *Br J Surg* 1994;81:1632–1634.

306. Martens MA, Hansen L, Mulier JC. Adductor tendinitis and musculus rectus abdominis tendonopathy. *Am J Sports Med* 1987;15:353–356.

307. Zimmerman G. Groin pain in athletes. *Aust Fam Physician* 1988;17:1046–1052.

308. Bounameaux H, Reber-Wasem MA. Superficial thrombophlebitis and deep vein thrombosis: A controversial association. *Arch Intern Med* 1997;157:1822–1824.

309. Markovic MD, et al. Acute superficial thrombophlebitis: Modern diagnosis and therapy. *Srp Arch Celok Lek* 1997;125:261–266.

310. Wiener SL. Unilateral and bilateral upper and lower leg pain references. In: Wiener SL, ed. *Differential Diagnosis of Acute Pain by Body Region*. New York, NY: McGraw-Hill; 1993:559–570.

311. Orava S, Kujala UM. Rupture of the ischial origin of the hamstring muscles. *Am J Sports Med* 1995;23:702–705.

312. Owen CA. Gluteal compartment syndromes. *Clin Orthop* 1978;132:57.

313. Schmalzried TP, Neal WC, Eckardt JJ. Gluteal compartment and crush syndromes. *Clin Orthop* 1992;277:161.

314. Clark JL, Tatum NO, Noble SL. Management of genital herpes. *Am Fam Physician* 1995;51:175–182, 187–188.

315. Tariq A, Ross JD. Viral sexually transmitted infections: Current management strategies. *J Clin Pharm Ther* 1999;24:409–414.

316. Swanson JM. The biopsychosocial burden of genital herpes: Evidence-based and other approaches to care. *Dermatol Nurs* 1999;11:257–268; quiz 269–270.

317. D'Ambrosia R. *Musculoskeletal Disorders: Regional Examination and Differential Diagnosis*. 2nd ed. Philadelphia, Pa: JB Lippincott; 1986.

318. Wiener SL. *Differential Diagnosis of Acute Pain by Body Region*. New York, NY: McGraw-Hill; 1993:1–4.

319. Fealy S, Paletta GA. Femoral nerve palsy secondary to traumatic iliacus muscle hematoma: Course after nonoperative management. *J Trauma* 1999;47:1150–1152.

320. Greenwood MJ, Erhard R, Jones DL. Differential diagnosis of the hip vs. lumbar spine: Five case reports. *J Orthop Sports Phys Ther* 1998;27:308–315.

321. Hillier SL, et al. Role of bacterial vaginosis-associated microorganisms in endometritis. *Am J Obstet Gynecol* 1996;175:435–441.

322. Rice VM. Conventional medical therapies for endometriosis. *Ann N Y Acad Sci* 2002;955:343–352; discussion 389–393,396–406.

323. Murphy AA. Clinical aspects of endometriosis. *Ann NY Acad Sci* 2002;955:1–10; discussion 34–36, 396–406.

324. Swiersz LM. Role of endometriosis in cancer and tumor development. *Ann NY Acad Sci* 2002;955:281–292; discussion 293–295, 396–406.

325. Parsons CL, Zupkas P, Parsons JK. Intravesical potassium sensitivity in patients with interstitial cystitis and urethral syndrome. *Urology* 2001;57:428–433.

326. Fagerson TL. Hip. In: Wadsworth C, ed. *Current Concepts of Orthopedic Physical Therapy—Home Study Course*. La Crosse, Wis: Orthopaedic Section, American Physical Therapy Association; 2001.

327. Barnes R. Subcapital fractures of the femur. *J Bone Joint Surg* 1976;58B:2.

328. Connolly WB, Hedburg EA. Observations on fractures of the pelvis. *J Trauma* 1969;9:104.

329. Arnett FC. Reactive arthritis (Reiter's syndrome) and enteropathic arthritis. In: Klippel JH, ed. *Primer on the Rheumatic Diseases*. Atlanta, Ga: Arthritis Foundation; 1997:184–188.

330. McClusky OE, Lordon RE, Arnett FC Jr. HL-A 27 in Reiter's syndrome and psoriatic arthritis: A genetic factor in disease susceptibility and expression. *J Rheumatol* 1974;1:263–268.

331. Do TT. Transient synovitis as a cause of painful limps in children. *Curr Opin Pediatr* 2000;12:48–51.

332. Spiera H. Osteoarthritis as a misdiagnosis in elderly patients. *Geriatrics* 1987;42:37–42.

333. Schon L, Zuckerman JD. Hip pain the elderly: Evaluation and diagnosis. *Geriatrics* 1988;43:48–62.

334. Puppione AA, Schumann L. Management strategies for older adults with osteoarthritis: How to promote and maintain function. *J Am Acad Nurse Pract* 1999;11:167–171.

335. Kenzora JE. Symposium on idiopathic osteonecrosis: Foreword. *Orthop Clin North Am* 1985;16:593–594.

336. Kenzora JE, et al. Experimental osteonecrosis of the femoral head in adult rabbits. *Clin Orthop* 1978;130:8–46.

337. Guerra JJ, Steinberg ME. Distinguishing transient osteoporosis from avascular necrosis of the hip. *J Bone Joint Surg* 1995;77:616–624.

338. Pauli S, et al. Osteomyelitis pubis versus osteitis pubis: A case presentation and review of the literature. *Br J Sports Med* 2002;36:71–73.

339. Karkos CD, et al. Thigh compartment syndrome as a result of a false aneurysm of the profunda femoris artery complicating fixation of an intertrochanteric fracture. *J Trauma Inj Infect Crit Care* 1999;47:393–395.

340. Sawmiller CJ, et al. Extraarticular pigmented villonodular synovitis of the shoulder: A case report. *Clin Orthop Rel Res* 1997;335:262–267.

341. Schwartz H, Krishnan U, Pritchard D. Pigmented villonodular synovitis. *Clin Orthop* 1989;247:243–255.

342. Chae J, Yu D, Walker M. Percutaneous, intramuscular neuromuscular electrical stimulation for the treatment of shoulder subluxation and pain in chronic hemiplegia: A case report. *Am J Phys Med Rehabil* 2001;80:296–301.

343. Shearman CM, el-Khoury GY. Pitfalls in the radiologic evaluation of extremity trauma: Part I. The upper extremity. *Am Fam Physician* 1998;57:995–1002.

344. Urquhart BS. Emergency: Anterior shoulder dislocation. *Am J Nurs* 2001;101:33–35.

345. Paxinos A, et al. Advances in the management of traumatic anterior and atraumatic multidirectional shoulder instability. *Sports Med* 2001;31:819–828.

346. Curran J, Ellman M, Brown N. Rheumatologic aspects of painful conditions of the shoulder. *Clin Orthop Rel Res* 1983;173:27–37.

347. Corrigan AB, et al. Benign rheumatoid arthritis of the aged. *BMJ* 1974;1:446.

348. Deal CL, et al. The clinical features of elderly-onset rheumatoid arthritis. *Arthritis Rheum* 1985;28:987–994.

349. Daigneault J, Cooney LM Jr. Shoulder pain in older people. *J Am Geriatr Soc* 1998;46:1144–1151.

350. Baker GL, Oddis CV, Medsger TA Jr. Pasteurella multocida polyarticular septic arthritis. *J Rheumatol* 1987;14:355–357.

351. Armbuster TG, et al. Extraarticular manifestations of septic arthritis of the glenohumeral joint. *J Roentgenol* 1977;129:667–672.

352. Kraft SM, Panush RS, Longley S. Unrecognized staphylococcal pyarthrosis with rheumatoid arthritis. *Sem Arthritis Rheum* 1985;14:196–201.

353. Smith KL, Matsen FA. Total shoulder arthroplasty versus hemiarthroplasty: Current trends. *Orthop Clin North Am* 1998;29:491–506.

354. Bridgman JF. Periarthritis of the shoulder and diabetes mellitus. *Ann Rheum Dis* 1972;31:69–71.

355. Balsund B, Thomsen S, Jensen E. Frozen shoulder: Current concepts. *Scand J Rheumatol* 1990;19:321–325.

356. Steinbrocker O, Argyros TG. Frozen shoulder: Treatment by local injection of depot corticosteroids. *Arch Phys Med Rehabil* 1974;55:209–213.

357. Ombregt L, et al. The shoulder girdle: Disorders of the inert structures. In: Ombregt L, ed. *A System of Orthopaedic Medicine*. London, England: Saunders; 1995:282–286.

358. Stralka SW, Head PL. Musculoskeletal pattern I: Impaired joint mobility, motor function, muscle performance, and range of motion associated with joint arthroplasty. In: Tovin BJ, Greenfield BH, eds. *Evaluation and Treatment of the Shoulder: An Integration of the Guide to Physical Therapist Practice*. Philadelphia, Pa: FA Davis; 2001:264–291.

359. Cofield RH. Degenerative and arthritic problems of the glenohumeral joint. In: Rockwood CA, Matsen FA III, eds. *The Shoulder*. Philadelphia, Pa: Saunders; 1990:678–749.

360. Fenlin JM Jr. Total glenohumeral joint replacement. *Orthop Clin North Am* 1975;6:525.

361. Dich VQ, Nelson JD, Haltalin KC. Osteomyelitis in infants and children: A review of 163 cases. *Am J Dis Child* 1975;129:1273–1278.

362. Barrett-Connor E. Bacterial infection and sickle cell anemia: An analysis of 250 infectious in 166 patients and review of the literature. *Med Sci Sports Exerc* 1971;50:97–112.

363. Bass J, Vincent J, Person D. The expanding spectrum of Bartonella infections: II. Cat scratch disease. *Pediatr Infect Dis J* 1997;16:163–179.

364. Bradford DS, et al. Osteonecrosis in the transplant recipients. *Surg Gynecol Obstet* 1984;159:328–334.

365. Cruess RL. Corticosteroid-induced osteonecrosis of the humeral head. *Orthop Clin North Am* 1985;16:789–796.

366. Cruess RL. Steroid-induced avascular necrosis of the head of the humerus. *J Bone Joint Surg* 1976;58B:313–317.

367. Rossleigh MA, et al. Osteonecrosis in patients with malignant lymphoma. *Cancer* 1986;58:1112–1116.

368. Dwyer A, Aprill C, Bogduk N. Cervical zygpophysial joint pain patterns: A study from normal volunteers. *Spine* 1990;15:453.

369. Booth RE, Rothman RH. Cervical angina. *Spine* 1976;1:28–32.

370. Boissonnault WG. Pathological origins of trunk and neck pain, part 1: Pelvic and abdominal viscera disorders. *J Orthop Sports Phys Ther* 1990;12:192–207.

371. Contorni L. Il circolo collaterale vertebro-vertebrale nell' obliterazione dell'arteria succlavia alla sua origine. *Minerva Chir* 1960;15:268–271.

372. Reivich M, et al. Reversal of blood flow through the vertebral artery and its effects on cerebral circulation. *N Engl J Med* 1961;265:878–885.

373. Fisher CM. A new vascular syndrome: The subclavian steal syndrome. *N Engl J Med* 1961;265:912–913.

374. Webster MW, et al. The effect of arm exercise on regional cerebral blood flow in the subclavian steal syndrome. *Am J Surg* 1994;168:91–93.

375. Meissner I, et al. The natural history of drop attacks. *Neurology* 1986;36:1029–1034.

376. Dieter RA Jr, Kuzycz GB. Iatrogenic steal syndromes. *Int Surg* 1998;83:355–357.

377. Marshall WG Jr, Miller EC, Kouchoukos NT. The coronary-subclavian steal syndrome: Report of a case and recommendations for prevention and management. *Ann Thorac Surg* 1988;46:93–96.

378. Blumenthal RS, et al. Use of intravascular Doppler ultrasonography to assess the hemodynamic significance of the coronary-subclavian steal syndrome. *Am Heart J* 1995;129:622–625.

379. Thompson AJ. Multiple sclerosis: symptomatic management. *J Neurol* 1996;243:559–565.

380. Borasio GD, Miller RG. Clinical characteristics and management of ALS. *Sem Neurol* 2001;21:155–166.

381. Pascuzzi RM, Fleck JD. Acute peripheral neuropathy in adults. *Neurol Clin* 1997;15:529–547.

382. Levy WJ, Mason L, Hahn JF. Chiari malformation presenting in adults: A surgical experience in 127 cases. *Neurosurgery* 1983;12:377–390.

383. Pancoast HK. Superior pulmonary sulcus tumor: Tumor characterized by pain, Horner's syndrome, destruction of bone and atrophy of hand muscles. *JAMA* 1932;99:1391–1396.

384. Pancoast HK. Importance of careful roentgen-ray investigations of apical chest tumors. *JAMA* 1924;83:1407–1411.

385. Arcasoy SM, Jett JR. Superior pulmonary sulcus tumors and Pancoast's syndrome. *N Engl J Med* 1997;337:1370–1376.

386. McKellar H. Clay shoveller's fracture. *J Bone Joint Surg* 1940;12:63–75.

387. Herrick R. Clay-shoveller's fracture in power lifting. *Am J Sports Med* 1981;9:29–30.

388. Hyde GP, Postma GN, Caress JB. Laryngeal paresis as a presenting feature of idiopathic brachial plexopathy. *Otolaryngol Head Neck Surg* 2001;124:575–576.

389. Lee VK, Simpkins L. Herpes zoster and postherpetic neuralgia in the elderly. *Geriatr Nurs* 2000;21:132–135; quiz 136.

390. Woodward AH, Bianco AJ. Osteochondritis dissecans of the elbow. *Clin Orthop* 1975;110:35–41.

391. Field LD, Savoie FH. Common elbow injuries in sport. *Sports Med* 1998;26:193–205.

392. Botte MJ, Gelberman RH. Acute compartment syndrome of the forearm. *Hand Clin* 1998;14:391–403.

393. Benjamin A. The relief of traumatic arterial spasm in threatened Volkmann's ischemic contracture. *J Bone Joint Surg* 1957;39:711–713.

394. Wiener SL. Acute elbow and forearm pain. In: Wiener SL, ed. *Differential Diagnosis of Acute Pain by Body Region.* New York, NY: McGraw-Hill; 1993:509–520.

395. Bijlsma JWJ, et al. *Leerboek Reumatologie.* Bohn: Stafleu VanLoghum; 1992:210–223.

396. van Vugt RM, Bijlsma JWJ, van Vugt AC. Chronic wrist pain: Diagnosis and management. Development and use of a new algorithm. *Ann Rheum Dis* 1999;58:665–674.

397. Hausman MR, Lisser SP. Hand infections. *Orthop Clin North Am* 1992;23:171–186.

398. Viegas SF. Atypical causes of hand pain. *Am Fam Physician* 1987;35:167–172.

399. van Vugt RM, van Dalen A, Bijlsma JWJ. Ultrasound guided synovial biopsy of the wrist. *Scand J Rheumatol* 1997;26:212–214.

400. Buskila D, et al. Patients with rheumatoid arthritis are more tender than those with psoriatic arthritis. *J Rheumatol* 1992;19:1115–1119.

401. Gladman DD. Psoriatic arthritis. In: Kelley WN, et al, eds. *Textbook of Rheumatology* Philadelphia, Pa: Saunders; 1997:999–1005.

402. Gladman DD, et al. HLA antigens in psoriatic arthritis. *J Rheumatol* 1986;13:586–592.

403. Mayeaux EJ Jr. Nail disorders. *Dermatology* 2000;27:333–351.

404. Daniel CR. Paronychia. *Dermatology* 1985;3:461.

405. Lee SJ, Cutcliffe DA, Hurst LC. Infections of the upper extremity. In: Dee R, et al, eds. *Principles of Orthopaedic Practice.* New York, NY: McGraw-Hill; 1997:1193–1199.

406. Kienböck R. Concerning traumatic malacia of the lunate and its consequences: Degeneration and compression fractures. *Clin Orth Rel Res* 1980;149:4–5.

407. Waggy C. Disorders of the wrist. In: Wadsworth C, ed. *Orthopaedic Physical Therapy Home Study Course—The Elbow, Forearm, and Wrist.* La Crosse, Wis: Orthopaedic Section, American Physical Therapy Association; 1997.

408. Alexander AH, Lichtman DM. Kienbock's disease. In: Lichtman DM ed. *The Wrist and its Disorders.* Philadelphia, Pa: Saunders; 1988.

409. Beckenbaugh RD, et al. Kienböck's disease: The natural history of Kienböck's disease and consideration of lunate fractures. *Clin Orthop* 1980;149:98–106.

410. Salmon J, Stanley JK, Trail IA. Kienbock's disease: Conservative management versus radial shortening. *J Bone Joint Surg* 2000;82B:820–823.

411. Onieal ME. *Essentials of Musculoskeletal Care.* 1st ed. Rosemont, Ill: American Academy of Orthopaedic Surgeons; 1997.

412. Onieal ME. The hand: Examination and diagnosis. In: American Society for Surgery of the Hand. New York, NY: Churchill Livingstone; 1990.

413. Gunther SF. Dorsal wrist pain and the occult scapholunate ganglion. *J Hand Surg Am* 1985;10A:697–703.

414. Tham S. Intraosseous ganglion cyst of the lunate: Diagnosis and management. *J Hand Surg Am* 1992;17A:429–432.

415. Onieal ME. Common wrist and elbow injuries in primary care. *Prim Care Pract* 1999;3:441–450.

416. Bogumill GP, Sullivan DJ, Baker GI. Tumors of the hand. *Clin Orthop* 1975;108:214–222.

417. Shaffer B, Bradley JP, Bogumill GP. Unusual problems of the athlete's elbow, forearm, and wrist. *Clin Sports Med* 1996;15:425–438.

418. Wiener SL. Acute wrist, hand, and finger pain. In: Wiener SL, ed. *Differential Diagnosis of Acute Pain by Body Region.* New York, NY: McGraw-Hill; 1993:521–555.

419. Steen VD. Treatment of systemic sclerosis. *Am J Clin Dermatol* 2001;2:315–325.

420. Jackson AM. Anterior knee pain. *J Bone Joint Surg* 2001;83B:937–948.

421. Boyle A, Walton N. Malign anterior knee pain. *J R Soc Med* 2000;93:639-640.

422. Jacobson JA, et al. MR imaging of the infrapatellar fat pad of Hoffa. *Radiographics* 1997;17:675–691.

423. Gebhardt MC, Ready JE, Mankin HJ. Tumors about the knee in children. *Clin Orthop Rel Res* 1990;255:86–110.

424. Sadat-Ali M. Metachronous multicentric giant cell tumour: A case report. *Indian J Cancer* 1997;34:169–176.

425. Kransdorf MJ. Primary tumours of the patella. A review of 42 cases. *Skeletal Radiol* 1989;18:365–371.

426. Pavlovich RI, Day B. Anterior knee pain in the adolescent: An anatomical approach to etiology. *Am J Knee Surg* 1997;10:176–180.

427. Mochida H, Kikuchi S. Injury to the infrapatellar branch of saphenous nerve in arthroscopic knee surgery. *Clin Orthop* 1995;320:88–94.

428. Pinar H, et al. Traumatic prepatellar neuroma: An unusual cause of anterior knee pain. *Knee Surg Sports Traumatol Arthrosc* 1996;4:154–156.

429. Kankate RK, Selvan TP. Primary haematogenous osteomyelitis of the patella: A rare cause for anterior knee pain in an adult. *Postgrad Med J* 2000;76:707–709.

430. Roy DR. Osteomyelitis of the patella. *Clin Orthop Rel Res* 2001;389:30–34.

431. Mars M, Hadley GP. Raised intracompartmental pressure and compartment syndromes. *Injury* 1998;29:403–411.

432. Matsen FA, Winquist RA, Krugmire RB. Diagnosis and management of compartment syndromes. *J Bone Joint Surg* 1980;62A:286–291.

433. Perron AD, Brady WJ, Keats TE. Orthopedic pitfalls in the ED: Acute compartment syndrome. *Am J Emerg Med* 2001;19:413–416.

434. Windsor RE, Chambers K. Overuse injuries of the leg. In: Kibler BW, Herring JA, Press JM, eds. *Functional Rehabilitation of Sports and Musculoskeletal Injuries.* Gaithersburg, Md: Aspen; 1998:265–272.

435. Gubbay AJ, Isaacs D. Pyomyositis in children. *Pediatr Infect Dis J* 2000;19:1009–1012; quiz 1013.

436. Leach KL. Fractures of the tibia and fibular. In: Rockwood CA, Green DP, eds. *Fractures in Adults.* Philadelphia, Pa: JB Lippincott; 1984:1652.

437. Warren DK, Wiss DA, Ting A. Isolated fibular shaft fracture in a sprinter. *Am J Sports Med* 1990;18:209–210.

438. Mann RA, Hagy J. Biomechanics of walking, running, and sprinting. *Am J Sports Med* 1980;8:345–350.

439. Gorman WP, Davis KR, Donnelly R. ABC of arterial and venous disease. Swollen lower limb-1: General assessment and deep vein thrombosis. *BMJ* 2000;320:1453–1456.

440. Morganti CM, McFarland EG, Cosgarea AJ. Saphenous neuritis: A poorly understood cause of medial knee pain. *J Am Acad Orthop Surg* 2002;10:130–137.

441. Mader JT, Cripps MW, Calhoun JH. Adult posttraumatic osteomyelitis of the tibia. *Clin Orthop Rel Res* 1999;360:14–21.

442. Omey ML, Micheli LJ. Foot and ankle problems in the young athlete. *Med Sci Sports Exerc* 1999;31(suppl):S470–S486.

443. Brodsky AE, Khalil MA. Talar compression syndrome. *Am J Sports Med* 1986;14:472–476.

444. McDougall A. The os trigonum. *J Bone Joint Surg* 1955;37B:257–265.

445. Keene JS, Lange RH. Diagnostic dilemmas in foot and ankle injuries. *JAMA* 1986;256:247–251.

446. Kelikian H, Kelikian AS. *Disorders of the Ankle.* Philadelphia, Pa: Saunders; 1985.

447. Marotta JJ, Micheli LJ. Os trigonum impingement in dancers. *Am J Sports Med* 1992;20:533–536.

448. Ihle CL, Cochran RM. Fracture of the fused os trigonum. *Am J Sports Med* 1982;10:47–50.

449. Hedrick MR, McBryde AM. Posterior ankle impingement. *Foot Ankle* 1994;15:2–8.

450. Wredmark T, et al. Os trigonum syndrome: A clinical entity in ballet dancers. *Foot Ankle* 1991;11:404–406.

451. Ecker M, Rilter M. The symptomatic os trigonum. *JAMA* 1967;201:204–206.

452. Hamilton WG, Geppert MJ, Thompson FM. Pain in the posterior aspect of the ankle in dancers. *J Bone Joint Surg* 1996;78A:1491–1500.

453. Veazey BL, et al. Excision of ununited fractures of the posterior process of the talus: A treatment for chronic posterior ankle pain. *Foot Ankle* 1992;13:453–457.

454. Burkus JK, Sella EJ, Southwick WD. Occult injuries of the talus diagnosed by bone scan and tomography. *Foot Ankle* 1982;4:316–324.

455. McManama GB Jr. Ankle injuries in the young athlete. *Clin Sports Med* 1988;7:547.

456. Sullivan JA. Ankle and foot injuries in the pediatric athlete. In: *Pediatric and Adolescent Sports Medicine.* Philadelphia, Pa: Saunders; 1994:441–455.

457. Berndt AL, Harty M. Transchondral fractures (osteochondritis dissecans) of the talus. *J Bone Joint Surg* 1959;41A:988.

458. Roden S, Tillegard P, Unander-Scharin L. Osteochondritis dissecans and similar lesions of the talus. *Acta Orthop Scand* 1953;23:51.

459. Gregg J, Das M. Foot and ankle problems in preadolescent and adolescent athletes. *Clin Sports Med* 1982;1:131–147.

460. Mann RA. Pain in the foot. *Postgrad Med* 1987;82:154–162.

461. Lahita RG. The clinical presentation of systemic lupus erythematosus. In: Lahita RG, ed. *Systemic Lupus Erythematosus.* San Diego, Calif: Academic Press; 1999:325–336.

462. Tigner R. Handling a sickle cell crisis. *RN* 1998;61:32–35; quiz 36.

463. Rho RH, et al. Complex regional pain syndrome. *Mayo Clin Proc* 2002;77:174–180.

464. Koman LA, et al. Reflex sympathetic dystrophy in an adolescent. *Foot Ankle* 1993;14:273–277.

465. Goodall S. Peripheral vascular disease. *Nurs Standard* 2000;14:48–52; quiz 53–54.

466. Gauthier G, Elbaz R. A subchondral bone fracture: A new surgical treatment. *Clin Orthop* 1979;142:93–95.

467. Hoskinson J. Freiberg's disease: A review of long-term results. *Proc R Soc Med* 1974;67:106–107.

468. Katcherian DA. Treatment of Freiberg's disease. *Orthop Clin North Am* 1994;25:69–81.

469. Smillie IS. Freiberg's infraction (Koehler's second disease). *J Bone Joint Surg* 1955;39B:580.

470. Harris RI, Beath T. Hypermobile flatfoot with short tendo Achilles. *J Bone Joint Surg* 1948;30A:116.

471. Mann RA, Coughlin MJ. Keratotic disorders of the skin. In: Mann RA, Coughlin MJ, eds. *Surgery of the Foot and Ankle.* St Louis, Mo: Mosby-Yearbook; 1993:533–544.

472. Hockenbury RT. Forefoot problems in athletes. *Med Sci Sports Exerc* 1999;31(suppl):S448–S458.

473. Wu KK. Morton's interdigital neuroma: A clinical review of its etiology, treatment, and results. *J Foot Ankle Surg* 1996;35:112–119.

474. Sullivan JA. The child's foot. In: Morrissy RT, ed. *Lovell and Winter's Pediatric Orthopaedics.* Philadelphia, Pa: Lippincott; 1996:1077–1135.

475. Chen YJ, et al. Posterior tibial tendon tear combined with a fracture of the accessory navicular: A new subclassification? *J Trauma Inj Infect Critl Care* 1995;39:993–996.

476. Grogan DP, Gasser SI, Ogden JA. The painful accessory navicular: A clinical and histopathological study. *Foot Ankle* 1989;10:164.

477. Kidner FC. The prehallux in relation to flatfoot. *JAMA* 1933;101:1539.

478. Sullivan JA, Miller WA. The relationship of the accessory navicular to the development of the flatfoot. *Clin Orthop* 1979;144:233.

479. Bennett GL, Weiner DS, Leighley B. Surgical treatment of symptomatic accessory tarsal navicular. *J Pediatr Orthop* 1990;10:445.

480. Hunter-Griffin LY. Injuries to the leg, ankle, and foot. In: Sullivan JA, Grana WA, eds. *The Pediatric Athlete*. Park Ridge, Ill: American Academy of Orthopaedic Surgeons; 1990:187–198.

481. Veitch JM. Evaluation of the Kidner operation and treatment of symptomatic accessory tarsal scaphoid. *Clin Orthop* 1978;131:210.

482. Manusov EG, et al. Evaluation of pediatric foot problems: Part I. The forefoot and midfoot. *Am Fam Physician* 1996;54:592–606.

483. Sanders R. Current concepts review: Displaced intraarticular fractures of the calcaneus. *J Bone Joint Surg* 2000;82A:225–250.

484. Antoniou D, Conner AN. Osteomyelitis of the calcaneus and talus. *J Bone Joint Surg* 1974;56A:338–345.

485. Nixon GW. Hematogenous osteomyelitis of metaphyseal equivalent locations. *AJR Am J Roentgenol* 1978;130:123–129.

486. Keck C. The tarsal tunnel syndrome. *J Bone Joint Surg* 1962;44A:180–182.

487. Lam S. A tarsal tunnel syndrome. *Lancet* 1962;2:1354–1355.

488. Turan I, et al. Tarsal tunnel syndrome. Outcome of surgery in longstanding cases. *Clin Orthop Rel Res* 1997;343:151–156.

489. DeLisa JA, Saleed MA. The tarsal tunnel syndrome. *Muscle Nerve* 1983;6:664–670.

490. Chater EH. Tarsal-tunnel syndrome in rheumatoid arthritis. *Br Med J* 1970;3:406.

491. Cimino W. Tarsal tunnel syndrome. Review of the literature. *Foot Ankle* 1990;11:47–52.

492. Francis H, et al. Benign joint hypermobility with neuropathy: Documentation and mechanism of tarsal tunnel syndrome. *J Rheum* 1987;14:577–581.

493. Joubert MJ. Tarsal tunnel syndrome. *S Afr Med J* 1972;46:507–508.

494. Rask M. Medial plantar neurapraxia (jogger's foot). *Clin Orthop* 1978;134:193–195.

495. DiStefano V, et al. Tarsal tunnel syndrome: Review of the literature and two case reports. *Clin Orthop* 1972;88:76–79.

496. Edwards W, et al. The tarsal tunnel syndrome: Diagnosis and treatment. *JAMA* 1969;207:716–720.

497. Radin E. Tarsal tunnel syndrome. *Clin Orthop* 1983;181:167–170.

498. Jackson DL, Haglund BL. Tarsal tunnel syndrome in runners. *Sports Med* 1992;13:146–149.

499. Lam SJS. Tarsal tunnel syndrome. *J Bone Joint Surg* 1967;49B:87–92.

500. Van Wyngarden TM. The painful foot, part II: Common rearfoot deformities. *Am Fam Physician* 1997;55:2207–2212.

501. Linscheid R, Burton R, Fredericks E. Tarsal tunnel syndrome. *South Med J* 1970;63:1313–1323.

502. Stefko RM, Lauerman WC, Heckman JD. Tarsal tunnel syndrome caused by an unrecognized fracture of the posterior process of the talus. *J Bone Joint Surg* 1994;76A:116–118.

503. Wilberger JE. Lumbosacral radiculopathy secondary to abdominal aortic aneurysms. *J Neurosurg* 1983;58:965.

504. Chad DA, Bradley DM. Lumbosacral plexopathy. *Sem Neurol* 1987;7:97.

505. Bodack MP, Cole JC, Nagler W. Sciatic neuropathy secondary to a uterine fibroid: A case report. *Am J Phys Med Rehabil* 1999;78:157–159.

INTERVENTION PRINCIPLES

CHAPTER OBJECTIVES

► *At the completion of this chapter, the reader will be able to:*

1. Understand and describe the principles of a comprehensive rehabilitation program.

2. Discuss the various components of the intervention and their respective importance.

3. List the clinical tools that can be used to control pain, inflammation, and edema and the rationale for each.

4. Discuss the intrinsic and extrinsic stimuli that can be used to promote and progress healing.

5. Describe the benefits of each of the electrotherapeutic modalities.

6. Describe the benefits of each of the physical agents and mechanical modalities.

7. Understand the rationale for the therapeutic techniques used in each of the three stages of healing.

8. Describe each of the five types of heat transfer and the modalities that are involved with each.

9. Describe the physiological effects of a local heat application and of cryotherapy.

10. Describe some of the pharmacological agents that are used in the management of pain and inflammation.

11. Describe the importance of strengthening and flexibility exercises in the rehabilitation process.

12. Discuss the importance of postural correction and some of the techniques that can be used.

13. Understand the concept of the kinetic chain and how it relates to exercise.

14. Describe the importance of neuromuscular re-education and discuss ways in which it can be incorporated into the rehabilitation process.

15. Discuss the importance of functional training.

16. Describe methods to increase the physical activity level of a patient and the benefits of exercise and fitness training.

17. Understand the importance of patient education.

18. Describe the various types of learners and the instructional strategies for each.

OVERVIEW

According to the "Guide to Physical Therapist Practice,"[1] an intervention is "the purposeful and skilled interaction of the physical therapist and the patient/client and, when appropriate, with other individuals involved in the patient/client care, using various physical therapy procedures and techniques to produce changes in the condition consistent with the diagnosis and prognosis."

Three components comprise the physical therapy intervention (Box 10-1): coordination, communication, and documentation; patient/client related instruction; and direct interventions[1] (Table 10-1).

Box 10-1 COMPONENTS OF AN INTERVENTION[1]

Coordination, Communication and Documentation

These interventions may include case management, communication with other health care providers or insurers, and the coordination of care with the patient/client or significant others involved in the care of the patient/client. This is to ensure a continuum of care among health care providers. Other interventions may include documentation of care, discharge planning, education plans, patient care conferences, record reviews, and referrals to other professionals or resources.

Patient-related Instruction

Patient education can include, but is not limited to, verbal, written, or pictorial instructions, which may be part of a home program. Computer-assisted instruction and demonstrations by the patient/client, or caregivers are also examples of instructions that may be given. Audio-visual aides and demonstrations of exercises or functional activities may be used. This enables the patient/client to continue with the program when out of the clinic, either independently or with assistance.

Direct Interventions

Direct interventions are selected based on the findings in the evaluation and examination of the patient/client, diagnosis, prognosis, and anticipated outcomes and goals for the individual. The direct interventions are performed with or on the patient. This section encompasses the largest component of patient care. Examples of direct interventions include, but are not limited to, therapeutic exercise, aerobic exercise, functional training, manual therapy, and use of assistive devices and modalities.

TABLE 10-1   Direct Interventions

Therapeutic exercise (includes aerobic conditioning)
Functional training in self-care and home management (ADLs)
Functional training in community and work integration and reintegration (IADLs)
Manual therapy
Prescription, application, and fabrication of devices and equipment
Airway clearance techniques
Wound management
Electrotherapeutic modalities
Physical agents and mechanical modalities

ADLs, activities of daily living; IADLs, instrumental activities of daily living.

An intervention is most effectively addressed from a problem-oriented approach and is based on the patient's functional needs and on mutually agreed-upon goals.[1] Decisions about the intervention are made to improve the patient's ability to perform basic tasks, and to restore functional homeostasis. The most successful intervention programs are those that are custom designed from a blend of clinical experience and scientific data, with the level of improvement achieved related to goal setting and the attainment of those goals (Table 10-2).

Whether the identification of the specific structure or structures causing the dysfunction is necessary in order to proceed with an intervention remains controversial. Cyriax[3] designed his examination process to selectively stress specific tissues in order to identify the structure involved and its stage of pathology. In contrast, Maitland[4,5] and McKenzie[6] seldom identify the involved structure, believing it is not always possible, or even necessary, for the prescription and safe delivery of appropriate therapeutic interventions. Based on the Maitland and McKenzie philosophy, the therapeutic strategy is determined solely from the responses obtained from tissue loading and the effect that loading has on symptoms. Once these responses have been determined, the focus of the intervention is to provide sound and effective self-management strategies for patients that avoid

TABLE 10-2   Key Questions for Intervention Planning[1]

What is the stage of healing: acute, subacute, or chronic?
How long do you have to treat the patient?
What does the patient do for activities?
How compliant is the patient?
How much *skilled* physical therapy is needed?
What needs to be taught to prevent recurrence?
Are any referrals needed?
What has worked for other patients with similar problems?
Are there any precautions?
What is your skill level?

TABLE 10-3 Intervention Principles

Control pain and inflammation
Promote and progress healing
Strengthen or increase flexibility
Correct posture and movement impairment syndromes
Analyze and integrate the entire kinetic chain
Incorporate neuromuscular re-education
Improve functional outcome
Maintain or improve overall fitness
Patient education and self-management
Ensure a safe return to function

harmful tissue loading.[6] However, although self-management must be encouraged whenever feasible, these strategies have their limitations. One cannot realistically expect the majority of patients to fully rehabilitate themselves with a condition that requires the integration of a multitude of decision-making processes such as occurs with a total joint replacement or an anterior cruciate ligament reconstruction.

Many factors can contribute to the patient's resistance to improvement. In some cases, it may be an individual factor that, when eliminated, will allow the patient to respond well. In the majority of cases, the resistance to improvement is based on the interaction of multiple factors, which must be recognized and corrected.

The principles listed in Table 10-3 should be applied as part of a comprehensive intervention. These principles are not listed in order of importance or application, but reflect the sequence of discussion in the remainder of this chapter.

Principle 1: Control Pain and Inflammation

Soft tissue injuries of all types are extremely common in the general population. Studies have shown that there is a linear relationship between soft tissue injuries and aging, with fewer than 10 percent of individuals younger than 34 years being affected, in contrast to 32 to 49 percent of those older than 75.[7] Concomitant with most soft tissue injuries is pain, inflammation, and edema. Pain serves as a protective mechanism, allowing an individual to be aware of a situation's potential for producing tissue damage, and to minimize further damage. At the simplest level, the transmission of information relating to pain from the periphery to the cortex is critically dependent on integration at three levels within the central nervous system: the spinal cord, brain stem, and forebrain (see Chap. 2). Inflammation and edema occur as part of the healing process (see Chap. 5). The goals during the initial phase of intervention for an acute lesion, therefore, are to decrease pain, control the inflammation and edema, and protect the damaged structures from further damage, while attempting to increase range of motion (ROM) and function.

Several tools are at the clinician's disposal to help to control pain, inflammation, and edema. These include the application of electrotherapeutic and physical modalities, gentle (ROM) exercises, and graded manual techniques. During the acute stage of healing the principles of PRICEMEM (*p*rotection, *r*est, *i*ce, *c*ompression, *e*levation, *m*anual therapy, *e*arly motion, and *m*edications) are recommended.

Protection
Excessive tissue loading must be avoided. For example, in the lower extremity when ambulation is painful, crutches or other assistive devices are advocated until the patient can bear weight painlessly.[8]

Rest
Rest is defined as absence from abuse, rather than an absence from activity.[9] Prolonged immobilization can have a detrimental effect on muscles (see Chap. 4), ligaments, bones, collagen, and joint surfaces.

Ice
The therapeutic application of cold or cryotherapy has been used as a healing modality since the days of the ancient Greeks (refer to principle 2).[10]

Compression
The most common method of applying compression is via an elastic bandage.[11] Compression provided by a pneumatic device,[12,13] or by a felt pad incorporated into an elastic wrap or taping,[14] also has been demonstrated to be effective in decreasing effusion.

Elevation
Elevation of an extremity aids in venous return and helps minimize swelling. Garrick[8] recommends that ice be used until the swelling has ceased. Elevation and compression should be continued until the swelling has completely dissipated.[8]

Manual Therapy
The controlled application of a variety of manual techniques, described in Chapter 11, can have several therapeutic benefits. These benefits are theoretically achieved through[15,16]:

▶ Stimulation of the large-fiber joint afferents of the joint capsule, soft tissue, and joint cartilage, which aids in pain reduction.

▶ Stimulation of endorphins, which aids in pain reduction.

▶ Decrease of intra-articular pressure, which aids in pain reduction.

▶ Mechanical effect, which increases joint mobility.

▶ Remodeling of local connective tissue.

▶ Increase of the gliding of tendons within their sheaths.

▶ Increase in joint lubrication.

Early Motion

Early motion is advocated to:

▶ Reduce the muscle atrophy that occurs primarily in type I fibers.[17–19]

▶ Maintain joint function.

▶ Prevent ligamentous "creeping."

▶ Reduce the chance of arthrofibrosis or excessive scarring.[20–24]

▶ Enhance cartilage nutrition and vascularization, thereby permitting an early recovery and enhanced comfort.[19,25,26]

Research has demonstrated that joint motion stimulates the healing of torn ligaments around a joint,[27,28] and that early joint motion stimulates collagen bundle orientation in the lines of force, a kind of Wolff's law of ligaments.[27,29] Early ROM exercises may be performed actively or passively while protecting the healing tissues. For example, in the lower extremity, seated balance board activities may be performed early in the rehabilitative process. These are progressed to standing balance board activities as healing progresses.

Medications

Although not a physical therapy intervention, medications play an important role in the healing process. Nonsteroidal anti-inflammatory drugs (NSAIDs) currently are the medication of choice to help control the inflammatory process at initial presentation (see principle 2). It has not been proved that these agents have a specific effect on fibroblast function or on connective tissue healing.[9,30] However, the analgesic effects of the anti-inflammatory medications make it easier to rehabilitate injured structures, as well as the muscles in the surrounding kinetic chain, and can help curb further inflammatory response as patients increases their activity level.[31]

The injection of corticosteroids can be used to decrease the pain at the site of inflammation, at least temporarily. Leadbetter[32] reviewed the literature on the use of injections of corticosteroids for the intervention of sports-related injuries and concluded that such intervention should remain a form of adjunctive therapy and not the sole means of intervention.

Principle 2: Promote and Progress Healing

Tissue repair can be viewed as an adaptive life process in response to both intrinsic and extrinsic stimuli.[33] Physical therapy cannot accelerate the healing process, but with correct education and supervision, it can ensure that the healing process is not delayed or disrupted and that it occurs in an optimal environment.[6]

> **Clinical Pearl**
>
> The promotion and progression of tissue repair involves a delicate balance between protection and the application of controlled functional stresses to the damaged structure.

The rehabilitation procedures used to assist with this repair process differ, depending on type of tissue involved, extent of the damage, and stage of healing. Healing is related to the signs and symptoms present rather than the actual diagnosis. These signs and symptoms inform the clinician as to the stage of repair that the tissue is undergoing. Awareness of the various stages of healing is essential for determining the intensity of a particular intervention, if the clinician is to avoid doing any harm. Decisions to advance or change the rehabilitative process need to be based on the recognition of these signs and symptoms, and on an awareness of the time frames associated with each of the phases.[34,35]

Given the number of pathologic entities that can be evoked by the repair process, such a complex regional pain syndrome (CRPS) and myositis ossificans, it is clear that neurophysiologic processes are at work. Three healing stages are recognized: (1) inflammation, (2) migration and proliferation, and (3) remodeling (see Chap. 5). Although the intervention principles for these stages are described separately, they should be viewed as a continuum. Throughout the various chapters in this book, the phases of intervention are based on the acute phase and the functional phase. The acute phase is analogous to the inflammatory stage of healing. The functional phase is analogous to the migration and proliferation, and remodeling stages.

Inflammation (Stage 1)

Clinical findings during the inflammatory stage include swelling, redness, heat, and impairment or loss of function. Usually there is pain at rest or with active motion, or when specific stress is applied to the injured structure. The pain, if severe enough, can result in muscle guarding and loss of function. With passive mobility testing, pain is reported before tissue resistance is felt by the clinician.

Janda[36] introduced the concept of the direct and indirect affects of neural input on muscle activation, and noted the influence that pain and swelling can have on direct muscle inhibition.

> **Clinical Pearl**
>
> According to Janda,[36] muscular development cannot proceed in the presence of pain, because pain has the potential to create a high degree of muscle inhibition that can alter muscle-firing patterns.

During this stage, the intervention goals of controlling pain and reducing the degree of inflammation, and swelling, are achieved by using the principles of PRICEMEM. This approach results in decreased early bleeding and facilitation of the removal of the inflammatory exudates, which can prevent further damage and inflammation to the area. Limiting the effusion serves to hasten the healing process by minimizing the amount of extracellular fluid and hematoma to be reabsorbed.[37,38]

Electrotherapeutic and physical modalities can be used during this stage to help control pain, swelling, and muscle guarding. Heat, ultrasound, and phonophoresis are introduced once the acute stage is ebbing (see later discussion).

During the inflammatory stage, it is also important for the patient to function as independently as possible. The aims of this phase are to avoid painful positions, improve ROM, reduce muscle atrophy through gentle isometric muscle setting, and maintain aerobic fitness.[33,39,40]

The criteria for advancement from this phase include adequate pain control and tissue healing, near-normal ROM, and tolerance for strengthening.[41]

Manual techniques, which are discussed in Chapter 11, allow the clinician to choose the degree of specificity of an intervention. Although the goal is to be as specific as possible, there are many times when a general technique is appropriate. General techniques are typically less aggressive, are applied to the larger muscle groups or regions, and often can be performed by the patient as part of the home exercise program. General manual therapy techniques that can be used during this stage include *gentle* massage to increase blood flow. Specific manual techniques that can be used during this stage include passive joint distractions and glides (grade I or II).

Clinical Pearl

The benefits of early mobilization are to prevent the detrimental physiologic effects of immobilization, including loss of muscle, ligament, and bone strength,[42,43] formation of adhesions,[44] and the loss of proprioception.[45]

Migration and Proliferation (Stage 2)

Clinically, this stage is characterized by a decrease in pain and swelling and an increase in pain-free active and passive ROM. During passive ROM, the occurrence of pain is synchronous with tissue resistance.

Although the pain-free ROM may be increased in this phase, it is still not within normal limits, and stress applied to the injured structures still produces pain, although the pain experienced is lessened.[46,47]

It seems that the fibroblasts need to be guided during this recovery phase so that the replaced collagen fibers are laid along the lines of stress. Gentle movements to the area provide natural tensions for the healing tissues, and should commence at about the fifth day to help produce a stronger repair.[48]

Clinical Pearl

The intervention goals during this phase are to protect the forming collagen, direct its orientation to be parallel to the lines of force it must withstand, and prevent cross-linking and scar contracture. If these goals are achieved, the scar will be strong and extensible.

A progressive increase in movement should be encouraged so that full ROM is possible by the third or fourth week. Passive ROM is progressed to active assistive, and then to active ROM,

based on tissue and patient responses. Strengthening exercises during this stage are initially restricted to submaximal isometrics. The submaximal isometrics are initially performed in the early part of the range, before being performed at multiple angles of the pain-free ROM. As ROM and joint play improve, isotonic exercises are initiated, with the resistance being increased as tolerated.

Clinical Pearl

The criteria for advancement to the functional or remodeling stage of rehabilitation includes no complaints of pain; full, pain-free ROM; good flexibility and balance; and strength of 75 to 80 percent, or greater, compared with uninvolved side.[41]

Manual therapies during this stage include joint mobilizations (grade II) to help restore normal joint play, transverse friction massage, and gentle contract-relax techniques. It is important to emphasize to the patient that an overly aggressive approach during this stage can result in a delay or disruption in the repair process through an increase in the stimulation of the inflammatory chemical irritants and exudates.

Remodeling (Stage 3)

During this stage, pain typically is felt at the end of range with passive ROM, after the tissue resistance has been encountered. The only intervention that consistently appears beneficial across a wide spectrum of spinal and nonspinal musculoskeletal problems is the continued application of controlled stresses. The musculoskeletal tissues respond to the controlled stresses applied to them by adaptation. This response has been described as a specific adaptation to imposed demand (SAID) (see Chap. 6).[49]

Clinical Pearl

The SAID principle acknowledges that the human body responds to explicit demands placed upon it with a specific and predictable adaptation.

Understanding the SAID principle is especially important when designing an active approach to intervention. The application of inappropriate stresses can lead to various forms of tissue dysfunction, such as contracture, laxity, fibrosis, adhesion, diminished function, repeated structural failure, and an alteration in neurophysiologic feedback.[50,51]

In the instance of chronic conditions, a slight increase or worsening of symptoms is sometimes permissible,[52] because the desensitization of some of the structures may require a mechanical input via stimulation of the large A fibers (see Chap. 2). However, the increase in symptoms also may signal a retriggering of the inflammatory process.[52] To help prevent these pathologic changes, Liebenson[53] recommends the following:

▶ Patient education about how to identify and control external sources of biomechanical overload.

▶ Early identification of psychosocial factors of abnormal illness behavior.

▶ Identification and rehabilitation of the functional pathology.

Exercises during this phase should incorporate open (non–weight-bearing) and close chain (weight-bearing) activities (refer to Principle 5), and eccentric and concentric contractions. The progression to functional or sports-specific exercises may be made, depending on the patient's requirements.

> ### Clinical Pearl
>
> If the ROM and joint play are restricted, the patient continues with isometrics at various angles in the range. Otherwise, the patient is progressed through isotonic resisted exercises.

Manual techniques may be required in this stage to emphasize the restoration of joint motion and to increase the extensibility of soft tissues. Techniques to increase joint motion may include joint mobilizations (grades II through V). Techniques to increase soft tissue extensibility include passive stretching and myofascial release techniques.

Rehabilitation Modalities

Clinicians have at their disposal a battery of physical agents and electrotherapeutic modalities for use in the acute phase and once the acute stage of healing has subsided. The modalities used during the acute phase involve the application of cryotherapy, electrical stimulation, pulsed ultrasound, and iontophoresis. Modalities used during the later stages of healing include thermotherapy, phonophoresis, electrical stimulation, ultrasound, iontophoresis, and diathermy (Tables 10-4 and 10-5).

At present, with the exception of cryotherapy, there is simply insufficient evidence to support or reject the use of modalities.[55–57] However, the absence of evidence does not always mean that there is evidence of absence (of effect), and there is always the risk of rejecting therapeutic approaches that are valid.[58]

TABLE 10-4   Clinical Decision Making on the Use of Various Therapeutic Modalities in Treatment of Acute Injury[54]

Phase	Approximate Time Frame	Clinical Picture	Possible Modalities Used	Rationale for Use
Initial acute	Injury–day 3	Swelling, pain to touch, pain on motion	CRYO ESC IC LPL Rest	↓ Swelling, ↓ pain ↓ Pain ↓ Swelling ↓ Pain
Inflammatory response	Day 1–6	Swelling subsides, warm to touch, discoloration, pain to touch, pain on motion	CRYO ESC IC LPL Range of motion	↓ Swelling, ↓ pain ↓ Pain ↓ Swelling ↓ Pain
Fibroblastic repair	Day 4–10	Pain to touch, pain on motion, swollen	THERMO ESC LPL IC Range of motion Strengthening	Mildly ↑ circulation ↓ Pain-muscle pumping ↓ Pain Facilitate lymphatic flow
Maturation-remodeling	Day 7–recovery	Swollen, no more pain to touch, decreasing pain on motion	ULTRA ESC LPL SWD MWD Range of motion Strengthening Functional activities	Deep heating to ↑ circulation ↑ Range of motion, ↑ strength ↓ Pain ↓ Pain Deep heating to ↑ circulation Deep heating to ↑ circulation

CRYO, cryotherapy; ESC, electrical stimulating currents; IC, intermittent compression; LPL, low-power laser; MWD, microwave diathermy, SWD, short-wave diathermy; THERMO, thermotherapy; ULTRA, ultrasound; ↓, decrease; ↑, increase.

TABLE 10-5 Indications and Contraindications for Therapeutic Modalities[54]

Therapeutic Modality	Physiologic Responses (Indications for Use)	Contraindications and Precautions
Electrical stimulating currents High voltage	Pain modulation Muscle re-education Muscle pumping contractions Retard atrophy Muscle strengthening Increase ROM Fracture healing Acute injury	Pacemakers Thrombophlebitis Superficial skin lesions
Low voltage	Wound healing Fracture healing Iontophoresis	Malignancy Skin hypersensitivities Allergies to certain drugs
Interferential	Pain modulation Muscle re-education Muscle pumping contractions Fracture healing Increase ROM	Same as high voltage
Russian MENS	Muscle strengthening Fracture healing Wound healing	Pacemakers Malignancy Infections
Shortwave diathermy and microwave diathermy	Increase deep circulation Increase metabolic activity Reduce muscle guarding and spasm Reduce inflammation Facilitate wound healing Analgesia Increase tissue temperatures over a large area	Metal implants Pacemakers Malignancy Wet dressings Anesthetized areas Pregnancy Acute injury and inflammation Near eyes Areas of reduced blood flow Anesthetized areas
Cryotherapy (cold packs, ice massage)	Acute injury Vasoconstriction, decreased blood flow Analgesia Reduce inflammation Reduce muscle guarding/spasm	Allergy to cold Circulatory impairments Wound healing Hypertension
Thermotherapy (hot whirlpool, paraffin, hydrocollator, infrared lamps)	Vasodilation, increased blood flow Analgesia Reduce muscle guarding and spasm Reduce inflammation Increase metabolic activity Facilitate tissue healing	Acute and postacute trauma Poor circulation Circulatory impairments Malignancy
Low-power laser	Pain modulation (trigger points) Facilitate wound healing	Pregnancy Near eyes

TABLE 10-5   *(cont.)*

Therapeutic Modality	Physiologic Responses (Indications for Use)	Contraindications and Precautions
Ultraviolet	Acne Aseptic wounds Folliculitis Pityriasis rosea Tinea Septic wounds Sinusitis Increase calcium metabolism	Psoriasis Eczema Herpes Diabetes Pellagra Lupus erythematosus Hyperthyroidism Renal and hepatic insufficiency Generalized dermatitis Advanced atherosclerosis
Ultrasound	Increase connective tissue extensibility Deep heat Increased circulation Treatment of most soft tissue injuries Reduce inflammation Reduce muscle spasm	Infection Acute and postacute injury Epiphyseal areas Pregnancy Thrombophlebitis Impaired sensation Near eyes
Intermittent compression	Decrease acute bleeding Decrease edema	Circulatory impairment

---

> **Clinical Pearl**
>
> It is important that the clinician have an understanding of the principles that relate to a particular modality so that the modality is used when indicated, and the maximum therapeutic benefit may be derived from its use.

If modalities have a place in the clinic, it is during the acute phase of healing, when there is little the clinician can do in the form of manual techniques or therapeutic exercise. In the remodeling or functional phase, thermal modalities may be used to promote blood flow to the healing tissues and to prepare the tissues for exercise or manual techniques. However, at the earliest opportunity, the patient should be weaned away from these modalities, and the focus of the intervention should shift to the application of movement and the repeated and prolonged functional restoration of the involved structures.

Two categories of modalities are recognized:

1. Physical agents and mechanical modalities.

2. Electrotherapeutic modalities.

Physical Agents and Mechanical Modalities

Cryotherapy.   The use of ice, or cryotherapy, by itself[59] or in conjunction with compression,[12–14,60] has been demonstrated to be effective in minimizing the amount of exudate. Cryotherapy, which removes heat from the body, thereby decreasing the temperature of the body tissues, is the most commonly used modality for the intervention of acute musculoskeletal injuries.[59,61–63] Hocutt and colleagues[60] demonstrated that cryotherapy started within 36 hours of injury was statistically better than heat for complete and rapid recovery. Patients using cryotherapy within 36 hours of injury reached full activity in an average of 13.2 days compared with an average 30.4 days for those initiating cryotherapy more than 36 hours after injury. Individuals who used heat required 33.3 days for return to full activity.[60]

The physiologic effects of a local cold application are principally the result of vasoconstriction, reduced metabolic function,[64] and reduced motor and sensory conduction velocities.[65,66] These effects include:

▶ A decrease in muscle and intraarticular temperature. This decrease in muscle temperature[67] and intra-articular structures[68–70] occurs because of a decrease in local blood flow,[59,61,63,71,72] and appears to be most marked between the temperatures of 40° and 25°C.[73] Temperatures below 25°C, which typically occur after 30 minutes of cooling therapy, actually result in an increase blood flow,[73] with a consequent detrimental increase in hemorrhage and an exaggerated acute inflammatory response.[66] The decrease in muscle and intraarticular temperature is maintained for several hours after removal of the cooling agent.[74] A prolonged application of cold, however, can result in a sympathetically mediated reflex vasodilation in an attempt to rewarm the area, which may actually worsen the swelling.[74,75]

TABLE 10-6   Stages of Analgesia Induced by Cryotherapy[60]

Stage	Response	Time After Initiation of Cryotherapy (min)
1	Cold sensation	0–3
2	Burning or aching	2–7
3	Local numbness or analgesia	5–12
4	Deep tissue vasodilation without increase in metabolism	12–15

▶ Local analgesia.[57,59,61,76–79] The stages of analgesia achieved by cryotherapy are outlined in Table 10-6. It is worth remembering that the timing of the stages depends on the depth of penetration and varying thickness of adipose tissue.[80] The patient should be advised as to these various stages, especially in light of the fact that the burning or aching phase occurs before the therapeutic phases.

▶ Decreased muscle spasm.[13,57,81–83]

▶ Decrease in swelling.[10,57,84]

▶ Decrease in nerve conduction velocity.[85]

Several methods of applying cryotherapy have been examined in different studies. The use of ice chips in toweling has been shown to be more effective in decreasing skin temperature than ice chips in plastic bags, or cold gel packs.[70,86] Findings from another study[87] indicated that ice massage and ice bags are equally effective in decreasing intramuscular temperature and in maintaining the duration of temperature depression. That study also found that ice massage achieves maximal intramuscular temperature decreases sooner than the ice bag.[87]

Ice massage is recommended in all of the phases when any inflammation is present, but particularly in the acute phase, because of its effectiveness in reducing both pain and edema.[61,62,87–89] Ice that has been frozen in a paper cup is applied to the area in small, circular motions for 10 to 15 minutes before and after activity, up to six times a day.

Cold packs applied directly to the joint area are useful in decreasing pain.[79] Current recommendations are to apply ice for 20 to 30 minutes every 2 hours.[74]

The application of cold to an area is contraindicated over superficial nerves or healing wounds, in patients with Raynaud's disease or cold sensitivity, and in areas with poor circulation or sensation.[2]

Thermotherapy.   Thermotherapy is the therapeutic application of heat. Thermal modalities generally involve the transfer of thermal energy. Five types of heat transfer exist:

1. *Convection* occurs when a liquid or gas moves past a body part. An example of this type of heat transfer is the whirlpool.

2. *Evaporation* occurs when there is a change in state of a liquid to a gas and a resultant cooling takes place. An example of this type of heat transfer occurs during spray and stretch techniques.

3. *Conversion* occurs when one form of energy is converted into another form. Examples of this type of heat transfer include ultrasound, shortwave diathermy, and microwave diathermy.

4. *Radiation* occurs when there is a transmission and absorption of electromagnetic waves.

5. *Conduction* occurs when heat is transferred between two objects that are in contact with each other. An example of this type of heat transfer occurs with hydrocollator heating packs.

Thermotherapy is used in the later stages of healing, because the deep heating of structures during the acute inflammatory stage may destroy collagen fibers and accelerate the inflammatory process.[90] However, in the later stages of healing, an increase in blood flow to the injured area is beneficial.

The physiologic effects of a local heat application include[71,91–94]:

▶ Dissipation of body heat. This effect occurs through selective vasodilation and shunting of blood via reflexes in the microcirculation, and regional blood flow.[95]

▶ Decreased muscle spasm.[66,78,95,96] The muscle relaxation probably results from a decrease in neural excitability on the sensory nerves, and hence gamma input.

▶ Increased capillary permeability, cell metabolism, and cellular activity, which have the potential to increase the delivery of oxygen and chemical nutrients to the area, while decreasing venous stagnation.[92,97]

▶ Increased analgesia through hyperstimulation of the cutaneous nerve receptors.

▶ Increased tissue extensibility.[95] This effect has obvious implications for the application of stretching techniques. The best results are obtained if heat is applied during the stretch, and if the stretch is maintained until cooling occurs after the heat has been removed.

Clinical Pearl

For a heat application to have a therapeutic effect, the amount of thermal energy transferred to the tissue must be sufficient to stimulate normal function, without causing damage to the tissue.[98]

Although the human body functions optimally between 36°C and 38°C, an applied temperature of 40°C and 45°C is considered effective for a heat intervention. Commercial hot packs, or electric heating pads, are a conductive type of superficial moist heat and the temperature of the unit is set anywhere between 65°C and 90°C. The moist heat pack causes an increase in the local tissue temperature, reaching its highest point about 8 minutes after the application.[99] The depth of penetration for traditional heating pads (and cold packs) is about 1 cm, which results in changes in the cutaneous blood vessels and the cutaneous nerve receptors.[70]

Wet heat produces a greater rise in local tissue temperature compared with dry heat at a similar temperature.[100] However, at higher temperatures, wet heat is not tolerated as well as dry heat.

It is important to assess the patient's sensitivity to temperature, pain, and circulation status prior to the use of thermotherapy. Moist heat should not be applied to an area with decreased sensation, poor circulation, an open wound, or an acute injury.[2] The application of moist heat to an area of malignancy also is contraindicated because it can increase the temperature of the tumor and increase the rate of growth.[2] Hemophiliacs also are at risk with thermotherapy because of the increased blood flow.

Ultrasound. Ultrasound is primarily used for its ability to deliver heat to deep musculoskeletal tissues such as tendon, muscle, and joint structures. Ultrasound produces high-frequency alternating current. The waves are delivered through the transducer, which has a metal faceplate with a piezoelectric crystal cemented between two electrodes. This crystal can vibrate very rapidly, converting electrical energy to acoustical energy. This energy leaves the transducer in a straight line. As the energy travels further from the transducer, the waves begin to diverge. The depth of penetration depends on the absorption and scattering of the beam. Depth of penetration is a factor of the medium being used (gel or lotion), contact quality of the transducer, treatment surface, and tissue type (muscle, skin, fat, etc.).[101,102] Scar tissue, tendon, and ligament demonstrate the highest absorption. Tissues that demonstrate poor absorption include bone, tendinous and aponeurotic attachments of skeletal muscle, cartilaginous covering of joint surfaces, and peripheral nerves lying close to bone.[103] The portion of the sound head that produces the sound wave is referred to as the effective radiating area (ERA). The ERA is always smaller than the transducer.

Clinical units typically deliver ultrasound of 0.75 to 3 MHz, with duty cycles ranging from 20 to 100 percent. The depth of penetration of the ultrasound is roughly inversely related to its frequency.[104,105] A frequency of 3 MHz is more superficial, reaching a depth of approximately 2 cm, whereas 1 MHz is effective to a depth of 4 or 5 cm.[106] Duty cycles less than 100 percent are usually termed *pulsed ultrasound*, whereas a 100 percent duty cycle is referred to as *continuous ultrasound*. Continuous mode ultrasound produces a thermal effect. Pulsed ultrasound does not. The thermal effects of ultrasound are similar to those previously described for thermotherapy. The nonthermal or mechanical properties of ultrasound are less well defined, but are believed to alter cellular permeability and metabolism, and may be important in the promotion of wound healing by reducing edema, pain, and muscle spasms.[107–110]

The beam nonuniformity ratio (BNR) of ultrasound is the maximal/average intensity (W/cm^2) found in the ultrasound field. Each transducer produces sound waves in response to the vibration of the crystal. This vibration has different intensities at points on the transducer head, having peaks and valleys of intensity. The greater ratio difference in the BNR, the more likely the transducer will have *hot spots*. Hot spots are areas of high intensity. High intensities have been shown to cause unstable cavitational effects and to retard tissue repair.[110,111] Intensities of 0.1 to 0.3 W/cm^2 are recommended for acute lesions, whereas 0.4 to 0.8 W/cm^2 are recommended for chronic lesions.[112]

Treatment times for ultrasound are based on the principle of 1 minute of ultrasound per treatment head area, although account must be taken of the pulse ratio employed. The pulse ratio needs to be higher for more acute lesions (1:4) and lower for more chronic ones (1:1, or continuous).

One study[113] demonstrated that to achieve a tissue temperature of 4°C, using continuous ultrasound, the following parameters and application times are necessary:

▶ 1 MHz at 1.5 W/cm^2 for 13 minutes.

▶ 3 MHz at 1.5 W/cm^2 for 4.5 minutes.

It must be remembered that the effects of ultrasound are predominantly empirical and are based on reported biophysical effects within tissue,[114,115] and on anecdotal experience in clinical practice.[116–118] Despite the paucity of documented evidence in terms of randomized control studies,[119] many benefits have been ascribed to ultrasound. These include:

▶ Production of cellular excitation, enhancing cellular activity rather than dampening it, and enhancing the inflammatory cascade, thereby encouraging the tissues to move into their next phase.[103,120–122]

▶ Decreased swelling when applied in a pulsed format during the inflammatory stage of healing.[112,114,115,123–128]

▶ Stimulation of the active cells and a maximization of scar production activity and quality, if applied during the neurovascular phase.[128–130] During the later phase, ultrasound appears to enhance the remodeling of tissue.[111,126,129]

▶ An alteration of the parameters of ultrasound changes the intent of the intervention.[58]

Phonophoresis. Phonophoresis refers to a specific type of ultrasound application in which pharmacologic agents, such as corticosteroids, local anesthetics, and salicylates, are introduced.[124,131–137] Phonophoresis has been used clinically since the early 1960s in attempts to drive these drugs transdermally into subcutaneous tissues. Both the thermal and nonthermal (mechanical) properties of ultrasound have been cited as possible mechanisms for the transdermal penetration of the pharmacologic agents. Increases in cell permeability and local vasodilation accompanied by the acoustic pressure wave may result in increased diffusion of the topical agent.[124,131,133]

The efficacy of phonophoresis has not been conclusively established. Some early studies have shown drug penetration as deep as 10 cm,[137-139] but a more recent study has cast doubt on these findings.[140] Other studies have examined the effects of phonophoresis with different corticosteroid concentrations, compared with ultrasound alone, in the intervention of various musculoskeletal conditions. Recent papers have argued that many of the commonly used cream-based preparations do not allow adequate transmission of the acoustic wave.[101,102,127] Gel-based preparations appear to be superior with respect to the transmissivity of ultrasound. Consequently, gel-based corticosteroid compounds might be expected to be superior for phonophoresis applications.

Hydrotherapy

Whirlpool. A whirlpool may be used in an attempt to facilitate the resorption of effusion. A cold whirlpool is indicated in acute and subacute conditions in which gentle exercise of the injured part is permitted. The temperature for a cold whirlpool is in the range of 50°F to 60°F (10° to 16°C). A warm whirlpool is indicated in chronic conditions. During the treatment, the body part may be exercised. The temperature of a warm whirlpool is in the range of 100°F to 110°F (39°C to 45°C).

Contrast Bath. Contrast baths are an alternating cycle of warm and cold whirlpools that create a cycle of alternating vasoconstriction and vasodilation. Contrast baths are used most often in the management of extremity injuries.[141,142] In a study by Myer and colleagues,[143] contrast therapy of 20 minutes' duration had no impact on the intramuscular temperature of the gastrocnemius of their subjects 1 cm below the subcutaneous fat, as measured by a microprobe.

Prolotherapy. Prolotherapy, also known as proliferation therapy, is a relatively controversial pain management technique that may be used as an intervention for degenerative or chronic injury to ligaments, tendons, fascia, and joint capsular tissue. Although prolotherapy is not administered by physical therapists, patients seen in the clinic may have received a course of prolotherapy from their physician and is thus included for completeness.

Prolotherapy is purported to allow rapid production of new collagen and cartilage through stimulation of the immune system's healing mechanism using injections of mild chemical or natural irritants, such as dextrose sugar, manganese, and glucosamine sulfate.[140a] The number of injections required per intervention are based on the type of injury.

Electrotherapeutic Modalities

Electrical stimulation. Historically, many clinicians have advocated electrical stimulation as a means of edema and pain reduction, and to enhance an individual's functional level and independence in the acute phase.[84,144-148] Electrical stimulation is traditionally used to[54]:

▶ Produce a muscle contraction.

▶ Stimulate sensory nerves to help treat pain (transcutaneous electrical nerve stimulation).

▶ Create an electrical field within the tissues to stimulate or alter the healing process.

In addition to its use in the acute phase, electrical stimulation can be used in the other stages of healing for the reduction of pain and for neuromuscular re-education.

Electrical current that passes through tissue forces nerves to depolarize. The type of nerve influenced in this way, and the rate at which the fiber is depolarized will determine the physiologic and, therefore, therapeutic effect achieved.[149,150] Recent reports in the literature utilizing animal models have shown varied results based on the type of waveform, polarity used, and frequency of intervention.[151-157]

The limited studies on post-surgical or acutely injured patients seem to indicate that electrical muscle stimulation is either as effective as, or more effective than, isometric exercises at increasing muscle strength and bulk,[158-162] in both atrophied[163] and normal muscles.[164,165]

However, according to Taylor and colleagues,[157] the present regimens being used (i.e., one intervention per day or three times per week) may be insufficiently aggressive to provide benefit.

Transdermal Iontophoresis. Transdermal iontophoresis is the administration of ionic therapeutic agents through the skin by the application of a low level electrical current. Iontophoresis has proved to be valuable in the intervention of musculoskeletal disorders. Iontophoresis causes an increased penetration of drugs and other compounds into tissues by the use of an applied current through the tissue. The principle behind iontophoresis is that an electrical potential difference will actively cause ions in solution to migrate according to their electrical charge. Ionized medications or chemicals do not ordinarily penetrate tissues, and if they do, it is not normally at a rate rapid enough to achieve therapeutic levels.[166] This problem is overcome by providing a direct current energy source that provides penetration and transport.[166,167]

> ### Clinical Pearl
>
> Negatively charged ions are repelled from a negative electrode and attracted toward the positive electrode. In contrast, the positive ions are repelled from the positive electrode and attracted toward the negative electrode.[166,167]

Iontophoresis has, therefore, been used for the transdermal delivery of systemic drugs in a controlled fashion.[168] The factors affecting transdermal iontophoretic transport include pH; the intensity of the current, or current density, at the active electrode; ionic strength; concentration of drug; molecular size; and the duration of the current flow (continuous or pulse current). The proposed mechanisms by which iontophoresis increases drug penetration are as follows:

▶ The electrical potential gradient induces changes in the arrangement of the lipid, protein, and water molecules.[169]

▶ Pore formation occurs in the stratum corneum (SC), the outermost layer of the skin.[170] The exact pathway by which ionized drugs transit the SC has not been elucidated. The impermeability of the stratum corneum is the main barrier to cutaneous or transcutaneous drug delivery. If the integrity of the SC is disrupted, the barrier to molecular transit may be greatly reduced.

▶ Hair follicles, sweat glands, and sweat ducts act as diffusion shunts with reduced resistance for ion transport.[171] Skin and fat are poor conductors of electrical current and offer greater resistance to current flow.

Iontophoresis can be performed using a wide variety of chemicals (Table 10-7). For a chemical to be successful in iontophoresis, it must solubilize into ionic components.

Following the basic law of physics that *like poles repel*, the positively charged ions are placed under the positive electrode while the negatively charged ions are placed under the negative electrode. If the ionic source is in an aqueous solution, it is recommended that a low concentration be used (2 to 4 percent) to aid in the dissociation.[178] Although electrons flow from negative to positive, regardless of electrode size, having a larger negative pad than a positive one will help shape the direction of flow.

Current intensity is recommended to be at 5 mA or less for all interventions. The duration of the treatment may vary from 10 to 45 minutes. Longer durations have been shown to produce a decrease in the skin impedance, thus increasing the likelihood of burns from an accumulation of ions under the electrodes.[179] An accumulation of negative ions under the positive electrode produces hydrochloric acid. An accumulation of positive ions under the negative electrode produces sodium hydroxide.

Other complications have included prolonged erythema that resolved in 24 hours, tingling, burning, and pulling sensations that were especially apparent at the start of the current, or if the amperage was turned up too rapidly. The visible erythema demonstrates the clear increase of blood flow and the influence of the iontophoresis.

At present, research has been focused on the development of iontophoretic patches for the systemic delivery of drugs. The iontophoretic patch has the option to monitor and control the power supplied during use, thus permitting safer and more reliable operation. The system can also detect the number of times the patch has been used and records the date and time of use, and its microprocessor can detect when the medicament is exhausted. Furthermore, the controller can be rendered unusable to avoid abuse once the drug is exhausted.

Extracorporal Shock-wave Therapy. High-energy extracorporeal shock waves have been used in urology for the disintegration of stone concretion for almost 15 years. For the past 10 years this technology has emerged as a treatment modality for managing pain caused by a broad range of musculoskeletal conditions. These conditions include tendinopathies and nonunion and delayed union of fractures.[180–182] Currently, the therapeutic mechanisms of shock waves in musculoskeletal problems or their specific biologic effects on the various musculoskeletal tissues (bone, cartilage, tendon, ligament) are not fully understood.[183] The extracorporeal shock wave is an acoustic wave characterized by high positive pressures of more than 1000 bar (100 Mpa), which can be developed within an extremely short rise time (10^{-9} sec) and followed by a low pressure phase of tensile stress equivalent to 100 bar (10 Mpa).[183a] A clinically applicable shock wave represents nothing more than a controlled explosion producing a sonic pulse in much the same way as a fast flying aircraft may produce a sonic boom.[183] When the shock wave enters the tissue it may be dissipated and reflected so that the kinetic energy is absorbed according to the integral structure of the tissues or structures that are exposed to the shock waves.[183] However, because the duration of the shock wave is so short (3 to 5 μsec) and is generated at low frequencies, no thermal effect is generated.[182] For shock waves to be effective in the clinical situation, the maximally beneficial pulse energy

TABLE 10-7 Various Ions Used in Iontophoresis

Ion	Polarity	Solution	Purpose/Condition
Acetate	−	2–5% acetic acid	Calcium deposits[172]
Atropine sulfate	+	0.001–0.01%	Hyperhidrosis
Calcium	+	2% calcium chloride	Myopathy, muscle spasm
Chlorine	−	2% sodium chloride	Scar tissue, adhesions
Copper	+	2% copper sulfate	Fungus infection
Dexamethasone	+	4 mg/mL dexamethasone Na-P	Tendonitis, bursitis[173]
Lidocaine	+	4% lidocaine	Trigeminal neuralgia[174]
Hyaluronidase	+	Wyadase	Edema[175]
Iodine	−	Iodex ointment	Adhesions, scar tissue[176]
Magnesium	+	2% magnesium sulfate (Epsom salts)	Muscle relaxant,[177] bursitis
Mecholyl	+	0.25%	Muscle relaxant
Potassium iodide	−	10%	Scar tissue
Salicylate	−	2% sodium salicylate	Myalgia, scar tissue
Tap water	+/−	—	Hyperhidrosis

+, positive, −, negative.

must be concentrated at the point at which treatment is to be provided. There are three mechanisms by which extracorporeal shock wave therapy (ESWT) units generate the shock waves: electromagnetic, electrohydraulic, and piezoelectric. The electromagnetic and piezoelectric units tend to generate lower energy shock waves than the electrohydraulic units.[183a] Medically useful shock waves usually are generated through a fluid medium (water) and a coupling gel to facilitate transmission into biologic tissues. The energy flux density (ED) refers to the shock wave energy "flow" through an area perpendicular to the direction of propagation.[183a] 1000 to 2000 shock waves of an energy flux density (ED) from 0.01 to 0.4 mJ/mm² are usually applied two to three times at weekly intervals.[184] Pulse duration is usually fixed at 3 to 5 μsec and the calculation of dose (total energy delivered) depends on the choice of energy level and the total number of shock wave impulses delivered.[183a] Most patients report a sharp pain sensation during the application of ESWT, necessitating a skin sensation test prior to its use.

A meta-analysis by Ogden et al[184a] reported that, of various applications of ESWT on musculoskeletal conditions, the use of ESWT for treating chronic, recalcitrant heel pain syndrome was the most credible.

ESWT is contraindicated for use in patients suffering from hemophilia (because it may cause microvascular disruption) and malignancy, and ESWT should not be applied over growth plates or where exposure to lung tissue may occur (clavicle or first rib).[183,183a]

Transcutaneous Electrical Nerve Stimulation (TENS). Transcutaneous electrical nerve stimulation (TENS) has been used effectively as a safe, noninvasive, drug-free method of treatment for various chronic and acute pain syndromes for many years. TENS was first introduced in the early 1950s to determine the suitability of patients with pain as candidates for the implantation of dorsal column electrodes. Depending on the parameters of electrical stimuli applied, there are several modes of therapy, resulting in different contributions of hyperaemic, muscle-relaxing, and analgesic components of TENS. TENS has been shown to be effective in providing pain relief in the early stages of healing following surgery,[185,185a,186–189] and in the remodeling phase.[190–193]

The percentage of patients who benefit from short-term TENS pain intervention has been reported to range from 50 to 80 percent, and good long-term results with TENS have been observed in 6 to 44 percent of patients.[190,192,194,195] However, most of the TENS studies rely solely on subjects' pain reports to establish efficacy and rarely on other outcome measures such as activity, socialization, or medication use.

TENS units typically deliver symmetric or balanced asymmetric biphasic waves of 100- to 500-msec pulse duration, with zero net current to minimize skin irritation,[196] and may be applied for extended periods.

Three modes of action are theorized for the efficacy of this modality (see Chap. 2):

1. ***Gate control mechanism.*** Spinal gating control through stimulation of the large, myelinated A-alpha fibers inhibits transmission of the smaller pain transmitting unmyelinated C fibers, and myelinated A-delta fibers[188,197] (Fig. 10-1).

2. ***Endogenous opiate control.*** When subjected to certain types of electrical stimulation of the sensory nerves, there may be a release of enkephalin from local sites within the central nervous system, and the release of β-endorphin from the pituitary gland into the cerebrospinal fluid[196,198,199] (Fig. 10-2). A successful application can produce an analgesic effect that lasts for several hours.

3. ***Central biasing.*** Intense electrical stimulation, approaching a noxious level, of the smaller C or pain fibers, produces a stimulation of the descending neurons (Fig. 10-3).

Summary of Rehabilitation Modalities
The purpose of a rehabilitative intervention is to improve the tolerance of a tissue to tension and stress, and to ensure that the tissue has the capacity to tolerate the various stresses that are placed on it. For the contractile tissues, such as the muscles, this is accomplished through measured rest, rehabilitative exercise, high-voltage electrical stimulation, central (cardiovascular)

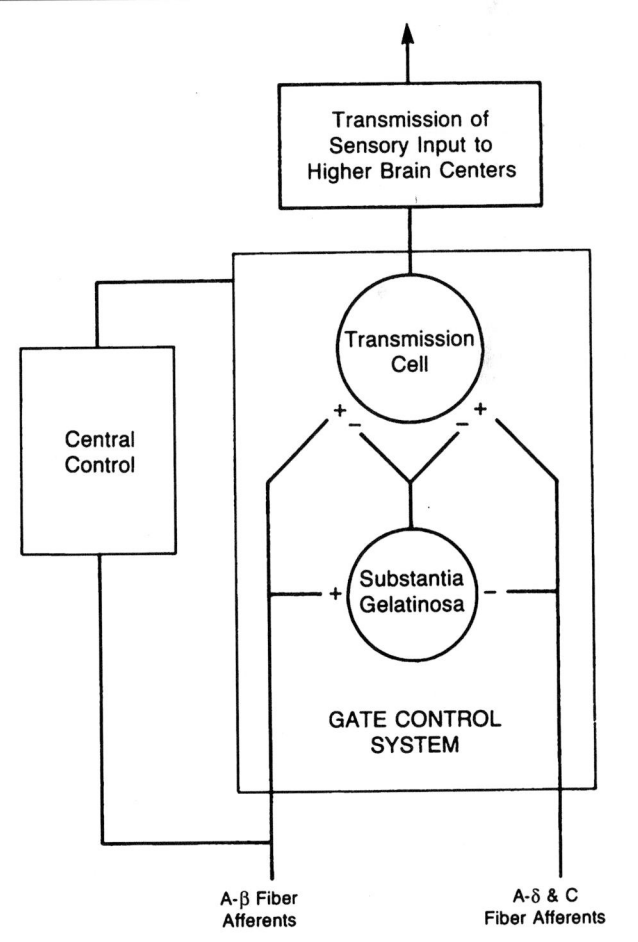

FIGURE 10-1 Modulation of pain by the gate control system. (Reproduced with permission from Dutton M. *Manual Therapy of the Spine: An Integrated Approach.* New York, NY: McGraw-Hill; 2002:58.)

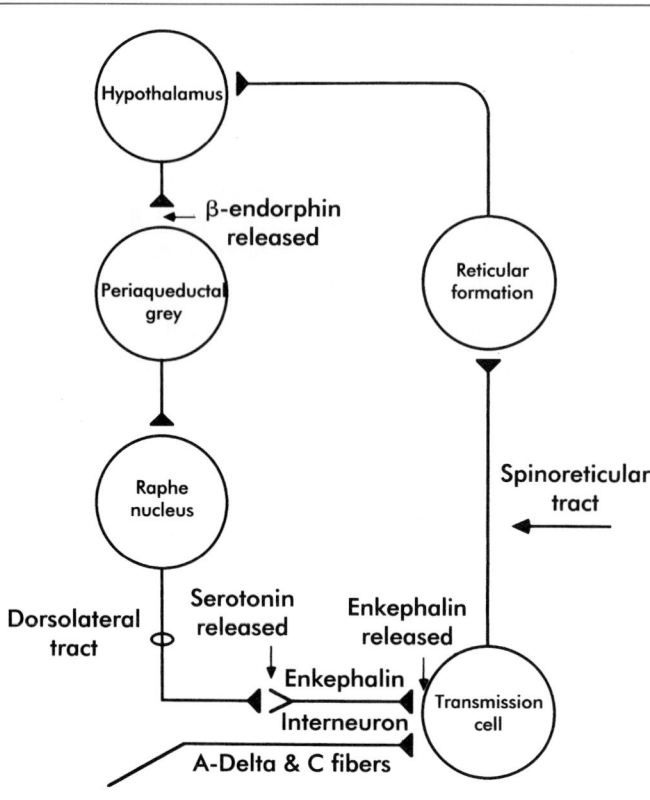

FIGURE 10-2 The endogenous opiate system of pain control. (Reproduced with permission from Dutton M. *Manual Therapy of the Spine: An Integrated Approach.* New York, NY: McGraw-Hill; 2002:59.)

aerobics, general conditioning, and absence from abuse.[9] The inert structures, such as ligaments and menisci, rely more on the level of tension and force placed on them for their recovery, which stimulates the fibroblasts to produce fiber and glycosaminoglycans.[200] Thus, the intervention chosen for these structures must involve the repetitive application of modified

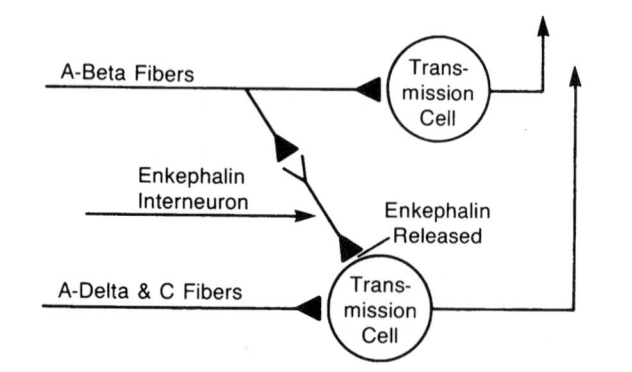

FIGURE 10-3 The descending analgesia system. (Reproduced with permission from Dutton M. *Manual Therapy of the Spine: An Integrated Approach.* New York, NY: McGraw-Hill; 2002:58.)

tension in the line of stress based on the stress of daily activities, or sporting activity.[200]

Restoration of normal ROM is essential to allow normal strength and mechanics to be regained.[31]

Misjudgments are sometimes made with the intervention. In general, the patient's pain should not last more than a couple of hours after an intervention. Pain that lasts longer than 2 hours is usually an indication that the intensity of the intervention, rather than the intervention itself, has been inappropriate. The clinician has to remove the notion that all pain is bad. In many respects, a slight increase in pain following an intervention is a more desirable finding than no change in pain, because it indicates that the correct structure is being stressed, albeit too aggressively.

Pharmacotherapy[201]

Pharmacologic intervention in the management of pain and inflammation is usually considered adjunctive to other interventions. Although physical therapists are not permitted by law to prescribe or dispense prescription drugs, an understanding of the potential effects of certain types of drugs commonly encountered during the rehabilitation process is essential. Drugs are widely used in the management of both acute and chronic pain and inflammation. The following discussion emphasizes drugs that are prescribed to control pain or inflammation. In the absence of data supporting a therapeutic benefit for a drug, toxicity associated with the drug can still occur. It is critical, therefore, for physicians to continually assess the balance between therapeutic benefit and safety.

Opioid Analgesics

Most of the narcotics used in medicine are referred to as *opioids*, because they are derived directly from opium or are synthetic opiates. Examples of these opioids include codeine, propoxyphene hydrochloride (Darvon), morphine, and meperidine (Demerol). Opioid receptors are present on the terminals of primary afferent nociceptive fibers that enter the spinal cord. Opioids block the potassium-evoked release of substance P and also act postsynaptically in the dorsal horn. Opioids typically are prescribed for patient populations with intractable pain, although there are many concerns with the use of these drugs. Most of the concern centers on the potential for addiction. The term *addiction* implies the development of physical dependence and tolerance requiring continued opioid use with increasing doses.

Nonopioid Analgesics

Nonopioid analgesics comprise a heterogeneous class of drugs, including the salicylates (aspirin and diflunisal), para-aminophenol derivatives (primarily acetaminophen), and the NSAIDs (Ibuprofen, Voltaren, Relafen, Naprosyn, Motrin, Indocin, Feldene, Lodine, Celebrex, Vioxx, and many others). Despite their diverse structures, nonopioid analgesics have similar therapeutic effects, oral efficacy, and side effect profiles. Nonopioid analgesics are better tolerated than opioids by ambulatory patients, have fewer sedative effects, and are much less likely to produce tolerance or dependence. Conversely, the hazards of long-term administration of these drugs are recognized.

NSAIDs have antipyretic, analgesic, and anti-inflammatory effects. The analgesic and anti-inflammatory activity of NSAIDs results primarily from the inhibition of arachidonic acid metabolism.[202] NSAIDs also seem to promote the inhibition of the release of cyclooxygenase-1 (COX-1) and cyclooxygenase-2 (COX-2) and the synthesis of prostaglandins at an injury site.[202] Inhibition of COX-1 also can produce gastrointestinal toxicity, including inflammation, ulceration, and bleeding, and can lead to perforation.[203] Suppression of prostaglandins is not limited to the site of injury and may result in alteration of normal function in the gastrointestinal mucosa and kidney blood flow. NSAIDs also may alter kidney blood flow by interfering with the synthesis of prostaglandins in the kidney that are involved in the autoregulation of blood flow and glomerular filtration.[204]

COX-2 inhibitors do not produce the same gastrointestinal effects as COX-1 inhibitors; therefore, they are safer to use in patients who are predisposed to gastric or kidney malfunctions. COX-2 drugs block only the COX-2 enzyme, which is responsible for triggering pain and inflammation.[202] Because COX-1 is not affected, the patient's stomach lining is protected and bleeding tendencies are avoided. Two COX-2 inhibitors currently available include celecoxib (Celebrex, Searle-Pharmacia) and rofecoxib (Vioxx, Merck).[202]

Corticosteroids

Corticosteroids are natural anti-inflammatory hormones produced by the adrenal glands under the control of the hypothalamus. Synthetic corticosteroids (cortisone, dexamethasone) commonly are used to treat a range of immunologic and inflammatory musculoskeletal conditions. Corticosteroids exert their anti-inflammatory effects by binding to a high-affinity intracellular cytoplasmic receptor present in all human cells.[205] As a result, these agents are capable of producing undesirable and sometimes severe systemic adverse effects that may offset clinical gains in many patients. The side effects from corticosteroids emulate from exogenous hypercortisolism, which is similar to the clinical syndrome of Cushing's disease. These side effects include[206]:

▶ *Cutaneous manifestations.* Cutaneous manifestations of hypercortisolism include delayed wound healing, acanthosis nigricans (a velvety, thickened, hyperpigmented plaque that usually occurs on the neck or in the axillary region), acne, ecchymoses after minor trauma, hyperpigmentation, hirsutism, petechia, and striae.

▶ *Hypokalemia.* Hypokalemia is a well-recognized side effect of corticosteroid therapy and is probably related to the mineralocorticoid effect of hydrocortisone, prednisone, and prednisolone. Dexamethasone has no mineralocorticoid effect.

▶ *Myopathy.* Two forms of corticosteroid-induced myopathy are recognized: acute and chronic. Acute myopathy may

be caused, in part, by hypokalemia, although corticosteroids (especially massive dosages) may have a direct effect on skeletal muscle. Both proximal and distal muscle weakness occur acutely, usually with an associated and significant elevation in serum creatinine phosphokinase, which is indicative of focal and diffuse muscle necrosis. In the more chronic form of myopathy, weakness is more insidious in onset and primarily involves proximal muscle groups.

▶ *Hyperglycemia.* Although it is not clear how corticosteroid use causes hyperglycemia, hyperglycemia, especially when combined with the immunosuppressive effect of corticosteroids, may significantly increase the risk for infection.

▶ *Neurologic impairments.* These impairments can include vertigo, headache, convulsions, and benign intracranial hypertension.

▶ *Osteoporosis.* Corticosteroids inhibit bone formation directly via inhibition of osteoblast differentiation and type I collagen synthesis and indirectly by inhibition of calcium absorption and enhancement of urinary calcium excretion.

▶ *Ophthalmologic side effects.* Corticosteroids increase the risk of glaucoma by increasing intraocular pressure, regardless of whether administered intranasally, topically, periocularly, or systemically.

▶ *Growth suppression.* Corticosteroids interfere with bone formation, nitrogen retention, and collagen formation, all of which are necessary for anabolism and growth.

Muscle Relaxants

Muscle relaxants, such as Robaxin and Soma, are thought to decrease muscle tone without impairment in motor function by acting centrally to depress polysynaptic reflexes. Because muscle guarding and spasm accompanies many musculoskeletal injuries, it was originally thought that these drugs, by eliminating the spasm and guarding, would facilitate the progression of a rehabilitation program. However, other drugs with sedative properties, such as barbiturates, also depress polysynaptic reflexes, making it difficult to assess whether centrally acting skeletal muscle relaxants actually are muscle relaxants as opposed to nonspecific sedatives.[207] There presently exists a discrepancy between the common clinical use of skeletal muscle relaxants and the results of controlled clinical trials evaluating their efficacy in comparison with placebo. Supporting evidence does not exist for their efficacy in pain of myogenic origin, nor is it clear if they provide an additive effect with exercises aimed at muscle relaxation.

Principle 3: Strengthen or Increase Flexibility

Therapeutic exercise is the foundation of physical therapy and a fundamental component of the vast majority of interventions. Prescribed accurately, therapeutic exercise can be used to restore, maintain, and improve a patient's functional status by increasing strength, endurance, and flexibility.

> **Clinical Pearl**
>
> The goal of the functional exercise progression is to identify the motion, or motions, that the patient is able to exercise into without eliciting symptoms other than postexercise soreness.[208]

Increasing Strength

Dosage

The dosage of an exercise refers to each particular patient's exercise capability, and is determined by a number of variables (see Chap. 6)[209] (Table 10-8). For these variables to be effective, the patient must be compliant and be able to train without exacerbating the condition.[200]

Exercise Hierarchy

A hierarchy exists for ROM and resistive exercises during the subacute (neovascularization) stage of healing, to ensure that any progression is done in a safe and controlled fashion. The hierarchy for the ROM exercises is as follows[210]:

1. Passive ROM.

2. Active assisted ROM.

3. Active ROM.

The hierarchy for the progression of resistive exercises is[210,211]:

1. Single-angle, submaximal isometrics performed in the neutral position.

2. Multiple-angle, submaximal isometrics performed at various angles of the range.

3. Multiple-angle maximal isometrics.

4. Small arc submaximal isotonics.

5. Full ROM submaximal isotonics.

6. Functional ROM submaximal isotonics.

Gentle resistance exercises can be introduced very early in the rehabilitative process. The various types of exercise progressions are described in Chapter 6 and in relevant chapters later in this book. Although some soreness can be expected, sharp pain should not be provoked.

At regular intervals, the clinician should ensure that:

▶ The patient is being compliant with their exercise program at home.

▶ The patient is aware of the rationale behind the exercise program.

▶ The patient is performing the exercise program correctly and at the appropriate intensity.

▶ The patient's exercise program is being updated appropriately based on clinical findings and patient response.

Flexibility

All clinicians would agree that restoration of, or improvement in, ROM is an important goal of the rehabilitation program.[212–214] ROM may be viewed as a combination of the amount of joint motion, termed *joint play*, and the degree of extensibility of the periarticular and connective tissues that cross the joint, termed *flexibility*. Some of the techniques used to restore joint play are described in Chapter 11. The principles concerning flexibility are discussed within this section.

> **Clinical Pearl**
>
> Optimum length-tension relationships and optimum force couple relationships ensure maintenance of normal joint kinematics.[215]

Restoration of normal length of the muscles may be accomplished using the following guidelines:

1. The muscle activity is inhibited and in the inhibitory period, the muscle should be stretched.
2. With true muscle shortness, stronger resistance is used to activate the maximum number of motor units, followed by vigorous stretching of the muscle.
3. Stretching should be performed at least three times a week using:
   a. Low force, avoiding pain.
   b. Prolonged duration.
   c. Rapid cooling of the muscle while it is maintained in the stretched position.
4. Heat should be applied to increase intramuscular temperature prior to, and during, stretching.[216,217] This heat can be achieved either through low-intensity warm-up exercise, or through the use of thermal modalities.[217] The application of a cold pack following the stretch is used to take advantage of the thermal characteristics of connective tissue, by lowering its temperature and thereby theoretically prolonging the length changes.[218]
5. Post-isometric relaxation techniques are advocated.

TABLE 10-8 Resistive Exercise Variables

Resistance (load or weight)
Duration
Frequency (weekly, daily)
Point of application
Bouts (timed sessions of exercise)
Sets and repetition
Mode (type of contraction)
Rests

Some areas of the body are difficult to stretch adequately using a lengthening technique. In these instances, techniques of localized manual release, using varying degrees of manual pressure along the length of the muscle and myofascial tissue, may be used[219] (see Chap. 11).

Principle 4: Correct Posture and Movement Impairment Syndromes

The focus of therapeutic intervention for posture and movement impairment syndromes is to alleviate symptoms and to play a significant role in educating the patient against habitual abuse. Therapeutic exercise programs for the correction of muscle imbalances should focus initially on regaining the normal length of a muscle, so that good movement patterns can be achieved. The intervention of any muscle imbalance is divided into three stages:

1. Restoration of normal length of the muscles. If the muscle activity is inhibited, the muscle should be stretched in the inhibitory period. If the muscle is hypertonic, muscle energy techniques may be used to produce minimal facilitation and a minimal stretch. With true adaptive shortening of the muscle, stronger resistance is used to activate the maximum number of motor units, followed by vigorous stretching of the muscle.

2. Strengthening of the muscles that have become inhibited and weak. Vigorous strengthening should be initially avoided to prevent substitutions and the reinforcement of poor patterns of movement.

3. Establishing optimal motor patterns to secure the best possible protection to the joints and the surrounding soft tissues.

In addition to using muscle energy techniques to stretch and strengthen muscles (see Chap. 11), and the techniques described under principle 3, earlier, other techniques may be used in the intervention of postural dysfunction and impairment. These include the Alexander technique, Feldenkrais method, Trager psychophysical integration, Pilates, and tai chi chuan.

Alexander Technique

The Alexander technique[220] is commonly viewed as a series of breathing and posture techniques. However, the purpose of the technique is to make patients more aware of structural imbalances, different ways of moving, and the excessive tensions that can be produced in activities of daily living. Although it is not within the scope of this text to fully describe the Alexander technique, some of its principles are outlined here, and the reader is encouraged to learn more about this technique through further reading.

The Alexander technique uses re-education to change the thought processes, as well as the postural and movement habits, that are theorized to provoke pain. According to this theory, the main reflex in the body, termed the *primary control*, which is situated in the area of the neck, controls all of the other reflexes of the body. Dysfunction of this main reflex, resulting from increased tension in the neck, causes a pulling back of the head and changes the relationship of the neck and back, eventually causing tensions in other parts of the body.

Based on these assumptions, Alexander devised three *directions*[220]:

1. *Allow the neck to be free.* The purpose of this direction is to eliminate any excess tension in the muscles of the neck.

2. *Allow the head to go forward and upward.* When the neck muscles are released, the head goes slightly forward and upward.

3. *Allow the back to lengthen and widen.* As the head moves slightly forward and upward, the spine lengthens. Because an increase in the spine length can also narrow the spine, widening of the back, through a retraction of the shoulders and broadening of the rib cage, is encouraged.

Feldenkrais Method

The Feldenkrais method of somatic education is a self-discovery process using movement. It was developed by Dr Moshe Feldenkrais, a physicist and electronics engineer. The aim of the Feldenkrais method is for an individual to move through relaxation and self-awareness, with minimum effort and maximum efficiency. The method teaches that many pains and movement restrictions are the result not of an actual physical defect or the inevitable deteriorations of age, but of habitual poor use.[221] Over time, this causes fatigue, disability, and pain.

The antidote, according to Feldenkrais, is to relearn certain functional movements and postures using a so-called organic learning style, based on the way humans learn to perform as they develop during early childhood. During this growth period, some of the movements are learned correctly, others are not. Incorrect movement patterns may result in inefficient movements or restrictions to movements. In humans, the premotor cortex relates to posture stability and the act of reaching. It is also the supplementary motor area for planning, programming, and initiating movement.[222] These latter components require correct sequencing and organization. The Feldenkrais method is seen as a way of reprogramming the nervous system and reteaching the body how to perform the functional movement patterns correctly.

Functional movement patterns involve the integration and sequencing of movement patterns while maintaining neuromuscular control. These patterns and postures are developed using the two aspects of the Feldenkrais method: awareness through movement (ATM) and functional integration (FI).[223] Although closely related, ATM and FI have fundamental differences[224]:

▶ ATM is usually done in a group, whereas FI involves one-on-one learning

▶ ATM involves the performance of gentle exploratory movements using verbal guidance. In contrast, FI uses guidance into nonhabitual movements, with tactile cueing by a trained practitioner

Both of the aspects work toward changing old movement patterns or creating new movement patterns. Individuals are led through a series of movement sequences. All movements are performed slowly, without pause and short of the range of discomfort and pain. The proponents of the Feldenkrais method claim that these movements promote improved attention and awareness.[225] It is also claimed that these movements refine the ability to detect information and make perceptual discriminations.[225] Regular use of such attentive explorations and integration of the skills lead to an automatic use of these motor abilities. An example of a Feldenkrais exercise is to move one's head in one direction and one's shoulder and eyes in the other.[223] These movement sequences are usually repeated a number of times.

Five key principles are involved in the development of the Feldenkrais method[224,225]:

1. Self-organization. Dynamic systems theorists believe that behaviors are assembled in the moment and context of the current movement task.

2. Behavior is dynamic and plastic.

3. Perturbation is the instrument of change.

4. Choice is necessary.

5. Human development follows a logical sequence.

The Feldenkrais method is both educational and experimental. It is process-, not goal-, oriented and is entirely pragmatic.[226] With acute conditions, the patient is started in the position of maximum comfort. The lesson then uses any movement, however small, within the limit of comfort. The patient is encouraged to become aware of the smoothness and clarity of the movement. The movement is repeated and practiced. Further movements within this framework are investigated and practiced. These movements are simple initially, becoming more complex as the patient gains confidence.[226]

Trager Psychophysical Integration[227]

Trager psychophysical integration (TPI) is a multifaceted intervention, consisting of light, gentle and painless movements to facilitate the release of deep-seated physical (and mental) patterns. TPI was designed at the beginning of the 20th century by Dr Milton Trager, and has been shown to be effective in promoting mobility and decreasing pain for patients with a wide variety of diagnoses, including cerebral palsy,[228] chronic spinal pain and dysfunction,[229] and arthritis.[227,230]

According to TPI philosophy, detrimental physical patterns are those developed by poor posture, trauma, stress, and poor movement habits.[231] Trager techniques serve to produce overall relaxation on the part of the patient, developing a sense of integration and effortless of movement through a series of guided movements and mental gymnastics.[232,233]

The Trager approach is broken down into two components: *tablework* and *mentastics*.

Tablework

Tablework consists of a series of gentle and painless movements that resemble general mobilization techniques. The body of the patient is passively moved by the clinician, who looks and feels for involvement of the tissue. The aim is to provoke a feeling of softness and freedom to motion throughout the body.[229] Using these movements, the entire body is mobilized. Rhythmic rocking motions are initiated during these movements to stimulate the vestibular and reticular activating systems of the patient. This is theorized to produce an overall sense of relaxation and well-being through an inhibition of the sympathetic system and the facilitation of the parasympathetic system.[234]

Mentastics

Mentastics is a system of active movements designed to enhance the feeling of well-being provided by the tablework exercises. Mentastics encourage the patient *not* to control the movement, as in traditional exercise, but to *let go* of the control.[229] The patient is taught to listen to signals of pain and fatigue and to change the symptoms by altering the movement. Over time, the patient learns how to move comfortably and to release tension.[233]

Pilates

The Pilates method of body conditioning (Pilates Inc) is a technique and apparatus developed in the 1940s by Joseph Pilates, who was prone to chronic illness as a child.

The Pilates method was first embraced by the dance community, but its inherent concept of core stabilization has since been used successfully in rehabilitation for the development of overall strength and fitness in patients with back pain, balance deficits, and urinary incontinence due to pelvic floor muscle weakness.

The Pilates method employs many of the concepts and techniques that physical therapists commonly employ, with an increased emphasis on neuromuscular control. As such, the Pilates method focuses on motor training, rather than motor strength, using precise and controlled exercises. The Pilates method stresses the importance of the so-called "powerhouse muscles" of the body, and the importance of deep, coordinated breathing. According to the Pilates method, the powerhouse muscles include the transversus abdominis, the lumbar multifidus, the pelvic floor muscles, and the diaphragm muscle. Approximately ten repetitions are needed for each exercise.

The Pilates exercises emphasize the maintenance of a neutral spine throughout machine and mat exercises. Many of the

Pilates exercises involve squeezing the inner thighs together in the Pilates stance, while simultaneously engaging the pelvic floor muscles in an effort to increase trunk stability. The *Pilates stance* involves slight external rotation in both hips and the lower extremities, while maintaining the thighs in firm contact. Other Pilates exercises include instructions on how to isolate a transversus abdominis contraction from the rest of the abdominal muscles. This is commonly achieved using the verbal cueing of "pull your belly button toward your spine". This contraction is then practiced in a variety of positions and techniques in order to enhance spinal, or core, stability. Pelvic stability is encouraged with such verbal cueing as "pull your sitting bones together" thereby producing a contraction of the ischiococcygeal muscle which provides support for the pelvic contents, in addition to contributing to sacroiliac joint stability.

Although many of the Pilates exercises can be performed on mats, specially designed Pilates equipment may also be used. Four basic machines comprise the Pilates equipment line:

1. *Reformer.* This is the basic machine of the Pilates method. It resembles a twin bed in size and frame and is equipped with handholds, pulleys, and cables that exercisers push or pull with their hands or feet. The reformer usually is used in the rehabilitation of hamstring tears, stress fractures, and lower back injuries.

2. *Cadillac, or trapeze table.* This piece of equipment is equipped with multiple bars and straps and features a pull-down bar. It is used for overall conditioning.

3. *Multi-chair.* The multi-chair is the equipment of choice for footwork and for ankle rehabilitation. It can be adapted for such activities as one-arm pushes, lunges, and dips.

4. *Ladder-barrel.* This piece of equipment consists of a sliding base and five rungs and is used for a variety of strengthening and flexibility exercises.

Tai Chi Chuan

Tai chi chuan (TCC) is a Chinese low-speed and low-impact conditioning exercise and is well known for its slow and graceful movements. During the practice, diaphragmatic breathing is coordinated with graceful motions to achieve mind tranquility.

Classical Yang TCC includes 108 postures, with some repeated sequences. Each training session includes 20 minutes of warm-up, 24 minutes of TCC practice, and 10 minutes of cool down.[235] Warm-up exercise is very important because it may enhance TCC performance and prevent injury. It usually includes ten movements (ROM exercises, stretching, and balance training), with 10 to 20 repetitions.[235]

The exercise intensity of TCC depends on training style, posture, and duration.[236,237] A high-squat posture and short training duration are suited to those with low levels of fitness or elderly participants; a low-squat posture and longer durations are suited to healthy or younger participants.[235]

Recent investigations have found that TCC is beneficial to cardiorespiratory function,[238] strength,[239] balance,[239,240] flexibility,[240] microcirculation,[241] and psychological profile.[236]

Hartman and colleagues[242] also reported that TCC could control fatigue and regulate pain during activities, and could improve walking speed and self-care activities in patients with osteoarthritis.

Principle 5: Analyze and Integrate the Entire Kinetic Chain

The expression *kinetic chain* is used to describe the function or activity of an extremity or trunk in terms of a series of linked chains. According to kinetic chain theory, each of the joint segments of the body involved in a particular movement constitutes a link along one of these kinetic chains. Because each motion of a joint is often a function of other joint motions, the efficiency of an activity can be dependent on how well these chain-links work together.[243]

> ### Clinical Pearl
>
> The number of links within a particular kinetic chain varies, depending on the activity. In general, the longer kinetic chains are involved with the more strenuous activities.

The concept of kinetic chains in rehabilitation originated from the work of Steindler.[244] Steindler[244] observed three types of *closed kinetic chain* (CKC) systems, noting an insurmountable load with no proximal or distal segment movement was the only "absolute" CKC. The second two types of CKC classifications observed by Steindler[244] involved segment movement and an external load on the distal segment in which (1) the load was overcome, or (2) the load was not overcome.[245] According to Steindler,[244] the open kinetic chain (OKC) system occurred when there was no load on the distal segment and the segment was free to move. Since Steindler originally proposed these definitions, the motion occurring at the distal segment has become a defining classification between OKC and CKC, whereby an OKC has a so-called free distal segment and a CKC has a fixed distal segment.[245]

Closed Kinetic Chain

A variety of definitions for a CKC activity have been proposed:

1. Palmitier defined an activity as closed if both ends of the kinetic chain are connected to an immovable framework, thus preventing translation of either the proximal, or distal joint center, and creating a situation whereby movement at one joint produces a predictable movement at all other joints.[246]
2. Gray[247] considered a closed-chain activity to involve fixation of the distal segment so that joint motion takes place in multiple planes, and the limb is supporting weight.
3. Dillman[248] described the characteristics of closed-chain activities to include relatively small joint movements, low joint accelerations, greater joint compressive forces, greater joint congruity, decreased shear, stimulation of joint proprioception, and enhanced dynamic stabilization through muscle co-activation.[249]

4. Kibler[249] defines a closed-chain activity as a sequential combination of joint motions that have the following characteristics:

   a. The distal segment of the kinetic chain meets considerable resistance.

   b. The movement of the individual joints, and translation of their instant centers of rotation, occurs in a predictable manner that is secondary to the distribution of forces from each end of the chain.

Examples of closed kinetic chain exercises (CKCEs) involving the lower extremities include the squat and the leg press. The activities of walking, running, jumping, climbing, and rising from the floor all incorporate closed kinetic chain components. An example of a CKCE for the upper extremities is the push-up, or when using the arms to rise out of a chair.

Clinical Pearl

In most activities of daily living, the activation sequence of the links involves a closed chain whereby the activity is initiated from a firm base of support and transferred to a more mobile distal segment.

Open Kinetic Chain

It is generally accepted that the difference between OKC and CKC activities is determined by the movement of the end segment. The traditional definition for an open-chain activity included all activities that involved the end segment of an extremity moving freely through space, resulting in isolated movement of a joint.

Examples of an open-chain activity include lifting a drinking glass and kicking a soccer ball. Open kinetic chain exercises (OKCEs) involving the lower extremity include the seated knee extension and prone knee flexion. Upper extremity examples of OKCE include the biceps curl and the military press.

OKCEs traditionally were deemed to be less functional in terms of many athletic movements, primarily serving a supportive role in strength and conditioning programs. As a result, the use of OKCE in clinical settings declined, and there was a shift in emphasis toward the use of CKCE.[246,250] This shift was initiated by the emergence of literature promoting the use of CKCE, particularly in knee rehabilitation following anterior cruciate ligament (ACL) reconstruction surgery (see Chap. 29).[246,250–256]

The benefit of CKCE over OKCE is based on the premise that CKCEs, particularly in the lower extremities, appear to replicate functional tasks better than OCKEs. This is because the CKCEs appear to allow the entire linkage system of the kinetic chain to be exercised together.[246,249,252,255,257–261] In addition, CKCEs have been shown to enhance joint congruency, decrease the shearing forces, and stimulate the articular mechanoreceptors using axial loading and increased compressive forces.[248,259,262–265] Thus, CKC activities are purported to

help reinforce the synchronization of the necessary muscle firing patterns for both antagonist and agonist muscle groups used during stabilization and ambulation.[246] However, there also appears to be much in the literature to suggest that OKCEs have a beneficial effect on function,[266–268] especially when combined with specific closed-chain exercises, or when used to strengthen individual muscles.[257]

The reason for this contradiction may be based on the terminology. For example, many activities, such as swimming and cycling, traditionally viewed as OKC activities, include a load on the end segment; yet the end segment is not "fixed" and restricted from movement. This ambiguity of definitions for CKC and OKC activities has allowed some activities to be classified in opposing categories.[248] Thus, there has been a growing need for clarification of OKC and CKC terminology, especially when related to functional activities.

The vast majority of functional activities involve a combination of the traditionally described open- and closed-chain actions, rather than one or the other. Thus, functional activities are best viewed as part of a continuum between open- and closed-chain actions. The work of Dillman and colleagues[248] and then Lephart and Henry[257] has attempted to address the confusion. Dillman and colleagues[248] proposed three classifications of activity because of the gray area between CKC and OKC activity. These classifications were based on the boundary condition, either moveable or fixed, and the presence or absence of a load on the end segment. An activity with a fixed boundary and no load does not exist, resulting in three classifications:

1. *Moveable no load (MNL).* These activities involve a moveable end with no load and closely resemble the extreme open-chain activity. An example of this type of activity is hitting a ball with a tennis racket.

2. *Moveable external load (MEL).* These activities involve a movable end with an external load and include a combination of open- and closed-chain actions, because they are characterized by co-contractions of the muscles around the joints. An example of this type of activity is the military press.

3. *Fixed external load (FEL).* These activities involve a fixed end with an external load (FEL), and closely resemble the extreme closed-chain activity. An example of this type of activity is the push-up.

Lephart and Henry suggested that a further definition could be made by analyzing the following characteristics of an activity:

▶ Direction of force.

▶ Magnitude of load.

▶ Muscle action.

▶ Joint motion.

▶ Neuromuscular function.

Under Lephart and Henry's classification, activities could be subdivided into four groups:

1. Activities that involve a fixed boundary with an external and axial load. An example of this type of activity is the use of a slide board.

2. Activities that involve a movable boundary with an external and axial load. An example of this type of activity is the bench press.

3. Activities that involve a movable boundary with an external and rotary load. An example of this type of activity is a resisted proprioceptive neuromuscular facilitation (PNF) motion pattern (see next section).

4. Activities that involve a moveable boundary with no load. An example of this type of activity is position training

Although both the Dillman and Lephart and Henry models appear to be describing the same concept, the Lephart and Henry model is distinct in that it incorporates diagonal or rotary components to the movements. Diagonal and rotary movements feature in the vast majority of functional activities.

In addition to the directions of motions and the magnitude of forces occurring, both open- and closed-chain activities rely heavily on neuromuscular input to control both the speed and the activation of the muscle contractions. This synchronization of motor activation is controlled by the various mechanoreceptors within the joint and muscle, which coordinate the relationship between the agonist and antagonist muscles. Another mechanoreceptor, the Golgi tendon organ, works to control the force generated during a particular activity, depending on the position of the joint (see Chap. 2). Several studies have concluded that the links within the system must be moving at their optimal velocity at the exact same moment, allowing for maximal velocity at the terminal segments, for the successful completion of an activity.[246,269] However, repetitive deviation from the correct movement pattern can result in an inefficient substitution patterning. A progression that includes slow unresisted activity, which is advanced to include quicker movements against resistance, theoretically results in central nervous system engram patterning, through repetition and precision of movement.[246]

Implications for a Rehabilitation Program

It should be clear that for a kinetic chain to operate efficiently, there must be an optimal sequential activation of the limb segments involved. This then allows for an efficient generation and transfer of force along the kinetic chain.[270] A number of studies have illustrated the importance of the sequential activation of these links.[271,272]

A comprehensive rehabilitation program thus should integrate the entire kinetic chain, using a blend of OKCEs and CKCEs. This integration must occur during functional exercises, with the emphasis determined by the activity to be restored.

> **Clinical Pearl**
>
> The rehabilitation of the kinetic chain should address the strength and flexibility of the kinetic chain, using the principle of specificity, with the specific elements of the rehabilitation program being determined by both the existing pathology and the functional goals of the patient.[257,273]

In addition, under the concept of specificity, rather than isolating OKCEs or CKCEs, it may be wise to emphasize functional positioning during the exercise training, while striking a balance between mobility and stability.[257,274]

Several objectives must be met if the rehabilitation of the functional kinetic chain is to be comprehensive[257]:

1. The first objective in the rehabilitation program, the healing phase, is the restoration of functional stability, which is the ability to control the translation of the joint during dynamic functional activities, through the integration of both the primary and secondary stabilizers.[275]

2. The second objective, the functional phase, is to restore sports-specific or functional-specific movement patterns. The functional phase begins once the patient has near full, pain-free ROM.

3. The final objective is assessing the readiness of the patient to return to his or her prior level of function or level of athletic performance.

Principle 6: Incorporate Neuromuscular Re-education

Neuromuscular re-education (NMR) has been defined as a method of training the enhancement of unconscious motor responses by stimulating both afferent signals and central mechanisms responsible for dynamic joint control.[276] The aims of NMR are to improve the ability of the nervous system to generate a fast and optimal muscle-firing pattern, to increase joint stability, to decrease joint forces, and to relearn movement patterns and skills.[276]

Many studies have evaluated the effect of injury to the neuromuscular system.[277–283] If muscle control is poor, joint strain and pain may result.[284,285] Trauma to tissues that contain mechanoreceptors may result in partial deafferentation, which can lead to proprioceptive deficits and alter joint function.[286,287] For example, in addition to the mechanical restraint provided by ligaments, it has been observed that ligaments provide neurologic feedback that directly mediates reflex muscle contractions about a joint.[286,288]

NMR is initiated with simple activities and progresses to more complex activities requiring proprioceptive and kinesthetic awareness, once the neuromuscular deficits are minimized.[257,273] It is recommended that NMR be initiated as early as possible in the rehabilitative process.[283]

The purposes of NMR are to:

▶ Decrease pain and spasm by reducing the tone.

▶ Restore mobility and control along the functional kinetic chain.

▶ Restore force-couple mechanisms to optimal efficiency.

▶ Restore functional movements away from the base of support.

▶ Restore functional movements against gravity.

Neuromuscular control is governed by the central nervous system via the integration of information from the vestibular, vision, and proprioceptive systems.

Proprioceptive Retraining

Because afferent input is altered after joint injury, proprioceptive training must focus on the restoration of proprioceptive sensibility to retrain these altered afferent pathways and enhance the sensation of joint movement.[283] Although ROM and progressive resistive exercises help reestablish joint proprioception, they are not as effective in restoring function as exercises that involve weight bearing (CKCEs). That is not to say that proprioceptive retraining cannot occur until the patient has achieved full weight-bearing status. On the contrary, these exercises can be performed within the confines of the weight-bearing status. According to Voight,[283,289] the standard progression for proprioceptive retraining involves:

1. *Static stabilization exercises with closed-chain loading and unloading* (**weight shifting**). This phase initially employs isometric exercises around the involved joint on solid and even surfaces, before progressing to unstable surfaces. The early training involves balance training and joint repositioning exercises and usually is initiated (in the lower extremities) by having the patient place the involved extremity on a 6- to 8-inch-high stool, so that the amount of weight bearing can be controlled more easily. The proprioceptive awareness of a joint can also be enhanced by using an elastic bandage or orthotic, or through taping.[286,290–294] As full weight bearing through the extremity is restored, a number of devices, such as a mini-trampoline, balance board, Swiss ball, and wobble board, can be introduced. Exercises on these devices are progressed from double limb support, to single leg support, to support while performing sports-specific skills.

2. *Transitional stabilization exercises.* The exercises during this phase involve conscious control of motion without impact and replace isometric activity with controlled concentric and eccentric exercises throughout a progressively larger range of functional motion. The physiologic rationale behind the exercises in this phase is to stimulate dynamic postural responses and increase muscle stiffness. Muscle stiffness has a significant role in improving

dynamic stabilization around the joint, by resisting and absorbing joint loads.[295]

3. *Dynamic stabilization exercises.* These exercises involve the unconscious control and loading of the joint, and introduce both ballistic and impact exercises to the patient.

A delicate balance between stability and mobility is achieved by coordination among muscle strength, endurance, flexibility, and neuromuscular control.[296] The neuromuscular mechanism that contributes to joint stability is mediated by the articular mechanoreceptors. These receptors provide information about joint position sense and kinesthesia.[280,286,294,297] The objective in NMR is to restore proximal stability, muscle control, and flexibility through a balance of proprioceptive retraining and strengthening.

Initially, CKCEs are performed within the pain-free ranges or positions. OKCEs, including mild plyometric exercises, may be built upon the base of the closed-chain stabilization to allow normal control of joint mobility.

The neuromuscular emphasis during these exercises is on functional positioning during exercise rather than isolating open- and closed-chain activities.[296] The activities should involve sudden alterations in joint positioning that necessitate reflex muscular stabilization coupled with an axial load.[286,296] Such activities include rhythmic stabilization performed in both a closed- and open-chain position,[298] and in the functional position of the joint.[296] The use of a stable, and then an unstable, base during CKCEs encourages co-contraction of the agonists and antagonists.[298]

Weight-shifting exercises are ideal for this. For example, the following weight-shifting exercises may be used for the upper extremity:

▶ Standing and leaning against a treatment table or object (Fig. 10-4).

▶ In the quadriped position, rocking forward and backward with the hands on the floor or on an unstable object (Fig. 10-5).

▶ Kneeling in the three-point position. A Body Blade can be added to this exercise to increase the difficulty (Fig. 10-6).

▶ Kneeling in the two-point position (Fig. 10-7).

▶ Weight shifting on a Fitter while in a kneeling position (Fig. 10-8).

▶ Weight shifting on a Swiss ball with the feet on a chair, in the push up position (Fig. 10-9).

▶ Slide board exercises in the quadruped position moving hands forward and backward, in opposite diagonals (Fig. 10-10) and in opposite directions.

Following treatment of any joint, re-training of the muscles must be carried out to re-establish coordination. PNF techniques are especially useful in this regard. PNF techniques require motions of the extremities in all three planes.[299] PNF techniques

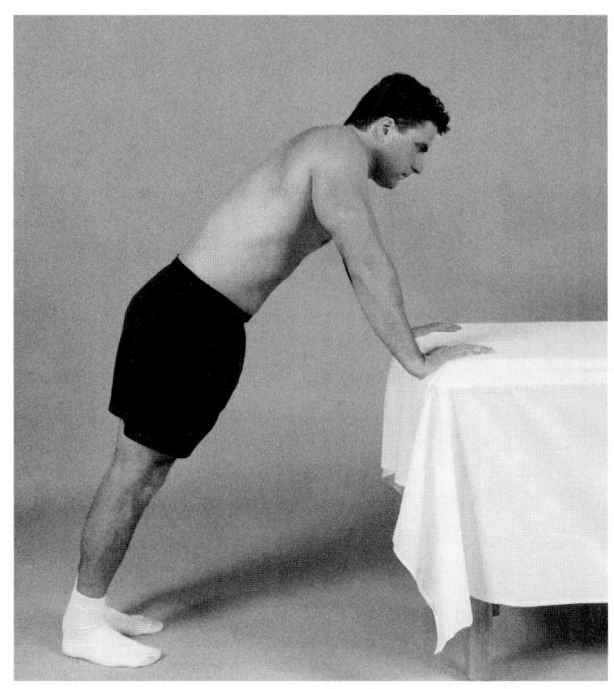

FIGURE 10-4   Joint compression and weight-shifting exercise.

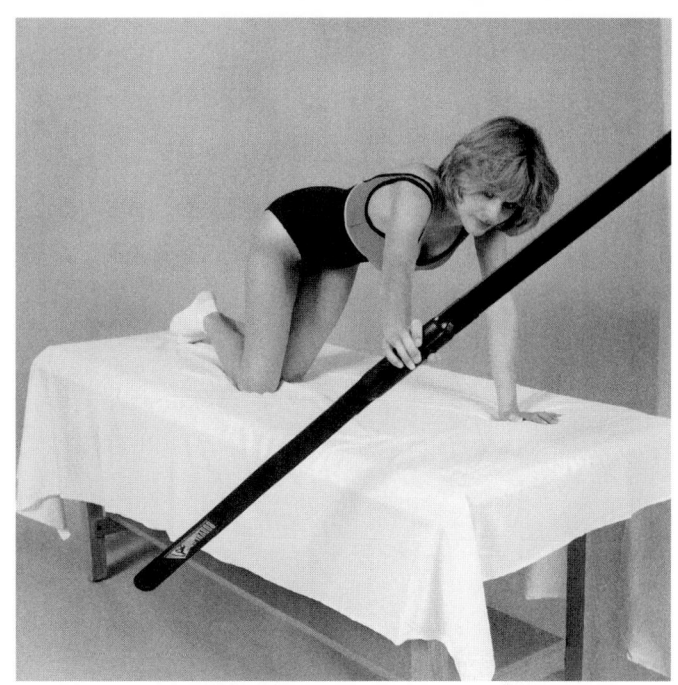

FIGURE 10-6   Three-point kneel with Body Blade.

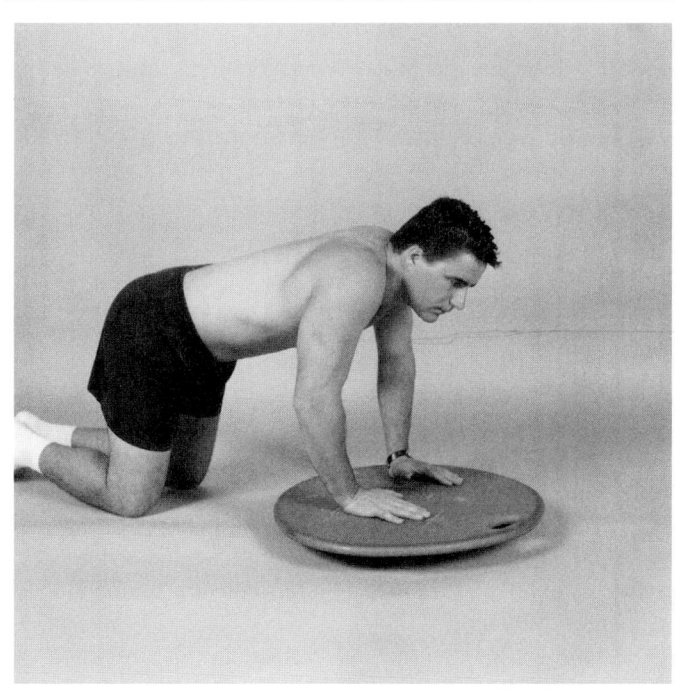

FIGURE 10-5   Quadriped rocking.

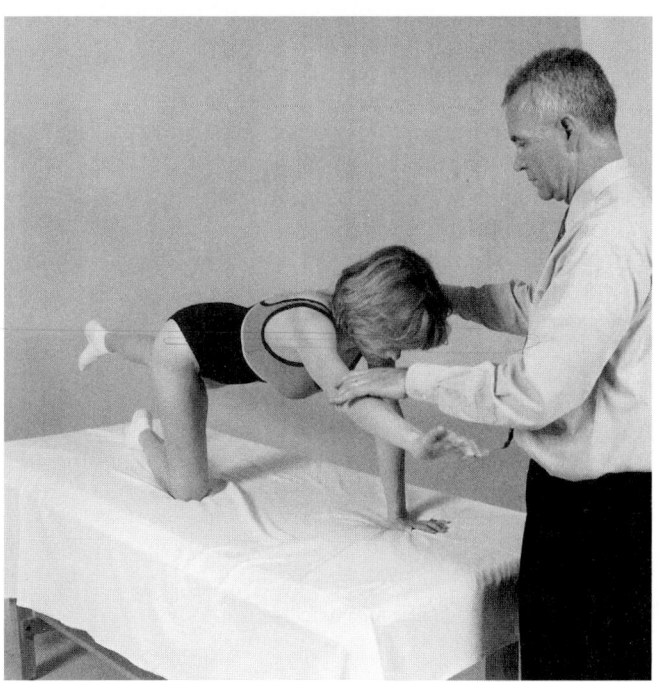

FIGURE 10-7   Two-point kneel.

that use combinations of spiral and diagonal patterns are designed to enhance coordination and strength.[300] The diagonal patterns 1 and 2 (see Chap. 11) are appropriate, with resistance being added as appropriate.

Balance Retraining

Balance retraining focuses on the ability to maintain a position through both conscious and subconscious motor control. Motor control of the extremities is dependent on afferent sensory and

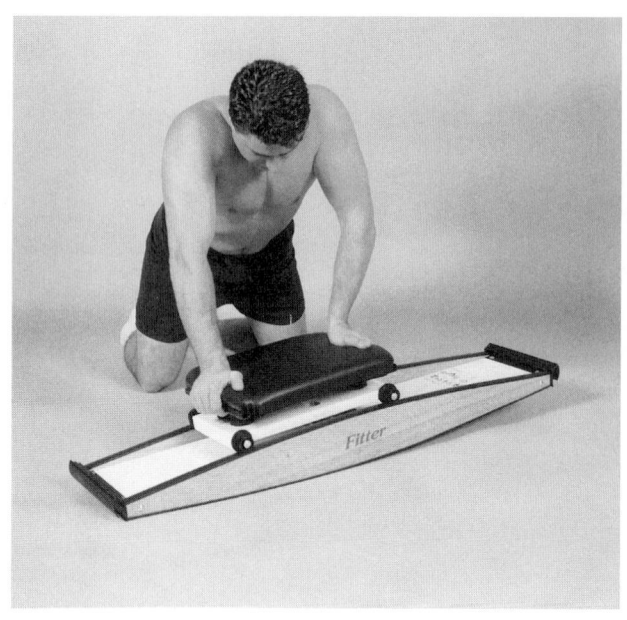

FIGURE 10-8 Weight shifting on a Fitter.

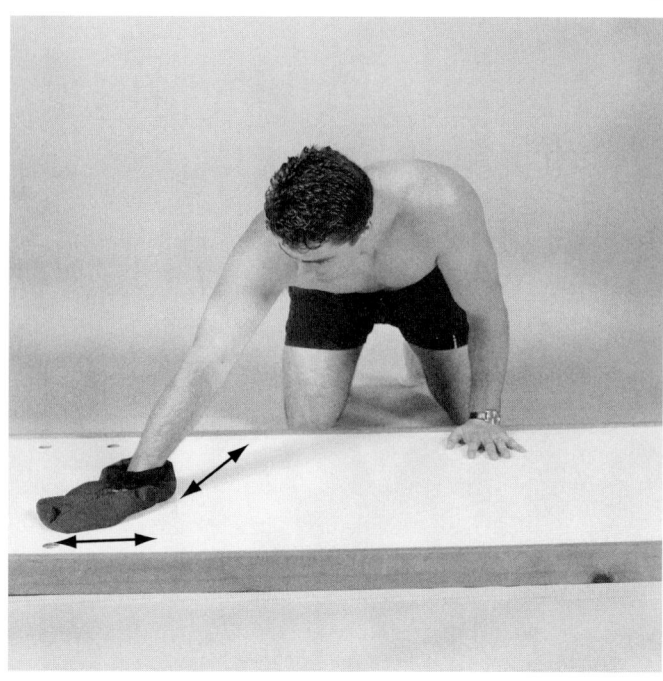

FIGURE 10-10 Slide board exercise.

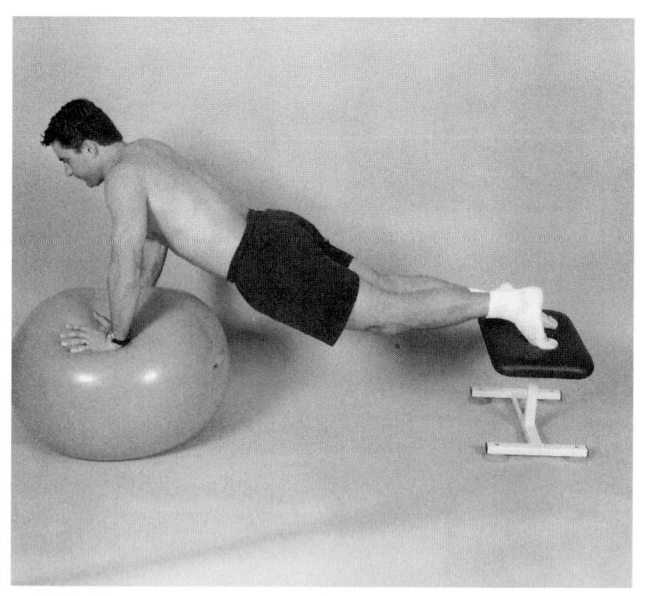

FIGURE 10-9 Weight shifting on a Swiss ball and chair.

proprioceptive mechanoreceptors, such as Golgi tendon units, muscle spindles, and joint receptors (see Chap. 2). It also is dependent on efferent reflexive and voluntary muscular response.[301]

Balance retraining is an important component of the rehabilitative process, particularly in the lower extremities. The usual progression employed involves a narrowing of the base of support while increasing the perturbation, and changing the weight-bearing surface from hard to soft, or from flat to uneven.

Principle 7: Improve Functional Outcome

Functional rehabilitation is an enhancement of the traditional concepts of rehabilitation of improving strength and ROM, and is related to agility, proprioception, pain level, and the severity of the injury.

Functional progression training should involve not merely the reproduction of an activity or task by an exercise. Instead, the ultimate goal of functional training is the restoration of the patient's confidence, which implies a return to normal of the neurovascular, neurosensory, and kinesthetic systems of the body, so that the reflex performance of a movement is not deliberate, hesitant, or dyskinetic.[302–304]

It should be obvious that the speed and extent by which the injured tissues heal determines both the speed and extent of the progression toward an optimum functional outcome. One of the keys to these progressions is a controlled and safe continuum, in which the patient can improve his or her functional status without harming the healing structures.

Functional progression training, as with exercise progressions, must be designed in a sequential, step-by-step manner, beginning with simple tasks and progressing to highly coordinated tasks, with each step in the process requiring greater skill than

TABLE 10-9 Sports Parameter Rating Scale[307]

Sport	Flexibility	Strength	Speed	Anaerobic	Aerobic
Football	3	4	4	3	2
Halfbacks	3	4	4	4	3
Basketball	3	3	4	4	4
Baseball	3	3	4	4	2
Tennis	4	2	4	4	3
Swimming	4	4	3	2	4
Sprinters	4	4	2	4	2
Long-distance running	3	2	2	2	4
Sprinting	3	3	2	4	2
Golf	3	4	3	2	1
Soccer	3	2	3	4	4
Bicycling	3	3	4	3	4
Ice skating	3	2	4	3	4
Skiing	3	3	4	3	2
Volleyball	3	2	4	4	2
Cheerleading	3	3	4	2	2

The scale (1–4) represents the relative importance of each parameter to the sport.

the last. The overriding principle of functional rehabilitation is to return patients to the functional level they desire, or at which they were previously functioning.[303]

Ideally, the functional progression should be based on the SAID (*specific adaptation to imposed demands*) principle, in order to prepare the patient to meet the specific demands of his or her vocation, ADLs, or recreation. Functional tasks can be designed to assess the speed, strength, agility, endurance, and power of the patient, which can then be equated with function.[305]

What is considered to be "normal" flexibility, strength, speed, and aerobic or anaerobic endurance for most patients in rehabilitation is inadequate for those patients returning to sport.[306] Kibler[307] advocates the use of a sports parameter scale in determining the relative contribution of these performance factors in various sporting activities (Table 10-9).

A number of functional progressions for athletes have been devised to guide the clinician. Most of these progressions originated from postsurgical protocols, in particular from ACL reconstructions and rotator cuff surgery, which deal with a variety of functional levels. Functional progressions that are specific to the lower or upper extremity are included in various chapters of this book. Functional progressions and their grading for the nonathlete also are included.[308]

Principle 8: Maintain or Improve Overall Fitness

Whenever possible, the clinician should address the impact on the patient resulting from the loss of physical activity. This loss of activity affects both the cardiovascular and the musculoskeletal systems and can occur very rapidly. Thus, it is important that the rehabilitation program includes exercises that maintain, or improve, the patient's cardiovascular endurance.

Physical activity has been defined as "any bodily movement produced by skeletal muscles that result in energy expenditure."[309] When a person undertakes work or exercise, a number of the body systems adapt to the demands of the required tasks, particularly the cardiorespiratory and neuromuscular systems.[310] The maximum work capacity of the cardiorespiratory system is a factor of the maximal amount of oxygen that can be taken in and used by the body, or VO_2 max, whereas the capacity of the neuromuscular system is a factor of the maximum tension that can be developed by the working muscle, or muscles—the maximal voluntary contraction. The maximum capacity of either of these systems can be sustained only for a very short period. The VO_2 max of an individual decreases by up to 25 percent after 3 weeks of bed rest.[311]

The basal metabolic rate (BMR) is the amount of energy required to sustain the body at rest in a supine position. Thus, physical activity is measured as a ratio between the BMR and the rate required to perform a particular task. This ratio is measured as a metabolic equivalent of the task (MET). Moderate physical activity is activity performed at an intensity of 3 to 6 METs, and is the equivalent of brisk walking at 3 to 4 mph for most healthy adults.[312]

Physical activity is closely related to, but distinct from, the subsets of exercise and physical fitness. Exercise is defined as "planned, structured, and repetitive bodily movement done to improve or maintain one or more components of physical fitness."[309] This differs from the definition of physical fitness, which is "a set of attributes that people have or achieve that relates to the ability to perform physical activity."[309]

Regular physical activity has long been regarded as an important component of a healthy lifestyle, and it is well established from controlled experimental trials that active individuals have high levels of cardiorespiratory fitness.[309] Intermittent activity, provided it is continued, also confers substantial benefits.[313-315] Studies have demonstrated that within a few weeks of discontinuing an endurance training program, the positive effects of exercise are almost completely lost, with approximately half of that loss occurring within the first 2 weeks.[316,317]

Clinical experience and limited studies suggest that people who maintain or improve their strength and flexibility may be better able to perform daily activities, may be less likely to develop pain, and may be better able to avoid disability, especially as they advance into older age.[309] Regular physical activity also may contribute to better balance, coordination, and agility, which in turn may help prevent falls in the elderly.[318]

Epidemiologic research has demonstrated protective effects of varying strength between physical activity and risk for several chronic diseases, including coronary heart disease,[313,319,320] hypertension,[321,322] non–insulin-dependent diabetes mellitus,[323,324] osteoporosis,[325,226] colon cancer,[327] and anxiety and depression.[328]

Patterns of physical activity appear to vary with demographic characteristics. Men are more likely than women to engage in regular activity,[329] vigorous exercise, and sports.[330] The total amount of time spent engaging in physical activity normally declines with age.[331,332] Adults at retirement age (65 years) show some increased participation in activities of light to moderate intensity, but, overall, physical activity declines continuously as age increases.[331,333] African Americans, and other ethnic minority populations, are less active than white Americans,[329,333,334] and this disparity is more pronounced for women.[334] People with higher levels of education participate in more leisure-time physical activity than do people with less education.[329] Differences in education and socioeconomic status account for most, if not all, of the differences in leisure-time physical activity associated with race and ethnicity.[335]

Cross-training exercises, including cycling, upper body ergonometer UBE, and water running, all increase cardiovascular endurance. However, it must be remembered that although cross training can produce a similar cardiovascular effort as the original sport, it does not necessarily produce the same musculoskeletal effects (Table 10-10).

Whenever exercise is performed, the body needs time to recover. Fatigue and recovery from fatigue are complex processes that depend on physiologic and psychological factors. The physiologic factors include the adequacy of the blood supply to the working muscle, and the maintenance of a viable chemical environment, whereas the psychological factors include motivation and incentive.[310]

The patient who is injured while performing an activity or exercise is likely to return to that activity once the symptoms subside.[312] Thus, the body needs to be prepared for a resumption of the stresses and demands that the activity or exercise will place upon it. If not, when the patient returns to competitive sports or functional and work activities, fatigue may result in alterations in efficient movements or make the individual susceptible to injury.

Aerobic conditioning is especially valuable for those who participate in sports that involve endurance.[337] Nirschl[9,338] recommends general body conditioning for patients, which provides the following benefits:

▶ Increased regional perfusion.

▶ Neurophysiologic synergy and overflow.

▶ Neurologic stimulation.

▶ Minimization of the domino effect of weakness of adjacent structures.

▶ Minimization of negative psychological effects.

▶ Obesity control.

A progressive program is recommended to condition the patient for a return to activity, and to prevent overload injuries. This program should address the following areas[22,249,339-342]:

▶ *Flexibility.* Attempts should be made to improve general body flexibility, with an emphasis on the specific activity or exercise. The general flexibility exercises should address the entire kinetic chain and not just the joint in question (shoulder rotation and elbow motion in the arm, low back, hip rotation, and hamstrings in the legs).

▶ *Strengthening.* The exercises to improve strength should be applied in appropriate amounts and locations to address sport-specific or functional-specific activities.

▶ *Power.* Power is incorporated through the use of rapid movements in appropriate planes with light weights and ballistic activities.

▶ *Endurance.* Endurance can be built up with anaerobic exercises.

If our sedentary society is to change to one that is more physically active, clinicians must play their role in communicating to their patients the amounts and types of physical activity that are needed to prevent disease and promote health, because patients respect their advice.[312,342] Patients should be routinely counseled to adopt and maintain regular physical activity.

Inadequate reimbursement, limited knowledge of the benefits of physical activity, and a lack of training in community physical activity counseling are barriers to achieving these goals. While policy makers work to improve reimbursement for preventive services, clinicians should develop effective ways to teach physical activity counseling.[312] The personal physical activity practices of health professionals should not be overlooked. Health professionals should be physically active, not only to benefit their own health but to make more credible their endorsement of an active lifestyle.[312]

TABLE 10-10 Comparison of Physiologic Adaptations to Resistance Training and Aerobic Training[336]

Variable	Result Following Resistance Training	Result Following Endurance Training
PERFORMANCE		
Muscle strength	Increases	No change
Muscle endurance	Increases for high power output	Increases for low power output
Aerobic power	No change or increases slightly	Increases
Maximal rate of force production	Increases	No change or decreases
Vertical jump	Ability increases	Ability unchanged
Anaerobic power	Increases	No change
Sprint speed	Improves	No change or improves slightly
MUSCLE FIBERS		
Fiber size	Increases	No change or increases slightly
Capillary density	No change or decreases	Increases
Mitochondrial density	Decreases	Increases
Fast heavy-chain myosin	Increases in amount	No change or decreases in amount
ENZYME ACTIVITY		
Creatine phosphokinase	Increases	Increases
Myokinase	Increases	Increases
Phosphofructokinase	Increases	Variable
Lactate dehydrogenase	No change or variable	Variable
METABOLIC ENERGY STORES		
Stored ATP	Increases	Increases
Stored creatine phosphate	Increases	Increases
Stored glycogen	Increases	Increases
Stored triglycerides	May increase	Increases
CONNECTIVE TISSUE		
Ligament strength	May increase	Increases
Tendon strength	May increase	Increases
Collagen content	May increase	Variable
Bone density	No change or increase	Increases
BONE COMPOSITION		
Percentage body fat	Decreases	Decreases
Fat-free mass	Decreases	No change

ATP, adenosine triphosphate.

Principle 9: Patient/Client-Related Instruction

Patient/client-related instruction forms the cornerstone of every intervention. During the physical therapy visits, the clinician and the patient work to alter the patient's perception of their functional capabilities. Together, the patient and clinician discuss the parts of the patient's life that he or she can and cannot control and then consider how to improve those parts that can be changed. It is imperative that the clinician spend time educating the patient about his or her condition, so that the patient can fully understand the importance of his or her role in the rehabilitation process and become an educated consumer. Educating the patient about strategies to adopt in order to prevent recurrences, and to self-manage his or her condition, is also very important. Discussions about intervention goals must continue throughout the rehabilitative process and must be mutually acceptable.

Oftentimes, the physician relies on the physical therapist to give a broader explanation about the condition, and to answer questions and concerns related to the rehabilitative process. The aim of patient education is to create independence, not dependence, and to foster an atmosphere of learning in the clinic. A detailed explanation should be given to the patient in a language that he or she can understand. This explanation should include:

▶ The name of the structure(s) involved, the cause of the problem, and the effect of the biomechanics on the area. Whenever possible, an illustration of the offending structure should be shown to the patient. Anatomic models can be used to explain biomechanical principles in lay person's terms.

▶ Information about tests, diagnosis, and interventions that are planned.

▶ The prognosis of the problem and a discussion about the patient's functional goals. An estimation of healing time is useful for the patient, so that he or she does not become frustrated at a perceived lack of progress.

▶ What patients can do to help themselves. This includes the allowed use of the joint or area, a brief description about the relevant stage of healing, and the vulnerability of the various structures during the pertinent healing phase. This information makes the patient aware and more cautious when performing ADLs, recreational activities, and the home exercise program. Emphasis should be placed on dispelling the myth of "no pain, no gain," and patients should be encouraged to respect pain. Patients often have misconceptions about when to use heat and ice, and it the role of the clinician to clarify such issues.

▶ Home exercise program. Before prescribing a home exercise program, the clinician should take into consideration the time that will be needed to perform the program. In addition, the level of tolerance and motivation for exercise varies among individuals, and is based on their diagnosis and stage of healing. A short series of exercises, performed more frequently during the day, should be prescribed for patients with poor endurance or when the emphasis is functional re-education. Longer programs, performed less frequently, are aimed at building strength or endurance. Each home exercise program needs to be individualized to meet the patient's specific needs. Although two patients may have the same diagnosis, the examination may reveal different positive findings and stages of healing both of which may alter the intervention.

There are probably as many ways to teach as there are to learn. The clinician needs to be aware that people may have very different preferences for how, when, where, and how often to learn. It is not within the scope of this text to discuss all of the theories on learning, but an overview of the major concepts is merited.

Litzinger and Osif[343] organized individuals into four main types of learners, based on instructional strategies:

1. *Accommodators.* This type looks for the significance of the learning experience. These learners enjoy being active participants in their learning and will ask many questions, such as, "What if?" and "Why not?"

2. *Divergers.* This type is motivated to discover the relevancy of a given situation and prefers to have information presented in a detailed, systematic, and reasoned manner.

3. *Assimilators.* This type is motivated to answer the question, "What is there to know?" These learners like accurate, organized delivery of information, and they tend to respect the knowledge of the expert. They are perhaps less instructor-intensive than some other types of learners and will carefully follow prescribed exercises, provided a resource person is clearly available and able to answer questions.

4. *Convergers.* This type is motivated to discover the relevancy, or "how," of a situation. The instructions given to this type of learner should be interactive, not passive.

Another way of classifying learners that frequently is used was devised by Taylor,[344] who proposed that there are three common learning styles:

1. *Visual.* As the name suggests, the visual learner assimilates information by observation, using visual cues and information such as pictures, anatomic models, and physical demonstrations.

2. *Auditory.* Auditory learners prefer to learn by having things explained to them verbally.

3. *Tactile.* Tactile learners, who learn through touch and interaction, are the most difficult of the three groups to teach. Close supervision is required with this group until they have demonstrated to the clinician that they can perform the exercises correctly, and independently. PNF techniques, with the emphasis on physical and tactile cues, often work well with this group.

A patient's learning style can be identified by asking how he or she prefers to learn. Some patients will prefer a simple handout with pictures and instructions; others will prefer to see the exercises demonstrated, and then be supervised while they perform the exercises. Some may want to know why they are doing the exercises, which muscles are involved, why they are doing three sets of a particular exercise, and so on. Others will require less explanation.

If the clinician is unsure about the patient's learning style, it is recommended that each exercise first be demonstrated by the clinician, and then by the patient. The rationale and purpose behind each of the exercises must be given, as well as the frequency and intensity expected.

Compliance is vitally important and varies from patient to patient. Various studies have found that average compliance with medication regimens only occurs in 50 to 60 percent of patients, and compliance with physical therapy programs is approximately 40 percent.[345]

Several factors have been outlined to improve compliance, among them[346–348]:

▶ Involving the patient in the intervention planning and goal setting.

▶ Realistic goal setting for both short- and long-term goals.

- Promoting high expectations regarding final outcome.
- Promoting perceived benefits.
- Projecting a positive attitude.
- Providing clear instructions and demonstrations with appropriate feedback.
- Keeping the exercises pain-free or with a low level of pain.
- Encouraging patient problem solving.

Principle 10: Ensure a Safe Return to Function

The purpose of the physical therapy intervention is to safely return a patient to their pre-injury state, with as little risk of re-injury as possible and with the minimum amount of patient inconvenience. Normally this is achieved with a gradual progression of strengthening and flexibility exercises while avoiding further damage to an already compromised structure.[349] For the athlete, the criteria for return to play include no pain, full pain free ROM, normal flexibility/strength/balance, good general fitness, normal sports mechanics, and demonstration of sports-specific skills.[350]

Most episodes of pain resolve on their own, provided that the condition is not exacerbated through constant re-injury, and that the injured tissue is allowed to progress through the natural stages of healing. If this natural progression does not occur, chronic pain can result. The prognosis for chronic pain syndromes is generally poor, and often requires a biopsychosocial approach. In these instances, the clinician may need to consider resources that will aid the patient both physically and emotionally. This can include referrals for counseling, pain-control, stress management, and self-help groups.

In the modern, cost-conscious health care environment, the stage at which the patient is ready to return to full function is not often played out in the clinic. Although patient education emphasizing a slow and gradual return to activity can, to some extent, prepare the subject for this phase, reinjury, or insufficient recovery, is a real possibility.

If the opportunity to supervise the return to full function presents itself, the clinician must focus on ensuring that the timing and dynamic control of muscular activity has returned. Activities to promote this goal include fast-alternating, weight-bearing co-contraction activities; quick changes of direction in a wide variety of weight-bearing postures; and simulation of activities broken down into smaller components.

Summary

Patient compliance and motivation in the rehabilitation program is paramount. Compliance and motivation are closely related to patient education, patient involvement, and patient encouragement. The focus of the intervention must include these factors,

and should also include an exercise program that emphasizes function and patient independence. Functional restoration is far more effective than seeking a technique to "repair" the problem.

It is important that the patient view his or her rehabilitative progression with a healthy respect for pain, combined with the importance of returning to normal levels of function as early as possible. Pain is, unfortunately, a necessary component of the healing process. However, the patient needs to be educated about what constitutes healing pain in comparison to injurious pain. Clear instructions must be given to the patient on how to recognize injurious pain, and how to avoid additional strain.

The frequency and duration of the patient's care need to be addressed. The common practice is to see patients two to three times per week; however, this is not always necessary, particularly with well-motivated patients. It is the duty of all clinicians to make the patient's visit meaningful. Clinic visits must include a level of skilled intervention that the patient cannot receive in the home environment. Placing the patient on a moist heating pad and then having him or her perform a routine rehabilitation program that is not constantly being updated or modified is a waste of the patient's time, and does little to foster public confidence in the profession.

Each session must have a purpose. The clinician should attempt to explain any gains or losses the patient has made since the previous session, and the possible reasons. New goals should be discussed at each session, and any changes to the intervention plan, and their rationale, discussed.

Documentation

Documentation of the examination and intervention process is an important part of any therapeutic regimen. As a record of client care, it provides useful information for the clinician, other members of the health-care team, and third-party payers. The American Physical Therapy Association (APTA) is committed to developing and improving the art and science of physical therapy, including practice, education, and research. To help meet these responsibilities, the APTA Board of Directors has approved a number of guidelines for physical therapy documentation. These guidelines are intended as a foundation for the development of more specific guidelines in specialty areas, while at the same time providing guidance across all practice settings. In all instances, it is the position of the APTA that the physical therapy examination, evaluation, diagnosis, prognosis and intervention shall be documented, dated, and authenticated by the physical therapist who performs the service.

REVIEW QUESTIONS*

1. What are the three components that comprise the intervention?
2. What is the pneumonic used to remember the principles utilized to control pain and inflammation?
3. Give five therapeutic benefits of the application of manual therapy in the early stages of healing.

4. With passive mobility testing, which stage of healing is indicated when pain is reported before tissue resistance is felt by the clinician?

5. What are the intervention goals during the inflammatory stage of healing?

---

* Additional questions to test your understanding of this chapter can be found in the Online Learning Center for *Orthopaedic Assessment, Evaluation, and Intervention* at www.duttononline.net.

REFERENCES

1. Guide to physical therapist practice. *Phys Ther* 2001;81:S13–S95.

2. Doucette SA, Goble EM. The effect of exercise on patellar tracking in lateral patellar compression syndrome. *Am J Sports Med* 1992;20:434–440.

3. Cyriax J. *Textbook of Orthopaedic Medicine, Diagnosis of Soft Tissue Lesions.* 8th ed. London, England: Bailliere Tindall; 1982.

4. Maitland GD. The hypothesis of adding compression when examining and treating synovial joints. *J Orthop Sports Phys Ther* 1980;2:7.

5. Maitland G. *Peripheral Manipulation.* 3rd ed. London, England: Butterworth; 1991.

6. McKenzie R, May S. Introduction. In: McKenzie R, May S, eds. *The Human Extremities: Mechanical Diagnosis and Therapy.* Waikanae, New Zealand: Spinal Publications New Zealand Ltd; 2000:1–5.

7. Bennett N, et al. *Results from the 1994 General Household Survey.* London, England: Office of Population Censuses and Surveys, HMSO; 1995.

8. Garrick JG. A practical approach to rehabilitation. *Am J Sports Med* 1981;9:67–68.

9. Nirschl RP. Prevention and treatment of elbow and shoulder injuries in the tennis player. *Clin Sports Med* 1988;7:289–308.

10. McMaster WC. Cryotherapy. *Phys Sports Med* 1982; 10:112–119.

11. Maadalo A, Waller JF. Rehabilitation of the foot and ankle linkage system. In: *The Lower Extremity and Spine in Sports Medicine.* St Louis, Mo: CV Mosby; 1986:560–583.

12. Quillen WS, Rouillier LH. Initial management of acute ankle sprains with rapid pulsed pneumatic compression and cold. *J Orthop Sports Phys Ther* 1981;4:39–43.

13. Starkey JA. Treatment of ankle sprains by simultaneous use of intermittent compression and ice packs. *Am J Sports Med* 1976;4:142–143.

14. Wilkerson GB. Treatment of ankle sprains with external compression and early mobilization. *Phys Sports Med* 1985; 13:83–90.

15. Cole AJ, Farrell JP, Stratton SA. Functional rehabilitation of cervical spine athletic injuries. In: Kibler BA, Herring JA, Press JM, eds. *Functional Rehabilitation of Sports and Musculoskeletal Injuries.* Gaithersburg, Md: Aspen; 1998:127–148.

16. Farrell JP. Cervical passive mobilization techniques: The Australian approach. *Phys Med Rehabil Rev* 1990;4:309–334.

17. Booth FW. Physiologic and biochemical effects of immobilization on muscle. *Clin Orthop Rel Res* 1987;219:15–21.

18. Booth FW, Kelso JR. The effect of hindlimb immobilization on contractile and histochemical properties of skeletal muscle. *Pflugers Arch* 1973;342:231–238.

19. Haggmark T, Eriksson E. Cylinder or mobile cast brace after knee ligament surgery. *Am J Sports Med* 1979;7:48–56.

20. Farmer JA, Pearl AC. Provocative issues. In: Leadbetter WB, Buckwalter JA, Gordon SL, eds. *Sports Induced Inflammation: Clinical and Basic Science Concepts.* Park Ridge, Ill: American Academy of Orthopaedic Surgeons; 1990:781–791.

21. Helminen HJ, et al. Effects of immobilization for 6 weeks on rabbit knee articular surfaces as assessed by the semi-quantitative stereomicroscopic method. *Acta Anat Nippon* 1983;115:327–335.

22. Kibler WB. Concepts in exercise rehabilitation of athletic injury. In: Leadbetter WB, Buckwalter JA, Gordon SL, eds. *Sports-Induced Inflammation: Clinical and Basic Science Concepts.* Park Ridge, Ill: American Academy of Orthopaedic Surgeons; 1990:759–769.

23. Salter RB, Field P. The effects of continuous compression on living articular cartilage. *J Bone Joint Surg* 1960;42A:31–49.

24. Woo SLY, Tkach LV. The cellular and matrix response of ligaments and tendons to mechanical injury. In: Leadbetter WB, Buckwalter JA, Gordon SL, eds. *Sports-Induced Inflammation: Clinical and Basic Science Concepts.* Park Ridge, Ill: American Academy of Orthopaedic Surgeons; 1990:189–202.

25. Cox JS. Surgical and nonsurgical treatment of acute ankle sprains. *Clin Orthop* 1985;198:118–126.

26. Eiff MP, Smith AT, Smith GE. Early mobilization versus immobilization in the treatment of lateral ankle sprains. *Am J Sports Med* 1994;22:83–88.

27. Akeson WH, et al. The chemical basis for tissue repair. In: Hunter LH, Funk FJ, eds. *Rehabilitation of the Injured Knee.* St Louis, Mo: CV Mosby; 1984:93–147.

28. Tipton CM, et al. Influence of exercise in strength of medial collateral knee ligaments of dogs. *Am J Physiol* 1970;218:894–902.

29. Noyes FR, et al. Biomechanics of ligament failure: II. An analysis of immobilization, exercise, and reconditioning effects in primates. *J Bone Joint Surg* 1974;56A:1406–1418.

30. Teitz CC, et al. Tendon problems in athletic individuals. *J Bone Joint Surg* 1997;79A:138–152.

31. Pease BJ, Cortese M. Anterior knee pain: Differential diagnosis and physical therapy management. In: *Orthopaedic Physical Therapy Home Study Course 92-1.* La Crosse, Wis: Orthopaedic Section, American Physical Therapy Association; 1992.

32. Leadbetter WB. Corticosteroid injection therapy in sports injuries. In: Leadbetter WB, Buckwalter JA, Gordon SL, eds. *Sports-Induced Inflammation: Clinical and Basic Science Concepts.* Park Ridge, Ill: American Academy of Orthopaedic Surgeons; 1990:527–545.

33. Dehne E, Tory R. Treatment of joint injuries by immediate mobilization based upon the spiral adaption concept. *Clin Orthop* 1971;77:218–232.

34. Hunt TK. Wound healing and wound infection: Theory and surgical practice. New York, NY: Appleton-Century-Crofts: 1980.

35. Singer AJ, Clark RAF. Cutaneous wound healing. *N Engl J Med* 1999;341:738–746.

36. Janda V. Muscle strength in relation to muscle length, pain and muscle imbalance. In: Harms-Ringdahl K, ed. *Muscle Strength.* New York, NY: Churchill Livingstone; 1993:83.

37. Hettinga DL. Inflammatory response of synovial joint structures. In: Gould JA, Davies GJ, eds. *Orthopaedic and Sports Physical Therapy.* St Louis, Mo: CV Mosby; 1985:87–117.

38. Thorndike A. *Athletic Injuries: Prevention, Diagnosis and Treatment.* Philadelphia, Pa: Lea and Febiger; 1962.

39. Bourne MH, et al. Anterior knee pain. *Mayo Clinic Proc* 1988;63:482–491.

40. Brody LT, Thein JM. Nonoperative treatment for patellofemoral pain. *J Orthop Sports Phys Ther* 1998;28:336–344.

41. Herring SA, Kibler BW. A framework for rehabilitation. In: Kibler BW, Herring JA, Press JM, eds. *Functional Rehabilitation of Sports and Musculoskeletal Injuries*. Gaithersburg, Md: Aspen; 1998:1–8.

42. Astrand PO, Rodahl K. *Textbook of Work Physiology*. New York, NY: McGraw-Hill; 1973:411–420.

43. Zarins B. Soft tissue injury and repair: Biomechanical aspects. *Int J Sports Med* 1982;3:9–11.

44. Frank G, et al. Medial collateral ligament healing. A multidisciplinary assessment in rabbits. *Am J Sports Med* 1983;11:379.

45. Leach RE. The prevention and rehabilitation of soft tissue injuries. *Int J Sports Med* 1982;3(suppl 1):18–20.

46. Safran MR, et al. Lateral ankle sprains: A comprehensive review: Part 2: Treatment and rehabilitation with an emphasis on the athlete. *Med Sci Sports Exerc* 1999;31(suppl):S438–S447.

47. Safran MR, et al. Lateral ankle sprains: A comprehensive review: Part 1: Etiology, pathoanatomy, histopathogenesis, and diagnosis. *Med Sci Sports Exerc* 1999;31(suppl):S429–S437.

48. Evans RB. Clinical application of controlled stress to the healing extensor tendon: A review of 112 cases. *Phys Ther* 1989; 69:1041–1049.

49. Klaffs CE, Arnheim DD. *Modern Principles of Athletic Training*. St Louis, Mo: CV Mosby; 1989.

50. Porterfield JA, DeRosa C. *Mechanical Low Back Pain*. 2nd ed. Philadelphia, Pa: WB Saunders; 1998.

51. Barlow Y, Willoughby J. Pathophysiology of soft tissue repair. *Br Med Bull* 1992;48:698–711.

52. McKenzie R, May S. Physical examination. In: McKenzie R, May S, eds. *The Human Extremities: Mechanical Diagnosis and Therapy*. Waikanae, New Zealand: Spinal Publications New Zealand Ltd; 2000:105–121.

53. Liebenson C. Integrating rehabilitation into chiropractic practice. In: Liebenson C, ed. *Rehabilitation of the Spine: A Practitioner's Manual*. Baltimore, Md: Lippincott Williams and Wilkins; 1996:13–43.

54. Prentice WE. Using therapeutic modalities in rehabilitation. In: Prentice WE, Voight ML, eds. *Techniques in Musculoskeletal Rehabilitation*. New York, NY: McGraw-Hill; 2001:289–303.

55. Chapman CE. Can the use of physical modalities for pain control be rationalized by the research evidence? *Can J Physiol Pharmacol* 1991;69:704–712.

56. Feine JS, Lund JP. An assessment of the efficacy of physical therapy and physical modalities for the control of chronic musculoskeletal pain. *Pain* 1997;71:5–23.

57. McMaster WC, Liddle S, Waugh TR. Laboratory evaluation of various cold therapy modalities. *Am J Sports Med* 1978; 6:291–294.

58. Watson T. The role of electrotherapy in contemporary physiotherapy practice. *Manual Ther* 2000;5:132–141.

59. Knight KL. *Cryotherapy: Theory, Technique, and Physiology*. Chattanooga, Tenn: Chattanooga Corp; 1985.

60. Hocutt JE, et al. Cryotherapy in ankle sprains. *Am J Sports Med* 1982;10:316–319.

61. Knight KL. *Cryotherapy in Sports Injury Management*. Champaign, Ill: Human Kinetics; 1995:38–98.

62. Meeusen R, Lievens P. The use of cryotherapy in sports injuries. *Sports Med* 1986;3:398–414.

63. Merrick MA, et al. The effects of ice and compression wraps on intramuscular temperatures at various depths. *J Athl Training* 1993;28:236–245.

64. Clarke R, Mellon R, Lind A. Vascular reactions of the human forearm to cold. *Clin Sci* 1958;17:165–179.

65. Fox RH. Local cooling in man. *Br Med Bull* 1961;17:14–18.

66. Kalenak A, et al. Athletic injuries: Heat vs cold. *Am Fam Phys* 1975;12:131–134.

67. Johnson DJ, et al. Effect of cold submersion on intramuscular temperature of the gastrocnemius muscle. *Phys Ther* 1979; 59:1238–1242.

68. Cobbold AF, Lewis OJ. Blood flow to the knee joint of the dog: Effect of heating, cooling and adrenaline. *J Physiol* 1956; 132:379–383.

69. Wakim KG, Porter AN, Krusen FH. Influence of physical agents and certain drugs on intra-articular temperature. *Arch Phys Med Rehab* 1951;32:714–721.

70. Oosterveld FGJ, et al. The effect of local heat and cold therapy on the intraarticular and skin surface temperature of the knee. *Arthritis Rheum* 1992;35:146–151.

71. Abramson DI, Bell B, Tuck S. Changes in blood flow, oxygen uptake and tissue temperatures produced by therapeutic physical agents: Effect of indirect or reflex vasodilation. *Am J Phys Med* 1961;40:5–13.

72. Knight KL, Londeree BR. Comparison of blood flow in the ankle of uninjured subjects during therapeutic applications of heat, cold, and exercise. *Med Sci Sports Exerc* 1980;12:76–80.

73. Pappenheimer SL, Eversole SL, Soto-Rivera A. Vascular responses to temperature in the isolated perfused hind-limb of a cat. *Am J Physiol* 1948;155:458–451.

74. Adamson C, Cymet T. Ankle sprains: Evaluation, treatment, rehabilitation. *Md Med J* 1997;46:530–537.

75. Irrgang JJ, Delitto A, et al. Rehabilitation of the injured athlete. *Orthop Clin North Am* 1995;26:561–578.

76. Daniel DM, Stone ML, Arendt DL. The effect of cold therapy on pain, swelling, and range of motion after anterior cruciate ligament reconstructive surgery. *Arthroscopy* 1994;10:530–533.

77. Konrath GA, et al. The use of cold therapy after anterior cruciate ligament reconstruction. A prospective randomized study and literature review. *Am J Sports Med* 1996;24:629–633.

78. Michlovitz SL. The use of heat and cold in the management of rheumatic diseases. In: Michlovitz SL, ed. *Thermal Agents in Rehabilitation*. Philadelphia, Pa: FA Davis; 1990.

79. Speer KP, Warren RF, Horowitz L. The efficacy of cryotherapy in the postoperative shoulder. *J Shoulder Elbow Surg* 1996; 5:62–68.

80. Kellett J. Acute soft tissue injuries: a review of the literature. *Med Sci Sports Exerc* 1986;18:5.

81. McMaster WC. A literary review on ice therapy in injuries. *Am J Sports Med* 1977;5:124–126.

82. Hartviksen K. Ice therapy in spasticity. *Acta Neurol Scand* 1962;3(suppl):79–84.

83. Basset SW, Lake BM. Use of cold applications in the management of spasticity. *Phys Ther Rev* 1958;38:333–334.

84. Lamboni P, Harris B. The use of ice, air splints, and high voltage galvanic stimulation in effusion reduction. *Athl Training* 1983; 18:23–25.

85. Waylonis GW. The physiological effects of ice massage. *Arch Phys Med Rehab* 1967;48:42–47.

86. Belitsky RB, Odam SJ, Hubley-Kozey C. Evaluation of the effectiveness of wet ice, dry ice, and cryogen packs in reducing skin temperature. *Phys Ther* 1987;67:1080–1084.

87. Zemke JE, et al. Intramuscular temperature responses in the human leg to two forms of cryotherapy: Ice massage and ice bag. *J Orthop Sports Phys Ther* 1998;27:301–307.

88. Fisher RL. Conservative treatment of patellofemoral pain. *Orthop Clin North Am* 1986;17:269–272.

89. Cwynar DA, McNerney T. A primer on physical therapy. *Prim Care Pract* 1999;3:451–459.

90. Feibel A, Fast A. Deep heating of joints: A reconsideration. *Arch Phys Med Rehab* 1976;57:513–514.

91. Clark D, Stelmach G. Muscle fatigue and recovery curve parameters at various temperatures. *Res Q* 1966;37:468–479.

92. Baker R, Bell G. The effect of therapeutic modalities on blood flow in the human calf. *J Orthop Sports Phys Ther* 1991;13:23.

93. Knight KL, et al. A re-examination of Lewis' cold induced vasodilation in the finger and ankle. *Athl Training* 1980; 15:248–250.

94. Zankel H. Effect of physical agents on motor conduction velocity of the ulnar nerve. *Arch Phys Med Rehab* 1994;47:197–199.

95. Frizzell LA, Dunn F. Biophysics of ultrasound. In: Lehman JF, ed. *Therapeutic Heat and Cold.* Baltimore, Md: Williams and Wilkins; 1982:353–385.

96. Lehman JF, et al. Effect of therapeutic temperatures on tendon extensibility. *Arch Phys Med Rehabil* 1970;51:481–487.

97. Barcroft H, Edholm OS. The effect of temperature on blood flow and deep temperature in the human forearm. *J Physiol* 1943; 102:5–20.

98. Griffin JG. Physiological effects of ultrasonic energy as it is used clinically. *J Am Phys Ther Assoc* 1966;46:18.

99. Lehmann JF, Silverman DR, et al. Temperature distributions in the human thigh produced by infrared, hot pack and microwave applications. *Arch Phys Med Rehabil* 1966;47:291.

100. Abramson DI, et al. Comparison of wet and dry heat in raising temperature of tissues. *Arch Phys Med Rehabil* 1967;48:654.

101. Benson HAE, McElnay JC. Transmission of ultrasound energy through topical pharmaceutical products. *Physiotherapy* 1988;74:587–589.

102. Cameron MH, Monroe LG. Relative transmission of ultrasound by media customarily used for phonophoresis. *Phys Ther* 1992;72:142–148.

103. Dyson M. Mechanisms involved in therapeutic ultrasound. *Physiotherapy* 1987;73:116–120.

104. Lehman JF, et al. Therapeutic temperature distribution produced by ultrasound as modified by dosage and volume of tissue exposed. *Arch Phys Med Rehabil* 1967;48:662–666.

105. Lehman JF, et al. Heating of joint structures by ultrasound. *Arch Phys Med Rehabil* 1968;49:28–30.

106. Goldman DE, Heuter TF. Tabulator data on velocity and absorption of high frequency sound in mammalian tissues. *J Acoust Soc Am* 1956;28:35.

107. Dyson M. Non-thermal cellular effects of ultrasound. *Br J Cancer* 1982;45:165–171.

108. Paaske WP, Hovind H, Sejrsen P. Influence of therapeutic ultrasound irradiation on blood flow in human cutaneous, subcutaneous and muscular tissue. *Scand J Clin Invest* 1973;31:388.

109. Warren CG, Koblanski JN, Sigelmann RA. Ultrasound coupling media: Their relative transmissivity. *Arch Phys Med Rehab* 1976;57:218–222.

110. Dyson M, Pond JB. The effect of pulsed ultrasound on tissue regeneration. *Physiotherapy* 1970;56:136.

111. Dyson M, Suckling J. Stimulation of tissue repair by therapeutic ultrasound: A survey of the mechanisms involved. *Physiotherapy* 1978;64:105–108.

112. Binder A, et al. Is therapeutic ultrasound effective in treating soft tissue lesions? *BMJ* 1985;290:512–514.

113. Draper DO, Castel JC, Castel D. Rate of temperature increase in human muscle during 1-MHz and 3-MHz continuous ultrasound. *J Orthop Sports Phys Ther* 1995;22:142–150.

114. Dyson M, et al. The stimulation of tissue regeneration by means of ultrasound. *Clin Sci* 1968;35:273–285.

115. Dyson M, Suckling J. Stimulation of tissue repair by ultrasound: A survey of the mechanisms involved. *Physiotherapy* 1978;64: 105–108.

116. Ebenbichler GR, Resch KL, Graninger WB. Resolution of calcium deposits after therapeutic ultrasound of the shoulder. *J Rheumatol* 1997;24:235–236.

117. Aldes JH, Klaras T. Use of ultrasonic radiation in the treatment of subdeltoid bursitis with and without calcareous deposits. *West J Surg* 1954;62:369–376.

118. Flax HJ. Ultrasound treatment for peritendinitis calcarea of the shoulder. *Am J Phys Med Rehabil* 1964;43:117–124.

119. Robertson VJ, Baker KG. A review of therapeutic ultrasound: Effectiveness studies. *Phys Ther* 2001;81:1339–1350.

120. Nussbaum EL, Biemann I, Mustard B. Comparison of ultrasound, ultraviolet C and laser for treatment of pressure ulcers in patients with spinal cord injury. *Phys Ther* 1994;74: 812–823.

121. Dyson M, Luke DA. Induction of mast cell degranulation in skin by ultrasound. *IEEE Trans Ultrason Ferroelectr Freq Control* 1986;33:194–201.

122. Nussbaum EL. Ultrasound: To heat or not to heat—that is the question. *Phys Ther Rev* 1997;2:59–72.

123. Makulolowe RTB, Mouzos GL. Ultrasound in the treatment of sprained ankles. *Practitioner* 1977;218:586–588.

124. Dinno MA, Crum LA, Wu J. The effect of therapeutic ultrasound on the electrophysiologic parameters of frog skin. *Med Biol* 1989;25:461–470.

125. Falconer J, Hayes KW, Chang RW. Therapeutic ultrasound in the treatment of musculoskeletal conditions. *Arthritis Care Res* 1990;3:85–91.

126. Maxwell L. Therapeutic ultrasound. Its effects on the cellular and molecular mechanisms of inflammation and repair. *Physiotherapy* 1992;78:421–426.

127. Ter Haar GR, Stratford IJ. Evidence for a non-thermal effect of ultrasound. *Br J Cancer* 1982;45:172–175.

128. Young SR, Dyson M. The effect of therapeutic ultrasound on angiogenesis. *Ultrasound Med Biol* 1990;16:261–269.

129. Dyson M, Niinikoski J. Stimulation of tissue repair by therapeutic ultrasound. *Infect Surg* 1982;12:37–44.

130. Young SR, Dyson M. Effect of therapeutic ultrasound on the healing of full-thickness excised skin lesions. *Ultrasonics* 1990;28:175–180.

131. Antich TJ. Phonophoresis: The principles of the ultrasonic driving force and efficacy in treatment of common orthopedic diagnoses. *J Orthop Sports Phys Ther* 1982;4:99–102.

132. Bommannan D, et al. Sonophoresis II: Examination of the mechanism(s) of ultrasound-enhanced transdermal drug delivery. *Pharm Res* 1992;9:1043–1047.

133. Bommannan D, et al. Sonophoresis. I: The use of high-frequency ultrasound to enhance transdermal drug delivery. *Pharm Res* 1992;9:559–564.

134. Byl NN. The use of ultrasound as an enhancer for transcutaneous drug delivery: Phonophoresis. *Phys Ther* 1995; 75:539–553.

135. Byl NN, et al. The effects of phonophoresis with corticos-teroids: A controlled pilot study. *J Orthop Sports Phys Ther* 1993; 18:590–600.

136. Ciccone CD, Leggin BG, Callamaro JJ. Effects of ultrasound and trolamine salicylate phonophoresis on delayed onset muscle soreness. *Phys Ther* 1991;71:39–51.

137. Davick JP, Martin RK, Albright JP. Distribution and deposition of tritiated cortisol using phonophoresis. *Phys Ther* 1988; 68:1672–1675.

138. Griffin JE, Touchstone JC. Effects of ultrasonic frequency on phonophoresis of cortisol into swine tissues. *Am J Phys Med* 1972;51:62–78.

139. Griffin JE, Touchstone JC, Liu ACY. Ultrasonic movement of cortisol into pig tissue: Movement into paravertebral nerve. *Am J Phys Med* 1965;44:20–25.

140. Munting E. Ultrasonic therapy for painful shoulders. *Physiotherapy* 1978;64:180–181.

140a. Reeves KD, Hassanein K., Randomized prospective double-blind placebo-controlled study of dextrose prolotherapy for knee osteoarthritis with or without ACL laxity. *Alternative Therapies Health Med* 2000;6:68–74,77–80.

141. Cox JS. The diagnosis and management of ankle ligament injuries in the athlete. *Athl Training* 1982;18:192–196.

142. Marino M. Principles of therapeutic modalities: implications for sports medicine. In: Nicholas JA, Hershman EB, eds. *The Lower Extremity and Spine in Sports Medicine*. St. Louis, Mo: CV Mosby; 195–244.

143. Myrer JW, Draper DO, Durrant E. Contrast therapy and intramuscular temperature in the human leg. *Athl Training* 1994;29:318–325.

144. Brown S. Ankle edema and galvanic muscle stimulation. *Phys Sportsmed* 1981;9:137.

145. Frank C, et al. Electromagnetic stimulation of ligament healing in rabbits. *Clin Orthop* 1983;175:263–272.

146. Ralston DJ. High voltage galvanic stimulation: can there be a state of the art? *Athl Training* 1985;21:291–293.

147. Tropp H. *Functional Instability of the Ankle Joint*. Likoping, Sweden: Linkoping University; 1985.

148. Voight ML. Reduction of post-traumatic ankle edema with high voltage pulsed galvanic stimulation. *Athl Training* 1984;20:278–279.

149. Scott O. Stimulative effects. In: Kitchen S, Bazin S, eds. *Clayton's Electrotherapy*. London, England: WB Saunders; 1996.

150. Low J, Reed A. *Electrotherapy Explained: Principles and Practice*. Oxford, England: Butterworth-Heinemann; 2000.

151. Bettany JA, Fish DR, Mendel FC. Influence of high voltage pulsed direct current on edema formation following impact. *Phys Ther* 1990;70:219–224.

152. Bettany JA, Fish DR, Mendel FC. High voltage pulsed direct current effect on edema formation following hyperflexion injury. *Arch Phys Med Rehabil* 1991;71:877–881.

153. Bettany JA, Fish DR, Mendel FC. Influence of cathodal high voltage pulsed current on acute edema. *J Clin Electrophysiol* 1990;2:5–8.

154. Fish DR, et al. Effect on anodal high voltage pulsed current on edema formation in frog hind limbs. *Phys Ther* 1991; 71:724–733.

155. Karnes JL, Mendel FC, Fish DR. Effects of low voltage pulsed current nonedema formation in frog hind limbs following impact injury. *Phys Ther* 1992;72:273–278.

156. Reed BV. Effect of high voltage pulsed electrical stimulation on microvascular permeability to plasma proteins: A possible mechanism of minimizing edema. *Phys Ther* 1988;68:491–495.

157. Taylor K, et al. Effect of a single 30 minute treatment of high voltage pulsed current on edema formation in frog hind limbs. *Phys Ther* 1992;72:63–68.

158. Delitto A, et al. Electrical stimulation versus voluntary exercise in strengthening thigh musculature after anterior cruciate ligament surgery. *Phys Ther* 1988;68:660–663.

159. Goth RS, et al. Electrical stimulation effect on extensor lag and length of hospital stay after total knee arthroplasty. *Arch Phys Med Rehab* 1994;75:957.

160. Laughman RK, et al. Strength changes in the normal quadriceps femoris muscle as a result of electrical stimulation. *Phys Ther* 1983;63:494–499.

161. McMiken DF, Todd-Smith M, Thompson C. Strengthening of human quadriceps muscles by cutaneous electrical stimulation. *Scand J Rehabil Med* 1983;15:25–28.

162. Snyder-Mackler L, et al. Strength of the quadriceps femoris muscle and functional recovery after reconstruction of the anterior cruciate ligament. A prospective, randomized clinical trial of electrical stimulation. *J Bone Joint Surg* 1995;77A:1166–1173.

163. Gould N, et al. Transcutaneous muscle stimulation as a method to retard disuse atrophy. *Clin Orthop* 1982;164:215–220.

164. Selkowitz DM. Improvement in isometric strength of quadriceps femoris muscle after training with electrical stimulation. *Phys Ther* 1985;65:186–196.

165. Currier DP, Mann R. Muscular strength development by electrical stimulation in healthy individuals. *Phys Ther* 1983; 63:915–921.

166. Gangarosa LP. *Iontophoresis in Dental Practice*. Chicago, Ill: Quintessence Publishing; 1982:13–20.

167. Coy RE. *Anthology of Craniomandibular Orthopedics*. Vol 2. 1993, Seattle, Wash: International College of Craniomandibular Orthopedics; 1993:41–85.

168. Burnette RR. Iontophoresis. In: Hadgraft J, Guy RH, eds. *Transdermal Drug Delivery: Developmental Issues and Research Initiatives*. New York, NY: Marcel Dekker; 1989:247–291.

169. Chien YW, et al. Direct current iontophoretic transdermal delivery of peptide and protein drugs. *J Pharm Sci* 1989;78:376–384.

170. Grimnes S. Pathways of ionic flow through human skin in vivo. *Acta Dermatol Venereol* 1984;64:93–98.

171. Lee RD, White HS, Scott ER. Visualization of iontophoretic transport paths in cultured and animal skin models. *J Pharm Sci* 1996;85:1186–1190.

172. Weider D. Treatment of traumatic myositis ossificans with acetic acid iontophoresis. *Phys Ther* 1992;72:133–137.

173. Banta C. A prospective nonrandomized study of iontophoresis, wrist splinting, and anti-inflammatory medication in the treatment of early mild carpal tunnel syndrome. *J Orthop Sports Phys Ther* 1995;21:120.

174. Gangarosa L. Iontophoresis in pain control. *Pain Digest* 1993;3:162–174.

175. Boone DC. Hyaluronidase iontophoresis. *J Am Phys Ther Assoc* 1969;49:139–145.

176. Tannenbaum M. Iodine iotophoresis in reduction of scar tissue. *Phys Ther* 1980;60:792.

177. Kahn J. Calcium iontophoresis in suspected myopathy. *Phys Ther* 1975;55:276.

178. O'Malley E, Oester Y. Influence of some physical chemical factors on iontophoresis using radioisotopes. *Arch Phys Med Rehabil* 1955;36:310–313.

179. Zeltzer L, et al. Iontophoresis versus subcutaneous injection: A comparison of two methods of local anesthesia delivery in children. *Pain* 1991;44:73–78.

180. Krischek O, et al. Shock-wave therapy for tennis and golfer's elbow—1 year follow-up. *Arch Orthop Trauma Surg* 1999; 119:62–66.

181. Rossouw P. Tennis elbow—is extracorporeal shock wave therapy (eswt) an alternative to surgery? *J Bone Joint Surg* 1999; 81B(suppl):306.

182. Rompe JD, et al. Chronic lateral epicondylitis of the elbow: A prospective study of low-energy shockwave therapy and low-energy shockwave therapy plus manual therapy of the cervical spine. *Arch Phys Med Rehab* 2001;82:578–582.

183. Ogden JA, Toth-Kischkat A, Schultheiss R. Principles of shock wave therapy. *Clin Orthop Rel Res* 2001;387:8–17.

183a. Cheing GLY, Chang H., Extracorporeal shock wave therapy. *J Orthop Sports Phys Ther* 2003;33:337–343.

184. Rompe JD. Differenzierte Anwendung extrakorporaler Stosswellen bei Tendopathien der Schulter und des Ellenbogens. *Electromedica* 1997;65:20.

184a. Ogden JA, Alvarez RG, Marlow M. Shockwave therapy for chronic proximal plantar fasciitis: a meta-analysis. *Foot Ankle Int* 2002;23:301–308.

185. Smith MJ. Electrical stimulation for the relief of musculoskeletal pain. *Phys Sports Med* 1983;11:47–55.

185a. Goth, R.S. and et al., *Electrical stimulation effect on extensor lag and length of hospital stay after total knee arthroplasty.* Arch Phys Med Rehab, 1994;75:957.

186. Magora F, et al. Treatment of pain by transcutaneous electrical stimulation. *Acta Anaesthesiol Scand* 1978;22:589–592.

187. Mannheimer JS, Lampe GN. *Clinical Transcutaneous Electrical Nerve Stimulation.* Philadelphia, Pa: FA Davis; 1984: 440–445.

188. Woolf CF. Segmental afferent fiber-induced analgesia: Transcutaneous electrical nerve stimulation (TENS) and vibration. In: Wall PD, Melzack R, eds. *Textbook of Pain.* New York, NY: Churchill Livingstone; 1989:884–896.

189. Smith MJ, Hutchins RC, Hehenberger D. Transcutaneous neural stimulation use in post-operative knee rehabilitation. *Am J Sports Med* 1983;11:75–82.

190. Long DM. Fifteen years of transcutaneous electrical stimulation for pain control. *Stereotact Funct Neurosurg* 1991;56:2–19.

191. Fried T, Johnson R, McCracken W. Transcutaneous electrical nerve stimulation: Its role in the control of chronic pain. *Arch Phys Med Rehabil* 1984;65:228–231.

192. Eriksson MBE, Sjölund BH, Nielzen S. Long-term results of peripheral conditioning stimulation as an analgesic measure in chronic pain. *Pain* 1979;6:335–347.

193. Fishbain DA, et al. Transcutaneous electrical nerve stimulation (TENS) treatment outcome in long term users. *Clin J Pain* 1996;12:201–214.

194. Ishimaru K, Kawakita K, Sakita M. Analgesic effects induced by TENS and electroacupuncture with different types of stimulating electrodes on deep tissues in human subjects. *Pain* 1995; 63:181–187.

195. Eriksson MBE, Sjölund BH, Sundbärg G. Pain relief from peripheral conditioning stimulation in patients with chronic facial pain. *J Neurosurg* 1984;61:149–155.

196. Murphy GJ. Utilization of transcutaneous electrical nerve stimulation in managing craniofacial pain. *Clin J Pain* 1990;6:64–69.

197. Melzack R. The gate theory revisited. In: LeRoy PL, ed. *Current Concepts in the Management of Chronic Pain.* Miami, Fla: Symposia Specialists; 1977.

198. Salar G. Effect of transcutaneous electrotherapy on CSF β-endorphin content in patients without pain problems. *Pain* 1981;10:169–172.

199. Clement-Jones V. Increased β endorphin but not metenkephalin levels in human cerebrospinal fluid after acupuncture for recurrent pain. *Lancet* 1980;8:946–948.

200. Grimsby O, Power B. Manual therapy approach to knee ligament rehabilitation. In: Ellenbecker TS, ed. *Knee Ligament Rehabilitation.* Philadelphia, Pa: Churchill Livingstone; 2000:236–251.

201. Dionne RA. Pharmacologic treatments for temporomandibular disorders. *Surg Oral Med Oral Pathol Oral Radiol Endodont* 1997;83:134–142.

202. Sperling RL. NSAIDs. *Home Healthcare Nurse* 2001;19:687–689.

203. Holvoet J, et al. Relation of upper gastrointestinal bleeding to non-steroidal anti-inflammatory drugs and aspirin: A case-control study. *Gut* 1991;32:730–734.

204. Clive DM, Stoff JS. Renal syndromes associated with nonsteroidal antiinflammatory drugs. *N Engl J Med* 1984;310:563 572.

205. Brattsand R, Linden M. Cytokine modulation by glucocorticoids: Mechanisms and actions in cellular studies. *Aliment Pharmacol Ther* 1996;10(suppl):81–90; discussion 1–2.

206. Buchman AL. Side effects of corticosteroid therapy. *J Clin Gastroenterol* 2001;33:289–294.

207. Elenbaas JK. Centrally acting oral skeletal muscle relaxants. *Am J Hosp Pharm* 1980;37:1313–1323.

208. Hyman J, Liebenson C. Spinal stabilization exercise program. In: Liebenson C, ed. *Rehabilitation of the Spine: A Practitioner's Manual.* Baltimore, Md: Lippincott Williams and Wilkins; 1996:293–317.

209. Albert M. Concepts of muscle training. In: Wadsworth C, ed. *Orthopaedic Physical Therapy: Topic—Strength and Conditioning Applications in Orthopaedics. Home Study Course 98A.* La Crosse, Wis: Orthopaedic Section, American Physical Therapy Association; 1998.

210. Ierna GF, Murphy DR. Management of acute soft tissue injuries of the cervical spine. In: Murphy DR, ed. *Conservative Management of Cervical Spine Disorders.* New York, NY: McGraw-Hill; 2000:531–552.

211. Davies GJ. *Compendium of Isokinetics in Clinical Usage and Rehabilitation Techniques.* 4th ed. Onalaska, Wis: S and S Publishers; 1992.

212. Harris ML. Flexibility. *Phys Ther* 1969;49:591–601.

213. Klinge K, et al. The effect of strength and flexibility on skeletal muscle EMG activity, stiffness and viscoelastic stress relaxation response. *Am J Sports Med* 1997;25:710–716.

214. American Orthopaedic Society for Sports Medicine. *Flexibility.* Chicago, Ill: AOSSM; 1988.

215. Clark MA. *Integrated Training for the New Millenium.* Thousand Oaks, Calif: National Academy of Sports Medicine; 2001.

216. Murphy P. Warming up before stretching advised. *Phys Sports Med* 1986;14:45.

217. Shellock F, Prentice WE. Warm-up and stretching for improved physical performance and prevention of sport-related injury. *Sports Med* 1985;2:267–278.

218. Sapega AA, et al. Biophysical factors in range of motion exercise. *Phys Sports Med* 1981;9:57–65.

219. Sucher BM. Thoracic outlet syndrome—A myofascial variant: Part 2. Treatment. *J Am Osteopath Assoc* 1990;90:810–823.

220. Brennan R. *The Alexander Technique: Natural Poise for Health.* New York, NY: Barnes and Noble Books; 1991.

221. Wanning T. Healing and the mind/body arts. *AAOHN J* 1993;41:349–351.

222. Ryverant J. *The Feldenkrais Method: Teaching by Handling.* New York, NY: KS Gringer; 1983.

223. Feldenkrais M. *The Elusive Obvious.* Cupertino, Calif: Meta Publications; 1981.

224. Nelson SH. Playing with the entire self: The Feldenkrais method and musicians. *Semin Neurol* 1989;9:97–104.

225. Buchanan PA, Ulrich BD. The Feldenkrais method: A dynamic approach to changing motor behavior. *Res Q Exerc Sport* 2001;72:315–323.

226. Lake B. Acute back pain: Treatment by the application of Feldenkrais principles. *Aust Fam Physician* 1985;14:1175–1178.

227. Ramsey SM. Holistic manual therapy techniques. *Prim Care* 1997;24:759–785.

228. Witt P, Parr C. Effectiveness of Trager psychophysical integration in promoting trunk mobility in a child with cerebral palsy, a case report. *Phys Occup Ther Pediatr* 1988;8:75–94.

229. Witt P. Trager psychophysical integration: An additional tool in the treatment of chronic spinal pain and dysfunction. *Trager J* 1987;2:4–5.

230. Savage FL. *Osteoarthritis: A Step-By-Step Success Story to Show Others How They Can Help Themselves.* Barrytown, NY: Station Hill Press; 1988.

231. Juhan D. *Multiple Sclerosis: The Trager Approach.* Mill Valley, Calif: Trager Institute; 1993.

232. Heidt P. Effects of therapeutic touch on the anxiety level of the hospital patient. *Nurs Res* 1991;30:32–37.

233. Stone A. The Trager approach. In: Davis C, ed. *Complementary Therapies in Rehabilitation; Holistic Approaches for Prevention and Wellness.* Thorofare, NJ: Slack; 1997.

234. Watrous I. The Trager approach: An effective tool for physical therapy. *Phys Ther For* 1992(April 10):12–14.

235. Lan C, Lai JS, Chen SY. Tai Chi Chuan: An ancient wisdom on exercise and health promotion. *Sports Med* 2002;32:217–224.

236. Brown DR, et al. Chronic psychological effects of exercise and exercise plus cognitive strategies. *Med Sci Sports Exerc* 1995;27:765–775.

237. Zhuo D, et al. Cardiorespiratory and metabolic responses during Tai Chi Chuan exercise. *Can J Appl Sport Sci* 1984;9:7–10.

238. Lai JS, et al. Cardiorespiratory responses of Tai Chi Chuan practitioners and sedentary subjects during cycle ergometry. *J Formos Med Assoc* 1993;92:894–899.

239. Jacobson BH, et al. The effect of T'ai Chi Chuan training on balance, kinesthetic sense, and strength. *Percept Mot Skills* 1997;84:27–33.

240. Hong Y, Li JX, Robinson PD. Balance control, flexibility, and cardiorespiratory fitness among older Tai Chi practitioners. *Br J Sports Med* 2000;34:29–34.

241. Wang JS, Lan C, Wong MK. Tai Chi Chuan training to enhance microcirculatory function in healthy elderly men. *Arch Phys Med Rehabil* 2001;82:1176–1180.

242. Hartman CA, et al. Effects of T'ai Chi Training on function and quality of life indicators in older adults with osteoarthritis. *J Am Geriatr Soc* 2000;48:1553–1559.

243. Marino M. Current concepts of rehabilitation in sports medicine. In: Nicholas JA, Herschman EB, eds. *The Lower Extremity and Spine in Sports Medicine.* St. Louis, Mo: Mosby; 1986:117–195.

244. Steindler A. *Kinesiology of the Human Body under Normal and Pathological Conditions.* Springfield, Ill: Charles C Thomas; 1955.

245. Blackard DO, Jensen RL, Ebben WP. Use of EMG analysis in challenging kinetic chain terminology. *Med Sci Sports Exerc* 1999;31:443–448.

246. Palmitier RA, et al. Kinetic chain exercises in knee rehabilitation. *Sports Med* 1991;11:402–413.

247. Gray GW. Closed chain sense. *Fitness Manage* 1992;31–33.

248. Dillman CJ, Murray TA, Hintermeister RA. Biomechanical differences of open and closed chain exercises with respect to the shoulder. *J Sport Rehabil* 1994;3:228–238.

249. Kibler BW. Closed kinetic chain rehabilitation for sports injuries. *Phys Med Rehabil North Am* 2000;11:369–384.

250. Shelbourne KD, Nitz P. Accelerated rehabilitation after anterior cruciate ligament reconstruction. *Am J Sports Med* 1990;18:292–299.

251. Henning CE, Lynch MA, Glick C. An in vivo strain gauge study of elongation of the anterior cruciate ligament. *Am J Sports Med* 1985;13:22–26.

252. Lutz GE, et al. Comparison of tibiofemoral joint forces during open-kinetic-chain and closed-kinetic-chain exercises. *Am J Bone Joint Surg* 1993;75:732–739.

253. More RC, et al. Hamstrings—an anterior cruciate ligament protagonist. An in vitro study. *Am J Sports Med* 1993;21:231–237.

254. Ohkoshi Y, et al. Biomechanical analysis of rehabilitation in the standing position. *Am J Sports Med* 1991;19:605–611.

255. Yack HJ, Collins CE, Whieldon TJ. Comparison of closed and open kinetic chain exercise in the anterior cruciate ligament-deficient knee. *Am J Sports Med* 1993;21:49–54.

256. Yack HJ, Washco LA, Whieldon T. Compressive forces as a limiting factor of anterior tibial translation in the ACL-deficient knee. *Clin J Sports Med* 1994;4:233–239.

257. Lephart SM, Henry TJ. Functional rehabilitation for the upper and lower extremity. *Orthop Clin North Am* 1995;26:579–592.

258. Witvrouw E, et al. Open versus closed kinetic chain exercises for patellofemoral pain. A prospective, randomized study. *Am J Sports Med* 2000;28:687–694.

259. Meglan D, Lutz G, Stuart M. Effects of closed chain exercises for ACL rehabilitation upon the load in the capsule and ligamentous structures of the knee. *Orthop Trans* 1993;17:719–720.

260. Irrgang JJ, Rivera J. Closed kinetic chain exercises for the lower extremity: Theory and application. *Sports Physical Therapy Section Home Study Course: Current Concepts in Rehabilitation of the Knee.* La Crosse, Wis: Orthopedic Section, APTA; 1994.

261. Blackburn JR, Morrissey MC. The relationship between open and closed kinetic chain strength of the lower limb and jumping performance. *J Orthop Sports Phys Ther* 1998;27:430–435.

262. Voight ML, Bell S, Rhodes D. Instrumented testing of tibial translation during a positive Lachman's test and selected closed chain activities in anterior cruciate deficient knees. *J Orthop Sports Phys Ther* 1992;15:49.

263. Clark FJ, et al. Role of intramuscular receptors in the awareness of limb position. *J Neurophysiol* 1985;54:1529–1540.

264. Grigg P. Peripheral neural mechanisms in proprioception. *J Sport Rehabil* 1994;3:1–17.

265. Doucette SA, Child DP. The effect of open and closed chain exercise and knee joint position on patellar tracking in lateral patellar compression syndrome. *J Orthop Sports Phys Ther* 1996;23:104–110.

266. Genuario SE, Dolgener FA. The relationship of isokinetic torque at two speeds to the vertical jump. *Res Q* 1980;51:593–598.

267. Pincivero DM, Lephart SM, Karunakara RG. Relation between open and closed kinematic chain assessment of knee strength and functional performance. *Clin J Sports Med* 1997;7:11–16.

268. Anderson MA, et al. The relationship among isokinetic, isotonic, and isokinetic concentric and eccentric quadriceps and hamstrings force and three components of athletic performance. *J Orthop Sports Phys Ther* 1991;14:114–120.

269. Bunn JW. *Scientific Principles of Coaching.* Englewood Cliffs, NJ: Prentice-Hall; 1972.

270. Kibler WB. Kinetic chain concept. In: Ellenbecker TS, ed. *Knee Ligament Rehabilitation.* Philadelphia, Pa: Churchill Livingstone; 2000:301–306.

271. Putnam CA. Sequential motions of body segments in stroking and throwing skills: Descriptions and explanations. *J Biomech* 1993;26:125–135.

272. Van Gheluwe B, Hebbelinck M. The kinematics of the serve movement in tennis. In: Winter D, ed. *Biomechanics.* Champaign, Ill: Human Kinetics; 1985:521–526.

273. Lephart SM, Borsa PA. Functional rehabilitation of knee injuries. In: Fu FH, Harner C, eds. *Knee Surgery.* Baltimore, Md: Williams and Wilkins; 1993:64–79.

274. Litchfield R, et al. Rehabilitation of the overhead athlete. *J Orthop Sports Phys Ther* 1993;2:433–441.

275. Youmans W. The so-called "isolated" ACL syndrome: A report of 32 cases with some observation on treatment and its effect on results. *Am J Sports Med* 1978;6:26–30.

276. Risberg MA, et al. Design and implementation of a neuromuscular training program following anterior cruciate ligament reconstruction. *J Orthop Sports Phys Ther* 2001;31:620–631.

277. Barrack RL, et al. Effect of articular disease and total knee arthroplasty on knee joint position sense. *J Neurophysiol* 1983;50:684–687.

278. Barrack RL, Skinner HB, Buckley SL. Proprioception in the anterior cruciate deficient knee. *Am J Sports Med* 1989;17:1–6.

279. Corrigan JP, Cashman WF, Brady MP. Proprioception in the cruciate deficient knee. *J Bone Joint Surg* 1992;74B:247–250.

280. Fremerey RW, et al. Proprioception after rehabilitation and reconstruction in knees with deficiency of the anterior cruciate ligament: A prospective, longitudinal study. *J Bone Joint Surg* 2000;82B:801–806.

281. Payne KA, Berg K, Latin RW. Ankle injuries and ankle strength, flexibility and proprioception in college basketball players. *J Athl Training* 1997;32:221–225.

282. Sell S, Zacher J, Lack S. Disorders of proprioception of arthrotic knee joint. *Z Rheumatol* 1993;52:150–155.

283. Voight M, Blackburn T. Proprioception and balance training and testing following injury. In: Ellenbecker TS, ed. *Knee Ligament Rehabilitation.* Philadelphia, Pa: Churchill Livingstone; 2000:361–385.

284. Panjabi MM. The stabilizing system of the spine. Part 1. Function, dysfunction adaption and enhancement. *J Spinal Disord* 1992;5:383–389.

285. Panjabi M, et al. Biomechanical studies in cadaveric spines. In: Jayson MIV, ed. *The Lumbar Spine and Back Pain.* New York, NY: Churchill Livingstone; 1992:133–135.

286. Lephart SM, et al. The role of proprioception in the management and rehabilitation of athletic injuries. *Am J Sports Med* 1997;25:130–137.

287. Schutte MJ, Happel RT. Joint innervation in joint injury. *Clin Sports Med* 1990;9:511–517.

288. Kennedy JC, Alexander IJ, Hayes KC. Nerve supply of the human knee and its functional importance. *Am J Sports Med* 1982;10:329–335.

289. Voight ML, Cook G. Impaired neuromuscular control: reactive neuromuscular training. In: Prentice WE, Voight ML, eds. *Techniques in Musculoskeletal Rehabilitation.* New York, NY: McGraw-Hill; 2001:93–124.

290. Jerosch J, Prymka M. Propriozeptive Fahigkeiten des gesunden Kniegelenks: Beeinflussung durch eine elastische Bandage. *Sportverletz. Sportsch* 1995;9:72–76.

291. Jerosch J, et al. The influence of orthoses on the proprioception of the ankle joint. *Knee Surg Sports Traumatol Arthrosc* 1995;3:39–46.

292. Perlau R, Frank C, Fick G. The effect of elastic bandages on human knee proprioception in the uninjured population. *Am J Sports Med* 1995;23:251–255.

293. Robbins S, Waked E, Rappel R. Ankle taping improves proprioception before and after exercise in young men. *Br J Sports Med* 1995;29:242–247.

294. Barrett DS. Proprioception and function after anterior cruciate ligament reconstruction. *J Bone Joint Surg* 1991;73B:833–837.

295. McNair PJ, Wood GA, Marshall RN. Stiffness of the hamstring muscles and its relationship to function in ACL deficient individuals. *Clin Biomech* 1992;7:131–137.

296. Borsa PA, et al. Functional assessment and rehabilitation of shoulder proprioception for glenohumeral instability. *J Sport Rehabil* 1994;3:84–104.

297. Lephart SM, et al. Proprioception of the shoulder joint in healthy, unstable and surgically repaired shoulders. *J Shoulder Elbow Surg* 1994;3:371–380.

298. Irrgang JJ, Whitney SL, Harner C. Nonoperative treatment of rotator cuff injuries in throwing athletes. *J Sport Rehabil* 1992;1:197–222.

299. Voss DE, Ionta MK, Myers DJ. *Proprioceptive Neuromuscular Facilitation: Patterns and Techniques.* Philadelphia, Pa: Harper and Row; 1985.

300. Janda DH, Loubert P. A preventative program focussing on the glenohumeral joint. *Clin Sports Med* 1991;10:955–971.

301. Johnston RB III, et al. Effect of lower extremity muscular fatigue on motor control performance. *Med Sci Sports Exerc* 1998;30:1703–1707.

302. Markey KL. Rehabilitation of the anterior cruciate deficient knee. *Clin Sports Med* 1985;4:513–526.

303. Markey KL. Functional rehabilitation of the anterior cruciate deficient knee. *Sports Med* 1991;12:407–417.

304. DeLorme TL. Restoration of muscle power by heavy resistance exercise. *J Bone Joint Surg* 1945;27:645–667.

305. Tippett SR, Voight ML. *Functional Progressions for Sports Rehabilitation.* Champaign, Ill: Human Kinetics; 1995.

306. Keggereis S. The construction and implementation of functional progressions as a component of athletic rehabilitation. *J Orthop Sports Phys Ther* 1985;5:14–19.

307. Kibler BW. *The Sports Preparticipation Fitness Examination.* Champaign, Ill: Human Kinetics; 1990.

308. Palmer ML, Epler M. *Clinical Assessment Procedures in Physical Therapy.* Philadelphia, Pa: Lippincott; 1990:68–73.

309. Caspersen CJ, Powell KE, Christenson GM. Physical activity, exercise and physical fitness. *Public Health Rep* 1985;100:125–131.

310. Kiser DM. Physiological and biomechanical factors for understanding repetitive motion injuries. *Semin Occup Med* 1987;2:11–17.

311. American College of Sports Medicine. *Guidelines for Exercise Testing and Prescription.* 4th ed. Philadelphia, Pa: Lea and Febiger; 1991.

312. Pate RR, et al. Physical activity and public health: a recommendation from the Centers for Disease Control and Prevention and the American College of Sports Medicine. *JAMA* 1995;273:402–407.

313. Paffenbarger RS, et al. Physical activity, all-cause mortality, and longevity of college alumni. *N Engl J Med* 1986;314:605–613.

314. Leon AS, et al. Leisure-time physical activity levels and risk of coronary heart disease and death: the Multiple Risk Factor Intervention trial. *JAMA* 1987;258:2388–2395.

315. DeBusk RF, et al. Training effects of long versus short bouts of exercise in healthy subjects. *Am J Cardiol* 1990;65:1010–1013.

316. Winter DA. Moments of force and mechanical power in jogging. *J Biomech* 1983;16:91–97.

317. Orlander J, et al. Low intensity training, inactivity and resumed training in sedentary men. *Acta Physiol Scand* 1977;101:351–362.

318. Parsons D, et al. Balance and strength changes in elderly subjects after heavy-resistance strength training. *Med Sci Sports Exerc* 1992;24(suppl):S21.

319. Powell KE, et al. Physical activity and the incidence of coronary heart disease. *Annu Rev Public Health* 1987;8:253–287.

320. Morris JN, et al. Incidence and prediction of ischemic heart disease in London busman. *Lancet* 1966;2:533–559.

321. Hagberg JM. Exercise, fitness, and hypertension. In: Bouchard C, et al, eds. *Exercise, Fitness, and Health*. Champaign, Ill: Human Kinetics; 1990:455–566.

322. Paffenbarger RS, et al. Physical activity and incidence of hypertension in college alumni. *Am J Epidemiol* 1983;117:245–257.

323. Helmrich SP, et al. Physical activity and reduced occurrence of non-insulin-dependent diabetes mellitus. *N Engl J Med* 1991;325:147–152.

324. Manson JE, et al. Physical activity and incidence of non-insulin-dependent diabetes mellitus in women. *Lancet* 1991;338:774–778.

325. Cummings SR, et al. Epidemiology of osteoporosis and osteoporotic fractures. *Epidemiol Rev* 1985;7:178–208.

326. Snow-Harter C, Marcus R. Exercise, bone mineral density, and osteoporosis. *Exerc Sport Sci Rev* 1991;19:351–388.

327. Lee I, Paffenbarger RS, Hsieh C. Physical activity and risk of developing colorectal cancer among college alumni. *J Natl Cancer Inst* 1991;83:1324–1329.

328. Taylor CB, Sallis JF, Needle R. The relationship of physical activity and exercise to mental health. *Public Health Rep* 1985;100:195–201.

329. Caspersen CJ, Christenson GM, Pollard RA. The status of the 1990 Physical Fitness Objectives—Evidence from NHIS 85. *Public Health Rep* 1986;101:587–592.

330. Stephens T, Jacobs DR, White CC. A descriptive epidemiology of leisure-time physical activity. *Public Health Rep* 1985;100:147–158.

331. Caspersen CJ, Pollard RA, Pratt SO. Scoring physical activity data with special consideration for elderly population. In: *Proceedings of the 21st National Meeting of the Public Health Conference on Records and Statistics: Data for an Aging Population*. Washington, DC: Dept Health Human Services; 1987.

332. Schoenborn CA. Health habits of US adults, 1985: The 'Alameda 7' revisited. *Public Health Rep* 1986;101:571–580.

333. Caspersen CJ, Merritt RK. Trends in physical activity patterns among older adults: The Behavioral Risk Factor Surveillance System, 1986-1990. *Med Sci Sports Exerc* 1992;24:S26.

334. DiPietro L, Caspersen C. National estimates of physical activity among white and black Americans. *Med Sci Sports Exerc* 1991;23(suppl):S105.

335. White CC, et al. The behavioral risk factor surveys, IV: The descriptive epidemiology of exercise. *Am J Prev Med* 1987;3:304–310.

336. Clancy WG. Specific rehabilitation for the injured recreational runner. *Instr Course Lect* 1989;38:483–486.

337. Kibler WB. Clinical implications of exercise: Injury and performance. In: *Instructional Course Lectures, American Academy of Orthopaedic Surgeons*. Rosemont, Ill: American Academy of Orthopaedic Surgeons; vol. 43 1994:17–24.

338. Nirschl RP. Elbow tendinosis: Tennis elbow. *Clin Sports Med* 1992;11:851–870.

339. Kibler WB, Livingston B, Bruce R. Current concepts in shoulder rehabilitation. *Adv Op Orthop* 1996;3:249–301.

340. Kibler WB, Livingston B, Chandler TJ. Shoulder rehabilitation: Clinical application, evaluation, and rehabilitation protocols. *Instr Course Lect* 1997;46:43–53.

341. Kibler WB. Shoulder rehabilitation: principles and practice. *Med Sci Sports Exerc* 1998;30(suppl):40–50.

342. Lewis BS, Lynch WD. The effect of physician advice on exercise behavior. *Prev Med* 1993;22:110–121.

343. Litzinger ME, Osif B. Accommodating diverse learning styles: Designing instruction for electronic information sources. In: Shirato L, ed. *What Is Good Instruction Now? Library Instruction for the 90s*. Ann Arbor, Mich: Pierian Press; 1993;27–42.

344. Taylor JA. A practical tool for improved communications. *Supervision* 1998;59:18–19.

345. Deyo RA. Compliance with therapeutic regimens in arthritis: Issues, current status, and a future agenda. *Sem Arthritis Rheum* 1982;12:233–244.

346. Blanpied P. Why won't patients do their home exercise programs? *J Orthop Sports Phys Ther* 1997;25:101–102.

347. Chen CY, et al. Factors influencing compliance with home exercise programs among patients with upper extremity impairment. *Am J Occup Ther* 1999;53:171–180.

348. Friedrich M, Cermak T, Madebacher P. The effect of brochure use versus therapist teaching on patients performing therapeutic exercise and on changes in impairment status. *Phys Ther* 1996;76:1082–1088.

349. Hungerford DS, Lennox DW. Rehabilitation of the knee in disorders of the patellofemoral joint: Relevant biomechanics. *Orthop Clin North Am* 1983;14:397–444.

350. Herring SA, Kibler BW. A framework for rehabilitation. In: *Functional Rehabilitation of Sports and Musculoskeletal Injuries*. Kibler BW, Herring JA, Press JM, eds. Aspen: Gaithersburg, Md; 1998:1–8.

MANUAL TECHNIQUES

CHAPTER OBJECTIVES

▶ *At the completion of this chapter, the reader will be able to:*

1. Summarize the various types of manual therapy.

2. Apply the knowledge of the various manual therapies in the planning of a comprehensive rehabilitation program.

3. Recognize the manifestations of abnormal tissue and develop strategies using manual techniques to treat these abnormalities.

4. Categorize the various affects of manual therapy on the soft tissues.

5. Make an accurate judgment when recommending a manual therapy technique to improve joint or muscle function.

6. Evaluate the effectiveness of a manual technique when used as a direct intervention.

OVERVIEW

Touch has always been and continues to be a primary healing modality. The first written records of massage go back to Ancient China, and wall paintings in Egypt depict hands-on healing techniques that go back 15,000 years.[1] From this early "laying on of hands" evolved many of the techniques used today.

A more common term for therapeutic touch is *manual therapy*. Manual therapy (MT) has become such an important component of the intervention for orthopedic and neurologic disorders that it is considered by many as an area of specialization within physical therapy.[2–5]

Several manual therapy approaches or techniques have evolved over the years. By their nature, many of these techniques have not been developed with the same scientific rigor as fields such as anatomy and physiology, and much of their use is based on clinical outcomes, rather than evidence-based proof. However, an absence of evidence does not always mean that there is evidence of absence (of effect), and there is always the risk of rejecting therapeutic approaches that are valid.[6]

Of the approaches commonly applied, the Cyriax,[7] Mennell,[8] and osteopathic techniques[9,10] originated from physicians (Table 11-1), whereas the Maitland,[14,15] Kaltenborn,[16] and McKenzie[17] approaches were derived by physical therapists[5,18,29] (Table 11-2).

Within these major philosophies, a number of subsets have also emerged, including myofascial release, positional release techniques, neurodynamic mobilization techniques (see Chap. 12), manually resisted exercise, proprioceptive neuromuscular facilitation, joint mobilization, and manipulation.

Manual Techniques

MT techniques have traditionally been used to produce a number of therapeutic alterations in pain and soft tissue extensibility through the application of specific external forces.[14,15,20,21] Although it is generally agreed that manual techniques are beneficial for specific impairments such as a restricted joint glide and adaptively shortened connective tissue, there is less agreement on which technique is best. The decision about which approach or technique to use has traditionally been based on the clinician's belief, level of expertise, and decision-making processes. This has led to widespread opinions on which tools to use to measure outcome; how to apply a particular technique in terms of patient setup, intensity, and duration; and how to gauge an individual's response to a technique.

Unfortunately, the therapeutic efficacy of manual therapy remains undetermined. However, there are many theories about why manual therapy produces improvement in a patient's condition.[22–26]

Part of the problem in determining the efficacy of manual therapy is that the selection of a particular technique is typically made on an ad hoc basis. Clear-cut definitions as to when one technique is more efficacious than another are lacking.

TABLE 11-1   Manual Therapy Approach: Physician Generated[2]

	Cyriax[7] (Orthopaedic Medicine) Contentions	Mennell[11] Contentions	Osteopathic Contentions[12,13]
Philosophical basis	All pain has an anatomic source All treatment must reach that anatomic source If diagnosis is correct, all treatment will benefit source	Dysfunction is a sign of serious pathologic process or joint disease Loss of normal joint movement or joint play can lead to dysfunction Joint manipulation can restore normal joint-play movements	Body is a total unit, and neuromusculoskeletal system is connected with other systems; therefore, disease processes can be visible in musculoskeletal system Structure of body governs function: abnormality in structure can lead to abnormal function Somatic dysfunction is impaired function of related components Manipulative therapy can restore and maintain normal structure and function relationships
Key concepts	Diagnosis of soft tissue lesions Categorization of referred pain Differentiation of contractile and noncontractile lesions	Assessment of joint play	Diagnosis of somatic dysfunction Clinical examination focuses on presence of asymmetry, restriction of movement, and palpation of soft tissue texture changes (i.e., palpation of skin, muscle, and other connective tissue for feeling of thickness, swelling, tightness, or temperature change)

Evaluation framework history	Observation, history
	  Age and occupation
	  Symptoms (site and spread, onset and duration, behavior)
	  Medical considerations
	  Inspection
		Present complaint
		  Onset
		  Nature of pain
		  Localization of pain
		  Loss of movement
		Past history
		Family history
		Medical systems review
			History
			  Knowledge of physical trauma, past history of visceral, and soft tissue problems
			Present Complaint
			  Establish relationship between adaptation, decompensation, trauma, and time from patient's history

Physical	Physical examination
	  Active movements
	  Passive movements
	  Resisted movements
	  Neurologic examination
	  Palpation
		Physical examination
		  Inspection
		  Palpation
		  Examination of voluntary movements
		  Muscle examination
		  Special tests (e.g., roentgenography)
		  Examination of joint-play movements
			Physical examination
			  Postural analysis
			Regional screening functional units
			  Pelvic girdle
			  Foot
			  Vertebral column
			  Shoulder girdle
			  Hand
			Detailed evaluation of regions in dysfunction

Interpretation of evaluation	Identification of anatomic structure associated with lesion	Joint dysfunction	Positional fault Restriction fault Segmental or multisegmental

TABLE 11-1   *(cont.)*

	Cyriax[7] (Orthopaedic Medicine) Contentions	Mennell[11] Contentions	Osteopathic Contentions[12,13]
Treatment strategies	Friction massage Injection Manipulation Mobilization Physical therapy (e.g., exercise, modalities) Patient education	Manipulation Mobilization Physical therapy (e.g., exercise, modalities) Patient education	Manipulation Mobilization Muscle energy Myofascial techniques Counterstrain Exercise therapy Patient education

TABLE 11-2   Manual Therapy Approach: Physical Therapist Generated[2]

	Maitland[14,15] (Australian) Contentions	Kaltenborn[16] (Norwegian) Contentions	McKenzie[17] Contentions
Philosophical basis	Personal commitment to understand patient Consideration and application of theoretical (e.g., pathology, anatomy) and clinical thinking (e.g., signs and symptoms) Continual assessment and reassessment of data	Biomechanical assessment of joint movements Pain, joint dysfunction, and soft tissue changes are found in combination	Predisposing factors of sitting posture, loss of extension range, and frequency of flexion contribute to spinal pain Patients should be involved in self-treatment
Key concepts	Examination, technique, and assessment are interrelated and interdependent Grades of movement (I–V) Strong emphasis on use of passive movement testing (testing accessory and physiologic joint movements) Differential assessment to prove or disprove clinical working hypothesis	Somatic dysfunction Application of principles from arthrokinematics (e.g., concave-convex rule, close- and loose-packed positions) Grades of movement (I–III)	During movements of spine, positional change to nucleus pulposus takes place Strong emphasis on use of active motions Flexed lifestyle leads to a more posterior position of nucleus Intervertebral disk is common source of back pain
Evaluation framework	Subjective examination (as defined by Maitland)[14,15] 　Establish kind of disorder 　Area of symptoms 　Behavior of symptoms 　Irritability 　Nature 　Special questions 　History Planning objective examination (as defined by Maitland)[14,15] Physical examination 　Observation 　Functional tests 　Active movements 　Isometric tests 　Other structures in plan 　Passive movements (e.g., special tests, physiologic and accessory joint movements, relevant adverse neural tissue tension tests)	History ("five by five scheme") 　Immediate case history (e.g., assess symptoms for localization, time, character, etc.) 　Previous history (e.g., assess for kind of treatment, relief of symptoms, presence of similar symptoms or related symptoms) 　Social background 　Medical history 　Family history Patient's assessment of cause of complaint Physical examination 　Inspection 　Function (active and passive movements; testing with traction, compression, and gliding; resisted tests) 　Palpation	History 　Interrogation (e.g., where did pain begin, how, constant or intermittent, what makes it better or worse, previous episodes, further questions?) Physical examination 　Posture (sitting, standing) 　Examination of movement (flexion, extension, side gliding) 　Movements in relation to pain 　Repeated movements 　Test movements 　Other tests (e.g., neurologic, other joints)

TABLE 11-2 *(cont.)*

	Palpation Neurologic examination Highlight main findings	Neurologic tests Additional tests	
Interpretation of evaluation	Initial assessment relates examination findings to: Behavior of patient's symptoms—pain or stiffness (somewhat analogous to McKenzie's derangement and dysfunction syndrome, respectively) Diagnosis, although no specific structure designated Stage of disorder Stability of disorder Irritability of disorder	Biomechanical assessment (i.e., restriction of joint mobility) and assessment of soft tissue changes	Diagnosis according to syndrome, as opposed to specific structure Postural syndrome (end range strain on normal tissues) Dysfunction syndrome (adaptive shortening of structure) Derangement syndrome (disturbance of normal anatomic relationship)
Treatment strategies	Based on continual assessment of subjective and objective findings Focus on treating pain or stiffness Mobilization Manipulation Adverse neural tissue mobilization Traction Exercise using movements that have positive influence on symptoms Patient education	Mobilization Exercise (emphasis on proprioceptive neuromuscular facilitation) Traction/distraction Soft tissue mobilization Manipulation Patient education	Patient self-treatment using repeated active movements Exercise using movements that have positive influence on symptoms Mobilization or manipulation (if needed) Strong emphasis on patient education and self treatment

It is unlikely that manual techniques alone can improve the function of a patient. Research studies seem to suggest that the best approach is a combination of manual techniques with other interventions, such as progressive exercises, the use of therapeutic modalities, and patient education about proper body mechanics, positions, and postures.[27–29]

Correct Application of Manual Techniques

Despite the varied approaches and rationales, there is general agreement concerning criteria that are important for the correct application of a manual technique. These include[30]:

▶ *Knowledge of the relative shapes of the joint surfaces (concave or convex).*[14–16,31] If the joint surface is convex relative to the other surface, the slide occurs in the direction opposite to the bone movement (angular motion). If, on the other hand, the joint surface is concave, the slide occurs in the same direction as the bone movement (angular motion).

▶ *Duration, type, and irritability of symptoms*[14,15] (Table 11-3). This information can provide the clinician with some

general guidelines in determining the intensity of the application of a selected technique (see "Indications for Manual Therapy" later in this chapter).

▶ *Patient and clinician position.* Correct positioning of the patient is essential both to help the patient relax and to ensure safe body mechanics from the clinician. When patients feel relaxed, their muscle activity is decreased, reducing the amount of resistance encountered during the technique.

▶ *Position of joint to be treated.* The position of the joint to be treated must be appropriate for the stage of healing and the skill of the clinician. It is recommended that the resting position of the joint be used when the patient has an acute condition or the clinician is inexperienced. The resting position in this case refers to the position that the injured joint adopts, rather than the classic resting (open-packed) position for a normal joint. Other positions for starting the mobilization may be used by a skilled clinician in patients with nonacute conditions.

▶ *Hand placement.* Wherever possible, contact with the patient should be maximized. The hand should conform to the area being treated so that the forces are spread over a

TABLE 11-3 Indications for Selection of Manual Technique Based on Duration of Symptoms[34]

	Acute	Subacute	Chronic
Muscle energy	Strongly indicated	Strongly indicated	Use to prepare tissue for joint manipulation and prevent recurrence of dysfunction
Joint mobilization	Grades I and II	Grades II and III	Grades III and IV
Joint manipulation	Rarely indicated	Moderate to strong indication if muscle energy technique unsuccessful	Strong indication if muscle energy technique ineffective

larger area. A gentle and confident touch inspires confidence from the patient. Accurate hand placement is essential for efficient stabilization and for the accurate transmission of force.

▶ *Specificity.* Specificity refers to the exactness of the procedure, based on its intent. Whenever possible, the forces imparted by a technique should occur at the point where they are needed.

▶ *Direction of force.* The direction of the force can either be *direct,* which is toward the motion barrier or restriction,[32] or *indirect,* which is away from the motion barrier.[12,33] Although the rationale for a direct technique is easy to understand, the rationale for using an indirect technique is more confusing. A good analogy is the stuck drawer. Often the movement that eventually frees the drawer is an inward motion followed by a pull.[30]

▶ *Amount of force.* The amount of force used depends on the intent of the manual procedure and a number of other factors, including but not limited to:

• Age, sex, and general health status of the patient.

• Barrier to motion and end-feel (stage of healing) (Table 11-4).

• Type and severity of the movement disorder.

▶ *Reinforcement of any gains made.* It has been demonstrated that movement gained by a specific manual technique performed in isolation will be lost within 48 hours.[35] Thus, motion gained by a manual technique must be reinforced by both the mechanical and neurophysiologic benefits of active movement.[36] These active movements must be as local and precise as possible to the involved segment or myofascial structure.

Reassessment is an integral part of any intervention. The clinician must be able to gauge how effective a technique has been so that necessary modifications can be made. Measurement

TABLE 11-4 Appropriate Technique Based on Barrier to Motion and End-feel

Barrier	End-feel	Technique
Pain	Empty	None
Pain	Spasm	None
Pain	Capsular	Oscillations
Joint adhesions	Early capsular	Passive articular motion stretch
Muscle adhesions	Early elastic	Passive physiologic motion stretch
Hypertonicity	Facilitation	Hold-relax
Bone	Bony	None

procedures used by the clinician to determine the effectiveness of a manual intervention must adequately reflect changes in pain level, impairments and functional ability. Although measurements of range of motion, pain, and strength are valid and reliable,[37–39] the functional measurement selected should be related to the particular functional limitation that the clinician is expected to change with the intervention.[40] Complicating the measurement of outcome and the effectiveness of a technique is the placebo effect (a response resulting from the suggestion that something is beneficial, even though it may be inert). Although manual therapy is not alone in its use of the placebo effect, it is increasingly important that clinicians determine the specific effects of everything they do.[41]

Indications for Manual Therapy

MT is indicated in the following cases:

▶ Mild pain.

▶ A nonirritable condition, demonstrated by pain that is provoked by motion but that disappears very quickly.

▶ Intermittent musculoskeletal pain.

▶ Pain reported by the patient that is relieved by rest.

▶ Pain reported by the patient that is relieved or provoked by particular motions or positions.

▶ Pain that is altered by postural changes.

Contraindications to Manual Therapy

Contraindications to manual therapy include those that are absolute contraindications, and those that are relative.[42,43]

Absolute

▶ Bacterial infection.

▶ Malignancy.

▶ Systemic localized infection.

▶ Sutures over the area.

▶ Recent fracture.

▶ Cellulitis.

▶ Febrile state.

▶ Hematoma.

▶ Acute circulatory condition.

▶ An open wound at the treatment site.

▶ Osteomyelitis.

▶ Advanced diabetes.

▶ Hypersensitivity of the skin.

▶ Inappropriate end-feel (spasm, empty, bony).

▶ Constant, severe pain, including pain that disturbs sleep, indicating that the condition is likely to be in the acute stage of healing.

▶ Extensive radiation of pain.

▶ Pain unrelieved by rest.

▶ Severe irritability (pain that is easily provoked, and that does not go away within a few hours).

Relative

▶ Joint effusion or inflammation.

▶ Rheumatoid arthritis.

▶ Presence of neurologic signs.

▶ Osteoporosis.

▶ Hypermobility.

▶ Pregnancy, if technique is to be applied to the spine.

▶ Dizziness.

▶ Steroid or anticoagulant therapy.

Soft Tissue Techniques

Transverse Friction Massage

Transverse friction massage (TFM) is a technique devised by Cyriax whereby repeated cross-grain massage is applied to muscle, tendons, tendon sheaths, and ligaments. TFM has long been used by physical therapists to increase the mobility and extensibility of individual musculoskeletal tissues such as muscles, tendons, and ligaments, and to help prevent and treat inflammatory scar tissue.[7,44–49]

> **Clinical Pearl**
>
> TFM is indicated for acute or subacute ligament, tendon, or muscle injuries; chronically inflamed bursae; and adhesions in ligament or muscle, or between tissues. TFM also can be applied before performing a manipulation or a strong stretch to desensitize and soften the tissues.

TFM is contraindicated for acute inflammation, hematomas, debilitated or open skin, peripheral nerves, and in patients who have diminished sensation in the area.

TFM is purported to have the following therapeutic effects:

▶ *Traumatic hyperemia.*[7] According to Cyriax, longitudinal friction to an area increases the flow of blood and lymph, which in turn removes the chemical irritant by-products of inflammation. In addition, the increased blood flow reduces venous congestion, thereby decreasing edema and hydrostatic pressure on pain-sensitive structures.

▶ *Pain relief.* The application of TFM stimulates type I and II mechanoreceptors, producing presynaptic anesthesia. This presynaptic anesthesia is based on the gate theory of pain control (see Chap. 2). However, if the frictions are too vigorous in the acute stage, the stimulation of nociceptors will override the effect of the mechanoreceptors, causing the pain to increase. Occasionally, the patient may feel an exacerbation of symptoms following the first two or three sessions of the massage, especially in the case of a chronically inflamed bursa.[50] In these cases it is important to forewarn the patient to apply ice at home.

▶ *Decreasing scar tissue.* The transverse nature of the friction assists with the orientation of the collagen in the appropriate lines of stress and also helps produce hypertrophy of the new collagen. Given the stages of healing for soft tissue (see Chap. 5), light TFM should only be applied in the early stages of a subacute lesion, so as not to damage the granulation tissue. These gentle movements theoretically serve to minimize cross-linking and so enhance the extensibility of the new tissue. Following a ligament sprain, Cyriax recommends immediate use of TFM to prevent adhesion formation between the tissue and its neighbors, by moving the ligamentous tissue over the underlying bone.[7]

The application of the correct amount of tension to a healing structure is very important. The tissue undergoing TFM should, whenever possible, be positioned in a moderate but not painful stretch. The exception to this rule is when applying TFM to a muscle belly, which is usually positioned in its relaxed position.[7,51] Lubricant is not typically used with the application of TFM. However, ultrasound can be applied to a tissue before TFM.

Beginning with light pressure, and using a reinforced finger (i.e., middle finger over the index finger), or thumb, the clinician moves the skin over the site of the identified lesion back and forth in a direction perpendicular to the normal orientation of its fibers. It is important that the patient's skin move with the clinician's finger to prevent blistering.

> ### Clinical Pearl
>
> The application of TFM is condition and patient dependent. The intensity of the application is based on the stage of healing. The pain induced by TFM should be kept within the patient's tolerance. Light pressure should be used in the early stages, before building up the pressure over a few minutes to allow for accommodation.

The amplitude of the massage should be sufficient to cover all of the affected tissue, and the rate should be at two to three cycles per second, applied in a rhythmical manner.

The duration of the friction massage is usually gauged by when desensitization occurs (normally within 3 to 5 minutes). Tissues that do not desensitize within 3 to 5 minutes should be treated using some other form of intervention. If the condition is chronic or in the remodeling stage of healing, then the frictions are continued for a further 5 minutes after the desensitization, in an effort to enhance the mechanical effect on the cross-links and adhesions. Following the application of TFM, the involved tissue is either passively stretched, or actively exercised, taking care not to cause pain.

Most conditions amenable to TFM should resolve in six to ten sessions over 2 to 8 weeks. Tissues that do not show signs of improvement after three treatment sessions should be treated using some other form of intervention.

Specific TFM Techniques[52,53]
Shoulder.   Deep TFM is a good treatment adjunct for tendon and ligament injuries of the shoulder. Because the procedure needs to be performed at a specific area, the examination must accurately determine which structure is involved.

Biceps.   The patient is positioned with the shoulder abducted to 30 degrees and the elbow flexed. The clinician stands at the patient's side and supports the arm (Fig. 11-1). The clinician

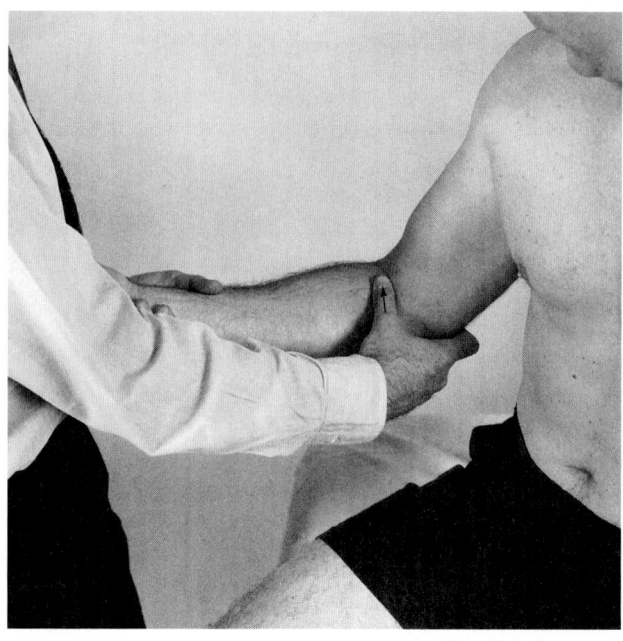

FIGURE 11-1   Transverse friction to the biceps tendon.

places his or her thumb on the biceps tendon and alternately applies a medial and lateral glide motion to the tendon to create gentle friction.

Supraspinatus.   The supraspinatus tendon is located just distal to the anterolateral corner of the acromion. It can become more discernible by positioning the patient's arm in slight extension behind the back (Fig. 11-2). The massage is applied perpendicular to the tendon at the point of relative hypovascularity, which is located approximately 1 cm proximal to its insertion on the greater tuberosity of the humerus[54] (see Fig. 11-2).

Elbow.   TFM is used to treat a number of soft tissue structures around the elbow.

Strain or Overuse of the Brachialis Muscle Belly.   Although uncommon, lesions of the brachialis muscle belly are most often seen in long-distance cross-country skiers with inadequate training. In the following example, the right brachialis is treated.

The patient is positioned next to the short side of the treatment table, sitting, with the elbow in 90 degrees of flexion and the forearm resting on the table in maximal supination. The clinician sits next to the long side of the treatment table diagonally facing the patient. The clinician locates the site of the lesion by palpation. In most cases, the affected site is directly in the middle (between medial and lateral) of the muscle belly, at the level of the biceps musculotendinous junction. The clinician places the left thumb just lateral to the musculotendinous junction of the biceps. The other hand holds the patient's forearm in maximal supination. The biceps musculotendinous junction is

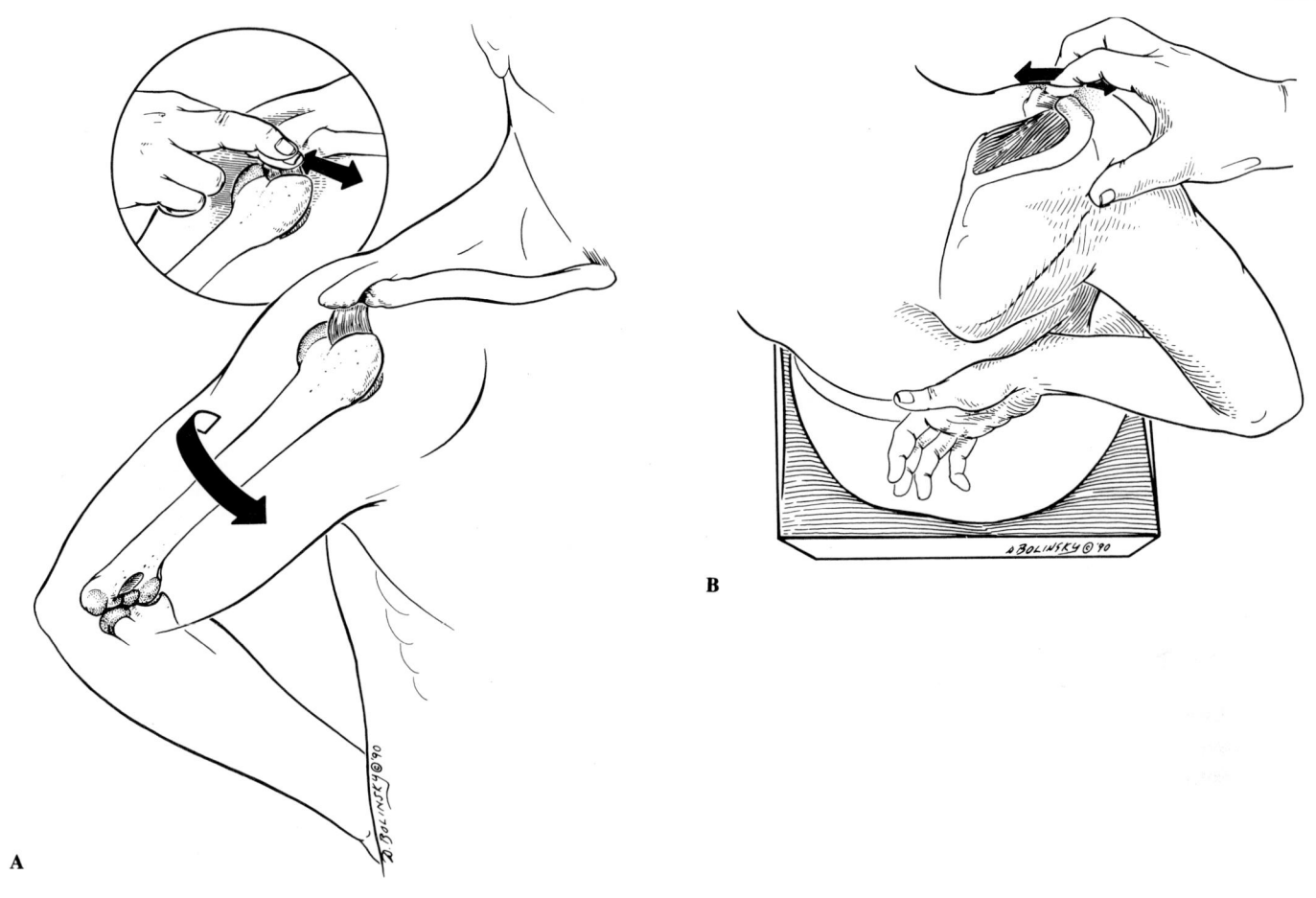

FIGURE 11-2   Transverse friction to the supraspinatus tendon. (*A*) The tendon is brought into a more sagittal position just below the anterior acromion. (*B*) Superior view of the supraspinatus tendon beneath the anterior acromion with the shoulder internally rotated. The forefinger should be between the anterior acromion and the greater tuberosity. (Reproduced with permission from Hammer WI. *Functional Soft Tissue Examination and Treatment by Manual Methods*. Gaithersburg, Md: Aspen; 1991:238. Copyright © 1990 by David Bolinsky.)

passively moved medially as far as possible with the thumb. After exerting pressure posteriorly, the clinician performs TFM in a lateral direction.

Strain or Overuse of the Muscle Belly–Musculotendinous Junction of the Biceps.   Lesions of the biceps muscle belly or musculotendinous junction can occur as a result of carrying a heavy object or from forceful throwing activities. In the following example, the right biceps tendon is treated.

The patient is positioned next to the short side of the treatment table, sitting, with the elbow in 90 degrees of flexion and the forearm resting on the table in supination. The clinician sits next to the long side of the treatment table diagonally facing the patient. The clinician locates the site of the lesion by palpation. This is done by means of a pinch grip between the clinician's thumb and index finger of the right hand, which grasps the posterior aspect of the muscle belly, while the other hand fixes the patient's forearm in supination. The transverse friction occurs through a "flat" pinching together of the thumb and index finger

with simultaneous extension of the wrist. This pulls the muscle belly fibers transversely through the fingers.

The biceps musculotendinous junction is treated in much the same way.

Insertion Tendonopathy of the Triceps.   Transverse friction is indicated for lesions in the musculotendinous junction (rare), the tendon, or the teno-osseous insertion of the triceps. Insertion tendonopathy of the triceps can occur as a result of chronic abuse or macrotrauma. Objective findings for this condition typically include pain with resisted elbow extension.

The patient is positioned prone on the treatment table with the upper arm resting on the table and the forearm hanging over the edge of the table. The clinician sits next to the patient at the patient's involved side. The exact site of the lesion is confirmed by palpation. With one hand, the clinician holds the patient's elbow in slightly more than 90 degrees of flexion. The thumb of the other hand is placed at the site of the lesion, while the fingers of this hand grasp the patient's forearm.

Static stretching of the triceps is combined with the transverse friction.

Insertion Tendonopathy at the Medial Humeral Epicondyle (Golfer's Elbow). The patient sits against the inclined head of the table with the affected arm elevated sideways to just below the horizontal. The elbow is extended and the forearm, supinated. The clinician sits on a chair or stool next to the patient. If the right elbow is to be treated, the clinician positions the patient's hand between the upper arm and thorax. The right hand grasps the patient's forearm just distal to the elbow and holds the elbow in extension. To determine the most painful site of the lesion, the tip of the left thumb carefully palpates the anterior plateau of the medial humeral epicondyle. The tip of the thumb is positioned in slight flexion. During the friction, the joint position of the thumb does not change. The friction motion consists of minimal wrist extension and an even smaller amount of adduction of the arm.

Tendonitis of the Extensor Carpi Radialis Brevis. The patient is positioned, sitting, next to the short end of the treatment table. The upper arm is positioned in 45 degrees of abduction, with the elbow in approximately 80 degrees of flexion and the forearm in pronation. The clinician sits next to the long side of the treatment table, diagonally facing the patient. To treat the right side, the clinician uses the left thumb. The tendon of the extensor carpi radialis brevis is located. In the pronated forearm, the extensor carpi radialis brevis tendon runs over the radial head (Fig. 11-3). In most cases, the tendon felt is, in fact, the common tendon of the extensor carpi radialis brevis and the extensor digitorum. Sometimes two tendons are palpated; the medial

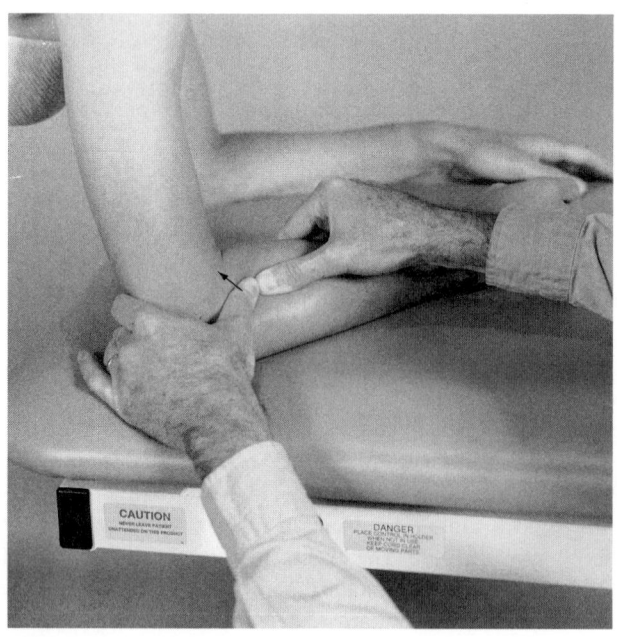

FIGURE 11-3 Transverse friction to the extensor carpi radialis brevis.

one is the extensor carpi radialis brevis. TFM is performed by moving the thumb in a medial to lateral direction over the tendon.

Wrist and Hand
Wrist Extensors. Transverse friction can be applied at the insertions of the extensor carpi radialis brevis (see Fig. 11-3), extensor carpi radialis longus, and extensor carpi ulnaris. The wrist is positioned in flexion, and TFM is applied as shown (see Fig. 11-3).

Wrist Flexors. Transverse friction can be applied at the insertions of the flexor carpi ulnaris, flexor carpi radialis, and tendons of the finger flexors.

Common Sheath of Abductor Pollicis Longus and Extensor Pollicis Brevis. Transverse friction can be applied to the common shared sheath of the abductor pollicis longus and extensor pollicis brevis, or at the point where the tendons pass over the wrist extensors.

Augmented Soft Tissue Mobilization[55]
Augmented soft tissue mobilization (ASTM) is a form of deep massage that uses specially designed handheld devices to assist the clinician in the mobilization of poorly organized scar tissue in and around muscles, tendons, and myofascial planes. ASTM originated from and expanded on the concepts of TFM.[56–58] The instruments used are solid, with angled edges, which are guided with the assistance of a lubricant such as cocoa butter. Longitudinal strokes are applied parallel to the fiber alignment in a stroking motion along the skin to mobilize the underlying soft tissues.

As the instruments move over an area with an underlying fibrotic lesion, a change in texture is palpable. The initial strokes, which are used for screening purposes, are smooth and flowing, but become shorter and more concentrated to increase the pressure per unit area once the fibrosis is located. The pressure exerted needs to be firm enough to locate the fibrosis and cause microtrauma, but not so hard that macrotrauma occurs. The microvascular trauma and capillary hemorrhage induces a localized inflammatory response and stimulates the body's healing cascade and immune-reparative system.[58]

The clinician assesses the effectiveness of the treatment by feeling for changes in the underlying soft tissue texture and making adjustments in the intensity and frequency of the treatment accordingly. The stroking motion is sustained for approximately 5 to 10 minutes. Usually, upon completion of the ASTM, there is immediate erythema and the potential for some transient ecchymosis. Following an application of ASTM, the tissue undergoes a stretching and strengthening program to maintain flexibility and reestablish muscular balance around the area that is being treated, as well as to influence the structural alignment of the remodeling collagen fibers and soft tissue matrix. Subsequently, cryotherapy is applied to the treated area for approximately 5 to 10 minutes to limit any post-treatment soreness.

Myofascial Release

Myofascial release (MFR) is a series of techniques designed to release restrictions in the myofascial tissue and is used for the treatment of soft tissue dysfunction. The development of a holistic and comprehensive approach for the evaluation and treatment of the myofascial system of the body is credited to John Barnes, who was strongly influenced by the teachings of Mennell[11] and Upledger.[59]

> ### Clinical Pearl
>
> Fascia is a tough connective tissue, composed of collagen, elastin, and a viscous gel, that exists in the body in the form of a continuous three-dimensional web of connective tissue, organized along the lines of tension imposed on the body (see Chap. 1).[60]

According to myofascial theory, the collagen provides strength to the fascia, the elastin gives it its elastic properties, and the gel functions to absorb the compressive forces of movement.[43] Three types of fascia are considered to exist[43,60]:

1. Superficial, lying directly below the dermis.

2. Deep, surrounding and infusing with muscle, bone, nerve, blood vessels, and organs to the cellular level.

3. Deepest, comprising the dura of the craniosacral system, which encases the central nervous system and brain.

The theory of MFR is based on the principle that trauma or structural abnormalities may create inappropriate fascial strain, because of an inability of the fascia to absorb or distribute the forces.[60] These strains to the fascia can result in a slow tightening of the fascia, causing the body to lose its physiologic adaptive capacity.[60] Over time, the fascial restrictions begin to pull the body out of its three-dimensional alignment, causing biomechanically inefficient movement and posture.[60] In addition, because of the association of fascia at the cellular level, it is theorized that trauma to or malfunction of the fascia can lead to poor cellular efficiency, disease, and pain throughout the body.[43,60] Three theoretical models for the manifestation of myofascial dysfunction are contraction, contracture, and cohesion-congestion (Table 11-5).

Thus, the purpose of MFR techniques is to apply a gentle sustained pressure to the fascia, in order to release fascial restrictions, thereby restoring normal pain-free function.[43] MFR relies entirely on the feedback received from the patient's tissues, with the clinician interpreting and responding to the feedback. This feedback is based on the Upledger concept of the natural body rhythm, called the craniosacral rhythm.[59] It is this rhythm that is theorized to guide the clinician as to the direction, force, and the duration of the technique.

It is not unusual for a patient to experience muscle soreness following MFR techniques. This soreness is thought to result from postural and alignment changes or from the techniques themselves.

Myofascial Stroking

The soft tissue techniques used in MFR are purported to break up cross-restrictions of the collagen of the fascia. Three of the more commonly used techniques involve stroking maneuvers.[43]

▶ *J stroke.* This technique is used to increase skin mobility. Counterpressure is applied with the heel of the hand, while a stroke in the shape of the letter J is applied in the direction of the restriction, with two or three fingers, which creates some torque at the end of the stroke.

▶ *Vertical stroke.* The purpose of vertical stroking is to open up the length of vertically oriented superficial fascia. As in the J stroke, counterpressure is applied with one hand, while the stroking is performed with the other.

▶ *Transverse stroke.* As its name suggests, the transverse stroke is applied in a transverse direction to the body. Force is applied downward into the muscle with the fingertips of both hands, and the force is applied slowly and perpendicular to the muscle fibers.

▶ *Cross-hands technique.* The cross-hands technique is used for the release of deep fascial tissues. The clinician places crossed hands over the site of restriction. The elastic component of the fascia is then stretched until the barrier is met. At this point, the clinician maintains consistent gentle pressure at the barrier for approximately 90 to 120 seconds. Once the release is felt, the clinician reduces the pressure.

TABLE 11-5 Theoretical Models for the Manifestation of Myofascial Disorders[34]

Model	Manifestation	End-feel
Contraction	Muscle hypertonicity or spasm	Reactive, firm, and painful end-feel
Contracture	Inert or noncontractile tissues that have undergone fibrotic alteration	Abrupt, firm, stiff, or hard end-feel
Cohesion-Congestion	Fluidochemical changes in microcellular transport systems, resulting in impaired lymphatic flow, vascular stasis, or ischemia	Boggy, stiff, or reactive end-feel

It is important to remember that the claimed benefits and effectiveness of MFR techniques are largely anecdotal, because at the time of writing there is no scientific experimental research to validate these claims.[61]

Soft Tissue Mobilization

Soft tissue mobilizations (STMs) are used in many of the manual techniques described within this chapter, including MFR, muscle energy, and proprioceptive neuromuscular facilitation. The techniques of STM described in this section are based on the concept that tissue restrictions occur at different layers, ranging from superficial to deep.

The general principles behind STM are that the superficial layers are treated before deep layers, with the force used applied in the direction of the maximum restriction, and where the choice of technique is dependent on the extent of the restriction, amount of discomfort, and degree of irritability. Deep tissue massage is recommended to reduce spasm[62] and promote pain reduction.[63] Several well-recognized STM techniques are described next.[64]

Sustained Pressure

This technique is applied to the center of the restricted tissue at the exact depth, direction, and angle of the maximal restriction. Applying a force in either a clockwise or counterclockwise direction, while the sustained pressure is maintained, can modify the technique of sustained pressure. This spiral motion increases the tissue tension in one direction, while easing it in the other. Sustained pressure also can be applied perpendicular to or parallel to the restriction.

Ischemic Compression

Ischemic compression is a similar technique to sustained pressure that can be used on both active and inactive trigger points. It is believed that the ischemic compression deprives the trigger points of oxygen, rendering them inactive and breaking the cycle of pain–spasm–pain. Usually the pressure is applied for 8 to 12 seconds. If the patient reports a lessening of local and referred pain, the therapist can repeat the treatment. However, if the pain does not lessen, the clinician may need to adjust the pressure or choose an alternative technique.

General Massage

Massage can be defined as the systematic, therapeutic, and functional stroking and kneading of the body.[65] The French are credited with the introduction of massage into Europe, and many of the terms associated with massage still bear French names.[66] Massage has long been a central part of the physical therapy curriculum. Studies have demonstrated that deep massage increases the circulation and skin temperature of the massaged area as a result of dilation of the capillaries.[67–70] A number of traditional massage techniques are used, including:

► *Effleurage.* This is a general stroking technique applied to the muscles and soft tissues in a centripetal direction (from distal to proximal) to enhance relaxation and increase venous and lymphatic drainage. The clinician applies a firm contact with the patient using the palms of the hand and, at the end of the stroke, lifts the hands from the patient's skin and replaces them at the starting position.[71] Oil or cream can be used to aid the stroking.

► *Stroking.* Stroking techniques are applied superficially along the whole length of a surface. These techniques are typically applied before the deeper techniques of massage to enhance relaxation.[70]

► *Petrissage.* This term is used to describe a group of techniques that involve the compression of soft tissue structures, and include kneading, wringing, rolling, and picking-up techniques to release areas of muscle fibrosis and to "milk" the muscles of waste products that collect from trauma or abnormal inactivity.[72]

► *Strumming.* The technique of perpendicular strumming involves the application of repeated, rhythmic deformations of a muscle belly in a strumming fashion.

Acupressure

Acupressure is based on the ancient arts of shiatsu and acupuncture, involving manual pressure over the acupuncture points of the body to improve the flow of the body's energy, known as *Qi*. This energy is thought to circulate throughout the body along a series of channels, called *meridians*. Traditional Eastern medicine is based on the concept that all disorders are reflected at specific points, either on the skin surface or just beneath it, along these channels. By careful manipulation of these points, the clinician can theoretically strengthen, disperse, or calm the Qi, enabling it to flow smoothly.[73] Modern acupressurists use traditional meridian acupuncture points; nonmeridian or extrameridian acupuncture points, which are fixed points not necessarily associated with meridians; and trigger points, which have no fixed locations and are found by eliciting tenderness at the site of most pain.[74] When acupressure is applied successfully, the patient is supposed to experience a sensation known as *teh chi,* defined as a subjective feeling of fullness, numbness, tingling, and warmth with some local soreness and a feeling of distention around the acupuncture point.[74] Western scientific research has proposed a number of mechanisms for the effect of acupressure in relieving pain, as follows:

► The gate control theory of pain.[75,76]

► Diffuse noxious inhibitory control. This theory implies that noxious stimulation of heterotopic body areas modulates the pain sensation originating in areas where a subject feels pain.[74]

► Stimulation of the production of endorphins, serotonin, and acetylcholine in the central nervous system, which enhances analgesia.[77–85]

Muscle Energy

The origin of muscle energy techniques is credited to Fred Mitchell, Sr.[86] Muscle energy techniques combine the precision of passive mobilization with the effectiveness, safety, and specificity of reeducation therapies and therapeutic exercise.[87]

> ### Clinical Pearl
>
> Muscle energy techniques require the active participation of the patient and are thus viewed as mobilization techniques, which utilize muscular facilitation and inhibition.[88]

Muscle energy techniques, which involve positioning a restricted muscle-joint complex at its restricted barrier, can be used to mobilize joints, strengthen weakened muscles, and stretch adaptively shortened muscles and fascia.[89] Optimal success with these techniques is more likely in the acute or subacute stages of healing, before prolonged joint changes have had the opportunity to occur.

According to the teachings of muscle energy, muscles function as flexors, extensors, rotators, and side benders of joints, as well as restrictors or barriers to movement. In other words, muscles both produce and control motion. Although it is obvious that muscles produce motion, it is easy to forget that they also resist motion. This resistance to motion is related to muscle tone, a complex neurophysiologic state governed by both cortical and spinal reflexes, and by the afferent activity from the articular and muscle systems. Afferent input from type I and II mechanoreceptors located in the superficial and deep aspects of the joint capsule is projected to the motor neurons.[90,91] Exaggerated spindle responses are provoked by any motions that attempt to lengthen the muscle, creating an increase in resistance to those motions. Stretching or lengthening of the muscle also stimulates the Golgi tendon organs, which have an inhibitory influence on muscle tension, leading to muscle relaxation. In addition, it has been demonstrated that cutaneous stimulation of certain areas of the body can produce inhibition or excitation of specific motor neuron pools.[92]

It is theorized that the neuromuscular system is "scarred" by pain and impairment, producing asymmetry in the musculoskeletal system and resulting in a disruption of the harmony and rhythm of the body, referred to as somatic dysfunction.[87] Somatic dysfunctions can be described or named in one of three ways[32]:

1. The direction of increased freedom of motion.

2. The position in lesion.

3. The direction of limitation of motion.

In the presence of a somatic dysfunction, there is usually an asymmetric pattern of motion, with restriction in one direction and increased freedom in the opposite direction.[32] The triad of ART (*a*symmetry, *r*ange of motion restriction or barrier, and *t*issue texture)[12] helps to describe the characteristics of somatic dysfunction. Primary somatic dysfunctions, which may result from trauma, are reversible as long as they are treated correctly and do not become chronic in terms of abnormal fibrosis or adhesions. Secondary somatic dysfunctions result from the consequences of visceral pathology, or from the adaptations made by somatic structures in response to forces or stresses imposed on them.

The consequence of a somatic dysfunction can be a change in the length of the tissues that surround a joint. Some of these tissues adaptively shorten, whereas others adaptively lengthen. These changes in length are theorized to produce changes in the neurophysiologic makeup of the muscle, affecting tension development, as well as changes in the angle of pull.

There is some commonality between muscle energy and several procedures used in orthopedic manual therapy, such as proprioceptive neuromuscular facilitation.[93] Greenman[12] summarizes the requirements for the correct application of muscle energy techniques to be control, balance, and localization.

▶ The technique, which involves a controlled effort in a controlled direction, commences from a controlled position. Eccentric, concentric, and isometric contractions, at varying levels of effort, are used in muscle energy within a range of movement controlled by the clinician.

▶ The clinician balances the degree of force used, depending on the intention.

▶ The force used is localized as much as possible to the joint in question. The localization of force is more important than the intensity of the force.

The intent of muscle energy is to treat somatic dysfunctions by restoring the muscles around a joint to their normal neurophysiologic state, through either stretching or strengthening the agonist and antagonist. Somatic dysfunctions include those in which the motion barrier is encountered before the physiologic barrier is reached.[87] The type of motion barrier is determined by the end-feel.

> ### Clinical Pearl
>
> A hard, capsular end-feel indicates pericapsular hypomobility, whereas a jammed or pathomechanical end-feel indicates hypomobility. An elastic end-feel indicates the presence of hypertonus, whereas an inelastic end-feel indicates fibrosis.[87]

A normal end-feel would indicate normal range, whereas an abnormal end-feel would suggest abnormal range, either hypomobile or hypermobile, with the latter characterized by a loss of end-feel resiliency and an abrupt approach to the anatomic barrier. All muscle energy techniques are classed as direct techniques because they engage the barrier.[33] Indirect techniques form the basis for the strain-counterstrain (positional release) techniques,[94] and the functional techniques,[95–97] both of which are discussed later.

The position of the clinician during the performance of the technique must allow easy access to the structures involved, while maintaining proper body mechanics. In each of the following recognized methods of muscle energy, the setup is identical. The clinician positions the bone or joint so that the muscle group to be used is at its resting length. The patient is then given specific instructions about the direction in which to move, the intensity of the contraction, and the duration of the contraction.[89,93,98,99] The amounts of force and counterforce are governed by the length and strength of the muscle group involved, as well as by the patient's symptoms.[89] The clinician's force can match the effort of the patient, thus producing an isometric contraction and allowing no movement to occur, or it may overcome the patient's effort, thus moving the area or joint in the direction opposite to that in which the patient is attempting to move it, thereby using an isotonic or isolytic contraction.[93] There appears to be no consensus as to whether to use the relaxation of the agonist or the antagonist to gain motion.[12,88,100–102]

Lewit's Postisometric Relaxation[88,103]

A commonly used technique in the field of muscle energy is postisometric relaxation (PIR). PIR refers to the effect of the subsequent reduction in tone experienced by a muscle, or group of muscles, after brief periods during which an isometric contraction has been performed.[93] The basis for PIR is related to the theory that light, brief isometric contractions of a hypertonic muscle externally stretch the nuclear bag fibers of the muscle spindles. This stretching, in turn, allows a lengthening of muscle during the postisometric phase, without stimulating myostatic reflexes.[87] Phasic muscles that have become adaptively shortened are treated using more forceful isometric contractions.

Clinical Pearl

PIR techniques are ideal as an initial technique to gain the patient's trust, especially in cases of reflex contraction or trigger point hypertonicity.[99] These techniques also can be used for joint mobilizations when a manipulation is not desirable.[103]

PIR techniques are performed as follows. The hypertonic muscle is taken to a length just short of pain, or to the point where tissue resistance is first felt. At this point, the patient is asked to contract the affected muscle away from the barrier for 5 to 10 seconds, using the agonist and using about 20 percent of maximum effort, while the clinician resists the movement isometrically. After the contraction, the patient is asked to relax, and the clinician gently takes the muscle to the new barrier, thereby avoiding the stretch reflex. The process is repeated two to three more times, and the muscle is reassessed for length.

Janda's Postfacilitation Stretch[102]

This method is well suited for the segmental and muscle tightness types of muscular hypertonicity.[99] Postfacilitation stretches are performed as follows. The hypertonic muscle is placed in its mid-range position, about halfway between the fully relaxed and fully stretched positions. The patient is asked to perform an isometric contraction using a maximum amount of effort for 5 to 10 seconds, while the clinician resists the

movement completely. When the patient relaxes, the clinician applies a rapid stretch to the muscle and holds the stretch for at least 10 seconds. The patient relaxes for about 20 seconds, and the procedure is repeated two to five more times.

Reciprocal Inhibition

The techniques of reciprocal inhibition are used mainly in acute settings, where tissue damage or pain prevents the use of the more usual agonist contraction. Reciprocal inhibition techniques are also commonly used to conclude a muscle energy session.[93,104]

Reciprocal inhibition techniques are performed as follows. The involved muscle is placed in its mid-range position, and the patient is instructed to contract firmly toward the restriction barrier, while the clinician either completely resists the motion or allows a movement toward it. The contraction is held for about 5 to 8 seconds, after which the patient completely relaxes and the clinician passively lengthens the muscle.

Strengthening

ME techniques can be used to strengthen muscles using isometric, concentric, eccentric, or isokinetic contractions.

▶ *Isometric.* The clinician applies resistance to joint motion that is equal to that of the patient, such that no motion occurs. The contraction is held for approximately 30 to 60 seconds to increase the tone and strength of the muscle, or muscle group.

▶ *Concentric.* The clinician applies resistance to joint motion such that it is less than that of the patient, so that the patient moves the joint in the desired direction and through the desired range at a speed controlled by the clinician. This is repeated five times, and serves to increase the concentric strength of the agonist muscles, and relaxation of the antagonists.

▶ *Eccentric.* The clinician applies resistance to joint motion such that it is greater than that of the patient. Thus, the patient is not only unable to move the joint in the desired direction, but is also unable to fully resist that of the clinician. As a result, even with maximum effort, the joint moves in the opposite direction of the desired movement. This is repeated five times and serves to increase the eccentric strength, and length, of the agonist muscles.

▶ *Isokinetic.* The patient begins with a weak contraction of the muscle against the clinician's resistance, but quickly increases the force to a maximal contraction in about 4 seconds. These contractions can be accompanied by mobilizations of the restricted ranges.[93]

Isolytic Contraction

This method involves the use of a contraction by the clinician to overcome the resistance of the patient's contraction (an isotonic eccentric contraction), in order to stretch and sometimes break down any fibrotic tissue that might be present in the involved muscle. These techniques can be uncomfortable for the patient, and the clinician should explain this before performing the techniques. Needless to say, these techniques are not to be used in the acute or subacute phases of healing.

Technique Examples

Some examples of muscle energy stretching techniques are outlined next. Other examples of these techniques are included in the later chapters of this book.

Hamstrings

Lower Hamstrings. The patient is positioned supine with the knee extended and with the opposite knee bent to 90 degrees. The clinician flexes the hip to the resistance barrier. The patient is asked to actively extend the hip and to plantar flex the ankle while clinician provides an equal and opposite resistance for 10 seconds. The patient then actively flexes the hip and dorsiflexes the ankle to the new range of motion with assistance from the clinician. This technique can be performed with abduction/internal rotation (medial hamstrings) and adduction/external rotation (lateral hamstrings). Three to five repetitions of the exercise are performed.

Upper Hamstrings. The patient is positioned supine with the opposite knee bent to 90 degrees. The hip and knee of the involved leg are flexed to 90/90 degrees. The patient is asked to flex the knee and plantar flex the ankle while the clinician provides equal and opposite resistance for 10 seconds. The patient then actively extends the knee and dorsiflexes the ankle to the new resistance barrier with assistance from the clinician. This technique can be performed with the tibia positioned in internal rotation (to stretch the bicep femoris) and external rotation (to stretch the semitendinosus and membranosus). Three to five repetitions of the exercise are performed.

Hip Adductors. The patient is positioned supine or side lying with the leg abducted. If the two-joint adductors are to be stretched, the knee is extended. If the one-joint adductors are to be stretched, the knee is flexed. The patient's leg is taken into abduction to the resistance barrier. The patient is instructed to attempt adduction against the clinician's equal and opposite force for 10 seconds. Three to five repetitions of the exercise are performed.

Gastrocnemius. The patient is positioned supine with the knee extended. The subtalar joint is positioned in neutral. The patient's foot and ankle are passively dorsiflexed to the point of first resistance. The patient is asked to actively plantar flex the foot against clinician's equal resistance. The contraction is held for 10 seconds. The patient is then asked to actively dorsiflex the ankle to the new point of resistance. Three to five repetitions of the exercise are performed.

Soleus. The patient is positioned prone with knee flexed to 90 degrees. The subtalar joint is positioned in neutral. The patient's foot and ankle are passively dorsiflexed to the point of first resistance. The patient is asked to actively plantar flex the foot against clinician's equal resistance. The contraction is held for 10 seconds. The patient is then asked to actively dorsiflex the ankle to the new point of restriction. Three to five repetitions of the exercise are performed.

Upper Trapezius. The patient is positioned supine with the head flexed, rotated toward and side bent away from the side of the intended stretch. The clinician stabilizes the patient's head with one hand, while the other hand is placed on the patient's shoulder. The patient is instructed to elevate the shoulder toward the ear against equal and opposite resistance from the clinician for 10 seconds. The clinician then moves the head and neck to the new resistance barrier. Three to five repetitions of the exercise are performed.

Levator Scapulae. The patient is positioned supine with the cervical spine flexed, side bent away and rotated away from the side of the intended stretch. The clinician stabilizes the head with one hand, while the other hand contacts the patient's shoulder. The patient is instructed to elevate the shoulder complex against equal and opposite resistance from the clinician for 10 seconds. Three to five repetitions of the exercise are performed.

Strain-Counterstrain (Positional Release)

The techniques of strain-counterstrain (positional release) involve a gentle and simple indirect manipulative approach for the treatment of somatic dysfunction, using passive positioning of the body in a position of ease (rather than into motion restriction) to evoke a therapeutic effect.[94,105] According to strain-counterstrain theory, so-called myofascial tender points are associated with specific somatic dysfunctions and can be used to both diagnose and guide the intervention for these dysfunctions.[106]

Positional release is an attempt by the body at self-mobilization, and occurs when the patient is passively positioned at what is termed the *position of ease* (mobile point), and maintained there for 90 to 120 seconds.[94] The mobile point corresponds to the point of maximum relaxation, from which any movement produces an increase in tissue tension under the monitoring hand at the selected tender point site.[94,105,106]

A possible neurophysiologic explanation of how and why these techniques work was first suggested by Korr,[107] who postulated that an injured segment behaved differently from an uninjured segment in that the γ motor neuron activity in the former became increased. Bailey[108] later refined the theory by suggesting that an inappropriate high "gainset" of the muscle spindle resulted in changes characteristic of somatic dysfunction.[109] Thus, the techniques of strain-counterstrain serve to effect the muscle spindle–γ loop, by allowing the extrafusal muscle fibers to lengthen to their normal relaxed state, thereby decreasing spindle output and interrupting the pain-spasm cycle.[109–111]

Strain-counterstrain is also thought to improve blood flow to the area through a circulatory flushing of previously ischemic tissues.[110,112]

The first step in the examination procedure for the spine is modification of the sagittal posture of the patient to produce a flattening of the lordosis-kyphosis in the region to be examined.[109] In the extremities, the body part is placed in a position of relaxation. Tissue texture abnormalities and areas of tenderness are then sought. The position of greatest resistance and pain is usually the position that is directly related to that of the original mechanism of injury; thus, the position of ease is usually opposite to that direction. In most cases, the tender point will be in, or near, the area of discomfort. Once the tender point is located, the involved muscle is passively shortened while the tender point is monitored for changes in discomfort. For example, if the biceps is being treated, the tender point is monitored while the elbow is flexed and the forearm is simultaneously supinated. If the muscle is being moved in the correct direction, the tenderness should lessen. Slight adjustments from the recommended positions in this text may be needed. If there is more than one tender point, the clinician treats each one at a time, until the dominant one is found.

Once the correct position is found, the position is maintained for 90 to 120 seconds, before the patient returns slowly to the normal position. Once the tender point has been successfully removed, the clinician should focus on lengthening and strengthening the involved muscle.

Strain-Counterstrain Technique Examples[113]
Shoulder

Anterior Acromioclavicular: Anterior Surface of Distal Clavicle. To treat the anterior acromioclavicular tender point (Fig. 11-4), the patient is positioned supine. The clinician stands at the side of the table opposite the tender point. The tender point is monitored as the clinician adducts the arm across the patient's chest and applies traction by pulling on the arm at the wrist.

Long Head of Biceps: Over Tendon. The technique for the tender point of the long head of the biceps (see Fig. 11-4) includes positioning the patient supine, with the clinician at the side of the table, next to the tender point and facing the patient's head. The clinician flexes the patient's arm to 90 degrees at the elbow and shoulder and applies downward pressure at the elbow along the humerus to the monitoring finger.

Short Head of Biceps: Inferior-lateral to Coracoid Process. The technique for the tender point of the short head of the biceps (see Fig. 11-4) is similar to that described for the long head. However, fine-tuning into adduction is needed.

Posterior Acromioclavicular: Behind Lateral End of Clavicle. The posterior acromioclavicular tender point (see Fig. 11-4) is

treated by positioning the patient prone. The clinician is positioned at the side of the table opposite the tender point. The clinician adducts the patient's arm across the back, before applying traction to the arm by pulling at the wrist.

Supraspinatus. This tender point is located in the supraspinatus fossa, beneath the trapezius, just above the spine of the scapula and approximately 1 inch lateral to the vertebral border at the midpoint of the muscle belly[85] (see Fig. 11-4). The supraspinatus tender point is treated by positioning the patient supine, with the clinician sitting on the involved side. The clinician places the index finger of one hand on the tender point, passively flexes the arm at the shoulder toward the ceiling 45 degrees, abducts it 45 degrees, and markedly rotates it externally with the other hand.[94,114]

Elbow.[113] These tender points are depicted in Figure 11-4.

Radial Head and Lateral Epicondyle Tender Points. The patient is positioned supine, and the elbow is positioned in full extension over the clinician's knee. From this position, the clinician supinates, extends, and abducts the forearm until the point of ease is found. The position is maintained for 90 seconds. The arm is then returned slowly to a neutral position.

Medial Epicondyle Tender Points. The patient is positioned sitting. The elbow is positioned in full flexion, and the wrist is positioned in full flexion, with the palm facing down. From this position, the clinician adjusts the amount of wrist flexion, and radial and ulnar deviation, until the point of ease is found. The position is maintained for 90 seconds. The arm is then returned slowly to a neutral position.

Coronoid Tender Points. The patient is positioned supine, and the elbow is positioned in full flexion. From this position, the clinician gently pronates and abducts the forearm until the point of ease is found. The position is held for 90 seconds. The arm is then returned slowly to a neutral position.

Wrist and Hand

Thumb. A tender point of the first carpometacarpal joint (see Fig. 11-4) that is associated with pain and weakness of the thumb is treated by markedly rotating the thumb toward the palm, with a slight amount of flexion.

Interossei. The interossei tender points (see Fig. 11-4) are treated by flexing the joint and applying some traction. An extension carpometacarpal tender point is treated by extending the joint and applying traction.

Hip[115]

Posterolateral Trochanteric Tender Point. The tender point is located on the posterolateral surface of the greater trochanter (see Fig. 11-4). The patient is positioned prone, with the clinician standing or seated beside the table. The clinician positions the patient's hip into extension and abduction. Hip external rotation may be needed.

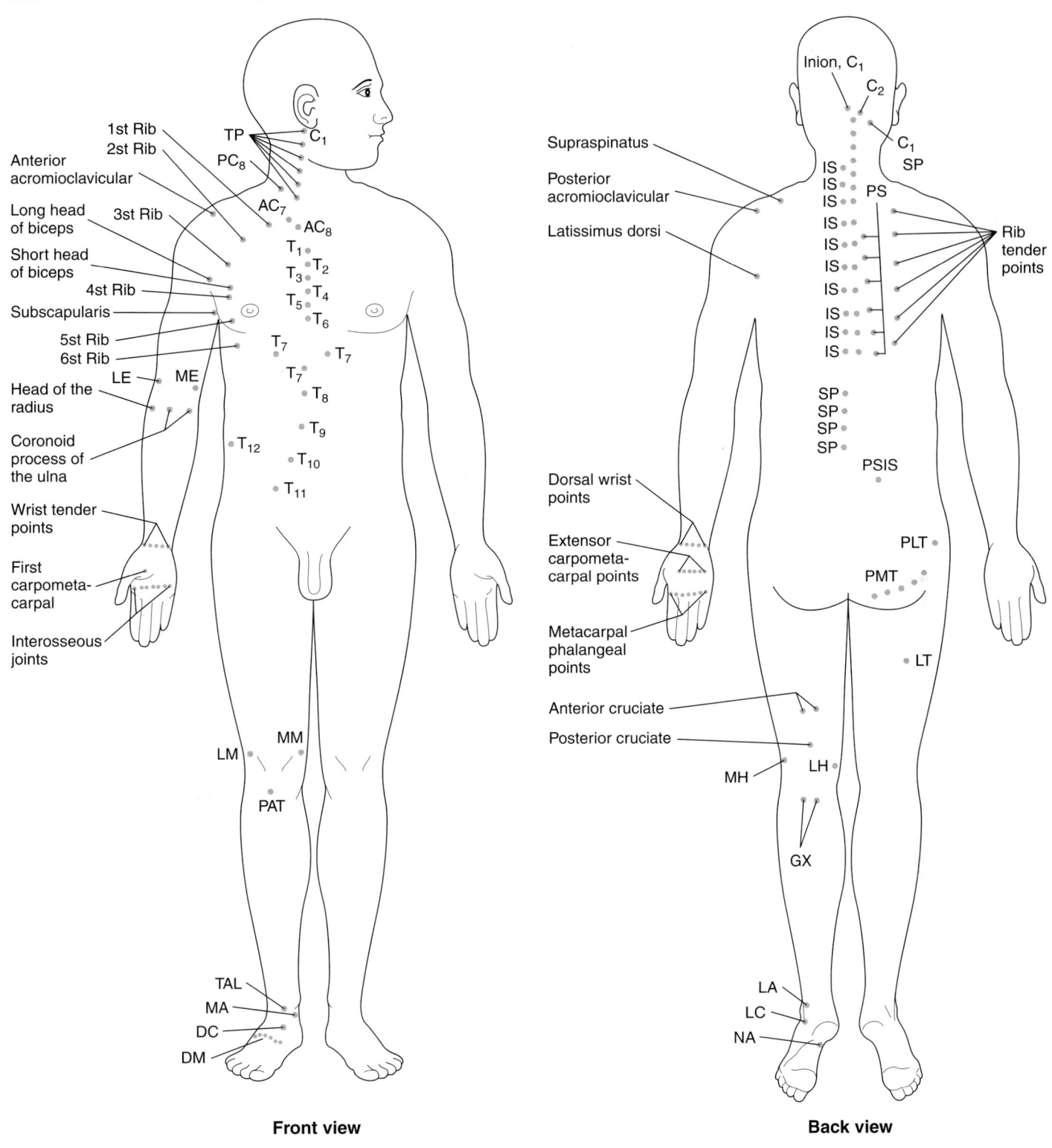

FIGURE 11-4 Strain-counterstrain tender points of the body. AC, anterior cervical; PC, posterior cervical; LH, lateral hamstring; MH, medial hamstring; GX, gastrocnemius; LA, lateral ankle; LC, lateral calcaneal; NA, navicular; LT, lateral trochanter; SP, spinous process; TP, transverse process; PS, paraspinal; LE, lateral epicondyle; ME, medial epicondyle; LM, lateral meniscus; MM, medial meniscus; PAT, patella; TAL, talus; MA, medial ankle; DC, dorsal cuboid; DM, dorsal metatarsal; IS, interspinal; PSIS, posterior superior iliac spine; PLT, posterolateral trochanteric; PMT, posteromedial trochanteric.

Lateral Trochanteric Tender Point. The tender point is located 5 to 6 inches below the trochanter on the lateral thigh (see Fig. 11-4). The patient is positioned prone, with the clinician standing or seated beside the table. The clinician positions the patient's hip into abduction. Some flexion may be introduced.

Posteromedial Trochanteric Tender Points. The tender point is located 2 to 3 inches below the trochanter along posterior shaft of femur, over to the ischial tuberosity (see Fig. 11-4). The patient is positioned prone, with the clinician standing beside the table opposite the tender point. The clinician positions the patient's hip into extension, adduction, and external rotation.

Knee. The tender points for the knee are depicted in Figure 11-4.

Anterior Tender Points. The major anterior tender point is the patellar tendon point, located just below the patella. The patient is positioned supine, with the clinician standing beside the table. A rolled pillow is placed beneath the patient's calf. The knee is hyperextended by the clinician, by pressing down on the anterior thigh just above the patella, with a fair amount of force. The foot is placed in internal rotation.

Anterior Cruciate Tender Point. The patient is positioned supine, with the clinician standing beside the table. A rolled pillow is placed under the thigh of the involved leg. The clinician presses down on the lower leg just below the joint, with a large amount of force. This technique shortens the anterior cruciate ligaments.

Posterior Cruciate Tender Point. The patient is positioned supine, with the clinician standing beside the table. A rolled pillow is placed behind the knee below the joint. The clinician presses down on the dorsum of the ankle with a large amount of force. The foot is internally rotated. This maneuver shortens the posterior cruciate ligament.

Gastrocnemius Tender Points. The patient is positioned prone, and the clinician stands beside the table with his foot on the table. The patient's foot is hyperextended over the clinician's knee by a downward force on the posterior ankle. This maneuver shortens the gastrocnemius muscle.

Medial Meniscus Tender Point. The patient is positioned supine, with the involved leg off the table. The clinician sits beside the table. The clinician grasps the patient's foot and internally rotates the lower leg, keeping the knee slightly flexed. The knee is adducted slightly against the edge of the table.

Medial Hamstring Tender Point. The patient is positioned supine, with the clinician standing beside the table. The knee is flexed to about 60 degrees, and the leg is externally rotated with a slight amount of adduction. This may be accomplished by grasping the patient's foot or ankle to use as a lever.

Lateral Meniscus Tender Point. The patient is positioned supine, with the leg off the table and the knee slightly flexed, while the clinician sits beside the table. The clinician grasps the patient's foot and internally rotates the tibia. The lower leg is slightly abducted. Occasionally external rotation may be needed.

Lateral Hamstring Tender Point. The patient is positioned supine, with the leg off the table and the knee slightly flexed, while the clinician sits beside the table. The clinician grasps the patient's foot and externally rotates the tibia. The knee is flexed about 30 degrees, and an abduction force is applied to the leg.

Leg, Foot, and Ankle
First Metatarsophalangeal Joint Pain. The tender point for this joint is typically located on the ball of the foot. The patient is positioned supine. The clinician grasps the forefoot and twists it into internal rotation (toward the center of the sole of the foot) until the point of ease is found. The position is maintained for 90 seconds, and then the foot is returned slowly to a neutral position.

Plantar Fasciitis Heel Pain. The tender point for plantar fasciitis is typically located at the attachment site for the plantar fascia on the calcaneus. The patient is positioned prone, with the knee flexed. The clinician grasps the forefoot with one hand and the calcaneus with the other hand. The clinician then simultaneously pushes the forefoot toward the heel and the heel toward the forefoot, thereby shortening the plantar fascia. The point of ease is found and the position is maintained for 90 seconds. Then the foot is returned slowly to a neutral position.

Dorsal Metatarsal Tender Points (see Fig. 11-4). The patient is positioned prone, with the knee flexed to 90 degrees, while the clinician stands beside the table. The foot and ankle are strongly dorsiflexed using a downward pressure.

Medial Ankle Tender Point (see Fig. 11-4). The patient is positioned lying on the side, with the involved leg uppermost. The clinician is seated beside the table. The patient's foot is brought off the table, and a rolled towel is placed under the anterior ankle. The clinician inverts the foot by pressing forcefully on the lateral side of the foot.

Lateral Ankle Tender Point (see Fig. 11-4). This technique is the same as for the medial ankle tender point, except that the ankle is forcefully everted.

Talar Tender Point. This tender point is on the anteromedial ankle, deep to the talus (see Fig. 11-4). The patient is positioned prone, with the foot up. The clinician is seated at the foot of the table. The patient's foot is dorsiflexed, inverted, and internally rotated.

Dorsal Cuboid Tender Point (see Fig. 11-4). The patient is positioned prone, with the clinician standing beside the table. The clinician grasps the patient's foot and inverts it by applying pressure on the lateral side.

Navicular Tender Point (see Fig. 11-4). The patient is positioned in prone position, with the clinician seated or standing beside the table. The clinician places his or her thumb or two fingers over the navicular bone to cause an inversion of the navicular. A slight amount of flexion is added.

Functional Techniques

Functional techniques are indirect techniques that use positional placement away from the restrictive barrier, similar to the techniques previously described for strain-counterstrain. The functional techniques were developed in the osteopathic profession in the 1950s, and much credit is given to Dr Andrew Taylor Still[116] for identifying the dysfunctions that are treated with these techniques.[95,117] Still considered the somatic lesion to be a mechanical involvement of the structure, and his teachings placed primary emphasis on pertinent anatomy, with palpation used to identify the position and arrangement of a particular structure.[96]

Although the term *functional technique* is itself somewhat of a misnomer, the criterion that distinguishes functional techniques from most manual techniques is the emphasis on moving the joint being treated away from, rather than toward, the restrictive barrier. As in the case of strain-counterstrain techniques, the joint in question is moved toward the normal physiologic barrier, at the opposite end of the range of motion to that of the restriction.

According to functional technique theory, there is a dynamic balance point located between the restrictive barrier and the opposite physiologic barrier, which is the joint position in which the tensions in the soft tissues around the joint become balanced equally in all three planes.[13] If this balance is achieved, the clinician can detect a sense of "ease" under his or her palpating fingers. It is the deep segmental tissues, which support and position the bones of a segment, and their reaction to normal motion demands, that are at the heart of functional technique specificity.[118] If motion in any plane is initiated away from the dynamic balance point, the soft tissue tension around the treated segment increases, and there will be an increased sense of palpatory tension, or "bind."[13]

Two theories have been proposed to explain the beneficial effects of these techniques[13]:

1. The afferent input from the proprioceptors is inhibited, which, in turn, suppresses the local protective cord reflexes.

2. The techniques stimulate the mechanoreceptors sufficiently to inhibit the pain receptors, allowing the tissues to relax.

Once the patient has been positioned correctly, the clinician can use one of two intervention options:

1. *Active.* In this method, the clinician initiates movement along the path of least resistance through the sequential release of any soft tissue tension that occurs, until the restrictive barrier is no longer detectable and normal motion is regained.

2. *Passive.* In this method, the clinician follows the articular unwinding through sequential releases of the treated joint to the point of full soft tissue release, until the restrictive barrier is no longer detectable and normal motion is regained.

Functional Techniques of the Shoulder

The following functional techniques are recommended for the shoulder.[94]

Stage One. The patient is positioned supine, while the clinician sits beside the patient on the same side as the shoulder to be treated. The clinician places one hand over the upper chest so that the fifth finger is along the axis of the clavicle with the fingertips of the fourth and fifth fingers palpating over the sternoclavicular area. The hypothenar eminence of the same hand is used to palpate in the region of the acromioclavicular joint. With the other hand, the clinician abducts the patient's arm to approximately 90 degrees, by either grasping the arm above or below the elbow. Fine adjustments to this position can be made on the basis of the monitoring hand, by slightly abducting and adducting, internally and externally rotating, or compressing and decompressing along the long axis of the humerus.

Stage Two. The patient is positioned supine. The clinician monitors with one hand, which is placed over the glenohumeral area with thumb over the posterior aspect of the shoulder and the fingers over the anterior aspect. This hand position permits the clinician to apply slight compression to the glenohumeral joint medially and slightly inferiorly, to assist in the relaxation of the rotator cuff muscles. Using the hand, with the same placement as previously described, the arm is again abducted to approximately 80 to 90 degrees, with further localization occurring through abduction and adduction, internal and external rotation, and compression and decompression.

Stage Three. The patient is positioned supine, with the clinician sitting beside the patient on the same side as the involved shoulder. The clinician places one hand over the chest region and along the axis of the pectoralis minor, while the other hand supports the arm either above or below the elbow. The patient's shoulder is abducted to a point where the long axis of the arm is approximately along the long axis of the pectoralis minor. Compression and decompression, abduction and adduction, or internal and external rotation, is introduced.

Functional Technique to Improve Scapular Motion

The patient is positioned supine, with the clinician sitting at the side to be treated. The clinician places one hand under the patient's scapula and the other hand on the anterior aspect of the rib cage, directly above the inferiorly placed hand. The clinician applies a slight compression force simultaneously to the rib cage and scapula. While stabilizing with the superior hand, the clinician uses the inferior hand to begin gentle motion testing of the scapula in six directions: superior-inferior glide; medial-lateral glide; and clockwise-counterclockwise rotation.[59,114]

Joint Mobilizations

Joint mobilization techniques include a broad spectrum, from the general passive motions performed in the physiologic cardinal planes at any point in the joint range, to the semispecific and specific accessory (arthrokinematic) joint glides, or joint distractions, initiated from the open-packed position of the joint.

These techniques form the cornerstone of most rehabilitative programs and involve low-high velocity passive movements within or at the limit of joint range of motion to restore any loss of accessory joint motion as the consequence of joint injury.[2]

> ### Clinical Pearl
>
> Mobilization techniques that utilize accessory movements and distractions are used primarily on inert tissues, and physiologic movements are used to mobilize both contractile and noncontractile tissues.[119]

Joint mobilizations are applied in a direction that is either parallel or perpendicular to the treatment plane to restore the physiologic articular relationship within a joint, and to decrease pain.[120] Additional benefits attributed to joint mobilizations include decreasing muscle guarding, lengthening the tissue around a joint, neuromuscular influences on muscle tone, and increased proprioceptive awareness.[121,122]

Three types of mobilizations are recognized, based on the level of participation by the clinician and patient:

1. Active, in which the patient exerts the force.

2. Passive, in which the clinician exerts the force.

3. Combined, in which the clinician and patient work together.

To apply joint mobilizations, the components can be utilized in a variety of ways, depending on the method employed.

▶ *Direct method.* An engagement is made against a barrier in several planes.

▶ *Indirect method.* Maigne[123] postulated "the concept of painless and opposite motion" in which disengagement from the barrier occurs, and a balance of ligamentous tension is sought.

▶ *Combined method.* Disengagement is followed by direct retracing of the motion.

Several other schools of thought have been put forward to address the concepts of increasing joint range of motion. Kaltenborn[16] introduced the Nordic program of manual therapy, which utilizes Cyriax's[7] method to evaluate, and the specific osteopathic techniques of Mennell[8] for intervention. Further influence from Stoddard,[9] an osteopath, cemented the foundations of the Nordic system of manual therapy.

Evjenth,[104] who joined Kaltenborn's group, brought a greater emphasis on muscle stretching, strengthening, and coordination training.

Kaltenborn Techniques

Kaltenborn refers to the amount of joint play at a joint as *slack*. Each joint interface has a plane of motion, an imaginary line lying across the joint surfaces. According to Kaltenborn, all joint mobilizations, when performed correctly, should be made parallel or at right angles to this plane of motion.[16] Kaltenborn's techniques use a combination of traction and mobilization to reduce pain and mobilize hypomobile joints. Three grades of traction are defined:

▶ *Grade I—piccolo (loosen).* This grade involves a traction force that neutralizes pressure in the joint without producing any actual separation of the joint surfaces. Grade I traction is used to reduce the compressive forces on the articular surfaces, both in the initial intervention session and with all of the mobilization grades.

▶ *Grade II—slack (take up the slack).* This grade of traction separates the articulating surfaces and eliminates the play in the joint capsule.

▶ *Grade III—stretch.* This grade of traction actually stretches the joint capsule and the soft tissues surrounding the joint to increase mobility. Grade III traction is used in conjunction with mobilization glides according the convex-concave rules to treat joint hypomobility in the remodeling stage of healing.[16]

Australian Techniques

The Australian approach was introduced primarily by Maitland,[15] whose grading system is used throughout this text. Under this system, the range of motion is defined as the available range, not the full range, and is usually in one direction, only (Fig. 11-5). Each joint has an anatomic limit, which is determined by the configuration of the joint surfaces and the surrounding soft tissues. The point of limitation is that point in the range that is short of the anatomic limit and is reduced by either pain or tissue resistance.

Maitland advocated five grades of joint mobilization or oscillations, each of which falls within the available range of motion that exists at the joint—a point somewhere between the beginning point and the anatomic limit (see Fig. 11-5). Although the relationship that exists between the five grades in terms of their positions within the range of motion is always constant, the point of limitation shifts further to the left as the severity of the motion limitation increases.

Grades I through IV are often performed as oscillatory-type movements during treatment. Grade I occurs at the beginning of range, grade II occurs in midrange, grade III is a large-amplitude movement toward the end of range, and grade IV is a small amplitude movement at the end of range. Many clinicians use a combination of Kaltenborn's grade III traction with Maitland's grade IV oscillations to decrease pain and increase joint mobility.

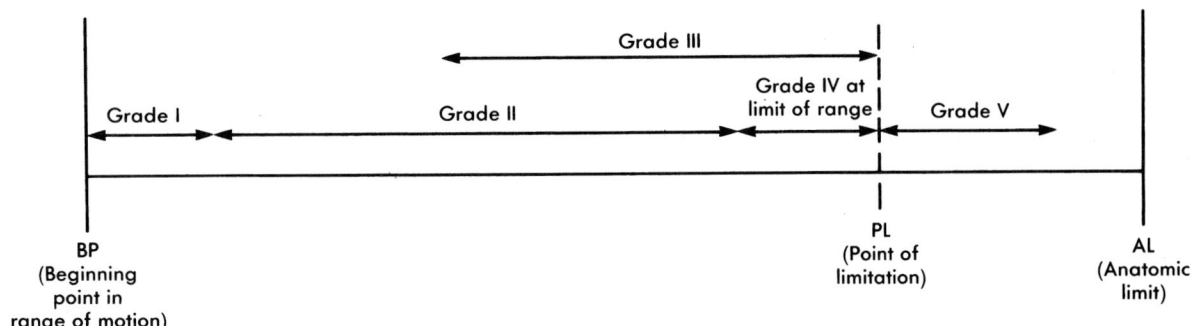

FIGURE 11-5 Maitland's five grades of motion. (Reproduced with permission from Dutton M. *Manual Therapy of the Spine: An Integrated Approach.* New York, NY: McGraw-Hill; 2002:44.)

Maitland's grades I and II are used solely for pain relief and have no direct mechanical effect on the restricting barrier, although they do have a hydrodynamic effect. Mobilization-induced analgesia has been demonstrated in a number of studies in humans,[124–126] and is characterized by a rapid onset and a specific influence on mechanical nociception. Grade I and II joint mobilizations are theoretically effective in pain reduction by improving joint lubrication and circulation in tissues related to the joint.[119,127] Rhythmic joint oscillations also possibly activate articular and skin mechanoreceptors that play a role in pain reduction.[91,128]

Maitland's grades III and IV (or at least III+ and IV+) do stretch the barrier and have a mechanical, as well as a neurophysiologic, effect. Grade III and IV joint distractions and stretching mobilizations may, in addition to the above-stated effects, activate inhibitory joint and muscle spindle receptors, which aid in reducing restriction to movement.[91,119,127,128]

When joint motion is less than 50 percent but joint resistance to movement is the dominant dysfunction, a progression from the use of physiologic movements (grade IV; see Fig. 11-5) to stretch the joint limitation, to use of accessory movement at the limit of the joint, is advocated.[15,119] Grades III and IV have been further subdivided into III+ (++) and IV+ (++), indicating that once the end of the range has been reached, a further stretch to impart a mechanical force to the movement restriction is given.[129] A grade V mobilization, defined as the skilled passive movement of a joint, is a short-duration, small-amplitude, high-velocity thrust that is applied at the physiologic limit of joint range (see Fig. 11-5).

The direction of the glide incorporated is determined by the concave-convex rule, and the joint to be mobilized is initially placed in its open-packed position. For example, if extension of the tibiofemoral joint is restricted, either the femur (convex) can be stabilized and the tibia (concave) glided anteriorly, or the tibia can be stabilized and the femur glided posteriorly. However, if mobilizing in the appropriate direction according to the convex-concave rule appears to exacerbate the patient's symptoms, the clinician should apply the technique in the opposite direction until the patient can tolerate the appropriate direction.[130]

> ### Clinical Pearl
>
> If the joint surface is convex relative to the other surface, the slide occurs in the opposite direction to the bone movement (angular motion). If, on the other hand, the joint surface is concave, the slide occurs in the same direction as the bone movement (angular motion).

The concave-convex rule cannot be applied to every situation. Exceptions include movements at plane joints, movements for which the axis of rotation passes through the articulating surfaces, and movements at joints in which the concave side of the joint forms a deep socket.[131]

Physiologic movement mobilizations and accessory and distraction mobilizations may be performed at any grade indicated. The mobilizations are performed both at the site of pain and to joints proximal to the site of pain to produce analgesia.[132]

The selection of the mobilization technique will depend on the barrier to movement felt by the clinician (the end-feel) and the acuteness of the condition (see Table 11-3). Muscle is usually the first barrier and is treated with light hold-relax techniques. Often some pain follows this initial mobilization, which is treated with grade III or IV oscillations.[129] As the pain is reduced, the real barrier to movement is approached. If this barrier is periarticular tissue, then grade IV+ rhythmical oscillations are used to stretch the tissue; if the joint is subluxed, erratic, jerky grade III+ are applied.[129]

Whichever technique or grade is employed, a number of further considerations help guide the clinician.

▶ The patient and clinician should be relaxed.

▶ One half of the joint should be stabilized while the other half is mobilized. Both the stabilizing and mobilizing hands should be placed as close as possible to the joint line. The other parts of the clinician involved in the mobilization should make maximum contact with the patient's body to spread the forces over a larger area and reduce pain from contact of bony prominences. The maximum contact also results in more stability and increased confidence from the patient. An alternative technique, which produces the desired results, must be sought if the contact between opposite sexes is uncomfortable to either the patient or the clinician.

▶ The direction of the mobilization is almost always parallel or perpendicular to a tangent across adjoining joint surfaces.

▶ The mobilization should not move into or through the point of pain.

▶ The velocity and amplitude of movement is carefully considered and is based on the goal of the intervention, to restore the joint motion or to alleviate the pain, or both.

▶ Slow stretches are used for large capsular restrictions.

▶ Fast oscillations are used for minor restrictions.

▶ One movement is performed at a time, at one joint at a time.

▶ The patient is reassessed regularly.

Muscle re-education is essential after mobilization or manipulation and often produces a noticeable reduction in post-treatment soreness. While the joint is maintained in the new range, five to six gentle isometric contractions are asked for from the agonists and antagonists of the motion mobilized.[129] Recently, the emphasis has shifted from mobilization of the joint in straight planes to mobilizations that incorporate the combined or congruent rotations that occur with normal motion (see Chap. 3), in order to take up all of the slack in the capsule.

Mobilizations with Movements

The concept of mobilizations with movements (MWMs) was introduced by Mulligan.[133,134] MWMs are based on the principles of joint mobilization originated by Kaltenborn.[16]

Clinical Pearl

The techniques of MWM combine a sustained manual gliding force to a joint with concurrent physiologic motion of the joint, either actively performed by the patient or passively performed by the clinician, with the intent of causing a repositioning of so-called bony positional faults.[133,134]

With few exceptions, Mulligan's mobilization techniques are applied parallel to the plane of motion and are sustained throughout the movement until the joint returns to its starting position, with the intention of producing no pain when applied.[134] Indeed, the golden rule of MWMs is that if pain is produced with an MWM, the techniques are contraindicated. The most common cause of pain with these techniques occurs when the mobilization is not sustained throughout the whole motion.[134]

The movements used with MWMs are patient dependent and can include active, passive, and resisted movements. Their

success is based on the theory that bony positional faults can contribute substantially to painful joint restrictions, which is similar to the theory behind the success of joint manipulations.[134]

Mulligan's MWM techniques were originally designed for the cervical spine but have since been expanded to include virtually every joint in the body.[133] Several studies[135–138,138a,138b] that looked at the effects of MWM concluded that MWM is a promising intervention.

Mulligan has devised a number of guidelines when applying these techniques[133,134]:

▶ The patient is placed in weight-bearing position.

▶ Other interventions should be used in conjunction with these techniques.

▶ When treating hinge joints, the sustained glide or mobilization should be at right angles to the glide that usually occurs with movement. For example, in the case of finger flexion, the glide-mobilization of the distal facet is applied in a medial or lateral direction.

▶ When joint movements involve adjacent long bones, as in the case at the wrist or ankle, it is often necessary for the clinician to adjust the relative positions of the long bones to enable pain-free joint movement to occur.

▶ The glide-mobilization is always successful in one direction only. The successful glide-mobilization is applied ten times before re-assessing the joint motion.

▶ Overpressure should be applied at the end range of the available active range of motion.

Mulligan techniques are described in detail in the relevant chapters of this text.

Joint Manipulations

The earliest physicians to use manipulations were English, and books on the subject were published in the early 1900s.[11,139–141] Therapeutic manipulation has been used since at least that time as a treatment modality for an array of musculoskeletal conditions.

Compared with the four grades of joint mobilization (I through IV), manipulation techniques are given the designation grade V. Recently, manipulative therapy has been broadly defined to include all procedures in which the hands are used to massage, stretch, mobilize, adjust, or manipulate musculoskeletal tissues for therapeutic reasons.[142] However, in this text, manipulative or thrust techniques refer to grade V techniques. Although the grade V technique shares similarities with the grade IV mobilization in terms of amplitude and position in the joint range, grade V differs in the velocity of delivery. The terms *velocity* and *amplitude* are used to describe the nature of the final activating force or thrust used with joint mobilizations. Most joint mobilizations of grades I through IV use varying degrees of amplitude, whereas grade V techniques generally employ a high-velocity (quick) and low amplitude-(short distance) thrust.

> ### Clinical Pearl
>
> Unlike mobilizations, which are applied singularly or repetitively within or at the physiologic range of joint motion,[143] joint manipulations involve a thrust to a joint so that the joint is briefly forced beyond the restricted range of motion.[2]

Manipulations may consist of long-lever techniques that exert forces on a point of the body some distance from the treatment area, or short-lever techniques that comprise forces directed specifically at an isolated joint.[144] The plane or direction of joint restriction determines the type and direction of manipulative technique to be used. A manipulative lesion may be defined by movement restriction and pain, especially a joint restriction that elicits pain on provocation. Manipulations are thus applied after first identifying the restriction through the end-feel, and then engaging the barrier, before applying the thrust. Engaging the barrier, which requires a high level of skill, ensures that the force will be applied to the restriction, thereby localizing the force.

When a specific force is applied to the bodily joints, to distract them, clicking or popping sounds, called *cavitations,* may be heard. The cavitations or clicks are thought to result from a sudden release of synovial gas during the manipulation. The gas is then reabsorbed by the joint over a period of about 30 minutes, which may explain why joints can only be re-cracked every 20 to 30 minutes.[145] However, the goal of thrust techniques is not to produce a cavitation, but to produce a temporary hypermobility that restores normal joint play.

Excessive force or failure to localize the force of a technique results in a dissipation of physical forces, and unless the patient is able to absorb these forces, they may prove to be harmful, especially in the spinal regions.[32] These harmful effects can include fracture, spinal cord compression, vertebral artery occlusion (see Chap. 21), cerebral ischemia, and even death.[146]

The evaluation of the effectiveness of manipulation interventions is difficult because the number of scientific studies on the subject is extremely limited.[147] It appears evident that manipulation does cause an immediate relief of low back pain in patients with acute low back pain,[148,149] although the degree of improvement varies between individuals. Some patients respond immediately to a manipulation; however, this population cannot be identified in advance, and there are no strong reasons for recommending manipulation instead of mobilizations.[147]

The mechanism behind the pain relief provided by manipulation is not yet understood, although attempts have been made to explain the possible effects, including the freeing of an entrapped meniscoid or discal element,[150] an alteration in muscle tone,[151] and a mechanical disruption of intra-articular adhesions.[152–154] Certainly, it is known that restriction of motion at a joint produces joint adhesions, soft tissue contracture, and degenerative joint disease.[155–158] Therefore, by increasing the

motion at a joint, a manipulation is thought to reverse the aforementioned detrimental effects. It is also possible that a manipulation may produce outcomes directly associated with a variety of psychological influences.[159]

Cervical manipulations have been linked to vertebrobasilar complications. In a review of the 58 cases in the English language literature of vertebrobasilar complications following cervical manipulation, Grant found the average age to be 37.3 years with a range of 7 to 63 years.[160] It was estimated from a study by Hosek[161] that 1 in 1 million cervical manipulations will result in a serious vertebrobasilar effect, whereas Dvorak and Orelli[162] estimated a much higher incidence of 1 in 400,000. This latter figure would indicate that a clinician performing cervical manipulations on 15 patients each day for 30 years (allowing for vacations) stands a little better than one in four chance of causing a serious stroke in the course of a career. Put another way, one in four clinicians, manipulating at the same rate, will run into a serious problem from the vertebral artery.

Neurophysiologic Techniques

Proprioceptive Neuromuscular Facilitation

Proprioceptive neuromuscular facilitation (PNF) was developed at the Kabat Kaiser Institute by Herman Kabat and Margaret Knott during the late 1940s and early 1950s. Initially, the approach was developed as a method of treatment for neurologically weak muscles. The techniques were later expanded for use in joint mobilizations and the stretching of adaptively shortened muscles, using active muscular relaxation techniques that incorporate muscle facilitation and inhibition to hasten the response of the neurophysiologic mechanisms involved in the stretch reflex.[163] Two fundamental neurophysiologic principles are credited for the neuromuscular inhibition that occurs during the performance of these techniques.

1. *Post-contraction inhibition.* This principle, states that after a muscle contracts, it is automatically relaxed for a brief, latent period. This concept is based on the Sherrington principle of successive induction.[119,164,165] According to the principle of successive induction, following a maximal contraction, the tight muscle is maximally relaxed (inhibited) upon the manifestation of the inverse stretch reflex.[163] Greater length following contraction of the tight muscle allows improved range of active or passive movement in the opposite direction.[119]

2. *Reciprocal inhibition.* This principle states that when one muscle is contracted, its antagonist is automatically inhibited. This concept is based on Sherrington's law of reciprocal inhibition.

Whenever a muscle is stretched, the frequency of the impulses transmitted to the spinal cord from the muscle spindle increases, which in turn increases the frequency of the motor nerve impulses returning to that muscle. This causes a reflex contraction of the muscle, resulting in an increased resistance to the stretch, and takes the stretch off the spindle. The increase in tension in the muscle is detected by the Golgi tendon organ (Fig. 11-6), whose subsequent volley of impulses reaches the spinal cord, resulting in an inhibitory effect on those motor impulses returning to the muscle and causing the muscle to relax.

PNF techniques, which are very complex, are used to increase strength, flexibility, and coordination, with the emphasis placed on the facilitation of an optimal structural and neuromuscular state, and the selective re-education of individual motor elements. Each movement is learned and then reinforced through repetition.[166] Manual contacts, patient prepositioning, and verbal commands are all used to initiate and control movement.

The patient is first taught the PNF pattern from starting position to terminal position, using brief and simple verbal cues, such as "push," "pull," and "hold," as well as visual and tactile input. A quick stretch applied to a muscle before contraction facilitates a muscular response of greater force, although care must be used in its application to avoid exceeding the extensibility limits of the musculotendinous unit.

PNF techniques provide the clinician with an efficient means for examining and treating structural and neuromuscular dysfunctions.[165,167,168] Structural dysfunctions (myofascial and articular hypermobilities and hypomobilities) affect the body's capacity to assume and perform optimal postures and motions.[169] Neuromuscular dysfunctions (inability to coordinate and efficiently perform purposeful movements) cause repetitive, abnormal, and stressful usage of the articular and myofascial system, often precipitating structural dysfunctions and symptoms.[169–171]

The key to the success of PNF is the ability of the clinician to apply manual contact with appropriate pressure and exact positioning, which allows for a smooth, coordinated motion throughout the pattern. Appropriate pressure is the amount of resistance that facilitates the desired motor response of a smooth, coordinated, and optimal muscle contraction.[166,167] If a dysfunction is identified in any of these characteristics, appropriate resistance applied in conjunction with various PNF techniques facilitates the relearning and rehabilitative process.[165–169] For example, the clinician can apply maximal resistance at specific points in the range to promote overflow to the weaker components of the movement pattern.

Stretching Techniques

Several PNF stretches have been demonstrated, including stretch-relax, contract-relax, and agonist contract-relax. In the following descriptions, the goal of the stretch is to increase the length of the hamstrings. The reader is expected to be able to extrapolate the principles and apply them to other agonist-antagonist muscle groups.

Stretch-relax. This technique involves the patient concentrating on relaxing the antagonist during the passive stretch. For example, the patient relaxes the hamstrings as the knee is passively moved into extension to the point of restriction.[104,167,168] This technique is believed to reduce antagonist muscle activation over time via an increased effect of neural inhibition.[169,172]

Contract and Hold-relax. The techniques of contract and hold-relax are designed to facilitate relaxation and increase range through neuromuscular relaxation and stretching of the intrinsic connective tissue elements of the muscle.[167] The techniques involve the patient contracting the agonist (hamstrings) for 5 seconds against manual resistance, after which the agonist is relaxed as it is passively stretched.[104] The contract-relax technique uses either a concentric or a maintained isotonic contraction, whereas the hold-relax uses an isometric contraction.[169] Hold-relax is the technique of choice in the presence of pain or when the concentric contraction is overpowering the clinician.[169]

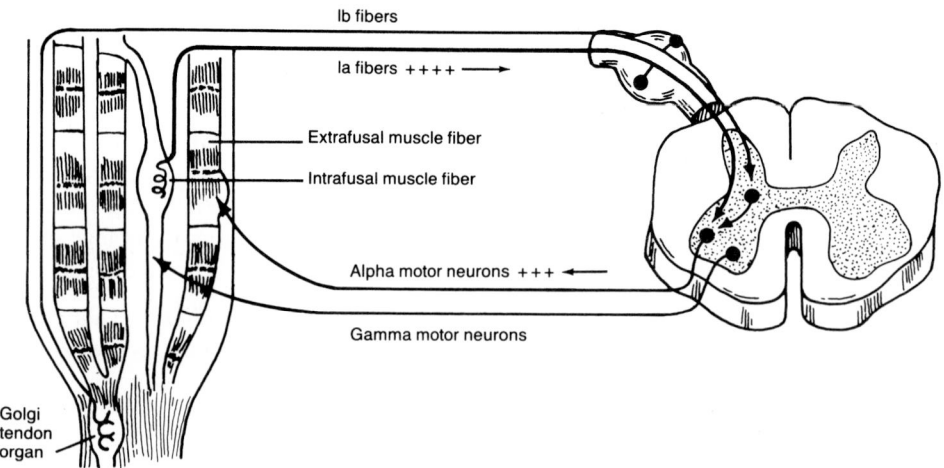

FIGURE 11-6 The muscle spindle and Golgi tendon apparatus. (Reproduced with permission from Wilk KE, Voight ML, Keirns MA, et al. Stretch-shortening drills for the upper extremities: Theory and clinical application. *J Orthop Sports Phys Ther* 1993;17:227.)

To perform this technique, the joint is placed at the point of limitation within the movement pattern. Resistance is applied to a concentric contraction of either the restricted agonist (direct contraction) or the antagonist (quadriceps—reciprocal relaxation).[169] The former technique relies on autogenic inhibition, which occurs more readily in a muscle following an intense contraction.[172] Autogenic inhibition of a muscle is controlled by the Golgi tendon organ, the role of which is to monitor tension within a muscle. The stimulation of the Golgi tendon organ by a muscle contraction causes the inhibition or relaxation of the muscle in which it is located.[163]

Strengthening Techniques

The following PNF techniques can be used for the development of muscular strength, endurance, and coordination.

Rhythmic Initiation. The rhythmic initiation technique is used to teach a patient a movement pattern, or with patients who are unable to initiate movement or those who have a limited range of motion because of increased tone.

The application of the technique involves a progression through the agonist pattern of passive, then active, assistive and then active movement. This technique is applied slowly against resistance through the available range of motion, while avoiding activation of a quick stretch.

Repeated Contraction. Repeated contraction is a useful technique for patients who have weakness, either at a specific point or throughout the entire range, and to correct imbalances that occur within the range. The patient is asked to push repeatedly by using the agonist concentrically and eccentrically against maximal resistance until fatigue occurs in the weaker ranges of the motion. The amount of resistance to motion given by the clinician is modified to accommodate the strength of the muscle group. A stretch can be applied at the weakest point in the range to facilitate the weaker muscles and promote a smoother, more coordinated motion.

Slow Reversal. The slow reversal technique, also known as an *isotonic reversal,* can be used for developing active range of motion of the agonists, while also developing the normal reciprocal timing between the antagonists and agonists that occurs during functional movements. The technique involves an isotonic contraction of the agonist followed immediately by an isotonic contraction of the antagonist, with the initial agonist push contraction facilitating the pull contraction of the antagonist muscles.

Slow Reversal-hold. The slow reversal-hold technique, which can be especially useful in developing strength at a specific point in the range of motion, utilizes the application of an isotonic contraction of the agonist followed immediately by an isometric contraction, with a hold command given at the end of each active movement. The direction of the pattern is then reversed by using the same sequence of contraction, but with no relaxation before shifting to the antagonistic pattern.

Rhythmic Stabilization. The techniques of rhythmic stabilization, also called *stabilizing reversals,* emphasize the co-contraction of agonists and antagonists, which results in an increase in the holding power to a point where the position cannot be broken. This effect is achieved by alternating isometric contraction of the agonist with isometric contraction of the antagonist to produce co-contraction of the two opposing muscle groups. The command "hold" is always given before movement is resisted in each direction. The goals of this technique are to improve stability around a joint, increase positional neuromuscular awareness, improve posture and balance, and enhance strength or stretch sensitivity of the tonic muscles in their functional range.[169]

Facilitating Techniques

PNF techniques also include the reinforcement or facilitation of movement patterns. These patterns, which are performed in spiral-diagonal combinations of movements, are designed to encourage the stronger synergistic muscle groups to assist the weaker ones during functional movements, and are concerned with gross motions as opposed to specific motions. The patterns, which integrate the motions of sport and daily living, are based on the infant developmental sequences such as rolling, crawling, and walking.

There are two diagonal patterns for the lower extremity (Table 11-6), and two diagonal patterns for the upper extremity and scapula (Table 11-7), which are referred to as the diagonal 1 (D1) and diagonal 2 (D2) patterns. These patterns are subdivided into D1 and D2 patterns that move into flexion and D1 and D2 patterns that move into extension. In addition to the upper and lower extremity patterns, patterns exist for the upper trunk, lower trunk, and cervical spine.

The components for each of these patterns include combinations of flexion-extension, abduction-adduction, and internal-external rotation (see Tables 11-6 and 11-7), because most human movement involves rotational movements rather than straight-plane movements.

The exercise pattern is initiated after positioning the patient so that the muscle groups are in the lengthened position. The muscle groups are then moved through their full range to their shortened position.

Figures 11-7 and 11-8 illustrate the starting and terminal positions, respectively, for the D2 lower extremity movement pattern moving into flexion.

Figure 11-9 illustrates the starting position for the D1 lower extremity movement pattern moving into extension.

Figure 11-10 illustrates the starting position for the D2 lower extremity movement pattern moving into flexion. Figure 11-11 illustrates the terminal position for the D2 lower extremity movement pattern moving into flexion.

The lower extremity patterns can be performed with both legs simultaneously to strengthen the trunk muscles. Figure 11-12 illustrates a lower trunk pattern into extension to the left.

Trunk patterns may also be performed using the upper extremities. Figures 11-13 through Figure 11-16 illustrate the upper extremity trunk patterns.

TABLE 11-6 Lower Extremity Proprioceptive Nuclear Facilitation Patterns

Start Position for D1 Pattern	
Moving into Extension	Moving into Flexion
Hip flexed, adducted, and externally rotated	Hip extended, abducted, and internally rotated
Knee flexed	Knee extended
Tibia internally rotated	Tibia externally rotated
Ankle and foot dorsiflexed and inverted	Ankle and foot plantarflexed and everted
Toes extended	Toes flexed
Start Position for D2 Pattern	
Moving into Extension	Moving into Flexion
Hip extended, adducted, and externally rotated	Hip flexed, abducted, and internally rotated
Knee extended	Knee flexed
Tibia externally rotated	Tibia internally rotated
Ankle and foot plantarflexed and inverted	Ankle and foot dorsiflexed and everted
Toes flexed	Toes extended

D1, diagonal 1; D2, diagonal 2.

Figures 11-17 through 11-20 illustrate several of the PNF patterns for the cervical spine.

Myofascial Trigger Point Therapy

Myofascial pain syndromes (see Chap. 9) are closely associated with tender areas that have come to be known as myofascial trigger points (MTrPs). Dysfunctional joints are also associated with trigger points and tender attachment points.[98] The term *myofascial trigger point* is a bit of a misnomer, because trigger points also can be cutaneous, ligamentous, periosteal, and fascial.[173]

The major goals of MTrP therapy are to relieve pain and tightness of the involved muscles, improve joint motion, improve circulation, and eliminate perpetuating factors. When treating a patient for a specific muscle syndrome, it is important to explain the function of the involved muscle and to describe or

TABLE 11-7 Upper Extremity and Scapular Proprioceptive Nuclear Facilitation Patterns

Start Position for D1 Pattern	
Moving into Extension	Moving into Flexion
Scapula elevated and abducted	Scapula depressed and adducted
Shoulder flexed, adducted, and externally rotated	Shoulder extended, abducted, and internally rotated
Elbow extended	Elbow extended
Forearm supinated	Forearm pronated
Wrist flexed and radially deviated	Wrist extended and ulnarly deviated
Fingers adducted and flexed	Fingers abducted and extended
Thumb flexed and adducted	Thumb extended and abducted
Start Position for D2 Pattern	
Moving into Flexion	Moving into Extension
Scapula depressed and abducted	Scapula elevated and adducted
Shoulder extended, adducted, and internally rotated	Shoulder flexed, abducted, and externally rotated
Elbow extended	Elbow extended
Forearm pronated	Forearm supinated
Wrist flexed and ulnarly deviated	Wrist extended and radially deviated
Fingers adducted and flexed	Fingers extended and abducted
Thumb flexed and abducted	Thumb extended and adducted

D1, diagonal 1; D2, diagonal 2.

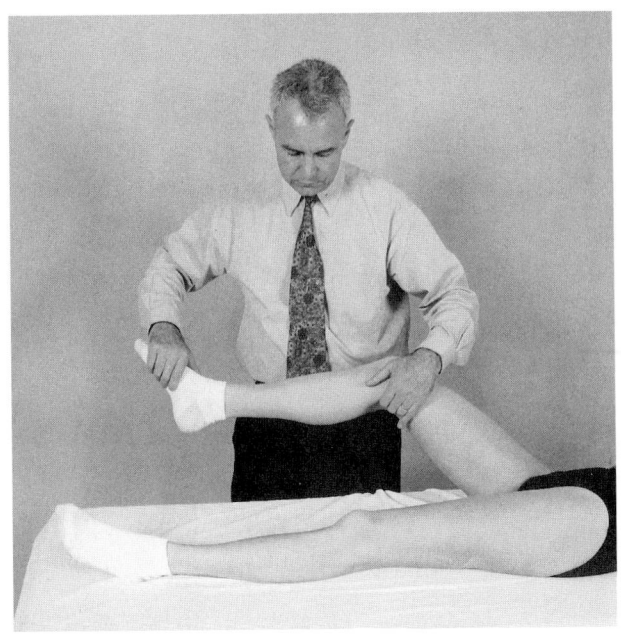

FIGURE 11-7 The starting position for D1 lower extremity movement pattern moving into flexion.

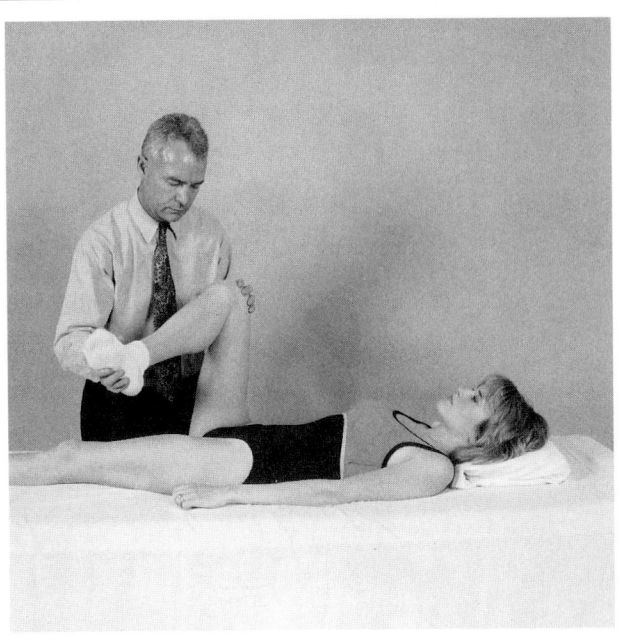

FIGURE 11-9 The starting position for D1 lower extremity movement pattern moving into extension.

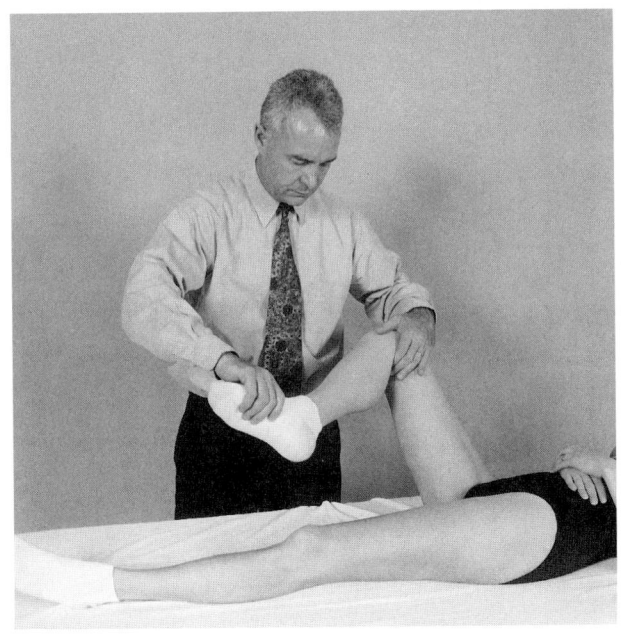

FIGURE 11-8 The terminal position for D1 lower extremity movement pattern moving into flexion.

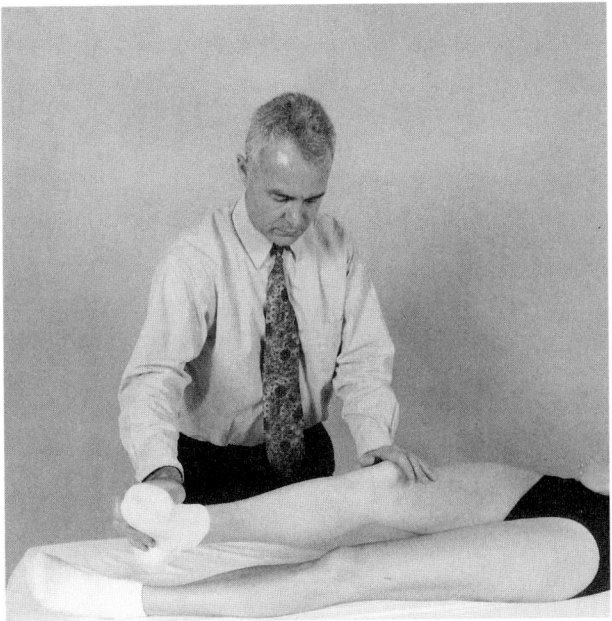

FIGURE 11-10 The starting position for the D2 lower extremity movement pattern moving into flexion.

demonstrate a few of the activities or postures that might overstress it, so that the patient can avoid such activities or postures.

A number of manual interventions for MTrPs are available; these include[82,174–176]:

Stretch and Spray, or Stretch and Ice[83,173]

Although not technically a manual technique, the spray-and-stretch technique involves a manual stretch during its application.

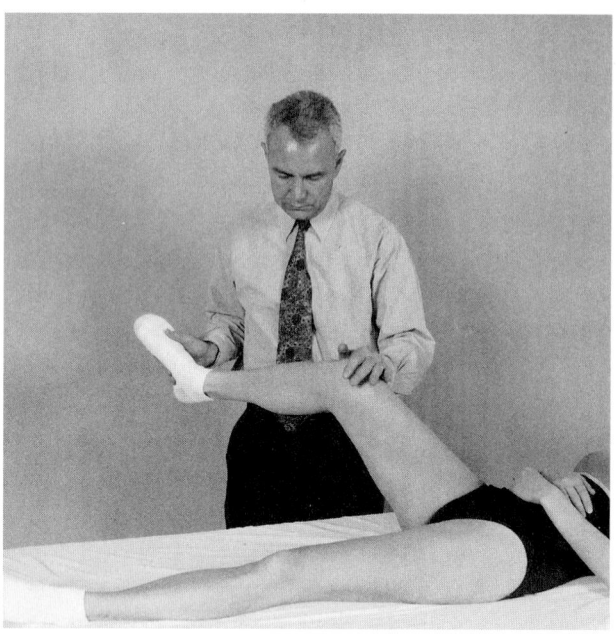

FIGURE 11-11   The terminal position for the D2 lower extremity movement pattern moving into flexion.

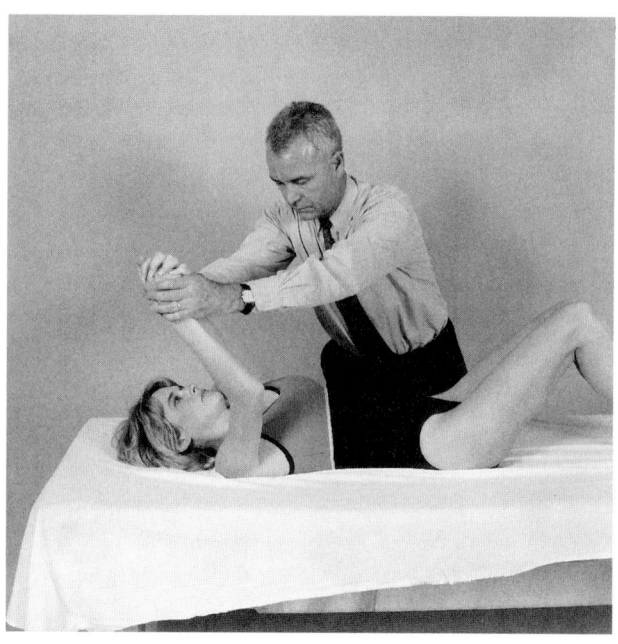

FIGURE 11-13   Upper trunk pattern moving into extension: starting position.

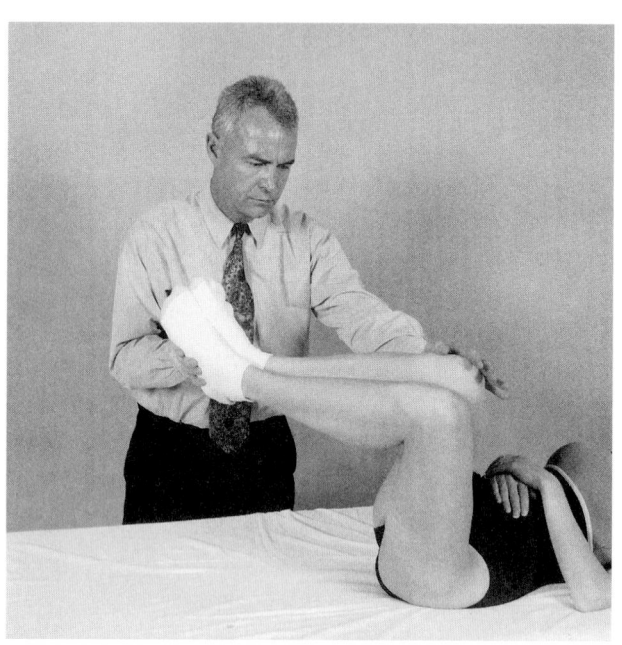

FIGURE 11-12   Lower trunk pattern into extension to the left.

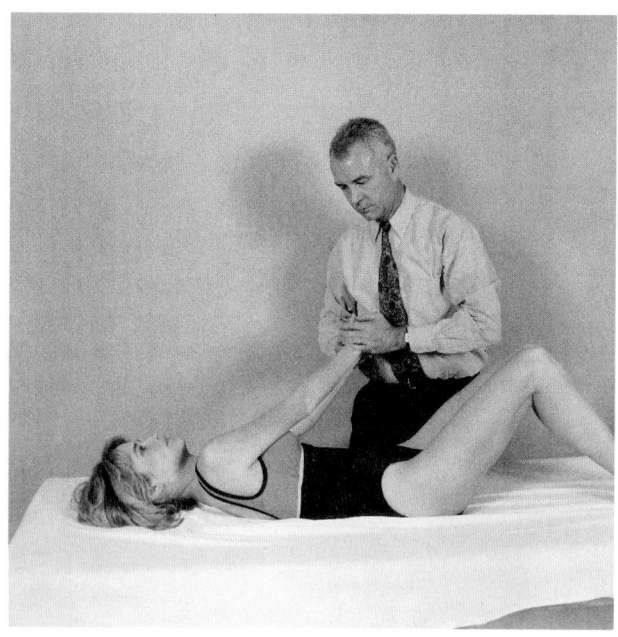

FIGURE 11-14   Upper trunk pattern moving into extension: terminal position.

The patient is placed in a position of maximum comfort to enhance muscle relaxation. The part of the body affected is then positioned so that a mild stretch is exerted specifically on the taut band. Parallel sweeps of the vapocoolant spray or ice are applied unidirectionally; then, while one of the clinician's hands anchors the base of the muscle, the other stretches the muscle to its full length.[177] The spray is held approximately 18 inches away from the skin to allow for sufficient cooling of the spray. One or two sweeps of coolant are sprayed over the area of the involved muscle to reduce any pain. As the muscle is passively stretched, successive parallel sweeps of the spray are applied over the skin from the MTrP to the area of referred pain, covering as much of the

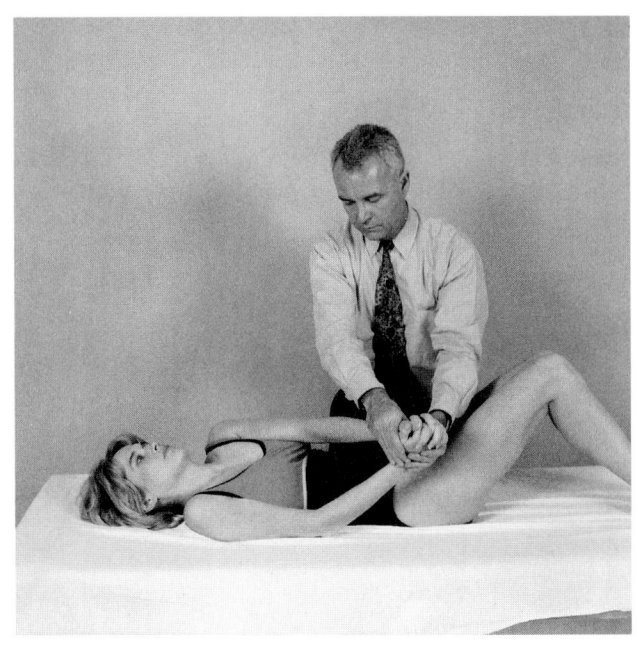

FIGURE 11-15   Upper trunk pattern moving into flexion: starting position.

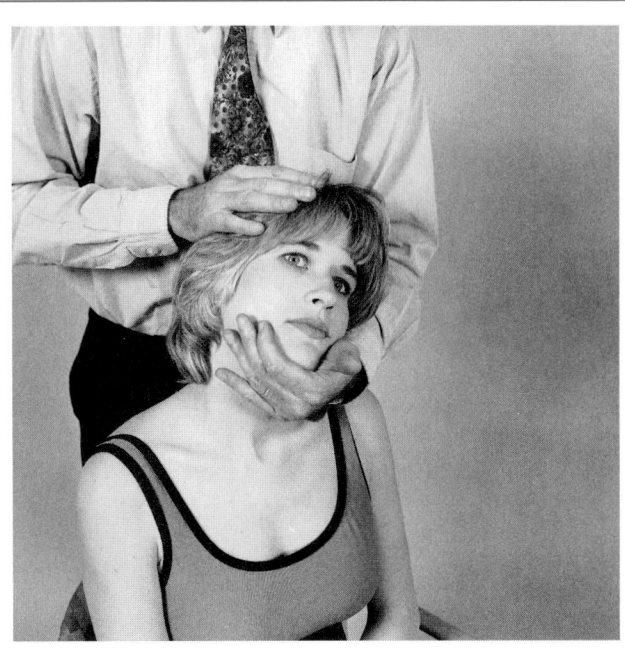

FIGURE 11-17   Neck flexion and right rotation pattern: starting position.

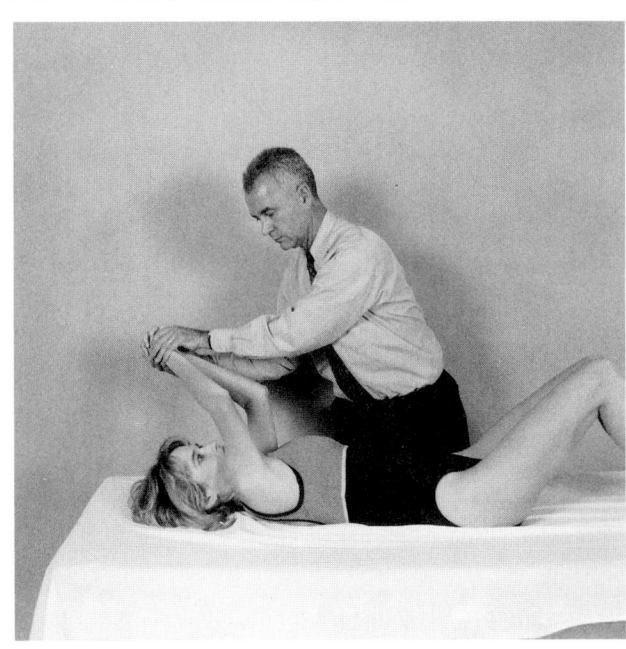

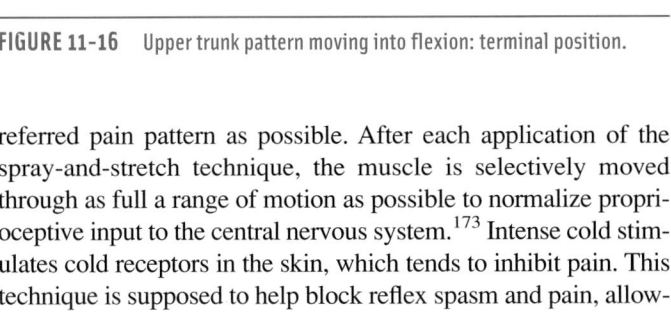

FIGURE 11-16   Upper trunk pattern moving into flexion: terminal position.

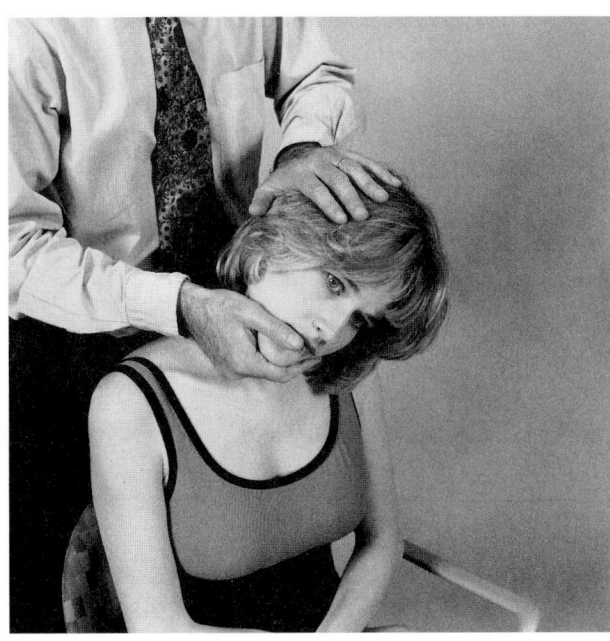

FIGURE 11-18   Neck extension and left rotation pattern: starting position.

referred pain pattern as possible. After each application of the spray-and-stretch technique, the muscle is selectively moved through as full a range of motion as possible to normalize proprioceptive input to the central nervous system.[173] Intense cold stimulates cold receptors in the skin, which tends to inhibit pain. This technique is supposed to help block reflex spasm and pain, allow-

ing for a gradual passive stretch of the muscle, which decreases muscle tension. Several treatments may be needed to eliminate the pain syndrome, and results should be seen after four to six treatments.[173] If vaporized coolants are not available, ice may be used in their place, taking care to prevent chilling of the underlying muscles, which is less likely with the use of vaporized coolants.[173]

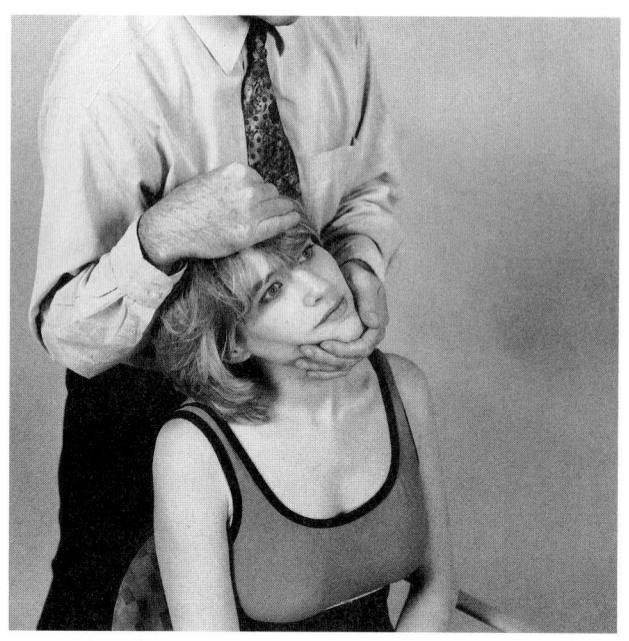

FIGURE 11-19   Neck flexion and left rotation pattern: starting position.

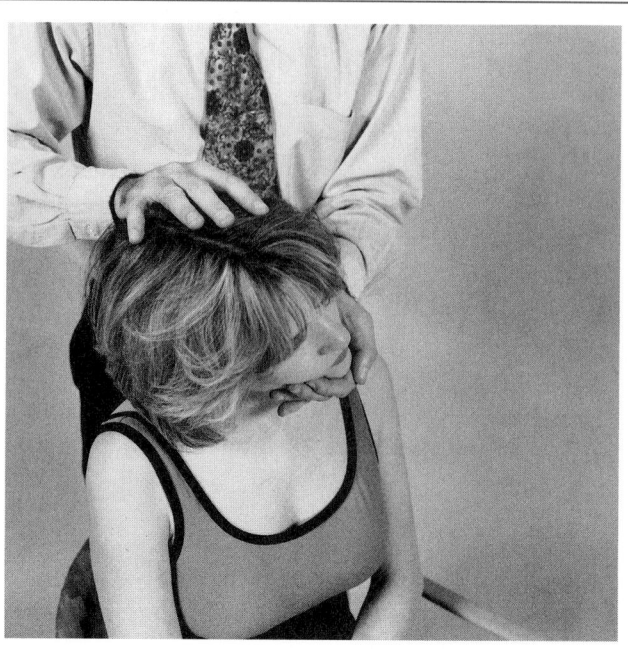

FIGURE 11-20   Neck extension and right rotation pattern: starting position.

Muscle Stripping

Muscle stripping is applied after first applying a lubricant to the skin. The technique involves the slow sliding of the thumb, knuckle, or elbow along the edge of a taut band with firm pressure, while at the same time attempting to bow it out.[173] This technique has the effect of applying brief ischemic compression as the thumb slowly slides over the MTrPs and of passively lengthening the taut band. Muscle stripping is as effective as the spray-and-stretch technique, although it is somewhat more painful.[173]

Massage Therapy

Deep massage mechanically helps break up the fibrous bands of MTrPs. The application of deep pressure produces local ischemia. When the pressure is released, a reactive hyperemia occurs, improving circulation and releasing energy to the area.[178]

Myofascial Release

These techniques, discussed in a previous section, combine massage with deep stretch techniques to relax muscle and break up the MTrPs.[60,83]

Ischemic Compression[173]

Compression can be applied with a thumb, knuckle, or elbow. The compression serves as the hyperstimulant, and the pain is usually relieved within 20 to 60 seconds. The technique involves the application of pressure directly on the trigger point, within the patient's tolerance. As the pain subsides, the clinician slowly increases the pressure until, ideally, the painful stimulus is eliminated and a softening of the area is felt.

Stretching

Lengthening of the taut band is an effective form of intervention. It is theorized to disengage the actin and myosin filaments of the skeletal muscle (see Chap. 1), allowing more normal muscle length and increased range of motion, and results in normal, patterned proprioceptive input to the central nervous system, which may prevent the resumption of pain.[173] Lengthening can be accomplished with gentle stretching of the involved muscles.

Joint Mobilizations

Typically, treatment of a dysfunctional joint leads to spontaneous resolution of soft tissue tension and the restoration of normal muscle lengths around the joint, thereby allowing the hypertonic muscles to relax.[11,98,102,103]

Nonmanual Interventions

The nonmanual interventions for MTrPs are included here for completeness.[82,174–176]

▶ *Thermotherapy.*   Moist heat, ultrasound, or a hot tub session of 5 to 15 minutes' duration helps relax underlying muscles and increase circulation, thereby improving the supply of nutrients and decreasing tension on the MTrPs.[83] Pain relief is theorized to be related to washout of pain mediators by increased blood flow, changes in nerve conduction, or alterations in cell membrane permeability that decrease inflammation.[179,180]

▶ *Cryotherapy.*   Brief, intense cold stimulation of the skin overlying the trigger point and its pain referral area is effective in releasing taut bands and inactivating trigger points, particularly when done in combination with a passive stretch.[173]

▶ *Trigger point injections.* Trigger point injections using various techniques have been widely used to inactivate MTrPs by disrupting the fibrous banding, although the injected local anesthetic agent seems less important for inactivation of the trigger point than the needling itself.[80,181,182] Trigger point injections should be followed by stretching and the application of heat.[83] The effectiveness of ultrasound therapy is comparable to trigger point injections and should be offered as a noninvasive treatment of choice to those patients who want to avoid injections.[180]

▶ *Elimination of causative or perpetuating factors, if any.* Mechanical and metabolic disorders need to be corrected to prevent further stress and strain on the muscles. Although many people have some degree of imbalanced body structure, structural imbalance is an extremely common contributing factor to myofascial constrictions and trigger points.[79,174,175,183,184] In addition, patients should be encouraged to limit caffeine intake to less than two caffeinated beverages per day and avoid smoking, both of which directly and indirectly aggravate MTrPs.[83] Nutrition deficiencies may require correction, and supplements of vitamins C, B_1, B_6, B_{12}, and folic acid have been advocated because of their essential role in normal muscle metabolism.[173]

▶ *Biofeedback and muscle relaxation.* Biofeedback and muscle relaxation techniques can be used to avoid chronic muscle tension.

▶ *Exercise.* Exercise is important in limiting recurrences of MTrPs.[184]

▶ *Counterirritation.* This very old method of controlling pain has been used for centuries. Its success relates to the fact that it breaks the pain-spasm-pain cycle that so often perpetuates a painful condition through the gate control mechanism of pain control.

▶ *Combination therapy.* One study,[180] that looked at the combined intervention of ultrasound, trigger point injections, and stretching, found that the combination of these three interventions were effective in the reduction of pain, and improving range of motion, independent of the severity or duration of pain present before the treatment. Another study, which examined a combined intervention of ultrasound, massage, and exercise, found that patients who had massage and exercise had a reduction in the number and intensity of MTrPs, whereas ultrasound gave no pain reduction.[185]

▶ *Electrotherapy.* Electrotherapy also has been found to be an effective therapeutic modality to relieve pain from myofascial trigger points,[78,186,187] although electrotherapy alone is reported not as effective as thermotherapy or intermittent cold with stretching.[186] Electrotherapy is thought to

work by producing muscle contractions, which squeeze out the edema from needling, increase blood flow to the area, and relax the muscles.[79] Two major types of electrical stimulation therapy used for soft tissue lesions are electrical nerve stimulation (ENS) and electrical muscle stimulation (EMS).

• ENS is the application of electrical current on the peripheral nerve by applying lower intensity of electrical current. In general, ENS, such as transcutaneous nerve stimulation (TENS), is used in reducing pain intensity and increasing the pain threshold of MTrPs (no matter how severe the initial pain).[188,189]

• EMS is the application of electrical current with stronger intensity directly to the involved muscle. EMS can be used to enhance muscle circulation, reduce muscle spasm, eliminate muscle pain, and increase muscle strength.[183,187,189]

▶ According to one study, ENS was found to be more effective than EMS for immediate pain relief, whereas EMS was more effective than ENS for improving range of motion.[189]

REVIEW QUESTIONS*

1. Give five indications for the use of manual therapy.
2. Give five absolute contraindications to manual therapy.
3. Give the three purported benefits of transverse friction massage.
4. Which manual technique uses the passive positioning of the body in a position of ease (rather than motion restriction) to evoke a therapeutic effect?
5. Which manual techniques involve low-velocity passive movements within or at the limit of joint range of motion to restore any loss of accessory joint motion as the consequence of joint injury?

---

* Additional questions to test your understanding of this chapter can be found in the Online Learning Center for *Orthopaedic Assessment, Evaluation, and Intervention* at www.duttononline.net.

REFERENCES

1. Sucher BM. Myofascial release of carpal tunnel syndrome. *J Am Osteopath Assoc* 1993;93:92–101.
2. Di Fabio RP. Efficacy of manual therapy. *Phys Ther* 1992; 72:853–864.
3. Cochrane CG. Joint mobilization principles: Considerations for use in the child with central nervous dysfunction. *Phys Ther* 1987;67:1105–1109.
4. Brooks SC. Coma. In: Payton OD, ed. *Manual of Physical Therapy.* New York, NY: Churchill Livingstone; 1989:215–238.
5. Farrell JP, Jensen GM. Manual therapy: A critical assessment of role in the profession of physical therapy. *Phys Ther* 1992;72:843–852.

6. Watson T. The role of electrotherapy in contemporary physiotherapy practice. *Manual Ther* 2000;5:132–141.

7. Cyriax J. *Textbook of Orthopaedic Medicine, Diagnosis of Soft Tissue Lesions.* 8th ed. London, England: Bailliere Tindall; 1982.

8. Mennell JM. *Back Pain. Diagnosis and Treatment Using Manipulative Techniques.* Boston, Mass: Little, Brown; 1960.

9. Stoddard A. *Manual of Osteopathic Practice.* New York, NY: Harper and Row; 1969.

10. DiGiovanna EL, Schiowitz S. *An Osteopathic Approach to Diagnosis and Treatment.* Philadelphia, Pa: JB Lippincott; 1991.

11. Mennell JB. *The Science and Art of Joint Manipulation.* London, England: J and A Churchill; 1949.

12. Greenman PE. *Principles of Manual Medicine.* 2nd ed. Baltimore, Md: Williams and Wilkins; 1996.

13. Bourdillon JF. *Spinal Manipulation.* 3rd ed. London, England: Heinemann Medical Books; 1982.

14. Maitland G. *Vertebral Manipulation.* Sydney, Australia: Butterworth; 1986.

15. Maitland G. *Peripheral Manipulation.* 3rd ed. London, England: Butterworth; 1991.

16. Kaltenborn FM. *Manual Mobilization of the Extremity Joints: Basic Examination and Treatment Techniques.* 4th ed. Oslo, Norway: Olaf Norlis Bokhandel, Universitetsgaten; 1989.

17. McKenzie RA. The Lumbar Spine: Mechanical Diagnosis and Therapy. Waikanae, New Zealand: Spinal Publications New Zealand Ltd; 1981.

18. Cookson JC. Orthopedic manual therapy—an overview. Part 2: The spine. *Phys Ther* 1979;59:259–267.

19. Cookson JC, Kent B. Orthopedic manual therapy—an overview. Part 1: The extremities. *Phys Ther* 1979;59:136–146.

20. Threlkeld AJ. The effects of manual therapy on connective tissue. *Phys Ther* 1992;72:893–902.

21. Jull GA, Janda V. Muscle and motor control in low back pain. In: Twomey LT, Taylor JR, eds. *Physical Therapy of the Low Back: Clinics in Physical Therapy.* New York, NY: Churchill Livingstone; 1987:258.

22. Goldberg J. The effect of two intensities of massage on H-reflex amplitude. *Phys Ther* 1992;72:449–457.

23. Kukulka CG, Beckman SM, Holte JB, Hoppenworth PK. Effects of intermittent tendon pressure on alpha motoneuron excitability. *Phys Ther* 1986;66:1091–1094.

24. Guissard N, Duchateau J, Hainaut K. Muscle stretching and motoneuron excitability. *Eur J Appl Physiol* 1988;58:47–52.

25. Zusman M. Prolonged relief from articular soft tissue pain with passive joint movement. *Manual Med* 1988;3:100–102.

26. Newham DJ, Lederman E. Effect of manual therapy techniques on the stretch reflex in normal human quadriceps. *Disabil Rehabil* 1997;19:326–331.

27. Nwuga VCB. Relative therapeutic efficacy of vertebral manipulation and conventional treatment in back pain management. *Am J Phys Med* 1982;61:273–278.

28. Nicholson GG. The effects of passive joint mobilization on pain and hypomobility associated with adhesive capsulitis of the shoulder. *J Orthop Sports Phys Ther* 1985;6:238–246.

29. Anderson M, Tichenor CJ. A patient with de Quervain's tenosynovitis: A case report using an Australian approach to manual therapy. *Phys Ther* 1994;74:314–326.

30. Nyberg R. Manipulation: Definition, types, application. In: Basmajian JV, Nyberg R, eds. *Rational Manual Therapies.* Baltimore, Md: Williams and Wilkins; 1993:21–47.

31. Nitz AJ. Physical therapy management of the shoulder. *Phys Ther* 1986;66:1912–1919.

32. Kappler RE. Direction action techniques. *J Am Osteopath Assoc* 1981;81:239–243.

33. Mitchell FL, Moran PS, Pruzzo NA. *An Evaluation and Treatment Manual of Osteopathic Muscle Energy Procedures.* Manchester, Mo: Mitchell, Moran and Pruzzo Assoc; 1979.

34. Ellis JJ, Johnson GS. Myofascial considerations in somatic dysfunction of the thorax. In: Flynn TW, ed. *The Thoracic Spine and Rib Cage: Musculoskeletal Evaluation and Treatment.* Boston, Mass: Butterworth-Heinemann; 1996:211–262.

35. Nansel D, Peneff A, Cremata E, Carlson J. Time course considerations for the effects of unilateral cervical adjustments with respect to the amelioration of cervical lateral flexion passive end-range asymmetry. *J Manipulative Physiol Ther* 1990;13:297–304.

36. Jull GA. Physiotherapy management of neck pain of mechanical origin. In: Giles LGF, Singer KP, eds. *Clinical Anatomy and ManageSment of Cervical Spine Pain.* London, England: Butterworth-Heinemann; 1998:168–191.

37. Riddle DL, Rothstein JM, Lamb RL. Goniometric reliability in a clinical setting: shoulder measurements. *Phys Ther* 1987;67:668–673.

38. Price DD, McGrath PA, Rafii A, Buckingham B. The validation of visual analogue scales as ratio scale measures for chronic and experimental pain. *Pain* 1983;17:46–56.

39. Youdas JW, Carey JR, Garrett TR. Reliability of measurements of cervical spine range of motion: Comparison of three methods. *Phys Ther* 1991;71:98–104.

40. Fitzgerald GK, McClure PW, Beattie P, Riddle DL. Issues in determining treatment effectiveness of manual therapy. *Phys Ther* 1994;74:227–233.

41. Basmajian JV. Introduction: A plea for research validation. In: Basmajian JV, Nyberg R, eds. *Rational Manual Therapies.* Baltimore, Md: Williams and Wilkins; 1993:1–6.

42. Kessler RM, Hertling D. *Management of Common Musculoskeletal Disorders.* 2nd ed. Philadelphia, Pa: Harper and Row; 1983.

43. Ramsey SM. Holistic manual therapy techniques. *Prim Care* 1997;24:759–785.

44. Johnson GS. Soft tissue mobilization. In: Donatelli RA, Wooden MJ, eds. *Orthopaedic Physical Therapy.* New York, NY: Churchill Livingstone; 1994.

45. Cyriax JH, Cyriax PJ. *Illustrated Manual of Orthopaedic Medicine.* London, England: Butterworth; 1983.

46. Gersten JW. Effect of ultrasound on tendon extensibility. *Am J Phys Med* 1955;34:662.

47. Hunter SC, Poole RM. The chronically inflamed tendon. *Clin Sports Med* 1987;6:371.

48. Palastanga N. The use of transverse frictions for soft tissue lesions. In: Grieve GP, ed. *Modern Manual Therapy of the Vertebral Column.* London, England: Churchill Livingstone; 1986:819–826.

49. Walker JM. Deep transverse friction in ligament healing. *J Orthop Sports Phys Ther* 1984;6:89–94.

50. Hammer WI. The use of transverse friction massage in the management of chronic bursitis of the hip or shoulder. *J Manipulative Physiol Ther* 1993;16:107–111.

51. Forrester JC, Zederfeldt BH, Hayes TL, Hunt TK. Wolff's law in relation to the healing skin wound. *J Trauma* 1970;10:770–779.

52. Hammer WI. Friction massage. In: Hammer WI, ed. *Functional Soft Tissue Examination and Treatment by Manual Methods.* Gaithersburg, Md: Aspen; 1991:235–249.

53. Chamberlain G. Cyriax's friction massage; A review. *J Orthop Sports Phys Ther* 1984;4:16.

54. Codman EA. *The Shoulder, Rupture of the Supraspinatus Tendon and Other Lesions in or About the Subacromial Bursa.* Boston, Mass: Thomas Todd Co; 1934.

55. Melham TJ, Sevier TL, Malnofski MJ, Wilson JK, Helfst RH Jr. Chronic ankle pain and fibrosis successfully treated with a new noninvasive augmented soft tissue mobilization technique (ASTM): A case report. *Med Sci Sports Exerc* 1998;30:801–804.

56. Buckley PD, Grana WA, Pascale MS. The biomechanical and physiologic basis of rehabilitation. In: Grana WA, Kalenak A, eds. *Clinical Sports Medicine.* Philadelphia, Pa: Saunders; 1991:233–250.

57. Harrelson GL. Physiologic factors of rehabilitation. In: Andrews JR, Harrelson GL, eds. *Physical Rehabilitation of the Injured Athlete.* Philadelphia, Pa: Saunders; 1991:13–39.

58. Stauber WT. Repair models and specific tissue responses in muscle injury. In: Leadbetter WB, Buckwalter JA, Gordon SL, eds. *Sports-Induced Inflammation: Clinical and Basic Science Concepts.* Park Ridge, Ill: American Academy of Orthopedic Surgeons; 1990:205–213.

59. Upledger JE, Vredevoogd JD. *Craniosacral Therapy.* Chicago, Ill: Eastland Press; 1983:48–49.

60. Barnes J. *Myofascial Release: A Comprehensive Evaluatory and Treatment Approach.* Paoli, Pa: MFR Seminars; 1990.

61. Morton T. Panel debates the pros and cons of myofascial release approach. *APTA Progress Report* 1988:10–12.

62. Sullivan SJ, Williams LR, Seaborne DE, Morelli M. Effects of massage on alpha motoneuron excitability. *Phys Ther* 1991;71:555–560.

63. Roy S, Irvin R. *Sports Medicine—Prevention, Evaluation, Management, and Rehabilitation.* Englewood Cliffs, NJ: Prentice-Hall; 1983.

64. Johnson GS. Soft tissue mobilization. In: Donatelli RA, Wooden MJ, eds. *Orthopaedic Physical Therapy.* Philadelphia, Pa: Churchill Livingstone; 2001:578–617.

65. Grodin AJ, Cantu RI. Soft tissue mobilization. In: Basmajian JV, Nyberg R, eds. *Rational Manual Therapies.* Baltimore, Md: Williams and Wilkins; 1993:199–221.

66. Licht S. *Massage, Manipulation and Traction.* Melbourne, Fla: E Licht; 1960.

67. Kamenetz HL. History of massage. In: Basmajian JV, ed. *Manipulation, Traction and Massage.* Baltimore, Md: Williams and Wilkins; 1985:5–21.

68. Wakim KG. The effects of massage on the circulation of normal and paralyzed extremities. *Arch Phys Med Rehabil* 1949;30:135.

69. Crosman LJ, Chateauvert SR, Weisberg J. The effects of massage to the hamstring muscle group on range of motion. *J Orthop Sports Phys Ther* 1984;6:168.

70. Beard G, Wood E. *Massage Principles and Techniques.* Philadelphia, Pa: Saunders; 1965.

71. Palastanga N. Soft-tissue manipulative techniques. In: Palastanga N, Boyling JD, eds. *Grieve's Modern Manual Therapy: The Vertebral Column.* Edinburgh, Scotland: Churchill Livingstone; 1994:809–822.

72. Hollis M. *Massage for Therapists.* Oxford, England: Blackwell; 1987.

73. Jarmey C, Tindall T. *Acupressure for Common Ailments.* New York, NY: Simon and Schuster; 1991.

74. van Tulder MW. The effectiveness of acupuncture in the management of acute and chronic low back pain: A systematic review within the framework of the Cochrane Collaboration Back Review Group. *Spine* 1999;24:1113.

75. Melzack R. The gate theory revisited. In: LeRoy PL, ed. *Current Concepts in the Management of Chronic Pain.* Miami, Fla: Symposia Specialists; 1977.

76. Melzack R, Wall PD. On the nature of cutaneous sensory mechanisms. *Brain* 1962;85:331–356.

77. Haldeman S. Manipulation and massage for the relief of pain. In: Wall PD, Melzack R, eds. *Textbook of Pain.* Edinburgh, Scotland: Churchill Livingstone; 1989:942–951.

78. Kahn J. Electrical modalities in the treatment of myofascial conditions. In: Rachlin ES, ed. *Myofascial Pain and Fibromyalgia, Trigger Point Management.* St Louis, Mo: Mosby; 1994:473–485.

79. Krause H, Fischer AA. Diagnosis and treatment of myofascial pain. *Mt Sinai J Med* 1991;58:235–239.

80. Lewit K. The needle effect in the relief of myofascial pain. *Pain* 1979;6:83–90.

81. Magora F, Aladjemoff L, Tannenbaum J, Magora A. Treatment of pain by transcutaneous electrical stimulation. *Acta Anaesthesiol Scand* 1978;22:589–592.

82. Sola AE, Bonica JJ. Myofascial pain syndromes. In: Bonica JJ, Loeser JD, Chapman CR, Fordyce WE, et al, eds. *The Management of Pain.* Philadelphia, Pa: Lea and Febiger; 1990:352–367.

83. Travell JG, Simons DG. *Myofascial Pain and Dysfunction—The Trigger Point Manual.* Baltimore, Md: Williams and Wilkins; 1983.

84. Vecchiet L, Giamberardino MA, Saggini R. Myofascial pain syndromes: Clinical and pathophysiological aspects. *Clin J Pain* 1991;7(suppl):16–22.

85. Stux G, Pomeranz B. *Basics of Acupuncture.* Berlin, Germany: Springer-Verlag; 1988.

86. Mitchell FL Sr. Structural pelvic function. *Academy of Applied Osteopathy Yearbook* 1958:71–89.

87. Mitchell FL Jr. Elements of muscle energy techniques. In: Basmajian JV, Nyberg R, eds. *Rational Manual Therapies.* Baltimore, Md: Williams and Wilkins; 1993:285–321.

88. Lewit K, Simons DG. Myofascial pain: Relief by post-isometric relaxation. *Arch Phys Med Rehabil* 1984;65:452–456.

89. Goodridge JP. Muscle energy technique: Definition, explanation, methods of procedure. *J Am Osteopath Assoc* 1981;81:249–254.

90. Wyke BD. The neurology of joints: A review of general principles. *Clin Rheum Dis* 1981;7:223–239.

91. Wyke BD. The neurology of joints. *Ann R Coll Surg Engl* 1967;41:25–50.

92. Hagbarth K. Excitatory inhibitory skin areas for flexor and extensor motoneurons. *Acta Physiol Scand* 1952;94:1–58.

93. Chaitow L. An introduction to muscle energy techniques. In: Chaitow L, ed. *Muscle Energy Techniques.* London, England: Churchill Livingstone; 2001:1–18.

94. Jones LH. *Strain and Counterstrain.* Colorado Springs, Co: American Academy of Osteopathy; 1981.

95. Bowles CH. Musculo-skeletal segment as a problem solving machine. *Yearbook of the Academy of Applied Osteopathy* 1964:157–183.

96. Johnston WL. Segmental behavior during motion. I. A palpatory study of somatic relations. II. Somatic dysfunction, the clinical distortion. *J Am Osteopath Assoc* 1972;72:352–361.

97. Johnston WL. Segmental behavior during motion. III. Extending behavioral boundaries. *J Am Osteopath Assoc* 1973;72:462–475.

98. Liebenson C. Active muscular relaxation techniques (part 2). *J Manipulative Physiol Ther* 1990;13:2–6.

99. Liebenson C. Active muscular relaxation techniques (part 1). *J Manipulative Physiol Ther* 1989;12:446–451.

100. Janda V. Muscles, motor regulation and back problems. In: Korr IM, ed. *The Neurological Mechanisms in Manipulative Therapy*. New York, NY: Plenum; 1978:27.

101. Janda V. *Muscle Function Testing*. London, England: Butterworth; 1983:163–167.

102. Janda V. Muscle strength in relation to muscle length, pain and muscle imbalance. In: Harms-Ringdahl K, ed. *Muscle Strength*. New York, NY: Churchill Livingstone; 1993:83.

103. Lewit K. *Manipulative Therapy in Rehabilitation of the Motor System*. 3rd ed. London, England: Butterworth; 1999.

104. Evjenth O, Hamberg J. *Muscle Stretching in Manual Therapy, A Clinical Manual*. Alfta, Sweden: Alfta Rehab Forlag; 1984.

105. Lewis C, Flynn TW. The use of strain-counterstrain in the treatment of patients with low back pain. *J Man Manipulative Ther* 2001;9:92–98.

106. Kusunose R. Strain and counterstrain. In: Basmajian JV, Nyberg R, eds. Rationale Manual Therapies. Baltimore, Md: Williams and Wilkins; 1993:chap 13.

107. Korr IM. Proprioceptors and somatic dysfunction. *J Am Osteopath Assoc* 1975;74:638–650.

108. Bailey HW. Some problems in making osteopathic spinal manipulative therapy appropriate and specific. *J Am Osteopath Assoc* 1976;75:486–499.

109. Schiowitz S. Facilitated positional release. *J Am Osteopath Assoc* 1990;90:145–155.

110. Chaitow L. Associated techniques. In: Chaitow L, ed. *Modern Neuromuscular Techniques*. New York, NY: Churchill Livingstone; 1996:109–135.

111. Carew TJ. The control of reflex action. In: Kandel ER, Schwartz JH, eds. *Principles of Neural Science*. New York, NY: Elsevier; 1985:464.

112. Rathbun JB, Macnab I. The microvascular pattern of the rotator cuff. *J Bone Joint Surg* 1970;52B:540–553.

113. DiGiovanna EL. Diagnosis and treatment of the upper extremity. In: DiGiovanna EL, Schiowitz S, eds. *An Osteopathic Approach to Diagnosis and Treatment*. Philadelphia, Pa: JB Lippincott; 1991.

114. Jacobson EC, Lockwood MD, Hoefner VC Jr, Dickey JL, Kuchera WL. Shoulder pain and repetition strain injury to the supraspinatus muscle: Etiology and manipulative treatment. *J Am Osteopath Assoc* 1989;89:1037–1045.

115. Schiowitz S. Diagnosis and treatment of the lower extremity—The hip. In: DiGiovanna EL, Schiowitz S, eds. *An Osteopathic Approach to Diagnosis and Treatment*. Philadelphia, Pa: JB Lippincott; 1991:325–330.

116. Still AT. *Osteopathy. Research and Practice*. Kirksville, Mo: AT Still; 1910.

117. Hoover HV. Collected papers. *Academy of Applied Osteopathy Year Book* 1969:16–68.

118. Bowles CH. Functional technique: A modern perspective. *J Am Osteopath Assoc* 1981;80:326–331.

119. Yoder E. Physical therapy management of nonsurgical hip problems in adults. In: Echternach JL, ed. *Physical Therapy of the Hip*. New York, NY: Churchill Livingstone; 1990:103–137.

120. Mennel J. *Joint Pain and Diagnosis Using Manipulative Techniques*. New York, NY: Little, Brown; 1964.

121. Tanigawa MC. Comparison of hold-relax procedure and passive mobilization on increasing muscle length. *Phys Ther* 1972;52:725–735.

122. Barak T, Rosen E, Sofer R. Basic concepts of orthopedic manual therapy. In: Gould J, Davies G, eds. *Orthopedic and Sports Physical Therapy*. St Louis, Mo: Mosby; 1990:195–212.

123. Maigne R. *Orthopedic Medicine*. Springfield, Ill: Charles C Thomas; 1972.

124. Vicenzino B, Collins D, Benson H, Wright A. An investigation of the interrelationship between manipulative therapy-induced hypoalgesia and sympathoexcitation. *J Manipulative Physiol Ther* 1998;21:448–453.

125. Vicenzino B, Collins D, Wright A. The initial effects of a cervical spine manipulative physiotherapy treatment on the pain and dysfunction of lateral epicondylalgia. *Pain* 1996;68:69–74.

126. Vicenzino B, Gutschlag F, Collins D, Wright A, et al. An investigation of the effects of spinal manual therapy on forequarter pressure and thermal pain thresholds and sympathetic nervous system activity in asymptomatic subjects. In: Schachloch MO, ed. *Moving in on Pain*. Adelaide, Australia: Butterworth-Heinemann; 1995.

127. Grieve GP. Manual mobilizing techniques in degenerative arthrosis of the hip. *Bull Orthop Section APTA* 1977;2:7.

128. Freeman MAR, Wyke BD. An experimental study of articular neurology. *J Bone Joint Surg* 1967;49B:185.

129. Meadows JTS. The principles of the Canadian approach to the lumbar dysfunction patient. In: *Management of Lumbar Spine Dysfunction—Independent Home Study Course*. La Crosse, Wis: Orthopaedic Section, American Physical Therapy Association; 1999.

130. Wadsworth C. *Manual Examination and Treatment of the Spine and Extremities*. Baltimore, Md: Williams and Wilkins; 1988.

131. Loubert P. A qualitative biomechanical analysis of the concave-convex rule. In: Proceedings of the Fifth International Conference of the International Federation of Orthopaedic Manipulative Therapists; 1992; Vail, Colorado.

132. Sluka KA, Wright A. Knee joint mobilization reduces secondary mechanical hyperalgesia induced by capsaicin injection into the ankle joint. *Eur J Pain* 2001;5:81–87.

133. Mulligan BR. *Manual Therapy: "NAGS", "SNAGS", "PRP'S"* etc. Wellington, New Zealand: Plane View Series; 1992.

134. Mulligan BR. Manual therapy rounds: Mobilisations with movement (MWMs). *J Man Manipulative Ther* 1993;1:154–156.

135. Abbott JH, Patla CE, Jensen RH. The initial effects of an elbow mobilization with movement technique on grip strength in subjects with lateral epicondylalgia. *Manual Ther* 2001;6:163–169.

136. Vicenzino B, Wright A. Effects of a novel manipulative physiotherapy technique on tennis elbow: A single case study. *Manual Ther* 1995;1:30–35.

137. Stephens G. Lateral epicondylitis. *J Man Manipulative Ther* 1995;3:50–58.

138. Miller J. Mulligan concept—management of tennis elbow. *Orthop Div Rev* 2000;May-June:45–46.

138a. Konstantinou K, Foster N, Rushton A, Baxter D. The use and reported effects of mobilization with movement techniques in low back pain management; a cross-sectional descriptive survey of physiotherapists in Britain. *Man Ther* 2002;7(4):206–214.

138b. Exelby L. The locked lumbar facet joint: Intervention using mobilizations with movement. *Man Ther* 2001;6(2):116–121.

139. Fisher AGT. *Treatment by Manipulation.* 5th ed. New York, NY: Paul B Hoeber; 1948.

140. Marlin T. *Manipulative Treatment for the General Practitioner.* London, England: Edward Arnold; 1934.

141. Mixter WJ, Barr JS Jr. Rupture of the intervertebral disc with involvement of the spinal canal. *N Engl J Med* 1934;211:210–215.

142. Haldeman S. Spinal manipulative therapy in sports medicine. *Clin Sports Med* 1986;5:277–293.

143. Gatterman MI. Glossary. In: Gatterman MI, ed. *Foundations of Chiropractic.* St Louis, Mo: Mosby; 1995:474.

144. Gatterman MI. Introduction. In: Gatterman MI, ed. *Chiropractic Management of Spine Related Disorders.* Baltimore, Md: Williams and Wilkins; 1990:xv–xx.

145. Unsworth A, Dowson D, Wright V. "Cracking joints": A bio-engineering study of cavitation in the metacarpophalangeal joint. *Ann Rheum Dis* 1971;30:348–358.

146. Kleynhans AM. Complications of and contraindications to spinal manipulative therapy. In: Haldeman S, ed. *Modern Developments in the Principles and Practice of Chiropractic.* New York, NY: Appleton-Century-Crofts; 1980.

147. Moritz U. Evaluation of manipulation and other manual therapy: Criteria for measuring the effect of treatment. *Scand J Rehabil Med* 1979;11:173–179.

148. Glover JR, Morris JG, Khosla T. A randomized clinical trial of rotational manipulation of the trunk. *Br J Indust Med* 1974;31:59–64.

149. Glover JR, Morris JG, Khosla T. A randomized clinical trial of rotational manipulation of the trunk. In: Buerger AA, Tobis JS, eds. *Approaches to the Validation of Manipulation Therapy.* Springfield, Ill: Charles C Thomas; 1977:271–283.

150. Bogduk N, Engel R. The menisci of the lumbar zygapophysial joints: A review of their anatomy and clinical significance. *Spine* 1984;9:454–460.

151. Lantz CA. The vertebral subluxation complex. In: Gatterman MI, ed. *Foundations of Chiropractic: Subluxation.* St Louis, Mo: Mosby; 1995:149–174.

152. Enneking WF, Horowitz M. The intra-articular effects of immobilization on the human knee. *J Bone Joint Surg* 1972;54A:973–985.

153. Terrett ACJ, Vernon H. Manipulation and pain tolerance. A controlled study of the effects of spinal manipulation on paraspinal cutaneous pain tolerance levels. *Am J Phys Med* 1980;63:217–225.

154. Vernon HT, Dhami MSI, Annett R. Abstract. Symposium on low back pain; Canadian Foundation for Spinal Research; 1985; Vancouver, Canada.

155. Akeson WH, Woo SL, Amiel D, Coutts RD, Daniel D. The connective tissue response to immobility: Biochemical changes in periarticular connective tissue of the immobilized rabbit knee. *Clin Orthop* 1973;93:356–362.

156. Akeson WH, Woo SL, Amiel D, Matthews JV. Biomechanical and biochemical changes in the periarticular connective tissue during contracture development of the immobilized rabbit knee. *Connect Tissue Res* 1974;2:315–323.

157. Akeson WH, Amiel D, Woo SLY. Immobility effects on synovial joints: The pathomechanics of joint contracture. *Biorheology* 1980;17:95–110.

158. Akeson WH, Amiel D, Abel MF, Garfin SR, Woo SL. Effects of immobilization on joints. *Clin Orthop* 1987;219:28–37.

159. Gross AR, Aker PD, Quartly C. Manual therapy in the treatment of neck pain. *Rheum Dis Clin North Am* 1996;22:579–598.

160. Grant ER. Clinical testing before cervical manipulation—can we recognise the patient at risk? In: Proceedings of the Tenth International Congress of the World Confederation for Physical Therapy; 1987; Sydney, Australia.

161. Hosek RS, Schram SB, Silverman H. Cervical manipulation. *JAMA* 1981;245:922.

162. Dvorak J, von Orelli F. The frequency of complications after manipulation of the cervical spine: Case report and epidemiology [in German; author's trans]. *Schweiz Rundsch Med Prax* 1982;71:64–69.

163. Pollard H, Ward G. A study of two stretching techniques for improving hip flexion range of motion. *J Manipulative Physiol Ther* 1997;20:443–447.

164. Griffin J. Use of proprioceptive stimuli in therapeutic exercise. *Phys Ther* 1974;54:1072.

165. Kabat H. Proprioceptive facilitation in therapeutic exercises. In: *Therapeutic Exercises.* Baltimore, Md: Waverly Press; 1965:327–343.

166. Saliba V, Johnson G, Wardlaw C. Proprioceptive neuromuscular facilitation. In: Basmajian JV, Nyberg R, eds. *Rational Manual Therapies.* Baltimore, Md: Williams and Wilkins; 1993: 68–92.

167. Knott M, Voss DE. *Proprioceptive Neuromuscular Facilitation.* 2nd ed. New York, NY: Harper and Row; 1968.

168. Sullivan PE, Markos PD, Minor MAD. *An Integrated Approach to Therapeutic Exercise.* Reston, Va: Reston Publishing; 1982.

169. Johnson GS, Johnson VS. The application of the principles and procedures of PNF for the care of lumbar spinal instabilities. *J Man Manipulative Ther* 2002;10:83–105.

170. Smidt, GL. Trunk muscle strength and endurance in the context of low-back dysfunction. In: Grieve G, ed. *Modern Manual Therapy of the Vertebral Column.* London, England: Churchill Livingstone; 1994:211–226.

171. Lewit K. The contribution of clinical observation to neurobiological mechanisms in manipulative therapy. In: Korr IM, ed. *The Neurobiological Mechanisms in Manipulative Therapy.* New York, NY: Plenum Press; 1977.

172. Prentice WE. A comparison of static stretching and PNF stretching for improving hip joint flexibility. *Athl Training* 1983;18:56–59.

173. Smolders JJ. Myofascial pain and dysfunction syndromes. In: Hammer WI, ed. *Functional Soft Tissue Examination and Treatment by Manual Methods—The Extremities.* Gaithersburg, Md: Aspen: 1991:215–234.

174. Rosen NB. The myofascial pain syndrome. *Phys Med Rehabil Clin North Am* 1993;4:41–63.

175. Simons DG. Myofascial pain syndromes. In: Foley KM, Payne RM, eds. *Current Therapy of Pain.* New York, NY: Churchill Livingstone; 1989:368–385.

176. Meisekothen-Auleciems L. Myofascial pain syndrome: A multidisciplinary approach. *Nurse Pract* 1995;20:18–31.

177. Simons DG. Muscular pain syndromes. In: Fricton JR, Awad E, eds. *Advances in Pain Research and Therapy.* New York, NY: Raven; 1990:1–41.

178. Goldman LB, Rosenberg NL. Myofascial pain syndrome and fibromyalgia. *Sem Neurol* 1991;11:274–280.

179. Falconer J, Hayes KW, Chang RW. Therapeutic ultrasound in the treatment of musculoskeletal conditions. *Arthritis Care Res* 1990;3:85–91.

180. Esenyel M, Caglar N, Aldemir T. Treatment of myofascial pain. *Am J Phys Med Rehabil* 2000;79:48–52.

181. Hong CZ. Lidocaine injection versus dry needling to myofascial trigger point: The importance of the local twitch response. *Am J Phys Med Rehabil* 1994;73:256–263.

182. Wreje U, Brorsson B. A multi-center randomized controlled trial of sterile water and saline for chronic myofascial pain syndromes. *Pain* 1995;61:441–444.

183. Chen SH, Wu YC, Hong CZ. Current management of myofascial pain syndrome. *Clin J Pain* 1996;6:27–46.

184. Kine GD, Warfiend CA. Myofascial pain syndrome. *Hosp Pract* 1986;9:194–196.

185. Gam AN, Warming S, Larsen LH, et al. Treatment of myofascial trigger-points with ultrasound combined with massage and exercise—a randomised controlled trial. *Pain* 1998;77:73–79.

186. Simons DG. Myofascial pain syndromes. In: Foley KM, Payne RM, eds. *Current Therapy of Pain*. Philadelphia, Pa: BC Decker; 1989:251–266.

187. Lee JC, Lin DT, Hong CZ. The effectiveness of simultaneous thermotherapy with ultrasound and electrotherapy with combined AC and DC current on the immediate pain relief of myofascial trigger point. *J Musculoskel Pain* 1997;5:81–90.

188. Woolf CF. Segmental afferent fiber-induced analgesia: Transcutaneous electrical nerve stimulation (TENS) and vibration. In: Wall PD, Melzack R, eds. *Textbook of Pain*. New York, NY: Churchill Livingstone; 1989:884–896.

189. Hsueh TC, Cheng PT, Kuan TS, Hong CZ. The immediate effectiveness of electrical nerve stimulation and electrical muscle stimulation on myofascial trigger points. *Am J Phys Med Rehabil* 1997;76:471–476.

NEURODYNAMIC MOBILIZATIONS

CHAPTER OBJECTIVES

▶ **At the completion of this chapter, the reader will be able to:**

1. Summarize the various types of neurodynamic examination and mobilization techniques.

2. Describe the proposed mechanisms behind the neurodynamic examination and mobilization techniques.

3. Apply knowledge of the various neurodynamic mobilization techniques in the planning of a comprehensive rehabilitation program.

4. Recognize the manifestations of abnormal nervous tissue tension and develop strategies using neurodynamic mobilization techniques to treat these abnormalities.

5. Evaluate the effectiveness of a neurodynamic mobilization technique when used as a direct intervention.

OVERVIEW

The nervous system is an electrical, chemical, and mechanical structure with continuity between its two subdivisions: the central and peripheral nervous systems. In addition to permitting inter- and intra-neural communication throughout the entire network, the nervous system is capable of withstanding mechanical stress as a result of its unique mechanical characteristics. Nervous tissue, a form of connective tissue, is viscoelastic. This viscoelasticity allows for the transfer of mechanical stress throughout the nervous system. These mechanical stresses may occur during trunk or limb movements. An early study by Inman and Saunders[1] found the spinal canal to be from 5 to 9 cm longer in flexion than extension. Later studies by Millesi[2,3] demonstrated that the peripheral nerves have the capacity to adapt to different positions by passive movement relative to the surrounding tissue via a gliding apparatus around the nerve trunk. Three mechanisms would appear to play an important role in this adaptability:[2]

▶ The ability of the nerve to elongate against elastic forces.

▶ Longitudinal movement of the nerve trunk in the longitudinal direction.

▶ An increase and decrease of tissue relaxation at the level of the nerve trunk.

According to Millesi,[2] the efficiency of this mechanism partially depends on the ability of the nerve to move against the surrounding tissue. This ability is provided by the loose connective tissue around the nerve (adventitia, conjunctiva nervorum, perineurium), which allows any traction forces to be distributed over the whole length of the nerve.[2] Conversely, if adhesions of the nerve trunk occur, this equal distribution of forces is prevented and can lead to an unfavorable rise of traction forces at certain segments, according to the anatomic site.[2] These adverse traction forces and the role that tension on the neural tissue plays in pain and dysfunction have been studied for over a century. During this time, a number of specific tests have been designed to examine the neurological structures for adaptive shortening and inflammation of the neural structures.[4–6] The more common of these neurodynamic mobility tests are described in this chapter.

Proposed Mechanisms for Neurodynamic Dysfunction

The spinal dura forms a loose sheath around the spinal cord from the foramen magnum to the level of the second sacral tubercle. From there, it continues as the filum terminale to end at the coccyx (Fig. 12-1). Laterally, the dura surrounds the exiting spinal nerve roots at the level of the intervertebral foramen. There are three areas, called *tension sites*, in which the dura is tethered to the bony canal, providing stability to the spinal cord. These tension sites are found at the segmental levels of C6, T6, and L4; the elbow; the shoulder; and the knee.[6a,6b] As a result of these sites of tension, the neurologic tissues move in different directions, depending on where the stress is applied and in which order it is applied.[6c]

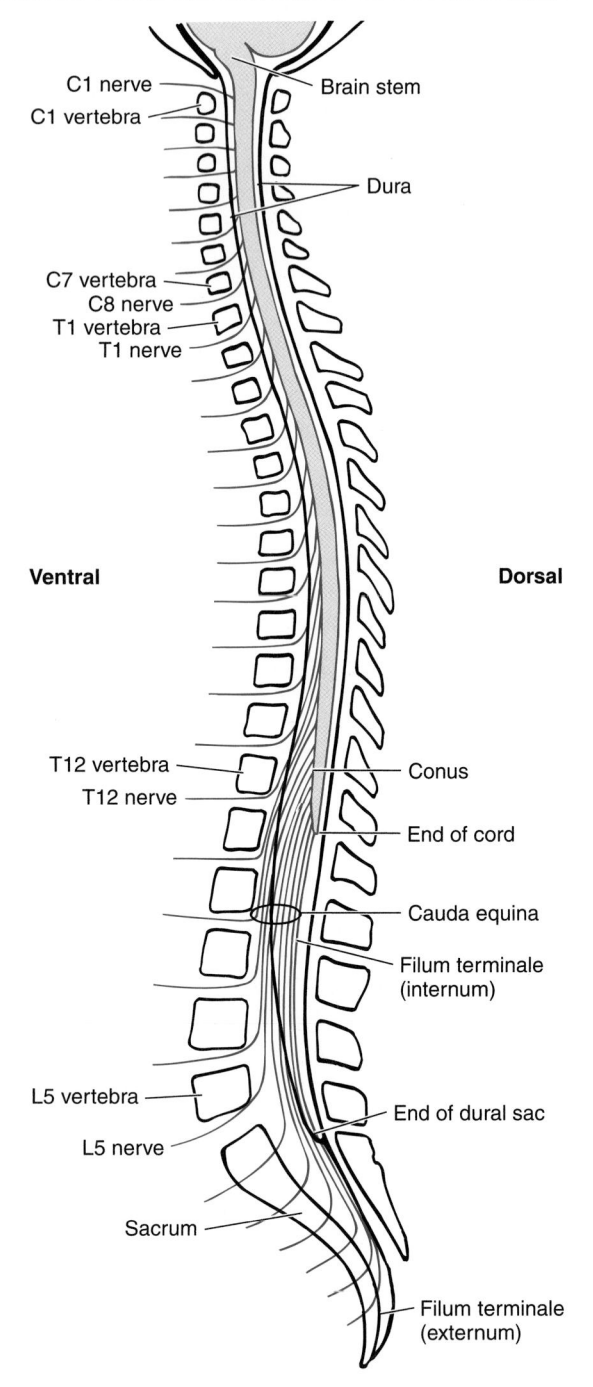

FIGURE 12-1 The spinal dura. (Reproduced with permission from Waxman SG. *Correlative Neuroanatomy.* 24th ed. New York, NY: McGraw-Hill; 1996.)

Various studies have demonstrated excursion of the nerve complex during movements of the extremity.[6a,6d,7–10] Under normal circumstances, the tension sites are not abnormally affected by motion of the extremities. However, if the dura becomes adherent, excessive stress may be produced in the areas of adhesion, increasing the length of the dura beyond its normal limit of tension.[10a] Theoretically, increased dural

tension may be felt throughout the neuromeningeal system and, potentially, it may affect the range of motion available to the trunk and to an extremity. Pathomechanically, a decrease in the mobility of a nerve along its entire length makes the nerve more vulnerable to additional injuries during repetitive movements.[10a,11]

Clinical Pearl

Neural tissue responds to trauma in the same way that a ligament or tendon does, by evoking the cascade of the inflammatory process, resulting in pain when stressed.[12,13] In addition to the effect that the inflammatory process can have on the nerve tissue, fibrous tissue formation can develop within the nerve root sheath, causing adhesions between the sheath and the nerve root.[13,14]

The nerves and their microcirculation are vulnerable to tension, friction, and compressive forces at multiple sites along their routes.[11] A number of mechanisms are hypothesized to contribute to an injury of the peripheral nerve trunk. These include[15]:

▸ *Posture.* Most abnormal postures result in a shortening of the distance traveled by the peripheral nerve trunk. Correction of this posture, after sufficient time has elapsed for adaptive shortening of structures to have taken place, may produce a stretching of the neural tissues.

▸ *Direct trauma.* Orthopaedic injuries account for some of the injuries to peripheral nerves. For example, the radial nerve is injured through orthopedic trauma more than any other major nerve.[16] These injuries can occur as the result of a direct blow to the nerve or secondary to damage of an adjacent structure, such as a fracture,[17,18] joint dislocation,[19] or tendon rupture.[20] Other causes of direct nerve trauma have included injections,[21] joint manipulation,[22] and surgical procedures.[23]

▸ *Extremes of motion.* Given the course of many of the peripheral nerve trunks, it is not difficult to envision movements of the extremities that could place a traction force on these trunks. Indeed, those very same movements are exploited in some of the neurodynamic mobility tests.

▸ *Electrical injury.* In a 17-year review of burn unit admissions, permanent nerve injuries were found in 22 percent of electrocuted patients.[24] The upper limb was most commonly involved, with the median and ulnar nerves most commonly injured.[24] Postneurologic symptoms in such cases can vary from neuropathy to reflex sympathetic dystrophy.

▸ *Compression.* Compression to a nerve can occur during muscle contraction and as a result of tight fascia, osteochondroma, ganglia, lipomas and other benign neoplasms, and bony protuberances.

Double-crush Injuries

The concept that many entrapment neuropathies result from a so-called double-crush along the peripheral nerve fibers was proposed by Upton and McComas in 1973.[25]

Theoretically, two focal lesions along the same axon could be related in that, if the axoplasmic flow is partially reduced at the proximal site of injury, further reduction can occur at the distal compression site. If this axoplasmic flow is reduced to the point that it drops below the safety margin, denervation can result.[25] Thus, a cervical radiculopathy, manifesting as little more than neck pain and stiffness, could still precipitate a distal focal entrapment neuropathy.[25] The term *double-crush syndrome* (DCS) is used to describe this mechanism of nerve injury: serial compromise of axonal transport along the same nerve fiber, causing a subclinical lesion at the distal site to become symptomatic.

At least eight other etiologic mechanisms have been proposed to explain the relationship between the proximal and distal nerve fiber lesions[25–29]:

1. A proximal nerve lesion renders the distal nerve segment more vulnerable to compression because of serial constraints of axoplasmic flow.

2. The peripheral nerves possess an underlying susceptibility to pressure.

3. Interruption of lymphatic and venous drainage at the proximal nerve lesion site renders the distal nerve segment more vulnerable.

4. Endoneurial edema at one lesion site compromises neural circulation, rendering nerve fibers at the other site more vulnerable.

5. A connective tissue abnormality common to both sites along the nerve fibers.

6. Tethering of the nerve at one site causes injurious shear forces at the other site.

7. Entrapment of the nerve at one site causes decreased use of the muscle pump, which creates a slight, generalized edema of limb. This increases tissue pressure in certain anatomic passages, which causes an additional entrapment nerve lesion.

8. The initial nerve lesion releases a metabolite that passes through the free intraneural circulation and increases the vulnerability of other segments of the nerve.

Since its introduction, the double-crush hypothesis has been invoked to explain a great number of coexisting proximal and distal nerve impairments. In fact, it has been expanded in various ways (i.e., to triple-crush, quadruple-crush, and multiple-crush syndromes, as well as the reversed double-crush syndrome).[27,30,31] Despite its acceptance, however, the double-crush hypothesis has anatomic and pathophysiologic restrictions that should severely limit its use, and render it inapplicable in many clinical situations.[32] For the DCS to occur, there must be anatomic continuity of nerve fibers between the two (or more) lesions sites. If this is lacking, then sequential impairment of axoplasmic flow obviously cannot occur. Consequently, two focal nerve disorders along the same neural pathway (e.g., cervical root lesions, and carpal tunnel syndrome) do not automatically fulfill this anatomic criterion of DCS, unless the same axons are compromised at both sites.[32] This requirement is the major impediment to acknowledging as authentic most of the reported clinical examples of DCS.

Experimental studies of the double-crush hypothesis have shown that successive lesions along a peripheral nerve can summate.[28,33] However, studies that have attempted to demonstrate the existence of DCS have proved inconclusive.[34]

For example, Golovchinsky[35] performed a retrospective analysis of results of electromyography and nerve conduction velocity in 169 patients with lower back pain, mostly caused by trauma. A total 289 peroneal, 280 posterior tibial, and 301 sural nerves were included in statistical analysis. Statistical analysis of these data showed significantly higher than random overlap of peripheral entrapment syndromes and signs of proximal nerve damage of the corresponding nerves (partial muscle denervation or abnormalities of F-wave). Golovchinsky feels that this higher-than-random coincidence of the two conditions strongly suggests a cause-and-effect relationship of damage of the proximal stretch of motor nerve fibers and development of peripheral entrapment syndromes in the same nerves.[35] However, these results are far from conclusive.

Richardson and colleagues,[36] in a 1999 study, analyzed cases of C6, C7, and C8 radiculopathy, and concluded that although median mononeuropathy was unexpectedly common (22.1 percent) among cases of cervical radiculopathy, they could identify no evidence to support a neurophysiologic explanation for the double-crush hypothesis.

Similarly Bednarik and colleagues[37] studied the association between spondylotic cervical myelopathy (SCM) and median nerve mononeuropathy (MNM) in 60 consecutive patients and a control group of 100, to examine the validity of the double-crush hypothesis by means of nerve conduction studies, electromyography, and median nerve somatosensory evoked potentials. Although the authors demonstrated a statistically significant association between SCM and MNM, they were unable to find any evidence of an etiologic relationship between these two conditions, and the electrophysiologic signs of MNM failed anatomic (segmental level and side) and pathophysiologic (axonal type of lesion) requirements of the double-crush hypothesis in most of the patients.[37]

Neurodynamic Mobility Examinations

Both Elvey[38] and Butler[1] have been credited with the development of the examination techniques for neurodynamic mobility. Elvey[38] developed what he named the *brachioplexus tension test,* which was later called the *upper limb tension test*

(ULTT). Similar tests, such as the straight leg raise and prone knee flexion tests, have been designed for the lower extremity. The slump test is considered to be a general test of neurodynamic mobility. The tension tests are designed to apply controlled mechanical and compressive stresses to the dura and other neurologic tissues, both centrally and peripherally.[39] These neurodynamic tests are designed to assess the contribution of the spinal nerve roots and peripheral nerves to extremity pain by employing a sequential and progressive stretch to the dura. The tests place tensile stresses on the dura of spinal nerve roots and peripheral nerves using a longitudinal traction force of the nerve until the patient's symptoms are reproduced.[40]

The examination of neural adhesions is by no means an exact science, but the principles are based on sound anatomic theory. Knowledge of the course of each of the peripheral nerves is thus essential in order to put a sequential and adequate tension through each of them (see Chap. 2).

Breig's tissue-borrowing phenomenon offers a plausible explanation for the neurodynamic tests.[41] Breig observed that tension produced in a lumbosacral nerve root results in displacement of the neighboring dura, nerve roots, and lumbosacral plexus toward the site of tension.[1,41–43] In effect, a borrowing of the resting slack in neighboring meningeal tissues occurs as neural structures are pulled toward the site of increased tension. This results in a decrease in the available slack and potential mobility of the neural tissues throughout the region.[5,41–45] This stretching and displacement of the nerve roots plexi reduces the available mobility of the peripheral nerves.[5,41–45]

Positive symptoms for the presence of neuropathic dysfunction include pain, paresthesia, and spasm.[15] Unfortunately, these signs and symptoms are also associated with a host of musculoskeletal injuries. Asbury and Fields[46] hypothesized that the type of pain that results from an injury to a peripheral nerve is characteristic and has two varieties:

1. *Dysesthetic pain.* This type of pain is felt in the peripheral sensory distribution of a sensory or mixed nerve and results from nociceptive afferent fibers.

2. *Nerve trunk pain.* This type of pain results from the nociceptors within the nerve sheaths and exhibits a pain distribution following the course of the nerve trunk.[15]

However, relying on the reproduction of a type of pain (a subjective issue at the best of times) is not sufficient to make the diagnosis of neural tissue dysfunction.

Because the subject of neural provocation tests and the intervention of neurodynamic mobilization remains controversial, the clinician should ensure that the results of these tests are always used in conjunction with findings from a complete neuromusculoskeletal examination, including[15,39,47,48]:

▶ *Observation.* An injury to a peripheral nerve trunk may result in visible atrophy within its motor distribution.

▶ *Palpation.* The clinician should carefully palpate along each of the nerve trunks in the region where they are superficial.

Physical deformation of an irritated nerve should reproduce pain with palpation.

▶ *Range of motion.* In areas of decreased neural mobility, both active and passive range of motion may be diminished in the same direction. However, a lesion to the musculotendinous unit would also reproduce pain with the same maneuver, particularly in muscles that cross two joints.

▶ *Resistive testing.* Resistive tests can be used to examine for the presence of weakness in the distribution of a peripheral nerve, and to help differentiate between pain reproduced with active or passive range of motion that indicates damage to the musculotendinous unit and pain that results from neural tension. For example, pain reproduced in the posterior thigh with the straight leg raise may indicate a lesion of the hamstring muscle belly or a lesion to the sciatic nerve. If resisted knee flexion does not reproduce pain, the musculotendinous unit is unlikely to be at fault, leaving the sciatic nerve as the likely cause. However, one study[49] found that a positive neural tension test (slump test) was recorded in 57 percent of subjects with apparent repetitive grade I hamstring strains, suggesting some form of relationship between the hamstrings and the sciatic nerve.

The purpose of the physical examination is to determine which tissue is at fault. This is accomplished by isolating (where possible) each tissue that has the potential to produce those symptoms and selectively stressing that tissue. Part of the problem with this approach lies in the fact that a positive finding for many of the techniques designed to assess the integrity of a neural structure may just be the result of a sensitive movement, rather than a stretch of the dura.[50] For example, when wrist extension is performed with the elbow in extension and the shoulder abducted, in addition to placing stress through the elbow and wrist joints, wrist flexors, and elbow flexors, the loading of the nervous system is continued proximally, at least up to the level of the axilla.[51]

Some of the so-called dural symptoms could also result from the imparted stretch on the dura during the various maneuvers, producing changes in the axoplasmic flow inside the nerves, provoking the firing of abnormal impulses, and decreasing the vascular supply to the nerve.[52–54]

Neurodynamic Mobility Interventions

The rationale behind the use of neural mobilization techniques is the theoretical assumption that the techniques can improve axonal transport, thereby improving nerve conduction velocity.[4,39]

The detrimental affects of immobilization on musculoskeletal structures is well documented, as are the benefits of early mobilization protocols.[55–64] By applying early mobilization to the neural system, it seems possible that similar benefits should occur. However, an important distinction needs to be made between techniques that lengthen or stretch the dura and techniques that stretch the anatomic structures that surround the involved neural tissue.

Elvey[15] recommends an initial intervention of passive, gentle, and controlled oscillatory movements to the anatomic structures that surround the neural tissue, before progressing to the techniques that stretch both the surrounding tissues and the neural tissues together. Using this approach, the treatment barrier is represented by the onset of muscle activity.[65] For example, in the cervical spine, the sequence of neurodynamic mobilizations is initiated with shoulder depression with the neck in neutral and the arm by the side, followed by shoulder depression with fixation of the cervical spine, then shoulder depression, cervical fixation, and arm traction with the arm by the side. Once this progression has been performed without any adverse affects, the more specific movements used to isolate the nerve are employed.

Evidence for the efficacy of this gradual approach has been demonstrated in subjects with low back pain and radiculopathy,[66–68] lateral epicondylalgia,[69] and chronic cervicobrachial pain.[15,70]

Lower Extremity Tension Tests

Sciatica is defined as pain along the course of the sciatic nerve or its branches and is most commonly caused by a herniated disk or by spinal stenosis.[71] Characteristically, patients with sciatica report gluteal pain radiating down the posterior thigh and leg, paresthesia in the calf or foot, and varying degrees of motor weakness. Extraspinal entrapment of the sciatic nerve (i.e., along its course within the pelvis or the lower extremity), although infrequent, is difficult to diagnose because its symptoms are similar to those of the more frequent causes of sciatica.[72–74]

Straight Leg Raise Test

The straight leg raise (SLR) test is recognized as the first neural tissue tension test to appear in the literature. It was first described by Lasègue well over 100 years ago.[75]

The SLR test places a tensile stress on the sciatic nerve and exerts a caudal traction on the lumbosacral nerve roots from L4 to S2.[5,6,76–78] During the SLR, the L4 to L5 and S1 to S2 nerve roots are tracked inferiorly and anteriorly, pulling the dura mater caudally, laterally, and anteriorly. Tension in the sciatic nerve, and its continuations, occurs in a sequential manner, developing first in the greater sciatic foramen, then over the ala of the sacrum, next in the area where the nerve crosses over the pedicle, and finally in the intervertebral foramen.

The inferior and anterior pull on the nerve root, and the relative fixation of the dural investment at the anterior wall, produces a displacement that pulls the root against the posterior-lateral aspect of the disk and vertebra. In addition, any space-occupying lesions situated at the anterior wall of the vertebral canal at the fourth and fifth lumbar and first and second sacral segments may interfere with the dura mater or nerve root structures.

The evaluation of the findings from the SLR test requires that the range of motion measured, and the symptoms produced, are compared with the contralateral side and with expected norms.[5,78–81] Because sitting knee extension and the SLR culminate in essentially identical positions, symptomatic responses to the two types of maneuvers should be similar, although the angle at which pain is elicited may vary.[82]

> ### Clinical Pearl
>
> Confounding the results from the SLR test, are the non-neural structures, such as the lumbar zygapophysial joints, muscles, and connective tissue. These structures may limit leg elevation and provoke patient discomfort during testing.[5,78,80,81,83]

When the SLR is severely limited, it is considered diagnostic for a disk herniation.[84] The following caveats are important for accurate assessment of the SLR:

▶ The patient must have the necessary available range of hip flexion (30 to 70 degrees).

▶ The SLR produces a posterior shear and some degree of rotation in the lumbar spine, a region not well suited to shearing or rotational forces. Thus, back pain alone with the SLR is not a positive test. The test is positive when buttock, thigh, or leg pain, or a combination, along the appropriate dermatomal distribution is reproduced.[82]

Performing the Classic Straight Leg Raise Test

The patient is positioned supine, with no pillow under their head. Each leg is tested individually (uninvolved side first). To ensure that there is no undue stress on the dura, the tested leg is placed in slight internal rotation and adduction of the hip, and extension of the knee. The classic SLR test has the clinician holding the patient's ankle and raising the straight leg until complaints of pain or tightness in the posterior thigh are elicited.[1] At this point, the range of motion is noted and the clinician then lowers the straight leg slightly until the patient reports a decrease in symptoms.

Deyo and colleagues[85] noted a sensitivity of 80 percent and a specificity of 40 percent for the classic SLR in the diagnosis of low lumbar disk herniation. Van den Hoogen and colleagues[86] reported a sensitivity of 88 to 100 percent and a specificity of 11 to 44 percent for the SLR in the diagnosis of lumbar disk herniation.

It is generally agreed that the first 30 degrees of the SLR serve to take up the slack or crimp in the sciatic nerve and its continuations. Using symptom reproduction below 40 degrees as a criterion for a positive SLR test result has been found to decrease the sensitivity to 72 percent and increase the sensitivity to 72 percent.[87]

Pain in the 0-to-30-degree range may indicate the presence of:

▶ Acute spondylolisthesis.

▶ Tumor of the buttock.

▶ Gluteal abscess.

▶ Very large disk protrusion or extrusion.[88]

▶ Acute inflammation of the dura.

▶ Malingering patient.

▶ The sign of the buttock (see Chap. 17).

Between 30 and 70 degrees, the spinal nerves, their dural sleeves, and the roots of the L4, L5, S1, and S2 segments are stretched with an excursion of 2 to 6 mm.[89] After 70 degrees, although these structures undergo further tension, other structures also become involved. These additional structures include the hamstrings, gluteus maximus, and hip, lumbar, and sacroiliac joints. An SLR test is positive if:

▶ The range is limited by spasm to less than 70 degrees.

▶ There is a reproduction of leg and back pain.

▶ The pain reproduced is neurologic in nature. This pain should be accompanied by other signs and symptoms, such as pain with coughing, tying of shoe laces, and so on, but not necessarily by muscle weakness.

Variations to the classic SLR include:

▶ *Soto-Hall test.* In this test, the straight leg is passively raised to a point just before the onset of symptoms, and the patient's head and neck are passively flexed.

▶ *Braggard's test.* This test involves raising the lower limb to a similar level as the Soto-Hall test, at which point, the patient's ankle is passively dorsiflexed.

Dorsiflexion of the ankle and cervical flexion may be used as sensitizers for the SLR test (Fig. 12-2). In addition, further internal rotation or extreme adduction of the hip may also be added to the SLR. These additional maneuvers increase the

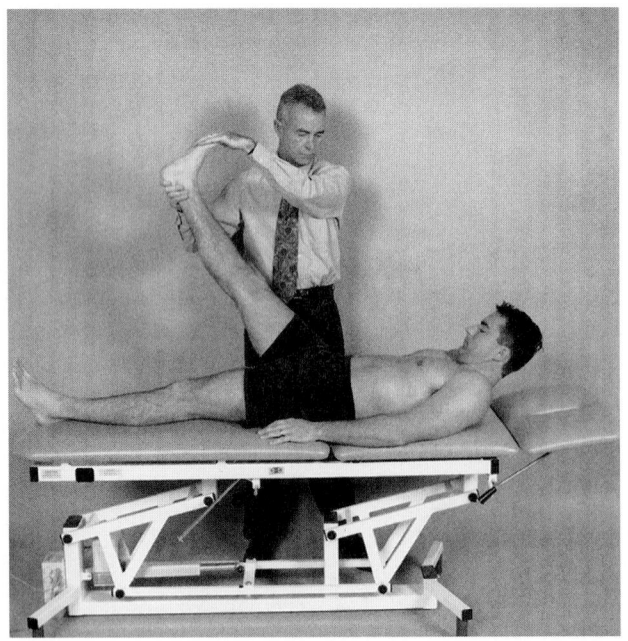

FIGURE 12-2 The straight leg raise with cervical flexion and passive ankle dorsiflexion.

tension exerted on the spinal cord, spinal dura, and lumbosacral nerve roots.[1,5,41–43,45,90] Research studies[41–44,90,91] have demonstrated that cervical flexion lengthens the spinal cord and dura. This action may provoke radicular symptoms without stressing non-neural tissues in the lower extremity.[1,66,92]

Thus, the dura can be pulled from below, using dorsiflexion, or from above, using cervical flexion. Further modifications can be incorporated to place stress through different branches of the sciatic and common peroneal nerves by adjusting the ankle and foot position, as follows:

▶ Dorsiflexion, foot eversion, and toe extension stress the tibial branch.

▶ Dorsiflexion and inversion stress the sural nerve.

▶ Plantar flexion and inversion stresses the common peroneal nerve (deep and superficial).

Crossed Straight Leg Raise Sign

The crossed SLR sign, or well leg raising test of Fajersztajn,[78] is associated with the SLR test, whereby a lifting of the asymptomatic leg produces pain in the symptomatic leg. There are three recognized types:

1. SLR that produces pain in the contralateral leg, but not when the contralateral leg is raised.

2. SLR that produces pain in both legs.

3. SLR of either leg that produces pain in the contralateral limb. For example, SLR of the right leg produces pain in the left leg, and SLR of the left leg produces pain in the right leg.

There are many theories as to the cause and significance of the crossover sign. One theory suggests that the neuromeninges are pulled caudally, resulting in compression of the dural sleeve against a large or medially displaced disk herniation. The crossover sign is thought to be more significant than the SLR test in terms of its diagnostic powers to indicate the presence of a large disk protrusion.[93] One study goes so far as to recommend using the combined results from the SLR and crossed SLR for a more accurate diagnosis.[86]

The following findings are strongly predictive of disk herniation.[88,93,94]

▶ Severely limited SLR.

▶ Positive crossover SLR.

▶ Severely restricted and painful trunk movements.

Bilateral Straight Leg Raise

Once the unilateral SLR test is completed, the clinician should test both legs simultaneously (Fig. 12-3). A limitation of the unilateral SLR is that it may not highlight the presence of a central disk protrusion, particularly a soft disk protrusion.[80] By performing a bilateral SLR and incorporating both neck flexion and dorsiflexion, central protrusions may be detected.[95]

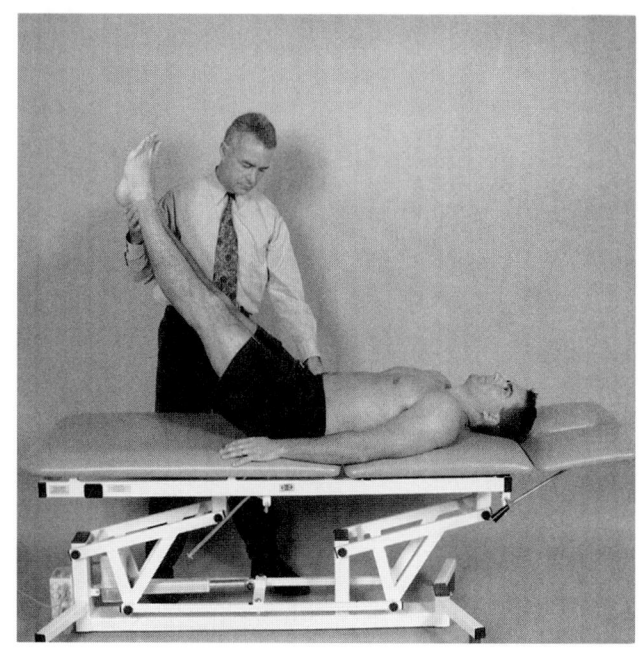

FIGURE 12-3 The bilateral straight leg raise.

Because a central protrusion may mimic a lateral recess stenosis, a differentiation test is needed. The bicycle test of van Gelderen[96] is advocated. The patient is appropriately positioned on a bicycle and asked to pedal against resistance.

▶ A patient with lateral spinal stenosis tolerates this position well.

▶ A patient with intermittent claudication of the lower extremities typically experiences an increase in symptoms with continued exercise, regardless of the position of the spine.

▶ A patient with intermittent cauda equina compression typically has an increase of symptoms with an increase in lumbar lordosis.

▶ A patient with a disk herniation usually fairs well if the lumbar spine remains extended.

Bowstring Tests

The bowstring tests are named after the technique applied to the nerve under examination. Both the tibial and common peroneal nerves can be tested, and although the tests impart an insufficient stretch of the dura to detect chronic adhesions, they can be used to make a prognosis about acute disk herniations. A positive bowstring test is a strong indicator for surgery, but it need only be performed if the SLR is positive with the addition of dorsiflexion.[95]

Cram's Tibial Nerve Test

The tibial nerve travels down the middle of the posterior thigh between the femoral condyles and down the back and middle of the calf, entering the foot under the medial malleolus of the ankle (see Chap. 2). The nerve is put on stretch with the addition of

dorsiflexion to the SLR. Once the reproduction of symptoms has occurred using the SLR, the clinician places the patient's leg over one shoulder, and the patient's knee is gently flexed until the symptoms fade. The clinician then places a thumb behind the patient's knee, between the femoral condyles and presses into the popliteal fossa, thereby deforming the tibial nerve. If the symptoms return with this maneuver, the test is considered positive.

Common Peroneal Test

Typically, the common peroneal nerve travels with the tibial branch to the posterior distal thigh region (see Chap. 2). It then wraps itself around the fibular head and has strong attachments to the tendon of the biceps femoris. The procedure for this test is similar to that of the tibial version of the test except that, after the knee is slightly flexed, the clinician pulls the biceps femoris tendon at the fibular head, medially and laterally. If this maneuver reproduces the symptoms, it is considered a positive test.

Slump Test

Despite refinements made to the SLR test, it remains inadequate to detect neural tension in some cases.[66,67,97] A neural tension test performed in a sitting position is necessary to simulate the extremes of spinal motion associated with symptom-provoking activities, such as slouched sitting or entering and exiting a car.[66,67,97]

The slump test, popularized by Maitland,[67] is a combination of other neuromeningeal tests; namely, the seated SLR, neck flexion, and lumbar slumping. In the slump test, the patient is seated in full flexion of the thoracic and lumbar regions of the spine.[98] Sensitizing maneuvers are then systematically applied and released to the cervical spine and lower extremities, while the tester maintains the patient's trunk position. The slump test assesses the excursion of neural tissues within the vertebral canal and intervertebral foramen[66] and detects impairments to neural tissue mobility from a number of sources as identified by Macnab[99] and Fahrni.[76] Maitland asserted that the slump test enables the tester to detect adverse nerve root tension caused by spinal stenosis, extraforaminal lateral disk herniation, disk sequestration, nerve root adhesions, and vertebral impingement.[66,97]

Several studies[41,45,91,100] have demonstrated the effects of trunk and head position on neural structures within the vertebral canal and intervertebral foramen during slump testing. These studies reported that full spinal flexion, or flexion of the cervical, thoracic, and lumbar regions of the spine, produces lengthening of the vertebral canal. This elongation of the vertebral canal stretches the spinal dura and transmits tension to the spinal cord, lumbosacral nerve root sleeves, and nerve roots.[41,45,91,100,101] During full spinal flexion, the cauda equina becomes taut and the lumbosacral nerve roots and root sleeves are pulled into contact with the pedicle of the superior vertebra.[41,77,91,100]

When extension of the cervical spine is introduced, the dura and the nerve roots slacken as the vertebral canal begins to shorten.[41,77,91,100–102] Extending the thoracic and lumbar spine increases the slack in the neural tissues as the vertebral canal continues to shorten.[41,77,91,100–102]

Because the slump test is a combination of other tests, a choice as to its use needs to be made. Either the classic SLR test or its variations should be performed; or the slump test should be used.[95] The only advantage of the slump test over the SLR test is that it increases the compression forces through the disk and will highlight the presence of dural adhesions.[95] Depending on the text used, there are a wide variety of progressive steps to the slump test; particularly when the lumbar kyphosis stage is introduced. Although the specific order of implementation remains controversial, it is important that the clinician consistently use the same sequence with each patient.

As soon as symptoms are reproduced during these tests, the test should be terminated. It is worth remembering that during a dural tension test, the dura itself does not move. It is merely stressed; hence, the name for the tests. One such method of sequencing is described next.

The patient is positioned sitting with the hands behind the back, and a slight arch in the back (Fig. 12-4), which will help to ensure that the lumbar spine is maintained in neutral. This initial position is then followed by a slump of the lumbar and thoracic spine as the clinician maintains the patient's neck in neutral (Fig. 12-5). This maneuver has the effect of tightening the entire dura, including the thorax dura. If the test is still negative, the patient is asked to flex the neck by first applying a chin tuck and placing the chin on the chest, and then to straighten the knee as much as possible. The test is repeated using the other leg and again with both legs at the same time. If the patient is unable to straighten the knee because of a reproduction of pain, he or she is asked to actively extend the neck. Following extension of the neck, if the patient cannot straighten the knee further, the test can be considered positive.

If symptoms have yet to occur, active dorsiflexion is added (Fig. 12-6). Passive over pressure can be applied to each of

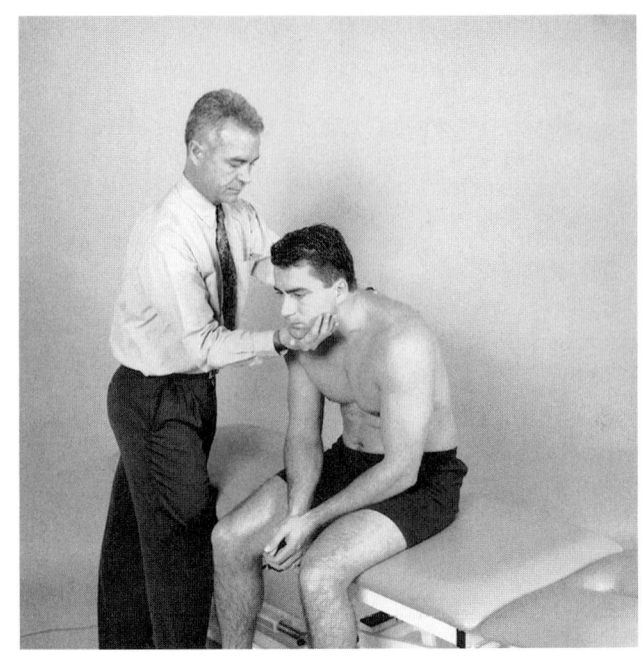

FIGURE 12-5 Thoracic and lumbar slump component of the slump test.

these moves. If the patient experiences positive symptoms with leg extension, the knee is slightly flexed and dorsiflexion is reapplied passively in an attempt to reproduce the symptoms. Throughout the entire slump test, each time a positive symptom is reproduced, the last movement applied is reduced slightly, to take the stress off the dura, and tension is applied from the opposite end of the dura. The test should also be performed in reverse (because a positive response may occur in one direction but not the other) and can be made more objective

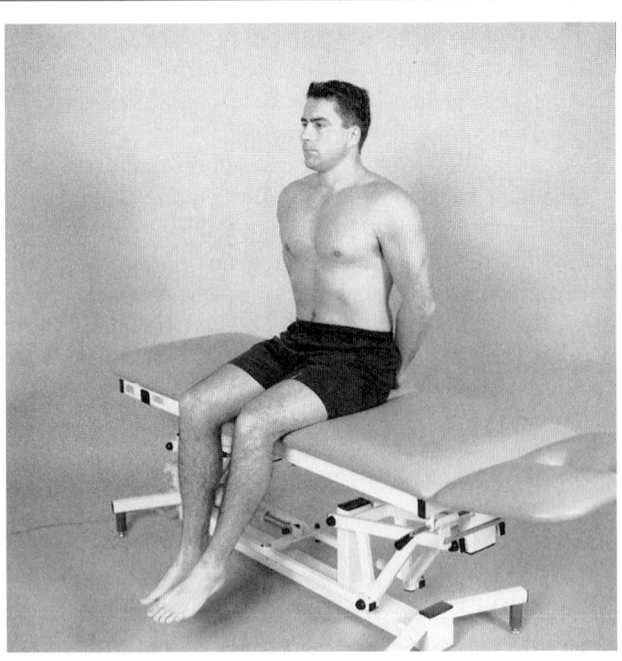

FIGURE 12-4 Starting position for the slump test.

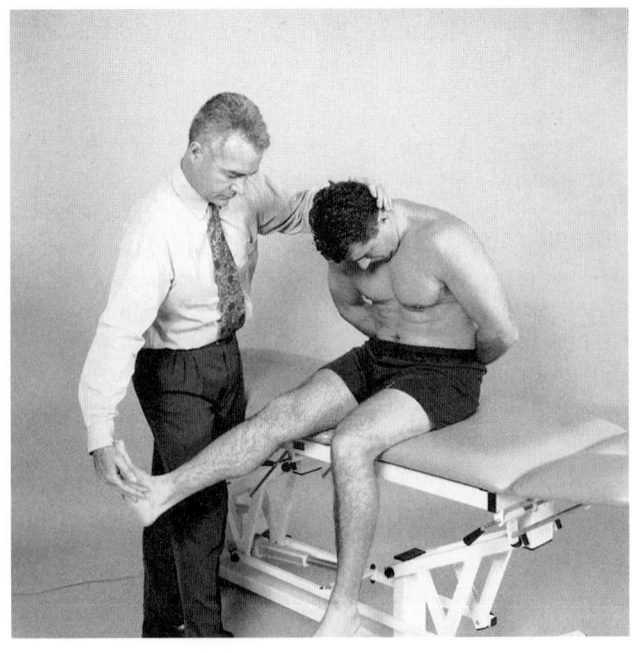

FIGURE 12-6 The full slump test.

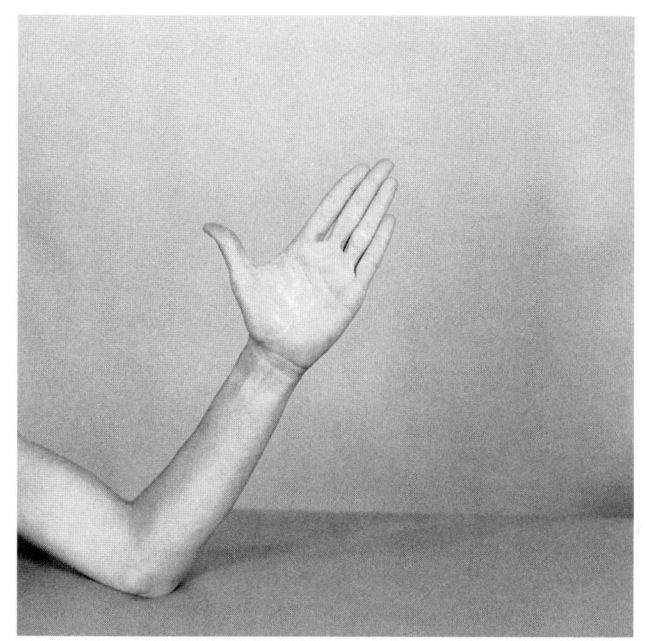

FIGURE 12-10 Median nerve gliding at the wrist.

▶ Reducing tenosynovial edema by a milking action.

▶ Improving venous return from the nerve bundles.

▶ Reducing pressure inside the carpal tunnel.

Six positions are used for mobilization of the median nerve at the wrist:

1. The wrist in neutral, with the fingers and thumb in flexion.

2. The wrist in neutral, with the fingers and thumb extended (Fig. 12-10).

3. The wrist and fingers extended, with the thumb in neutral.

4. The wrist, fingers, and thumb extended.

5. The wrist, fingers, and thumb extended, with the forearm supinated.

6. The wrist, fingers, and thumb extended, with the forearm supinated, and the other hand gently stretching the thumb.

Each position is held for 7 seconds and is repeated five times per session.[112] All of the exercises performed in the clinic should be performed by the patient at home whenever possible.

ULTT 2 (Radial Nerve Dominant)

The patient is positioned supine. The clinician depresses, abducts, and internally rotates the shoulder, pronates the forearm, extends the elbow, and flexes the wrist and thumb (Fig. 12-11). The sensitizers for this test are cervical spine side flexion, either toward or away from the involved side. The test is repeated on the contralateral extremity, and the results are compared.

FIGURE 12-11 Radial nerve stretch. (Reproduced with permission from Butler DS. The upper limb tension test revisited. In: Grant R, ed. *Physical Therapy of the Cervical and Thoracic Spine.* New York, NY: Churchill Livingstone; 1994:232.)

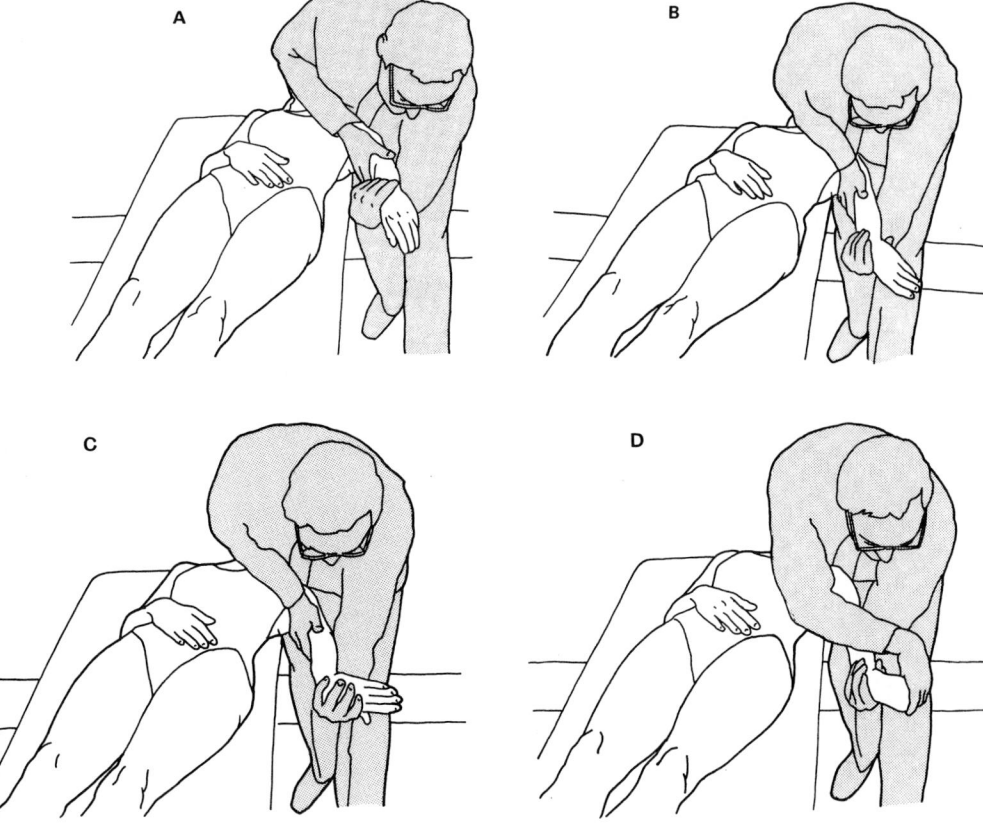

ULTT 3 (Ulnar Nerve Dominant)

The patient is positioned supine. The clinician extends the wrist, supinates the forearm, fully flexes the elbow, and depresses and abducts the shoulder (Fig. 12-12). The sensitizers for this test are side flexion of the head and neck, both toward and away from the test side. The test is repeated on the contralateral extremity, and the results are compared.

Evans[113] described a modification of the basic ULTT 3. The patient actively abducts the humerus with the elbow straight, stopping just short of the onset of symptoms. The patient then externally rotates the shoulder just short of symptoms, and the clinician holds this position. Finally, the patient flexes the elbows so that the hand is placed behind the head. Reproduction of the symptoms with elbow flexion is considered a positive test.

Musculocutaneous Nerve

The patient is positioned supine, with the head unsupported by a pillow. The clinician, facing the patient's feet, supports the patient's arm in about 80 degrees of elbow flexion. The shoulder is placed in full external rotation and approximately 10 degrees of abduction. Shoulder depression is then applied followed by glenohumeral extension (the "sensitizer"), elbow extension, and wrist ulnar deviation.

Axillary Nerve

The patient is positioned supine, with the head unsupported by a pillow. The clinician places one hand on top of the patient's shoulder and depresses the shoulder. The glenohumeral joint is then externally rotated, and the patient side flexes the head

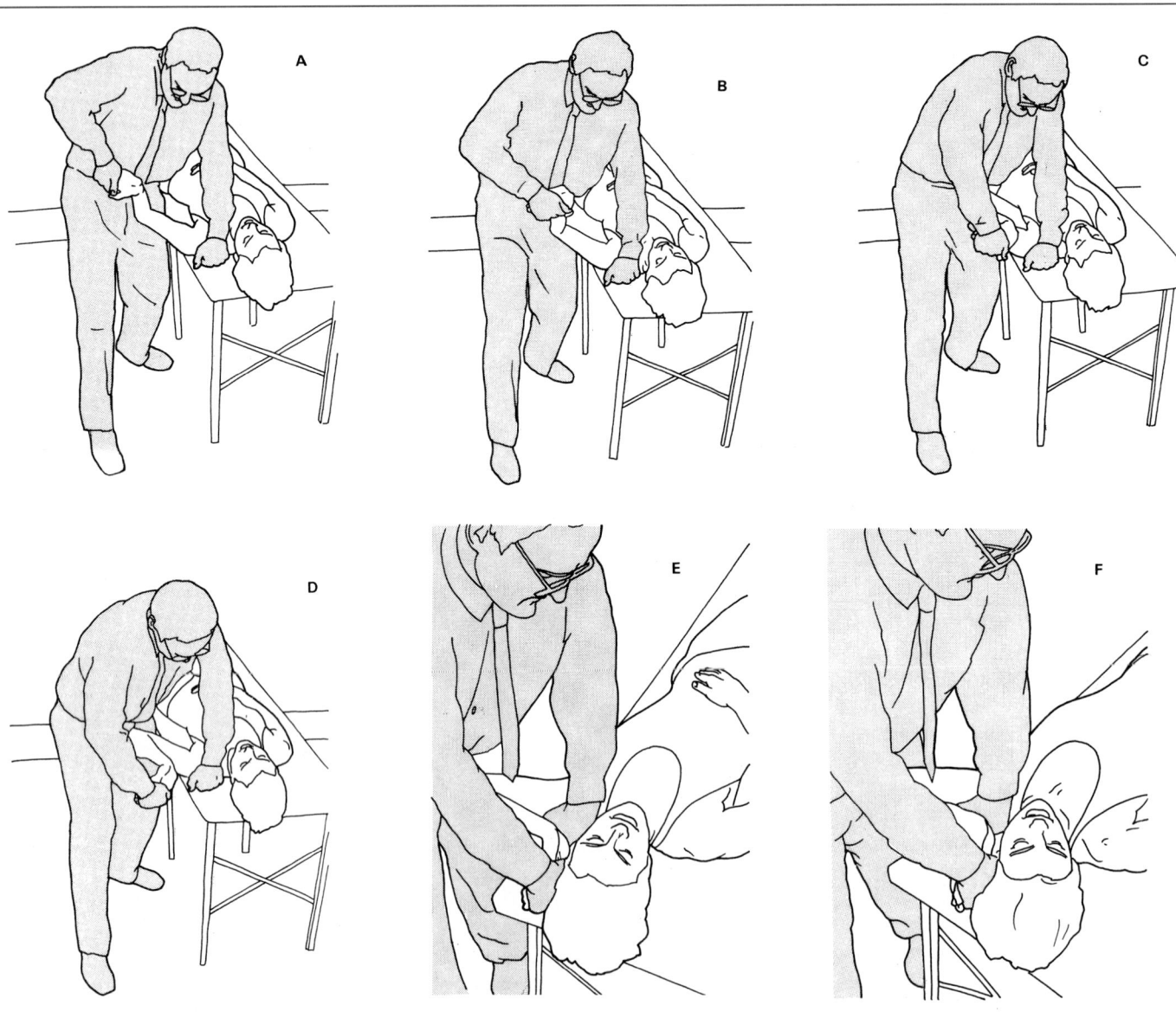

FIGURE 12-12　Ulnar nerve stretch. (Reproduced with permission from Butler DS. The upper limb tension test revisited. In: Grant R, ed. *Physical Therapy of the Cervical and Thoracic Spine*. New York, NY: Churchill Livingstone; 1994:234.)

away from the tested side. The shoulder is then abducted to approximately 40 degrees.

Suprascapular Nerve

The patient is positioned supine, with the head unsupported by a pillow. The clinician places a hand on top of the patient's shoulder. The patient's arm is placed in internal rotation and shoulder girdle protraction. The arm is then moved into horizontal adduction, followed by the patient side bending the head away from the test side. The clinician now depresses the shoulder.

Home Exercise Program to Improve Adaptive Shortening of the Upper Extremity Nerves[63]

The recommended home stretching exercise to improve tissue mobility and neural extensibility of the median nerve throughout the upper extremity is performed in four phases or positions, as follows.

1. The patient stands with the involved side close to a wall. The patient places the hand against the wall at a point slightly posterior and superior to the shoulder. The patient extends the fingers, pointing them backward. The elbow is slightly flexed (Fig. 12-13).

2. Keeping the palm of the hand flat against the wall, the patient moves away from the wall and attempts to straighten the elbow. When a gentle stretch is felt, the position is held for 10 to 15 seconds.

3. When the patient is able to maintain the previous stretch for 30 to 60 seconds, trunk rotation away from the involved side is added.

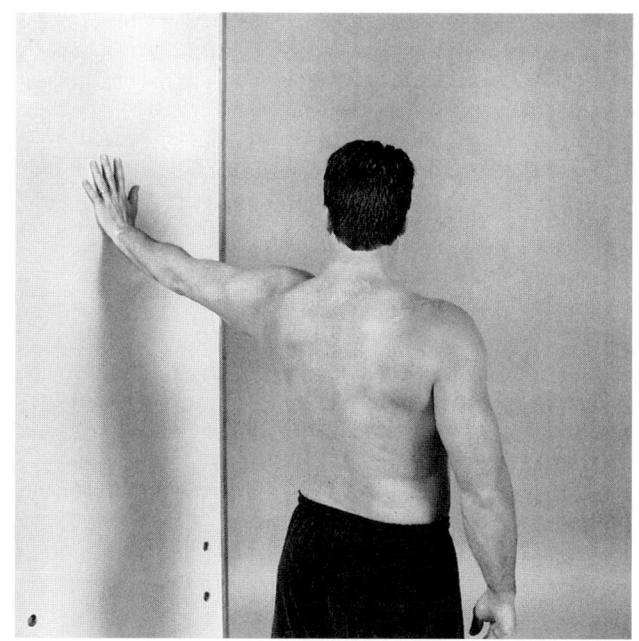

FIGURE 12-13   Upper extremity flexor stretch.

4. Once full trunk rotation is achieved and the elbow is maintained in an extended position, the patient can add cervical side flexion away from the involved side.

Each position is held for 7 seconds and is repeated five times per session. The radial and ulnar nerves can be stretched in a similar fashion:

Radial Nerve

1. The patient stands with the involved side close to a wall. The patient places the back of the hand against the wall with the fingers pointing down and the shoulder abducted to approximately 40 degrees. The patient flexes the fingers and the elbow is flexed.

2. Keeping the back of the hand flat against the wall and the fingers flexed, the patient moves away from the wall and attempts to straighten the elbow, while maintaining the shoulder abduction. When a gentle stretch is felt, the position is held for 10–15 seconds.

3. When the patient is able to maintain the previous stretch for 30–60 seconds, trunk rotation away from the involved side is added.

4. Once full trunk rotation is achieved and the elbow is maintained in an extended position, the patient can add cervical side flexion away from the involved side.

Ulnar Nerve

1. The patient stands with the involved side close to a wall. The patient places the palm of the hand against the wall with the fingers pointing toward the floor, and the hand at a point slightly posterior and inferior to the shoulder. The patient extends the fingers and the wrist. The elbow is slightly flexed.

2. Keeping the palm of the hand flat against the wall, the patient moves toward the wall and attempts to flex the elbow. When a gentle stretch is felt, the position is held for 10–15 seconds.

3. When the patient is able to maintain the previous stretch for 30–60 seconds, trunk rotation away from the involved side is added.

4. Once full trunk rotation is achieved and the elbow is maintained in a flexed position, the patient can add cervical side flexion away from the involved side.

REVIEW QUESTIONS*

1. List the number of mechanisms that are hypothesized to contribute to an injury of the peripheral nerve trunk.
2. Which term is used to describe a serial compromise of axonal transport along the same nerve fiber, causing a subclinical lesion at the distal site to become symptomatic?

3. In addition to complaints of pain, what other signs and symptoms are likely to be present with a diagnosis of neurodynamic tension?

4. The straight by raise (SLR) test exerts a caudal traction on which of the lumbosacral nerve roots?

5. Within which range of the SLR are positive findings more significant for a decrease in neurodynamic mobility?

---

* Additional questions to test your understanding of this chapter can be found in the Online Learning Center for *Orthopaedic Assessment, Evaluation, and Intervention* at www.duttononline.net.

REFERENCES

1. Inman V, Saunders J. The clinico-anatomical aspects of the lumbosacral region. *Radiology* 1942;38:669–678.
2. Millesi H. The nerve gap. Theory and clinical practice. *Hand Clinics* 1986;2:651–663.
3. Millesi H, Zoch G, Rath T. The gliding apparatus of peripheral nerve and its clinical significance. *Annales de Chirurgie de la Main et du Membre Superieur* 1990;9:87–97.
4. Butler DS. *Mobilization of the Nervous System.* New York, NY: Churchill Livingstone; 1992.
5. Butler DS. The upper limb tension test revisited. In: Grant R, ed. *Physical Therapy of the Cervical and Thoracic Spine.* Churchill Livingstone: Edinburgh, Scotland; 1994:217–244.
6. Slater H, Butler DS, Shacklock MD. The dynamic central nervous system: Examination and assessment using tension tests. In: *Grieve's Modern Manual Therapy,* Boyling JD, Palastanga N. eds. Churchill Livingstone: Edinburgh; 1994.
6a. Brieg A, Troup J. Biomechanical considerations in the straight leg raising test. *Spine* 1979;4:242–250.
6b. Butler DL, Gifford L. The concept of adverse mechanical tension in the nervous system: Part 1: Testing for "dural tension". *Physiotherapy* 1989;75:622–629.
6c. Slater H, Butler DS, Shacklock MD. The dynamic central nervous system: Examination and assessment using tension tests. In: Boyling JD, Palastanga N, eds. *Grieve's Modern Manual Therapy.* Edinburgh, Scotland: Churchill Livingstone; 1994.
6d. Goddard MD, Reid JD. Movements induced by straight leg raising in the lumbosacral roots, nerves and plexus and in the intrapelvic section of the sciatic nerve. *J Neurol Neurosurg Psychiatry* 1965;28:12–17.
7. Inman V, Saunders J. The clinico-anatomical aspects of the lumbosacral region. *Radiology* 1942;38:669–678.
8. McLellan DL, Swash M. Longitudinal sliding of the median nerve during movements of the upper limb. *J Neurol Neurosurg Psychiatry* 1976;39:566–570.
9. Elvey RL. Peripheral neuropathic disorders and neuromusculoskeletal pain. In: Schachloch MO, ed. *Moving in on Pain.* Oxford, England: Butterworth-Heinemann; 1995;115–123.
10. Wilgis EF, Murphy R. The significance of longitudinal excursion in peripheral nerves. *Hand Clin* 1986;2:761–766.
10a. Butler DS. *Mobilization of the Nervous System.* New York, NY: Churchill Livingstone; 1992.
11. Keller K, Corbett J, Nichols D. Repetitive strain injury in computer keyboard users: Pathomechanics and treatment principles in individual and group intervention. *J Hand Ther* 1998; 11:9–26.
12. Smyth MJ, Wright V. Sciatica and the intervertebral disc. An experimental study. *J Bone Joint Surg* 1958;40A:1401–1418.

13. Elvey RL. Treatment of arm pain associated with abnormal brachial plexus tension. *Aust J Physiother* 1986;32:225–230.
14. Murphy RW. Nerve roots and spinal nerves in degenerative disc disease. *Clin Orth Rel Res* 1977;129:46–60.
15. Elvey RL, Hall TM. Nerve trunk pain: Physical diagnosis and treatment. *Manual Ther* 1999;4:63–73.
16. Omer G Jr. Results of untreated peripheral nerve injuries. *Clin Orthop* 1982;163:15.
17. Boerger TO, Limb D. Suprascapular nerve injury at the spinoglenoid notch after glenoid neck fracture. *J Shoulder Elbow Surg* 2000;9:236–237.
18. Shim JS, Lee YS. Treatment of completely displaced supracondylar fracture of the humerus in children by cross-fixation with three Kirschner wires. *J Ped Orthop* 2002;22:12–16.
19. Cornwall R, Radomisli TE. Nerve injury in traumatic dislocation of the hip. *Clin Orthop Rel Res* 2000;377:84–91.
20. Fletcher MD, Warren PJ. Sural nerve injury associated with neglected tendo Achilles ruptures. *Br J Sports Med* 2001;35:131–132.
21. Choi HR, et al. Axillary nerve injury caused by intradeltoid muscular injection: A case report. *J Shoulder Elbow Surg* 2001;10:493–495.
22. Schram DJ, Vosik W, Cantral D. Diaphragmatic paralysis following cervical chiropractic manipulation: Case report and review. *Chest* 2001;119:638–640.
23. Yavuzer G, Tuncer S. Accessory nerve injury as a complication of cervical lymph node biopsy. *J Phys Med Rehabil* 2001;80A:622–623.
24. Moran KT, Kotowski MP, Munster AM. Long-term disability following high-voltage electric hand injuries. *J Burn Care Rehabil* 1986;7:526.
25. Upton RM, McComas AJ. The double crush in nerve entrapment syndromes. *Lancet* 1973;2:359–362.
26. Massey EW, Riley TL, Pleet AB. Coexistent carpal tunnel syndrome and cervical radiculopathy (double crush syndrome). *South Med J* 1981;74:957–959.
27. Dahlin LB, Lundborg G. The neurone and its response to peripheral nerve compression. *J Hand Surg* 1990;15B:5–10.
28. Dellon AL, Mackinnon SE. Chronic nerve compression model for the double crush hypothesis. *Ann Plast Surg* 1991;26B:259–264.
29. Saplys R, Mackinnon SE, Dellon LA. The relationship between nerve entrapment versus neuroma complications and the misdiagnosis of de Quervain's disease. *Contemp Orthop* 1987;15:51.
30. Narakas AO. The role of thoracic outlet syndrome in double crush syndrome. *Ann Chir Main Memb Super* 1990;9:331–340.
31. Wood VE, Biondi J. Double-crush nerve compression in thoracic-outlet syndrome. *J Bone Joint Surg* 1990;72A:85–88.
32. Wilbourn AJ, Gilliatt RW. Double-crush syndrome: A critical analysis. *Neurology* 1997;49:21–29.
33. Nemoto K, Matsumoto N, Tazaki K, Horiuchi Y, Uchinishi K, Mori Y. An experimental study on the "double crush" hypothesis. *J Hand Surg* 1987;12B:552–559.
34. Swensen RS. The 'double crush' syndrome. *Neurol Chronicle* 1994;4:1–6.
35. Golovchinsky V. Double crush syndrome in lower extremities. *Electromyogr Clin Neurophysiol* 1998;38:115–120.
36. Richardson JK, Forman GM, Riley B. An electrophysiological exploration of the double crush hypothesis. *Muscle Nerve* 1999;22:71–77.
37. Bednarik J, Kadanka Z, Vohanka S. Median nerve mononeuropathy in spondylotic cervical myelopathy: Double crush syndrome? *J Neurol Neurosurg Psychiatry* 1999;246:544–551.

38. Elvey RL. Brachial plexus tension tests and the pathoanatomical origin of arm pain. In: Glasgow EF, Twomey LT, eds. *Aspects of Manipulative Therapy*. Melbourne, Australia: Lincoln Institute of Health Sciences; 1979:105–110.

39. Shacklock M. Neurodynamics. *Physiotherapy* 1995;81:9–16.

40. Butler DS. The upper limb tension test revisited. In: Grant R, ed. *Physical Therapy of the Cervical and Thoracic Spine*. Edinburgh, Scotland: Churchill Livingstone; 1994:217–244.

41. Breig A. *Adverse Mechanical Tension in the Central Nervous System*. Stockholm, Sweden: Almqvist and Wiskell; 1978.

42. Breig A, Troup JDG. Biomechanical considerations in the straight leg raising test. *Spine* 1979;4:242–250.

43. Breig A, Marions O. Biomechanics of the lumbosacral nerve roots. *Acta Radiol* 1963;1:1141–1160.

44. Reid JD. Effects of flexion-extension. Movements of the head and spine upon the spinal cord and nerve roots. *J Neurol Neurosurg Psychiatry* 1960;23:214–221.

45. Smith CG. Changes in length and posture of the segments of the spinal cord with changes in posture in the monkey. *Radiology* 1956;66:259–265.

46. Asbury AK, Fields HL. Pain due to peripheral nerve damage: An hypothesis. *Neurology* 1984;34:1587–1590.

47. Coppieters MW, Stappaerts KH. The immediate effects of manual therapy in patients with cervicobrachial pain of neural origin: A pilot study. In: Singer K, ed. *Proceedings of the Seventh Scientific Conference*. Perth, Australia: International Federation of Orthopaedic Manipulative Therapists; 2000:113–117.

48. Di Fabio RP. Neural mobilization: The impossible editorial. *J Orthop Sports Phys Ther* 2001;31:224–225.

49. Turl SE, George KP. Adverse neural tension: A factor in repetitive hamstring strain? *J Orthop Sports Phys Ther* 1998;27:16–20.

50. Butler DS. Commentary—adverse mechanical tension in the nervous system: A model for assessment and treatment. In: Maher C, ed. *Adverse Neural Tension Reconsidered*. Melbourne, Australia: Australian Physiotherapy Association; 1999:33–35.

51. Kleinrensink GJ, Stoeckart R, Vleeming A, Snijders CJ, Mulder PG. Mechanical tension in the median nerve. The effects of joint positions. *Clin Biomech* 1995;10:240–244.

52. Devor M, Seltzer Z. Pathophysiology of damaged nerves in relation to chronic pain. In: Wall PD, Melzack R, eds. *Textbook of Pain*. Edinburgh, Scotland: Churchill Livingstone; 1999:129–161.

53. Lundborg G, Rydevik B. Effects of stretching the tibial nerve of the rabbit. *J Bone Joint Surg* 1973;55B:390–401.

54. Ogato K, Naito M. Blood flow of peripheral nerves: Effects of dissection, stretching and compression. *J Hand Surg* 1986;11:10.

55. Akeson WH, Amiel D, Abel MF, Garfin SR, Woo SL. Effects of immobilization on joints. *Clin Orthop* 1987;219:28–37.

56. Amiel D, Woo SLY, Harwood FL. The effect of immobilization on collagen turnover in connective tissue: A biochemical-biomechanical correlation. *Acta Orthop Scand* 1982;53:325–332.

57. Behrens F, Kraft EL, Oegema TR Jr. Biochemical changes in articular cartilage after joint immobilization by casting or external fixation. *J Orthop Res* 1989;7:335–343.

58. Booth FW, Kelso JR. The effect of hindlimb immobilization on contractile and histochemical properties of skeletal muscle. *Pflugers Arch* 1973;342:231–238.

59. Eiff MP, Smith AT, Smith GE. Early mobilization versus immobilization in the treatment of lateral ankle sprains. *Am J Sports Med* 1994;22:83–88.

60. Enneking WF, Horowitz M. The intra-articular effects of immobilization on the human knee. *J Bone Joint Surg* 1972;54A:973–985.

61. Giebel GD, Edelmann M, Huser R. Sprain of the cervical spine: Early functional vs. immobilization treatment [in German]. *Zentralbl Chir* 1997;122:512–521.

62. Jurvelin J, Kiviranta I, Tammi M, Helminen JH. Softening of canine articular cartilage after immobilization of the knee joint. *Clin Orthop* 1986;207:246–252.

63. Olson VL. Connective tissue response to injury, immobilization, and mobilization. In: Wadsworth C, ed. *Current Concepts in Orthopedic Physical Therapy—Home Study Course*. La Crosse, Wis: Orthopaedic Section, American Physical Therapy Association; 2001.

64. Woo SLY, Gomez MA, Woo YK, Akeron WH. Mechanical properties of tendons and ligaments. II. The relationships of immobilization and exercise on tissue remodeling. *Biorheology* 1982;19:397–408.

65. Elvey RL, Hall T. Neural tissue evaluation and treatment. In: Donatelli RA, ed. *Physical Therapy of the Shoulder*. New York, NY: Churchill Livingstone; 1997:131–152.

66. Maitland GD. Movement of pain sensitive structures in the vertebral canal and intervertebral foramina in a group of physiotherapy students. *S Afr J Physiother* 1980;36:4–12.

67. Maitland GD. The slump test: Examination and treatment. *Aust J Physiother* 1985;31:215–219.

68. Stoddard A. *Manual of Osteopathic Practice*. New York, NY: Harper and Row; 1969.

69. Vicenzino B, Collins D, Wright A. The initial effects of a cervical spine manipulative physiotherapy treatment on the pain and dysfunction of lateral epicondylalgia. *Pain* 1996;68:69–74.

70. Hall T, Elvey RL, Davier N, et al. Efficacy of manipulative physiotherapy for the treatment of cervicobrachial pain. In: *Tenth Biennial Conference of the MPAA*. Melbourne, Australia: Manipulative Physiotherapists Association of Australia; 1997:73–74.

71. Bianco AJ. Low back pain and sciatica. Diagnosis and indications for treatment. *J Bone Joint Surg* 1968;50A:170.

72. Bickels J, Kahanovitz N, Rubert CK, et al. Extraspinal bone and soft-tissue tumors as a cause of sciatica. Clinical diagnosis and recommendations: Analysis of 32 cases. *Spine* 1999;24:1611–1616.

73. Odell RT, Key JA. Lumbar disc syndrome caused by malignant tumors of bone. *JAMA* 1955;157:213–216.

74. Paulson EC. Neoplasms of the bony pelvis producing the sciatic syndrome. *Minn Med* 1951;11:1069–1074.

75. Lasègue C. Considérations sur la sciatique. *Arch Gen Med Paris* 1864;2:258.

76. Fahrni WH. Observations on straight leg raising with special reference to nerve root adhesions. *Can J Surg* 1966;9:44–48.

77. Inman VT, Saunders JB. The clinicoanatomical aspects of the lumbosacral region. *Radiology* 1941;38:669–678.

78. Woodhall B, Hayes GJ. The well leg raising test of Fajersztajn in the diagnosis of ruptured lumbar intervertebral disc. *J Bone Joint Surg* 1950;32A:786–792.

79. Cyriax J. *Textbook of Orthopaedic Medicine, Diagnosis of Soft Tissue Lesions*. 8th ed. London, England: Bailliere Tindall; 1982.

80. Smith C. Analytical literature review of the passive straight leg raise test. *S Afr J Physiother* 1989;45:104–107.

81. Urban LM. The straight leg raising test: A review. In: Grieve GP, ed. *Modern Manual Therapy of the Vertebral Column*. Edinburgh, Scotland: Churchill Livingstone; 1986:567–575.

82. Cocciarella L, Andersson GBJ, eds. *American Medical Association, Guides to the Evaluation of Permanent Impairment*. 5th ed. Chicago, Ill: AMA; 2001.

83. Gajdosik RL, Barney FL, Bohannon RW. Effects of ankle dorsi-flexion on active and passive unilateral straight leg raising. *Phys Ther* 1985;65:1478–1482.

84. Harada Y, Nakahara S. A pathologic study of lumbar disc herniation in the elderly. *Spine* 1989;14:1020.

85. Deyo RA, Rainville J, Kent DL. What can the history and physical examination tell us about low back pain? *JAMA* 1992;268:760–765.

86. van den Hoogen HJ, Koes BW, van Eijk JT, Bouter LM, Deville W. On the course of low back pain in general practice: A one year follow up study. *Ann Rheum Dis* 1998;57:13–19.

87. Andersson GBJ, Deyo RA. History and physical examination in patients with herniated lumbar discs. *Spine* 1996;21:10S–18S.

88. Vucetic N, Svensson O. Physical signs in lumbar disc herniation. *Clin Orthop* 1996;333:192.

89. Scham SM, Taylor TKF. Tension signs in lumbar disc prolapse. *Clin Orthop* 1971;75:195–204.

90. Lew PC, Morrow CJ, Lew MA. The effect of neck and leg flexion and their sequence on the lumbar spinal cord. *Spine* 1994;19:2421–2424.

91. Louis R. Vertebroradicular and vertebromedullar dynamics. *Anat Clin* 1981;3:1–11.

92. Cyriax J. Perineuritis. *Br Med J* 1942;1:578–580.

93. Supic LF, Broom MJ. Sciatic tension signs and lumbar disc herniation. *Spine* 1994;19:1066.

94. Hakelius A, Hindmarsh J. The comparative reliability of preoperative diagnostic methods in lumbar disc surgery. *Acta Orthop Scand* 1972;43:234.

95. Meadows J. *Orthopedic Differential Diagnosis in Physical Therapy*. New York, NY: McGraw-Hill; 1999.

96. Dyck P, Doyle JB. "Bicycle test" of van Gelderen in diagnosis of intermittent cauda equina compression syndrome. *J Neurosurg* 1977;46:667–670.

97. Maitland GD. Negative disc exploration: Positive canal signs. *Aust J Physiother* 1979;25:129–134.

98. Maitland G. *Vertebral Manipulation*. Sydney, Australia: Butterworth; 1986.

99. Macnab I. Negative disc exploration. *J Bone Joint Surg* 1971;53A:891–903.

100. Breig A. *Biomechanics of the Central Nervous System*. Stockholm, Sweden: Almqvist and Wiskell; 1960.

101. Penning L, Wilmink JT. Biomechanics of lumbosacral dural sac. A study of flexion-extension myelography. *Spine* 1981;6:398–408.

102. White AA, Punjabi MM. *Clinical Biomechanics of the Spine*. 2nd ed. Philadelphia, Pa: JB Lippincott; 1990.

103. Dyck P. The femoral nerve traction test with lumbar disc protrusions. *Surg Neurol* 1976;6:136.

104. Estridge MN, Rouhe SA, Johnson NG. The femoral stretching test: A valuable sign in diagnosing upper lumbar disc herniations. *J Neurosurg* 1982;57:813.

105. Christodoulide AN. Ipsilateral sciatica on femoral nerve stretch test is pathognomic of an L 4-5 disc protrusion. *J Bone Joint Surg* 1989;21:1584.

106. Davidson S. Prone knee bend: An investigation into the effect of cervical flexion and extension. In: *Fifth Biennial Proceedings of the MTAA*. Melbourne, Australia: Manipulative Therapy Association of Australia; 1987:234–235.

107. Kenneally M, Rubenach H, Elvey R. The upper limb tension test: The SLR of the arm. In: Grant R, ed. *Physical Therapy of the Cervical and Thoracic Spine*. New York, NY: Churchill Livingstone; 1988.

108. Yaxley GA, Jull GA. Adverse tension in the neural system. A preliminary study of tennis elbow. *Aust J Physiother* 1993;39:15–22.

109. Quintner J. Stretch-induced cervicobrachial pain syndrome. *Aust J Physiother* 1990;36:99–104.

110. Selvaratnam PJ, Matyas TA, Glasgow EF. Non-invasive discrimination of brachial plexus involvement in upper limb pain. *Spine* 1994;19:26–33.

111. Hack GD, Koritzer RT, Robinson WL, Hallgren RC, Greenman PE. Anatomic relation between the rectus capitis posterior minor muscle and the dura mater. *Spine* 1995;20:2484–2486.

112. Rozmaryn LM, Dovelle S, Rothman ER, Gorman K, Olvey KM, Bartko JJ. Nerve and tendon gliding exercises and the conservative management of carpal tunnel syndrome. *J Hand Ther* 1998;11:171–179.

113. Evans RC. *Illustrated Essentials in Orthopedic Physical Assessment*. St. Louis, Mo: Mosby-Year Book; 1994.

GAIT ANALYSIS

▶ *At the completion of this chapter, the reader will be able to:*

1. Summarize the various components of the gait cycle.

2. Apply the knowledge of gait components to gait analysis.

3. Recognize the manifestations of abnormal gait and develop strategies to counteract these abnormalities.

4. Categorize the various compensations of the body and their influences on gait.

5. Perform a comprehensive gait analysis.

6. Describe and demonstrate a number of abnormal gait syndromes.

7. Make an accurate judgment when recommending an assistive device to improve gait and function.

8. Describe and demonstrate the various gait patterns used with assistive devices.

9. Evaluate the effectiveness of an intervention for a gait dysfunction.

OVERVIEW

For most individuals, gait is an innate characteristic, as much a part of their personality as their smile. Indeed many people can be recognized in a moving group by their gait alone. It is not clear whether gait is learned or is preprogrammed at the spinal cord level. However, once mastered, gait allows us to move around our environment in an efficient manner, requiring little in the way of conscious thought, at least in familiar surroundings.

Although gait appears to be a simple process, it is prone to breakdown. Pain, weakness, and disease can all cause a disturbance in the normal rhythm of gait. However, except in obvious cases, abnormal gait does not always equate with impairment.

The purpose of this chapter is to describe the various components of gait and provide the clinician with the necessary tools for its analysis.

Gait Cycle

Normal human gait is a method of bipedal locomotion involving the complex synchronization of the neuromuscular and cardiovascular systems. The fall that occurs at the initiation of gait so that an individual can lift one foot off the ground and take the first step is controlled by the central nervous system.[9] The central nervous system computes in advance the required size and direction of this fall of the body toward the supporting foot. In addition, gait relies on the control of the limb movements by reflexes. Two such reflexes include the stretch reflex and the extensor thrust. The stretch reflex is involved in the extremes of joint motion, whereas the extensor thrust may facilitate the extensor muscles of the lower extremity during weight bearing.[11]

Walking involves the alternating action of the two lower extremities. The walking pattern is studied as a gait cycle. The *gait cycle* is defined as the interval of time between any of the repetitive events of walking. Such an event could include the point when the foot initially contacts the ground, to the point when the same foot contacts the ground again.[12] The gait cycle consists of two periods (Fig. 13-1):

1. *Stance.* This period constitutes approximately 60 percent of the gait cycle[13,14] and describes the entire time the foot is in contact with the ground and the limb is bearing weight. The stance period begins with the initial contact of the foot on the ground and concludes when the ipsilateral foot leaves the ground. The stance period takes about 0.6 seconds during an average walking speed.

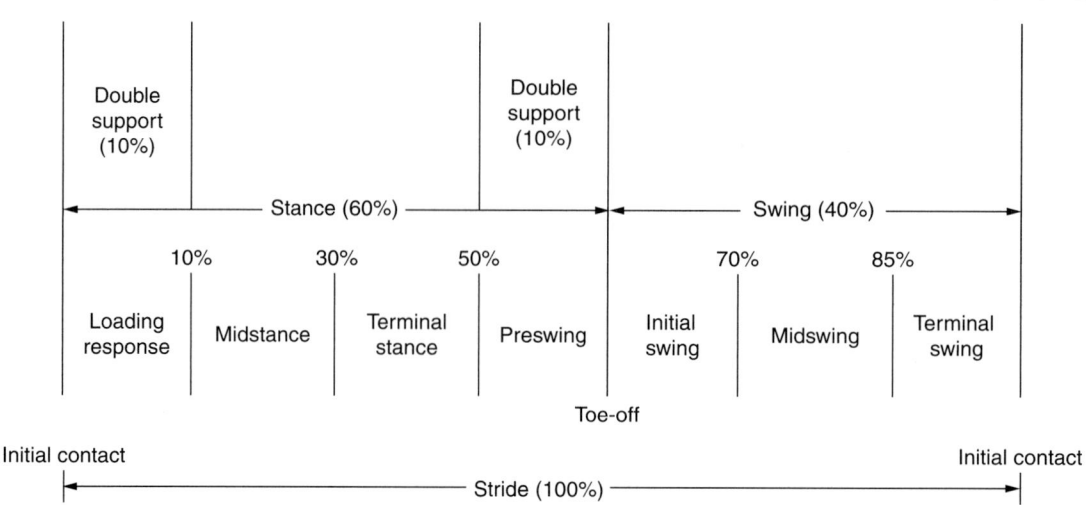

FIGURE 13-1   Approximate values for the two phases of gait.

2. **Swing.** The swing period constitutes approximately 40 percent of the gait cycle[13,14] and describes the period when the foot is not in contact with the ground. The swing period begins as the foot is lifted from the ground and ends with initial contact of the ipsilateral foot.[12]

Stance Period

Within the stance period, two tasks and four intervals are recognized.[13,15,16] The two tasks are weight acceptance and single limb support. The four intervals are loading response, midstance, terminal stance, and preswing[16] (see Fig. 13-1). Initial contact and toe-off are instantaneous events. The initial contact, which occurs when one foot makes contact with the ground, takes place at the beginning of the stance period and represents the first 0 to 2 percent of the gait cycle. As the initial contact of one foot is occurring, the contralateral foot is preparing to come off the floor.

Weight Acceptance
The weight acceptance task occurs during the first 10 percent of the stance period. The *loading response* interval begins as one limb bears weight while the other leg begins to go through its swing period. This interval may be referred to as the *initial double stance* period and consists of the first 0 to 10 percent of the gait cycle.[16]

Single Leg Support
The middle 40 percent of the stance period is divided equally into midstance and terminal stance.

The *midstance* interval, representing the first half of the single limb support task, begins as one foot is lifted and continues until the body weight is aligned over the forefoot.[16] The midstance interval comprises the 10- to 30-percent phase of the gait cycle.[16]

The *terminal stance* interval is the second half of the single limb support task. It begins when the heel of the weight-bearing foot lifts off the ground and continues until the contralateral

foot strikes the ground. Terminal stance comprises the 30- to 50-percent phase of the gait cycle.[16]

Limb Advancement
The *preswing* interval represents the 50- to 60-percent phase of the gait cycle. The preswing interval refers to the last 10 percent of the stance period. This interval begins with initial contact of the contralateral limb and ends with ipsilateral toe-off. Because both feet are on the floor at the same time during this interval, double support occurs for the second time in the gait cycle. This last portion of the stance period is, therefore, referred to as the *terminal double stance.* Each interval of double stance lasts about 0.11 seconds. Timing for the phases of stance is 10 percent for each double stance interval, and 40 percent for single limb support, so that the period of single limb support of one limb equals the period of swing for the other.[16]

Swing Period

Gravity and momentum are the primary sources of motion for the swing period.[11] Within the swing period, one task and four intervals are recognized.[13,15,16] The task involves limb advancement. The four intervals are preswing, initial swing, midswing, and terminal swing.[16]

Limb Advancement
The swing period involves the forward motion of the non–weight-bearing foot. The four intervals of the swing period include[16]:

1. **Preswing.** In addition to representing the final portion of the stance period and single limb support task, the preswing interval is considered part of the swing period.

2. **Initial swing.** This interval begins with lifting of the foot from the floor and ends when the swinging foot is opposite the stance foot. It represents the 60- to 73-percent phase of the gait cycle.[16]

3. *Midswing.* This interval begins as the swinging limb is opposite the stance limb, and ends when the swinging limb is forward and the tibia is vertical. It represents the 73- to 87-percent phase of the gait cycle.[16]

4. *Terminal swing.* This interval begins with a vertical tibia of the swing leg with respect to the floor, and ends the moment the foot strikes the floor. It represents the last 87 to 100 percent of the gait cycle.

The precise duration of the gait cycle intervals depends on a number of factors, including age, impairment, and the patient's walking velocity. Velocity is defined as the distance a body moves in a given time and is thus calculated by dividing the distance traveled by the time taken. Normal free gait velocity on a smooth and level surface averages about 62 m/min for adults, with men being about 5 percent faster than women.[17] As gait speed increases, it develops into jogging and then running, with changes in each of the intervals. For example, as speed increases, the stance period decreases and the terminal double stance phase disappears altogether. This produces a double unsupported phase.[18]

Determinants of Gait Velocity

The primary determinants of gait velocity are the repetition rate (cadence), physical conditioning, and the length of the person's stride.[17]

Cadence. Cadence is defined as the number of separate steps taken in a certain time. Normal cadence is between 90 and 120 steps per minute.[19,20] The cadence of women is usually 6 to 9 steps per minute slower than that of men.[20] Cadence is also affected by age, decreasing from the age of 4 to the age of 7 years, and then again in advancing years.[21]

Stride Length. Step length is measured as the distance between the same point of one foot on successive footprints (ipsilateral to the contralateral foot fall). Stride length, on the other hand, is the distance between successive points of foot-to-floor contact of the same foot. A stride is one full lower extremity cycle. Two step lengths added together make the stride length.

The average stride length for normal individuals is 1.41 m.[17] Typically, the stride length does not vary more than a few centimeters between tall and short individuals. Men typically have longer stride lengths than women.

Stride length decreases with age, pain, disease, and fatigue.[22] It also decreases as the speed of gait increases.[23] A decrease in stride length may also result from a forward head posture, a stiff hip, or a decrease in the availability of motion at the lumbar spine. The decrease in stride length that occurs with aging is thought to be the result of the increased likelihood of falling during the swing period of ambulation, caused by diminished control of the hip musculature.[24] This lack of control prevents the aged person from being able to intermittently lose and recover the same amount of balance that the younger adult can lose and recover.[24]

TABLE 13-1   Gait Parameters[12]

Cadence (steps/min) = velocity (m/s) × 120/stride length (m)
Stride length (m) = velocity (m/s) × 120/cadence (steps/min)
Velocity (m/s) = cadence (steps/min) × stride length (m)/120

Clinical Pearl

A mathematical relationship exists between cadence, stride length, and velocity, such that if two of them are directly measured, the third may be derived by calculation[12] (Table 13-1).

Characteristics of Normal Gait

Much has been written about the criteria for normal and abnormal gait.[12,14,25–32] Although the presence of symmetry in gait appears to be important, asymmetry in of itself does not guarantee impairment. It must be remembered that the definition of what constitutes so-called normal gait is elusive. Unlike posture, which is a static event, gait is dynamic and as such is protean.

Gait involves the displacement of body weight in a desired direction utilizing a coordinated effort between the joints of the trunk and extremities and the muscles that control or produce these motions. Any interference that alters this relationship may result in a deviation or disturbance of the normal gait pattern. This, in turn, may result in increased energy expenditure or functional impairment.

Perry[19] lists four *priorities* of normal gait:

1. Stability of the weight-bearing foot throughout the stance period.

2. Clearance of the non–weight-bearing foot during the swing period.

3. Appropriate prepositioning (during terminal swing) of the foot for the next gait cycle.

4. Adequate step length.

Gage[21] added a fifth priority, energy conservation. The typical energy expended in normal gait (2.5 kcal/min) is less than twice that spent while sitting or standing (1.5 kcal/min).[21] Two-dimensional kinetic data has revealed that approximately 85 percent of the energy for normal walking comes from the plantar flexors of the ankle, and 15 percent from the flexors of the hip.[33] For gait to be efficient and to conserve energy, the center of gravity (COG) must undergo minimal displacement. The COG of the body is located approximately midline in the frontal plane and slightly anterior to the second sacral vertebra in the sagittal plane. To minimize the energy costs of walking, the body uses a number of biomechanical mechanisms. The three-dimensional excursion of the COG-body mass is minimized through the intricate interactions of the segments of the lower extremity, especially at the knee and pelvis.[21]

> ### Clinical Pearl
>
> The COG in men is at a point that corresponds to 56.18 percent of their height. In women, the COG is at a point that corresponds to 55.44 percent of their height.[34]

During the gait cycle, the COG is displaced both vertically and laterally.

▶ *Vertical displacement.* Displacement of the whole trunk vertically occurs twice during each cycle through a total distance of 50 mm. This vertical displacement is at its lowest in double support and at its highest around midstance and midswing.[12] This vertical displacement of the COG is minimized through pelvic rotation, flexion and extension movements at the hip and knee, and rotation of the tibia and subtalar joint. Under normal conditions, the vertical displacement of the COG occurs in a sinusoidal manner and totals approximately 5 cm.[35]

▶ *Lateral displacement.* The lateral displacement of the COG occurs during the left and right stance periods. The whole trunk also moves side to side about 50 mm once each cycle, being over each leg during the stance period.[12] Under normal conditions, the lateral displacement of the COG occurs in a sinusoidal manner.

Joint Motions

Trunk and Upper Extremities

During the gait cycle, the swing of the arms is out of phase with the legs. As the upper body moves forward, the trunk twists about a vertical axis. The thoracic spine and the pelvis rotate in opposite directions to each other to enhance stability and balance. In contrast, the lumbar spine tends to rotate with the pelvis. The shoulders and trunk rotate out of phase with each other during the gait cycle.[35] Unless they are restrained, the arms tend to swing in opposition to the legs, the left arm swinging forward as the right leg swings forward, and vice versa.[11] When the arm swing is prevented, the upper trunk tends to rotate in the same direction as the pelvis, producing an ungainly gait.

Maximum flexion of both the elbow and shoulder joints occurs at initial contact interval of the opposite foot, and maximum extension occurs at initial contact of the foot on the same side.[36]

Although the majority of the arm swing results from momentum, the pendular actions of the arms are also produced by gravity and muscle action.[11,37]

▶ The posterior deltoid and teres major appear to be involved during the backward swing.

▶ The posterior deltoid serves as a braking mechanism at the end of the forward swing.

▶ The middle deltoid is active in both the forward and backward swing, perhaps to prevent the arms from brushing against the sides of the body during the swing.

Pelvis

The pelvis serves the double function of weight transfer and of acetabulum placement during gait. For normal gait to occur, the pelvis must both rotate and tilt. This combination of rotation and tilting serves to prevent excessive motion of the trunk. The rotation of the pelvis normally occurs about a vertical axis in the transverse plane toward the weight-bearing limb. The total pelvic rotation is approximately 4 degrees to each side.[21] In addition to decreasing the lateral deviation of the COG, the pelvic rotation also results in a relative lengthening of the femur, and thus step length, during the termination of the swing period.[16]

During the swing period, there is a slight pelvic tilt to the unsupported leg. The downward tilting of the pelvis occurs in the frontal plane on the contralateral side of the stance limb. The pelvic tilt is approximately 5 degrees to each side and results in a relative adduction of the weight-bearing limb and a relative abduction of the non–weight-bearing limb.[16,35] The pelvic tilting, produced by an eccentric contraction of the hip abductors, serves to reduce excessive elevation of the COG. The amount of lateral tilting may be accentuated in the presence of a leg length discrepancy, or hip abductor weakness, the latter of which results in a Trendelenburg sign. A positive Trendelenburg sign is indicated when the pelvis lists toward the non–weight-bearing side during single limb support.

Sacroiliac Joint[38]

In the following description, the right leg is used as a reference. As the right leg moves through the swing period, the position of the right innominate changes from one of extreme anterior rotation at the point of preswing to a position of posterior rotation at the point of initial contact. The hip flexion that occurs during the swing period initiates the posterior iliac rotation, while the initial contact and the loading response accentuates it. As the right extremity moves through the loading response to midstance, the ilium on that side begins to convert from a posteriorly rotated position to a neutrally rotated position. From midstance to terminal stance, the ilium rotates anteriorly, achieving maximum position at terminal stance.[39] The sacrum rotates forward around a diagonal axis (see Chap. 27) during the loading response, reaching its maximum position at midstance (e.g., right rotation on a right oblique axis at right midstance), and then begins to reverse itself during terminal stance.

A loss of sacroiliac joint mobility on one side of the joint may result in compensatory mechanisms occurring in the lumbar spine, or the contralateral joint. Compensatory changes may also occur distally in the kinetic chain.

Hip

Hip motion occurs in all three planes during the gait cycle.

▶ Hip rotation occurs in the transverse plane. The hip rotates approximately 40 to 45 degrees in the sagittal plane during a normal stride.[40] The hip begins in internal rotation during the loading response. Maximum internal rotation is reached near midstance. The hip externally rotates during the swing period, with maximal external rotation occurring in terminal swing.[29]

▶ The hip flexes and extends once during the gait cycle, with the limit of flexion occurring at the middle of the swing period, and the limit of extension being achieved before the end of the stance period (Table 13-2). At the point of initial

TABLE 13-2   Joint Motions and Muscle Activity at the Hip, and Knee, and Joint Positions and Motions of the Tibia, Foot, and Ankle During Gait

Phase	Hip	Knee	Tibia	Ankle	Foot
Heel strike	Gluteus maximus and hamstrings work eccentrically to resist flexion moment at hip Erector spinae working eccentrically to control trunk flexion Hip begins to extend from a position of 20–40 degrees of flexion Reaction force anterior to hip joint creating flexion moment Hip positioned in slight adduction and external rotation	Positioned in full extension before heel contact, but flexing as heel makes contact Reaction force behind knee causing flexion moment Quadriceps femoris contracting eccentrically to control knee flexion	Slight external rotation	Moving into plantarflexion	Supination
Foot flat	Gluteus maximus and hamstrings contract concentrically to move hip toward extension Hip moving into extension, adduction, and internal rotation	In 20 degrees of knee flexion, moving toward extension Flexion moment After foot is flat, quadriceps femoris activity becoming concentric to bring femur over tibia	Internal rotation	Plantarflexion to dorsiflexion over fixed foot	Pronation, adapting to support surface
Midstance	Hip moves through neutral position Pelvis rotates posteriorly Reaction force now posterior to hip joint creating extension moment Iliopsoas contracting eccentrically to resist hip extension Gluteus medius creating reverse action to stabilize opposite pelvis	In 15 degrees of flexion, moving toward extension Maximum flexion moment Quadriceps femoris activity decreasing	Neutral rotation	3 degrees of dorsiflexion	Neutral
Heel-off	Hip positioned in 10–15 degrees of hip extension, abduction, and external rotation Iliopsoas activity continuing Extension moment decreases after double-limb support begins	In 4 degrees of flexion, moving toward extension Maximum flexion moment Quadriceps femoris activity decreasing	External rotation	15 degrees dorsiflexion toward plantarflexion Maximum dorsiflexion moment	Supination as foot becomes rigid for push-off
Toe-off	Hip moving towards 10 degrees of extension, abduction, and external rotation Continued decrease of extension moment Iliopsoas activity continuing Adductor magnus working eccentrically to control pelvis	Moving from near full extension to 40 degrees of flexion Reaction forces moving posterior to knee as knee flexes Flexion moment Quadriceps femoris contracting eccentrically	External rotation	20 degrees of plantarflexion Dorsiflexion moment	Supination

contact, the hip is in approximately 35 degrees of hip flexion, where it begins to extend. Maximum hip flexion of 30 to 35 degrees occurs in late swing period at about 85 percent of the gait cycle; maximum extension of approximately 10 degrees is reached near toe-off at approximately 50 percent of the cycle[29,40,41] (Fig. 13-2).

▶ In the coronal plane, hip adduction occurs throughout early stance and reaches a maximum at 40 percent of the cycle.[41] Hip adduction totaling 5 to 7 degrees occurs in early swing period, which is followed by slight hip abduction at the end of the swing phase, especially if a long stride is taken[11,40,41] (Fig. 13-3). Perry reports the total transverse plane motion is 8 degrees.[40]

The movements of the thigh and lower leg occur in conjunction with the rotation of the pelvis. The pelvis, thigh, and lower leg normally rotate toward the weight-bearing limb at the beginning of the swing period.[35]

Knee

During weight-bearing activities such as gait, the tibiofemoral joint is subject to constant large muscular loads, bending, and rotational moments. These forces become particularly significant during sports activities, which place additional stresses on the joint (see Chap. 18).

During walking, the tibiofemoral joint reaction force has two peaks, the first immediately following initial contact (two to three times body weight) and the second during preswing (three to four times body weight).[42] Tibiofemoral joint reaction forces increase to five to six times body weight for running and stair climbing, and eight times body weight with downhill walking.[42–44]

The knee flexes twice and extends twice during each gait cycle: once during weight bearing and once during non–weight bearing.

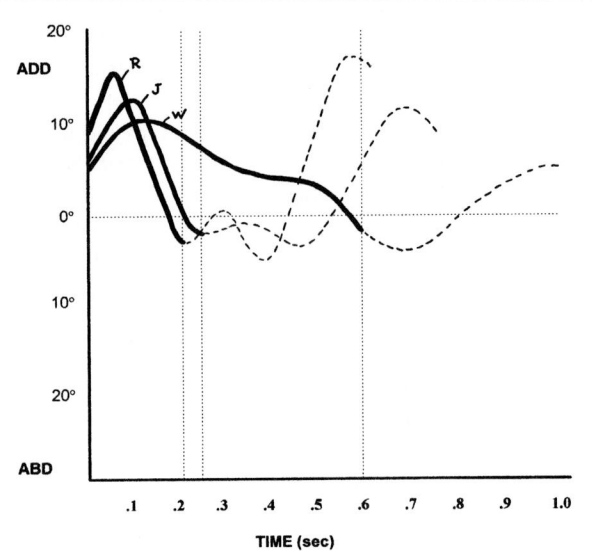

FIGURE 13-3   Hip abduction and adduction during walking (W), jogging (J), and running (R). (Reproduced with permission from Shamus E, Shamus J. *Sports Injury: Prevention and Rehabilitation.* New York, NY: McGraw-Hill; 2001:246.)

The knee flexes to about 20 degrees during the loading response interval, and this acts as a shock-absorbing mechanism. The knee then begins to extend and, as the heel rises during the terminal stance interval, it is almost fully extended, but flexes again as the swing period begins. The flexion occurs so that the lower limb can be advanced during the swing period with minimum vertical displacement of the COG. The knee then continues to flex as the leg moves into the swing period, before extending again prior to initial contact[12] (Fig. 13-4). In normal walking, about 60 degrees of knee motion is required

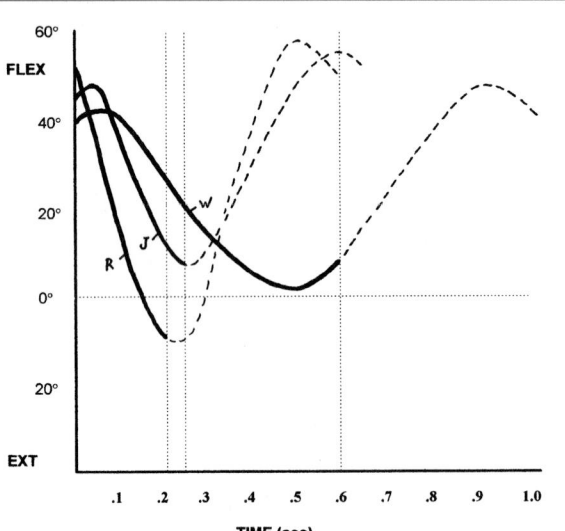

FIGURE 13-2   Hip flexion and extension during walking (W), jogging (J), and running (R). (Reproduced with permission from Shamus E, Shamus J. *Sports Injury: Prevention and Rehabilitation.* New York, NY: McGraw-Hill; 2001:245.)

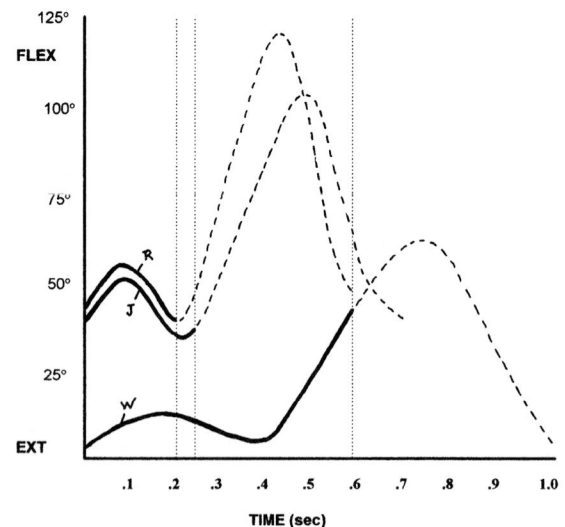

FIGURE 13-4   Knee flexion and extension during walking (W), jogging (J), and running (R). (Reproduced with permission from Shamus E, Shamus J. *Sports Injury: Prevention and Rehabilitation.* New York, NY: McGraw-Hill; 2001:247.)

for adequate clearance of the foot in the swing period. The peak flexion is required during initial swing, right after toe-off, because at that point in the gait cycle, the toe is still pointed toward the ground.[21]

The arthrokinematics involved during the loading response include an anterior gliding of the femoral condyles, which serves to "unlock" the knee. This forward gliding is controlled by the passive restraint of the posterior cruciate ligament, and by the active contraction of the quadriceps muscles.

> ### Clinical Pearl
>
> Anterior cruciate ligament (ACL) strain increases dramatically during the last 30 degrees of knee extension[45] and is minimized during isometric quadriceps exercises between 60 and 90 degrees.[46] However, patellofemoral contact pressures can increase dramatically with increased knee flexion.[47–49] As a result, patellofemoral pain is exacerbated but can be avoided and treated by strengthening the quadriceps in the 0- to 30-degree knee flexion range.[50] Because ACL-reconstructed patients, especially those with patellar tendon autografts, may experience patellofemoral pain,[51–53] it is important to prescribe exercises that decrease ACL strain through increased flexion and minimize patellofemoral pain by exercising with the knee near full extension.[54] This has been recognized as a paradox[45,55]; however, exercises performed between the two extremes, at approximately 30 to 60 degrees of knee flexion, may avoid excessive ACL strain and limit patellofemoral pain.[54]

A loss of knee extension, which can occur with a flexion deformity, results in the hip being unable to extend fully, which can alter the gait mechanics. Patients with patellofemoral dysfunction demonstrate less knee flexion than normal in the stance period of gait, combined with increased external rotation of the femur during the swing period.[28] Excessive compensatory internal rotation of the femur of the weight-bearing leg during the stance period may result in abnormal stresses being placed on the patellofemoral joint.[28]

Foot and Ankle

Ankle joint motion during the gait cycle occurs primarily in the sagittal plane (Fig. 13-5). During normal gait, the initial contact with the ground is made by the heel. In individuals with poor control of dorsiflexion (e.g., hemiplegics), the initial contact is made with the low part of the heel and forefoot simultaneously. This is usually accompanied by a toe drag during the swing period.

The ankle is usually within a few degrees of the neutral position at the time of initial contact, with the heel slightly inverted and the subtalar joint slightly supinated.[56] The initial impact is taken through the lateral tubercle of the calcaneus, a structure unique to humans and designed to tolerate the shock of heel strike via the calcaneal fat pad. As the heel contacts the ground, its forward momentum comes to an abrupt halt. During the loading response interval, plantar flexion occurs at the talocrural joint, with pronation occurring at the subtalar joint.[56]

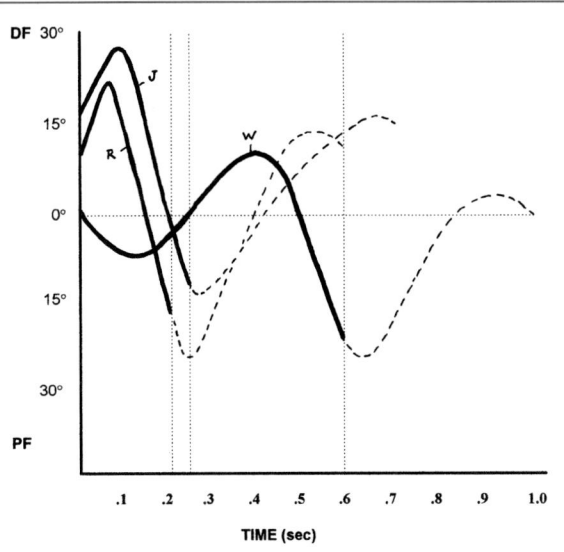

FIGURE 13-5 Ankle dorsiflexion and plantar flexion during walking (W), jogging (J), and running (R). (Reproduced with permission from Shamus E, Shamus J. *Sports Injury: Prevention and Rehabilitation.* New York, NY: McGraw-Hill; 2001:247.)

The pronation of the subtalar joint unlocks the foot and allows maximal range of motion of the midtarsal joint, which brings the articulating surfaces of the cuboid and navicular to a position relatively parallel to the weight-bearing surface and allows the forefoot to become supple.[57,58] This increase in midtarsal joint mobility enhances the foot's ability to adapt to uneven terrain.

At the end of the midstance interval, the talocrural joint is maximally dorsiflexed, and the subtalar joint begins to supinate. During the latter part of the stance period, the foot must become a rigid lever. From the midstance to the terminal stance interval, the foot is in supination (plantar flexion of the ankle, external rotation of the tibia, dorsiflexion and abduction of the talus, and inversion of the calcaneus).[57] Supination at the subtalar joint locks the foot into a rigid lever[56,59] by promoting supination at the midtarsal joint, which results in the articulating surfaces of the cuboid and calcaneus adopting a position that is perpendicular to one another, thus stabilizing their articulation.[58] The fixed cuboid acts as a fulcrum for the peroneus longus muscle, facilitating plantar flexion of the first metatarsal in push-off.[57]

Once the ankle is fully close packed, the heel is lifted by a combination of passive force and contraction from the taut gastrocnemius and the soleus. The lifting of the heel accentuates the force applied to the mid- and forefoot, and reinforces the close packing of this area, while simultaneously un–close packing the ankle joint.

As ankle plantar flexion reaches its peak at the end of the terminal stance interval, the first metatarsophalangeal (MTP) joint is extended. The dorsiflexion of the first MTP places tension on the plantar fascia and helps to elevate the medial longitudinal arch through the windlass mechanism of the plantar fascia (see Chap. 19). This windlass mechanism creates a dynamic stable arch and, hence, a more rigid lever for push-off.[57]

While the forefoot is on the ground and the heel is off, the heel is inverted, and the foot is supinated.[56] The heel rise coincides with the opposite leg swinging by the stance leg.[60] Approximately 40 percent of the body weight is borne by the toes in the final stages of foot contact.[61,62] Muscle activity during push-off is designed to initiate propulsion.[57]

Bojsen-Möller[63] describes the heel rise and the push-off as taking place at the MTP joints around two primary axes: one oblique and one transverse. The heel rise occurs first around the oblique axis, which passes through the MTP joints of the second through the fifth toes.

This is followed by the push-off around the transverse axis passing through the MTP joints of the first and second toes. The resistance arm offered against the force arm of the triceps surae during the push-off varies and is 20 percent longer when the push-off is being performed along the transverse axis. Bojsen-Möller characterizes the motion around the oblique MTP joint axis as a low-gear motion and the motion around the transverse axis as a high-gear motion.[62–64] High-gear motion is used for sprinting and low-gear motion is used for uphill walking with loads and in the first step of a sprint.

> ### Clinical Pearl
>
> An adaptively shortened gastrocnemius muscle may produce movement impairment by restricting normal dorsiflexion of the ankle from occurring during the midstance to heel raise portion of the gait cycle. This motion is compensated for by increased pronation of the subtalar joint, increased internal rotation of the tibia, and resultant stresses to the knee joint complex.

From initial contact to early midstance, the tibia moves anteriorly, internally rotating within the ankle mortise, and producing talar adduction and plantar flexion, and calcaneal eversion (weight-bearing pronation of the subtalar joint).[57] The forward tibial advancement requires approximately 10 degrees of ankle joint dorsiflexion to prevent excessive pronation at the subtalar and oblique midtarsal joints.[14,58,65]

During the swing period, the ankle must dorsiflex in order for the forefoot to clear the ground. The ankle adopts a neutral position in terms of dorsiflexion and plantar flexion prior to the next initial contact.

Muscle Actions

The ankle and hip muscles are responsible for the majority of positive work performed during walking (54 percent of the hip and 36 percent of the ankle).[66] The knee contributes the majority of the negative work (56 percent).[66] The muscle actions that occur during the stance period of gait are depicted in Tables 13-2 and 13-3.[67]

Spine and Pelvis

During the swing period, the semispinalis, rotatores, multifidus, and external oblique muscles are active on the side toward which the pelvis rotates.[11] The erector spinae and internal oblique abdominal muscles are active on the opposite side. The psoas major and quadratus lumborum help to support the pelvis on the side of the swinging limb, while the contralateral hip abductors also provide support.

Hip

During the early to midportion of the swing phase, the iliopsoas is the prime mover, with assistance from the rectus femoris,

TABLE 13-3 Muscle Functions of the Lower Leg During the Stance Phase of Gait[67]

Muscle	Action
HEEL STRIKE TO WEIGHT ACCEPTANCE	
Anterior tibialis	Eccentric—controls pronation of subtalar joint
Extensor hallucis longus, extensor digitorum	Eccentric—decelerate plantar flexion and posterior shear of tibia on talus
Posterior tibialis, soleus, gastrocnemius	Eccentric—decelerate pronation of subtalar joint and internal rotation of the tibia
MIDSTANCE	
Posterior tibialis, soleus, flexor hallucis longus, flexor digitorum longus	Eccentric—decelerate forward movement of tibia
Posterior tibialis, soleus, gastrocnemius	Concentric—supinate subtalar and midtarsal joints
PUSH-OFF AND PROPULSION	
Peroneus longus, abductor hallucis	Concentric—plantarflexion of first ray
Peroneus brevis	Antagonist to supinators of subtalar and midtarsal joints
Flexor digitorum longus	Concentric—stabilize toes against ground
Extensor hallucis longus and brevis	Concentric—stabilize first metatarsophalangeal joint
Abductor hallucis, abductor digit quinti, flexor hallucis brevis, flexor digitorum brevis, extensor digitorum brevis, interossei, lumbricals	Concentric—stabilize midtarsal and forefoot, raise medial arch of foot in push-off

sartorius, gracilis, adductor longus, and possibly the tensor fascia latae, pectineus, and short head of the biceps femoris during the initial swing interval.[11] Perry notes the adductor longus muscle to be "the first and most persistent hip flexor."[40] In terminal swing, there is no appreciable action of the hip flexors when ambulating on level ground. Instead, the hamstrings and gluteus maximus are strongly active to decelerate hip flexion and knee extension.[40,41] Both these superficial muscles and their deeper counterparts, such as the hip adductors, gemelli, and short rotators, certainly contribute.[31] In rapid walking, there is increased activity of the sartorius and the rectus femoris during the swing period.[11]

During initial contact, the gluteal muscles and the hamstrings contract isometrically with moderate intensity. The passive hip extension moment at initial contact has been calculated to be approximately 60 to 100 percent of the total moment occurring during the stance period, suggesting that passive elastic energy is stored and released during gait.[68] The loading response interval is accompanied by hamstring and gluteus maximus activity, which aids hip extension.[40,41,69] The adductor magnus muscle supports hip extension and also rotates the pelvis externally toward the forward leg. In midstance, coronal plane muscle activity is greatest as the abductors stabilize the pelvis.[70–74] The muscle activity initially is eccentric as the pelvis shifts laterally over the stance leg. The gluteus medius and minimus remain active in terminal stance for lateral pelvic stabilization. The iliacus and anterior fibers of the tensor fasciae latae are also active in the terminal stance and preswing intervals.[40,41] Notable, but inconsistent, muscle activity of the rectus femoris is described by several authors.[40,41,69] The only muscles of the hip that contract significantly during the last part of the stance period are the adductor magnus, longus, and possibly brevis.[11]

Knee

During the swing period, there is very little activity from the knee flexors. The knee extensors contract slightly at the end of the swing period prior to initial contact. During level walking, the quadriceps achieve peak activity during the loading response interval (25 percent maximum voluntary contraction) and are relatively inactive by midstance as the leg reaches the vertical position and locks, making quadriceps contraction unnecessary.[25,75–77] In graded exercise, Brandell[78] examined the effect of speed and grade on electromyographic (EMG) activity of the quadriceps and calf musculature. The author concluded that increases in speed and grade resulted in a relative increase in EMG activity of the vasti compared with the calf. Recently Ciccotti and colleagues[79] noted similar magnitudes and profiles of EMG activity in the quadriceps during level walking (1.5 m/s) and ascending a ramp of 10 percent grade at the same speed as level walking. Although minimal data were presented for comparison, the authors did note a decrease in vastus lateralis activity from 16 percent to less than 10 percent of maximum manual muscle test with addition of grade. Therefore, it remains questionable whether graded walking actually facilitates quadriceps activity.[54]

Hamstring involvement is also important to normal knee function. The hamstrings provide dynamic stability to the knee by resisting both mediolateral and anterior translational forces on the tibia.[43] The coactivation of the antagonist muscles about the knee during the loading response aids the ligaments in maintaining joint stability by equalizing the articular surface pressure distribution and controlling tibial translation.[80,81] EMG activity of the hamstrings during level walking has shown that the hamstrings decelerate the leg prior to heel contact and then act synergistically with the quadriceps during the stance period to stabilize the knee.[76,82] The hamstrings also demonstrate activity at the end of the stance period. Hamstring activity during graded walking and increased speed demonstrates increased activity and for a longer duration.[11]

Clinical Pearl

Not only is quadriceps and hamstrings training important in knee rehabilitation, but proper range of motion must also be considered.[54]

Foot and Ankle

During the beginning of the swing period, the tibialis anterior, extensor digitorum longus, extensor hallucis longus, and possibly the peroneus tertius contract concentrically with slight to moderate intensity, tapering off during the middle of the swing period.[11,83,84] As the swing period begins, the peroneus longus also contracts concentrically to evert the entire foot and bring the sole of the foot parallel with the substrate. At the point where the leg is perpendicular to the ground during the swing period, the tibialis anterior, extensor digitorum longus, and extensor hallucis longus group of muscles contract concentrically to dorsiflex and invert the foot in preparation for the initial contact.[11,83,84] There is very little activity, if any, from the plantar flexors during the swing period.

Following initial contact, the anterior tibialis works eccentrically to lower the foot to the ground during the loading response interval.[83,84] Calcaneal eversion is controlled by the eccentric activity of the posterior tibialis, and the anterior movement of the tibia and talus is limited by the eccentric action of the gastrocnemius and soleus muscle groups as the foot moves toward midstance.[67] Pronation occurs in the stance period to allow for shock absorption, ground terrain changes, and equilibrium.[58,85] The triceps surae become active again from midstance to the late stance period, contracting eccentrically to control ankle dorsiflexion as the COG continues to move forward. In late stance period, the Achilles tendon is stretched as the triceps surae contracts and the ankle dorsiflexes.[86] At this point, the heel rises off the ground and the action of the plantar flexors changes from one of eccentric contraction to one of concentric contraction. The energy stored in the stretched tendon helps to initiate plantar flexion and the initiation of propulsion.[86] The peroneus longus provides important stability to the forefoot during propulsion.

Clinical Pearl

During the stance period, three ankle rocker periods are recognized.

1. The first rocker occurs between the initial contact and when the foot is flat on the floor. This rocker involves the ankle dorsiflexors working eccentrically to gradually permit the foot to come into full contact with the ground.

2. During the second rocker, the foot remains flat on the ground while the tibia advances. This motion results from the plantar flexors working eccentrically to control the ankle dorsiflexion that occurs.

3. The third rocker is the push-off required for advancement of the limb. This is the period of power generation.

Thus, the first two rockers are deceleration rockers, in which the perspective muscles are working eccentrically by undergoing a lengthening contraction with energy absorption. The third rocker is an acceleration rocker and aids in propulsion.

Influences on Gait

Pain

Refer to section entitled "Abnormal Gait Syndromes" later in this chapter.

Posture

Good alignment of the weight-bearing segments of the body:

▶ Reduces the likelihood of strain and injury by reducing joint friction and tension in the soft tissues.

▶ Improves the stability of the weight-bearing limb and the balance of the trunk. The stability of the body is directly related to the size of the base of support. In order to be stable, the intersection of the line of gravity with the base of support should be close to the geometric center of the base.[87]

▶ Reduces excess energy expenditure.

Flexibility and the Amount of Available Joint Motion

A decrease in flexibility or joint motion, or both, may result in an increase in both "internal resistance" and the energy expenditure required.

Endurance: Economy of Mobility

It has been proposed that the type of gait selected is based on metabolic energy considerations.[83] Current commonly used parameters used to measure walking efficiency include oxygen consumption, heart rate, and comfortable speed of walking.[89–91]

Economy of mobility is a measurement of submaximal oxygen uptake (submax VO_2) for a given speed.[92,93] A decline in functional performance may be evidenced by an increase in submax VO_2 for walking.[94] This change in economy of mobility may be indicative of an abnormal gait pattern.[94] Some researchers have reported no gender differences for economy of mobility,[95–97] whereas others suggest that men are more economical, or have lower energy costs than women at the same absolute work.[98–100]

Age-related declines in economy of mobility also have been reported in the literature, with differing results. Some researchers reported that older adults were less economical than younger adults while walking at various speeds.[92,101,102] Conversely, economy of mobility appears to be unaffected by aging for individuals who maintain higher levels of physical activity.[103–105]

Clinical Pearl

The cardiovascular benefits derived from increases in gait speed may be acceptable for a normal population or advanced rehabilitation but should be used cautiously with postsurgical patients.[54]

Base of Support

The size of the base of support and its relation to the COG are important factors in the maintenance of balance and, thus, the stability of an object. The COG must be maintained over the base of support if equilibrium is to be maintained. The base of support includes the part of the body in contact with the supporting surface and the intervening area.[106] The normal base of support is considered to be between 5 and 10 cm. Larger than normal bases of support are observed in individuals who have muscle imbalances of the lower limbs and trunk, as well as those who have problems with overall static dynamic balance.[107] As the COG moves forward with each step, it briefly passes beyond the anterior margin of the base of support, resulting in a temporary loss of balance.[106] This temporary loss of equilibrium is counteracted by the advancing foot at initial contact, which establishes a new base of support.

The base width should decrease to around zero with increased speed. If the base width decreases to a point below zero, crossover occurs, whereby one foot lands where the other should, and vice versa. The presence of crossover can lead to alterations in gait.[108]

Assistive devices, such as crutches or walkers, can be prescribed to increase the base of support and, therefore, enhance stability.

Interlimb Coordination

Different patterns of interlimb coordination between arms and legs have been observed within the human walking mode.[109,110] At lower walking speeds, the arms are synchronized to the stepping frequency (2:1 ratio of arm to leg), whereas at higher walking velocities, the arms are synchronized to the stride frequency (1:1 ratio of arm to leg). These results also suggest that at lower speeds, the resonant frequency of the arms dominates the interlimb coupling, whereas at higher speeds, the resonant frequency of the legs is dominant.[111]

Leg Length

Limb-length discrepancy is a common clinical finding, with one study finding as many as 70 percent of 1000 consecutive, non-selected adult men with some degree of discrepancy.[112] Some authors have claimed that a limb-length discrepancy leads to mechanical and functional changes in gait[113] and increased energy expenditure.[114]

Intervention has been advocated for discrepancies of less than 1 cm to discrepancies greater than 5 cm,[113–115] but the rationale for these recommendations has not been well defined, and the literature contains little substantive information regarding the functional significance of these discrepancies.[116]

For example, Gross found no noticeable functional or cosmetic problems in a study of 74 adults who had less than 2 cm of discrepancy and 35 marathon runners who had as much as 2.5 cm of discrepancy.[115]

Gender

Most authorities agree that men and women walk differently, and the literature is replete with information regarding temporal gait parameter differences between men and women. Compared with men, women generally have narrower shoulders, greater valgus at the elbow, greater varus at the hip, and greater valgus at the knee.[117] Women also have a smaller Achilles tendon, a narrower heel in relationship to the forefoot, and a foot that is narrower than a man's in length. As the body attempts to maintain its COG, the wider female pelvis may contribute to an increase in varus at the hip, which in turn leads to increased pronation at the hindfoot.[117] As women get older, their feet become larger, flatter, and stiffer.[117] The intrinsic muscles of the feet, which are important for balance, can become weak and atrophic from years of wearing constricting shoewear. Other conditions, such as peripheral neuropathy, poor vision, arthritis, and general deconditioning, also can cause gait changes.[117]

On average, women walk at a higher cadence than men (6 to 9 steps higher), but at lower speeds.[32,118–121] Women also have slightly shorter stride lengths,[32,118,120–124] although when normalized for height, women tend to have the same or slightly greater stride lengths.[121–123]

Because leg length in women is 51.2 percent of total body height compared with 56 percent in men, women must strike the ground more often to cover the same distance.[125] Furthermore, because their feet are shorter, women complete the heel-to-toe gait in a shorter time than men do. Therefore, the cumulative ground reaction forces may be greater in women.[117]

Pregnancy

Substantial hormonal and anatomic changes occur during pregnancy that dramatically alter body mass, body-mass distribution, and joint laxity. During pregnancy, musculoskeletal disorders are common and may cause problems ranging from mild discomfort to serious disability. It is widely presumed that pregnant women exhibit marked gait deviations. The results of a recent study appear to refute that notion.[126] The study concluded that velocity, stride length, and cadence during the third trimester of pregnancy were similar to those measured 1 year postpartum, and that only small deviations in pelvic tilt and hip flexion, extension, and adduction were observed during pregnancy.[126] The study found significant increases ($p<.05$) in hip extensor, hip abductor, and ankle plantar flexor kinetic gait parameters, which suggests an increased use of hip extensor, hip abductor, and ankle plantar flexor muscles to compensate for increases in body mass and changes in body-mass distribution during pregnancy. These increases keep speed, stride length, cadence, and joint angles relatively unchanged.[126] These compensations may result in overuse injuries to the muscle groups about the pelvis, hip, and ankle, including low back, pelvic, and hip pain; calf cramps; and other painful lower extremity musculoskeletal conditions associated with pregnancy.[126] It was unclear from this study whether the women examined had gained normal amounts of weight associated with pregnancy. It would seem obvious that obesity associated with pregnancy may have differing affects on gait.

Obesity

Obesity is reaching epidemic proportions in the United States and is a growing problem in developed countries. It is associated with a number of comorbidities, such as coronary artery disease, type 2 diabetes, gall bladder disease, and sleep apnea. Given a normal body-mass index (defined as the weight in kilograms divided by the square of the height in meters) ranging from 18.5 to 24.9, 34 percent of the adult population is overweight (body-mass index of 25 to 29.9), and another 27 percent is obese (body-mass index of 30 or more).[127]

The gait deviations caused by obesity are perhaps clinically insignificant compared with its associated health risks. However, as obesity is becoming more common, the clinician needs to be aware of its effects on the normal gait pattern to help discriminate compensatory patterns as opposed to pathologic manifestations. The gait used by the obese patient is often described as a waddling gait. Depending on the degree of obesity, the waddling gait is characterized by increased lateral displacement, pelvic obliquity, hip circumduction, increased knee valgus, external foot progression angle, overpronation, and increases in the normalized dynamic base of support. The changes in the natural alignment of the weight-bearing segments may result in musculoskeletal dysfunction, including overuse injuries such as tendonitis and bursitis and eventual osteoarthritis of the hip or knee, or both.

Age

Age may be a factor in gait variations. As the body ages, there may be some decrease in both strength and flexibility. As vision may also diminish, balance may become a concern. Consequently, although the cadence of gait may remain unchanged, the step length typically is shorter, the width of the base of support wider, and the time spent in the double support phase increased.

Lateral and Vertical Displacement of the Center of Gravity

Rotation of the trunk may be excessive or lacking. Excessive trunk rotation may result from a restricted or exaggerated arm swing. A pelvic drop (excessive descent of the ipsilateral or contralateral pelvis) may occur on one side. The reasons for this differ according to whether the drop is ipsilateral or contralateral, as follows[128]:

▶ *Ipsilateral.* Occurs as a result of a short ipsilateral limb (including a leg length discrepancy, or a knee flexion contracture), contralateral hip abductor weakness, calf muscle weakness, and scoliosis.

▶ *Contralateral.* Occurs as a result of gluteus medius insufficiency, hip adductor contracture or spasticity, contralateral hip abductor contracture, and scoliosis.

A pelvic hike (excessive elevation of the ipsilateral side of the pelvis) may result during the swing period to help with foot clearance in the presence of inadequate hip or knee flexion, or excessive planter flexion of the ankle.[128]

As previously discussed, an increase in lateral displacement also may occur with obesity.

Properly Functioning Reflexes

Diseases that interfere with the normal reflexes of gait can result in disturbances in gait. Muscle weakness and reduced walking capacity are among several functional deficits associated with a lumbar herniated nucleus pulposus.[129] Weakness of the gastrocnemius is a clinical sign associated with involvement of the L5 to S1 disk (neurologic level S1), whereas weakness of the extensor hallucis longus is a positive sign for involvement of the L4 to L5 disk (neurologic L5). One study demonstrated that joint moments during gait are reduced in patients with lumbar disk herniations, and that the changes in moments are related to the level of the lesion.[129]

Vertical Ground Reaction Forces

Newton's third law states that for every action there is an equal and opposite reaction. During gait, vertical ground reaction forces are created by a combination of gravity, body weight, and the firmness of the ground. Under normal conditions, we are mostly unaware of these forces. However, in the presence of joint inflammation or tissue injury, the significance of these forces becomes apparent.

Vertical ground reaction force begins with an impact peak of less than body weight and then exceeds body weight at the end of the initial contact interval, dropping during midstance, and rising again to exceed body weight, reaching its highest peak during the terminal stance interval. Thus, there are two peaks of ground reaction force during the gait cycle: the first at maximum limb loading during the loading response, and the second during terminal stance (Fig. 13-6).

The ground reaction force vector changes from anterior to the hip joint at initial contact to migrate progressively posteriorly until late stance, when the ground reaction force is posterior to the hip.[29,40] Peak flexion torque occurs at initial contact

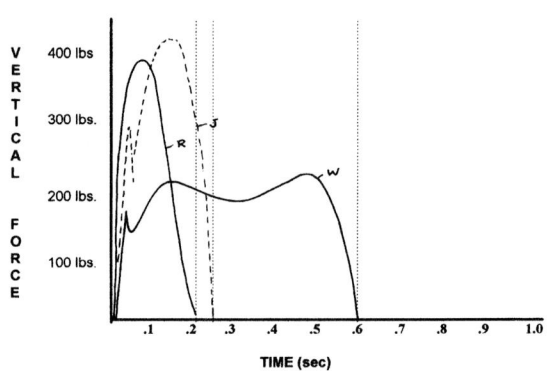

FIGURE 13-6   Vertical ground reaction forces J, jogging; R, running; W, walking. (Reproduced with permission from Shamus E, Shamus J. *Sports Injury: Prevention and Rehabilitation.* New York, NY: McGraw-Hill; 2001:244.)

but gradually declines, changing to an extension torque in midstance. The extension torque remains until terminal stance.[29,40]

It is well established that joint angles and ground reaction force components increase with walking speed.[130] This is not surprising, because the dynamic force components must increase as the body is subject to increasing deceleration and acceleration forces when walking speed increases.

Mediolateral Shear Forces

Mediolateral shear in walking gait begins with an initial medial shear (occasionally lateral) after initial contact, followed by lateral shear for the remainder of the stance period[29,40] (Fig. 13-7). At the end of the stance period, the shear shifts to a medial direction because of propulsion forces.

Anteroposterior Shear Forces

Anteroposterior shear forces in walking gait begin with an anterior shear force at initial contact and the loading response intervals, and a posterior shear at the end of the terminal stance interval (Fig. 13-8).

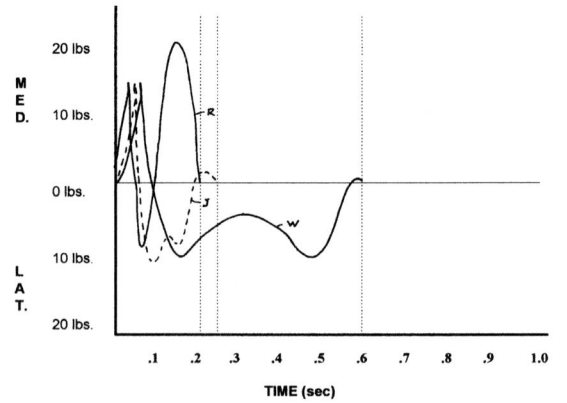

FIGURE 13-7   Mediolateral shear forces J, jogging; R, running; W, walking. (Reproduced with permission from Shamus E, Shamus J. *Sports Injury: Prevention and Rehabilitation.* New York, NY: McGraw-Hill; 2001:244.)

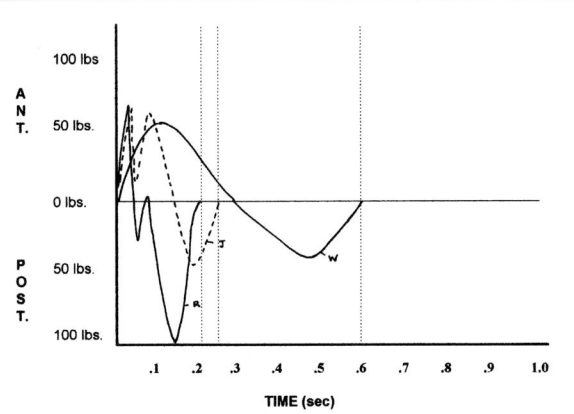

FIGURE 13-8 Anterior-posterior forces. J, jogging; R, running; W, walking. (Reproduced with permission from Shamus E, Shamus J. *Sports Injury: Prevention and Rehabilitation.* New York, NY: McGraw-Hill; 2001:245.)

Specific Deviations of Individual Joints[21]

Hip

The major problems that occur at the hip during gait are inadequate power, inadequate or inappropriate range of motion, and malrotation.

Inadequate Power

Weakness of the hip flexors is best seen during the preswing and initial swing intervals. Weakness of the hip abductors is noted during the single support phase of stance, because the hip abductors are required to prevent collapse of the pelvis toward the unsupported side. Weakness of the hip extensors is usually seen at initial contact and during loading response.

Inadequate or Inappropriate Range of Motion

As the flexors, adductors, and internal rotators of the hip are dominant over their antagonists, flexion, adduction, and internal rotation deformities tend to be the rule.

Malrotation

Malrotation of the hip usually results from conditions such as femoral anteversion.

Knee

The common problem at the knee during the stance period is excessive flexion. During the swing period, the most common error results from inadequate motion.

If excessive flexion at the knee occurs in midstance, the ground reaction force moves posteriorly to the knee and generates a flexion rather than an extension moment. This change in the moment requires the quadriceps and, to some degree, the hip extensors to maintain stability.

Excessive flexion at the knee results in excessive flexion occurring at the hip. This, in turn, increases the magnitude of the load on both the hip and knee joints.[131]

Foot and Ankle

There are three broad types of errors of the foot and ankle in the stance and swing periods:

1. Malrotation.

2. Varus or valgus deformity.

3. Abnormal muscle moments.

In the stance period, these deviations may interfere with the first and fourth of Perry's priorities of gait (stability in stance, and adequate step length). In the swing period, these deviations may interfere with priorities 2 and 3 (clearance of the foot in swing, and prepositioning of the foot in terminal swing).

The malrotation in stance rotates the plane of the foot outside of the plane of progression, resulting in the COG prematurely passing outside of the base of support. This alteration, in turn, results in a shortening of the contralateral step length. In addition, if the foot is malrotated significantly into external rotation, a valgus moment and an external rotation moment are introduced at the knee.

Varus and valgus deformities produce a loss of stability throughout the stance period because they introduce large external moments in the coronal plane that must be balanced by large muscle moments if stability is to be maintained.

Abnormal muscle moments during the stance period can manifest as weakness of the tibialis anterior, resulting in a "foot slap" at initial contact during the first rocker. Weakness of the triceps surae allows the tibia to progress too rapidly during the second rocker, causing the ground reaction force to fall behind the knee, and induces knee flexion. Abnormal muscle moments during the swing period include excessive activity of the plantar flexors and insufficient strength of the dorsiflexors, resulting in foot drop and poor foot clearance.

Abnormal Gait Syndromes[132]

Each of the attributes of normal gait described earlier under "Characteristics of Normal Gait" are subject to compromise by disease states, particularly neuromuscular conditions.[66] In general, gait deviations fall under four headings: those caused by weakness, those caused by abnormal joint position or range of motion, those caused by muscle contracture, and those caused by pain.[21]

► Weakness implies that there is an inadequate internal joint moment or loss of the natural force–couple relationship. Neuromuscular conditions may be associated with abnormalities of muscle tone, timing of muscle contractions, and proprioceptive and sensory disturbances, the latter of which can profoundly affect reflex postural balance.

► Abnormal joint position can be caused by an imbalance of flexibility and strength around a joint or by contracture.

► Contractures, changes in the connective tissue of muscles, ligaments, and the joint capsule, may produce changes in gait. If the contracture is elastic, the gait changes are apparent in the swing period only. If the contractures are rigid, the gait changes are apparent during the swing and the stance periods.

▶ Pain can alter gait as the patient attempts to use the position of minimal articular pressure (see the discussion of antalgic gait following). Pain also may produce muscle inhibition and eventual atrophy.

Antalgic Gait

The antalgic gait pattern can result from numerous causes (Table 13-4). This pain may result from a joint inflammation or an injury to the muscles, tendons, and ligaments of the lower extremity. The antalgic gait is characterized by a decrease in the stance period on the involved side in an attempt to eliminate the weight from the involved leg and use of the injured body part as much as possible. In the case of joint inflammation, attempts may be made to avoid positions of maximal intra-articular pressure and to seek the position of minimum articular pressure[134]:

▶ Minimum articular pressure occurs at the ankle at 15 degrees of plantar flexion.

▶ Minimum articular pressure occurs at the knee at 30 degrees of flexion. With a painful knee, the gait is characterized by a decrease in knee flexion at initial contact and the loading

TABLE 13-4   Some Causes of Antalgic Gait[133]

Cause	Examples
Bone disease	Fracture
	Infection
	Tumor
	Avascular necrosis (Legg-Calvé-Perthes disease, Osgood Schlatter disease, Köhler's bone disease)
Muscle disorder	Traumatic rupture, contusion
	Cramp secondary to fatigue, strain, malposition, or claudication
	Inflammatory myositis
Joint disease	Traumatic arthritis
	Infectious arthritis
	Rheumatoid arthritis
	Crystalline arthritis (gout, pseudogout)
	Hemarthrosis
	Bursitis
Neurologic disease	Lumbar spine disease with nerve root irritation or compression
Other	Hip, knee, or foot trauma
	Corns, bunions, blisters, or ingrown toenails

response interval, and an increase in knee extension during the remainder of the stance period.

▶ Minimum articular pressure occurs at the hip at 30 degrees of flexion.

Equinus Gait

Spastic diplegia is the most common pattern of motor impairment in patients with cerebral palsy.[135] In these patients, motor impairment occurs as a result of a number of deficits, including poor muscle control, weakness, impaired balance, hypertonicity, and spasticity.[136] However, reduced joint motion as a consequence of spasticity is perhaps the most noticeable and recorded impairment. As a consequence, muscle-tendon units frequently become contracted over time, contributing to malalignment of the extremity during gait.

Equinus gait (toe-walking), one of the more common abnormal patterns of gait in patients with spastic diplegia, is characterized by forefoot strike to initiate the cycle and premature plantar flexion in early to midstance.[137] Toe-walking may be a primary gait deviation, which is the consequence of excessive myostatic contracture of the triceps surae, excessive dynamic contraction of the ankle plantar flexors, or a combination of both factors. Additionally, toe-walking may be a compensatory deviation for myostatic deformity or dynamic overactivity of the ipsilateral hamstring muscles, which directly limit knee alignment and secondarily compromise foot and ankle position during stance phase.

Associated gait deviations are frequently seen at the knees, hips, and pelvis in children with cerebral palsy who are walking on their toes.[138]

▶ Deviations seen at the knees include increased flexion in stance phase at initial contact and in midstance, and delayed and diminished peak knee flexion in swing phase.

▶ The hips often show diminished extension in the sagittal plane at terminal stance.

▶ A common deviation seen at the pelvis in children with cerebral palsy who are toe-walking is increased anterior tilt.

Gluteus Maximus Gait

The gluteus maximus gait, which results from weakness of the gluteus maximus, is characterized by a posterior thrusting of the trunk at initial contact in an attempt to maintain hip extension of the stance leg. The hip extensor weakness also results in forward tilt of the pelvis, which eventually translates into hyperlordosis of the spine to maintain posture.

Plantar Flexor Gait

This type of gait is characterized by walking on the toes. The plantar flexor gait demonstrates premature firing of the calf muscle in the swing phase of gait with EMG.[139] A toe-walking gait pattern describes dynamic ankle deviations that include[138]:

▶ A loss of heel strike at initial contact, with disruption of the first ankle rocker.

▶ Inversion of the second rocker, with ankle plantar flexion (instead of dorsiflexion) occurring at midstance.

▶ Variable disruption of the third rocker in terminal stance.

▶ Variable ankle alignment during swing phase.

This type of gait is a common gait deviation in children with cerebral palsy. For the clinician, the challenge is to distinguish between changes that are the direct consequence of such an underlying neuromuscular disorder and are, therefore, primary, and those changes that follow from biomechanical constraints of toe-walking and are, therefore, secondary or compensatory. It is not unusual for normal children to display intermittent tiptoe gait when they first begin to walk; however, a more mature heel-toe gait pattern should become consistent by the age of 2 years.[140] Older children with persistent tiptoe gait are often labeled idiopathic toe walkers. Toe-walking that begins after a mature heel-toe gait pattern has been established may signify muscular dystrophy, diastematomyelia, peroneal muscular atrophy, or spinal cord tumor. Toe-walking has been associated with premature birth, developmental delay, schizophrenia, autism, and various learning disorders.[141]

Quadriceps Gait

Quadriceps weakness can result from peripheral nerve lesion (femoral), spinal nerve root lesion, trauma, or disease (muscular dystrophy). Quadriceps weakness requires that forward motion be propagated by circumducting each leg. The patient leans the body toward the other side to balance the COG, and the motion is repeated with each step.

Spastic Gait

A spastic gait may result from either unilateral or bilateral upper motor neuron lesions.

Spastic Hemiplegic (Hemiparetic) Gait

This type of gait results from a unilateral upper motor neuron lesion. Spastic hemiplegic gait frequently is seen following a completed stroke. Spasticity of all muscles on the involved side is noted, but it is more marked in some muscle groups. During gait the leg tends to circumduct in a semicircle, rotating outward, or is pushed ahead, with the foot dragging and scraping the floor. The upper limb typically is carried across the trunk for balance.

Spastic Paraparetic Gait

This type of gait results from bilateral upper motor neuron lesions (e.g., cervical myelopathy in adults and cerebral palsy in children). Spastic paraparetic gait is characterized by slow, stiff, and jerky movements. Spastic extension occurs at the knees with adduction at the hips (scissors gait).

Ataxic Gait

The ataxic gait is seen in two principal disorders: cerebellar disease (cerebellar ataxic gait) and posterior column disease (sensory ataxic gait).

Cerebellar Ataxic Gait

The nature of the gait abnormality with a cerebellar lesion is determined by the site of the lesion. In vermal lesions, the gait is broad based, unsteady, and staggering, with an irregular sway. The patient is unable to walk in tandem or in a straight line. The ataxia of gait worsens when the patient attempts to stop suddenly or to turn sharply, resulting in a tendency to fall.

In hemispheral lesions, the ataxia tends to be less severe, but there is persistent lurching or deviation toward the involved side.

Sensory Ataxic Gait

With this type of ataxia, because the patient is unaware of the position of the limbs, the gait is broad based, and the patient tends to lift the feet too high and slap on the floor in an uncoordinated and abrupt manner. The patient tends to watch the floor and the feet to maximize attempts at visual correction and may have difficulty walking in the dark.

Steppage Gait

This type of gait occurs in patients with a foot drop. A foot drop is the result of weakness or paralysis of the dorsiflexor muscles resulting from an injury to the muscles, their peripheral nerve supply, or the nerve roots supplying the muscles.[129] The patient lifts the leg high enough to clear the flail foot off the floor by flexing excessively at the hip and knee, and then slaps the foot on the floor.

Trendelenburg Gait

This type of gait results from weakness of the hip abductors (gluteus medius and minimus). The normal stabilizing effect of these muscles is lost, and the patient demonstrates an excessive lateral list in which the trunk is thrust laterally in an attempt to keep the COG over the stance leg. A positive Trendelenburg sign is also present.

Parkinsonian Gait

The parkinsonian gait is characterized by a flexed and stooped posture, with flexion of the neck, elbows, metacarpophalangeal joints, trunk, hips, and knees. The patient has difficulty initiating movements and walks using short steps, with the feet barely clearing the ground. This results in a shuffling type of gait with rapid steps. As the patient gets going, he or she may lean forward and walk progressively faster as though chasing the COG (propulsive or festinating gait). Less commonly, deviation of the COG backward may cause retropulsion. There is also a lack of associated arm movement during the gait, because the arms are held stiffly.

Hysterical Gait

The hysterical gait is nonspecific and bizarre. It does not conform to any specific organic pattern, with the abnormality varying from moment to moment and from one examination to another. There may be ataxia, spasticity, inability to move, or other types of abnormality. The abnormality is often minimal or absent when the patient is unaware of being watched or when distracted. However, although all hysterical gaits are bizarre, all bizarre gaits are not hysterical.

Clinical Examination of Gait

The clinical examination of gait can be performed using methods ranging from observation to computerized analysis. Computerized gait analysis measures gait parameters more precisely than is possible with clinical observation alone[142,143] and is used in the evaluation and treatment planning for patients with gait abnormalities.[144] However, computerized gait analysis is often cost-prohibitive and, thus, not practical for most clinicians, who must therefore rely on their powers of observation. The reliability and agreement both between and within raters for gait problems detected by observation alone has been reported. Krebs and colleagues[143] found moderate reliability within and between physical therapists observing children's gait from videotape. Eastlack and associates[145] found only slight to moderate reliability between raters in the assessment of deviations at a single joint from a videotape.[144]

Perhaps the most commonly used gait analysis chart is the one designed by the Rancho Los Amigos Medical Center (Fig. 13-9), which allows the clinician to determine deviations and their effect on gait in a user-friendly format.

Several other examination tools are available. Some of these tools are specific to a particular population. For example, the modified version of the Gait Abnormality Rating Scale (GARS-M; Table 13-5) can be used with community-dwelling, frail older persons to help predict individuals who are at high risk for falling.[146]

FIGURE 13-9 Rancho Los Amigos gait analysis chart.

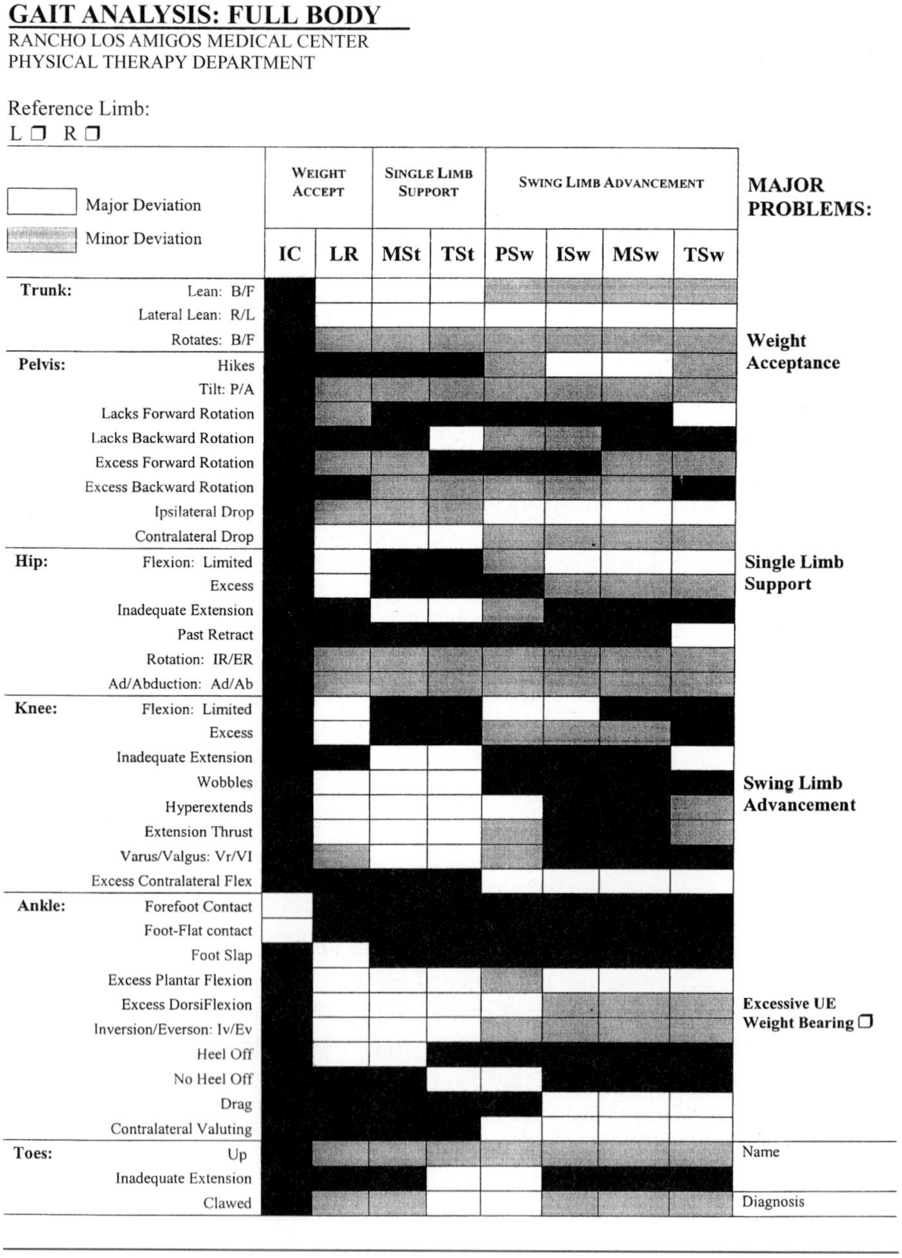

GAIT ANALYSIS: FULL BODY
RANCHO LOS AMIGOS MEDICAL CENTER
PHYSICAL THERAPY DEPARTMENT

TABLE 13-5   Modified Gait Abnormality Rating Scale (GARS-M)

NAME_____ NO._____ VISIT_____ DATE_____

1. VARIABILITY–A MEASURE OF INCONSISTENCY AND ARRHYTHMICITY OF STEPPING AND OF ARM MOVEMENTS.

0 = fluid and predictably paced limb movements.

1 = occasional interruptions (changes in velocity), approximately 25% of time.

2 = unpredictability of rhythm approximately 25–75% of time.

3 = random timing of limb movements.

2. GUARDEDNESS–HESITANCY, SLOWNESS, DIMINISHED PROPULSION, AND LACK OF COMMITMENT IN STEPPING AND ARM SWING.

0 = good forward momentum and lack of apprehension in propulsion.

1 = center of gravity of head, arms, and trunk (HAT) projects only slightly in front of push-off, but still good arm-leg coordination.

2 = HAT held over anterior aspect of foot, and some moderate loss of smooth reciprocation.

3 = HAT held over rear aspect of stance-phase foot, and great tentativity in stepping.

3. STAGGERING–SUDDEN AND UNEXPECTED LATERALLY DIRECTED PARTIAL LOSSES OF BALANCE.

0 = no losses of balance to side.

1 = a single lurch to side.

2 = two lurches to side.

3 = three or more lurches to side.

4. FOOT CONTACT–THE DEGREE TO WHICH THE HEEL STRIKES THE GROUND BEFORE THE FOREFOOT.

0 = very obvious angle of impact of heel on ground.

1 = barely visible contact of heel before forefoot.

2 = entire foot lands flat on ground.

3 = anterior aspect of foot strikes ground before heel.

5. HIP ROM–THE DEGREE OF LOSS OF HIP RANGE OF MOTION SEEN DURING A GAIT CYCLE.

0 = obvious angulation of thigh backward during double support (10 degrees).

1 = just barely visible angulation backward from vertical.

2 = thigh in line with vertical projection from ground.

3 = thigh angled forward from vertical at maximum posterior excursion.

6. SHOULDER EXTENSION–A MEASURE OF THE DECREASE OF SHOULDER ROM.

0 = clearly seen movement of upper arm anterior (15 degrees) and posterior (20 degrees) to vertical axis of trunk.

1 = shoulder flexes slightly anterior to vertical axis.

2 = shoulder comes only to vertical axis, or slightly posterior to it during flexion.

3 = shoulder stays well behind vertical axis during entire excursion.

7. ARM–HEEL STRIKE SYNCHRONY–THE EXTENT TO WHICH THE CONTRALATERAL MOVEMENTS OF AN ARM AND LEG ARE OUT OF PHASE.

0 = good temporal conjunction of arm and contralateral leg at apex of shoulder and hip excursions all of the time.

1 = arm and leg slightly out of phase 25% of the time.

2 = arm and leg moderately out of phase 25–50% of time.

3 = little or no temporal coherence of arm and leg.

ROM, range of motion.

Observational Analysis

Observational analysis of gait should focus on one gait interval at a time. For example, the clinician should observe the pattern of initial contact with the floor and then, in turn, study the actions throughout the initial contact at the ankle, knee, hip, pelvis, trunk, and upper extremities.

A paper walkway, approximately 25 feet long, on which the patient's footprints can be recorded, is very useful for gait analysis.[27,147] To assess gait, knowledge of what is deemed abnormal and the reasons for those abnormalities is a prerequisite (Table 13-6).

Gait is assessed by having the patient walk barefoot, and with footwear. Barefoot walking provides information about foot function without support and can highlight compensations, such as excessive pronation, and foot deformities, such as claw toes.[149] Having the patient walk with footwear can provide information about the effectiveness of the footwear to counteract the compensations. The patient should be asked to walk on the toes, and then on the heels. An inability to perform either of these actions could be the result of pain, weakness, or a motion restriction. Metatarsalgia is indicated if the metatarsal heads are made more painful with barefoot walking. Pain at initial contact may indicate a heel spur, bone contusion, calcaneal fat pad injury, or bursitis.

TABLE 13-6 Some Gait Deviations and Their Causes[12,19,30,31,101,107,116,148]

Gait Deviations	Reasons
Slower cadence than expected for person's age	Generalized weakness Pain Joint motion restrictions Poor voluntary motor control
Shorter stance phase on involved side and decreased swing phase on uninvolved side Shorter stride length on uninvolved side Decrease lateral sway over involved stance limb Decrease in cadence Decrease in velocity Use of assistive device	Antalgic gait, resulting from painful injury to lower limb and pelvic region
Stance phase longer on one side	Pain Lack of trunk and pelvic rotation Weakness of lower limb muscles Restrictions in lower limb joints Poor muscle control Increased muscle tone
Lateral trunk lean Purpose is to bring center of gravity of trunk nearer to hip joint	Ipsilateral lean—hip abductor weakness (gluteus medius/Trendelenburg gait) Contralateral lean—decreased hip flexion in swing limb Painful hip Abnormal hip joint (congenital dysplasia, coxa vara, etc.) Wide walking base Unequal leg length
Anterior trunk leaning Occurs at initial contact to move line of gravity in front of axis of knee	Weak or paralyzed knee extensors or gluteus maximus Decreased ankle dorsiflexion Hip flexion contracture
Posterior trunk leaning Occurs at initial contact to bring line of external force behind axis of hip	Weak or paralyzed hip extensors, especially gluteus maximus (gluteus maximus gait) Hip pain Hip flexion contracture Inadequate hip flexion in swing Decreased knee range of motion
Increased lumbar lordosis Occurs at end of stance period	Inability to extend hip, usually due to flexion contracture or ankylosis
Pelvic drop during stance	Contralateral gluteus medius weakness Adaptive shortening of quadratus lumborum on swing side Contralateral hip adductor spasticity
Excessive pelvic rotation	Adaptively shortened/spasticity of hip flexors on same side Limited hip joint flexion
Circumducted hip Ground contact by swinging leg can be avoided if it is swung outward for natural walking to occur, leg that is in its stance phase needs to be longer than leg that is in its swing phase to allow toe clearance of swing foot	Functional leg-length discrepancy Arthrogenic stiff hip or knee

TABLE 13-6 *(cont.)*

Hip hiking Pelvis is lifted on side of swinging leg, by contraction of spinal muscles and lateral abdominal wall	Functional leg-length discrepancy Inadequate hip flexion, knee flexion, or ankle dorsiflexion Hamstring weakness Quadratus lumborum shortening
Vaulting Ground clearance of swinging leg will be increased if subject goes up on toes of stance period leg	Functional leg-length discrepancy Vaulting occurs on shorter limb side
Abnormal internal hip rotation Produces "toe-in" gait	Adaptive shortening of iliotibial band Weakness of hip external rotators Femoral anteversion Adaptive shortening of hip internal rotators
Abnormal external hip rotation Produces "toe-out" gait	Adaptive shortening of hip external rotators Femoral retroversion Weakness of hip internal rotators
Increased hip adduction (scissors gait) Results in excessive hip adduction during swing (scissoring), decreased base of support, and decreased progression of opposite foot	Spasticity or contracture of ipsilateral hip adductors Ipsilateral hip adductor weakness Coxa vara
Inadequate hip extension/excessive hip flexion Results in loss of hip extension in mid stance (forward leaning of trunk, increased lordosis, and increased knee flexion and ankle dorsiflexion) and late stance (anterior pelvic tilt), and increased hip flexion in swing	Hip flexion contracture Iliotibial band contracture Hip flexor spasticity Pain Arthrodesis (surgical or spontaneous ankylosis) Loss of ankle dorsiflexion
Inadequate hip flexion Results in decreased limb advancement in swing, posterior pelvic tilt, circumduction, and excessive knee flexion to clear foot	Hip flexor weakness Hip joint arthrodesis
Decreased hip swing through (psoatic limp) Manifested by exaggerated movements at pelvis and trunk to assist hip to move into flexion	Legg-Calvé-Perthes disease Weakness or reflex inhibition of psoas major muscle
Excessive knee extension/inadequate knee flexion Results in decreased knee flexion at initial contact and loading response, increased knee extension during stance, and decreased knee flexion during swing	Pain Anterior trunk deviation/bending Weakness of quadriceps, hyperextension is a compensation and places body weight vector anterior to knee Spasticity of the quadriceps; noted more during the loading response and during initial swing intervals Joint deformity
Excessive knee flexion/inadequate knee extension At initial contact or around midstance; results in increased knee flexion in early stance, decreased knee extension in midstance and terminal stance, and decreased knee extension during swing	Knee flexion contracture, resulting in decreased step length and decreased knee extension in stance Increased tone/spasticity of hamstrings or hip flexors Decreased range of motion of ankle dorsiflexion in swing period Weakness of plantar flexors, resulting in increased dorsiflexion in stance Lengthened limb
Inadequate dorsiflexion control ("foot slap") during initial contact to midstance	Weak or paralyzed dorsiflexors Lack of lower limb proprioception

TABLE 13-6 *(cont.)*

Gait Deviations	Reasons
Steppage gait during the acceleration through deceleration of the swing phase Exaggerated knee and hip flexion are used to lift foot higher than usual, for increased ground clearance resulting from foot drop	Weak or paralyzed dorsiflexor muscles Functional leg-length discrepancy
Increased walking base (> 20 cm)	Deformity such as hip abductor muscle contracture Genu valgus Fear of losing balance Leg-length discrepancy
Decreased walking base (< 10 cm)	Hip adductor muscle contracture Genu varum
Excessive eversion of calcaneus during initial contact through midstance	Excessive tibia vara (refers to frontal plane position of the distal one third of leg as it relates to supporting surface) Forefoot varus Weakness of tibialis posterior Excessive lower extremity internal rotation (due to muscle imbalances, femoral anteversion)
Excessive pronation during midstance through terminal stance	Insufficient ankle dorsiflexion (< 10 degrees) Increased tibial varum Compensated forefoot or rearfoot varus deformity Uncompensated forefoot valgus deformity Pes planus Long limb Uncompensated medial rotation of tibia or femur Weak tibialis anterior
Excessive supination during initial contact through midstance	Limited calcaneal eversion Rigid forefoot valgus Pes cavus Uncompensated lateral rotation of tibia or femur Short limb Plantar flexed first ray Upper motor neuron muscle imbalance
Excessive dorsiflexion	Compensation for knee flexion contracture Inadequate plantar flexor strength Adaptive shortening of dorsiflexors Increased muscle tone of dorsiflexors Pes calcaneus deformity
Excessive plantar flexion	Increased plantar flexor activity Plantar flexor contracture
Excessive varus	Contracture Overactivity of muscles on medial aspect of foot
Excessive valgus	Weak invertors Foot hypermobility
Decreased or absence of propulsion (plantar flexor gait)	Inability of plantar flexors to perform function, resulting in a shorter step length on involved side

The patient's footwear is examined for patterns of wear. The greatest amount of wear on the sole of the shoe should occur beneath the ball of the foot, and in the area corresponding to the first, second, and third MTP joints, and slight wear to the lateral side of the heel. The upper portion of the shoe should demonstrate a transverse crease at the level of the MTP joints. A stiff first MTP joint can produce a crease line that runs obliquely, from forward and medial to backward and lateral.[150] Scuffing of the shoe might indicate tibialis anterior weakness or adaptively shortened heel cords.[149]

The patient's foot also is examined for callus formation, blisters, corns, and bunions. Callus formation on the sole of the foot is an indicator of dysfunction and provides the clinician with an index to the degree of shear stresses applied to the foot, and a clear outline of abnormal weight-bearing areas.[151] Adequate amounts of calluses may provide protection, but in excess amounts they may cause pain. Callus formation under the second and third metatarsal heads could indicate excessive pronation in a flexible foot, or Morton's neuroma if just under the former. A callus under the fifth, and sometimes the fourth, metatarsal head may indicate an abnormally rigid foot.

The patient is asked to walk in his or her usual manner and at the usual speed. The clinician begins the gait assessment with an overall look at the patient while they walk and noting the cadence, stride length, step length, and velocity. The arm swing during gait also should be observed. If an individual has a problem with the foot or ankle on one side, the opposite arm swing often is decreased.[60]

The patient is observed from head to toe and then back again, from the side, from the front, and then from the back.

In addition to observing the patient walking at his or her normal pace, the clinician should observe the patient walking at varying speeds. This can be achieved on a treadmill by adjusting speed, or by asking the patient to change walking speed.

Once an overall assessment has been made of the patient's gait, the clinician can focus attention on the various segments of the kinetic chain of gait, including the trunk, pelvis, lumbar spine, hip, knee, and ankle and foot (see Table 13-2).

Attempts are made to determine the primary cause of any gait deviations or compensations (see Table 13-6).

Anterior View

When observing the patient from the front, the clinician can note the following:

▶ Head position. The subject's head should not move too much during gait in a lateral or vertical direction and should remain fairly stationary during the gait cycle.

▶ Amount of lateral tilt of the pelvis.

▶ Amount of lateral displacement of the trunk and pelvis.

▶ Whether there is excessive swaying of the trunk or pelvis.

▶ Amount of vertical displacement. Vertical displacement can be assessed by observing the patient's head. A "bouncing"

gait is characteristic of adaptively shortened gastrocnemii, or increased tone of the gastrocnemius and soleus.

▶ Reciprocal arm swing. Movements of the upper trunk and limbs usually occur in the opposite directions to the pelvis and the lower limbs.

▶ Whether the shoulders are depressed, retracted, or elevated.

▶ Whether the elbows are flexed or extended.

▶ Amount of hip adduction or abduction that occurs. Causes of excessive adduction include an excessive angle of the coxa vara, hip abductor weakness, hip adductor contracture or spasticity, and contralateral hip abduction contracture. Excessive hip abduction may be caused by an abduction contracture, a short leg, obesity, impaired balance, or hip flexor weakness.[152]

▶ Amount of valgus or varus at the knee. During gait, there may be an obvious varus-extension thrust. According to Noyes and colleagues, this gait pattern is characteristic of chronic injuries to the posterolateral structures of the knee.[1]

▶ Width of the base of support.

▶ *Degree of "toe-out."* The term *toe-out* refers to the angle formed by the intersection of the line of progression of the foot and the line extending from the center of the heel through the second metatarsal. The normal toe-out angle is approximately 7 degrees, and this angle decreases as the speed of gait increases.[123]

▶ Whether any circumduction of the hip occurs. Hip circumduction can indicate a leg-length discrepancy, decreased ability of the knee to flex, or hip abductor shortening or overuse.

▶ Whether any hip hiking occurs. Hip hiking can indicate a leg-length discrepancy, hamstring weakness, or shortening of the quadratus lumborum.

▶ Evidence of thigh atrophy.

▶ Degree of rotation of the whole lower extremity. Because positioning the lower extremity in external rotation decreases the stress on the subtalar joint complex, an individual with a foot or ankle problem often adopts this position during gait.[60] Excessive internal or external rotation of the femur can indicate adaptive shortening of the medial or lateral hamstrings, respectively, resulting in anteversion or retroversion, respectively.

Lateral View

When observing the patient from the side, the clinician can note the following:

▶ *Amount of thoracic and shoulder rotation.* Each shoulder and arm should swing reciprocally, with equal motion.

▶ *Orientation of trunk.* The trunk should remain erect and level during the gait cycle as it moves in the opposite direction to the pelvis. Compensation can occur in the lumbar spine for a loss of motion at the hip. A backward lean of the trunk may result from weak hip extensors or inadequate hip flexion. A forward lean of the trunk may result from pathology of the hip, knee, or ankle; abdominal muscle weakness; decreased spinal mobility; or hip flexion contracture. Forward leaning during the loading response and early midstance intervals may indicate hip extensor weakness.[128]

► *Orientation of the pelvic tilt.* An anterior pelvic tilt of 10 degrees is considered normal. Excessive anterior tilting can be caused by weak hip extensors, hip flexion contracture, or hip flexor spasticity. Excessive posterior pelvic tilting during gait usually occurs in the presence of hip flexor weakness.

► *Degree of hip extension.* Causes of inadequate hip extension and excessive hip flexion include hip flexion contracture, iliotibial band contracture, hip flexor spasticity, or pain.[152] Causes of inadequate hip flexion may include hip flexor weakness or hip joint arthrodesis.[152]

► *Knee flexion and extension.* The knee should be extended during the initial contact interval, followed by slight flexion during the loading response interval. During the swing period, there must be sufficient knee flexion. Causes of excessive knee flexion and inadequate knee extension include inappropriate hamstring activity, knee flexion contracture, soleus weakness, and excessive ankle plantar flexion. Causes of inadequate flexion and excessive extension at the knee include quadriceps weakness, pain, quadriceps spasticity, excessive ankle plantar flexion, hip flexor weakness, and knee extension contractures.[153] Individuals with genu recurvatum may have a functional strength deficit in the quadriceps muscle or gastrocnemius that allows knee hyperextension.[154]

► *Ankle dorsiflexion and plantar flexion.* During midstance, the ankle dorsiflexes and the body pivots over the stationary foot. At the end of the stance period, the ankle should be seen to plantar flex to raise the heel. At the beginning of the swing period, the ankle is plantar flexed, moving into dorsiflexion as the swing period progresses and reaching a neutral position at the time of heel contact at the termination of the swing. Excessive plantar flexion in midswing, initial contact, and loading response may be caused by pretibial (especially the anterior tibialis) weakness. Excessive plantar flexion also may be caused by plantar flexion contracture, soleus and gastrocnemius spasticity, or weak quadriceps.[155] Excessive dorsiflexion may be caused by soleus weakness, ankle fusion, or persistent knee flexion during the midstance period.[128]

► *Stride length of each limb.*

► *Cadence.* The cadence should be normal for the patient's age (see Table 13-6).

► *Heel rise.* An early heel rise indicates an adaptively shortened Achilles tendon.[60] Delayed heel rise may indicate a weak gastrocnemius-soleus complex.

► *Heel contact.* A low heel contact during initial contact may be caused by plantar flexion contracture, tibialis anterior weakness, or premature action by the calf muscles.[155]

► *Preswing.* An exaggerated preswing is manifested by the patient walking on the toes. Causes include pes equines deformity, adaptive shortening or increased tone of the triceps surae, weakness of the dorsiflexors, and knee flexion occurring at midstance. A decreased preswing is often characterized by a lack of plantar flexion at terminal stance and preswing. Causes for this can include ankle or foot pain or weakness of the plantar flexor muscles.

Posterior View

When observing the patient from the back, the clinician can note the following:

► Amount of subtalar inversion (varus) or eversion (valgus). Excessive inversion and eversion usually relate to abnormal muscular control. Generally speaking, varus tends to be the dominant dysfunction in spastic patients, whereas valgus tends to be more common with flaccid paralysis.[155]

► Base of support.

► Pelvic list.

► Degree of hip rotation. As in standing, excessive femoral internal rotation past the midstance of gait will accentuate genu recurvatum. Causes of excessive external hip rotation may include gluteus maximus overactivity and excessive ankle plantar flexion.[152] Causes of excessive internal hip rotation include medial hamstring overactivity, hip adductor overactivity, anterior abductor overactivity, and quadriceps weakness.[152]

► Amount of hip adduction or abduction.

► Amount of knee/tibial rotation.

Assistive Devices

The most common cause for the breakdown of the normal gait cycle is an injury to one or both of the lower extremities. Such an injury usually results in an antalgic gait. If the injury is severe enough, an assistive device is needed. Assistive devices are used to make ambulation as safe and as painless as possible.

In essence, an assistive device is an extension of the upper extremity, used to provide support, balance, and weight bearing normally provided by an intact functioning lower extremity.[156] Assistive devices function to reduce ground reaction forces, with the size of the base of support that they provide being proportional to the amount of reduction in these forces.

Assistive devices, in order of the stability they provide, include a walker, crutches, walker cane, quad cane, straight cane, and bent cane, with the walker providing the most stability.

The indications for using an assistive device include[157]:

▶ Decreased ability to bear weight through the lower extremities.

▶ Muscle weakness or paralysis of the trunk or lower extremities.

▶ Decreased balance and proprioception in the upright posture.

Correct fitting for an assistive device is important to ensure for the safety of the patient and to allow for minimal energy expenditure. Once fitted, the patient should be taught the correct walking technique with the device. The fitting depends on the device chosen:

▶ *Walkers, hemiwalking canes, quad canes, and standard canes.* The height of the device handle should be adjusted to the level of the greater trochanter of the patient's hip.

▶ *Standard crutches.* A number of methods can be used for determining the correct crutch length for axillary crutches. The crutch tip should be vertical to the ground and positioned approximately 15 cm (6 in.) lateral and 15 cm (6 in.) anterior to the patient's foot. The handgrips of the crutch are adjusted to the height of the greater trochanter of the hip of the patient. There should be a 5–8 cm (2–3 in.) gap between the tops of the axillary pads and the patient's axilla. Bauer and colleagues[158] found that the best calculation of ideal crutch length was either 77 percent of the patient's height, or the height minus 40.6 cm (16 in.).

▶ *Forearm/Loftstrand crutches.* The crutch is adjusted so that the handgrip is level with the greater trochanter of the patient's hip, and the top of the forearm cuff just distal to the elbow.

▶ *Canes.* Using a cane to aid walking is perhaps as old as the history of humankind. In ancient times, canes were used for support, defense, and the procurement of food.[159] Later, canes became a symbol of power and aristocracy.[160] Currently, canes are used to provide support and protection, to reduce pain in the lower extremities, and to improve balance during ambulation.[161] It is common practice to instruct patients with lower extremity pain to use the cane in the hand contralateral to the symptomatic side.[162] The use of a cane in the contralateral hand helps preserve reciprocal motion and a more normal pathway for the center of gravity.[163] Use of a cane in this fashion also helps to decrease forces at the hip, as estimated by external kinematics and kinetics.[164–166] Use of a cane can transmit 20 to 25 percent of body weight away from the lower extremities.[168,169] The cane also allows the subject to increase the effective base of support, thereby decreasing the hip abductor force exerted.

Gait Training With Assistive Devices

The clinician must always provide adequate physical support and instruction while working with a patient using an assistive gait device. The clinician positions himself or herself on the involved side of the patient, to be able to assist the patient on the side where the patient will most likely have difficulty. In addition, a gait belt should be fitted around the patient's waist to enable the clinician to assist the patient. When ambulating with a patient, the clinician should be just behind the patient, standing toward the involved side.

The selection of the proper gait pattern to instruct the patient is dependent on the patient's balance, strength, cardiovascular status, coordination, functional needs, and weight-bearing status. Several gait patterns are recognized.

Two-Point Pattern

The two-point gait pattern, which closely approximates the normal gait pattern, requires the use of an assistive gait device (canes or crutches) on each side of the body. This pattern requires the patient to move the assistive gait device and the contralateral lower extremity at the same time.

Three-Point Gait Pattern

The three-point gait pattern involves the use of two crutches or a walker. This pattern is used when the patient is permitted to bear weight through only one lower extremity. The three-point gait pattern requires good upper body strength, good balance, and good cardiovascular endurance. The pattern is initiated with the forward movement of the assistive gait device. Next, the involved lower extremity is advanced. The patient then presses down on the assistive gait device and advances the uninvolved lower extremity. If the uninvolved lower extremity is advanced to a point at which it is parallel to the involved lower extremity, this is a "swing to" pattern. If the uninvolved lower extremity is advanced ahead of the uninvolved lower extremity, then this is a "swing through" pattern.

A modification of the three-point gait pattern requires two crutches or a walker. This pattern is used when the patient can bear full weight with one lower extremity but is only allowed to touch the involved lower extremity to the floor. This is known as *touchdown weight bearing.* In *partial weight bearing,* only part of the patient's weight is allowed to be transferred through the involved lower extremity. It must be remembered that most patients have difficulty replicating a prescribed weight-bearing restriction, and will need constant reinforcement.[170]

The pattern is initiated with the forward movement of one of the assistive gait devices and then the involved lower extremity is advanced forward. The patient presses down on the assistive gait device and advances the uninvolved lower extremity using either a "swing to" or a "swing through" pattern.

Four-Point Pattern

The four-point gait pattern, which requires the use of an assistive gait device (canes or crutches) on each side of the body, is used when the patient requires maximum assistance with balance and stability. The pattern is initiated with the forward movement of one of the assistive gait devices, and then the contralateral lower extremity, the other assistive gait device, and finally the opposite lower extremity (e.g., right crutch, then left foot; left crutch, then right foot).

Sit-to-Stand Transfers

Before the patient can begin ambulation, he or she must first learn to safely transfer from a sitting position to a standing position. The wheels of the bed or wheelchair are locked, and the patient is reminded of any weight-bearing restrictions. The patient is asked to slide to the front edge of the chair or bed, and the weight-bearing foot is placed underneath the body so that the COG is closer to the base of support, which will make it easier for the patient to stand.

The patient is then instructed to lean forward and push up with the hands from the bed or armrests.

▶ If the patient is being instructed on the use of a walker, he or she should grasp the handgrips of the walker only after becoming upright, and should not be permitted to try to pull up to a standing position using the walker, because this can cause the walker to tip over, and increase the potential for falls.

▶ If the patient is using crutches, he or she is instructed to hold both crutches with the hand on the same side as the involved lower extremity. The patient then presses down on the handgrips of the crutches, the armrest or bed, and with the uninvolved lower extremity, to stand. Once standing, and with adequate balance, the patient moves the crutches into position and begins to ambulate.

▶ If the patient is using one or two canes, he or she is instructed to push up with the hands from the bed or armrests. Once standing, the patient should grasp the handgrip(s) of the cane(s) with the appropriate hand and begin to ambulate.

Stand-to-Sit Transfers

The stand-to-sit transfer is essentially the reverse of the sit-to-stand transfer. In order to sit down using an assistive device, the patient must first back up against the front edge of the bed or chair. If the patient has difficulty bending the knee of the involved lower extremity, he or she is instructed to slowly advance this extremity forward. Once in position:

▶ The patient using a walker reaches for the bed or armrest with both hands and slowly sits down.

▶ The patient using crutches moves both crutches to the hand on the side of the involved lower extremity. With that hand holding onto both handgrips of the crutches, the patient reaches back for the bed or armrest with the other hand before slowly sitting down.

▶ The patient using one or two canes, places the handgrip of the cane(s) against the edge of the chair or bed. Next, the patient reaches back for the bed or armrest and slowly sits down.

Stair Negotiation

Ascending Stairs. To ascend steps, the patient must first move to the front edge of the step. The walker will have to be turned toward the opposite side of the handrail or wall. Ascending more than two to three stairs with a walker is not recommended.

▶ To ascend stairs using a walker, the patient is instructed to grasp the stair handrail with one hand, and to turn the walker sideways so that the two front legs of the walker are placed on the first step. When ready, the patient pushes down on the walker handgrip and the handrail, and advances the uninvolved lower extremity onto the first step. The patient then advances the uninvolved lower extremity to the first step, and moves the legs of the walker to the next step. This process is repeated as the patient moves up the steps.

▶ To ascend steps or stairs with crutches, the patient should use grasp the stair handrail with one hand, and grasp both crutches by the handgrips with the other hand. If the patient is unable to grasp both crutches with one hand, or if the handrail is not stable, then the patient should use both crutches only, although this is not recommended if there are more than two to three steps. When in the correct position at the front edge of the step, the patient pushes down on the crutches and handrail, if applicable, and advances the uninvolved lower extremity to the first step. The patient then advances the involved lower extremity, and finally the crutches. This process is repeated for the remaining steps.

▶ To ascend steps or stairs with one or two canes, the patient should use the handrail and the cane(s). If the handrail is not stable, then the patient should use the cane(s), only. The patient pushes down on the cane(s) or handrail, if applicable, and advances the uninvolved lower extremity to the first step. The patient then advances the involved lower extremity. This process is repeated for the remaining steps.

Descending Stairs. In order to descend steps, the patient must first move to the front edge of the top step. Descending more than two to three stairs with a walker is not recommended.

▶ To descend stairs using a walker, the walker is turned sideways so that the two front legs of the walker are placed on the lower step. One hand is placed on the rear handgrip, and the other hand grasps the stair handrail. When ready, the patient lowers the involved lower extremity down to the first step. Then the patient pushes down on the walker and handrail, and advances the uninvolved lower extremity down the first step. This process is repeated as the patient moves down the steps.

▶ To descend steps or stairs with crutches, the patient should use one hand to grasp the stair handrail and the other to grasp both crutches and handrail. If the patient is unable to grasp both crutches with one hand, or if the handrail is not stable, then the patient should use both crutches only, although this is not recommended if there are more than two to three steps. When ready, the patient lowers the involved lower extremity down to the first step. Next, the patient pushes down on the crutches and handrail, if applicable, and advances the uninvolved lower extremity down to the first step. This process is repeated for the remaining steps.

▶ To descend steps or stairs with one or two canes, the patient should use the cane(s) and handrail. If the handrail is not stable, then the patient should use the cane(s) only. When ready, the patient lowers the involved lower extremity down to the first step. Next, the patient pushes down on the cane(s) and handrail, if applicable, and advances the uninvolved lower extremity down to the first step. This process is repeated for the remaining steps.

Instructions

Whichever gait pattern is chosen, it is important that the patient receive verbal and illustrated instructions for use of the assistive gait device to negotiate stairs, curbs, ramps, doors, and transfers. These instructions should include any weight-bearing precautions pertinent to the patient, the appropriate gait sequence, and a contact number at which to reach the clinician if questions arise.

REVIEW QUESTIONS*

1. List the two periods and three tasks of the gait cycle.
2. List, in order of occurrence, the eight intervals of the gait cycle.
3. As speed increases, what effect is there on the stance period and the double stance phase?
4. True or false: The thoracic spine and the pelvis rotate in opposite directions to each other during the gait cycle.
5. From midstance to terminal stance, in which direction should the ilium rotate?

---

* Additional questions to test your understanding of this chapter can be found in the Online Learning Center for *Orthopaedic Assessment, Evaluation, and Intervention* at www.duttononline.net.

REFERENCES

1. Noyes FR, Dunworth LA, Andriacchi TP, Andrews M, Hewett TE. Knee hyperextension gait abnormalities in unstable knees. *Am J Sports Med* 1996;24:35–45.
2. Schwartz RP, Heath AL. The pneumographic method of recording gait. *J Bone Joint Surg* 1932;14:783–794.
3. Steindler A. *Mechanics of Normal and Pathological Locomotion in Man*. London, England: Bailliere, Tindall and Cox; 1936.
4. Rasch PJ, Burke RK. *Kinesiology and Applied Anatomy*. Philadelphia, Pa: Lea and Febiger; 1971.
5. Tully PD. *Locomotion, Walking and Gait and the Clinical Evaluation of Gait by Use of Two Force Plates*. Guildford, England: University of Surrey; 1973.
6. Weber EH. Anatomisch-physiologische Untersuchung über einige Einrichtungen im Mechanismus der Menschlichen Wirbelsäule. *Archiv Anat Physiol* 1827;240–271.
7. Weber W. Sechster Band. *Mechanik der Menschlichen Gehwerkzenge*. Berlin, Germany: Verlag von Julius Springer; 1894.
8. Steindler A. An historical review of the studies and investigations made in relation to human gait. *J Bone Joint Surg* 1953;35A:540–542.
9. Mann RA, Hagy JL, White V, Liddell D. The initiation of gait. *J Bone Joint Surg* 1979;61A:232–239.
10. Burnett CN, Johnson EW. Development of gait in children; I. Method; II. Results. *Dev Med Child Neurol* 1971;13:196.
11. Luttgens K, Hamilton N. Locomotion: Solid surface. In: Luttgens K, Hamilton N, eds. *Kinesiology: Scientific Basis of Human Motion*. Dubuque, Iowa: McGraw-Hill; 1997:519–549.
12. Levine D, Whittle M. Gait analysis: The lower extremities. In: *Orthopaedic Physical Therapy Home Study Course—The Lower Extremity*. Vol. 92-1. La Crosse, Wis: Orthopaedic Section, American Physical Therapy Association; 1992.
13. Mann RA, Hagy J. Biomechanics of walking, running, and sprinting. *Am J Sports Med* 1980;8:345–350.
14. Murray MP. Gait as a total pattern of movement. *Am J Phys Med* 1967;46:290.
15. Scranton J, Rutkowski R, Brown TD. Support phase kinematics of the foot. In: Bateman JE, Trott AW, eds. *The Foot and Ankle*. New York, NY: BC Decker; 1980:195–205.
16. Perry J. Gait cycle. In: Perry J, ed. *Gait Analysis: Normal and Pathological Function*. Thorofare, NJ: Slack; 1992:3–7.
17. Perry J. Stride analysis. In: Perry J, ed. *Gait Analysis: Normal and Pathological Function*. Thorofare, NJ: Slack; 1992: 431–441.
18. Mann RA, Moran GT, Dougherty SE. Comparative electromyography of the lower extremity in jogging, running and sprinting. *Am J Sports Med* 1986;14:501–510.
19. Perry J. *Gait Analysis: Normal and Pathological Function*. Thorofare, NJ: Slack; 1992.
20. Rogers MM. Dynamic foot mechanics. *J Orthop Sports Phys Ther* 1995;21:306–316.
21. Gage JR, Deluca PA, Renshaw TS. Gait analysis: Principles and applications with emphasis on its use with cerebral palsy. *Inst Course Lect* 1996;45:491–507.
22. Ostrosky KM, VanSwearingen JM, Burdett RG, Gee Z. A comparison of gait characteristics in young and old subjects. *Phys Ther* 1994;74:637–646.
23. Adelaar RS. The practical biomechanics of running. *Am J Sports Med* 1986;14:497–500.
24. Basmajian JV. *Therapeutic Exercise*. 3rd ed. Rehabilitation Medicine Library. Baltimore, Md: Williams and Wilkins; 1979.
25. Arsenault AB, Winter DA, Marteniuk RG. Is there a "normal" profile of EMG activity in gait? *Med Biol Eng Comput* 1986;24:337–343.
26. Berchuck M, Andriacchi TP, Bach BR, Reider B. Gait adaptations by patients who have a deficient anterior cruciate ligament. *J Bone Joint Surg* 1990;72A:871–877.
27. Boeing DD. Evaluation of a clinical method of gait analysis. *Phys Ther* 1977;57:795–798.
28. Dillon P, Updyke W, Allen W. Gait analysis with reference to chondromalacia patellae. *J Orthop Sports Phys Ther* 1983;5:127–131.
29. Giannini S, et al. Terminology, parameterization and normalization in gait analysis. In: *Gait Analysis: Methodologies and Clinical Applications*. Washington, DC: IOS Press; 1994:65–88.
30. Hunt GC, Brocato RS. Gait and foot pathomechanics. In: Hunt GC, ed. *Physical Therapy of the Foot and Ankle*. Edinburgh, Scotland: Churchill Livingstone; 1988.
31. Krebs DE, Robbins CE, Lavine L, Mann RW. Hip biomechanics during gait. *J Orthop Sports Phys Ther* 1998;28:51–59.
32. Oberg T, Karsznia A, Oberg K. Basic gait parameters: Reference data for normal subjects, 10–79 years of age. *J Rehabil Res Dev* 1993;30:210–223.

33. Winter DA. Biomechanical motor patterns in normal walking. *J Motor Behav* 1983;15:302–329.

34. Croskey MI, et al. The height of the center of gravity in man. *Am J Physiol* 1922;61:171–185.

35. Richardson JK, Iglarsh ZA. Gait. In: Richardson JK, Iglarsh ZA, eds. *Clinical Orthopaedic Physical Therapy*. Philadelphia, Pa: Saunders; 1994:602–625.

36. Murray MP, Sepic SB, Barnard EJ. Patterns of sagittal rotation of the upper limbs in walking. *Phys Ther* 1967;47:272–284.

37. Hogue RE. Upper extremity muscular activity at different cadences and inclines during normal gait. *Phys Ther* 1969;49:963–972.

38. Voorn R. Case report: Can sacroiliac joint dysfunction cause chronic Achilles tendinitis? *J Orthop Sports Phys Ther* 1998;27:436–443.

39. Alderink GJ. The sacroiliac joint: Review of anatomy, mechanics, and function. *J Orthop Sports Phys Ther* 1991;13:71–84.

40. Perry J. The hip. In: Perry J, ed. *Gait Analysis: Normal and Pathological Function*. Thorofare, NJ: 1992:111–129.

41. Oatis CA. Role of the hip in posture and gait. In: Echternach J, ed. *Clinics in Physical Therapy: Physical Therapy of the Hip*. New York, NY: Churchill Livingstone; 1983:165–179.

42. Reinking MF. Knee anatomy and biomechanics. In: Wadsworth C, ed. *Disorders of the Knee—Home Study Course*. LaCrosse, Wis: Orthpedic Section, American Physical Therapy Association; 2001.

43. Norkin C, Levangie P. *Joint Structure and Function: A Comprehensive Analysis*. Philadelphia, Pa: FA Davis; 1992:355–358.

44. Kuster MS, Wood GA, Stachowiak GW, Gachter A. Joint load considerations in total knee replacement. *J Bone Joint Surg* 1997;79B:109–113.

45. Paulos LE, Noyes FR, Grood ES. Knee rehabilitation after anterior cruciate ligament reconstruction and repair. *Am J Sports Med* 1981;9:140–149.

46. Renstrom P, Arms SW, Stanwyck TS, Johnson RJ, Pope MH. Strain within the anterior cruciate ligament during hamstring and quadriceps activity. *Am J Sports Med* 1986;14:83–87.

47. Ahmed AM, Burke DL. In vitro measurement of static pressure distribution in synovial joints: I. Tibial surface of the knee. *J Biomed Eng* 1983;105:216–225.

48. Huberti HH, Hayes WC. Contact pressures in chondromalacia patellae and the effects of capsular reconstructive procedures. *J Orthop Res* 1988;6:499–508.

49. Matthews LS, Sonstegard DA, Henke JA. Load bearing characteristics of the patello-femoral joint. *Acta Orthop Scand* 1977;48:511–516.

50. Bourne MH, Hazel WA Jr, Scott SG, Sim FH. Anterior knee pain. *Mayo Clinic Proc* 1988;63:482–491.

51. Hejgaard RJ, Sandberg H, Hede A, Jacobsen K. The course of differently treated isolated ruptures of the anterior cruciate ligament as observed by prospective stress radiography. *Clin Orthop* 1984;182:236–241.

52. Johnson RJ, Eriksson E, Haggmark T, Pope MH. Five to ten year follow-up evaluation after reconstruction of the anterior cruciate ligament. *Clin Orthop* 1984;83:122–140.

53. Straub T, Hunter RE. Acute anterior cruciate ligament repair. *Clin Orthop* 1988;227:238–250.

54. Lange GW, Hintermeister RA, Schlegel T, Dillman CJ, Steadman JR. Electromyographic and kinematic analysis of graded treadmill walking and the implications for knee rehabilitation. *J Orthop Sports Phys Ther* 1996;23:294–301.

55. Palmitier RA, An KN, Scott SG, Chao EY. Kinetic chain exercises in knee rehabilitation. *Sports Med* 1991;11:402–413.

56. Hunt GC. Functional biomechanics of the subtalar joint. In: *Orthopaedic Physical Therapy Home Study Course 92-1: Lower Extremity*. La Crosse, Wis: Orthopedic Section, American Physical Therapy Association; 1992.

57. Donatelli R. Normal anatomy and pathophysiology of the foot and ankle. In Wadsworth C, ed. Contemporary Topics on the Foot and Ankle. La Crosse, Wis: Orthopedic Section, American Physical Therapy Association 2000.

58. Root M, Orien W, Weed J. *Clinical Biomechanics: Normal and Abnormal Function of the Foot*. Vol. II. Los Angeles, Calif: Clinical Biomechanics Corp; 1977.

59. Inman VT, Ralston HJ, Todd F. *Human Walking*. Baltimore, Md: Williams and Wilkins; 1981.

60. Mann RA. Biomechanical approach to the treatment of foot problems. *Foot Ankle* 1982;2:205–212.

61. Mann RA, Hagy JL. The function of the toes in walking, jogging and running. *Clin Orthop* 1979;142:24.

62. Bojsen-Möller F, Lamoreux L. Significance of dorsiflexion of the toes in walking. *Acta Orthop Scand* 1979;50:471–479.

63. Bojsen-Möller F. Normal and pathologic anatomy of metatarsals German. *Orthopade* 1982;11:148–153.

64. Bojsen-Möller F. Calcaneocuboid joint and stability of the longitudinal arch of the foot at high and low gear push off. *J Anat* 1979;129:165–176.

65. Perry J. The mechanics of walking: A clinical interpretation. In: Perry J, Hislop HJ, eds. *Principles of Lower Extremity Bracing*. New York, NY: American Physical Therapy Association; 1967:9–32.

66. Dee R. Normal and abnormal gait in the pediatric patient. In: Dee R, et al, eds. *Principles of Orthopaedic Practice*. New York, NY: McGraw-Hill; 1997:685–692.

67. Donatelli RA. Normal anatomy and biomechanics. In: Donatelli RA, ed. *Biomechanics of the Foot and Ankle*. Philadelphia, Pa: Saunders; 1990:3–31.

68. Yoon YS, Mansour JM. The passive elastic moment at the hip. *J Biomech* 1982;15:905–910.

69. Lehmkuhl LD, Smith LK. *Brunnstrom's Clinical Kinesiology*. Phildelphia, Pa: Davis; 1983:361–390.

70. Neumann DA, Cook TM. Effects of load and carry position on the electromyographic activity of the gluteus medius muscles during walking. *Phys Ther* 1985;65:305–311.

71. Neumann DA, et al. An electromyographic analysis of hip abductor activity when subjects are carrying loads in one or both hands. *Phys Ther* 1992;72:207–217.

72. Neumann DA, Hase AD. An electromyographic analysis of the hip abductors during load carriage: Implications for joint protection. *J Orthop Sports Phys Ther* 1994;19:296–304.

73. Neumann DA, Soderberg GL, Cook TM. Comparisons of maximal isometric hip abductor muscle torques between sides. *Phys Ther* 1988;68:496–502.

74. Neumann DA, Soderberg GL, Cook TM. Electromyographic analysis of the hip abductor musculature in healthy right-handed persons. *Phys Ther* 1989;69:431–440.

75. Adler N, Perry J, Kent B, Robertson K. Electromyography of the vastus medialis oblique and vasti in normal subjects during gait. *Electromyogr Clin Neurophysiol* 1983;23:643–649.

76. Battye CK, Joseph J. An investigation by telemetering of the activity of some muscles in walking. *Med Biol Eng Comput* 1966;4:125–135.

77. Dubo HI, Peat M, Winter DA, et al. Electromyographic temporal analysis of gait: Normal human locomotion. *Arch Phys Med Rehabil* 1976;57:415–420.

78. Brandell BR. Functional roles of the calf and vastus muscles in locomotion. *Am J Phys Med Rehabil* 1977;56:59–74.

79. Ciccotti MG, Kerlan RK, Perry J, Pink M. An electromyographical analysis of the knee during functional activities—I. The normal profile. *Am J Sports Med* 1994;22:645–650.

80. Baratta R, Solomonow M, Zhou BH, Letson D, Chuinard R, D'Ambrosia R. Muscular coactivation: The role of the antagonist musculature in maintaining knee stability. *Am J Sports Med* 1988;16:113–122.

81. Draganich LF, Jaeger RJ, Fralj AR. Coactivation of the hamstrings and quadriceps during extension of the knee. *J Bone Joint Surg* 1989;71A:1076–1081.

82. Molbech S. On the paradoxical effect of some two-joint muscles. *Acta Morphol Neerl Scand* 1965;6:171.

83. Basmajian JV, Deluca CJ. *Muscles Alive: Their Functions Revealed by Electromyography.* Baltimore, Md: Williams and Wilkins; 1985.

84. Rose J, Gamble JG. *Human Walking.* Baltimore, Md: Williams and Wilkins; 1994.

85. Mann RA. Biomechanics of running. In: *AAOS Symposium on the Foot and Leg in Running Sports.* St Louis, Mo: Mosby; 1982:30–44.

86. Teitz CC, Garrett WE Jr, Miniaci A, Lee MH, Mann RA. Tendon problems in athletic individuals. *J Bone Joint Surg* 1997; 79A:138–152.

87. Luttgens K, Hamilton N. The standing posture. In: Luttgens K, Hamilton N, ed. *Kinesiology: Scientific Basis of Human Motion.* Dubuque, Iowa: McGraw-Hill; 1997:445–459.

88. Hoyt DF, Taylor CF. Gait and the energetics of locomotion in horses. *Nature* 1981;292:239–240.

89. Corcoran PJ, Brengelmann G. Oxygen uptake in normal and handicapped subjects in relation to the speed of walking beside a velocity-controlled cart. *Arch Phys Med Rehabil* 1970; 51:78–87.

90. Gonzalez EG, Corcoran PJ, Reyes RL. Energy expenditure in below-knee amputees: Correlation with stump length. *Arch Phys Med Rehabil* 1974;55:111–119.

91. Waters RL, Hislop HJ, Perry J, Antonelli D. Energetics: Application to the study and management of locomotor disabilities. *Orthop Clin North Am* 1978;9:351–377.

92. Martin PE, Rothstein DE, Larish DD. Effects of age and physical activity status on the speed-aerobic demand relationship of walking. *J Appl Physiol* 1992;73:200–206.

93. Prampero PE. The energy cost of human locomotion on land and in the water. *Int J Sports Med* 1986;7:55–72.

94. Davies MJ, Dalsky GP. Economy of mobility in older adults. *J Orthop Sports Phys Ther* 1997;26:69–72.

95. Daniels J, Krahenbuhl G, Foster C, Gilbert J, Daniels S. Aerobic responses of female distance runners to submaximal and maximal exercise. *Ann N Y Acad Sci* 1977;301:726–733.

96. Pate RR, Barnes CG, Miller CA. A physiological comparison of performance-matched female and male distance runners. *Res Q Exerc Sport* 1985;56:245–250.

97. Wells CL, Hecht LH, Krahenbuhl GS. Physical characteristics and oxygen utilization of male and female marathon runners. *Res Q Exerc Sport* 1981;52:281–285.

98. Bransford DR, Howley ET. Oxygen cost of running in trained and untrained men and women. *Med Sci Sports Exerc* 1977;9:41–44.

99. Daniels J, Daniels N. Running economy of elite male and females runners. *Med Sci Sports Exerc* 1992;24:483–489.

100. Howley ET, Glover ME. The caloric costs of running and walking one mile for men and women. *Med Sci Sports Exerc* 1974;6:235–237.

101. Larish DD, Martin PE, Mungiole M. Characteristic patterns of gait in the healthy old. *Ann N Y Acad Sc* 1987;515:18–32.

102. Waters RL, Hislop HJ, Perry J, Thomas L, Campbell J. Comparative cost of walking in young and old adults. *J Orthop Res* 1983;1:73–76.

103. Allen W, Seals DR, Hurley BF, Ehsani AA, Hagberg JM. Lactate threshold and distance running performance in young and older endurance athletes. *J Appl Physiol* 1985;58:1281–1284.

104. Trappe SW, Costill DL, Vukovich MD, Jones J, Melham T. Aging among elite distance runners: A 22-year longitudinal study. *J Appl Physiol* 1996;80:285–290.

105. Wells CL, Boorman MA, Riggs DM. Effect of age and menopausal status on cardiorespiratory fitness in masters women runners. *Med Sci Sports Exerc* 1992;24:1147–1154.

106. Luttgens K, Hamilton N. The center of gravity and stability. In: Luttgens K, Hamilton N, eds. *Kinesiology: Scientific Basis of Human Motion.* Dubuque, Iowa: McGraw-Hill; 1997: 415–442.

107. Epler M. Gait. In: Richardson JK, Iglarsh ZA, eds. *Clinical Orthopaedic Physical Therapy.* Philadelphia, Pa: Saunders; 1994:602–625.

108. Subotnick SI. Variations in angles of gait in running. *Phys Sportsmed* 1979;7:110–114.

109. Craik R, Herman RM, Finley FR. The human solutions for locomotion: Interlimb coordination. In: Herman RM, Grillner S, Stein PS, eds. *Neural Control of Locomotion.* New York, NY: Plenum; 1976:51–63.

110. Wagenaar RC, Van Emmerik RE. Dynamics of pathological gait: Stability and adaptability of movement coordination. *Hum Mov Sci* 1994;13:441–471.

111. Van Emmerik RE, Wagenaar RC, Van Wegen EE. Interlimb coupling patterns in human locomotion: Are we bipeds or quadrupeds? *Ann N Y Acad Sci* 1998;860:539–542.

112. Rush WA, Steiner HA. A study of lower extremity length inequality. *Am J Roentgenol* 1946;56:616–623.

113. Moseley CF. Leg-length discrepancy. In: Morrissy RT, ed. *Lovell and Winter's Pediatric Orthopaedics.* Philadelphia, Pa: JB Lippincott; 1990:767–813.

114. Beaty JH. Congenital anomalies of lower extremity. In: Crenshaw AH, ed. *Campbell's Operative Orthopaedics.* St Louis, Mo: Mosby-Year Book; 1992:2126–2158.

115. Gross RH. Leg length discrepancy: How much is too much? *Orthopedics* 1978;1:307–310.

116. Song KM, Halliday SE, Little DG. The effect of limb-length discrepancy on gait. *J Bone Joint Surg* 1997;79A:1690–1698.

117. Frey C. Foot health and shoewear for women. *Clin Orthop Rel Res* 2000;372:32–44.

118. Molen NH, Rozendal RH, Boon W. Fundamental characteristics of human gait in relation to sex and location. *Proc Koninklijke Ned Akad Wetenschap Biol Med Sci* 1972;45:215–223.

119. Finley FR, Cody KA. Locomotive characteristics of urban pedestrians. *Arch Phys Med Rehabil* 1970;51:423–426.

120. Sato H, Ishizu K. Gait patterns of Japanese pedestrians. *J Hum Ergol (Tokyo)* 1990;19:13–22.

121. Richard R, Weber J, Majjad O, et al. Spatiotemporal gait parameters measured using the Bessou gait analyzer in 79 healthy

subjects: Influence of age, stature, and gender. *Rev Rhum Engl Ed* 1995;62:105–114.

122. Murray MP, Kory RC, Sepic SB. Walking patterns of normal women. *Arch Phys Med Rehabil* 1970;51:637–650.

123. Murray MP, Drought AB, Kory RC. Walking patterns of normal men. *J Bone Joint Surg*1964;46A:335–360.

124. Bhambhani Y, Singh M. Metabolic and cinematographic analysis of walking and running in men and women. *Med Sci Sports Exerc* 1985;17:131–137.

125. Corrigan J, Moore D, Stephens M. The effect of heel height on forefoot loading. *Foot Ankle* 1991;11:418–422.

126. Foti T, Davids JR, Bagley A. A biomechanical analysis of gait during pregnancy. *J Bone Joint Surg* 2000;82A:625–632.

127. National Center for Health Statistics. *Prevalence of Overweight and Obesity Among Adults: United States.* Hyattsville, Md: NCHS; 2000.

128. Perry J. Pelvis and trunk pathological gait. In: Perry J, ed. *Gait Analysis: Normal and Pathological Function.* Thorofare, NJ: Slack; 1992:265–279.

129. Morag E, Hurwitz DE, Andriacchi TP, Hickey M, Andersson GB. Abnormalities in muscle function during gait in relation to the level of lumbar disc herniation. *Spine* 2000; 25:829–833.

130. Andriacchi TP, Ogle JA, Galante JO. Walking speed as a basis for normal and abnormal gait measurements. *J Biomech* 1977;10:261–268.

131. Gage JR. *Gait Analysis in Cerebral Palsy.* London, England: MacKeith Press; 1991.

132. Rengachary SS. Gait and station; examination of coordination. In: Wilkins RH, Rengachary SS, eds. *Neurosurgery.* New York, NY: McGraw-Hill; 1996:133–137.

133. Judge RD, Zuidema GD, Fitzgerald FT. Musculoskeletal system. In: Judge RD, Zuidema GD, Fitzgerald FT, eds. *Clinical Diagnosis.* Boston, Mass: Little, Brown; 1982:365–403.

134. Eyring EJ, Murray W. The effect of joint position on the pressure of intra-articular effusion. *J Bone Joint Surg* 1965;47A: 313–322.

135. Blair E, Stanley F. Issues in the classification and epidemiology of cerebral palsy. *Mental Retard Devel Disab Res Rev* 1997; 3:184–193.

136. Baddar A, Granata K, Damiano DL, Carmines DV, Blanco JS, Abel MF. Ankle and knee coupling in patients with spastic diplegia: Effects of gastrocnemius-soleus lengthening. *J Bone Joint Surg* 2002;84A:736–744.

137. Abel MF, Daminao DL, Pannunzio M, Bush J. Muscle-tendon surgery in diplegic cerebral palsy: Functional and mechanical changes. *J Pediatr Orthop* 1999;19:366–375.

138. Davids JR, Foti T, Dabelstein J, Bagley A. Voluntary (normal) versus obligatory (cerebral palsy) toe-walking in children: A kinematic, kinetic, and electromyographic analysis. *J Pediatr Orthop* 1999;19:461–469.

139. Griffin PP, Wheelhouse WW, Shiavi R, Bass W. Habitual toe walkers: A clinical and electromyographic gait analysis. *J Bone Joint Surg* 1977;59A:97–101.

140. Statham L, Murray MP. Early walking patterns of normal children. *Clin Orthop* 1971;79:8–24.

141. Stricker SJ, Angulo JC. Idiopathic toe walking: A comparison of treatment methods. *J Pediatr Orthop* 1998;18:289–293.

142. Kadaba MP, Ramakrishnan HK, Wootten ME, Gainey J, Gorton G, Cochron GV. Repeatability of kinematic, kinetic, and elec-

tromyographic data in normal adult gait. *J Orthop Res* 1989; 7:849–860.

143. Krebs DE, Edelstein JE, Fishman S. Reliability of observational kinematic gait analysis. *Phys Ther* 1985;65:1027–1033.

144. Skaggs DL, Rethlefsen SA, Kay RM, Dennis SW, Reynolds RA, Tolo VT. Variability in gait analysis interpretation. *J Ped Orthop* 2000;20:759–764.

145. Eastlack ME, Arvidson J, Snyder-Mackler L, Danoff JV, McGarvey CL. Interrater reliability of videotaped observational gait-analysis assessments. *Phys Ther* 1991;71:465–472.

146. VanSwearingen JM, Paschal KA, Bonino P, Yang JF. The modified Gait Abnormality Rating Scale for recognizing the risk of recurrent falls in community-dwelling elderly adults. *Phys Ther* 1996;76:994–1002.

147. McPoil TG, Schuit D, Knecht HG. A comparison of three positions used to evaluate tibial varum. *J Am Podiat Med Assoc* 1988;78:22–28.

148. Giallonardo LM. Clinical evaluation of foot and ankle dysfunction. *Phys Ther* 1988;68:1850–1856.

149. Appling SA, Kasser RJ. Foot and ankle. In: Wadsworth C, ed. *Current Concepts of Orthopedic Physical Therapy—Home Study Course.* La Crosse, Wis: Orthopaedic Section, American Physical Therapy Association; 2001.

150. Hertling D, Kessler RM. *Management of Common Musculoskeletal Disorders: Physical Therapy Principles and Methods.* 3rd ed. Philadelphia, Pa: Lippincott Williams and Wilkins; 1996.

151. Reid DC. *Sports Injury Assessment and Rehabilitation.* New York, NY: Churchill Livingstone; 1992.

152. Perry J. Hip gait deviations. In: Perry J, ed. *Gait Analysis: Normal and Pathological Function.* Thorofare, NJ: Slack; 1992:245–263.

153. Perry J. Knee abnormal gait. In: Perry J, ed. *Gait Analysis: Normal and Pathological Function.* Thorofare, NJ: Slack; 1992:223–243.

154. Stauffer RN, Chao EYS, Gyory AN. Biomechanical gait analysis of the diseased knee joint. *Clin Orthop* 1977;126:246–255.

155. Perry J. Ankle and foot gait deviations. In: Perry J, ed. *Gait Analysis: Normal and Pathological Function.* Thorofare, NJ: Slack; 1992:185–220.

156. Hoberman M. Crutch and cane exercises and use. In: Basmajian JV, ed. *Therapeutic Exercise.* Baltimore, Md: Williams and Wilkins; 1979:228–255.

157. Duesterhaus MA, Duesterhaus S. *Patient Care Skills.* 2nd ed. East Norwalk, Conn: Appleton and Lange; 1990.

158. Bauer DM, Finch DC, McGough KP, Benson CJ, Finstuen K, Allison SC. A comparative analysis of several crutch-length-estimation techniques. *Phys Ther* 1991;71:294–300.

159. Lyu SR, Ogata K, Hoshiko I. Effects of a cane on floor reaction force and center of force during gait. *Clin Orthop Rel Res* 2000;375:313–319.

160. Blount WP. Don't throw away the cane. *J Bone Joint Surg* 1956;38A:695–708.

161. Joyce BM, Kirby RL. Canes, crutches and walkers. *Am Fam Phys* 1991;43:535–542.

162. Deaver GG. What every physician should know about the teaching of crutch walking. *JAMA* 1950;142:470–472.

163. Baxter ML, Allington RO, Koepke GH. Weight-distribution variables in the use of crutches and canes. *Phys Ther* 1969;49:360–365.

164. Edwards BG. Contralateral and ipsilateral cane usage by patients with total knee or hip replacement. *Arch Phys Med Rehabil* 1986;67:734–740.

165. Oatis CA. Biomechanics of the hip. In: Echternach J, ed. *Clinics in Physical Therapy: Physical Therapy of the Hip*. New York, NY: Churchill Livingstone; 1990:37–50.

166. Olsson EC, Smidt GL. Assistive devices. In: Smidt G, ed. *Gait in Rehabilitation*. New York, NY: Churchill Livingstone; 1990:141–155.

167. Vargo MM, Robinson LR, Nicholas JJ. Contralateral vs. ipsilateral cane use: Effects on muscles crossing the knee joint. *Am J Phys Med Rehabil* 1992;71:170–176.

168. Jebsen RH. Use and abuse of ambulation aids. *JAMA* 1967; 199:5–10.

169. Kumar R, Roe MC, Scremin O. Methods for estimating the proper length of a cane. *Arch Phys Med Rehabil* 1995;76:1173–1175.

170. Li S, Armstrong CW, Cipriani D. Three-point gait crutch walking: Variability in ground reaction force during weight bearing. *Arch Phys Med Rehabil* 2001;82:86–92.

PERIPHERAL JOINTS: THE UPPER EXTREMITIES

CHAPTER 14

THE SHOULDER COMPLEX

CHAPTER OBJECTIVES

▶ *At the completion of this chapter, the reader will be able to:*

1. Describe the anatomy of the joints, ligaments, muscles, blood, and nerve supply that comprise the shoulder complex.

2. Describe the biomechanics of the shoulder complex, including the open and close packed positions, muscle force couples, and the static and dynamic stabilizers.

3. Describe the relationship between muscle imbalance and functional performance of the shoulder.

4. Describe the purpose and components of the tests and measures for the shoulder complex.

5. Perform a comprehensive examination of the shoulder complex, including history, systems review, palpation of the articular and soft tissue structures, specific passive mobility tests, passive articular mobility tests, and special tests.

6. Evaluate the key findings from the examination data to establish a diagnosis and prognosis.

7. Summarize the various causes of shoulder dysfunction.

8. Describe and demonstrate intervention strategies and techniques based on clinical findings and established goals.

9. Evaluate the intervention effectiveness in order to determine progress and modify an intervention as needed.

10. Plan an effective home program, and instruct the patient in its use.

OVERVIEW

The shoulder is the most rewarding joint in the body because when a limited or painful movement is found, the finding is seldom ambiguous and often implicates the offending structure.

JAMES CYRIAX, MD (1904–1985)

The primary function of the shoulder complex is to position the hand in space thereby allowing an individual to interact with his or her environment and to perform fine motor functions. An inability to position the hand results in profound impairment of the entire upper extremity.[1]

Secondary functions of the shoulder complex include:

▶ to suspend the upper limb.

▶ to provide sufficient fixation so motion of the upper extremity can occur.

▶ to serve as a fulcrum for arm elevation. Arm elevation in this text, unless otherwise specified, indicates upward motion in the scapular plane, rather than in the coronal plane (*abduction*), or sagittal plane (*flexion*). Another term for this motion is *scaption*.

The shoulder is endowed with a unique blend of mobility and stability. The degree of mobility is contingent upon a healthy articular surface, intact muscle-tendon units, and supple capsuloligamentous restraints. The degree of stability is dependent upon intact capsuloligamentous structures, the proper function of the muscles, and the integrity of the osseous articular structures.[1]

Anatomy

The shoulder complex functions as an integrated unit involving a complex relationship between its various components. The components of the shoulder joint complex consist of:

▶ Three bones (the humerus, the clavicle, and the scapula).

▶ Three joints [the sternoclavicular (S-C), the acromioclavicular (A-C), and the glenohumeral (G-H) joints].

▶ One "pseudojoint" (the articulation between the scapula and the thorax).

▶ One physiological area (the suprahumeral or subacromial space).

For optimal function to occur at the shoulder, motion also has to be available at the cervicothoracic junction and at the connections between the first three ribs and the sternum and spine.

Glenohumeral Joint

The glenohumeral (G-H) joint is a true synovial-lined diarthrodial joint that connects the upper extremity to the trunk, as part of the upper kinetic chain. The G-H joint is formed by the humeral head and the glenoid fossa of the scapula. The head of the humerus faces medially, posteriorly, and superiorly, with the axis of the head forming an angle of 130 to 150 degrees with the long axis of the humerus.[2] In the frontal plane, the head of the humerus is angled posteriorly (retroverted) by 30 to 40 degrees.[3,4] The significance of the head version angle and its relationship to shoulder pathology including instability patterns has yet to be correlated.

The glenoid fossa of the scapula faces laterally, superiorly, and anteriorly at rest and inferiorly and posteriorly when the arm is in the dependent position.[5] The G-H joint is described as a ball and socket joint—the humeral head forms roughly half a ball or sphere (Fig. 14-1), while the glenoid fossa forms the socket. The glenoid fossa is flat and covers only one third to one fourth of the surface area of the humeral head. This arrangement allows for a great deal of mobility but little in the way of articular stability.

However, the glenoid fossa is made approximately 50 percent deeper and more concave by a ring of fibrocartilage called a labrum,[6] which forms part of the articular surface and is attached to the margin of the glenoid cavity and the joint capsule. The labrum enhances joint stability by increasing the humeral head contact areas to 75 percent vertically and 56 percent transversely.[5,6] The humeral and glenoid contact area provides two primary functions[7]: it spreads the joint loading over a broad area, and it permits movement of opposing joint surfaces with

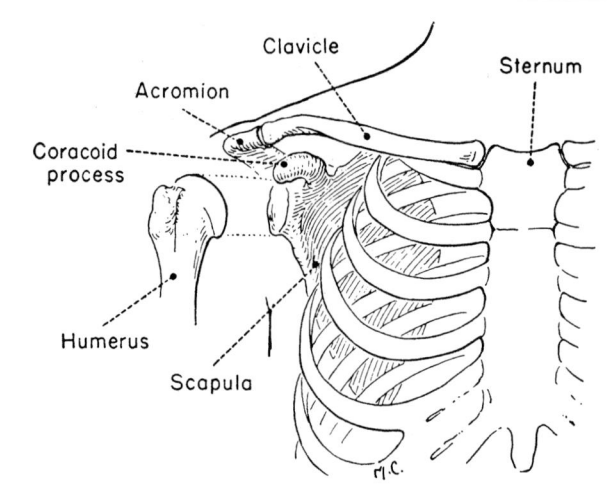

FIGURE 14-1 Bony anatomy of the shoulder. (Reproduced with permission from Luttgens K, Hamilton K. *Kinesiology: Scientific Basis of Human Motion.* New York: McGraw-Hill; 1997.)

minimal friction and wear.[8] Contact between the humeral head and glenoid fossa is significantly reduced when the humerus is positioned in[9–11]:

▶ adduction, flexion, and internal rotation.

▶ abduction and elevation.

▶ adducted at the side, with the scapula rotated downwards.

While the labrum provides some stability for the glenohumeral joint, additional support is provided by a number of other mechanisms. These mechanisms are both dynamic and static. The dynamic mechanisms include the muscles of the rotator cuff (supraspinatus, infraspinatus, teres minor, and subscapularis), and a number of muscle force couples which are described later. The static mechanisms, which include reinforcements of the joint capsule, joint cohesion and geometry, and ligamentous support, are also described later.

The scapula (Fig. 14-2) functions as a stable base from which glenohumeral mobility can occur. The scapula is a flat blade of bone that lies along the thoracic cage at 30 degrees to the frontal plane, 3 degrees superiorly relative to the transverse plane, and 20 degrees forward in the sagittal plane.[12–14] This orientation results in arm elevation occurring in a plane that is 30 to 45 degrees anterior to the frontal plane. When elevation of the arm occurs in this plane, the motion is referred to as scapular plane abduction or scaption. The scapula's wide and thin configuration allows for its smooth gliding along the thoracic wall, and provides a large surface area for muscle attachments both distally and proximally.[15] In all, 16 muscles gain attachment to the scapula (Table 14-1). Six of these muscles, including the trapezius, rhomboids, levator scapulae, and serratus anterior, support and move the scapula, while nine of the others are concerned with G-H motion.[16–18]

Posteriorly, the scapula is divided by the elevated scapula spine into two unequal sized muscle compartments. The

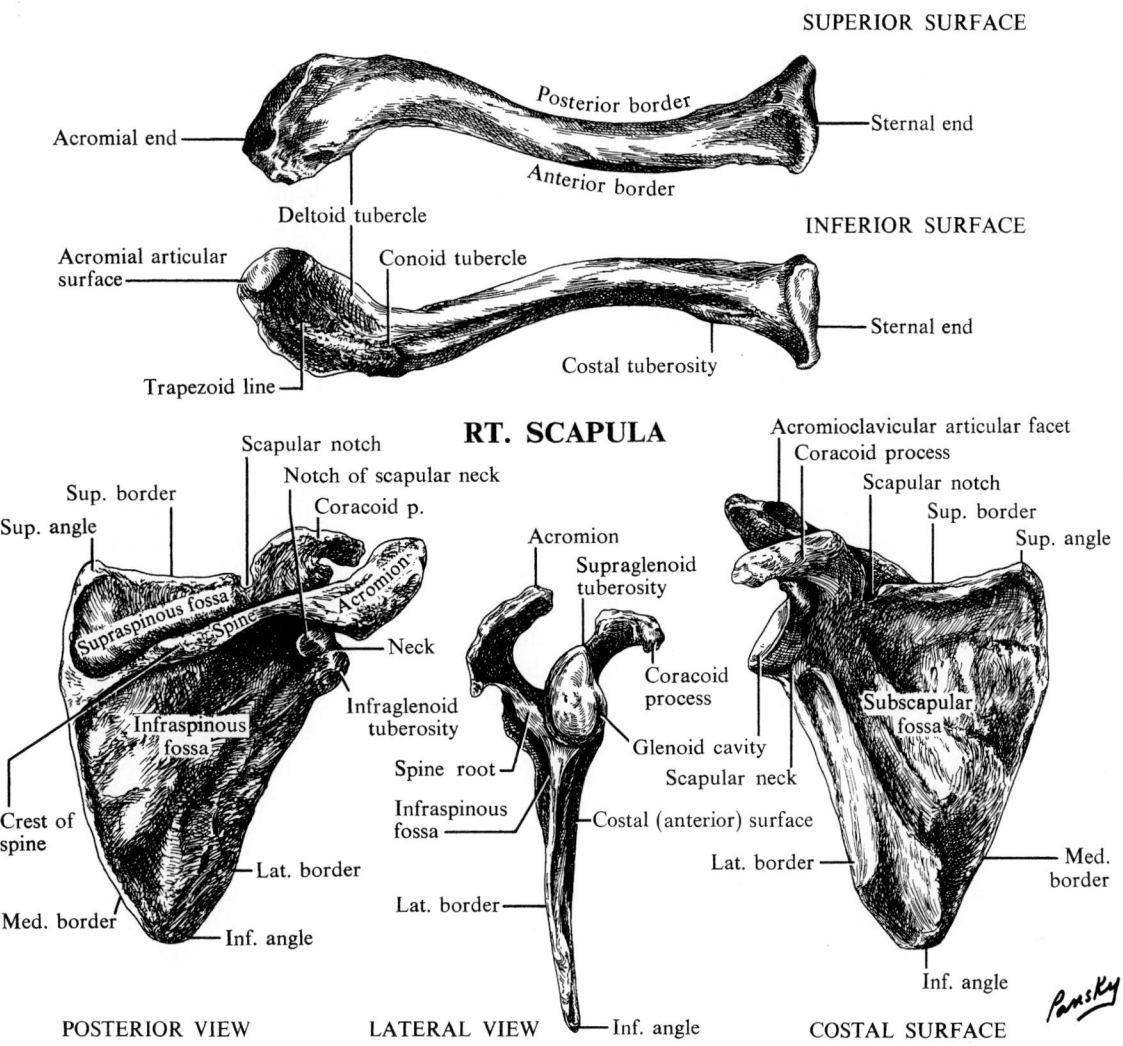

RT. CLAVICLE

SUPERIOR SURFACE

Posterior border

Acromial end

Sternal end

Anterior border

Deltoid tubercle

INFERIOR SURFACE

Acromial articular surface

Conoid tubercle

Sternal end

Trapezoid line

Costal tuberosity

RT. SCAPULA

Scapular notch

Notch of scapular neck

Coracoid p.

Sup. border

Sup. angle

Supraspinous fossa

Spine

Acromion

Neck

Infraspinous fossa

Infraglenoid tuberosity

Crest of spine

Med. border

Lat. border

Inf. angle

Acromion

Supraglenoid tuberosity

Coracoid process

Glenoid cavity

Spine root

Scapular neck

Infraspinous fossa

Costal (anterior) surface

Lat. border

Lat. border

Inf. angle

Acromioclavicular articular facet

Coracoid process

Scapular notch

Sup. border

Sup. angle

Subscapular fossa

Lat. border

Med. border

Inf. angle

POSTERIOR VIEW   LATERAL VIEW   COSTAL SURFACE

FIGURE 14-2 The scapula and clavicle. (Reproduced with permission from Pansky B. *Review of Gross Anatomy*, 6th ed. New York: McGraw-Hill; 1996.)

supraspinous fossa is small and serves as the site of origin for the supraspinatus muscle (see Fig. 14-2). The infraspinous fossa gives attachment for the downward acting infraspinatus and teres minor muscles, important muscles for the stabilization of the humeral head (see "Muscles of the Shoulder Complex" later).

TABLE 14-1   Muscles of the Scapula

Trapezius	Subscapularis
Levator scapulae	Coracobrachialis
Long and short head of the biceps	Pectoralis minor
Rhomboid major (C4,5)	Serratus anterior
Rhomboid minor (C4,5)	Long head of triceps
Supraspinatus	Teres major
Infraspinatus	Teres minor
Deltoid	Omohyoid

The spine of the scapula (see Fig. 14-2) provides a continuous line of attachments for the supporting trapezius muscle along its upper border, while the deltoid muscle, which suspends the humerus, gains origin from its lower border (see Fig. 14-2)[18a]. A prominent feature of the scapula is the large overhanging acromion (see Fig. 14-2), which, along with the coracoacromial ligament and the previously mentioned labrum, functionally enlarges the glenohumeral socket. The position of the acromion also places the deltoid muscle in a dominant position to provide strength during elevation of the arm. Three types of acromion morphology have been described:[14]

▶ Type I has a relatively flat undersurface.

▶ Type II is slightly convex.

▶ Type III is hooked; this anomaly can predispose the shoulder to rotator cuff pathology.[14]

The undersurface of the scapula is covered by the subscapularis muscle, which also assists in stabilizing the humeral head against the glenoid fossa.

The distance, or angle, between the scapula and the clavicle is variable and depends on function. While the shoulder is protracted the angle is 50 degrees. At rest the angle is approximately 60 degrees, and with retraction the angle increases to 70 degrees.[3]

Along the medial border of the scapula arise three muscles: the two rhomboid muscles, and the serratus anterior, all of which aid with scapular stability during arm elevation (see later). The coracoid process (see Fig. 14-2) projects forward like a crow's beak, for which it is named. This forward position provides an efficient lever whereby the small pectoralis muscle can help to stabilize the scapula. In addition, the process serves as a point of origin for the coracobrachialis and the short head of the biceps muscle.

The voluminous joint capsule of the glenohumeral joint allows for large amounts of motion to occur at the G-H joint.[19] The lateral attachment of the glenohumeral joint capsule attaches to the anatomical neck of the humerus. Medially, the capsule is attached to the periphery of the glenoid and its labrum. The overall strength of the joint capsule bears an inverse relationship to the patient's age; the older the patient, the weaker the joint capsule. The fibrous portion of the capsule is very lax and has several recesses, depending on the position of the arm. At its inferior aspect, the capsule forms an axillary recess, which is both loose and redundant. The recess permits normal elevation of the arm, although it can also be the site of adhesions. The tendons of the rotator cuff (supraspinatus, infraspinatus, teres minor and subscapularis) reinforce the superior, posterior, and anterior aspects of the capsule, as does the long head of the biceps tendon. The anterior aspect of the joint capsule is reinforced by three ligaments (Z ligaments), which are described in the next section. An inner synovial membrane lines the fibrous capsule and secretes synovial fluid into the joint cavity. The synovium typically lines the joint capsule and extends from the glenoid labrum down to the neck of the humerus. It also forms variously sized bursae, the largest of which, the subacromial or subdeltoid bursa, lies on the superior aspect of the joint.

The greater and lesser tuberosities, which serve as attachment sites for the tendons of the rotator cuff muscles, are located on the lateral aspect of the anatomical neck of the humerus. The lesser tuberosity serves as the attachment for the subscapularis. The greater tuberosity serves as the attachment for the supraspinatus, infraspinatus, and teres minor. The greater and lesser tuberosities are separated by the intertubercular groove, through which passes the tendon of the long head of the biceps on its route to attach on the superior rim of the glenoid fossa. This groove has wide variance in the angle of its walls, but 70 percent fall within a 60- to 75-degree range.[20] Certain shoulder disorders, including rotator cuff and bicipital tendonitis, have been associated with anomalies of this groove.[21] As the tendon of the long head of the biceps passes over the humeral head from its origin, it makes a right angle turn to lie in the anterior aspect of the humerus. This abrupt turn may permit abnormal wearing of the tendon at this point. The roof of this groove is formed by the transverse ligament. The transverse humeral ligament, which runs perpendicular over the biceps tendon, was once thought to function as a restraint to the biceps tendon within the intertubercular groove. However, this appears to be the role of the coracohumeral ligament.[21]

The region below the greater and lesser tuberosities, where the upper margin of the humerus joins the shaft of the humerus, is referred to as the surgical neck. The axillary nerve and posterior humeral circumflex artery lie in close proximity to the medial aspect of the surgical neck.

Ligaments

A number of ligaments function during motion of the arm to reciprocally tighten and loosen, thereby limiting translation and rotation of the G-H joint in a load-sharing fashion.[25] In the midrange of rotation, these structures are relatively lax and stability is maintained primarily by the action of the rotator cuff muscle group compressing the humeral head into the conforming glenoid articulation (Table 14-2).[25]

At the anterior portion of the outer fibers of the joint capsule, three local reinforcements are present: the superior, middle, and inferior G-H ligaments (Z ligaments) (Fig. 14-3). These ligaments are closely fused to the joint capsule, so that on dissection a thin and sometimes perforated capsule is left. The orientation of these ligaments is described as though looking at the glenoid cavity and picturing an analogue clock superimposed over the cavity.

Superior Glenohumeral Ligament. The superior glenohumeral ligament (see Fig. 14-3) arises from the glenoid rim from approximately 12 or 1 o'clock and runs inferiorly and laterally to insert on the anatomical neck near the medial ridge of the intertubercular groove. It serves to limit external rotation and inferior translation of the humeral head with the arm at the side (0 degrees of abduction) (Tables 14-3 and 14-4). This ligament is present in 90 percent of individuals.[26]

Middle Glenohumeral Ligament. The middle glenohumeral ligament is poorly developed and is often absent. It arises from the glenoid rim from approximately 2 or 3 o'clock and runs inferiorly and laterally to insert on the anatomical neck, medial to the lesser tuberosity. It serves to limit external rotation (see Table 14-4) and anterior translation of the humeral head with the arm in 0 and 45 degrees of abduction (see Fig. 14-3).[27] The middle G-H ligament is present in 70 percent of individuals.[26]

Inferior Glenohumeral Ligament Complex. The inferior glenohumeral ligament (IGHLC), present in 80 percent of individuals,[26] is actually a ligament complex. It consists of an anterior band, which arises from the glenoid between 2 and 4 o'clock and inserts on the humerus below the lesser tuberosity, a posterior band that arises from the glenoid rim between 7 and 9 o'clock,[26] and an axillary pouch. The anterior band of the IGHLC restrains external rotation and inferior translation of the humeral head

TABLE 14-2   Restraints about the Glenohumeral Joint[a]

Passive (Static)	Active (Dynamic)	
Joint capsule and labrum Geometry of humeral and glenoid articular surface Coracohumeral ligament Superior glenohumeral ligament	Supraspinatus Infraspinatus Subscapularis Teres minor	Humeral stabilizers
Middle glenohumeral ligament Inferior glenohumeral ligament Coracoacromial ligament Joint cohesion	Pectoralis major Latissimus dorsi Biceps (long head) Triceps Deltoid Teres major	Movers of glenohumeral joint
	Serratus anterior Latissimus dorsi Trapezius Rhomboids Levator scapulae Pectoralis minor	Movers of scapula

[a] From Magee DJ, Reid DC: Shoulder injuries. In Zachazewski JE, Magee DJ, Quillen WS (eds) Athletic Injuries and Rehabilitation. Philadelphia, WB Saunders, 1996;509–542

FIGURE 14-3   The Z ligaments of the glenohumeral joint. (Reproduced with permission from Skinner HB. *Current Diagnosis and Treatment in Orthopedics*, 2d ed. New York: McGraw-Hill; 2000.)

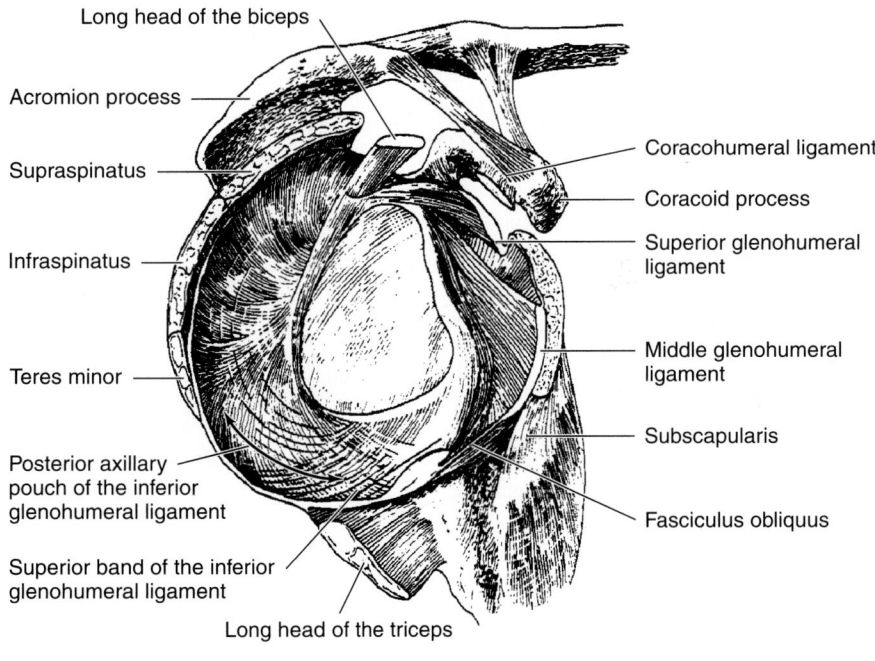

with the arm abducted to 90 degrees (see Tables 14-3, 14-4 and 14-5).[27,28] The posterior band restrains against internal rotation with the arm in all positions of abduction (Table 14-5). The anterior and posterior bands restrain against anterior translation at 90 degrees of abduction.[27] The axillary pouch and then the posterior band become taut in a sequential fashion as the glenohumeral joint moves into the terminal degrees of external rotation from the 90 degrees abducted position.[26]

Other ligaments help provide stability to the G-H joint (see Table 14-2). These include:

▶ The coracohumeral ligament. The coracohumeral ligament (Fig. 14-4) arises from the lateral end of the coracoid process and runs laterally, where it splits into two bands by the presence of the biceps tendon. The posterior band blends with the supraspinatus tendon to insert near the

TABLE 14-3   Static Restraints to Inferior Translation (Dependent on the Position of the Arm)[29,151]

Degrees of Glenohumeral Abduction	Restraining Structures
0	Superior glenohumeral and coracohumeral ligaments
90	Inferior glenohumeral ligament (posterior band in external rotation, anterior band in internal rotation)

TABLE 14-4   Dynamic and Static Restraints to External Rotation (Dependent on the Position of the Arm)[29,152]

Degrees of Glenohumeral Abduction	Restraining Structures
0	Subscapularis, superior glenohumeral and coracohumeral ligaments
45	Subscapularis, middle glenohumeral ligament, superior fibers of the inferior glenohumeral ligament
90	Inferior glenohumeral ligament

TABLE 14-5   Static Restraints to Internal Rotation (Dependent on the Position of the Arm)[29,151]

Degrees of Glenohumeral Abduction	Restraining Structures
0	Posterior band of inferior glenohumeral ligament, teres minor, posterior capsule (superior)
45	Anterior and posterior bands of the inferior glenohumeral ligament
90	Posterior band of the inferior glenohumeral ligament, posterior capsule (inferior)

greater tuberosity, and the anterior band blends with the subscapularis tendon to insert near the lesser tuberosity. The coracohumeral ligament covers the superior G-H ligament anterosuperiorly, and fills the space between the tendons of the supraspinatus and subscapularis muscle, uniting these tendons to complete the rotator cuff in this area. Tears of the cuff usually extend longitudinally between the supraspinatus and coracohumeral ligament, so that the hood action of the cuff is lost. It is generally agreed that the posterior band of the coracohumeral ligament limits flexion, while the anterior band limits extension of the G-H joint.[29] Both

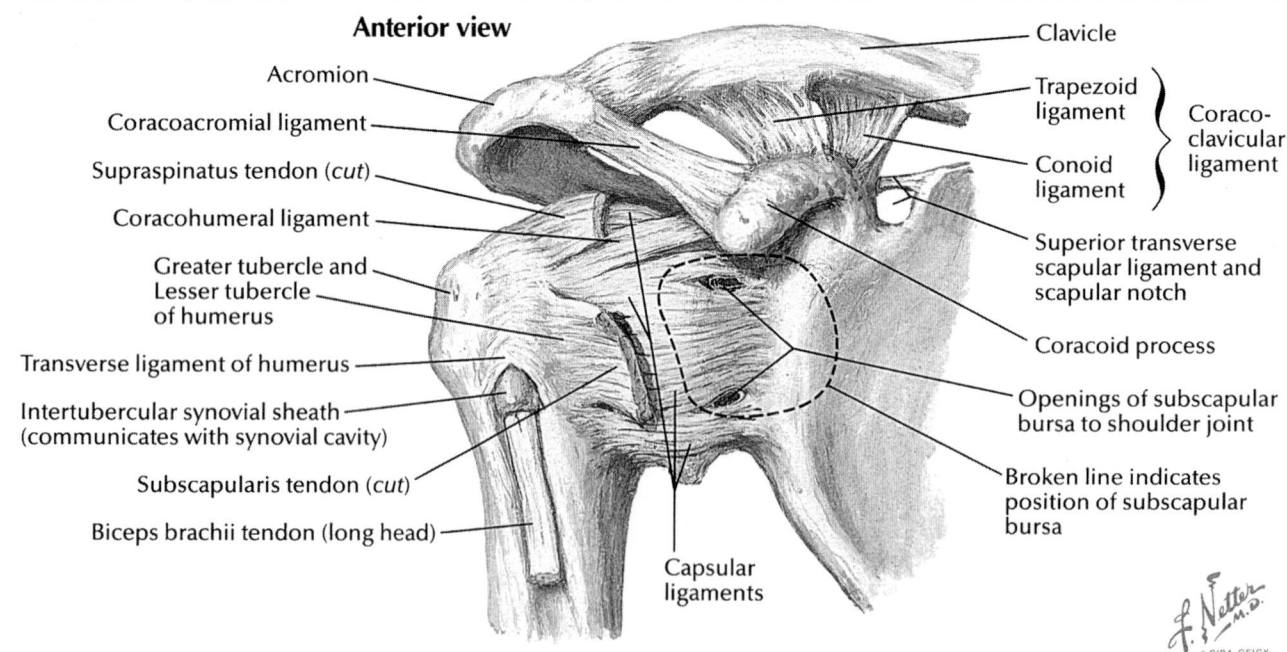

Anterior view

Acromion
Coracoacromial ligament
Supraspinatus tendon (*cut*)
Coracohumeral ligament
Greater tubercle and Lesser tubercle of humerus
Transverse ligament of humerus
Intertubercular synovial sheath (communicates with synovial cavity)
Subscapularis tendon (*cut*)
Biceps brachii tendon (long head)
Capsular ligaments
Clavicle
Trapezoid ligament
Conoid ligament
} Coraco-clavicular ligament
Superior transverse scapular ligament and scapular notch
Coracoid process
Openings of subscapular bursa to shoulder joint
Broken line indicates position of subscapular bursa

FIGURE 14-4   Shoulder complex ligaments. (Reproduced with permission from Netter FH. *Atlas of Human Anatomy*, 4th ed., New Jersey: CIBA-GEIGY; 1992.)

bands also limit inferior and posterior translation of the humeral head, strengthening the superoanterior aspect of the capsule.[29,30]

▶ The coracoacromial ligament. The coracoacromial ligament (see Fig. 14-4) is often described as the roof of the shoulder. It is a very thick structure which runs from the coracoid process to the anteroinferior aspect of the acromion, with some of its fibers extending to the A-C joint. The ligament consists of two bands that join near the acromion, and it is ideally suited, both anatomically and morphologically, to prevent separation of the A-C joint surfaces. The coracoclavicular ligaments and the costoclavicular ligament, are described in the acromioclavicular joint section and the sternoclavicular joint section, respectively.

Coracoacromial Arch

The coracoacromial arch (Fig. 14-5) is formed by the anteroinferior aspect of the acromion process, coracoacromial ligament, and inferior surface of the A-C joint.[31–33] During overhead motion in the plane of the scapula, the supraspinatus tendon, the region of the cuff most involved in overuse syndromes of the shoulder, can pass directly underneath the coracoacromial arch. If the arm is elevated while internally rotated, the supraspinatus tendon passes under the coracoacromial ligament, whereas if the arm is externally rotated, the tendon passes under the acromion itself.[34]

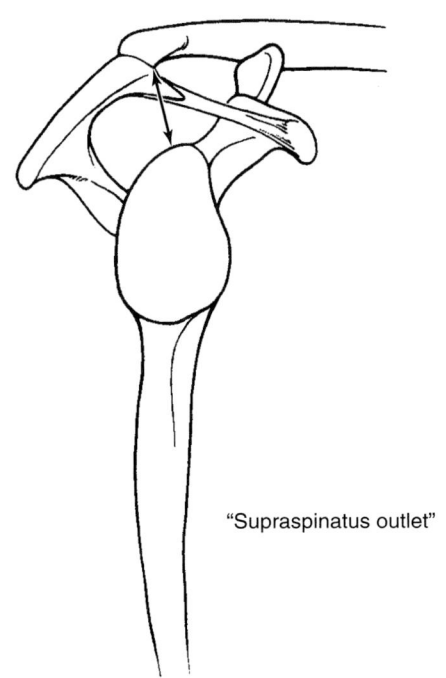

"Supraspinatus outlet"

FIGURE 14-5 Coracoacromial arch. (Reproduced with permission from Skinner HB. *Current Diagnosis and Treatment in Orthopedics*, 2d ed. New York: McGraw-Hill; 2000.)

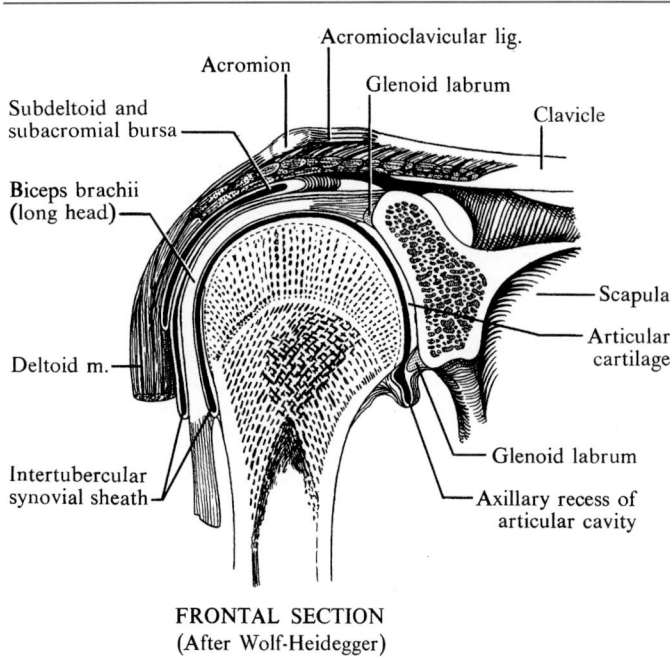

FRONTAL SECTION
(After Wolf-Heidegger)

FIGURE 14-6 Anterior aspect of the shoulder and suprahumeral space. (Reproduced with permission from Pansky B. *Review of Gross Anatomy*, 6th ed. New York: McGraw-Hill; 1996.)

Suprahumeral/Subacromial Space

As the name suggests, the suprahumeral space is an area located on the superior aspect of the G-H joint (Fig. 14-6). The boundaries of the space are formed by:

▶ The tuberosity of the humeral head, inferiorly.

▶ The coracoid process, anteromedially.

▶ The coracoacromial arch, superiorly.

The structures that are located within the suprahumeral space include (from inferior to superior):

▶ The head of the humerus.

▶ The long head of biceps tendon (intra-articular portion).

▶ The superior aspect of the joint capsule.

▶ The supraspinatus and upper margins of subscapularis and infraspinatus.

▶ The subdeltoid-subacromial bursae.

▶ The inferior surface of coracoacromial arch.

In normal individuals, the suprahumeral space averages 10 to 11 mm in height with the arm adducted to the side.[35,36] Elevating the arm decreases the distance between the acromion and the humerus to 5.7 mm at 90 degrees of scaption. The space is at its narrowest between 60 and 120 degrees of scaption.[37] Muscle imbalances or capsular contractures can cause an increase in superior translation of the humeral head, further narrowing the space (see "Subacromial Impingement Syndrome," later).

Bursae

The subdeltoid-subacromial bursae are collectively referred to as the subacromial bursa because they are often continuous in nature. The subacromial bursa is one of the largest bursa in the body and provides two smooth serosal layers, one of which adheres to the overlying deltoid muscle and the other to the rotator cuff lying beneath. This bursa is also connected to the acromion, greater tuberosity, and coracoacromial ligament. As the humerus elevates, it permits the rotator cuff to slide easily beneath the deltoid muscle. There are also smaller bursae interposed between most of the muscles in contact with the joint capsule:

► the subcoracoid bursa. This bursa is located under the coracoid process.

► the subscapular bursa is also significant. It lies between the subscapular muscle tendon and the anterior neck of the scapula, and protects the tendon as it passes under the coracoid process.

Neurology

The shoulder complex is embryologically derived from C5 to C8, except the A-C joint, which is derived from C4.[18a] The sympathetic nerve supply to the shoulder originates primarily in the thoracic region from T2 down as far as T8.[38]

A recent study[39] attempted to determine the variability of the course and the pattern of these nerves, and found that the peripheral nerves contributing to the anterior shoulder joint included the axillary (C5–6), subscapular (C5–6), and lateral pectoral (C5–6). The same study found that the nerves contributing articular branches to the posterior joint structures are the suprascapular nerve (C5–6) and small branches of the axillary nerve.[39] The pathways of these nerves are described in Chap. 2.

Other nerves innervate the muscles that act upon the shoulder. These include the long thoracic nerve (C5–7) which innervates the serratus anterior, the spinal accessory nerve (cranial nerve XI and C3–4) which innervates the sternocleidomastoid and trapezius muscles, and the musculocutaneous nerve (C5–6,7) which innervates the coracobrachialis, biceps brachii, and brachialis, before dividing into its cutaneous branches.

Clinical Pearl

Shoulder pain that persists despite extensive conservative approaches could be of neural origin, as the peripheral nerves that innervate the ligaments, capsule, and bursae of the shoulder joint may have been subject to damage, either at the time of initial trauma or through subsequent surgical intervention.[39–41]

Vascularization

The glenohumeral joint receives its blood supply from the anterior and posterior circumflex humeral as well as the suprascapular and circumflex scapular vessels.[41a] The microvasculature of the rotator cuff has been the subject of much discussion. The vascular supply to the rotator cuff muscles of the shoulder consists of three main sources: the thoracoacromial, suprahumeral, and subscapular arteries.[41a] The supraspinatus receives its primary supply from the thoracoacromial arteries. The subscapularis receives its supply from the anterior humeral circumflex and the thoracoacromial arteries. The posterior rotator cuff muscles, the infraspinatus and teres minor, receive their blood supply from the posterior humeral circumflex and suprascapular artery.

The brachial artery provides the dominant arterial supply to each of the two heads of the biceps. The artery travels in the medial intermuscular septum and is bordered by the biceps muscle anteriorly, the brachialis muscle medially, and the medial head of the triceps muscle posteriorly.[42]

The supraspinatus and biceps tendons appear to be particularly vulnerable to areas of relative avascularity, referred to as *critical zones*. (see "Subacromial Impingement Syndrome" later). The vascular compromise of the supraspinatus is thought to be due to a number of factors:

► it can be directly compressed by the subacromial structures.

► its blood vessels travel parallel to the tendon fibers, which make them vulnerable to stretch.[43]

► the presence of a critical zone just proximal to the supraspinatus insertion point.[44]

Close Packed Position

The close packed position for the G-H joint is 90 degrees of glenohumeral abduction and full external rotation; or full abduction and external rotation, depending on the source.

Open Packed Position

Without internal or external rotation occurring, the open packed position of the G-H joint has traditionally been cited as 55 degrees of semi-abduction and 30 degrees of horizontal adduction.[45] More recently, a cadaver study which examined the point in the range at which maximal capsular laxity occurred in seven subjects, determined the open packed position to be 39 degrees of abduction in the scapular plane, or at the point which is 45 percent of the maximal available abduction range of motion.[46] This finding suggests that the open packed position may be closer to neutral and that the joint mobility testing and joint mobilizations of the G-H joint should be initiated according to a smaller angle of abduction than the traditional open packed position.[46]

The zero position for the G-H joint is the arm relaxed by the side, which relative to the scapula averages about 0 degrees of abduction, 12 degrees of flexion, and 10 degrees of external rotation.[47]

Capsular Pattern

According to Cyriax,[48] the capsular pattern for the G-H joint is that external rotation is the most limited, abduction the next most limited, and internal rotation the least limited in a 3:2:1 ratio, respectively. However, this pattern only appears to be consistent with adhesive capsulitis of the shoulder. Internal rotation, rather than external rotation or abduction, appears to be the most limited motion in conditions with selected capsular hypomobility.[49]

The Acromioclavicular Joint

The acromioclavicular (A-C) joint is a diarthrodial joint, formed by the acromion and the lateral end of the clavicle. The joint serves as the main articulation that suspends the upper extremity from the trunk, and it is at this joint about which the scapula moves. The clavicle also serves as an attachment site for many soft tissues. These include the costoclavicular, conoid, and trapezoid ligaments, and the pectoralis major, sternocleidomastoid, deltoid, and trapezius muscles (see Fig. 14-4).[24,50] When viewed from above the clavicle is convex anteriorly in the medial two thirds, and convex posteriorly in the lateral one third (see Fig. 14-2). The clavicle serves as the lever by which the upper extremity acts on the torso.[50,51] The A-C joint is predisposed to chronic stress injury, especially in the situation in which it is subjected to repetitive high demand.[51,52] The joint can also be affected by direct trauma and by nontraumatic factors such as degenerative arthritis, and inflammatory arthropathies.[50]

In the early stages of development, the articular surfaces of the A-C joint are lined with hyaline cartilage, which changes to fibrocartilage toward the end of adolescence.[51] The shape of the articulating surface of the lateral end of the clavicle can be either convex or concave and corresponds with the articulating surface of the acromion. Consequently, although the joint is described as a planar joint, there is often a male-female relationship. Within the A-C joint, there is variable presence of a thumbtack shaped intra-articular fibrous disk that projects superiorly into, and incompletely divides, the A-C joint. This disk is subject to tearing.[51] Variability in the inclination of the joint is common and can be anywhere from 10 to 50 degrees, but the anteromedial border of the acromion usually faces anteriorly, medially, and superiorly.[53]

The joint has a thin capsule lined with synovium, which is strengthened inferiorly and superiorly by capsular ligaments (see Fig. 14-4). Superiorly, the A-C ligament (see Fig. 14-4) gives support to the capsule and serves as the primary restraint to posterior translation and posterior axial rotation at the joint.[51]

The motions available at this joint occur around three axes:

▶ Rotation in an anterior/posterior direction around a longitudinal axis that projects through the A-C and S-C joints (Fig. 14-7), and rotation in a superoinferior (vertical) direction. The anterior/posterior rotation occurs during arm elevation. The superoinferior rotation, which occurs around the costoclavicular ligament, is involved during protraction (anterior movement of the acromial end of the clavicle and retraction (posterior motion of the acromial end). The anteroposterior rotation of the clavicle on the scapula is three times greater than that of the superoinferior rotation. The clavicle can rotate approximately 30–50 degrees in the anteroposterior direction, most of which is contributed by the mobile sternoclavicular joint. The A-C joint only contributes approximately 5 to 8 degrees to the rotation.[54] The type of glide and rotation that occurs with clavicular motion depends on the shoulder motion and the shape of the articular surfaces. If the lateral end of the clavicle presents a concave surface, an anterior glide is combined with an anterior rotation. If the lateral end presents a convex surface, an anterior glide is combined with a posterior rotation.

▶ Pure spin/rotation. A pure spin occurs during abduction/adduction (lateral and medial rotation of inferior scapula angle) motions.

▶ Glides. Glides of the clavicle can occur in an anteroposterior and superoinferior direction.

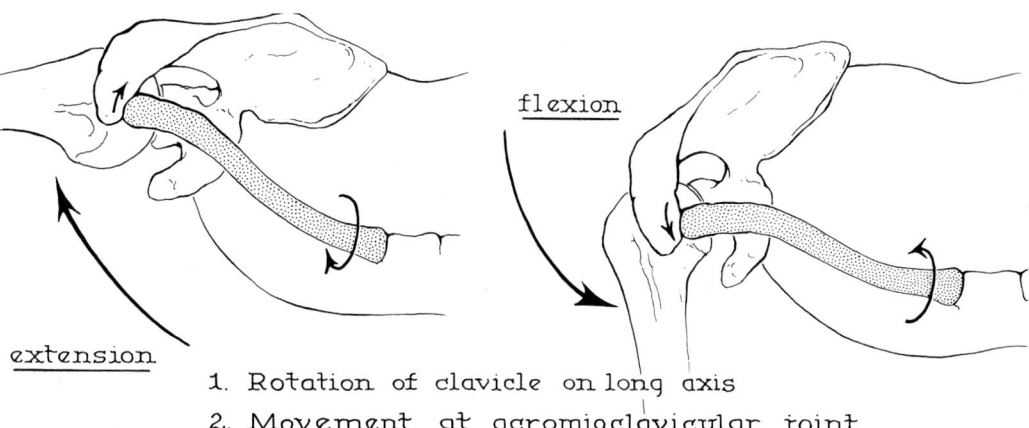

FIGURE 14-7 Clavicular motions. (Reproduced with permission from Bateman JE. *The Shoulder and Neck.* Philadelphia: WB Saunders; 1972.)

extension

flexion

1. Rotation of clavicle on long axis
2. Movement at acromioclavicular joint

Ligaments

The coracoclavicular ligaments (conoid and trapezoid) (see Fig. 14-4) are the primary support for the A-C joint and run from the coracoid process to the inferior surface of the clavicle. These ligaments provide mainly vertical stability, with control of superior and anterior translation as well as anterior axial rotation.[51,55,56]

The conoid ligament (see Fig. 14-4) is fan-shaped with its apex pointing inferiorly. It lies in the frontal plane and is the more medial of the two ligaments. This ligament functions to block coracoid movement away from the clavicle inferiorly.[55]

The trapezoid ligament (see Fig. 14-4) arises from the medial border of the upper surface of the coracoid process and runs superiorly and laterally to insert on the inferior surface of the clavicle. It is larger, longer, and stronger than the conoid, and forms a quadrilateral sheet that lies in a plane that is at right angles to the plane formed by the conoid ligament. The function of this ligament is unclear, although its orientation suggests that it may block medial movement of the coracoid,[55] or act as a restraint to superior or posterior displacement of the clavicle.[57]

In addition, the superior and inferior A-C ligaments (see Fig. 14-4) resist anterior and posterior translation, and provide support to the relatively thin joint capsule.

Neurology

Innervation to this joint is provided by the suprascapular, lateral pectoral, and axillary nerves.[58]

Vascularization

The A-C joint receives its blood supply from branches of the suprascapular and thoracoacromial arteries.[18a]

Capsular Pattern

Joints like the A-C joint, which are not controlled by muscles, lack true capsular patterns. However, anecdotal clinical evidence suggests that the capsular pattern for the A-C joint is pain at the extremes of range of motion, especially horizontal adduction and full elevation.

Close Packed Position

The close pack position for this joint is probably only achievable in the under-30 age group, and clinically seems to correspond to 90 degrees of G-H joint abduction.

Open Packed Position

The open packed position for this joint is undetermined, although it is likely to be when the arm is by the side. This positions the clavicle in approximately 15 to 20 degrees of retraction relative to the coronal plane and elevated about 2 degrees from the horizontal plane.[59]

Sternoclavicular (S-C) Joint

The S-C joint represents the articulation between the medial end of the clavicle, the clavicular notch of the manubrium of the sternum, and the cartilage of the first rib, which forms the floor of the joint (Fig. 14-8). The articulating surfaces of the S-C joint are covered with fibrocartilage. Some confusion seems to exist about classification of the S-C joint—it has been classified as a ball and socket joint,[58] a plane joint,[60] and as a saddle joint.[58] The S-C joint is angulated slightly upward approximately 20 degrees in a posterior and lateral direction. The clavicle presents with an irregularly shaped surface to the meniscus and this lateral part of the joint acts as an ovoid (see Fig. 14-8). If held vertically the proximal end of the clavicle is convex while the manubrium surface is concave (see Fig. 14-8). If held antero-posteriorly, the proximal end of the clavicle is concave and the

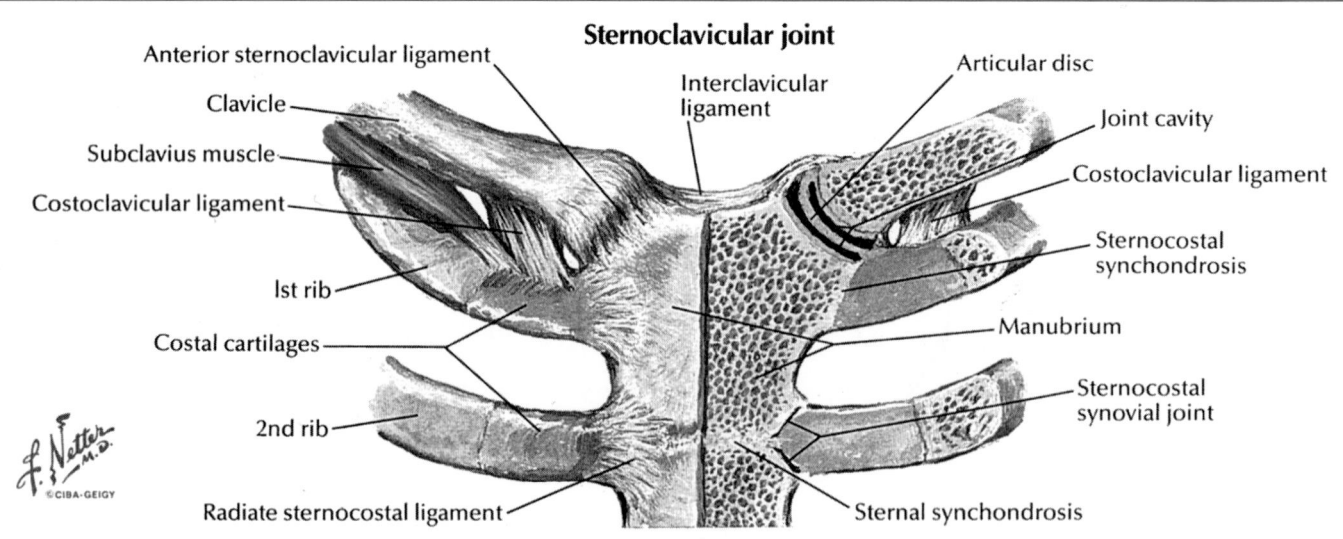

Sternoclavicular joint

Anterior sternoclavicular ligament
Interclavicular ligament
Articular disc
Clavicle
Joint cavity
Subclavius muscle
Costoclavicular ligament
Costoclavicular ligament
Sternocostal synchondrosis
1st rib
Costal cartilages
Manubrium
Sternocostal synovial joint
2nd rib
Sternal synchondrosis
Radiate sternocostal ligament

FIGURE 14-8 The sternoclavicular joint. (Reproduced with permission from Hollinshead WH. *Anatomy for Surgeons*, 2d ed., Vol. 3. New York: Harper & Row; 1969.)

manubrium is convex. A very thick meniscus is the key to the joint curvature. The disk is attached to the upper and posterior margin of the clavicle, and to the cartilage of the first rib (see Fig. 14-8), and functions to help prevent medial displacement of the clavicle. It is thicker peripherally than it is centrally, and completely divides the joint into two cavities: a larger one that is above and lateral to the disk, and a smaller one that is medial and below the disk.[18a] Greater movement occurs between the clavicle and the disk than between the disk and the manubrium.

Ligaments
A number of ligaments provide support to this joint.

Capsular-Ligamentous Structures
Anterior Sternoclavicular Ligament (see Fig. 14-8). This ligament covers the anterior aspect of the joint, running obliquely from the proximal end of the clavicle to the sternum in a downward and medial direction.

Posterior Sternoclavicular Ligament. This ligament covers the posterior aspect of the joint. It is weaker than the anterior ligament, and runs obliquely from the proximal end of the clavicle to the sternum in a downward and medial direction.

Interclavicular (see Fig. 14-8). This ligament connects the superomedial sternal ends of each clavicle with the capsular ligaments and the upper sternum, producing a bilateral depression force.

Costoclavicular (rhomboid ligament) (see Fig. 14-8). This short and strong ligament runs from the upper border of the first rib to the inferior surface of the clavicle and serves as the primary restraint for the S-C joint. The ligament consists of two laminae: fibers of the anterior lamina run upwards and laterally and check elevation and lateral movement (upward rotation) of the clavicle. The posterior lamina fibers run upwards and medially and check downward rotation of the clavicle.

Thus the S-C joint is very stable and trauma to the clavicle usually results in a fracture rather than a joint dislocation.[61] Gross motions occur here as with the A-C joint. The sternocleidomastoid, which can be seen clearly with rotation of the head, has a tendinous sternal and clavicular insertion. The subclavius (C5–6) has a questionable function, but may function as a dynamic ligament, which contracts and pulls the clavicle towards the manubrium. Two types of translation also occur at this joint: anterior to posterior and superior to inferior, with the former exceeding the latter motion by 2:1.[62] These translations allow for three degrees of freedom: the movements of elevation, depression; protrusion, retraction; and upward (backward) and downward (forward) motion.

▶ *Protraction/retraction.* Approximately 15–20 degrees of protraction and retraction of the clavicle are available.

　With protraction, the concave surface of the medial clavicle moves on the convex sternum, producing an ante-

rior glide of the clavicle, and an anterior rotation of the lateral clavicle.[62]

　With retraction to the neutral position, the medial clavicle articulates with a flat surface and tilts/swings, causing an anterolateral gapping, and a posterior rotation at the lateral end.[62]

▶ *Elevation/depression of the clavicle.* There are 35 to 40 degrees of elevation, and approximately 15 degrees of depression available,[3,62,63] involving the convex clavicle gliding on the concave sternum.

As the clavicle elevates and rolls upward on the manubrium, an inferior glide is produced, with the reverse occurring with depression. Elevation and depression movements at the S-C joint are associated with reciprocal motions of the scapula because of the lateral attachment of the clavicle to the scapula at the A-C joint.[24]

Rotation around the long axis produces a spin of the clavicle on the manubrium. Approximately 40 degrees of upward rotation and 5 degrees of downward rotation is available.[3,63]

Close Packed Position
The close packed position for the S-C joint is maximum arm elevation and protraction.

Open Packed Position
The open packed position for the S-C joint has yet to be determined, but is likely to be when the arm is by the side.

Capsular Pattern
Similarly to the A-C joint, the S-C joint is not controlled by muscles and therefore lacks a specific capsular pattern. One possibility, seen clinically, is pain at the extreme ranges of motion, especially full arm elevation and horizontal adduction.

Neurology
Pain can be referred from this joint to the throat, anterior chest, and axillae. The neural supply to this joint is primarily from[64]:

▶ The anterior supraclavicular nerve.

▶ The nerve to the subclavius (medial accessory phrenic) C5–6.

▶ The T1 spinal nerve root.

Vascularization
The S-C joint receives its blood supply from the internal thoracic and suprascapular arteries.[18a]

Scapulothoracic Joint

This articulation is functionally a joint but it lacks the anatomic characteristics of a true synovial joint. A lack of ligamentous support at this "joint" delegates the function of stability fully to the muscles that attach the scapula to the thorax.

An altered position of the scapula has been linked with shoulder complex dysfunction.[15,65–67] Motions at this joint are described according to the movement of the scapula relative to the thorax. Available motion consists of approximately 60 degrees of upward rotation of the scapula, 40 to 60 degrees of internal/external rotation, and 30 to 40 degrees of anterior and posterior tipping of the scapula.[68] Other motions occurring here include elevation and depression and adduction and abduction of the scapula (Fig. 14-9).

Close Packed and Capsular Pattern

Because the scapulothoracic joint is not a true joint, it does not have a close packed position or a capsular pattern.

Open Packed Position

Relative to the thorax, when the arm is by the side, the scapula is in an average of 30 to 45 degrees of internal rotation, and slight upward rotation, and approximately 5 to 20 degrees of anterior tipping.[47,68]

Bursae

There are a number of bursae located in and around the scapulothoracic articulation. The scapulothoracic bursa is located between the thoracic cage and the deep surface of the serratus anterior.[69] The subscapular bursa (see Fig. 14-4) is most often located between the superficial surface of the serratus anterior and the subscapularis.[69]

The scapulotrapezial bursa, lies between the middle and lower trapezius fibers and the superomedial scapula.[69] The purpose and clinical significance of the scapulotrapezial bursa are not known. It may encourage smooth gliding of the superomedial angle of the scapula against the undersurface of the trapezius during scapular rotation in the same manner that the scapulothoracic bursa (between the serratus attachment at

FIGURE 14-9 Movements of the shoulder girdle. a. Elevation. b. Abduction (combined with lateral tilt and upward rotation). c. Upward rotation. d. Upward tilt. (Reproduced with permission from Luttgens K, Hamilton K. *Kinesiology: Scientific Basis of Human Motion*. New York: McGraw-Hill; 1997.)

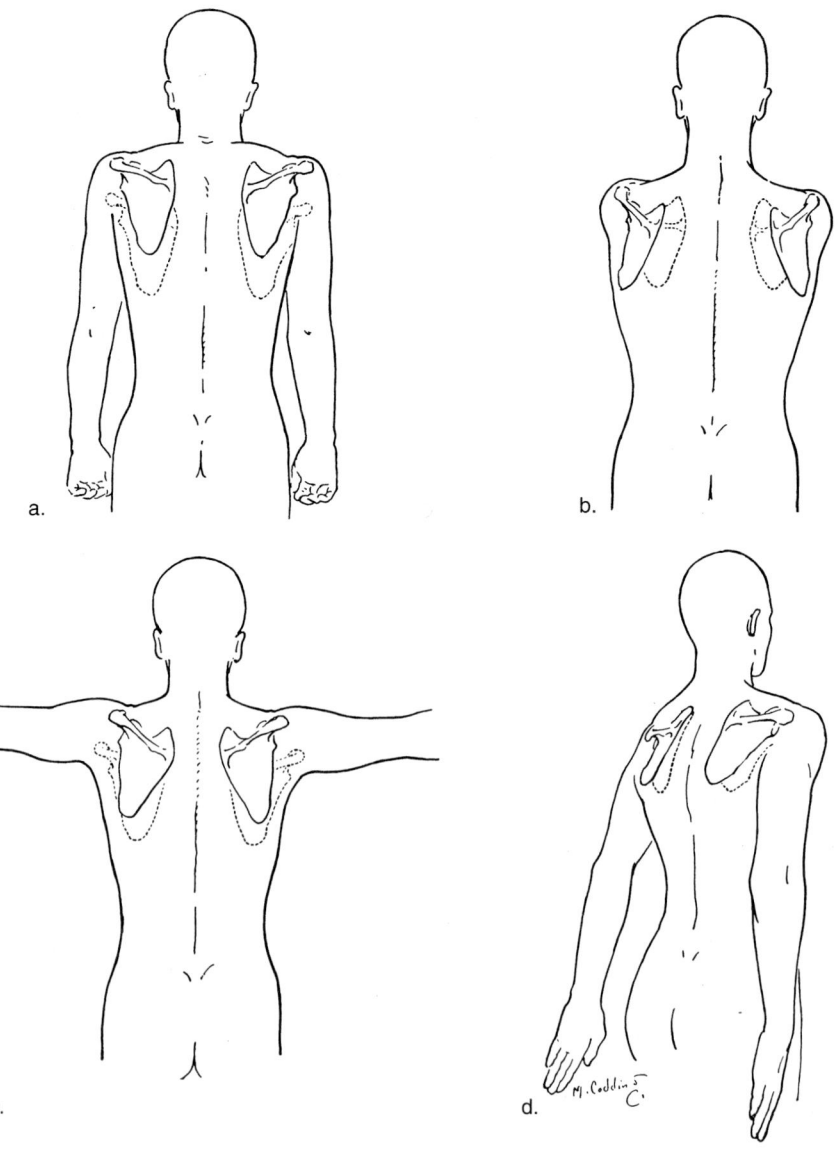

the anteromedial surface of the superior angle) encourages smooth gliding against the underlying ribs.[69] It is possible that inflammation of either of these bursae, directly or as a consequence of injury, may result in painful clicking at the superomedial angle of the scapula.[69]

The relationship of the spinal accessory nerve to the scapulotrapezial bursa also may have clinical importance, especially as it is closely applied to the superficial wall of the scapulotrapezial bursa.[69] The spinal accessory nerve receives afferent fibers from C3 and C4, which are thought to be proprioceptive, before reaching the deep surface of the trapezius.[69,70] As a consequence of their proximity, inflammation and fibrosis within the bursa may cause irritation and pain of the nerve, or interference with the normal proprioceptive feedback mechanism provided by the nerve.[69]

Muscles of the Shoulder Complex

A number of significant muscles control motion at the shoulder (Table 14-6). For simplicity, the muscles acting at the shoulder may be described in terms of their functional roles: scapular pivoters, humeral propellers, humeral positioners, and shoulder protectors.[71]

Scapular Pivoters

The scapular pivoters comprise the trapezius, serratus anterior, levator scapulae, rhomboid major, and rhomboid minor.[71] As a group, these muscles are involved with motions at the scapulothoracic articulation, and their proper function is vital to the normal biomechanics of the whole shoulder complex.

Trapezius. The trapezius muscle (Fig. 14-10) originates from the medial third of the superior nuchal line, the external occipital protuberance, the ligamentum nuchae, the apices of the seventh cervical vertebra, all the thoracic spinous processes, and the supraspinous ligaments of the cervical and thoracic vertebrae. The upper fibers descend to attach to the lateral third of the posterior border of the clavicle. The middle fibers of the trapezius run horizontally to the medial acromial margin and superior lip of the spine of the scapula. The inferior fibers ascend to attach to an aponeurosis gliding over a smooth triangular surface at the medial end of the spine of the scapula to a tubercle at the scapular lateral apex.

It has been suggested that the upper fibers of this muscle have a different motor supply than the middle and lower portions.[72,73] Recent clinical and anatomical evidence seems to

TABLE 14-6 Muscles of the Shoulder Complex According to Their Actions on the Scapula and at the Glenohumeral Joint

Scapular abductors	*Shoulder abductors*
Trapezius	Supraspinatus
Serratus anterior (upper fibers)	Deltoid
Scapular adductors	*Shoulder adductors*
Levator scapulae	Subscapularis
Rhomboids	Pectoralis major
	Latissimus dorsi
Scapular flexors	Teres major
Serratus anterior (lower fibers)	Teres minor
Scapular extensors	*Shoulder internal rotators*
Pectoralis minor	Pectoralis major and minor
	Serratus Anterior
Scapular external rotators	Subscapularis
Trapezius	Pectoralis major
Rhomboids	Latissimus dorsi
	Teres major
The shoulder flexors	
Coracobrachialis	*Shoulder external rotators*
Short head biceps	Infraspinatus
Long head biceps	Supraspinatus
Pectoralis major	Deltoid
Anterior deltoid	Teres minor
The shoulder extensors	
The triceps	
Posterior deltoid	
Teres minor	
Teres major	
Latissimus dorsi	

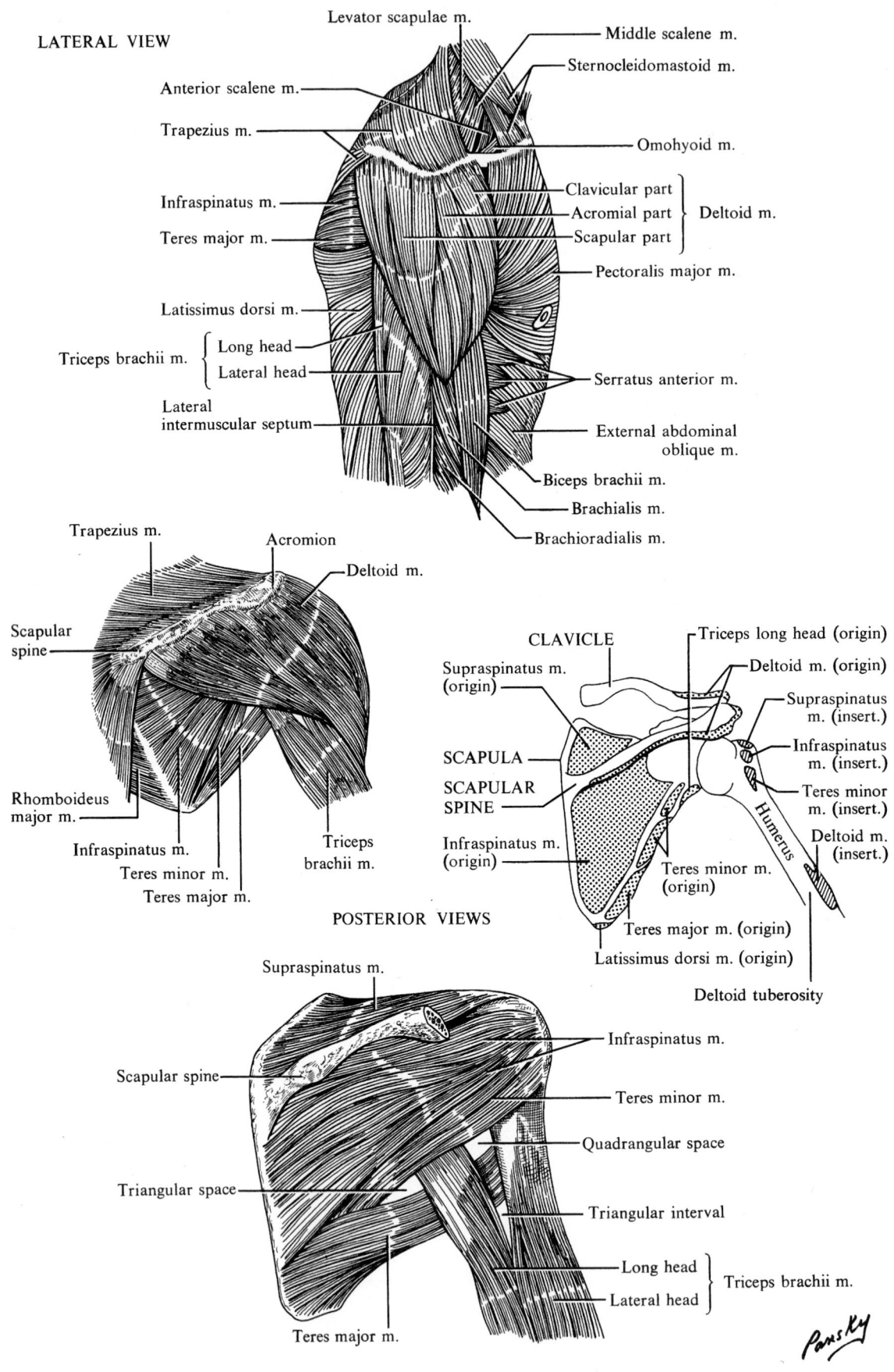

LATERAL VIEW

Levator scapulae m.

Middle scalene m.

Sternocleidomastoid m.

Anterior scalene m.

Trapezius m.

Omohyoid m.

Infraspinatus m.

Clavicular part
Acromial part — Deltoid m.
Scapular part

Teres major m.

Pectoralis major m.

Latissimus dorsi m.

Triceps brachii m. { Long head / Lateral head

Serratus anterior m.

Lateral intermuscular septum

External abdominal oblique m.

Biceps brachii m.

Brachialis m.

Brachioradialis m.

Trapezius m.

Acromion

Deltoid m.

Scapular spine

CLAVICLE

Triceps long head (origin)

Supraspinatus m. (origin)

Deltoid m. (origin)

Supraspinatus m. (insert.)

SCAPULA

Infraspinatus m. (insert.)

SCAPULAR SPINE

Teres minor m. (insert.)

Rhomboideus major m.

Infraspinatus m. (origin)

Deltoid m. (insert.)

Infraspinatus m.

Teres minor m.

Teres major m.

Triceps brachii m.

Teres minor m. (origin)

Humerus

Teres major m. (origin)

Latissimus dorsi m. (origin)

Deltoid tuberosity

POSTERIOR VIEWS

Supraspinatus m.

Scapular spine

Infraspinatus m.

Teres minor m.

Quadrangular space

Triangular space

Triangular interval

Long head
Lateral head } Triceps brachii m.

Teres major m.

FIGURE 14-10   The muscles of the shoulder complex. (Reproduced with permission from Pansky B. *Review of Gross Anatomy*, 6th ed. New York: McGraw-Hill; 1996.)

suggest that the spinal accessory nerve provides the most important and consistent motor supply to all portions of the trapezius muscle, and that although the C2–4 branches of the cervical plexus are present, no particular elements of innervation within the trapezius have been determined.[74]

One of the functions of the trapezius is to produce shoulder girdle elevation on a fixed cervical spine. For the trapezius to perform its actions, the cervical spine must be stabilized by the anterior neck flexors to prevent simultaneous occipital extension from occurring. Failure to prevent this occipital extension would allow the head to translate anteriorly, resulting in a decrease in the length, and therefore the efficiency, of the trapezius,[75] and an increase in the cervical lordosis.

Serratus Anterior. The muscular digitations of the serratus anterior (see Fig. 14-10), originate from the upper 8 to 10 ribs and fascia over the intercostals. The muscle is composed of three functional components.[76,77]

▶ The upper component originates from the first and second ribs and inserts on the superior angle of the scapula.

▶ The middle component arises from the second, third, and fourth ribs, and inserts along the anterior aspect of the medial scapular border.

▶ The lower component is the largest and most powerful, originating from the fifth through ninth ribs. It runs anterior to the scapula, and inserts on the medial border of the scapula.

The serratus anterior is activated with all shoulder movements, but especially during shoulder flexion and abduction.[77] Working in synergy with the trapezius, as part of a force couple (see later), the main function of the serratus anterior is to protract and upwardly rotate the scapula,[78,79] while providing a strong, mobile base of support to position the glenoid optimally for maximum efficiency of the upper extremity.[80] Its lower fibers draw the lower angle of the scapula forward to rotate the scapula upward while maintaining the scapula on the thorax during arm elevation.[81] This moves the coracoacromial arch out of the path of the advancing greater tuberosity, and opposes the excessive elevation of the scapula by the levator scapulae and trapezius muscles.[82] Dysfunction of serratus anterior muscle causes winging of the scapula as the patient attempts to elevate the arm.[4,83] Without upward rotation and protraction of the scapula by the serratus anterior, full glenohumeral elevation is not possible. In fact, in patients with complete paralysis of the serratus anterior, Gregg and colleagues[80] reported that abduction is limited to 110 degrees.

Scapulothoracic dysfunction can also contribute to glenohumeral instability, as the normal stable base of the scapula is destabilized during abduction or flexion.[4,84,85]

The serratus anterior muscle is innervated by the long thoracic nerve (C5–7).

Levator Scapulae. The levator scapulae muscle (see Fig. 14-11) originates by tendonous strips from the transverse processes of the atlas, axis, C3 and C4 vertebrae, and descends diagonally to insert on the medial superior angle of the scapula.

The levator scapulae can act on the cervical spine (see Chap. 23) and on the scapula. If it acts on the cervical spine, it can produce extension, side flexion, and rotation of the cervical spine to the same side.[86] When acting on the scapula during upper extremity flexion or abduction, the levator scapula muscle acts as an antagonist to the trapezius muscle, and provides eccentric control of scapular upward rotation in the higher ranges of motion.[87]

Both the trapezius and levator scapulae muscles are activated with increased upper extremity loads.[75,77,88]

The levator scapulae muscle is innervated by the dorsal scapular nerve (C3–5).

Rhomboids. The rhomboid major muscle (Fig. 14-11) originates from the 2nd–5th thoracic spinous processes and the overlying supraspinous ligaments. The fibers descend to insert on the medial scapular border between the root of the scapular spine and the inferior angle of the scapula.

The rhomboid minor muscle (see Fig. 14-11) originates from the lower ligamentum nuchae, and the 7th cervical and first thoracic spinous processes, and attaches to the medial border of the scapula at the root of the spine of the scapula.

The rhomboid muscles help control scapular positioning, particularly with horizontal flexion and extension of the shoulder complex.[87]

The rhomboid muscles are innervated by the dorsal scapular nerve (C4–5).

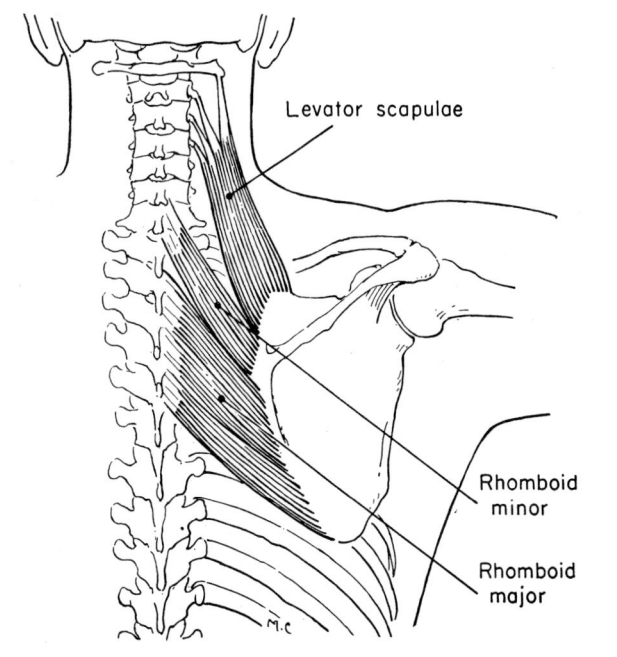

FIGURE 14-11 Rhomboid major and minor. (Reproduced with permission from Luttgens K, Hamilton K. *Kinesiology: Scientific Basis of Human Motion.* New York: McGraw-Hill; 1997.)

Humeral Propellers

Latissimus Dorsi.   The latissimus dorsi muscle (see Fig. 14-10) originates from the spinous processes of the last six thoracic vertebrae, the lower three or four ribs, the lumbar and sacral spinous processes through the thoracolumbar fascia, the posterior third of the external lip of the iliac crest, and a slip from the inferior scapular angle. The scapular slip allows the latissimus dorsi to act at the scapulothoracic articulation. The latissimus dorsi inserts on the intertubercular sulcus of the humerus. The muscle functions as an extensor, adductor, and powerful internal rotator of the shoulder, and also assists in scapular depression, retraction, and downward rotation.[89] It is innervated by the thoracodorsal nerve (C6–8).

Pectoralis Major.   The pectoralis major (see Fig. 14-10) originates from the sternal half of the clavicle, half of the anterior surface of the sternum to the level of the sixth or seventh costal cartilage, the sternal end of the sixth rib, and the aponeurosis of the obliquus externus abdominis. The fibers of the pectoralis major converge to form a tendon that inserts on the lateral lip of the intertubercular sulcus of the humerus. Although this muscle does not insert on the scapula, it does act upon the scapulothoracic articulation through its insertion on the humerus.

The pectoralis major is innervated by the medial and lateral pectoral nerves (C5–T1).

Clinical Pearl

The pectoralis major and latissimus dorsi muscles are referred to as *humeral propeller* muscles as they have been shown to be the only muscles in the upper extremity to have a positive correlation between peak torque and pitching velocity, and during the propulsive phase of the swim stroke.

Pectoralis Minor.   The pectoralis minor (see Fig. 14-10) originates from the outer surface of the upper margins of the third to fifth ribs near their cartilage. The fibers of the pectoralis minor ascend laterally, converging to a tendon that inserts on the coracoid process of the scapula.

The pectoralis minor muscle is innervated by the medial pectoral nerve (C6–8).

Humeral Positioners

Deltoid.   The deltoid muscle originates from the lateral third of the clavicle, the superior surface of the acromion, and the spine of the scapula (see Fig. 14-10). It inserts into the deltoid tuberosity of the humerus. The deltoid can be described as three separate muscles, anterior, middle, and posterior, all of which function as humeral positioners, positioning the humerus in space.[71]

The deltoid muscle is innervated by the axillary nerve (C5–6).

Shoulder Protectors

Rotator Cuff.   The rotator cuff muscles (see Fig. 14-10), which consist of the supraspinatus, infraspinatus, teres minor, and

subscapularis, are commonly involved with shoulder pathology. The anatomy of these muscles was described previously (see Glenohumeral Joint). These muscles are referred to as the protectors of the shoulder since they fine-tune the humeral head position during arm elevation.[71] The rotator cuff muscles have an important role in the function of the shoulder and serve to:

▶ Assist in the rotation of the shoulder and arm.

▶ Reinforce the glenohumeral capsule. For example, firing of the rotator cuff muscles increases the tension of the middle glenohumeral ligament when the arm is abducted to 45 degrees and externally rotated.[29]

▶ Hold the humeral head securely in the glenoid cavity, which provides stability to the joint, and also maintains a mechanically efficient fulcrum for elevation of the arm.

The rotator cuff muscles function as contractile ligaments together with the coracohumeral ligament, and the long head of the biceps (often referred to as the fifth rotator cuff muscle).

Biceps Brachii.   The biceps brachii muscle is a large fusiform muscle in the anterior compartment of the upper extremity, which has two tendinous origins from the scapula. The medial head and long head originate from the coracoid process and supraglenoid tubercle of the scapula, respectively. The two heads join and insert into the radial tuberosity by a common tendon.[90] The medial tendon is interarticular, lying inside the glenohumeral capsule.[31–33] This tendon is not as common a source of shoulder pain as the long tendon, and rarely ruptures.[31–33]

The function of the biceps as a forearm supinator and secondarily as an elbow flexor is well known.[91] At the shoulder joint, however, the function of this muscle is less clear.[92] Compounding this question is the theory that the majority of bicipital symptoms occur secondary to other shoulder pathologies such as bursitis, impingement, instability, and labral pathology.[32] Cadaveric studies have suggested that at the shoulder the biceps functions as a humeral head depressor, an anterior stabilizer, a posterior stabilizer, a limiter of external rotation, a lifter of the glenoid labrum, and a humeral head compressor of the shoulder.[93–96]

The biceps brachii muscle is innervated by the musculocutaneous nerve.

Biomechanics

The G-H joint has three degrees of freedom: flexion/extension, abduction/adduction, and internal/external rotation. Available ranges of motion *at the glenohumeral joint* are approximately as follows:

▶ *Flexion and abduction.*   Approximately 100–120 degrees are available, with females demonstrating more motion than males

▶ *External rotation.*   Approximately 60–80 degrees are available, with females demonstrating more motion than males

▶ *Internal rotation.* Approximately 80–90 degrees are available, with females demonstrating more motion than males

▶ *Extension.* Great variability exists with extension, with ranges existing from 10 to 90 degrees.

Glenohumeral motions (Tables 14-7 and 14-8) consist of a combination of glides and rolls based on the concave-convex rule (see Chap. 11). At the G-H joint, the concave-convex rule dictates the articulating surface to move in the opposite direction of the shoulder motion (Table 14-9). Motions at this joint do not occur in isolation, but rather as coupled motions.[102a] For example, external rotation and abduction occur with flexion, and external rotation and adduction accompanies extension.[102b]

Complete movement at the shoulder girdle involves a complex interaction between the glenohumeral, A-C, sternoclavicular, scapulothoracic, upper thoracic, costal, and sternomanubrial joints, and the lower cervical spine. Within the joints of the shoulder complex, there appear to be no well-defined points within the range where one joint's motion ends and another begins. Rather, they all blend into a smooth harmonious movement during elevation.

During shoulder rotation and arm activities, the scapula invariably acts as a platform upon which the activities are based. It is worth noting that the supporting structures of the glenohumeral joint are only effective if the scapula can maintain its range of motion with the humerus (see The Scapulohumeral Rhythm, later).

The G-H joint has been described as being similar to a golf ball on a tee due to the size relationships. A more accurate biomechanical description is that the G-H joint is like a ball on a seal's nose.[22] As the ball or humeral socket moves, the seal's nose, or the scapula, needs to move to maintain the position of the ball on the glenoid. The orientation of the G-H joint causes motions at this joint to occur in the scapular plane (approximately 30 to 45 degrees anterior to the frontal plane). The shoulder has the greatest range of motion of any joint, with a vast array of muscles producing those motions.[1] The correct function of these muscles is dependent on length-tension relationships, and coordinated activation.[97] Over 1,600 different positions in three-dimensional space can be assumed by the shoulder.[98,99] Due to this wide range of motion, the G-H joint is faced with the task of maintaining equilibrium between functional mobility and adequate stability.[100]

The complex kinematics of this region probably account for the fact that strains and sprains may remain symptomatic for much longer than in other joints.[1]

Full elevation of the arm occurs through an arc of approximately 180 degrees, and can occur in an infinite number of body planes.[101] Locally, this motion is a result of abduction of the G-H joint and upward rotation of the scapulothoracic joint. During abduction of the shoulder, the G-H joint is reported to contribute up to 120 degrees of the total arc of motion, with the remaining 60 degrees occurring at the scapulothoracic joint (see scapulohumeral rhythm, later). Arm elevation beyond 90 degrees requires motion in other, more distal joints such as the A-C, and S-C joint, and the vertebral joints of the upper thorax and lower cervical spine (Tables 14-7 and 14-8).

Glenohumeral Joint Arthrokinematics

Flexion at the glenohumeral joint involves a pure spin. However, although flexion involves a pure spin, elevation of the arm in the scapular plane involves a combination of flexion, abduction, and external rotation. Thus, at the joint surface of the glenohumeral joint during arm elevation, the head of the humerus spins (flexion component), glides inferiorly (abduction component), and glides anteriorly (external rotation component) (Table 14-9).

Functional Movements

Depending on the type of function performed, motions of the shoulder complex involve both local motions and motions at other joints.

Kibler[102] labels the motions that occur in other joints of the body during an activity such as throwing (i.e., trunk and hip rotation) as *distant functions*. In contrast, those motions occurring at the shoulder during the same activity (i.e., glenohumeral external rotation) are termed *local functions*.

Distant Functions[102]

The majority of shoulder motions involve a series of sequentially activated links in a kinetic chain of body segments.[99,103] For those motions requiring more force, the number of links in the kinetic chain increases. The sequence of activation starts as a ground reaction force and moves up through the knees and hips to the trunk, and into the shoulder. Approximately 50 percent of the total kinetic energy and force occurring at the G-H joint originates from a combination of the ground reaction force and the forces from the legs and hips.[99,103,104] At the shoulder, glenohumeral, A-C, S-C, and scapulothoracic motion occurs simultaneously, as a result of muscle action and ligamentous tension in these joints. The specific sequence of muscle activation in the upper extremity depends on the activity, although the direction of activation is usually from proximal to distal as this is the most efficient method for producing large forces and accelerations to the arm. As part of this activation sequence, specific muscle activation patterns and joint positions are developed depending on the activity. Any changes to this sequence of activation can produce an abnormal movement pattern, involving substitution or compensation from the more distal links.[105,106] For example, a throwing athlete with decreased trunk rotation due to stiffness has to rely more on the shoulder to provide the force for the throw. These adaptive patterns eventually result in either decreased performance, or increased injury risk.

Local Functions

The G-H joint accounts for approximately two thirds of all shoulder motions with the remainder provided by the scapulothoracic joint.[63] For full motion at these joints to occur, a complex interaction between the deltoid, rotator cuff, long head of the biceps, glenohumeral capsule, glenoid articulating cartilage, and scapular pivoters (trapezius, serratus anterior, levator scapulae, and rhomboids) is required.[102]

TABLE 14-7   Contributors to Glenohumeral Abduction

Degree of Abduction	Biomechanics Involved
0–90	The concerted action of the active stabilizers (deltoid, biceps, and rotator cuff muscles) and the passive restraints (articular surfaces, osseous structures, and ligaments) is necessary for the purposeful function of the shoulder articulation. The supraspinatus contracts to initiate abduction of the glenohumeral joint.[a] The remaining rotator cuff muscles also contract to pull the humeral head into the glenoid fossa. At approximately 20 degrees of humeral abduction, scapular upward rotation begins with concurrent clavicular elevation and axial rotation.[b,c] At approximately 90°, or a little more in females, the upper extreme of glenohumeral abduction is reached, and clavicular elevation ceases due to tension of the costoclavicular ligament.[d] Continued abduction of the humerus requires continued upward rotation of the scapula, which by this point has rotated through a range of approximately 30 degrees.[e]
90–150	As the scapula upwardly rotates on the posterior chest wall, the glenoid fossa faces upwards and laterally, and its inferior angle moves laterally through about 60°. The scapular contribution peaks between 90 and 140 degrees.[f] The scapular upward rotation is accommodated at both the sternoclavicular and A-C joints by a posterior axial rotation of the clavicle of 30–40 degrees and a clavicular elevation of approximately 30–36 degrees.[c] The muscles producing this movement are the serratus anterior and trapezius, acting as a couple on the scapulothoracic joint. The movement is limited by the acromion and sternoclavicular joints, and by the scapular and humeral adductors (notably latissimus dorsi and pectoralis major).
150–180	Abduction beyond 150 degrees requires adequate motion at the vertebral joints of the upper thorax and cervical spine.[g] Bilateral abduction demands that the thoracic spine extend and the lumbar lordosis increase.

[a] Poppen NK, Walker PS: Forces at the glenohumeral joint in abduction. *Clin Orthop* 1978;135;165–170.
[b] Poppen NK, Walker PS: Normal and abnormal motion of the shoulder. *J Bone Joint Surg* 1976;58A:195–201.
[c] Saha AK: Mechanisms of shoulder movements and a plea for the recognition of "Zero Position" of the glenohumeral joint. *Clin Orthop* 1983;173:3–10.
[d] Freedman L, Munro RR: Abduction of the arm in the scapular plane: Scapular and glenohumeral movements. *J Bone Joint Surg* 1966;48A:1503–1510.
[e] Abelew T: Kinesiology of the shoulder. In: Tovin BJ, Greenfield B, eds. *Evaluation and Treatment of the Shoulder—An Integration of the Guide to Physical Therapist Practice*. Philadelphia: FA Davis; 2001:25–44.
[f] Doody SG, Freedman L, Waterland JC: Shoulder movements during abduction in the scapular plane. *Arch Phys Med Rehabil* 1970;51:595–604.
[g] Kapandji IA: *The Physiology of the Joints, Upper Limb*. New York: Churchill Livingstone; 1991.

Clinical Pearl

During approximately the first 150 degrees of arm elevation through flexion:

- The upper and lower fibers of the trapezius contract concentrically.
- The fibers of the lower serratus anterior contract concentrically.
- The levator scapulae contracts eccentrically.
- The rhomboids contract eccentrically.

From approximately 150 to 180 degrees:

- The lower fibers of the serratus anterior contract isometrically.
- The lower fibers of the trapezius contract concentrically.
- The pectoralis minor contracts eccentrically.
- The upper fibers of the serratus anterior contract eccentrically.

Stabilization of the Static Shoulder.   The dependent shoulder requires very little muscular support with only the trapezius and supraspinatus being active. Its vertical stability is a result of the inferior-lateral projection and upward inclination of the glenoid fossa, which is maintained by a mild contraction of the fibers of the trapezius. It was traditionally theorized that the humeral head was prevented from rolling off of this lateral projection by a moderate contraction of the supraspinatus and the deltoid.[95,107] More recent studies have demonstrated that the muscle tone of the rotator cuff is not a significant contributor to the static inferior stability of the dependent shoulder with light loads, but that maintenance of the intra-articular pressure, and the adhesion and cohesion properties of the articular surfaces are far more significant.[108,109] However, the rotator cuff does provide a passive restraint to translation, especially to posterior translation, during the early to midranges of elevation.[110]

During the midranges and end ranges of motion, a combination of several different static restraints create a vector that keeps the humerus securely seated at the glenoid, through concavity-compression (see Tables 14-2, 14-3, 14-4, and 14-5).[98,102,108,111–113] Static restraints include the anatomic curvature of the humerus and glenoid, the extra depth of the

TABLE 14-8 Contributors to Glenohumeral Elevation

Degree of Elevation and Main Contributor	Biomechanics Involved
0–60°—Glenohumeral elevation	A combined motion of flexion, abduction, and lateral rotation occurs at the glenohumeral joint, produced by the anterior deltoid, coracobrachialis, and the clavicular fibers of pectoralis major. Motion is limited by the increasing tension in the posterior coracohumeral ligament and the stretching of the shoulder extensors, adductors, and external rotators.[a]
60–120°—Sternoclavicular and acromioclavicular elevation	The scapula depresses, protracts, and abducts on the posterior thoracic wall, such that the glenoid fossa faces anteriorly and superiorly and its inferior angle faces laterally and anteriorly. This motion is accommodated by the S-C and A-C joints. The scapulothoracic motion is produced in the same manner as with abduction, by the serratus anterior and trapezius, and is limited by the ligaments of the two joints and the tension in the shoulder extensor and adductor musculature.[a]
120–180°—Costospinal elevation	Kapandji[b] states that the extreme of flexion is the same as the extreme of abduction. That is, during unilateral elevation, the lateral displacement is produced by the contralateral spinal muscles while bilateral abduction requires an exaggeration of the lumbar lordosis to bring the arms vertical. In addition, the medial attachments of the 1st and 2nd ribs descend while those of the 4–6th ascend and the 3rd acts as the axis.[a] Bilateral abduction demands that the thoracic spine extends and the lumbar lordosis increase.

[a] Pettman E: *Level III Course Notes*. Berrien Springs, Michigan: North American Institute of Manual Therapy, Inc.; 2003.
[b] Kapandji IA: *The Physiology of the Joints, Upper Limb*. New York: Churchill Livingstone; 1991.

labrum, a negative articular pressure, and ligamentous restraints.[114] The ligamentous restraints contribute especially at the end ranges of motion,[115] and are assisted with concomitant muscle activity (see Table 14-2).

Stabilization of the Dynamic Shoulder. Dynamic stability of the shoulder complex is dependent upon a variety of mechanisms including the optimal alignment of the scapula, correct glenohumeral orientation, and the quality of the length-tension relationship of the scapular pivoters, the rotator cuff, and the biceps and triceps (Table 14-2). The long head of the biceps (see later) and the triceps muscles are major dynamic stabilizers of the glenohumeral joint predominately functioning as "shunt" muscles

(muscles that produce a compression at the joint surfaces of the joints they cross) during high velocity activities. Indeed, the glenohumeral joint, like the temporomandibular joint, enjoys the benefit of the fact that all of its prime movers compress the joint surface, thus optimizing joint stability.

As motion occurs at the glenohumeral joint, the glenoid cavity of the scapular adopts a diverse number of reciprocal positions. It is likely that these scapular positions are based on both the functional task and the placement of the hand.

The function of the rotator cuff in normal and pathologic conditions has been the subject of several studies.[7,116–120] Until recently, electromyography (EMG), or cadaver studies have been the primary method of evaluating the contribution of each

TABLE 14-9 Glenohumeral Joint Motions and Their Appropriate Axis and Accessory Motions

Plane/Axis of Motion	Physiologic Motion	Accessory Motion
Sagittal/mediolateral	Flexion/extension	Spin
Coronal/anteroposterior	Abduction Adduction	Inferior glide Superior glide
Transverse/longitudinal	Internal rotation External rotation	Posterior glide Anterior glide

rotator cuff and shoulder muscle to a particular motion or exercise.[7,116,117,121–124] Using cadavers, Keating and colleagues[125] determined that the subscapularis contributes 53 percent of the cuff moment and believed it to be the most important muscle in humeral head stabilization.

Magnetic resonance imaging (MRI) is now being used to show increases in muscle signal intensity detected immediately following exercise, although few studies have looked at the muscles of the shoulder.[126–128] Based on the level of signal intensity, this so-called exercise-induced enhancement seen on MR images can determine which muscles are used for a given exercise.[119,126,127,129–131] For example, one study[128] demonstrated that side lying abduction produced the greatest signal intensity in the supraspinatus, infraspinatus, and subscapularis. Surprisingly, scaption with internal rotation, previously associated with isolation of the supraspinatus muscle, did not provide the highest increase in any muscle of the rotator cuff.[128] However, caution must be used in drawing conclusions from single studies, and further research is certainly warranted in this area.

The Scapulohumeral Rhythm. The angle between the glenoid and the moving humeral head has to be maintained within a safe zone of 30 degrees of angulation during activities to decrease shear and translatory forces.[132] The scapula must be actively positioned muscularly in relation to the moving humerus. The scapula must also act as a stable base of muscle origin for the rotator cuff muscles for stabilization. If the scapula cannot be controlled, the glenoid cannot be positioned correctly to allow for the optimal length-tension relationships within the shoulder complex.[82,84,114,133]

The combination and synchronization of the motions that occur between the scapula and the humerus during elevation is termed *scapulohumeral rhythm*. Proper rhythm involves a rotation of the scapula during arm elevation, which serves to significantly decrease the shearing effect between the humeral head and the glenoid. By allowing the glenoid to stay centered under the humeral head, the strong tendency for a downward dislocation of the humerus is resisted and the glenoid is maintained within a physiologically tolerable range (Fig. 14-12). At full abduction, the glenoid completely supports the humerus.

Several studies have examined the scapulohumeral rhythm three-dimensionally.[16,17,63,134,135] An early study by Inman[63] determined that a 2:1 ratio existed between the motion occurring at the G-H joint and scapula, respectively. For example, for each 3 degrees of arm elevation, 2 degrees of motion occurs at the G-H joint, and 1 degree is due to rotation of the scapula on the thorax (see Fig. 14-12). After 90 degrees of elevation, 60 degrees of the motion has occurred at the G-H joint, with the remaining 30 degrees consisting of scapular motion. After the first 90 degrees, the rest of the elevation occurs at a 2:1 glenohumeral:scapula ratio. This ratio is not consistent throughout the range of motion, with early abduction (0 to 80 degrees) involving more humeral motion, the midrange (80 to 140 degrees) involving more scapular motion, and the end ranges (140 to 170 degrees) involving motion at neighboring joints.[16,87,134]

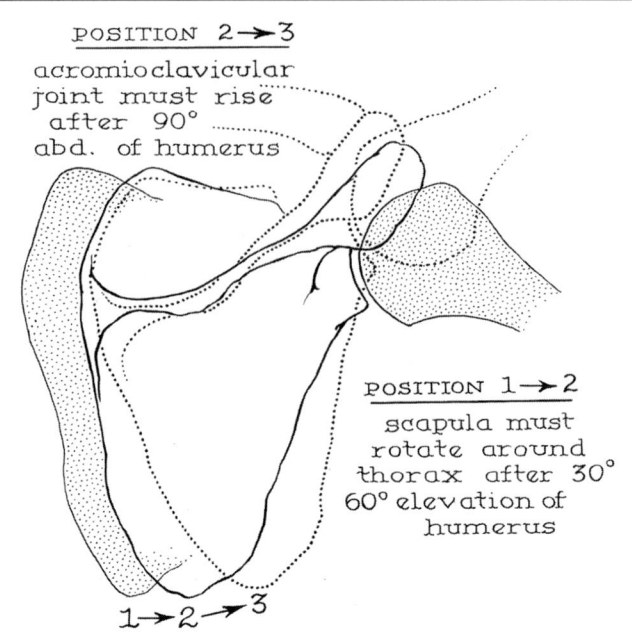

FIGURE 14-12   Scapulohumeral rhythm. (Reproduced with permission from Bateman JE. *The Shoulder and Neck.* Philadelphia: WB Saunders; 1972.)

A more recent study[135] described the scapulohumeral rhythm consisting of five phases, with each of the phases representing 20 percent increments of the subject range of motion for arm elevation. For example, if a patient has a maximum range of motion of 175 degrees, the five increments would be 0 to 35 degrees (20 percent of maximum range), 36 to 70 degrees (40 percent of maximum range), 71 to 105 degrees (60 percent of maximum range), 106 to 140 degrees (80 percent of maximum range), and 141 to 175 degrees (100 percent of maximum range). The same study described a 3:1 ratio of humeral elevation and scapular upward rotation relative to the trunk. In this scenario, for every 1 degree of scapular upward rotation, 3 degrees of humeral elevation occurs relative to the trunk, a finding that is comparable to Inman's study.[135]

It is worth noting that the scapulohumeral rhythm has been found to change with external loading of the arm, with increasing ratios of humeral elevation to scapular rotation occurring, depending on which of the five phases is assessed (3.2:1 for the first two phases, 3.6:1 for the third phase, 4.0:1 for the fourth phase, and 4.3:1 for the final phase.)[135]

Movement of the scapula requires rotation about an axis that travels through the A-C joint and S-C joint.[51] There is a total of 40 to 50 degrees of clavicle rotation with only 5 to 8 degrees occurring at the A-C joint, the remainder being supplied by the mobile S-C joint.[50,136] The rotation of the scapula helps to maintain an effective length-tension relationship between the three groups (force couples) of muscles that attach to the scapula.

Scapular rotation about an axis that passes through the base of the spine of the scapula during arm elevation occurs in various phases (see Tables 14-7 and 14-8). In the normal abduction mechanism, the scapula moves laterally in the first 20 to 50 degrees of glenohumeral abduction.[15]

During the first 30 degrees of upward rotation of the scapula, the serratus anterior muscle and the upper and lower divisions of the trapezius muscle are considered the principal upward rotators of the scapula. Together these muscles form two force couples; one formed by the upper trapezius and the upper serratus anterior muscles (Fig. 14-13), the other formed by the lower trapezius and lower serratus anterior muscles.[19,63,137] A *force couple* is defined as two forces that act in opposite directions to rotate a segment around its axis of motion.[60,138]

The trapezius appears to be more critical for abduction, whereas the serratus is more critical during flexion.[63,139] The lower trapezius also contributes during this phase by preventing tipping of the scapula and assisting in the stabilization of the scapula through eccentric control of the scapula during scapular upward rotation. It is primarily active with heavy resistance activities through 90 to 120 degrees of abduction.[87,134]

Elevation of the distal end of the clavicle allows further upward rotation of the scapula. From 0 to 150 degrees of arm elevation, the prime movers are the rotator cuff muscles, the deltoid muscle, the upper and lower fibers of the trapezius and the middle, and lower fibers of serratus anterior.[140] The middle trapezius and rhomboids may also contribute to the scapular motions involved during arm elevation.[140] The antagonists are the pectoralis major, teres major, latissimus dorsi, and coracobrachialis, all working eccentrically. At approximately 150 to 160 degrees of arm elevation, the lower fibers of serratus anterior reach their maximally short position and now continue to contract isometrically, effectively fixating the inferior angle of the scapular to the chest wall. This sets up a new axis within the shoulder girdle, an oblique axis which goes between the S-C joint and the fixed inferior angle of the scapular around which the clavicle and scapula may move as one in an arcuate swing across the thorax. Normal motion of the scapula on the thorax is believed to include consistent contact between the thoracic wall and the medial border and inferior angle of the scapula.[137,140] Loss of this contact has been clinically implicated as evidence of abnormal scapular kinematics. These abnormal scapular kinematics may result in additional stress on the anterior shoulder stabilizers.[121,141,142]

Motion at the A-C joint is controlled by tension in the coracoclavicular ligaments. Elevation of the acromion occurs due to the upward rotation of the scapula (see Fig. 14-12). The final 30 to 60 degrees of upward rotation of the scapula is essentially the result of 30 to 45 degrees of posterior rotation around the long axis of the clavicle (Fig. 14-7) and an elevation of the acromion.[143] It is, as yet, unclear whether this posterior rotation occurs at the S-C or at the A-C joint. The rotation of the clavicle though is controlled by tension in the coracoclavicular ligaments and the clavipectoral fascia. The elevation of the acromion during arm elevation allows the subacromial structures to pass under the coracoacromial arch.[143a] The appropriate force couples for acromial elevation are the lower trapezius and serratus muscles working together, paired with the upper trapezius and rhomboid muscles (Fig. 14-13).[143a] For each 10 degrees of arm elevation, there are approximately 2 degrees of clavicular elevation,[62] with the maximum elevation occurring at approximately 130 degrees.[144]

The EMG activity of the levator scapula muscle, upper and lower trapezius muscles, and serratus anterior muscle during arm elevation increase progressively as the humeral angle increases.[47] Activities which maintain an upwardly rotated scapula while accentuating scapular protraction, such as a push-up plus, elicit the greatest serratus anterior EMG activity.[24]

The last few degrees of shoulder elevation consist of upper thoracic movement once full G-H joint and shoulder girdle motion have been completed.[145] As the arm continues to elevate beyond the 150-degree mark, the thorax begins to extend and ipsilaterally rotate and side flex.

The scapula also functions during retraction and protraction along the thoracic wall (see Fig. 14-9).[15] Protraction occurs as the serratus anterior at the scapula, and the pectoralis major at the humerus, contract simultaneously. Retraction is produced by the combined action of the trapezius and rhomboids.[146] A 15 to 18 cm translation of the scapula around the thoracic wall occurs during retraction and protraction, depending on the size of the individual and the vigorousness of the activity.[15,104] This retraction and protraction is used during such activities as the setting phase and acceleration phases in throwing and serving, respectively.[15]

Lastly, the scapula functions to transfer the large forces and energy from the legs, hips, back and trunk, to the actual delivery mechanism, the arm and hand.[15,103,147,148]

Muscular Mechanisms. In addition to the muscle co-activation force couples previously mentioned, other force couple mechanisms are found at the shoulder and include the long head of the biceps,[29,96,149–151] the supraspinatus, and the deltoid and rotator cuff mechanism.[152]

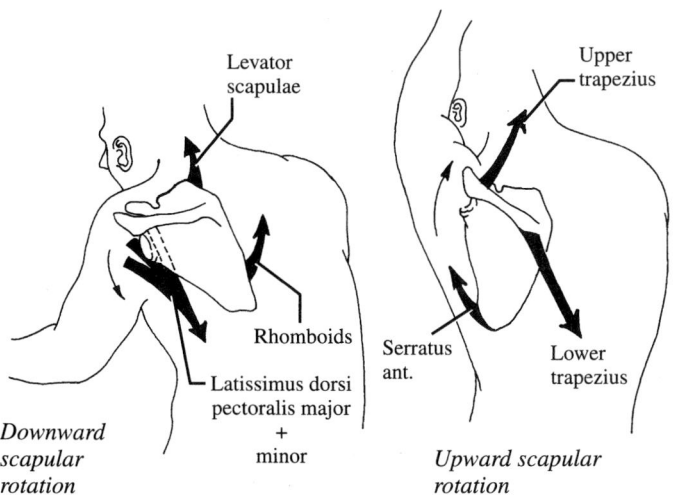

FIGURE 14-13 The force couples involved with scapular rotation. (Reproduced with permission from Pansky B. *Review of Gross Anatomy*, 6th ed. New York: McGraw-Hill; 1996.)

Long Head of the Biceps Mechanism. In the anatomical position, the biceps has no ability to elevate the humerus. If the arm is rotated 90 degrees externally, the tendon of the long head lines up with the muscle belly to form a straight line across the humeral head. As the biceps contracts in this position, the humeral head rotates beneath the tendon, resisting external rotation of the humeral head and increasing the anterior stability of the G-H joint.[60,150,153] Contraction of the long head of the biceps when the arm is abducted and externally rotated fixes the humeral head snugly against the glenoid cavity, as the resultant force passes obliquely through the center of rotation of the humeral head and at right angles to the glenoid.[150] The humeral head is prevented from moving upwards by the hood-like action of the biceps tendon (Fig. 14-14), which exerts a downward force and assists the depressor function of the cuff.[154–156] Interestingly, the biceps tendon was found to be wider in cuff-deficient shoulders in one study.[157]

Supraspinatus Mechanism. This is another pulley mechanism similar to the biceps. However, the muscle motor is located at the scapula and the tendinous insertion is at the greater tuberosity. The supraspinatus is responsible for approximately 50 percent of the torque occurring with shoulder abduction and flexion, with the deltoid responsible for the remaining 50 percent.[133,158] As the weight of the arm pulls downwards, the force of the supraspinatus pulls slightly above horizontal, helping to steer the humeral head[60] and producing abduction of the arm. Initially it was thought that the only function of the supraspinatus was to help in the initiation of abduction.[12,159,160] More recent EMG studies have found that the supraspinatus muscle contracts throughout the entire phase of abduction of the arm, with maximal activity occurring at 100 degrees, where it contributes to stability by drawing the humeral head toward the glenoid.[7,117] Despite its apparent importance with abduction, it has been shown that abduction of the humerus can be accomplished without the supraspinatus, providing that the deltoid and remaining rotator cuff muscles are intact.[161]

Deltoid and Rotator Cuff Mechanism. A force couple develops between the rotator cuff, serving to stabilize and depress the humeral head, and the deltoid muscle, serving to elevate the humerus (Fig. 14-15). The deltoid muscle is substantially more massive than the muscles forming the rotator cuff.

"After electrical stimulation of the deltoid alone, I observed that during the elevation of the arm caused by the contraction of the muscle, the humeral head subluxated downward and tended to leave the cavitas glenoidalis. It is of course necessary to keep the head up, facing the cavitas glenoidalis: such it is the function of the supraspinatus."[162]

This is how Duchenne de Boulogne described the effect of electrical stimulation on the deltoid.[163] This description contrasted with later models of the effect of the deltoid on the humerus,[63,164] which found that during low levels of elevation (< 90 degrees), the deltoid force vector acts tangentially to the glenoid face, which encourages superior migration. This is counteracted by the cuff vector that compresses the humeral head into the glenoid (see Fig. 14-15).[37,165–167]

However, in clinical practice, shoulders having large cuff tears and good function are frequently encountered. This would indicate that the deltoid alone can stabilize the humeral head. One study found that at the beginning of elevation, the middle part of the deltoid supplies all of the strength required, because the anterior and posterior parts provide only adduction to the humerus.[163] In addition, the resultant force of the deltoid has a horizontal component that causes the humeral head to press against the glenoid (see Fig. 14-15).[163] This suggests that one of the deltoid's functions is to prevent the upward migration of the humeral head and compress it against the glenoid, even in the presence of a large cuff tear.[163]

Electromyography studies have shown that during casual elevation of the arm in normal shoulders, the deltoid and the rotator cuff act continuously throughout the motion of abduction, each reaching a peak of activity between 120 and 140 degrees

FIGURE 14-14 The biceps apparatus. (Reproduced with permission from Bateman JE. *The Shoulder and Neck.* Philadelphia: WB Saunders; 1972.)

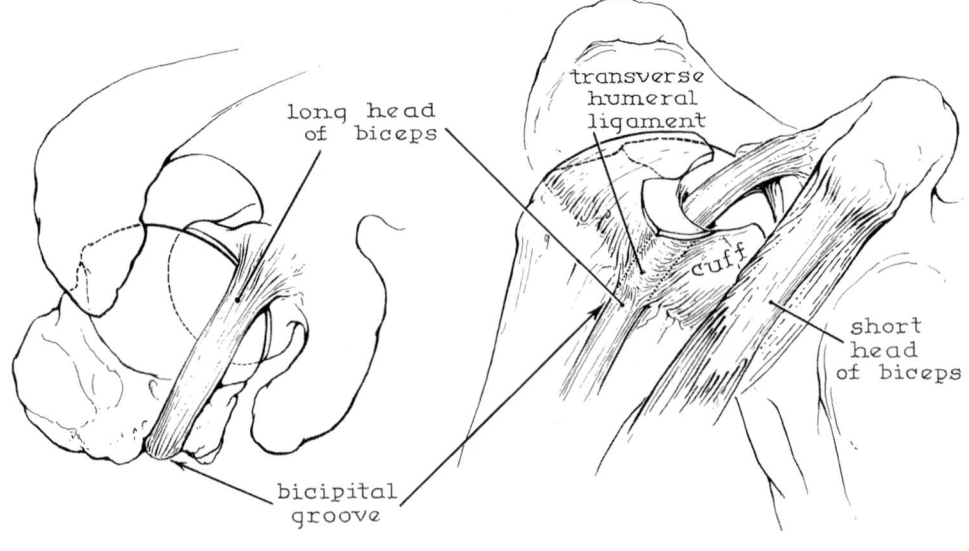

FIGURE 14-15 The deltoid and rotator cuff force couple. (Reproduced with permission from Bateman JE. *The Shoulder and Neck.* Philadelphia: WB Saunders; 1972.)

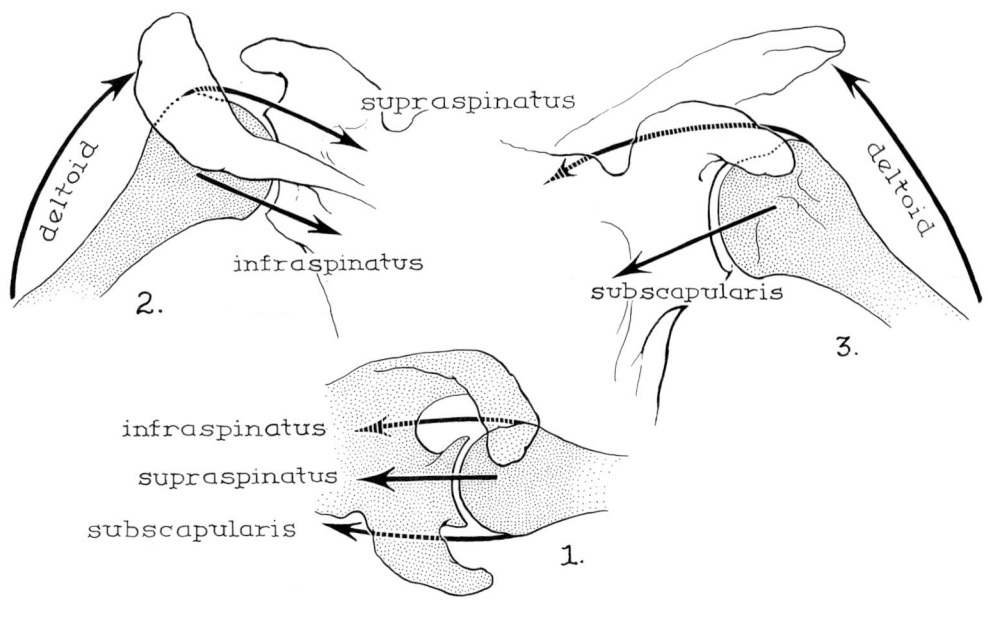

of abduction.[7,117] However, during more rapid and precise movements such as those involved with throwing, a more selective pattern emerges with specific periods of great intensity.[168] Weakening of the rotator cuff appears to allow the deltoid to elevate the proximal part of the humerus in the absence of an adequate depressor effect from the rotator cuff. A decrease in the subacromial space is created and impingement of the rotator cuff on the anterior aspect of the acromion occurs (see Fig. 14-15).[169,170]

At the G-H joint, elevation through abduction of the arm requires that the greater tuberosity of the humerus pass under the coracoacromial arch. For this to occur, the humerus must externally rotate, and the acromion must elevate.[171] External rotation of the humerus is produced actively by a contraction of the infraspinatus and teres minor, and by a twisting of the joint capsule. The importance of the external rotation can be demonstrated clinically. If the humerus is held in full internal rotation, only about 60 degrees of glenohumeral abduction is passively possible before the greater tuberosity impinges against the coracoacromial arch and blocks further abduction. This helps explain why individuals with marked internal rotation contractures cannot abduct fully, but can elevate the arm in the forward plane.

Subacromial Impingement Syndrome (SIS). Subacromial impingement syndrome (SIS) as a pathologic entity is described in detail in the Intervention Strategies section. However, SIS is mentioned here because the development of this syndrome is closely related to biomechanical dysfunction of the shoulder complex.

In the presence of a normal rotator cuff, normal scapular pivoters, and no capsular contractures, the humeral head translates less than 3 mm superiorly during the mid ranges of active

elevation, whereas at the end ranges, anteroposterior and superoinferior translations of 4 to 10 mm do occur, all of which are coupled with specific motions of internal or external rotation.[12,97,102,165,166,172–175] An increase in superior translation with active elevation may result in encroachment of the coracoacromial arch.[32,165] This encroachment produces a compression of the suprahumeral structures against the anteroinferior aspect of the acromion and coracoacromial ligament. Repetitive compression of these structures, coupled with other predisposing factors, results in a condition called subacromial impingement syndrome (SIS). SIS was first recognized by Jarjavay[176] in 1867, and the term *impingement syndrome* was popularized by Neer[32] in the 1970s.

Both intrinsic and extrinsic factors have been implicated as etiologies of the impingement process, and a number of impingement types have evolved. Two of those types include the outlet (intrinsic) impingement, and the nonoutlet (extrinsic) impingement.

Outlet (Intrinsic) Impingement. Neer[32] proposed that a tight or crowded subacromial space (e.g., one in which the space is compromised by an anterior acromial osteophyte) could cause a mechanical abrasion of the rotator cuff against the acromion with abduction above 80 to 90 degrees without concomitant external rotation.

This abrasion of the soft tissue structures located between the head of the humerus and the roof of the shoulder during elevation of the arm produces an irritation, inflammation, and tearing of the rotator cuff muscles, an irritation of the long head of the biceps and the subacromial bursitis.[177–179]

This type of impingement is known as an *outlet impingement,* because it occurs at the supraspinatus outlet formed by the coracoid process, the anterior acromion, the A-C joint, and the coracoacromial ligament (Fig. 14-5). It clinically manifests as a "painful arc." A painful arc describes a region of pain in a particular motion, which has pain free areas on either side of it.[180] For example, during abduction the patient may feel an onset of pain at 80 degrees, which then disappears at 100 degrees. The general cause of a painful arc is impingement of a tender subacromial structure during motion, although loose bodies and instabilities may also cause a painful arc.

Although Neer and Poppen[181] reported that 90 to 95 percent of rotator cuff tears were the result of the outlet subacromial impingement, the role of age-related or senescent degeneration and tensile overload has been emphasized more recently (see later).[178,179,182–186]

Nonoutlet (Extrinsic) Impingement.   Nonoutlet impingement, in which the subacromial space appears to be normal, occurs in the younger patient performing repetitive overhead motions. The mechanism in this condition appears to be an impingement of the rotator cuff against the posterior superior glenoid labrum and the humeral head during forced humeral elevation and internal rotation. This can eventually result in posterior superior tears in the glenoid labrum, and lesions in the posterior humeral head (Bankart lesion).

Primary and Secondary Impingement.   Jobe[187] and Jobe and Pink[71] proposed two other types of impingement, which relate to chronic disorders of the rotator cuff, with four subclassifications (Table 14-10):

▶ Primary impingement occurs when the superior aspect of the rotator cuff is compressed and abraded by the surrounding bony and soft tissues due to a decreased subacromial space.[188] This type of impingement is the same as the outlet impingement proposed by Neer.

▶ Secondary impingement is a condition found in both older and younger individuals with varying levels of activity. This type results from glenohumeral instability and/or tensile overload of the rotator cuff resulting in poor control of the humeral head during overhead activities.[71,187,189] Patients in this group are usually younger than 35 years, have a

traumatic anterior instability, posterior defect of the humeral head, and damage to the posterior glenoid labrum.

Thus the pathophysiology of SIS and rotator cuff disorders may have both intrinsic and extrinsic factors. These intrinsic and extrinsic factors include[31,33,190–192]:

1. ***The shape and form of the acromion.***   Acromial morphology is a strong predictor of rotator cuff impingement. The mechanical effect of the acromion is considered as the extrinsic theory for impingement. Bigliani[193] has described three acromial shapes (Fig. 14-16). Cadaveric studies have confirmed a 70 percent incidence of rotator cuff tears in patients with a Type III acromial shape and only a 3 percent incidence in patients with a Type I acromion.[193,194]

2. ***The amount of vascularization to the cuff.***   The circulation of the rotator cuff is unidirectional with no flow traversing the tide mark at the insertion of the supraspinatus.[192] With the arm adducted to the side, the vessels within the supraspinatus tendon are unperfused (Fig. 14-17).[44] Other arm positions, such as raising the arm above 30 degrees, have been shown to increase intramuscular pressure in the supraspinatus muscle to an extent that may impair normal blood perfusion.[44,177] Avascularity appears to increase with age beginning as early as 20 years of age.[195] Two early studies noted a critical zone that lies slightly proximal to the supraspinatus insertion point.[196,197] Since then it has been determined that the critical zone is more likely a zone of anastomoses between the vessels supplying the bone and the tendon, and is not less vascular except in certain positions.[44,190,198] While it is possible that sustained isometric contractions, prolonged adduction of the arm, or increases in subacromial pressure[199] may reduce the microcirculation, it is unlikely that frequent abduction or elevation of the arm would produce selective avascularity of the supraspinatus or biceps tendon.[31]

3. ***The correct functioning of the dynamic stabilizers.***   If the dynamic stabilizers are weak or injured, increased translation occurs between the humeral head and glenoid labrum.[149] This increase in translation may lead to increased wear on

TABLE 14-10   Jobe and Pink's Classification of Shoulder Dysfunction in the Overhead Athlete[71]

- Group I. This group, typically found in the older population, encompasses those patients with pure and isolated impingement and no instability

- Group II. Patients in this group, who are usually young overhead athletes, demonstrate instability with impingement secondary to microtrauma that comes from overuse

- Group III. Patients in this group, who are also typically young overhead athletes, demonstrate generalized ligamentous laxity

- Group IV. Patients in this group are those who have experienced a traumatic event, resulting in instability in the absence of impingement

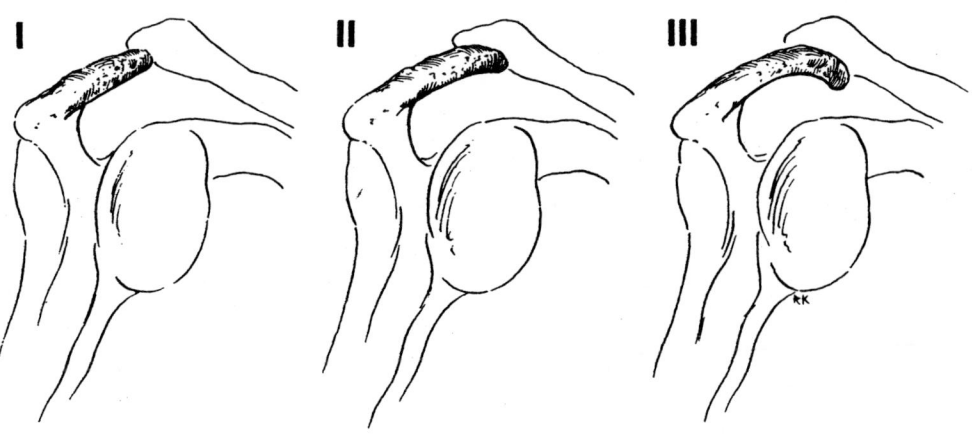

FIGURE 14-16 Acromion morphology. (Reproduced with permission from Zachazewski JE, Magee DJ, Quillen WS. *Athletic Injuries and Rehabilitation*. Philadelphia: WB Saunders; 1996.)

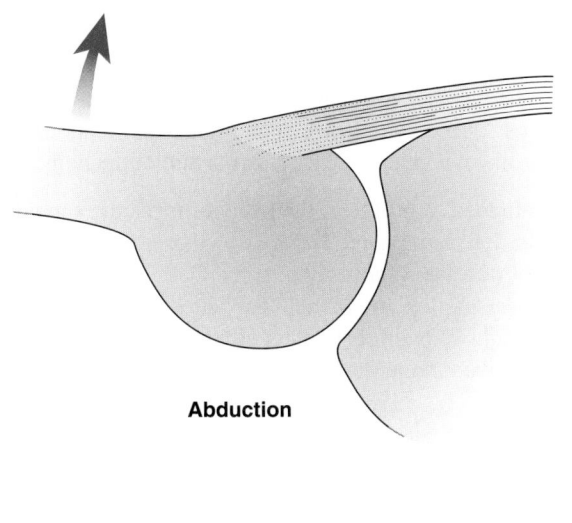

Abduction

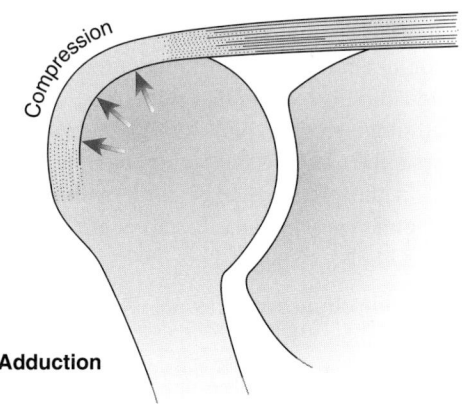

Adduction

FIGURE 14-17 Vascularity of the supraspinatus tendon in various arm positions.

the labrum, increased reliance on the static restraints, and eccentric overloading of the dynamic restraints, which in turn can result in instability and/or impingement.[97,106]

4. ***Condition of the A-C joint.*** Degenerative changes of the A-C joint, including narrowing of the joint space and the

formation of inferior osteophytes, also can accompany impingement syndrome.[33,200,201]

5. ***Age.*** The age of the patient appears to be an important etiologic factor in the development of subacromial impingement in association with repetitive motion.[202–206] In the absence of repetitive motion as a mitigating factor, SIS is more common after the third decade of life, and is uncommon in individuals younger than 30 years.[31,32] In addition, there is a normal age-related increase in asymptomatic rotator cuff defects.[202–204,206,207] Constant and Murley[208] also have shown that there is an age-related decrease in shoulder function in healthy volunteers.

6. ***Position of the arm during activities.*** The arm position adopted during work activities may contribute to the development of subacromial impingement significantly.[209] Because of the tangential vector of deltoid contraction, the tendency for superior translation of the humeral head is greatest between 60 and 90 degrees of elevation.[37,165,210] Thus repetitive activities in this range of elevation place a high demand on the rotator cuff to counteract this tendency. In addition, repetitive activities that occur during higher levels of elevation of the arm bring the greater tuberosity and supraspinatus insertion into close proximity to the coracoacromial arch.[37,165,210]

7. ***Poor endurance of scapular pivoters.*** Sustained or repetitive overhead activity requires endurance from the scapular pivoters to maintain appropriate scapular rotation.[31,84,170] Fatigue of the scapular pivoters may lead or contribute to relative subacromial impingement because of poor or asymmetric scapular rotation.[31,84,170] Secondary impingement can occur because of serratus anterior dysfunction, resulting in the forward and downward movement of the coracoacromial arch. This reduces available clearance for the rotator cuff and greater tuberosity as the shoulder is flexed forward (Fig. 14-18).[4,84] Scapular lag from dysrhythmic scapulothoracic motion also can contribute to subacromial impingement because the acromion fails to

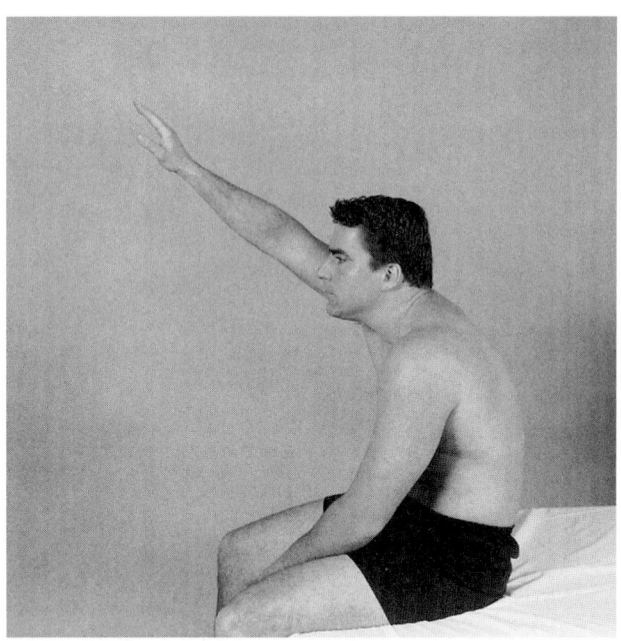

FIGURE 14-18   Forward head and arm elevation.

rotate with the humerus, thereby producing a relative decrease in the acromiohumeral interval.[31,84]

8. ***Capsular tightness.***[211] Capsular tightness appears to be a common mechanical problem in primary impingement syndrome and has been reported to occur at the posterior,[84] anterior,[37] and inferior[212,213] portions of the capsule. Individuals who avoid painful overhead activity, or who are predisposed to motion imbalances because of their work or sport, can develop capsular tightness.[214] During the period of pain avoidance or unbalanced movement, the capsular connective tissue may lose the ability to lengthen due to decreased critical fiber distance and abnormal collagen fiber cross-linking. This in turn can lead to capsular tightness, joint stiffness, painful or limited function and to an earlier onset or greater degree of subacromial compression, particularly in elevated planes of movement.[31,215–217] This is particularly true with a posterior capsular contracture, which commonly coexists with SIS and rotator cuff disease. Posterior capsular contracture may add to the abnormal subacromial contact by producing an anterosuperior translation during active elevation.[30,31] Tightness of the posterior capsule can also cause a decrease in internal rotation of the G-H joint, which leads to an increase in the anterior and superior migration of the humeral head. In contrast, tightness of the anteroinferior capsule results in limited external rotation, preventing the greater tuberosity from sufficient external rotation to "clear" the coracoacromial arch.[171] Thus the restoration of capsular mobility is an important component in the rehabilitation process.

9. ***Postural imbalance.***   Postural imbalance, particularly scapulothoracic dysfunction, has been implicated as an etiologic factor in secondary impingement syndrome (Fig. 14-18).[31,218] The likely cause of this are the resultant changes in the activation patterns of the length-dependent force couples. Postural imbalance can also occur as a secondary development in primary shoulder impingement syndrome.[211]

10. ***Repetitive activities*** that involve humeral flexion have been reported to predispose individuals to rotator cuff disorders.[33,174] In fact, any repetitive elevation beyond 90 degrees has the potential to provoke rotator cuff disorders.[37]

11. ***Structural asymmetry.***   Scapular asymmetry and its role in impingement has been widely reported by investigators of upper extremity pathology.[84,219–221] Warner and colleagues[221] determined that 57 percent of their subjects with impingement syndrome demonstrated static scapular postural asymmetry, and all demonstrated weakness of the scapular pivoters (rhomboids, serratus anterior, lower trapezius, deltoid, and rotator cuff).

12. ***The position of the humerus at rest*** can affect the healing process of patients with primary shoulder impingement syndrome. The work of Rathburn and Macnab[44] illustrated the deleterious "wringing out" effect on rotator cuff tendon vascularity with an adducted dependent posture of the humerus.

If SIS is allowed to progress, the patient moves the shoulder less frequently due to the pain. The lack of movement increases the potential of developing a condition called adhesive capsulitis (frozen shoulder), particularly in the older patient. This idiopathic condition of insidious painful shoulder stiffness and loss of joint mobility is described in the Intervention Strategies section.

Examination

The intervention strategies for the common pathologies of the shoulder complex are detailed after the examination section. An understanding of both is necessary. As mention of the various pathologies occurs with reference to the examination and vice versa, the reader is encouraged to alternate between the two.

In the presence of shoulder girdle dysfunction (assuming systemic or orthopaedic causes have been ruled out) there are three likely causes:

▶ Compromise of the passive restraint components of the shoulder girdle.

▶ Compromise of the neuromuscular system's production or control of shoulder girdle motion.

▶ Compromise to one or more of the neighboring joints that contribute to shoulder girdle motion, including:

  • The acromioclavicular joint.

  • The sternoclavicular joint.

  • The joints of the upper thoracic spine and ribs.

  • The joints of the lower cervical spine.

Due to this complexity, all of the above joints must be selectively tested in a specific sequence before proceeding with a more detailed examination of the suspected joint or joints.

History

A good history is the cornerstone of proper diagnosis, especially since shoulder pain has a broad spectrum of patterns and characteristics. A body chart can be used to record the patient's symptom distribution (see Chap. 8). The body chart is a symptomatic representation of a patient's complaints and can be an important element in guiding both the history and the tests and measures.

The history should begin with a brief outline of the patient's profile including age, occupation, hand dominance, recreational pursuits, work requirements, and activities of daily living.[222] Age is occasionally significant[223]:

▶ Children and adolescents may have an epiphysitis of the humerus, or an osteogenic sarcoma.

▶ Calcific deposits in the shoulder are more common between 20 and 40 years of age.

▶ Chondrosarcomas usually occur after age 30.

▶ Rotator cuff degeneration usually occurs in the 40s and 50s.

▶ A frozen shoulder is more common in those aged 45 to 60 years, and is associated with medical conditions such as diabetes mellitus and ischemic heart disease.[222]

The exact mechanism of injury should be determined as it can help with a preliminary diagnosis[224]:

▶ Overhead exertion involving repetitive motions is a common mechanism for subacromial disease, encompassing subacromial bursitis,[196] impingement syndrome,[32] rotator cuff tendonitis,[32,225] and rotator cuff tear.[226]

▶ A fall on an outstretched hand ("FOOSH" injury) can result in a sprain or strain injury to the wrist, elbow, and shoulder. More serious injuries include fractures of the wrist and elbow, A-C separations, clavicular fractures, and glenohumeral fractures and dislocations.

▶ A fall on the tip of the shoulder is a common mechanism for A-C separation. In addition, this mechanism can result in a compression periostitis (bone contusion) or a cervical spine injury, both of which appear remarkably similar to an A-C separation especially in the early stages.

▶ Forced horizontal extension of the abducted, externally rotated arm is a common mechanism for anterior dislocation.

It is important to establish the patient's chief presenting complaint (which is not always pain) as well as defining their other symptoms. The most common complaints associated with shoulder pathology include pain, instability, stiffness, deformity, locking, and swelling.[222] Patients will sometimes complain of catching, clunking, grinding, or popping of the shoulder with various movements. These sounds and sensations may be asymptomatic and nonpathologic. However, they may also indicate pathology including labral disorders, rotator cuff tears, snapping scapular, subacromial bursitis, or biceps tendon disorders, especially if the sound or sensation is associated with pain or instability.[222] Periscapular pain is often associated with local muscle strain but may be referred.[1]

Common complaints with a rotator cuff tear include difficulty with elevation of the arm in abduction, as well as external rotation, when patients attempt to put their hand behind their head.[227] Patients who report difficulty tucking in their shirts may have limited internal rotation from posterior capsular stiffness.[228] The hallmark of posterior capsular contracture is symmetric loss of active and passive internal rotation. Posterior capsular stiffness may occur independent of rotator cuff disease. Stiffness or loss of motion at the shoulder may be the chief complaint in conditions such as adhesive capsulitis.[222]

Weakness may be the chief complaint, leading to some diagnostic confusion. It is important to distinguish true weakness from weakness secondary to pain, both in terms of history and examination findings.[229] Painless weakness is usually due to neurological problems or myopathies, although peripheral nerve injuries can be painful (Table 14-11). Shoulder weakness may be caused by a rotator cuff tear or nerve injury (suprascapular, axillary, long thoracic, or thoracodorsal nerves, or cervical nerve root injury) (see Table 14-11).[83]

Symptoms that are not associated with movement should alert the clinician to a more serious condition (see "Systems Review"). Pain that is worse at night, but increased when rolling onto the shoulder, points to periarticular mechanical problems.[227]

Determining the location of pain is important. Posterior neck pain may be indicative of a cervical radiculopathy, as neither the A-C joint or a subacromial irritation refers pain to this area.[50,230]

Clinical Pearl

Pain due to rotator cuff pathology and impingement is usually felt over the anterior or lateral part of the shoulder, is characterized by radiation down the upper arm, and is aggravated with overhead activities.[222,231] Pain that radiates beyond the elbow is far less likely to be due to shoulder pathology, particularly if it is associated with any sensory disturbance in the limb such as distal radiation of pain, numbness, or paresthesias.[222] In such cases the clinician should rule out thoracic outlet syndrome, cervical radiculopathy, or referred pain from neighboring areas.

Pain due to A-C joint pathology is usually well localized to the region of the joint, but there is often a clear history of injury to this region. Severe pain on top of the shoulder with an associated deformity could indicate an A-C joint sprain.

The clinician should determine which positions or movements relieve the pain, as these can provide helpful information:[224]

▶ Pain relieved with arm elevation overhead could indicate a cervicogenic cause.[232]

▶ Pain relieved with the elbow supported is suggestive of A-C separation and rotator cuff tears.

TABLE 14-11   Peripheral Nerve Tests

Spinal accessory nerve	Inability to abduct the arm beyond 90°
	Pain in shoulder with abduction
Musculocutaneous nerve	Weak elbow flexion with forearm supinated
Long thoracic nerve	Pain on flexing fully extended arm
	Inability to flex fully extended arm
	Winging of scapula at 90° of forward flexion
Suprascapular nerve	Increased pain on forward shoulder flexion
	Pain increased with scapular abduction
	Pain increased with cervical rotation to opposite side
Axillary nerve	Inability to abduct arm with neutral rotation

► Pain relieved by circumduction of the shoulder with an accompanying click or clunk could indicate an internal derangement or subluxation.

► Pain relieved with arm distraction is suggestive of bursitis or rotator cuff tendonitis.

A general inquiry about general health, any existing medical conditions, medications, and allergies should be made. Corticosteroid use causes osteoporosis, tendon atrophy, and affects wound healing; therefore a history of its use will alter the differential diagnosis.[222,227] The use of anticoagulant medication should be noted. Patients who are undergoing renal dialysis are at increased risk for tendon tears as are patients who are 80 years of age or older.[227] Bilateral shoulder involvement is not uncommon in these groups.

Past physical therapy interventions, previous injections, and previous surgery are important to document, as are previous shoulder injuries and what relationship, if any, they have with the present symptomatology.[222]

Systems Review

The clinician should be able to determine the suitability of the patient for physical therapy. If the clinician is concerned with any signs or symptoms of a visceral, vascular, neurogenic, psychogenic, spondylogenic, or systemic disorder (see Chap. 9) that is out of the scope of physical therapy, the patient should be referred back to their physician or another appropriate health care provider.

Scenarios related to the shoulder that warrant further investigation by the clinician include an insidious onset of symptoms, and complaints of numbness or paresthesia in the upper extremity.

The most common causes of numbness in the shoulder and arm are due to cervical or upper thoracic involvement, with either the segmental roots involved, or the brachial plexus. The patient should be questioned about recent changes in work requirements or environment, and the presence of neck pain.[31–33,209] In studies in which normal cervical ligaments and muscles,[233] cervical zygapophysial joints,[234] and disks[235] have been stimulated, subjects have reported pain in the head, anterior and posterior chest wall, shoulder girdle, and upper limb, depending on the cervical level stimulated.[87]

The Cyriax scanning examination (see Chap. 9) may demonstrate the presence of subtle weakness of cervical root or peripheral nerve innervated muscles. Depressed or absent upper extremity reflexes are also frequently noted. Finally, reproduction of the patient's pain with cervical motion and not with shoulder movement is a strong indicator of cervical origin.

In addition to the cervical and upper thoracic spine, the related joints referring symptoms to the shoulder require clearing. These include the temporomandibular joint, costosternal joint, costovertebral and costotransverse joint, thoracic spine, and the elbow and forearm.[49,231]

Systemic causes of insidious shoulder pain include rheumatoid arthritis. Rheumatoid arthritis often affects the shoulders and hips in older individuals and can be difficult to distinguish from polymyalgia rheumatica. Morning stiffness lasting for more than 1 hour, constitutional signs, and physical signs of joint inflammation are all indicative of an inflammatory disease.[227] Other systemic sources of shoulder pain include lupus erythematosus and gallbladder and liver disease.[49] These latter conditions are associated with other signs and symptoms which are not related to movement and are systemic in nature. Chronic respiratory and cardiovascular conditions must also come into consideration.[222] The shoulder is very close to the chest and its viscera, so reference of pain to the shoulder from these structures is common (see Chap. 9). It is vital that questions be asked that would reveal a relationship between the onset of symptoms and stress different from that which could be considered as local (apex of lung, heart, and diaphragm).

> **Clinical Pearl**
>
> Severe progressive pain not affected by movement, persistent throughout the day and night, and associated with systemic signs, may indicate referred pain from a malignancy. The exception to this may be adhesive capsulitis (frozen shoulder), which is often characterized by boring, unrelenting, aching pain, even at rest.[236]

Tests and Measures

Observation

Observation of the patient begins when the patient enters the clinic. The clinician observes how the patient holds the arm, the overall position of the upper extremity, and the willingness of the patient to move the arm. Once in the treatment room, the patient is appropriately disrobed, and the shoulder is systematically inspected from anterior, lateral, and posterior positions. Total body alignment is examined for overall posture, the relative rotation of the humerus, structural malalignment such as kyphosis, and the presence of scars, color changes, and swelling.[222] The relative heights of the shoulder girdles should be assessed. The height of the shoulder may or may not be significant. If the shoulders are elevated, the neck appears short. If they are depressed, the A-C joint is seen to be lower than the S-C joint.[237] Elevation of the shoulder can be due to shortness of the upper trapezius, such that the lateral end of the clavicle appears appreciably higher than its medial aspect.[237] A low shoulder can result from[224]:

- Adaptive laxity of the shoulder.

- Leg length discrepancy.

- Scoliosis.

- Soft tissue hypertonicity.

- Mechanical dysfunction of the pelvis.

- *Hand dominance.* The shoulder on the dominant side may be slightly lower than the nondominant side. This is a normal finding.

Deformity is a common complaint with injuries of the A-C joint and fractures of the clavicle. For example, a second- or severe first-degree sprain of the A-C joint can be seen as a high-riding lateral clavicle (elevation of the distal end) causing a step-off to form between the clavicle and acromion.[11,238] It is frequently referred to as a tent-pole deformity. Other causes of deformity include an anterior dislocation of the shoulder, which may produce a squaring of the shoulder, as the deltoid is no longer rounded out over the humeral head.

Observation of muscle symmetry should be noted. Specific atrophy can imply certain diagnoses. For example, muscle weakness or atrophy, especially post-trauma, might indicate peripheral nerve damage[239]:

- Atrophy of the deltoid from axillary nerve neuropathy can result in a squared appearance of the lateral shoulder,[238,239] which is best observed from the front.[11]

- Atrophy of the posterior deltoid can occur in patients with multidirectional instability.[239]

- Atrophy at the infraspinatus or supraspinatus fossa is a hallmark of a rotator cuff tear,[11] or suprascapular nerve entrapment. Wasting of the supraspinati and infraspinati can be determined by pushing the examining finger into the respective muscle bellies.

- Atrophy of the trapezius may indicate compromise of the spinal accessory nerve. Atrophy of the trapezius is characterized by the appearance of a shoulder girdle that droops in association with a protracted inferior border of the scapula and an elevated acromion.[15,82,240]

- Atrophy of the serratus anterior muscle can create a prominent superior medial border of the scapula and a depressed acromion.

A balled up muscle may indicate a muscle rupture, the most common of which are of biceps and infraspinatus. Rupture of the long head of biceps can be noticed by the change in contour of the anterior arm with bunching of the muscle (the "Popeye" appearance).[222]

Observable swelling in the shoulder may indicate a serious problem or damage.

The position and attitude of the scapula, both statically and dynamically, should be noted (see later). In standing with their arms by their sides, the patient's medial (vertebral) border of the scapula should be 5 to 9 cm lateral to thoracic spinous processes,[223,241] the medial border of the spine of the scapula should be level with the T3 spinous process, and the inferior angle of the scapula should be level with the T7 spinous process. The medial border of the scapula should be seen to extend from the spinous process of T2 to the level of the spinous process of T7. Excessive prominence of the scapular spine may indicate atrophy of the infraspinatus and supraspinatus.[239] Two conditions, which may present with deformity of the scapula as their main symptom are Sprengel's deformity and winging of the scapula.[222]

Sprengel's deformity is the most common congenital abnormality affecting the shoulder. It is characterized by the presence of a hypoplastic, incorrectly rotated scapula, which sits abnormally high on the posterior chest wall. The condition results from a failure of the normal descent of the scapula, which occurs in utero, and is commonly associated with other significant musculoskeletal and visceral congenital abnormalities.[222]

Winging of the scapula (Fig. 14-19) is due to a loss of the normal scapular stability. Subtle forms of scapular winging, usually evident at the inferior border, occur commonly with many shoulder disorders such as G-H joint stiffness and shoulder instability.[84] In cases of G-H joint stiffness, there is passive limitation of glenohumeral motion, while with instability there is evidence of excessive movements or positive apprehension signs. Scapular winging may occur as the result of serratus anterior weakness, trapezius palsy,[240] excessive shortening of the pectoralis minor muscle,[2] or myopathies.[222,242–244] Scapular winging may also be caused by G-H joint stiffness, shoulder instability, and rotator cuff disease (see "Analysis of the Static Shoulder," later).

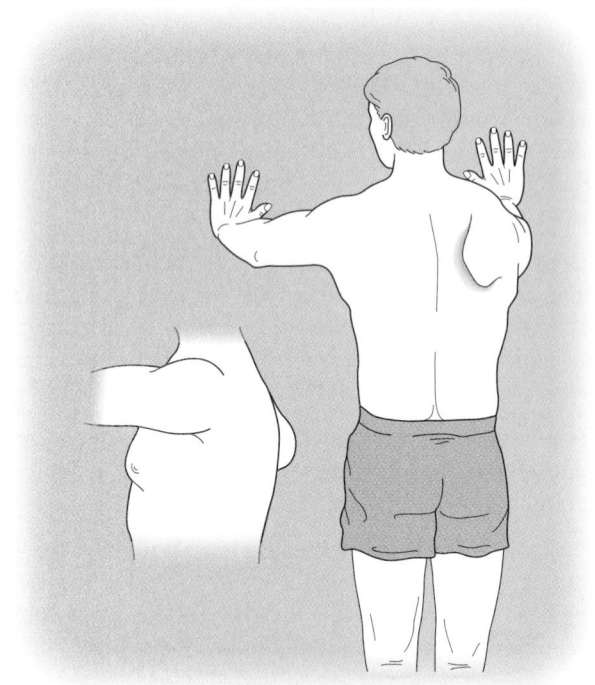

FIGURE 14-19   Scapular winging.

Gait.   Gait is evaluated to observe freedom of arm swing, reciprocal upper extremity movement, position of the arms and scapulae, and motion of the trunk and lower extremities (see Chap. 13).[49,231]

Posture.   An analysis of posture prompts the clinician as to the area of movement disturbance or excessive stresses. Postural dysfunctions of the upper quarter are a common cause of shoulder pain. A wide variety of structural changes can produce shoulder pain.[141,245,246] Poor positioning of the cervical or thoracic spine may alter the position of the shoulder girdle.[247,248] For example, thoracic kyphosis, scoliosis, or neck lordosis can result in excessive protraction of the scapula, producing interscapular pain.[15,249] In the older patient (over 50), an increased thoracic kyphosis may be related to a decrease in shoulder elevation.[250]

The relationship of the humeral head to the acromion should be observed. One third of the humeral head should be anterior to the acromion. A finding of less than one third may indicate a tight posterior capsule, or adaptive shortening of the external rotators.[251]

The patient's hands and arms should also be observed. Normally, the thumb faces anterior, or slightly medial. If the dorsum of the hand faces anteriorly, there may be excessive adaptive shortening of the internal rotators.[251]

Muscle balances in the upper quadrant can cause a characteristic postural pattern of the forward head position.[252] The most common muscle imbalances are outlined in Table 14-12. The clinician should observe the trunk and neck positions in sitting and standing, as well as the relationship of the scapulae relative to the trunk, and the humerus relative to the acromion. Any change in the scapular position has an impact on the A-C and S-C joint, and can also alter the length-tension relationship of the scapular muscles.

The forward head and rounded shoulder posture includes an abducted and elevated position of the scapula and a medially rotated humerus,[15,75,248,253] and is more common in patients presenting with shoulder pain[219] and interscapular pain.[249] A forward head posture in the presence of an abducted scapula and protracted shoulders results in a decrease in the size of the subacromial space, which may predispose the patient to rotator cuff disorders.[254] This posture results in an adaptive shortening of the upper trapezius, levator scapulae, and pectoralis, with weakening and lengthening of the deep neck flexors and lower scapular stabilizers (Fig. 14-18).[75,219,255]

If the pectoralis major is tight or strong, the muscle will be prominent. If there is an imbalance present, it will lead to rounded and protracted shoulders and a slight internal rotation of the humerus.[256,257] The altered position of the scapulae can distort the course of the suprascapular nerve, placing it at risk for a traction injury during upper extremity movements.[258–260]

Normally, the insertion of the sternocleidomastoid (SCM) is barely visible. If the clavicular insertion is prominent, it may indicate adaptive shortening of the SCM.[256] A groove along the SCM is an early sign of weakness of the deep neck flexors. A weakening and atrophy of the deep neck flexors has been proposed as a sign to estimate biological age.[261] The change in the anatomical relationship of the clavicle associated with this weakness and atrophy decreases the width of the thoracic inlet, rendering the brachial plexus vulnerable to compression (refer to Chap. 23).[258,262,263]

A loss of bulk in the interscapular muscles may indicate tightness in the trapezius and levator scapula.

TABLE 14-12   Common Muscle Imbalances of the Shoulder Complex

Muscles Prone to Tightness	Muscles Prone to Inactivity or Lengthening
Upper trapezius	Middle and lower trapezius
Levator scapulae	Rhomboids
Pectoralis major and minor	Serratus anterior
Upper cervical extensors	Deep neck flexors
Sternocleidomastoid	Subscapularis
Scalenes	Supraspinatus
Teres major and minor	Infraspinatus

Analysis of the Static Scapula. An abnormal position of the scapula at rest is common in patients with shoulder overuse injuries.[75,219,237,255] The scapular position is initially examined with the arms by the side. The clinician notes any signs of winging, elevation, depression, adduction, abduction, and rotation of the scapula. Abnormalities in alignment include a flattening of the interscapular area and an increase in the distance between the thoracic spinous processes and the medial border of the scapula. When the scapula is abducted (more than 8 cm from the midline of the thorax), it is also rotated more than 30 degrees anterior to the frontal plane and produces a medial rotation of the humerus.[237]

Tipping of the scapula, in which the inferior angle protrudes away from the rib cage, often results from a weakness of the lower trapezius, and positions the glenoid fossa so that it faces a more inferior direction.[87] This alignment is often associated with shortness of the pectoralis minor muscle, or biceps brachii muscle.[237]

Adaptive shortening of the rhomboids and levator scapulae muscles in the presence of a lengthened upper trapezius and serratus anterior, results in an elevation of the scapulae at the superior angle, and a downward rotation of the scapula. This causes the G-H joint to move into a position of abduction.[237,264] In addition, if the levator scapula adaptively shortens, both cervical and shoulder motions occur sooner than normal because the starting position of the scapula is changed. This modification to the starting position of the scapula for shoulder-elevated tasks presumably has an effect on the timing of the scapular muscles responsible for upward rotation. This results in an end position of arm elevation which is lower than usual (see Examination of the Dynamic Scapula, later).[87]

Extremity dominance can affect the orientation of the scapula, with the greater degree of unilateral activity producing the greater changes. A bilateral comparison should be made and allowances made for the dominance. Bilateral comparisons do not always highlight dysfunctions. For example, the symmetrical effects of an adaptive shortening of the anterior chest and shoulder musculature and lengthening of the posterior musculature that occurs in the forward head and rounded shoulder posture, will be confirmed during the mobility tests.

A number of static tests for the scapular position exist. The amount of scapular protraction available can be measured clinically using the method described by Diveta and colleagues,[265] who advocate two linear measurements with a piece of string. The distance in centimeters between the root of the scapular spine and the inferior angle of the acromion (scapular width) is divided into the distance from the third thoracic spinous process to the inferior angle of the acromion (scapular protraction). The resulting ratio provides a measurement of scapular protraction corrected for scapular size (normalized scapular protraction). This method of measurement of scapular protraction has been found to be both reliable and valid when compared to radiographic measurements.[219,265,266]

The lateral scapular slide test (LSST) is an objective method to quantitatively measure scapular stabilizer strength by comparing the position of the scapula on each side with varying degrees of loads, in three different positions.[11,15] This test has been found to have acceptable intratester reliability, but inconsistent intertester reliability.[266] The first position is with the arm relaxed by the side. The second is with the hands on the hips with the fingers anterior and the thumb posterior with about 10 degrees of shoulder extension (Fig. 14-20). The third position is with the arms at or below 90 degrees of arm elevation (Fig. 14-21). The inferior-medial angle of the scapula is palpated and marked on

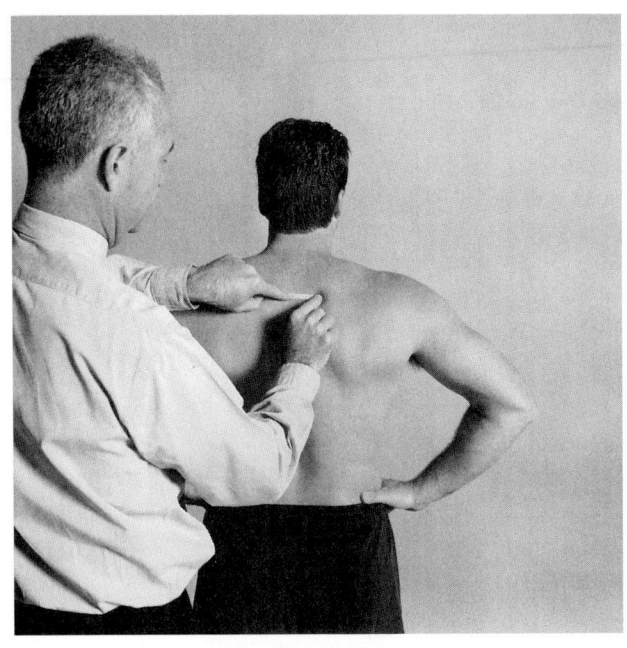

FIGURE 14-20 Lateral slide test: second position.

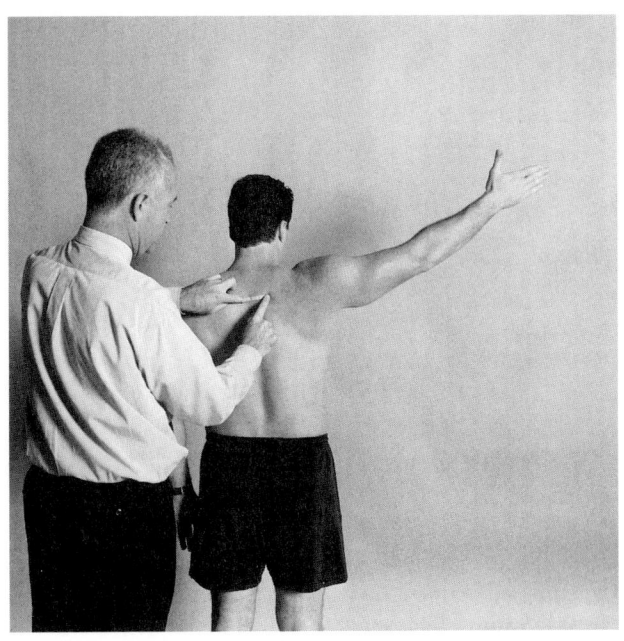

FIGURE 14-21 Lateral slide test: third position.

both the involved and noninvolved sides. The nearest spinous process to this point is marked with an "X" and becomes the reference point. The distance between the reference point and the inferior-medial angle mark are measured on both sides. In the second position, the new position of the inferior-medial border of the scapula is marked, and the new distance is measured on both sides between the reference point and the inferior-medial border. The same protocol is used for the third position. The degree of asymmetry between the involved and noninvolved sides is calculated. In the injured population, the degree of asymmetry increases when going from the first to third position.

Kibler[15] established a threshold of 1.5 cm asymmetry between the injured and noninjured sides in any of the three positions as the point of significant asymmetry, indicating the presence of shoulder dysfunction.[67,266a] However, a recent study by Koslow et al[266a] which examined the specificity of the LSST in 71 asymptomatic competitive athletes, found the scapular position to be asymmetrical in 52 of the subjects. The same study found the LSST to have a specificity of 26.8% and did not recommend its use for determining shoulder dysfunction in competitive athletes.[266a] In the injured population, Gibson et al.[266] found the LSST to have acceptable intratester reliability, but inconsistent intertester reliability.

Palpation

Palpation must be performed in a systematic manner and focus on specific anatomical structures. Traditionally palpation has been viewed as a static process. However, palpation is a dynamic process and should be performed along with other aspects of the examination. The optimal methods of palpating the shoulder tendons occur in regions where there is the least amount of overlying soft tissue.[267]

It is best to divide the shoulder complex into compartments for palpation as symptoms reproduced by palpation in these compartments are frequently associated with a specific underlying pathology.

Anterior and Superior Compartment. The clinician should begin anteriorly, with palpation of the contours of the clavicle. The anterior and superior aspects of the clavicle are covered by the platysma muscle. The sternal end of the clavicle, which projects cranially over the border of the manubrium, is covered by the sternocleidomastoid (SCM). The following areas related to the clavicle should be palpated for tenderness, swelling, or symptom reproduction:

▶ The supraclavicular fossa, bordered medially by the SCM and laterally by the omohyoid.

▶ The infraclavicular fossa, between the pectoralis major, deltoid, and clavicle. The coracoid process is located in the infraclavicular fossa, especially if the shoulder is placed in extension. Several palpable ligaments and muscles attach here including the coracoclavicular, on the conoid tubercle, the coracoacromial ligament, the pectoralis minor, the coracobrachialis, and the short head of the biceps. A prominent coracoid could indicate a posterior dislocation of the shoulder.

▶ The subclavius and costoclavicular ligament.

▶ *The suprasternal (jugular) notch.* This indentation on the superior border of the sternal manubrium is an important reference point. Three centimeters above the notch is the caudal border of the larynx, while the sternal bellies of the SCM form the sides of the notch. The interclavicular ligament is located within the notch. Disruption of the normal contours of the notch are associated with S-C dislocations.

▶ *The S-C joint and joint line.* Arthrotic changes of the S-C joint are evidenced by crepitus at the joint during internal/external rotation of the humerus with the arm abducted to 90 degrees. The contours of the S-C joint are palpated and a comparison should be made with the contralateral side. Thickening of the S-C, or an S-C dislocation produces an inability to abduct the arm.

▶ *The A-C joint.* Injuries and arthritis of this joint are common, and focal tenderness is an important sign of A-C pathology.[222] Changes in the size and shape of the joint may indicate past or present separation, fracture, or osteoarthritis.

With the arm hanging by the side and the palm facing the body, the greater tuberosity lies laterally and the lesser tuberosity lies anteriorly with respect to each other. They are separated by a bicipital groove. The bicipital groove is made more accessible for palpation with internal rotation of the arm of 15–20 degrees.[267,268] Within this groove lies the biceps tendon, which should be palpated for tenderness. If the arm at rest appears slightly abducted and externally rotated, an anterior dislocation might be present. An adducted and internally rotated arm suggests many shoulder conditions, including a posterior dislocation.

The lesser tuberosity (shaped like an inverted teardrop), is palpated during passive internal and external rotation of the humerus at a point lateral to the coracoid process. The subscapularis can be palpated deep in the deltopectoral triangle at its insertion to the lesser tuberosity. This is accomplished by positioning the arm by the side in neutral rotation, and palpating just lateral to the coracoid.[267]

The greater tuberosity is located directly anterior to the acromion while the shoulder is internally rotated. It is best located when the patient is in side lying, facing the clinician, with their upper arm in front of them in approximately 60 degrees of shoulder flexion. The clinician palpates laterally along the spine of the scapula until contact is made with the superior facet of the greater tuberosity. The supraspinatus and posterior coracohumeral ligament insert on the superior facet, the infraspinatus on its middle facet, and the teres minor on its inferior facet. The supraspinatus, located just distal to the anterolateral corner of the acromion, can be made more discernible by positioning the patient's arm behind the back in slight extension.[267,269]

The subacromial-subdeltoid bursa can be palpated by positioning the patient in prone, and passively stretching the arm into extension before palpating anterior to the A-C joint. Tenderness reported with shoulder extension and relieved with shoulder flexion is indicative of an inflammation of this bursa.

The anterior joint capsule can be located by palpating one fingerbreadth lateral to the coracoid process with the arm by the side. Persistent tenderness at this point with internal and external rotation of the arm suggests capsular involvement.[270]

The muscle bellies, origins, and insertions of the upper trapezius, supraspinatus, and levator scapula should be palpated for tenderness or asymmetries.

Lateral Compartment.   The deltoid muscle belly and insertion should be palpated for tenderness or atrophy.

Posterior Compartment.   The spine of the scapula should be located. The clinician should be able to locate the inferior pole of the scapula, the medial border of the scapula, and the posterior angle of the acromion.

The infraspinatus can be palpated just distal to the posterolateral acromion with the arm in 90 degrees flexion, 10 degrees adduction (Fig. 14-22).[267] The teres minor is isolated and palpated using the same patient position.[267] To help locate the teres minor, the long head of the triceps is palpated by placing the patient's arm in 90 degrees of abduction followed by extension. Once the long head of the triceps is located, the patient is repositioned and the teres minor, now cranial to the long head of the triceps, can be palpated. Tenderness of the posterior capsule suggests capsular laxity.

Inferior Compartment.   The lymph nodes in the axilla are palpated for swelling or tenderness. Also located in the inferior

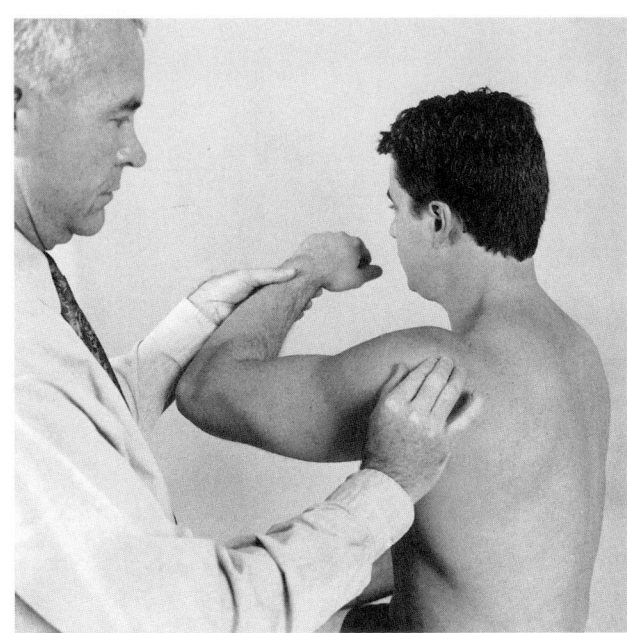

FIGURE 14-22 Palpation of infraspinatus.

compartment are the anterior coracohumeral ligament, glenohumeral ligament, transverse humeral ligament, and pectoralis major. The latissimus dorsi tendon can be palpated deep in the axilla.

The teres major tendon is palpated medial to the cranial part of the latissimus dorsi tendon insertion. It can be differentiated from the latissimus dorsi by using a combination of isometric internal rotation and adduction with the patient's shoulder positioned in 90 degrees of abduction and maximum external rotation.

The subscapularis tendon is palpable between the serratus anterior and the latissimus dorsi while the patient's arm is elevated.

Active and Passive Range of Motion

Due to the complex nature of the arthrokinematics, osteokinematics, and myokinetics of this region, the results from the active and passive movements can be misleading. Active motion testing provides the clinician with information regarding:

▶ Overall functional capacity of the shoulder.

▶ Painful or hesitant initiation or ending of movement. Such a hesitation may be a subtle sign of instability or rotator cuff dysfunction.[271]

▶ Quantity of movement (Table 14-13).

▶ Developed trick movements or modifications to the movement, such as an altered plane, the use of trunk movements, or abnormal recruitment of muscles.

▶ Associated signs and symptoms not reproduced with nonfunctional motion testing.

▶ Presence of a capsular pattern (Table 14-14).

▶ Detection of a "painful arc."

▶ End-feels (see Table 14-13), if passive overpressure is applied.

McClure and Flowers[272] classify limited shoulder motion into two categories:

▶ Decreased ROM secondary to changes in the periarticular structures, including shortening of the capsule, ligaments, or muscles as well as adhesion formation. Clinical findings for this category include a history of trauma,[217,273,274] immobilization,[217,273,274] presence of a capsular pattern,[275] capsular end-feel,[275] and no pain with the isometric testing.[275]

▶ Decreased ROM due to nonstructural problems, including the presence of pain, protective muscle spasm, or a loose body within the joint space.[276] Clinical findings for this patient include a history of trauma or overuse, and the presence of a noncapsular pattern of motion restriction.

The patient is asked to bring the arm actively through the ranges of motion. These motions include flexion, extension,

TABLE 14-13 Normal Ranges for Movements of the Shoulder Complex and Potential Causes of Pain[27,29,49,152,166,281]

Motion	Range Norms (Degrees)	End-Feel	Potential Source of Pain
Elevation-flexion	160–180	Tissue stretch	• Suprahumeral impingement • Stretching of glenohumeral, acromioclavicular, sternoclavicular joint capsule • Triceps tendon if elbow flexed
Extension	50–60	Tissue stretch	• Stretching of glenohumeral joint capsule • Severe suprahumeral impingement • Biceps tendon if elbow extended
Elevation-abduction	170–180	Tissue stretch	• Suprahumeral impingement • Acromioclavicular arthritis at terminal abduction
External rotation	80–90	Tissue stretch	• Anterior glenohumeral instability
Internal rotation	60–1000	Tissue stretch	• Suprahumeral impingement • Posterior glenohumeral instability

TABLE 14-14 Close Packed, Open Packed and Capsular Patterns of the Shoulder Complex

	Close Packed	Open Packed	Capsular Pattern
Glenohumeral	90° of glenohumeral abduction and full external rotation; or full abduction and external rotation	55° abduction, 30° horizontal adduction	External rotation, abduction, internal rotation
Acromioclavicular	90° abduction	Arm resting by side	Pain at extremes of range, especially horizontal adduction and full elevation
Sternoclavicular	Full arm elevation and shoulder protraction	Arm resting by side	Pain at extremes of range, especially horizontal adduction and full elevation

abduction, internal rotation (Fig. 14-23), external rotation, horizontal adduction, and shrugging of the shoulders.

Arm Elevation. The clinician should view the patient carefully as he or she attempts arm elevation. Elevation in the frontal plane and scapular plane is assessed. Typically, 170 to 180 degrees of elevation is possible in both of these planes, with the upper portion of the arm able to be placed adjacent to the head. If the patient is unable to achieve 170–180 degrees, the clinician must determine where and why movement is not occurring. If there is an arc of pain, the point in the range where the arc of pain occurs can be diagnostic in implicating the cause.

> ### *Clinical Pearl*
>
> Pain that occurs between 70 and 110 degrees of abduction is deemed a "painful arc" and may indicate rotator cuff impingement, or tearing, or subacromial bursitis.[200] Pain that occurs in the 120–160/160–180 degree range, may indicate involvement of the A-C joint.[200]

One study attempted to differentiate various types of painful arcs and proposed that adding external rotation to the painful range indicated subscapularis involvement, or possibly supraspinatus and/or infraspinatus involvement when the pain was increased.[200] The same study suggested that the addition of

FIGURE 14-23A Shoulder active range of motion. Range of arm movement on trunk (involving both shoulder joint and shoulder girdle) a. Rotation with arm at side. b. Rotation with arm in abduction. c. Internal rotation posteriorly. (Reproduced with permission from Luttgens K, Hamilton K. *Kinesiology: Scientific Basis of Human Motion.* New York: McGraw-Hill; 1997.)

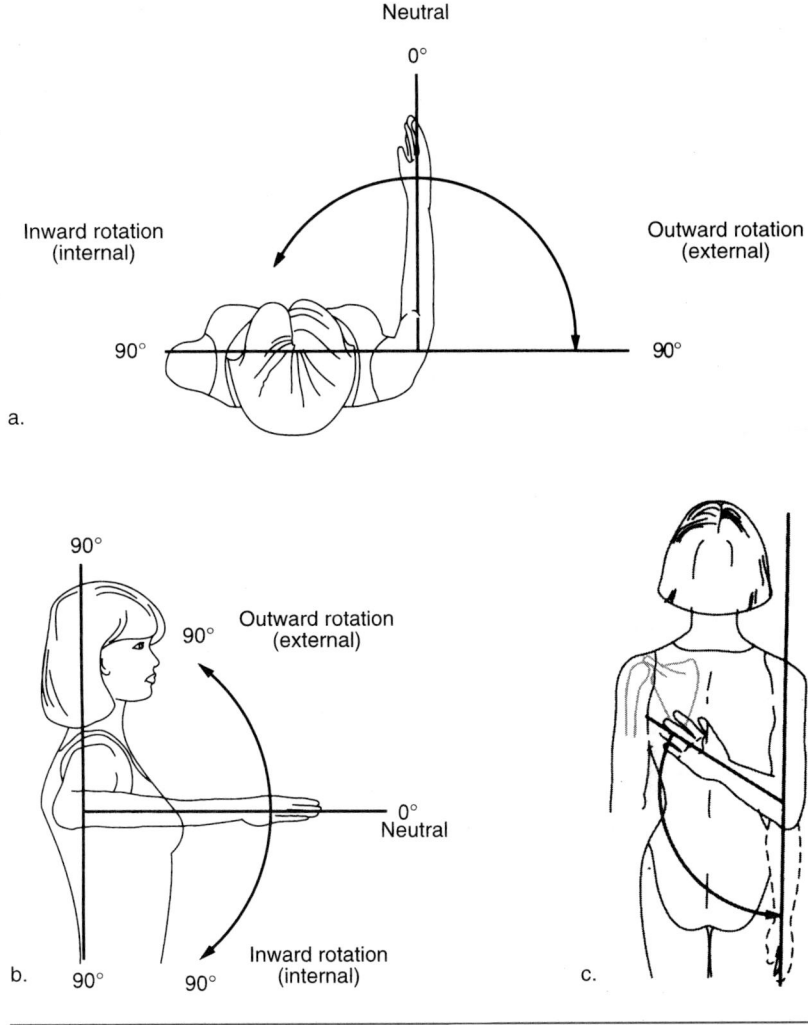

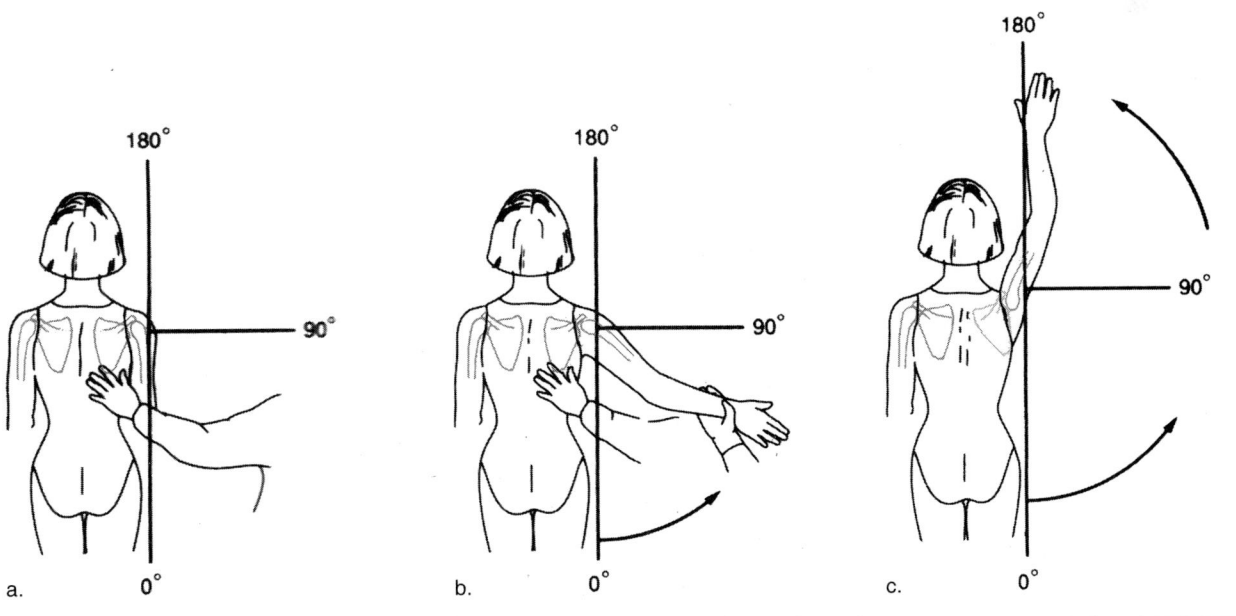

FIGURE 14-23B Shoulder active range of motion. Range of shoulder joint (glenohumeral) motion. a. Starting position. b. Abduction. c. Sideward-upward elevation of arm (combining abduction of arm and upward rotation of scapula). (Reproduced with permission from Luttgens K, Hamilton K. *Kinesiology: Scientific Basis of Human Motion.* New York: McGraw-Hill; 1997.)

internal rotation to the painful range indicated that the supraspinatus and/or infraspinatus was more likely the source of involvement when the pain was increased.[200]

Kibler[15] advocates the use of the "muscle assistance" test to assess scapular motion and position during elevation and lowering of the arm to see if impingement may be due to a lack of acromial elevation or poor scapular control (Fig. 14-24). The clinician pushes laterally and superiorly on the inferior-medial border of the scapula during arm elevation to simulate the action of the serratus anterior/lower trapezius force couple. If the impingement symptoms are abolished with this maneuver, muscle inhibition should be suspected.[15]

Weakness of the serratus anterior muscle, due to palsy or disuse, produces winging of the scapula as the patient attempts to elevate the arm.[4,83,85] In addition to winging, serratus anterior dysfunction presents with a loss of scapular protraction during attempted shoulder elevation and an increase in the prominence of the inferior tip of the scapula.[82] Differentiating between active shoulder abduction and active shoulder flexion can often help highlight the cause of dysfunction.

Abduction of the shoulder requires a greater utilization of the upper and lower trapezius muscles, whereas shoulder flexion is more likely to recruit the serratus anterior muscle.[63,139]

While lesions to the deltoid are rare, imbalances of the deltoid and the rotator cuff are common. When the deltoid becomes dominant, the humeral head will be seen to glide superiorly during arm elevation because the downward pull of the rotator cuff muscles are insufficient to counterbalance the upward pull of the deltoid (humeral superior glide syndrome).[237] This alteration in the glenohumeral force couple usually occurs during the middle phase of elevation[134] (between 80 and 140 degrees), because the upward translation force of the

deltoid peaks during this phase, requiring more compressive and depressive forces from the rotator cuff muscles.[174,277]

An anterior glide of the humeral head, which occurs during arm elevation (humeral anterior glide syndrome)[237] suggests that the posterior deltoid has become the dominant external rotator.[237] This syndrome should be expected if the pain is located in the anterior or anteromedial aspect of the shoulder and is increased glenohumeral internal rotation, shoulder hyperextension, and by horizontal abduction, and is decreased when the humeral head is prevented from moving anteriorly during shoulder rotation and flexion movements.[237]

When compared, the range achieved for unilateral arm elevation should be greater than that achieved when bilateral arm elevation is attempted. This is because the joints of the cervicothoracic junction have to be permitted to rotate towards the elevating arm and arc prevented from doing so during bilateral arm elevation. The clinician should observe the smoothness of the scapulohumeral rhythm during elevation and the ratio between the scapular upward rotation and glenohumeral elevation (refer to Examination of the Dynamic Scapula).

Compressive forces across the A-C joint occur mainly in the terminal 60 degrees of abduction. This often causes pain during this range if pathology exists at this joint.[222]

Rotation. The loss of external rotation at the shoulder is often associated with adhesive capsulitis. The following arm positions can be used to assess internal and external rotation:

▶ The arm at shoulder level (at 90 degrees of abduction) (i.e., as in an attempt to throw a baseball). Normal external rotation is to 90 degrees or beyond. Internal rotation is then carried out, rotating the hand towards the hip, as if positioning it behind the body. Normal internal rotation approaches 90 degrees. However, this position is often uncomfortable, and is not very functional, except for pitchers.

▶ The arm to the side, and the elbow flexed to 90 degrees. Again, it is important to assess active and passive range, because a loss of active motion alone may indicate muscular weakness.

▶ The arm at the side and the forearm behind the back. This measurement for internal rotation is assessed by the position reached with the extended thumb up the dorsal aspect of the spine using the spinous processes as landmarks (Fig. 14-25).[278] This is the more functional test, and the thumb tip of normal subjects will reach the T5–T10 level.[222] Loss of motion with this test affects the patient's ability to perform toileting duties, hook bras behind the back, reach into a back pocket, and tuck in shirts.[279] The examination is made relative to the opposite side, as there is quite a large variation in range among normal subjects.

Horizontal Adduction. Pain with horizontal adduction may indicate A-C joint pathology.

The patient then completes the motions of shoulder girdle elevation (shrug) and depression, and shoulder protraction and retraction. An inability to shrug the shoulder may indicate a trape-

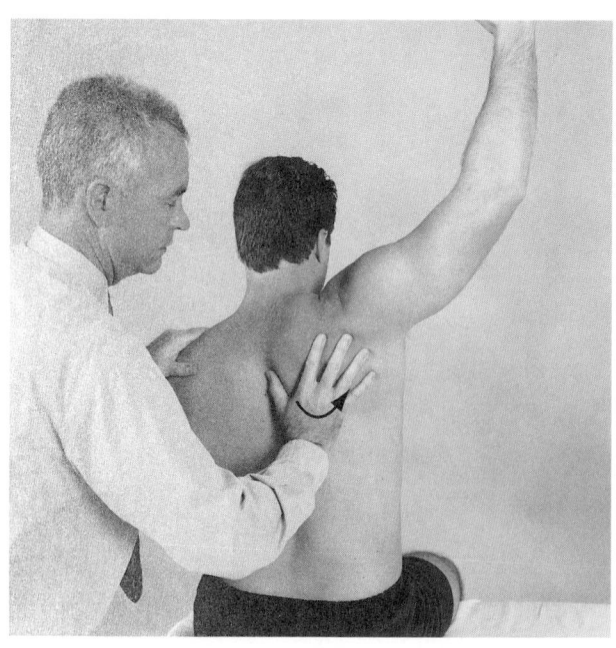

FIGURE 14-24   Scapular assist.

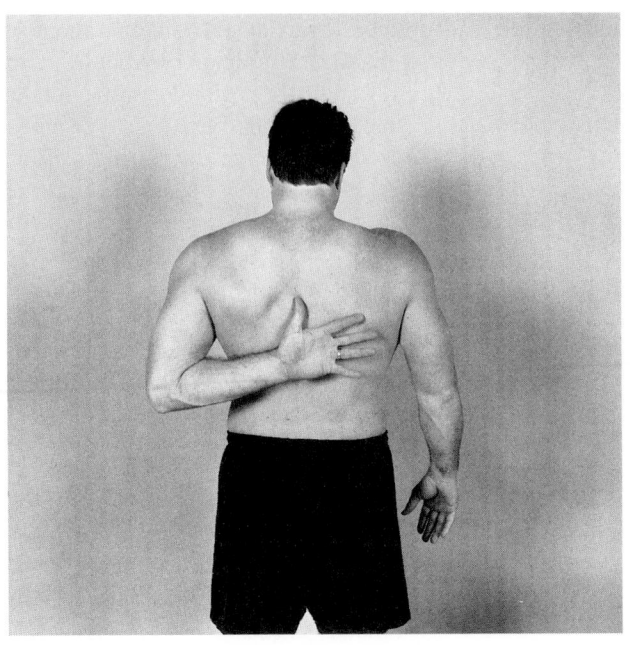

FIGURE 14-25 Shoulder internal rotation.

zius palsy.[82] Hiking of the shoulder and the scapular during arm elevation is often seen in patients with large rotator cuff tears.[227]

Movement combinations are assessed.

> ### Clinical Pearl
>
> If pain is reproduced when internal rotation and extension are combined from a position of 90 degrees abduction, the A-C joint, subcoracoid bursa, or subscapularis tendon may be implicated.
>
> If the pain is reproduced with extension with the humerus in 90 degrees of flexion, the shoulder abductors, external rotators, and suprascapular nerve may be implicated. A jammed end-feel with this maneuver may indicate a thoracic dysfunction.
>
> An isolated limitation of passive external rotation may indicate subcoracoid bursitis, which is aggravated by the pectoralis major muscle being stretched over it.[277]

Passive range of motion is performed if there is a deficiency in active motion to determine the end-feel.[275] Traditionally passive range of motion has been performed with the patient positioned in supine. Given the importance of scapular motion during humeral elevation, care must be taken that the scapular is not being prevented from rotating during these tests.

A discrepancy between active and passive motion may indicate a painful periarticular condition.[227] Loss of active motion with preservation of passive motion is likely caused by rotator cuff tear,[196] or rarely, suprascapular nerve injury.[209,280] A severely restricted active abduction pattern with no pain is suggestive of a rupture of the supraspinatus or deltoid. Loss of both active and passive motion is usually caused by adhesive capsulitis.[236]

A loss of passive or active range of motion may be associated with a loss of flexibility in the passive restraints to motion. This can occur with both single plane motions and combined motions.[27,29,152,166,281] For example, if both internal and external rotations are restricted and muscle tightness has been ruled out as a cause, an adhesion of the middle glenohumeral ligament is implicated.[166]

Examination of the Dynamic Scapula

Given the importance of the scapulothoracic joint to overall shoulder function, it is important to examine the scapulothoracic joint arthrokinematics, and muscle power.[282]

A number of muscles play an important role in the kinematics of the scapula, including the trapezius and serratus anterior. Increased activity of the upper trapezius muscle, or imbalances between the upper and lower trapezius muscle during shoulder elevation may have adverse effects on the kinematics of the scapula.[66,87,141,218]

According to Sahrmann[237] four abnormal clinical findings exist for the scapula:

▶ The scapular alignment is correct but its movement is impaired.

▶ The scapula alignment is impaired and its movement is impaired.

▶ The scapula alignment is impaired and its movement is of normal range, but does not correct or compensate for the impaired start position.

▶ The scapula alignment is impaired but its movement is sufficient to compensate for the impaired start position.

Kibler[15] recommends the use of the isometric "scapular pinch" test to examine the strength of the medial scapular muscles. This involves the patient squeezing their shoulder blades together. Normally, the scapula can be held in this position for 15 to 20 seconds without difficulty. If a burning pain occurs in less than 15 seconds, Kibler suggests that scapular muscle weakness may be the cause.[15]

Observation of the scapulohumeral rhythm should reveal that the scapula stops its rotation when the arm has been elevated to approximately 140 degrees. Upon completion of the elevation, the inferior angle of the scapula should be in close proximity to the mid-line of the thorax, and the vertebral border of the scapular should be rotated 60 degrees. Movement beyond these points may indicate excessive scapular abduction.[237] At the end range of elevation, the scapula should slightly depress, posteriorly tilt, and adduct.[237] The scapulothoracic rhythm should be assessed carefully in patients with suspected multidirectional instability. A scapulothoracic dyskinesia (decrease in scapular abduction and external rotation with progressive arm abduction) is often observed in patients with anteroinferior instability.[283] Posteroinferior instability is characterized by excessive scapular retraction.[268] An inferior instability is characterized by a drooping of the lateral scapula or "scapular dumping."[268]

Positioning the patient in prone with their arm abducted to 90 degrees and external rotation tests the ability of the scapula to remain in its correct position rather than abducting due to excessive lengthening of the thoracoscapular muscles (trapezius and rhomboids) and shortening of the scapulohumeral muscles.[237]

Resistive Tests

In addition to pain, shoulder dysfunction is often caused or exacerbated by loss of motion or weakness. The resistive tests assess function in the important muscle groups of the upper kinetic chain (Tables 14-15 and 14-16).

TABLE 14-15   Muscle Groups Tested in the Shoulder Examination[49]

Trunk flexors, extensors, and obliques
Scapulothoracic elevators
Scapulothoracic depressors
Scapulothoracic protractors
Scapulothoracic retractors
Scapulothoracic upward rotators
Scapulothoracic downward rotators
Glenohumeral flexors
Glenohumeral extensors
Glenohumeral abductors
Glenohumeral adductors
Glenohumeral internal rotators
Glenohumeral external rotators
Glenohumeral horizontal flexors
Glenohumeral horizontal extensors
Elbow flexors
Elbow extensors
Forearm supinators
Forearm pronators
Wrist flexors
Wrist extensors
Hand intrinsics

Localized, individual isometric muscle tests around the shoulder girdle can give the clinician information about patterns of weakness other than from spinal nerve root or peripheral nerve palsies, e.g., instabilities, postural dysfunction, and also help to isolate the pain generators. Weakness on isometric testing needs to be analyzed for the type (increasing weakness with repeated contractions of the same resistance indicating a palsy versus consistent weakness with repeated contractions which could suggest a deconditioned muscle, or a significant muscle tear), and the pattern of weakness (spinal nerve root, nerve trunk, or peripheral nerve). A painful weakness is invariably a sign of serious pathology, and depending on the pattern, could indicate a fracture or a tumor. However, if a single motion is painfully weak this could indicate muscle inhibition due to pain.

> ### Clinical Pearl
>
> Pain with isometric muscle testing is generally considered a sign of first or second degree musculotendinous lesion. According to Cyriax,[275] pain that occurs during a muscle contraction is more likely to indicate a lesion within a muscle belly, whereas pain that occurs upon release of the contraction is more likely to indicate a lesion within a tendon.[277] However, because of the large amount of accessory joint gliding that occurs in the girdle joints with isometric contraction, the tests for inert tissue involvement must be negative before coming to the conclusion that the musculotendinous structure is at fault.

Cyriax[275] believed that supraspinatus tendonitis is the most common cause of a painful arc. The supraspinatus can be tested using the Jobe test or empty can position (Fig. 14-26). The

TABLE 14-16   Shoulder Girdle Muscle Function and Innervation

Muscles	Peripheral Nerve	Nerve Root	Motions
Pectoralis major	Pectoral	C5–C8	Adduction, horizontal adduction, and internal rotation Clavicular fibers: forward flexion Sternocostal fibers: extension
Latissimus dorsi	Thoracodorsal	C7(C6,C8)	Adduction, extension, and internal rotation
Teres major	Subscapular	C5–C8	Adduction, extension, horizontal abduction, and internal rotation
Teres minor	Axillary	C5(6)	Horizontal abduction (also a weak external rotator)
Deltoid	Axillary	C5(6)	Anterior: forward flexion, horizontal adduction Middle: abduction Posterior: extension, horizontal abduction
Supraspinatus	Suprascapular	C5(6)	Abduction
Subscapularis	Subscapular	C5–C8	Adduction, and internal rotation
Infraspinatus	Suprascapular	C5(C6)	Abduction, horizontal abduction, and external rotation

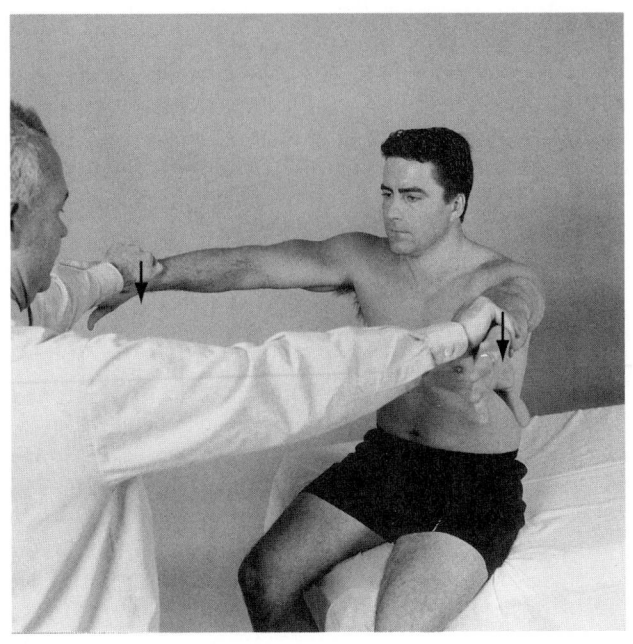

FIGURE 14-26 Jobe or empty can test for supraspinatus.

patient's arm is positioned in the scaption plane—internal rotation and approximately 90 degrees of shoulder flexion. Manual resistance is then applied by the clinician in a direction toward the floor. The Jobe test can also be performed similarly with the humerus externally rotated (full can test). One study[284] found the empty can test to have a high sensitivity of 86 percent and a low specificity of 50 percent in diagnosing supraspinatus tendon tears in a series of 55 patients. However, in another study,[285] the full can test had higher specificity (74 versus 68 percent) and an equal sensitivity of 77 percent when compared with the empty can test in a series of 136 patients.

A partial rupture of the supraspinatus tendon will result in abduction that is both weak and painful.[48] The tendon of the supraspinatus can be passively stretched by positioning it in adduction and internal rotation to see if this increases the pain.[286] A painless weakness with abduction could indicate a complete rupture of the supraspinatus tendon.[48]

It has been documented that if coracohumeral pain decreases during resisted abduction with the addition of arm traction, subacromial-subdeltoid bursitis or an A-C joint lesion should be suspected.[287] However, this was not found to be the case with ultrasonography.[288] Similar claims have been reported that if the pain increases with arm traction, the supraspinatus may be implicated. However, this has yet to be substantiated.

The test position for the *infraspinatus* and *teres minor* muscles is 90 degrees of glenohumeral flexion and one-half full external rotation.[289] If the pain is isolated to external rotation, then the infraspinatus is at fault. If external rotation and resisted adduction are painful, the teres minor is at fault, although isolated involvement of the teres minor is not common. To test the teres minor further, the muscle is placed on stretch by

positioning the patient in prone with their upper arms vertical, adducted, and externally rotated to approximately 20 degrees. The patient is asked to lean towards the tested side to increase the adduction.

The *teres major* muscle can be tested by positioning the patient in prone with their hand resting on their lower back. The patient is asked to adduct and extend the humerus while the clinician applies resistance at the elbow into shoulder abduction.

To assess for *rhomboid* dominance, the patient positions their arm by their side with their elbow flexed to about 90 degrees. Resisted external rotation in this position should not result in any scapular adduction, unless there is rhomboid dominance and poor control of glenohumeral external rotation.[237] There should also be no superior or anterior gliding of the humerus during this test, unless deltoid dominance is occurring.[237]

Conditions to be ruled out if there is a painless weakness of external rotation include, but are not limited to:

▶ A complete rupture of the infraspinatus tendon.

▶ A C5 nerve root palsy.

▶ A suprascapular nerve palsy.

▶ Neuralgic amyotrophy.

The *subscapularis* is best assessed using the lift-off test as described by Gerber and Krushell, who found the tests had a sensitivity of 80 percent and a specificity of 100 percent for a tear of the subscapularis.[290] The lift-off test is performed with the arm internally rotated so that the posterior surface of the hand rests on the lower back. Actively lifting the hand away from the back (Fig. 14-27) and providing a resisting force suggests integrity of the subscapularis.

Resisted adduction is tested with the arm at 0 degrees of abduction so that the subscapularis is not facilitated.[290] Pain with resisted adduction tends to be fairly rare, but could implicate the pectoralis major, latissimus dorsi, teres major, and teres minor.

> **Clinical Pearl**
>
> A patient with subacromial-subdeltoid bursitis, in the absence of a rotator cuff tear, will often demonstrate weakness of the rotator cuff secondary to pain if tested with the arm positioned in the arc of impingement. It will, however, show good strength if tested with the arm out of abduction. A patient with a significant cuff tear usually demonstrates profound weakness of the rotator cuff in various arm positions.

Testing of *deltoid* function is best done with resisted abduction with the arm in 90 degrees of abduction and neutral rotation.[222] A painful arc cannot be produced by a lesion to the deltoid muscle due to its anatomical position.

Differential diagnosis will be needed to rule out several neurological disorders, which may provoke painless weakness

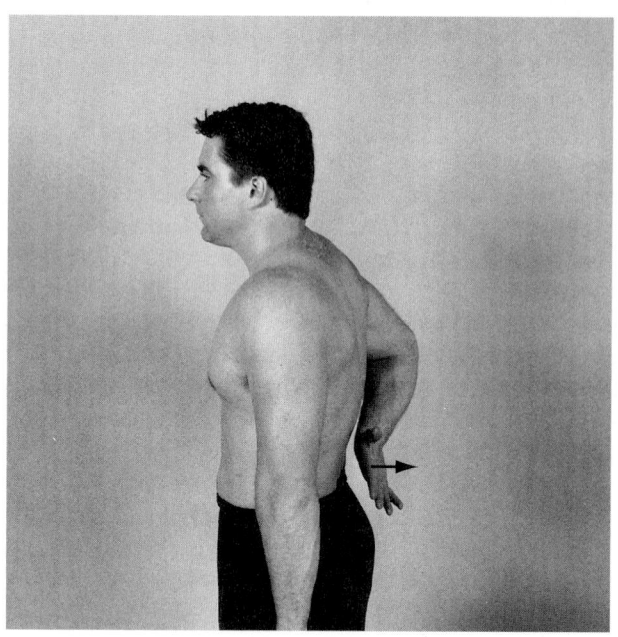

FIGURE 14-27   Lift-off test.

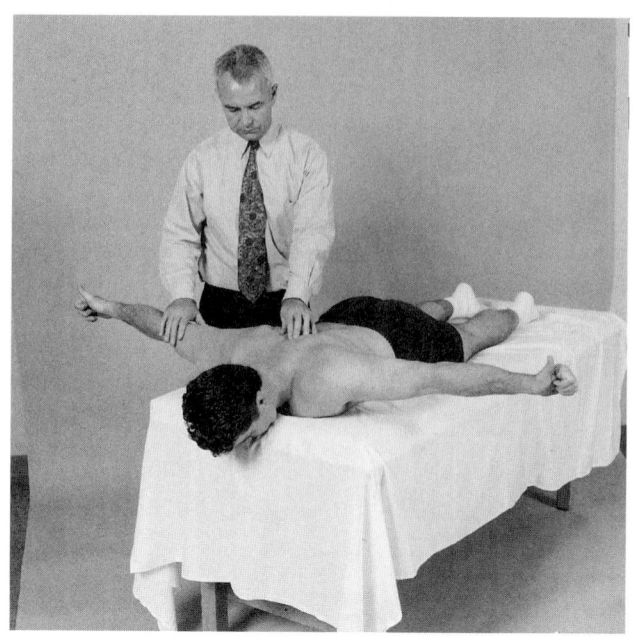

FIGURE 14-28   Middle trapezius test.

on resisted abduction. These include an axillary nerve palsy, a suprascapular nerve palsy, or a fifth cervical root palsy.

The three components of the *trapezius* are assessed as follows:

▶ *Upper trapezius (and levator scapulae).*   Usually both sides are tested simultaneously. The patient is asked to shrug the shoulders to the ears. If the patient is unable to perform this action, he or she is positioned in supine to eliminate the effect of gravity, and asked to repeat the test. Resistance is applied by the clinician in an attempt to depress the shoulders. Unilateral resistance can be applied to the posterior lateral aspect of the head while stabilizing the shoulder.

▶ *Middle trapezius.*   The patient is positioned in prone with the shoulder joint abducted to 90 degrees, elbow extended, and the forearm in maximum supination so that the thumb is pointing to the ceiling (Fig. 14-28). The clinician applies pressure on the humerus by pushing towards the floor.

▶ *Lower trapezius.*   The patient is positioned in prone, with the upper limb supported in the elevated position, and aligned in the direction of the lower trapezius muscle fibers (Fig. 14-29). The grades of 0 to 2 are determined by the firmness of the muscle contraction. Grades 2+ and 3− are based on how far the limb is lifted from the table. Grades 3 to 5 require the application of resistance by the clinician.

The *serratus anterior* can be assessed in a number of ways, including using the wall push-up. A more sensitive test involves positioning the patient in supine with their shoulder flexed to 90 degrees, and their elbow flexed. The patient is asked to protract the shoulder by lifting the elbow to the ceiling. Resistance

is applied by the clinician at the elbow pushing downwards (Fig. 14-30).

Finally, resisted elbow flexion and extension, as well as forearm supination, are examined to assess *biceps*, *brachialis* and *triceps* function. Isometric elbow extension and flexion with the muscles in a stretched position will help exclude the biceps and

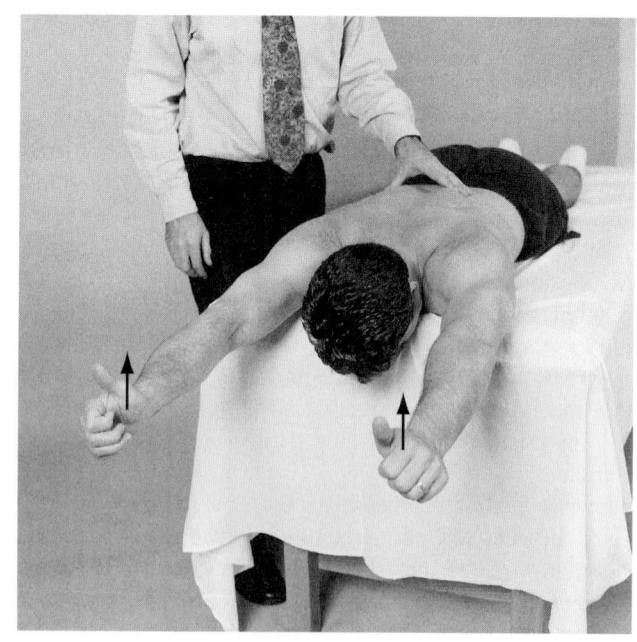

FIGURE 14-29   Lower trapezius test.

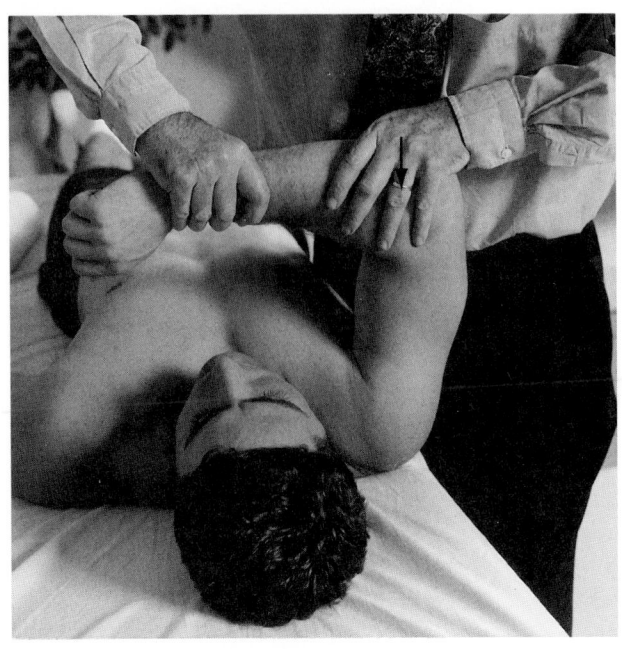

FIGURE 14-30 Serratus anterior test.

triceps muscles. Pain reproduced with resisted elbow flexion could indicate a lesion to one or more of the elbow flexors, such as an intra-articular lesion of the long head of the biceps or a lesion in the sulcus of the long head of the biceps. The sulcus lesion can be tested with the patient side lying, facing away from the clinician, their arm hanging behind them. The clinician stabilizes the scapula, and applies a longitudinal force along the humerus in a superior direction, to drive the humerus superiorly. A positive sign is pain reproduced with this maneuver.

A painless weakness of elbow flexion can result from a fifth cervical root palsy, or a sixth cervical root palsy. (A complete rupture of all of the elbow flexors is an extremely unlikely event.)

The wrist and hand are also evaluated for motor function (see Chap. 16).

Examination of Movement Patterns[237]

These tests are concerned with the coordination, timing, or sequence of activation of the muscles during movement.

Serratus Anterior. The patient is positioned in prone and is asked to perform a push-up and then return to the start position extremely slowly. The clinician checks for the quality of scapula stabilization. If the stabilizers are weak, the scapula on the side of impairment will shift outward and upward with a resultant winging of the scapula.

Shoulder Abduction. The patient is positioned in sitting with their elbow flexed to control the humeral rotation. The patient is asked to slowly abduct the arm. Three components are evaluated:

▶ Abduction at the G-H joint.

▶ Rotation of the scapula.

▶ Elevation of the whole shoulder girdle. The abduction movement is stopped at the point at which the shoulder begins to elevate. This typically occurs at about 60 degrees of glenohumeral abduction.

Functional Testing

The assessment of shoulder function is an integral part of the examination of the shoulder complex. Functional testing of the shoulder complex can include tests designed to detect a biomechanical dysfunction or tests designed to assess the patient's ability to perform the basic functions of activities of daily living.

Biomechanical Function. There are only two functional motions within the shoulder girdle: arm elevation using a combination of flexion and abduction, and arm extension with adduction. All other motions of the shoulder are parts or composites of these two basic functional sets.

Basic Function Testing. By referring to Table 14-17, the clinician can determine the functional status of the shoulder for basic functions simply by measuring the amount of available range of motion. For example, humeral motions necessary for eating and drinking have been reported at 5 to 45 degrees of

TABLE 14-17   Range of Motion Necessary at the Shoulder for Functional Activities[322,505]

Activity	Necessary Range of Motion
Eating	70–100° horizontal adduction 45–60° abduction
Combing hair	30–70° horizontal adduction 105–120° abduction 90° external rotation
Reach perineum	75–90° horizontal adduction 30–45° abduction 90° or greater internal rotation
Tuck in shirt	50–60° horizontal adduction 55–65° abduction 90° internal rotation
Position hand behind head	10–15° horizontal adduction 110–125° forward flexion 90° external rotation
Put an item on a shelf	70–80° horizontal adduction 70–80° forward flexion 45° external rotation
Wash opposite shoulder	60–90° forward flexion 60–120° horizontal adduction

TABLE 14-18 Functional Testing of the Shoulder[a]

Starting Position	Action	Functional Test
Sitting, cuff weight attached to wrist	Forward flex arm to 90°, elbow extended	Raise 1- to 3-lb weight: functionally fair Raise arm without weight: functionally poor Cannot raise arm: nonfunctional
Sitting, cuff weight attached to wrist	Extend shoulder, elbow extended	Raise 4- to 5-lb weight: functional Raise 3- to 4-lb weight: functional fair Raise arm without weight: functionally poor Cannot extend arm: nonfunctional
Sitting with hand behind low back	Shoulder internal rotation	Raise 5-lb weight: functional Raise 1- to 3-lb weight: functional fair Raise arm without weight: functionally poor Cannot raise arm: nonfunctional
Side lying, cuff weight attached to wrist	Shoulder external rotation	Raise 5-lb weight: functional Raise 3- to 4-lb weight: functional fair Raise arm without weight: functionally poor Cannot raise arm: nonfunctional
Sitting, cuff weight attached to wrist	Shoulder abduction to 90°	Raise 5-lb weight: functional Raise 3- to 4-lb weight: functional fair Raise arm without weight: functionally poor Cannot raise arm: nonfunctional
Sitting, arm abducted to 145°	Shoulder adduction	Pull 5-lb weight: functional Pull 3- to 4-lb weight: functional fair Pull 1- to 2-lb weight: functionally poor Cannot pull 1 lb: nonfunctional
Sitting	Shoulder elevation (Shoulder shrug)	5 Repetitions: functional 3 to 4 Repetitions: functional fair 1 to 2 Repetitions: functionally poor 0 Repetitions: nonfunctional
Sitting	Scapular depression	5 Repetitions: functional 3 to 4 Repetitions: functional fair 1 to 2 Repetitions: functionally poor 0 Repetitions: nonfunctional

[a] From Magee DJ: Shoulder. In: Magee DJ, ed, Orthopedic Physical Assessment. Philadelphia: WB Saunders; 1992:90–142.

flexion, 5 to 35 degrees of abduction, and 5 to 25 degrees of internal rotation relative to the trunk.[291] Combing hair has been found to require 112 degrees of arm elevation.[115]

The assessment tools outlined in Tables 14-18 and 14-19 can also be used as functional tests of the shoulder.

Simple Shoulder Test. Lippitt and colleagues[292] advocate the use of the Simple Shoulder Test (Table 14-20). The Simple Shoulder Test is a standardized self-assessment of shoulder function consisting of 12 yes/no questions. The Simple Shoulder Test has high test and retest reproducibility, and is sensitive to a wide variety of shoulder disorders.[292] In addition, the Simple Shoulder Test has been shown to be a practical tool for documenting the efficacy of treatment for shoulder conditions. Patients without rotator cuff disease or other shoulder disorders are able to do all 12 functions of the Simple Shoulder Test.[228,293–295]

When compared with other available shoulder self-assessment questionnaires, the Simple Shoulder Test has the highest test/retest reliability, takes the shortest amount of time for a patient to complete, is the easiest to score, and has satisfactory responsiveness.[296,297] The questions can be asked at the initial visit and then at subsequent visits to track progress.

TABLE 14-19   Athletic Rating Scale[619]

Athletic Shoulder Outcome Rating Scale

Name _____   Age _____   Sex _____
Dominant Hand (R) _____ (L) _____ (Ambidextrous)
Date of Examination _____   Position Played
Surgeon _____   Years Played
Type of Sport _____   Prior Injury

Activity Level
1. Professional (Major League)
2. Professional (Minor League)
3. College
4. High School
5. Recreational (Full Time)
6. Recreational (Occasionally)

Diagnosis
1. Anterior Instability
2. Posterior Instability
3. Multidirectional Instability
4. Recurrent Dislocations
5. Impingement Syndrome
6. Acromioclavicular Separation
7. Acromioclavicular Arthrosis
8. Rotator Cuff Repair (Partial)
9. Rotator Cuff Tear (Complete)
10. Biceps Tendon Rupture
11. Calcific Tendonitis
12. Fracture

Subjective (90) Points

I. Pain	Points
No pain with competition	10
Pain after competing only	8
Pain while competing	6
Pain preventing competing	4
Pain with ADLs	2
Pain at rest	0

II. Strength/Endurance	Points
No weakness, normal competition fatigue	10
Weakness after competition, early competition fatigue	8
Weakness during competition, abnormal competition fatigue	6
Weakness or fatigue preventing competition	4
Weakness or fatigue with ADLs	2
Weakness or fatigue preventing ADLs	0

III. Stability	Points
No looseness during competition	10
Recurrent subluxations while competing	8
Dead-arm syndrome while competing	6
Recurrent subluxations prevent competition	4
Recurrent subluxations during ADLs	2
Dislocation	0

IV. Intensity	Points
Pre-injury versus post-injury hours of competition (100%)	10
Pre-injury versus post-injury hours of competition (less than 75%)	8
Pre-injury versus post-injury hours of competition (less than 50%)	6
Pre-injury versus post-injury hours of competition (less than 25%)	4
Pre-injury and post-injury hours of ADLs (100%)	2
Pre-injury and post-injury hours of ADLs (less than 50%)	0

V. Performance	Points
At the same level, same proficiency	50
At the same level, decreased proficiency	40
At the same level, decreased proficiency, not acceptable to athlete	30
Decreased level with acceptable proficiency at that level	20
Decreased level, unacceptable proficiency	10
Cannot compete, had to switch sport	0

Objective (10 Points)
Range of Motion

	Points
Normal external rotation at 90°-90° position: Normal Elevation	10
Less than 5° loss of external rotation: Normal Elevation	8
Less than 10° loss of external rotation: Normal Elevation	6
Less than 15° loss of external rotation: Normal Elevation	4
Less than 20° loss of external rotation: Normal Elevation	2
Greater than 20° loss of external rotation, or any loss of elevation	0

Overall Results

Excellent:	90–100 points
Good:	70–89 points
Fair:	50–69 points
Poor:	Less than 50 points

TABLE 14-20   The Simple Shoulder Test[295]

1. Is your shoulder comfortable with your arm at rest by your side?

2. Does your shoulder allow you to sleep comfortably?

3. Can you reach the small of your back to tuck in your shirt with your hand?

4. Can you place your hand behind your head with the elbow straight out to the side?

5. Can you place a coin on a shelf at the level of your shoulder without bending your elbow?

6. Can you lift 1 lb (a full pint container) to the level of your shoulder without bending your elbow?

7. Can you lift 8 lb (a full gallon container) to the level of the top of your head without bending your elbow?

8. Can you carry 20 lb at your side with the affected extremity?

9. Do you think you can toss a softball underhand 10 yards with the affected extremity?

10. Do you think you can throw a softball overhand 20 yards with the affected extremity?

11. Can you wash the back of your opposite shoulder with the affected extremity?

12. Would your shoulder allow you to work full time at your usual job?

Disabilities of the Arm, Shoulder, and Hand (DASH). The acronym DASH was chosen to describe an outcome measure that reflects the impact on function of a variety of musculoskeletal diseases and injuries in the upper extremity.[298] Items covered by the DASH questionnaire are symptoms and functional status. The components included under the concept of symptoms are pain, weakness, stiffness, and tingling/numbness.[298] There are three dimensions under functional status: physical, social, and psychological status. Two versions of the DASH are available: a 30-item questionnaire that has optional 3-question modules for sport/music and heavy work activities (Table 14-21), and a 15- to 20-item questionnaire suitable for office use.

One-Arm Hop Test. The one-arm hop test is a functional performance test for athletes, which can be used in preseason screens or to assist in return-to-play decisions. The test requires the patient to be in a one-arm push-up position on the floor (Fig. 14-31). The patient uses his arm to hop onto a 10.2-cm (4-inch) step and back to the floor. The time required to perform five repetitions of this movement as quickly as possible is recorded and compared with the uninvolved arm. With sufficient training, a time of under 10 seconds is considered normal.[299]

The one-arm hop test requires concentric and eccentric muscle strength and coordination while the distal portion of the upper extremity has a significant load placed upon it.[299]

Muscle Length Tests

Pectoralis Major. The patient is positioned in supine with the trunk stabilized. The clinician passively abducts the patient's arm and differentiates between the different bands of the pectoralis major.

Clavicular portion: The patient's arm hangs loosely down over the edge of the table. The clinician moves the patient's shoulder down towards the floor. A slight barrier to the motion is normal; a hard barrier is abnormal.

Sternal portion: With the patient supine on a mat table, they actively abduct their arm fully. Their arm should maintain contact with the table throughout the range.

Pectoralis Minor. The patient is positioned in supine with the trunk stabilized. Adaptive shortening of the pectoralis minor is demonstrated if the lateral border of the spine of the scapula is more than 1 inch off the table.[237]

Latissimus Dorsi. The patient is positioned in supine with the trunk stabilized. The patient is asked to perform bilateral shoulder flexion. Under normal circumstances the patient should be able to perform complete shoulder flexion without any increase in lumbar lordosis occurring.[237] Shoulder flexion that requires an increase in lumbar lordosis to complete is indicative of an adaptively shortened latissimus dorsi.

External Rotators. The patient is positioned in supine with the trunk stabilized. The shoulder is positioned in 90 degrees of abduction with the elbow flexed to approximately 90 degrees. The patient is then asked to allow the shoulder to passively internally rotate. Internal rotation accompanied by an anterior tilt of the scapula, rather than the range of internal rotation increasing is indicative of adaptive shortness of the external rotators.[237] This is confirmed by having the patient perform the maneuver again while the clinician prevents the anterior tilt of the scapula from occurring. With the second test there should be a decrease in the amount of passive internal rotation available.

Passive Physiologic Motion Tests of the Glenohumeral Joint

To ensure that the passive physiological tests are accurate, scapula fixation is essential. For all of these tests, the patient is positioned in supine, with their head supported on a pillow, while the clinician is standing facing the patient. It is assumed that the techniques are performed on the patient's right side, and in these examples the clinician uses the right hand to stabilize the clavicle and scapula, and the left hand to move the

TABLE 14-21   The DASH Questionnaire

Please rate your ability to do the following activities in the last week by circling the number below the appropriate response.

	No Difficulty	Mild Difficulty	Moderate Difficulty	Severe Difficulty	Unable
1. Open a tight or new jar.	1	2	3	4	5
2. Write.	1	2	3	4	5
3. Turn a key.	1	2	3	4	5
4. Prepare a meal.	1	2	3	4	5
5. Push open a heavy door.	1	2	3	4	5
6. Place an object on a shelf above your head.	1	2	3	4	5
7. Do heavy household chores (e.g., wash walls, wash floors).	1	2	3	4	5
8. Garden or do yard work.	1	2	3	4	5
9. Make a bed.	1	2	3	4	5
10. Carry a shopping bag or briefcase.	1	2	3	4	5
11. Carry a heavy object (over 10 lbs).	1	2	3	4	5
12. Change a light bulb overhead.	1	2	3	4	5
13. Wash or blow dry your hair.	1	2	3	4	5
14. Wash your back.	1	2	3	4	5
15. Put on a pullover sweater.	1	2	3	4	5
16. Use a knife to cut food.	1	2	3	4	5
17. Recreational activities which require little effort (e.g., cardplaying, knitting, etc.)	1	2	3	4	5
18. Recreational activities in which you take some force or impact through your arm, shoulder or hand (e.g., golf, hammering, tennis, etc.).	1	2	3	4	5
19. Recreational activities in which you move your arm freely (e.g., playing frisbee, badminton, etc.).	1	2	3	4	5
20. Manage transportation needs (getting from one place to another).	1	2	3	4	5
21. Sexual activities.	1	2	3	4	5

DISABILITIES OF THE ARM, SHOULDER, AND HAND

	Not at All	Slightly	Moderately	Quite a Bit	Extremely
22. During the past week, *to what extent* has your arm, shoulder, or hand problem interfered with your normal social activities with family, friends, neighbors or groups? (*circle number*)	1	2	3	4	5

	Not Limited At All	Slightly Limited	Moderately Limited	Very Limited	Unable
23. During the past week, were you limited in your work or other regular daily activities as a result of your arm, shoulder or hand problem? (*circle number*)	1	2	3	4	5

Please rate the severity of the following symptoms in the last week. (*circle number*)

	None	Mild	Moderate	Severe	Extreme
24. Arm, shoulder, or hand pain.	1	2	3	4	5
25. Arm, shoulder, or hand pain when you performed any specific activity.	1	2	3	4	5
26. Tingling (pins and needles) in your arm, shoulder, or hand.	1	2	3	4	5
27. Weakness in your arm, shoulder, or hand.	1	2	3	4	5
28. Stiffness in your arm, shoulder, or hand.	1	2	3	4	5

TABLE 14-21   *(cont.)*

DISABILITIES OF THE ARM, SHOULDER, AND HAND

	No Difficulty	Mild Difficulty	Moderate Difficulty	Severe Difficulty	So Much Difficulty That I Can't Sleep
29. During the past week, how much difficulty have you had sleeping because of the pain in your arm, shoulder or hand? *(circle number)*	1	2	3	4	5

	Strongly Disagree	Disagree	Neither Agree nor Disagree	Agree	Strongly Agree
30. I feel less capable, less confident or less useful because of my arm, shoulder, or hand problem. *(circle number)*	1	2	3	4	5

Scoring DASH function/symptoms: Add up circled responses (items 1–30); subtract 30; divide by 1.20 = DASH score.
SPORTS/PERFORMING ARTS MODULE (Optional)
The following questions relate to the impact of your arm, shoulder, or hand problem on playing *your musical instrument or sport.* If you play more than one sport or instrument (or play both), please answer with respect to that activity which is most important.

Please indicate the sport or instrument which is most important to you: _____
    I do not play a sport or an instrument. (You may skip this section.)

Please circle the number that best describes your physical ability in the past week. Did you have any difficulty:

	No Difficulty	Mild Difficulty	Moderate Difficulty	Severe Difficulty	Unable
1. Using your usual technique for playing your instrument or sport?	1	2	3	4	5
2. Playing your musical instrument or sport because of arm, shoulder, or hand pain?	1	2	3	4	5
3. Playing your musical instrument or sport as well as you would like?	1	2	3	4	5
4. Spending your usual amount of time practicing or playing your instrument or sport?	1	2	3	4	5

WORK MODULE (Optional)

The following questions ask about the impact of your arm, shoulder, or hand problem on your ability to work (including homemakers if that is your main work role).
    I do not work. (You may skip this section.)

Please circle the number that best describes your physical ability in the past week. Did you have any difficulty:

	No Difficulty	Mild Difficulty	Moderate Difficulty	Severe Difficulty	Unable
1. Using your usual technique for your work?	1	2	3	4	5
2. Doing your usual work because of arm, shoulder, or hand pain?	1	2	3	4	5
3. Doing your work as well as you would like?	1	2	3	4	5
4. Spending your usual amount of time doing your work?	1	2	3	4	5

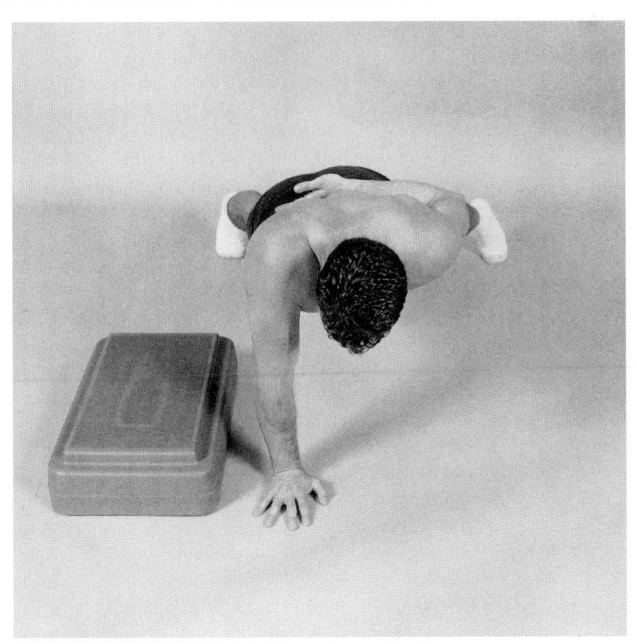

FIGURE 14-31 One-arm hop test.

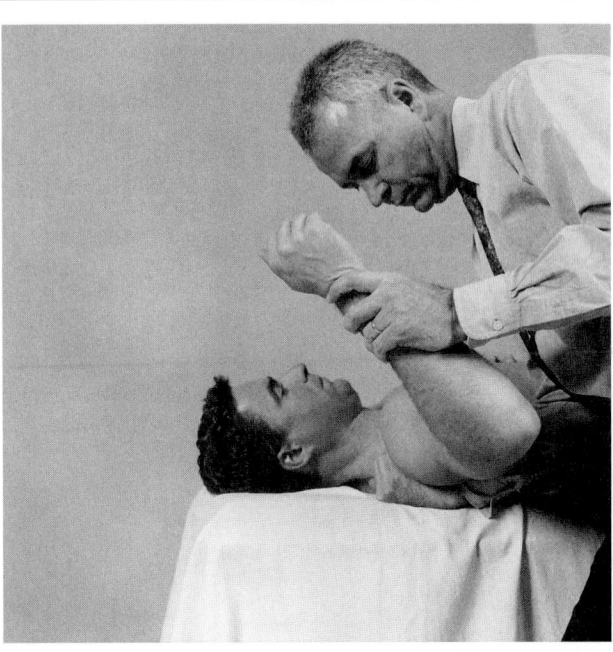

FIGURE 14-32 Clinician and patient position for mobility testing of the shoulder. Note: The clinician's left hand is holding the patient's forearm rather than the elbow so that the stabilizing hand can be viewed.

humerus (Fig. 14-32). As with all tests involving the extremity, both sides must be assessed and comparisons made between the quantity and quality of the motion as well as the end-feel.

The neutral or start position for the techniques is established by positioning the patient's arm against their body, with their forearm vertical. From this position, the clinician pushes the patient's arm into the patients' thorax and allows it to rebound. The joint is now in the start position.

Flexion. Full elevation involves a combination of flexion, abduction, and a conjunct rotation of external rotation. While preventing any internal rotation at the glenohumeral joint from occurring, the clinician flexes the humerus about the appropriate axis. The end-feel is assessed and should be capsular. The normal range for flexion varies depending on general mobility, age, and gender.

Extension. The clinician extends the humerus about the appropriate axis through the glenohumeral joint. The end-feel is assessed and should be capsular. The normal range varies between the genders. For females, it is approximately 90 degrees, while for males it is approximately 50 to 60 degrees.[287]

Abduction/Adduction. The clinician abducts the humerus until the end-feel is perceived. The end-feel should be capsular. The normal range for abduction varies between 70 and 120 degrees, depending on general mobility, age, and gender.[287]

To assess adduction, the clinician pushes along the line of the humerus in a cranial direction to elevate the shoulder girdle, slightly flexes the humerus, and then adducts the humerus.

External Rotation. The humerus is moved into the end range of external rotation. The end-feel should be capsular. The normal range for external rotation varies between 60 and 110 degrees, depending on general mobility, age, and gender.[287]

Internal Rotation. The humerus is moved into the end range of internal rotation. The end-feel should be capsular. The normal range for internal rotation varies depending on general mobility, age, and gender.

Passive Accessory Motion (PAM) Tests

The passive accessory motion tests are performed at the end of the patient's available range to determine if the joint itself is responsible for the loss of motion. For all of these tests, the patient is positioned in supine, with their head supported on a pillow, while the clinician is standing facing the patient.

Distraction/Compression of the G-H Joint. The clinician palpates and stabilizes the shoulder girdle and the anterior thorax. With the other hand, the clinician gently grasps the proximal third of the humerus. The clinician distracts/compresses the G-H joint perpendicular to the plane of the glenoid fossa (30 degrees off the sagittal plane) (Fig. 14-33). The quantity of motion is noted and compared with the other side.

Inferior Glide of the G-H Joint. The clinician palpates and stabilizes the coracoid process of the scapula and the lateral clavicle. With the other hand, the clinician gently grasps proximal to the patient's elbow. The humerus is glided inferiorly at the G-H joint, parallel to the superoinferior plane of the glenoid fossa

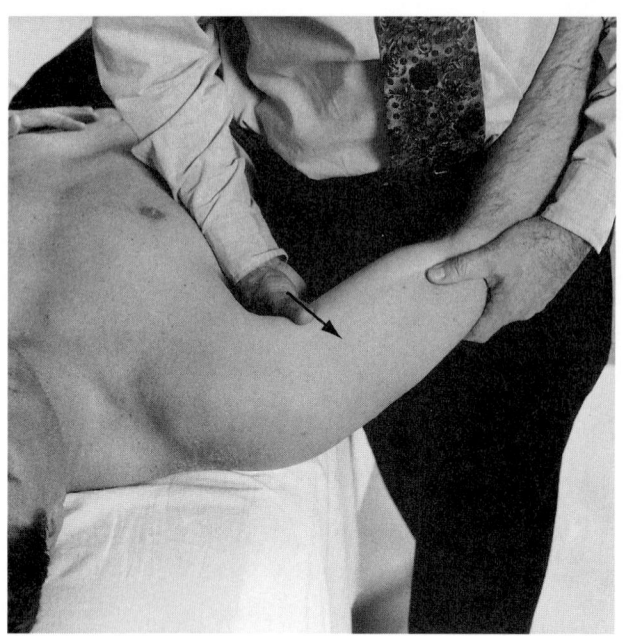

FIGURE 14-33　Glenohumeral distraction.

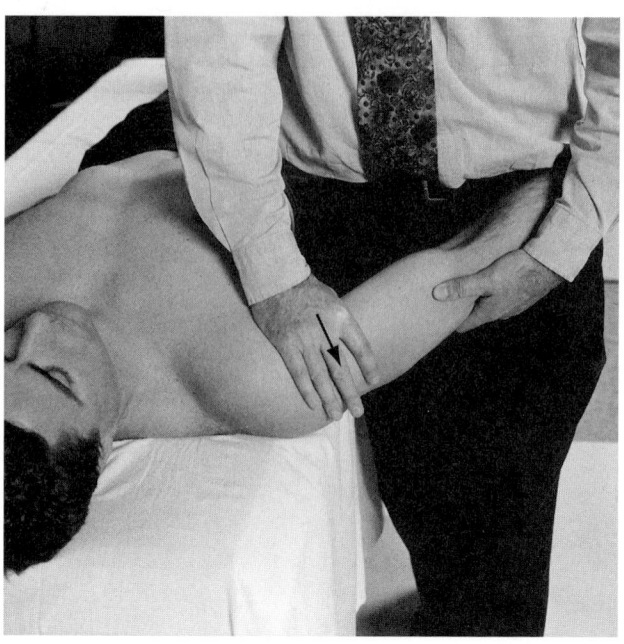

FIGURE 14-35　Posterior glide.

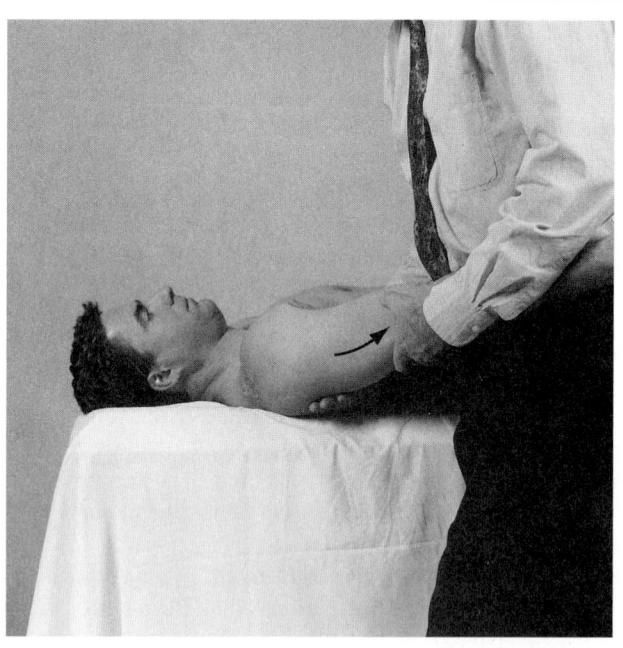

FIGURE 14-34　Inferior glide.

(Fig. 14-34). The quantity of motion is noted and compared with the other side.

Posterior Glide of the G-H Joint.　The clinician palpates and stabilizes the coracoid process and the lateral third of the clavicle. With the thenar eminence of the same hand, the clinician

palpates the anterior aspect of the humeral head (Fig. 14-35). With the other hand, the clinician gently grasps the distal end of the humerus. From this position, the clinician glides the humerus posteriorly at the G-H joint, parallel to the anteroposterior plane of the glenoid fossa. The quantity of motion is noted and compared with the other side.

The intervention for joint glide restrictions uses similar techniques and positioning as for the assessment except that:

▶ Grade I and II oscillations are used for pain, and are graded depending on the stage of healing.

▶ Grade III–V techniques are used to increase range.

Passive Accessory Motion Testing of the Acromioclavicular Joint
Anterior and Posterior Rotation of the Clavicle.　During glenohumeral abduction, or shoulder elevation, the lateral end of the clavicle moves superiorly, the medial end slides and rolls inferiorly, and the clavicle rotates anteriorly (Table 14-22).[60] During glenohumeral adduction, or shoulder depression, the lateral end of the clavicle moves inferiorly, while the medial end rolls and slides superiorly.[60] During this motion, the clavicle rotates posteriorly (see Table 14-22).[60]

The patient is positioned in side lying. The clinician stabilizes the humerus with one hand and grasps the anterior and posterior aspects of the clavicle with the other hand, using the thumb, index, and middle fingers, so that the fingers are hooked around the lateral aspect of the clavicle (Fig. 14-36). The clinician passively pulls the clavicle into the limit of anterior rotation and assesses the end-feel (see Fig. 14-36). The clinician then passively pushes the clavicle into the limit of posterior rotation and assesses the end-feel (see Fig. 14-36).

TABLE 14-22 Clavicle Motions in Relation to Other Motions

Moving Bone	Motion	Rotation
Ribs	Inspiration	Posterior
	Expiration	Anterior
Scapula	Protraction	Anterior
	Retraction	Posterior
	Elevation	Anterior
	Depression	Posterior
Head/neck	Ipsilateral rotation	Posterior
	Contralateral rotation	Anterior
	Ipsilateral flexion	Posterior
	Contralateral flexion	Anterior
	Flexion	Anterior
	Extension	Posterior

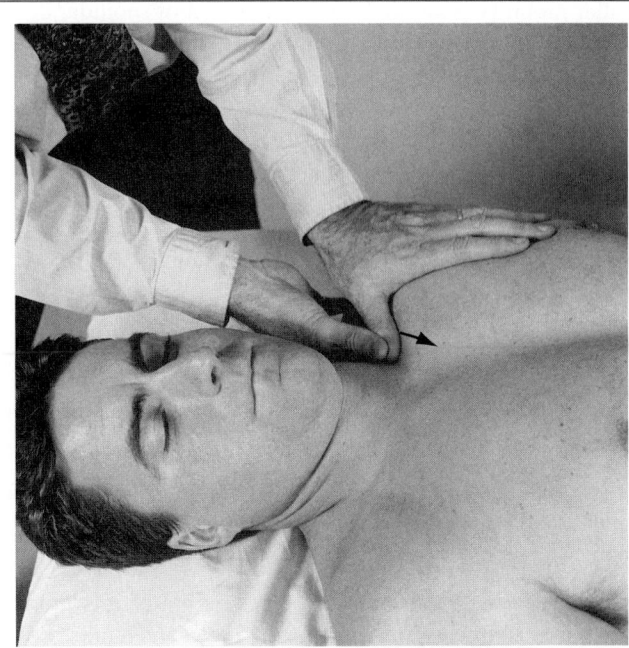

FIGURE 14-37 Anterior and inferior glide of sternoclavicular joint.

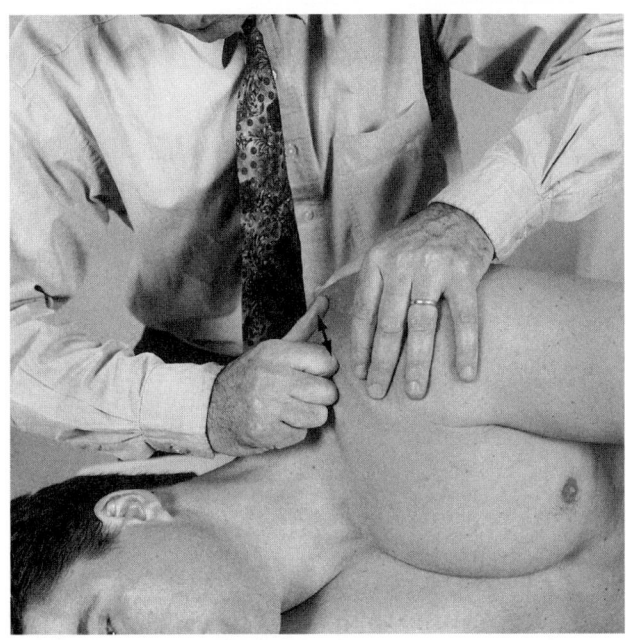

FIGURE 14-36 Anterior and posterior glides of acromioclavicular joint.

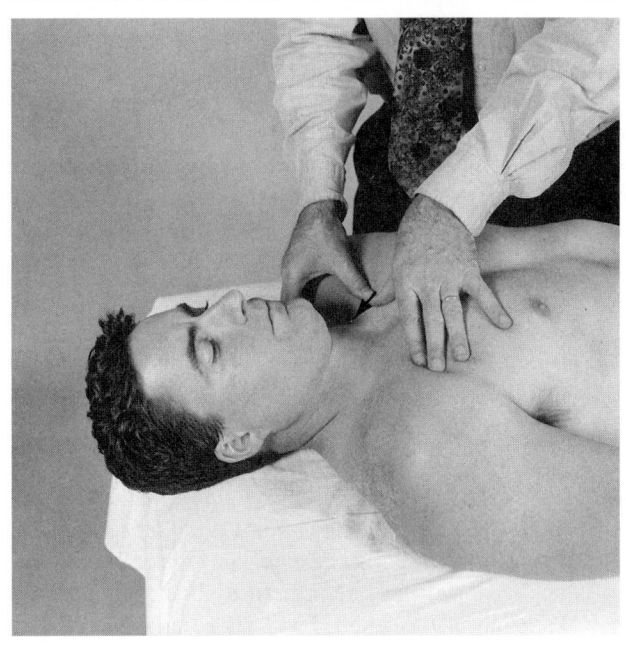

FIGURE 14-38 Superior glide of sternoclavicular joint.

Passive Accessory Motion Testing of the Sternoclavicular Joint
The patient is positioned in supine. It is assumed that the techniques are performed on the patient's left side.

Anterior and Inferior Glide. With the thumbs superimposed on one another, the clinician palpates the superior aspect of the medial end of the clavicle and the S-C joint and applies an anteroinferior glide to the S-C joint (Fig. 14-37). The quantity and quality of motion is noted.

Superior Glide. With the thumbs superimposed on one another, the clinician palpates the inferior aspect of the medial end of the

clavicle and the S-C joint and applies a posterosuperior glide to the S-C joint (Fig. 14-38). The quantity and quality of motion is noted.

Passive Accessory Motion Testing of the Scapulothoracic Joint. These tests are not "true" accessory motion tests as the scapulothoracic joint is not considered a true joint. However, adequate scapular mobility is an important component of shoulder complex function. The patient is positioned in side lying. Their head is sufficiently supported to maintain the cervical spine in neutral. The clinician stands in front of the patient. Using one hand the clinician grasps the inferior and medial border of the uppermost scapula. The other hand grasps the anterior aspect of the shoulder. The clinician gently brings both hands together, lifting the scapula. This position is held until the muscles are felt to relax. Once the muscle relaxation has occurred, the clinician moves the scapula into the PNF patterns for the scapula:

▶ *Elevation with protraction.* A restriction of this motion indicates adaptive shortening or hypertonicity of the latissimus dorsi.

▶ *Elevation with retraction.* A restriction of this motion indicates adaptive shortening or hypertonicity of the mid and lower fibers of the serratus anterior.

▶ *Depression with retraction.* A restriction of this motion indicates adaptive shortening of the pectoralis minor.

▶ *Depression with protraction.* A restriction of this motion indicates adaptive shortening or hypertonicity of the levator scapula.

If protraction is restricted in both elevation and depression of the shoulder girdle, adaptive shortening or hypertonicity of the rhomboids should be suspected. To test the strength of these muscles, the patient is asked to maintain the position by isometrically holding the scapula at the end range of each of these diagonals and to then attempt to control the scapular motion as the clinician attempts to return the scapula to the start position.

Special Tests of the Shoulder Complex

The special tests for the shoulder are divided into diagnostic categories. Selection for their use is at the discretion of the clinician and is based on a complete patient history, and the findings from the physical examination.

Rotator Cuff Integrity and Subacromial Impingement Tests

Subacromial Impingement Tests. Patients with subacromial impingement syndrome usually perceive pain when a compressing force is applied on the greater tuberosity and rotator cuff region.[300] Pain may also be elicited with shoulder abduction in internal or external rotation.[300] These maneuvers constitute the basis of the Hawkins-Kennedy and Neer tests.[301]

Neer Impingement Test. While scapular rotation is prevented by one hand of the clinician, the arm of the patient is passively forced into elevation at an angle between flexion and abduction by the clinician's other hand. Overpressure is applied with the glenohumeral joint in neutral, internal rotation, and then external rotation (Fig. 14-39). Post and Cohen[302] found the Neer test to have a sensitivity of 93 percent in the confirmation of subacromial impingement.

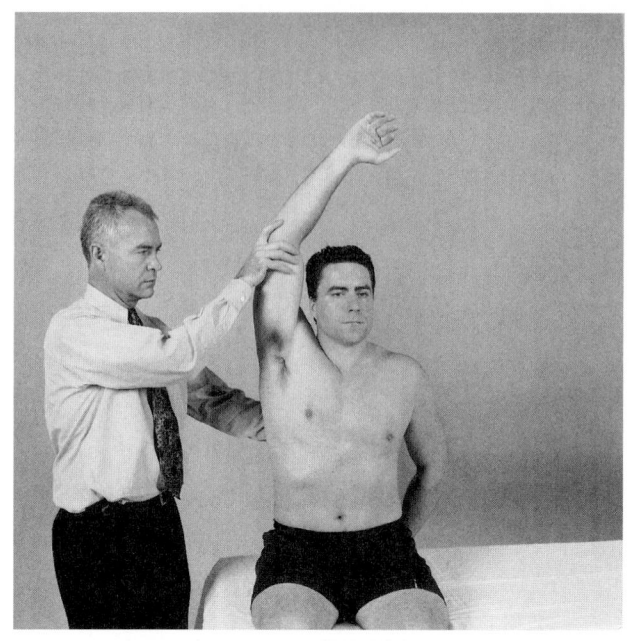

FIGURE 14-39   Neer impingement test.

Hawkins-Kennedy Impingement Test.[303] The arm of the patient is passively flexed up to 90 degrees in the plane of the scapula. The elbow is stabilized and the arm is forced into internal rotation (Fig. 14-40).

In a cadaver study, Pink and Jobe[304] found that rotator cuff tendons were impinged under the acromion with the Hawkins-Kennedy test, and that the lower surface of the same tendons

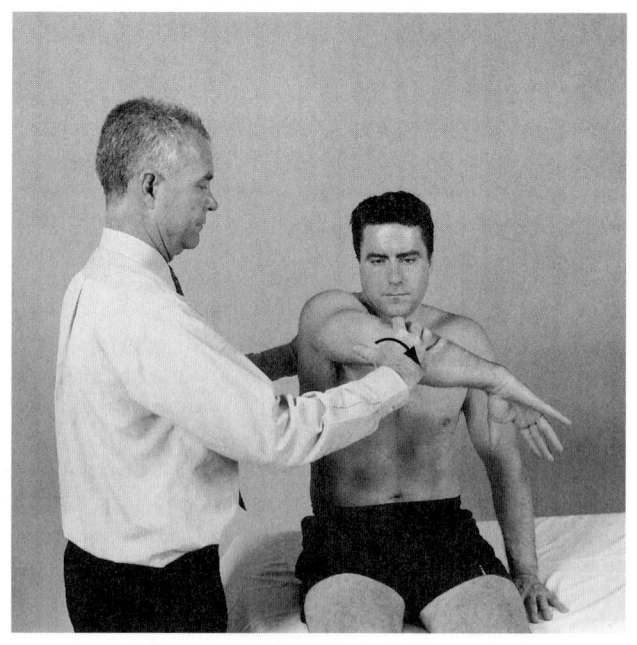

FIGURE 14-40   Hawkins-Kennedy Impingement test.

were impinged in the anterosuperior part of the glenoid margin with the Neer test. Ure and colleagues[305] found that the sensitivity of the Hawkins-Kennedy test was 62 percent and the sensitivity of the Neer test was 46 percent in 45 patients with stage II subacromial impingement syndrome, as determined using arthroscopy.

Another study[306] found that the Hawkins-Kennedy test was more accurate than the Neer test in a series of 44 shoulders, with the former having a sensitivity of 78 percent and the latter a sensitivity of 0 percent.

Yocum Test.   The Yocum test is performed by having the patient lift the elbow to shoulder height while resting the hand on the opposite shoulder (Fig. 14-41). A study[284] comparing the Neer, Hawkins-Kennedy, and Yocum tests found all three to demonstrate a high sensitivity for diagnosing subacromial impingement.

Patte Test.[307,308]   The Patte test, also known as the "hornblower's sign" (Fig. 14-42) is performed with the patient in sitting or standing. The patient's arm is supported in 90 degrees of abduction in the scapular plane, with the elbow flexed to 90 degrees. The patient is then asked to rotate the forearm externally against the resistance of the clinician's hand. If the patient is unable to externally rotate the shoulder in this position, the hornblower's sign is said to be present.

This test was found to have 100 percent sensitivity and 93 percent specificity in the diagnosis of irreparable degeneration of the teres minor muscle when compared with CT arthrography findings in a series of 54 shoulders scheduled for rotator cuff repair.[309] The loss of integrity of the teres minor was confirmed at the time of surgery.

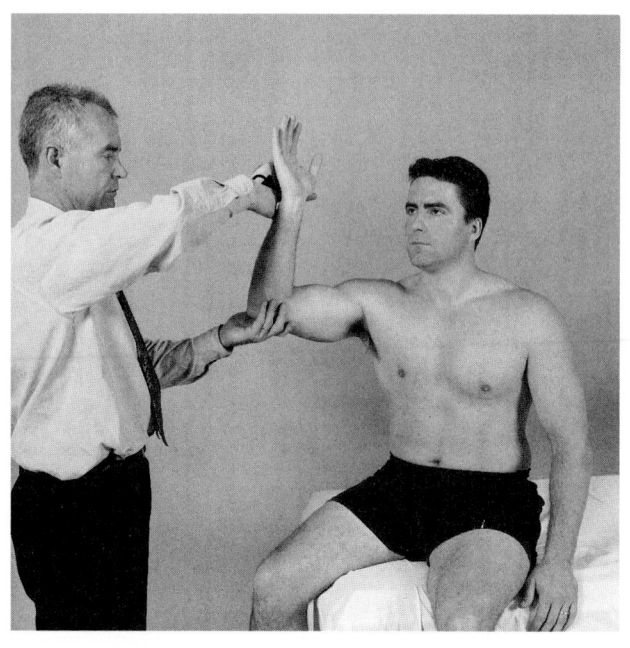

FIGURE 14-42   Patte test.

One study[284] attempted to determine the diagnostic value of three impingement tests (Yocum, Neer, and Hawkins-Kennedy), and four tests used to determine the location of the specific rotator cuff lesion (Jobe empty can [see resisted tests], Gerber lift-off [see resisted tests], Patte test, and Speed's test [see later]), by comparing the clinical findings from the tests with the operative findings in a series of 55 patients with chronic shoulder pain and functional impairment.[310] The Neer test (89 percent), the Hawkins-Kennedy test (87 percent), and the Yocum test (78 percent) all demonstrated a high sensitivity for diagnosing subacromial impingement. Both the Jobe empty can test (86 percent) and the Patte test (92 percent) demonstrated high sensitivity, but poor specificity (50 percent and 30 percent, respectively). Both the Gerber lift-off and the Speed's test demonstrated poor sensitivity (0 percent and 63 percent, respectively), and poor specificity (61 percent and 35 percent, respectively).[310]

Painful Arc Test.   The patient actively abducts the arm. Pain occurs between the angles of 60 and 120 degrees of shoulder abduction. Hermann and colleagues[180] found that the painful arc test was positive in 48.9 percent of 50 patients with degenerative impingement. Akgün and colleagues[311] observed 57.5 percent positive results with the test in stage II subacromial impingement syndrome patients.

Cross-Over Impingement/Horizontal Adduction Test.   The patient's arm is positioned in 90 degrees of glenohumeral flexion. The clinician passively moves the patient's arm into horizontal adduction, and applies overpressure (Fig. 14-43). Although the cross-over impingement/horizontal adduction test provokes compressing forces on rotator cuff tendons that are localized

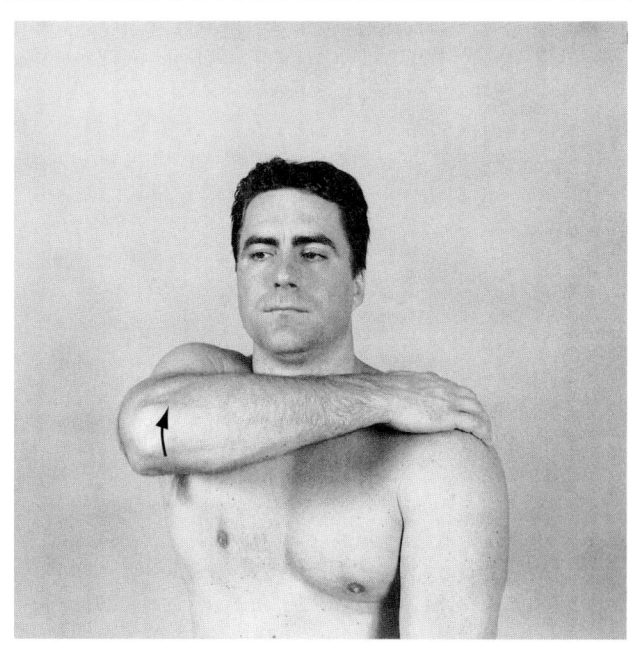

FIGURE 14-41   Yocum test.

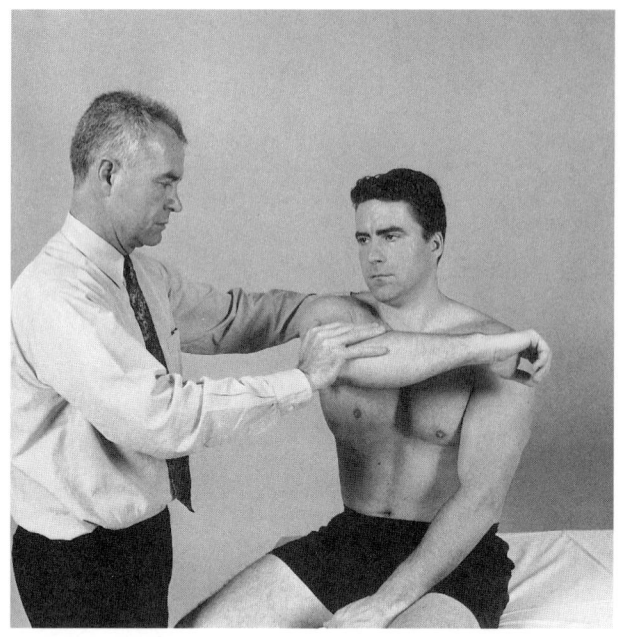

FIGURE 14-43   Cross-over impingement test.

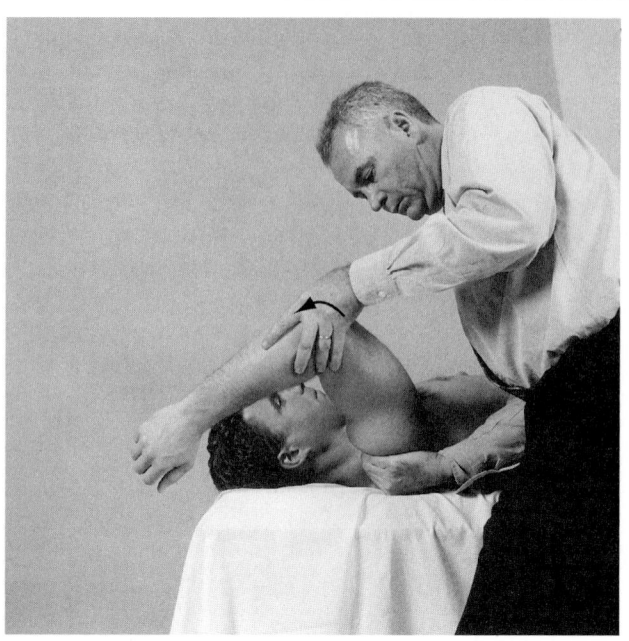

FIGURE 14-44   Lock test.

under the A-C joint, it is a test more likely to be used to investigate A-C joint dysfunction.[180,311–313]

Lock Test.[314,315]   The Lock test is used to help differentiate the cause of symptoms when the patient complains of localized catching shoulder pain and pain or restricted movement when attempting to place the hand behind the back. Since the clinician controls the motion, this test can be a very sensitive test to help confirm the presence of an impingement of the supraspinatus tendon. It is assumed that the techniques are performed on the patient's right side.

The patient is positioned in supine with the right shoulder at the edge of the table, positioned in 45 degrees abduction, 30 degrees internal rotation, and the elbow positioned 10 degrees posterior to the frontal plane (Fig. 14-44). The clinician places their right hand under the scapula with the fingertips stabilizing the trapezius, and with the thumb on the vertebral border of the scapula. The clinician's left hand is placed on the patient's right elbow.

After assessing the resting symptoms, the clinician slowly glides the patient's elbow anteriorly by performing a weight shift to their front leg, noting the location of onset of resistance and/or pain in the available range. The end position for the test is achieved when the patient's right shoulder is in maximal humeral abduction with overpressure, and neither the patient nor clinician can externally rotate the arm further while at this end range.

In the locking position, the greater tuberosity and its rotator cuff attachments are caught within the subacromial space. Further motion into external rotation, flexion, or abduction is not possible, unless the arm is allowed to move forward. Positive

findings for this test include reproduction of the patient's symptoms and a decrease in range of motion compared to the uninvolved shoulder.

Dropping Sign.[316]   The "dropping sign" is performed with the patient sitting or standing. The clinician places the patient's elbow in 90 degrees of flexion with the arm by the side. The shoulder is externally rotated to 45 degrees and the patient is then asked to externally rotate the shoulder against resistance. If the patient is unable to maintain the externally rotated position, the arm drops back to the neutral position of shoulder rotation. This is called the dropping sign.

This test was found to have a 100 percent sensitivity and 100 percent specificity for irreparable degeneration of the infraspinatus muscle.[309] This loss of integrity was confirmed at the time of surgery.

Rotator Cuff Rupture Tests
Drop Arm Test.   The clinician passively raises the patient's arm to an overhead position. The patient is asked to lower their arm with their palm down. If at any point in the descent, the patient's arm drops, this is indicative of a full thickness tear.

Biceps and Superior Labral Tears.   The long head of the biceps tendon runs up the bicipital groove under the transverse ligament, through the shoulder joint and attaches to the superior glenoid via the superior labrum. The biceps tendon and superior labrum can be involved in various pathological processes including bicipital tendonitis, biceps rupture, biceps tendon subluxation or dislocation, and tears of the superior labrum.[222]

Clunk Test. The Clunk test is the traditional test for diagnosing labral tears. The patient is positioned in supine. One hand of the clinician is placed on the posterior aspect of the shoulder over the humeral head, while the other hand grasps the humerus above the elbow. The clinician fully abducts the arm over the patient's head. Using the hand placed posterior to the humeral head, the clinician pushes anteriorly while the other hand externally rotates the humerus. A clunk-like sensation may be felt if a free labral fragment is caught in the joint.[222] Clinical studies have found that a click on manipulation of the G-H joint was a common finding in patients with labral tears, even in the absence of joint instability.[317,318]

The sensitivity of this test was found to be low (15 percent) in one study[319] when it was used to detect labral tears in a series of 96 arthroscopic surgery patients.

Crank Test. The crank test[320] is performed with the patient positioned in supine. Their arm is elevated to 160 degrees in the scapular plane of the body and is in maximal internal or external rotation. The clinician then applies an axial load along the humerus. A positive test is indicated by the reproduction of a painful click in the shoulder during the maneuver. This test was found to have a high sensitivity (91 percent) and specificity (93 percent) for diagnosing labral tears in a series of 62 patients who presented with shoulder pain that was refractory to 3 months of conservative management.[320]

The crank test has been found to have a higher sensitivity (90 percent) than MRI (59 percent) and equal specificity (85 percent) to MRI in diagnosing labral tears.[318]

Speed's Test. The patient's arm is positioned in shoulder flexion, full external rotation, full elbow extension, and full forearm supination (Fig. 14-45). Manual resistance is applied by the clinician. The test is positive if localized pain at the bicipital groove is reproduced.

A positive Speed's test suggests a superior labral tear when resisted forward flexion of the shoulder causes bicipital groove pain.[1,321] Speed's test is also used to detect bicipital tendonitis (see Yergason's test).[180,322]

Yergason's Test.[323] The patient's arm is positioned in 90 degrees of elbow flexion. The patient is asked to supinate their forearm, and externally rotate their arm against the manual resistance of the clinician (Fig. 14-46).

Speed's and Yergason's tests probably discriminate bicipital tendon disorders.[300] However, irritation and edema may occur in the long head of biceps in any stage of subacromial impingement syndrome. Biceps tendons may be thickened by fibrinoid degeneration in the subacromial impingement syndrome.[311] This may lead to inappropriate diagnosis as primer bicipital tendonitis and subsequent tenodesis.[300] In a number of studies, the sensitivity of the Speed's test in biceps tendon disorders was found to be higher than that of the Yergason's test.[300,322,324] The higher tendon mobilization capability out of the bicipital groove of this test was suggested as a possible reason for this.[322,324]

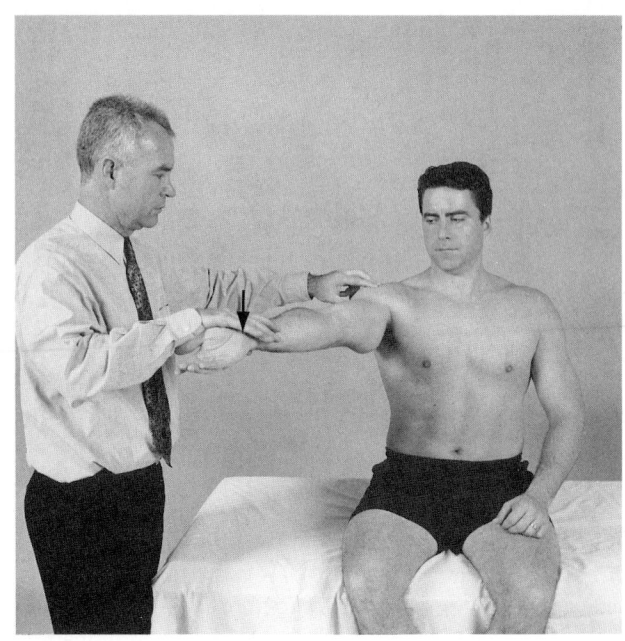

FIGURE 14-45 Speed's test.

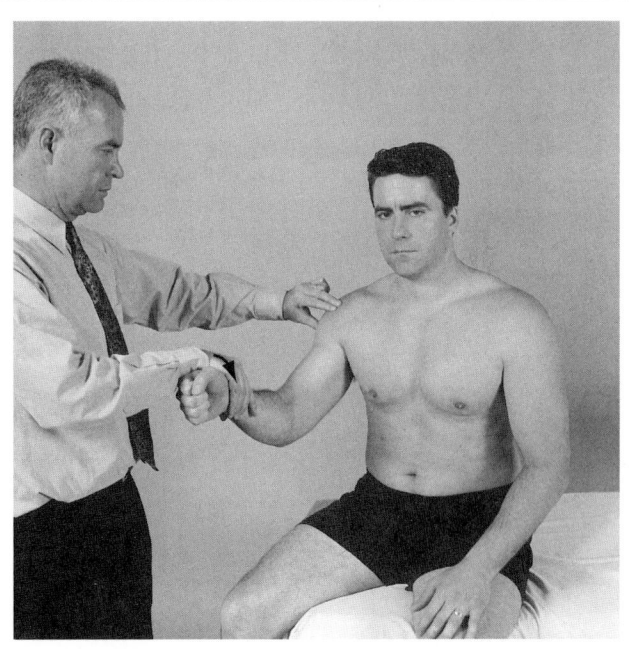

FIGURE 14-46 Yergason's test.

O'Brien Test. The O'Brien test, which has a sensitivity of 100 percent and a specificity of 98.5 percent for detecting a labral abnormality,[325] is a two-part active compression test. The test is performed with the patient's arm adducted 10 degrees in the front of the chest with the shoulder flexed to 90 degrees and fully internally rotated and the elbow fully extended. In this position, the arm is flexed upward against the clinician's downward-directed force. The test is then repeated in the same manner except that the arm is positioned in maximum external rotation. Pain with this maneuver is typical in patients with superior labral tears.[1]

Anterior Slide Test.   The anterior slide test[326] is another clinical test designed to stress the superior labrum.[222] The patient stands with hands on the hips such that the thumbs are positioned posteriorly. One of the clinician's hands is placed over the patient's shoulder and the other hand behind the elbow (Fig. 14-47). A force is then applied anteriorly and superiorly, and the patient is asked to push back against the force. The test is considered positive if pain is localized to the anterosuperior aspect of the shoulder, if there is a pop or a click in the anterosuperior region, or if the maneuver reproduces the symptoms.[222]

The anterior slide test has demonstrated good sensitivity (78 percent) and high specificity (92 percent) when used to detect glenoid labrum tears.[326]

Other Tests.   The remaining tests are reserved for when the clinician needs to differentiate the structure causing the symptoms, when the provocation of symptoms during the examination has been minimal, or to rule out the possibility of instability.

Acromioclavicular Tests

Acromioclavicular Shear Test.   The clinician cups their hands together and applies a compressive force with the hands over the A-C joint, creating a posterior to anterior glide (shear) of the A-C joint (Fig. 14-48).

Examination of the Passive Restraint System

If following the range of motion, strength, and functional movement tests, the clinician is unable to determine a working

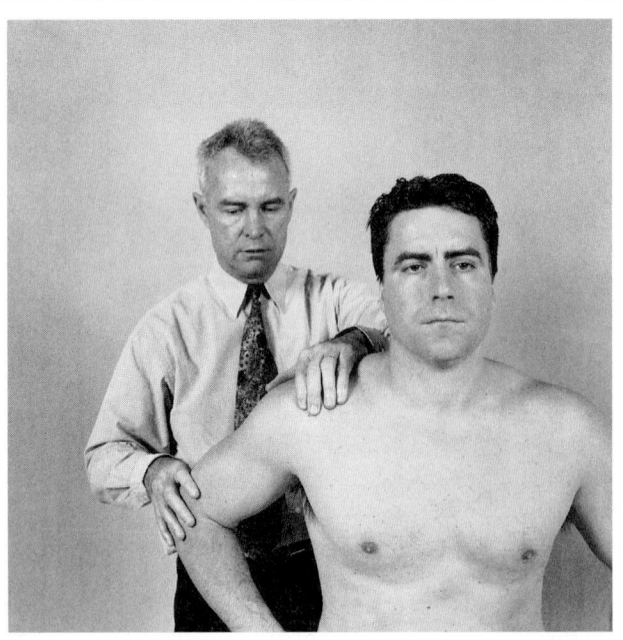

FIGURE 14-47   Anterior slide test.

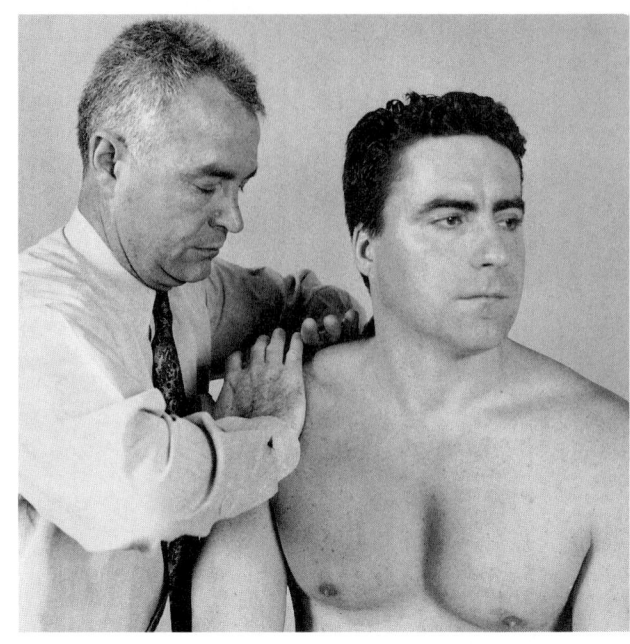

FIGURE 14-48   Acromioclavicular shear test.

hypothesis from which to treat the patient, further examination is required. This more detailed examination involves the assessment of the mobility and stability of the passive restraint systems of the shoulder girdle.

Stability Testing.   It is important to remember that there is no correlation between the amount of joint laxity/mobility and joint instability at the shoulder.[327] Joint stability is more likely a function of connective tissue support and an intact neuromuscular system.[264]

Many provocative maneuvers including anterior and posterior apprehension tests, the sulcus test,[328–330] and load and shift test have been described previously. The reproduction of symptoms is important because laxity alone does not indicate instability. Side-to-side translational asymmetry often has been taken as being representative of disease, but it is useful to realize that healthy shoulders may also have asymmetry up to grade II laxity.[331,332]

Pain and muscle spasm can make the examination challenging. Rarely is examination with the patient under anesthesia useful for anything other than fine-tuning the amount of capsular shift required at surgery.[333]

Glenohumeral: Load and Shift Test.   The patient is seated on the treatment table with their arm supported in their lap. The clinician sits beside the patient with the inside of the hand over the patient's shoulder and their forearm stabilizing the scapula to the thorax. The clinician places their thumb across the posterior G-H joint line and humeral head, and the web space across the patient's acromion. The clinician's index finger is placed across the anterior G-H joint line and humeral head, and the long finger over the coracoid process (Fig. 14-49). The clinician

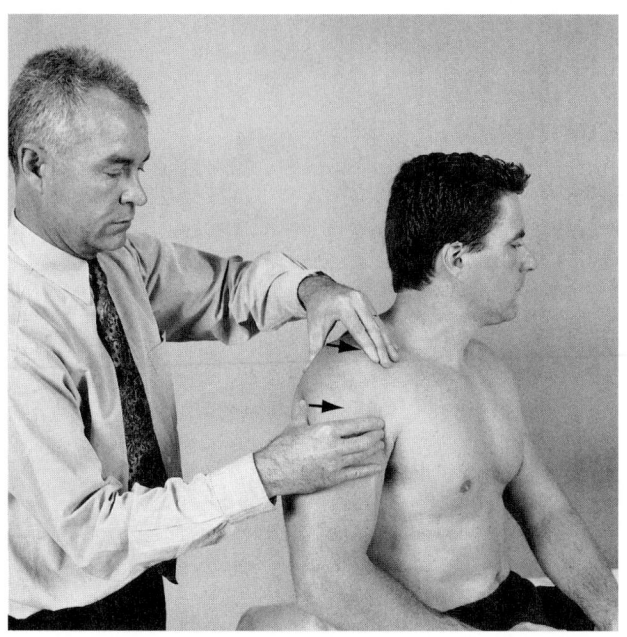

FIGURE 14-49 Load and shift test.

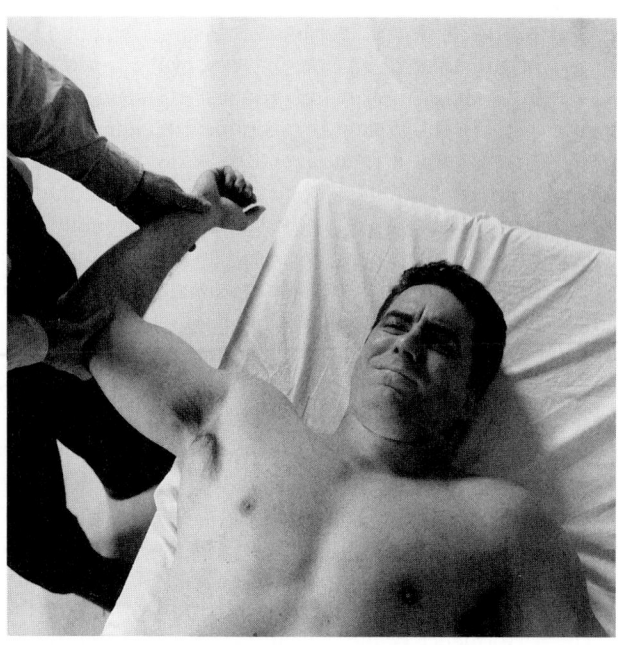

FIGURE 14-50 Apprehension test.

then applies a "load and shift" of the humeral head across the stabilized scapula in an anteromedial direction to assess anterior stability, and in a posterolateral direction to assess posterior instability. The normal motion anteriorly is half of the distance of the humeral head. Although attempts have been made to grade or quantify the degree of instability more specifically, the literature supports no consistency in the grading to date.[132,334–337] This test has been reported to be 100 percent sensitive for the detection of instability in patients with recurrent dislocation, but not in cases of recurrent subluxation.[335]

Apprehension Test. The patient is positioned in supine with the arm in 90 degrees of abduction and full external rotation. The clinician holds the patient's wrist with one hand, while the other hand stabilizes the patient's elbow (Fig. 14-50). The clinician applies overpressure into external rotation. Patient apprehension from this maneuver, rather than pain, is considered a positive test for anterior instability. Pain with this maneuver, but without apprehension, may indicate pathology other than instability, such as posterior impingement of the rotator cuff.[24] This test has been demonstrated to have a specificity of 61 percent and a sensitivity of 63 percent.[338]

Sulcus Sign for Inferior Instability. The sulcus sign was described by Neer[329] and is used to detect inferior instability due to a laxity of the superior glenohumeral and coracohumeral ligaments. The patient's arm is positioned in 20 to 50 degrees of abduction and neutral rotation.[101,339] A positive test results in the presence of a sulcus sign (a depression greater than a fingerbreadth between the lateral acromion and the head of the humerus) (Fig. 14-51) when longitudinal traction is applied to the dependent arm in more than one position.[340]

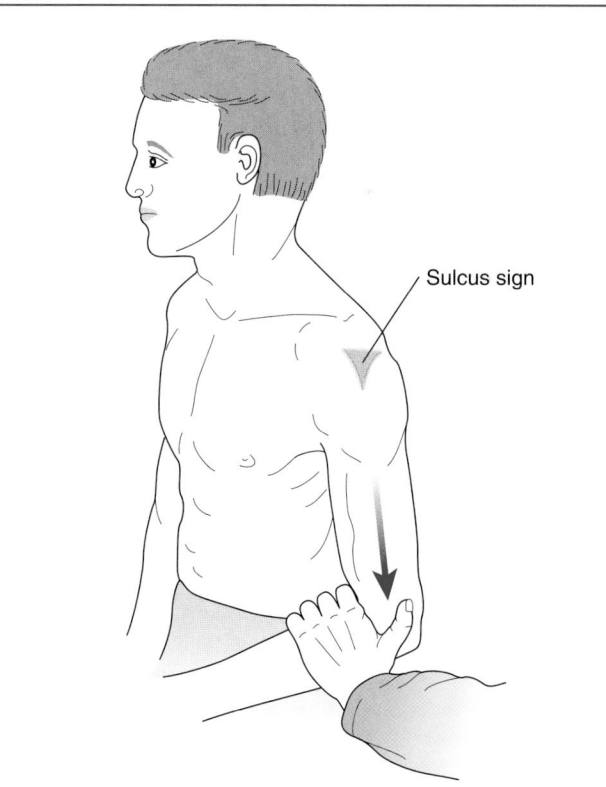

Sulcus sign

FIGURE 14-51 Sulcus sign.

The sulcus sign can be graded by measuring the distance from the inferior margin of the acromion to the humeral head. A distance of less than 1 cm is graded as 1+ sulcus, 1 to 2 cm as a 2+ sulcus, and greater than 2 cm as a grade 3+ sulcus.[329]

Jobe Subluxation/Relocation Test. This test is similar to the apprehension test, except that manual pressure is applied anteriorly by the clinician in an attempt to provoke a subluxation, before using manual pressure in the opposite direction to relocate the subluxation. The patient is positioned in supine with their arm in 90 degrees of abduction and full external rotation. The clinician grasps the patient's forearm with one hand to maintain the testing position, and grasps the humeral head with the other hand (Fig. 14-52). The clinician gently applies an anterior push to the posterior aspect of the subluxed humeral head. Pain and apprehension from the patient indicate a positive test for a superior labral tear.[1] After pushing the humeral head anteriorly and demonstrating pain and apprehension, the clinician should then push the humeral head posteriorly while maintaining the shoulder in the same position (the relocation part of the test). Reduction of pain and apprehension further substantiates the clinical finding of anterior instability and may indicate a positive test. The sensitivity and specificity of the relocation test is reported to be low when assessing pain response only, but very high when assessing the apprehension response only.[341]

The performance of the relocation part of the test (based on operative findings and manual examination under anesthesia) was compared between two groups of patients: those with anterior instability and those with rotator cuff disease.[341] The study found that it is not possible to discriminate between anterior instability and rotator cuff disease using the relocation test for assessing pain response only.

Rockwood Test for Anterior Instability.[342] The patient is positioned sitting with the clinician standing behind. With the arm by the patient's side, the clinician passively externally rotates the shoulder. The patient then abducts the arm to approximately

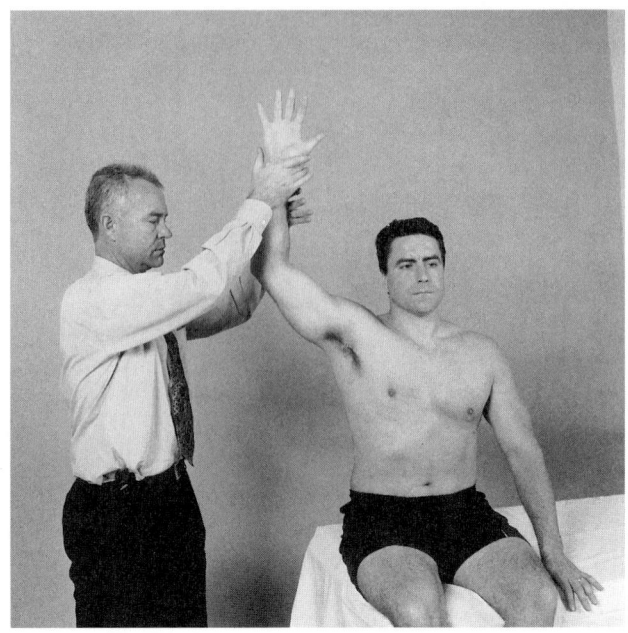

FIGURE 14-53 Rockwood test for anterior instability.

45 degrees and the test is repeated. The same maneuver is again repeated with the arm abducted to 90 degrees and then 120 degrees (Fig. 14-53), in order to assess the different stabilizing structures. A positive test is indicated when apprehension is noted in the latter three positions (45, 90, and 120 degrees).

Anterior Release Test. The anterior release test[343] is performed with the patient in supine and their shoulder positioned in 90 degrees of abduction and maximally externally rotated while a posteriorly directed force is applied to the proximal humerus (Fig. 14-54). A positive test produces an increase or reproduction in the patient's symptoms upon release of the posteriorly directed force on the humerus. The test was found to have high sensitivity (92 percent) and high specificity (89 percent) for detecting anterior instability in a series of 100 athletes.[343]

Thoracic Outlet Syndrome Tests. These tests are described in the Special Test section of Chap. 23.

Diagnostic Studies

The conclusions on the radiology reports concerning single-plane views (anteroposterior [A-P] view with the humerus in internal rotation and a second A-P view with the humerus in external rotation) should be treated with caution as they have been well documented to result in misdiagnosis.[344]

The "scapular-Y" view, obtained by tilting the x-ray beam approximately 60 degrees relative to the A-P view, provides good visualization of the glenohumeral alignment.[345] Arthrography aids in the diagnosis of full thickness rotator cuff tears.[346] Bone scans are rarely used in the diagnosis of shoulder pain, but a computed tomographic (CT) scan report can be useful in confirming the clinical findings in some cases.[1] The MRI is very reliable in

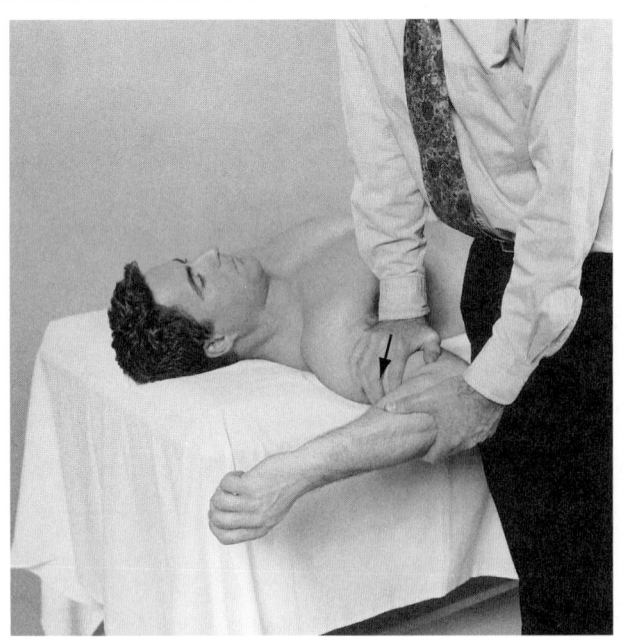

FIGURE 14-52 Jobe subluxation/relocation test.

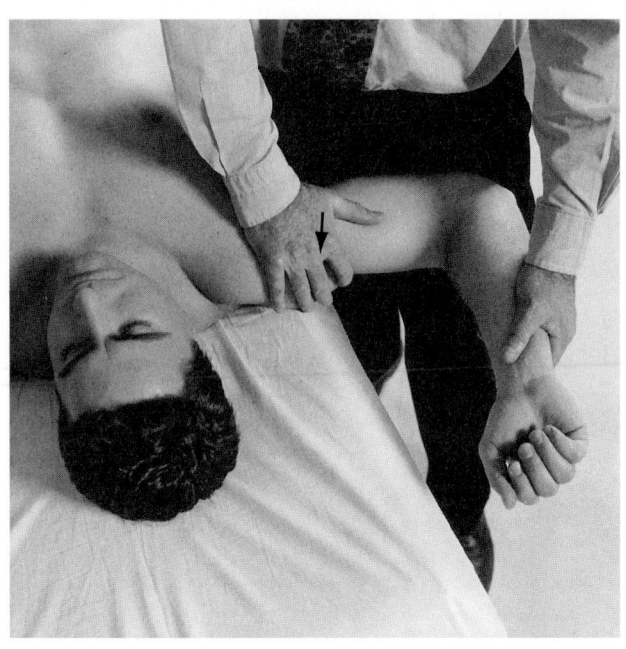

FIGURE 14-54 Anterior release test.

detecting lesions of the capsule and labrum, as well as associated rotator cuff tears. It can generally indicate the approximate size of a rotator cuff tear, and may also indicate whether the critically important subscapularis tendon is torn.[1,347,348]

In a limited number of studies, a comparison has been made as to the accuracy of physical diagnostic tests versus arthroscopic examination. One such study found that the physical therapists were unable to differentiate between a partial and complete tear of the rotator cuff tendons.[349] However, a later study showed that physical therapists were able to discern subacromial disorders and passive restraint disorders with an agreement of 85 percent and 67 percent, respectively.[350]

Intervention Strategies

With the possible exceptions of acute traumatic shoulder dislocation and acute traumatic inability to raise the arm (acute massive rotator cuff tear), an initial minimum 6-week period of conservative empiric intervention is normally indicated for shoulder injuries. A number of principles can be used to guide the clinician in the conservative rehabilitation of the shoulder:[351]

► Rehabilitate the shoulder according to the stage of healing and degree of irritability. The degree of irritability of each condition can often indicate the stage of healing to the clinician. The degree of irritability can be determined by inquiring about the vigor, duration, and intensity of the pain. Greater irritability is associated with very acutely inflamed conditions. The characteristic sign for an acute

inflammation of the shoulder is pain at rest, which is diffuse in its distribution and often referred from the site of the primary condition.[314] Pain above the elbow indicates less severity than pain below the elbow. Chronic conditions usually have low irritability, but have an associated loss of active and passive ROM. The degree of movement and the speed of progression are both guided by the signs and symptoms.

► Rehabilitate the shoulder in scapular planes rather than in the straight planes of flexion, extension, and abduction. Exercises performed in the scapular plane, rather than the straight planes, are more functional.

► Short lever arms should be used with exercises initially, thereby decreasing the torque at the shoulder. This can be achieved by flexing the elbow, or by exercising with the arm closer to the body.

► Obtain a stable scapular platform as early as possible.

► Achieve the closed pack position at the earliest opportunity. By definition, the close pack position of the shoulder is that position which provides the joint with the maximum amount of passive stability through the inert structures. All range of motion exercises for the shoulder are typically initiated in the early ranges of flexion with the goal of achieving full elevation. Given the protection afforded the joint by the passive restraint system of inert tissues, perhaps thought should be given to providing range of motion exercises initiated at the end ranges of elevation. Exceptions to this would be the patient whose condition precluded such exercises, i.e., following shoulder surgery, adhesive capsulitis, or instability.

► Reproduce the forces and loading rates that will approach the patient's functional demands as the rehabilitation progresses.

The manual techniques to increase joint mobility and the techniques to increase soft tissue extensibility are described in the Therapeutic Techniques section.

Acute Phase

The goals of the acute phase include:

► Protection of the injury site.

► Restoration of pain-free range of motion in the entire kinetic chain.

► Improve patient comfort by decreasing pain and inflammation.

► Retard muscle atrophy.

► Minimize detrimental effects of immobilization and activity restriction.[217,273,352–355]

► Maintain general cardiovascular fitness.

► Independence with home exercise program.

During the early stages of the acute phase, the principles of PRICEMEM (protection, rest, ice, compression, elevation, manual therapy, early motion, and medication) are applied as appropriate. Icing for 20 to 30 minutes, 3 to 4 times a day, concurrent with nonsteroidal anti-inflammatory drugs (NSAIDs) or aspirin can aid in reducing pain and swelling.

Early active assisted and passive exercises are performed in all planes of shoulder movement to nourish the articular cartilage and assist in collagen tissue synthesis and organization.[356–360] These exercises are initiated in pain-free arcs, below 90 degrees of abduction. Recommended ROM exercises for the acute phase include:

▶ Codman's or other pendulum exercises (Fig. 14-55).

▶ Active assisted range-of-motion exercises. These may include wand or cane exercises into functional planes incorporating combinations of forward flexion, extension, abduction, internal rotation, and external rotation (Fig. 14-56). Over-the-door pulley exercises (Fig. 14-57) are performed later in the acute phase as tolerated.

Strengthening exercises are introduced as tolerated using isometric exercises, with the arm positioned below 90 degrees of abduction and 90 degrees of flexion. Specific scapular rehabilitation exercises are typically initiated with the isometric exercises. Patterns of scapular retraction and protraction are started in single planes and then progress to elevation and depression of the entire scapula. It is important to remember that to improve backward reaching the patient must first learn correct retraction procedures.

Jobe and Pink[71] believe that the order of strengthening in the rehabilitation process is important. They advocate strengthening the glenohumeral *protectors* (rotator cuff muscles) and scapular *pivoters* (trapezius, levator scapulae, serratus anterior,

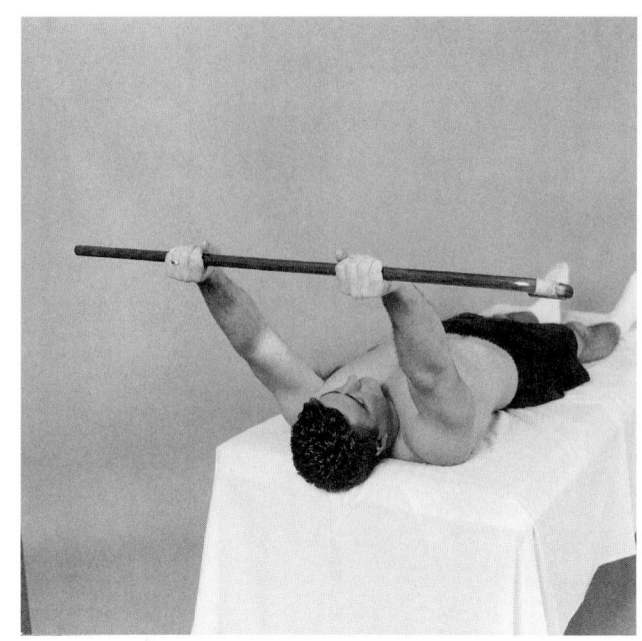

FIGURE 14-56   Wand exercises.

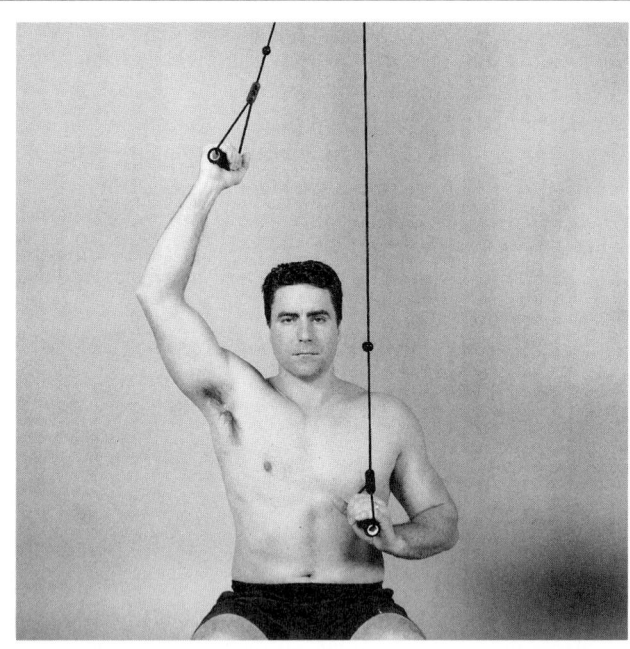

FIGURE 14-57   Over-the-door pulley exercise.

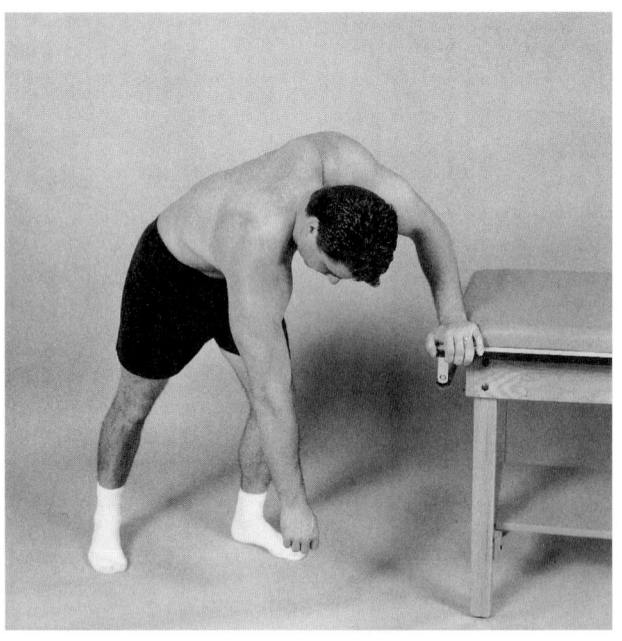

FIGURE 14-55   Codman's pendulum.

and rhomboids) initially because of the role they play in providing stability. Exercises for the humeral "positioners" (deltoid) and the humeral "propellers" (latissimus dorsi and pectoralis major) are introduced in the "Functional Phase," see later. Exercises for the glenohumeral *protectors* include the wand exercises, progressing to active range of motion in the pain-free ranges in functional planes. In addition, the integration of scapular retraction and scapular elevation exercises with gleno-humeral movements will help stimulate a co-contraction of the glenohumeral protectors and allow for a more normal physiologic pattern to redevelop. Scapular *pivoter* exercises can be performed early in the rehabilitation process. These include the *scapular pinch*, which is an isometric activity involving scapula retraction toward the midline (Fig. 14-58), and scapular elevation (Fig. 14-59).[102,105] Once the arm can be safely raised and

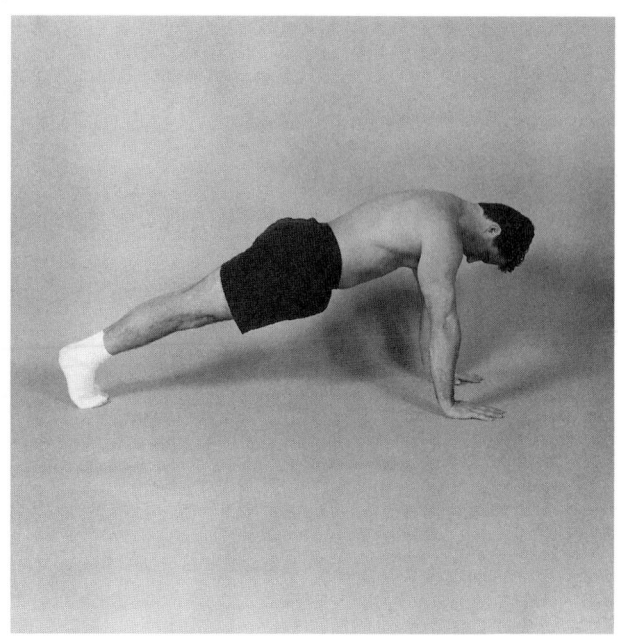

FIGURE 14-60   Push-up plus.

held in the position of 90 degrees abduction while standing or sitting, the patient is positioned in supine and the arm is actively raised as high as the pain-free range will allow (from 90 to 150 degrees depending on tolerance). From this position, the patient performs a serratus punch with a "plus." At the end of each push up as the arm is fully straightened, an extra push is applied. This extra push with the push-up is termed a push-up plus (Fig. 14-60). This exercise strengthens the pectoralis minor, and the lower and middle serratus anterior.[7,117]

The application of joint compression with contraction through the application of closed chain exercises is important, as closed chain activities help to balance compression and shear forces at the shoulder. These activities also encourage the correct sequencing of muscle contraction around the shoulder girdle and emphasize the co-contraction of force couples at the scapulothoracic and G-H joints.[63] This results in a correct scapular position and stabilization.[102] Closed chain exercises may be done early in the rehabilitation phase as they do not put shear on the joint. They also allow the rotator cuff muscles to be activated without being inhibited by pain or deltoid overactivity. The closed chain exercises can be initiated with the hand stabilized on the wall, or on a ball on the wall (Fig. 14-61), superimposing specific scapular maneuvers such as elevation (see Fig. 14-59), depression, retraction, and protraction. These exercises are started at elevations of 60 degrees or less and are moved up to 90 degrees of flexion, and then abduction, as tolerated to allow for healing of the tissues.[15,98,102,105] Other closed-chain exercises for the rotator cuff include clock exercises (Fig. 14-62) and scapular retraction.[361]

Weight-bearing exercises are introduced by placing both hands on a table and flexing the shoulder to <60 degrees and abducted to 45 degrees. Progression is made to weight bearing

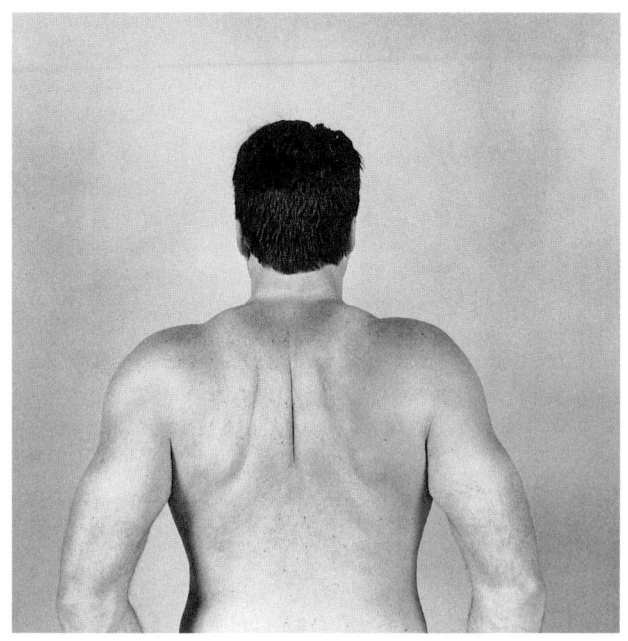

FIGURE 14-58   Scapular pinch.

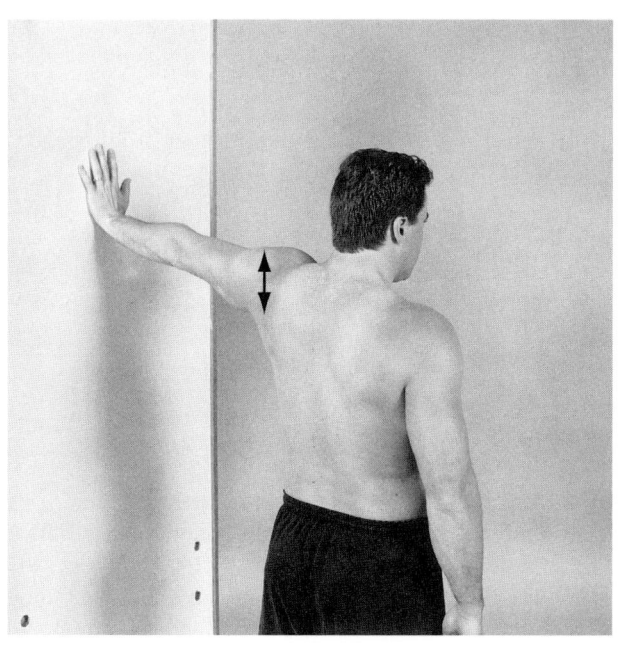

FIGURE 14-59   Scapular elevation.

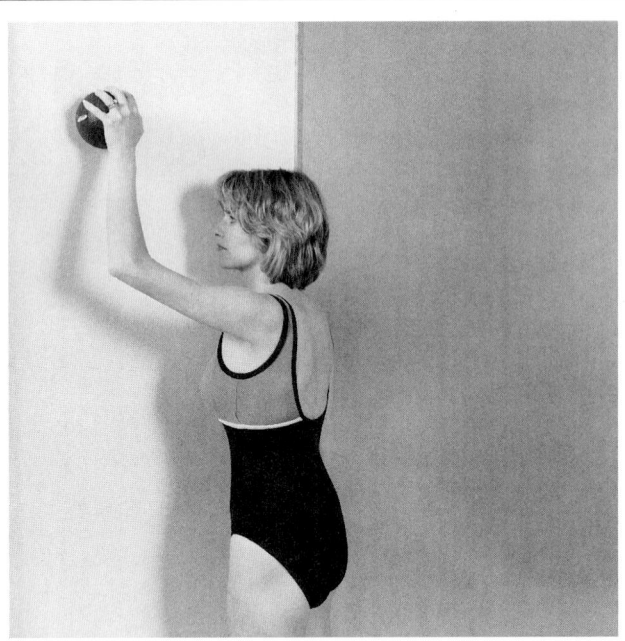

FIGURE 14-61   Compression.

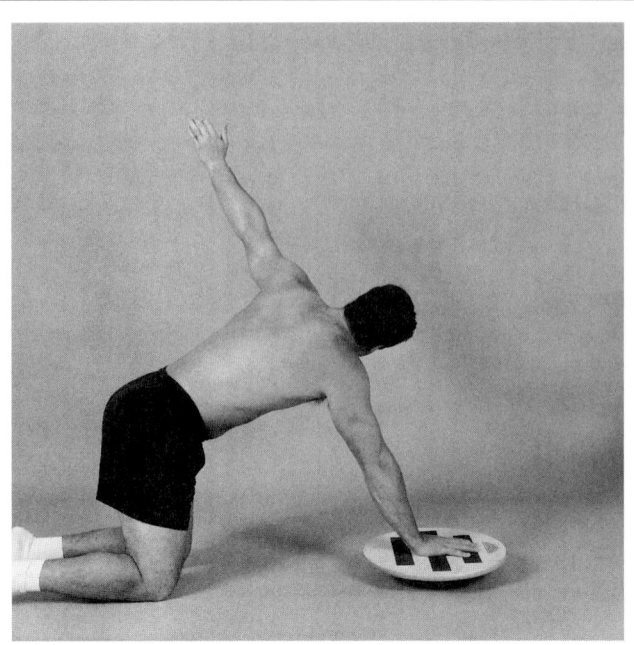

FIGURE 14-63   Tilt board weight-bearing exercise.

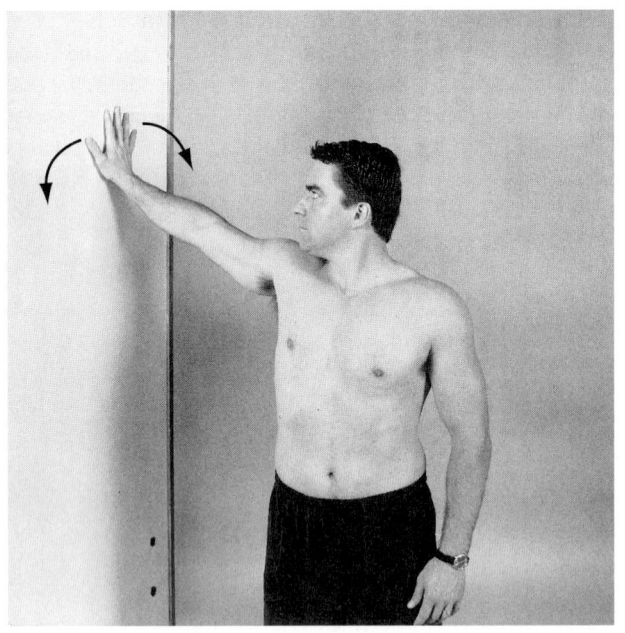

FIGURE 14-62   Clock exercise.

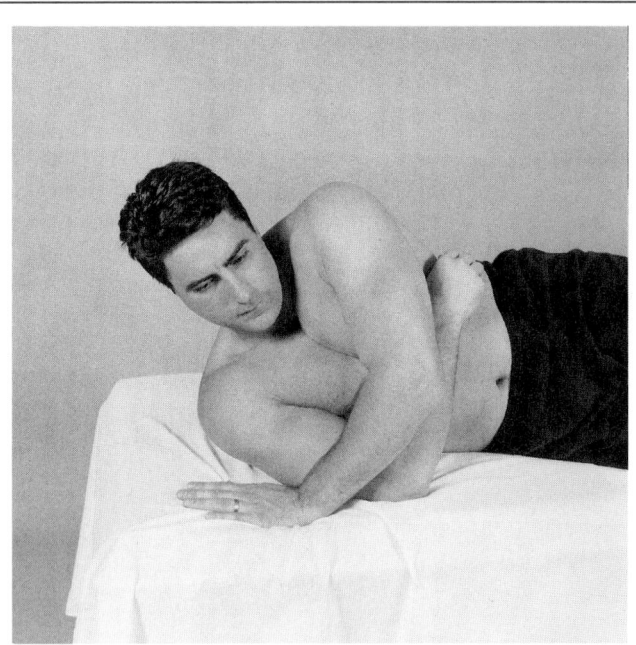

FIGURE 14-64   Side-lying to sit transfer.

on a tilt board or a circular board (Fig. 14-63) within tolerance. Other exercises that provide joint compression include:

▶ *Side-lying to sit transfers* (Fig. 14-64).

▶ *Elbow rest.* The patient supine in a semi-reclined position, leaning on the elbows, with the humerus in a neutral or extended position (Fig. 14-65).

▶ *Chair press up.* The patient is seated on a chair or bed. The patient then raises and lowers the buttocks off the chair by straightening the elbow (Fig. 14-66). This works the triceps muscles, the pectoralis major and minor, and the latissimus dorsi muscles.[7] This exercise can be progressed to include pushing and pulling exercises and quadruped and tripod balancing (Fig. 14-67).

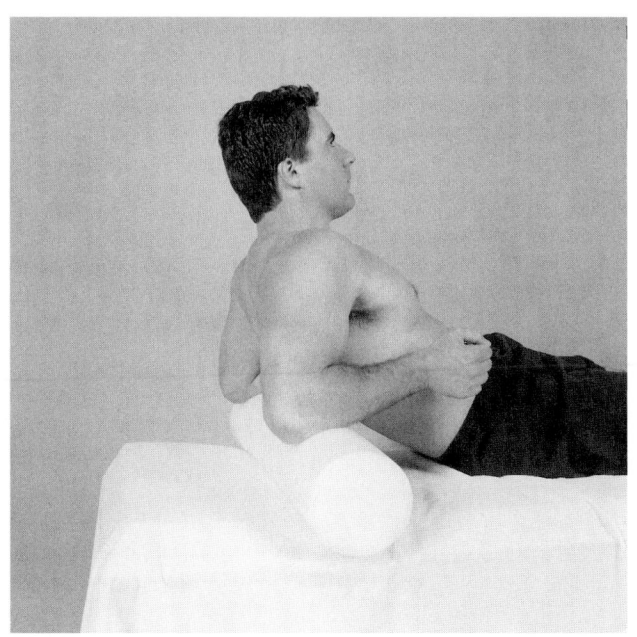

FIGURE 14-65   Elbow recline.

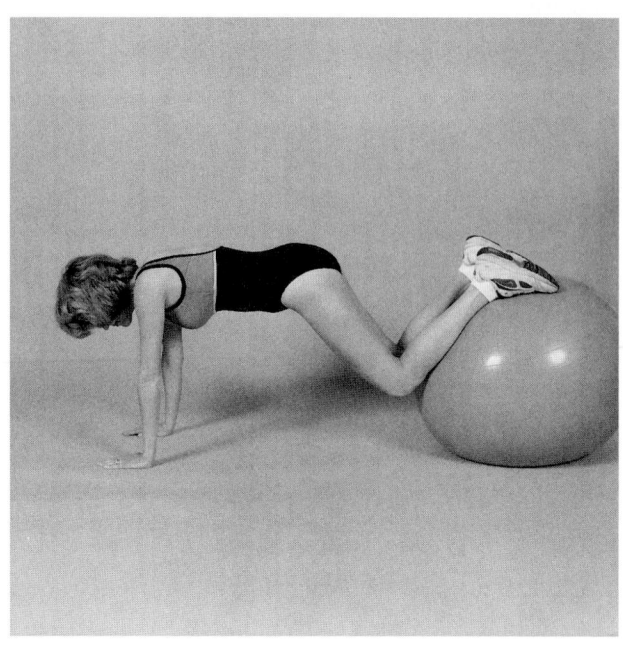

FIGURE 14-67   Quadruped balancing.

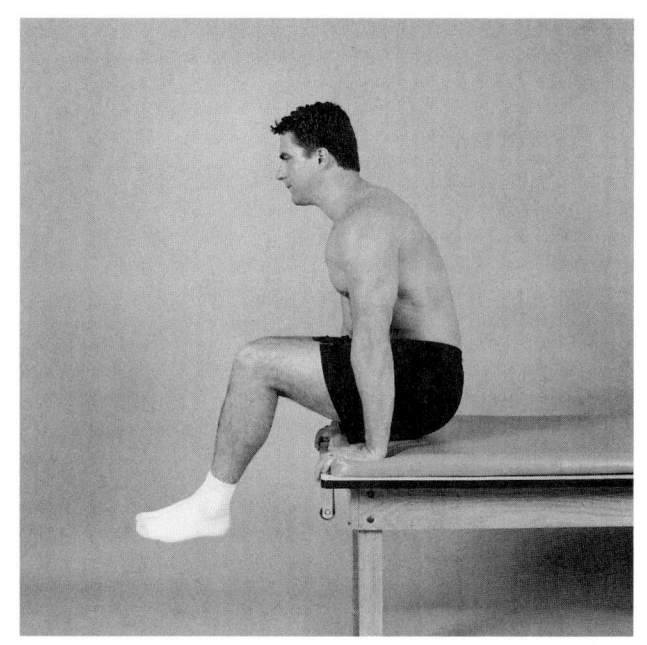

FIGURE 14-66   Chair push up.

Flexibility exercises to stretch both the joint capsule and the shoulder girdle muscles are a vital component of the rehabilitation process. Gentle grade I or II capsular stretches are performed by the clinician as tolerated. To supplement the stretches applied by the clinician, a number of techniques can be used by the patient to maintain and improve the range-of-motion gains achieved in the clinic (see Therapeutic Techniques section).

Kinetic chain preparation can begin in the early stages while the shoulder is recovering from the injury or surgery. The length of the kinetic chain required depends on the needs of the patient and the goals of the rehabilitative process. Longer kinetic chains are associated with the more active patients, and may include the entire lower kinetic chain and the trunk in addition to the upper extremity (see Biomechanics section). Kinetic chain preparation will allow for the normal sequencing of velocity and force when the patient returns to their normal activities or recreational pursuits.[102,105]

According to Kibler,[102] progression to the functional phase of the rehabilitative process requires that the following criteria be met:

▶ Progression of tissue healing (healed or sufficiently stabilized for active motion and tissue loading).

▶ Pain-free range of motion of at least 120° elevation.

▶ Manual muscle strength in nonpathologic areas 4+/5.

▶ Scapular control, with dominant side/nondominant side scapular asymmetry <1.5 cm with lateral slide test.

Functional Phase

The functional phase addresses any tissue overload problems and functional biomechanical deficits. The goals of the functional phase include:

▶ Attain full range of pain-free motion.

▶ Restore normal joint kinematics.

▶ Improve muscle strength to within normal limits.

▶ Improve neuromuscular control.

▶ Restore normal muscle force couples.

During the functional phase, the closed chain exercises introduced in the earlier phase of the rehabilitation process are progressed. Closed chain exercises in this phase may include:

▶ Modified push-ups (Fig. 14-68) and regular push-ups are added as tolerated.

▶ Medicine ball catch-and-throw (Fig. 14-69).

Scapular isolation exercises are introduced. The patient is positioned in side lying with their involved hand placed on the table to create a closed kinetic chain. While the clinician applies pressure to the scapula in random directions, the patient moves the scapula isotonically into the direction of the resistance (Fig. 14-70).

Dynamic weight shifting exercises are introduced during this phase. With the patient weight bearing on all fours in the quadruped position, and while keeping their hands stationary in the same position, the patient can rock the body forwards and backwards, and side to side (Fig. 14-71). Alternatively, the patient can slide their hands, or one hand, forwards, backwards, and side to side while maintaining their trunk still.

Open chain exercises designed to further strengthen the rotator cuff muscles are emphasized. These exercises may include:

▶ Proprioceptive neuromuscular facilitation (PNF) exercises with elastic tubing (Fig. 14-72).

▶ PNF exercises with the Bodyblade (Fig. 14-73).

The open chain exercises should also include resisted internal and external (Fig. 14-74) rotation with the arm in increasing amounts of abduction to strengthen the infraspinatus/teres

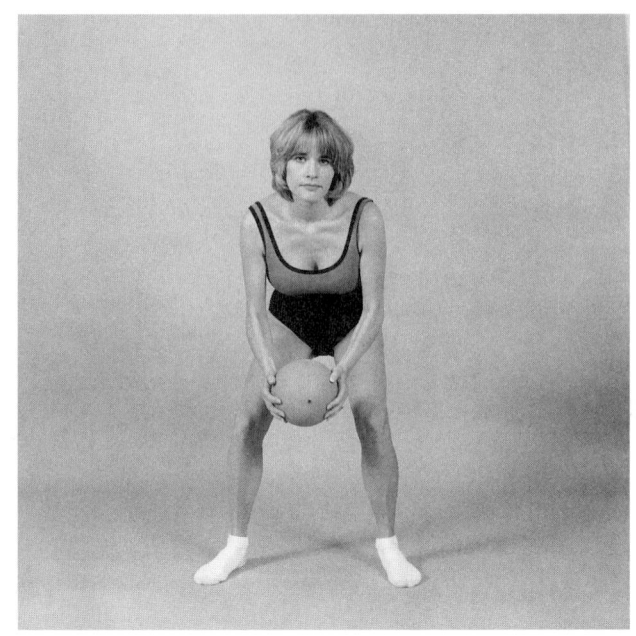

FIGURE 14-69 Medicine ball catch-and-throw.

minor and subscapularis muscles respectively. To avoid concurrent strengthening of the deltoid during the earlier phases of strengthening, the patient is instructed to hold a magazine or towel roll between the extremity and the trunk while strengthening the rotator cuff muscles (see Fig. 14-74). This forced adduction relaxes the deltoid and isolates the oblique muscles of the rotator cuff. By strengthening the infraspinatus, teres minor, and subscapularis (relative to the supraspinatus and the deltoid),

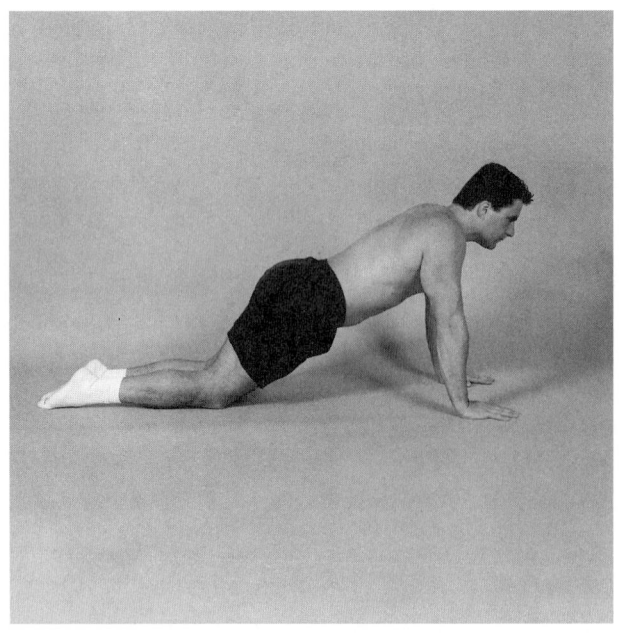

FIGURE 14-68 Modified push-ups.

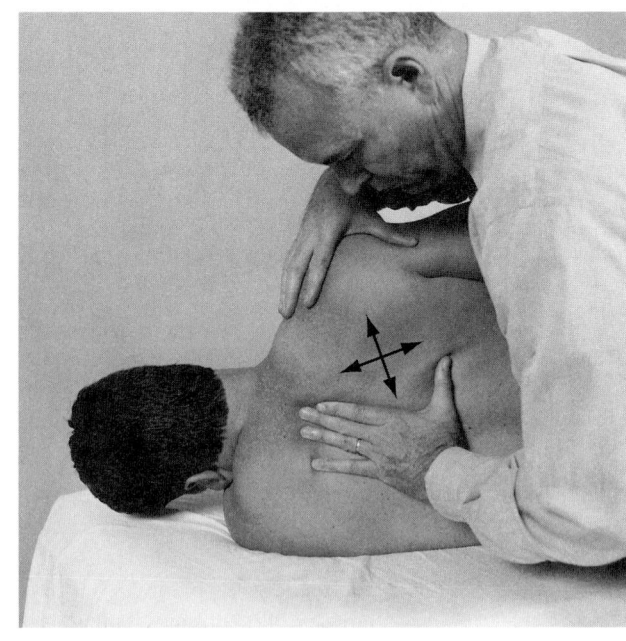

FIGURE 14-70 Resisted scapular exercises.

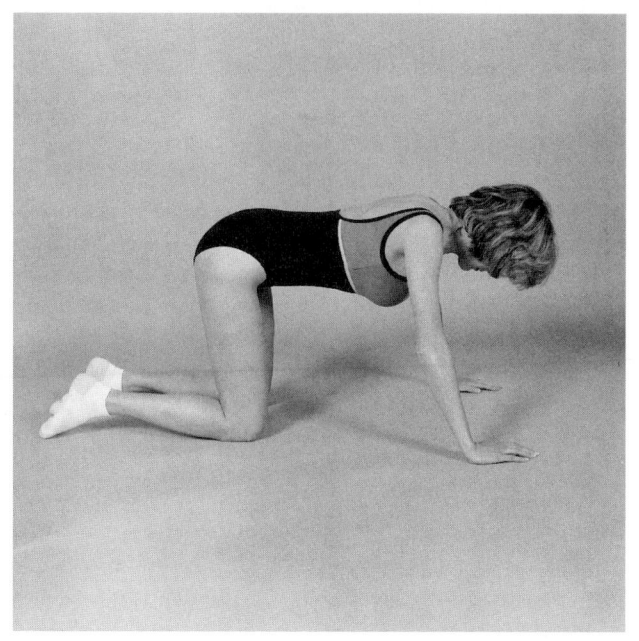

FIGURE 14-71   Quadriped rocking.

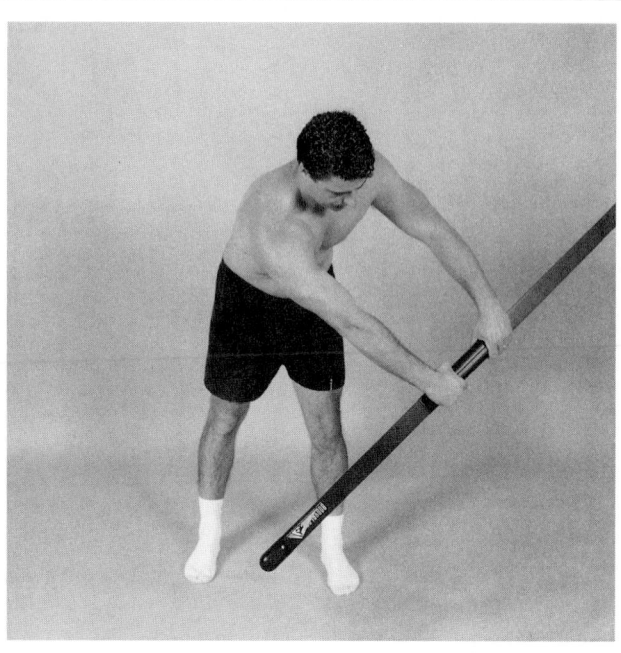

FIGURE 14-73   Bodyblade exercises.

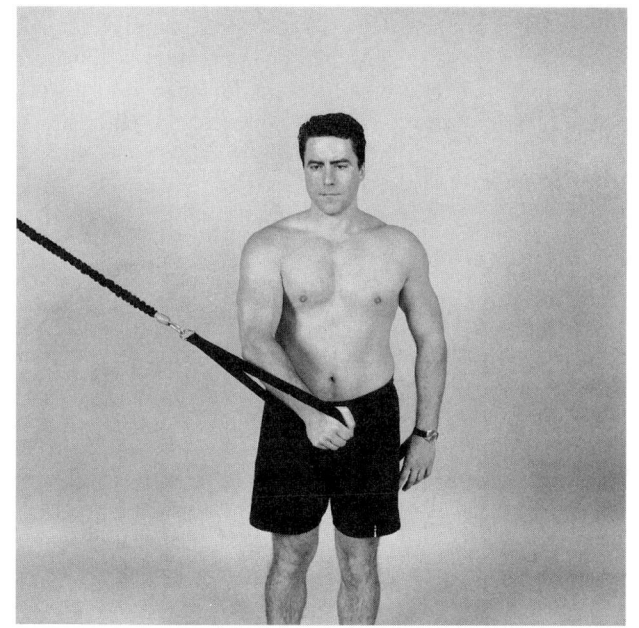

FIGURE 14-72   Proprioceptive neuromuscular facilitation (PNF) exercises with tubing.

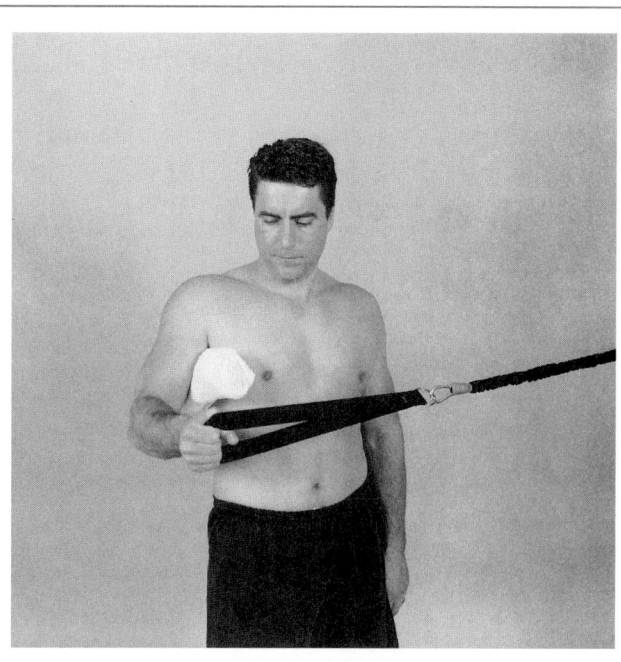

FIGURE 14-74   Resisted external rotation.

it may be possible to re-establish the normal balance and force couple during elevation of the G-H joint.[4,31,216]

The exercises are performed slowly at first and then progress to higher functional speeds. Three sets of the strengthening exercises should be performed daily using weights of 1 to 10 pounds. The number of repetitions is determined by tissue response (pain, fatigue, and compensatory patterns).

Once the rotator cuff strengthening exercises are tolerated well, open chain exercises for the scapular pivoters are progressed, and exercises for the humeral positioners (deltoid) are initiated. As with the exercises for the rotator cuff muscles, the exercises for the deltoid are performed slowly at first and then progress to higher functional speeds. Three sets of the strengthening exercises should be performed daily using weights of 1 to

10 pounds. The number of repetitions is determined by tissue response (pain, fatigue, and compensatory patterns).

Proper strengthening of the scapular pivoters assures that the scapula follows the humerus, providing dynamic stability and assuring synchrony of scapulohumeral rhythm. As the scapulothoracic muscles are not required to contract powerfully over short periods, or produce large amounts of force, it could be hypothesized that the scapulothoracic muscles serve a primarily postural function. Thus in the rehabilitation of the scapulothoracic muscles, their postural function should be addressed and retrained. This can be accomplished in the form of endurance exercises by training the muscles with low weights and high repetitions.[277]

Exercises for the scapular pivoters, the rotator cuff, and the deltoid during this phase include:

▶ Elevation in the plane of the scapula (scaption) in internal rotation (Fig. 14-75). This exercise strengthens the anterior and middle deltoids and subscapularis, and to a lesser extent the supraspinatus.[7,123] The scaption with internal rotation (SIR) (also known as "empty the can," "supraspinatus exercise," "supraspinatus fly," and "Jobe's exercise") is defined to be abduction in the plane of the scapula (90 degrees combined with 30 degrees of flexion) and internal rotation.[122]

▶ Elevation in the plane of the scapula (scaption) in external rotation. This exercise strengthens the scapula pivoters.[7,117,123]

▶ *Military press.* This exercise, which is performed by raising both hands from shoulder height straight up towards the ceiling, strengthens the supraspinatus, subscapularis, upper trapezius,[128] anterior deltoid, middle serratus anterior, lower serratus anterior, and middle deltoid.[7,117] As the military press can cause impingement, care must be taken with its use. This exercise is probably better used in a prevention program.

▶ Scapula retraction with horizontal abduction of the externally rotated shoulder, done in prone. Blackburn and colleagues[117] demonstrated that externally rotating the humerus during prone exercise increased EMG activity to the highest levels. Horizontal abduction (90 degrees or 100 degrees) in external rotation strengthens the infraspinatus and to a lesser extent, the teres minor and posterior deltoid (Table 14-23).[7,117,123,277] The patient lies prone on the table with both arms abducted to 90 degrees (Fig. 14-76) or 100 degrees and thumbs pointing towards the ceiling. With or without a weight in the hand, the patient then raises their thumbs towards the ceiling. Prone horizontal abduction with the arm externally rotated and abducted to 90 degrees in the frontal plane also strengthens the middle trapezius. If the arm is abducted to 100 degrees in the frontal plane, the lower trapezius is exercised.[117]

▶ Scapular retraction with horizontal abduction of the internally rotated shoulder, performed in prone; this is similar to the previous exercise, but the patient now has the thumbs pointing down towards the ground. They are again prone and their arms are abducted to approximately 90 degrees. They then raise their hypothenar eminences towards the ceiling. This exercise strengthens in order of effectiveness the posterior deltoid, middle trapezius, rhomboids, middle deltoid, levator scapulae, infraspinatus, teres minor, upper trapezius, and lower trapezius.[7,117,123]

▶ Shoulder shrugs (periscapular—trapezius, levator scapula). Resistance can be added to this exercise by having the patient hold dumbbells in the hands.

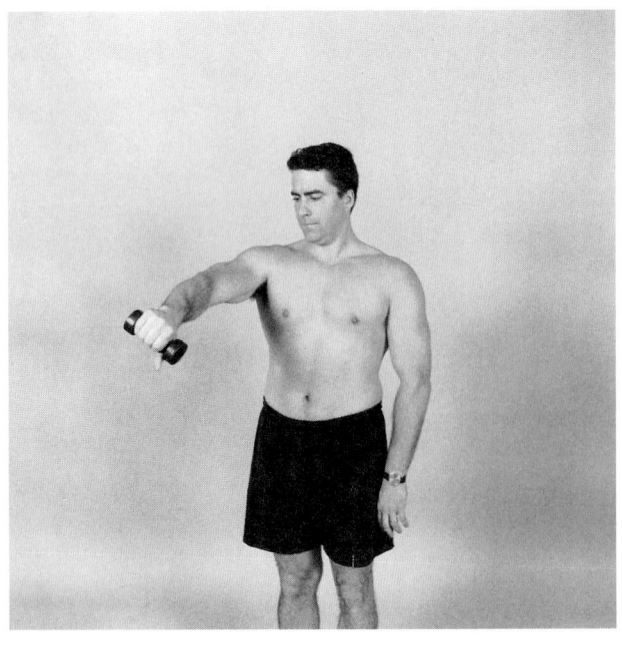

FIGURE 14-75   Scaption exercise.

TABLE 14-23   Scapular and Humeral Control Exercises

Scapular Control	Humeral Control
Bent-over rowing	Prone horizontal abduction
Push-ups with a plus (maximum shoulder protraction)	Scaption in internal rotation (thumbs down)
Press-ups	Scaption with external rotation (thumbs up)
Forward punch-outs	Prone extension
Scapular squeezes	Side-lying internal and external rotation Prone 90°/90° (90° abduction, 90° elbow flexion) external rotation

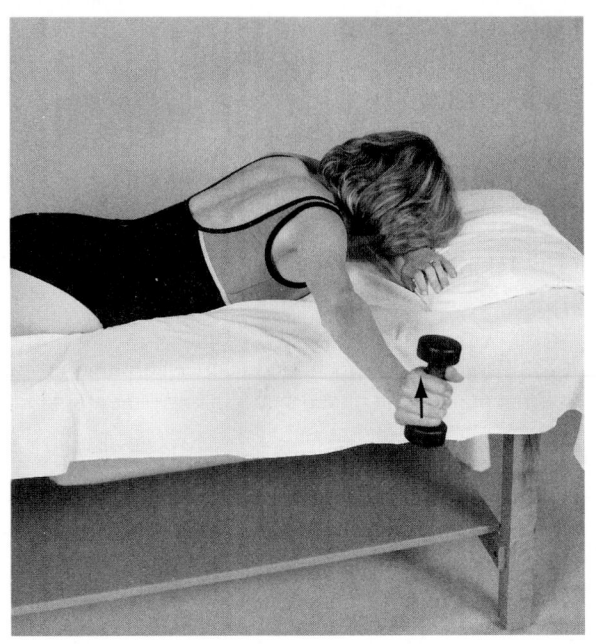

FIGURE 14-76 Horizontal abduction.

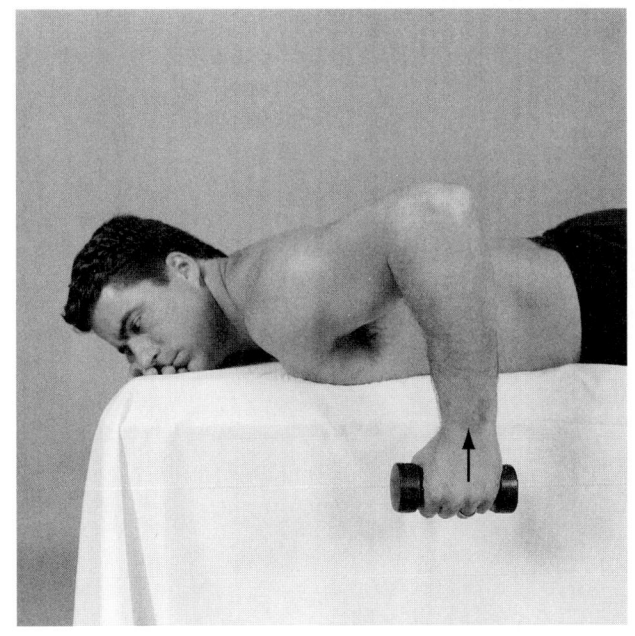

FIGURE 14-77 Prone rowing.

▶ Prone rowing. The patient lies prone on the table with weight in the hand. With the elbow flexed to approximately 90 degrees, the patient raises the elbow to the ceiling (Fig. 14-77). This exercise strengthens the upper trapezius, levator scapulae, lower trapezius, posterior deltoid, and to a lesser extent, the middle trapezius, rhomboids, and middle deltoid.[7,117,123]

▶ Push-up plus (see Fig. 14-60).

▶ Side-lying abduction exercises are performed with the subject lying on his or her side and moving into 45 degrees abduction in a neutral rotation position from a neutral or adducted position. Using MRI, side-lying abduction has been shown to produce the greatest signal intensity increase in three muscles of the rotator cuff: supraspinatus, infraspinatus, and subscapularis, as well as the deltoid.[128]

Eccentric exercises for all muscle groups (pivoters, positioners, and protectors) are introduced as tolerated, especially for those patients where tensile overloading is suspected to be the cause. Special emphasis on eccentric strengthening must be employed for the overhead athlete population.[351,362]

Lastly, the glenohumeral *propellers* (the latissimus dorsi and pectoralis major) are strengthened for functional performance.

In addition to addressing the musculature of the shoulder complex, the clinician must address the whole kinetic chain involved in an activity to which the patient is planning to return. This may include rehabilitation of the legs and hips to focus on the generation of appropriate activity-specific force and velocity from the lower extremity.[102,105] Examples include exercises that develop normal agonist-antagonist force couples in the legs such as squats, plyometric depth jumps, lunges, and hip extensions. Most shoulder activities involve rotation and diagonal patterns.[98,105] Thus the exercises must incorporate trunk rotation exercises (using medicine ball or tubing), which integrate leg and trunk stabilization (Fig. 14-78). Trunk rotations involving diagonal patterns from hip to shoulder, and medicine ball throws (Fig. 14-79) are added as tolerated. These exercises are

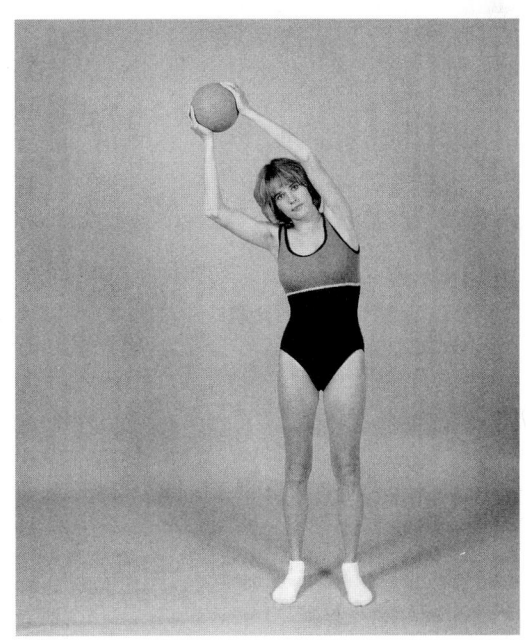

FIGURE 14-78 Weighted ball exercises.

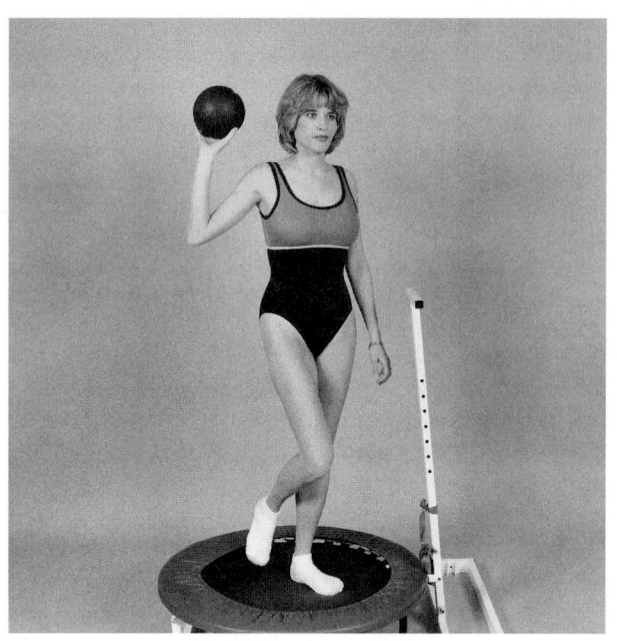

FIGURE 14-79 Integration of kinetic chains.

progressed to incorporate combined patterns of hip and trunk rotation in both directions, and hip and shoulder diagonal patterns from the left hip to the right shoulder and from the right hip to the left shoulder.[98,105]

Endurance activities in the legs should also be emphasized. Both aerobic endurance for recovery from exercise bouts and anaerobic endurance for agility and power work should also be advocated. These can be done using mini-trampoline exercises, agility drills with running and jumping, jumping jacks, and slider or Fitter boards.[102]

Activity-specific progressions must be completed before full return to function is allowed. This is done to test all of the working parts involved in the activity. Very few deviations from normal parameters of arm motion, arm position, force generation, smoothness of all of the kinetic chain, and from preinjury form should be allowed. Most of these adaptations will be biomechanically inefficient.[98,102,105,361,363]

The reader is referred to Table 14-24 for a typical program given for a pitcher returning to full function. This program can and should be modified as needed by the clinician. Each phase may take a longer or shorter time than that listed, and the program should be monitored closely.

Pattern 4D: Impaired Joint Mobility, Motor Function, Muscle Performance, Range of Motion with Connective Tissue Dysfunction

The primary impairment in pattern 4D, when applied to the shoulder, is hypomobility due to capsular restriction. In addition to limited joint movement and decreased range of motion associated with pain, the impairments in this pattern include decreased motor control and muscle performance.

The clinical findings in this pattern include but are not limited to pain, limited range of motion in a capsular pattern of restriction, an alteration in the scapulohumeral rhythm, crepitus, and a positive impingement sign.

Arthritis

Traumatic Arthritis of the G-H Joint. Traumatic or primary glenohumeral arthritis is an entity that has been well described and documented by Neer and colleagues,[316,364] who highlighted the presence of significant posterior glenoid erosion causing static posterior subluxation of the humeral head. Traumatic arthritis of the G-H joint rarely occurs in individuals under the age of 45. The condition is characterized by pain, progressive functional impairment, and reports of instability.[365] Passive horizontal adduction is usually the most limited and painful motion.

Conservative intervention consists of rest, modification of activity, and NSAIDs. Electrotherapeutic modalities and physical agents may be used to control pain and the active inflammation. Joint mobilizations of grade I or II may also be used to decrease pain. Once pain and inflammation is under control, the rehabilitation progresses to strengthening of the shoulder protectors and scapular pivoters, as described in the Intervention Strategies section.

Immobilization. Postsurgical immobilization occurs at any age, although it is more common in the elderly. The clinical

---

TABLE 14-24 Thrower's Ten Program[356]

1. Dumbbell exercises for the deltoid and supraspinatus muscles
2. Prone horizontal shoulder abduction
3. Prone shoulder extension
4. Internal rotation at 90 degrees abduction of the shoulder with elastic tubing
5. External rotation at 90 degrees abduction of the shoulder with elastic tubing
6. Elbow flexion/extension exercises with elastic tubing
7. Serratus anterior strengthening: progressive push-ups
8. Diagonal D_2 pattern for shoulder flexion and extension with elastic tubing
9. Press-ups
10. Dumbbell wrist extension/flexion and pronation/supination

progression is similar to that of traumatic arthritis. This condition should ideally be treated by prophylaxis.

Rheumatoid Arthritis. Rheumatoid arthritis is described in Chap. 9. Conservative intervention for this population includes patient education on how they can influence their disease process by alleviating the impairments, functional limitations, and disability. Electrotherapeutic modalities and cryotherapy can be used to help control pain and inflammation. Thermal modalities may also be used in the nonacute phases. Therapeutic exercise can be beneficial for the patients who are weak and stiff prior to the onset of end-stage arthritis, where the range of motion and strength can be regained, or at least maintained.[366] However, caution must be used with those patients with end-stage arthritis who have stiffness secondary to joint incongruity, as they may actually have their symptoms exacerbated with aggressive stretching exercises.[366]

When pain becomes too severe and conservative intervention is unable to relieve this pain and restore function, surgical measures are considered. These measures may include synovectomy, glenohumeral arthrodesis, or total joint arthroplasty (see Chap. 28).

Septic Arthritis. See Chap. 9.

Avascular Necrosis of the Humeral Head
Avascular necrosis of the humeral head is described in Chap. 9.

Hemorrhagic Shoulder (Milwaukee Shoulder)
L'épaule sénile hémorragique (the hemorrhagic shoulder of the elderly) was first described in 1968. It consisted of recurrent, blood-streaked effusions of the shoulder along with radiographic findings of severe degenerative glenohumeral arthritis and a chronic tear of the rotator cuff.[367] The term *Milwaukee shoulder* was not introduced until 1981.[368–370]

The condition generally affects a subset of the elderly population who has glenohumeral arthritis in conjunction with a complete rotator cuff tear.

One theory to explain the Milwaukee shoulder states that a hydroxyapatite-mineral phase develops in the altered capsule, synovial tissue, or degenerative articular cartilage. This releases basic calcium phosphate crystals into the synovial fluid.[368–370] These crystals are phagocytized by synovial cells and form calcium phosphate crystal microspheroids. These induce the release of activated enzymes from these cells, causing destruction of the periarticular tissues and articular surfaces.[371]

Another theory is the cuff tear theory. In 1983, Neer and colleagues[372] postulated that untreated chronic, massive tears would lead to a degenerated G-H joint. The mechanism of destruction of the articular cartilage was said to include mechanical and nutritional alterations in the shoulder with a rotator cuff tear.[372] The mechanical factors include anteroposterior instability of the humeral head resulting from a massive tear of the rotator cuff, and rupture or dislocation of the long head of the biceps which leads to proximal migration of the humeral head and acromial impingement.[371] Glenohumeral articular wear

was thought to occur as a result of repetitive trauma from the altered biomechanics associated with the loss of primary and secondary stabilizers of the G-H joint.[371] Changes in the composition of the articular cartilage follows because of inadequate diffusion of nutrients and the diminished quantity of synovial fluid.[371] Degenerative arthritis and subchondral collapse eventually develops.[371]

If the resultant rotator cuff tear arthropathy causes relatively mild symptoms, intervention should consist of mild antiinflammatory medication and gentle stretching exercises to maintain or regain a functional ROM.[371] A strengthening program should follow to improve the active use of the arm for activities of daily living. If conservative management fails, a humeral hemiarthroplasty is the procedure of choice to provide reliable relief of pain and functional improvement.[371]

Frozen Shoulder/Adhesive Capsulitis
Because this condition also involves an inflammation of the capsule, a patient with this condition could also be classified under preferred practice pattern 4E.

The frozen shoulder syndrome was first described by Duplay in 1872,[373] who used the term *peri-arthritis scapulo-humerale*. It wasn't until 1934 that Codman[196] used the term *frozen shoulder* to describe this condition. In 1945, Neviaser coined the term *adhesive capsulitis* to reflect his findings of a chronic inflammatory process at surgery and autopsy in patients treated for a painful, stiff shoulder.[374]

Although the etiology of frozen shoulder remains elusive, the understanding of the pathophysiology has recently improved. Factors associated with adhesive capsulitis include female gender,[375] age older than 40 years,[376] trauma,[376] diabetes,[253,272,377–380] prolonged immobilization,[381] thyroid disease,[382–384] stroke or myocardial infarction,[378,385] certain psychiatric conditions,[386,387] and the presence of autoimmune diseases.[388,389]

The prevalence of frozen shoulder in the general population is slightly greater than 2 percent,[375,390] and 11 percent of the adult diabetic population.[377] Approximately 70 percent of patients with adhesive capsulitis are women, and 20 to 30 percent of those affected subsequently will have adhesive capsulitis develop in the opposite shoulder.[391]

Nash and Hazelman[392] have described the concept of primary and secondary frozen shoulder, with the former idiopathic in origin, and the latter either traumatic in origin or related to a disease process, neurologic, or cardiac condition.

Primary Adhesive Capsulitis. Primary adhesive capsulitis is characterized by an idiopathic, progressive, and painful loss of active and passive shoulder motion, particularly external rotation, which causes the individual to gradually limit the use of the arm. Difficulty is reported with putting on a jacket or coat, putting objects in back pockets, or hooking garments in the back.[227,393–395] Inflammation and pain can cause muscle guarding of the shoulder muscles, without true fixed contracture of the joint capsule. Disuse of the arm results in a loss of shoulder mobility, whereas continued use of the arm through pain can result in development of subacromial impingement.[391] Over a period of weeks, compensatory movements of the shoulder girdle develop in order to minimize pain.[391] With time, there is resolution of pain and the individual is left with a stiff shoulder with severe limitation of function.

Secondary or Idiopathic Adhesive Capsulitis.   Zuckerman and Cuomo[396] defined idiopathic adhesive capsulitis as a condition characterized by substantial restriction of both active and passive shoulder motion that occurs in the absence of a known intrinsic shoulder disorder. Two clinical forms are recognized.

1. One form is defined as when the pain is more noticeable than the motion restriction. This condition is self-limiting, and the patient spontaneously recovers within 6 months to a year. Two studies[397,398] of patients with idiopathic adhesive capsulitis found that the vast majority of patients with this condition were successfully treated with a specific shoulder-stretching exercise program.

2. The other form is defined as when the pain, which can radiate below the elbow, is as noticeable as the restriction. The patient complains of pain at rest and is unable to sleep on the involved side. External rotation of the G-H joint is usually affected more than abduction or flexion.[227] The initial phase of this condition is characterized by pain and progressive loss of motion lasting 2 to 6 months. This form responds well to a series of corticosteroid injections or local anesthetic (distension therapy).

To formulate a logical approach to the intervention of patients with adhesive capsulitis, the clinician needs to determine the degree of inflammation and irritability. To help in this determination, it is necessary to have a better understanding of the underlying cellular and biochemical pathophysiology of this disease.

There is disagreement as to whether the underlying pathologic process is an inflammatory condition[399–401] or a fibrosing condition.[402] Significant evidence exists[388,389,401,403] in support of the hypothesis that the underlying pathologic changes in adhesive capsulitis are synovial inflammation with subsequent reactive capsular fibrosis, making adhesive capsulitis an inflammatory and a fibrosing condition, dependent on the stage of the disease. The initial biological trigger in this cascade of inflammation and subsequent fibrosis is unknown, although it is likely to involve multiple factors. In some areas, there seems to be a seasonal variation in patients presenting with adhesive capsulitis, suggesting that a virus is responsible.[391]

Stages of Progression.   Adhesive capsulitis is suggested by Neviaser[374] to pass through four stages based on pathologic changes in the synovium and subsynovium, with each stage having an individual intervention strategy, although there is controversy about this idea.[24]

Stage I.   In stage I patients present with mild signs and symptoms of less than 3 months' duration, which are often described as achy at rest, and sharp at extremes of range of motion. The symptoms often mimic those of an impingement syndrome, where restriction of motion is minimal and pain that appears to be due to a rotator cuff tendonitis has been present for less than 3 months. However, the patient reports a progressive loss of motion, and intervention protocols for rotator cuff tendonitis fail. A capsular pattern of motion (loss of external rotation and abduction) is present, and a more subtle loss of internal rotation in adduction. In adhesive capsulitis due to type 1 diabetes mellitus, the capsular pattern is typically equal limitation of external rotation and internal rotation, which is greater than the limitation of abduction.

In this early stage, the majority of motion loss is secondary to the painful synovitis, rather than a true capsular contraction.

Stage II.   Patients presenting with stage I and stage II adhesive capsulitis have pain on palpation of the anterior and posterior capsules and describe pain radiating to the deltoid insertion. An intra-articular injection of steroid and local analgesic given by a physician can be extremely useful in the diagnosis and intervention of adhesive capsulitis.[391] After the injection, passive glenohumeral ROM is reevaluated. If the patient has significant improvement in pain and normalization of motion, the diagnosis of stage I adhesive capsulitis is confirmed.[391] If the patient has a significant improvement in pain but no significant improvement in ROM, then by definition he or she has stage II adhesive capsulitis, although it must be emphasized that these stages represent a continuum of the inflammatory and scarring processes.[399]

In stage II, symptoms have been present for 3 to 9 months with progressive loss of ROM and persistence of the pain pattern described above. The motion loss in stage II adhesive capsulitis reflects a loss of capsular volume and a response to the painful synovitis. The patient demonstrates a loss of motion in all planes, as well as pain in all parts of the range. Evaluation of active and passive range of motion (PROM) should be performed because documenting the initial ROM, especially passive motion, is critical in determining the efficacy of the intervention plan. The causes of the restricted PROM need to be assessed and a differentiation must be made between protective muscle guarding, adaptive changes in musculotendinous structures, or capsular adhesions and contracture.

Stage III.   In stage III, patients present with a history of painful stiffening of the shoulder, and a significant loss of ROM. Symptoms have been present for 9 to 14 months and have been observed to change with time. Patients often report a history of an extremely painful phase that has resolved, resulting in a relatively pain-free but stiff shoulder.

Poor scapulohumeral rhythm is observed during elevation of the arm. There is a dominance of the upper trapezius resulting in hiking of the shoulder girdle. This is attributed to decreased inferior glide of the G-H joint, which prevents glenohumeral abduction.[213]

Stage IV.   Stage IV, also known as the "thawing stage" for adhesive capsulitis, is characterized by the slow, steady recovery of some of the lost ROM resulting from capsular remodeling in response to use of the arm and shoulder. Although many people feel less restricted in this phase, objective measurement shows only minor improvement.[404] No arthroscopic or histologic data are available for patients with stage IV adhesive capsulitis because these patients rarely undergo surgery. Patients who present with stages III and IV adhesive capsulitis often report a history of long-standing pain at rest and pain at night that have resolved spontaneously.[405] The objective findings typically include a stiff shoulder, with striking alteration of scapulohumeral mechanics and limited use of the arm during activities of daily living. A capsular pattern of motion is a characteristic finding. Resistance in the form of a capsular end-feel is felt before pain is reached as the G-H joint is taken through passive ROM.

Other pathological conditions that can create a painful restriction of glenohumeral motion should be ruled out. Typically, the physician has used a routine radiographic evaluation to rule out other causes for a stiff, painful shoulder including glenohumeral arthritis, calcific tendonitis, or long-standing rotator cuff disease.[391] Radiographs usually are negative in patients with frozen shoulder, although there may be evidence of disuse osteopenia.[391] Magnetic resonance imaging has been used for investigation purposes in patients with adhesive capsulitis and has shown an increased blood flow to the synovium in frozen shoulder.[406]

Intervention. The primary goal of conservative intervention is the restoration of the range of motion and focuses on the application of controlled tensile stresses to produce elongation of the restricting tissues.[217,272,391,407–409] The patient with capsular restriction and low irritability may require aggressive soft tissue and joint mobilization, whereas patients with high irritability may require pain-easing manual therapy techniques.[410] In contrast, the emphasis on intervention of limited ROM due to nonstructural changes is aimed at addressing the cause of the pain.[276,390,396,403,411–414]

The trust and confidence of the patient is necessary, and it is important to ensure that no harm is caused or that the clinician does not indicate any frustration.

Earlier studies have indicated that a gradual return of full mobility occurs within 18 months to 3 years in most patients, even without specific intervention.[411,415,416] More recent studies have documented persistent pain and stiffness beyond 3 years.[375,395,417] At 7 years, Shaffer noted that 30 percent of patients had restricted mobility on objective measurements and 50 percent complained of pain or stiffness.[397] However, major function limitation is rarely noted in these studies.

A number of questions are often raised by the patient with regard to corticosteroid injections. While these questions are best answered by the appropriate physician, there is extensive information regarding the efficacy of intra-articular corticosteroid in the intervention of patients with adhesive capsulitis.[418–422] Hazelman[423] summarized numerous studies on the use of intra-articular corticosteroid and reported that the success of intervention is dependent on the duration of symptoms.

▶ Patients treated within 1 month of onset of symptoms recovered in an average of 1.5 months.

▶ Patients treated within 3 months of the onset of symptoms reported a significant improvement in symptoms.

▶ Patients treated within 2 to 5 months of onset of symptoms recovered within 8.1 months of onset of symptoms.

▶ Patients treated after 5 or more months of onset of symptoms had a more delayed recovery, with the time necessary for full recovery reported to be dependent on the duration of symptoms.

▶ Patients treated 6 to 12 months after onset of symptoms required an average of 14 months for full recovery.

These data and along with others support the hypothesis that adhesive capsulitis is an inflammatory and fibrotic condition.[399,401,402, 418,424] Early intervention with intra-articular corticosteroid may provide a chemical ablation of the synovitis, thus limiting the subsequent development of fibrosis and shortening the natural history of the disease.[399] With resolution of the synovitis and loss of the cytokine stimulus to the capsular fibroblasts, capsular remodeling and recovery of ROM take place.[399]

Surgical intervention is reserved for those patients that do not respond to conservative intervention. Historically, arthroscopy has been of little diagnostic and therapeutic value in patients with adhesive capsulitis of the shoulder,[376] and closed manipulation appears to be the operation of choice if conservative methods fail. However, closed manipulation is contraindicated in patients with significant osteopenia, recent surgical repair of soft tissues about the shoulder, or in the presence of fractures, neurologic injury and instability.[391]

Acromioclavicular Joint Arthrosis

Acromioclavicular joint arthrosis may be degenerative or posttraumatic. It is most commonly seen in middle-aged patients, either as an isolated entity or in combination with rotator cuff tendonitis and impingement syndrome.[50,51]

Acromioclavicular joint arthrosis is diagnosed by the history and physical examination. Patients typically complain of pain locally or distributed to the anterolateral neck, the trapezius-supraspinatus region, and the anterolateral deltoid.[425] This pain is usually exacerbated with overhead and/or flexed and adducted positions of the arm.[51] Direct palpation to the A-C joint will sometimes reproduce the patient's pain. Impingement of the rotator cuff must be ruled out. The selective use of cortisone injections into the A-C joint or the subacromial space can be used to help differentiate acromioclavicular pain from rotator cuff tendonitis and help treat both of these conditions.[50,51]

Conservative intervention consists of rest, modification of activity, and NSAIDs. Electrotherapeutic modalities and cryotherapy may be used to control pain and the active inflammation. Joint mobilizations of grade I or II may also be used to decrease pain. Once pain and inflammation is under control, the rehabilitation progresses to strengthening of the dynamic restraints of the A-C joint (primarily the deltoid, trapezius, and pectorals).[50,230] Any activities involving raising the arm above the level of the shoulder or reaching across the chest should be avoided as these will tend to aggravate the A-C joint.[227]

Selective Hypomobility

A generalized decrease in shoulder range of motion may be due to a number of reasons such as arthritis or adhesive capsulitis. Selective hypomobility is usually the result of a restriction of the joint capsule. An asymmetrical restriction of the capsule causes a translation away from the side of the joint where the tightness is located. For example, a posterior capsule restriction results in an increase in anterior translation of the humeral head during cross-arm adduction and with flexion of the gleno-humeral joint.[149] The posterior capsule restriction also results in a superior translation of the humeral head with flexion of the glenohumeral joint.

Passive movement testing may be used to detect the direction of the hypomobility by examining the end-feel, and the amount of translation that occurs. Such tests include the load and shift test, the anterior release test, and the sulcus sign test. Range-of-motion tests are used to determine the amount of internal and external rotation. There is a close association between internal rotation of the G-H joint and posterior shoulder capsule tightness.[426]

The intervention for this impairment includes a warm-up phase using a moist heating pad or upper body ergonometer. The patient is then taught the position to adopt in order to stretch the restricted portion of the capsule. The maximum stretch position is then maintained for approximately 20 minutes, or as long as the patient can tolerate. The patient is instructed to perform the warm-up and stretch at home. The duration of the stretch is gradually increased until the patient is able to tolerate the stretch position for 60 minutes per day.

The patient performs multiple angle isometrics or short arc exercises in the newly acquired range to improve neuromuscular dynamic control. When full range of motion has been restored, the patient performs full range resistive exercises and combinations of arm and trunk exercises, such as proprioceptive neuromuscular facilitation (PNF).

According to Sahrmann, correction of resting scapular malalignment is always indicated, particularly when the passive range of motion is not restricted by more than 20 degrees.[237]

Downwardly Rotated Scapula.[237] The G-H joint becomes the site of compensation because the scapula does not fully upwardly rotate. The scapula should be supported in its correct position constantly by providing support for the arm. Exercise intervention should include strengthening for the serratus anterior and the trapezius. Stretching exercises are prescribed for those muscles found to be shortened in the examination. Those muscles usually include the rhomboid and levator scapulae.

Scapular Depression.[237] This syndrome is characterized by weakness and lengthening of the upper trapezius. It is often accompanied by shortness of the latissimus dorsi, pectoralis major, and pectoralis minor. When the scapula fails to elevate sufficiently during glenohumeral flexion or abduction, the lower trapezius becomes more dominant than its upper counterpart. The intervention should focus on providing support for the shoulder so that it does not become depressed. The patient is instructed to perform shoulder shrugs with the G-H joint in its anatomic position and with the shoulder flexed above 120 degrees. A mirror can be used to teach the patient to correct the depression of the shoulder girdle during arm elevation. Stretching exercises are prescribed for those muscles found to be shortened in the examination.

Scapular Abduction Syndrome.[237] This syndrome is characterized by excessive scapular abduction during glenohumeral flexion or abduction. It is also associated with a lengthening of the trapezius and possible lengthening of the rhomboid muscles and shortening of the serratus anterior, resulting in poor control of the scapula. Shortness of the deltoid or supraspinatus muscles can also indirectly hold the scapula in an abducted position. Intervention should focus on stretching the short glenohumeral and thoracohumeral muscles and improving the performance of the adductor components of the lower and middle trapezius muscles.

Scapular Winging Syndrome. This syndrome is characterized by an inability to elevate and/or lower the arm without the scapula winging or its inferior angle tilting. This syndrome results from a weakness and shortness of the serratus anterior, with accompanying shortness of the pectoralis minor and scapulohumeral muscles.

Intervention should focus on stretching the pectoralis minor to correct the tilting and serratus anterior for strengthening and retraining.

Humeral Anterior Glide Syndrome.[237] This syndrome is characterized by a humeral head that is positioned more than one third anteriorly to the acromion, and which moves anteriorly during glenohumeral abduction. Other findings typically include relative tightness of the posterior capsule when compared to the anterior, weak or lengthened subscapularis, shortness of the scapulohumeral external rotators, and shortness of the pectoralis major.

Intervention should shorten and strengthen the subscapularis, and stretch the humeral external rotators.

Humeral Superior Glide Syndrome.[237] This syndrome is characterized by an excessive movement of the humeral head in a superior direction during glenohumeral flexion, abduction, or elevation. Clinical findings usually include shortness of the deltoid, weakness of the rotator cuff muscles, and shortness of the humeral internal and/or external rotators. Intervention focuses on the deltoid; increasing its length if shortened, and diminishing its activity if dominant. The patient should be instructed to avoid performing activities that involve external rotation in adduction, as well as abduction exercises and resisted shoulder flexion with the elbow extended, as these can exacerbate the condition.

Glenohumeral Instability

In the early years of life, the G-H joint remains fairly stable due to the active mechanisms stabilizing the joint. However, if the person begins to decondition with time, the dynamic mechanisms can no longer support the joint. The joint becomes involved in a self-perpetuating cycle of more instability, less use, more shoulder dysfunction, and more instability. In addition to shoulder capsular redundancy, underlying causes of glenohumeral instability can include genetic, biochemical (collagen), and biomechanical factors.[333]

Characteristic of this pattern is the complaint of the shoulder "slipping" or "popping out" during overhead activities. As previously described in the Biomechanics section, a number of structures are involved in the maintenance of shoulder stability, including muscles and the capsuloligamentous structures.[29] These structures also provide neurological feedback which mediates reflex stabilization around the joint.[427,428]

Laxity is the physiologic motion of the G-H joint that allows a normal ROM. It is normally asymptomatic.[333] Laxity is not always synonymous with instability.[429] It is a necessary attribute of the shoulder that permits motion. Instability is the abnormal symptomatic motion of the G-H joint that affects normal joint kinematics and results in pain, subluxation, or dislocation of the shoulder.[22,427,430,431]

There is considerable variation in the amount of translation normally elicited in an asymptomatic shoulder.[331,332,336,432] Shoulder laxity tests show that translations in the asymptomatic shoulder as compared with the contralateral symptomatic shoulder can be as large as 11 mm in one direction.[332,433] Although it has been shown that healthy shoulders can have asymmetric translation in at least one direction, no healthy shoulder is asymmetric in all three directions.[332] When a motion becomes symptomatic, the distinction between laxity and instability is made.[333]

Instability of the shoulder can be classified by frequency, magnitude, direction, and origin.[24] The frequency of occurrence is classified as acute or chronic. Acute traumatic instability with dislocation of the shoulder is the most dramatic variety, and often requires manipulative reduction. Unilateral dislocations occurring from acute traumatic events include the Bankart lesion or Hill-Sachs lesion. The Bankart lesion is an avulsion of the anterior inferior labrum from the glenoid rim and requires surgical stabilization (*T*raumatic, *U*nidirectional instability with *B*ankart lesion requiring *S*urgery or TUBS). This is done using the Bankart procedure, which addresses the lesion without significant loss of external rotation,[434] or a capsular reconstruction procedure (refer to Chap. 28). The Hill-Sachs lesion is a compression fracture on the posterior humeral head at the site where the humeral head impacted the inferior glenoid rim.

Most patients presenting with hypermobility or instability of the G-H joint are athletic adolescents or young adults with joint laxity.[333,435] Such individuals may have pain with overhead movements due to an inability to control their laxity by means of their muscles. They may develop enough instability directed superiorly that they present with impingement-like symptoms (instability-impingement overlap), especially in positions of abduction and external rotation.[436] In general, the patients have had normal asymptomatic shoulder function until some event precipitates symptoms. The event is usually

relatively minor trauma when compared with traumatic causes of unidirectional instability, or repetitive microtrauma as occurs in patients who participate in swimming and gymnastics.[281] The most common presenting complaint is pain.[437,438]

Dislocation of the G-H joint is not uncommon in older people, although the incidence is less after 50 years of age.[227] Chronic recurrent dislocations of the shoulder can lead to degenerative arthritis. An older person who dislocates a shoulder is likely to have concurrently torn the rotator cuff and should be examined with this idea in mind.[439–441] Lesser traumatic injuries can cause subluxation of the shoulder to such a degree that recurrent subluxation rather than dislocation becomes a source of dysfunction.[22]

Shoulder instability is also classified according to the direction of the subluxation. These instabilities can be unidirectional (anterior, posterior, or inferior), bidirectional, or multidirectional. Recently, both multidirectional instability and its hallmark, inferior glenohumeral instability, have been scrutinized much more closely.[95,109,442]

The predominant pattern of instability is best determined from the patient's medical history and provocative maneuvers on physical examination.[333] The mechanism for a subluxation or recurrent dislocation usually involves a fall on an outstretched hand (FOOSH injury), whereby the arm is forced into abduction, extension, and external rotation. Due to the potential for nerve injury with these dislocations, a thorough neurovascular examination is essential.[24]

Loss of internal rotation in young patients may be an important finding suggestive of posterior capsular contracture that is often associated with subtle instability.[229] Symptoms also include varying degrees of instability, transient neurologic symptoms, and easy fatigability.[438] A brief period of sling immobilization is usually necessary for comfort. Prolonged immobilization should be avoided because of the tendency of the shoulder to stiffen quickly in older people.[227]

Anterior Instability. Anterior instability of the G-H joint is the most common direction of instability. Repetitive overhead activities such as throwing can lead to microtrauma at the shoulder, leading to eventual breakdown of both the static and dynamic stabilizers of the joint, or glenohumeral instability. Once the stability of the G-H joint has been compromised, the structures of the rotator cuff can become injured, resulting in a tear of one or more of the muscles. Patients who describe symptoms occurring in the abducted and externally rotated position have chronic anteroinferior instability.

The mechanism for an anterior dislocation is abduction, external rotation, and extension and is common in throwing and racquet sports, gymnastics, and swimming. Following an acute trauma, the patient typically complains of severe pain and a sense that the shoulder is "out." Radiographs confirm the dislocation and reduction is often necessary. Frank anterior subluxation and dislocation of the G-H joint is rare in children but common in adolescents.[443] Severe pain causes the patient to immobilize the involved arm, in a slightly abducted and externally rotated position with the other hand. Spasm will occur to stabilize the joint. The humeral head will be palpable anteriorly and the posterior shoulder will exhibit a hollow beneath the acromion (see Special Tests section). In younger age groups (about 25 years and younger), the chance of recurrent anterior dislocation after the initial event is greater than 95 percent.[444] Recurrences are rare in patients more than 50 years of age.[431]

When anterior instability is suspected, the clinician should assess for tightness of the posterior capsule. Posterior capsule tightness has been shown to accentuate anterior translation and superior migration.[337] A loss of internal rotation can indicate tightness of the posterior capsule. The posterior joint glide is also restricted.

SLAP Lesions. Athletes performing overhead movements, particularly baseball pitchers, may develop a "dead arm" syndrome[445] in which they have a painful shoulder with throwing and can no longer throw a baseball with their preinjury velocity. The main problem is usually a tear of the superior labrum, the so-called SLAP lesion.[1] SLAP lesions are defined as *Superior Labral* lesions that are both *Anterior* and *Posterior*.[446] During a dislocation, tears to the glenoid labrum occur in isolation or in combination. The superior aspect of the labrum is more mobile and prone to injury due to its close attachment to the long head of the biceps tendon.[24] The lesion typically results from a fall on an outstretched hand (FOOSH injury), sudden deceleration or traction forces such as catching a falling heavy object, and anterior and posterior instability.[446,447]

Traumatic SLAP lesions can also develop in the nonathletic population.[447] This occurs as the result of a fall or motor vehicle accident (e.g., drivers who have their hands on the wheel and sustain a rear-end impact).

SLAP lesions can be classified by signs and symptoms into four main types:[447]

▶ *Type I.* This type involves a fraying and degeneration of the edge of the superior labrum. The patient loses the ability to horizontally abduct or externally rotate with the forearm pronated without pain.[448]

▶ *Type II.* This type involves a pathologic detachment of the labrum and biceps tendon anchor, resulting in a loss of the stabilizing effect of the labrum and the biceps.[449]

▶ *Type III.* This type involves a vertical tear of the labrum, similar to the bucket-handle tear of the meniscus, although the remaining portions of the labrum and biceps are intact.[24]

▶ *Type IV.* This type involves an extension of the bucket-handle tear into the biceps tendon, with portions of the labral flap and biceps tendon displaceable into the G-H joint.[24]

Diagnosis of a SLAP lesion can often be difficult as the symptoms are very similar to those of instability and rotator cuff disease. The patient typically complains of pain with overhead activities and symptoms of catching or locking.[450]

Several special tests can be used to help identify the presence of a SLAP lesion, including the clunk test,[317,318] the crank test,[320] the Speed's test,[447] and the anterior slide test.[326]

Conservative intervention should address the underlying hypermobility or instability of the shoulder using dynamic stabilization exercises of the G-H joint to effectively return function and symptomatic relief to the patient (see "Intervention" section, later).[452]

Arthroscopic labral debridement is not an effective long-term solution for labral pathology.[451]

Studies of surgical labral repairs are generally good to excellent in terms of returning patients to their prior level of activity, whether sports or work.[24,450,453,454]

Posterior Instability. Posterior instabilities are rare, and comprise approximately 2 percent of all shoulder dislocations.[112] Posterior dislocations are often associated with seizure, electric shock, diving into a shallow pool, or motor vehicle accidents. Patients who have symptoms with the arm in a forward flexed, adducted position, such as when pushing open heavy doors, have a posterior instability pattern. These dislocations are classified as subacromial (posterior and inferior to the acromion process), subglenoid (posterior and inferior to the glenoid rim), and subspinous (medial to the acromion and inferior to the scapular spine), with the former being the more common for posterior dislocations.[24]

The classic sign for a posterior dislocation is a loud clunk as the shoulder is moved from a forward flexed position to an abducted and externally rotated position,[112] a positive finding often associated and confused with an anterior dislocation. The findings for a posterior dislocation are usually severe pain, limited external rotation, often to less than 0 degrees, and limited elevation to less than 90 degrees. There is usually a posterior prominence and rounding of the shoulder compared to the opposite side and a flattening of the anterior aspects of the shoulder. Looking down at the patient's shoulders from behind can best assess these asymmetries.

Inferior Instability. Inferior dislocations are uncommon. Inferior instability is elicited by carrying heavy objects at one's side (i.e., grocery bags or a suitcase), or by hyperabduction forces that cause a levering of the humeral neck against the acromion.[430,451]

The diagnosis for this type of dislocation is relatively straightforward, as the patient's arm is typically locked in abduction.[24] The sulcus sign can be used to assess inferior stability.

Multidirectional Instability. Multidirectional instability is symptomatic glenohumeral instability in more than one direction.[430] Multidirectional instability is often described using the abbreviation AMBRII (*A*traumatic onset of *M*ultidirectional instability that is accompanied by *B*ilateral laxity or hypermobility. *R*ehabilitation is the primary course of intervention to restore glenohumeral stability. However, if an operation is necessary, a procedure such as a capsulorraphy is performed to tighten the *I*nferior capsule and the rotator *I*nterval).[455]

It is commonly believed that females have more joint laxity than males, a fact propagated by the medical literature and medical training.[333] In describing multidirectional instability of the shoulder, a typical patient is presented, as "an adolescent female who can habitually and reproducibly sublux one or both shoulders."[442] However, with the exception of a few articles, there are inadequate data to confirm this view. One of the exceptions was a recent study by Borsa and colleagues,[456] which demonstrated that healthy women have significantly more anterior joint laxity and less anterior joint stiffness than do men. Another study by Huston and Wojtys[457] used an instrumented arthrometer to assess knee joint laxity in athletic and nonathletic men and women. Overall, they found women to have significantly more knee joint laxity than men. Interestingly, they found that athletic women had significantly less knee joint laxity than nonathletic women did, and athletic men had significantly less knee joint laxity than nonathletic men. These findings imply that physical training and conditioning may decrease joint laxity.[456]

The AMBRII patient is difficult to diagnose as there is usually no associated traumatic event or mechanism of injury. Rotator cuff pain is often the first presenting symptom.

Intervention. Intervention goals for glenohumeral instability or hypermobility are similar regardless of the instability classification. The goal is to restore dynamic stability to the shoulder using rehabilitation exercises that address motor control or surgery.

Little is provided in the way of dynamic stability from the capsular or ligamentous structures. Consequently, dynamic control of the shoulder using the dynamic stabilizers to contain the humeral head within the glenoid is critical.[12,89,112,436,458]

Warner and colleagues[221] reported a lower internal rotation:external rotation ratio for peak torque and total work in the dominant shoulder of patients with instability as compared with healthy controls. This suggests that an association exists between relative internal rotation weakness and anterior instability.[333] Patients with multidirectional instability also have scapulothoracic dyskinesia that contributes to the instability.[283]

Lephart and colleagues[459] showed that patients with multidirectional instability have deficits in shoulder proprioception. Therefore intervention of patients with instability should begin with a rehabilitation program aimed at improving the dynamic stabilizers, neuromuscular coordination, and proprioception of the glenohumeral and scapulothoracic joints.[15,333,458]

Range-of-motion exercises for the G-H joint should emphasize posterior capsule stretching to decrease the accentuation of the anterior translation and superior migration. The positions and exercises to modify or avoid are illustrated in Table 14-25.[460]

Scapular stability exercises can be started early and include the scapular pinch (see Fig. 14-58) and shoulder shrug exercises.[15] In this early stage, the control of the scapula position can be aided by taping the scapular in a retracted or elevated position, or by the use of a figure-eight collar, both of which help to normalize the scapular muscle firing pattern.[15]

Close chain exercises, normally performed with the hand stabilized on a wall or object, simulate normal functional patterns and reorganize and reestablish normal motor firing patterns.[15,98,99,282] All of the movements of the scapula and shoulder are coupled and are predictable based on arm position.[134,461] Similarly to the lower extremity, close chain exercises should involve integration of all of the joints in the appropriate kinetic chain with the specific scapular maneuvers of elevation, depression, retraction, and protraction.[15]

Early exercises to rehabilitate scapular dyskinesis include modified push-ups, and progress to facilitation patterns that include hip extension, trunk extension, and scapular retraction.[361] Clock exercises, in which the scapula is rotated in elevation/depression and retraction/protraction, also develop coordinated patterns for scapular control (see Fig. 14-62).[361]

Open chain exercises follow the isometric and closed-chain activities as these exercises are more strenuous.[15] Open chain exercises include PNF patterns, diagonals, upright rows, and external rotation and scapular retraction activities, as well as machine exercises consisting of lat pull-downs.[15]

Progression of the scapular rehabilitation can be evaluated using the scapular slide measurements, and once the lateral slide asymmetry is less than 1 cm, specific strengthening for the rotator cuff can commence.[15]

Besides rehabilitation, activity modifications to avoid any arm positioning that provokes symptoms can be helpful.[333]

TABLE 14-25   Exercise Modification According to the Direction of Glenohumeral Instability[460]

Direction of Instability	Position to Avoid	Exercises to Modify or Avoid
Anterior	Combined position of external rotation and abduction	Fly, pull-down, push-up, bench press, military press
Posterior	Combined position of internal rotation, horizontal adduction, and flexion	Fly, push-up, bench press, weight-bearing exercises
Inferior	Full elevation, dependent arm	Shrugs, elbow curls, military press

Sprained Conoid and Trapezoid Ligaments

A sprain of these ligaments can result from a clavicular fracture. But it can also be found in sports that require the arm to be pulled into the extremes of extension or external rotation. Pain here is felt at the extreme of all passive arm and scapula movements. However, no limitation of shoulder range is usually found and resistive movements are painless. However, forced external rotation with the arm in horizontal abduction will usually be the most painful test, and differentiation between the two structures is made by palpation of the coracoid process.

Interventions for these ligament sprains include electrotherapeutic modalities and physical agents, transverse friction massage, and progression of range of motion of the shoulder complex and strengthening of the glenohumeral and scapular pivoters.

Sternoclavicular Joint Sprain

The S-C joint is less involved with osteoarthritis or mechanical conditions than is the A-C joint.[227] The joint can sustain sprains, dislocations, or physeal injuries, usually secondary to a fall on an outstretched arm with the arm in either a flexed and adducted position, or extended and adducted position.[436] The joint can also be injured through motor vehicle accidents and sports.[64] The well-developed interarticular meniscus can be torn and can lead secondarily to degenerative changes. Irritation of this joint may also occur in inflammatory conditions, such as rheumatoid arthritis or repetitive microtrauma.[224] Infection of this joint usually indicates a systemic source, such as bacterial endocarditis.[227]

S-C sprains are graded according to severity.[45]

▶ *Type I:*   sprain of sternoclavicular ligament.

▶ *Type II:*   subluxation, partial tear of capsular ligaments, disk, or costoclavicular ligaments.

▶ *Type IIA:*   anterior subluxation; this is the most common grade.

▶ *Type IIB:*   posterior subluxation; posterior subluxations have the potential to result in circulatory vessel compromise, nerve tissue impingement, and difficulty swallowing.[224]

▶ *Type IIIA:*   anterior dislocation.

▶ *Type IIIB:*   posterior dislocation.

▶ *Type IV:*   habitual dislocation (rare).

S-C dislocations, while rare, are frequently delayed in their diagnosis. Any trauma to the shoulder girdle may cause a S-C dislocation, which is more common and more obvious when it occurs in the anterior direction.[222]

The conservative intervention for these injuries needs to address the function of the shoulder complex, particularly the end ranges. Following reduction, a shoulder sling or figure-8 strap is worn for 6 weeks and then the arm is protected for a further two weeks. Following reduction, the figure-8 strap serves to minimize stress on the joint. ROM exercises are initiated early, and care is taken to avoid excessive movement at the S-C

joint. Any hypomobilities of the neighboring joints are addressed using specific mobilizations of an appropriate grade. In cases with residual ligamentous laxity, stabilization exercises should focus on strengthening those muscles that attach to the clavicle (pectoralis major and upper trapezius), using seated press-ups (see Fig. 14-66) and shoulder shrugs done within ranges that do not stress the joint. The scapular pivoters should also be strengthened.

Acromioclavicular Joint Sprain

Disorders of the A-C joint are commonly seen in the athletic population. Injuries to this joint can be categorized as either acute traumatic or chronic injuries.[51] The chronic disorder may be atraumatic or post-traumatic, with the former being attributed to generalized osteoarthritis, inflammatory arthritis, or mechanical problems of the meniscus of this joint.[227] The majority of traumatic injuries occur from a fall onto the shoulder with the arm adducted at the side. The ground reaction force produces displacement of the scapula in relation to the distal clavicle.[51] Injuries to the A-C joint were originally classified by Tossy and colleagues[462] and Allman[61] as incomplete (grades I and II) and complete (grade III). This classification has been expanded to include six types of injuries based on the direction and amount of displacement (Table 14-26)[144,463–465]:

▶ *Type I:*   Tenderness and mild pain at the A-C joint. Sometimes there is a high, painful arc (160 to 180 degrees), and resisted adduction is painful. Passive anteroposterior joint gliding is painful, especially in patients over 50 years of age.[466]

▶ *Type II:*   Moderate to severe local pain with tenderness in the coracoclavicular space. The clavicle may appear to be slightly higher than the acromion, although in reality the opposite is true. All passive motions are painful at the end range of motion, and usually both resisted adduction and abduction are painful. Passive posteroanterior translation at the A-C joint is greater than that of the opposite joint.

▶ *Type III:*   The patient usually holds the arm against the body in a slightly adducted position, and exerts an upward axial pressure through the humerus. An obvious gap is visible between the acromion and the clavicle. All active motions are painful, especially abduction. The piano key phenomenon is present; after pushing the clavicle inferiorly, it springs back to its original position.

▶ *Type IV:*   Similar findings as those of type III, except the pain is severe and the clavicle is displaced posteriorly.

▶ *Type V:*   This is the worst form of type III injury. There is a large distance between the clavicle and coracoid process and tenderness to palpation over the entire lateral half of the clavicle.

▶ *Type VI:*   The superior aspect of the affected shoulder is flatter than the nonaffected side. Often there are associated fractures of the clavicle and upper ribs, as well as injury to the brachial plexus.

TABLE 14-26 Classification of A-C Injuries and Clinical Findings[a,b]

Type I	Isolated sprain of acromioclavicular ligaments
	Coracoclavicular ligaments intact
	Deltoid and trapezoid muscles intact
	Tenderness and mild pain at A-C joint
	High (160–180°) painful arc
	Resisted adduction is often painful
	Intervention is with TFM, ice and pain-free AROM
Type II	A-C ligament is disrupted
	Sprain of coracoclavicular ligament
	A-C joint is wider; may be a slight vertical separation when compared to the normal shoulder
	Coracoclavicular interspace may be slightly increased
	Deltoid and trapezoid muscles intact
	Moderate to severe local pain
	Tenderness in coracoclavicular space
	PROM all painful at end range with horizontal adduction being the most painful
	Resisted abduction and abduction are often painful
	Intervention initiated with ice and pain-free AROM/PROM; TFM introduced on day 4
Type III	A-C ligament is disrupted
	A-C joint dislocated and the shoulder complex displaced inferiorly
	Coracoclavicular interspace 25–100% greater than normal shoulder
	Coracoclavicular ligament is disrupted
	Deltoid and trapezoid muscles are usually detached from the distal end of the clavicle
	A fracture of the clavicle is usually present in patients under 13 years of age
	Arm held by patient in adducted position
	Obvious gap visible between acromion and clavicle
	AROM all painful; PROM painless if done carefully
	Piano key phenomenon (clavicle springs back after being pushed caudally) present
Type IV	A-C ligament is disrupted
	A-C joint dislocated and the clavicle anatomically displaced posteriorly into or through the trapezius muscle
	Coracoclavicular ligaments completely disrupted
	Coracoclavicular interspace may be displaced but may appear normal
	Deltoid and trapezoid muscles are detached from the distal end of the clavicle
	Clavicle displaced posteriorly; Surgery indicated for types IV–VI
Type V	A-C ligaments disrupted
	Coracoclavicular ligaments completely disrupted
	A-C joint dislocated and gross disparity between the clavicle and the scapula (300–500% greater than normal)
	Deltoid and trapezoid muscles are detached from the distal end of the clavicle
	Tenderness over entire lateral half of the clavicle
Type VI	A-C ligaments disrupted
	Coracoclavicular ligaments completely disrupted
	A-C joint dislocated and the clavicle anatomically displaced inferiorly to the clavicle or the coracoid process
	Coracoclavicular interspace reversed with the clavicle being inferior to the acromion or the coracoid process
	Deltoid and trapezoid muscles are detached from the distal end of the clavicle
	Cranial aspect of shoulder is flatter than opposite side; Often accompanied with clavicle or upper rib fracture and/or brachial plexus injury

AROM, active range of motion; PROM, passive range of motion; TFM, transverse friction massage.
[a] Allman FL. Fractures and ligamentous injuries of the clavicle and its articulation. *J Bone Joint Surg (Am)* 1967;49:774–784.
[b] Rockwood CA, Jr, Young DC. Disorders of the acromioclavicular joint. In: Rockwood CA, Jr, Matsen FA III, eds. *The Shoulder*. Philadelphia: WB Saunders; 1990: 413–468.

Types I, II, III, and V all involve inferior displacement of the acromion with respect to the clavicle. They differ in the severity of injury to the ligaments and the amount of resultant displacement.[136]

Types I and II usually result from a fall or a blow to the point on the lateral aspect of the shoulder, or a fall on an outstretched hand (FOOSH), producing a sprain.

Types III and IV usually involve a dislocation (commonly called A-C separations) and a distal clavicle fracture, both of which commonly disrupt the coracoclavicular ligaments.[51] In addition, damage to the deltoid and trapezius fascia, and rarely the skin, can occur.[51]

Type IV injuries are characterized by posterior displacement of the clavicle. Type VI injuries have a clavicle inferiorly displaced into either a subacromial or subcoracoid position. These types (IV, V, VI) also have complete rupture of all the ligament complexes and are much rarer injuries than types I through III.[51]

In the immature athlete, A-C sprains are usually grade I or II and may occur without clavicular fracture.[443] Grade III sprains in this population commonly rupture the dorsal clavicular periosteum. However, the coracoclavicular ligaments and acromioclavicular ligaments remain intact.[443]

The joint is quite superficial and direct palpation is accomplished easily. The patient may report that the arm feels better with a superiorly directed support on the arm, such as a sling. Pain is typically reproduced at the end range of passive elevation, passive external and internal rotation, and passive horizontal adduction, across the chest. This cross-arm test compresses the A-C joint and is highly sensitive for A-C joint pathology.[50,51,144,467] The range of motion available depends on the stage of healing and severity. In the very acute stage, range may be limited by pain, whereas the less acute stage will be painful at the end of range in full elevation or horizontal adduction. Pain, crepitus, or hypermobility may be encountered with mobility testing. Resistive movements are usually painless.

A complete radiographic examination including a 15-degrees-superior anteroposterior view, a lateral Y view, and an axillary film should confirm the diagnosis.[51]

The intervention for these patients depends on the severity of the injury, the age of the patient, and the physical demands of the patient.

▶ *Types I and II:* These patients will usually recover full painless function with conservative intervention.[50] Although adhesive taping devices and orthotics have been used in the early phase after injury to attempt reduction of the clavicle in the type II injury, they have not demonstrated efficacy in any good experimental trials.[51] Ice, nonsteroidal anti-inflammatories, and analgesics should be used judiciously. Most physicians prescribe a sling for 1 to 2 weeks. Gentle range-of-motion exercises and functional rehabilitation are started immediately after the period of immobilization, followed by isometric exercises to those muscles with clavicular attachments. The exercises are progressed to progressive resistive exercises (PREs) for the muscles that attach to the clavicle and the scapular pivoters. A graduated return to full

activity is very important. Most patients will be back to full sport participation within 12 weeks, although they may have a slight cosmetic deformity.[51]

▶ *Type III:* The intervention for type III injuries is controversial.[51] A survey of orthopaedic residency programs in 1992 revealed that 86.4 percent preferred conservative intervention.[468] The natural history of this injury with conservative intervention suggests that patients have no long-term difficulty with pain or loss of function.[469–473] A more recent study[474] found no strength deficits at follow-up, although discomfort at higher levels of activity was more pronounced. There is a reported high complication rate with attempts at surgical stabilization.[475,476] Citing the concern regarding greater displacement, some authors have proposed surgical intervention. But there have been several controlled comparative studies[467,475,476] that suggest that conservative intervention gave results comparable to those of surgically treated patients, but without surgical complications.[51]

A reasonable approach would be to initially treat patients conservatively with sling immobilization, followed by supervised rehabilitation.[51] Once the sling is removed, pendulum exercises can be initiated. PROM in the extremes of motion are avoided for the first 7 days, but the goal should be for full PROM after 2 to 3 weeks. A graduated resistance exercise program is initiated once pain is improved and active range of motion is full. These exercises should emphasize strengthening of the deltoid and upper trapezius muscles and promote dynamic stabilization of the shoulder complex.[230] Full return to sport is expected by 6 to 12 weeks.[51] If patients are still functionally limited after more than 3 months, a secondary reconstructive procedure may be necessary.[51]

▶ *Types IV, V, and VI:* These more unusual types of displacement all require surgical intervention.[50] Care should be taken to accurately identify these injuries and refer them early to a surgical specialist.[51] The greater displacement and injury includes damage to the deltoid and trapezius muscle and fascia. Failure to reduce these and repair them may lead to chronic pain and dysfunction.[51] The postsurgical progression involves gaining pain-free range of motion prior to advancing to exercises to regain strength, manual techniques to normalize arthrokinematics, and functional training to improve neuromuscular control of the shoulder complex.

Late complications including degenerative change of the distal clavicle can develop with a subluxed clavicle.[51] Symptoms may be treated with the selective use of modalities and steroid injections. If this conservative approach fails, then the patient should be considered a surgical candidate.[51]

Pattern 4E: Impaired Joint Mobility, Motor Function, Muscle Performance, Range of Motion with Localized Inflammation

In addition to those conditions producing impaired range of motion, motor function, and muscle performance attributed to inflammation, this pattern includes conditions that cause pain and muscle guarding without the presence of structural changes. Such conditions include rotator cuff tears, tendonitis, bursitis, capsulitis, and tenosynovitis.

Rotator Cuff Pathology

Rotator cuff tendon problems are the most frequent cause of shoulder problems. Fifty to seventy percent of shoulder problems seen by clinicians are related to conditions of the rotator cuff.[477,478] The frequency of rotator cuff problems is not surprising. These structures play an essential role in supporting the shoulder capsule and holding the humeral head in proper alignment in the glenoid cavity. Problems occur because of trauma, attrition, and the anatomical structure of the subacromial space. The supraspinatus is the tendon most often affected because of its precarious location beneath the anterior acromion, and has extensions into the infraspinatus tendon which may also become involved if the problem persists.[479,480] Massive tears of the rotator cuff rarely involve the subscapularis tendon.[479,480]

A number of mechanisms are recognized and include compression, tensile overload, and macrotrauma.

▶ *Compression.* Compression of the cuff can either be primary due to a reduction in the size of the subacromial space, or secondary, due to a decrease in joint stability. Both of these mechanisms result in direct trauma to the rotator cuff and its eventual deterioration.

▶ *Tensile overload.* Tension overload can occur to the rotator cuff when it attempts to resist horizontal adduction, internal rotation, anterior translation, and distraction forces. These forces typically occur during such activities as throwing (the deceleration phase) and hammering.

▶ *Macrotrauma.* Macrotrauma and subsequent tearing of the tendon, results when the forces generated by the trauma exceed the tensile strength of the tendon. Rotator cuff tears are not as common in the skeletally immature athlete as in the older athlete. Indeed, the incidences of rotator cuff tear increases with age. Approximately 50 percent of individuals older than 55 years demonstrated an arthrographically detectable rotator cuff tear.[481] Although cadaver studies of individuals older than 40 years have generally shown a prevalence of full-thickness rotator cuff tears between 5 and 20 percent,[33,482,483] the prevalence of partial-thickness rotator cuff tears has been shown to be in the 30 to 40 percent range in adult cadavers.[482,483]

The patient complains initially of a dull ache radiating into the upper and lower arm. This ache is worse after activity, at night, and with actions such as reaching above the head or putting on a coat. The characteristic physical finding is the painful arc. The pain may begin around 50 to 60 degrees of abduction in patients with shoulder immobility.

The clinician can often determine the involved tendon by resisting the active range of motion of each tendon.

Palpable anterior tenderness over the coracoacromial ligament is common with impingement.[193,484] Tenderness of the biceps tendon and at the supraspinatus insertion is also commonly found.

Patients with a painful arc and the above history, but no pain to resisted shoulder movements, are likely to have subacromial-subdeltoid bursitis.[227]

Subacromial Impingement Syndrome. Subacromial impingement syndrome (SIS) is a recurrent and troublesome condition closely related to rotator cuff disease.[485]

Neer[33] divided the impingement process into three stages, although the condition is a continuum of symptoms with overlap at the margins of each stage.[24] Each impingement stage is managed based on the specific findings and the intrinsic or extrinsic factors contributing to the problem, whether they result from compression, tensile overload, or macrotrauma.

Stage I. This stage consists of localized inflammation, slight bleeding, and edema of the rotator cuff. This stage is typically observed in patients under 25 years of age, although it can also be seen in older populations due to overuse. The patient reports pain in the shoulder and a history of acute trauma or repetitive microtrauma.

The physical examination reveals tenderness at the supraspinatus insertion and anterior acromion, a painful arc, and weakness of the rotator cuff secondary to pain, particularly when tested at 90 degrees abduction or flexion. Acromial elevation and scapular stabilization are often jeopardized early in the injury process due to pain-based inhibition of the serratus anterior and lower trapezius, and due to subclinical adaptations altering the position of the scapula to accommodate injury patterns in subluxation or impingement.[102,105] Stage I is a reversible condition.

The emphasis during the intervention of this phase is to control the pain and inflammation. The pain from subacromial impingement usually resolves with a period of rest and activity modification. Rest is advocated to prevent further trauma to the area and reduce excessive scar formation.[486] In addition to the rest and modification of activities, pain and inflammation may be controlled with the use of electrotherapeutic modalities, cryotherapy, and NSAIDs prescribed by the physician. ROM exercises that avoid irritating the tendon are introduced as tolerated.

The progression outlined in the Intervention Strategies section is followed for the acute and functional stages. Jobe and Bradley[121] describe a program of kinesiologic repair that strengthens the rotator cuff (in order to increase the depressor effect on the humeral head) and the scapular pivoters, but avoids any increase in the elevating effect of the deltoid. The mainstays of this strengthening program for the rotator cuff are the internal and external rotation exercises (Table 14-27).[277] These are initially performed as isometric exercises at various parts of the range. Once these are tolerated well, isotonic exercises of the scapular pivoters are introduced beginning with manual resistance and progressing to free weights (see Intervention Strategies). Care should be taken with exercises that involve the use of weights with the arm flexed or abducted away, or

TABLE 14-27 Specific Strengthening Exercises for the Shoulder Girdle[100,117,123,124,132,246,620,621]

Muscle	Exercise
Middle trapezius	Prone horizontal abduction in neutral rotation Prone horizontal abduction in external rotation Prone extension Rowing (prone with dumbbell)
Supraspinatus	Prone horizontal abduction at 100° abduction in external rotation Scaption in external rotation Scaption in internal rotation (Fig. 14-75) Flexion Abduction
Lower trapezius	Abduction Rowing (prone with dumbbell) Prone horizontal abduction in external rotation Flexion Prone horizontal abduction in neutral rotation
Infraspinatus	Prone horizontal abduction in external rotation Side lying external rotation in 0° abduction Prone horizontal abduction in neutral rotation Flexion Abduction
Rhomboids	Prone horizontal abduction in neutral rotation Scaption in external rotation Abduction Rowing (prone with dumbbell)
Teres minor	Side lying external rotation in 0° abduction Prone horizontal abduction in external rotation Prone horizontal abduction in neutral rotation
Middle serratus anterior	Flexion Abduction Scaption in external rotation Push-up with plus (Fig. 14-60)
Subscapularis	Lift-off Scaption in internal rotation (Fig. 14-75) Flexion Abduction
Lower serratus anterior	Scaption in external rotation Abduction Flexion Push-up with plus (Fig. 14-60)
Anterior deltoid	Scaption in internal rotation (Fig. 14-75) Scaption in external rotation Flexion Abduction

TABLE 14-27 *(cont.)*

Muscle	Exercise
Middle deltoid	Scaption in internal rotation (Fig. 14-75) Prone horizontal abduction in neutral rotation Prone horizontal abduction in external rotation Flexion Scaption in external rotation Abduction
Posterior deltoid	Prone horizontal abduction in neutral rotation Prone horizontal abduction in external rotation Rowing (prone with dumbbell) Prone extension Side lying external rotation in 0° abduction
Pectoralis major	Press-up Push-up with hands apart
Latissimus dorsi	Press-up

overhead, as these may exacerbate supraspinatus impingement and tendonitis symptoms if performed in the early stages of rehabilitation. The exercises prescribed should be as specific as possible, and tailored to the patient's functional and recreational goals. The lower extremity and trunk muscles that provide core stability should also be strengthened. Deficits in strength, strength balance, and flexibility in the legs, hips, and trunk should be addressed. This is particularly so in throwing athletes, where restrictions of the hip and back motion are common.[97,98,104,487]

Manual techniques can be used to address any tightness in the capsule (usually the posterior and inferior aspects) or motion restrictions of the S-C or A-C joints (see Therapeutic Techniques section).

Stage II. Stage II represents a progressive process in the deterioration of the tissues of the rotator cuff. This stage is generally seen in the 26- to 40-year-old age group. Irritation of the subacromial structures continues as a result of the abnormal contact with the acromion. The subacromial bursa loses its ability to lubricate and protect the underlying rotator cuff, and tendonitis of the cuff develops. The patient often reports that a specific activity brings on their symptoms, especially an overhead activity. Pain is generally located on the top of the shoulder and will radiate to the mid-brachium in the region of the deltoid insertion. The physical examination reveals crepitus or catching at approximately 100 degrees and restriction of passive range of motion (due to fibrosis). This stage is no longer reversible with just rest. Although this stage often responds to long-term conservative care, it can progress to a partial thickness tear. If the level of symptoms is severe enough, surgery is often required. Conservative intervention during this stage involves a progressive strengthening program as described in the Intervention Strategies section.[488,489] During this stage, the patient should be exercising with free weights, with an emphasis on eccentric exercises of the rotator cuff. Concentric exercises for the upper trapezius and deltoid are added. These include shoulder flexion, and reverse flys. The serratus anterior is strengthened using push-ups and the push-up plus (see Fig. 14-60). Neuromuscular retraining exercises for the shoulder complex include rocking on all fours, the Fitter board, and Bodyblade (see Fig. 14-73) as appropriate. Plyometric exercises using small medicine balls and push-ups with a hand clap are also included during this stage as appropriate. Neuromuscular techniques can also be applied manually and include quick reversals during PNF patterns. Other manual techniques include stretching of the capsule and any other pericapsular structures that appear tight. A number of studies[218,490,491] have examined the efficacy of passive joint mobilization and/or passive range of motion. They found this mode of intervention to be effective for enhancing range of motion in the patient with SIS. A study by Bang and Deyle determined that a combination of manual therapy applied by experienced clinicians and supervised exercise was better than exercise alone to increase strength, decrease pain, and improve function in patients with SIS.[492]

Fifteen to twenty-eight percent of those patients diagnosed with shoulder impingement syndrome may eventually require surgery.[216,493] Surgical intervention is usually reserved for those who have failed to make satisfactory improvement over a period of 6 months. However, at least two randomized controlled clinical trials that examined the efficacy of conservative intervention with SIS have found that exercise supervised by a physical therapist was superior to placebo, and was as effective as surgical subacromial decompression combined with postoperative rehabilitation in the intervention of patients with stage II primary impingement.[492,494] Another randomized controlled study[495] reported improved ROM, decreased pain, and increased function in patients with shoulder pain who underwent a program of individualized muscle stretching, strengthening, and retraining versus surgery.[492]

Stage III.   Stage III is the end stage, common in the over-40 age group, where destruction of the soft tissue and rupture, or macrotrauma of the rotator cuff is seen. Localized atrophy can occur with this stage. Osteophytes of the acromion and A-C joint develop. The wear of the anterior aspect of the acromion on the greater tuberosity and the supraspinatus tendon eventually results in a full-thickness tear of the rotator cuff. The physical examination reveals atrophy of the infraspinatus and supraspinatus, and more limitation in active and passive range of motion than the other stages. Rotator cuff tears are described by size, location, direction and depth.

Weakness to some extent always accompanies rotator cuff tears. The amount of weakness is directly related to the size of the tear.[1] For example, with small tears, the weakness may not be detected and the patient may have full range of motion, although there may be a painful arc. Massive tears of the rotator cuff present with sudden profound weakness with an inability to raise the arm overhead, and exhibit a positive "drop arm" sign (see Special Tests).[496] In this situation, infiltration of the subacromial space with a local anesthetic may eliminate the pain and allow more accurate testing of the muscle-tendon unit.

Acute massive tears require prompt evaluation for surgical repair because little is known about the efficacy of conservative intervention.[1,212,493,497–503] However, the patient may decide against surgery for various reasons, include concerns about a successful repair, surgical risks, or lack of functional improvement.[504] The conservative program for full-thickness rotator cuff tears is directed toward stretching and strengthening the remaining rotator cuff, deltoid, pectoralis major, and trapezius muscles.[478,505]

The conservative intervention for patients with a partial tear varies. If the symptomatic tear is partial, then a period of conservative intervention should be attempted.[466,478,506,507]

The use of corticosteroid injections for rotator cuff tears to promote healing is controversial because of their association with weakening the integrity of tendons with repeated use. Some studies have supported this belief,[31,508–510] although only one case of rotator cuff rupture following steroid injection has been reported in the literature.[508] Two recent studies have demonstrated that corticosteroid injections are more effective than anti-inflammatory drugs in the management of rotator cuff problems.[511,512] However, if the patient has not responded to 1 to 2 well-placed injections, either other intervention modalities should be considered or the diagnosis questioned.

Posterior Superior Glenoid Impingement.   Posterior superior glenoid impingement is newly recognized as a source of rotator cuff pathology in athletes. This type of impingement is thought to result from an impingement of the rotator cuff between the greater tuberosity and the posterior superior glenoid labrum, although the actual cause has yet to be determined.[513,514]

Periarticular Syndromes

The historical features of all of these syndromes are similar. Pain is increased after exercise and is usually worse at night, often waking the patient from sleep. Certain movements, such

as reaching above the head or putting on a coat, will produce pain. External and internal rotation motions are usually within normal limits when compared to the uninvolved side, but abduction and flexion are painful between 70 and 110 degrees. Disorders of the periarticular inert structures, such as the bursae, are characterized by a noncapsular pattern. These can be divided into two subgroups. One group has a restricted range of passive movement, and the other has an unrestricted range. Two common periarticular syndromes that affect the shoulder in older patients are subacromial-subdeltoid bursitis and bicipital tendonitis.

According to Neviaser,[515] primary shoulder bursitis is seen only in gout, rheumatoid arthritis, pyogenic infections, and tuberculosis.[516] Secondary bursitis, due to their proximity to an inflamed tendon, is far more common.

Calcified Bursitis.   Etiology of this condition is a result of decreased vascularization, cuff degeneration, and/or increased levels of the HLA 1 antigen. There are three recognized stages:

▶ *Precalcific:*   calcium deposits in matrix of vesicles.

▶ *Calcific:*   continued calcium deposition and increased pressure.

▶ *Postcalcific:*   the body decreases its blood supply to the area in an attempt to get rid of the calcium producing severe pain (comparable to kidney stones).

The condition produces a limitation of range of motion in all directions and the area is very tender to touch or compression.

Conservative intervention consists of an intramuscular steroid injection to decrease pain and inflammation, ice applications, and Codman's exercises to relieve pressure. Typically, the pain decreases with an increase in ROM in 48 to 72 hours. After 72 hours, the bursitis is treated as a traumatic bursitis (see below).

Traumatic Bursitis and Hemorrhagic Bursitis.   Traumatic bursitis is the result of direct trauma. But it can also be secondary to a degenerative rotator cuff. The patient often complains of pain at night. Pain is typically felt over the deltoid and its insertion, with the arm in extension. The patient demonstrates limited active and passive ROM in a noncapsular pattern, and an empty end-feel at approximately 70 to 80 degrees with glenohumeral abduction.

The condition responds well to a conservative regimen of pain and inflammation control, capsular stretching (especially posteriorly), Codman's exercises, manual techniques to increase the acromiohumeral interval (scapula down and back, inferior glide), postural re-education, restoration of normal synergy patterns for the glenohumeral depressors, and functional restoration.[515]

Calcific Tendonitis.   Calcific tendonitis, more accurately termed calcific tendinopathy, is characterized by a reactive calcification that affects the rotator cuff tendons. It is a common cause of shoulder pain.[517] Frequently, such calcifications are incidental radiographic findings in asymptomatic patients.[518] Approximately 50 percent of patients with calcific tendonitis have shoulder pain,[519,520] with associated acute or chronic painful restrictions of the range of motion of the shoulders that limits activities of daily living.

The cause and pathogenesis of calcifications of the rotator cuff are unclear.[44,521] Ischemia as a result of hypovascularization in the so-called critical zone of the rotator cuff,[44] degeneration of the tendons,[521] and metabolic disturbances[522] have all been suggested as possible causes. According to Uhthoff and colleagues,[523,524] fibrocartilaginous transformation of the tendon tissue leads to calcium deposits. The course of the disease may be cyclic, with spontaneous resorption and reconstitution of the tendon.[523,524] The factor that triggers metaplasia has not yet been determined, although tissue hypoxia is thought to be the primary factor.[522] Clearly, degeneration of the rotator cuff tendons is a precursor for calcification.[227] Both shoulders are involved in 20 to 30 percent of patients with calcific tendonitis of the shoulder.[519,520] Calcific tendonitis is observed infrequently in people under age 40.[227] The prevalence of calcific tendonitis has been reported to be between 3 percent[519] and 7 percent.[525] Calcific tendonitis can be acute or chronic.[524] In general, the condition is found more frequently in women than men.[519] A relationship to occupation must be considered because there is a high incidence among clerical workers.[524]

The course of calcific tendinopathy is variable. In most cases, the deposits are located 1 to 2 cm from the insertion of the supraspinatus tendon on the greater tuberosity.[518] In some patients, the deposits are absorbed spontaneously with limited pain. Chronic calcific tendonitis generally presents with impingement symptoms of pain with overhead motion. Other patients have persistent and recurring episodes of severe pain.

Uhthoff[524] suggests dividing calcific tendonitis into four stages, namely a precalcific phase, a formative phase, a resorptive phase, and a postcalcific phase. The precalcific phase is not normally associated with symptoms. In the formative phase, calcium deposits crystallize with minimal inflammation. Pain is usually mild and self-limited during this phase. In the later, resorptive phase, the calcific material changes consistency from a solid to a paste or liquid. Shoulder pain is seen more often in this phase. This pain can be severe and develop abruptly. During these acute episodes of shoulder pain, the physical examination is often difficult due to pain limiting active and passive range of motion. The final phase is characterized by a general subsidence in symptoms.[524]

Management of calcific tendonitis is often conservative, consisting of ice applications and pendulum exercises (prescribed in the acute phase) to prevent the development of adhesive capsulitis.[24]

Promising results have been reported for shock-wave therapy.[526,527] Ultrasound therapy using a wide intensity range is commonly used as an intervention for painful musculoskeletal disorders.[528] The way in which ultrasound stimulates resorption of calcium deposits has not been established.[518] It may stimulate the accumulation of peripheral blood mononuclear cells by activating endothelial cells. It may also act indirectly by increasing intracellular calcium levels.[529] At higher intensities, ultrasound may trigger or accelerate the disruption of apatite-like microcrystals. The appearance of these smaller calcium crystals may then stimulate macrophages to remove calcifications by phagocytosis.[530,531] Finally, the increases in the temperature of tissue exposed to ultrasound may increase blood flow (i.e., induce hyperemia) and metabolism, thus facilitating the disintegration of calcium deposits.[518]

Invasive interventions directed at the calcium deposits, such as open surgical removal of the deposits, percutaneous needle aspiration, and closed lavage of the deposits with lidocaine, reduce pain and restore shoulder function in some patients, but not in all.[227,520,532–534]

Acute Subacromial-Subdeltoid Bursitis

This is an extremely uncomfortable condition. Active elevation is very painful and greatly restricted, and can be accompanied by a painful arc. While most patients with subacromial-subdeltoid bursitis describe a mechanical origin as a mechanism, bilateral bursitis is often seen in patients with inflammatory arthritis.[227] A differential diagnosis should be made between gouty arthritis, septic arthritis, a pathologic fracture, or a dislocation of the shoulder, and these can be differentiated from one another by their accompanying symptoms. Regardless of the severity of the pain, other conditions need to be ruled out. These include subscapular tendonitis, a pectoralis major lesion, a sprain of the conoid-trapezoid ligament, or early glenohumeral arthritis. The pain of bursitis usually reproduced with passive abduction at 180 degrees, passive internal rotation, and passive horizontal adduction. Resistive testing may also produce pain. Associated and predisposing findings may also be noted. These include winging of the scapula, and forward head and rounded shoulder posture.

With the shoulder positioned in extension to expose more of the bursa, palpation of the shoulder region can elicit tenderness of the rotator cuff tendons and tenderness of the subacromial-subdeltoid bursa over the anterior humeral head.

Conservative intervention for this condition involves the use of modalities to help control the pain and inflammation, and patient education to avoid exacerbation.

Primary Chronic Subacromial-Subdeltoid Bursitis.

Two types of primary chronic bursitis are defined:

1. The type caused by degenerative changes, especially of the supraspinatus and A-C joint. This can produce a reduced space for the bursa and cause an inflammatory reaction of the bursa.

2. The type caused by a systemic disease such as rheumatoid arthritis.

With primary chronic bursitis, pain develops gradually. The pain is usually localized to the shoulder and lateral deltoid area, but it can spread into the upper arm. Findings from the objective examination include a positive painful arc into abduction or forward flexion, but full movement in other directions. One or more resisted tests are often painful, but may be negative if repeated with an inferior pull on the arm.

The intervention of choice is a course of local anesthetic injections.

Secondary Chronic Subacromial-Subdeltoid Bursitis.

Secondary chronic bursitis is more common than the primary type, and results from other shoulder pathologies, including a rupture of the medial coracohumeral ligament. Similar to primary chronic bursitis, the pain develops gradually in the shoulder and lateral deltoid region, but can radiate into the upper arm.

The objective findings are the same as those for the primary chronic bursitis. However, the exception is that other pathologies are present and make a specific diagnosis more difficult.

The intervention of choice is similar to primary chronic bursitis, although the primary lesion should be sought and treated.

Bicipital Tendonitis[227]

Tendonitis of the long head of the biceps occurs more often as a secondary condition related to an impingement syndrome.[394,515] Because the tendon passes beneath the anterior edge of the acromion, impingement can cause biceps tendinopathy as well as rotator cuff problems. In addition, the biceps tendon sheath is a direct extension of the G-H joint, and inflammatory conditions such as rheumatoid arthritis can involve the biceps tendon.

The pain associated with inflammation of the long head of the biceps is typically felt along the anterior lateral aspect of the shoulder with radiation into the biceps muscle, and tenderness is noted directly over the bicipital groove.

Objective findings for this condition include:

▶ Full active and passive ROM, although pain is often reported at the end range of flexion and abduction.

▶ Normal accessory glides at the G-H joint (negating the need to use joint mobilizations).[394,515]

▶ Pain upon palpation of the bicipital groove while the arm is in 10 degrees of internal rotation.

▶ Pain with resisted elbow flexion or resisted forward flexion of the shoulder.

▶ Pain on passive stretch of the biceps tendon.

▶ Positive Speed's test.

The conservative intervention for biceps tendonitis secondary to chronic impingement is similar to that described for rotator cuff tendonitis. These include electrotherapeutic modalities, physical agents, NSAIDs, transverse friction massage (TFM), and gentle stretching of the contractile tissues. Care must be taken with the TFM not to exacerbate the acutely or chronically inflamed tissue. Once the pain and inflammation is under control, the patient is progressed through range-of-motion exercises within the pain-free ranges. Intensive strengthening is initiated when full pain-free active range of motion has been restored.

Subluxing Biceps Tendon

The long head of the biceps tendon, with its proximal point of exit at a 30- to 40-degree angle from the straight line of the tendon and the tunnel, swings from one side of the groove to the other during the motions of internal and external rotation of the humerus.[20] If the groove is shallow, the tendon may force its way over the lesser or greater tuberosity, tearing the transverse humeral ligament in the process. Repeated subluxation wears down the tuberosity and increases the frequency of the subluxation.

If the groove is narrow and tight, the constant pressure of the tendon has the potential to cause tendonitis or even rupture of the tendon.[20]

The pain, not often severe, has the same referral pattern as that of bicipital tendonitis. A click is typically felt during abduction and external rotation motions, with reduction of the tendon occurring with adduction and internal rotation. There is tenderness over the bicipital groove, which follows the groove as the arm is rotated. On internal rotation the groove is under the coracoid, and during external rotation it is at the anteromedial line.[20]

The intervention depends largely on how important athletics is to the participant. Conservative intervention involves the temporary avoidance of the pain and click-provoking movements, and the application of transverse friction massage. In severe cases surgical intervention may be indicated, which offers excellent results.[20]

Rupture of the Long Head of Biceps

A total rupture of the biceps is usually seen in middle-aged patients. The condition usually results from repeated injections of steroid into the bicipital groove or in cases of chronic impingement.[227] The tendon is avascular, and as it weakens, it tears with a minimal amount of force.

Patients usually report hearing or feeling a "snap" at the time of the injury. Typically, rupture is followed by a few weeks of mild to moderate pain, followed by resolution of the pain and restoration of normal function.[227] When attempts are made to contract the biceps, the muscle belly rolls down over the distal humerus, producing a swelling close to the elbow instead of in the middle of the arm: the so-called "Popeye" sign. Functional limitations are unusual after this rupture, especially in the older population, because the short head of the biceps remains intact.[535] Typically, there is a negligible loss of elbow flexion and supination strength.

Surgical repair is rarely indicated except in the younger, active population (<50 years). With or without surgery, a rupture of the long head of the biceps increases the risk of developing a subacromial impingement syndrome. This results from the short head of the biceps pulling the humeral head upward, without the presence of the long head to hold the humeral head downward.

Pattern 4G: Impaired Joint Mobility, Motor Function, Muscle Performance, Range of Motion with Fractures

Atraumatic Osteolysis of the Distal Clavicle[51]

Atraumatic osteolysis of the distal clavicle (AODC) was first described in 1959 by Ehricht.[536]

The etiology is thought to be stress failure of the distal clavicle due an initial stress fracture, followed by cystic and erosive changes secondary to bone resorption. Subsequent bone formation and remodeling cannot occur because of continued stress on the joint.

It is most common in athletes involved in prolonged weight training and appears to be on the increase. The recent increase in incidence may be due to the emphasis on strength training regimens in sport. In a group of Danish weightlifters, the prevalence was found to be 27 percent compared with a normal (non–weight-lifting) control group.[537]

The symptoms usually begin insidiously. They are usually described as a painful, dull ache localized to the A-C joint. The ache, which tends to be worse at the beginning of exercise, may radiate into the deltoid and trapezius. Bench presses, dips, and push-ups are usually the most painful exercises. Abduction of the arm beyond 90 degrees causes pain. Throwing is also painful. On examination, there is point tenderness and pain at the A-C joint and forced arm adduction across the chest. Symptoms are bilateral in 20 percent of cases.

The most common differential diagnoses to be considered are cervical spondylosis and rotator cuff disease. AODC can be distinguished from rotator cuff tendonitis by selective injection of anesthetic into the A-C joint. An abolishment of the pain with the provocative maneuvers subsequent to the injection helps confirm the diagnosis.

The majority of patients with this condition respond to conservative management and activity modification, with most improving by reducing or eliminating their strength training activities.[537] However, even after several years' layoff, if strength training is reinstituted at the same level, the symptoms will commonly recur.[538,539] Other aspects of conservative intervention involve heat, NSAIDs, range of motion, and stretching and strengthening exercises. The exercises should be performed below 90 degrees of abduction. Ultrasound has also been advocated.[537] Although a consideration, intra-articular injection of steroid does not provide long-lasting success. It is more helpful to aid in the diagnosis and predicting surgical success.

Conservative intervention failure is an indication for surgical management. This consists of resection of the distal clavicle, either open or arthroscopically.

Clavicle Fractures

Fractures of the clavicle usually result from a fall on the outstretched hand (FOOSH), a fall or blow to the point of the shoulder, or less commonly from a direct blow.[61]

Patients with a clavicle fracture demonstrate guarded shoulder motions and have difficulty elevating the arm beyond 60 degrees. A clavicular deformity is usually observable. There is also exquisite tenderness to palpation or percussion (bony tap) over the fracture site. Horizontal adduction is painful. The diagnosis is confirmed by radiograph.

The intervention for clavicle fractures includes approximation of the fracture ends followed by immobilization with a sling and figure-8 strap for 6 to 8 weeks. Using pain as a guide, active (AROM) and passive range-of-motion (PROM) exercises for the shoulder can be initiated 1 week after the fitting of the figure-8 strap. Joint mobilizations are started immediately after the period of immobilization, and strengthening exercises for the deltoid and upper trapezius muscles are prescribed when appropriate.

Proximal Humeral Fractures

A proximal humeral fracture is the most common fracture of the humerus. Proximal humeral fractures involve the proximal third of the humerus and result from a direct blow to the anterior, lateral, or posterolateral aspect of the humerus, or a fall on an outstretched hand (FOOSH injury).[54]

The majority of proximal humeral fractures are stable with no significant displacement of the fracture. This type is typically treated conservatively, with an emphasis on controlling distal edema and stiffness, and early motion at the shoulder to prevent the development of arthrofibrosis secondary to prolonged immobilization.[541]

The arm is usually immobilized in a sling until pain and discomfort subsides, often after 2 weeks. AROM exercises for the wrist and hand are initiated immediately. Typically, passive and active assisted exercises for the shoulder can be initiated about 1 week after injury. Clinical unity of the fracture usually occurs after 1 to 4 weeks. This can be tested by having the patient stand with the involved arm at their side with the elbow flexed. The clinician places one hand on the humeral head, and then gently rotates the humerus with the other. Clinical unity is established when the fracture fragments move in unison and the movement is free of crepitation. At this point, gentle AROM exercises are initiated for the shoulder and elbow. Once clinical union is confirmed by radiograph (usually at around 6 weeks), full PROM exercises to the shoulder and elbow are performed, with progressive resistive exercises typically initiated at 6 to 8 weeks.

Integration of Patterns 4B and 4D: Impaired Joint Mobility, Motor Function, Muscle Performance, Range of Motion Secondary to Impaired Posture and Connective Tissue Dysfunction

Snapping Scapular

The term *snapping scapula* has been used to describe the clinical scenario of tenderness at the superomedial angle of the scapula, painful scapulothoracic motion, and scapulothoracic crepitus.[69,542–545] Infrequently, an underlying cause for the scapulothoracic dyskinesia is identified. The uncommon etiologies of snapping scapula include scapular exostoses, malunited scapular or rib fractures and Sprengel's deformity[543,546–548] Pain is usually reported at the superomedial angle of the scapula, with or without scapulothoracic crepitus.

The intervention for this condition is based on the cause. Common causes for this condition are an inflammation of the bursa between the scapula and thorax (scapulothoracic bursitis), prominence of the superomedial angle of the scapula, and muscular imbalance of the scapular pivoters.[69,543–545,549–552]

Integration of Patterns 4B, 4C, 4F, and 5F: Impaired Joint Mobility, Motor Function, Muscle Performance, Range of Motion Secondary to Impaired Posture, Spinal Disorders, Myofascial Pain Dysfunction, Thoracic Outlet Syndrome, Complex Regional Pain Syndrome (CRPS), Peripheral Nerve Entrapment

Impaired Posture

Patients with impaired posture have functional limitation associated with muscle imbalances, repetitive altered joint mobility, and pain. Impaired posture is commonly associated with referred pain to the shoulder. The most common posture referring pain to the shoulder is a forward head and rounded shoulders. This posture is characterized by hypertrophy of the anterior chest and cervical musculature (including the pectoralis minor muscle and the anterior and medial scalene muscles). The position adopted in the forward head posture can compromise the space in the scalene triangle and cause compression of the neurovascular structures, resulting in a condition called thoracic outlet syndrome (see Chap. 23).[410]

This posture can also lead to soft tissue restrictions of the anterior shoulder muscles, suboccipital muscles, and shoulder rotators.[410]

The intervention includes a conservative regime of postural re-education and exercises to restore the normal synergy patterns for glenohumeral depressors, to increase shoulder stability, and facilitate functional restoration (see Chap. 23). Cervical and thoracic stabilization exercises may be introduced in addition to the correction of any muscle imbalances.

Referred Pain

See Chapter 9.

Scapulocostal Syndrome (SCS)

Although this syndrome has been documented,[553–555] it is poorly understood. SCS is an enthesopathy of the origin of the serratus posterior superior muscle (an enthesopathy is a disorder of the attachment of a ligament, tendon, joint capsule, or muscle to bone). Clinically, it appears that SCS is a distinct variety of fibromyalgia.[555]

SCS has been postulated to have many causes including[555]:

▶ Ischemia.[556]

▶ Trigger point.[553]

▶ Postural degeneration.[557,558]

▶ Physical sloth.[559]

Clinical findings for this syndrome include[555]:

▶ Pain of a cervicobrachial nature, which is described as burning and aching, is the most common presenting symptom.

▶ Active and passive motions of the shoulder girdle are usually full and pain-free.

▶ Poor overall physical conditioning.

Conservative intervention, which includes intralesional injections and physical rehabilitation involving range of motion, strengthening, and conditioning exercises, was shown in one study[555] to be successful in 95.9 percent of 201 patients.

Subclavian Steal Syndrome

See Chapter 9.

Myofascial Pain Syndrome

Shoulder pain can often be caused by myofascial dysfunction. The following muscles are most commonly involved. The intervention strategies for myofascial trigger points are described in Chapter 11.

Infraspinatus. The infraspinatus is a frequent cause of myofascial shoulder pain, with the trigger points in this muscle commonly referring pain deep into the shoulder joint. Due to the severity of the referred pain from this muscle's trigger points, it is often misdiagnosed as subdeltoid bursitis or supraspinatus tendonitis.

Pain can also be felt in the anterior shoulder and anterior upper arm. In extreme cases, the pain may refer to the extensor area of the forearm and into the hand.

Clinical findings can include[560]:

▶ A history of sleeping difficulty on the involved side because of pressure on trigger points. Sleeping on the uninvolved side can also produce pain because of stretching of the muscle. Supporting the involved arm on a pillow while sleeping on the uninvolved side is a significant help.

▶ Limited internal rotation and adduction of the shoulder, including horizontal adduction in severe cases.

▶ Shoulder girdle muscle fatigue rather than weakness. Pain is elicited on resisted testing of the infraspinatus and middle and posterior deltoid muscles.

▶ Decreased grip strength.

▶ Positive signs of subacromial impingement due to dysfunction of the infraspinatus.

Anterior Deltoid. Anterior deltoid trigger points typically refer pain and tenderness in the area of the muscle itself. Clinical findings include decreased external rotation and extension of the shoulder.

Posterior Deltoid. Trigger points in this muscle (located posterior to the humeral head) and in the levator scapulae are the most frequent cause of myogenic posterior shoulder pain.[560] Pain is elicited on resisted testing, reaching across to the opposite shoulder anteriorly and towards the end of external rotation while the arm is abducted at 90 degrees because of the shortening reaction in the muscle.[560]

Levator Scapulae. This muscle is one of the most frequent myofascial sources of shoulder and neck pain. Pain reference is to the base of the neck, the posterior shoulder joint over the area of the humeral head, and along the medial scapular border.

Clinical findings include:

▶ Painful ipsilateral rotation of the neck.

▶ A limitation of full shoulder abduction accompanied by reproduction of posterior shoulder pain.[560]

These trigger points are activated by holding a telephone receiver between the shoulder and ear; sleeping on a sofa with the head on the armrest, which causes prolonged stretching deformation of the muscle; postural stress due to shoulder girdle asymmetry; and psychologic distress.[560]

Scalenes. The pain pattern is similar for all three scalenes, and can include the anterior chest, the upper arm both anterolaterally and posteriorly, the thumb and index finger, and the medial scapular area.[560] Tenderness is referred to the infraclavicular fossa and disappears immediately after inactivation of trigger points.

Supraspinatus. Rarely occurring in isolation, supraspinatus trigger points refer pain around the shoulder area, particularly to the mid-deltoid region, and the lateral epicondyle of the humerus. When the muscle is less severely involved, the patient will have difficulty fully abducting the shoulder.

As described previously, supraspinatus dysfunction can have wide-ranging consequences in shoulder biomechanics.

Subscapularis. Pain for subscapular trigger points is felt at rest or on motion over the posterior shoulder. The pain may also extend over the scapula and posteromedial arm as far as the wrist.

Clinical findings include:

▶ Painful and limited shoulder abduction, especially if external rotation of the arm is added to the movement.

▶ Painful resisted shoulder adduction and internal rotation.

▶ Decreased posterior glide of the G-H joint.

▶ Positive subacromial impingement signs.

Trapezius. The trigger points of the trapezius are usually found in the upper trapezius near the distal clavicle and in the lower border of the lower trapezius near the medial scapular border. Both areas refer pain and tenderness to the top of the shoulder over the acromion.[560] These trigger points may cause tenderness of the A-C joint ligaments. Trigger points in the lower trapezius can refer pain into the ipsilateral posterior neck and suboccipital region.[560]

Thoracic Outlet Syndrome (TOS)

The chief complaint of TOS is one of diffuse arm and shoulder pain, especially when the arm is elevated beyond 90 degrees. Potential symptoms include pain localized in the neck, face, head, upper extremity, chest, shoulder, or axilla; and upper extremity paresthesias, numbness, weakness, heaviness, fatigability, swelling, discoloration, ulceration, or Raynaud's phenomenon. Thoracic outlet syndrome is described in Chap. 23.

Crutch Palsy

Brachial plexus compressive neuropathy following the use of axillary crutches is rare but well-recognized. There are a number of documented reports of compressive neuropathies stemming from the incorrect use of axillary crutches, the so-called "crutch palsy."[561–563] The diagnosis of crutch palsy is usually made clinically by taking a careful history and performing a physical examination. This includes observation of the patient during ambulation using crutches, and looking at the axilla for such signs of chronic irritation as hyperpigmentation and skin hypertrophy. A detailed neurologic examination is usually sufficient to determine the cord or terminal branch(es) involved and the level of the involvement.[561]

The incorrect use of axillary crutches, with excessive weight bearing on the axillary bar leads to a sevenfold increase in force on the axilla.[564]

Complex Regional Pain (Shoulder/Hand) Syndrome

This condition is described in detail in Chapter 16.

Cervical Radiculitis

The onset of cervical radiculitis (see Chap. 20) can be insidious or traumatic, or secondary to shoulder disease such as adhesive capsulitis.[238,565]

The patient reports a wide range of symptoms. These range from mild discomfort to severe pain which is associated with neck motion restrictions, particularly hyperextension and rotation.[53,566]

Objectively, there may be a loss of cervical lordosis with associated paravertebral muscle spasm. Palpation may reveal tenderness over the posterior aspect of the neck, which can exacerbate the radicular symptoms in the arm.[567] The testing of muscle strength, sensation, and deep tendon reflexes should help confirm the diagnosis.

Conservative intervention consists of control of pain and inflammation through rest and activity modification. The patient is educated on positions to avoid, including rotation toward the involved side and neck extension. Once the pain is controlled, the program is progressed to cervical range-of-motion and strengthening exercises, postural education, and general strengthening and conditioning of the upper extremities.

Peripheral Nerve Entrapment

There are a number of common peripheral nerve neuropathies in the shoulder region (Tables 14-11 and 14-28).

Quadrilateral Space Syndrome. Idiopathic quadrilateral space syndrome, a compression of the axillary nerve as it passes with the posterior circumflex artery through the quadrilateral space, is rare.

The typical clinical presentation includes[568]:

▶ Vague, poorly localized shoulder discomfort.

▶ Pain with fatigue when the patient attempts to maintain the arm above shoulder level.

▶ Paresthesias in a nondermatomal pattern.

▶ Tenderness to palpation in the quadrilateral space.[568]

TABLE 14-28 Peripheral Neuropathies about the Shoulder[622]

Involved Nerve Root	Muscle Weakness	Sensory Alteration	Reflexes Involved	Mechanism
Suprascapular nerve (C5–C6)	Supraspinatus, infraspinatus (external rotation)	Superior aspect of shoulder from the clavicle to spine of scapula Pain in posterior aspect of shoulder radiating into arm	None	Compression Traction (scapular protraction plus horizontal adduction) Direct blow Space-occupying lesion
Axillary (circumflex) nerve (posterior cord; C5–C6)	Deltoid, teres minor (abduction)	Deltoid area Anterior shoulder pain	None	Anterior glenohumeral dislocation Fracture of surgical neck of humerus Forced abduction
Radial nerve (C5–C8, T1)	Triceps, wrist extensors, finger extensors (shoulder, wrist, and hand extension)	Dorsum of hand	Triceps	Fracture of humeral shaft Direct pressure (e.g., crutch palsy)
Long thoracic nerve (C5–C6, C7)	Serratus anterior (scapular control)			Direct blow Traction Compression against internal chest wall (backpack injury) Heavy effort above shoulder height Repetitive strain
Musculocutaneous nerve (C5–C7)	Coracobrachialis, biceps, brachialis (elbow flexion)	Lateral aspect of forearm	Biceps	Compression Muscle hypertrophy Direct blow Fracture (clavicle and humerus) Dislocation (anterior) Shoulder surgery
Spinal accessory nerve (cranial nerve XI: C3–C4)	Trapezius (shoulder elevation)	Brachial plexus symptoms possible because of drooping of shoulder Shoulder aching	None	Direct blow Traction (shoulder depression and neck rotation to opposite side)
Subscapular nerve (posterior cord; C5–C6)	Subscapularis, teres major (internal rotation)	None	None	Direct blow Traction
Dorsal scapular nerve (C5)	Levator scapulae, rhomboid major, rhomboid minor (scapular retraction and elevation)	None	None	Direct blow Compression
Lateral pectoral nerve (C5–C6)	Pectoralis major, pectoralis minor	None	None	Direct blow
Thoracodorsal nerve (C6–C7, C8)	Latissimus dorsi	None	None	Direct blow
Supraclavicular nerve	—	Mild clavicular pain Sensory loss over anterior shoulder		Compression

The initial intervention is conservative and includes rest, muscle relaxants, and NSAIDs. Surgery may be required if there is no improvement in 3 to 6 months.[568]

Suprascapular Nerve Lesion. There are several ways the suprascapular nerve may be injured. These include compression traction, and laceration.[569] A direct blow at Erb's point can cause a compression type injury.[569] Compression neuropathy of the suprascapular nerve often occurs in the scapular notch under the transverse scapular ligament or at the spinoglenoid notch. This compression occurs through extraneural inflammation, lipoma or cyst development, scarring following distal clavicle resection, and ligament entrapment.[570–573]

Due to the location of this entrapment, entrapment of this nerve may be misdiagnosed as rotator cuff tendonitis, a tear of the rotator cuff, or cervical disk disease.[574,575]

The cause for this entrapment can be acute trauma resulting from a fall on the outstretched hand (FOOSH), scapular fracture, or overuse injuries involving repetitive overhead motions.[571,575,576]

The suprascapular nerve is a mixed nerve. Thus the patient presentation usually includes:

▶ A dull, deep ache at the posterior and lateral aspects of the shoulder, which may have a burning quality.

▶ Muscle atrophy and weakness of the supraspinatus and infraspinatus.

▶ Changes in glenohumeral biomechanics with an increase of scapula elevation occurring during arm elevation. This may produce impingement-like findings and complicate the diagnosis.

▶ Full external rotation of the G-H joint and passive horizontal adduction is painful.[260] EMG is the definitive test for suprascapular neuropathy.[577]

Conservative intervention includes rest, ice, analgesics, and a series of perineural injections of corticosteroid to help reduce neural inflammation. A home exercise program of scapular pivoter strengthening, scapulohumeral coordination, and activity-specific training may be indicated.[572]

Surgical intervention, involving neurolysis, cyst removal, or the excision of the transverse scapular ligament is indicated if symptoms persist.

Accessory Nerve Lesion. The accessory nerve is formed by the union of cranial nerve XI and the spinal nerve roots of C3 and C4, and innervates the trapezius and sternocleidomastoid (SCM) muscle. Thus dysfunction of the nerve causes paralysis of the SCM and trapezius muscles.

Isolated lesions to this nerve result from forces acting across the G-H joint. Combined lesions of the axillary nerve result from forces acting broadly across the scapulothoracic joint. These lesions are associated with fractures of the clavicle and/or scapula and subclavian vascular lesions.[578]

The superficial course of the nerve makes it susceptible to injury during operative procedures or blunt trauma.[579] The accessory nerve is also vulnerable to stretch type injuries,[580,581] such as during a manipulation of the shoulder under anesthesia.[408] However, stretch type injuries do not always involve the SCM.[582] Accessory nerve paresis can also result from serious pathology such as a tumor at the base of the skull, or from surgery.[45]

Clinical findings for this condition include:

▶ Neck, shoulder, and medial scapular pain.

▶ Decreased cervical lordosis.

▶ A downwardly rotated scapula.

▶ Winging of the scapula.

▶ Trapezius weakness, especially with active arm elevation.

A confirmatory test includes resisted adduction of the scapula while the clinician applies counterpressure at the medial border of the inferior scapular angle. This will highlight weakness on the affected side.

Conservative intervention for this condition involves patient education to avoid traction to the nerve, specific upper, middle, and lower trapezius strengthening, neuromuscular electrical stimulation (NMES) to the upper and lower trapezius, cervical PNF, scapular PNF, prone-on-elbows scapular stabilization exercises (Fig. 14-80), and shoulder elevation strengthening. McConnell taping is also used to facilitate the middle and lower trapezius muscle.[408]

Long Thoracic Nerve Lesion. Lesions of the long thoracic nerve are common and are the single most common peripheral nerve lesion at the shoulder. The two most common causes of long thoracic nerve injury are trauma resulting from carrying a heavy

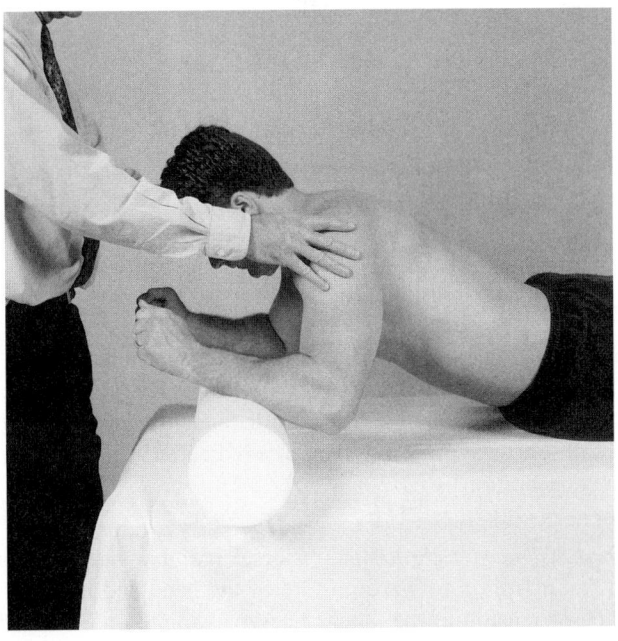

FIGURE 14-80 Scapular stabilization.

object on the shoulder, or idiopathic change. Other causes include postinfection, postinjection, postpartum and postoperative.[583] Similarly to other peripheral nerve injury, trauma can be a direct blow or a traction force to the nerve. The traction injury can occur when concurrent head rotation away, side bending away, and flexion, are coupled with the arm positioned overhead.[80,572,584] Other mechanisms that have been attributed to long thoracic nerve dysfunction include lifting weights overhead, driving a golf ball, and serving a tennis ball.[79]

The typical clinical presentation includes:

▶ Vague pain in the neck and scapula region

▶ An inability to fully elevate the arm overhead

▶ Shoulder flexion and abduction are weak and limited in active range of motion due to the loss of the trapezius-serratus anterior force couple. The clinician should note winging of the scapula when testing the serratus anterior.

Conservative intervention includes protection of the serratus anterior with a brace or restraint,[80,82,583] galvanic stimulation to the serratus anterior, muscle taping,[585] and strengthening exercises for the rhomboids, pectoralis, trapezius, and serratus anterior muscles.[79,572,586] The average rate of return ranges from 3 to 7 months[583,587] to 2 years.[79]

Axillary Nerve Lesion. Axillary nerve lesions may result from acute glenohumeral dislocation, surgery to the glenohumeral complex, blunt trauma to the axilla, secondary hematoma and fibrous formation, entrapment, and tractioning.[572,588–590]

The typical clinical presentation includes:

▶ Deep pain in the axilla, or in the anterior shoulder in the case of a glenohumeral dislocation.

▶ Tingling in the deltoid aspect of the shoulder.

▶ Atrophy may be seen in the deltoid and teres minor.

▶ Weakness when elevating the arm in flexion and abduction.[572]

▶ Manual muscle testing will reveal weakness of the deltoid and teres minor.

▶ Sensory testing should highlight a loss of sensation at the lateral deltoid region.

The diagnostic test for this lesion is to ask the patient to abduct the arm to 90 degrees and to bring it back into horizontal extension. A patient with an axillary lesion cannot accomplish this.[591] Intervention for this lesion is initially conservative and consists of thermal modalities, protection, and strengthening exercises.[572] Surgical exploration may be indicated in cases of complete denervation.

Dorsal Scapular Nerve Lesion. Dorsal scapular nerve lesions can result from a forward posture of the head and neck. This increases tension in the anterior cervical spine, producing the potential for hypertonicity and hypertrophy of the medial scalene.[570]

The chief complaint is usually one of scapular pain radiating to the lateral shoulder and arm.

Musculocutaneous Nerve Lesion. Although rare, an isolated lesion to the musculocutaneous nerve can result in weakness of the biceps, coracobrachialis, and brachialis. Injury to this nerve can result from demanding physical work involving shoulder flexion and repetitive elbow flexion with a pronated forearm.[588,592,593]

The typical clinical presentation includes:

▶ Reports: muscle wasting and sensory changes to the lateral side of the forearm.

▶ Weakness of the biceps, brachialis, and coracobrachialis.

▶ Diminished biceps reflex.

▶ Decreased sensation at the lateral forearm.

▶ Positive EMG study.

Conservative intervention includes cessation of the strenuous activity and a gradual return to activity with resolution of symptoms.[593]

Adverse Neural Tension. An abnormal response to mechanical stimuli of neural tissue is termed *adverse neural tension* (see Chap. 12).[594,595] The G-H joint can be the source of neurologic tension due to multidirectional instability, direct trauma, or poor posture and resultant tension on the brachial plexus.[238,596] The movements of external rotation and depression stretch the brachial plexus. Side flexion of the cervical spine away from the tested side also stretches the brachial plexus. Often the patient adopts postures to compensate for tight neurologic structures and relieve the tension on the brachial plexus. One of the most common of these adaptive postures is elevation of the shoulder girdle.

Adhesions of the brachial plexus can be detected using the upper limb tension tests (ULTT) 1 and 2 (refer to Chap. 12).[595]

Therapeutic Techniques

Techniques to Increase Joint Mobility

With some slight variations, the same techniques that are used to examine the joint glides of the shoulder complex can be used to mobilize the joints, with the clinician varying the intensity of the mobilizations based on patient response and the stage of tissue healing.

Joint mobilization may be preferable to stretching because it provides a precise stretch to a specific part of the capsule. It also can be performed with less pain, reduced load on other periarticular structures, and less compressive force on articular structures[390,597] as compared with physiologic stretching.[1] Investigators have suggested that joint mobilization, especially posterior gliding, may have an important role in restoring capsular extensibility in primary shoulder impingement syndrome[213,221] by preventing or stretching abnormal collagen cross-linkage,[273] rupturing adhesions,[598] reducing edema,[599] or reducing pain.[600] In addition to the G-H joint, the clinician should also ensure that the mobility at the A-C, S-C, and scapulothoracic joints are normal.

Kaltenborn[286] stressed the importance of promoting joint glides for increasing capsular mobility and prevention of joint compression and periarticular soft tissue injury that may occur with long lever angular mobilizations.[399] Sustained manual capsule stretches are particularly effective in regaining motion.[1,601,602] Low load, prolonged stretching produces plastic elongation of tissues as opposed to the high tensile resistance seen in high load, brief stretching[409,603] (i.e., the arm is brought to end range, pushed slightly beyond that range, and held in that position for 10 to 20 seconds).

Specific Passive Physiologic Mobilization: Humerus and Scapula

Quadrant Technique

The quadrant technique previously described as the Lock test (special tests of the shoulder) can also be utilized as mobilization techniques. This is done by adjusting the intensity according to the irritability of the condition. If the pain is severe, grade IV (small oscillatory techniques just into the tissue resistance) are used. If this technique decreases the pain, the technique is reapplied and reassessed. If the intervention produces no change in the symptoms, the clinician increases the grade slightly or increases the vigor and reassesses. If the intervention produces an increase in pain, the clinician continues with the same intervention but at a lesser grade.

The patient is positioned in supine with their head supported on a pillow. Using a hook grip, the clinician palpates and stabilizes the shoulder girdle both posteriorly and anteriorly with one hand, while holding the elbow with the other hand (see Fig. 14-32). From this position, the clinician passively extends, abducts, and internally rotates the humerus at the glenohumeral joint while maintaining the fixed position of the scapula and the clavicle. A "hump" will be encountered, necessitating slight horizontal adduction and external rotation of the humerus.[604] The clinician continues to elevate the humerus through abduction and external rotation until the limit of the physiologic range of motion has been reached.

Once repetitions of the technique have been completed, the clinician performs flexion/abduction (large amplitude, short of resistance) to ease intervention soreness.

Specific Passive/Active Physiologic Mobilization of the Shoulder[604]

Elevation through Abduction

The patient is positioned in supine with their head supported on a pillow. Their upper extremity is adducted across their abdomen. The clinician palpates the posterior aspect of the patient's wrist with one hand and the proximal forearm with the other. The motion barrier is localized by instructing the patient to elevate the arm in the scaption plane to the limit of the physiologic range of motion. From this position, the patient is instructed to hold still while the clinician applies a gentle resistance into further elevation. The contraction is held for 3 to 5 seconds, after which the patient is instructed to relax completely. The new barrier of elevation/abduction is located and the mobilization repeated.

Elevation through Adduction

The technique is identical to the one described above with the exception that the abduction component is replaced by one of adduction, so that the patient performs a combination of elevation and adduction.

Mobilizations with Movement[605]

Decreased Elevation

The patient is seated and the clinician stands behind the patient on their uninvolved side. The clinician places one hand over the scapula of the involved side. Using the other hand, the clinician reaches around the front of the patient to place the thenar eminence or a belt as in the figure on the anterior aspect of the head of the humerus of the involved shoulder (Fig. 14-81). The patient is asked to elevate their arm while the clinician applies a posterior glide to the humeral head (avoiding pressure over the sensitive coracoid process). If this technique is successful, the patient is asked to hold a weight while elevating the arm.

Decreased Internal Rotation

The patient is seated with their hand as far behind the back as possible. The clinician stands facing the patient on the involved side. The clinician places one hand in the crease of the patient's elbow and the web space of other hand in the patient's axilla to stabilize the scapula by using a lumbrical grip (Fig. 14-82). While maintaining the stabilization of the scapula, the clinician glides the humerus inferiorly in the glenoid fossa using the hand at the

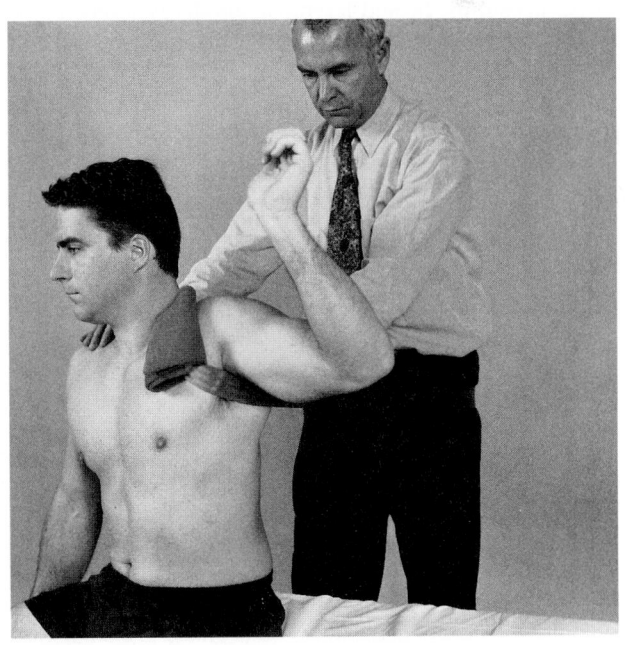

FIGURE 14-81 Mobilization with movement to increase elevation.

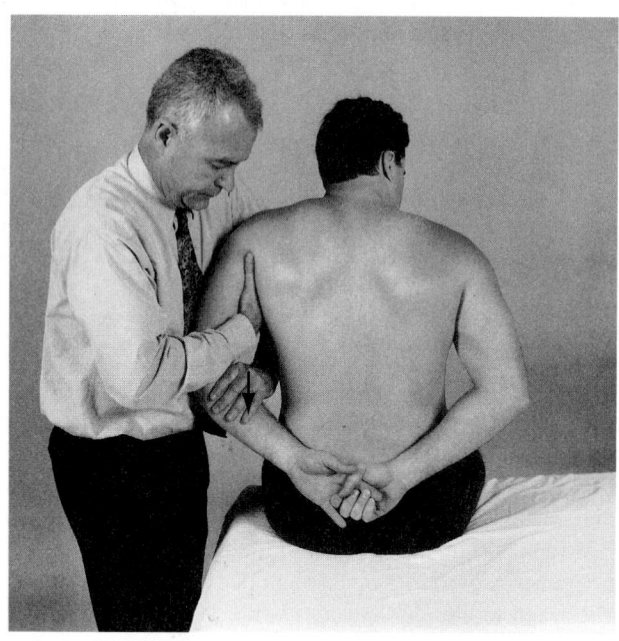

FIGURE 14-82 Mobilization with movement to increase internal rotation.

elbow and applies an adduction force by pressing their abdomen against the patient (see Fig. 14-82) as the patient internally rotates the shoulder (using their other hand to help if necessary).

Techniques to Increase Soft Tissue Extensibility

Spencer Techniques[606]

The Spencer techniques are a series of gentle stretching techniques. They are used to increase shoulder motion in situations in which the restriction is the result of hypertonic muscles, early adhesive capsulitis, healed fractures and dislocations, or other traumatic or degenerative conditions.[606] The general guidelines for all of the techniques follows.

The patient is positioned in side lying, involved side up, with the head supported and their knees and hips flexed. The clinician stands facing the patient. The clinician grasps the patient's forearm with one hand and flexes the patient's elbow, and places the other hand on top of the patient's shoulder to stabilize the shoulder girdle.

▶ To increase extension, the clinician moves the patient's arm in a horizontal plane, extending the shoulder, yet maintaining the elbow flexion before returning it to its neutral position.

▶ To increase flexion, the clinician flexes the patient's shoulder and extends the elbow until the arm is over the patient's ear. This motion is gently repeated in a rhythmic motion with the shoulder returned to a neutral position each time.

▶ To increase circumduction, the patient's elbow is fully flexed and the shoulder is abducted to 90 degrees. The clinician stabilizes the patient's shoulder girdle in this position, and using the patient's elbow as a pivot, gently rotates the humerus in

gradually increasing circles (clockwise and then counter-clockwise) (Fig. 14-83). A traction force can be superimposed on the circumduction maneuver by extending the patient's elbow and maintaining a traction force at the patient's wrist.

▶ To increase abduction, the clinician places one hand on the patient's shoulder while the other hand flexes the patient's elbow (Fig. 14-84). By grasping the point of the patient's

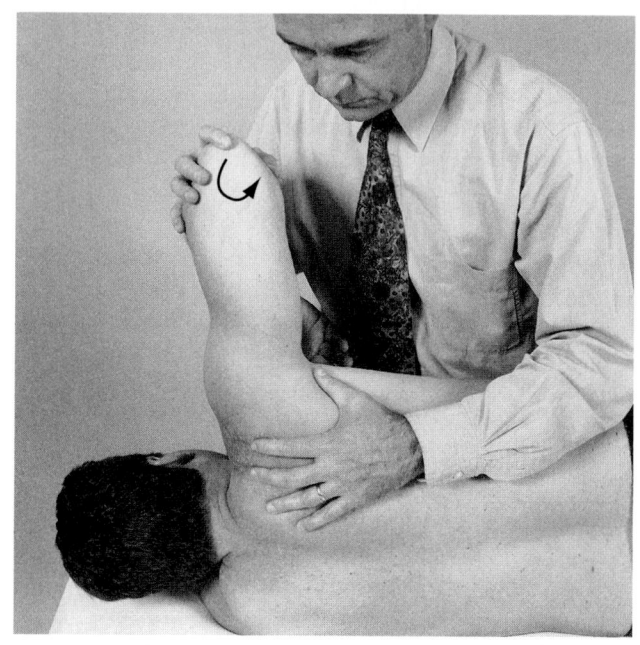

FIGURE 14-83 Spencer technique to increase circumduction.

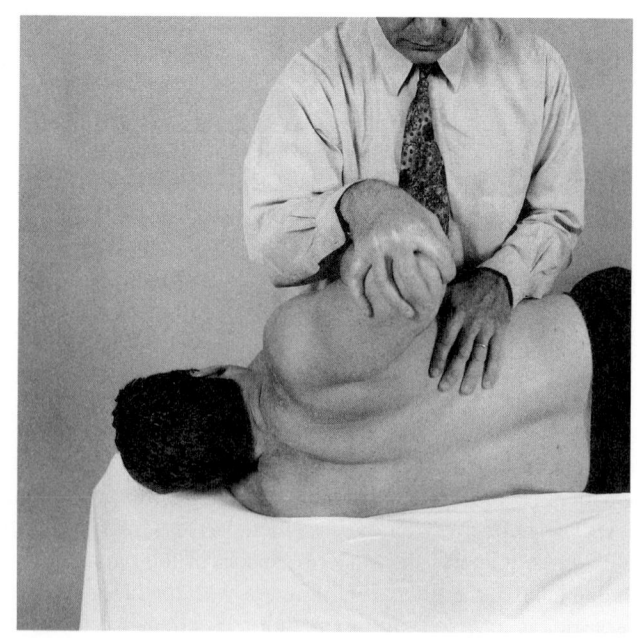

FIGURE 14-84 Spencer technique to increase abduction.

elbow, the clinician gently moves the patient's arm into abduction.

▶ To increase internal rotation, the patient is positioned so that their hand, with the elbow flexed, is placed behind the lower ribs. The clinician stabilizes the shoulder with one hand, and gently draws the patient's elbow forward and down using the other hand. An external rotation force may also be used in this position.

Each technique is repeated 6 to 8 times and attempts are made to gain more motion each time. The technique is stopped if pain arises. With each movement the clinician tries to exceed the point reached in the previous excursion.

The positions used in the Spencer techniques may also be used with hold-relax and contract-relax techniques to treat the shoulder by moving the arm and shoulder to the barrier. For example, in the case of restricted motion in extension, the patient assumes a position of maximum comfortable extension and then tries to move his arm into flexion while the clinician applies a mild isometric resistive force. This position is held for 3–5 seconds. The patient relaxes and the clinician increases the patient's arm extension to the new barrier.

Indirect Techniques

These gentle techniques are used with the acutely painful shoulder. They use trunk movements to obtain motion at the shoulder.

The patient is positioned in sitting on the treatment table, with the hand of the involved side resting on a pillow or towel roll. The patient leans toward the involved side slightly. While maintaining the hand against the support, the patient is then asked to gently:

▶ Turn at the waist, first towards and then away from the involved side, using pain as a guide.

▶ Side-glide the trunk both towards and away from the involved side.

▶ Turn their head both towards and away from the involved side.

▶ Lift the thigh off the table.

Muscle Energy

Restricted Scapulothoracic Motion

The patient is positioned in side lying. Their head is sufficiently supported to maintain the cervical spine in neutral. The clinician stands in front of the patient. Using one hand the clinician grasps the inferior and medial border of the uppermost scapula. The other hand grasps the anterior aspect of the shoulder. The clinician gently brings both hands together, lifting the scapula. This position is held until the muscles are felt to relax. Once the muscle relaxation has occurred, the clinician moves the scapula into the PNF patterns for the scapula:

▶ Elevation with protraction.

▶ Elevation with retraction.

▶ Depression with retraction.

▶ Depression with protraction.

At the end range of each of these diagonals, the patient is asked to maintain the position by isometrically holding the scapula. The patient is then asked to resist the clinician as they attempt to return the scapula to the start position.

Myofascial Techniques[607]

Arm Pull

The patient is supine, lying close to the edge of the table. The clinician stands on the involved side, facing the patient's head. The clinician grasps the fingers of the patient with both hands and leans gently backwards to exert a longitudinal traction force to the patient's arm, which is in about 30 degrees of flexion. By moving their feet, the clinician induces abduction to the arm while maintaining the traction force (Fig. 14-85). At 90 degrees of abduction, the clinician begins to externally rotate the arm. The arm is brought over the patient's head to the opposite side of the body until it lies across the patient's chest. The entire motion is then reversed.

Self Stretches

The "Saw." This exercise can be used to stretch the anterior capsule when motion above 90 degrees is restricted. The patient can be positioned in standing or sitting. Maintaining their arm in approximately 90 degrees of elbow flexion, the patient is asked to perform a sawing motion as though cutting through wood.

Wall Walking. Wall walking can be used when attempting to regain full range elevation. Clock exercises are a variation of wall walking. The hand is moved to the various positions on an

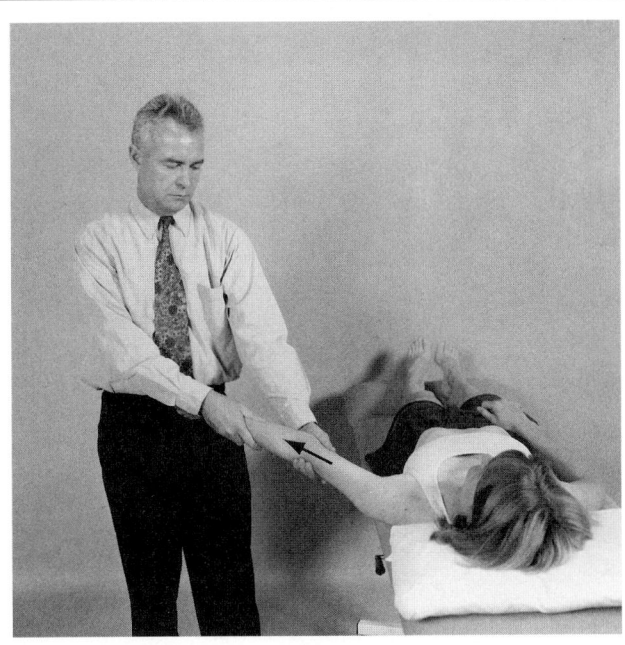

FIGURE 14-85 Arm pull.

imaginary clock face on the wall, ranging from 8 o'clock, through 12 o'clock, to 4 o'clock (see Fig. 14-62). This allows for rotation of the humerus throughout varying degrees of flexion or abduction to replicate rotator cuff activity. This exercise is first performed against fixed resistance such as a wall or a countertop, and then can be moved to moveable resistance such as a ball or some other moveable implement.

Pulleys.   Pulley exercises are commonly used as an active-assistive exercise to help regain full overhead motion. However, it is recommended that pulley exercises not be used until the patient has at least 120 degrees of elevation, and then only used in a pain-free arc to decrease the potential for impingement.

Wall Corner Stretch.   This stretch is used to increase the flexibility of the anterior joint capsule, pectoralis major and minor, anterior deltoid, and coracobrachialis. The patient stands in a corner and places both hands on the wall, level with the shoulders. The stretch is applied by moving the trunk toward the wall, while keeping it perpendicular to the floor. The exercise can be modified to stretch one shoulder by performing the exercise in a doorway.

Horizontal Abductors.   The horizontal abductors (posterior deltoid, infraspinatus, teres minor, rhomboids, and middle trapezius) and the posterior joint capsule are stretched by having the patient pull the arm across the front of their body (Fig. 14-86). This exercise should be used with caution for those patients with an impingement syndrome or A-C dysfunction.

Inferior Capsule.   The inferior capsule stretch is performed by placing the arm in the fully elevated overhead position (Fig. 14-87).

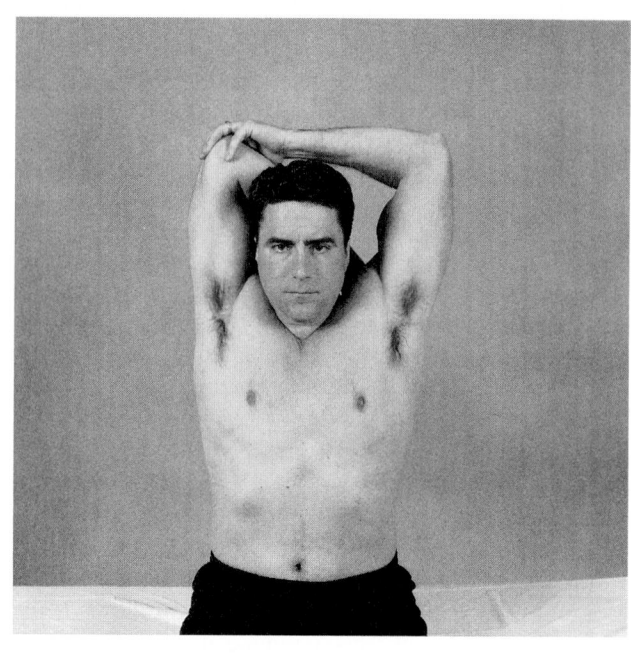

FIGURE 14-87   Inferior capsule stretch.

Shoulder Flexors.   A T-bar or L-bar is used for this exercise. Two positions are used depending on the intent of the stretch.

To stretch the latissimus dorsi, teres major and minor, the posterior deltoid, triceps, and inferior joint capsule, the patient is positioned in supine with the arm overhead (Fig. 14-88). Overpressure can be applied with the bar.

To stretch the anterior deltoid, coracobrachialis, pectoralis major, biceps, and anterior joint capsule, the patient's arm is

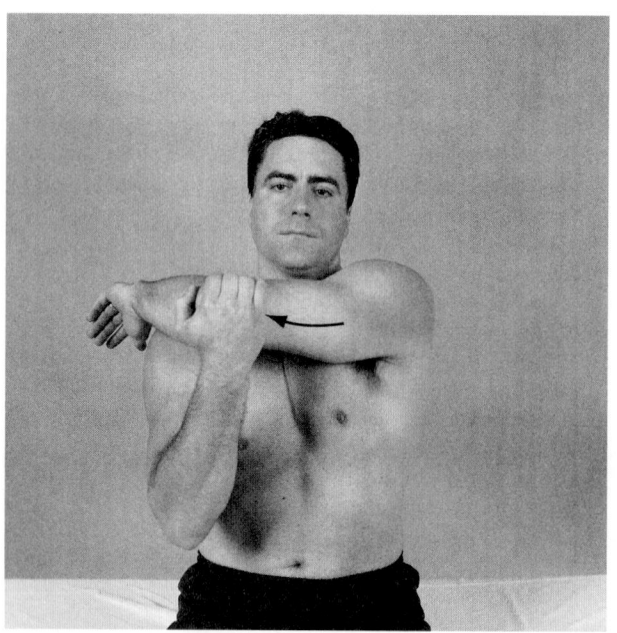

FIGURE 14-86   Horizontal adduction and posterior capsule stretch.

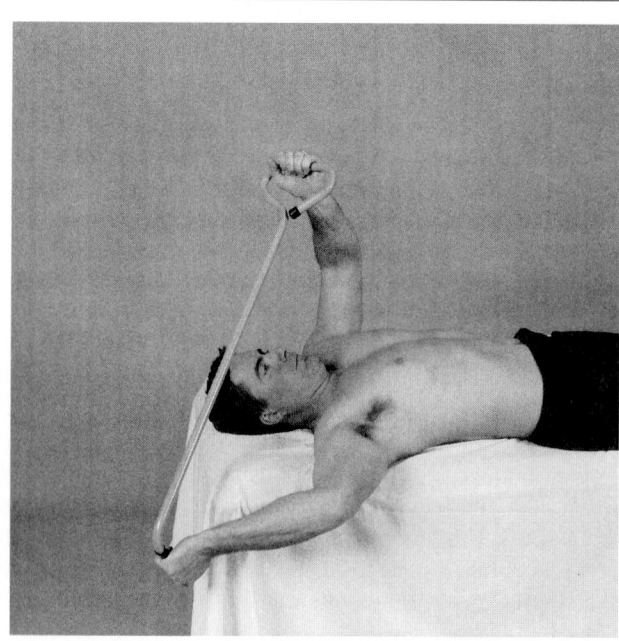

FIGURE 14-88   T bar exercise.

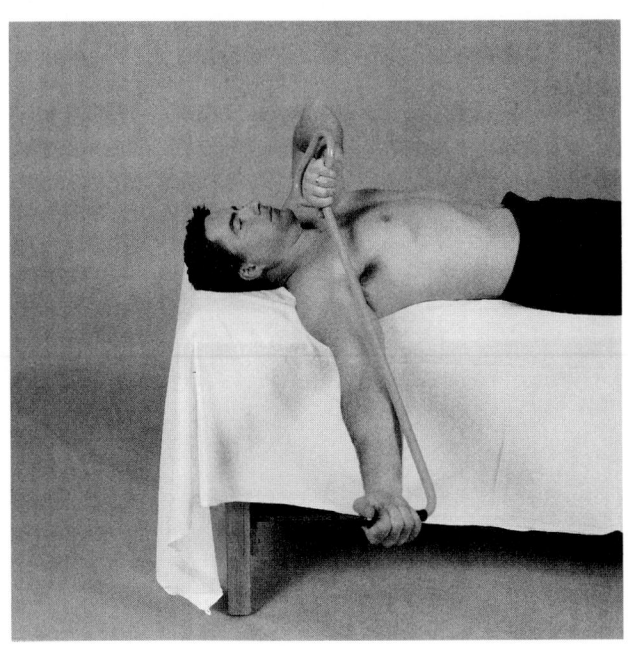

FIGURE 14-89   T bar exercise.

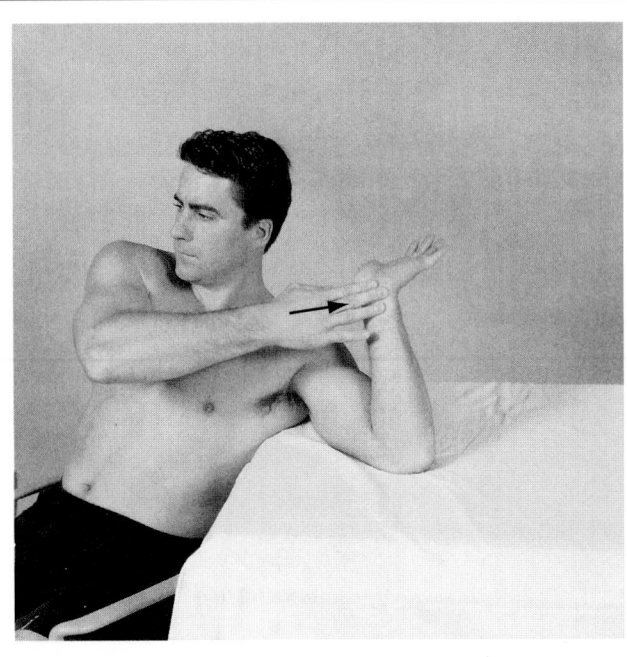

FIGURE 14-90   Passive external rotation.

positioned out to the side in approximately 90 degrees of abduction. The patient extends the arm as far as is comfortable (Fig. 14-89). The bar can be used to apply overpressure into further shoulder extension.

Shoulder Horizontal Adductors.   A T-bar or L-bar is used for this exercise. The patient is positioned in supine with the arm positioned in approximately 120 degrees of abduction. The bar can be used to apply pressure into shoulder extension. This exercise stretches the latissimus dorsi, teres major and minor, posterior deltoid, coracobrachialis, pectoralis major and minor, triceps, and inferior joint capsule.

Shoulder Internal Rotators.   A T-bar or L-bar is used for this exercise. The patient is positioned in supine. The arm is flexed at the elbow and in one of three positions of abduction at the shoulder: 0 degrees, 90 degrees (see Fig. 14-88), and 130 degrees. For each of the three positions the shoulder is externally rotated as far as is comfortable. Overpressure is then applied by the bar to stretch the subscapularis, pectoralis major, anterior deltoid, latissimus dorsi, and the anterior joint capsule.

Alternatively, the patient can sit sideways to a table. The entire upper arm is placed on the table top, bending the trunk as necessary. The elbow is flexed to approximately 90 degrees (Fig. 14-90). Using the other arm, the patient grasps the forearm of the involved arm and moves the arm into external rotation as far as is comfortable. Rhythmic oscillations or hold-relax techniques can be applied at the end of range.

Shoulder External Rotators.   A T-bar or L-bar is used for this exercise. The patient is positioned in supine. The elbow is flexed

and the arm is abducted into one of three positions at the shoulder: 0 degrees, 90 degrees, and 130 degrees. For each of the three positions, the shoulder is internally rotated as far as is comfortable. Overpressure can then be applied using the bar to stretch the infraspinatus, teres minor, posterior deltoid, and posterior joint capsule.

Alternatively, the patient can sit sideways to a table. The entire upper arm is placed on the table top, bending the trunk as necessary. The elbow is flexed to about 90 degrees. Using the other arm, the patient grasps the forearm of the involved arm and moves it into internal rotation as far as is comfortable. Rhythmic oscillations, or hold-relax techniques, can be applied at the end of range.

Towel Stretch.   The towel stretch exercise (Fig. 14-91) combines the motions of external rotation, and internal rotation, and stretches the capsule accordingly.

Automobilization Techniques[608]

Inferior Distraction
The patient is positioned in sitting with their arm draped over a high-back chair, and a towel placed in their axilla (Fig. 14-92). Using the opposite hand, the patient grasps the involved arm either just proximal to the humeral epicondyles or by the forearm. From this position, the patient applies an inferior glide to the G-H joint as they pull the involved arm downward toward the floor and use rhythmic oscillations (see Fig. 14-92). For a sustained inferior distraction, a weight or bag can be placed in the hand.

Inferior Distraction with Adduction
The patient is positioned in standing, or sitting on a stool. A towel roll is placed under the axilla, and the arm to be mobilized

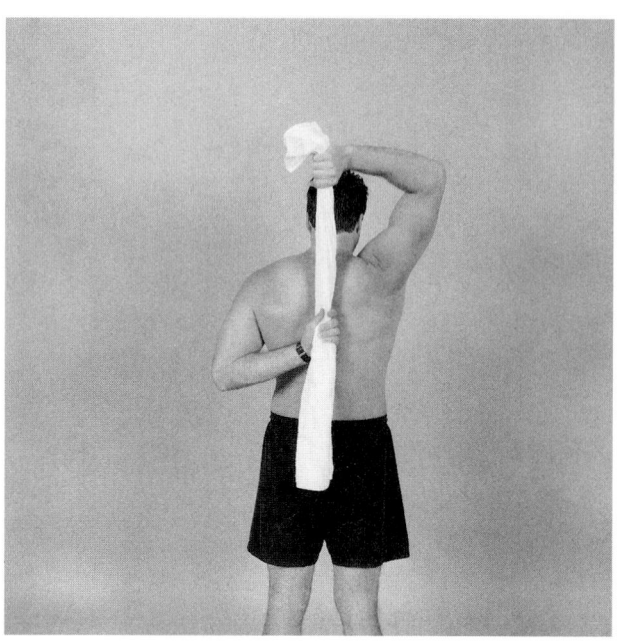

FIGURE 14-91   Towel stretch.

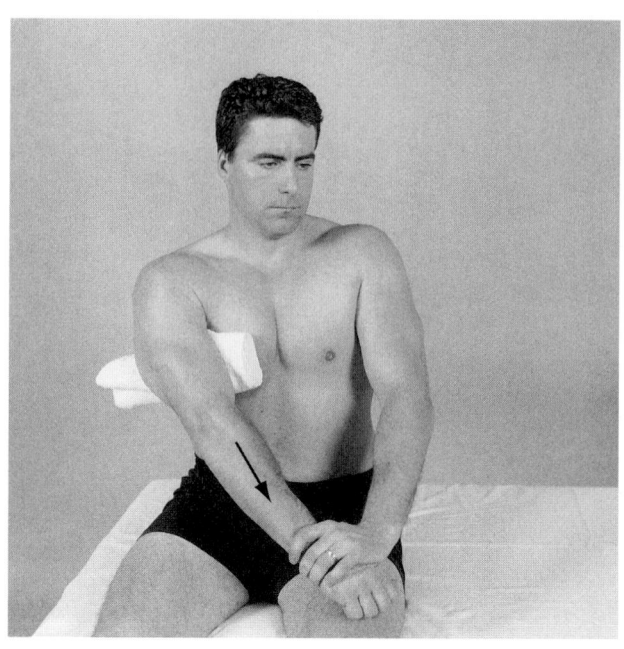

FIGURE 14-93   Inferior distraction with adduction.

Inferior Glide

This is a good technique if the patient's shoulder abduction range is limited to below 90 degrees. The patient sits sideways next to a table. The involved arm is comfortably positioned on the table in as much abduction as can be tolerated painlessly. The elbow is in full extension (Fig. 14-94). Using the uninvolved hand, or a towel wrapped around the humerus, the

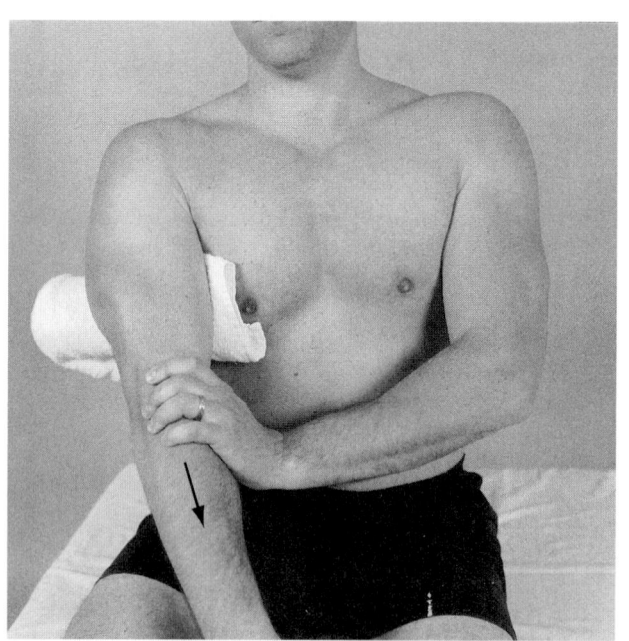

FIGURE 14-92   Self inferior distraction.

is positioned across the chest. Using the uninvolved hand, the patient grasps the involved forearm just above the styloid processes and pulls the arm rhythmically across the chest into glenohumeral adduction, and downward toward the floor (Fig. 14-93).

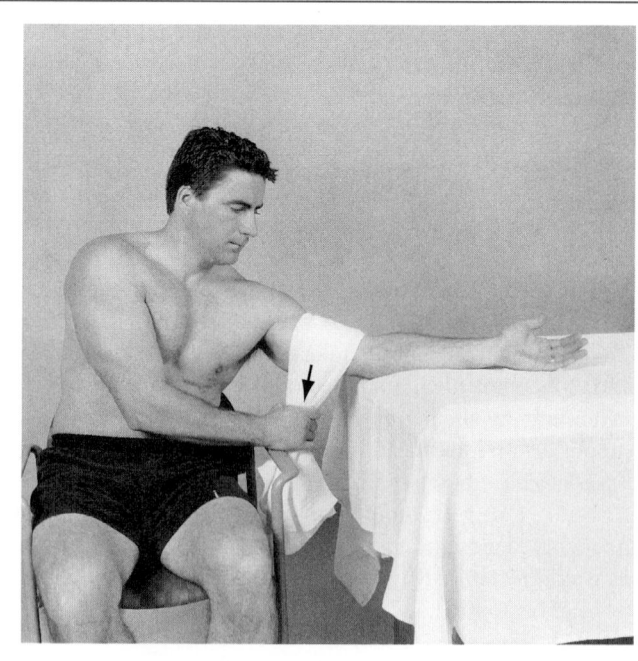

FIGURE 14-94   Inferior glide.

patient grasps the superoanterior aspect of the proximal humerus of the involved arm (see Fig. 14-94). From this position, an inferior glide is produced by pushing the humerus directly downward, or pulling the towel toward the floor. Rhythmic oscillations can be used.

If the patient has more than 90 degrees of abduction, another technique is preferable. The patient stands against a wall with the involved shoulder positioned comfortably into abduction. The elbow is flexed to approximately 90 degrees and the fleshy part of the forearm rests against a wall. The other hand grasps the superoanterior aspect of the proximal humerus of the involved arm and applies an inferior glide by pushing the humerus downward toward the floor.

CASE STUDY SHOULDER PAIN WITH CERTAIN MOTIONS

HISTORY AND SYSTEMS REVIEW

General Demographics

The patient is a 22-year-old male who lives at home with his parents.

History of Current Condition

Insidious onset of intermittent left shoulder pain began 2 weeks ago, with a report of occasional referral of pain into upper left arm. The patient denies numbness or tingling into the left upper extremity. Pain increased sufficiently this past week to prompt patient to see a physician, who diagnosed the condition as rotator cuff impingement, and prescribed physical therapy and NSAIDs. Patient also placed on work restrictions; maximum lift limited to 10 lbs.

Past History of Current Condition

No past history of left shoulder pain.

Past Medical and Surgical History

Unremarkable.

Medications

800 mg of ibuprofen daily.

Functional Status and Activity Level

The patient reported stiffness and soreness of the left shoulder upon arising in the morning and again at the end of the day after working. Difficulty was also reported with putting on a jacket, driving to work which takes 45 minutes, and the use of a hedge trimmer. The patient reported that the shoulder pain interrupts his sleep 2 to 3 times every night, and that he was having difficulty combing his hair, brushing his teeth, or lifting his arm without pain. He also reported that he enjoyed swimming but cannot swim the crawl or backstroke because of the pain. The patient described "cracking" and "popping" of the shoulder with activity.

Health Status (self-report)

Generally in good health but pain interferes with tasks at home and at work.

QUESTIONS

1. What structure(s) do you suspect to be involved in this patient?
2. What could the history of pain with certain overhead movements indicate?
3. Why do you think the patient's symptoms are worsened with certain functional and recreational activities?
4. What additional questions would you ask to help rule out cervical involvement or pain referred from a visceral structure?
5. What is your working hypothesis at this stage? List the various diagnoses that could present with these signs and symptoms, and the tests you would use to rule out each one.
6. Does this presentation/history warrant a Cyriax upper quarter/quadrant scanning examination (see Chap. 9)? Why or why not?

TESTS AND MEASURES

The physical examination of the patient included an inspection for muscle atrophy, palpation for areas of tenderness and crepitation, muscle testing of all major muscles about the shoulder, measurement of active and passive range of motion, observation of symmetry of scapulothoracic motion, and specific testing for superior labral tear. Further questioning indicated that the symptoms were mechanical in nature rather than referred. The cervical spine was also examined to determine whether neck pathology was causing pain referred to the shoulder.

Aerobic Capacity and Endurance

Not tested.

Community and Work Reintegration

Patient reports that he cuts grass, trims hedges, and performs leaf blowing. His job also requires carrying buckets of compost and lifting a lawnmower off the back of a truck.

Gait, Locomotion, and Balance

Functional use of arm during gait.

Range of Motion (Including Muscle Length)

A markedly positive impingement test, with the range of motion in the left shoulder at only 85 degrees for active forward flexion, and 80 degrees for active abduction; left thumb at L4 for internal rotation with significant pain limiting motion at that point. Passive forward flexion was measured at 150 degrees. When overpressure is applied at the end range, the same local pain was elicited. Active external rotation and horizontal flexion were full and pain free, but pain was elicited with overpressure.

Active right upper extremity ROM was within normal limits.

Joint Integrity and Mobility

- Palpation revealed slight tenderness of the anterior and posterior portions of the glenohumeral capsule, supraspinatus, and infraspinatus insertions. There was no pain with direct palpation of the A-C joint or S-C joint.
- Passive physiologic motions of the shoulder revealed anterior shoulder pain at 150 degrees flexion, and anterior and superior

shoulder pain at 85 degrees abduction. Anterior shoulder pain was provoked with 90 degrees external rotation and at 60 degrees of internal rotation.
- Positive Lock test for anterior shoulder pain at top of hill.
- Lock test produced pain with overpressure in the superior acromiohumeral area.
- With the exception of a restricted posterior glide, the passive accessory motions were within normal limits as compared contralaterally.
- Tenderness in the anterior shoulder region with the anterior stability test at 115 degrees of abduction.

Motor Performance: Strength, Power, Endurance
The physical examination revealed the following findings:

- The cervical spine examination was negative.
- Antalgic movement pattern with dressing activities.
- Pain with resisted abduction and external rotation, and resisted elbow flexion.
- Weakness of serratus anterior and decreased ability in performing posterior depression and anterior elevation at the end of the scapula's available range.
- Asymmetry of the left scapular motion, described as dysfunctional scapulothoracic motion, accompanied by palpable and audible crepitus.
- Positive lateral scapular slide test.
- Left upper extremity strength: deltoid 4/5, lats 4/5, rhomboids 4/5, serratus 4/5, biceps and triceps 4/5, supraspinatus 3+/5, other rotator cuff muscles at 4/5.

Special Tests
- Positive rotator cuff impingement tests of Neer and Hawkins-Kennedy.
- Negative apprehension test.

Pain
Pain rated at 5 to 6 out of 10 on a visual analogue scale.

Posture
Forward head position, rounded shoulders, flattening of thoracic spine. Shoulder girdle asymmetry manifested by winging of the scapula, a depressed clavicular position, and an anterior humeral head in relation to the acromion.

EVALUATION (CLINICAL JUDGMENT)

The patient is a young sedentary male with joint and soft tissue mobility restrictions, and impaired left shoulder and scapular muscle performance, which results in functional limitations both at home and at work.

DIAGNOSIS BY PHYSICAL THERAPIST

Although pain with overhead motion might suggest an impingement syndrome, the description of possible instability symptoms raises the question of instability-impingement overlap,[436] a condition in which multidirectional instability permits enough superior migration of the humerus that impingement of the humerus under

the acromion results. The impingement is not a primary phenomenon but is secondary to the instability. From a rehabilitation viewpoint, it is more important to know the extent of the alterations in the tissues or in the biomechanics than to know a specific anatomy-based diagnosis.[102]

For example, the anatomic "diagnosis" of impingement does not convey enough information to allow a successful rehabilitation program.[609] Impingement is a clinical sign or symptom associated with many tissue alterations that may create the impingement syndrome.[98,187,609] Some of these alterations, such as glenohumeral instability or scapular dyskinesis, have little relationship to subacromial pathology.[102]

QUESTIONS

1. Having made the provisional diagnosis, what will be your intervention?
2. How would you describe this condition to the patient?
3. What would you tell the patient about your intervention?
4. How will you determine the intensity of your intervention?
5. Estimate this patient's prognosis
6. What electrotherapeutic modalities and physical agents could you use in the intervention of this patient? Why?
7. Which manual techniques would be appropriate for this patient, and what is your rationale?
8. What exercises would you prescribe? Why?

PROGNOSIS

Predicted Optimal Level of Improvement in Function
Over the course of 2 months, patient will demonstrate a return to normal home activities and to full work duty without restrictions.

Predicted Interval Levels of Improvement in Function
Within 6 to 8 weeks, patient will:

- Improve left shoulder range of motion equal to other extremity in forward flexion, abduction, external rotation, and T4 for internal rotation allowing easy donning/doffing of jacket in 6 weeks.
- Report pain at 2 out of 10 with resisted activity or following functional activity.
- Improve strength of scapular stabilizers to equal that of the other side.
- Demonstrate normal scapulohumeral rhythm and negative lateral scapular slide test.
- Demonstrate independence with progressive home exercise program.
- Be able to drive to work without pain for 45 minutes in 5 weeks.
- Be able to reach into back pocket without pain.
- Be able to comb hair without pain.
- Be able to lift 55 lbs from chest height to floor, demonstrating proper body mechanics and controlled speed in 6 weeks so he can meet job requirements.

PLAN OF CARE

Frequency and Duration

Two times per week for 4 weeks.

Re-examination

Perform selected tests and measures to evaluate patient's progress toward goals in order to modify or redirect intervention if patient fails to show progress.

Criteria for Discharge

Patient to be discharged when he reaches established functional goals, decline further intervention, is unable to progress towards goals because of complications, or PT determines that patient will no longer benefit from PT services.

INTERVENTION

Addressing the tendonitis as an inflammatory process without considering the underlying degeneration or biomechanical deficits will lead to certain failure. Intervention approaches should be based on functional criteria, which are based on stages of tendon healing.[610]

PHASE I (0 TO 2 WEEKS)

This phase typically involves 1 to 4 visits of physical therapy. The intervention in the acute stage can include any one of the following: rest and activity modification, anti-inflammatory medications, exercises, and corticosteroid injections. The patient is given an explanation as to the importance of compliance with the home exercise program and receives instruction in the use of cryotherapy at home.

Goals

- Pain at 5 out of 10 with resistive motion, 2 out of 10 at rest.
- Pain-free ROM for flexion to 90 degrees, extension to 25 degrees, internal rotation to 45 degrees, and external rotation to 45 degrees.
- Correct upper extremity motion with gait.
- Independence and compliance with home exercise program.

Electrotherapeutic Modalities and Physical Agents

Physical modalities such as iontophoresis, pulsed ultrasound, and cold have been suggested for control of pain and inflammation. Anti-inflammatory medication, ice, and pulsed ultrasound have been shown to be effective in the intervention of impingement syndrome.[33,98,611]

Therapeutic Exercise and Home Program

Exercises during this phase should be kept within pain-free arcs as control of pain is being obtained.

- AROM for elbow, wrist, and hand.
- AROM for cervical spine.
- PROM of shoulder using wand or pulley.
- Pain-free AROM using exercises with high repetition and low resistance to promote vascularization. Exercises should include flexion, internal and external rotation with the elbow

supported, supraspinatus isolation exercise (internal rotation of the shoulder, thumb pointing down, and arm raised in the scapular plane), and abduction of the arm to 90 degrees, maintaining a position 30 degrees anterior to the mid-frontal plane. Early exercises should be performed in a range avoiding the impingement position. They are usually followed by a progression of isometric contractions and isotonic contractions. The isometrics can be performed by squeezing a tennis ball in various positions of elevation/abduction, or against a firm object such as a wall or Swiss ball. Isotonic exercises are accomplished with elastic tubing, beginning with slow mid-range exercises. Progression is made to fast mid-range exercises and fast full-range exercises.[612]

- Scapular retraction/depression.
- Postural correction exercises.
- The kinetic chain needs to be restored early in the rehabilitation process as a basis for shoulder activity and shoulder strength.[102] Inflexibilities of the hamstrings, hip, and trunk, and strength, weakness, or imbalances of the rotators of the trunk, flexors, and extensors of the trunk and hip, and any subclinical adaptations of stance patterns or gait pattern, should be corrected before starting formal strength rehabilitation.[1,211]
- A walking program and use of a stationary bike are initiated to maintain or improve the patient's cardiovascular fitness.

Manual Therapy

- Assisted stretching in pain-free ranges. Stretching exercises are performed by the patient at home and with the clinician until a normal range of motion is achieved. Then a strengthening program is initiated.
- Manually resisted exercises in the pain-free ranges.
- Joint mobilizations[314] and physiologic stretching.[613]
- Transverse friction massage is applied perpendicular to the involved fibers, slightly distal or proximal to the site of maximum tenderness. Intervention time is usually 7 to 9 minutes.
- Left shoulder quadrant mobilization is performed just into the pain (where symptom reproduction is most significant).
- Manual PNF patterns of the scapula.
- Scapula mobilizations.
- Soft tissue techniques to the rotator cuff muscles and scapular stabilizers.
- Myofascial release techniques as appropriate.
- Upper limb tension test (ULTT) stretches as appropriate.

PHASE II (WEEKS 3 TO 8)

This phase typically involves 2 to 6 visits.

Goals

- Decrease pain to 2 out of 10 with resisted motion, 0 out of 10 at rest.
- Performance of functional activities including reaching into back pocket, fastening undergarments, combing hair, lift and reach overhead, and perform weight- and repetition-specific work and ADL tasks.
- Shoulder AROM to be within 90 percent of uninvolved side.

- Strength at 4 out of 5 for shoulder girdle musculature.
- Independence with expanded home exercise program.

Electrotherapeutic Modalities and Physical Agents

Continue use of effective modalities with increased emphasis on use as needed at home.

Therapeutic Exercise and Home Program

- Cardiovascular conditioning using walking program, upper body ergonometer (UBE), NordicTrack.
- Flexibility exercises for the internal rotators and pectoralis minor.
- Progressive strengthening exercises using surgical tubing, free weights, and pulleys. Eccentric exercises are introduced as tolerated.[614,615]
- An attempt must be made to balance the ratio of strength between the internal rotators/adductors and the external rotators/abductors.[102]
- Rotator cuff strengthening. The rotator cuff muscles, together with the deltoid, are important in creating concavity/compression to maintain the humeral head in the glenoid socket.[1] The rotator cuff muscles do not work in isolation in shoulder function—they act as a unit in functional shoulder activities, and should thus be rehabilitated as an integrated unit, rather than as individual muscles. Closed chain rotator cuff strengthening exercises are an extremely efficient way of redeveloping composite rotator cuff strength.[98,102,105,361,363] A useful clinical sign for deficiencies in rotator cuff rehabilitation is exacerbation of clinical symptoms when rotator cuff exercises are started. If rotator cuff exercises increase clinical symptoms, further evaluation of the kinetic chain should be done. Then the exercises should be directed to the source of weakness, usually the scapular stabilizers.[1]

Manual Therapy

- Continue use of effective soft tissue techniques.
- Continue mobilization to areas of hypomobility.
- Rhythmic stabilization exercises.
- Progression of passive stretches in pain-free range.

Neuromuscular Re-education

Neuromuscular re-training involves:

- Hand knee rocking.
- Three-point rocking.
- Push-up progression.
- Push-ups off a Swiss ball.
- Body blade.
- Plyometrics. Plyometric exercises develop the athlete's ability to generate power. These exercises develop a large amount of strain in the eccentric phase of the activity and force in the concentric phase of the activity. Thus they should be done when complete anatomic healing has occurred.[102] Similarly, because large ranges of motion are required, full range of motion should be obtained before the plyometrics are started.[102]

PHASE III (WEEK 9 +)

This phase involves sport-specific or activity-specific training and is typically completed as a home exercise program.

Coordination, Communication, and Documentation

Communicate with the physician, patient, work manager, and work comp case management regarding patient's status (direct or indirect). Documentation will include all elements of patient/client management, including therapeutic intervention. Discharge planning will be provided.

Patient-Related Instruction

Patient is given basic instruction in relation to the anatomy of the shoulder muscles and tendons, and the joint structure. Information to be provided on pathology of tendonitis, relationship of posture to current condition, and the importance of adequate lower extremity and trunk performance.

Periodic re-examination and reassessment of the home program is performed, utilizing written instruction and illustrations. Educate patient in proper postures, and positions and motions to avoid during home and work activities. Educate patient in the benefits of an ongoing conditioning program to prevent re-occurrence of impairments. Educate the patient on the use of physical agents, transverse friction, and massage at home.

Criteria for Discharge

Patient will be discharged when all rehabilitation goals have been achieved. Instruct patient to call for advice should progression plateau or decline. Review of home exercise program.

Outcome

The patient's outcome depends on their level of adherence to the recommended home exercise program and intervention plan, as well as recommended lifestyle changes. It is anticipated that the patient will return to preinjury work level in 2 months, without recurrence of left shoulder pain in the following year. Patient understands the strategies to self-manage any minor recurrences.

Secondary prevention will include awareness of factors indicating need for re-examination.

CASE STUDY   STIFF AND PAINFUL SHOULDER

HISTORY AND SYSTEMS REVIEW

General Demographics

The patient is a 55-year-old female who lives alone.

History of Current Condition

The patient reports a 7-month history of unilateral shoulder girdle stiffness, pain, and weakness with a diagnosis from the physician of "right frozen shoulder." There was no history of trauma, but the patient reported an abrupt onset of very severe pain 7 months prior. Within several days, she also had right forearm and thumb pain of lesser severity, and weakness of the right shoulder.

The forearm and thumb pain had since resolved, and although there was some restricted motion of the shoulder, the more marked painful stiffness of the shoulder did not occur until 2 or 3 months after the onset of symptoms. After 3 months, she was having difficulties performing her job functions and sought medical attention. Thus far she had been treated with a series of two corticosteroid injections, both of which had given her short-term relief.

Past History of Current Condition

Non-work-related right shoulder injury 5 years ago, which resolved in 2 months with a course of physical therapy, including ROM and strengthening exercises, which she followed for 1 month after discharge from PT.

Past Medical and Surgical History

Unremarkable. Gallbladder surgery 2 years ago.

Medications

800 mg ibuprofen daily, and blood pressure medication.

Other Tests and Measures

None.

Occupational, Employment, and School

Patient was a mail reception clerk for the postal service, and her job involved monitoring incoming mail, which required the repeated opening and lifting of mail packages.

Functional Status and Activity Level

Stiffness/soreness occurs first hour in morning, again at end of day after working. Pain interferes with sleep two times per night, especially with rolling in bed or driving to work (which takes 30 minutes). Patient discontinued her normal three-times-a-week aerobic workout and upper and lower body resistance exercises approximately 3 months ago.

Health Status (Self-Report)

In general, the patient is in good health, except for minor heart problem (congestive heart failure) and high blood pressure.

QUESTIONS

1. At this point in the examination, is it possible to determine the patient's diagnosis? Why or why not?
2. What does the history of pain with sleeping on the shoulder, and pain/stiffness in the morning tell the clinician?
3. Why do you think the patient's symptoms are related to time of day?
4. What additional questions would you ask to help rule out pain referred from a visceral structure given the patient's past medical history?
5. Do you have a working hypothesis at this stage? List the various diagnoses that could present with these signs and symptoms, and the tests you would use to rule out each one.
6. Does this presentation/history warrant a scan? Why or why not?
7. Do you think the patient's age is a factor?

PHYSICAL THERAPY TESTS AND MEASURES

Based on the insidious onset, a Cyriax upper quarter/quadrant scan was performed on the patient to help rule out any serious pathology or cervical involvement. The scan indicated no signs and symptoms of serious pathology, or cervical involvement.

Community and Work Reintegration

Patient reports numerous repetitive motions at work. The job also requires some lifting.

Posture

The patient demonstrated a forward-head position. There was also a postural deficit of increased thoracic convexity, which altered the resting position of the scapula. This causes the head of the humerus to move into internal rotation to maintain its resting position in the glenoid, which affects the balance of shoulder girdle musculature.[75]

Range of Motion (Including Muscle Length)

It is worth remembering that the stages of capsulitis of the shoulder do not depend on the degree of motion that is limited. In acute lesions or Stage I lesions, ROM may be severely limited. In Stage III conditions, ROM may not necessarily be as limited. Findings included:

- Marked loss of active and passive shoulder motion in a capsular pattern with external rotation most limited (greater than a 50 percent loss) followed by abduction, then internal rotation.
- Pain reported at the extremes of all active motions.
- Hiking of the shoulder girdle was evident with elevation of the arm as a result of capsular contracture and inhibition of the rotator cuff musculature.
- Passive range of motion assessment reveals an "empty" end-feel, where pain stops passive movement before resistance is felt by the clinician.[48]

Joint Integrity and Mobility

Anterior translation of the humeral head on the involved side, probably as a result of a decrease in capsular volume.[616]

Globally limited glenohumeral translations with a rigid, capsular end-feel.

Motor Performance: Strength, Power, Endurance

No significant deficits in resisted movements are seen.

Pain

Pain rated at 6 to 7 out of 10 on a visual analogue scale. Pain on palpation of the anterior and posterior capsules and describe pain radiating to the deltoid insertion.

EVALUATION (CLINICAL JUDGMENT)

The patient is a deconditioned, obese woman with joint and soft tissue mobility restrictions, and impaired shoulder function.

DIAGNOSIS BY PHYSICAL THERAPIST

Pattern 4D: Impaired joint mobility, motor function, muscle performance, and range of motion associated with capsular restriction of the right shoulder: right shoulder adhesive capsulitis.

PROGNOSIS

Predicted Interval Levels of Improvement in Function

Within 6 to 8 weeks, the patient will:

- Improve shoulder range of motion to WNL as compared to the other side in order to perform work duties and return to exercise regime.
- Report pain at 2 out of 10 or less with activity or 0 out of 10 at rest.
- Drive to work without pain.
- Be able to comb hair without pain.
- Be independent with progressive home exercise program emphasizing function.
- Perform repetitive activities with right shoulder, simulating work activities and functions.

PLAN OF CARE

Frequency and Duration

2 to 3 times per week for 4 weeks.

Re-examination

Perform selected tests and measures to evaluate patient's progress toward goals in order to modify or redirect intervention if patient fails to show progress.

Criteria for Discharge

Patient reaches established functional goals, patient declines further intervention, is unable to progress towards goals because of complications, or PT determines that patient will no longer benefit from PT services.

QUESTIONS

1. Having made the provisional diagnosis, outline your intervention in terms of the phases of healing?
2. How would you describe this condition to the patient?
3. What would you tell the patient about your intervention?
4. How will you determine the intensity of your intervention?
5. Estimate this patient's prognosis.
6. What modalities could you use in the intervention of this patient? Why?
7. Which manual techniques would be appropriate for this patient, and what is your rationale?
8. What exercises would you prescribe? Why?

INTERVENTION

Adhesive capsulitis appears to worsen with rest, but arm movement results in improvement.[227] While certain basic principles apply to all stages, patients presenting with different stages of primary adhesive capsulitis should have individualized intervention.[391] The patient should be made aware that this condition, depending on which stage, may last from 6 to 9 months to as long as 1 to 3 years.

Phase I (Weeks 0 to 2)

This phase typically involves 2 to 6 visits of physical therapy.

Goals

- Decrease pain to 5 out of 10 or less.
- Control inflammation.
- Strength at 4 out of 5 on manual muscle test for shoulder girdle musculature.
- Shoulder ROM to be within 60 percent of uninvolved side.
- Increased duration of uninterrupted sleep.

Electrotherapeutic Modalities and Physical Agents

The major objective in the intervention of individuals with adhesive capsulitis is to restore function by decreasing the inflammatory response and pain. The following can be used to reduce pain[414]:

- High-voltage galvanic stimulation.
- Transcutaneous electrical nerve stimulation.[617]
- Iontophoresis.
- Cryotherapy.

   Inflammation can be reduced using[414]:

- Iontophoresis.
- Phonophoresis.
- Cryotherapy.

   Relaxation can be promoted using[414]:

- Moist heat.
- Ultrasound.
- Hydrotherapy can be used to cause a "glove effect" that stimulates the proprioceptors of the skin and generates a biofeedback-like effect.[383] The recommended water temperature is tepid to neutral. Basic exercises including flexion in the plane of the scapula and horizontal abduction and adduction along the surface of the water are performed.[391]

Therapeutic Exercise and Home Program

- Gentle exercises such as the pendulum, circumduction, pulleys, and active assisted wand exercises are advocated within the pain-free range.
- AROM in pain-free ranges, including scapular retraction/depression.
- Postural correction exercises. Postural training is incorporated to discourage thoracic kyphosis and a forward humeral head position during forward elevation.
- Education on sleeping postures. An understanding of the diagnosis through patient education will encourage patient compliance and decrease patient frustration. The optimal resting position of the arm in comfortable abduction for improved vascularization of the cuff[44] is demonstrated to the patient.[391]
- Closed chain exercises can be performed early during the rehabilitation process. This permits the rotator cuff to work as a glenohumeral compressor.[102] This exercise also reduces the shearing effect of the deltoid, causes co-contraction of force couples around the shoulder, and creates an axial load through the joint.

- Training of the scapular pivoters should be initiated as soon as tolerated by the patient to provide a stable base for distal mobility.
- Flexibility exercises. A stretching program which addresses the shortened internal rotators and adductors such as the subscapularis is initiated before attempting to strengthen the weakened external rotators and abductors.[607] The individual is encouraged to use pain as a guide to limit activities of daily living because inflammation and pain can alter shoulder mechanics. The patient is instructed to stretch the shoulder to the point of tolerable discomfort five times each day.
- Cardiovascular exercises including stationary bike and walking program. These must be monitored closely given the patient's past medical history of congestive heart failure and high blood pressure.
- AROM exercises for elbow, wrist, and hand.
- Gripping exercises.

Manual Therapy

- Gentle joint mobilizations and physiologic movements that use the opposite extremity within a pain-free ROM will assist in reducing pain by stimulating the joint mechanoreceptors and decreasing nociceptive input.[413] The joint mobilization grades used depend on the intent of the intervention. Grades I and II are used for pain relief, while grades III and IV are used to address any painless hypomobilities due to the forward head posture.
- Soft tissue techniques to the cervical, thoracic, and shoulder musculature as appropriate.
- Myofascial techniques as appropriate.

Phase II (Weeks 2 to 6)

This phase typically involves 4 to 6 visits of physical therapy.

Goals

- Decrease pain to 2 out of 10 or less.
- Minimize capsular restriction thereby minimizing loss of motion.[399]
- Strength at 4+ out of 5 or equal to uninvolved extremity.
- Shoulder AROM to be within 80 percent of uninvolved extremity.
- Performance of functional activities including reaching into back pocket, fastening undergarments, combing hair, lift and reach overhead, and perform weight- and repetition-specific work and ADL tasks.

Electrotherapeutic Modalities and Physical Agents

Continue use of effective modalities with increased emphasis on use as needed at home. In this phase, modalities are used to decrease pain and inflammation and to increase tissue extensibility.[399]

Heat may be used to promote muscle relaxation, ultrasound may be used to promote tissue extensibility in the axillary fold, and cryotherapy may be used to reduce discomfort after stretching.[399] The ultrasound is applied prior to mobilization techniques with the shoulder positioned in abduction and external rotation, and the ultrasound applied to the anterior, inferior capsule, or posterior capsule as indicated.[218]

An active warm-up to increase soft tissue circulation is preferred over passive intervention.[399]

Therapeutic Exercise and Home Program

It is important to educate the patient regarding their improvement in ROM because the patient will continue to perceive pain at the end of the range and may not recognize the objective improvement in function.[399]

Because ROM is improved, active exercise is performed in the plane of the scapula at an angle 30 to 45 degrees anterior to the coronal plane.[12,399] Exercises using wands, pulleys, and Codman exercises with cuff weights are performed in straight planes as well as diagonals.

As the ROM improves, and if rotator cuff weakness persists, isolation of the cuff can be initiated to address strength and endurance.[399]

The home exercise program should emphasize frequent ROM exercises including pendulums, cane exercises for improving internal rotation and external rotation, and elevation.[399]

Manual Therapy

Passive range-of-motion exercises including passive joint mobilizations are used to restore joint glide and separation.[399] The goal is to stretch the capsule sufficiently to allow restoration of normal glenohumeral biomechanics.[399]

Neuromuscular Re-education

Neuromuscular re-training involves:

- Hand knee rocking in single planes and then multidirections.
- Three-point rocking.
- Push-up progression.
- Push-ups off a Swiss ball.
- Body blade.

Although most patients will have significant improvement by 12 to 16 weeks, some patients do not improve and may worsen. The options then include continued physical therapy or surgical intervention, which could include closed manipulation, arthroscopy, or capsular release and manipulation.[399] The decision to proceed with operative versus nonoperative intervention is dependent on the degree of functional disability and the patient's response to a rehabilitative program.[391]

Coordination, Communication, and Documentation

Communicate with MD regarding the patient's status (direct or indirect) every 2 weeks. Discharge planning will be provided. Documentation of therapeutic interventions will be provided for each episode of care. Additional communication will depend on the patient's home, work, and recreational situation.

Patient-Related Instruction

The patient is given an explanation about the physiologic changes that occur with soft tissues and the joint capsule and their relationship to adhesive capsulitis. The clinician performs a periodic re-examination and reassessment of the home program, utilizing written instructions and illustrations. Educate patient in positions and motions to avoid during home and work, including the avoidance of sleeping on the involved shoulder. Educate patient in the benefits of an ongoing conditioning program to prevent re-occurrence. Educate the patient on the use of cryotherapy at home, and the importance of maintaining good posture throughout the day.

Patients are encouraged to begin using the arm in a normal fashion for reaching and other daily activities, in a controlled and progressive manner.

Criteria for Discharge

Patient will be discharged when all rehabilitation goals have been achieved. Instruct patient to call for advice should progression plateau or decline. Review home exercise program. Additional visits may be required if current vocational demands exacerbate the symptoms.

Outcomes

The outcome of the patient depends on their level of compliance to the recommended intervention plan, as well as other recommended lifestyle changes. The patient should return to a preinjury pain level in 2 months, without recurrence of shoulder pain over the next year. The patient understands the strategies to self-manage any minor recurrences.

REVIEW QUESTIONS*

1. What is the capsular pattern of the G-H joint?
2. The shoulder joint is capable of much motion, but sacrifices some stability to achieve this degree of motion. The weakest portion of the shoulder joint capsule is located:
   A. anteriorly
   B. posteriorly
   C. laterally
   D. inferiorly
   E. superiorly
3. Name four muscles that internally rotate the shoulder.
4. Name three muscles that externally rotate the shoulder.
5. Name four muscles that attach to the greater tuberosity of the humerus.

*Additional questions to test your understanding of this chapter can be found in the Online Learning Center for *Orthopaedic Assessment, Evaluation, and Intervention* at www.duttononline.net.

REFERENCES

1. Burkhart SS. A 26-year-old woman with shoulder pain. *JAMA* 2000;284:1559–1567.
2. Kapandji IA. *The Physiology of the Joints, Upper Limb.* New York: Churchill Livingstone; 1991.
3. Inman VT, Saunders JB. Observations on the function of the clavicle. *Calif Med* 1946;65:158.
4. Perry J. Biomechanics of the shoulder. In: Rowe CR, ed. *The Shoulder.* New York: Churchill Livingstone; 1988:1–15.
5. Saha AK. Dynamic stability of the glenohumeral joint. *Acta Orthop Scand* 1971;42:491–505.
6. Howell SM, Galinat BJ. The glenoid-labral socket: a constrained articular surface. *Clin Orthop* 1989;243:122–125.
7. Bradley JP, Tibone JE. Electromyographic analysis of muscle action about the shoulder. *Clin Sports Med* 1991;4:789–805.
8. Bradley JP, Perry J, Jobe FW. The biomechanics of the throwing shoulder. *Perspect Orthop* 1990;1:49–59.
9. Answorth AA, Warner JJP. Shoulder instability in the athlete. *Orthop Clin North Am* 1995;26:487–504.
10. Alcheck DW, Dines DM. Shoulder injuries in the throwing athlete. *J Am Acad Orthop Surg* 1995;3:159–165.
11. Boublik M, Hawkins RJ. Clinical examination of the shoulder complex. *J Orthop Sports Phys Ther* 1993;18:379–385.
12. Poppen NK, Walker PS. Normal and abnormal motion of the shoulder. *J Bone Joint Surg* 1976;58A:195–201.
13. Saha AK. Mechanisms of shoulder movements and a plea for the recognition of "Zero Position" of the glenohumeral joint. *Clin Orthop* 1983;173:3–10.
14. Warner JJP. The gross anatomy of the joint surfaces, ligaments, labrum, and capsule. In: Matsen FA, Fu FH, Hawkins RJ, eds. *The Shoulder: A Balance of Mobility and Stability.* Rosemont, Ill: American Academy of Orthopedic Surgeons; 1993:7–29.
15. Kibler BW. The role of the scapula in athletic shoulder function. *Am J Sports Med* 1998;26:325–337.
16. Doody SG, Freedman L, Waterland JC. Shoulder movements during abduction in the scapular plane. *Arch Phys Med Rehabil* 1970;51:595–604.
17. Freedman L, Munro RR. Abduction of the arm in the scapular plane: Scapular and glenohumeral movements. *J Bone Joint Surg* 1966;48A:1503–1510.
18. Jobe FW, Moynes DR, Brewster CE. Rehabilitation of shoulder joint instabilities. *Orthop Clin North Am* 1987;18:473–482.
18a. Gray H: Gray's Anatomy. Philadelphia, Pa: Lea & Febiger; 1995.
19. Perry J. Normal upper extremity kinesiology. *Phys Ther* 1978;58:265–278.
20. O'Donoghue, DH. Subluxing biceps tendon in the athlete. *Clin Orthop* 1982;164:26–29.
21. Petersson CJ. Spontaneous medial dislocation of the long head of the biceps brachii in its causation. *Clin Orthop* 1986;211:224.
22. Rowe CR, Zarins B. Recurrent transient subluxation of the shoulder. *J Bone Joint Surg Am* 1981;63:863–872.
23. Terry GC, et al. The stabilizing function of passive shoulder restraints. *Am J Sports Med* 1991;19:26–34.
24. Brody LT. Shoulder. In: Wadsworth C, ed. *Current Concepts of Orthopedic Physical Therapy—Home Study Course.* La Crosse, Wis: Orthopaedic Section, APTA; 2001.
25. Gerber A, Warner JJ. Thermal capsulorrhaphy to treat shoulder instability. *Clin Orthop* 2002;400:105–116.
26. O'Brien SJ, et al. The anatomy and histology of the inferior glenohumeral complex of the shoulder. *Am J Sports Med* 1990;18:449.
27. O'Connell PW, et al. The contribution of the glenohumeral ligaments to anterior stability of the shoulder joint. *Am J Sports Med* 1990;18:579–584.
28. Ferrari DA. Capsular ligaments of the shoulder. *Am J Sports Med* 1990;18:20–24.
29. Turkel SJ, et al. Stabilizing mechanisms preventing anterior dislocation of the glenohumeral joint. *J Bone Joint Surg Am* 1981;63:1208–1217.

30. Harryman DT III, et al. The role of the rotator interval capsule in passive motion and stability of the shoulder. *J Bone Joint Surg* 1992;74A:53–66.

31. Matsen FA III, Arntz CT. Subacromial impingement. In: Rockwood CA Jr, Matsen FA III, eds. *The Shoulder.* Philadelphia, Pa: WB Saunders; 1990:623–648.

32. Neer CS II. Anterior acromioplasty for the chronic impingement syndrome in the shoulder: a preliminary report. *J Bone Joint Surg Am* 1972;54:41–50.

33. Neer C. Impingement lesions. *Clin Orthop* 1983;173:71–77.

34. Wickiewicz TL. The impingement syndrome. Postgraduate Advances in Sports Medicine—NATA Home Study Course, 1986.

35. Petersson CJ, Redlund-Johnell I. The subacromial space in normal shoulder radiographs. *Acta Orthop Scand* 1984;55:57–58.

36. Weiner DS, Macnab I. Superior migration of the humeral head: a radiological aid in the diagnosis of the tears of the rotator cuff. *J Bone Joint Surg Br* 1970;52:524–527.

37. Flatow EL, et al. Excursion of the rotator cuff under the acromion. Patterns of subacromial contact. *Am J Sports Med* 1994;22:779–788.

38. Keele CA, Neil E. *Samson Wright's Applied Physiology*, 12th ed. London: Oxford University Press; 1971.

39. Aszmann OC, et al. Innervation of the human shoulder joint and its implications for surgery. *Clin Orthop* 1996;330:202–207.

40. Bosley RC. Total acromionectomy. A twenty-year review. *J Bone Joint Surg* 1991;73A:961–968.

41. Ellman H, Kay SP. Arthroscopic subacromial decompression for chronic impingement: 2- to 5-year results. *J Bone Joint Surg Br* 1991;73:395–401.

41a. de la Garza O, Lierse W, Steiner D. Anatomical study of the blood supply in the human shoulder region. *Acta Anatomica* 1992;145(4):412–415.

42. Willcox TM, et al. The biceps brachii muscle flap for axillary wound coverage. *Plast Reconstr Surg* 2002;110:822–826.

43. Taylor GI, Palmer JH. The vascular territories (angiosomes) of the body: experimental study and clinical implications. *Br J Plast Surg* 1987;40:113.

44. Rathbun JB, Macnab I. The microvascular pattern of the rotator cuff. *J Bone Joint Surg Br* 1970;52:540–553.

45. Winkel D, Matthijs O, Phelps V. Pathology of the shoulder. In: *Diagnosis and Treatment of the Upper Extremities*. Maryland, Md: Aspen; 1997:68–117.

46. Hsu A-T, Chang J-H, Chang CH. Determining the resting position of the glenohumeral joint: A cadaver study. *J Orthop Sports Phys Ther* 2002;32:605–612.

47. Ludewig PM. Alterations in shoulder kinematics and associated muscle activity in persons with shoulder impingement symptoms. Iowa City: The University of Iowa; 1998.

48. Cyriax J. *Examination of the Shoulder. Limited Range Diagnosis of Soft Tissue Lesions*, 8th ed. Vol. 1. London: Balliere Tindall; 1982:127–142.

49. Davies GJ, DeCarlo MS. Examination of the shoulder complex. In: Bandy WD, ed. *Current Concepts in the Rehabilitation of the Shoulder.* Sports Physical Therapy Section—Home Study Course, 1995.

50. Gladstone JN, Rosen AL. Disorders of the acromioclavicular joint. *Curr Opin Orthop* 1999;10:316–321.

51. Turnbull JR. Acromioclavicular joint disorders. *Med Sci Sports Exerc* 1998;30(4 Suppl):S26–32.

52. Norfray JF, et al. The clavicle in hockey. *Am J Sports Med* 1977;5:275–280.

53. DePalma AF. *Surgery of the Shoulder*, 2nd ed. Philadelphia: Lippincott; 1973.

54. Butters KP. Fractures of the clavicle. In: Rockwood CA, Matsen FA, eds. *The Shoulder*. Philadelphia: WB Saunders; 1990:432.

55. Fukuda K, et al. Biomechanical study of the ligamentous system of the acromioclavicular joint. *J Bone Joint Surg* 1986;68A:434–439.

56. Urist MR. Complete dislocation of the acromioclavicular joint: the nature of the traumatic lesion and effective methods of treatment with an analysis of 41 cases. *J Bone Joint Surg* 1946;28:813–837.

57. Lee K, et al. Functional evaluation of the ligaments at the acromioclavicular joint during anteroposterior and superoinferior translation. *Am J Sports Med* 1997;25:858–862.

58. Moore KL, Dalley AF. Upper Limb. In: Moore KL, Dalley AF, eds. *Clinically Oriented Anatomy*, Philadelphia, Pa: Williams & Wilkins; 1999:664–830.

59. Karduna AR, et al. Dynamic measurements of three-dimensional scapular kinematics: a validation study. *J Biomech Eng* 2001;123:184–190.

60. Norkin C, Levangie P. *Joint Structure and Function: A Comprehensive Analysis.* Philadelphia: FA Davis; 1992:355–358.

61. Allman FL Jr. Fractures and ligamentous injuries of the clavicle and its articulation. *J Bone Joint Surg* 1967;49A:774–784.

62. Conway AM. Movements at the sternoclavicular and acromioclavicular joints. *Phys Ther Rev* 1961;41:421–432.

63. Inman T, Saunders JR, Abbott LC. Observations on the function of the shoulder joint. *J Bone Joint Surg* 1944;26:1–18.

64. Omer GE. Osteotomy of the clavicle in surgical reduction of anterior sternoclavicular dislocations. *J Trauma* 1967;7:584–590.

65. Steindler A. *Kinesiology of the Human Body under Normal and Pathological Conditions.* Springfield, Ill: Charles C Thomas; 1955.

66. Paine RM, Voight M. The role of the scapula. *J Orthop Sports Phys Ther* 1993;18:386–391.

67. Kibler WB, Chandler TJ, Livingston BP. Correlation of lateral scapular slide measurements with x-ray measurements. *Med Sci Sports Exerc* 1999;31(5 Suppl):S237.

68. Ludewig PM. *Functional Shoulder Anatomy and Biomechanics.* Home Study Course—Solutions to Shoulder Disorders. La Crosse, Wis: Orthopaedic Section, APTA, Inc.; 2001.

69. Williams GR Jr, et al. Anatomy of the scapulothoracic articulation. *Clin Orthop* 1999;359:237–246.

70. Hollinshead WH. *Anatomy for Surgeons—The Back and Limbs.* Harper and Row: Philadelphia; 1982:300–308.

71. Jobe FW, Pink M. Classification and treatment of shoulder dysfunction in the overhead athlete. *J Orthop Sports Phys Ther* 1993;18:427–431.

72. Haymaker W, Woodhall B. *Peripheral Nerve Injuries. Principles of Diagnosis.* London: WB Saunders; 1953.

73. Brodal A. *Neurological Anatomy.* London: Oxford University Press; 1981.

74. Mercer S, Campbell AH. Motor innervation of the trapezius. *J Man Manip Ther* 2000;8:18–20.

75. Ayub E. Posture and the upper quarter. In: Donatelli RA, ed. *Physical Therapy of the Shoulder.* New York: Churchill Livingstone; 1991:81–90.

76. White SM, Witten CM. Long thoracic nerve palsy in a professional ballet dancer. *Am J Sports Med* 1993;21:626–629.

77. Jobe CM. Gross anatomy of the shoulder. In: Rockwood CA, Matsen FA, eds. *The Shoulder.* Philadelphia, Pa: WB Saunders; 1998:35–97.

78. Connor PM, et al. Split pectoralis major transfer for serratus anterior palsy. *Clin Orthop* 1997;341:134–142.

79. Schultz JS, Leonard JA. Long thoracic neuropathy from athletic activity. *Arch Phys Med Rehab* 1992;73:87–90.

80. Gregg JR, et al. Serratus anterior paralysis in the young athlete. *J Bone Joint Surg* 1979;61A:825–832.

81. Marks PH, Warner JJP, Irrgang JJ. Rotator cuff disorders of the shoulder. *J Hand Ther* 1994;7:90–98.

82. Warner JJ, Navarro RA. Serratus anterior dysfunction. Recognition and treatment. *Clin Orthop* 1998;349:139–148.

83. Leffert RD. Neurological problems. In: Rockwood CA Jr, Matsen FR III, eds. *The Shoulder*. Philadelphia: WB Saunders; 1990:750–773.

84. Warner JJP, et al. Scapulothoracic motion in normal shoulders and shoulders with glenohumeral instability and impingement syndrome. A study using Moire topographic analysis. *Clin Orthop* 1992;285:191–199.

85. Post M. Pectoralis major transfer for winging of the scapula. *J Shoulder Elbow Surg* 1995;4:1–9.

86. Kapandji IA. *The Physiology of Joints*, Vol. 3. New York: Churchill Livingstone; 1974:54–71.

87. Dunleavy K. Relationship between the shoulder and the cervicothoracic spine. Independent Home Study Course: Solutions to Shoulder Disorders. La Crosse, Wis: Orthopedic Section, APTA; 2001:1–25.

88. Porterfield J, De Rosa C. *Mechanical Neck Pain: Perspectives in Functional Anatomy*. Philadelphia: WB Saunders; 1995:38–91.

89. Perry J. Muscle control of the shoulder. In: Rowe CR, ed. *The Shoulder*. New York: Churchill Livingstone; 1988:17–34.

90. Mathes SJ, Nahai F. Biceps brachii. In: Mathes SJ, Nahai F, eds. *Clinical Atlas of Muscle and Musculocutaneous Flaps*. St. Louis: Mosby; 1979:426–432.

91. Lucas DB. Biomechanics of the shoulder joint. *Arch Surg* 1973;107:425–432.

92. Levy AS, et al. Function of the long head of the biceps at the shoulder: electromyographic analysis. *J Shoulder Elbow Surg* 2001;10:250–255.

93. Andrews JR, Carson WG, McLeod WD. Glenoid labrum tears related to the long head of the biceps. *Am J Sports Med* 1985;13:337–341.

94. Basmajian JV, Deluca CJ. *Muscles Alive: Their Functions Revealed by Electromyography*. Baltimore: Williams & Wilkins; 1985.

95. Basmajian JV, Bazant FJ. Factors preventing downward dislocation of the adducted shoulder joint: an electromyographic and morphological study. *J Bone Joint Surg* 1959;41A:1182–1186.

96. Itoi E, et al. Stabilising function of the biceps in stable and unstable shoulders. *J Bone Joint Surg Am* 1993;75B:546–550.

97. Kibler BW. Normal shoulder mechanics and function. *Instructional Course Lectures*. 1997;46:39–42.

98. Kibler WB, Livingston B, Bruce R. Current concepts in shoulder rehabilitation. *Adv Op Orthop* 1996;3:249–301.

99. Pink MM, Screnar PM, Tollefson KD. Injury prevention and rehabilitation in the upper extremity. In: Jobe FW, ed. *Operative Techniques in Upper Extremity Sports Injuries*. St. Louis: Mosby; 1996:3–15.

100. Jobe FW, et al. An EMG analysis of the shoulder in pitching and throwing: A preliminary report. *Am J Sports Med* 1983;11:3–5.

101. Pagnani MJ, Galinat BJ, Warren RF. Glenohumeral instability. In: *Orthopaedic Sports Medicine: Principles and Practice*. DeLee JC, Drez D, eds. Philadelphia: WB Saunders; 1993.

102. Kibler WB. Shoulder rehabilitation: principles and practice. *Med Sci Sports Exerc* 1998;30(4 Suppl 1):40–50.

102a. Terry GC, Hammon D, France P, et al: The stabilizing function of passive shoulder restraints. *Am J Sports Med* 1991;19:26–34.

102b. Brody LT: Shoulder. In: Wadsworth C, ed. *Current Concepts of Orthopedic Physical Therapy—Home Study Course*, Vol. 11.2.6. La Crosse, Wis: Orthopaedic Section, APTA; 2001.

103. Kibler WB. Biomechanical analysis of the shoulder during tennis activities. *Clin Sports Med* 1995;14:79–85.

104. Kibler WB. Evaluation of sports demands as a diagnostic tool in shoulder disorders. In: Matsen FA, Fu F, Hawkins RJ, eds. *The Shoulder: A Balance of Mobility and Stability*. Rosemont, Ill: American Academy of Orthopedic Surgeons; 1994:379–399.

105. Kibler WB, Livingston B, Chandler TJ. Shoulder rehabilitation: clinical application, evaluation, and rehabilitation protocols. *AAOS Instruct Course Lect* 1997;46:43–53.

106. Nichols TR. A biomechanical perspective on spinal mechanisms of coordinated muscular action. *Acta Anat Nippon* 1994;15:1–13.

107. Ovesen J, Nielsen S. Experimental distal subluxation in the glenohumeral joint. *Arch Orthop Trauma Surg* 1985;104:78–81.

108. Gibb TD, et al. The effect of capsular venting on glenohumeral laxity. *Clin Orthop* 1991;268:120–127.

109. Itoi E, et al. The static rotator cuff does not affect inferior translation of the humerus at the glenohumeral joint. *J Trauma* 1999;47:55–59.

110. Debski RE, et al. Contribution of the passive properties of the rotator cuff to glenohumeral stability during anterior-posterior loading. *J Shoulder Elbow Surg* 1999;8:324–329.

111. Lee S-B, et al. Dynamic glenohumeral stability provided by the rotator cuff muscles in the mid-range and end-range of motion. *J Bone Joint Surg* 2000;82A:849–857.

112. Matsen FA, Harryman DT, Sidles JA. Mechanics of glenohumeral instability. *Clin Sports Med* 1991;10:783–788.

113. Habermeyer PU, Schuller U, Wiedemann E. The intra-articular pressure of the shoulder: an experimental study on the role of the glenoid labrum in stabilizing the joint. *J Arthrosc* 1992;8:166–172.

114. Warner JJP, Schulte KR, Imhoff AB. Current concepts in shoulder instability. In: *Advances in Operative Orthopedics*. St Louis, Mo: CV Mosby; 1995:217–248.

115. Pearl ML, et al. A system for describing positions of the humerus relative to the thorax and its use in the presentation of several functionally important arm positions. *J Shoulder Elbow Surg* 1992;1:113–118.

116. Birac D, Andriacchi TP, Bach BR Jr. Time related changes following ACL rupture. *Trans Orthop Res Soc* 1991;16:231.

117. Blackburn TA, et al. EMG analysis of posterior rotator cuff exercises. *Athl Training* 1990;25:40–45.

118. Brewster C, Moynes-Schwab DR. Rehabilitation of the shoulder following rotator cuff injury or surgery. *J Orthop Sports Phys Ther* 1993;18:422–426.

119. Fleckenstein JL, Shellock FG. Exertional muscle injuries: magnetic resonance imaging evaluation. *Top Magn Reson Imaging* 1991;3:50–70.

120. Fleckenstein JL, et al. Sports-related muscle injuries: MR imaging. *Radiology* 1989;172:793–798.

121. Jobe FW, Bradley JP. Rotator cuff injuries in baseball: prevention and rehabilitation. *Sports Med* 1988;6:378–387.

122. Jobe FW, Moynes DR. Delineation of diagnostic criteria and a rehabilitation program for rotator cuff injuries. *Am J Sports Med* 1982;10:336–339.

123. Townsend J, et al. Electromyographic analysis of the gleno-humeral muscles during a baseball rehabilitation program. *Am J Sports Med* 1991;3:264–272.

124. Worrell TW, et al. An analysis of supraspinatus EMG activity and shoulder isometric force development. *Med Sci Sports Exerc* 1992;7:744–748.

125. Keating JF, et al. The relative strength of rotator cuff muscles: A cadaver study. *J Bone Joint Surg* 1993;75B:137–140.

126. Fisher MJ, et al. Direct relationship between proton T2 and exercise intensity in skeletal muscle MR images. *Invest Radiol* 1990;25:480–485.

127. Fleckenstein JL, et al. Acute effects of exercise on MR imaging of skeletal muscle in normal volunteers. *Am J Roentgenol* 1988;151:231–237.

128. Horrigan JM, et al. Magnetic resonance imaging evaluation of muscle usage associated with three exercises for rotator cuff rehabilitation. *Med Sci Sports Exerc* 1999;31:1361.

129. Fleckenstein JL, et al. Exercise enhanced MR imaging of variations in forearm muscle anatomy and use: importance in MR spectroscopy. *Am J Roentgenol* 1989;153:693–698.

130. Fleckenstein JL, et al. Skeletal muscle size as a determinant of exercise performance: a new application of MRI. *Soc Magn Reson Med* 1988;1:192–196.

131. Fleckenstein JL, et al. Finger-specific flexor recruitment in humans: depiction by exercise enhanced MRI. *J Appl Physiol* 1992;72:1974–1977.

132. Glousman R, Jobe FW, Tibone JE. Dynamic EMG analysis of the throwing shoulder with glenohumeral instability. *J Bone Joint Surg* 1988;70:220–226.

133. Babyar SR. Excessive scapular motion in individuals recovering from painful and stiff shoulders: causes and treatment strategies. *Phys Ther* 1996;76:226–247.

134. Bagg SD, Forrest WJ. A biomechanical analysis of scapular rotation during arm abduction in the scapular plane. *Am J Phys Med* 1988;67:238–245.

135. McQuade KJ, Smidt GL. Dynamic scapulohumeral rhythm: the effects of external resistance during elevation of the arm in the scapular plane. *J Orthop Sports Phys Ther* 1998;27:125–133.

136. Rockwood CA. *Rockwood and Green's Fractures in Adults.* Philadelphia: Lippincott; 1991:1181–1239.

137. Dvir Z, Berme N. The shoulder complex in elevation of the arm: a mechanism approach. *J Biomech* 1978;11:219–225.

138. Schenkman M, De Cartaya VR. Kinesiology of the shoulder complex. In: Andrews J, Wilk KE, eds. *The Athlete's Shoulder.* New York: Churchill Livingstone; 1994:15–35.

139. Laumann U. Kinesiology of the shoulder: electromyographic and stereophotogrammetric studies. In: *Surgery of the Shoulder.* Philadelphia: BC Decker Co; 1984.

140. Van Der Helm FCT. Analysis of the kinematic and dynamic behavior of the shoulder mechanism. *J Biomech* 1994; 27:527–550.

141. Kuhn JE, Plancher KD, Hawkins RJ. Scapular winging. *J Am Acad Orthop Surg* 1995;3:319–325.

142. Jobe FW, Bradley JP, Pink M. Treatment of impingement syndrome in overhand athletes: A philosophical basis: I. *Surg Rounds Orthop* 1990;4:19–24.

143. Rockwood CA Jr, Young DC. Disorders of the acromioclavicular joint. In: Rockwood CA, Matsen FA, eds. *The Shoulder.* Philadelphia: WB Saunders; 1990:413–468.

143a. Kibler BW: The role of the scapula in athletic shoulder function. *Am J Sports Med* 1998;26(2):325–337.

144. Morrey BF, An K-N. Biomechanics of the shoulder. In: Rockwood CA, Matsen FA, eds. *The Shoulder.* Philadelphia: WB Saunders; 1990:208–245.

145. Lee DG. Biomechanics of the thorax. In: Grant R, ed. *Physical Therapy of the Cervical and Thoracic Spine.* New York: Churchill Livingstone; 1988:47–76.

146. Campos GER, Freitas VD, Vitti M. Electromyographic study of the trapezius and deltoideus in elevation, lowering, retraction and protraction of the shoulders. *Electromyog Clin Neurophysiol* 1994;34:243–247.

147. Elliott BC, Marshall R, Noffal G. Contributions of upper limb segment rotations during the power serve in tennis. *J Appl Biomech* 1995;11:433–442.

148. Kennedy K. Rehabilitation of the unstable shoulder. *Oper Tech Sports Med* 1993;1:311–324.

149. Harryman DT III, Sidles JA, Clark JM. Translation of the humeral head on the glenoid with passive glenohumeral motion. *J Bone Joint Surg* 1990;72A:1334–1343.

150. Rodosky MW, Harner CD, Fu FH. The role of the long head of the biceps muscle and superior glenoid labrum in anterior stability of the shoulder. *Am J Sports Med* 1994;22:121–130.

151. Warner JJP, et al. Static capsuloligamentous restraints to superior-inferior translation of the glenohumeral joint. *Am J Sports Med* 1992;20:675–685.

152. Warner JJP, et al. Dynamic capsuloligamentous anatomy of the glenohumeral joint. *J Shoulder Elbow Surg* 1993;2:115–133.

153. Pagnani M, et al. Effect of lesions of the superior portion of the glenoid labrum on glenohumeral translation. *J Bone Joint Surg* 1995;77A:1002–1010.

154. Payne LZ, et al. The combined dynamic and static contributions to subacromial impingement. *Am J Sports Med.* 1997;25:801–808.

155. Warner JJP, McMahon PJ. The role of the long head of the biceps brachii in superior stability of the glenohumeral joint. *J Bone Joint Surg* 1995;77A:366–372.

156. Kido T, et al. The depressor function of biceps on the head of the humerus in shoulders with tears of the rotator cuff. *J Bone Joint Surg* 2000;82B:416–419.

157. Itoi E, et al. Morphology of the torn rotator cuff. *J Anat* 1995;186:429–434.

158. Howell SM, et al. Clarification of the role of the supraspinatus muscle in shoulder function. *J Bone Joint Surg* 1986; 68A:398–404.

159. Colachis SC, Strohm BR. Effects of suprascapular and axillary nerve blocks in muscle force in the upper extremity. *Arch Phys Med Rehab* 1971;52:22–29.

160. VanLinge B, Mulder JD. Function of the supraspinatus muscle and its relationship to the supraspinatus syndrome. *J Bone Joint Surg Am* 1963;45B:750–759.

161. Thompson WO, et al. A biomechanical analysis of rotator cuff deficiency in a cadaveric model. *Am J Sports Med* 1996; 24:286–292.

162. Duchenne de Boulogne GB. Physiologie des Mouvements. Paris: JB Baillière et Fils; 1867:53–72.

163. Gagey O, Hue E. Mechanics of the deltoid muscle. A new approach. *Clin Orthop* 2000;375:250–257.

164. Comtet JJ, Auffray Y. Physiologie des muscles élévateurs de l'épaule. *Rev Chir Orthop* 1970;56:105–117.

165. Deutsch A, et al. Radiologic measurement of superior displacement of the humeral head in the impingement syndrome. *J Shoulder Elbow Surg* 1996;5:186–193.

166. Karduna AR, et al. Kinematics of the glenohumeral joint: Influences of muscle forces, ligamentous constraints, and articular geometry. *J Orthop Res* 1996;14:986–993.

167. Kuechle DK, et al. Rotator cuff function during humeral elevation in 4 planes. The relevance of moment arm of shoulder muscles with respect to axial rotation of the glenohumeral joint in four positions. *Clin Biomech* 2000;15:322–329.

168. Perry J, Glousman, RE. Biomechanics of throwing. In: Nicholas JA, Hershman EB, eds. *The Upper Extremity in Sports Medicine.* St Louis: CV Mosby; 1990:727–751.

169. Sharkey NA, Marder RA. The rotator cuff opposes superior translation of the humeral head. *Am J Sports Med* 1995;23:270–275.

170. Sharkey NA, Marder RA, Hanson PB. The role of the rotator cuff in elevation of the arm. *Trans Orthop Res Soc* 1993;18:137.

171. Culham E, Peat M. Functional anatomy of the shoulder complex. *J Orthop Sports Phys Ther* 1993;18:342–350.

172. Kelkar R, et al. The effects of articular congruence and humeral head rotation on glenohumeral kinematics. *Adv Bioeng* 1994; 28:19–20.

173. Kelkar R, et al. Glenohumeral kinematics. *J Shoulder Elbow Surg* 1993;2(Suppl):S28.

174. Poppen NK, Walker PS. Forces at the glenohumeral joint in abduction. *Clin Orthop* 1978:135:165–170.

175. Howell SM. Normal and abnormal mechanics of the glenohumeral joint in the horizontal plane. *J Bone Joint Surg* 1988;70:227–235.

176. Jarjavay JF. Sur la luxation du tendon de la longue portion du muscle biceps humeral; sur la luxation des tendons des muscles peroniers latercux. *Gaz hebd med chir* 1867;21:325.

177. Jarvholm U, et al. Intramuscular pressure and muscle blood flow in the supraspinatus. *Eur J Appl Physiol* 1988;58:219–224.

178. Stenlund B, et al. Shoulder tendinitis and its relation to heavy manual work and exposure to vibration. *Scand J Work Environ Health* 1993;19:43–49.

179. Andersen JH, Gaardboe O. Musculoskeletal disorders of the neck and upper limb among sewing machine operators: a clinical investigation. *Am J Ind Med* 1993;24:689–700.

180. Hermann B, Rose DW. Stellenwert von Anamnese und klinischer Untersuchung beim degenerativen Impingement Syndrom im Vergleich zu operativen Befunden-eine prospektive Studie. *Z Orthop Ihre Grenzgeb* 1996;134:166–170.

181. Neer CS, Poppen NK. Supraspinatus outlet. *Orthop Trans* 1987;11:234.

182. Brewer BJ. Aging of the rotator cuff. *Am J Sports Med* 1979;17:102–110.

183. Ogata S, Uhthoff HK. Acromial enthesopathy and rotator cuff tears: A radiographic and histologic postmortem investigation of the coracoacromial arc. *Clin Orthop* 1990;254:39–48.

184. Uhthoff HK, Loehr J. The effect of aging on the soft tissues of the shoulder. In: Matsen FA, Fu FA, Hawkins R, eds. *The Shoulder: A Balance of Mobility and Stability.* Rosemont, Ill: American Academy of Orthopaedic Surgeons; 1993:269–278.

185. Ohlsson K, et al. Disorders of the neck and upper limbs in women in the fish processing industry. *Occup Environ Med* 1994;51:826–832.

186. Checkoway H, Pearce N, Dement JM. Design and conduct of occupational epidemiology studies: I. design aspects of cohort studies. *Am J Ind Med* 1989;15:363–373.

187. Jobe FW, Kvitne RS, Giangarra CE. Shoulder pain in the overhand and throwing athlete: the relationship of anterior instability and rotator cuff impingement. *Orthop Rev* 1989;18:963–975.

188. Mohr KJ, Moynes Schwab R, Tovin BJ. Musculoskeletal pattern F: Impaired joint mobility, motor function, muscle performance, and range of motion associated with localized inflammation. In: Tovin BJ, Greenfield B, eds. *Evaluation and Treatment of the Shoulder: An Integration of the Guide to Physical Therapist Practice.* Philadelphia: FA Davis; 2001:210–230.

189. Jobe CM, et al. Anterior shoulder instability, impingement and rotator cuff tear. In: Jobe FW, ed. *Operative Techniques in Upper Extremity Sports Injuries.* St. Louis: Mosby-Year Book; 1996.

190. Moseley HF, Goldie I. The arterial pattern of the rotator cuff of the shoulder. *J Bone Joint Surg* 1963;45-B:780–789.

191. Neer CS II, Welsh RP. The shoulder in sports. *Orthop Clin North Am* 1977;8:583–591.

192. Rothman RH, Parke WW. The vascular anatomy of the rotator cuff. *Clin Orthop* 1965;41:176–186.

193. Bigliani LU, Morrison D, April EW. The morphology of the acromion and its relationship to rotator cuff tears. *Orthop Trans* 1986;10:228.

194. Bigliani LU, et al. The relationship of acromial architecture to rotator cuff disease. *Clin Sports Med* 1991;4:823–838.

195. Ling SC, Chen SF, Wan RX. A study of the vascular supply of the supraspinatus tendon. *Surg Radiol Anat* 1990;12:161.

196. Codman EA. *The Shoulder, Rupture of the Supraspinatus Tendon and Other Lesions in or about the Subacromial Bursa.* Boston: Thomas Todd Co; 1934.

197. Lindblom K. On pathogenesis of ruptures of the tendon aponeurosis of the shoulder joint. *Acta Radiol* 1939;20:563.

198. Chansky, HA, Ianotti JP: The vascularity of the rotator cuff. *Clin Sports Med* 1991;10(4)807–822.

199. Sigholm G, et al. Pressure recording in the subacromial bursa. *J Orthop Res* 1988;6:123–128.

200. Kessel L, Watson M. The painful arc syndrome: Clinical classification as a guide to management. *J Bone Joint Surg Br* 1977;59:166–172.

201. Neer CS II. Impingement lesions. *Clin Orthop* 1983 Mar; (73):70–77.

202. DePalma AF, Gallery G, Bennett CA. Variational Anatomy and Degenerative Lesions of the Shoulder Joint. In: Blount W, ed. American Academy of Orthopaedic Surgeons Instructional Course Lectures. Ann Arbor, Mich: JW Edwards; 1949:255–281.

203. DePalma AF, Gallery G, Bennett CA. Degenerative Lesions of the Shoulder Joint at Various Age Groups Which are Compatible with Good Function. In: Blount W, ed. American Academy of Orthopaedic Surgeons Instructional Course Lectures. Ann Arbor, Mich: JW Edwards; 1950:168.

204. Ozaki J, et al. Tears of the rotator cuff on the shoulder associated with pathological changes in the acromion: a study in cadavera. *J Bone Joint Surg Am* 1988;70-A:1224–1230.

205. Petterson G. Rupture of the tendon aponeurosis of the shoulder joint in anterior inferior dislocation. *Acta Chir Scand* 1942;99(Suppl):1–184.

206. Sher J, et al. Abnormal findings on magnetic resonance images of symptomatic shoulders. *J Bone Joint Surg* 1995;77A:10–15.

207. Cotton RE, Rideout DF. Tears of the humeral rotator cuff: A radiological and pathological necropsy survey. *J Bone Joint Surg* 1964;46B:314–328.

208. Constant CR, Murley AHG. A clinical method of functional assessment of the shoulder. *Clin Orthop* 1987;214:160–164.

209. Cohen RB, Williams GR Jr. Impingement syndrome and rotator cuff disease as repetitive motion disorders. *Clin Orthop* 1998;351:95–101.

210. Soslowsky LJ, et al. Subacromial contact (impingement) on the rotator cuff in the shoulder. *Trans Orthop Res Soc* 1992;17:424.

211. Conroy DE, Hayes KW. The effect of joint mobilization as a component of comprehensive treatment for primary shoulder impingement syndrome. *J Orthop Sports Phys Ther* 1998;28:3–14.

212. Cofield RH. Current concepts review: Rotator cuff disease of the shoulder. *J Bone Joint Surg* 1985;67A:974–979.

213. Hjelm R, Draper C, Spencer S. Anterior-superior capsular length insufficiency in the painful shoulder. *J Orthop Sports Phys Ther* 1996;23:216–222.

214. Donatelli RA. Mobilization of the shoulder. In: Donatelli RA, ed. *Physical Therapy of the Shoulder.* New York: Churchill Livingstone; 1991:271–292.

215. Cofield RH, Simonet WT. Symposium on sports medicine: part 2. The shoulder in sports. *Mayo Clin Proc* 1984;59:157–164.

216. Morrison DS, Frogameni AD, Woodworth P. Nonoperative treatment of subacromial impingement syndrome. *J Bone Joint Surg Am* 1997;79:732–737.

217. Akeson WH, Amiel D, Woo SL-Y. Immobility effects on synovial joints: The pathomechanics of joint contracture. *Biorheology* 1980;17:95–110.

218. Kamkar A, Irrgang JJ, Whitney S, Non-operative management of secondary shoulder impingement syndrome. *J Orthop Sports Phys Ther* 1993;17:212–224.

219. Greenfield B, et al. Posture in patients with shoulder overuse injuries and healthy individuals. *J Orthop Sports Phys Ther* 1995;21:287–295.

220. Ruwe P, et al. The normal and the painful shoulders during the breast stroke: Electromyographic and cinematographic analysis of twelve muscles. *Am J Sports Med* 1994;22:789–796.

221. Warner JJP, et al. Patterns of flexibility, laxity, and strength in normal shoulders and shoulders with instability and impingement. *Am J Sports Med* 1990;18:366–375.

222. Clarnette RG, Miniaci A. Clinical exam of the shoulder. *Med Sci Sports Exerc* 1998;30(4 Suppl):1–6.

223. Magee DJ. *Orthopedic Physical Assessment,* 2nd ed. Philadelphia: WB Saunders; 1992.

224. Souza TA. History and examination of the shoulder. In: Souza TA, ed. *Sports Injuries of the Shoulder—Conservative Management.* New York: Churchill Livingstone; 1994:167–219.

225. Burkhart SS. A stepwise approach to arthroscopic rotator cuff repair based on biomechanical principles. *Arthroscopy* 2000;16:82–90.

226. Buckle P. Musculoskeletal disorders of the upper extremities: the use of epidemiological approaches in industrial settings. *J Hand Surg Am* 1987;12:885–889.

227. Daigneault J, Cooney LM Jr. Shoulder pain in older people. *J Am Geriatrics Soc* 1998;46:1144–1151.

228. Matsen FA III, et al. Shoulder motion. In: Matsen FA III, et al, eds. *Practical Evaluation and Management of the Shoulder.* Philadelphia: WB Saunders; 1994:19–58.

229. Miniaci A, Salonen D. Rotator cuff evaluation: imaging and diagnosis. *Orthop Clin North Am* 1997;28:43–58.

230. Gladstone J, Wilk KE, Andrews J. Nonoperative treatment of acromioclavicular joint injuries. *Op Tech Sports Med* 1998;5:78–87.

231. Cappel K, et al. Clinical examination of the shoulder. In: Tovin BJ, Greenfield B, eds. *Evaluation and Treatment of the Shoulder—An Integration of The Guide to Physical Therapist Practice.* Philadelphia: FA Davis; 2001:75–131.

232. Foreman SM, Croft AC. *Whiplash Injuries: The Cervical Acceleration/Deceleration Syndrome.* Baltimore: Williams & Wilkins; 1988.

233. Feinstein B, et al. Experiments on referred pain from deep somatic tissues. *J Bone Joint Surg Am* 1954;36:981–997.

234. Dwyer A, Aprill C, Bogduk N. Cervical zygapophyseal joint pain patterns: a study from normal volunteers. *Spine* 1990;15:453.

235. Cloward RB. Cervical discography: a contribution to the etiology and mechanism of neck, shoulder and arm pain. *Ann Surg* 1959;150:1052–1064.

236. Cuomo F. Diagnosis, classification, and management of the stiff shoulder. In: Iannotti JP, Williams GR, eds. *Disorders of the Shoulder: Diagnosis and Management.* Philadelphia: Lippincott Williams & Wilkins; 1999:397–417.

237. Sahrmann SA. Movement impairment syndromes of the shoulder girdle. In: Sahrmann SA, ed. Movement Impairment Syndromes. St. Louis: Mosby; 2001:193–261.

238. Hawkins RJ, Bokor DJ. Clinical evaluation of shoulder problems. In: Rockwood CA, Matsen FA, eds. *The Shoulder.* Philadelphia: WB Saunders; 1990.

239. Silliman FJ, Hawkins RJ. Clinical examination of the shoulder complex. In: Andrews JR, Wilk KE, eds. *The Athlete's Shoulder.* New York: Churchill Livingstone; 1994.

240. Barron OA, Levine WN, Bigliani LU. Surgical management of chronic trapezius dysfunction. In: Warner JJP, Iannotti JP, Gerber C, eds. *Complex and Revision Problems in Shoulder Surgery.* Philadelphia: Lippincott-Raven; 1997:377–384.

241. Hoppenfeld S. *Physical Examination of the Spine and Extremities.* East Norwalk, CT: Appleton-Century-Crofts; 1976.

242. Miniaci A, Fowler PJ. Impingement in the athlete. *Clin Sports Med* 1993;12:91–110.

243. Miniaci A, Froese WG. Rotator cuff pathology and excessive laxity or instability of the glenohumeral joint. *Sports Med Arthrosc Rev* 1995;3:26–29.

244. Ketenjian AY. Scapulocostal stabilization for scapular winging in fascioscapulohumeral muscular dystrophy. *J Bone Joint Surg* 1978;60A:476–480.

245. Bagg SD, Forrest WJ. Electromyographic study of the scapular rotators during arm abduction in the scapular plane. *Am J Phys Med* 1986;65:111–124.

246. Moseley JB, et al. EMG analysis of the scapular muscles during a shoulder rehabilitation program. *Am J Sports Med* 1992;20:128–134.

247. Bowling RW, Rockar PA, Erhard R. Examination of the shoulder complex. *Phys Ther* 1986;66:1886–1893.

248. Kendall FP, McCreary EK, Provance PG. *Muscles: Testing and Function.* Baltimore: Williams & Wilkins; 1993.

249. Griegel-Morris P, et al. Incidence of common postural abnormalities in the cervical, shoulder, and thoracic regions and their association with pain in two age groups of healthy subjects. *Phys Ther* 1992;72:426–430.

250. Crawford HJ, Jull GA. The influence of thoracic posture and movement on range of arm elevation. *Physiother Theory Pract* 1993;9:143–148.

251. Sahrmann SA. *Diagnosis and Treatment of Movement Impairment Syndromes.* St Louis: Mosby; 2001.

252. Lewit K. *Manipulative Therapy in Rehabilitation of the Motor System,* 3rd ed. London: Butterworths; 1999.

253. Janda DH, Hawkins RJ. Shoulder manipulation in patients with adhesive capsulitis and diabetes mellitus. A clinical note. *J Shoulder Elbow Surg* 1993;2:36–38.

254. Solem-Bertoft E, Thuomas KA, Westerberg CE. The influence of scapular retraction and protraction on the width of the sub-acromial space. *Clin Orthop* 1993;296:99–103.

255. Turner M. Posture and pain. *Phys Ther* 1957;37:294.

256. Jull GA, Janda V. Muscle and motor control in low back pain. In: Twomey LT, Taylor JR, eds. *Physical Therapy of the Low Back: Clinics in Physical Therapy.* New York: Churchill Livingstone; 1987:258.

257. Greenfield B. Upper quarter evaluation: structural relationships and interindependence. In: Donatelli R, Wooden M, eds. *Orthopedic Physical Therapy.* New York: Churchill Livingstone; 1989:43–58.

258. Keller K, Corbett J, Nichols D. Repetitive strain injury in computer keyboard users: pathomechanics and treatment principles in individual and group intervention. *J Hand Ther* 1998;11:9–26.

259. Pratt NE. Neurovascular entrapment in the regions of the shoulder and posterior triangle of the neck. *Phys Ther* 1986; 66:1894–1899.

260. Pecina M, Krmpotic-Nemanic J, Markiewitz A. *Tunnel Syndromes.* Boca Raton, Fla: CRC; 1991.

261. Bourliere F. The assessment of biological age in man. *Public Health Papers,* Vol. 37. 1979, Geneva: WHO.

262. Rayan GM, Jensen C. Thoracic outlet syndrome: provocative examination maneuvers in a typical population. *J Shoulder Elbow Surg* 1995;4:113–117.

263. Sucher BM. Thoracic outlet syndrome—A myofascial variant: Part 2. Treatment. *JAOA* 1990;90:810–823.

264. Jenkins WL. Relationship of overuse impingement with subtle hypomobility or hypermobility. Home Study Course—Solutions to Shoulder Disorders. La Crosse, Wis: Orthopaedic Section, APTA, Inc.; 2001.

265. Diveta J, Walker ML, Skibinski B. Relationship between performance of selected scapular muscles and scapular abduction in standing subjects. *Phys Ther* 1990;70:470–479.

266. Gibson MH, Goebel GV, Jordan TM, et al. A reliability study of measurement techniques to determine static scapular position. *J Orthop Sports Phys Ther* 1995;21:100–106.

266a. Koslow PA, Prosser LA, Strony GA, et al. Specificity of the lateral scapular slide test in asymptomatic competitive athletes. *J Orthop Sports Phys Ther* 2003;33:331–336.

267. Mattingly GE, Mackarey PJ. Optimal methods for shoulder tendon palpation: a cadaver study. *Phys Ther* 1996;76:166–174.

268. Matsen FA, et al. *Practical Evaluation and Management of the Shoulder.* Philadelphia: WB Saunders; 1994.

269. Jackson D, Einhorn A. Rehabilitation of the shoulder. In: Jackson DW, ed. *Shoulder Surgery in the Athlete.* Rockville, Md: Aspen; 1985.

270. Kulund DN. *The Injured Athlete.* Philadelphia: JB Lippincott; 1982.

271. Andrews JR, Gillogly S. Physical examination of the shoulder in throwing athletes. In: Zarin B, Andrews JR, Carson WG, eds. *Injuries to the Throwing Arm.* WB Saunders: Philadelphia; 1985.

272. McClure PW, Flowers KR. Treatment of limited shoulder motion: A case study based on biomechanical considerations. *Phys Ther* 1992;72:929–936.

273. Woo SL-Y, et al. Connective tissue response to immobility: A correlative study of biochemical and biomechanical measurements of normal and immobilized rabbit knee. *Arthritis Rheum* 1975;18:257–264.

274. Akeson WH, et al. The connective tissue response to immobility: biochemical changes in periarticular connective tissue of the immobilized rabbit knee. *Clin Orthop* 1973;93:356–362.

275. Cyriax J. *Textbook of Orthopaedic Medicine, Diagnosis of Soft Tissue Lesions,* 8th ed. London: Bailliere Tindall; 1982.

276. Neviaser RJ, Neviaser TJ. The frozen shoulder. Diagnosis and management. *Clin Orthop* 1987;223:59–64.

277. Johanson MA. Solutions to shoulder disorders. Home Study Course. La Crosse, Wis: Orthopaedic Section, APTA; 2001:1–25.

278. Brems JJ. Rehabilitation following shoulder arthroplasty. In: Friedman RJ, ed. *Arthroplasty of the Shoulder.* New York: Thieme; 1994:99–112.

279. Brown DD, Friedman RJ. Postoperative rehabilitation following total shoulder arthroplasty. *Orthop Clin North Am* 1998;29:535–547.

280. Post M, Mayer J. Suprascapular nerve entrapment: diagnosis and treatment. *Clin Orthop* 1987;223:126–130.

281. Pagnani MJ, Warren RF. Stabilizers of the glenohumeral joint. *J Shoulder Elbow Surg* 1994;3:173–190.

282. Davies GJ, Dickhoff-Hoffman S. Neuromuscular testing and rehabilitation of the shoulder complex. *J Orthop Sports Phys Ther* 1993;18:449–458.

283. Ozaki J. Glenohumeral movements of the involuntary inferior and multidirectional instability. *Clin Orthop* 1989;238:107–111.

284. Leroux JL, et al. Diagnostic value of clinical tests for shoulder impingement. *Rev Rheum* 1995;62:423–428.

285. Itoi E, et al. Which is more useful, the "full can test" or the "empty can test" in detecting the torn supraspinatus tendon? *Am J Sports Med* 1999;27:65–68.

286. Kaltenborn FM. *Manual Mobilization of the Extremity Joints: Basic Examination and Treatment Techniques,* 4th ed. Oslo, Norway: Olaf Norlis Bokhandel, Universitetsgaten; 1989.

287. Winkel D, Matthijs O, Phelps V. Examination of the shoulder. In: *Diagnosis and Treatment of the Upper Extremities.* Aspen: Maryland; 1997:42–67.

288. Pfund R, et al. Manual test for specific structural differentiation in the subacromial space: correlation between specific manual testing and ultrasonography. In: Proceedings of the Tenth Biennial Conference of the Manipulative Physiotherapists Association of Australia. Melbourne: 1997.

289. Jenp Y, et al. Activation of the rotator cuff in generating isometric shoulder rotation torque. *Am J Sports Med* 1996;24:477–485.

290. Gerber C, Krushell RJ. Isolated rupture of the tendon of the subscapularis muscle: clinical features in 16 cases. *J Bone Joint Surg* 1991;73B:389–394.

291. Safee-Rad R, et al. Normal functional range of motion of upper limb joints during performance of three feeding activities. *Arch Phys Med Rehab* 1990;71:505–509.

292. Lippitt SB, Harryman DT III, Matsen FA III. A practical tool for evaluating function. The simple shoulder test. In: Matsen FA III, Fu FH, Hawkins RJ, eds. *The Shoulder: A Balance of Mobility and Stability.* Rosemont, Ill: American Academy of Orthopaedic Surgeons; 1993:501–518.

293. Fuchs B, Jost B, Gerber C. Posterior-inferior capsular shift for the treatment of recurrent, voluntary posterior subluxation of the shoulder. *J Bone Joint Surg* 2000;82A:16–25.

294. Harryman DT II, Matsen FA III, Sidles JA. Arthroscopic management of refractory shoulder stiffness. *Arthroscopy* 1997;13:133–147.

295. Matsen FA, et al. Evaluating the Shoulder. In: Matsen FA, et al, eds. *Practical Evaluation and Management of the Shoulder.* Philadelphia: WB Saunders; 1994:1–17.

296. Beaton DE, Richards RR. Measuring function of the shoulder. A cross-sectional comparison of five questionnaires. *J Bone Joint Surg* 1996;78A:882–890.

297. Beaton DE, Richards RR. Assessing the reliability and responsiveness of five shoulder questionnaires. *J Shoulder Elbow Surg* 1998;7:565–572.

298. Hudak PL, et al. Development of an upper extremity outcome measure: the DASH (Disabilities of the Arm, Shoulder, and Hand). *Am J Ind Med* 1995;29:602–608.

299. Falsone SA, et al. One-arm hop test: reliability and effects of arm dominance. *J Orthop Sports Phys Ther* 2002;32:98–103.

300. Calis M, et al. Diagnostic values of clinical diagnostic tests in subacromial impingement syndrome. *Ann Rheum Dis* 2000; 59:44–47.

301. Frieman BG, Albert TJ, Fenlin JM. Rotator cuff disease: a review of diagnosis, pathophysiology and current trends in treatment. *Arch Phys Med Rehabil* 1994;75:604–609.

302. Post M, Cohen J. Impingement syndrome: a review of late stage II and early stage III lesions. *Clin Orthop* 1986;207:127–132.

303. Hawkins RJ, Kennedy JC. Impingement syndrome in athletics. *Am J Sports Med* 1980;8:151–163.

304. Pink MM, Jobe FW. Biomechanics of swimming. In: Zachazewski JE, Magee DJ, Quillen WS, eds. *Athletic Injuries and Rehabilitation*. Philadelphia: WB Saunders; 1996:317–331.

305. Ure BM, et al. Zuverlassigkeit der klinischen untersuchung der schulter im vergleich zur arthroskopie. *Unfallchirurg* 1993;96:382–386.

306. Rupp S, Berninger K, Hopf T. Shoulder problems in high level swimmers—impingement, anterior instability, muscular imbalance. *Int J Sports Med* 1995;16:557–562.

307. Patte D, et al. Over-extension lesions. *Rev Chir Orthop* 1988;74:314–318.

308. Arthuis M. Obstetrical paralysis of the brachial plexus I. diagnosis: clinical study of the initial period. *Rev Chir Orthop Reparatrice Appar Mot* 1972;58:124–136.

309. Walch G, et al. The "dropping" and "hornblower's" signs in evaluation of rotator-cuff tears. *J Bone Joint Surg Br* 1998; 80:624–628.

310. Tomberlin J. Physical diagnostic tests of the shoulder: An evidence-based perspective. Home Study Course—Solutions to Shoulder Disorders. La Crosse, Wis: Orthopedic Section, APTA, Inc.; 2001.

311. Akgün K. Kronik subakromiyal sikisma sendromunun konservatif tedavisinde ultrasonun etkinligi. [Proficiency Thesis]. Istanbul: University of Istanbul; 1993.

312. Warren RF. Shoulder pain. In: Paget S, Pellicci P, Beary JF, eds. *Manual of Rheumatology and Outpatient Orthopaedic Disorders*. Boston: Little, Brown; 1993;99–109.

313. Akgün K, et al. Subakromiyal sikisma sendromu klinik tanisinda sikisma (Neer) testinin önemi. *Fizik Tedavi ve Rehabilitasyon Dergisi* 1997;22:5–7.

314. Maitland G. *Peripheral Manipulation,* 3rd ed. London: Butterworth; 1991.

315. Mullen F. Locking and quadrant of the shoulder: relationships of the humerus and scapula during locking and quadrant. In: Proceedings of the Sixth Biennial Conference, Manipulative Therapist Association of Australia. Adelaide, Australia: 1989.

316. Neer CS. Anatomy of shoulder reconstruction. In: Neer CS, ed. *Shoulder Reconstruction*. Philadelphia: WB Saunders; 1990:1–39.

317. Glascow S, et al. Arthroscopic resection of glenoid labral tears in the athlete. *Arthroscopy* 1992;8:48–54.

318. Liu SH, et al. Diagnosis of glenoid labral tears: a comparison between magnetic resonance imaging and clinical examinations. *Am J Sports Med* 1996;24:149–154.

319. Hurley JA, Andersen TE. Shoulder arthroscopy: its role in evaluating shoulder disorders in the athlete. *Am J Sports Med* 1990;18:480–483.

320. Liu SH, Henry MH, Nuccion SL. A prospective evaluation of a new physical examination in predicting glenoid labral tears. *Am J Sports Med* 1996;24:721–725.

321. Field LD, Savoie FH. Arthroscopic suture repair of superior labral detachment lesions of the shoulder. *Am J Sports Med* 1993;21:783–791.

322. Magee DJ. Shoulder. In: *Orthopedic Physical Assessment.* Philadelphia: WB Saunders; 1992:90–142.

323. Yergason RM. Rupture of biceps. *J Bone Joint Surg* 1931; 13:160.

324. Bak K, and Faunl P. Clinical findings in competitive swimmers with shoulder pain. *Am J Sports Med* 1997;25:254–260.

325. O'Brien SJ, et al. The active compression test; a new and effective test for diagnosing labral tears and acromioclavicular abnormality. *Am J Sports Med* 1998;26:610–613.

326. Kibler WB, Specificity and sensitivity of the anterior slide test in throwing athletes with superior glenoid labral tears. *Arthroscopy* 1995;11:296–300.

327. Engebretsen L, Craig EV. Radiographic features of shoulder instability. *Clin Orthop* 1993;291:29–44.

328. Neer CSI. Involuntary inferior and multidirectional instability of the shoulder: Etiology, recognition, and treatment. *Instr Course Lect* 1985;34:232–238.

329. Neer CSI. Foster CR. Inferior capsular shift for involuntary inferior and multidirectional instability of the shoulder. *J Bone Joint Surg* 1980;62A:897–908.

330. Pollock RG. Multidirectional and Posterior Instability of the Shoulder. In: Norris TR, ed. *Orthopaedic Knowledge Update: Shoulder and Elbow.* American Academy of Orthopaedic Surgeons: Rosemont, Ill; 1997:85–94.

331. Emery RJH, Mullaji AB. Glenohumeral joint instability in normal adolescents: Incidence and significance. *J Bone Joint Surg* 1991;73B:406–408.

332. Lintner SA. et al. Glenohumeral translation in the asymptomatic athlete's shoulder and its relationship to other clinically measurable anthropometric variables. *Am J Sports Med* 1996; 24:716–720.

333. Brown, GA, JL. Tan, and Kirkley A. The lax shoulder in females. Issues, answers, but many more questions. *Clinical Orthopaedics & Related Research,* 2000;372:110–22.

334. Bigliani LU. The unstable shoulder. Rosemont, Ill: *Amer Acad Orthop Surg* 1995.

335. Gerber C, Ganz R. Clinical assessment of instability of the shoulder. *J Bone Joint Surg* 1984;66B:551.

336. Hawkins RJ, et al. Translation of the glenohumeral joint with the patient under anesthesia. *J Shoulder Elbow Surg* 1996; 5:286–292.

337. Hanyman DT, et al. Translation of the humeral head on the glenoid with passive glenohumeral motion. *J Bone and Joint Surg* 1990;72A:1334.

338. Mok DWH, et al. The diagnostic value of arthroscopy in glenohumeral instability. *J Bone Joint Surg* 1990;72B: 698–700.

339. Callanan M, et al. Shoulder instability. Diagnosis and management. *Australian Family Physician* 2001;30:655–61.

340. Jobe FW, Bradley JP. The diagnosis and nonoperative treatment of shoulder injuries in athletes. *Clin Sports Med* 1989; 8:419–439.

341. Speer KP, et al. An evaluation of the shoulder relocation test. *Am J Sports Med* 1994;22:177–183.

342. Rockwood CA, Subluxations and dislocations about the shoulder. In: Rockwood CA, Green DP, eds. *Fractures in Adults–I.* Philadelphia: JB Lippincott; 1984.

343. Gross ML, Distefano MC. Anterior release test: a new test for occult shoulder instability. *Clin Orth Rel Res* 1997;339: 105–108.

344. Rockwood CA, Jr, et al. X-ray evaluation of shoulder problems. In: Rockwood CA, Jr. and Matsen FA, III, eds. *The Shoulder.* Philadelphia, Pa: WB Saunders Co; 1990:178–207.

345. Rubin SA, Gray RL, Green WR. The scapular "Y" view: a diagnostic aid in shoulder trauma. A technical note. *Radiology* 1974;110:725–726.

346. Swen WA, et al. Is sonography performed by the rheumatologist as useful as arthrography executed by the radiologist for the assessment of full thickness rotator cuff tears? *J Rheum* 1998;25: 1800–1806.

347. Kneeland JB. Magnetic resonance imaging: general principles and techniques. In: Iannotti JP, Williams GR. eds. *Disorders of the Shoulder: Diagnosis and Management.* Philadelphia, Pa: Lippincott Williams & Wilkins; 1999:911–925.

348. Tirman PF, et al. Association of glenoid labral cysts with labral tears and glenohumeral instability: radiologic findings and clinical significance. *Radiology* 1994;190:653–658.

349. Magarey ME, Hayes MG, Trott PH. The accuracy of manipulative physiotherapy diagnosis of shoulder complex dysfunction: a pilot study. In: *Proceedings of the Sixth Biennial Conference.* Adelaide: Manipulative Physiotherapists Association of Australia; 1989.

350. Magarey ME, et al. The shoulder complex: a preliminary analysis of diagnostic agreement reached from a physiotherapy clinical examination and an arthroscopic evaluation. In: *Clinical Solutions: Proceedings of the Ninth Biennial Conference.* Gold Coast: Manipulative Physiotherapists Association of Australia; 1995.

351. Litchfield R, et al. Rehabilitation of the overhead athlete. *J Orthop Sports Phys Ther* 1993;2:433–441.

352. Booth F.W. Physiologic and biochemical effects of immobilization on muscle. *Clin Orthop Relat Res* 1987;219:15–21.

353. Eiff MP, Smith AT, Smith GE. Early mobilization versus immobilization in the treatment of lateral ankle sprains. *Am J Sports Med* 1994;22:83–88.

354. Akeson WH, et al. Collagen cross-linking alterations in the joint contractures: changes in the reducible cross-links in periarticular connective tissue after 9 weeks immobilization. *Connect. Tissue Res* 1977;5:15.

355. Akeson WH, et al. Effects of immobilization on joints. *Clin Orthop* 1987;219:28–37.

356. Wilk KE, Arrigo C, Andrews JR. Rehabilitation of the elbow in the throwing athlete. *J Orthop Sports Phys Ther* 1993;17: 305–317.

357. Coutts RD. Continuous passive motion in the rehabilitation of the total knee patient. It's role and effect. *Orthop Rev* 1986;15:27.

358. Dehne E, Tory R. Treatment of joint injuries by immediate mobilization based upon the spiral adaption concept. *Clin Orthop* 1971;77:218–232.

359. Haggmark T, Eriksson E. Cylinder or mobile cast brace after knee ligament surgery. *Am J Sports Med* 1979; 7:48–56.

360. Noyes FR, Mangine RE, Barber S. Early knee motion after open and arthroscopic anterior cruciate ligament reconstruction. *Am J Sports Med* 1987;15:149–160.

361. Kibler BW. Closed kinetic chain rehabilitation for sports injuries. *Phys Med Rehab No Amer* 2000;11(2):369–384.

362. Dillman CJ, Murray TA, Hintermeister RA. Biomechanical differences of open and closed chain exercises with respect to the shoulder. *J Sport Rehabil* 1994;3:228–238.

363. Kibler WB. Concepts in exercise rehabilitation of athletic injury. In: Leadbetter WB, Buckwalter JA, and Gordon SL, eds. *Sports-Induced Inflammation: Clinical and Basic Science Concepts.* Park Ridge, Ill: American Academy of Orthopaedic Surgeons; 1990:759–769.

364. Neer CSI, Watson KC, Stanton FJ. Recent experience in total shoulder replacement. *J Bone and Joint Surg* 1982;64: 319–337.

365. Walch G, et al. Static posterior subluxation of the humeral head: an unrecognized entity responsible for glenohumeral osteoarthritis in the young adult. *J Shoulder Elbow Surg* 2002;11:309–314.

366. Hayes PRL, Flatow EL. Total shoulder arthroplasty in the young patient. *AAOS Instr Course Lect* 2001;50:73–88.

367. DeSeze M, *L'épaule sénile hémorragique. L'actualité rhumatologique.* Paris: Expansion Scientifique Française; 1968: 107–115.

368. Garancis JC, et al. "Milwaukee shoulder"—association of microspheroids containing hydroxyapatite crystals, active collagenase, and neutral protease with rotator cuff defects. III. Morphologic and biochemical studies of an excised synovium showing chondromatosis. *Arthrit Rheumat* 1981;24: 484–491.

369. Halverson PB, et al. "Milwaukee shoulder"—association of microspheroids containing hydroxyapatite crystals, active collagenase, and neutral protease with rotator cuff defects. II. Synovial fluid studies. *Arthrit Rheumat* 1981;24:474–483.

370. McCarty DJ, et al. "Milwaukee shoulder"—association of microspheroids containing hydroxyapatite crystals, active collagenase, and neutral protease with rotator cuff defects. I. Clinical aspects. *Arthrit Rheumat* 1981;24:464–473.

371. Jensen KL, et al. Rotator Cuff Tear Arthropathy. *J Bone Joint Surg—Amer* 1999;81-A(9):1312–1324.

372. Neer CS, II, Craig EV, Fukuda H. Cuff-tear arthropathy. *J Bone Joint Surg* 1983;65-A:1232–1244.

373. Duplay S, De la péri-arthrite scapulo-humérale et des raideurs de l'épaule qui en sont la consequénce. *Arch Gen Med* 1872; 20:513–542.

374. Neviaser JS. Adhesive capsulitis of the shoulder. Study of pathological findings in periarthritis of the shoulder. *J Bone Joint Surg* 1945;27:211–222.

375. Binder AI, et al. Frozen shoulder: A long-term prospective study. *Ann Rheum Dis* 1984;43:361–364.

376. Lloyd-Roberts, GG. and PR. French, Periarthritis of the shoulder: A study of the disease and its treatment. *Br Med J* 1959;1: 1569–1574.

377. Bridgman JF. Periarthritis of the shoulder and diabetes mellitus. *Ann Rheum Dis* 1972;31:69–71.

378. Miller MD, Rockwood CA, Jr. Thawing the frozen shoulder: The "patient" patient. *Orthopedics,* 1997;19:849–853.

379. Pal B, Anderson JJ, Dick WC. Limitations of joint mobility and shoulder capsulitis in insulin and noninsulin dependent diabetes mellitus. *Br J Rheumatol* 1986;25:147–151.

380. Fisher L, Kurtz A, Shipley M. Relationship of cheiroarthropathy and frozen shoulder in patients with insulin dependent diabetes mellitus. *Br J Rheum* 1986;25:141.

381. DePalma AF. Loss of scapulohumeral motion (frozen shoulder). *Ann Surg* 1952;135:193–197.

382. Bowman CA, Jeffcoate WJ, Patrick M. Bilateral adhesive capsulitis, oligoarthritis and proximal myopathy as presentation of hypothyroidism. *Br J Rheumatol* 1988;27:62–64.

383. Speer KP, et al. A role for hydrotherapy in shoulder rehabilitation. *Am J Sports Med* 1993;21:850–853.

384. Wohlgethan JR. Frozen shoulder in hyperthyroidism. *Arthritis Rheum* 1987;30:936–939.

385. Mintner WT. The shoulder-hand syndrome in coronary disease. *J Med Assoc GA* 1967;56:45–49.

386. Coventry MB. Problem of the painful shoulder. *JAMA* 1953;151:177.

387. Tyber MA. Treatment of the painful shoulder syndrome with amitriptyline and lithium carbonate. *Can Med Assoc J* 1974;111:137.

388. Bulgen DY, Binder A, Hazelman BL. Immunological studies in frozen shoulder. *J Rheumatol* 1982;9:893–898.

389. Rizk TE, Pinals RS. Histocompatibility type and racial incidence in frozen shoulder. *Arch Phys Med Rehabil* 1984;65:33–34.

390. Lundberg BJ. The frozen shoulder. *Acta Orthop Scand* 1969;119(Suppl):1–5.

391. Hannafin JA, Chiaia TA. Adhesive capsulitis. A treatment approach. *Clin Orthop* 2000;372:95–109.

392. Nash P, Hazelman BD. Frozen shoulder. *Baillieres Clin Rheumatol* 1989;3:551–566.

393. Neviaser JS. Adhesive capsulitis and the stiff and painful shoulder. *Orthop Clin North Am* 1980;11:327–331.

394. Neviaser RJ. Painful conditions affecting the shoulder. *Clin Orthop* 1983;173:63–69.

395. Reeves B. The natural history of the frozen shoulder syndrome. *Scand J Rheumatol* 1975;4:193–196.

396. Zuckerman JD, Cuomo F. Frozen shoulder. In: Matsen FA, Fu FH, Hawkins RJ, eds. *The Shoulder: A Balance of Mobility and Stability.* Rosemont, Ill: American Academy of Orthopaedic Surgeons; 1993:253–267.

397. Shaffer B, Tibone JE, Kerlan RK. Frozen shoulder: A long-term follow-up. *J Bone Joint Surg Am* 1992;74:738–746.

398. Griggs SM, Ahn A, Green A. Idiopathic adhesive capsulitis: A prospective functional outcome study of nonoperative treatment. *J Bone Joint Surg Am* 2000;82-A(10):1398–1407.

399. Hannafin JA, et al. Adhesive capsulitis: Capsular fibroplasia of the glenohumeral joint. *J Shoulder Elbow Surg* 1994;3(Suppl):5.

400. Rodeo SA, et al. Immunolocalization of cytokines and their receptors in adhesive capsulitis of the shoulder. *J Orthop Res* 1997;15:427–436.

401. Wiley AM. Arthroscopic appearance of frozen shoulder. *Arthroscopy* 1991;7:138–143.

402. Bunker, T.D. and P.P. Anthony, The pathology of frozen shoulder. A Dupuytren-like disease. *J Bone Joint Surg* 1995;77B:677–683.

403. Grubbs N. Frozen shoulder syndrome: A review of literature. *J Orthop Sports Phys Ther* 1993;18:479–487.

404. Uhthoff HK, Sarkar K. An algorithm for shoulder pain caused by soft tissue disorders. *Clin Orthop* 1990;254:121.

405. Boyle-Walker KL, et al. A profile of patients with adhesive capsulitis. *J Hand Ther* 1997;10:222–228.

406. Tamai K, Yamato M. Abnormal synovium in the frozen shoulder: A preliminary report with dynamic magnetic resonance imaging. *J Shoulder Elbow Surg* 1997;6:534–543.

407. McClure PW, Flowers KR. Treatment of limited shoulder motion using an elevation splint. *Phys Ther* 1992;72:57.

408. Laska T, Hannig K. Physical Therapy for spinal accessory nerve injury complicated by adhesive capsulitis. *Phys Ther* 2001;81(3):936–944.

409. Rizk TE, et al. Adhesive capsulitis (frozen shoulder): A new approach to its management and treatment. *Arch Phys Med Rehabil* 1983;64:29–33.

410. Tovin BJ, Greenfield BH. Impairment-based diagnosis for the shoulder girdle. In: *Evaluation and Treatment of the Shoulder: An Integration of the Guide to Physical Therapist Practice.* Philadelphia: F.A. Davis; 2001:55–74.

411. Haggart GE, Digman RJ, Sullivan TS. Management of the "frozen" shoulder. *JAMA* 1956;161:1219–1222.

412. Leffert RD. The frozen shoulder. *Instructional Course Lectures* 1985;34:199–203.

413. Owens-Burkhart H, Management of Frozen Shoulder. In: Donatelli RA. ed. *Physical Therapy of the Shoulder,* New York: Churchill Livingstone; 1991:91–116.

414. Wadsworth CT. Frozen shoulder. *Phys Ther* 1986;(66):1878–1883.

415. Grey RG. The natural history of "idiopathic" frozen shoulder. *J Bone Joint Surg Am* 1978;60:564.

416. Withers RJW. The painful shoulder: Review of one hundred personal cases with remarks on the pathology. *J Bone Joint Surg* 1949;31:414–417.

417. Clarke GR, et al. Preliminary studies in measuring range of motion in normal and painful stiff shoulder. *Rheumatol Rehabil* 1975;14:39–46.

418. Bulgen DY, et al. Frozen shoulder: Prospective clinical study with an evaluation of three treatment regimens. *Ann Rheum Dis* 1984;43:353–360.

419. D'Acre JE, Beeney N, Scott DL. Injections and physiotherapy for the painful stiff shoulder. *Ann Rheum Dis* 1989; 48:322–325.

420. DeJong BA, et al. Intraarticular triamcinolone acetonide injection in patients with capsulitis of the shoulder: A comparative study of two dose regimes. *Clin Rehab* 1998;12:211–215.

421. Quigley TB. Indications for manipulation and corticosteroids in the treatment of stiff shoulder. *Surg Clin North Am* 1975;43:1715–1720.

422. Steinbrocker O, Argyros TG. Frozen shoulder: Treatment by local injection of depot corticosteroids. *Arch Phys Med Rehabil* 1974;55:209–213.

423. Hazelman BD. The painful stiff shoulder. *Rheumatol Phys Med* 1972;11:413–421.

424. Binder A, et al. A controlled study of oral prednisone in frozen shoulder. *Br J Rheumatol* 1986;25:288–292.

425. Gerber C, Galantay R, Hersche O. The pattern of pain produced by irritation of the acromioclavicular joint and the subacromial space. *J Shoulder Elbow Surg* 1998;7:352–355.

426. Tyler TF, et al. Reliability and validity of a new method of measuring posterior shoulder tightness. *J Orthop Sports Phys Ther* 1999;29:262–274.

427. Kennedy JC, Alexander IJ, Hayes KC. Nerve supply of the human knee and its functional importance. *Am J Sports Med* 1982;10:329–335.

428. Baxendale RA, Ferrell WR, Wood L. Responses of quadriceps motor units to mechanical stimulation of knee joint receptors in decerebate cat. *Brain Res* 1988;453:150–156.

429. Lippitt SB, et al. In vivo quantification of the laxity of normal and unstable glenohumeral joints. *J Shoulder Elbow Surg* 1994; 3:215–223.

430. Flatow EL, Warner JJP. Instability of the shoulder: Complex problems and failed repairs: Part I. Relevant biomechanics, multidirectional instability, and severe glenoid loss. *Instr Course Lect* 1998;47:97–112.

431. Rowe CR, and Sakellarides HT. Factors related to recurrences of anterior dislocations of the shoulder. *Clin Orthop* 1961;20:40.

432. Maki NJ. Cineradiographic studies with shoulder instabilities. *Am J Sports Med* 1988;16:362–364.

433. Sidles JA, et al. In vivo quantification of glenohumeral stability. *Trans Orthop Res Soc* 1991;16:646.

434. Gill TD, et al. Bankhart repair for anterior instability of the shoulder: long term outcomes. *J Bone and Joint Surg* 1997; 79A:850–857.

435. Garth WP, Allman FL, Armstrong WS. Occult anterior subluxations of the shoulder in noncontact sports. *Am J Sports Med* 1987;15:579–585.

436. Jobe FW, et al. The shoulder in sports. In: Rockwood CA Jr. Matsen FA. III, ed. *The Shoulder;* Philadelphia, Pa: WB Saunders Co; 1990:963–967.

437. Schenk TJ, Brems JJ. Multidirectional instability of the shoulder: Pathophysiology, diagnosis, and management. *J Am Acad Orthop Surgeons* 1998;6:65–72.

438. Hawkins RJ, Abrams JS, Schutte J. Multidirectional instability of the shoulder—An approach to diagnosis. *Orthop Trans* 1987;11:246.

439. Berbig R, et al. Primary anterior shoulder dislocation and rotator cuff tears. *J Shoulder Elbow Surg* 1999;8:220–225.

440. Sonnabend DH. Treatment of primary anterior shoulder dislocation in patients older than 40 years of age. *Clin Orthop* 1994; 304:74–77.

441. Tijimes J, Loyd HM, Tullos HS. Arthrography in acute shoulder dislocations. *South Med J* 1979;72:564–567.

442. Arendt EA. Multidirectional shoulder instability. *Orthopedics* 1988;11:113–120.

443. Ireland ML. Andrews JR. Shoulder and elbow injuries in the young athlete. *Clin Sports Med* 1988;7:473–494.

444. Hovelius L, et al. Recurrences after initial dislocation of the shoulder. *J Bone Joint Surg Am* 1983;65:343–349.

445. Burkhart SS, Morgan CD, Kibler WB. Shoulder injuries in overhead athletes: the "dead arm" revisited. *Clin Sports Med* 2000;19:125–158.

446. Snyder SJ, et al. SLAP lesions of the shoulder. *Arthoscopy* 1990;6:274.

447. Morgan CD. et al. Type II SLAP lesions: three subtypes and their relationship to superior instability and rotator cuff tears. *Arthroscopy* 1998;14:553–565.

448. Berg EE, DeHoll D. Radiography of the medial elbow ligaments. *J Shoulder Elbow Surg* 1997;6:528–533.

449. Urban WP, Babom DNM. Management of superior labral anterior posterior lesions. *Oper Tech Orthop* 1995;5:223.

450. Mileski RA, Snyder SJ. Superior labral lesions in the shoulder: Pathoanatomy and surgical management. *J Am Acad Orthop Surgeons* 1998;6:121–131.

451. Cordasco FA, Bigliani LU. Multidirectional Shoulder Instability: Open Surgical Treatment. In: Warren RF, Craig EV, Altchek DW, eds. *The Unstable Shoulder.* Philadelphia: Lippincott-Raven Publishers; 1999;249–261.

452. Altchek DW, et al. Arthroscopic labral debridement: A three year follow-up study. *Am J Sports Med* 1992;20:702.

453. Snyder SJ, Banas MP, Karzel RP. An analysis of 140 injuries to the superior glenoid labrum. *J Shoulder Elbow Surg* 1995;4:243–248.

454. Berg EE, Ciullo JV. The SLAP lesion: a cause of failure after distal clavicle resection. *Arthroscopy* 1997;13:85–89.

455. Lippitt SB, et al. Diagnosis and management of AMBRII syndrome. *Tech Orthop* 1991;6:61.

456. Borsa PA, Sauers EL, Herling DE. Patterns of glenohumeral joint laxity and stiffness in healthy men and women. *Med Sci Sports Exerc* 2000;32:1685–1690.

457. Huston LJ, Wojtys EM. Neuromuscular performance characteristics in elite female athletes. *Am J Sports Med* 1996;24:427–436.

458. Burkhead WZ Jr, Rockwood CA Jr. Treatment of instability of the shoulder with an exercise program. *J Bone Joint Surg* 1992;74A:890–896.

459. Lephart SM, et al. Proprioception of the shoulder joint in healthy, unstable and surgically repaired shoulders. *J Shoulder Elbow Surg* 1994;3:371–380.

460. Schneider R, Prentice WE. Rehabilitation of the shoulder. In: Prentice WE, Voight ML, eds. *Techniques in Musculoskeletal Rehabilitation.* New York: McGraw-Hill; 2001:411–456.

461. Happee R, Van Der Helm FCT. The control of shoulder muscles during goal directed movements. *J Biomech* 1995; 28:1179–1191.

462. Tossy JD, Mead MC, Simond HM. Acromioclavicular separations: Useful and practical classification for treatment. *Clin Orthop* 1963;28:111–119.

463. Rockwood CA Jr. Injuries to the acromioclavicular joint. In: Rockwood CA Jr, Green DP, eds. *Fractures in Adults.* Philadelphia: JB Lippincott; 1984:860–910.

464. Williams GR, Nguyen VD, Rockwood CA Jr. Classification and radiographic analysis of acromioclavicular dislocations. *Appl Radiol* 1989;28:29–34.

465. Wirth MA, Rockwood CA Jr. Chronic Conditions of the acromioclavicular and sternoclavicular joints. In: Chapman MW, ed. *Operative Orthopaedics.* Philadelphia: JB Lippincott; 1993:1673–1683.

466. Gordon EJ. Diagnosis and treatment of common shoulder disorders. *Med Trial Tech Q* 1981;28:25–73.

467. Bannister GC, et al. The management of acute acromioclavicular dislocation: a randomized prospective controlled trial. *J Bone Joint Surg* 1989;71B:848–850.

468. Cox JS. Current method of treatment of acromioclavicular joint dislocations. *Orthopedics* 1992;15:1041–1044.

469. Bjerneld H, Hovelius L, Thorling J. Acromioclavicular separations treated conservatively: a five year follow-up study. *Acta Orthop Scand* 1983;54:743–745.

470. Dias JJ, et al. The conservative treatment of acromioclavicular dislocation: review after five years. *J Bone Joint Surg* 1987; 69B:719–722.

471. Glick JM, et al. Dislocated acromioclavicular joint: follow-up study of thirty-five unreduced acromioclavicular dislocations. *Am J Sports Med* 1977;5:264–270.

472. Rawes ML, Dias JJ. Long-term results of conservative treatment for acromioclavicular dislocation. *J Bone Joint Surg* 1996; 78B:410–412.

473. Sleeswijk-Viser SV, Haarsma SM, Speeckaert MTC. Conservative treatment of acromioclavicular dislocation: Jones strap versus mitella. *Acta Orthop Scand* 1984;55:483.

474. Tibone J, Sellers R, Tonino P. Strength testing after third-degree acromioclavicular dislocations. *Am J Sports Med* 1992;20:328–331.

475. Larsen E, Bjerg-Nielsen A, Christensen P. Conservative or surgical treatment of acromioclavicular dislocation: a prospective, controlled randomized study. *J Bone Joint Surg* 1986;68A:552–555.

476. Taft TN, Wilson FC, Oglesby JW. Dislocation of the acromioclavicular joint: an end-result study. *J Bone Joint Surg* 1987;69A:1045–1051.

477. Van der Windt DA, et al. Shoulder disorders in general practice: Incidence, patient characteristics, and management. *Ann Rheum Dis* 1995;54:959–964.

478. Goldberg BA, Nowinski RJ, Matsen FA III. Outcome of nonoperative management of full-thickness rotator cuff tears. *Clin Orthop* 2001;1:99–107.

479. Kunkel SS, Hawkins RJ. Open repair of the rotator cuff. In: Andrews JR, Wilk KE, eds. *The Athlete's Shoulder.* New York: Churchill Livingstone; 1994:141–151.

480. Leffert RD, Rowe CR. Tendon ruptures. In: Rowe CR, ed. *The Shoulder.* New York: Churchill Livingstone; 1988:131–154.

481. Pettersson G. Rupture of the tendon aponeurosis of the shoulder joint in anterior inferior dislocation. *Acta Chir Scand* 1942;77(suppl):1–184.

482. Yamanaka K, et al. Incomplete thickness tears of the rotator cuff. *Orthop Traumatol Surg [Tokyo]* 1983;26:713–717.

483. Uhtoff HK, Loehr J, Sarkar K. The pathogenesis of rotator cuff tears. In: Proceedings of the Third International Conference on Surgery of the Shoulder. Fukuoka, Japan: October 27, 1986.

484. Cuillo J. Swimmer's shoulder. *Clin Sports Med* 1984;5:115.

485. Chard M, Sattele L, Hazleman B. The long-term outcome of rotator cuff tendinitis—A review study. *Br J Rheum* 1988;27:385–389.

486. Evans P. The healing process at cellular level: A review. *Physiotherapy* 1980;66:256–260.

487. Wilk KE, Arrigo C, Andrews JR. Current concepts in rehabilitation of the athlete's shoulder. *J South Orthop Assoc* 1994;3:216–231.

488. Davies GJ. Compendium of isokinetics In: *Clinical Usage and Rehabilitation Techniques,* 4th ed. Onalaska, Wis: S & S Publishers; 1992.

489. Dvir Z. Isokinetics: muscle testing, interpretation and clinical applications. New York: Churchill Livingstone; 1995.

490. Nitz AJ. Physical therapy management of the shoulder. *Phys Ther* 1986;66:1912–1919.

491. Nicholson GG. The effects of passive joint mobilization on pain and hypomobility associated with adhesive capsulitis of the shoulder. *J Orthop Sports Phys Ther* 1985;6:238–246.

492. Bang MD, Deyle GD. Comparison of supervised exercise with and without manual physical therapy for patients with shoulder impingement syndrome. *J Orthop Sports Phys Ther* 2000;30:126–137.

493. Bartolozzi A, Andreychik D, Ahmad S. Determinants of outcome in the treatment of rotator cuff disease. *Clin Orthop* 1994;308:90–97.

494. Brox JI, et al. Arthroscopic surgery compared with supervised exercises in patients with rotator cuff disease (stage II impingement syndrome). *Br Med J* 1993;307:899–903.

495. Ginn KA, et al. A randomized controlled clinical trial of a treatment for shoulder pain. *Phys Ther* 1997;77:802–811.

496. Norwood LA, Barrack RL, Jacobson KE. Clinical presentation of complete tears of the rotator cuff. *J Bone Joint Surg Am* 1989;71:499–505.

497. Bateman JE. Diagnosis and treatment of rupture of the rotator cuff. *Surg Clin North Am* 1963;43:1523–1530.

498. Ellman H, Hanker G, Bayer M. Repair of the rotator cuff: End results of factors influencing reconstruction. *J Bone Joint Surg* 1986;68A:1136–1142.

499. Essman JA, Bell RH, Askew M. Full-thickness rotator-cuff tear. Analysis of results. *Clin Orthop* 1991;265:170–177.

500. Hawkins RJ. Surgical management of rotator cuff tears in surgery of the shoulder. In: Bateman JE, Welsh RP, eds. *Surgery of the Shoulder.* New York: Dekker; 1984:161–175.

501. Bokor DJ, et al. Results of nonoperative management of full-thickness tears of the rotator cuff. *Clin Orthop* 1993;294:103–110.

502. Hawkins RH, Dunlop R. Nonoperative treatment of rotator cuff tears. *Clin Orthop* 1995;321:178–188.

503. Itoi E, Tabata S. Conservative treatment of rotator cuff tears. *Clin Orthop* 1992;275:165–173.

504. Matsen FA III, Arntz CT, Lippitt SB. Rotator cuff. In: Rockwood CA, Matsen FA III, eds. *The Shoulder.* Philadelphia: WB Saunders; 1998:810–813.

505. Matsen FH III, et al. *Practical Evaluation of Management of the Shoulder.* Philadelphia: WB Saunders; 1994:19–150.

506. Nixon JE, DiStefano V. Ruptures of the rotator cuff. *Orthop Clin North Am* 1975;6:423–445.

507. Ellman H. Diagnosis and treatment of incomplete rotator cuff tears. *Clin Orthop* 1990;254:64–74.

508. Ford LT, DeBender J. Tendon rupture after local steroid injection. *South Med J* 1979;72:827–830.

509. Watson M. Major ruptures of the rotator cuff: The results of surgical repair in 89 patients. *J Bone Joint Surg Br* 1985;67:618–624.

510. Kennedy JD, Willis RB. The effects of local steroid injections on tendons: A biomechanical and microscopic correlative study. *Am J Sports Med* 1976;4:11–21.

511. Adebago A, Nash P, Hazleman BL. A prospective double-blind dummy placebo controlled study comparing triamcinolone hexacetomide injection with oral diclofenac 50 mg TDS in patients with rotator cuff tendinitis. *J Rheum* 1990;17:1207–1209.

512. Hollingworth GR, Ellis RM, Hattersley TS. Comparison of injection techniques for shoulder pain: Results of a double-blind, randomized study. *BMJ* 1983;287:1339–1341.

513. Jobe CM. Posterior superior glenoid impingement: expanded spectrum. *Arthroscopy* 1995;11:530–539.

514. Paley KJ, et al. Arthroscopic findings in the overhand throwing athletes: evidence of posterior internal impingement of the rotator cuff. *Arthoscopy* 2000;16:35–40.

515. Neviaser TJ. The role of the biceps tendon in the impingement syndrome. *Orthop Clin North Am* 1987;18:383–386.

516. Hammer WI. The use of transverse friction massage in the management of chronic bursitis of the hip or shoulder. *J Man Physiol Ther* 1993;16:107–111.

517. Uhthoff HK, Sarkar K. Calcifying tendinitis. In: Rockwood CA Jr, Matsen FA III, eds. *The Shoulder.* Philadelphia: WB Saunders Co; 1990:774–788.

518. Ebenbichler GR, et al. Ultrasound therapy for calcific tendinitis of the shoulder. *New Engl J Med* 1999;340:1533–1538.

519. Bosworth BM. Calcium deposits in the shoulder and subacromial bursitis: a survey of 12,122 shoulders. *JAMA* 1941;116:2477–2482.

520. McKendry RJR, et al. Calcifying tendinitis of the shoulder: prognostic value of clinical, histologic, and radiologic features in 57 surgically treated cases. *J Rheumatol* 1982;9:75–80.

521. Booth RE Jr, Marvel JR Jr. Differential diagnosis of shoulder pain. *Orthop Clin North Am* 1975;6:353–379.

522. Chard MD, et al. Rotator cuff degeneration and lateral epicondylitis: a comparative histological study. *Ann Rheum Dis* 1994;53:30–34.

523. Uhthoff HK. Calcifying tendinitis. *Ann Chir Gynaecol* 1996; 85:111–115.

524. Uhtoff HK, Sarkar K, Maynard JA. Calcifying tendinitis. *Clin Orthop* 1976;118:164–168.

525. Wefling J, Kahn MF, Desroy M. Les calcifications de l'epaule, II: la maladie des calcifications tendineuses multiples. *Rev Rheum* 1965;32:325–334.

526. Loew M, et al. Treatment of calcifying tendinitis of rotator cuff by extracorporeal shock waves: a preliminary report. *J Shoulder Elbow Surg* 1995;4:101–106.

527. Rompe JD, et al. Extracorporal shock wave therapy for calcifying tendinitis of the shoulder. *Clin Orthop* 1995;321:196–201.

528. Ter Haar G, Dyson M, Oakley EM. The use of ultrasound by physiotherapists in Britain, 1985. *Ultrasound Med Biol,* 1987;13:659–663.

529. Mortimer AJ, Dyson M. The effect of therapeutic ultrasound on calcium uptake in fibroblasts. *Ultrasound Med Biol* 1988;14:499–506.

530. Naccache PH, et al. Crystal-induced neutrophil activation. I. Initiation and modulation of calcium mobilization and superoxide production by microcrystals. *Arthritis Rheum* 1991;34:333–342.

531. Terkeltaub R, et al. Monocyte-derived neutrophil chemotactic factor/interleukin-8 is a potential mediator of crystal-induced inflammation. *Arthritis Rheum* 1991;34:894–903.

532. Ark JW, et al. Arthroscopic treatment of calcific tendinitis of the shoulder. *Arthroscopy* 1992;8:183–188.

533. Klein W, Gassen A, Laufenberg B. Endoskopische subacromiale Dekompression und Tendinitis calcarea. *Arthoskopie* 1992;5:247–251.

534. Gartner J. Tendinosis calcarea—Rehandlungsergebnisse mit dem needling. *Z Orthop Ihre Grenzgeb* 1993;131:461–469.

535. Warren RF. Lesions of the long head of the biceps tendon. *AAOS Instr Course Lect* 1985;34:204–209.

536. Ehricht HG. Die osteolyse im lateralen claviculaende nach pressluftschaden. *Arch Orthop Unfallchir* 1959;50:576–582.

537. Scavenius M, Iverson BF. Nontraumatic clavicular osteolysis in weight lifters. *Am J Sports Med* 1992;20:463–467.

538. Cahill BR. Atraumatic osteolysis of the distal clavicle: a review. *Sports Med* 1992;13:214–222.

539. Cahill BR. Osteolysis of the distal part of the clavicle in male athletes. *J Bone Joint Surg* 1982;64A:1053–1058.

540. Bigliani LU, Craig EV, Butters KP. Fractures of the shoulder. In: Rockwood CA, Green DP, Bucholz RW, eds. *Fractures in Adults*. Philadelphia: Lippincott; 1991.

541. Cornell CN, Schneider K. Proximal humerus fractures. In: Koval KJ, Zuckerman JD, eds. Fractures in the elderly. Philadelphia: Lippincott-Raven; 1998.

542. Boinet J. Snapping scapula. *Societe Imperiale de Chirurgie* (2nd series) 1867;8:458.

543. Butters KP. The scapula. In: Rockwood CA, Matsen FA, eds. *The Shoulder*. Philadelphia: WB Saunders; 1990:335–336.

544. Milch H. Partial scapulectomy for snapping in the scapula. *J Bone Joint Surg* 1950;32A:561–566.

545. Milch H. Snapping scapula. *Clin Orthop* 1961;20:139–150.

546. Alvik I. Snapping scapula and Sprengel's deformity. *Acta Orthop Scand* 1959;29:10–15.

547. Cooley LH, Torg JS. Pseudowinging of the scapula secondary to subscapular osteochondroma. *Clin Orthop* 1982; 162:119–124.

548. Parsons TA. The snapping scapula and subscapular exostoses. *J Bone Joint Surg* 1973;55B:345–349.

549. Bristow WR. A case of snapping shoulder. *J Bone Joint Surg* 1924;6:53–55.

550. Cameron HU. Snapping scapulae: A report of three cases. *Eur J Rheum Inflam* 1984;7:66–67.

551. Cobey MC. The rolling scapula. *Clin Orthop* 1968;60:193–194.

552. Edelson JG. Variations in the anatomy of the scapula with reference to the snapping scapula. *Clin Orthop* 1996;322:111–115.

553. Travell J, Rinzler S, Herman M. Shoulder pain: pain and disability of the shoulder and arm. *JAMA* 1942;120:417–422.

554. Michele AA, et al. Scapulocostal syndrome (fatigue-postural paradox). *NY State J Med* 1950;50:1353–1356.

555. Fourie LJ. The scapulocostal syndrome. *S Afr Med J* 1991; 79:721–724.

556. Bazett HC, McGlone B. Note on the pain sensations which accompany deep punctures. *Brain* 1928;51:18–23.

557. Todd TW. Posture and the cervical rib syndrome. *Ann Surg* 1922;75:105–109.

558. Naffziger HC, Grant WC. Neuritis of the brachial plexus, mechanical in origin: the scalenus syndrome. *Surg Gynecol Obstet* 1938;67:722–730.

559. Halliday JL. Psychosomatic medicine and the rheumatism problem. *Practitioner* 1944;152:6–15.

560. Smolders JJ. Myofascial pain and dysfunction syndromes. In: Hammer WI, ed. *Functional Soft Tissue Examination and Treatment by Manual Methods—The Extremities*. 1991, Gaithersburg, Md: Aspen; 1991:215–234.

561. Raikin S, Froimson MI. Bilateral brachial plexus compressive neuropathy (crutch palsy). *J Orthop Trauma* 1997;11:136–138.

562. Rudin LN. Bilateral compression of radial nerve (crutch paralysis). *Phys Ther* 1951;31:229.

563. Poddar SB, et al. Bilateral predominant radial nerve crutch palsy: a case report. *Clin Orthop* 1993;297:245–246.

564. Ang EJ, Goh JC, Bose K. A biofeedback device for patients on axillary crutches. *Arch Phys Med Rehabil.* 1989;70:644–647.

565. Hawkins RJ, Bilco T, Bonutti P. Cervical spine and shoulder pain. *Clin Orthop* 1990;258:142–146.

566. Manifold SG, McCann PD. Cervical radiculitis and shoulder disorders. *Clin Orthop* 1999;368:105–113.

567. DePalma AF. Shoulder-arm-pain of mesodermal, neurogenic, and vascular origin. In: DePalma AF, ed. *Surgery of the Shoulder*. Philadelphia: JB Lippincott; 1983:571–580.

568. Lubahn JD, Cermak MB. Uncommon nerve compression syndromes of the upper extremity. *J Am Acad Orthop Surg* 1998;6:378–386.

569. Drye C, Zachazewski JE. Peripheral nerve injuries. In: Zachazewski JE, Magee DJ, Quillen WS, eds. *Athletic Injuries and Rehabilitation*. Philadelphia: WB Saunders; 1996:441–463.

570. Koppell HP, Thompson WAL. *Peripheral Entrapment Neuropathies*, 2nd ed. New York: R.E. Kreiger; 1976.

571. Ringel SP, et al. Suprascapular neuropathy in pitchers. *Am J Sports Med* 1990;18:80–86.

572. Miller T. Peripheral nerve injuries at the shoulder. *J Manual Manipulative Ther* 1998;6:170–183.

573. Mallon WJ. et al. Suprascapular neuropathy after distal clavicle resection. *Clin Orthop* 1996;329:207–211.

574. Fabre T, et al. Entrapment of the suprascapular nerve. *J Bone Joint Surg* 1999;81B:414–419.

575. Drez DJ, Jr. Suprascapular neuropathy in the differential diagnosis of rotator cuff injuries. *Am J Sports Med* 1976;4:43–45.

576. Ferretti A, Cerullo G, Russo G. Suprascapular neuropathy in volleyball players. *J Bone Joint Surg* 1987;69A:260–263.

577. Clein L. Suprascapular entrapment neuropathy. *J Neurosurg* 1975;43:337–342.

578. Bonnard C, et al. Isolated and combined lesions of the axillary nerve: A review of 146 cases. *J Bone Joint Surg* 1999; 81B:212–217.

579. Wright TA. Accessory spinal nerve injury. *Clin Orthop* 1975; 108:15–18.

580. Wright PE II, Jobe MT. Peripheral nerve injuries. In: Canale ST, Daugherty K, Jones L, eds. *Campbell's Operative Orthopaedics.* St. Louis, Mo: Mosby Year Book; 1998: 3827–3894.

581. Cohn BT, Brahms MA, Cohn M. Injury to the eleventh cranial nerve in a high school wrestler. Orthop Rev 1986; 15:590–595.

582. Petersen CM. Spinal accessory nerve palsy. *J Man Manip Ther* 1996;4:65–69.

583. Johnson JTH, Kendall HO. Isolated paralysis of the serratus anterior muscle. *J Bone Joint Surg* 1955;37A:567–574.

584. Martin JT. Postoperative isolated dysfunction of the long thoracic nerve: A rare entity of uncertain etiology. *Anesth Analg* 1989;69:614–619.

585. Brecker LR. Jenny McConnell offers new technique for problem shoulders. *ADVANCE for Physical Therapists* 1993(November 1):11–12.

586. Goodman CE, Kenrick MM, Blum MV. Long thoracic nerve palsy: a follow-up study. *Arch Phys Med Rehab* 1975; 56:352–355.

587. Dumestre G. Long thoracic nerve palsy. *J Man Manip Ther* 1995;3:44–49.

588. Mendoza FX, Main K. Peripheral nerve injuries of the shoulder in the athlete. *Clin Sports Med* 1990;9:331–341.

589. Paladini D, et al. Axillary neuropathy in volleyball players: report of two cases and literature review. *J Neurol Neurosurg Psychiatry* 1996;60:345–347.

590. Loomer R, Graham B. Anatomy of the axillary nerve and its relation to inferior capsular shift. *Clin Orthop* 1993; 291:103–106.

591. Ombregt L, et al. Nerve lesions and entrapment neuropathies of the upper limb. In: Ombregt L, ed. *A System of Orthopaedic Medicine.* London: WB Saunders; 1995:378–401.

592. Braddom RL, Wolf C. Musculocutaneous nerve injury after heavy exercise. *Arch Phys Med Rehab* 1978;59:290–293.

593. Kim SM, Goodrich JA. Isolated proximal musculocutaneous nerve palsy. *Arch Phys Med Rehab* 1984;65:735–736.

594. Butler DL, Gifford L. The concept of adverse mechanical tension in the nervous system: part 1: testing for "dural tension." *Physiotherapy* 1989;75:622–629.

595. Butler DS. *Mobilization of the Nervous System.* New York: Churchill Livingstone; 1992.

596. Brown JT. Nerve injuries complicating dislocation of the shoulder. *J Bone Joint Surg Br* 1952;34:562.

597. Johns R, Wright V. Relative importance of various tissues in joint stiffness. *J Appl Physiol* 1962;17:824–830.

598. Enneking WF, Horowitz M. The intra-articular effects of immobilization on the human knee. *J Bone Joint Surg* 1972; 54-A:973–985.

599. Randall T, Portney L, Harris B. Effects of joint mobilization on joint stiffness and active motion of the metacarpophalangeal joint. *J Orthop Sports Phys Ther* 1992;16:30–36.

600. Wyke BD. The neurology of joints. *Ann R Coll Surg Engl* 1967;41:25–50.

601. Arem A, Madden J. Effects of stress on healing wounds: Intermittent non-cyclical tension. *J Surg Res* 1971;42:528–543.

602. Warren CG, Lehmann JF, Koblanski JN. Elongation of rat tail: Effect of load and temperature. *Arch Phys Med Rehabil* 1971;52:465–474.

603. Light KE, Nuzik S. Low-load prolonged stretch vs high-load brief stretch in treating knee contractures. *Phys Ther* 1984;64:330–333.

604. Lee DG. *A Workbook of Manual Therapy Techniques for the Upper Extremity,* 2nd ed. Delta, B.C.: Delta Orthopedic Physiotherapy Clinic; 1991:58–79.

605. Mulligan BR. *Manual Therapy: "NAGS," "SNAGS," "PRP'S" etc.* Wellington, New Zealand: Plane View Series; 1992.

606. DiGiovanna EL. Diagnosis and treatment of the upper extremity. In: DiGiovanna EL, Schiowitz S, eds. *An Osteopathic Approach to Diagnosis and Treatment.* Philadelphia: JB Lippincott; 1991.

607. Seidel-Cobb D, Cantu R. Myofascial treatment. In: Donatelli RA, ed. *Physical Therapy of the Shoulder.* New York: Churchill Livingstone; 1997:383–401.

608. Rohde J. Die automobilisation der extremitatengelenke (III). *Zschr Physiother* 1975;27:121–134.

609. Seltzer DG, Wirth MA, Rockwood CA. Complications and failures of open and arthroscopic arthroplasties. *Op Tech Sports Med* 1994;2:136–150.

610. Reid DC. *Sports Injury Assessment and Rehabilitation.* New York: Churchill Livingstone; 1992.

611. Neviaser RJ, Neviaser TJ. Observations on impingement. *Clin Orthop* 1990;254:60–63.

612. Souza TA. Impingement syndrome, tendinopathies, and degenerative joint disease. In: Souza TA, ed. *Sports Injuries of the Shoulder—Conservative Management.* New York: Churchill Livingstone; 1994:371–408.

613. Pink M, Jobe FW. Shoulder injuries in athletes. *J Clin Management* 1991;11:39–47.

614. Stanish WD, Rubinovich RM, Curwin S. Eccentric exercise in chronic tendinitis. *Clin Orthop* 1986;208:65–68.

615. Curwin S, Stanish WD. *Tendinitis, Its Etiology and Treatment.* Lexington, MA: Collamore Press; 1984.

616. Roubal PJ, Dobritt D, Placzek JD. Glenohumeral gliding manipulation following interscalene brachial plexus block in patients with adhesive capsulitis. *J Orthop Sports Phys Ther* 1996;24:66–77.

617. Rhind V, et al. Naproxen and indomethacin in periarthritis of the shoulder. *Rheumatol Rehabil* 1982;21:51–53.

618. Palmer ML, Epler M. *Clinical Assessment Procedures in Physical Therapy.* Philadelphia: JB Lippincott; 1990:68–73.

619. Tibone JE, Bradley JP. Athletic shoulder outcome rating scale. In: Matsen FA, Fu FH, Hawkins RJ, eds. *The Shoulder: A Balance of Mobility and Stability.* Rosemont, IL: American Academy of Orthopedic Surgeons; 1993:526–527.

620. Greis PE, et al. Validation of the lift-off test and analysis of subscapularis activity during maximal internal rotation. *Am J Sports Med* 1996;24:589–593.

621. Jobe FW, et al. An EMG analysis of pitching—a second report. *Am J Sports Med* 1984;12:218–220.

622. Magee DJ. *Orthopedic Physical Assessment.* Philadelphia: WB Saunders; 1997.

THE ELBOW COMPLEX

CHAPTER OBJECTIVES

▶ *At the completion of this chapter, the reader will be able to:*

1. Describe the anatomy of the joints, ligaments, muscles, and blood and nerve supply comprising the elbow complex.

2. Describe the biomechanics of the elbow complex, including open and close packed positions, normal and abnormal joint barriers, force couples, and stabilizers.

3. Describe the purpose and components of the tests and measures for the elbow complex.

4. Perform a comprehensive examination of the elbow complex, including palpation of the articular and soft tissue structures, specific passive mobility and passive articular mobility tests, and stability tests.

5. Evaluate the total examination data to establish a prognosis.

6. Describe the relationship between muscle imbalance and functional performance of the elbow.

7. Outline the significance of the key findings from the tests and measures and establish a diagnosis.

8. Summarize the various causes of elbow dysfunction.

9. Develop self-reliant intervention strategies based on clinical findings and established goals.

10. Develop a working hypothesis.

11. Describe and demonstrate intervention strategies and techniques based on clinical findings and established goals.

12. Evaluate the intervention effectiveness in order to progress or modify an intervention.

13. Plan an effective home program, and instruct the patient in same.

OVERVIEW

The elbow complex is an inherently strong and stable compound joint, which is enclosed within the capsule of the cubital articulation. The stability of the elbow complex allows little in the way of compensatory adjustments, making it prone to overuse injuries.

The primary function of the elbow complex is to work together with the shoulder to position the hand for functional activities.

Anatomy

The elbow complex is comprised of three distinct articulations: the humeroulnar joint, the humeroradial joint, and the proximal radioulnar joint (Fig. 15-1).

Humeroulnar Joint

The proximal ulna consists of the trochlear notch, which articulates with the spool-shaped trochlea of the humerus to form a uniaxial hinge joint, consisting of incongruent saddle-shaped joint surfaces (see Fig. 15-1). The articular surface of the

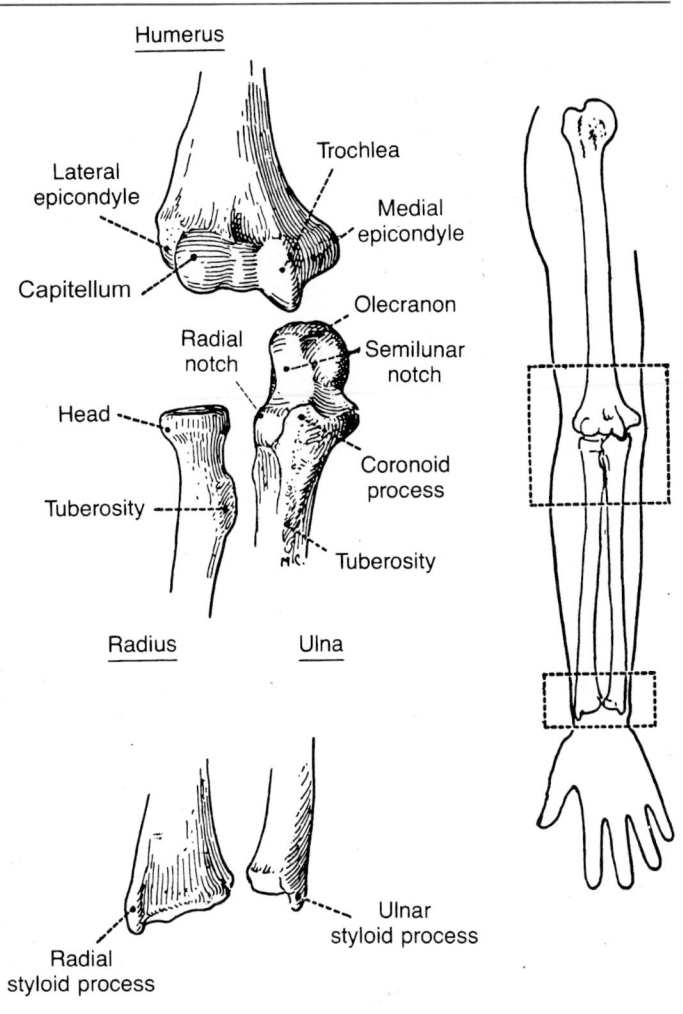

FIGURE 15-1 The bony structures of the elbow complex. (Reproduced with permission from Luttgens K, Hamilton K. *Kinesiology: Scientific Basis of Human Motion.* New York: McGraw-Hill; 1997.)

trochlea extends posteriorly into the olecranon fossa, its medial portion extending further distal than the lateral portion. Anteriorly, the humeral trochlear groove is vertical and parallel to the longitudinal groove, while posteriorly, the groove runs obliquely lateral and distal, forming an acute angle of about 15 degrees with the longitudinal axis of the humerus.[1] This valgus angulation is referred to as the "carrying angle" of the elbow.

Clinical Pearl

The carrying angle serves to direct the ulna laterally during extension, and increase the potential for elbow flexion motion, as the offset allows room anteriorly for approximation of the muscles of the arm and forearm. The carrying angle is approximately 11 to 14 degrees in males and 13 to 16 degrees in females.[2–4]

Humeroradial Joint

The humeroradial joint is a uniaxial hinge joint formed between the spherical capitellum of the humerus, and the concave head of the radius (see Fig. 15-11). The design of this joint allows the elbow to flex and extend, and for the radius to rotate. The superior surface of the proximal end of the radius is biconcave, while the head of the radius is slightly oval. The radial tuberosity (see Fig. 15-1) serves as a site of attachment for the biceps brachii. The humerus widens at the elbow and forms the medial and lateral epicondyles (see Fig. 15-1).

Proximal Radioulnar Joint

The radius and ulna lie side by side, with the radius being the shorter and more lateral of the two forearm bones. The proximal or superior radioulnar joint is a uniaxial pivot joint. It is formed between the periphery of the convex radial head, and the fibrous osseous ring formed by the concave radial notch of the ulna (see Fig. 15-11), which lies distal to the trochlear notch, and the annular ligament.

The proximal and distal radioulnar joints together form a bicondylar joint. An interosseous membrane located between the radius and ulna serves to help distribute forces throughout the forearm, and provide muscle attachment.

The annular ligament (Fig. 15-2) forms 80 percent of the articular surface of the proximal radioulnar joint.

Joint Capsule

The joint capsule of the elbow complex is thin but strong. The capsule of the joint does not respond well to injury or prolonged immobilization, and often forms thick scar tissue, which may result in flexion contractures of the elbow.[5–7]

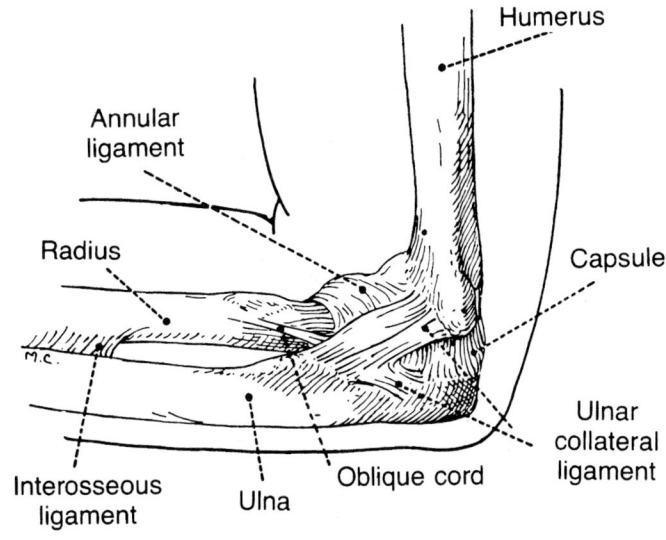

FIGURE 15-2 Medial aspect of the elbow. (Reproduced with permission from Luttgens K, Hamilton K. *Kinesiology: Scientific Basis of Human Motion.* New York: McGraw-Hill; 1997.)

Ligaments

Support for the elbow complex is provided through strong ligaments (Table 15-1).

Medial (Ulnar) Collateral Ligament

The medial collateral ligament (MCL) extends from the central two thirds of the anteroinferior surface of the medial epicondyle to the proximal medial ulna, from just posterior to the axis of the elbow medial epicondyle[8–10] to just distal to the tip of the coronoid (see Fig. 15-2).[11,12]

The fan-shaped MCL is functionally the most important ligament in the elbow for providing stability against valgus stress, particularly in the range of 20 to 130 degrees of flexion and extension,[13] with the humeroradial joint functioning as a secondary stabilizer to valgus loads.[14,15] The MCL achieves this stability through almost the total range of flexion and extension due to its eccentric location with respect to the axis of elbow motion.[16–19] In full elbow extension, valgus stability of the elbow is provided equally by the MCL, the joint capsule, and the joint relationships.[6]

There are three distinct components of the MCL[8,11,20,21]: the anterior bundle, the transverse bundle, and the posterior bundle.

Anterior Bundle. The anterior bundle of the MCL is the strongest and stiffest of the elbow collateral ligaments, with an average load to failure of 260 newtons (N).[13] The anterior bundle of the MCL inserts an average of 18 mm distal to the coronoid tip, and is composed of two other components, the anterior band and the posterior band, which perform reciprocal functions[11,16,20]:

▶ The anterior band of the anterior bundle is the most important component of the ligamentous complex, because it primarily stabilizes the elbow against valgus stress in the ranges of 20 to 120 degrees of flexion, and becomes a secondary restraint with further flexion.[8,11,14–16,18,20,22,23] Recently, Ochi and colleagues[9] determined that the deep middle portion of the anterior band, previously described as the "guiding bundle,"[21] is a prime limiting factor in humeroulnar motion.[16,24]

▶ The posterior band is taut beyond 55 degrees of elbow flexion, and is a secondary restraint to valgus stress at lesser degrees of flexion. The posterior band functions as an equal co-restraint with the anterior band at terminal elbow flexion,[13,16,20,22,23] and also acts as a primary restraint to passive elbow extension. In the higher degrees of flexion,

TABLE 15-1 Articular and Ligamentous Contributions to Elbow Stability

Stabilization	Elbow Extended	Elbow Flexed 90°
Valgus stability	Anterior capsule MCL and bony articular (proximal half of sigmoid notch) *equally divided*	MCL provides 55% 0% anterior capsule and bony articulation (proximal half of sigmoid notch)
Varus stability	Anterior capsule (32%) Joint articulation (55%) RCL (14%)	Joint articulation (75%) Anterior capsule (13%) RCL (9%)
Anterior displacement	Anterior oblique ligament Anterior joint capsule Trochlea-olecranon articulation (minimal)	
Posterior displacement	Anterior capsule Radial head against capitellum Coracoid against trochlea	
Distraction	Anterior capsule (85%) RCL (5%) MCL (5%) Triceps, biceps, brachial, brachioradial, forearm muscles	RCL 10% MCL 78% Capsule 8%

MCL, Medial collateral ligament; RCL, radial collateral ligament.
From Sobel J, Nirschl RP. Elbow injuries. In: Zachazewski JE, Magee DJ, Quillen WS, eds. *Athletic Injuries and Rehabilitation*. Philadelphia: WB Saunders; 1996:543–583.

the posterior band is nearly isometric and is thus functionally important in the overhead athlete in counteracting valgus stresses.[25]

Transverse Bundle. The transverse bundle, also known as Cooper's ligament, is variably present.[8,11,26] It does not cross the elbow joint, and is comprised of fibers running along the medial joint capsule from the tip of the olecranon to the medial ulna, just distal to the coronoid.[8,27] The transverse fibers have little role in elbow stability due to the fact that they both originate and insert on the ulna.

Posterior Bundle. The posterior bundle of the MCL originates from the medial epicondyle and inserts onto the medial margin of the semilunar notch. This bundle appears to be a thickening of the posterior elbow capsule.[27,28] Being thinner and weaker than the anterior bundle, the posterior bundle provides only secondary restraint to valgus stress at flexion beyond 90 degrees.[16,17]

Lateral (Radial) Collateral Ligament

The lateral collateral ligament (LCL) complex (Fig. 15-3) consists of the annular ligament and the accessory collateral ligament.[13] The LCL courses distally and forms a broad conjoint insertion onto the proximal ulna.[29,30] The proximal margin of this conjoined insertion begins at the proximal margin of the radial head. The insertion attaches just inferior to the radial notch and progresses along a rough ridge in line with the supinator crest of the ulna.[13] The LCL is closely associated with the insertions of the extensor carpi radialis brevis and the supinator,

with the latter muscle crossing this ligament complex obliquely from distal to proximal at its ulnar attachment, and becoming confluent with the underlying annular ligament and LCL more proximally at its humeral origin.[13]

As the axis for rotation passes through the origin of the LCL, the various fibers of this ligament maintain consistent patterns of tension whether varus, valgus, or no force is applied to the elbow throughout the arc of flexion.[8,23] The LCL functions to maintain the ulnohumeral and radiohumeral joints in a reduced position when the elbow is loaded in supination.[13] The LCL contributes only 9 percent of the restraint to varus stress at 90 degrees of flexion. In extension the LCL contributes 14 percent of this restraint.[23]

Insufficient lateral support of the elbow complex results in lateral gapping at the ulnohumeral joint and posterior translation of the radial head in relation to the capitellum.[13] However, the proximal radioulnar relationship remains undisturbed.

Secondary restraints of the lateral elbow consist of the bony articulations, the joint capsule, and the extensor muscles with their fascial bands and intermuscular septa. These independently support the forearm unit from laterally rotating away from the humerus by virtue of their anatomic arrangement, and provide a secondary static and dynamic vector supporting the lateral joint.[30]

Annular Ligament

The annular ligament, which is wider proximally and distally, runs around the radial head from the anterior and posterior margin of the radial notch, to approximate the radial head to the radial notch and enclose the radial circumference. The ligament functions to maintain the relationship between the head of the radius and the humerus and ulna.

Bursae

There are numerous bursae in the elbow region.[17] The olecranon bursa is the main bursa of the elbow complex and lies posteriorly between the skin and the olecranon process. Under normal conditions the bursa does not communicate with the elbow joint, although its superficial location puts it at high risk for injury from direct trauma to the elbow.

Other bursae in the posterior elbow region include the deep intratendinous bursa, and a deep subtendinous bursa, which are present between the triceps tendon and olecranon. Anteriorly, the bicipitoradial bursa separates the biceps tendon from the radial tuberosity. Along the medial and lateral aspects of the elbow are the subcutaneous medial epicondylar bursa and the subcutaneous lateral epicondylar bursa.[31]

Muscles

The forearm consists of three major fascial compartments, the anterior forearm, the posterior forearm, and the compartment referred to as the mobile wad (Tables 15-2 and 15-3).

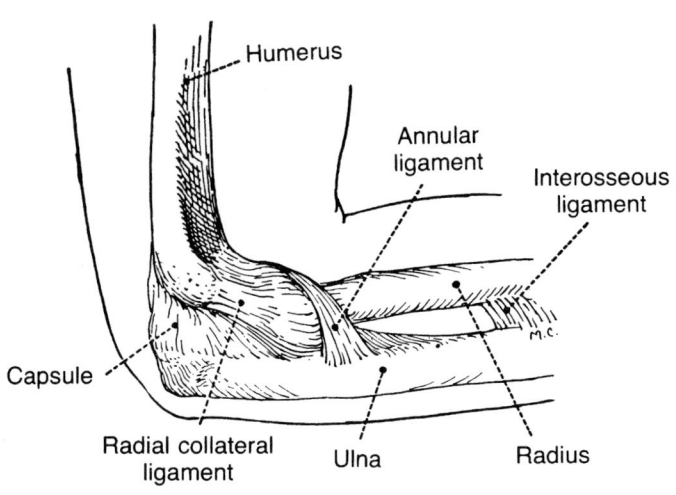

FIGURE 15-3 Lateral aspect of the elbow. (Reproduced with permission from Luttgens K, Hamilton K. *Kinesiology: Scientific Basis of Human Motion.* New York: McGraw-Hill; 1997.)

TABLE 15-2   Muscle Compartments of the Forearm

Compartment	Principal Muscles
Anterior	Pronator teres
	Flexor carpi radialis
	Palmaris longus
	Flexor digitorum superficialis
	Flexor digitorum profundus
	Flexor pollicis longus
	Flexor carpi ulnaris
	Pronator quadratus
Posterior	Abductor pollicis longus
	Extensor pollicis brevis
	Extensor pollicis longus
	Extensor digitorum communis
	Extensor digitorum proprius
	Extensor digiti quinti
	Extensor carpi ulnaris
Mobile wad	Brachioradialis
	Extensor carpi radialis longus
	Extensor carpi radialis brevis

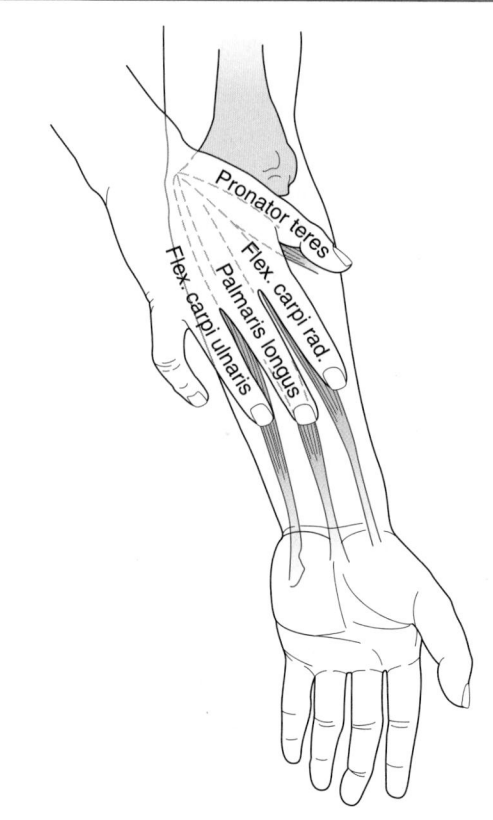

FIGURE 15-4   The flexor-pronator group.

Elbow Flexors

The prime movers of elbow flexion are the biceps, brachialis, and brachioradialis (see Table 15-3).[32] The pronator teres, flexor carpi radialis (FCR), and flexor carpi ulnaris (FCU) (Fig. 15-4), and the extensor carpi radialis longus (ECRL) muscles are considered to be weak flexors of the elbow.[31]

Biceps Brachii.   The biceps is a two-headed muscle that spans two joints. The short head of the biceps arises from the tip of the coracoid process of the scapula, whereas the long head arises

TABLE 15-3   Muscles of the Forearm, Wrist, and Hand: Their Actions, Nerve Supply, and Nerve Root Derivation[335]

Action	Muscles Acting	Nerve Supply	Nerve Root Derivation
Supination of the forearm	Supinator	Posterior interosseous (radial)	C5–C6
	Biceps brachii	Musculocutaneous	C5–C6
Pronation of the forearm	Pronator quadratus	Anterior interosseous (median)	C8, T1
	Pronator teres	Median	C6–C7
	Flexor carpi radialis	Median	C6–C7
Extension of the wrist	Extensor carpi radialis longus	Radial	C6–C7
	Extensor carpi radialis brevis	Posterior interosseous (radial)	C7–C8
	Extensor carpi ulnaris	Posterior interosseous (radial)	C7–C8
Flexion of the wrist	Flexor carpi radialis	Median	C6–C7
	Flexor carpi ulnaris	Ulnar	C7–C8
Ulnar deviation of the wrist	Flexor carpi ulnaris	Ulnar	C7–C8
	Extensor carpi ulnaris	Posterior interosseous (radial)	C7–C8

TABLE 15-3 *(cont.)*

Radial deviation of the wrist	Flexor carpi radialis	Median	C6–C7
	Extensor carpi radialis longus	Radial	C6–C7
	Abductor pollicis longus	Posterior interosseous (radial)	C7–C8
	Extensor pollicis brevis	Posterior interosseous (radial)	C7–C8
Extension of the fingers	Extensor digitorum communis	Posterior interosseous (radial)	C7–C8
	Extensor indicis	Posterior interosseous (radial)	C7–C8
	Extensor digiti minimi	Posterior interosseous (radial)	C7–C8
Flexion of the fingers	Flexor digitorum profundus	Anterior interosseous (median)	C8, T1
		Anterior interosseous (median)	C8, T1
		lateral two digits	C8, T1
	Flexor digitorum superficialis	Ulnar: medial two digits	C7–C8, T1
	Lumbricals	Median	C8, T1
		First and second: median	C8, T1
	Interossei	Third and fourth: Ulnar (deep terminal branch)	C8, T1
	Flexor digiti minimi	Ulnar (deep terminal branch)	
		Ulnar (deep terminal branch)	C8, T1
Abduction of the fingers (with fingers extended)	Dorsal interossei	Ulnar (deep terminal branch)	C8, T1
	Abductor digiti minimi	Ulnar (deep terminal branch)	C8, T1
Adduction of the fingers (with fingers extended)	Palmar interossei	Ulnar (deep terminal branch)	C8, T1
Extension of the thumb	Extensor pollicis longus	Posterior interosseous (radial)	C7–C8
	Extensor pollicis brevis	Posterior interosseous (radial)	C7–C8
	Abductor pollicis longus	Posterior interosseous (radial)	C7–C8
Flexion of the thumb	Flexor pollicis brevis	Superficial head: median (lateral terminal branch)	C8, T1
			C8, T1
	Flexor pollicis longus	Deep head ulnar	C8, T1
	Opponens pollicis	Anterior interosseous (median)	C8, T1
		Median (lateral terminal branch)	
Abduction of the thumb	Abductor pollicis longus	Posterior interosseous (radial)	C7–C8
	Abductor pollicis brevis	Median (lateral terminal branch)	C8, T1
Adduction of the thumb	Adductor pollicis	Ulnar (deep terminal branch)	C8, T1
Opposition of the thumb and little finger	Opponens pollicis	Median (lateral terminal branch)	C8, T1
	Flexor pollicis brevis	Superficial head: median (lateral terminal branch)	C8, T1
	Abductor pollicis brevis	Median (lateral terminal branch)	C8, T1
	Opponens digiti minimi	Ulnar (deep terminal branch)	C8, T1

from the supraglenoid tuberosity of the scapula (Fig. 15-5). The biceps has two insertions: the radial tuberosity, and by the lacertus fibrosus (see Fig. 15-5).

At the elbow, the biceps is the dominant flexor, but its secondary function is supination of the forearm.[33] The supination action of the biceps increases the more the elbow is flexed and is maximal at 90 degrees. It diminishes again when the elbow is fully flexed. No,[34] or limited[35] biceps muscle activity has been demonstrated during elbow flexion with the forearm pronated.[31] The biceps, via its long head, also functions as a shoulder flexor (see Chap. 14).

FIGURE 15-5   The biceps. (Reproduced with permission from Luttgens K, Hamilton K. *Kinesiology: Scientific Basis of Human Motion*. New York: McGraw-Hill; 1997.)

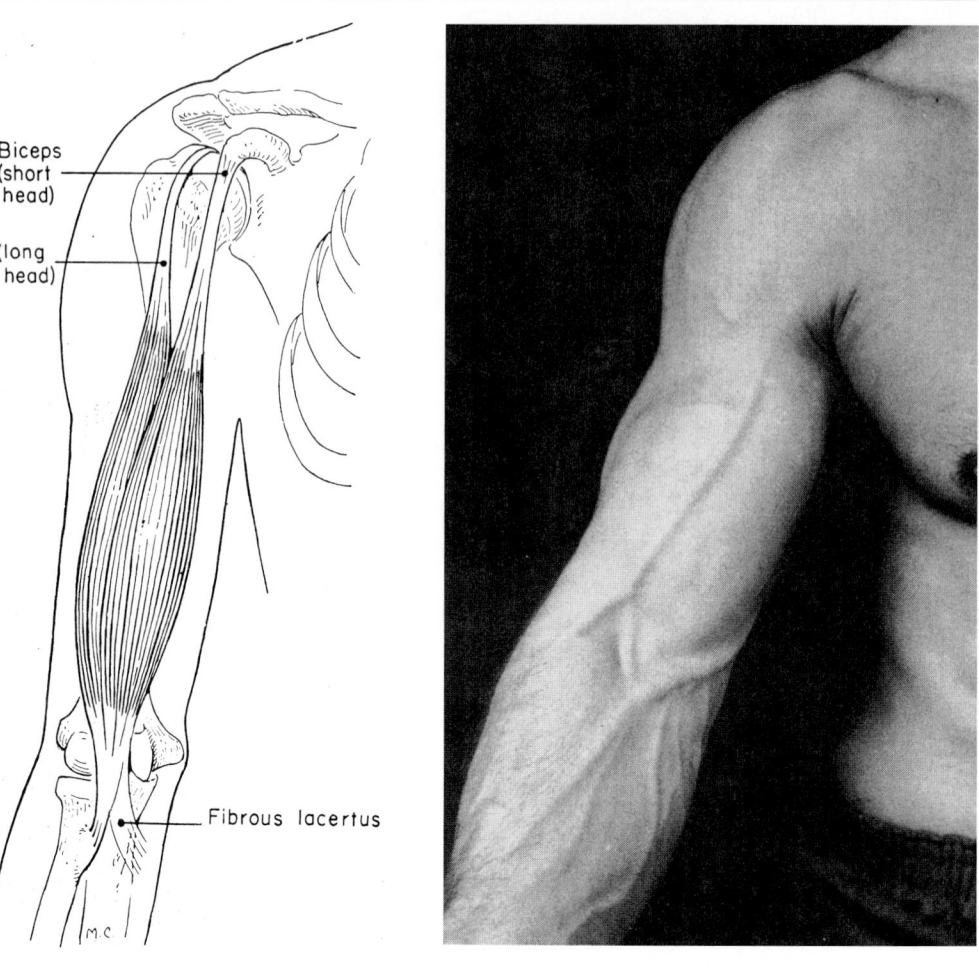

Brachialis.   The brachialis (Fig. 15-6) originates from the lower two thirds of the anterior surface of the humerus, and inserts on the ulnar tuberosity and the coronoid process. The brachialis is the workhorse of the elbow, and functions to bend the elbow regardless of the degree of pronation and supination of the forearm.[35] It is the most powerful flexor of the elbow when the forearm is pronated.[36]

Brachioradialis.   The brachioradialis (Fig. 15-7) arises from the proximal two thirds of the lateral supracondylar ridge of the humerus, and the lateral intermuscular septum. It travels down the forearm and inserts on the lateral border of the styloid process on the distal aspect of the radius.

The brachioradialis appears to have a number of functions, two of which occur with rapid movements of elbow flexion. Initially it functions as a shunt muscle, overcoming centrifugal forces acting on the elbow, and then by adding power to increase the speed of flexion.[33]

The brachioradialis also functions to bring a pronated or supinated forearm back into the neutral position of pronation and supination. In the neutral or pronated position, the muscle acts as a flexor of the elbow, an action that diminishes when the forearm is held in supination.[35,37]

Pronator Teres.   The pronator teres (see Fig. 15-7) has two heads of origin, a humeral head and an ulnar head. The humeral head arises from the medial epicondylar ridge of the humerus and common flexor tendon, whereas the ulnar head arises from the medial aspect of the coronoid process of the ulna. The pronator teres inserts on the anterolateral surface of the midpoint of the radius. The muscle functions predominantly to pronate the forearm, but can also assist with elbow flexion.[6,36,37]

Extensor Carpi Radialis Longus.   The extensor carpi radialis longus (ECRL) arises from a point superior to the lateral epicondyle of the humerus on the lower third of the supracondylar ridge, just distal to the brachioradialis. It travels down the forearm to insert on the posterior surface of the base of the second metacarpal. The muscle functions as a weak flexor of the elbow, as well as providing wrist extension and radial deviation.

Flexor Carpi Radialis.   The flexor carpi radialis (FCR) (see Fig. 15-4) arises from the common flexor tendon on the medial epicondyle of the humerus, and inserts on the base of the second and third metacarpal bones. The FCR functions to flex the

superoposterior surface of the olecranon and deep fascia of the forearm. The triceps has its maximal force in movements that combine both elbow extension and shoulder extension. Like the biceps, it is a two-joint muscle.

Anconeus. The anconeus arises from the lateral epicondyle of the humerus, and inserts on the lateral aspect of the olecranon and posterior surface of the ulna. The exact function of the anconeus in humans has yet to be determined. It has been suggested that in addition to assisting with elbow extension, it functions to stabilize the ulnar head in all positions (except radial deviation) and to pull the subanconeus bursa and the joint capsule out of the way during extension, thus avoiding impingement.[6,38] The anconeus has also been found to be active during forearm pronation and supination.[35]

> ### Clinical Pearl
>
> Tendonitis of the anconeus can mimic tennis elbow, while hypertrophy of the anconeus muscle can compress the ulnar nerve.[39]

Forearm Pronators

Pronator Teres (See Above)

Pronator Quadratus. The pronator quadratus (Figure 16-12) arises from the anteromedial surface of the distal quarter of the ulna, and inserts on the slightly more distal anterolateral surface of the radius. As its name suggests, the function of the pronator quadratus is to pronate the forearm, but it also serves to maintain the opposition of the radius and ulna.

The pronator quadratus (Fig. 16-12) is the main pronator of the forearm.

Flexor Carpi Radialis (See Above)

Forearm Supinators

Biceps (See Above)

Supinator. The supinator (see Fig. 15-8) originates from the lateral epicondyle of the humerus, lateral collateral ligament, the annular ligament, the supinator crest, and the ulnar fossa. It inserts on the superior third of the anterior and lateral surface of the radius. The supinator functions to supinate the forearm in any elbow position, while the previously mentioned extensor carpi radialis longus and brevis work as supinators during fast movements, and against resistance.

Cubital Tunnel

The cubital tunnel (Fig. 15-9), a fibro-osseous canal, was originally described by Feindel and Stratford.[40] The ulnar nerve passes through this tunnel. The floor of the tunnel is formed by the MCL, whereas the roof is formed by an aponeurosis, the arcuate ligament, or Osborne's band, which extends from the medial epicondyle to the olecranon, and arises from the origin of the two heads of the FCU.[41–44] The medial head of the triceps constitutes the posterior border of the tunnel, and its anterior and lateral borders are formed by the medial epicondyle and olecranon, respectively.[25]

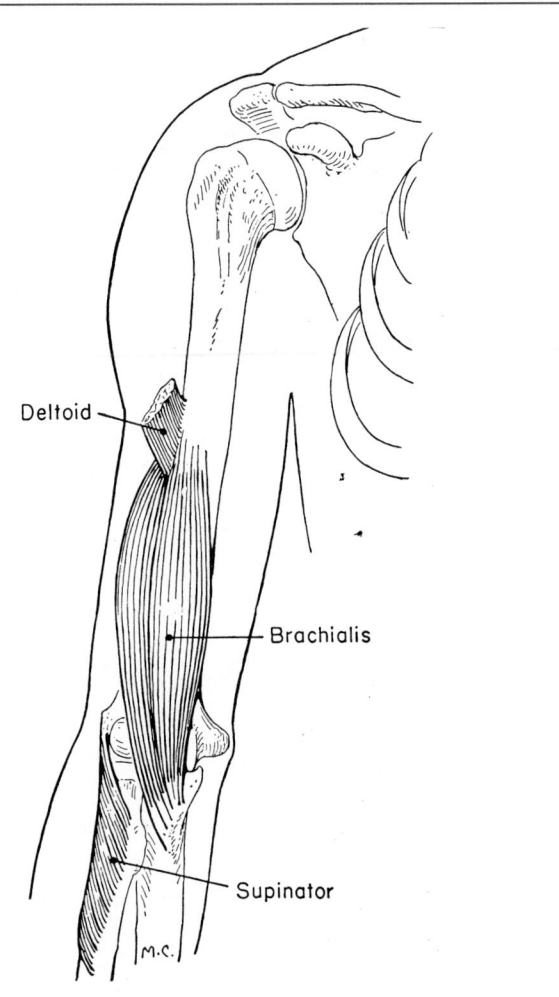

FIGURE 15-6 The brachialis and supinator. (Reproduced with permission from Luttgens K, Hamilton K. *Kinesiology: Scientific Basis of Human Motion.* New York: McGraw-Hill; 1997.)

elbow and wrist, but also assists in pronation and radial deviation of the wrist.

Flexor Carpi Ulnaris. The flexor carpi ulnaris (FCU) (see Fig. 15-4) has two heads of origin. The humeral head arises from the common flexor tendon on the medial epicondyle of the humerus. It inserts on the pisiform, hamate, and fifth metacarpal bones. The FCU functions to assist with elbow flexion in addition to flexion and ulnar deviation of the wrist.

Elbow Extensors

There are two muscles that extend the elbow: the triceps and the anconeus (see Table 15-3).

Triceps Brachii. The triceps brachii (Fig. 15-8) has three heads of origin. The long head arises from the infraglenoid tuberosity of the scapula, the lateral head from the posterior and lateral surface of the humerus, and the medial head from the lower posterior surface of the humerus. The muscle inserts on the

FIGURE 15-7 The brachioradialis and pronator teres. (Reproduced with permission from Luttgens K, Hamilton K. *Kinesiology: Scientific Basis of Human Motion.* New York: McGraw-Hill; 1997.)

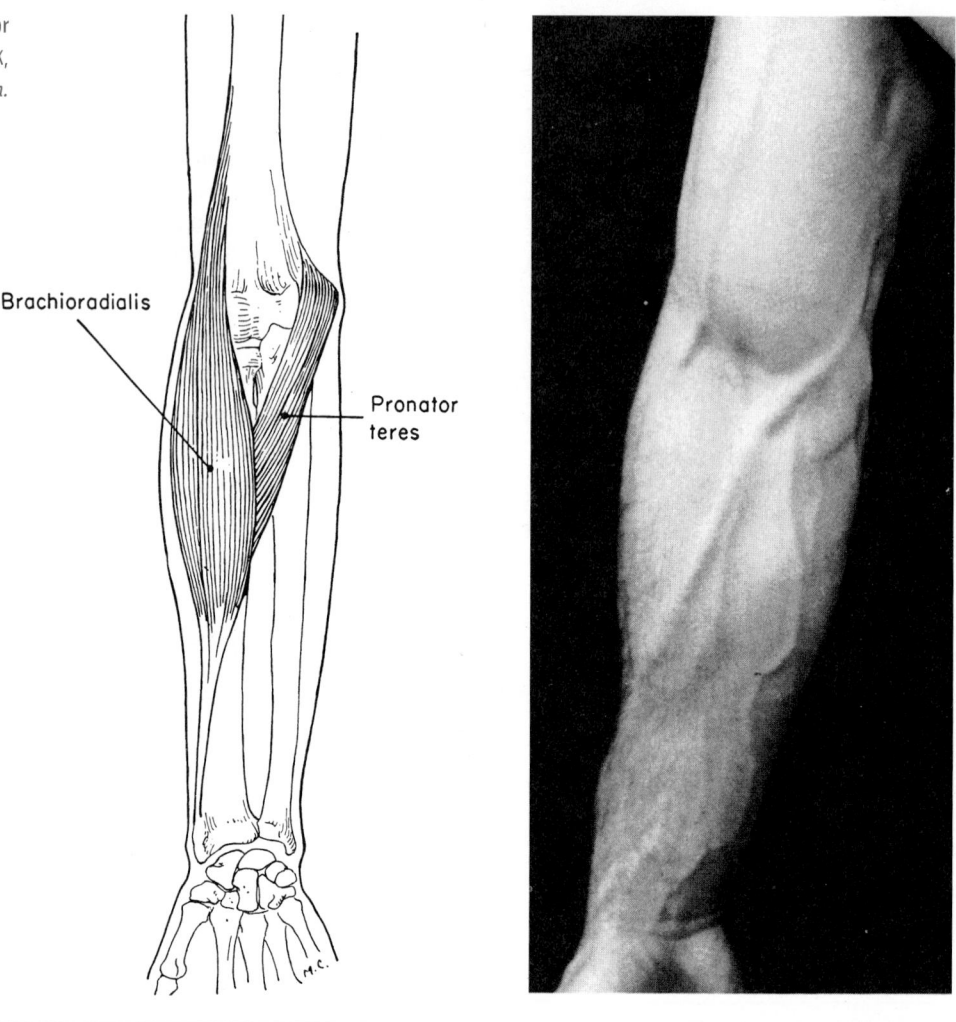

The volume of the cubital tunnel is greatest with the elbow held in extension.[45] As the elbow is brought into full flexion there is a 55 percent decrease in canal volume.[41] Vanderpool and colleagues[46] reported that with each 45 degrees of flexion of the elbow there was a concomitant 5-mm increase in distance between the ulnar and humeral attachments of the arcuate ligament. At full elbow flexion there was a 40 percent elongation of the ligament and a decrease in canal height of approximately 2.5 mm.

A few other factors have been associated with a decrease in the size of the cubital tunnel. These include space-occupying lesions, osteoarthritis, rheumatoid arthritis, heterotopic bone formation, or trauma to the nerve.[45] Patients with systemic conditions such as diabetes mellitus, hypothyroidism, alcoholism, and renal failure also may have a predisposition.[47]

Bulging of the MCL has also been described as a factor.[46] More than 40 percent of athletes with valgus instability develop ulnar neuritis secondary to irritation from inflammation of the MCL.[48,49]

O'Driscoll and coworkers[44] reported that the groove on the inferior aspect of the medial epicondyle was not as deep as the groove posteriorly, and the floor of the canal seems to rise with elbow flexion.[44] These changes lead to an alteration of the cross sectional area of the cubital tunnel from a rounded surface to a triangular or elliptic surface with elbow flexion.[41,45]

> **Clinical Pearl**
>
> The volume of the cubital tunnel is greatest with the elbow held in extension.

Cubital Fossa

The cubital fossa (Fig. 15-10) represents the triangular space, or depression, which is located over the anterior surface of the elbow joint, and which serves as an "entrance" to the forearm, or antebrachium. The boundaries of the fossa are:

▶ *Lateral:* brachioradialis and extensor carpi radialis longus muscles.

▶ *Medial:* pronator teres muscle.

FIGURE 15-8 The triceps and supinator. (Reproduced with permission from Luttgens K, Hamilton K. *Kinesiology: Scientific Basis of Human Motion*. New York: McGraw-Hill; 1997.)

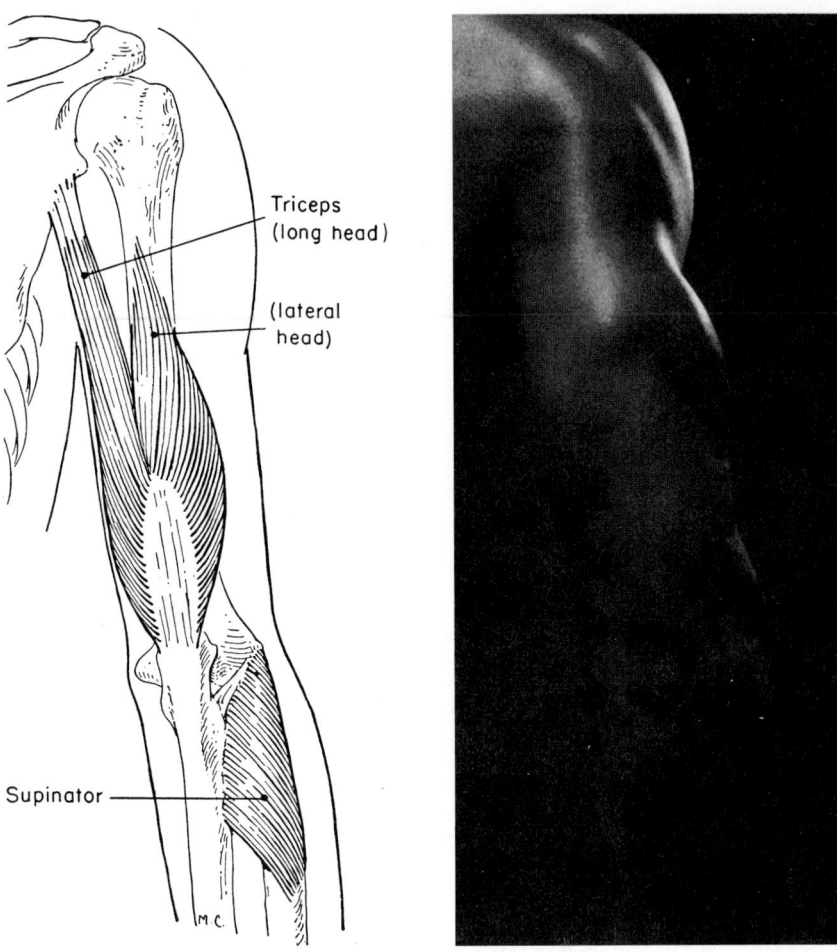

- ▶ *Proximal:* an imaginary line that passes through the humeral condyles.

- ▶ *Floor:* brachialis muscle.

  The contents of the fossa include (see Fig. 15-10):

- ▶ The tendon of the biceps brachii lies as the central structure in the fossa.

- ▶ The median nerve runs along the lateral edge of the pronator teres muscle.

- ▶ The brachial artery enters the fossa just lateral to the median nerve and just medial to the biceps brachii tendon.

- ▶ The radial nerve (not shown) runs along the medial edge of the brachioradialis and ECRL muscles, and is vulnerable to injury here.

- ▶ The median cubital or intermediate cubital cutaneous vein crosses the surface of the fossa.

Nerves

The neurologic supply of the bones, joints, muscles, and skin of the lateral forearm is derived from the C5 through C8 nerve roots, which exit from the intervertebral foramina of C4 to C5 through C7 to T1.[50]

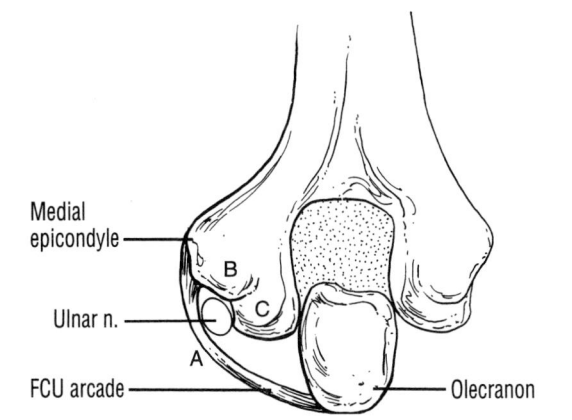

FIGURE 15-9 Cross-sectional anatomy of the cubital tunnel that demonstrates three borders. A. Medial. B. Anterior. C. Lateral. Cubital decompression concerns the medial border; medial epicondylectomy concerns the medial and anterior borders. If abnormalities exist involving the tunnel itself or lateral border, anterior transposition is required. (Reproduced with permission from Herndon JH. *Surgical Reconstruction of the Upper Extremity*. Stamford, CT: Appleton & Lange; 1999.)

FIGURE 15-10 The cubital fossa. (Reproduced with permission from Cipriano JJ. *Photographic Manual of Regional Orthopaedic and Neurological Tests*, 3rd ed. Baltimore: Williams & Wilkins; 1997.)

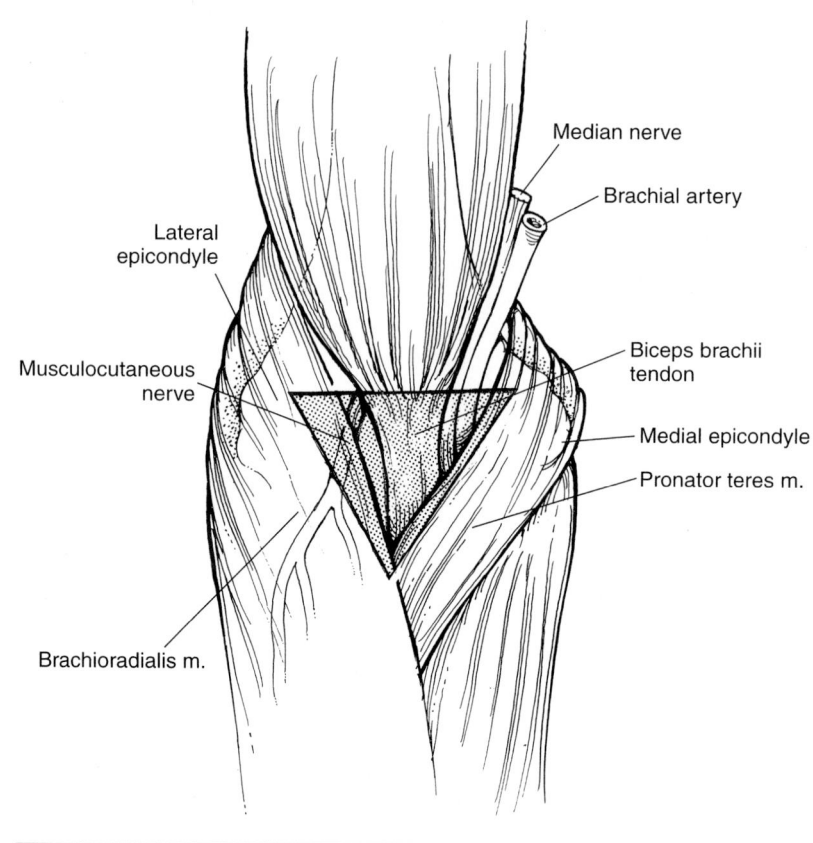

Ulnar Nerve (C8–T1)

From its origin as the largest branch of the medial cord of the brachial plexus, the ulnar nerve continues along the anterior compartment of the arm before passing through the medial intermuscular septum at the level of the coracobrachialis insertion.

At the level of the elbow, the ulnar nerve passes posterior to the medial epicondyle, where it enters the cubital tunnel. Ulnar nerve compression in the cubital tunnel is a common entrapment neuropathy of the upper extremity, second only to carpal tunnel syndrome.[51] After leaving the cubital tunnel, the ulnar nerve passes between the two heads of the FCU origin and traverses the deep flexor-pronator aponeurosis.[52,53]

Median Nerve (C5–T1)

The median nerve extends medially down the upper arm across the anterior aspect of elbow joint. The ligament of Struthers (Fig. 15-11) arises from an abnormal spur on the shaft of the humerus, and runs to the medial supracondylar process.[43] The supracondylar process with its ligamentous extension encloses a foramen bounded medially by the medial intermuscular septum, and the distal anterior surface of the medial epicondyle, through which the brachial artery and median nerve pass.[54]

As the median nerve passes through the cubital fossa, the anterior interosseous nerve branches off the median nerve as it passes through the two heads of the pronator teres muscle. The anterior interosseous nerve supplies the motor innervation to the index and middle flexor digitorum profundus (FDP), the flexor pollicis longus (FPL), and the pronator quadratus.

Radial Nerve (C5–T1)

The radial nerve sits superiorly and medially in the upper arm, winds around humeral shaft, and extends over the lateral epicondyle. At a point approximately 10 to 12 cm proximal to the elbow joint, the radial nerve passes from the posterior compartment of the arm by piercing the lateral intermuscular septum.[55] The nerve travels in the anterior distal arm between the brachialis muscle and the biceps tendon medially, and the brachioradialis, extensor carpi radialis longus (ECRL), and extensor carpi radialis brevis (ECRB) muscles laterally.[55] Within an area approximately 3 cm proximal or distal to the elbow joint, the radial nerve branches into a deep mixed nerve (posterior interosseous nerve) and a superficial sensory branch.[56,57] After dividing, the two terminal divisions usually follow the same course, sharing a single epineurium for several centimeters, before the superficial radial nerve moves anteriorly to lie on the undersurface of the brachioradialis, and the deep branch travels posteriorly to enter the radial tunnel/supinator canal, distal to the origin of the ECRB, at the level of the radiohumeral joint.[55] Entering the canal, the deep branch supplies the ECRB then passes deep to the superficial head of the supinator, where the arcade of Fröhse* can impinge on the nerve (see later).[58,59]

---

* The arcade of Fröhse is an inverted arched structure that lies within 1 cm distal of the fibrous edge of the ECRB and approximately 2 to 4 cm distal to the radiohumeral joint. It represents the proximal border of the superficial head of the supinator, through which the radial nerve passes. See ref. 55 for more information.

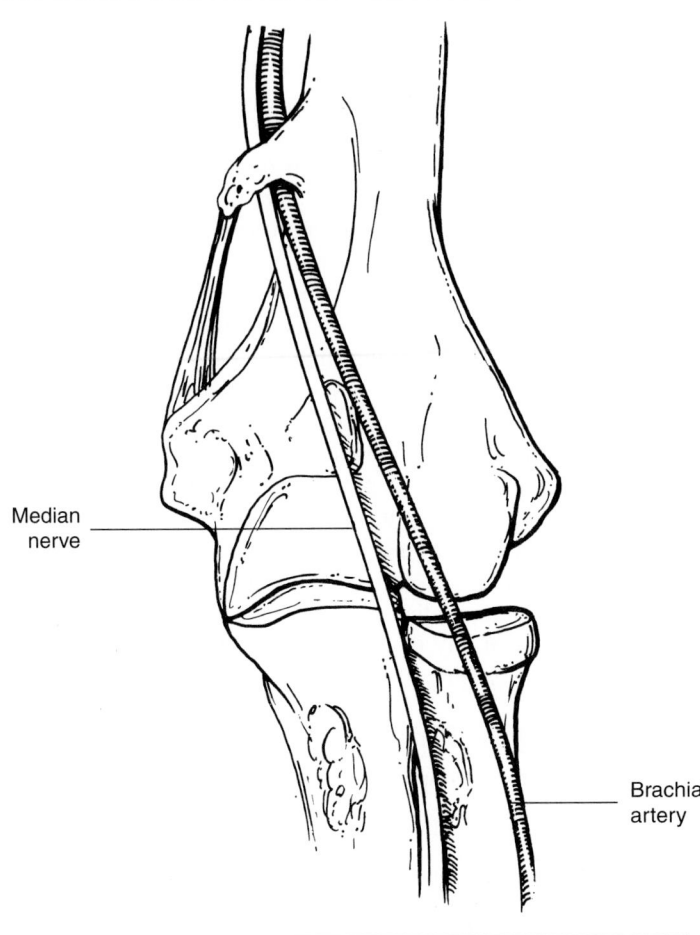

Median
nerve

Brachial
artery

FIGURE 15-11 Ligament of Struthers. (Reproduced with permission from Herndon JH. *Surgical Reconstruction of the Upper Extremity.* Stamford, CT: Appleton & Lange; 1999.)

The nerve continues between the two heads of the supinator and innervates this muscle during its passage to the posterolateral aspect of the radius. On emerging from the supinator, a motor division (supplying the abductor pollicis longus, extensor pollicis brevis, extensor indicis proprius, and extensor pollicis longus muscles) and a mixed lateral branch (supplying the extensor carpi ulnaris, extensor digitorum communis, and extensor digiti minimis muscles) are recognized. The lateral branch continues along the posterior radial border of the radius to the wrist as the sensory branch of the posterior interosseous nerve, which innervates the dorsal capsule of the wrist and intercarpal joints (see Chap. 16).[55,58]

The Radial Tunnel/Supinator Canal. The radial tunnel lies on the anterior aspect of the radius, and is approximately three to four fingerbreadths long, beginning just proximal to the radiohumeral joint, and ending at the site where the nerve passes deep to the superficial part of the supinator muscle.[60] The lateral wall of the tunnel is formed by the brachioradialis, ECRL, and ECRB. These muscles cross over the nerve to form the anterior wall of the radial tunnel as well, while the floor of the tunnel is

formed by the capsule of the humeroradial joint, and the medial wall is composed of the brachialis and biceps tendon.[55]

Vascular Supply

The vascular supply to the elbow includes the brachial artery, the radial and ulnar arteries, the middle collateral artery laterally, and the anterior and posterior ulnar recurrent arteries.[31]

Biomechanics

There is still controversy in the literature as to the precise biomechanics of the elbow,[61] and how the axes of motion relate to the anatomy of the joint. Biomechanically, the elbow predominantly functions as an important link in the upper extremity kinetic chain, allowing the generation and transfer of forces that occur in the upper extremity. These forces produce repetitive tensile loads on the ligamentous and muscular support systems around the elbow, and compressive and shear loads on the bony constraints.[62] Truly impressive loads can be placed through the elbow during such activities as throwing or pitching (Fig. 15-12; see later).

Humeroulnar Joint

The motions that occur at the humeroulnar joint involve impure flexion and extension, which are primarily the result of rotation of the ulna about the trochlea. The range of flexion-extension is from 0 to 150 degrees, with about 10 degrees of hyperextension being available. Full active extension in the normal elbow is some 5 to 10 degrees short of that obtainable by forced extension, due to passive muscular restraints (biceps, brachialis, and supinator).[63,64] Passive extension is limited by the impact of the olecranon process on the olecranon fossa, and tension on the ulnar collateral ligament and anterior capsule.[65] Passive flexion is limited by bony structures (the head of the radius against the radial fossa, and the coronoid process against the coronoid fossa), tension of the posterior capsular ligament, soft tissue approximation and passive tension in the triceps[65] (see Table 15-3).

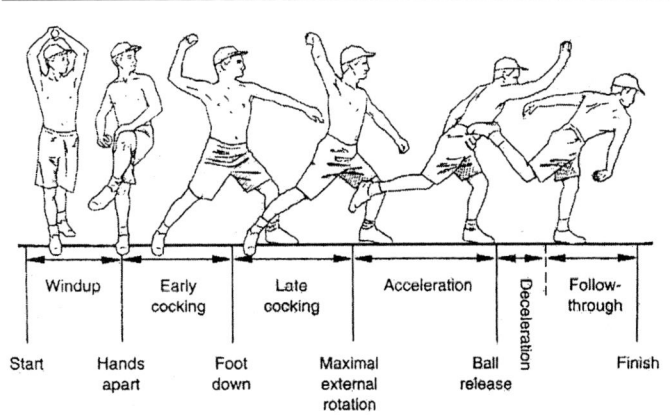

| Windup | Early cocking | Late cocking | Acceleration | Deceleration | Follow-through |

| Start | Hands apart | Foot down | Maximal external rotation | Ball release | Finish |

FIGURE 15-12 The baseball pitch.

The resting, or open-packed, position for the humeroulnar joint is 70 degrees of flexion with 10 degrees of forearm supination. The close-packed position is full extension and maximum forearm supination. The capsular pattern is much more limitation in flexion than extension.[66]

Humeroradial Joint

During flexion and extension of the elbow, the humeroradial joint follows the pathway dictated by the anatomy of the ulnohumeral joint to which it is firmly attached by the annular and interosseous ligaments (Chap. 16).[50] Some supination and pronation also occurs at this joint due to a spinning of the radial head. The axis for pronation and supination passes from the center of the radial head to the pit adjacent to the styloid process of the ulna distally.

The resting, or open-packed, position of the humeroradial joint is extension and forearm supination. The close-packed position is approximately 90 degrees of elbow flexion and 5 degrees of supination. There is no true capsular pattern at this joint, although clinically an equal limitation of pronation and supination is observed.

Proximal Radioulnar Joint

At the proximal radioulnar joint, 1 degree of freedom exists, permitting pronation and supination. Pronation and supination involve the articulations at the elbow as well as the distal radioulnar joint and the radiocarpal articulation. Both the fascia and musculature of the forearm depend on the integrity of the interosseous radioulnar relationship for their mechanical efficiency.[50]

The proximal radioulnar joint is structurally an ovoid, with very little swing available to it due to its ligamentous constraints. As a consequence, its movement is confined to accommodating the osteokinematic spin of the radius. As the radial head forms the convex partner, there is a tendency for the radial head to move posterolaterally during pronation and anteromedially during supination, but these movements are strongly curtailed by the annular and interosseous ligaments.

The resting, or open-packed, position for the proximal radioulnar joint is 70 degrees of flexion and 35 degrees of forearm supination. The close-packed position is 5 degrees of forearm supination. The capsular pattern is minimal to loss of motion, with pain at the end ranges of pronation and supination.[66]

Coupled Motions

Conjunct rotations occur at the elbow complex with all motions. In addition, the elbow motions of flexion and extension are associated with adduction and abduction motions. The ability to abduct and adduct can easily be observed during pronation and supination. In the fully supinated position, the ulna is much nearer the midline of the body than it is in full pronation. Therefore abduction occurs with pronation, and adduction occurs with supination.

The abduction that occurs with extension occurs at the humeroulnar joint, and is more apparent than real. An increase in the carrying angle of the forearm during extension must not be confused with abduction of the ulna, which occurs because of the unequal ranges of extension between the ulna and the humerus, and the radius and the humerus (the capitellum being orientated more anteriorly than the trochlear). This inequity produces a conjunct humeral adduction with flexion, and conjunct humeroulnar abduction with extension, both of which are controlled by the radial and ulnar collateral ligaments.[50]

Thus it is apparent that pronation-supination and flexion-extension are interdependent, and each a conjunct motion of the other, at least at the extremes of range. Because pronation and supination involve the proximal and distal radioulnar joints, the humeroulnar, humeroradial, and the radiocarpal joints, mechanical dysfunction of any of these joints may become apparent, especially in the extremes of elbow flexion or extension.[50]

Force Couples of the Elbow

The important force couples of the elbow include[67]:

► The triceps/biceps during arm extension and flexion.

► Pronator teres, pronator quadratus/supinator during forearm pronation and supination.

► Flexor carpi radialis (FCR), flexor carpi ulnaris (FCU), flexor digitorum communis (FDC)/extensor carpi radialis longus (ECRL), extensor carpi radialis brevis (ECRB), extensor communis (EC) during wrist flexion and extension.

► Triceps/biceps, brachioradialis; pronator teres/supinator; FCR, FCU/ECRB, ECRL during activities requiring elbow stabilization.

Examination

The interventions for the common pathologies of the elbow complex and their interventions are detailed after the examination is described. An understanding of both is obviously necessary. As mention of the various pathologies occurs with reference to the tests and measures and vice versa, the reader is encouraged to switch between the two.

History

Elbow injuries are common in sports as well as from cumulative overuse in the athlete and nonathlete. During the history, the clinician must determine the chief complaint. The patient's chief complaint can often afford clues as to the underlying pathology. Twinges of pain, or locking of the elbow, could indicate a loose body within the joint. An inability to fully extend the elbow may indicate a number of conditions including synovitis of the elbow,[68] especially if it is accompanied by pain and fullness of the paraolecranon grooves.[68a] A chief complaint of pain upon leaning on the point of the elbow is usually associated with olecranon bursitis. In addition to the chief complaint, answers to the following questions must be obtained.

▶ Was there a mechanism of injury or any antecedent trauma? Traumatic elbow injuries often occur with a fall on the outstretched hand (FOOSH injury). This type of fall can result in a number of upper extremity and neck injuries. At the elbow the FOOSH injury can result in a hyperextension injury of the joint. If the fall was on the tip of the elbow, or there was blunt trauma to the olecranon process, this may indicate an olecranon bursitis, ulnar nerve lesion, or olecranon fracture.[68]

▶ Is the patient right or left hand dominant? This may have an impact on the ability of the elbow to rest, or on the functional status of the patient.

▶ Is there a history of pain following overuse or repetitive activities? Repetitive hyperextension, accompanied by pronation of the elbow can stress the distal biceps and lacertus fibrosis in the cubital fossa.[69]

  • Are the symptoms related to the patient's occupation? The improper use or unaccustomed use of tools such as hammers, saws, and screwdrivers can cause lateral or medial elbow pain.

  • Is the patient an athlete? A history of a "pop" followed by pain and swelling on the medial aspect of the elbow in a throwing athlete may indicate an ulnar collateral ligament sprain.[69a,69b] Individuals involved in racket sports commonly develop lateral elbow pain suggesting lateral epicondylitis (tennis elbow). In these situations it is well worth investigating recent changes in equipment (e.g., tennis racket head size, string tension, grip size).

▶ How long has the patient had the symptoms and are the symptoms improving or worsening? Such information can give clues as to the stage of healing or seriousness of the condition.

▶ Where is the pain located?

  • *Lateral elbow pain.* Epicondylitis should be suspected if there is tenderness over a bony prominence.

  • *Medial elbow pain.* This is usually due to a tendinopathy at the site of the attachment of the superficial forearm flexors and the pronator teres muscle to the medial epicondyle.[69c] However, it may also indicate a medial collateral ligament sprain, or an ulnar nerve compression.

  • *Posterior elbow pain* suggests olecranon bursitis, triceps tendonosis, or a valgus extension overload.[70]

  • *Cubital fossa pain.* This is most likely to result from a tear of the brachialis muscle at the musculotendinous junction, and is a common injury in rock climbers,[71] or a biceps brachii lesion. Cubital fossa pain may also be

associated with a compression of the posterior interosseous nerve, or a capsular injury.[72]

  • *Left arm and elbow pain* precipitated by physical exertion and relieved by rest should suggest angina.[68]

▶ Are there any associated joint noises or crepitus? A snapping elbow is synonymous with the relatively common recurrent dislocation of the ulnar nerve. However, the medial head of the triceps muscle or tendon also may dislocate over the medial epicondyle and result in snapping either as the elbow is flexed or as it is extended from a flexed position.[73] Dislocation of the medial head of the triceps can occur in combination with dislocation of the ulnar nerve, producing the clinical finding of at least two snaps at the elbow, with or without discomfort on the medial side of the elbow and with or without ulnar neuropathy. Joint crepitus may also indicate the presence of a loose body or synovitis. Catching or locking sensations are suggestive of joint instability or a loose joint body.

▶ Which activities or arm positions appear to aggravate the condition? Grasping and twisting activities tend to stress the elbow structures.

▶ Is the pain constant or intermittent? A visual analog scale can be used to record the patient's pain level.

▶ Is there any associated pain in the neck or shoulder? Intrinsic pain of the elbow structures is exacerbated by movement of the elbow joint, whereas referred pain is usually independent of elbow activity (see "Systems Review," later).[68,74]

▶ Are there any other joints that appear to be painful? This finding may suggest a systemic or infectious component.

▶ Are the symptoms better or worse at particular times of day or night?

▶ Are there any sensory changes, paresthesia, and muscle weakness in the ipsilateral limb? Such neurological findings are suggestive of a spinal nerve root or peripheral nerve lesion.

▶ Is there any underlying joint disease? Several types of arthritides or osteochondrosis dissecans develop in the elbow region without a known cause.[75]

▶ How old is the patient? Some elbow conditions are age related. Dislocation of the radiohumeral and radioulnar joint is seen in children up to the age of about 8 years. In toddlers, a dislocation of the radial head is common following a forceful tug on the arm. Panner's disease is seen up to age 10. From ages 15 to 20, osteochondrosis dissecans is found, whereas tennis elbow is seen in the 35- to 60-year age group.

▶ How is the condition affecting the patient's function in activities of daily living and recreational pursuits?

▶ Has the patient had this condition before and, if so, how was it treated and what was the outcome?

▶ Is the patient taking any medications? What conditions in addition to the present condition are the medications for?

▶ How is the patient's general health?

Systems Review

Following the history and systems review, the clinician may be able to determine the suitability of the patient for physical therapy. Signs or symptoms of a visceral, vascular, neurogenic, psychogenic, spondylogenic, or systemic disorder that may be local or referred are described in Chapter 9. Conditions that are out of the scope of physical therapy require that the patient be referred to an appropriate health care provider. Scenarios related to the elbow that warrant further investigation include an insidious onset of symptoms and complaints of numbness or paresthesia in the upper extremity. The Cyriax scanning examination can help highlight the presence or absence of neurological complications including spinal nerve root and peripheral nerve palsies. The scanning examination includes strength testing of the key muscles (see "Resistive Testing"), sensation testing and reflex testing. The sensory nerves supplying the elbow include branches of C5, C6, C8, and T1.[76] Sensory testing may include Semmes-Weinstein sensibility, and two-point discrimination. The three major deep tendon reflexes of the elbow are the biceps, brachioradialis, and the triceps. The biceps reflex, a function of C5, is elicited by placing a thumb over the biceps tendon in the cubital fossa and striking it with a reflex hammer while the patient's arm is relaxed and partially flexed. The biceps muscle should be felt or seen to jerk slightly. The brachioradialis reflex is a radial jerk elicited by tapping the brachioradialis tendon at the distal end of the radius. The triceps reflex can be elicited with the arm in the same position of partial, relaxed flexion. The triceps muscle should jerk when the triceps tendon is tapped where it crosses the olecranon fossa. Depressed, exaggerated, or absent upper extremity reflexes are noted and compared with reflex testing at the other elbow.

Reproduction of the patient's elbow symptoms with cervical motion, rather than elbow movement, is a strong indicator of a cervical and upper thoracic source for the symptoms, with either the segmental roots involved, or the brachial plexus.[76a–76d] In studies where normal cervical ligaments and muscles,[76e] cervical zygapophysial joints,[76f] and disks[76g] have been stimulated, subjects have reported pain in the head, anterior and posterior chest wall, shoulder girdle, and upper limb depending on the cervical level stimulated.[76h]

In addition to the cervical and upper thoracic spine, the related joints referring symptoms to the elbow require clearing, especially the shoulder.[76i,76j]

Systemic causes of insidious elbow pain include gout, infective arthritis, polyarthritis and vascular disorders, such as Volkmann's ischemia (see Chap. 9). Morning stiffness lasting for more than 1 hour, constitutional signs, and physical signs of joint inflammation are all indicative of an inflammatory disease.[76k] Systemic conditions are typically associated with other signs and symptoms which are not related to movement and that are systemic in nature (fever, chills, etc.). Respiratory

and cardiovascular conditions must also come into consideration when examining the elbow.[76l] The upper arm is very close to the chest and its viscera, so reference of pain to the elbow from these structures can occur.

Clinical Pearl

Severe progressive pain not affected by movement, persistent throughout the day and night, and associated with systemic signs, may indicate referred pain from a malignancy.[76m]

Tests and Measures

Observation

For an accurate and thorough examination of the elbow, the clinician must be able to visualize both arms. The affected elbow should be inspected for scars, deformities, and swelling. The earliest sign of elbow effusion is a loss of the elbow dimples. Most swelling appears beneath the lateral epicondyle. Even minor swelling or effusion prevents full extension of the elbow. Anterior joint effusion is evidence of significant swelling. Gradual swelling over the posterior tip of the elbow, which can be golf ball–sized and is often not tender to palpation, is usually olecranon bursitis. The clinician should observe for normal soft tissue and bony contours. Hypertrophy of the dominant forearm is common in tennis players and pitchers.

Clinical Pearl

Sudden swelling in the absence of trauma suggests infection, inflammation, or gout.

The triangular relationship of the epicondyles and the olecranon at 90 degrees of elbow flexion (Fig. 15-13) and full extension is often disrupted in the presence of a fracture, dislocation, or degeneration. At 90 degrees of flexion the three bony landmarks form an isosceles triangle, and when the arm is extended they form a straight line.[71,76n]

The clinician should observe the "carrying angle" of the affected elbow and compare it to the other side. The carrying angle varies from 13 to 16 degrees for females, and 11 to 14 degrees for males.[4,6] Any difference in the carrying angle of the elbow is obvious when the elbow is in extension. An increased carrying angle is called cubitus valgus. Cubitus varus, or "gunstock deformity" is the term used to describe a decreased carrying angle. The most common causes of an altered carrying angle are past trauma or epiphyseal growth disturbances. For example, a cubitus valgus can be caused by a lateral epicondylar fracture, whereas a cubitus varus is frequently the result of a supracondylar fracture.

Excessive tension at the elbow can be produced in occupations that place the elbows in sustained positions of flexion and adduction (e.g., keyboard operators). The tension increases resistance to movement and joint play at the elbow.[77,78] Elbow flexion also increases tension at the fibrous arch that connects the two heads of the flexor carpi ulnaris, which can lead to compression of the ulnar nerve.[79]

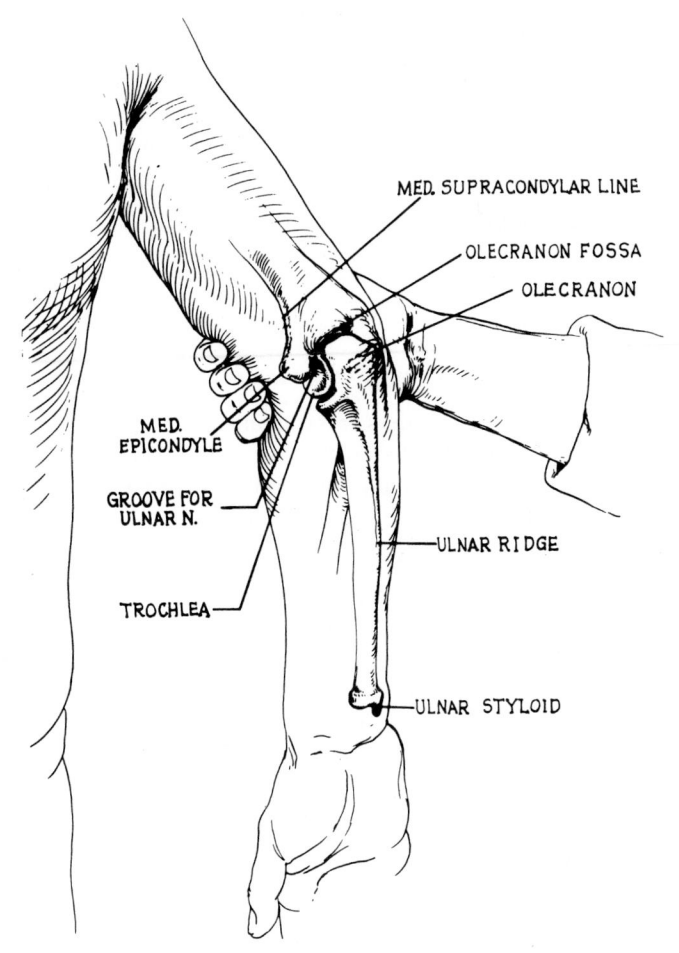

FIGURE 15-13 Palpation points of the elbow. (Reproduced with permission from Hoppenfeld S. *Physical Examination of the Spine and Extremities.* East Norwalk, CT: Appleton-Century-Crofts; 1976.)

A combination of sustained flexion and a restriction in joint play decreases the overall volume within the cubital tunnel, which can further increase the potential of ulnar nerve compression.[79,80]

Clinical Pearl

The pronated forearm position, combined with elbow flexion, wrist extension, and cyclic finger flexion and extension, creates shearing and compressive forces at several soft tissue interfaces in the forearm.[81,82] The pronators and extensor digitorum communis adaptively shorten over time because of prolonged contractions in their most shortened positions.[77,81]

Palpation

Because they are superficial, most of the elbow structures are easily palpable, making it easier for the clinician to pinpoint the specific area of pain. However, in cases in which the pain is more diffuse, the diagnosis becomes somewhat more difficult.

Palpation of the elbow complex is best performed with the patient seated or supine so they are able to relax. A logical sequence based on surface anatomy is outlined below.

Bony Structures. Bony structures feel hard, whereas ligamentous structures feel firm. Bony palpation of the elbow should start with assessment for crepitus during flexion and extension of the elbow. The presence of pain, swelling, or temperature elevation should also be appreciated.

▶ *Medial and lateral epicondyle (Figs. 15-13 and 15-14).* The lateral and medial epicondyles should be palpated for tenderness or effusion. The medial epicondyle can be palpated on the medial aspect of the distal humerus, while the lateral epicondyle is more difficult to palpate.

▶ *The joint line.* The joint line is located at a point approximately 2 cm down from an imaginary line joining the two epicondyles, which passes medially and inferiorly. The joint lines are firm on palpation, and lie between two structures that are harder.[75]

▶ *Supracondylar ridge (see Fig. 15-13).* By asking the patient to make a fist with the wrist in slight extension, the

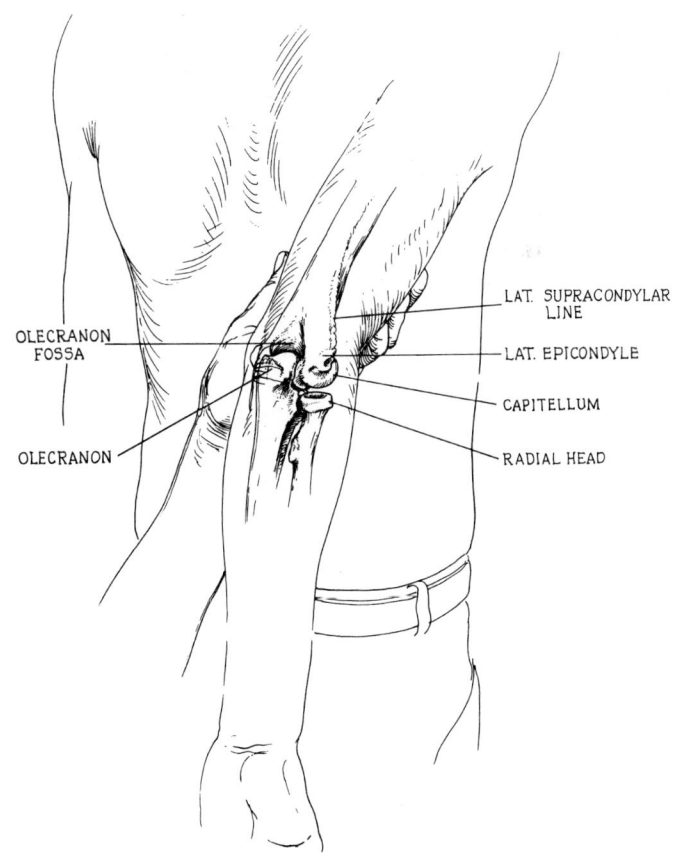

FIGURE 15-14 Lateral view of the elbow. (Reproduced with permission from Hoppenfeld S. *Physical Examination of the Spine and Extremities.* East Norwalk, CT: Appleton-Century-Crofts; 1976.)

extensor carpi radialis longus (ECRL) can be felt on the supracondylar ridge, which is just superior to the lateral epicondyle.[75]

▶ *Olecranon.* The olecranon (see Fig. 15-14) should be easy to locate. The olecranon ends distally in a point. Just distal to this point, the posterior border of the ulna can be palpated along its entire length (see Fig. 15-13).

▶ *Head of the radius.* The radial head is located in the skin depression immediately distal to the lateral epicondyle. To palpate the radial head (see Fig. 15-14) at the humeroradial joint, the clinician places the index finger on the lateral humeral epicondyle. From here, the index finger slides posteriorly and distally between the humerus and the radial head (see Fig. 15-14).[75] A traumatically dislocated radius will appear out of position and tender to palpation.

After examining the elbow's bony components, attention should be turned to the elbow's soft tissue structures, which may be divided into four clinical zones: medial, posterior, lateral, and anterior.[82a] The elbow's soft tissue structures are best appreciated in 90 degrees of flexion. Swelling of the elbow can be localized as in a swollen olecranon bursa, or diffuse as in a supracondylar fracture.

The medial aspect of the elbow contains the ulnar nerve, the wrist flexor-pronator muscle groups, and the medial collateral ligament (MCL). The ulnar nerve can be felt as a soft tubule coursing through the groove between the medial epicondyle and the olecranon process. Secondary damage to the ulnar nerve can occur in supracondylar or epicondylar injuries.[82a] The four muscles of the wrist flexor-pronator muscle group, pronator teres, flexor carpi radialis, palmaris longus and flexor carpi ulnaris (see Fig. 15-4), originate from the medial epicondyle before diverging into separate paths down the forearm (see "Muscles," later). The fan-shaped MCL connects the medial epicondyle to the medial margin of the ulna's trochlear notch. Tenderness in this area can be due to MCL sprain. The valgus stress test is performed to assess MCL stability (see later).

Within the lateral aspect of the elbow are the wrist extensors, the lateral collateral ligament (LCL), and the annular ligament. The three muscles of the wrist extensor group, brachioradialis, extensor carpi radialis longus, and extensor carpi radialis brevis, are palpated as a unit with the forearm in a neutral position and the wrist at rest (see "Muscles," later). These three muscles are commonly involved in lateral epicondylitis or "tennis elbow."[82a] The LCL extends from the lateral epicondyle to the side of the annular ligament, a ring-shaped band, cupping the radial head and neck. Disruption of either the LCL or the annular ligament can be assessed by palpation of the area and by the varus stress test (see later).

Muscles

▶ *Biceps.* The short head of the biceps is located at the coracoid process (together with the coracobrachialis muscle).[75] The long head of the biceps cannot be palpated at its origin, but it is palpable in the intertubercular groove of the proximal

humerus. The muscle belly of the biceps is easily identifiable, especially with resisted elbow flexion and forearm supination.

▶ *Brachialis.* The origin of the brachialis can be palpated posterior to the deltoid tuberosity. Its insertion can be palpated at a point medial to the musculotendinous junction of the biceps, at the proximal border of the bicipital aponeurosis.[75]

▶ *Brachioradialis.* The brachioradialis can be palpated from the radial border of the cubital fossa distally to the radial styloid process.

▶ *Common flexor origin at the medial epicondyle.*

▶ *Common extensor origin at the lateral epicondyle.*

▶ *Supinator.* The borders of the supinator within the cubital fossa are formed by the brachioradialis (radially), pronator teres (ulnarly), and tendon of the biceps (proximally) (see Fig. 15-10).[75]

▶ *Triceps.* Palpation of the triceps can be simplified by having the patient abduct the arm to 90 degrees. The lateral head of the triceps borders directly on the brachial muscle, whereas the medial head runs underneath both the long and lateral heads of the triceps. These two heads of the triceps can be palpated until their common insertion at the olecranon (see Fig. 15-13).[75]

▶ *Anconeus.* This small muscular triangle can be palpated between the olecranon, the posterior border of the ulna, and the lateral epicondyle (see Fig. 15-14). If crepitus is felt at full elbow extension, the clinician can manually push the sub-anconeus bursa superiorly during elbow extension. If the crepitus decreases, a dysfunction of the anconeus should be suspected, which can be treated with electrical stimulation, and mobilization of the olecranon in a medial or lateral direction.

Active Range of Motion with Passive Overpressure

Range of motion can be assessed with the patient seated, although elbow extension is better evaluated with the patient standing. The patient is asked to perform active flexion and extension of the elbow, pronation and supination of the forearm, and wrist flexion and extension (Fig. 15-15). The ranges are recorded. Wrist flexion and extension and forearm supination and pronation should be tested with the elbow flexed to 90 degrees and then fully extended. Capsular or noncapsular patterns should be determined. The capsular pattern at the elbow is characterized by limitation of more flexion than extension. If motion restrictions are present, the nature and location of the motion barrier, and the relationship of pain to the motion barrier should be noted.[5]

The end-feels of elbow motion should be classified as either compliant, suggesting soft tissue restriction, or rigid, suggesting a mechanical bony limit. Pain that occurs at the limit(s) of motion suggests bony impingement. The clinician should also note the degree of ulnar adduction or abduction that occurs with the elbow motions.

Passive pronation and supination are applied by grasping the proximal aspect of the forearm. Passive overpressure is

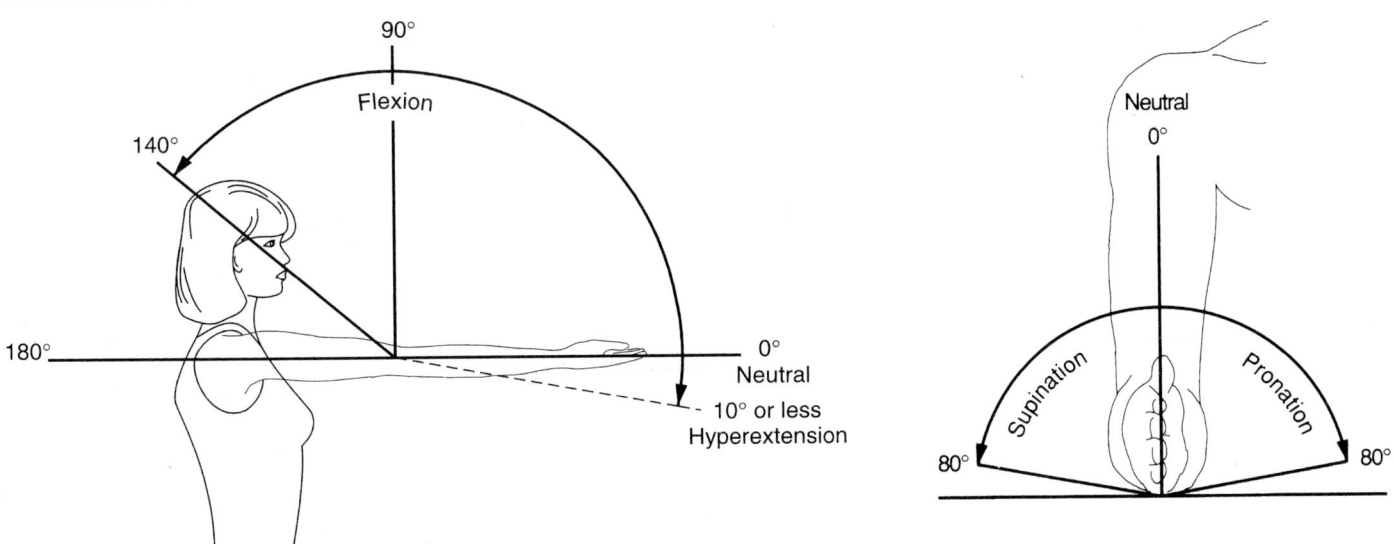

FIGURE 15-15 Elbow flexion and extension, and elbow pronation and supination. (Reproduced with permission from Luttgens K, Hamilton K. *Kinesiology: Scientific Basis of Human Motion.* New York: McGraw-Hill; 1997.)

superimposed at the end of the available ranges of flexion and extension, using the appropriate conjunct rotations. Internal rotation of the forearm (pronation) is the conjunct rotation associated with elbow extension; external rotation of the forearm (supination) is the conjunct rotation associated with elbow flexion[83]. Normal values for elbow pronation and supination are 75 degrees pronation and 85 degrees supination.[5]

> ### Clinical Pearl
>
> Decreased supination and pronation are frequent sequelae of a Colles' fracture, advanced degenerative changes, dislocations, and fractures of the forearm and elbow.

If there is a gross loss of pronation and supination post-trauma, a fractured radial head is a possibility. Of particular interest is the acute limitation of supination and extension in children, which likely results from a "pulled elbow" (see "Intervention Strategies" section).

Passive elbow flexion (Fig. 15-16) should have an end-feel of soft tissue approximation. Elbow flexion combined with supination should have a capsular end-feel, whereas elbow flexion combined with pronation should have a bony end-feel. Passive flexion may aggravate an ulnar nerve neuropathy.[65] Loss of normal elbow flexion (approximately 140 degrees) may be caused by osteophytic arthritis, intra-articular loose bodies, posterior capsule tightness, or possibly triceps tendonosis.[5]

Passive elbow extension (Fig. 15-17) should have a bony end-feel. A springy end-feel may indicate a loose body. Elbow extension is usually the first motion to be limited and the last to be restored with intrinsic joint problems.[65,69] The clinician should be particularly careful of the elbow that has lost a gross amount of extension post-trauma, especially if accompanied by

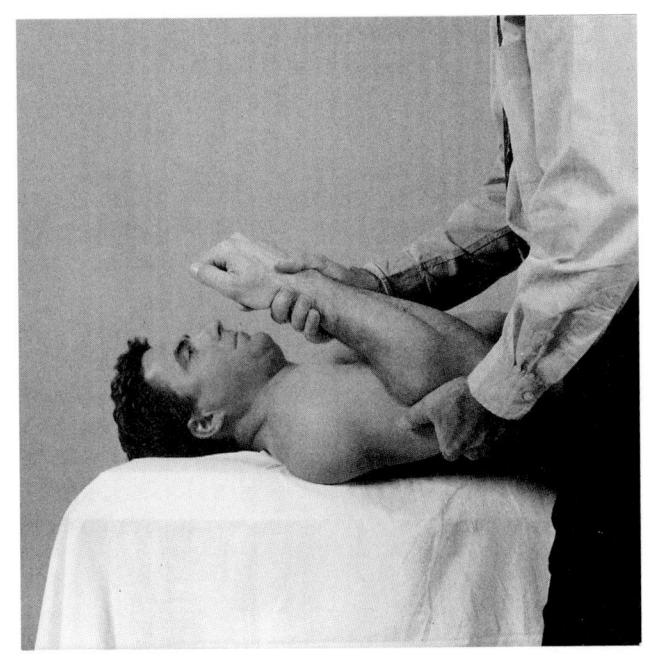

FIGURE 15-16 Elbow flexion.

a painful weakness of elbow extension, as this may indicate an olecranon fracture. A significant loss of motion, with no accompanying weakness, could indicate myositis ossificans.

> ### Clinical Pearl
>
> Pain throughout the central arc of flexion and extension, or pronation and supination, implies degeneration of the humeroulnar or proximal radioulnar joints, respectively.

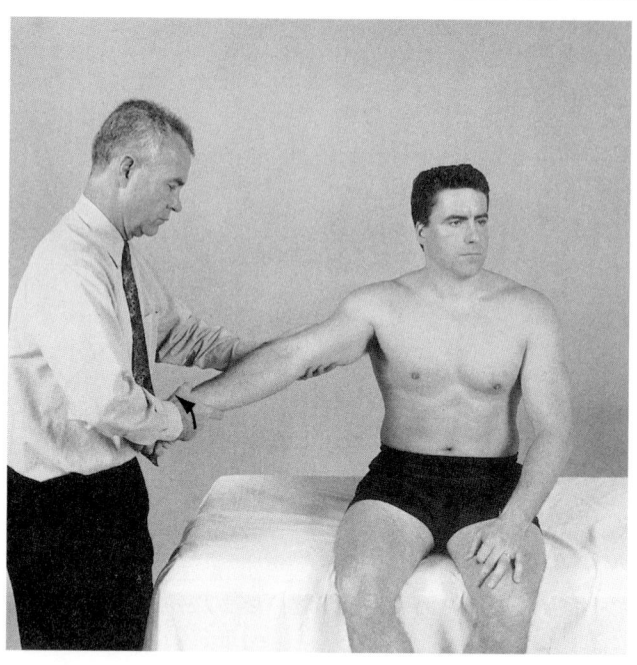

FIGURE 15-17   Elbow extension.

Combined Motions.   Combined movement testing is used to assess the patient who has full range of motion, but still has complaints of pain. The following combinations are assessed:

▶ Elbow flexion, adduction, and forearm pronation (Fig. 15-18).

▶ Elbow flexion, abduction, and forearm supination (see Fig. 15-16).

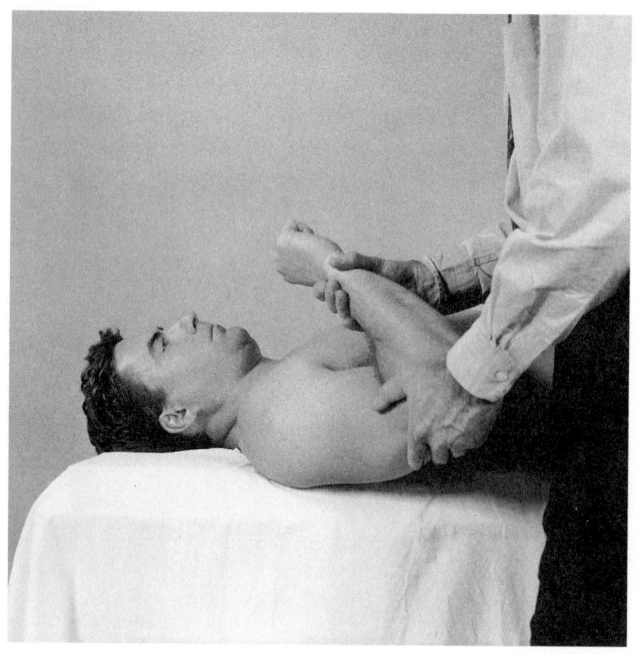

FIGURE 15-18   Combined motion of elbow flexion and pronation.

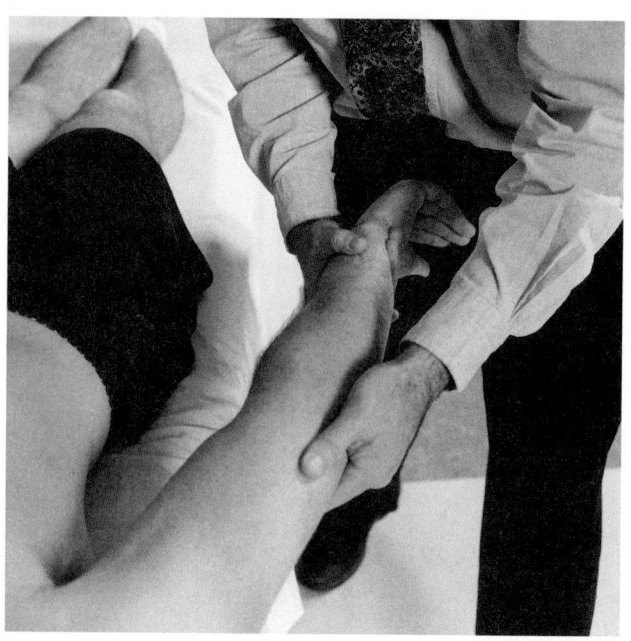

FIGURE 15-19   Combined motion of elbow extension and pronation.

▶ Elbow extension, abduction, and forearm pronation (Fig. 15-19).

▶ Elbow extension, adduction, and forearm supination (see Fig. 15-17).

Resistive Testing

In addition to all of the shoulder muscles that insert at or near the elbow (biceps, brachialis, triceps), the clinician must also test the other muscles responsible for elbow flexion and extension, and the muscles involved with forearm supination, pronation, and wrist flexion and extension.

Elbow Flexion (C5–6).   Resisted elbow flexion is tested with the elbow flexed to 90 degrees with the forearm in pronation, then supination, and then neutral rotation (Fig. 15-20). Pain with resisted elbow flexion most frequently implicates the biceps, especially if resisted supination is also painful. The brachialis is implicated if resisted elbow flexion with the forearm in full pronation is painful. The brachioradialis is rarely involved. Both sides are tested for comparison.

Elbow Extension (C7).   Resisted elbow extension is tested with forearm pronation, supination, and neutral. Both sides are tested for comparison. Pain with resisted elbow extension implicates the triceps muscle, although the anconeus muscle could also be involved.

Forearm Pronation/Supination (C5–7).   The clinician should test the strength of the forearm muscles by grasping the patient's hand in a handshake. The patient should be asked to exert maximum pressure to turn the palm first up (using supinators) then

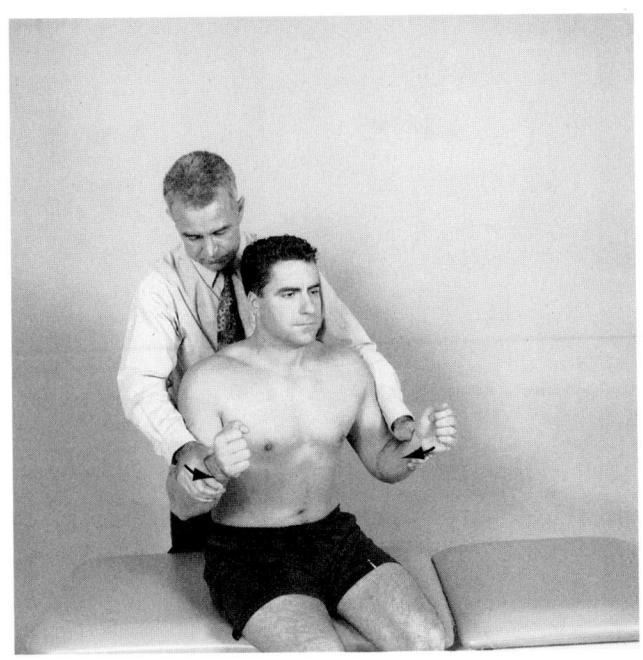

FIGURE 15-20   Resisted elbow flexion.

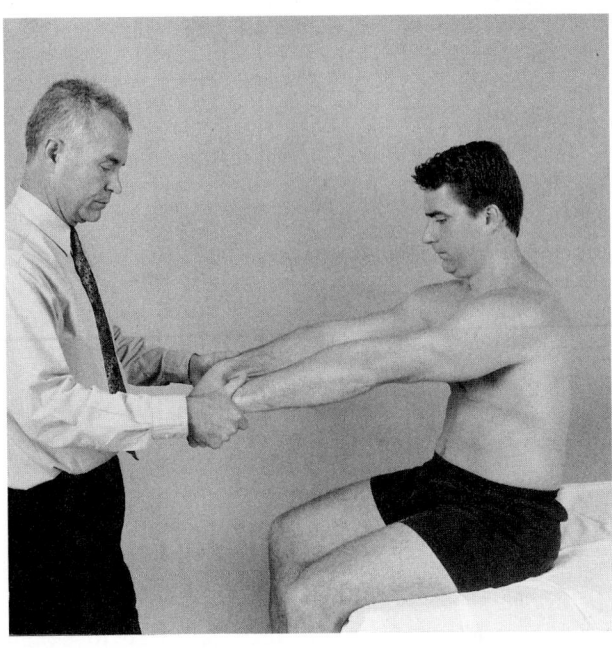

FIGURE 15-21   Resisted wrist flexion.

down (using pronators). Weakness in the supinators may indicate tendonitis, a rupture, or a subluxation of the biceps tendon at the shoulder. It may also indicate a C5 through C6 nerve root lesion, radial nerve lesion (supinator), or musculocutaneous nerve lesion (biceps). The supinator muscle is rarely injured.

Pronator weakness is associated with rupture of the pronator teres from the medial epicondyle, fracture of the medial elbow, and lesions of the C6 through C7 or median nerve roots. Pronator quadratus weakness, which is tested with the elbow held in a flexed position to neutralize the humeral head of the pronator teres muscle, could indicate a lesion of the anterior interosseous nerve. The pronator teres or quadratus muscles are rarely injured. Individuals with medial or lateral epicondylitis will also find the aforementioned maneuvers painful, and resisted wrist flexion and extension can be used to help differentiate the former and latter, respectively.

Wrist Flexion.   The flexor carpi ulnaris is the strongest wrist flexor. To test the flexors, the clinician stabilizes the patient's mid-forearm with one hand while placing the fingers of the other hand in the patient's palm, with the palm facing the patient (Fig. 15-21). The patient attempts to flex the wrist with the elbow flexed and then extended. Weakness is evident in rupture of the muscle origin, lesions involving the ulnar (C8, T1) or median nerve (C6, C7), or tendonitis at the medial elbow.

Wrist Extension.   The most powerful wrist extensor is the extensor carpi ulnaris. To test the wrist extensors, the clinician's hands are placed in the same position as in the preceding test, with the patient's palm facing the clinician. The patient is asked to extend the wrist with the elbow flexed and then extended (Fig. 15-22).

Rupture of the extensor origin, lesions of the C6 through C8 nerve root, or lateral epicondylitis can cause weakness.

Radial Deviation.   Resisted radial deviation is tested with the elbow at 90 degrees of elbow flexion, and at full elbow extension. Pain with resisted radial deviation is usually the result of lateral epicondylitis.

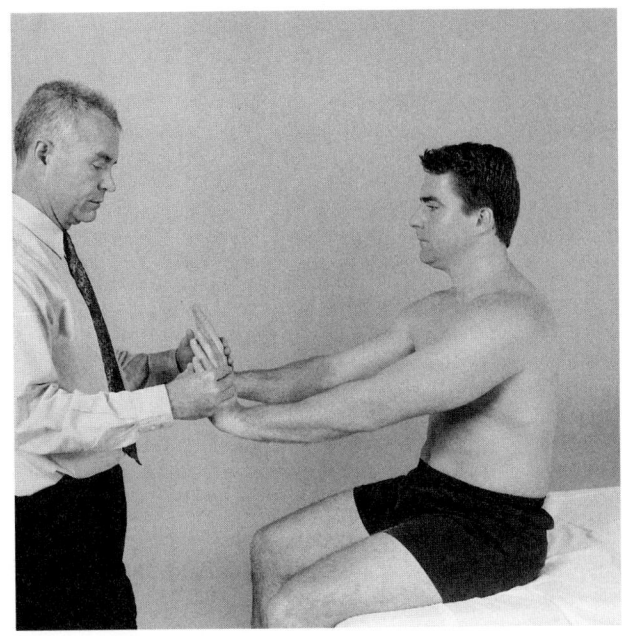

FIGURE 15-22   Resisted wrist extension.

Ulnar Deviation. Resisted ulnar deviation, although rarely affected, is tested with the fingers in full flexion, and then in full extension.

Extension of Fingers 2–5. For resisted extension of fingers 2 through 5, the elbow is positioned in full extension, the wrist in neutral, and the metacarpophalangeal (MCP) joints at 90 degrees of flexion. Pain here is usually the result of extensor digitorum tendonitis, or lateral epicondylitis.

Extension of Fingers 2–3. For resisted extension of fingers 2 through 3, the patient is positioned as above. Pain with resistance implicates lateral epicondylitis.

Functional Assessment

Like the shoulder, the elbow serves to position the hand for functional activities. A number of tests have been designed to assess elbow function (Table 15-4).

Passive Articular Motion Testing

The passive articular mobility tests are used to examine the arthrokinematic, or accessory motions of a joint (see Chap. 8).

Ulnohumeral Joint. The patient is positioned in supine with their head supported on a pillow. The clinician sits or stands facing the patient.

Distraction/Compression. The clinician wraps the fingers around the proximal third of the forearm (Fig. 15-23). The clinician applies a longitudinal force through the proximal

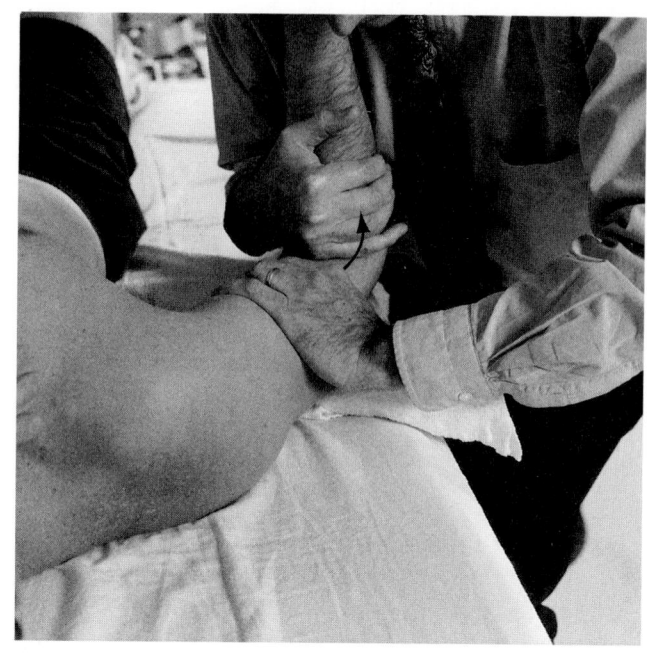

FIGURE 15-23 Ulnohumeral distraction/compression.

forearm, and along the line of the humerus to distract the ulnohumeral joint. The quality and quantity of motion is noted. The test is repeated on the opposite extremity and the findings compared.

Medial Glide. The clinician, using the medial aspect of the MCP joint of the index finger of the medial hand, palpates and

TABLE 15-4 Functional Testing of the Elbow[336]

Starting Position	Action	Functional Test
Sitting, cuff weight attached to wrist	Elbow flexion	5-lb weight: Functional 3- to 4-lb weight: Functionally fair Active flexion (0 lb): Functionally poor Cannot flex elbow: Nonfunctional
Standing	Elbow extension with wall push-up	5 reps: Functional 3–4 reps: Functionally fair 1–2 reps: Functionally poor 0 reps: Nonfunctional
Standing facing door	Turning door knob into supination	5 reps: Functional 3–4 reps: Functionally fair 1–2 reps: Functionally poor 0 reps: Nonfunctional
Standing facing door	Turning door knob into pronation	5 reps: Functional 3–4 reps: Functionally fair 1–2 reps: Functionally poor 0 reps: Nonfunctional

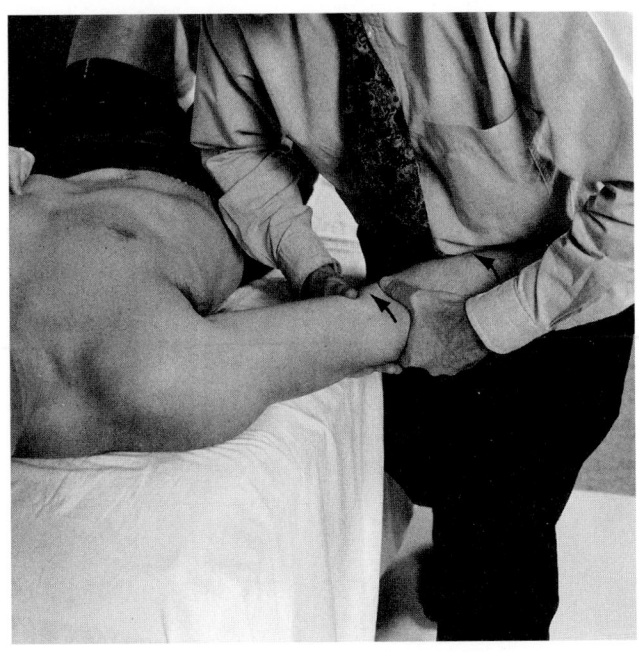

FIGURE 15-24   Medial glide of ulnohumeral joint.

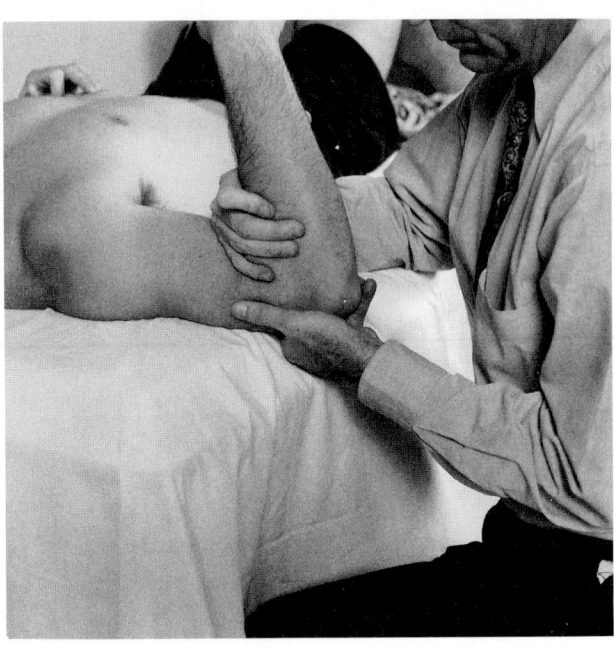

FIGURE 15-25   Lateral glide of ulnohumeral joint.

stabilizes the medial aspect of the distal humerus (Fig. 15-24). Using the other hand, the clinician palpates the lateral aspect of the olecranon with the lateral aspect of the MCP joint of the index finger (see Fig. 15-24). The elbow is extended to the limit of physiologic range of motion. From this position, the clinician glides the ulna medially on the fixed humerus along the mediolateral plane of the joint line. The quality and quantity of motion is noted. The test is repeated on the opposite extremity and the findings compared.

Lateral Glide.   Using the lateral aspect of the MCP joint of the little finger of the medial hand, the clinician palpates and stabilizes the lateral aspect of the distal humerus (Fig. 15-25). Using the other hand, the clinician palpates the medial aspect of the olecranon with the MCP joint of the index finger (see Fig. 15-25). The elbow is flexed to the limit of physiologic range of motion. From this position, the clinician glides the ulna laterally on the fixed humerus along the mediolateral plane of the joint line. The quality and quantity of motion is noted. The test is repeated on the opposite extremity and the findings compared.

Radiohumeral Joint.   The joint glides for the radiohumeral joint are performed with the elbow positioned in 70 degrees of flexion and 35 degrees of supination. The patient is positioned in sitting with their hand resting on the table. The following tests are performed.[84,85]

Anterior Glide.   The clinician stabilizes the humerus and applies an anterior glide of the radius (Fig. 15-26) to assess the accessory glide that accompanies flexion.

Posterior Glide.   The clinician stabilizes the humerus and applies a posterior glide of the radius (see Fig. 15-26) to assess the accessory glide that accompanies extension.

Distraction.   The clinician stabilizes the radial head and the lateral epicondyle. With the other hand, the clinician grasps the radius and applies a longitudinal distraction force along

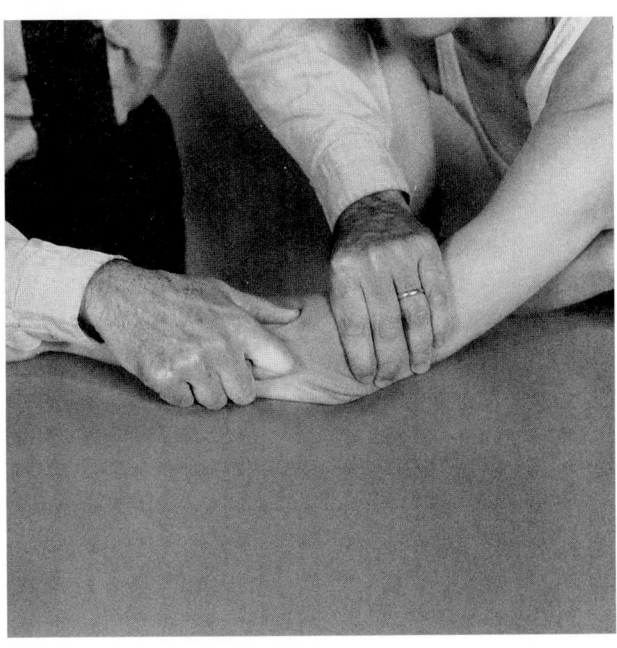

FIGURE 15-26   Radiohumeral joint glides.

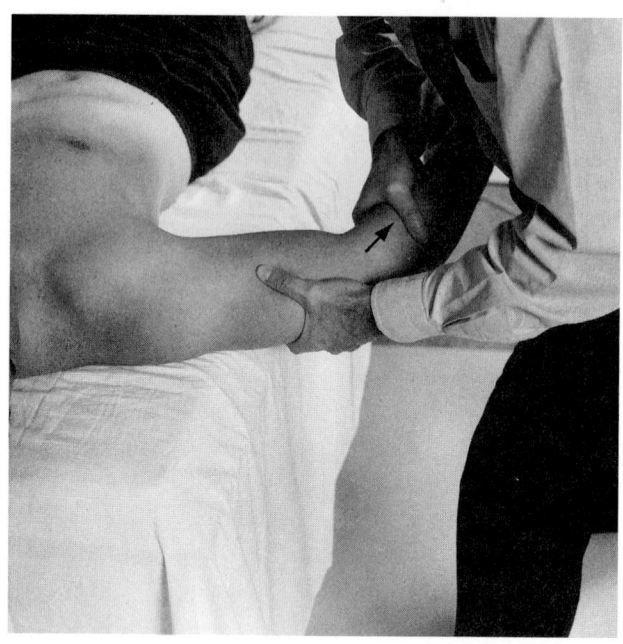

FIGURE 15-27   Distraction of the radius.

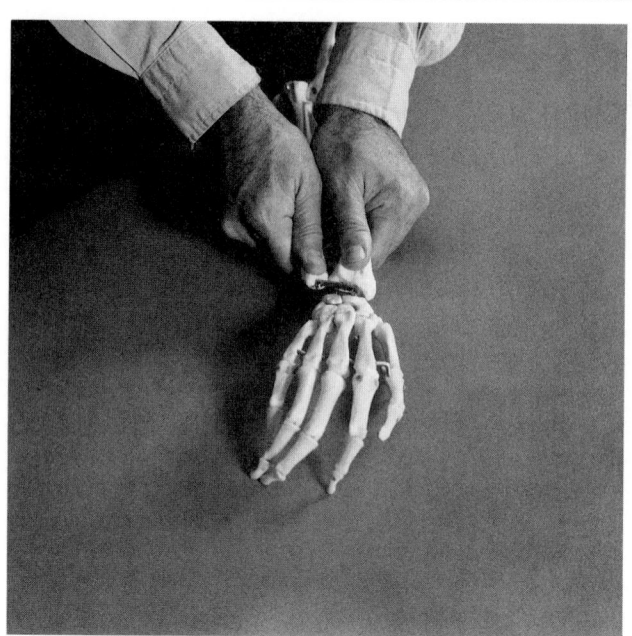

FIGURE 15-28   Anterior-posterior glide of the distal radioulnar joint.

the length of the radius (Fig. 15-27). A longitudinal compression force can be applied using the same patient-clinician position.

Motion Testing of the Radial Head.   The patient is positioned in sitting or supine, with the clinician facing the patient. The radial head is located by flexing and extending the elbow. Once located, the radial head is grasped by the clinician between the thumb and index finger (see Fig. 15-26). The radial head is moved in an anterior and posterior direction, and any restriction of motion is noted. The posterior glide of the radius is coupled with pronation/extension, and anterior glide is coupled with supination/flexion. The most common dysfunction of the radial head is a posterior radial head, which is accompanied by a loss of the anterior glide.

Proximal Radioulnar Joint

Anterior-Posterior Glide.   The patient is positioned in sitting or in supine with their head resting on a pillow. The clinician palpates and stabilizes the proximal third of the ulna with one hand. With a pinch grip of the index finger and thumb, the clinician palpates the head of the radius in a posterolateral plane with the other hand (see Fig. 15-26). From this position, the clinician glides the head of the radius anteroposteriorly at the proximal radioulnar joint, in an obliquely anteromedial/posterolateral direction. The quality and quantity of motion is noted. The test is repeated on the opposite extremity and the findings compared.

Distal Radioulnar Joint

Anterior-Posterior Glide.   The patient is positioned in supine with their head resting on a pillow. The clinician palpates and stabilizes the distal third of the ulna with one hand. With a pinch

grip of the fingers and thenar eminence of the other hand, the clinician palpates the distal third of the radius (Fig. 15-28). From this position, the clinician glides the radius anterorposteriorly at the distal radioulnar joint, in an obliquely anteromedial/posterolateral direction. The quality and quantity of motion is noted. The test is repeated on the opposite extremity and the findings compared.

Stress Tests

Medial (Ulnar) Collateral Ligament (Valgus Test).   The patient is positioned in supine with their head supported on a pillow. The clinician stabilizes the distal humerus with one hand, and palpates the distal forearm with the other. The anterior band of the MCL tightens in the range of 20 to 120 degrees of flexion, becoming lax in full extension, before tightening again in hyperextension. The posterior bundle is taut in flexion beyond 55 degrees.[8,17,22,69]

The anterior band is tested by flexing the elbow to between 20 and 30 degrees to unlock the olecranon from its fossa as a valgus stress is applied continuously (Fig. 15-29).[19,48]

The posterior band is best tested using a "milking" maneuver. The patient is seated and their arm is positioned in shoulder flexion, elbow flexion beyond 55 degrees, and forearm supination. The clinician pulls downward on the patient's thumb (Fig. 15-30).[19] This maneuver generates a valgus stress on the flexed elbow. A positive sign is indicated by the reproduction of pain.

The tests are repeated on the opposite extremity and the findings compared.

Lateral Pivot Shift Apprehension Test.   The lateral pivot shift test is used in the diagnosis of posterolateral rotatory instability. The patient is positioned in supine with the involved extremity

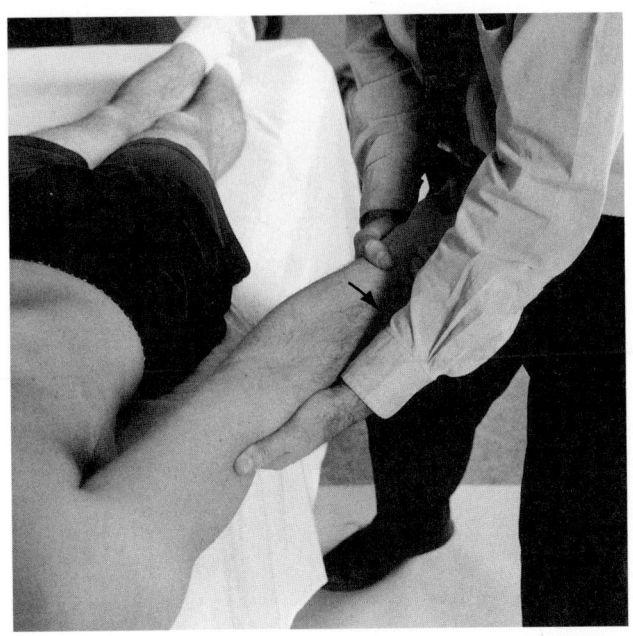

FIGURE 15-29 Medial collateral ligament stress test.

overhead. The clinician grasps the patient's wrist and elbow. The elbow is supinated with a mild force at the wrist, and a valgus moment and compressive force is applied to the elbow during flexion.[86] This results in a typical apprehension response with reproduction of the patient's symptoms and a sense that the elbow is about to dislocate. Reproducing the actual subluxation, and the clunk that occurs with reduction,

usually can only be accomplished with the patient under general anesthesia or occasionally after injecting local anesthetic into the elbow.

Lateral (Radial) Collateral Ligament (Varus Test). The LCL is tested with the elbow positioned in 5 to 30 degrees short of full extension. The clinician stabilizes the humerus and adducts the ulna, producing a varus force at the elbow (Fig. 15-31). The end-feel is noted.

Special Tests
Tennis Elbow. A number of tests exist for tennis elbow (lateral epicondylitis). Two are described here.

Cozen's Test. The clinician stabilizes the patient's elbow with one hand and the patient is asked to pronate the forearm, and extend and radially deviate the wrist against the manual resistance of the clinician (Fig. 15-32). A reproduction of pain in the area of the lateral epicondyle indicates a positive test.

Mill's Test. The clinician palpates the patient's lateral epicondyle with one hand, while pronating the patient's forearm, fully flexing the wrist, and extending the elbow (Fig. 15-33). A reproduction of pain in the area of the lateral epicondyle indicates a positive test.

Golfer's Elbow (Medial Epicondylitis). The clinician palpates the medial epicondyle with one hand, while supinating the forearm and extending the wrist and elbow with the other hand. A reproduction of pain in the area of the medial epicondyle indicates a positive test.

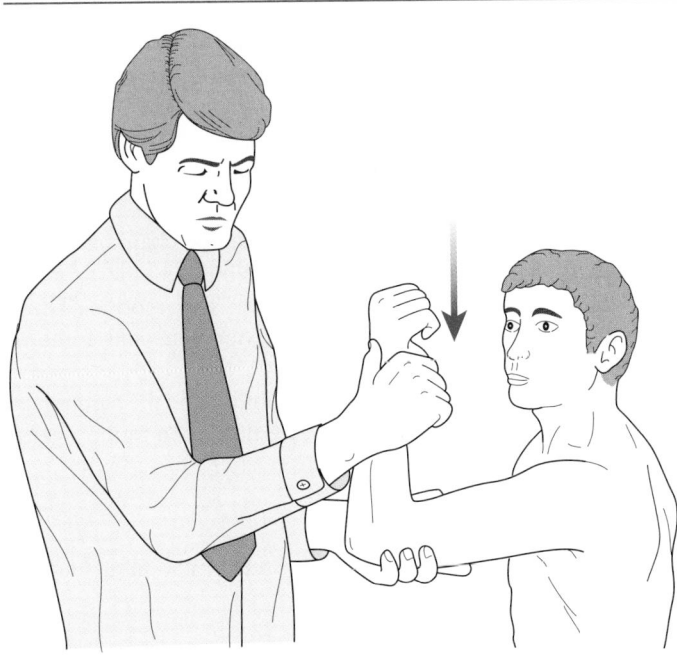

FIGURE 15-30 Milking maneuver.

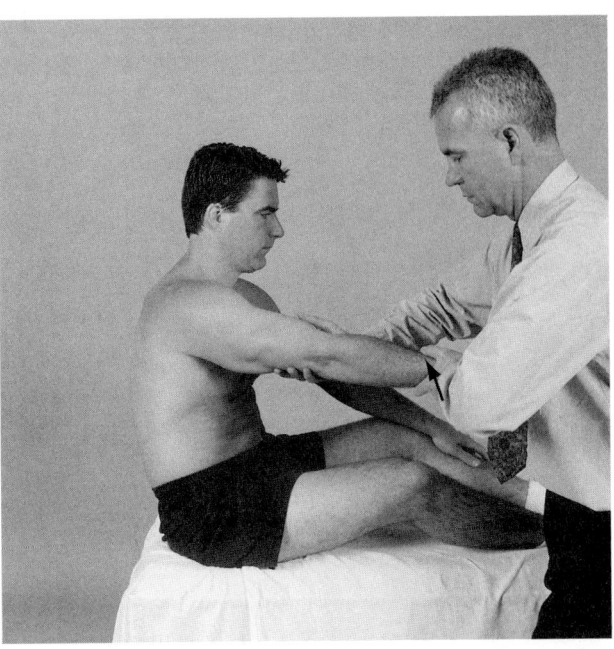

FIGURE 15-31 Lateral collateral ligament stress test.

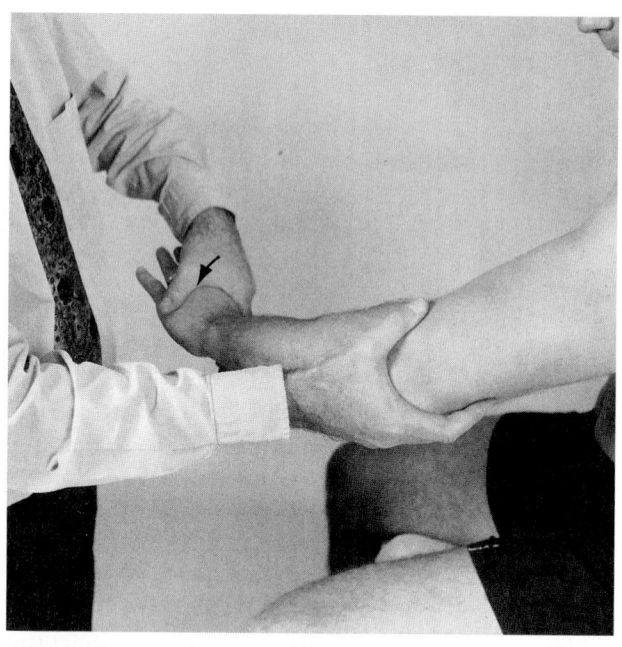

FIGURE 15-32　Cozen's test.

Elbow Flexion Test for Cubital Tunnel Syndrome. The patient is positioned in sitting. The patient is asked to depress both shoulders, flex both elbows maximally, supinate the forearms, and extend the wrists (Fig. 15-34).[87] This position is maintained for 3 to 5 minutes. Tingling or paresthesia in the ulnar distribution of the forearm and hand indicates a positive test.

Pressure Provocative Test for Cubital Tunnel Syndrome. Pressure is applied by the clinician, proximal to the cubital tunnel, with

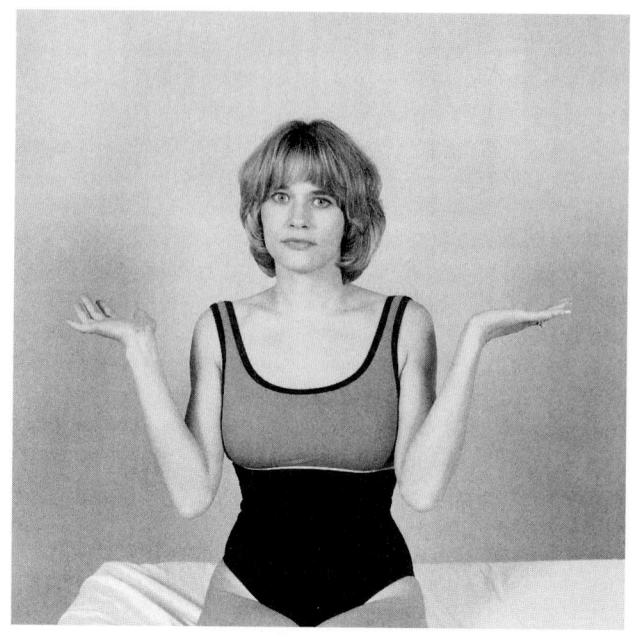

FIGURE 15-34　Elbow flexion test.

the elbow held in 20 degrees of flexion and the forearm in supination.[88]

Tinel's Sign (at the Elbow). The clinician locates the groove between the olecranon process and the medial epicondyle through which the ulnar nerve passes. This groove is tapped by the index finger of the clinician. A positive sign is indicated by a tingling sensation in the ulnar distribution of the forearm and hand distal to the tapping point.

Intervention Strategies

Due to the unique orientation of the elbow complex, the clinician is faced with multiple clinical challenges to successfully rehabilitate the injured elbow.[1]

The elbow is the central link in the kinetic chain of the upper extremity. It is important that the elbow is able to move freely and painlessly throughout its available motion. These motions include elbow flexion and extension, and forearm pronation and supination.

The techniques to increase joint mobility and the techniques to increase soft tissue extensibility are described in the Therapeutic Techniques section.

Acute Phase

The goals of the acute phase of elbow rehabilitation include:

▶ Protection of the injury site.

▶ Restoration of pain-free range of motion in the entire kinetic chain.

▶ Improve patient comfort by decreasing pain and inflammation.

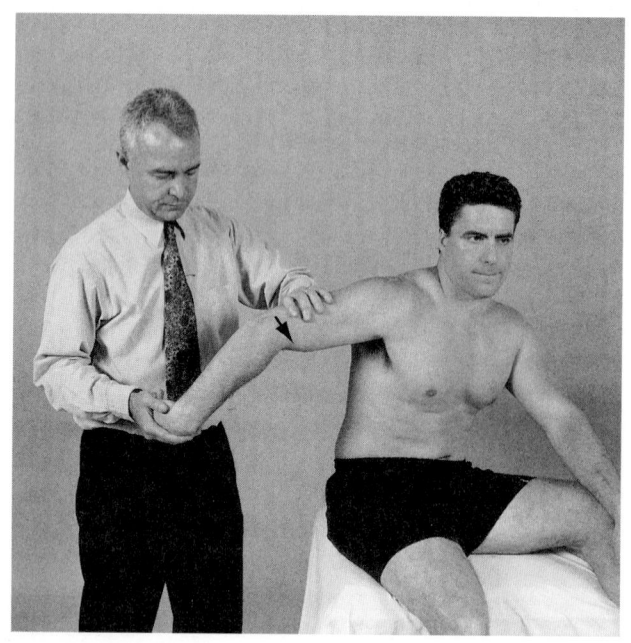

FIGURE 15-33　Mill's test.

► Retard muscle atrophy.

► Minimize detrimental effects of immobilization and activity restriction.[89–94]

► Maintain general fitness.

► Allow the patient to be independent with a home exercise program.

During the early stages of the acute phase, the principles of PRICEMEM (protection, rest, ice, compression, elevation, manual therapy, early motion, and medication) are applied as appropriate. Icing for 20 to 30 minutes, three to four times a day, concurrent with nonsteroidal anti-inflammatory drugs (NSAIDs) or aspirin can aid in reducing pain and swelling.

Early active assisted and passive exercises are performed in all planes of shoulder, elbow, and wrist motions to nourish the articular cartilage and assist in collagen tissue synthesis and organization.[1,95–98] As the available range at the elbow occurs at the humeroulnar, humeroradial and proximal and distal radioulnar joints, restrictions or laxities at any of these joints can affect the eventual outcome of the rehabilitative process.

> ### *Clinical Pearl*
>
> Corticosteroid injections have been advocated for elbow injuries to promote and progress healing. Although the use of local injections increases the risks of disrupting tissue planes, fenestration of the area of tendonosis may be beneficial because of the bleeding that occurs in the new channels, which has the potential for transforming a failed intrinsic healing process into an extrinsic response.[99,100]

The formation of an elbow flexion contracture must be avoided, as this contracture can place abnormal stresses on the elbow complex, especially during athletic activities.[101] One of the most common causes of joint contracture at the elbow is scar formation at the anterior capsule, and at the insertion site of the brachialis.[1] This scarring can be minimized by performing joint mobilizations to the humeroulnar and humeroradial joints. A posterior glide of the ulna on the humerus is used to help restore elbow extension. The anterior capsule can be stretched using long-duration, low-intensity stretching to produce a plastic response of the collagen tissue.[1,102,103] This can be accomplished by positioning the patient in supine, with a towel roll placed posterior to the elbow joint, and the forearm hanging over the edge of the bed (Fig. 15-35). A light weight (2 to 4 lb) is placed in the hand, and the elbow is extended as far as is comfortable. The passive stretch is maintained for 5 to 7 minutes, avoiding pain or a protective muscle response. This exercise becomes an important component of the patient's home exercise program.

Initially, the patient is advised to decrease the level of activity with use of pain as the limiting factor, but without immobilizing the injured part completely.

Once full range of pain-free motion has been achieved, the patient's strengthening program is progressed. The resistance-based exercise program is the mainstay of nonoperative inter-

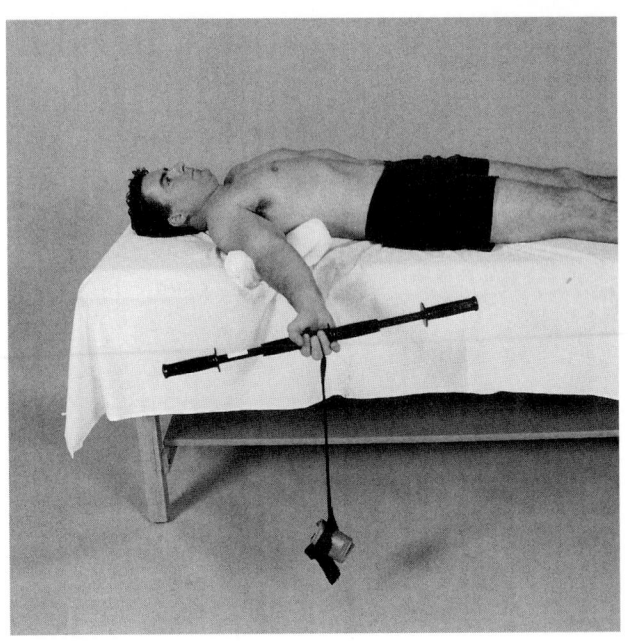

FIGURE 15-35   Passive elbow flexion.

vention for the elbow, and serves to retard muscle atrophy of the elbow and wrist musculature. Patients are advanced in concordance with their ability to participate in the program. Patients should be taught how to perform these exercises independently at the earliest opportunity.

Patients are initially instructed to perform submaximal isometric exercises at multiple angles for the elbow flexors and extensors, the forearm supinators and pronators, and the wrist flexors and extensors. The exercise program is progressed from the multiple angle isometrics to isotonic progressive resistive exercises using dumbbells or surgical tubing for the biceps, triceps, pronators, and supinators, the wrist flexors and extensors, and the shoulder musculature. Low resistance is used initially with 1 to 2 sets of 10 repetitions, progressing as tolerated to 5 sets of 10 repetitions. Once 5 sets of 10 repetitions can be performed without pain and in a slow and controlled manner, additional resistance is added in 1- to 3-lb increments.[1]

Exercises to increase strength should include:

► Concentric exercises to the wrist flexors and extensors, elbow flexors and extensors, and radial and ulnar deviators, performed at varying speeds.

► Mechanical resistance using a small bar with asymmetrically placed weight for strengthening the pronators (Fig. 15-36) and supinators (Fig. 15-37).

► Exercises for wrist flexors and extensors. The broom-handle exercise is recommended. A weight is tied to a rope or piece of string approximately 3 feet in length, which is then tied to a broom-handle or dowel. The broom-handle is held out in front of the patient with the palms down (for wrist extensors, see Fig. 15-38) or palms up (for wrist flexors). The patient then rolls the string onto the handle/dowel to raise and then lower the weight.

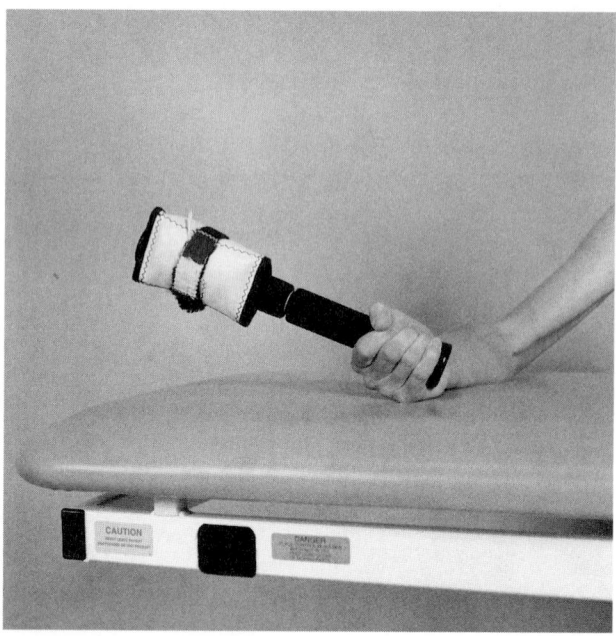

FIGURE 15-36 Strengthening exercise for pronators.

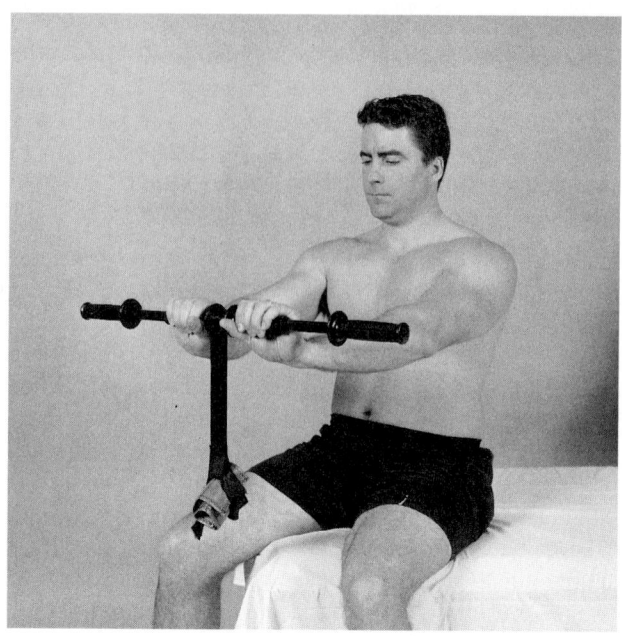

FIGURE 15-38 Broom-handle exercise.

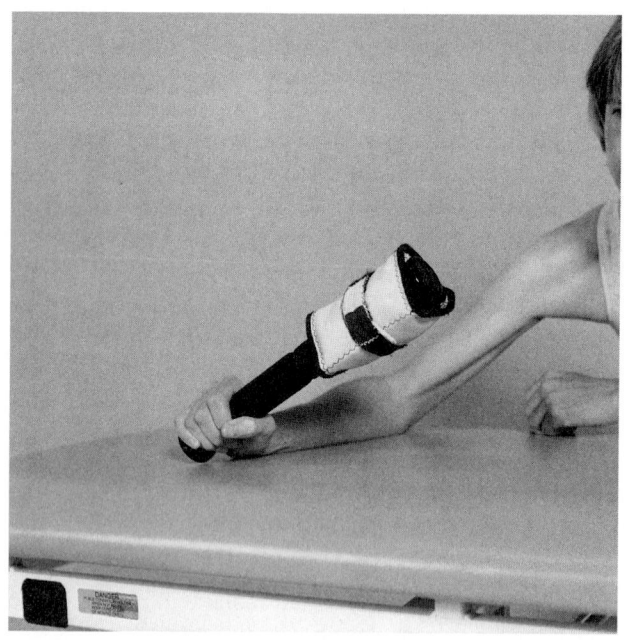

FIGURE 15-37 Strengthening exercise for supinators.

▶ Tennis ball squeezes to improve grip strength (once symptoms have subsided).

▶ Exercises to increase the strength in opposing muscles, such as the flexors of the wrist and digits, in order to balance the force couple.

Shoulder exercises should also be introduced as early as possible, although caution should be used with shoulder external

rotation exercises because of the potential for valgus stress to the elbow.[1,100,104,105] In the earlier phases of pain, modification of activity may involve alternating between low- and high-intensity workouts.[106,107] Endurance is developed over time as the patient becomes able to tolerate more repetitions and sustained activities. If endurance is not developed and the muscle-tendon unit becomes fatigued, the muscular portion can no longer absorb the stresses and greater stresses are absorbed by the tendon.[108] Throughout all phases of rehabilitation and exercise, training should be within physiologic limits for cellular response and homeostasis.[109] Therefore, relative rest is sometimes advised during painful periods.

Stability at the shoulder and the elbow is extremely important for those patients returning to overhead sports, and can be addressed using proprioceptive neuromuscular facilitation (PNF) patterns with increasing resistance.

Once the functional tests are pain free, an eccentric strengthening program based on the principles of healing can be initiated. These exercises are an essential component of the rehabilitation program with conditions such as medial or lateral epicondylitis. Cryotherapy should be used immediately following these exercises.

In the presence of joint laxity that is not controllable with adequate exercise or ergonomic modifications, bracing can be effective.

Functional Phase

The functional phase addresses any tissue overload problems and functional biomechanical deficits. The goals of the functional phase include:

▶ Attain full range of pain-free motion in the upper kinetic chain.

► Restore normal joint kinematics.

► Improve muscle strength to within normal limits.

► Improve neuromuscular control.

► Restore normal muscle force couples.

If the feet and trunk are stabilized during an activity, the upper quarter kinetic chain involves the cervical spine, thoracic outlet, thoracic spine, shoulder, elbow, wrist, and hand. The upper quarter operates as a mechanical unit whose links are functionally interdependent on one another.

Athletes instinctively modify their techniques of play to avoid motions involving painful, injured tissues, and prevent further abuse of the overused tissues.[107,109] For example, in order to adapt to weakness of the muscles of the shoulder, a tennis player will attempt to generate force with the muscles of the forearm, thereby predisposing to tendonosis of the elbow. The application of kinetic-chain exercises to the treatment of the elbow involves strengthening of the muscles of the rotator cuff and those around the scapula. Weakness of the muscles about the shoulder, especially the external rotators, must be treated in patients who have sustained tendonosis of the elbow while participating in racquet or throwing sports.[100,106]

The patient begins concentric exercises with elastic tubing to simulate the upper extremity activity (Fig. 15-39), initially with use of low speeds and resistance; the speed and the intensity of resistance are then gradually increased.

Co-contraction of the muscles around the elbow can be produced with closed chain exercises such as the push-up, quadruped exercises, and dips, incorporating a wide range of equipment such as gymnastic balls, BAPS boards, mini-tramp, and slide board.

Training can also involve dynamic muscle co-contractions in an open kinetic chain by using high-speed ballistic movement patterns with elastic tubing incorporating PNF diagonals. These rapid ballistic movements result in synchronous activation of agonists and antagonists.[110–112]

The function of the biceps is integral to the stability of the elbow complex and must be exercised emphasizing slow and fast muscular contractions in both concentric and eccentric modes.[1] Wilk and colleagues[1] advocate the following drill to enhance the dynamic stability of the elbow:

► The patient flexes the elbow against resistance provided by elastic tubing.

► The patient holds a position isometrically while the clinician employs rhythmic stabilization resistance anteriorly and posteriorly.

The procedure is repeated for the wrist flexors-extensors and the forearm pronators-supinators.

Plyometric exercises are also used at the elbow using elastic tubing.[113] The patient grasps the elastic tubing and fully flexes the elbow, with the shoulder flexed to about 60 degrees. This position is maintained briefly. The patient then releases the isometric hold, allowing the elbow to extend rapidly. As full extension is reached, the movement is quickly reversed back into full elbow flexion.[113] The forearm pronators-supinators can all be exercised in a similar fashion.

The shoulder stabilizers, triceps, and the wrist flexors-extensors can all be trained using Swiss ball exercises (Fig. 15-40), medicine ball soccer throw (Fig. 15-41), diagonal pass (Fig. 15-42), side throw (Fig. 15-43), ball squeeze (Fig. 15-44), and modified push-up (Fig. 15-45).

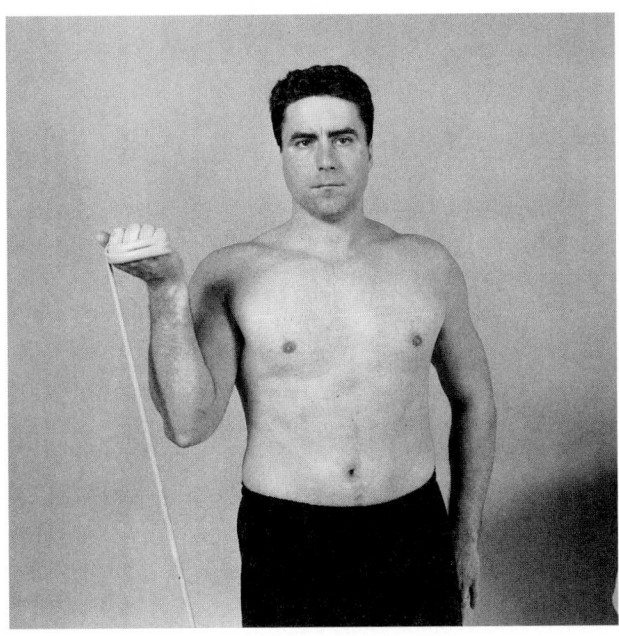

FIGURE 15-39 Exercise with elastic tubing.

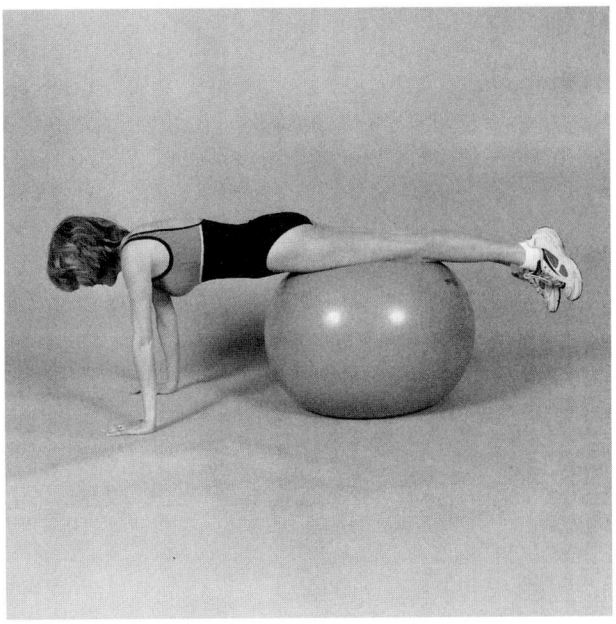

FIGURE 15-40 Stabilization exercises with Swiss ball.

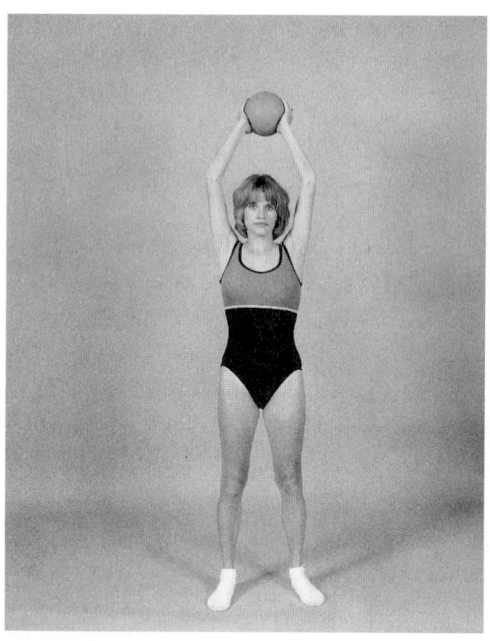

FIGURE 15-41   Medicine ball soccer throws.

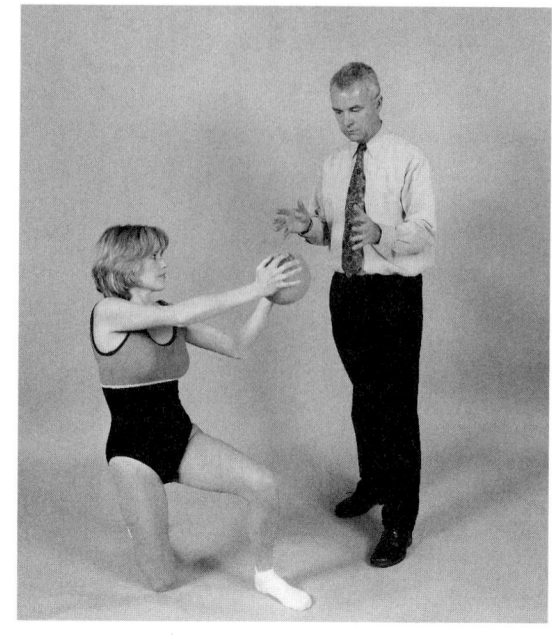

FIGURE 15-43   Side pass.

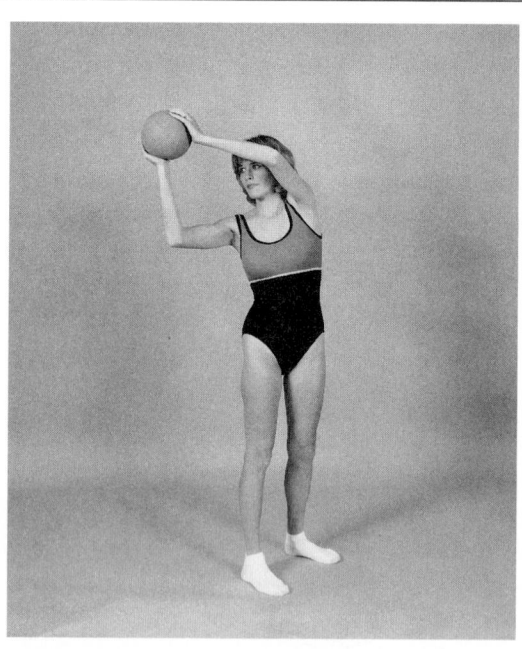
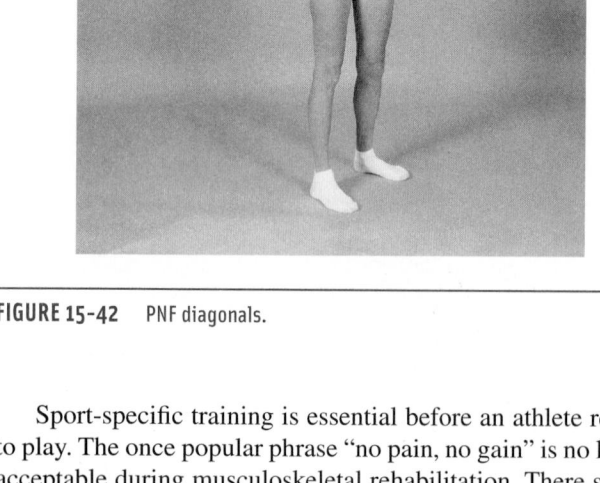

FIGURE 15-42   PNF diagonals.

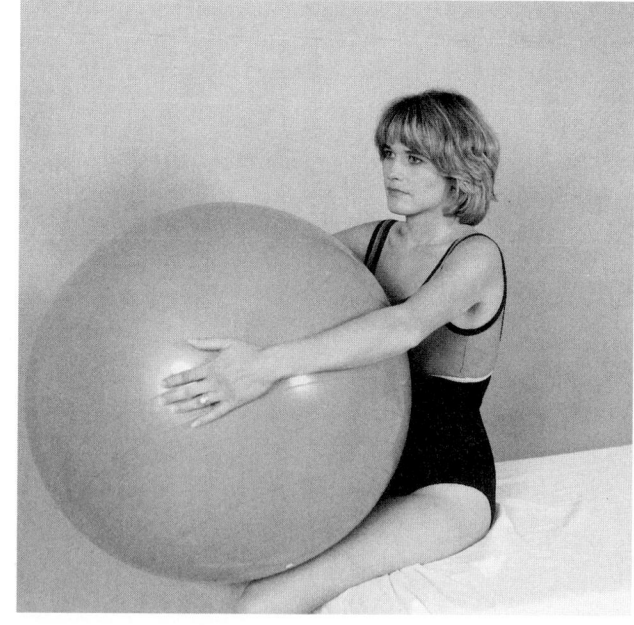

FIGURE 15-44   Ball squeeze.

Sport-specific training is essential before an athlete returns to play. The once popular phrase "no pain, no gain" is no longer acceptable during musculoskeletal rehabilitation. There should be a gradual transition back to sports activities and other strenuous activities of daily living, depending on the recovery of the involved tissues, and on the restoration of the athletic skills required to perform the activity. Too often, patients return to full activity prematurely, with resulting reinjury. This is both frustrating and discouraging for the patient.

In order for the athlete to begin the return to sporting activities, the elbow must have full, pain-free range of motion, no pain or tenderness on physical examination, and adequate muscle strength, power, and endurance that is 70 percent of the uninvolved side.[1]

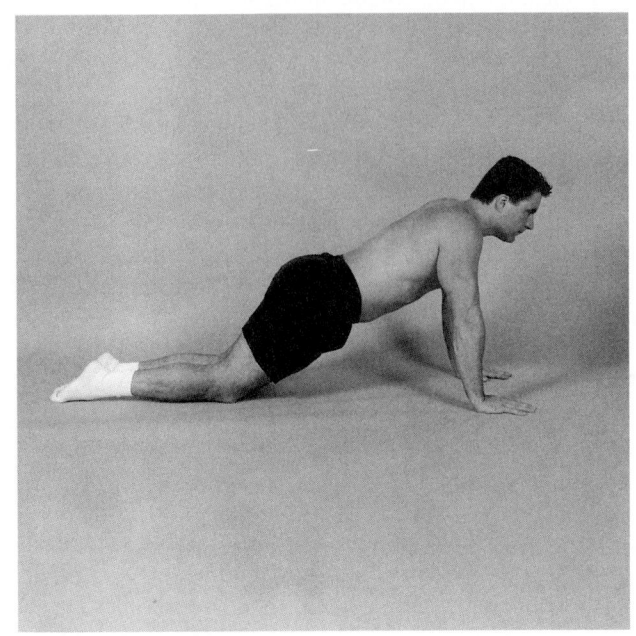

FIGURE 15-45 Modified push-up.

Those athletes that are returning to throwing can undergo a strength comparison through isokinetic testing. This can be achieved with the patient in the seated position. Speeds of 180 degrees per second and 300 degrees per second are used. A bilateral comparison should indicate the overhead athlete's elbow flexors are 10 to 20 percent stronger, the elbow extensors are 5 to 15 percent stronger when compared to the uninvolved side, and that the flexor : extensor ratio should be 70 to 80 percent at 180 degrees per second, and 63 to 69 percent at 300 degrees per second.[1]

Advanced strengthening exercises specific for the patient's activity/position are emphasized during the later part of this phase. These include high-speed/high-energy strengthening, and eccentric muscular contractions performed in functional positions.[1]

Practice Pattern 4D: Impaired Joint Mobility, Motor Function, Muscle Performance, Range of Motion Associated with Connective Tissue Dysfunction

Impairments involving capsular restriction include every form of arthritis. It is important that the clinician establish the cause of the arthritis using the history, the tests and measures, results from imaging studies, and findings from any laboratory tests before initiating treatment.

Traumatic Arthritis

The trauma involved at the elbow that has the potential to produce a traumatic arthritis is a hyperextension injury, resulting in a sprain of the anterior capsule and the anterior band of the medial (ulnar) collateral ligament. The patient complains of diffuse elbow pain, especially on the medial aspect. Upon examination, the capsular pattern of passive flexion more limited than extension is present, whereas the motions of pronation and supination are unaffected. Traumatic arthritis at the elbow is usually treated with a corticosteroid injection in adults, whereas in children a brief period of immobilization in a sling, followed by gentle passive and active range of motion is recommended.

Arthrosis
See Chap. 9.

Osteochondritis Dissecans
See Chap. 9.

Posterior Elbow Impingement
Posterior elbow impingement results from mechanical abutment of bone and soft tissues in the posterior compartment of the elbow. Pathologic processes such as fibrous tissue deposits in the olecranon fossa, chondral injury, osteophytes, and loose bodies are sometimes responsible.[114] Medial collateral ligament insufficiency may also be present.

Radiography may show posterior or posteromedial osteophytes and loose bodies.

Surgical removal of osteophytes and loose bodies is indicated if symptoms do not resolve with conservative treatment of range of motion and strengthening exercises.

Malpositioning of the Elbow
Abducted Ulna Lesion. This lesion usually results from a fall on an outstretched arm (FOOSH injury), forcing the ulna medially into full extension and abduction. Clinical findings include[115]:

▶ An increased carrying angle and apparent longer radius which is forced to glide distally. Initially, the hand is held in slight ulnar deviation due to a relative distal shift of the radius. However, this usually adapts, producing an ulnar carpal shift due to the pull of the radial deviators and wrist extensors.

▶ Elbow flexion may be decreased, but usually only an abnormal hard end-feel is detected.

▶ Forearm supination may be decreased, but usually only an abnormal hard end-feel is detected.

▶ The lateral glide at the elbow is decreased with an abnormally hard end-feel (the ulna is unable to adduct).

▶ Decreased wrist extension.

There are potentially many and varied consequences of this lesion, including[115]:

▶ The development of tennis elbow symptoms as the radial deviators overwork to correct the ulnar deviation.

▶ An ulnar nerve traction injury, medial ligament sprain, and medial epicondylitis due to the increased carrying angle.

▶ Carpal dysfunction due to the abnormal wrist biomechanics because of the distally displaced radius.

▶ Medial collateral ligament laxity due to the adaptation occurring to correct the ulnar deviation.

▶ Hypertonicity and overuse of the radial deviators and extensors as the hand attempts to adopt a neutral position by attempting to radially deviate or extend.

The intervention for these conditions includes a correction of the malposition with either joint mobilizations or a high-velocity thrust. These techniques are described in the Therapeutic Techniques section.

Adducted Ulna Lesions. In the adducted ulna lesion, there is no involvement of the wrist. In fact, the head of the radius impacts the capitellum, resulting in decreased extension and pronation, and clinical findings that are exactly the opposite of those described above. The consequences of this lesion are less severe than with the abducted ulna, as the shift of the wrist is less due to the accommodation by the ulnar meniscus, but they include[115]:

▶ The development of tennis elbow symptoms due to the prolonged stretch on the common extensor tendon.

▶ Lateral collateral ligament laxity.

▶ Minor carpal dysfunction.

▶ Ulnar meniscus tearing due to continuous compression.

Posterior Radial Head (External Rotation of the Ulna) Lesion. With this lesion, the radial head shifts posteriorly into extension on the humerus and the ulna. There is typically a history involving forced or excessive supination. Range-of-motion testing demonstrates decreased elbow extension and forearm pronation. Passive accessory motion testing reveals a decreased medial radial glide and decreased gapping space between the ulna and the radius.

Anterior Radial Head (Internal Rotation of the Ulna) Lesion. With this lesion, the radial head shifts anteriorly into flexion on the humerus and the ulna. There is typically a history involving forced or excessive pronation. Range-of-motion testing demonstrates decreased elbow flexion and forearm supination. Passive accessory motion testing reveals a decreased lateral radial glide.

Medial (Ulnar) Collateral Ligament Sprain

The most common mechanisms of MCL insufficiency are a chronic attenuation of valgus and external rotation forces,[16,26,48,116,117] as seen in the tennis serve or in the baseball throwing pitch,[118,119] and post-traumatic, usually after a FOOSH injury.[13] Associated injuries after trauma may include fractures of the radial head, olecranon, or medial humeral epicondyle.[16,26] Medial collateral ligament injury also can be iatrogenic, secondary to excessive medial epicondylectomy for cubital tunnel syndrome.[120,121] Irritation of the ulnar nerve, with symptoms of ulnar neuritis may be present secondary to inflammation of the ligamentous complex.[48,122,123]

The most common complaint from the patient is medial elbow pain at the ligament's origin,[124] or at the insertion site if there is an acute avulsion.[13] As the primary restraint to valgus stress is the anterior bundle of the MCL,[8,14–18,23] the physical examination of an individual with presumed medial joint insufficiency should focus on palpation of the course of the MCL.[13] Valgus stress testing of the elbow should be performed.

An important secondary stabilizer of the elbow is the articular geometry of the joint complex.[15,22] Repetitive stress to the joint can lead to osteophyte formation and degenerative changes, which can produce medial elbow pain.

The intervention for early symptoms of MCL injury in the throwing athlete includes rest and activity modification or restriction for about 2 to 4 weeks, physical therapy modalities, and nonsteroidal anti-inflammatory medications.[25]

Strengthening and stretching of the flexor carpi ulnaris, pronator teres, and flexor digitorum superficialis is initiated once the acute inflammatory stage has subsided, and are performed in the pain-free mid-range of motion.[118,125–127] In addition, strengthening of the shoulder and elbow muscles may help prevent or minimize injury, and may facilitate rehabilitation.[124,125] A well-supervised throwing and conditioning program is initiated at approximately 3 months, once the athlete has regained full range of motion and strength.[25]

Operative repair of the MCL typically is required only in competitive throwing athletes or those involved in heavy manual labor,[13] as valgus laxity has been shown to cause minimal functional impairment with normal activities of daily living.[26] The surgical repair or reconstruction (see Chap. 28) can be performed with or without ulnar nerve transposition.[128] The palmaris longus tendon, which has been found to have a tensile strength of 357 N, is the most frequently used graft for elbow reconstruction,[129] although the plantaris and toe extensor tendons can also be used.[116]

Lateral Collateral Ligament Sprain

Posterolateral rotatory instability results from insufficiency of the lateral soft tissue support of the elbow, especially the LCL complex.[29,86,130] This condition typically involves a combination of axial compression, external rotation, and valgus force applied to the elbow.[131,132] It also may have an iatrogenic origin, and has been reported after overly aggressive debridement of the lateral soft tissues for patients with recalcitrant tennis elbow.[130,133]

Instability

Both the humeroulnar and the humeroradial articulations provide approximately 50 percent of the overall stability of the elbow.[15,18,19] Additional support is supplied by ligaments and muscles. The flexor and pronator muscles, which originate at the medial epicondyle, provide additional static and dynamic support to the medial elbow,[6] with the flexor carpi ulnaris and flexor digitorum superficialis being the most effective in this regard.[125]

Although elbow instability has been documented for decades, the mechanism by which an elbow becomes recurrently unstable was only described in the last decade, as were the clinical tests for making the diagnosis of elbow instability.[86,131]

A simple classification system for elbow instability, consisting of five criteria, is necessary for correct diagnosing and treatment decision making[134–136]:

1. *The timing (acute, chronic, or recurrent).*
2. *The articulation(s) involved.* Because the elbow is a complex joint, there are two categories of elbow instability, according to the articulation(s) involved, although the instability can involve both joints in a combined fashion[134]:
   a. *The hinge joint (ulnohumeral joint).* The instability can be congenital or acquired, although the former is rare. It is most commonly the hinge joint that is predisposed to recurrent instability.
   b. *The proximal radioulnar joint.* This involves a subluxation or dislocation of the radial head from the ulna, which can be congenital or acquired. Dislocation of the radial head from the ulna is usually traumatic and often part of a Monteggia fracture-subluxation.
3. *The direction of displacement (valgus, varus, anterior, or posterolateral rotatory).*
   a. *Valgus displacement.* As in the knee, the medial stabilizers of the elbow are the strongest. The mechanism is usually a FOOSH injury (can also be from using a sledgehammer, etc), and occurs in athletes who perform overhead movements such as baseball pitchers and javelin throwers.[117] The instability is characterized by pain in the anteromedial aspect of the arm, moderate to severe flexion limitation (acute), and positive valgus test at 20 degrees of flexion. Valgus instability is seen in one of two varieties: post-traumatic or chronic overload.[134]
      (1) *Post-traumatic valgus instability implies rupture of the MCL.*[137] This type of instability may be associated with disruption of the other soft tissues on the medial side of the elbow, including the common flexor and pronator origin. Valgus instability usually is found in patients with radial head fractures that are associated with tears of the MCL, or in patients with severe elbow instability such as occurs after a dislocation that has disrupted the lateral ligament complex.
      (2) *Valgus instability also can occur from repetitive microtrauma or overload, resulting in attenuation or rupture of the anterior band of the MCL.*
   b. *Varus displacement.* Because of the anatomic alignment, the forces across the elbow are principally valgus. Thus a pure varus mechanism of injury is uncommon.[114] More common is a combined varus and external rotation rotatory mechanism of injury as occurs from a FOOSH injury. However, lateral instability can occur acutely in patients with elbow dislocations and in many patients with recurrent or chronic instability when the lateral collateral ligament fails to heal.[134] Patients with a varus instability are unlikely to complain

of symptoms except perhaps those patients who use their arms as weight-bearing extremities (patients who use crutches to walk).[134]
   c. *Anterior displacements of the elbow are rare.*[138] These injuries usually occur from a blow to the flexed elbow, which drives the olecranon anteriorly. Associated injuries include fractures of the olecranon, with tearing of the collateral ligaments and damage to vessels and nerves around the joint. On examination the arm appears shorter, while the forearm appears elongated and held in supination. The elbow is usually held in extension.
   d. *Posterior displacements.* With posterior displacements, the ulna is displaced posteriorly in relation to the distal humerus. The patient's arm is held in 45 degrees of flexion. These are subdivided into three types: posterior, posterior-medial and posterior-lateral.[130,136] The most common is usually posterior-lateral rather than direct posterior, so that the coronoid can pass inferior to the trochlea, and the ulnar displacement on the humerus is three-dimensional (the radius moving with the ulna), such that the ulna supinates (externally rotates) away from the trochlea.[134] The lateral ulnar collateral ligament is the primary static restraint against posterolateral rotatory instability.[131] The most common mechanism for a posterolateral instability involves proximal attenuation or avulsion of the ligamentous and muscular origins from the lateral epicondyle during a traumatic event.[28,29,137,139–141] The lateral pivot shift test, also called the posterolateral rotatory instability test, is the best physical examination finding.[114] The surgical intervention for posterolateral rotatory instability involves a repair of this common tendon and ligament origin to the lateral epicondyle to reestablish lateral elbow stability.[13]
4. *The degree of displacement (subluxation or dislocation).* Posterolateral rotatory instability can be considered as a spectrum consisting of three stages, each of which has specific clinical, radiographic, and pathologic features that are predictable and have implications for treatment[134]:
   a. *Stage 1.* The elbow subluxates in a posterolateral rotatory direction and the patient has an associated positive lateral pivot shift test.
   b. *Stage 2.* The elbow dislocates incompletely so that the coronoid is perched under the trochlea.
   c. *Stage 3.* The elbow dislocates fully so that the coronoid rests behind the humerus.
5. *The presence or absence of associated fractures.* Elbow subluxations and dislocations can be associated with fractures about the elbow. Fracture-dislocations most commonly involve the coronoid and/or radial head, an injury so difficult to treat and prone to unsatisfactory results that it has been termed the "terrible triad" of the elbow.[142] When the radial head and coronoid are fractured in a dislocated elbow, the elbow is stable to valgus when holding the forearm pronated.

The diagnosis for elbow instability is made by the history and a careful physical examination. Patients typically present with a history of recurrent painful clicking, snapping, clunking, or locking of the elbow. Careful examination reveals that this occurs in the extension portion of the arc of motion with the forearm in supination.[134] The clinician must also perform an examination of the peripheral nerves and distal pulses to help determine the severity of the instability. Swelling may make the diagnosis of elbow instability difficult. However, if the clinician palpates the two epicondyles and the tip of the olecranon, the following findings help determine the diagnosis:

▶ If the three points are on the same plane, a supracondylar fracture is suspected.

▶ If the olecranon is displaced from the plane of the epicondyles, a posterior dislocation is suspected.

The diagnosis of a dislocation can be confirmed by radiograph.

With patients presenting with a history of dislocation, the diagnosis of recurrent elbow instability is to be suspected. This diagnosis should also be considered when there has been trauma without dislocation. Recurrent instability may also be caused by surgery. Examples include tennis elbow surgery or surgery on the radial head caused by violation of the ulnar part of the lateral collateral ligament complex with inadequate attention to its repair.[86,130,133,134]

Conservative intervention should focus on the entire kinetic chain, including the lower extremities and trunk.[143,144] Included in the strengthening program are[144,145]:

▶ Leg and pelvis exercises with emphasis on strengthening of the gluteus muscle group.

▶ Trunk strengthening, particularly into rotation.

▶ Scapulothoracic control exercises.

▶ Rotator cuff strengthening, with a focus on eccentric training.

▶ Elbow flexion and extension exercises.

▶ Forearm pronation and supination exercises.

▶ Wrist strengthening.

Posterior capsular tightness in the shoulder must be addressed, and the clinician should ensure that the throwing athlete has 180 degrees of glenohumeral joint motion.[146]

Proprioceptive neuromuscular facilitation, rhythmic stabilization, and plyometric exercises are used to improve functional stabilization of the joint, beginning with two-handed exercises in the nonprovocative ranges with the elbow close to the body, and progressing to one-handed activities with the involved arm in the throwing position.[31]

Surgical intervention is reserved for those patients in whom conservative measures fail.

Practice Pattern 4E: Impaired Joint Mobility, Motor Function, Muscle Performance, Range of Motion Associated with Localized Inflammation

Olecranon Bursitis

Because of its location, the olecranon bursa is easily bruised through direct trauma, or is irritated through repetitive grazing and weight bearing, causing bursitis. Olecranon bursitis is common in students and wrestlers, as well as those athletes who play basketball, football, indoor soccer, and hockey, where the potential for falling and striking an elbow on hard playing surfaces is high.[147]

Acute bursitis presents as a swelling over the olecranon process that can vary in size from a slight distension to a mass as large as 6 cm in diameter.[148] An inflamed bursa can occasionally become infected, requiring differentiation between septic and nonseptic bursitis.[149]

Pain and swelling can be gradual as in the chronic cases, or sudden as in acute injury or an infection.[148] Redness and heat suggest infection, whereas exquisite tenderness indicates trauma or infection as the underlying cause. Patients often note a decreased range of motion or an inability to don a long-sleeved shirt.[150] While the simple post-traumatic bursitis can be treated with the principles of PRICEMEM, the infected bursa needs prompt medical attention.[150]

In the differential diagnoses of these cases, acute fractures, rheumatoid arthritis, gout, and synovial cysts should be considered.[148] If the patient is experiencing significant pain or discomfort with movement of the elbow, a sling helps to reduce these symptoms and quiet the joint.[148] In cases of marked swelling, or to distinguish between a septic and nonseptic bursitis, aspiration is the appropriate management. Aspiration also helps to reduce the level of discomfort and restriction of movement. The aspirated fluid is cultured and evaluated for crystals to rule out infection or gout. After aspiration, the elbow should be maintained in a splint and sling and reevaluated in 1 week. Bursitis that recurs despite three or more repeated aspirations, or infection that does not respond to antibiotics, require evaluation for surgical excision.[148,150]

Injection of corticosteroids is used to manage chronic bursitis once the diagnosis of infection has been excluded.[148]

Tendon Injuries of the Elbow

Tendon injuries of this region can be divided into several categories on the basis of the nature of their onset and the tissues involved. While acute tendon injuries, such as laceration of the flexor tendons of the fingers, are traumatic in nature, chronic overuse injuries are the result of multiple microtraumatic events that cause disruption of the internal structure of the tendon, and produce tendonitis or tendonosis.

Bicipital Tendonitis. Bicipital tendonitis usually results from repetitive hyperextension of the elbow with pronation, or repetitive stressful pronation-supination.[69] Typically there are complaints of pain located at the anterior aspect of the distal part of the arm. There is tenderness to palpation of the distal biceps belly, the musculotendinous portion of the biceps, or the bicipital insertion of the radial tuberosity.[65,69] Other findings include pain on resisted elbow flexion and supination, and pain with passive shoulder and elbow extension.

Intervention at the source involves electrotherapeutic and thermal modalities, transverse friction massage, trigger point assessment, correction of muscle imbalances, and specific elbow joint mobilizations.

Biceps Tendon Rupture. The biceps brachii may be injured either at the musculotendinous junction or at the radial tuberosity, being avulsed partially or completely. These distal injuries account for 3 to 10 percent of all biceps tendon ruptures, with the remainder occurring at the shoulder.[151] Avulsions of the biceps tendon at the elbow occur almost exclusively in males.[152] Most typical is the dominant elbow of a muscular male in his fifth decade of life.[114] Biceps ruptures that typically involve a sudden contracture of the biceps against significant load with the elbow in 90 degrees of flexion are common in competitive weight lifters.[153]

Clinical findings vary depending on whether the rupture is partial or complete. The history may include either a report of a sharp, tearing-type pain coincident with an acute injury, or swelling and activity-related pains in the antecubital fossa from chronic injury.[114] The physical examination may reveal ecchymosis in the antecubital fossa (and sometimes also in the distal ulnar part of the arm), a palpable defect of the distal biceps, loss of strength of elbow flexion and grip, but especially a loss of forearm supination strength.[154]

In active individuals, primary repair of the acute tendon avulsion is recommended. If not repaired, a 30 percent loss of elbow flexion and a 40 percent loss of supination strength can be expected.[154] Postoperatively, the elbow is protected for 6 to 8 weeks, after which unrestricted range of motion and gentle strengthening exercises are initiated. Return to unrestricted activity is usually not allowed until nearly 6 months of healing has passed.[114]

Triceps Tendon Rupture. Triceps tendon ruptures usually occur with a deceleration force during extension or an uncoordinated contraction of the triceps muscle against the flexing elbow.[155] As with rupture of the biceps tendon, the physical findings depend on whether the avulsion is partial or complete. Loss of elbow extension strength, inability to extend overhead against gravity, and a tendon defect are findings if the tear is complete.[114]

Primary repair is the treatment of choice in acute complete ruptures. Partial injury may be treated conservatively with immobilization for about 3 weeks followed by a gradual progression of range of motion and strengthening.

Brachialis Strain. A strain to the brachialis is relatively rare, but can occur from overuse in activities such as weight lifting. The brachialis is also prone to myositis ossificans, a pathologic bone formation, due to the fact that it is likely to hemorrhage when injured (see later).

As in the lesion of the biceps, the pain is felt on the anterior aspect of the distal part of the arm. There is palpable tenderness in the muscle belly of the brachialis, at the level of the musculotendinous junction of the biceps. Resisted supination is not painful, although resisted elbow flexion with the forearm pronated is.

The conservative intervention involves electrotherapeutic and thermal modalities, transverse friction massage, trigger point assessment, correction of muscle imbalances, and specific elbow joint mobilizations.

Epicondylitis

Defined literally, epicondylitis suggests an inflammation at one of the epicondyles of the elbow. Two types of epicondylitis are commonly described: tennis elbow and golfer's elbow (see below). Both types of epicondylitis are common in persons who frequently overuse the upper arm, particularly with activities that involve rotation of the arm with flexion and extension. However, lateral epicondylitis has been found to be from four to seven times more common than medial epicondylitis.[156]

Lateral Epicondylitis (Tennis Elbow). Lateral epicondylitis, more commonly known as tennis elbow, represents a pathologic condition of the common extensor muscles at their origin on the lateral humeral epicondyle. Specifically, the condition involves the tendons of the muscles that control wrist extension and radial deviation resulting in pain on the lateral side of the elbow with contraction of these muscles.[124]

The first description of tennis elbow is attributed to Runge,[157] but the name derives from Lawn Tennis Arm described by Morris in the *Lancet* in 1882.[158] This was followed in 1883 by Dr H.P. Major describing his own affliction in 1883.[159] In Runge's original description he called it writer's cramp (Schreibekrampf) and attributed it to a periostitis of the lateral humeral epicondyle.[157] Since then it has been referred to by a number of names including epicondylalgia,[160–163] epicondyle pain,[164] musician's palsy (Musikerlähmung),[165] and tennis pain (Tennisschmerz),[165] although most authors have used the terms epicondylitis, or tennis elbow.

Tennis elbow affects between 1 and 3 percent of the population, and occurs most commonly between the ages 35 and 50 years of age with a mean age of 45,[166] is seldom seen in those under 20 years of age, and usually affects the dominant arm.[167–169] Cyriax[170] noted that the origin of the extensor carpi radialis brevis (ECRB) was the primary site of this injury, and pathologic changes have been consistently documented at this location,[171–174] although findings are also found in the extensor carpi radialis longus, and extensor carpi ulnaris.[124] One third of patients also have involvement of the origin of the extensor digitorum communis.[170,173,174]

The proposed presence of macro- or microtears in the ECRB tendon was based upon findings extrapolated from abnormal physical and intraoperative examinations showing gross alterations in the ECRB tendon.[170–172,175] However, a recent study involving gross and microscopic dissections found that it was not possible to separate the origin of the ECRB from that of the common extensor tendon, and that at times the two tendons appeared to interdigitate, indicating that any pathology believed to be isolated to the ECRB must be common to both.[176]

Over 25 conditions have been suggested as causes of tennis elbow,[170] including periostitis,[157,167,170,177] infection,[178,179] bursitis,[162,167,170,180–183] fibrillation of the radial head,[184] radioulnar joint disease,[185] annular ligament lesion,[159,186,187] nipped synovial fringe,[188–193] calcific tendonitis,[194] neurogenic causes,[195,196] osteochondritis dissecans, and radial nerve entrapment.[59,60,195,197–199]

Capsular and ligamentous lesions have been mentioned by a number of authors. Landelius[161] regarded the pull of the radial head on the orbicular ligament and the capsule to be the cause. Bosworth[187] considered the impingement of the orbicular ligament on the head of the radius to be the sole problem.[200,201]

Dysfunction of the cervical spine has been speculated to cause tennis elbow. A frank radiculopathy may weaken the extensor muscles to the point at which normal use is traumatic and induces a grade I tear in the muscle belly or tendon. Less definite compression of the nerve root may compromise axoplasmic transportation, producing a trophic malnutrition of the muscle, resulting in damage. A facilitated segment at C5 through C6, with its resulting hypertonicity, might lead to a chronic overuse syndrome, or poor coordination. Wright and colleagues[202] found that neuronal changes within the spinal cord may be more important than peripheral nociceptor sensitization in the development of such disorders as tennis elbow. Gunn and Milbrandt[203] discussed a reflex localization of pain from radiculopathy at the cervical spine in patients with a intervention-resistant tennis elbow who had hypomobility of the lower cervical motion segments.[204] Maitland[205] has also reported improving the symptoms of lateral epicondylitis with a program of heat, mobilization, and traction of the cervical segments.[204]

The shoulder has also been speculated to be a cause of tennis elbow, due to the effect of an abnormal tension in the clavi-pectoral fascia on the brachial plexus. This fascia is attached to the clavicle around the subclavius muscle. From there it passes down to the upper border of the pectoralis minor and extends from the anterior intercostal membrane to the coracoid process. The fascia encloses the pectoralis minor and becomes the suspensory ligament of the axilla. It is speculated that if the fascia is distorted due to clavicular malposition, the traction exerted on the brachial plexus could lead to similar problems as those encountered with a cervical lesion. In these cases, altering the position of the shoulder girdle (protracting, retracting, elevating, and depressing it) would alter the symptoms produced during the isometric tests.

Whatever the source of the symptoms, tennis elbow is usually the result of overuse, but can be traumatic in origin. One possible etiology is the fact that the hand does not have a supportive function during activities, but is functioning predominantly to grasp some object. Individuals who perform repetitive wrist extension against resistance are particularly at risk. The tendons involved in locomotion and ballistic performance, which transmit loads under elastic and eccentric conditions, are susceptible to injury. Some tendons, such as those that wrap around a convex surface or the apex of a concavity, those that cross two joints, those with areas of scant vascular supply, and those that are subjected to repetitive tension, are particularly vulnerable to overuse injuries.[206–211] Participants of tennis,

baseball, javelin, golf, squash, racquetball, swimming, and weight lifting are all predisposed to this condition.[114]

While the terms *epicondylitis* and *tendonitis* are commonly used to describe tennis elbow, histopathologic studies have demonstrated that tennis elbow is often not an inflammatory condition; rather, it is a degenerative condition, a tendonosis.[156,173]

Nirschl previously categorized the stages of repetitive microtrauma[212]:

▶ A stage 1 injury is probably inflammatory, is not associated with pathologic alterations, and is likely to resolve.

▶ A stage 2 injury is associated with pathologic alterations such as tendonosis or angiofibroblastic degeneration. It is this stage that is most commonly associated with sports-related tendon injuries such as tennis elbow, and with overuse injuries in general. Within the tendon, there is a fibroblastic and vascular response (tendonosis) rather than an immune blood-cell response (inflammation).

▶ A stage 3 injury is associated with pathologic changes (tendonosis) and complete structural failure (rupture).

▶ A stage 4 injury exhibits the features of a stage 2 or 3 injury and is associated with other changes such as fibrosis, soft matrix calcification, and hard osseous calcification. The changes that are associated with a stage 4 injury also may be related to the use of cortisone.

Nirschl[213] postulates that some patients who have tennis elbow may have a genetic predisposition that makes them more susceptible to tendonosis at multiple sites. He terms this condition *mesenchymal syndrome* on the basis of the stem-cell line of fibroblasts and the presence of a potentially systemic abnormality of cross-linkage in the collagen produced by the fibroblasts. Patients may have mesenchymal syndrome if they have two or more of the following conditions[208,213]:

▶ Bilateral lateral tennis elbow.

▶ Medial tennis elbow.

▶ Cubital tunnel syndrome.

▶ Carpal tunnel syndrome.

▶ De Quervain tenosynovitis.

▶ Trigger finger.

▶ Rotator cuff tendonosis.

Clinical Presentation.   Three types of tennis elbow are recognized based on the mode of onset.

▶ The acute onset (indirect) type of tennis elbow is associated with a recognizable mechanism with acute pain, associated bruising on occasion,[214] and a feeling of something giving way within the elbow.[170]

▶ Rupture of the ECRL with tenderness in the muscles.[215,216] This type is associated with direct trauma to the lateral side of the elbow, but with no tearing of the ligaments.[167,217]

▶ The chronic type that is associated with a gradual onset, and is occasionally termed occupational neuralgia (Beschaftigung-ensneuralgie).[218]

The pain of tennis elbow is often related to activities that involve wrist extension/grasp, as it is the wrist extensors that must contract during grasping activities to stabilize the wrist. Diffuse achiness and morning stiffness are also common complaints.[124] Occasionally the pain is experienced at night and the patient may report frequent dropping of objects, especially if they are carried with the palm facing down.

The exact location of the pain is revealed by palpation, and tenderness is usually found over the ECRB and ECRL, especially at the lateral epicondyle. The site of maximum tenderness is most commonly over the anterior aspect of the lateral epicondyle,[124] the next most common site is tenderness over the radial head, or where the lateral part of the common extensor tendon arises from the bone.[170] Tenderness can be found in other sites as well, in addition to swelling, but not consistently.[170] Differentiation between the various tendons is obviously important. Five types of tendon lesions of the elbow are recognized:

▶ A lesion of the muscle origin of the extensor carpi radialis longus (ECRL), which is usually located just proximal to the lateral epicondyle (type 1).

▶ An insertion tendonopathy of the extensor carpi radialis brevis (ECRB) (type 2). This is the most common site and is usually associated with type 5. As the ECRB also originates from the radial collateral ligament, involvement of the tendon can produce pain here, or at the radial head (type 3).

▶ An ECRB muscle belly strain (type 4).

▶ Inflammation at the origin of the extensor digitorum (type 5).

The range-of-motion tests typically reveal the following:

▶ Active motions are usually painless, although there may be pain with wrist flexion with elbow extension.

▶ Passive motion can produce pain, especially with passive wrist flexion with the forearm pronated and the elbow extended.

The resisted tests typically reproduce symptoms with resisted wrist extension and radial deviation with the elbow extended. Pain on resisted finger extension has also been reported. Cozen's or Mill's special tests are typically positive.

The cervical spine, shoulder, and wrist must also be examined. As a large number of tennis elbows appear to be secondary either to a dysfunction of the cervical spine or shoulder, testing isometric wrist extension in varying positions of the cervical spine or shoulder will help differentiate the cause. If the primary cause is remote, the amount of discomfort on testing will vary with changes of the head or shoulder girdle position. If the pain disappears entirely during these maneuvers, there can be no symptomatic pathologic changes at the elbow and no local treatment is required. However, usually the pain is reduced rather than being eliminated, indicating that the cause may be remote and local pathologic changes have since supervened.

Tennis elbow is normally a self-limiting complaint; without intervention, the symptoms will usually resolve within 8 to 12 months.

Intervention. The lack of agreement in the literature regarding the pathogenesis of tennis elbow has led to a proliferation of interventions, both medical and surgical.[219] In fact, more than 40 treatments have been suggested, indicating that the ideal remedy has yet to be found, although there is agreement that management of the patient who presents for the first time with tennis elbow should be conservative. Many studies of the use of physical therapy in the management of tennis elbow are poorly designed and statistically weak.[220,221] The effectiveness of ultrasound for tennis elbow is undetermined. One study[222] found ultrasound to be effective in a placebo-controlled, double-blind trial,[223] but another study[224] found no difference. A recent randomized pilot study by Struijs et al.[224a] of 31 patients diagnosed with tennis elbow found that manipulation of wrist was more effective at a follow-up of 3 and 6 weeks than ultrasound, friction massage, and muscle stretching and strengthening exercises. The wrist manipulation used was a ventral manipulation of the scaphoid (refer to Chap. 16), which was repeated 15 times, two times a week, with a maximum of nine intervention sessions. However, the authors admit that replication of these results is needed in a large-scale randomized clinical trial with a control group and a longer-term follow-up before any meaningful conclusions can be drawn. Other forms of physical therapy including electrotherapy and thermotherapy have not been proven to be effective.[222]

The benefits of tennis elbow braces remains unproven. Snyder-Mackler and colleagues reported on a comparison of a "standard" tennis elbow brace and one with an air-filled bladder,[225] but it is not possible to extrapolate from their findings to the efficacy of tennis elbow braces in the management of tennis elbow. Counterforce bracing[175] (such as the Count-R-Force brace from Medical Sports, Arlington, Virginia) has been shown to:

▶ Have a beneficial effect on the force couple imbalances, and altered movements associated with tennis elbow.[104,226,227]

▶ Decrease elbow angular acceleration.[228]

▶ Decrease electromyographic activity.[228]

However, contrary to popular belief, tennis elbow braces have been shown to have little effect in vibrational dampening.[229] As an alternative to elbow bracing, Gellman[230] recommends a protective 20-degree wrist extension splint for tennis elbow to help offload the ECRB.[124]

Cyriax recommends the Mill's manipulation (see Intervention section) to treat true tennis elbow, which is intended to maximally stretch the extensor carpi radialis brevis tendon in order to try to pull apart the two surfaces of the painful scar.[170] Manipulation of this kind has also been advocated in other studies.[231–233]

Nirschl[100] has attempted to determine whether the presenting symptoms are helpful in both diagnosing and in directing the intervention. This information was previously published in the form of a table.[100]

▶ *Type 1 and 2.*   Benign (nonharmful) pain: Type 1 pain is characterized by stiffness or mild soreness after activity and resolves within 24 hours. Type 2 pain is marked by stiffness or mild soreness after exercise, lasts more than 48 hours, is relieved with warm-up exercises, is not present during activity, and resolves within 72 hours after the cessation of activity. The pain associated with types 1 and 2 may be due to peritendinous inflammation.

▶ *Type 3.*   Semi-benign (likely nonharmful) pain: Type 3 pain is characterized by stiffness or mild soreness before activity and is partially relieved with warm-up exercises. The pain does not prevent participation in activity and is mild during activity. However, minor adjustments in the technique, intensity, and duration of activity are needed to control the pain. Type 3 pain may necessitate the use of nonsteroidal anti-inflammatory medications.

▶ *Type 4.*   Semi-harmful pain: Type 4 pain is more intense than type 3 pain and produces changes in the performance of a specific sport- or work-related activity. Mild pain accompanies the activities of daily living. Type 4 pain may reflect tendon damage.

▶ *Type 5, 6, and 7.*   Harmful pain: Type 5 pain, which is characterized as moderate or severe before, during, and after exercise, greatly alters or prevents performance of the activity. Pain accompanies but does not prevent the performance of activities of daily living. Complete rest controls the pain. Type 5 pain reflects permanent tendon damage. Type 6 pain, which is similar to type 5 pain, prevents the performance of activities of daily living and persists despite complete rest. Type 7 pain is a consistent, aching pain that intensifies with activity and that regularly interrupts sleep.

The pain of type 1 and 2 is usually self-limiting when proper precautions are taken. Type 3 and 4 pain usually responds to nonoperative medical therapy. The pain types of 5, 6, and 7, are more likely to necessitate operative treatment.[100]

An exercise regimen consisting of progressive resistance exercise to the wrist extensors, with the elbow flexed to 90 degrees and also with the elbow straight is recommended.[234] This should be performed as a ten-repetition maximum, morning and night. Gradually the weight must be increased so that the ten-repetition maximum is always maintained. Pain will be increased for the first week or two or three, but by the fifth or sixth weeks, the elbow pain will be better. An ice pack or heating pad can be a mitigating modality during the painful period.[234]

If the symptoms are not controlled with the above measures, local injection of corticosteroid may be helpful. It was not until the 1950s that the injection of corticosteroids was first reported.[163,193,235] Freeland and Gribble found that hydrocortisone was neither more nor less effective than procaine and

concluded that the short-term relief of pain was a nonspecific response that may be due to the volume of fluid injected or to the trauma of introducing the needle.[235] Subsequently a number of studies have shown steroids to be beneficial, and this has remained one of the mainstays of conservative treatment.[236–238]

Poor technique, particularly with racket sports, is the cause of many elbow problems. Emphasis should be placed on recruiting the whole of the shoulder and trunk when hitting the ball, so as to dissipate the forces as widely as possible. It is important to hit strokes with a firm wrist and not by means of wrist movements to return the ball. A late backhand in tennis should be corrected as this stroke is the most common cause of stress to the elbow if performed incorrectly.[107,156,212] Whereas the forehand demonstrates good weight transfer, the faulty backhand has no forward weight transfer, and the front shoulder is usually elevated.[150] The trunk leans away from the net at the time of impact, and the racket head is down.[150] The elbow and wrist extend before impact, and the power source is forearm extension in the pronated position, resulting in a stroke that is nonrhythmic and jerky and with sharp pronation at follow through.[150] Sometimes the use of a two-handed backhand may be helpful. One theory to support this is that the one-handed backhand links five body parts prior to impact (hips to trunk to shoulder to elbow to wrist), while the two-handed backhand only links two body parts (hips to trunk) prior to impact with the ball.[124]

The ball should be hit with the center point of the strings, or "sweet spot." When the ball is hit incorrectly, the forces are transmitted as an acute strain up and along the muscle mass to the extensor origin at the elbow.[212]

In addition to correcting poor technique, patient education should address racket size, grip size, and string tension. A fiberglass, graphite, or wood racket is more forgiving than a metal one. Tennis racquets with larger head sizes reduce arm vibration.[239] Tennis rackets should be strung with gut, as it is more resilient than nylon strings, to 52 to 55 pounds to allow the impact to be spread over slightly more time and decrease the forces transmitted to the forearm muscles.[240,241] Currently, the use of a mid-sized medium-flex, graphite tennis racquet with loosely strung nylon monofilament is recommended. The grip size should not be too large or too small,[242] and an increased racket handle diameter is helpful for players with relatively weak wrist extensors.

Operative Intervention.   Surgery is indicated if the symptoms do not resolve despite properly performed nonoperative treatments lasting 6 months.[114] A simple handshake test can help to determine whether surgical intervention is required.[243] The patient is asked to perform a firm handshake with the elbow extended, and then supinate the forearm against resistance. The clinician notes whether the patient reports having pain at the origin of the extensors of the wrist. The elbow is then flexed to 90 degrees, and the same maneuver is performed. If pain is decreased in the flexed position, operative treatment is less likely to be needed. If the pain is equally severe with the elbow flexed and extended, then operative intervention is more likely to be needed.[243]

The goals of operative treatment of tendonosis of the elbow are to resect pathologic material, to stimulate neovascularization by producing focused local bleeding, and to create a healthy scar while doing the least possible structural damage to surrounding tissues. Postoperatively, a carefully guided resistance-based rehabilitation program is recommended.

Medial Epicondylitis (Golfer's Elbow). Medial epicondylitis is only one third as common as lateral epicondylitis.[244] It primarily involves a tendinopathy of the common flexor origin, specifically the flexor carpi radialis and the humeral head of the pronator teres.[125,166,244] To a lesser extent the palmaris longus, flexor carpi ulnaris, and flexor digitorum superficialis may also be involved.[212]

The mechanism for medial epicondylitis is not usually related to direct trauma, but rather to overuse. This commonly occurs for three reasons:

▶ The flexor-pronator tissues fatigue in response to repeated stress.

▶ There is a sudden change in the level of stress that predisposes the elbow to medial ligamentous injury.[245]

▶ The ulnar collateral ligament fails to stabilize the valgus forces sufficiently.[246]

Similar to lateral epicondylitis, medial epicondylitis usually begins as a microtear. The microtear in medial epicondylitis frequently occurs at the interface between the pronator teres and FCR origins with subsequent development of fibrotic and inflammatory granulation tissue.[25] In an attempt to speed up tissue production to compensate for the increased rate of microdamage caused by increased use and decreased recovery time, an inflammation develops.[247] Chronic symptoms result from a loss of extensibility of the tissues, leaving the tendon unable to attenuate tensile loads.

Clinical Presentation. The typical clinical presentation for medial epicondylitis is pain and tenderness over the flexor-pronator origin, slightly distal and anterior to the medial epicondyle. The symptoms are typically reported to be exacerbated with either resisted wrist flexion and pronation, or passive wrist extension and supination.[25,244]

Differential diagnosis for medial elbow symptoms includes[248]:

▶ Medial ulnar collateral ligament injury or insufficiency.[16,249,250]

▶ Ulnar nerve entrapment.

▶ Medial elbow intra-articular pathology.[251]

Intervention. Conservative intervention for medial epicondylitis has been shown to have success rates as high as 90 percent.[244] The conservative intervention for this condition initially involves rest, activity modification, and local modalities. Complete immobilization is not recommended, even in the acute phase, as it eliminates the stresses necessary for maturation of new collagen tissue, resulting in healed tissue that is not strong enough to withstand the stresses associated with a return to activity. Once the acute phase has passed, the focus is to restore the range of motion, and correct imbalances of flexibility and strength. The strengthening program is progressed to include concentric and eccentric exercises of the flexor pronator muscles.

Splinting or the use of a counterforce brace may be a useful adjunct.[25]

Integration of Practice Patterns 4F and 5F: Impaired Joint Mobility, Motor Function, Muscle Performance, and Range of Motion, or Reflex Integrity Secondary to Spinal Disorders, Peripheral Nerve Entrapments, Compartment Syndrome, Myofascial Pain Dysfunction

Compressive Neuropathies

In the region of the elbow, there are a multitude of sites where the peripheral nerves can be entrapped or compressed (Table 15-5), with involvement of the ulnar and median and radial nerves and their branches being by far the most common.[55]

Ulnar Nerve Entrapment (Cubital Tunnel Syndrome). Although the ulnar nerve is well protected above the elbow, the nerve can be compressed or entrapped at a number of locations (see Fig. 15-9), including the cubital tunnel and in the medial intermuscular septum, which slopes from a thick wide base at the medial epicondyle, to a weak and thin edge more proximal on the humeral shaft.[47,53]

It has been suggested that because of the superficial location of the ulnar nerve, repetitive motion may initiate a cycle of inflammation and edema that inhibits the normal gliding of the nerve.[42,252] Additional injury occurs when traction forces caused by elbow flexion produce an additional compressive force on the internal architecture of the nerve.[45,253] The severity of nerve injury will be dependent on the magnitude, duration, and character of the applied forces.[42,252]

The anconeus has also been reported as a cause of cubital tunnel syndrome, and has been found to occur in 3 to 28 percent of human anatomic specimen elbows,[44,254] and as many as 9 percent of patients undergoing surgical treatment for cubital tunnel syndrome.[255]

The clinical findings for an ulnar nerve entrapment in the upper extremity depend on the location of the lesion and may include[256]:

▶ Activity-related pain or paresthesias involving the fourth and fifth digits, accompanied by pain that may extend proximally or distally in the medial aspect of the elbow.

▶ Pain or paresthesias worse at night.

▶ Decreased sensation in the ulnar distribution of the hand.

▶ Progressive inability to separate the fingers.

▶ Loss of grip power and dexterity.

▶ Atrophy or weakness of the ulnar intrinsic muscles of the hand (late sign).

▶ Clawing contracture of the ring and little fingers (late sign).[257]

TABLE 15-5　　Nerve Injuries about the Elbow[335]

Nerve	Motor Loss	Sensory Loss	Functional Loss
Median nerve (C6–C8, T1)	Pronator teres Flexor carpi radialis Palmaris longus Flexor digitorum superficialis Flexor pollicis longus Lateral half of flexor digitorum profundus Pronator quadratus Thenar eminence Lateral two lumbricals	Palmar aspect of hand with thumb, index, middle, and lateral half of ring finger Dorsal aspect of distal third of index, middle, and lateral half of ring finger	Pronation weakness Wrist flexion and abduction weakness Loss of radial deviation at wrist Inability to oppose or flex thumb Thumb abduction weakness Weak grip Weak or no pinch (ape hand deformity)
Anterior interosseous nerve (branch of median nerve)	Flexor pollicis longus Lateral half of flexor digitorum profundus Pronator quadratus Thenar eminence muscles Lateral two lumbricals	None	Pronation weakness, especially at 90° elbow flexion Weakness of opposition and thumb flexion Weak finger flexion Weak pinch (no tip-to-tip)
Ulnar nerve (C7–C8, T1)	Flexor carpi ulnaris Medial half of flexor digitorum profundus Palmaris brevis Hypothenar eminence Adductor pollicis Medial two lumbricals All interossei	Dorsal and palmar aspect of little and medial half of ring finger	Weak wrist flexion Loss of ulnar deviation at wrist Loss of distal flexion of little finger Loss of abduction and adduction of fingers Inability to extend second and third phalanges of little and ring fingers (benediction hand deformity) Loss of thumb adduction
Radial nerve (C5–C8, T1)	Anconeus Brachioradialis Extensor carpi radialis longus and brevis Extensor digitorum Extensor pollicis longus and brevis Abductor pollicis longus Extensor carpi ulnaris Extensor indicis Extensor digiti minimi	Dorsum of hand (lateral two thirds) Dorsum and lateral aspect of thumb Proximal two thirds of dorsum of index, middle, and half of ring finger	Loss of supination Loss of wrist extension (wrist drop) Inability to grasp Inability to stabilize wrist Loss of finger extension Inability to abduct thumb
Posterior interosseous nerve (branch of radial nerve)	Extensor carpi radialis and brevis Extensor digitorum Extensor pollicis longus and brevis Abductor pollicis longus Extensor carpi ulnaris Extensor indicis Extensor digiti minimi	None	Weak wrist extension Weak finger extension Difficulty stabilizing wrist Difficulty with grasp Inability to abduct thumb

▶ Positive elbow flexion and pressure provocative test.

▶ Positive Wartenberg's sign and Froment's sign (see Chap. 16).

▶ Positive Tinel's sign at the elbow.

Conservative intervention is recommended for patients with intermittent symptoms and without changes in two-point discrimination or muscle atrophy. Activity modification with avoidance of pressure over the cubital tunnel and limiting repetitive elbow flexion and extension is recommended, and night splinting at 40 to 60 degrees may be helpful.[45] In severe cases the splint is worn during the day, or the elbow is casted at about 45 degrees. Elbow pads, placed on the medial-posterior aspect, can be used to protect the ulnar nerve within the ulnar groove from direct pressure or trauma.[256]

A number of surgical options are available for patients with muscle atrophy, persistent sensory changes, or persistent symptoms despite nonoperative care.[53]

Median Nerve Entrapment (Humeral Supracondylar Process Syndrome).

Median nerve entrapment at the elbow is relatively rare, although it is often misdiagnosed as carpal tunnel syndrome.[80] The most proximal site at which the median nerve can be compressed is in the distal arm by the ligament of Struthers, an anatomic variant present in 0.7 to 2.7 percent of the population.[258] Very few cases of a ligament of Struthers neuropathy are described in the literature.[54,259,260] The patient may complain of pain in the wrist or medial forearm, which is exacerbated with full elbow extension or pronation of the forearm.[54,260] The patient may also report paresthesias in the index or long finger.[54]

In the antecubital area, there are three sites of potential median nerve entrapment.[80] One site is as the nerve passes under the lacertus fibrosus, or bicipital aponeurosis, a fascial band extending from the biceps tendon to the forearm fascia.[261] The second site is at the level of the pronator muscle, after the nerve crosses the elbow. The third potential site is as the median nerve travels under the flexor digitorum superficialis (FDS). Compression of the median nerve at any one of these three sites constitutes what is described in the literature as the pronator syndrome.

Pronator Syndrome. The patient with the pronator syndrome typically complains of an insidious onset of pain that is usually felt on the radial side of the palm, and the palmar side of the first, second, third, and half of the fourth digits. There is often associated "heaviness" of the forearm.[80] Unlike carpal tunnel syndrome, there is no Tinel's sign at the wrist, and there are no nocturnal symptoms.[262,263] Pain can be reproduced with[51]:

▶ Direct pressure applied over the pronator teres 4 cm distal to the cubital crease with concurrent resistance against pronation, elbow flexion, and wrist flexion.[264]

▶ Resisted supination due to compression of the lacertus fibrosus (Fig. 15-46).

▶ Resistance of the long finger flexors due to compression by the flexor digitorum superficialis arch (Fig. 15-46).

Pronator syndrome typically responds well to activity modification, and surgery is rarely required.[262]

Anterior Interosseous Syndrome. Anterior interosseous syndrome was first described by Tinel in 1918, and was further delineated by Kiloh and Nevin in 1952.[262]

Potential sources of entrapment of the anterior interosseous nerve (AIN) include the Gantzer's muscle (an accessory head of the flexor pollicis longus [FPL]), the palmaris profundus muscle, and the flexor carpi radialis muscle.[80,261,265]

Compression of the AIN results in forearm pain, and motor loss of the flexor pollicis longus, pronator quadratus, and lateral half of flexor digitorum profundus, such that the patient is unable to perform the "OK" sign with the index finger and thumb. This must be differentiated from a rupture of the muscle or its tendon. No sensory changes occur, even though the AIN carries sensory information from the distal radioulnar joint, radiocarpal joint, and intercarpal joints.[266]

Pain and weakness is typically provoked with resisted flexion of the interphalangeal joint of the thumb, and with the distal interphalangeal joint of the index finger.

The differential diagnosis includes neuralgic amyotrophy, FPL tendon rupture, and index finger FDP rupture. Most cases of AIN syndrome typically resolve spontaneously.[267]

Radial Nerve Entrapment. The radial nerve is the most commonly injured peripheral nerve. Because of the radial nerve's spiral course across the back of the mid-shaft of the humerus, and its relatively fixed position in the distal arm as it penetrates the lateral intermuscular septum, it is the most frequently injured nerve associated with fractures of the humerus. Radial nerve injuries usually involve a contusion or a mild stretch, and full recovery can generally be expected.

A number of radial nerve entrapments are recognized, and are named according to the location at which they occur. Four radial nerve entrapments are commonly cited: high radial nerve palsy, posterior interosseous nerve palsy, radial tunnel syndrome, and superficial radial nerve palsy. The various symptoms of these entrapments can aid the clinician to determine the level of entrapment.

Clinical Pearl

There is motor and sensory involvement with the high radial nerve palsy, motor involvement with the posterior interosseous nerve palsy (PINS), pain with the radial tunnel syndrome (RTS), and sensory disturbances with the superficial radial nerve palsy.[268] Symptoms of pain, cramping, and tenderness in the proximal dorsal forearm, without muscle weakness, are associated with RTS, whereas PINS involves the loss of motor function of some or all of the muscles innervated by the posterior interosseous nerve, and is thus characterized by weakness.[268]

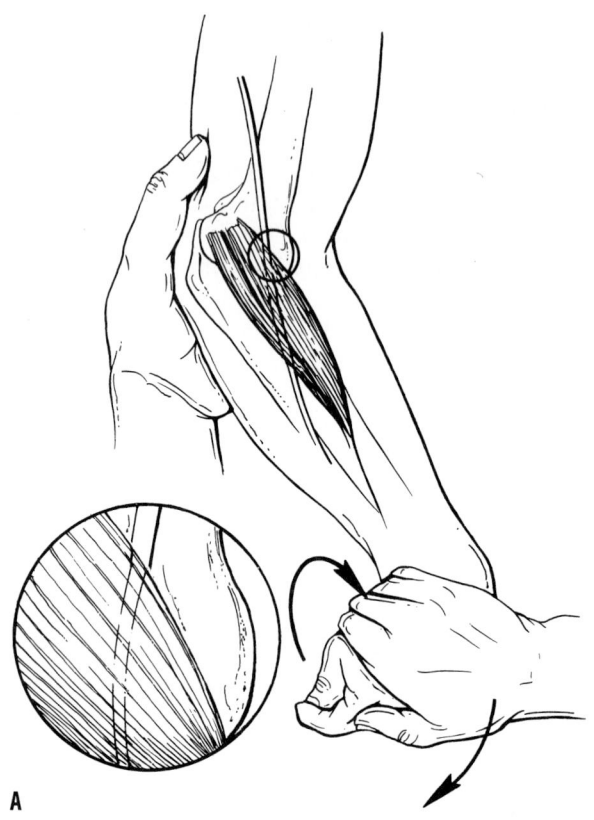

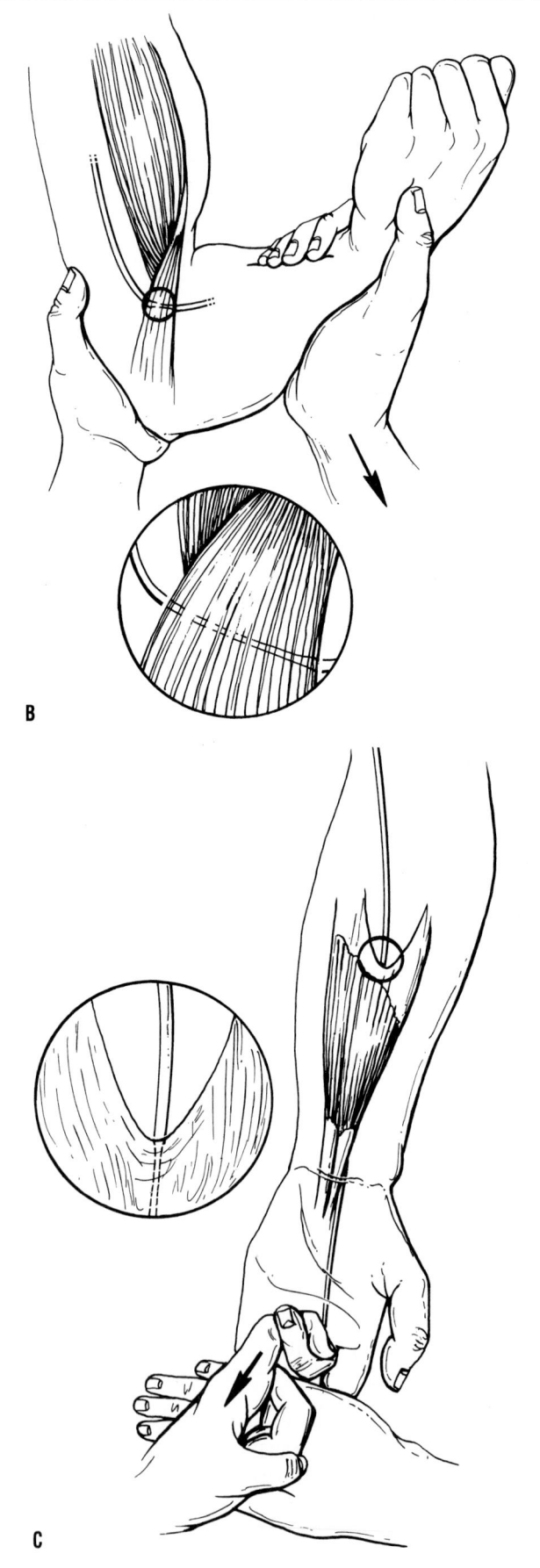

FIGURE 15-46 Pronator syndrome tests. A. Proximal forearm pain increased by resistance to pronation and elbow flexion as well as flexion of the wrist. B. Pain in the proximal forearm increased by resistance to supination is suggestive of compression by the lacertus fibrosus. C. Resistance of the long finger flexor produces pain in the proximal forearm when compression of the median nerve occurs at the flexor digitorum superficialis arch. (Reproduced with permission from Herndon JH. *Surgical Reconstruction of the Upper Extremity*. Stamford, CT: Appleton & Lange; 1999.)

High Radial Nerve Compression.   A spontaneous nerve compression may occur in the midarm at the level of the lateral head of the triceps due to strenuous muscular exercise.[269] A midshaft humerus fracture can result in a radial neuropathy at the spiral groove of the humerus in 14 percent of humeral fractures.[270] Regardless of the cause, a high radial nerve palsy will result in a loss of wrist extension, an inability to extend the fingers and thumb, and a decrease in sensibility of the first dorsal web space.[268] Involvement of the triceps muscle is dependent on the level of compression. A cervical radiculopathy and thoracic outlet syndrome (TOS) must be considered in the differential diagnosis.

Posterior Interosseous Nerve Syndrome (PINS).   The first reported case of PINS was in 1863, when Agnew[271] described muscle weakness in the wrist and finger extensors.[268] There are five potential sites of compression of the PIN as it traverses through the radial tunnel (Fig. 15-47)[55,59,196,268]:

▶ The fibrous bands that connect the brachialis to the brachio-radialis.[60,272]

FIGURE 15-47 Compression sites for the posterior interosseous nerve. (Reproduced with permission from Herndon JH. *Surgical Reconstruction of the Upper Extremity.* Stamford, CT: Appleton & Lange; 1999.)

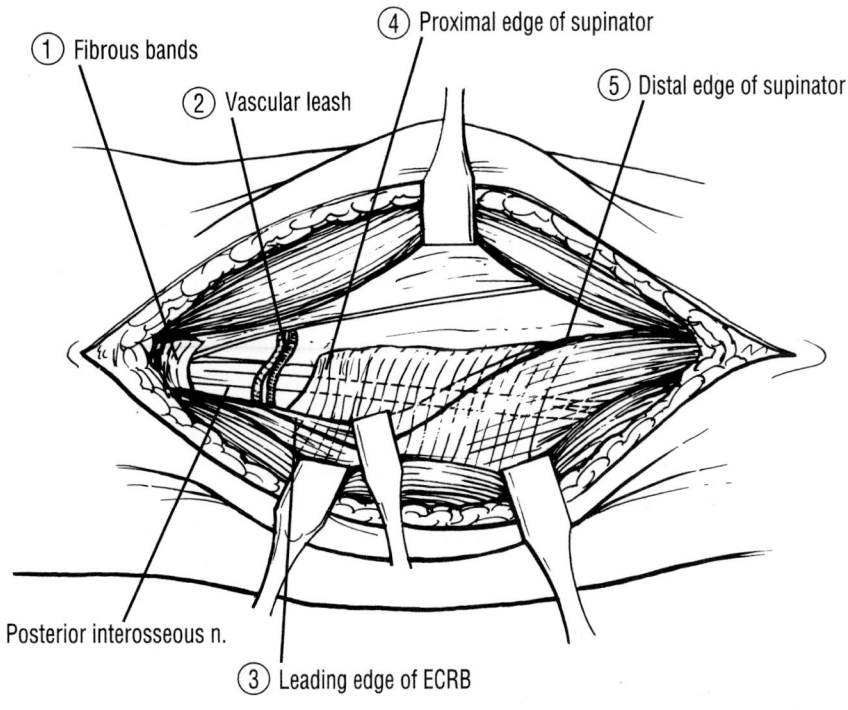

① Fibrous bands
④ Proximal edge of supinator
② Vascular leash
⑤ Distal edge of supinator
Posterior interosseous n.
③ Leading edge of ECRB

▶ The vascular leash of Henry, a fan of blood vessels that cross the nerve at the level of the radial neck.[59,60,273]

▶ Medial proximal portion (leading edge) of the ECRB.[59,60]

▶ Between fibrous bands at the proximal and distal edge of the supinator.[276] The proximal border of the supinator, through which the radial nerve passes, is referred to as the Arcade of Fröhse.

PIN palsy produces an inability to extend the metacarpophalangeal joints of the thumb, index, long, ring, or small fingers either individually or in combination.[277,278] Additionally, there is a loss of thumb interphalangeal extension and radial abduction of the thumb.[268] Because the PIN can innervate the ECRB prior to the nerve's entrance into the radial tunnel, this muscle may not be involved in the PIN palsy. Thus when compression within the radial tunnel is sufficient to cause paralysis but there is no palsy, the condition is termed posterior interosseous nerve syndrome.[262]

Initial conservative intervention includes rest, activity modification, and the use of a cock-up splint. Regular gentle stretching of the wrist extensor muscles with the elbow held in full extension is begun after a spontaneous recovery.[262]

Radial Tunnel Syndrome. Radial tunnel syndrome involves compression of the deep branch of the radial nerve. Michele and Krueger[279] have been credited with recognizing RTS as a distinct entity and gave it the name radial pronator syndrome. The term radial tunnel syndrome was introduced by Roles and Maudsley,[60] who suggested that RTS was the cause of resistant tennis elbow pain.

The same structures implicated in PIN compression syndrome can cause radial tunnel syndrome, although RTS is often thought of as a dynamic compression syndrome.[198] This is because compression of the nerve occurs during elbow extension, forearm pronation, and wrist flexion, which causes the ECRB and the fibrous edge of the superficial part of the supinator to tighten around the nerve. The symptoms from this compression can mimic those of tennis elbow, namely tenderness over the lateral aspect of the elbow, pain on passive stretching of the extensor muscles, and pain on resisted extension of the wrist and fingers.[60,198] Men and women are equally affected, and the compression appears to be common in the fourth to sixth decades of life.[59]

Pain, which is poorly localized over the radial aspect of the proximal forearm, is the most common primary presenting symptom in RTS. In fact it is the only nerve compression syndrome in which the signs and symptoms are not based on the nerve distribution.[280]

Upon palpation, maximal tenderness is usually elicited over the radial tunnel, some 5 cm distal to the lateral epicondyle, anterior to the radial neck (see Fig. 15-47). Resisted middle finger extension,[60] which tightens the fascial origin of the ECRB, and resisted supination of the forearm with the elbow fully extended[59] should reproduce the pain at the point of maximal tenderness. Positioning the arm in elbow extension, forearm pronation, and wrist flexion produces significant compression of the radial nerve.[262]

Conservative intervention should focus on education to avoid the provocative positioning of the arm into forceful extension and supination of the wrist and forearm, and should include rest, stretching, and splinting.[60,281]

If a wrist immobilization splint is used, it is fitted in 45 degrees of extension for continual wear.

Surgical intervention is reserved for patients whose symptoms are not relieved by conservative intervention.

Radial Sensory Nerve Entrapment.   The terms *Wartenberg's syndrome*[282] or *Cheiralgia Paresthetica* are used to describe a mononeuritis of the superficial radial nerve, which can become entrapped where it pierces the fascia between the brachioradialis and extensor carpi radialis longus tendons.[261,268] Symptoms include shooting or burning pain along the posterior-radial forearm, wrist, and thumb, associated with wrist flexion and ulnar deviation.[268] These symptoms can lead the clinician to believe that the first carpometacarpal joint and/or tendons of the anatomic snuffbox are involved, and that DeQuervain's disease is present.

Musculocutaneous Nerve Entrapment.   The brachialis is a pure elbow flexor, whereas the biceps brachii is an elbow flexor and supinator of the forearm.[36,283] With complete loss of motor function of these two muscles due to a lesion of the musculocutaneous nerve, functional elbow flexion strength can still be obtained with contraction of the brachioradialis and pronator teres.[284] The extensor carpi radialis longus, flexor carpi ulnaris, flexor carpi radialis, and palmaris longus may also assist with flexing the elbow.[285] The brachioradialis has a better mechanical advantage when the elbow is flexed to 90 degrees and is more active when the forearm is in the pronated or neutral position.[285] The pronator teres can produce full elbow flexion, but this is accompanied by forearm pronation.[284,286] Thus with a complete musculocutaneous nerve palsy, full antigravity elbow flexion can still be obtained and is strongest with the elbow flexed at 90 degrees and the forearm pronated.

Acute Compartment Syndrome

See Chapter 9.

Myofascial Pain Dysfunction

Elbow pain, when not related to the joint or to microtearing of the common flexor or extensor tendons, is commonly referred into the elbow from a number of sources, including myofascial. Even if microtearing is present, trigger points can also be present in the relevant muscles, placing a chronic strain on that tendon.

Supinator.   This muscle refers pain and tenderness primarily to the lateral epicondyle of the elbow, but also to the dorsal web space between the thumb and index finger. According to Travell and Simons,[287] each of the common sites for tennis elbow can be accounted for by trigger points in the supinator, extensor carpi radialis longus, and triceps muscles.

Supinator pain referral is activated by playing tennis with an extended elbow, which does not allow the biceps brachii to take part in the supination required to control the head of the tennis racket.[288]

Triceps Brachii.   A trigger point in the medial head of the triceps is a common cause of lateral elbow pain from the lateral side of this muscle or of medial elbow pain from the medial side of this muscle.[288]

Integration of Practice Patterns 4G and 4I: Impaired Joint Mobility, Motor Function, Muscle Performance, and Range of Motion, Associated with Fractures and Bony or Soft Tissue Surgical Procedures

Monteggia Fracture

Monteggia lesions are a combination of injuries involving a fracture of the ulna and a dislocation of the proximal end of the radius, which typically result from a direct blow to the forearm or a FOOSH injury with the arm positioned in either hyperextension or hyperpronation. Although relatively rare, they can present with serious problems and poor functional outcomes if mismanaged.[201,289] The complications include damage to the posterior branch of the radial nerve, anterior interosseous nerve, and ulnar nerve, as well as nonunion and poor active range of motion (AROM).[201]

Following the surgery, the elbow is immobilized for about 4 weeks in 90 to 120 degrees of elbow flexion, after which AROM exercises for elbow flexion and forearm supination are initiated. AROM into extension beyond 90 degrees begins 4 to 6 weeks postoperatively.

Essex-Lopresti Fractures

This type of fracture is defined as a fracture of the radial head with proximal radius migration and disruption of the distal radioulnar joint and interosseous membrane,[290] which typically results from a FOOSH injury.[291]

Gentle AROM for forearm rotation is initiated about 6 weeks after surgery and immobilization in a Muenster cast.

Panner's Disease

Panner's disease (osteochondrosis deformans or osteochondritis) is an aseptic or avascular necrosis of the epiphysis.[292] Although related to direct trauma or to changes in the circulation, the actual etiology is unknown. Panner's disease is rarely seen before the age of 5 years and after the age of 16, and it almost exclusively (90 percent) affects boys. The main presenting symptoms are pain to the lateral aspect of the elbow, swelling, and a limitation of elbow movement in a noncapsular pattern. If a displaced fragment is present, there is often a painless limitation of elbow extension, with a soft end-feel, but a hard end-feel when flexion is limited.[66]

Conservative intervention involves rest from throwing or impact-loading stress, with a short period of splint immobilization sometimes necessary. The exercise progression is based on clinical findings and patient tolerance.

Olecranon Fracture

An olecranon process fracture is not uncommon due to its subcutaneous position, and may be caused by either a high- or low-energy injury.[293,294] The high-energy mechanism is usually a fall backwards onto the elbow or a FOOSH injury, which produces passive elbow flexion combined with a sudden powerful contraction of the triceps muscle, resulting in an avulsion fracture of the olecranon.

Recognition of an avulsion fracture involving the triceps is through loss of active extension, a palpable gap, pain and swelling at the fracture site, and a large hematoma developing into diffuse ecchymosis.[295]

The focus on the intervention for the nondisplaced or minimally displaced fractures is to allow restoration of the articular surfaces and maintaining triceps function, while allowing early range of motion.

All other fractures require open reduction with internal fixation (ORIF) or excision of the bone fragments with repair of the extensor mechanism.[201,293,294,296] Rehabilitation following surgery is dependent upon the extent of the surgery and the length of the immobilization, although the emphasis on regaining early motion remains the same.

Radial Head Fractures

Radial head fractures present several challenges during the rehabilitative process, as the radial head is a secondary stabilizer for valgus forces at the elbow, and resists longitudinal forces along the forearm.[297] Compromise of the medial (ulnar) collateral ligament makes the radial head a more important stabilizer of the elbow.[6,297,298]

The most common cause of radial head fracture is a FOOSH injury, due to the axial loading through the radial head. The presenting symptoms are pain and tenderness over the lateral aspect of the elbow, followed by a decreased range of motion. Dislocations often occur with the radial head fracture.[148]

Three classifications define these fractures: type I (nondisplaced), type II (at the margin of the radial head with displacement), and type III (comminuted, involving the entire radial head). In the type I fracture, the pain usually subsides about 30 minutes after the injury, but recurs as a result of bleeding into the joint.

Use of a splint or a sling for 3 days is indicated in type I fractures, with active elbow flexion exercises being initiated immediately. As much early mobilization as the patient can tolerate is the key to a favorable outcome. Strengthening, initially involving isometric exercises, begins at 3 weeks and progresses to isotonic exercises at 5 to 6 weeks. Heavy resistance is not performed until after 8 weeks, or when adequate healing is demonstrated on radiographs.

Most type II fractures follow a similar rehabilitative course, providing the fracture fragment does not exceed 30 percent of the radial head surface.[148]

Fractures with radial head surface involvement of more than 30 percent, fracture fragment displacement, and type III characteristics require management by an orthopaedic surgeon.[148]

Rehabilitation following elbow fractures that undergo internal fixation usually lasts for 12 weeks. Immediately following the immobilization of elbow fractures, active and passive motion exercises are initiated. The goal is to achieve 15 to 105 degrees of motion by the end of week 2. Isometric exercises for elbow flexion and extension, and forearm pronation/supination are started within the first week. Active assistive pronation/

supination exercises do not begin until week 6. Isotonic exercises are given for the shoulder and the wrist and hand. Joint mobilizations, which begin if needed in the second week, are used to help regain elbow extension.

By the third week, the patient should be performing light-weight isotonic exercises for elbow flexion and extension, and beginning at week 7, eccentric and plyometric exercises are prescribed. At about the same time, neuromuscular re-education exercises and functional training exercises are added.

Pathologic Bone Formation[299]

Pathologic bone formation about the elbow occurs in several distinct forms, which include heterotopic ossification, myositis ossificans, periarticular calcification, and ectopic ossification.

Heterotopic ossification is defined as the formation of mature lamellar bone in nonosseous tissues.

Myositis ossificans refers to heterotopic ossification that forms in inflammatory muscle. Although heterotopic ossification and myositis ossificans are radiographically and histologically similar, these processes are distinguished by their anatomic locations.[300]

Periarticular calcification refers to collections of calcium pyrophosphates within soft tissues such as the collateral ligaments or joint capsule.

The term ectopic ossification includes heterotopic ossification and myositis ossificans. Because most cases of pathologic bone formation about the elbow consist of heterotopic ossification and myositis ossificans, ectopic ossification is the most appropriate descriptive term for this process.

Ectopic ossification about the elbow can result from direct injury, neural axis trauma, burns, and genetic disorders,[301] although direct elbow trauma is the most common cause.[302] Although elbow ectopic ossification may be asymptomatic, it frequently causes severe elbow stiffness or even ankylosis, and a resultant loss of function.[69,83]

Regan and Reilly[303] outlined three factors that predispose the elbow to post-traumatic stiffness:

▶ the high degree of articular congruity.

▶ the conformity of the elbow joint.

▶ the covering of the anterior joint capsule by the brachialis, predisposing it to post-traumatic ectopic ossification. Post-traumatic elbow ectopic ossification typically begins to form 2 weeks after trauma, surgery, burn, or neurologic insult,[303–305] resulting in localized tissue swelling and tenderness, hyperemia, and pain.

Mobilization after elbow injury often is delayed, because it is difficult to achieve rigid internal fixation of comminuted elbow fractures. Furthermore, post-traumatic elbow stiffness may occur despite early aggressive motion and prophylactic measures.

Elbow stiffness may develop 1 to 4 months after an initial phase of motion recovery after injury.[306] The patient's chief complaint may be pain, stiffness, instability, sensory loss, weakness, or locking. If pain is present, it is located anteriorly, in the middle third of the arm.

Limited active and passive elbow flexion and extension are characteristic of ectopic ossification formation about the elbow. However, in some patients, active and passive elbow motion may remain normal, especially in the early phase. However, even with aggressive intervention, including static and dynamic splinting and frequent active and passive ROM exercises, elbow motion may diminish. Strength testing reveals weak and painful elbow flexion and extension, and the end-feels of elbow ROM become rigid or abrupt. Once the ectopic ossification matures, usually at 3 to 9 months after injury, elbow ROM remains stable as long as an active and passive ROM program is continued.

Ectopic ossification about the elbow may lead to delayed nerve palsy. The ulnar nerve is most commonly affected; however, tardy median and radial palsies also have been reported.[307–309] This complication may occur several months or many years after the formation of ectopic bone.

Plain radiographs establish the diagnosis of ectopic ossification, define its location, and show its maturity. Radiographs show ectopic ossification as early as 2 weeks after injury, and joint incongruity, osteophytes, and/or malunion will also be apparent.

Nearly all patients who present with elbow stiffness and ectopic ossification should be started on an aggressive active motion program to combat the progressive loss of motion that occurs during ectopic ossification maturation. In some patients, elbow motion may improve; however, in others, loss of motion occurs and ankylosis may result. Active exercises, passive exercises, continuous passive motion, dynamic splinting, and static splinting have all been advocated, although some authors suggest that passive elbow exercises enhance elbow ectopic ossification formation and exacerbate elbow stiffness,[310] even though there is little evidence to support this belief. Until there is a prospective study comparing patients with elbow injuries treated with passive stretching with patients treated without passive stretching, the relationship between passive elbow motion and ectopic ossification formation will remain unclear. However, the passive force should be applied slowly and progressively so as not to cause any damage to the soft tissues and thereby provoke an exacerbation.

Unless there is a contraindication, all patients are started on an active and active-assisted ROM program.

Splinting is also commonly used to restore elbow ROM. Spring-loaded hinged dynamic splints may be used to counteract flexion and extension contractures. Patients are instructed to wear these splints for six 1-hour sessions daily and while they sleep. If flexion and extension are limited, the patient is issued a dynamic flexion splint and a dynamic extension splint, and instructed to alternate use of them. Turnbuckle splints also are available, and are typically used for rigid contractures. This splint allows the patient to impart a static constant stretch to the soft tissues by tightening the turnbuckle.[302]

Elbow ectopic ossification can be prevented in many cases with prophylactic measures. Patients who sustain an elbow injury and have a risk factor for ectopic ossification should be treated to prevent this complication. Two forms of prophylaxis are available:

▶ *Chemotherapeutic agents.* These include nonsteroidal anti-inflammatory drugs. NSAIDs have been shown to decrease the incidence and severity of ectopic ossification about the hip. No studies exist regarding its effect on elbow ectopic ossification.

▶ *Low-dose external beam radiation.* Clinical studies showed that this modality inhibits ectopic ossification formation after total hip arthroplasty.[311,312]

Pediatric Pathology

Little Leaguer's Elbow

Little leaguer's elbow is a common term, credited to Brogden,[313] for an avulsion lesion to the medial apophysis. The term has since been used to describe a variety of pathoanatomic lesions in the immature athlete, all of which relate to the mechanics of throwing. Additional factors that influence its development include age, skeletal maturity, individual susceptibility, competitive level, and geographic location.[314]

The act of baseball pitching has been described in five stages (see Fig. 15-12)[25,32,118,119]:

▶ *Wind-up.* This stage involves the initial preparation as the elbow is flexed and the forearm is slightly pronated, and is characterized by low load to the arm. Elbow flexion is maintained by an isometric contraction of the elbow flexors. During the stride of the wind-up phase, the biceps contract to isometrically and eccentrically control the elbow angle, while the wrist and finger extensors concentrically move the wrist from slight flexion to hyperextension.[5,315]

▶ *Early cocking.* This stage begins when the ball leaves the nondominant gloved hand and ends when the forward foot comes into contact with the ground. The shoulder begins to abduct and externally rotate, and valgus stress to the elbow begins.

▶ *Late cocking.* This stage is characterized by further shoulder abduction and maximal external rotation. At the elbow, flexion of between 90 and 120 degrees and increasing forearm pronation to approximately 90 degrees occurs. Dynamic stability is provided by the flexor-pronator muscle mass, and the triceps contracts isometrically to limit elbow flexion.[5]

▶ *Acceleration.* This phase is characterized by the generation of a significant anteriorly-directed force on the upper extremity by the shoulder musculature, resulting in internal rotation and adduction of the humerus, accompanied by rapid elbow extension. The period from the late cocking stage through the acceleration phase is the time when the elbow is subjected to maximum valgus stresses.[316]

▶ *Follow-through.* This phase is characterized by the dissipation of all excess kinetic energy as the elbow reaches full extension and ends when all motion is complete. McLeod further divides this phase into release and deceleration.[317]

The repetitive motions involved in the various phases of throwing place enormous strains on the elbow, particularly during the late cocking and acceleration phases, which can result in inflammation, scar formation, loose bodies, ligament sprains or ruptures, and the more serious conditions of osteochondritis or an avulsion fracture.[32,318] Little leaguer's elbow may start insidiously or suddenly. Usually a sudden onset of pain is secondary to fracture at the site of the lesion.

Clinical findings include a history of pain on the medial side of the elbow, with and without throwing. Physical findings relate to the specific lesion, but are commonly a persistent elbow discomfort or stiffness due to aggravation by the injury. A locking or "catching" sensation indicates a loose body.

Management is conservative, involving rest and elimination of the offending activity for 3 to 6 weeks. If osteochondritis dissecans is present, the joint needs protection for several months.[148] The patient cannot return to pitching until full and normal motion has returned.

To prevent elbow disorders young athletes should adhere to the rules of Little League, which limit the number of pitches per game, per week, and per season, and the number of days of rest between pitching.[68] The pitch count is the most important of these statistics.

Surgical intervention is reserved for those patients with symptoms of a loose body, osteochondritis, or who fail to respond to conservative therapy.

Avulsion of Medial Epicondyle

Before epiphyseal closure, a rapid strong contraction of the forearm flexors is capable of avulsing the medial epicondyle. This lesion can be associated with a posterior dislocation of the elbow, where the fragment dislocates posteriorly, but is reduced when the elbow joint is reduced.

The conservative intervention typically involves splinting of the elbow for 2 weeks if the medial stability is intact, and open reduction if the fragment is widely displaced.

Supracondylar Fracture of Humerus

This is a common and serious elbow injury, where the flat and flared distal metaphysis of the humerus is injured by hyperextension or a fall on a flexed elbow. The forces are transmitted through the elbow joint to the distal humerus, producing a fracture just proximal to the elbow. Sometimes, a "follow-through" of fragments results in a proximal fragment piercing the anterior periosteum, brachialis muscle, and possibly the brachial artery and median nerve.

The patient presents with an obvious deformity and swelling. Due to the nature of this condition, peripheral circulation and nerve function must be assessed.

The intervention is dependent upon severity. Nondisplaced fractures are immobilized with the elbow flexed for 3 weeks, whereas displaced fractures require closed reduction and immobilization in a cast that does not constrict circulation, for 3 weeks. During the period of immobilization, the patient is closely monitored for changes in peripheral circulation.

Following the period of immobilization, active range-of-motion exercises are initiated in an effort to regain extension.

Pulled Elbow

The term *pulled elbow* refers to a common minor soft tissue injury of the radiohumeral joint in children of preschool age, caused by sudden traction on the pronated wrist and extended elbow.[319,320] A pulled elbow results from the radial head slipping through the annular ligament, causing the fibers of the annular ligament to become interposed between the radius and the capitellum of the humerus.[321,322]

The incidence of pulled elbow is 3 percent in children under the age of 8 years,[323] and it comprises 5.6 percent of all injuries involving the upper extremity in children under the age of 10.[322,324] The disorder is more common in boys than in girls, and the left elbow is more commonly affected than the right.[325]

These are common causes of pulled elbow[322]:

▶ The child's forearm or hand is being held firmly by a parent as the child attempts to walk away.

▶ The child is lifted by an adult from the ground by his hands.

▶ A mother snatches the hand of a child to prevent a fall as he wanders towards the edge of the pavement.

▶ The young child may be lifted by the hand from a lying or sitting position, or may even be swung around by the hands several times during the course of play.

▶ The child actually does the pulling, either as he or she stumbles and falls, or while trying to escape the grasping hand of an adult.

The child presents with a painful and dangling arm, which hangs limply with the elbow extended and the forearm pronated.[322] There is usually no obvious swelling or deformity. The common sites of pain are (in order of occurrence) the forearm and wrist, the wrist alone, and the elbow alone.[321] In all cases the child resists attempted supination of the elbow.

The intervention of choice is manipulation.[322] Before attempting the manipulation, it is important to explain the procedure to the parents, and to win the confidence of the child, by gently supporting the injured arm before manipulation. During the procedure, the clinician holds the child's wrist with one hand while the other hand supports the elbow and palpates the radial head. The child's attention is diverted and the forearm is forcibly supinated with one quick motion, together with application of downward pressure on the radial head. A click in the region of the radial head (palpable and sometimes audible) is indicative of a successful reduction. Sometimes the forearm has to be pronated after forcible supination to reduce the pulled elbow. The click results from release of the trapped annular ligament. Soon after the manipulation, the child usually begins to use the arm again, but sometimes there is a delay of a day or two. In such cases a sling can be used to both give comfort and protect the arm from being pulled again.

An important aspect in the management is to advise the parents to avoid longitudinal traction strain on the child's arm—the parents should not pull on the hands or wrists of the child.[322]

Therapeutic Techniques

Techniques to Increase Joint Mobility

With some slight variations, the same techniques that are used to examine the joint glides of the elbow complex can be used to mobilize the joints, with the clinician varying the intensity of the mobilizations based on patient response and the stage of tissue healing.

Passive Accessory Mobilization: Superior Radioulnar Joint
The patient is positioned in supine with their head supported on a pillow. The clinician faces the patient.

Anteromedial/Posterolateral Glide. The clinician palpates and stabilizes the proximal third of the ulna with one hand, while palpating the head of the radius in the posteroanterior plane with a pinch grip of the index finger and thumb of the other hand (see Fig. 15-26). The clinician glides the radial head anteromedially/posterolaterally at the superior radioulnar joint. The amplitude and the velocity of the technique (i.e., grade) are varied according to the irritability of the joint.

Passive Accessory Mobilization: Inferior Radioulnar Joint
Anteroposterior Glide. The patient is positioned in supine or sitting with the clinician facing the patient. Using one hand, the clinician palpates and stabilizes the distal third of the ulna. With a pinch grip of the fingers and thumb of the other hand, the clinician palpates the distal third of the radius. The clinician glides the radius anteroposteriorly at the inferior radioulnar joint in an obliquely anteromedial/posterolateral plane. The intensity of the technique (i.e., grade) is varied according to the irritability of the joint.

Mobilizations with Movements[326,327]
To Increase Motion at the Elbow. The patient is positioned in supine with the involved arm on the bed and the forearm supinated. A belt is wrapped around the posterior aspect of the clinician and around the patient's forearm so the belt edge is level with the elbow joint (Fig. 15-48). Using one hand, the clinician stabilizes the patient's humerus, while the other hand supports the patient's forearm and wrist (see Fig. 15-48). From this position, the ulna is glided laterally as the clinician gently moves their hips backwards. Adjustments in the direction of the mobilization glide are made with respect to the carrying angle of the elbow. If there is no pain, the patient actively flexes or extends their elbow while the mobilization force is maintained. The active motion can be progressed to resisted wrist extension, or resisted gripping performed during the mobilization.

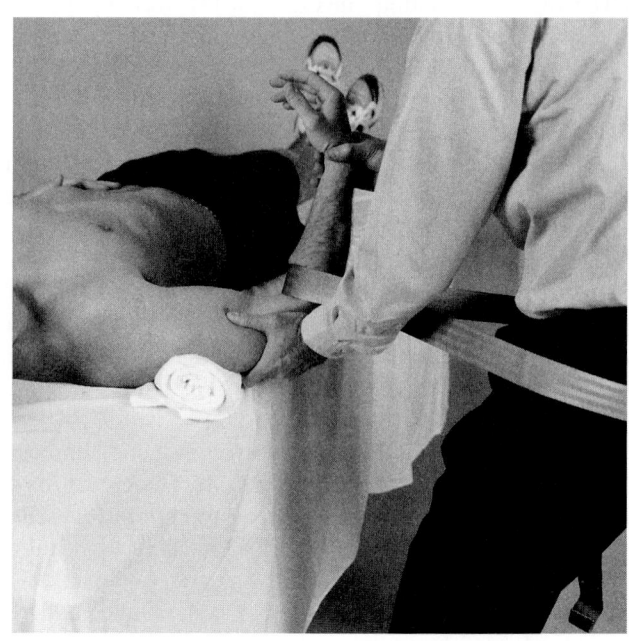

FIGURE 15-48   Mobilizations with movement to increase elbow motion.

Automobilizations
Mediolateral Glide of the Ulnohumeral Joint. The patient can be sitting or standing in a doorway with the involved forearm and hand stabilized against the wall, and the elbow in slight flexion, close to full extension. Using the other hand, the patient grasps the humerus of the involved arm by the humeral epicondyles, and applies a medial and lateral glide at the involved elbow, producing a medial and lateral tilt at the humeroulnar joint.

Distraction. The patient sits in a chair, with the shoulder abducted to 90 degrees, and the elbow flexed over a firm pillow or towel roll. Using the other hand, the patient grasps the wrist of the involved upper extremity and applies slow oscillatory mobilizations in the direction of further elbow flexion, using pain as a guide.

Techniques to Increase Soft Tissue Extensibility
An increase in flexibility is achieved through a routine stretching program that may be instituted early in the course of treatment, with emphasis on stretching the entire hand, forearm, and shoulder complex. Stretching should follow the application of local heat such as that afforded by ultrasound or transverse friction massage. Patients should be taught how to perform these techniques on themselves at the earliest opportunity.

In each of the following techniques, the left arm is being treated.

Biceps. The patient stands by a table, and places the back of the hand on the tabletop with the forearm supinated. The elbow is gradually extended and the forearm is moved into further supination (Fig. 15-49).

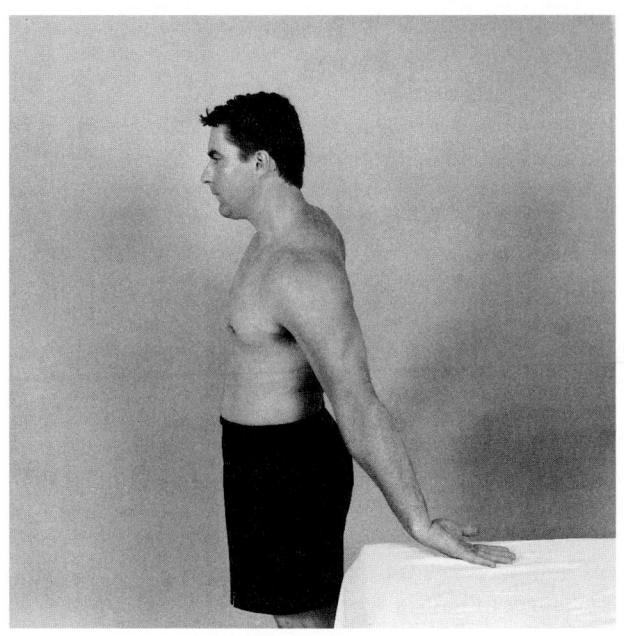

FIGURE 15-49   Biceps stretch.

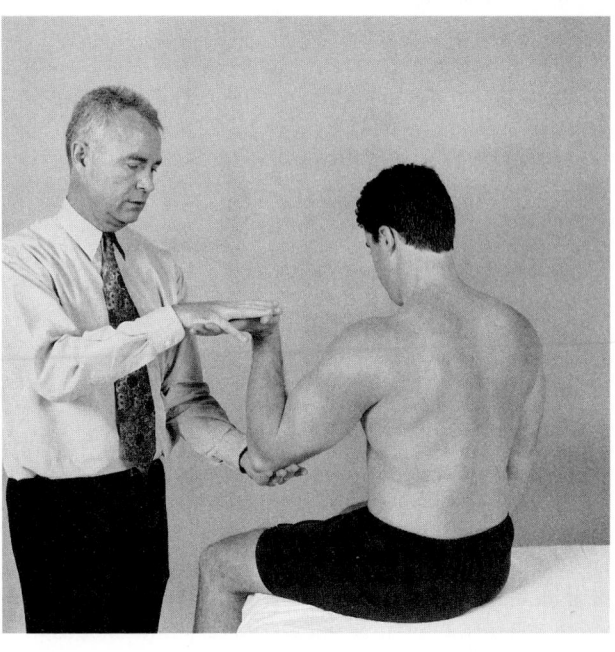

FIGURE 15-50   Stretch for golfer's elbow.

Wrist and Finger Extensors.   Stretching of the extensor carpi radialis brevis is always combined with stretching of the extensor carpi radialis longus and extensor digitorum, and is indicated in all types of tennis and golfer's elbow.

The patient is positioned in sitting. The upper arm is held horizontally, with the elbow flexed 90 degrees, the forearm pronated, and the wrist flexed. The patient uses the right hand to grasp their left hand and positions the wrist in maximal flexion and ulnar deviation, with the forearm in maximal pronation. The elbow is brought very slowly into extension.

Stretch for Golfer's Elbow.   The function of the long wrist flexors is flexion of the elbow, pronation of the forearm, and flexion of the wrist. The patient sits on a chair with the affected arm elevated approximately 60 degrees. The elbow is slightly flexed, the forearm supinated, and the wrist extended (Fig. 15-50). The patient uses the right hand to bring the wrist and fingers into as much extension as possible (see Fig. 15-50). While holding the wrist in maximal extension, the clinician very slowly extends the patient's elbow. As soon as pain or muscle guarding occurs, the motion is stopped and the elbow is brought slightly back into more flexion. If the pain disappears after a few seconds, the elbow can be brought further into extension.

Weight-Bearing Wrist Flexor Stretch.   This stretch is performed by asking the patient to position their hand palm side down on a table, and to position their elbow in slight flexion, their wrist into maximal ulnar deviation and extension, and the forearm in maximal pronation. Being careful to avoid pain and muscle splinting, the patient slowly straightens the elbow. The stretch should be held for approximately 40 seconds. At this point,

the patient can gently pull the fingers up from the table to stretch the flexor muscles of the palm. Against very slight resistance (performed by the other hand), the arm is then brought back to the original position. This stretching procedure is repeated six times before repeating the entire procedure on the uninvolved side.

Muscle Energy Treatment

Adduction (Supination) Restriction of the Ulnohumeral Joint.[328] The patient is positioned in supine with their forearm positioned into full supination, with the clinician standing at the side of the table. The patient is asked to gently try and pronate their forearm against the clinician's equal restraining isometric force. This position is held for 4 seconds, and then the patient relaxes. The technique is repeated.

Abduction (Pronation) Restriction.[328]   To treat an abduction restriction, the position of the forearm and the direction of the isometric contraction is reversed.

Supination/Pronation.   The patient is positioned in supine, their head supported on a pillow. The clinician stands or sits facing the patient. Using one hand, the clinician palpates the distal third of the patient's forearm while palpating the proximal ulna with the other hand. The clinician supinates/pronates the forearm to the end range, around the appropriate oblique axis. From this position the patient is instructed to hold still while the therapist applies a gentle resistance to further supination/pronation. The contraction is held for 3 to 5 seconds, after which the patient is instructed to completely relax. The new barrier of supination/pronation is localized and the mobilization repeated.

High-Velocity, Low-Amplitude Thrusting

***Mill's Manipulation.*[66]** This technique is designed to break adhesions of the common extensor tendon, and let the orbicular ligament slip back to its normal position. The Mill's manipulation is used instead of slowly stretching the tissues during the last few degrees of maximal elbow extension.

This manipulation is indicated only for certain patients, namely those:

▶ Who demonstrate full active and passive elbow extension with a normal end-feel.

▶ Whose elbow demonstrates only a slight limitation of motion with a myofascial end-feel.

Prior to the manipulation, transverse frictions should be applied to the site in order to soften the scar.

The patient is positioned in sitting, with the clinician standing behind the patient's shoulder (see Fig. 15-33). The patient's wrist is flexed. Maintaining the position of the patient's wrist, the clinician extends the elbow. The Mill's maneuver involves a forcible extension of the elbow, while simultaneous digital pressure is exerted over the point of maximum tenderness. If the wrist flexion is not maintained, the force will be through the elbow joint. Mills stressed the need to elicit an audible click during the procedure, although in practice many normal elbows can be made to click by the same maneuver,[329] indicating that the click is probably coincidental.

A modification to the patient position can be used for this manipulation. The patient is positioned in supine with their arm off the edge of the table. The clinician adjusts the table height so the patient's elbow joint can be rested on their thigh while the clinician's foot is in contact with the floor. The patient's arm is then placed in slight shoulder extension and full internal rotation (palm down). In this position the various tendons can be tested as to their level of involvement by having each one contract. The involved tendon is then softened up using transverse friction before the manipulation is applied using the aforementioned positions. The patient's elbow is then slightly raised off the clinician's thigh and then dropped quickly back onto the thigh.

Following the manipulation, exercises to stretch the scar should be carried out.

***Technique for Abduction/Adduction Restriction of the Ulnohumeral Joint.*[328]** The patient is positioned in sitting, while the clinician stands facing the patient. The clinician grasps the patient's elbow and places the fingers of the monitoring hand on either side of the olecranon. The other hand is used to hold and stabilize the patient's forearm in supination/extension. The radioulnar joint motion is tested in both adduction and abduction.

If a restriction of motion is noted in abduction, the clinician places the patient's elbow into abduction and full extension (see Fig. 15-17), and exerts a hyperabduction corrective thrust.

If a restriction of motion is noted in adduction, the clinician places the patient's elbow into adduction and full extension (see Fig. 15-17) and exerts a hyperadduction corrective thrust. A muscle energy assist of the biceps can be used to take up the slack into adduction. In addition to applying a manipulation thrust, the clinician can also perform active mobilizations to restore the end range of adduction.

***Technique for the Anterior Radial Head.*[328]** The patient is positioned in sitting, while the clinician stands facing the patient. The clinician grasps the patient's dysfunctional arm, flexing it at the elbow and pronating it at the wrist (see Fig. 15-18). The clinician places the second and third digits of their other hand into the crease of the patient's elbow, directly over the radial head. From this position the clinician exerts a rapid hyperflexion force on the elbow while simultaneously thrusting the radial head posteriorly with the fingers of the other hand.

***Posterior Radial Head Somatic Dysfunction.*[328]** The patient is positioned in sitting, while the clinician stands facing the patient. The clinician encircles the patient's dysfunctional elbow with both hands and extends it. From this position, the clinician places both thumbs over the head of the radius anteriorly, and the phalanges of both index fingers over the radial head posteriorly. The clinician then exerts a rapid hyperextension force on the patient's elbow, while simultaneously inducing a anterior counterforce through the radial head.

CASE STUDY LATERAL ELBOW PAIN

HISTORY

History of Current Condition

A 43-year-old female patient presents who complains of left elbow pain which she reported having for about a year. The patient described the onset of elbow pain as gradual and attributed it to her work as an electronics assembler, where she spent the day pulling out plugs. Over time the pain had worsened to the point where it hurt all of the time. Although the patient had tried a course of anti-inflammatories, they had been discontinued due to an adverse reaction. The patient was placed on light duty at work with a lifting restriction of 10 lb.

Past History of Current Condition

No past history of left elbow pain.

Past Medical and Surgical History

Unremarkable.

Medications

None.

Living Environment

Lives in a two-story house.

Occupational, Employment, and School

Assembly line worker. High school education.

Functional Status and Activity Level

The patient's goals were to decrease pain with activities of daily living and to be able to return to work without pain.

Health Status (Self-Report)

In general good health, but pain interferes with tasks at home and at work.

QUESTIONS

1. What is the most common diagnosis characterized by lateral elbow pain?
2. What can a history of gradual onset tell the clinician?
3. What can a history of repetitive activity tell the clinician?
4. What findings do you expect to note in the physical examination in terms of palpation, resistive tests, and special tests?
5. What additional questions would you ask to help rule out referral of pain from the cervical spine or shoulder?
6. List the various diagnoses that could present with these signs and symptoms, and the tests you would use to rule out each one.
7. Does this presentation and history warrant an upper quarter scanning examination? Why or why not?

PHYSICAL THERAPY TESTS AND MEASURES

The physical examination of the patient included an inspection for muscle atrophy, palpation for areas of tenderness and crepitation, muscle testing of all major muscles about the elbow, measurement of active and passive range of motion, observation of symmetry of carrying angle, and specific testing for tennis elbow and instability.[99] The cervical spine and shoulder were also examined.

Motor Performance: Strength, Power, and Endurance

Although no strength deficits were noted in either upper extremity, pain was elicited with resistive testing for all motions except wrist flexion and elbow pronation. Cozen's test for tennis elbow reproduced the patient's pain at the left lateral epicondyle.

Manual muscle testing of C6 and C7 key muscles were within normal limits (WNL) as compared to the uninvolved side.

Strength testing of grip was WNL compared to the uninvolved side, except pain was elicited.

Orthotic, Protective, or Supportive Devices

Patient does not use any device, and has not tried a tennis elbow brace.

Pain

Palpation revealed extreme tenderness, warmth, and slight edema on and around the left lateral epicondyle. Pain was reported at 6 of 10 at rest after a day of work.

Posture

Forward head position, kyphotic dorsal spine, and protracting shoulders.

Range of Motion (Including Muscle Length)

Active range of motion of both upper extremities was within normal limits for all elbow and shoulder motions. The right elbow demonstrated full AROM, but the left elbow, although it demonstrated normal ranges for flexion, extension, pronation, and supination, exhibited pain associated with all motions. Active range of motion for the left wrist was painful for radial deviation, but was otherwise normal.

Special Tests

- AROM with overpressure of cervical spine did not reproduce symptoms.
- Shoulder motions were WNL and pain free.
- Negative quadrant compression of the cervical spine (Spurling's test).
- Specific length test for the extensor mechanism (wrist flexion, elbow extension, and forearm pronation) reproduced the patient's pain.
- No pain with specific length test for flexor mechanism (wrist extension, elbow extension, supination, and finger extension).
- Upper limb tension tests (ULTT) for median, radial, and ulnar nerves were negative.

EVALUATION (CLINICAL JUDGMENT)

Patient is a moderately obese, sedentary female with soft tissue mobility restrictions and impaired left elbow performance, which results in functional limitations both at home and at work.

DIAGNOSIS BY PHYSICAL THERAPIST

A provisional diagnosis of lateral epicondylitis is made. Given the ambiguity of this diagnosis, it is often more important to know the extent of the alterations in the tissues or in the biomechanics than to know a specific anatomy-based diagnosis.[330]

QUESTIONS

1. Having made a provisional diagnosis, what will be your intervention?
2. How would you describe this condition to the patient?
3. How would you explain the rationale behind your intervention to the patient?
4. What activities and positions would you advise the patient to avoid? Why?
5. How will you determine the intensity of your intervention?
6. Estimate this patient's prognosis.
7. What modalities could you use in the intervention of this patient? Why?
8. Which manual techniques would be appropriate for this patient, and what is your rationale for each?
9. What exercises would you prescribe? Why?
10. What therapeutic device would you recommend for this patient? Why?

PROGNOSIS

Predicted Optimal Level of Improvement in Function

Over the course of 4 to 6 weeks the patient will demonstrate:

- A return to normal home activities and to full work duty without restrictions.

- Grip strength at 90 percent as compared with the uninvolved side.
- Independence with home exercise program and prevention strategies.

Predicted Interval Levels of Improvement in Function

- Patient will be able to drive to work without pain for 45 minutes in 5 weeks.
- Return to work for a full shift with no restrictions in 6 weeks.

PLAN OF CARE

Frequency and Duration

Two to three times per week for 4 weeks.

Criteria for Discharge

Patient to be discharged when she reaches established functional goals, declines further treatment, is unable to progress towards goals because of complications, or PT determines that patient will no longer benefit from PT services.

INTERVENTION

Addressing the tendonosis as an inflammatory process without considering the underlying degeneration or biomechanical deficits will lead to certain failure. The intervention should be based on functional criteria which are based on stages of tendon healing.[331]

PHASE I (WEEKS 1–3)

This phase typically involves 2 to 4 physical therapy visits. Instructions were given with regard to rest positions and the avoidance of aggravating motions and activities.

Goals

The goals for this phase of the intervention are:

- To control pain and preserve motion.
- Decrease pain to 5 out of 10 or less with activity, and 2 out of 10 or less at rest.
- Decrease inflammation as evidenced by reduced edema and tenderness to palpation.
- Increased flexibility of wrist extensors to 90 percent as compared with the uninvolved side.
- Pain-free ability to make a fist.
- Promote the development of endurance and normal vascularization and collagen production.[99]
- Independence with home exercise program and home cryotherapy.

Electrotherapeutic Modalities

Any of the following could be attempted:

- Ice packs are applied to the left lateral epicondyle after the exercises and at the end of each day.
- High-voltage galvanic stimulation was applied to help relieve pain.
- Iontophoresis with dexamethasone.
- Shock-wave therapy.[245,332]

- Pulsed ultrasound with a 20 percent duty cycle, 3-MHz frequency, and an intensity of 1.2 W/cm² was applied to the lateral epicondyle for 5 minutes.

Therapeutic Exercise and Home Program

- Submaximal isometrics to the wrist extensors are performed in the pain-free ROM following the transverse friction massage.
- AROM exercise involving simultaneous wrist flexion, forearm pronation, and elbow extension, to promote extensibility of muscle and tendon.
- High-repetition pain-free active wrist flexion/extension to help vascularize involved tendon and to promote alignment of collagen fibers.
- The patient is instructed on stretches for the extensor-supinator group, as well as stretches for the shoulder, hand, and forearm.

Manual Therapy

- Lateral mobilization of the left forearm at the elbow was performed during active wrist extension and forearm supination.
- A dorsal glide of the hand was performed at the wrist during radial deviation.
- Tape was initially applied at the elbow to maintain the lateral mobilization, but was discontinued following an adverse reaction to the tape. Instead, the patient was issued a tennis elbow brace.
- Transverse friction massage was applied to the specific area of affected tendon to induce hyperemia. The patient was instructed in the technique as part of her home exercise program.
- Gentle stretches were applied to the wrist extensors and flexors in the pain-free ROM. The patient was instructed in the techniques as part of her home exercise program.
- Soft tissue mobilization was applied to patient tolerance.
- Myofascial release techniques were initiated.
- Acupressure can be introduced if applicable.
- Joint mobilizations can be applied to any areas of hypomobility in the cervical spine, shoulder, or elbow.

PHASE II (WEEKS 4–6)

This phase typically involves 2 to 6 physical therapy visits.

Goals

- Decrease pain to 2 out of 10 or less with activity, and 0 out of 10 at rest.
- Increase ROM to achieve pain-free simultaneous full flexion of wrist and hand with pronation of forearm and extension of elbow.
- Increase muscle performance to achieve manual muscle test of 4 out of 5 for all muscle groups.
- Grip strength at 80 percent as compared to uninvolved side.
- Gradual resumption of activities with use of an orthosis as needed.

Electrotherapeutic Modalities

Continued use of effective modalities as in acute phase, with increased emphasis on use at home as needed.

Therapeutic Exercises and Home Program

- All exercises of the wrist extensor-supinator group were started with the elbow in flexion.
- Perform slow and gentle stretches to extensor mechanism 3 to 5 times a day into wrist flexion, ulnar deviation, forearm pronation, and elbow extension.
- The patient is instructed in concentric as well as eccentric exercises for wrist extension and forearm supination, initially without resistance, and then with progressively more resistance using surgical tubing, ensuring that the patient worked to fatigue with each set.[1,113]
- Introduction of broom-handle exercise to strengthen wrist extensors. A weight is tied to a rope or piece of string approximately 3 feet in length, which is then tied to a broom handle or dowel. The broom handle is held out in front of the patient with the palms down, and she then rolls the string onto the handle/dowel to raise and lower the weight.
- In order to help balance the force couple, the patient was also instructed on a course of exercises to increase the strength in opposing muscles—the flexors of the wrist and digits.
- Squeezing exercises using theraputty or bags of rice.
- AROM of horizontal shoulder abduction while holding a weight in the hand.
- Strengthening exercises for biceps, triceps, latissimus dorsi.
- Upper body ergometer (UBE) progression.

Manual Therapy

- Continue with use of effective soft tissue techniques.
- Continue with progressive graded mobilizations for persistent hypomobilities.
- Cyriax manipulation as indicated (contraindicated in the presence of elbow osteoarthritis and loss of full elbow extension).
- Assisted stretching to the muscle bellies of the extensor mechanism to decrease tension of involved tendons.

PHASE III (WEEK 7+)

This phase typically involves 2 to 4 physical therapy visits.

Goals

- A return to normal home and recreational activities and to full work duty without restrictions.
- Pain at 0 out of 10 with activity.
- Grip strength at 90 to 100 percent as compared with the uninvolved side.
- Independence with home exercise program and prevention strategies.

Therapeutic Exercise and Home Program

All of the following exercises are performed at varying velocities, beginning with slow speeds, before gradually increasing the speed as tolerated.

- Activities and exercises incorporating the shoulder, wrist, and elbow were introduced. These included PNF patterns with wall pulleys and the Fitter board.
- Strength and endurance of the upper kinetic chain was addressed with resisted PNF diagonals and the use of a grip dynamometer.
- Sport- or activity-specific training.
- Plyometrics are introduced.[1,113]
- A gradual return to normal activity is predicated upon normal restoration of strength, flexibility, and range of motion without pain.

Operative intervention, which is reserved for patients who fail to respond to a well-structured program of rehabilitation, is intended to revitalize, debride, and bypass the area of tendonosis.[206,208,209,333,334]

Coordination, Communication, and Documentation

Communicate with MD, patient, work manager, and work comp case management regarding patient's status (direct or indirect). Documentation will include all elements of patient/client management. Discharge planning will be provided.

Patient-Related Instruction

Periodic re-examination and evaluation of the home program utilizing written instruction and illustrations. Educate patient in proper postures, and positions and motions to avoid at home and at work. Educate patient in the benefits of an ongoing conditioning program to prevent re-occurrence of impairments.

CASE STUDY MEDIAL ELBOW PAIN

HISTORY

History of Current Condition

A 23-year-old apprentice carpenter was seen in the clinic with complaints of right elbow pain, which he reported having for the last few months. The patient described the onset of elbow pain as gradual and attributed it to his work, where he spends most of the day using carpentry tools. Over time the pain had worsened to the point where it hurt all of the time. The patient went to see his physician who prescribed a course of anti-inflammatory medications and physical therapy, and placed the patient on light duty at work.

Past History of Current Condition

No past history of elbow pain.

Past Medical and Surgical History

Unremarkable.

Medications

Ibuprofen, 800 mg a day.

Functional Status and Activity Level

The patient's goals were to decrease pain with activities of daily living and recreational sports, and to be able to return to work without pain.

Health Status (Self-Report)

In general good health, but pain interferes with tasks at home and at work.

QUESTIONS

1. What structure(s) do you suspect to be at fault with complaints of medial elbow pain?
2. What is the probable mechanism of injury for this patient?
3. What type of activities would you expect to exacerbate this condition?
4. What additional questions would you ask?
5. List the various diagnoses that could present with these signs and symptoms, and the tests you would use to rule out each one.

PHYSICAL THERAPY TESTS AND MEASURES

The physical examination of the patient included[99]:

- Palpation for areas of tenderness and crepitation.
- An inspection for muscle atrophy and posture.
- Muscle testing of the major muscles, including grip and the key muscles of C6 and C7.
- Measurement of active and passive range of motion of the elbow, wrist, and forearm.
- Observation of symmetry of carrying angle, and specific testing for golfer's elbow and elbow instability.
- The cervical spine was also examined to determine whether neck pathology was causing pain referred to the elbow.

Motor Performance: Strength, Power, and Endurance

Although no strength deficits were noted in either upper extremity, pain was elicited with resistive testing for all motions except wrist extension and elbow supination. The special test for golfer's elbow reproduced the patient's pain at the right medial epicondyle.

Manual muscle testing of C6 and C7 key muscles were WNL as compared to the uninvolved side.

Strength testing of grip was WNL as compared to the uninvolved side, except pain was elicited.

Orthotic, Protective, and Supportive Devices

Patient does not use any brace.

Pain

Palpation revealed extreme tenderness, warmth, and slight edema on and around the left lateral epicondyle. Pain reported at 5 out of 10 at rest after a day of work.

Posture

Forward head position, kyphotic dorsal spine, and protracting shoulders.

Range of Motion (Including Muscle Length)

Active range of motion of both upper extremities was within normal limits for all elbow and shoulder motions. The left elbow demonstrated full AROM, but in the right elbow, although it too demonstrated normal ranges for flexion, extension, pronation, and supination, there was pain associated with all of the motions. Wrist motion on the right was limited to 50 degrees extension compared to 60 degrees on the left.

Special Tests

- AROM with overpressure of cervical spine did not reproduce symptoms.
- Negative quadrant compression of the cervical spine (Spurling's test).
- Specific length test for the extensor mechanism (wrist and finger flexion, elbow extension, and forearm pronation) reproduced no pain.
- Pain elicited with specific length test for flexor mechanism (wrist extension, elbow extension, forearm supination, and wrist and finger extension).
- Upper limb tension tests for median, radial, and ulnar nerves were negative (see Chap. 12).

EVALUATION (CLINICAL JUDGMENT)

Patient is a young, athletic male with soft tissue mobility restrictions and impaired right elbow performance, which results in functional limitations both at home and at work.

DIAGNOSIS BY PHYSICAL THERAPIST

Medial epicondylitis.

PROGNOSIS

Predicted Optimal Level of Improvement in Function

Over the course of 4 to 6 weeks the patient will demonstrate:
- Pain at 0 out of 10 at rest, 2 out of 10 with activity.
- Pain-free AROM of simultaneous wrist extension, forearm supination, and elbow extension.
- A return to normal home activities and to full work duty without restrictions.
- Grip strength at 80 percent as compared with the uninvolved side.
- Independence with home exercise program and prevention strategies.

Predicted Interval Levels of Improvement in Function

Return to work for a full shift with no restrictions in 6 weeks.

PLAN OF CARE

Frequency and Duration

Two to three times per week for 6 weeks.

INTERVENTION

Addressing the tendonosis as an inflammatory process without considering the underlying degeneration or biomechanical deficits will lead to certain failure.[62] The intervention should be based on functional criteria that are based on stages of tendon healing.[331]

PHASE I (WEEKS 1–3)

This phase typically involves 2 to 4 physical therapy visits. Instructions were given with regard to rest positions and the avoidance of aggravating motions and activities.

Goals

The goals for this phase of the intervention are:

- To control pain and preserve motion.
- Decrease pain to 3 out of 10 or less with activity, and 1 out of 10 or less at rest.
- Decrease inflammation as evidenced by reduced edema and tenderness to palpation.
- Increased flexibility of wrist flexors to 90 percent as compared with the uninvolved side.
- Pain-free ability to make a fist, and for wrist flexion/extension.
- Promote the development of endurance, normal vascularization, and collagen production.[99]
- Independence with home exercise program and home cryotherapy.

Electrotherapeutic Modalities

Any of the following could be used:

- Ice packs are applied to the right medial epicondyle after the exercises, and at the end of each day.
- High-voltage galvanic stimulation was applied to help relieve pain.
- Iontophoresis with dexamethasone.
- Shock-wave therapy.[245,332]
- Pulsed ultrasound with a 20 percent duty cycle, 3-MHz frequency, and an intensity of 1.2 W/cm^2 was applied to the medial epicondyle for 5 minutes.

Therapeutic Exercise and Home Program

- Submaximal isometrics to the wrist flexors are performed in the pain-free ROM following the transverse friction massage.
- Active wrist extension to inhibit wrist flexors.
- Submaximal resistive wrist flexion exercises involving both concentric and eccentric exercises in the pain-free ranges.
- High-repetition pain-free active wrist flexion/extension to help vascularize involved tendon and to promote alignment of collagen fibers.
- The patient is instructed on stretches for the wrist flexor-forearm pronator group, as well as stretches for the shoulder, hand, and forearm.

Manual Therapy

- Medial mobilization of the right forearm at the elbow was performed during active wrist flexion and forearm pronation.
- A ventral glide of the hand was performed at the wrist during ulnar deviation.
- Tape was initially applied at the elbow to maintain the medial mobilization.
- Transverse friction massage was applied to the specific area of affected tendon to induce hyperemia. The patient was instructed in the technique as part of his home exercise program.
- Gentle stretches were applied to the wrist extensors and flexors in the pain-free ROM. The patient was instructed in the techniques as part of his home exercise program.

- Soft tissue mobilization techniques are applied to patient tolerance.
- Myofascial release techniques are initiated.
- Acupressure can be introduced if applicable.
- Joint mobilizations can be applied to any areas of hypomobility in the cervical spine, shoulder, or elbow.

PHASE II (WEEK 4–6)

This phase typically involves 2 to 6 physical therapy visits.

Goals

- Decrease pain to 2 out of 10 or less with activity and 0 out of 10 at rest.
- Increased ROM to achieve pain-free simultaneous full flexion of wrist and hand with pronation of forearm and extension of elbow.
- Increased muscle performance to achieve manual muscle test of 4 or 5 for all muscle groups.
- Grip strength at 80 percent as compared to uninvolved side.
- Gradual resumption of activities with use of an orthosis as needed.

Electrotherapeutic Modalities

Continued use of *effective* modalities as in acute phase, with increased emphasis on use at home as needed.

Therapeutic Exercises and Home Program

All exercises of the wrist flexor-pronator group were started with the elbow in flexion.

- Slow and gentle stretches performed to flexor mechanism 3 to 5 times a day into wrist extension, radial deviation, forearm supination, and elbow extension.
- AROM of simultaneous wrist extension, forearm supination, and elbow extension.
- The patient is instructed in concentric as well as eccentric exercises for wrist flexion and forearm pronation, initially without resistance, and then with progressively more resistance using surgical tubing, ensuring that the patient worked to fatigue with each set.[1,113]
- Introduction of wrist flexor broom-handle exercise (Fig. 15-38). A weight is tied to a rope or piece of string approximately 3 feet in length, which is then tied to a broom handle or dowel. The broom handle is held out in front of the patient with the palms up, who then rolls the string onto the handle/dowel to raise and lower the weight.
- In order to help balance the force couple, the patient was also instructed on a course of exercises to increase the strength in opposing muscles—the extensors of the wrist and digits.
- Squeezing exercises using theraputty or bags of rice for grip strength.
- AROM of horizontal shoulder abduction while holding a weight in the hand.
- Strengthening exercises for biceps, triceps, and latissimus dorsi.

- Pulley program for strength and ROM of upper extremity and trunk.
- Upper body ergonometer progression.

Manual Therapy
- Continue with use of effective soft tissue techniques.
- Continue with progressive graded mobilizations for persistent hypomobilities.
- Assisted stretching to the muscle bellies of the flexor mechanism to decrease tension of involved tendons.

PHASE III (WEEK 7+)

This phase typically involves 2 to 4 physical therapy visits.

Goals
- A return to normal home and recreational activities, and to full work duty without restrictions.
- Pain at 0 out of 10 with activity.
- Grip strength at 90 to 100 percent as compared with uninvolved side.
- Independence with home exercise program and prevention strategies.

Therapeutic Exercise and Home Program
All of the following exercises are performed at varying velocities, beginning with slow speeds, before gradually increasing the speed as tolerated.

- Activities and exercises incorporating the shoulder, wrist, and elbow were introduced. These included PNF patterns with wall pulleys and the Fitter board.
- Strength and endurance of the upper kinetic chain was addressed with resisted PNF diagonals and the use of a grip dynamometer.
- Plyometrics are introduced.[1,113]
- Sport- or activity-specific training.
- A gradual return to normal activity is predicated upon normal restoration of strength, flexibility, and range of motion without pain.

Criteria for Discharge
Patient to be discharged when he reaches established functional goals, declines further treatment, is unable to progress towards goals because of complications, or PT determines that patient will no longer benefit from PT services.

Coordination, Communication, and Documentation
Communicate with MD, patient, work manager, and work comp case management regarding patient's status (direct or indirect). Documentation will include all elements of patient/client management. Discharge planning will be provided.

Patient-Related Instruction
Periodic re-examination and reassessment of the home program, utilizing written instruction and illustrations. Educate patient in proper postures, and positions and motions to avoid at home and at work. Educate patient in the benefits of an ongoing conditioning program to prevent re-occurrence of impairments.

REVIEW QUESTIONS*

1. True/False: The primary restraint to valgus stress at the elbow is bony congruity.
2. What is the maximal close-packed position of the humeroulnar joint?
3. Which muscles are involved with forearm pronation?
4. In which direction do most elbow dislocations occur?
5. Which muscle could flex the elbow if the three major elbow flexors were *not* available?
   - A. The pronator teres.
   - B. The flexor pollicis longus.
   - C. The supinator.
   - D. The pronator quadratus.

---

*Additional questions to test your understanding of this chapter can be found in the Online Learning Center for *Orthopaedic Assessment, Evaluation, and Intervention* at www.duttononline.net.

REFERENCES

1. Wilk KE, Arrigo C, Andrews JR. Rehabilitation of the elbow in the throwing athlete. *J Orthop Sports Phys Ther* 1993;17:305–317.
2. Potter HP. The obliquity of the arm of the female in extension. The relation of the forearm with the upper arm in flexion. *J Anat Physiol* 1895;29:488–491.
3. Atkinson WB, Elftman H. The carrying angle of the human arm as a secondary sex character. *Anat Rec* 1945;91:42–49.
4. An K-N, Morrey BF, Chao EY. The carrying angle of the human elbow joint. *J Orthop Res* 1984;1:369–378.
5. Sobel J, Nirschl RP. Elbow injuries. In: Zachazewski JE, Magee DJ, Quillen WS, eds. *Athletic Injuries and Rehabilitation.* Philadelphia: WB Saunders; 1996:543–583.
6. An KN, Morrey BF. Biomechanics of the elbow. In: Morrey BF, ed. *The Elbow and Its Disorders.* Philadelphia: WB Saunders; 1993:53–73.
7. O'Driscoll SW, Morrey BF, An K-N. Intraarticular pressure and capacity of the elbow. *J Arthrosc Rel Surg* 1990;6:100–103.
8. Morrey BF, An KN. Functional anatomy of the ligaments of the elbow. *Clin Orthop* 1985;201:84–90.
9. Ochi N, et al. Anatomic relation between the medial collateral ligament of the elbow and the humero-ulnar joint axis. *J Shoulder Elbow Surg* 1999;8:6–10.
10. O'Driscoll SW, et al. Origin of the medial ulnar collateral ligament. *J Hand Surg Am* 1992;17A:164–168.
11. Floris S, et al. The medial collateral ligament of the elbow joint: Anatomy and kinematics. *J Shoulder Elbow Surg* 1998;7:345–351.
12. Neill-Cage DJ, et al. Soft tissue attachments of the ulnar coronoid process: An anatomic study with radiographic correlation. *Clin Orthop* 1995;320:154–158.
13. Cohen MS, Bruno RJ. The collateral ligaments of the elbow: Anatomy and clinical correlation. *Clin Orthop* 2001;1:123–130.
14. Hotchkiss RN, Weiland AJ. Valgus stability of the elbow. *J Orthop Res* 1987;5:372–377.

15. Morrey BF, Tanaka S, An KN. Valgus stability of the elbow: A definition of primary and secondary constraints. *Clin Orthop* 1991;265:187–195.

16. Schwab GH, et al. Biomechanics of elbow instability: The role of the medial collateral ligament. *Clin Orthop* 1980;146:42–52.

17. Morrey BF. Applied anatomy and biomechanics of the elbow joint. *Inst Course Lect* 1986;35:59–68.

18. Sojbjerg JO, Ovesen J, Nielsen S. Experimental elbow instability after transection of the medial collateral ligament. *Clin Orthop* 1987;218:186–190.

19. Jobe FW, Kvitne RS. Elbow instability in the athlete. *Inst Course Lect* 1991;40:17–23.

20. Callaway GH, et al. Biomechanical evaluation of the medial collateral ligament of the elbow. *J Bone Joint Surg* 1997;79A:1223–1231.

21. Fuss FK. The ulnar collateral ligament of the human elbow joint. Anatomy, function and biomechanics. *J Anat* 1991;175: 203–212.

22. Morrey BF, An KN. Articular and ligamentous contributions to the stability of the elbow joint. *Am J Sports Med* 1983;11: 315–319.

23. Regan WD, et al. Biomechanical study of ligaments around the elbow joint. *Clin Orthop* 1991;271:170–179.

24. Guterieriez L. A contribution to the study of limiting factors of elbow extension. *Acta Anat* 1964;56:145.

25. Chen FS, Rokito AS, Jobe FW. Medial elbow problems in the overhead-throwing athlete. *J Am Acad Orthop Surg* 2001;9: 99–113.

26. Kuroda S, Sakamaki K. Ulnar collateral ligament tears of the elbow joint. *Clin Orthop* 1986;208:266–271.

27. Berg EE, DeHoll D. Radiography of the medial elbow ligaments. *J Shoulder Elbow Surg* 1997;6:528–533.

28. Josefsson PO, Johnell O, Wendeberg B. Ligamentous injuries in dislocations of the elbow joint. *Clin Orthop* 1987;221:221–225.

29. Cohen MS, Hastings H. Diagnosis and surgical management of the acute elbow dislocation. *J Am Acad Orthop Surg* 1998;6:16–23.

30. Cohen MS, Hastings H. Rotatory instability of the elbow: The role of the lateral stabilizers. *J Bone Joint Surg* 1977;79A:225–233.

31. Ryan J. Elbow. In: *Current Concepts of Orthopedic Physical Therapy—Home Study Course*. Wadsworth C, ed. La Crosse, WI: APTA, Orthopaedic Section: 2001.

32. Jobe FW, Nuber G. Throwing injuries of the elbow. *Clin Sports Med* 1986;5:621.

33. Pauly JE, Rushing JL, Schering LE. An electromyographic study of some muscles crossing the elbow joint. *Anat Rec* 1967;1:42.

34. Basmajian JV, Latif A. Integrated actions and functions of the chief flexors of the elbow: a detailed electromyographic analysis. *J Bone Joint Surg* 1957;39A:1106–1118.

35. Funk DA, et al. Electromyographic analysis of muscles across the elbow joint. *J Orthop Res* 1987;5:529–538.

36. Basmajian JV, Deluca CJ. *Muscles Alive*. Baltimore: Williams & Wilkins; 1985:268–269.

37. Thepaut-Mathieu C, Maton B. The flexor function of the muscle pronator teres in man: a quantitative electromyographic study. *Eur J Appl Physiol* 1985;54:116–121.

38. Reid DC. *Functional Anatomy and Joint Mobilization*, 2nd ed. Edmonton: University of Alberta Press; 1975.

39. Hirasawa Y, Sawamura H, Sakakida K. Entrapment neuropathy due to bilateral epitrochlearis muscles: A case report. *J Hand Surg Am* 1979;4:181–184.

40. Feindel W, Stratford J. The role of the cubital tunnel in tardy ulnar palsy. *Can J Surg* 1958;1:287.

41. Apfelberg DB, Larson SJ. Dynamic anatomy of the ulnar nerve at the elbow. *Plast Reconstr Surg* 1973;51:76–81.

42. Idler RS. General principles of patient evaluation and nonoperative management of cubital syndrome. *Hand Clin* 1996;12:397–403.

43. Khoo D, Carmichael SW, Spinner RJ. Ulnar nerve anatomy and compression. *Orthop Clin North Am* 1996;27:317–338.

44. O'Driscoll SW, et al. The cubital tunnel and ulnar neuropathy. *J Bone Joint Surg* 1991;73B:613–617.

45. Bozentka DJ. Cubital tunnel syndrome pathophysiology. *Clinical Orthop* 1998;351:90–94.

46. Vanderpool DW, et al. Peripheral compression lesions of the ulnar nerve. *J Bone Joint Surg* 1968;50B:792–803.

47. Folberg CR, Weiss APC, Akelman E. Cubital tunnel syndrome. Part I: Presentation and diagnosis. *Orthop Rev* 1994;23:136–144.

48. Conway JE, et al. Medial instability of the elbow in throwing athletes: Treatment by repair or reconstruction of the ulnar collateral ligament. *J Bone Joint Surg* 1992;74A:67–83.

49. Gabel GT, Morrey BF. Operative treatment of medial epicondylitis: Influence of concomitant ulnar neuropathy at the elbow. *J Bone Joint Surg* 1995;77:1065–1069.

50. Lee DG. "Tennis elbow": A manual therapist's perspective. *J Orthop Sports Phys Ther* 1986;8:134–142.

51. Spinner M, Linscheid RL. Nerve entrapment syndromes. In: Morrey BF, ed. *The Elbow and Its Disorders*. Philadelphia: WB Saunders; 1985:691–712.

52. Amadio PC, Beckenbaugh RD. Entrapment of the ulnar nerve by the deep flexor-pronator aponeurosis. *J Hand Surg Am* 1986;11A:83–87.

53. Gabel GT, Amadio PC. Reoperation for failed decompression of the ulnar nerve in the region of the elbow. *J Bone Joint Surg*. 1990;72A:213–219.

54. Smith RV, Fisher RG. Struthers ligament: A source of median nerve compression above the elbow. *J Neurosurg* 1973;38:778–779.

55. Barnum M, et al. Radial tunnel syndrome. *Hand Clin* 1996;12:679–689.

56. Hrayama T, Takemitsu Y. Isolated paralysis of the descending branch of the posterior interosseous nerve. *J Bone Joint Surg* 1988;70A:1402–1403.

57. Spinner M. Injuries to the major branches of the peripheral nerves of the forearm. Philadelphia: WB Saunders;1978.

58. Carr D, Davis P. Distal posterior interosseous nerve syndrome. *J Hand Surg Am* 1985;10(6 Pt 1):873–878.

59. Lister GD, Belsoe RB, Kleinert HE. The radial tunnel syndrome. *J Hand Surg Am* 1979;4:52–59.

60. Roles NC, Maudsley RH. Radial tunnel syndrome: Resistant tennis elbow as a nerve entrapment. *J Bone Joint Surg Br* 1972;54B:499–508.

61. Morrey BF, Chao EY. Passive motion of the elbow joint. *J Bone Joint Surg Am* 1976;58:501–508.

62. Kibler, BW. Clinical biomechanics of the elbow in tennis: implications for evaluation and diagnosis. *Med Sci Sports Exerc* 1994;26:1203–1206.

63. Cummings GS. Comparison of muscle to other soft tissue in limiting elbow extension. *J Orthop Sports Phys Ther* 1984;5:170.

64. Kapandji IA. *The Physiology of the Joints, Upper Limb*. New York: Churchill Livingstone; 1991.

65. Hammer WI. *Functional Soft Tissue Examination and Treatment by Manual Methods*. Gaithersburg, MD: Aspen; 1991.

66. Cyriax J. *Textbook of Orthopaedic Medicine, Diagnosis of Soft Tissue Lesions*, 8th ed. London: Bailliere Tindall; 1982.

67. Kibler BW, Press JM. Rehabilitation of the elbow. In: Kibler BW, Herring JA, Press JE, eds. *Functional Rehabilitation of Sports and Musculoskeletal Injuries*. Gaithersburg, MD: Aspen; 1998.

68. Watrous BG, Ho G Jr. Elbow pain. *Prim Care* 1988;15:725–735.

68a. Polley HF, Hunder GG. *Physical Examination of the Joints*. Philadelphia: WB Saunders; 1978:81–89.

69. Morrey BF, An KN, Chao EYS. Functional evaluation of the elbow. In: Morrey BF, ed. *The Elbow and Its Disorders*. Philadelphia: WB Saunders; 1993:86–97.

69a. Azar FM, Andrews JR, Wilk KE, Groh D. Operative treatment of ulnar collateral ligament injuries of the elbow in athletes. *Am J Sports Med* 2000;28:16–23.

69b. Wilson FD, Andrews JR, Blackburn TA, McClusky GM: Valgus extension overload in the pitching elbow. *Am J Sports Med* 1983;11:83–88.

69c. Hochholzer T, Keinath C. Soweit die hande greifen (4). Wenn die arme knarren. *Rotpunkt*. 1991;2:62–65.

70. Sobel J, Nirschl RP: Elbow injuries. In: Zachazewski JE, Magee DJ, Quillen WS, eds. *Athletic Injuries and Rehabilitation*. Philadelphia: WB Saunders; 1996:543–583.

71. Bollen SR. Soft tissue injury in extreme rock climbers. *Br J Sports Med* 1988;22:145–147.

72. Hochholzer T, Keinath C. Soweit die hande greifen (3). Wenn die finger kribbeln. *Rotpunkt*. 1991;1:46–49.

73. Spinner RJ, Goldner RD: Snapping of the medial head of the triceps and recurrent dislocation of the ulnar nerve: Anatomic and dynamic factors. *J Bone Joint Surg* 1998;80A:239–247.

74. Katz WA. *Rheumatic Diseases, Diagnosis and Management*. Philadelphia: JB Lippincott; 1977:71–77.

75. Winkel D, Matthijs O, Phelps V. Examination of the elbow. In: *Diagnosis and Treatment of the Upper Extremities*. Maryland, MD: Aspen; 1997:207–233.

76. Yen KL, Metzl JD. Sports-specific concerns in the young athlete: baseball. *Ped Emerg Care* 2000;16:215–220.

76a. Cohen RB, Williams GR, Jr. Impingement syndrome and rotator cuff disease as repetitive motion disorders. Clin Orthop Rel Res 1998;351:95–101.

76b. Matsen FA III, Arntz CT. Subacromial impingement. In: Rockwood CA, Jr., Matsen FA III, eds. *The Shoulder*. Philadelphia: WB Saunders, 1990:623–648.

76c. Neer CS II. Anterior acromioplasty for the chronic impingement syndrome in the shoulder: A preliminary report. *J Bone Joint Surg Am* 1972;54:41–50.

76d. Neer C. Impingement lesions. *Clin Orthop* 1983;173:71–77.

76e. Feinstein B, Langton JBK, Jameson RF, Schiller F. Experiments on referred pain from deep somatic tissues. *J Bone Joint Surg [Am]* 1954;36:981–997.

76f. Dwyer A, Aprill C, Bogduk N. Cervical zygapophyseal joint pain patterns: a study from normal volunteers. *Spine* 1990;15:453.

76g. Cloward RB. Cervical discography: a contribution to the etiology and mechanism of neck, shoulder and arm pain. *Ann Surg* 1959;150:1052–1064.

76h. Dunleavy K. Relationship between the shoulder and the cervicothoracic spine. La Crosse, WI: Orthopedic Section, APTA, Independent Home Study Course: Solutions to Shoulder Disorders; 2001.

76i. Cappel K, Clark MA, Davies GJ, Ellenbecker TS. Clinical Examination of the Shoulder. In: Tovin BJ, Greenfield B, eds. *Evaluation and Treatment of the Shoulder—An Integration of the Guide to Physical Therapist Practice*. Philadelphia: FA Davis; 2001;75–131.

76j. Davies GJ, DeCarlo MS. Examination of the shoulder complex. In: Bandy WD, ed. *Current Concepts in the Rehabilitation of the Shoulder: Sports Physical Therapy Section*. Home Study Course, American Physical Therapy Association; 1995.

76k. Daigneault J, Cooney LM, Jr. Shoulder pain in older people. *J Am Ger Soc* 1998;46(9):1144–1151.

76l. Clarnette RG, Miniaci A. Clinical exam of the shoulder. *Med Sci Sports Exer* 1998;30(4,Suppl):1–6.

76m. Cuomo F. Diagnosis, classification, and management of the stiff shoulder. In: Iannotti JP, Williams GR, eds. *Disorders of the Shoulder: Diagnosis and Management*. Philadelphia: Lippincott Williams & Wilkins; 1999:397–417.

76n. American Academy of Orthopaedic Surgeons. Orthopedic knowledge update 4: home study syllabus. Rosemont, IL: The Academy; 1992.

77. Kiser DM. Physiological and biomechanical factors for understanding repetitive motion injuries. *Semin Occup Med* 1987; 2:11–17.

78. Lewit K. Manipulative therapy. In: *Rehabilitation of the Motor System*, 3rd ed. London: Butterworths; 1999.

79. Pecina M, Krmpotic-Nemanic J, Markiewitz A. *Tunnel Syndromes*. Boca Raton: CRC; 1991.

80. Vennix MJ, Werstsch JJ. Entrapment neuropathies about the elbow. *J Back Musculoskel Rehabil* 1994;4:31–43.

81. Keller K, Corbett J, Nichols D. Repetitive strain injury in computer keyboard users: pathomechanics and treatment principles in individual and group intervention. *J Hand Ther* 1998; 11:9–26.

82. Anderson M, Tichenor CJ. A patient with de Quervain's tenosynovitis: A case report using an Australian approach to manual therapy. *Phys Ther* 1994;74:314–326.

82a. Yen KL, Metzl JD: Sports-specific concerns in the young athlete: baseball. *Pedi Emerg Care* 2000;16:215–220.

83. Morrey BF, Askew LJ, Chao EYS. A biomechanical study of normal functional elbow motion. *J Bone Joint Surg* 1981; 63A:872–877.

84. Kaltenborn FM. *Manual Mobilization of the Extremity Joints: Basic Examination and Treatment Techniques*, 4th ed. Oslo, Norway: Olaf Norlis Bokhandel, Universitetsgaten; 1989.

85. Maitland G. *Peripheral Manipulation*, 3rd ed. London: Butterworth; 1991.

86. O'Driscoll SW, Bell DF, Morrey BF. Posterolateral rotatory instability of the elbow. *J Bone Joint Surg* 1991;73A:440–446.

87. Buehler MJ, Thayer DT. The elbow flexion test: A clinical test for cubital tunnel syndrome. *Clin Orthop* 1988; 233:213–216.

88. Novak CB, et al. Provocative testing for cubital tunnel syndrome. *J Hand Surg Am* 1994;19:817–820.

89. Booth FW. Physiologic and biochemical effects of immobilization on muscle. *Clin Orthop* 1987;219:15–21.

90. Eiff MP, Smith AT, Smith GE. Early mobilization versus immobilization in the treatment of lateral ankle sprains. *Am J Sports Med* 1994;22:83–88.

91. Akeson WH, et al. Collagen cross-linking alterations in the joint contractures: changes in the reducible cross-links in periarticular connective tissue after 9 weeks immobilization. *Conn Tissue Res* 1977;5:15.

92. Akeson WH, et al. Effects of immobilization on joints. *Clin Orthop* 1987;219:28–37.

93. Akeson WH, Amiel D, Woo SL-Y. Immobility effects on synovial joints: The pathomechanics of joint contracture. *Biorheology* 1980;17:95–110.

94. Woo SL-Y, et al. Connective tissue response to immobility: A correlative study of biochemical and biomechanical measurements of normal and immobilized rabbit knee. *Arthritis Rheum* 1975;18:257–264.

95. Coutts RD. Continuous passive motion in the rehabilitation of the total knee patient. Its role and effect. *Orthop Rev* 1986; 15:27.

96. Dehne E, Tory R. Treatment of joint injuries by immediate mobilization based upon the spiral adaption concept. *Clin Orthop* 1971;77:218–232.

97. Haggmark T, Eriksson E. Cylinder or mobile cast brace after knee ligament surgery. *Am J Sports Med* 1979;7:48–56.

98. Noyes FR, Mangine RE, Barber S. Early knee motion after open and arthroscopic anterior cruciate ligament reconstruction. *Am J Sports Med* 1987;15:149–160.

99. Kraushaar BS, Nirschl RP. Tendinosis of the elbow (tennis elbow). Clinical features and findings of histological, immunohistochemical, and electron microscopy studies. *J Bone Joint Surgery Am* 1999;81:259–278.

100. Nirschl RP, Sobel J. *Arm Care. A Complete Guide to Prevention and Treatment of Tennis Elbow.* Arlington, VA: Medical Sports; 1996.

101. Andrews JR, Frank W. Valgus extension overload in the pitching elbow. In: Andrews JR, Zarins B, Carson WG, eds. *Injuries to the Throwing Arm.* Philadelphia: WB Saunders; 1985: 250–257.

102. Kottke FJ. Therapeutic exercise to maintain mobility. In: Kottke FJ, Stillwell GK, Lehman JF, eds. *Krusen's Handbook of Physical Medicine and Rehabilitation.* Baltimore: WB Saunders; 1982:389–402.

103. Warren CG, Lehmann JF, Koblanski JN. Elongation of rat tail: Effect of load and temperature. *Arch Phys Med Rehabil* 1971;52:465–474.

104. Kibler WB. Concepts in exercise rehabilitation of athletic injury. In: Leadbetter WB, Buckwalter JA, Gordon SL, eds. *Sports-Induced Inflammation: Clinical and Basic Science Concepts.* Park Ridge, IL: American Academy of Orthopaedic Surgeons; 1990:759–769.

105. Kibler WB, Chandler TJ, Pace BK. Principles of rehabilitation after chronic tendon injuries. *Clin Sports Med* 1992; 11:661–671.

106. Kibler WB. Clinical implications of exercise: injury and performance. In: Instructional Course Lectures. Rosemont, IL: American Academy of Orthopaedic Surgeons; 1994:17–24.

107. Leadbetter WB. Corticosteroid injection therapy in sports injuries. In: Leadbetter WB, Buckwalter JA, Gordon SL, eds. *Sports-Induced Inflammation: Clinical and Basic Science Concepts.* Park Ridge, IL: American Academy of Orthopaedic Surgeons; 1990:527–545.

108. Woo SL-Y, Tkach LV. The cellular and matrix response of ligaments and tendons to mechanical injury. In: Leadbetter WB, Buckwalter JA, Gordon SL, eds. *Sports-Induced Inflammation: Clinical and Basic Science Concepts.* Park Ridge, IL: American Academy of Orthopaedic Surgeons; 1990:189–202.

109. Novacheck TF. Running injuries: a biomechanical approach. *J Bone Joint Surg* 1998;80-A:1220–1233.

110. Freund HJ, Budingen HJ. The relationship between speed and amplitude of the fastest voluntary contractions of human arm muscles. *Exp Brain Res* 1978;35:407–418.

111. Marsden CD, Obeso JA, Rothwell JC. The function of the antagonist muscle during fast limb movements in man. *J Physiol* 1983;335:1–13.

112. Wierzbicka MM, Wiegner AW, Shahani BT. Role of agonist and antagonist muscles in fast arm movements in man. *Exp Brain Res* 1986;63:331–340.

113. Wilk KE, et al. Stretch-shortening drills for the upper extremities: theory and clinical application. *J Orthop Sports Phys Ther* 1993;17:225–239.

114. Kandemir U, Fu FH, McMahon PJ. Elbow injuries. *Curr Opin Rheumatol* 2002;14:160–167.

115. Fryette HH. *Principles of Osteopathic Technique.* Carmel, Ca: Academy of Osteopathy; 1980.

116. Azar FM, et al. Operative treatment of ulnar collateral ligament injuries of the elbow in athletes. *Am J Sports Med* 2000;28:16–23.

117. Jobe FW, Stark H, Lombardo SJ. Reconstruction of the ulnar collateral ligament in athletes. *J Bone Joint Surg* 1986;68A:1158–1163.

118. Jobe FW, et al. An EMG analysis of the shoulder in pitching and throwing: A preliminary report. *Am J Sports Med* 1983;11:3–5.

119. Jobe FW, et al. An EMG analysis of pitching—a second report. *Am J Sports Med* 1984;12:218–220.

120. Froimson AI, et al. Ulnar nerve decompression with medial epicondylectomy for neuropathy at the elbow. *Clin Orthop* 1991;265:200–206.

121. Heithoff SJ, et al. Medial epicondylectomy for the treatment of ulnar nerve compression at the elbow. *J Hand Surg Am* 1990;15A:22–29.

122. Glousman RE. Ulnar nerve problems in the athlete's elbow. *Clin Sports Med* 1990;9:365–370.

123. Ciccotti MG, Jobe FW. Medial collateral ligament instability and ulnar neuritis in the athlete's elbow. *Instr Course Lect* 1999;48:383–391.

124. Field LD, Savoie FH. Common elbow injuries in sport. *Sports Med* 1998;26:193–205.

125. Davidson PA, et al. Functional anatomy of the flexor pronator muscle group in relation to the medial collateral ligament of the elbow. *Am J Sports Med* 1995;23:245–250.

126. Glousman R, Jobe FW, Tibone JE. Dynamic EMG analysis of the throwing shoulder with glenohumeral instability. *J Bone Joint Surg* 1988;70:220–226.

127. Sisto DJ, et al. An electromyographic analysis of the elbow in pitching. *Am J Sports Med* 1987;15:260–263.

128. Smith GR, et al. A muscle splitting approach to the ulnar collateral ligament of the elbow: Neuroanatomy and operative technique. *Am J Sports Med* 1996;24:575–580.

129. Wright PE. Flexor and extensor tendon injuries. In: Crenshaw AH, ed. *Campbell's Operative Orthopaedics.* St Louis: Mosby-Year Book; 1992:3003–3054.

130. Nestor BJ, O'Driscoll SW, Morrey BF. Ligamentous reconstruction for posterolateral rotatory instability of the elbow. *J Bone Joint Surg* 1992;74A:1235–1241.

131. O'Driscoll SW, et al. Elbow subluxation and dislocation: A spectrum of instability. *Clin Orthop* 1992;280:186–197.

132. Sojbjerg JO, Helmig P, Kjaersgaard-Andersen P. Dislocation of the elbow: an experimental study of the ligamentous injuries. *Orthopedics* 1989;12:461–463.

133. Morrey BF. Reoperation for failed surgical treatment of refractory lateral epicondylitis. *J Shoulder Elbow Surg* 1992;1:47–49.

134. O'Driscoll SW. Classification and evaluation of recurrent instability of the elbow. *Clin Orthop* 2000;370:34–43.

135. O'Driscoll SW. Classification and spectrum of elbow instability: Recurrent instability. In: Morrey BF, ed. *The Elbow and Its Disorders*. Philadelphia: WB Saunders; 1993:453–463.

136. O'Driscoll SW. Elbow instability. *Hand Clin* 1994;10:405–415.

137. Josefsson PO, et al. Surgical vs. non-surgical treatment of ligamentous injuries following dislocation of the elbow. *J Bone Joint Surg* 1987;69A:605–608.

138. Torchia M, DiGiovine N. Anterior dislocation of the elbow in an arm wrestler. *J Shoulder Elbow Surg* 1998;7:539–541.

139. Doria A, et al. Recurrent dislocation of the elbow. *Int Orthop* 1990;14:41–55.

140. Durig M, et al. The operative treatment of elbow dislocation in the adult. *J Bone Joint Surg* 1979;61A:239–244.

141. Josefsson PO, et al. Dislocations of the elbow and intraarticular fractures. *Clin Orthop* 1989;246:126–130.

142. Hotchkiss RN. Fractures and dislocations of the elbow. In: Rockwood CA, et al, eds. *Fractures in Adults*. Philadelphia: Lippincott Raven; 1996:980–981.

143. Wilson FD, et al. Valgus extension overload in the pitching elbow. *Am J Sports Med* 1983;11:83–88.

144. Azar FM, Wilk KE. Nonoperative treatment of the elbow in throwers. *Oper Tech Sports Med* 1996;4:91–99.

145. Pappas AM, Zawacki RM, Sullivan TJ. Biomechanics of baseball pitching: a preliminary report. *Am J Sports Med* 1985;13:216–222.

146. Burkhart SS, Morgan CD, Kibler WB. Shoulder injuries in overhead athletes: the "dead arm" revisited. *Clin Sports Med* 2000;19:125–158.

147. Reilly J, Nicholas JA. The chronically inflamed bursa. *Clin Sports Med* 1987;6:345–370.

148. Onieal M-E. Common wrist and elbow injuries in primary care. *Lippincott's Primary Care Practice. Musculoskeletal Conditions*, 1999;3:441–450.

149. Shell D, Perkins R, Cosgarea A. Septic olecranon bursitis: Recognition and treatment. *J Am Board Fam Pract* 1995; 8:217–220.

150. Reid DC, Kushner S. The elbow region. In: Donatelli RA, Wooden MJ, eds. *Orthopaedic Physical Therapy*. New York: Churchill Livingstone; 1994:203–232.

151. Hempel K, Schwencke K. About avulsions of the distal insertion of the biceps brachii tendon. *Arch Orthop Unfallchir* 1974;79:313–319.

152. McReynolds IS. Avulsion of the insertion of the biceps brachii tendon and its surgical treatment. *J Bone Joint Surg* 1963;45A:1780–1781.

153. D'Alessandro DF, et al. Repair of distal biceps tendon ruptures in athletes. *Am J Sports Med* 1993;21:114–119.

154. Morrey BF, et al. Rupture of the distal tendon of the biceps brachii: a biomechanical study. *J Bone Joint Surg* 1985;67A:418–421.

155. Farrar EL, Lippert FG. Avulsion of triceps tendon. *Clin Orthop* 1981;161:242–246.

156. Nirschl RP. Elbow tendinosis: Tennis elbow. *Clin Sports Med* 1992;11:851–870.

157. Runge F. Zur genese und behandlug des schreibekrampfs. *Berliner klinische Wochenschrift* 1873;12:245–246.

158. Morris H. The rider's sprain. *Lancet* 1882;29:133–134.

159. Major HP. Lawn-tennis elbow. *BMJ* 1883;15:557.

160. Féré C. Note sur l'épicondylalgie. *Rev Méd* 1897;17:144–150.

161. Landelius ESK. Tennisarmbåge eller epicondylalgi. *Nord Med* 1941;10:1176–1177.

162. Osgood RB. Radiohumeral bursitis, epicondylitis, epicondylalgia (tennis elbow): A personal experience. *Arch Surg* 1922; 4:420–433.

163. Quin CE, Binks FA. Tennis elbow (Epicondylalgia externa): Treatment with hydrocortisone. *Lancet* 1954;2:221–222.

164. Brandesky W. Über den Epicondylusschmerz. *Dtsch Zeitschr Chir* 1929;219:246–255.

165. Bähr F. Aus der ärztlichen Praxis. Tennisschmerzen, Musikerlähmung. Ein kleiner Beitrag zur Pathologie des Radio-Humeral-Gelenkes. *Dtsch Med Wochenschr* 1900;26:713.

166. Nirschl RP. Muscle and tendon trauma: tennis elbow. In: Morrey BF, ed. *The Elbow and Its Disorders*. Philadelphia: WB Saunders; 1993:681–703.

167. Fischer AW. Ueber die Epicondylus: und Styloidesneuralgie, ihre Pathogenese und zweckmäβige therapie. *Archiv Klin Chir* 1923;125:749–775.

168. Fischer E. Zur Röntgenbehandlung der Epikondylitis und verwandter Krankheitszustände. *Münch Med Wochenschr* 1936; 83:149.

169. Wiesner H. Die Epicondylitis humeri lateralis und ihre Behandlung unter besonderer Berücksichtigung der Hohmannschen Operation. *Zentralbl Chir* 1952;77:787–791.

170. Cyriax JH. The pathology and treatment of tennis elbow. *J Bone Joint Surg* 1936;18:921–940.

171. Coonrad RW, Hooper WR. Tennis elbow: its course, natural history, conservative and surgical management. *J Bone and Joint Surg* 1973;55-A:1177–1182.

172. Goldie I. Epicondylitis lateralis humeri (epicondylalgia or tennis elbow). *Acta Chir Scand* 1964;32:339–345.

173. Nirschl RP. Tennis elbow tendinosis: pathoanatomy, nonsurgical and surgical management. In: Gordon SL, Blair SJ, Fine LJ, eds. *Repetitive Motion Disorders of the Upper Extremity*. Rosemont, IL: American Academy of Orthopaedic Surgeons; 1995: 467–479.

174. Regan W, et al. Microscopic histopathology of chronic refractory lateral epicondylitis. *Am J Sports Med* 1992;20:746–749.

175. Nirschl RP, Pettrone FA. Tennis elbow. *J Bone Joint Surg Am* 1979;61-A:832–839.

176. Greenbaum B, et al. Extensor carpi radialis brevis. An anatomical analysis of its origin. *J Bone Joint Surg Br* 1999;81:926–929.

177. Vulliet H. Die Epicondylitis humeri. *Zentralbl Chir* 1910; 40:1311–1312.

178. Franke F. Ueber Epicondylitis humeri. *Dtsch Med Wochenschr* 1910;36:13.

179. Elmslie RC. Tennis elbow. *Proc Royal Soc Med* 1929;23 (Part 1):328.

180. Gruber W. Monographie der Bursae Mucosae Cubitales. St Petersburg: Mém. de l'Acad. Imp. d. Science de St Petersburg: 1866.

181. Schmitt J. Bursitis calcarea am Epicondylus externus humeri: Ein beitrag zur Pathogenese der epicondylitis. *Archiv für Orthopädie und Unfall-Chirurgie* 1921;19:215–221.

182. Crawford HD. Discussion to epicondylitis humeri (Hansson). *NY State J Med* 1943;43:32–33.

183. Swensen L. Tennis elbow. *J Mich State Med Soc* 1949;48:997.

184. Neuman JH, Goodfellow JW. Fibrillation of head of radius as one cause of tennis elbow. *BMJ* 1975;2:328–330.

185. Preiser G. Ueber 'Epicondylitis humeri.' *Dtsch Med Wochenschr* 1910;36:712.

186. Mills PG. The treatment of 'Tennis Elbow.' *BMJ* 1928;1:12–13.
187. Bosworth DM. The role of the orbicular ligament in tennis elbow. *J Bone Joint Surg Am* 1955;37A:527–533.
188. Trethowan WH. Tennis elbow. *BMJ* 1929;2:1218.
189. Trethowan WH. Minor injuries of the elbow joint. *BMJ* 1929;2:1109.
190. Ogilvie WH. Tennis elbow. In: *Proceedings of the Royal Society of Medicine*: 1929.
191. Bell Allen JC. Epicondylitis: Traumatic radio-humeral synovitis. *Med J Aust* 1944;1:273–274.
192. Moore M. Radiohumeral synovitis, a cause of persistent elbow pain. *Surg Clin North Am* 1953;33:1363–1371.
193. Murley AHG. Tennis elbow: Treated with hydrocortisone acetate. *Lancet* 1954;2:223–225.
194. Paul NW. Radio-humeral bursitis—Is it traumatic? Analysis and report of 314 cases. *Ind Med Surg* 1957;26:383–390.
195. Winkworth CE. Lawn-tennis elbow. *BMJ* 1883;6:708.
196. Kaplan EB. Treatment of tennis elbow (epicondylitis) by denervation. *J Bone Joint Surg Am* 1959;41A:147–151.
197. O'Sullivan S. Tennis-elbow. *BMJ* 1883;8:1168.
198. Moss SH, Switzer HE. Radial tunnel syndrome: a spectrum of clinical speculations. *J Hand Surg* 1983;8:414–418.
199. Morrison DL. Tennis elbow and radial tunnel syndrome: differential diagnosis and treatment. *JAOA* 1981;80:823–826.
200. Bosworth DM. Surgical treatment of tennis elbow: a followup study. *J Bone Joint Surg* 1965;47A:1533–1536.
201. Crenshaw AH. Shoulder and elbow injuries. In: Crenshaw AH, ed. *Campbell's Operative Orthopaedics*. St. Louis: Mosby-Year Book;1992.
202. Wright A, et al. Hyperalgesia in tennis elbow patients. *J Musculoskeletal Pain* 1994;2:83–96.
203. Gunn C, Milbrandt W. Tennis elbow and the cervical spine. *Can Med Assoc J* 1976;114:803–809.
204. Rompe JD, et al. Chronic lateral epicondylitis of the elbow: A prospective study of low-energy shockwave therapy and low-energy shockwave therapy plus manual therapy of the cervical spine. *Arch Phys Med Rehab* 2001;82:578–582.
205. Maitland G. Vertebral manipulation. Sydney: Butterworth; 1986.
206. Curwin S, Stanish WD. *Tendinitis, Its Etiology and Treatment*. Lexington, MA: Collamore Press; 1984.
207. Leadbetter WB. Cell-matrix response in tendon injury. Clin Sports Med 1992;11:533–578.
208. Nirschl RP. Patterns of failed tendon healing in tendon injury. In: Leadbetter WB, Buckwalter JA, Gordon SL, eds. *Sports-Induced Inflammation: Clinical and Basic Science Concepts*. American Academy of Orthopaedic Surgeons: Park Ridge, Ill; 1990:609–618.
209. Teitz CC, et al. Tendon problems in athletic individuals. *J Bone Joint Surg* 1997;79-A:138–152.
210. Woo SL-Y, et al. Mechanical properties of tendons and ligaments. II. The relationships of immobilization and exercise on tissue remodeling. *Biorheology* 1982;19:397–408.
211. Woo SL-Y, et al. Anatomy, biology, and biomechanics of tendon, ligament, and meniscus. In: Simon SR, ed. *Orthopaedic Basic Science*. American Academy of Orthopaedic Surgeons: Rosemont, Ill; 1994:45–87.
212. Nirschl RP. Prevention and treatment of elbow and shoulder injuries in the tennis player. *Clin Sports Med* 1988;7:289–308.
213. Nirschl RP. Mesenchymal syndrome. *Virginia Med Monthly* 1969;96:659–662.
214. Clado GR. Tennis-arm. *Le Progrès Médical* 1902;16:273–277.
215. Rosenburg G. Tennisellenbogen und Muskelriß. *Med Klin* 1925;21:771–773.
216. Heald CB. *Injuries and Sport: A General Guide for the Practitioner*. London: Humphrey Milford and Oxford University Press; 1931.
217. von Goeldel W. Beitrag zum Wesen und der Behandlung der Epikondylitis. *Münch Med Wochenschr* 1920;67:1147–1148.
218. Bernhardt M. Ueber eine wenig bekannte Form der Beschäftigungsneuralgie. *Neurolog Centralbl* 1896;15:13–17.
219. Friedlander HL, Reid RL, Cape RF. Tennis elbow. *Clin Orthop* 1967;51:109–116.
220. Foley AE. Tennis elbow. *Am Fam Physician* 1993;48:281–288.
221. Labelle H, et al. Lack of scientific evidence for the treatment of lateral epicondylitis of the elbow: An attempted meta-analysis. *J Bone Joint Surg* 1992;74B:646–651.
222. Ernst E. Conservative therapy for tennis elbow. *Br J Clin Pract* 1992;46:55–57.
223. Binder A, et al. Is therapeutic ultrasound effective in treating soft tissue lesions? *BMJ* 1985;290:512–514.
224. Lundeberg T, Abrahamsson P, Haker E. A comparative study of continuous ultrasound, placebo ultrasound and rest in epicondylalgia. *Scand J Rehabil* 1988;20:99–101.
224a. Struijs PA, et al. Manipulation of the wrist for management of lateral epicondylitis: A randomized pilot study. *Phys Ther Rev* 2003;83:608–616.
225. Snyder-Mackler L, Epler M. Effect of standard and Aircast tennis elbow bands on integrated electromyography of forearm extensor musculature proximal to the bands. *Am J Sports Med* 1989;17:278–281.
226. Froimson A. Treatment of tennis elbow with forearm support. *J Bone Joint Surg* 1961;43:100–103.
227. Ilfeld FW, Field SM. Treatment of tennis elbow: use of special brace. *JAMA* 1966;195:67–71.
228. Groppel J, Nirschl RP. A biomechanical and electromyographical analysis of the effects of counter force braces on the tennis player. *Am J Sports Med* 1986;14:195–200.
229. Chiumento AB, Bauer JA, Fiolkowski P. A comparison of the dampening properties of tennis elbow braces. *Med Sci Sports Exerc* 1997;29(5 Suppl):123.
230. Gellman H. Tennis elbow (lateral epicondylitis). *Orthop Clin North Am* 1992;23:75–79.
231. Marlin T. Treatment of 'Tennis elbow': With some observations on joint manipulation. *Lancet* 1930;1:509–511.
232. Bryce A. A case of 'tennis elbow' treated by luminous heat. *Br J Actinother Physiother* 1930;5:55.
233. Kininmonth DA. (Discussion on manipulation.) Tennis elbow. *Ann Phys Med* 1953;1:144.
234. Johnson EW. Tennis elbow. Misconceptions and widespread mythology. *Am J Phys Med Rehabil* 2000;79:113.
235. Freeland DE, Gribble M de G. Hydrocortisone in tennis-elbow. *Lancet* 1954;2:225.
236. Clarke AK, Woodland J. Comparison of two steroid preparations to treat tennis elbow using the hypospray. *Rheumatol Rehabil* 1975;14:47–49.
237. Day BH, Govindasamy N, Patnaik R. Corticosteroid injections in the treatment of tennis elbow. *Practitioner* 1978;220: 459–462.
238. Hughes GR, Currey HL. Hypospray treatment of tennis elbow. *Ann Rheum Dis* 1969;28:58–62.
239. Hennig EM, Rosenbaum D, Milani TL. Transfer of tennis racket vibrations onto the human forearm. *Med Sci Sports Exerc* 1992;24:1134–1138.

240. Legwold G. Tennis elbow: joint resolution by conservative treatment and improved technique. *Phys Sportsmed* 1984; 12:168.

241. Liu YK. Mechanical analysis of racquet and ball during impact. *Med Sci Sports Exerc* 1983;15:388.

242. Hatze H. The effectiveness of grip bands in reducing racquet vibration transfer and slipping. *Med Sci Sports Exerc* 1992; 24:226–229.

243. Kraushaar BS, Nirschl RP. Pearls: handshake lends epicondylitis cues. *Phys Sportsmed* 1996;24:15.

244. Jobe FW, Ciccotti MG. Lateral and medial epicondylitis of the elbow. *J Am Acad Orthop Surg* 1994;2:1–8.

245. Krischek O, et al. Shock-wave therapy for tennis and golfer's elbow—1 year follow-up. *Arch Orthop Trauma Surg* 1999; 119:62–66.

246. Glousman RE, et al. An electromyographic analysis of the elbow in normal and injured pitchers with medial collateral ligament insufficiency. *Am J Sports Med* 1992;20:311–317.

247. Bauer M, et al. Osteochrondritis dissecans of the elbow: a long-term follow-up study. *Clin Orthop* 1992;284:156–162.

248. Balasubramaniam P, Prathap K. The effect of injection of hydrocortisone into rabbit calcaneal tendons. *J Bone Joint Surg* 1972;54:729–736.

249. Baumgard SH, Schwartz DR. Percutaneous release of the epicondylar muscles for humeral epicondylitis. *Am J Sports Med* 1982;10:233–238.

250. Barry NN, McGuire JL. Overuse syndromes in adult athletes. *Rheum Dis Clin North Am* 1996;22:515–530.

251. Bennett JB. Articular injuries in the athlete. In: Morrey BF, ed. *The Elbow and Its Disorders*. Philadelphia: WB Saunders; 1993:803–831.

252. Lundborg G. Surgical treatment for ulnar nerve entrapment at the elbow. *J Hand Surg Am* 1992;17B:245–247.

253. Wilgis EF, Murphy R. The significance of longitudinal excursion in peripheral nerves. *Hand Clin* 1986;2:761–766.

254. Dellon AL. Musculotendinous variations about the medial humeral epicondyle. *J Hand Surg Am* 1986;11B:175–181.

255. Macnicol MF. The results of operation for ulnar neuritis. *J Bone Joint Surg* 1979;61B:159–164.

256. Piligian G, et al. Evaluation and management of chronic work-related musculoskeletal disorders of the distal upper extremity. *Am J Ind Med* 2000;37:75–93.

257. Preston D, Shapiro B. Electromyography and neuromuscular disorders. In: *Clinical Electrophysiologic Correlations*. Boston, MA: Butterworth-Heinemann; 1998.

258. Terry RJ. A study of the supracondyloid process in the living. *Am J Phys Anthropol* 1921;4:129–139.

259. Gross PT, Jones HR. Proximal median neuropathies: Electromyographic and clinical correlation. *Muscle Nerve* 1992; 15:390–395.

260. Symeonides PP. The humerus supracondylar process syndrome. *Clin Orthop* 1972;82:141–143.

261. Anto C, Aradhya P. Clinical diagnosis of peripheral nerve compression in the upper extremities. *Orthop Clin North Am* 1996;27:227–245.

262. Lubahn JD, Cermak MB. Uncommon nerve compression syndromes of the upper extremity. *J Am Acad Orthop Surg* 1998;6:378–386.

263. Werner CO, Rosen I, Thorngren KG. Clinical and neurophysiological characteristics of the pronator syndrome. *Clin Orthop* 1985;197:231–236.

264. Gainor BJ. The pronator compression test revisited—a forgotten physical sign. *Orthop Rev* 1990;19:888–892.

265. Mangini V. Flexor pollicis longus: Its morphology and clinical significance. *J Bone Joint Surg* 1960;42A:467–470.

266. Spinner M. The anterior interosseous nerve syndrome with special attention to its variations. *J Bone Joint Surg* 1970;52A:84–94.

267. Nakano KK, Lundergran C, Okihiro MM. Anterior interosseous nerve syndromes: Diagnostic methods and alternative treatments. *Arch Neurol* 1977;34:477–480.

268. Plate A-M, Green SM. Compressive radial neuropathies. *AAOS Instr Course Lect* 2000;49:295–304.

269. Manske PR. Compression of the radial nerve by the triceps muscle. *J Bone Joint Surg* 1977;59A:835–836.

270. Wright PE II, Jobe MT. Peripheral nerve injuries. In: Canale ST, Daugherty K, Jones L, eds. *Campbell's Operative Orthopaedics*. St. Louis, MO: Mosby Year Book;1998:3827–3894.

271. Agnew DH. Bursal tumour producing loss of power of forearm. *Am J Med Sci* 1863;46:404–405.

272. Sharrard WJW. Posterior interosseous neuritis. *J Bone Joint Surg* 1966;48B:777–780.

273. Thompson WAL, Kopell HP. Peripheral entrapment neuropathies of the upper extremity. *N Engl J Med* 1959; 260:1261–1265.

274. Fröhse F, Frankel M. *Die Muskeln des Menschlichen*. Arms: Jena G Fischer; 1908.

275. Fuss FK, Wurzl GH. Radial nerve entrapment at the elbow: Surgical anatomy. *J Hand Surg Am* 1991;16A:742–747.

276. Derkash RS, Niebauer JJ. Entrapment of the posterior interosseous nerve by a fibrous band in the dorsal edge of the supinator muscle and erosion of a groove in the proximal radius. *J Hand Surg Am* 1981;6:524–526.

277. Steichen JB, Christensen AW. Posterior interosseous nerve compression syndrome. In: Gelberman RH, ed. *Operative Nerve Repair and Reconstruction*. Philadelphia: JB Lippincott; 1991:1005–1022.

278. Hirayama T, Takemitsu Y. Isolated paralysis of the posterior interosseous nerve: Report of a case. *J Bone Joint Surg* 1988;70A:1402–1403.

279. Michele AA, Krueger FJ. Lateral epicondylitis of the elbow treated by fasciotomy. *Surgery* 1956;39:277–284.

280. Verhaar J, Spaans F. Radial tunnel syndrome: An investigation of compression neuropathy as a possible cause. *J Bone Joint Surg* 1991;73:539–544.

281. Eaton CJ, Lister GD. Radial nerve compression. *Hand Clin* 1992;8:345–357.

282. Wartenberg R. Cheiralgia paresthetica (isolierte neuritis des ramus superficialis nervi radialis). *Ztschr Ges Neurol Psychiatr* 1932;141:145–155.

283. Sunderland S. The musculocutaneous nerve. In: Sunderland S, ed. *Nerves and Nerve Injuries*. Edinburgh: Churchill Livingstone; 1978:796–801.

284. Sunderland S. Voluntary movements and the deceptive action of muscles in peripheral nerve lesions. *Aust N Z J Surg* 1944;13:160–183.

285. Kendall FP, McCreary EK, Provance PG. *Muscles: Testing and Function*. Baltimore: Williams & Wilkins; 1993.

286. Bartosh RA, Dugdale TW, Nielen R. Isolated musculocutaneous nerve injury complicating closed fracture of the clavicle: A case report. *Am J Sports Med* 1992;20:356–359.

287. Travell JG, Simons DG. *Myofascial Pain and Dysfunction—The Trigger Point Manual*. Baltimore: Williams & Wilkins;1983.

288. Smolders JJ. Myofascial pain and dysfunction syndromes. In: Hammer WI, ed. *Functional Soft Tissue Examination and Treatment by Manual Methods—The Extremities.* Gaithersburg, MD: Aspen; 1991:215–234.

289. Bado JL. The Monteggia lesion. *Clin Orthop* 1967;50:71.

290. Bowers WH. The distal radioulnar joint. In: Green DP, Hotchkiss RN, eds. *Operative Hand Surgery.* New York: Churchill Livingstone; 1993:995.

291. Morgan WJ, Breen TF. Complex fractures of the forearm. *Hand Clin* 1994;10:375.

292. Panner HJ. A peculiar affection of the capitellum humeri resembling Calve-Perthes' disease of the hip. *Acta Radiol* 1929;10:234.

293. Rettig AC, Waugh TR, Evanski PM. Fracture of the olecranon: a problem of management. *J Trauma* 1979;19:23–28.

294. Horne JG, Tanzer TL. Olecranon fractures: a review of 100 cases. *J Trauma* 1981;21:469–472.

295. Bach BR, Warren RF, Wickiewicz TL. Triceps rupture. A case report and literature review. *Am J Sports Med* 1987;15:285–289.

296. O'Driscoll SW. Technique for unstable olecranon fracture-subluxations. *Oper Tech Orthop* 1994;4:49–53.

297. Hotchkiss RN. Displaced fractures of the radial head: internal fixation or excision. *J Am Acad Orthop Surg* 1997;5:1–10.

298. King GJW, Morrey BF, An K-N. Stabilizers of the elbow. *J Shoulder Elbow Surg* 1993;2:165–170.

299. Viola RW, Hastings H II. Treatment of ectopic ossification about the elbow. *Clin Orthop* 2000;370:65–86.

300. Ackerman LV. Extra-osseous localized non-neoplastic bone and cartilage formation (so-called myositis ossificans). *J Bone Joint Surg* 1958;40A:279–298.

301. Connor JM, Evans DA. Fibrodysplasia ossificans progressiva: The clinical features and natural history of 34 patients. *J Bone Joint Surg* 1982;64B:76–83.

302. Green DP, McCoy H. Turnbuckle orthotic correction of elbow-flexion contractures after acute injuries. *J Bone Joint Surg* 1979;61A:1092–1095.

303. Regan WD, Reilly CD. Distraction arthroplasty of the elbow. *Hand Clin* 1993;9:719–728.

304. Hastings H. Elbow contractures and ossification. In: Peimer CA, ed. *Surgery of the Hand and Upper Extremity.* New York: McGraw-Hill; 1996:507–534.

305. Hastings H, Graham TJ. The classification and treatment of heterotopic ossification about the elbow and forearm. *Hand Clin* 1994;10:417–437.

306. Thompson HC, Garcia A. Myositis ossificans: Aftermath of elbow injuries. *Clin Orthop* 1967;50:129–134.

307. Garland DE, O'Hollaren RM. Fractures and dislocations about the elbow in the head-injured adult. *Clin Orthop* 1982;168:38–41.

308. Keenan MA, et al. Late ulnar neuropathy in the brain-injured adult. *J Hand Surg Am* 1988;13A:120–124.

309. Wainapel SF, Rao PU, Schepsis A. Ulnar nerve compression by heterotopic ossification in a head-injured patient. *Arch Phys Med Rehabil* 1985;66:512–514.

310. Stover SL, Hataway CJ, Zeiger HE. Heterotopic ossification in spinal cord-injured patients. *Arch Phys Med Rehabil* 1975;56:199–204.

311. Ritter MA, Seiber JM. Prophylactic indomethacin for the prevention of heterotopic bone following total hip arthroplasty. *Clin Orthop* 1985;196:217–225.

312. Schmidt SA, et al. The use of indomethacin to prevent the formation of heterotopic bone after total hip replacement: A randomized, double-blind clinical trial. *J Bone Joint Surg* 1988;70A:834–838.

313. Brogden BG, Cros NW. Little leaguer's elbow. *Am J Radiol* 1960;83:671.

314. Leffers D, Greene TL, Germaine BF. The elbow region. In: Leek JC, Gershwin ME, Fowler WM Jr, eds. *Principles of Physical Medicine and Rehabilitation in the Musculoskeletal Diseases.* New York: Grune and Stratton; 1986:369–392.

315. DiGiovine NM, et al. An electromyographical analysis of the upper extremity in pitching. *J Shoulder Elbow Surg* 1992;1:15–25.

316. Bowyer BL, Gooch JL, Geringer SR. Sports medicine 2: upper extremity injuries. *Arch Phys Med Rehab* 1993;74:437.

317. McLeod WD. The pitching mechanism. In: Zarins B, Andrews J, Carson WG, eds. *Injuries to the Throwing Arm.* Philadelphia: WB Saunders; 1985:22–29.

318. Cabrera JM, McCue FC. Nonosseous athletic injuries of the elbow, forearm, and hand. *Clin Sports Med* 1986;5:681–700.

319. Salter RB, Zaltz C. Anatomic investigations of the mechanism of injury and pathologic anatomy of pulled elbow in young children. *Clin Orthop* 1971;77:134–143.

320. Dee R, Carrion W. Pulled elbow. In: *Principles of Orthopaedic Practice.* New York: McGraw-Hill; 1997:579.

321. Hagroo GA, et al. Pulled elbow—not the effect of hypermobility of joints. *Injury* 1995;26:687–690.

322. Sai N. Pulled elbow. *J Royal Soc Med* 1999;92:462–464.

323. Corrigan AB. The pulled elbow. *Med J Aust* 1965;2:1.

324. Amir D, Frankl U, Pogrund H. Pulled elbow and hypermobility of joints. *Clin Orthop* 1990;257:94.

325. Matles AL, Eliopoulous K. Internal derangement of the elbow in children. *Int Surg* 1967;48:259–263.

326. Mulligan BR. *Manual Therapy: "NAGS," "SNAGS," "PRP'S" etc.* Wellington: Plane View Series; 1992.

327. Mulligan BR. Manual therapy rounds: Mobilisations with movement (MWM's). *J Man Manip Ther* 1993;1:154–156.

328. DiGiovanna EL. Diagnosis and treatment of the upper extremity. In: DiGiovanna EL, Schiowitz S, eds. *An Osteopathic Approach to Diagnosis and Treatment.* Philadelphia: JB Lippincott; 1991.

329. Lahz JRS. Concerning the pathology and treatment of tennis elbow. *Med J Aust* 1947;2:737–742.

330. Kibler WB. Shoulder rehabilitation: principles and practice. *Med Sci Sports Exerc* 1998;30(4 Suppl 1):40–50.

331. Reid DC. *Sports Injury Assessment and Rehabilitation.* New York: Churchill Livingstone; 1992.

332. Rossouw P. Tennis elbow—is extracorporeal shock wave therapy (eswt) an alternative to surgery? *J Bone Joint Surg Br* 1999;81-B(Suppl III):306.

333. Nirschl RP. Rotator cuff tendinitis: basic concepts of pathoetiology. In: Barr JS Jr, ed. *Instructional Course Lectures, American Academy of Orthopacdic Surgeons.* Park Ridge, IL: American Academy of Orthopaedic Surgeons; 1989:439–445.

334. Stanish WD, Rubinovich RM, Curwin S. Eccentric exercise in chronic tendinitis. *Clin Orthop* 1986;208:65–68.

335. Magee DJ, ed. *Orthopedic Physical Assessment.* Philadelphia: WB Saunders; 2002.

336. Palmer ML, Epler M. *Clinical Assessment Procedures in Physical Therapy.* Philadelphia: JB Lippincott; 1990:68–73.

THE FOREARM, WRIST, AND HAND

▶ **At the completion of this chapter, the reader will be able to:**

1. Describe the anatomy of the joints, ligaments, muscles, blood and nerve supply that comprise the forearm, wrist, and hand.

2. Describe the biomechanics of the forearm, wrist, and hand, including open- and close-packed positions, normal and abnormal joint barriers, and stabilizers.

3. Describe the purpose and components of the tests and measures for the forearm, wrist, and hand.

4. Perform a comprehensive examination of the forearm, wrist, and hand, including palpation of the articular and soft tissue structures, specific passive mobility and passive articular mobility tests, and stability tests.

5. Evaluate the total examination data to establish a diagnosis.

6. Describe the relationship between muscle imbalance and functional performance of the forearm, wrist, and hand.

7. Outline the significance of the key findings from the tests and measures and establish a diagnosis.

8. Summarize the various causes of forearm, wrist, and hand dysfunction.

9. Develop self-reliant intervention strategies based on clinical findings and established goals.

10. Develop a working hypothesis.

11. Describe and demonstrate intervention strategies and techniques based on clinical findings and established goals.

12. Evaluate the intervention effectiveness in order to progress or modify an intervention.

13. Plan an effective home program, and instruct the patient in same.

OVERVIEW

"A hand is a very personal thing. It is the interface between the patient and his or her world. It is an emblem of strength, beauty, skill, sexuality and sensibility. When it is damaged it becomes a symbol of vulnerability of the whole patient."

PAUL W. BRAND (1914–)

In a sense, the shoulder, elbow, and wrist joints are merely mechanical devices that contribute to the usefulness of the hand.[1] The correct synchronization of these biological devices, coupled with patient motivation, produce a remarkable level of dexterity and precision.

The carpus, or wrist, represents a highly complex anatomic structure, comprising a core structure of 8 bones, more than twenty radiocarpal, intercarpal, and carpometacarpal joints, 26 named intercarpal ligaments, and the 6 or more parts of the triangular fibrocartilage complex (TFCC).[2]

While these structures can be differentiated anatomically, they are functionally interrelated with movement in one joint having an effect on the motion of neighboring joints. This relationship extends as far as the elbow.

The hand accounts for about 90 percent of upper limb function.[3] The thumb, which is involved in 40 to 50 percent of hand function, is the more functionally important of the digits.[3] The index finger, involved in about 20 percent of hand function, is the second most important, and the ring finger the least important. The middle finger, which accounts for about 20 percent of all hand function, is the strongest finger, and is important for both precision and power functions.[3]

The following sections describe the respective bones, joints, soft tissues, and nerves, detailing both their individual and collective functions. For simplicity's sake, the forearm, wrist, and hand are separated into their various compartments.

Anatomy

Distal Radioulnar Joint

The distal radioulnar joint (DRUJ) plays an important role in wrist and forearm function. The DRUJ is a double pivot joint that unites the distal radius and ulna and an articular disk (Fig. 16-1). The articular disk, known as the triangular fibrocartilage complex (TFCC), assists in binding the distal radius and is the main stabilizer of the distal radioulnar joint (see next section).[4]

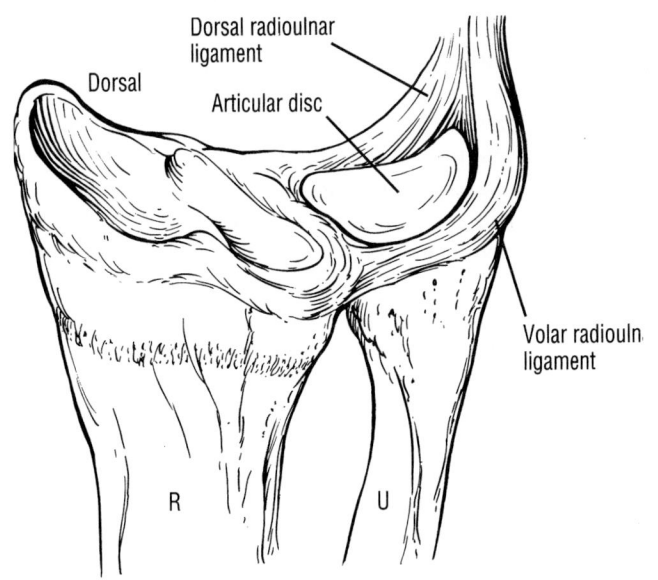

FIGURE 16-1 Triangular fibrocartilage complex. R, radius; U, ulna. (Reproduced with permission from Herndon JH. *Surgical Reconstruction of the Upper Extremity*. Stamford, CT: Appleton & Lange; 1999.)

At its distal end, the radius widens to form a broad concave articular surface. The articular surface has an ulnar inclination in the frontal plane, which averages 23 degrees, and a palmar inclination in the sagittal plane, that averages 11 degrees.[5] The distal end of the ulna expands slightly laterally into a rounded head, and medially into an ulnar styloid process (see Fig. 16-1). The rounded head of the ulnar head contacts both the ulnar notch of the radius laterally, and the TFCC distally.[6] The ulnar styloid process is approximately one-half inch shorter than the radial styloid process, resulting in more ulnar deviation than radial deviation.[6] The articular capsule, which attaches to the articular margins of the radius and ulna and to the disk enclosing the inferior radioulnar joint is lax. Palmar and dorsal radioulnar ligaments strengthen the capsule anteriorly and posteriorly. Supination tightens the anterior capsule and pronation tightens the posterior part, adding to the overall stability of the wrist.[7]

The DRUJ functions to transmit the loads from the hand to the forearm.

Triangular Fibrocartilage Complex (TFCC)

The TFCC is essentially comprised of a fibrocartilage disk interposed between the medial proximal row and the distal ulna within the medial aspect of the wrist.[8] The primary function of the TFCC is to enhance joint congruity and to cushion against compressive forces. Indeed the TFCC transmits about 20 percent of the axial load from the hand to the forearm.[7] The broad base of the disk is attached to the medial edge of the ulnar notch of the radius, and its apex is attached to the lateral aspect of the base of the ulnar styloid process. The disk's anterior and posterior borders are thickened.

A number of ligaments originate from the TFCC and provide support to it. These include the ulnolunate and ulnotriquetral ligaments, the ulnar collateral, and the radioulnar ligaments. Other structures that lend support to the TFCC include:

► The ulnocarpal ligaments

► The sheath of the extensor carpi ulnaris tendon, which is the only wrist tendon that broadly connects to the TFCC

Both the superior and inferior articular surfaces of the TFCC are smooth and concave.[8] The disk separates the distal ulna from direct contact with the carpals, but allows gliding between the carpals, disk, and ulna during pronation and supination.[8,8a]

The TFCC is innervated by branches of the posteriorinterosseous, ulnar, and dorsal sensory ulnar nerves.[9]

The Wrist

The wrist joint is comprised of the distal radius and ulna, eight carpal bones, and the bases of five metacarpals. The carpal bones lie in two transverse rows. The proximal row contains (lateral to medial) the scaphoid (navicular), lunate, triquetrum, and pisiform. The distal row holds the trapezium, trapezoid, capitate, and hamate.

Radiocarpal Joint

The radiocarpal joint is formed by the large articular concave surface of the distal end of the radius, the scaphoid and lunate of the proximal carpal row, and the TFCC. A radial styloid process projects distally from the lateral side of the radius. A cartilage-covered ulnar notch occupies the distal medial side of the radius.[10] Posteriorly, a dorsal (Lister's) tubercle arises near the center of the radius, forming a pulley around which the extensor pollicis longus (EPL) tendon passes.[10]

> **Clinical Pearl**
>
> The Lister's tubercle is a common site of attritional changes and potential tendon rupture.[18]

The Carpals

Scaphoid. The scaphoid (Fig. 16-2) is the largest of the proximal carpal row bones, and its shape resembles that of a boat or canoe (thus the old term *navicular*).[8a] The scaphoid bone links the proximal and distal carpal rows and helps provide stability to the wrist joint.

The scaphoid is tethered to the proximal carpal row by a number of strong ligamentous attachments, and two thirds of its

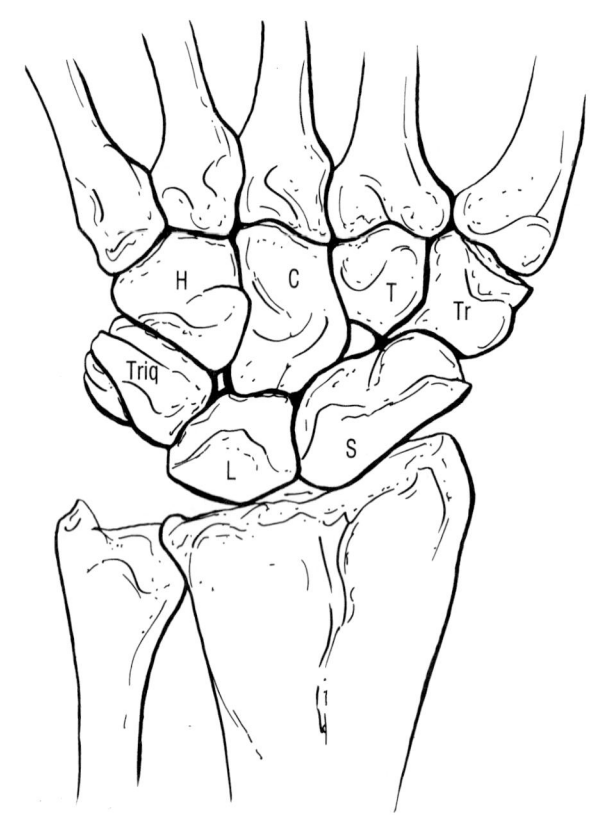

FIGURE 16-2 The carpals. H, hamate; C, capitate; T, trapezoid; Tr, trapezium; Triq, triquetrum; S, scaphoid; L, lunate. (Reproduced with permission from Herndon JH. *Surgical Reconstruction of the Upper Extremity.* Stamford, CT: Appleton & Lange; 1999.)

surface area is articular. The proximal surface of the scaphoid is convex and articulates with the radius. The medial surface is concave and articulates with the capitate.[10] The articulating surface for the lunate is flat. The distal surface consists of two convex facets for articulation with the trapezium and trapezoid (the scaphotrapeziotrapezoid [STT] joint).[8a] The round tubercle on the inferolateral part of its palmar surface serves as the attachment of the flexor retinaculum and the abductor pollicis brevis.[10]

The blood vessels to this bone enter the scaphoid at or distal to the wrist. This configuration predisposes a fracture on the proximal aspect to aseptic necrosis.[11]

Lunate. The lunate (see Fig. 16-2) articulates between the scaphoid and triquetrum in the proximal carpal row. Its smooth convex proximal surface articulates with the radius and the TFCC at the lunate fossa.[10] Its lateral surface contains a flat semilunar facet for the scaphoid. The medial surface articulates with the triquetrum. The distal surface is deeply concave and articulates with the edge of the hamate in adduction, and the medial aspect of the capitate.[10]

Triquetrum. The triquetrum (see Fig. 16-2) is a pyramid-shaped bone. It articulates with the pisiform on its distal palmar surface at the pisiform-triquetral joint.[10] The almost square distal-medial surface of the triquetrum articulates with the concavo-convex surface of the hamate. The ulnar collateral ligament attaches to the medial and dorsal surfaces of the triquetrum.[10] The proximal surface of the triquetrum articulates with the TFCC in full adduction.[8a] The lateral surface of the triquetrum articulates with the lunate.

Pisiform. The pisiform (see Fig. 16-2), as its name implies, is shaped like a "P" with a dorsal flat articular facet for the triquetrum.[10] The pisiform is formed within the tendon of the flexor carpi ulnaris, and serves as an attachment for the flexor retinaculum, abductor digiti minimi, ulnar collateral ligament, pisohamate ligament, and pisometacarpal ligament. The pisiform is a sesamoid bone that functions to increase the flexion moment of the flexor carpi ulnaris.[8a]

As mentioned, the pisiform articulates with the palmar surface of the triquetral, and is thus separated from the other carpal bones, all of which articulate with their neighbors. The pisiform is closely related to the ulnar artery and nerve on its radial border, the nerve being the closer.[12]

Trapezium. The trapezium has a groove on its medial palmar surface which contains the tendon of the flexor carpi radialis.[10] To its margins are attached two layers of the flexor retinaculum. The opponens pollicis is between the flexor pollicis brevis distally, and the abductor pollicis brevis proximally.[10] The lateral surface serves as an attachment site for the radial collateral ligament and capsular ligament of the first carpometacarpal joint. The distal articulating surface of the trapezium is saddle-shaped. Medially, its concave surface articulates with the trapezoid, while more distally its convex surface articulates with the second metacarpal base.[10] Proximally, its concave surface articulates with the scaphoid.

Trapezoid. The trapezoid (see Fig. 16-2) is small and irregular. The distal surface articulates with the grooved second metacarpal base. The medial surface articulates by a concave facet with the distal part of the capitate. The lateral surface of the trapezoid articulates with the trapezium and its proximal surface articulates with the scaphoid bone.[10]

Capitate. The capitate (see Fig. 16-2) is the most central and the largest of the carpal bones. Its distal aspect articulates with the third metacarpal base. Its lateral border articulates with the medial side of the second metacarpal base.[10] The convex proximal head of the capitate articulates with the lunate and scaphoid. The medial surface of the head articulates with the lunate and the lateral aspect of the head articulates with the scaphoid.[10] Medially, the capitate articulates with the hamate.

With its central location, the capitate serves as the keystone of the proximal transverse arch. This arch is important to prehensile activity of the hand.[8a,13,14]

Hamate. The hamate (see Fig. 16-2) is a cuneiform bone and contributes to the medial wall of the carpal tunnel. To the hook (hamulus) of the hamate is attached the flexor retinaculum. The hamate articulates with three carpal bones and two metacarpals.[8a] The medial surface articulates with the triquetrum and by association with the pisohamate ligament, the pisiform. The lateral surface articulates with the capitate.[10] On its distal aspect the hamate articulates with the fourth and fifth metacarpal heads.

Midcarpal Joints

The midcarpal joint lies between the two rows of carpals. It is referred to as a 'compound' articulation because each row has both a concave and convex segment. Wrist flexion, extension, and radial deviation are mainly midcarpal joint motions. Approximately 50 percent of the total arc of wrist flexion and extension occur at the midcarpal level with more flexion (66 percent) occurring than extension (34 percent).[15]

The proximal row of the carpals is convex laterally and concave medially. The scaphoid, lunate, trapezium trapezoid, and triquetrum present with a concave surface to the distal row of carpals. The scaphoid, capitate, and hamate present a convex surface to a reciprocally arranged distal row.

Carpal Ligaments

Excessive migration of the carpal bones is prevented by strong ligaments, and by the ulnar support provided by the TFCC (Table 16-1). The major ligaments of the wrist include the palmar intrinsic ligaments (Fig. 16-3), the volar extrinsic (Fig. 16-4) and the dorsal extrinsic and intrinsic ligaments (Fig. 16-5).

The ligaments of the wrist provide support for the region. These ligaments can be divided into two types: extrinsic and intrinsic (see Table 16-1). The extrinsic palmar ligaments provide the majority of the wrist stability. The intrinsic ligaments serve as rotational restraints, binding the proximal row into a unit of rotational stability.[16] The proximal row of carpals has no muscle insertions. Its stability depends entirely on the capsular and interosseous ligaments between the scaphoid, lunate, and triquetrum.[17] The ligaments between the proximal and distal carpal rows provide support, centering especially on the capitate.[10] The midcarpal ligaments, which are longer than the interosseous ligaments, cross the midcarpal joint and connect bones of the distal and proximal rows on both the dorsal and palmar surfaces.[8a] No midcarpal ligaments directly attach to the lunate.

TABLE 16-1 Ligaments of the Wrist

Intrinsic		Extrinsic
Interosseous	Midcarpal	Radiocarpal/ulnocarpal
Distal row Trapezium-trapezoid Trapezoid-capitate Capitohamate	*Dorsal* Scaphotriquetral Dorsal intercarpal	*Dorsal* Dorsal radiocarpal
Proximal row Scapholunate Lunotriquetral	*Palmar* Scaphotrapeziotrapezoid Scaphocapitate Triquetrocapitate Triquetrohamate	*Palmar* Radioscaphocapitate Long radiolunate Short radiolunate Radioscapholunate Ulnolunate Ulnotriquetral Ulnocapitate

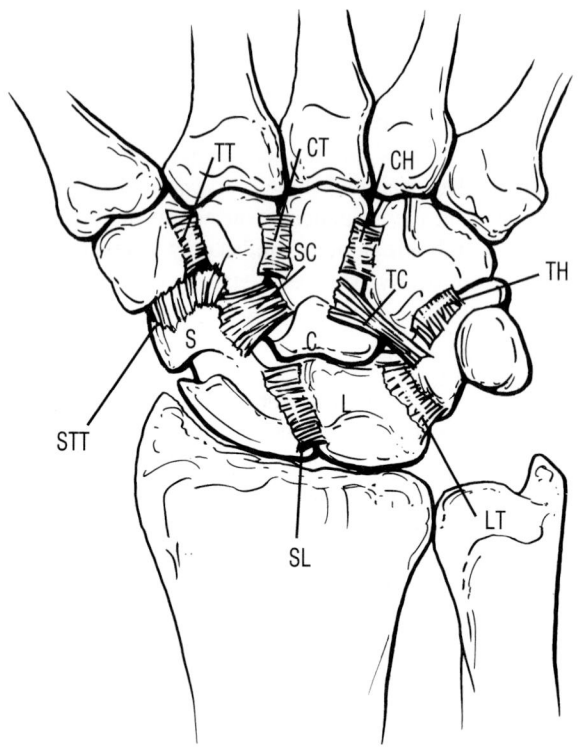

FIGURE 16-3 Palmar intrinsic ligaments. S, scaphoid; L, lunate; C, capitate; SL, scapholunate ligament; LT, lunotriquetral ligament; STT, scaphotrapeziotrapezoidal ligament; SC, scaphocapitate ligament; TC, triquetrocapitate ligament; TH, triquetrohamate ligament; TT, trapeziotrapezoid ligament; CT, capitotrapezoid ligament; CH, capitohamate ligament. (*Reproduced with permission from Herndon JH. Surgical Reconstruction of the Upper Extremity.* Stamford, CT: Appleton & Lange; 1999.)

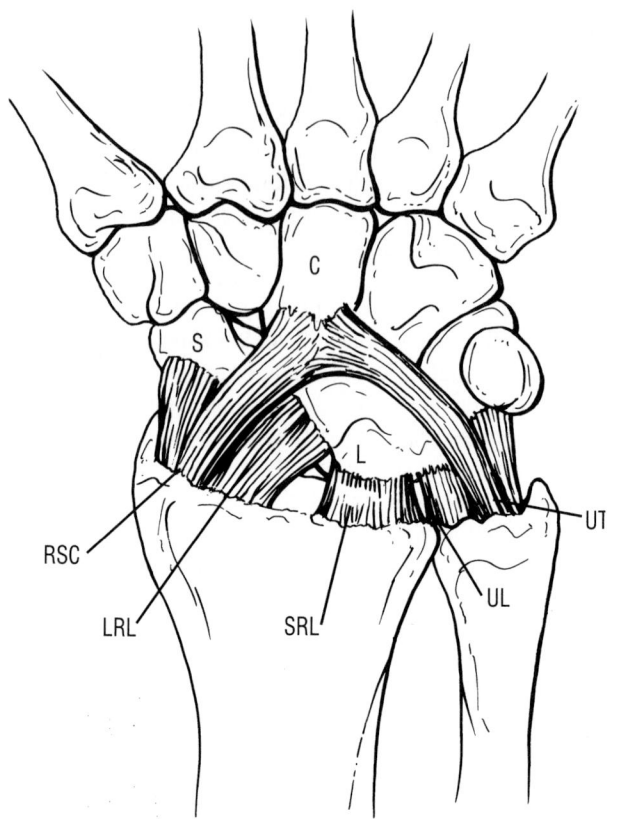

FIGURE 16-4 Volar extrinsic ligaments. S, scaphoid; C, capitate; L, lunate; RSC, radioscaphocapitate ligament; SRL, short radiolunate ligament; LRL, long radiolunate ligament; UT, ulnotriquetral ligament; UL, ulnolunate ligament. (*Reproduced with permission from Herndon JH. Surgical Reconstruction of the Upper Extremity.* Stamford, CT: Appleton & Lange; 1999.)

Antebrachial Fascia

The antebrachial fascia is a dense connective tissue "bracelet" that encases the forearm and maintains the relationships of the tendons that cross the wrist. The fascia is firmly attached to the subcutaneous border of the ulna, from which it sends a septum to the radius. This septum divides the forearm into an anterior compartment and a posterior compartment (see later).

The Extensor Retinaculum

Where the tendons cross the wrist, a ligamentous structure called a retinaculum appears to lay over the tendons and their sheaths. This retinaculum serves to prevent the tendons from "bow-stringing" when the tendons turn a corner at the wrist.[19] The extensor retinaculum extends from the lateral border of the distal radius across the dorsal surface of the distal forearm onto the posterior surface of the distal ulna and ulnar styloid process. It then wraps part way around the ulna to attach to the triquetrum and pisiform bones. The tunnel-like structures formed by the retinaculum and the underlying bones are called fibro-osseous compartments. There are six fibro-

osseous compartments, or tunnels, on the dorsum of the wrist (Fig. 16-6). The compartments, from lateral to medial, contain the tendons of:

1. Abductor pollicis longus and extensor pollicis brevis

2. Extensor carpi radialis longus and brevis

3. Extensor pollicis longus

4. Extensor digitorum (four tendons) and extensor indicis (not shown)

5. Extensor digiti minimi

6. Extensor carpi ulnaris

Clinical Pearl

The mnemonic 2 2 1 2 1 1 can be used to remember the number of tendons in each compartment.[9]

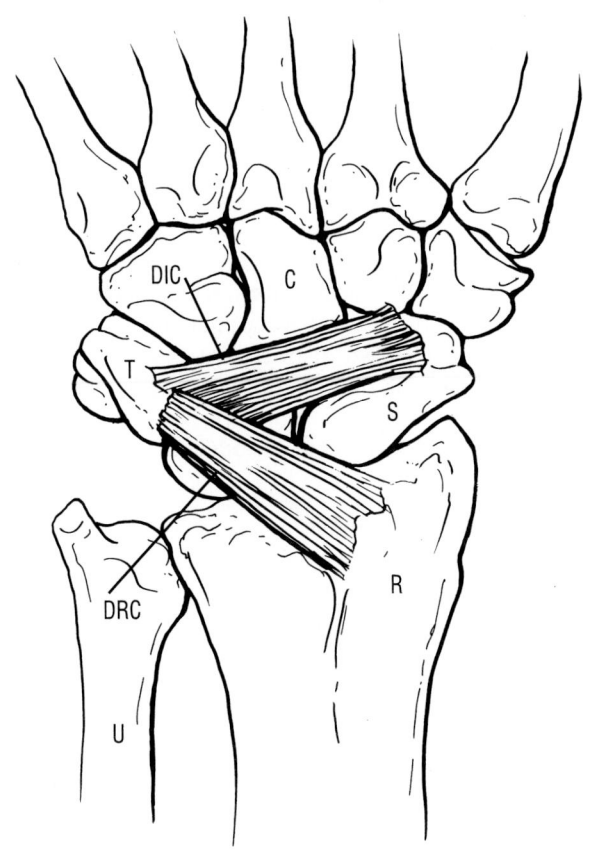

FIGURE 16-5 Dorsal extrinsic and intrinsic ligaments. R, radius; U, ulna; S, scaphoid; C, capitate; T, triquetrum; DRC, dorsal radiocarpal ligament (radiotriquetral); DIC, dorsal intercarpal ligament (scaphotriquetral). (Reproduced with permission from Herndon JH. *Surgical Reconstruction of the Upper Extremity.* Stamford, CT: Appleton & Lange; 1999.)

As these tendons pass through the compartments, they are invested with synovial sheaths.

The dorsal compartments serve to enhance the efficiency and effectiveness of the wrist and finger extensors (see Extensor Hood). Proximal to the metacarpal heads, juncturae tendinae connect the four tendons of the extensor digitorum (ED) muscles, limiting their independent motion.[6] For example, flexion of the middle and little fingers restricts extension of the ring finger metacarpophalangeal (MCP) joint because the juncturae tendinae pull the ring finger extensor tendon distally. Conversely, extension of the ring finger exerts an extensor force upon its neighbors, such that they can be actively extended even if the middle and little finger extensor tendons are severed proximal to the juncturae.[6]

The Flexor Retinaculum

The flexor retinaculum (transverse carpal ligament) spans the area between the pisiform, hamate, scaphoid, and trapezium. It transforms the carpal arch into a tunnel, through which pass the median nerve and some of the tendons of the hand. Proximally, the retinaculum attaches to the tubercle of the scaphoid and the pisiform. Distally it attaches to the hook of the hamate and the tubercle of the trapezium. The retinaculum also[6]:

► serves as an attachment site for the thenar and hypothenar muscles.

► helps maintain the transverse carpal arch.

► acts as a restraint against bowstringing of the extrinsic flexor tendons.

► protects the median nerve.

In the condition known as carpal tunnel syndrome, the median nerve is compressed in this relatively unyielding space (see "Intervention Strategies" section). The tendons that pass *deep* to the flexor retinaculum (see Fig. 16-6) include:

► flexor digitorum superficialis (FDS).

► flexor digitorum profundus (FDP).

► flexor pollicis longus (FPL).

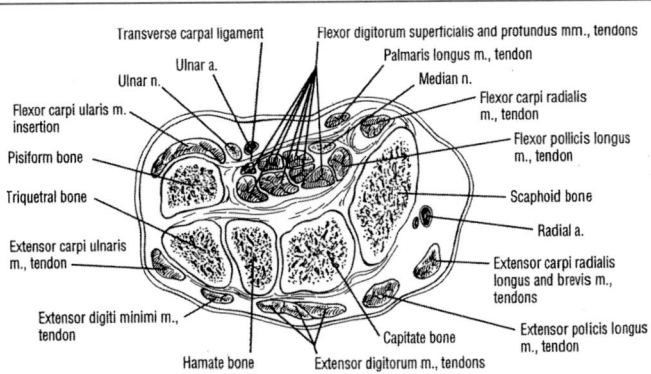

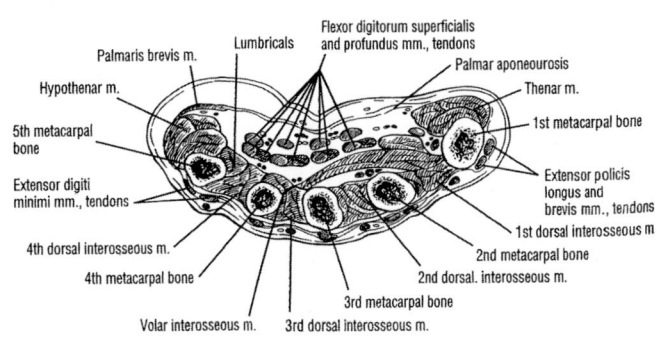

FIGURE 16-6 Distal cross section of the left hand at the level of the pisiform and the midshaft level of the metacarpal bones. (Reproduced with permission from Herndon JH. *Surgical Reconstruction of the Upper Extremity.* Stamford, CT: Appleton & Lange; 1999.)

▶ flexor carpi radialis (FCR).

Structures that pass *superficial* to the flexor retinaculum (see Fig. 16-6) include the:

▶ ulnar nerve and artery.

▶ the tendon of the palmaris longus.

▶ the sensory branch (palmar branch) of the median nerve (not shown).

Fibrous sheaths between the distal palmar crease and the proximal interphalangeal (PIP) joints bind the flexor tendons to the fingers. Some surgeons refer to the area where the sheaths contain two tendons as "no man's land."[6]

Carpal Tunnel

The carpal tunnel serves as a conduit for the median nerve and nine flexor tendons. The palmar radiocarpal ligament and the palmar ligament complex form the floor of the canal. As mentioned previously, the roof of the tunnel is formed by the flexor retinaculum (transverse carpal ligament). The ulnar and radial borders are formed by carpal bones (trapezium and hook of hamate, respectively). Within the tunnel, the median nerve divides into a motor branch and distal sensory branches.

Tunnel of Guyon

The tunnel of Guyon (Fig. 16-7) is a depression superficial to the flexor retinaculum, located between the hook of the hamate

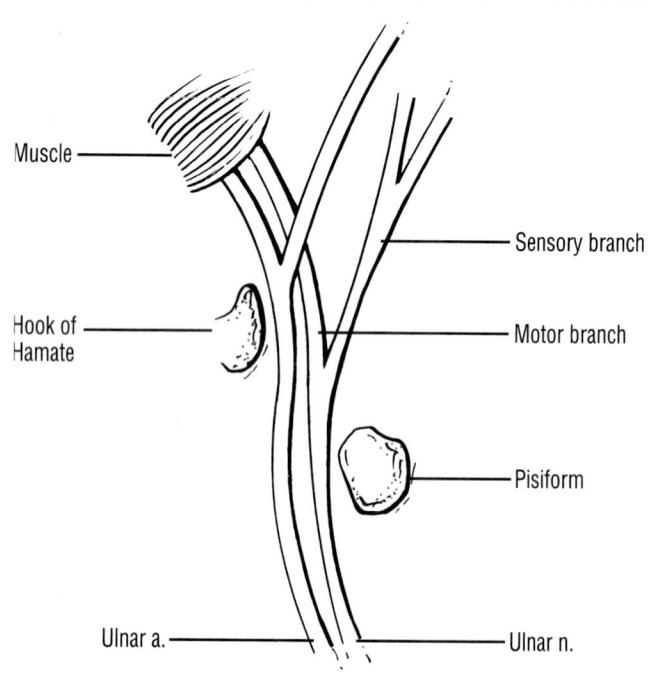

Muscle

Hook of Hamate

Sensory branch

Motor branch

Pisiform

Ulnar a.

Ulnar n.

FIGURE 16-7 Coronal anatomy. Guyon's canal. (Reproduced with permission from Herndon JH. *Surgical Reconstruction of the Upper Extremity.* Stamford, CT: Appleton & Lange; 1999.)

and the pisiform bones. The palmar (volar) carpal ligament, palmaris brevis muscle, and the palmar aponeurosis form its roof. Its floor is formed by the flexor retinaculum (transverse carpal ligament), pisohamate ligament, and pisometacarpal ligament.[6] The tunnel serves as a passageway for the ulnar nerve and artery into the hand.

Phalanges

The fourteen phalanges each consist of a base, shaft, and head (Fig. 16-8). Two shallow depressions, which correspond to the pulley-shaped heads of the adjacent phalanges, mark the concave proximal bases. Two distinct convex condyles produce the pulley-shaped configuration of the phalangeal heads.[6]

Metacarpophalangeal Joints of the Second through Fifth Fingers

The five metacarpals resemble miniature versions of the long bones of the body, with elongated shafts and expanded ends. The second through fifth metacarpals articulate with the respective proximal phalanges in biaxial joints. Their widened, proximal bases articulate with the carpals and with one another in plane joints.[10] Their biconvex distal heads are broader anteriorly than posteriorly, the significance of which is discussed later.

The metacarpophalangeal (MCP) joints allow flexion-extension and medial-lateral deviation associated with a slight degree of axial rotation. The design of the MCP joint allows for a great amplitude of movement, at the expense of stability.

Approximately 90 degrees of flexion is available at the second MCP. The amount of available flexion progressively increases towards the fifth MCP. Active extension at these joints is 25 to 30 degrees, while 90 degrees is obtainable passively. A loss of flexion and extension at the carpometacarpal (CMC) joint of the little finger reduces the amount of opposition available, resulting in dysfunction of the prehensile pattern and difficulty in making a fist.[6] Approximately 20 degrees of abduction/adduction can occur in either direction, with more being available in extension than in flexion.

> **Clinical Pearl**
>
> Abduction-adduction movements of the MCP joints are restricted in flexion and freer in extension.[21]

> **Clinical Pearl**
>
> The goal of function for the MCP joint flexion is 75 degrees for the index finger and middle finger, 80 degrees for the ring finger, and 85 degrees for the little finger.

The joint capsules are attached to the articular margins of the metacarpals and phalanges and surround the MCP joints. The joint capsule of these joints is relatively lax and redundant, endowed with collateral ligaments that pass posterior to the joint axis for flexion/extension of the MCP joints (see Fig. 16-8).

WRIST AND HAND BONES

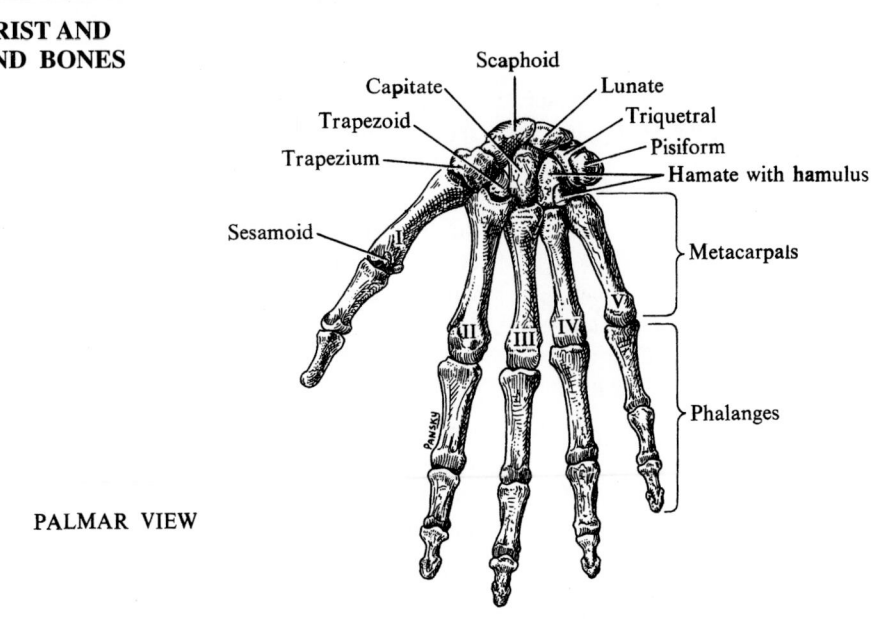

PALMAR VIEW

- Capitate
- Scaphoid
- Lunate
- Trapezoid
- Triquetral
- Trapezium
- Pisiform
- Hamate with hamulus
- Sesamoid
- Metacarpals
- Phalanges

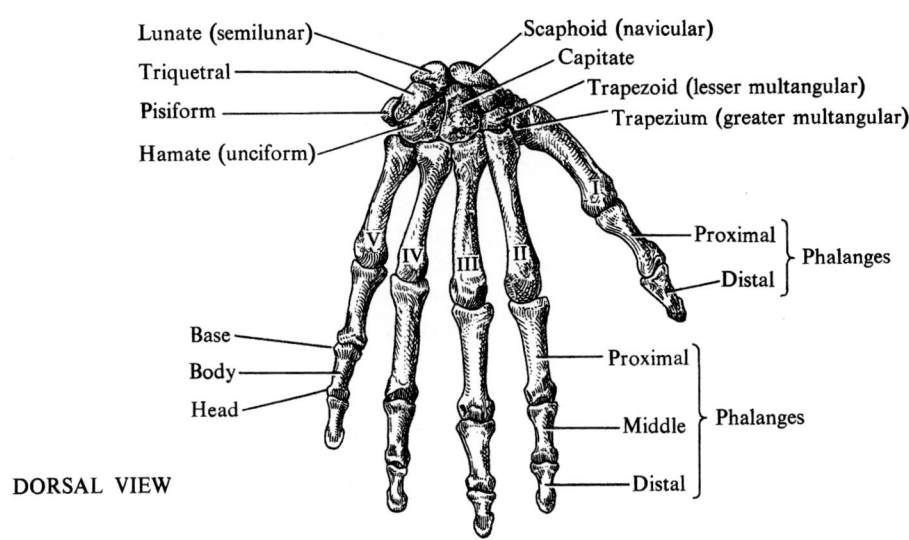

DORSAL VIEW

- Lunate (semilunar)
- Scaphoid (navicular)
- Capitate
- Triquetral
- Trapezoid (lesser multangular)
- Pisiform
- Trapezium (greater multangular)
- Hamate (unciform)
- Proximal
- Distal
- Phalanges
- Base
- Body
- Head
- Proximal
- Middle
- Distal
- Phalanges

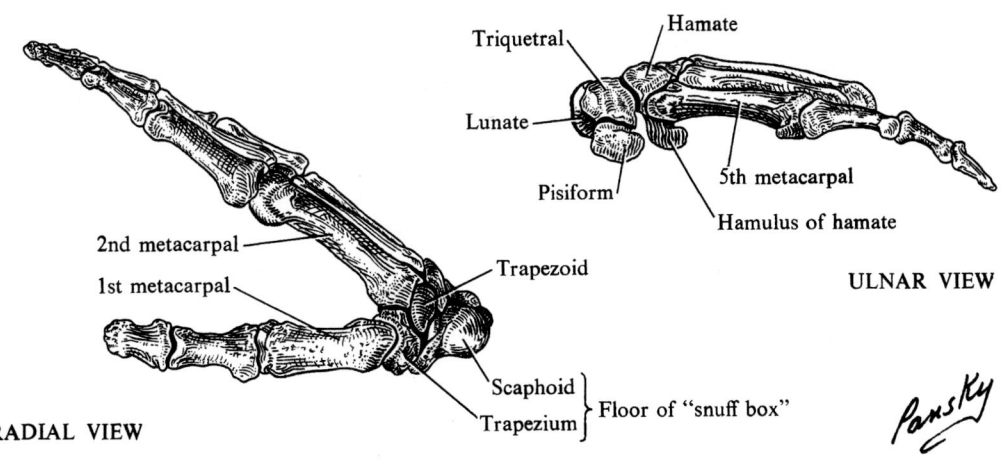

RADIAL VIEW

- 2nd metacarpal
- 1st metacarpal
- Trapezoid
- Scaphoid
- Trapezium
- Floor of "snuff box"

ULNAR VIEW

- Triquetral
- Hamate
- Lunate
- Pisiform
- 5th metacarpal
- Hamulus of hamate

FIGURE 16-8 Wrist and hand bones. (Reproduced with permission from Pansky B. *Review of Gross Anatomy*, 6th ed. New York: McGraw-Hill; 1996.)

Although lax in extension, these collateral ligaments become taut in approximately 70 to 90 degrees of flexion of the MCP joint.[20]

The dorsal hood apparatus reinforces (or replaces) the dorsal joint capsules. The fibrocartilaginous volar plates reinforce the palmar aspects of the joints (Fig. 16-9). The volar plates attach firmly to the phalangeal bases, but connect only loosely to the metacarpal heads by membranous fibers. Their dorsal surface contributes to the joint area, while their palmar surface channels the finger flexor tendons.[21]

The asymmetry of the metacarpal heads as well as the difference in length and direction of the collateral ligaments also explains the rotational movement of the proximal phalanx during flexion-extension and why the ulnar deviation of the digits normally is greater than the radial deviation.[21] The rotary movements that occur are called conjunct rotations. The index finger has a conjunct rotation of internal rotation with abduction and flexion, whereas the ring and little finger each have a conjunct rotation of external rotation with abduction and flexion. The middle finger is not thought to have a conjunct rotation.

Carpometacarpal Joints

The distal borders of the distal carpal row bones articulate with the bases of the metacarpals, thereby forming the carpometacarpal (CMC) joints. The CMC joints progress in mobility from the second to the fifth.

Stability for the CMC joints is provided by the palmar and dorsal carpometacarpal and intermetacarpal ligaments. While the trapezoid articulates with only one metacarpal, all of the other members of the distal carpal row combine one carpal bone with two or more metacarpals (see Fig. 16-8).

First Carpometacarpal Joint

The thumb is the most important digit of the hand and greatly magnifies the complexity of human prehension.[21a] Functionally, the sellar (saddle-shaped) carpometacarpal (CMC) joint is the most important joint of the thumb and consists of the articulation between the base of the first metacarpal and the distal aspect of the trapezium.

The articular surfaces of the trapezium and the proximal end of the first metacarpal are reciprocally shaped. Three other adjacent articulations are functionally related to this joint, which include the joints between the trapezium and the scaphoid, the trapezium and the trapezoid, and the base of the first metacarpal and the radial side of the base of the second metacarpal.[21a]

Motions that can occur at this joint include flexion/extension, adduction/abduction, and opposition, which includes varying amounts of flexion, internal rotation, and palmar adduction (see "Biomechanics" section and Fig. 16-10). Although the joint capsule of the first CMC joint is large and relatively loose, motions at the joint are controlled and supported by muscle actions, and by at least five ligaments: anterior oblique, ulnar collateral, intermetacarpal, posterior oblique, and radial collateral. In general, most of the thumb ligaments are placed on tension with abduction, extension, and opposition.[21a]

Metacarpophalangeal Joint of the Thumb

The metacarpophalangeal (MCP) joint of the thumb is a hinge joint. Its bony configuration, which resembles the interphalangeal joints, provides it with some inherent stability. In addition, support for the joint is provided by palmar and collateral ligaments. The MCP joint of the thumb consists of a convex surface on the head of the metacarpal, and a concave surface on the base of the phalanx. The area of the articulating surface is increased by the presence of a volar plate, which allows greater range of motion than would be available otherwise. Approximately 75 to 80 degrees of flexion is available at this joint. The extension movements as well as the abduction and adduction motions are negligible. Traction, gliding, and rotatory accessory movement are also present.

Interphalangeal Joints

Adjacent phalanges articulate in hinge joints that allow motion in only one plane. The congruency of the interphalangeal (IP) joint surfaces contributes greatly to finger joint stability. In addition, the IP joints are surrounded by joint capsules that are attached to the articular margins of the phalanges.

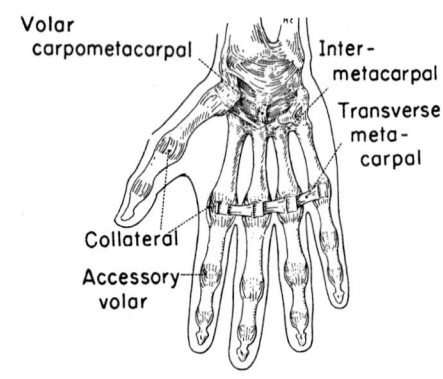

FIGURE 16-9 Volar plates. (Reproduced with permission from Luttgens K, Hamilton K. *Kinesiology: Scientific Basis of Human Motion.* New York: McGraw-Hill; 1997.)

FIGURE 16-10 Movements of the thumb. (Reproduced with permission from Luttgens K, Hamilton K. *Kinesiology: Scientific Basis of Human Motion.* New York: McGraw-Hill; 1997.)

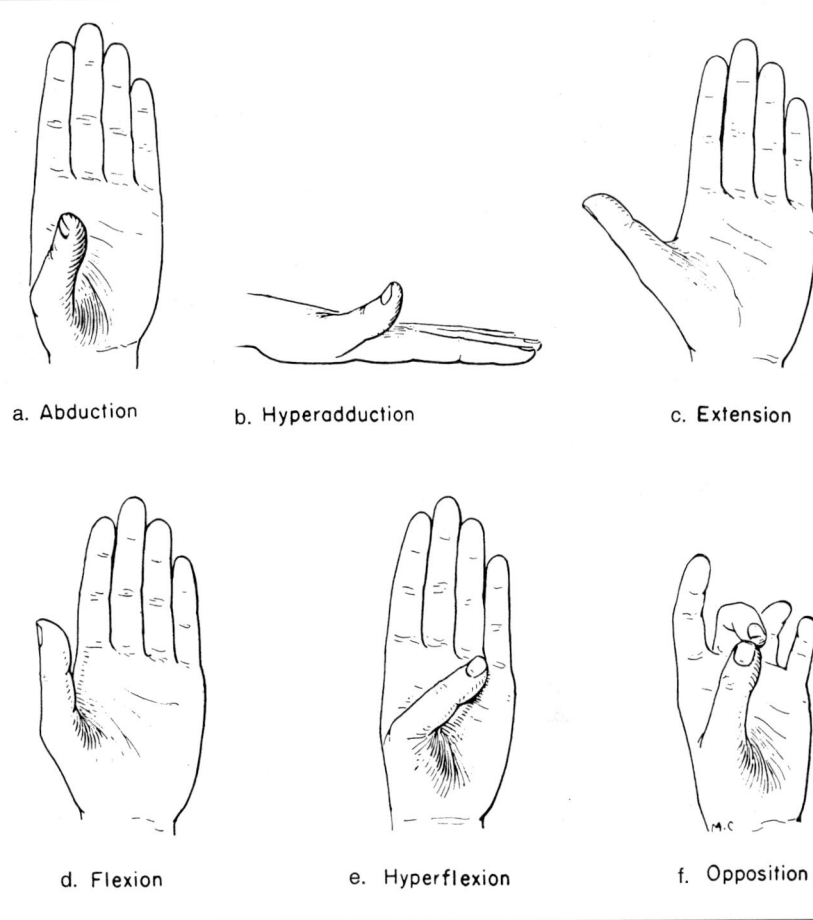

a. Abduction   b. Hyperadduction   c. Extension

d. Flexion   e. Hyperflexion   f. Opposition

Proximal Interphalangeal Joint (PIP)

The PIP joint is a hinged joint capable of flexion and extension. The supporting ligaments and tendons provide the bulk of the static and dynamic stability of this joint as it travels through a normal range of 110 degrees.[20,22–25] The capsule surrounding the articular surface of the joint is composed of the volar plate, lateral and accessory collateral ligaments, and extensor expansion.

The proximal interphalangeal joint is stable in all positions. The configuration of the volar plate allows it to function as a static restraint to hyperextension, and to influence the mechanical advantage of the flexor tendons at the initiation of PIP joint flexion.[20] The volar plate also increases the surface area. This allows for a greater range of motion than would be available otherwise.

The thick collateral ligaments (true and accessory) of the PIP joint combine with the volar plate to provide lateral stability: the collateral ligaments of the PIP joints are maximally taut at 25 degrees of finger flexion.[20] For this reason the IP joints are usually splinted in 25 degrees of flexion following surgery to prevent joint contractures. The splinting position is changed as the patient resumes function.

The flexor tendon system at the level of the PIP joint is less complex than the extensor mechanism and contributes very little to injuries about the PIP joint.[20]

The phalangeal bases effectively form a sellar surface, with bone projections allowing for a wide range of accessory movements to accommodate the gripping of a large array of irregular surfaces.

The motions available at these joints consist of approximately 110 degrees of flexion at the PIP joints and 90 degrees at the thumb interphalangeal (IP) joint. Extension reaches 0 degrees at the PIP joints, and 25 degrees at the thumb IP joint. Traction, gliding, and accessory movement also occur at the IP joints.

Distal Interphalangeal Joints (DIP)

The distal interphalangeal joint has similar structures but less stability and allows some hyperextension. The motions available at these joints consist of approximately 90 degrees of flexion and 25 degrees of extension. Traction, gliding, and accessory movement also occur at the DIP joints.

Palmar Aponeurosis

The palmar aponeurosis is located just deep to the subcutaneous tissue. It is a dense fibrous structure continuous with the palmaris longus tendon and fascia covering the thenar and hypothenar muscles. The aponeurosis travels distally to attach to the transverse metacarpal ligaments and flexor tendon sheaths.

The aponeurosis offers some protection for the ulnar artery and nerve, and digital vessels and nerves. From the central region of the palm, the aponeurosis continues toward the fingers and splits into four slips. As these slips approach the MCP joints, they split and wrap around the tendons of their respective digit. Dupuytren's contracture is a fibrotic condition of the palmar aponeurosis that results in nodule formation or scarring of the aponeurosis, and which may ultimately cause finger flexion contractures (see "Intervention Strategies" section).

Extensor Hood

At the level of the MCP joint, the tendon of the extensor digitorum fans out to cover the dorsal aspect of the joint in a hood-like structure. A complex tendon that covers the dorsal aspect of the digits is formed from a combination of the tendons of insertion from the extensor digitorum (ED), extensor indicis, and extensor digiti minimi. The distal portion of the hood receives the tendons of the lumbricals and interossei over the proximal phalanx. The tendons of the intrinsic muscles pass palmar to the MCP joint axes, but dorsal to the PIP and DIP joint axes. Between the MCP and PIP joints, the complete, complex ED tendon (after all contributions have been received) splits into three parts: a central slip, and two lateral bands[6]:

▶ *A central band.* This band inserts into the proximal dorsal edge of the middle phalanx.

▶ *The lateral bands.* These bands rejoin over the middle phalanx into a terminal tendon, which inserts into the proximal dorsal edge of the distal phalanx. Rupture of the tendon insertion into the distal phalanx produces a "mallet" finger (see "Intervention Strategies" section). The lateral bands, comprised of fibers from both extrinsic and intrinsic tendons, are prevented from dislocating dorsally by the transverse retinacular ligaments, which link them to the volar plates of the PIP joints.[6]

The arrangement of the muscles and tendons in this expansion hood, creates a cable-like system that provides a mechanism for extending the MCP and IP joints, and allows the lumbrical and possibly interosseous muscles to assist in the flexion of the MCP joints.

Stretching or laxity of these supporting structures allows "bowstringing" of the lateral bands, which transmit excessive extension force to the PIP joint.[6]

The oblique retinacular ligament (Landsmeer's ligament) assists in the extensor hood mechanism. The ligament attaches between the PIP volar plate, where it is palmar to the PIP joint axis, and the terminal tendon, where it is dorsal to the DIP joint axis. This relationship to the PIP and DIP joints is essentially the same as that of the intrinsic muscles (lumbricals and interosseous) to the MP and PIP joints—when the PIP joint extends, the oblique retinacular ligament exerts a passive extensor force on the DIP joint, and when the PIP joint flexes, it allows the DIP joint to flex.[26]

Proximal interphalangeal joint position also may influence DIP joint position through lateral band action. The lateral bands normally slip palmarly upon PIP joint flexion, decreasing the excursion required for full DIP joint flexion. If scar tissue tethers the lateral bands so that they do not move palmarly, then a person cannot fully flex both the PIP and DIP joints at the same time.[6]

Synovial Sheaths

Synovial sheaths can be thought of as long narrow balloons filled with synovial fluid, which wrap around a tendon so that one part of the balloon wall (visceral layer) is directly on the tendon, while the other part of the balloon wall (parietal layer) is separate.[18] During wrist motions, the sheaths move longitudinally, reducing friction.

At the wrist, the tendons of both the flexor digitorum superficialis and flexor digitorum profundus are essentially covered by a synovial sheath and pass dorsal (deep) to the flexor retinaculum. The flexor digitorum profundus tendons are dorsal to those of the flexor digitorum superficialis.

In the palm, the flexor digitorum superficialis and flexor digitorum profundus tendons are covered for a variable distance by a synovial sheath.

At the base of the digits, both sets of tendons enter a "fibro-osseous tunnel" formed by the bones of the digit (head of the metatarsals and phalanges) and a fibrous digital tendon sheath on the palmar surface of the digits.

Flexor Pulleys

Annular (A) and cruciate (C) pulleys (Fig. 16-11) restrain the flexor tendons to the metacarpals and phalanges and contribute to fibro-osseous tunnels through which the tendons travel.[17] The A1 pulley arises from the MP joint and volar plate; A2 from the proximal phalanx; A3 from the PIP joint volar plate; A4 from the middle phalanx; and A5 from the DIP joint volar plate.[17] The C1 pulley originates near the head of the proximal phalanx; C2 near the base of the middle phalanx; and C3 near the head of the middle phalanx.[17]

The pulley system of the thumb includes the A1 arising from the MP joint palmar plate, A2 from the IP joint palmar plate, and the oblique pulley from the proximal phalanx.[17]

Muscles of the Wrist and Forearm

The muscles of the forearm, wrist, and hand (Table 16-2) can be subdivided into the 19 intrinsic muscles that arise and insert within the hand, and the 24 extrinsic muscles that originate in the forearm and insert within the hand.[4] The flexors, which are located in the anterior compartment, flex the wrist and digits while the extensors, located in the posterior compartment, extend the wrist and the digits.

The extrinsic group, whose muscle bellies lie proximal to the wrist, join with intrinsic muscles located entirely within the hand. This design provides for a large number of muscles to act on the hand without excessive bulkiness. The extrinsic tendons enhance wrist stability by balancing flexor and extensor forces and compressing the carpals.

The amount of tendon excursion determines the available range of motion at a joint. To calculate the amount of tendon

FIGURE 16-11 Flexor pulleys. (Reproduced with permission from Herndon JH. *Surgical Reconstruction of the Upper Extremity.* Stamford, CT: Appleton & Lange; 1999.)

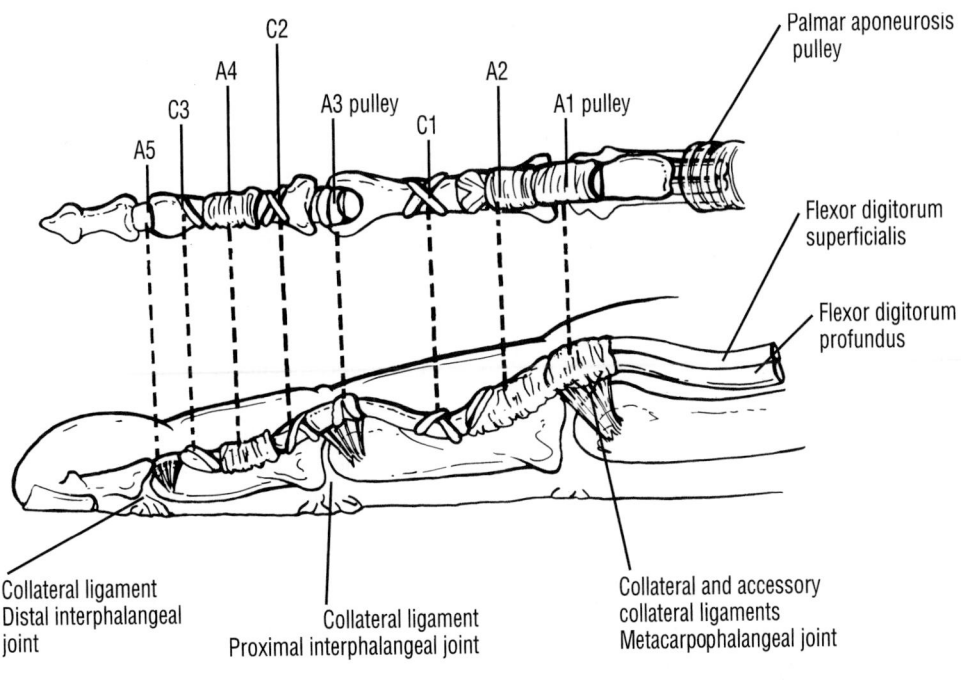

Collateral ligament Distal interphalangeal joint

Collateral ligament Proximal interphalangeal joint

Collateral and accessory collateral ligaments Metacarpophalangeal joint

Palmar aponeurosis pulley

Flexor digitorum superficialis

Flexor digitorum profundus

excursion needed to produce a certain number of degrees of joint motion involves an appreciation of geometry. A circle's radius equals approximately 1 radian (57.29 degrees). The mathematical radius, which is equivalent to the moment arm, represents the amount of tendon excursion required to move the joint through 1 radian.[27] For example, if a joint's moment arm is 10 mm, the tendon must glide 10 mm to move the joint 60 degrees (approximately 1 radian) or 5 mm to move the joint 30 degrees (½ radian).[17]

Anterior Compartment of the Forearm
Superficial Muscles
Pronator Teres. The pronator teres is described in Chapter 15.

Flexor Carpi Radialis (FCR). The FCR (Fig. 16-12) originates from the medial humeral epicondyle as part of the common flexor tendon. It inserts on the ventral surface and base of the second metacarpal, possibly providing a slip to the third metacarpal. The FCR is innervated by the median nerve, and functions to flex and radially deviate the wrist.

Palmaris Longus. The inconsistent palmaris longus (see Fig. 16-12) arises from the medial humeral epicondyle as part of the common flexor tendon, and inserts on the transverse carpal ligament and palmar aponeurosis. It receives its innervation from the median nerve. The function of the palmaris longus is to flex the wrist, and it may play a role in thumb abduction in some people.[14]

Flexor Carpi Ulnaris (FCU). The FCU (Fig. 16-12) arises from two heads. The humeral head arises from the medial humeral epicondyle as part of the common flexor tendon, while the ulnar head arises from the proximal portion of the subcutaneous bor-

der of the ulna. The FCU inserts directly onto the pisiform, the hamate via the pisohamate ligament, and onto the ventral surface of the base of the fifth metacarpal, via the pisometacarpal ligament. The FCU is innervated by the ulnar nerve and functions to flex and ulnarly deviate the wrist.

Intermediate Muscle
Flexor Digitorum Superficialis (FDS). The FDS (see Fig. 16-12) has a three-headed origin. The humeral head arises from the medial humeral epicondyle as part of the common flexor tendon. The ulnar head arises from the coronoid process of the ulna. The radial head arises from the oblique line of the radius. The FDS inserts on the middle phalanx of the medial four digits via a split, "sling" tendon. This muscle is innervated by the median nerve and serves to flex the proximal and middle interphalangeal joints of the medial four digits, and assist with elbow flexion and wrist flexion. The FDS possesses tendons that are capable of relatively independent action at each finger.

Deep Muscles
Flexor Pollicis Longus (FPL). The FPL (see Fig. 16-12) has its origin on the ventral surface of the radius, medial border of the coronoid process of the ulna, and the adjacent interosseous membrane. It inserts on the distal phalanx of the thumb. The FPL is innervated by the anterior interosseous branch of the median nerve, and it functions to flex the thumb.

Flexor Digitorum Profundus (FDP). The FDP (see Fig. 16-12) arises from the medial and ventral surfaces of the proximal ulna, the adjacent interosseous membrane, and the deep fascia of the forearm. The FDP inserts on the base of the distal phalanges of the medial 4 digits. The FDP has a dual nerve supply:

TABLE 16-2   Muscles of the Wrist, and Hand: Their Actions and Nerve Supply

Action	Muscles	Nerve Supply
Wrist extension	Extensor carpi radialis longus	Radial
	Extensor carpi radialis brevis	Posterior interosseous
	Extensor carpi ulnaris	Posterior interosseous
Wrist flexion	Flexor carpi radialis	Median
	Flexor carpi ulnaris	Ulnar
Ulnar deviation of wrist	Flexor carpi ulnaris	Ulnar
	Extensor carpi ulnaris	Posterior interosseous
Radial deviation of wrist	Flexor carpi radialis	Median
	Extensor carpi radialis longus	Radial
	Abductor pollicis longus	Posterior interosseous
	Extensor pollicis brevis	Posterior interosseous
Finger extension	Extensor digitorum communis	Posterior interosseous
	Extensor indicis	Posterior interosseous
	Extensor digiti minimi	Posterior interosseous
Finger flexion	Flexor digitorum profundus	Anterior interosseous, lateral two digits
		Ulnar, medial two digits
	Flexor digitorum superficialis	Median
		First and second: median
	Lumbricals	Third and fourth: ulnar
	Interossei	Ulnar
	Flexor digiti minimi	Ulnar
Abduction of fingers	Dorsal interossei	Ulnar
	Abductor digiti minimi	Ulnar
Adduction of fingers	Palmar interossei	Ulnar
Thumb extension	Extensor pollicis longus	Posterior interosseous
	Extensor pollicis brevis	Posterior interosseous
	Abductor pollicis longus	Posterior interosseous
Thumb flexion	Flexor pollicis brevis	Superficial head: median
		Deep head: ulnar
	Flexor pollicis longus	Anterior interosseous
	Opponens pollicis	Median
Abduction of thumb	Abductor pollicis longus	Posterior interosseous
	Abductor pollicis brevis	Median
Adduction of thumb	Adductor pollicis	Ulnar
Opposition of thumb and little finger	Opponens pollicis	Median
	Flexor pollicis brevis	Superficial head: median
	Abductor pollicis brevis	Median
	Opponens digiti minimi	Ulnar

FIGURE 16-12 Flexor muscles. (Reproduced with permission from Marble HC. *The Hand: A Manual and Atlas for the General Surgeon.* Philadelphia: WB Saunders; 1961.)

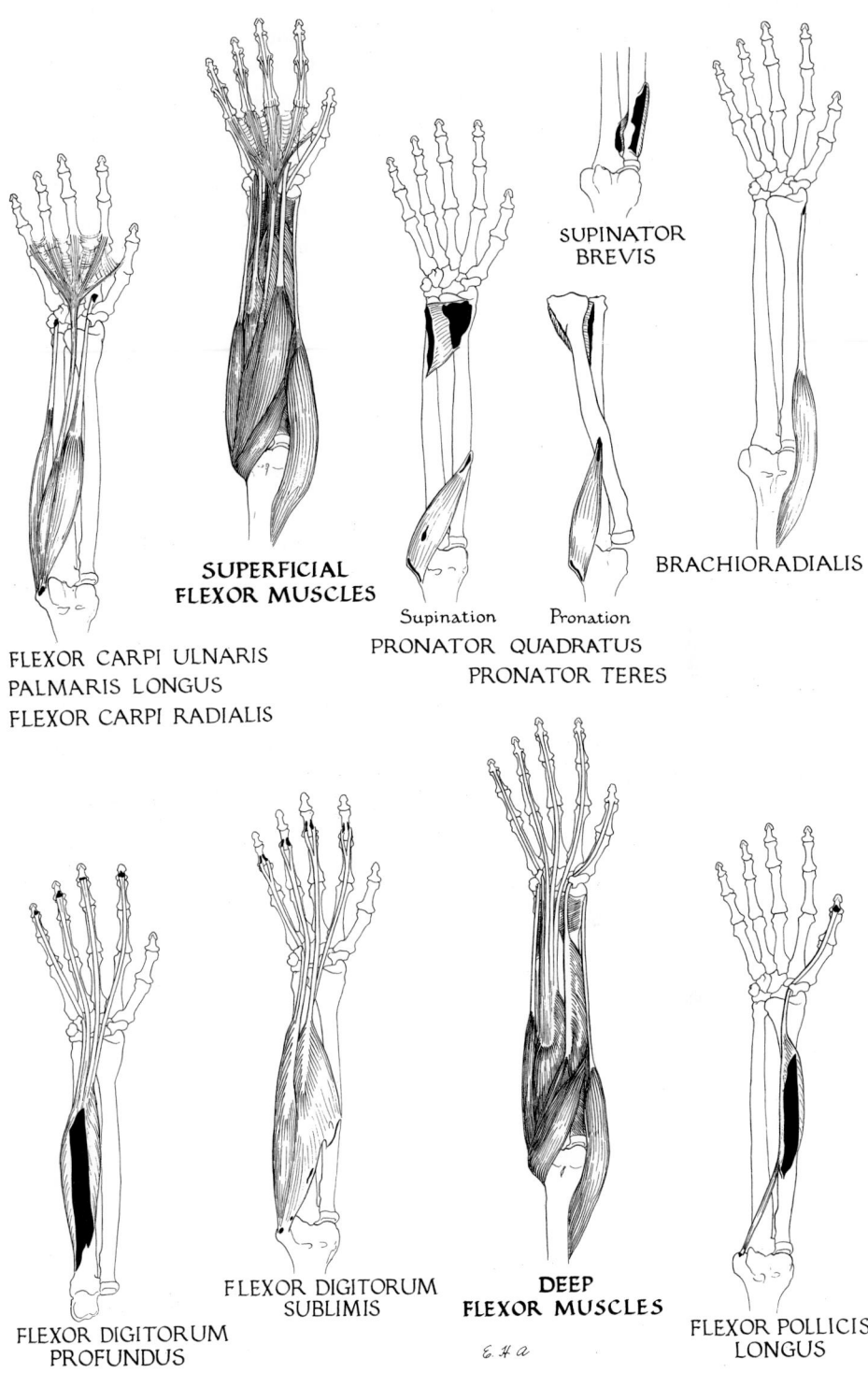

SUPINATOR BREVIS

SUPERFICIAL FLEXOR MUSCLES

BRACHIORADIALIS

Supination   Pronation
PRONATOR QUADRATUS
PRONATOR TERES

FLEXOR CARPI ULNARIS
PALMARIS LONGUS
FLEXOR CARPI RADIALIS

FLEXOR DIGITORUM PROFUNDUS

FLEXOR DIGITORUM SUBLIMIS

DEEP FLEXOR MUSCLES

FLEXOR POLLICIS LONGUS

the medial two heads are supplied by the ulnar nerve, while the lateral two heads are supplied by the anterior interosseous branch of the median nerve. The FDP functions to flex the distal interphalangeal (DIP) joints, after the FDS flexes the second phalanges, and assists with flexion of the wrist. The tendons of the FDS and FDP are held against the phalanges by a fibrous sheath. At strategic locations along the sheath, five dense annular pulleys (designated A1, A2, A3, A4, and A5) and three thinner cruciform pulleys (designated C1, C2, and C3) prevent tendon bowstringing (see Fig. 16-11).[28]

Unlike the FDS tendons, the FDP tendons cannot act independently. To isolate the PIP joint flexor function of these two muscles, a clinician holds the adjoining finger(s) in extension while the patient attempts to flex the finger being tested. This anchors the profundus muscle of the finger being tested distally, and allows the superficialis muscle to act alone at the PIP joint.

Tendinous connections between the FDP and the FPL is a common anatomic anomaly, which has been linked to a condition causing chronic forearm pain, called Linburg syndrome,[29] although the association is by no means conclusive.[30]

Pronator Quadratus. The pronator quadratus (see Fig. 16-12) arises from the ventral surface and distal quarter of the ulna, and inserts on the ventral surface and distal quarter of the radius.

The muscle functions to pronate the forearm and it is innervated by the anterior interosseous branch of the median nerve.

Posterior Compartment of the Forearm
Superficial Muscles

Extensor Carpi Radialis Longus (ECRL). The ECRL (Fig. 16-13) takes its origin at the supracondylar ridge of the humerus about 4 to 5 cm proximal to the epicondyle, and the thickest part of the muscle is proximal to the elbow joint. The ECRL inserts on the base of the second metacarpal, and functions to extend and

FIGURE 16-13 Extensor muscles. (Reproduced with permission from Marble HC. *The Hand: A Manual and Atlas for the General Surgeon.* Philadelphia: WB Saunders; 1961.)

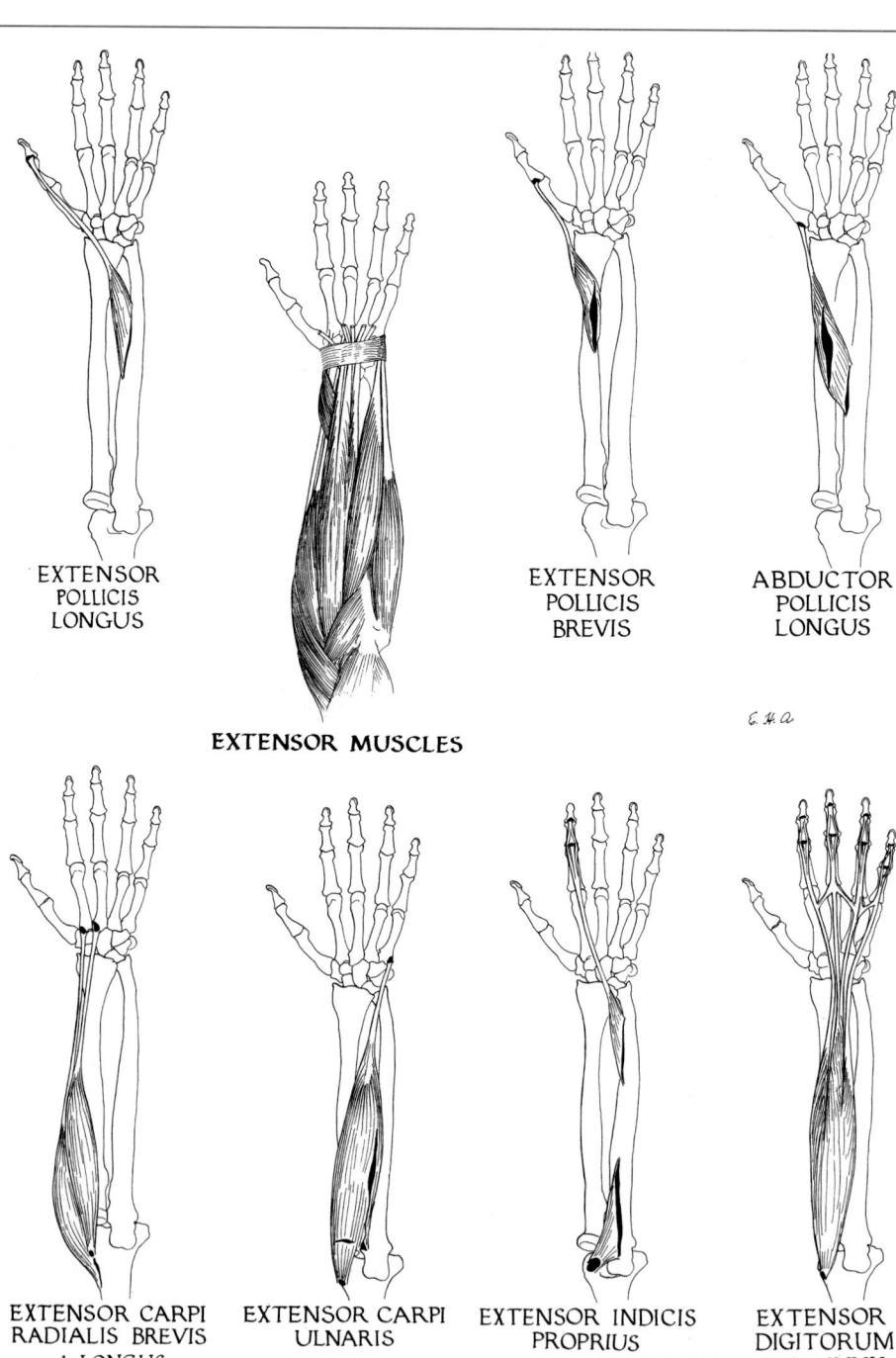

EXTENSOR
POLLICIS
LONGUS

EXTENSOR
POLLICIS
BREVIS

ABDUCTOR
POLLICIS
LONGUS

EXTENSOR MUSCLES

EXTENSOR CARPI
RADIALIS BREVIS
and LONGUS

EXTENSOR CARPI
ULNARIS

EXTENSOR INDICIS
PROPRIUS
ANCONAEUS

EXTENSOR
DIGITORUM
COMMUNIS

radially deviate the wrist. It also plays a role in elbow flexion, losing a part of its wrist action when the elbow is flexed.[21]

Extensor Carpi Radialis Brevis (ECRB). The extensor carpialis brevis (ECRB) (see Fig. 16-13) arises from the common extensor tendon on the lateral epicondyle of the humerus, and from the radial collateral ligament. It inserts on the posterior surface of the base of the third metacarpal bone, and receives its nerve supply from the posterior interosseous branch of the radial nerve. The muscle stretches across the radial head during pronation, resulting in increased tensile stress when the forearm is pronated, the wrist is flexed, and the elbow is extended. The more medial location of the ECRB compared to the ECRL makes it the primary wrist extensor, but it has also a slight action of radial deviation.

Extensor Digitorum and Extensor Digiti Minimi. The extensor digitorum (see Fig. 16-13) arises from the lateral humeral epicondyle, part of the common extensor tendon, while the extensor digiti minimi (EDM) arises from a muscular slip from the ulnar aspect of the extensor digitorum muscle. The extensor digitorum inserts on the lateral and dorsal aspect of the medial 4 digits, while the EDM inserts on the proximal phalanx of the 5th digit. Both muscles are innervated by the posterior interosseous branch of the radial nerve. While the extensor digitorum functions to extend the medial 4 digits, the EDM extends the fifth digit.

Extensor Carpi Ulnaris (ECU). The extensor carpi ulnaris (ECU) arises from the common extensor tendon on the lateral epicondyle of the humerus and the posterior border of the ulna. It inserts on the medial side of the base of the fifth metacarpal bone (see Fig. 16-13). It is innervated by the posterior interosseous branch of the radial nerve. The ECU is an extensor of the wrist in supination, and primarily causes ulnar deviation of the wrist in pronation, working in synergy with the FCU to prevent radial deviation during pronation.[21]

Extension of the wrist is dependent on three muscles:

▶ Extensor carpi radialis longus (ECRL).

▶ Extensor carpi radialis brevis (ECRB).

▶ Extensor carpi ulnaris (ECU).

The ECRB and ECRL are commonly considered to be similar muscles, but in fact they differ in many respects.[31] The ECRB, because of its origin on the epicondyle, is not affected by the position of the elbow, so that all of its action is on the wrist.[21] Taken together, both ECR tendons comprise about 10 percent of the muscle mass of the forearm and 76 percent of the muscle mass of the extensors of the wrist.[32] The ECRL has longer muscular fibers, mostly at the level of the elbow. The ECRL only becomes a wrist extensor after radial deviation is balanced against the ulnar forces of the ECU.

The ECU, the antagonist of extensor pollicis longus (EPL), has the weakest moment of extension, which becomes zero when the wrist is in complete pronation.

Thus the three wrist extensors have very different moment arms of extension. The ECRB is the most effective extensor of the wrist, because it has the greatest tension and the most favorable moment arm.[21]

Deep Muscles

Abductor Pollicis Longus (APL). The APL (see Fig. 16-13) arises from the dorsal surface of the proximal portion of the radius, ulna, and interosseous membrane, and inserts on the ventral surface of the base of the first metacarpal. The APL is innervated by the posterior interosseous branch of the radial nerve and functions in abduction, extension, and external rotation of the first metacarpal.

Extensor Pollicis Brevis (EPB). The EPB (see Fig. 16-13) arises from the dorsal surface of the radius and interosseous membrane, just distal to the origin of the APL. It inserts on the dorsal surface of the proximal phalanx of the thumb via the extensor expansion. The EPB is innervated by the posterior interosseous branch of the radial nerve and functions in extension of the proximal phalanx of the thumb.

Extensor Pollicis Longus (EPL). The EPL (see Fig. 16-13) arises from the dorsal surface of the midportion of the ulna and interosseous membrane. It inserts on the dorsal surface of the distal phalanx of the thumb via the extensor expansion. The EPL is innervated by the posterior interosseous branch of the radial nerve. It functions in extension of the distal phalanx of the thumb, and is thus involved in extension of the middle phalanx, and the metacarpophalangeal (MCP) joint of the thumb.

Extensor Indicis (EI). The EI (see Fig. 16-13) arises from the dorsal surface of the ulna, distal to the other deep muscles, and inserts on the extensor expansion of the index finger. It is innervated by the posterior interosseous branch of the radial nerve and is involved in extension of the proximal phalanx of the index finger.

Muscles of the Hand

The muscles of the hand are those that originate and insert within the hand, and are responsible for the fine finger movements.

Short Muscles of the Thumb

Abductor Pollicis Brevis (APB). The APB (Fig. 16-14) arises from the flexor retinaculum and the trapezium bone and inserts on the radial aspect of the proximal phalanx of the thumb. It is innervated by the median nerve, and functions to abduct the first metacarpal and proximal phalanx of the thumb.

Flexor Pollicis Brevis (FPB). The FPB (see Fig. 16-14) arises from two heads. The superficial head arises from the flexor retinaculum and the trapezium bone, while the deep head arises from the floor of the carpal canal. The FPB inserts on the base of the proximal phalanx of the thumb. The superficial head receives its innervation from the median nerve, while the deep

FIGURE 16-14 Hand intrinsic muscles. (Reproduced with permission from Marble HC. *The Hand: A Manual and Atlas for the General Surgeon.* Philadelphia: WB Saunders; 1961.)

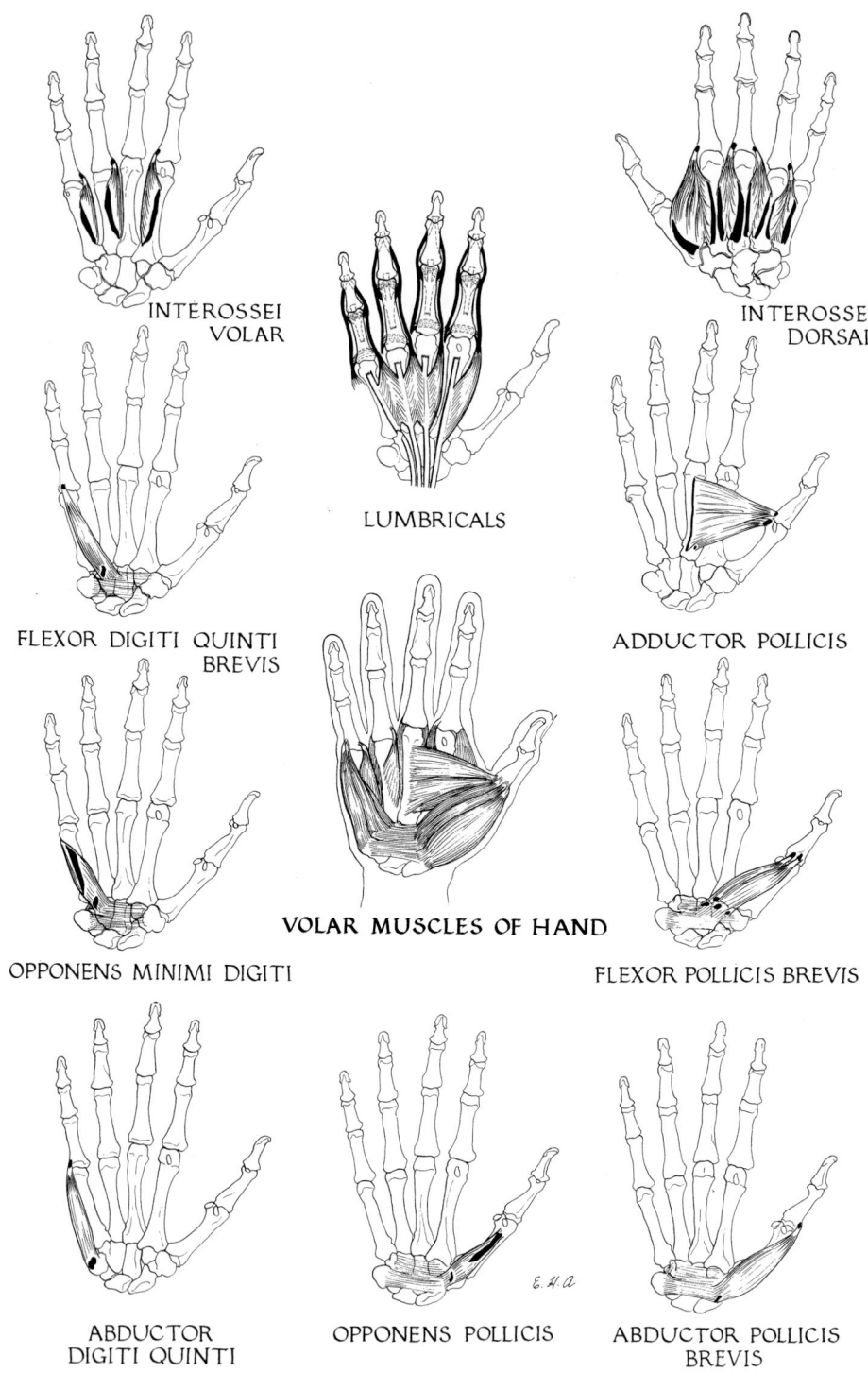

INTEROSSEI VOLAR

INTEROSSEI DORSAL

LUMBRICALS

FLEXOR DIGITI QUINTI BREVIS

ADDUCTOR POLLICIS

VOLAR MUSCLES OF HAND

OPPONENS MINIMI DIGITI

FLEXOR POLLICIS BREVIS

ABDUCTOR DIGITI QUINTI

OPPONENS POLLICIS

ABDUCTOR POLLICIS BREVIS

head is innervated by the ulnar nerve. The FPB functions to flex the proximal phalanx of the thumb.

Opponens Pollicis (OP). The OP (see Fig. 16-14) arises from the flexor retinaculum and the trapezium bone and inserts along the radial surface of the first metacarpal. The OP is innervated by the median nerve, and functions to flex, rotate, and slightly abduct the first metacarpal across the palm to allow for opposition to each of the other digits.

Adductor Pollicis (AP). The AP (see Fig. 16-14) arises from two heads. The transverse head originates from the ventral surface of the shaft of the third metacarpal, while the oblique head originates from the trapezium, trapezoid, and capitate bones, and the base of the second and third metacarpal bone. The AP inserts on the ulnar side of the base of the proximal phalanx of the thumb, and is innervated by the deep branch of the ulnar nerve. The AP functions to adduct the thumb and aids in thumb opposition.

Short Muscles of the Fifth Digit

Abductor Digiti Minimi (ADM). The ADM (see Fig. 16-14) arises from the pisiform bone and the tendon of the flexor carpi ulnaris. It inserts on the ulnar aspect of the base of the proximal phalanx of the fifth digit, together with the flexor digiti minimi brevis. It is innervated by the deep branch of the ulnar nerve and functions to abduct the fifth digit.

Flexor Digiti Minimi (FDM). The FDM (see Fig. 16-14) originates from the flexor retinaculum and the hook of the hamate bone. It inserts on the ulnar aspect of the base of the proximal phalanx of the fifth digit, together with the abductor digiti minimi. It is innervated by the deep branch of the ulnar nerve and functions to flex the proximal phalanx of the fifth digit.

Deep branches of the ulnar artery and nerve enter the thenar mass, and course into the deep region of the hand by passing between the ABD and the FDM.

Opponens Digiti Minimi (ODM). The ODM (see Fig. 16-14) arises from the flexor retinaculum and the hook of the hamate bone, and inserts on the ulnar border of the shaft of the fifth metacarpal bone. It is innervated by the deep branch of the ulnar nerve, and functions to provide a small amount of flexion and external rotation of the fifth digit.

Interosseous Muscles of the Hand

The interossei muscles of the hand are divided by anatomy and function into palmar and dorsal interossei.

Palmar Interossei. The three palmar interossei (see Fig. 16-14) have a variety of origins and insertions. The first interosseus originates from the ulnar surface of the second metacarpal bone and inserts on the ulnar side of the proximal phalanx of the second digit. The second palmar interosseus arises from the radial side of the fourth metacarpal bone, and inserts into the radial side of the proximal phalanx of the fourth digit. The third palmar interosseus originates from the radial side of the fifth metacarpal bone and inserts into the radial side of the proximal phalanx of the fifth digit. The palmar interossei are innervated by the deep branch of the ulnar nerve, and each muscle functions to adduct the digit to which it is attached toward the middle digit. The palmar interossei also function to extend the distal and then the middle phalanges.

Dorsal Interossei. The four dorsal interossei (see Fig. 16-14) have a similar varied origin and insertion as their palmar counterparts. The dorsal interossei originate via two heads from adjacent sides of the metacarpal bones. The first dorsal interosseus

muscle inserts into the radial side of the proximal phalanx of the second digit. The second inserts into the radial side of the proximal phalanx of the third digit. The third inserts into the ulnar side of the proximal phalanx of the third digit, and the fourth inserts into the ulnar side of the proximal phalanx of the fourth digit. The dorsal interossei receive their innervation from the deep branch of the ulnar nerve. The dorsal interossei abduct the index, middle, and ring fingers from the midline of the hand.

Lumbricals

The lumbrical muscles are usually four small intrinsic muscles of the hand that originate from the flexor digitorum profundus (FDP) tendons and insert into the dorsal hood apparatus. Occasionally, more than four lumbricals are found in one hand.[33]

During contraction, they pull the FDP tendons distally, thus possessing the unique ability to relax their own antagonist.[6] They function to perform the motion of interphalangeal joint extension with the MCP joint held in extension, and can assist in MCP flexion.[21]

The lumbrical muscles also serve an important role in the proprioception of the hand, providing feedback about the position and movement of the hand and finger joints.[6]

In instances of lumbrical spasm or contracture, attempts to flex the fingers via the profundus result in transmission of force through the lumbricals into the extensor apparatus, producing extension rather than flexion.[6] A "lumbrical plus" deformity occurs if there is excessive lumbrical force, or if there is imbalance of opposing forces, which produces exaggerated lumbrical action (i.e., MCP joint flexion and IP joint extension).[6]

The lumbricals have dual innervation. Lumbricals I and II are innervated typically by the median nerve, while the third and fourth lumbricals are innervated by the ulnar nerve.

Anatomic Snuffbox

The anatomic snuffbox (Fig. 16-15) is represented by a depression on the dorsal surface of the hand at the base of the thumb, just distal to the radius. This structure can be observed during active radial abduction of the thumb. The radial border of the snuffbox is formed by the tendons of the APL and EPB, while the ulnar border is formed by the tendon of the EPL. Along the floor of the snuffbox is the deep branch of the radial artery and the tendinous insertion of the ECRL. Underneath these structures, the scaphoid and trapezium bones are found.

> ### Clinical Pearl
>
> Tenderness with palpation in the anatomic snuffbox suggests a scaphoid fracture, but also can present in minor wrist injuries or other conditions.[4]

Mobile Arch Systems

The bones and soft tissues of the hand form a number of functional arches of the hand that provide a perfect balance of force distribution in an equiangular spiral. The arches of the hand,

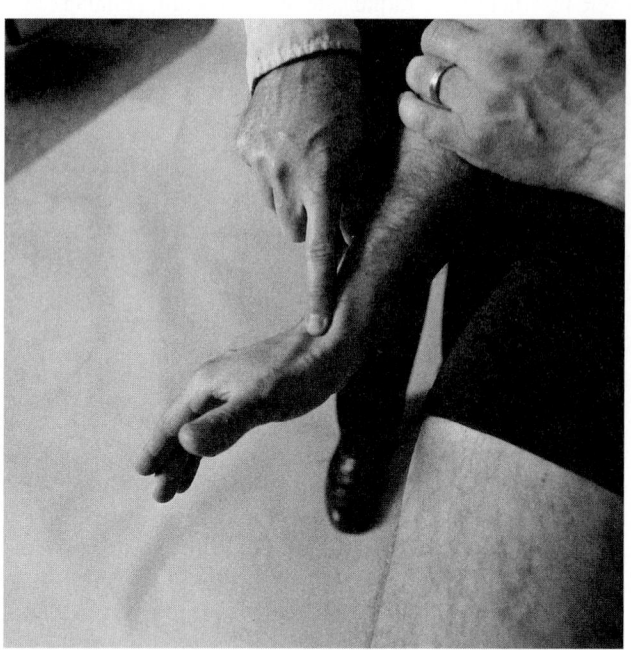

FIGURE 16-15   Anatomic snuffbox.

which are all concave palmarly, serve to enhance prehensile function. This prehensile function is best illustrated by the ability of the human hand to grasp an egg. A number of arches are commonly recognized:

▶ *The transverse arch.*   The proximal, relatively immobile transverse arch is formed within the palmar concavity of the carpal bones.[6] This carpal arch, deepened by the palmar projections of the scaphoid and trapezium laterally and the pisiform and hamate medially, should correspond to the concavity of the wrist. The distal transverse arch is more mobile, and is defined by the alignment of the metacarpals. This arch allows the hand to adapt to objects held in the palm.[17]

▶ *The metacarpal arch.*   This arch is formed by the metacarpal heads is a relatively mobile transverse arch.

▶ *The longitudinal arch.*   This is particularly the arch of the middle finger and the arch of the index finger. The longitudinal arch, which contributes to powerful gripping, spans the hand lengthwise, with its keystone at the MCP joints.[6]

▶ *The oblique arches.*   These arches are formed by the thumb in opposition to the other fingers.

Neurology

The three peripheral nerves that supply the skin and muscles of the wrist and hand include the median, ulnar, and radial nerves.

Median Nerve

The median nerve (Fig. 16-16), which originates from two large roots—the medial cord and the lateral cord—of the brachial plexus, enters the forearm by coursing ventrally through the medial aspect of the cubital fossa and passing deep to the lacertus fibrosis, between the heads of the pronator teres muscle.

Below the elbow, muscular branches leave the nerve and innervate the flexor carpi radialis, palmaris longus, and pronator teres muscles. The anterior interosseous branch comes off at the proximal aspect of the forearm, at the level of the pronator teres, and passes distally along the ventral surface of the interosseous membrane in the groove between the flexor digitorum profundus and flexor pollicis longus muscles. The anterior interosseous branch innervates the pronator quadratus, flexor pollicis longus, and the flexor digitorum profundus to the index finger and middle fingers and sometimes the ring finger.

Approximately 8 cm proximal to the wrist, the median nerve gives off a sensory branch, the palmar cutaneous nerve that passes superficial to the flexor retinaculum and remains outside the carpal tunnel. This nerve innervates the skin in the central aspect of the palm, over the thenar eminence. The rest of the median nerve passes distally to the wrist, where it enters the carpal tunnel, which passes deep to the flexor retinaculum.

The nerve enters the hand through the carpal tunnel, deep to the tendon of the palmaris longus, and in between the tendons of the flexor pollicis longus and flexor digitorum superficialis (more radial of the two). From this point, the nerve divides into two branches, a motor branch which passes dorsal to the flexor retinaculum, and a sensory branch.

Motor Branch.   This short branch enters the thenar eminence, where it usually supplies the abductor pollicis brevis and opponens pollicis muscles, the flexor pollicis brevis (occasionally), and the first and second lumbrical muscles.

Sensory Branch.   The sensory palmar digital branch innervates the palmar surface and dorsal aspect of the distal phalanges of the thumb, second and third fingers, and the radial half of the forefinger.

A number of median nerve entrapment syndromes exist (refer to "Peripheral Nerve Entrapment" section), each with their own clinical features and functional implications. For example, entrapment of the median nerve in the carpal tunnel may result in numbness, pain, or paresthesia of the fingers and may severely hinder a patient's ability to perform precision maneuvers due to loss of critical sensory and motor function in the thumb, index, and middle fingers.

Ulnar Nerve

The ulnar nerve has been referred to as the nerve of fine movements of the hand. The ulnar nerve originates from the inferior roots of the brachial plexus (C 8-T 1). Two branches of the ulnar nerve arise in the midforearm:

1. The palmar cutaneous branch. The palmar cutaneous branch supplies a portion of the skin over the hypothenar eminence.

2. The dorsal cutaneous branch. Eight to 10 cm proximal to the ulnar styloid process, the dorsal cutaneous branch of

FIGURE 16-16 Nerves of the hand. (Reproduced with permission from Marble HC. *The Hand: A Manual and Atlas for the General Surgeon.* Philadelphia: WB Saunders; 1961.)

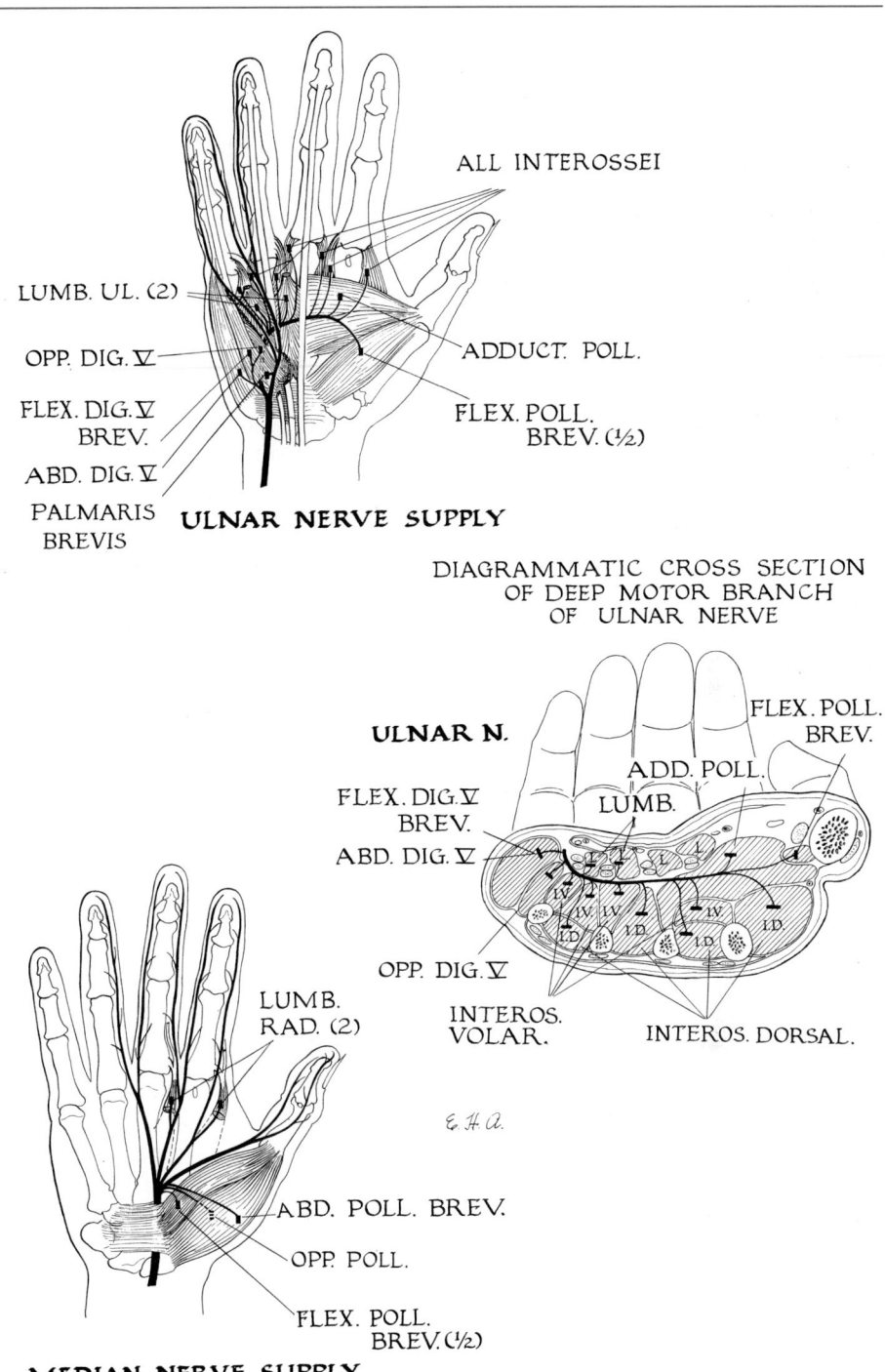

the ulnar nerve splits from the main trunk. The dorsal cutaneous branch terminates into two dorsal digital branches that supply sensation to the dorsal and ulnar aspect of the middle phalanx of the ring and little fingers.[34]

Before reaching the wrist, the ulnar nerve branches to innervate the flexor digitorum profundus and the flexor carpi ulnaris.

At the wrist, the ulnar nerve (see Fig. 16-16) emerges just lateral to the tendon of the flexor carpi ulnaris as it passes superficial to the flexor retinaculum. The ulnar nerve passes into the hand via the tunnel of Guyon, where it divides into its superficial and deep terminal branches. The deep (motor) branch supplies the flexor digiti minimi, abductor digiti minimi, opponens digiti minimi, adductor pollicis, palmaris brevis, third and fourth lumbricals, deep head of the flexor pollicis brevis, and the interossei. The superficial branch, which is primarily sensory with the exception of its innervation to the palmaris brevis, divides into three branches.[34] The first of these three branches is a sensory branch to the ulnar aspect of the little finger, and the second is a sensory branch to the central ulnar palmar area. The third branch, often referred to as the common digital nerve, innervates the fourth intermetacarpal space. The common digital nerve further divides into two proper digital nerves supplying the ulnar portion of the ring finger and the radial portion of the little finger.[34]

A number of ulnar nerve entrapment syndromes exist (refer to "Peripheral Nerve Entrapment" section), each with their own clinical features and functional implications. For example, entrapment of the ulnar nerve in the cubital tunnel may result in numbness, pain, or paresthesia of the little and ring fingers and dorsal-ulnar aspect of the hand and may severely hinder a patient's ability to perform activities that require forceful grasping due to loss of critical motor function in the little finger and hand intrinsic muscles.

Radial Nerve

As the radial nerve enters the cubital fossa, it typically splits into a superficial and deep branch. The superficial branch typically courses distally along the lateral border of the forearm under cover of the brachioradialis muscle and tendon. At the wrist this branch divides into four to five digital branches, which provide cutaneous and articular innervation. The cutaneous innervation includes the lateral two thirds of the dorsum of the hand and the dorsal lateral 2½ fingers to the proximal phalanx.

All of the motor branches of the radial nerve are located in the forearm. The deep branch (posterior interosseous nerve) (see Fig. 16-16) typically penetrates the ventral surface of, and passes through, the supinator muscle. It reaches the deep region of the posterior forearm by passing through the arcade of Fröhse. The nerve courses subcutaneously from the midportion of the forearm to an area adjacent to the styloid process of the radius, and terminates on the dorsum of the wrist.

Clinical Pearl

Radial nerve entrapment (refer to "Peripheral Nerve Entrapment" section) may result in a loss of extension at the wrist and MCP joints of the fingers, and thumb extension and abduction. Since the wrist extensor muscles are synergists and stabilizers for the finger flexor muscles during gripping, this loss can significantly hamper hand function.

Vasculature of the Wrist and Hand

The brachial artery bifurcates at the elbow into radial and ulnar branches, which are the main arterial branches to the hand.

Radial Artery

The radial artery (Fig. 16-17) is formed from the lateral branch of the bifurcation of the brachial artery. The artery gives off branches in the proximal portion of the forearm that form an anastomosis around the elbow joint. It runs distally under the cover of the brachioradialis muscle. Just proximal to the wrist, it is located between the brachioradialis and flexor carpi radialis tendons. A small branch called the superficial palmar artery leaves the radial artery 5 to 8 mm proximal to the tip of the radial styloid, passes between the flexor carpi radialis and brachioradialis, and continues distally to contribute to the superficial palmar arch, which supplies the thenar mass. The radial artery has seven major carpal branches: three dorsal, three palmar, and a final branch that continues distally (see below).

Ulnar Artery

The ulnar artery (see Fig. 16-17) originates as the medial branch from the bifurcation of the brachial artery. It too gives off branches in the proximal portion of the forearm that form an anastomosis around the elbow joint. The artery passes dorsal to the ulnar head of the pronator teres and courses distally deep to the flexor digitorum superficialis, at which point it passes distally in the groove between the flexor carpi ulnaris and flexor digitorum profundus, in the company of the ulnar nerve. In the proximal portion of the forearm, the artery gives off a common interosseous branch. The artery bifurcates, giving rise to the anterior and posterior interosseous arteries, which provide blood to structures in the deep anterior and posterior compartments of the forearm. The artery emerges at the wrist, just lateral to the tendon of the flexor carpi ulnaris. It then passes through the tunnel of Guyon, and enters the superficial compartment of the hand. At the level of the carpus, the ulnar artery gives off a latticework of fine vessels that span the dorsal and palmar aspects of the medial carpus. Proximal to the end of the ulna, there are three branches: a branch to the dorsal radiocarpal arch, one to the palmar radiocarpal arch, and one to the proximal pole of the pisiform and to the palmar aspect of the triquetrum.[35]

Vascular Arches of the Hand

Dorsal Arches.   The dorsal arches are connected longitudinally at their medial and lateral aspects by the ulnar and radial arteries. They are connected centrally by the dorsal branch of the anterior interosseous artery. There are three dorsal transverse arches: the radiocarpal, the intercarpal, and the basal metacarpal transverse arches[35]:

▶ *Dorsal radiocarpal.*   The radiocarpal arch is supplied by branches of the radial and ulnar arteries and the dorsal branch of the anterior interosseous artery.

▶ *Dorsal intercarpal.*   The dorsal intercarpal arch has a variable supply, which can include the radial, ulnar, and anterior interosseous arteries.

▶ *Basal metacarpal.*   The basal metacarpal arch is supplied by perforating arteries from the second, third, and fourth interosseous spaces. It contributes to the vascularity of the distal carpal row through anastomoses with the intercarpal arch.

Palmar Arches.   Similar to the dorsal vascularity, the palmar vascularity is composed of three transverse arches: the palmar radiocarpal, the palmar intercarpal, and the deep palmar arch[35]:

▶ *Palmar radiocarpal.*   This arch supplies the palmar surface of the lunate and triquetrum.

FIGURE 16-17 Vascular supply to the hand. (Reproduced with permission from Marble HC. *The Hand: A Manual and Atlas for the General Surgeon.* Philadelphia: WB Saunders; 1961.)

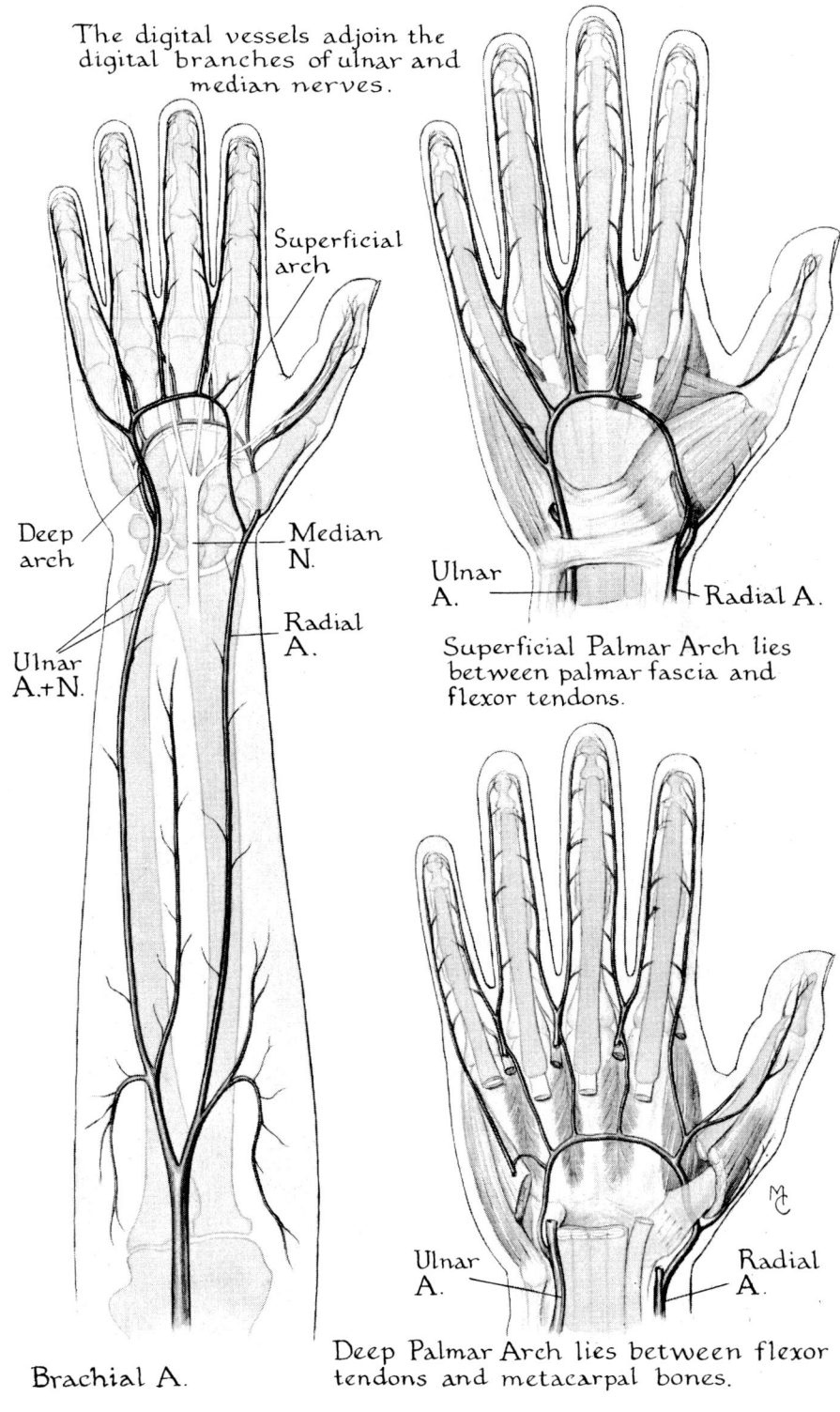

The digital vessels adjoin the digital branches of ulnar and median nerves.

Superficial arch

Deep arch

Median N.

Radial A.

Ulnar A.+N.

Brachial A.

Ulnar A.

Radial A.

Superficial Palmar Arch lies between palmar fascia and flexor tendons.

Ulnar A.

Radial A.

Deep Palmar Arch lies between flexor tendons and metacarpal bones.

▶ *Palmar intercarpal.* This arch is small and is not a major contributor of nutrient vessels to the carpus.

▶ *Deep palmar.* This arch contributes to the radial and ulnar recurrent arteries and sends perforating branches to the dorsal basal metacarpal arch and to the palmar metacarpal arteries.

Biomechanics

The wrist contains several segments whose combined movements create a total range of motion that is greater than the sum of its individual parts.[21]

A number of studies have examined the necessary range of motion at the wrist to perform functional activities. These studies report that at least 5 degrees of wrist flexion, 35 degrees of wrist extension, 10 degrees of radial deviation, and 15 degrees of ulnar deviation are needed to perform common personal care activities comfortably.[36,37] Less motion is required for 90 percent of personal care activities: 5 degrees of flexion, 6 degrees of extension, 7 degrees of radial deviation, and 6 degrees of ulnar deviation.[38]

Pronation and Supination

Approximately 90 degrees of forearm pronation is available. During pronation, the concave ulnar notch of the radius glides around the peripheral surface of the relatively fixed convex ulnar head. Pronation is limited by the bony impaction between the radius and the ulna.

Approximately 85 to 90 degrees of forearm supination is available. Supination is limited by the interosseous membrane and the bony impaction between the ulnar notch of the radius and the ulnar styloid process.

During pronation-supination, the distal ulna moves in a small circle, which is opposite in direction to the movement.[39] Thus the true axis for this motion may be situated anywhere between the radial and ulnar styloid, resulting in not one, but many pronation-supination axes.[40]

Congruency of the DRUJ surfaces is maximal at mid-range of motion, although the joint is not considered to be truly locked in this position.[6] At this position, the triangular cartilage is maximally stretched and the interosseous membrane is relatively lax.

The proximal and distal radioulnar joints are intimately related biomechanically, with the function and stability of both joints dependent on the configuration of and distance between the two bones. This configuration and distance maintains ligament and muscle tension.[41] A change in the length of the ulna of as little as 2 mm results in a change in the transmission of forces of 5 to 40 percent.[42]

Movement of the Hand on the Forearm

Due to the morphology of the wrist, movement at this joint complex involves a coordinated interaction between a number of articulations. These include the radiocarpal joint, the proximal row of carpals, and the distal row of carpals. All of these joints permit motion to occur around two axes: anterior-posterior in flexion-extension and transverse in lateral deviation. Wrist extension is accompanied by a slight radial deviation and pronation of the forearm. Wrist flexion is accompanied by a slight ulnar deviation and supination of the forearm.

A number of concepts have been proposed over the years to explain the biomechanics of wrist motion. The traditional concept viewed the wrist as two transverse functional rows of carpals, with both rows moving with respect to each other at the midcarpal joint. In addition, the proximal row moved on the radius and ulnar disk at the radiocarpal joint.[43] In this "fixed-row" concept, the proximal and distal rows were each thought to rotate as a rigid group around fixed axes, in both wrist flexion

and extension, and radioulnar deviations.[44] However, because this concept only related to movements between the hand and forearm, it was found to be inadequate, especially in situations in which the examination of intercarpal motion and carpal bone malalignment were considered.[45,46]

A more recent concept viewed the mechanism of the carpus motions as being related to that of longitudinal parallel chains.[45,47–50] The chains consist of a radial chain, middle chain, and ulnar chain.

▶ The radial chain is composed of the radius, scaphoid, trapezoid, trapezium, and the column of the thumb.

▶ The middle chain comprises the radius, lunate, capitate, and the third metacarpal.

▶ The ulnar chain, formed by the triquetrum and the hamate, constitutes the axis of pronation-supination, and has been called the column of rotation.[51] This chain strongly supports the movements in the central chain, while simultaneously anchoring the wrist to the radius.[52]

Under the chain concept, the radial and ulnar chains are proposed to move with the central chain due to mutual displacements between the proximal facets of the scaphoid and lunate. In addition, the proximal carpals are considered to move at the radiocarpal and midcarpal levels.[21,44]

Flexion and Extension Movements of the Wrist

"The wrist is the key joint of the hand."[53] Wrist movements occur around a combination of three functional axes: longitudinal, transverse, and anteroposterior. In a neutral wrist position, the scaphoid contacts the radius, and the lunate contacts the radius and disk.

The movements of flexion and extension of the wrist are shared between the radiocarpal articulation and the intercarpal articulation in varying proportions.[19]

During wrist flexion, most of the motion occurs in the midcarpal joint (60 percent or 40 degrees, versus 40 percent or 30 degrees at the radiocarpal joint), and is associated with slight ulnar deviation and supination of the forearm.[19]

During wrist extension, most of the motion occurs at the radiocarpal joint (66.5 percent or 40 degrees versus 33.5 percent or 20 degrees at the midcarpal joint), and is associated with slight radial deviation and pronation of the forearm.[19]

Flexion

According to Kapandji,[54] wrist flexion is limited by the dorsal radiocarpal ligaments. During flexion of the wrist, the triquetrum is moved towards the radial articular surface of the hamate and the capitate is flexed more than the lunate.[55]

Extension

When the wrist is extended, the radiolunotriquetral and radiocapitate ligaments are stretched. The stretch results in a simultaneous extension of the scaphoid and capitate. This effect is transmitted through the scapholunate ligament and brings the lunate into extension.

Loss of active extension in the wrist constitutes a considerable functional impairment, including the following[21]:

▶ A reduction in grip strength.

▶ Loss of active movement in the wrist, which has serious implications when considering the action of the extrinsic muscles of the hand. For example, the strength of the thumb and finger flexors requires normal motion and function of wrist extension.

Frontal Lateral Movements of the Wrist

There is a physiological ulnar deviation at rest, which is easily demonstrated clinically and radiographically. The amount of deviation is approximately 40 degrees of ulnar deviation and 15 degrees of radial deviation.

Radial Deviation
Radial deviation occurs primarily between the proximal and distal rows of the carpal bones. The motion of radial deviation is limited by impact of the scaphoid onto the radial styloid, and the ulnar collateral ligament. The abductor pollicis longus and extensor pollicis brevis are best suited to produce radial deviation of the wrist.[21]

Ulnar Deviation
Ulnar deviation occurs primarily at the radiocarpal joint.[54] Ulnar deviation is limited by the radial collateral ligament.[54]

Although ulnar deviation brings the triquetrum into contact with the disk, the lack of direct ulnar-triquetral articulation permits a greater range of ulnar deviation. The muscle with the best biomechanical advantage to produce ulnar deviation of the wrist in pronation is the extensor carpi ulnaris.[21]

Extension of the wrist is accompanied by radial deviation, and flexion of the wrist is accompanied by ulnar deviation. The wrist also allows relatively extensive traction and gliding accessory movement.

The open-packed and close-packed positions of the wrist and hand articulations, in addition to the capsular patterns of each joint, are depicted in Table 16-3.

Wrist Movements and the Digits

The position of the wrist in flexion or extension influences the tension of the long or "extrinsic" muscles of the digits.

The position of the wrist has important repercussions on the position of the thumb and fingers. Neither the flexors nor the extensors of the fingers are long enough to allow maximal range of motion at the wrist and the fingers simultaneously.[21] In fact, due to the restraining action of the long antagonistic muscles, complete flexion of the fingers is possible only if the wrist is in approximately 20 degrees of extension, which corresponds to the optimal position for hand function.[21] Thus the movements of the wrist reinforce the action of the extrinsic muscles of the fingers and are synergistic with the more powerful digital

TABLE 16-3 The Open-Packed and Close-Packed Positions, and Capsular Patterns for the Articulations of the Wrist and Hand

Joint	Open-Packed	Close-Packed	Capsular Pattern
Distal radioulnar	10° of supination	5° of supination	Minimal to no limitation with pain at the end ranges of pronation and supination
Radiocarpal (wrist)	Neutral with slight ulnar deviation	Extension	Equal limitation of flexion and extension
Intercarpal	Neutral or slight flexion	Extension	None
Midcarpal	Neutral or slight flexion with ulnar deviation	Extension with ulnar deviation	Equal limitation of flexion and extension
Carpometacarpal	*Thumb:* Midway between abduction and adduction and midway between flexion and extension *Fingers:* Midway between flexion and extension	*Thumb:* Full opposition *Fingers:* Full flexion	*Thumb:* Abduction then extension *Fingers:* Equal limitation in all directions
Metacarpophalangeal	Slight flexion	*Thumb:* Full opposition *Fingers:* Full flexion	Flexion then extension
Interphalangeal	Slight flexion	Full extension	Flexion, extension

flexors. As the wrist position changes, the functional lengths of the digital flexor tendons change and the resultant forces in finger flexion vary. In order for grip to be effective and have maximal force, the wrist must be stable, and positioned in slight extension and ulnar deviation.[21]

Studies have evaluated the effect of wrist position on the force generated at the middle and distal phalanges, and found that the greatest force is exerted in ulnar deviation and then extension, with the least force being generated in flexion.[56]

Articulations of the Fingers

There are notable differences between the interphalangeal and MCP articulations of the digits and even between the articulations at the same level for each digit.[21] These differences are produced by:

▶ The shape of the articulations.

▶ The orientation of the articular surface.

▶ The synovial insertion.

▶ The disposition of the collateral ligaments.

▶ The degree of play in the volar plate.

These elements determine the degree of mobility and stability of these articulations and the orientation of the distal segments. As the thumb pulp pronates in opposition, the pulps of the fingers supinate in external rotation when the MCP joints flex, or when the index finger moves radially. These variations in orientation allow for optimal use of the finger pulps for functional tasks of the hand (see later).[21]

Thumb Movements

The first CMC joint is a saddle joint. The characteristic feature of a saddle joint is that each articular surface is concave in one dimension and convex in the other. Within the first CMC joint, the longitudinal diameter of the articular surface of the trapezium is generally concave from a palmar to dorsal direction, while the transverse diameter is generally convex along a medial to lateral direction. The proximal articular surface of the first metacarpal is reciprocally shaped to that of the trapezium. This articular relationship produces the following:[21a]

▶ Thumb flexion and extension occur around an anterior-posterior axis in the frontal plane (Fig. 16-10) that is perpendicular to the sagittal plane of finger flexion and extension. In this plane, the metacarpal surface is concave, and the trapezium surface is convex. Flexion occurs with a conjunct rotation of internal rotation of the metacarpal. Extension occurs with a conjunct rotation of external rotation of the metacarpal. A total range of 50–70° is available.

▶ Thumb abduction and adduction occur around a medial-lateral axis in the sagittal plane (Fig. 16-10) that is perpendicular to the frontal plane of finger abduction and adduction. During thumb abduction and adduction, the convex metacarpal surface moves on the concave trapezium. Abduction occurs with a conjunct rotation of internal rotation.

Adduction occurs with a conjunct rotation of external rotation. A total range of 40–60° is available.

▶ Opposition of the thumb involves a wide arc motion comprised of sequential palmar abduction and flexion from the anatomic position, accompanied by internal rotation of the thumb. Retroposition of the thumb returns the thumb to the anatomic position, a motion that incorporates elements of adduction with extension and external rotation of the metacarpal.

Normal Ulnar Inclination of the Fingers

A normal ulnar inclination of the fingers occurs at the MCP joints due to a number of factors[21]:

▶ Asymmetry of the metacarpal heads and the collateral ligaments.

▶ Tendon factors: the extrinsic tendons, extensors, and flexors cross into the hand on the ulnar side of its longitudinal axis.

▶ Muscle factors: the intrinsic muscles have a predominantly ulnar inclination and predominate over those with a radial inclination.

▶ The physiologic action of the thumb, which in lateral grip pushes the fingers in an ulnar direction.

The inclination is most marked in the index finger, less in the middle and little fingers, and almost nonexistent in the ring finger. The ulnar inclination is normally limited by the capsuloligamentous resistance at the MCP joints and by the action of the interosseous muscles, which act in a radial direction.[21] The weakness of these stabilizing elements, particularly in rheumatoid arthritis, allows the ulnar inclination to be accentuated, resulting in pathologic ulnar deviation.

Functional Position of the Hand

The hand serves many important functions that allow us to interact with others and the environment. In addition to providing a wealth of sensory information, the hand functions to grasp objects. A loss of grip is a measurable factor used in the determination of permanent disability by compensation boards in some states.[57] The grip is typically divided into stages[58,59]:

▶ Opening of the hand.

▶ Positioning and closing of the fingers to grasp an object and adapt to the object's shape.

▶ Controlled approach and purposeful closing of the fingers and/or palm. The amount of force exerted is determined by the weight, surface characteristics, and fragility of the object.[60]

▶ Maintenance and stabilization of the grip. This phase is not used in precision tasks.

▶ The release of the object.

A number of grips have been recognized. These include the fist grip, the cylindrical grip, the ball grip, the hook grip, the ring grip, the pincer grip, and the pliers grip (Fig. 16-18).[61,62]

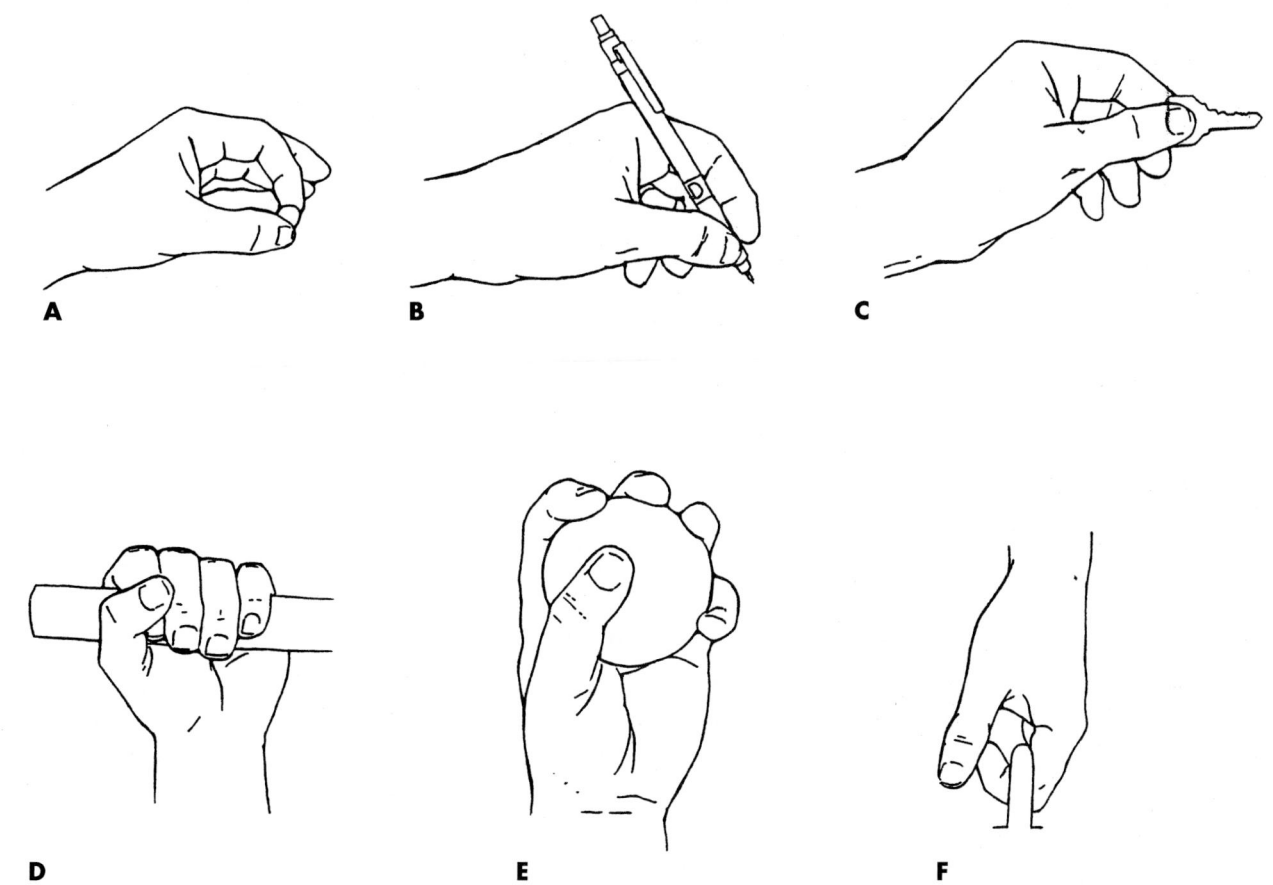

FIGURE 16-18 Prehension grips. *Pinch:* (*A*) Tip. (*B*) Palmar (three-jaw chuck). (*C*) Lateral. *Grasp:* (*D*) Cylindrical. (*E*) Spherical. *Hook:* (*F*) Hook. (Reproduced with permission from Prentice WE, Voight ML, *Techniques in Musculoskeletal Rehabilitation.* New York: McGraw-Hill; 2001.)

Hand functions have been further categorized by adding the terms *grasp* and *prehension*. These terms are used to describe functions of power or precision.[63,64]

Power Grip

The power grip involves the use of force to stabilize an object in the hand. The strength and power of a grip comes from a combination of:

▶ thumb adduction.

▶ isometric flexion.

▶ an approximation of the thenar and hypothenar eminences.

▶ intact function of the ulnar side of the hand.

Participation of the intrinsic muscles follows specific patterns in the various power grips.

▶ The hook grip involves the fourth dorsal interosseus, fourth lumbrical, and the abductor digiti minimi.

▶ The spherical grip involves all of the interossei (except the second), the abductor digiti minimi, and the fourth lumbrical.[61,65]

Precision Grip

In the precision grip, the muscles primarily function isotonically to provide exact control of finger and thumb position, so the position of the handled object can be changed either in space or about its own axis.[58,61] Due to the higher levels of sensory input required during these tasks, the areas with the most sensory receptors are used. A number of precision grips are recognized[21,54]:

▶ *Pulp-to-pulp pinch,* in which the pad of the thumb is opposed to the pad of one or more fingers.

▶ *Lateral prehension,* where the palmar aspect of the thumb presses against the radial aspect of the first phalanx of the index finger.

▶ *Tip prehension,* in which the extreme tip of the thumb pad is opposed to the tip of the index or middle finger.

▶ *Three-fingered pinch* (thumb, index finger, and middle finger), as in sprinkling herbs.

▶ *Five-fingered pinch,* as in picking up a face towel.

The radial side of the hand and the MCP joints are involved more in the precision or prehensile types of grips.[21,54]

TABLE 16-4 Estimated Use of Grips for Activities of Daily Living[1]

Type of Grip	Estimated Use (%)
Pulp-to-pulp pinch	20
Lateral pinch	20
Five-finger pinch	15
Fist grip	15
Cylinder grip	14
Three-fingered pinch	10
Spherical grip	4
Hook grip	2

Different grip patterns are used regularly during daily functional activities (Table 16-4).[1,66]

Examination

Elucidating the cause of forearm, wrist, and hand pain can be challenging. The examination of the forearm, wrist, and hand requires a sound knowledge of differential diagnosis, and must incorporate an examination of the entire upper kinetic chain, including the cervical and thoracic spine.

The common pathologies for the forearm, wrist, and hand and their interventions are detailed after the examination section. An understanding of both is obviously necessary. As mention of the various pathologies occurs with reference to the tests and measures and vice versa, the reader is encouraged to switch between the two.

History

The assessment of the forearm, wrist, and hand begins by recording a detailed history. The history helps focus the examination. All relevant information must be gathered about the site, nature, behavior, and onset of the current symptoms. This should include information about the patient's age, hand dominance, avocational activities, and occupation.

> **Clinical Pearl**
>
> The non-neutral position of the hand is extension, flexion, or ulnar deviation.[67,68] Sustained non-neutral positions of the hand and wrist subject nerves to prolonged stretch and periods of high pressure.[69] In addition, these positions place muscles in inefficient length-tension relationships,[68] resulting in decreased transmission of contractile forces to the fingers.[68,70]

The following questions should be asked:

▶ *Are there any local areas of tenderness?* Localized tenderness may indicate a carpal fracture, particularly of the scaphoid. Scaphoid fractures are associated with a load applied to the radial side of the palm when the wrist is in extreme extension,[71] and can be ongoing sources of pain and dysfunction (refer to "Intervention Strategies" section). The patient's perception of their pain can be measured using a visual analog scale.

▶ *When did the injury occur?* The date of injury is particularly important, especially as simple traumatic arthritis of the wrist does not last more than a few days if the wrist is rested.

The mechanism of injury should be thoroughly explored. If the problem is trauma related, the clinician should ascertain:

▶ The forces applied.

▶ Where and when the injury occurred.

▶ The position of the wrist and hand at the time of the trauma.

▶ Whether the conditions were clean or dirty (if a wound is present).

▶ Whether there was an accompanying "pop" or "click."

▶ Whether swelling occurred.

If the problem is non-trauma related, the onset of pain or sensory change, swelling, or contracture should be ascertained. The clinician should note the sequence of symptoms, the level of functional impairment, the progression of symptoms, the time of day the symptoms are worse, and whether the symptoms appear to be posture- or work-related.

It is important to obtain information regarding the use of medications as well as determining whether radiologic films were taken. Knowledge of the past behavior of previous wrist, hand, and finger disorders and their interventions can help in assessing the nature of the patient's current problem.

The patient's goals should be ascertained. Dysfunction of the hand can be very disabling, so inquiries concerning the functional demands of the patient must be made, and the intervention tailored accordingly.

Systems Review

A complete review of the medical history and general health of the patient should be included along with a review of systems, and the presence of other orthopaedic, neurologic, or cardiopulmonary conditions. An upper quarter scanning examination is performed to provide an overview of the upper extremity, the direction for a more detailed examination, and to rule out referral from the cervical, thoracic, shoulder girdle, and elbow joints.

The clinician should be able to determine the suitability of the patient for physical therapy. All inflammatory conditions, whether infectious or not, are accompanied by diffuse pain or tenderness with movement. Rheumatoid arthritis (RA) often affects this region with more severity and frequency than elsewhere. Therefore questions concerning other joint involvement and general debility must be asked. The presence of carpal tunnel syndrome, which is usually felt at night, may also indicate RA.

If the clinician is concerned with any signs or symptoms of a visceral, vascular, neurogenic, psychogenic, spondylogenic, or systemic disorder that is out of the scope of physical therapy (see Chap. 9), the patient should be referred back to their physician.

Tests and Measures

Observation

The physical examination should begin with a general observation of the patient's posture—especially the cervical spine, the thoracic spine, and the position of the hand in relation to the body. For example, is the arm held against the chest in a protec-tive manner, does the arm swing during the gait pattern, or does it just hang loosely?

The patient's hands can be highly informative (Table 16-5). The posture and alignment of the wrist is examined. Wrist angulation into ulnar deviation increases shearing in the first dorsal compartment. This angulation can predispose the patient to De Quervain's syndrome (see "Intervention Strategies" section).[72] A prominence of the distal ulna may indicate distal radioulnar joint instability.[73] The posture of the hand should be analyzed. The clinician should observe how the patient appears to relate to the involved hand, and how the patient attempts to use the hand.[17] The contour of the palmar surface, including the arches, should be

TABLE 16-5 Outline of Physical Findings of the Hand[75,325]

I. Variations in size and shape of hand
  A. Large, blunt fingers (spade hand)
    1. Acromegaly
    2. Hurler's disease (gargoylism)
  B. Gross irregularity of shape and size
    1. Paget's disease of bone
    2. Maffucci's syndrome
    3. Neurofibromatosis
  C. Spider fingers, slender palm (arachnodactyly)
    1. Hypopituitarism
    2. Eunuchism
    3. Ehlers-Danlos syndrome, pseudoxanthoma elasticum
    4. Tuberculosis
    5. Asthenic habitus
    6. Osteogenesis imperfecta
  D. Sausage-shaped phalanges
    1. Rickets (beading of joints)
    2. Granulomatous dactyliltis (tuberculosis, syphilis)
  E. Spindliform joints (fingers)
    1. Early rheumatoid arthritis
    2. Systemic lupus erythematosus
    3. Psoriasis
    4. Rubella
    5. Boeck's sarcoidosis
    6. Osteoarthritis
  F. Cone-shaped fingers
    1. Pituitary obesity
    2. Frohlich's dystrophy
  G. Unilateral enlargement of hand
    1. Arteriovenous aneurysm
    2. Maffucci's syndrome
  H. Square, dry hands
    1. Cretinism
    2. Myxedema
  I. Single, widened, flattened distal phalanx
    1. Sarcoidosis

J. Shortened fourth and fifth metacarpals (bradymetacarpalism)
K. Shortened, incurved fifth finger (symptom of DuBois)
    1. Mongolism
    2. "Behavioral problem"
    3. Gargoylism (broad, short, thick-skinned hand)
L. Malposition and abduction, fifth finger
    1. Turner's syndrome (gonadal dysgenesis, webbed neck, etc.)
M. Syndactylism
    1. Congenital malformations of the heart, great vessels
    2. Multiple congenital deformities
    3. Laurence-Moon-Biedl syndrome
    4. In normal individuals as an inherited trait
N. Clubbed fingers
    1. Subacute bacterial endocarditis
    2. Pulmonary causes
      a. Tuberculosis
      b. Pulmonary arteriovenous fistula
      c. Pulmonic abscess
      d. Pulmonic cysts
      e. Bullous emphysema
      f. Pulmonary hyperthrophic osteoarthropathy
      g. Bronchogenic carcinoma
    3. Alveolocapillary block
      a. Interstitial pulmonary fibrosis
      b. Sarcoidosis
      c. Beryllium poisoning
      d. Sclerodermatous lung
      e. Asbestosis
      f. Miliary tuberculosis
      g. Alveolar cell carcinoma

    4. Cardiovascular causes
      a. Patent ductus arteriosus
      b. Tetralogy of Fallot
      c. Taussig-Bing complex
      d. Pulmonic stenosis
      e. Ventricular septal defect
    5. Diarrheal states
      a. Ulcerative colitis
      b. Tuberculous enteritis
      c. Sprue
      d. Amebic dysentery
      e. Bacillary dysentery
      f. Parasitic infestation (gastrointestinal tract)
    6. Hepatic cirrhosis
    7. Myxedema
    8. Polycythemia
    9. Chronic urinary tract infections (upper and lower)
      a. Chronic nephritis
    10. Hyperparathyroidism (telescopy of distal phalanx)
    11. Pachydermoperiostosis (syndrome of Touraine, Solente, and Gole)
O. Joint disturbances
    1. Arthritides
      a. Osteoarthritis
      b. Rheumatoid arthritis
      c. Systemic lupus erythematosus
      d. Gout
      e. Psoriasis
      f. Sarcoidosis
      g. Endocrinopathy (acromegaly)
      h. Rheumatic fever
      i. Reiter's syndrome
      j. Dermatomyositis
    2. Anaphylactic reaction-serum sickness
    3. Scleroderma

TABLE 16-5 *(cont.)*

II. Edema of the hand
- A. Cardiac disease (congestive heart failure)
- B. Hepatic disease
- C. Renal disease
  1. Nephritis
  2. Nephrosis
- D. Hemiplegic hand
- E. Syringomyelia
- F. Superior vena caval syndrome
  1. Superior thoracic outlet tumor
  2. Mediastinal tumor or inflammation
  3. Pulmonary apex tumor
  4. Aneurysm
- G. Generalized anasarca, hypoproteinemia
- H. Postoperative lymphedema (radical breast amputation)
- I. Ischemic paralysis (cold, blue, swollen, numb)
- J. Lymphatic obstuction
  1. Lymphomatous masses in axilla
- K. Axillary mass
  1. Metastatic tumor, abscess, leukemia, Hodgkin's disease
- L. Aneurysm of ascending or transverse aorta, or of axillary artery
- M. Pressure on innominate or subclavian vessels
- N. Raynaud's disease
- O. Myositis
- P. Cervical rib
- Q. Trichiniasis
- R. Scalenus anticus syndrome

III. Neuromuscular effects
- A. Atrophy
  1. Painless
     a. Amyotrophic lateral sclerosis
     b. Charcot-Marie-Tooth peroneal atrophy
     c. Syringomyelia (loss of heat, cold, and pain sensation)
     d. Neural leprosy
  2. Painful
     a. Peripheral nerve disease
        1. Radial nerve (wrist drop)
           a. Lead poisoning, alcoholism, polyneuritis, trauma
           b. Diphtheria, polyarteritis, neurosyphilis, anterior poliomyelitis
        2. Ulnar nerve (benediction palsy)
           a. Polyneuritis, trauma
        3. Median nerve (claw hand)
           a. Carpal tunnel syndrome
              1. Rheumatoid arthritis
              2. Tenosynovitis at wrist
              3. Amyloidosis
              4. Gout
              5. Plasmacytoma
              6. Anaphylactic reaction
              7. Menopause syndrome
              8. Myxedema
- B. Extrinsic pressure on the nerve (cervical, axillary, supraclavicular, or brachial)
  1. Pancoast tumor (pulmonary apex)
  2. Aneurysms of subclavian arteries, axillary vessels, or thoracic aorta
  3. Costoclavicular syndrome
  4. Superior thoracic outlet syndrome
  5. Cervical rib
  6. Degenerative arthritis of cervical spine
  7. Herniation of cervical intervertebral disk
- C. Shoulder-hand syndrome
  1. Myocardial infarction
  2. Pancoast tumor
  3. Brain tumor
  4. Intrathoracic neoplasms
  5. Discogenic disease
  6. Cervical spondylosis
  7. Febrile panniculitis
  8. Senility
  9. Vascular occlusion
  10. Hemiplegia
  11. Osteoarthritis
  12. Herpes zoster
- D. Ischemic contractures (sensory loss in fingers)
  1. Tight plaster cast applications
- E. Polyarteritis nodosa

- F. Polyneuritis
  1. Carcinoma of lung
  2. Hodgkin's disease
  3. Pregnancy
  4. Gastric carcinoma
  5. Reticuloses
  6. Diabetes mellitus
  7. Chemical neuritis
     a. Antimony, benzene, bismuth, carbon tetrachloride, heavy metals, alcohol, arsenic lead, gold, emetine
  8. Ischemic neuropathy
  9. Vitamin B deficiency
  10. Atheromata
  11. Arteriosclerosis
  12. Embolic
- G. Carpodigital (carpopedal spasm) tetany
  1. Hypoparathyroidism
  2. Hyperventilation
  3. Uremia
  4. Nephritis
  5. Nephrosis
  6. Rickets
  7. Sprue
  8. Malabsorption syndrome
  9. Pregnancy
  10. Lactation
  11. Osteomalacia
  12. Protracted vomiting
  13. Pyloric obstruction
  14. Alkali poisoning
  15. Chemical toxicity
     a. Morphine, lead, alcohol
- H. Tremor
  1. Parkinsonism
  2. Familial disorder
  3. Hypoglycemia
  4. Hyperthyroidism
  5. Wilson's disease (hepatolenticular degeneration)
  6. Anxiety
  7. Ataxia
  8. Athetosis
  9. Alcoholism, narcotic addiction
  10. Multiple sclerosis
  11. Chorea (Sydenham's, Huntington's)

examined. If a finger is involved, its attitude should be observed. Digital deformities are the hallmark of rheumatoid arthritis.[74]

A visual inspection of the involved wrist and hand is made and is compared with the uninvolved side. The clinician inspects for lacerations, surgical scars, masses, localized swelling, or erythema. Scars should be examined for degree of adherence, degree of maturation, hypertrophy (excess collagen within the boundary of the wound), and keloid (excess collagen that no longer conforms to wound boundaries). The location and type of edema should be noted. A determination is made as to whether the swelling is generalized or localized, hard or soft. Anterior effusion over the flexor tendons at the wrist may indicate rheumatoid tenovaginitis. Swelling that persists more than a few days following trauma probably suggests a carpal fracture. Localized swelling accompanied with redness and tenderness may indicate an infection.

Clinical Pearl

The normal physiologic angles for relaxed hand posture are 14 to 15 degrees of ulnar deviation for the index finger, 13 degrees for the middle finger, 4 degrees for the ring finger, and 7 to 8 degrees for the little finger.

The swan-neck deformity is one of the most frequently encountered deformities (see "Intervention Strategies" section).[74]

The nails should be inspected to see if they are healthy and pink (Table 16-6). Local trauma to the nails seldom involves more than one or two digits. The nails should be checked for hangnail infection, or whether they appear ridged, which could indicate a rheumatoid arthritis dysfunction. Clubbed nails are an indication of hypertrophy of underlying structures. The presence of a paronychia or a pale paronychia should prompt the clinician to probe the axilla and neck lymph nodes for tenderness and swelling. Beau's lines are transverse furrows that begin at the lunula and progress distally as the nail grows. They result from a temporary arrest of growth of the nail matrix occasioned by trauma or systemic stress.[75] With the knowledge that nails grow about 0.1 mm/day, by measuring the distance between the Beau's lines and the cuticle, one may be able to approximately determine the date of the stress. For example, if the distance is 5 mm, the stress event occurred approximately 50 days before. Spoon nails (koilonychias) may occur in a form of iron deficiency anemia, coronary disease, and with the use of strong detergents.[75] Clubbing of the nails, characterized by a bulbous enlargement of the distal portion of the digits, may occur in association with cardiovascular disease, subacute endocarditis, advanced cor pulmonale, and pulmonary disease.[75]

Finger color should be observed. Fingers that are white in appearance might indicate Raynaud's disease. Blotchy or red fingers might indicate liver disease. Blue fingers may indicate a circulatory problem.

Any other finger deformities such as mallet finger and boutonniere are noted (Table 16-7).

Intrinsic muscle fibrosis is characterized by stiffness at the interphalangeal (IP) joints. On flexion of the MCP joint, extension

TABLE 16-6   Glossary of Nail Pathology[75,326]

Condition	Description	Occurrence
Beau's lines	Transverse lines or ridges marking repeated disturbances of nail growth	Systemic diseases, toxic or nutritional deficiency states of many types, trauma (from manicuring)
Defluvium unguium (onychomadesis)	Complete loss of nails	Certain systemic diseases such as scarlet fever, syphilis, leprosy, alopecia areata, and exfoliative dermatitis; dermatoses such as nail infection, psoriasis, eczema; arsenic poisoning.
Diffusion of lunula unguis	Spreading of lunula	Dystrophies of the extremities
Eggshell nails	Nail plate thin, semitransparent bluish-white, with a tendency to curve upward at the distal edge	Syphilis
Fragilitas unguium	Friable or brittle nails	Dietary deficiency, local trauma
Hapalonychia	Nails very soft, split easily	Following contact with strong alkalis; endocrine disturbances, malnutrition, syphilis, chronic arthritis
Hippocratic nails	"Watch-glass nails associated with drumstick fingers"	Chronic respiratory and circulatory diseases, especially pulmonary tuberculosis; hepatic cirrhosis
Koilonychia	"Spoon nails"; nails are concave on the outer surface	Dysendocrinisms (acromegaly), trauma, dermatoses, syphilis, nutritional deficiencies, hypothyroidism

TABLE 16-6   *(cont.)*

Condition	Description	Occurrence
Leukonychia	White spots or striations or rarely the whole nail may turn white (congenital type)	Local trauma, hepatic cirrhosis, nutritional deficiencies, and many systemic diseases
Mees' lines	Transverse white bands	Hodgkin's granuloma, arsenic and thallium toxicity, high fevers, local nutritional derangement
Moniliasis of nails	Infections (usually paronychial) caused by yeast forms (*Candida albicans*)	Occupational (common in food-handlers, dentists, dishwashers, and gardeners)
Onychatrophia	Atrophy or failure of development of nails	Trauma, infection, dysendocrinism, gonadal aplasia, and many systemic disorders.
Onychauxis	Nail plate is greatly thickened	Mild persistent trauma, systemic diseases such as peripheral stasis, peripheral neuritis, syphilis, leprosy, hemiplegia, or at times may be congenital
Onychia	Inflammation of the nail matrix causing deformity of the nail plate	Trauma, infection, many systemic diseases
Onychodystrophy	Any deformity of the nail plate, nail bed, or nail matrix	Many diseases, trauma, or chemical agents (poisoning, allergy)
Onychogryposis	"Claw nails"; extreme degree of hypertrophy, sometimes with horny projections arising from the nail surface	May be congenital or related to many chronic systemic diseases (see onychauxis)
Onycholysis	Loosening of the nail plate beginning at the distal or free edge	Trauma, injury by chemical agents, many systemic diseases
Onychomadesis	See defluvium unguium.	
Onychophagia	Nail biting	Neurosis
Onychorrhexis	Longitudinal ridging and splitting of the nails	Dermatoses, nail infections, many systemic diseases, senility, injury by chemical agents, hyperthyroidism
Onychoschizia	Lamination and scaling away of nails in thin layers	Dermatoses, syphilis, injury by chemical agents
Onychotillomania	Alteration of the nail structures caused by persistent neurotic picking of the nails	Neurosis
Pachyonychia	Extreme thickening of all the nails; the nails are more solid and more regular than in onychogryposis	Usually congenital and associated with hyperkeratosis of the palms and soles
Pterygium unguis	Thinning of the nail fold and spreading of the cuticle over the nail plate	Associated with vasospastic conditions such as Raynaud's phenomenon and occasionally with hypothyroidism

TABLE 16-7   Hand and Finger Deformities and Their Possible Causes

Deformity	Possible Cause
MCP joint flexion	Rupture of the extensor tendon just proximal to the MCP joint
Hyperextension of the MCP joint	Paralysis of the interossei
Deepening of the palmar gutter and an inability to fully stretch out the palm	Tightness of the palmar aponeurosis
Wasting of the hypothenar eminence and a clawed hand with flexion of the fourth and fifth digits (hand of benediction)	Ulnar nerve palsy
Wrist drop with increased flexion of the wrist, flexion of the MCP joint and extension of the DIP joints	Radial nerve lesion
Isolated thenar atrophy	Arthritis of the carpometacarpal joint Median nerve lesion C8 or T1 nerve root lesion
Ape-hand deformity with a wasting of the thenar eminence, and an inability to oppose or flex the thumb or abduct it in its own plane[110]	Median nerve palsy
Z-deformity of the wrist	Pattern of deformity in the rheumatoid hand[327]
Atrophy of the hand intrinsics	Pancoast tumor
Claw-hand deformity	Loss of ulnar nerve motor innervation to the hand, with resultant paralysis of the interosseous muscles, and muscle atrophy of the hypothenar eminence; this deformity is more severe in lesions distal to innervation of the FDP muscle, as this muscle adds to the flexion force upon the IP joints[6]
PIP hyperextension and slight flexion of the DIP	Rupture or paralysis of the flexor digitorum superficialis (FDS)
A fixed flexion deformity of the MCP and PIP joints, especially in the ring or little finger	Dupuytren's contracture
A hook-like contracture of the flexor muscles, which is worse with wrist extension as compared to flexion	Volkmann's ischemic contracture

DIP, distal interphalangeal; FDP, flexor digitorum profundus; MCP, metacarpophalangeal; PIP, proximal interphalangeal

of the fingers becomes tight and flexion is restricted. On extension of the MCP joint, flexion of the IP joints is possible.

▶ Adhesions proximal to the MCP joint allow lumbrical action (i.e., MCP flexion and PIP and DIP joint extension).

▶ Adhesions distal to the MCP joints result in the ability to extend the MCP and flex the PIP and DIP joints, but there is no extension possible in the fingers.

Active Range of Motion (AROM), Then Passive Range or Motion (PROM) with Overpressure

The gross motions of wrist, hand, finger, and thumb flexion, extension, and radial and ulnar deviation are tested, first actively and then passively (Table 16-8). Any loss of motion compared with the contralateral, asymptomatic wrist and hand should be noted. Palpation may be performed with the range-of-motion tests.

TABLE 16-8   Active Range of Motion Norms for the Forearm, Wrist, and Hand

Motion	Degrees
Forearm pronation	85–90
Forearm supination	85–90
Radial deviation	15
Ulnar deviation	30–45
Wrist flexion	80–90
Wrist extension	70–90
Finger flexion	MCP: 85–90; PIP: 100–115; DIP: 80–90
Finger extension	MCP: 30–45; PIP: 0; DIP: 20
Finger abduction	20–30
Finger adduction	0
Thumb flexion	CMC: 45–50; MCP: 50–55; IP: 85–90
Thumb extension	MCP: 0; IP: 0–5
Thumb adduction	30
Thumb abduction	60–70

CMC, carpometacarpal; DIP, distal interphalangeal; IP, interphalangeal; MCP, metacarpophalangeal; PIP, proximal interphalangeal.

During flexion of the fingers, the overall area of the fingers should converge to a point on the wrist corresponding to the radial pulse. This can only occur if the index finger flexes in a sagittal plane and all the others in an increasingly oblique plane. A skyline view of the knuckles is made. In full flexion, a dorsally subluxed capitate may be seen as a local swelling on the back and middle of the flexed wrist.

During measurement of motion, one must be aware that finger joint positions may affect wrist joint ranges (and vice versa) due to the constant length of the extrinsic tendons that cross multiple joints. For example, greater wrist flexion occurs with finger extension than with finger flexion because the extensor digitorum tendons are not stretched maximally. Thus during the examination, the clinician should maintain all joints in a consistent position (usually neutral), except the one being measured. In addition, the clinician should identify wrist and finger joint position when measuring the strength of related muscles.

Somatic dysfunction of the wrist permits motion toward the dysfunction; motion away from the dysfunction will be restricted.

Fanning and folding of the hand is performed by palpating the palmar surface of the pisiform, scaphoid, hamate, and trapezium with the index and middle fingers, and the dorsal surface of the capitate with the thumbs as the hand is alternately fanned and folded (Fig. 16-19A and 16-19B). During these motions, the clinician should note the quantity and quality of the conjunct rotations. An absence of the conjunct rotations may indicate an intercarpal dysfunction.

The uninvolved joint should always be examined first. This allows for a determination of the normal function, allays the patient's anxiety, and allows for a true comparison of function.[4] During palpation, the clinician should be on the alert for any thickening over tendons, tenderness, or areas of fluctuation.[4] During active and passive testing, the presence of crepitus must be determined. The presence of crepitus with motion may indicate a tendon sheath synovitis or vaginitis.

Clinical Pearl

Crepitus usually accompanies a particularly acute tendonitis.

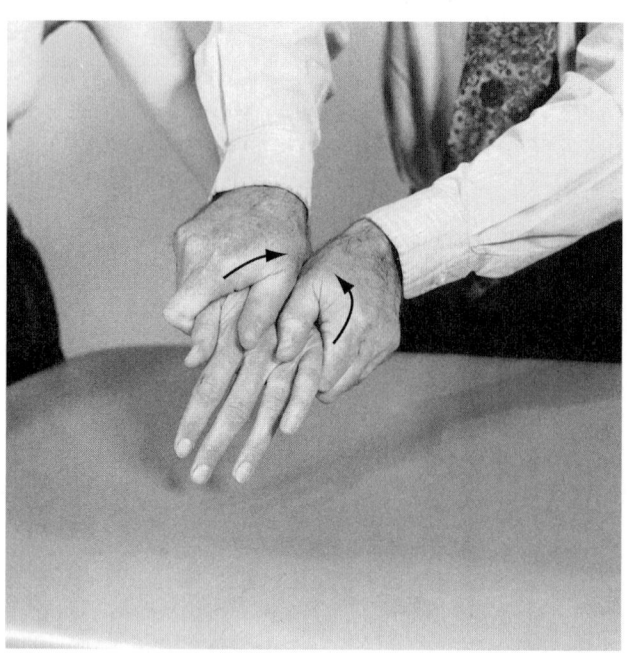

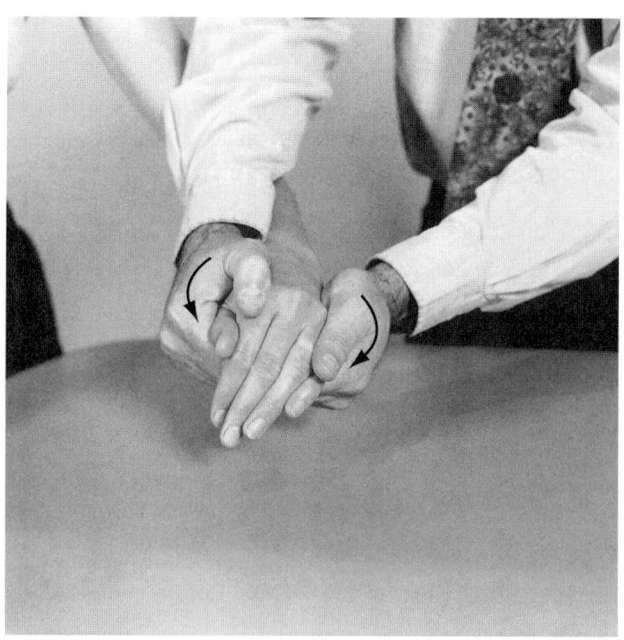

A   **B**

FIGURE 16-19   (A) Fanning of the hand. (B) Folding of the hand.

Wrist

Pronation and supination of the wrist on the forearm will provisionally test the TFCC and the proximal and distal radioulnar joints. Full forced pronation-supination without evoking pain eliminates the DRUJ and the TFCC as potential sources of the patient's complaints.[2]

Wrist flexion, extension, ulnar deviation, and radial deviation are assessed. According to Watson,[2] any loss of passive wrist flexion is a sign of underlying organic carpal pathology.

If the single-plane motions do not provoke symptoms, combined motions can be used. These include wrist extension with ulnar and then radial deviation, and wrist flexion with ulnar and radial deviation.

Thumb

The following motions are tested in varying degrees of wrist flexion and extension:

▶ First CMC abduction, adduction, flexion, extension, and opposition. During opposition, the clinician should observe for the conjunct rotation component of the motion.

▶ First MCP and IP flexion and extension.

Fingers

It should never be assumed that lack of full active flexion or extension of the PIP is merely secondary to joint pain or fusion, because closed rupture of the middle slip of the extensor hood is easily missed until the appearance of a boutonniere deformity.[20] Total active motion of the fingers is the sum of all angles formed by the MP, PIP, and DIP joints in simultaneous maximum active flexion, minus the total extension deficit at the MP, PIP, and DIP joints (including hyperextension at the IP joints) in maximum active extension.

A normal value for total active range of motion in the absence of a normal contralateral digit for comparison is 260 degrees, based on 85 degrees of MP flexion, 110 degrees of PIP motion, and 65 degrees of DIP motion.[76]

A comparison of active and passive motion indicates the efficiency of flexor and extensor excursion and/or degree of muscle strength within the available passive range of motion.[76] Instances of greater passive than active motion may indicate a limited tendon glide due to adherence of the tendon to surrounding structures, or relative lengthening of the tendon due to injury or surgery, weakness, or pain.[76]

Due to the multitude of joints and multiarticular muscles found in the hand, the clinician may need to differentiate between various structures in order to determine the cause of a motion restriction. The soft tissue structures that may contribute to a motion restriction include[76]:

▶ *Hand intrinsics.* The Bunnell-Littler test is used to determine whether flexion restriction of the PIP is due to tightness of the intrinsic muscles, or to a restriction of the MCP joint capsule. The MCP joint is held by the clinician in a few degrees of extension with one hand, while the other hand attempts to flex the PIP joint. If the joint cannot flex, tightness of the intrinsics or a joint capsular contraction

should be suspected.[77] From this position, the clinician now slightly flexes the MCP joint, thereby relaxing the intrinsics, and attempts to flex the PIP joint. If the joint can now flex, the intrinsics are tight. If the joint still cannot flex, the restriction is probably due to a capsular contraction of the joint. This test is also called the intrinsic-plus test.[21]

▶ *Oblique retinacular (Landsmeer's) ligament.* The Haines-Zancolli test is used to determine whether restricted flexion in the DIP joints is due to a restriction of the proximal interphalangeal joint capsule, or tightness of the oblique retinacular ligament. The test for a contracture of this ligament is the same as the Bunnell-Littler test, only at the PIP and DIP joints. The clinician positions and holds the PIP joint in a neutral position with one hand, and attempts to flex the DIP joint with the other hand. If no flexion is possible, it can be due to either a tight retinacular ligament or capsular contraction. The PIP joint is then slightly flexed to relax the retinacular ligament. If the DIP can now flex, the restriction is due to tightness in the retinacular ligament. If the DIP cannot flex, then the restriction is due to a capsular contraction.

▶ *Extrinsic flexor and extensor tendons.* Adherence of the extrinsic flexors is tested by passively maintaining the fingers and thumb in full extension while passively extending the wrist. In the presence of flexor tightness, the increasing flexor tension that develops as the wrist is passively extended will pull the fingers into flexion. Adherence of the extensor tendons is simply a reverse process. The digits are passively maintained in full flexion while the wrist is passively flexed. If tension pulling the fingers into extension is detected by the clinician's hand as the wrist is brought into flexion, extrinsic extensor tightness exists.

Functional Screen

A number of motions can be used to quickly assess hand function, including:

1. Opposition of the thumb and little finger.
2. Pad to pad mobility of the thumb and other fingers. The majority of the functional activities of the hand require at least 5 cm of opening of the fingers and thumb.[78]
3. The ability to make three different fists:
   a. The hook fist (placing fingertips onto MCP joints) (Fig. 16-20).
   b. Standard fist (Fig. 16-21).
   c. Straight fist (placing fingertips on the thenar and hypothenar eminences) (Fig. 16-22). The ability to flex the fingers to within 1 to 2 cm of the distal palmar crease is an indication of functional range of motion for many hand activities.[78]

Palpation and Pain Provocation Tests

The palpation and pain provocation tests are integral components of the physical examination, as they can help define the areas of tenderness by systematically palpating the bony and

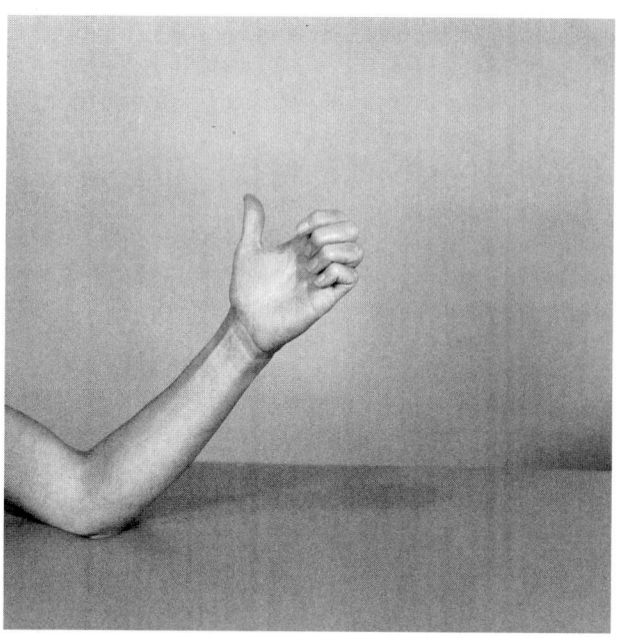

FIGURE 16-20   Hook fist.

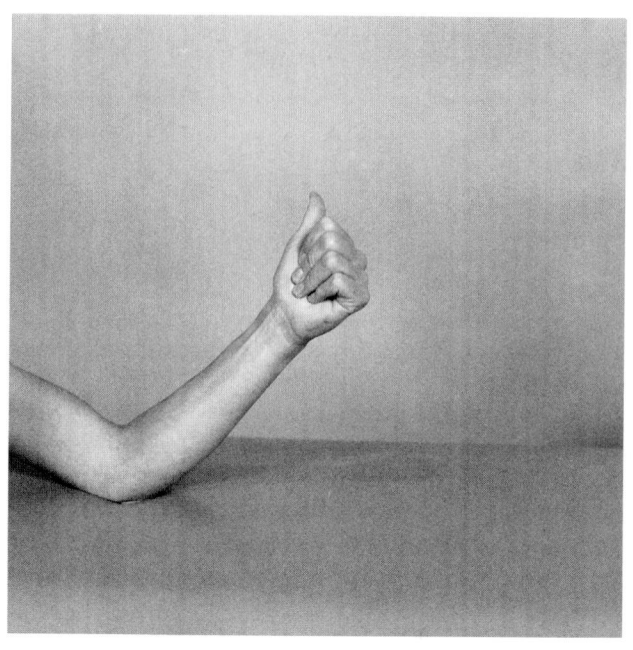

FIGURE 16-22   Straight fist.

soft tissue anatomy, while testing the ability of these structures to withstand stresses.

Palpation.   Palpation of the following muscles, tendon, insertions, ligaments, capsules, and bones should occur as indicated, and be compared with the uninvolved side.

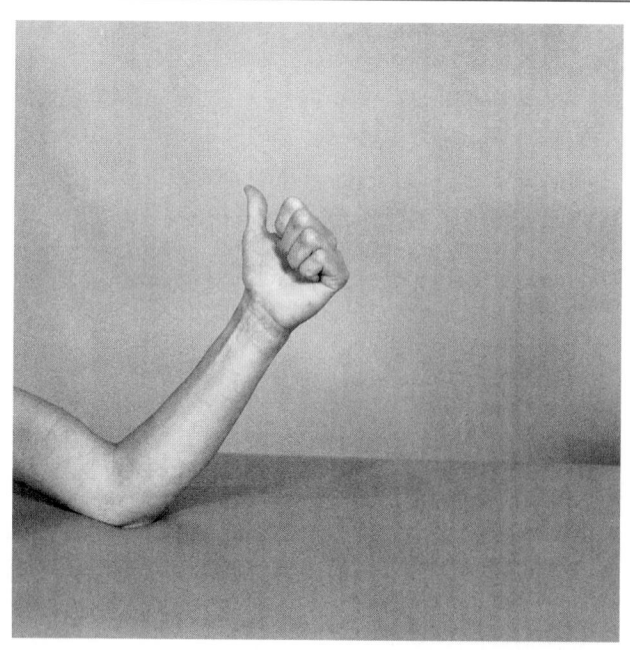

FIGURE 16-21   Standard fist.

Radial Styloid Process.   The radial styloid process (Fig. 16-23) is larger and rounder than the ulnar styloid process. It is best palpated at the most proximal point of the anatomic snuffbox (see below), during radial abduction of the thumb. With simultaneous radial deviation of the wrist, this prominence becomes visible. Tenderness over the styloid, especially with radial deviation, may indicate contusion, fracture, or radioscaphoid arthritis.[79]

Scaphoid.   The scaphoid is palpated just distal to the radial styloid in the anatomic snuffbox (see Fig. 16-15). The neck of the scaphoid is located on the floor of the anatomic snuffbox. Palpation can be made easier by positioning the wrist in ulnar deviation. The scaphoid may be grasped and moved passively by firm pressure between an opposed index finger and thumb applied to the palmar surface and anatomic snuffbox simultaneously. In most individuals, the scaphoid is mildly tender to palpation, but those with scaphoid fracture, nonunion, or scaphoid instability have severe discomfort (see "Special Tests" section).[2,80]

Trapezium.   The trapezium is located immediately proximal to the base of the first metacarpal bone, just distal to the scaphoid (see Fig. 16-23). The tubercle of the trapezium lies anteriorly at the base of the thenar eminence. It can be made more prominent by opposing the thumb to the little finger, and ulnarly deviating the wrist. Tenderness over this carpal may indicate scaphotrapezial arthritis secondary to scaphoid instability.[81]

Thumb CMC Joint.   To examine the thumb CMC joint, the clinician palpates carefully along the shaft of the thumb metacarpal down to its proximal flare. Just proximal to this flare is a small depression where the CMC joint is located (see Fig. 16-23). By

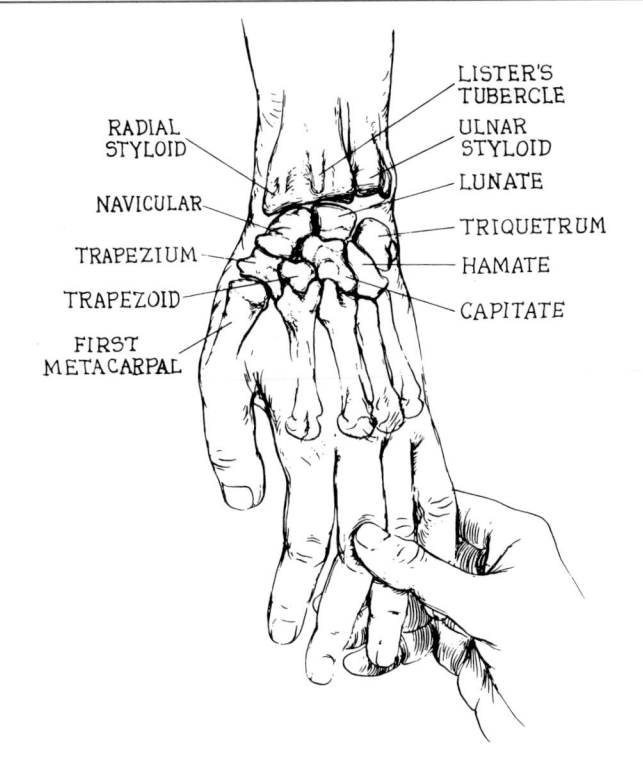

FIGURE 16-23 Palpation of bony landmarks. (Reproduced with permission from Hoppenfeld S. *Physical Examination of the Spine and Extremities.* East Norwalk, CT: Appleton-Century-Crofts; 1976.)

applying direct radial and ulnar stresses to the joint, the clinician can determine the overall stability of the joint as compared to the other thumb. Tenderness here is usually indicative of degenerative arthritis.

EPB and APL Tendons. The EPB and APL tendons make up the first extensor compartment on the dorsum of the wrist, and together form the radial border of the anatomic snuffbox. Prominence of these tendons can be enhanced by extending and radially abducting the thumb. Tenderness over these tendons may indicate De Quervain's tenosynovitis.

Lister's Tubercle. This is a small bony prominence on the dorsal and distal end of radius. It is found by sliding a finger proximally from a point between the index and middle finger (see Fig. 16-23). Just distal to Lister's tubercle is the joint line of the scaphoid and radius. The ECRL and ECRB tendons travel radial to Lister's tubercle, and insert on the base of the second and third metacarpals. The EDC tendon travels ulnarly to Lister's tubercle.

Lunate. The lunate is located just distal and ulnar to Lister's tubercle with the wrist flexed, and is immediately proximal to, and in line with, the capitate (see Fig. 16-23). The mobile lunate can be felt to glide dorsally with extension. It is the most commonly dislocated carpal and the scapholunate articulation is the most common area for carpal instability. Scapholunate

synovitis (dorsal wrist syndrome) or a scapholunate ligament injury presents with tenderness or fullness in this region.[2] Tenderness specific to the lunate can indicate Kienböck's disease or avascular necrosis of the lunate.[82,83]

Capitate. The capitate is localized by palpating proximally over the dorsal aspect of the third metacarpal until a small depression is felt. While palpating in this depression, as the wrist is flexed, the clinician should feel the capitate, the central bone of the carpus, move dorsally. Tenderness in this depression may indicate scapholunate or lunotriquetral instability, or capitolunate degenerative joint disease.

Second and Third Metacarpals. The base of the second and third metacarpals and the CMC joints are localized by palpating proximally along the dorsal surfaces of the index and long metacarpals to their respective bases (see Fig. 16-23).[73] A bony prominence found at the base of the second or third metacarpal may be a carpal boss, a variation found in some individuals due to hypertrophic changes of traumatic origin.[73]

Ulnar Head and Styloid Process. The ulnar head forms a rounded prominence on the ulnar side of the wrist, which is easily palpated with the forearm in pronation (see Fig. 16-23).[73] The ulnar styloid process is ulnar and distal to the head of the ulna. It is best located with the forearm in supination.

Triangular Fibrocartilage Complex (TFCC). The TFCC is located distal to the ulnar styloid, and proximal to the triquetrum (see Fig. 16-1). Tenderness over this structure indicates an injury to the TFCC.[4]

Hamate. The hook of the hamate is palpated just distal and radial (in the direction of the thumb web space) to the pisiform on the palmar aspect (see Fig. 16-23). Locating the hamate can be made easier if the clinician places the middle of the distal phalanx of the thumb on the pisiform, with the thumb pointing between the web space between the index and long finger. The clinician flexes the IP joint of the thumb and presses into the hypothenar eminence to feel the firm hook. The hook of the hamate is concave laterally, and the ulnar nerve's superficial division can be rolled on it. Tenderness over this carpal is common, and so the clinician should compare findings with the other side. Severe tenderness could indicate a fracture of the hamate, especially if associated with a fall on the outstretched hand (FOOSH injury) or a missed hit swing of a racket or bat.[84]

Triquetrum. The triquetrum is located by radially deviating the wrist while palpating just distal to the ulnar styloid (see Fig. 16-23). With ulnar deviation, the triquetrum articulates with the TFCC, which functions as a buffer between the styloid and the triquetrum. Tenderness and swelling in the triquetral hamate region are often present with midcarpal instability, which occurs when the palmar triquetral-hamate-capitate ligament is ruptured or sprained.[85]

Pisiform. The pisiform is located on the flexor aspect of the palm, on top of the triquetrum, at the distal crease (see Fig. 16-23). Tenderness of this structure may indicate pisotriquetral arthritis or inflammation of the flexor carpi ulnaris tendon.[4]

Tunnel of Guyon. The tunnel of Guyon is located in the space between the hamate and pisiform.[6]

Carpal Tunnel. The distal wrist crease marks the proximal edge of the carpal tunnel. The boundaries of the carpal tunnel are:

- ▶ Radial: palmar scaphoid tubercle and trapezium.

- ▶ Ulnar: pisiform and hamate.

- ▶ Dorsal: the carpal bones.

- ▶ Palmar: transverse carpal ligament.

- ▶ Proximal: palmar antebrachial fascia.

- ▶ Distal: distal edge of the retinaculum at the CMC level, FCR, and scaphoid tubercle.

Flexor Retinaculum. The flexor retinaculum transforms the carpal arch into the carpal tunnel. It is attached laterally to the tubercle of the scaphoid and tubercle of the trapezium, and attached medially to the pisiform and hook of the hamate. Its proximal edge is at the distal crease of the wrist.

Proximal Interphalangeal (PIP) Joints. Palpation of the PIP joint offers important information. Palpation of the joint over four planes (dorsal, palmar, medial, and lateral) allows assessment of point tenderness over ligamentous origins and insertions that is highly suggestive of underlying soft-tissue disruption.[20] In cases in which the joint is grossly swollen and tender, this part of the examination may provide more accurate information several days after the injury.[20]

Pain Provocation Tests

Pain with Wrist Flexion. To determine whether painful wrist flexion is due to a problem between the scaphoid and radius, or the scaphoid and the trapezium and trapezoid, the wrist is placed in full flexion, with the dorsal surface of the hand resting on the treatment table. The clinician pushes on the scaphoid and second metacarpal in a dorsal direction. An increase in pain with this maneuver may indicate a problem at the scaphoid-radius articulation.

If there is no increase in pain with this maneuver, the wrist is placed in a neutral position with regard to flexion and extension. The clinician stabilizes the trapezium and trapezoid and pushes the scaphoid dorsally. An increase in pain with this maneuver may indicate a problem at the trapezium/trapezoid-scaphoid articulation.

To determine whether the painful wrist flexion is due to a problem between the capitate and the lunate, or the lunate and the radius, the wrist is placed in full flexion. The clinician pushes the lunate in a palmar direction. An increase in pain with this maneuver may indicate a problem at the capitate-lunate

articulation. If the pain is not increased with this maneuver, the wrist is placed in full flexion and the clinician pushes the lunate in a dorsal direction. An increase in pain with this maneuver may indicate a problem at the lunate-radius articulation. A decrease in pain with this maneuver may indicate a problem at the capitate-lunate articulation.

Pain with Wrist Extension. To determine whether the pain with wrist extension is due to a problem between the scaphoid and the radius, or the scaphoid and the trapezium/trapezoid, the wrist is positioned in full extension with the palm positioned on the table. The clinician pushes on the radius in a palmar direction, thus increasing the amount of wrist extension. An increase in pain with this maneuver may indicate a problem at the scaphoid-radius articulation. If this maneuver does not increase pain, the wrist is positioned as before. The clinician now pushes on the radius in a dorsal direction. A decrease in pain with this maneuver may indicate a problem at the scaphoid-radius articulation. An increase in pain with this maneuver may indicate a problem at the scaphoid and trapezium/trapezoid articulation.

This is confirmed by placing the wrist as before in full extension and pushing on the scaphoid in a dorsal direction. A decrease in pain with this maneuver indicates a problem between the scaphoid and radius, whereas an increase in pain with this maneuver indicates the problem is between the scaphoid and the trapezium/trapezoid.

The clinician fixes the scaphoid and pushes the trapezium/trapezoid in a palmar direction. A decrease in pain with this maneuver may indicate a problem at the scaphoid-trapezium/trapezoid articulation. If the pain remains unchanged with this maneuver, the problem is likely to be at the scaphoid-radius articulation. To confirm this hypothesis, the scaphoid can be pushed in a palmar direction while the wrist is maintained in the position of full extension. This should increase the pain if the hypothesis is correct.

To determine whether pain is due to a problem between the capitate and lunate, or the lunate and radius, the wrist is positioned in full extension, with the palm of the hand on the table. The clinician pushes on the radius in a palmar direction. An increase in pain with this maneuver indicates a problem at the capitate-lunate articulation.

If the pain is increased by pushing the lunate and capitate in a palmar direction, this may indicate a problem at the lunate-radius articulation.

If fixing the lunate and pushing the capitate in a palmar direction (a relative motion of the lunate dorsally in relation to the capitate) increases the pain, the problem is likely at the capitate-lunate articulation.

Thumb CMC Grind Test. The grind test is used to assess the integrity of the thumb CMC joint by axially loading the thumb metacarpal into the trapezium.[9,86] The clinician grasps the thumb metacarpal using the thumb and index finger of one hand, and the proximal aspect of the thumb CMC joint with the other hand. An axial compressive force, combined with rotation, is applied to the thumb CMC joint. Reproduction of the patient's pain and crepitus is a positive test for arthrosis and synovitis.

Lichtman Test. The Lichtman test is a provocative test for midcarpal instability.[9] The patient's forearm is positioned in pronation and the hand is held relaxed and supported by the clinician. The clinician gently moves the patient's hand from radial to ulnar deviation while compressing the carpus into the radius. A positive test is when the midcarpal row appears to jump or snap from a palmarly subluxed position to the height of the proximal row.[9]

Linscheid Test. The Linscheid test is used to detect ligamentous injury and instability of the second and third CMC joints. The test is performed by supporting the metacarpal shafts and pressing distally over the metacarpal heads in a palmar and dorsal direction.[73] A positive test produces pain localized to the CMC joints.[87]

Scapholunate Provocation Tests

Scapholunate Shear (Ballottement) Test. The patient is positioned in sitting with their forearm pronated. With one hand, the clinician places an index finger on the scaphoid tuberosity and the thumb on the dorsal aspect of the scaphoid. With the other hand, the clinician grasps the lunate between the thumb and index finger. The lunate and scaphoid are then sheared in a palmar and then dorsal direction.[2] Laxity and reproduction of the patient's pain are positive signs for this test.[9]

Watson's Test (Scaphoid Shift) for Carpal Instability. As the scaphoid plays a critical role in coordinating and stabilizing movements between the proximal and distal rows of the carpals, damage to the intrinsic and extrinsic ligaments that support the scaphoid can result in persistent pain and dysfunction with loading activities.[81,88,89]

The scaphoid shift maneuver examines the dynamic stability of the wrist, in particular the integrity of the scapholunate ligament.[81]

The patient is positioned with their elbow resting in their lap in approximately 90 degrees of flexion. The forearm is slightly pronated, and the wrist ulnarly deviated. The clinician stabilizes the scaphoid tubercle with the thumb, and the dorsal aspect of the scaphoid with the index finger. As the wrist is brought passively into radial deviation, the normal flexion of the proximal row forces the scaphoid tubercle into a palmar direction (into the clinician's thumb). The clinician attempts to prevent the palmar motion of the scaphoid. When the scaphoid is unstable, its proximal pole is forced to sublux dorsally.[9] Pain at the dorsal wrist or a clunk suggests instability.[16,24] The results are compared with the other hand.

The results from the scaphoid shift test should be used with caution, as the test can be positive in up to one third of uninjured individuals,[88] and has been found to have a sensitivity of 69 percent and a specificity of between 64 and 68 percent.[90,91]

Finger Extension Test. This test is used to demonstrate dorsal wrist syndrome, a localized scapholunate synovitis.[81] The

clinician instructs the patient to fully flex the wrist, and then actively extend the digits at both the IP and MCP joints. The clinician then applies pressure on the fingers into flexion at the MCP joints while the patient continues to actively extend. A positive test occurs when there is production of central dorsal wrist pain, and indicates the possibility of Kienböck's disease, carpal instability, joint degeneration, or synovitis (see "Intervention Strategies" section).[9]

Strength Testing

Isometric tests are carried out in the extreme range, and if positive, in the neutral range. These isometric tests must include the interossei and lumbricals. The straight plane motions of wrist flexion, extension, and ulnar and radial deviation are tested initially. Pain with any of these tests requires a more thorough examination of the individual muscles. The clinician should be able to extrapolate hand placements for these tests by noting the anatomy of these muscles from the figures.

Wrist

Flexor Carpi Radialis/Flexor Carpi Ulnaris. During the testing of these muscles, substitution by the finger flexors should be avoided by not allowing the patient to make a fist. The clinician applies the resistive force into extension and radial deviation for the FCU, and extension and ulnar deviation for the FCR.

Extensor Carpi Radialis Longus/Brevis. Any action of the EDC should be ruled out by having the patient make a fist while extending the wrist. The clinician applies the resistive force on the dorsum of the second and third metacarpals, with the force directed into flexion and ulnar deviation.

Extensor Carpi Ulnaris. The ECU is tested by having the patient make a fist in wrist extension, while the clinician applies resistance on the ulnar dorsum of hand, with the force directed into flexion and radial deviation.

Thumb

Abductor Pollicis Longus/Brevis. The forearm is positioned midway between pronation and supination, or in maximal supination. The MCP and IP joints are positioned in flexion. The muscles are tested with palmar abduction of the thumb in the frontal plane for the longus and in the sagittal plane for the brevis.

Opponens Pollicis. The forearm is positioned in supination and the dorsal aspect of the hand rests on the table. The patient is asked to touch the finger pads of the thumb and little finger together. Using one hand, the clinician stabilizes the first and fifth metacarpals and the palm of the hand. With the other hand, the clinician applies a force to the distal end of the first metacarpal in the opposite direction of opposition (retroposition).

Flexor Pollicis Longus/Brevis. The forearm is positioned in supination and supported by the table, and the hand is positioned so that the dorsal aspect rests on the table. The thumb is adducted. The longus is tested by resistance applied to the distal phalanx, whereas both heads of the brevis are tested by resistance applied to the proximal phalanx.

Adductor Pollicis.   This muscle is tested by having the patient hold a piece of paper between the thumb and radial aspect of the index finger's proximal phalanx while the clinician attempts to remove it. If weak or nonfunctioning, the IP joint of the thumb flexes during this maneuver due to substitution by the flexor digitorum profundus (FDP) (Froment's sign).

Extensor Pollicis Longus (EPL)/Brevis (EPB).   Both of these muscles can be tested with the patient's hand flat on the table, palm down, and asking the patient to lift only the thumb off the table. To test each individually, resistance is applied to the dorsal aspect of the distal phalanx for the EPL while stabilizing the proximal phalanx and metacarpal, and to the dorsal aspect of the proximal phalanx for the EPB while stabilizing the first metacarpal.

Intrinsics

Lumbricals.   The four lumbricals are tested by applying resistance to the dorsal surface of the middle and distal phalanges, while stabilizing under the proximal phalanx of the finger being tested.

Palmar Interossei.   The palmar and dorsal interossei act with the lumbricals to achieve MCP flexion coupled with PIP and DIP extension. The three palmar interossei also adduct the second, fourth, and fifth fingers to midline. Resistance is applied by the clinician to the radial aspect of the distal end of the proximal phalanx of the second, fourth, and fifth fingers, after first stabilizing the hand and fingers not being tested.

Dorsal Interossei/Abductor Digiti Minimi.   The four dorsal interossei abduct the second, third, and fourth fingers from midline. The abductor digiti minimi abducts the fifth finger from midline.

The intrinsic muscles are tested in the frontal plane to avoid substitution by the extrinsic flexors and extensors. Resistance is applied by the clinician to the ulnar aspect of the distal end of the proximal phalanx of each of the four fingers, after first stabilizing the hand and fingers not being tested.

Fingers

Flexor Digitorum Profundus (FDP).   This muscle is tested with DIP flexion of each digit, while the MCP and PIP are stabilized in extension and wrist neutral. Due to the variability of nerve innervation for this muscle group, each of the fingers can be tested to determine if a peripheral nerve lesion is present. The index finger is served by the anterior interosseous nerve, the middle finger by the main branch of the median nerve, and the ring and little finger by the ulnar nerve.

Flexor Digitorum Superficialis.   There is normally one muscle-tendon unit for each finger; however, an absent flexor digitorum superficialis to the little finger is common. The clinician should only allow the finger to be tested to flex by firmly blocking all joints of the nontested fingers, with the wrist in neutral.

Extensor Digitorum (EDM)/Extensor Indicis Proprius (EIP).   There is only one muscle belly for this four-tendon unit. These three muscles are the sole MP joint extensors. With the wrist in neutral, the strength is tested with the metacarpals in extension and the PIP/DIP flexed. The EIP can be isolated by positioning the index finger and hand in the "number one" position—the index finger in extension with other fingers clenched in a fist. The EDM muscle is tested with resistance of little finger extension with the other fingers maintained in a fist.

To isolate intrinsic muscle function, the patient is asked to actively extend the MP joint and then to attempt to actively extend the PIP joint. Because the ED, EI, and EDM tendons are "anchored" at the MP joint by active extension, only the intrinsic muscles can now extend the PIP joint.[17] To test the terminal extensor tendon function, the clinician stabilizes the middle phalanx and asks the patient to extend the DIP joint.[17]

Flexor Digiti Minimi.   The forearm is positioned in supination and the dorsal aspect of the hand rests on the table. The clinician stabilizes the fifth metacarpal and the palm with one hand, and then applies resistance to the palmar surface of the proximal phalanx of the fifth digit with the other hand.

Opponens Digiti Minimi.   The forearm is positioned in supination and the dorsal aspect of the hand rests on the table. The patient is asked to touch the finger pads of the thumb and little finger together. Using one hand, the clinician stabilizes the first and fifth metacarpals and palm of the hand. With the other hand, the clinician applies a force to the distal end of the fifth metacarpal in the opposite direction of opposition (retroposition).

Grip Strength.   A patient's grip strength is commonly used to assess hand function. A number of protocols using a sealed hydraulic dynamometer, such as the Jamar dynamometer (Fig. 16-24) (Asimow Engineering Co., Santa Monica, CA), have been shown to be accurate, reliable, and valid in measuring grip strength.[92] These dynamometers register force in pounds per square inch, and have adjustable handles to accommodate any sized hand, or any hand that may have a limitation of finger joint motion.[93]

Studies have demonstrated that the second handle setting of the Jamar dynamometer allows for the maximum grip strength from the patient.[93,94] The widest grip uses mostly the profundus muscles. At the narrowest grip, the profundus and superficialis muscle excursion are fully used, preventing much in the way of their contribution to the overall grip strength.[57,93]

Unfortunately, these tests are not purely objective, as they rely on the sincerity of effort from the patient.[95] Thus a number of tests have been introduced in an attempt to aid in the detection of insincerity of effort:

▶ ***The five-position grip strength test.***[57]   This test uses the Jamar dynamometer and uses the five handle settings to

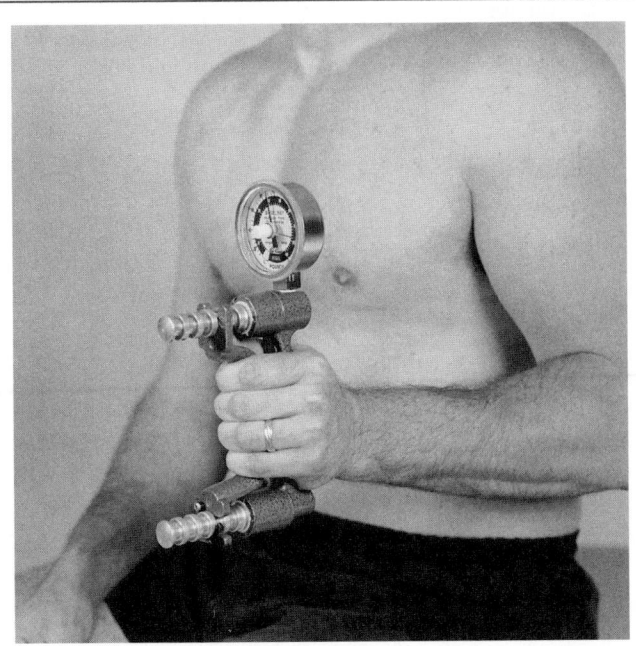

FIGURE 16-24 Measuring grip strength.

TABLE 16-9 Average Strength of Pulp Pinch with Separate Digits (100 Subjects) Using a Hydraulic Dynamometer[328]

	Pulp-to-Pulp Pinch (kg)			
	Male Hand		Female Hand	
Digit	Major	Minor	Major	Minor
II	5.3	4.8	3.6	3.3
III	5.6	5.7	3.8	3.4
IV	3.8	3.6	2.5	2.4
V	2.3	2.2	1.7	1.6

It is probably wise to combine the results of different grip strength tests before making any decisions.[100]

The assessment of pinch strength is also used to assess function of the hand, using a pinch meter. Average values for the pulp-to-pulp pinch of each finger with the thumb are given in Table 16-9.

Functional Assessment

The *functional position* of the wrist is the position in which optimal function is likely to occur.[54,101] This position involves wrist extension of between 20 and 35 degrees, ulnar deviation of 10 to 15 degrees, slight flexion of all of the finger joints, midrange thumb opposition, and slight flexion of the thumb MCP and IP joints.[54] In this position, which minimizes the restraining action of the long extensor tendons, the pulps of the index finger and thumb are in contact.

The *functional range of motion* for the hand is the range in which the hand can perform most of its grip and other functional activities (Table 16-10).

The percentage losses of digital function are as follows: thumb, 40 to 50 percent; index finger, 20 percent; long finger, 20 percent; ring finger, 10 percent; little finger, 5 percent. Loss of the hand is 90 percent of the upper extremity and 54 percent of the whole person.

measure grip strength at the five different grip widths. In normal and motivated patients, maximum grip strength occurs at the second or third grip width. The maximum grip strength, recorded at the first or fifth width setting, is supposed to be indicative of an insincerity of effort, although the reliability of the five-position grip strength test has been questioned.[94,96]

▶ *The rapid exchange grip test, rapid simultaneous grip strength tests.* The first test was developed by Lister.[97] Both of these tests use the Jamar dynamometer, and compare the maximum grip strength during a five-position static grip strength test, with the maximum grip strength recorded when gripping the dynamometer repeatedly at a fast rate (80 times per minute).[98,99] In normal and motivated patients the static measure of grip strength of grip strength should be approximately 15 percent greater than the dynamic measure, while in patients demonstrating insincerity of effort, the dynamic measure is equal to or greater than the initial static measure.[99] The rapid exchange and the rapid simultaneous grip strength tests are time consuming and frequently performed erroneously in the clinical setting.[95]

▶ *The rapid repeat test.* The patient is seated with their arm by their side, the elbow in 90 degrees of flexion, and the forearm and wrist in neutral. The dynamometer, set at the second handle setting, is supported by the clinician and the patient alternately grips with both right and left hands on ten occasions, or until the patient has to stop due to fatigue or discomfort. This test has been found to be an unreliable discriminator of true and faked hand weakness.[95]

TABLE 16-10 Functional Range of Motion of the Hand and Wrist[21,36,37,54,78,329,330]

Joint Motion	Functional Range of Motion (Degrees)
Wrist flexion	5–40
Wrist extension	30–40
Radial deviation	10–20
Ulnar deviation	15–20
MCP flexion	60
PIP flexion	60
DIP flexion	40
Thumb MCP flexion	20

DIP, distal interphalangeal; MCP, metacarpophalangeal; PIP, proximal interphalangeal.

Function of the digits is related to nerve distribution. Flexion and sensation of the radial digits, important in precision grips, are controlled mainly by the median nerve, whereas flexion and sensation of the ulnar digits, important to the power grip, are controlled by the ulnar nerve. The muscles of the thumb, used in all forms of gripping, are controlled by both the median and ulnar nerve. The release of a grip or opening of the hand is controlled by the radial nerve. A loss of the relationship between the thumb and index finger results in an inability to perform fine motor skills that involve pulp-to-pulp pinch, as well as functions that require power.

Hand Disability Index.[102]   The patient is asked to rate the following seven questions on a scale of zero to three, with three being the most difficult.

Unable to perform task = 0

Able to complete task partially = 1

Able to complete task but with difficulty = 2

Able to perform task normally = 3

Are you able to:

1. Dress yourself, including tying shoelaces and doing buttons?
2. Cut your meat?
3. Lift a full cup or glass to your mouth?
4. Prepare your own meal?
5. Open car doors?
6. Open jars that have previously been opened?
7. Turn taps on and off?

A variety of evaluation tools have been devised for the hand, and they can be categorized into assessments of the neurovascular system, range of motion, sensibility, and function (Table 16-11).[78]

Grip and pinch measurements were outlined under "Grip Strength." Dexterity tests include the following:

Minnesota Rate of Manipulation Test (MRMT).   This test, which primarily measures gross coordination and dexterity, consists of five functions:

TABLE 16-11   Functional Testing of the Wrist and Hand[331]

Starting Position	Action	Functional Test
1. Forearm supinated, resting on table	Wrist flexion	Lift 0 lb: Nonfunctional Lift 1 to 2 lb: Functionally poor Lift 3 to 4 lb: Functionally fair Lift 5+ lb: Functional
2. Forearm pronated, resting on table	Wrist extension lifting 1 to 2 lb	0 Repetitions: Nonfunctional 1 to 2 Repetitions: Functionally poor 3 to 4 Repetitions: Functionally fair 5+ Repetitions: Functional
3. Forearm between supination and pronation, resting on table	Radial deviation lifting 1 to 2 lb	0 Repetitions: Nonfunctional 1 to 2 Repetitions: Functionally poor 3 to 4 Repetitions: Functionally fair 5+ Repetitions: Functional
4. Forearm between supination and pronation, resting on table.	Thumb flexion with resistance from rubber band around thumb	0 Repetitions: Nonfunctional 1 to 2 Repetitions: Functionally poor 3 to 4 Repetitions: Functionally fair 5+ Repetitions: Functional
5. Forearm resting on table, rubber band around thumb and index finger	Thumb extension against resistance of rubber band	0 Repetitions: Nonfunctional 1 to 2 Repetitions: Functionally poor 3 to 4 Repetitions: Functionally fair 5+ Repetitions: Functional
6. Forearm resting on table, rubber band around thumb and index finger	Thumb abduction against resistance of rubber band	0 Repetitions: Nonfunctional 1 to 2 Repetitions: Functionally poor 3 to 4 Repetitions: Functionally fair 5+ Repetitions: Functional

TABLE 16-11 *(cont.)*

7. Forearm resting on table	Thumb adduction, lateral pinch of piece of paper	Hold 0 s: Nonfunctional Hold 1 to 2 s: Functionally poor Hold 3 to 4 s: Functionally fair Hold 5+ s: Functional
8. Forearm resting on table	Thumb opposition, pulp-to-pulp pinch of piece of paper	Hold 0 s: Nonfunctional Hold 1 to 2 s: Functionally poor Hold 3 to 4 s: Functionally fair Hold 5+ s: Functional
9. Forearm resting on table	Finger flexion, patient grasps mug or glass using cylindrical grasp and lifts off table	0 Repetitions: Nonfunctional 1 to 2 Repetitions: Functionally poor 3 to 4 Repetitions: Functionally fair 5+ Repetitions: Functional
10. Forearm resting on table	Patient attempts to put on rubber glove keeping fingers straight	21+ s: Nonfunctional 10 to 20 s: Functionally poor 4 to 8 s: Functionally fair 2 to 4 s: Functional
11. Forearm resting on table	Patient attempts to pull fingers apart (finger abduction) against resistance of rubber band and holds	Hold 0 s: Nonfunctional Hold 1 to 2 s: Functionally poor Hold 3 to 4 s: Functionally fair Hold 5+ s: Functional
12. Forearm resting on table	Patient holds piece of paper between fingers while examiner pulls on paper	Hold 0 s: Nonfunctional Hold 1 to 2 s: Functionally poor Hold 3 to 4 s: Functionally fair Hold 5+ s: Functional

1. Placing.

2. Turning.

3. Displacing.

4. One-hand turning and placing.

5. Two-hand turning and placing.

The activities are timed and compared with the time taken by the other hand, and then compared with normal values.[78,103]

Jebsen-Taylor Hand-Function Test.[104] This test, which requires the least amount of extremity coordination, measures prehension and manipulative skills, and consists of seven subtests:

1. Writing.

2. Card turning.

3. Picking up small objects.

4. Simulated feeding.

5. Stacking.

6. Picking up large, light objects.

7. Picking up large, heavy objects.

The subtests are timed and compared with the time taken by the other hand. The results are also compared with normal values.[78,103]

Nine-Hole Peg Test. This test was designed to assess finger dexterity of each hand.[105] The patient is asked to use one hand to place nine 3.2-cm (1.3-inch) pegs in a 12.7 by 12.7 cm (5 by 5 inch) board, and is then asked to remove them. The task is timed and compared with the time taken by the other hand. The results are compared with normal values.[78,103]

Purdue Pegboard Test.[106,107] This test evaluates finer coordination, requiring prehension of small objects, with measurement categories divided into:

1. Right hand.

2. Left hand.

3. Both hands.

4. Right, left, and both hands.

5. Assembly.

The subtests are timed and compared with normal values based on gender and occupation.[78,103]

Crawford Small Parts Dexterity (CSPD) Test.[108]   The CSPD test involves the use of tweezers and a screwdriver, and requires patients to control not only their hands, but also small tools. This test correlates positively with vocational activities that demand fine coordination skills.[78]

The problem with most of these tests and others is that the critical measure of function used is time, even though time is not an accurate measure of function.

Although not standardized, a few other simple tests can be used to assess hand dexterity. These include writing in a straight line, buttoning and unbuttoning different sized buttons, and zipping and unzipping using a variety of zipper sizes (Fig. 16-25). The following scale can be used to grade these activities:

Unable to perform task = 0.

Able to complete task partially = 1.

Able to complete task but with difficulty = 2.

Able to perform task normally = 3.

Passive Physiologic Mobility Testing

In the following tests, the patient is positioned in sitting, and the clinician is standing or sitting, facing the patient. In each of the tests, the clinician notes the quantity of motion as well as the joint reaction. The tests are always repeated on, and compared to, the same joint in the opposite extremity.

The Wrist.   Using one hand, the clinician palpates and stabilizes the distal aspect of the forearm, while using the other hand to grasp the patient's hand, distal to the wrist.

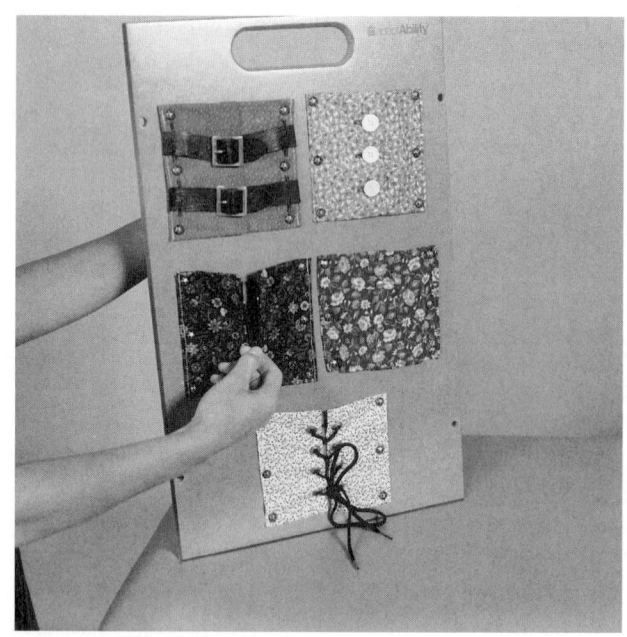

FIGURE 16-25   Dexterity tests.

Flexion/Extension.   The carpal bones are flexed and extended about the appropriate coronal axis through the midcarpal and radiocarpal joints.

Radial/Ulnar Deviation.   The clinician radially and ulnarly deviates the carpal bones about the appropriate sagittal axis through the midcarpal and radiocarpal joints.

Fanning/Folding: Metacarpal.   Using both hands, the clinician grasps the palmar and dorsal aspects of the thenar and hypothenar eminence, and then fans and folds the metacarpal bones about a longitudinal axis (see Figs. 16-18 and 16-19). This technique can also be used as a passive/active mobilization technique.

Phalanges.   Using one hand, the clinician palpates and stabilizes the distal end of the metacarpal/phalanx close to the joint line, while using the other hand to palpate the proximal end of the adjacent phalanx.

Flexion/Extension.   The clinician flexes and then extends the phalanx about the appropriate coronal axis through the MCP/interphalangeal joint.

Abduction/Adduction.   The clinician abducts, and then adducts the phalanx about the appropriate sagittal axis through the MCP joint.

Passive Accessory Mobility Tests

In the following tests, the patient is positioned in sitting, and the clinician is standing or sitting, facing the patient. In each of the tests, the clinician notes the quantity of joint motion as well as the joint reaction. The tests are always repeated on, and compared to, the same joint in the opposite extremity.

Carpal Motion
The Atkinson Method
Lateral Column.   The clinician assesses the motion of the scaphoid in relation to the:

▶ Radius.

▶ Capitate.

▶ Lunate.

▶ Trapezium.

▶ Trapezoid.

Central Column.   The clinician assesses the motion of the lunate in relation to the:

▶ Radius.

▶ Capitate.

Medial Column.   The clinician assesses the motion of the hamate in relation to the:

▶ Ulna.

▶ Lunate.

▶ Triquetrum.

Carpometacarpal Joints. Using one hand, the clinician uses a pinch grip of the index finger and thumb to palpate and stabilize the carpal bone that articulates with the metacarpal bone being tested (Fig. 16-26). With a pinch grip of the index finger and thumb of the other hand, the clinician palpates the metacarpal.

Posterior-Anterior Glide. The first through fifth carpometacarpal joints are tested. The carpal bone is stabilized and the metacarpal is glided posteroanteriorly along the plane of the carpometacarpal joint (see Fig. 16-26).

Metacarpophalangeal/Interphalangeal Joints. Using a pinch grip of the index finger and thumb of one hand, the clinician palpates and stabilizes the metacarpal/phalanx. With a pinch grip of the index finger and thumb of the other hand, the clinician palpates the adjacent phalanx (Fig. 16-27).

Posterior-Anterior Glide. The clinician stabilizes the proximal bone, and then glides the phalanx posteroanteriorly along the plane of the joint (see Fig. 16-27).

Medial-Lateral Glide. The clinician stabilizes the proximal bone, and then glides the phalanx mediolaterally along the plane of the joint.

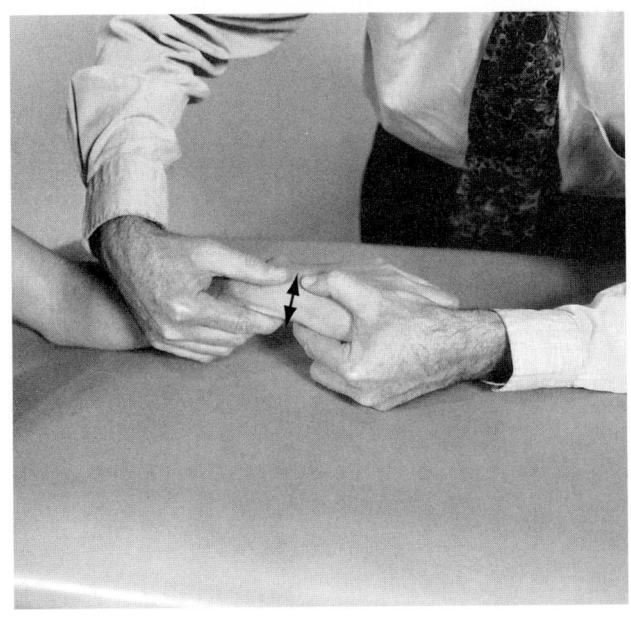

FIGURE 16-26 Carpometacarpal joint testing.

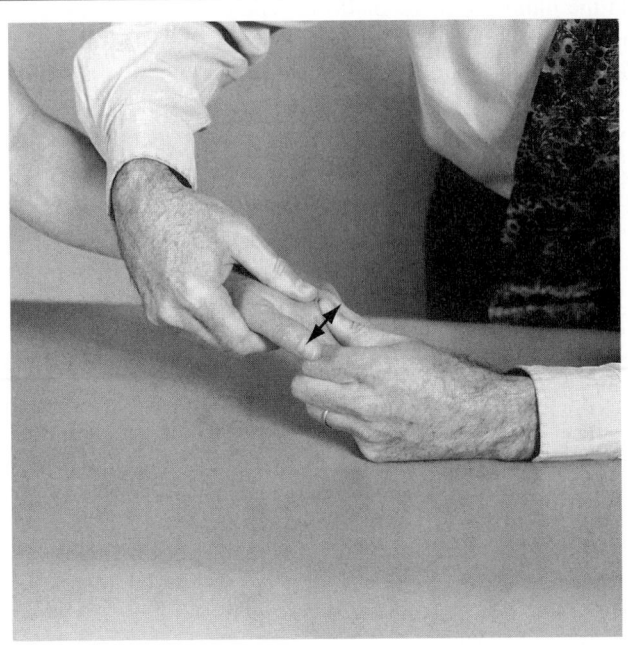

FIGURE 16-27 MCP joint mobility testing.

Ligament Stability

A number of tests are available to evaluate the ligamentous stability of the forearm, wrist, hand, and finger joints. In the following tests, the patient is positioned in sitting, and the clinician is standing or sitting, facing the patient. The clinician must remember to perform these tests on the uninvolved sides to provide a basis for comparison.

Piano Key Test. The piano key test evaluates the stability of the distal radioulnar joint.[4] The clinician firmly stabilizes the distal radius with one hand and grasps the head of the ulna between the thumb and index fingers of the other hand. The ulnar head is depressed in an anterior direction (as in depressing a key on a piano).[9] The test is positive if there is excessive movement in a palmar direction, or if upon release of the ulna, the bone springs back into its high dorsal position. There may also be discomfort reported during the test.[73]

The Lunotriquetral Shear (Reagan's) Test. The lunotriquetral shear maneuver, or Reagan's test,[109] assesses the stability of the lunotriquetral interosseous ligament.[4] The lunate is moved dorsally with the thumb of one hand, while the triquetrum is pushed palmarly by the index finger of the other hand. The wrist is placed in either radial or ulnar deviation. Stress is created between these two bones in the anteroposterior plane. Crepitation, clicks, or discomfort in this area suggests injury to the ligament.[9,110]

The Pisotriquetral Shear Test. The pisotriquetral shear test assesses the integrity of the pisotriquetral articulation.[9] The clinician stabilizes the wrist with the fingers dorsal to the triquetrum, and the thumb over the pisiform. The pisiform is rocked back and forth in a medial and lateral direction. A positive test is manifested with pain during this maneuver.

Pivot Shift Test of the Midcarpal Joint.   The patient is positioned in sitting with the elbow flexed to 90 degrees, resting on a firm surface, and the forearm supinated. The clinician uses one hand to stabilize the forearm, while using the other hand to take the patient's hand into full radial deviation while maintaining the wrist in neutral with regard to flexion and extension. The patient's hand is then taken into full ulnar deviation. A positive test results if the capitate is felt to shift away from the lunate and indicates an injury to the anterior capsule and interosseous ligaments.[21]

Triangular Fibrocartilage Complex (TFCC) Load Test.   This test can be used to detect an injury to the TFCC. It is performed by ulnarly deviating and axially loading the wrist and moving it dorsally and palmarly, or by rotating the forearm. A positive test elicits pain, clicking, or crepitus.[73]

Neurovascular Status

A number of tests can be used to document the neurovascular status of the wrist and hand.

Allen Test.   The Allen test is used to determine the patency of the vessels supplying the hand. The clinician compresses both the radial and ulnar arteries at the wrist (Fig. 16-28), and then asks the patient to open and clench the fist three to four times to drain the venous blood from the hand. The patient is then asked to hold the hand open while the clinician releases the pressure on the ulnar artery, and then the radial artery. The fingers and palm should be seen to regain their normal pink color. This

procedure is repeated with the radial artery released and compression on the ulnar artery maintained. Normal filling time is usually less than 5 seconds. A distinct difference in the filling time suggests the dominance of one artery filling the hand.[110]

Tinel's Test for Carpal Tunnel Syndrome.   The Tinel test is used to assist in the diagnosis of carpal tunnel syndrome. The area over the median nerve is tapped gently at the palmar surface of the wrist (Fig. 16-29). If this produces tingling in the median distribution, then the test is positive.[111] Tinel's sign has a sensitivity of 60 percent and a specificity of 67 percent.[112] The reliability and validity of Tinel's test is moderately acceptable for use in clinical practice.[113–116]

Sensibility Testing

Sensation is the conscious perception of basic sensory input. Sensibility describes the neural events occurring at the periphery, nerve fibers, and nerve receptors. Sensation is what clinicians reeducate, whereas sensibility is what clinicians assess.[117]

The assessment of sensibility of the hand is an important component of every hand examination because sensation is essential for precision movements and object manipulation. Altered sensory perceptions can result from injuries to peripheral nerves or from spinal nerve root compression. The sensory system is described in Chapter 2. Two types of sensibility can be assessed[118]:

▶ *Protective.*   This is evidenced by the ability to perceive pinprick, touch, and temperature.

▶ *Functional.*   This is evidenced by a return of sensibility to a level that enables the hand to engage in full activities of daily living.

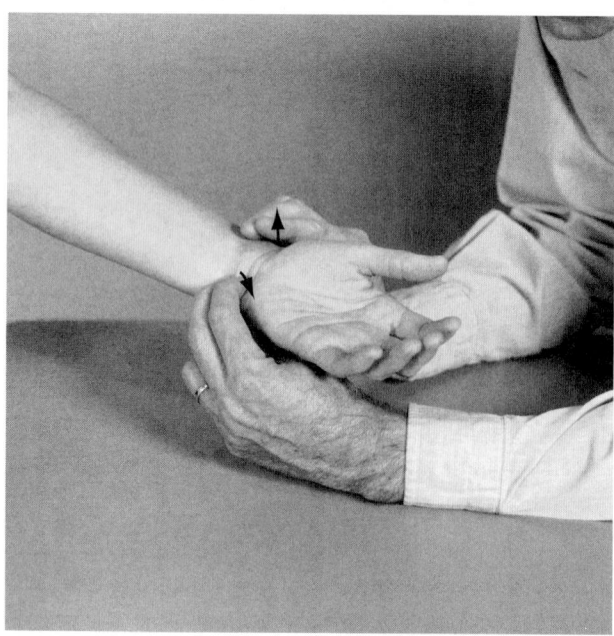

FIGURE 16-28   Allen test.

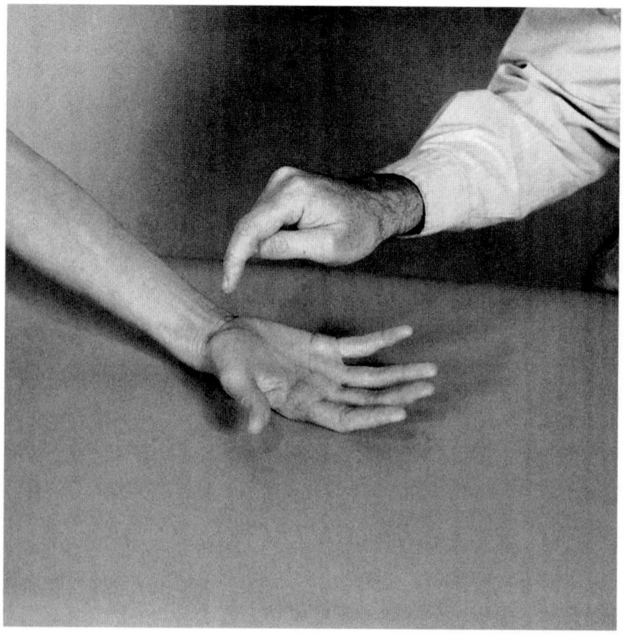

FIGURE 16-29   Tinel's test at the wrist.

There exists a hierarchy of sensibility capacity[118,119]:

▶ *Detection.* This is the simplest level of function and requires that the patient be able to distinguish a single-point stimulus from normally occurring atmospheric background stimulation.

▶ *Innervation density or discrimination.* This represents the ability to perceive that stimulus A differs from stimulus B.

▶ *Quantification.* This involves organizing tactile stimuli according to degree, texture, etc.

▶ *Recognition.* This is the most complicated level of function, and involves the identification of objects with the vision occluded.

Based on this hierarchy, sensibility testing is classified neurophysiologically into four types: threshold tests, stress tests, innervation density tests, and sensory nerve conduction studies.[120]

Threshold Tests. Threshold tests measure the intensity of the stimulus necessary to depolarize the cell membrane and produce an action potential—the ability to detect. Threshold tests are helpful in assessing diminished sensibility in nerve compressions and in monitoring nerve recovery after surgical decompression.[120,121] Examples of threshold tests include vibratory testing and Semmes-Weinstein monofilament testing.

Vibratory Testing. Vibration testing is performed using a 128-Hz tuning fork applied to a bony prominence such as the ulna or radius. The patient is asked to report the perception of both the start of the vibration sensation and the cessation of vibration on dampening. The time (in seconds) at which vibration sensation diminished beyond the clinician's perception is then recorded and compared with the uninvolved side. Alternatively, a vibrometer, such as the Bio-Thesiometer can be used.[120] The Bio-Thesiometer is an electrically controlled testing instrument that produces vibration at a fixed frequency (120 Hz) with a variable amplitude. The vibrating head is applied to the patient's fingertip and the amplitude is slowly and gradually increased. The threshold is recorded as the voltage required to perceive the vibratory stimulus.[120]

Semmes-Weinstein Monofilament Testing. The assessment of cutaneous sensibility was first described in 1899, using horse hairs of varying thickness.[122] In 1960 Semmes and Weinstein[123] made the testing procedure more exacting when they introduced the use of pressure-sensitive nylon monofilaments mounted onto Lucite rods. These monofilaments, which are graded according to thickness, are calibrated to exert specific pressures. Each kit consists of 20 probes, each numbered from 1.65 to 6.65, a number that represents the logarithm of 10 multiplied by the force in milligrams required to bow the filaments.[21]

For the purposes of this test, the palm of the hand is divided into several areas, and only one point (usually in the center) is tested in each area.

▶ Between the fingertip and DIP joint.

▶ Between the DIP joint and PIP joint.

▶ Between the PIP joint and finger web.

▶ Between the finger web and distal palmar crease.

▶ Between the distal palmar crease and central palm.

▶ Base of palm and wrist.

The patient is blindfolded, or turns away during the examination and the clinician applies each filament perpendicular to the finger until the filament bends, starting with the filament with the lowest number and gradually moving up the scale until the patient feels one before or just as it bends.[78,124] The test is repeated three times for confirmation.[125] Normal values are depicted in Table 16-12.

Stress Tests. Stress tests are those that combine the use of sensory tests with activities that provoke the symptoms of nerve compression. These tests are helpful in cases of patient reports of mild nerve compression when no abnormalities are detected by baseline sensory testing. Examples of stress tests include the Phalen's test, the reverse Phalen's test, and the hand elevation test.

Phalen's Test for Carpal Tunnel Syndrome. For Phalen's test,[126,127] the patient sits comfortably with the wrists and elbows flexed (Fig. 16-30). The test is positive if the patient experiences numbness or tingling within 45 seconds. For some patients, performance of this test recreates their wrist, thumb, or forearm ache.[128] Phalen's sign has a sensitivity of 75 percent and a specificity of 47 percent. The reliability and validity of Phalen's test is moderately acceptable for use in clinical practice.[114–116]

Reverse Phalen's Test for Carpal Tunnel Syndrome. For the reverse Phalen's test, the patient sits comfortably with the wrists extended and elbows flexed.[129] Wrist extension has demonstrated a larger increase in intracarpal canal pressure when compared to wrist flexion.[111,130]

Hand Elevation Test for Carpal Tunnel Syndrome. The patient is seated or standing and is asked to elevate both arms above the

TABLE 16-12 Light Touch Testing Using Semmes-Weinstein Monofilaments[119]

Monofilament Number	Pressure (g/mm²)	Interpretation
2.44–2.83	3.25–4.86	Normal light touch
3.22–4.56	11.1–47.3	Diminished light touch
4.74–6.10	68.0–243.0	Minimal light touch
6.10–6.65	243.0–439.0	Sensation intact, but no localization

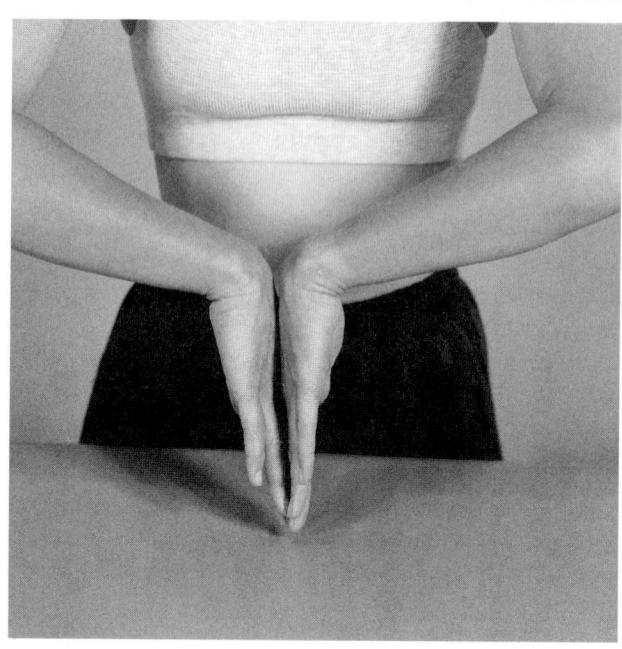

FIGURE 16-30   Phalen's test.

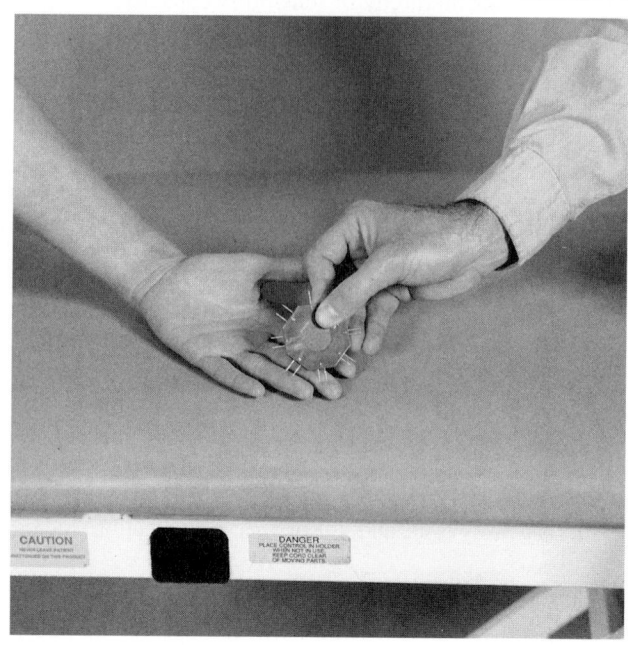

FIGURE 16-31   Disk-Criminator.

head, and maintain them in this position for 2 minutes, or until the patient feels paresthesia or numbness in the hands.[131] In one study, this test was found to be more specific than Phalen's and Tinel's tests.[131]

Innervation Density Tests.   These are a class of sensory tests that test the ability to discriminate between two identical stimuli placed close together on the skin. These tests are helpful in assessing sensibility after nerve repair and during nerve regeneration.[132]

Weber's (Moberg's) Two-Point Discrimination Test.   The two-point discrimination tests were first introduced by Weber in 1953 using calipers, and by Moberg in 1958[132] using a paper clip.

Today it is recommended that a tool such as a Disk-Criminator (Fig. 16-31) be used. The instrument is explained and demonstrated to the patient until an appreciation can be made between one and two points in an area of normal sensibility. The instrument is applied, in a perpendicular fashion, to all of the fingertips in a mixed series of two and one points for five consecutive applications. The patient should be able to recognize at least four out of the five, or seven out of ten.[21] The clinician repeats the tests in an attempt to find the minimal distance at which the patient can distinguish between the two stimuli, decreasing or increasing the distance between the points depending on the response by the patient.[21] This distance is called the threshold for discrimination. Normal discrimination distance is less than 6 mm, although this can vary between individuals (Tables 16-12 and Table 16-13), and in the area of the hand, with normal fingertip scores

between 2 and 5 mm, and finger surface scores between 3 and 7 mm.[125]

Sensory Nerve Conduction Studies.   Sensory nerve conduction studies are electrophysiologic tests that assess the conduction of sensory action potentials along a nerve trunk.[120] These tests require only passive cooperation of the patient, not subjective interpretation of a stimulus. A slowing of nerve conduction velocity or an alteration in potential amplitudes indicates a compression or partial laceration of the nerve.[133]

Neural Tension and Neural Mobility
The Median Nerve.   The patient is positioned in supine lying or sitting. The cervical spine is side bent and rotated to the opposite

TABLE 16-13   Two-Point Discrimination Normal Values and Discrimination Distances Required for Certain Tasks[118]

Grade/Task	Distance
Normal	Less than 6 mm
Fair	6–10 mm
Poor	11–15 mm
Protective	1 point perceived
Anesthetic	0 points perceived
Sewing	6–8 mm
Handling precision tools	12 mm
Handling gross tools	> 15 mm

side. The shoulder girdle is positioned in retraction, depression, extension, and external rotation. The elbow is positioned in extension, the forearm in supination, and the wrist in extension. The fingers are positioned in extension. Nerve irritation is suspected if:

► With the cervical spine in the resting position, the upper extremity position described above results in symptoms in the palmar/radial side of the hand.

► If the symptoms increase with cervical side bending and rotation away from the tested extremity.

► If the symptoms decrease with side bending and rotation towards the tested extremity.

If adherence of the nerve is suspected at the wrist, the cervical spine is positioned in the resting position and the extremity is positioned as before. Neural involvement should be suspected if:

► With wrist flexion the symptoms decrease, but increase when the cervical spine is side bent and rotated away from the tested extremity.

► With wrist extension and the cervical spine side bent and rotated to the tested extremity, the symptoms decrease.

Radial Nerve. The patient is positioned in a supine or sitting position and the shoulder is positioned in retraction, depression, extension, and medial rotation. The elbow is positioned in extension, the forearm in pronation, the wrist in flexion and ulnar deviation, and the fingers in flexion. If a nerve adhesion is suspected at the wrist, the procedure is as for the median nerve, except that the wrist is placed in extension and then taken back into flexion.

The dorsal sensory nerve, which can become implicated (Wartenberg's syndrome; see "Intervention Strategies" section) in a variety of radial-sided injuries because of its superficial location, can be stretched with a combination of wrist flexion and ulnar deviation.

Ulnar Nerve. The shoulder girdle positioning used to describe the test for the median nerve is used. The elbow is flexed and supinated, the wrist is extended and radially deviated, and the fingers extended. If a nerve adhesion at the wrist is suspected, the procedure is as for the median nerve.

Special Tests

Carpal Shake Test. This test is used if intercarpal synovitis is suspected.[9] The clinician grasps the patient's distal forearm (Fig. 16-32). The patient is asked to relax and the clinician shakes the wrist (see Fig. 16-32). Pain or resistance to this test indicates a positive test.

Sit to Stand Test. This test is used if synovitis of the wrist is suspected.[9] The patient is instructed to place both hands on the armrests of a chair and attempt to lift their body slightly off the chair. Pain or resistance to this test indicates a positive test.

Ulnar Impaction Test. This test is used to assess the articulation between the ulnar carpus and the triangular fibrocartilage.[9] The

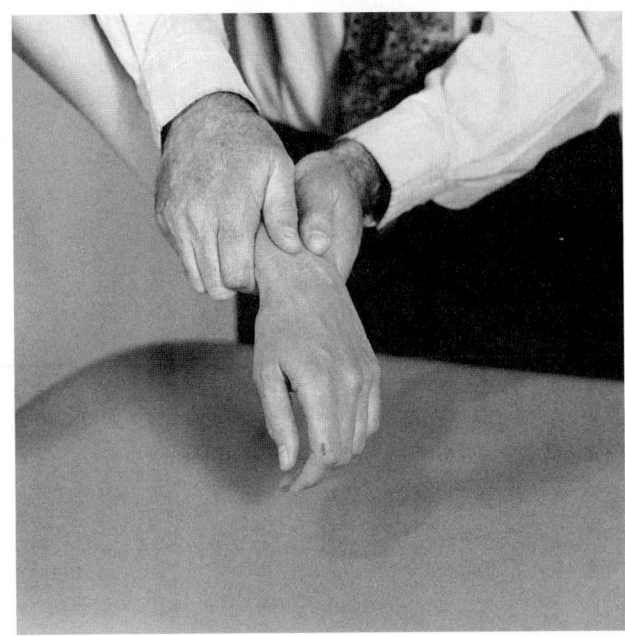

FIGURE 16-32 Carpal shake test.

patient is positioned in sitting, with the elbow flexed to about 90 degrees and the wrist positioned in ulnar deviation, and the fingers positioned in a slight fist. The clinician loads the wrist by applying a compressive force through the ring and small metacarpals (Fig. 16-33). Pain with this test indicates a possible tear of the triangular fibrocartilage or ulnar impaction syndrome (see "Intervention Strategies" section).

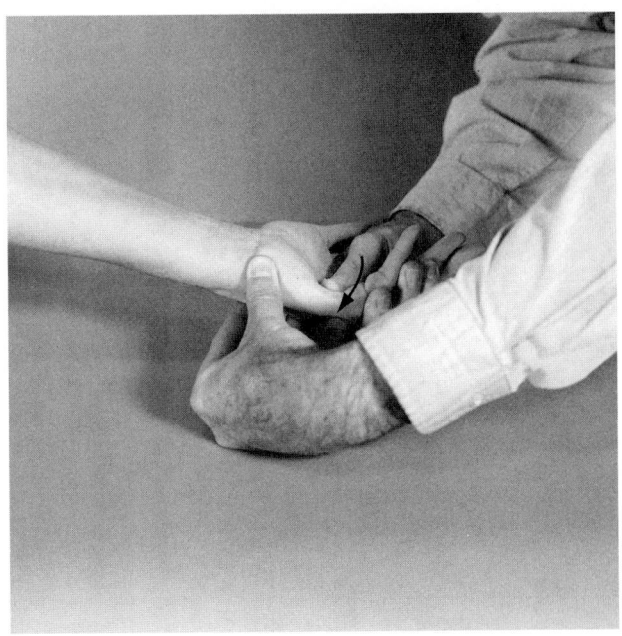

FIGURE 16-33 Ulnar impaction test.

Finkelstein's Test.[134]   This test is used to detect stenosing tenosynovitis of the abductor pollicis longus (APL) and extensor pollicis brevis (EPB). The clinician grasps the patient's thumb, stabilizes the forearm with one hand, then deviates the wrist to the ulnar side with the other hand (Fig. 16-34).

Flexor Digitorum Superficialis (FDS) Test.   This test is used to test the integrity of the FDS tendon. The clinician holds the patient's fingers in extension except for the finger being tested (this isolates the FDS tendon). The patient is instructed to flex the finger at the PIP joint. If this is possible, the FDS tendon is intact. Since this tendon can act independently because of the position of the finger, it is the only functioning tendon at the PIP joint. The DIP joint, motored by the FDP, has no power of flexion when the other fingers are held in extension.

Flexor Digitorum Profundus Test.   These tendons work only in unison. To test the FDP, stabilize the PIP joint and the MCP joint in extension. Instruct the patient to flex this finger at the DIP joint. If flexion occurs, the FDP is intact. If no flexion is possible, the tendon is severed or the muscle denervated.

Extensor Hood Rupture.   Elson[135] describes this test: From 90 degrees of PIP flexion, the patient tries to extend the PIP joint

against resistance. The absence of extension force at the PIP joint, and fixed extension at the distal joint, indicate complete rupture of the central slip.[20]

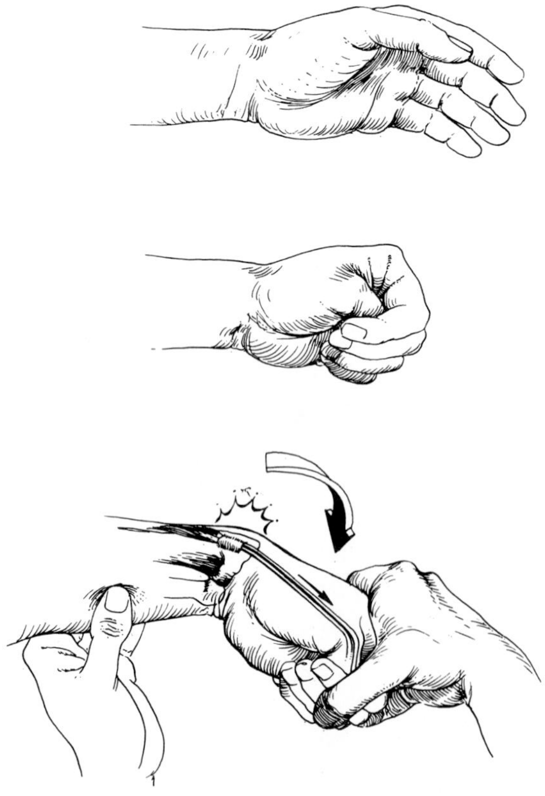

Froment's Sign.   This is more of a sign than a test, and may present as a complaint from the patient who reports an inability to pinch between the index finger and thumb without flexion at the DIP joint occurring.[136] A positive Froment's sign, which results from a weakness in the adductor pollicis and short head of the FPB muscles, indicates an ulnar nerve entrapment at the elbow or at the wrist.

Murphy's Sign.   The patient is asked to make a fist. If the head of the third metacarpal is level with the second and fourth metacarpals, the sign is positive for the presence of a lunate dislocation.[137]

Diagnostic Testing

Diagnostic testing of the forearm, wrist, and hand is limited to plain radiographs for most patients. Bony tenderness with a history of trauma or a suspicion of bone or joint disruption indicates a need for radiographs. Standard projections for the wrist are the posteroanterior, lateral, and oblique. For the patient with a suspicion of a scaphoid injury, a scaphoid view should be added.[4] Wrist conditions rarely require computed tomography (CT) scans and magnetic resonance imaging (MRI) scans.[110]

FIGURE 16-34   Finkelstein's test. (Reproduced with permission from Hoppenfeld S. *Physical Examination of the Spine and Extremities.* East Norwalk, CT: Appleton-Century-Crofts, 1976.)

Intervention Strategies

"To restore the balance and beauty and power to a disabled hand is an adventure. The stakes are high. The rewards are exciting. The penalties of failure are grievous."

PAUL W. BRAND (1914–)

Functional rehabilitation of the upper extremity emphasizes the restoration of functional use of the hand.[78] Hand functions can range from activities that require a strong gripping action to those that require fine precision and gentle touch. Stability of the wrist and hand is provided by a combination of muscular effort and ligamentous support. Motion of the hand and wrist is provided by a vast array of muscles and tendons and several articulated linkages. The hand and wrist can be involved in both open and closed kinetic chain activities.

Pain is perhaps the most common complaint with wrist and hand injuries, with stiffness following closely behind.

The techniques to increase joint mobility and the techniques to increase soft tissue extensibility are described in the "Therapeutic Techniques" section.

Acute Phase

The goals of the acute phase include:

▶ Protection of the injury site to allow healing.

▶ Control pain and inflammation.

► Control and then eliminate edema.

► Restoration of pain-free range of motion in the entire kinetic chain.

► Improve patient comfort by decreasing pain and inflammation.

► Retard muscle atrophy.

► Minimize detrimental effects of immobilization and activity restriction.[138–143]

► Scar management if appropriate.

► Maintain general fitness.

► Patient to be independent with home exercise program.

Pain and inflammation control is the major focus of the intervention program in the acute phase. This may be accomplished using the principles of PRICEMEM (protection, rest, ice, compression, elevation, manual therapy, early motion, and medication). Icing for 20 to 30 minutes, three to four times a day, concurrent with nonsteroidal anti-inflammatory drugs (NSAIDs) or aspirin can aid in reducing pain and swelling.

One of the most significant problems a clinician faces with a hand-injured patient is the control and elimination of edema. Edema can increase the risk of infection, decrease motion, and inhibit arterial, venous, and lymphatic flow.[144] Methods to control edema include elevation of the extremity and hand above the level of the heart, active exercise, retrograde massage, intermittent compression, continuous compression wrapping, and contrast baths.

Therapeutic exercises are performed with the goal of adequate soft tissue rebalancing of the wrist to restore the alignment of the extensor and flexor tendons as near to normal as possible, and to prevent scarring or soft tissue contractures by influencing the physiologic process of collagen formation. Movement is the activity necessary to maintain joint mobility and gliding tendon function. Range-of-motion exercises are introduced as early as tolerated. These may be passive, active assisted, or active, as appropriate. If protected motion is necessary, it can be provided with taping, bracing, or in extreme cases, casting. Passive range-of-motion exercises are performed through the available range of motion to maintain joint and soft tissue mobility, or a passive stretch can be applied at the end range of motion to lengthen pathologically shortened soft tissue structures, thereby increasing motion. Depending on the focus of the intervention, the passive range-of-motion exercises may include:

► MP flexion and extension (Fig. 16-35).

► Proximal interphalangeal (PIP) flexion and extension (Fig. 16-36).

► Distal interphalangeal (DIP) flexion and extension (Fig. 16-37).

Active range-of-motion exercises are performed throughout the available range. Active exercises should include specific and

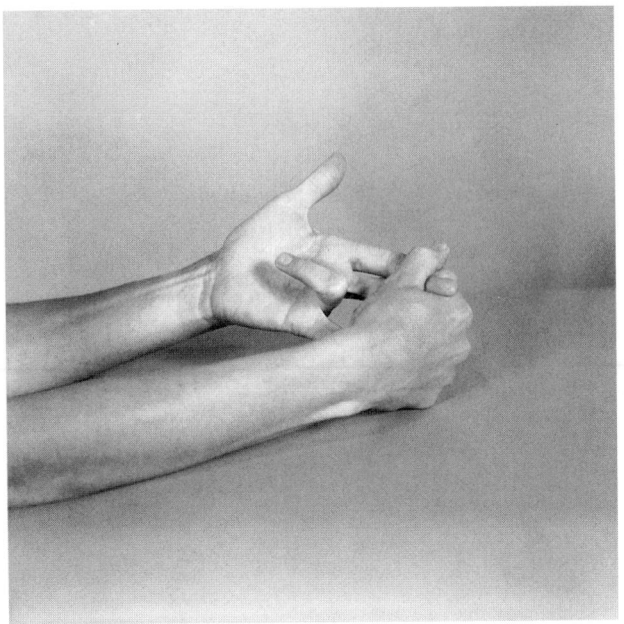

FIGURE 16-35   Isolated MP flexion.

composite exercises. Composite exercises, which reproduce normal functional activities, include fisting and thumb opposition to each digit in addition to exercises involving the wrist, elbow, and shoulder. When active exercises are used to restore mobility in the presence of increasing tissue resistance, fast

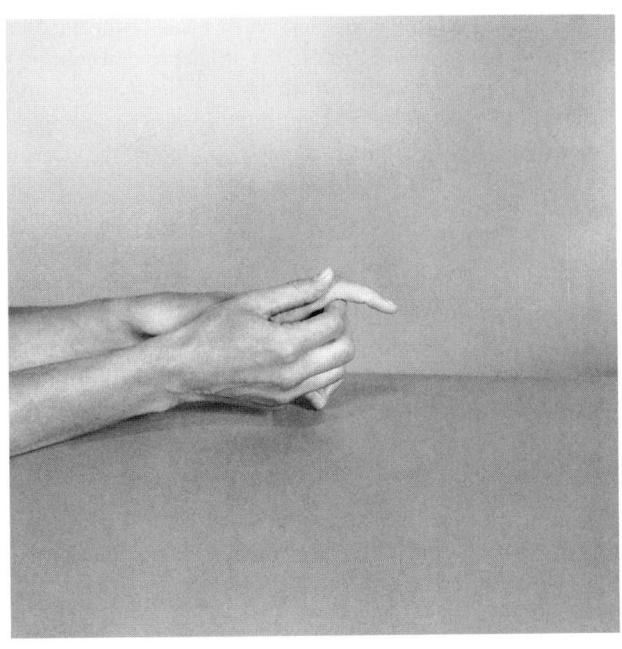

FIGURE 16-36   Isolated PIP flexion and extension.

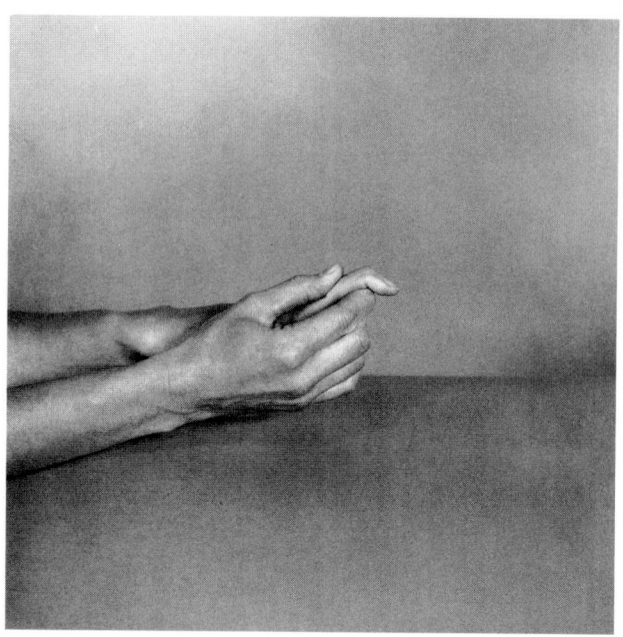

FIGURE 16-37   Isolated DIP flexion and extension.

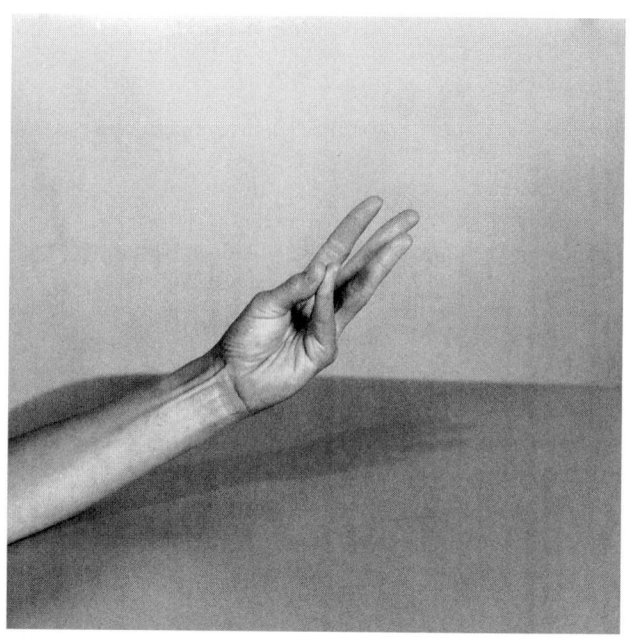

FIGURE 16-38   Thumb opposition.

ballistic movements are discouraged.[145] Examples of active range-of-motion exercises include:

▶ Active wrist and finger flexion and extension, wrist ulnar and radial deviation, finger adduction and abduction, and thumb opposition (Fig. 16-38), flexion, extension, abduction, and adduction. The wrist and hand muscles are usually exercised as a group if their strength is similar. If one muscle is weaker, the clinician should exercise that muscle in isolation, in a similar fashion as that used when isolating the muscle for manual muscle testing. Protected range-of-motion exercises are performed to selectively mobilize joints and tendons while minimizing stress on repairing structures. As their name suggests, protected range-of-motion exercises are accomplished by placing the repaired structure in a protected position while adjacent tissues are carefully mobilized. An example of protective exercise can be seen following a radial nerve injury, where tendon transfers of the pronator teres, flexor carpi ulnaris, and flexor digitorum superficialis may be performed.[145] Following the surgery the hand is immobilized with the wrist, MCP joints, and thumb in extension. At approximately 4 weeks, protective active motion exercises are introduced. These include MCP joint flexion, and then PIP and DIP joint flexion with the MCP joint maintained in extension.[145]

▶ Active exercises of forearm pronation and supination.

The active range-of-motion exercises are progressed to submaximal isometrics and muscle co-contractions. Isometric exercise allows for strengthening early in the rehabilitative process without the stress to joints and soft tissue produced by other forms of exercise. These early strengthening exercises are

performed initially in the available pain-free ranges and are gradually progressed so that they are performed throughout the entire range.

Scar tissue management focuses on the control of stresses placed on healing tissues. Early active and passive motion provides controlled stress, encouraging optimal remodeling of scar tissue.[144] Methods to control scarring include the use of thermal agents, transverse friction massage (see Chap. 11), mechanical vibration, compressive techniques, and splinting.

Splinting of the wrist and hand may be necessary. It is not within the scope of this text to provide comprehensive detail with regard to splinting. Entire texts are devoted to the subject.[146–149] However, splinting can often be an integral part of the rehabilitation program, and the clinician needs to be aware of the purposes of splinting as well as some of the options available. Creative splinting can provide a useful adjunct to exercise. The general purposes of a splint are to[150,151]:

▶ *Prevent deformity.*   Maintain normal tissue length, balance, and excursion.

▶ *Immobilize/stabilize.*   Splinting is especially useful for stabilizing mobile joints so the corrective exercise force can be directed to the stiff joint or adherent tendon.[145]

▶ *Protect.*   Static splints have no moveable parts and maintain joints in one position to promote healing and minimize friction.

▶ *Correct deformity or dysfunction.*   Re-establish normal tissue length, balance, and excursion.

▶ *Control/modify scar formation.*

▶ *Substitute for dysfunctional tissue.*

▶ *Exercise.* *Drop-out* splints block joint motion in one direction but allow motion in another. Drop-out splints are commonly used with elbow flexion contractures. Articulated splints contain at least two static components and are connected in such a way as to allow motion in one plane at a joint. *Dynamic splints* are used to provide active resistance in the direction opposite their line of pull to increase muscle strength, as well as to apply a corrective passive stretch to tendon adhesions and joint contractures.[145] *Static-progressive* splints involve the use of inelastic components such as hook-and-loop tapes, Dacron line, turnbuckles, and screws, to allow progressive changes in joint position as PROM changes without changing the structure of the splint. *Serial static* splints differ from static progressive splints in that they require the clinician to remold the splint to accommodate increases in mobility.

Functional Phase

The functional phase of rehabilitation usually commences when normal wrist positions and co-contractions of the wrist flexors and extensors can be performed. The goals of the functional phase include:

▶ Attain full range of pain-free motion.

▶ Restore normal joint kinematics.

▶ Improve muscle strength to within normal limits.

▶ Improve neuromuscular control.

▶ Restore normal muscle force couple relationships.

The AROM exercises, initiated during the acute phase, are progressed until the patient demonstrates they have achieved the maximum range anticipated.

Normal joint kinematics are restored using joint mobilization techniques. Joint mobilization techniques refer to passive traction and/or gliding movements to joint surfaces that maintain or restore the joint play normally allowed by the capsule. The joint mobilization techniques for the forearm, wrist, and hand are described in the "Therapeutic Techniques" section at the end of this chapter.

Resistive exercises not only increase muscle strength and endurance, but also improve the ability of the patient to actively mobilize stiff joints.[145] Resistance exercises for the hand and wrist can be classified as either static (isometric) or dynamic (concentric, eccentric, or isokinetic). Strengthening of the muscles of the wrist and hand begins with specific exercises and progresses to exercises that involve the entire upper kinetic chain. Isometric exercises may be continued from the acute phase when the available range of motion remains restricted. Wherever possible, resistance exercises that strengthen functional muscle groups rather than individual muscles should be selected.[145] Specific exercises for the wrist and hand include:

▶ Resisted exercises into pronation (Fig. 16-39) and supination (Fig. 16-40).

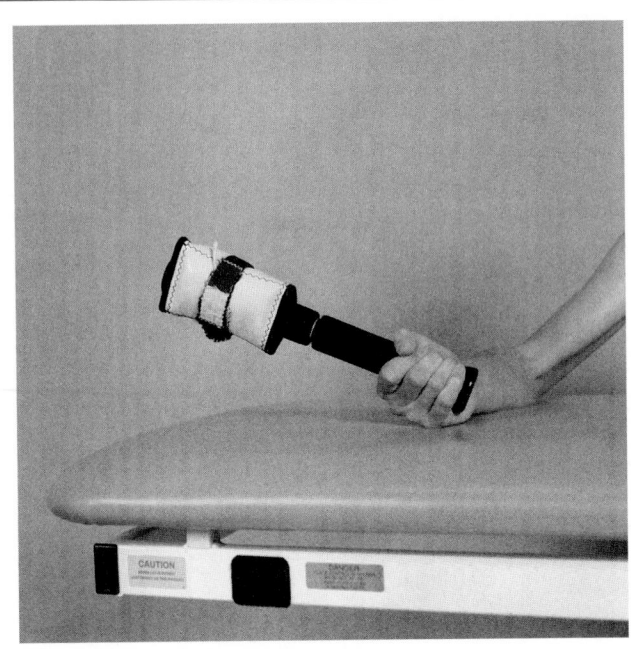

FIGURE 16-39 Resisted pronation.

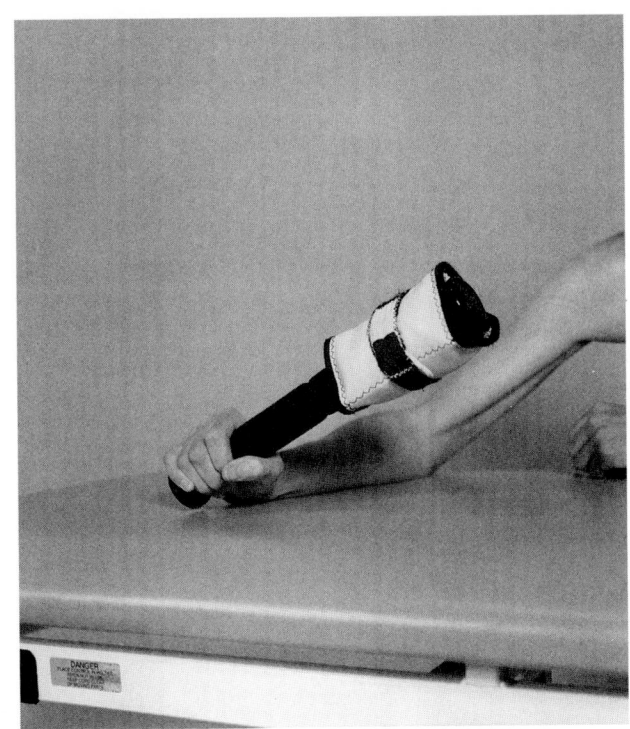

FIGURE 16-40 Resisted supination.

▶ Hand and finger dexterity exercises including the nine-peg board (Fig. 16-41), or stroking exercises.

▶ Manually resisted exercises (Fig. 16-42). These are performed by the clinician initially, before becoming part of the patient's home exercise routine.

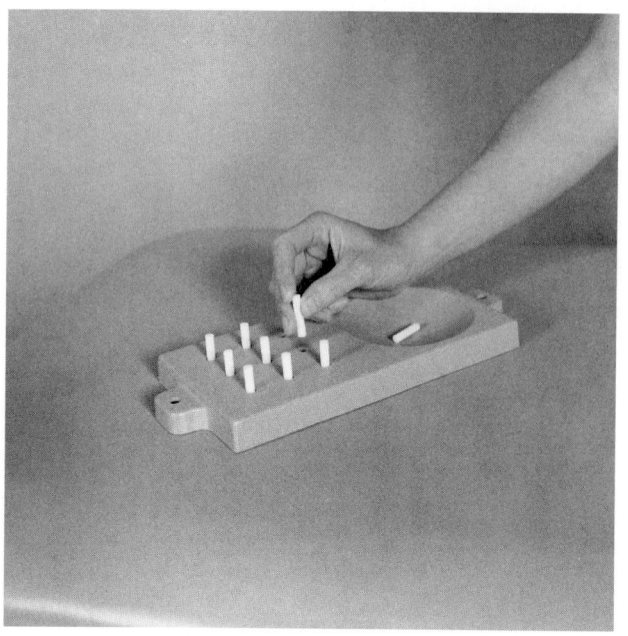

FIGURE 16-41   Nine-peg board.

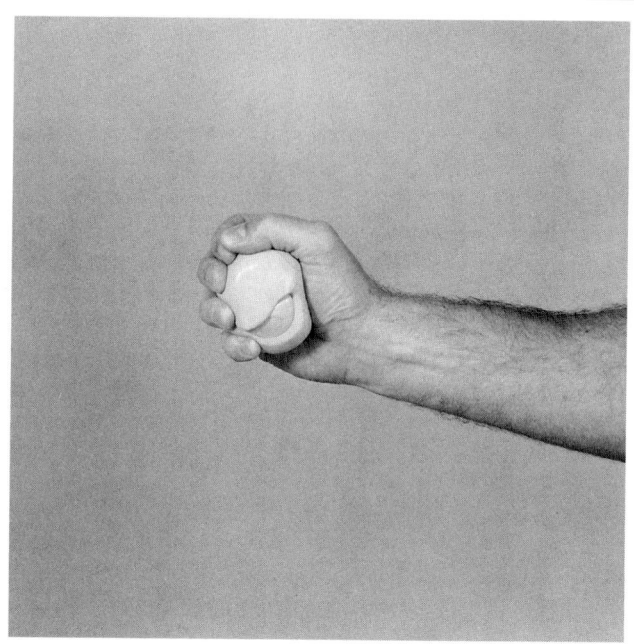

FIGURE 16-43   Putty exercises.

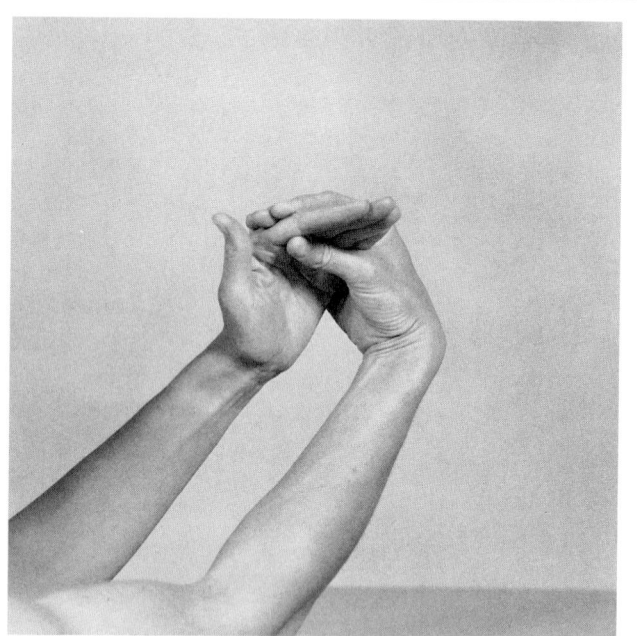

FIGURE 16-42   Manually resisted exercises.

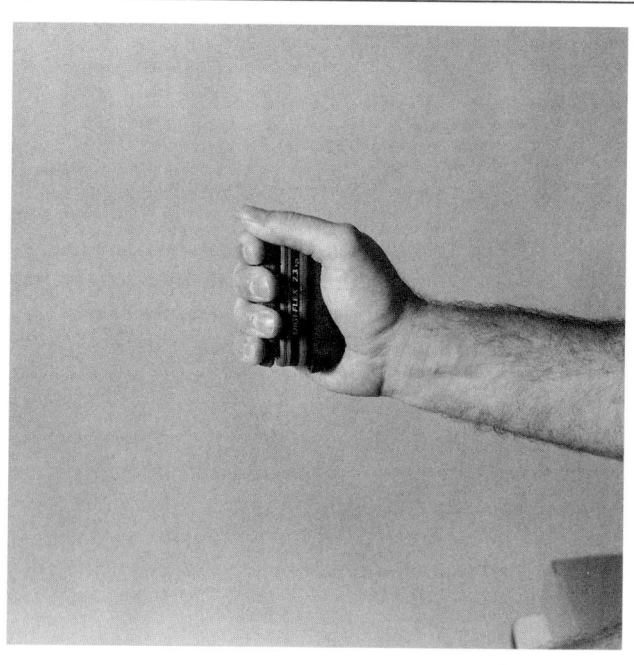

FIGURE 16-44   Hand exerciser.

▶ Resisted exercises can be performed using gripping with light resistive putty (Fig. 16-43), or a hand exerciser (Fig. 16-44). Care must be taken with gripping or squeezing exercises because they typically restrict the use of the full range of motion.

▶ Resisted exercises can also be performed using elastic resistance (Fig. 16-45), or dumbbells (Fig. 16-46).

▶ Wrist extension should be done in pronation to work against gravity, or in neutral forearm rotation to eliminate gravity. This exercise encourages the involvement of the ECRL, ECRB, and ECU. MCP flexion can be employed to eliminate any contribution from the ECU, thereby isolating the wrist musculature.

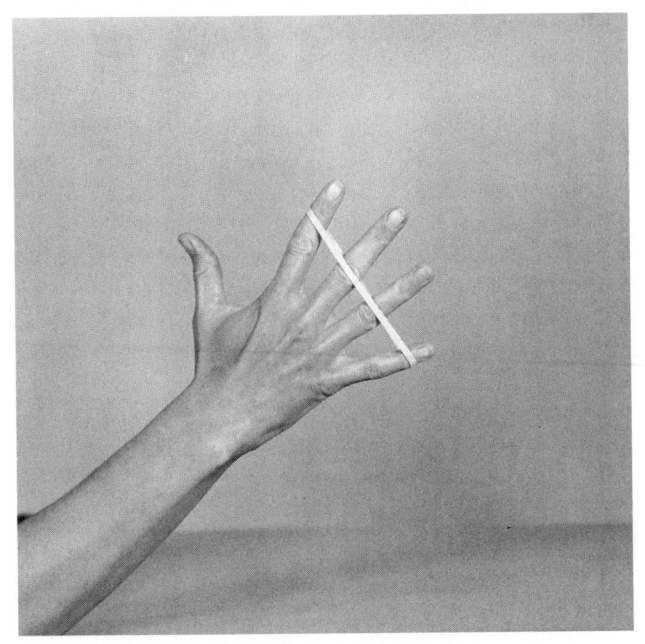

FIGURE 16-45 Resisted finger abduction.

▶ Wrist flexion should be done in supination to work against gravity, or in neutral forearm rotation to eliminate gravity. Wrist flexion works the FCU and FCR.

▶ Proprioceptive neuromuscular facilitation (PNF) patterns of the upper extremity are performed actively and then with re-

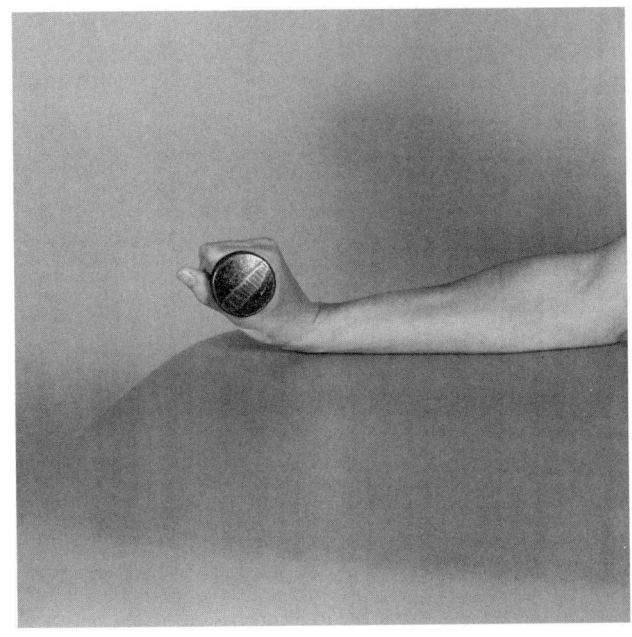

FIGURE 16-46 Resisted wrist extension.

sistance. These patterns incorporate the conjunct rotations involved with finger, hand, and wrist motions.

▶ Wall push-ups encourage full wrist extension, while full push-ups require full, or close to full, wrist extension.

The exercises for the other joints of the upper extremity are outlined in Chapters 14 and 15.

Practice Pattern 4D: Impaired Joint Mobility, Motor Function, Muscle Performance, Range of Motion Associated with Connective Tissue Dysfunction

Rheumatoid Arthritis[152]

Rheumatoid arthritis is a disease that affects the entire body and the whole person. It is a lifelong disease, which in the majority of people is only modified somewhat by intervention.[153] The cycle of stretching, healing, and scarring that occurs as a result of the inflammatory process seen in patients with rheumatoid arthritis causes significant damage to the soft tissues and periarticular structures.[154] As a consequence, these events may lead to pain, stiffness, joint damage, instability, and ultimately deformity. Many common deformities can be seen,[155] such as ulnar deviation of the MCP joints,[156] boutonnière deformity,[157] and swan-neck deformities of the digits.[158]

Ulnar Drift.   The deformity of the ulnar drift and palmar subluxation (Fig. 16-47A) is a result of a complex interaction of forces and damage to collateral ligaments and extensor mechanisms. Clinically, ulnar drift of the MCP articulations often precedes the wrist deformities.[21] The ulnar drift results in an imbalance that has the resultant effect of pulling the fingers into ulnar deviation, pronation, and palmar subluxation. The list of causes includes[155,159]:

▶ Subcollateral synovitis and weakening of the radial collateral ligament.

▶ Distortion and attenuation of the sagittal fibers of the extensor hood.

▶ A natural displacement of the extensor tendons to the ulnar side.

▶ Radial deviation of the wrist.

▶ Secondary contracture of the ulnar side intrinsic muscles.

▶ Dysfunction of the radial side intrinsics.

▶ Displacement of the flexor tendons to the ulnar side.

▶ Appositional pinch (i.e., key pinch).

▶ Gravity.

▶ The natural anatomic shape of the metacarpal head.

Boutonnière Deformity.   The boutonnière or buttonhole deformity (Fig. 16-47B) occurs when the common extensor tendon that inserts on the base of the middle phalanx is damaged. Damage to the central slip insertion requires extra effort to extend

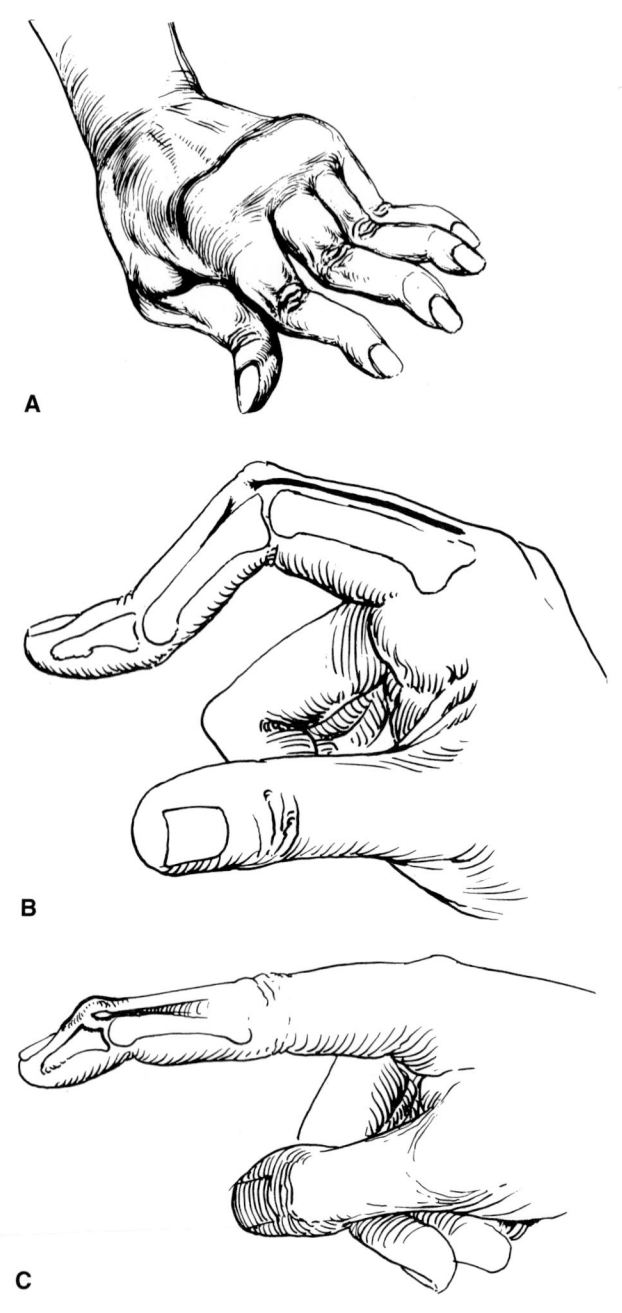

FIGURE 16-47 Finger deformities. (Reproduced with permission from Hoppenfeld S. *Physical Examination of the Spine and Extremities.* East Norwalk, CT: Appleton-Century-Crofts; 1976.) (*A*) Ulnar drift and swan-neck deformity. (*B*) Boutonnière deformity. (*C*) Mallet finger.

The realignment of the extensor mechanism, coupled with the loss of certain muscle influence, produces a deformity of extension of the MCP and DIP joints, and flexion of the PIP joint (see Fig. 16-47). This is the classic boutonnière deformity.[158] The causes, namely synovitis, central slip rupture, and displaced lateral bands, are treatable by synovectomy,[160] repair, or reconstruction of the central slip and relocation of the lateral bands.

Other causes of boutonnière deformity include injuries caused by division, rupture, avulsion, or closed trauma to the common extensor tendon. The boutonnière deformity is the second most common closed tendon injury in sports.[24] In sports, the mechanism of injury is either a severe flexing force to the PIP joint, or a direct blow to the dorsal aspect of the PIP joint, which results in damage to the common extensor tendon. If traumatic in origin, this condition can be difficult to diagnose due to the degree of swelling, but if more than a 30-degree extension lag is present at the PIP joint, a boutonnière lesion should be suspected.[24]

The presence of a mobile correctable deformity requires little more than immobilizing the PIP in full extension for 6 to 8 weeks, with the DIP and MCP joints held free. Gentle AROM exercises can begin for flexion and extension of the PIP joint at 4 to 8 weeks, with the splint being re-applied between exercises. General strengthening usually begins at 10 to 12 weeks. For a return to competition an additional 2 months is required.[24]

Swan-Neck (Recurvatum) Deformity. The swan-neck deformity is characterized by a flexion deformity at the DIP, and hyperextension of the PIP joint. This deformity is the least functional of all of the deformities that exist within the hand. In addition to rheumatologic diseases, other etiologies include extensor terminal tendon injuries, spastic conditions, fractures to the middle phalanx that heal in hyperextension, and generalized ligamentous laxity.[158] Destruction of the oblique retinacular ligament of the extensor mechanism leads to dorsal displacement of the lateral bands of the extensor mechanism. This rearrangement leads to an increased extensor force across the PIP joint with a resulting hyperextension of the PIP joint. The extended position of the PIP joint stretches the FDS and FDP tendons. The pull on the FDP tendon causes a passive flexion of the DIP joint. The resultant loss of function includes an inability to bring the tips of the fingers into grasp. The hypertrophy of rheumatoid synovitis displaces the tendon of the extensor carpi ulnaris forward. An alteration in posture at one joint leads to the reverse posture of the adjacent joint.[74]

Clinical findings include a hyperextended PIP joint with a flexed DIP joint of the same digit (Fig. 16-47A).

The intervention for swan-neck deformity depends on the etiological status of the PIP joint and its related anatomic structures. The intervention for a swan-neck deformity with no loss of PIP joint flexion is usually conservative, with a Silver Ring splint used for the correction of the PIP hyperextension.[74]

Other Deformities Produced by Rheumatoid Arthritis
Radial Deviation of the Carpometacarpal Block. This deformity is the result of the predominant action of the radial tendons

the joint, causing hyperextension at the DIP joint. The failure of the lateral bands to be connected to the central slip allows these bands to drift forward. Eventually they pass the axis of rotation of the PIP joint, and instead of extending this joint, they act as flexors while still hyperextending the distal joint. Such destruction also results in the loss of the influence of the interosseous muscles, extensor digitorum longus, and lumbrical muscles on the PIP joints. Simultaneous with the loss of this muscle influence, the lateral bands of the extensor mechanism slide ventrally.

(i.e., the flexor carpi radialis and the extensors carpi radialis longus and brevis), which radially deviate the carpometacarpal block. This deviation increases the angle between the radial border of the second metacarpal and the lower border for the distal radius, resulting in an important loss of muscular power in the flexors.[21,56]

The deviation of the wrist can involve an opposite deviation of the MCP joint, when the stabilizing elements of these joints (lateral ligament and volar plate) are weakened. The radial deviation of the carpometacarpal block may produce ulnar deviation of the MCP joints because of the interdependence of various articulations in the longitudinal chains.[21,161,162]

Effects of Rheumatoid Arthritis

The end result of the above-mentioned deformities is a reduction in the function of the hand and upper limb. Although humans are capable of significant compromise and adaptation, the loss of function that occurs with RA progressively accumulates to a point at which simple tasks become more difficult. The decreased excursion of tendons, weakness of muscles, and reduction of range of motion in joints multiplies the overall effects. Even when the muscle power is available, it may not be applied in the most effective direction. Joint laxity, which has been precipitated by synovitis and recurrent effusion, is progressively aggravated. Eventually the individual cannot cope with the resulting difficulties with doing activities of daily living. This is the characteristic end point of this progressive disease.

Interventions for Rheumatoid Arthritis of the Hand and Wrist

Because pain and instability of the wrist prevent much of the power from the forearm muscles from being transmitted to the wrist to the hand, some stabilization at the wrist level is necessary. The assessment of the thumb and finger problems involves careful evaluation of grasp and pinch. Based on the pathomechanics of the rheumatoid process, the following concepts form the foundation of any intervention to manage RA of the hand[163]:

1. Control the inflammation.
2. Focus on joint systems rather than isolated joints.
3. Consider the status of all tissues in the hand.
4. Consider the type of rheumatoid disease. The intervention is related to the type of rheumatoid disease:
   a. The type in which scarring outweighs the articular damage. Patients with stiff joints because of scarring do poorly after soft tissue surgery. Patients in this group require aggressive and sustained therapy, often for 3 to 4 months.
   b. The type in which joint laxity and tissue laxity become difficult to stabilize after soft tissue procedures. The patients in this group require careful intervention and control of the ROM and the direction of motion by the use of splints for many months after surgery.

The components of the intervention for patients with RA of the hand include:

1. *Exercises.* A combination of active exercises and isometric exercises are recommended to maintain muscle strength and improve range of motion. Range-of-motion exercises that encourage excursion of the long flexors are emphasized. The hand intrinsics are stretched by placing the MP joints in extension and radial deviation, while simultaneously flexing the PIP and DIP joints. Resistive exercises need to be introduced carefully due to the inflammatory nature of RA. Squeezing exercises using a sponge in a tub of warm water are recommended. Bony and soft tissue surgery will be less than successful in restoring function if there is residual severe imbalance in the forces acting across the joint.

2. *Joint protection/energy conservation.* Joint protection is the process of reducing internal and external stresses on the joints during functional activity and to help prevent poor use and abuse of the hand and wrist. Joint protection techniques include:
   a. Patient education to increase awareness of those activities that are stressful to the joints. In particular, tight and prolonged grasping should be avoided.
   b. The reduction of forces through the use of adaptive equipment and the avoidance of repetitive activities, positions of deformity, and the lifting of heavy weights. Many excellent self-help devices are available. Unless there is a reasonable use of the hand, any remaining imbalance will cause failure as shown in the secondary cycle of rheumatoid disease.
   c. The use of the larger/stronger and more proximal joints and muscles when available.
   d. The balance of rest and activity by planning ahead and using paced rests. Stress, rest, and sleep can have a significant effect on symptoms.
   e. The use of energy conservation techniques and labor-saving devices. Energy conservation involves sitting when able, organizing workspace and storage for accessibility, resting during activities when able, and using time-savers such as prepared foods. Many different merchants offer adaptive equipment such as zipper pulls, kitchen utensils with enlarged handles, jar openers, and pens with a large grip.
   f. Elimination of some activities.
   g. Work simplification.

3. *Splinting.* Static splinting can be used to immobilize painful joints and prevent further deformity through positioning.

4. *Pain management.* The clinician should encourage the patient to investigate alternatives to pain medication, such as relaxation techniques, yoga, adopting a positive outlook, and the use of thermo- or cryotherapy.

Triangular Fibrocartilage (TFCC) Lesions

Injuries to the triangular fibrocartilage complex (TFCC) typically occur following a fall on the supinated outstretched wrist, or as the result of chronic repetitive rotational loading.

Patients with lesions of the TFCC complain of medial wrist pain just distal to the ulna, which is increased with end range forearm pronation/supination and with forceful gripping. Often there is a painful click during wrist motions. Tenderness is clearly localized to the dorsal anatomic depression, which is immediately distal to the ulnar head.[164] Passive mobilization of the carpal condyle against the head of the ulna, with the wrist in passive or active ulnar deviation, will frequently elicit a painful crepitus or roughness, or more rarely, an actual snap (McMurray's test for the wrist). Passive supination combined with ulnar deviation can also reproduce the pain.

Initial radiographs are usually negative, but can provide information as to whether an ulna-plus variance coexists with the triangular fibrocartilage tear (ulnocarpal impingement syndrome).[164] This condition is diagnosed on radiographs showing cystic or erosive changes in the ulnar head and along the proximal contour of the lunate.[165]

Injuries to the central, avascular portion of the disk are not amenable to spontaneous repair, whereas injuries to the vascularized periphery are.[164]

Conservative invention for TFCC injuries includes a long arm cast or splint fitted with the elbow in 90 degrees of flexion, and the forearm and wrist in ulnar deviation and extension for 6 weeks, if the TFCC is unstable.

While the wrist is in a cast or splint, the intervention should include proximal range-of-motion and strengthening exercises.

Active and active assisted exercises are initiated to the wrist and forearm after cast removal, with emphasis on flexion and extension initially, followed by pronation/supination, and radial/ulnar deviation. Two weeks after cast removal, assuming the patient is asymptomatic, progressive strengthening is initiated to the hand and wrist, taking care to prevent torsional loads to the wrist.

Osteoarthritis

Osteoarthritis (OA) is the most common joint disease. This condition can be primary or secondary, depending on the presence of a pre-existing condition. While primary OA commonly involves the first CMC joint or sometimes the scaphotrapeziotrapezoid (STT) joint, it is uncommon in other parts of the joint.[164]

Secondary OA of the wrist attributable to an old trauma or infection is very common. In the case of malalignment of the scaphoid, degenerative arthritis will progress according to a very specific pattern that leads to an SLAC (scapholunate advanced collapse) wrist.[164] Degeneration occurs between the radius and the scaphoid and then between the lunate and capitate. The radiolunate joint is almost never involved. Finally, a scapholunate diastasis develops and the capitate slides in between the lunate and scaphoid.[166]

Patients with first CMC joint arthritis typically present with joint pain at the base of the thumb which is increased with use, restricted ROM in a capsular pattern, and joint crepitus.[164] First CMC arthritis is more common in women than men, and is typically found in those 45 years and older.

Conservative intervention includes splinting, thermal modalities (moist heat or paraffin), and patient education.

Splinting. The splint should position the CMC joint in palmar abduction, to maximize the stability and anatomic alignment of the joint, with the IP joint free.[164]

Patient Education. The patient should be advised to:

▶ Minimize or avoid mechanical stresses including sustained pinching.

▶ Avoid sleeping on the hands as this forces the thumb into adduction.

▶ Use self-help devices such as jar lid openers and ergonomic scissors.

Gout
See Chapter 9.

Dupuytren's Contracture (Palmar Fasciitis)
Population studies have shown that Dupuytren's disease nearly always affects Caucasian races, particularly those of northern European descent.[167,168] The incidence increases with advancing age and it is exceedingly rare in children.[169] Men are 7 to 15 times more likely to have a clinical presentation requiring surgery than women, who tend to develop a more benign form of the disease that appears later in life.[170,171]

The etiology of Dupuytren's disease is thought to be multifactorial. There is a higher incidence in the alcoholic population, the diabetic population, and the epileptic population.[171–173] Because of the association between smoking and microvascular changes in the hand, some believe that tobacco may also play a role in this disease.[171] Although not usually related to hand trauma, Dupuytren's disease occasionally develops after significant hand injuries, including surgery.[174]

Dupuytren's disease, an active cellular process in the fascia of the hand, is characterized by the development of nodules in the palmar and digital fascia. These nodules occur in specific locations along longitudinal tension lines.[167,171] The appearance of the nodules is followed by the formation of tendon-like cords, which are due to the pathologic change in normal fascia.[175–177] The thickening and shortening of the fascia causes contracture, which behaves similarly to the contracture and maturation of wound healing.[171] The contractures form at the MCP joint, the PIP joint, and occasionally the DIP joint.[178]

The diagnosis of Dupuytren's disease in its early stages may be difficult, and is based on the palpable nodule, characteristic skin changes, changes in the fascia, and progressive joint contracture. The skin changes are caused by a retraction of the skin, resulting in dimples or pits.

Dupuytren's disease can be classified into three biologic stages[176]:

▶ ***First stage.*** The first stage is the proliferative stage, characterized by an intense proliferation of myofibroblasts (the cells believed to generate the contractile forces responsible for tissue contraction) and the formation of nodules.

▶ ***Second stage.*** The second, involutional stage, is represented by the alignment of the myofibroblasts along lines of tension.

▶ ***Third stage.*** During the third, residual stage, the tissue becomes mostly acellular and devoid of myofibroblasts, and only thick bands of collagen remain.[179]

The disease is usually bilateral, with one hand being more severely involved. However, there appears to be no association with hand dominance. The patient may have one, two, or three rays involved in the more severely affected hand. The most commonly involved digit is the little finger, which is involved in approximately 70 percent of patients.

Conservative interventions have not yet proven to be clinically useful or of any long-term value in the treatment of established contractures.[180] Some surgeons feel that any amount of proximal interphalangeal (PIP) joint contracture warrants surgery, whereas others feel that 15 degrees or greater is an indication.[167,181] Surgery is the intervention of choice when the MCP joint contracts to 30 degrees and the deformity becomes a functional problem.[181]

Studies have shown that 50 percent of operative results depend on the postoperative management of effective splinting and exercise.[171,182] The intervention should be directed toward promoting wound healing, which in turn minimizes scarring and maximizes scar mobility so that hand function can be restored.[171]

Scar management and splinting are an important part of the postoperative management. The initial splint is positioned to provide slight MCP joint flexion of 10 to 20 degrees with PIP joint extension to allow maximal elongation of the wound.[171] Active, active assisted, and passive exercises are usually initiated at the first treatment session.

Wrist Sprains

Wrist sprains are more common than wrist fractures, with the most common wrist sprain resulting from a downward force to the wrist exceeding its normal range of motion. In ligament injuries, the injury usually is to the middle of the ligament.[183]

In the common presentation of a wrist injury, forced movement of the joint is followed immediately by intense pain that subsides and then returns.[4] Swelling occurs within 1 to 2 hours of the injury. The degree of joint swelling indicates the degree of injury. Ecchymosis develops in severe injuries in 6 to 12 hours. Differential diagnosis includes a carpal fracture, particularly the scaphoid and lunate, traumatic instability, or a ligament tear.[184]

Conservative intervention includes immobilization of the wrist, depending on the degree of the sprain, to avoid exacerbating the injury. Custom splints made from casting material allow for proper hand and wrist contouring, and should cover the palm, allowing the fingers to move freely, and extend to about midforearm.[4] Cocking the wrist up about 10 degrees puts the wrist in a position of rest.

Slight sprains should remain splinted for 3 to 5 days. Icing for 20 to 30 minutes, three to four times a day, concurrent with nonsteroidal anti-inflammatory drugs (NSAIDs) or aspirin can aid in reducing pain and swelling. More severe sprains take longer to recover, but should still be removed from the splint in 3 to 5 days to avoid stiffness.[4]

After splint removal, a rehabilitation program of wrist curls without weights should be started. Until the pain and swelling subside, wrist curls can be done in water to reduce muscle effort.[183] The clinician should consider taping the wrist to provide support and help decrease pain. Once the patient can do three sets of ten curls twice a day without pain, sports activities can be gradually resumed.

Perilunate Dislocation

Most carpal dislocations are of the perilunate variety with the lunate dislocating in a palmar direction. This is accompanied by damage to both of the interosseous ligaments of the proximal row, and possible injury to the median nerve.[9]

The usual mechanism of injury is hyperextension of the wrist. The dislocation is easily reduced if the intervention occurs soon after the injury. The reduction involves placing the wrist in extension and putting pressure on the lunate, after which the wrist is moved into flexion and immobilized.

Kienböck's Disease

Kienböck's disease is an aseptic necrosis of the lunate. When the disease becomes advanced, carpal collapse, joint incongruity, and osteoarthritis develop (see Chap. 9 for the description of this disease). The choice of treatment for patients with symptomatic Kienböck's disease depends largely on the severity of the disease. Surgical intervention can include excision arthroplasty, limited intercarpal arthrodesis, revascularization, arthrodesis between the radius and the lunate, and vascular bundle implantation.[185] Conservative management of Kienböck's disease involves immobilization in a short arm cast. Upon cast removal at 6 to 10 weeks, AROM exercises are initiated for the wrist, forearm, and thumb. Within 1 to 2 weeks following cast removal, PROM exercises are initiated. A wrist and thumb static splint is fitted with the wrist in neutral and the thumb midway between radial and palmar abduction, and is worn between exercise sessions and at night.

Intercarpal Instabilities

The integrity of the carpal relationship depends on the stability provided by both the interosseous ligaments and the midcarpal ligaments.[9] This relationship ensures that the carpal bones move as a unit. Conversely, disruption of this relationship allows abnormal independent motion of one or two carpal bones. Instability patterns are divided into those that are static and those that are dynamic. Static instability is the more severe of the two, and usually involves a complete tear of one of the supporting ligaments, or a fracture.[9] Dynamic instability patterns typically occur when the wrist is stressed. Carpal instability patterns that occur within the same row are classified as dissociative, while those that occur across different rows are classified as nondissociative.

Dissociative. Two types of dissociative instability have been recognized[46]:

1. ***DISI (dorsal intercalated segment instability).*** The most common dissociated instability is the scapholunate dissociation, in which the scapholunate angle is greater than 70 degrees when viewed on radiograph. Scapholunate instability usually follows a fall on the outstretched hand (FOOSH injury) where the primary forces are transferred

through the wrist in extension and ulnar deviation. As the scaphoid and lunate become disassociated, the lunate no longer follows the scaphoid into flexion, instead migrating with the triquetrum into a dorsal angulation.[9] The patient with this type presents with difficulties and weakness with grasping, and complains of chronic, vague wrist pain. The examination reveals tenderness over the scaphoid and/or lunate, laxity between the scaphoid and lunate, and a positive scaphoid-shift test.

2. ***VISI (ventral intercalated segment instability).*** The second most common dissociative instability is the lunatotriquetrum dissociation. Ventral refers to the ventral tilt of the distal end of the lunate. The signs and symptoms for this instability are similar to those of the scapholunate instability, except for the location. In this type, the lunate remains tethered to the scaphoid by the interosseous ligament, but not necessarily to the triquetrum.[9] During wrist motions, the lunate follows the scaphoid into a flexed posture, but the triquetrum does not. A scapholunate angle of less than 30 degrees indicates a VISI lesion.

Nondissociative. This is the most common dynamic instability of the wrist, and usually results from an insufficiency of the dorsal intercarpal ligaments. The nondissociative instability may not be symptomatic, and the patient may be able to sublux and reduce the joint at will.[9] A clunk can be felt to occur as the distal row jumps back into place at the extreme of ulnar deviation.[186]

Conservative intervention for carpal instabilities usually involves a trial period of cast immobilization. Surgery is reserved for chronic cases.

Ulnar Collateral Ligament Sprain of the Thumb

Ulnar collateral joint ligament (UCL) injuries, also known as *gamekeeper's thumb, skier's thumb,*[187] and *breakdancer's thumb,* involve injury to the MCP joint of the thumb, and are the most common ligament injury of the hand.[188]

The patient typically complains of pain or tenderness on the ulnar aspect of the MCP joint.

For the purposes of intervention, these injuries can be divided into two categories:

▶ Grade I and II sprains, in which the majority of the ligament remains intact. The stability of the joint is tested in full extension, and at 30 degrees of flexion, which stress the accessory collateral ligament and the ulnar collateral ligament, respectively. An angulation of greater than 35 degrees or 15 degrees greater than the uninvolved side indicates instability and the need for surgical intervention. The intervention for grade I and II tears is immobilization in a thumb spica cast for 3 weeks, with additional protective splinting for 2 weeks. Thumb spica splints, which are a forearm-based splint fabricated from a palmar or radial approach, are designed to immobilize the wrist, carpometacarpal, and MCP joints of the thumb, thereby permitting the radial wrist extensors and the proximal thumb to rest. Thumb spicas can

be used for the intervention of a number of conditions including de Quervain's disease and CMC arthritis.

When applying these splints, it is very important to ensure that the superficial radial nerve and the ulnar digital nerve of the thumb are not compromised. The splint is worn at all times except for removal for hygiene and exercise. AROM of flexion and extension begins at 3 weeks, and progresses to strengthening exercises by 8 weeks, taking care not to apply any abduction stress to the MCP joint during the first 2 to 6 weeks.

▶ Grade III tears and displaced bony avulsions are treated with surgery and immobilization. If the ligament is completely torn, there is concern for a Stener lesion, in which the torn UCL protrudes beneath the adductor aponeurosis.[189] Postsurgical rehabilitation involves wearing a thumb spica cast or splint for 3 weeks with an additional 2 weeks of splinting, except during the exercises of active flexion and extension. Otherwise the exercise progression is the same as for the grade I and II sprains.

Radial collateral sprains are classified and treated in a similar manner.

Ulnar Impaction Syndrome

The ulnar impaction syndrome can be defined as excessive impaction of the ulnar head against the triangular fibrocartilage complex and ulnar carpus. This results in a progressive degeneration of those structures.[190]

The patient presents with ulnar wrist pain and a limitation of motion. Upon physical examination, a combined motion of ulnar deviation and compression reproduces the pain (see "Special Tests").

The differential diagnosis includes ulnar impingement syndrome and arthrosis or incongruity of the distal radioulnar joint.[190]

It is important to remember that in the absence of obvious structural abnormalities, the ulnar impaction syndrome may result from daily activities that result in excessive intermittent loading of the ulnar carpus.

Conservative intervention includes the use of an ulnar gutter splint if there is evidence of wrist overloading.

Ganglia

See Chapter 9.

Chondromalacia

Chondromalacia of the ulnar head is usually seen in young patients after a fall on the dorsiflexed wrist with the impact predominantly hypothenar, or repeated episodes of stressful pronation and supination (work or leisure activity).[164] The pain is localized to the dorsal distal radioulnar area and manipulation of the ulnar head can elicit crepitation or a painful snap.[165]

Racquet Player's Pisiform

Racquet player's pisiform is a condition involving a minor subluxation of the pisiform, with occasional chondromalacia of the articular cartilage of the pisotriquetral joint.[12] The probable mechanism is a torsional stress upon the capsule of the pisotriquetral joint by the powerful and rapid pronation and supination movements at the wrist seen when wielding a racquet, particularly in badminton, racquetball, and squash players.

The typical clinical presentation is one of pain, disability, and swelling on the ulnar aspect of the wrist or proximal palm. The pain is reproduced with passive movement of the pisiform upon the triquetrum with the relaxed wrist flexed and ulnarly deviated.[12]

The typical intervention for this condition is surgical excision of the pisiform.[12]

Practice Pattern 4E: Impaired Joint Mobility, Motor Function, Muscle Performance, Range of Motion Associated with Localized Inflammation

Tendonitis and Tenosynovitis

Tendonitis is a term that clearly indicates an inflammation of the tendon or tendon-muscle attachment, whereas tenosynovitis involves an inflammation of the tendon sheath.

Overuse syndromes are a common cause of tendonitis, particularly in the "weekend warrior." As a rule, the tendons of the abductor pollicis longus and extensor pollicis brevis are involved. There are, however, some uncommon locations and types of tendonitis. There has been a marked increase in reports of the so-called repetitive strain injury of the upper extremity.[164] One of the difficulties in evaluating this disorder is the establishment of a diagnosis in the absence of objective physical findings or confirmatory diagnostic images or laboratory data. These issues become more complicated when insurers and attorneys ask physicians to establish a causal relation between the job and the complaints.[191,192]

Tenosynovitis is frequently seen in inflammatory rheumatic diseases, diabetes mellitus, or hypothyroid conditions.

Patients are typically considered for surgery when a tenosynovitis has persisted for a period of 3 months despite reasonable conservative treatment in the form of medication, rest, steroid injections, and therapy.

DeQuervain's Disease. De Quervain's disease[193] is a progressive stenosing tenosynovitis, which affects the tendon sheaths of the first dorsal compartment of the wrist, resulting in a thickening of the extensor retinaculum, a narrowing of the fibro-osseus canal, and an eventual entrapment and compression of the tendons, especially during radial deviation.[194]

In most circumstances, the first dorsal compartment is a single compartment, which contains the tendons and synovial sheaths of the abductor pollicis longus (APL) and the extensor pollicis brevis (EPB) tendons. These tendons allow the thumb to flex, extend, and grip objects. Overuse, repetitive tasks which involve overexertion of the thumb, and arthritis are the most common predisposing factors, as they cause the greatest stresses on the structures of the first dorsal compartment.[72,134] Such activities include golf, fly fishing, typing, sewing, knitting, cutting, and any activity which involves repetitive finger-thumb gripping combined with radial deviation.[72,195–198]

Frequently, patients report a gradual and insidious onset[72,134,199] of a dull ache over the radial aspect of the wrist made worse by turning doorknobs or keys.[4] Patients also may note a "creaking" in the wrist as the tendon moves.

Examination of the wrist may reveal:

▶ A localized swelling and tenderness in the region of the radial styloid process[134,199] and wrist pain radiating proximally into the forearm and distally into the thumb.[134,199–201]

▶ Severe pain[134,199] with wrist ulnar deviation and thumb flexion and adduction.[202] A reproduction of the pain can also be reported with thumb extension and abduction.[203]

▶ Crepitus of the tendons moving through the extensor sheath.[202,204]

▶ Palpable thickening of the extensor sheath and of the tendons distal to the extensor tunnel.[205]

▶ A loss of abduction of the carpometacarpal (CMC) joint of the thumb.

▶ A positive Finkelstein's test (see Fig. 16-34).[134] The results of this test must be interpreted with caution,[206] as it may also be positive in Wartenberg's syndrome (entrapment of the superficial radial sensory nerve),[202,207,208] basilar thumb arthrosis, or intersection syndrome (see later).[208] Deviating the wrist using pressure over the index metacarpal avoids confusion with thumb conditions.[209] A variation of Finkelstein's test can be used to rule out an incomplete release of previous de Quervain's disease.[210] If the usual Finkelstein's test is positive, full abduction of the APL followed by flexion of the thumb's MCP joint will isolate the action of the EPB. Pain with this test will occur if the EPB lies in a separate sheath and was not released.[210]

Although the diagnosis is mostly clinical, posteroanterior and lateral radiographs of the wrist can be obtained to rule out any bony pathology, such as a scaphoid fracture, radioscaphoid, or triscaphoid arthritis; and Kienböck's disease.[4]

The intervention can be conservative or surgical. Conservative intervention includes rest, continuous immobilization through splinting with a thumb spica for 3 weeks, and anti-inflammatory medication. The splint is fabricated with the wrist in 15 degrees of extension, the thumb midway between palmar and radial abduction, and the thumb MP joint in 10 degrees of flexion. When fitting the splint it is important that the thumb is able to oppose the index and long finger to aid with hand function. Following the removal of the splint, ROM exercises are prescribed, with a gradual progression to strengthening.

The more invasive intervention begins with cortisone injections. If two to three injections do not give relief, surgical tendon sheath release is an option.[4]

Intersection Syndrome. Intersection syndrome is a tenosynovitis of the radial wrist extensors (ECRL and ECRB), where they cross under the more obliquely oriented APL and EPB.[192] The cause is typically repetitive wrist flexion and extension[211] and is common in rowers, weightlifters, and canoeists.[209]

Although similar to de Quervain's, differentiation is made with the pain distribution. With the intersection syndrome, the pain is located over the distal forearm, 4 to 8 cm proximal to Lister's tubercle.[192]

Intervention, in addition to NSAIDs, involves[192,212]:

▶ Splint immobilization of the wrist and thumb with the wrist in 15 to 20 degrees of extension.

▶ Iontophoresis/phonophoresis.

▶ Deep transverse friction massage followed by exercises for stretching and strengthening.

▶ Patient education to emphasize the importance of avoiding repetitive wrist flexion and extension in combination with a power grip.

Extensor Pollicis Longus Tendonitis. This condition is rare except in rheumatoid arthritis, but occurs when the EPL muscle extends into a tight third compartment.[213] Overuse (drummer boy palsy), direct trauma, forced wrist extension, and distal radius fractures may cause EPL tendonitis, which presents with the clinical signs and symptoms of decreased thumb flexion, pain, swelling, and crepitus at Lister's tubercle.[192]

Extensor Indicis Proprius Syndrome. An increase in muscle size of the extensor indices, caused by swelling or hypertrophy from repetitive exercise, may cause stenosis of the fourth dorsal compartment, and resultant tenosynovitis.[192]

A simple test of a resistance applied to active index finger extension while holding the wrist in a flexed position is a reliable provocative test.[214]

Extensor Carpi Ulnaris Tendonitis. ECU tendonitis, a tenosynovitis of the sixth dorsal compartment, usually presents as chronic dorsoulnar wrist pain, which is aggravated with forearm supination and ulnar deviation, which causes the tendon to sublux palmarly.[192,215]

Flexor Carpi Ulnaris Tendonitis. The FCU is the most common wrist flexor tendon to become inflamed, and is often associated with repetitive trauma and racquet sports.[12] The clinical signs and symptoms include pain and swelling localized just proximal to the pisiform, which is aggravated with wrist flexion and ulnar deviation.[192]

Flexor Carpi Radialis Tendonitis. FCR tendonitis usually develops due to stenosis and tenosynovitis in the FCR fibro-osseous tunnel within the transverse metacarpal ligament. FCR tendonitis usually produces localized pain and swelling, and painful deviation of the wrist.[192] FCR tendonitis frequently coexists with other conditions including fracture or arthritis around the CMC joint of the thumb.[192]

Digital Flexor Tendonitis and Trigger Digits. Painful snapping or triggering of the fingers and thumb is due to a disproportion between the flexor tendon and its tendon sheath. The condition invariably occurs at the metacarpal head level, and at the A1 pulley, with the result that the tendon is pulled through too narrow a canal.[192,216–218] The condition is more common in the fibrous flexor sheath of the thumb or ring finger.

The etiology for this condition is unknown, although it shows a predilection for young children and menopausal women. Trigger finger also commonly coexists with rheumatic changes of the hand and may be the earliest sign of rheumatoid arthritis.[219]

The first sign is usually the trigger phenomenon. Over time the condition becomes very painful, and in some cases locking occurs.[220]

Conservative intervention involves the fitting of a hand-based MP flexion block splint for the involved digit only, with the MP joint only immobilized in full extension, for up to 6 weeks.[221] This immobilization theoretically alters the mechanical forces on the proximal pulley system and encourages maximal differential tendon gliding.

Medical intervention usually involves one or a series of steroid injections,[222] with surgical release of the trigger finger reserved for the recalcitrant cases.[192]

Tendon Ruptures

Mallet Finger Deformity. Mallet finger deformity is a traumatic disruption of the terminal tendon resulting in a loss of active extension of the DIP joint. This is one of the most common hand injuries sustained by the athletic population, and is especially common in the baseball catcher and football receiver. The deformity usually results from the delivery of a longitudinal force to the tip of the finger.[24] The sudden acute flexion force which is produced results in a rupture of the extensor tendon just proximal to its insertion into the third phalanx, or a fracture at the base of the distal phalanx.

The physical examination reveals a flexion deformity of the distal interphalangeal (DIP) joint (see Fig. 16-47C), which can be extended passively but not actively. This lack of active extension at the DIP joint is due to the zero tension being provided by the extensor digitorum communis (EDC), in addition to the resulting increased tone in the flexor digitorum profundus (FDP).

The primary goal of treatment is to promote healing of the tendon so as to maximize function and range of motion of the involved DIP joint. Conservative intervention involves 6 weeks of immobilization. Mallet deformities with an associated large fracture fragment are typically treated with 6 weeks of immobilization following open reduction and internal fixation, usually with K-wires.[24] Closed reduction is used for other types, followed by 6 weeks of continuous dorsal splinting of the DIP in 0 degrees of extension to 15 degrees of hyperextension.[24] The PIP joint should be free to move. If splinted, the splint is removed once a day while simultaneously holding the DIP joint in extension to allow air to reach the palmar aspect of the middle and distal phalanx. Following the period of immobilization, the splint or fixators are removed and the terminal tendon is evaluated. If the tendon is unable to maintain extension of the DIP joint, a splint is reapplied and the tendon is retested periodically. Once the tendon has healed sufficiently to perform active extension of the DIP, AROM exercises to 20 to 35 degrees are initiated to the DIP joint. The clinician should continue to monitor for an extensor lag, and it is recommended that the patient continues to wear the splint between exercise sessions, at night, and when competing. Gentle progressive resistive exercises (PREs) using putty or a hand exerciser are initiated at week 8. Usually the splint is discontinued at 9 weeks if the DIP extension remains at 0 to 5 degrees and there is no extensor lag. Unrestricted use usually occurs after 12 weeks.

Rupture of the Terminal Phalangeal Flexor (Jersey Finger). The rupture of the FDP tendon from its insertion on the distal phalanx (Jersey finger) is often misdiagnosed as a sprained or "jammed" finger, as there is no characteristic deformity associated with it.[24]

The injury is typically caused by forceful passive extension while the flexor digitorum profundus muscle is contracting. A common example is in football when the flexed finger is caught in a jersey while the athlete is attempting to make a tackle, hence the term jersey finger.

Three types are recognized:

▶ In Type I the tendon retracts into the palm with or without a bony fragment.

▶ Type II is the most common. The tendon retracts to the proximal interphalangeal joint and the long vinculum remains intact. As in type I, type II injuries may have a small bony avulsion.

▶ Type III injuries involve a large bony fragment.

Although this condition can occur in any finger, the most commonly injured is the ring finger.[223] The injury usually occurs with forced passive extension of a flexed finger.

To test the integrity of the tendon, isolate the FDP by holding the MCP and PIP joints of the affected finger in full extension, and have the patient attempt to flex the DIP. If it flexes, it is intact. If not, it is ruptured.

The intervention can involve doing nothing if function is not seriously affected, or surgical reattachment of the tendon, which requires a 12-week course of rehabilitation.

Integration of Practice Patterns 4F and 5F: Impaired Joint Mobility, Motor Function, Muscle Performance, and Range of Motion, or Reflex Integrity Secondary to Referred Pain, Spinal Disorders, Peripheral Nerve Entrapment, Myofascial Pain Syndrome, Complex Regional Pain Syndrome

Referred Pain

A number of structures can refer pain to the wrist and hand, and include visceral structures, neurologic structures, and the more proximal joints (see Chap. 9). The most common joints, which refer pain to the wrist and hand, include the cervical, thoracic, shoulder, and elbow joints.

Tumors
See Chapter 9.

Peripheral Nerve Entrapment
Peripheral nerve entrapments are common in the forearm and wrist. Neurogenic syndromes are usually incomplete, indicating the absence of severe motor or sensory deficits, but in the typical case they are accompanied by a history of pain or vague sensory disturbances.[224] As a result, nerve injuries are frequently overlooked as a source of acute, or more commonly chronic, symptomatology.[164] Loss of vibration sensibility has been suggested as an early indicator of peripheral compression neuropathy.[130] Nerve conduction studies may be performed, focusing on the sites of interest. Diabetes, with its associated neuropathies or cheiroarthropathy, may be an underlying cause of chronic wrist pain.[164]

Radial Nerve. The posterior interosseous nerve, the terminal branch of the radial nerve, ends distal to Lister's tubercle in a bulbous expansion over the dorsal wrist joint. Repetitive dorsiflexion maneuvers compress the nerve as it enters the dorsal wrist capsule, inciting symptomatic inflammation.[225]

The major disability associated with radial nerve injury is weak wrist and finger extension, with the wrist and fingers adopting a position termed "wrist drop." The hand grip is weakened as a result of poor stabilization of the wrist and finger joints, and the patient typically demonstrates an inability to extend the thumb, proximal phalanges, wrist, and elbow, depending on the level. Supination of the forearm and adduction of the thumb are also affected. There is also decreased or impaired sensation on the dorsal surface of the first interosseous space.

Wartenberg's Syndrome. Wartenberg's syndrome is a compression of the superficial sensory radial nerve. Inflammation of the tendons of the first dorsal compartment can result in superficial radial neuritis. This results in pain, paresthesias, and numbness of the radial aspects of the hand and wrist.[226] In addition, the tendons of the brachioradialis and extensor carpi radialis longus (ECRL) muscles can press on the nerve in a scissor-like fashion when the forearm is pronated, causing a proximal tethering on the distal segment of the nerve at the wrist.[227]

Wartenberg's sign is described wherein the patient is asked to extend the fingers and abduction or clawing of the little finger occurs.[136]

Median Nerve Compression at the Wrist. Carpal tunnel syndrome (CTS) is a cause of chronic wrist pain and functional impairment of the hand. It results from an ischemic compression of the median nerve at the wrist as it passes through the carpal tunnel. Compression of the nerve in the carpal tunnel is compounded by an increase in synovial fluid pressure and tendon tension, which decreases the available volume.

Moersch[228] provided the first description of spontaneous median nerve compression in 1938 and is credited with coining the term *carpal tunnel syndrome*.[229] A study of the syndrome in Rochester, Minnesota, which examined medical records, included symptoms compatible with the syndrome, and excluded other illnesses, found an incidence of 125 per 100,000 population for the period 1976 through 1980.[230]

The compression of the median nerve may result from a wide variety of factors, several of which can easily be remembered using the mnemonic PRAGMATIC:

▶ *P*regnancy secondary to fluid retention.[231]

▶ *R*enal dysfunction.

▶ *A*cromegaly.

▶ *G*out and pseudogout.[232]

▶ *M*yxedema or mass.

▶ *A*myotrophy. Neuralgic amyotrophy is the most likely diagnosis in patients who suddenly develop arm pain followed within a few days by arm paralysis in the distribution of single or multiple nerves or extending over multiple myotomes.[233]

▶ *T*rauma (repetitive or direct). About half of the cases of CTS are related to repetitive and cumulative trauma in the workplace, making it the occupational epidemic syndrome of our time.[234,235] Frequent repetitive wrist flexion and extension or motions that cause repeated palmar trauma may be a factor in the development of carpal tunnel syndrome. Forceful and repetitive contraction of the finger flexors can also provoke CTS, as demand for tendon lubrication overwhelms the ability of the sheath to respond, producing an inflammatory reaction.[236] Acute wrist trauma has also been associated with CTS. A fall onto the outstretched hand (FOOSH injury) or other trauma can cause a palmar subluxation of the lunate,[237] or a distal radius fracture.[238,239] The degree of compression can be so great that profound neurologic deficit can rapidly follow, and if not treated appropriately, it can become permanent due to the decrease in capillary blood flow producing ischemia of the nerve.[240] A manipulative reduction should be carried out. If manipulation fails, the patient should be referred to a surgeon for immediate decompression.

▶ *I*nfection.[241,242]

▶ *C*ollagen disorders. The incidence of carpal tunnel syndrome in patients with polyarthritis is high; 60 to 70 percent of patients at some time have a significant carpal tunnel syndrome.[243,244] This usually is seen in association with a flexor tenosynovitis.[245]

Other causes include rheumatoid arthritis,[246] diabetes, hypothyroidism, and hemodialysis.[247] Less common causes include incursion of the lumbrical muscles within the tunnel during finger movements,[248,249] and hypertrophy of the lumbricales.[250]

Although it occurs in all age groups, CTS more commonly occurs between the fourth and sixth decades. CTS is the most common compression neuropathy, with a prevalence of 9.2 percent in women and 0.6 percent in men.[251,252]

Carpal tunnel pressure appears to be an important factor in the pathophysiology of CTS, as increased pressure on the median nerve can produce short term sensory and motor nerve

conduction deficits and elicit symptoms of median nerve neuropathy.[240] Extreme wrist and finger postures can increase the tunnel pressure.[253] In addition, the angle of the MCP joint has been found to have a significant effect on carpal tunnel pressure during active wrist flexion and extension and radioulnar maneuvers. Motions performed in 0 degrees MCP flexion exhibit the highest pressures, followed by an MCP angle of 90 degrees.[254] This information should be considered in the design of splints for CTS patients. Fingertip loading has also been found to increase pressure in the carpal tunnel.[255]

The diagnosis of carpal tunnel syndrome is most reliably made by an experienced clinician after a review of the patient's history and a physical examination.[256] The clinical features of this syndrome include intermittent pain and paresthesias in the median nerve distribution of the hand, which can become persistent as the condition progresses.[243,257–259] Muscle weakness and paralysis can occasionally occur. The symptoms are typically worse at night, exacerbated by strenuous wrist movements, and can be associated with morning stiffness. The pain may radiate proximally into the forearm and arm.

Differential diagnosis for this condition includes cervical radiculitis,[260] thoracic outlet syndrome, pronator syndrome,[261] coronary artery ischemia, tendonitis, fibrositis, and wrist joint arthritis.[262,263] Cervical radiculopathy may be identified by the occurrence of proximal radiation of pain above the shoulder, paresthesias with coughing or sneezing, or a pattern of motor or sensory disturbances outside of the territory of the median nerve.[257] Ulnar neuropathy must be considered since no more than half of patients with carpal tunnel syndrome can reliably report the location of their paresthesias.[264] Thoracic outlet syndrome is occasionally a concern. Transient cerebral ischemia, not a rare occurrence, can be recognized by the absence of pain during an episode of numbness.

The physical assessment focuses on an examination of the motor and sensory functions of the hand as compared to the uninvolved hand and includes Phalen's test, and Tinel's sign.[116,257,265] A study[266] that examined the effect of upper extremity position on median nerve tension, found the upper limb tension test (ULTT) for the median nerve to be specific.

Another study[267] described a maneuver that abolishes paresthesias in the carpal tunnel. The authors of this study suggest that this maneuver could be useful in the diagnosis of the syndrome, as well as providing a means of relieving symptoms and providing the basis for the design of a splint. With the involved hand positioned palm up, the clinician gently squeezes the distal metacarpal heads together.[267] If the basic maneuver does not relieve the symptoms, it may also be necessary to pronate the forearm while simultaneously stretching digits three and four.[267]

A number of medical tests can be used to help diagnose CTS. These include the median nerve conduction study and EMG study. Median nerve conduction studies have been found to be normal in 5 percent of patients with symptoms.[128] The EMG study was found in one study[268] to confirm a diagnosis of CTS in only 61 percent of cases. However, radiculopathy due to disease of the cervical spine, diffuse peripheral neuropathy, or proximal median neuropathy can pose clinical questions that electrodiagnostic testing can settle.[257]

A carpal tunnel view radiograph may be the only view that shows abnormalities within the carpal tunnel.[16]

The conservative intervention for mild cases typically includes the use of splints, activity modification, diuretics, and NSAIDs.[269] The rationale for splints was originally based on observations that CTS symptoms improve with rest and worsen with activity.[270] However, prescription parameters for the type of splint are not standardized,[271] with some advocating neutral positioning,[272] and some recommending 0 to 15 degrees of wrist extension. The length of time for wearing the splint is also undetermined, with some recommending day and night use,[273] while others instruct patients to wear the brace at night and during activities stressful to the wrist.[274] Still others recommend only night use.[272] Rigid splints have been found to be superior to flexible ones in controlling carpal tunnel pressure,[275] although the softer flexible ones enhance compliance in rheumatoid arthritis patients.[276]

Night splints appear to help reduce the nocturnal symptoms and allow the wrist to rest fully, although one study found that night splints did not significantly reduce intracarpal pressure when compared to controls who did not wear them.[277] Splints during the day are helpful only if they do not interfere with normal activity. The positioning of the splint may be significant.

Yoga that focuses on upper body postures was found to be of benefit in one study,[278] although the sample size was small and the results were not conclusive.

Ergonomic modifications can help reduce the incidence of carpal tunnel syndrome and alleviate symptoms in the already symptomatic patient. Patient education is also important to avoid sustained pinching or gripping, repetitive wrist motions, and sustained positions of full wrist flexion.

Isolated tendon excursion exercises are performed. These include isolated tendon gliding of the FDS and FDP of each digit.

Contrast baths can be used in 10-minute sessions to assist in the reduction of inflammation and edema.

Evaluation for surgical management is necessary for patients with atrophy of the thenar muscles, decreased sensation, and persistent symptoms that are intolerable despite conservative therapy.[247]

Ulnar Nerve. Entrapment of the ulnar nerve can occur at the elbow in the cubital tunnel (see Chap. 15). Entrapment of the ulnar nerve at the wrist can occur at Guyon's canal. The clinical features of an ulnar nerve entrapment at the wrist include[279]:

▶ Claw hand resulting from unopposed action of the extensor digitorum communis in the fourth and fifth digits.

▶ An inability to extend the second and distal phalanges of any of the fingers.

▶ An inability to adduct or abduct the fingers, or to oppose all the fingertips, as in making a cone with the fingers and thumb.

▶ An inability to adduct the thumb.

▶ Positive Froment's sign.

▶ Atrophy of the interosseous spaces (especially the first) and of the hypothenar eminence.

▶ A loss of sensation on the ulnar side of the hand, the ring finger, and most markedly over the entire little finger. The dorsal ulnar aspect of the hand should be normal as that is innervated by the dorsal cutaneous branch.

If ulnar neuropathy at Guyon's canal is suspected, it is often helpful to evaluate the pisotriquetral joint and the hook of the hamate. Abnormalities may be present at either site, resulting in secondary ulnar neuropathy.[280] In addition, the clinician must ask the patient whether they have any medical history involving diabetes and peripheral neuropathies.

The intervention for ulnar nerve compression can be surgical or conservative depending on the severity. Indications for surgical intervention include preventing deformity and increasing functional use of the hand. Conservative intervention for mild compression involves the application of a protective splint and patient education to avoid positions and postures that could compromise the nerve.

Hand-Arm Vibration Syndrome (HAVS)

Vibration is a physical stressor to which many people are exposed at work, in the home, or in their social activities. Humans respond characteristically to certain critical vibration frequencies at which there is maximum energy transfer from source to receiver.[281]

HAVS is frequently underdiagnosed and misdiagnosed as carpal tunnel syndrome since the two entities typically coexist.[282] HAVS is associated with occupations involving exposure to sources of vibration including air-compressed drilling, grinding, and electric drills and saws.[283]

The pathophysiology of HAVS is poorly understood, but chronic exposure to vibration produces circulatory, neurologic-sensory-motor, and musculoskeletal disturbances. Khilberg[284] has studied the acute effects and symptoms of work with vibrating hand-held power tools. He found that workers using nonimpact tools (grinders) had a lower prevalence of elbow and shoulder symptoms than those using low-frequency impact tools (chipping hammers), but did not differ in this respect from workers using high-frequency impact tools. Work with impact tools in general was associated with a higher prevalence of pain in the wrist than work with nonimpact tools.[281]

The diagnosis of HAVS is based on a history of HAV exposure and sensorineural or vascular signs and symptoms, which include[203]:

▶ Episodic tingling and numbness. The numbness or tingling can be graded.

▶ Mild to severe sensory deficits.

▶ Blanching white fingers (Raynaud's phenomenon). This is the most common symptom, and it occurs on exposure to cold. Its extent and frequency of occurrence determines the severity of the vascular grading.[281]

▶ Swelling of the digits and forearm tissue.

▶ Trophic skin changes.

The intervention for HAVS includes maintaining central body temperature, avoiding exposure to cold and vibrating tools, job modification, and splinting at night.[203]

Myofascial Pain Syndrome

The most frequent cause of wrist, hand, and finger pain is myofascial referral from the forearm flexors and especially from the forearm extensors. Trigger points in these muscles increase tendon tension and therefore relative compression of the carpal joints, which causes cracking and crepitus at the wrist due to abnormal joint glide.[285] The patient often reports a sense of stiffness in the wrist and hand, and pain exacerbated with wrist and finger flexion, which stretches these muscles, and on full wrist extension, which shortens these muscles.[285]

Complex Regional Pain Syndrome (CRPS)

The term CRPS refers to a classification of disorders, which can occur even after minor injury to a limb, and which is a major cause of disability.[286]

Complex regional pain syndrome, originally termed *causalgia*, has since been referred to by a number of names including post-traumatic osteoporosis, Sudeck's atrophy, transient osteoporosis, algoneurodystrophy, shoulder-hand syndrome, gardenalic rheumatism, neurotrophic rheumatism, reflex neurovascular dystrophy, and reflex sympathetic dystrophy (RSD).[287]

Two types of CRPS are recognized by the International Association for the Study of Pain:

▶ *CRPS 1.* This type refers to the pain syndrome, previously termed RSD, which involves a pain syndrome triggered by a noxious event that is not limited to a single peripheral nerve.

▶ *CRPS 2.* This type refers to the pain syndrome, previously termed causalgia, which involves a pain syndrome that involves direct partial or complete injury to a nerve or one of its major branches.

The signs and symptoms for both types include pain, edema, stiffness, skin temperature changes, and sweating.[288]

Type I CRPS. The pain of type I CRPS is classified as sympathetically maintained pain (SMP) or sympathetically independent pain (SIP), where SMP is characterized by an abnormal reaction of the sympathetic nervous system.[288]

The edema, which can be pitting or nonpitting, is often present throughout all stages of CRPS and may be the result of vasomotor instability coupled with a lack of motion.[287]

The stiffness is one of the components of CRPS 1 that increases with time, and is due to increased fibrosis in the ligamentous structures and adhesion formation around the tendons.[287]

The reported incidence of CRPS 1 is 1 to 2 percent after various fractures,[289] from 2 to 5 percent after peripheral nerve injury,[290] and 7 to 35 percent in prospective studies of Colles' fracture.[291] In 10 to 26 percent of cases no precipitating factor can be found.[292] A number of psychological components have been proposed, including:

1. A significant period of stress, anxiety, or depression.
2. Childhood experiences.
   a. Sexual abuse.
   b. Physical abuse.
   c. Emotional abuse.
   d. Abandonment.
   e. Family history of drug or alcohol abuse.
3. Adult experiences.
   a. Care provider for aging or ill parent(s) or other relative.
   b. Problem children, parents, or siblings.
   c. Unhappy marriage.
   d. Alcoholism.
   e. Grief.
   f. Abuse of any type.
4. A low self-esteem.
5. A negative outlook on life.

However, there has been no evidence to support such notions. Instead, it is thought that the emotional and behavioral changes noted are a result, rather than a cause, of the prolonged pain and disability.[293]

The diagnosis of CRPS is made from the physical examination and the patient's medical history, which may include past events of trauma, persistent pain, hyperalgesia, allodynia (perception of a nonpainful stimulus as painful), edema, and diminished function of the area.

The type of pain and its duration are perhaps the most important diagnostic signs. The pain is typically burning in nature, and is of a much longer duration than would be expected from the injury.[293]

A number of other conditions need to be ruled out before establishing a diagnosis of CRPS 1, and these include, but are not limited to:

▶ Rheumatoid and septic arthritis.

▶ Gout.

▶ Disk herniation.

▶ Peripheral neuropathy.

▶ Peripheral nerve entrapment.

▶ Peripheral vascular disease.

Classically, CRPS 1 has been subdivided into three progressive clinical phases[294,295]:

▶ An acute inflammatory phase that can last from 10 days to 2 to 3 months. The acute stage of CRPS lasts from 1 to 3 months. This stage is reversible if the patient is treated. The affected limb becomes flushed, warm, and dry because regional blood vessels are relaxed, and stimulation of the sweat glands is reduced.[288] The pain is diffuse, severe, and constant with a burning, throbbing, or aching quality. Edema and increased hair and nail growth can also occur. By the end of this stage, the limb turns cold, sweaty, and cyanotic from vasoconstriction caused by paradoxical sympathetic stimulation.[288]

▶ A phase of vasomotor instability that can last for several months. This is the dystrophic stage, which lasts another 3 to 6 months. Constricted blood vessels can cool limb temperature by nearly 10 degrees.[288] The area will be pale, mottled, edematous, and sweaty. Pain remains continuous, burning, or throbbing, but is more severe.[288] Nails may crack or become brittle and heavily grooved. Limb movement is limited by muscle wasting and joint stiffness. Osteoporosis and contractures can develop.[288]

▶ A cold end phase. The atrophic stage is characterized by irreversible damage to muscles and joints. Over the next 2 to 3 months the bones atrophy and the joints become weak, stiff, or even ankylosed.[288] The pain lessens and may become spasmodic or breakthrough, but is no longer mediated by the sympathetic nervous system.[288] The skin is cool and looks glossy and pale or cyanotic.

No prospective studies are available in which this staging is confirmed. However, a prospective study of 829 patients[287] indicated that:

▶ In its early phase, reflex sympathetic dystrophy is characterized by regional inflammation and not of a disturbance of the sympathetic nervous system. The regional inflammation increases after muscular exercise.

▶ Tremor was found in 49 percent and muscular incoordination in 54 percent of patients.

▶ Sympathetic signs such as hyperhidrosis are infrequent.

These data support the concept of an exaggerated regional inflammatory response to injury or operation in reflex sympathetic dystrophy.[287,296]

The most effective intervention for CRPS 1 is disputed. However, most agree that the intervention requires a team approach, in which the physical therapist plays a pivotal role, and that the earlier the intervention is instituted, the better the prognosis. Immobilization and overprotecting the affected limb may produce or exacerbate demineralization, vasomotor changes, edema, and trophic changes.[297]

Physical therapy is the first line of intervention, whether it be the sole intervention or performed immediately following a nerve block.[293,298]

The most important rule is to minimize pain while employing physical therapy. When excessive pain is created, sympathetically mediated pain may worsen.[293] It is vital to not reinjure the region or aggravate the problem with aggressive physical rehabilitation.[299]

The patient's involved limb must be elevated as often as possible, and actively mobilized several times per day.[293]

Recovery from muscle dysfunction, swelling, and joint stiffness requires appropriate physical activity and exercise, and pressure and motion are necessary to maintain joint movement and prevent stiffening.[293] The progression should occur slowly and gently with strengthening, active assisted range-of-motion, and active range-of-motion exercises.

Weight-bearing exercises and active stress loading exercises should also be incorporated.

Sensory threshold techniques including fluidotherapy, vibration desensitization, transcutaneous electrical nerve stimulation (TENS), contrast baths, and desensitization using light and heavy pressure of various textures over the sensitive area should be used.

Affected joints should be rested and elevated to counteract the vascular stasis, but the joint also should be mobilized gently several times per day.[300] Physical therapy is advised as long as the patient works within his or her pain threshold.[293] Complete rest to the affected region, particularly immobilization in a cast, is harmful.[299,300]

Topical capsaicin is helpful, as are nonsteroidal anti-inflammatory medications.

Integration of Practice Patterns 4G and 4I: Impaired Joint Mobility, Motor Function, Muscle Performance, Range of Motion Associated with Fractures and Bony or Soft Tissue Surgical Procedures

Distal Radius Fractures

Fracture of the distal radius is the most common wrist injury for all age groups. The older patient usually sustains an extra-articular metaphyseal fracture, whereas the younger patient experiences the more complicated intra-articular fracture.[184]

Colles' Fracture.[4] Colles' fracture is defined as a complete fracture of the distal radius with dorsal displacement of the distal fragment. The typical mechanism of injury is a fall on an outstretched hand (FOOSH). The fracture displacement and angulation are evident on the lateral film—the Colles' fracture has the characteristic dorsiflexion or "silver fork" deformity. Radiographs of the anteroposterior view show the usual comminuted fracture.

Management of this fracture requires an accurate reduction of the fracture and maintenance of the normal length of the radius. The method of reduction, as well as the position of immobilization, is quite variable. In most cases closed reduction and a cast are effective. In other cases, open reduction and external fixation is necessary.[301] Loss of full rotation of the forearm is a common sequelae of this fracture.

Smith Fracture. A Smith fracture, sometimes called a reverse Colles' fracture, is a complete fracture of the distal radius with palmar displacement of the distal fragment.[302] The usual mechanism for this type of fracture is a fall on the back of a flexed hand. Smith's fractures are classified into three types[303]:

▶ *Type I.* This is described as a transverse fracture through the distal radial shaft.

▶ *Type II.* This is an oblique fracture through the distal shaft starting at the dorsal articulating lip.

▶ *Type III.* This type (also referred to as a reverse Barton's fracture) is an oblique fracture beginning further down on the articular surface of the radius.

Customary management for a Smith's fracture is with closed reduction and long arm casting in supination for 3 weeks, followed by 2 to 3 weeks in a short-arm cast.[302] Types II and III are frequently unstable, however, and thus require an open reduction and internal fixation (ORIF).

Barton's Fracture. A Barton's fracture involves a dorsal or volar articular fracture of the distal radius resulting in a subluxation of the wrist.[302] The mechanism of injury for this type of fracture usually includes some form of direct and violent injury to the wrist, or from a sudden pronation of the distal forearm on a fixed wrist. Seventy percent of these fractures occur in young men. A technique to reduce these dislocations under anesthesia has been described in the literature.[304] The technique involves applying traction to the wrist and then placing the patient's wrist in full supination, mid-extension and ulnar deviation, which closes the diastasis by reducing the scaphoid to its correct anatomic plane. An above-elbow cast is then applied for 4 weeks, followed by a forearm cast for a further 3 weeks with the wrist in ulnar deviation. Other techniques describe using an ORIF with 16 weeks being the average healing time.

Buckle Fracture. A buckle fracture is an incomplete, undisplaced fracture of the distal radius commonly seen in children. Immobilization for 3 to 4 weeks in a short-arm cast or palmar splint is adequate.[128] The possibility of abuse should be considered in the child with a fracture. Consultation with an orthopaedist is advisable for fractures in the pediatric population.

The fracture is treated with a cast, ORIF, or external fixation. The fracture site is immobilized for 6 weeks if casted, 8 weeks with an external fixator, or 2 weeks if an ORIF with plate and screws is performed. If the fracture is nondisplaced, rehabilitation may last 2 to 6 weeks, whereas displaced fractures typically require 8 to 12 weeks.

Conservative intervention can begin while the fracture is immobilized, and involves AROM of the shoulder in all planes, elbow flexion and extension, and finger flexion and extension. The finger exercises must include isolated MCP flexion, composite flexion (full fist), and intrinsic minus fisting (MCP extension with IP flexion). If a fixator or pins are present, pin site care should be performed according to physician preference.

Following the period of immobilization, an immobilization capsular pattern will initially be present. Extension and supination are commonly limited and need to be mobilized. AROM exercises of wrist flexion and extension and ulnar and radial deviation are initiated. Wrist extension exercises are performed with the fingers flexed, especially at the MCP joints. PROM is performed according to physician preference, either immediately or after 1 to 2 weeks.

The AROM exercises of the wrist and forearm are progressed to strengthening exercises, using light weights and tubing. Putty can be used to increase grip strength if necessary.

Plyometrics and neuromuscular re-education exercises are next, followed by return to function or sports activities.

Fractured Scaphoid

Of all the wrist injuries encountered in the emergency department, fracture of the scaphoid is one of the most commonly missed.[305,306] This is unfortunate given that the scaphoid is the most commonly fractured carpal bone due to its location, and is the only bone fractured in approximately 70 percent of all carpal fracture cases.[110,128,183,231] Accurate early diagnosis of scaphoid fracture is critical as the morbidity associated with a missed or delayed diagnosis is significant, and can result in long-term pain, loss of mobility, and decreased function.[11] This degree of morbidity is related to the scant blood supply to the scaphoid, which results in a high incidence of delayed healing or nonunion, and the fact that scaphoid fractures are inherently unstable.

Although a fracture can occur in any part of the scaphoid, the common areas are at the waist and at the proximal pole.

Classically, the injury results from a fall on an outstretched hand (FOOSH) with the wrist pronated. Patients typically complain of dorsal wrist pain and have tenderness over the anatomic snuffbox. On physical examination, little swelling may be noted, although loss of the concavity of the anatomic snuffbox is frequently seen.[306] Many investigators feel a reliable test for scaphoid injury is axial compression of the thumb along its longitudinal axis.[307,308] Described by Chen,[307] this test translates force directly across the scaphoid, and should elicit pain if there is a fracture. It may be good practice to treat all cases of wrist sprain that are accompanied with pain and swelling in the anatomic snuffbox as a scaphoid fracture until proven otherwise. Even with appropriate radiographs, fractures of the scaphoid can be subtle and difficult to visualize.[306] In cases in which there is a high clinical suspicion, a scaphoid view of the wrist is usually obtained. This is a clenched fist view with the wrist held in ulnar deviation. This view reduces the foreshortening of the scaphoid that occurs on a normal PA view, and clearly displays the entire length of the scaphoid.[306]

Conservative management of a scaphoid fracture is controversial. There is no agreement on the optimum position for immobilization. Current management is immobilization in a long-arm or short-arm thumb spica cast, with the wrist position and length of immobilization dependent on the location of the fracture:

▶ *Proximal pole.* Immobilization is for 16 to 20 weeks in a long-arm or short-arm thumb spica, with the wrist in slight extension and radial deviation.

▶ *Central third.* Immobilization is for 6 weeks in a long-arm thumb spica, followed by a further 6 weeks in a short-arm thumb spica. Some physicians advocate splinting the wrist in radial deviation and mild flexion for the 6 weeks.[71,128,231] After 6 weeks, if healing is evident on radiographs, a short-arm thumb spica cast is applied for 2 to

4 weeks. If after 6 weeks the fracture line seems greater or the fracture appears displaced, evaluation for possible surgery is in order.[128,309]

▶ *Distal third.*   Immobilization is for 6 to 8 weeks in a short-arm thumb spica.

▶ *Tuberosity.*   Immobilization is for 5 to 6 weeks in a long-arm or short-arm thumb spica.

For the patient with pain over the anatomic snuffbox but normal initial radiographs, application of a thumb spica cast for 3 weeks followed by repeat radiographs is indicated. If the radiographs remain normal but pain persists, a bone scan is the next step. If the bone scan is positive, management is continued as for an acute fracture. Chronic pain, loss of motion, and decreased strength from prolonged immobilization or early arthritis is common following a scaphoid fracture.

Following the removal of the splint, a capsular pattern of the wrist will dominate. In addition, there will be a painful weakness of the thumb and/or wrist extension/radial deviation and compression of the first metacarpal on the scaphoid will be painful. AROM exercises for wrist flexion and extension, and radial and ulnar deviation are initiated as early as possible after the splint removal, with PROM to the same motions beginning after 2 weeks. A wrist and thumb immobilization splint can be fabricated to wear between exercises and at night for comfort and protection.

At about the same time as the PROM exercises, gentle strengthening exercises are begun with 1- to 2-lb weights or putty. Over a period of several weeks, the exercise program is progressed to include weight-bearing activities, plyometrics, open and closed chain exercises, and neuromuscular reeducation, before finally progressing to functional and sport-specific exercises and activities.

The most common complication of scaphoid fracture is nonunion. Missed and therefore untreated scaphoid fractures often progress to nonunions. Because of the precarious nature of the blood supply and potential for movement at the fracture line, nonunion can occur in 8 to 10 percent of cases.[305,310] The rate of nonunion varies with the actual fracture site. Nonunion complicates up to 20 to 30 percent of proximal third fractures, and 10 to 20 percent of middle third fractures.[306] Nonunion of distal third fractures is relatively rare.[305,310]

Scapholunate advanced collapse (SLAC) wrist is a late complication of scaphoid fracture, scapholunate dissociation, Kienböck's disease, fracture of the distal radius, Preiser's disease, and deposition of crystals of calcium pyrophosphate dehydrate.[311] The SLAC wrist is thought to result from a loss of the stabilizing effect of the scaphoid, with the development of an arthrosis at the radioscaphoid articulation. When the injury has progressed to this state, proximal row carpectomy or wrist fusion is the only option for the hand surgeon.[312]

Carpal Boss

A carpal boss is a rounded bony prominence that presents between the base of second and third metacarpal and the trapezoid and capitate, resulting from repetitive forced extension of the wrist and subsequent irritation of soft tissues. The ECRL and ECRB are commonly involved. This prominence resembles a ganglion, and is not necessarily pathologic, although it can cause pain and irritation of the local soft tissues.[313] Confirmation is through radiographs.

Conservative intervention includes a wrist immobilization splint with the wrist positioned in slight extension (10 to 15 degrees) to reduce tension on the radial wrist extensors.

Finger Fractures

Phalangeal fractures represent approximately 46 percent of fractures of the hand and wrist, and are more common than those of metacarpal or carpal fractures.[314] These fractures can be divided into base, shaft, and neck and head fractures. Unstable displaced articular fractures require surgical intervention. Conservative intervention of the more stable fractures involves closed reduction in as near normal a position as possible with an appropriate cast or splint[315]:

Distal Phalanx Fractures.   A protective splint is worn for 2 to 4 weeks until the fracture site is nontender. AROM begins at 2 to 4 weeks, or earlier if the fracture is stable enough. PROM begins at 5 to 6 weeks. PREs normally begin at 7 to 8 weeks.

Middle Phalanx Fractures.   If nondisplaced, these fractures are splinted in the intrinsic plus position for approximately 3 weeks. Buddy splinting, the taping of a neighboring finger to the involved finger, may also be an option. AROM is initiated when pain and edema subsides. PROM begins at 4 to 6 weeks, with PREs normally beginning at 6 to 8 weeks.

Proximal Phalanx Fractures.   Nondisplaced extra-articular fractures are splinted with buddy tape. AROM is initiated immediately, with PROM being initiated at 6 to 8 weeks. Nondisplaced intra-articular fractures are splinted in the intrinsic plus position for 2 to 3 weeks. AROM begins at 2 to 3 weeks, with PROM being initiated at 4 to 8 weeks. PREs normally begin at clinical union (8 to 12 weeks).

Therapeutic Techniques

Myofascial Release

Carpal Tunnel Release

A number of myofascial techniques can be used to treat carpal tunnel syndrome.

Opening the Canal.   The patient is positioned in sitting or supine lying with their palms facing upwards. The clinician applies pressure centrally from the dorsal surface of the carpal bones simultaneously with pressure applied from the ventral edges of the carpal bones, using a three-point-opposing-pressure technique.[316]

Abductor Brevis Release. The patient is positioned in sitting or supine lying with their palm facing upwards. The clinician grasps the thumb with one hand and pulls it back into hyperextension with abduction, while simultaneously performing the opening canal technique described above.[316]

Carpal Tunnel Stretch. The patient is positioned in sitting or supine lying with their palm facing upwards. The clinician stabilizes the patient's wrist with one hand and simultaneously hyperextends the digits and wrist of the patient with the other hand.[316]

Techniques to Increase Joint Mobility

The majority of the mobility tests described in the tests and measures section can also be utilized as mobilization techniques. For each of the following techniques, the patient is positioned in sitting with their forearm and wrist in a neutral position, with the clinician positioned to the side of the patient. The amplitude and the velocity of each of the techniques (i.e., grade) is varied according to the stage of healing and the irritability of the joint.

The clinician must be cognizant of the joints that are responsible for the individual motions that occur at the wrist and hand in order to deliver the most specific technique.

▶ Supination-pronation occurs primarily at the ulnomeniscotriquetral joint and the proximal and inferior radioulnar joints.

▶ Wrist flexion occurs primarily at the radiocarpal joint (distal radius and the articulating surfaces of the navicular and lunate).

▶ Wrist extension occurs primarily at the mid-carpal joints (articulating surface of the scaphoid, lunate, and triquetral bones proximally, and the trapezium, trapezoid, capitate, and hamate bones distally).

Passive Accessory Mobilizations[317]
Radiocarpal, Ulnocarpal, Midcarpal, Carpometacarpal, Metacarpophalangeal, and Interphalangeal Joints
Distraction. Using a pinch grip of the index finger and thumb of one hand, the clinician palpates and stabilizes the proximal bone of the joint being distracted. With a pinch grip of the index finger and thumb of the other hand, the clinician palpates and mobilizes the distal bone longitudinally (Fig. 16-48).

Posterior-Anterior Glide (Flexion/Extension). Using a pinch grip of the index finger and thumb of one hand, the clinician palpates and stabilizes the proximal bone of the joint being mobilized in a dorsal-palmar plane. With a pinch grip, the clinician glides the distal bone along the dorsal-palmar plane of the corresponding joint (Fig. 16-49). The appropriate conjunct rotation of the bone may be added. For example, to restore flexion at the radioscaphoid joint, the clinician rotates the scaphoid toward

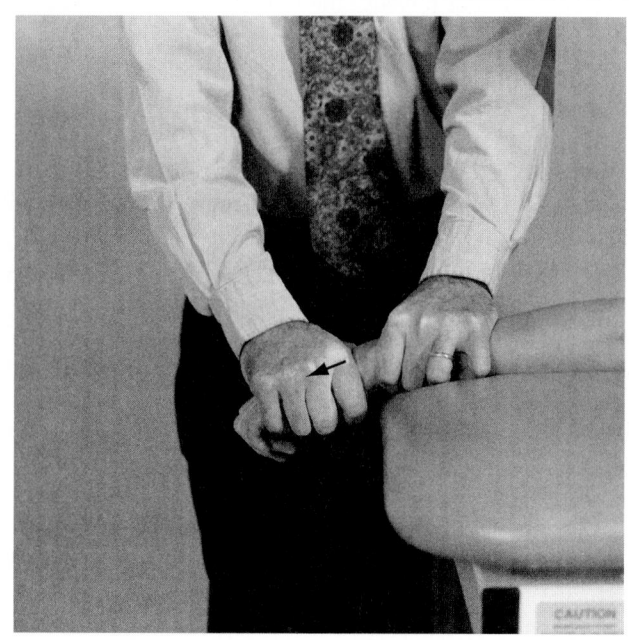

FIGURE 16-48 Joint distraction.

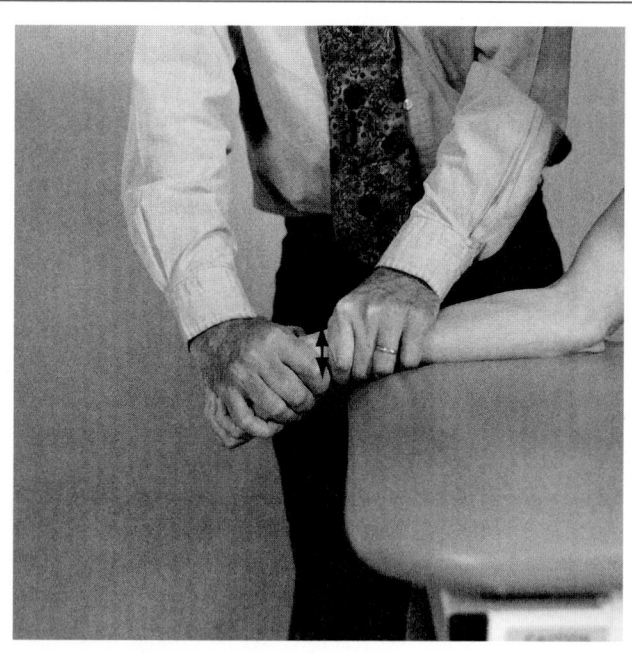

FIGURE 16-49 Posterior-anterior glide.

the center of the palm, while simultaneously gliding the scaphoid in a dorsal direction.

The clinician can make the technique patient-assisted by flexing/extending the distal bone about the appropriate intra-articular axis to the limit of the physiologic range of motion. From this position, the patient is instructed to perform an isometric contraction against the clinician's equal resistance.

The contraction is held for 3 to 5 seconds, following which the patient is instructed to completely relax. The new barrier of flexion/extension is localized and the mobilization repeated.

First Carpometacarpal and Metacarpophalangeal Joints

Medial-Lateral Glide (Abduction/Adduction). Using a pinch grip of the index finger and thumb of one hand, the clinician palpates and stabilizes the proximal bone of the joint being mobilized in a medial-lateral plane. With a pinch grip of the index finger and thumb of the other hand, the clinician glides the distal bone along the medial-lateral plane of the corresponding joint (Fig. 16-50). The appropriate conjunct rotation of the bone may be added.

The clinician can make the technique patient-assisted by abducting/adducting the distal bone about the appropriate intraarticular axis to the limit of the physiologic range of motion. From this position, the patient is instructed to perform an isometric contraction against the clinician's equal resistance. The contraction is held for 3 to 5 seconds, following which the patient is instructed to completely relax. The new barrier of motion is localized and the mobilization repeated.

Intermetacarpal Articulations. Using a pinch grip of the index finger and thumb of one hand, the clinician palpates and stabilizes one metacarpal. With the thumb and index finger of the other hand, the clinician mobilizes the neighboring metacarpal into an anterior or posterior glide, with the appropriate conjunct rotation (Fig. 16-51).

Metacarpophalangeal Joints. Using a pinch grip of the index finger and thumb of one hand, the clinician palpates and stabi-

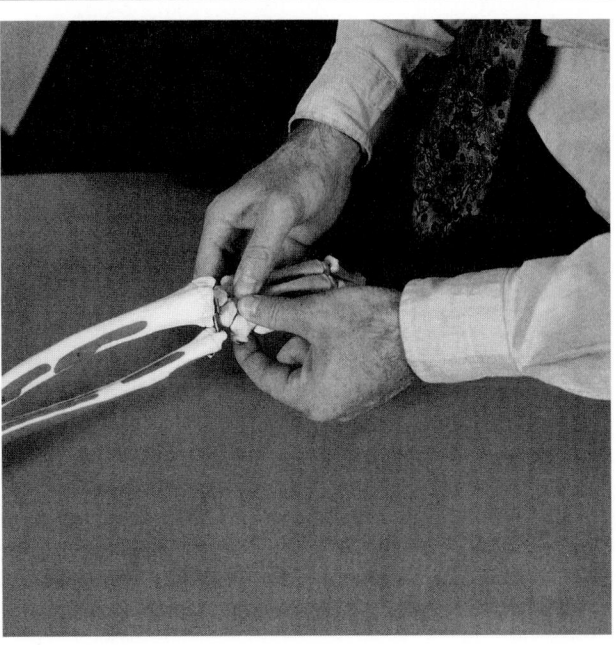

FIGURE 16-51 Intermetacarpal joint mobilizations.

lizes one metacarpal. The clinician places the thumb of the other hand on the dorsum of the corresponding phalanx and the index finger on the palmar surface of the same phalanx. While applying a long-axis extension (straight-line traction), the clinician mobilizes the phalanx in a palmar or dorsal direction with the appropriate conjunct rotation.

Mobilizations with Movements[318]

Technique for Pain and/or Loss of Pronation/Supination at the Distal Radioulnar Joint. The patient is positioned in sitting. The clinician grasps the distal end of the radius with one hand and the distal end of the ulna with the other hand (Fig. 16-52). The clinician applies a palmar glide of the ulna on the radius while the patient simultaneously actively moves in the painful and/or restricted direction (pronation or supination). If this is found to be painful, the clinician glides the ulna dorsally while the patient simultaneously actively moves in the painful and/or restricted direction. The successful mobilization procedure is repeated several times and the joint is reassessed

Technique for a Loss of and Pain with Wrist Flexion and/or Extension. The patient is positioned in sitting. Using one hand, the clinician grasps the distal ends of the radius and ulna, so that the web space between the index finger and thumb lies over the distal end of the radius. The clinician places the web space of the other hand medially, over the proximal row of carpals, so that the index finger and thumb are not in contact with the patient. The carpals are glided laterally and the patient is asked to actively move in the restricted direction (flexion or extension) while the mobilization is sustained. If the lateral glide is unsuccessful, the clinician rotates the proximal row of carpals on the

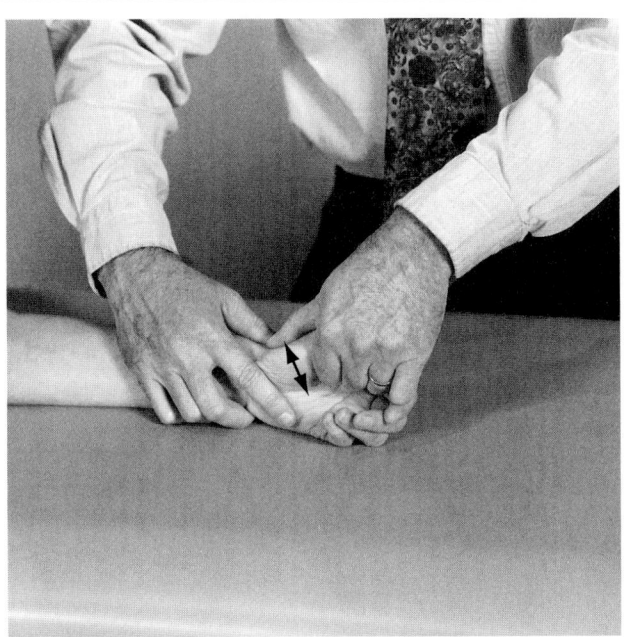

FIGURE 16-50 Medial-lateral glide of first CMC.

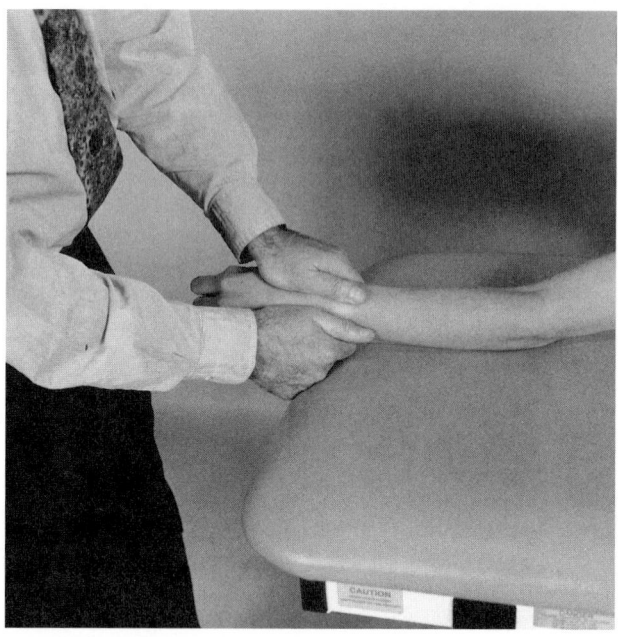

FIGURE 16-52 Mobilization with movement to increase pronation/supination.

radius and ulna in either a medial or lateral direction, depending on which elicits the optimal result.

High Velocity, Low Amplitude Thrusting

Intercarpal Manipulations

High velocity thrust techniques can be used with any of the carpals. The following example describes the technique for a dorsally displaced scaphoid:

> The patient is positioned in sitting with the forearm of their affected side resting on a table with the palmar side facing down. The clinician sits or stands at right angles to the patient's affected side. The clinician grips the patient's scaphoid bone between their thumb and index finger. The clinician reinforces this grip by placing the thumb and index of the other hand on top of them. The patient's wrist is then passively extended to the end range. At the end of available range, the scaphoid is thrusted ventrally while passively extending the wrist slightly.

Techniques to Increase Soft Tissue Extensibility

A number of techniques can be used to increase the extensibility of the soft tissues of the wrist, hand, and forearm. These include passive or active range-of-motion exercises into:

▶ Wrist and finger flexion and extension.

▶ Wrist ulnar and radial deviation.

▶ Finger adduction and abduction.

▶ Thumb opposition, flexion, extension, abduction, and adduction.

CASE STUDY PAINFUL LEFT THUMB

HISTORY

History of Current Condition
A 23-year-old female patient complained of left thumb pain following a home do-it-yourself project that involved a lot of hammering of nails. The patient described a gradual onset of pain about 2 months ago, and described the pain as burning located at the base of the left thumb. The patient also reported some swelling at the wrist. The patient attributed the pain to the hammering of nails as subsequent attempts to use the hammer reproduced the pain. Over time, the pain had worsened to the point where it hurt all of the time, even at night. The NSAIDs prescribed by the physician 2 weeks ago appeared to be helping.

Past History of Current Condition
No past history of left elbow, wrist, or hand pain.

Past Medical/Surgical History
Unremarkable except for removal of ganglion cysts from her right wrist/hand about 1 year ago.

Growth and Development
Right-hand dominant.

Medications
None, except for the prescribed NSAIDs.

Occupational/Employment/School
Office worker. College education.

Functional Status/Activity Level
The patient experienced pain with vacuuming and lifting heavy pots and pans. The patient's goals were to decrease pain with activities of daily living.

Health Status (Self-Report)
In general good health, but pain interferes with gripping tasks at home and at work.

QUESTIONS

1. What are some of the more common diagnoses characterized by thumb pain?
2. What does the history of the gradual onset and of repetitive activity tell the clinician?
3. What findings do you expect to note in the physical examination in terms of palpation, resistive tests, and special tests?
4. What additional questions would you ask to help rule out referral of pain from the cervical spine or shoulder?

5. List the tests you would use to rule out the various diagnoses that you listed in question 1.
6. Does this presentation/history warrant an upper quarter scanning examination? Why or why not?

TESTS AND MEASURES

The physical examination of the patient included an inspection for muscle atrophy, palpation for areas of tenderness and crepitation, muscle testing of all major muscles about the elbow, forearm and wrist, measurement of active and passive range of motion, and specific testing for carpal tunnel and de Quervain's. The cervical spine and the other joints of the upper extremity were also examined to determine whether the pain was being referred.

Joint Integrity and Mobility

Passive accessory motions of the lunate and capitate were reduced as compared with the other side.

Motor Performance: Strength, Power, and Endurance

- The left wrist displayed weakness (4 out of 5) throughout the range of motion of flexion and extension.
- All resisted thumb movements were painful, so muscle grading was deferred. All other fingers tested normal. The special test for de Quervain's disease reproduced the patient's pain.

Orthotic, Protective, and Supportive Devices

Patient does not use any device.

Pain

Palpation revealed point tenderness at the base of the left thumb. Fine crepitus was noted over the length of the tendons in the anatomic snuffbox. Pain was reported across the carpal joints (6 out of 10) with gripping.

Range of Motion (Including Muscle Length)

- Patient demonstrated a decrease in axial extension of the cervical spine to neutral because of "stiffness" and pain located over the spinous process of C6.
- Active cervical rotation was 70 degrees to the left and 90 degrees to the right. Overpressure into right rotation revealed a stiff end-feel.
- All left shoulder motions were full and pain-free, although the quadrant test of the right glenohumeral joint (see Chap. 14) produced a "pulling sensation" at the right elbow.
- All left elbow motions were full and pain-free.
- Active motion of the left wrist was 60 degrees of extension and 50 degrees of flexion with end-range pain reported with both motions.
- Active range of motion of the left thumb was grossly within functional limits, although touching the tips of the thumb and small finger was slow and painful.
- Pain reproduced with passive left thumb extension and abduction beyond midrange.
- No deficits noted in the other fingers.

Reflex Integrity

The patient's upper extremities were neurologically intact. Normal and symmetrical biceps and triceps reflexes bilaterally.

Sensory Integrity

Intact to light touch throughout C5 to T1 distributions bilaterally.

Special Tests

- Phalen's test was deferred secondary to the limitation of wrist motion.
- Finkelstein's test was positive for pain.
- Tinel's testing at the right wrist produced a tingling sensation into the hand.
- ULTT tests for the radial and median nerve were positive for pain and reduced motion.

EVALUATION (CLINICAL JUDGMENT)

Patient is a young active female with soft tissue mobility restrictions and impaired left thumb performance, which results in difficulties with gripping and pain at night.

DIAGNOSIS BY PHYSICAL THERAPIST

Practice Pattern E: Impaired joint mobility, motor function, muscle performance, and range of motion associated with localized inflammation of the left thumb; most likely de Quervain's disease.

From a rehabilitation standpoint, it is often more important to know the extent of the alterations in the tissues or in the biomechanics than to know a specific anatomy-based diagnosis.[319]

QUESTIONS

1. Having made a provisional diagnosis, what will be your intervention?
2. How would you describe this condition to the patient?
3. How would you explain the rationale behind your intervention to the patient?
4. What activities and positions would you advise the patient to avoid? Why?
5. How will you determine the intensity of your intervention?
6. Estimate this patient's prognosis.
7. What modalities could you use in the intervention of this patient? Why?
8. Which manual techniques would be appropriate for this patient, and what is your rationale for each?
9. What exercises would you prescribe? Why?
10. What therapeutic device would you recommend for this patient? Why?

PROGNOSIS

Predicted Optimal Level of Improvement in Function

Over the course of 4 to 6 weeks, the patient will demonstrate a return to normal home activities.

Predicted Interval Levels of Improvement in Function

Patient will be able to use a hammer for 15 minutes without pain in 6 weeks.

PLAN OF CARE

Frequency and Duration

Two to three times per week for 4 weeks.

Re-examination

Perform selected tests and measures to evaluate the patient's progress toward goals in order to modify or redirect intervention if patient fails to show progress.

Criteria for Discharge

Patient to be discharged when she reaches established functional goals, declines further treatment, is unable to progress towards goals because of complications, or PT determines that the patient will no longer benefit from PT services.

INTERVENTION

The intervention should be based on functional criteria which are based on stages of tendon healing.[320]

PHASE I (WEEKS 1–3)

This phase typically involves 2 to 6 visits of physical therapy.

Goals

The goals of treatment for this patient are[321]:

- To control pain to 2 out of 10 with activity and 0 out of 10 at rest.
- Edema to be within 20 percent of uninvolved side.
- To preserve motion, flexibility, and strength.
- To promote the development of endurance and normal vascularization and collagen production.
- Increase cervical mobility to within normal limits for rotation to the left.
- Independence with home exercise program.

Electrotherapeutic Modalities

- A combination of rest and ice massage to the first dorsal compartment can be applied in the initial stage.
- High-voltage galvanic stimulation can be applied to help relieve pain.
- Pulsed ultrasound with a 20 percent duty cycle, 3-MHz frequency, and an intensity of 1.2 W/cm² is applied to the base of the left thumb once the severe pain had subsided for 5 minutes, three times a week.
- A course of iontophoresis with dexamethasone was also initiated.
- A forearm-based thumb spica splint was issued to the patient with the following positioning: wrist in 15 to 20 degrees of extension, carpometacarpal joint in 40 to 50 degrees of palmar abduction, and the MCP joint in 5 to 10 degrees of flexion. The thumb IP is free. The splint is to be worn at all times for 3 to 6 weeks, except for exercises or hygiene.

- The patient was taught about the avoidance of aggravating motions and activities.

Therapeutic Exercise and Home Program

1. Gentle active range-of-motion exercises for short periods lasting 10 to 20 minutes within the pain-free ranges are initiated, to prevent joint stiffness and adhesion formation. ROM exercises include:
   a. Digit abduction/adduction.
   b. Intrinsic-plus position (MP flexion, PIP and DIP extension).
   c. Fisting.
   d. Guarded thumb MP and IP flexion with the thumb initially held in a protected abduction position, progressing to full thumb flexion as tolerated.
   e. Thumb radial and palmar abduction.
   f. Opposition of thumb, beginning with opposition to index finger only and progressing to other fingers as tolerated.
   g. Wrist flexion and extension.
   h. Wrist radial and ulnar deviation to neutral only, progressing to full ulnar deviation as tolerated.
   i. Forearm pronation and supination.

2. The patient was progressed to grasping and releasing small objects emphasizing a wide variety of prehensile patterns that avoid overuse of the first dorsal compartments.

   The home exercise program complemented the exercise program completed in the clinic.

Manual Therapy

- Soft tissue mobilizations to the forearm musculature.
- Transverse friction massage to the involved tendons (APL and EPB).
- Manual therapy techniques to increase cervical rotation to the left.
- ULTT techniques as appropriate.

PHASE II (WEEKS 4–8)

This phase involves 6 to 8 visits of physical therapy.

Goals

- Pain at 0 out of 10 with activity.
- Edema within 10 percent as compared with uninvolved side.
- Strength at 5 out of 5 on wrist/hand manual muscle tests and grip motor performance equal to uninvolved side.

Electrotherapeutic Modalities

Continued use of effective modalities as in phase I, with increased emphasis on use as needed at home.

Therapeutic Exercise and Home Program

- ROM and stretching exercises.
- Wrist progressive resistive exercises (PREs) in all planes, beginning with ¹/₂-lb weight.
- Graded therapy putty, Hand-Helper, and Digi-Flex.

- The strengthening program is progressed to isometrics, such as activities and exercises incorporating the shoulder, wrist, and elbow. Depending on the patient's physical demands, they can include PNF patterns with wall pulleys and the Fitter board.
- Upper extremity plyometrics are introduced.
- Strength and endurance of the upper kinetic chain was addressed with resisted PNF diagonals and the use of a grip dynamometer.

Manual Therapy
- Manual resistive exercise of the wrist, finger, and thumb extensors.
- Passive stretching.

PHASE III (WEEKS 9–12)
This phase typically involves 2 to 4 physical therapy visits.

Goals
- Full return to sports and recreational activities.

Therapeutic Exercises and Home Program
- Continued progression of exercises from phase II with emphasis on varying speed and intensity of exercises.
- Reproduction of sport- and activity-specific movements using progressive resistance.

Coordination, Communication, and Documentation
Communicate with MD, patient, work manager, and work comp case management regarding patient's status (direct or indirect). Documentation will include all elements of patient/client management. Discharge planning will be provided.

Patient-Related Instruction
Periodic re-examination and reassessment of the home program, utilizing written instruction and illustrations. Educate patient in proper postures, proper neutral wrist posture, and positions and motions to avoid during home and work. Educate patient in the benefits of an ongoing conditioning program to prevent recurrence of impairments.

Ensure a Safe Return to Function
A gradual return to normal activity is predicated upon normal restoration of strength, flexibility, and range of motion without pain.

CASE STUDY PAIN, WEAKNESS, AND NUMBNESS OF THE HAND

HISTORY

History of Current Condition
A 49-year-old female secretary complains of insidious onset of right hand numbness and pain, which began about 5 weeks previously. The symptoms are felt mainly in the right index finger, especially when working at her computer at work, but also in her right thumb and middle finger after a day at work. The symptoms are also reported to be worse during the night and early morning. The patient has also noted a slight decrease in her grip strength, which prompted her to see a MD, who prescribed PT, ibuprofen, vitamin B_6, and a short course of diuretics. The patient denies any neck pain.

Past Medical/Surgical History
No history of previous symptoms or of diabetes mellitus reported by the patient.

Medications
800 mg of ibuprofen daily.

Other Tests and Measures
None. X-rays 1 year ago were unremarkable (per patient). Physician mentioned that further testing may be warranted (nerve conduction velocity, EMG).

Social Habits (Past and Present)
Smoker (1/2 pack per day).

Growth and Development
Right-hand dominant.

Occupational/Employment/School
Full-time secretary at local community hospital for last 6 years. Recently promoted which has meant an increase in computer work.

Functional Status/Activity Level
Symptoms interfering with work and at home with her needle craft. Symptoms also interfering with sleep approximately 2 times per night.

QUESTIONS

1. What are some of the more common diagnoses characterized by symptoms in this distribution?
2. What does the history of the gradual onset and of repetitive activity tell the clinician?
3. What findings do you expect to note in the physical examination in terms of palpation, resistive tests, and special tests?
4. What additional questions would you ask to help rule out referral of pain from the cervical and thoracic spine?
5. What additional questions would you ask to help rule out referral of pain from the shoulder or elbow?
6. List the tests you would use to rule out the various diagnoses that you listed in question 1.
7. Does this presentation/history warrant a scan? Why or why not?

PHYSICAL THERAPY TESTS AND MEASURES

Anthropometric Characteristics

- Height 5′5″; weight 200 lb.
- Evidence of slight atrophy of thenar eminence.
- No deformity of right hand present.
- No swelling is evident.

Integumentary Integrity

No scarring present. Good capillary refilling.

Joint Integrity and Mobility

No deficits noted.

Motor Performance: Strength, Power, and Endurance

- Grip and pinch strength diminished in right hand to 75 percent as compared with uninvolved hand.
- 4+ out of 5 with manual testing of right thumb for opposition and abduction, compared to 5 out of 5 for left thumb.
- All other resistive testing negative.

Orthotic, Protective, and Supportive Devices

Patient has never used any device such as a night splint.

Pain

Pain rated at 7 to 8 out of 10 with activity, 5 out of 10 at rest on an analog scale. No tenderness elicited with palpation.

Posture

Forward head position, kyphotic dorsal spine and protracting shoulders.

Range of Motion (Including Muscle Length)

Range of motion within normal limits for right upper extremity as compared to uninvolved extremity.

Reflex Integrity

Normal and symmetrical biceps and triceps reflexes.

Sensory Integrity

Intact to light touch and vibration to all fingertips except for the index finger. Two-point discrimination diminished to 8 mm in right hand per Semmes-Weinstein monofilament test.

Special Tests

The following special tests were positive:

- Phalen's.
- Tinel's.
- ULTT 1 (median nerve bias).

EVALUATION (CLINICAL JUDGMENT)

Patient demonstrating clinical signs and symptoms of carpal tunnel syndrome (Practice Pattern F): Impaired motor function, muscle performance, and range of motion associated with localized inflammation.

QUESTIONS

1. Having made a provisional diagnosis, what will be your intervention?
2. How would you describe this condition to the patient?
3. How would you explain the rationale behind your intervention to the patient?
4. What activities and positions would you advise the patient to avoid? Why?
5. How will you determine the intensity of your intervention?
6. Estimate this patient's prognosis.
7. What modalities could you use in the intervention of this patient? Why?
8. Which manual techniques would be appropriate for this patient, and what is your rationale for each?
9. What exercises would you prescribe? Why?
10. What therapeutic device would you recommend for this patient? Why?

PROGNOSIS

Predicted Optimal Level of Improvement in Function

Within 2 months, the patient will demonstrate a return to normal home activities and to full work duty. The following objective improvements will be achieved:

- Full pain-free AROM of right wrist and forearm as compared to the uninvolved extremity.
- Pain at 3 out of 10 or less with activity, 0 out of 10 at rest.
- Restoration of strength/endurance of forearm/wrist complex to restore functional use of involved extremity.
- Grip and pinch strength to be at 90 percent as compared with uninvolved side.
- 5 out of 5 on manual muscle testing for wrist, forearm, and elbow, or equal to uninvolved extremity.
- Return to prior functional status and activity level as identified by patient.
- Independence and compliance with home exercise program and progression.

PLAN OF CARE

Frequency and Duration

2 times per week for 4 weeks.

Re-examination

Perform selected tests and measures to evaluate patient's progress toward goals in order to modify or redirect intervention if patient fails to show progress.

Criteria for Discharge

Patient reaches established functional goals, patient declines further treatment, is unable to progress toward goals because of complications, or PT determines that patient will no longer benefit from PT services.

INTERVENTION
PHASE I (WEEKS 1–5)

This phase typically involves 6 to 9 visits of physical therapy.

Goals

- Decrease inflammation to allow healing.
- Pain at 5 out of 10 with activity, 3 out of 10 at rest.
- Sensory: 7 mm on two-point discrimination test.
- Increase in functional activity to include light work.

Electrotherapeutic Modalities

- Iontophoresis.
- TENS.
- Fluidotherapy for desensitization.
- Hydrotherapy.
- Cryotherapy.

Therapeutic Exercise and Home Program

- Postural exercises.
- Strengthening of the forearm, elbow, and shoulder girdle is initiated.
- Advice on modification of work conditions and habits, and wrist posture.
- Tendon gliding exercises.
  - IP flexion or "hook fist."
  - MP flexion, followed by PIP flexion "straight fist."
  - Full fisting: active-assisted/gentle.
  - Patient performs thumb flexion, extension, and opposition.
  - Patient performs digit abduction/adduction.
  - Patient performs isometrics in the neutral wrist position for wrist extension and flexion.

Manual Therapy

- Soft tissue mobilization techniques to the thenar eminence and the carpal tunnel region.
- Manual lymphatic drainage using a light retrograde massage.
- ULTT 1 gentle stretching.

Therapeutic Devices

Patient issued wrist support positioned in neutral or slight wrist extension, to be worn routinely for approximately 4 to 6 weeks, with gradual decreased use over 4 weeks.[322]

Sensory Retraining

Patient performs desensitization including the use of a mini-vibrator, gripping of different textured materials, and rubbing the fingers with different textured materials.[323] Rice gripping can also be used.

PHASE II (WEEKS 6 TO 8)

This phase typically involves 4 to 6 visits of physical therapy.

Goals

- Full pain-free AROM as compared with the uninvolved extremity.
- Pain at 3 out of 10 with activity, 0 out of 10 at rest.
- Grip strength at 90 percent as compared with other side.
- Increased tolerance for repetitive functional activities.
- Sensory: 6 mm or less on two-point discrimination test.

Electrotherapeutic Modalities

Moist heat is applied before the exercises and ice is applied after the intervention sessions. Overall decrease in reliance on modalities and increased emphasis on use at home as needed.

Therapeutic Exercise and Home Program

- The isometric exercises initiated in phase I are progressed to isotonic strengthening.
- Resisted gripping with light resistive putty is initiated, and is limited to two 3-minute sessions every day. The progression of the theraputty grade is determined by motor performance and pinch assessment results.
- Progressive resisted exercises of the wrist are added when pain and neurologic symptoms are controlled.[324] Resistance begins with ½ lb, and is progressed to 5 lb as tolerated.

Manual Therapy

- Median nerve glide as needed.
- Proprioceptive neuromuscular facilitation (PNF) patterns, performed gently and focusing on the hand component.

Coordination, Communication, and Documentation

Possible referral to smoking cessation and nutrition and weight loss programs. Communicate with MD, patient, work manager, and work comp case management regarding patient's status (direct or indirect). Documentation will include all elements of patient/client management. Discharge planning will be provided.

Patient-Related Instruction

Periodic re-examination and reassessment of the home program, utilizing written instruction and illustrations. Educate patient in proper body mechanics and postures, and in positions and motions to avoid at home and at work. Educate patient in the benefits of an ongoing conditioning program to prevent functional decline, and to prevent recurrence of impairments. Modeling/demonstration or use of audiovisual aids will be used for teaching.

REVIEW QUESTIONS*

1. Which two carpal bones does the radius articulate with?
2. Name the carpal bones in the distal row.
3. Which structures run through Guyon's canal?
4. Which combination of symptoms indicates injury to the median nerve?
   A. The middle and index fingers lose the ability to flex and the thumb cannot adduct or extend.

B. The ring and little fingers lose the ability to flex, and the little finger cannot abduct or oppose.

C. The inability of the wrist and fingers to extend interferes with grasp.

D. The middle and index fingers lose their ability to flex, and the thumb cannot oppose.

5. Finkelstein's test is designed to assess involvement of which of the following contractile structures?

A. Extensor pollicis longus and abductor pollicis brevis muscles.

B. Extensor pollicis brevis and abductor pollicis longus muscles.

C. Extensor pollicis longus and abductor pollicis longus muscles.

D. Extensor pollicis brevis and abductor pollicis brevis muscles.

---

*Additional questions to test your understanding of this chapter can be found in the Online Learning Center for *Orthopaedic Assessment, Evaluation, and Intervention* at www.duttononline.net.

REFERENCES

1. McPhee SD. Functional hand evaluations: A review. *Am J Occup Ther* 1987;41:158–163.

2. Watson HK, Weinzweig J. Physical examination of the wrist. *Hand Clin* 1997;13:17–34.

3. Hume MC, et al. Functional range of motion of the joints of the hand. *J Hand Surg* 1990;15A:240–243.

4. Onieal M-E. Common wrist and elbow injuries in primary care. *Lippincott's Primary Care Practice. Musculoskeletal Conditions*. 1999;3:441–450.

5. Frykman GK, Kropp WE. Fractures and traumatic conditions of the wrist. In: Hunter JM, Mackin EJ, Callahan AD, eds. *Rehabilitation of the Hand: Surgery and Therapy*. St. Louis: Mosby-Year Book; 1995:315–336.

6. Wadsworth CT. Anatomy of the hand and wrist. In: *Manual Examination and Treatment of the Spine and Extremities*. Baltimore, Md: Williams & Wilkins; 1988:128–138.

7. Ward LD, et al. The role of the distal radioulnar ligaments, interosseous membrane, and joint capsule, in distal radioulnar joint stability. *J Hand Surg Am* 2000;25:341–351.

8. Palmer AK, Werner FW. The triangular fibrocartilage complex of the wrist—anatomy and function. *J Hand Surg* 1981;6:153–162.

8a. Waggy C. Disorders of the wrist. In: Wadsworth C, ed. *Orthopaedic Physical Therapy Home Study Course—The Elbow, Forearm, and Wrist*. La Crosse, WI: Orthopaedic Section, APTA, Inc; 1997.

9. Gupta R, Nelson SD, Baker J, Jones NF, Meals RA. The innervation of the triangular fibrocartilage complex: Nitric acid maceration rediscovered. *Plast Reconstr Surg* 2001;107:135–139.

10. Gray H. *Gray's Anatomy*. Philadelphia: Lea & Febiger; 1995.

11. Wackerle JF. A prospective study identifying the sensitivity of radiographic findings and the efficacy of clinical findings in carpal navicular fractures. *Ann Emerg Med* 1987;16:733–737.

12. Helal B. Racquet player's pisiform. *Hand* 1978;10:87.

13. Chase RA. Anatomy and kinesiology of the hand. In: Hunter DM, Mackin E, Callaghan M, eds. *Rehabilitation of the Hand*. Mosby: St Louis; 1995.

14. Kaplan EB. Anatomy and kinesiology of the hand. In: *Hand Surgery*. Flynn JE, ed. Williams & Wilkins: Baltimore; 1975.

15. Sarrafian SK, Melamed JL, Goshgarian GM. Study of wrist motion in flexion and extension. *Clin Orthop* 1977;126:153–159.

16. Culver JE. Instabilities of the wrist. *Clin Sports Med* 1986;5:725–740.

17. Taleisnik J. Classification of carpal instability. In: Taleisnik J, ed. *The Wrist*. New York: Churchill Livingstone; 1985:229–238.

18. Wadsworth C. Wrist and hand. In: Wadsworth C, ed. *Current Concepts of Orthopedic Physical Therapy—Home Study Course*. La Crosse, WI: Orthopaedic Section, APTA; 2001.

19. Moore JS. De Quervain's tenosynovitis: Stenosing tenosynovitis of the first dorsal compartment. *J Occup Environ Med* 1997;39:990–1002.

20. Freiberg A, et al. Management of proximal interphalangeal joint injuries. *J Trauma-Injury Infection Crit Care* 1999;46:523–528.

21. Tubiana R, Thomine J-M, Mackin E. *Examination of the Hand And Wrist*. London: Mosby; 1996.

21a. Neumann DA, Bielfeld T. The carpometacarpal joint of the thumb: stability, deformity, and therapeutic intervention. *J Orthop Sports Phys Ther* 2003;33:386–399.

22. Kuczymski K. The proximal interphalangeal joint: anatomy and causes of stiffness in the fingers. *J Bone Joint Surg Br* 1968;50:656–663.

23. Eaton RG. *Joint Injuries in the Hand*. Springfield, IL: Charles C Thomas; 1971:15–32.

24. Burton RI, Eaton RG. Common hand injuries in the athlete. *Orthop Clin North Am* 1973;4:809–838.

25. Bowers WH, et al. The proximal interphalangeal joint volar plate. I. An anatomical and biochemical study. *J Hand Surg Am* 1980;5:79–88.

26. Zancolli E. *Structural and Dynamic Basis of Hand Surgery*, 3rd ed. Philadelphia: JB Lippincott; 1979.

27. Brand PW, Hollister AM, Agee JM. Transmission. In: Brand PW, Hollister AM, eds. *Clinical Mechanics of the Hand*. St Louis: Mosby Inc; 1999:61–99.

28. Holtzhausen L-M, Noakes TD. Elbow, forearm, wrist, and hand injuries among sport rock climbers. *Clin J Sports Med* 1996;6:196–203.

29. Linburg RM, Conmstock BE. Anomalous tendon slips from the pollicis longus to the flexor digitorum profundus. *J Hand Surg* 1979;4:79–83.

30. Rennie WRJ, Muller H. Linburg syndrome. *Can J Surg* 1998;41:306–308.

31. Brand PW. *Clinical Mechanics of the Hand*. St. Louis: CV Mosby; 1985.

32. Ketchum LD, Thompson DE. An experimental investigation into the forces internal to the human hand. In: Brand PW, ed. *Clinical Mechanics of the Hand*. St. Louis: CV Mosby; 1985.

33. Hollinshead WH. *Anatomy for Surgeons*, 2nd ed. Vol. 3. New York: Harper & Row; 1969.

34. Bowers WH, Tribuzi SM. Functional anatomy. In: Stanley BG, Tribuzi SM, eds. *Concepts in Hand Rehabilitation*. Philadelphia: FA Davis; 1992:3–34.

35. Freedman DM, Botte MJ, Gelberman RH. Vascularity of the carpus. *Clin Orthop* 2001;383:47–59.

36. Brumfield RH, Champoux JA. A biomechanical study of normal functional wrist motion. *Clin Orthop* 1984;187:23–25.

37. Palmer AK, et al. Functional wrist motion: A biomechanical study. *J Hand Surg* 1985;10A:39–46.

38. Nelson DL. Functional wrist motion. *Hand Clin* 1997;13:83–92.

39. Carpener N. The hand in surgery. *J Bone Joint Surg* 1956; 38B:128.

40. Kapandji AI. *Physiologie articulaire*. Vol. 1. Paris: Librairie Maloine; 1963.

41. Bonnel F, Allieu Y. Les articulations radio cubito carpienne et medio carpienne: organisation anatomique et bases biomechaniques. *Ann Chir Main* 1984;3:287–296.

42. Palmer AK. The distal radioulnar joint. *Hand Clin* 1987;3:31.

43. Fick R. Allgemeine Gelenk- und Muskelmechanik. In: von Bardeleben K, ed. *Handb. Anat. d. Menschen*. Jena: Verlag von Gustav Fischer; 1910.

44. De Lange A, Kauer JM, Huiskes R. Kinematic behaviour of the human wrist joint: a rontgenstereophotogrammetric analysis. *J Orthop Res* 1985;3:56–64.

45. Gilford WW, Bolton RH, Lambrinudi C. The mechanism of the wrist joint with special reference to fractures of the scaphoid. *Guy's Hosp Rep* 1943;92:52–59.

46. Linscheid RL, Dobyns JH, Beabout J. Traumatic instability of the wrist: Diagnosis, classification and pathomechanics. *J Bone Joint Surg* 1972;54A:1612–1632.

47. Navarro A. Anatomia y fisiologie del carpo. *Ann Inst Clin Quir Chir Exp* 1937;1:162–250.

48. Landsmeer JMF. Les coherences spatiales et l'equilibre spatial dans la region carpienne. *Acta Anat* 1968;70(Suppl 54):1–84.

49. Landsmeer JMF. *Atlas of Anatomy of the Hand*. Edinburgh: Churchill Livingstone; 1976.

50. Kauer JMG. Een analyse van de carpale flexie. Leiden: Med Diss, 10.6; 1964.

51. Taleisnik J. The ligaments of the wrist. *J Hand Surg Am* 1976;2:110–118.

52. Kauer JMG. The mechanism of the carpal joint. *Clin Orthop* 1986;202:16–26.

53. Bunnell S. Boyes JH. Bunnell's *Surgery of the Hand*. Philadelphia: JB Lippincott; 1956.

54. Kapandji IA. *The Physiology of the Joints, Upper Limb*. New York: Churchill Livingstone; 1991.

55. Kuhlmann JN, et al. Stability of the normal wrist. In: Tubiana R, ed. *The Hand*. Philadelphia: WB Saunders; 1985:934–944.

56. Hazelton FT, et al. The influence of wrist position on the force produced by the finger flexors. *J Biomech* 1975;8:301–306.

57. Stokes HM. The seriously uninjured hand—weakness of grip. *J Occup Med* 1983;25:683–684.

58. Landsmeer JMF. The anatomy of the dorsal aponeurosis of the human finger and its functional significance. *Anat Rec* 1949; 104:31–45.

59. Bendz P. Systematization of the grip of the hand in relation to finger motion systems. *Scand J Rehabil Med* 1974;6:158–165.

60. Magee DJ. *Orthopedic Physical Assessment*, 2nd ed. Philadelphia: WB Saunders; 1992.

61. Long C, Conrad DW, Hall EA. Intrinsic-extrinsic muscle control of the hand in power grip and precision handling. *J Bone Joint Surg* 1970;52A:853–867.

62. Griffiths HE. Treatment of the injured worker. *Lancet* 1943;1:729–731.

63. Tylor C, Schwartz R. The anatomy and mechanics of the human hand. *Artificial Limbs* 1955;2:49–62.

64. Napler JR. The prehensile movements of the human hand. *J Bone Joint Surg* 1956;38B:902–913.

65. Landsmeer JMF. Power grip and precision handling. *Ann Rheum Dis* 1962;21:164–170.

66. Sollerman C, Sperling L. Evaluation of activities of daily living function—especially hand function. *Scand J Rehabil Med* 1978;10:139–145.

67. Armstrong TJ. Ergonomics and cumulative trauma disorders. *Hand Clin* 1986;2:553–565.

68. Kiser DM. Physiological and biomechanical factors for understanding repetitive motion injuries. *Semin Occup Med* 1987;2:11–17.

69. Butler DS. *Mobilization of the Nervous System*. New York: Churchill Livingstone; 1992.

70. Keller K, Corbett J, Nichols D. Repetitive strain injury in computer keyboard users: pathomechanics and treatment principles in individual and group intervention. *J Hand Ther* 1998;11:9–26.

71. Weber ER, Chao EY. An experimental approach to the mechanism of scaphoid waist fractures. *J Hand Surg* 1978;3:142–153.

72. Muckart RD. Stenosing tendovaginitis of abductor pollicis brevis at the radial styloid (de Quervain's disease). *Clin Orthop* 1964;33:201–208.

73. Skirven T. Clinical examination of the wrist. *J Hand Ther* 1996;9:96–107.

74. Nalebuff EA. The rheumatoid swan-neck deformity. *Hand Clin* 1989;5:214–215.

75. Judge RD, Zuidema GD, Fitzgerald FT. General appearance. In: Judge RD, Zuidema GD, Fitzgerald FT, eds. *Clinical Diagnosis*. Boston: Little, Brown and Co; 1982:29–47.

76. Nicholson B. Clinical evaluation. In: Stanley BG, Tribuzi SM, eds. *Concepts in Hand Rehabilitation*. Philadelphia: FA Davis; 1992:59–91.

77. Hoppenfeld S. *Physical Examination of the Spine and Extremities*. East Norwalk, CT: Appleton-Century-Crofts; 1976.

78. Blair SJ, et al. Evaluation of impairment of the upper extremity. *Clin Orthop* 1987;221:42–58.

79. Whipple TL. Preoperative evaluation and imaging. In: Whipple TL, ed. *Arthroscopic Surgery: The Wrist*. Philadelphia: JB Lippincott; 1992:11–36.

80. Osterman AL, Mikulics M. Scaphoid nonunion. *Hand Clin* 1988;14:437–455.

81. Watson HK, Ashmead D, Makhlouf MV. Examination of the scaphoid. *J Hand Surg* 1988;13A:657–660.

82. Alexander AH, Lichtman DM. Kienbock's disease. In: Lichtman DM, ed. *The Wrist and its Disorders*. Philadelphia: WB Saunders; 1988.

83. Kienböck R. Concerning traumatic malacia of the lunate and its consequences: degeneration and compression fractures. *Clin Orthop* 1980;149:4–5.

84. Polivy KD, et al. Fractures of the hook of the hamate—a failure of clinical diagnosis. *J Hand Surg* 1985;10A:101–104.

85. Rao SB, Culver JE. Triquetralhamate arthrodesis for midcarpal instability. *J Hand Surg* 1995;20A:583–589.

86. Swanson A. Disabling arthritis at the base of the thumb: treatment by resection of the trapezium and flexible implant arthroplasty. *J Bone Joint Surg* 1972;54A:456.

87. Beckenbaugh RD. Accurate evaluation and management of the painful wrist following injury. *Orthop Clin* 1984;15:289–306.

88. Wolfe SW, Gupta A, Crisco JJ III. Kinematics of the scaphoid shift test. *J Hand Surg* 1997;22A: 801–806.

89. Taleisnik J. Scapholunate dissociation. In: Taleisnik J, ed. *The Wrist*. New York: Churchill Livingstone; 1985:239–278.

90. LaStayo P, Howell J. Clinical provocative tests used in evaluating wrist pain: a descriptive study. *J Hand Surg* 1995;8:10–17.

91. Easterling KJ, Wolfe SW. Scaphoid shift in the uninjured wrist. *J Hand Surg* 1994;19A:604–606.

92. Mathiowetz V, et al. Reliability and validity of grip and pinch strength evaluations. *J Hand Surg* 1984;9A:222–226.

93. Bechtol CO. Grip test: the use of a dynamometer with adjustable hand spacings. *J Bone Joint Surg* 1954;36A:820–824.

94. Tredgett MW, Pimble LJ, Davis TRC. The detection of feigned hand weakness using the five position grip strength test. *J Hand Surg* 1999;24B:426–428.

95. Tredgett MW, Davis TRC. Rapid repeat testing of grip strength for detection of faked hand weakness. *J Hand Surg* 2000; 25B:372–375.

96. Niebuhr BR, Marion R. Voluntary control of submaximal grip strength. *Am J Phys Med Rehabil* 1990;69:96–101.

97. Lister G. *The Hand: Diagnosis and Indications*, 2nd ed. New York: Churchill Livingstone; 1984.

98. Joughin K, et al. An evaluation of rapid exchange and simultaneous grip tests. *J Hand Surg* 1993;18A:245–252.

99. Hildreth DH, et al. Detection of submaximal effort by use of the rapid exchange grip. *J Hand Surg* 1989;14A:742–745.

100. Stokes HM, et al. Identification of low effort patients through dynamometry. *J Hand Surg* 1995;20A:1047–1056.

101. Norkin C, Levangie P. *Joint Structure and Function: A Comprehensive Analysis*. Philadelphia: FA Davis; 1992:355–358.

102. Eberhardt K, Malcus Johnson P, Rydgren L. The occurrence and significance of hand deformities in early rheumatoid arthritis. *Br J Rheum* 1991;30:211–213.

103. Fess EE. The need for reliability and validity in hand assessment instruments. *J Hand Surg* 1986;11A:621–623 (editorial).

104. Jebsen RH, et al. An objective and standardized test for hand function. *Arch Phys Med Rehab* 1969;50:311.

105. Beckenbaugh RD, et al. Kienböck's disease: The natural history of Kienböck's disease and consideration of lunate fractures. *Clin Orthop* 1980;149:98–106.

106. *Purdue Pegboard Test of Manipulative Dexterity*. Chicago: Service Research Associates; 1968.

107. Tiffin J, Asker E. The Purdue pegboard: Norms and studies of reliability and validity. *J Appl Psychol* 1948;32:324.

108. Crawford J. Crawford small parts dexterity test (CSPDT). In: Psychological Corp. (catalog): Tests, products and services for business, industry, and government. Cleveland: Harcourt Brace Jovanovich; 1985:32.

109. Reagan DS, Linscheid RL, Dobyns JH. Lunotriquetral sprains. *J Hand Surg* 1984;9A:502–514.

110. Onieal M-E. The hand: Examination and diagnosis. In: *American Society for Surgery of the Hand*. New York: Churchill Livingstone; 1990.

111. Werner CO, Elmqvist D, Ohlin P. Pressure and nerve lesion in the carpal tunnel. *Acta Orthop Scand* 1983;54:312–316.

112. Stewart JD, Eisen A. Tinel's sign and the carpal tunnel syndrome. *BMJ* 1978;2:1125–1126.

113. Gellman H, et al. Carpal tunnel syndrome. An evaluation of the provocative diagnostic tests. *J Bone Joint Surg* 1986; 68A:735–737.

114. Marx RG, et al. The reliability of physical examination for carpal tunnel syndrome. *J Hand Surg* 1998;23B:499–502.

115. Golding DN, Rose DM, Selvarajah K. Clinical tests for carpal tunnel syndrome: an evaluation. *Br J Rheum* 1986;25:388–390.

116. Heller L, et al. Evaluation of Tinel's and Phalen's signs in diagnosis of the carpal tunnel syndrome. *Eur Neurol* 1986;25:40–42.

117. Mackinnon SE, Dellon AL. Sensory rehabilitation after nerve injury. In: Mackinnon SE, Dellon AL, eds. *Surgery of the Peripheral Nerve*. New York: Thieme Medical Publishers; 1988:521.

118. Anthony MS. Wounds. In: Clark GL, et al, eds. *Hand Rehabilitation: A Practical Guide*. Philadelphia: Churchill Livingstone; 1998:1–15.

119. Fess EE. Documentation: essential elements of an upper extremity assessment battery. In: Hunter JM, Mackin EJ, Callahan AD, eds. *Rehabilitation of the Hand: Surgery and Therapy*. St. Louis: Mosby; 1995:185.

120. Tan AM. Sensibility testing. In: Stanley BG, Tribuzi SM, eds. *Concepts in Hand Rehabilitation*. Philadelphia: FA Davis; 1992:92–112.

121. Gelberman RH, et al. Sensibility testing in peripheral nerve compression syndromes. An experimental study in humans. *J Bone Joint Surg* 1983;65A:632–638.

122. von Frey M, Kiesow F. Uber die Function der Tastkorperchen Yeit. *Ztschr Psychol Physiol Sinnesorg* 1899;20:126–163.

123. Semmes J, et al. Somatosensory changes after penetrating brain wounds in man. Cambridge, MA: Harvard University Press; 1960.

124. Callahan AD. Sensibility testing. In: Hunter J, et al, eds. *Rehabilitation of the Hand: Surgery and Therapy*. St Louis: CV Mosby; 1990:605.

125. Omer GE. Report of committee for evaluation of the clinical result in peripheral nerve injury. *J Hand Surg* 1983;8:754–759.

126. Phalen GS. The carpal tunnel syndrome: Clinical evaluation of 598 hands. *Clin Orthop* 1972;83:29–40.

127. Phalen GS. Spontaneous compression of the median nerve at the wrist. *JAMA* 1951;145:1128–1133.

128. Onieal ME. *Essentials of Musculoskeletal Care*, 1st ed. Rosemont, IL: American Academy of Orthopaedic Surgeons; 1997.

129. Robert AW, Cynthia B, Thomas JA. Reverse Phalen's maneuver as an aid in diagnosing carpal tunnel syndrome. *Arch Phys Med Rehab* 1994;75:783–786.

130. Brain WR, Wright AD, Wilkinson M. Spontaneous compression of both median nerves in the carpal tunnel: six cases treated surgically. *Lancet* 1947;1:277–282.

131. Duck-Sun A. Hand elevation: A new test for carpal tunnel syndrome. *Ann Plast Surg* 2001;46:120–124.

132. Moberg E. Objective methods for determining the functional value of sensibility in the hand. *J Bone Joint Surg* 1958;40A:454–476.

133. Sunderland S. *Nerves and Nerve Injuries*. Edinburgh: E & S Livingstone, Ltd; 1968.

134. Finkelstein H. Stenosing tenovaginitis at the radial styloid process. *J Bone Joint Surg* 1930;12A:509.

135. Elson RA. Rupture of the central slip of the extensor hood of the finger: a test for early diagnosis. *J Bone Joint Surg Br* 1986;68:229–231.

136. Preston D, Shapiro B. *Electromyography and Neuromuscular Disorders. Clinical Electrophysiologic Correlations*. Boston: Butterworth-Heinemann; 1998.

137. Booher JM, Thibodeau GA. *Athletic Injury Assessment*. St. Louis: CV Mosby; 1989.

138. Booth FW. Physiologic and biochemical effects of immobilization on muscle. *Clin Orthop* 1987;219:15–21.

139. Eiff MP, Smith AT, Smith GE. Early mobilization versus immobilization in the treatment of lateral ankle sprains. *Am J Sports Med* 1994;22:83–88.

140. Akeson WH, et al. Collagen cross-linking alterations in the joint contractures: changes in the reducible cross-links in periarticular connective tissue after 9 weeks immobilization. *Conn Tissue Res* 1977;5:15.

141. Akeson WH, et al. Effects of immobilization on joints. *Clin Orthop* 1987;219:28–37.

142. Akeson WH, Amiel D, Woo SL-Y. Immobility effects on synovial joints: The pathomechanics of joint contracture. *Biorheology* 1980;17:95–110.

143. Woo SL-Y, et al. Connective tissue response to immobility: A correlative study of biochemical and biomechanical measurements

of normal and immobilized rabbit knee. *Arthritis Rheum* 1975;18:257–264.

144. Walsh M, Muntzer E. Wound management. In: Stanley BG, Tribuzi SM, eds. *Concepts in Hand Rehabilitation*. Philadelphia: FA Davis; 1992:153–177.

145. Stanley BG. Therapeutic exercise: Maintaining and restoring mobility in the hand. In: Stanley BG, Tribuzi SM, eds. *Concepts in Hand Rehabilitation*. Philadelphia: FA Davis; 1992:178–215.

146. Fess EE, Phillips CA. *Hand Splinting: Principles and Methods*, 2nd ed. St. Louis: CV Mosby; 1987.

147. Malick MH. *Manual on Static Hand Splinting*. Pittsburgh: Harmarville Rehabilitation Center; 1972.

148. Lohman H, Schultz-Johnson K, Coppard BM. *Introduction to Splinting: A Clinical-Reasoning & Problem-Solving Approach*. St. Louis: Mosby; 2001.

149. Cannon NM. *Manual of Hand Splinting*. New York: Churchill Livingstone; 1985.

150. Gribben MG. Splinting principles for hand injuries. In: Moran CA, ed. *Hand Rehabilitation: Clinics in Physical Therapy*. New York: Churchill Livingstone; 1986:166.

151. Schultz-Johnson K. Splinting—A problem-solving approach. In: Stanley BG, Tribuzi SM, eds. *Concepts in Hand Rehabilitation*. Philadelphia: FA Davis; 1992:238–271.

152. Stanley JK. Soft tissue surgery in rheumatoid arthritis of the hand. *Clin Orthop* 1999;366:78–90.

153. Brewerton DA. The rheumatoid hand. *Proc R Soc Med* 1966; 59:225–228.

154. Wynn-Parry CB, Stanley JK. Synovectomy of the hand. *Br J Rheumatol* 1993;32:1089–1095.

155. Flatt AE. Some pathomechanics of ulnar drift. *Plast Reconstr Surg*. 1966;37:295–303.

156. Shapiro JS. The etiology of ulnar drift: A new factor. *J Bone Joint Surg* 1968;50A:634.

157. Ferlic DC. Boutonniere deformities in rheumatoid arthritis. *Hand Clin* 1989;5:215–222.

158. Kiefhaber TR, Strickland JW. Soft tissue reconstruction for rheumatoid swan-neck and boutonniere deformities: Long-term results. *J Hand Surg Am* 1993;18A:984–989.

159. Hastings DE, Evans JA. Rheumatoid wrist deformities and their relation to ulnar drift. *J Bone Joint Surg* 1975;57A:930–934.

160. Pahle J. Die Synovektomie der Proximalen Interphalangealgelenke. *Orthopaede* 1973;2:13–17.

161. Pahle JA, Raunio P. The influence of wrist position on finger deviation in the rheumatoid hand. *J Bone Joint Surg* 1969;51B:664.

162. Stack GH, Vaughan-Jackson OJ. The zig-zag deformity in the rheumatoid hand. *Hand* 1971;3:6267.

163. Marx H. Rheumatoid arthritis. In: Stanley BG, Tribuzi SM, eds. *Concepts in Hand Rehabilitation*. Philadelphia: FA Davis; 1992:395–418.

164. van Vugt RM, Bijlsma JWJ, van Vugt AC. Chronic wrist pain: diagnosis and management. Development and use of a new algorithm. *Ann Rheum Dis* 1999;58:665–674.

165. Taleisnik J. Pain on the ulnar side of the wrist. *Hand Clin* 1987;3:51–68.

166. Watson HK, Brenner LH. Degenerative disorders of the wrist. *J Hand Surg Am* 1985;10A:1002–1006.

167. McFarlane RM, Albion U. Dupuytren's disease. In: Hunter JM, et al, eds. *Rehabilitation of the Hand*. St. Louis: CV Mosby; 1990:867.

168. Sladicka MS, et al. Dupuytren's contracture in the black population: A case report and review of the literature. *J Hand Surg Br* 1996;21:898.

169. Urban M, et al. Dupuytren's disease in children. *J Hand Surg Br* 1996;21:112.

170. Ross DC. Epidemiology of Dupuytren's disease. *Hand Clin* 1999;15:53.

171. Saar JD, Grothaus PC. Dupuytren's disease: An overview. *Plast Reconstructive Surg* 2000;106:125–136.

172. Noble J, et al. The association between alcohol, hepatic pathology and Dupuytren's disease. *J Hand Surg Br* 1992;17:71.

173. Yi IS, Johnson G, Moneim MS. Etiology of Dupuytren's disease. *Hand Clin* 1999;1543–1551.

174. Lanzetta M, Morrison WA. Dupuytren's disease occurring after a surgical injury to the hand. *J Hand Surg Br* 1996;21:481.

175. Hill NA, Hurst LC. Dupuytren's contracture. In: Doyle JR, ed. *Landmark Advances in Hand Surgery*. Philadelphia: WB Saunders; 1989:349.

176. Luck JV. Dupuytren's contracture: A new concept of the pathogenesis correlated with surgical management. *J Bone Joint Surg Am* 1959;41:635.

177. Rayan GM. Clinical presentation and types of Dupuytren's disease. *Hand Clin* 1999;15:87.

178. Strickland JW, Leibovic SJ. Anatomy and pathogenesis of the digital cords and nodules. *Hand Clin* 1991;7:645.

179. Tomasek JJ, Vaughan MB, Haaksma CJ. Cellular structure and biology of Dupuytren's disease. *Hand Clin* 1999;15:21.

180. Hurst LC, Badalamente MA. Nonoperative treatment of Dupuytren's disease. *Hand Clin* 1999;15:97.

181. Eckhaus D. Dupuytren's disease. In: Clark GL, et al, eds. *Hand Rehabilitation*. Edinburgh: Churchill Livingstone; 1993:37–42.

182. Gosset J. Dupuytren's disease and the anatomy of the palmodigital aponeuroses. In: Hueston JT, Tubiana R, eds. *Dupuytren's Disease*. Edinburgh: Churchill Livingstone; 1985.

183. Onieal M-E. Common wrist and ankle injuries. *ADVANCE for Nurse Practitioners* 1996;4:31–36.

184. Chin HW, Visotsky J. Wrist fractures in the hand in emergency medicine. *Emerg Med Clin North Am* 1993;11:703–735.

185. Takase K, Imakiire A. Lunate excision, capitate osteotomy, and intercarpal arthrodesis for advanced Kienbock disease. Long-term follow-up. *J Bone Joint Surg* 2001;83-A:177–183.

186. Ambrose L, Posner MA. Lunate-triquetral and midcarpal joint instability. *Hand Clin* 1992;8:653–668.

187. Husband JB, McPherson SA. Bony skier's thumb injuries. *Clin Orthop* 1996;327:79–84.

188. Rettig AC. Current concepts in management of football injuries of the hand and wrist. *J Hand Ther* 1991;4:42–50.

189. Stener B. Displacement of the ruptured ulnar collateral ligament of the metacarpophalangeal joint of the thumb. *J Bone Joint Surg* 1962;44B:869–879.

190. Friedman SL, Palmer AK. The ulnar impaction syndrome. *Hand Clin* 1991;7:295–310.

191. Kasdan ML, Millender LH. Occupational soft-tissue and tendon disorders. *Orthop Clin North Am* 1996;27:795–803.

192. Thorson E, Szabo RM. Common tendinitis problems in the hand and forearm. *Orthop Clin North Am* 1992;23:65–74.

193. de Quervain F. Uber eine Form von chronischer Tendovaginitis. *Cor-Bl f schweiz Aertze* 1895;25:389–394.

194. Lapidus PW, Fenton R. Stenosing tenovaginitis at the wrist and fingers: report of 423 cases in 269 patients. *Arch Surg* 1952;64:475–487.

195. Patterson DC. DeQuervain's disease: stenosing tendovaginitis at the radial styloid. *N Engl J Med* 1936;214:101–102.

196. Cotton FJ, Morrison GM, Bradford CH. DeQuervain's disease: radial styloid tendovaginitis. *N Engl J Med* 1938;219:120–123.

197. Diack AW, Trommald JP. DeQuervain's disease: a frequently missed diagnosis. *West J Surg* 1939;47:629–633.

198. Wood CF. Stenosing tendovaginitis at the radial styloid. *South Surgeon* 1941;10:105–110.

199. Lamphier TA, Crooker C, Crooker JL. DeQuervain's disease. *Ind Med Surg* 1965;34:847–856.

200. Lamb DW, Hooper G, Kuczynski K. *Practice of Hand Surgery.* London: Blackwell Scientific Publications Ltd; 1989.

201. Reid DAC, McGrouther DA. *Surgery of the Thumb.* London: Butterworth & Co. Ltd; 1986.

202. Arons MS. De Quervain's release in working women: report of failures, complications, and associated diagnoses. *J Hand Surg Am* 1987;12:540–544.

203. Piligian G, et al. Evaluation and management of chronic work-related musculoskeletal disorders of the distal upper extremity. *Am J Ind Med* 2000;37:75–93.

204. Harrington JM, et al. Surveillance case definitions for work related upper limb pain syndrome. *Occup Environ Med* 1998;55:264–271.

205. Anderson M, Tichenor CJ. A patient with de Quervain's tenosynovitis: A case report using an Australian approach to manual therapy. *Phys Ther* 1994;74:314–326.

206. Elliot BG. Finkelstein's test: a descriptive error that can produce a false positive. *J Hand Surg Am* 1992;17B:481–482.

207. Belsole J. De Quervain's tenosynovitis diagnostic and operative complications. *Orthopedics* 1981;12A:899.

208. Saplys R, Mackinnon SE, Dellon LA. The relationship between nerve entrapment versus neuroma complications and the misdiagnosis of de Quervain's disease. *Contemp Orthop* 1987;15:51.

209. Williams JG. Surgical management of traumatic noninfective tenosynovitis of the wrist extensors. *J Bone Joint Surg* 1977;59B:408.

210. Louis DS. Incomplete release of the first dorsal compartment—a diagnostic test. *J Hand Surg* 1987;12A:87.

211. Grundberg AB, Reagan DS. Pathologic anatomy of the forearm: intersection syndrome. *J Hand Surg* 1985;10A:299.

212. Hunter SC, Poole RM. The chronically inflamed tendon. *Clin Sports Med* 1987;6:371.

213. Mogensen BA, Mattson HS. Stenosing tenovaginitis of the third compartment of the hand. *Scand J Plast Reconstr Surg* 1980;14:127.

214. Spinner M, Olshansky K. The extensor indicis proprius syndrome. *Plast Reconstr Surg* 1973;51:134.

215. Hajj AA, Wood MB. Stenosing tenosynovitis of the extensor carpi ulnaris. *J Hand Surg* 1986;11A:519.

216. Hueston JT, Wilson WF. The aetiology of trigger finger. *Hand* 1972;4:257.

217. Kolin-Sorensen V. Treatment of trigger fingers. *Acta Orthop Scand* 1970;41:428.

218. Lipscomb PR. Tenosynovitis of the hand and wrist: Carpal tunnel syndrome, de Quervain's disease, trigger digit. *Ann Surg* 1951;134:110.

219. Pulvertaft RG. *Clinical Surgery of the Hand.* London: Butterworths; 1966.

220. Kolind-Sorensen V. Treatment of trigger fingers. *Acta Orthop Scand* 1970;41:428–432.

221. Evans BE, Hunter JM, Burkhalter WE. Conservative management of the trigger finger: a new approach. *J Hand Ther* 1988;1:59–68.

222. Newport ML, Lane LB, Stuchin SA. Treatment of the trigger finger by steroid injection. *J Hand Surg* 1990;15A:748.

223. Lubahn JD, Hood JM. Fractures of the distal interphalangeal joint. *Clin Orthop* 1996;327:12–20.

224. Weinstein SM. Nerve problems and compartment syndromes in the hand. *Clin Sports Med* 1992;11:161–188.

225. Carr D, Davis P. Distal posterior interosseous nerve syndrome. *J Hand Surg Am* 1985;106 (Pt 1):873–878.

226. Rask MR. Superficial radial neuritis and de Quervain's disease. *Clin Orthop* 1979;131:176–178.

227. MacKinnon EJ, Dellon AL. *Surgery of the Peripheral Nerve.* New York: Thieme Medical Publishers; 1988.

228. Moersch FP. Median thenar neuritis. *Proc Surg Meetings Mayo Clin* 1938;13:220–222.

229. Slater RR Jr, Bynum DK. Diagnosis and treatment of carpal tunnel syndrome. *Orthop Rev* 1993;22:1095–1105.

230. Stevens JC, et al. Carpal tunnel syndrome in Rochester, Minnesota, 1961 to 1980. *Neurology* 1988;38:134–138.

231. Gates SJ, Mooar PA. *Orthopaedics and Sports Medicine for Nurses: Common Problems in Management.* Baltimore: Williams & Wilkins; 1999.

232. Ogilvie C, Kay NRM. Fulminating carpal tunnel syndrome due to gout. *J Hand Surg* 1988;13:42–43.

233. Rosenbaum R. Disputed radial tunnel syndrome. *Muscle Nerve* 1999;22:960–967.

234. Center for Disease Control. Occupational diseases surveillance: carpal tunnel syndrome. *JAMA* 1989;77:889.

235. Rempel DM, Harrison RJ, Barnhart S. Work-related cumulative trauma disorders of the upper extremity. *JAMA* 1992;267:838–842.

236. Rowe L. The diagnosis of tendon and tendon sheath injuries. *Semin Occup Med* 1987;1:1–6.

237. Robbins H. Anatomical study of the median nerve in the carpal canal and etiologies of the carpal tunnel syndrome. *J Bone Joint Surg* 1963;45:953–956.

238. Bauman TD, et al. The acute carpal tunnel syndrome. *Clin Orthop* 1981;156:151–156.

239. Paley D, McMurtry RY. Median nerve compression by volarly displaced fragments of the distal radius. *Clin Orthop* 1987;215:139–147.

240. Gelberman R, et al. Tissue pressure threshold for peripheral nerve viability. *Clin Orthop* 1983;178:285–291.

241. Flynn JM, Bischoff R, Gelberman RH. Median nerve compression at the wrist due to intracarpal canal sepsis. *J Hand Surg* 1995;20A:864–867.

242. Gerardi JA, Mack GR, Lutz RB. Acute carpal tunnel syndrome secondary to septic arthritis of the wrist. *JAOA* 1989;89:933–934.

243. Barnes CG, Curry HLE. Carpal tunnel syndrome in rheumatoid arthritis: A clinical and electrodiagnostic survey. *Ann Rheum Dis* 1970;26:226–233.

244. Stanley JK. Conservative surgery in the management of rheumatoid disease of the hand and wrist. *J Hand Surg Am* 1992;17B:339–342.

245. Vainio K. Carpal canal syndrome caused by tenosynovitis. *Acta Rheumatoid Scand* 1957;4:22–27.

246. Gelberman RH. Carpal tunnel syndrome. In: Gelberman RH, ed. *Operative Nerve Repair.* Philadelphia: JB Lippincott; 1991:939–948.

247. Von Schroeder HP, Botte MJ. Carpal tunnel syndrome. *Hand Clin* 1996;12:643–655.

248. Cobb TK, et al. Lumbrical muscle incursion into the carpal tunnel during finger flexion. *J Hand Surg* 1994;19B:434–438.

249. Yii NW, Elliot D. A study of the dynamic relationship of the lumbrical muscles and the carpal tunnel. *J Hand Surg* 1994;19B:439–443.

250. Robinson D, Aghasi M, Halperin N. The treatment of carpal tunnel syndrome caused by hypertrophied lumbrical muscles. *Scand J Plast Reconstr Surg* 1989;23:149–151.

251. DeKrom MC, et al. Carpal tunnel syndrome: prevalence in the general population. *J Clin Epidemiol* 1992;45:373–376.

252. Stevens JC, et al. Carpal tunnel syndrome in Rochester, Minnesota, 1961–1980. *Neurology* 1988;38:134–138.

253. Szabo RM, Chidgey LK. Stress carpal tunnel pressures in patients with carpal tunnel syndrome and normal patients. *J Hand Surg* 1989;14A:624–627.

254. Keir PJ, Bach JM, Rempel DM. Effects of finger posture on carpal tunnel pressure during wrist motion. *J Hand Surg* 1998;23A:1004–1009.

255. Rempel D, et al. Effects of static fingertip loading on carpal tunnel pressure. *J Orthop Res* 1997;15:422–426.

256. Katz JN, et al. The carpal tunnel syndrome: diagnostic utility of the history and physical examination findings. *Ann Intern Med* 1990;112:321–327.

257. D'Arcy CA, McGee S. Does this patient have carpal tunnel syndrome? *JAMA* 2000;283:3110–3117.

258. Feuerstein M, et al. Clinical management of carpal tunnel syndrome: a 12 year review of outcomes. *Am J Ind Med* 1999;35:232–245.

259. Szabo RM. Carpal tunnel syndrome—general. In: Gelberman RH, ed. *Operative Nerve Repair and Reconstruction*. Philadelphia: JB Lippincott; 1991:882–883.

260. Bowles AP Jr, Asher SW, Pickett JB. Use of Tinel's sign in carpal tunnel syndrome [letter]. *Ann Neurol* 1983;13:689–690.

261. Hartz CR, et al. The pronator teres syndrome: compressive neuropathy of the median nerve. *J Bone Joint Surg* 1981; 63:885–890.

262. Anto C, Aradhya P. Clinical diagnosis of peripheral nerve compression in the upper extremities. *Orthop Clin North Am* 1996;27:227–245.

263. Cambell WW. Diagnosis and management of common compression and entrapment neuropathies. *Neurol Clin* 1997; 15:549–567.

264. Loong SC. The carpal tunnel syndrome: a clinical and electrophysiological study of 250 patients. *Proc Aust Assoc Neurol* 1977;14:51–65.

265. Kenneally M, Rubenach H, Elvey R. The upper limb tension test: the SLR of the arm. In: Grant R, ed. *Physical Therapy of the Cervical and Thoracic Spine*. Churchill Livingstone: New York; 1988.

266. Kleinrensink GJ, et al. Mechanical tension in the median nerve. The effects of joint positions. *Clin Biomech* 1995;10:240–244.

267. Manente G, et al. A relief maneuver in carpal tunnel syndrome. *Muscle Nerve* 1999;22:1587–1589.

268. Buch-Jaeger N, Foucher G. Correlation of clinical signs with nerve conduction tests in the diagnosis of carpal tunnel syndrome. *J Hand Surg Br* 1994;19:720–724.

269. Chang MH, et al. Oral drug of choice in carpal tunnel syndrome. *Neurology* 1998;51:390–393.

270. Roaf R. Compression of median nerve in carpal tunnel [letter to the editor]. *Lancet* 1947;1:387.

271. Sailer SM. The role of splinting and rehabilitation in the treatment of carpal and cubital tunnel syndromes. *Hand Clin* 1996;12:223–241.

272. Burke DT, et al. Splinting for carpal tunnel syndrome: In search of the optimal angle. *Arch Phys Med Rehab* 1994;75:1241–1244.

273. Kruger VL, et al. Carpal tunnel syndrome: Objective measures and splint use. *Arch Phys Med Rehab* 1991;72:517–520.

274. Dolhanty D. Effectiveness of splinting for carpal tunnel syndrome. *Can J Occup Ther* 1986;53:275–280.

275. Rempel D, et al. The effect of wearing a flexible wrist splint on carpal tunnel pressure during repetitive hand activity. *J Hand Surg* 1994;19:106–110.

276. Callinan NJ, Mathiowetz V. Soft versus hard resting hand splints in rheumatoid arthritis: pain relief, preference and compliance. *Am J Occup Ther* 1995;50:347–353.

277. Luchetti R, et al. Serial overnight recordings of intracarpal canal pressure in carpal tunnel syndrome patients with and without wrist splinting. *J Hand Surg* 1994;19:35–37.

278. Garfinkel MS, et al. Yoga-based intervention for carpal tunnel syndrome: a randomized trial. *JAMA* 1998;280:1601–1603.

279. Chusid JG. *Correlative Neuroanatomy & Functional Neurology*. Norwalk, CT: Appleton-Century-Crofts; 1985:144–148.

280. Chidgey LK. Chronic wrist pain. *Orthop Clin North Am* 1992;23:49–64.

281. Pelmear P, Wills M. Impact vibration and hand-arm vibration syndrome. *J Occup Environmental Med* 1997;39:1092–1096.

282. Miller RF, et al. An epidemiologic study of carpal tunnel syndrome and hard-arm vibration in relation to vibration syndrome. *J Hand Surg* 1994;19A:99–105.

283. Pelmear P. Vibration-related occupational injuries. In: Herrington TN, Morse LH, eds. *Occupational Injuries—Evaluation, Management, Prevention*. St. Louis: Mosby; 1995:411–421.

284. Khilberg S. Acute effects and symptoms of work with vibrating hand-held powered tools exposing the operator to impact and reaction forces [Thesis]. *Arbete och Hälsa* 1995;10:1–50.

285. Smolders JJ. Myofascial pain and dysfunction syndromes. In: Hammer WI, ed. *Functional Soft Tissue Examination and Treatment by Manual Methods—The Extremities*. Gaithersburg, MD: Aspen; 1991:215–234.

286. Subarrao J, Stillwell GK. Reflex sympathetic dystrophy syndrome of the upper extremity: analysis of total outcome of management of 125 cases. *Arch Phys Med Rehab* 1981;62:549–554.

287. Veldman PHJM, et al. Signs and symptoms of reflex sympathetic dystrophy: prospective study of 829 patients. *Lancet* 1993;342:1012–1016.

288. Metules TJ. When a simple fall turns into years of pain. *RN* 2000;63:65–66.

289. Bohm E. Das Sudecksche Syndrom. *Hefte zur Unfallheilkunde* 1985;174:241–250.

290. Omer GC, Thomas MS. Treatment of causalgia. *Tex Med* 1971;67:93–96.

291. Atkins RM, Duckworth T, Kanis JA. Features of algodystrophy after Colles' fracture. *J Bone Joint Surg* 1990;72:105–110.

292. Acquaviva P, et al. Les algodystrophies: terrain et facteurs pathogeniques. Resultats d'une enquete multicentrique portant sur 765 observations (Rapport). *Rev Rhum Mal Osteoartic* 1982;49:761–766.

293. Dunn D. Chronic regional pain syndrome, Type 1: Part I. *AORN J* 2000;72:421–424, 426, 428–432, 435, 437–442, 444–449, 452–458.

294. Maurer G. Umbau, Dystrophie und Atrophie an den Gliedmassen (Sogenannte Sudecksche Knochenatrophie). *Erg Chir* 1940;33:476–531.

295. Steinbrocker O. The shoulder-hand syndrome. Associated painful homolateral disability of the shoulder and hand with swelling and atrophy of the hand. *Am J Med* 1947;3:402–407.

296. Sudeck P. Ueber die acute entzundliche Knochenatrophie. *Arch Klin Chir* 1900;62:147–156.

297. Walker SM, Cousins MJ. Complex regional pain syndromes: Including "reflex sympathetic dystrophy" and "causalgia." *Anaesthesia Intensive Care* 1997;25:113–125.

298. Kingery WS. A critical review of controlled clinical trials for peripheral neuropathic pain and complex regional pain syndromes. *Pain* 1997;73:123–139.

299. Wilson PR. Post-traumatic upper extremity reflex sympathetic dystrophy: Clinical course, staging, and classification of clinical forms. *Hand Clinics* 1997;13:367–372.

300. Gordon N. Review article: Reflex sympathetic dystrophy. *Brain Development* 1996;18:257–262.

301. McLatchie GR. *Essentials of Sports Medicine*, 2nd ed. Edinburgh: Churchill Livingstone; 1993.

302. Wilson RL, Carter MS. Management of hand fractures. In: Hunter J, et al, eds. *Rehabilitation of the Hand*. St. Louis: CV Mosby; 1990:284.

303. Sorenson MK. Fractures of the wrist and hand. In: Moran CA, ed. *Hand Rehabilitation: Clinics in Physical Therapy*. New York: Churchill Livingstone; 1986:191–225.

304. King RJ. Scapholunate diastasis associated with a Barton fracture treated by manipulation or Terry-Thomas and the wine waiter. *J Royal Soc Med* 1983;76:421–423.

305. Ring D, Jupiter JB, Herndon JH. Acute fractures of the scaphoid. *J Am Acad Orthop Surg* 2000;8:225–231.

306. Perron AD, et al. Orthopedic pitfalls in the ED: scaphoid fracture. *Am J Emerg Med* 2001;19:310–316.

307. Chen SC. The scaphoid compression test. *J Hand Surg* 1989;14:323–325.

308. Waizenegger M, et al. Clinical signs in scaphoid fractures. *J Hand Surg* 1994;19B:743–747.

309. Onieal M-E. *Athletic Training and Sports Medicine*, 2nd ed. Park Ridge, IL: American Academy of Orthopaedic Surgeons; 1991.

310. Ritchie JV, Munter DW. Emergency department evaluation and treatment of wrist injuries. *Emerg Med Clin North Am* 1999;17:823–842.

311. Watson HK, Kao SD. Degenerative disorders of the carpus. In: Lichtman DM, Alexander AH, eds. *The Wrist and Its Disorders*. Philadelphia: WB Saunders; 1997:583–591.

312. Watson HK, Weinzweig J, Zeppieri J. The natural progression of scaphoid instability. *Hand Clin* 1997;13:39–49.

313. Joseph RB, et al. Chronic sprains of the carpometacarpal joints. *J Hand Surg* 1981;6:172–180.

314. Hove LM. Fractures of the hand. Distribution and relative incidence. *Scand J Plast Reconstr Surg Hand Surg* 1993;27:317–319.

315. Hritcko G. Finger fracture rehabilitation. In: Clark GL, et al, eds. *Hand Rehabilitation: A Practical Guide*. Philadelphia: Churchill Livingstone; 1998:319–327.

316. Sucher BM. Myofascial release of carpal tunnel syndrome. *JAOA* 1993;93:92–101.

317. Lee DG. *A Workbook of Manual Therapy Techniques for the Upper Extremity*, 2nd ed. Delta, BC: Delta Orthopedic Physiotherapy Clinic; 1991:58–79.

318. Mulligan BR. *Manual Therapy: "NAGS," "SNAGS," "PRP'S" etc*. Wellington: Plane View Series; 1992.

319. Kibler WB. Shoulder rehabilitation: principles and practice. *Med Sci Sports Exerc* 1998;30(4 Suppl 1):40–50.

320. Reid DC. *Sports Injury Assessment and Rehabilitation*. New York: Churchill Livingstone; 1992.

321. Kraushaar BS, Nirschl RP. Tendinosis of the elbow (tennis elbow). Clinical features and findings of histological, immunohistochemical, and electron microscopy studies. *J Bone Joint Surg Am* 1999;81:259–278.

322. Lillegard WA, Rucker KS. *Handbook of Sports Medicine: A Symptom-Oriented Approach*. Boston: Andover Medical Publishers; 1993.

323. Waylett-Rendall J. Use of therapeutic modalities in upper extremity rehabilitation. In: Hunter JM, Mackin EJ, Callahan AS, eds. *Rehabilitation of the Hand: Surgery and Therapy*. Mosby: St. Louis; 1995.

324. Kasch M. Therapists evaluation and treatment of upper extremity cumulative trauma disorders. In: Hunter JM, Mackin EJ, Callahan AD, eds. *Rehabilitation of the Hand: Surgery and Therapy*. Mosby: St. Louis; 1995.

325. Berry TJ. *The Hand as a Mirror of Systemic Disease*. Philadelphia: FA Davis; 1963:193–204.

326. Berry TJ. *The Hand as a Mirror of Systemic Disease*. Philadelphia: FA Davis; 1963:79–191.

327. Feldon P, Millender LH, Nalebuff EA. Rheumatoid arthritis in the hand and wrist. In: Green DP, ed. *Operative Hand Surgery*. New York: Churchill Livingstone; 1993:1587–1690.

328. Hunter J, et al. Evaluation of impairment of hand function. In: Hunter J, et al, eds. *Rehabilitation of the Hand: Surgery and Therapy*. CV Mosby: St. Louis; 1990:115.

329. Lamereaux L, Hoffer MM. The effect of wrist deviation on grip and pinch strength. *Clin Orthop* 1995;314:152–155.

330. Ryu J, et al. Functional ranges of motion of the wrist joint. *J Hand Surg* 1991;16A:409–420.

331. Palmer ML, Epler M. *Clinical Assessment Procedures in Physical Therapy*. Philadelphia: JB Lippincott; 1990:68–73.

PERIPHERAL JOINTS: THE LOWER EXTREMITIES

THE HIP JOINT

CHAPTER OBJECTIVES

▶ *At the completion of this chapter, the reader will be able to:*

1. Describe the anatomy of the joint, ligaments, muscles, and blood and nerve supply that comprise the hip joint complex.

2. Describe the biomechanics of the hip joint, including open- and close-packed positions, normal and abnormal joint barriers, force couples, and stabilizers of the joint.

3. Describe the purpose and components of the examination of the hip joint.

4. Perform a comprehensive examination of the hip joint, including palpation of the articular and soft tissue structures, specific passive mobility, passive articular mobility tests, and stability stress tests.

5. Evaluate the total examination data to establish a diagnosis.

6. Describe the relationship between muscle imbalance and functional performance of the hip.

7. Summarize the various causes of hip dysfunction.

8. Develop self-reliant intervention strategies based on clinical findings and established goals.

9. Develop a working hypothesis.

10. Describe and demonstrate intervention strategies and techniques based on clinical findings and established goals.

11. Evaluate the intervention effectiveness in order to progress or modify an intervention.

12. Plan an effective home program, and instruct the patient in same.

OVERVIEW

The hip articulation is formed between the head of the femur and the acetabulum of the pelvic bone (Fig. 17-1). The primary function of the hip is to support the weight of the head, arms, and trunk during the static erect posture and during dynamic activities such as ambulation, running, and stair climbing. In addition, the hip joint provides a pathway for the transmission of forces between the pelvis and the lower extremities. The hip joint transmits truly impressive loads, both tensile and compressive. For example, during walking, the hip supports 1.3 to 5.8 times the body weight, and 4.5 times the body weight while running.[1] Finally, the hip joint functions to provide a wide range of lower limb movement.

The hip joint is well designed to provide such an important service, provided that it is permitted to grow and develop normally.

Normal hip joint growth and development occur due to a genetically determined balance of growth of the acetabulum, and the presence of a strategically located spherical femoral head.[1–5]

▶ Absence of a normal femoral head during growth, such as in developmental dysplasia of the hip, causes the acetabulum to have a flat shape.

▶ A deformed head stimulates the formation of a correspondingly deformed acetabulum if the deformation occurs at a young enough age.[1]

Anatomy

Bony Anatomy

The os coxa (hip bone) initially begins life as three individual bones: the ilium, ischium, and pubis.

Ilium

The ilium (see Fig. 17-1) is the largest of these three bones. It is composed of a large fan-like wing (ala), and an inferiorly positioned body. The body of the ilium forms the superior two fifths of the acetabulum.

▶ The wing of the ilium spans superiorly from the posterior superior iliac spine (PSIS) to the anterior superior iliac spine (ASIS). The wing serves as the insertion for the gluteus minimus, medius, and maximus.

▶ The anterior surface of the ilium forms a fossa and serves as the proximal attachment of the iliacus muscle.

Ischium

The ischium (see Fig. 17-1) is composed of a body, which contributes to the acetabulum, and a ramus. The ischium forms the posterior two fifths of the acetabulum. Together, the ischium and the ramus form the ischial tuberosity. The ischial tuberosity is an important landmark for palpation as it serves as the attachment for several muscles (Table 17-1), and the sacrotuberous ligament. The ischial spine, located on the body

TABLE 17-1 Muscles That Attach to the Ischial Tuberosity

Semimembranosus
Semitendinosus
Long head of the biceps femoris
Adductor magnus
Quadratus femoris
Gemellus inferior

of the ischium, serves as the attachment for the sacrospinous ligament.

Pubis

The pubis (see Fig. 17-1) is the smallest of the three bones, and consists of a body and inferior and superior rami. The pubis forms the anterior fifth of the acetabulum.

Acetabulum

The ilium, ischium, and pubis fuse together within the acetabulum. While the majority of acetabular development is determined by the age of 8,[6–8] the depth of the acetabulum increases additionally at puberty, due to the development of three secondary centers of ossification.[1,2,9]

The acetabulum is angled laterally, inferiorly, and anteriorly (see Fig. 17-1). The acetabular rim, or labrum, deepens the acetabulum thereby increasing the stability of the hip joint. The acetabular labrum has a triangular cross section and improves the mobility of the hip by providing an elastic alternative to the bony rim. The whole of the acetabulum is covered with hyaline cartilage, except for the fovea capitis (see Fig. 17-1), the area occupied by the ligamentum teres and obturator artery.

FIGURE 17-1 Bones of the hip joint. (Reproduced with permission from Luttgens K, Hamilton K. *Kinesiology: Scientific Basis of Human Motion.* New York: McGraw-Hill; 1997.)

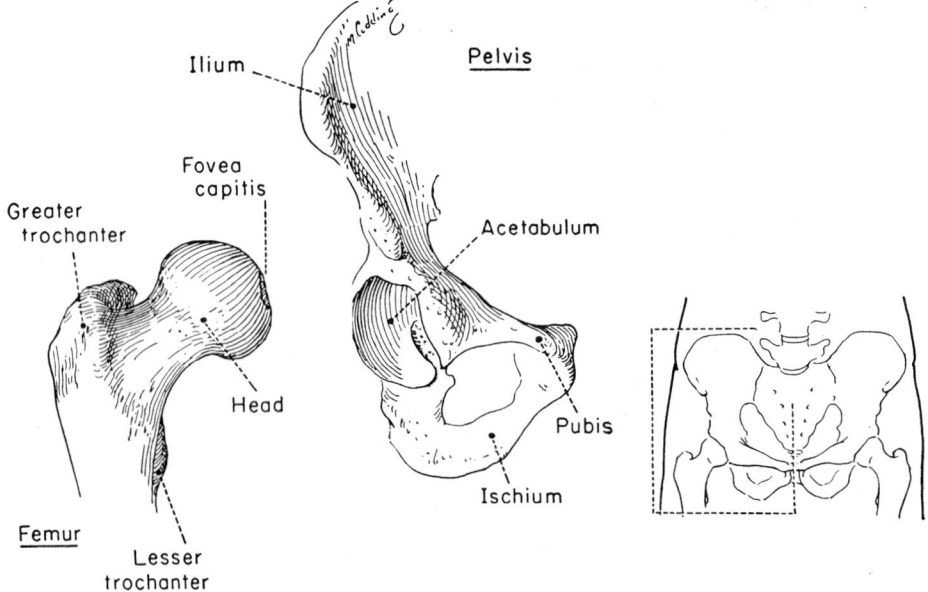

Femur

The femur is the strongest and the longest bone in the body. The proximal end of the femur consists of a head, a neck, and a greater and lesser trochanter (see Fig. 17-1). Approximately two thirds of the femoral head is covered with a smooth layer of cartilage except for a depression, the aforementioned fovea capitis. The fovea capitis serves as the attachment of the ligamentum teres. It is from this attachment that the femoral head receives its blood supply from a tiny posterior branch of the internal iliac artery. This artery is a significant source of blood to the femoral head in infants and children,[10] but becomes less significant in adulthood, due to collateral circulation from the circumflex arteries (see "Vascular Supply").[11] Interruption to this artery has been linked to avascular necrosis of the femoral head, although it is likely that other vascular supplies would also have to be interrupted for this to occur.

The trabecular bone in the femoral neck and head is specially designed to withstand high loads. The design incorporates both primary and secondary compressive and tensile patterns. However, within this trabecular system, there is a point of weakness called the Ward triangle, which is a common site of osteoporotic fracture.[12]

The neck of the femur is located between the shaft of the femur and its head. On the anterior surface of the femoral neck is the rough intertrochanteric line. A large ridge of bone, the intertrochanteric crest, marks the posterior junction between the neck and the shaft of the femur. The greater trochanter serves as the insertion site for several muscles that act on the hip joint (Table 17-2). The lesser trochanter, located on the posteromedial junction of the neck and shaft of the femur, is created from the pull of the iliopsoas muscle.

The head of the femur is angled anteriorly, superiorly, and medially. The femoral neck is externally rotated with respect to the shaft. The angle that the femoral neck makes with the acetabulum is called the angle of anteversion/declination (see "Biomechanics" section).

Joint Capsule

The joint capsule of the hip is a cylindrical sleeve running from the acetabular rim to the base of the femoral neck (Fig. 17-2). Both the articular cartilage and the joint capsule are thicker anterosuperiorly, where maximal stress occurs, and thinnest posteroinferiorly. The joint capsule is supported by intra-articular and extra-articular ligaments and by muscles.

TABLE 17-2 Muscles That Attach to the Greater Trochanter

Piriformis
Gluteus medius
Gluteus minimus
Obturator internus
Gemellus superior
Gemellus inferior

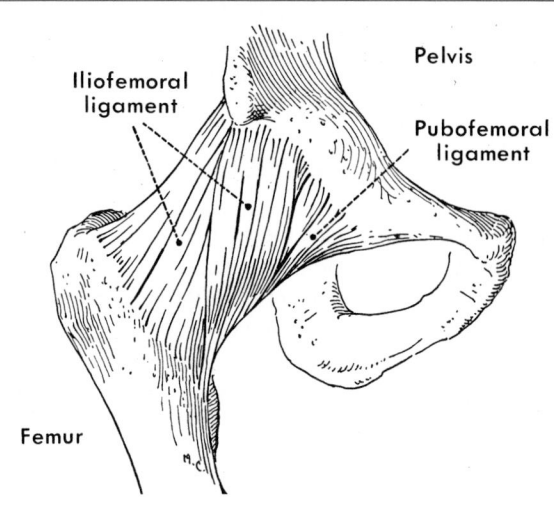

FIGURE 17-2 Anterior view of right hip. (Reproduced with permission from Luttgens K, Hamilton K. *Kinesiology: Scientific Basis of Human Motion*. New York: McGraw-Hill; 1997.)

Intra-articular Ligaments

The Transverse Acetabular Ligament

The transverse acetabular ligament is a fibrous tissue link spanning the inferior acetabular notch that connects the anteroinferior and posteroinferior horns of the semilunar surface of the acetabulum. The posterior aspect of the ligament attaches to the bone beneath the lunate surface, and the anterior aspect attaches to the labrum.[12a] The transverse acetabular ligament contains no cartilage cells.[12b] The function of this ligament in the hip is currently unknown.

The Acetabular Labrum

The acetabular labrum is a fibrocartilaginous rim that is attached to the acetabular margin and deepens the acetabular cup.[12c] The labrum varies greatly in form and thickness. It has three surfaces: an internal articular surface, an external surface contacting the joint capsule, and a basal surface attached to the acetabular bone and transverse ligaments.[12b] Most of the labrum is composed of thick, type I collagen fiber bundles principally arranged parallel to the acetabular rim, with some fibers scattered throughout this layer running obliquely to the predominant fiber orientation.[12d] Other histological examinations of the labrum have shown free nerve-endings and sensory end organs in its superficial layers.[12e] These nerve-endings may participate in nociceptive and proprioceptive mechanisms.[12c] The normal microvasculature of the acetabular labrum consists of a group of small vessels located in the substance of the labrum traveling circumferentially around the labrum at its attachment site on the outer surface of the bony acetabular extension.[12f] In addition, the labrum is surrounded by highly vascularized synovium that is present in the capsular recess.[12f]

The acetabular labrum functions to deepen the hip socket in a fashion that is similar to the way that the glenoid labrum deepens the shoulder socket (see Chap. 14). However, in contrast to the glenoid in the glenohumeral joint, the osseous acetabulum in the hip is much deeper and provides substantial static stability to the hip joint.[12e] Deepening of the socket that is provided by the labrum would therefore appear to be less important at the hip. Some research does indicate, however, that the labrum may enhance stability by providing negative intra-articular pressure in the hip joint.[12g]

Konrath et al[12c] examined the role of the acetabular labrum in load transmission in a biomechanical study. The distribution of contact area and pressure between the acetabulum and the femoral head was measured in cadaver hips before and after removal of the acetabular labrum. No appreciable changes with regard to contact area, load, and mean pressure were noted after removal of the labrum.[12c]

Extra-articular Ligaments

Three extra-articular ligaments help provide stability at the hip joint: the fan-shaped iliofemoral ligament of Bertin/Bigelow (see Fig. 17-2), the pubofemoral ligament (see Fig. 17-2) and the ischiofemoral ligament (Fig. 17-3).

▶ The iliofemoral ligament consists of two parts: an inferior (medial) portion and a superior (lateral) portion. The iliofemoral ligament is the strongest ligament in the body. The ligament is oriented superior-laterally and blends with the iliopsoas muscle.

▶ The pubofemoral ligament blends with the inferior band of the iliofemoral, and with the pectineus muscle. The orientation of the pubofemoral ligament is more inferior-medial.

▶ The ischiofemoral ligament winds posteriorly around the femur and attaches anteriorly, strengthening the capsule. This ligament is more commonly injured than the other hip ligaments.

All of the extra-articular ligaments are taut in hip extension, especially the inferior portion of the iliofemoral ligament. Conversely, all of the ligaments are relaxed in hip flexion. In ex-

ternal rotation of the hip, the superior portion of the iliofemoral ligament and the pubofemoral ligament are both taut. The ischiofemoral ligament is taut with hip internal rotation. Hip abduction tightens the pubofemoral and ischiofemoral ligaments. Hip adduction tightens the superior portion of the iliofemoral ligament.

Because of their inherent strength, the hip ligaments are only usually compromised with severe macrotrauma involving a fracture/dislocation of the hip.

Muscles

The hip joint is surrounded by a large number of muscles, which enable the joint to move through a wide range of motion, but which are prone to strains. The origin, insertion, and innervation of these muscles are outlined in Table 17-3.

Iliopsoas

The iliopsoas muscle, formed by the iliacus and psoas major muscles (see Fig. 17-4), is the most powerful of the hip flexors. This muscle also functions as a weak adductor and external rotator of the hip. The iliopsoas attaches to the hip joint capsule, thereby affording it some support.

Pectineus

The pectineus (see Fig. 17-4) is an adductor, flexor, and internal rotator of the hip. Like the iliopsoas, the pectineus attaches to, and supports, the joint capsule of the hip.

Rectus Femoris

The reflected head of the rectus femoris (Fig. 17-5) attaches to the hip capsule, therefore an injury to it can cause a capsular adhesion of the hip. The rectus femoris combines movements of flexion at the hip and extension at the knee. It functions more effectively as a hip flexor when the knee is flexed, as when a person kicks a ball.[13]

Tensor Fascia Latae

The tensor fascia latae (TFL) (see Fig. 17-5) envelops the muscles of the thigh. The TFL counteracts the backward pull of the gluteus maximus on the iliotibial band (ITB). The TFL also assists in flexing, abducting, and internally rotating the hip. The trochanteric bursa is found deep to this muscle as it passes over the greater trochanter (see later).[14]

Sartorius

The sartorius muscle (see Fig. 17-5) is the longest muscle in the body. The sartorius is responsible for flexion, abduction, and external rotation of the hip, and some degree of knee flexion.[15]

Gluteus Maximus

The gluteus maximus (Fig. 17-6) is the largest and most important hip extensor and external rotator of the hip. The muscle consists of a superficial and deep portion. The larger, superficial portion of this muscle inserts at the proximal part of the ITB, while the deep portion inserts into the gluteal tuberosity of the femur. The inferior gluteal nerve, which innervates the muscle, is located on the deep portion.

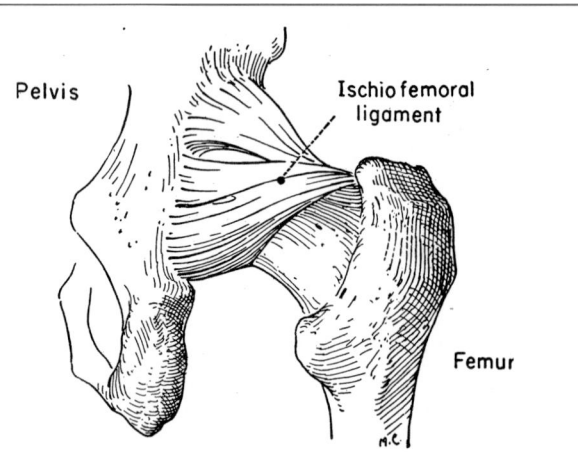

FIGURE 17-3 Posterior view of the right hip joint. (Reproduced with permission from Luttgens K, Hamilton K. *Kinesiology: Scientific Basis of Human Motion.* New York: McGraw-Hill; 1997.)

TABLE 17-3 Muscles Acting Across the Hip Joint

Muscle	Origin	Insertion	Innervation
Adductor brevis	External aspect of the body and inferior ramus of the pubis	The line from the greater trochanter of the linea aspera of the femur	Obturator nerve
Adductor longus	In angle between pubic crest and symphysis	The middle third of the linea aspera of the femur	Obturator nerve
Adductor magnus	Inferior ramus of pubis, ramus of ischium and the inferolateral aspect of the ischial tuberosity	To the linea aspera and adductor tubercle of the femur	Obturator nerve and tibial portion of the sciatic nerve
Biceps femoris	Long head arises from the sacrotuberous ligament and posterior aspect of the ischial tuberosity. Short head does not act across the hip.	On the lateral aspect of the head of the fibula, the lateral condyle of the tibial tuberosity, the lateral collateral ligament, and the deep fascia of the leg	Tibial portion of the sciatic nerve, S1
Gemelli (superior and inferior)	Superior-dorsal surface of the spine of the ischium, inferior-upper part of the tuberosity of the ischium	Superior and inferior-medial surface of the greater trochanter	Sacral plexus
Gluteus maximus	Posterior gluteal line of the ilium, iliac crest, aponeurosis of the erector spinae, dorsal surface of the lower part of the sacrum, side of the coccyx, sacrotuberous ligament, and intermuscular fascia	Iliotibial tract of the fascia latae, gluteal tuberosity of the femur	Inferior gluteal nerve
Gluteus medius	Outer surface of the ilium between the iliac crest and the posterior gluteal line, anterior gluteal line, and fascia.	Lateral surface of the greater trochanter	Superior gluteal nerve
Gluteus minimus	Outer surface of the ilium between the anterior and inferior gluteal lines, and the margin of the greater sciatic notch	On the anterior surface of the greater trochanter	Superior gluteal nerve
Gracilis	The body and inferior ramus of the pubis	The superior medial surface of the proximal tibia, just proximal to the tendon of the semitendinosus	Obturator nerve
Iliacus	Superior two thirds of the iliac fossa, upper surface of the lateral part of the sacrum	Fibers converge with tendon of the psoas major to lesser trochanter	Femoral nerve
Obturator externus	Rami of the pubis, ramus of the ischium, medial two thirds of the outer surface of the obturator membrane	Trochanteric fossa of the femur	Obturator nerve

TABLE 17-3   *(cont.)*

Muscle	Origin	Insertion	Innervation
Obturator internus	Internal surface of the antero-lateral wall of the pelvis, and obturator membrane	Medial surface of the greater trochanter	Sacral plexus
Pectineus	Pectineal line	Along a line extending from the lesser trochanter to the linea aspera	Femoral or obturator or accessory obturator nerves
Piriformis	Pelvic surface of the sacrum, gluteal surface of the ilium, capsule of the sacroiliac joint, and sacrotuberous ligament	Upper border of the greater trochanter of femur	Sacral plexus
Psoas major	Transverse processes of all the lumbar vertebrae bodies and intervertebral disks of the lumbar vertebrae	Lesser trochanter of the femur	Lumbar plexus
Quadratus femoris	Ischial body next to the ischial tuberosity	Quadrate tubercle on femur	Nerve to quadratus femoris
Rectus femoris	By two heads, from the anterior inferior iliac spine, and a reflected head from the groove above the acetabulum	Upper border of the patella	Femoral nerve
Sartorius	Anterior superior iliac spine and notch below it	Upper part of the medial surface of the tibia in front of the gracilis	Femoral nerve
Semimembranosus	Ischial tuberosity	The posterior-medial aspect of the medial condyle of the tibia	Tibial nerve
Semitendinosus	Ischial tuberosity	Upper part of the medial surface of the tibia behind the attachment of the sartonus and below that of the gracilis	Tibial nerve
Tensor fascia latae	Anterior part of outer lip of the iliac crest and the lateral surface of the anterior superior iliac spine	Iliotibial tract	Superior gluteal nerve

The gluteus maximus is usually active only when the hip is in flexion, as during stair climbing or cycling, or when extension of the hip is resisted.[13]

Gluteus Medius
The gluteus medius (see Fig. 17-6) is the main abductor of the hip, and a primary stabilizer of the hip and pelvis. Due to its shape and function, the gluteus medius is known as the deltoid of the hip. On the deep surface of this muscle is located the superior gluteal nerve, and the superior and inferior gluteal vessels.

The muscle can be divided into two functional parts: an anterior portion and a posterior portion. The anterior portion works to flex, abduct, and internally rotate the hip. The posterior portion extends and externally rotates the hip.

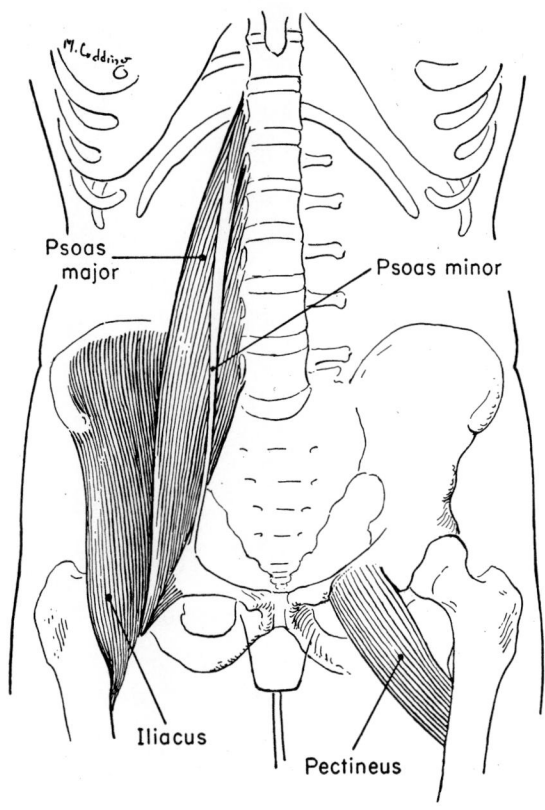

FIGURE 17-4 The psoas major and minor and pectineus. (Reproduced with permission from Luttgens K, Hamilton K. *Kinesiology: Scientific Basis of Human Motion.* New York: McGraw-Hill; 1997.)

The muscle also functions to provide pelvic support during one-legged stance.[16] In addition to its role as a stabilizer, the gluteus medius also functions as a decelerator of hip adduction.

Gluteus Minimus

The gluteus minimus (see Fig. 17-6) is a rather thin muscle situated between the gluteus medius muscle and the external surface of the ilium. The muscle is the major internal rotator of the femur. It receives assistance from the tensor fascia latae, semitendinosus, semimembranosus, and gluteus medius.[13] The gluteus minimus also abducts the thigh, as well as helping the gluteus medius with pelvic support.

Piriformis

The piriformis (see Fig. 17-6) is the most superior of the external rotators of the hip. The piriformis is an external rotator of the hip at less than 60 degrees of hip flexion. At 90 degrees of hip flexion, the piriformis reverses its muscle action, becoming an internal rotator and abductor of the hip.[17] The piriformis with its close association with the sciatic nerve can be a common source of buttock and leg pain.[18–21]

Obturator Internus

The obturator internus (see Fig. 17-6) is normally an external rotator of the hip and an internal rotator of the ilium, but becomes an abductor of the hip at 90 degrees of hip flexion.[22]

Obturator Externus

The obturator externus (see Fig. 17-6), named for its location external to the pelvis, is an adductor and external rotator of the hip.[23]

Gemelli

The superior and inferior gemelli muscles (see Fig. 17-6) are considered accessories to the obturator internus tendon. The superior gemellus is the smaller of the two. Both of the gemelli function as minor external rotators of the hip.[23]

Quadratus Femoris

The quadratus femoris muscle (see Fig. 17-6) is a flat, quadrilateral muscle, located between the inferior gamellus and the superior aspect of the adductor magnus. The quadratus femoris is an external rotator of the hip. The quadratus femoris and the inferior gemellus share the same innervation (L4–L5).[23] The obturator internus and superior gemellus also share the same innervation (L5–S1).[23]

Hamstrings

The hamstrings muscle group consists of the biceps femoris, the semimembranosus, and the semitendinosus.

Biceps Femoris. The biceps femoris (see Fig. 17-6) arises by way of a long and short head. Only the long head acts on the hip. The long head is active during conditions that require lower amounts of force, such as decelerating the limb at the end of the swing phase, and during forceful hip extension.[24] The biceps femoris extends the hip, flexes the knee, and externally rotates the tibia.

Semimembranosus. The semimembranosus (see Fig. 17-6) gains its name from its membranous origin at the ischial tuberosity.

Semitendinosus. The semitendinosus (see Fig. 17-6) arises from the ischial tuberosity and inserts as part of the pes anserinus on the superior and medial aspect of the tibia, and deep fascia of the leg.

The semimembranosus and semitendinosus extend the hip, flex the knee, and internally rotate the tibia.[25]

Hip Adductors

The adductors of the hip (Fig. 17-7) are found on the medial aspect of the joint.

Adductor Magnus. The adductor magnus is the most powerful adductor, and it is active to varying degrees in all hip motions except abduction. The posterior portion of the adductor magnus is sometimes considered functionally as a hamstring due to its anatomic alignment. Due to its size the adductor magnus is less likely to be injured than the other hip adductors.[26]

Adductor Longus. During resisted adduction, the adductor longus is the most prominent muscle of the adductors and forms

FIGURE 17-5 Muscles of the anterior thigh. (Reproduced with permission from Luttgens K, Hamilton K. *Kinesiology: Scientific Basis of Human Motion.* New York: McGraw-Hill; 1997.)

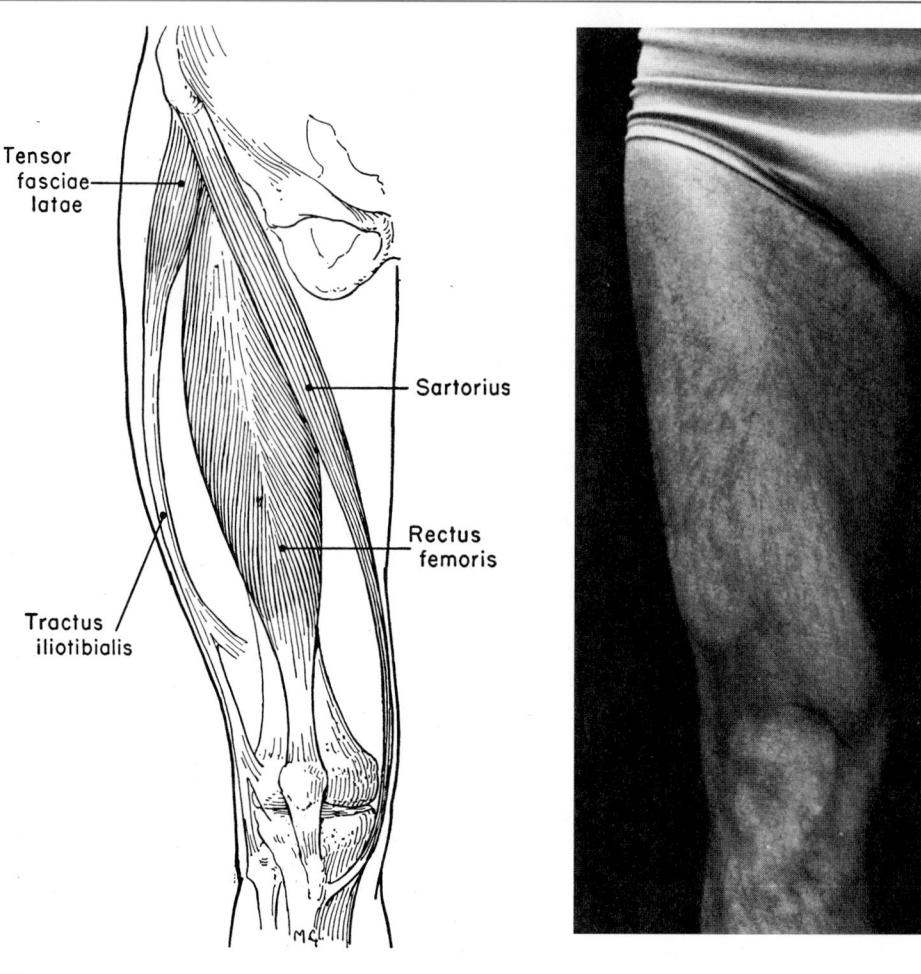

Tensor fasciae latae

Sartorius

Rectus femoris

Tractus iliotibialis

FIGURE 17-6 Posterior thigh muscles. (Reproduced with permission from Pansky B. *Review of Gross Anatomy*, 6th ed. New York: McGraw-Hill; 1996.)

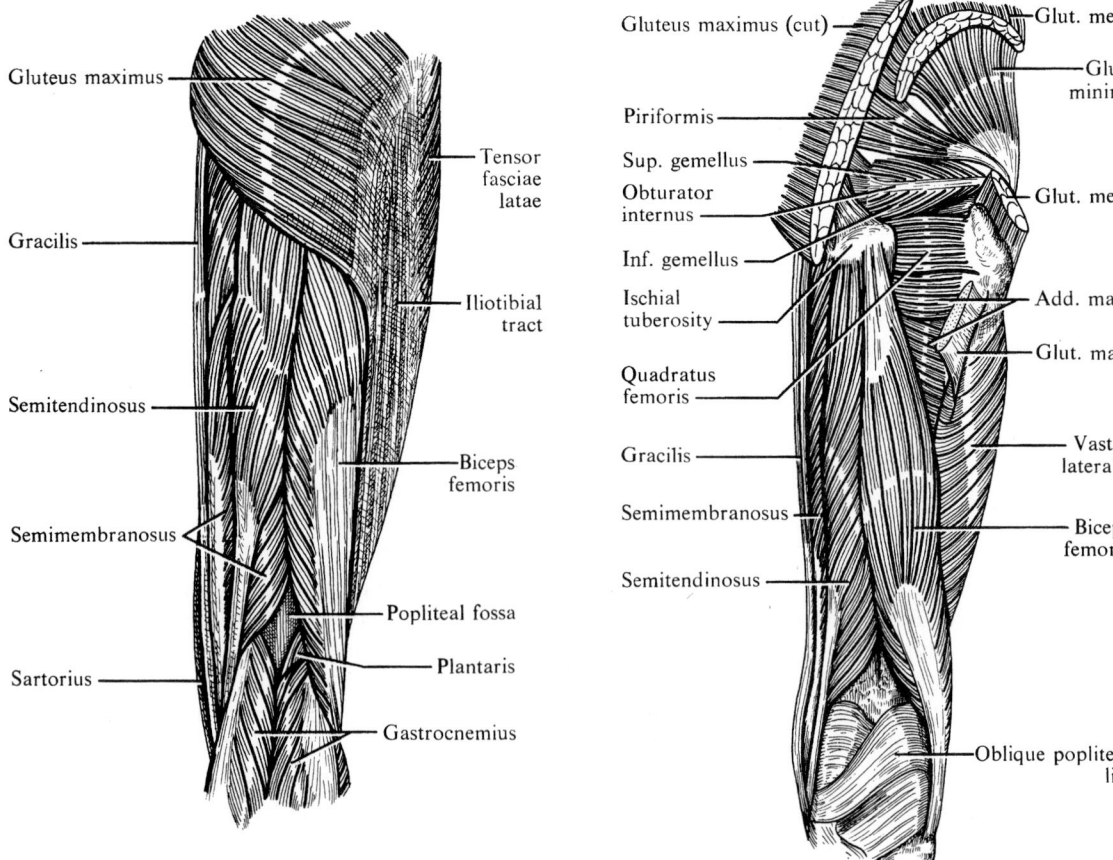

Gluteus maximus

Gracilis

Semitendinosus

Semimembranosus

Sartorius

Tensor fasciae latae

Iliotibial tract

Biceps femoris

Popliteal fossa

Plantaris

Gastrocnemius

Gluteus maximus (cut)

Glut. med.

Glut. minim.

Piriformis

Sup. gemellus

Obturator internus

Inf. gemellus

Glut. med.

Ischial tuberosity

Add. mag.

Glut. max.

Quadratus femoris

Gracilis

Vastus lateralis

Semimembranosus

Biceps femoris

Semitendinosus

Oblique popliteal lig.

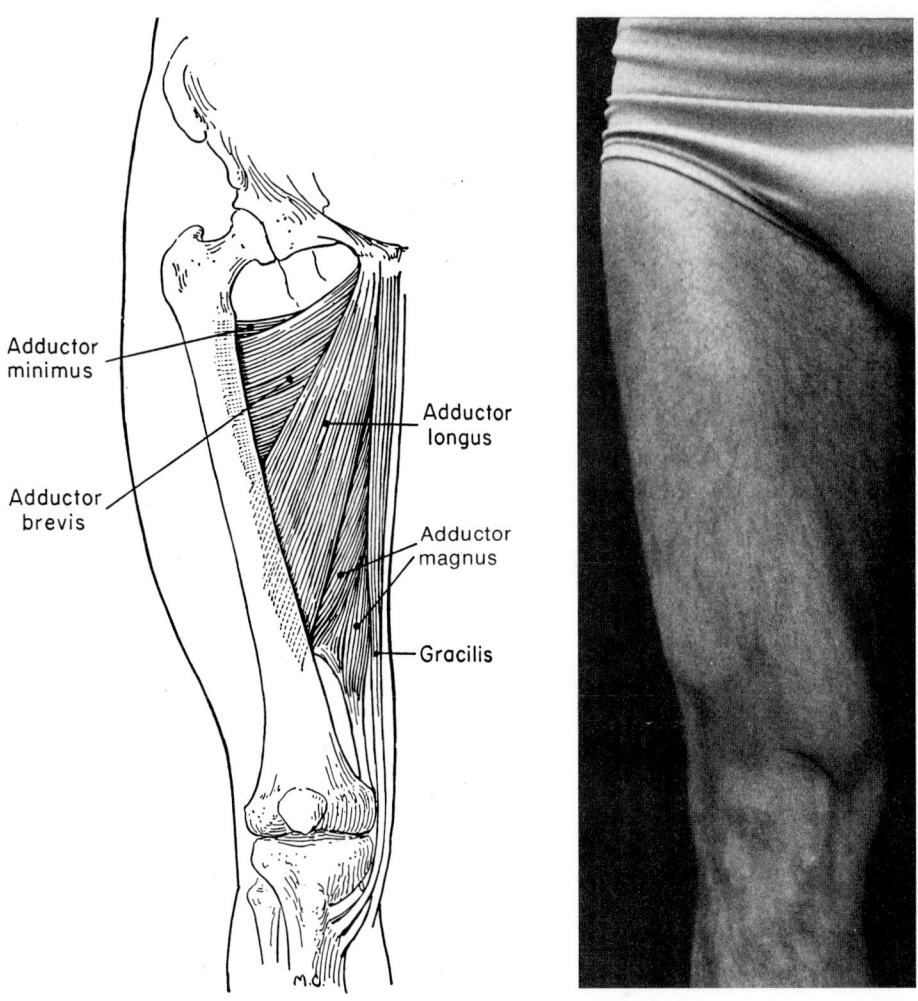

FIGURE 17-7 Hip adductor muscles. (Reproduced with permission from Luttgens K, Hamilton K. *Kinesiology: Scientific Basis of Human Motion.* New York: McGraw-Hill; 1997.)

the medial border of the femoral triangle. The adductor longus also assists with external rotation, in extension, and internal rotation in other positions. The adductor longus is commonly strained.[27]

Gracilis. The gracilis (see Fig. 17-7) is the most superficial and medial of the hip adductor muscles. It is also the longest. The gracilis functions to adduct and flex the thigh, and flex and internally rotate the leg.

The other adductors of the hip include the adductor brevis and the pectineus muscles.

Bursa

There are more than a dozen bursae in this region.[28] The more clinically significant ones are described below.

Iliopsoas Bursa

Many names have been used to describe the iliopsoas bursa (IPB), including the iliopsoas, iliopectineal, iliac, iliofemoral, and subpsoas bursa.[28a] The IPB (Fig 17-8) is the largest and most constant bursa about the hip, present in 98 percent of normal adult individuals, usually bilaterally.[28b] The IPB is situated deep to the iliopsoas tendon and serves to cushion the tendon from the structures on the anterior aspect of the hip joint capsule. Its dimensions may be up to 7 cm in length and 4 cm in width.[28b] Anatomic boundaries of the bursa include the iliopsoas muscle anteriorly, the pectineal eminence and the hip joint capsule posteriorly, the iliofemoral ligament laterally, and the acetabular labrum medially.[28c]

In 15% of patients, the IPB communicates with the hip joint via a 1 mm to 3 cm point of relative capsular thinning between the iliofemoral and pubofemoral ligaments.[28a,28d] While this connection may occur on a congenital basis,[28a] this number rises to 30–40 percent in patients with hip joint pathology.[28e]

As with other bursae, the IPB can become inflamed and distended. Inflammation and distension of this bursa is most commonly associated with rheumatoid arthritis, but it is also seen in association with athletic activity, overuse and impingement syndromes, osteoarthrosis, pigmented villonodular synovitis, synovial chondromatosis, infection, pseudogout, metastatic bone disease, and in rare cases after total hip arthroplasty (see "Interventions" section).[28f]

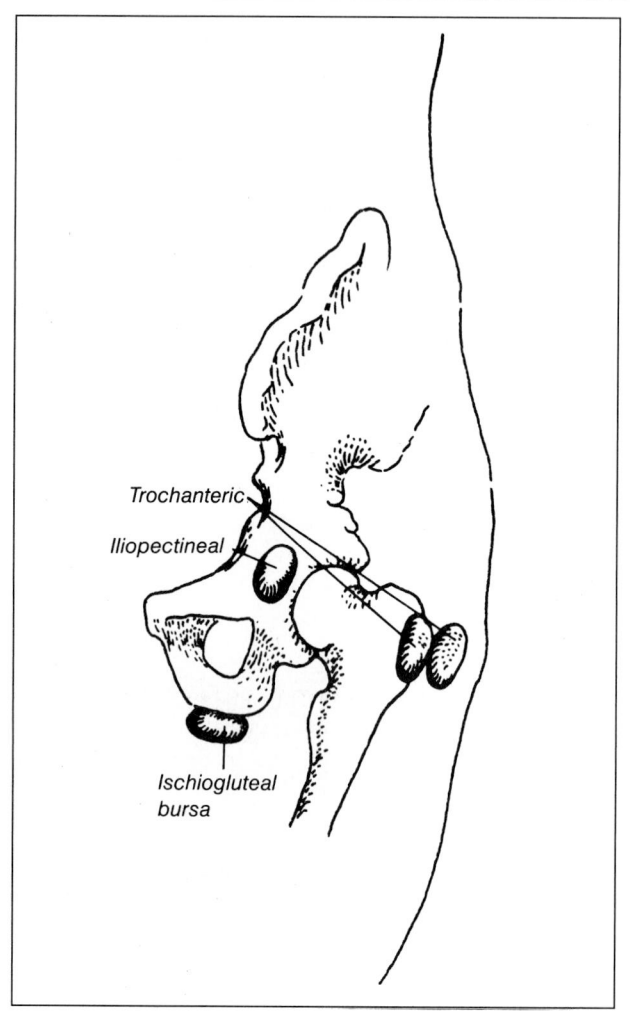

FIGURE 17-8 The bursae of the hip. (Reproduced with permission from Simon RR, Koenigsknecht SJ. *Emergency Orthopedics: The Extremities*, 4th ed. New York: McGraw-Hill; 2001.)

Trochanteric Bursa

There are two clinically significant trochanteric bursae: one between the gluteus medius and minimus, and a superficial one (see Fig. 17-8). The superficial (subtrochanteric) bursa is located between the greater trochanter and the tensor fascia latae. Compression and friction of the bursa from an adaptively shortened tensor fascia latae can result in trochanteric bursitis.

Ischiogluteal Bursa

The ischiogluteal bursa (see Fig. 17-8) is located between the ischium and the gluteus maximus muscle. It can be painfully squeezed between the ischial tuberosity and the hard surface of a chair during sitting, producing an ischial bursitis. This condition is often referred to as *weaver's bottom.*

Femoral Triangle

For topographic reasons, it is important to have an understanding of the anatomy of the femoral triangle (Fig. 17-9). The

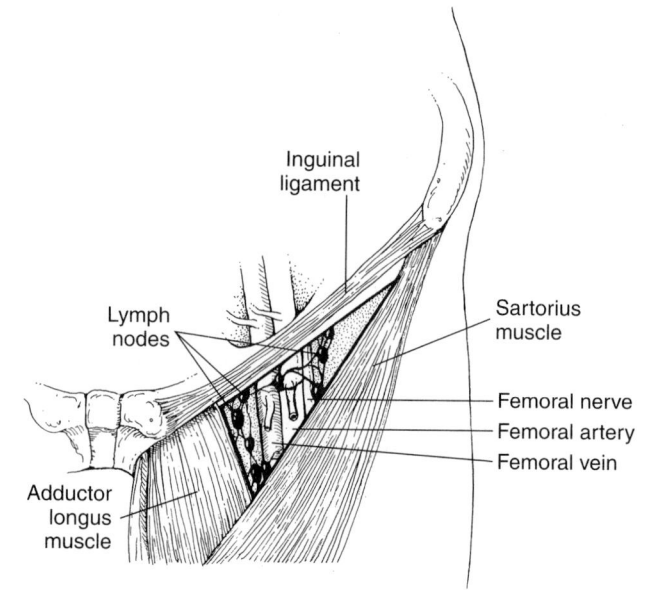

FIGURE 17-9 Femoral triangle. (Reproduced with permission from Cipriano JJ. *Photographic Manual of Regional Orthopaedic and Neurological Tests*, 3rd ed. Baltimore: Williams & Wilkins; 1997.)

femoral triangle is defined superiorly by the inguinal ligament, medially by the adductor longus, and laterally by the sartorius. The floor of the triangle is formed by portions of the iliopsoas on the lateral side, and by the pectineus on the medial side. A number of neurovascular structures pass through this triangle. These include (from medial to lateral) the femoral vein, artery, and nerve. Thus the clinician should use caution when palpating in this area, or when applying soft tissue techniques.

Neurology

The posterior gluteal region receives cutaneous innervation by way of the subcostal nerve, the iliohypogastric nerve, the dorsal rami of L1, L2, and L3, and the dorsal primary rami (cluneal nerves) of S1, S2, and S3.[29]

The anterior region of the hip has its cutaneous supply divided around the inguinal ligament. The area superior to the ligament is supplied by the iliohypogastric nerve. The area inferior to the ligament is supplied by the subcostal nerve, the femoral branch of the genitofemoral nerve, and the ilioinguinal nerve (see Chap. 2).[29]

The nerves of the muscles that cross the hip joint (femoral, obturator, superior gluteal, and the nerve to the quadratus femoris) also supply the joint capsule and the joint. Therefore pain referred from the hip joint may be felt anywhere in the thigh, leg, or foot.

Vascular Supply

The external iliac artery becomes the femoral artery as it passes underneath the inguinal ligament. The femoral artery forms two branches. The anterior portion of the femoral neck and the anterior portion of the capsule of the hip joint are supplied by the lateral femoral circumflex artery (LFCA). The medial femoral circumflex artery (MFCA) perforates and supplies the posterior hip joint capsule and the synovium.[29] The deep branch of the MFCA gives rise to two to four superior retinacular vessels, and occasionally to inferior retinacular vessels.[30,31]

Most of the femoral head, comprising its upper one half or upper two thirds, is supplied by the lateral epiphyseal artery, a terminal branch of the MFCA.[11] The inferior epiphyseal artery, a branch of the lateral circumflex artery, contributes to the vascularization of the lower area of the femoral head. The supply to the femoral head from the ligamentum teres artery is extremely variable.[32] The blood supply to the weight bearing portion of the head of the femur is derived from the MFCA.[33]

Two other branches are formed from the internal iliac artery: the inferior and superior gluteal arteries. These arteries supply the superior portion of the capsule and the gluteus maximus muscle.

Biomechanics

The hip joint is classified as an unmodified ovoid (ball and socket) joint. This arrangement permits motion in three planes: sagittal (flexion and extension around a transverse axis), frontal (abduction and adduction around an anteroposterior axis), and transverse (internal and external rotation around a vertical axis). All three of these axes pass through the center of the femoral head.

Active range of motion of the hip is variable. Hip flexion averages 110 to 120 degrees, extension 10 to 15 degrees, abduction 30 to 50 degrees, and adduction 25 to 30 degrees. Hip external rotation averages 40 to 60 degrees and internal rotation averages 30 to 40 degrees (Table 17-4). Motions about the hip joint can occur independently; however, the extremes of motion require motion at the pelvis.[34]

> ### Clinical Pearl
>
> End-range hip flexion is associated with a posterior rotation of the ilium bone. The end-range of hip extension is associated with an anterior rotation of the ilium. Hip abduction/adduction are associated with an upward/downward tilting of the pelvis (see Table 17-11).

The structure and design of the hip allows for both mobility and stability. The stability is particularly important for weight bearing and ambulation.

The relationship between the proximal femur, the greater trochanter, and the overall femoral neck width is affected by muscle pull and the forces transmitted across the hip joint. In addition, normal joint nutrition, circulation, and muscle tone during development play an important role.[1,35–37]

In the anatomic position, the orientation of the femoral head causes the contact force between the femur and acetabulum to be high in the anterosuperior region of the joint.[38] Because the anterior aspect of the femoral head is somewhat exposed in this position, the joint has more flexibility in flexion than extension.[39]

The angle between the femoral shaft and the neck is called the collum/inclination angle. This angle is approximately 125 to 130 degrees (Fig. 17-10),[17] but can vary with body types. In a tall person the collum *angle* is larger (valga). The opposite is true with a shorter individual. The collum angle has an important influence on the hips. An increase in the collum angle causes the femoral head to be directed more superiorly in the acetabulum, and is known as coxa valga. Coxa valga has the following effects at the hip joint:

► It changes the orientation of the joint reaction force from the normal vertical direction, to one that is almost parallel to the femoral shaft.[40,41] This lateral displacement of the joint reaction force reduces the weight-bearing surface, resulting in an increase in stress applied across joint surfaces not specialized to sustain such loads.

► It shortens the moment arm of the hip abductors, placing them in a position of mechanical disadvantage.[41] This causes the abductors to contract more vigorously to stabilize the pelvis, producing an increase in the joint reaction force.[39]

► It increases the overall length of the lower extremity, affecting other components in the kinetic chain. Coxa valga has the effect of decreasing the normal physiologic angle at the knee. This places an increased mechanical stress on the medial aspect of the knee joint and more tensile stress on the lateral aspect of the joint.

If the collum angle is reduced, it is known as coxa vara. The mechanical effects of coxa vara are for the most part the opposite of those found in coxa valga, although they appear to be less deleterious than those of coxa valga.[42]

Femoral alignment in the transverse plane also influences the mechanics of the hip joint. Anteversion (Fig. 17-11) is

TABLE 17-4 Normal Ranges and End-Feels at the Hip[221]

Motion	Range of Motion (Degrees)	End-Feel
Flexion	110–120	Tissue approximation or tissue stretch
Extension	10–15	Tissue stretch
Abduction	30–50	Tissue stretch
Adduction	25–30	Tissue approximation or tissue stretch
External rotation	40–60	Tissue stretch
Internal rotation	30–40	Tissue stretch

FIGURE 17-10 Neck shaft angles. (Reproduced with permission from Richardson JK, Iglarsh ZA. *Clinical Orthopaedic Physical Therapy*. Philadelphia: WB Saunders; 1994.)

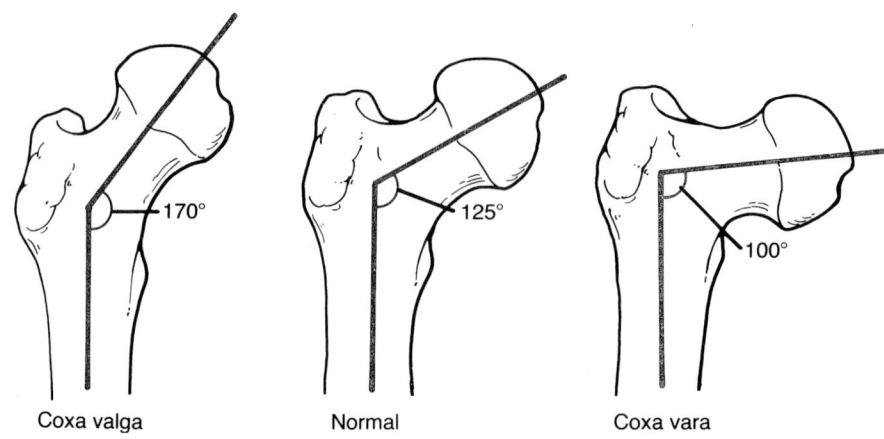

Coxa valga   Normal   Coxa vara

defined as the anterior position of the axis through the femoral condyles.[43,44] Retroversion is defined as a femoral neck axis that is parallel or posterior to the condylar axis (see Fig. 17-11).[39] The normal range for femoral alignment in the transverse plane in adults is 12 to 15 degrees of anteversion.[44,45] Subjects with excessive anteversion usually have more hip internal rotation range of motion than external rotation, and gravitate to the typical "frog-sitting" posture as a position of comfort. There is also associated in-toeing while weight bearing.[39]

Excessive anteversion directs the femoral head toward the anterior aspect of the acetabulum when the femoral condyles are aligned in their normal orientation. Some studies have supported the hypothesis that a persistent increase in femoral anteversion predisposes to osteoarthritis of the hip,[42,46–49] and knee,[50–52] although other studies have refuted this.[53–55]

The most stable position of the hip is the normal standing position: hip extension, slight abduction, and slight internal rotation.[23,59,60] The commonly cited open-packed (resting) positions of the hip are between 10 and 30 degrees of flexion,

FIGURE 17-11 The femoral anteversion angle. (Reproduced with permission from Richardson JK, Iglarsh ZA. *Clinical Orthopaedic Physical Therapy*. Philadelphia: WB Saunders; 1994.)

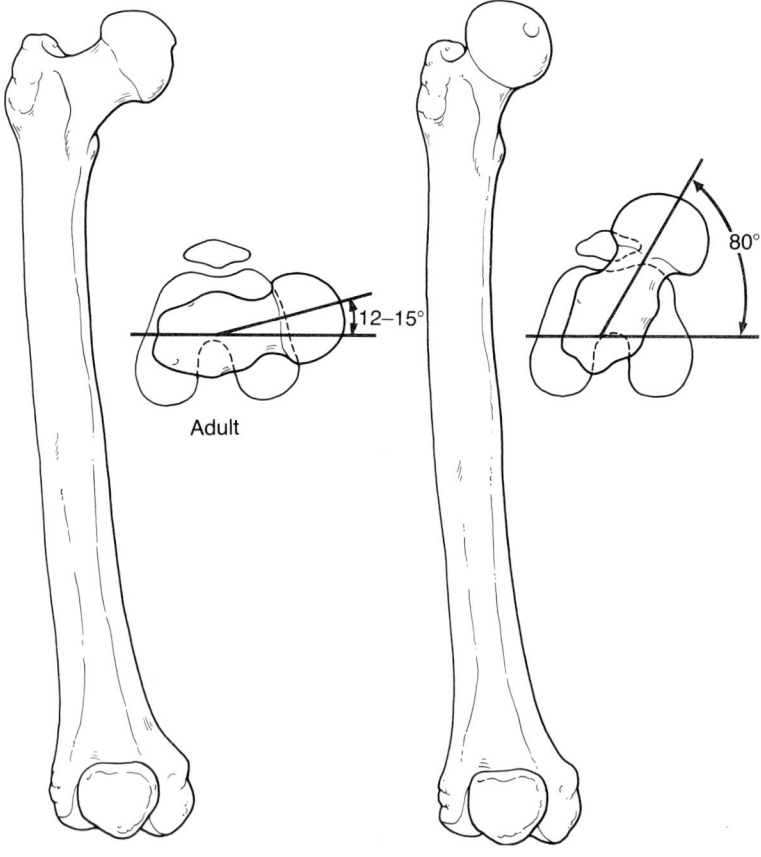

Adult

10 to 30 degrees of abduction, and 0 to 5 degrees of external rotation.

When body weight is evenly distributed across both legs during upright standing, the weight supported at each hip is one half the weight of the body segments above the hip, or about one third of the total body weight.[63] The simple act of lifting one leg transfers the body weight to the weight-bearing hip.

During gait, because of muscle tension, compression on the hip is approximately the same as body weight during the swing phase.[64] However, during the support phase, peak joint forces can range from 300 to 400 percent of body weight at normal walking speed, to 550 percent of body weight during fast walking and jogging, and as high as 870 percent of body weight during stumbling.[13,65] Stair climbing and descending increase the loads on the hip by approximately 10 percent and 20 per-

cent, respectively.[13,66] The use of a cane or crutch in the hand contralateral to the involved hip can be used to decrease pressure on the hip joint.[67]

According to Cyriax,[61,62] the capsular pattern of the hip is a marked limitation of flexion, abduction, and internal rotation. Kaltenborn[59] considers the capsular pattern of the hip to be extension more limited than flexion, internal rotation more limited than external rotation, and abduction more limited than adduction.

Examination

The common pathologies and the interventions for the hip joint are detailed after the examination. Table 17-5 outlines the clinical findings, differential diagnosis, and intervention

TABLE 17-5   History, Clinical Findings, Differential Diagnosis, and Intervention Strategies of Some Hip Conditions[167]

Diagnosis	History	Physical Findings	Differential Diagnosis
Legg-Calvé-Perthes disease	Insidious onset (1 to 3 months) of limp with hip or knee pain	Limited hip abduction, flexion, and internal rotation	Juvenile arthritis, other inflammatory conditions of the hip
Slipped capital femoral epiphysis	Acute (<1 month) or chronic (up to 6 months) presentation, pain may be referred to knee or anterior thigh	Pain and limited internal rotation, leg more comfortable in external rotation; chronic presentation may have leg length discrepancy	Muscle strain, avulsion fracture
Avulsion fracture	Sudden, violent muscle contraction; may hear or feel a "pop"	Pain on passive stretch and active contraction of involved muscle; pain on palpation of involved apophysis	Muscle strain, slipped capital femoral epiphysis
Hip pointer	Direct trauma to iliac crest	Tenderness over iliac crest, may have pain on ambulation and active abduction of hip	Contusion, fracture
Contusion	Direct trauma to soft tissue	Pain on palpation and motion, ecchymosis	Hip pointer, fracture, myositis ossificans
Myositis ossificans	Contusion with hematoma approximately 2 to 4 weeks earlier	Pain on palpation, firm mass may be palpable	Contusion, soft tissue tumors, callus formation from prior fracture
Femoral neck stress fracture	Persistent groin discomfort increasing with activity, history of endurance exercise, female athlete triad (eating disorder, amenorrhea, osteoporosis)	ROM may be painful, pain on palpation of greater trochanter	Trochanteric bursitis, osteoid osteoma, muscle strain
Osteoid osteoma	Vague hip pain present at night and increased with activities	Restricted motion, quadriceps atrophy	Femoral neck stress fracture, trochanteric bursitis

TABLE 17-5   *(cont.)*

Diagnosis	History	Physical Findings	Differential Diagnosis
Iliotibial band syndrome	Lateral hip, thigh, or knee pain, snapping as iliotibial band passes over the greater trochanter	Positive Ober's test	Trochanteric bursitis
Trochanteric bursitis	Pain over greater trochanter on palpation, pain during transitions from standing to lying down to standing	Pain on palpation of greater trochanter	Iliotibial band syndrome; femoral neck stress fracture
Avascular necrosis of the femoral head	Dull ache or throbbing pain in groin, lateral hip or buttock, history of prolonged steroid use, prior fracture, slipped femoral capital epiphysis	Pain on ambulation, abduction, internal and external rotation	Early degenerative joint disease
Piriformis syndrome	Dull posterior pain, may radiate down the leg mimicking radicular symptoms, history of track competition or prolonged sitting	Pain on active external rotation, passive internal rotation of hip and palpation of sciatic notch	Nerve root compression, stress fractures
Iliopsoas bursitis	Pain and snapping in medial groin or thigh	Reproduce symptoms with active and passive flexion/ extension of hip	Avulsion fracture
Meralgia paresthetica	Pain or paresthesia of anterior or lateral groin and thigh	Abnormal distribution of lateral femoral cutaneous nerve on sensory examination	Other causes of peripheral neuropathy
Degenerative arthritis	Progressive pain and stiffness	Reduction in internal rotation early, in all motion later, pain on ambulation	Inflammatory arthritis

Diagnosis	Special Tests	Intervention	Referral
Legg-Calvé-Perthes Disease	Normal CBC and ESR, plain films positive (early with changes in the epiphysis, later with flattening of the femoral head)	Maintain ROM, follow position of femoral head in relation to acetabulum radiographically	Orthopaedic surgery if unresolved
Slipped capital femoral epiphysis	Plain films show widening of epiphysis early, later slippage of femur under epiphysis	Non-weight bearing, surgical pinning	Urgent orthopaedic surgery with acute, large slips
Avulsion fracture	Plain films; if these are negative, CT or MRI	Rehabilitation program of progressive increase in ROM and strengthening	Orthopaedic surgery of >2 cm displacement
Hip pointer	Plain films if suspect fracture	Rest, ice, NSAIDs, local steroid and anesthetic injection for severe pain, gradual return to activities with protection of site	PT appropriate

TABLE 17-5 *(cont.)*

Contusion	Plain films negative	Rest, ice, compression, static stretch, NSAIDs	PT appropriate
Myositis ossificans	Radiograph or ultrasound examination reveals typical calcified, intramuscular hematoma	Ice, stretching of involved structure, NSAIDs; surgical resection after 1 year if conservative treatment fails	PT appropriate; orthopaedic surgery if resection needed
Femoral neck stress fracture	Plain films may show cortical defects in femoral neck (superior or inferior surface); bone scan, MRI, CT may also be used if plain films are negative and diagnosis is suspected	Inferior surface fracture; no weight bearing until evidence of healing (usually 2 to 4 weeks) with gradual return to activities; superior surface fracture: ORIF	Orthopaedic surgery for ORIF
Osteoid osteoma	Plain films, if these are negative and symptoms persist, MRI or CT	Surgical romoval if unresponsive to medical therapy with aspirin or NSAIDs	Orthopaedic surgery
Iliotibial band syndrome	Positive Ober's test	Modification of activity, footwear; stretching program, ice massage, NSAIDs	PT appropriate
Trochanteric bursitis	Plain films, bone scan, MRI negative for bony involvement	Ice, NSAIDs, stretching of iliotibial band, protection from direct trauma, steroid injection	PT appropriate
Avascular necrosis of the femoral head	Plain films, MRI	Protected weight bearing, exercises to maximize soft tissue function (strength and support), total hip replacement	PT trial appropriate, orthopaedic surgery
Piriformis syndrome	EMG studies may be helpful, MRI of lumbar spine if nerve root compression is suspected	Stretching, NSAIDs, relative rest, correction of offending activity	PT appropriate
Iliopsoas bursitis	Plain films are negative	Iliopsoas stretching, steroid injection	PT appropriate
Meralgia paresthetica	Nerve conduction velocity testing may be helpful	Avoid external compression of nerve (clothing, equipment, pannus)	—
Degenerative arthritis	Plain films help with diagnosis and prognosis	Maximizing support and strength of soft tissues, ice, NSAIDs, modification of activities, cane, total hip replacement	PT trial appropriate, orthopaedic surgery

CBC, complete blood count; CT, computed tomography; EMG, electromyelography; ESR, erythrocyte sedimentation rate; MRI, magnetic resonance imaging; NSAIDs, nonsteroidal anti-inflammatory drugs; ORIF, open reduction with internal fixation; PT, physical therapy; ROM, range of motion.

strategies of some hip conditions. An understanding of the pathology and the clinical findings is obviously necessary. As mention of the various pathologies occurs with reference to the examination and vice versa, the reader is encouraged to switch between the two.

History

The history should determine the mechanism of injury, if any, and the patient's chief complaint. Falls on the outside of the hip are a common cause of trochanteric bursitis. Macrotraumatic forces applied along the femur such as those that occur with dashboard injuries and falls on the knee can result in damage to the articular cartilage, an acetabular labrum tear, or a subluxation. An immediate loss of movement following direct trauma to this area usually indicates the presence of a hip or pelvic fracture, or a dislocation. If the patient is unable to recall a specific mechanism, the clinician should suspect a systemic (see

"Systems Review") or biomechanical cause. The hip is a region that is prone to overuse injuries. Walking or running can aggravate trochanteric bursitis, iliotibial band friction syndrome, hamstring and adductor strains, or a femoral neck stress fracture.

The hip and pelvic areas are also common sites for pain referral (Table 17-6). The referred sources of hip pain are described in Chapter 9. To help determine the symptom distribution, a pain diagram should be completed by the patient (see Chap. 8). Following its completion, the patient should be encouraged to describe the type of symptoms experienced for each of the areas highlighted on the diagram, as well as the motions or positions that increase the symptoms. The location of the pain can provide the clinician with some useful information (Table 17-6). Groin pain can result from local and referred sources (Table 17-7). One of the more common causes of groin pain in the older patient is osteoarthritis of the hip. However, osteoarthritis (OA) of the hip may also cause pain behind the greater trochanter, anterior thigh,

TABLE 17-6   Differential Diagnosis for Pain in the Hip or Buttock Area[221]

Pain Distribution	Potential Cause
Groin area	Stress fractures of the pelvis and femur
	Crystal-induced synovitis (gout)
	An inguinal/femoral hernia
	Muscle calcification
	Hip adductor strain
	Iliopectineal bursitis
	Iliopsoas strain or avulsion fracture of the lesser trochanter
	Arthritis of the hip
	Hip arthrosis
	Femoral neck fracture
	Osteonecrosis of the femoral head
	Pubic symphysis dysfunction
	• Osteitis pubis
	• Osteomyelitis pubis
	• Pyogenic arthritis
	• Pubic fracture
	• Pubic osteolysis
	• Postpartum symphyseal pain
	Sacroiliac joint lesion
	Tumor
	Ureteral stone
	Hernia
	Inflammatory synovitis (e.g., rheumatoid arthritis, ankylosing spondylitis, systemic lupus erythematosus)
	Subluxation
	Dislocation
	Transient synovitis
	Infection
	Loosened prosthesis
	Inflamed lymph nodes
	Lower abdominal muscle strain
	Referred pain from viscera or spinal nerve

TABLE 17-6   *(cont.)*

Pubic area	Sprain of pubic symphysis
	Osteitis pubis
	Abdominal muscle strain
	Bladder infection
Lateral buttock area	Trochanteric bursitis
	Tendonitis of abductors or external rotators
	Apophysitis of greater trochanter
	Referred pain from mid or lower lumbar spine
	Thrombosis of gluteal arteries
Anterior and lateral thigh	Strain of quadriceps
	Meralgia paresthetica
	Entrapment of femoral nerve
	Thrombosis of femoral artery or great saphenous vein
	Stress fracture of femur
	Referred pain from hip or mid lumbar spine
Medial thigh	Strain of adductor muscles
	Entrapment of obturator nerve
	Referred pain from hip or knee
Anterior superior iliac spine	Apophysitis or sartorius or rectus femoris
Iliac crest	Strain of gluteal, oblique abdominals, tensor fascia latae, quadratus lumborum
	Entrapment of iliohypogastric nerve
	Referred pain from upper lumbar spine

and knee due to the various nerves that cross the hip.[67a] It is important to identify patients with symptomatic OA correctly and to exclude conditions that may be mistaken for or coexist with OA.[67b,67c] Periarticular pain that is not reproduced by passive motion and direct joint palpation suggests an alternate etiology such as bursitis, tendonitis, or periostitis. The distribution of painful joints is also helpful to distinguish OA from other types of arthritis because MCP, wrist, elbow, ankle, and shoulder arthritis are unlikely locations for OA except after trauma.

Lateral and posterior hip (buttock) pain may be referred from the lumbar spine. It may also be the result of trochanteric bursitis, or a strain of the gluteus medius muscle.

The time of day that appears to change the pain for better or worse can provide some clues. Hip joint pathology is usually associated with stiffness of the hip in the morning upon arising. Such pathologies include:

▶ Osteoarthritis of the hip joint.

▶ Rheumatoid arthritis of the hip joint. Prolonged morning stiffness (greater than 1 hour) should raise suspicion for this type of inflammatory arthritis.

▶ Avascular necrosis of the femoral head.

Reports of twinges of pain with weight-bearing activities may indicate the presence of a loose body within the joint. Noises in and around the joint can result from many causes. One of the more common causes is a "snapping" hip, especially if the snapping consistently occurs at approximately 45 degrees of hip flexion. This type of snapping hip is thought to be due to the iliopsoas tendon riding over the greater trochanter or anterior acetabulum. The other types of snapping hip are described in the "Interventions" section.

Information must be gathered with regard to the activities or positions that appear to aggravate or lessen the symptoms. For example, prolonged sitting on a hard surface may aggravate the ischial bursa, whereas buttock pain with prolonged sitting on a soft surface is more likely to be the result of a lumbar disk lesion. As the hip is a weight-bearing joint, it is very important to gather information concerning the role of weight bearing in pain activities, particularly whether the patient has pain at rest as well as during weight bearing, or whether specific weight-bearing activities (e.g., stair climbing and walking) are the cause of increased pain.[67d] Weight bearing tends to aggravate articular pathologies.

Finally, the clinician should determine the impact that the patient's condition has on their activities of daily living.

TABLE 17-7 Differentiation of Hip Pathologies

Factor	Congenital Hip Dislocation	Septic Arthritis	Legg-Calvé-Perthes Disease	Transient Synovitis	Slipped Femoral Capital Epiphysis	Avascular Necrosis	Degenerative Joint Disease	Fracture
Age	Birth	Less than 2y; rare in adults	2–13 y	2–12 y	Males 10–17 y; females 8–15 y	30–50 y	>40 y	Older adults
Incidence	Female>male; left>right; blacks<whites		Male>female; rare in blacks; 15% bilateral	Male>female; unilateral	Male>female; blacks>whites	Male>female	Female>male	Female>male
Observation	Short limb, associated with torticollis	Irritable child; motion-less hip; prominent greater trochanter; mild illness	Short limb; high greater trochanter; quad atrophy; adductor spasm	Decreased flexion, abduction, external rotation; thigh atrophy; muscle spasm	Short limb; obese; quad-riceps atrophy; adductor spasm		Frequently obese; joint crepitus; atrophy of gluteal muscles	Ecchymosis; may be swelling; short limb
Position	Flexed and abducted	Flexed; abducted; externally rotated			Flexed, abducted, externally rotated			External rotation
Pain		Mild pain with palpation and passive motion; often referred to knee	Gradual onset; aching in hip, thigh and knee	Acute: severe pain in knee. Moderate: pain in thigh and knee; tenderness over hip	Vague pain in knee, supra-patellar area, thigh and hip; pain in extreme motion	50% sharp pain, 50% insidious and intermittent pain in extreme ends of range	Insidious onset, pain with fall in barometric pressure	Severe pain in groin area

History	May be breech birth	Steroid therapy; fever	20–25% familial; low birth weight; growth delay	Low-grade fever	May be trauma		May be prolonged trauma, faulty body mechanics	May be trauma, fall
Range of motion	Limited abduction	Decreased (capsular pattern)	Limited abduction, extension	Decreased flexion; limited extension, internal rotation	Limited internal rotation, abduction, flexion; increased external adductor spasm	Decreased range of motion	Decreased motion, external, internal rotation, and extreme flexion	Limited
Special tests	Galeazzi's sign; Ortolani's sign; Barlow's sign;	Joint aspiration						
Gait		Refuses to walk	Antalgic gait after activity	Refuses to walk; antalgic limp	Acute: antalgic Chronic: Trendelenberg external rotation	Coxalgic limp	Limp	
Radiologic findings	Upward and lateral displacement, delayed development of acetabulum	CT scan: localized abscess; increased separation of ossification center	In stages: increased density, fragmentation, flattening of epiphysis	Normal at first, widened medial joint space	Displacement of upper femoral epiphysis; especially in frog position	Flattening followed by collapse of femoral head	Increased bone density, osteophytes, subarticular cysts; degenerated articular cartilage	Fracture line, possible displacement; short femoral neck

(From Richardson JK, Iglarsh ZA, ed. *Clinical Orthopaedic Physical Therapy*. Philadelphia: Saunders; 1994:367–368.)

Systems Review

Pain may be referred to the hip region from a number of sources (see Chap. 9). These include:

- Pubic symphysis dysfunction.
- Sacroiliac joint dysfunction.
- Lumbar and low thoracic disk degenerative disease.
- Lumbar facet dysfunctions and spine nerve root impingements.
- Lumbar stenosis with neurogenic claudication.
- Peripheral nerve entrapments (lateral femoral cutaneous).
- Systemic dysfunctions.
- Myofascial pain syndrome.
- Spondyloarthropathy.

Complaints associated with referred pain include:

- Thigh pain, knee pain, and leg pain with or without hip pain may be indicative of lumbar radiculopathy.
- Pain that is decreased with walking up stairs may indicate that the patient has lumbar spine stenosis.

The Cyriax lower quarter scanning examination can be used to screen for the presence of upper motor neuron or lower motor neuron lesions, or the referral of symptoms from the spine.

Evidence of intense inflammation on examination suggests infectious or microcrystalline processes such as gout or pseudogout. Weight loss, fatigue, fever, and loss of appetite should be sought out because these are clues to a systemic illness such as polymyalgia rheumatica, rheumatoid arthritis, lupus, or sepsis.

If following the history and systems review, the clinician is concerned with any signs or symptoms of a visceral, vascular, or systemic disorder, the patient should be referred to the appropriate health care professional.

Tests and Measures

Observation

The clinician observes the hip region, noting any scars, bruising, swelling, etc. The patient is observed from the front, back, and sides for general alignment of the hip, pelvis, spine, and lower extremities.

Both pain and musculotendinous dysfunction can produce movement and postural dysfunctions at the hip joint.[71a] According to Kendall,[57] the ideal alignment of the pelvis is indicated when the anterior superior iliac spine (ASIS) is on the same vertical plane as the symphysis pubis. The degree of pelvic tilt, which is measured as the angle between the horizontal plane and a line connecting the ASIS with the posterior superior iliac spine, varies from 5 to 12° in normal individuals.[71b] Both a low ASIS in women, and a structurally flat back in men, can cause structural variations in pelvic alignment, which can be misinterpreted as acquired postural impairments.[71a] According to Sahrmann, all of the following are necessary to indicate the presence of a postural impairment of the hip[71a]:

- An increase or decrease in the depth of the normal lumbar curve.
- A marked deviation from the horizontal line between the ASIS and PSIS.
- An increase or decrease in the hip joint angle in the anterior-posterior plane, with neutral knee joint alignment.

The following should be examined[56]:

- The glutei should be symmetrical and well rounded, not hanging loosely. The pelvic crossed syndrome (see Chap. 25) demonstrates weakness and inhibition of the glutei muscles.[72] This syndrome can be easily identified by having the patient perform a partial bridge with single leg support. This maneuver results in cramping of the hamstrings within a few seconds if the pelvic crossed syndrome is present. Atrophy of one buttock cheek compared with the other side may also indicate a superior or inferior gluteal nerve palsy. A balling-up of the gluteal muscle typically indicates a grade III tear of the gluteal muscles. Buttock swelling occurs with the sign of the buttock.[61]

> **Clinical Pearl**
>
> The pelvic crossed syndrome is exhibited by adaptively shortened hip flexors and hamstrings, and inhibited glutei muscles and lumbar erector spinae.

- Swelling over the greater trochanter could indicate trochanteric bursitis.
- Adaptive shortening of the short hip adductors is indicated by a distinct bulk in the muscles of the upper third of the thigh.[72]
- The bulk of the tensor fascia latae should not be distinct. A visible groove passing down the lateral aspect of the thigh may indicate that the tensor fascia latae is overused, and both it and the iliotibial band are adaptively shortened.[72]

The architecture and position of the hip joint and lower extremity is observed.

- In acute arthritis and gross osteoarthrosis, the hip joint is usually held in flexion and external rotation. This may be compensated for by an anterior tilt of the pelvis, together with an increased lordosis of the lumbar spine.
- Excessive external rotation of the leg, accompanied with toeing-out, occurs in extreme femoral neck retroversion or a slipped upper femoral epiphysis.
- Increased hip flexion in standing can result from weakness of excessive lengthening of the external oblique or rectus abdominis muscles. Increased hip flexion may also be due to a hip flexion contracture.
- Increased hip extension in relaxed standing is indicative of a swayback posture. This is characterized by a posterior pelvic tilt and hyperextension of the knees. This results in a

stretch on the anterior joint capsule of the hip and stress on the iliopsoas muscle and tendon.

▶ Lateral asymmetry in relaxed standing is characterized by a high iliac crest on one side. The difference in height between the two crests must be greater than one-half inch to have clinical significance. Lateral asymmetry may indicate a positive Trendelenburg sign (see "Special Tests"), which indicates hip abductor weakness.

Observation of the lower components of the kinetic chain includes:

▶ The degree of genu varum/valgus (see Chap. 18).

▶ The degree of tibial torsion (see Chap. 18).

▶ The amount of calcaneal inversion/eversion (see Chap. 19).

Functional Tests

The functional weight-bearing tests of the hip can include gait analysis (see Chap. 13) and weight-bearing tests. Quantitative and qualitative analysis of the generation of compressive forces at the hip and the muscular mechanisms during weight-bearing have been thoroughly documented.[60,73–79]

Gait. Analysis of both the stance and swing phases of gait is essential to determine the problems that must be dealt with during the intervention. Determinants of stance-phase gait involve interaction between the pelvis and hip and distal limb joints (knee and ankle).[80,81] The clinician should note whether[60]:

▶ The patient is using an assistive device. If they are, is it fitted at the correct height and do they use it correctly?

▶ There is a lack of hip motion, particularly extension. A lack of hip extension can have an impact on gait (see Chap. 13).

▶ There is a lateral horizontal shift of the pelvis and trunk over the stance leg during the swing phase. This may indicate a positive Trendelenburg sign (see "Special Tests"). Activation of the abductor mechanism on weight bearing is necessary to stabilize the hip and pelvis and prevent excessive lateral tilting of the pelvis to the contralateral side during the swing phase.

Strong activation of the hip extensors (with the abductors) is necessary at heel strike into early stance, from 30 degrees initial flexion to approximately 10 degrees of extension at heel off.[80] If the hip flexors are short or stiff in relation to the abdominal muscles, there may be an exaggeration in the anterior pelvic tilt and increased lumbar extension during this phase.[56]

Joint Loading Tests. Pain on weight bearing is a common complaint in some patients with hip joint pathology, including rheumatoid arthritis and osteoarthritis.[60] Depending on the capability of the patient, the following weight-bearing tests may produce pain.

▶ *High step.* The patient places one foot on a chair, and then leans onto it (Fig. 17-12). This maneuver flexes the raised hip and extends the other. The test is repeated on the other side. This test gives the clinician an indication as to the range of flexion and extension at the hip.

▶ *Unilateral standing.* The patient stands on one leg (Fig. 17-13). An inability to maintain the pelvis in a horizontal position during unilateral standing is called a positive Trendelenburg (see "Special Tests").

Palpation

Hoppenfeld[82] advocates an approach to palpation that is organized by region. Under this system, the palpation of bony

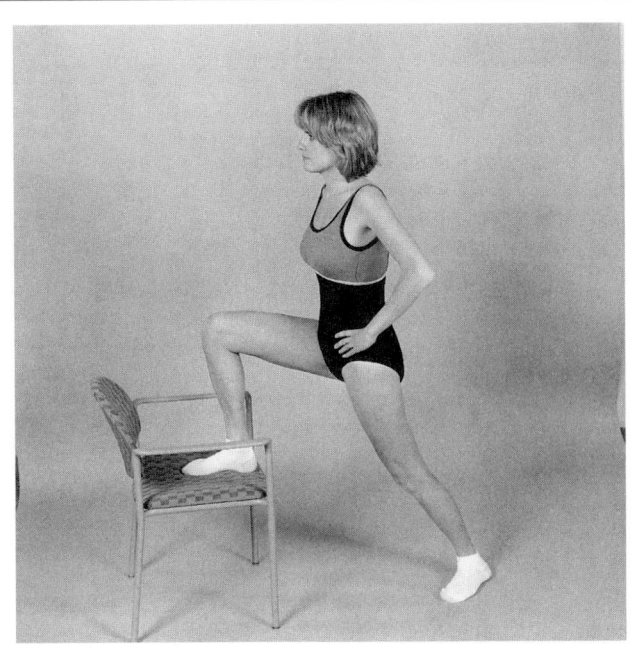

FIGURE 17-12   The high step.

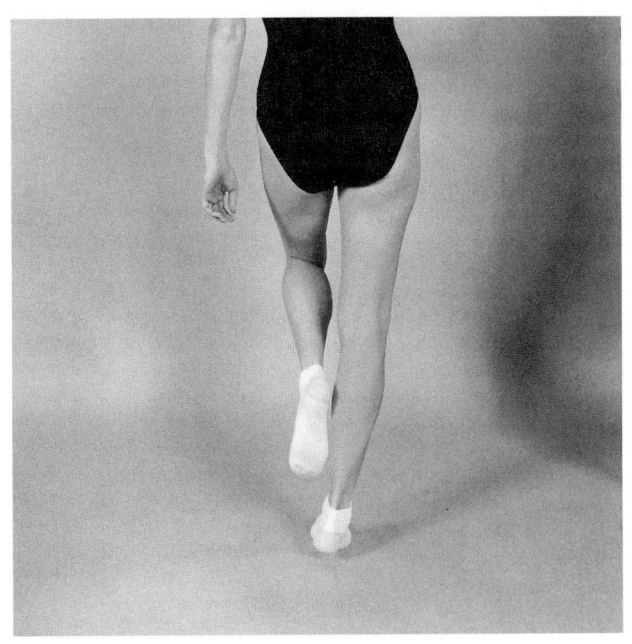

FIGURE 17-13   Unilateral standing.

structures occurs separately from the palpation of the soft tissues. While this may be helpful to the clinician, time constraints often dictate that the two are examined concurrently.

> ### Clinical Pearl
>
> The following are useful landmarks to use when locating the hip joint center of rotation.[12]

▶ The midpoint between the ASIS and pubic symphysis, over the femoral pulse.

▶ The superior tip of the greater trochanter is in line with the center of rotation.

Anterior Aspect of Hip and Groin

Anterior Superior Iliac Spine (ASIS). The anterior iliac spine serves as the origin for the sartorius muscle and the tensor fascia latae (TFL). Both can be located by flexing and abducting the patient's hip, which produces a groove that resembles an inverted V close to the ASIS. The lateral side of the inverted V is formed by the TFL, while the medial side is formed by the tendon of the sartorius.

Anterior Inferior Iliac Spine (AIIS). The anterior inferior iliac spine (Fig. 17-14) can be palpated in the space formed by the sartorius and the TFL during passive flexion of the hip in the space known as the *lateral femoral triangle*. The lateral femoral cutaneous nerve passes through this triangle. Compression of this nerve produces a condition called *meralgia paresthetica* (see Chap. 9). The AIIS serves as the origin for the rectus femoris tendon.

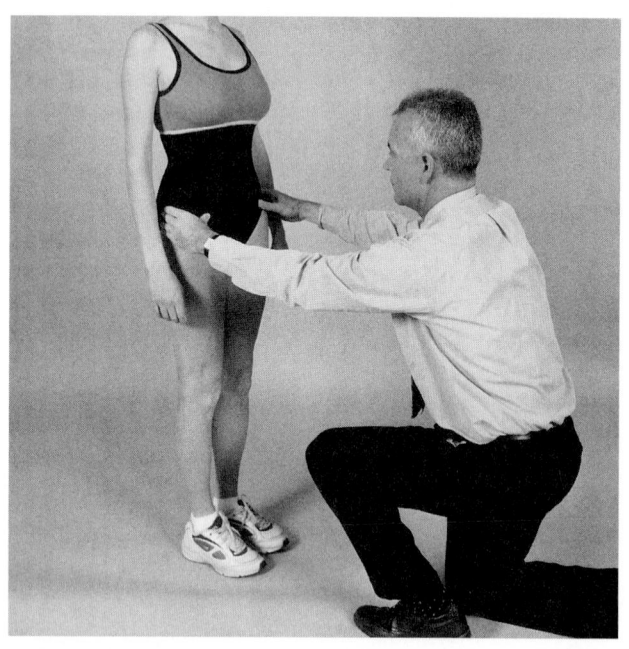

FIGURE 17-14 Palpation of ASIS.

Pubic Tubercle. The pubic tubercle is located by finding the groin crease and then traveling in an inferomedial direction, or by following the tendon of the adductor longus proximally. In males, the spermatic cord runs directly over the tubercle and can be tender to palpation in normal individuals. Inguinal hernias are usually found cranial and medial to the tubercle, while femoral hernias are located lateral to the tubercle.

Adductor Magnus. The adductor magnus is palpable in a small triangle in the distal thigh, posterior to the gracilis muscle and anterior to the semimembranosus.

Rectus Femoris. The rectus femoris has its origin at the AIIS, which is located just distal to the ASIS, between the TFL and sartorius.

Iliopsoas Bursa. At the iliopectineal eminence, the iliopsoas muscle makes an angle of about 30 degrees in a posterolateral direction. To palpate this bursa, the patient is positioned in supine with their hip positioned in approximately 40 degrees of flexion and external rotation, and resting on a pillow. At the proximal end of the femur, the clinician palpates the adductor tubercle and then moves to the anterior superior iliac spine (ASIS). From there, the clinician proceeds to the inguinal ligament, under the fold of the external oblique, and into the femoral triangle. The psoas bursa is located under the floor of the triangle, close to the pubic ramus.

Femoral Triangle. The femoral artery lies superficial and medial to the iliopsoas muscle and is easily located by palpation of the pulse. The femoral nerve is the most lateral structure in the femoral triangle. To examine the femoral triangle, the patient is positioned in supine, and if it is possible for the patient to do this, the heel of the leg resting upon the opposite knee. This places the patient in a position of flexion-abduction and external rotation.

Inguinal Ligament. The inguinal ligament is located in the fold of the groin, running from the ASIS to the pubic tubercle. It can be located by using transverse palpation.

Adductor Longus. Together with the gracilis, the adductor longus forms the medial border of the femoral triangle. The gracilis is located medial and posterior to the adductor longus. The adductor longus is best viewed during resisted adduction, when it forms a cord-like structure just distal to the pubic tubercle, before crossing under the sartorius. It is often tender in dancers, cheerleaders, and others who perform strenuous activity requiring abduction at the hip.

Lateral Aspect of the Hip. The patient is positioned in side lying.

Iliac Crest. The iliac crest is easy to locate. The cluneal nerves are superficial structures and can be located just superior to the crest.

Greater Trochanter. The superior border of the greater trochanter represents the transverse axis of hip, and when the leg is abducted, an obvious depression appears above the greater trochanter. The gluteus medius inserts into the upper portion of the trochanter and can be palpated on the lateral aspect.[68]

Palpation of the greater trochanter is also used to assess the angle of anteversion and retroversion using the Craig test (see "Special Tests").

Lesser Trochanter. The lesser trochanter, covered as it is with the iliopsoas and adductor magnus, is very difficult to palpate directly, but it can be located on the dorsal aspect if the hip is placed in extension and internal rotation, and the palpation is performed deeply lateral to the ischial tuberosity.

Piriformis Attachment. The origin of the piriformis can be found on the medial aspect of the superior point of the greater trochanter. Moving inferiorly from this point and the quadratus femoris, on the quadrate tubercle the following tendon insertions can be palpated: superior gemellus, obturator internus, and inferior gemellus.

Psoas. The insertion for the psoas is located on the inferior aspect of the greater trochanter, and can be found by placing the patient's leg in maximum internal rotation of the hip. Once the superior aspect of the greater trochanter is located, the clinician moves in a posterior/medial/inferior direction to locate the inferior aspect of the greater trochanter.

Subtrochanteric Bursa. The subtrochanteric bursa cannot be palpated directly. However, it can be tested by positioning the patient's leg in hyperadduction. At this point, the patient is asked to abduct the hip isometrically against the clinician's resistance. The contraction of the hip abductors compresses the bursa and may cause pain if the bursa is inflamed.

Posterior Aspect of the Hip. The patient is positioned in side lying.

Quadratus Lumborum. Palpation of the quadratus lumborum is best accomplished with the patient in side lying with the arm abducted overhead to open the space between the iliac crest and the 12th rib.

Ischial Tuberosity. A number of structures have their attachments on the ischial tuberosity. These include the ischial bursa, the semimembranosus tendon, the sacrotuberous ligament, the biceps femoris and semitendinosus tendons, and the tendons of the quadratus femoris, adductor magnus, and inferior gemellus. The ischial tuberosity is best palpated in the side lying position with the hip flexed to 90 degrees (see Chap. 27). This position moves the gluteus maximus upwards, permitting direct palpation at the tuberosity. The *ischial bursa* is located on the inferior and medial aspect of the ischial tuberosity. A diagnosis of ischial bursitis is usually based on a history of pain with sitting on a hard surface, and finding tenderness with palpation of the ischial tuberosity.

Sciatic Nerve. One of the most important structures to palpate in this area is the sciatic nerve. It can be located for palpation at a point halfway between the greater trochanter and ischial tuberosity. Tenderness of this nerve can be produced by a piriformis muscle spasm or by direct trauma.

Active, Passive, and Resistive Tests

During the examination of the range of motion, the clinician should note which portions of the range of motion are pain free, and which portion causes the patient to feel pain. The capsular pattern of the hip is variable but usually involves a loss of flexion, abduction, and internal rotation. Twinges of pain with active motions may indicate the presence of a loose body within the joint. At the end of available active range of motion, passive overpressure is applied to determine the end-feel. The normal ranges and end-feels for the various hip motions are outlined in Table 17-4. Abnormal end-feels common in the hip are firm capsular end-feel before expected end range, empty end-feel from severe pain, as in the Sign of the Buttock, and bony block in cases of advanced osteoarthritis.[12] Horizontal abduction and adduction of the femur occur when the hip is in 90 degrees of flexion. Because these actions require simultaneous, coordinated actions of several muscles, they can be used to assess the overall strength of the hip muscles.

Resisted testing is performed to provide the clinician with information about the integrity of the neuromuscular unit, and to highlight the presence of muscle strains.[82]

If the history indicates that repetitive motions or sustained positions cause the symptoms, the clinician should have the patient reproduce these motions or positions.[83]

> **Clinical Pearl**
>
> In the child, pain and loss of range at the hip joint should always alert the clinician to the possibility of transient synovitis, Legg-Calvé-Perthes disease, or a slipped femoral capital epiphysis.

In addition to reports of pain and overall range of motion, the clinician also notes information about weakness, joint end-feel, palpation of the moving joint, and muscle tightness.

Flexion. The six muscles primarily responsible for hip flexion are the iliacus, psoas major, pectineus, rectus femoris, sartorius, and tensor fascia latae (Table 17-8). The primary hip flexor is the iliopsoas muscle.

Hip flexion motion can be tested in sitting or supine, first with the knee flexed (Fig. 17-15), and then with the knee extended. With the hip flexed, the range of motion should be approximately 110 to 120 degrees. More hip flexion should be available with the knee flexed.

Resisted tests are then performed.

▶ To test the strength of the iliopsoas, the patient is seated with the thigh raised off the bed and resistance is applied by the clinician.

▶ The action of the sartorius muscle, which flexes, abducts, and externally rotates the hip, is tested by asking the patient to bring the plantar aspect of the foot toward the opposite knee. The clinician applies resistance at the medial malleolus and at the lateral aspect of the thigh to resist flexion, abduction, and external rotation.

TABLE 17-8   Muscle Actions at the Hip

Hip flexion	Psoas
	Iliacus
	Rectus femoris
	Sartorius
	Pectineus
	Adductor longus
	Adductor brevis
	Gracilis
Hip extension	Biceps femoris
	Semimembranosus
	Semitendinosus
	Gluteus maximus
	Gluteus medius (posterior fibers)
	Adductor magnus (ischiocondylar portion)
Hip adduction	Adductor longus
	Adductor brevis
	Adductor magnus (ischiofemoral portion)
	Gracilis
	Pectineus
Hip abduction	Tensor fascia latae
	Gluteus medius
	Gluteus minimus
	Gluteus maximus
	Sartorius
Hip internal rotation	Adductor longus
	Adductor brevis
	Adductor magnus
	Gluteus medius (anterior fibers)
	Gluteus minimus (anterior fibers)
	Tensor fascia latae
	Pectineus
	Gracilis
Hip external rotation	Gluteus maximus
	Obturator internus
	Obturator externus
	Quadratus femoris
	Piriformis
	Gemellus superior
	Gamellus inferior
	Sartorius
	Gluteus medius (posterior fibers)

A painless weakness of hip flexion is rarely a good sign. Although it may indicate a disk protrusion at the L1 or L2 level, these protrusions are not common. A more likely scenario is compression of the nerves by a neurofibroma or a metastatic invasion. Pain with the active motion or resisted tests should prompt the clinician to examine the contractile tissues individually. Passive stretching can also produce pain in a contractile structure.

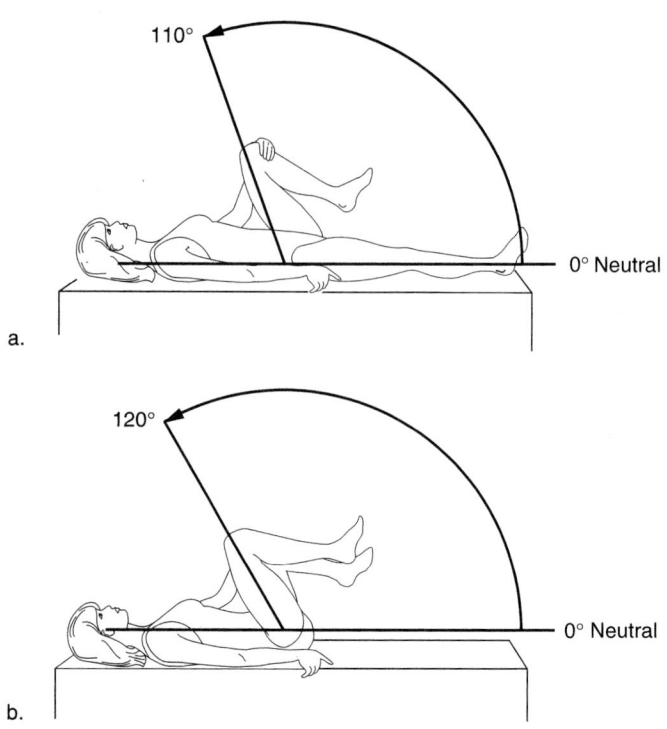

FIGURE 17-15   Hip flexion. a. Starting position. b. Maximal flexion without rotating pelvis. (Reproduced with permission from Luttgens K, Hamilton K. *Kinesiology: Scientific Basis of Human Motion*. New York: McGraw-Hill; 1997.)

Extension.   The primary hip extensor is the gluteus maximus (Table 17-8). The hamstrings also serve as hip extensors. Hip extension also involves assistance from the adductor magnus, gluteus medius and minimus, and indirect assistance from the abdominals and the erector spinae.[84]

The patient is positioned in prone over the end of a table. As the clinician palpates the buttock mass and stabilizes the sacrum to prevent the lumbar spine from extending, the patient is asked to lift the thigh toward the ceiling (Fig. 17-16). With a normal recruitment pattern, the order of firing should be gluteus maximus, opposite erector spinae, and then the ipsilateral erector spinae and hamstrings.[72] Poor recruitment patterns are demonstrated by:

1. An initial activation of the hamstrings and erector spinae with a delayed contraction of the gluteus maximus. The biceps femoris has a tendency to become shortened and overactive, resulting in delayed activation of the gluteus maximus.[85]

2. The erector spinae initiate the movement with a delayed activity of the gluteus maximus. This would lead to little if any extension of the hip joint, as the leg lift would be achieved by an anterior pelvic tilt and a hyperextension of the lumbar spine. This is a very poor movement pattern.

The normal range of motion for hip extension is approximately 10 to 15 degrees. Reduced hip extension with the knee extended can be the result of a number of reasons, including:

▶ Adaptive shortening of the iliopsoas. This is characterized by an increased lumbar lordosis, and externally rotated

FIGURE 17-16 Hip extension, internal and external rotation, and abduction. a. Hyperextension. b. Inward and outward rotation. c. Abduction. (Reproduced with permission from Luttgens K, Hamilton K. *Kinesiology: Scientific Basis of Human Motion.* New York: McGraw-Hill; 1997.)

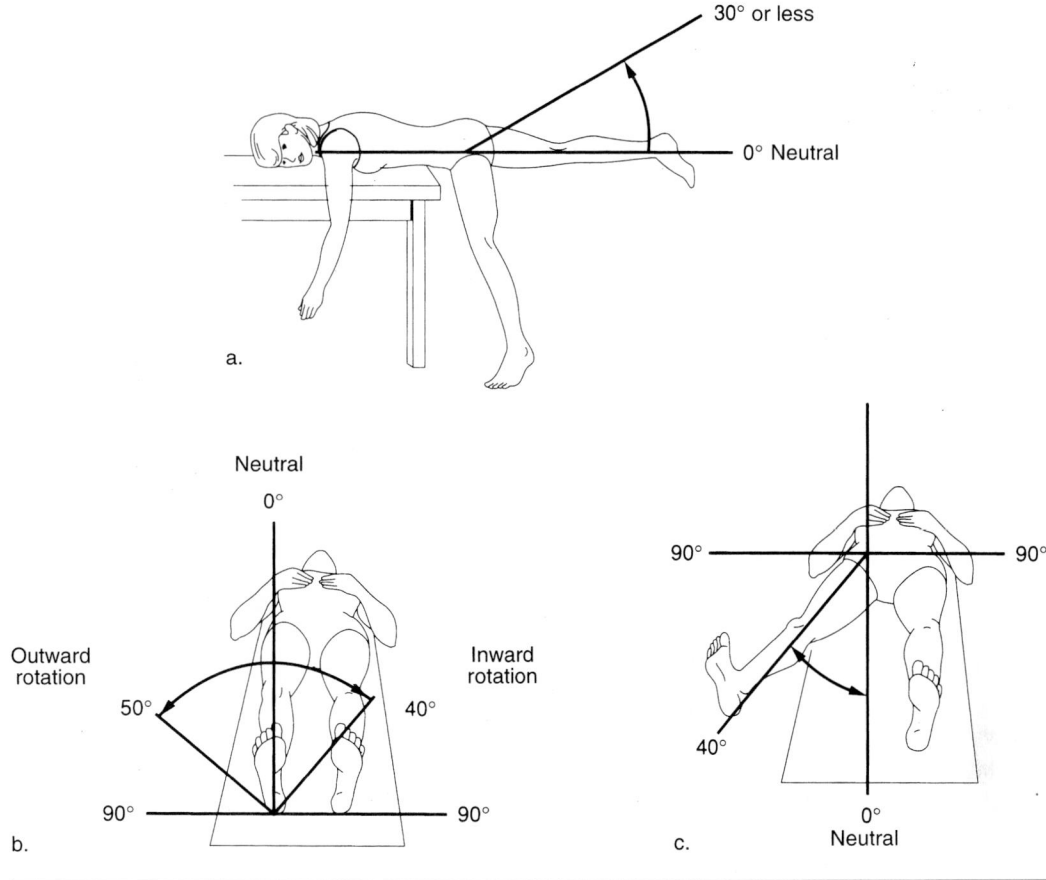

lower extremity, and a noticeable groove in the iliotibial band in standing.[86]

▶ A hip flexion contracture.

As before, the sacrum is stabilized and the patient is asked to raise the thigh off the table. The strength of the gluteus maximus is tested with the knee flexed. The hamstrings can be tested with the knee extended. By observing the patient's shoulder during this test, the recruitment pattern can be analyzed. The opposite shoulder should be seen to raise off the bed. With the abnormal pattern, the same shoulder raises off the bed. Patients who use this abnormal recruitment pattern will often have well-developed thoracic musculature on the dorsal aspect, and as a result develop problems at the thoracolumbar junction.[72]

Resistance is then applied by the clinician. A strong and painful finding with resisted hip extension may indicate a grade I muscle strain of the gluteus maximus or hamstrings. It may also indicate a gluteal bursitis or a lumbosacral strain.

Abduction/Adduction. Hip adduction and abduction range of motion can be tested in supine, making sure that both ASIS are level, and the legs are perpendicular to a line joining the ASIS (Fig. 17-16).

Abduction. The patient is supine or sidelying. The clinician monitors the ipsilateral ASIS, and the patient is asked to abduct the leg. The abduction motion is stopped when the ASIS is felt to move. The prime movers for this movement are the gluteus medius/minimus and the tensor fascia latae (TFL). The quadratus lumborum functions as the stabilizer of the pelvis. The correct sequence of firing for hip abduction in sidelying should be gluteus medius, followed by the quadratus lumborum and tensor fascia latae after approximately 15 degrees of hip abduction. Altered patterning demonstrates:

1. External rotation of the leg during the upward movement, indicating an initiation and dominance of the movement by the tensor fascia latae, accompanied by a weakness of the gluteus medius/minimus. The tensor fascia latae has a tendency to become shortened and overactive.[85]

2. Full external rotation of the leg occurs during the leg lift, indicating a substitution of hip flexion and iliopsoas activity for the true abduction movement. If the piriformis is shortened and overactive, the external rotation of the leg is reinforced.[85]

3. A lateral pelvic tilt at the initiation of movement indicates that the quadratus lumborum, which has a tendency to become shortened and overactive, is stabilizing the pelvis and is initiating the movement.[85] This is indicative of a very poor movement pattern.

Adduction. Hip adduction is tested with the patient supine, and with the uninvolved leg adducted over the other leg or held in flexion. As before, the ASIS is monitored for motion, indicating the end of range for adduction. The primary hip adductor is the adductor longus. Adaptive shortening of the hip adductors can theoretically result in inhibition of the gluteus medius, a decrease in frontal stability, ITB tendonitis, and anterior knee pain. Pain can be referred from the hip adductors into the anterolateral hip, groin, medial thigh, the anterior knee, and medial tibia. Pain in these regions with passive abduction, or active adduction, may indicate a strain of one of the adductors. The cause of the pain can be differentiated between the two-joint gracilis and the other hip adductors (longus, brevis, and pectineus) in the following manner. The patient is positioned in side lying with the tested leg supported by the clinician. The clinician places the hip into the fully abducted position and the knee is flexed (Fig. 17-17). If no pain is reproduced with this maneuver, the patient is asked to extend the knee (Fig. 17-18), thereby bringing in the gracilis, and implicating it if the pain is now reproduced. This can be confirmed with resisted hip adduction and knee flexion. If the other adductors are implicated, this can be confirmed with resisted adduction (longus and brevis) or resisted hip adduction and hip flexion (pectineus).

The strength of the hip adductor muscle group is tested in side lying, by flexing the uninvolved leg over the tested leg, or by supporting the upper leg and then applying resistance. This position also stretches the hip abductors, and can be a source of pain in the case of an iliotibial band syndrome.

The strength of the gluteus medius and minimus is tested with the patient in side lying. The patient is asked to perform hip abduction of the uppermost leg without any flexion or external rotation occurring. The clinician applies resistance to the distal thigh.

A strong and painful finding with resisted adduction is usually the result of an adductor longus lesion, whereas a painless weakness with resisted abduction is often found in a palsy of the fifth lumbar root due to a disk herniation of the same level.

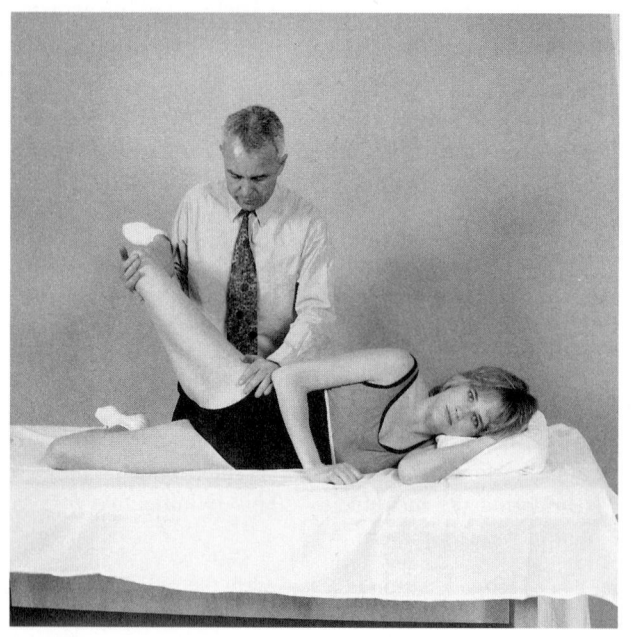

FIGURE 17-17   Hip abduction and knee flexion.

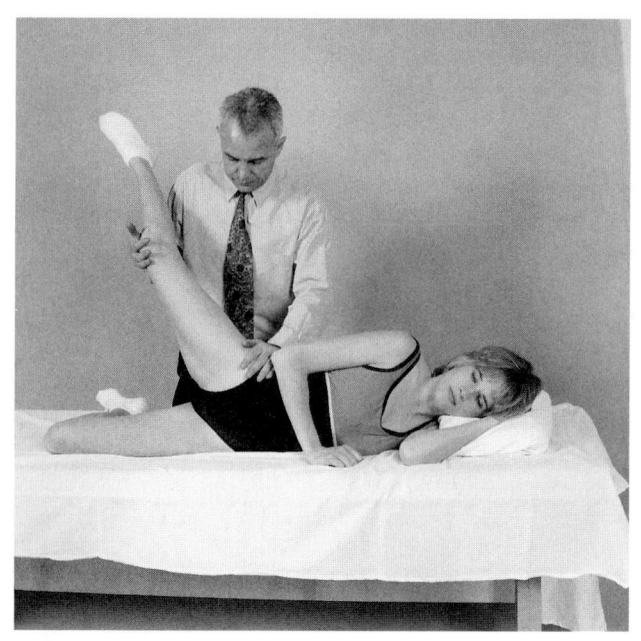

FIGURE 17-18   Hip abduction and knee extension.

Internal and External Rotation.   Although a number of muscles contribute to external rotation of the femur (see Table 17-8), six muscles function solely as external rotators.[13] These are the piriformis, gemellus superior, gemellus inferior, obturator internus, obturator externus, and quadratus femoris. Normal range of motion for hip external rotation is approximately 40 to 60 degrees. Excessive external rotation of the hip may indicate hip retroversion.

The major internal rotator of the femur is the gluteus minimus, assisted by the gluteus medius, tensor fascia latae, semitendinosus, and semimembranosus. The internal rotators of the femur are estimated to be only approximately one third the strength of the external rotators.[63] Normal range of motion for hip internal rotation is approximately 30 to 40 degrees. Excessive internal rotation of the hip may indicate hip anteversion.

If an asymmetry exists between the two positions such that more range of motion is available in the prone position compared with supine, a muscle restriction is likely present.[87] When the asymmetry of internal rotation range of motion is much greater than the external rotation range in both the hip flexed and extended positions, structural anteversion may be present.[87] If retroversion is present, the range of external rotation is greater than the range of internal rotation in both the flexed and extended positions of the hip.[87]

To assess the range of motion of the hip rotators, the patient is positioned in supine with the leg in 90 degrees of hip flexion and 90 degrees of knee flexion. Alternatively, the patient can be positioned in prone, with the knee flexed to 90 degrees and the hip in neutral (Fig. 17-19).

Functional Assessment

Table 17-9 outlines a functional assessment tool for the hip.[88] An assessment of the patient's functional status can also be made through observation or through use of a self-report measure, which allow a patient to rate his or her capacity to perform activities of daily living.

The Harris Hip Rating Scale (Table 17-10) is the most commonly used functional outcome assessment for the hip, and can be used to assess patient status following the onset of traumatic arthritis, and a variety of hip disorders.

Examination of Movement Patterns

Some of the movement patterns were assessed in the "Active, Passive, and Resistive Tests" section. One further test is described here.

Trunk Curl Up. This test assesses the patient's ability to sit up from a supine position, and assesses the relationship between the abdominal and iliopsoas muscles. The patient is positioned in supine with the hips and knees flexed, both feet flat on the bed.

During the patient's attempt to sit up from the supine position, little flexion of the trunk will be evident if the iliopsoas is dominant, as most of the flexion occurs at the hip. The patient is then asked to perform a sit-up while actively plantar flexing their ankles, thus removing the effect of the

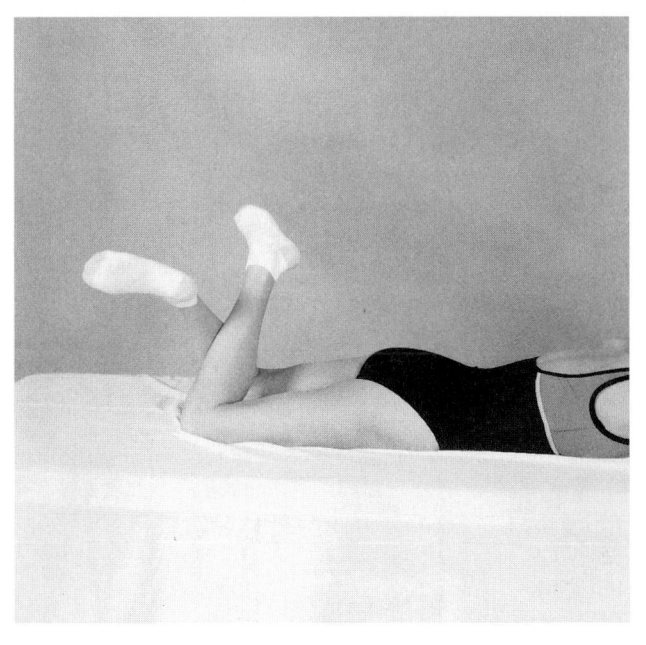

FIGURE 17-19 Hip external rotation.

TABLE 17-9 Functional Tests of the Hip

Starting Position	Action	Functional Test
Standing	Hip flexion: lift foot onto an 8-inch / 20-cm step and return	5–6 repetitions: Functional 3–4 repetitions: Functionally fair 1–2 repetitions: Functionally poor 0 repetitions: Nonfunctional
Standing	Hip extension: sit in a chair and return to standing	5–6 repetitions: Functional 3–4 repetitions: Functionally fair 1–2 repetitions: Functionally poor 0 repetitions: Nonfunctional
Standing	Hip abductors: lift leg to balance on one leg while keeping pelvis level	Hold 1–1.5 minutes: Functional Hold 30–59 seconds: Functionally fair Hold 1–29 seconds: Functionally poor Cannot hold: Nonfunctional
Standing	Hip adductors: walk sideways 6 m	6–8 m one way: Functional 3–6 m one way: Functionally fair 1–3 m one way: Functionally poor 0 m: Nonfunctional
Standing	Hip internal rotation: test leg off floor (holding onto object for balance if necessary) internally rotate non–weight-bearing hip	10–12 repetitions: Functional 5–9 repetitions: Functionally fair 1–4 repetitions: Functionally poor 0 repetitions: Nonfunctional
Standing, facing closed door	Hip external rotation: test leg off floor (holding onto object for balance if necessary) externally rotate non–weight-bearing hip	10–12 repetitions: Functional 5–9 repetitions: Functionally fair 1–4 repetitions: Functionally poor 0 repetitions: Nonfunctional

TABLE 17-10   Harris Hip Rating Scale[222]

Harris Hip Function Scale

(Circle one in each group)

Pain (44 points maximum)

None/ignores	44
Slight, occasional, no compromise in activity	40
Mild, no effect on ordinary activity, pain after unusual activity, uses aspirin	30
Moderate, tolerable, makes concessions, occasional codeine	20
Marked, serious limitations	10
Totally disabled	0

Function (47 points maximum)

Gait (walking maximum distance)(33 points maximum)

1. Limp:

None	11
Slight	8
Moderate	5
Unable to walk	0

2. Support:

None	11
Cane, long walks	7
Cane, full time	5
Crutch	4
Two canes	2
Two crutches	0
Unable to walk	0

3. Distance walked:

Unlimited	11
Six blocks	8
Two to three blocks	5
Indoors only	2
Bed and chair	0

Functional activities (14 points maximum)

1. Stairs:

Normally	4
Normally with banister	2
Any method	1
Not able	0

2. Socks and tie shoes:

With ease	4
With difficulty	2
Unable	0

3. Sitting:

Any chair, 1 hour	5
High chair, ½ hour	3
Unable to sit ½ hour any chair	0

4. Enter public transport:

Able to use public transportation	1
Not able to use public transportation	0

Absence of deformity (requires all four) (4 points maximum)

1. Fixed adduction <10°	4
2. Fixed internal rotation in extension <10°	0
3. Leg length discrepancy less than 1¼″	
4. Pelvic flexion contracture <30°	

Range of motion (5 points maximum)

Instructions

Record 10° of fixed adduction as "−10° abduction, adduction to 10°"

Similarly, 10° of fixed external rotation as "−10° internal rotation, external rotation to 10°"

Similarly, 10° of fixed external rotation with 10° further external rotation as "−10° internal rotation, external rotation to 20°"

Permanent flexion (1)_____°	Range	Index Factor	Index Value*
A. Flexion to	_____°		
(0–45°)		1.0	
(45–90°)		0.6	
(90–120°)		0.3	
(120–140°)		0.0	
B. Abduction to	_____°		
(0–15°)		0.8	
(15–30°)		0.3	
(30–60°)		0.0	
C. Adduction to	_____°		
(0–15°)		0.2	
(15–60°)		0.0	
D. External rotation in extension to	_____°		
(0–30°)		0.4	
(30–60°)		0.0	
E. Internal rotation in extension to	_____°		
(0–60°)		0.0	

*Index Value = Range × Index Factor

Total index value (A + B + C + D + E) ___

Total range of motion points ___

(multiply total index value × 0.05)

Pain points: ____

Function points: _____

Absence of deformity points: ____

Range of motion points: ____

Total points: _____

(100 points maximum)

Comments:

iliopsoas.[84] The patient progressively flexes the spine, starting at the cervical region, until the lumbar region is flexed. As soon as the iliopsoas becomes involved in the motion, the patient's feet will lift from the bed. Normally, the patient should be able to curl up so that the thoracic and lumbar spines are clear of the bed before the feet lift. A patient in excellent condition can complete a full sit-up without the feet lifting from the bed.

Passive Accessory Movements

Due to the extreme congruency of the joint partners at the hip joint, this is a difficult area to assess with any degree of accuracy, especially as the glides that occur are very slight. Thus only one accessory motion, lateral distraction, is examined.

The patient is positioned in supine with the hip and knee flexed to 90 degrees, with the knee placed on the clinician's shoulder (Fig. 17-20). The clinician places one hand over the greater trochanter and the other close to the superior aspect of the medial thigh (see Fig. 17-20). A distraction force and then a compression force are applied in line with the femoral neck. The test is positive if excessive movement is detected.

Neurological Tests

Hoppenfeld[82] advocates the conventional use of manual muscle testing and sensation testing for the neurological examination of the hip.

For sensation testing, the clinician should be aware of the dermatomal pattern as well as the areas supplied by the peripheral nerves (inferior femoral cutaneous, lateral femoral cutaneous, and posterior femoral cutaneous nerves).

Paresthesia or anesthesia is not commonly found in the buttock, hip, or groin region because of the degree of dermatome overlap. However, paresthesia in the "saddle" region should be considered indicative of a sign of cauda equina compression.

Special Tests

Special tests are merely confirmatory tests and should not be used alone to form a diagnosis. The results from these tests are used in conjunction with the other clinical findings to help guide the clinician. To assure accuracy with these tests, both sides should be tested for comparison.

Quadrant (Scour) Test. The quadrant or scour test is a dynamic test of the inner quadrant and outer quadrant of the hip joint surface.[89]

The patient is positioned in supine, close to the edge of the bed, with their hip flexed and foot resting on the bed. The clinician places one hand over the top of the patient's knee. The patient's hip is placed in 90 degrees of flexion with the knee allowed to flex comfortably. From this point, the clinician adducts the hip to the point at which the patient's pelvis begins to lift on the bed to assess the inner quadrant (Fig. 17-21). The position of flexion and adduction of the hip has the potential to compress or stress a number of structures including[89]:

► The articular surfaces of the hip joint.

► The insertion of the tensor fascia latae and the sartorius.

► The iliopsoas muscle.

► The iliopsoas bursa and neurovascular bundle.

► The insertion of the pectineus.

► The insertion of the adductor longus.

► The femoral neck.

Thus care must be taken when interpreting the results from this test. At the end range of flexion and adduction, a compression force is applied at the knee along the longitudinal axis of

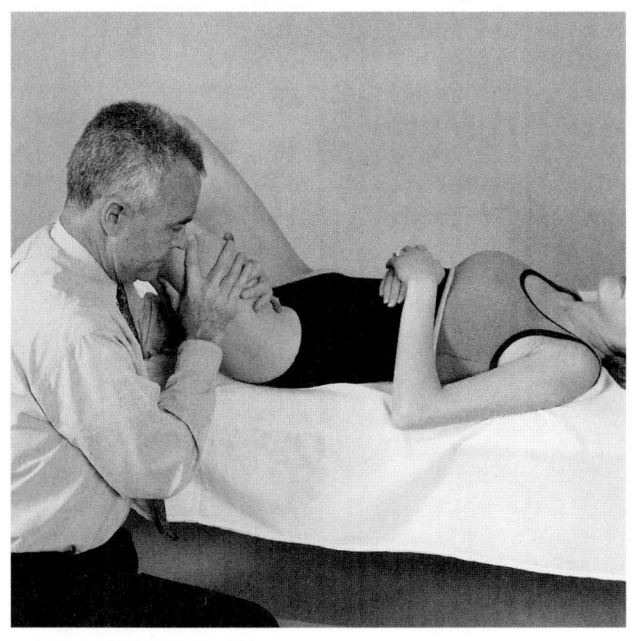

FIGURE 17-20 Hip joint distraction.

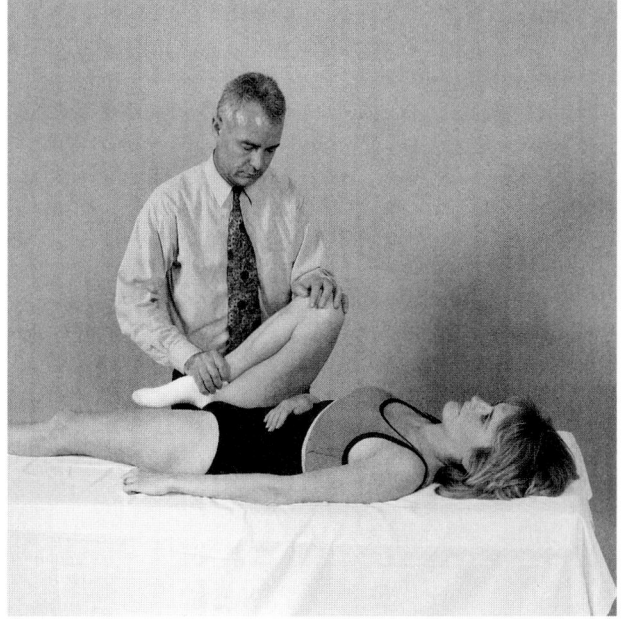

FIGURE 17-21 The scour test.

the femur. From this point, the clinician moves the hip into a position of flexion and abduction to examine the outer quadrant. Throughout the entire movement, the femur is held midway between internal and external rotation, and the movement at the hip joint should follow the smooth arc of a circle. An abnormal finding is resistance felt anywhere during the arc. The resistance may be caused by capsular tightness, an adhesion, a myofascial restriction, or a loss of joint congruity.

FABER (Flexion, Abduction, External Rotation) or Patrick's Test. The FABER test (Fig. 17-22) is a screening test for hip, lumbar, or sacroiliac joint dysfunction, or an iliopsoas spasm.

The patient is positioned in supine. The clinician places the foot of the test leg on top of the knee of the opposite leg (see Fig. 17-22) (placing the sole of the test leg foot against the medial aspect of the opposite thigh may be more comfortable for the patient with knee pathology). The clinician then slowly lowers the test leg into abduction, in the direction toward the examining table. A positive test results in pain and/or loss of motion as compared with the uninvolved side.

Having the patient demonstrate where the pain is with this test may assist with the interpretation of this test.

SI Provocation Tests. A number of tests can be used to examine the sacroiliac joint (see Chap. 27). Unless the patient history or the physical examination highlights the presence of a sacroiliac dysfunction, the clinician relies on two simple stress tests to rule out sacroiliac pathology, the anterior gapping (Fig. 17-23) and posterior gapping (Fig. 17-24) tests.

In addition to the provocative tests, the passive motions of the hip can be examined with the innominate stabilized. The hip motions and their respective innominate motions in parenthesis are outlined in Table 17-11.

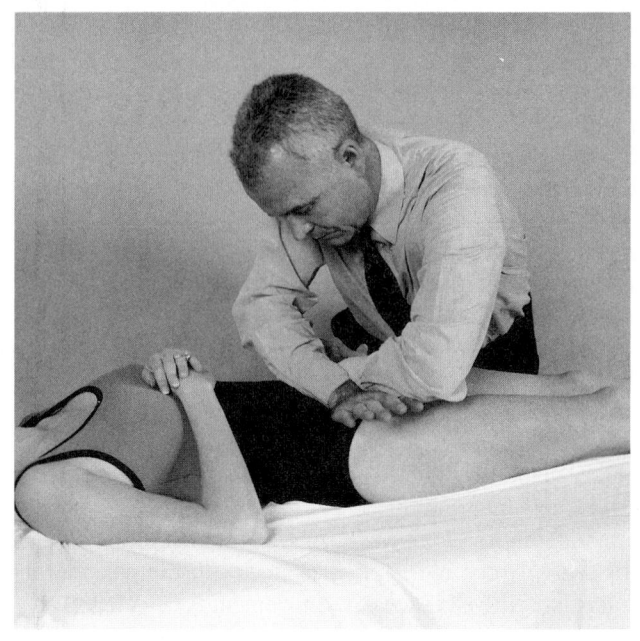

FIGURE 17-23   Anterior gapping of SI joint.

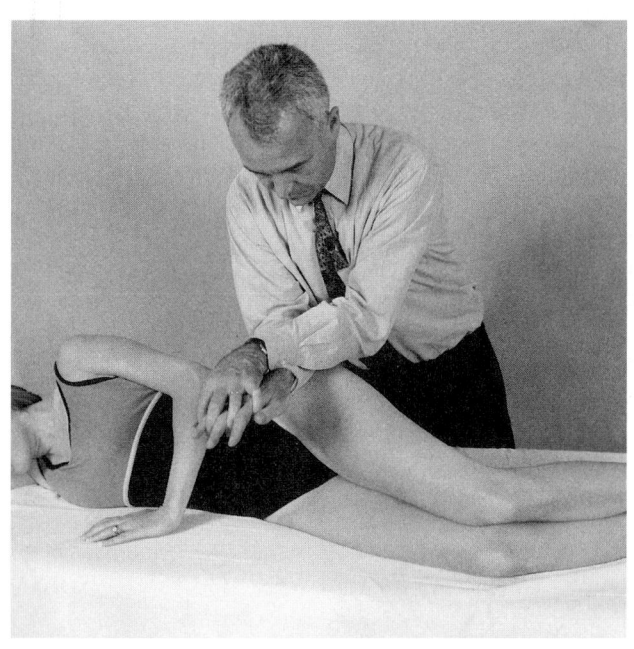

FIGURE 17-24   Posterior gapping of SI joint.

TABLE 17-11   Hip Motion and Associated Innominate Motions

Flexion (posterior rotation)
Extension (anterior rotation)
Abduction (upward)
Adduction (downward)
Internal rotation (IR)
External rotation (ER)

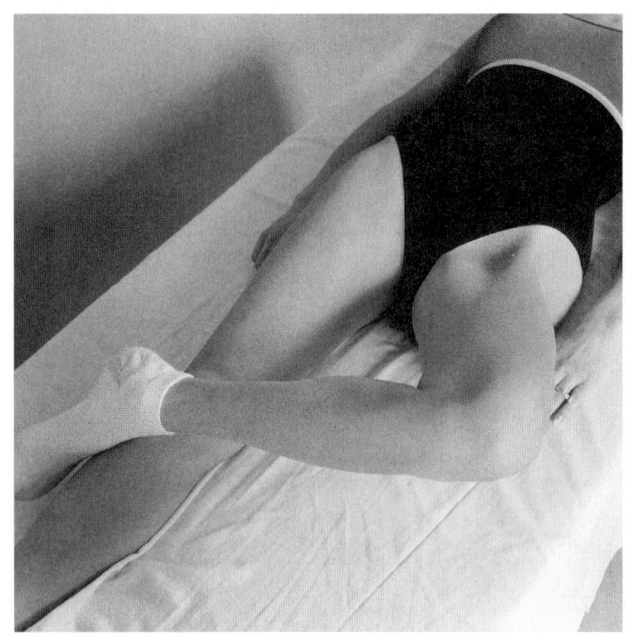

FIGURE 17-22   The FABER test.

Craig Test. The Craig test is used to assess femoral anteversion/retroversion. The patient is positioned in prone with the knee flexed to 90 degrees. The clinician rotates the hip through the full ranges of hip internal and external rotation while palpating the greater trochanter and determining the point in the range at which the greater trochanter is the most prominent laterally. If the angle is greater than 8 to 15 degrees in the direction of internal rotation when measured from the vertical and long axis of the tibia, the femur is considered to be in anteversion.[43,48,87,90]

One study[90] showed this test to be accurate to within 4 degrees of intraoperative measurements, for the assessment of femoral anteversion/retroversion, and was more accurate than radiographic measurement techniques.

Flexion-Adduction Test. This test is used as a screening test for early hip pathology.[91] The patient is positioned in supine and the hip is passively flexed to 90 degrees and in neutral rotation. From this position the clinician stabilizes the pelvis and the hip is passively adducted. The resultant end-feel, restriction, discomfort, or pain is noted and compared with the normal side.

Trendelenburg Sign. The Trendelenburg sign indicates weakness of the gluteus medius muscle during unilateral weight bearing. This position produces a strong contraction of the gluteus medius, which is powerfully assisted by the gluteus minimus and tensor fascia latae, in order to keep the pelvis horizontal. For example, when the body weight is supported by the right foot, the right hip abductors contract isometrically and eccentrically to prevent the left side of the pelvis from being pulled downward.

The clinician crouches or kneels behind the patient with their eyes level with the patient's pelvis, and ensures that the patient does not lean to one side during the testing. The patient is asked to stand on one limb for approximately 30 seconds and the clinician notes whether the pelvis remains level. If the hip remains level, the test is negative. A positive Trendelenburg sign is indicated if during unilateral weight bearing the pelvis drops toward the unsupported limb (Fig. 17-25). A number of dysfunctions can produce the Trendelenburg sign. These include a superior gluteal nerve palsy, a lumbar disk herniation, weakness of the gluteus medius, and advanced degeneration of the hip.

Pelvic Drop Test.[92] The patient is asked to place one foot on a 20-cm (8-inch) stool or step and to stand up straight. The patient then lowers the non–weight bearing leg to the floor. On lowering the leg there should be no arm abduction, anterior or pelvic motion, or trunk flexion, nor should there be any hip adduction or internal rotation of the weight-bearing hip. These compensations are indications of an unstable hip or weak external rotators.

Sign of the Buttock. To test for the presence of this syndrome (refer to Chap. 9), the patient is positioned in supine. The clinician performs a passive unilateral straight leg raise. If there is a unilateral restriction, the clinician flexes the knee and notes whether the hip flexion increases. If the restriction was due to the lumbar spine or hamstrings, hip flexion increases. If the hip flexion does not increase when the knee is flexed, it is a positive sign of the buttock

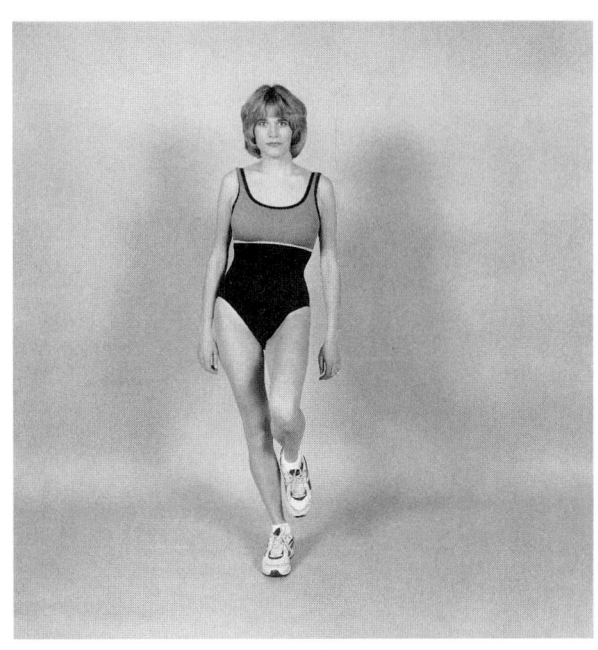

FIGURE 17-25 Positive Trendelenburg.

test. If the sign of the buttock is encountered, the patient must be immediately returned to the physician for further investigation.

Muscle Length Tests

Thomas Test and Modified Thomas Test. The original Thomas test was designed to test the flexibility of the iliopsoas complex, but has since been modified and expanded to assess a number of other soft tissue structures.

The original test involved positioning the patient in supine, with one knee held to the chest at the point when the lumbar spine begins to flex (Fig. 17-26). The clinician assesses whether the thigh of the extended leg maintains full contact with the surface of the bed. If the thigh is raised off the surface of the treatment table, the test is positive. A positive test indicates a decrease in flexibility in the rectus femoris or iliopsoas muscles or both.

A modified version to this test is commonly used. For the modified version, the patient is positioned in sitting at the end of the bed. From this position the patient is asked to lie down, while bringing both knees against the chest. Once in this position, the patient is asked to perform a posterior pelvic tilt. While the contralateral hip is held in maximum hip flexion with the arms, the tested limb is lowered over the end of the bed towards the floor (Fig. 17-27). In this position, the thigh should be parallel with the bed, in neutral rotation, and neither abducted nor adducted, with the lower leg perpendicular to the thigh and in neutral rotation. There should be 100 to 110 degrees of knee flexion present with the thigh in full contact with the table.

If the thigh is raised off the treatment table, a decrease in the flexibility of the iliopsoas muscle complex should be suspected. If the rectus femoris is adaptively shortened, the amount of knee extension should increase with the application of overpressure into hip extension.[84] If the decrease in flexibility lies with the

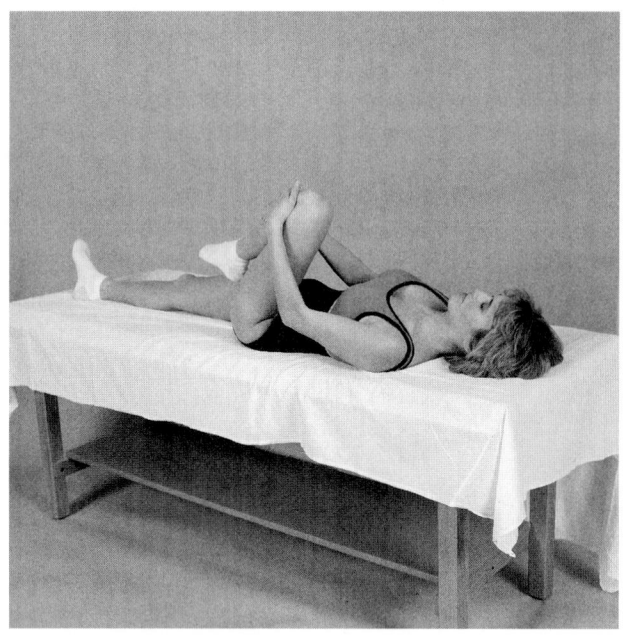

FIGURE 17-26   Thomas test.

iliopsoas, attempts to correct the hip position should result in an increase in the external rotation of the thigh.[84]

The application of overpressure into knee flexion can also be used. If the increase in knee flexion produces an increase in hip flexion (the thigh rises higher off the bed), the rectus femoris is implicated, whereas if the overpressure produces no change in the degree of hip flexion, the iliopsoas is implicated.

This test can also be used to assess the flexibility of the tensor fascia latae, if the hip of the tested leg is maximally

adducted while monitoring the ipsilateral ASIS for motion. There should be 20 degrees of hip adduction available.

Two things must be remembered when interpreting the results of this test.

▶ The criteria are arbitrary and have been shown to vary between genders, limb dominance, and depend on the types and the levels of activity undertaken by the individual.[93]

▶ The apparent tightness might simply be normal tissue tension producing a deviation of the leg due to an increased flexibility of the antagonists.

As always, the cause of the asymmetry must be found (or at least looked for) and addressed.

Ely's Test.   This is a test to assess the flexibility of the rectus femoris. The patient is positioned in prone and the knee is flexed. If the rectus is tight, the pelvis is observed to anteriorly rotate early in the range of knee flexion, and the hip flexes.

Ober's Test.   The Ober's test is used to evaluate tightness of the iliotibial band and tensor fascia latae (see also Thomas test).[94] The patient is placed in the side lying position, and with the hip extended and abducted and the knee flexed, the proximal part of the leg is allowed to drop passively onto the contralateral limb (Fig. 17-28). The test is considered positive when the leg fails to lower. There have been some doubts expressed as to the reliability of Ober's test as a measure for ITB tightness.[95]

Straight Leg Raise Test for Hamstring Length.   The patient is positioned in supine with the legs together and extended. The clinician stands on the side of the leg to be tested and grasps the

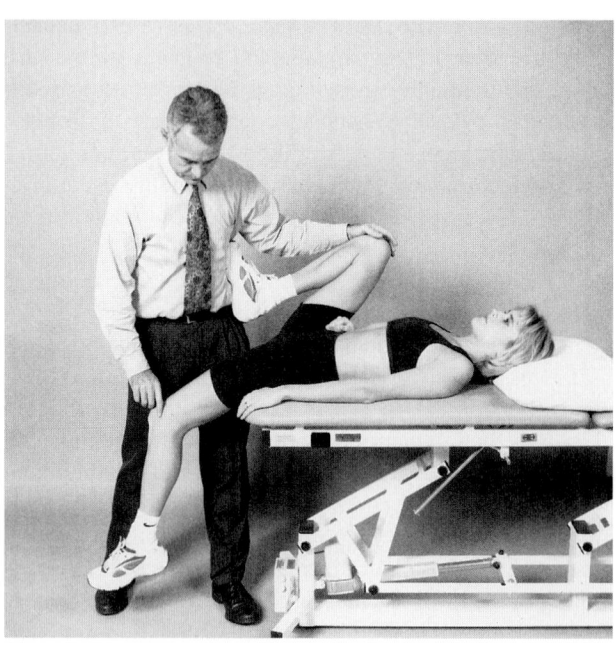

FIGURE 17-27   Modified Thomas test.

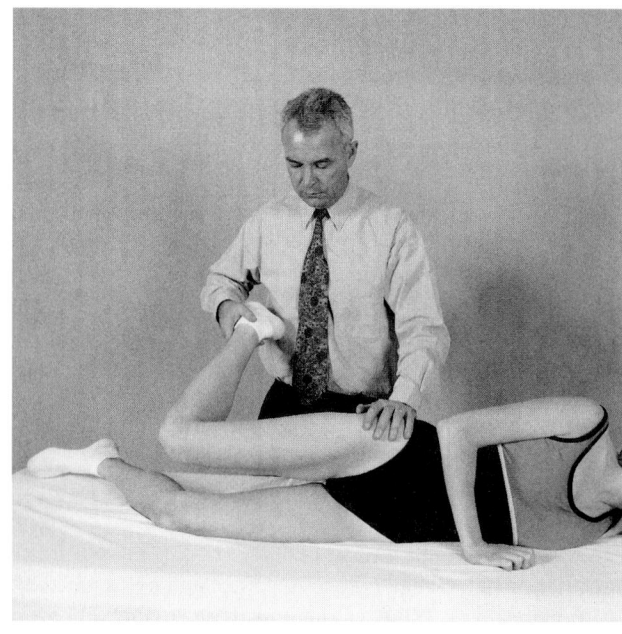

FIGURE 17-28   Ober's test.

patient's ankle with one hand, while placing the other hand on the patient's opposite anterior superior iliac spine. With the patient's knee extended, the clinician lifts the patient's leg, flexing the hip until motion is felt at the opposite anterior superior iliac spine. The angle of flexion from the treatment table is measured. The clinician returns the leg to the table and repeats the maneuver from the other side of the table with the other leg. The hamstrings are considered shortened if a straight leg cannot be raised to an angle of 80 degrees from the horizontal, while the other leg is straight.[72] Any limitation of flexion is interpreted as being caused by adaptively shortened hamstring muscles.

This straight leg raise test may also be used as a screen for adverse neural tension, particularly of the sciatic nerve (see Chap. 12).

90-90 Straight Leg Raise.   The hamstring length can also be assessed with the patient positioned in supine and the tested leg flexed at the hip and knee to 90 degrees. From this position, the patient is asked to extend the knee of the involved side without extending the hip (Fig. 17-29). The measurement is taken at the first resistance barrier.

Piriformis.   The patient is positioned in supine. The clinician flexes the involved hip to 60 degrees. After stabilizing the patient's pelvis, the clinician applies a downward pressure through the femur, and maximally adducts the involved hip. From this position, the hip is moved into internal rotation and then external rotation. Internal rotation stresses the superior fibers, while external rotation stresses the inferior fibers. Normal range of motion should be 45 degrees into either rotation.

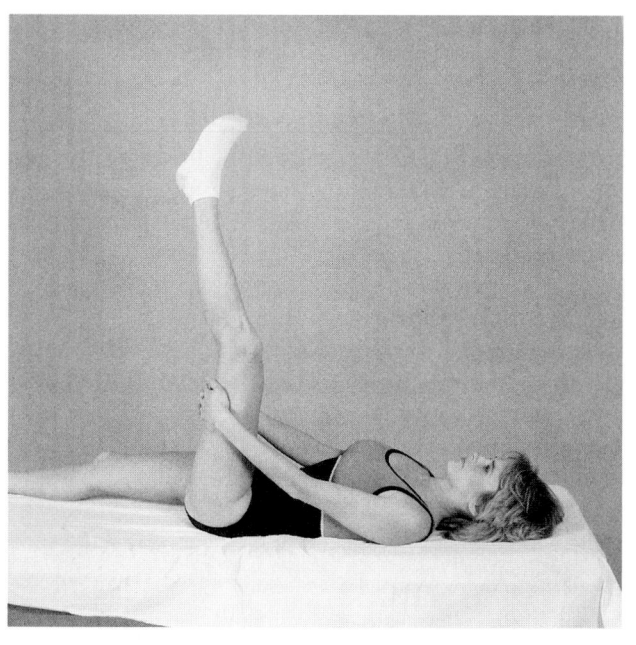

FIGURE 17-29 90-90 straight leg raise.

Hip Adductors.   The patient is positioned supine with the leg to be tested close to the edge of the mat table. The leg not to be tested is 15 to 25 degrees abducted at the hip joint with the heel over the end of the mat table. Maintaining the tested knee in extension, the clinician passively abducts the tested leg. The normal range is 40 degrees. When the full range is reached, the knee of the tested leg is passively flexed and the leg abducted further. If the maximum range does not increase when the knee is flexed, the one-joint adductors (pectineus, adductor magnus, adductor longus, adductor brevis) are shortened. If the range does increase with the knee passively flexed, the two-joint adductors (gracilis, biceps femoris, semimebranosus, and semitendinosus) are shortened.

Leg Length Discrepancy.   The test for a leg length discrepancy is best performed radiographically. However, the following clinical test can be used to highlight the more significant discrepancies.

The patient is positioned in supine and the clinician palpates the anterior superior iliac spine. From this point, the clinician slides distally into the depression and then measures from this point to the tip of the malleolus, making sure that the course of the tape follows the same route for both legs.

Fulcrum Test.   The fulcrum test[96] is used to test for the presence of a stress fracture of the femoral shaft. The patient is positioned in sitting with their knees bent over the edge of the bed and feet dangling. A firm towel roll is placed under the involved thigh, and is moved proximal to distal as gentle pressure is applied to the dorsum of the knee with the clinician's hand. A positive test is when the patient reports sharp pain or expresses apprehension when the fulcrum arm is placed under the fracture site.

Pediatric Screening Tests for Congenital (CHD) or Developmental (DDH) Dysplasia of the Hip.   The value of the neonatal hip screening examination remains controversial.[97] At present, tests including the ones outlined below are currently used to examine the infant. The examination requires patience and skill and the newborn must be relaxed on a firm surface.

The examiner attempts to reduce the dislocation or subluxation using the Ortolani (Fig. 17-30) and Barlow (see Fig. 17-30) maneuvers.[97]

With the newborn supine, the clinician places the tips of the long and index fingers over the greater trochanter, with the thumb along the medial thigh. The infant's leg is positioned in neutral rotation with 90 degrees of hip flexion, and is gently abducted while lifting the leg anteriorly.[97] With abduction one can feel a clunk as the femoral head slides over the posterior rim of the acetabulum and into the socket (see Fig. 17-30). This is the clunk originally described by Ortolani.[98] This is called the sign of entry, as the hip relocates with this maneuver. Maintaining the same position, the leg is then gently adducted while gentle pressure is directed posteriorly on the knee, and a palpable clunk is noted as the femoral head slides over the posterior rim of the acetabulum and out of the socket.[97] This clunk was

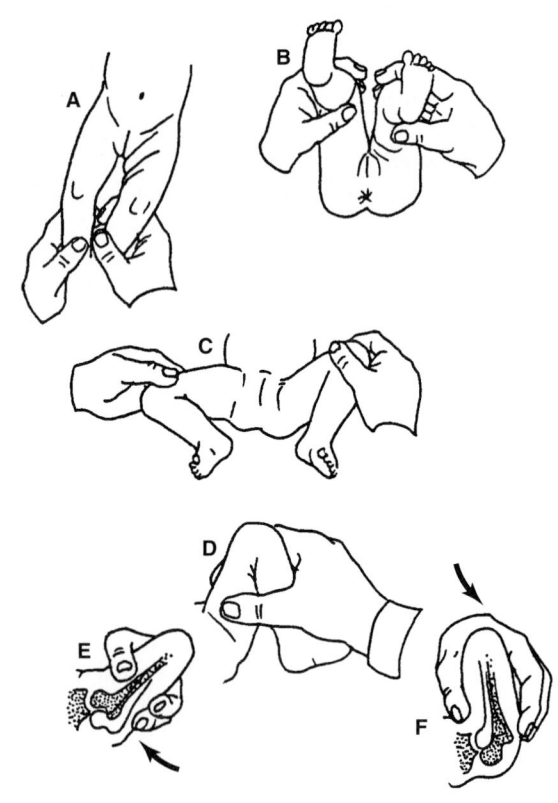

FIGURE 17-30 Screening tests for developmental dislocation. A. Asymmetric skin folds. B. Galeazzi's test. C. Limitation of abduction. D, E, F. Ortolani's and Barlow's tests. (Reproduced with permission from Skinner HB. *Current Diagnosis and Treatment in Orthopedics*, 2nd ed. New York: McGraw-Hill; 2000.)

originally described by Barlow,[99] and it is called the sign of exit, as the hip dislocates with this maneuver. Both tests are designed to detect motion between the femoral head and the acetabulum.[97] The reproducibility of these tests is dependent on ligamentous or capsular laxity, which usually disappears by 10 to 12 weeks of age.[97]

In the 3- to 12-month-old infant, the best physical finding is a limitation of hip abduction. In the supine position, with the hip in 90 degrees of flexion and one hand stabilizing the pelvis, each hip should easily abduct to 75 degrees and adduct to 30 degrees past the midline.[97]

In addition to the special tests, the clinician looks for asymmetry between the lower extremities. Asymmetric thigh folds, a short leg appearance, or a prominent greater trochanter may be significant findings.[97]

Once a child is ambulatory the physical signs are more noticeable. There is a typical limp and the child often toe-walks on the affected side. If both hips are dislocated, increased lumbar lordosis, prominent buttocks, and a waddling gait pattern are noted.[97] When the patient is asked to stand on the affected leg, the pelvis drops to the opposite side and the trunk leans toward the affected side (positive Trendelenburg test).[97]

In addition to the clinical tests, both CHD and DDH can be detected with radiographs or ultrasound (see "Intervention").

Intervention Strategies

The hip joint and surrounding tissues is prone to soft tissue injuries, impingement syndromes, muscle imbalances of strength and flexibility, and joint dysfunctions. It is also an area of symptom referral from other regions. The intervention of the hip joint must take into account the influences that the lumbar spine, pelvis, and lower extremities can have on this area. It is imperative that the clinician views the hip as part of a kinetic chain extending from the foot to the lumbar spine. A dysfunction in any part of this kinetic chain can have either a direct or indirect affect on hip function and symptoms.

The techniques to increase joint mobility and soft tissue extensibility are described in the "Therapeutic Techniques" section.

Acute Phase

During the acute phase, the principles of PRICEMEM (protection, rest, ice, compression, elevation, manual therapy, early motion, and medication) are applied as appropriate. Elevation of the hip joint is usually not applicable or possible. The goals of the acute phase include:

► Protection of the injury site.

► Restoration of pain-free range of motion in the entire kinetic chain.

► Improve patient comfort by decreasing pain and inflammation.

► Retard muscle atrophy.

► Minimize detrimental effects of immobilization and activity restriction.[100–105]

► Maintain general fitness.

► Patient to be independent with home exercise program.

The promotion and progression of healing may involve decreasing the weight-bearing function of the hip through rest, modification of activity, or by using an assistive device. Assistive devices may be necessary to offset the load through the hip joint and promote a symmetric gait pattern.[60,106] Use of a walker for maximum functional ambulation and safety may be required for other patients.[60]

The use of shoes with specially made cushion heels may further aid in diminishing pain on initiation of weight bearing.

According to patient tolerance, the clinician should also attempt to remove any other stresses to the hip joint such as joint restrictions in the lumbar spine or sacroiliac joint, and any muscle imbalances.

The approach during this phase may depend on the specific tissue involved:

► Contractile tissue lesions are treated with rest, gentle friction massage, gentle isometric exercises, pain-free range-of-motion exercises, and appropriate modalities.

▶ Articular lesions are best treated with positioning in the open-packed position (flexion, abduction and external rotation) and grade I and II joint mobilizations.

A progressive stretching program is initiated for those muscles that are prone to adaptive shortening. These include the hip flexors, short hip adductors, sartorius, piriformis, rectus femoris, hamstrings, tensor fascia latae, and iliotibial band. The stretches can be performed using postisometric relaxation techniques, myofascial release, and other manual techniques (see "Techniques" section). Self-stretching is taught to the patient (Fig. 17-31). The stretching is performed in conjunction with facilitation and re-education techniques to the muscles that are prone to be weak or inhibited. These include the glutei muscles and the lumbar erector spinae.

Once the muscle imbalances are addressed, the patient may progress to sensorimotor stimulation through balance and coordination retraining. These activities are usually performed in weight bearing, provided there are no contraindications (pain or instability) to weight bearing and resistance.[60] Wherever possible, active exercises are performed within a functional context. Simultaneous contraction of hip extensors and abductors in weight bearing is the normal co-activation pattern used in early stance-phase gait.[60,80] Exercises and balance training in standing can be used to reinforce this pattern. Initially the balance exercises are performed with double limb support and then progressed to single leg support as the patient progresses. Once the static weight-bearing exercises in double limb support can be performed, gait activities are introduced. Gait involves the integration of the entire lower kinetic chain. Dysfunctions of gait are typically related to biomechanical alterations occurring during the swing and/or stance phases of gait.[60] Such dysfunctions include pain on weight bearing or move-

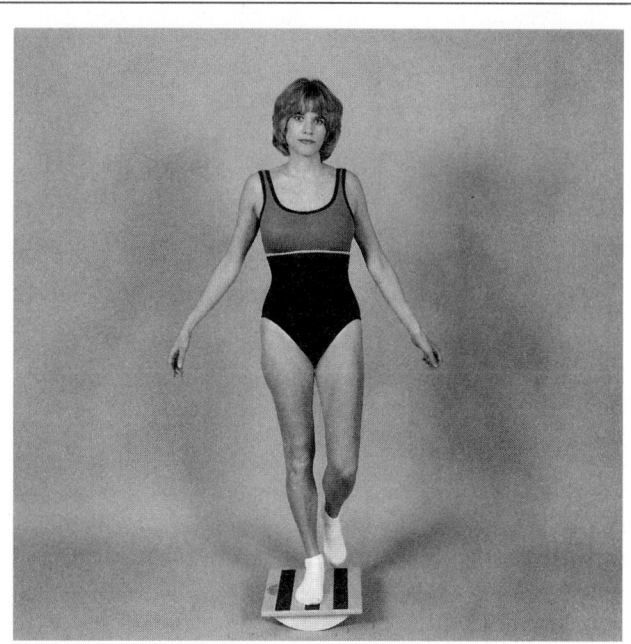

FIGURE 17-32 Weight shift and balance exercise.

ment, joint range restrictions, functional muscle weakness, leg length discrepancy, or deformity (see Chap. 13).[60] Gait-training procedures[107,108] for the stance phase involve the use of manual contacts at the pelvis to guide and stretch, and to apply joint approximation or resistance. These exercises promote the development of appropriate patterns of neuromuscular control. A balance board can be used for weight shift practice (Fig. 17-32). Unilateral stance activities may also be performed (Fig. 17-33).

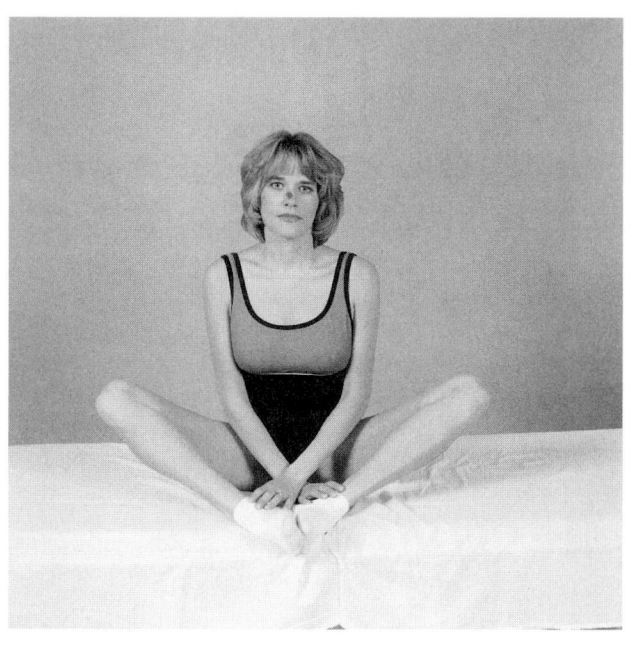

FIGURE 17-31 Self-stretch for hip joint.

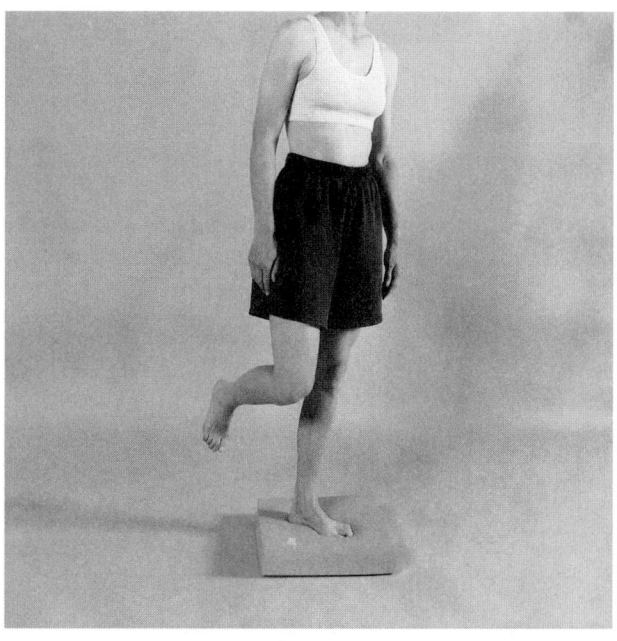

FIGURE 17-33 Unilateral stance exercise.

The essential components of normal swing-phase gait[80,108] to develop are:

▶ Forward rotation of the pelvis on swing-phase flexion of the hip.

▶ Pelvic dip (drop) of approximately 5 degrees on the side of swing limb.

▶ Flexion of the hip to a maximum of 30 degrees (activation of hip flexors) with kinematic knee flexion and dorsiflexion.

Active hip flexion with adduction, knee flexion, and dorsiflexion in standing simulates the normal swing phase of gait and promotes balance control in weight bearing on the contralateral stance leg.[60] A multi-hip machine can be introduced as the hip muscles become stronger.

Functional exercises such as sit-stand-sit require simultaneous activation of hip muscles coordinated with other trunk and limb patterns normally used to accomplish the activity.[60] Likewise, task-oriented exercise programs (work hardening) should be instituted for the patient who intends to resume a type of employment that requires a predetermined level of work performance.

Cardiovascular fitness can be maintained during this phase using an upper body ergonometer. If tolerated, a stationary bicycle can be used.

Functional Phase

The patient progresses to the functional stage once there is no pain and when the range of motion is equal to that of the uninvolved limb. The patient should also be able to perform normal walking and daily activities without pain. The goals of the functional phase include:

▶ Attain full range of pain-free motion.

▶ Restore normal joint kinematics.

▶ Improve muscle strength to within normal limits.

▶ Improve neuromuscular control.

▶ Restore normal muscle force couple relationships.

The following exercises are recommended during this phase:

▶ Quadruped exercises incorporating rocking forwards and backwards. These exercises help to stretch the joint capsule and apply joint compression.

▶ Lunging, squatting, and hip circumduction. These exercises simulate weight bearing while increasing range of motion and stretching the capsule.

▶ Open chain exercises using cuff weights or tubing may be used to develop strength and endurance of all of the hip musculature. The exercises are initially performed using concentric contractions and then advanced to eccentric contractions.

▶ Bridging. Bridging utilizes body weight as a resistance force to the hip extensors and abductors.[60] Manually applied resistance can be superimposed on the pelvis or thighs to generate maximal muscular tension in the contracting muscles.

▶ Strengthening of the gluteus medius muscle is often an important component of the hip rehabilitation program. The gluteus medius can be strengthened in side lying, with the upper leg in slight hip extension and external rotation (Fig. 17-34), or in standing with the pelvic drop exercise (Fig. 17-35). The pelvic drop exercise involves standing on a step with the involved leg, and lowering the uninvolved leg off the step while keeping both knees locked.

▶ The stationary bicycle is used to increase lower extremity strength, endurance, and range during repetitive reciprocal movements of the lower extremities.[60] Electromyographic analysis of lower limb muscles during pedaling has shown that the highest peak of activity for the gluteus maximus and biceps femoris muscles as hip extensors occurred during the pedal downstroke.[109] Stationary bicycling has also been found to be as effective for increasing range of motion at the hip joint as static stretching.[110] The stationary bicycle is a convenient mode of exercise for home use; however, the use of vigorous protocols should be carefully monitored for cardiac effects, especially in light of the fact that both blood pressure and heart rates have been found to increase markedly during this type of exercise.[60,111]

▶ Pool walking, swimming, and kicking may also be incorporated.

Neuromuscular re-education exercises for the hip are prescribed to emphasize specific movement patterns and sequencing of muscle contractions. These exercises demand a high level of control and coordination.[112–115] Ambulation activities can be used initially, progressing to more difficult unilateral extremity exercises.

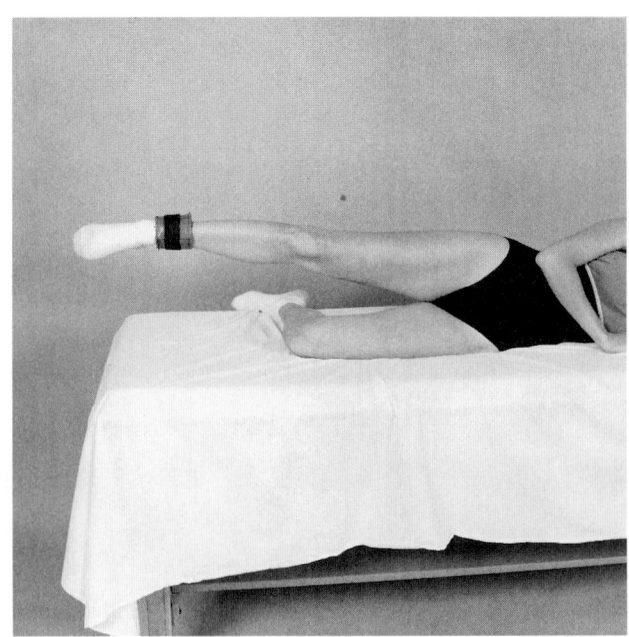

FIGURE 17-34   Hip abductor strengthening.

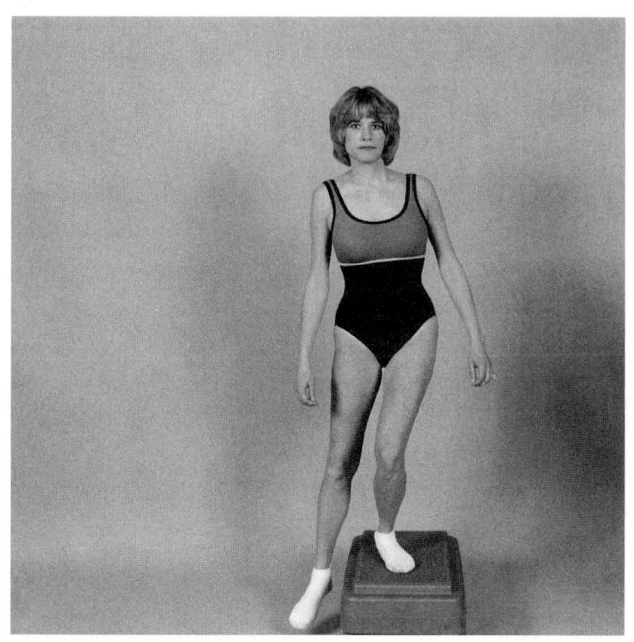

FIGURE 17-35   Pelvic drop exercise.

The following exercises are recommended to help correct the muscle sequence patterns.

Hip Extension
Method 1.   This exercise focuses on the gluteus maximus and the lumbar paraspinals. The patient is positioned in prone with two pillows under their abdomen to position the hip joint in slight flexion. The patient is asked to perform a unilateral gluteal set and to slowly lift the ipsilateral leg off the mat table. The opposite hand of the patient can be placed over the lumbar paraspinals to palpate for contraction of the contralateral paraspinal muscles prior to the ipsilateral muscle. Once the patient is able to perform the correct sequence, concentric and eccentric progressions are added.

Method 2.   This exercise focuses on the latissimus dorsi, multifidus, and gluteal group. The patient is positioned in standing and leaning over a table edge, with a pillow under the abdomen. The patient positions their pelvis in the functional neutral position and maintains this while performing a pivot-prone shoulder retraction movement, as though trying to put their elbow in their back pocket. While this movement is sustained, the patient adds hip extension of the contralateral hip to facilitate the gluteal group. The exercise is repeated for as long as the control and quality can be maintained.

Hip Abduction
Method 1.   This exercise focuses on the gluteus medius, minimus, and tensor fascia latae. The patient is positioned in the side lying position and a pillow is placed under the contralateral hip. While maintaining the pelvis perpendicular to the floor, the patient lifts the uppermost leg toward the ceiling, making sure that their pelvis does not roll backwards and introduce substitution by the hip flexors.

Method 2.   This exercise focuses on the gluteus medius and minimus. The patient stands with a length of tubing around one ankle. The patient maintains a functional neutral position while the patient steps outward with the leg with the surgical tubing on it (Fig. 17-36), thereby performing a combination of open- and closed-chain abduction.

Once the patient is able to demonstrate a high level of control and coordination with a specific movement, further resistance is added.

Proprioceptive neuromuscular facilitation (PNF) patterns performed as maximally resisted isotonic motions can be considered as a manual isokinetic exercise. The clinician uses varying amounts of resistance throughout the range of movement to match the patient's maximal effort. Optimal patterns for application of stretch, resistance, and proprioceptive joint stimuli have been outlined for each of the hip muscles. The PNF patterns can also be performed isometrically against resistance at any point in the range of joint motion.

A more aggressive protocol needs to be adopted for the returning athlete. These exercise programs attempt to incorporate activities that simulate the actual circumstances and patterns of contraction used in the sport.[60,116] Examples of two such protocols are outlined in Table 17-12 and 17-13.

Practice Pattern 4A: Primary Prevention/Risk Factor Reduction for Skeletal Demineralization

Idiopathic Transient Osteoporosis of the Hip
Osteoporosis is the most prevalent bone disease among the aging population, and osteoporotic hip fractures account for substantial morbidity, mortality, and health care costs.[117] Two

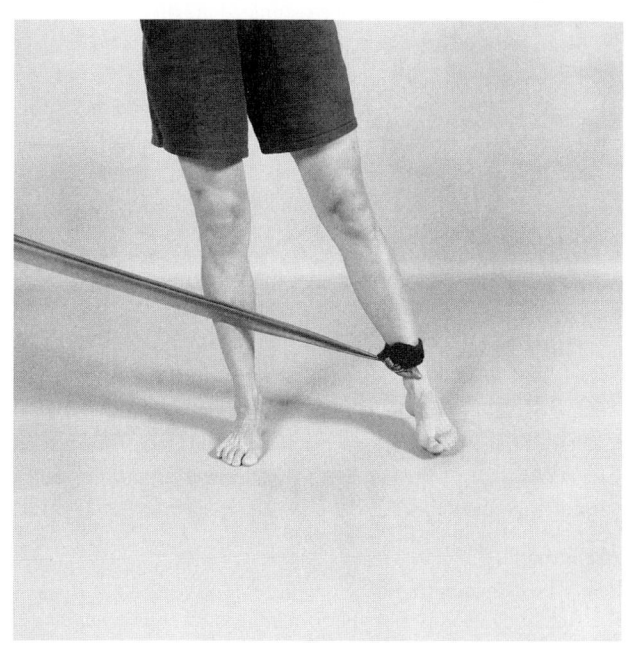

FIGURE 17-36   Closed- and open-chain hip exercise.

TABLE 17-12   Return to Sport for Runners Following Soft Tissue Injury[223]

Aerobic Capacity and Endurance

Cycling

- Incorporating appropriate warm-up and cool-down intervals, cardiovascular conditioning may be performed on stationary or regular bicycle as symptoms permit.
- Attention to proper bike fit is important, as hip and back pain may result from improper biking biomechanics.
- If biking has not been used as a cross-training method in the past, an appropriate base building period is necessary:
  - 3 to 5 minute warm-up at 70 to 90 rpm, at 55 to 65% of age-estimated maximum heart rate.
  - 10 to 15 minutes at 80 to 90 rpm, at 70 to 75% of age-estimated maximum heart rate, building this phase at no more than 3 to 5 minutes per session as symptoms and cardiovascular condition permit.
  - 3 to 5 minute cool-down at 70 rpm, at 55 to 65% of age-estimated maximum heart rate.

Aqua jogging

- Deep-water jogging has been shown to be an effective mode of cross-training for runners, with good specificity of carryover.
- Use of a flotation device (Wet Vest) will enhance the comfort of beginners.
- Appropriate warm-up and cool-down intervals should be incorporated, as well as a base building period if this is an unfamiliar activity.

Running

As soon as symptoms permit, a return to running should be initiated. This should consist of level-ground or treadmill running at first, at a speed that brings the heart rate no higher than 60% of age-estimated maximum (warm-up pace), for durations that do not exacerbate symptoms (generally less than 15 minutes). As symptoms permit, duration (mileage) should be increased by no more than 10% per week. Once a substantial base of mileage has been built with no return of symptoms, the addition of speed-specific training may be incorporated. This may consist of "fartlek" (short bursts of acceleration within a longer run) or "tempo" (runs of longer duration at or near race pace), or it may be more regimented intervals using a track and stopwatch.

- For marathoners, the distance covered on any interval may range from 400 meters at 10K race pace to 3 to 5 miles at marathon race pace.
- For shorter-distance runners, the intervals would be relatively shorter. For example, a 10K racer may do intervals of 100 to 400 meters at 5K-race pace and 400 meters up to 2 miles at 10K-race pace.

Speed-specific intervals should be performed no more than once per week initially and should be pursued cautiously. Total speedwork distance should make up no more than 10% of total weekly mileage.

Additional strengthening may be obtained with the incorporation of hill repeats.

Specific hill training should be performed no more than twice per week and pursued cautiously.

- Monitoring of heart rate will assist in avoiding excessive speed on the uphill.
- Maintaining proper form on the downhill will reduce risk of impact injuries.
- To avoid overuse injury, periodization of mileage, terrain, interval training, proper footwear, etc., is crucial. For example, the following beginning marathon training schedule demonstrates good periodization of intensity, duration, and terrain:
  - Sun: 10 miles at 70% of age-estimated maximum heart rate on rolling trails
  - Mon: 3 miles at 70% of age-estimated maximum heart rate on rolling hills.
  - Tues: 6 miles at 70% of age-estimated maximum heart rate on rolling hills.
  - Wed: Off, or alternate form of training (e.g., swimming, biking)
  - Thur: 5 miles, consisting of 1-mile warm-up, 2 to 3 miles of interval work at 80 to 85% of age-estimated maximum heart rate, and 1-mile cool-down (track).
  - Fri: 3 miles at 70% of age-estimated maximum heart rate on flat pavement.
  - Sat: Off, or alternate form of training.

Balance/Proprioceptive Re-education

Balance/Reach drills

The following exercises are performed at 3 to 5 sets of 10 to 15 reaches.

- Unilateral stance balancing, reaching one or both arms in various directions to maximum distance, avoiding use of other leg for counterbalance. Additional challenges can be added by holding a light weight or medicine ball or by using resistive tubing.
- Anterior reach. The anterior reach stimulates hamstrings, soleus, gastrocnemius, and hip/back extensors (depending on height of reach).
- Posterior overhead reach. The posterior overhead reach stimulates the gluteals, quadriceps, hip/back extensors.
- Rotational reach to side. This reaching exercise stimulates the gluteals, quadriceps, trunk stabilizers, hip abductors, and abdominals.

Strengthening

Open-kinetic chain exercises

The following exercises are performed using weight machines, cuff weights, or resistive tubing: 3 to 5 sets of 15 to 18 repetitions.

- Hip flexion
- Hip extension

TABLE 17-12 *(cont.)*

- Hip abduction
- Hip adduction

Closed-kinetic chain functional exercises

The following exercises are performed: 3 to 5 sets of 15 to 18 repetitions, observing for deterioration of proper form due to fatigue.

Squats. Progression is made from mini-squats to deeper squats as symptoms permit, with additional challenges from additional weight.

Lunges. Progression is made from straight anterior/posterior and lateral lunges to rotational lunges as appropriate, increasing distance lunged or using additional weight as appropriate.

Step-ups/step-downs. Variations are made with step height and direction of step (lateral, anterior, posterior, or rotational) as appropriate, with additional challenges of increasing distance from step or use of additional weight as appropriate.

Flexibility

Flexibility exercises

These exercises are performed once the athlete has warmed-up. For example, after walking at least 3 to 5 minutes, or after a warm shower or bath. Emphasis should be on proper technique and form. The stretch should be held for at least 15 to 30 seconds.

The patient performs 3 to 5 repetitions of each stretch on both sides on a regular basis.

- Gastrocnemius/soleus
- Hamstrings
- Quadriceps
- Gluteals
- Psoas

TABLE 17-13 Return to Sport Following Osteitis Pubis[173]

Phase I

1. Static adduction against soccer ball placed between feet when lying supine; each adduction is held for 30 seconds and is repeated ten times.
2. Abdominal sit-ups performed both in straight direction and in oblique direction. The patient performs five sets to fatigue.
3. Combined abdominal sit-up and hip flexion (crunch). The patient starts from supine position and with a soccer/basketball placed between knees. The patient performs five sets to fatigue.
4. Balance training on wobble board for 5 min.
5. One-foot exercises on sliding board, with parallel feet as well as with a 90 degree angle between feet. Five sets of 1-minute continuous work are performed with each leg, and in both positions.

Phase II (from third week)

1. Leg abduction and adduction exercises in side lying on side. The patient performs five series of ten repetitions of each exercise.
2. Low-back extension exercises while in prone over the end of treatment table. The patient performs five series of ten repetitions.
3. One-leg weight-pulling abduction/adduction standing. The patient performs five series of ten repetitions of the exercise for each leg.
4. Abdominal sit-ups both in straight forward direction and in oblique direction. The patient performs five sets to fatigue.
5. One-leg coordination exercise flexing and extending knee and swinging arms in same rhythm (cross-country skiing on one leg). The patient performs five sets of ten repetitions for each leg.
6. Skating movements on sliding board. This is performed five times for 1 min continuous work.

---

types of osteoporosis are distinguished on the basis of age of presentation[118] and differing rates of loss of cortical or trabecular bone.[119] Type I is characterized by vertebral fractures in postmenopausal women at about the age of 65 years; type II may occur in both sexes at about 75 years of age and produces mainly osteoporotic hip fractures.[119]

Men with osteoporosis of the hip are likely to have an underlying metabolic abnormality contributing to bone loss. The most common etiologies in men are hypogonadism, alcohol and corticosteroid use, anticonvulsant use, malabsorption syndromes, hyperthyroidism, and neoplasias.[120] Many factors have been cited for women, including decreased bone mass with an accelerated loss after menopause, parity, smoking, alcohol consumption, various medications, and diet. Although the reasons are unclear, in male patients either hip may be involved, whereas in women, the left hip is involved much more frequently.[121]

Hip pain begins spontaneously, without an antecedent history of trauma. The condition is aggravated by weight bearing. The symptoms may become severe enough to result in a limp. The clinical findings are self-limited and resolve in 2 to 6 months without permanent sequelae.[121] Biopsy of the synovium reveals normal findings or slight (mild, minimal, or equivocal) chronic inflammation.[122]

Radiographic findings are characteristic and become apparent within weeks or months of the onset of clinical findings. Progressive and marked osteoporosis of the femoral head is identified on plain radiographs.[122] Osteoporosis is not usually found in the acetabulum, but may be seen in the femoral neck. The joint space is normal and the femoral subchondral bone is usually intact.

The differential diagnosis includes avascular necrosis, osteoarthritis, septic arthritis, and rheumatoid arthritis.[122] The intervention for osteoporosis is discussed in Chap. 9.

Practice Pattern 4D: Impaired Joint Mobility, Motor Function, Muscle Performance, Range of Motion Associated with Connective Tissue Dysfunction

Osteoarthritis

Osteoarthritis is defined as focal loss of articular cartilage with variable subchondral bone reaction. The prevalence of hip osteoarthritis ranges from 7 to 25 percent in adults aged 55 years and older in the white European population.[122a] Studies of the natural history of hip osteoarthritis clearly demonstrate heterogeneity of disease progression, and the lack of a universal agreement as to the definition of progression of hip osteoarthritis. Most define progression by radiological features such as loss of joint space, osteophytes, and sclerosis.[122b,122c] However, the demonstration of a correlation between radiographic features and clinical symptoms is not easy in osteoarthritis: factors differentiating symptomatic osteoarthritis from asymptomatic disease are unknown.[122d] The two clinical sequelae of osteoarthritis that are most relevant to epidemiological studies are joint pain and functional impairment.

The start of symptomatic hip osteoarthritis is usually insidious, although in a few cases pain starts abruptly. The development of osteoarthritis at any joint site depends upon a generalized predisposition to the condition, and abnormalities of biomechanical loading which act at specific joints.[122e] Individual risk factors which may be associated with a generalized susceptibility to the disorder include obesity, a family history, and hypermobility.[122d] Those that reflect local biomechanical insults include minor trauma to an already diseased joint, abnormalities of joint shape, and physical activity.[122d]

The pain of hip osteoarthritis can vary greatly in both its site and nature, sometimes making early diagnosis difficult.[122f] The pain may be felt in the area of the buttock, groin, thigh, or knee and varies in character from a dull ache to sharp stabbing pains. The discomfort is generally related to activity and exercise may induce bouts of pain that last for several hours.[122f] As the disease process progresses, the patient begins to have difficulty climbing stairs with the involved leg, and may have difficulty in putting on socks or stockings.[122g] In advanced disease a decline in the participation of recreational activities occurs and the patient may complain of severe pain that is present at night or during rest. Stiffness of the hip is usual, particularly after inactivity, and can be the presenting feature.

Early physical signs include restriction of internal rotation and abduction of the affected hip, with pain at the end of the range.[122f] The diagnosis can usually be confirmed by radiography; joint space width of 2.5 mm or less indicates substantial loss of cartilage in the hip joint, and osteophytes, subchondral bone sclerosis, or cysts are usually present.[122f] As mentioned, though, radiographs can be misleading due to the relative insensitivity of the their findings with clinical signs and symptoms.

The narrowing of the joint space associated with osteoarthritis could potentially slacken the supporting ligaments, rendering them less effective, and producing changes in proprioceptive input. Indeed, osteoarthritis of the hip has been associated with deficits in a patient's proprioception and balance.[122h,122i] The joint space narrowing may also result in a relative decrease in the length of the muscles that cross the hip joint, which could feasibly result in a mechanical disadvantage of the muscles that act on the hip joint. In addition, osteoarthritis of the hip can have many manifestations in neighboring joints, particularly the lumbar spine and the foot. This is likely because the joint stiffness associated with the disease diminishes the amount of rotation available at the hip, forcing the lumbar spine and foot to compensate for this loss.

The intervention goals include relieving symptoms, minimizing disability and handicap, and reducing the risk of disease progression.[122f] Intervention in the earlier stages includes:

▶ Education and empowerment. Giving advice about what patients can do for themselves is of immense value.

▶ Modalities for muscle relaxation, pain relief and anti-inflammation.

▶ Modification of activities of daily living and self-care is one of the most important components. Patients are often frightened that use will "wear out" a damaged hip joint and need "permission" to use it.[122f] Evidence suggests that while the affected joint will benefit from regular loading to help maintain its integrity, prolonged or heavy activity may cause further damage.[122j] Patients need to learn an appropriate balance and intersperse periods of activity with rest.

▶ It is important to maintain a full range of hip movement, if possible. In addition to specific exercises for hip range of motion, recreations such as swimming or cycling may help. Contact sports and activities such as jogging, which can cause repetitive high impact loading of the hip, are probably best avoided.[122j]

▶ Diet and weight. There is no evidence for the involvement of any dietary factor in the etiopathogenesis of hip osteoarthritis.[122f] However, it is possible that obesity may accelerate progression or cause more pain. A reduction in weight can significantly improve a patient's symptoms, increase mobility, and improve health status.[122k]

▶ Many people with arthritis of the spine or legs are more comfortable wearing trainers or other shoes with good shock absorbing properties than they are in regular footwear. Sorbithane and other shock absorbing insoles, which are available in sports and shoe shops, may be helpful.[122f]

▶ A simple walking stick can make a big difference, reducing loading on a hip by 20–30 percent, but attention must be given to its length, characteristics, and use. In most cases it will be most beneficial if it is held on the unaffected side of the body and if it comes to the top of the pelvis and has a good ferrule and a comfortable handle.[122f]

The patient should be advised to:

▶ Engage in adequate warm-ups before exercising.

▶ Pay attention and respect the limitations of their body and not exercise if in discomfort.

▶ Not use medication to cover up pain from exercising.

Other measures include:

▶ Manual techniques to stretch the capsule and maintain mobility, particularly distractive techniques, are helpful. Following these distractions, a fairly vigorous stretching program into flexion, abduction, and external rotation should be initiated. The FABER position, or cross-legged sitting, is ideal for this. Stretching the hip joint capsule involves maintaining the stretch for as long as an hour.

▶ Strengthening exercises are performed for the major muscle groups of the hip region, especially the gluteus medius.

The surgical intervention for advanced osteoarthritis of the hip is addressed in Chap. 29.

Rheumatoid Arthritis

Rheumatoid arthritis is a systemic, inflammatory, and chronic disorder of unknown etiology, which is characterized with periods of exacerbation and remission, which eventually result in destruction of the joint surfaces and progressive disability.[142]

In the early phases of the disease, systemic manifestations such as malaise, weight loss, and ability fatigue are seen.[142] The patient typically experiences vague pain and stiffness in the hip, especially when arising from bed in the morning. With time the stiffness and pain becomes more severe and persistent and is accompanied by protective muscle spasms. Eventually, a hip flexion contracture develops.

Conservative intervention involves pharmacologic management, and active exercises of the hip within the limits of pain to preserve joint motion and maintain good muscle tone.[142] The activity modifications outlined for osteoarthritis of the hip are also advocated. The patient is instructed on joint protection skills, and to take frequent breaks.

Ankylosing Spondylitis

Ankylosing spondylitis (AS), also known as Marie-Strümpell disease or rheumatoid spondylitis, is a form of inflammatory arthritis usually characterized by initial involvement of the sacroiliac joints, later involvement of the spinal joints, and occasional involvement of the hip joints and other joints of the body (refer to Chap. 9).[142] The patient is usually between 15 and 40 years and AS affects 1 to 3 per 1000 people. Although males and females are affected evenly, mild courses of ankylosing spondylitis are more common in the latter.[143] Clinical findings in the hip include an early capsular pattern of motion restriction.

An exercise program is particularly important for these patients to maintain functional outcomes (see Chap. 9).[144] The goal of exercise therapy is to maintain the mobility of the involved joints for as long as possible and to prevent stiffening. A strict regime of daily exercises, which include positioning and spinal extension exercises, breathing exercises, and exercises for the peripheral joints must be followed. Several times a day the patient should lie prone for 5 minutes and they should be encouraged to sleep on a hard mattress and avoiding side lying. Swimming is the best routine sport.

Avascular Necrosis of the Femoral Head

Avascular necrosis of the femoral head is a condition in which there is progressive ischemia and secondary death of osteocytes or bone cells of the femoral head, resulting in the collapsing of bone of the femoral head and the later development of degenerative arthritis.[142] Avascular necrosis of the femoral head is described in more detail in Chap. 9.

Acetabular Labral Tear

In the last 15 years, there have been numerous studies on the location and anatomical features of acetabular labral tears, including cadaver, arthroscopic, and magnetic resonance imaging (MRI) studies.[144a] These tears represent the most common cause for mechanical hip symptoms—in a recent study, they were found to be the cause of groin pain in more than 20 percent of athletes presenting with groin pain.[144b]

Labral tears can be classified according to location, etiology:[144c]

▶ *Location.* With respect to location, tears can be anterior, posterior, or superior (lateral), although anterior tears appear to be the most common.[144c] Anterior labral tears also are common in patients with degenerative hip disease or acetabular dysplasia.

▶ *Etiology.* With respect to etiology, tears can be degenerative, dysplastic, traumatic, or idiopathic. Degenerative tears also can be seen in association with inflammatory arthropathies.

Seldes et al.[144d] classified acetabular labral tears into type 1 and type 2 on the basis of their anatomical and histological features. Type 1 tears consist of detachment of the labrum from the articular cartilage surface. These tears tend to occur at the transition zone between the fibrocartilaginous labrum and the articular hyaline cartilage.[144d] They are perpendicular to the articular surface and, in some cases, extend to the subchondral bone. Type 2 tears consist of one or more cleavage planes of variable depth within the substance of the labrum.[144d] Both types of tear are associated with chondrocyte proliferation and hyalinization of the labral fibrocartilage along the edges of the defect. All labral tears are associated with increased microvascularity within the substance of the labrum at the base of the tear adjacent to the labrum's attachment to bone.[144e] Osteophyte formation is also sometimes seen within the labral tears.

The diagnosis of an acetabular labral tear can be made on the basis of the history and physical examination. However, it must be remembered that labral tears can have a variety of clinical presentations associated with a wide degree of clinical findings.[144e]

▶ *History.*   There may or may not be a history of trauma. In the presence of a recalled incident, the trauma can vary from severe to very mild such as twisting or falling.[144e] The injury is usually caused by the hip joint being stressed in rotation. The pain is mainly in the groin, but could be in the trochanteric and buttock region.[144e] It could have an acute onset or be gradual. It is common for it to be sharp with a clicking, catching, or locking sensation.[144e] Activities that involve forced adduction of the hip joint in association with rotation in either direction tend to aggravate the pain.[144e]

▶ *Physical examination.*   On examination, range of motion may not be limited but there may be pain at the extremes.[144e] Generally speaking the combined movement of flexion and rotation causes pain in the groin. More precisely, the specific maneuvers that may cause pain in the groin include:[144f]

• Flexion, adduction, and internal rotation of the hip joint (with anterior superior tears)

• Passive hyperextension, abduction, and external rotation (with posterior tears)

• Acute flexion of the hip with external rotation and full abduction, followed by extension, abduction, and internal rotation (anterior tears)[144g]

• Extension, abduction, and external rotation brought to a flexed, adducted, and internally rotated position (posterior tears)[144g]

The diagnosis is typically confirmed with arthrography, magnetic resonance imaging with intravenous or intra-articular administration of contrast medium, or arthroscopy.[144h]

Conservative intervention includes bed rest with or without traction followed by a period of protected weight bearing and use of nonsteroidal anti-inflammatory medication. Operative treatment consists of arthrotomy or arthroscopy with resection of the entire labrum or the portion of the labrum that is torn.

Loose Bodies

In advanced cases of osteoarthritis, the hip joint becomes susceptible to loose bodies within the joint. The loose body can be a piece of cartilage or bone. If the loose body is large enough, it will cause a distraction in the joint, which will produce muscle inhibition and problems with gait.

The patient typically reports sudden leg pain twinges with weight bearing and periodic giving way of the leg. Clinical findings include a springy end feel in the hip, which is often painless. This springy end feel is often found during passive hip extension, as this is the close-packed position of the joint.

Confirmation and intervention usually involves arthroscopic techniques to identify and then remove the loose body.

The Limping Child

Limping is a common reason for children to present to accident and emergency departments. A proportion will have a preceding history of injury, but often this is absent. The main concerns are not to miss serious pathology and to begin appropriate management for the underlying condition. Potentially serious diseases include bone or joint sepsis, primary or metastatic tumors of the bone, Legg-Calvé-Perthes disease, and slipped femoral capital epiphysis (SFCE) (Table 17-14). A more benign cause for the limp is "irritable hip"/transient synovitis.

The flexion-adduction test can provide an early indication of underlying hip disease, often before any noticeable or measurable change in abduction, internal rotation, or total flexion arc.[91] It is often the first quadrantric movement to be restricted.[145,146]

Legg-Calvé-Perthes Disease (Osteochondritis Dissicans).   Legg-Calvé-Perthes disease, a disorder of the hip in young children, was described around the turn of the century independently by Legg, Calvé, Perthes, and Waldenström.[1] The incidence of Perthes disease varies considerably from place to place. Low rates of around 5 or 6 per 100,000 have been reported from British Columbia, Massachusetts, and rural Wessex, England, whereas rates of between 11 and 15.6 per 100,000 have been found in Liverpool, England.

There is considerable epidemiologic, histologic, and radiographic evidence to support the theory that Legg-Calvé-Perthes disease is probably a localized manifestation of a generalized disorder of epiphyseal cartilage manifested in the proximal femur because of its unusual and precarious blood supply.[147,148]

The definitive cause of Legg-Calvé-Perthes disease remains unknown. Many etiologic theories have been proposed. Most current etiologic theories involve vascular embarrassment, with repeated episodes of infarction and ensuing abnormalities.[149]

The onset is usually insidious and the course is prolonged over a period of several years. The initial sign is a limp. There may also be a slight dragging of the leg and slight atrophy of the thigh muscles. The patient complains of a vague ache in the groin that radiates to the medial thigh and inner aspect of the knee. Muscle spasm is another common complaint in the early stages of the disease.

The intervention for Legg-Calvé-Perthes disease remains controversial. There is lack of agreement regarding whether operative or nonoperative intervention is beneficial.[1] In reviewing long-term studies, it is apparent that the results improve with time.[150,151] Most patients (70 to 90 percent) are active and pain free regardless of intervention. The prognosis is much improved

TABLE 17-14 Differentiation of Pediatric Hip Pathologies

	Congenital Hip Dislocation	Septic Arthritis	Legg-Calvé-Perthes Disease	Transient Synovitis	Slipped Femoral Capital Epiphysis
Age	Birth	Less than 2 y; rare in adults	2–13 y	2–12 y	Males: 10–17 y; females 8–15 y
Incidence	Female>male; left>right; blacks<whites		Male>female; rare in blacks; 15% bilateral	Male>female; unilateral	Male>female; blacks>whites
Observation	Short limb, associated with torticollis	Irritable child; motionless hip; prominent greater trochanter; mild illness	Short limb; high greater trochanter; quad atrophy; adductor spasm	Decreased flexion, abduction, external rotation; thigh atrophy; muscle spasm	Short limb; obese; quadriceps atrophy; adductor spasm
Position	Flexed and abducted	Flexed; abducted; externally rotated			Flexed; abducted; externally rotated
Pain		Mild pain with palpation and passive motion; often referred to knee	Gradual onset; aching in hip, thigh, and knee	Acute: severe pain in knee; moderate: pain in thigh and knee; tenderness over hip	Vague pain in knee, suprapatellar area, thigh and hip; pain in extreme motion
History	May be breech birth	Steroid therapy; fever	20–25% familial; low birth weight; growth delay	Low-grade fever	May be trauma
Range of motion	Limited abduction	Decreased (capsular pattern)	Limited abduction, extension	Decreased flexion; limited extension, internal rotation	Limited internal rotation, abduction, flexion, increased external adductor spasm
Special tests	Galeazzi's sign, Ortolani's sign, Barlow's sign	Joint aspiration			
Gait		Refuses to walk	Antalgic gait after activity	Refuses to walk; antalgic limp	Acute: antalgic; chronic: Trendelenberg external rotation
Radiologic findings	Upward and lateral displacement, delayed development of acetabulum	CT scan: localized abscess; increased separation of ossification center	In stages: increased density, fragmentation, flattening of epiphysis	Normal at first; widened medial joint space	Displacement of upper femoral epiphysis, especially in frog position

(From Richardson JK, Iglarsh ZA, ed. *Clinical Orthopaedic Physical Therapy*. Philadelphia: Saunders; 1994:367–368.)

if there is no collapse of the femoral head. An important aspect in the intervention is the containment of the femoral head in the acetabulum. This is ensured by maintaining the hip in abduction and mild internal rotation for an extended period, using a Scottish-Rite brace. Although the brace maintains the hip in abduction, it does permit approximately 90 degrees of hip flexion. This allows the patient to run and ride a bicycle while wearing the brace.[152]

Congenital or Developmental Dysplasia of the Hip. Up to 10 percent of infants in the United States are born with congenital dislocation of the hip.[153] The acronym CDH (congenital dysplasia of the hip) is confusing and has been used synonymously with congenital dislocation or congenital disease of the hip. A dislocated hip is a physical sign, not a diagnosis, and the term *congenital* means present at birth.[97]

Thus the acronym DDH (developmental dysplasia of the hip) is replacing CDH. The word *developmental* invokes the dimension of time, acknowledging that the dysplasia or dislocation may occur before or after birth, while *dysplasia* means an abnormality of development and encompasses a wide spectrum of hip problems.[97]

DDH includes hips that are unstable, malformed, subluxated, or dislocated. Instability is the inability of the hip to resist an externally applied force without developing a subluxation or dislocation.[97] A subluxation is an incomplete dislocation with some residual contact between the femoral head and acetabulum, whereas a dislocation indicates complete displacement of the femoral head from the acetabulum.[97]

In utero, the hip is in a position of flexion and abduction that results in a tightened iliopsoas tendon and anterior-lateral orientation of the acetabulum.[154] The tight iliopsoas may push the femoral head out posteriorly with hip extension during kicking. The labrum (cartilaginous rim of the acetabulum) becomes everted and flattened.

If the hip reduces spontaneously within a few days, hip development usually proceeds normally. In contrast, if a subluxation or dislocation persists, the femoral head becomes flattened on the posteromedial surface, the acetabulum becomes shallow and dysplastic, and femoral anteversion gradually increases.

Prolonged dislocation makes it difficult to return the femoral head to the acetabulum and is associated with a higher incidence of osteoarthritis and impaired hip function in adulthood.[153]

Clinical screening programs are important in reducing the incidence of surgery. The early neonatal assessment for hip dislocation includes an examination using the Barlow and Ortolani tests.[155,156] However, there are dislocations that are not detected or that occur late, after a normal neonatal screening examination.[157–159] Later examinations include assessment of gluteal folds, knee height, and the degree of hip abduction.[156] In the older child, a limp, toe-walking, in-toeing, or out-toeing may be secondary to DDH.[97]

The goal of intervention is to safely obtain and maintain a concentric reduction of the hip to provide an environment for normal bony development. The preferred intervention is use of the Pavlik harness, an outpatient intervention regimen that provides effective reduction in 90 percent of the cases.[156] The harness uses flexion and free abduction to direct the femoral head into the acetabulum, using time, gravity, and motion to return the hip to a reduced position. The harness requires 3 to 6 months of continuous wear for the hip to become radiographically stable. However, if the condition is not detected until after the infant is 6 weeks old, or the harness is ineffective after 3 weeks, skin traction, closed reduction and spica-cast application may be needed.[156] Open reduction and recasting are also options. In rare cases, total hip replacement is necessary in later life.

Slipped Capital Femoral Epiphysis (SCFE). Slipped capital femoral epiphysis is the most common disorder of the hip in adolescents. The average age for girls in whom slipped capital femoral epiphyses develop is 12.1 ± 1 years, and for boys 14.4 ± 1.3 years.[160] The disorder is characterized by a sudden or gradual anterior displacement of the femoral neck from the capital femoral epiphysis. The effects of coxa vara and valga demonstrate the principles underlying the mechanism of this condition. While the adult femur has a collum angle of approximately 125 degrees, the developing femur demonstrates considerably more coxa valga initially.[161] Failure of the epiphyseal plate occurs as a result of shear forces, which are forces applied parallel to the surface of the growth plate.[39,162]

The traumatic episode may be as minimal as turning over in bed. If the patient can walk, it is with difficulty and with a limp. Patients with chronic slipped capital femoral epiphysis generally have a history of groin or medial thigh pain for months to years.[1] Approximately 45 percent will have knee or lower thigh pain as their initial symptom.[163]

The term slipped capital femoral epiphysis is actually a misnomer in that the head is held in the acetabulum by the ligamentum teres. Thus it is actually the neck that comes upward and outward while the head remains in the acetabulum.[1] The natural history of slipped capital femoral epiphysis is that the capital femoral epiphysis eventually will fuse with the femoral neck at the end of adolescence. Two devastating complications that can affect the result adversely are avascular necrosis and chondrolysis. These complications are uncommon sequelae in the untreated slip, but are serious complications in the operative and nonoperative management of slipped capital femoral epiphysis.[164]

On the basis of the patient's history, physical examination, and radiographs, slipped capital femoral epiphysis can be classified as a stable or unstable hip.[164,165] In the stable hip, weight bearing is possible with or without crutches. In the unstable hip, the patient presents more with fracture-like symptoms with pain so severe that weight bearing is impossible.[1]

The goals of intervention are relief of symptoms, containment of the femoral head, and restoration of a range of motion.[166] Intervention for the relief of symptoms includes the use of traction, at home or in the hospital, for periods ranging from 1 or 2 days to several weeks; partial weight bearing with use of crutches in order to rest an inflamed, painful joint; and the use of anti-inflammatory medication.[166] The goal of containment is to maintain the sphericity of the femoral head.

Transient Synovitis.   This is the most common cause of hip pain in young children. The child usually presents with a limp of acute onset, and may refuse to move the affected leg in any direction due to pain. This condition should resolve in 2 to 3 days, unless there is a more serious condition such as septic arthritis or juvenile rheumatoid arthritis present.[167]

The watershed age for prognosis of pediatric hip conditions is 8 years old. This is the age when most acetabular development is complete.[1] In children younger than 8 years of age, deformities in the femoral head as a result of a disease process such as Perthes disease or aseptic necrosis secondary to the intervention of developmental dysplasia of the hip may be accommodated for by secondary changes in acetabular development.[1] After 8 years of age, accommodation of acetabular shape to a deformed femoral head may not be possible.

Integration of Practice Patterns 4C and 4D: Impaired Joint Mobility, Motor Function, Muscle Performance, Range of Motion Associated with Muscle Performance Due to Impaired Muscle Performance and Connective Tissue Dysfunction

Snapping Hip (Coxa Saltans)

Multiple etiologies for snapping hip (coxa saltans) exist. The etiologies are categorized as internal, external, and intra-articular.[123,124]

1. The internal type has been attributed to:
   a. The iliopsoas snapping over structures just deep to it, namely the femoral head, proximal lesser trochanter, pectineus fascia, and iliopectineal eminence, which produces a snapping in the anterior groin region.[125–128]
   b. Stenosing tenosynovitis of the iliopsoas insertion.[129]
2. The external causes include snapping of the iliotibial band or gluteus maximus over the greater trochanter.[125,127,128,130–132] This condition is more common in females with a wide pelvis and prominent trochanters, and is exacerbated with running on banked surfaces.[133]
3. The intra-articular causes have included synovial chondromatosis, loose bodies, fracture fragments, and labral tears.[134–136] Snapping of the iliofemoral ligament over the anterior femoral head also has been described,[126,137,138] as has snapping of the long head of biceps origin over the ischium.[139]

Despite the availability of various diagnostic tests, the actual etiology often remains elusive. When no cause can be identified, as in most patients, the condition is classified as a myopathy of idiopathic origin.

The intervention is based on etiology. If an imbalance of the tensor fascia latae or iliopsoas is producing the symptoms, the intervention is focused on reconditioning and prevention. This includes increasing the flexibility of the soft tissues, and the correction of any strength imbalances. If the iliotibial band is tight, the emphasis is on stretching the iliotibial band.

Flexion Contracture

A flexion contracture at the hip is a common occurrence. Hip flexion contractures can result from:

► Adaptive shortening of the iliopsoas muscle or rectus femoris muscles.

► Contracture of the anterior hip capsuloligamentous complex.

These changes to the soft tissue and connective tissues around the hip can result from osteoarthritis, injury, or sustained postures involving hip flexion.

The resulting anterior rotation of the pelvis shifts the weight bearing of the hip to a thinner region of hyaline cartilage, in both the femur and acetabulum, and places the hip extensors in a state of low-level tension.[12]

Flexion contractures can be diagnosed using the Thomas test.

The intervention for the contracture is based on the cause. Adaptive shortening of the contractile tissues may be addressed using muscle energy, passive stretching, and myofascial techniques. Stretching of the capsuloligamentous complex is accomplished by grade III distraction mobilizations and by prolonged stretching.

Movement Impairment Syndromes of the Hip[56]

Three of the movement impairment syndromes detailed by Sahrmann in her excellent book, *Movement Impairment Syndromes*,[56] are described. The intervention for these syndromes focuses on the correction of muscle imbalances. The adaptively shortened structures are stretched and the weak muscles are strengthened.

Femoral Anterior Glide Syndrome.   The characteristic findings for this condition result from an insufficient posterior glide of the femoral head during hip flexion. Typically, the patient complains of groin pain, particularly during hip flexion, gait, and running. The consequences of this syndrome are:

► Stretching of the anterior joint capsule and tightening of the posterior structures resulting in excessive hip extension range of motion.

► An increase or decrease in the length of the hip external rotators.

► Decreased posterior glide of femoral head.

► Decreased length of the tensor fascia latae on the involved side.

► Weakness and lengthening of the iliopsoas on the involved side.

► Dominance of hamstring activity over gluteus maximus activity, both of which are shortened.

Hip Extension with Knee Extension Syndrome.   The characteristic findings for this condition result from an insufficient participation of the gluteus maximus during hip extension or the quadriceps during knee extension. Typically, the patient complains of pain at the hamstring insertion site on the ischial tuberosity and along the muscle belly, particularly during resisted hip extension, knee flexion, or both. The consequences of this syndrome are:

▶ A decrease in hip flexion due to the hypertrophy of the hamstrings.

▶ Dominance of hamstring activity over gluteus maximus activity.

▶ Weakness of the gluteus maximus and hip external rotators.

▶ Decreased length of the hamstrings.

▶ Increased frequency of hamstring strains.

Femoral Accessory Motion Hypermobility. The characteristic findings for this condition result from early degenerative changes in the hip joint and increased compression into the hip joint due to stretching forces on the rectus femoris and hamstrings. Typically, the patient complains of pain deep in the hip joint and in the anterior groin that may extend along the medial and anterior thigh, particularly during gait. The consequences of this syndrome are:

▶ A slight antalgic gait.

▶ Internal rotation of the hip during single leg stance.

▶ External rotation of the hip with passive knee flexion in prone.

▶ Medial rotation of the femur with knee extension in sitting.

▶ Rectus femoris and hamstrings are stiffer than the iliopsoas and intrinsic hip internal rotators.

▶ Anterior hip joint pain with FABER test.

Practice Pattern 4E: Impaired Joint Mobility, Motor Function, Muscle Performance, Range of Motion Associated with Localized Inflammation

In addition to those conditions producing impaired range of motion, motor function, and muscle performance attributed to inflammation, practice pattern E includes conditions that cause pain and muscle guarding without the presence of structural changes. Such conditions include:

▶ Sprains of the hip ligaments.

▶ Strains of the hip muscles.

▶ Internal derangements of the hip joint, including labral tears.

▶ Periarticular syndromes: tendonitis, bursitis, capsulitis, and tenosynovitis.

▶ Pubalgia.

Hip Joint Sprains

The classic history of a hip joint sprain is a vigorous twisting of the lower extremity or trunk.[168] Clinical findings include an inability to circumduct the leg due to pain.[169]

Conservative intervention includes an ACE wrap hip spica. Crutches are used for partial weight-bearing ambulation. The crutch walking continues until the patient is able to ambulate without pain.[170] The patient is progressed to strengthening and flexibility exercises, and functional tests of hopping, sprinting, running backwards, cutting, and pivoting in the athlete must be satisfactorily passed prior to return of play.[168]

Muscle Strains

Muscle strains at the hip can occur insidiously or be incurred traumatically, although first- and second-degree muscle strains are frequent injuries in sports activities.[60] The adductors, iliopsoas, rectus abdominis, gluteus medius, and hamstrings muscles are commonly involved.

Adductor. The hip adductor muscles, including the gracilis, pectineus, and adductor longus, brevis, and magnus are the most frequent cause of groin region pain, with the adductor longus being the most commonly injured.[27,171] Adductor strains have been known to cause long-standing problems.[172]

There are a number of causative factors for an adductor strain, including a muscular imbalance of the combined action of the muscles stabilizing the hip joint, resulting from fatigue or an abduction overload.[173] Laboratory studies have shown that strengthening exercises can protect these muscles from injury.[174]

Adductor strains are associated with jumping, running, and twisting activities, particularly when external rotation of the affected leg is an added component of the activity.[169] Soccer players involved with forceful kicking that is stopped by an opponent's foot, or by a sliding tackle with an abducted leg are particularly vulnerable to an adductor strain. In fact, the incidence of groin pain among male soccer players is 10 to 18 percent per year.[175–177]

The signs and symptoms are easily recognizable[178]:

▶ Twinging or stabbing pain in the groin area with quick starts and stops.

▶ Edema or echemosis several days postinjury.

▶ Pain with manual resistance to hip adduction when tested in different degrees of hip flexion (0 degrees [gracilis], 45 degrees [adductor longus and brevis], 90 degrees [if combined with adduction, pectineus]).

▶ Possibly a palpable defect in severe ruptures.

▶ Muscle guarding.

The differential diagnosis includes abdominal muscle strains, inguinal hernia, osteitis pubis, and referred pain from the hip joint or lumbar spine.

Conservative intervention involves the principles of PRICEMEM in the acute stage (see Chap. 10). This is followed by heat applications, hip adductor isometrics, and gentle stretching during the subacute phase, progressing to a graded resistive program and then a gradual return to full activity. As part of the rehabilitation program, any imbalance between the adductors and the abdominals needs to be addressed. In addition, the clinician should examine the patient's technique in their required activity as poor technique can overload and fatigue the adductors.

Iliopsoas. As the strongest flexor of the hip, the iliopsoas is one of the more frequently strained muscles of this region.[179] The mechanism of injury is forced extension of the hip while it is being actively flexed. Clinical findings include:

▶ Complaints of pain with attempts at acceleration and high-stepping activities.

▶ Increased pain with resisted flexion, adduction, and external rotation.[168]

Conservative intervention involves rest, ice, and compression during the acute phase, progressing to prone lying, heat, a graded resistive exercise program, and specific instructions on proper warm-up and cool-down. Recovery from this condition can be lengthy, and recurrences are frequent.

Rectus Abdominis. Rectus abdominis strains usually occur when the muscle is strongly contracting as it is being moved into a stretched and lengthened position. These strains are common in such sports as tennis, wrestling, pole vaulting, weight lifting, and soccer. Abdominal strains are primarily the result of inadequate abdominal strength and/or incorrect technique.[168] As it may be difficult to differentiate this condition from an inflammation of one of the internal abdominal organs, a physician should be consulted whenever there is any doubt.[179]

These are difficult injuries to heal. Although mild strains may only take 2 to 3 weeks to heal, premature return to play can create large muscle ruptures, leading to hernia formation in the abdominal wall.[168]

Conservative intervention is that of all muscle strains, and involves rest, ice, and compression during the acute phase, progressing to heat and gentle stretching, a graded resistive exercise program, and specific instructions on proper warm-up and cool-down. Training and retraining of the rectus abdominis should include half sit-ups, done slowly with the knees bent, to eliminate compensation by the iliopsoas.[168,179]

Hamstrings. The hamstrings are the most commonly strained muscles of the hip, especially in runners and joggers.[169] Strain is most likely to occur in the hamstrings during two stages of the running cycle: late forward swing and takeoff (toe-off).[60,116,180] A hamstring strain has a varied list of potential causes including poor posture, decreased flexibility, strength imbalance between the hamstrings and the quadriceps, inadequate warm-up, fatigue, and poor coordination.[170]

The patient usually reports a distinctive mechanism of injury with immediate pain during full stride running or while decelerating quickly.[168] Clinical findings include:

▶ Tenderness with stretching of the hamstrings.

▶ Posterior thigh pain with resisted knee flexion.

With grade I strains, gait appears normal and there is only pain with extreme range of a straight leg raise.

A patient with a grade II strain normally ambulates with an antalgic gait, or may ambulate with a flexed knee. Resisted knee flexion and hip extension is both painful and weak.

A grade III strain usually requires the use of crutches for ambulation. In severe cases ecchymosis, hemorrhage, and a muscle defect may be visible several days postinjury.[168]

The differential diagnosis for posterior thigh pain includes neoplasms, overt disk protrusions with definite signs of nerve root impingement or ischial tuberosity apophysitis, or an avulsion fracture.

Conservative management of hamstring strains during the acute stage involves the principles of PRICEMEM. Improper management of this condition may lead to recurrent tears or hamstring syndrome, an entrapment of the sciatic nerve.[168] To prevent this from occurring, it is recommended that scar massage, gentle stretching, and phonophoresis be initiated early.

Patients with a grade I strain may continue activities as much as possible. A grade II strain typically requires 5 to 21 days for rehabilitation, whereas a patient with a grade III strain might require 3 to 12 weeks of rehabilitation.

Muscle imbalances of strength and flexibility must be addressed, and proper techniques to stretch the hamstrings should be taught. Because there is a great deal of variability in the rehabilitation time, anywhere from 2 to 3 weeks to 2 to 6 months, an athlete should not be permitted to return to full participation in sports until flexibility and strength ratios have been restored, and before plyometric and functional exercises are able to be performed pain free.[168,170]

Tendonitis

Rectus Femoris. Rectus femoris tendonitis is typically sport related, from acute or chronic overuse. The pain is usually located at the origin (ASIS), or just distal to it. The patient often complains of groin pain during sprinting or lifting the knee. In most cases, the cause is adaptive shortening of the rectus. Intervention involves stretching and transverse friction massage (TFM).

Iliopsoas. Tendonitis of the iliopsoas complex almost always involves an overstretching of the muscle belly. The patient complains of groin pain, which can radiate into the anterior thigh. Resisted hip flexion and external rotation are often painful. In addition passive hip flexion or passive hip extension/internal rotation are painful. The involved site is almost always just distal to the inguinal ligament, and just medial to the sartorius muscle. Conservative intervention involves TFM and stretching.

Quadriceps Contusion

The term *charley horse* is synonymous with a contusion of the quadriceps muscle. These contusions are quite common and can vary in their degree of discomfort. They are usually due to a direct blow to the anterior thigh, with the vastus lateralis and intermedius the most frequently involved.

The patient usually describes a specific mechanism and complains of a dull aching pain over the thigh. Clinical findings include:

▶ Palpable tenderness over the anterior lateral aspect of the thigh.

▶ Variable swelling. Extreme swelling should alert the clinician to the possibility of an injury to major vessels.

▶ Pain increased with knee flexion sometimes accompanied by spasm.

▶ There may be a palpable hematoma.

Quadriceps contusions can be graded according to functional loss[181]:

▶ *Grade I.* In a mild contusion, the patient has localized tenderness with no alteration of gait. Knee motion can be performed without pain up to at least 90 degrees of flexion.

▶ *Grade II.* In a moderate contusion, the patient displays swelling and a tender muscle mass. Knee flexion motion is restricted to less than 90 degrees and an antalgic gait is present. The patient is unable to climb stairs or arise from a chair without considerable discomfort.

▶ *Grade III.* In a severe contusion, the patient cannot bend their knee beyond approximately 45 degrees. The patient is unable to walk unaided. Marked tenderness and swelling are present.

Conservative intervention involves a gradual progression of range of motion and strengthening exercises.

Hip Pointer

A hip pointer is a subcutaneous contusion of the iliac crest resulting from a direct blow, usually at or near the anterior superior iliac spine (ASIS). The contusion is graded from I to III depending on the extent of damage. Grade I hip pointers functionally limit the patient for about 5 to 14 days, while grade II and III hip pointers can functionally limit the patient for 14 to 21 days.

Usually the patient reports point tenderness over the ASIS. The pain is increased with active trunk motions, and with such activities as laughing, coughing, or sneezing.[168]

Early intervention within 2 to 4 hours is critical to avoid severe pain and limited trunk motion. The early intervention includes ice, compression, rest, and anti-inflammatory measures. Early motion exercises, which emphasize trunk side flexion to the side opposite the injury, should be initiated when tolerated, and can be accompanied with transcutaneous electrical nerve stimulation (TENS). As the symptoms subside, gentle graded stretching exercises are added in addition to trunk-strengthening exercises.

Prophylactic prevention of the injury with adequate padding of the iliac crest using materials such as high-density foam and orthoplast is recommended.

Pubalgia

Pubalgia is a collective term for all disorders that cause chronic pain in the region of the pubic tubercle and the structures attached to the pubic bone (inguinal region). Pubalgia typically results from a sports injury. It usually results from a unipodal movement, where the weight-bearing leg is rotated as the other leg performs a movement such as kicking, or during activities such as sprinting and pivoting. During this kind of motion, small shearing movements occur in the pubic symphysis. The condition is rarely found in women—this may be due to variations in pelvis anatomy between men and women, strength differences between genders, or participation levels.

Pubalgia typically presents as lower abdominal pain with exertion, minimal to no pain at rest, and increased pain with activities that involve resisted hip adduction. After the initial pain, the pain disappears when the patient is warmed up, only to return, often more intensely, after the activity. Eventually the pain will increase with exertion and only slightly diminish with rest.

In most cases, the pain is unilateral at onset, with progression to bilateral pain in about 40% of cases.[181a] Examination findings include:

▶ Pain with passive hip flexion, when combined with hip adduction.

▶ Painful passive abduction with a straight or bent knee.

Groin pain is a common complaint and can be ascribed to various disorders (see Table 17-6) necessitating a thorough knowledge of differential diagnosis. Palpation of the relevant structures should help in locating the cause, as will resistive testing of the various abdominal muscles.

Once the diagnosis has been established, the conservative intervention should be causal:

▶ Transverse friction massage (TFM) can be applied locally.

▶ Ultrasound, electrical stimulation, thermotherapy, and cryotherapy.

▶ Stretching as tolerated to the muscles surrounding the injured area:

　• The short and long adductors.

　• Hip flexors (iliopsoas and rectus femoris).

　• Hip internal rotators.

　• Abdominals.

　• Gluteal muscles.

▶ Strengthening of the same muscle groups. The strengthening exercises are performed isometrically initially and then concentrically and eccentrically, and finally isokinetically as appropriate.

▶ Core stability training.

▶ Proprioception training.

Effective warm ups and preparation before the sporting activity can play an important preventative role.

In cases of failed conservative intervention, which is common, surgical intervention (pelvic floor repair) or cessation from the offending activity becomes the patient's only choice. Postsurgical rehabilitation uses many of the same exercises and modalities as in the traditional rehabilitation program outlined above.

Bursitis

Trochanteric/Subtrochanteric. Trochanteric bursitis is the collective name given to inflammation of any one of the trochanteric bursae. The bursae become inflamed through either friction or direct trauma, such as a fall on the side of the hip. Trochanteric bursitis is the second most frequent cause of lateral hip pain.[182]

The history may reveal complaints of lateral thigh, groin, and gluteal pain, especially when lying on the involved side.[183] Although the pain is typically local to the hip region, it can radiate distally to the knee and the lower leg.

Objectively, the clinical findings include:

▶ The reproduction of pain with palpation, or with stretching of the iliotibial band (ITB) across the trochanter with hip adduction or the extremes of internal or external hip rotation.[184]

▶ Resisted abduction, extension, or external rotation of the hip are also painful.

▶ There is often associated tightness of the hip adductors, which cause the patient's feet to cross the midline, resulting in increased stress on the trochanteric bursae.

Differential diagnosis should include[14,185]:

▶ Tendopathy of the gluteus medius or maximus muscles, with or without calcification.

▶ Inguinal and femoral hernia.

▶ An irritation of the L4 to L5 nerve root.

▶ Meralgia paresthetica.

▶ A "snapping" hip.

▶ Lower spinal neoplasm.

▶ Pelvic tumor.

▶ Hip infection.

▶ Avascular necrosis.

▶ Stress fracture of the femur.

▶ Bone or soft tissue tumor.

There is very little research evidence on physical therapy intervention for trochanteric bursitis.[186] The intervention usually consists of the removal of the causative factors by stretching the soft tissues of the lateral thigh, especially the tensor fascia latae and iliotibial band. Other interventions include heat and ultrasound. Transverse friction massage has also been advocated.[187] Orthotics may be prescribed if there is a biomechanical fault in the kinetic chain due to an ankle/foot dysfunction.

Iliopsoas/Iliopectineal. The iliopsoas bursa is located between the anterior side of the joint capsule of the hip and the musculotendinous junction of the iliopsoas. Although iliopsoas bursitis seems to be under recognized by the medical community, reports continue to be published. This may be because the entity often exists for years without being identified. The usual complaint is one of anterior hip or groin pain, which is aggravated by lumbar or hip hyperextension, or power walking. In the older populations, psoas bursitis can mimic such conditions as hip joint pathology, an L2 to L3 nerve root pathology, and meralgia paresthetica.

Objective findings are few, and they include:

▶ Pain with passive hip flexion and adduction at the end range.

▶ Pain with passive hip extension and external rotation, which is increased if the hip flexors are resisted in this position.

▶ Palpable tenderness of the involved bursa.

Conservative intervention consists of a stretching and strengthening program of the hip rotators and hip flexors. Johnston and colleagues[188] have published a conservative approach to iliopsoas bursitis, based on a retrospective study of nine patients with the condition. The recommended protocol consists of the following exercises:

▶ Seated hip internal and external resisted exercises using elastic resistance.

▶ Side-lying abduction/external rotation resisted exercises using elastic resistance.

▶ Mini-squats, weight bearing on the affected leg.

▶ Stretching of the hip flexor, quadriceps, and lateral hip/ piriformis, and hamstring muscles.

Ischial. An ischial bursitis (Weaver's bottom) involves two different bursae, one between the ischial tuberosity and the inferior part of the gluteus maximus belly, and the other between the tendons of the biceps femoris and semimembranosus. Inflammation of these bursae usually results from chronic compression or direct trauma.

With ischial bursitis, the patient typically reports pain with sitting in a firm chair, almost as soon as the buttocks touch the chair. Ischial bursitis tends to affect thinner people more than obese individuals and women more than men.

Differential diagnosis should include lumbar nerve root impingement, hamstring syndrome, piriformis syndrome, and hamstring insertion tendopathy. These can be differentiated between using the history, palpation, and resistive testing.

Conservative intervention should be causal. This involves the use of a padded seat cushion, anti-inflammatory measures such as ice massage, and ultrasound.

Gluteal. Inflammation of the gluteal bursa (located above and behind the greater trochanter, underneath the gluteus maximus and medius) is one of the most frequent causes of pseudo-radicular pain in the lower limb. The patient is usually in their fourth or fifth decade and complains of pain in the gluteal or trochanteric area. The pain may spread to the outer or posterior thigh, and down to the calf muscles and the malleolus. Unlike the pain caused by a disk lesion, the symptoms are not related to sitting, but only to walking and going up stairs. A typical pattern is pain on passive internal rotation and abduction, and resisted external rotation or abduction.

Conservative intervention should be causal. This involves the use of a padded seat cushion, anti-inflammatory measures such as ice massage, and ultrasound.

Integration of Practice Patterns 4C, 4F, and 5F: Impaired Joint Mobility, Motor Function, Muscle Performance, Range of Motion Associated with Spinal Disorders, Sign of the Buttock, Myofascial Pain Dysfunction (Referred Pain Patterns), Peripheral Nerve Entrapments

If the tests and measures of the hip are negative for a hip disorder or a dysfunction of the lower kinetic chain, the clinician should examine the lumbar spine and sacroiliac joint, both of which can refer pain to this region.

Many internal disorders such as femoral and inguinal hernias, pelvic inflammatory disease, prostatitis, and nephrolithiasis can produce pain in the lower abdomen and groin region (see Chap. 9). These are all out of the scope of practice for the physical therapist and a proper referral to an internist, urologist, or gynecologist should be sought.

Sign of the Buttock

The sign of the buttock is a collection of signs that indicate the presence of serious pathology posterior to the axis of flexion and extension in the hip. Among the causes of the syndrome are osteomyelitis, fracture of the sacrum/pelvis, infections, sacroiliitis, gluteal hematoma, septic bursitis, ischiorectal abscess, tumor, and rheumatic bursitis. Typical findings include gross hip weakness with empty end-feel. The involved buttock looks larger. The seven signs of the buttock are:

▶ A limited straight leg raise.

▶ Limited hip flexion.

▶ Limited trunk flexion.

▶ A noncapsular pattern of hip restriction.

▶ Painful and weak hip extension.

▶ Gluteal swelling.

▶ An empty end-feel on hip flexion.

Meralgia Paresthetica

Patients with meralgia paresthetica typically describe burning, coldness, lightning-type pain, deep muscle achiness, and tingling or frank anesthesia in the anterolateral thigh (see Chap. 9). There may also be local hair loss in the anterolateral thigh.[189] The symptoms may be exacerbated when the hip is extended, as in prone lying, or when standing erect. Sitting may relieve the symptoms in some patients but exacerbate them in others. Eventually, there may be no position that provides relief.[189]

The initial intervention of meralgia paresthetica is conservative, and patients may benefit from analgesics, nonsteroidal anti-inflammatory drugs, looser clothing, and weight loss.

Piriformis Syndrome

Piriformis syndrome is the result of entrapment of the sciatic nerve by the piriformis muscle as it passes through the sciatic notch (see Chap. 9). Clinical findings include[190]:

▶ Restriction in range of motion of hip adduction and internal rotation.

▶ Positive FABER test.

▶ Weak gluteus maximus, gluteus medius, and biceps femoris.

▶ Neurologic symptoms in the posterior lower limb if the peroneal nerve is involved.

▶ Ipsilateral short leg.

Conservative intervention for this condition includes gentle, pain-free static stretching of the piriformis muscle, strain-counterstrain techniques, ice massage to the gluteal region, and spray and stretch techniques.[168,191]

Entrapment of the Obturator Nerve

Compression of the anterior division of the obturator nerve in the thigh has been described recently as one possible cause for adductor region pain, and entrapment of this nerve has been documented by nerve conduction studies.[192] The fascia over the nerve is thought to contribute to compression of the nerve, or perhaps allow for the development of a compartment syndrome.[192]

Myofascial Pain Dysfunction

Myofascial pain is referred into the hip from the following muscles: quadratus lumborum, piriformis, gluteus minimus, and adductor longus.

Quadratus Lumborum. This muscle is perhaps one of the most overlooked sources of hip pain. The more superficial trigger points of this muscle refer pain to the lateral ilium and greater trochanter and may also refer pain into the groin in the region of the inguinal ligament. The tenderness in the trochanteric region can be misdiagnosed as trochanteric bursitis.

Clinical findings can include:

▶ Restriction of hip joint movements by lumbar spasm.

▶ Trochanteric and buttock tenderness.

▶ A contralateral short leg.

▶ An ipsilateral flexed innominate.

Conservative intervention includes gentle, pain-free static stretching of the muscle, soft tissue techniques, and progressive strengthening.

Gluteus Minimus.   Trigger points may be located in the posterior and anterior portions of this muscle. The posterior trigger point refers pain to the medial lower buttock and into the posterior thigh and calf. These trigger points have the potential to increase the tone in the hamstring and calf muscles. Stretching the gluteus minimus before hamstring and calf stretching allows these two muscles to lengthen much more readily. The anterior trigger point refers symptoms to the lower buttock, and down the lateral thigh and leg as far as the lateral malleolus on occasion.

Conservative intervention includes gentle, pain-free static stretching of the muscle, soft tissue techniques, and progressive strengthening.

Adductor Longus.   Trigger points in this muscle strongly refer to the anterior hip and anterior knee. Clinical findings include:

▶ Pain with resisted strength testing.

▶ Positive FABER test for pain.

▶ Marked restriction of hip abduction.

Conservative intervention includes gentle, pain-free static stretching of the muscle, soft tissue techniques, and progressive strengthening.

Practice Pattern 4G: Impaired Joint Mobility, Motor Function, Muscle Performance, Range of Motion Associated with Fractures

Avulsions

Apophyseal avulsions of the pelvis and proximal femur occur most commonly to male athletes 10 to 20 years old, usually as the direct result of vigorous or uncoordinated activities such as kicking, jumping, hurdling, sprinting, and punting, involving the sartorius or tensor fascia latae.[168,193] The anterior iliac spine is a common site for the injury, especially during the middle to late teenage years when the iliac crest unites with the ilium. Clinical findings can include[194]:

▶ Point tenderness.

▶ Crepitus.

▶ Hematoma.

▶ Limited hip motion.

▶ Pain with resisted hip flexion and passive hip extension increase pain at the site.

Conservative intervention includes ice and hip spica compression, followed by bed rest, progressing to crutch ambulation and activity modification. Return to normal activity follows a period of strength, flexibility, and functional training.[168]

Stress Fracture

Stress fractures of the femoral neck are seen in military recruits and fervent joggers. The fracture typically occurs on the superior side (tension-side fractures) or the inferior side (compression-side fractures) of the femoral neck.[195] These fractures may develop into a complete and displaced fracture if left untreated.

The most frequent early symptom is the onset of sudden hip pain. The earliest and most frequent symptom is pain in the inguinal or anterior groin area.[195] Pain can also occur in the lateral aspect or anteromedial aspect of the thigh. The pain usually occurs with weight bearing or at the extremes of hip motion. Less severe cases may only have pain following a long run. Night pain may occur if the fracture progresses.

The physical examination is often negative, although there may be pain at the extremes of hip internal or external rotation or with resisted hip external rotation.[196]

Differential diagnosis includes osteoarthritis of the hip, referred symptoms from the spine, trochanteric bursitis, or septic arthritis.

Radiographs taken soon after the symptoms begin have been reported to be positive in only 20 percent of cases.[195] Diagnosis is best confirmed with bone scintigraphy (scan), although these have also been shown to be prone to false negatives.[197] The intervention varies according to the bone scintigraphy findings.[195]

▶ If there is a positive scan only, or sclerosis and no fracture line on the radiographs, the intervention ranges from modified bed rest to non-weight bearing with crutches until symptoms subside. Once pain free, weight bearing is progressed. When significant partial weight bearing is pain free, cycling and swimming may be permitted. Weekly radiographs are obtained until the athlete is full weight bearing without pain. Water running and water walking are progressed. If these remain pain free, running on land is commenced, with the initial run being no further than one quarter mile.

▶ If there is an overt fracture line on the radiographs with no displacement, and provided that only the cortex is involved, an initial period of either bed rest or complete non-weight bearing is necessary. The patient is progressed to partial and then full weight bearing on crutches as symptoms permit. Roentgenograms every 2 to 3 days during the first week are necessary to detect any widening of the fracture line. If healing does not occur, internal fixation with some form of hip pin is indicated.

An overt fracture with radiographic evidence of opening or displacement is significant and requires surgical intervention, usually in the form of a hip screw and plate. Displaced fractures must be treated as an orthopaedic emergency.

Therapeutic Techniques

Techniques to Increase Joint Mobility

Passive Articular Mobilization Techniques

Mobilizations of this joint are typically performed using a sustained stretch to decrease a hip joint capsular restriction, with the stretch governed by the direction of the restriction, rather than by the concave-convex rule. For example, if hip joint extension is restricted, the distal femur is moved into the direction of hip extension.[146]

The joint is initially positioned in its neutral position and is progressively moved closer to the end of range. Rotations can be combined with any sustained stretch performed in a cardinal plane. Distraction or compression techniques can be used alone or combined with rotations.

Distraction. Joint distractions are indicated for pain and any hypomobility at the hip joint, as in the case when pain is reported by the patient before tissue resistance is felt by the clinician.

The patient is positioned in supine and the hip is placed in its resting position. The patient's thigh is grasped by the clinician as proximal as possible, and a distraction force is applied along the line of the femoral neck (see Fig. 17-20). A belt can also be used for this technique.

A caudal distraction can be used for temporary relief of joint pain and for stretching capsular adhesion that is pronounced in the inferior portion of the joint capsule.[60,73] During this distraction, the clinician passively rotates the patient's hip using the arm/hand around the midthigh and the clinician's body.

Leg Traction (Inferior Glide). The patient is positioned in supine with the hip in its resting position. The clinician grasps the patient's ankle and applies a series of oscillations along the length of the leg. An assistant or a belt (Fig. 17-37) may be necessary to provide stabilization at the hip.

Quadrant (Scouring) Mobilizations. Quadrant mobilizations involve flexion and adduction of the hip, combined with simul-

taneous joint compression through the femur.[60,146,198,199] The flexed and adducted thigh is swept through a 90 to 140 degree arc of flexion while maintaining joint compression. This arc of motion should feel smooth, and should be pain free. In an abnormal joint, pain or an obstruction to the arc occur during the movement. In selected nonacute cases, the procedure may be used as an effective mobilizing procedure where grade II to III mobilizations are applied perpendicular to the arc throughout.[60,198]

Mobilizations with Movement[200,201]

To Restore Internal Rotation of the Hip.[202] This is a good technique to employ when the patient presents with early signs of hip joint degeneration as indicated by minor capsular signs, and slight degenerative changes on radiographs. A belt that can be altered in length is required for the technique.

The patient is positioned in supine with the involved hip and knee flexed, and the foot just off the edge of the bed, with the clinician standing on the involved side, facing the patient's head. A belt is placed around the back of the clinician, just below the hip joints, and around the patient's thigh as proximal as possible, and so that the belt is approximately horizontal. Using the hand closest to the patient's head, the clinician grasps the lateral iliac crest of the involved side, with the elbow in the crease of the clinician's groin to stabilize the pelvis during the maneuver. The clinician wraps the other hand around the patient's mid-thigh. From this position, the clinician slowly extends their own hips to apply a distraction force to the patient's hip joint while maintaining the fixation of the ilium.

If the maneuver produces any pain, it should be discontinued. This should be differentiated from discomfort, which might be caused by inappropriate placement of the belt.

To Restore Flexion of the Hip.[202] The technique to restore flexion of the hip is identical to the one described above, except that during the distraction, the clinician passively flexes the patient's hip into flexion by side flexing at the waist.

Techniques to Increase Soft Tissue Extensibility

The efficacy of manual techniques for improving hip range of motion has been reported in the literature. Crosman and colleagues[203] studied the effects of hamstring massage (effleurage, petrissage, friction) on hip flexion range in normal individuals and noted significant range improvements after the soft tissue massage (STM).[60] Godges and colleagues[204] reported improved hip flexion and hip extension ranges in normal individuals after the application of manual stretches to muscle groups opposing each respective motion, combined with exercise of agonistic muscles.

Myofascial Therapy

The onset of myofascial pain is often associated with acute overload stress or a chronic muscle overload. In addition to those manual techniques outlined below, spray and stretch can also be applied.

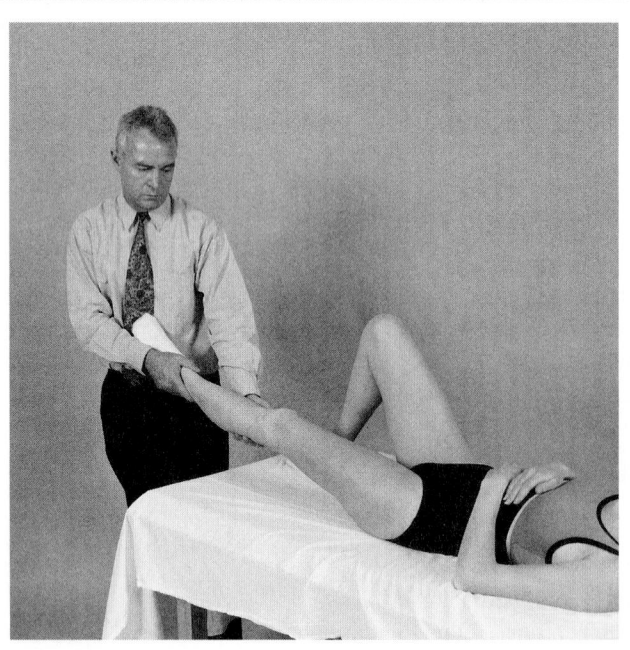

FIGURE 17-37   Leg traction.

The patient is positioned comfortably to allow stretch of the involved muscle during simultaneous spray of the involved area with a vapocoolant spray.[205] The spray is directed at a 30 degree angle to the skin and applied in parallel unidirectional sweeps at a distance of 18 inches from the body surface.[205] Precautions against spray inhalation and skin tissue damage from the vapocoolant must be observed.[60]

Myofascial Stretch: Passive and Active.[206] The patient is positioned in supine with the hips and knees flexed, with the clinician standing on the side of dysfunction, facing the table. The clinician places both hands on the posterior aspect of the patient's thigh, near the popliteal region, and applies an increasing force to the patient's thigh in the direction of limitation of motion, to the point of creating pain. This position is held for 3 seconds. From this position, the patient pushes their thigh against the clinician's resisting hands, creating an isometric contraction in the direction opposite to the passive motion. This position is held for 3 seconds. The clinician relaxes all force and returns the hip to the starting position. The patient rests for 3 seconds, then the procedure is repeated. This maneuver is performed three times, with each repetition allowing greater freedom of motion. The technique can be repeated in another direction of limited motion.

Passive Myofascial Release: Combined Hip and Knee.[206] The patient is positioned in supine with the hips and knees flexed to 90 degrees if possible, and the clinician stands on the side of dysfunction, facing the table. From this position, the patient's hip is placed into abduction and external rotation to the end point of pain-free motion. Using one hand, the clinician palpates the medial aspect of the patient's knee, and stabilizes the limb in its abduction-external rotation position. With the other hand, the clinician grasps the patient's foot or shin and externally rotates the tibia to its maximum pain-free position. This position is maintained for 3 seconds, while the clinician increases the motion pressure of both hands until the muscles relax. While maintaining pressure with both hands, the clinician slowly returns the patient's hip and knee to full extension on the table, releasing the pressure of both hands only at the last 5 degrees of full extension. The patient rests, and the technique is repeated.

This procedure can also be performed with the patient's hip in adduction and internal rotation, where the clinician places one hand on the lateral aspect of the patient's knee and moves the tibia into internal rotation.

Myofascial Release with Traction of the Hip Joint.[206] The patient is positioned in supine with the clinician sitting beside the table on the side of the dysfunction, facing toward the patient's head. The patient's ankle and shin are placed in the clinician's axilla and maintained in position by firm adduction of the arm. The clinician grasps the patient's extended leg above the knee and rotates the hip internally and externally, testing for ease of motion. The hip is placed into its position of ease and is firmly held there. From this position, the clinician then applies traction to the entire leg by leaning back, creating a pull on the leg that is grasped by the axilla and gradually increasing rotation into the freedom of motion. This position is held for 3 seconds, then the clinician quickly rotates the hip fully in the opposite direction. This position is held for 3 seconds. The clinician releases the leg and relaxes the position. The patient rests for 3 seconds, then the technique is repeated.

Muscle Energy

Muscle energy techniques can be used to treat a wide variety of contractile and noncontractile tissue dysfunctions about the hip, including muscle spasm, adaptive shortening, and fibrous adhesions. These techniques can produce an increased blood flow and decongestion, and improve proprioceptive awareness.[207]

Hamstrings

Lower. The patient is positioned in supine, with the clinician beside the table on the involved side, facing toward the patient's head. The patient's ankle is placed on the clinician's shoulder, and the clinician places a hand on the anterior aspect of the patient's knee to maintain the leg in full extension (Fig. 17-38). The clinician raises the extended leg further into hip flexion and ankle dorsiflexion, to the point of pain onset, at which point the leg is maintained. The patient is asked to press that leg down onto the clinician's shoulder and to plantarflex the ankle for 3 to 5 seconds (internal and external rotation of the lower leg can be superimposed on the knee flexion to emphasize the medial and lateral hamstrings, respectively). The patient relaxes for 3 seconds, and the technique is repeated.

Upper. The patient is positioned in supine, with the clinician beside the table on the involved side, facing toward the patient's head. The hip and knee are flexed to 90 degrees. The patient

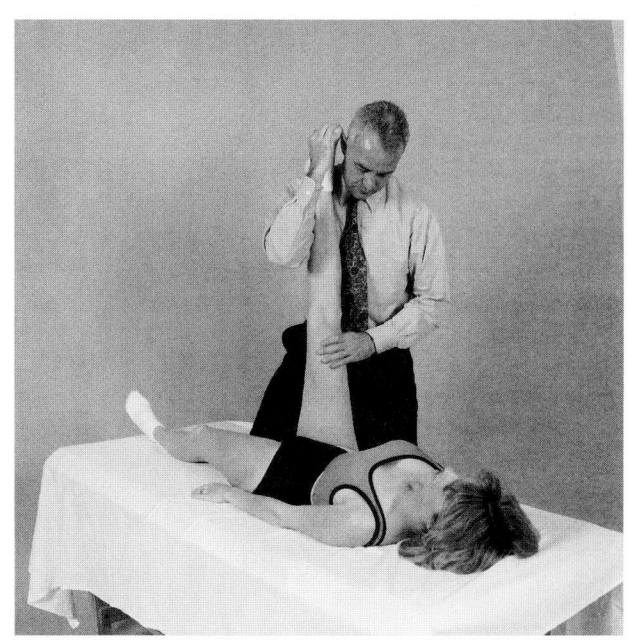

FIGURE 17-38 Hamstring and gastrocnemius stretch.

flexes the knee and simultaneously plantarflexes the ankle to the motion barrier. At this point, the clinician asks the patient to contract isometrically while the clinician provides an equal and opposite force for 10 seconds. The patient then actively extends the knee and dorsiflexes the ankle to the new resistance barrier.

Hip Adductor Stretch. The patient is positioned in supine with both legs straight, with the clinician beside the table on the involved side, facing toward the patient's head. The patient flexes the involved leg at the hip and knee and places that foot on the table beside the other knee as in the FABER position (see Fig. 17-22). The patient then abducts and externally rotates the flexed hip, so that the plantar aspect of the foot lies beside the medial aspect of the extended knee. The clinician places one hand on the anterior superior iliac spine of the uninvolved side, and the other hand on the medial aspect of the patient's flexed knee, holding it in its position of flexion, hip abduction-external rotation. From this position, the patient exerts a gentle force upward into adduction, internal rotation-flexion, against the clinician's equal and opposite force. The contraction is held for 3 to 5 seconds. The patient relaxes, and the procedure is repeated.

Piriformis. The patient is positioned in supine with the involved leg flexed and adducted over the noninvolved leg. The clinician stabilizes the pelvis at the ASIS while applying longitudinal compression into the femur (Fig. 17-39). The patient attempts to abduct and externally rotate the lower leg while the clinician applies equal and opposite resistance for 10 seconds. The patient then adducts and internally rotates the femur with assistance from the clinician. The procedure is repeated 3 to 5 times.

Automobilization and Self-Stretching

Anterior-Inferior Capsule. The patient places one foot on a chair in front of them (see Fig. 17-12). While maintaining the spine in a functional neutral position, the patient slowly leans toward the chair, thereby stretching the anterior-inferior aspect of the hip joint of the standing leg. The position is held for about 30 seconds.

Posterior Capsule and Piriformis Stretch. The patient is positioned in the quadruped position. The automobilization is performed by the patient by having them perform oscillatory sit back motions in the direction of the hip joint to be mobilized (Fig. 17-40).

The hip internal rotators can be stretched in a similar fashion as above except that the lateral aspect of the foot and lower leg rests on the stool or hi-lo table. In order to stretch the internal rotators and to increase external rotation, the patient allows gravity to move the knee of the involved leg toward the floor, or can apply pressure with the hands.

Distraction. The patient is positioned in side lying, close to the edge of the table, with the involved side uppermost. A firm pillow may be placed between the patient's thighs, and the involved hip is extended so that the lower part of the leg is over the edge of the bed (Fig. 17-41). An ankle weight is placed around the ankle of the involved leg. The patient can actively raise the involved leg against the pull of the ankle weight, hold the position for a few seconds, and then allow the leg to move further into adduction at the hip, by relaxing the contraction.

Abdominal Stretch. The patient is positioned supine with their legs hanging over the end of the bed (Fig. 17-42). The technique can be

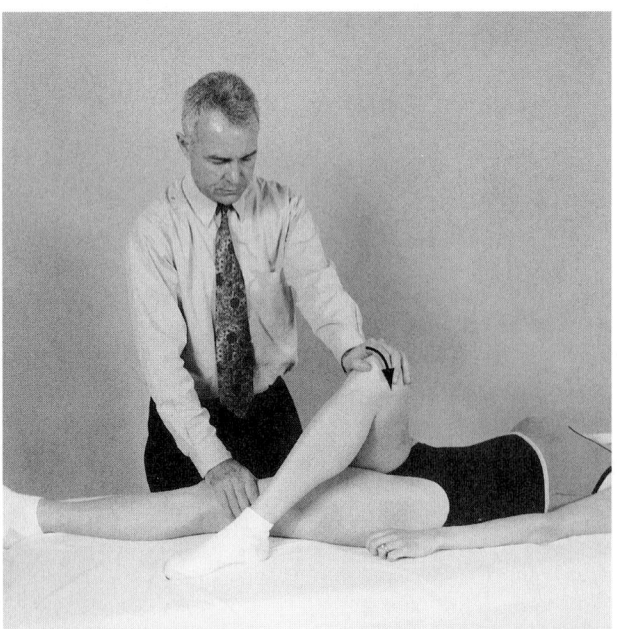

FIGURE 17-39 Piriformis stretch.

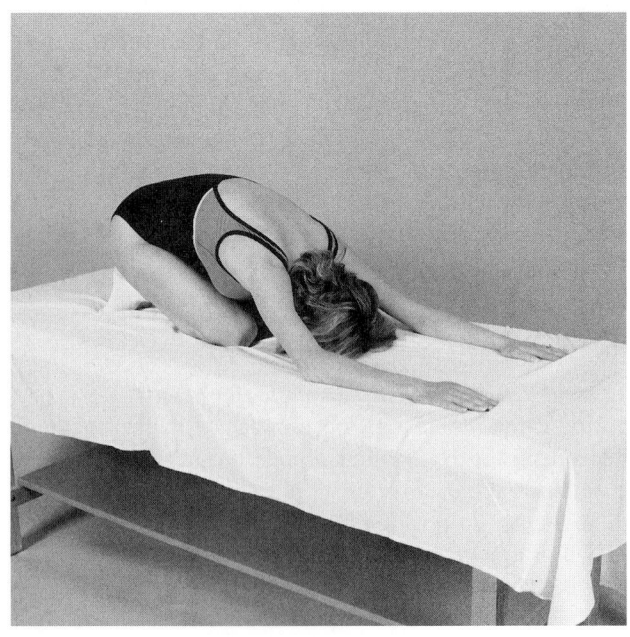

FIGURE 17-40 Posterior capsule stretch.

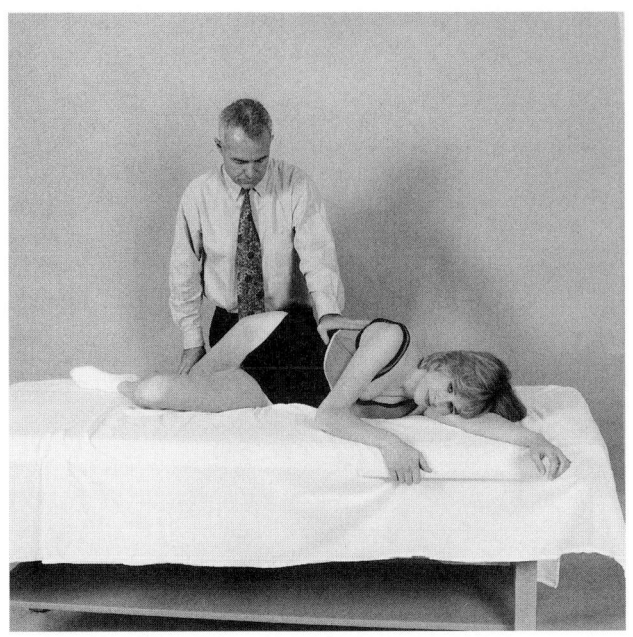

FIGURE 17-41 Passive and gravity-assisted joint capsule distraction.

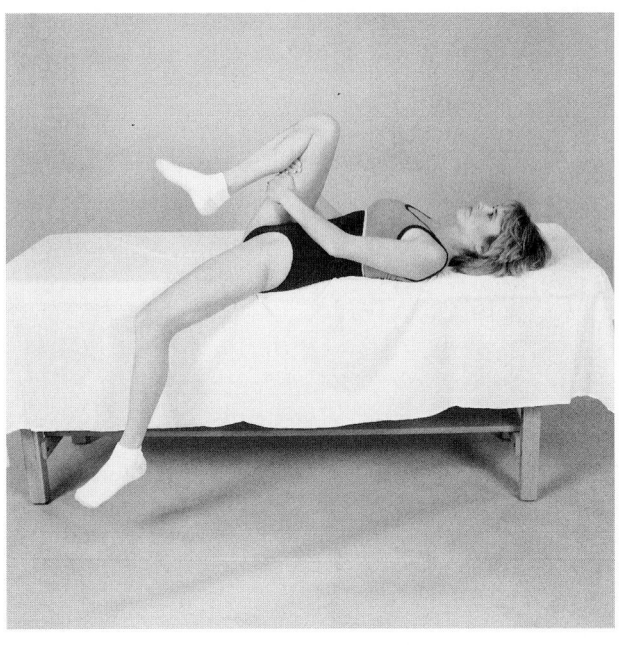

FIGURE 17-43 Unilateral abdominal and hip flexor stretch.

performed unilaterally by hanging the uninvolved extremity over the edge of the bed (Fig. 17-43).

Iliopsoas and Rectus Femoris.   Although a number of exercises have been advocated to stretch these muscle groups, because of their potential to increase the anterior shear of the lumbar vertebrae either directly or indirectly, the standing/kneeling position is preferred.

A pillow is placed on the floor and the patient kneels down on the pillow with the other leg placed out in front in the typical lunge position (Fig. 17-44). The patient is asked to perform a posterior pelvic tilt and to maintain an erect position with respect to the trunk. From this starting position, the patient glides the trunk anteriorly, maintaining the trunk in the near vertical position. A stretch on the upper aspect of the anterior thigh of the kneeling leg should be felt. The rectus femoris can be stretched

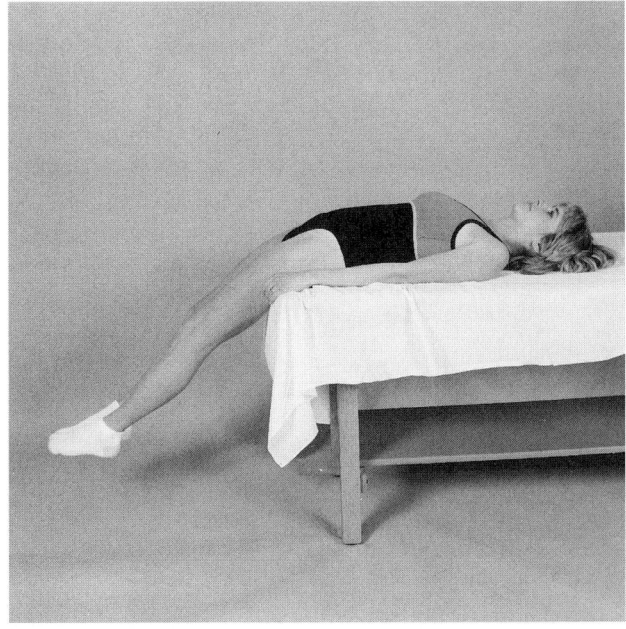

FIGURE 17-42 Abdominal stretch.

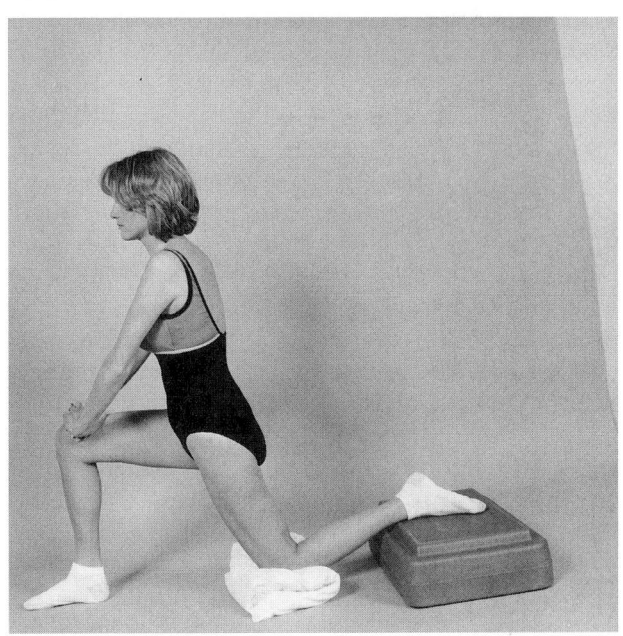

FIGURE 17-44 Psoas stretch.

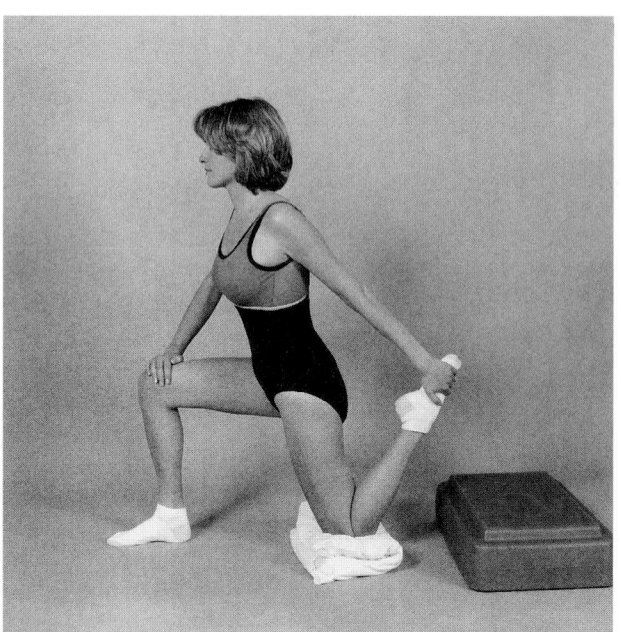

FIGURE 17-45　Psoas and rectus femoris stretch.

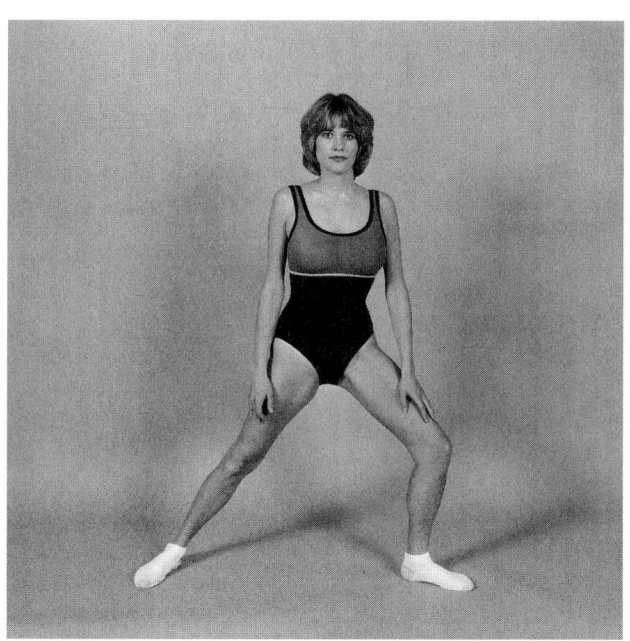

FIGURE 17-46　Standing hip adductor stretch.

further from this position by grasping the ankle of the kneeling leg, and raising the foot toward the buttock (Fig. 17-45).

Hamstrings. A number of techniques have evolved over the years to stretch the hamstrings. The problem with most of these techniques is that they do not afford the lumbar spine much protection while performing the stretch.

The hamstring stretch should be taught with the patient in a supine position. The lumbar spine is protected by placing a small towel roll under the lumbar spine to maintain a slight lordosis, or by having the patient sustain a pelvic tilt opposite to the lordosis during the stretch. The uninvolved leg is kept straight while the patient flexes the hip of the side to be tested to about 90 degrees (see Fig. 17-29). From this position, the patient extends the knee on the tested leg until a stretch is felt on the posterior aspect of the thigh. This position is maintained for about 30 seconds before allowing the knee to flex slightly.

Hip Adductors. The patient stands facing a table with their feet spread apart, and their toes pointing forward. The pelvis is tilted to adopt a functional neutral position of the spine. To stretch the left adductor muscle, the patient lunges to the right while keeping the left knee extended (Fig. 17-46).

Gluteus Maximus and Short Hip Extensors. This stretch is performed in supine by pulling one or both knees to the chest (see Fig. 17-26), or in the lunge position, depending on patient ability and tolerance.

Tensor Fascia Latae. The patient is positioned supine with the legs straight. The foot of the leg to be stretched is placed on the table on the outside of the uninvolved straight leg. The patient

reaches and grasps the knee of the involved leg and pulls the knee across and over the straight leg. Both shoulders should be kept flat against the table. At the point the stretch is felt, the position is maintained for approximately 30 seconds. The stretch is repeated ten times (Fig. 17-47).

Iliotibial Band. The patient stands close to a bed with the uninvolved side closer to the bed, and the balance supported. Both

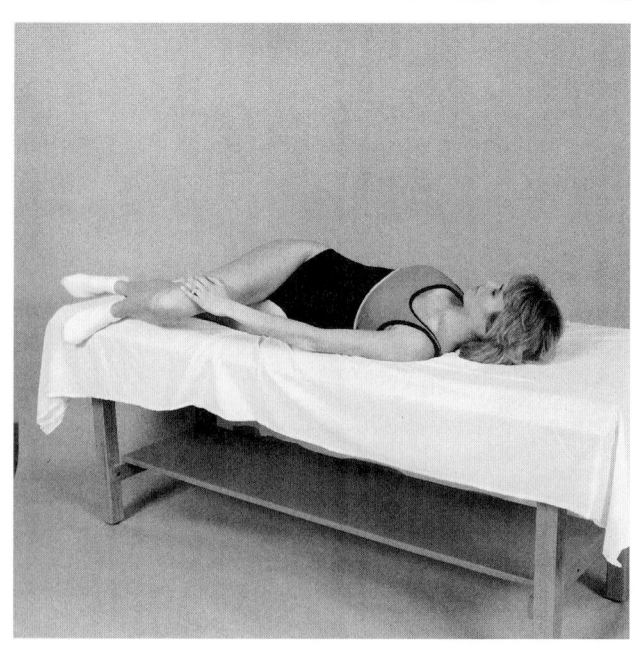

FIGURE 17-47　Tensor fascia latae stretch.

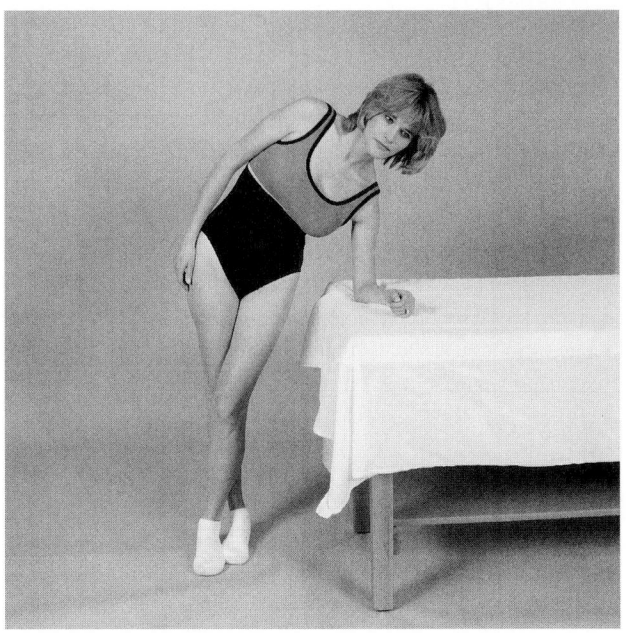

FIGURE 17-48 Iliotibial band stretch.

legs are crossed, and the hip is translated away from the bed while the trunk is leaned towards the bed until a stretch is felt on the outside of the hip and thigh (Fig. 17-48).[208]

CASE STUDY RIGHT GROIN PAIN

HISTORY

General Demographics
A 62-year-old English speaking male.

History of Current Condition
The patient presented with complaints of aching pain in the right groin that varies in severity and extends down the anterior thigh to the knee. The pain began gradually about 3 months before. Initially the patient felt stiffness whenever he sat for prolonged periods of time or after a night's sleep. The patient reports that he can no longer walk as far as he once did, and that negotiating stairs was especially painful.

Past History of Current Condition
A long history of osteoarthritis of the spine and occasional twinges of pain in the right groin. The patient also has history of right-sided sciatica.

Past Medical/Surgical History
Patient had a total joint replacement of the right knee approximately 4 months ago.

Medications
Celecoxib.

Other Tests and Measures
Radiographs of right hip are negative for loose bodies, tumors, and fracture. Advanced osteoarthritis of right hip noted.

Social Habits (Past and Present)
Nonsmoker. Drinks occasionally. Active life style.

Social History
Married. Two children, both live close by.

Family History
No relevant history of hip problems in family.

Growth and Development
Normal development; left-handed.

Living Environment
Lives in an apartment. One flight of stairs to negotiate.

Occupational/Employment/School
Retired railroad laborer. High school education.

Functional Status/Activity Level
The patient demonstrates difficulty rising from a chair, and transferring from bed to chair.

Health Status (self-report)
In general good health, but pain interferes with tasks at home and with helping his sick wife.

Systems Review
Unremarkable

QUESTIONS

1. List the possible structure(s) that can produce groin pain.
2. What might the history of pain with early morning stiffness and pain with stair negotiation tell the clinician?
3. What other activities might increase the patient's symptoms? Why?
4. To help rule out the various causes of groin pain, what other questions can you ask?
5. What is your working hypothesis at this stage? List the various diagnoses that could present with these signs and symptoms, and the tests you would use to rule out each one.
6. Does this presentation/history warrant a Cyriax lower quarter scanning examination? Why or why not?

TESTS AND MEASURES

Due to the insidious nature of the patient's pain, a lower quarter scanning examination was performed but failed to elicit any signs and symptoms of serious pathology or overt neurologic compromise. The physical examination of the patient included an inspection for muscle atrophy, palpation for areas of tenderness and crepitus, muscle testing of all major muscles about the hip, measurement of active and passive range of motion, and special tests.

Community and Work Integration/Reintegration

Patient is retired.

Environment, Home, and Work Barriers

Difficulties experienced looking after spouse.

Gait, Locomotion, and Balance

Excessive hyperextension of the left knee is noted during stance, especially during the push-off phase as the patient ambulates by circumducting the right hip. A shorter stride length and decreased heel strike is noted on the right. The patient also demonstrated a lack of hip extension, and ankle plantar flexion at the end of single leg stance.[209]

Integumentary Integrity

Not tested.

Joint Integrity and Mobility

Negative compression and distraction tests of the sacroiliac joint (see Chap. 27). Negative pubic stress tests (see Chap. 27). Positive scour test and FABER test of right hip. Abnormal capsular end-feel noted at right hip. A 5-degree flexion contracture is noted in the left knee.

Motor Performance: Strength, Power, and Endurance

Strength of the right thigh musculature is at 4 out of 5 compared with the contralateral extremity, particularly in the gluteus medius, maximus, and hamstring muscles. Weakness of left hip adductors noted.

Orthotic, Protective, and Supportive Devices

Patient ambulating with cane.

Pain

Pain rated at 8 out of 10 with ascending stairs and after arising in the morning.

Posture

In standing, a pelvic obliquity of the higher right pelvis was noted. The right lower extremity is held in relative abduction, while the left lower extremity is held in relative adduction at the hip. The right knee is slightly flexed. Scoliotic curves of the low back and cervical spine are noted. A slight leg length discrepancy of 3 centimeters is noted, with the left leg shorter than the right.

Range of Motion (Including Muscle Length)

Capsular pattern of motion noted at the right hip with extension, abduction, and internal rotation markedly diminished. Seventy degrees of straight leg raising is available on the left, whereas 55 degrees is available on the right. Hip adduction limited on the left. Hip abduction limited on the right.

Reflex Integrity

Normal and symmetrical patellar and Achilles reflexes bilaterally.

Self-Care and Home Management

Patient has a sick wife who is unable to perform any domestic duties.

Sensory Integrity

The distal right limb is intact neurovascularly.

EVALUATION (CLINICAL JUDGMENT)

The patient is an elderly, moderately obese male with suspected advanced osteoarthritis of the right hip, with pain with weight-bearing activities including ascending stairs, which results in functional limitations at home.

DIAGNOSIS BY PHYSICAL THERAPIST

Impaired joint mobility, motor function, muscle performance, and range of motion associated with capsular restriction, localized inflammation, and impaired posture.

PROGNOSIS

Predicted Optimal Level of Improvement in Function

Over the course of 6 weeks, a trial course of conservative physical therapy intervention will be performed in an attempt to achieve the highest possible functional outcome for the patient.

QUESTIONS

1. What will be your intervention?
2. How would you describe this condition to the patient?
3. What would you tell the patient about your intervention?
4. How will you determine the intensity of your intervention?
5. Estimate this patient's prognosis
6. Given the physical therapy diagnosis, why is it not possible to plan the intervention based on the phases of healing?
7. What modalities could you use in the intervention of this patient? Why?
8. Which manual techniques would be appropriate for this patient, and what is your rationale?
9. What exercises would you prescribe? Why?

PLAN OF CARE

Direct Intervention

PAIN AND INFLAMMATION CONTROL. Modalities such as moist heat, hydrotherapy, and TENS can be used to minimize swelling and decrease pain.[210,211] While cold is most effective in the acute stage, heat is more effective in the subacute or chronic stages.

PROMOTION AND PROGRESSION OF HEALING. Loss of excess weight may reduce the load assumed by the right hip joint and can be accomplished with a combination of diet and exercise. Joint protection plays a significant role in daily activities. The use of an assistive device can decrease the weight-bearing function of the hip. A cane, used correctly on the uninvolved side, can reduce the forces on the affected side to just slightly more than body weight, decreasing the magnitude of the resultant force on the joint.[212–216]

SPECIFIC MANUAL TECHNIQUES. A variety of specific manual stretching techniques can be used to stretch the iliopsoas, hamstrings, quadriceps, piriformis, and gastrocnemius. The focus is initially placed on the hip flexors and hamstrings, as the decreased mobility of this patient forces him to spend more time in the seated position, which places the hip flexors and hamstrings in an adaptively shortened position.

ANALYSIS AND INTEGRATION OF THE OPEN AND CLOSED KINETIC CHAINS INTO REHABILITATION. Strengthening exercises are advocated in the anterior and posterior thigh musculature, the hip adductors and abductors, the gastrocnemius, and the abdominals. Concentric exercises in both the open-chain and closed-chain modes are recommended.

CONTROLLING ABUSE AND FORCE LOADS. Specific strengthening exercises are used to complement the stretching regimen to provide better shock-absorbing capabilities to the joint, thereby diminishing the magnitude of concussive forces to the joint. The previously mentioned muscle groups are strengthened with emphasis on the exercises simulating functional activities. For example, the triceps can be strengthened, simulating rising up from a chair by pushing down with the arms.

One of the goals with the patient with osteoarthrosis of the hip is to regain muscle extensibility of the hip flexors, abductors, internal rotators, and extensors. Various stretching or soft tissue techniques can be used.

- A sustained stretch for the inner quadrant of flexion.
- Stretch in the FABER position while stabilizing the ilium. The home program for this involves sitting cross-legged on a stool or pile of newspapers, progressively lowering the height until seated on the floor. Progress to lying supine with legs in this position (soles touching).
- Stretch into extension and internal rotation.
- Stretching of the adductors in the prone FABER position.
- Sling suspension (axial and off-set) of involved extremity.
- Hip pendulum. The patient stands on a step and swings the involved leg like a pendulum.

Other exercises to regain muscle extensibility include:

1. The patient is positioned in good sitting posture, with their hips flexed, abducted, and externally rotated. The patient is asked to rotate the trunk to the left, and then to bring their left knee to the chest. The exercise is repeated on the other side.
2. Side lying extension. The patient is positioned in side lying with the uninvolved thigh held against the chest. The clinician passively extends the involved hip, ensuring that no motion occurs at the lumbar spine.
3. Climb extension. The patient raises one leg and places the foot on a chair. While keeping the other leg extended, the patient leans into the chair to increase flexion of the raised hip, and extension of the lower hip. This is repeated on the other side. This is an excellent exercise for the older population and can be used as part of a functional weight-bearing progression into a full squat.
4. Gluteus maximus sets with electrical stimulation in prone lying. The patient is positioned in prone lying. The pads are placed on the hip extensors (buttocks), with a moist heat pad placed on top to apply some compression.
5. Side-stepping.
6. Walking. If there is no antalgia with gait, the patient should be encouraged to walk. Pain-free walking is an excellent method of joint mobilization. If full weight bearing without pain is not possible, the patient should be educated on how to walk in a pool with a life jacket on.

All of the above exercises should be done frequently and the stretches should be held for sustained periods.

GENERAL STRENGTH AND FITNESS. The patient's general level of fitness must be maintained during the intervention period. This is particularly important in patients with osteoarthritis due to decreased activity levels.[217] This can be accomplished in a safe manner through low-impact exercises using an upper body ergonometer or a stationary bike, avoiding the painful ranges by adjusting the seat height. Walking through water can also be used with a water temperature of 86 degrees F.[218,219]

EDUCATION. The patient is instructed to avoid low chairs, sustained weight bearing, and deep knee bends. The patient is advised to sit in a high chair and elevated toilet seat. The importance of compliance with the home exercise program is explained, as is the importance of losing weight to reduce the forces through the joint.

RETURN TO FUNCTION. A gradual return to function is recommended. Exercises to continue strengthening, flexibility, and endurance training are maintained, and the patient should avoid deep-knee squatting or knee-bending activities in the immediate future.[220]

Frequency and Duration
2 to 3 times per week for 6 weeks.

Re-examination
Perform selected tests and measures to evaluate patient's progress toward goals in order to modify or redirect intervention if the patient fails to show progress.

Criteria for Discharge
Patient to be discharged when they reach established functional goals, decline further intervention, is unable to progress towards goals because of complications, or PT determines that patient will no longer benefit from PT services.

Coordination, Communication, and Documentation
Communicate with MD and patient regarding patient's status (direct or indirect). Documentation will include all elements of patient/client management. Discharge planning will be provided.

Patient-Related Instruction
Periodic re-examination and reassessment of the home program, utilizing written instruction and illustrations. Educate patient in proper postures, and positions and motions to avoid at home and at

work. Educate patient in the benefits of an ongoing conditioning program to prevent recurrence of impairments.

CASE STUDY THIGH PAIN

HISTORY

History of Current Condition

A 22-year-old male sustained a kick to the right thigh approximately 2 weeks ago while playing college soccer. He complains of a dull ache on the anterior aspect of his thigh. The pain is worse with activities that involve attempting to squat or kick. The patient also reports feeling a lump on the front of his thigh. The patient saw his physician who diagnosed the condition as a deep quadriceps contusion, and prescribed 8 weeks of physical therapy.

Past History of Current Condition

No previous history of thigh pain.

Past Medical/Surgical History

- No history of previous knee or hip injury.
- No back pain/surgery reported.
- No knee surgeries reported.
- History of chronic ankle sprains.

Medications

None.

Other Tests and Measures

Radiograph results pending.

Occupational/Employment/School

Full-time student at local college for the past 2 years.

Functional Status/Activity Level

Very active. In addition to soccer, the patient also plays tennis and racquetball.

Health Status (Self-Report)

In general good health.

QUESTIONS

1. Given the specific mechanism of injury, list all of the structures you suspect could be injured and will require a specific examination.
2. What condition could be present with the history of pain in a muscle belly following a contusion?
3. What other activities do you suspect would increase the patient's symptoms? Why?
4. In a patient with an insidious onset of pain, what questions would you ask to help rule out the various causes of anterior thigh pain?
5. What is your working hypothesis at this stage?
6. Does this presentation/history warrant a lower quarter scan? Why or why not?

TESTS AND MEASURES

Community and Work Integration/Reintegration

Patient reports having difficulty getting to and from dorm room, which involves negotiating two flights of stairs.

Gait, Locomotion, and Balance

Gait examination revealed:

- A decrease in right leg stance phase, a decrease in right stride length, and slight positive right Trendelenburg.
- The patient demonstrated difficulty with unilateral lower extremity balance-reach testing. This test involves standing on the involved leg and reaching in various directions and at various heights with the uninvolved extremity.
- The patient also demonstrated diminished ability with unilateral upper extremity balance-reach testing. This test involves standing on the involved leg and reaching in various directions and at various heights with the upper extremities.

Integumentary Integrity

No signs of redness or streaking noted around the contusion. Swelling appears to extend down to right knee. The palpable mass is approximately 4×8 cm in the anterior lateral right thigh and is tender to palpation.

Motor Performance: Strength, Power, and Endurance

- Pain with attempted squatting. Patient able to perform mini-squat.
- Pain with isometric and resistive right knee extension.
- Pain with resistive hip flexion with hip placed in extreme hip extension.
- Strength at 5 out of 5 for all muscle groups except right hip flexion and right knee extension, which were graded at 4 out of 5, due more to pain than apparent weakness.

Pain

Pain rated at 7 out of 10 on visual analog scale.

Range of Motion (Including Muscle Length)

- Range of motion of the right hip decreased to 5 degrees in hip extension due to pain, and 100 degrees in hip flexion when the knee is flexed.
- Range of motion of the right knee decreased due to pain to 85 degrees in flexion.
- Range of motion of other joints were within normal limits.
- Positive Thomas test in right lower extremity.
- Positive Ober test, indicating adaptive shortening of iliotibial band in right lower extremity.

Reflex Integrity

Normal and symmetrical Achilles and patellar reflexes bilaterally.

Sensory Integrity

Intact to light touch L2 to S1 bilaterally.

EVALUATION (CLINICAL JUDGMENT)

This is a young, healthy and physically active male, who has sustained a grade II contusion to the thigh, and is experiencing difficulty with stair negotiation due to pain and loss of knee ROM.

DIAGNOSIS BY PHYSICAL THERAPIST

Impaired joint mobility, motor function, muscle performance, and range of motion associated with muscle performance; localized inflammation of the soft tissues of the thigh.

QUESTIONS

1. Having made the provisional diagnosis, outline the three phases of your intervention.
2. How would you describe this condition to the patient?
3. How would you explain the rationale of your intervention to the patient?
4. How will you determine the intensity of your intervention?
5. Estimate this patient's prognosis.
6. Which modalities would be appropriate for this patient? Why?
7. Which manual techniques would be appropriate for this patient, and what is your rationale?
8. What exercises would you prescribe? Why?

PROGNOSIS

Predicted Optimal Level of Improvement in Function

Over the course of 8 weeks or less, the patient will demonstrate a return to normal sporting activities and will be able to negotiate stairs without pain or difficulty. Patient will be able to:

- Attain full and pain-free AROM of the right hip and knee as compared to the uninvolved side.
- Report pain at 2 out of 10 or less with activity 0 out of 10 at rest.
- Demonstrate strength of right hip flexion and right knee extension at 5 out of 5 with manual muscle testing and closed chain functional testing as compared with the uninvolved extremity.
- Demonstrate a pain-free and normal gait pattern on all surfaces.
- Demonstrate independence and compliance with home exercise program and will demonstrate a knowledge of progression to return to sport.

PLAN OF CARE

Frequency and Duration

2 times per week for 8 weeks.

Re-examination

Perform selected tests and measures to evaluate patient's progress toward goals in order to modify or redirect intervention if patient fails to show progress.

Criteria for Discharge

Patient reaches established functional goals, declines further intervention, is unable to progress toward goals because of complications, or PT determines that patient will no longer benefit from PT services.

INTERVENTION
PHASE I (0 TO WEEK 3)

This phase typically involves 2 to 6 visits of physical therapy.

Goals

- Pain at 5 out of 10 or less with activity.
- Normal gait pattern.
- Pain-free AROM of right hip and knee flexion to be within 20 degrees of normal. Right hip extension to be within normal limits with knee extended
- Strength at 4 out of 5 on manual muscle testing on areas of weakness detected in examination.

Electrotherapeutic Modalities

- Iontophoresis.
- Electrical stimulation.
- Cryotherapy.
- Ultrasound.
- Phonophoresis.

Therapeutic Exercise and Home Program

- Flexibility exercises for hamstrings, quadriceps, iliotibial band, hip flexors, and hip adductors.
- Weight-bearing exercises in the pain-free range, including squats, weight shifts, lunges (anterior, posterior, and lateral), and step-ups/downs.
- Non-weight bearing chain exercises including pain-free AROM, and strengthening exercises with emphasis on the gluteus maximus, gluteus medius, and hip adductors.
- Cardiovascular training using UBE (upper body ergometer).

Manual Therapy

- Soft tissue techniques of myofascial release, and soft tissue mobilizations as indicated.
- Gentle passive stretching to right quadriceps, iliotibial band, and right hip flexors. Care taken with quadriceps stretching to avoid provoking myositis ossificans.

Neuromuscular Re-education

- Balance and reach drills.
- Gait drills.
- BAPS (biomechanical ankle platform system).

PHASE II (WEEKS 4–8)

This phase typically involves 4 to 8 visits of physical therapy.

Goals

- Pain at 2 out of 10 or less with activity.
- Pain-free, normal AROM of right hip and knee.
- Return to previous functional level for ADL.

Electrotherapeutic Modalities

Continued use of those modalities that are beneficial.

Therapeutic Exercise and Home Program

- Progression of flexibility exercises.
- Progression of strengthening exercises.
- Progression of previous weight-bearing exercises and addition of pulley and tubing exercises for four-way hip exercises.

Manual Therapy

- Proprioceptive neuromuscular facilitation (PNF) patterns.
- Soft tissue techniques as appropriate.
- Continuation of passive stretches as needed.

Neuromuscular Re-education

- Continuation of previous drills.
- Introduction of plyometric activities as tolerated.

PHASE III (RETURN TO SPORT)

Coordination, Communication, and Documentation

Communicate with MD and patient. Documentation will include all elements of patient/client management. Discharge planning will be provided.

OUTCOMES

Patient's outcome depends on adherence to the recommended home exercise program and intervention plan.

REVIEW QUESTIONS*

1. What is the close-packed position of the hip?
2. In which direction is the acetabulum angled?
3. Which ligament contains the blood supply to the femoral head?
4. The pubofemoral ligament is taut in which three directions?
5. Which muscle is known as the deltoid of the hip?

* Additional questions to test your understanding of this chapter can be found in the Online Learning Center for *Orthopaedic Assessment, Evaluation, and Intervention* at www.duttononline.net.

REFERENCES

1. Bergmann G, Graichen F, Rohlmann A. Hip joint loading during walking and running measured in two patients. *J Biomech* 1993;26:969–990.
1a. Weinstein, SL. Natural history and treatment outcomes of childhood hip disorders. *Clin Orthop* 1997;344:227–242.
2. Ponseti IV. Growth and development of the acetabulum in the normal child. Anatomical, histological, and roentgenographic studies. *J Bone Joint Surg* 1978;60A:575–585.
3. Skirving AP, Scadden WJ. The African neonatal hip and its immunity from congenital dislocation. *J Bone Joint Surg Br* 1979;27:339–341.
4. Coleman CR, Slager RF, Smith WS. The effect of environmental influence on acetabular development. *Surg Forum* 1958;9:775–780.
5. Harrison TJ. The influence of the femoral head on pelvic growth and acetabular form in the rat. *J Anat* 1961;95:127–132.
6. Harris NH. Acetabular growth potential in congenital dislocation of the hip and some factors upon which it may depend. *Clin Orthop* 1976;119:99–106.
7. Harris NH, Lloyd-Roberts GC, Gallien R. Acetabular development in congenital dislocation of the hip with special reference to the indications of acetabuloplasty and pelvic or femoral realignment osteotomy. *J Bone Joint Surg* 1975;57B:46–52.
8. Lindstrom, JR, Ponseti IV, Wenger DR. Acetabular development after reduction in congenital dislocation of the hip. *J Bone Joint Surg* 1979;61A:112–118.
9. Harrison TJ. The growth of the pelvis in the rat—A mensural and morphological study. *J Anat* 1958;92:236–260.
10. Agus H, et al. Evaluation of the risk factors of avascular necrosis of the femoral head in developmental dysplasia of the hip in infants younger than 18 months of age. *J Pediatr Orthop* 2002;11:41–46.
11. Trueta I, Harrison MHM. The normal vascular anatomy of the femoral head in adult man. *J Bone Joint Surg* 1953;35B:442–461.
12. Fagerson TL. Hip. In: Wadsworth C, ed. *Current Concepts of Orthopedic Physical Therapy—Home Study Course.* La Crosse, WI: Orthopaedic Section, APTA; 2001.
12a. Maquet PG, Van de Berg AJ, Simonet JC. Femorotibial weight-bearing areas. Experimental determination. *J Bone Joint Surg,* 1975;57A:766–771.
12b. Williams PL. *Gray's Anatomy,* 38 ed. Williams PL, ed. New York: Churchill Livingstone; 1995.
12c. Konrath, GA, et al. The role of the acetabular labrum and the transverse acetabular ligament in load transmission in the hip. *J Bone Joint Surg* 1998;80A:1781–1788.
12d. Narvani AA, et al. Acetabular labrum and its tears. *Brit J Sports Med* 2003;37:207–211.
12e. Kim YT, Azuma H. The nerve endings of the acetabular labrum. *Clin Orthop* 1995;320:176–181.
12f. Seldes R, et al. Anatomy, histologic features, and vascularity of the adult acetabular labrum. *Clin Orthop Rel Res* 2001; 382:232–240.
12g. Takechi H, Nagashima H, Ito S. Intra-articular pressure of the hip joint outside and inside the limbus. *J Japanese Orthop Assn* 1982;56:529–536.
13. Hall SJ. The biomechanics of the human lower extremity. In: *Basic Biomechanics.* New York: McGraw-Hill: 1999:234–281.
14. Gordon, EJ. Trochanteric bursitis and tendinitis. *Clin Orthop* 1961;20:193–202.
15. Johnson CE, Basmajian JV, Dasher W. Electromyography of the sartorius muscle. *Anat Rec* 1972;173:127–130.
16. Janda V. On the concept of postural muscles and posture in man. *Aust J Physiother* 1983;29:83–84.
17. Kapandji IA. *The Physiology of the Joints, Lower Limb.* New York: Churchill Livingstone; 1991.
18. Durrani Z, Winnie AP. Piriformis muscle syndrome: an underdiagnosed cause of sciatica. *J Pain Symptom Manag* 1991; 6:374–379.
19. Julsrud ME. Piriformis syndrome. *J Am Podiat Med Assn* 1989;79:128–131.
20. Pace JB, Nagle D. Piriformis syndrome. *West J Med* 1976; 124:435–439.
21. Steiner C, et al. Piriformis syndrome: pathogenesis, diagnosis, and treatment. *J Am Osteopath Assn* 1987;87:318–323.
22. Harvey G, Bell S. Obturator neuropathy. An anatomic perspective. *Clin Orthop* 1999;363:203–211.

23. Williams PL, et al. *Gray's Anatomy*, 37th ed. London: Churchill Livingstone; 1989.

24. Anderson MA, et al. The relationship among isokinetic, isotonic, and isokinetic concentric and eccentric quadriceps and hamstrings force and three components of athletic performance. *J Orthop Sports Phys Ther* 1991;14:114–120.

25. More RC, et al. Hamstrings—an anterior cruciate ligament protagonist. An in vitro study. *Am J Sports Med* 1993;21:231–237.

26. Holmich P. Adductor related groin pain in athletes. *Sports Med Arth Rev* 1998;5:285–291.

27. Hasselman CT, Best TM, Garrett WE. When groin pain signals an adductor strain. *Physician Sports Med* 1995;23:53–60.

28. Shbeeb MI, Matteson EL. Trochanteric bursitis (greater trochanter pain syndrome). *Mayo Clin Proc* 1996;71:565–569.

28a. Melamed A, Bauer C, Johnson H. Iliopsoas bursal extension of arthritic disease of the hip. *Radiology* 1967;89:54–58.

28b. Armstrong P, Saxton H, Ilio-psoas bursa. *Br J Radiol* 1972;45:493–495.

28c. Chandler SB. The iliopsoas bursa in man. *Anat Rec* 1934;58:235–240.

28d. Fagerson TL. Hip. In: *Current Concepts of Orthopedic Physical Therapy—Home Study Course.* Wadsworth C, ed. La Crosse, Wis: Orthopaedic Section. APTA, 2001.

28e. Sartoris DJ, et al. Synovial cysts of the hip joint and iliopsoas bursitis: a spectrum of imaging abnormalities. *Skeletal Radiol* 1985;14:85–94.

28f. Yamamoto T, et al. Dumbbell-shaped iliopsoas bursitis penetrating the pelvic wall: a rare complication of hip arthrodesis. A case report. *J Bone Joint Surg* 2003;85A:343–345.

29. Croley TE. Anatomy of the Hip. In: Echternach JL, ed. *Physical Therapy of the Hip.* New York: Churchill Livingstone: 1990:1–16.

30. Bruce J, Walmsley R, Ross JA. *Manual of Surgical Anatomy.* Edinburgh: Churchill Livingstone; 1964.

31. Sevitt S, Thompson RG. The distribution and anastomoses of arteries supplying the head and neck of the femur. *J Bone Joint Surg Br* 1965;47B:560–573.

32. Bachiller FG, Caballer AP, Portal LF. Avascular necrosis of the femoral head after femoral neck fracture. *Clin Orthop* 2002;399:87–109.

33. Gautier E, et al. Anatomy of the medial femoral circumflex artery and its surgical implications. *J Bone Joint Surg Br* 2000;82:679–683.

34. Cibulka MT, et al. Unilateral hip rotation range of motion asymmetry in patients with sacroiliac joint regional pain. *Spine* 1998;23:1009–1015.

35. Gage JR, Camy JM. The effects of trochanteric epiphysiodesis on growth of the proximal end of the femur following necrosis of the capital femoral epiphysis. *J Bone Joint Surg* 1980;62A:785–794.

36. Osborne D, et al. The development of the upper end of the femur with special reference to its internal architecture. *Radiology* 1980;137:71–76.

37. Schofield CB, Smibert JG. Trochanteric growth disturbance after upper femoral osteotomy for congenital dislocation of the hip. *J Bone Joint Surg* 1990;72B:32–36.

38. Afoke NYP, Byers PD, Hutton WC. Contact pressures in the human hip joint. *J Bone Joint Surg Am* 1987;69B:536.

39. Oatis CA. Biomechanics of the hip. In: Echternach J, ed. *Clinics in Physical Therapy: Physical Therapy of the Hip.* New York: Churchill Livingstone; 1990:37–50.

40. Pauwels F. *Biomechanics of the Normal and Diseased Hip.* Berlin: Springer-Verlag; 1976.

41. Maquet PGJ. *Biomechanics of the Hip as Applied to Osteoarthritis and Related Conditions.* Berlin: Springer-Verlag; 1985.

42. Menke W, et al. Transversale Skelettachsen der unteren Extremitat bei Coxarthrose. *Zeitschr Orthop* 1991;129:255–259.

43. Pizzutillo PT, MacEwen GD, Shands AR. Anteversion of the femur. In: Tonzo RG, ed. *Surgery of the Hip Joint.* Springer-Verlag: New York; 1984.

44. Lausten GS, Jorgensen F, Boesen J. Measurement of anteversion of the femoral neck, ultrasound and CT compared. *J Bone Joint Surg Am* 1989;71B:237.

45. Gross MT. Lower quarter screening for skeletal malalignment—suggestions for orthotics and shoewear. *J Orthop Sports Phys Ther* 1995;21:389–405.

46. Giunti A, et al. The importance of the angle of anteversion in the development of arthritis of the hip. *Italian J Orthop Traumatol* 1985;11:23–27.

47. Reikeras O, Hoiseth A. Femoral neck angles in osteoarthritis of the hip. *Acta Orthop Scand* 1982;53:781–784.

48. Reikeras O, Bjerkreim I, Kolbenstvedt A. Anteversion of the acetabulum and femoral neck in normals and in patients with osteoarthritis of the hip. *Acta Orthop Scand* 1983;54:18–23.

49. Terjesen T, et al. Increased femoral anteversion and osteoarthritis of the hip. *Acta Orthop Scand* 1982;53:571–575.

50. Eckhoff DG. Femoral anteversion in arthritis of the knee [letter]. *J Pediat Orthop* 1995;15:700.

51. Eckhoff DG, et al. Femoral morphometry and anterior knee pain. *Clin Orthop* 1994;302:64–68.

52. Aranow S, Zippel H. Untersuchung zur femoro-tibialen Torsion bei Patellainstabilitaten. Ein Beitrag zur Pathogenese rezidivierender und habitueller Patelluxationen. *Beitr Orthop Traumat* 1990;37:311–326.

53. Swanson AB, Greene PW Jr, Allis HD. Rotational deformities of the lower extremity in children and their clinical significance. *Clin Orthop* 1963;27:157–175.

54. Hubbard DD, et al. Medial femoral torsion and osteoarthritis. *J Pediat Orthop* 1988;8:540–542.

55. Kitaoka HB, et al. Relationship between femoral anteversion and osteoarthritis of the hip. *J Pediat Orthop* 1989;9:396–404.

56. Sahrmann SA. Movement impairment syndromes of the hip. In: Sahrmann SA, ed. *Movement Impairment Syndromes.* St. Louis: Mosby; 2001:121–191.

57. Kendall FP, McCreary EK, Provance PG. *Muscles: Testing and Function.* Baltimore: Williams & Wilkins; 1993.

58. Deusinger R. Validity of pelvic tilt measurements in anatomical neutral position. *J Biomech* 1992;25:764.

59. Kaltenborn FM. *Manual Mobilization of the Extremity Joints: Basic Examination and Treatment Techniques,* 4th ed. Oslo, Norway: Olaf Norlis Bokhandel, Universitetsgaten; 1989.

60. Yoder E. Physical therapy management of nonsurgical hip problems in adults. In: Echternach JL, ed. *Physical Therapy of the Hip.* New York: Churchill Livingstone; 1990:103–137.

61. Cyriax J. *Textbook of Orthopaedic Medicine, Diagnosis of Soft Tissue Lesions,* 8th ed. London: Bailliere Tindall; 1982.

62. Cyriax JH, Cyriax PJ. *Illustrated Manual of Orthopaedic Medicine.* London: Butterworth; 1983.

63. Johnston RC. Mechanical considerations of the hip joint. *Arch Surg* 1973;107:411.

64. Paul JP, McGrouther DA. Forces transmitted at the hip and knee joint of normal and disabled persons during a range of activities. *Acta Orthop Belg* 1975;41(Suppl):78.

65. Bergmann G, Graichen F, Rohlmann A. Hip joint loading during walking and running, measured in two patients. *J Biomech* 1993;26:969.

66. Bergmann G, Graichen F, Rohlmann A. Is staircase walking a risk for the fixation of hip implants? *J Biomech* 1995;28:535.

67. Norkin C, Levangie P. *Joint Structure and Function: A Comprehensive Analysis*. Philadelphia: FA Davis; 1992:355–358.

67a. Wroblewski BM. Pain in osteoarthrosis of the hip. *Practitioner* 1978;1315:140–141.

67b. Spiera H. Osteoarthritis as a misdiagnosis in elderly patients. *Geriatrics* 1987;42:37–42.

67c. Schon L, Zuckerman JD. Hip pain in the elderly: Evaluation and diagnosis. *Geriatrics* 1988;43:48–62.

67d. Echternach JL. Evaluation of the hip. In: Echternach JL, ed. *Physical Therapy of the Hip*. New York: Churchill Livingstone; 1990:17–32.

68. Echternach JL. Evaluation of the hip. In: Echternach JL, ed. *Physical Therapy of the Hip*. New York: Churchill Livingstone; 1990:17–32.

69. Wroblewski BM. Pain in osteoarthrosis of the hip. *Practitioner* 1978;1315:140–141.

70. Spiera H. Osteoarthritis as a misdiagnosis in elderly patients. *Geriatrics* 1987;42:37–42.

71. Schon L, Zuckerman JD. Hip pain in the elderly: Evaluation and diagnosis. *Geriatrics* 1988;43:48–62.

71a. Sahrmann SA. Movement impairment syndromes of the hip. In: *Movement Impairment Syndromes,* Sahrmann SA, ed. Mosby: St. Louis; 2001:121–191.

71b. Deusinger R. Validity of pelvic tilt measurements in anatomical neutral position. *J Biomech* 1992;25:764.

72. Jull GA, Janda V. Muscle and motor control in low back pain. In: Twomey LT, Taylor JR, eds. *Physical Therapy of the Low Back: Clinics in Physical Therapy.* New York: Churchill Livingstone; 1987:258.

73. Turek SL. *Orthopaedics—Principles and Their Application,* 4th ed. Vol. 2. Philadelphia: JB Lippincott; 1984.

74. Cailliet R. *Soft Tissue Pain and Disability.* Philadelphia: FA Davis; 1980.

75. Yamomoto S, et al. Quantitative gait evaluation of hip diseases using principal component analysis. *J Biomech* 1983;16:717.

76. Neumann DA, Cook TM. Effects of load and carry position on the electromyographic activity of the gluteus medius muscles during walking. *Phys Ther* 1985;65:305–311.

77. Clark JM, Haynor DR. Anatomy of the abductor muscles of the hip as studied by computed tomography. *J Bone Joint Surg* 1987;69A:1021.

78. Isacson J, Brostrom LA. Gait in rheumatoid arthritis: An electromyographic investigation. *J Biomech* 1988;21:451.

79. Neumann DA, Soderberg GL, Cook TM. Electromyographic analysis of the hip abductor musculature in healthy right-handed persons. *Phys Ther* 1989;69:431–440.

80. Inman VT, Ralston HJ, Todd F. *Human Walking.* Baltimore: Williams & Wilkins; 1981.

81. Lehmkuhl LD, Smith LK. *Brunnstrom's Clinical Kinesiology.* Philadelphia: FA Davis; 1983.

82. Hoppenfeld S. Physical examination of the hip and pelvis. In: *Physical Examination of the Spine and Extremities.* East Norwalk, CT: Appleton-Century-Crofts; 1976:143.

83. McKenzie R, May S. History. In: McKenzie R, May S, eds. *The Human Extremities: Mechanical Diagnosis and Therapy.* Waikanae, New Zealand: Spinal Publications New Zealand Ltd; 2000:89–103.

84. Janda V. *Muscle Function Testing.* London: Butterworth; 1983: 163–167.

85. Vasilyeva LF, Lewit K. Diagnosis of muscular dysfunction by inspection. In: Liebenson C, ed. *Rehabilitation of the Spine: A Practitioner's Manual.* Baltimore: Lippincott Williams & Wilkins; 1996:113–142.

86. Clark MA. *Integrated Training for the New Millenium.* Thousand Oaks, CA: National Academy of Sports Medicine; 2001.

87. Gelberman RH, et al. Femoral anteversion. *J Bone Joint Surg* 1987;69B:75.

88. Palmer ML, Epler M. *Clinical Assessment Procedures in Physical Therapy.* Philadelphia: JB Lippincott; 1990:68–73.

89. Maitland GD. *The Peripheral Joints: Examination and Recording Guide.* Adelaide, Australia: Virgo Press; 1973.

90. Ruwe PA, et al. Clinical determination of femoral anteversion: a comparison with established techniques. *J Bone Joint Surg* 1992;74:820.

91. Woods D, Macnicol M. The flexion-adduction test: an early sign of hip disease. *J Pediatr Orthop* 2001;10:180–185.

92. Zimney NJ. Clinical reasoning in the evaluation and management of undiagnosed chronic hip pain in young adult. *Phys Ther* 1998;78:62–73.

93. Harvey D. Assessment of the flexibility of elite athletes using the modified Thomas test. *Br J Sports Med* 1998;32:68–70.

94. Grelsamer RP, McConnell J. *The Patella: A Team Approach.* Gaithersburg, Maryland: Aspen; 1998.

95. Melchione WE, Sullivan MS. Reliability of measurements obtained by the use of an instrument designed to indirectly measure ilio-tibial band length. *J Orthop Sports Phys Ther* 1993;18:511–515.

96. Johnson AW, Weiss CB, Wheeler DL. Stress fractures of the femoral shaft in athletes—more common than expected: A new clinical test. *Am J Sports Med* 1994;22:248–256.

97. Aronsson DD, et al. Developmental dysplasia of the hip. *Pediatrics* 1994;94(2 Pt 1):201–208.

98. Ortolani M. Un segno poco noto e sue importanza per la diagnosi precoce di prelussazione congenita dell'anca. *Pediatria* 1937;45:129–136.

99. Barlow TG. Early diagnosis and treatment of congenital dislocation of the hip. *J Bone Joint Surg Br* 1962;44:292–301.

100. Booth FW. Physiologic and biochemical effects of immobilization on muscle. *Clin Orthop* 1987;219:15–21.

101. Eiff MP, Smith AT, Smith GE. Early mobilization versus immobilization in the treatment of lateral ankle sprains. *Am J Sports Med* 1994;22:83–88.

102. Akeson WH, et al. Collagen cross-linking alterations in the joint contractures: changes in the reducible cross-links in periarticular connective tissue after 9 weeks immobilization. *Conn Tissue Res* 1977;5:15.

103. Akeson WH, et al. Effects of immobilization on joints. *Clin Orthop* 1987;219:28–37.

104. Akeson WH, Amiel D, Woo SL-Y. Immobility effects on synovial joints: The pathomechanics of joint contracture. *Biorheology* 1980;17:95–110.

105. Woo SL-Y, et al. Connective tissue response to immobility: A correlative study of biochemical and biomechanical measurements of normal and immobilized rabbit knee. *Arthritis Rheum* 1975;18:257–264.

106. Mennet P, Egger B, *Hüftdisziplin.* Rheinfelden, Switzerland: Solbadklink Rheinfelden; 1986.

107. Rothstein JM. Muscle biology: Clinical considerations. *Phys Ther* 1982;62:1823.

108. Carr JH. A Motor Relearning Programme for Stroke. Rockville, MD: Aspen; 1987.

109. Mohr TM, Allison JD, Patterson R. Electromyographic analysis of the lower extremity during pedalling. *J Orthop Sports Phys Ther* 1981;2:163.

110. Hubley CL, Kozey JW, Stanish WD. The effects of static stretching exercises and stationary cycling on range of motion at the hip joint. *J Orthop Sports Phys Ther* 1984;6:104.

111. Negus RA, et al. Heart rate, blood pressure, and oxygen consumption during orthopaedic rehabilitation exercise. *J Orthop Sports Phys Ther* 1987;8:346.

112. Knott M, Voss DE. *Proprioceptive Neuromuscular Facilitation*, 2nd ed. New York: Harper & Row; 1968.

113. Malone T, et al. Neuromuscular concepts. In: Ellenbecker TS, ed. *Knee Ligament Rehabilitation.* Philadelphia: Churchill Livingstone; 2000:399–411.

114. Risberg MA, et al. Design and implementation of a neuromuscular training program following anterior cruciate ligament reconstruction. *J Orthop Sports Phys Ther* 2001; 31:620–631.

115. Saliba V, Johnson G, Wardlaw C. Proprioceptive neuromuscular facilitation. In: Basmajian JV, Nyberg R, eds. *Rational Manual Therapies.* Baltimore: Williams & Wilkins; 1993.

116. Stanton PE. Hamstring injuries in sprinting—the role of eccentric exercise. *J Orthop Sports Phys Ther* 1989;10:343.

117. Bukata SV, Rosier RN. Diagnosis and treatment of osteoporosis. *Curr Opin Orthop* 2000;11:336–340.

118. Gallagher JC. The pathogenesis of osteoporosis. *Bone Miner* 1990;9:215–217.

119. Riggs BL, et al. Differential changes in bone mineral density of the appendicular and axial skeleton with aging: relationship to spinal osteoporosis. *J Clin Invest* 1981;67:328–335.

120. Kelepouris N, et al. Severe osteoporosis in men. *Ann Intern Med* 1995;123:452–460.

121. Wilson A, et al. Transient osteoporosis: transient bone marrow edema? *Radiology* 1988;167:757–760.

122. Major NM, Helms CA. Idiopathic transient osteoporosis of the hip. *Arthritis Rheum* 1997;40:1178–1179.

122a. Tepper S, Hochberg MC. Factors associated with hip osteoarthritis: Data from the first National Health and Nutrition Examination Survey (NHANES-I). *Am J Epidemiol,* 1993; 137:1081–1088.

122b. Danielsson, L., Incidence and prognosis of coxarthrosis. *Acta Orthop Scand* 1964;66(Suppl):9–87.

122c. Seifert MH, Whiteside CG, Savage O. A 5-year follow-up of fifty cases of idiopathic osteoarthritis of the hip. *Ann Rheum Dis* 1969;28:325–326.

122d. Cooper C, et al. Occupational activity and the risk of hip osteoarthritis. *Ann Rheum Dis* 1996;55:680–682.

122e. Felson DT. Epidemiology of hip and knee osteoarthritis. *Epidemiol Rev* 1988;10:1–28.

122f. Dieppe P. Management of hip osteoarthritis. *BMJ* 1995; 311:853–857.

122g. Spear CV. Common pathological problems of the hip. In: *Physical Therapy of the Hip.* Echternach JL, ed. Churchill Livingstone: New York; 1990:51–69.

122h. Guralnik J, et al. Lower-extremity function in persons over the age of 70 years as a predictor of subsequent disability. *N Engl J Med* 1995;332:556–560.

122i. Fried LP, Guralnik JM. Disability in older adults: Evidence regarding significance, etiology, and risk. *J Am Geriatr Soc* 1997;45:92–100.

122j. Minor MA, et al. Efficacy of physical conditioning exercise in patients with rheumatoid arthritis and osteoarthritis. *Arthritis Rheum* 1989;32:1396–1405.

122k. Felson DT. The epidemiology of osteoarthritis: Prevalence and risk factors. In: *Osteoarthritic Disorders.* Keuttner KE, Goldberg VM, eds. Rosemont, Ill: American Academy of Orthopaedic Surgeons; 1995:13–24.

123. Allen WC, Cope R. Coxa saltans: The snapping hip revisited. *J Am Acad Orthop Surg* 1995;3:303–308.

124. Teitz CC, et al. Tendon problems in athletic individuals. *J Bone Joint Surg* 1997;79-A:138–152.

125. Jacobson T, Allen WC. Surgical correction of the snapping iliopsoas tendon. *Am J Sports Med* 1990;18:470–474.

126. Lyons JC, Peterson LFA. The snapping iliopsoas tendon. *Mayo Clin Proc* 1984;59:327–329.

127. Sammarco GJ. The dancer's hip. *Clin Sports Med* 1983; 2:485–498.

128. Schaberg JE, Harper MC, Allen WC. The snapping hip syndrome. *Am J Sports Med* 1984;12:361–365.

129. Micheli LJ. Overuse injuries in children's sports. *Orthop Clin North Am* 1983;14:337–360.

130. Binnie JF. The snapping hip. *Ann Surg* 1913;58:59–66.

131. Mayer L. Snapping hip. *Surg Gynecol Obstet* 1919;29:425–428.

132. Brignall CG, Brown RM, Stainsby GD. Fibrosis of the gluteus maximus as a cause of snapping hip. A case report. *J Bone Joint Surg Am* 1993;75:909–910.

133. Faraj AA, Moulton A, Sirivastava VM. Snapping iliotibial band: Report of ten cases and review of the literature. *Acta Orthop Belg* 2001;67:19–23.

134. Altenberg AR. Acetabular labrum tears: A cause of hip pain and degenerative arthritis. *South Med J* 1977;70:174–175.

135. Dorrell JH, Catterall A. The torn acetabular labrum. *J Bone Joint Surg* 1986;68B:400–403.

136. Ikeda T, Awaya G, Suzuki S. Torn acetabular labrum in young patients: Arthroscopic diagnosis and management. *J Bone Joint Surg* 1988;70B:13–16.

137. Howse AJG. Orthopaedists aid ballet. *Clin Orthop* 1972; 89:52–63.

138. Quirk R. Ballet injuries: The Australian experience. *Clin Sports Med* 1983;2:507–514.

139. Rask MR. "Snapping bottom": Subluxation of the tendon of the long head of the biceps femoris muscle. *Muscle Nerve* 1980; 3:250–251.

140. Guralnik J, et al. Lower-extremity function in persons over the age of 70 years as a predictor of subsequent disability. *N Engl J Med* 1995;332:556–560.

141. Fried LP, Guralnik JM. Disability in older adults: Evidence regarding significance, etiology, and risk. *J Am Geriatr Soc* 1997;45:92–100.

142. Spear CV. Common pathological problems of the hip. In: Echternach JL, ed. *Physical Therapy of the Hip.* New York: Churchill Livingstone; 1990:51–69.

143. Haslock I. Ankylosing spondylitis. *Baillieres Clin Rheumatol* 1993;7:99.

144. Kraag G, et al. The effects of comprehensive home physiotherapy and supervision on patients with ankylosing spondylitis: an 8-month follow-up. *J Rheumatol* 1994;21:261–263.

144a. Byrd JW. Labral lesions: An elusive source of hip pain case reports and literature review. *Arthroscopy* 1996;12:603–612.

144b. Narvani AA, et al. Prevalence of acetabular labrum tears in sports patients with groin pain. *Knee Surg Sports Traumatol Arthrosc* 2003; in press.

144c. McCarthy J, et al. Anatomy, pathologic features, and treatment of acetabular labral tears. *Clin Orthop Rel Res* 2003; 406:38–47.

144d. Seldes R, et al. Anatomy, histologic features, and vascularity of the adult acetabular labrum. *Clin Orthop Rel Res* 2001; 382:232–240.

144e. Narvani AA, et al. Acetabular labrum and its tears. *Br J Sports Med* 2003;37:207–211.

144f. Leunig M, et al. Evaluation of the acetabulum labrum by MR arthrography. *J Bone Joint Surg* 1997;79B:230–234.

144g. Fitzgerald RH. Acetabular labrum tears. Diagnosis and treatment. *Clin Orthop* 1995;311:60–68.

144h. Konra GA, et al. The role of the acetabular labrum and the transverse acetabular ligament in load transmission in the hip. *J Bone Joint Surg* 1998;80A:1781–1788.

145. Lesquesne M. Diseases of the hip in adult life. *Folia Rheumatol* 1967;17A:5–24.

146. Maitland G. *Peripheral Manipulation,* 3rd ed. London: Butterworth; 1991.

147. Barker DJP, Hall AJ. The epidemiology of Perthes' disease. *Clin Orthop* 1986;209:89–94.

148. Ponseti IV, et al. Legg-Calvé-Perthes disease. Histochemical and ultrastructural observations of the epiphyseal cartilage and the physis. *J Bone Joint Surg* 1983;65A:797–807.

149. Martinez AG, Weinstein SL. Recurrent Legg-Calvé-Perthes disease. *J Bone Joint Surg* 1991;73A:1081.

150. Catterall A. Legg-Calvé-Perthes disease. In: *Legg-Calvé-Perthes Disease.* Edinburgh: Churchill Livingstone; 1982.

151. Herring JA, et al. Evolution of femoral head deformity during the healing phase of Legg-Calvé-Perthes disease. *J Pediatr Orthop* 1993;13:14–45.

152. Wenger DR, Ward WT, Herring JA. Current concepts review. Legg-Calvé-Perthes disease. *J Bone Joint Surg* 1991;73A:778.

153. Churgay CA, Caruthers BS. Diagnosis and treatment of congenital dislocation of the hip. *Am Family Physician* 1992;45:1217–1228.

154. McKibbin B. Anatomical factors in the stability of the hip joint in the newborn. *J Bone Joint Surg Br* 1970;52:148–159.

155. Boeree NR, Clarke NMP. Ultrasound imaging and secondary screening for congenital dislocation of the hip. *J Bone Joint Surg Br* 1994;76-B:525–533.

156. Curry LC, Gibson LY. Congenital hip dislocation: the importance of early detection and comprehensive treatment. *Nurse Practitioner* 1992;17:49–55.

157. Williamson J. Difficulties of early diagnosis and treatment of congenital dislocation of the hip in Northern Ireland. *J Bone Joint Surg Br* 1972;54:13–17.

158. Davies SJ, Walker G. Problems in the early recognition of hip dysplasia. *J Bone Joint Surg Br* 1984;66:479–484.

159. Galasko CS, Galley S, Menon TJ. Detection of congenital dislocation of the hip by an early screening program, with particular reference to false negatives. *Isr J Med Sci* 1980; 16:257–259.

160. Loder RT, et al. Narrow window of bone age in children with slipped capital femoral epiphysis. *J Pediatr Orthop* 1993; 13:290–293.

161. Goss CM. *Anatomy of the Human Body by Henry Gray, FRS.* Philadelphia: Lea & Febiger; 1973.

162. Chung SMK, Hirata TT. Multiple pin repair of the slipped capital femoral epiphysis. In: Black J, Dumbleton JH, eds. *Clinical Biomechanics. A Case History Approach.* New York: Churchill Livingstone; 1981.

163. Carney BT, Weinstein SL. Long term follow up slipped capital femoral epiphysis. *J Bone Joint Surg (Am)* 1991;73:667–674.

164. Aronsson DD, Loder RT. Treatment of the unstable acute slipped capital femoral epiphysis. *Clin Orthop* 1996; 322:99–110.

165. Loder RT, et al. Acute slipped capital epiphysis: The importance of physeal stability. *J Bone Joint Surg* 1993;75A:134–140.

166. Herring JA. The treatment of Legg-Calvé-Perthes disease. A critical review of the literature. *J Bone Joint Surg Am* 1994; 76:448–458.

167. Adkins SB, Figler RA. Hip pain in athletes. *Am Fam Phys* 2000;61:2109–2118.

168. Lambert SD. Athletic injuries to the hip. In: Echternach J, ed. *Physical Therapy of the Hip.* New York: Churchill Livingstone; 1990:143–164.

169. Klaffs CE, Arnheim DD. *Modern Principles of Athletic Training.* St Louis: CV Mosby; 1989.

170. Ellison AE, et al. *Athletic Training and Sports Medicine.* Chicago: American Academy of Orthopaedic Surgery; 1984.

171. Lovell G. The diagnosis of chronic groin pain in athletes: a review of 189 cases. *Aust J Sci Med Sport* 1995;27:76–79.

172. Renstrom P, Peterson L. Groin injuries in athletes. *Br J Sports Med* 1980;14:30–36.

173. Holmich P, et al. Effectiveness of active physical training as treatment for long-standing adductor-related groin pain in athletes: randomised trial. *Lancet* 1999;353:439–443.

174. Garrett WEJ, et al. Biomechanical comparison of stimulated and nonstimulated skeletal muscle pulled to failure. *Am J Sports Med* 1987;15:448–454.

175. Ekstrand J, Gillquist J. Soccer injuries and their mechanisms: a prospective study. *Med Sci Sports Exerc* 1983;15:267–270.

176. Nielsen AB, Yde J. Epidemiology and traumatology of injuries in soccer. *Am J Sports Med* 1989;17:803–807.

177. Engstrom B, et al. Does a major knee injury definitely sideline an elite soccer player? *Am J Sports Med* 1990;18:101–105.

178. Casperson PC, Kauerman D. Groin and hamstring injuries. *Athletic Training* 1982;17:43.

179. Peterson L, Renstrom P. *Sports Injuries—Their Prevention and Treatment.* Chicago: Year Book Medical; 1986.

180. Sutton G. Hamstrung by hamstring strains: A review of the literature. *J Orthop Sports Phys Ther* 1984;5:184–195.

181. Jackson DW. Quadriceps contusions in the young athlete. *J Bone Joint Surg* 1973;55:95.

181a. Meyers WC, Foley DP, Garrett WE, et al. Management of severe lower abdominal or inguinal pain in high-performance athletes. *Am J Sports Med* 2000;28:2–8.

182. Roberts WN, Williams RB. Hip pain. *Primary Care* 1988; 15:783–793.

183. Traycoff RB. Pseudotrochanteric bursitis: the differential diagnosis of lateral hip pain. *J Rheumatol* 1991;18:1810–1812.

184. Hammer WI. The use of transverse friction massage in the management of chronic bursitis of the hip or shoulder. *J Man Physiol Ther* 1993;16:107–111.

185. Buckingham RB. Bursitis and tendinitis. *Compr Ther* 1981; 7:52–57.

186. Cibulka MT, Delitto A. A comparison of two different methods to treat hip pain in runners. *J Orthop Sports Phys Ther* 1993;17:172–176.

187. Hammer WI. Friction massage. In: Hammer WI, ed. *Functional Soft Tissue Examination and Treatment by Manual Methods.* Gaithersburg, MD: Aspen; 1991:235–249.

188. Johnston CAM, Kindsay DM, Wiley JP. Treatment of iliopsoas syndrome with a hip rotation strengthening program: a retrospective case series. *J Orthop Sports Phys Ther* 1999;29:218–224.

189. Ivins GK. Meralgia paresthetica, the elusive diagnosis: clinical experience with 14 adult patients. *Ann Surg* 2000;232:281–286.

190. Smolders JJ. Myofascial pain and dysfunction syndromes. In: Hammer WI, ed. *Functional Soft Tissue Examination and Treatment by Manual Methods—The Extremities.* Gaithersburg, MD: Aspen; 1991;215–234.

191. Roy S, Irvin R. *Sports Medicine—Prevention, Evaluation, Management, and Rehabilitation.* Englewood Cliffs, NJ: Prentice-Hall; 1983.

192. Bradshaw C, et al. Obturator neuropathy a cause of chronic groin pain in athletes. *Am J Sports Med* 1997;25:402–408.

193. Miller ML. Avulsion fractures of the anterior superior iliac spine in high school track. *Athletic Training* 1982;17:57.

194. Andersen JL, et al. *Year Book of Sports Medicine.* Chicago: Year Book Medical; 1982.

195. Fullerton LR Jr, Snowdy HA. Femoral neck stress fractures. *Am J Sports Med* 1988;16:365–367.

196. Jones DL, Erhard RE. Diagnosis of trochanteric bursitis versus femoral neck stress fracture. *Phys Ther* 1997;77:58–67.

197. Keene JS, Lash EG. Negative bone scan in a femoral neck stress fracture. *Am J Sports Med* 1992;20:234–236.

198. Grieve GP. The hip. *Physiotherapy* 1983;69:196.

199. Maitland GD. The hypothesis of adding compression when examining and treating synovial joints. *J Orthop Sports Phys Ther* 1980;2:7.

200. Mulligan BR. Manual Therapy: "NAGS," "SNAGS," "PRP'S" etc. Wellington, New Zealand: Plane View Series; 1992.

201. Mulligan BR. Manual therapy rounds: Mobilisations with movement (MWM's). *J Man Manip Ther* 1993;1:154–156.

202. Mulligan BR. Mobilisations with movement (MWMS) for the hip joint to restore internal rotation and flexion. *J Man Manip Ther* 1996;4:35–36.

203. Crosman LJ, Chateauvert SR, Weisberg J. The effects of massage to the hamstring muscle group on range of motion. *J Orthop Sports Phys Ther* 1984;6:168.

204. Godges JJ, et al. The effects of two stretching procedures on hip range of motion and gait economy. *J Orthop Sports Phys Ther* 1989;10:350.

205. Travell JG, Simons DG. *Myofascial Pain and Dysfunction—The Trigger Point Manual.* Baltimore: Williams & Wilkins; 1983.

206. Schiowitz S. Diagnosis and treatment of the lower extremity—the hip. In: DiGiovanna EL, Schiowitz S, eds. *An Osteopathic Approach to Diagnosis and Treatment.* Philadelphia: JB Lippincott; 1991;325–330.

207. Spoerl, JJ, Benner EK, Mottice M. *Soft Tissue Mobilization.* Ohio: JEMD Company; 1994.

208. Kisner C, Colby LA. *Therapeutic Exercise. Foundations and Techniques.* Philadelphia: FA Davis; 1997.

209. Morrison JB. The mechanics of the knee joint in relation to normal walking. *J Biomech* 1970;3:51.

210. Haralson K. Physical modalities. In: Banwell BF, Gall V, eds. *Physical Therapy Management of Arthritis.* New York: Churchill Livingstone; 1987.

211. Michlovitz SL. The use of heat and cold in the management of rheumatic diseases. In: Michlovitz SL, ed. *Thermal Agents in Rehabilitation.* Philadelphia: FA Davis; 1990.

212. Baxter ML, Allington RO, Koepke GH. Weight-distribution variables in the use of crutches and canes. *Phys Ther* 1969;49:360–365.

213. Blount WP. Don't throw away the cane. *J Bone Joint Surg* 1956;38A:695–708.

214. Joyce BM, Kirby RL. Canes, crutches and walkers. *Am Fam Phys* 1991;43:535–542.

215. Kumar R, Roe MC, Scremin OU. Methods for estimating the proper length of a cane. *Arch Phys Med Rehabil* 1995;76:1173–1175.

216. Vargo MM, Robinson LR, Nicholas JJ. Contralateral vs. ipsilateral cane use: Effects on muscles crossing the knee joint. *Am J Phys Med Rehabil* 1992;71:170–176.

217. Panush RS, Lane NE. Exercise and the musculoskeletal system. *Baillieres Clin Rheumatol* 1994;8:79–102.

218. Gerber LH, Hicks JH. Exercises in the rheumatic diseases. In: Basmajian JV, Wolf SL, eds. *Therapeutic Exercise.* Baltimore: Williams & Wilkins; 1990.

219. Golland A. Basic hydrotherapy. *Physiotherapy* 1981;67:258.

220. Bourne MH, et al. Anterior knee pain. *Mayo Clinic Proc* 1988;63:482–491.

221. Beattie P. The hip. In: Malone TR, McPoil T, Nitz A, eds. *Orthopaedic and Sports Physical Therapy.* St. Louis: CV Mosby Co; 1996:506.

222. Harris WH. Traumatic arthritis of the hip after dislocation and acetabular fractures. Treatment by mold arthroplasty: an end-result study using a new method of result evaluation. *J Bone Joint Surg* 1969;51:737–755.

223. Schunk C, Reed K. *Clinical Practice Guidelines.* Gaithersburg, MD: Aspen; 2000.

THE KNEE JOINT COMPLEX

CHAPTER OBJECTIVES

► *At the completion of this chapter, the reader will be able to:*

1. Describe the anatomy of the joint, ligaments, muscles, and blood and nerve supply that comprise the knee joint complex.

2. Describe the biomechanics of the tibiofemoral and patellofemoral joint, including the forces involved with closed-chain and open-chain activities, the open- and close-packed positions, normal and abnormal joint barriers, force couples, and joint stabilizers.

3. Describe the purpose and components of an examination for the knee joint complex.

4. Perform a detailed examination of the knee joint complex, including palpation of the articular and soft tissue structures, specific passive and active mobility tests, stability tests, and special tests.

5. Understand the purpose of muscle function testing and extrapolate information from the findings.

6. Describe the significance of muscle imbalance in terms of functional muscle performance.

7. Outline the significance of the key findings from the history and the tests and measures of the knee complex, and establish a diagnosis.

8. Describe the common pathologies of the knee joint complex and their relationship to impairment.

9. Develop self-reliant intervention strategies based on clinical findings and established goals.

10. Apply active and passive techniques to the knee joint complex and its surrounding structures, using the correct intensity and duration.

11. Evaluate intervention effectiveness in order to progress or modify the intervention.

12. Plan an effective home program, and instruct the patient in this program.

13. Help the patient to develop self-reliant intervention strategies.

OVERVIEW

The knee joint complex is extremely elaborate and includes three articulating surfaces, which form two distinct joints contained within a single joint capsule: the patellofemoral and tibiofemoral joint. Despite its proximity to the tibiofemoral joint, the patellofemoral joint can be considered as its own entity, in much the same way as the craniovertebral joints are when compared with the rest of the cervical spine. In 15 to 20 percent of the population, an accessory sesamoid bone occurring in the gastrocnemius, the fabella, is present as part of the knee joint complex.[1,2] The fabella, when present, articulates with the lateral femoral condyle and is hence an articular sesamoid.

The knee is one of the most commonly injured joints in the body. The types of knee injuries seen clinically can be generalized into the following categories:

▶ Unspecified sprains or strains, and other minor injuries, including overuse injuries.

▶ Contusions.

▶ Meniscal or ligamentous injuries.

It is important that the clinician be familiar with the diagnostic and therapeutic procedures appropriate for all of the categories of injury. It is also important that the clinician have a good understanding of differential diagnosis as thigh, knee, and calf pain can result from a broad spectrum of conditions.

Anatomy

Tibiofemoral Joint

The tibiofemoral joint consists of the distal end of the femur and the proximal end of the tibia. The tibiofemoral joint has great demands placed upon it in terms of both stability and mobility. The femur is the largest bone in the body and represents approximately 25 percent of a person's height.[3] Its distal aspect (Fig. 18-1) is composed of two femoral condyles that are separated by an intercondylar notch. The intercondylar notch serves to accept the anterior cruciate ligament (ACL) and the posterior cruciate ligament (PCL).

> ### Clinical Pearl
>
> A narrow intercondylar notch has been associated with an increase in injuries to the ACL.[4]

The femoral condyles (see Fig. 18-2) project posteriorly from the femoral shaft. The smaller lateral femoral condyle is ball-shaped and faces outward, whereas the elliptical-shaped medial femoral condyle faces inward. The lateral condyle serves as the origin of the popliteus. The lateral epicondyle serves as the origin for the lateral head of the gastrocnemius and the lateral collateral ligament (LCL). The medial epicondyle (see Fig. 18-2) serves as the insertion site for the adductor magnus, the medial head of the gastrocnemius, and the medial collateral ligament (MCL).

The anteroposterior length of the adult medial femoral condyle is on average 1.7 cm greater than that of its lateral counterpart, resulting in an increased length of the articular surface on the medial femoral condyle as compared to that of the lateral femoral condyle.[5] Thus, the articulating surfaces are asymmetric, yet work in unison.[2] The distal and the posterior portion of the femoral condyles articulate with the tibia.

The proximal tibia (see Fig. 18-2) is composed of two plateaus separated by the intercondylar eminence, including the medial and lateral tibial spines.[6] The tibial plateaus are concave in a mediolateral direction. In the anteroposterior direction, the medial tibial plateau is also concave, while the lateral is convex, producing more asymmetry and an increase in lateral mobility. The medial plateau has a surface area that is approximately 50 percent greater than that of the lateral plateau, and its articular surface is three times thicker.[7] The concavity of the tibial plateaus is accentuated by the presence of the menisci (see later).

Patellofemoral Joint

The patellofemoral joint is a complex articulation, dependent on both dynamic and static restraints for its function and stability.

The patella (Fig. 18-3), a ubiquitous sesamoid bone found in birds and mammals, plays an important role in the biomechanics of the knee. Its articular anatomy is uncomplicated: it is a very hard, triangular-shaped bone, situated in the intercondylar notch and embedded in the tendon of the quadriceps femoris muscle above and the patellar tendon below. The posterior

FIGURE 18-1 Anterior and posterior views of the bones of the tibiofemoral joint. (Reproduced with permission from Luttgens K, Hamilton K. *Kinesiology: Scientific Basis of Human Motion.* New York, NY: McGraw-Hill; 1997:207.)

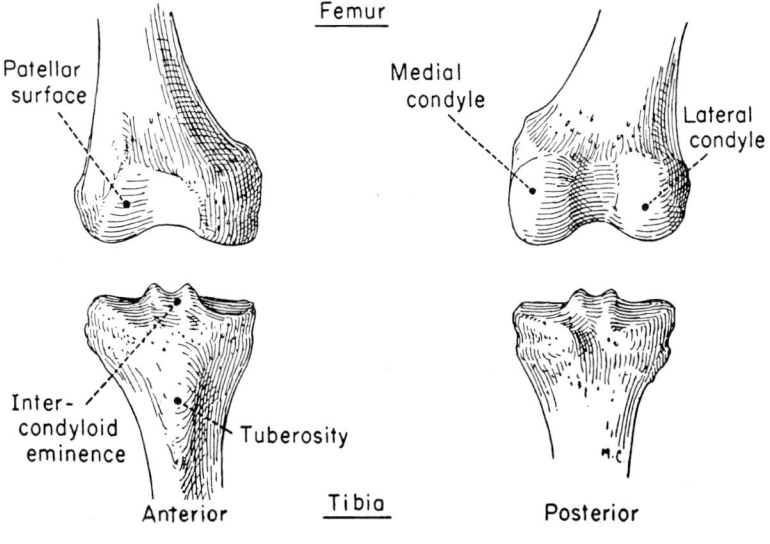

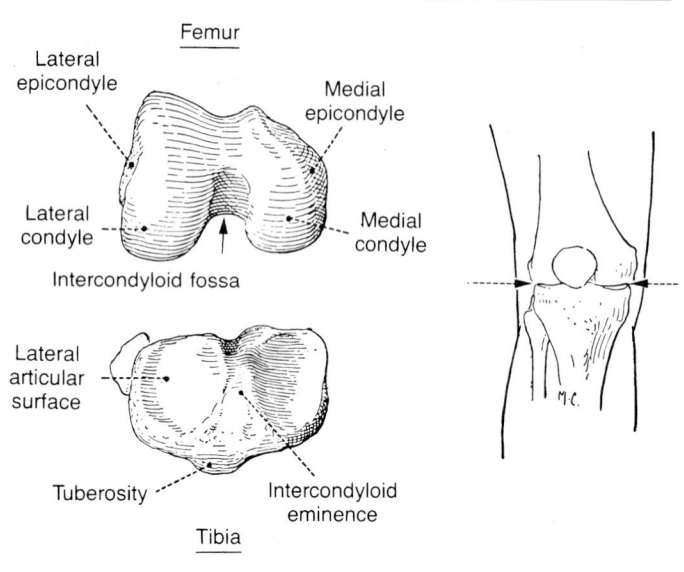

FIGURE 18-2   Articulating surfaces of the knee. (Reproduced with permission from Luttgens K, Hamilton K. *Kinesiology: Scientific Basis of Human Motion.* New York, NY: McGraw-Hill; 1997:206.)

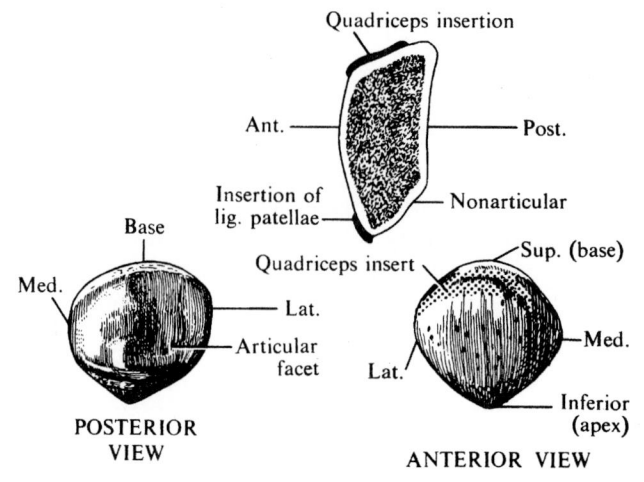

FIGURE 18-3   The patella. (Reproduced with permission from Pansky B. *Review of Gross Anatomy.* 6th ed. New York, NY: McGraw-Hill; 1996:539.)

surface of the patella can include up to seven facets (Fig. 18-4C). These concave medial and lateral facets are separated by a vertical ridge.[8] A smaller facet, known as the odd facet, exists medially and is delineated by a second vertical ridge[9] (see Fig. 18-4). Radiographic and cadaver studies have classified the patella into four types based on the size and shape of these lateral and medial facets[10] (Table 18-1, Fig. 18-5).

The posterior surface of the patella, especially the central portion, is covered with a layer of hyaline cartilage. The articular cartilage of the patella is the thickest in the body (up to 7 mm thick) and is unique in its lack of conformity with the underlying bone.[11] The hyaline cartilage, here as elsewhere, functions

to minimize the friction that occurs at the functional contact areas of the joint surfaces.

The patellar surface of the femur is divided into medial and lateral facets that closely correspond to those on the posterior surface of the patella.[12] The patellofemoral joint functions to[13]:

▶ Provide an articulation with low friction.

▶ Protect the distal aspect of the femur from trauma, and the quadriceps from attritional wear.

▶ Improve the cosmetic appearance of the knee.

▶ Improve the moment arm (distance between the center of gravity and the center of rotation) of the quadriceps. This is achieved by elevating the quadriceps femoris muscle from the center of knee rotation. This increases the efficiency of

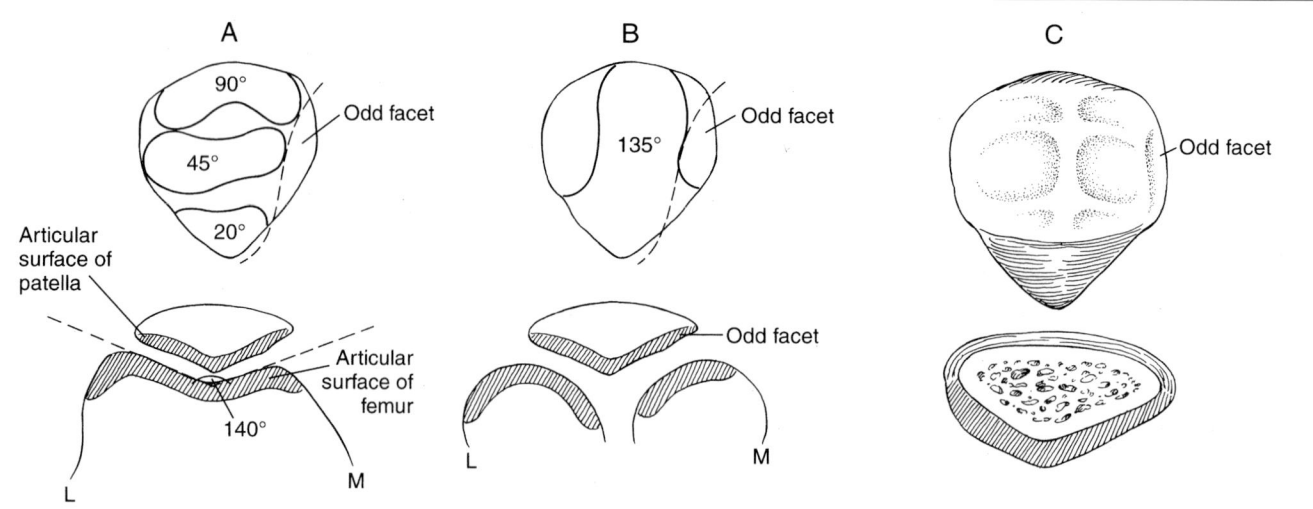

FIGURE 18-4   Articulating surfaces of the patella. L, lateral; M, medial. (Reproduced with permission from Zachazewski JE, Magee DJ, Quillen WS. *Athletic Injuries and Rehabilitation.* Philadelphia, Pa: Saunders; 1996.)

TABLE 18-1   Classification of Patella Types

Type	Facet Size	Facet Shape
I	Equal	Concave
II	Medial < lateral	Concave
III	Medial < lateral	Medial convex, lateral concave
IV	Medial < lateral	Medial flat or narrow

(From Zachazewski JE, Magee DJ, Quillen WS. *Athletic Injuries and Rehabilitation.* Philadelphia, Pa: Saunders; 1996:695.)

the quadriceps muscle and provides it with leverage for extending the leg. The patellar contribution to increasing the knee extensor moment arm increases with increasing amounts of knee extension.

▶ Decrease the amount of anteroposterior tibiofemoral shear stress placed on the knee joint.

Joint Capsule and Synovium

The capsule of the knee joint complex is composed of a thin, strong fibrous membrane and is the largest synovial capsule in the body. The capsule ascends anteriorly about two fingerbreadths above the patella to form the suprapatellar pouch. Posteriorly, it ascends to the origins of the gastrocnemius (Fig. 18-6). Inferiorly, the capsule attaches along the edges of the articulating surfaces of the tibial plateaus, with the exception of the intercondylar eminence, and a small portion of the anterior intercondylar region.[14] A synovial membrane lines the inner portion of the knee joint capsule. By lining the joint capsule, the synovial membrane excludes the cruciate ligaments from the interior portion of the knee joint, making them extrasynovial yet intra-articular.

The articularis genu, located superior to the patella, is thought to function to retract the knee capsule during knee extension. Thus, it serves a similar function as the anconeus in the elbow.

Proximal Tibiofibular Joint

The proximal tibiofibular joint is an almost plane joint with a slight convexity on the oval tibial facet and a slight concavity of the fibular head.[15] The joint is located below the tibial plateau on the lateral condyle of the tibia. The tibial articulating facet faces laterally, posteriorly, and inferiorly. Although the joint is often described as a simple, synovial, modified ovoid, it functions as a modified sellar when combined with the inferior tibiofibular joint.[15]

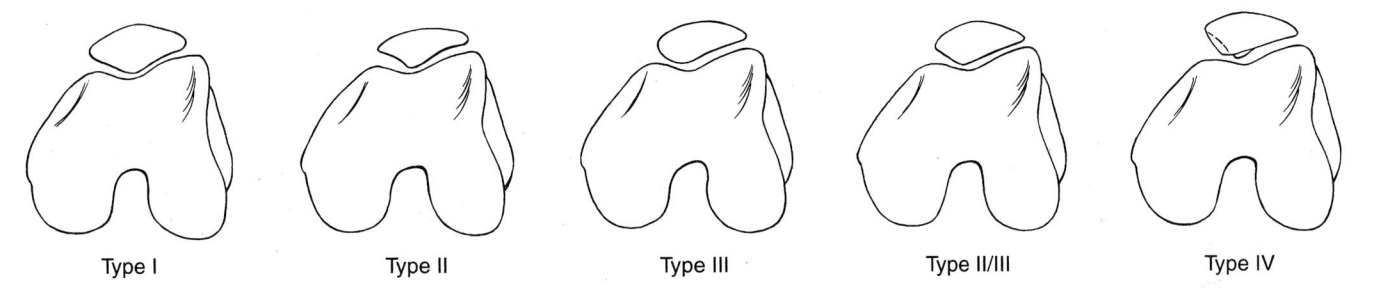

Type I   Type II   Type III   Type II/III   Type IV

FIGURE 18-5   Patella shapes. (Reproduced with permission from Zachazewski JE, Magee DJ, Quillen WS. *Athletic Injuries and Rehabilitation.* Philadelphia, Pa: Saunders; 1996.)

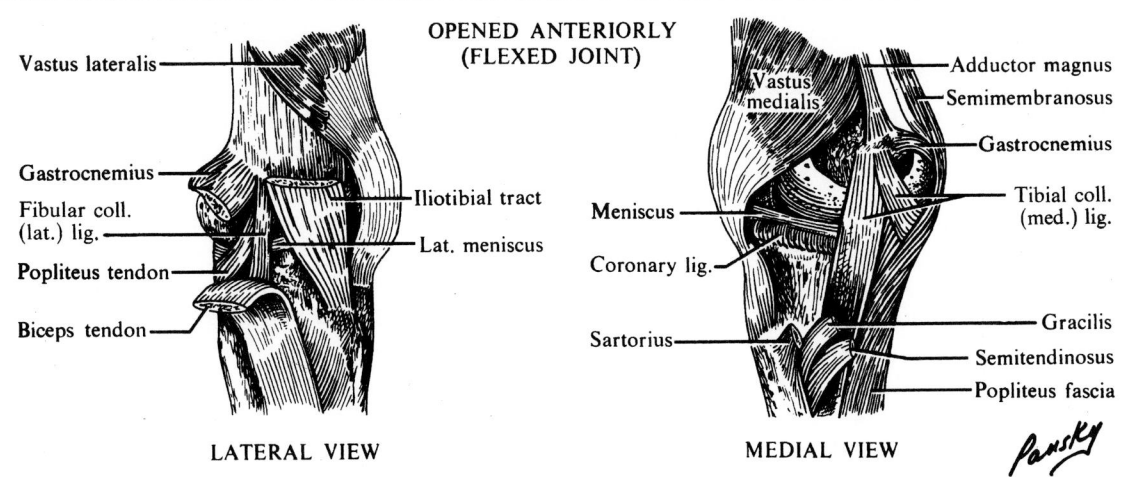

FIGURE 18-6   Opened anteriorly flexed joint. (Reproduced with permission from Pansky B. *Review of Gross Anatomy.* 6th ed. New York, NY: McGraw-Hill; 1996:537.)

The joint capsule of the proximal tibiofibular joint complex is thicker anteriorly than posteriorly and, in 10 percent of the population, the synovium is continuous with that of the knee joint.[15] The joint receives support from anterior and posterior ligaments, and an interosseous membrane. The interosseous membrane attaches between the medial border of the fibular and the lateral border of the tibia, providing attachment to the deep anterior and posterior muscles of the leg. The majority of its fibers pass obliquely in an inferior and lateral direction.

The proximal tibiofibular joint has more motion than its distal partner. The motion occurring at the proximal joint consists of two glides, one in a superoinferior direction and the other in an anteroposterior direction.[7] These motions are possible because of the orientation of the joint line, which also facilitates an osteokinematic spin of the fibula. The motion at this joint can be decreased by articular fibrosis or by soft tissue restraints; the biceps femoris can pull or hold it posteriorly, whereas the anterior tibialis can pull or hold it anteriorly.

Although the capsular pattern of restriction for this joint is unclear, it is probably indicated by pain during an isometric contraction of the biceps femoris with the knee at 90 degrees of flexion. The close-packed position for this joint, equally debatable, is probably weight-bearing ankle dorsiflexion.

Both the tibia and fibula are vulnerable to fracture at the lower third of their shaft. Anterior joint subluxations occur at this joint as a result of medial knee joint strain or an inversion sprain of the ankle. Posterior joint subluxations can occur as a result of lateral knee joint strain. The latter lesion is often missed because of the more serious ligament damage to the knee.

The nerve supply for this joint is provided by the common peroneal and recurrent articular nerves.[16] The joint receives its blood supply from a perforating branch of the peroneal artery, and the anterior tibial artery.[16]

Ligaments

The static stability of the knee joint complex depends on four major knee ligaments, which provide a primary restraint to abnormal knee motion (Table 18-2):

► Anterior cruciate (Fig. 18-7).

► Posterior cruciate (see Fig. 18-7).

► Medial (tibial) collateral (see Fig. 18-7).

► Lateral (fibular) collateral (see Fig. 18-7).

Cruciate Ligaments

The cruciate ligaments are intra-articular and extrasynovial because of the posterior invagination of the synovial membrane. These ligaments differ from those of other joints in that they restrict normal, rather than abnormal, motion.

The two central intra-articular cruciate ligaments derive their name from the Latin word *crucere* (cross) because they cross one another. Both the anterior cruciate ligament (ACL) and the posterior cruciate ligament (PCL) lie in the center of the joint (see Fig. 18-8), and each are named according to their attachment sites on the tibia.[15] These two ligaments are the main stabilizing ligaments of the knee and restrain against anterior (the ACL) and posterior (the PCL) translations of the tibia on the femur. They also restrain against excessive internal and external rotation and varus movement of the tibia.[16] One study[17] analyzed the coupled internal-external rotation of the tibia, finding that when an anterior force was applied to the tibia of a knee with intact ligaments, internal rotation occurred, whereas a posterior force produced external rotation of the tibia. These movements, rotations with coupled anterior and posterior translation, were found to be greater in flexion than near extension.[18] Another study[19] found this increase to be more marked at an angle of 20 degrees of flexion than at full extension or at 90 degrees of flexion.

The cruciate ligaments are innervated by the posterior articular nerve, a branch of the posterior tibial nerve.[20] In addition, the cruciate ligaments contain mechanoreceptors, suggesting

TABLE 18-2　Primary and Secondary Restraints of the Knee[14a]

Tibial Motion	Primary Restraints	Secondary Restraints
Anterior translation	ACL	MCL, LCL; middle third of mediolateral capsule, popliteus corner, semimembranosus corner, iliotibial band
Posterior translation	PCL	MCL, LCL; posterior third of mediolateral capsule, popliteus tendon, anterior and posterior meniscofemoral ligaments
Valgus rotation	MCL	ACL, PCL; posterior capsule when knee fully extended, semimembranosus corner
Varus rotation	LCL	ACL, PCL; posterior capsule when knee fully extended, popliteus corner
Lateral rotation	MCL, LCL	Popliteus corner
Medial rotation	ACL, PCL	Anteroposterior meniscofemoral ligaments, semimembranosus corner

ACL, anterior cruciate ligament; LCL, lateral collateral ligament; MCL, medial collateral ligament; PCL, posterior cruciate ligament.

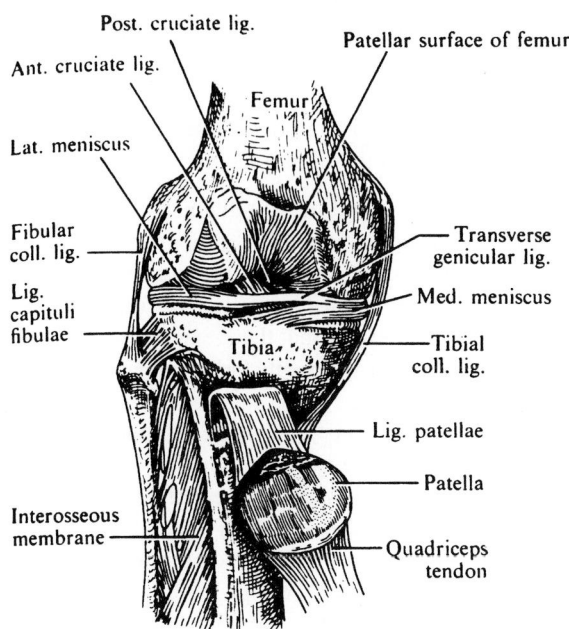

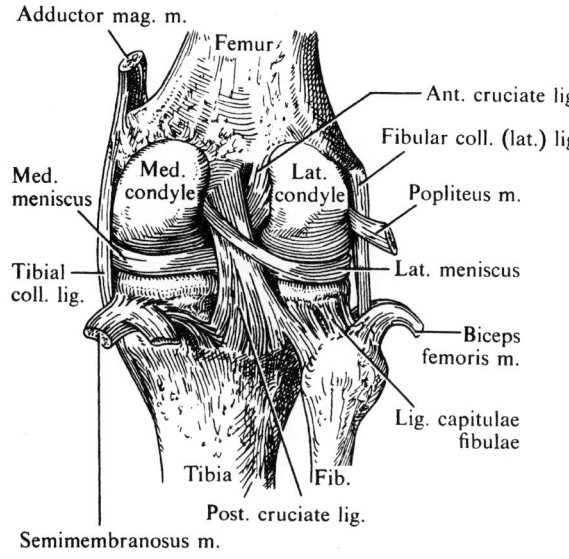

FIGURE 18-7 Anterior and posterior views of the knee. (Reproduced with permission from Pansky B. *Review of Gross Anatomy*. 6th ed. New York, NY: McGraw-Hill; 1996:539.)

that disruption of the ligament structure can produce partial deafferentation of the joint.[21] Evidence of a proprioceptive function of the ACL comes from extensive histologic observations demonstrating that the ACL appears to contain proprioceptive nerve endings.[22–24] Indeed, Krauspe and colleagues,[20] in single-fiber studies, identified a total of 26 mechanoreceptors of the cruciate ligament among 13 animals.

Although these ligaments function together, they are described separately.

Anterior Cruciate Ligament. The ACL is a unique structure and is one of the most important ligaments to knee stability, serving as a primary restraint to anterior translation of the tibia relative to the femur, and a secondary restraint to both internal and external rotation in the non–weight-bearing knee.[25–28] An injury to this ligament has terminated many a promising sports career.[29,30]

The ACL (see Fig. 18-8) is composed of a vast array of individual fascicles. These, in turn, are composed of numerous interlacing networks of collagen fibrils. The fascicles originate on the inner aspect of the lateral femoral condyle (see Fig. 18-8) in the intercondylar notch and travel obliquely and distally through the knee joint. They insert on the anterior intercondylar surface of the tibial plateau, where they partially blend with the lateral meniscus.[16] As the fascicles of the ACL course through the knee joint and attach to their insertion sites, they fan out and give a slight spiral appearance to the ligament, a phenomenon that is more pronounced during knee flexion.[31,32]

The synovial tissue that enfolds the ACL consists of an intimal layer, facing the joint cavity, and a subsynovial layer.[16] The subsynovial layer is in direct contact with the ACL and contains neurovascular structures.

The posterior articular nerve is the major nerve for the ACL, although afferent fibers have also been demonstrated in the medial and lateral articular nerves.[33]

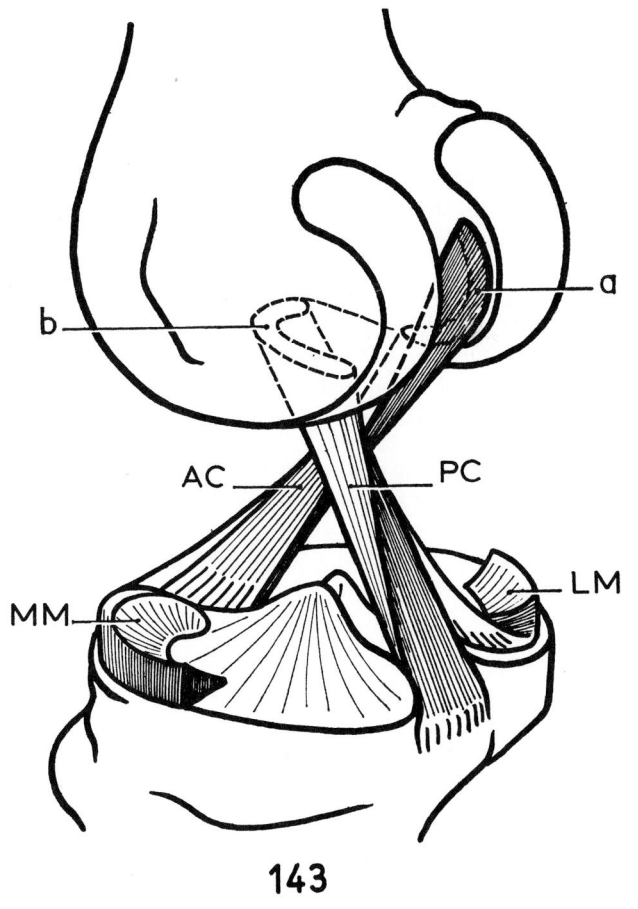

FIGURE 18-8 The cruciform appearance of the two cruciate ligaments. AC, anterior cruciate; LM, lateral meniscus; MM, medial meniscus; PC, posterior cruciate. (Reproduced with permission from Kapandji IA. *The Physiology of the Joints, Lower Limb*. New York, NY: Churchill Livingstone; 1991:119.)

Like all ligaments, the ACL behaves as a viscoelastic structure, allowing it to dissipate energy and to adjust its length and internal load distribution as a function of load history.[34,35] This means that the normal ACL is capable of microscopic adjustments to internal stresses over time, thus influencing the laxity, stresses, and kinematics of the joint in subtle but potentially important ways.[36] One anatomic factor that contributes to selective fiber recruitment during tensile loading is the specific location of the insertions of the ACL on the femur and the tibia. These differing insertion sites allow different fibers of the ACL to be recruited with every subtle three-dimensional change in the position of the joint.[31,36–38]

Butler and colleagues[39] have shown that whatever the angle of knee flexion, the ACL absorbs nearly 90 percent of the force causing anterior translation. The anteromedial bundle of the ACL is taut in flexion whereas in extension, the posterolateral fibers are stretched. These unique properties not only make the ACL the "crucial" ligament of the knee joint, but also increase its potential for injury.[28,40,41] The observation about the varying orientation and tensions of the ACL has clinical importance in a number of ways, and can help to define[36]:

▶ *Mechanism of injury.* Because the posterolateral portion of the ligament is taut when the knee is in extension, it is the most commonly injured portion.[36]

▶ *How diagnostic tests are performed.* When the ACL is tested for torn fibers, the knee joint should be assessed for stability in various positions, especially in slight flexion.

▶ *Operative reconstruction.* Reconstruction should be aimed at replacing the damaged portions of the ACL at the relevant angles of the joint.

The tensile strength of the ACL is equal to that of the knee collaterals, but is half that of the PCL.[42] Because its fibers are unyielding, forcing the ACL more than 5 percent beyond its resting length may result in rupture.[28] Several factors can influence the amount of tension on the ACL.

▶ Compressive loading of the tibiofemoral joint, such as occurs during weight bearing, has been shown to reduce anteroposterior laxity and stiffen the joint when compared with the non–weight-bearing position.[43] These changes appear to reflect the increased strain borne by the ACL during the transition from non-weight bearing to weight bearing.[44] Thus, the popular belief in the beneficial effects of early weight bearing and closed kinetic chain exercises following anterior cruciate reconstruction may be open to question[44] (Table 18-3).

▶ Stair-climbing exercises using exercise equipment such as the Stairmaster 4000PT (Randall Sports Medicine, Kirkland, WA) have been shown to produce moderate strain on the ACL compared with other rehabilitation activities[45] (see Table 18-3).

▶ The circumstances that cause the highest loads and strains on the ACL during daily function are[36]:

• Quadriceps-powered extension of the knee, moving it from approximately 40 degrees of flexion to full extension.

• Hyperextension of the knee.

• Excessive internal tibial rotation; or excessive varus or valgus stress on the tibia if a collateral ligament is torn.

Both estimates[46,47] and measurements[25,26] have shown that the maximum measured strain differential in the ACL is approximately 5 percent during any rehabilitation exercise.[36,48] This strain represents only about one quarter of the failure strain of the normal ACL, suggesting that these exercises load the normal ACL to only a small fraction of its failure capacity.[34,36,38]

Posterior Cruciate Ligament. The PCL attaches posteriorly to the insertion of the posterior horns of the lateral and medial menisci on the posterior part of the posterior intercondylar fossa of the tibia.[49] From here the PCL extends obliquely medially, anteriorly, and superiorly, to attach to the lateral surface of the medial femoral condyle (see Fig. 18-8).

Information regarding the biomechanical function of the PCL is scant compared with that of the ACL. It is known that the PCL is 50 percent thicker and has twice the tensile strength of the ACL.[50] Like the ACL, the PCL consists of two bundles: anterolateral and posteromedial. The anterolateral bundle is taut in flexion, whereas the posteromedial bundle is taut in extension. According to Butler and colleagues,[36] the PCL provides 90 to 95 percent of the total restraint to posterior translation of the tibia on the femur, with the remainder being provided by the collateral ligaments, the posterior portion of the medial and lateral capsules, and the popliteus tendon. The PCL is significantly loaded if a posteriorly directed force is applied to the tibia when the knee is flexed to 90 degrees or greater while in neutral rotation.[51] If the same force is applied to the tibia when the knee is in terminal extension, the load on the PCL is not increased.[51] This is contrary to the popular belief that hyperextension of the knee is the mechanism of injury of the PCL. The PCL also restrains internal rotation of the tibia on the femur and helps prevent posteromedial instability at the knee.[52]

A significant force is needed to tear the PCL. Thus, tears of the PCL are usually the result of severe contact injuries that often occur in traumatic situations, such as a dashboard injury during a motor vehicle accident.

Medial Collateral Ligament

Both the MCL and the LCL are considered to be extra-articular ligaments.

The MCL, or tibial collateral ligament (see Fig. 18-7) develops as a condensation of the joint capsule.[53] It can be subdivided into a superficial band and a deep band.

▶ The superficial band is a thick, flat band, and has a fanlike attachment proximally on the medial femoral condyle, just distal to the adductor tubercle, from which it extends to the medial surface of the tibia approximately 6 cm below the joint line, covering the medial inferior genicular artery and nerve.[54] The superficial band blends with the posteromedial

TABLE 18-3 Rank Comparison of Peak ACL Strain Values During Commonly Prescribed Rehabilitation Activities[44a]

Rehabilitation Activity	Peak Strain (Mean ± ISD)	No. of Subjects
Isometric quads contraction at 15 degrees (30 Newton meters [Nm] of extension torque)	4.4 (0.6)%	8
Squatting with sport cord	4.0 (1.7)%	8
Active flexion-extension of the knee with 45-N weight boot	3.8 (0.5)%	9
Lachman test (150 N of anterior shear load: 30 degrees of flexion)	3.7 (0.8)%	10
Squatting	3.6 (1.3)%	8
Active flexion-extension (no weight boot) of the knee	2.8 (0.8)%	18
Simultaneous quadriceps and hamstring contraction at 15 degrees	2.8 (0.9)%	8
Isometric quadriceps contraction at 30 degrees (30 Nm of extension torque)	2.7 (0.5)%	18
Stair climbing	2.7 (2.9)%	5
Anterior drawer (150 N of anterior shear load: 90 degrees of flexion)	1.8 (0.9)%	10
Stationary bicycling	1.7 (1.9)%	8
Isometric hamstring contraction at 15 degrees (to −10 Nm of flexion torque)	0.6 (0.9)%	8
Simultaneous quadriceps and hamstring contraction at 30 degrees	0.4 (0.5)%	8
Passive flexion-extension of the knee	0.1 (0.9)%	10
Isometric quads contraction at 60 degrees (30 Nm of extension torque)	0.0%	8
Isometric quadriceps contraction at 90 degrees (30 Nm of extension torque)	0.0%	18
Simultaneous quadriceps and hamstring contraction at 60 degrees	0.0%	8
Simultaneous quadriceps and hamstring contraction at 90 degrees	0.0%	8
Isometric hamstring contraction at 30 degrees, 60 degrees, and 90 degrees to −10 Nm of flexion torque)	0.0%	8

ACL, anterior cruciate ligament; ISD, implied standard deviation.

corner of the capsule and, when combined, is referred to as the posterior oblique ligament.[55] The superficial band is separated from the deep layer of the ligament by a bursa.

▶ The deep band (medial capsular ligament) is a continuation of the capsule. It blends with the medial meniscus and consists of an upper meniscofemoral portion and a lower meniscotibial portion.

The anterior fibers of the MCL are taut in flexion, and can be palpated easily in this position. The posterior fibers, which are taut in extension, blend intimately with the capsule and with the medial border of the medial meniscus, making them difficult to palpate.

Information regarding the biomechanical function of the collateral ligaments is quite scarce compared with that of the ACL. It would appear that the MCL is the primary stabilizer of the medial side of the knee against valgus forces and external rotation of the tibia, especially when the knee is flexed.[56] Grood and colleagues[57] determined that the MCL was the primary restraint, providing 57 and 78 percent of the total restraining moment against valgus force at 5 and 25 degrees of flexion.[58]

Lateral Collateral Ligament

The LCL, or fibular collateral ligament (see Figure 18-7) arises from the lateral femoral condyle and runs distally and posteriorly to insert into the head of the fibula. The LCL forms part of the so-called arcuate-ligamentous complex. This complex also comprises the biceps femoris tendon, iliotibial tract, and the popliteus.

The cordlike LCL develops independently, and remains completely free, from the joint capsule and the lateral meniscus. It is separated from these structures by the popliteus tendon, and straddled by the split tendon of the biceps femoris. The LCL can be divided into three parts:

1. *Anterior.* This part consists of the joint capsule.

2. *Middle.* This part is considered to be part of the iliotibial band and covers the capsular ligament.

3. *Posterior.* This Y-shaped portion of the ligament is part of the arcuate ligamentous complex, which supports the posterior capsule.[59,60]

The main function of the LCL is to resist varus forces. It offers the majority of the varus restraint at 25 degrees of knee flexion,[61,62] and in full extension.

Other Restraints

Some structures in the knee clearly augment the functions of the ACL and PCL. These structures are known as secondary restraints[33] (see Table 18-2). The secondary restraints include the structures in the posterolateral and posteromedial corners of the knee, which serve to control anterior tibial translation relative to the femur.[33,51,63,64]

Dynamic stability synergistic to the PCL is provided by unopposed contraction of the quadriceps complex, which increases anterior tibial translation. Conversely, an isolated contraction of the hamstrings results in a posterior translation of

the tibia, which is synergistic to the ACL. Co-contraction of the hamstrings and the quadriceps has been theorized to minimize tibial translation in either direction.[33]

The knee joint also is strengthened externally by the patellar ligament, oblique popliteal ligaments, and the fabella.

▶ The patellar ligament, or patellar tendon, lies in the thickened portion of the quadriceps femoris tendon between the top of the patella and the tibia. The patellar ligament strengthens the anterior portion of the knee joint and prevents the lower leg from being flexed excessively.

▶ The oblique popliteal ligament, located on the posterior surface of the knee joint, is a dense thickening in the posterior capsule made up of a continuation of the popliteal tendon and part of the insertion of the semimembranosus.[57] It arises posterior to the medial condyle of the tibia and extends superomedially to attach to the posterior fibrous capsule. The oblique popliteal ligament provides reinforcement to the lateral capsule, limits anteromedial rotation of the tibia, and prevents hyperextension of the knee.[16]

▶ The fabella is located in the posterolateral corner of the knee and may be osseous or cartilaginous in makeup. When the fabella is present, there is a fabellofibular ligament, which courses superiorly and obliquely from the lateral head of the gastrocnemius to the fibular styloid.[60] The fabellofibular ligament helps prevent excessive internal rotation of the tibia and adds further ligamentous support on the lateral and posterolateral aspects of the knee.[65] Seebacher and colleagues found through dissection that the arcuate ligament was quite large in the absence of a fabella.[1]

Clinical Pearl

Purists classify the patellar tendon as a ligament, because it serves as the connection between two bones (tibia and patella). However, because this structure attaches the quadriceps unit to the tibia, it functions as a tendon.

Menisci

The crescent-shaped lateral and medial menisci (Fig. 18-9), attached on top of the tibial plateaus, are pieces of fibrocartilage material that lie between the articular cartilage of the femur

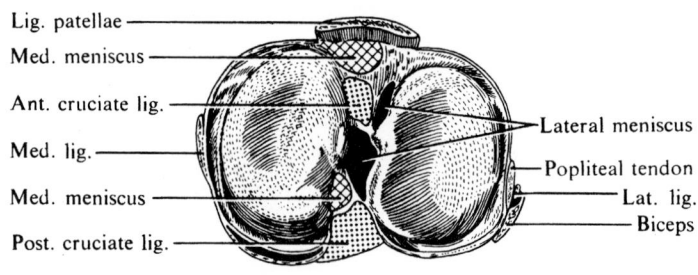

FIGURE 18-9 Superior surface of the tibia. (Reproduced with permission from Pansky B. *Review of Gross Anatomy.* 6th ed. New York, NY: McGraw-Hill; 1996:539.)

and the tibia. The meniscus is composed of 75 percent water, collagen fibers (more than 90 percent type I; smaller amounts of types II, III, V, and VI), noncollagenous proteins, and fibrochrondrocytes.[66] The collagen fibers of the menisci are arranged parallel to the peripheral border in the deeper areas, and are more radially oriented in the superficial region. The radially oriented fibers provide structural rigidity, and the deep fibers resist tension.

Menisci tend to be found in noncongruent joints. The knee menisci, once described as "the functionless remains of leg muscles,"[67] are now recognized as being integral to normal knee function. The blood supply for the menisci comes from the perimeniscal capsular arteries, which are branches of the lateral, medial, and middle genicular arteries.[16] The outer 25 percent of the lateral meniscus (with the exception of the posterolateral corner of the lateral meniscus adjacent to the popliteus tendon) and the outer 30 percent of the medial menisci are vascularized, giving these areas the potential for healing.[68] The remaining inner portions of the menisci are considered avascular. Despite the lack of vascularity to the inner portions, tears involving the avascular zone may heal. This healing capacity may be improved with the addition of a fibrin clot, or with such techniques as trephination.[66,69]

Medial Meniscus

The semilunar or C-shaped medial meniscus (see Fig. 18-9) is larger and thicker than its lateral counterpart and sits in the concave medial tibial plateau. The medial meniscus is wider posteriorly than anteriorly. It is attached to the anterior and posterior tibial plateau by coronary ligaments. These ligaments connect the outer meniscal borders with the tibial edge and restrict movement of the meniscus. The medial meniscus also has an attachment to the deeper portion of the MCL and the knee joint capsule. The horns of the medial meniscus are further apart than those of the lateral, which makes the former nearly semilunar and the latter almost circular (see Fig. 18-9). The posterior horn of the medial meniscus receives a piece of the semimembranosus tendon.

The transverse genicular ligament serves as a link between the lateral and medial menisci.

Lateral Meniscus

The rounder, O-shaped lateral meniscus sits atop the convex lateral tibial plateau (see Fig. 18-9). It is smaller and thinner than its medial counterpart. It is also more mobile.

The lateral meniscus has an interesting relationship with the popliteus tendon, which supports it during knee extension and separates it from the joint (see later discussion).[70]

The periphery of the lateral meniscus attaches to the tibia, the capsule, and the coronary ligament, but not to the LCL. Two meniscofemoral ligaments, the ligaments of Humphrey and Wrisberg attach to the lateral meniscus.[5]

▶ The Ligament of Humphrey runs anteriorly from the lateral meniscus to the PCL.

▶ The Ligament of Wrisberg extends from the medial femoral condyle and attaches to the posterior horn of the lateral meniscus, posterior to the PCL.[71]

Gray[54] describes these structures as giving support to the capsule during rotational movement of the tibia and stabilization of the meniscus.

The lateral meniscus often is associated with the appearance of synovial filled cysts, which may occur following a minor injury to the meniscus and produce a small internal tear. As fluid begins to congregate within this tear, it is pushed deeper and deeper into the meniscus. The swelling eventually produces a small bulge on the lateral aspect of the meniscus.

Menisci Function

The menisci assist in a number of functions, including load transmission, shock absorption, joint lubrication, joint stability, and the guiding of movements.[72]

Load Transmission. The meniscus is viscoelastic, with greater stiffness at higher deformation rates. Many studies have confirmed the role of the menisci in load transmission by showing decreased contact area and increased peak articular stresses following partial or total meniscectomy.[73–75] In fact, the menisci have been shown to transmit 50 to 60 percent of the compressive loads at the knee joint in weight bearing.[76–81] This transmission increases to 85 percent at 90 degrees of flexion.[76–81] The lateral meniscus transmits a greater percentage of the compressive load in the lateral compartment than the medial meniscus does in the medial compartment.[78,80,81]

The mechanism by which the menisci transmit loads is related to their circumferentially oriented collagen structure and viscoelastic nature.[79,82–84] These properties are important in protecting articular cartilage during the prolonged stresses of weight bearing.[85]

Shock Absorption. Because of their viscoelastic nature, the menisci are able to assist in shock absorption. Compressive forces at the tibiofemoral joint have been found to be slightly greater than three times body weight during the stance phase of gait, increasing up to four times body weight during stair climbing.[86] The medial tibial plateau bears most of this load during stance when the knee is extended, with the lateral tibial plateau bearing more of the much smaller loads imposed during the swing phase.[86] This is compensated for by the fact that the medial tibial plateau has a surface area roughly 50 percent larger than the lateral plateau, and articular cartilage that is approximately three times thicker than the lateral articular cartilage.[87]

Clinical Pearl

A meniscectomy can reduce the shock-absorbing capacity of the knee by 20 percent.[88]

Joint Lubrication. The menisci assist in joint lubrication by helping to compress synovial fluid into the articular cartilage, which reduces frictional forces during weight bearing. A meniscectomy increases the coefficient of friction within the knee, thereby increasing the stresses on the articular surfaces.[89]

Joint Stability. The menisci deepen the tibial socket. This increases the stability of the knee, especially during axial rotation and valgus-varus stresses.[89–93]

If the ACL is intact, the menisci do not significantly contribute to anteroposterior stability.[94–97] However, in an ACL-deficient knee, the posterior horn of the medial meniscus functions as a secondary restraint to anteroposterior translation by wedging between the femur and tibia.[95,98] In contrast, the increased mobility of the lateral meniscus prevents it from contributing to anteroposterior stability.[94] This difference helps to explain the higher incidence of medial meniscus tears seen in ACL-deficient knees.[99]

Guiding Movement. The lateral meniscus has greater mobility because it does not attach to the LCL, and, as mentioned previously, its capsular attachment is interrupted by the passage of the popliteus tendon.[70,100] During knee motion, the menisci move on the tibial plateau with the femoral condyles to maintain joint congruence.[100] The femur, accompanied by the menisci, rolls anteriorly on the tibia during extension, and posteriorly during flexion.[89,100,101] Thompson and colleagues[102] demonstrated that the mean anteroposterior excursion of the menisci during a 120-degree arc of motion was 5.1-mm at the medial meniscus, and 11.2-mm at the lateral. The inner sides of the menisci, which are attached by their horns to the tibial plateau, move with the tibia. As the body of each meniscus is fixed around the femoral condyle, they move with the femur. Therefore, during movements between tibia and femur, distortion of the menisci is inevitable.

▶ During flexion of the knee, the menisci move posteriorly. The medial meniscus is moved about 5 mm by the pull of the semimembranosus tendon, and the lateral meniscus is pulled about 11 mm by the popliteus, resulting in an external rotation of the tibia.

▶ During extension, the menisci move anteriorly.

▶ During external rotation of the tibia, the menisci will follow the displacement of the femoral condyles, which means that the medial meniscus is pushed posteriorly and the lateral meniscus is pulled anteriorly. During internal rotation, the opposite occurs. These rotations are conjunct, integral with flexion and extension, but can also be adjunct and independent, best demonstrated with the knee semi-flexed. Conjunct external rotation of the tibia on the femur during the last stages of knee extension is part of a locking mechanism called the *"screw home" mechanism,* described later.

▶ The medial coronary ligament is stretched during external rotation of the tibia, whereas the lateral coronary ligament is stretched during internal rotation of the tibia.

Bursae

There are a number of bursae situated in the soft tissues around the knee joint (Fig. 18-10). The bursae serve to reduce friction, and to cushion the movement of one body part over another.

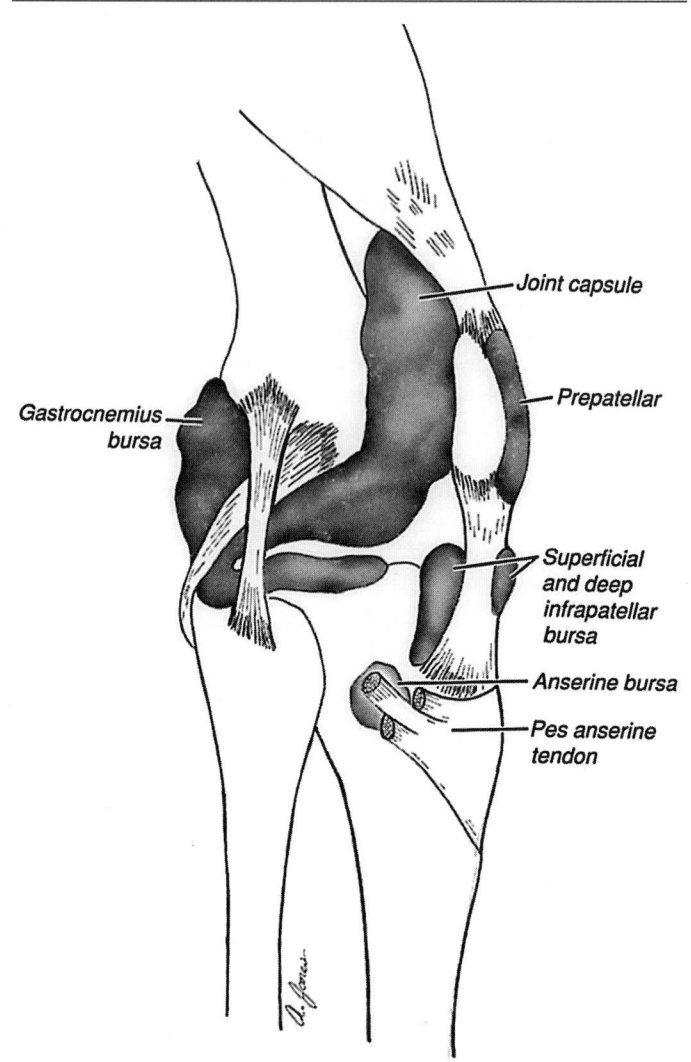

FIGURE 18-10 Bursae of the knee. (Reproduced with permission from Simon RR, Koenigsknecht SJ. *Emergency Orthopedics: The Extremities.* 4th ed. New York, NY: McGraw-Hill; 2001:452.)

Superficial and Deep Infrapatellar Bursae

The superficial infrapatellar bursa is located between the patellar tendon and the skin, whereas the deep infrapatellar bursa is located between the patellar tendon and the tibia (see Fig. 18-10).

Prepatellar Bursa

The prepatellar bursa is located between the skin and the anterior aspect of the patella (see Fig. 18-10).

Tibiofemoral Bursa

The tibiofemoral bursae consist of a bursa between the head of the gastrocnemius muscle and the joint capsule on both sides, a bursa between the LCL and both the biceps femoris and popliteus, and a bursa between the MCL and the femoral condyle. There are also a number of bursae between the various tendons of the pes anserinus and between the medial collateral ligament and the superficial pes anserinus (see Fig. 18-10).

The bursae around the knee can have contact with each other and with the knee joint capsule.

> ### Clinical Pearl
>
> A "Baker's cyst" (see Fig. 18-11) may occur with fluid accumulation when there is a natural connection between the semimembranosus bursa and the knee joint.

Plica

Synovial plicae of the knee were first described in the beginning of the last century.[103,104] Postmortem studies have shown plica to be present in 20 to 50 percent of knees,[10,105,106] with the highest prevalence in individuals of Japanese descent.[104,107–110]

Synovial plica represents a remnant of the three separate cavities in the synovial mesenchyme of the developing knee. These cavities are supposed to coalesce into one cavity at the 12-week stage of fetal growth.[111,112] The size and extent of this remnant depends on the degree of reabsorption.[113]

The three joints involved in the developing knee from which the remnants evolve are[111]:

1. The joint between the fibular and the femur.

2. The joint between the tibia and the femur.

3. The joint between the patella and the femur.

The most common plica in the knee is called the anterior or inferior plica, or mucous ligament.[111,114] This plica is represented by tapelike fold running from the fat pad to the intercondylar notch of the femur and overlying the ACL. The plicae to the medial and lateral sides of the patella, which run in a horizontal plane from the fat pad to the side of the patellar retinaculum, are referred to as the superomedial or superolateral plicae or the suprapatellar membrane, or the medial or lateral synovial shelf.[111]

It has been suggested that symptomatic synovial plicae are one of the causes of anterior pain in the knee in children and adolescents.[115–117]

Retinacula

The winglike retinacula of the knee are formed from structures in the first and second layers of the knee joint. The retinacula can be subdivided into the medial and the lateral retinacula for clinical examination and intervention purposes (Fig. 18-12).[118,119] The retinacula serve to connect the patella to a number of structures, including the femur, menisci, and tibia, both medially and laterally.[9]

The lateral retinaculum is the stronger and thicker of the two. It consists of two distinct layers of fibrous connective tissue: the superficial and deep retinacula. These structures are oriented longitudinally with the knee extended.[119]

▶ The superficial retinaculum consists of fibers from the vastus lateralis and the iliotibial band.[120]

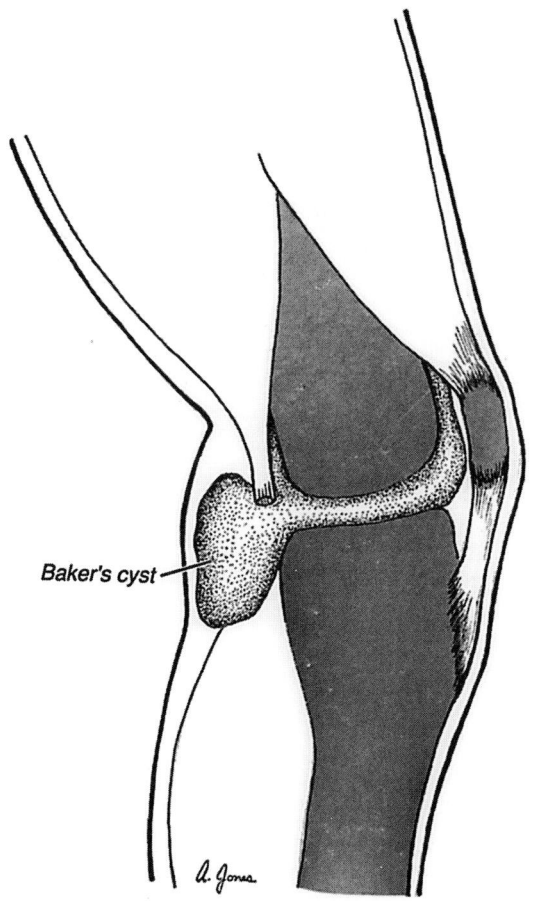

FIGURE 18-11 Baker's cyst. (Reproduced with permission from Simon RR, Koenigsknecht SJ. *Emergency Orthopedics: The Extremities.* 4th ed. New York, NY: McGraw-Hill; 2001:452.)

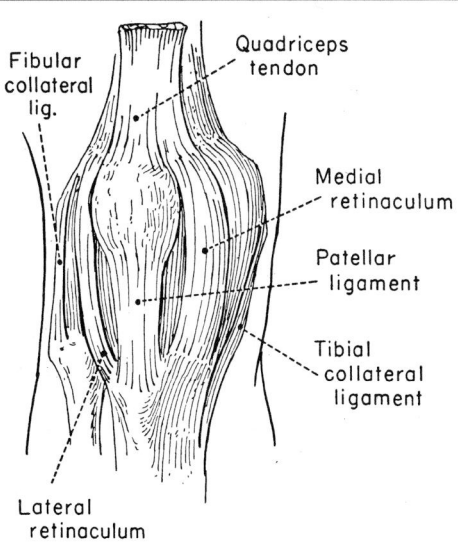

FIGURE 18-12 Retinaculum of the knee. (Reproduced with permission from Luttgens K, Hamilton K. *Kinesiology: Scientific Basis of Human Motion.* New York, NY: McGraw-Hill; 1997:208.)

▶ The deep retinaculum consists of the lateral patellofemoral ligament, the deep fibers of the iliotibial band, and the lateral patellotibial ligament.[120]

Although partially located deep to the iliotibial band, the lateral retinaculum is blended with the biceps femoris to form the so-called conjoint tendon.[1,119] This relationship may explain why adaptively shortened hamstrings can lead to patellofemoral symptoms.[9] It is also well established that adaptive shortening of the lateral retinaculum is a common finding in patellofemoral dysfunction.[121–125]

Given the fact that the medial retinaculum is thinner than the lateral retinaculum, it is not thought to be as significant to patella position and tracking as its lateral counterpart.

Muscles

The major muscles that act on the knee joint complex are the quadriceps, the hamstrings (semimembranosus, semitendinosus, and biceps femoris), the gastrocnemius, the popliteus, and the hip adductors (Table 18-4).

Quadriceps

The quadriceps muscles can act to extend the knee when the foot is off the ground, although more commonly, they work as decelerators, preventing the knee from buckling when the foot strikes the ground.[126,127] The four muscles that make up the quadriceps are the rectus femoris, the vastus intermedius, the

vastus lateralis, and the vastus medialis (Fig. 18-13). The quadriceps tendon represents the convergence of all four muscles tendon units, and it inserts at the anterior aspect of the superior pole of the patella. The quadriceps muscle group is innervated by the femoral nerve.

Rectus Femoris. The rectus femoris (see Fig. 18-13) is the only quadriceps muscle that crosses the hip joint. It originates at the anterior inferior iliac spine. The other quadriceps muscles originate on the femoral shaft. This gives the hip joint considerable importance with respect to the knee extensor mechanism in the examination and intervention.[127] The line of pull of the rectus femoris, with respect to the patella, is at angle of about 5 degrees with the femoral shaft[127] (see Fig. 18-13).

Vastus Intermedius. The vastus intermedius (see Fig. 18-13) has its origin on the proximal part of the femur, and its line of action is directly in line with the femur.

Vastus Lateralis. The vastus lateralis is composed of two functional parts: the vastus lateralis (VL) and the vastus lateralis oblique (VLO)[126] (see Fig. 18-13). The VL has a line of pull of about 12 to 15 degrees to the long axis of the femur in the frontal plane, whereas the VLO has a pull of 38 to 48 degrees[127] (see Fig. 18-13).

TABLE 18-4   Muscles of the Knee: Actions, Nerve Supply, and Nerve Root Derivation

Action	Muscles Involved	Nerve Supply	Nerve Root Derivation
Flexion of knee	Biceps femoris	Sciatic	L5, S1–2
	Semimembranosus	Sciatic	L5, S2–2
	Semitendinosus	Sciatic	L5, S1–2
	Gracilis	Obturator	L2–3
	Sartorius	Femoral	L2–3
	Popliteus	Tibial	L4–5, S1
	Gastrocnemius	Tibial	S1–2
	Tensor fascia latae	Superior gluteal	L4–5
Extension of knee	Rectus femoris	Femoral	L2–4
	Vastus medialis	Femoral	L2–4
	Vastus intermedius	Femoral	L2–4
	Vastus lateralis	Femoral	L2–4
	Tensor fascia latae	Superior gluteal	L4–5
Internal rotation of flexed leg (non–weight bearing)	Popliteus	Tibial	L4–5
	Semimembranosus	Sciatic	L5, S1–2
	Semitendinosus	Sciatic	L5, S1–2
	Sartorius	Femoral	L2–3
	Gracilis	Obturator	L2–3
External rotation of flexed leg (non–weight bearing)	Biceps femoris	Sciatic	L5, S1–2

(From Magee DJ. *Orthopedic Physical Assessment*. Philadelphia, Pa: Saunders; 2002:679.)

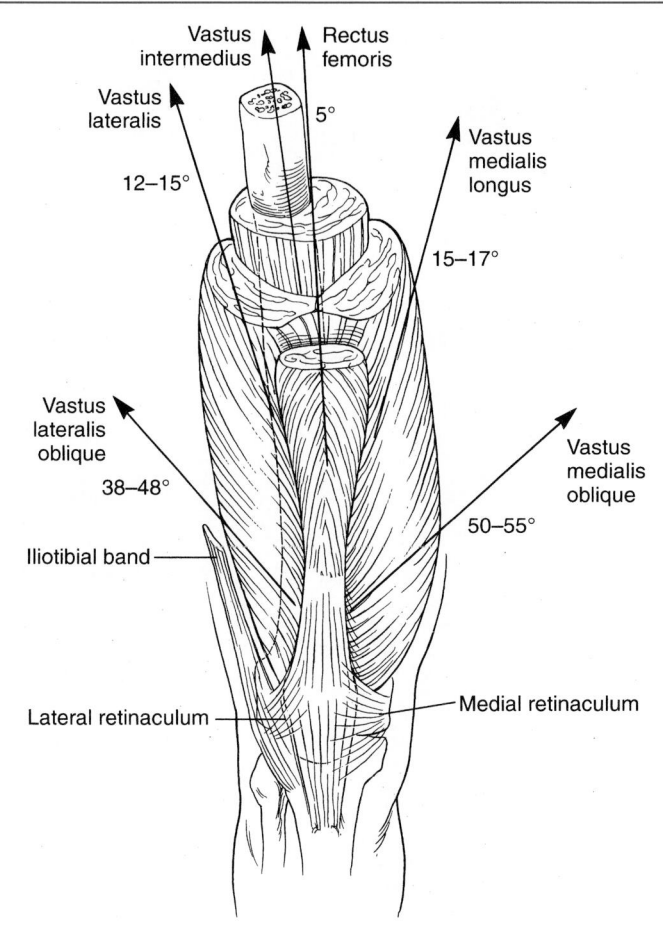

FIGURE 18-13 The quadriceps. (Reproduced with permission from Zachazewski JE, Magee DJ, Quillen WS. *Athletic Injuries and Rehabilitation.* Philadelphia, Pa: Saunders; 1996:697.)

Vastus Medialis.   The vastus medialis is composed of two functional parts which are anatomically distinct[126]: the vastus medialis obliquus (VMO) and the vastus medialis proper, or longus (VML).[128]

Vastus Medialis Obliquus.   The VMO arises from the adductor magnus tendon.[129] The insertion site of the normal VMO is the medial border of the patella, approximately one third to one half of the way down from the proximal pole. If the VMO remains proximal to the proximal pole of the patella and does not reach the patella, there is an increased potential for malalignment.[11]

The vector of the VMO is medially directed, and it forms an angle of 50 to 55 degrees with the mechanical axis of the leg.[126,129–131] The VMO is least active in the fully extended position,[132–134] and plays little role in extending the knee, acting instead to realign the patella medially during the extension maneuver. It is active in this function throughout the whole range of extension.

According to Fox,[135] the vastus medialis is the weakest of the quadriceps group and appears to be the first muscle of the quadriceps group to atrophy and the last to rehabilitate.[136] The

normal VMO/VL ratio of electromyographic activity in standing knee extension from 30 to 0 degrees is 1:1,[137] but in patients who have patellofemoral pain, the activity in the VMO decreases significantly; instead of being tonically active, it becomes phasic in action.[138] The presence of swelling also inhibits the VMO, and it requires almost half of the volume of effusion to inhibit the VMO as it does the rectus femoris and VL muscles.[139]

The VMO is frequently innervated independently from the rest of the quadriceps by a separate branch from the femoral nerve.[126]

Vastus Medialis Longus.   The vastus medialis longus (VML) originates from the medial aspect of the upper femur and inserts anteriorly into the quadriceps tendon, giving it a line of action of approximately 15–17 degrees off the long axis of the femur in the frontal plane.[127]

Because the quadriceps group is aligned anatomically with the shaft of the femur and not with the mechanical axis of the lower extremity, a dynamic lateral force is applied to the patella during extension of the knee.[140]

Hamstrings

As a group, the hamstrings primarily function to extend the hip and to flex the knee. The hamstrings are innervated by branches of the sciatic nerve.

Semimembranosus.   The semimembranosus muscle (Fig. 18-14) originates from the lateral facet of the ischial tuberosity and receives slips from the ischial ramus. This muscle inserts on the posterior medial aspect of the medial condyle of the tibia and has an important expansion that reinforces the posteromedial corner of the knee capsule. The semimembranosus pulls the meniscus posteriorly, and internally rotates the tibia on the femur, during knee flexion, although its primary function is to extend the hip and flex the knee.

Semitendinosus.   The semitendinosus (see Fig. 18-14) originates from the upper portion of the ischial tuberosity via a shared tendon with the long head of the biceps femoris. It travels distally, becoming cordlike about two thirds of the way down the posteromedial thigh. Passing over the MCL, it inserts into the medial surface of the tibia and deep fascia of the lower leg, distal to the attachment of the gracilis, and posterior to the attachment of the sartorius. These three structures are collectively called the *pes anserinus* ("goose's foot") at this point. Like the semimembranosus, the semitendinosus functions to extend the hip, flex the knee, and internally rotate the tibia.

Biceps Femoris.   The biceps femoris (see Fig. 18-14) muscle is a two-headed muscle. The longer of the two heads originates from the inferomedial facet of the ischial tuberosity, whereas the shorter head arises from the lateral lip of the linea aspera of the femur. The muscle inserts on the lateral condyle of the tibia, and the head of the fibula. The biceps femoris functions to extend the hip, flex the knee, and externally rotate the tibia. The

FIGURE 18-14 Hamstring muscles. (Reproduced with permission from Luttgens K, Hamilton K. *Kinesiology: Scientific Basis of Human Motion,* New York, NY: McGraw-Hill; 1997:216.)

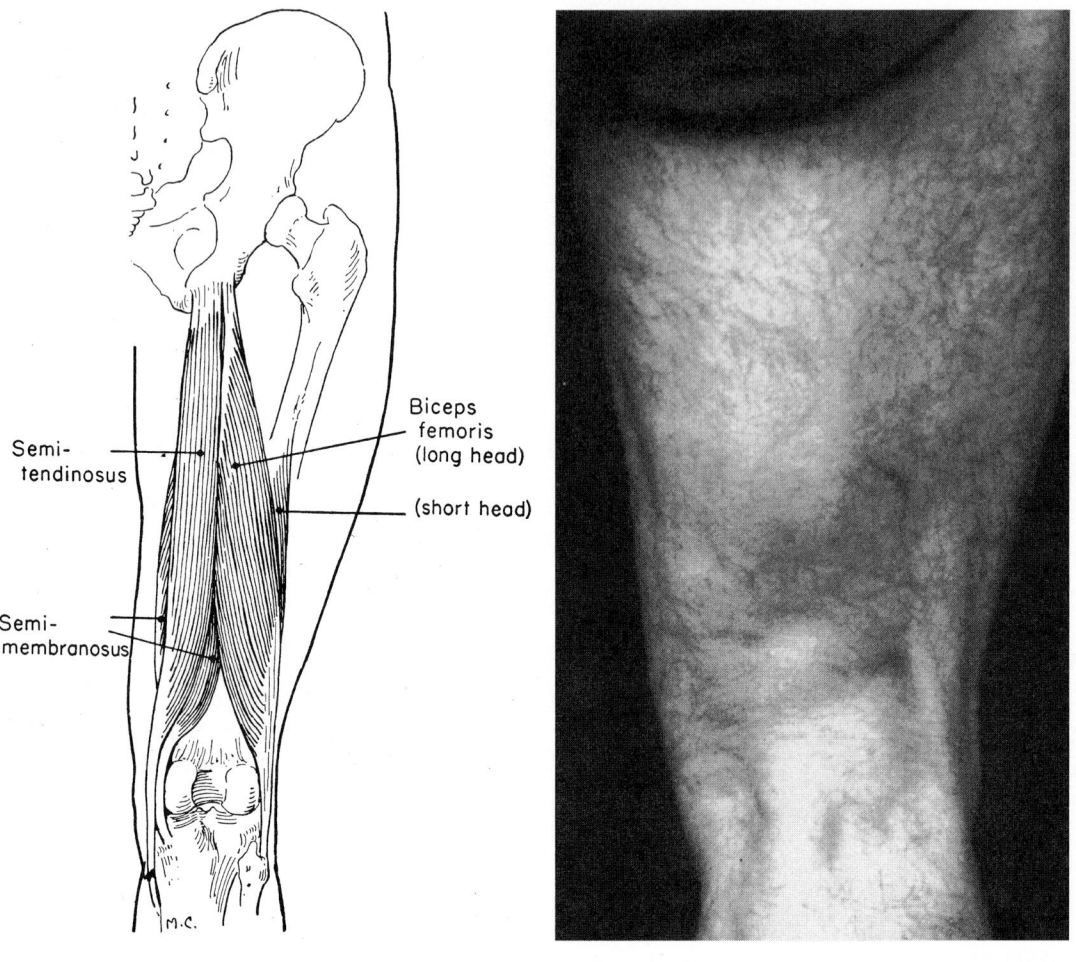

superficial layer of the common tendon has been identified as the major force creating external tibial rotation and controlling internal rotation of the femur.[141] The pull of the biceps on the tibia retracts the joint capsule and pulls the iliotibial tract posteriorly, keeping it taut throughout flexion.

Gastrocnemius

The gastrocnemius originates from above the knee by two heads, each head connected to a femoral condyle and to the joint capsule. Approximately halfway down the leg the gastrocnemius muscles blend to form an aponeurosis. As the aponeurosis progressively contracts, it accepts the tendon of the soleus, a flat broad muscle deep to the gastrocnemius. The aponeurosis and the soleus tendon end in a flat tendon, called the *Achilles tendon,* that attaches to the posterior aspect of the calcaneus. The two heads of the gastrocnemius and the soleus are collectively known as the *triceps surae* (see Chap. 19).

Although the primary function of the gastrocnemius-soleus complex is to plantar flex the ankle and supinate the subtalar joint, the gastrocnemius also functions to flex or extend the knee, depending on whether the lower extremity is weight bearing or not. Kendall and colleagues[142] have proposed that a weakness of the gastrocnemius may cause knee hyperextension.

In addition, it has been proposed that the gastrocnemius acts as an antagonist of the ACL, exerting an anteriorly directed pull on the tibia throughout the range of knee flexion-extension motion, particularly when the knee is near extension.[143,144]

Popliteus

The popliteus is classified as an arcuival muscle because its function is one of rotation. The muscle has several attachments, including the lateral aspect of the lateral femoral condyle, the posterior-medial aspect of the head of the fibula, and the posterior horn of the lateral meniscus.[145] The larger base of this triangular muscle inserts obliquely into the posterosuperior part of the tibia above the soleal line. The muscle has several important functions, including the reinforcement of the posterior third of the lateral capsular ligament,[59] and the unlocking of the knee during flexion from terminal knee extension. It performs this latter task by internally rotating the tibia on the femur, preventing impingement of the posterior horn of the lateral meniscus by drawing it posteriorly, and, with the PCL, preventing a posterior glide of the tibia.[59,146–148] Attached to the popliteus tendon is the popliteofibular ligament, which forms a strong attachment between the popliteal tendon and the fibula. This ligament adds to posterolateral stability.[149–152] A medial portion of the popliteus penetrates the joint, becoming intracapsular with the lateral meniscus. This part of the popliteus tendon is pain-sensitive, and an injury here can often mimic a meniscal injury on the lateral aspect of the joint line.[70] Differentiation between these two lesions can be elucidated with the reproduction of pain with resisted flexion in an extended and externally rotated position of the tibia if the popliteus is involved.

Hip Adductors

Although some of the hip adductors play an indirect role in the medial stability of the knee (Table 18-5), they are primarily movers of the hip, and thus are described in Chapter 17. The exception to this is the two-joint gracilis muscle, which in addition to adducting and flexing the hip, assists in flexion of the knee and internal rotation of the lower leg. The gracilis is the third member of the pes anserinus group.

Tensor Fascia Latae

The tensor fascia latae (TFL) arises from the outer lip of the iliac crest and the lateral surface of the anterior superior iliac spine. Over the flattened lateral surface of the thigh, the fascia latae thickens to form a strong band, the iliotibial tract.[16] When the hip is flexed, the TFL is anterior to the greater trochanter and helps maintain the hip in flexion. As the hip extends the TFL moves posteriorly over the greater trochanter to assist in hip extension. The TFL is also a weak extensor of the knee, but only when the knee is already extended. The muscle is innervated by the superior gluteal nerve, L4 to L5.

Iliotibial Band (Tract)

The iliotibial band or tract begins as a wide covering of the superior and lateral aspects of the pelvis and thigh in continuity with the fascia latae. It inserts distal and lateral to the patella at the tubercle of Gerdy on the lateral condyle of the tibia. Anteriorly, it attaches to the lateral border of the patellar. Posteriorly, it is attached to the tendon of the biceps femoris. Laterally, it blends with an aponeurotic expansion from vastus lateralis.[153] (see Chap. 17).

Like the patella tendon, the iliotibial band can be viewed as a ligament or a tendon. Its location adjacent to the center of rotation of the knee allows it to function as an anterolateral stabilizer of the knee in the frontal plane,[154] and to both flex and extend the knee.[127,155] During static standing, the primary function of the iliotibial band is to maintain knee and hip extension, providing the thigh muscles an opportunity to rest. While walking or running, the iliotibial band helps maintain flexion of the hip and is a major support of the knee in squatting from full extension until 30 degrees of flexion. In knee flexion greater than 30 degrees, the iliotibial tract becomes a weak knee flexor, as well as an external rotator of the tibia.

Major Nerves and Blood Vessels

The posterior structure of the knee joint is a complex of nerves and blood vessels. The major blood supply to this area comes from the femoral, popliteal, and genicular arteries.[16]

Femoral Nerve

The course and distribution of the femoral nerve is described in Chapter 2.

Saphenous Nerve. The saphenous nerve is the largest cutaneous branch of the femoral nerve (L2–4). It leaves the subsartorial canal about 8 to 10 cm above the medial condyle of the knee and gives off branches to the medial aspect of the knee. Entrapment of the saphenous nerve during its course here can occur because of direct trauma, genu valgus, or knee instability, resulting in saphenous neuritis.

Sciatic Nerve

The sciatic nerve (see Chap. 2) provides motor branches to the hamstrings and all muscles below the knee.[156] It also provides the sensory innervation to the posterior thigh and entire leg and foot below the knee (except the medial aspect, which is innervated by the saphenous nerve).[156] The tibial and peroneal divisions of the sciatic nerve serve the posterior aspect of the knee. The common peroneal nerve is formed by the upper four

TABLE 18-5 Hip Adductors Involved in Knee Stability

Muscle	Proximal Attachment	Distal Attachment	Innervation
Adductor longus	Pubic crest and symphysis	By an aponeurosis to middle third of linea aspera of femur	Obturator nerve, L3
Adductor magnus	Inferior ramus of pubis, ramus of ischium, and inferolateral aspect of ischial tuberosity	By an aponeurosis to linea aspera and adductor tubercle of femur	Obturator nerve and tibial portion of sciatic nerve, L2–4
Gracilis	Thin aponeurosis from medial margins of lower half of body of pubis, whole of inferior ramus, and joining part of ramus of ischium	Upper part of medial surface of tibia, below tibial condyle and just proximal to tendon of semitendinosus	Obturator nerve, L2

posterior divisions (L4,5, and S1,2) of the sacral plexus, and the tibial nerve, is formed from all five anterior divisions (L4,5, and S1,2,3).

Common Peroneal Nerve. The common peroneal nerve is a component of the sciatic nerve as far as the upper part of the popliteal space. At the apex of the popliteal fossa, the common peroneal begins its independent course, descending along the posterior border of the biceps femoris, before traveling diagonally across the dorsum of the knee joint to the upper external portion of the leg near the head of the fibula.[16] Sensory branches are given off in the popliteal space. These include the superior and inferior articular branches to the knee joint, and the lateral sural cutaneous nerve.[16] The latter nerve joins the medial calcaneal nerve (from the tibial nerve) to form the sural nerve, supplying the skin of the lower dorsal aspect of the leg, the external malleolus, and the lateral side of the foot and fifth toe.[16]

The common peroneal nerve curves around the lateral aspect of the fibula toward the anterior aspect of the bone, before passing deep to the two heads of the peroneus longus muscle, where it divides into three terminal branches: the recurrent articular, and the superficial and deep peroneal nerves. The recurrent articular nerve accompanies the anterior tibial recurrent artery, supplying branches to the tibiofibular and knee joints, and a twig to the tibialis anterior muscle.

Tibial Nerve. The tibial nerve, the larger of the two branches of the sciatic nerve, begins its own course in the upper part of the popliteal space. It descends vertically through this space, passing between the heads of the gastrocnemius muscle to the dorsum of the leg, and to the posteromedial aspect of the ankle, where its terminal branches serve the foot and ankle (see Chap. 19).

The tibial nerve supplies the gastrocnemius, plantaris, soleus, popliteus, tibialis posterior, flexor digitorum longus pedis, and flexor hallucis longus muscles. Articular branches pass to the knee and ankle joints.

Biomechanics

Tibiofemoral Joint

The tibiofemoral joint, or knee joint, is a ginglymoid, or modified hinge joint, which has six degrees of freedom. The bony configuration of the knee joint complex is geometrically incongruous and lends little inherent stability to the joint. Joint stability is therefore dependent on the static restraints of the joint capsule, ligaments, and menisci, and the dynamic restraints of the quadriceps, hamstrings, and gastrocnemius.[33,157] Because the ligaments share tensile load-carrying functions with the musculotendinous units, these structures can be considered to complement each other's functions directly.[33]

The motions that occur about the knee consist of flexion and extension, coupled with other motions such as varus and valgus

motions, and external and internal rotation. This is because the longitudinal axis of the knee is not perpendicular to the sagittal plane, but lies along a line that connects the origins of the collateral ligaments on the medial and lateral femoral epicondyles.[12,158]

All of the motions about the tibiofemoral joint consist of a rolling, gliding, and rotation between the femoral condyles and the tibial plateaus. This rolling, gliding, and rotation occurs almost simultaneously, albeit in different directions, and serves to maintain joint congruency.[5,159]

▶ Flexion and extension occurs with a mediolateral translation around a mediolateral axis. In the relaxed standing position, with the knee straight or slightly flexed, the vector force is behind the knee, so there is a tendency for further knee flexion unless the quadriceps contracts.[100]

▶ A varus-valgus angulation occurs with anteroposterior translation around an anteroposterior axis.

▶ External and internal rotation of the joint occurs with superoinferior translation around a superoinferior axis, and transverse plane. The available range of motion in rotation is dependent on the flexion-extension position of the knee.[160] The amount of rotation progressively increases from no rotation at terminal extension to 70 degrees of rotation (40 degrees of external rotation and 30 degrees of internal rotation) available at 90 degrees of flexion. The amount of available rotation decreases as further flexion occurs.[5,101]

For flexion to be initiated from a position of full extension, the knee joint must first be "unlocked." As mentioned previously, the service of locksmith is provided by the popliteus muscle, which acts to internally rotate the tibia with respect to the femur, enabling flexion to occur.[87]

During flexion of the knee, the femur rolls posteriorly and glides anteriorly, with the opposite motion occurring on extension of the knee. This arrangement resembles a twin wheel, rolling on a central rail. Between 120 and 160 degrees of knee flexion are available, depending on the position of the hip and the girth of the soft tissues around the leg and the thigh.

In the last 30 to 5 degrees of weight-bearing knee extension, the lateral condyle of the femur, together with the lateral meniscus, become congruent, moving the axis of movement more laterally. The tibial glide now becomes much greater on the medial side, which produces internal rotation of the femur, and the ligaments, both extrinsic and intrinsic, start to tighten near terminal extension. At this point, the cruciates become crossed and are tightened.

In the last 5 degrees of extension, rotation is the only movement accompanying extension. This rotation is referred to as the "screw home" mechanism and is a characteristic motion in the normal knee, in which the tibia externally rotates and the femur internally rotates as the knee approaches extension. This motion is known to be a complex function of surface geometry, tension in ligamentous structures, and the action of muscles,[161,162] and has been described both in vivo[163–166] and in vitro.[167,168]

From 0 to 15 degrees of knee hyperextension is usually available.[169] During knee hyperextension, the femur does not continue to roll anteriorly but instead tilts forward. This creates anterior compression between the femur and tibia.[142] In the normal knee, bony contact does not limit hyperextension as it does at the elbow. Rather, hyperextension is checked by the soft tissue structures. When the knee hyperextends, the axis of the thigh runs obliquely inferiorly and posteriorly, which tends to place the ground reaction force anterior to the knee. In this position, the posterior structures are placed in tension, which helps to stabilize the knee joint, negating the need for quadriceps muscle activity.[146]

> ### Clinical Pearl
>
> The transition from non–weight bearing to weight bearing has been found to produce a threefold increase of anterior translation of the tibia relative to the femur in the ACL deficient knee compared with the contralateral normal knees.[170]

The normal capsular pattern of the knee joint is gross limitation of flexion and slight limitation of extension. The ratio of flexion to extension is roughly 1:10; thus, 5 degrees of limited extension corresponds to a 45- to 60-degree limitation of flexion. The causes of a capsular pattern in the knee are the same as for any other joint. These include traumatic arthritis, rheumatoid and reactive arthritis, osteoarthrosis, monarticular and steroid-sensitive arthritis, crystal synovitis or gout, hemarthrosis, and septic arthritis.

Patellofemoral Joint

The patella is a passive component of the knee extensor mechanism, in which the static and dynamic relationships of the underlying tibia and femur determine the patellar-tracking pattern. To assist in the control of the forces around the patellofemoral joint, there are a number of static and dynamic restraints. The static restraints include:

▶ *Medial retinaculum.* Although not as robust as its lateral counterpart, the medial retinaculum is the primary static restraint to lateral patellar displacement at 20 degrees of knee flexion, contributing 60 percent of the total restraining force.[171]

▶ *Bony configuration of the trochlea.* The patellofemoral joint is intrinsically unstable because the tibial tubercle lies lateral to the long axis of the femur and the quadriceps muscle, and the patella is therefore subject to a laterally directed force.[172] If the patella fails to engage securely in the patellar groove at the start of flexion, it slips laterally, and as flexion continues, it can dislocate completely or slip back medially to its correct position.[172] The causes of insufficient engagement include:

- An abnormally high patella.
- Patellar dysplasia.
- A poorly developed patellar groove (trochlea).

▶ *Medial patellomeniscal ligament and lateral retinaculum.* These structures contribute 13 percent and 10 percent of the restraint to translation of the patella, respectively.

▶ *Passive restraints.* The passive restraints to translation of the patella are provided by the structures that form the superficial and deep lateral retinaculum.

The primary dynamic restraints to patellar motion are the quadriceps muscles, particularly the VMO. The activity of the VMO increases as the torque around the knee increases, and it provides the only dynamic medial stability for the patella.[134,139] However, the muscle vector of the VMO is more vertical than normal when a patellar malalignment is present, making it less effective as a dynamic stabilizer.[173,174] The timing of the VMO contractions relative to those of other muscles, especially the VL, also appears to be critical, and has been found to be abnormal with patellar malalignment.[126,175–178]

Deficits in the timing of muscle activity have been identified in other musculoskeletal conditions such as lower back pain, in which the electromyographic (EMG) activity of transversus abdominus has been shown to be delayed compared with a control group[177,179] (see Chap. 25).

A study by Cowan and colleagues,[177] which found that on average the onset of EMG activity of the VL occurred before that of VMO in subjects with patellofemoral pain syndrome, appears to lend support to this theory. Thus, specific retraining of the VMO is believed to improve patellar tracking.[177]

Quadriceps Angle

The quadriceps (Q) angle can be described as the angle formed by the bisection of two lines, one line drawn from the anterior superior iliac spine (ASIS) to the center of the patella, and the other line drawn from the center of the patella to the tibial tubercle[180] (Fig. 18-15). The angle is a measure of the tendency of the patella to move laterally when the quadriceps muscles are contracted.[181,182]

The Q angle was originally described by Brattström,[183] although many authors had previously described the importance of genu valgus and its relationship to patellofemoral instability. Brattström described the Q angle as the angle formed by the resultant vector of the quadriceps force and the patellar tendon with the knee in an "extended, end-rotated" position.

Various normal values for the Q angle have been reported in the literature.[116,180,184–187] The most common ranges cited are 8 to 14 degrees for males and 15 to 17 degrees for females. The discrepancy between males and females supposedly results from the wider pelvis of the female, although this has yet to be proven. Indeed, it is not even clear that, on average, women have a significantly greater Q angle.[185,188] Angles of greater than 20 degrees are considered abnormal (Fig. 18-15) and may be indicative of potential displacement of the patella.[189–191]

The Q angle can vary significantly with the degree of foot pronation and supination, and when compared with measurements made in the supine position.[187,192] Confusing this issue is that the Q angle is increased in patients with a lateralized tibial

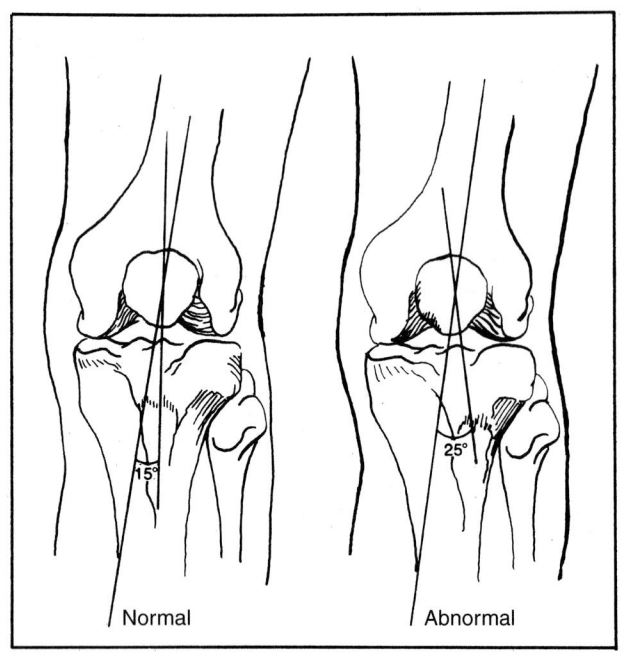

FIGURE 18-15 The Q angle. (Reproduced with permission from Simon RR, Koenigsknecht SJ. *Emergency Orthopedics: The Extremities.* 4th ed. New York, NY: McGraw-Hill; 2001:469.)

tuberosity, but it can be falsely normal when the patella is laterally displaced.[11]

> ### Clinical Pearl
>
> Although an increased Q angle is traditionally associated with valgus knees, some of the highest Q angles are found in patients with a combination of genu varus and proximal tibial torsion.[182,193]

Patella-Femur Contact and Loading

In view of the frequent problems associated with the patellofemoral joint, it is remarkable that, for much of the time, the articulating surfaces of this joint are not even in contact.[194] Indeed, there is no bone-to-bone contact with the femur in full knee extension, or during standing or walking on level ground[11,195,196] (Table 18-6).

The amount of contact between the patella and the femur appears to vary according to a number of factors, including (1) the angle of knee flexion, (2) the location of contact, (3) the surface area of contact, and (4) the patellofemoral joint reaction force.[194] Each of these factors is discussed separately.

Angle of Knee Flexion. As knee flexion proceeds, the quadriceps vector becomes more perpendicular, and the force on the patella gradually increases.[197] This increasing force is somewhat dissipated by the increased patellofemoral contact with increasing flexion (see later discussion).[136] However, because the

TABLE 18-6 Patella-Femur Contact During Range of Knee Flexion[195,196]

Knee Range of Flexion (degrees)	Facet Contact
0	No contact
15–20	Inferior pole
45	Middle pole
90	All facets
Full flexion (135)	Odd facet and lateral aspect

force increases more rapidly than the surface area, the stress on the patella increases significantly with flexion.[195] Any muscle imbalance between the lateral and medial quadriceps muscles can affect the patellar alignment and distribution of pressure in the lower flexion angles of less than 60 degrees.[194] This can produce a rotation of the patella in the coronal plane.[198] At higher flexion angles, imbalances are likely to produce a tilt of the patella in the sagittal plane.[198]

Location of Contact. In the normal knee, as the knee flexes from 10 to 90 degrees, the contact area shifts gradually from the distal to the proximal pole of the patella.[196,199–201] At full extension, the patella is not in contact with the femur, but rests on the supratrochlear fat pad.[198] From full extension to 10 degrees of flexion, the tibia internally rotates, allowing the patella to move into the trochlea.[194] This brings the distal third of the patellar into contact with the femur. From 10 to 20 degrees of flexion, the patella contacts the lateral surface of the femur on the inferior patellar surface.[196,202] The middle surfaces of the inferior aspect of the patellar come into contact with the femur at around 30 to 60 degrees of flexion, at which point the patella is well seated in the groove.[196,202] As the knee continues to flex to 90 degrees, the patella moves laterally, and the area of patella contact moves proximally.[194] At 90 degrees of knee flexion, the entire articular surface of the patella (except the odd facet) is in contact with the femur.[196,202] Beyond 90 degrees, the patella rides down into the intercondylar notch. At this point, the medial and lateral surfaces of the patella are in contact with the femur, and the quadriceps tendon articulates with the patellar groove of the femur.[194] At approximately 120 degrees of knee flexion, there is no contact between the patella and the medial femoral condyle.[174,203] At 135 degrees of knee flexion, the odd facet of the patella makes contact with the medial femoral condyle.[196,202]

Surface Area of Contact.[199] From 0 to 60 degrees of flexion, the magnitude of the patellofemoral contact area increases as flexion proceeds. Some authors have proposed that the contact area quadruples as the knee flexes from 10 to 60 degrees.[81,178] From 0 to 30 degrees of flexion, the medial ridge of the patella lies lateral to the center of the patellar groove.[194] Between 30 and 60 degrees of flexion, the patella moves medially to become centered in the groove. Contact between the quadriceps tendon and the femur begins at more than 70 degrees of flexion.[199]

When the knee is flexed beyond 90 degrees, the patella tilts so that its medial facet articulates with the medial femoral condyle.[194] As knee flexion approaches 120 degrees, the contact area moves back toward the center of the patella. This is the point of maximum contact area between the patella and the femur.[200]

Patellofemoral Joint Reaction Force (PJRF). The PJRFs cause compression of the patellofemoral joint. These forces are caused by the increase in patellar and quadriceps tendon tension and the increase in the acuity of the Q angle that occurs during knee flexion.[178,201,204,205] Maximum force in the quadriceps muscle and patellar tendon is generated at 60 degrees of flexion with values approaching 3000 newtons (N).[201] Forces in the patellar tendon are 30 percent greater than those in the quadriceps muscle at 30 degrees of flexion, whereas the converse is true at 90 and 120 degrees of flexion.[201] Any imbalance of the quadriceps that produces a decrease in the magnitude or direction of the tension of the VMO may result in a significant displacement of the patella laterally, placing the PJRF almost entirely on the lateral patellar facet.[194]

This imbalance is felt more acutely during an eccentric load. For example, during activities such as walking, the patellar surface is subjected to forces that are one and a half times the normal body weight, three times body weight for stairs, and up to seven to eight times the normal body weight with squatting.[190,200,206–208]

Given the forces that are generated within the normal patellofemoral joint, it is easy to see that an increase in these shearing and compression forces has the potential to contribute to patellofemoral pain.[180,209,210] These forces are readily accentuated by physical activity, and this can ultimately lead to articular cartilage changes and eventual loss of articular cartilage attributable to excessive pressure on the lateral patella facet.[211] In particular, the distal central aspect of the patella may undergo degeneration related to abnormal shear stress and deficient contact early in knee flexion. This process may result in pain from the articular cartilage changes and resulting subchondral bone irritation, from synovitis and inflammatory response within the knee.[211,212]

Patellar Stability

Once engaged, the patella is held in place as flexion proceeds by two mechanisms:

1. ***Static restraints.*** The primary static restraints for this joint are the medial and lateral retinacula and the contact of the patella with the lateral edge of the patellar groove.
   a. Appropriate tension within the retinacula assures patellar tracking through the groove. Inappropriate tensioning may result in excessive pressure on the lateral patellofemoral joint surfaces (lateral patellofemoral pressure syndrome) or medial subluxation of the patella from the groove.
   b. The trochlea acts as a lateral buffer to the patella. Sometimes the patella engages correctly at the start of the flexion but subluxes or dislocates as flexion proceeds.[172]

This disengagement may be the result of a defective lateral trochlear margin, an unusually shallow groove, or malalignment (if excessive genu valgus is present, the laterally directed force applied to the patella is greater).

2. ***Dynamic restraints.*** The dynamic restraints of the patellofemoral joint are the quadriceps muscle and the extensor mechanism in general. The tension provided by these soft tissues can prevent the patella from slipping laterally. However, excessively tight lateral structures or deficient medial structures may increase the laterally directed force. This may result in maltracking of the patella or possible subluxation.[135] The lateral structures (VL, lateral retinaculum, and iliotibial band) may be tight from fibrosis of the VL[213] or adaptively shortened for no obvious reason.[172] The medial structures (medial retinaculum) may be loose after injury to the medial retinaculum, from stretching after repeated dislocations, or from severe wasting of the vastus medialis.[172]

Patellar Tracking

Patellar tracking, specifically patella maltracking, continues to be the subject of much study.[174,178,214–216] In the normal knee, the patella glides in a sinuous path inferiorly and superiorly during flexion and extension, respectively, covering a distance of 5 to 7 cm with respect to the femur.[217] A concave, lateral, C-shaped curve is produced by the patella as it moves from approximately 120 degrees of knee flexion toward approximately 30 degrees of knee extension. The lateral curve produces a gradual medial glide of the patella in the frontal plane and a medial tilt in the sagittal plane.[178,215] Further extension of the knee (between 30 and 0 degrees) produces a lateral glide of the patella in the frontal plane and a lateral tilt in the sagittal plane.[178,215]

One proposed mechanism for abnormal patellar tracking is an imbalance in the activity or tension of the medial and lateral restraints.[176,177,218]

The cause of the imbalance tends to be hypertonus of the VL, or an excessively tight tensor fascia latae or iliotibial band.[194] Other joints within the lower kinetic chain also can influence the tracking of the patella.

Open and Closed Kinetic Chain Activities

In relation to the lower kinetic chain, which includes the lumbar spine, pelvic joints, hip, knee, foot, and ankle joints, the motions that occur during activities can be described as closed-chain or open-chain motions.

> **Clinical Pearl**
>
> A closed-chain motion at the knee joint complex occurs when the knee bends or straightens while the lower extremity is weight bearing, or when the foot is in contact with any firm surface. An open-chain motion occurs when the knee bends or straightens when the foot is not in contact with any surface.

Because the knee joint complex is an integral part of the lower kinetic chain, movement at any member of the kinetic chain will influence knee joint mechanics, necessitating an examination of both as part of a comprehensive assessment. An understanding of the forces generated and the muscle activity employed by different exercises is essential for determining how to achieve optimal balance of muscle force, ligament tension, and joint compression. In 1955, Steindler[219] first noted differences in muscle recruitment and joint biomechanics during closed kinetic chain exercises (CKCEs) compared with open kinetic chain exercises (OKCEs).[220]

Kinetic chain exercises need to be monitored carefully to detect the influence of any abnormal motion that occurs in one portion of the segment, on the remaining portions of the kinetic chain.[221] For example, normal biomechanics dictate that the tibiofemoral joint extends during midstance as the body traverses the fixed foot. Excessive pronation in either magnitude or duration prevents the knee joint from acquiring the external rotation of the tibia (or internal rotation of the femur) needed for extension, which in turn may affect patella tracking.[139,222]

Another example occurs during the descending phase of a squat, which requires simultaneous flexion at the hip and knee, and dorsiflexion at the ankle. If ankle dorsiflexion motion is limited, subtalar joint pronation will increase to compensate for the lack of dorsiflexion.[221,222] This increased pronation, which is coupled with internal rotation of the lower extremity, results in an increase in the functional Q angle and may contribute to patellofemoral pain.[221]

Whether the motion occurring at the knee joint complex occurs as a closed or open kinetic chain has implications for the biomechanics and the joint compressive forces induced. A significant number of studies[39,223–235] have examined the biomechanics of the knee during open-chain and closed-chain activities and have attempted to quantify and compare cruciate ligament tensile forces, tibiofemoral compressive forces, and muscle activity about the knee during these activities.

Closed-chain Motion

Tibiofemoral Joint. During closed-chain knee flexion, as the femur rolls posteriorly, the distance between the tibial and femoral insertions of the ACL increases. Because the ACL cannot lengthen, it guides the femoral condyles anteriorly.[169] In contrast, during closed-chain extension of the knee, the distance between the femoral and tibial insertions of the PCL increases. Because the PCL cannot lengthen, the ligament pulls the femoral condyles posteriorly as the knee extends.[169]

It has been suggested by some studies that the closed-chain exercise, with its axial loading of the joint, and resultant joint compressive forces and minimization of shear forces exerted across the knee, may protect the anterior cruciate-graft during quadriceps exercises through use of the contours of the joint, thereby providing greater stabilization to the knee.[236,237] Other studies have shown that CKCEs such as squatting do not necessarily protect the ACL any more than open-chain flexion and extension exercises[238] (see Table 18-3). However, increasing the resistance during the CKCEs does not produce a significant

increase in ACL strain values, unlike increased resistance during open-chain flexion-extension exercises.[238]

It would appear that closed-chain exercises are only beneficial if performed in a restricted range, with some studies demonstrating that these exercises performed at greater than 30 degrees of knee flexion can exacerbate patellofemoral problems.[225,227]

Thus, a "paradox of exercise"[226] is encountered, whereby the patient risks excessive ACL strain if these exercises are performed at less than 30 degrees of knee flexion, but patellofemoral joint complications if the exercises are performed at greater than 60 degrees of knee flexion.[228] Consequently, patients undergoing ACL rehabilitation who are susceptible to patellofemoral pain should be forewarned about potential patellofemoral joint complications when performing these exercises. These patients also should be advised to inform the clinician of any anterior knee pain that develops during their rehabilitative process.

Patellofemoral Joint. During CKCEs, the flexion moment arm increases as the angle of knee flexion increases. In addition, the joint-reaction force increases proportionately more during knee flexion than the magnitude of the contact area.[174] Thus, the articular pressure gradually increases as the knee flexes, with maximum values occurring at 90 degrees of flexion.[200] However, because this increasing force is distributed over a larger patellofemoral contact area, the contact stress per unit area is minimized. Changes in the Q angle of 10 degrees can increase patellofemoral contact pressures by 45 percent at 20 degrees of flexion.[200] As the Q angle increases, the patella tends to track more laterally.[136] A 50 percent decrease in tension in the VMO can displace the patella laterally by up to 5 mm.[198]

From 90 to 120 degrees of flexion, the articular pressure remains essentially unchanged because the quadriceps tendon is in contact with the patellar groove, which effectively increases the contact area.[239]

Thus, for the patellofemoral joint, CKCEs are performed in the 0-to-45-degree range of flexion, with caution used when exercising between 90 and 50 degrees of knee flexion, where the patellofemoral joint reaction forces can be significantly greater.[239]

Open-chain Motion

Tibiofemoral Joint. During open-chain flexion, the tibia rolls and glides posteriorly on the femur, whereas during extension the opposite occurs. Open-chain knee extension involves a conjunct external rotation of the tibia, whereas open-chain knee flexion involves a conjunct internal rotation of the tibia.

Open-chain activities produce shear forces at the tibiofemoral joint in the direction of tibial movement. For example, open kinetic chain knee extension produces anterior shear stresses.[240] Because the ACL provides 85 percent of the restraining force to this tibial shear,[36] open-chain knee extension may compromise a repaired or reconstructed ACL,[241] especially in the last 45 degrees of knee extension,[240,242,243] although at full extension, the ACL is under no tension.[23,224,241,244–246] However, if resistance is applied to the lower leg during

OKCEs, an increase in strain on the ACL is demonstrated,[23] particularly in the last few degrees of extension.[33] OKCE is preferred over CKCE if minimal PCL tensile force is desired. Because PCL tension generally increases with knee flexion, knee ranges of motion that are less than 60 degrees will minimize PCL tensile force.[228] The higher compressive forces that occur during the beginning and end ranges of knee flexion in OKCE may serve to unload some of the tensile force in these respective cruciate ligaments.[228]

Both OKCEs and CKCEs appear equally effective in minimizing ACL tensile force, except during the final 25 degrees of knee extension in OKCEs.

Open-chain knee flexion resulting from an isolated contraction of the hamstrings reduces ACL strain throughout the range of motion,[23] but increases the strain on the PCL as flexion increases from 30 to 90 degrees.[244]

> ### Clinical Pearl
>
> It may be prudent to exclude the final 25 degrees of knee extension range for the patient using OKCE for rehabilitation immediately following an ACL injury.[228]

Patellofemoral Joint. In an open-chain activity, the forces across the patella are their lowest at 90 degrees of flexion. As the knee extends from this position, the flexion moment arm (contact stress-unit) for the knee increases, peaking between 35 and 40 degrees of flexion, while the patella contact area decreases.[208,225] This produces an increase in the PJRF at a point when the contact area is very small. At 0 degrees of flexion (full knee extension), the quadriceps force is high, but the contact stress-unit is low.

Thus OKCEs for the patellofemoral joint should be performed in the ranges of 25 to 90 degrees of flexion (60 to 90 degrees, if there are distal patellar lesions), or at 0 degrees of extension (or hyperextension) from a point of view of cartilage stress.[239] OKCEs are not recommended for the patellofemoral joint between 0 and 45 degrees of knee flexion, especially if there are proximal patellar lesions, because the PJRF are significantly greater.[239]

> ### Clinical Pearl
>
> Increased tension in the PCL occurs at greater than 65 degrees of knee flexion in CKCE, and at greater than 30 degrees with OKCEs.[228] Therefore, it may be prudent to limit knee flexion during both OKCE and CKCE to knee angles of less than 30 degrees following a PCL injury.[228]

Examination

The common pathologies for the knee joint complex are detailed after the examination section. An understanding of both is obviously necessary. Because mention of the various pathologies occurs with reference to the examination, and vice versa, the reader is encouraged to switch between the two discussions.

History

With the larger number of specific tests available for the knee joint complex, it is tempting to overlook the important role of the history, which can detail both the chronology, and mechanism, of events. Questions about the onset of symptoms (traumatic versus insidious) are, as with any joint, important. The diagnosis of tibiofemoral and patellofemoral joint disorders often can be made on the basis of history and physical examination alone.

The mechanism of the injury is one of the most important aids in making a diagnosis.[247] The position of the joint at the time of the traumatic force dictates which anatomic structures are at risk for injury; hence, an important aspect of obtaining the patient's history for acute injuries is to allow him or her to describe the position of the knee and direction of forces at the time it was injured.[248] The primary mechanisms of injury in the knee are direct trauma, a varus or valgus force (with or without rotation), hyperextension, flexion with posterior translation, a twisting force, and overuse.[56]

▶ *Direct trauma.* A direct blow to the anterior aspect of the knee may cause a patellar injury. Repetitive microtrauma to the patella may also be a factor. Bloom[249] describes a condition called *airplane knee,* in which the frequent flyer in coach class gets repetitive knee bumps from the passenger in front when the seat is dropped back suddenly.

▶ *Valgus force.* A history of a valgus force to the knee without rotation could indicate damage to the medial meniscus, collateral ligament, epiphyseal plate, or patellar dislocation-subluxation.[247] A history of a valgus force with rotation could indicate damage to the ACL, or the posteromedial capsule (the so-called unholy triad).

▶ *Varus force.* A history of a varus force with rotation can involve the LCL, the posterolateral capsule, and the PCL.[247]

▶ *Hyperextension.* A hyperextension force can result in ACL injuries and associated medial meniscal tears.

▶ *Flexion.* During flexion, as the tibia is rotated internally, the posterior horn of the medial meniscus is pulled toward the center of the joint. If excessive, this movement can produce a traction injury of the medial meniscus, tearing it from its peripheral attachment and producing a longitudinal tear of the substance of the meniscus.[248]

▶ *Flexion with a posterior translation.* This mechanism can result in a PCL injury.

▶ *Twisting force.* Meniscal injuries are usually associated with a torsional force that combines compression and rotation, often in activities that require cutting maneuvers.[249] In addition, the ACL often is injured during traumatic twisting injuries in which the tibia moves forward with respect to the femur, often accompanied by valgus stress.[248] No direct blow to the knee or leg is required, but the foot is usually planted and the patient may remember a "popping" sensation at the time of the injury. Similar to the ACL, PCL injuries often occur during twisting with a planted foot in which the force of the injury is directed posteriorly against the tibia with the knee flexed.[248]

▶ *Overuse.* Patellar injury is most often a result of overuse.[249] Typically, there is an associated 4- to 6-week training program change. These changes can include (1) increasing a training load more than 10 percent per week; (2) not allowing a 15 percent decrease for a week off; (3) not using an alternate-day or hard-easy pattern; (4) changing quickly from flat to hill training; (5) running in one direction on a canted road; (6) running in worn-out shoes; or (7) biking in cleated shoes that fix the tibial rotation relative to the pedal.[249]

The location of the pain may afford the clinician clues as to the cause. Medial meniscal lesions frequently result in posterior medial joint line pain and mild medial joint line pain.[247] Medial knee pain also may suggest a medial collateral ligament injury. Medial collateral injury can produce pain at the medial femoral condyle, medial joint line, or proximal tibia.[247] Lateral joint line pain may be caused by a lateral collateral ligament injury. Localized swelling over specific knee structures, such as the MCL or LCL, also may accompany the pain. Midlateral joint line pain often is caused by a lateral meniscal lesion. Patellofemoral joint pain usually is anterior, radiating medially and laterally, but primarily in, around, or under the patella.[249] Posterior knee pain may be secondary to joint effusion producing distention of the posterior capsule, a mild strain of one of the gastrocnemius muscles, or a PCL tear.[247] Posterior knee pain accompanied by snapping could indicate a Baker's cyst (see Fig. 18-11).

Pain that is not alleviated with rest could indicate a nonmechanical source, or a chemically induced source, such as an inflammatory reaction. A hot and swollen joint without a history of trauma should provoke suspicions about hemophilia, rheumatoid arthritis, an infection, or gout.

The quality of the pain can provide the clinician with some information. Deep knee pain may indicate damage to one of the cruciate ligaments. Generalized pain in the knee region is characteristic of referred pain, or pain from a contusion or partial tear of a muscle or ligament.[250]

In the presence of trauma, the main thrust of the history should be to establish whether the patient experienced an effusion or hemarthrosis. (The assessment of swelling is described later under "Observation.") An effusion is the method by which the joint reacts to all stress, and usually takes several hours to accumulate. The effusion can result from blood filling the joint, or from an increased production of synovial fluid. The time frame of onset provides the clinician with clues as to the nature of the effusion. Synovial effusion usually takes 6 to 12 hours to develop and produces a dull, aching pain as the joint capsule is distended. By contrast, an acute hemarthrosis is usually well formed after 1 to 2 hours, leaving a very tense and inflamed

knee. The two diagnoses that represent over 80 percent of the causes of an acute tense hemarthrosis are ACL tear and patellar dislocation.[251] Other causes of an intra-articular effusion include MCL rupture and intra-articular fracture. Patients with meniscal lesion often report repetitive episodes of effusion.[249]

Reports of grinding, popping, and clicking in the knee with a particular maneuver are common but may not be related to a pathologic process.[155] However, reports of a "pop" involving sudden rotation of the femur or tibia may indicate damage to the ACL, MCL, coronary ligament, or meniscus, or an osteochondral fracture.[155] Sprains to the ligaments of the knee are often more painful than complete ruptures, because the latter have no intact fibers from which pain of a mechanical origin can occur. Instability of the knee often is described as a sensation of "giving way," sliding, or buckling. Sharp, catching pain usually indicates a mechanical problem.

Complaints of locking or pseudo-locking during active or passive flexion and extension can highlight a dysfunctional structure. True locking of the knee is rare; however, loose bodies can cause recurrent locking or the sensation of something catching or getting in the way of movement. "Locking" that occurs with extension could indicate a lesion of the meniscus, a hamstring muscle spasm, or an entrapment of the cruciate ligament. "Locking" that occurs with flexion could indicate a lesion to the posterior horn of the medial meniscus. With patellar irritability, there is no true mechanical blocking, although there may be stiffness, grating, or rapid movement inhibition.[249]

The clinician should determine which functional activities reproduce the pain or exacerbate the symptoms. The following statements should be viewed as generalizations, as there are always exceptions.

▶ Weight-bearing activities involving a twisting weight-bearing load (e.g., getting in and out of a car with low seats) tend to aggravate a meniscal lesion.

▶ Patellofemoral joint pain often develops as a result of extended activity, such as in the middle of a long run or bike ride, continues into the evening or night, and can disturb sleep.[249]

▶ Walking upstairs or downstairs is usually difficult for patients with knee pathology. Usually, patients with a meniscal lesion complain of increased pain with stair climbing, whereas patients with a patellofemoral joint lesion complain of increased pain when descending stairs.

▶ Patients with a meniscal lesion or patellofemoral pain rarely can do a full squat without pain.

▶ Complaints of pain with kneeling activities are more likely to indicate a patellofemoral lesion than a meniscal lesion.

▶ Sitting tends to provoke more symptoms in patients with patellofemoral dysfunction than it does in those with meniscal or ligamentous lesions.

A gradual, nontraumatic onset of knee pain could indicate patellofemoral joint dysfunction or symptomatic degenerative joint disease of the knee joint complex. The characteristic clinical features in an uncomplicated osteoarthritis of the knee joint are a dull and aching pain that occurs at the end of the day, or after prolonged periods of standing or walking.[252] As the disease progresses, there is pain and stiffness on rising in the morning, which eases with activity or rest, and a limitation of movement in the capsular pattern.

Anterior Knee Pain

Anterior knee pain is most commonly associated with patellofemoral dysfunction, which is a frequent source of impairment.[253] There is a significant temptation to cut corners with a patient who presents with anterior knee pain, and to proceed directly to the diagnosis of patellofemoral pain.[136] However, this should be avoided, especially in light of the fact that the literature is replete with descriptions of physical examination techniques for the evaluation of the patellofemoral joint.[122,217,254–259]

> **Clinical Pearl**
>
> The differential diagnosis of anterior knee pain (see Chap. 9) should include tears of the menisci, medial synovial plica syndrome, inflammatory or degenerative arthritis, tumors of the joint, ligament injuries that mimic patellar instability, osteochondritis dissecans of the medial femoral condyle, prepatellar bursitis, patellar tendonitis, inflammation of the patellar fat pad, and Sindig-Larsen-Johansson syndrome.[8,136,260–262]

Pain from patellofemoral joint dysfunction can be misleading. Classically, the pain is anterior, but it also can be medial,[182,263] lateral,[182,263] or popliteal.[180] Particular activities can help with differential diagnosis. Complaints of pain that occur when a patient arises from a seated position, negotiates stairs, or squats are associated with patellofemoral dysfunction. The so-called movie-theater sign[182]—pain with prolonged sitting—traditionally has been associated with patellar pain from any source. Venous congestion and stretching of painful tissues are potential explanations for this symptom.[239] Activities that involve eccentric loading of the knee, and increased hill work with running, tend to provoke patellar tendonitis, whereas inferior patellar pain following vigorous kicking, flip turns in swimming, or delivery of a fast ball in cricket would tend to implicate the fat pad.[264] The fat pad also may be irritated with the straight leg raise exercise.[257]

Edema rarely is reported with insidious onset overuse injuries, except in the case of plical irritation, iliotibial band friction syndrome, irritation of the pes anserine, or Osgood-Schlatter's disease.[155]

Systems Review

Knee pain can be referred to the knee from the lumbosacral region (L3 to S2 segments), or from the hip. For example, anteromedial pain can be referred from the L2 and L3 spinal levels, whereas posterolateral knee pain can be referred from the L4,

L5 and S1 to S2 levels. The peripheral nerves are also capable of referring pain to this area. Medial knee pain having a burning quality could indicate saphenous nerve neuritis. Pain that is constant and burning in nature should alert the clinician to the possibility of reflex sympathetic dystrophy, gout, or radicular pain. Intermittent pain usually indicates a mechanical problem (meniscus). Chapter 9 describes some of the more common causes of referred knee pain, and causes of a more serious nature.

Tests and Measures

Observation

The observation component of the examination begins as the clinician meets the patient and ends as the patient is leaving. This informal observation should occur at every visit.

As mentioned, diffuse swelling indicates fluid in the joint or synovial swelling, or both. An effusion can be detected by noticing the loss of the peripatellar groove and by palpation of the fluid. A perceptible bulge on the medial aspect suggests a small effusion; this sign may not be present with larger effusions. The swelling is examined with the patient positioned supine, in the following manner[265]:

▶ *Patellar ballottement (maximal effusion).* Ballottement of the patella also may be a useful technique for detecting an effusion. Using one hand, the clinician grasps the patient's thigh at the anterior aspect about 10 cm above the patella, placing the fingers medial and the thumb lateral (Fig. 18-16). The patient's knee is extended. With the other hand, the clinician grasps the patient's lower leg about 5 cm distal to the patella, placing the fingers medial and the thumb lateral. The proximal hand exerts compression against the anterior, lateral, and medial aspects of the thigh and, while maintaining this pressure, slides distally. The distal hand exerts compression in a similar way and slides proximally. Using the index finger of the distal hand, the clinician now taps the patella against the femur. In the normal knee joint with minimal free fluid, the patella moves

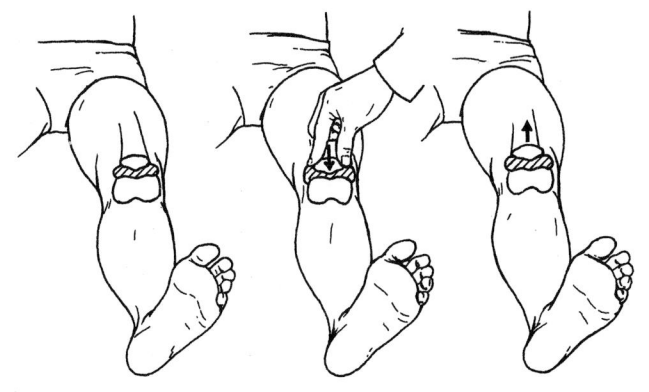

FIGURE 18-16 Patellar ballottement. (Reproduced with permission from Palmer ML, Epler M. *Clinical Assessment Procedures in Physical Therapy.* Philadelphia, Pa: JB Lippincott; 1990:282.)

directly into the femoral condyle and there is no tapping sensation underneath the clinician's fingertips. However, in the knee with excess fluid, the patella is "floating"; thus, ballottement causes the patella to tap against the femoral condyle. This sensation is transmitted to the clinician's fingertips. A positive test is indicative of a significant synovial effusion or hemarthrosis in the knee joint. Sometimes, this test can produce false-positive results. When this is the case, the uninvolved side usually tests positive as well.

▶ *Test for moderate effusion.*   Using one hand, the clinician grasps the patient's thigh at the anterior aspect about 10 cm above the patella, placing the fingers medial and the thumb lateral. The patient's knee is extended. The clinician places the index and middle fingers of the other hand at the level of the medial joint space and the thumb at the lateral joint space. Fingers and thumb exert slight pressure. The proximal hand now slides distally, exerting moderate pressure, until the superior edge of the patella is reached. This test is positive when the thumb and fingers are pushed away from each other by the moderate amount of fluid in the joint.

▶ *Test for minimal effusion.*   Applying moderate pressure with the dorsal aspect of the fingers of one hand, the clinician strokes from just distal to the medial joint space over the medial side of the knee, to the midline at the anterior aspect of the thigh, about 10 cm proximal to the patella. In so doing, the medial side of the patella is followed from its medial-distal edge to its medial-proximal edge. This movement is repeated two or three times. Directly afterward, the same movement is performed against the lateral aspect of the knee. The test is positive when, at the end of the movement of the clinician's hand at the lateral side of the knee, the small indentation at the medial side of the knee temporarily fills with fluid. This indicates a slight synovial effusion in the knee.

If there is no swelling but there is evidence of bruising or bleeding into the tibial area, disruption to the joint capsule may be present, or a slipped capital epiphysis, if the patient is an adolescent. Popliteal swelling, which can compress the tibial or common peroneal nerves, or both, can produce complaints of paresthesia and anesthesia.

The formal observation of the patient is divided into three sections: standing, seated, and lying examinations.

Standing.   The patient is asked to stand with the feet slightly apart and aligned straight ahead. This position can be used to assess overall limb alignment as well as to identify possible foot abnormalities. A careful physical examination of the hip, knee, and ankle is performed, observing for both static restraints, and, to a great degree, dynamic restraints.[117] Following this position, the patient is asked to stand with the feet shoulder-width apart. The entire trunk and lower extremities are observed. Areas of atrophy should be noted and correlated with other findings. Common areas include the medial aspect of the quadriceps following trauma, nerve injury or knee surgery.

Degree of Femoral Retroversion or Anteversion.   Femoral retroversion-anteversion is indicated by whether the feet are rotated outward or inward, respectively, in the relaxed standing position. The position of the patella is examined to see whether it looks inward (so-called squinting patella), which could indicate femoral anteversion. Femoral anteversion results in internal rotation of the femoral sulcus, and an increase in the Q angle. Femoral anteversion has been associated with abnormal patellofemoral mechanics.[136,266] Even if the patella looks straight in the presence of femoral anteversion, it may be held there by tight lateral structures.[257]

Leg-length Discrepancy.   Compensations for leg-length discrepancies include excessive foot pronation, toeing-out (forefoot abduction), and a flexed knee gait or stance.[267,268]

Degree of Genu Varus.   Genu varus can be the result of bowing of the tibia or varus at the knee joint. An increased varus moment can contribute to early degeneration of the knee and, when exaggerated, is most often an indication of advanced degenerative joint disease.[269] Based on the relationship between the proximal and distal aspects of the femur, a change in the orientation between the shaft and neck will change the orientation of the tibiofemoral joint, thereby altering the weight-bearing forces through the knee joint. For example, an increase in the normal angle of inclination at the hip (coxa valga), will redirect the femoral shaft more laterally than normal, resulting in a decrease in the normal physiologic valgus angle of the knee (genu varus). This results in a shifting of the mechanical axis to the medial compartment of the knee, increasing the compression forces medially.[58]

Degree of Genu Valgus.   Genu valgus can result from a change of angulation of the femur caused by femoral anteversion, tibial torsion, or excessive foot pronation. A valgus knee increases the Q angle by displacing the tibial tuberosity laterally and can be associated with patellofemoral pain.[270]

Degree of Knee Flexion.   A flexed knee in the relaxed standing position is often indicative of arthritic changes of the knee.

Degree of Genu Recurvatum or Hyperextension.   Knee recurvatum may be an expression of a generalized ligamentous laxity or may be associated with patella alta.[191] Hyperextension of knee produces stress on the posterior capsule, slackening of the ACL, and alterations in the compressive forces acting on the anterior articulating surface of the tibia.[269] The anterior compressive forces can cause the inferior pole of the patella to be driven posteriorly into the fat pad, producing an irritation.

Q-Angle Assessment.   A properly measured Q angle can contribute significantly to the evaluation of patellofemoral malalignment. However, relying solely on the Q-angle measurement to determine patellofemoral alignment is an oversimplification. As with other clinical signs, an abnormal value does not necessarily identify the source of pain. The Q angle itself is not pathologic and is increased in only a small percentage of patients with patellar pain.[271]

The Q angle should be assessed dynamically and statically. It is important that this angle be measured in a consistent fashion.

▶ *Dynamically.* The preferred position for this test is the one-legged standing position without shoes. Hyperpronation of the feet can be masked unless the foot and ankle are placed in a subtalar neutral position[272] (see Chap. 19). A measurement is then taken using an imaginary line drawn from the ASIS to the center of the patella, and a second line from the tibial tuberosity to the center of the patella (see Fig. 18-15). The weight-bearing position can be simulated in a supine patient by dorsiflexing the ankles, extending the knees, and pointing the toes to the ceiling.

▶ *Statically.* The preferred position for the static test is the supine position. The measurement is first taken with the limb in a relaxed position. If the knee is passively flexed to approximately 20 degrees, the Q angle will be seen to increase by a few degrees. Passive external rotation of the foot and tibia will then further increase the angle to 25 to 30 degrees in ligamentously lax individuals.[272] The clinician also can measure the position of the tibial tubercle with respect to the midline of the patellar groove. With the knee flexed to 90 degrees, the tibial tubercle should lie less than 20 mm lateral to the midline of the femur at the upper edge of the femoral condyles; a distance of more than 20 mm indicates an abnormally lateral tubercle.[11]

Degree of Tibial Torsion.[273] This measurement is indicated by the position of the feet in relation to the patella. External tibial torsion increases the Q angle, whereas internal torsion decreases it.[136] The vast majority of the studies focusing on anterior knee pain have examined the coronal relationships at the knee (Q angle, patellar tilt, patellar subluxation). Few studies have addressed the rotational relationships, specifically the rotational orientation of the tibia to the femur.[274] This rotational relationship of the tibia to the femur in the transverse plane is referred to as *knee version.* Knee version often is recognized as a factor in the context of the osteoarthritic knee.[275–277] The significance of this rotational characteristic of the knee with anterior pain is that the patella is tethered to the tibia by the infrapatellar tendon and retinaculum, and if the tibia is rotated externally with respect to the femur, the patella will be pulled laterally by virtue of this attachment.[274] If the patella is not free to translate laterally, because of its soft tissue attachments and its conformity with the patellar groove, increased pressure may be placed on the lateral facet. This pressure may produce a condition called a *lateral patellar compression syndrome.*[274,278]

Tibia-to-Floor Angle. If the tibia-to-floor angle is 10 degrees or greater, the extremity requires an excessive amount of subtalar joint pronation to produce a plantigrade foot.[191]

Patella Tendon-to-Patella Height Ratio. This measurement is best performed radiographically. The patella tendon length should

be equal, or slightly longer than the height of the patella.[279] If a ratio of greater than 15 to 20 percent exists, patella alta should be suspected. If the ratio is less than 15 to 20 percent, patella baja should be suspected.

Subtalar Neutral. An often-neglected feature, which directly impacts the patellofemoral joint, is that of foot alignment. The normal weight-bearing foot exhibits a mild amount of pronation. If the foot pronates excessively, a compensatory internal rotation of the tibia may occur. This produces an increased amount of rotatory stress and dynamic abduction movement at the knee that has to be absorbed through the peripatellar soft tissues at the knee joint.[191,217,266,280] These stresses can force the patella to displace laterally.[281,282] In addition, a change in the position of the talus can affect the functional leg length. Subtalar supination may cause the leg to lengthen, whereas subtalar pronation shortens the leg.

Gait. The purpose of the gait assessment is to identify deviations of the foot, ankle, knee, or hip joint, such as excessive subtalar and midtarsal joint pronation, limited ankle dorsiflexion, tibial or femoral torsion abnormalities, and excessive varus or valgus at the knee, all of which could place the knee structures at risk for further microtrauma.[155]

During normal gait, the knee should be observed to flex to approximately 15 degrees at initial contact before extending to the neutral position at terminal stance.[269] An increase in 5 degrees of pronation at midstance, a period where the foot should be in supination, holds more potential for producing pain than if the 5 degrees occurs during the contact phase.[222]

Because the joint reaction forces are reported to increase with the magnitude of quadriceps contraction and the knee-flexion angle,[283] patients with patellofemoral pain often adopt compensatory gait strategies to reduce the muscular demands at the knee. Evidence in support of this premise was reported by Dillon and colleagues,[284] who found that subjects with patellofemoral pain limited the amount of stance phase knee flexion during level and ramp walking.

An injury to the ACL produces distinct changes in lower extremity biomechanics during gait.[285] Whereas healthy individuals demonstrate an extensor torque at the knee for 10 to 45 percent of the stance phase,[286–288] gait analysis of individuals with recent ACL deficiency shows functional adaptations in a high proportion of patients, with an extensor torque that lasts for nearly the entire stance phase.[286] Other analysis has also shown a decrease in the flexion moment of the knee in the range of 0 to 40 degrees of flexion in patients who have a chronic tear of the ACL.[289,290]

When the normal limb moves into the midstance phase, gravity and inertia generate a moment that tends to flex the knee. Because the quadriceps muscles balance this moment, a decrease in the flexion moment suggests a decrease in the quadriceps muscle moment.[291] Such a decrease has been noted in both limbs of patients who had only one knee with a torn ACL.[290]

Andriacchi[291] termed this finding the *quadriceps-avoidance gait,* although not all patients who have a torn ACL have such a gait, and its prevalence appears to be partly related to the time since the injury.[292] In activities that involve knee-flexion angles of less than 30 degrees (i.e., those involving normal gait), the quadriceps-avoidance gait is most effective in preventing anterior tibial translation.[291,293,294] In activities that involve knee-flexion angles of 40 degrees or more (e.g., jumping or sharp changes in running direction), increased contraction of the hamstrings is effective in preventing anterior tibial translation.[143,294–296]

Gait adaptations in individuals with ACL injury who have reconstruction surgery are less clear for two reasons[285]:

1. Very few comprehensive gait analyses have been conducted on this population.

2. The large variation in surgical and rehabilitation procedures and patient characteristics, and in patient compliance with rehabilitation, limit the generalization of these potential results.

Gait also can be affected by genu recurvatum, because during the loading response in gait, an individual with genu recurvatum transfers body weight directly from the femur to the tibia without the usual muscle energy absorption and cushioning a flexed knee provides. This may lead to pain in the medial tibiofemoral joint (compression) and posterolateral ligamentous structures (tensile). In individuals with quadriceps weakness, compensation may occur by hyperextending the knee to provide greater knee stability.

Gait analysis is described in Chapter 13.

Seated

Active Knee Extension. Although formally assessed as part of the active range of motion with passive overpressure (see later), active knee extension may be used during the observation phase of the examination. The patient should fully extend the knee from a flexed position. Normally, the patella follows a straight line, or a slight and smooth, gradual, lateral concave "C" curve as the knee extends. The presence of a "J sign," in which the patella slips off laterally as the knee approaches extension, or apprehension with motion involving lateral or medial stress, is necessary to confirm patellar instability.[11]

The patella may be compressed with the palm of the hand through the full range of motion, as ulcerated lesions can be tender with this provocative test.[11] However, care should be taken with this maneuver, because it can provoke pain in otherwise asymptomatic patients.

Distal patellar lesions are often tender with this test in the early degrees of knee flexion, whereas proximal lesions are tender at approximately 90 degrees.[11] This information can help guide the clinician with the intervention. Crepitus at the knee is a nonspecific finding and can be associated with both cartilaginous and synovial lesions.[11] Although often a concern to patients, because they believe it to be indicative of arthritis, crepitus often is a result of tight, deep, lateral retinacular structures and can be improved with retinacular stretching techniques.[257]

Lying

Hip Screening. With the patient supine and then prone, the hip is flexed and rotated as the clinician checks for a source of

referred pain.[182] Because patellar malalignment can be associated with adaptive shortening, the following structures (in decreasing order of frequency) are assessed[173,182]:

▶ *Lateral retinaculum (see "Special Tests," later).* A tight lateral retinaculum may pull the patella laterally.

▶ *Hamstrings (see "Special Tests," later).* When an individual with tight hamstrings runs, there is a decrease in stride length and a potential for the quadriceps to fatigue in an effort to overcome the passive resistance of the hamstrings.[297] Tightness of the hamstrings also produces an increase in knee flexion at heel strike. Because the knee cannot straighten, an increased dorsiflexion is required to position the body over the planted foot.[257] If the range of full dorsiflexion has already occurred at the talocrural joint, further range is achieved by subtalar pronation. This has the effect of increasing the valgus vector force and the dynamic Q angle.[257,298]

▶ *Iliotibial band (see "Special Tests," later).* The iliotibial band is maximally taut at 20–30 degrees of flexion. Adaptive shortening of this band can cause a lateral tracking and tilting of the patella, and often a stretching of the medial retinaculum.[222]

▶ *Tensor fascia latae and rectus femoris (see "Special Tests," later).* Adaptive shortening of these structures can increase the amount of compression of the patella on the femur.[222]

▶ *Hip rotators.* The hip rotators can accentuate anteversion or retroversion.[222]

Achilles–Soleus Length. A decrease in talocrural joint dorsiflexion range of motion may result in a compensatory subtalar pronation during ambulation and weight bearing.[299] Soft tissue tightness is particularly prevalent during the adolescent growth spurt, in which the long bones are growing faster than the surrounding soft tissues.[300]

Active Range of Motion with Passive Overpressure

Normal knee motion (Table 18-7) has been described as 0 degrees of extension to 135 degrees of flexion, although hyperextension is frequently present to varying degrees.[301] In general, however, the best way to ascertain normal motion is to examine the contralateral knee, provided that it has no abnormal conditions.

Clinical Pearl

Full range of knee motion requires:

- Congruent articular surfaces.

- Adequate muscle function.

- An articular capsule with suitable capacity and flexibility.

- Effective space in the medial and lateral articular recesses, intercondylar notch, and suprapatellar pouch.

- Sufficient meniscal motion.[302]

TABLE 18-7 Normal Ranges and End-feels at the Knee

Motion	Range of Motion (degrees)	End-Feel
Flexion	0–135	Tissue approximation or tissue stretch
Extension	0–15	Tissue stretch
External rotation of tibia on femur	30–40	Tissue stretch
Internal rotation of tibia on femur	20–30	Tissue stretch

Passive movements, as elsewhere, can determine the amount of available motion and the end-feel. For example, passive hyperextension of the knee with overpressure (Fig. 18-17) is performed to assess (from the end-feel) whether the knee extension is limited as a result of an articular disorder. Articular disorders include arthritis or arthrosis, a lesion of one of the menisci, or a loose body involvement. In diagnosing motion limitations, differentiation is made between capsular and noncapsular patterns. However, any motions that provoke symptoms are carefully noted.

According to the osteopathic theories of somatic dysfunction,[303] the following guidelines are used:

▶ If the restriction to movement is opposite to the direction that the bone seems to have traveled (e.g., the tibia has a

reduced joint glide), a mobilization or a manipulation is the intervention of choice.

▶ If the restriction to movement is in the same direction that the bone seems to have moved, and the opposite movement seems to be excessive (a change has occurred in the overall starting position), a muscle imbalance should be suspected, and a muscle energy technique used.

▶ If the patient demonstrates normal range but pain with movement, the joint cannot be at fault.

▶ If a muscle is very hypertonic, a spinal dysfunction may be present (unless trauma is involved), producing a hypermobility.

Even minor losses of knee motion may have adverse effects. It is common to lose both flexion and extension; however, loss of extension is usually more debilitating.[304] A loss of extension of more than 5 degrees may cause patellofemoral pain and a limp during walking,[305] whereas restricted flexion does not severely affect gait as long as the knee can be flexed to at least 60 degrees.[306] Diminished running speed is associated with loss of flexion of 10 degrees or more,[307] whereas an extension deficit of more than 10 degrees is poorly tolerated by active people.[308] A loss of more than 20 degrees of extension may cause a significant functional limb-length discrepancy.[307]

Patellar Motion Tests. Probably the most important part of the patellofemoral examination is the observation of the dynamics of patellar tracking in weight bearing and non–weight bearing.

A unilateral squat (Waldron test) can be used to assess patellofemoral function.[309] The patient stands on the affected leg, and the clinician sits or squats next to the patient. Using the entire surface of the palm, the clinician exerts slight pressure in an anteroposterior direction against the patient's patella (Fig. 18-18). From this position, the patient is asked to bend the knee slowly, if possible, to about 90 degrees, while the clinician palpates for crepitus and locking of the patella and assesses the

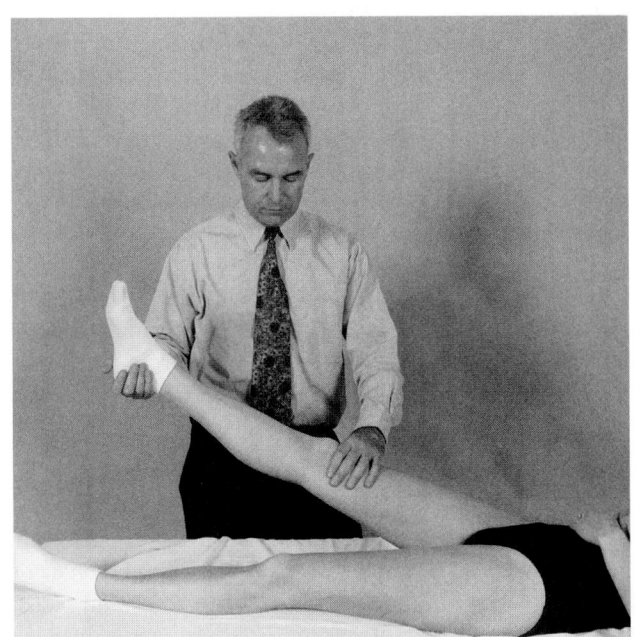

FIGURE 18-17 Passive overpressure of knee extension.

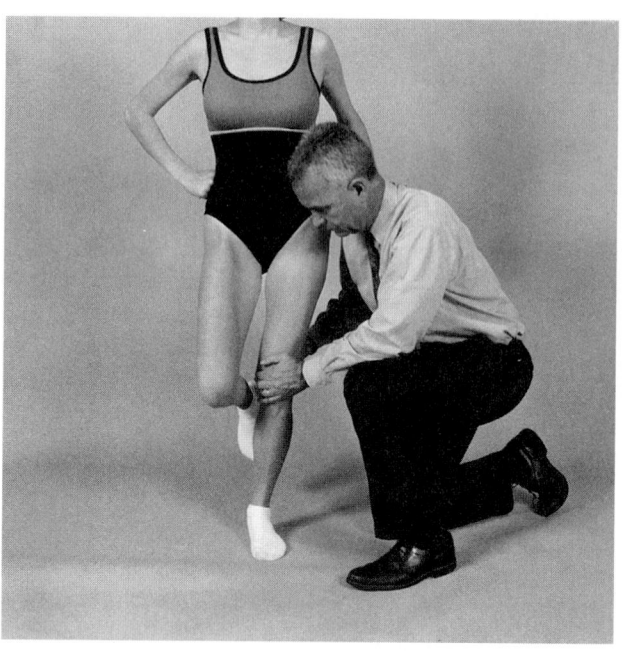

FIGURE 18-18   Waldron test.

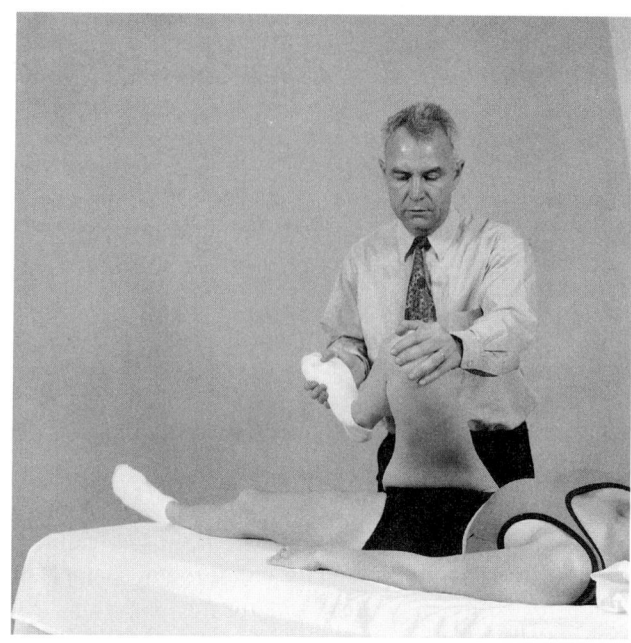

FIGURE 18-19   Passive overpressure into knee flexion.

course of movement of the patella. Crepitus or locking can in-dicate the presence of patellofemoral chondropathy or patellofemoral arthrosis. In patellar malalignment or patholo-gies of the corresponding femoral joint surface, movement of the patella can be disturbed. The patella is observed while the patient initiates flexion of the knee to see if it engages smoothly at the proximal end of the trochlea, or more distally than normal. Lateralization of the patella can occur during flexion, particularly when the Q angle is excessive.

The passive mobility tests for the patella are outlined in the discussion of "Patellar Stability Tests," later.

Flexion.   The amount of knee flexion should be assessed to see if the motion is restricted by tight structures. If no restriction is suspected, tests are required for generalized ligament laxity and for abnormally loose patellar retinacula (see later discussion).

The primary flexors of the knee are the three hamstring muscles, assisted by the gracilis, sartorius, popliteus, and gas-trocnemius muscles, and the tensor fascia latae (in 45 to 145 de-grees of flexion; see Table 18-4). The patient is positioned supine. Using one hand, the clinician grasps the anterior aspect of the patient's lower leg, just proximal to the malleoli, while the other hand grasps the anterior aspect of the patient's thigh, just above the patella. The patient's hip is flexed to about 90 de-grees and stabilized with one hand, while the clinician flexes the knee with the other hand (Fig. 18-19). At the end of the range of motion, the clinician exerts slight overpressure. The normal end-feel is usually one of soft tissue approximation. A flexion limitation other than soft tissue approximation is usually the result of an articular lesion, such as arthritis or arthrosis (capsular pattern), a lesion of one of the menisci, or a loose body.[265]

Rotation of the tibia relative to the femur is possible when the knee is flexed and non–weight bearing, with rotational capability greatest at approximately 90 degrees of flexion.[87]

Extension.   The primary extensors of the knee are the quadri-ceps muscles, consisting of the rectus femoris, vastus lateralis, vastus medialis, and vastus intermedius (see Table 18-4). Also assisting with knee extension in the 0-to-30-degree flexion range is the iliotibial band and tensor fascia latae.

The patient extends the knee, and the clinician applies over-pressure by stabilizing the thigh and pulling the ankle up to the ceiling (see Fig. 18-17), while allowing the conjunct external rotation of the tibia. Under normal conditions, the end-feel is usually hard.

A limitation of active knee motion can have a number of causes. The patient may have a neurologic deficit from a lumbar intervertebral disk herniation, with loss of knee motion as the primary symptom. Any acute injury causing pain may limit ac-tive knee motion as a result of muscle inhibition.[310] Quadriceps reflex inhibition has been well documented throughout the liter-ature and is thought to result from pain or effusion, or both, al-though the exact etiology has yet to be determined.[251,310–315] Some of the proposed causes for this reflex inhibition include:

▶ The result of capsular stretching.[314]

▶ The result of increased intra-articular pressure.[310]

In the presence of various pain syndromes, such as complex regional pain syndrome,[311] additional muscle inhibition can oc-cur. In most patients, limitations of motion resolve as the pain and effusion dissipate. However, this quadriceps inhibition may allow scar tissue to form while the knee is held in a flexed position.

Atrophy of the quadriceps muscle and flexion contracture usually results, and activities of daily living become more difficult to perform. Joint immobilization can complicate all of these factors. Disuse may induce abnormal cross-links between collagen fibers at abnormal locations,[316,317] decreasing their extensibility[318] and promoting intra-articular and extra-articular scarring.

Passive Tibial External Rotation. The patient is positioned supine. Using one hand, the clinician grasps the posteromedial aspect of the patient's foot and brings the ankle into maximal plantar flexion. The other hand is positioned on the anterior aspect of the patient's thigh, just proximal to the patella, so that the index and middle fingers can palpate the medial joint space[265] (Fig. 18-20). The patient's knee is flexed to 90 degrees and the hip to about 45 degrees. The distal hand performs an external rotation of the tibia, while maintaining the ankle in maximum plantar flexion (see Fig. 18-20). At the end of the range of motion, the clinician exerts slight overpressure. Under normal conditions, the end-feel is firm. The clinician notes whether pain is provoked or whether there is a hypermobility or hypomobility[265]:

▶ Pain with passive external rotation of the tibia can be the result of a lesion of the medial meniscotibial ligament, medial meniscus, MCL, or the posteromedial capsuloligamentous complex.

▶ Hypermobility with this maneuver can be the result of a lesion of the posteromedial capsuloligamentous complex, often in combination with lesions of the MCL and the ACL. Hypermobility may also be seen in ballet dancers.

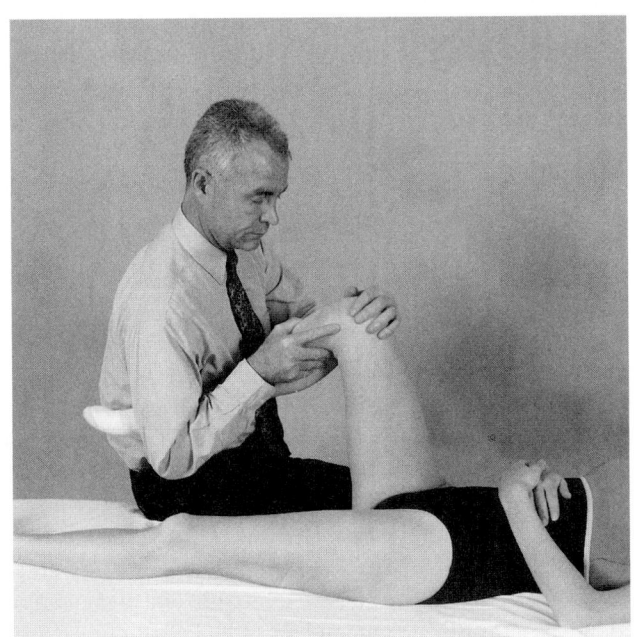

FIGURE 18-20 Passive external rotation of tibia.

▶ Hypomobility of passive tibial external rotation is seen only in severe articular disorders with significant capsular limitations of motion.

Passive Tibial Internal Rotation. The patient is positioned supine. Using the ipsilateral hand, the clinician grasps the posteromedial aspect of the patient's foot and brings the ankle into maximal plantar flexion. The contralateral hand is positioned on the anterior aspect of the patient's thigh, just proximal to the patella, so that the index and middle fingers can palpate the medial joint space (Fig. 18-20). The patient's knee is flexed to 90 degrees and the hip to about 45 degrees. The distal hand performs an internal rotation of the tibia while maintaining the ankle in maximum plantar flexion. At the end of the range of motion, the clinician exerts slight overpressure. Under normal conditions, the end-feel is firm. The clinician notes whether pain is provoked or whether there is hypermobility or hypomobility[265]:

▶ Pain can be the result of a lesion of the lateral meniscotibial ligament, lateral meniscus, or posterolateral capsuloligamentous complex.

▶ Hypermobility can be the result of a lesion of the posterolateral capsuloligamentous complex.

▶ Hypomobility is seen only in severe articular disorders with significant capsular limitations of motion.

Ankle Motions. Ankle motions are tested because a number of structures share a common relationship with the foot, ankle, and knee joint complex (refer to Chap. 19). Adaptive shortening of the gastrocnemius, particularly in the presence of adaptively shortened hamstring muscles, may produce increased knee flexion at initial contact and during the stance phase of gait.[198] Additionally, passive dorsiflexion can cause motions at the proximal tibiofibular joint and tibiofemoral joint.

Hip Motions. Several muscles cross both the hip and the knee. These include the rectus femoris, gracilis, sartorius, and hamstrings. Adaptive shortening of any of these structures may cause alterations in postural mechanics and gait. The hip rotators can also influence other aspects of the lower kinetic chain. Sahrmann advocates the testing the length-strength relationship of the hip external rotators because of their closed kinetic chain function of decelerating lower extremity internal rotation.[155,319]

Strength Testing

Gross muscle testing is useful in checking for deficits in the lower extremities. Strength testing involves the performance of resisted isometric tests. The joint is placed in its resting position to minimize any joint compression forces.

Knee Flexion. The strength of the knee flexors (the hamstrings) can be assessed by positioning the patient prone with the knee flexed to about 80–90 degrees. By internally rotating the tibia (Fig. 18-21) and resisting knee flexion, the clinician can theoretically assess the integrity of the medial hamstrings

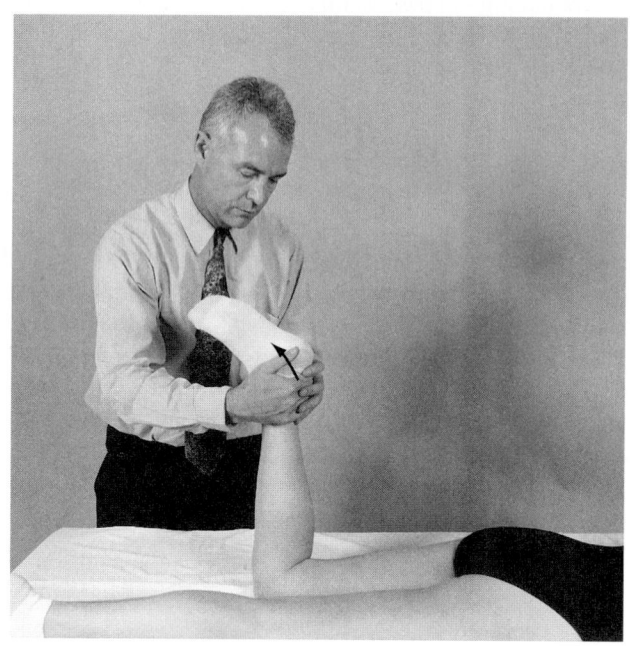

FIGURE 18-21　Strength testing: medial hamstrings.

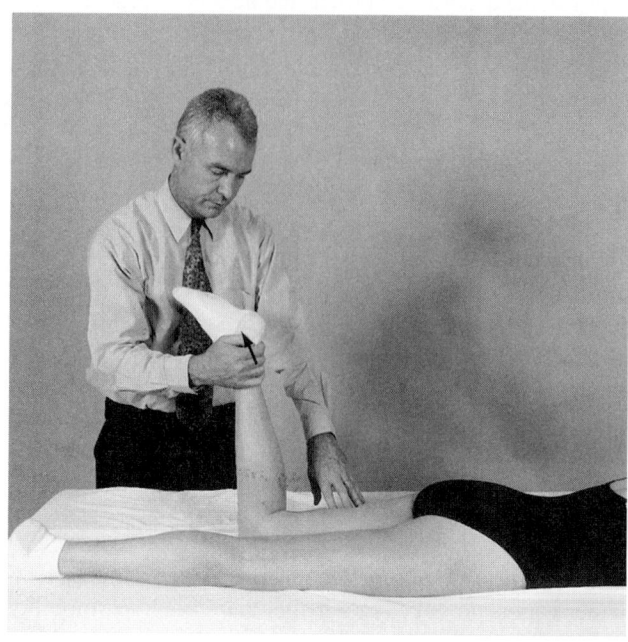

FIGURE 18-22　Strength testing: biceps femoris.

(semimembranosus and semitendinosus). The biceps femoris is assessed similarly by externally rotating the tibia and resisting knee flexion (Fig. 18-22).

Knee Extension.　Pain may be reproduced, and localized, with multiple angle isometric testing of the quadriceps, as described by McConnell.[175] Thus, the strength of the knee extensors (the quadriceps) is tested in 0, 30, 60, 90, and 120 degrees of knee flexion and held for 1 second with the femur externally rotated, to see if the pain can be reproduced or localized. The reproduction of pain with these tests suggests excessive pain from patellar compression. Any abnormal tibial movement with these tests may suggest ligamentous instability.[320] If pain is noted during this testing, McConnell suggests returning the knee to full extension, producing and maintaining a medial glide of the patella, and then returning the knee to the painful position to retest. This action should reduce the pain if it is of a patellofemoral origin.[175]

The final 15 degrees of knee extension require a 60 percent increase in muscle firing.[321] An extension lag (passive knee extension that is greater than active knee extension) indicates a slight loss of quadriceps muscle function.[155,257,322]

Plantar Flexion.　The strength of the gastrocnemius muscle is tested because of its intimate relationship to the knee. This can be achieved by having the patient perform 10–20 unilateral heel raises (depending on age and physical ability) while standing.

Palpation

For palpation to be reliable, the clinician must have a sound knowledge of surface anatomy, and the results from the palpation

examination should be correlated with other findings. A logical sequence should be employed by the clinician. The skin, retinacula, quadriceps tendon, and patellar tendon are palpated to rule out soft tissue sources of pain. Differences in temperature between the knees suggest inflammation in the warmer of the two. The following structures should be identified and palpated.

Posterior Aspect.　The patient is positioned prone. The clinician locates the popliteal fossa. The semimembranosus and semitendinosus form the proximal medial border of the fossa. Just deep to this, if it is present, is the location of a Baker's cyst. With the knee in a slightly flexed position, the thin round tendon of the semitendinosus should be easy to palpate. Medial and lateral to this tendon are the deeper parts of the semimembranosus. The popliteal pulse can be located just below the crease of the knee, more to the lateral side than medial side, and posterior to the tibial plateau. Medial to the pulse is the tendon of semimembranosus. At this point, if the thumb is pushed deeper, the attachment of the PCL can be located as it arises from the back of the tibia. Under normal circumstances, this attachment will be tender. A little lateral to this is the attachment of the meniscofemoral ligament. The PCL and meniscofemoral ligament curve inward, to attach on the inner aspect of the medial condyle of the femur.

At the proximal lateral part the fossa, the biceps tendon is found. This tendon is palpable together with the common peroneal nerve. The tendon of the gracilis is medial and anterior to the medial part of the semimembranosus. Palpation performed medially and anteriorly to this point leads to the sartorius muscle. The tendons of the sartorius, gracilis, and semitendinosus form the pes anserinus. The sartorius and gracilis muscles can be differentiated as follows: the gracilis contracts during hip adduction, while the sartorius contracts during hip abduction. Palpation more anteriorly leads to the medial femoral condyle and the adductor tubercle. Tenderness at the anterior aspect of the medial femoral condyle, associated with a snapping sensation as the knee is flexed, can indicate a symptomatic plica.[323] The adductor tubercle serves as the attachment site for the patellar retinaculum and the medial patellofemoral ligament, and is a hallmark site of tenderness with lateral patellar dislocation.[265] The adductor tubercle is also the attachment site of the adductor magnus, and the origin of the MCL. The distal borders of the popliteal fossa are palpated by positioning the patient's knee in slight flexion. The medial head of the gastrocnemius can be palpated deep and medial to the fossa, while the lateral head can be found deep and medial to the tendon of the biceps femoris muscle.

Anterior Aspect. The patient lies supine with the hip and thigh positioned in extension. The clinician palpates the medial and lateral edges of the patella. Palpation of the rectus femoris insertion on the superior aspect of the patella is only possible with the patella tipped slightly forward.[265] Complaints of pain distal to the patella during extension of the knee may indicate a patella tendon–ligament lesion at the inferior pole. In some individuals, the continuation of the tendon of the VL muscle, the lateral patellar retinaculum, can be palpated at the lateral side of the patella.[265]

Palpation of the joint space is made easier when the tibia is rotated internally and externally while in the flexed position. The anterior part of the medial meniscus is palpable in the medial joint space with the tibia externally rotated, between the patellar tendon–ligament and the anterior edge of the MCL. Under normal circumstances, the medial meniscus is not palpable beyond 30 degrees of flexion.[265] The medial meniscotibial or coronary ligament, which attaches the medial meniscus to the tibia, is palpable anteriorly with the knee positioned in 90 degrees of flexion and the tibia maximally externally rotated, proximal to the tibia (passive external rotation of the knee will provoke the patient's pain, if the ligament is damaged).[265]

Clinical Pearl

Joint line tenderness usually is associated with a tibiofemoral injury, such as a meniscal or collateral ligament tear; it can be associated with patellar pathology, although the reasons are probably multifactorial.[191,260,263]

Other structures to palpate for tenderness on the anterior aspect of the knee include:

▶ *Base (inferior pole) of patella.* Tenderness at the inferior tip of the patella indicates patellar tendonitis.

▶ *Infrapatellar fat pad (Hoffa's fat pad).* This structure is located between the patella ligament (anteriorly) and the anterior joint capsule (posteriorly).

▶ *Lateral retinaculum.*

▶ *Apex of patella.*

▶ *Accessory retinaculum from the iliotibial tract.*

▶ *Medial retinaculum.*

▶ *Medial and lateral patellar facets.* These facets can be tested for tenderness, as can the overhang of the lateral facet over the patellar groove, by pushing the patella to one side and then the other, and then curling the fingers around and under the borders of the patella. The clinician should be able to palpate under one third of the patella.

▶ *Dynamic restraints.* The patient is asked to contract the quadriceps. In patients with malalignment, the VMO typically cannot be identified by sight or palpation; it inserts no farther distally than the proximal pole of the patella and it remains soft, even with maximal quadriceps contraction.[182] In the normal knee, the VMO should be felt to contract simultaneously with the VL.

Lateral Aspect. The fibula head can be palpated by following the tendon of the biceps femoris distally. It is often more distal and posterior than imagined. On the lateral side, the highest point on the lateral femoral condyle is the lateral epicondyle, which serves as the origin of the LCL. The LCL is best palpated when the hip is maximally externally rotated and the knee is flexed to 90 degrees in the "figure-four" cross-legged stance.[265] If the LCL is followed down to the fibular head, it will be felt to blend with the biceps femoris. On the posterolateral aspect of the condyle is the attachment for the lateral head of the gastrocnemius. Anterior to this, there is a small circular groove, which is where the tendon of the popliteus sets in on the lateral condyle. Tenderness in this location, just behind the LCL, either anterior or posterior to it, would suggest damage to the popliteus muscle.[265] On the anterolateral aspect of the knee is Gerdy's tubercle, the largest bony prominence medial to the apex of the fibular head, which serves as the attachment site for the iliotibial band.

The lateral joint space is palpated starting at a point just lateral to the patellar tendon–ligament. The anterior part of the lateral meniscus is best palpated with the knee in an extended position.

Medial Aspect. The highest point of the medial aspect of the femur is the medial epicondyle, which serves as the origin for the MCL. Superior to this point is the adductor tubercle, and superior to that is the supracondylar ridge, which is the attachment for the VMO. Very localized tenderness at the medial aspect of the knee, away from the joint line, may indicate a neuroma.[322]

Functional Tests
Functional outcome following knee injury must consider the patient's perspective, and not just objective measurements of instability. Functional motion requirements of the knee vary according to the specific task. In normal level ground walking,

60 to 70 degrees of knee flexion is required. This requirement increases to 80 to 85 degrees for stair climbing, and to 120 to 140 degrees for running.[3] Approximately 120 degrees of knee flexion are necessary for activities such as squatting to tie a shoelace or to don a sock.[324] Table 18-8 outlines the amounts of knee range of motion that must be available for common activities of daily living.

Subjective Tests.   A number of commonly used rating scales are used to assess function in the knee. These include:

WOMAC Index.   The Western Ontario and McMaster Universities Osteoarthritis Index (WOMAC) (Table 18-9) is a widely used measure of symptoms and physical disability, originally developed for people with osteoarthritis of the hip or knee.[325] The measure was developed to evaluate clinically important, patient-relevant changes in health status as a result of intervention.[326] Evidence of the reliability (test-retest), validity, and responsiveness of the WOMAC has been provided in osteoarthritis patients undergoing total knee or hip arthroplasty,[325] and in osteoarthritis patients receiving nonsteroidal anti-inflammatory drugs (NSAIDs).[327] The WOMAC evaluates three dimensions: pain, stiffness, and physical function with 5, 2, and 17 questions, respectively[328] (see Table 18-9). Each subscale is summated to a maximum score of 20, 8, and 68, respectively. There is also an index score or global score, which is most commonly calculated by summating the scores for the three subscales.[328]

Lysholm Knee Scoring Scale.   The Lysholm Knee Scale[329] is commonly used as a subjective-report scoring system designed to evaluate the intervention outcome and postsurgical result of knee patients. The scale consists of eight items related to limping; the need for an assistive device; ability to squat or climb stairs; and the presence of pain, swelling, locking, or "giving way," and leg atrophy.[330] Points are given for each level of ability or disability reported, with the perfect score being 100 (Table 18-10). The designers of this scale found that patients suffering from knee instability scored significantly lower than

patients with minimal or no instability (average = 75.6 and 93.6, respectively).

Irrgang Activities of Daily Living Scale.   The Activities of Daily Living Scale (Table 18-11) assesses the full spectrum of symptoms and functional limitations that may occur as a result of knee disorders.[330] The test-retest reliability of this scale is 0.97.[332]

Patellar Joint Evaluation Scale.   This scale assesses seven components of patellofemoral joint function (Table 18-12).

Objective Functional Tests.   The functional tests for the knee are introduced once the patient is able to perform active and resisted motions without pain.

Heel Raise.   The heel raise can be used to assess the strength of the gastrocnemius. The patient is positioned standing, leaning against a wall, with the knees extended. One foot is tested at a time as the patient rises up on the toes for 10–20 repetitions depending on age and physical ability.

▶ The patient everts the foot and raises up on the toes to test the lateral head.

▶ The patient inverts the foot and raises up on the toes to test the medial head.

The soleus muscle can be tested similarly by having the patient perform a unilateral heel raise with the knee flexed.

Full Squat or Semi-squat.   The simplest functional weight-bearing test for the knee is the squat position. The patient should be able to perform this maneuver without pain.

Duck Walk/Childress Sign.   The patient squats with the toes pointing outward and walks forward. This maneuver is similar to the McMurray test for meniscal lesion (although more stressful). Pain, or crepitus, with this test indicates a lesion of the posterior horn of the meniscus or the MCL.[333] Patients with a patellofemoral lesion can duck walk without difficulty, but experience difficulty coming up out of the squat.[249]

Advanced Functional Tests.   More advanced functional tests for the knee include the vertical jump, functional hop, single-leg squat, and running tests.[330]

Vertical Jump.   Vertical jumping is an explosive movement, in which the vertical velocity of the trunk is of decisive importance for jump height. The vertical jump test is commonly used in sports medicine, and investigators have found it to be significantly related to athletic performance.[334-340] The vertical jump is performed in the following manner. A baseline measurement is made of the highest point that the patient can reach while remaining flat-footed. The patient's fingertips are covered in chalk, and he or she is then asked to jump as high as possible, marking the wall with the chalk on the fingertips. The patient is

TABLE 18-8   Approximate Range of Motion Required for Common Activities of Daily Living[324]

Activity	Required Flexion Range of Motion (degrees)
Running	120–140
Squatting	120
Tying shoelace	120
Donning a sock	120
Climbing downstairs	110
Sitting and rising	85
Climbing upstairs	80
Swing phase of gait	70
Stance phase of gait	20

TABLE 18-9   Western Ontario and McMaster Universities Osteoarthritis Index (WOMAC)

Name: _____

Primary Care Physician: _____

This survey asks for your views about the amount of pain, stiffness, and disability you are experiencing. Please answer every question by filling in the appropriate response. If you are unsure about how to answer a question, please give the best answer you can. (Please mark your answers with an "X")

SECTION A: PAIN

The following questions concern the amount of pain you are currently experiencing due to arthritis in your hips and/or knees. For each situation, please enter the amount of pain recently experienced.

Question: **How much pain do you have?**

	None	Mild	Moderate	Severe	Extreme
1. Walking on a flat surface.	☐	☐	☐	☐	☐
2. Going up or down stairs.	☐	☐	☐	☐	☐
3. At night while in bed.	☐	☐	☐	☐	☐
4. Sitting or lying.	☐	☐	☐	☐	☐
5. Standing upright.	☐	☐	☐	☐	☐

SECTION B: JOINT STIFFNESS

The following questions concern the amount of joint stiffness (not pain) you are currently experiencing in your hips and/or knees. Stiffness is a sensation of restriction or slowness in the ease with which you move your joints.

	None	Mild	Moderate	Severe	Extreme
1. How severe is your stiffness after first wakening in the morning?	☐	☐	☐	☐	☐
2. How severe is your stiffness after sitting, lying, or resting later in the day?	☐	☐	☐	☐	☐

SECTION C: PHYSICAL FUNCTION

The following questions concern your physical function. By this we mean your ability to move around and to look after yourself. For each of the following activities, please indicate the degree of difficulty you are currently experiencing due to arthritis in your hips and/or knees. (Please mark your answers with an "X")

Question: **What degree of difficulty do you have with:**

	None	Mild	Moderate	Severe	Extreme
1. Descending stairs.	☐	☐	☐	☐	☐
2. Ascending stairs.	☐	☐	☐	☐	☐
3. Rising from sitting.	☐	☐	☐	☐	☐
4. Standing.	☐	☐	☐	☐	☐
5. Bending to floor.	☐	☐	☐	☐	☐
6. Walking on flat.	☐	☐	☐	☐	☐
7. Getting in/out of car.	☐	☐	☐	☐	☐
8. Going shopping.	☐	☐	☐	☐	☐
9. Putting on socks/stockings.	☐	☐	☐	☐	☐
10. Rising from bed.	☐	☐	☐	☐	☐
11. Taking off socks/stockings.	☐	☐	☐	☐	☐
12. Lying in bed.	☐	☐	☐	☐	☐
13. Getting in/out of bath.	☐	☐	☐	☐	☐
14. Sitting.	☐	☐	☐	☐	☐
15. Getting on/off toilet.	☐	☐	☐	☐	☐
16. Heavy domestic duties.	☐	☐	☐	☐	☐
17. Light domestic duties.	☐	☐	☐	☐	☐

TABLE 18-10   Lysholm Knee Scoring Scale[331]

Category	Score
LIMP	
None	5
Slight or periodic	3
Serve and constant	0
SUPPORT	
None	5
Stick or crutch	3
Weight bearing impossible	0
LOCKING	
No locking and no catching sensations	5
Catching, but no locking sensation	4
Locking	
Occasionally	2
Frequently	3
Locked joint on examination	0
INSTABILITY	
Never giving way	30
Rarely during athletics or other severe exertion	25
Frequently during athletics or other severe exertion (incapable of participation)	20
Occasionally in daily activities	10
Often in daily activities	5
With every step	0
PAIN	
None	30
Inconstant and slight during severe exertion	25
Marked on giving way	20
Marked during severe exertion	15
Marked on or after walking more than 2 km	10
Marked on or after walking less than 2 km	5
Constant	0
SWELLING	
None	10
With giving way	7
On severe exertion	5
On ordinary exertion	2
Constant	0
STAIR CLIMBING	
No problems	10
Slightly impaired	6
One step at a time	2
Impossible	0
SQUATTING	
No problems	5
Slightly impaired	4
Not beyond 90 degrees	2
Impossible	0

allowed three jumps, after which the clinician subtracts the baseline reach from the maximum vertical jump to obtain the vertical jump distance.

Functional Hop Tests

▶ *Hop for distance.* This test has good test-retest reliability (0.79 to 0.99),[337,338,340–345] although its correlation with power and isokinetic strength testing is unclear.[305,336,338,345–348] The patient stands on the involved leg, with the toes as close to the starting position as possible. The hands are placed behind the back or on the hips. The patient then tries to hop as far as possible, landing on the same extremity. Three attempts are permitted. The distance is measured from the take-off toe to the landing heel and is compared with the hop distance of the uninvolved leg, and scored as a percentage. The distances hopped are influenced by age and sex.[344] Norms for this test in high school athletes are an average of 155 cm for boys and an average of 121 cm for girls.[349] The sensitivity of this test has been found to be 52 percent, and the specificity, 97 percent.[350] Barber and colleagues[338] found a significant relationship between the one-leg hop and the subjective limitations of sprinting, jumping, and landing.

▶ *Triple hop.*[337,351] The triple-hop test is similar to the hop-for-distance test, except that the patient hops for three consecutive hops, and the score is the distance measured from the take-off toe to the landing heel of the third jump. One study reported a high correlation between concentric isokinetic strength of the quadriceps muscle and the triple hop for distance.[348]

▶ *Timed 6-m hop.*[338,340,342] This test is reliable, with an intraclass correlation coefficient (ICC) ranging from 0.66 to 0.77,[337,341] and is considered to be one of the best indicators of function.[346] The clinician marks off a distance of 6 m, and the patient performs single-leg hops over the distance. The time taken is measured to the nearest 0.01 second and compared with the uninvolved leg. This functional test evaluates the strength, endurance, proprioception, balance, and power of the various knee structures. The test is recommended for use with athletes returning to sport. The sensitivity of this test has been found to be 49 percent, and the specificity, 94 percent.[350]

▶ *Crossover hop.* The crossover hop has an ICC of 0.96 for test-retest reliability.[337] The results of this test have a relationship with the isokinetic parameter of acceleration range, and are considered to be the best indicator of knee function.[346] The test is performed as follows: The patient places his or her feet behind the start line, and a tape measure is laid perpendicular to that line. The patient is asked to stand on one leg to the right of the tape measure. The patient is then asked to jump, on one leg, to the left side of the tape, back to the right, and then back to the left, attempting to propel himself or herself forward as far as possible with each hop. The score is the distance measured from the

TABLE 18-11   Patient Reported Measure of Knee Function

ACTIVITIES OF DAILY LIVING SCALE

Instructions: The following questionnaire is designed to determine the symptoms and limitations that you experience because of your knee while you perform your usual daily activities. Please answer each question by checking the statement that best describes you over the last 1 to 2 days. For a given question, more than one of the statements may describe you, but please mark ONLY the statement that best describes you during your usual daily activities.

SYMPTOMS

1. To what degree does pain in your knee affect your daily activity level?
   5   I never have pain in my knee.
   4   I have pain in my knee, but it does not affect my daily activity.
   3   Pain affects my activity slightly.
   2   Pain affects my activity moderately.
   1   Pain affects my activity severely.
   0   Pain in my knee prevents me from performing all daily activities.

2. To what degree does grinding or grating of your knee affect your daily activity level?
   5   I never have grinding or grating in my knee.
   4   I have grinding or grating in my knee, but it does not affect my daily activity.
   3   Grinding or grating affects my activity slightly.
   2   Grinding or grating affects my activity moderately.
   1   Grinding or grating affects my knee slightly.
   0   Grinding or grating in my knee prevents me from performing daily activities.

3. To what degree does stiffness in your knee affect your daily activity level?
   5   I never have stiffness in my knee.
   4   I have stiffness in my knee, but it does not affect my daily activity.
   3   Stiffness affects my activity slightly.
   2   Stiffness affects my activity moderately.
   1   Stiffness affects my activity severely.
   0   Stiffness in my knee prevents me from performing all daily activities.

4. To what degree does swelling in your knee affect your daily activity level?
   5   I never have swelling in my knee.
   4   I have swelling in my knee, but it does not affect my daily activity.
   3   Swelling affects my activity slightly.
   2   Swelling affects my activity moderately.
   1   Swelling affects my activity severely.
   0   Swelling in my knee prevents me from performing all daily activities.

5. To what degree does slipping of your knee affect your daily activity level?
   5   I never have slipping of my knee.
   4   I have slipping of my knee, but it does not affect my daily activity.
   3   Slipping affects my activity slightly.
   2   Slipping affects my activity moderately.
   1   Slipping affects my activity severely.
   0   Slipping of my knee prevents me from performing all daily activities.

6. To what degree does buckling of your knee affect your daily activity level?
   5   I never have buckling of my knee.
   4   I have buckling of my knee, but it does not affect my daily activity level.
   3   Buckling affects my activity slightly.
   2   Buckling affects my activity moderately.
   1   Buckling affects my activity severely.
   0   Buckling of my knee prevents me from performing all daily activities.

TABLE 18-11 *(cont.)*

SYMPTOMS

7. To what degree does weakness or lack of strength of your leg affect your daily activity level?

   5 My leg never feels weak.

   4 My leg feels weak, but it does not affect my daily activity.

   3 Weakness affects my activity slightly.

   2 Weakness affects my activity moderately.

   1 Weakness affects my activity severely.

   0 Weakness of my leg prevents me from performing all daily activities.

FUNCTIONAL DISABILITY WITH ACTIVITIES OF DAILY LIVING

8. How does your knee affect your ability to walk?

   5 My knee does not affect my ability to walk.

   4 I have pain in my knee when walking, but it does not affect my ability to walk.

   3 My knee prevents me from walking more than 1 mile.

   2 My knee prevents me from walking more than ½ mile.

   1 My knee prevents me from walking more than 1 block.

   0 My knee prevents me from walking.

9. Because of your knee, do you walk with crutches or a cane?

   3 I can walk without crutches or a cane.

   2 My knee causes me to walk with 1 crutch or a cane.

   1 My knee causes me to walk with 2 crutches.

   0 Because of my knee, I cannot walk even with crutches.

10. Does your knee cause you to limp when you walk?

   2 I can walk without a limp.

   1 Sometimes my knee causes me to walk with a limp.

   0 Because of my knee, I cannot walk without a limp.

11. How does your knee affect your ability to go up stairs?

   5 My knee does not affect my ability to go up stairs.

   4 I have pain in my knee when going up stairs, but it does not limit my ability to go up stairs.

   3 I am able to go up stairs normally, but I need to rely on use of a railing.

   2 I am able to go up stairs one step at a time with use of a railing.

   1 I have to use crutches or a cane to go up stairs.

   0 I cannot go up stairs.

12. How does your knee affect your ability to go down stairs?

   5 My knee does not affect my ability to go down stairs.

   4 I have pain in my knee when going down stairs, but it does not limit my ability to go down stairs.

   3 I am able to go down stairs normally, but I need to rely on use of a railing.

   2 I am able to go down stairs one step at a time with use of railing.

   1 I have to use crutches or a cane to go down stairs.

   0 I cannot go down stairs.

13. How does your knee affect your ability to stand?

   5 My knee does not affect my ability to stand. I can stand for unlimited amounts of time.

   4 I have pain in my knee when standing, but it does not limit my ability to stand.

   3 Because of my knee I cannot stand for more than 1 hour.

   2 Because of my knee I cannot stand for more than ½ hour.

   1 Because of my knee I cannot stand for more than 10 minutes.

   0 I cannot stand because of my knee.

14. How does your knee affect your ability to kneel on the front of your knee?

   5 My knee does not affect my ability to kneel on the front of my knee. I can kneel for unlimited amounts of time.

   4 I have pain when kneeling on the front of my knee, but it does not limit my ability to kneel.

   3 I cannot kneel on the front of my knee for more than 1 hour.

TABLE 18-11 *(cont.)*

    2 I cannot kneel on the front of my knee for more than ½ hour.

    1 I cannot kneel on the front of my knee for more than 10 minutes.

    0 I cannot kneel on the front of my knee.

15. How does your knee affect your ability to squat?

    5 My knee does not affect my ability to squat. I can squat all the way down.

    4 I have pain when squatting, but I can still squat all the way down.

    3 I cannot squat more than ¾ of the way down.

    2 I cannot squat more than ½ of the way down.

    1 I cannot squat more than ¼ of the way down.

    0 I cannot squat at all.

16. How does your knee affect your ability to sit with your knee bent?

    5 My knee does not affect my ability to sit with my knee bent. I can sit for unlimited amounts of time.

    4 I have pain when sitting with my knee bent, but it does not limit my ability to sit.

    3 I cannot sit with my knee bent for more than 1 hour.

    2 I cannot sit with my knee bent for more than ½ hour.

    1 I cannot sit with my knee bent for more than 10 minutes.

    0 I cannot sit with my knee bent.

17. How does your knee affect your ability to rise from a chair?

    5 My knee does not affect my ability to rise from a chair.

    4 I have pain when rising from the seated position, but it does not affect my ability to rise from the seated position.

    3 Because of my knee I can only rise from a chair if I use my hands and arms to assist.

    0 Because of my knee I cannot rise from a chair.

TABLE 18-12 Patellofemoral Joint Evaluation Scale[332a]

Function	Points	Function	Points
LIMP		**INSTABILITY (GIVING WAY)**	
None	5	Never	20
Slight or episodic	3	Occasionally with vigorous activities	10
Severe	0	Frequently with vigorous activities	8
		Occasionally with daily activities	5
ASSISTIVE DEVICES		Frequently with daily activities	2
None	5	Every day	0
Cane or brace	3		
Unable to bear weight	0	**SWELLING**	
		None	10
STAIR CLIMBING		After vigorous activities only	5
No problem	20	After walking or mild activities	2
Slight impairment	15	Constant	0
Very slowly	10		
One step at a time, always same leg first	5	**PAIN**	
Unable	0	None	35
		Occasionally with vigorous activities	30
CREPITATION		Marked with vigorous activities	20
None	5	Marked after walking 1 mile or mild or	
Annoying	3	moderate rest pain	15
Limits activities	2	Marked with walking < 1 mile	10
Severe	0	Constant and severe	0

Scoring: 90–100 points = excellent; 80–90 points = good; 60–79 points = fair; < 60 points = poor.

take-off toe to the landing heel of the third jump. Three attempts are permitted, and two sides are compared as a percentage of each other.

▶ *Stairs hop.* The patient is timed as he or she hops up and down several steps (20 to 25 steps are recommended), first on the uninvolved leg, and then on the involved leg.[351]

▶ *Side-to-side hop.* Steadman[352] advocates the use of the side-to-side Heiden hop. The Heiden hop involves the patient jumping from side to side, to a line placed approximately 5 to 6 feet (1.5 to 1.8 m) apart. The landing is controlled with a soft flexion of the knee, balancing the body on the foot closest to the line. The patient then leaps sideways to the other line, landing on the opposite foot in a controlled fashion, gently assuming a semi-squat position on the single leg.[353] This exercise is performed side to side for 5 to 10 minutes. Evidence of an ungraceful landing, loss of balance, or shaking muscles on the involved side indicates weakness of the quadriceps.[353]

Single-leg Squat Test. The patient is asked to balance on one leg, and then to squat down on that leg while keeping the trunk erect. The amount of flexion at the knee is measured with a goniometer and is compared with a similar measure of the uninvolved leg. If a hand or the opposite extremity touches the ground, the measurement is retaken. Although seemingly a static test, this is a test of the dynamic ability of the quadriceps, hamstring, gluteal, and gastrocnemius muscles to maintain eccentric control, and for the patient to maintain balance.

Running Tests
▶ *Figure-of-eight.* Two cones are positioned 10 m apart. The patient is asked to run around the cones in a figure-of-eight pattern, for a certain number of rotations, rounding the turns rather than planting and cutting, while the clinician times the run. The time ratio of figure-of-eight running to straight running is one of the most definitive ways to compare patients with an ACL-deficient knee to those with normal knees.[354]

▶ *Carioca.* The carioca test involves the patient running laterally with a crossover of the legs and a weaving of the feet, beginning with the trailing leg in front, then trailing the leg in back of the leading leg, for a distance of either 8 feet,[355] or 24.4 m.[356]

▶ *Shuttle run.*[347,357] The shuttle run involves having the patient run between cones or varying distances.

Stress Testing
The stress tests are used to determine the integrity of the joint, ligaments, and menisci. Serious functional instability of the knee appears to occur unpredictably. The reasons for such discrepancies are unknown, but they may be a result of[33]:

▶ Varying definitions of instability.

▶ Varying degrees of damage of the ACL.[358,359]

▶ Different combinations of injuries.[63]

▶ Different mechanisms of compensation for the loss of the ACL.

▶ Differences in rehabilitation.

▶ The diverse physical demands and expectations of different populations.

One Plane Medial Instability: Abduction Valgus Stress. The patient is positioned supine, with the involved knee extended. The clinician applies a strong valgus force, with a counterforce applied at the lateral femoral condyle (Fig. 18-23). Normally, there is little or no valgus movement in the knee, and, if present, it should be less than the amount of varus motion. Under normal conditions, the end-feel is firm. With degeneration of the medial or lateral compartments, varus and valgus motions may be increased, while the end-feels will be normal.

With the knee tested in full extension, any demonstrable instability is usually very significant. Pain with this maneuver is caused by an increase in tension of the medial collateral structures or the connection of these structures with the medial meniscus. If pain or an excessive amount of motion is detected compared with the other extremity, a hypermobility or instability, should be suspected. The following structures may be implicated:

▶ Superficial and deep fibers of the MCL.

▶ Posterior oblique ligament.

▶ Posteromedial capsule.

▶ Medial capsular ligament.

▶ ACL.

▶ PCL.

The test is then repeated at 10 to 30 degrees of flexion (see Fig. 18-23) to further assess the MCL, posterior oblique ligament, and PCL. One plane valgus instability in 30 degrees of flexion usually denotes a tearing, of at least a second degree, of the middle third of the capsular ligament and the parallel fibers of the MCL.

The posterior fibers of the MCL can be isolated, by placing the knee in 90 degrees of flexion with full external rotation of the tibia.[265] The femur is prevented from rotating by the clinician's shoulder. The clinician places one hand on the dorsum of the foot and the other on the heel, and an external rotation force is applied using the foot as a lever (see Fig. 18-23).

One Plane Lateral Instability. The patient is positioned supine, with the involved knee in full extension. The clinician applies a strong varus force, with a counterforce applied at the medial femoral condyle (see Fig. 18-23). To be able to assess the amount of varus movement, the clinician should repeat the maneuver several times, applying slight overpressure at the end of the range of motion. Under normal conditions, the end-feel is firm, after slight movement.

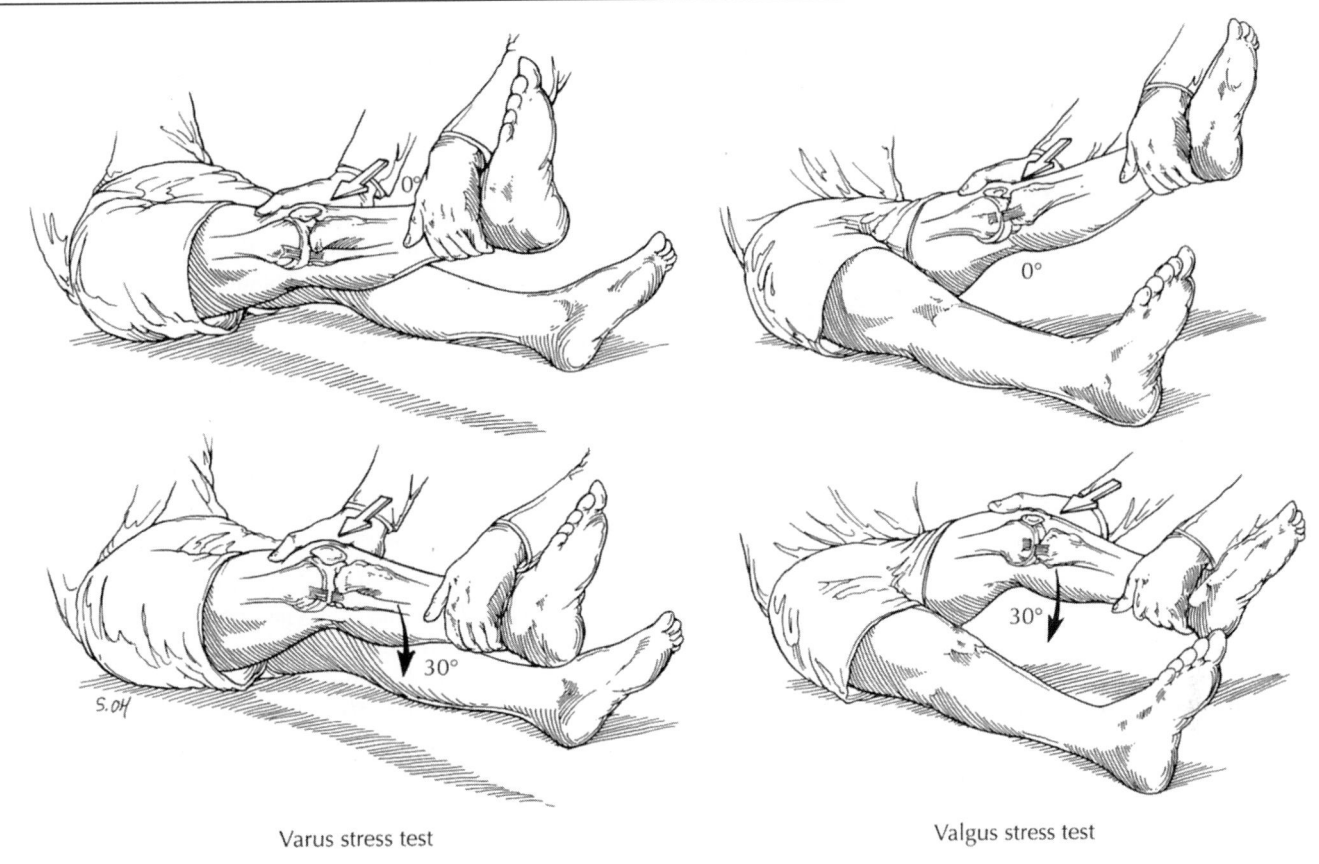

Varus stress test   Valgus stress test

FIGURE 18-23   Varus and valgus test. (Reproduced with permission from Smith BW, Green GA. Acute knee injuries: Part I. History and physical examination. *Am Fam Phys* 1995;51:615–621.)

If this test is positive for pain or excessive motion compared with the other extremity, the following structures may be implicated:

► LCL.

► Lateral capsular ligament.

► Arcuate-popliteus complex.

► ACL.

► PCL.

If the instability is gross, one or both cruciate ligaments may be involved as well as, occasionally, the biceps femoris tendon and the iliotibial band, leading to a rotary instability if not in the short term, certainly over a period of time.[148]

The test is then repeated at 10 to 30 degrees of flexion with the tibia in full external rotation (see Fig. 18-23) to further assess the LCL, posterolateral capsule, and arcuate-popliteus complex.

One Plane Anterior Instability.   Ensuring the integrity of the ACL is crucial for maintaining the normal biomechanical properties of the knee joint, protecting its periarticular structures, and preventing premature osteoarthritis. Knee joints with ACL

deficiencies have rotary instabilities that expose supporting ligaments and menisci adjacent to the ACL to further damage and degenerative joint disease.[25] Signs and symptoms of chronic rotary knee instabilities from ACL deficiencies include swelling, pain, a "giving way" of patients' knee joints, arthritis, and possible subsequent meniscal injuries.

Several tests have been advocated for testing the integrity of the ACL. Two of the more commonly used ones are the Lachman test, and the anterior drawer test.

Lachman Test.   The Lachman test (Fig. 18-24) is one of the easiest and most accurate diagnostic measures used to assess ACL injuries.[360] Torg and colleagues[361] were the first to publish a description of the Lachman test, whereby the knee is held in 30 degrees of flexion while the tibia is anteriorly translated with respect to the femur (Fig. 18-24).

In the hands of the experienced clinician, accuracy of this test has been found to be 81.8 percent sensitive and 96.8 percent specific,[362] increasing to 100 percent if the patient is anesthetized.[363,364] A number of factors can influence the results of the Lachman test. These include:

► An inability of the patient to relax.

► The degree of knee flexion.

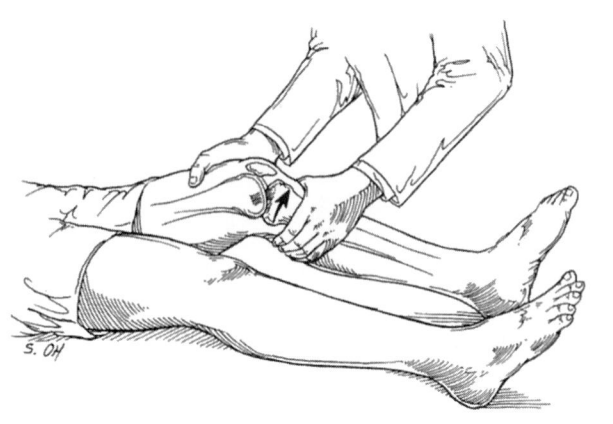

FIGURE 18-24 Lachman test. (Reproduced with permission from Smith BW, Green GA. Acute knee injuries: Part I. History and physical examination. *Am Fam Phys* 1995;51:615–621.)

▶ The size of the clinician's hand.

▶ The stabilization (and thus relaxation) of the patient's thigh.

According to Weiss and colleagues,[365] these factors can be minimized by the use of the modified Lachman test. In this modification, the patient is positioned supine, with the feet resting firmly on the end of the table and the knees flexed 10 to 15 degrees. The clinician stabilizes the distal end of patient's femur using the thigh rather than the hand, as in the Lachman test, and then attempts to displace patient's tibia anteriorly. If the tibia moves forward, and the concavity of the patellar tendon-ligament becomes convex, the test is considered positive.

The grading of knee instability is as follows[52,366,367]:

1+ (mild): 5 mm or less.

2+ (moderate): 5 to 10 mm.

3+ (serious): more than 10 mm.

False-negatives with this test can occur. False-negatives may be caused by a significant hemarthrosis, protective hamstring spasm, or tear of the posterior horn of the medial meniscus.[361]

Anterior Drawer Test. The aforementioned Lachman test is a modification of the anterior drawer test, of which there are a number of variations, all of which involve positioning the patient supine.[265]

▶ *Anterior drawer test in 80 degrees of flexion without rotation.*[265] The clinician grasps the lower leg of the patient just distal to the joint space of the knee. The patient's knee is flexed 80 degrees, and the lower leg is not rotated. The clinician fixates the patient's leg by sitting on the foot. The clinician can place the thumbs either in the joint space or just distal to it to assess mobility. The clinician tests the tension in the musculature. It is important that all muscles

around the knee be relaxed to allow any translatory movement to occur. With both hands, the clinician now abruptly pulls the lower leg forward. This test is positive when an abnormal anterior movement of the tibia occurs compared with the other extremity.

▶ *Anterior drawer test in 80 degrees of flexion and maximal external rotation.*[265] The initial positions of the patient and clinician are the same as in the anterior drawer test in 80 degrees of flexion without rotation, except that the lower leg is positioned in maximum external rotation. For the performance, refer to the preceding description. The ACL and the medial and posteromedial capsuloligamentous structures are tested in this position. If this test is positive, there is likely to be an anteromedial rotatory instability. The specific medial and posteromedial structures that are affected can be further differentiated by the abduction (valgus) stress tests previously described.

▶ *Anterior drawer test in 80 degrees of flexion and 50 percent internal rotation.*[265] The initial positions of the patient and clinician are the same as in the anterior drawer test in 80 degrees of flexion without rotation, except that the lower leg is placed in 50 percent internal rotation. For the performance, refer to the description of that test. The ACL and the posterolateral capsuloligamentous structures are tested in this position. If the test is positive, there is likely to be an anterolateral rotatory instability. The adduction (varus) tests (one plane lateral instability) allow for further determination as to which of the lateral and posterolateral structures are affected.

▶ *Anterior drawer test in 80 degrees of flexion and maximal internal rotation.*[265] The initial positions of the patient and clinician are the same as in the anterior drawer test in 80 degrees of flexion without rotation, except that the lower leg is now maximally internally rotated. Performance of the test is the same as described earlier for that test. When in maximal internal rotation, the PCL can completely restrict anterior translation of the tibia. Thus, for this test to demonstrate excessive anterior translation, the PCL, ACL, and lateral or posterolateral capsuloligamentous structures have to be affected.

The anterior drawer test has been found to be 40.9 percent sensitive and 96.8 percent specific.[362] False-negatives may occur with this test for the same reasons as those in the Lachman test.

Comparison of the Lachman and Anterior Drawer Tests. The Lachman test has two advantages over the anterior drawer test in 90 degrees of knee flexion. First, all parts of the ACL are more or less equally taut. Second, in acute lesions it is often impossible to position the knee in 90 degrees flexion because of a hemarthrosis. In a study of patients with an ACL rupture, the Lachman test was positive in 80 percent of nonanesthetized patients and 100 percent of anesthetized patients. In comparison, the anterior drawer sign was positive in 9 percent of nonanesthetized patients and 52 percent of anesthetized patients.[368]

Jonsson and colleagues[369] compared both the Lachman and anterior drawer tests in 45 patients with an acute ACL injury and 62 patients with a chronic knee injury. Patients were tested while nonanesthetized and anesthetized, and the diagnosis was verified by arthroscopy. The Lachman test results for the acute injury group was 87 percent (conscious) and 100 percent (anesthetized). The anterior drawer test results were 33 percent and 98 percent, respectively. The chronic injury group scored a positive Lachman test by 97 percent (conscious) and 99 percent (anesthetized). The anterior drawer test was positive in 92 percent and 100 percent, respectively.

According to Larson,[370] the Lachman test proved to be the most sensitive test for an ACL rupture. However, this article lacked statistical data to verify this assertion. Another study[364] that compared the two tests reported a sensitivity of 99 percent for the Lachman test and a sensitivity of 70 percent for the anterior drawer sign.

One Plane Posterior Instability.   The PCL is very strong and is rarely completely torn. It is typically injured in a dashboard injury or in knee flexion activities (kneeling on the patella). Several tests have been advocated to test the integrity of the PCL.[265]

Gravity (Godfrey) Sign.   The patient is positioned supine, with the knee flexed to about 90 degrees. The clinician assesses the contour of the tibial tuberosities. If there is a rupture (partial) of the PCL, the tibial tuberosity on the involved side will be less visible than that on the noninvolved side (Fig. 18-25). This discrepancy is caused by an abnormal posterior translation, resulting from a rupture of the PCL. In cases of doubt, the patient can be asked to contract the hamstrings slightly by pushing the heels into the clinician's hands. This maneuver usually results in an increase in the posterior translation of the tibia and is often performed as a quick test of the integrity of the PCL.

Posterior Drawer Test.   The patient is positioned supine, with the knee flexed to 90 degrees. The clinician attempts a posterior displacement of the tibia on the femur (Fig. 18-26).

Rotary Instabilities.   Rotary or complex instabilities occur when the abnormal or pathologic movement is present in two or more planes. The ligamentous laxities present at the knee joint in these situations allow motion to take place around the sagittal, coronal, and horizontal axes.

Posterolateral Instability.   This type of instability is relatively rare, because it requires complete posterior cruciate laxity. It occurs when the lateral tibial plateau subluxes posteriorly on the femur, with the axis shifting posteriorly and medially to the medial joint area. With a hyperextension test, this posterior displacement is obvious and has been labeled the *external rotation recurvatum sign.*

Active Posterolateral Drawer Test.[371]   The patient sits with the foot on the floor in neutral rotation and the knee flexed to 80 to 90 degrees. The patient is asked to isometrically contract the hamstrings while the clinician stabilizes the foot. A positive result for the test is a posterior subluxation of the lateral tibial plateau.

Hughston's Posterolateral Drawer Test.[52,367]   The patient is positioned supine with the involved leg flexed at the hip to 45 degrees, the knee flexed to 80 to 90 degrees, and the lower leg in slight external rotation.[372] The clinician pushes the lower leg posteriorly. If the tibia rotates posteriorly during the test, the test is positive for posterolateral instability, indicating that the following structures may have been injured:

▶ PCL.

▶ Arcuate-popliteus complex.

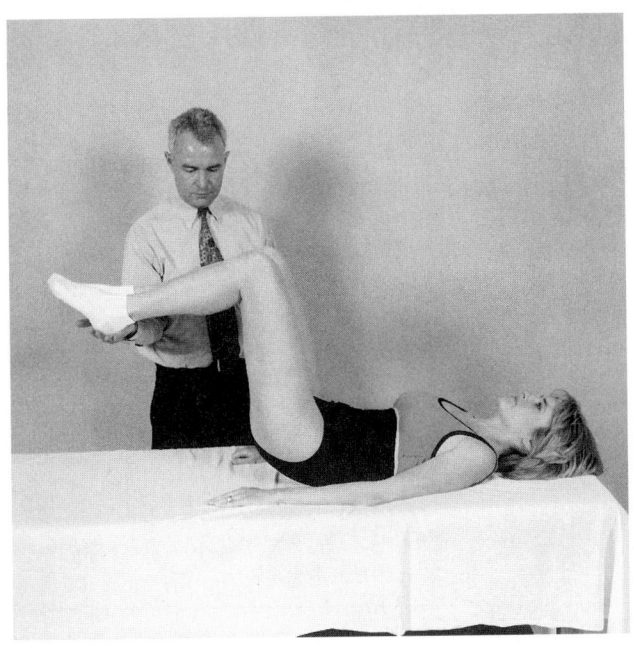

FIGURE 18-25   Godfrey sign.

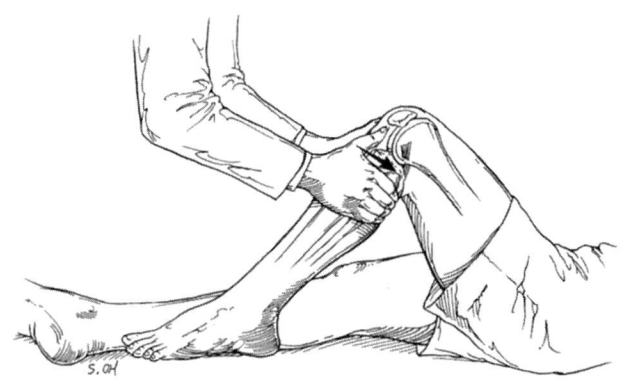

FIGURE 18-26   Posterior drawer test. (Reproduced with permission from Smith BW, Green GA. Acute knee injuries: Part I. History and physical examination. *Am Fam Phys* 1995;51:615–621.)

► LCL.

► Posterolateral capsule.

The one plane medial and lateral stability tests, described earlier, can be used to further differentiate which lateral and posterolateral structures are affected.

Hughston's External Rotational Recurvatum Test.[52,367] This test is used to detect an abnormal relationship between the femur and tibia in knee extension. The patient is positioned supine, with the legs straight, and the clinician stands at the foot of the table. The clinician gently grasps the great toes of both of the patient's feet at the same time, and lifts the feet from the table, while focusing on the tibial tuberosities of both legs. The patient must be completely relaxed. In the presence of a posterolateral rotary instability, the knee moves into relative hyperextension at the lateral side of the knee and the tibia externally rotates.[372]

Posteromedial Rotary Instability: Hughston's Posteromedial Drawer Test. The patient is positioned supine, with the involved leg flexed at the hip to 45 degrees, the knee flexed to 80 to 90 degrees, and the lower leg in slight internal rotation.[372] The clinician pushes the lower leg posteriorly. If the tibia rotates posteriorly during the test, the test is positive for posteromedial instability, indicating that the following structures may have been injured:

► PCL.

► Posterior oblique ligament.

► MCL.

► Posteromedial capsule.

► ACL.

The one plane medial and lateral stability tests, described earlier, can be used to further differentiate which medial and posteromedial structures are affected.

Anterolateral Rotary Instability. The pathology for this condition almost certainly involves the ACL and, clinically, the instability allows the medial tibial condyle to sublux posteriorly, because the axis of motion has moved to the lateral joint compartment.[148]

The diagnosis of anterolateral instability is based on the demonstration of a forward subluxation of the lateral tibial plateau as the knee approaches extension and the spontaneous reduction of the subluxation during flexion, in the lateral pivot shift test.[148] This form of instability usually occurs when the individual is either decelerating or changing direction, and the sudden shift of the lateral compartment is experienced as a "giving way" phenomenon, often associated with pain.[148]

Pivot-shift Test. This test was first described by Galway and colleagues[373] in 1972 and has been described since by a number of authors.[374–377]

The pivot shift is the anterior subluxation of the lateral tibial plateau that occurs when the lower leg is stabilized in (almost) full extension, whereby further flexion produces a palpable

springlike reduction.[378] The pivot shift is the most widely recognized dynamic instability of the knee, and it has been shown to correlate with reduced sports activity,[379] degeneration of the cartilage,[380,381] reinjury, meniscal damage,[382] joint arthritis,[382] and a history of instability symptoms.[383,384]

Because the majority of patients with an ACL rupture complain of a "giving way" sensation, the pivot-shift test is regarded in current literature as capable of identifying rotational instability.[374,375,377]

There are two main types of clinical tests to determine the presence of the pivot shift: the reduction test and the subluxation test.

► *Reduction test.* In this test, the knee is flexed from full extension under a valgus moment.[384] A sudden reduction of the anteriorly subluxed lateral tibial plateau is seen as the pivot shift.[373]

► *Subluxation test.* This test is effectively the reverse of the reduction test.[52] However, only 35 to 75 percent of patients whose knees pivot while the patient is under anesthesia will experience such a pivot when awake.[364,385–387] The test begins with patient's knees extended. The clinician internally rotates the patient's tibias with one hand and applies a valgus stress to the knee joint with the other hand (Fig. 18-27). As the clinician gradually flexes the patient's ACL-deficient

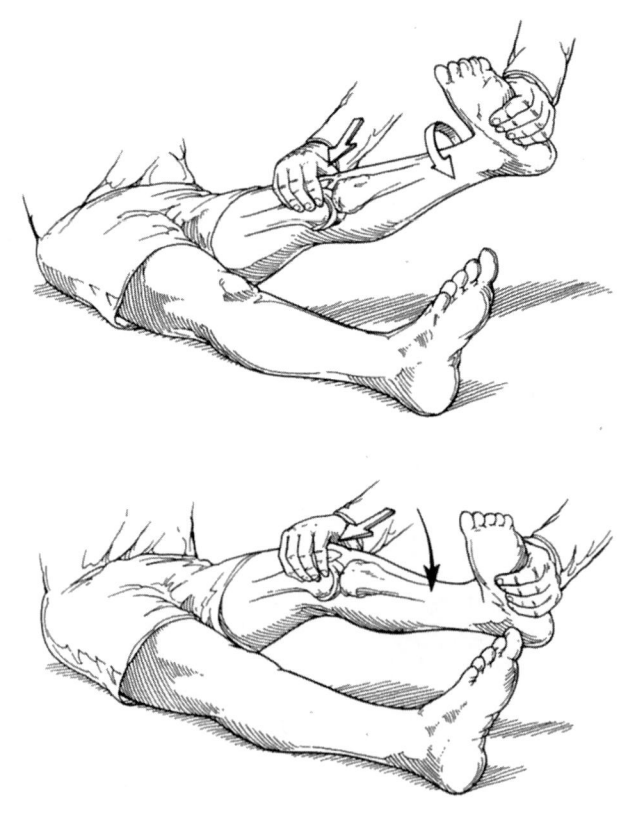

FIGURE 18-27 Pivot-shift test. (Reproduced with permission from Smith BW, Green GA. Acute knee injuries: Part I. History and physical examination. *Am Fam Phys* 1995;51:615–621.)

knee joint, the subluxated anterior tibia snaps back into normal alignment at 20 to 40 degrees of flexion.[374]

There is little agreement in the literature with regard to the sensitivity of the pivot-shift test, which varies between 0 and 98 percent.[364,368,388]

The pivot-shift test can be positive with an isolated ACL injury[364,389] or a tear or stretching of the lateral capsule,[376,390] although an injury to the MCL reduces the likelihood of a pivot shift even with ACL injury.[364,391]

MacIntosh (True Pivot-shift) Test. The MacIntosh test[392] is the most frequently used test to detect anterolateral instability, although Hughston,[52] Slocum, and Losee[390] have all described variations, with the latter author having received credit for describing the instability simultaneously, and independently, from MacIntosh.

The clinician picks up the patient's relaxed leg by grasping the ankle, and flexes the leg by placing the heel of the other hand over the lateral head of the gastrocnemius. The knee is then extended, and a slight valgus stress is applied to its lateral aspect to support the tibia. Under the influence of gravity, the femur falls backward and, as the knee approaches extension, the tibial plateau subluxes forward. This subluxation can be accentuated by internally rotating the tibia gently with the hand that is cradling the foot and ankle. At this point, a strong valgus force is placed on the knee by the upper hand, thereby impinging the subluxed tibial plateau against the lateral femoral condyle by jamming the two joint surfaces together. This position prevents easy reduction, because the tibia is then flexed on the femur. At approximately 30 to 40 degrees of flexion, the displaced tibial plateau suddenly reduces, often in a dramatic fashion.

Anteromedial Instability. Patients who demonstrate excessive anteromedial tibial condylar displacement during the anterior drawer test are exhibiting anteromedial instability, because the axis of motion has moved to the lateral joint compartment.[148] The pathology involves the ACL, MCL, and posterior medial capsule, which, along with its reinforcing fibers, is termed the posterior oblique ligament.[148]

Slocum Test. The Slocum test consists of two parts designed to assess for rotary and anterior instabilities.[393] The patient is positioned supine, with the knee flexed to 80 to 90 degrees and the hip flexed to 45 degrees.

For the first part of the test, the foot of the involved leg is first placed in 30 degrees of internal rotation. Excessive internal rotation results in a tightening of the remaining structures and can lead to a false-negative result. The clinician sits on the foot to maintain its position, and pulls the tibia forward (Fig. 18-28). A positive test results from movement occurring primarily on the lateral side of the knee and indicates a lesion to one or more of the following structures:

▶ ACL.

▶ Posterolateral capsule.

▶ Arcuate-popliteus complex.

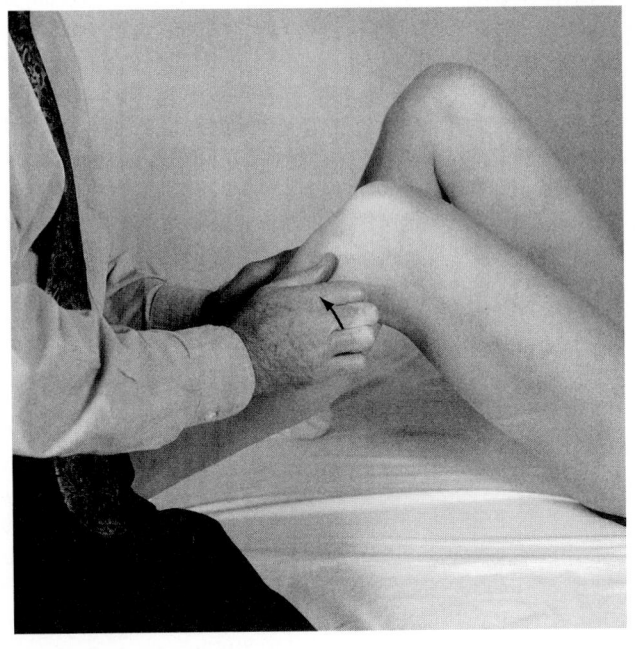

FIGURE 18-28 Slocum test.

▶ LCL.

▶ PCL.

If this initial test is positive, the second part of the test, which assesses anteromedial rotary instability, is less reliable.[394]

The second part of the test is similar to the first, except that the patient's foot is placed in about 15 degrees of external rotation. Again, by placing the foot in too much external rotation, the clinician runs the risk of a false-negative result during testing. Movement occurring primarily on the medial side of the knee during testing is a positive result and indicates a lesion to one or more of the following structures:

▶ MCL.

▶ Posterior oblique ligament.

▶ Posteromedial capsule.

▶ ACL.

Patellar Stability Tests

Patellar stability is assessed by gently pushing the patella medially and laterally while the knee is in a position of 90 degrees of flexion. This position is used because it places all of the retinacula on stretch. If this test is positive for laxity, further testing is performed by applying medial and lateral patellar glides, tilts, and rotations, with the knee in relaxed extension, and noting any limitations of motion or excessive excursion.[257]

▶ *Glide.* The glide component determines the amount of lateral deviation of the patella in the frontal plane. A 5-mm lateral displacement of the patella causes a 50 percent decrease in VMO tension.[395] In the normal knee when fully extended and relaxed, the patella can be passively displaced medially and laterally approximately 1 cm in each direction, or approximately one third of the width of the patella.[173] Displacement of more than half the patella over the medial or lateral aspect is considered abnormal.[9] If the patient is apprehensive as the glide maneuver is being performed, the problem is likely to be one of poor patellar engagement. A decreased medial glide of the patella has been found to be related to iliotibial band and/or lateral retinaculum tightness.[396]

▶ **Tilt.** The degree of patellar tilt is assessed by comparing the height of the medial patellar border with the height of the lateral border, which helps to determine the degree of tightness in the deep retinacular fibers. A slight lateral tilt of patella is normal. An increased medial tilt results from a tight lateral retinaculum. If the passive lateral structures are too tight, the patella will tilt so that the medial border is higher than the lateral border (lateral tilt), making the posterior edge of the lateral border difficult to palpate.[257] A posterior tilt results in fat pad irritation.

▶ **Rotation.** The rotation component determines whether there is any deviation of the long axis of the patella from the long axis of the femur. If the inferior pole is sitting lateral to the long axis of the femur, the patient has an externally rotated patella, whereas if the inferior pole is sitting medial to the long axis, the patient has an internally rotated patella.

If the patient has one or more of these components present, the clinician needs to determine which of them if any is abnormal.

Meniscal Lesion Tests

Modified McMurray's Test.[265] The McMurray test was originally developed to diagnose posterior horn lesions of the medial meniscus. By modifying this test, it is possible to diagnose other meniscal lesions as well.

The patient is positioned supine, and the clinician maximally flexes the hip and knee. This is accomplished by grasping the patient's foot in such a way that the thumb is lateral, the index and middle fingers are medial, and the ring and little fingers hold the medial edge of the foot (Fig. 18-29). The thumb of one hand is placed against the lateral aspect of the patient's knee (see Fig. 18-29). By rotating the patient's lower leg several

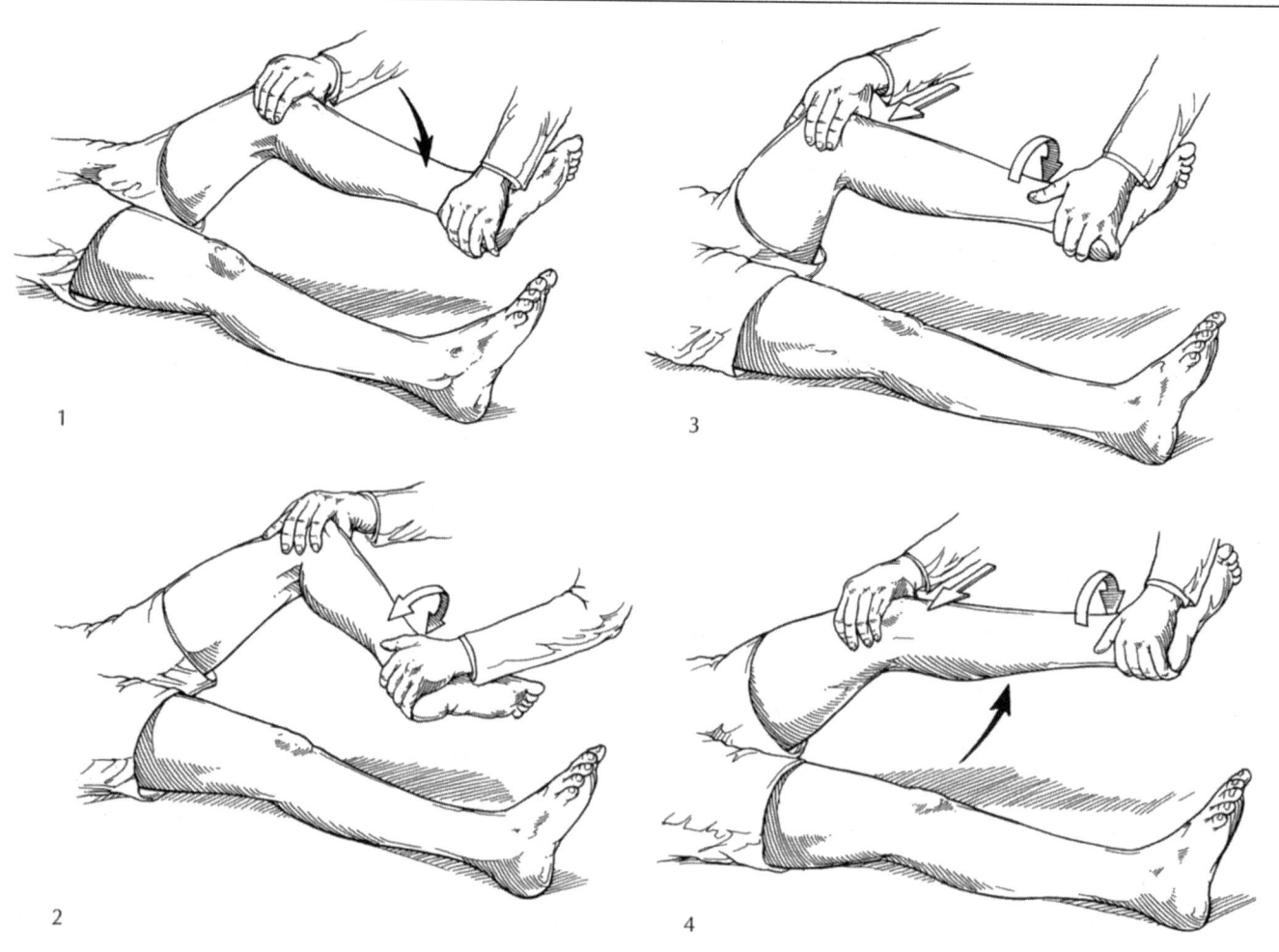

FIGURE 18-29 McMurray's test. (Reproduced with permission from Smith BW, Green GA. Acute knee injuries: Part I. History and physical examination. *Am Fam Phys* 1995;51:615–621.)

times, the clinician can assess whether the patient is fully relaxed. While the lower leg is slightly externally rotated, the clinician's ipsilateral hand moves the patient's foot in a varus direction. The knee is flexed as far as is comfortable, after which the foot is brought into a valgus direction with simultaneous internal rotation of the lower leg. The clinician then gently extends the knee to about 120 degrees, and at the same time exerts valgus pressure on the knee with the hand. This test is positive when a palpable click, or audible thump, is elicited that is also painful. It is thought that pain with passive external rotation implicates lesions of the posterior horn of the lateral meniscus, whereas pain with passive internal rotation implicates lesions of the posterior horn of the medial meniscus; however, false-positives are common.

When the test is positive, the lesion can be located in the posterior horn, or elsewhere in the medial meniscus. A lesion of the lateral meniscus also may provoke pain during this test.

If the test is negative, a meniscal lesion may still be present. One after another, similar maneuvers can be repeated, first with valgus pressure and external rotation, then with varus pressure and external rotation, and finally with varus pressure and internal rotation.

Apley's Test.[397] The patient is placed in the prone position, with the knee flexed to 90 degrees. The patient's thigh is stabilized by the clinician's knee. The clinician applies internal and external rotation with compression to the lower leg, noting any pain and the quality of motion (Fig. 18-30). Pain with this maneuver may indicate a meniscal lesion.

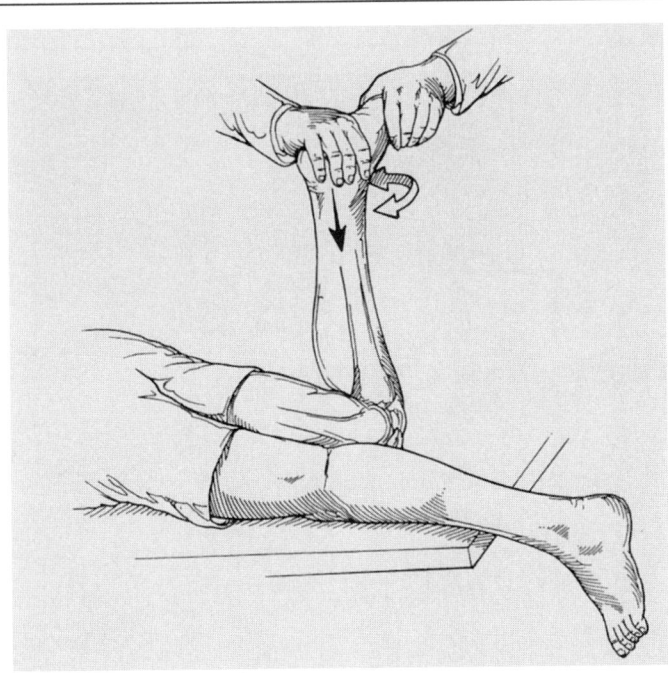

FIGURE 18-30 Apley's test. (Reproduced with permission from Smith BW, Green GA. Acute knee injuries: Part I. History and physical examination. *Am Fam Phys* 1995;51:615–621.)

Steinmann's Tenderness Displacement Test.[265] Steinmann's test can be used to diagnose meniscal lesions. The patient is positioned supine, while the clinician stands to the side. Using one hand, the clinician grasps the patient's lower leg just proximal to the malleolus. The other hand grasps the lateral side of the patient's lower leg as proximal to the knee as possible, while also palpating the medial joint space with the thumb. The knee is extended, and the joint line between the patellar tendon and the MCL is palpated. After the painful site is located with the thumb, pressure against this site is maintained while the knee is flexed. After several degrees of motion, the pain disappears, and the painful site can sometimes again be palpated more posteriorly in the joint space. If the most painful site is found in the joint space at the level of the MCL, the test is less reliable, because both the medial meniscus and the ligament move posteriorly during flexion.

Anderson Mediolateral Grind Test. The Anderson mediolateral grind test[398] can be used to detect meniscal lesions. The patient is positioned supine, and the clinician grasps the uninvolved leg between the trunk and arm. The clinician places the index finger and thumb of the other hand over the anterior knee joint line. With the patient's knee flexed at 45 degrees, a valgus stress is applied as the knee is simultaneously slightly flexed, followed by a varus component while the knee is extended, producing a circular motion of the knee. The maneuver is repeated, increasing the valgus and varus stresses with each rotation.

In one study that examined 100 knees with the Anderson mediolateral grind test, as well as arthroscopically, the test was found to have an accuracy of 68 percent.[398]

O'Donahue's Test. The patient is positioned supine, with the knee flexed to 90 degrees. The clinician stabilizes the thigh and rotates the tibia medially and laterally twice, and then fully flexes and rotates the tibia both ways again. Pain in either or both of the positions is a positive sign for capsular irritation or a meniscal tear.

Special Tests
Plical Irritation. Plical irritation has a characteristic pattern of presentation. The anterior pain in the knee is episodic and associated with painful clicking, "giving way," and the feeling of something catching in the knee. Careful palpation of the patellar retinaculum and fat pad, with the knee extended and then flexed, can be used to detect tender plicae, and to differentiate tenderness within the fat pad from tenderness over the anterior horn of the menisci.

▶ *Patellar bowstring test.* This test can also be used to detect plical irritation. The patient lies on his or her side, with the tested side uppermost. Using the heel of the cranial hand, the clinician pushes the patella medially and maintains it there. While the patella is maintained in this position, the clinician flexes the patient's knee and internally rotates the tibia with the other hand. The knee is then extended from the flexed position while the clinician palpates for any clunks.

▶ *Medial shift at about 30 degrees of knee flexion (Mital-Hayden test).*   The patient is supine on the bed, with the knee supported in about 30 degrees of flexion by either a towel roll or the clinician's thigh, which rests on the table. The clinician places both thumbs together at the lateral aspect of the patella and pushes the patella medially. If a painful click is elicited during this test, there is likely to be a symptomatic mediopatellar synovial plica.

Suprapatellar or Infrapatellar Tendonitis.   The patient is positioned supine, with the lower extremity extended.

▶ *Infrapatellar test.*   The clinician pushes down on the suprapatellar aspect, palpates under the inferior pole of the patella, and checks for tenderness, which may indicate infrapatellar tendonitis.

▶ *Suprapatellar test.*   The clinician pushes on the infrapatellar aspect of the patella, palpates under the superior pole of the patella, and checks for tenderness, which may indicate suprapatellar tendonitis.

Integrity of Patellofemoral Articulating Surfaces.   These tests involve the application of manual compression to the patella in an attempt to elicit pain.

The McConnell Test.   This test involves manual compression to the patella with the palm of the hand at various angles of knee flexion to compress the articulating facets.[257] Although the findings have little bearing on the overall intervention, they can guide the clinician as to which knee flexion angles to avoid during exercise.

Zohler's Test.   The patient is supine on the bed, with the knee extended and resting on the table. The clinician pushes the patient's patella in a distal direction. While continuing to exert pressure in a distal direction, the clinician instructs the patient to contract the quadriceps muscle. If this test is painful, there is likely to be a symptomatic patellar chondromalacia, although this test may be positive in a large proportion of asymptomatic individuals.

Clarke's Test.   This test is similar to Zohler's test, except that the clinician applies an increasing compressive force to the base of the patella while the patient actively contracts the quadriceps. Like Zohler's test, this test may be positive in a large proportion of asymptomatic individuals.

Waldron Test.   Refer to Patella Motion Tests.

Patellar Mobility and Retinaculum Tests.   Patellar glides can be used to examine retinacular mobility. The patella should be able to translate at least 33 percent of its width both medially and laterally. Inability to do this indicates tightness of the retinacula. Hypermobility of the patella is demonstrated if the patella can be translated 100 percent of its width medially or laterally.

The lateral retinaculum is assessed by way of a patellar tilt and a mediolateral displacement (glide).[175,399–401] A number of patient positions can be used to assess the flexibility of the retinacular tissue.

▶ *Medial shift.*[265]   The patient is supine, with the knee extended. The clinician places both thumbs together at the lateral aspect of the patella and pushes the patella medially (Fig. 18-31). The amount of motion and the end-feel are assessed. Often the patella is found to have less range of motion medially than laterally. Whether this condition is pathologic is best determined by comparison to the noninvolved side. This patellar movement often is limited after surgery and after immobilization.

▶ *Lateral shift.*   The patient is supine, with the knee extended. The clinician places the fingertips of both hands against the medial aspect of the patella and pushes the patella laterally (Fig. 18-31). The amount of motion and the end-feel are assessed. Usually the patella has more range of motion laterally than medially. When there are instabilities of the patella, the lateral mobility is usually abnormally increased. This patellar movement often is limited after surgery and after immobilization.

▶ *Distal shift.*   The patient is supine, with the knee extended. With the thenar and hypothenar eminences placed against the base of the patient's patella, the clinician pushes the patella in a distal direction. As with the previous two shift tests, the amount of motion and end-feel are assessed. The motion usually is limited in instances of patella alta (a high position of the patella), after surgery, and after immobilization.

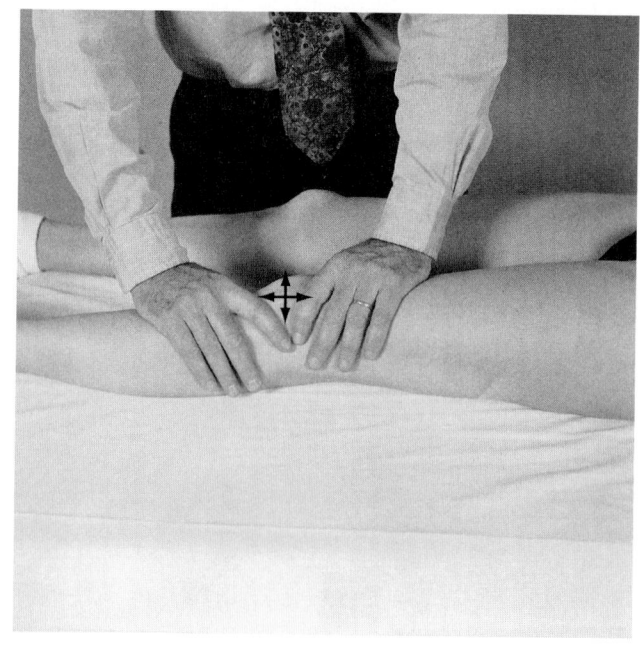

FIGURE 18-31   Patellar mobility testing.

▶ *Prone technique.* The clinician passively flexes the patient's knee to 90 degrees and internally rotates the tibia. The lower extremity is then moved into hip adduction. The test is positive for tightness of the lateral structures if the hip cannot be fully adducted. This test also can be performed in the side-lying position, with the involved side uppermost.

▶ *Lateral tilt of the patella.* The patient is positioned supine, with the knee extended and relaxed. The clinician attempts to lift the lateral border of the patella. An inability to lift the lateral border of the patella above the horizontal plane is an indication of tightness of the lateral retinaculum.

▶ *Side-lying technique.*[257] With the knee of the uppermost leg flexed to 20 degrees, the patella is moved in a medial direction toward the treatment table. The clinician should be able to expose the lateral femoral condyle, unless the tissues of the superficial lateral retinacula are tight. To test the deep fibers, the clinician places a hand on the middle of the patella, takes up the slack of the glide, and applies an anteroposterior pressure on the medial border of the patella. The lateral femoral condyle should move freely away from the femur. This test also can be used as an intervention technique.[257]

Fairbank's Apprehension Test for Patellar Instability. The Fairbank test[402] is best performed with the patient supine and the patient's leg supported at approximately 30 degrees of knee flexion. The clinician applies a laterally directed force to the medial aspect of the patella, attempting to sublux it laterally while applying a small amount of passive flexion to the knee.[191]

Wilson Test for Osteochondritis Dissecans. The following accessory test can be performed when osteochondritis dissecans of the knee is suspected. The patient is supine. The clinician flexes the patient's hip and knee to 90 degrees. Axial compression is exerted at the knee by pushing proximally, in line with the tibia, with the distal hand. The lower leg is held in internal rotation as the knee is slowly extended, maintaining the axial compression. In many cases of osteochondritis dissecans, the patient experiences pain because the pressure on the medial cartilaginous surfaces is increased significantly with this maneuver.

Hamstring Flexibility. The popliteal angle is the most popular method reported in the literature for assessing hamstring tightness, especially in the presence of a knee flexion contracture.[403] The patient is positioned supine, and the opposite hip is extended. The popliteal angle is determined by measuring the angle that the tibia subtends with the extended line of the femur when the ipsilateral hip is flexed to 90 degrees and the knee of the limb under examination is maximally passively extended to initial tissue resistance.[404] The popliteal angle is at the maximum of 180 degrees from birth to age 2 years.[403] This angle then decreases to an average of 155 degrees by age 6 years and remains steady thereafter.[403] An angle less than 125 degrees suggests significant hamstring tightness.[403]

Hamstring flexibility also can be assessed with a passive straight leg raise, while ensuring that the lumbar spine is flattened on the treatment table and the pelvis is stabilized. However, this method may be used only if there is full extension at the knee of the leg being examined. Normal hamstring length should allow 80 to 85 degrees of hip flexion when the knee is extended and the lumbar spine is flattened.[257]

Iliotibial Band Flexibility. The cardinal sign of iliotibial contracture is the presence in a supine patient of an abduction contracture when the hip and knee are extended, which is eliminated when the hip and knee are flexed.[405] Other tests include the following.

Retinacula Test. The patient is placed in the side-lying position, and the knee is fully flexed. This position tightens the iliotibial band. The clinician applies a medial and oblique force to the patella with the thumbs. Approximately 0.5 to 1 cm of patella motion should be available.

Ober's Test. The Ober test for iliotibial band length is described in Chapter 17.

Prone Lying Test. This relatively new test can be used to estimate the degree of contracture of the iliotibial band.[405] The patient is positioned prone on a flat surface. The clinician stands on the side opposite to the leg being tested. With one hand, the clinician grasps the ankle of the involved leg, placing it in maximum abduction at the hip, as the other hand applies pressure to the buttock of the involved leg to flatten the pelvis and correct any flexion deformity at the hip. The hip is maintained in neutral rotation, with the knee flexed at 90 degrees. The hip is then gradually adducted until a firm end-feel is reached. The angle of abduction of the thigh relative to the vertical axis of the body is measured, and compared with the measurement of the other side.[405]

Tests for Iliotibial Tendonitis. Iliotibial band tendonitis may be classified into four grades, based on pain and activity limitation[406]:

▶ *Grade I.* Pain beginning after activity that neither restricts distance nor speed of athletic activity.

▶ *Grade II.* Pain beginning during activity that neither restricts distance or speed.

▶ *Grade III.* Pain beginning during activity that may restrict either distance or speed.

▶ *Grade IV.* Pain so severe as to preclude athletic participation.

Renne's Test.[153] The patient stands on the affected leg and flexes the knee to 30 to 40 degrees. A positive test is indicated when a palpable "creak" is produced as the maneuver brings the iliotibial band into tight contact with the lateral femoral condyle.

Noble's Compression Test.[407]   The patient is positioned supine, with the affected knee flexed to 90 degrees. Pressure is applied over the proximal, prominent part of the lateral femoral condyle as the knee is gradually extended. A positive test is indicated when pain is reproduced at 30 to 40 degrees.

Creak Test.   The patient stands on the involved leg. As the patient flexes the knee to approximately 30 degrees, a "creak" will occur over the lateral femoral condyle.[408]

Quadriceps Flexibility.   Quadriceps flexibility is examined by placing the patient prone and passively flexing the knee, bringing the heel toward the buttocks. The lumbar spine is monitored and stabilized if necessary to prevent motion. The heel should touch the buttocks. An adaptively shortened rectus femoris is usually the structure that prevents this motion (see later discussion).

Intervention Strategies

Acute knee injuries are a common occurrence. One study[409] demonstrated, perhaps not surprisingly, that the most common type of acute knee injuries were sports related, occurred in men younger than 35 years of age, and were of moderate severity. Studies[409-411] that compare the two sexes, report higher rates of sports injuries in men. This finding could be a result of the greater numbers of men participating in sports activities, or the greater frequency of injuries in men who do participate in sports.

Of particular interest are non–sports-related falls, which are experienced two to three times more frequently in women than in men, except in the group older than 55 years, for whom the incidence of falls is equal in both sexes.[409]

Most knee pain of nontraumatic origin diminishes with conservative intervention.[412] Different approaches have been emphasized over the years, including patient education,[413-415] modification of activity,[136,414,416,417] progressive muscle stretching and strengthening (particularly the vastus medialis for the patellofemoral joint),[125,136,413,415-420] functional lower extremity training,[421] external patellar supports and braces,[136,413,415,422,423] foot orthotics,[423,424] and taping to improve patella tracking.[413,416,419,425,426]

This wide range of interventions raises the question of whether any of them are efficacious, or whether a combination of some is to be recommended. What is clear is that the impairments and functional limitations found during the examination must guide the intervention. The successful intervention requires detailing the factors that influence these impairments and functional limitations, and determining the stage of healing.

Whatever the cause of the knee injury, the goal of the rehabilitation program is to return the patient to the optimum level of function. Emphasis during knee rehabilitation must focus on achieving a balance between permitting the healing of damaged structures improving the strength of the controlling musculature, and increasing the efficiency of the static restraints. In addition, consideration must be given to the various forces placed on the knee during closed and open-chain exercises, so that the healing process is allowed to proceed.

The techniques to increase joint mobility and the techniques to increase soft tissue extensibility are described under "Therapeutic Techniques," later.

Acute Phase

Every attempt is made to protect the joint to promote and progress the healing. The goals during the acute phase are to:

► Reduce pain and swelling.

► Control inflammation.

► Regain range of motion.

► Minimize muscle atrophy and weakness.

► Attain early neuromuscular control.

► Maintain or improve the patient's general fitness.

The reduction of pain and the control of swelling are extremely important. Pain and swelling can both inhibit normal muscle function and control. Pain, swelling, and inflammation are minimized by using the principles of PRICEMEM (protection, rest, ice, compression, elevation, manual therapy, early motion, and medication). Icing for 20 to 30 minutes, three to four times a day, concurrent with NSAIDs or aspirin, can aid in reducing pain and swelling.

Once the pain, swelling, and inflammation are under control, early controlled range-of-motion exercises are initiated. In the acute phase of healing, the interventions focus on decreased loading of the joint complex, which might include postural correction, activity modification, or the use of an assistive device. Bracing may be needed to provide adequate protection (see the discussion under "Functional Phase," later). Exercises prescribed for the knee joint complex must include those that promote neuromuscular control, timing, balance, and proprioception.

Exercises recommended for this phase include isometric muscle setting (quadriceps sets, hamstring sets, gluteal sets), active knee flexion (heel slides), straight leg raises (if appropriate) (Fig. 18-32), and patellar mobilizations (see Fig. 18-31). Proprioceptive neuromuscular facilitation (PNF) activities may be initiated with slow-speed, low-force, controlled exercises. Electrical stimulation can be used to facilitate muscle activity and to promote muscle reeducation.[427] The training of the vastus medialis obliquus (VMO) should be regarded as a motor skill acquisition rather than a strengthening procedure,[139,428] with the goal of the training to produce a modification of the length-tension relationship between the VMO, and its antagonist, the vastus lateralis (VL). This may result in a change of the equilibrium point, which will enable the appropriate alignment of the patella.[429] If the muscle control of the VMO is poor, biofeedback can be used to augment the hip adductor training.[430] Taping can be used as an adjunct (see later discussion).

Once the muscle control is achieved, gentle closed-chain exercises are initiated. Contractions of the quadriceps should be

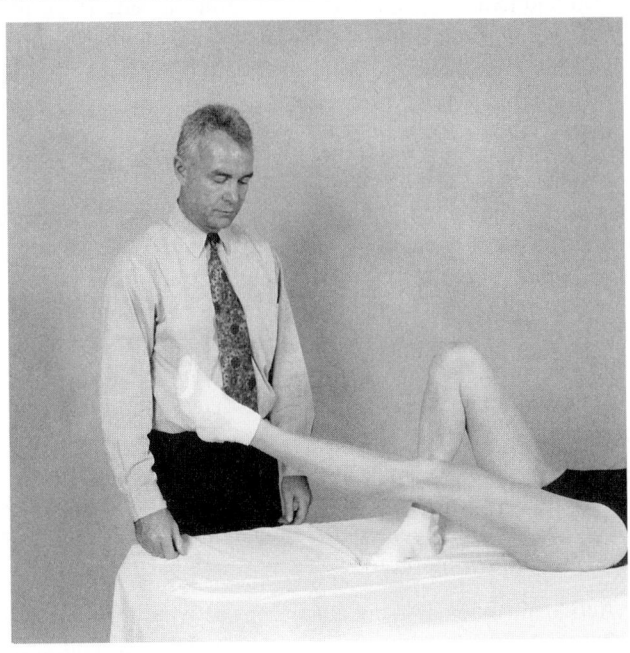

FIGURE 18-32 Straight leg raise.

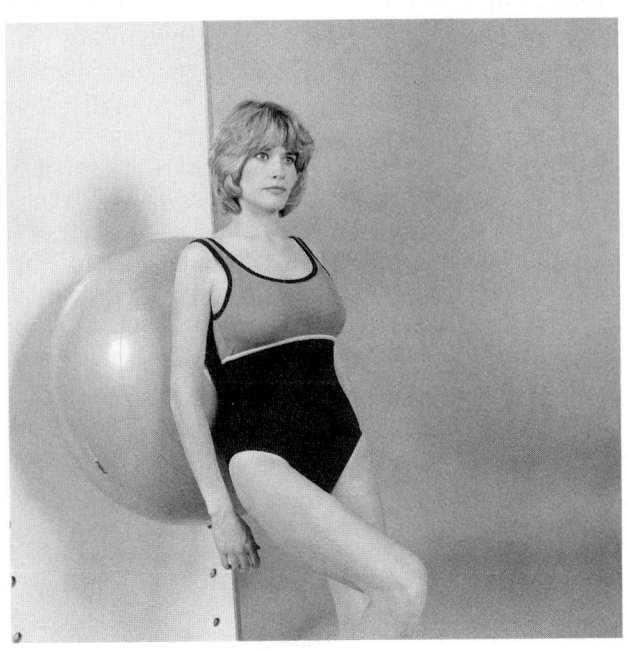

FIGURE 18-33 Wall slide with Swiss ball.

encouraged in the functional knee positions that provoke pain, such as sitting, and stair negotiation. The benefit of closed kinetic chain exercises (CKCEs) is that they decrease shear forces and emphasize co-contractions.[431,432] General recommendations for closed-chain exercise at the knee (e.g., mini-squats, step-ups, leg press) are from 0 to 20 degrees,[433] or 0 to 40 degrees of flexion.[227] All of the exercises performed in the clinic should be performed by the patient at home whenever possible.

Tibiofemoral Joint

Closed-chain exercises should be initiated as tolerated.[224] Closed-chain exercises initially include wall slides and heel raises. These exercises are progressed to include the leg press, the hip sled, and the squat.[434] The exercises are performed bilaterally initially and then unilaterally once there is evidence of good dynamic stability.

Co-contraction exercises for the hamstrings and quadriceps, which further reduce tibiofemoral shear forces,[236,237,296,435,436] can be achieved by having the patient perform single leg bridges by leaning back on a Swiss ball (see Chap. 25) and raising the uninvolved leg off the floor, while the involved leg is used to maintain balance. Co-contraction also can be accomplished by single-leg wall slides using the Swiss ball (Fig. 18-33), with the involved leg supporting the body weight.

Stationary bicycling has long been recognized as a useful therapeutic exercise for knee rehabilitation to control the range of motion and impact forces at the knee.

▶ The range of motion at the knee can be controlled by adjusting the seat height.

▶ The impact forces can be adjusted on most exercise bicycles by varying the resistance at the pedal-foot interface.

The amount of strain on the ACL during stationary bicycling is relatively low compared with other rehabilitation activities[437] (see Table 18-3).

Patellofemoral Joint

Exercises for the patellofemoral joint initially include range-of-motion exercises performed in the pain-free ranges. These exercises are usually performed in the non–weight-bearing position. Strengthening exercises are initiated when there is minimal swelling, pain, and inflammation. During the early stages of healing, the patient must be warned against jumping, squatting, prolonged sitting with the knee flexed beyond 40 degrees, prolonged kneeling, prone lying, or standing in genu recurvatum.[9,136] In the presence of biomechanical dysfunctions of the foot, including pronation, correct footwear must be worn. If the malalignment of the lower extremity is severe, a foot orthosis can be prescribed.[422,429] The type of orthosis used is dependent on the diagnosis. Most commonly, an orthosis is used to correct a flat foot so that the patella no longer squints. Foot pronation imparts internal torsion to the tibia and a valgus moment at the knee. Klingman and colleagues[438] have shown that medial rearfoot-posted orthoses result in a more medial position of the patella during static weight-bearing radiographs. In the presence of genu recurvatum, a heel raise can be issued for use during exercise. It is therefore reasonable, for selected patients, to prescribe an orthotic device for the shoe.[174,439]

It remains unclear to what extent there are specific exercises to strengthen the VMO.[11,135,440] Wilk and colleagues[297] believe that a focus on strengthening of the VMO should only occur if the fibers of the VMO attach onto the patella in a position that can prevent lateralization of the patella dynamically (50 to 55 degrees). The VMO does not extend the knee and is not, therefore, activated by traditional straight leg raises,[441] even with the addition of adduction.[442] However, because of the relationship of the VMO to the adductor magnus, and its separate nerve supply in most cases,[126] the clinician should still emphasize adduction of the thigh, while minimizing internal rotation of the hip, to facilitate a VMO contraction.[430] According to Hodges and Richardson,[443] activation of the adductor magnus significantly improves the VMO contraction in weight-bearing, but maximum contraction of adductor magnus in non–weight-bearing is required before facilitating VMO activity.

Exercises during this phase include:

▶ Isometric quadriceps sets at 20 degrees of flexion, progressing to multiple angle isometrics.

▶ Heel slides with the tibia positioned in internal and then external rotation.

▶ Straight leg raises performed with the thigh externally rotated and the knee flexed to 20 degrees. Performing the exercise in this fashion is reported to allow the least amount of patellofemoral contact force while maximally stressing the vastus medialis component of the quadriceps muscle.[200,225,444] The resistance is progressed from 0 to 5 lb.

▶ Low-resistance terminal knee extension (short-arc quadriceps) exercises performed with the leg externally rotated from 50 to 20 degrees (Fig. 18-34). The resistance is progressed from 0 to 5 lb.

▶ Hip adduction exercises performed in the side-lying position on the involved side, with the hip internally rotated and the knee flexed to 20 degrees[129,445] (Fig. 18-35). This position of knee flexion places the patella midway between the two femoral condyles.

In addition to the hip adductors, attention must also be paid to the ability of the other hip joint muscles to control the forces applied to the patellofemoral joint. For example, weakness of the hip external rotators, may allow uncontrolled and excessive pronation of the foot to occur along with excessive femoral internal rotation, both contributing to an increase in the valgus alignment of the knee, thereby increasing the Q angle.[155] Strengthening of the hip rotators may need to be initiated in the open kinetic chain, but should be advanced to strengthening in the closed kinetic chain as soon as functional muscular control is present.[155]

Functional exercises that incorporate the entire lower kinetic chain are implemented as soon as tolerated. Kibler[220] advocates the following protocol:

▶ Active hip extension and quadriceps activation with the foot flat on the floor or stepping on or off a flat step. This reactivates the normal sequencing pattern for the entire leg.

▶ Isolation and maximal activation of the quadriceps in a closed-chain position by working with the foot on a slant board, effectively removing the hip and ankle from full activation, but placing maximal load on the slightly flexed knee. Care must be taken not to exercise through pain, as this may indicates that muscle control is insufficient.[139]

▶ Unilateral stance with hip extension, slight knee flexion, and hip and trunk rotation.

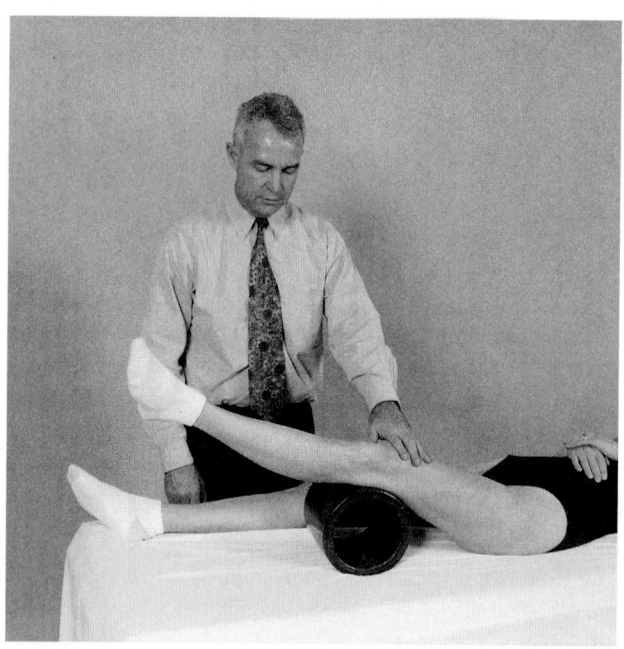

FIGURE 18-34 Short arc quadriceps exercise in external rotation.

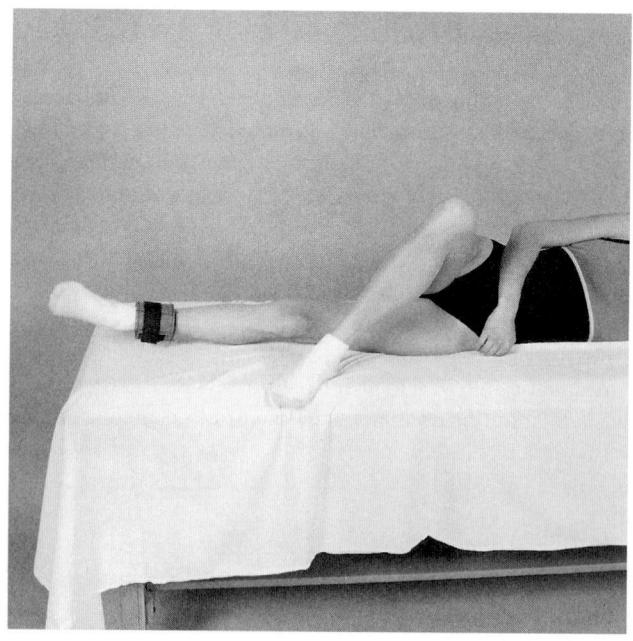

FIGURE 18-35 Straight leg raise in side lying into adduction.

The correction of muscle inflexibilities is very important in the rehabilitative process. Stretching of the hip flexors, iliotibial band, lateral retinaculum, hamstrings, and gastrocnemius are usually initiated during this phase. The rationale for stretching the iliotibial band and lateral retinaculum is well recognized.[119,413,446] Adaptive shortening in the hamstrings and gastrocnemii has been associated with a compensatory pronation.[298] In addition, adaptively shortened hamstrings may cause increased flexion of the knee and increased patellofemoral compression forces, especially during the stance phase of gait.[288] Correction of muscle imbalances is based on a full analysis as to the effect that these interventions will have on the pathologic process, or on other structures within the kinetic chain. For example, stretching the hamstrings of an elderly patient to relieve the stresses at the knee may exacerbate the symptoms of lateral recess stenosis, because the adaptively shortened hamstrings may be helping to maintain the pelvis in a posterior pelvic tilt.[447]

Functional Phase

Patients progress to this phase when terminal knee extension exercises can be done with 25- to 30-lb weights.[9] The functional phase of the knee rehabilitation program addresses any tissue overload problems and functional biomechanical deficits. Among the goals for this phase are to:

▶ Attain full range of pain-free motion.

▶ Restore normal joint kinematics.

▶ Improve muscle strength.

▶ Improve neuromuscular control.

▶ Restore normal muscle force-couple relationships.

Range-of-motion exercises during this phase include flexion and extension exercises; stationary cycling, progressing to moderate resistance; and supine and wall slides (see Fig. 18-33). The stationary bike exercises are initially performed with a high seat (providing about 15 degrees of knee flexion in the extended leg).

There is controversy about whether knee exercises should be performed in an open-chain or closed-chain manner.[227] CKCEs, such as the squat, leg press, dead lift, and power-clean, have long been used as core exercises by athletes to enhance performance in sport.[448,449] These multijoint exercises develop the largest and most powerful muscles of the body and have biomechanical and neuromuscular similarities to many athletic movements, such as running and jumping.[228] Open kinetic chain exercises (OKCEs) appear to be less functional in terms of many athletic movements and primarily serve a supportive role in strength and conditioning programs. However, it is advised that a combination of the open-chain and closed-chain exercises be used.

Closed-chain Exercises

CKCEs during this phase include a progression of those exercises introduced during the acute phase. In addition, other exercises are introduced. These include one quarter step-ups and step-downs, single knee dips and squats,[413] the seated leg press, front and side lunges (Fig. 18-36), plyometric exercises (Fig. 18-37), slide board exercises (Fig. 18-38), weight-bearing resisted walking with leg pulls in all four planes (flexion, extension, abduction, and adduction) using elastic tubing (Figs. 18-39

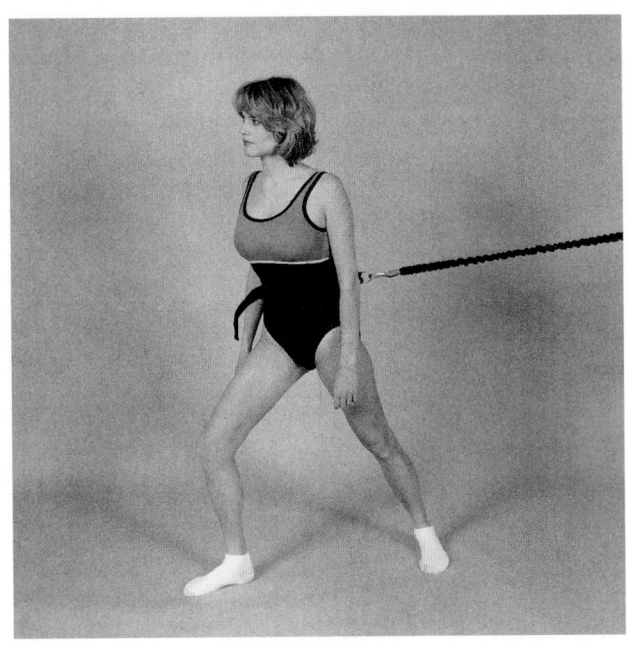

FIGURE 18-36   Resisted side lunges.

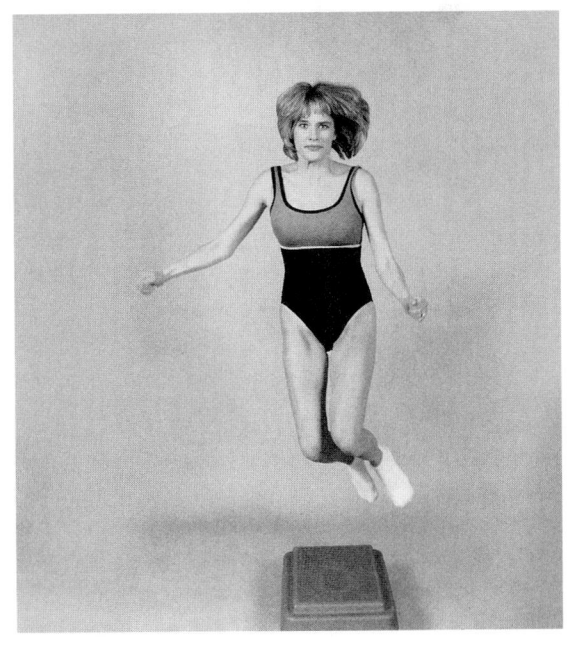

FIGURE 18-37   Plyometric exercise.

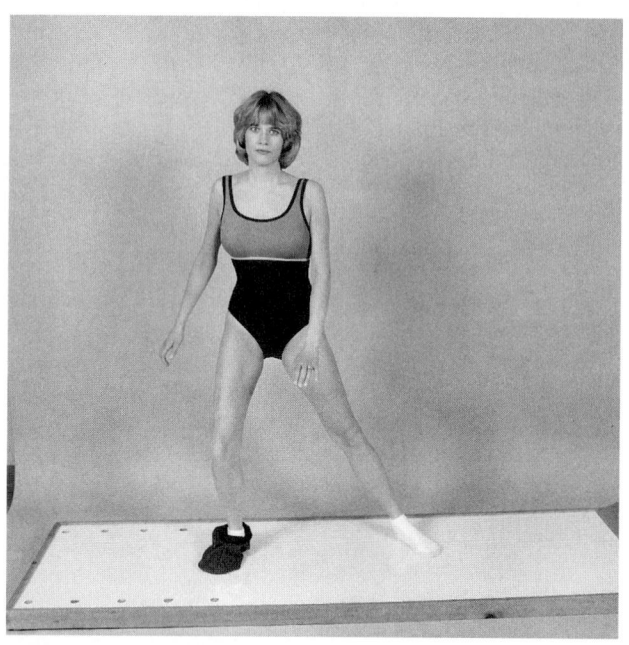

FIGURE 18-38   Slide board exercises.

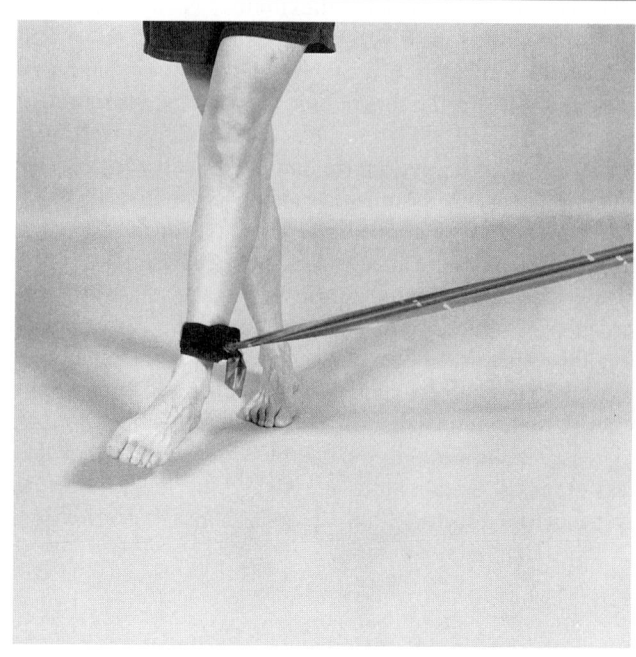

FIGURE 18-40   Surgical tubing exercise, example 2.

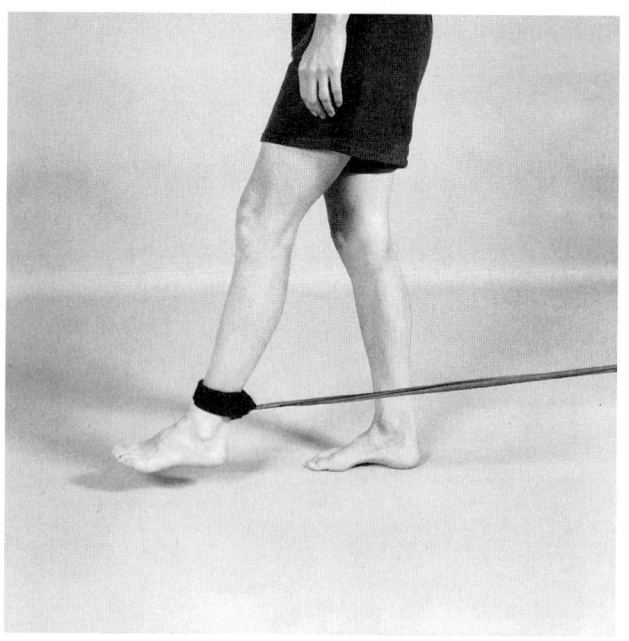

FIGURE 18-39   Surgical tubing exercise, example 1.

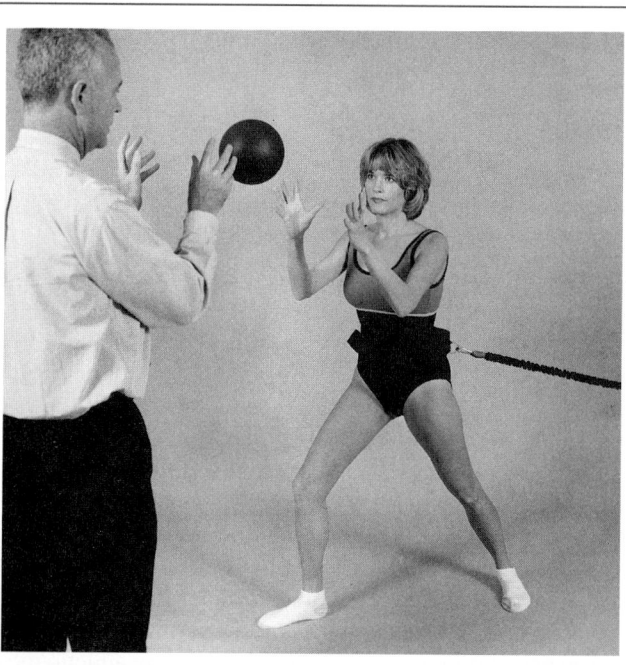

FIGURE 18-41   Agility drills.

and 18-40), balance board activities for the foot supinators and pronators, and agility drills[450] (Fig. 18-41).

In the presence of knee version, an adjunct to the usual exercise regimen may be strengthening of the internal tibial rotators (semimembranosus, gracilis, semitendinosus, sartorius), with greater emphasis placed on hamstring stretching, particularly the biceps femoris, while adding stretching of the iliotibial band.[274] CKCEs to strengthen the hamstrings, gastrocnemii, and quadriceps in a functional manner include a variety of exercises on a stair climber. The patient stands on the machine backward for the quadriceps, and forward for the hamstrings. The use of an inclined treadmill also can be used to selectively exercise the hamstrings, gastrocnemii, and quadriceps, as follows:

▶ Walking or running downhill works the quadriceps eccentrically.

▶ Walking or running uphill works the gastrocnemii and hamstrings concentrically.

▶ Walking or running downhill backward works the gastrocnemii and hamstrings eccentrically.

▶ Walking backward uphill uses the quadriceps concentrically.

The interplay between the VMO and the VL during this phase of the rehabilitation continues to be of great interest.[174,451,452] A study by Mirzabeigi and colleagues[453] attempted to isolate the VMO from the VL, vastus intermedius, and vastus medialis longus, using nine sets of strengthening exercises. These exercises included isometric knee extension with the hip in neutral, 30 degrees of external rotation, and 30 degrees of internal rotation; isokinetic knee extension through full range; isokinetic knee extension in the terminal 30-degree arc; side-lying ipsilateral and contralateral full knee extension; and stand and jump from full squat. Although the study concluded that isometric exercises in neutral and external rotation of the hip challenged both the VMO and VL, none of the exercises demonstrated isolation of the VMO.[453] Other studies have reported that certain closed-chain activities strengthen the VMO. These include bicycling, and uphill and retrotreadmill walking.[255,413,440,444,445,454] Uphill and retrotreadmill walking have been found to produce less patellofemoral joint restrictive forces than forward walking.[455]

Open-chain Exercises

OKCEs during this phase include seated knee extension and knee flexion exercises, and are viewed as single-joint, single-muscle-group exercises.[228] Using the knowledge of the compressive forces at the joint, open-chain exercises (e.g., short-arc quadriceps, multiple-angle isometrics) should be performed in the 50 to 90-degree, or 90 to 50-degree range of knee flexion.[227,441] Other exercises include:

▶ Straight leg raises in all four planes (flexion, extension, abduction, and adduction), progressing to about 10 percent of body weight in resistance.

▶ Supine leg lowering.

▶ Seated leg lowering.

▶ Short-arc quadriceps progression to about 10 percent of body weight in resistance.

Swenson and colleagues[456] recommend the use of the 4-minute open-chain exercise for patellofemoral pain. The exercise protocol was developed by Glen Porter, ATC, a basketball trainer at Michigan State University, and Alan Glock, MD, an orthopaedic surgeon in Richmond, Indiana. The exercise is performed as follows:

The patient sits on the edge of a chair, with the upper leg supported. The patient is asked to contract the quadriceps muscle with the knee in full extension. The contraction is held for 1 minute, after which the leg is flexed to 45 degrees for 30 seconds. Four cycles of extension and flexion constitute the 4-minute VMO program. Initially, the exercise is performed four to six times a day. Ankle weights are added after 1 to 2 weeks, and the number of sets is decreased.[456]

For some patients, a return to sports may be a goal. Because strenuous activities may exert five times more force than is imparted with the various ligament stress tests,[457] the clinician cannot rely on the results from the ligament stress tests as a means to assess a patient's readiness to return to sport. Once strength and endurance have reached at least 70 percent of the uninvolved extremity with isokinetic testing, the more advanced (PNF) exercises involving high-speed, high-force, uncontrolled movements are initiated, stopping short of cutting, jumping, and twisting maneuvers if symptoms of instability develop.[458,459] Running, jumping, and twisting activities must be included in the clinical examinations of such patients to enable true assessment.[351] Criteria for progression into the return to sport phase include:

▶ Full active and passive range of motion compared with the uninvolved knee. It has been suggested that the patient should have 8 to 118 degrees of knee motion, demonstrate a normal gait pattern, ascend and descend stairs, and demonstrate no gait deviation when running, before participating in athletic activity.[353,460]

▶ A quadriceps-to-hamstring ratio of 2:3, and equal to or greater than 75 percent of the uninvolved leg.

▶ Ability to perform a one-leg squat for 15 to 20 repetitions.

▶ Normal joint kinematics.

A return to cutting sports at the competition level is permitted when the quadriceps strength index is 85 to 90 percent of the uninvolved leg at 60 degrees per second with isokinetic testing. Sport-specific drills are added late in the functional phase as the athlete approaches return to play. Activity-specific progressions must be completed in order to test all of the working parts involved in the activity before full return to function is advised.

Bracing

Patellofemoral Bracing. External patellar supports, which range in complexity from simple straps across the patellar tendon to complex supports, are commonly employed in the management of patellofemoral pain as an adjunct to other intervention methods. Although they relieve symptoms in many patients, their mode of action remains speculative and their effectiveness is unpredictable.[258]

Theoretically, the purpose of the brace is to centralize the patella within the patellar groove, thereby reducing symptoms and improving function.[422,461] The various commercially available patellofemoral braces use a number of methods to improve patellar tracking, including patellar cut-outs, lateral buttresses, air bladders, and positioning straps.

Despite the wide use of patellofemoral bracing, only a few studies have attempted to document their effectiveness in correcting patellar alignment. Using magnetic resonance imaging, Koskinen and Kujala[462] reported a quantitative decrease in lateral patellar displacement using the Safety brace (Axini, Boliden, Sweden), while Worrell and colleagues[463] found that the Palumbo brace (Dynorthotics LP, Vienna, VA) reduced lateral patellar displacement and increased patellofemoral congruence at 10 degrees of flexion. These studies, however, used static imaging techniques and, therefore, actual patellar tracking was not assessed. This is an important limitation because patellar tracking is considered to be a dynamic entity. Studies comparing active and passive procedures have shown that patellar motion is significantly influenced by the degree of quadriceps contraction.[201,258,464,465] Finestone and colleagues[466] found that some braces were less effective and more harmful to the skin than conservative therapy (i.e., maintaining activity and avoiding pain-causing activity, or no therapy, or simple muscle stretching and strengthening).[467]

Although it can be debated whether bracing can influence patellar tracking, it appears that external supports must, in some way, interact mechanically with the patellofemoral joint because many patients report significant clinical improvements.

Tibiofemoral Bracing. Functional knee braces are commonly prescribed following an ACL injury or reconstruction to promote healing, by reducing anterior translation of the tibia with respect to the femur and thereby restoring normal joint kinematics.[21,468,469]

The efficacy of knee bracing with regard to providing adequate protection is controversial, because the compliance of the soft tissues around the thigh decreases the ability of the brace to function correctly, particularly at high loads.[469,470]

A study by Fleming and colleagues[469] using the Legend brace (dj Orthopaedics LLC, Vista, CA) indicated that a functional knee brace can protect the ACL during anteroposterior shear loading in the non–weight-bearing and weight-bearing knee and during internal torques in the non–weight-bearing knee. However, this study used only one brace and one knee flexion angle (20 degrees).

Risberg and colleagues,[471] who used randomized, prospective clinical trials of bracing after ACL injury or reconstruction, found no difference in joint laxity, pain, muscle strength, and functional knee tests between patients who wore a functional knee brace and those who did not wear a functional brace during postsurgical rehabilitation.

Several studies have indicated that subjects with chronic ACL-deficient knees have impaired proprioception.[472–474] Whether functional knee braces enhance proprioception in ACL-deficient knees remains unclear. Although a few studies have addressed the relationship between proprioception and functional outcome measures,[472,473] the studies that have compared the effect of functional braces on proprioception between ACL reconstructed knees and the contralateral uninvolved knee have as yet demonstrated no improvement in proprioception with the wearing of such braces,[475] and no effect on long-term outcome.[21]

Interestingly, bandaging of the knee, or the use of a neoprene brace, have been shown to improve proprioception in both normal individuals and those with different types of knee disorders, including knee osteoarthritis and an ACL tear.[21,476]

Taping

The use of tape in the management of patellofemoral disorders was originally proposed by McConnell, whose initial success rate in an uncontrolled study was 96 percent.[413]

The primary goal of taping[175,477] is to pull the patella away from a painful area, thereby unloading it and reducing pain.[413,478,479] The extent to which this is possible and the amount of displacement required to provide pain relief varies from patient to patient.[11] Indeed, the displacement does not need to be perceptible to effect improvement. Bockrath and colleagues[478] found that taping did affect perceived pain but was not associated with patellar position changes. A recent computed tomography (CT) study,[480] involving 16 female patients (aged 16 to 25 years) who had anterior knee pain related to patellofemoral incongruence, evaluated the effect of patellar taping on patellofemoral incongruence. The subjects underwent CT examination with their quadriceps muscles relaxed and contracted, both before and after patellar taping. The study found that patellar taping did not significantly affect patellofemoral lateralization, or tilt, and concluded that although patellar taping may well be effective in controlling anterior knee pain, it does not do so by medializing the patella.[480] Another study found that McConnell taping was effective in moving the patella medially but ineffective in maintaining this difference after exercise.[481]

A secondary goal of taping is to inhibit muscle firing by taping perpendicular to the direction of the muscle fibers.[482,483] Grabiner and colleagues[484] have postulated that the VMO needs time to develop force, relative to the VL, to optimally track the patella. This lag time can cause the patella to track laterally. By applying tape across an overly powerful VL, the clinician may be able to change the relative excitation of the VMO and VL, diminishing the pull of the VL,[11,175,477] although the mechanisms by which this works are unknown.

The final goal of taping for malalignment of the patella is to position the patella in the optimal position so that the area of contact between the patella and femur is maximized.[257] This position places the patella parallel to the femur in the frontal and sagittal planes, and the patella is midway between the two condyles when the knee is flexed to 20 degrees.[257]

Once the tape is applied, the clinician assesses:

▶ The overall limb alignment. This includes an assessment of the dynamic alignments when walking normally, on the heels, and with the feet in the inverted and everted positions; stair climbing; and squatting.

▶ The effect on functional painful and pain-free ranges.

From this information, the patellar position is adjusted by taping. The more obvious deviation is always corrected first. Often, repositioning of the patella involves positioning the patella so that it is approximately midway between the two femoral condyles and parallel with the long axis of the femur.

The glide component can be corrected by firmly gliding the patella medially and taping the lateral patellar border (Fig. 18-42). The tilt component can be corrected by firm taping from the middle of the patella medially, which lifts the lateral border and provides a passive stretch to the lateral structures (Fig. 18-43). To correct external rotation of the patella, firm taping from the middle inferior pole upward and medially is required. For correction of internal rotation, firm taping from the middle superior pole downward and medially is needed.

In addition to the taping, biofeedback, stretching of the lateral structures, and a home exercise program are recommended.[139] For a more detailed description of the application of the tape, the reader is referred to an excellent book, *The Patella: A Team Approach*.[174]

Taping also can be used with patients who have patellar osteoarthritis. A controlled clinical trial[485] found that patients achieved significant reduction in pain after medial knee taping to realign the patella.

Walking Poles

Results from a number of studies[486–488] have demonstrated that walking poles reduce the forces on the lower extremity during level walking when walking velocity is controlled. Schwameder and colleagues[489] reported 12 to 25 percent reduction in peak and average ground reaction force, knee joint moments, and tibiofemoral compressive and shear forces walking down a 25-degree gradient.

A study by Willson and colleagues[486] found that the use of the poles tended to reduce the vertical joint reaction forces at the knee over the no poles condition. Differences of 4.4 percent were found in vertical joint reaction forces at the knee between the no poles, pole back, and pole front conditions.[486] However, knee extensor angular impulse was greater

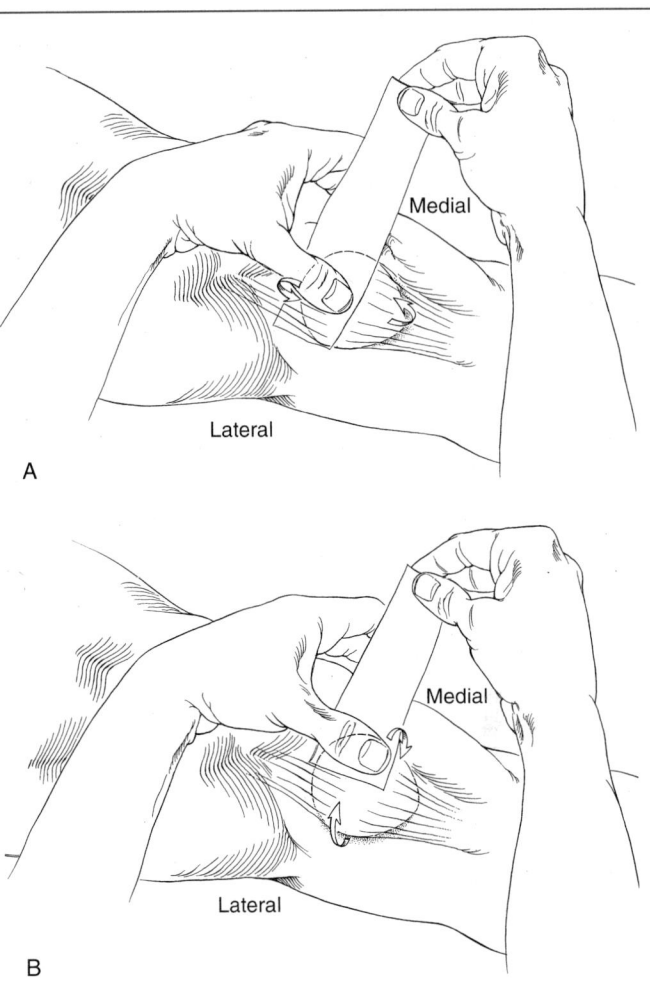

FIGURE 18-43 **A** and **B.** Patellar taping for correction of tilt. (Reproduced with permission from Zachazewski JE, Magee DJ, Quillen WS. *Athletic Injuries and Rehabilitation.* Philadelphia, Pa: Saunders; 1996.)

with all pole conditions compared with no poles. Thus, walking with poles caused a more flexed knee position through stance, reducing the vertical bone-on-bone forces and increasing the internal (muscular) knee extensor kinetics.[486] This reduction of lower extremity stress during a faster walking velocity may symbolize a less harmful mode of exercise for healthy and pathologic populations alike. Thus, the use of walking poles may lead to an increased training stimulus as a result of the greater walking velocity and reduced lower extremity loading conditions compared with a self-selected walking velocity.[486]

Preferred Practice Pattern 4C: Impaired Muscle Performance

The conditions in pattern C include those that produce patellofemoral pain as a result of malalignment of the patellar tracking mechanisms, but are not accompanied by episodes of instability. The term *malalignment* implies that the static or

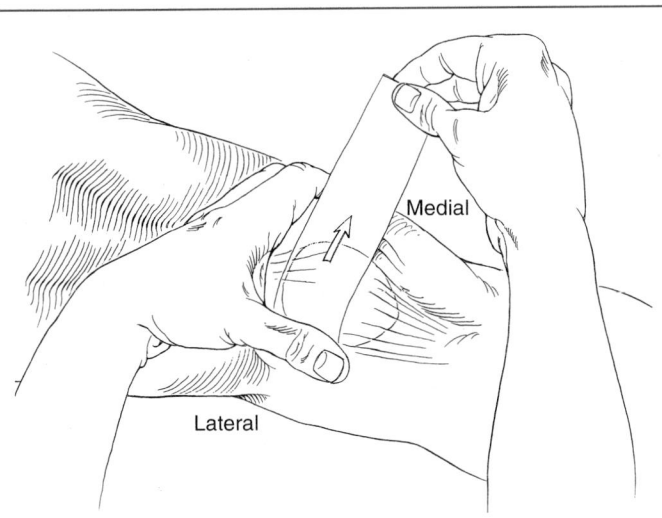

FIGURE 18-42 Patellar taping for correction of glide. (Reproduced with permission from Zachazewski JE, Magee DJ, Quillen WS. *Athletic Injuries and Rehabilitation.* Philadelphia, Pa: Saunders; 1996:715.)

dynamic restraints of the patellofemoral joint are insufficient to allow normal patellar tracking. Malalignment appears to be a necessary but not sufficient condition for the onset of anterior knee pain. Symptoms seem to be set off by a trigger, or combination of structural and dynamic factors, the nature of which varies from patient to patient. The structural factors include the size of the lateral femoral condyle, the depth of the patellar groove, and the angle of pull between the pull of the quadriceps and the pull of the patellar tendon (refer to Anterior Knee Pain—Practice Pattern 4E).[272]

Coordinated firing of the dynamic stabilizing muscles is important in the normal functioning of the patellofemoral joint. Electromyographic evidence of poorly coordinated muscle activation has been documented in other joints, such as the shoulder.[490] At the knee, the VMO may be proximally positioned and abnormally oriented, and the timing of its contractions may be poorly synchronized with those of the surrounding muscles.[135,182,413,442,445,491]

The intervention for a maltracking patella must seek to restore the balance of force production of the medial and lateral stabilizers of the patellofemoral joint, and to attempt the reestablishment of functional control of the VMO (see "Intervention Strategies," earlier).[174,175,272,413,416,425,426,477]

Preferred Practice Pattern 4D: Impaired Joint Mobility, Motor Function, Muscle Performance, Range of Motion Associated with Connective Tissue Dysfunction

Tibiofemoral Osteoarthritis

Osteoarthritis has been identified as the most common cause of disability in the United States.[492,493] Thirty-three percent of persons aged 63 to 94 years are affected by osteoarthritis of the knee, which often limits the ability to rise from a chair, stand comfortably, walk, and use stairs.[494,495]

Osteoarthritis may affect one or more of the three compartments of the knee: medial tibiofemoral, lateral tibiofemoral, and patellofemoral.

For many years, osteoarthritis has been regarded as a "wear-and-tear" or "degenerative" condition, a view supported by epidemiologic surveys that demonstrated associations with certain occupations and life choices, and its increased prevalence with advancing age.[496] Established risk factors include physically demanding occupations,[304,497–505] particularly in jobs that involve kneeling or squatting,[304,499,506–508] certain sports,[509,510] older age, female sex, evidence of osteoarthritis in other joints, obesity,[511] and previous injury or surgery of the knee.[512]

The clinical findings of osteoarthritis at the knee include swelling, which can vary from minimal to severe, depending on the clinical stage and severity. The joint can also be warm to touch, although that again depends on the stage and severity. Usually, the patient complains of pain with weight-bearing activities and, occasionally, pain at rest. The loss of motion, if present, is typically in a capsular pattern. Muscle weakness is probably the longest recognized and best established correlate of functional limitation in individuals with osteoarthritis, particularly of the knee.[506,513–515]

The conservative intervention for osteoarthritis of the knee has involved NSAIDs, cortisone injections, patient education, weight loss, therapeutic exercise, thermal modalities, and shoe inserts.[516,517] The use of shoes with a well-cushioned sole is recommended, as are frequent rest periods during the day. Wedged insoles with an angle of 5 to 10 degrees on a frontal section have been shown to be helpful for osteoarthritis of the medial compartment.[518,519] The patient is instructed in principles of joint protection, and advised to seek alternatives to prolonged standing, kneeling, and squatting.[517]

Exercises to strengthen the quadriceps, such as quad-setting exercises and isometric exercises, are becoming accepted as useful conservative treatment for osteoarthritis of the knee.[517] Isokinetic and isotonic exercises must be prescribed carefully to avoid excessive compressive forces or shear forces at the knee. Puett and Griffin[520] reviewed 15 controlled trials of conservative intervention for hip and knee osteoarthritis from 1966 through 1993 and concluded that exercise reduces pain and improves function in patients with osteoarthritis of the knee, but that the optimal exercise regimen had yet to be determined.[520] Fitness walking, aerobic exercise, and strength training have all been reported to result in functional improvement in patients with osteoarthritis of the knee.[520–526] Unweighted treadmill walking has not been shown to decrease pain associated with osteoarthritis of the knee.[527]

Another study by Deyle and colleagues[516] found that patients with osteoarthritis of the knee who were treated with manual physical therapy and exercise experienced clinically and statistically significant improvements in self-perceptions of pain, stiffness, and functional ability, and the distance walked in 6 minutes. The beneficial effects of intervention, which were achieved in eight clinic visits, persisted at 4 weeks and 1 year after the conclusion of clinical treatment.[516]

Patellofemoral Osteoarthritis

Patellofemoral osteoarthritis is diagnosed by correlating patellofemoral pain with radiographic changes consistent with joint degeneration. Differentiation of idiopathic and post-traumatic subtypes is based on the history. Intervention for patellofemoral osteoarthritis is usually conservative unless it coexists with severe tibiofemoral degenerative joint disease, in which case a total knee replacement may be warranted.

The term *chondromalacia patella* has long been a catch-all category of anterior and, specifically, retropatellar knee pain. The term *chondromalacia* was first used by Aleman in 1928.[528] He used the term "chondromalacia post-traumatica patellae" to describe lesions of the patella found at surgery and thought to be caused by prior trauma. With time, "chondromalacia" became an all-inclusive term with no agreed-on classification system or definitions of terms.[272]

True chondromalacia refers to a softening of the cartilage on the posterior aspect of the patella and is estimated to occur in fewer than 20 percent of persons who present with anterior knee pain.[190] The syndrome is most common in the 12- to 35-year-old-age-group, and most studies show a predominance in females.[115,189,190,420,456,529]

Two types of chondromalacia have been described. One type involves surface degeneration of the patella that is age-dependent and most often asymptomatic. The other type involves basal degeneration. This type results from trauma and abnormal tracking of the patella and is symptomatic.[196]

Chondromalacia is classified into four grades, according to the degree of degeneration noted arthroscopically.[530]

▶ *Grade 1.* Closed disease. This grade is characterized by an intact joint surface that is spongy. The softening is reversible. A blister or raised portion of the articular surface is seen.

▶ *Grade 2.* Open disease. This grade is characterized by fissures that may or may not be obvious initially.

▶ *Grade 3.* Severe exuberant fibrillation or "crabmeat" appearance.

▶ *Grade 4.* The fibrillation is full-thickness and the erosive changes extend down to bone, which may be exposed. This is, in effect, osteoarthritis and its extent depends on the size of the lesion.

Because cartilage has no nerve supply, chondral lesions themselves are usually asymptomatic,[531] although cartilage that is worn down to bone remains a potential source of pain due to irritation of, or abnormal pressure on, the richly innervated subchondral bone.[456]

The conservative intervention for patellofemoral osteoarthritis includes the removal of any muscle imbalances of flexibility or strength. Occasionally, surgical realignment may prove beneficial when the articular degeneration is isolated to the lateral patellofemoral joint.

Arthrofibrosis

The term *arthrofibrosis* has been used to describe a spectrum of knee conditions in which loss of motion is the major finding.[449,532–536] It is perhaps best defined as a condition of restricted knee motion characterized by dense proliferative scar formation, in which intra-articular and extra-articular adhesions can progressively spread to limit joint motion.[537] This dense scar tissue can obliterate the parapatellar recesses, suprapatellar pouch, intercondylar notch, and eventually the articular surfaces.[307] Patella infera and chronic patellar entrapment also may develop as a consequence of this process.[307]

Arthrofibrosis may occur as the result of the inflammatory cascade after injury or operative treatment. Although inflammation is undoubtedly present in a large number of individuals, it is not clear why an aggressive form of this condition may develop in some patients.

In order to diagnose arthrofibrosis accurately, other causes of restricted active and passive motion of the knee must first be eliminated. Mechanical causes include loss of articular congruency (e.g., as a result of fracture, meniscal tear, or loose body), interruption of the extensor or flexor mechanism, substantial effusion,[538,539] or nonisometric placement of the graft during reconstruction of the ACL.[308,316,534] Some investigators believe

that an ACL reconstruction performed within 3 weeks after an injury may increase the likelihood of arthrofibrosis[540,541] although others disagree.[542] Poor or unsupervised rehabilitation[316] preoperatively or postoperatively, with delayed motion protocols, may further increase the risk.[543]

Symptoms vary and often do not correlate with the severity of the condition. Because arthrofibrosis usually occurs after trauma or an operative procedure, pain and stiffness may be the initial symptoms.

▶ The presence of pain may complicate preexisting knee stiffness.[307,544] Although pain can be present early, it often becomes more prominent when joint degeneration and arthritis occur because of long-standing arthrofibrosis. Pain also may be constant, especially when it is associated with complex regional pain syndrome.[307,544]

▶ Stiffness is usually the primary symptom and is often worse in the morning hours.[537] Patients may complain of a warm, swollen knee that is painful with attempted motion.

Global arthrofibrosis of the knee manifests as marked limitation of flexion, extension, and patellar glide associated with widespread joint inflammation as well as intra-articular formation of fibrous tissue. This can progress to chondrification and ossification of soft tissues.[537]

Quadriceps function can be decreased or absent because of pain.[544] As function of the quadriceps muscle decreases, the ability of the muscle to act as a shock absorber is lessened, which may lead to additional articular degeneration. Often, the knee is held in a flexed position, which encourages tightening of the posterior part of the capsule and the hamstrings.

Crepitus and weakness are frequently present with swelling following prolonged standing or walking. Even when the patient does not have pain, loss of motion and quadriceps weakness can be substantial impediments to the performance of activities of daily living. An antalgic, flexed-knee gait is often seen.[308] Although effusion may be present, swelling is more often a result of inflamed, thickened capsular and pericapsular tissues.

Active and passive knee flexion and extension often are restricted in a capsular pattern, and the mediolateral and superoinferior patellar glides are reduced. This restriction of passive motion often has a springlike end-feel, reflecting the density and stiffness of the thickened, inflamed, or scarred peripatellar tissue.

Intervention includes range-of-motion exercises and the stretching of specific structures. When a plateau has been reached during rehabilitative efforts to restore motion or when there is progressive loss of motion, additional intervention of a gentle manipulation of the knee under anesthesia may result in improvement. Closed manipulation or vigorous attempts to gain passive motion may cause indiscriminate tearing of intra-articular tissue,[533] excessive tibiofemoral and patellofemoral compression with the risk of chondral damage or fracture,[302,533,545] rupture of the patellar ligament,[533,545] and even femoral fracture.[533] Manipulation also has been noted to initiate complex regional pain syndrome.[545]

Anteroposterior Slide Dysfunction: Tibia on Femur[303]

In this condition, the tibia demonstrates a restricted anterior or posterior joint glide. This motion is coupled to knee flexion-extension. Movement of the tibia on the femur into extension is coupled with an anterior glide. Movement of the tibia on the femur into flexion is coupled with a posterior glide. The initial complaints or findings are restrictions of flexion or extension movements.

The technique used to treat this dysfunction is a modification of the anterior drawer test. The patient is positioned supine, with the involved knee flexed and the foot flat on table, while the clinician sits on the patient's foot, anchoring it to the table. The clinician wraps both hands around the proximal tibia, placing the thumbs in front of the medial and lateral condyles and pressing on them. The clinician's hand encircles the leg and grasps it firmly below the popliteal space. The clinician creates a direct anteroposterior translatory glide of the tibia on the femur by first pulling the tibia forward with both hands, before pushing it backward with both thumbs.

Tibiofemoral Instability

Both intrinsic and extrinsic trauma to the knee occurs frequently. Several factors can predispose an individual to knee joint laxity:

▶ Repetitive microtrauma.

▶ Severe macrotrauma.

▶ Genetics.[546]

▶ Gender.[546]

▶ Ethnic factors.[546]

Knee laxity may contribute to the development and progression of knee osteoarthritis. It also may be a consequence of moderate to severe osteoarthritis, although some knees become more stable with time because of the formation of osteophytes. Laxity is associated with more abrupt joint motion, large displacements, and suboptimal distribution of larger forces over the articular cartilage.[547,548] Because significant instability or damage to the internal structures of the knee joint can damage the articular surfaces and lead to degenerative changes, it is imperative that these injuries be treated as soon as possible.[148]

There is no typical clinical presentation for knee instability in terms of the history. However, a history of "giving way" should always be taken seriously, as well as any evidence of locking or "catching" within the joint.[148]

The examination may reveal laxity. The direction of the laxity will determine the intervention. The intervention usually consists of muscle strengthening, correcting muscle imbalances, and the use of passive restraints, such as orthotics.

Anterior Cruciate Ligament Tear

More than 250,000 athletes are diagnosed with ACL injuries each year, making the management of sports-related ACL injuries the most widely discussed subject in the field of sports medicine.[549] This emphasis could be a result of the increasing frequency of the problem, and the controversy surrounding its management. ACL injury factors have been divided into intrinsic and extrinsic factors.[550]

▶ Intrinsic factors include a narrow intercondylar notch, weak ACL, generalized overall joint laxity, and lower extremity malalignment.

▶ Extrinsic factors include abnormal quadriceps and hamstring interactions, altered neuromuscular control, shoe-to-surface interface, playing surface, and athlete's playing style.

Gender has also been implicated. ACL injury rates are two to eight times higher in women than in men participating in the same sports.[550,551] Speculation about the possible etiology of ACL injuries in women has centered on[552]:

▶ *Anatomic alignment and structural differences.* Differences in pelvic width and tibiofemoral angle between males and females may affect the entire lower extremity.[553] The magnitude of the quadriceps femoris angle (Q-angle) and the width of the femoral notch are thought to be anatomic factors that have contributed to the disparity of ACL injury rates between males and females.[552] Theoretically, larger Q-angles increase the lateral pull of the quadriceps femoris muscle on the patella and put medial stress on the knee.[553] This increased Q-angle also decreases the functional effectiveness of the quadriceps as a knee extensor and of the hamstrings—the antagonist muscle group responsible for exerting a posterior force on the proximal tibia to protect the ACL.

▶ *Femoral notch.* A narrow intercondylar notch may be a predictive factor for ACL ruptures.[554] In a cadaver study, Norwood and Cross[555] showed that the ACL impinges on the anterior intercondylar notch with the knee in full extension.[552] The shape of the femoral notch may vary with gender and may contribute to the incidence of ACL injury.[556] A small, A-shaped notch may not be actually pinching a normal-size ACL, but it may be a sign of a congenitally smaller ACL.[556]

▶ *Joint laxity.* Several studies have shown that joint laxity tends to be greater in women than in men,[557–559] although the relationship between ligamentous laxity and injury is not clear.

▶ *Hormonal influence.* Hormones, especially estrogen, estradiol, and relaxin, may be involved indirectly in increased ACL injury in females.[560,561]

▶ *ACL size.* Females typically have a smaller ACL than males, which would tend to increase the risk of tissue failure.[561a]

▶ *Muscular strength and muscular activation patterns.* Several researchers have documented that women have significantly less muscle strength in the quadriceps and hamstrings compared with men, even when muscle strength is normalized for body weight.[559,562–565]

It is impossible to say that any one mechanism is responsible for ACL injuries. The multitude of intrinsic and extrinsic factors that come into play make focusing on one variable difficult.[4]

All ACL tears (i.e., sprains) are categorized as grade I, II, or III injuries. Ligament tears are classified according to the degree of injury, which ranges from overstretched ligament fibers (i.e., partial or moderate tears) to ligament ruptures (i.e., complete tears or disruptions). The term *midsubstance tear* refers to the site of the ACL injury and indicates a central ligament tear as opposed to a tear at one of the ligament's bony attachment sites. Almost all ACL tears are complete midsubstance tears.[37,38] Young athletes may sustain growth plate injuries (e.g., avulsion fractures) rather than midsubstance tears because the epiphyseal cartilage in their growth plates is structurally weaker than their ligaments, collagen, or bones. In the past, research has shown that tears in ACL complexes of young athletes usually resulted in avulsion fractures, not midsubstance tears. Recent studies, however, now suggest that young athletes may sustain midsubstance tears similar to those in adult athletes.[2,566]

Symptomatic ACL deficiencies in young athletes' knee joints are subject to the same long-term detrimental effects that occur in adult athletes.[567] Young athletes also may be more predisposed to more long-term degenerative knee conditions as the result of more years of chronic rotary knee instabilities from ACL deficiencies.[568]

Associated Knee Injuries. Isolated ACL injuries are rare, because the ACL functions in conjunction with other structures of the knee. When the outer aspect of the knee receives a direct blow that causes valgus stress, the MCL often is torn first, followed by the ACL, which becomes the second component of a sports-related ACL injury.[25] Meniscal injuries also can occur in conjunction with ACL tears. Approximately 49 percent of patients with sports-related ACL injuries have meniscal tears.[569]

Transection of the ACL leads to slight degenerative changes in the cartilage, but additional deafferentation of the knee joint produces severe degenerative changes.[570,571] This suggests that sensory input from the joint may play a role in adapting movement strategies so that potentially harmful positions and loads are prevented.

Mechanism of Injury. Most published studies of the ACL are directed toward the basic mechanics of the ligament, method of surgical repair, and rehabilitation.[240,572–575] Unfortunately, little is known about the actual mechanism of injury during sport activity, although one sport that has been studied in some detail is alpine (downhill) skiing,[576,577] in which three common causes of ACL injury have been discussed.

▶ The first is referred to as the "phantomfoot" mechanism.[577] This mechanism occurs when a skier falls backward with the knee flexed and the tibia internally rotated. The combination of a strong quadriceps contraction (to maintain balance) with a rigid boot that fails to release may lead to an ACL disruption.[578] As a result, the ligament disruption occurs during a hard landing when the skier is off-balance.

▶ In the second mechanism, when the skier lands on the ski's tail, the stiff posterior shell of the boot combined with a strong quadriceps contraction to maintain balance slides the tibia anteriorly, leading to an anterior drawer maneuver.

▶ The third mechanism, valgus rotation, seems to be more common in men who participate in downhill or cross-country skiing. It occurs when the inside (medial) edge of the front of the ski becomes caught in the snow. The leg is abducted and externally rotated while the skier is driven forward by momentum. High-speed skiing and poorly groomed ski slopes also are factors that contribute to this type of injury.

Regrettably, little attention has been directed to the mechanism of ACL injuries in other sports, although sudden deceleration, an abrupt change of direction, and a fixed foot have all been cited as key elements of an ACL injury.[578] For example, a common mechanism of injury to the ACL occurs when excessive lateral force (i.e., valgus stress) is applied to the outer aspect of the knee joint. This type of injury often is seen in contact sports activities (e.g., football, soccer, and rugby), resulting from tackles or blows to the lateral side of the knee. A twisting injury to the ACL occurs when the knee is in full extension and the femur is rotated externally on a fixed tibia. This mechanism of injury usually occurs because of abrupt changes in speed, direction, or velocity that torque the knee. Maneuvers often seen in sports activities, such as football, basketball, and soccer, can cause twisting injuries to the ACL. Snowboarders also may experience the same mechanism of injury when their feet and ankles are locked in ski boots and their knees are torqued. A less common mechanism of injury to the ACL occurs with extreme hyperflexion or hyperextension of the knee joint.[25]

Examination. Diagnoses of sports-related ACL injuries can be difficult, and clinicians must consider many factors when determining the best treatment options for patients with ACL injuries. Thorough patient histories and physical examinations are essential for accurate diagnoses of ACL injuries. Patients commonly describe the sensation of their knee "popping" or "giving out" as the tibia subluxes anteriorly. Other signs and symptoms of ACL injuries include pain, immediate dysfunction, and instability in the involved knee, and the inability to walk without assistance. In rare instances, when patients have isolated ACL injuries that do not involve related collateral or meniscal tears, local tenderness around the knee joint may be absent.[568]

A classic sign of ACL injuries is acute hemarthrosis (i.e., extravasation of blood into a joint or synovial cavity).[360] The signs and symptoms of hemarthrosis (i.e., pain, edema, and joint stiffness) make clinical examinations more difficult for clinicians and very uncomfortable for patients.

Atrophy of the quadriceps is an almost constant finding with patients who have a torn ACL.[579–583] Several authors found a decrease in extensor torque that was larger than would be expected on the basis of the decrease in the volume of the quadriceps as measured with CT,[580,581,584–586] whereas the hamstring muscles do not have a comparable force deficit. It would appear that even specific conservative intervention can only partially correct the deficit.[587] The difference in torque has been reported to persist after reconstruction of the ACL with use of autogenous grafts or allografts from the patellar ligament,[587,588] or with use of semitendinosus grafts.[589,590]

During the examination, it is important for the clinician to examine the patient's contralateral knee for baseline comparisons. This especially is true in children who have inherent or congenital laxities, such as knock-knee (genu valgum) or saber legs (genu recurvatum). It also is important to remember that the pain the patient experiences during the examination may affect the accuracy of the test results. Common manual tests to assess the ACL include the anterior drawer and the Lachman (see "Stress Testing").

Arthrometer. An arthrometer, such as a KT-1000, is a mechanical testing device for measuring anteroposterior knee ligament instability. This noninvasive device assesses the amount of displacement between the femur and the tibia at a given force in millimeters.

Although most patients who have a complete tear of the ACL have increased tibial translation on instrumented testing,[591] it is not known exactly how many of these patients will have "giving way" of the knee or how many knees will have overt or latent damage of the cartilage within a few years.[33,592,593]

Imaging Studies. Radiographs can identify arthritic changes that may be associated with chronic rotary instability from ACL deficiencies. They also can demonstrate avulsion fractures of the tibial spine, or hypoplastic intracondylar notches with diminished tibial spines, which indicate a congenital absence of the cruciate ligaments.[24]

Magnetic resonance imaging (MRI) scans are useful for diagnosing ACL injuries, although their use in discriminating between complete and partial ACL tears is limited. Diagnostic MRI scans, however, can detect associated meniscal tears that routine radiographs cannot show.[2] Both MRI scans and radiographs are necessary to assess whether young athletes' growth plates are closed or open, a factor that may affect treatment decisions.

Genu Recurvatum ("Saber Legs")[594]

Genu recurvatum is a position of the knee joint complex in which the range of motion occurs beyond neutral or 0 degrees of extension.[146] Genu recurvatum appears to be more common in females than males and may exist due to postural habit, increased joint laxity, or knee injury.

Traditionally, rehabilitation has only been used to address this condition when poor muscle control of the knee exists, such as occurs following trauma or a cerebral vascular accident. However, one might question whether genu recurvatum predisposes an individual to knee injury. Certainly, the posterior structures of the knee (the capsular and noncapsular soft tissue structures, including the arcuate complex, posterior capsule, lateral meniscus, fabellofibular ligament, and biceps femoris muscle)

are likely to be stressed with genu recurvatum. The posterior capsule forms two pouches that extend over the articular surface of the femoral condyle and tibial plateaus.[145] The capsule is thin over the posterior aspect of the femoral condyles but is supported by the two heads of the gastrocnemius and reinforced by the oblique popliteal ligament. The arcuate ligament also reinforces the capsule laterally. Stability is further enhanced internally by the lateral meniscus, which forms a concave articular surface for articulation with the convex lateral femoral condyle.[5]

A thorough history will guide the clinician to suspect genu recurvatum as a contributing factor in knee or other lower leg injury. Individuals with genu recurvatum may present with one of a variety of lower extremity diagnoses. It is doubtful that their primary diagnosis is genu recurvatum. Patients may have a history of an injury that forced them into hyperextension. Examples include landing from a jump on an extended knee; a blow to the anteromedial aspect of the proximal tibia, forcing the knee into hyperextension; and a noncontact external rotation hyperextension injury. From the anatomic and biomechanical review, it appears that the possible consequence of genu recurvatum in the active individual may be an increase in stress placed on the ACL, the anterior joint, or the posterolateral corner of the knee. Symptoms attributable to genu recurvatum include:

▶ *Anteromedial joint pain.* This pain results from the compressive forces at the medial tibiofemoral compartment. This pain may be accentuated if a varus alignment is present.

▶ *Posterolateral knee pain.* This pain results from the tension placed on the posterior structures and is aggravated by stepping or forceful knee extension in weight bearing.[90]

The patient also may complain of knee instability during activities of daily living. Noyes and colleagues have described the posterolateral syndrome as an injury to the posterolateral structures in conjunction with a torn ACL.[595] This syndrome is usually characterized by no history of injury and a gradual onset of knee pain. Loudon and colleagues[596] found a positive correlation between genu recurvatum and ACL injury in female athletes. Hutchison and Ireland[597] attributed the recurvatum posture and laxity in the posterior capsule to habitual posture.

Patients with genu recurvatum are easily identified during static standing. The sagittal view best demonstrates this posture. Individuals also may present with excessive femoral internal rotation, genu varum or valgum, tibial varum, or excessive subtalar joint pronation, which is more noticeable in the frontal plane.

When performing activities such as step-ups, patients will use momentum to straighten the lower extremity, and they will be unable to control weight-bearing terminal knee extension. Kendall and colleagues[142] report that the hyperextension posture of the knee is caused from weakness in the gastrocnemius.

Proprioception in individuals with genu recurvatum may be deficient, especially near the end range of extension. One study[596] demonstrated that individuals who stood in hyperextension and without knee injury were unable to reproduce knee joint angles in the last 15 degrees of extension compared with other knee angles of 45 and 60 degrees on a leg press machine. Individuals may perceive the hyperextended knee position as "normal" and, when they are introduced to a more vigorous activity, they may have a tendency to stay in hyperextension, putting the knee at risk for injury.[596,597]

If genu recurvatum is suspected as contributing to the patient's symptoms, special attention is needed to identify posterolateral instability. This can be achieved using the posterolateral drawer test and the varus stress test at 30 degrees. If the recurvatum is unilateral, the clinician should assess the lumbar spine and pelvis for obliquity or muscle imbalance. In addition, the hip should be evaluated for excessive internal rotation, which contributes to genu recurvatum, and the subtalar and midfoot joints should be checked for excessive pronation, which allows excessive internal rotation of the tibia (see Chap. 19).

Patients with genu recurvatum need to learn that 0 degrees of knee extension is the normal knee position, and that hyperextension is to be avoided.[598] The patient is taught to keep the knee in the same plane as the foot. Verbal cueing is helpful, but other strategies, such as the temporary use of posterior knee taping, can give the patient direct sensory feedback. This neutral position should then be carried over to dynamic strengthening exercises.

Muscle sequencing is the key, with the hamstrings and gastrocnemius firing in conjunction with the quadriceps to guide the knee into extension rather than using the passive force of gravity.[559] Patients should progress through weight-bearing exercises that require sequential use of eccentric and concentric control of the lower extremity, such as resistive terminal extension, single leg balance, mini-dips, squats, forward and backward step-ups, lunges, and jump landings.

Knee control during gait can be taught in conjunction with the previously mentioned exercises. Noyes and colleagues recommend that the patient maintain knee flexion of 5 degrees throughout the stance phase of gait.[595] A 1- to 2-inch elevated heel may be used in the initial training to create a flexion moment at the knee, and the trunk should be maintained in an upright position versus a forward lean or flexed hip during midstance to avoid an anterior shift of body weight.[595] Excessive internal femoral rotation also should be controlled during this phase of gait.[595]

Continued training of the patient with genu recurvatum should focus on functional tasks. These include stair climbing and sit-to-stand transfers, such as stair climbing. During the pull-up phase of stair climbing, patients should be trained to refrain from thrusting into knee extension. Individuals may have a tendency to hyperextend their knees with other daily activities, such as bending forward to brush their teeth or prolonged standing.

The final phase of rehabilitation focuses on more complex activities and sports-specific skills. It is important that athletes involved in jumping and cutting sports master a flexed knee position. Henning and colleagues[224] have suggested that extreme loads are placed on the ACL when the knee is straight or near-straight during planting and cutting, landing from jumps, and sudden stops while running. Emphasis should thus be placed on flexing the knee during these sports activities to prevent injuries to the ACL. Hamstrings that are adaptively shortened offer protection to these joints and should not be stretched.

Meniscal Tears

Because of the interrelationship of the menisci with other structures of the knee, a torn meniscus is the most common cause of mechanical symptoms in the knee. Knee injuries may result in isolated or combined meniscal lesions. Meniscal lesions usually occur when the patient attempts to turn, twist, or change direction when weight bearing, but they also can occur from contact to the lateral or medial aspect of the knee while the lower extremity is planted.[58]

A number of meniscal tears are recognized (Fig. 18-44). With aging, the meniscal tissue degenerates and can delaminate, thus making it more susceptible to splitting from shear stress, resulting in horizontal cleavage tears.[599] Without the menisci, the loads on the articular surfaces are increased significantly, leading to a greater potential for degenerative arthritis. Because the menisci are without pain fibers, it is the tearing and bleeding into the peripheral attachments as well as traction on the capsule that most likely produce a patient's symptoms.[248] In fact, 16 percent of asymptomatic patients have meniscal tears demonstrated on MRI, with the incidence increasing to 36 percent for patients older than 45 years.[600]

Patients with meniscal injuries typically present with a history of swelling, popping, or clicking, and pain along the joint line. With posterior horn tears, the meniscus may return to its anatomic position with extension. If the tear extends anteriorly beyond the MCL, creating a bucket-handle tear, then the unstable meniscus fragment cannot always move back into an anatomic position.[248] Such a meniscal tear can result in locking of the knee in a flexed position. The lateral meniscus, being more mobile, is less likely to be associated with locking when torn. The patient may also note a "clicking" sensation while walking as a result of traction against a torn medial or lateral meniscus.[600] Locking of the knee is more common in younger patients with meniscal tears, because older patients are more likely to have degenerative meniscal tears with less mechanical symptoms and an insidious onset.[248]

The joint line pain is thought to result from capsular irritation. Meniscal tears are symptomatic as they render a portion of the meniscus abnormally mobile.[601] The shape and location of the meniscal tear determines the symptoms and clinical findings.

At the time of writing, four conservative approaches exist for the intervention of meniscal injuries: rehabilitation, meniscectomy, meniscus repair, and allograft transplantation.[58] The choice of intervention depends on the several factors, including age, activity demands, size and location of the tear, and collateral tissue damage.[602]

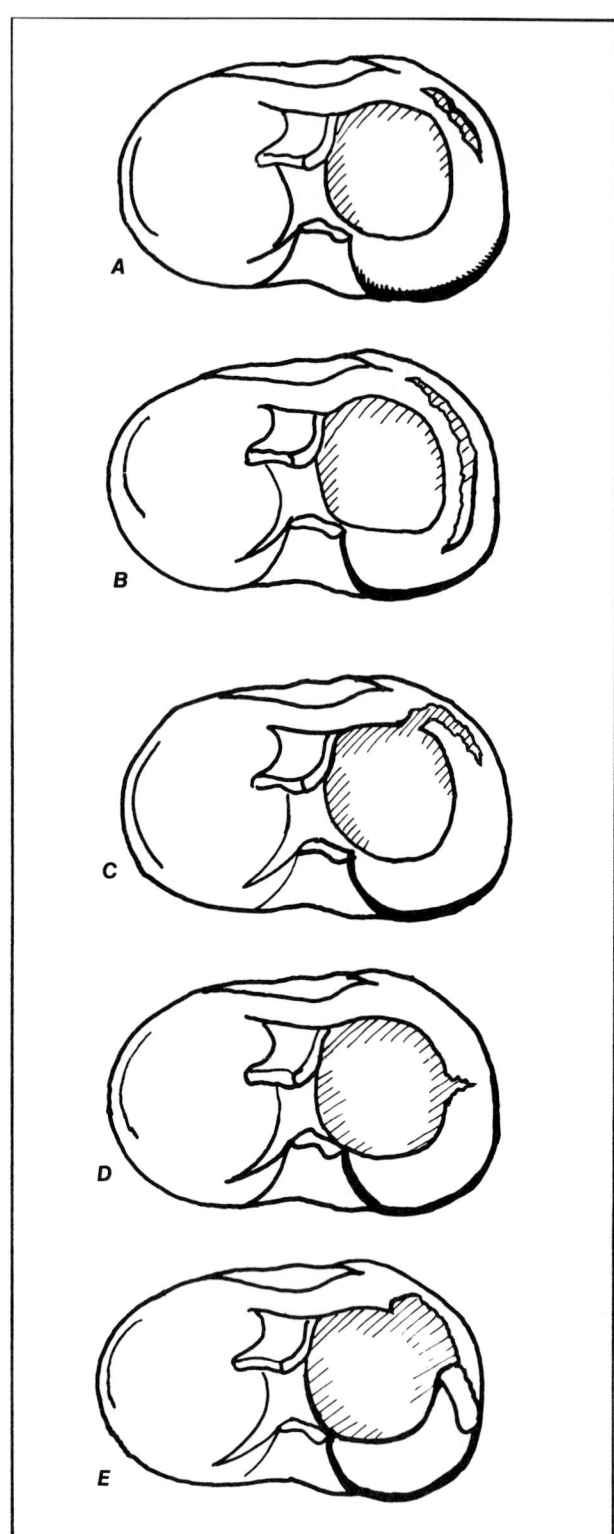

FIGURE 18-44 Meniscal tears. **A.** Partial longitudinal tear of the medial meniscus. **B.** "Bucket-handle" tear. **C.** Anterior horn tear. **D.** An uplifted fragment, which can produce locking of the knee. **E.** Transverse tear of the meniscus. (Reproduced with permission from Simon RR, Koenigsknecht SJ. *Emergency Orthopaedics: The Extremities.* 4th ed. New York, NY: McGraw-Hill; 2001:462.)

Meniscal lesions that can be treated conservatively include the diffusely degenerative meniscus. Unless a tear is acute, peripheral, and stable, the relative avascularity of the middle third and inner third of both menisci indicates a poor healing potential in these areas.

If the knee is locked or cannot be fully extended, the torn meniscal fragment is displaced and must be treated surgically. Although most peripheral tears are successfully repaired because of the healing capabilities of the meniscus, tears to the inner third of the meniscus are usually treated by meniscectomies[58] (see Chap. 29).

Approximately one third of meniscal tears can be treated with conservative intervention that focuses on the resolution of impairments such as swelling, restricted range of motion, and strength, using exercises, bracing, and oral medications.[603]

Posterior Cruciate Ligament Tear

Injury to the PCL is thought to account for 3 to 20 percent of all knee injuries depending on the source, which suggests that many go undiagnosed.[604,605] Because of its inherent strength, damage to the PCL usually only occurs with significant trauma such as a motor vehicle accident,[606] or when landing in a hyperflexed knee position from a jump.[607]

Many isolated PCL injuries heal with conservative intervention, especially in light of the fact that many PCL-deficient patients do not experience functional instability.[608] However, the long-term follow-up studies of PCL injuries reveal a progressive development of pain and degeneration of the medial compartment of the tibiofemoral joint.[609]

Clinical findings for a PCL tear include pain in the posterior aspect of the knee joint that may be aggravated with kneeling. Instability may or may not be present, depending on the severity of the tear.

The focus of the intervention is to restore range of motion and to strengthen the quadriceps. Quadriceps strengthening is performed to help reduce posterior tibial translation.[610] Hamstring strengthening is delayed for approximately 6 to 8 weeks following the injury to decrease the potential for PCL stress. A combination of OKCEs and CKCEs are initiated to promote dynamic stability of the knee. Heavy resistance open kinetic chain knee extension exercises through a range of 45 to 20 degrees of flexion are avoided to protect the patellofemoral joint.[208,225]

Important exercises include squats, lunges, and closed-chain knee extensions. Balance and proprioceptive exercises also are performed. Plyometrics are introduced for appropriate patients such as athletes.

Return to sport may occur in as little as 6 to 8 weeks, but on average takes 12 to 16 weeks, providing that there are no complicating factors. These complicating factors include significant varus or valgus alignment, or damage to additional tissues.

The management of patients who have PCL injuries combined with other ligament or capsular injuries is less definitive.

Patellofemoral Instability

Patella instability can be produced by:

▶ *A small patella.* A smaller patella decreases the stability of the patella during its tracking.[11,611,612]

▶ *A shallow patellar groove.* The term *dysplastic femoral trochlea* implies a shallow intercondylar sulcus, especially at the lateral ridge, which often contributes to instability, although it can also be seen in painful knees without episodes of instability.[11,611,612]

▶ *An abnormal patellar position.* The patella may lie too far proximally or distally relative to the trochlea, conditions called *patella alta* and *patella baja* (or patella infera), respectively.[218,613,614] Patella alta, as a separate entity, does not necessarily contribute to knee pain, but it can certainly contribute to lateral maltracking by causing the patella to enter into the patellar groove late in knee flexion. Patella baja occurs rarely in otherwise normal individuals. It is seen in achondroplastic dwarfs, who seldom have anterior knee pain, and as a postoperative complication of knee surgery.[308,615,616] Several radiographic methods for diagnosis of patella alta and baja have been reported in the literature.[614,617-619]

▶ *A muscle imbalance between the VMO and VL.*[122,135,419] These imbalances are discussed under "Biomechanics," earlier.

▶ *Generalized ligamentous laxity or complex malalignments of the entire extremity (genu recurvatum).*[173,273,620]

Instability is usually identified through the history, with the patient reporting either dislocation or subluxation episodes. A subluxation needs to be differentiated from "giving way," as this can be simply a reflex inhibition of the quadriceps secondary to pain. The direction of instability is usually lateral, with medial instability almost always secondary to iatrogenic causes.[272] On palpation, medial retinacular and distal patellar pole tenderness or distal quadriceps tenderness may be elicited.[297]

The number of episodes is important, because patients who are first-time dislocators and infrequent subluxators should have a trial of conservative intervention or limited arthroscopic evaluation for documented osteochondral lesions,[173] whereas, recurrent instability is an indication for surgical intervention.[272] Once the instability and its direction have been established, the anatomic cause of the instability is determined.

Cruciate ligament instabilities can lead to secondary patellofemoral pain through increased patellofemoral contact pressures and abnormal joint loading patterns.

Symptomatic Plica

The plica syndrome has been associated with anterior pain as well as clicking, catching, locking, or pseudolocking of the knee, and it may even mimic acute internal derangement of the knee.[109,323,621-626]

There is some controversy regarding the prevalence of the plica syndrome, with some reports suggesting that it does not exist.[627-629] Jackson and colleagues,[109,629] Dandy,[628] and others[105,106,218,323,630-633] have stated that although plicae may

indeed cause symptoms, the syndrome is overdiagnosed and many normal synovial plicae are removed. Conversely, other authors consider the plica syndrome to be a common cause of anterior pain in the knee that is often misdiagnosed, and believe that a suprapatellar membrane is virtually never asymptomatic.[114,634,635]

Sherman and Jackson[636] proposed a set of criteria for the diagnosis of symptomatic synovial plica:

▶ History of the appropriate clinical symptoms.

▶ Failure of non-operative intervention.

▶ Arthroscopic finding of a plica with an avascular fibrotic edge that impinges on the medial femoral condyle during flexion of the knee. This is often a diagnosis of exclusion and can only be confirmed at arthroscopy.

▶ No other abnormality in the knee that would explain the symptoms. It has also been suggested that a localized area of chondromalacia at the site of impingement by a plica on the femoral condyle is evidence that a plica is the cause of the symptoms.

Clinical Findings. The mediopatellar plica (also termed *Lino's shelf*), although the least present, is often the cause of problems if it becomes thickened, resulting in pain with palpation over the medial parapatellar area. The severity of symptoms is not proportional to the size or breadth of the synovial plica.[109] There also appears to be no correlation between the duration of symptoms and the presence of pathologic changes in the plica.[637]

A palpable band or snapping, especially over the medial femoral condyle, should be sought. In one study of plicae in the knee, clicking was reported in 64 percent, "giving way" in 59 percent, and pseudolocking in 45 percent of the patients.[323] A number of special tests exists for the detection of plical irritation (see "Special Tests").

Plicae are not visualized well on plain radiographs, but a double-contrast arthrogram may demonstrate a suprapatellar plica or an anterior plica.[632,638-642] A skyline radiograph may demonstrate a synovial shelf.[622,643,644]

The conservative intervention for plica syndrome involves stretching of the quadriceps, hamstrings, and gastrocnemius as well as isometric strengthening, cryotherapy, ultrasound, patellar bracing, anti-inflammatory medication, and an altered sports-training schedule.[106,621,645-648] In an uncontrolled study,[649] this type of intervention resulted in an improvement in 40 percent of patients over a 1-year period.

Injection of the synovial plicae with corticosteroids and a local anesthetic in another uncontrolled study[650] was reported to have an excellent result in 73 percent of patients.

When patients are truly symptomatic, or when conservative measures have failed, surgical excision is usually curative.

Patellar Compression Syndromes

Patellar compression syndromes result from an overconstrained patella whose motion is severely restricted by surrounding soft tissues.

Lateral Patellar Compression Syndrome.[135,173,396,651] A tight lateral retinaculum may be responsible for patellar tilt and excessive pressure on the lateral patellar facet, producing the excessive lateral pressure syndrome as described by Ficat and Hungerford.[256] The patient typically complains of pain over the lateral retinaculum.[173,212,652] The diagnosis is confirmed clinically by a decreased medial patellar glide and evidence of a lateral patellar tilt.

The medial stabilizers play a role in the lateral pressure syndrome, and the VMO frequently becomes atrophied, probably as a result of the new patellar position, the associated pain, and the resultant inflammation.[297] The presence of nerve-fiber changes in the lateral retinaculum[119,173] raises the possibility that these changes might be a catalyst for pain, although it is not clear whether the malalignment precedes the nerve changes or vice versa. The major long-term problem with excessive lateral pressure syndrome is a chronic imbalance of facet loading and the subsequent effect on the articular cartilage and surrounding soft tissue.

Fortunately, this condition seems to respond well to a conservative approach consisting of[297]:

▶ Stretching of the lateral retinacular structures.

▶ Patellar taping to correct the excessive lateral tilt and to apply a long duration, low-load stretch of the lateral retinaculum.

▶ Stretching of the hamstrings, quadriceps, and iliotibial band.

▶ Strengthening of the VMO.

▶ Anti-inflammatory measures.

▶ Activity modification through minimization of stair ambulation and deep knee squats.

Infrapatellar Contracture Syndrome.[653] The term *infrapatellar contracture syndrome (IPCS)* was first coined by Paulos et al. in 1987.[308] This condition is characterized by a restriction of patellar movement because both the medial and lateral retinaculum are excessively tight. This restriction may result in a decrease in knee flexion and extension. Another term for this condition, *global patellar pressure syndrome,* was proposed by Wilk and colleagues.[297]

The development of this condition appears to be related to direct trauma and subsequent pathologic fibrous hyperplasia in the peripatellar tissues, or secondary to prolonged immobilization after surgery.[308]

IPCS has been described as having three progressive stages: a prodromal stage, an active stage, and a residual stage.[654]

Prodromal Stage. The first, prodromal, stage begins between 2 and 8 weeks after trauma to the knee. Knee range of motion is painful, there is a decrease in patellar mobility, and an extensor lag is present. This scenario is usually noted with patients who fail routine postoperative rehabilitation. Without recognition, patients can progress to the second stage within 6 to 20 weeks. Early detection of IPCS is important because only stage 1 is amenable to non-surgical intervention. Rehabilitation should be initiated with early patellar mobilization, stretching of the hamstrings, hip flexors, quadriceps, gastrocnemius, and iliotibial band, with the emphasis on restoring full knee extension. Other components in the prodromal stage should include active range of motion, multi-angle isometric strengthening of the quadriceps, neuromuscular stimulation, transcutaneous electrical nerve stimulation, and NSAIDs. When performing the patella mobilizations, the glides should be held for a long duration (1 to 12 minutes) to enhance the remodeling of the soft tissue.[297,655] Activities such as bicycling, resisted knee extensions, deep knee bends, or deep squats (beyond 60 degrees) should not be initiated until patellar mobility is restored, to prevent excessive patellar compression and patellofemoral joint contact pressures.[297]

Active Stage. In the second stage, there is loss of the extensor lag because of the restriction of passive and active knee range of motion. There are also tissue texture changes in the patella tendon. This creates a positive shelf sign: an abrupt step-off or "shelf" from the patellar tendon to the tibial tubercle.[308] Patients who progress to stage 2 require surgery, with open intraarticular and extra-articular debridement. Immediate daily rehabilitation with continuous passive motion, full active range of motion, and extension splints at night also can be used.

Residual Stage. The third stage is notable for significant patellofemoral arthrosis and a residual low-riding patella at 8 months or even years after the onset of IPCS. Additional classifications distinguish whether the patellar entrapment is primary, caused by infrapatellar contracture (see separate section), or secondary, as a result of surgical intervention or postoperative immobilization. The patient history typically includes complaints of knee pain and stiffness, swelling, crepitus, and "giving way" may also be reported. On physical examination, the diagnosis may be made by a 10-degree or greater loss of extension, a 25-degree or greater loss of flexion, and significantly reduced patellar mobility as demonstrated by decreased patellar glide. Additional findings include atrophy of the quadriceps femoris, palpable patellofemoral crepitus, diffuse synovitis, and an antalgic or flexed knee gait.

Patients presenting in stage 3 of IPCS usually fail to respond to all attempts of physical therapy.

Preferred Practice Pattern 4E: Impaired Joint Mobility, Motor Function, Muscle Performance, Range of Motion Associated with Localized Inflammation

Tendonitis

Patellar tendonitis (jumper's knee) and quadriceps tendonitis are overuse conditions that are frequently associated with eccentric overloading during deceleration activities (e.g., repeated jumping and landing, downhill running). The association of patellar tendonitis with jumping was first described by Maurizio,[656] but the term *jumper's knee* originated from Blazina and colleagues.[657] Some authors feel that the term *patellar tendonitis* is a misnomer because the patellar "tendon," which connects two bones, is in fact a ligament.[658,659]

The high stresses placed on these areas during closed kinetic chain functioning place them at high risk for overuse injuries. Overuse is simply a mismatch between stress on a given structure and the ability of that structure to dissipate the forces, resulting in inflammatory changes.[660]

The diagnosis of tendonitis is based on a detailed history, and careful palpation of the tendon in both flexion and extension. Pain on palpation near the patellar insertion is present in both patellar and quadriceps tendonitis. These are usually self-limiting conditions that respond to rest, stretching, eccentric strengthening,[661–663] bracing, and other conservative techniques. When treating overuse injuries, it is essential that the clinician limit both the chronic inflammation and degeneration by working on both sides of the problem: tissue strength should be maximized through proper training, and adequate healing time must be allowed before returning to full participation.[660]

Several protocols have been advocated for the conservative intervention of patellar tendonitis. Stanish and colleagues[663] proposed the following strengthening program of eccentric exercise for chronic patellar tendonitis.

A 5-minute warm-up period consisting of a series of three to five static stretches held for 15 to 30 seconds each is performed. Next, the patient, from a standing position, flexes the knees, abruptly drops to a squatting position, and then recoils to the standing position. The velocity of the drop is increased until the patient is able to perform it as quickly as possible without pain. At this point, sandbags are added to the patient's shoulders to increase the load on the tendon. Apart from some minor discomfort during the exercises and some postexercise muscle soreness, the procedures should be performed without pain.[663]

Reid[664] proposes a protocol based on the severity of the lesion. Grade I lesions, which are characterized by no undue functional impairment and pain only after the activity, are addressed with adequate warm-up before training and ice massage after. With grade II to III strains, activity modification, localized heating of the area, a detailed flexibility assessment, and an evaluation of athletic techniques are recommended. In addition, a concentric-eccentric program for the anterior tibialis muscle group is prescribed, which progresses into a purely eccentric program as the pain decreases.[665]

The patient starts with the foot in full plantar flexion. The clinician applies overpressure on the dorsum of the foot, placing the foot into further plantar flexion and stretching the anterior tibialis. The patient is asked to perform a concentric contraction into full dorsiflexion, which is resisted by the clinician. An eccentric contraction is then performed by the patient as the clinician resists the motion from full dorsiflexion to full plantar flexion. This maneuver is repeated to the point of fatigue of the anterior tibialis.[665] As soon as possible, the eccentric loading program is added.

It is not clear why a program initially directed at the anterior tibialis muscle group should be therapeutic for the infrapatellar tendon and ligament, but it is theorized that the program may stretch the infrapatellar ligament, change the

quadriceps-to-foreleg strength ratio, or alter the biomechanics of take-off and landing.[664]

Surgical intervention is usually required only if significant tendonosis develops and is successful in the majority of patients.[666]

Iliotibial Band Friction Syndrome

As its name suggests, iliotibial band friction syndrome (ITBFS) is a repetitive stress injury that results from friction of the iliotibial band as it slides over the prominent lateral femoral condyle at approximately 30 degrees of knee flexion[667] (Fig. 18-45). The friction has been found to occur at the posterior edge of the band, which is felt to be tighter against the lateral femoral condyle than the anterior fibers.[667,668] The friction causes a gradual development of a reddish-brown bursal thickening at the lateral femoral condyle.

ITBFS is the most common overuse syndrome of the knee, being particularly common in long-distance runners (20 to 40 miles/week). In addition, long-distance runners who train on hilly terrain, graded slopes, or road cambers are also at risk, especially if their runs include downhill running,[668,669] which positions the knee in significantly less flexion than normal at initial contact. Finally, running on canted surfaces can result in a leg-length inequality and a change in the Q angle, which can increase the stress on the iliotibial band.

Although most cases of ITBFS have been reported in distance runners, anyone engaging in activity that requires repetitive knee flexion and extension, such as downhill skiing, circuit training, weight lifting, and jumping sports, is prone to developing this pathology.[446] ITBFS is also common in cyclists.[406,670,671] This is thought to be due to the pedaling stroke, which causes the iliotibial band to be pulled anteriorly on the downstroke and posteriorly on the upstroke. Extrinsic factors

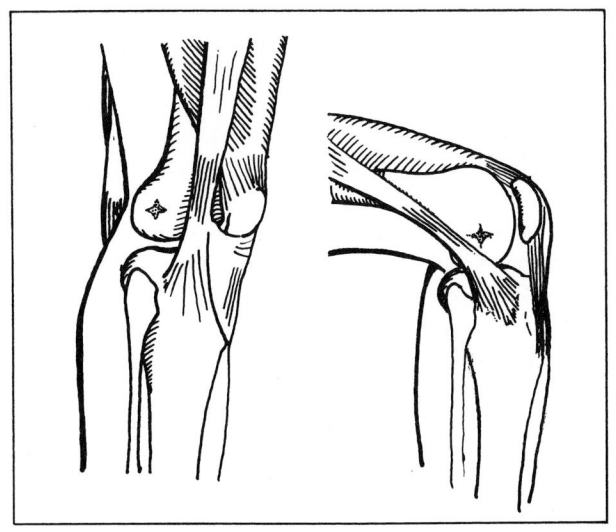

FIGURE 18-45 Iliotibial band friction syndrome. (Reproduced with permission from Simon RR, Koenigsknecht SJ. *Emergency Orthopedics: The Extremities.* 4th ed. New York, NY: McGraw-Hill; 2001:451.)

include excessive bike seat height or cleat position on the pedal. If the cleats are excessively internally rotated on the pedal, the tibia also internally rotates, resulting in a valgus force on the knee and increased tension of the iliotibial band.

A study of six cadavers by Muhle and colleagues[672] found that, in four of six individuals, some fibers of the iliotibial tendon remained in contact with the lateral femoral condyle during extension. With further flexion, the iliotibial tendon moves posteriorly and contacts the lateral femoral epicondyle and lateral collateral ligament, indicating a phase during knee flexion during which an impingement of the band occurs. In runners, this impingement phase occurs predominantly during the early stance phase, very soon after initial contact.[446] In general, the faster the speed of running, the less the time spent in the impingement zone, because the knee flexion angle at initial contact increases with speed of running.[673–675]

Subjectively, the patient reports pain with the repetitive motions of the knee. There is rarely a history of trauma. Although walking on level surfaces does not generally reproduce symptoms, especially if a stiff-legged gait is used,[153,668] climbing or descending stairs often aggravates the pain.[676] Patients do not usually complain of pain during sprinting, squatting, or during such stop-and-go activities as tennis, racquetball, or squash.[668] The progression of symptoms is often associated with changes in training surfaces, increased mileage, or training on crowned roads. The lateral knee pain is described as diffuse and hard to localize.

Objectively, there is localized tenderness to palpation at the lateral femoral condyle or Gerdy's tubercle on the anterolateral portion of the proximal tibia. The resisted tests are likely to be negative for pain. The special tests for the iliotibial band (Ober's test, Noble compression test, and creak test) should be positive for pain, or crepitus or both, especially at 30 degrees of weight-bearing knee flexion. There also may be associated biomechanical changes. In addition to a tight iliotibial band, the following findings have all been associated with iliotibial band friction problems, although they have yet to be substantiated: cavus foot (calcaneal varus) structure,[677] leg-length difference (with the syndrome developing on the shorter side),[678,679] fatigue,[680] internal tibial torsion (increased lateral retinaculum tension), anatomically prominent lateral femoral epicondyle, and genu varum.[681]

A study by Fredericson and colleagues[682] found that long-distance runners with ITBFS have weaker hip abduction strength in the involved leg compared with the uninvolved leg, and that symptoms improved with a successful return of hip abductor strength. To control coronal plane movement during stance phase, the gluteus medius and tensor fascia latae must exert a continuous hip abductor movement. Fatigued runners or those with weak gluteus medius muscles are prone to increased thigh adduction and internal rotation at midstance. This, in turn, leads to an increased valgus vector at the knee and increased tension on the iliotibial band, making it more prone to impingement.[682]

Conservative intervention for ITBFS consists of activity modification to reduce the irritating stress (decreasing mileage, changing the bike seat position, and changing the training surfaces), using new running shoes,[683] heat or ice applications, strengthening of the hip abductors, and stretching of the iliotibial band.[189] Surgical intervention, consisting of a resection of the posterior half of the iliotibial band at the level that passes over the lateral femoral condyle, is reserved for the more recalcitrant cases.[671]

Bursitis

Several types of bursitis are differentiated:

▶ *Superficial and deep infrapatellar bursitis.* Inflammation of these bursae usually results from a mechanical irritation during such activities as kneeling ("nun's knee"), or direct trauma.

▶ *Prepatellar bursitis ("housemaid's knee").* Inflammation of this bursa is seen in patients who experience recurrent minor trauma of the anterior knee. Those whose occupations require long periods of kneeling are particularly at risk. Diagnosis is straightforward, with pain and possibly swelling present on palpation of the prepatellar bursa.

▶ *Superficial pes anserinus bursitis.* This condition can involve any of the bursae lying between the various tendons of the superficial pes anserinus, or a bursa between the medial collateral ligament and the superficial pes anserinus. Inflammation of these bursae is common in novice swimmers and long-distance runners. Clinical findings may include medial knee pain just distal to the joint line, and an externally rotated tibia, compared with the uninvolved side.

▶ *Medial collateral ligament bursitis.*[653] MCL bursitis was first described by Brantigan and Voshell[684] as inflammation of the bursae deep to the MCL.[684–686] Because of the proximity of this bursa to the medial meniscus or medial meniscotibial ligament, this condition is often misdiagnosed. Patients describe pain along the medial joint line, confirmed on physical examination by a tender palpable mass that can be exacerbated by placing the knee under a valgus load. Because of the proximity of the semimembranosus tendon to the bursa, internal and external rotation can also impinge on the bursa and cause pain.[684] Imaging is not essential, but an MRI scan may show the inflamed bursa.[250]

The intervention for bursitis includes the removal of the irritation. This may involve the stretching of adaptively shortened structures or joint mobilizations to help correct alignment.

Sindig-Larson-Johansson Syndrome and Osgood-Schlatter Disease

This condition is an apophysitis of the tibial tubercle (Osgood-Schlatter disease) and inferior pole of the patella (Sinding-Larsen-Johanssen syndrome) that occurs in skeletally immature individuals, especially those involved in sports requiring repetitive-loaded knee flexion.

Osgood-Schlatter's disease presents between the ages of 8 and 13 years in females and 10 and 15 years in males, who are affected about three times as often.[664] In 25 to 33 percent of the cases, there is bilateral involvement.[687] The condition is the result of a retrograde ossification of the tibial tubercle, producing an apophysitis. Although usually self-limiting, it can progress to an avascular necrosis.

Sinding-Larsen-Johanssen syndrome usually occurs prior to the growth spurt. Fragmentation of the tibial tubercle or irregular calcification of the inferior patellar pole may be seen on radiographs. Pain is usually reported with use of the knee in such activities as athletics, cycling, or resisted knee extension. The involved area is tender and usually prominent on physical examination.

The intervention for these conditions is usually symptomatic, including short courses of anti-inflammatory medications, a focus on hamstring flexibility, and moderate-intensity quadriceps strengthening. The traditional approach of activity limitations is no longer considered necessary. Rarely, individuals will require excision of symptomatic ossicles or degenerated tendons for persistent symptoms at skeletal maturity. More persistent cases may require immobilization for 6 to 8 weeks.[664]

Quadriceps Contusion

Quadriceps contusions, resulting from a direct blow, can be very disabling.[688] Contusions of the anterior portion of the muscle are usually more serious than those involving the lateral portion of the muscle because of the differences in muscle mass present in the two areas.

As elsewhere in the body, contusions are graded according to severity. A grade I contusion produces only mild discomfort, with no swelling and no detrimental effect on gait. The patient with a grade II contusion may or may not have a normal gait cycle. Grade III contusions in this muscle are very rare due to the lack of muscle belly tissue.

These are frustrating injuries for the clinician and the patient, because there are often few clinical and radiographic findings to establish the diagnosis, resulting in a diagnosis made by way of exclusion. MRI may be helpful in the acute phase, but this remains a diagnosis that is largely based on the history.

If the intervention for these contusions occurs too early, or is too aggressively, myositis ossificans can develop. Myositis ossificans is a pathologic bone formation resulting from muscle tissue damage, bleeding, and damage to the periosteum of the femur, and resulting in ectopic bone formation.[689,690]

The intervention includes ice and 24-hour compression applied immediately, which should be continued until all of the signs and symptoms are absent. Gentle pain-free quadriceps stretching exercises are begun on the first day, progressing to resistive exercises as tolerated, usually on the second day. If an abnormal gait is present, the patient may be issued crutches until the normal gait returns.

Patients with a grade I contusion can continue with normal activities as tolerated. A patient with a grade II contusion may require 3 to 21 days for rehabilitation. Grade III contusions may require 3 weeks to 3 months to fully heal.

Turf Knee or Wrestler's Knee

Turf knee, or wrestler's knee, is an injury to the soft tissue overlying the knee. It is caused by a shearing mechanism within the subcutaneous tissues. Swelling and tenderness are present, but the swelling is present in the extra-articular tissues and should be differentiated from a true joint effusion. A joint effusion is characterized by a ballotable patella, and the intra-articular fluid is mobile and can be pushed to and from the suprapatellar pouch. With turf knee, these signs are absent, but there is boggy swelling in the soft tissue, and a sense of subcutaneous fluid is present on palpation. This injury usually responds well to rest and avoidance of the aggravating trauma.

Hoffa's (Fat Pad) Syndrome

The infrapatellar fat pad may be a cause of anterior knee pain. This syndrome was first described by Hoffa[691] in 1904. It is thought to represent hypertrophy and inflammation of the infrapatellar fat pad secondary to impingement between the femoral condyles and tibial plateau during knee extension. Direct trauma and overuse have also been attributed as causes. Irritation also can be produced by a posterior tilt of the inferior pole of patella.

Symptoms include anterior knee pain that is inferior to the pole of the patella. Pain is exacerbated by knee extension, particularly hyperextension, but not by knee flexion.[297] Inspection may reveal inferior patellar edema and associated tenderness of the fat pad when palpated through the tendon. Direct palpation of the fat pad on either side of the patellar tendon as the knee is brought from flexion into full extension is painful if the fat pad is inflamed. A diagnostic test, termed the *bounce test* (eliciting pain with passive knee hyperextension), is sometimes useful.[250] One must be careful to look for other causes of inflammation, such as osteoarthritis, before concluding that the fat pad is the primary source of pain.[272] Plain radiographs are invariably negative, but abnormalities of the fat pad can be noted on MRI.[692]

Conservative intervention includes rest, ice, anti-inflammatory medications, and iontophoresis or phonophoresis. Local corticosteroid injections into the fat pad are preferred by some physicians because they can be both diagnostic and therapeutic.

Biomechanical interventions include addressing the causes of hyperextension through orthotic interventions, such as heel lifts, or taping the superior pole posteriorly and holding the patella in a superior glide with tape.

In recalcitrant cases, surgical resection of portions of the fat pad is indicated.

Medial Retinaculitis

Medial retinaculitis is a rare condition seen almost exclusively in runners. It probably represents a fatigue tear in the medial capsular insertion into the patella. A positive bone scan in the medial edge of the patella confirms this diagnosis.

Baker's Cyst

Usually a Baker's cyst is asymptomatic, but in the presence of a synovial effusion, the cyst can swell up with fluid and become painful. On occasion, the cyst can become so large that it protrudes through the soft tissues, just proximal to the popliteal fossa, between the heads of the gastrocnemius. Ruptures of the cyst can occur, and these can mimic the symptoms of a tear of the gastrocnemius.

Clinical findings with the larger cysts include pain with active and passive knee flexion and extension, and with weight bearing, and pain and an increased prominence of the swelling with resisted knee flexion.

The conservative intervention for this condition normally involves treating the articular disorder that caused the cyst to swell. The medical management includes aspiration or surgical resection.

Popliteus Tendonitis

Popliteus tendonitis is common in runners who used banked surfaces, which produce oblique lateral rotary stresses to the knee, or who run downhill frequently. The condition typically manifests as point tenderness in the lateral aspect of the knee corresponding to the popliteus insertion site, which is exacerbated with eccentric loading.

Popliteus tendonitis can be diagnosed by having the patient sit so that the leg is in the figure-four position, with the lateral aspect of the ankle resting on the contralateral knee.

Intervention involves a modification in the training regimen, ultrasound, and transverse friction massage.

Breaststroker's Knee

This condition of pain and tenderness localized on the medial aspect of the knee is often associated with performance of the whip-kick, the kick used with breaststroke.[87] The forceful whipping together of the lower legs often forces the lower leg into slight abduction at the knee, with subsequent irritation and inflammation to the MCL of the knee.

In a study of breaststroke kinematics,[693] it was found that angles of hip abduction of less than 37 degrees, or greater than 42 degrees at the initiation of the kick, resulted in a dramatic increase in the incidence of knee pain.[87]

Anterior Knee Pain

Anterior knee pain, or patellofemoral pain syndrome, is a commonly recognized symptom complex characterized by pain in the vicinity of the patella that is worsened by sitting and climbing stairs,[136,694] inclined walking, and squatting.[695] It is a common reason for referral to physical therapy.[416] A British sports injury clinic study showed that 5.4 percent of the total injuries seen, and 25 percent of all knee problems, treated for a 5-year period were attributed to this syndrome.[696] Although anterior knee pain can occur in anyone, particularly athletes, women who are not athletic appear to be more prone to this problem than men who are not athletic.[697]

Patients presenting with various patellofemoral conditions invariably report similar symptoms, which have previously led to the indiscriminate use of such terms as *anterior knee pain* and *chondromalacia patellae*. Numerous authors have proposed classification systems using various clinical, radiographic, etiologic, and pathologic criteria to categorize patients.[123,273,697–702] Until recently, probably the best and most comprehensive classification system for patellofemoral disorders was that developed by Merchant,[273] who used a medical model based on etiology and consisting of five major categories, as follows:

1. Trauma.

2. Patellofemoral dysplasia.

3. Idiopathic chondromalacia patellae.

4. Osteochondritis dissecans.

5. Synovial plicae.

With the shift in the physical therapy profession from a medical model to an impairment-based model, Merchant's model is no longer as useful. The purpose of a physical therapy classification system is to aid in proper diagnosis and intervention based on impairment. To help in the determination of the classification, the clinician must answer the following questions:

▶ Is the problem truly related to the patellofemoral joint or its related structures?

▶ Is a muscle imbalance present?

▶ Is inflammation present?

▶ Is instability present?

Determining the classification gives significant guidance to intervention options. Patellofemoral instability, especially recurrent, usually requires surgical intervention, whereas patellofemoral pain resulting from inflammation or a muscle imbalance usually responds well to conservative intervention.[272]

The impairments resulting from patellofemoral dysfunction have been related to problems that cannot be improved by physical therapy, and those that can.

Anatomic Variance. A number of anatomic features can have an impact on the function of the patellofemoral joint and subsequent dysfunction:

▶ Femoral trochlear dysplasia.[183,703]

▶ Patellar morphology and the amount of congruence of the patellofemoral joint.

▶ The natural positioning of the patella (alta or baja).[180,210,279,704,705]

Gender.[211] A commonly cited reason as to why women have more anterior knee pain than men is the difference in the orientation and alignment of the lower extremity. The broader pelvis of the female moves the hip joints farther lateral relative to the midline. This produces an increased valgus angle from the hip to the knee and then to the ground. Females also have a higher prevalence of increased femoral anteversion, which also increases the valgus angle.[706] Although the increased valgus thrust on the patella is not necessarily a problem, it increases the tendency of excessive lateral pressure on the patella, which then can lead to retinacular stress around the patella and, in some people, concavity of the lateral facet and anterior knee pain.

Preferred Practice Pattern 4G: Impaired Joint Mobility, Muscle Performance, Range of Motion Associated with Fracture

Tendon Ruptures or Fractures

Quadriceps and patellar tendon ruptures, and patellar fractures, usually result from eccentric overload of the extensor mechanism or direct trauma. These are usually easy to diagnose, because the patient is unable to actively extend the knee, and there is a palpable defect at the site of injury. Radiographs will confirm fractures or avulsions. In skeletally immature individuals, fractures involving the proximal tibial epiphysis can occur. These are usually evident on radiographs and often require surgical intervention.

Integration of Preferred Patterns 4F and 5F: Impaired Joint Mobility, Motor Function, Muscle Performance, and Range of Motion Secondary to Complex Regional Pain Syndrome (Reflex Sympathetic Dystrophy), Myofascial Pain Syndromes (Referred Pain Syndromes), Peripheral Nerve Entrapment

Peripheral Nerve Entrapment

Compression Neuropathy of the Saphenous Nerve.[653] Saphenous nerve palsy is an impingement of the large cutaneous branch of the femoral nerve by the fascia of its three bordering muscles (anterolaterally by the vastus medialis, posterolaterally by the adductor longus, and medially by the sartorius) as it exits the adductor canal.[685,707–709] Occasionally, branches of the femoral vessels also may impinge on the nerve. The onset can be insidious or secondary to trauma or surgery about the knee.

Entrapment of the saphenous nerve often results in marked pain at the medial aspect of the knee. Patients describe a burning sensation in the nerve's sensory distribution, which typically worsens at night and is exacerbated by lower limb activity. The pain can be confused with an internal derangement of the knee or an anserine bursitis.

Physical examination reveals a Tinel's sign at the adductor canal. Often there is associated local tenderness. Sensory changes may be seen within the sensory distribution of the nerve. There is no motor weakness. Confirmation of a saphenous lesion can be made using resisted flexion of the knee or resisted adduction of the thigh, which should increase the pain, or pressure over the saphenous opening, in the sub-sartorial fascia, producing a radiation of the pain. Active flexion of the knee beyond 60 degrees also can reproduce the pain.

Electromyography and nerve conduction studies can help eliminate L-3 and L-4 radiculopathies, and aid in the diagnosis.[707] Diagnostic peripheral nerve blocks with lidocaine also may be performed. Mild to moderate cases can be treated with rest, anti-inflammatory medications, ice, ultrasound, and transcutaneous electrical nerve stimulation.[685,709,710] Second-line interventions include therapeutic nerve blocks with phenol.[708] Cases refractory to these interventions can be managed with surgical release of fascial bands and neurectomy.[709]

Compression Neuropathy of Superficial Peroneal Nerve. This nerve can be entrapped as a result of fibrosis following a direct blow[711,712] or surgery. Symptoms typically include pain over the lateral distal aspect of the leg and ankle, mimicking symptoms of a disk herniation, with irritation of the L5 nerve root. However, differentiation can be made with percussion or pressure over the nerve at its point of exit, which will cause reproduction of the symptoms in this syndrome.[713]

Myofascial Pain Dysfunction: Vastus Medialis

This muscle refers pain deep to the patella, and patients typically complain of knee joint stiffness and loud cracking noises as the patella suddenly releases during knee flexion.[714] Dysfunction of the vastus medialis, which counters the lateral pull of the other three quadriceps muscles and ensures proper patellar tracking, can lead to patellofemoral dysfunction and pain. Structural deformities, such as valgus deviation of the knee or overpronation of the foot, put additional strain on this muscle and perpetuate trigger point activity.[714]

Complex Regional Pain Syndrome (Reflex Sympathetic Dystrophy)

This condition is characterized by intractable knee pain of considerable duration. The patient may appear severely disabled, often using crutches, and may appear anxious and depressed. The presence of cyanosis or mottling indicates autonomic dysfunction. There also may be a noticeable difference in temperature between the involved area and the contralateral limb. In late cases, trophic changes of the skin occur. In addition, wasting of the quadriceps and stiffness of the joint may be evident.

Early diagnosis is the key to a successful intervention. The intervention should include a comprehensive team approach involving the physician and physical therapist. The most important rule is to avoid excessive pain.[715] Complete rest to the affected region, particularly immobilization in a cast, is harmful.[716,717]

It is important to not reinjure the region or aggravate the problem with aggressive physical rehabilitation.[717] Thus, the progression should occur slowly and gently.

► Exercises are prescribed for strengthening, active assistive range of motion, and active range of motion. Weight-bearing exercises and active stress loading exercises also should be incorporated.

► Sensory threshold techniques, including fluidotherapy, vibration desensitization, transcutaneous electrical nerve stimulation, contrast baths, and desensitization using light and heavy pressure of various textures over the sensitive area, should be used.

▶ Affected joints should be rested and elevated to counteract the vascular stasis, but the joint also should be mobilized gently several times per day.[716]

Therapeutic Techniques

Techniques to Increase Joint Mobility

Mobilizations

The mobilizations described in this section should always be complimented with exercises or automobilization techniques performed at home by the patient.

Posterior Glide of the Tibia on the Femur. This technique is used to increase the joint glide associated with flexion of the tibiofemoral joint. The technique used is identical to the passive physiologic articular mobility test used to assess the joint (Fig. 18-46). The emphasis of the mobilization technique at the tibiofemoral joint varies according to the range of motion being treated.

In the midranges of flexion, the posterior glide of the tibia is applied along the plane of the joint, whereas in the last few degrees of flexion, the posterior glide is applied with the congruent rotation of internal rotation of the tibia. Active mobilization also can be employed by positioning the patient's foot and leg into internal rotation, and asking the patient to pull isometrically with the hamstrings.

Posterior Glide of the Femur on the Tibia. This technique is used to increase the joint glide associated with extension of the

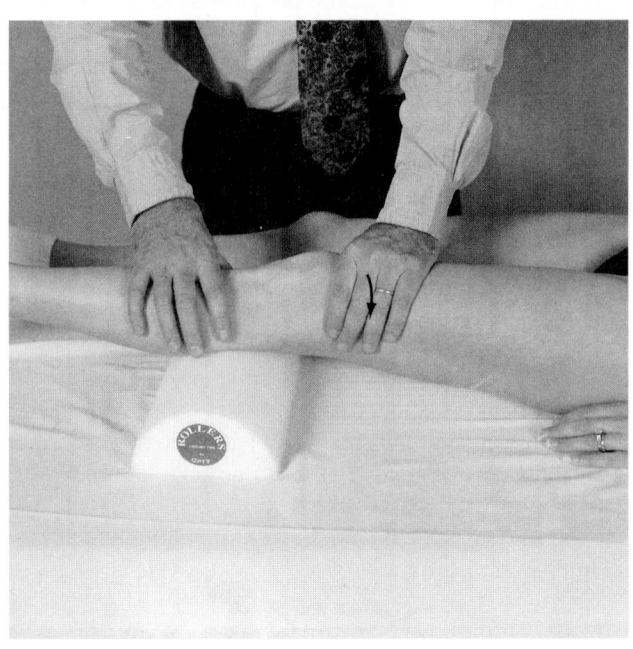

FIGURE 18-47   Posterior glide of the femur.

tibiofemoral joint. The technique used is identical to the passive physiologic articular mobility test used to assess the joint (Fig. 18-47).

If the clinician is attempting to regain the last 10 to 30 degrees of extension, the emphasis is placed on positioning the tibia in external rotation, and applying a posterior glide of the femur, thereby addressing the conjunct rotation.

Proximal Tibiofibular Joint. The mobilizations for this joint are identical to the techniques used to assess the joint, which are described in the passive physiologic articular mobility tests of the examination.

Myofascial restrictions of this joint present with the fibular head in an anterior or posterior position, and in the absence of adaptive shortening, the passive mobility tests will be normal. The intervention should be aimed at the cause of the muscle imbalance, but if direct treatment is attempted, active mobilization (muscle energy) techniques are used.

▶ To increase the posterior movement, the patient is asked to contract the hamstrings. The biceps femoris is attached to the fibular head and will help draw the fibular posteriorly.

▶ To increase the anterior glide, the patient is asked to contract the anterior tibialis, whose attachment will pull the fibula anteriorly.

Pericapsular hypomobility restrictions also present with the fibular head positioned anteriorly or posteriorly. The passive mobility test demonstrates reduced motion with a capsular end-feel. Treatment is by anterolateral (foot in plantar flexion; Fig. 18-48) or posteromedial (foot in dorsiflexion) capsular stretches.

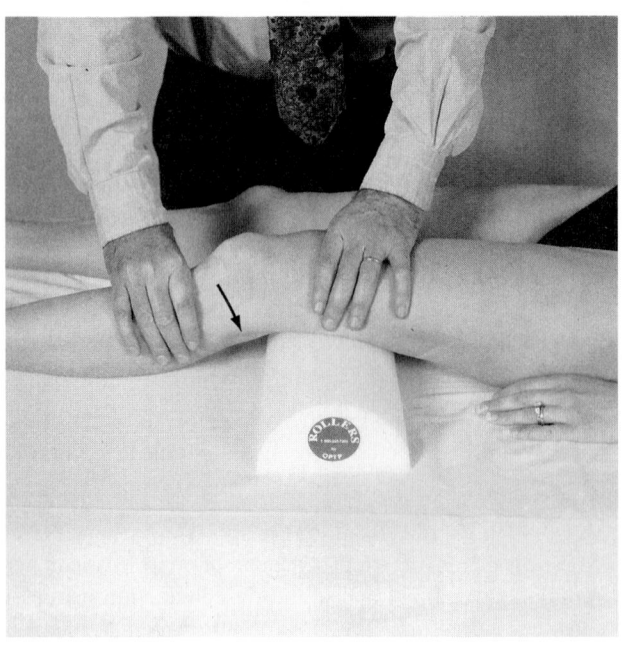

FIGURE 18-46   Posterior glide of the tibia.

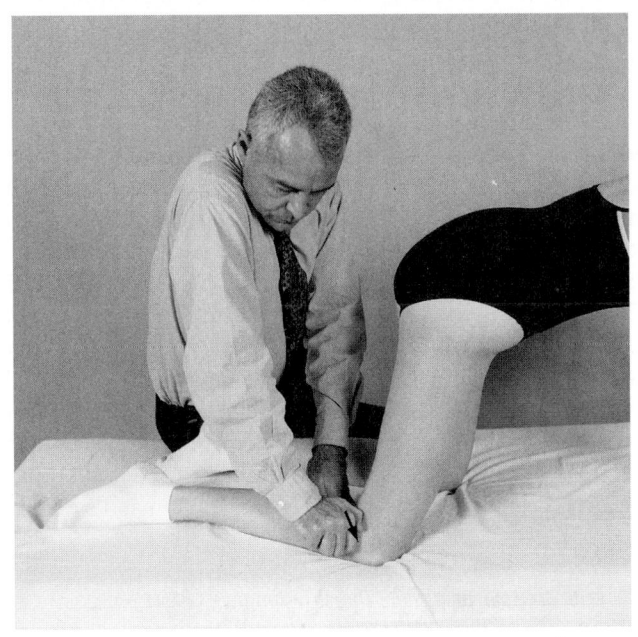

FIGURE 18-48 Mobilization of the proximal tibiofibular joint.

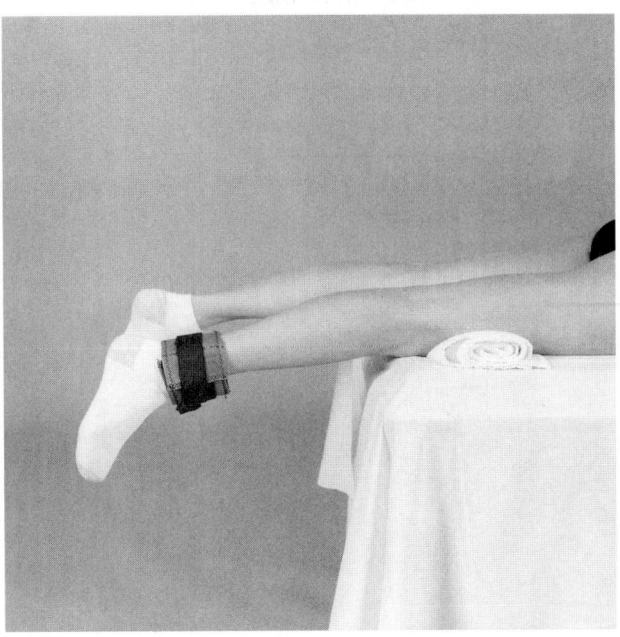

FIGURE 18-50 Prone hangs.

Automobilizations
To Increase Extension

▶ Towel hyperextensions. A towel of sufficient height to elevate the calf and thigh off the table is placed under the heel (Fig. 18-49). A weight can be added to the anterior tibia or femur to assist in regaining hyperextension at the knee.

▶ Prone hangs (Fig. 18-50).

▶ Quadriceps setting. These exercises are done repeatedly during the day, and can also be performed during the towel extension exercise.

▶ Standing extension (Fig. 18-51) with foot placed on a stool or chair.

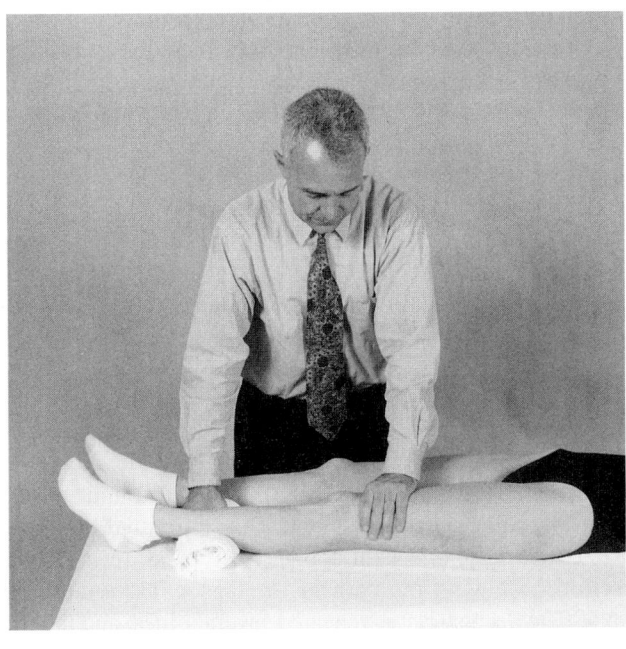

FIGURE 18-49 Towel hyperextensions.

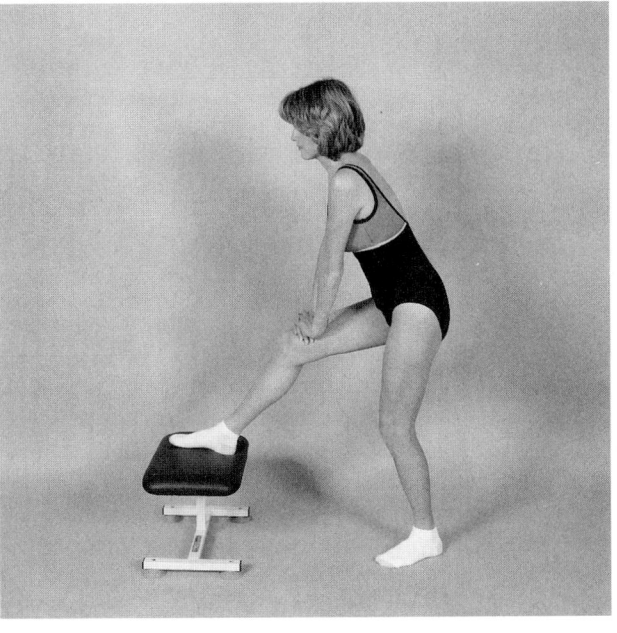

FIGURE 18-51 Standing extension.

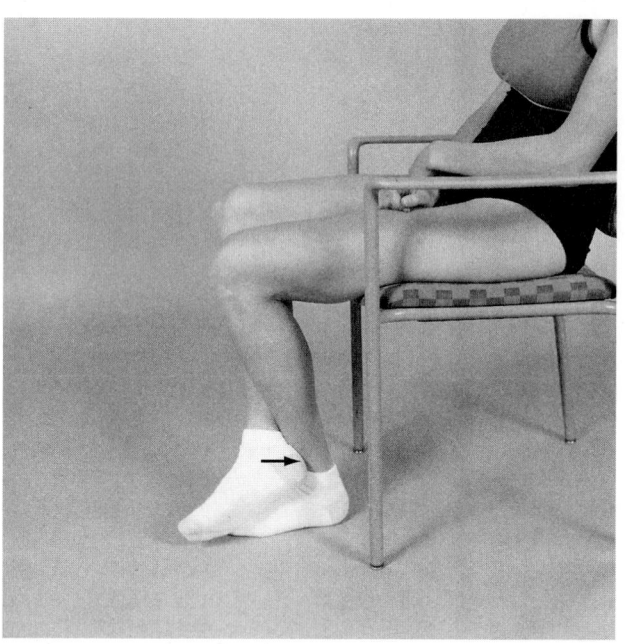

FIGURE 18-52   Seated heel slides with passive overpressure.

To Increase Flexion

▶ Wall slides in supine are performed until 90 degrees of flexion is obtained, and then seated heel slides with passive overpressure are initiated (Fig. 18-52).

▶ The patient is positioned supine, or sitting, with the hip flexed slightly above 90 degrees over a firm pillow or towel roll, which acts as the fulcrum. Using both hands, the patient grasps the anterior aspect of the lower leg, and interlaces the fingers. By gently pulling the lower leg posteriorly, flexion of the knee can be increased.

▶ The patient is positioned on all fours with the knee over a padded surface and with the foot positioned in inversion and plantarflexion. The patient attempts to hold the heel down with the right hand while trying to bring the buttock to the heel, at the same time maintaining the internal rotation.

Mobilizations With Movements[718]

Technique to Improve Knee Flexion.   The general rule when using mobilization with movement techniques (see Chap. 11) for knee pain is that the clinician glides medially for medial knee pain, and laterally for lateral knee pain.[718]

The patient is in the prone lying position, and the clinician stands on the contralateral side to the involved joint. A belt is placed around the clinician's waist and the patient's lower leg. The clinician stabilizes the patient's thigh with one hand, while the other hand supports the lower leg. The clinician glides the knee medially using the belt, while the patient is asked to flex the knee.

To apply a lateral glide, the clinician stands on the involved side and uses the belt in a similar fashion. A dorsal glide also can be attempted, if the medial or lateral glide is unsuccessful.

Alternative Technique.   The patient is positioned supine, with the involved knee flexed so that the foot is resting on the bed. The clinician stands on the involved side. A belt is placed around the patient's ankle and held by the patient. The clinician grasps the involved knee with both hands by interlacing the fingers and placing the heels of one hand over the tibial plateau and the heel of the other hand over the distal end of the femur. From this position, the clinician approximates the heels of the hands, thereby gliding the tibia in a posterior direction, while the patient attempts to actively flex the involved knee and apply overpressure into further flexion with the belt. The technique is repeated several times, and the range of motion and symptoms are reassessed.

High-velocity, Low-amplitude Thrust Techniques

Correction for a Posterior Fibular Head.[719]   The patient is positioned supine, with the clinician standing beside the table, opposite the dysfunction. The clinician grasps the patient's foot and ankle on the side of the dysfunction with the nonthrusting hand, and flexes the patient's hip and knee to 90 degrees. The clinician first places the index finger of his or her thrusting hand into the patient's popliteal crease, monitoring the dysfunctional fibular head. Next, the clinician locks the patient's foot on the side of the dysfunction in his or her armpit. The clinician then exerts a rapid downward thrust on the distal tibia and fibula while simultaneously pulling the fibular head anteriorly with his or her index finger.

Techniques to Increase Soft Tissue Extensibility

Increasing soft tissue extensibility is the hallmark of the functional knee rehabilitation protocol, and includes stretching of the iliotibial band, hamstring muscles, quadriceps, hip flexors, and Achilles tendon[175,297] (Table 18-13). The stretching techniques for the iliotibial band, hamstring muscles, quadriceps, and hip flexors are described in Chapter 17. The technique for the Achilles tendon is described in Chapter 19.

Patients with marked internal rotation of the hip may require stretching of the anterior hip structures to increase the available external rotation and to help the gluteal muscles work in the inner range.[430]

Soft Tissue Mobilization Technique for Tensor Fascia Latae

The patient is placed in the side-lying position, with the uppermost leg flexed at the hip to approximately 80 degrees, facing away from the clinician (Fig. 18-53). Using the thumbs of both hands, the clinician places them at the proximal end of the tensor fascia latae and then applies deep pressure in a caudal direction, following the path of the tensor fascia latae (Fig. 18-53). The deep stroke is repeated several times, and the flexibility of the tensor fascia latae is reassessed. The clinician also

TABLE 18-13 Muscle Stretching: Positions of Maximal Elongation and Stretch

Muscle	Maximal Elongation	Stretch
Gastrocnemius	Subtalar joint neutral, knee extension	Ankle dorsiflexion
Soleus	Subtalar joint neutral, knee flexion	Ankle dorsiflexion
Medial hamstrings	Hip external rotation, abduction, and flexion	Knee extension
Lateral hamstrings	Hip internal rotation and flexion	Knee extension
Rectus femoris	Hip extension	Knee flexion
Tensor fascia lata	Knee flexion, hip extension and external rotation	Hip adduction
Iliotibial band	Hip extension, neutral hip rotation, slight knee flexion	Hip adduction

can use the knuckle of the middle finger or the point of the elbow to apply the deep pressure, although care should be taken to avoid applying too much force.

Soft Tissue Mobilization of the Hamstring Area

The patient is positioned prone, with the knee supported in a flexed position. Using one hand, the clinician stabilizes the patient's upper hamstring area. The clinician uses the heel of the other hand while using the knuckle to apply a series of vertical strokes (Fig. 18-54). The clinician also can use the knuckle of the middle finger or point of the elbow to apply the deep pressure.

Myofascial Release Techniques

In each of the following techniques, the applied sustained pressure follows the tissues three-dimensionally, and is held for a minimum of 3 to 5 minutes, or until a softening or release occurs.

Myofascial Release of the Suprapatellar and Quadriceps Area. The patient is positioned supine. Using one hand, the clinician gently pushes the patella in a caudal direction, while pulling the quadriceps area cranially with the other hand.

Myofascial Release of the Infrapatellar Area. The patient is positioned supine. Using one hand, the clinician gently pushes the patella in a cranial direction, while pulling the posterior aspect of the lower leg caudally with the other hand.

Myofascial Release of the Triceps Surae Area. The patient is positioned prone, with the involved leg flexed at the knee and the foot resting on the clinician's shoulder. Using both hands, the

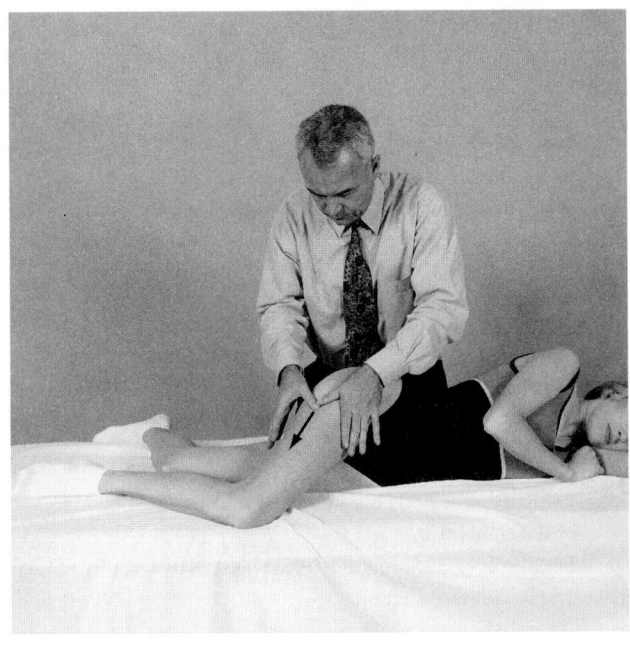

FIGURE 18-53 Soft tissue mobilization to the tensor fascia latae.

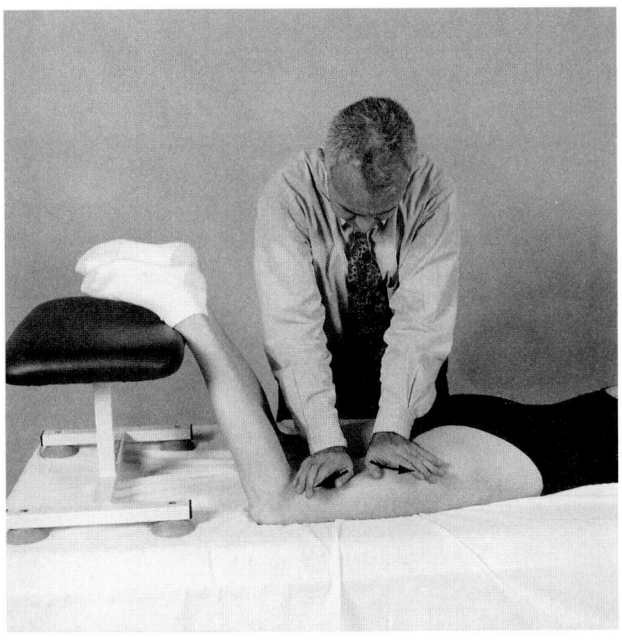

FIGURE 18-54 Soft tissue mobilization to the hamstrings.

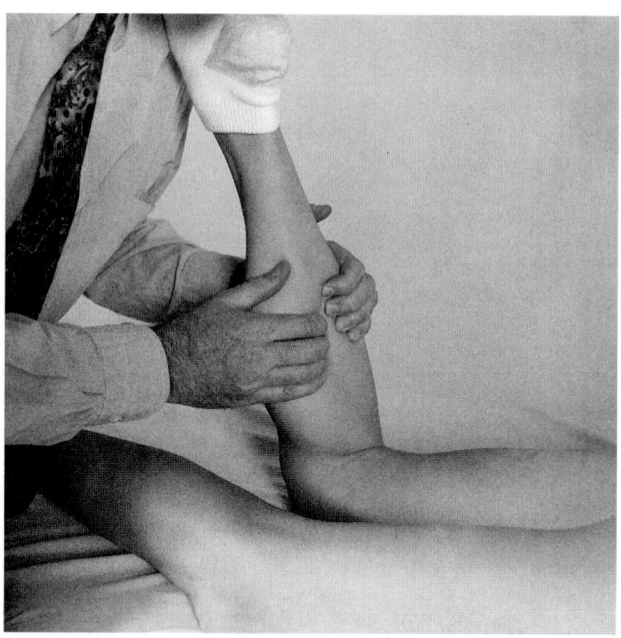

FIGURE 18-55   Myofascial release of the triceps surae.

clinician presses the fingers deep into the gastrocnemius area and spreads laterally (Fig. 18-55).

CASE STUDY MEDIAL KNEE PAIN

HISTORY

History of Current Condition

A 27-year-old man presented at the clinic with a sudden onset of intermittent right knee pain that began 2 weeks ago when the patient felt his right knee twist while descending stairs. The patient reported the sensation of "giving way," particularly when negotiating stairs, and occasional feelings of "locking" at the right knee. The pain was reportedly increased with activities involving bending of the right knee. The patient saw his physician, who ordered radiographs, diagnosed the condition as a possible medial meniscal tear, and prescribed a trial course of physical therapy. The patient also was issued a pair of crutches.

Past History of Current Condition

No past history of knee pain or problems.

Past Medical/Surgical History

Unremarkable.

Medications

None.

Imaging Studies

Radiographs were negative for loose bodies, tumors, and fracture.

Social Habits (past and present)

Nonsmoker and drinker; active lifestyle.

Social History

Single; living alone.

Family History

No relevant history of knee problems in family.

Living Environment

Single-story apartment.

Occupational/Employment/School

Full-time laborer; high school education.

Functional Status/Activity Level

Stiffness and soreness of the right knee were present on arising in the morning, although there was minimal swelling. Pain was increased with weight bearing, especially when walking on inclines or stairs. Swelling was increased by the end of the day, and after working.

Health Status (self-report)

The patient reported being in generally good health, but pain interfered with tasks at home and at work.

TESTS AND MEASURES

The physical examination of the patient included an inspection for muscle atrophy, palpation for areas of tenderness and crepitus, muscle testing of all major muscles, measurement of active and passive ranges of motion, and specific testing for medial meniscal tear (modified McMurray's, McIntosh, Apley's, Steinmann's tests) and instability (Lachman, pivot-shift tests).

Anthropometric Characteristics

The patient was 5 ft, 11 in, 180 lb. Girth measurements for the right quadriceps and vastus medialis obliquus were normal, compared with the other side. Minimal swelling was observed at the medial joint line.

Community and Work Integration/Reintegration

The patient reported working in a construction job that involved a lot of climbing, heavy lifting, and squatting.

Gait, Locomotion, and Balance

The patient was ambulating well on crutches, using weight bearing as tolerated.

Joint Integrity and Mobility

- Palpation revealed point tenderness along the medial joint line of the right knee.
- Passive accessory motions were decreased into flexion, compared with the other side.

Motor Performance: Strength, Power, Endurance

The physical examination revealed that the patient was only able to actively flex the knee to 60 degrees (see below). Normal strength was found between the ranges of 0 and 60 degrees of knee flexion.

Pain

Pain was rated at 8/10 with certain knee positions and with weight bearing.

Posture

Overall posture was good.

Range of Motion (including muscle length)

Active range of motion (ROM) for the right knee was 0 to 60 degrees of flexion. Passive knee flexion was measured at 70 degrees. When overpressure was applied at the end range, the same local pain was elicited, and a springy end-feel was detected. Active extension of the knee was full and pain free.

Active left lower extremity ROM was within normal limits.

Reflex Integrity

Normal and symmetric patellar and Achilles reflexes, bilaterally.

Sensory Integrity

Intact to light touch at L2 to S2, bilaterally.

EVALUATION

The patient was a young, active male with slight joint effusion, medial joint point tenderness, joint "locking" of the right knee, and pain with weight bearing, which resulted in functional limitations both at home and at work.

DIAGNOSIS BY PHYSICAL THERAPIST

Impaired joint mobility, motor function, muscle performance, and ROM associated with ligament or other connective tissue disorders of the right knee. Clinical findings indicated a possible medial meniscal tear of the right knee.

INTERVENTION

A trial course of conservative intervention was performed in an attempt to improve the patient's tolerance of normal home activities and work duty. The patient was instructed to avoid closed kinetic chain exercises and to restrict weight bearing during ambulation for 3 to 5 weeks.

Unfortunately, the patient did not respond well to the conservative approach. He was referred back to his physician and underwent a meniscectomy and meniscal repair (see Chap. 29 for discussion of these procedures).

CASE STUDY LEFT ANTERIOR KNEE PAIN

HISTORY

History of Current Condition[653]

A 30-year-old woman presented with a 2-month history of progressive anterior left knee pain. The pain had started insidiously 3 months after she began playing field hockey. She denied any traumatic inciting mechanism. The pain was increased with hyperflexion and weight-bearing activities, abated with rest, but seemed aggravated with prolonged sitting. The patient also noted difficulty achieving full knee extension and had intermittent swelling and stiffness. Previous trials of oral anti-inflammatories had only mildly improved her pain.

Past History of Current Condition

No previous history of knee surgery or injury.

Past Medical/Surgical History

Unremarkable.

Medications

None.

Other Tests and Measures

Radiographs were negative for loose bodies, tumors, and fracture.

Social Habits (Past and Present)

Nonsmoker and drinker; active lifestyle.

Social History

Single; living alone.

Family History

No relevant history of knee problems in family.

Growth and Development

Normal development; right-handed.

Living Environment

Two-story house.

Occupational/Employment/School

Full-time laborer; high school education.

Functional Status/Activity Level

The patient denied any locking of her left knee, although there had been occasions when she felt the knee give way because of pain. Pain increased with stair negotiation, particularly ascending stairs, and with prolonged sitting.

Health Status (Self-Report)

The patient reported being in generally good health, but pain interfered with tasks at home and at work.

QUESTIONS

1. What structure(s) do you suspect to be at fault in this patient and to require a specific examination?
2. What might the history of pain with prolonged sitting and stair negotiation tell the clinician?
3. What other activities do you suspect would increase the patient's symptoms? Why?

4. To help rule out the various causes of anterior knee pain, what other questions can you ask?
5. What is your working hypothesis at this stage? List the various diagnoses that could present with these signs and symptoms, and the tests you would use to rule out each one.
6. Does this presentation/history warrant a scan? Why or why not?

TESTS AND MEASURES

Because of the insidious nature of the patient's pain, a lower quarter scanning examination was performed that did not elicit any signs and symptoms of serious pathology, or overt neurologic compromise. The physical examination of the patient included an inspection for muscle atrophy, palpation for areas of tenderness and crepitus, muscle testing of all major muscles about the knee, measurement of active and passive ranges of motion (ROMs), and special tests.

Anthropometric Characteristics

The patient was 5 ft, 9 in, 165 lb. Girth measurements for the left quadriceps and vastus medialis obliquus revealed mild vastus medialis oblique atrophy compared with the other side. Inspection of the left knee revealed a 1+ effusion.

Community and Work Integration/Reintegration

The patient stated she worked at a desk job.

Gait, Locomotion, and Balance

The patient was ambulating with slight antalgic gait pattern, and an increased stance phase on the left.

Integumentary Integrity

Not tested.

Joint Integrity and Mobility

- Patella baja was noted.
- There was no crepitus.
- Special tests (including Lachman, anterior drawer, and varus and valgus stress testing at near 0 and 30 degrees of flexion, each) were negative. The McMurray test was positive on the left.

Motor Performance: Strength, Power, Endurance

There was weakness of the gluteus medius on the left. Hip external rotation was weaker on the left than on the right.

Pain

The left patellar tendon was contracted and tender. Tenderness also was noted over the medial and lateral patellar facets, anterior medial joint line, and popliteal fossa. The collateral ligaments, lateral structures, and hamstrings were not painful. Pain was rated at 8/10 with ascending stairs and after prolonged sitting.

Posture

Overall posture was good.

Range of Motion (including muscle length)

The left knee lacked 3 degrees of full extension and 10 degrees of full flexion. The left knee exhibited a positive J sign. Active right

lower extremity ROM was within normal limits. Bilateral flexibility deficits were found in the iliotibial band, gastrocnemius, and rectus femoris, but they were more marked on the left.

Reflex Integrity

Normal and symmetric patellar and Achilles reflexes, bilaterally.

EVALUATION

The patient was a young, active female with slight joint effusion, point tenderness, and pain with weight-bearing activities, including ascending stairs, which resulted in functional limitations both at home and at work.

DIAGNOSIS BY PHYSICAL THERAPIST

This patient appeared to have impairments of motor function, muscle performance, joint mobility, localized inflammation, and ROM. More specifically, the patient appeared to fall into the category of patellar pain with malalignment, with the presence of mild instability.

PROGNOSIS

Predicted Optimal Level of Improvement in Function

Over the course of 6 weeks, a trial course of conservative intervention was planned in an attempt to improve the patient's tolerance of normal home activities and work duty.

QUESTIONS

1. Having made the provisional diagnosis, what will be your intervention?
2. How would you describe this condition to the patient?
3. How would you explain the rationale behind your intervention to the patient?
4. What activities would you advise the patient to avoid? Why?
5. How will you determine the intensity of your intervention?
6. Estimate this patient's prognosis.
7. What modalities could you use in the intervention of this patient? Why?
8. Which manual techniques would be appropriate for this patient, and what is your rationale?
9. What exercises would you prescribe? Why?

Pain and Inflammation Control

Moist heat was applied to the knee prior to each session, and a cold pack was applied to the knee at the end of each session. Ice massage could also have been performed before and after activity.

Promotion and Progression of Healing

The malalignment and maltracking were addressed initially with taping, muscle stabilization, and electrical stimulation. Bracing would then have been used if these did not provide relief.

Exercise modification is one of the keys to a successful rehabilitation program, and the identification of the specific triggering mechanism is important. The ROM through which resistance did not promote discomfort was identified, and a strengthening program utilizing this pain-free range was devised.[139]

Specific Manual Techniques

A variety of specific manual stretching techniques were used to stretch the rectus femoris, iliotibial band, and gastrocnemius. Patellar mobilizations were used at the end ranges of flexion and extension.

Stretching of the lateral retinaculum was performed manually, following an application of ultrasound, and the patient was instructed in the stretching techniques to be performed at home.

Analysis and Integration of Open and Closed Kinetic Chains into Rehabilitation

The atrophy of the vastus medialis obliquus and strength deficit in the gluteus medius were both addressed. Both closed- and open-chain exercises were included in the protocol, making sure to stay in the safe ranges. Eccentric loading was encouraged during the rehabilitation process and incorporated into functional exercises of the five basic patterns of quadriceps activity[139]:

1. Isometric straight leg quadriceps setting and leg raising.
2. Isometric or isokinetic concentric knee extension.
3. Extensor thrust (squatting) pattern concentric work.
4. Isotonic eccentric work in a leg extension pattern.
5. Eccentric quadriceps work in an extensor thrust squatting pattern.

Control of Abuse and Force Loads: Stabilization and Flexibility

The intervention was initiated without an orthosis; if progress had not been made, the orthosis would have served as a second line of supplemental therapy.[139] Home exercises to stretch the iliotibial band, rectus femoris, and gastrocnemius were prescribed to complement the manual stretching program. Proximal and distal segment stretches were both included.

Maintenance of General Strength and Fitness

To maintain the patient's general level of fitness during the intervention period, use of an upper body ergometer was prescribed. Alternately, a stationary bike could have been used, avoiding the painful ranges by adjusting the seat height.

Neuromuscular Re-education

The specific control of the vastus medialis obliquus and the gluteus medius were addressed.

Patient Education

The patient was instructed in the use of moist heat and ice, and taping. The reasons for not exercising through the pain were discussed, and the patient was instructed to avoid deep-knee squatting or knee-bending activities in the immediate future.[9] Exercising of the vastus medialis obliquus was designed to occur in frequent but short exercise sessions spread throughout the day. A program of home stretching was also included.

Return to Function

A gradual return to function was implemented, based on the development of the specific neuromuscular skills for the patient's sports activities. Exercises to continue strengthening, flexibility,

and endurance training were maintained, and the patient was instructed to continue to use ice after activities.[9]

Frequency and Duration

Sessions were scheduled two to three times per week for 4 weeks.

Re-examination

Selected tests and measures were performed to evaluate patient's progress toward goals, in order to modify or redirect intervention if she failed to show progress.

Criteria for Discharge

Patient to be discharged when she reaches established functional goals, declines further intervention, is unable to progress toward goals because of complications, or when the clinician determines that she will no longer benefit from physical therapy services.

Coordination, Communication, and Documentation

The patient's status was communicated to the patient and her physician. Documentation included all elements of patient/client management. Discharge planning was provided.

Patient-related Instruction

Periodic reexamination and reassessment of the home program were scheduled, utilizing written instruction and illustrations. The patient was educated in proper postures, and in positions and motions to avoid at home and at work. The patient was also instructed in the benefits of an ongoing conditioning program to prevent reoccurrence of impairments.

CASE STUDY LATERAL KNEE PAIN WITH RUNNING

HISTORY

History of Current Condition

A 22-year-old male runner complained of lateral right knee pain that radiated from the lateral aspect of the knee, up the lateral thigh, and down to the proximal aspect of the lateral tibia. The pain was aggravated with running, especially on hills, and had begun about 6 weeks ago when he began training for a triathlon. The patient reported no pain with walking. The patient saw his physician, who prescribed a course of nonsteroidal anti-inflammatory drugs (NSAIDs) and recommended physical therapy.

Past History of Current Condition

No previous history of lower extremity pain.

Past Medical/Surgical History

Unremarkable.

Medications

Ibuprofen, 800 mg daily.

Functional Status/Activity Level

Pain was interfering with training for a triathlon. The patient also experienced pain with stair climbing.

Health Status (self-report)

The patient reported being in generally good health.

QUESTIONS

1. What structure(s) could be at fault with complaints of lateral knee pain aggravated with running?
2. What might the history of a gradual onset of pain related to a change in training tell the clinician?
3. Why do you think the patient's symptoms are worsened with running on hills, but not affected with walking?
4. What additional questions would you ask to help rule out referred pain from the lumbar spine?
5. What is your working hypothesis at this stage? List the various diagnoses that could present with these signs and symptoms, and the tests you would use to rule out each one.
6. Does this presentation/history warrant a scan? Why or why not?

TESTS AND MEASURES

The physical examination of the patient revealed an area of mild swelling over the left lateral femoral condyle. A slight dimpling of the skin was noted along the midline of the lateral length of the left thigh.

Gait, Locomotion, and Balance

Patient ambulated with evidence of a heel whip. The feet were held in slight external rotation throughout gait, with the right side more noticeable than the left. Excessive pronation was noted with gait and weight bearing, right side greater than left.

There was decreased static and dynamic balance on the right leg as evidenced by unilateral balance activities.

Motor Performance: Strength, Power, Endurance

- Lower extremity strength was rated at 5/5 for the major lower extremity muscles.
- Pain was elicited with resisted hip abduction.
- Hamstring dominance over the gluteus maximus was noted.

Orthotic, Protective, and Supportive Devices

The patient had never used any device but had been told that he had a leg-length discrepancy. Footwear analysis revealed excessive compression wear of the midsole.

Pain

- Pain was rated at 7/10 with running.
- Pain was elicited with resisted palpation of the lateral knee, tensor fascia lata, and gluteus medius.
- Slight crepitus was felt over the right femoral condyle with knee motion.
- There was a positive Noble compression test for pain.

Posture

- The patient's posture was very erect.
- The iliac crest on the right was lower by 1 inch.

- Relaxed calcaneal position demonstrated pronation bilaterally, with the right greater than the left.
- There was slight genu valgus, bilaterally.

Range of Motion (including muscle length)

Active right knee range of motion was within normal limits, compared with the uninvolved side. A painful arc was elicited at approximately 30 degrees of flexion with active knee extension. Other findings included:

- Decreased flexibility of the gastrocnemius, with active dorsiflexion limited to 0 degrees bilaterally when the foot was positioned in subtalar neutral and the knee extended.
- Decreased flexibility of the quadriceps bilaterally using Ely's test at 90 degrees of knee flexion.
- Decreased flexibility of the hamstrings bilaterally, as demonstrated with a straight leg raise of 70 degrees.
- A positive Thomas test with 20 degrees of hip flexion, and knee flexion at 40 degrees.
- A positive Ober test for decreased flexibility and pain, with the adducted leg measured at 5 inches from the table.

Reflex Integrity

Normal and symmetric Achilles and patellar reflexes, bilaterally.

Sensory Integrity

Intact to light touch at L2 to S1, bilaterally.

DIAGNOSIS BY PHYSICAL THERAPIST

Integration of Practice Patterns 4D and 4E: Impaired joint mobility, motor function, muscle performance, and range of motion associated with a ligament or other connective tissue disorder and with localized inflammation, specifically iliotibial band syndrome.

QUESTIONS

1. Having made the provisional diagnosis, what will be your intervention?
2. How would you describe this condition to the patient?
3. Why do you think the patient has the symptoms in one leg only?
4. How would you explain the rationale behind your intervention to the patient?
5. What activities would you advise the patient to avoid? Why?
6. How will you determine the intensity of your intervention?
7. Estimate this patient's prognosis.
8. What modalities could you use in the intervention of this patient? Why?
9. Which manual techniques would be appropriate for this patient, and what is your rationale?
10. What exercises would you prescribe? Why?

PROGNOSIS

Predicted Optimal Level of Improvement in Function

Over the course of 6 weeks, the patient was expected to demonstrate:

- Pain at 2/10 with activity.
- Active ankle dorsiflexion to at least 10 degrees.
- Ober test motion increased versus initial testing.
- Straight leg raise increased by 15 degrees versus initial evaluation.
- Return to prior functional level with stair negotiation.
- Normalized gait pattern with possible use of orthotics to correct pronation and leg-length discrepancy.
- Independence and compliance with the home exercise program.

PLAN OF CARE

Frequency and Duration

Sessions were scheduled two times per week for 4 weeks.

Re-examination

Selected tests and measures were performed to evaluate the patient's progress toward goals, in order to modify or redirect intervention if he failed to show progress.

Criteria for Discharge

Patient to be discharged when he reaches established functional goals, declines further intervention, is unable to progress toward goals because of complications, or when the clinician determines that he will no longer benefit from physical therapy services.

PHASE I (WEEKS 1 TO 3)

This phase typically involves two to four physical therapy sessions.

Goals

- Decreased inflammation, as evidenced by reduction of swelling, normalization of skin temperature, or decreased tenderness to palpation.
- Pain to be at 5/10 or less with activity.
- Increased flexibility, with the Thomas test showing 10 degrees of hip flexion and at least 50 degrees of knee flexion, and active ankle dorsiflexion demonstrated to at least 5 degrees in subtalar neutral, with the knee extended.
- Ober test showing adduction of the leg to within 3 inches of the table.
- Straight leg raise to be at 75 degrees.

Electrotherapeutic and Thermal Modalities

- Cryotherapy, as needed after activity.
- Deep or superficial thermal modalities used as needed prior to stretches and manual techniques.
- Iontophoresis.
- Pulsed or continuous ultrasound.

Therapeutic Exercise and Home Program

- Sustained stretching exercises for hamstrings, quadriceps, gastrocnemius, and iliotibial band.

- Strengthening exercises, to include partial squats, strides, and lunges in anterior and lateral directions.
- Walking, as tolerated.
- Use of an upper body ergonometer (UBE).

Manual Therapy

- Soft tissue techniques to tensor fascia latae and iliotibial band.
- Gentle passive stretching of hamstrings, quadriceps, gastrocnemius, and iliotibial band.

Neuromuscular Re-education

- Patient was issued a half-inch heel lift and instructed on its use.
- BAPS (Biomechanical Ankle Platform System) training was provided in the standing position, alternating speed and direction of rotation.
- Unilateral standing and reaching activities were taught, using the uninvolved leg to reach, as well as the upper extremities.
- Gait drills were performed, including walking backward; forward and backward balance beam walking; and cariocas.

PHASE II (WEEKS 4 TO 6)

This phase typically involves two to four physical therapy sessions.

Goals

- Resolution of inflammatory process, as evidenced by the elimination of tenderness to palpation.
- Pain to be at 0/10 with activity.
- Flexibility to be within 90 percent of accepted norms for straight leg raise, Ober, and Thomas tests.
- Static and dynamic balance to be equal to uninvolved side.
- Return to prior functional status and ready for progression of return to running.

Electrotherapeutic Modalities

Effective electrotherapeutic modalities were continued.

Therapeutic Exercise and Home Program

- Sustained static stretching of the muscles outlined in phase I.
- Dynamic stretching of hamstrings and gluteals using high marching drills and high-kicking drills.
- Squats to 90 degrees, as tolerated.
- Lateral rotation; posterior and posterolateral lunges.
- Step-ups and step-downs, progressing to jump-ups and jump-downs using appropriate step heights, ranging from 4 to 12 inches.
- Leg press.
- Leg extension.
- Leg curl.
- Agility drills, including shuttle runs, carioca on stairs, running and cutting drills in all directions, skipping, and backward running.

- Cardiovascular conditioning, including UBE, stationary bike, and stair-stepper, using multiple approaches and foot positions with the latter.
- Fitness walking progressing from level ground to hills and uneven terrain.

Manual Therapy

- Deep myofascial release to tensor fascia latae and iliotibial band.
- Continued stretching of muscles, as outlined in phase I.

Neuromuscular Re-education

- BAPS progression, including challenges of throwing and catching, ball dribbling, eyes closed, and speed and direction changes.
- Unilateral stance balance-and-reach drills.

OUTCOMES

The patient's outcome depends on adherence to the recommended home exercise program and intervention plan, as well as other recommended lifestyle changes. It is anticipated the patient will return to preinjury level in 6 weeks, without recurrence in the following year. The patient understands the strategies to prevent further functional limitations and to self-manage any minor recurrences.

CASE STUDY KNEE INJURY WITH RAPID SWELLING

HISTORY

History of Current Condition

A 22-year-old man experienced the sudden onset of right knee pain 2 weeks ago, when his right heel was planted while the rest of his body twisted to the left. The patient heard a loud pop and fell to the ground. The pain was excruciating and localized to the posterolateral aspect of the proximal tibia. The patient was initially unable to stand without assistance, and was seen by an orthopaedic surgeon the next day. A right anterior cruciate ligament (ACL) reconstruction has been scheduled. The patient had been seen at the clinic last week for a preoperative assessment; today's session was his second visit.

Past History of Current Condition

No past history of knee pain or problems.

Past Medical/Surgical History

Unremarkable.

Medications

Ibuprofen as needed for pain.

Social Habits (past and present)

Nonsmoker and drinker; active lifestyle.

Family History

No relevant history of knee problems in family.

Living Environment

Ranch-style house.

Occupational/Employment/School

College student.

Functional Status/Activity Level

Mild stiffness and soreness of the right knee on arising in the morning, with minimal swelling.

Health Status (self-report)

The patient reported being in generally good health.

TESTS AND MEASURES

The physical examination of the patient included an inspection for muscle atrophy, palpation for areas of tenderness and crepitus, muscle testing of all major muscles about the right knee, and measurements of active and passive ranges of motion (ROMs).

Gait, Locomotion, and Balance

The patient was ambulating well on crutches, using weight bearing as tolerated.

Integumentary Integrity

Not tested.

Joint Integrity and Mobility

- Positive Lachman test.
- Positive pivot-shift test.
- Positive anterior drawer test.
- Negative reverse pivot-shift, McMurray, Apley, and Slocum tests.
- Negative varus and valgus stress tests.

Motor Performance: Strength, Power, Endurance

The strength examination revealed overall strength of involved knee to be at 3+/5, although results may have been affected by pain.

Pain

Pain was rated at 7/10 with simple functional activities.

Posture

Overall posture was good.

Range of Motion (including muscle length)

ROM of the involved knee was grossly limited to the flexed open-packed position for the knee. The patient was unable to achieve terminal extension. Muscle lengths were not assessed secondary to pain.

DIAGNOSIS BY PHYSICAL THERAPIST

Pattern D: Impaired joint mobility, motor function, muscle performance, and range of motion associated with ligament or other connective tissue disorders of the right knee. Anterior cruciate ligament tear suspected.

INTERVENTION

Recent studies suggest that patients should undergo preoperative physical therapy, directed by experienced physical therapists, for a minimum of 3 to 4 weeks to obtain full ROM and knee strength, and to decrease the patient's postoperative knee joint stiffness and immobility.[540,720,721] During the preoperative sessions, the clinician should pay particular attention to the patient's gait, lower extremity strength, and ROM.

The primary healing potential of the ACL has been reported to be extremely poor in both clinical and experimental studies.[382,722–725] This is probably due to its minimal blood supply and the presence of joint fluid, both of which contribute to a reduced healing potential.[725–727] One study[727] did report two rare cases of spontaneous healing of an acute tear of the ACL, although the injuries were either near the origin, or near the insertion, of the ACL.

Patients with either partial (grades I and II) ACL tears (negative pivot shifts), or "isolated" ACL tears, who lead a less active lifestyle, and participate in linear, nondeceleration activities are considered to be candidates for conservative intervention.[458] To return to normal preinjury activity levels, however, patients must be thoroughly rehabilitated, and protective measures (e.g., knee bracing, and activity restrictions) must be taken to prevent further knee injuries. For these patients, a well-planned regimen of physical therapy is necessary, with the recovery period being approximately 20 weeks.

Conservative intervention for these patients does not mean "nonintervention," because these patients require aggressive treatment to decrease pain and swelling, protect the joint from further injury, regain motion, increase strength and endurance, and return to function.[458] Numerous lower extremity rehabilitation protocols following injury or surgery have been reported in the literature.[206,226,259,352,543,728–737] For the middle-aged and older athlete, physical therapy often is the treatment of choice, unless the patient plans to participate in sports activities that expose the knees to vigorous twisting forces. Certain sports activities, however, must be avoided, especially those involving jumping, quick starts and stops, and abrupt lateral movements (e.g., soccer, basketball).

ROM exercises, which are initiated as early as possible, must be performed carefully, so as not to further aggravate soft tissue injury, and prolong pain and effusion. Failure of the pain and effusion to resolve, and ROM to improve, should arouse suspicion of a displaced torn meniscus.[458]

Most authors stress the importance of strengthening the quadriceps, gastrocnemius-soleus, and hamstrings muscles to prevent, or minimize, atrophy and maintain or improve strength.[206,226,259,543,728–731,733,735,736,738] The strengthening exercises should be performed through a limited ROM, determined by patient tolerance and response to the exercises.[224,226,352,729,730,735,736] Others recommend closed-chain exercises,[236,543,729,735] to promote co-contraction of the thigh musculature and limit anterior tibial translation. A comprehensive knee rehabilitation protocol should include all of these factors.

PHASE I/PREOPERATIVE PHASE

Goals

- Control postinjury swelling.
- Obtain full active range of motion (AROM).
- Achieve normal gait pattern.

Electrotherapeutic Modalities

Cryotherapy is used to control inflammation and swelling.

Range of Motion Exercises and Home Program

ROM should be restored by the end of the acute phase, which typically lasts between 1 and 3 weeks.

Gait Training

Crutches are used until the patient is able to ambulate without a limp. Patients are encouraged to progress their weight bearing as tolerated. Once this is achieved, the clinician focuses on normalizing the gait pattern.

Gait analysis studies have demonstrated adaptive gait patterns that reflect "quadriceps avoidance" and "hamstring overuse."[290,458]

Strengthening Exercises and Home Program

Strength training begins once the patient has decreased swelling and has regained full AROM and a normal gait pattern. Exercises that cause anterior tibial translation (open-chain quadriceps femoris exercises) should be avoided to prevent undue stress on the secondary restraints, and to avoid patellofemoral symptoms.[458]

Neuromuscular retraining is an important component of the rehabilitative process, so that the patient can enhance neuromuscular control and dynamic stability of the joint.[739]

Education

It is extremely important that patients learn their activity limits so that a modification in lifestyle will avoid damaging activities.[458] Athletes are allowed to resume sports activities when they can perform all sports-specific skills required to the satisfaction of therapists and physicians.[740] Functional knee braces can be prescribed. Although studies seem to indicate that these braces provide little mechanical stability, they appear to improve confidence and proprioceptive awareness. If patients continue to experience knee instability or secondary knee injuries occur, patients may be required to modify their participation in sports activities or undergo surgical repairs to stabilize their knee joints.

REVIEW QUESTIONS*

1. Name a structure of the knee joint that is extra-articular and extrasynovial.
2. List three functions of the menisci.
3. Which peripheral nerve is primarily responsible for knee extension?
4. Anteversion of the hip may result in which knee deformity?
5. Which facet of the patella is likely to be involved if pain is reproduced at 20 to 30 degrees of knee flexion?

---

* Additional questions to test your understanding of this chapter can be found in the Online Learning Center for *Orthopaedic Assessment, Evaluation, and Intervention* at www.duttononline.net.

REFERENCES

1. Seebacher JR, et al. The structure of the posterolateral aspect of the knee. *J Bone Joint Surg* 1982;64A:536–541.

2. Clasby L, Young MA. Management of sports-related anterior cruciate ligament injuries. *AORN J* 1997;66:609–625, 628, 630; quiz 632–636.

3. Reinking MF. Knee anatomy and biomechanics. In: Wadsworth C, ed. *Disorders of the Knee: Home Study Course*. La Crosse, WI: Orthopaedic Section, American Physical Therapy Association; 2001.

4. Kirkendall DT, Garrett WEJ. The anterior cruciate ligament enigma. Injury mechanisms and prevention. *Clin Orthop* 2000;372:64–68.

5. Kapandji IA. *The Physiology of the Joints, Lower Limb*. New York, NY: Churchill Livingstone; 1991.

6. Tortora GJ, Anagnostakos NP. *Principles of Anatomy and Physiology*. 5th ed. New York, NY: Harper and Row; 1987:186–193.

7. Nordin M, Frankel VH. *Basic Biomechanics of the Musculoskeletal System*. 2nd ed. Philadelphia, Pa: Lea and Febiger; 1989.

8. Reider B, et al. The anterior aspect of the knee joint: an anatomical study. *J Bone Joint Surg* 1981;63A:351–356.

9. Bourne MH, et al. Anterior knee pain. *Mayo Clin Proc* 1988;63:482–491.

10. Wiberg G. Roentgenographic and anatomic studies on the femoropatellar joint. *Acta Orthop Scand* 1941;12:319–410.

11. Grelsamer RP. Patellar malalignment. *J Bone Joint Surg* 2000;82A:1639–1650.

12. Yoshioka Y, Siu D, Cooke TDV. The anatomy and functional axes of the femur. *J Bone Joint Surg* 1987;69A:873–879.

13. Brick GW, Scott RD. The patellofemoral component of total knee arthroplasty. *Clin Orthop* 1988;231:163–178.

14. Jouanin T, Dupont JY, Lassau FP. The synovial folds of the knee joint: Anatomical study. *Anat Clin* 1983;4:47.

14a. Irrgang JJ, Safran MC, Fu FH. The knee: Ligamentous and meniscal injuries. In: Zachazewski JE, Magee DJ, Quillen WS, eds. *Athletic Injuries and Rehabilitation*. Philadelphia, Pa: Saunders; 1996:623–692.

15. Gray H. The joints: Articulation of the lower limb. In: Clemente CD, ed. *Anatomy of the Human Body*. Philadelphia, Pa: Lea and Febiger; 1985:309–310, 397, 401.

16. Pick TP, Howden R. *Gray's Anatomy*. 15th ed. New York, NY: Barnes and Noble Books; 1995.

17. Gollehon DL, Torzilli PA, Warren RF. The role of the posterolateral and cruciate ligaments in the stability of the human knee. *J Bone Joint Surg* 1987;69A:233–242.

18. Lerat JL, et al. Knee instability after injury to the anterior cruciate ligament. Quantification of the Lachman test. *J Bone Joint Surg* 2000;82:42–47.

19. Markolf KL, Kochan A, Amstutz HC. Measurement of knee stiffness and laxity in patients with documented absence of the anterior cruciate ligament. *J Bone Joint Surg* 1984;66A:242–253.

20. Krauspe R, Schmidt M, Schaible HG. Sensory innervation of the anterior cruciate ligament. An electrophysiological study of the response properties of single identified mechanoreceptors in the cat. *J Bone Joint Surg* 1992;74A:390–397.

21. Beynnon BD, Good L, Risberg MA. The effect of bracing on proprioception of knees with anterior cruciate ligament injury. *J Orthop Sports Phys Ther* 2002;32:11–15.

22. Biedert RM, Stauffer E, Friederich NF. Occurrence of free nerve endings in the soft tissue of the knee joint. A histologic investigation. *Am J Sports Med* 1992;2:430–433.

23. Haus J, Halata Z, Refior HJ. Proprioception in the human anterior cruciate ligament. Basic morphology. A light microscopic, scanning and transmission electron microscopic study. *Zeitschr Orthop* 1992;130:484–494.

24. Johansson H, Sjolander P, Sojka P. Receptors in the knee joint ligaments and their role in the biomechanics of the joint. *Crit Rev Biomed Eng* 1991;18:341–368.

25. Beynnon B, et al. The measurement of anterior cruciate ligament strain in vivo. *Int Orthop* 1992;16:1–12.

26. Beynnon BD, et al. Anterior cruciate ligament strain behavior during rehabilitation exercises in vivo. *Am J Sports Med* 1995;23:24–34.

27. Canale ST, Tolo VT. Fractures of the femur in children. *Instr Course Lect* 1995;44:255–273.

28. Stanish WD, Lai A. New concepts of rehabilitation following anterior cruciate reconstruction. *Clin Sports Med* 1993;12:25–58.

29. Erikson E. Acute sports injuries: An introduction and brief overview. In: Harries M, et al, eds. *Oxford Textbook of Sports Medicine*. New York, NY: Oxford University Press; 1994:341.

30. Johnson RJ. Acute knee injuries: An introduction. In: Harries M, et al, eds. *Oxford Textbook of Sports Medicine*. New York, NY: Oxford University Press; 1994:342–344.

31. Arnoczky SP, et al. Anatomy of the anterior cruciate ligament. In: Jackson DW, et al, eds. *The Anterior Cruciate Ligament. Current and Future Concepts*. New York, NY: Raven Press; 1993:5–22.

32. Samuelson TS, Drez D, Maletis GB. Anterior cruciate ligament graft rotation: Reproduction of normal graft rotation. *Am J Sports Med* 1996;24:67–71.

33. Gomez-Barrena E, Munuera L, Martinez-Moreno E. Neural pathways of anterior cruciate ligament traced to the spinal ganglia. *Trans Orthop Res Soc* 1992;17:503.

34. Haut RC. The mechanical and viscoelastic properties of the anterior cruciate ligament and of ACL fascicles. In: Jackson DW, et al, eds. *The Anterior Cruciate Ligament. Current and Future Concepts*. New York, NY: Raven Press; 1993:63–73.

35. Kwan MK, Lin TH, Woo SLY. On the viscoelastic properties of the anteromedial bundle of the anterior cruciate ligament. *J Biomech* 1993;26:447–452.

36. Frank CB, Jackson DW. The science of reconstruction of the anterior cruciate ligament. *J Bone Joint Surg* 1997;79:1556–1576.

37. Takai S, et al. Determination of the in situ loads on the human anterior cruciate ligament. *J Orthop Res* 1993;11:686–695.

38. Butler DL, et al. Location-dependent variations in the material properties of the anterior cruciate ligament. *J Biomech* 1992;25:511–518.

39. Butler DL, Noyes FR, Grood ES. Ligamentous restraints to anterior posterior drawer in the human knee: A biomechanical study. *J Bone Joint Surg* 1980;62A:259–270.

40. Arnoczky SP. Anatomy of the anterior cruciate ligament. In: Urist MR, ed. *Clinical Orthopaedics and Related Research* Philadelphia, Pa: JB Lippincott; 1983:19–25.

41. Cabaud HE. Biomechanics of the anterior cruciate ligament. In: Urist MR, ed. *Clinical Orthopaedics and Related Research*. Philadelphia, Pa: JB Lippincott; 1983:26–30.

42. Kennedy JC, Hawkins RJ, Willis RB. Strain gauge analysis of knee ligaments. *Clin Orthop* 1977;129:225–229.

43. Bargar WL, et al. In vivo stability testing of post meniscectomy knees. *Clin Orthop* 1980;150:247–252.

44. Fleming BC, et al. The effect of weightbearing and external loading on anterior cruciate ligament strain. *J Biomech* 1999;34:163–170.

44a. Beynnon BD, Fleming BC. Anterior cruciate ligament strain invivo: A review of previous work. *J Biomech* 1998;31:519–525.

45. Fleming BC, et al. The strain behavior of the anterior cruciate ligament during stair climbing: An in vivo study. *J Arthrosc Rel Surg* 1999;15:185–191.

46. O'Connor JJ, Zavatsky A. Anterior cruciate ligament function in the normal knee. In: Jackson DW, et al, eds. *The Anterior Cruciate Ligament, Current and Future Concepts.* New York, NY: Raven Press; 1993:39–52.

47. O'Connor JJ, Zavatsky A. Anterior cruciate ligament forces in activity. In: Jackson DW, et al, eds. *The Anterior Cruciate Ligament, Current and Future Concepts.* New York, NY: Raven Press; 1993:131–140.

48. Beynnon BD, Johnson RJ, Fleming BC. The mechanics of anterior cruciate ligament reconstruction. In: Jackson DW, et al, eds. *The Anterior Cruciate Ligament Current and Future Concepts.* New York, NY: Raven Press; 1993:259–272.

49. Noyes FR, et al. Clinical biomechanics of the knee: Ligamentous restraints and functional stability. In: Funk FJ, Jr, ed. *American Academy of Orthopaedic Surgeon's Symposium on the Athlete's Knee.* St Louis, Mo: Mosby; 1980:1–35.

50. Kennedy JC, et al. Tension studies of human knee ligaments, yield point, ultimate failure, and disruption of the cruciate and tibial collateral ligaments. *J Bone Joint Surg* 1976;58A:350.

51. Markolf KL, Wascher DC, Finerman GAM. Direct in vitro measurement of forces in the cruciate ligaments. Part II: The effect of section of the posterolateral structures. *J Bone Joint Surg* 1993;75A:387–394.

52. Hughston JC, et al. Classification of knee ligament instabilities. Part 1. *J Bone Joint Surg* 1976;58A:159–172.

53. Merida-Velasco JA, et al. Development of the human knee joint ligaments. *Anat Rec* 1997;248:259–268.

54. Gray H. *Gray's Anatomy.* Philadelphia, Pa: Lea and Febiger; 1995.

55. Hughston JC, Jacobson KE. Chronic posterolateral rotatory instability of the knee. *J Bone Joint Surg* 1985;67A:351–359.

56. Tria AJ. *Ligaments of the Knee.* New York, NY: Churchill Livingstone; 1995.

57. Grood ES, et al. Ligamentous and capsular restraints preventing medial and lateral laxity in intact human cadaver knees. *J Bone Joint Surg* 1981;63A:1257–1269.

58. Greenfield B, Tovin BJ, Bennett JG. Knee. In: Wadsworth C, ed. *Current Concepts of Orthopaedic Physical Therapy.* La Crosse, Wis: Orthopaedic Section, American Physical Therapy Association; 2001.

59. Sudasna S, Harnsiriwattanagit K. The ligamentous structures of the posterolateral aspect of the knee. *Bull Hosp Joint Dis Orthop Inst* 1990;50:35–40.

60. Kaplan EB. The fabellofibular and short lateral ligaments of the knee joint. *J Bone Joint Surg* 1961;43A:169–179.

61. DeLee JC, Riley MD. Acute straight lateral instability of the knee. *Am J Sports Med* 1983;11:404–411.

62. Nicholas JA. Lateral instability of the knee. *Orthop Rev* 1977;6:33–44.

63. Terry GC, et al. How iliotibial tract injuries of the knee combine with acute anterior cruciate ligament tears to influence abnormal anterior tibial displacement. *Am J Sports Med* 1993;21:55–60.

64. Wroble RR, et al. The role of the lateral extraarticular restraints in the anterior cruciate ligament-deficient knee. *Am J Sports Med* 1993;21:257–262.

65. Watanabe Y, et al. Functional anatomy of the posterolateral structures of the knee. *J Arthrosc Rel Surg* 1993;9:57–62.

66. Barber FA, Click SD. Meniscus repair rehabilitation with concurrent anterior cruciate reconstruction. *Arthroscopy* 1997; 13:433.

67. Sutton JB. *Ligaments: Their Nature and Morphology.* London, England: MK Lewis; 1897.

68. Arnoczky SP, Warren RF. Microvasculature of the human meniscus. *Am J Sports Med* 1982;10:90–95.

69. Arnoczky SP, Warren RF, Spivak JM. Meniscal repair using an exogenous fibrin clot: An experimental study in dogs. *J Bone Joint Surg* 1988;70A:1209–1217.

70. Last RJ. The popliteus muscle and the lateral meniscus. *J Bone Joint Surg* 1950;32B:93–99.

71. Wallace LA, Mangine RE, Malone T. The knee. In: Gould JA, Davies GJ, eds. *Orthopaedic and Sports Physical Therapy.* St. Louis, Mo: Mosby; 1985:342–363.

72. Fritz JM, Irrgang JJ, Harner CD. Rehabilitation following allograft meniscal transplantation: A review of the literature and case study. *J Orthop Sports Phys Ther* 1996;24:98–106.

73. Jackson DW, et al. Meniscal transplantation using fresh and cryopreserved allografts. *Am J Sports Med* 1992;20:644–656.

74. Baratz ME, Fu FH, Mengato R. Meniscal tears: The effect of meniscectomy and of repair on intraarticular contact areas and stress in the human knee. A preliminary report. *Am J Sports Med* 1986;14:270–275.

75. Radin EL, Delamotte F, Maquet P. The role of the menisci in the distribution of stress in the knee. *Clin Orthop* 1984; 185:290–294.

76. Fukubayashi T, Kurosawa H. The contact area and pressure distribution pattern of the knee: A study of normal and osteoarthritic knee joints. *Acta Orthop Scand* 1980;51:871–879.

77. Kettlekamp DB, Jacobs AW. Tibiofemoral contact area: Determination and implications. *J Bone Joint Surg* 1972;54A: 349–356.

78. Seedholm BB, Hargreaves DJ. Transmission of the load in the knee joint with special reference to the role of the menisci—Part II. *Med Eng* 1979;8:220–228.

79. Shrive NG, O'Connor JJ, Goodfellow JW. Load bearing in the knee joint. *Clin Orthop* 1978;131:279–287.

80. Walker PS, Erkman MJ. The role of the menisci in force transmission across the knee. *Clin Orthop* 1975;109:184–192.

81. Ahmed AM, Burke DL. In vitro measurement of static pressure distribution in synovial joints: I. Tibial surface of the knee. *J Biomed Eng* 1983;105:216–225.

82. Anderson DR, et al. Viscoelastic shear properties of the equine medial meniscus. *J Orthop Res* 1991;9:550–558.

83. Arnoczky SP, et al. Meniscus. In: Woo SLY, Buckwalter JA, eds. *Injury and Repair of the Musculoskeletal Soft Tissues.* Chicago, Ill: American Academy of Orthopaedic Surgeons; 1987:487–537.

84. Bullough PG, Vosburgh F, Arnoczky SP. The menisci of the knee. In: Insall, JN, ed. *Surgery of the Knee.* New York, NY: Churchill Livingstone; 1984:135–146.

85. Rosenberg LC, et al. Articular cartilage. In: Woo SLY, Buckwalter JA, eds. *Injury and Repair of the Musculoskeletal Soft Tissues.* Chicago, Ill: American Academy of Orthopaedic Surgeons; 1988:401–482.

86. Morrison JB. The mechanics of the knee joint in relation to normal walking. *J Biomech* 1970;3:51.

87. Hall SJ. The biomechanics of the human lower extremity. In: *Basic Biomechanics*. New York, NY: McGraw-Hill; 1999:234–281.

88. Voloshin AS, Wosk J. Shock absorption of meniscectomized and painful knees. A comparative in vivo study. *J Biomed Eng* 1983;5:157–193.

89. Renstrom P, Johnson RJ. Anatomy and biomechanics of the menisci. *Clin Sports Med* 1990;9:523–538.

90. Markloff KL, et al. The role of joint load in knee stability. *J Bone Joint Surg* 1981;63A:570–585.

91. Smillie IS. *Injuries of the Knee Joint*. London, England: Churchill Livingstone; 1971.

92. Shields CL, et al. Evaluation of residual instability after arthroscopic meniscectomy in anterior cruciate deficient knees. *Am J Sports Med* 1987;15:129–131.

93. Wang CJ, Walker PS. Rotational laxity of the human knee. *J Bone Joint Surg* 1974;56A:161–170.

94. Levy M, et al. The effect of lateral meniscectomy on the motion of the knee. *J Bone Joint Surg* 1989;71A:401–406.

95. Levy M, Torzelli PA, Warren RF. The effect of medial meniscectomy on anterior-posterior motion of the knee. *J Bone Joint Surg* 1982;64A:883–888.

96. Bargar WL, et al. In-vivo stability testing of post-meniscectomy knees. *Clin Orthop* 1980;150:247–252.

97. Hsieh HH, Walker PS. Stabilizing mechanisms of the loaded and unloaded knee joint. *J Bone Joint Surg* 1976;58A:87–93.

98. Sullivan D, et al. Medial restraints to anterior-posterior motion of the knee. *J Bone Joint Surg* 1984;66A:930–936.

99. Thompson WO, Fu FH. The meniscus in the cruciate-deficient knee. *Clin Sports Med* 1993;12:771–796.

100. Kapandji IA. *The Physiology of Joints, Lower Limb*. 2nd ed. Vol. 2. New York, NY: Churchill Livingstone; 1970.

101. Norkin C, Levangie P. *Joint Structure and Function: A Comprehensive Analysis*. Philadelphia, Pa: FA Davis; 1992:355–358.

102. Thompson WO, et al. Tibial meniscal dynamics using three-dimensional reconstruction of magnetic resonance imaging. *Am J Sports Med* 1991;19:210–215.

103. Fullerton A. The surgical anatomy of the synovial membrane of the knee-joint. *Br J Surg* 1916;4:191–200.

104. Mayeda P. Ueber das Strangartige Gebilde in der Knigel—Enkhoehle (Chordi Cavi Artioularis Genu). Mitt Med. Fak, Kaisert University, Tokyo, 1918;21:507–553.

105. Hardaker WT, Whipple TL, Bassett FH III. Diagnosis and treatment of the plica syndrome of the knee. *J Bone Joint Surg* 1980;62A:221–225.

106. Zanoli S, Piazzai E. The synovial plica syndrome of the knee. Pathology, differential diagnosis and treatment. *Ital J Orthop Traumatol* 1983;9:241–250.

107. Aoki T. The "ledge" lesion in the knee. In: *Proceedings of the Twelfth Congress of Orthopaedic Surgery and Traumatology*. Amsterdam, Holland: Excerpta Medica; 1972:462.

108. Iino S. Normal arthroscopic findings in the knee joint in adult cadavers. *J Jpn Orthop Assoc* 1939;14:467–523.

109. Jackson RW, Marshall DJ, Fujisawa Y. The pathologic medial shelf. *Orthop Clin North Am* 1982;13:307–312.

110. Sakakibara J. Arthroscopic study on Iino's band (plica synovialis mediopatellaris). *J Jpn Orthop Assoc* 1976;50:513–522.

111. Johnson DP, Eastwood DM, Witherow PJ. Symptomatic synovial plicae of the knee. *J Bone Joint Surg* 1993;75A:1485–1496.

112. Gray DJ, Gardner E. Prenatal development of the human knee and superior tibiofibular joints. *Am J Anat* 1950;86:235–287.

113. Ogata S, Uhthoff HK. The development of synovial plica in human knee joints: An embryologic study. *Arthroscopy* 1990;6:315–321.

114. Johnson LL. *Diagnostic and Surgical Arthroscopy: The Knee and Other Joints*. St Louis, Mo: Mosby; 1981.

115. Dugdale TW, Barnett PR. Historical background: Patellofemoral pain in young people. *Orthop Clin North Am* 1986;17:211–219.

116. Fairbank JCT, et al. Mechanical factors in the incidence of knee pain in adolescents and young adults. *J Bone Joint Surg* 1984;66B:685–693.

117. Cox JS, Cooper PS. Patellofemoral instability. In: Fu FH, Harner, CD, Vince KG, eds. *Knee Surgery*. Baltimore, Md: Williams and Wilkins; 1994:959–962.

118. Warren LF, Marshall JL. The supporting structures and layers on the medial side of the knee. *J Bone Joint Surg* 1979;61:56–62.

119. Fulkerson JP, Gossling HR. Anatomy of the knee joint lateral retinaculum. *Clin Orthop* 1980;153:183–188.

120. Terry GC, Hughston JC, Norwood LA. The anatomy of the iliopatellar band and iliotibial tract. *Am J Sports Med* 1986;14:39–44.

121. Fulkerson JP. The etiology of patellofemoral pain in young, active patients: A prospective study. *Clin Orthop* 1983;179:129–133.

122. Fulkerson JP. Disorders of the patellofemoral joint: Evaluation and treatment. In: *Evaluation and Treatment of Injured Athletes Course*. Cape Cod, Mass: Boston University; 1993.

123. Insall JN. Chondromalacia patellae: Patellar malalignment syndrome. *Orthop Clin North Am* 1979;10:117–127.

124. Kramer P. Patellar malalignment syndrome: Rationale to reduce excessive lateral pressure. *J Orthop Sports Phys Ther* 1986;8:301–309.

125. Paulos L, et al. Patellar malalignment: A treatment rationale. *Phys Ther* 1980;60:1624–1632.

126. Lieb F, Perry J. Quadriceps function. *J Bone Joint Surg* 1968;50:1535.

127. Grelsamer RP, McConnell J. Normal and abnormal anatomy of the extensor mechanism. In: Grelsamer RP, McConnell J, eds. *The Patella: A Team Approach*. Gaithersburg, Md: Aspen; 1998:11–24.

128. Hallisey MJ, et al. Anatomy of the junction of the vastus lateralis tendon and the patella. *J Bone Joint Surg* 1987;69:545–549.

129. Bose K, Kanagasuntheram R, Osman MBH. Vastus medialis oblique: An anatomic and physiologic study. *Orthopaedics* 1980;3:880–883.

130. Koskinen SK, Kujala UM. Patellofemoral relationships and distal insertion of the vastus medialis muscle: A magnetic resonance imaging study in nonsymptomatic subjects and in patients with patellar dislocation. *Arthroscopy* 1992;8:465–468.

131. Raimondo RA, et al. Patellar stabilization: A quantitative evaluation of the vastus medialis obliquus muscle. *Orthopaedics* 1998;21:791–795.

132. Nakamura Y, Ohmichi H, Miyashita M. EMG relationship during maximum voluntary contraction of the quadriceps. Paper presented at Ninth Congress of the International Society of Biomechanics; 1983; Waterloo, Ontario.

133. Knight KL, Martin JA, Londerdee BR. EMG comparison of quadriceps femoris activity during knee extensions and straight leg raises. *Am J Phys Med* 1979;58:57–69.

134. Brownstein BA, Lamb RL, Mangine RE. Quadriceps torque and integrated electromyography. *J Orthop Sports Phys Ther* 1985;6:309–314.

135. Fox TA. Dysplasia of the quadriceps mechanism: Hypoplasia of the vastus medialis muscle as related to the hypermobile patella syndrome. *Surg Clin North Am* 1975;55:199–226.

136. Tria AJ, Palumbo RC, Alicia JA. Conservative care for patellofemoral pain. *Orthop Clin North Am* 1992;23:545–554.

137. Reynolds L, et al. EMG activity of the vastus medialis oblique and the vastus lateralis in their role in patellar alignment. *Am J Sports Med* 1983;62:62–70.

138. Moller BN, et al. Isometric contractions in the patellofemoral pain syndrome. *Arch Orthop Trauma Surg* 1986;105:24.

139. Reid DC. Anterior knee pain and the patellofemoral pain syndrome. In: Reid, DC, ed. *Sports Injury Assessment and Rehabilitation*. New York, NY: Churchill Livingstone; 1992: 345–398.

140. Larson RL, Jones DC. Dislocations and ligamentous injuries of the knee. In: Rockwood CA, Green DP, eds. *Fractures in Adults*. Philadelphia, Pa: JB Lippincott; 1984:1480–1591.

141. Gill DM, Corbacio EJ, Lauchle LE. Anatomy of the knee. In: Engle RP, ed. *Knee Ligament Rehabilitation*. New York, NY: Churchill Livingstone; 1991:1–15.

142. Kendall FP, McCreary EK, Provance PG. *Muscles: Testing and Function*. Baltimore, Md: Williams and Wilkins; 1993.

143. O'Connor JJ. Can muscle co-contraction protect knee ligaments after injury or repair? *J Bone Joint Surg* 1993;75B:41–48.

144. Fleming BC, et al. The gastrocnemius muscle is an antagonist of the anterior cruciate ligament. *J Orthop Res* 2001; 19:1178–1184.

145. Timm KE. Knee. In: Richardson JK, Iglarsh ZA, eds. *Clinical Orthopaedic Physical Therapy*. Philadelphia, Pa: Saunders; 1994:399–482.

146. Brownstein B, et al. Anatomy and biomechanics. In: Mangine, RE, ed. *Physical Therapy of the Knee*. New York, NY: Churchill Livingstone; 1988:1–30.

147. Magee DJ. *Orthopaedic Physical Assessment*. 2nd ed. Philadelphia, Pa: Saunders; 1992.

148. Reid DC. Knee ligament injuries, anatomy, classification, and examination. In: Reid DC, ed. *Sports Injury Assessment and Rehabilitation*. New York, NY: Churchill Livingstone; 1992:437–493.

149. Veltri DM, et al. The role of the cruciate and posterolateral ligaments in stability of the knee. A biomechanical study. *Am J Sports Med* 1995;23:436–443.

150. Veltri DM, et al. The role of the popliteofibular ligament in stability of the human knee. A biomechanical study. *Am J Sports Med* 1996;24:19–27.

151. Maynard MJ, et al. The popliteofibular ligament. Rediscovery of a key element in posterolateral stability. *Am J Sports Med* 1996;24:311–316.

152. Veltri DM, et al. Current status of allographic meniscal transplantation. *Clin Orthop* 1994;306:155–162.

153. Renne JW. The iliotibial band friction syndrome. *J Bone Joint Surg* 1975;57:1110–1111.

154. Evans P. The postural function of the iliotibial tract. *Ann R Coll Surg Engl* 1979;61:271–280.

155. Pease BJ, Cortese M. Anterior knee pain: Differential diagnosis and physical therapy management. In: *Orthopaedic Physical Therapy Home Study Course 92-1*. La Crosse, Wis: Orthopaedic Section, American Physical Therapy Association; 1992.

156. Vloka JD, et al. The division of the sciatic nerve in the popliteal fossa: Anatomical implications for popliteal nerve blockade. *Anesth Analg* 2001;92:215–217.

157. Wojtys EM, Huston LJ. Neuromuscular performance in normal and anterior cruciate ligament-deficient lower extremities. *Am J Sports Med* 1994;22:89–104.

158. Hollister AM, et al. The axes of rotation of the knee. *Clin Orthop* 1993;290:259–268.

159. Goodfellow J, O'Connor J. The mechanics of the knee and prothesis design. *J Bone Joint Surg* 1978;60B:358.

160. Boeckmann RR, Ellenbecker TS. Biomechanics. In: Ellenbecker TS, ed. *Knee Ligament Rehabilitation*. Philadelphia, Pa: Churchill Livingstone; 2000:16–23.

161. Blankevoort L, Huiskes R, De Lange A. The envelope of passive knee joint motion. *J Biomech* 1988;21:705–720.

162. Ishii Y, et al. Screw home motion after total knee replacement. *Clin Orthop* 1999;358:181–187.

163. Asai O. The combination method for diagnosis of meniscus lesion in the knee [O Asai, trans]. *Nippon Seikeigeka Gakkai Zasshi* 1981;7:625–633.

164. Kuriwaka Y. A biomechanical study of osteoarthritis of the knee with special reference to the rotatory movement of the knee joint [Y Kunuaka, trans]. *Nippon Seikeigeka Gakkai Zasshi* 1982;56:713–726.

165. Lafortune MA, et al. Three-dimensional kinematics of the human knee during walking. *J Biomech* 1992;25:347–357.

166. Tasker T, Waugh W. Articular changes associated with internal derangement of the knee. *J Bone Joint Surg* 1982;64B:486–488.

167. Eckhoff DG, et al. Automatic rotation (screw-home) in the cruciate deficient and prosthetic knee. *Trans Orthop Res Soc* 1996;21:216.

168. Schlepckow P. Experimental studies of the kinematics of the stable and unstable human knee joint [in German]. *Z Orthop Ihre Grenzgeb* 1989;127:711–715.

169. McGinty G, Irrgang JJ, Pezzullo D. Biomechanical considerations for rehabilitation of the knee. *Clin Biomech* 2000; 15:160–166.

170. Beynnon BD, et al. Chronic anterior cruciate ligament deficiency is associated with increased translation of the tibia during the transition from non-weightbearing to weightbearing. *J Orthop Res* 2002;20:332–337.

171. Desio SM, Burks RT, Bachus KN. Soft tissue restraints to lateral patellar translation in the human knee. *Am J Sports Med* 1998;26:59–65.

172. Dandy DJ. Chronic patellofemoral instability. *J Bone Joint Surg* 1996;78B:328–335.

173. Fulkerson JP. *Disorders of the Patellofemoral Joint*. Baltimore, Md: Williams and Wilkins; 1997.

174. Grelsamer RP, McConnell J. *The Patella: A Team Approach*. Gaithersburg, Md: Aspen; 1998.

175. McConnell J. Conservative management of patellofemoral problems. In: Grelsamer RP, McConnell J, eds. *The Patella: A Team Approach*. Gaithersburg, Md: Aspen; 1998:119–136.

176. Voight M, Weider D. Comparative reflex response times of the vastus medialis and the vastus lateralis in normal subjects and subjects with extensor mechanism dysfunction. *Am J Sports Med* 1991;10:131–137.

177. Cowan SM, et al. Delayed onset of electromyographic activity of vastus medialis obliquus relative to vastus lateralis in subjects with patellofemoral pain syndrome. *Arch Phys Med Rehab* 2001;82:183–189.

178. Ahmed AM, Burke DL, Hyder A. Force analysis of the patellar mechanism. *J Orthop Res* 1987;5:69–85.

179. Hodges PW, Richardson CA. Inefficient muscular stabilization of the lumbar spine associated with low back pain. *Spine* 1996;21:2640–2650.

180. Insall JN, Falvo KA, Wise DW. Chondromalacia patellae. A prospective study. *J Bone Joint Surg* 1976;58A:1–8.

181. Grana WA, Kriegshauser LA. Scientific basis of extensor mechanism disorders. *Clin Sports Med* 1985;4:247–257.

182. Hughston JC, Walsh WM, Puddu G. Patellar subluxation and dislocation. In: *Saunders Monographs in Clinical Orthopaedics.* Philadelphia, Pa: Saunders; 1984.

183. Brattström H. Shape of the intercondylar groove normally and in recurrent dislocation of the patella. *Acta Orthop Scand Suppl* 1964;68:1–48.

184. Aglietti P, Insall JN, Cerulli G. Patellar pain and incongruence. *Clin Orthop* 1983;176:217–224.

185. Horton MG, Hall TL. Quadriceps femoris muscle angle: Normal values and relationships with gender and selected skeletal measures. *Phys Ther* 1989;69:897–901.

186. Hsu RWW, et al. Normal axial alignment of the lower extremity and load-bearing distribution at the knee. *Clin Orthop* 1990;255:215–227.

187. Woodland LH, Francis RS. Parameters and comparisons of the quadriceps angle of college aged men and women in the supine and standing positions. *Am J Sports Med* 1992;20: 208–211.

188. Kernozek TW, Greer NL. Quadriceps angle and rearfoot motion: Relationships in walking. *Arch Phys Med Rehab* 1993;74: 407–410.

189. Cox JS. Patellofemoral problems in runners. *Clin J Sports Med* 1985;4:699–715.

190. Percy EC, Strother RT. Patellalgia. *Phys Sportsmed* 1985; 13:43–59.

191. Carson WG. Diagnosis of extensor mechanism disorders. *Clin Sports Med* 1985;4:231–246.

192. Olerud C, Berg P. The variation of the quadriceps angle with different positions of the foot. *Clin Orthop* 1984;191:162–165.

193. Harrison MM, et al. Patterns of knee arthrosis and patellar subluxation. *Clin Orthop* 1994;309:56–63.

194. Rand JA. The patellofemoral joint in total knee arthroplasty. *J Bone Joint Surg* 1994;76A:612–620.

195. Aglietti P, et al. A new patella prosthesis. *Clin Orthop* 1975;107:175–187.

196. Goodfellow JW, Hungerford DS, Woods C. Patellofemoral joint mechanics and pathology: I and II. *J Bone Joint Surg* 1976; 58B:287–299.

197. Kaufer H. Patellar biomechanics. *Clin Orthop* 1979;144: 51–54.

198. McConnell J, Fulkerson JP. The knee: Patellofemoral and soft tissue injuries. In: Zachazewski JE, Magee DJ, Quillen WS, eds. *Athletic Injuries and Rehabilitation.* Philadelphia, Pa: Saunders; 1996:693–728.

199. Hehne HJ. Biomechanics of the patellofemoral joint and its clinical relevance. *Clin Orthop* 1990;258:73–85.

200. Huberti HH, Hayes WC. Patellofemoral contact pressures. The influence of Q-angle and tendofemoral contact. *J Bone Joint Surg* 1984;66A:715–724.

201. Huberti HH, et al. Force ratios in the quadriceps tendon and ligamentum patellae. *J Orthop Res* 1984;21:49–54.

202. Fujikawa K, Seedholm BB, Wright V. Biomechanics of the patellofemoral joint. Parts 1 and 2. Study of the patellofemoral compartment and movement of the patella. *Eng Med* 1983; 12:3–21.

203. Kwak SD, et al. Anatomy of the human patellofemoral joint articular cartilage: Surface curvature analysis. *J Orthop Res* 1997;15:468–472.

204. Bishop RED, Denham RA. A note on the ratio between tensions in the quadriceps tendon and infrapatellar ligament. *Eng Med* 1977;6:53–54.

205. Buff HU, Jones JC, Hungerford DS. Experimental determination of forces transmitted through the patello-femoral joint. *J Biomech* 1988;21:17–23.

206. Pevsner DN, Johnson JRG, Blazina ME. The patellofemoral joint and its implications in the rehabilitation of the knee. *Phys Ther* 1979;59:869–874.

207. McDonald DA, Hutton JF, Kelly IG. Maximal isometric patellofemoral contact force in patients with anterior knee pain. *J Bone Joint Surg* 1989;71B:296–299.

208. Reilly DT, Martens M. Experimental analysis of the quadriceps muscle force and patello-femoral joint reaction force for various activities. *Acta Orthop Scand* 1972;43:126–137.

209. Heywood WB. Recurrent dislocation of the patella. *J Bone Joint Surg* 1961; 43B:508–517.

210. Hvid I, Andersen L, Schmidt H. Chondromalacia patellae: The relation to abnormal patellofemoral joint mechanics. *Acta Orthop Scand* 1981;52:661–666.

211. Fulkerson JP, Arendt EA. Anterior knee pain in females. *Clin Orthop* 2000;372:69–73.

212. Fulkerson JP, et al. Histologic evidence of retinacular nerve injury associated with patellofemoral malalignment. *Clin Orthop* 1985;197:196–205.

213. Lloyd-Robert GC, Thomas TG. The etiology of quadriceps contracture in children. *J Bone Joint Surg* 1964;46B:498–502.

214. Heegaard J, et al. Influence of soft structures on patellar three-dimensional tracking. *Clin Orthop* 1994;299:235–243.

215. Van Kampen A, Huiskes R. The three-dimensional tracking pattern of the human patella. *J Orthop Res* 1990;8:372–382.

216. Ateshian GA, et al. A stereophotogrammetric method for determining in situ contact areas in diarthrodial joints, and a comparison with other methods. *J Biomech* 1994;27:111–124.

217. Carson WG, et al. Patellofemoral disorders: Physical and radiographic examination. Part I. Physical examination. *Clin Orthop* 1984;185:178–186.

218. Insall JN. Patellar pain: Current concepts review. *J Bone Joint Surg* 1982;64A:147–152.

219. Steindler A. *Kinesiology of the Human Body under Normal and Pathological Conditions.* Springfield, Ill: Charles C Thomas; 1955.

220. Kibler BW. Closed kinetic chain rehabilitation for sports injuries. *Phys Med Rehabil North Am* 2000;11:369–384.

221. Irrgang JJ, Rivera J. Closed kinetic chain exercises for the lower extremity: Theory and application. *Sports Physical Therapy Section Home Study Course: Current Concepts in Rehabilitation of the Knee.* LaCrosse, WI: The Sports Physical Therapy Section; 1994.

222. Tiberio D. The effect of excessive subtalar joint pronation on patellofemoral mechanics: A theoretical model. *J Orthop Sports Phys Ther* 1987;9:160–165.

223. Arms SW, et al. The biomechanics of anterior cruciate ligament rehabilitation and reconstruction. *Am J Sports Med* 1984;12:8–18.

224. Henning CE, Lynch MA, Glick C. An in vivo strain gauge study of elongation of the anterior cruciate ligament. *Am J Sports Med* 1985;13:22–26.

225. Hungerford DS, Barry M. Biomechanics of the patellofemoral joint. *Clin Orthop* 1979;144:9–15.

226. Paulos LE, Noyes FR, Grood ES. Knee rehabilitation after anterior cruciate ligament reconstruction and repair. *Am J Sports Med* 1981;9:140–149.

227. Steinkamp LA, et al. Biomechanical considerations in patellofemoral joint rehabilitation. *Am J Sports Med* 1993; 21:438–444.

228. Escamilla RF, et al. Biomechanics of the knee during closed kinetic chain and open kinetic chain exercises. *Med Sci Sports Exerc* 1998;30:556–569.

229. Ariel BG. Biomechanical analysis of the knee joint during deep knee bends with heavy loads. In: Nelson R, Morehouse C, eds. *Biomechanics IV*. Baltimore, Md: University Park Press; 1974:44–52.

230. Dahlkvist NJ, Mayo P, Seedhom BB. Forces during squatting and rising from a deep squat. *Eng Med* 1982;11:69–76.

231. Nisell R, Nemeth G, Ohlsen H. Joint forces in extension of the knee. Analysis of a mechanical model. *Acta Orthop Scand* 1986;57:41–46.

232. Meglan D, Lutz G, Stuart M. Effects of closed chain exercises for ACL rehabilitation upon the load in the capsule and ligamentous structures of the knee. *Orthop Trans* 1993; 17:719–720.

233. Andrews JG, Nay JG, Vaughan CL. Knee shear forces during a squat exercise using a barbell and a weight machine. In: Matsui H, Kobayashi K, eds. *Biomechanics VIII-B*. Champaign, Ill: Human Kinetics; 1983:923–927.

234. Harttin HC, Pierrynowski MR, Ball KA. Effect of load, cadence, and fatigue on tibio-femoral joint force during a half squat. *Med Sci Sports Exerc* 1989;21:613–618.

235. Stuart MJ, et al. Comparison of intersegmental tibiofemoral joint forces and muscle activity during various closed kinetic chain exercises. *Am J Sports Med* 1996;24:792–799.

236. Palmitier RA, et al. Kinetic chain exercises in knee rehabilitation. *Sports Med* 1991;11:402–413.

237. Ohkoshi Y, et al. Biomechanical analysis of rehabilitation in the standing position. *Am J Sports Med* 1991;19:605–611.

238. Beynnon BD, et al. The strain behavior of the anterior cruciate ligament during squatting and active flexion and extension: A comparison of an open and a closed kinetic chain exercise. *Am J Sports Med* 1997;25:823–829.

239. Grelsamer RP, McConnell J. Applied mechanics of the patellofemoral joint. In: Grelsamer RP, McConnell J, eds. *The Patella: A Team Approach*. Gaithersburg, Md: Aspen; 1998:25–41.

240. Grood ES, et al. Biomechanics of the knee extension exercise. *J Bone Joint Surg* 1984;66A:725–734.

241. Yasuda K, Sadaki T. Exercise after anterior cruciate ligament reconstruction: The force exerted on the tibia by the separate isometric contractions of the quadriceps of the hamstrings. *Clin Orthop* 1987;220:275–283.

242. Kaufman KR, et al. Dynamic joint forces during knee isokinetic exercise. *Am J Sports Med* 1991;19:305–316.

243. Yack HJ, Collins CE, Whieldon TJ. Comparison of closed and open kinetic chain exercise in the anterior cruciate ligament-deficient knee. *Am J Sports Med* 1993;21:49–54.

244. Lutz GE, et al. Comparison of tibiofemoral joint forces during open-kinetic-chain and closed-kinetic-chain exercises. *J Bone Joint Surg* 1993;75A:732–739.

245. Nisell R, Ekholm J. Joint load during the parellel squat in powerlifting and force analysis of in vivo bilateral quadriceps tendon rupture. *Scand J Sports Sci* 1986;8:63–70.

246. Sawhney R, et al. Quadriceps exercise following anterior cruciate ligament reconstruction without anterior tibial translation. Paper presented at American Conference of the American Physical Therapy Association; 1990; Anaheim, Calif.

247. Clancy WG. Evaluation of acute knee injuries. In: Finerman G, ed. *American Association of Orthopaedic Surgeons, Symposium on Sports Medicine: The Knee*. St Louis, Mo: Mosby; 1985:185–193.

248. Solomon DH, et al. The rational clinical examination. Does this patient have a torn meniscus or ligament of the knee? Value of the physical examination. *JAMA* 2001;286:1610–1620.

249. Bloom MH. Differentiating between meniscal and patellar pain. *Phys Sports Med* 1989;17:95–108.

250. Safran MR, Fu FH. Uncommon causes of knee pain in the athlete. *Orthop Clin North Am* 1995;26:547–559.

251. Fahrer H, et al. Knee effusion and reflex inhibition of the quadriceps. *J Bone Joint Surg* 1988;70B:635–638.

252. Dieppe P. The classification and diagnosis of osteoarthritis. In: Kuettner KE, Goldberg WM, eds. *Osteoarthritic Disorders*. Rosemont, Ill: American Academy of Orthopaedic Surgeons; 1995:5–12.

253. Sisk TD. Knee injuries. In: Crenshaw AH, ed. *Campbell's Operative Orthopaedics*. St Louis, Mo: Mosby; 1987:2283–2496.

254. Boden BP, et al. Patellofemoral instability: evaluation and management. *J Am Acad Orthop Surg* 1997;5:47–57.

255. Brody LT, Thein JM. Nonoperative treatment for patellofemoral pain. *J Orthop Sports Phys Ther* 1998;28:336–344.

256. Ficat P, Hungerford DS. *Disorders of the Patellofemoral Joint*. Baltimore, Md: Williams and Wilkins; 1977.

257. Grelsamer RP, McConnell J. Examination of the patellofemoral joint. In: Grelsamer RP, McConnell J, eds. *The Patella: A Team Approach*. Gaithersburg, Md: Aspen; 1998:109–118.

258. Shellock FG, et al. Patellofemoral joint: Identification of abnormalities using active movement, "unloaded" vs "loaded" kinematic MR imaging techniques. *Radiology* 1993;188:575–578.

259. Zappala FG, Taffel CB, Scuderi GR. Rehabilitation of patellofemoral joint disorders. *Orthop Clin North Am* 1992; 23:555–565.

260. Bentley G, Dowd G. Current concepts of etiology and treatment of chondromalacia patella. *Clin Orthop* 1984;189:209.

261. Insall JN. Patella pain syndromes and chondromalacia patellae. *Inst Course Lect* 1981;30:342–356.

262. Kummel B. The treatment of patellofemoral problems. *Prim Care* 1980;7:217–229.

263. Karlson S. Chondromalacia patellae. *Acta Chir Scand* 1940;83:347–381.

264. McConnell J. Fat pad irritation: A mistaken patellar tendinitis. *Sports Health* 1991;9:7–9.

265. Winkel D, Matthijs O, Phelps V. *Examination of the Knee. Diagnosis and Treatment of the Lower Extremities*. Gaithersburg, Md: Aspen; 1997:166–197.

266. James SL. Chondromalacia patella. In: Kennedy JC, ed. *The Injured Adolescent Knee*. Baltimore, Md: Williams and Wilkins; 1979:46–60.

267. Wallace L. *Lower Quarter Pain: Mechanical Evaluation and Treatment*. Cleveland, Ohio: Western Reserve Publishers; 1984.

268. Wallace L. Rehabilitation following patellofemoral surgery. In: Davies GJ, ed. *Rehabilitation of the Surgical Knee*. Ronkonkoma, NY: Cypress; 1984:60–62.

269. Sahrmann SA. Movement impairment syndromes of the hip. In: Sahrmann SA, ed. *Movement Impairment Syndromes*. St Louis, Mo: Mosby; 2001:121–191.

270. Larson RL. Subluxation-dislocation of the patella. In: Kennedy JC, ed. *The Injured Adolescent Knee*. Baltimore, Md: Williams and Wilkins; 1979.

271. Post WR. Clinical evaluation of patients with patellofemoral disorders. *Arthroscopy* 1999;15:841–851.

272. Holmes SWJ, Clancy WGJ. Clinical classification of patellofemoral pain and dysfunction. *J Orthop Sports Phys Ther* 1998;28:299–306.

273. Merchant AC. Classification of patellofemoral disorders. *Arthroscopy* 1988;4:235–240.

274. Eckhoff DG, et al. Knee version associated with anterior knee pain. *Clin Orthop* 1997;339:152–155.

275. Eckhoff DG, et al. Version of the osteoarthritic knee. *J Arthroplasty* 1994;9:73–80.

276. Takai S, et al. Rotational alignment of the lower limb in osteoarthritis of the knee. *Int Orthop (SICOT)* 1985;9:209–216.

277. Yagi T, Sasaki T. Tibial torsion in patients with medial-type osteoarthritic knee. *Clin Orthop* 1986;213:177–182.

278. Ficat P, Ficat C, Bailleux A. Syndrome d'hyperpression externe de la rotule (S.H.P.E.). *Rev Chir Orthop* 1975;61:39–59.

279. Insall JN, Goldberg V, Salvati E. Recurrent dislocation and the high-riding patella. *Clin Orthop* 1972;88:67–69.

280. James SL, Bates BT, Osternig LR. Injuries to runners. *Am J Sports Med* 1978;6:40–49.

281. Sammarco GJ, Hockenbury RT. Biomechanics of the foot and ankle. In: Frankel VH, Nordin M, eds. *Basic Biomechanics of the Musculoskeletal System*. Baltimore, Md: Williams and Wilkins; 2000.

282. Wright DG, Desai SM, Henderson WH. Action of the subtalar and ankle joint complex during stance phase of walking. *J Bone Joint Surg* 1964;46A:361–382.

283. Maquet PG. *Biomechanics of the Knee*. New York, NY: Springer-Verlag; 1984.

284. Dillon P, Updyke W, Allen W. Gait analysis with reference to chondromalacia patellae. *J Orthop Sports Phys Ther* 1983;5:127–131.

285. DeVita P, Hortobagyi T, Barrier J. Gait biomechanics are not normal after anterior cruciate ligament reconstruction and accelerated rehabilitation. *Med Sci Sports Exerc* 1998;30:1481–1488.

286. DeVita P, et al. Gait adaptations before and after anterior cruciate ligament reconstruction surgery. *Med Sci Sports Exerc* 1997;29:853–859.

287. DeVita P, et al. A functional knee brace alters joint torque and power patterns during walking and running. *J Biomech* 1996;29:583–588.

288. Winter DA. Biomechanical motor patterns in normal walking. *J Motor Behav* 1983;15:302–329.

289. Andriacchi TP, Birac D. Functional testing in the anterior cruciate ligament-deficient knee. *Clin Orthop* 1993;288:40–47.

290. Berchuck M, et al. Gait adaptations by patients who have a deficient anterior cruciate ligament. *J Bone Joint Surg* 1990;72A:871–877.

291. Andriacchi TP. Dynamics of pathological motion: Applied to the anterior cruciate deficient knee. *J Biomech* 1990;23(suppl 1):99–105.

292. Birac D, Andriacchi TP, Bach BR Jr. Time related changes following ACL rupture. *Trans Orthop Res Soc* 1991;16:231.

293. Mikosz RP, Andriacchi TP, Andersson GBJ. Model analysis of factors influencing the prediction of muscle forces at the knee. *J Orthop Res* 1988;6:205–214.

294. Mikosz RP, Wu CD, Andriacchi TP. Model interpretation of functional adaptations in the ACL-deficient patient. *Proc North Am Congr Biomech* 1992;2:441.

295. More RC, et al. Hamstrings: An anterior cruciate ligament protagonist. An in vitro study. *Am J Sports Med* 1993;21:231–237.

296. Renstrom P, et al. Strain within the anterior cruciate ligament during hamstring and quadriceps activity. *Am J Sports Med* 1986;14:83–87.

297. Wilk KE, et al. Patellofemoral disorders: A classification system and clinical guidelines for nonoperative rehabilitation. *J Orthop Sports Phys Ther* 1998;28:307–322.

298. Root M, Orien W, Weed J. *Clinical Biomechanics*. Vol. 2. Los Angeles, Calif: Clinical Biomechanics Corp; 1977.

299. Powers CM, Maffucci R, Hampton S. Rearfoot posture in subjects with patellofemoral pain. *J Orthop Sports Phys Ther* 1995;22:155–160.

300. Subotnick SI. The foot and sports medicine. *J Orthop Sports Phys Ther* 1980;2:53–54.

301. Barber-Westin SD, Noyes FR, Andrews M. A rigorous comparison between the sexes of results and complications after anterior cruciate ligament reconstruction. *Am J Sports Med* 1997;25:514–526.

302. Enneking WF, Horowitz M. The intra-articular effects of immobilization on the human knee. *J Bone Joint Surg* 1972;54A:973–985.

303. Schiowitz S. Diagnosis and treatment of the lower extremity: The knee. In: DiGiovanna EL, Schiowitz S, eds. *An Osteopathic Approach to Diagnosis and Treatment*. Philadelphia, Pa: JB Lippincott; 1991:330–346.

304. Cooper C, et al. Occupational activity and osteoarthritis of the knee. *Ann Rheum Dis* 1994;53:90–93.

305. Sachs RA, et al. Patellofemoral problems after anterior cruciate ligament reconstruction. *Am J Sports Med* 1989;17:760–765.

306. Benum P. Operative mobilization of stiff knees after surgical treatment of knee injuries and posttraumatic conditions. *Acta Orthop Scand* 1982;53:625–631.

307. Cosgarea AJ, DeHaven KE, Lovelock JE. The surgical treatment of arthrofibrosis of the knee. *Am J Sports Med* 1994;22:184–191.

308. Paulos LE, et al. Infrapatellar contracture syndrome. An unrecognized cause of knee stiffness with patella entrapment and patella infera. *Am J Sports Med* 1987;15:331–341.

309. Waldron VD. A test for chondromalacia patella. *Orthop Rev* 1983;12:103.

310. DeAndrade JR, Grant C, Dixon ASJ. Joint distension and reflex muscle inhibition in the knee. *J Bone Joint Surg* 1965;47A:313–322.

311. Stanton-Hicks M, et al. Reflex sympathetic dystrophy: Changing concepts and taxonomy. *Pain* 1995;63:127–133.

312. Jensen K, Graf BK. The effects of knee effusion on quadriceps strength and knee intraarticular pressure. *Arthroscopy* 1993;9:52–56.

313. Jones DW, Jones DA, Newham DJ. Chronic knee effusion and aspiration: The effect on quadriceps inhibition. *Br J Rheumatol* 1987;26:370–374.

314. Snyder-Mackler L, et al. Reflex inhibition of the quadriceps femoris muscle after injury or reconstruction of the anterior cruciate ligament. *J Bone Joint Surg* 1994;76A:555–560.

315. Stratford P. Electromyography of the quadriceps femoris muscles in subjects with normal knees and acutely effused knees. *Phys Ther* 1981;62:279–283.

316. Sprague NF III. Motion-limiting arthrofibrosis of the knee: The role of arthroscopic management. *Clin Sports Med* 1987;6:537–549.

317. Steadman JR, et al. Surgical treatment of arthrofibrosis of the knee. *J Orthop Tech* 1993;1:119–127.

318. Akeson WH, et al. The connective tissue response to immobility: Biochemical changes in periarticular connective tissue of the immobilized rabbit knee. *Clin Orthop* 1973;93:356–362.

319. Sahrmann SA. Diagnosis and treatment of muscle imbalances associated with regional pain syndromes. In: *Lecture Outline*. New Brunswick, NJ; 1991.

320. Segal P, Jacob M. *The Knee*. Chicago, Ill: Year Book; 1983.

321. Lieb F, Perry J. Quadriceps function: An anatomical and mechanical study using amputated limbs. *J Bone Joint Surg* 1968;50A:1535–1547.

322. Grelsamer RP, McConnell J. The history and physical examination. In: Grelsamer RP, McConnell J, eds. *The Patella: A Team Approach*. Gaithersburg, Md: Aspen; 1998:43–55.

323. Broom HJ, Fulkerson JP. The plica syndrome: A new perspective. *Orthop Clin North Am* 1986;17:279–281.

324. Laubenthal KN, Smidt GL, Kettelkamp DB. A quantitative analysis of knee motion for activities of daily living. *Phys Ther* 1972;52:34–42.

325. Bellamy N, et al. Validation study of WOMAC: A health status instrument for measuring clinically important patient-relevant outcomes following total hip or knee arthroplasty in osteoarthritis. *J Orthop Rheumatol* 1988;1:95–108.

326. Bellamy N. Outcome measurement in osteoarthritis clinical trials. *J Rheumatol* 1995;43(suppl):49–51.

327. Bellamy N, et al. Validation study of WOMAC: A health status instrument for measuring clinically important patient relevant outcomes to antirheumatic drug therapy in patients with osteoarthritis of the hip or knee. *J Rheumatol* 1988;15:1833–1840.

328. McConnell S, Kolopack P, Davis AM. The Western Ontario and McMaster Universities Osteoarthritis Index (WOMAC): A review of its utility and measurement properties. *Arthritis Rheum* 2001;45:453–461.

329. Lysholm J, Gilquist J. Evaluation of knee ligament surgery results with special emphasis on the use of a scoring scale. *Am J Sports Med* 1982;10:150–154.

330. Manske R, Vequist SW. Examination of the knee with special and functional testing. In: Wadsworth C, ed. *Disorders of the Knee—Home Study Course*. La Crosse, Wis: Orthopaedic Section, American Physical Therapy Association; 2001.

331. Tegner Y, Lysholm J. Rating systems in the evaluation of knee ligament injuries. *Clin Orthop* 1985;198:43–49.

332. Irrgang JJ, et al. Development of a patient-reported measure of function of the knee. *J Bone Joint Surg* 1998;80A:1132–1145.

332a. Karlson J, Thomee R, Sward L. Eleven year follow-up of patellofemoral pain syndromes. *Clin J Sports Med* 1996;6:23.

333. Strobel M, Stedtfeld HW. *Diagnostic Evaluation of the Knee*. Berlin, Germany: Springer-Verlag; 1990.

334. Wilson G, Murphy A. The efficacy of isokinetic, isometric and vertical jump tests in exercise science. *Aust J Sci Med Sport* 1995;27:20–24.

335. Curl WW, Markey KL, Mitchell WA. Agility training following anterior cruciate ligament reconstruction. *Clin Orthop* 1983; 172:133–136.

336. Delitto A, et al. Relationship of isokinetic quadriceps peak torque and work to one-legged hop and vertical jump in ACL reconstructed subjects. *Phys Ther* 1993;73:S85.

337. Bolga LA, Keskula DR. Reliability of lower extremity functional performance tests. *J Orthop Sports Phys Ther* 1997;26:138.

338. Barber SD, et al. Quantitative assessment of functional limitations in normal and anterior cruciate ligament-deficient knees. *Clin Orthop* 1990;255:204–214.

339. Blackburn JR, Morrissey MC. The relationship between open and closed kinetic chain strength of the lower limb and jumping performance. *J Orthop Sports Phys Ther* 1998;27:430–435.

340. Fitzgerald GK, et al. Hop tests as predictors of dynamic knee stability. *J Orthop Sports Phys Ther* 2001;31:588–597.

341. Booher LD, et al. Reliability of three single hop tests. *J Sports Rehabil* 1993;2:165–170.

342. Daniel D, et al. Quantification of knee instability and function. *Contemp Orthop* 1982;5:83–91.

343. Hu HS, et al. Test-retest reliability of the one-legged vertical jump test and the one-legged standing hop test. *J Orthop Sports Phys Ther* 1992;15:51.

344. Ageberg E, Zatterstrom R, Moritz U. Stabilometry and one-leg hop test have high test-retest reliability. *Scand J Med Sci Sports* 1998;8:198–202.

345. Sekiya I, et al. Significance of the single-legged hop test to the anterior cruciate ligament-reconstructed knee in relation to muscle strength and anterior laxity. *Am J Sports Med* 1998;26:384–388.

346. Wilk KE, et al. The relationship between subjective knee scores, isokinetic testing, and functional testing in the ACL-reconstructed knee. *J Orthop Sports Phys Ther* 1994;20:60–73.

347. Tegner Y, et al. A performance test to monitor rehabilitation and evaluate anterior cruciate ligament injuries. *Am J Sports Med* 1986;14:156–159.

348. Shaffer SW, et al. Relationship between isokinetic and functional tests of the quadriceps. *J Orthop Sports Phys Ther* 1994;19:55.

349. DeCarlo MA, Snell KE. Normative data for range of motion and single-leg hop in high school athletes. *J Sport Rehabil* 1997;6:246–255.

350. Noyes FR, Barber SD, Mangine RE. Abnormal lower limb asymmetry determined by function hop tests after anterior cruciate ligament rupture. *Am J Sports Med* 1991;19:513–518.

351. Risberg MA, Ekeland A. Assessment of functional tests after anterior cruciate ligament surgery. *J Orthop Sports Phys Ther* 1994;19:212.

352. Steadman JR. Rehabilitation of acute injuries of the anterior cruciate ligament. *Clin Orthop* 1983;172:129–132.

353. Markey KL. Functional rehabilitation of the anterior cruciate deficient knee. *Sports Med* 1991;12:407–417.

354. Fonseca ST, et al. Validation of a performance test for outcome evaluation of knee function. *Clin J Sports Med* 1992; 2:251–256.

355. Lephart SM, et al. Functional performance tests for the anterior cruciate ligament insufficient athlete. *Athl Train* 1991;26: 44–50.

356. Lephart SM, et al. Relationship between selective physical characteristics and functional capacity in the anterior cruciate ligament-deficient athlete. *J Orthop Sports Phys Ther* 1992;16:174–181.

357. Barber SD, et al. Rehabilitation after ACL reconstruction: Function testing. *Sports Med Rehabil Series* 1992;8:969–974.

358. Rauch G, et al. Is conservative treatment of partial or complete anterior cruciate ligament rupture still justified? An analysis of the recent literature and a recommendation for arriving at a decision. *Zeitschr Orthop* 1991;129:438–446.

359. Sommerlath K, Odensten M, Lysholm J. The late course of acute partial anterior cruciate ligament tears. A nine to 15-year follow-up evaluation. *Clin Orthop* 1992;281:152–158.

360. Liu SH, et al. The diagnosis of acute complete tears of the anterior cruciate ligament. *J Bone Joint Surg* 1995;77:586.

361. Torg JS, Conrad W, Kalen V. Clinical diagnosis of anterior cruciate ligament instability in the athlete. *Am J Sports Med* 1976;4:84–93.

362. Katz JW, Fingeroth RJ. The diagnostic accuracy of ruptures of the anterior cruciate ligament comparing the Lachman's test, the anterior drawer sign, and the pivot-shift test in acute and chronic knee injuries. *Am J Sports Med* 1986;14:88–91.

363. DeHaven K. Arthroscopy in the diagnosis and management of the anterior cruciate deficient knee. *Clin Orthop* 1983;172:52–56.

364. Donaldson WF, Warren RF, Wickiewicz TL. A comparison of acute anterior cruciate ligament examinations. *Am J Sports Med* 1985;13:5–10.

365. Weiss JR, et al. A functional assessment of anterior cruciate ligament deficiency in an acute and clinical setting. *J Orthop Sports Phys Ther* 1990;11:372–373.

366. Hanten WP, Pace MB. Reliability of measuring anterior laxity of the knee joint using a knee ligament arthrometer. *Phys Ther* 1987;67:357–359.

367. Hughston JC, et al. Classification of knee ligament instabilities. Part 2. *J Bone Joint Surg* 1976;58A:173–179.

368. DeHaven KE. Diagnosis of acute knee injuries with hemarthrosis. *Am J Sports Med* 1980;8:9–14.

369. Jonsson T, et al. Clinical diagnosis of ruptures of the anterior cruciate ligament. *Am J Sports Med* 1982;10:100–102.

370. Larson RL. Physical examination in the diagnosis of rotatory instability. *Clin Orthop* 1983;172:38–44.

371. Shino K, Horibe S, Ono K. The voluntary evoked posterolateral drawer sign in the knee with posterolateral instability. *Clin Orthop* 1987;215:179–186.

372. Hughston JC, Norwood LA. The posterolateral drawer test and external rotation recurvatum test for posterolateral rotary instability of the knee. *Clin Orthop* 1980;147:82–87.

373. Galway HR, Beaupre A, MacIntosh DL. Pivot shift: A clinical sign of symptomatic anterior cruciate deficiency. *J Bone Joint Surg* 1972;54B:763–764.

374. Jensen K. Manual laxity tests for anterior cruciate ligament injuries. *J Orthop Sports Phys Ther* 1990;11:474–481.

375. Jakob RP, Stäubli HU, Deland JT. Grading the pivot shift. *J Bone Joint Surg* 1987;69B:294–299.

376. Losee RE. Concepts of the pivot shift. *Clin Orthop* 1983;172:45–51.

377. Noyes FR, et al. An analysis of the pivot shift phenomenon. *Am J Sports Med* 1991;19:148–155.

378. Neeb TB, et al. Assessing anterior cruciate ligament injuries: the association and differential value of questionnaires, clinical tests, and functional tests. *J Orthop Sports Phys Ther* 1997;26:324–331.

379. Kaplan N, Wickiewicz TL, Warren RF. Primary surgical treatment of anterior cruciate ligament ruptures. A long-term follow-up study. *Am J Sports Med* 1990;18:354–358.

380. Conteduca F, et al. Chondromalacia and chronic anterior instabilities of the knee. *Am J Sports Med* 1991;19:119–123.

381. Tamea CD, Henning CE. Pathomechanics of the pivot shift maneuver. *Am J Sports Med* 1981;9:31–37.

382. Noyes FR, et al. The symptomatic anterior cruciate-deficient knee. Part I. The long-term functional disability in athletically active individuals. *J Bone Joint Surg* 1983;65A:154–162.

383. Kujala UM, Nelimarkka O, Koskinen SK. Relationship between the pivot shift and the configuration of the lateral tibial plateau. *Arch Orthop Trauma Surg* 1992;111:228–229.

384. Bull AM, et al. Incidence and mechanism of the pivot shift. An in vitro study. *Clin Orthop* 1999;363:219–231.

385. Bach BR Jr, et al. Arthroscopy-assisted anterior cruciate ligament reconstruction using patellar tendon substitution. Two- to four-year follow-up results. *Am J Sports Med* 1994;22:758–767.

386. Daniel DM, Stone ML, Riehl B. Ligament surgery: The evaluation of results. In: Daniel DM, Akeson WH, O'Connor JJ, eds. *Knee Ligaments, Structure, Function and Repair.* New York, NY: Raven Press; 1990:521–534.

387. Norwood LA, et al. Acute anterolateral rotatory instability of the knee. *J Bone Joint Surg* 1979;61A:704–709.

388. Otter C, Aufdemkampe G, Lezeman H. Diagnostiek van knieletsel en relatie tussen de aanwezigheid van knieklachten en de resultaten van functionele testen en Biodex-test. In: *Jaarboek 1994 Fysiotherapie Kinesitherapie.* Bonn, Germany: Stafleu, van Loghum; 1994:195–228.

389. Harilainen A, et al. Prospective preoperative evaluation of anterior cruciate ligament instability of the knee joint and results of reconstruction with patellar ligament. *Clin Orthop* 1993;297:17–22.

390. Losee RE, Johnson TR, Southwick WO. Anterior subluxation of the lateral tibial plateau. A diagnostic test and operative repair. *J Bone Joint Surg* 1978;60A:1015–1030.

391. Gerber C, Matter P. Biomechanical analysis of the knee after rupture of the anterior cruciate ligament and its primary repair. An instant-centre analysis of function. *J Bone Joint Surg* 1983;65B:391–399.

392. MacIntosh DL, Galway RD. The lateral pivot shift. A symptomatic and clinical sign of anterior cruciate insufficiency. Paper presented at 85th Annual Meeting of American Orthopaedic Association; 1972; Tucker's Town, Bermuda.

393. Slocum DB, Larson RL. Rotary instability of the knee. *J Bone Joint Surg* 1968;50A:211–225.

394. Slocum DB, et al. A clinical test for anterolateral rotary instability of the knee. *Clin Orthop* 1976;118:63–69.

395. Ahmed AM, et al. The effect of quadriceps tension characteristics on the patellar tracking pattern. In: *Transactions of the 34th Orthopaedic Research Society.* Atlanta, Ga: 1988.

396. Puniello MS. Iliotibial band tightness and medial patellar glide in patients with patellofemoral dysfunction. *J Orthop Sports Phys Ther* 1993;17:144–148.

397. Apley AG. The diagnosis of meniscus injuries: Some new clinical methods. *J Bone Joint Surg* 1947;29B:78–84.

398. Anderson AF. Clinical diagnosis of meniscal tears: Description of a new manipulation test. *Am J Sports Med* 1982;14:291–296.

399. Fithian DC, et al. Instrumented measurement of patellar mobility. *Am J Sports Med* 1995;23:607–615.

400. Kolowich PA, et al. Lateral release of the patella: Indications and contraindications. *Am J Sports Med* 1990;18:359–365.

401. Teitge RA, et al. Stress radiographs of the patellofemoral joint. *J Bone Joint Surg* 1996;78A:193–203.

402. Fairbank HA. Internal derangement of the knee in children. *Proc R Soc Med* 1937;3:11.

403. Kuo L, et al. The hamstring index. *J Pediatr Orthop* 1997; 17:78–88.

404. Thompson NS, et al. Musculoskeletal modelling in determining the effect of botulinum toxin on the hamstrings of patients with crouch gait. *Dev Med Child Neurol* 1998;40:622–625.

405. Gautam VK, Anand S. A new test for estimating iliotibial band contracture. *J Bone Joint Surg* 1998;80B:474–475.

406. Holmes JC, Pruitt AL, Whalen NJ. Iliotibial band syndrome in cyclists. *Am J Sports Med* 1993;21:419–424.

407. Noble HB, Hajek MR, Porter M. Diagnosis and treatment of iliotibial band tightness in runners. *Phys Sports Med* 1982;10:67–74.

408. Lehman WL Jr. Overuse syndromes in runners. *Am Fam Phys* 1984;29:152–161.

409. Yawn BP, et al. Isolated acute knee injuries in the general population. *J Trauma* 2000;48:716–723.

410. Kannus P, Jarvinen M. Incidence of knee injuries and the need for further care: A one-year prospective follow-up study. *J Sports Med Phys Fitness* 1989;29:321–325.

411. Nielsen AB, Yde J. Epidemiology of acute knee injuries: A prospective hospital investigation. *J Trauma* 1991; 31:1644–1648.

412. Henry JH, Crosland JW. Conservative treatment of patellofemoral subluxation. *Am J Sports Med* 1979;7:12–14.

413. McConnell J. The management of chondromalacia patellae: a long-term solution. *Aust J Physiother* 1986;32:215–223.

414. Reid DC. The myth, mystic and frustration of anterior knee pain [editorial]. *Clin J Sports Med* 1993;3:139–143.

415. Shelton GL. Conservative management of patellofemoral dysfunction. *Prim Care* 1992;19:331–350.

416. Hilyard A. Recent advances in the management of patellofemoral pain: The McConnell programme. *Physiotherapy* 1990; 76:559–565.

417. Kujala UM. Patellofemoral problems in sports medicine. *Ann Chir Gynaecol* 1991;80:219–223.

418. Garrick JG. Anterior knee pain (chondromalacia patella). *Phys Sportsmed* 1989;17:75–84.

419. Fulkerson JP, Shea KP. Current concepts review: Disorders of patellofemoral alignment. *J Bone Joint Surg* 1990; 72A:1424–1429.

420. Levine J. Chondromalacia patellae. *Phys Sportsmed* 1979; 7:41–49.

421. O'Neill DB. Arthroscopically assisted reconstruction of the anterior cruciate ligament. *J Bone Joint Surg* 1996;78A:803–813.

422. Palumbo PM. Dynamic patellar brace: a new orthosis in the management of patellofemoral pain. *Am J Sports Med* 1981;9:45–49.

423. Walsh WM, Helzer-Julin M. Patellar tracking problems in athletes. *Prim Care* 1992;19:303–330.

424. Whitelaw GP, et al. A conservative approach to anterior knee pain. *Clin Orthop* 1989;246:234–237.

425. Gerrard B. The patello-femoral pain syndrome: A clinical trial of the McConnell programme. *Aust J Physiother* 1989;35:71–80.

426. Gilleard W, McConnell J, Parsons D. The effect of patella taping on the onset of vastus medialis obliquus and vastus lateralis muscle activity in persons with patellofemoral pain. *Phys Ther* 1998;78:25–32.

427. Bohannon RW. The effect of electrical stimulation to the vastus medialis muscle in a patient with chronically dislocating patella. *Phys Ther* 1983;63:1445–1447.

428. Mariani P, Caruso I. An electromyographic investigation of subluxation of the patella. *J Bone Joint Surg* 1979;61B:169.

429. Villar RN. Patellofemoral pain and the infrapatellar brace: A military view. *Am J Sports Med* 1985;13:313.

430. Grelsamer RP, McConnell J. Conservative management of patellofemoral problems. In: Grelsamer RP, McConnell J, eds. *The Patella: A Team Approach.* Gaithersburg, Md: Aspen; 1998:109–118.

431. Chu DA. Rehabilitation of the lower extremity. *Clin Sports Med* 1995;14:205–222.

432. Lehman RC, Host JV, Craig R. Patellofemoral dysfunction in tennis players. A dynamic problem. *Clin J Sports Med* 1995;14:177–205.

433. Doucette SA, Child DP. The effect of open and closed chain exercise and knee joint position on patellar tracking in lateral patellar compression syndrome. *J Orthop Sports Phys Ther* 1996; 23:104–110.

434. Griffin LY. Ligamentous injuries. In: Griffen LY, ed. *Rehabilitation of the Injured Knee.* St Louis, Mo: Mosby; 1995:149–164.

435. Baratta R, et al. Muscular coactivation: The role of the antagonist musculature in maintaining knee stability. *Am J Sports Med* 1988;16:113–122.

436. Hawkins RJ, Misamore GW, Merritt TR. Follow-up of the acute nonoperated isolated anterior cruciate ligament tear. *Am J Sports Med* 1986;14:205–210.

437. Fleming BC, Beynnon BD, Renstrom PA. The strain behavior of the anterior cruciate ligament during bicycling: An in vivo study. *Am J Sports Med* 1998;26:109–118.

438. Klingman RE, Liaos SM, Hardin KM. The effect of subtalar joint posting on patellar glide position in subjects with excessive rearfoot pronation. *J Orthop Sports Phys Ther* 1997;25:185–191.

439. Pedowitz WJ, Kovatis P. Flatfoot in the adult. *J Am Acad Orthop Surg* 1995;3:293–302.

440. LeVeau BF, Rogers C. Selective training of the vastus medialis muscle using EMG biofeedback. *Phys Ther* 1980;60:1410–1415.

441. Soderberg G, Cook T. An electromyographic analysis of quadriceps femoris muscle settings and straight leg raising. *Phys Ther* 1983;63:1434.

442. Karst GM, Jewett PD. Electromyographic analysis of exercises proposed for differential activation of medial and lateral quadriceps femoris muscle components. *Phys Ther* 1993;73:286–295.

443. Hodges P, Richardson C. An investigation into the effectiveness of hip adduction in the optimization of the vastus medialis oblique contraction. *Scand J Rehabil Med* 1993;25:57–62.

444. Doucette SA, Goble EM. The effect of exercise on patellar tracking in lateral patellar compression syndrome. *Am J Sports Med* 1992;20:434–440.

445. Hanten WP, Schulthies SS. Exercise effect on electromyographic activity of the vastus medialis oblique and the vastus lateralis muscles. *Phys Ther* 1990;70:561–565.

446. McNicol K, Taunton JE, Clement DB. Iliotibial band friction syndrome in athletes. *Can J Appl Sport Sci* 1981;6:76–80.

447. Laus M, et al. Degenerative spondylolisthesis: Lumbar stenosis and instability. *Chir Organi Mov* 1992;77:39–49.

448. Cahill BR, Griffith EH. Effect of preseason conditioning on the incidence and severity of high school football knee injuries. *Am J Sports Med* 1978;6:180–184.

449. Klein W, Shah N, Gassen A. Arthroscopic management of postoperative arthrofibrosis of the knee joint: Indication, technique, and results. *Arthroscopy* 1994;10:591–597.

450. Thomeé R. A comprehensive treatment approach for patellofemoral pain syndrome in young women. *Phys Ther* 1997; 77:1690–1703.

451. Witvrouw E, et al. Reflex response times of vastus medialis oblique and vastus lateralis in normal subjects and subjects with patellofemoral pain syndrome. *J Orthop Sports Phys Ther* 1996;24:160–165.

452. Kasman GS, Cram JR, Wolf SL. *Clinical Applications in Surface Electromyography: Chronic Musculoskeletal Pain.* Gaithersburg, Md: Aspen; 1998.

453. Mirzabeigi E, et al. Isolation of the vastus medialis oblique muscle during exercise. *Am J Sports Med* 1999;27:50–53.

454. Lange GW, et al. Electromyographic and kinematic analysis of graded treadmill walking and the implications for knee rehabilitation. *J Orthop Sports Phys Ther* 1996;23:294–301.

455. Flynn TW, Soutas-Little RW. Patellofemoral joint compressive forces in forward and backward running. *J Orthop Sports Phys Ther* 1995;21:277–282.

456. Swenson EJ Jr, Hough DO, McKeag DB. Patellofemoral dysfunction: How to treat, when to refer patients with problematic knees. *Postgrad Med* 1987;82:125–141.

457. Noyes FR, et al. Knee ligament tests: What do they really mean? *Phys Ther* 1980;60:1578–1581.

458. Williams JS, Bernard RB. Operative and nonoperative rehabilitation of the ACL-injured knee. *Sports Med Arth Rev* 1996;4:69–82.

459. Engle RP, Canner GC. Proprioceptive neuromuscular facilitation (PNF) and modified procedures for anterior cruciate ligament (ACL) instability. *J Orthop Sports Phys Ther* 1989;11:230.

460. Lephart SM, Borsa PA. Functional rehabilitation of knee injuries. In: Fu FH, Harner C, eds. *Knee Surgery.* Baltimore, Md: Williams and Wilkins; 1993.

461. Hunter LY. Braces and taping. *Clin Sports Med* 1985;4:439–454.

462. Koskinen SK, Kujala UM. Effect of patellar bracing on patellofemoral relationships. *Scand J Med Sci Sports* 1991;1:119–122.

463. Worrell T, et al. Effect of patellar taping and bracing on patellar position as determined by MRI in patients with patellofemoral pain. *Athl Train* 1998;33:16–20.

464. Brossmann J, et al. Patellar tracking patterns during active and passive knee extension: evaluation with motion-triggered cine MR imaging. *Radiology* 1993;187:205–212.

465. Sasaki T, Yagi T. Subluxation of the patella. *Int Orthop* 1986;10:115–120.

466. Finestone A, et al. Treatment of overuse patellofemoral pain: Prospective randomized controlled clinical trial in a military setting. *Clin Orthop* 1993;293:208–210.

467. Arroll B, et al. Patellofemoral pain syndrome: A critical review of the clinical trials on nonoperative therapy. *Am J Sports Med* 1997;25:207–212.

468. Branch TP, Hunter R, Donath M. Dynamic EMG analysis of anterior cruciate deficient legs with and without bracing during cutting. *Am J Sports Med* 1989;17:35–41.

469. Fleming BC, et al. The influence of functional knee bracing on the anterior cruciate ligament strain biomechanics in weight-bearing and nonweightbearing knees. *Am J Sports Med* 2000;28:815–824.

470. Liu SH, Daluiski A, Kabo JM. The effects of thigh soft tissue stiffness on the control of anterior tibial displacement by functional knee orthoses. *J Rehabil Res Dev* 1995;32:135–140.

471. Risberg MA, et al. The effect of knee bracing after anterior cruciate ligament reconstruction: A prospective, randomized study with two years' follow-up. *Am J Sports Med* 1999;27:76–83.

472. Borsa PA, et al. The effects of joint position and direction of joint motion on proprioceptive sensibility in anterior cruciate ligament-deficient athletes. *Am J Sports Med* 1997;25:336–340.

473. Barrett DS. Proprioception and function after anterior cruciate ligament reconstruction. *J Bone Joint Surg* 1991;73B:833–837.

474. Corrigan JP, Cashman WF, Brady MP. Proprioception in the cruciate deficient knee. *J Bone Joint Surg* 1992;74B:247–250.

475. Risberg MA, et al. Proprioception after anterior cruciate ligament reconstruction with and without bracing. *Knee Surg Sports Traumatol Arthrosc* 1999;7:303–309.

476. Barrett DS, Cobb AG, Bentley G. Joint proprioception in normal, osteoarthritic and replaced knees. *J Bone Joint Surg* 1991;73B:53–56.

477. McConnell J. Promoting effective segmental alignment. In: Crosbie J, McConnell J, eds. *Key Issues in Musculoskeletal Physiotherapy.* Boston, Mass: Butterworth Heinemann; 1993:172–194.

478. Bockrath K, et al. Effects of patella taping on patella position and perceived pain. *Med Sci Sports Exerc* 1993;25:989–992.

479. Gerrard B. The patellofemoral pain syndrome in young, active patients: A prospective study. *Clin Orthop* 1989;179:129–133.

480. Gigante A, et al. The effects of patellar taping on patellofemoral incongruence. A computed tomography study. *Am J Sports Med* 2001;29:88–92.

481. Larsen B, et al. Patellar taping: A radiographic examination of the medial glide technique. *Am J Sports Med* 1995;23:465–471.

482. Marumoto JM, Jordan C, Akins R. A biomechanical comparison of lateral retinacular releases. *Am J Sports Med* 1995;23:151–155.

483. Masse Y. "La trochléoplastie." Restauration de la gouttière trochléene dans les subluxations et luxations de la rotule. *Rev Chir Orthop* 1978;64:3–17.

484. Grabiner M, Koh T, Draganich L. Neuromechanics of the patellofemoral joint. *Med Sci Sports Exerc* 1994;26:10–21.

485. Cushnaghan J, McCarthy C, Dieppe P. Taping the patella medially: A new treatment for osteoarthritis of the knee joint? *BMJ* 1994;308:753–755.

486. Willson J, et al. Effects of walking poles on lower extremity gait mechanics. *Med Sci Sports Exerc* 2001;33:142–147.

487. Brunelle EA, Miller MK. The effects of walking poles on ground reaction forces. *Res Q Exerc Sport* 1998;69(suppl):A30.

488. Neureuther G. Ski poles in the summer. *Landesarszt Bayerischen Bergwacht Munich Med Wacherts* 1981;13:123.

489. Schwameder H, et al. Knee joint forces during downhill walking with hiking poles. *J Sport Sci* 1999;17:969–978.

490. Rowe CR, Pierce DS, Clark JG. Voluntary dislocation of the shoulder: A preliminary report on a clinical, electromyographic, and psychiatric study of 26 patients. *J Bone Joint Surg* 1973;55A:445–460.

491. Wise HH, Fiebert IM, Kates JL. EMG biofeedback as treatment for patellofemoral pain syndrome. *J Orthop Sports Phys Ther* 1984;6:95–103.

492. Prevalence of disabilities and associated health conditions—United States, 1991–1992. *JAMA* 1994;272:1735–1736.

493. Panush RS, Lane NE. Exercise and the musculoskeletal system. *Baillieres Clin Rheumatol* 1994;8:79–102.

494. Felson DT, et al. The prevalence of knee osteoarthritis in the elderly. The Framingham Osteoarthritis Study. *Arthritis Rheum* 1987;30:914–918.

495. Felson DT. The epidemiology of knee osteoarthritis: Results from the Framingham Osteoarthritis Study. *Sem Arthritis Rheum* 1990;20:42–50.

496. Peyron JG, Altman RD. The epidemiology of osteoarthritis. In: Moskowitz RW, et al, eds. *Osteoarthritis: Diagnosis and Medical/Surgical Management.* Philadelphia, Pa: Saunders; 1992:15–37.

497. Genti G. Occupation and osteoarthritis. *Clin Rheumatol* 1989; 3:193–204.

498. Felson DT. Do occupation-related physical factors contribute to arthritis? In: Panush RSLN. *Bailliere's Clinical Rheumatology: Exercise and Rheumatic Disease.* Philadelphia, Pa: Bailliere Tindall; 1994:63–77.

499. Maetzel A, et al. Osteoarthritis of the hip and knee and mechanical occupational exposure: A systematic overview of the evidence. *J Rheum* 1997;24:1599–1607.

500. Kellgren JH, Lawrence JS. Rheumatism in miners. Part II. X-ray study. *Br J Ind Med* 1952;9:197–207.

501. Partridge REH, Duthie JJR. Rheumatism in dockers and civil servants: A comparison of heavy manual and sedentary workers. *Ann Rheum Dis* 1968;27:559–567.

502. Lindberg H, Montgomery F. Heavy labor and the occurrence of gonarthrosis. *Clin Orthop* 1987;214:235–236.

503. Kohatsu ND, Schurman DJ. Risk factors for the development of osteoarthrosis of the knee. *Clin Orthop* 1990;261:242–246.

504. Vingård E, et al. Disability pensions due to musculo-skeletal disorders among men in heavy occupations. *Scand J Soc Med* 1992;20:31–36.

505. Vingård E, et al. Occupation and osteoarthrosis of the hip and knee: A register-based cohort study. *Int J Epidemiol* 1991;20: 1025–1031.

506. Anderson JJ, Felson DT. Factors associated with osteoarthritis of the knee in the first National Health and Nutrition Examination Survey. *Am J Epidemiol* 1988;128:179–189.

507. Felson DT, Hannan MT, Naimark A. Occupational physical demands, knee bending and knee osteoarthritis: Results from the Framingham study. *J Rheumatol* 1991;18:1587–1592.

508. Jensen LK, Eenberg W. Occupation as a risk factor for knee disorders. *Scand J Work Environ Health* 1996;22:165–175.

509. Kujala UM, Kaprio J, Sarna S. Osteoarthritis of weight bearing joints of lower limbs in former elite male athletes. *BMJ* 1994;308:231–234.

510. Kujala UM, et al. Knee osteoarthritis in former runners, soccer players, weight lifters, and shooters. *Arthritis Rheum* 1995;38:539–546.

511. Felson DT, et al. Risk factors for incident radiographic knee osteoarthritis in the elderly: The Framingham Study. *Arthritis Rheum* 1997;40:728–733.

512. Felson DT. Epidemiology of hip and knee osteoarthritis. *Epidemiol Rev* 1988;10:1–28.

513. Baker K, McAlindon T. Exercise for knee osteoarthritis. *Curr Opin Rheumatol* 2000;12:456–463.

514. Wessel J. Isometric strength measurements of knee extensors in women with osteoarthritis of the knee. *J Rheumatol* 1996;23:328–331.

515. Slemenda C, et al. Quadriceps weakness and osteoarthritis of the knee. *Ann Intern Med* 1998;127:97–104.

516. Deyle GD, et al. Effectiveness of manual physical therapy and exercise in osteoarthritis of the knee. A randomized, controlled trial. *Ann Intern Med* 2000;132:173–181.

517. Brandt KD. Nonsurgical management of osteoarthritis, with an emphasis on nonpharmacologic measures. *Arch Fam Med* 1995;4:1057–1064.

518. Yasuda K, Sasaki T. The mechanics of treatment of the osteoarthritic knee with a wedged insole. *Clin Orthop* 1985;215:162–172.

519. Yasuda K, Sasaki T. Clinical evaluation of the treatment of osteoarthritic knees using a newly designed wedged insole. *Clin Orthop* 1985;221:181–187.

520. Puett DW, Griffin MR. Published trials of nonmedicinal and noninvasive therapies for hip and knee osteoarthritis. *Ann Intern Med* 1994;121:133–140.

521. Fisher NM, et al. Muscle rehabilitation: its effect on muscular and functional performance of patients with knee osteoarthritis. *Arch Phys Med Rehabil* 1991;72:367–374.

522. Fisher NM, Gresham GE, Pendergast DR. Effects of a quantitative progressive rehabilitation program applied unilaterally to the osteoarthritic knee. *Arch Phys Med Rehabil* 1993; 74:1319–1326.

523. Fisher NM, et al. Quantitative effects of physical therapy on muscular and functional performance in subjects with osteoarthritis of the knees. *Arch Phys Med Rehabil* 1993; 74:840–847.

524. Kovar PA, et al. Supervised fitness walking in patients with osteoarthritis of the knee. A randomized, controlled trial. *Ann Intern Med* 1992;116:529–534.

525. Ettinger WH Jr, et al. A randomized trial comparing aerobic exercise and resistance exercise with a health education program in older adults with knee osteoarthritis. The Fitness Arthritis and Seniors Trial. *JAMA* 1997;277:25–31.

526. Lane NE, Buckwalter JA. Exercise: A cause of osteoarthritis? *Rheum Dis Clin North Am* 1993;19:617–633.

527. Mangione KK, Axen K, Haas F. Mechanical unweighting effects on treadmill exercise and pain in elderly people with osteoarthritis of the knee. *Phys Ther* 1996;76:387–394.

528. Aleman O. Chondromalacia post-traumatica patellae. *Acta Chir Scand* 1928;63:149–190.

529. Beck JL, Wildermuth BP. The female athlete's knee. *Clin J Sports Med* 1985;4:345–366.

530. Outerbridge RE. The aetiology of chondromalacia patellae. *J Bone Joint Surg* 1961;43B:752–757.

531. Dye SF, Vaupel GL. The pathophysiology of patellofemoral pain. *Sports Med Arthrosc Rev* 1994;2:203–210.

532. Gillespie MJ, Friedland J, DeHaven K. Arthrofibrosis: Etiology, classification, histopathology, and treatment. *Oper Tech Sports Med* 1998;6:102–110.

533. Parisien JS. The role of arthroscopy in the treatment of postoperative fibroarthrosis of the knee joint. *Clin Orthop* 1988;229:185–192.

534. Richmond JC, Assal M. Arthroscopic management of arthrofibrosis of the knee, including infrapatellar contraction syndrome. *Arthroscopy* 1991;7:144–147.

535. Sebastianelli WJ, et al. The histopathology of arthrofibrosis. *Arthroscopy* 1993;9:359–360.

536. Shelbourne KD, Johnson GE. Outpatient surgical management of arthrofibrosis after anterior cruciate ligament surgery. *Am J Sports Med* 1994;22:192–197.

537. Lindenfeld TN, Wojtys EM, Husain A. Operative treatment of arthrofibrosis of the knee. *J Bone Joint Surg* 1999;81A: 1772–1784.

538. Delcogliano A, et al. Light and scan electron microscopic analysis of cyclops syndrome: Etiopathogenic hypothesis and technical solutions. *Knee Surg Sports Traumatol Arthrosc* 1996; 4:194–199.

539. Jackson DW, Schaefer RK. Cyclops syndrome: Loss of extension following intra-articular anterior cruciate ligament reconstruction. *Arthroscopy* 1990;6:171–178.

540. Shelbourne KD, et al. Arthrofibrosis in acute anterior cruciate ligament reconstruction. The effect of timing of reconstruction and rehabilitation. *Am J Sports Med* 1991;19: 332–336.

541. Wasilewski SA, Covall DJ, Cohen S. Effect of surgical timing on recovery and associated injuries after anterior cruciate ligament reconstruction. *Am J Sports Med* 1993;21:338–342.

542. Hunter RE, et al. The impact of surgical timing on postoperative motion and stability following anterior cruciate ligament reconstruction. *Arthroscopy* 1996;12:667–674.

543. Shelbourne KD, Nitz P. Accelerated rehabilitation after anterior cruciate ligament reconstruction. *Am J Sports Med* 1990; 18:292–299.

544. Lindenfeld TN, Bach BR Jr, Wojtys EM. Reflex sympathetic dystrophy and pain dysfunction in the lower extremity. *J Bone Joint Surg* 1996;78A:1936–1944.

545. Christel P, et al. A comparison of arthroscopic arthrolysis and manipulation of the knee under anaesthesia in the treatment of postoperative stiffness of the knee. *French J Orthop Surg* 1988;2:348–355.

546. Silman AJ, Day SJ, Haskard DO. Factors associated with joint mobility in an adolescent population. *Ann Rheum Dis* 1987;46:209–212.

547. Woo SLY, et al. Acute injury to ligament and meniscus as inducers of osteoarthritis. In: Kuettner KE, Goldberg VM, ed. *Osteoarthritic Disorders*. Rosemont, Ill: American Academy of Orthopaedic Surgeons; 1995:185–196.

548. Buckwalter JA, Lane NE, Gordon SL. Exercise as a cause for osteoarthritis. In: Kuettner KE, Goldberg VM, eds. *Osteoarthritic Disorders*. Rosemont, Ill: American Academy of Orthopaedic Surgeons; 1995:405–417.

549. Johnson DL. Acute knee injuries: An introduction. *Clin Sports Med* 1993;12:344.

550. Arendt E, Dick R. Knee injury patterns among men and women in collegiate basketball and soccer. NCAA data and review of literature. *Am J Sports Med* 1995;23:694–701.

551. Bjordal JM, et al. Epidemiology of anterior cruciate ligament injuries in soccer. *Am J Sports Med* 1997;25:341–345.

552. Huston LJ, Greenfield ML, Wojtys EM. Anterior cruciate ligament injuries in the female athlete. Potential risk factors. *Clin Orthop* 2000;372:50–63.

553. Shambaugh JP, Klein A, Herbert JH. Structural measures as predictors of injury in basketball players. *Med Sci Sports Exerc* 1991;23:522–527.

554. Muneta T, Takakuda K, Yamomoto H. Intercondylar notch width and its relation to the configuration of cross-sectional area of the anterior cruciate ligament. *Am J Sports Med* 1997;25:69–72.

555. Norwood LA, Cross MJ. The intercondylar shelf in the anterior cruciate ligament. *Am J Sports Med* 1977;5:171–176.

556. Ireland ML. Special concerns of the female athlete. In: Fu FH, Stone DA, eds. *Sports Injuries: Mechanism, Prevention, and Treatment*. Baltimore, Md: Williams and Wilkins; 1994:153–162.

557. Grana WA, Moretz JA. Ligamentous laxity in secondary school athletes. *JAMA* 1978;240:1975–1976.

558. Hutchinson MR, Ireland ML. Knee injuries in female athletes. *Sports Med* 1995;19:288–302.

559. Huston LJ, Wojtys EM. Neuromuscular performance characteristics in elite female athletes. *Am J Sports Med* 1996;24:427–436.

560. Liu SH, et al. Estrogen affects the cellular metabolism of the anterior cruciate ligament. A potential explanation for female athletic injury. *Am J Sports Med* 1997;25:704–709.

561. Slauterbeck JR, et al. Effects of estrogen level on the tensile properties of the rabbit anterior cruciate ligament. *J Orthop Res* 1999;17:405–408.

561a. Ireland ML. The female ACL: why is it more prone to injury? *Orthop Clin N Amer*. 2002;33:637–651.

562. Griffin JW, et al. Eccentric muscle performance of elbow and knee muscle groups in untrained men and women. *Med Sci Sports Exerc* 1993;25:936–944.

563. Hakkinen K, Kraemer WJ, Newton RU. Muscle activation and force production during bilateral and unilateral concentric and isometric contractions of the knee extensors in men and women at different ages. *Electromyogr Clin Neurophysiol* 1997;37:131–142.

564. Kanehisa H, et al. Sex difference in force generation capacity during repeated maximal knee extensions. *Eur J Appl Physiol* 1996;73:557–562.

565. Miller AEJ, et al. Gender differences in strength and muscle fiber characteristics. *Eur J Appl Physiol* 1993;66:254–262.

566. Mizuta H, et al. The conservative treatment of complete tears of the anterior cruciate ligament in skeletally immature patients. *J Bone Joint Surg* 1995;77:890.

567. Parker AW, Drez D, Cooper JL. Anterior cruciate injuries in patients with open physes. *Am J Sports Med* 1994;22:47.

568. Micheli LJ, Jenkins M. Knee injuries. In: Micheli LJ, ed. *The Sports Medicine Bible*. Scranton, Pa: Harper and Row; 1995:130.

569. Daniel DM, et al. Fate of the ACL-injured patient. *Am J Sports Med* 1994;22:642.

570. O'Connor BL, et al. Neurogenic acceleration of osteoarthrosis. The effects of previous neurectomy of the articular nerves on the development of osteoarthrosis after transection of the anterior cruciate ligament in dogs. *J Bone Joint Surg* 1992;74A:367–376.

571. Vilensky JA, et al. Serial kinematic analysis of the canine hindlimb joints after deafferentation and anterior cruciate ligament transection. *Osteoarthritis Cartilage* 1997;5:173–182.

572. Gillquist J, Messner K. Anterior cruciate ligament reconstruction and the long-term incidence of gonarthrosis. *Sports Med* 1999;27:143–156.

573. Hoher J, Moller HD, Fu FH. Bone tunnel enlargement after anterior cruciate ligament reconstruction: Fact or fiction? *Knee Surg Sports Traumatol Arthrosc* 1998;6:231–240.

574. Howell SM. Principles for placing the tibial tunnel and avoiding roof impingement during reconstruction of a torn anterior cruciate ligament. *Knee Surg Sports Traumatol Arthrosc* 1998;6(suppl 1):S49–S55.

575. Kumar PJ, et al. Rehabilitation after total knee arthroplasty: A comparison of 2 rehabilitation techniques. *Clin Orthop* 1996; 331:93–101.

576. Elmqvist LG, Johnson RJ. Prevention of cruciate ligament injuries. In: Feagin JA, ed. *The Crucial Ligaments: Diagnosis and Treatment of Ligamentous Injuries About the Knee*. New York, NY: Churchill Livingstone; 1994:495–505.

577. Ettlinger CF, Johnson RJ, Shealy JE. A method to help reduce the risk of serious knee sprains incurred in alpine skiing. *Am J Sports Med* 1995;23:531–537.

578. Feagin JA Jr, Lambert KL. Mechanism of injury and pathology of anterior cruciate ligament injuries. *Orthop Clin North Am* 1985;16:41–45.

579. Gerber C, et al. The lower-extremity musculature in chronic symptomatic instability of the anterior cruciate ligament. *J Bone Joint Surg* 1985;67A:1034–1043.

580. Kariya Y, et al. Magnetic resonance imaging and spectroscopy of thigh muscles in cruciate ligament insufficiency. *Acta Orthop Scand* 1989;60:322–325.

581. Lorentzon R, et al. Thigh musculature in relation to chronic anterior cruciate ligament tear: Muscle size, morphology, and mechanical output before reconstruction. *Am J Sports Med* 1989;17:423–429.

582. Noyes FR, Mangine RE, Barber S. Early knee motion after open and arthroscopic anterior cruciate ligament reconstruction. *Am J Sports Med* 1987;15:149–160.

583. Yasuda K, et al. Quantitative evaluation of knee instability and muscle strength after anterior cruciate ligament reconstruction using patellar and quadriceps tendon. *Am J Sports Med* 1992;20:471–475.

584. Elmqvist LG, et al. Knee extensor muscle function before and after reconstruction of anterior cruciate ligament tear. *Scand J Rehab Med* 1989;21:131–139.

585. Fink C, et al. (Neuro)Muskulare Veranderungen der kniegelenksstabilisierenden Muskulatur nach Ruptur des vorderen Kreuzbandes. *Sportverletz Sportsch* 1994;8:25–30.

586. Lopresti C, Kirkendall DT, Streete GM. Quadriceps insufficiency following repair of anterior cruciate ligament. *J Orthop Sports Phys Ther* 1988;9:245–249.

587. Snyder-Mackler L, et al. Strength of the quadriceps femoris muscle and functional recovery after reconstruction of the anterior cruciate ligament. A prospective, randomized clinical trial of electrical stimulation. *J Bone Joint Surg* 1995;77A:1166–1173.

588. Yahia LH, Newman N, Rivard CH. Neurohistology of lumbar spine ligaments. *Acta Orthop Scand* 1988;59:508–512.

589. Rosenberg TD, Pazik TJ, Deffner KT. Primary quadrupled semitendinosus ACL reconstruction: A comprehensive 2-year evaluation. In: *Proceedings of the Twentieth SICOT Congress.* Amsterdam, Holland: SICOT; 1996.

590. Kramer J, et al. Knee flexor and extensor strength during concentric and eccentric muscle actions after anterior cruciate ligament reconstruction using the semitendinosus tendon and ligament augmentation device. *Am J Sports Med* 1993;21:285–291.

591. Daniel DM, et al. Instrumented measurement of anterior laxity of the knee. *J Bone Joint Surg* 1985;67A:720–725.

592. Indelicato PA, Bittar ES. A perspective of lesions associated with ACL insufficiency of the knee. A review of 100 cases. *Clin Orthop* 1985;198:77–80.

593. Irvine GB, Glasgow MMS. The natural history of the meniscus in anterior cruciate insufficiency. Arthroscopic analysis. *J Bone Joint Surg* 1992;74B:403–405.

594. Loudon JK, Goist HL, Loudon KL. Genu recurvatum syndrome. *J Orthop Sports Phys Ther* 1998;27:361–367.

595. Noyes FR, et al. Knee hyperextension gait abnormalities in unstable knees. *Am J Sports Med* 1996;24:35–45.

596. Loudon JK, Jenkins WJ, Loudon KL. The relationship between static posture and ACL injury in female athletes. *J Orthop Sports Phys Ther* 1996;24:91–97.

597. Hutchison MR, Ireland ML. Knee injuries in female athletes. *Sports Med* 1995;19:288–302.

598. Rubinstein RA, et al. Effect on knee stability if hyperextension is restored immediately after autogenous bone-patellar tendon-bone anterior cruciate ligament reconstruction. *Am J Sports Med* 1995;23:365–368.

599. Egner E. Knee joint meniscal degeneration as it relates to tissue fiber structure and mechanical resistance. *Pathol Res Pract* 1982;173:310–324.

600. Boden SD, et al. A prospective and blinded investigation of magnetic resonance imaging of the knee: Abnormal findings in asymptomatic subjects. *Clin Orthop* 1992;282:177–185.

601. O'Connor RL. *Arthroscopy.* Philadelphia, Pa: JB Lippincott; 1977.

602. Diment MT, DeHaven KE, Sebastianelli WJ. Current concepts in meniscal repair. *Orthopaedics* 1993;16:973–977.

603. Tria AJ, Klein KS. *An Illustrated Guide to the Knee.* New York, NY: Churchill Livingstone; 1992.

604. Miyasaka KC, et al. The incidence of knee ligament injuries in the general population. *Am J Knee Surg* 1991;4:3–8.

605. Cooper DE, Warren RF, Warner JJP. The PCL and posterolateral structures of the knee: Anatomy, function and patterns of injury. *Inst Course Lect* 1991;40:249–270.

606. Trickey EL. Injuries to the PCL: Diagnosis and treatment of early injuries and reconstruction of late instability. *Clin Orthop* 1980;147:76–81.

607. Insall JN, Hood RW. Bone block transfer of the medial head of the gastrocnemius for posterior cruciate insufficiency. *J Bone Joint Surg* 1982;65A:691–699.

608. Harner CD, Hoher J. Evaluation and treatment of posterior cruciate ligament injuries. *Am J Sports Med* 1998;26:471–482.

609. Dejour H, et al. The natural history of rupture of the PCL. *French J Orthop Surg* 1988;2:112–120.

610. Tibone JE, et al. Functional analysis of untreated and reconstructed posterior cruciate ligament injuries. *Am J Sports Med* 1988;16:217–223.

611. Picard F, et al. Étude morphométrique de l'articulation fémoropatellaire à partir de l'incidence radiologique de profil. *Rev Chir Orthop* 1997;83:104–111.

612. Dejour H, et al. La dysplasie de la trochlée fémorale. *Rev Chir Orthop* 1990;76:45–54.

613. Brattström H. Patella alta in non-dislocating knee joints. *Acta Orthop Scand* 1970;41:578–588.

614. Blackburn J, Peel T. A new method of measuring patellar height. *J Bone Joint Surg* 1977;58B:241–245.

615. Noyes FR, Wojtys EM, Marshall MT. The early diagnosis and treatment of developmental patella infera syndrome. *Clin Orthop* 1991;265:241–252.

616. Paulos LE, Wnorowski D, Greenwald AE. Infrapatellar contracture syndrome. *Am J Sports Med* 1994;22:440–449.

617. Blumensaat C. Die Lageabweichungen und Verrunkungen der Kniescheibe. *Ergeb Chir Orthop* 1938;31:149–223.

618. Fulkerson JP, et al. Computerized tomography of the patellofemoral joint before and after release or realignment. *Arthroscopy* 1987;3:19–24.

619. Grelsamer RP, Meadows S. The modified Insall-Salvati ratio for assessment of patellar height. *Clin Orthop* 1992;282:170–176.

620. Turner MS. The association between tibial torsion and knee joint pathology. *Clin Orthop* 1994;302:47–51.

621. Amatuzzi MM, Fazzi A, Varella MH. Pathologic synovial plica of the knee. Results of conservative treatment. *Am J Sports Med* 1990;18:466–469.

622. De la Caffiniere JY, Mignot M, Bruch JM. Pli synovial interne et chondropathie rotulienne. *Rev Chir Orthop* 1981;67:479–484.

623. Hughston JC, et al. The role of the suprapatellar plica in internal derangement of the knee. *Am J Orthop* 1963;5:25–27.

624. Patel D. Arthroscopy of the plicae—synovial folds and their significance. *Am J Sports Med* 1978;6:217–225.

625. Pipkin G. Knee injuries: The role of suprapatellar plica and suprapatellar bursa in simulating internal derangements. *Clin Orthop* 1971;74:161–176.

626. Vaughan-Lane T, Dandy DJ. The synovial shelf syndrome. *J Bone Joint Surg* 1982;64B:475–476.

627. Dandy DJ. *Arthroscopic Surgery of the Knee.* New York, NY: Churchill Livingstone; 1981.

628. Dandy DJ. Arthroscopy in the treatment of young patients with anterior knee pain. *Orthop Clin North Am* 1986;17:221–229.

629. Jackson RW. The sneaky plicae [editorial]. *J Rheumatol* 1980;7:437.

630. Apple JS. Infrapatellar plica on lateral knee arthrograms. *AJR Am J Roentgenol* 1983;141:843.

631. Dupont JY. La place des replis synoviaux dans la pathologie du genou. *Rev Chir Orthop* 1985;71:401–403.

632. Lupi L, et al. Arthrography of the plica syndrome and its significance. *Eur J Radiol* 1990;11:15–18.

633. Patel D. Plica as a cause of anterior knee pain. *Orthop Clin North Am* 1986;17:273–277.

634. Fujisawa Y, Jackson R, Marshall DM. Problems caused by the medial and lateral synovial folds of the patella. *Kansetsukyo* 1976;1:40–44.

635. Reid GD, et al. Pathologic plicae of the knee mistaken for arthritis. *J Rheumatol* 1980;7:573–576.

636. Sherman RMP, Jackson RW. The pathological medial plica: Criteria for diagnosis and prognosis. *J Bone Joint Surg* 1989;71B:351.

637. Richmond JC, McGinty JB. Segmental arthroscopic resection of the hypertrophic retropatellar plica. *Clin Orthop* 1983;178:185–189.

638. Apple JS, et al. Synovial plicae of the knee. *Skeletal Radiol* 1982;7:251–254.

639. Aprin H, Shapiro J, Gershwind M. Arthrography (plica views). A noninvasive method for diagnosis and prognosis of plica syndrome. *Clin Orthop* 1984;183:90–95.

640. Brody GA, et al. Plica synovialis infrapatellaris: Arthrographic sign of anterior cruciate ligament disruption. *AJR Am J Roentgenol* 1983;140:767–769.

641. Pipkin G. Lesions of the suprapatellar plica. *J Bone Joint Surg* 1950;32A:363–369.

642. SanDretto MA, et al. Suprapatellar plica synovialis: A common arthrographic finding. *J Can Assoc Radiol* 1982;33:163–166.

643. Deutsch AL, et al. Synovial plicae of the knee. *Radiology* 1981;141:627–634.

644. Thijn CJP, Hillen B. Arthrography and the medial compartment of the patellofemoral joint. *Skeletal Radiol* 1984;11:183–190.

645. Fisher RL. Conservative treatment of patellofemoral pain. *Orthop Clin North Am* 1986;17:269–272.

646. Morrison RJ. Synovial plicae syndrome. *J Manipulative Physiol Ther* 1988;11:296–299.

647. Newell SG, Bramwell ST. Overuse injuries to the knee in runners. *Phys Sports Med* 1984;12:80–92.

648. Subotnick SI, Sisney P. The plica syndrome: A cause of knee pain in the athlete. *J Am Podiatr Med Assoc* 1986;76:292–293.

649. Rovere GD, Nichols AW. Frequency, associated factors, and treatment of breaststroker's knee in competitive swimmers. *Am J Sports Med* 1985;13:99–104.

650. Rovere GD, Adair DM. The medial synovial shelf plica syndrome. Treatment by intraplical steroid injection. *Am J Sports Med* 1985;13:382–386.

651. Jeffreys TE. Recurrent dislocation of the patella due to abnormal attachment of the ilio-tibial tract. *J Bone Joint Surg* 1963;45B:740–743.

652. Fulkerson JP, Schutzer SF. After failure of conservative treatment of painful patellofemoral malalignment: Lateral release or realignment? *Orthop Clin North Am* 1996;17:283–288.

653. Ellen MI, Jackson HB, DiBiase SJ. Uncommon causes of anterior knee pain: A case report of infrapatellar contracture syndrome. *Am J Phys Med Rehabil* 1999;78:376–380.

654. Paulos LE, Wnorowski DC, Greenwald AE. Infrapatellar contracture syndrome: Diagnosis, treatment, and long-term followup. *Am J Sports Med* 1994;22:440–449.

655. Woo SLY, Buckwalter JA. *Injury and Repair of the Musculoskeletal Tissue.* Park Ridge, Ill: American Academy of Orthopaedic Surgeons; 1988.

656. Maurizio E. La tendinite rotulea del giocatore di pallavolo. *Arch Soc Tosco Umbra Chir* 1963;24:443–445.

657. Blazina ME, et al. Jumper's knee. *Orthop Clin North Am* 1973;4:665–678.

658. Anderson JE. Grant's *Atlas of Anatomy.* 7th ed. Baltimore, Md: Williams and Wilkins; 1980.

659. Hollinshead WH, Rosse C. *Textbook of Anatomy.* Philadelphia, Pa: Harper and Row; 1985:434–435.

660. Fredberg U, Bolvig L. Jumper's knee. *Scand J Med Sci Sports* 1999;9:66–73.

661. Bennett JG, Stauber WT. Evaluation and treatment of anterior knee pain using eccentric exercise. *Med Sci Sports Exerc* 1986;18:526–530.

662. Fyfe I, Stanish WD. The use of eccentric training and stretching in the treatment and prevention of tendon injuries. *Clin J Sports Med* 1992;11:601–624.

663. Stanish WD, Rubinovich RM, Curwin S. Eccentric exercise in chronic tendinitis. *Clin Orthop* 1986;208:65–68.

664. Reid DC. Bursitis and knee extensor mechanism pain syndromes. In: Reid DC, ed. *Sports Injury Assessment and Rehabilitation.* New York, NY: Churchill Livingstone; 1992:399–437.

665. Black JE, Alten SR. How I manage infrapatellar tendinitis. *Phys Sports Med* 1984;12:86–90.

666. Popp JE, Yu SS, Kaeding CC. Recalcitrant patellar tendinitis, magnetic resonance imaging, histologic evaluation, and surgical treatment. *Am J Sports Med* 1997;25:218–222.

667. Noble CA. The treatment of iliotibial band friction syndrome. *Br J Sports Med* 1979;13:51–54.

668. Noble CA. Iliotibial band friction syndrome in runners. *Am J Sports Med* 1980;8:232–234.

669. Lindenberg G, Pinshaw R, Noakes TD. Iliotibial band friction syndrome in runners. *Phys Sportsmed* 1984;12:118–130.

670. Sutker AN, Jackson DW, Pagliano JW. Iliotibial band syndrome in distance runners. *Phys Sportsmed* 1981;9:69–73.

671. Biundo JJ Jr, Irwin RW, Umpierre E. Sports and other soft tissue injuries, tendinitis, bursitis, and occupation-related syndromes. *Curr Opin Rheumatol* 2001;13:146–149.

672. Muhle C, Ahn JM, Yeh L. Iliotibial band friction syndrome: MR imaging findings in 16 patients and MR arthrographic study of six cadaveric knees. *Radiology* 1999;212:103–110.

673. Mann RA, Hagy J. Biomechanics of walking, running, and sprinting. *Am J Sports Med* 1980;8:345–350.

674. Mann RA. Biomechanics of running. In: *AAOS Symposium on the Foot and Leg in Running Sports.* St Louis, Mo: Mosby; 1982:30–44.

675. Orchard JW, et al. Biomechanics of the iliotibial band friction syndrome in runners. *Am J Sports Med* 1996;24:375–379.

676. Barber FA, Sutker AN. Iliotibial band syndrome. *Sports Med* 1992;14:144–148.

677. Lineger JM, Christensen CP. Is iliotibial band syndrome often overlooked? *Phys Sportsmed* 1984;20:98–108.

678. Krissoff WB, Ferris WF. Runners' injuries. *Phys Sportsmed* 1979;7:55–63.

679. Krivickas LS. Anatomical factors associated with overuse sports injuries. *Sports Med* 1997;24:132–146.

680. Messier SP, Pittala KA. Etiologic factors associated with selected running injuries. *Med Sci Sports Exerc* 1988;20:501–505.

681. Schwellnus MP. Lower limb biomechanics in runners with the iliotibial band friction syndrome. *Med Sci Sports Exerc* 1993;25:S68.

682. Fredericson M, et al. Hip abductor weakness in distance runners with iliotibial band syndrome. *Clin J Sports Med* 2000; 10:169–175.

683. Pinshaw R, Atlas V, Noakes TD. The nature and response to therapy of 196 consecutive injuries seen at a runners' clinic. *S Afr Med J* 1984;65:291–298.

684. Brantigan OC, Voshell AF. The tibial collateral ligament: Its function, its bursae and its relation to the medial meniscus. *J Bone Joint Surg* 1943;25A:121–131.

685. Worth RM, et al. Saphenous nerve entrapment: a cause of medial knee pain. *Am J Sports Med* 1984;12:80–81.

686. Voshell AF, Brantigan OC. Bursitis in the region of the tibial collateral ligament. *J Bone Joint Surg* 1944;26:793–798.

687. Mital MA, Matza RA. Osgood-Schlatter's disease: The painful puzzler. *Phys Sports Med* 1977;5:60.

688. Ryan J, Wheeler J, Hopkinson W. Quadriceps contusion: West Point update. *Am J Sports Med* 1991;19:299–303.

689. Beauchesne RP, Schutzer SF. Myositis ossificans of the piriformis muscle: An unusual cause of piriformis syndrome. A case report. *J Bone Joint Surg* 1997;79A:906–910.

690. Thompson HC, Garcia A. Myositis ossificans: Aftermath of elbow injuries. *Clin Orthop* 1967;50:129–134.

691. Hoffa A. The influence of the adipose tissue with regard to the pathology of the knee joint. *JAMA* 1904;43:795–796.

692. Jacobson JA, et al. MR imaging of the infrapatellar fat pad of Hoffa. *Radiographics* 1997;17:675–691.

693. Vizsolyi P, et al. Breaststroker's knee. *Am J Sports Med* 1987;15:63.

694. Heng RC, Haw CS. Patellofemoral pain syndrome. *Curr Orthop* 1996;10:256–266.

695. Douchette SA, Goble EM. The effects of exercise on patellar tracking in lateral patellar compression syndrome. *Am J Sports Med* 1992;20:434–440.

696. Devereaux MD, Lachman SM. Patellofemoral arthralgia in athletes attending a sports injury clinic. *Br J Sports Med* 1984;18:8–21.

697. Hughston JC. Subluxation of the patella. *J Bone Joint Surg* 1968;50A:1003–1026.

698. Ficat P, Bizou H. Luxations récidivantes de la routle. *Rev Orthop* 1967;53:721.

699. Fulkerson JP, et al. Patellofemoral pain. *Am Acad Orthop Surg Instruct Course Lect* 1992;41:57–71.

700. Martinez S, et al. Diagnosis of patellofemoral malalignment by computed tomography. *J Comput Assist Tomogr* 1983; 7:1050–1053.

701. Merchant AC, et al. Roentgenographic analysis of patellofemoral congruence. *J Bone Joint Surg* 1974;56A:1391–1396.

702. Minkoff J, Fein L. The role of radiography in the evaluation and treatment of common anarthrotic disorders of the patellofemoral joint. *Clin Sports Med* 1989;8:203–260.

703. Malghem J, Maldague B. Depth insufficiency of the proximal trochlear groove on lateral radiographs of the knee: Relation to patellar dislocation. *Radiology* 1989;170:507–510.

704. Geenen E, Molenaers G, Martens M. Patella alta in patellofemoral instability. *Acta Orthop Belg* 1989;55:387–393.

705. Moller BN, Krebs B, Jurik AG. Patellar height and patellofemoral congruence. *Arch Orthop Trauma Surg* 1986; 104:380–381.

706. Hvid I, Andersen LI. The quadriceps angle and its relation to femoral torsion. *Acta Orthop Scand* 1982;53:577–579.

707. Kimura J. Diseases of the root and plexus in electrodiagnosis. In: Kimura J, ed. *Diseases of Nerve and Muscle: Principles and Practice*. Philadelphia, Pa: FA Davis; 1989:507.

708. Lippitt AB. Neuropathy of the saphenous nerve as a cause of knee pain. *Bull Hosp Joint Dis Orthop Inst* 1993;52:31–33.

709. Romanoff ME, et al. Saphenous nerve entrapment in the adducter canal. *Am J Sports Med* 1989;17:478–481.

710. Magora F, et al. Treatment of pain by transcutaneous electrical stimulation. *Acta Anaesthesiol Scand* 1978;22:589–592.

711. Sunderland S. Traumatized nerves, roots and ganglia: Musculoskeletal factors and neuropathological consequences. In: Knorr IM, Huntwork EH, eds. *The Neurobiologic Mechanisms in Manipulative Therapy*. New York, NY: Plenum Press; 1978: 137–166.

712. Tibrewall SB, Goodfellow JW. Peroneal nerve palsy at the level of the lower third of the leg. *J R Soc Med* 1984;77:72–73.

713. Sridhara CA, Izzo KL. Terminal sensory branches of the superficial peroneal nerve: An entrapment syndrome. *Arch Phys Med Rehab* 1985;66:789–791.

714. Smolders JJ. Myofascial pain and dysfunction syndromes. In: Hammer WI, ed. *Functional Soft Tissue Examination and Treatment by Manual Methods—The Extremities*. Gaithersburg, Md: Aspen; 1991:215–234.

715. Dunn D. Chronic Regional Pain Syndrome, Type 1: Part I. *AORN J* 2000;72:421–424, 426, 428–432, 435, 437–442, 444–449, 452–458.

716. Gordon N. Review article: Reflex sympathetic dystrophy. *Brain Devel* 1996;18:257–262.

717. Wilson PR. Post-traumatic upper extremity reflex sympathetic dystrophy: Clinical course, staging, and classification of clinical forms. *Hand Clin* 1997;13:367–372.

718. Mulligan BR. *Manual Therapy: "NAGS," "SNAGS," "PRP'S" etc*. Wellington, New Zealand: Plane View Series; 1992.

719. Schiowitz S. Diagnosis and treatment of the lower extremity: The foot and ankle. In: DiGiovanna EL, Schiowitz S, eds. *An Osteopathic Approach to Diagnosis and Treatment*. Philadelphia, Pa: JB Lippincott; 1991:338–346.

720. Graf BK, et al. Risk factors for restricted motion after anterior cruciate reconstruction. *Orthopaedics* 1994;17:909–912.

721. Mohtadi NH, Webster-Bogaert S, Fowler PJ. Limitation of motion following anterior cruciate ligament reconstruction. *Am J Sports Med* 1991;19:620–624.

722. Andersson C, et al. Surgical or non-surgical treatment of acute rupture of the anterior cruciate ligament. A randomized study with long-term follow-up. *J Bone Joint Surg* 1989;71A:965–974.

723. Hefti FL, et al. Healing of the transected anterior cruciate ligament in the rabbit. *J Bone Joint Surg* 1991;73A:373–383.

724. Kleiner JB, et al. Primary healing of the anterior cruciate ligament (ACL). *Trans Orthop Res Soc* 1986;11:131.

725. Nagineni CN, et al. Characterization of the intrinsic properties of the anterior cruciate and medial collateral ligament cells: an in vitro cell culture study. *J Orthop Res* 1992;10:465–475.

726. Andrish J, Holmes R. Effects of synovial fluid on fibroblasts in tissue culture. *Clin Orthop* 1979;138:279–283.

727. Kurosaka M, et al. Spontaneous healing of a tear of the anterior cruciate ligament. A report of two cases. *J Bone Joint Surg* 1998;80:1200–1203.

728. Antich TJ, Brewster CE. Rehabilitation of the nonreconstructed anterior cruciate ligament-deficient knee. *Clin Sports Med* 1988;7:813–826.

729. Bynum EB, Barrack RL, Alexander AH. Open versus closed kinetic chain exercises in rehabilitation after anterior cruciate ligament reconstruction: A prospective randomized study. Paper presented at Annual Conference of the American Academy of Orthopaedic Surgeons; 1994; New Orleans, La.

730. Frndak PA, Berasi CC. Rehabilitation concerns following anterior cruciate ligament reconstruction. *Sports Med* 1991; 12:338–346.

731. Mangine RE, Noyes FR, DeMaio M. Minimal protection program: Advanced weight bearing and range of motion after ACL reconstruction—Weeks 1 to 5. *Orthopaedics* 1992;15:504–515.

732. Seto JL, Brewster CE, Lombardo SJ. Rehabilitation of the knee after anterior cruciate ligament reconstruction. *J Orthop Sports Phys Ther* 1989;11:8–18.

733. Shelbourne KD, Wilckens JH. Current concepts in anterior cruciate ligament rehabilitation. *Orthop Rev* 1990;19:957–964.

734. Silfverskold JP, Steadman JR, Higgins RW. Rehabilitation of the anterior cruciate ligament in the athlete. *Sports Med* 1988;6:308–319.

735. Steadman JR, Forster RS, Silfverskold JP. Rehabilitation of the knee. *Clin Sports Med* 1989;8:605–627.

736. Steadman JR, Sterett WI. The surgical treatment of knee injuries in skiers. *Med Sci Sports Exerc* 1995;27:328–333.

737. Timm KE. Postsurgical knee rehabilitation. A five-year study of four methods and 5,381 patients. *Am J Sports Med* 1988;16:463–468.

738. Gryzlo SM, Patek RM, Pink M. Electromyographic analysis of knee rehabilitation exercises. *J Orthop Sports Phys Ther* 1994;20:36–43.

739. Lephart SM, et al. The role of proprioception in the management and rehabilitation of athletic injuries. *Am J Sports Med* 1997;25:130–137.

740. Janarv PM, et al. Anterior cruciate ligament injuries in skeletally immature patients. *J Pediatr Orthop* 1996;16:673.

CHAPTER 19

THE ANKLE AND FOOT

CHAPTER OBJECTIVES

▶ *At the completion of this chapter, the reader will be able to:*

1. Describe the anatomy of the joints, ligaments, muscles, and blood and nerve supply which comprise the foot and ankle complex.

2. Describe the biomechanics of the foot and ankle complex, including the open and closed pack positions, normal and abnormal joint end-feels, kinesiology, and the effects of open and closed chain activities.

3. Outline the purpose and components of the tests and measures of the foot and ankle complex.

4. Perform a detailed examination of the foot and ankle complex, including palpation of the articular and soft tissue structures, range-of-motion testing, passive articular mobility tests, and stability tests for the foot and ankle complex.

5. Discuss the significance of the key findings from the tests and measures.

6. Evaluate the total examination data to establish a physical therapy diagnosis.

7. Describe the significance of muscle imbalance in terms of functional muscle performance and the deleterious effects on the lower kinetic chain.

8. Develop self-reliant examination and intervention strategies.

9. Describe the intervention strategies based on clinical findings and established goals.

10. Apply manual techniques to the foot and ankle complex, using the correct grade, direction, and duration.

11. Incorporate appropriate therapeutic exercises into the intervention progression.

12. Evaluate intervention effectiveness in order to progress or modify the intervention.

13. Plan an effective home program and instruct the patient in same.

OVERVIEW

The ankle and foot is a complex structure comprised of 28 bones (including 2 sesamoid bones) and 55 articulations (including 30 synovial joints), interconnected by ligaments and muscles.

The foot has undergone a number of evolutionary adaptations, which makes it very well designed for bipedal loco-motion.[1] First, the foot has become plantigrade, which allows most of the sole to be a weight-bearing surface.[1] Second, the great toe has come to lie in a position with the other toes, and because of the relative immobility of the first metatarsal at the metatarsophalangeal (MTP) joint, is now relatively nonprehensile.[1] Third, the metatarsals and phalanges have progressively shrunk and become small in comparison to the hypertrophied tarsus.[1] Lastly, the medial side of the foot has become larger and stronger than that of any other primate.[1]

The ankle joint sustains the greatest load per surface area of any joint of the body.[2] The joints and ligaments of the ankle and foot complex act as stabilizers, and constantly adapt during weight-bearing activities. This is particularly true on uneven surfaces. The ankle and foot support loads that are truly impressive. Peak vertical forces reach 120 percent body weight during walking, and they approach 275 percent during running.[3] Five times the body weight is placed across the talocrural joint during initial contact while running.[3] As a consequence, it is estimated that an average 150-lb man absorbs 63.5 tons on each foot while walking 1 mile, and that the same man absorbs 110 tons per foot while running 1 mile.[4] About 60 percent of this weight-bearing load is carried out by the rearfoot, 8 percent by the midfoot, and 28 percent by the metatarsal heads,[5] with the second and third metatarsal heads bearing the greatest forefoot pressures.[6] Although the ankle and foot complex normally adapts well to the stresses of everyday life, sudden or unanticipated stresses to this region have the potential to produce dysfunction.[7–10]

Anatomy

The ankle and foot complex is a sophisticated musculoskeletal arrangement designed to facilitate numerous and various weight-bearing and non–weight-bearing functions.[11] Anatomically and biomechanically, the foot is often subdivided into the rearfoot or hindfoot (the talus and calcaneus), the midfoot (the navicular, cuboid, and the 3 cuneiforms), and the forefoot (the 14 bones of the toes, the 5 metatarsals, and the medial and lateral sesamoids) (Table 19-1 and Fig. 19-1).

Rearfoot

The function of the rearfoot is to:

▶ convert the torque of the lower limb.

▶ influence the function and movement of the midfoot and forefoot.

▶ convert the transverse rotations of the lower extremity into sagittal, transverse, and frontal plane movements.[12]

Midfoot

The midfoot transmits motion from the rearfoot to the forefoot and promotes stability, while the forefoot adapts to the terrain, adjusting to uneven surfaces.[12]

Forefoot

The bones of the forefoot may be divided into the tarsus, metatarsus, and phalanges. The seven tarsal bones occupy the proximal half of the foot (see Fig. 19-2). The proximal row of tarsals comprises the talus and calcaneus. The talus (astragalus) attaches the foot to the leg. Its long axis inclines anteromedially

TABLE 19-1 The Joints of the Foot and Ankle: Their Open-Packed, Close-Packed Positions, and Capsular Patterns

Joints of the Hind Foot	Open-Packed Position	Close-Packed Position	Capsular Pattern
Tibiofibular joint	Plantar flexion	Maximum dorsiflexion	Pain on stress
Talocrural joint	10 degrees of plantar flexion and midway between inversion and eversion	Maximum dorsiflexion	Plantar flexion, dorsiflexion
Subtalar joint	Midway between the extremes of range of motion	Supination	Varus, valgus
Joints of the Midfoot			
Midtarsal joints	Midway between the extremes of range of motion	Supination	Dorsiflexion, plantar flexion, adduction, internal rotation
Joints of the Forefoot			
Tarsometatarsal joints	Midway between the extremes of range of motion	Supination	None
Metatarsophalangeal joints	10 degrees of extension	Full extension	Great toe: extension, flexion 2nd–5th toes: variable
Interphalangeal joints	Slight flexion	Full extension	Flexion, extension

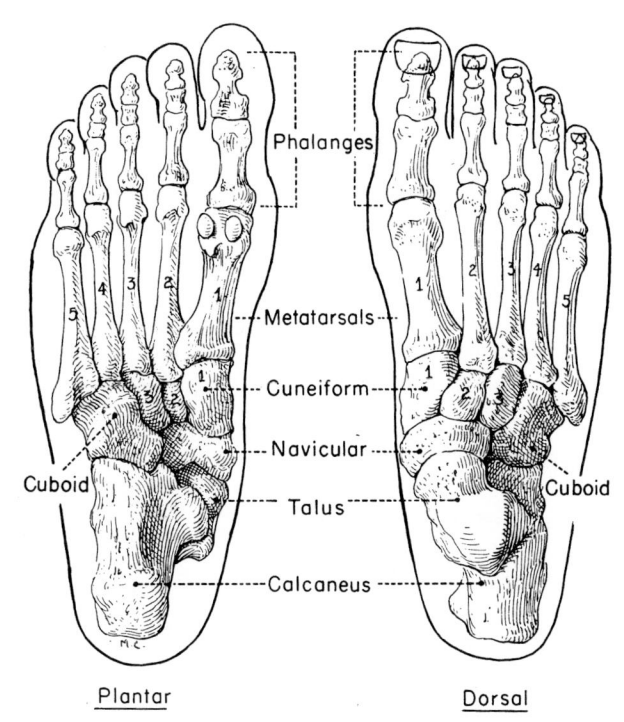

FIGURE 19-1 Bones of the foot: plantar and dorsal views. (Reproduced with permission from Luttgens K, Hamilton K. *Kinesiology: Scientific Basis of Human Motion.* New York: McGraw-Hill; 1997.)

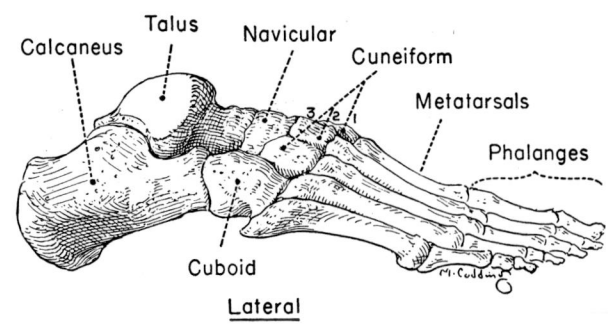

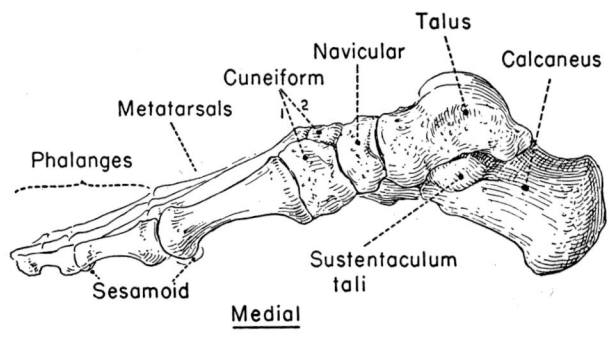

FIGURE 19-2 Bones of the foot: lateral and medial views. (Reproduced with permission from Luttgens K, Hamilton K. *Kinesiology: Scientific Basis of Human Motion.* New York: McGraw-Hill; 1997.)

and down, and its distal head is medial to the calcaneus and at a higher level (see Fig. 19-1). The calcaneus (or calcis) (see Fig. 19-2) is the largest tarsal bone, but is also the most frequently fractured. The calcaneus articulates with the talus superiorly, with the cuboid laterally, and with the navicular medially. The distal tarsal row contains, medial to lateral, the medial, intermediate, and lateral cuneiforms, and the cuboid, which is roughly in parallel with the proximal row, and which forms a transverse arch, dorsally convex (Fig. 19-2). Medially, the navicular is positioned between the talus and cuneiforms (see Fig. 19-2). Laterally, the cuboid is positioned between the calcaneus and the lateral cuneiform and fourth and fifth metatarsal (see Fig. 19-2). The first metatarsal is the shortest and strongest (see Fig. 19-1), while the second is the longest and least mobile, serving as the anatomic touchstone for abduction and adduction of the foot.[13] The phalanges of the foot, although similar in number and distribution to those in the hand, are shorter and broader than their counterparts.

Clinical Pearl

The midtarsal, or Chopart's joint, consists of the calcaneocuboid joint and talonavicular joint and connects the rearfoot to the midfoot. The midtarsal joint facilitates adduction and abduction of the forefoot.[11] The tarsometatarsal, or Lisfranc's joint, connects the midfoot and the forefoot.[11]

The shapes of the articulating surfaces of the leg and foot are outlined in Table 19-2. An appreciation of the shapes of the articulating surfaces is important when examining the joint glides and when performing joint mobilizations.

Most of the stability of the foot and ankle is provided by a vast array of ligaments (Table 19-3).

Distal Tibiofibular Joint

The distal tibiofibular joint (Fig. 19-3) is classified as a syndesmosis, except for about 1 mm of the inferior portion, which is covered in hyaline cartilage. The joint consists of a concave tibial surface and a convex or plane surface on the medial distal end of the fibula. There is an elongation into the joint by the synovium of the talocrural joint, the fibers of which are oriented inferiorly and laterally. The fibula serves as a site for muscular and ligamentous attachment, providing stability for the talus at the talocrural joint. The tibia is the second longest bone of the skeleton and is a major weight-bearing bone.

As at the proximal tibiofibular joint (see Chap. 18), support for this joint is provided primarily by ligaments. The joint is stabilized by four ligaments collectively known as the syndesmotic ligaments. These include the inferior interosseous ligament, the anterior inferior tibiofibular ligament, the posterior inferior tibiofibular ligament, and the inferior transverse ligament. Of these ligaments, the inferior interosseous ligament is the primary stabilizer.

TABLE 19-2 Shapes of the Articulating Surfaces of the Leg and Foot[9]

Joint	Proximal Bone and Shape of Its Joint Surface	Distal Bone and Shape of Its Joint Surface
Inferior tibiofibular	Tibia—concave	Fibula—convex
Talocrural	Tibia—concave in anterior-posterior direction and concave-convex-concave in mediolateral direction	Fibula—convex in anterior-posterior direction and convex-concave-convex in mediolateral direction
Talocalcaneal	Talus—posterior facet biconcave, middle facet biconvex, anterior facet convex	Calcaneus—posterior facet biconvex, middle facet biconcave, anterior facet concave
Talonavicular	Talus—biconvex	Navicular—biconcave
Calcaneocuboid	Calcaneus—convex in mediolateral direction and concave in superior-inferior direction (saddle-shaped)	Cuboid—concave in mediolateral direction and convex in superior-inferior direction (saddle-shaped)
Cuboideonavicular	Navicular—planar	Cuboid—planar
Cuneonavicular	Navicular—slightly convex	Cuneiforms—slight concave
Intercuneiform	Cuneiforms (medial and middle)—planar	Cuneiforms (middle and lateral)—planar
Cuneocuboid	Lateral cuneiform—planar	Cuboid—planar
Tarsometatarsal	Cuneiforms and cuboid—planar to slightly convex	Bases of metatarsals—planar to slightly concave
Metatarsophalangeal	Metatarsals—biconvex	Proximal phalanges—biconcave
Interphalangeal	Proximal phalanges—convex in superior-inferior and concave in medial-lateral direction	Middle phalanges—concave in superior-inferior and convex in a medial-lateral direction

TABLE 19-3 Ankle and Foot Joints and Associated Ligaments[9]

Joint	Associated Ligament	Fiber Direction	Motions Limited
Distal tibiofibular	Anterior tibiofibular	Distolateral	Distal and posterior glide of fibula
	Posterior tibiofibular	Distolateral	Distal and anterior glide of fibula
	Interosseous	Distolateral	Separation of tibia and fibula
Ankle	Deltoid (medial collateral) Superficial		
	Tibionavicular	Plantar-anterior	Lateral translation and external rotation of the talus
	Calcaneotibial	Plantar, plantar-posterior	Eversion (abduction of talus, calcaneus and navicular)
	Posterior talotibial	Plantar-posterior	Dorsiflexion, lateral translation and external rotation of the talus
	Deep		
	Anterior talotibial	Anterior	Abduction of the talus when in plantar flexion or eversion
	Lateral or fibular collateral		
	Anterior talofibular	Anterior-medial	Inversion and plantar flexion Anterior displacement of the talus Internal rotation of the talus
	Calcaneofibular	Posterior distal and medial	Inversion and dorsiflexion
	Posterior talofibular	Horizontal	Dorsiflexion Posterior displacement of foot Inversion

TABLE 19-3 *(cont.)*

Subtalar	Lateral (anterior) talocalcaneal	Distal anterolateral	Joint separation during inversion and dorsiflexion
	Deltoid	(See ankle)	
	Lateral collateral		
	Medial (posterior) talocalcaneal	Distal	Anterior translation of talus and inversion
	Cervical ligament	Distal-posterior-lateral	Inversion
	Interosseous	Distal and lateral	Joint separation
Main ligamentous support of longitudinal arches	Long plantar	Anterior, slightly medial	Eversion
	Short plantar	Anterior	Eversion
	Plantar calcaneonavicular	Dorsal-anterior-medial	Eversion
	Plantar aponeurosis	Anterior	Eversion
Midtarsal or transverse	Bifurcated		Joint separation
	Medial band	Longitudinal	Plantar flexion
	Lateral band	Horizontal	Inversion
	Dorsal talonavicular	Longitudinal	Plantar flexion of talus on navicular
	Dorsal calcaneocuboid	Longitudinal	Inversion, plantar flexion
	Ligaments supporting the arches		
Intertarsal	Dorsal and plantar ligaments		Joint motion in direction causing ligament tautness
	Interosseous ligaments connecting cuneiforms, cuboid, and navicular		Flattening of transverse or longitudinal arch
Tarsometatarsal	Dorsal, plantar, and interosseous		Joint separation
Intermetatarsal	Dorsal, plantar, and interosseous		Joint separation
	Deep transverse metatarsal		Joint separation / Flattening of transverse arch
Metatarsophalangeal	Fibrous capsule		
	Dorsal, thin—separated from extensor tendons by bursae		Flexion
	Plantar		
	Inseparable from deep surface of plantar and collateral ligaments		Extension
	Collateral	Plantar-anterior	Flexion, abduction, or adduction in flexion
Interphalangeal	Collateral		Flexion, abduction, or adduction in flexion
	Plantar		Extension

The Talocrural (Ankle) Joint

The talocrural joint is formed between the talus and the distal tibia. The saddle-shaped talus is the link between the foot and the leg through the ankle joint (see Fig. 19-3) and is considered as the mechanical keystone of the ankle as it serves to distribute the body weight backwards towards the heel, and forwards to the midfoot. This ability to distribute forces is due to the massive articulating surface of the talus that both spreads and focuses forces. The talus is divided into a head (anteriorly) and a neck and body (posteriorly).

▶ *Body.* The superior dome-shaped surface of the body articulates with the tibia. The body is convex in the A-P direction and slightly concave in the M-L and superior directions.[9] The shape of this articulating surface can be

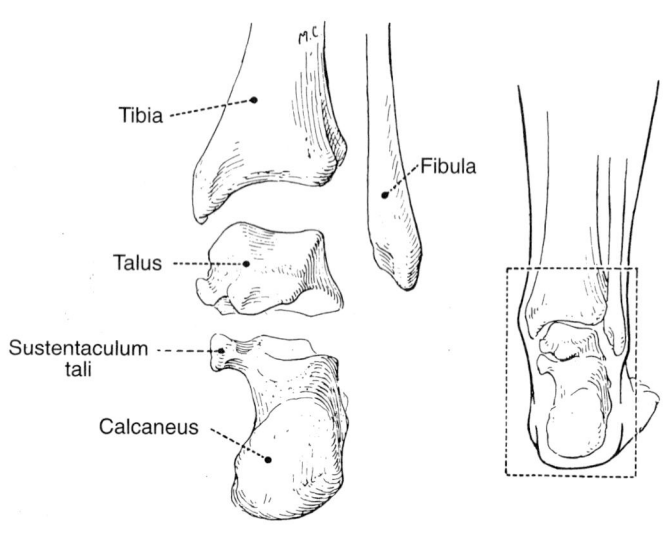

FIGURE 19-3 Distal tibiofibular joint. (Reproduced with permission from Luttgens K, Hamilton K. *Kinesiology: Scientific Basis of Human Motion.* New York: McGraw-Hill; 1997.)

compared to that of a cone, with the base of the cone facing laterally, and the apex medially. Because the superior aspect of the body of the talus is wedge-shaped with the wider portion anterior, no varus/valgus movement is possible when the ankle is positioned in maximum dorsiflexion unless the mortise or the tibiofibular ligaments are compromised.

▶ *Neck.*   The neck of the talus is a narrow region between the head and the body of the talus and it is medially inclined. Its rough surfaces serve as attachments for ligaments. Inferior to the neck of the talus is the sulcus tali, which when the talus and calcaneus are articulated, roofs the sinus tarsi, and is occupied by the talocalcaneal interosseous and cervical ligaments.

▶ *Head.*   The plantar surface of the head has three articular areas separated by smooth ridges. The most posterior and largest of the articular areas is oval, slightly convex, and rests on a shelf-like medial calcanean projection called the *sustentaculum tali.*[9] The other two articulating facets connect the talus with the navicular and the plantarcalcaneonavicular ligament.[9]

The medial malleolus extends distally to about one third of the height of the talus, whereas the lateral malleolus extends distally to about two thirds the height of the talus.[14]

The fibrous capsule of the ankle joint is relatively thin on its anterior and posterior aspects.[9] It is lined with synovial membrane and reinforced by the collateral ligaments (see later).

> ### Clinical Pearl
>
> No tendons, with the exception of a small slip from the posterior tibialis, attach to the talus. However, the talus serves as the attachment for many ligaments.

The talus receives its blood supply from the branches of the anterior and posterior tibial arteries (Fig. 19-4), and is very susceptible to aseptic necrosis, particularly with proximal fractures.[15]

Talocrural Ligaments

The major ligaments of the talocrural joint can be divided into two main groups: lateral collaterals and medial (deltoid) collaterals.

Lateral Collaterals.   The lateral collateral ligament complex consists of three separate bands, which function together as the static stabilizers of the lateral ankle. Each of the lateral ligaments has a role in stabilizing the ankle and/or subtalar joint, depending on the position of the foot. As such, these ligaments are commonly involved in ankle sprains.[16–20]

Anterior Talofibular Ligament (ATFL).   This thickening of the anterior capsule extends from the anterior surface of the fibular malleolus, just lateral to the articular cartilage of the lateral malleolus, to just anterior to the lateral facet of the talus and to the lateral surface of the talar neck (Fig. 19-5).[21]

The ATFL is an intracapsular structure and is approximately 2 to 5 mm thick and 10 to 12 mm long.[22] The ATFL functions to resist ankle inversion in plantar flexion. Regardless of ankle position, the ATFL is usually the first ankle ligament to be torn in an inversion injury.[22] The accessory functions of the ATFL include resistance to anterior talar displacement from the mortise, and resistance to internal rotation of the talus within the mortise.[23]

> ### Clinical Pearl
>
> The ATFL requires the lowest maximal load to produce failure of the lateral ligaments, though it has the highest strain to failure of that group.[24]

Calcaneofibular Ligament (CFL).   The CFL (see Fig. 19-5), an extra-articular structure covered by the peroneal tendons, is larger and stronger than the ATFL.[22] It fans out at 10 to 40 degrees from the tip of the fibular malleolus to the lateral side of the calcaneus, paralleling the horizontal axis of the subtalar joint. This ligament effectively spans the ankle and subtalar joints, which have markedly different axes of rotation.[25–28] Thus its attachment is designed so that it does not restrict motion in either joint, whether they move independently or simultaneously.[21,27,29] However, the CFL indirectly aids talofibular stability during dorsiflexion due to its anatomic location, where it can act as a true collateral ligament and prevent talar tilt into inversion.[14,21] As the ankle joint passes from dorsiflexion to plantar flexion, the calcaneofibular ligament is less able to resist talar tilt to inversion, although the anterior talofibular ligament is more able to resist this tilt.[21]

Posterior Talofibular Ligament (PTFL).   The PTFL (see Fig. 19-5) is the strongest of the lateral ligament complex.[22] As such, it is rarely injured except in severe ankle sprains. The ligament is coalescent with the joint capsule, and its orientation is relatively

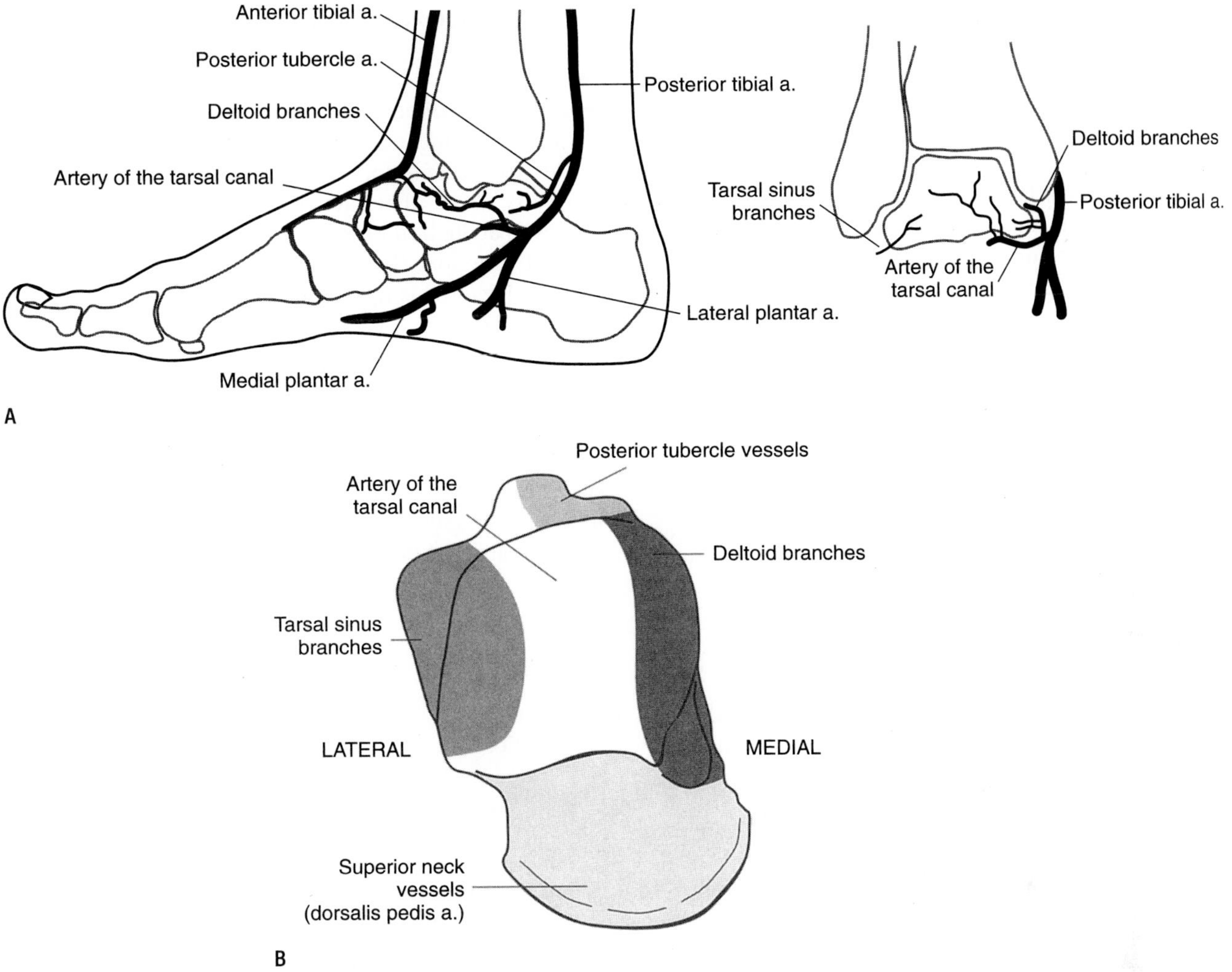

Anterior tibial a.

Posterior tubercle a.

Deltoid branches

Artery of the tarsal canal

Posterior tibial a.

Deltoid branches

Posterior tibial a.

Tarsal sinus branches

Artery of the tarsal canal

Lateral plantar a.

Medial plantar a.

A

Posterior tubercle vessels

Artery of the tarsal canal

Deltoid branches

Tarsal sinus branches

LATERAL

MEDIAL

Superior neck vessels (dorsalis pedis a.)

B

FIGURE 19-4 Vascular supply to the talus. A. Extraosseus blood supply to the talus. B. The regional blood supply to the talus. (Reproduced with permission from Kelikian AS. *Operative Treatment of the Foot and Ankle*. New York: Appleton-Lange; 1999.)

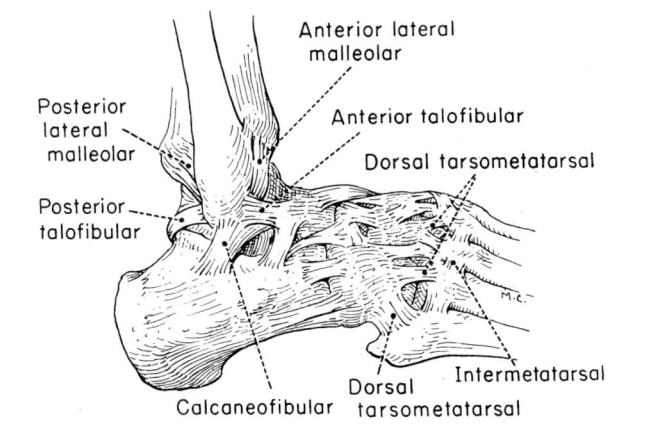

Anterior lateral malleolar

Posterior lateral malleolar

Anterior talofibular

Posterior talofibular

Dorsal tarsometatarsal

Posterior talofibular

Calcaneofibular

Dorsal tarsometatarsal

Intermetatarsal

FIGURE 19-5 Lateral ligaments of the ankle joint. (Reproduced with permission from Luttgens K, Hamilton K. *Kinesiology: Scientific Basis of Human Motion*. New York: McGraw-Hill; 1997.)

horizontal. Its attachment on the talus involves nearly the entire nonarticular portion of the posterior talus to the groove for the flexor hallucis longus tendon, and anteriorly to the digital fossa of the fibula, which transmits the vessels that supply the talus and the fibula.[30,31]

Lateral Talocalcaneal Interosseous. The lateral talocalcaneal interosseous (LTCIL) ligament is not traditionally included in this group, though it does play a role in lateral ankle and subtalar stability.[22,32] The ligament varies in configuration from a distinct rectangular structure spanning the subtalar joint, to a fan-shaped ligament contiguous with the calcaneofibular ligament inferiorly, which broadens to insert along the entire inferior portion of the anterior tibiofibular ligament.[21]

Its role in subtalar instability is not completely understood. It is possible that a CFL injury may result in greater relative symptomatic instability for an individual lacking a LTCIL as compared with an individual who has an intact LTCIL.[21,30]

Besides maintaining lateral ankle stability, the lateral ankle ligaments play a significant role in maintaining rotational ankle stability.[21] Significant compromise to the ATFL and/or CFL leads to a measurable increase in inversion without any tilting of the talus or subtalar gapping.[21] A loss of ATFL function permits an increase in external rotation of the leg, and unlocks the subtalar joint, allowing further inversion, which may lead to symptomatic instability.[21]

Medial Collaterals. Collectively the medial collateral ligaments form a triangular-shaped ligamentous structure known as the deltoid ligament (Fig. 19-6). Wide variations have been noted in the anatomic description of the deltoid ligament, but is generally agreed that it consists of both superficial and deep fibers.

The Superficial Fibers

▶ ***Tibionavicular (see Fig. 19-6).*** These fibers extend from the medial malleolus to the tuberosity of the navicular and serve to resist lateral translation and external rotation of the talus.

▶ ***Posterior talotibial (see Fig. 19-6).*** These fibers travel in a posterolateral direction from the medial malleolus to the medial side of the talus and medial tuberosity of the talus. These fibers resist ankle dorsiflexion and lateral translation and external rotation of the talus.

▶ ***Calcaneotibial (see Fig. 19-6).*** These thin fibers extend from the medial malleolus to the sustentaculum tali. The fibers are oriented in such a way that they resist abduction

of the talus, calcaneus, and navicular when the foot and ankle are positioned in plantar flexion and eversion.[26]

The Deep Fibers

▶ ***Anterior talotibial (see Fig. 19-6).*** The fibers of this strong ligament extend from the tip of the medial malleolus to the anterior aspect of the medial surface of the talus. These fibers are oriented in such a way that they resist abduction of the talus when it is in plantar flexion and eversion. Such is the strength of these fibers that an injury to this ligament is often associated with an avulsion fracture.

Whereas the calcaneotibial ligament is very thin and supports only negligible forces before failing, the talotibial ligaments are very strong.[36,37] Rasmussen and colleagues[38,39] found that the superficial fibers of the deltoid ligament specifically limited talar abduction or negative talar tilt, but that the deep layers of the deltoid ligament ruptured with external rotation of the leg without the superficial portion being involved.

Subtalar (Talocalcaneal) Joint

The subtalar joint (Fig. 19-7) is a synovial, bicondylar compound joint consisting of two separate, modified ovoid surfaces with their own joint cavities (one male and one female) (Fig. 19-7). The two surfaces, consisting of anterior and posterior articulations, are connected by an interosseous membrane.

▶ The anterior joint consists of a concave facet on the calcaneus, and a convex facet on the talus. The anterior component is situated more medial than the posterior, giving the plane of the joint an average 42 degrees (±9 degrees) superior from the transverse foot plane and 23 degrees (±11 degrees) medial from the sagittal foot plane.[41]

▶ The posterior joint consists of a convex facet on the calcaneus and a concave facet on the talus (see Fig. 19-7).

This relationship ensures that the anterior and posterior aspects can move in opposite directions to each other during functional movements (while the anterior aspect is moving medially, the posterior aspect is moving laterally).

The calcaneus, the largest tarsal bone, projects posterior to the tibia and fibula. It serves as a weight-bearing bone and as a short lever for muscles of the calf, which are attached to its posterior surface. The skin and fat over the distal-inferior area of the calcaneus are specialized for friction and shock absorption.[42]

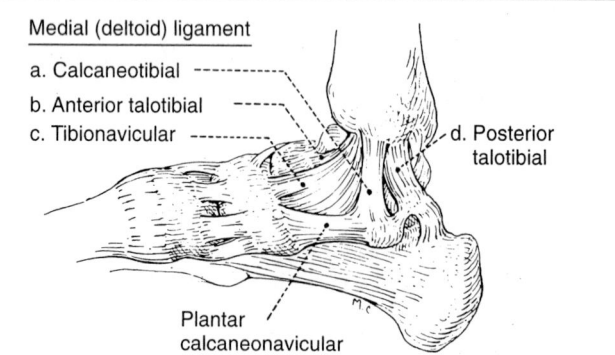

FIGURE 19-6 Medial ligaments of the ankle joint. (Reproduced with permission from Luttgens K, Hamilton K. *Kinesiology: Scientific Basis of Human Motion.* New York: McGraw-Hill; 1997.)

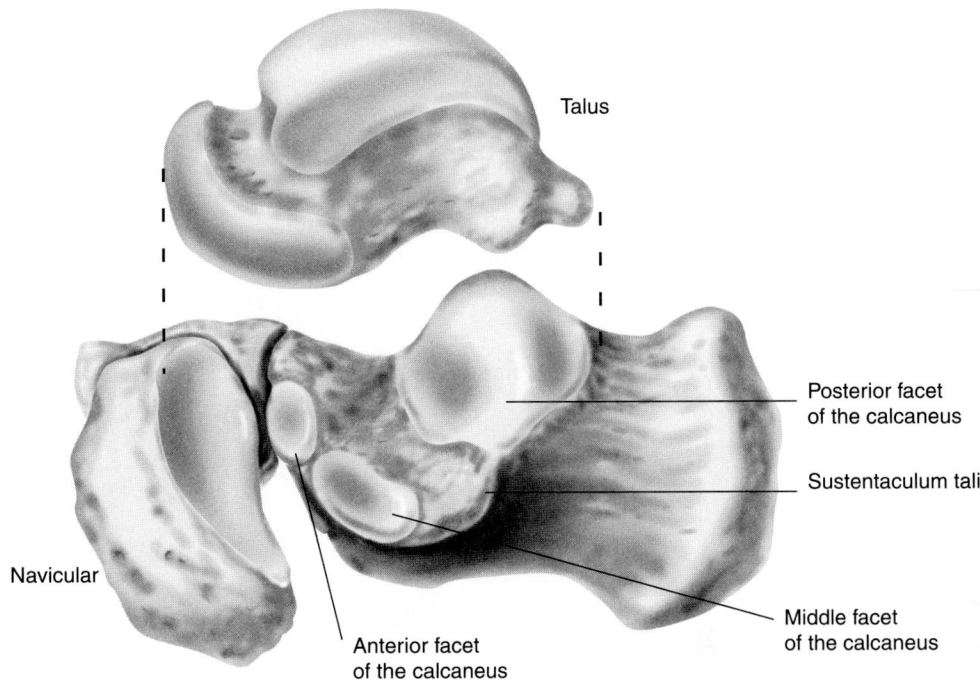

FIGURE 19-7 Subtalar joint. (Reproduced with permission from Kelikian AS. *Operative Treatment of the Foot and Ankle.* New York: Appleton-Lange; 1999.)

Talus

Posterior facet of the calcaneus

Sustentaculum tali

Middle facet of the calcaneus

Anterior facet of the calcaneus

Navicular

Clinical Pearl

The skin on the sole of the foot is thicker than anywhere else in the body. The heel area comprises a honeycombed pattern of subcutaneous fat globules in fibroelastic septae 13 to 21 mm thick, surrounded by the calcaneus and the skin.[43] This structure cushions initial contact by the heel and allows the skin to resist forces up to five times the body weight during running.[43] However, after the age of 40, the thickness of the subcutaneous fat decreases, with a resultant loss of shock absorbency.[44]

The retrocalcaneal bursa lies anterior to the posterosuperior calcaneal tuberosity of the calcaneus. It lubricates the Achilles tendon anteriorly as well as the superior aspect of the calcaneus.[45] The superior or proximal surface of the calcaneus is divisible into thirds.

▶ *The posterior third.* This is a roughened surface that is concavoconvex in extension, the convexity transverse. It supports fibroadipose tissue between the calcaneal tendon and the ankle joint. Distal to the posterior articular facet is a rough depression which narrows into a groove on the medial side—the sulcus calcanei—which completes the sinus tarsi with the talus.[9]

▶ *The middle third.* This surface carries the posterior talar facet, and is oval and convex anteroposteriorly.

▶ *The anterior third.* This surface is only partly articular.

Talocalcaneal Ligaments

A number of ligaments provide support to this joint, although some confusion exists in the descriptions and nomenclature of these ligaments. In relation to the sinus tarsi, the most medial ligament is the talocalcaneal interosseous ligament, which branches superiorly into medial and lateral bands (Figs. 19-8 and 19-9).[46] The cervical ligament and portions of the retinaculum are located more laterally. The talocalcaneal interosseous and cervical ligaments are often collectively referred to as the interosseous ligaments.

Medial (Posterior) Talocalcaneal Interosseous. The medial talocalcaneal interosseous ligament extends from the medial tubercle of the talus to the posterior aspect of the sustentaculum tali and the area of the calcaneus just posterior to the sustentaculum tali. It functions to stabilize against anterior translation of the talus (especially at the initial contact phase of the gait cycle) by producing passive eversion of the talus. This results in a close packing of the lateral foot and fibula. Damage to this ligament, which typically occurs with inversion sprains and rotational compression fractures of the calcaneus, can permit excessive anterior motion of the talus. This excessive motion may result in posterior tibialis tendonitis[47] and on occasion, Achilles tendonitis.[48]

Lateral (Anterior) Talocalcaneal Interosseous. The lateral talocalcaneal interosseous ligament originates from the roof of the sinus tarsi and extends in a posteroinferior direction from the lateral process of the talus to the lateral surface of the calcaneus, just anterior to the calcaneofibular ligament. This ligament functions to prevent the talus and calcaneus from separating during inversion movements. This highly innervated structure is typically injured with a dorsiflexion and inversion mechanism.[49]

FIGURE 19-8   Talocalcaneal ligaments.
(Reproduced with permission from Kelikian AS.
Operative Treatment of the Foot and Ankle.
New York: Appleton-Lange; 1999.)

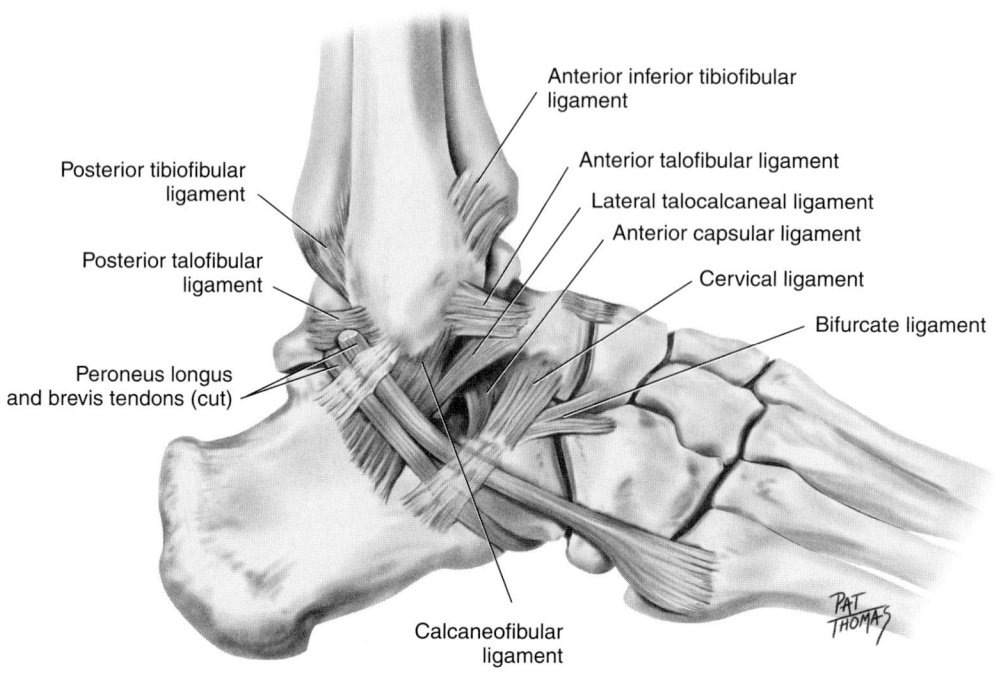

Midtarsal (Transverse Tarsal) Joint Complex

The midtarsal joint complex consists of the talonavicular and calcaneocuboid articulations.

Talonavicular

The talonavicular joint (see Fig. 19-2) is classified as a synovial, compound, modified ovoid joint.

The joint is actually formed by components of the talus, navicular, calcaneus, and plantar calcaneonavicular (spring) ligament. The rounded convex, anterior head of the talus fits into the concavity of the posterior navicular and the anterior component

of the subtalar joint, and rests on the dorsal surface of the spring ligament. The joint capsule is only well developed posteriorly, where it forms the anterior part of the interosseus ligament.

Calcaneocuboid

The calcaneocuboid joint (see Fig. 19-2) is classified as a simple, synovial modified sellar joint.

The anterior surface of the calcaneus, which articulates with the reciprocally shaped posterior surface of the cuboid, is relatively convex in an oblique horizontal direction, and relatively concave in an oblique vertical direction.[50]

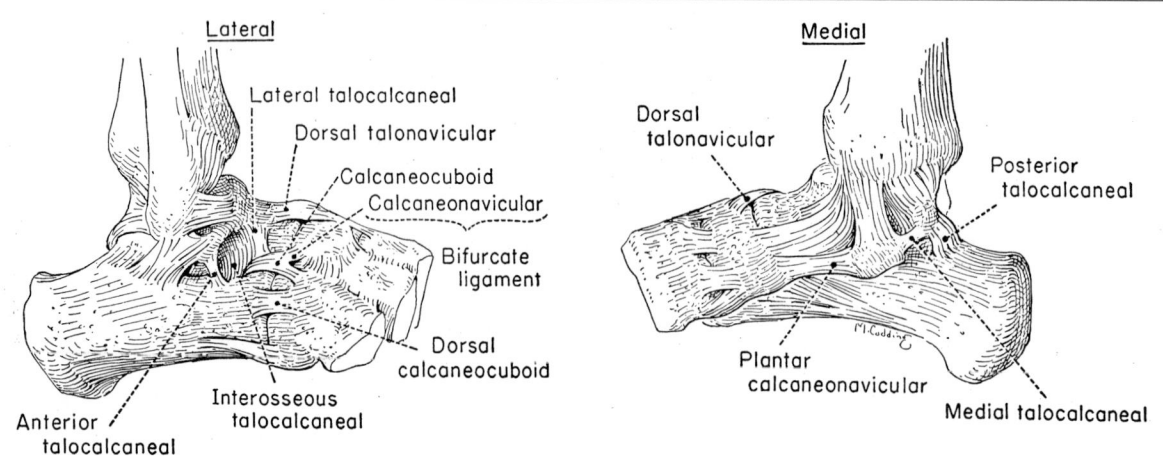

FIGURE 19-9   Ligaments of the tarsal joints. (Reproduced with permission from Luttgens K, Hamilton K. *Kinesiology: Scientific Basis of Human Motion.* New York: McGraw-Hill; 1997.)

The cuboid, most lateral in the distal tarsal row, is located between the calcaneus proximally and the fourth and fifth metatarsals distally. To the dorsal surface are attached dorsal calcaneocuboid, cubonavicular, cuneocuboid, and cubometatarsal ligaments, and to the proximal edge of the plantar ridge, deep fibers of the long plantar ligament.[9] To the projecting proximal-medial part of the plantar surface are attached a slip of the tendon of tibialis posterior and flexor hallucis brevis. To the rough part of the medial cuboidal surface are attached interosseous, cuneocuboid, and cubonavicular ligaments, and proximally the medial calcaneocuboid, which is the lateral limb of the bifurcated ligament.[9]

The capsule is thickened dorsally to form the dorsal calcaneocuboid ligament. The joint has a large plantar phalanx to provide additional support during weight bearing.

A number of ligaments help provide support to this region. The spring ligament (plantar calcaneonavicular; Fig. 19-9) connects the navicular bone to the sustentaculum tali on the calcaneus. The ligaments of the calcaneocuboid joint include the long plantar ligament and a portion of the bifurcate ligament (see Figs. 19-8 and 19-9) dorsally.

The long and strong plantar ligament attaches to the plantar surface of the calcaneus, the tuberosity on the plantar surface of the cuboid bone, and to the bases of the second, third, and fourth (and possibly fifth) metatarsals.[9] The plantar ligament functions to provide indirect plantar support to the joint, by limiting the amount of flattening of the lateral longitudinal arch of the foot.[50] Together with the groove in the cuboid bone, it forms a tunnel for the passage of the peroneus longus tendon across the plantar surface of the foot.[9]

The bifurcate ligament (see Fig. 19-9) functions to support the medial and lateral aspects of the foot when weight bearing in a plantar flexed position (twisted).

The plantar calcaneocuboid ligament (see Fig. 19-9), sometimes referred to as the short plantar ligament, is a relatively broad and strong strap-like structure that extends from the area of the anterior tubercle of the calcaneus to the adjacent plantar surface of the cuboid bone. It provides plantar support to the joint and possibly helps to limit flattening of the lateral longitudinal arch.

Cuneonavicular

The cuneonavicular joint is classified as a compound, synovial, modified ovoid joint. The navicular presents a convex surface to the concave surface of the combined cuneiforms. The wedge-like cuneiform bones articulate with the navicular proximally, and with the bases of the first to third metatarsals distally (see Fig. 19-1). The medial cuneiform is the largest, the intermediate the smallest. In the intermediate and lateral cuneiforms, the dorsal surface is the base of the wedge, but in the medial, the wedge is reversed, a prime factor in shaping the transverse arch. The wedge shape of these bones also provides a cavity for the neurovascular and musculotendinous structures of the foot.

The cuneiforms, together with articulations with the metatarsal bones, form Lisfranc's joint.[13] The proximal surface of all three cuneiforms form a concavity for the navicular. The ligament of Lisfranc runs between the medial cuneiform and second metatarsal base. Disruption to this ligament can lead to a dislocation of the medial aspect of the foot as the first metatarsal and medial cuneiform separate from the second metatarsal and intermediate cuneiform.

The joint cavity and capsule of the cuneonavicular joint is continuous with that of the intercuneiform and cuneocuboid joints, and the synovium is continuous with that of these joints, the second and third cuneometatarsal joints, and the intermetatarsal joints of each base except the fifth.

Intercuneiform and Cuneocuboid Joints

These joints (see Fig. 19-1) are classified as compound, synovial, modified ovoid joints. The joint capsule and synovium is contiguous between all of these joints and with that of the cuneonavicular joint.

Dysfunctions in the cuneocuboid joint result from a collapse of the plantar supporting structures or from direct trauma. Such dysfunctions may result in the cuboid subluxing in a plantar direction (medial border of cuboid moves inferiorly). At the intercuneiform joints, the third cuneiform may sublux on the second cuneiform.

Cubometatarsal

Laterally, the cuboid bone articulates with the fourth and fifth metatarsals distally and with the calcaneus proximally. When considered alone, the cubometatarsal joint is classified as a compound modified ovoid, synovial joint. When the cubometatarsal joints are considered together they form a modified sellar joint. The joint capsule and synovium of the fourth and fifth cubometatarsal joints is separated from the other tarsometatarsal joints by an interosseous ligament.

Cubonavicular

The cubonavicular joint (see Fig. 19-1) is classified as a syndesmosis, or a plane surfaced joint. If the joint is synovial, the capsule and synovium is continuous with the cuneonavicular joint.

Intermetatarsal

The first intermetatarsal joint (see Fig. 19-1) is classified as a simple, synovial, modified ovoid joint, while the second, third, and fourth are classified as compound joints. If the joint is synovial, the capsule and synovium is continuous with the cuneonavicular joint. Motion at these joints is confined to dorsal/plantar gliding, producing a fanning and folding motion of the foot. Proximally, the five metatarsals articulate with the tarsals and with themselves through broad concavities.[13]

Metatarsophalangeal

The metatarsophalangeal (MTP) joints (see Fig. 19-1) are classified as simple, synovial, modified ovoid joints. The capsule and synovium in each of these joints is confined to its own joint and dorsally is thin, while plantarly it is blended with the plantar and collateral ligaments. Rotation occurring in the early stages of development of the limbs results in the thumb being the most lateral digit in the hand, while the hallux (great toe) is the most medial digit in the foot.[51]

The concave bases of the proximal phalanges (see Fig. 19-1) articulate with the convex heads of the metatarsals. The first MTP joint, with its more extensive articular surface on the plantar aspect of the metatarsal than on the dorsal, allows for a greater freedom of motion,[52] and its plantar surface forms two grooves for articulation with the hallucal sesamoids (see next section). The fifth metatarsal has a lateral styloid process at its base, which serves as the insertion site for the tendon of the peroneus brevis. The styloid area is often avulsed during acute inversion injuries of the foot.[13]

Three types of forefoot are recognized based on the length of the metatarsal bones, although it is unclear whether these various types affect foot function in any way:[51]

▶ *Index plus.* This type is characterized by the first metatarsal being longer than the second, with the other three of progressively decreasing lengths, so that $1 > 2 > 3 > 4 > 5$.

▶ *Index plus-minus.* In this type, the first metatarsal is of the same length as the second, with the others progressively diminishing in length, so that $1 = 2 > 3 > 4 > 5$.

▶ *Index minus.* With this type, the second metatarsal is longer than the first and third metatarsals. The fourth and fifth metatarsals are progressively shorter than the third, so that $1 < 2 > 3 > 4 > 5$.

Stability of the MTP joints is primarily provided by a musculocapsular ligamentous complex plantarly, and medially and laterally by the medial and lateral collateral ligaments, respectively.[53]

First Metatarsophalangeal Joint

During normal gait, the first MTP joint dorsiflexes approximately 60 degrees.[53] During sprinting (running sports), squatting (football, baseball), and relevé (in dance), greater than 90 degrees of dorsiflexion is necessary.[54]

Although there is some anatomic variation from patient to patient, the first MTP joint is typically a cam-shaped, condylar hinged joint.[55] The joint is stabilized dorsally by the capsule and expansion of the extensor hallucis tendon, and laterally by collateral ligaments. The plantar surface of the capsule is reinforced by a fibrocartilaginous plate, called the plantar accessory ligament. It contains the medial and lateral sesamoid bones.

> ### Clinical Pearl
>
> The sesamoids are contained within the tendon of the flexor hallucis brevis, and serve to increase the lever arm for flexion of the MTP joint, analogous to the function of the patella in knee extension.[56]

The sesamoids are connected distally to the base of the proximal phalanx by extensions of the flexor hallucis brevis called the plantar plate. Typically, the sesamoids are plantar to the medial and lateral condyles of the metatarsal pad. The sesamoids are separated on the plantar aspect of the first metatarsal head by a cresta, which helps to stabilize the sesamoids, and are connected to one another by the intersesamoidal ligament. The abductor hallucis inserts into the medial sesamoid and the adductor hallucis inserts into the lateral sesamoid. The flexor hallucis longus (Fig. 19-10) pierces the two heads of the flexor hallucis brevis muscle to run just plantar to the intersesamoidal ligament. The sesamoids bear up to three times body weight during a normal gait cycle of which the medial sesamoid bears the majority of the force.[57–63]

FIGURE 19-10 Medial muscles of the ankle. (Reproduced with permission from Cipriano JJ. *Photographic Manual of Regional Orthopaedic and Neurological Tests*, 3rd ed. Baltimore: Williams & Wilkins; 1997.)

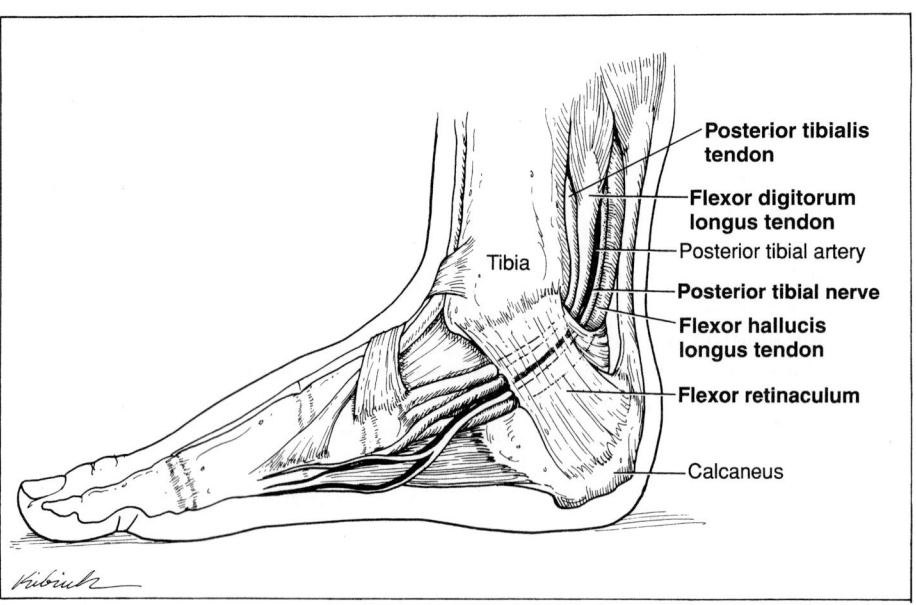

Posterior tibialis tendon

Flexor digitorum longus tendon

Posterior tibial artery

Posterior tibial nerve

Flexor hallucis longus tendon

Flexor retinaculum

Calcaneus

Tibia

Interphalangeal

The hallux has two phalanges, while each of the remaining toes have three (see Fig. 19-1). The interphalangeal (IP) joints are classified as simple, synovial modified sellar joints. The saddle-shaped articular fossa of the head of the proximal phalanx articulates with the base of the intermediate phalanx. This in turn receives the smaller and flatter distal phalanx.

Accessory Bones

Accessory bones are anomalous bones that fail to unite during developmental ossification. The accessory navicular is the most common accessory bone in the foot.[64] It occurs on the medial, plantar border of the navicular at the site of tibialis posterior tendon insertion.[65] The incidence in the general population has been reported to be 4 to 14 percent.[65,66]

The posterior aspect of the talus often exhibits a separate ossification center, appearing at 8 to 10 years of age in girls and 11 to 13 years of age in boys. Fusion usually occurs 1 year after its appearance.[67,68] When fusion does not occur, an os trigonum is formed. An os trigonum has been reported to be present in approximately 10 percent of the general population and is often unilateral.[67,69–71] The origin of this ossicle may be congenital or acquired. Congenitally, it can be a persistent separation of the secondary center of the lateral tubercle from the remainder of the posterior talus secondary to repeated microtrauma during development.[67,71] The acquired form may be secondary to an actual fracture that has not united.[67,71,72]

Plantar Fascia/Plantar Aponeurosis

The plantar fascia is the investing fascial layer of the plantar aspect of the foot that originates from the os calcis and inserts through a complex network to the plantar forefoot. It is a tough, fibrous layer, composed histologically of both collagen and elastic fibers. The terms *plantar fascia* and *plantar aponeurosis* are often used interchangeably, although strictly speaking only the central part of the plantar fascia is extensively aponeurotic.[46]

The plantar fascia is often regarded as being analogous to the palmar fascia of the hand. However, unlike the fascial layer of the palm, which is generally thin, the plantar fascia is a thick structure, and not only serves a supportive and protective role, but is also intricately involved with the weight bearing function of the foot.[72a] The plantar fascia is divided into three major areas: a central portion, and medial and lateral sections, each oriented longitudinally on the plantar surface of the foot.[72b]

▶ *Central portion.* The central portion is the major portion of the plantar fascia both anatomically and functionally.[72a] This portion is the thickest and strongest, and is narrowest proximally where it attaches to the medial process of the calcaneal tuberosity, proximal to the flexor digitorum brevis. This attachment site is often involved in a condition called plantar fasciitis (see "Intervention Strategies"); however, pain can occur anywhere along the structure. From its insertion, the central portion of the fascia fans out and becomes thinner distally. Its fibers are longitudinally oriented and adhere to the underlying flexor digitorum brevis muscle.[72a] The central portion envelops the flexor digitorum brevis muscle on both sides, forming the medial and lateral intermuscular septums, which anchor the plantar fascia to the deep planta pedis.[72a] At the midshaft of the second to fifth metatarsophalangeal joints, the body of the central portion branches into five superficial longitudinal tracts.[72a] All five superficial longitudinal tracts terminate by inserting into, and blending with, the overlying subcutaneous tissues and skin. Due to the anatomical connections of the central portion, dorsiflexion of the toe slides the plantar pads distally, placing tension on the plantar aponeurosis. The central portion of the fascia primarily functions as a dynamic stabilizer of the medial longitudinal arch during weight-bearing activities.

▶ *Lateral and medial portions.* The smaller and thinner lateral and medial portions are thin and cover the under surface of the abductor digiti minimi, and abductor hallucis muscles, respectively.

With standing and weight bearing, the plantar fascia plays a major role in the support of the weight of the body by virtue of its attachments across the longitudinal arch. During the different phases of gait, the plantar fascia assumes different biomechanical functions. For example, during the toe-off portion of the gait cycle, the windlass effect on the plantar fascia helps to reconstitute the arch and generates a more rigid foot for propulsion.*[72c,73] During heel strike, and during the first half of the stance phase of the gait cycle with the toes in neutral, the plantar fascia relaxes, flattening of the arch. This allows the foot to accommodate to irregularities in the walking surface and to absorb shock.[73] As the foot proceeds from foot flat to toe-off, the toes dorsiflex and, through its attachments to the toes via the plantar plate, the plantar fascia tightens. The plantar fascia is pulled over the metatarsal heads, causing the metatarsal heads to be depressed and the longitudinal arch to rise.[72a] During the swing phase of gait, the plantar fascia is under little tension and appears to serve no important functional role.

Retinacula

There are four important ankle retinacula, which function to tether the leg tendons as they cross the ankle to enter the foot (Figs. 19-11 and 19-12).[13]

▶ *Extensor retinaculum.* The extensor retinaculum consists of two parts, superior and inferior (Fig. 19-12). The superior part functions to contain the tendons of the extensor digitorum longus, extensor hallucis longus, tibialis anterior, and peroneus tertius. The Y-shaped inferior part consists of an upper and lower band which prevent "bowstringing" of the dorsal tendons.

▶ *Superio-peroneal retinacula (Fig. 19-11).* This firmly tethers the peroneus longus and brevis tendons behind the fibular malleolus.

---

* The orientation of the aponeurosis promotes inversion of the calcaneus, and supination of the subtalar joint when it is under tension, which raises the longitudinal arch, and provides a rigid lever for propulsion.

FIGURE 19-11 Lateral aspect of foot and ankle. (Reproduced with permission from Cipriano JJ. *Photographic Manual of Regional Orthopaedic and Neurological Tests*, 3rd ed. Baltimore: Williams & Wilkins; 1997.)

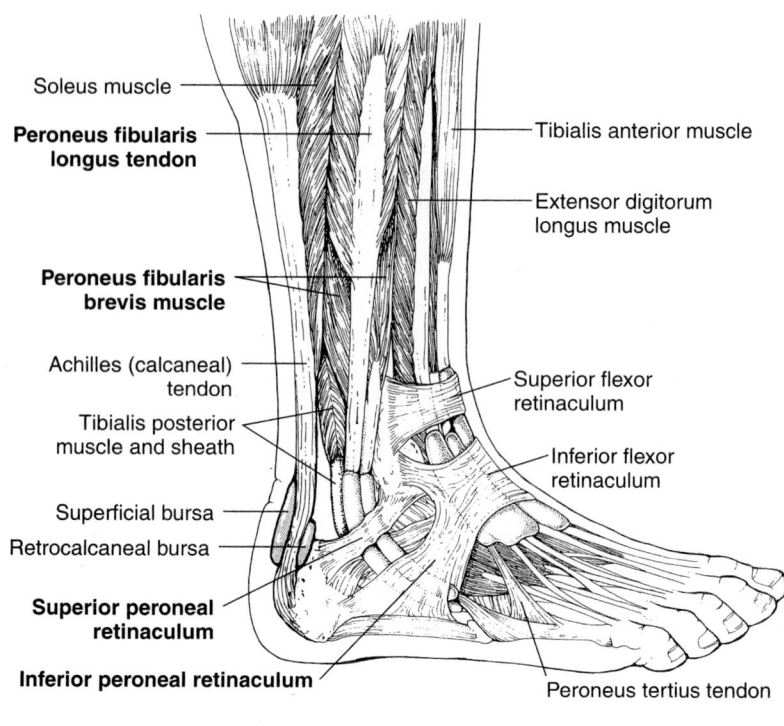

FIGURE 19-12 Tendons and retinacula of the anterior and dorsal foot and ankle. (Reproduced with permission from Cipriano JJ. *Photographic Manual of Regional Orthopaedic and Neurological Tests*, 3rd ed. Baltimore: Williams & Wilkins; 1997.)

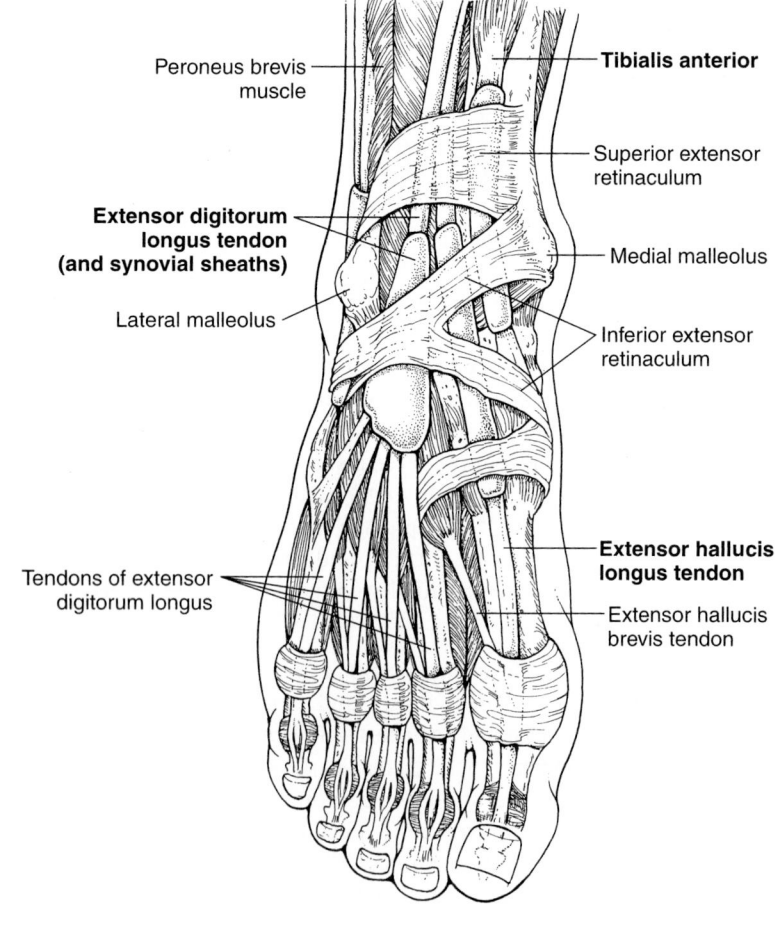

▶ *Flexor retinaculum (Fig. 19-11).* The flexor retinaculum provides a firm support structure for the flexor digitorum longus, flexor hallucis longus, tibialis posterior, and the neurovascular bundle.

Extrinsic Muscles of the Leg and Foot

The extrinsic muscles of the foot (Table 19-4) can be divided into anterior, posterior superficial, posterior deep, and lateral compartments.

Anterior Compartment

This compartment contains the dorsiflexors (extensors) of the foot. These include the tibialis anterior, extensor digitorum longus, extensor hallucis longus, and peroneus tertius (see Fig. 19-12).

Posterior Superficial Compartment

This compartment, located posterior to the interosseous membrane, contains the calf muscles which plantarflex (flex) the foot. These include the gastrocnemius, soleus, and the plantaris muscle (see Fig. 19-13).

Triceps Surae. The triceps surae comprises the two heads of the gastrocnemius, which arise from the posterior aspects of the distal femur, and the soleus, which arises from the tibia and fibula, which combine to form the Achilles tendon.[74]

TABLE 19-4 Extrinsic Muscle Attachments and Innervation[9]

Muscle	Proximal	Distal	Innervation
Gastrocnemius	Medial and lateral condyle of femur	Posterior surface of calcaneus through Achilles tendon	Tibial S2 (S1)
Plantaris	Lateral supracondylar line of femur	Posterior surface of calcaneus through Achilles tendon	Tibial S2 (S1)
Soleus	Head of fibula, proximal third of shaft, soleal line and midshaft of posterior tibia	Posterior surface of calcaneus through Achilles tendon	Tibial S2 (S1)
Tibialis anterior	Distal to lateral tibial condyle, proximal half of lateral tibial shaft, and interosseous membrane	First cuneiform bone, medial and plantar surfaces and base of first metatarsal	Deep peroneal L4 (L5)
Tibialis posterior	Posterior surface of tibia, proximal two thirds posterior of fibula, and interosseous membrane	Tuberosity of navicular bone, tendinous expansion to other tarsals and metatarsals	Tibial L4 and L5
Peroneus longus	Lateral condyle of tibia, head and proximal two thirds of fibula	Base of first metatarsal and first cuneiform, lateral side	Superficial peroneal L5 and S1 (S2)
Peroneus brevis	Distal two thirds of lateral fibular shaft	Tuberosity of fifth metatarsal	Superficial peroneal L5 and S1 (S2)
Peroneus tertius	Lateral slip from extensor digitorum longus	Tuberosity of fifth metatarsal	Deep peroneal L5 and S1
Flexor hallucis longus	Posterior distal two thirds fibula	Base of distal phalanx of great toe	Tibial S2 (S3)
Flexor digitorum longus	Middle three fifths of posterior tibia	Base of distal phalanx of lateral four toes	Tibial S2 (S3)
Extensor hallucis longus	Middle half of anterior shaft of fibula	Base of distal phalanx of great toe	Deep peroneal L5 and S1
Extensor digitorum longus	Lateral condyle of tibia proximal anterior surface of shaft of fibula	One tendon to each lateral four toes, to middle phalanx and extending to distal phalanges	Deep peroneal L5 and S1

The medial head of the gastrocnemius is by far the largest component, and according to electromyographic (EMG) studies, is the most active of the two during running.[77,78]

The soleus, because it does not cross the knee joint, is subject to early disuse atrophy with undertraining and/or immobilization.[77]

The fibers from the gastrocnemius and soleus interweave and twist as they descend, producing an area of high stress 2 to 6 cm above the distal tendon insertion.[79] A region of relative avascularity exists in the same area,[80] which correlates well with the site of some Achilles tendon injuries.[77,81,82]

The plantaris muscle (Fig. 19-13) has its own tendon, and contributes no fibers to the Achilles tendon.[83]

Achilles Tendon. The Achilles tendon is the thickest, strongest tendon in the body.[83a] As the Achilles tendon comes off the posterior calf muscles it courses distally to attach about three quarters of an inch below the superior portion of the os calcis, on the medial aspect of the calcaneus. Two bursae occur at the point of

insertion of the Achilles tendon onto the calcaneus. The retrocalcaneal bursa (Fig. 19-11) lies deep to the tendon, adjacent to the calcaneus. The superficial bursa of the tendo achillis (Fig. 19-11) lies superficial to the distal portion of the tendon, between the tendon itself and the subcutaneous tissues, but is not visible unless it is pathologically inflamed. Deeper to the Achilles tendon is the pre-Achilles fat pad, a triangular area of adipose tissue, also known as Kager's triangle. Further anterior to this fat pad are the deep flexor tendons of the calf, predominantly the flexor hallucis longus, which overlies the posterior tibia and talus.

There is no synovial sheath surrounding the Achilles tendon. The peritendon covers the endotendon and is composed of a thin sheath, called the epitenon, and another fine outer sheath, the peritenon, composed of fatty areola tissue, which fills the interstices of the fascial compartment in which the tendon is situated.[83b] The peritenon is able to stretch 2 to 3 cm with tendon movement, which allows the Achilles tendon to glide smoothly.[83c]

Posterior Deep Compartment

This compartment contains the flexors of the foot. These muscles course behind the medial malleolus. They include the posterior tibialis (Fig. 19-14), flexor digitorum longus (see Fig. 19-14), and flexor hallucis longus (see Fig. 19-15).

The primary function of the tibialis posterior muscle is to invert and plantarflex the foot. It also provides support to the medial longitudinal arch.[84]

The flexor digitorum longus functions to flex the phalanges of the lateral four toes, and assists with plantarflexion of the foot.

The flexor hallucis longus flexes the great toe and also assists with plantar flexion of the foot.

Lateral Compartment

This compartment contains the peroneus longus and brevis (see Fig. 19-11). The peroneal tendons lie behind the lateral malleolus in a fibro-osseous tunnel formed by a groove in the fibula and the superficial peroneal retinaculum. The peroneal retinaculum and the posterior calcaneofibular ligament form the posterior wall of this tunnel.

Clinical Pearl

The peroneal muscles serve as both plantar flexors and evertors of the foot.[85,86] The peroneus longus also abducts the forefoot in the transverse plane, thereby serving as a support for the medial longitudinal arch.[87]

Intrinsic Muscles of the Foot

Beneath the plantar aponeurosis-plantar fascia are the four muscular layers of the intrinsic muscles of the plantar foot (Table 19-5), as well as the plantar ligaments of the rearfoot and midfoot. The intrinsic muscles provide support to the foot during propulsion.[88]

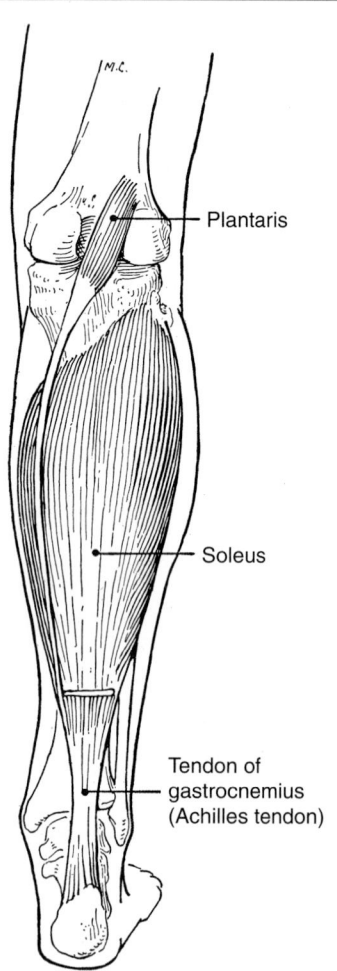

FIGURE 19-13 Plantaris muscle. (Reproduced with permission from Luttgens K, Hamilton K. *Kinesiology: Scientific Basis of Human Motion.* New York: McGraw-Hill; 1997.)

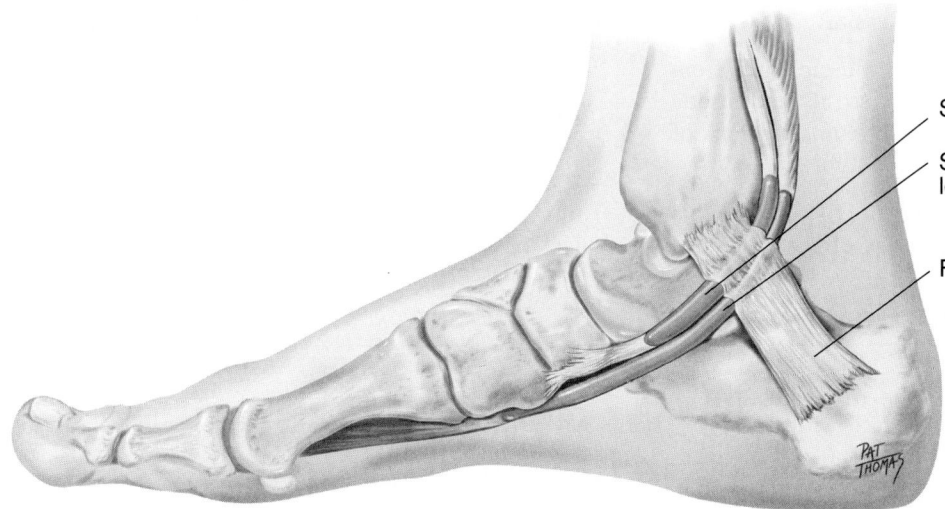

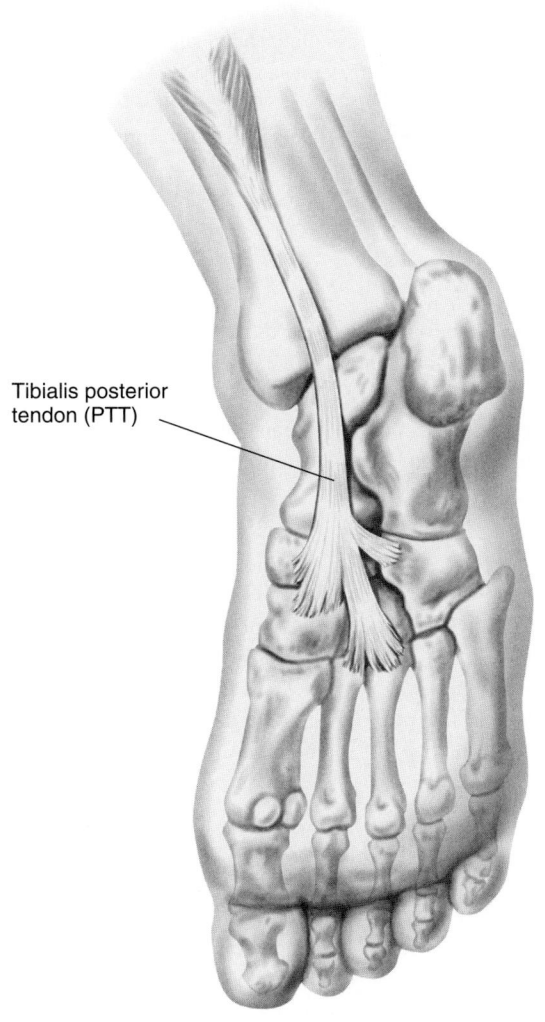

FIGURE 19-14   The posterior tibialis. (Reproduced with permission from Kelikian AS. *Operative Treatment of the Foot and Ankle.* New York: Appleton-Lange; 1999.)

First Layer

The first layer is the most plantar and consists of:

▶ *Abductor hallucis (Fig. 19-15).* This muscle arises from the medial process of the calcaneal tuberosity and inserts into the medial side of the base of the proximal phalanx of the great toe.

▶ *Abductor digiti minimi brevis (see Fig. 19-15).* This muscle arises from the lateral process of the calcaneal

tuberosity as well as the plantar aponeurosis and inserts into the lateral side of the base of the proximal phalanx of the little toe.

▶ *Flexor digitorum brevis (see Fig. 19-15).* This muscle arises from the medial process of the calcaneal tuberosity, lateral to the abductor hallucis and deep to the central portion of the plantar fascia, and inserts into the middle phalanx of the lateral four toes.

TABLE 19-5   Intrinsic Muscles of the Foot[9]

Muscle	Proximal	Distal	Innervation
Extensor digitorum brevis	Distal superior surface of calcaneus	Dorsal surface of second through fourth toes, base of proximal phalanx	Deep peroneal S1 and S2
Flexor hallucis brevis	Plantar surface of cuboid and third cuneiform bones	Base of proximal phalanx of great toe	Medial plantar S3 (S2)
Flexor digitorum brevis	Tuberosity of calcaneus	One tendon slip into base of middle phalanx of each of the lateral four toes	Medial and lateral plantar S3 (S2)
Extensor hallucis brevis	Distal superior and lateral surfaces of calcaneus	Dorsal surface of proximal phalanx	Deep peroneal S1 and S2
Abductor hallucis	Tuberosity of calcaneus and plantar aponeurosis	Base of proximal phalanx, medial side	Medial plantar L5 and S1 (L4)
Adductor hallucis	Base of second, third, and fourth metatarsals and deep plantar ligaments	Proximal phalanx of first digit lateral side	Medial and lateral plantar S1 and S2
Lumbricals	Medial and adjacent sides of flexor digitorum longus tendon to each lateral digit	Medial side of proximal phalanx and extensor hood	Medial and lateral plantar L5, S1, and S2 (L4)
Plantar interossei			
First	Base and medial side of third metatarsal	Base of proximal phalanx and extensor hood of third digit	
Second	Base and medial side of fourth metatarsal	Base of proximal phalanx and extensor hood of fourth digit	Medial and lateral plantar S1 and S2
Third	Base and medial side of fifth metatarsal	Base of proximal phalanx and extensor hood of fifth digit	
Dorsal interossei			
First	First and second metatarsal bones	Proximal phalanx and extensor hood of second digit medially	
Second	Second and third metatarsal bones	Proximal phalanx and extensor hood of second digit laterally	Medial and lateral plantar S1 and S2
Third	Third and fourth metatarsal bones	Proximal phalanx and extensor hood of third digit laterally	
Fourth	Fourth and fifth metatarsal bones	Proximal phalanx and extensor hood of fourth digit laterally	
Abductor digiti minimi	Lateral side of fifth metatarsal bone	Proximal phalanx of fifth digit	Lateral plantar S1 and S2

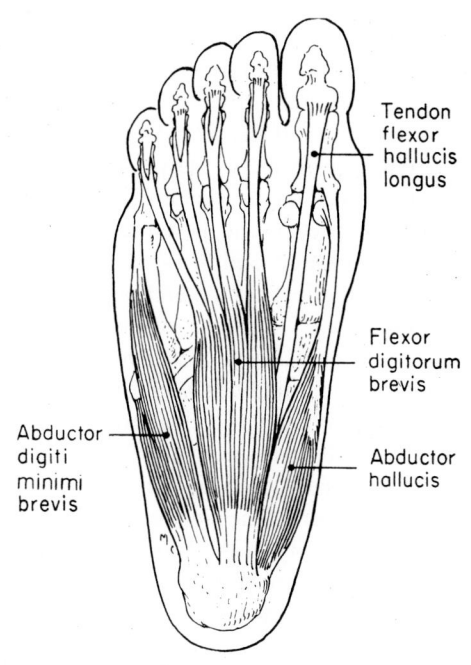

FIGURE 19-15 Plantar muscles—superficial layer. (Reproduced with permission from Luttgens K, Hamilton K. *Kinesiology: Scientific Basis of Human Motion.* New York: McGraw-Hill; 1997.)

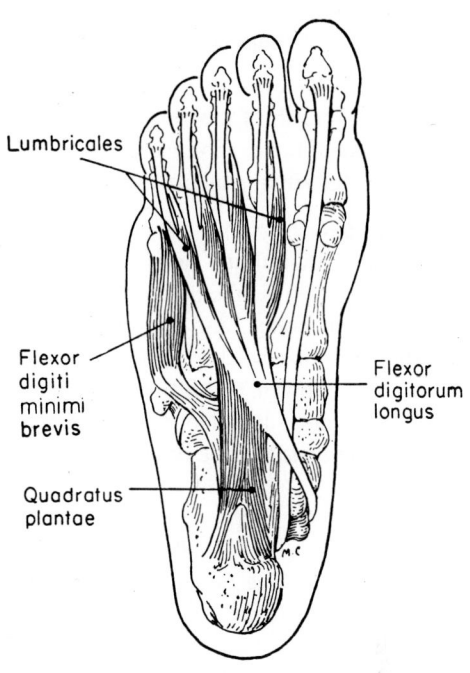

FIGURE 19-16 Plantar muscles—middle layer. (Reproduced with permission from Luttgens K, Hamilton K. *Kinesiology: Scientific Basis of Human Motion.* New York: McGraw-Hill; 1997.)

Second Layer

▶ *Flexor digitorum accessorius (quadratus plantae; Fig. 19-16).* This muscle arises from the calcaneal tuberosity via two heads. The medial head arises from the medial surface of the calcaneus and the medial border of the long plantar ligament, while the lateral head arises from the lateral border of the plantar surface of the calcaneus and the lateral border of the long plantar ligament. The muscle terminates in tendinous slips, joining the long flexor tendons to the second, third, fourth, and occasionally fifth toes.

▶ *Lumbricales.* There are four lumbricales (see Fig. 19-16), all of which arise from the tendon of the flexor digitorum longus. The first arises from the medial side of the tendon of the second toe, the second from adjacent sides of the tendons for the second and third toes, the third from adjacent sides of the tendons for the third and fourth toes, and the fourth from adjacent sides of tendons for the fourth and fifth toes. They insert with the tendons of the extensor digitorum longus and interossei into the bases of the terminal phalanges of the four lateral toes. The function of the lumbricales is to flex the MTP joint and extend the proximal IP joint.

Third Layer

▶ *Flexor hallucis brevis (Fig. 19-17).* This muscle arises from the medial part of the plantar surface of the cuboid bone, the adjacent portion of the lateral cuneiform, and the

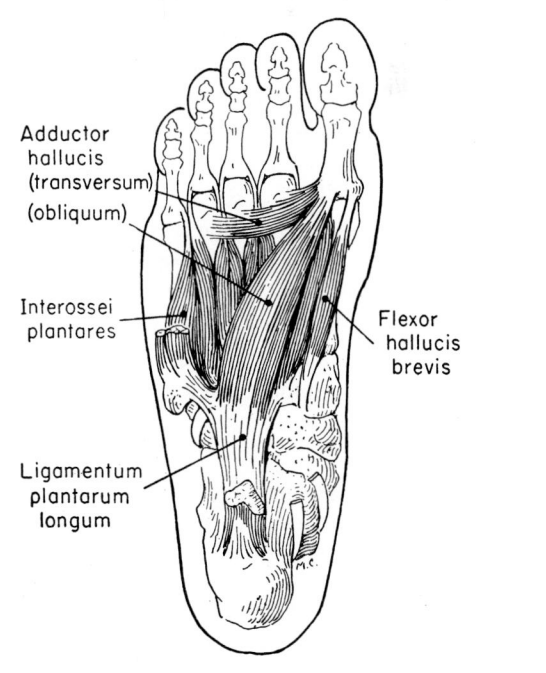

FIGURE 19-17 Plantar muscles—deep layer. (Reproduced with permission from Luttgens K, Hamilton K. *Kinesiology: Scientific Basis of Human Motion.* New York: McGraw-Hill; 1997.)

posterior tibialis tendon, and inserts on the medial and lateral side of the proximal phalanx of the great toe.

▶ *Flexor digiti minimi brevis (see Fig. 19-16).* This muscle arises from the sheath of the peroneus longus, the base of the fifth metatarsal bone, and inserts into the lateral side of the base of the proximal phalanx of the little toe.

▶ *Adductor hallucis (see Fig. 19-17).* This muscle arises via two heads, an oblique and a transverse head. The oblique head arises from the bases of the second, third, and fourth metatarsal bones, and the sheath of the peroneus longus. The transverse head arises from the joint capsules of the second, third, fourth, and fifth MTP heads, and the deep transverse metatarsal ligament. The adductor hallucis inserts on the lateral side of the base of the proximal phalanx of the great toe.

Fourth Layer

▶ *Dorsal interossei.* The four dorsal interossei are bipennate, and they arise from adjacent sides of the metatarsal bones. The first inserts into the medial side of the proximal phalanx of the second toe. The second inserts into the lateral side of the proximal phalanx of the second toe. The third inserts into the lateral side of the proximal phalanx of the third toe, and the fourth inserts into the lateral side of the proximal phalanx of the fourth toe. The dorsal interossei function to abduct the second, third, and fourth toes from an axis through the second metatarsal ray.

▶ *Plantar interossei (Fig. 19-17).* The three plantar interossei are unipennate, and arise from the bases and medial sides of the third, fourth, and fifth metatarsal bones. They insert into the medial sides of the bases of the proximal phalanges of the third, fourth, and fifth toes. The plantar interossei function to adduct the lateral three toes.

Dorsal Intrinsic Muscles

The dorsal intrinsic muscles of the foot are the extensor hallucis brevis (EHB) and extensor digitorum brevis (EDB). The EHB inserts into the base of the proximal phalanx of the great toe, while the EDB inserts into the base of the second, third, and fourth proximal phalanges. Both of these muscles are innervated by the lateral terminal branch of the deep peroneal nerve.

Arches of the Foot

No discussion about the anatomy of the foot could be complete without a mention of the various arches. The arches support the foot by three mechanisms:[89]

▶ The osseous relationship of the tarsal and metatarsal bones.

▶ Ligamentous support from the plantar aponeurosis and plantar ligaments.

▶ Muscle support.[90]

There are three main arches: the medial longitudinal and lateral longitudinal arches, and the transverse arch.

▶ The *medial longitudinal arch* is comprised of the calcaneus, talus, navicular, medial cuneiform, and first metatarsals (two sesamoids). While some of the integrity of the arch depends on the bony architecture, support is also provided by the ligaments and muscles, including the plantar calcaneonavicular (spring) ligament, the plantar fascia, the tibialis posterior, peroneus longus, flexor digitorum longus, flexor hallucis longus (FHL), and peroneus longus (PL).[87,91,92] The soleus and gastrocnemius muscle group has also been noted to have an effect on the arch and can flatten it with adaptive shortening.[87] Analysis of the medial longitudinal arch has long been used by clinicians to make determinations about foot abnormalities, with a high arch indicating a supinated foot, and a low or collapsed arch associated with a pronated or flat foot, respectively.[93] This has continued in spite of the fact that as long ago as 1907,[94] it was demonstrated that the height of the arch has no value on estimating the functional capacity of the foot. However, studies have found a higher incidence of stress fractures, plantar fasciitis, metatarsalgia, and lower extremity injuries, including knee strains and iliotibial band syndrome, in individuals with high arches, compared with those who have low arches.[95–97] This difference has always been attributed to the decreased shock-absorbing ability of the higher-arched foot,[98] although one study reported that arch height does not affect shock absorption.[99]

▶ The *lateral longitudinal arch*, which is more stable and less mobile than the medial longitudinal arch, consists of the calcaneus, cuboid, and fifth metatarsal. The superior and deep longitudinal plantar ligament supports the calcaneocuboid and cubometatarsal joints, together with the peroneus brevis, longus, and tertius, and the abductor digiti minimi and flexor digitorum brevis muscles.[100]

▶ The *transverse arch* forms the convexity of the dorsum of the foot, and consists of metatarsal heads 1 through 5, including the sesamoids (arch I); cuneiforms 1 through 3 and cuboid (arch II); and navicular and cuboid (arch III). The adductor hallucis, peroneus longus, posterior tibialis, and anterior tibialis all add dynamic support to this arch.

Nail Plate

The nail plate is composed of keratinized squamous cells, bordered by proximal and lateral nail folds.[101] The hyponychium lies between the distal portion of the nail bed and the distal nail fold, and marks the transition to normal finger epidermis.[101] Fingernail plates grow on average at a rate of 3 mm per month, and toenail plates grow at one half to one third that rate.[101]

Neurology

The saphenous nerve, the largest cutaneous branch of the femoral nerve, provides cutaneous distribution to the medial aspect of the foot. Branches of the sciatic nerve provide the sensory and motor innervation for the foot and leg (see Chap. 2). The branches are the common peroneal and tibial nerves. The common peroneal nerve in turn divides into the superficial peroneal and deep peroneal nerves (Fig. 19-18). The tibial nerve divides into the sural, medial calcaneal, medial plantar, and lateral plantar nerves.[102]

Vascular Supply

Two branches of the popliteal artery, the anterior tibial artery and the posterior tibial artery, form the main blood supply to the foot.

Anterior Tibial Artery

The anterior tibial artery supplies the anterior compartment of the leg, and enters the dorsum of the foot under the superior and inferior retinacula as the dorsal pedis artery. The dorsal pedis artery (Fig. 19-18) gives rise to the arcuate artery and the first dorsal and plantar metatarsal artery, which serve the dorsum of the foot and the digits.

Posterior Tibial Artery

The posterior tibial artery, which supplies the posterior and lateral compartments and 75 percent of the blood to the foot, enters the foot after traveling around the medial malleoli. At this point, the artery divides into the medial and lateral plantar arteries, which serve the plantar aspect of the foot. A main branch

of the posterior tibial artery, the peroneal artery, supplies the lateral compartment as well as many hindfoot structures.

Biomechanics

Terminology

Motions of the leg, foot, and ankle consist of single-plane and multiplane movements (Fig. 19-19). The single-plane motions include:

▶ *The frontal plane motions of inversion and eversion.* There is some confusion in the literature as to the terms *inversion* and *eversion*. In some anatomy or kinesiology texts, inversion is described as a combination of supination and adduction, while eversion is described as a combination of pronation and abduction.[8] In this text, eversion is a combination of pronation, abduction, and dorsiflexion, whereas inversion is a combination of supination, adduction, and plantar flexion (refer to triplanar motions later). Thus eversion can be described as frontal plane motion of the foot about an anteroposterior axis in which the medial aspect of the sole of the foot moves in a plantar direction. Inversion can be described as frontal plane motion of the foot about an anteroposterior axis in which the lateral aspect of the sole of the foot moves in a plantar direction.

▶ *The sagittal plane motions of dorsiflexion and plantar flexion.* These terms indicate movement at the ankle and at the midtarsal joint, which occur in the sagittal plane about a mediolateral axis.[9] Plantar flexion is movement of the foot downwards towards the ground, and dorsiflexion is a movement of the foot upwards towards the tibia.

▶ *The horizontal plane motions of adduction and abduction.* These terms describe motions of the forefoot in the horizontal plane about a superoinferior axis.[9] Abduction moves the forefoot laterally, whereas adduction moves the forefoot medially on the midfoot.

A triplane motion describes a movement about an obliquely oriented axis through all three body planes. Triplanar motions occur at the talocrural, subtalar, and midtarsal joints, and at the first and fifth rays.[10] Pronation and supination are considered triplanar motions (Fig. 19-20). The three body plane motions in pronation are abduction in the transverse plane, dorsiflexion in the sagittal plane, and eversion in the frontal plane (Fig. 19-21).[10] The three body plane motions in supination are a combined movement of adduction, plantar flexion, and inversion.[10] In pronation, the forefoot is rotated big toe downward and little toe upward, whereas in supination the reverse occurs.

Distal Tibiofibular Joint

The two tibiofibular joints (proximal and distal) are described as individual articulations, but in fact they function as a pair. The movements that occur at these joints are primarily a result of the ankle's influence.

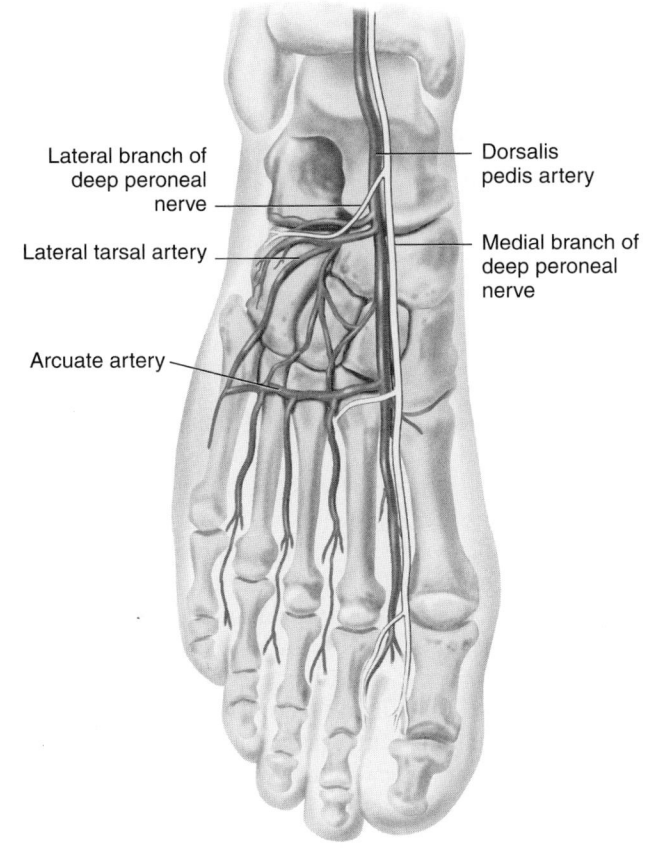

Lateral branch of deep peroneal nerve

Lateral tarsal artery

Arcuate artery

Dorsalis pedis artery

Medial branch of deep peroneal nerve

FIGURE 19-18 Deep peroneal nerve. (Reproduced with permission from Kelikian AS. *Operative Treatment of the Foot and Ankle*. New York: Appleton-Lange; 1999.)

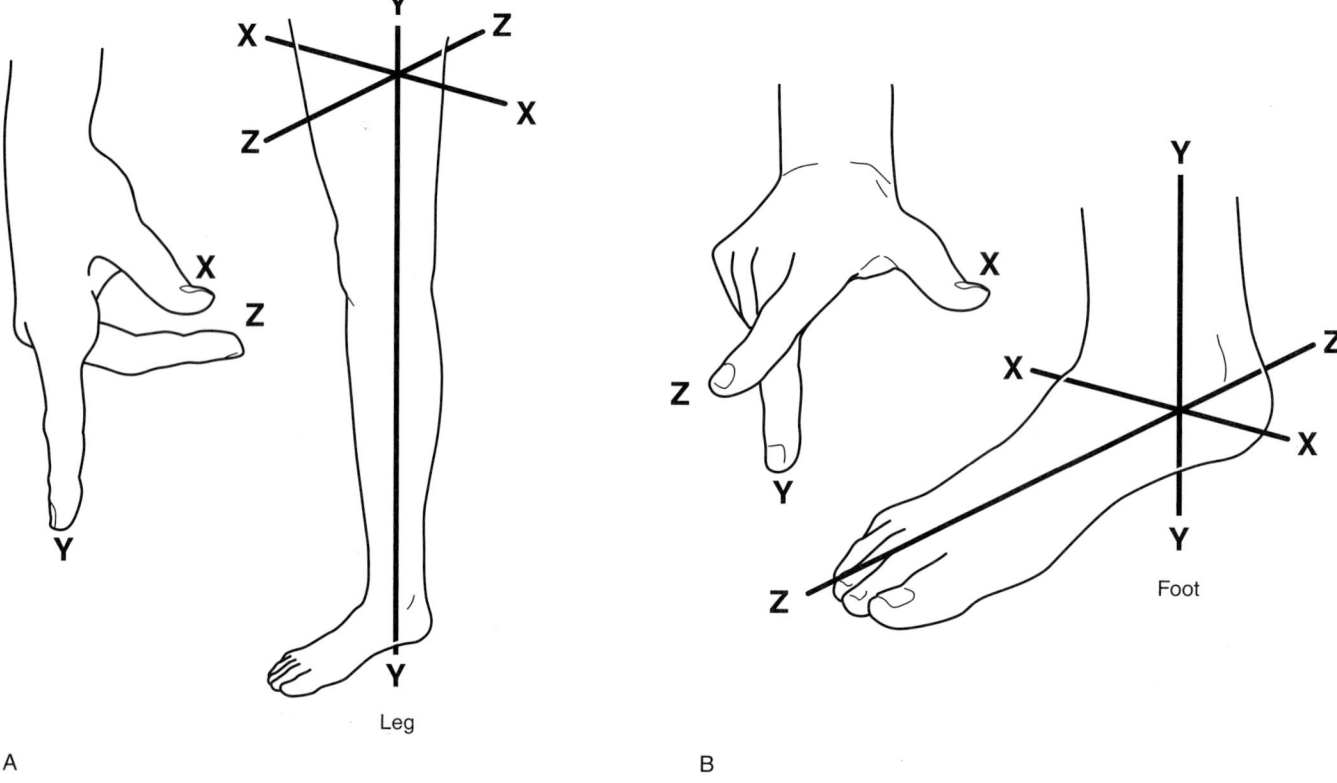

A   B

FIGURE 19-19   Single plane motions. *A.* The hand is pronated and the wrist is in neutral. The three fingers are all perpendicular to one another. The thumb represents the X axis through which flexion and extension occur. The index finger represents the Y axis through which internal and external rotation occur. The middle finger represents the Z axis through which abduction and adduction occur. *B.* If the wrist is extended, the coordinate system of the foot is represented. (Reproduced with permission from Kelikian AS. *Operative Treatment of the Foot and Ankle.* New York: Appleton-Lange; 1999.)

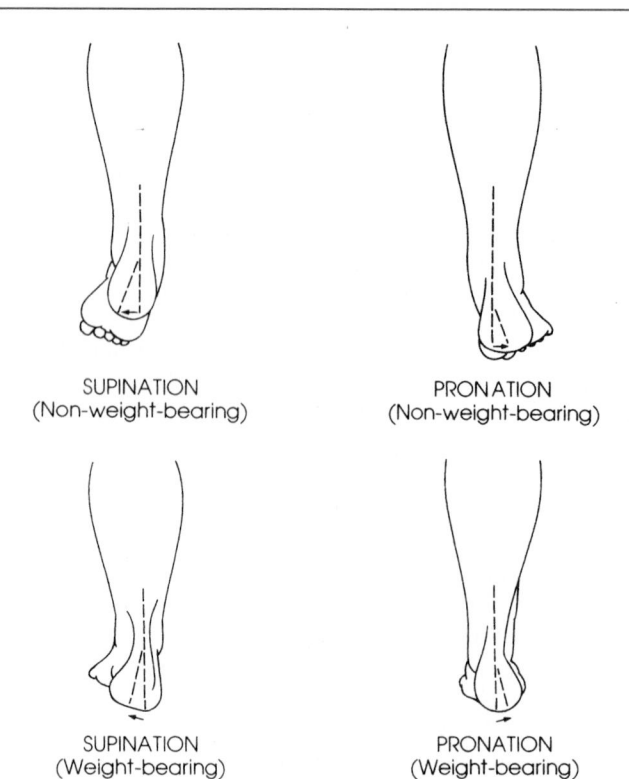

FIGURE 19-20   Pronation and supination. (Reproduced with permission from Magee DJ, ed. *Orthopedic Physical Assessment.* Philadelphia: WB Saunders; 2002.)

▶ Supination of the foot produces a distal and posterior glide of the head of the fibula.

▶ Pronation produces a proximal and anterior glide with an external rotation of the fibula.

▶ Plantar flexion of the foot produces a distal glide with a slight medial rotation of the fibula.

▶ Dorsiflexion of the ankle yields a proximal glide. The fibula rotates externally around its longitudinal axis.

During these movements, however, it is the tibia that performs the greatest amount of movement as it rotates around the fibula. This is probably a consequence of more body weight falling through the larger bone. During ipsilateral rotation, both the tibia and fibula rotate laterally, but in relative terms, the tibia moves more laterally than the fibula, causing a relative anterior and superior glide of the fibular head on the tibia at the superior joint. During contralateral rotation, the tibia rotates more medially, producing a relative posterior and inferior fibular glide at the joint.

The ligaments of the distal tibiofibular joint are more commonly injured than the anterior talofibular ligament.[103] Injuries to the ankle syndesmosis most often occur as a result of forced external rotation of the foot or during internal rotation of the tibia on a planted foot.[23] Hyperdorsiflexion may also be a contributing mechanism.[104]

The capsular pattern of this joint is probably pain with weight-bearing dorsiflexion of the ankle, as this produces the

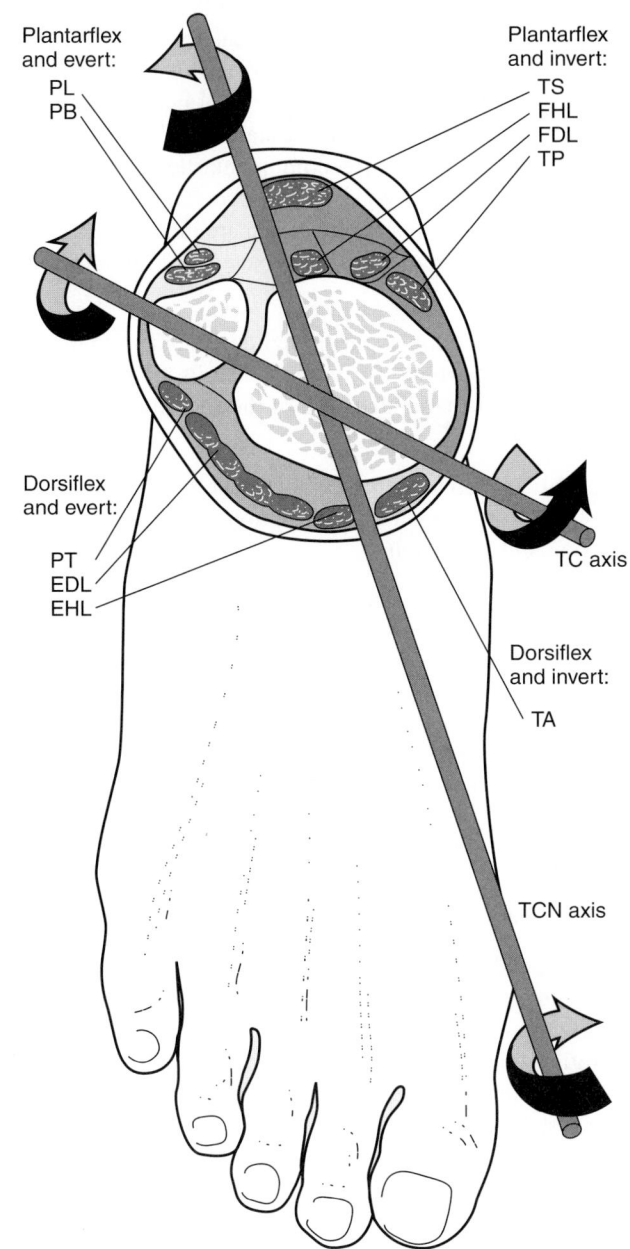

Plantarflex
and evert:
PL
PB

Plantarflex
and invert:
TS
FHL
FDL
TP

Dorsiflex
and evert:

PT
EDL
EHL

TC axis

Dorsiflex
and invert:

TA

TCN axis

FIGURE 19-21 Extrinsic muscles of the foot. TC, transcrural; TCN, talocalcaneo-navicular. (Reproduced with permission from Kelikian AS. *Operative Treatment of the Foot and Ankle.* Stamford, Conn: Appleton & Lange; 1999.)

greatest ligamentous tension (Table 19-1). For the same reason, the close-packed position is considered as weight-bearing dorsiflexion of the ankle.

Clinical Pearl

Because of the interaction between the proximal and distal tibiofibular joints with the knee and the ankle function, the clinician should always assess the functional mobility of both these complexes when treating one or the other.

Talocrural Joint

The talocrural joint is classified as a synovial hinge, or modified sellar joint. There is general agreement that motion between the tibia and the foot is a complex combination of talocrural and subtalar joint motion, which is limited by the shape of the articulations and soft tissue interaction.[21]

The primary motions at this joint are dorsiflexion and plantar flexion, with a total range of 70 to 80 degrees. The maximum amount of dorsiflexion necessary at the talocrural joint during human gait is approximately 10 degrees,[10,105,106] and occurs during the stance phase, just prior to heel rise.[107] The orientation of the talocrural joint axis, which is oriented on average 20 to 30 degrees posterior to the frontal plane as it passes posteriorly from the medial malleolus to the lateral malleolus (see Fig. 19-21),[29,92,108] can be estimated clinically as a line that passes inferiorly from the medial malleolus to the lateral malleolus (with a mean orientation of 10 degrees to the horizontal plane) with the adult distal leg oriented vertically.[92,108,109] Although talocrural motion occurs primarily in the sagittal plane, an appreciable amount of horizontal motion appears to occur in the horizontal plane, especially during internal rotation of the tibia, or pronation of the foot.[92,108]

Because of the fit of the talus within the mortise, the talus is able to produce a slight separation of the tibial and fibula malleoli during the extremes of dorsiflexion and plantarflexion.[110] In addition, because of the fit, the tibia follows the talus during weight bearing so that the talocrural joint externally rotates with supination, and internally rotates with pronation.[111] Therefore the tibia internally rotates during pronation and externally rotates during supination.[112]

Stability for this joint in weight bearing is provided by the articular surfaces, while in non–weight bearing, the ligaments appear to provide the majority of stability.[14]

Theoretically, the capsular pattern of the ankle joint is more restriction of plantarflexion than dorsiflexion, although clinically this appears to be reversed (Table 19-1). The close-packed position is weight-bearing dorsiflexion, while the open-packed position is midway between supination and pronation.

Subtalar Joint

The subtalar joint is responsible for inversion and eversion of the hindfoot. Approximately 50 percent of apparent ankle inversion observed actually comes from the subtalar joint.[113] The axis of motion for the subtalar joint is approximately 45 degrees from horizontal and 20 degrees medial to the midsagittal plane.[28,41,92] This axis, which moves during subtalar joint motion,[114–116] allows the subtalar joint to produce a triplanar motion that has been compared to a ship on the sea, or an oblique mitered hinge.[117] This triplanar motion is one of pronation/supination, and varies according to whether the joint is weight bearing (close chain), or non–weight bearing (open chain).[118]

▶ During weight-bearing activities, pronation involves a combination of calcaneal eversion, adduction, and plantar flexion of the talus, and internal rotation of the tibia (see Fig. 19-20), whereas supination involves a combination of calcaneal inversion, abduction and dorsiflexion of the talus, and external rotation of the tibia (see Fig. 19-20).[119]

▶ During non–weight-bearing activities, pronation involves a combination of calcaneal eversion and abduction and dorsiflexion of the talus (see Fig. 19-20), whereas supination involves a combination of calcaneal inversion and adduction and plantar flexion of the talus (see Fig. 19-20).[119]

The subtalar joint controls supination and pronation in close conjunction with the transverse tarsal joints of the midfoot. Subtalar joint supination and pronation are measured clinically by the amount of calcaneal or hindfoot inversion and eversion. In normal individuals, there is an inversion to eversion ratio of 2:3 to 1:3, which amounts to approximately 20 degrees of inversion and 10 degrees of eversion.[10,27,92,117] For normal gait, a minimum of 4 to 6 degrees of eversion, and 8 to 12 degrees of inversion are required.[116]

During normal gait, the foot needs to pronate and supinate 6 to 8 degrees from the neutral position.[120] If the foot pronates excessively, a compensatory internal rotation of the tibia may occur. This produces an increased amount of rotatory stress and dynamic abduction moment at the knee that has to be absorbed through the peripatellar soft tissues at the knee joint.[121–124] These stresses can force the patella to displace laterally and may result in patellofemoral dysfunction.[3,125] In addition, a change in the position of the talus can affect the functional leg length. Subtalar supination may cause the leg to lengthen, while subtalar pronation shortens the leg. Thus the mid-position of the subtalar joint, subtalar joint neutral, is considered the range at which the subtalar joint should act to prevent dysfunction. The subtalar joint neutral position is actually a measurement of the angle between a line that bisects the distal third of the lower leg and a line that bisects the calcaneus.[126] The bisection of the calcaneus represents the position of the plantar condyles because the calcaneus is almost perpendicular to the condyles. The angle between the bisections should be 0 degrees in the normal foot, but actually is 2 to 3 degrees of varus (inverted in most subjects).[127]

Clinical Pearl

Mathematically, the subtalar joint neutral position is that angle at which the ratio of calcaneal inversion to eversion is approximately 2:1.[10]

Stability for the subtalar joint is provided by the calcaneofibular ligament, the cervical ligament, the talocalcaneal interosseous ligaments, the fibulotalocalcaneal ligament (ligament of Rouviere), and the extensor retinaculum.[128]

The capsular pattern of this joint varies. In chronic arthritic conditions, there is an increasing limitation of inversion, but with traumatic arthritis, eversion appears most limited clinically. The close-packed position for this joint is full inversion, while the open-packed position is inversion/plantarflexion (Table 19-1).

Midtarsal (Transverse Tarsal) Joint Complex

The function of the midtarsal joint complex is to provide the foot with an additional mechanism for raising and lowering the arch, and to absorb some of the horizontal plane tibial motion that is transmitted to the foot during stance.[111,129] The midtarsal joints have two degrees of freedom: plantarflexion/dorsiflexion and inversion/eversion, with motion occurring around a longitudinal and oblique axis, both of which are independent of each other.[129] Motions around the two axes at the midtarsal joint involve:

▶ A rotational motion about a longitudinal axis into inversion and eversion, which can be observed in the elevation and depression of the medial arch of the foot during the stance phase of gait.[27,28]

▶ An oblique axis, producing the near sagittal motions of forefoot dorsiflexion and abduction, and forefoot plantar flexion and adduction.[27]

Both axes are dependent on the position of the subtalar joint.[27,116,129] When the subtalar joint is pronated, the two sets of axes are parallel to one another, allowing for the maximum amount of motion at the midtarsal joint. When the subtalar joint is supinated, the two sets of axes are in opposition, allowing little motion to occur.

During gait, the midtarsal joint has two functions:[129a]

▶ To permit adaptation of the foot to uneven terrain in the early stance.

▶ To provide a stable foot during terminal stance.

Theoretically, as a modified ovoid, the joint complex can sublux into dorsiflexion/plantarflexion, abduction/adduction, with or without rotation. In practice, the most commonly found subluxations may be considered as inversion/dorsiflexion or eversion/plantarflexion lesions.[129b] The capsular pattern of the midtarsal joint complex is a limitation of dorsiflexion, plantar flexion, adduction, and internal rotation (Table 19-1). The close-packed position for the midtarsal joint is supination (Table 19-1). The open-packed position is midway between the extremes of range of motion.

Cuneonavicular Joint

The cuneonavicular joint has one to two degrees of freedom: plantar/dorsiflexion, inversion/eversion. The capsular pattern of this joint is a limitation of dorsiflexion, plantar flexion, adduction and internal rotation. The close-packed position is supination. The open-packed position is considered to be midway between the extremes of range of motion (Table 19-1).

Intercuneiform and Cuneocuboid Joints

Due to their very plane curvature, these joints have only one degree of freedom: inversion/eversion. The close-packed position for these joints is supination. The open-packed position is considered to be midway between extremes of range of motion (Table 19-1).

Cubometatarsal Joint

The capsular pattern of this joint is a limitation of dorsiflexion, plantar flexion, adduction and internal rotation. The close-packed position is pronation. The open-packed position is considered to be midway between extremes of range of motion (Table 19-1).

Cubonavicular Joint

The close-packed position for this joint is supination. The open-packed position is midway between extremes of range of motion (Table 19-1).

Intermetatarsal Joints

The close-packed position for these joints is supination. The open-packed position is midway between extremes of range of motion (Table 19-1).

Metatarsophalangeal Joints

The MTP joints have 2 degrees of freedom: flexion/extension and abduction/adduction. Range of motion of these joints is variable, ranging from 40 degrees to 100 degrees dorsiflexion (with a mean of 84 degrees), 3 to 43 degrees (mean, 23 degrees) plantar flexion, and 5 to 20 degrees varus and valgus.[129c] The closed-packed position for the MTP joints is full extension. The capsular pattern for these joints is variable, with more limitation of extension than flexion. The open-packed position is 10 degrees of extension.

First Metatarsophalangeal Joint

The function of the great toe is to provide stability to the medial aspect of the foot, and to provide for normal propulsion during gait. Normal alignment of the first MTP joint varies between 5 degrees varus and 15 degrees valgus.[130]

The great toe is characterized by having a remarkable discrepancy between active and passive motion. Approximately 30 degrees of active plantar flexion is present, as is at least 50 degrees of active extension, which can frequently be increased passively to between 70 and 90 degrees.

Interphalangeal (IP) Joints

Each of the IP joints has one degree of freedom: flexion/extension. The capsular pattern is more limitation of flexion than of extension. The close-packed position is full extension (Table 19-1). The open-packed position is slight flexion.

Examination

The common pathologies for the foot and ankle complex are detailed after the examination. An understanding of both is obviously necessary. As mention of the various pathologies occurs with reference to the examination and vice versa, the reader is encouraged to switch between the two.

The examination is used to identify static and dynamic, and structural or mechanical foot abnormalities. The clinical diagnosis is based on an assessment of the changes in joint mobility and tissue changes at the foot and ankle, and the effect these have on the function of the foot and ankle and the remainder of the lower kinetic chain.

The exact form of the examination is very dependent on the acuteness of the condition.

Clinical Pearl

With an acute lesion, the purpose of the examination is to try to determine if a serious injury might have occurred, and whether there is a need to refer the patient back for further medical examination. Due to the acute pain and inflammatory state of the tissues in the acute stage, the physical examination may need to be modified and sometimes curtailed.

Weight-bearing tests cannot be done if the patient cannot bear weight, and most stress tests will prove impossible if the joints cannot be taken to their full range. In these cases, the clinician must rely heavily on the history.

History

The primary purposes of the history are to:

▶ Determine the mechanism of injury, if any.

▶ Determine the severity of the condition.

▶ Ascertain when the symptoms began.

▶ Determine the area, nature, and behavior of the symptoms.[131]

▶ Help determine the specific structure at fault.[132]

▶ Detect systemic conditions (eg, collagen disease, neuropathy, radiculopathy, and vascular problems) or the presence of serious pathology.

Information about the patient's chief complaint should include when, where, how, and if an injury occurred. Details about the mechanism of injury allow the clinician to infer the pathologic status and structures involved, although it must be remembered that the patient's recollection of the mechanism involved frequently does not correspond to the structures damaged.[22,133] Most ankle sprains occur when the foot is plantar flexed, inverted, and adducted. This same mechanism can also lead to a malleolar or talar dome fracture. A history involving sudden changes in training patterns may indicate an overuse injury. A dorsiflexion injury with associated snapping and pain on the lateral aspect of the ankle that rapidly diminishes may indicate a tear of the peroneal retinaculum.[134]

The site and severity of the pain can be measured using a body diagram and visual analogue scale, respectively. The distribution of pain is important and the clinician should determine whether the pattern is referred, associated with a structure, related to a dermatome or peripheral nerve, or is systemic in nature.[135] A stress fracture or tendonitis typically has a localized site of pain, whereas diffuse pain is associated with compartment syndromes.

Information should be gleaned about whether activities aggravate the symptoms and if so, which. For example, pain with forced dorsiflexion and eversion and with squatting activities may suggest ankle instability. Pain after activity suggests an overuse or chronic injury. Pain during an activity suggests stress on the injured structure.

Information about the time of injury, the time of the onset of swelling, and its location are important. Most often, the patient can point to the location of the pain. The patient may note hearing a "snap," "crack," or "pop" at the time of injury, which could indicate a ligamentous injury or a fracture. The patient may report that their ankle felt weak and/or unstable at the time of the initial trauma or sometime thereafter. An inability to bear weight, or presence of severe pain and rapid swelling indicate a serious injury such as a capsular tear, fracture, or grade III ligament sprain.[136–139]

If there is no traumatic event, the clinician must determine if there has been a change in exercise or activity intensity (eg, increased mileage with runners), training surface, or changes in body weight or shoe wear (causal agents).[22,133] In addition, the clinician must determine whether the symptoms vary with activity, type of terrain, or with changes in position. Complaints of cramping may accompany muscular fatigue or intermittent claudication from arterial insufficiency. Plantar fasciitis is typically associated with an insidious onset of heel pain. Achilles tendonitis is an overuse injury associated with an insidious onset of posterior calcaneal pain. Increased symptoms when walking or running on uneven terrain as compared with on even terrain may suggest ankle instability. Increased symptoms when walking or running on hard surfaces as compared to a softer surface may suggest a lack of shock absorbency of the foot or shoe. Pain that is related to a certain time of day may indicate an activity-related problem, or a condition such as plantar fasciitis if the pain is felt when first bearing weight in the morning.

Additionally, questions regarding previous ankle injury, goals of the patient regarding the functional results, level and intensity of sports involvement, and past medical history are important to individualize the intervention to the patient.

The impact of the injury on the patient's personal life, work, and athletic demands will largely direct the early intervention.[22,133]

▶ If painless ambulation is essential, then rigid immobilization (ie, a cast) may be appropriate.

▶ If rapid return to sports competition is of paramount importance, functional immobilization is preferred.

Systems Review

As symptoms can be referred distally to the leg, foot, and ankle from a host of other joints and conditions, the clinician must be able to differentially diagnose from the presenting signs and symptoms (see Chap. 9). The cause of the referred symptoms may be neurologic or systemic in origin. If a disorder involving a specific nerve root (L4, L5, S1, or S2) is suspected, the neces-

sary sensory, motor, and reflex testing should be performed. Peripheral nerve injuries may also occur in this region and often go unrecognized. These include Morton's neuroma, and entrapment of the tibial nerve or its branches, the deep peroneal nerve, superficial peroneal nerve, and sural and saphenous nerves.[70]

Systemic problems that may involve the leg, foot, and ankle include diabetes mellitus (peripheral neuropathy), osteomyelitis, gout and pseudogout, sickle cell disease, complex regional pain syndrome, peripheral vascular disease, and rheumatoid arthritis (refer to Chap. 9). A systemic problem such as rheumatoid arthritis may be associated with other signs and symptoms, including other joint pain, although the other joint pain may also be the result of overcompensation in the rest of the kinetic chain.

Warning signs at the ankle and foot that should alert the clinician to a more insidious condition include:

▶ Immediate and continuous inability to bear weight, which may indicate a fracture.

▶ Nocturnal pain, which may indicate a malignancy, hemarthrosis, fracture, or infection.

▶ Gross pain during ankle valgus and tenderness with pressure on the distal fibula, which may indicate a fractured fibula.

▶ Pain and weakness during resisted eversion, which may indicate fracture of the fifth metatarsal bases.

▶ Calf pain and/or tenderness, swelling with pitting edema, increased skin temperature, superficial venous dilatation, or cyanosis, which may indicate the presence of a deep vein thrombosis, requiring immediate medical attention (see Chap. 9).

▶ Feelings of warmth or coldness in the foot. An abnormally warm foot can indicate local inflammation, but can also originate from a tumor in the pelvic or lumbar region.[140] An abnormally cold foot usually indicates a vascular problem.[140]

Tests and Measures

Observation

Observation of the lower extremity is extensive. It is extremely important to observe the entire kinetic chain when assessing the leg, foot, and ankle. Weight-bearing and non–weight-bearing postures of the foot are compared.

Observing the patient while they move from sitting to standing and walk to the treatment area gives the clinician a sense of the patient's functional ability in weight bearing, and provides the first opportunity for gait analysis.[109] An important part of the examination of the foot and ankle is the gait assessment (see Chap. 13).

Clinical Pearl

Patients with an ankle injury usually avoid the normal heel-to-toe progression to decrease weight bearing and painful ankle dorsiflexion.[141] Instead, the patient is likely to adopt a toe-to-heel or toe-out progression with varying amounts of hip circumduction, or steppage gait to further unload the ankle.[142]

The following are assessed with the patient standing:

▶ *Shoulder and pelvic heights.*

▶ *Spinal curvature.*

▶ *Pelvic rotation.*

▶ *The degree of knee flexion or hyperextension.* A genu recurvatum places the talocrural joint in more plantar flexion than normal, and can often be a compensatory mechanism in the longer limb of individuals who have a leg length inequality.[143] An increase in knee flexion accomplishes the same compensation for a leg length inequality.[143]

▶ *The degree of hip rotation.* In the femur, anteversion and retroversion angles should be noted (refer to Chap. 17). Excessive internal rotation of the hip toward the opposite hip may result in a flattening of the medial longitudinal arch and toeing-in/internal torsion of the tibia (pigeon toes). Excessive external rotation of the hip away from the opposite hip may result in an elevation of the medial longitudinal arch.

▶ *Rearfoot to leg orientation (Fig. 19-22).* This can be an indicator of weight-bearing subtalar position. It is assessed by measuring the acute angle formed between a line representing the posterior aspect of the distal third of the leg, and a line approximately 1 cm distal to the first mark, representing the midline of the posterior aspect of the calcaneus (see Fig. 19-22).[143] The angle is assessed as the patient shifts weight onto the lower extremity to simulate single-limb support. If the lines are parallel or in slight varus (2 to 8 degrees), the leg-rearfoot orientation is considered normal.[144,145] Movement of

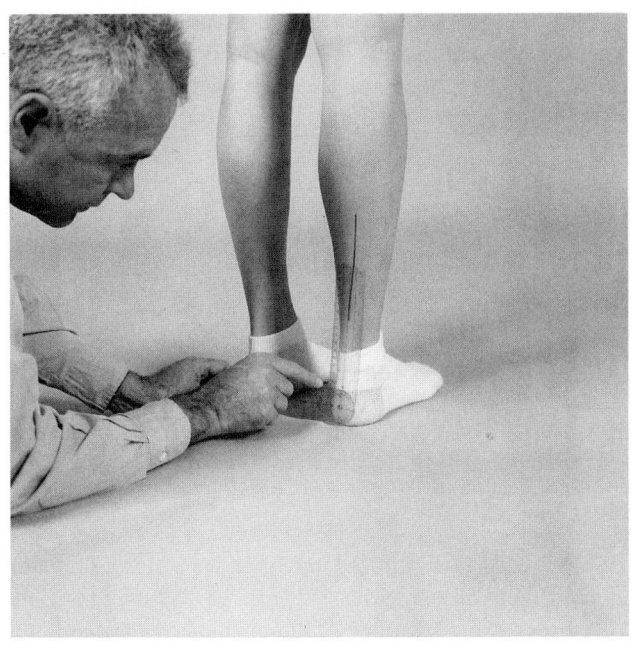

FIGURE 19-22 Rearfoot to leg orientation.

the rearfoot into eversion (rearfoot valgus) during this maneuver is indicative of subtalar pronation.[10] Pronation of the foot is manifested by eversion of the heel, abduction of the forefoot, a decrease in the medial longitudinal arch, internal rotation of the leg in relation to the foot, and dorsiflexion of the subtalar and midtarsal joints. If the heel is in too much valgus, the forefoot is excessively abducted, or there is excessive external rotation of the tibia, more toes can be seen on the affected side than the normal side when viewing the leg from behind ("Too-many-toes sign").[47] If the patient is asked to raise up on the toes, the calcaneus should be observed to move into a position of inversion. An inability of the calcaneus to invert with this maneuver could indicate the presence of an abnormality within the subtalar joint mechanism, or a weakness of the posterior tibialis.[47,145]

▶ *The degree of varus and valgus of the knee, tibia, and heel.* Excessive tibia varum, genu varus, or forefoot varus can increase the frontal angle of the talocrural joint, which promotes excessive weight bearing on the lateral aspect of the foot unless compensatory pronation is available within the foot to bring the medial aspect of the foot to the support surface.[143] Tibia varum refers to the frontal plane position of the distal one third of the leg as it relates to the supporting surface.[115] A number of methods to measure tibia varum have been proposed. The most reliable appears to be the measurement taken in the resting calcaneal stance,[146] which is measured as follows. The patient is asked to stand in a normal angle and base of support. The rearfoot to leg orientation is checked (see above). If the orientation is acceptable, the clinician measures the frontal plane relationship of the tibia to the transverse plane. Tibia varum is present when the distal end of the bisecting line of the leg is closer to the midsagittal plane than the proximal end (see Fig. 19-22). If the leg is angulated in the opposite direction, tibia valgum is present. Caution must be taken with the interpretation of these findings as static measurements have been found to have questionable validity in terms of predicting dynamic motion.[147–149]

▶ *Rotational components of the tibia.* Tibial torsion is assessed with the patient in sitting with their feet hanging over the end of the bed so that their knees are in about 90 degrees of flexion.[109] The thumb of one hand is placed over the apex of one malleolus, and the index finger of the same hand is placed over the apex of the other malleolus. A qualitative estimate of the direction and magnitude of tibial torsion can be made by envisioning a line that passes through the malleoli and estimating its orientation to the frontal plane of the proximal tibia.[143] Alternatively, tibial torsion can be measured with the patient in prone with the knee flexed to 90 degrees. The subtalar joint is positioned and stabilized in subtalar neutral.* To locate subtalar neutral, the patient is

---

* The subtalar neutral position refers to the position in which all bones of the subtalar joints and the talocrural joints line up optimally in their open-packed positions.

positioned in prone with the opposite hip flexed, abducted, and externally rotated. If evaluating the right ankle, the clinician uses the thumb and forefinger of the left hand to palpate the hollows over the neck of the talus on either side of the anterior portion of the ankle. Using the thumb and forefinger of the other hand, the clinician grasps the head of the fourth and fifth metatarsals and rocks the foot back and forth until the talus lies central between the fingers, which is approximately the midposition of movement for the subtalar joint. Once the subtalar neutral position has been established, a line is drawn on the sole of the foot parallel to the length of the femur. A second line is drawn in line with the foot. The angle between these lines is the tibial torsion angle.[150] There is normally an angle of 12 to 18 degrees to the frontal plane.[151] Tibial torsion is generally less in children. A position of relative internal rotation of the tibia produces an increase in rigidity to the subtalar joint prior to mid-stance due to premature stabilization of the longitudinal arch of the foot.[145] Excessive external rotation of the tibia places an increased strain along the longitudinal arch, as well as the first MTP joint.[145]

▶ *The weight-bearing foot.* The major components of the normal weight-bearing foot are:[127,152]

- Both planar condyles of the calcaneus are on the floor surface. An imaginary plane representing the ground surface is applied to the plantar surface of the calcaneus. The metatarsal heads should rest upon this plane. If the plane of the metatarsal heads is perpendicular to the bisection of the calcaneus, the forefoot-to-rearfoot relationship is normal, or neutral.

- All of the metatarsal heads lie in one plane, which is in the same plane as the plantar condyles of the calcaneus.[153]

- The ball of the foot is level with the plantar surface of the heel.

- A normal forefoot-to-rearfoot relationship (see below).

- The orientation of the distal third of the lower leg should be vertical, to position the foot properly for the stance phase.

- The midtarsal joint is maximally pronated, while the subtalar joint, MTP, and IP joints are in neutral.

- The presence of a well-formed static medial arch should be noted, as well as its dynamic formation with heel raising.

▶ *Forefoot-to-rearfoot relationship.* Neutral alignment of the forefoot relative to the rearfoot is present when a line representing the plantar aspect of the metatarsal heads is perpendicular to the line bisecting the rearfoot. The forefoot-to-rearfoot angle is approximately 10 to 12 degrees.[127,152] Forefoot varus is the term used to describe inversion of the forefoot away from this neutral position, while forefoot valgus describes an everted forefoot position.[143] The relationship can be assessed with the patient positioned in prone with their knee extended and their feet

over the end of the table. The subtalar neutral position is located using the method described previously. Slight pressure is applied to the metatarsal heads while maintaining subtalar neutral. This will determine the relationship of the forefoot to rearfoot, and both of these to the bisection of the lower leg. A varus or valgus tilt of the forefoot in relation to the hindfoot becomes significant when the first metatarsal is in a plantarflexed position, as this positions the hindfoot into an inverted position during weight bearing.[145]

▶ *Foot deviations in weight bearing.* These include pes planus (low inclined subtalar joint axis), pes cavus (high inclined subtalar joint axis), talipes equinus (plantarflexed foot), talipes equinovarus (supinated foot), and hallux valgus.[109]

▶ *Degree of foot pronation or supination in non–weight bearing.* The patient is positioned in prone with the foot extended over the edge of the table. The clinician holds the foot over the fourth and fifth metatarsal heads with one hand. Both sides of the talus are palpated on the dorsum of the foot using the thumb and index finger of the other hand. The clinician then passively dorsiflexes the foot until a resistance is felt. At this point, and while maintaining the dorsiflexed position, the clinician moves the foot back and forth through the arc of supination and pronation. During supination, the talus should be felt to bulge laterally, while during pronation, the talus should be felt to bulge medially.

▶ *Degree of toe-out.* The normal foot in relaxed standing adopts a slight toe-out position of about 12 to 18 degrees from the sagittal axis of the body (Fick angle).[70]

▶ *Forefoot equinus.* To assess for forefoot equinus, the clinician stabilizes the rearfoot with one hand, and applies pressure on the entire forefoot via pressure across the metatarsal heads, into dorsiflexion. If the plantar declination of the lateral structures cannot be reduced so that the plantarflexed attitude is no longer visible, a positive identification of forefoot equinus can be made.[152]

▶ *Presence of a talar bulge.* The patient is positioned in standing, and the clinician observes to see whether the talar head bulges excessively on the medial side of the midfoot, indicating excessive subtalar joint pronation in weight bearing. Tightness of the gastrocnemius/soleus group is indicated with a prominence of the soleus, particularly on the medial side of the teno-calcaneum.

Other areas that should be examined include:

▶ *The distal tibiofibular joint.* The distal tibiofibular joint is structurally and functionally an integral part of the ankle joint and must be examined with the ankle.

▶ *Condition of the nails.* When examining the nails a systematic approach is used, involving an inspection of the shape, contour, and color of the nails. The clinician should observe for the presence of subungual hematomas, subungual exostosis, onychocryptosis, onychia, onychauxis, onychomycosis, paronychia, tinea pedis, or blisters.

▶ *Toe deformities.* Contractions of the capsule of the IP or MTP joints of the toes in association with tendon shortening may produce a series of deformities, ranging from hammer toe to mallet toe to claw toe. *Hammer toe* (Fig. 19-23B) usually involves a flexion contracture of the plantar surface of the proximal interphalangeal joint (PIP), with a mild associated extension contracture of the MTP joint. *Mallet toe* (see Fig. 19-23C) results from a flexion deformity of the distal interphalangeal joint (DIP) with plantar contracture. Often a corn or callus is present on the dorsum of the affected joint. Corns are similar to calluses but have a central nidus. *Claw toe* deformity (see Fig. 19-23A) is a more advanced contracture of capsules and intrinsic musculature, which may also be associated with pes cavus and neurologic or primary muscle pathology to the lumbrical and interosseous muscles. The claw toe results in hyperextension of the MTP joints and flexion of the PIP and DIP joints.

▶ *Functional hallux limitus.* Clinically, the presence of functional hallux limitus, an inability of the first metatarsophalangeal (MTP) joint to extend, can be determined by assessing the range of motion available at the first metatarsophalangeal joint while the first ray is prevented from plantarflexing. The patient is positioned in standing, the feet shoulder-width apart. The patient is asked to actively raise the great toe off the floor while keeping the remaining toes and foot on the ground. The amount of hallux extension is measured; less than 10 degrees is considered limited.[153a] This test has been found to have a sensitivity of 0.72 and a specificity of 0.66.[153a]

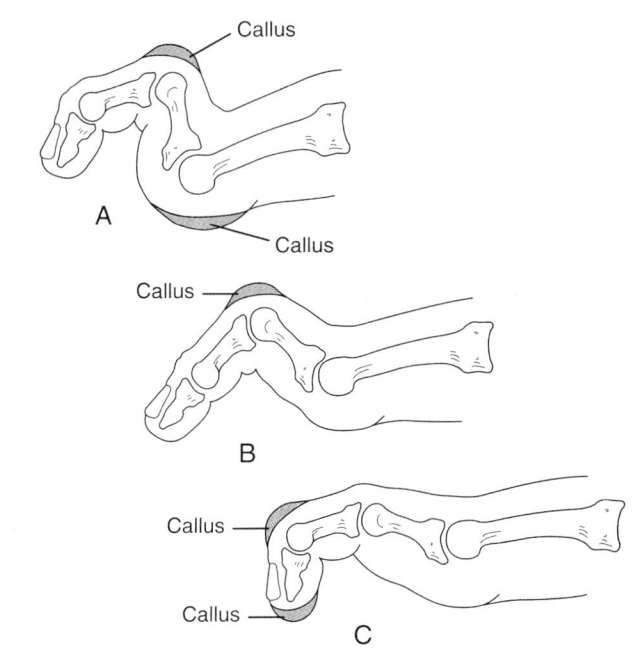

Callus

Callus

A

Callus

B

Callus

Callus

C

FIGURE 19-23 Toe deformities. A. Claw toe. B. Hammer toe. C. Mallet toe. (Reproduced with permission from Magee DJ, ed. *Orthopedic Physical Assessment*. Philadelphia: WB Saunders; 2002.)

▶ *The leg, foot, and ankle are examined for the presence of bruising, swelling, or unusual angulation.* Extracellular fluid pools on the dorsum of the foot and around the malleoli after injury or surgery.[109] Shortly after a lateral ligament sprain, the swelling is limited to the lateral ankle. Subsequently the swelling is diffuse, and the localization of tenderness may be difficult. Ecchymosis may be present, but the blood usually settles along the medial or lateral aspects of the heel.[22,133] The appearance of bluish-black plaques on the posterior and posterolateral aspect of one or both heels in a young distance runner is found in a condition called *black-dot heel*, which results from a shearing stress or a pinching of the heel between the counter and the sole of the shoe at heel strike during running.

▶ *Callus formation.* Calluses provide the clinician with an index to the degree of shear stresses applied to the foot, and clearly outline abnormal weight-bearing areas.[154] In adequate amounts calluses provide protection, but in excess they may cause pain. Callus formation under the second and third metatarsal heads could indicate excessive pronation in a flexible foot, or Morton's (interdigital) neuroma if under the second through fourth. A callus under the fifth and sometimes the fourth metatarsal head may indicate an abnormally rigid foot.

▶ *Any evidence of circulatory impairment or vasomotor changes.* Brick-red coloring or cyanosis when the leg is dependent is an indication of impairment, especially if the color changes when the leg is elevated. Vasomotor changes include toenail changes, changes in skin texture, abnormal skin moisture or dryness, and loss of hair on the foot. Vasomotor changes may be associated with complex regional pain syndrome (see Chap. 9).

▶ *The type of shoes.* High-heeled shoes have been associated with adaptive shortening of the gastrocnemius soleus complex, knee pain, and low back pain.[56,155] They have also been associated with an increased potential for ankle sprains, hallux valgus, bunions, metatarsalgia, interdigital neuromas, peripheral nerve compression, and stress fractures.[56,155] Shoes with a negative heel may result in hyperextension of the knees.

▶ *The weight-bearing and wear patterns of the shoe.* The greatest amount of wear on the sole of the shoe should occur beneath the ball of the foot, in the area corresponding to the first, second, and third MTP joints, and slight wear to the lateral side of the heel. Old running shoes belonging to patients who excessively pronate tend to display overcompression of the medial arch of the midsole and extensive wear of the lateral regions of the heel counter and medial forefoot. The upper portion of the shoe should demonstrate a transverse crease at the level of the MTP joints. A stiff first MTP joint can produce a crease line that runs obliquely, from forward and medial to backward and lateral.[156] The cup at the rear of the shoe, which is formed by the heel counter (Fig. 19-24), should be vertical and

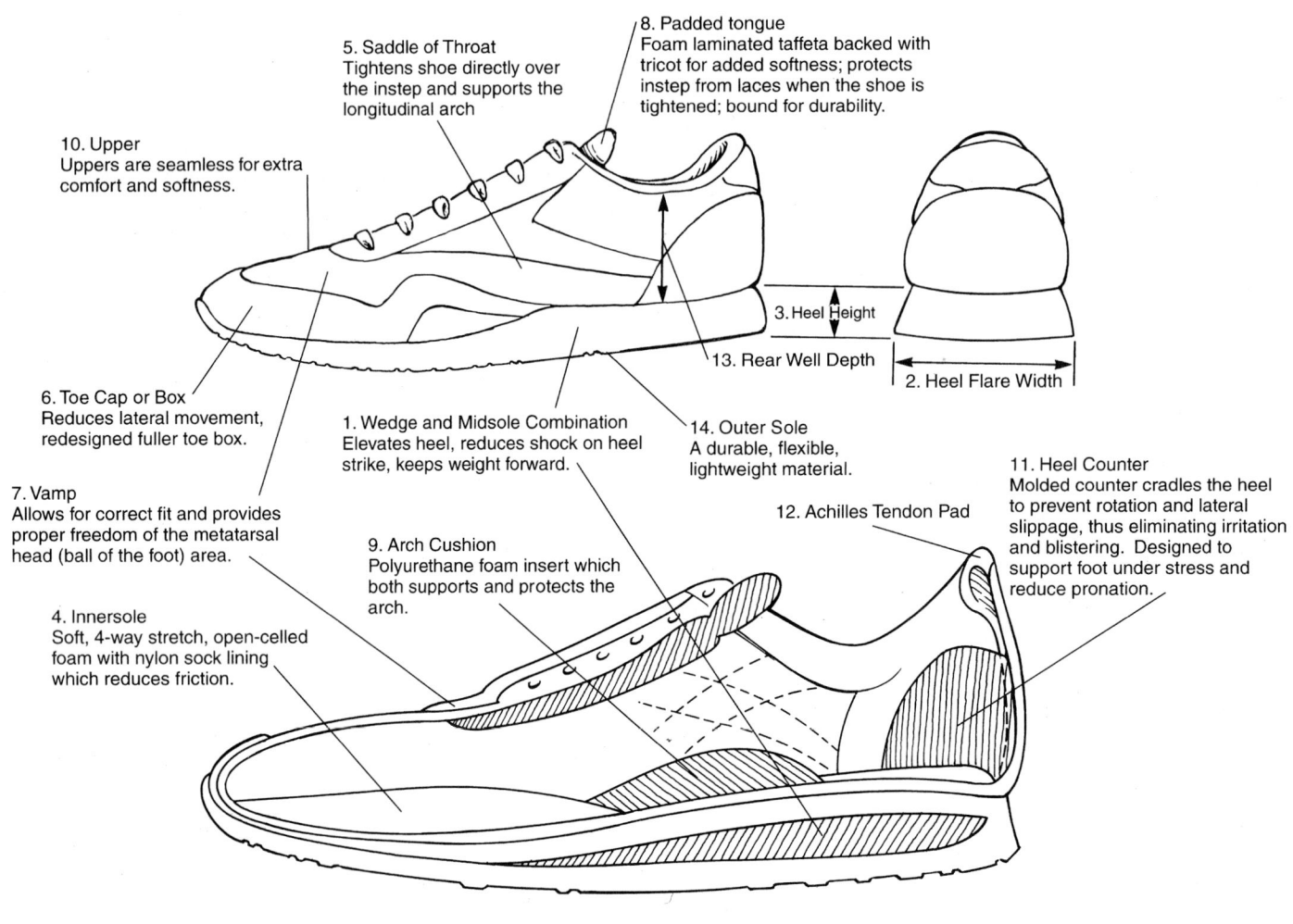

FIGURE 19-24   Shoe structure. (Reproduced with permission from Zachazewski JE, Magee DJ, Quillen WS, eds. *Athletic Injuries and Rehabilitation.* Philadelphia: WB Saunders; 1996.)

symmetrical with respect to the shoe, and should be of a durable enough material to hold the heel in place.[157] A medial inclination of the cup, with bulging of the lateral lip of the counter, indicates a pronated foot.[156] A lateral bulge of the heel counter indicates a supinated foot. Scuffing of the shoe might indicate tibialis anterior weakness.[89] The shape of the last influences the amount of motion that the shoe permits.[158] As the degree of curvature in the last increases, more foot mobility is available.

The non–weight-bearing component of the examination is initiated by having the patient seated on the edge of the bed, feet dangling. The feet should adopt an inverted and plantarflexed position. A mobile or nonstructural flat foot will take on a more normal configuration in non–weight bearing, whereas a fixed or structural flat foot will maintain its planus state. By placing one hand on the patella and the other hand on the tips of the malleoli, the clinician should note approximately 20 to 30 degrees of external rotation of the ankle in relation to the knee.[145]

Palpation

Careful palpation should be performed around the leg, foot, and ankle to differentiate tenderness of specific ligaments and other structures. Areas of localized swelling and ecchymosis over the ligaments on the medial or lateral aspects of the foot and ankle should be noted.

Posterior Aspect of Foot and Ankle

Achilles Tendon.   The Achilles tendon is inspected for contour changes such as swelling, erythema, and thickening. Any gaps or nodules in the tendon and specific sites of pain should be carefully examined. Palpable gaps in the tendon accompanied by an inability to rise up on the toes could indicate a rupture of the tendon.

Calcaneus.   At the distal end of the Achilles tendon is the calcaneal tuberosity. The posterior aspect of the calcaneus and surrounding soft tissue is palpated for evidence of exostosis ("pump bump" or Haglund's deformity), and associated swelling (retrocalcaneal bursitis). The inferior medial process of the cal-caneus, just distal to the weight-bearing portion of the calca-neus, serves as the attachment of the plantar fascia and is often tender with plantar fasciitis.

Anterior and Anteromedial Aspects of the Foot and Ankle. While reading the next section, the reader may find it helpful to re-move a shoe and sock and self-palpate.

Great Toe and the Phalanges. Beginning medially the clinician locates and palpates the great toe and its two phalanges. The first metatarsal bone is more proximal, the head of which should be palpated for tenderness on the lateral aspect (bunion), and inferior aspect (sesamoiditis).

Moving laterally from the phalanges of the great toe, the cli-nician palpates the phalanges and metatarsal heads of the other four toes.

Tenderness of the second metatarsal head could indicate the presence of Freiberg's disease, an osteochondritis of the second metatarsal head (see Chap. 9). A callus under the second and third metatarsal head may indicate a fallen metatarsal arch. Pal-pable tenderness in the region of the third and fourth metatarsal heads could indicate a Morton's neuroma, especially if the char-acteristic sharp pain between the toes of this condition is relieved by walking barefoot. Tenderness on the lateral aspect of the fifth metatarsal head could indicate the presence of a tailor's bunion.

Cuneiform. The first cuneiform is located at the proximal end of the first metatarsal (see Fig. 19-2), and is palpated for tenderness.

Navicular. The navicular is the most prominent bone on the medial aspect of the foot. The navicular tuberosity can be lo-cated by moving proximally from the medial aspect of the first cuneiform (see Fig. 19-2). The talonavicular joint line lies directly proximal to the navicular tuberosity. In addition, the posterior tibialis, which can be made more prominent with re-sisted plantar flexion, adduction, and supination, can be used as a reference as it inserts on the plantar surface of the navicular (see later). Tenderness of the navicular could indicate the pres-ence of a fracture, or osteochondritis of the navicular (Köhler's disease).

Second and Third Cuneiforms. These two bones can be palpated by moving laterally from the first cuneiform (see Fig. 19-1). Tenderness of these bones may indicate a cuneiform fracture.

Dorsal Pedis Pulse. The pulse of the dorsal pedis artery, a branch of the anterior tibial artery, can be palpated over the talus, cuneiform bones (Fig. 19-25), between the first and second cuneiform, or between the first and second metatarsal bones.

Medial Malleolus. The medial malleolus is palpated for swelling or tenderness. Moving proximally from the anterior aspect of the medial malleolus, the distal aspect of the tibia is palpated. Distal to that is the talus bone. Moving distal from the tibia, the clinician palpates the long extensor tendons (see Fig.

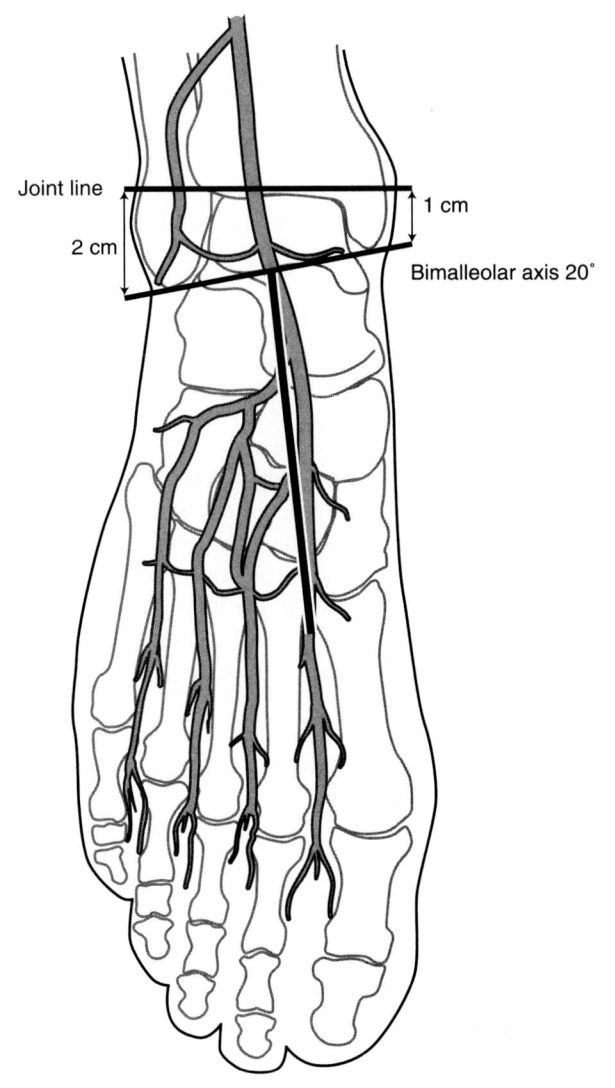

FIGURE 19-25 Topographic method for locating the dorsal pedis pulse. (Repro-duced with permission from Kelikian AS. *Operative Treatment of the Foot and Ankle.* New York: Appleton-Lange; 1999.)

19-12), the tibialis anterior (see Fig. 19-12), and the superior and inferior extensor retinaculum (Fig. 19-12). The tendon of the tibialis anterior is visible at the level of the medial cuneiform and the base of the first metatarsal bone, especially if the foot is positioned in dorsiflexion and supination.

Talus. The talus can be located by moving from the distal as-pect of the medial malleolus along a line joining the navicular tuberosity. It can be more easily located by everting and invert-ing the foot. Eversion causes the talar head to become more prominent while inversion causes the head to be less visible.

Sustentaculum Tali. Distal and inferior to the medial malleolus, a shelf-like bony prominence of the calcaneus, the sustentacu-lum tali (Fig. 19-3), can be palpated. At the dorsal aspect of the sustentaculum tali, the talocalcaneal joint line can be palpated.

Posterior Tibialis Tendon. This tendon (Fig. 19-14) is palpable at the level of the medial malleolus, especially with the foot held in plantar flexion and supination. Distal and medial to this tendon, the crossing of the flexor digitorum longus and flexor hallucis tendons can be felt.

Posterior Tibial Artery. The posterior tibial artery (Fig. 19-10) can be located posterior to the medial malleolus, and anterior to the Achilles tendon.

Deltoid Ligaments. The deltoid ligaments are very difficult to differentiate, so they are usually palpated as a group on the medial aspect of the ankle (see Fig. 19-6).

Anterior and Anterolateral Aspects of the Foot and Ankle

Tibial Crest. The tibial crest is palpated for tenderness, which may indicate the presence of shin splints. Swelling in this area may indicate the presence of anterior compartment syndrome. The muscles of the lateral compartment (peronei) and anterior compartment (tibialis anterior and the long extensors) are palpated here for swelling or tenderness. Swelling or tenderness of these structures usually indicates inflammation.

Lateral Malleolus. The lateral malleolus is located at the distal aspect of the fibula. Distal to the lateral malleolus is the calcaneus.

Peroneus Longus. The tendon of the peroneus longus (Fig. 19-11) runs superficially behind the lateral malleolus. Resisted pronation and plantar flexion of the foot makes the tendon more prominent.

Peroneus Brevis. The origin for the peroneus brevis is more distal to the peroneus longus and lies deeper (Fig. 19-12). It becomes superficial on the lateral aspect of the foot at its insertion at the tuberosity of the fifth metatarsal.

Anterior Talofibular Ligament (ATFL). The ATFL can be palpated two to three fingerbreadths anteroinferior to the lateral malleolus (see Fig. 19-5).[136] This is usually the area of most extreme tenderness following an inversion sprain. The anterior aspect of the distal tibiofibular syndesmosis may also be tender following this type of sprain.

Calcaneofibular Ligament (CFL). The CFL can be palpated one to two fingerbreadths inferior to the lateral malleolus (see Fig. 19-5).[136]

Posterior Talofibular Ligament (PTFL). The PTFL can be palpated posteroinferior to the posterior edge of the lateral malleolus (see Fig. 19-5).[136]

Sinus Tarsi. The sinus tarsi is visible as a concave space between the lateral tendon of the extensor digitorum longus muscle and the anterior aspect of the lateral malleolus. The origin of the extensor digitorum brevis is at the level of this tunnel.

Cuboid. The cuboid bone can be palpated by moving distally about one fingerbreadth from the sinus tarsi (see Fig. 19-2).

Active and Passive Range of Motion

Range-of-motion testing is divided into active range of motion (AROM), and passive range of motion (PROM) with overpressure superimposed at the end of available range to assess the end-feel. AROM tests are used to assess the patient's willingness to move and the presence of movement restriction patterns such as a capsular or noncapsular pattern. The end-feel may provide the clinician with information as to the cause of a motion restriction. The normal ranges of motion and end-feels for the lower leg, ankle, and foot are outlined in Table 19-6. The open- and close-packed positions and capsular patterns for the ankle and foot are outlined in Table 19-1.

TABLE 19-6 Normal Ranges of Motion and End-feels for the Lower Leg, Ankle, and Foot[34,560]

Motion	Normal Range (Degrees)	End-Feel
Plantar flexion	30–50	Tissue stretch
Dorsiflexion	20	Tissue stretch
Hind foot inversion (supination)	20	Tissue stretch
Hind foot eversion (pronation)	10	Tissue stretch
Toe flexion	Great toe: MTP, 45; IP, 90 Lateral four toes: MTP, 40; PIP, 35; DIP, 60	Tissue stretch
Toe extension	Great toe: MTP, 70; IP, 0 Lateral four toes: MTP, 40; PIP, 0; DIP, 30	Tissue stretch

General active range of motion of the foot and ankle in the non–weight-bearing position is assessed first, with painful movements being performed last. The hip and knee joints may also be examined as appropriate. Weight-bearing tests are usually performed after the non–weight-bearing tests.

If the symptoms are experienced during the general tests, then passive, active, and resisted tests of specific structures must be performed. If the general tests are negative, there is probably no immediate need to proceed with a more detailed examination, although this may have to be done if no other region appears to be the cause of the problem.

Distal Tibiofibular Joint. Although specific motions at this joint cannot be produced voluntarily, the function of this joint can be assessed indirectly by asking the patient to twist around both feet in each direction while weight bearing.

Dorsiflexion. The patient is positioned in supine, with the knee slightly flexed and supported by a pillow, while the clinician stands at the foot at the table, facing the patient.

Active dorsiflexion is initially performed with the knee flexed (Fig. 19-26). Care must be taken to prevent pronation at the subtalar and oblique midtarsal joint during dorsiflexion. The foot is slightly inverted to lock the longitudinal arch.[145] Passive overpressure is applied. With the knee flexed to approximately 90 degrees, the length of the soleus muscle is examined. Passive overpressure into dorsiflexion when the knee is flexed assesses the joint motion, as well as the soleus length. The soleus is implicated if pain is produced in this test, especially if resisted plantar flexion is painful or more painful with the knee flexed than with the knee extended. With the knee flexed, 20 degrees of dorsiflexion past the anatomic position (the foot at 90 degrees to the bones of the leg) is found in the normally flexible person.[159] The flexibility of the soleus muscle may also be assessed in standing in able-bodied individuals by asking the patient to perform a deep squat. If the muscle length is normal, the

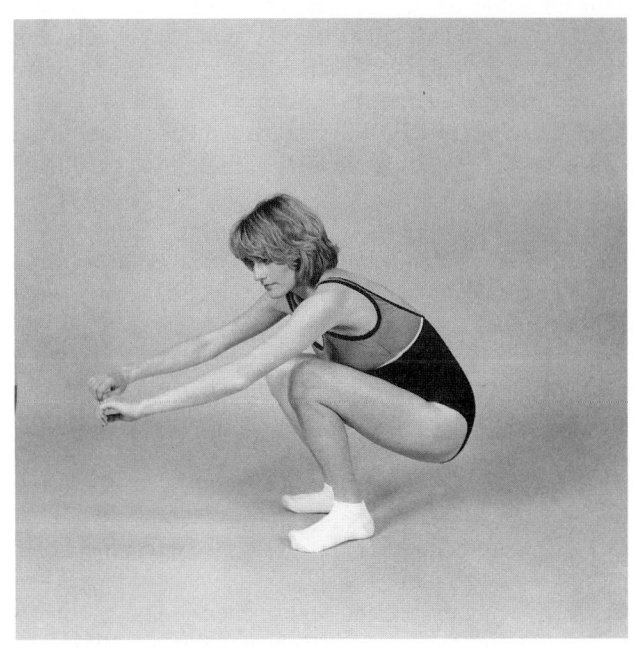

FIGURE 19-27 Soleus length test.

patient should be able to place the whole foot on the floor, including the heel, while in the full squat position (Fig. 19-27). If the soleus is short, the heel will not touch the floor.

Clinical Pearl

Chronic adaptive shortening of the soleus muscle can be caused by excessive running, a weak posterior tibialis, or a weak quadriceps. Adaptive shortening of the soleus can result in forefoot pronation and a valgus stress at the knee.

To assess the length of the gastrocnemius, the patient is positioned in supine with the knee extended, and the ankle positioned in subtalar neutral. The patient is then asked to dorsiflex the ankle. Passive overpressure into dorsiflexion is applied. The normal range is 20 degrees. If the gastrocnemius is shortened, dorsiflexion of the ankle will be reduced as the knee is extended and increased as the knee is flexed. A muscular end-feel should be felt with the knee extended, and a capsular end-feel should be felt with the knee flexed.

Clinical Pearl

A decrease in the flexibility of the gastrocnemius can result from a number of dysfunctions including dysfunction of the subtalar joint or transtarsal joint, an ankle sprain, high-heeled footwear, or poor gait/running mechanics.

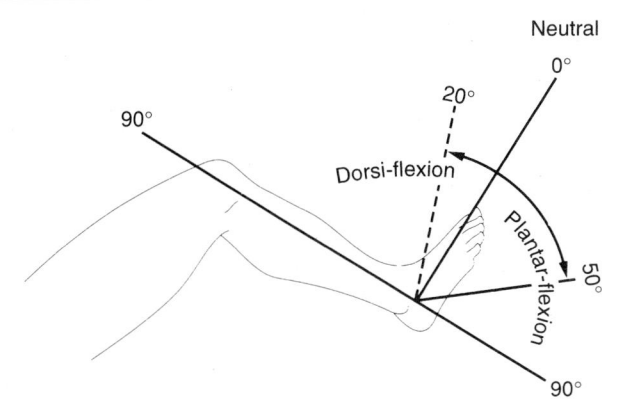

FIGURE 19-26 Range of ankle joint dorsiflexion and plantar flexion. (Reproduced with permission from Luttgens K, Hamilton K. *Kinesiology: Scientific Basis of Human Motion.* New York: McGraw-Hill; 1997.)

Plantar Flexion. The patient is positioned in supine with the leg supported by a pillow, while the clinician stands at the foot of the table facing the patient. The patient is asked to plantarflex the ankle. Plantar flexion of the ankle is approximately 30 to 50 degrees.[10] When tested in weight bearing with the unilateral heel raise, heel inversion should be seen to occur. Failure of the foot to invert may indicate instability of the foot/ankle, posterior tibialis dysfunction, or adaptive shortening.[160]

Hindfoot Inversion (Supination) and Hindfoot Eversion (Pronation).   The patient is positioned in prone, while the clinician stands at the foot at the table, facing the patient. Both hindfoot inversion (Fig. 19-28) and hindfoot eversion (Fig. 19-29) are tested by lining up the longitudinal axis of the leg and vertical axis of the calcaneus. Passive motion of hindfoot inversion (supination) is normally 20 degrees.[10] The amount of hindfoot eversion (pronation) is normally 10 degrees.[10]

Great Toe Motion.   The patient is positioned in supine with the leg supported by a pillow, while the clinician stands at the foot at the table, facing the patient. Active extension of the great toe is performed and assisted passively without dorsiflexing the first ray. Extension of the great toe occurs primarily at the MTP joint. Passive extension of the great toe at the MTP joint should demonstrate elevation of the medial longitudinal arch (windlass effect), and external rotation of the tibia.[161] Passive MTP joint extension of between 55 and 90 degrees is necessary at terminal stance,[52,162,163] depending on length of stride, shoe flexibility, and toe-in/toe-out foot placement angle.[143] Forty-five degrees of first MTP flexion and 90 degrees of IP joint flexion are considered normal.[145]

Strength Testing
Ankle
Gastrocnemius and Plantaris Muscles.   If no plantar flexion weakness is apparent in non–weight-bearing, a test is performed in the functional position, standing with the knee extended and the opposite foot off the floor. Technically, one heel raise through full range of motion while standing with support on one leg scores a 3/5 (Fair) with manual muscle testing with five single limb heel raises scoring a 4/5 (Good) and 10 single-limb heel raises scoring a 5/5 (Normal). From a functional viewpoint, a wider range of scoring can sometimes prove more useful. Table 19-7 outlines an alternative scoring method.

Soleus Muscle.   The soleus muscle produces plantar flexion of the ankle joint regardless of the position of the knee. To determine the individual functioning of the soleus as a plantar flexor, the knee is flexed to minimize the effect of the gastrocnemius muscle. To test the soleus, the patient stands with some degree of knee flexion, and then rises up on toes. Ability to perform 10 to 15 raises in this fashion is considered normal, 5 to 9 raises is graded as fair, 1 to 4 raises is graded as poor, and 0 repetitions is graded as nonfunctional.

Tibialis Anterior Muscle.   The tibialis anterior muscle produces the motion of dorsiflexion and inversion. The knee must remain flexed during the test to allow complete dorsiflexion. The patient's foot is positioned in dorsiflexion and inversion. The leg is stabilized, and resistance is applied to the medial dorsal aspect of the forefoot into plantar flexion and eversion.

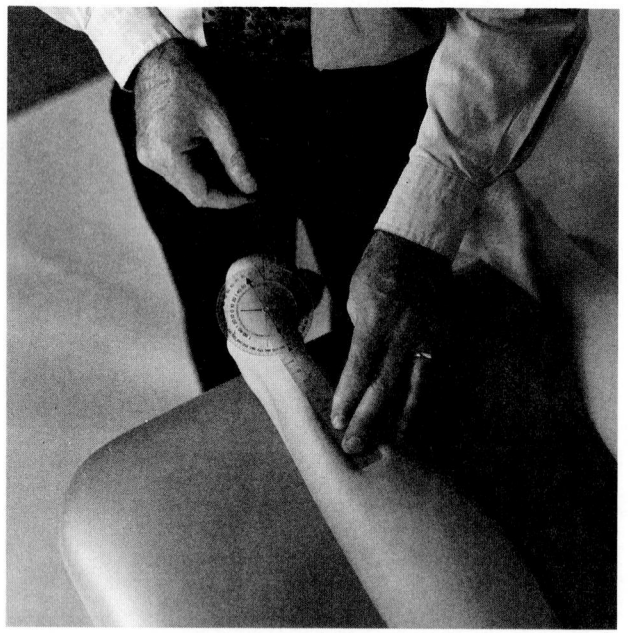

FIGURE 19-28   Ankle inversion.

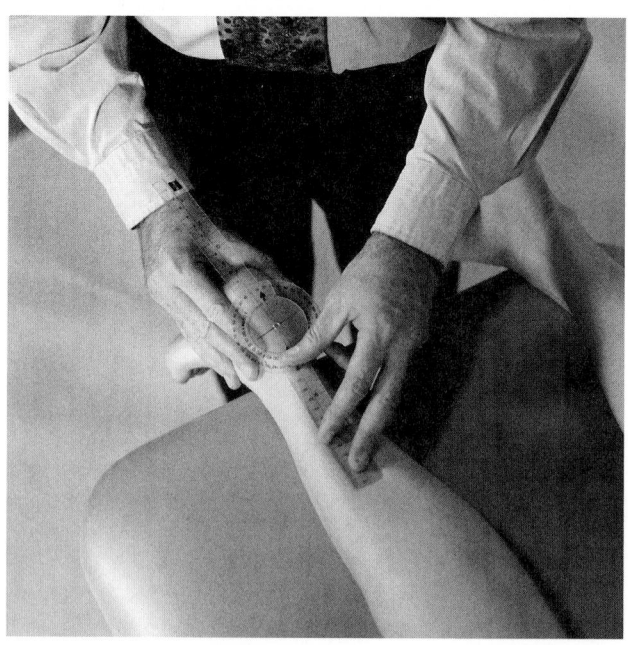

FIGURE 19-29   Ankle eversion.

TABLE 19-7   Functional Testing of the Foot and Ankle[184]

Starting Position	Action	Functional Test
Standing on one leg	Lift toes and forefeet off ground (dorsiflexion)	10 to 15 Repetitions: Functional 5 to 9 Repetitions: Functionally fair 1 to 4 Repetitions: Functionally poor 0 Repetitions: Nonfunctional
Standing on one leg	Lift heels off ground (plantar flexion)	10 to 15 Repetitions: Functional 5 to 9 Repetitions: Functionally fair 1 to 4 Repetitions: Functionally poor 0 Repetitions: Nonfunctional
Standing on one leg	Lift lateral aspect of foot off ground (ankle eversion)	5 to 6 Repetitions: Functional 3 to 4 Repetitions: Functionally fair 1 to 2 Repetitions: Functionally poor 0 Repetitions: Nonfunctional
Standing on one leg	Lift medial aspect of foot off ground (ankle inversion)	5 to 6 Repetitions: Functional 3 to 4 Repetitions: Functionally fair 1 to 2 Repetitions: Functionally poor 0 Repetitions: Nonfunctional
Seated	Pull small towel up under toes or pick up and release small object (ie, pencil, marble, cottonball) (toe flexion)	10 to 15 Repetitions: Functional 5 to 9 Repetitions: Functionally fair 1 to 4 Repetitions: Functionally poor 0 Repetitions: Nonfunctional
Seated	Lift toes off ground (toe extension)	10 to 15 Repetitions: Functional 5 to 9 Repetitions: Functionally fair 1 to 4 Repetitions: Functionally poor 0 Repetitions: Nonfunctional

Tibialis Posterior Muscle.   The tibialis posterior muscle produces the motion of inversion in a plantar flexed position. The leg is stabilized in the anatomic position, with the ankle in slight plantar flexion. Resistance is applied to the medial border of the forefoot into eversion and dorsiflexion.

Peroneus Longus, Peroneus Brevis, and Peroneus Tertius Muscles. The lateral compartment muscles and the peroneus tertius muscle produce the motion of eversion. The patient is positioned in supine with the foot over the edge of the table and the ankle in the anatomic position. Resistance is applied to the lateral border of the forefoot.

Digits.   Grades for the toes differ from the standard format because gravity is not considered a factor.

   0: No contraction.

   Trace or 1: Muscle contraction is palpated, but no movement occurs.

Poor or 2: Subject can partially complete the range of motion.

Fair or 3: Subject can complete the test range.

Good or 4: Subject can complete the test range, but is able to take less resistance on the test side than on the opposite side.

N or 5: Subject can complete the test range and take maximal resistance on the test side as compared with the normal side.

Flexor Hallucis Brevis and Longus Muscles.   The flexor hallucis brevis and flexor hallucis longus muscles produce MTP joint flexion and IP joint flexion. The foot is maintained in midposition. The first metatarsal is stabilized, and resistance is applied beneath the proximal and distal phalanx of the great toe into toe extension.

Flexor Digitorum Brevis and Longus Muscles.   The flexor digitorum longus and brevis muscles produce IP joint flexion. The motion is tested with the foot in the anatomic position. If the gastrocnemius muscle is shortened, preventing the ankle from assuming the anatomic position, the knee is flexed. The toes may be tested simultaneously.

The foot is held in the midposition and the metatarsals are stabilized. Resistance is applied beneath the distal and proximal phalanges.

Extensor Hallucis Longus and Brevis Muscles. The extensor hallucis longus and the extensor hallucis brevis muscles produce the motion of extension of the IP and MTP joints. The foot is maintained in midposition. Resistance is applied to the dorsum of both phalanges of the first digit into toe flexion.

Extensor Digitorum Longus and Brevis Muscles. The extensor digitorum longus and the extensor digitorum brevis muscles produce the motion of extension at the MTP and IP joints of the lateral four digits from a flexed position. Resistance is applied to the dorsal surface of the proximal and distal phalanges into toe flexion.

Intrinsic Muscles of the Foot. The intrinsic muscles of the foot are tested with the patient in either the supine or sitting position. Most subjects are unable to voluntarily contract the intrinsic muscles of the foot individually.

Abductor Hallucis Muscle. The metatarsals are stabilized and resistance is applied medially to the distal end of the first phalanx.

Adductor Hallucis Muscle. The metatarsals are stabilized and resistance is applied to the lateral side of the proximal phalanx of the first digit.

Lumbrical Muscles. The lateral four metatarsals are stabilized and resistance is applied to the middle and distal phalanges of the lateral four digits.

Plantar Interossei Muscles. The lateral three metatarsals are stabilized and resistance is applied to the middle and distal phalanges.

Dorsal Interossei and Abductor Digiti Minimi Muscles. The metatarsals are stabilized and resistance is applied:

▶ Dorsal interossei: Applied to the middle and distal phalanges.

▶ Abductor digiti minimi: Applied to the lateral side of the proximal phalanx of the fifth digit.

Functional Tests
Subjective Tests
The Ankle Joint Functional Assessment Tool. The Ankle Joint Functional Assessment Tool (AJFAT)[164] is composed of 12 questions rating the ankle's functional ability (Table 19-8). The AJFAT questions are based on assessment tools previously used for evaluating the functional level of the knee.[165–167]

TABLE 19-8 Ankle Joint Functional Assessment Tool (AJFAT)[164]

1. How would you describe the level of pain you experience in your ankle?
   _____(0) Much more than the other ankle
   _____(1) Slightly more than the other ankle
   _____(2) Equal in amount to the other ankle
   _____(3) Slightly less than the other ankle
   _____(4) Much less than the other ankle
2. How would you describe any swelling of your ankle?
   _____(0) Much more than the other ankle
   _____(1) Slightly more than the other ankle
   _____(2) Equal in amount to the other ankle
   _____(3) Slightly less than the other ankle
   _____(4) Much less than the other ankle
3. How would you describe the ability of your ankle when walking on uneven surfaces?
   _____(0) Much less than the other ankle
   _____(1) Slightly less than the other ankle
   _____(2) Equal in ability to the other ankle
   _____(3) Slightly more than the other ankle
   _____(4) Much more than the other ankle
4. How would you describe the overall feeling of stability of your ankle?
   _____(0) Much less stable than the other ankle
   _____(1) Slightly less stable than the other ankle
   _____(2) Equal in stability to the other ankle
   _____(3) Slightly more stable than the other ankle
   _____(4) Much more stable than the other ankle

TABLE 19-8 *(cont.)*

5. How would you describe the overall feeling of strength of your ankle?
_____(0) Much less strong than the other ankle
_____(1) Slightly less strong than the other ankle
_____(2) Equal in strength to the other ankle
_____(3) Slightly stronger than the other ankle
_____(4) Much stronger than the other ankle

6. How would you describe your ankle's ability when you descend stairs?
_____(0) Much less than the other ankle
_____(1) Slightly less than the other ankle
_____(2) Equal in amount to the other ankle
_____(3) Slightly more than the other ankle
_____(4) Much more than the other ankle

7. How would you describe your ankle's ability when you jog?
_____(0) Much less than the other ankle
_____(1) Slightly less than the other ankle
_____(2) Equal in amount to the other ankle
_____(3) Slightly more than the other ankle
_____(4) Much more than the other ankle

8. How would you describe your ankle's ability to "cut," or change direction, when running?
_____(0) Much less than the other ankle
_____(1) Slightly less than the other ankle
_____(2) Equal in amount to the other ankle
_____(3) Slightly more than the other ankle
_____(4) Much more than the other ankle

9. How would you describe the overall activity level of your ankle?
_____(0) Much less than the other ankle
_____(1) Slightly less than the other ankle
_____(2) Equal in amount to the other ankle
_____(3) Slightly more than the other ankle
_____(4) Much more than the other ankle

10. Which statement best describes your ability to sense your ankle beginning to "roll over"?
_____(0) Much later than the other ankle
_____(1) Slightly later than the other ankle
_____(2) At the same time as the other ankle
_____(3) Slightly sooner than the other ankle
_____(4) Much sooner than the other ankle

11. Compared with the other ankle, which statement best describes your ability to respond to your ankle beginning to "roll over"?
_____(0) Much later than the other ankle
_____(1) Slightly later than the other ankle
_____(2) At the same time as the other ankle
_____(3) Slightly sooner than the other ankle
_____(4) Much sooner than the other ankle

12. Following a typical incident of your ankle "rolling," which statement best describes the time required to return to activity?
_____(0) More than 2 days
_____(1) 1 to 2 days
_____(2) More than 1 hour and less than 1 day
_____(3) 15 minutes to 1 hour
_____(4) Almost immediately

TABLE 19-9 Foot Function Index Disability Subsection

The line to the right of each item represents the amount of difficulty you had during the past week performing an activity because of your foot condition. On the far left is "No difficulty" and on the far right is "So difficult unable." Place a vertical mark on the line to indicate how much difficulty you had performing each activity because of your feet during the past week. If you did not perform an activity during the past week, mark that item N/A.

How Much Difficulty Did You Have?

1. Walking around the house?   No difficulty _____ So difficult unable
2. Walking outside on   No difficulty _____ So difficult unable
   uneven ground?
3. Walking four or more blocks? No difficulty _____ So difficult unable
4. Climbing stairs?   No difficulty _____ So difficult unable
5. Descending stairs?   No difficulty _____ So difficult unable
6. Standing on tip toe?   No difficulty _____ So difficult unable
7. Getting out of a chair?   No difficulty _____ So difficult unable
8. Climbing up or down curbs? No difficulty _____ So difficult unable
9. Walking fast or running?   No difficulty _____ So difficult unable

Foot Function Index Pain Subsection

The line to the right of each item represents the amount of foot pain that you experienced during the last week relative to several questions. On the far left is "No pain" and on the far right is "Worst pain imaginable." Place a vertical mark on the line to indicate how bad your foot pain was during the last week in response to each of the questions. If a particular question does not apply, please mark that item N/A.

How Severe Is Your Foot Pain?

1. At its worst?   No pain _____ Worst pain imaginable
2. When you walked barefoot? No pain _____ Worst pain imaginable
3. When you stood barefoot? No pain _____ Worst pain imaginable
4. When you walked wearing   No pain _____ Worst pain imaginable
   shoes?
5. When you stood wearing   No pain _____ Worst pain imaginable
   shoes?
6. At the end of the day?   No pain _____ Worst pain imaginable

Score: _____   _____ /15 = _____ %

The Foot Function Index. The Foot Function Index (FFI)[168] is a functional outcome measure that consists of three subsections: pain, disability (Table 19-9), and activity. A study by Budiman-Mak and colleagues[168] examined test-retest reliability (Intraclass correlation coefficient, ICC = 0.87), internal consistency (0.96), and construct and criterion validity of the questionnaire.

Objective Tests. In weight bearing, with the feet fixed, the patient should be asked to perform the following while the clinician notes any reproduction of pain or abnormal motion:

▶ *Weight bearing on the foot borders.* The patient is asked to bear weight on the medial borders of the feet while keeping the knees extended. The patient is then asked to bear weight on the lateral borders of the feet while maintaining the knee extension.

▶ *Heel raising.* In addition to being a general screening test, heel raising also assesses the ability of the medial arch to increase and produce a supinated/inverted arch. Under normal conditions, the tibialis posterior tendon inverts the hindfoot as the patient raises their heel. With poor or absent

tibialis posterior function, the patient just rolls onto the outside of the foot and demonstrates a decreased ability to unilaterally raise the heel.

▶ *Twisting of the lower leg.* Twisting tests the ability of the foot to supinate on the ipsilateral side, and its ability to pronate on the contralateral side.

The results of these tests may not be helpful in forming an actionable diagnosis, but they may be the only way to reproduce the patient's symptoms, and will therefore be of use in the formation of a diagnosis.

Functional Examination
See Table 19-7.

Passive Articular Mobility
Passive articular mobility tests assess the accessory motions available between the joint surfaces. These include tests of the joint glides, joint compression, and joint distraction tests. As with any other joint complex, the quality and quantity of joint motion must be assessed to determine the level of joint involvement. The

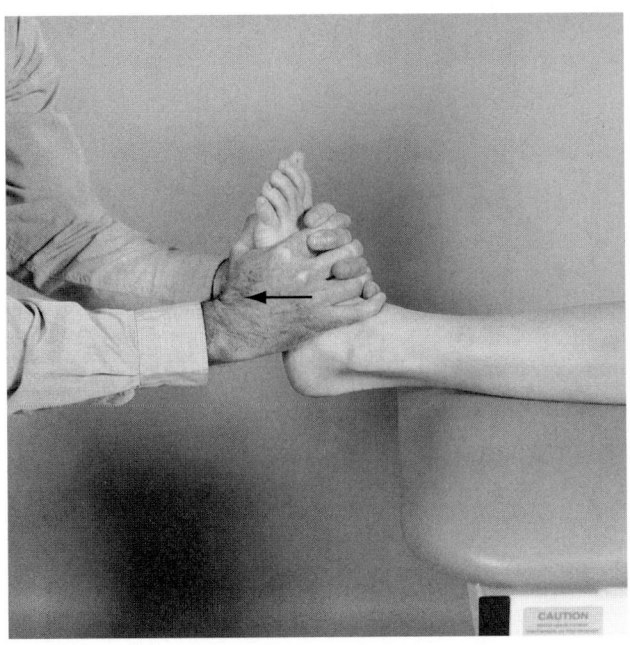

FIGURE 19-30   Long axis distraction of the talocrural joint.

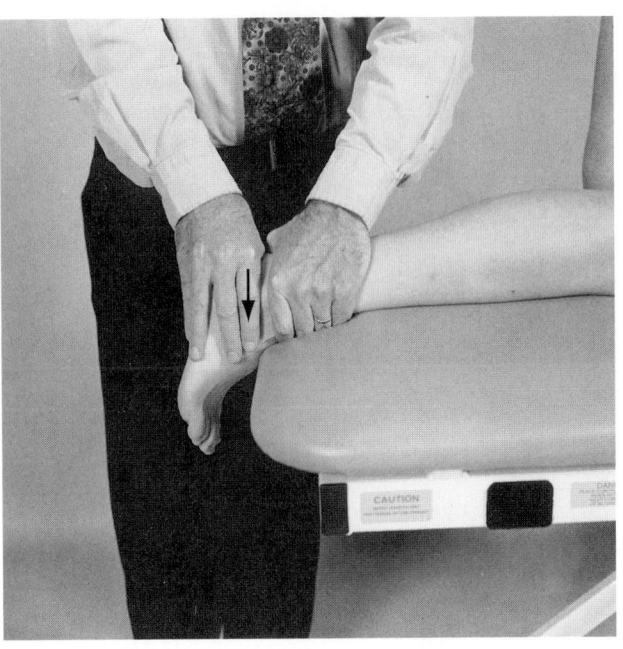

FIGURE 19-32   Anterior glide.

joint play movement tests must be performed on both sides so that comparisons can be made. The patient is positioned in lying.

Long-Axis Distraction.   The clinician stabilizes the proximal segment and applies traction to the distal segment. This test is performed at the talocrural joint (Fig. 19-30), the subtalar joint (Fig. 19-31), the MTP joints, and the IP joints.

Anterior-Posterior Glide.   To test the anterior movement, the clinician stabilizes the tibia and fibula and draws the talus and foot forward (Fig. 19-32). Pushing the talus and foot together in a posterior direction on the tibia and fibula (Fig. 19-33) tests the posterior movement.

The anterior-posterior glides can also be applied to the midtarsal, tarsometatarsal, MTP, and IP joints.

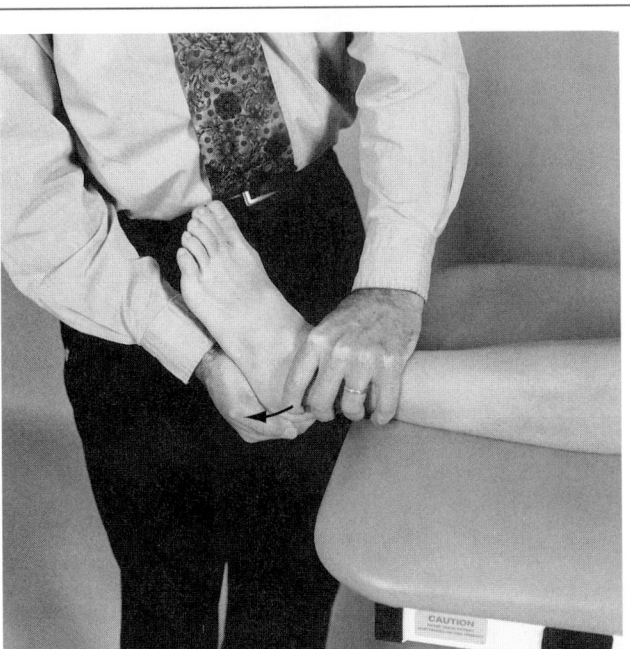

FIGURE 19-31   Long axis distraction of the subtalar joint.

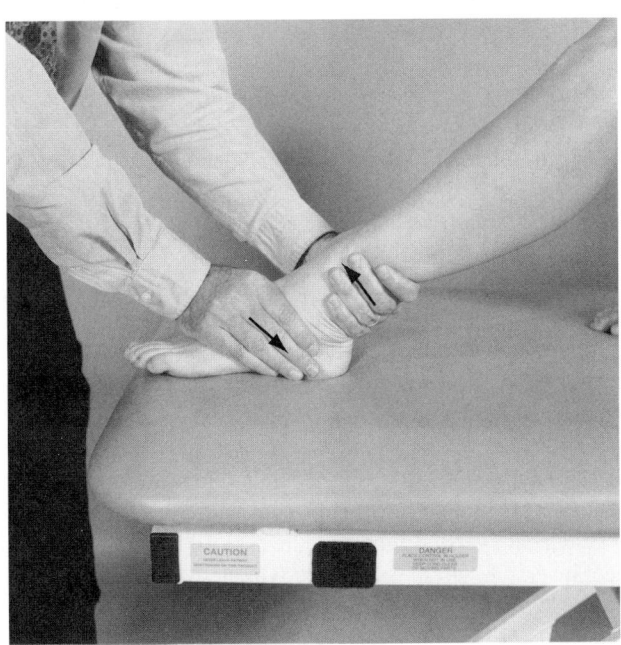

FIGURE 19-33   Posterior glide.

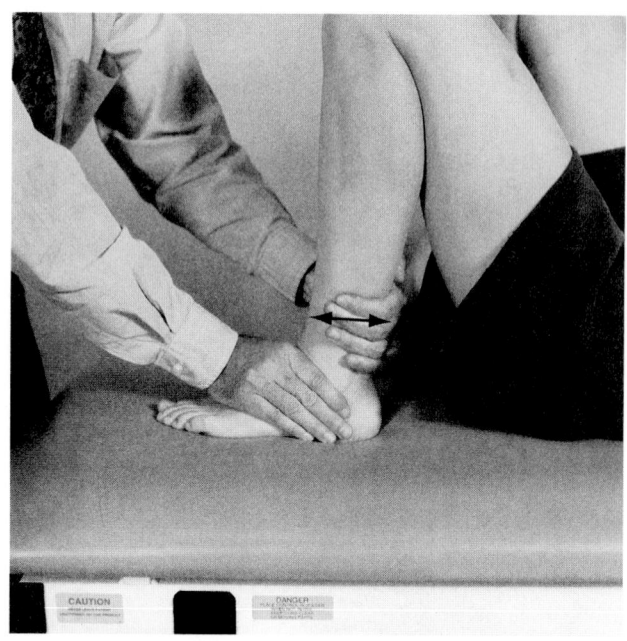

FIGURE 19-34   Tibial excursion.

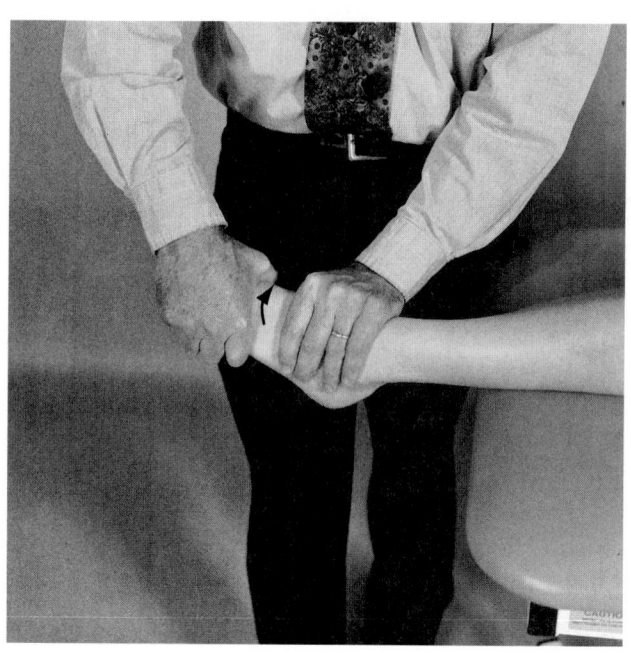

FIGURE 19-35   Forefoot adduction.

Tibial Excursion.   Tibial excursion in an anterior and posterior direction occurs during dorsiflexion and plantar flexion, respectively. This motion may be assessed in the non–weight-bearing position. The calcaneus and talus are fixed against a stable surface, and the tibia and fibula are glided in an anterior and posterior direction (Fig. 19-34).[93]

Abduction-Adduction (Subtalar).   The patient is positioned in supine, with the knee slightly flexed and supported by a pillow. The clinician stands at the foot of the table, facing the patient. The clinician grasps the forefoot and places it into adduction (Fig. 19-35) and abduction (Fig. 19-36). The amount and quality of the motions as compared with the other foot are compared. The range of adduction is generally twice that of abduction, approximately 30 degrees and 15 degrees, respectively.[137]

Calcaneal Inversion-Eversion.   Subtalar joint motion is extremely important to normal foot function. A loss of eversion causes weight bearing to occur along the lateral side of the ankle joint. The patient is positioned in supine, with the knee slightly flexed and supported by a pillow, while the clinician stands at the foot of the table, facing the patient. The clinician grasps the calcaneus in one hand, while the other hand locks the talus. The calcaneus is passively inverted (varus) and everted (valgus) on the talus (Fig. 19-37). The amount and quality of the motions as compared with the other foot are noted. Although some differences exist, generally calcaneal eversion will measure 5 to 10 degrees, while calcaneal inversion will measure approximately 20 degrees.[10,27,145]

Midtarsal Joint Motion.   The rotational movements of the midtarsal joint, which allow the forefoot to twist on the rearfoot,

can be observed in the non–weight-bearing position. The clinician stabilizes the calcaneus with one hand, while inverting and everting the foot with the other hand.[93]

Navicular Motion.   The patient is positioned in supine, with the clinician seated at the foot of the table facing away from the patient. The foot to be examined is positioned on a pillow or in the

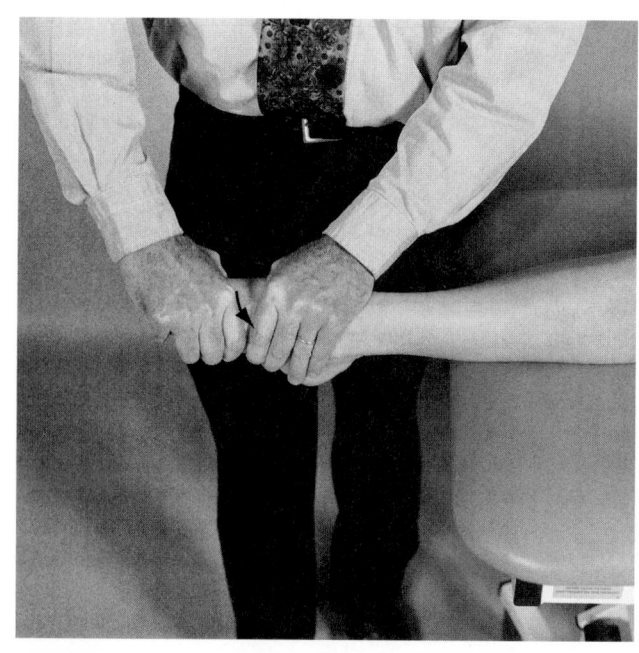

FIGURE 19-36   Forefoot abduction.

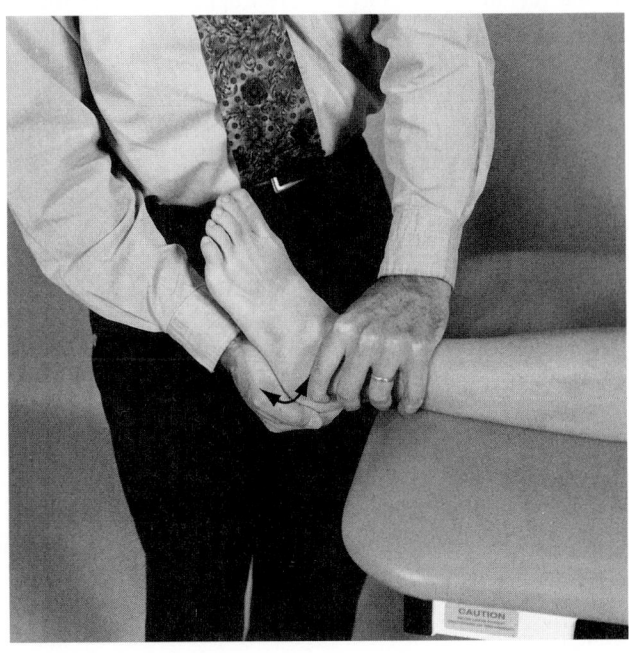

FIGURE 19-37 Calcaneal inversion and eversion.

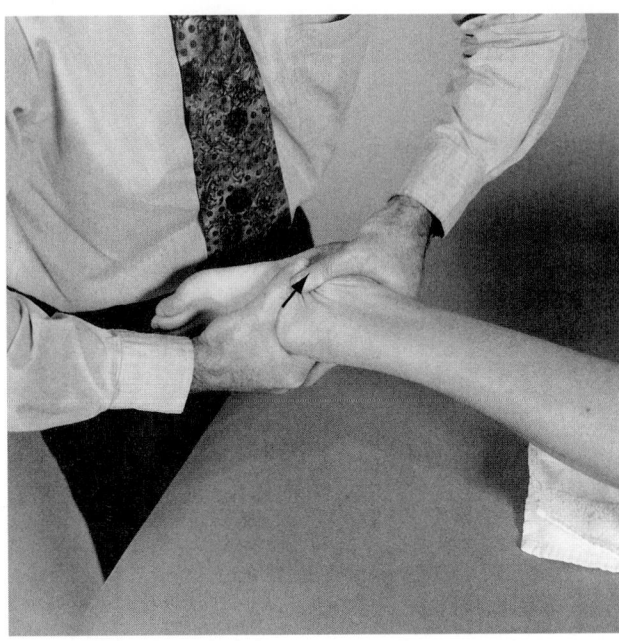

FIGURE 19-39 Cuboid motion.

clinician's lap. The clinician grasps the foot and talus with one hand, locking the latter. With the other hand, the clinician grasps the navicular and moves it dorsally and ventrally (Fig. 19-38). The quality and quantity of motion is noted and compared with the other side.

Cuneiform Motion. Cuneiform motion is assessed in a similar fashion to navicular motion. The patient is positioned in side lying,

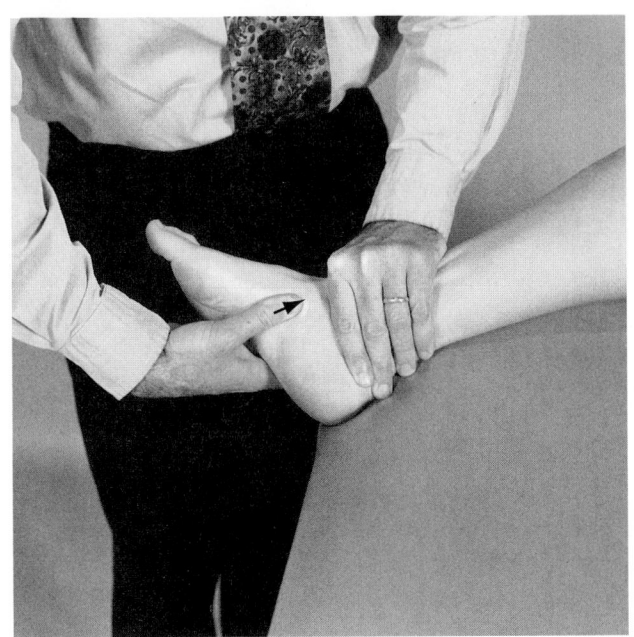

FIGURE 19-38 Navicular motion.

with the clinician seated at the foot of the table facing the patient. The clinician grasps and locks the navicular, and then moves the cuneiform on the navicular.

Cuboid Motion. The patient is positioned in prone with the clinician standing at the foot of the table. The patient's knee is flexed, and rested on a pillow. Using one hand, the clinician grasps the calcaneus, locking it, while with the thumb of the other hand, the clinician moves the cuboid plantarmedially (Fig. 19-39). The quality and quantity of motion is noted by the clinician.

First MTP Joint (First Ray) Motion. The patient is positioned in supine, with the clinician at the foot of the table facing away from the patient. The clinician grasps and locks the first MTP joint, before grasping the great toe first metatarsal joint and moving it into extension and flexion (dorsally and ventrally, respectively) (Fig. 19-40).

Limited range may result from a combination of biomechanical factors such as excessive pronation or joint glide restriction.[169] To examine the conjunct rotation of the metatarsals, the clinician locks the second metatarsal to evaluate the first, and locks the third to evaluate the second. The quantity and quality of motion is noted and compared to the other side.

Fifth Metatarsal Motion. The patient is positioned in prone, with the clinician standing beside the table. Using one hand, the clinician grasps the cuboid and stabilizes it. With the other hand, the clinician grasps the fifth metatarsal and moves it dorsally and ventrally (Fig. 19-41). To examine rotary motion of the metatarsal, the clinician locks the fourth metatarsal and examines motion of the fifth. To examine motion of the fourth

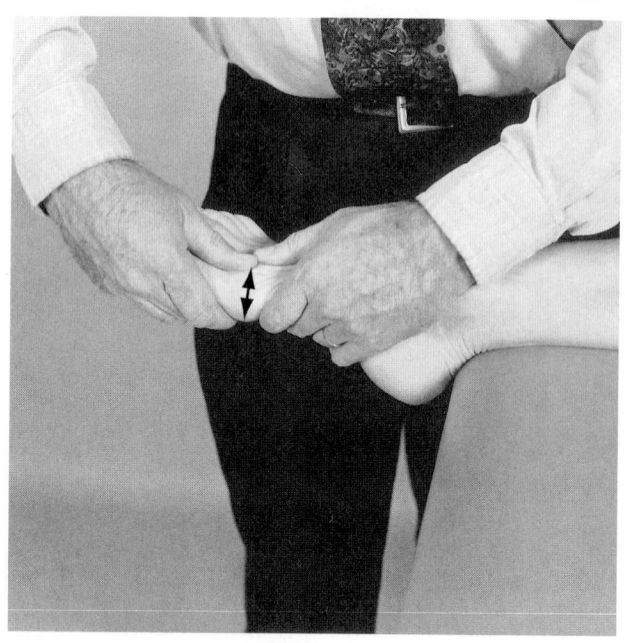

FIGURE 19-40   First MTP joint motion.

metatarsal, the third metatarsal is locked. The quality and quantity of motion is noted and compared with the other side.

Phalangeal Motion.   The patient is positioned in supine, with the clinician seated at the foot of the table facing away from the patient. The foot to be examined is positioned on a pillow in the clinician's lap. The clinician grasps the metatarsal and locks it with one hand. With the other hand the first phalanx articulating

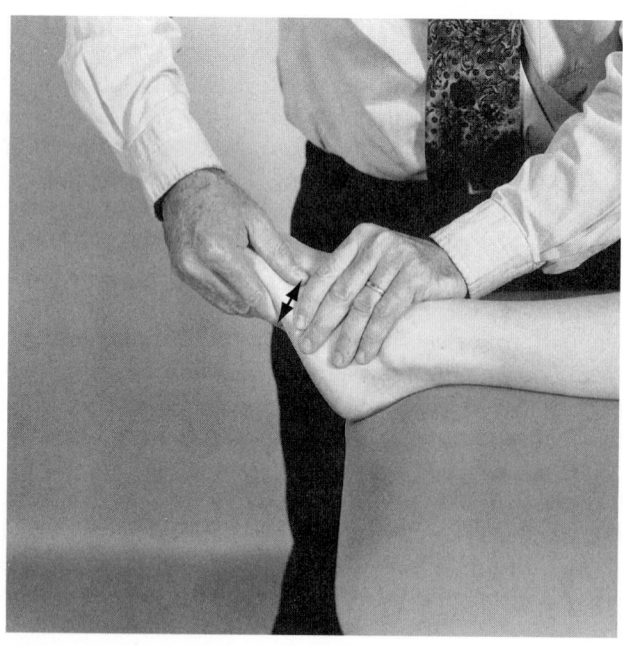

FIGURE 19-41   Fifth metatarsal motion.

with that metatarsal is grasped. After applying slight traction, the clinician examines the dorsal, ventral, abduction, adduction, and rotary motions. The quantity and quality of motion is noted and compared to the other side.

Special Tests

Special tests are merely confirmatory tests and should not be used alone to form a diagnosis. Selection for their use is at the discretion of the clinician and is based on a complete patient history. The results from these tests are used in conjunction with the other clinical findings and should not be used alone to form a diagnosis. To assure accuracy with these tests, both sides should be tested for comparison.

Ligamentous Stress Tests.   The examination of the ligamentous structures in the ankle and foot is essential, not only because of their vast array, but also because of the amount of stability that they provide. Positive results for the ligamentous stability tests include excessive movement as compared with the same test on the uninvolved extremity, pain (depending on the severity), or apprehension.

Mortise/Syndesmosis

Clunk (Cotton) Test.   The patient is positioned in supine with their foot over the end of the bed. One hand is used to stabilize the distal leg, while the clinician uses the other hand to grasp the heel and move the calcaneus medially and laterally (see Fig. 19-37).[170] A clunk can be felt as the talus hits the tibia and fibula if there has been significant mortise widening.[136]

Alternatively, the patient can be positioned in supine with their knee flexed to the point where the ankle is in the position of full dorsiflexion (see Fig. 19-34). The clinician applies overpressure into further dorsiflexion by grasping the femoral condyles with one hand and leaning down into the table. The clinician uses the other hand to pull the tibia (crura) anteriorly. Because the ankle is in its close-packed position, no movement should be felt.

Posterior Drawer Test.   The posterior drawer test can also be used to test for the presence of instability at the inferior tibiofibular joint. The patient is supine. The hip and knee are fully flexed to provide as much dorsiflexion of the ankle as possible. This drives the wide anterior part of the talus back into the mortise. An anterior stabilizing force is then applied to the cruris, and the foot and talus are translated posteriorly. If the inferior tibiofibular joint is stable, there will be no drawer available, but if there is instability, there will be a drawer.

Squeeze (Distal Tibiofibular Compression) Test.   In the squeeze test, the clinician squeezes the upper to middle third of the leg at a point about 6 to 8 inches below the knee (Fig. 19-42).[141] Pain felt in the distal third of the leg may indicate a compromised syndesmosis, if the presence of a tibia and/or fibula fracture, calf contusion, or compartment syndrome have been ruled out.[134,171]

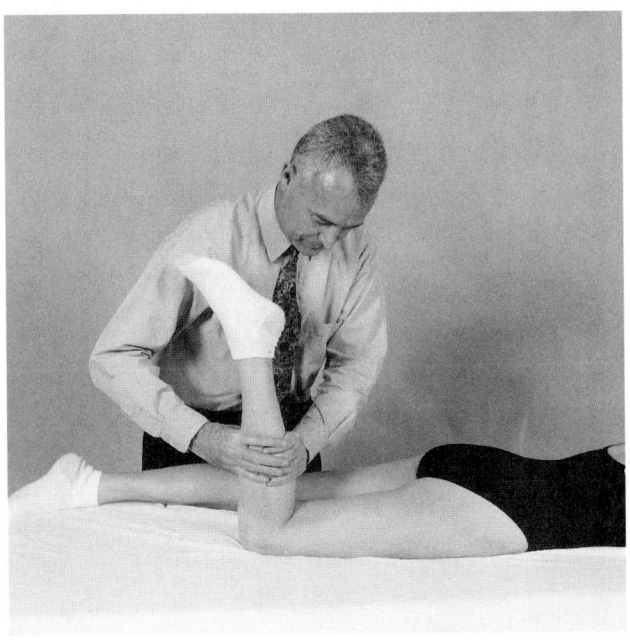

FIGURE 19-42 Squeeze test.

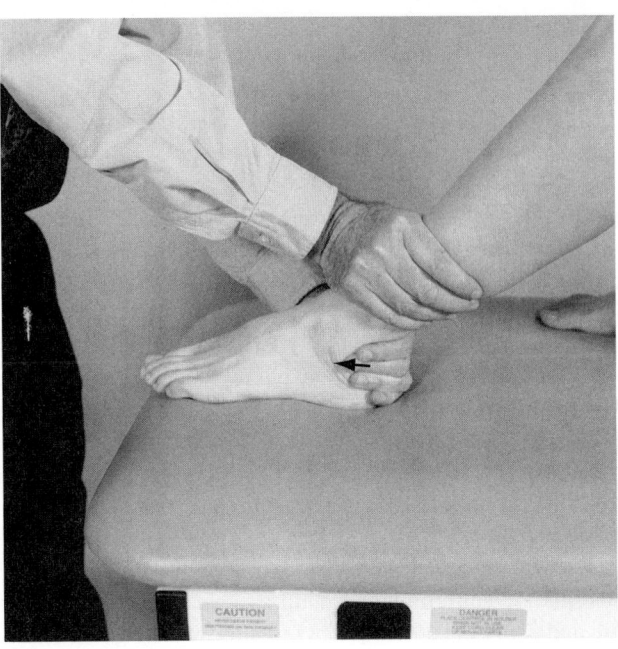

FIGURE 19-43 Anterior drawer test.

Lateral Collaterals. The lateral collaterals resist inversion and consist of the anterior talofibular, calcaneofibular, and posterior talofibular. An additional function of the lateral ligaments of the ankle is to prevent excessive varus movement, especially during plantar flexion. In extreme plantar flexion, the mortise no longer stabilizes the broader anterior part of the talus, and varus movement of the ankle is then possible.

Anterior Talofibular Ligament (ATFL). The patient is positioned in supine. The cruris is gripped with the stabilizing hand using a lumbrical grip, while the other hand grasps over the mortise and onto the neck of the talus, so that the index fingers are together at the point between fibular and talus. The clinician moves the patient's foot into plantar flexion and full inversion, and a force is applied in an attempt to adduct (distract) the calcaneus, thereby gapping the lateral side of the ankle. Pain on the lateral aspect of the ankle with this test, and/or displacement (depending on severity), may indicate a sprain of the ligament.

The Anterior Drawer Test. The anterior drawer stress test is performed to estimate the stability of the ATFL.[32,172,173] The test is performed with the patient sitting at the end of the bed or lying supine with their knee flexed to relax the gastrocnemius-soleus muscles and the foot supported perpendicular to the leg.[174,175] The clinician uses one hand to stabilize the distal aspect of the leg, while the other hand grasps the patient's heel and positions the ankle in 10 to 15 degrees of plantar flexion (Fig. 19-43). The heel is very gently pulled forward, and if the test is positive the talus, and with it the foot, rotates anteriorly out of the ankle mortise around the intact deltoid ligament, which serves as the center of rotation.

This test has limited reliability, particularly if it is negative, or if it is performed without anesthesia in the presence of muscle guarding.[176] It has been reported that 4 mm of laxity in the ATFL, resulting from post-traumatic attenuation or fibrosis, will give a clinically apparent anterior drawer (2 mm is normal).[177,178]

The Dimple Sign. Another positive sign for a rupture of the ATFL, if pain and spasm are minimal, is the presence of a dimple located just in front of the tip of the lateral malleolus during the anterior drawer test.[179] This results from a negative pressure created by the forward movement of the talus, which draws the skin inwards at the side of ligament rupture.[180] This dimple sign is also seen with a combined rupture of the ATFL and calcaneofibular ligaments.[179] However, the sign is only present within the first 48 hours after injury, due to organized hematoma and repair tissue blocking the communication between the joint and the subcutaneous tissues.[179]

Calcaneofibular Ligament (CFL). The inversion stress maneuver is a test that attempts to assess CFL integrity.[172] The patient is positioned supine. The cruris is gripped with the stabilizing hand while the moving hand cups the heel. The ankle is dorsiflexed via the calcaneus to a right angle (total dorsiflexion is impractical) and inverted. An adduction and anteromedial translation of the calcaneus is then applied, tending to gap the lateral side of the joint. Pain on the lateral aspect of the ankle with this test, and/or displacement (depending on severity), may indicate a sprain of the ligament.

Posterior Talofibular. The patient is either prone or supine, and the cruris is gripped or the fibular stabilized. The patient's leg is stabilized in internal rotation, and the foot is placed in full dorsiflexion. The clinician externally rotates the heel/calcaneus, thereby moving the talar attachment of the ligament away from the malleolus. Pain on the lateral aspect of the ankle with this test, and/or displacement (depending on severity), may indicate a sprain of the ligament.

Medial Collaterals (Deltoid Complex). The medial collaterals function to resist eversion. Given their strength, these ligaments are usually only injured as the result of major trauma.

Kleiger (External Rotation) Test. The Kleiger (external rotation) test[23,141,181] is a general test to assess the integrity of the deltoid ligament complex, but can also implicate the syndesmosis if pain is produced over the anterior or posterior tibiofibular ligaments and the interosseous membrane.[171,182] If this test is positive, further testing is necessary to determine the source of the symptoms.

The patient sits with their legs dangling over the end of the bed, with the knee flexed to approximately 90 degrees and the foot relaxed. The clinician stabilizes the lower leg with one hand, and using the other hand, grasps the foot and rotates it laterally (Fig. 19-44). Pain on the medial and lateral aspect of the ankle, and/or displacement of the talus from the medial malleolus (depending on severity) with this test may indicate a tear of the deltoid ligament.

Thompson Test for Achilles Tendon Rupture. In this test, the patient is positioned in prone, or in kneeling with the feet over the edge of the bed. With the patient relaxed, the clinician gently squeezes the calf muscle (Fig. 19-45) and observes for the production of plantar flexion. An absence of plantar flexion indicates a complete rupture of the Achilles tendon.[183]

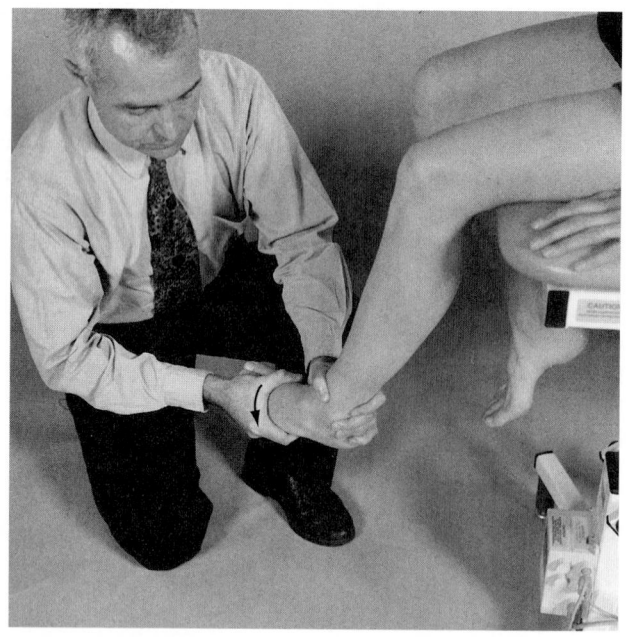

FIGURE 19-44 Kleiger test.

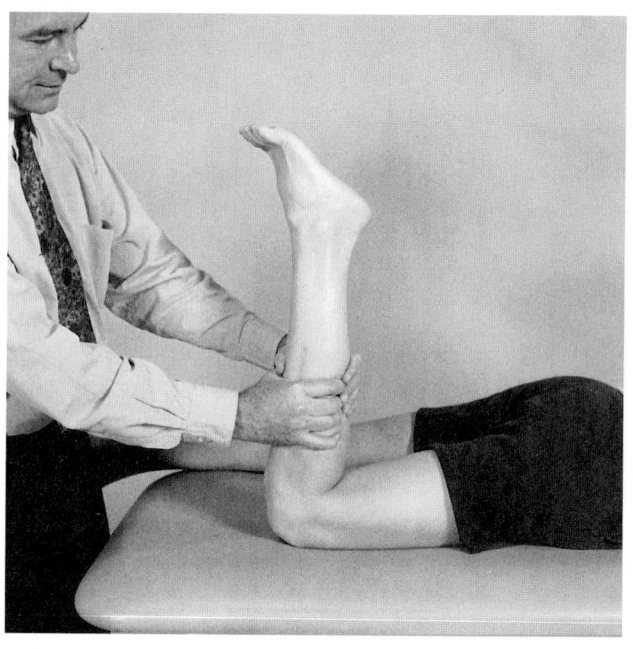

FIGURE 19-45 Thompson test.

Patla's Test for Tibialis Posterior.[160] The patient is positioned in prone with the knee flexed to 90 degrees. The clinician stabilizes the calcaneus in eversion and the ankle in dorsiflexion with one hand. With the other hand, the clinician contacts the plantar surface of the bases of the second, third, and fourth metatarsals with the thumb, while the index and middle fingers contact the plantar surface of the navicular. The clinician then pushes the navicular and metatarsal heads dorsally and compares the end-feel and patient response with the uninvolved side. A positive test is indicated with reproduction of the patient's symptoms.

Feiss Line.[184] The Feiss line test is used to assess the height of the medial arch, using the navicular position. With the patient non–weight bearing, the clinician marks the apex of the medial malleolus and the plantar aspect of the first MTP joint, and a line is drawn between the two points. The navicular is palpated on the medial aspect of the foot, and an assessment is made as to the position of the navicular relative to the imaginary line. The patient is then asked to stand with their feet about 3 to 6 inches apart. In weight bearing the navicular normally lies on or very close to the line. If the navicular falls one third of the distance to the floor, it represents a first-degree flatfoot; if it falls two thirds of the distance, it represents a second-degree flatfoot; and if it rests on the floor, it represents a third-degree flatfoot.

"Too Many Toes" Sign. The patient is asked to stand in a normal relaxed position while the clinician views the patient from behind. If the heel is in valgus, the forefoot abducted, or the tibia externally rotated more than normal, the clinician will observe more toes on the involved side than on the normal side.[185]

Articular Stability Tests

Navicular Drop Test. The navicular drop test is a method by which to assess the degree to which the talus plantarflexes in space on a calcaneus that has been stabilized by the ground, during subtalar joint pronation.[186,187]

The clinician palpates the position of the navicular tubercle as the patient's foot is non–weight bearing but resting on the floor surface with the subtalar joint maintained in neutral. The clinician then attempts to quantify inferior displacement of the navicular tubercle as the patient assumes 50 percent weight bearing on the tested foot.[143] A navicular drop which is greater than 10 mm from the neutral position to the relaxed standing position suggests excessive medial longitudinal arch collapse of abnormal pronation.[187,188]

This test has been found to have an intratester reliability which ranged from ICC = 0.61 to 0.79, and intertester reliability of ICC = 0.57.[143]

Talar Rock. The talar rock[189] is an articular stability test for the subtalar joint. The test is performed with the patient positioned in side lying, their hip and knee flexed (Fig. 19-46). The clinician sits on the table with their back to the patient, and places both hands around the ankle just distal to the malleoli. The clinician applies a slight distraction force to the ankle, before applying a rocking movement to the foot in a upward or downward direction (see Fig. 19-46). A "clunk" should be felt at the end of each of the movements.

Passive Foot Rotation. This test assesses the integrity of the midtarsal and tarsometatarsal joints. A rotational movement is applied to the midtarsal and tarsometatarsal joints. At the

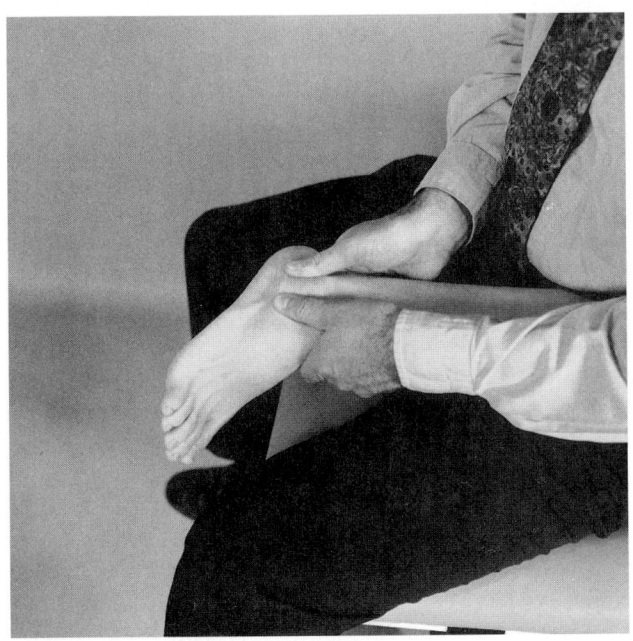

FIGURE 19-46 Talar rock test.

midtarsal joint, the proximal row of the tarsal bones (navicular, calcaneus, and talus) is stabilized, and the distal row (cuneiforms and cuboid) is rotated in both directions. At the tarsometatarsal joints, the distal row of the tarsals is stabilized and the metatarsals are rotated in both directions.

Vascular Status

Homans' Sign. The patient is positioned in supine with their knee extended. The clinician stabilizes the thigh with one hand, and passively dorsiflexes the patient's ankle with the other. Pain in the calf with this maneuver may indicate a positive Homans' sign for deep vein thrombophlebitis, especially if there are associated signs including pallor and swelling in the leg and a loss of the dorsal pedis pulse.

Buerger's Test. The patient is positioned in supine with the knee extended. The clinician elevates the patient's leg to about 45 degrees and maintains it there for at least 3 minutes. Blanching of the foot is positive for poor arterial circulation, especially if, when the patient sits with the legs over the end of the bed, it takes 1 to 2 minutes for the limb color to be restored.

Dorsal Pedis Pulse. The dorsal pedis pulse can be palpated just lateral to the tendon of the extensor hallucis longus over the dorsum of the foot (see Fig. 19-25).

Neurologic Tests. The applicable sensory, motor, and reflex testing should be performed if a disorder related to a spinal nerve root (L4–S2), or peripheral nerve is suspected. A neurogenic cause of foot pain must be considered in a patient, especially if the pain is refractory. The patient usually complains of pain that is poorly localized which is aggravated by activity, but may also occur at rest. Any difference in sensation between extremities should be noted and can be mapped out in more detail using a pinwheel. The segmental and peripheral nerve innervations are listed in Chap. 2. Common reflexes tested in this area are the Achilles reflex (S1–S2), and the posterior tibial reflex (L4–L5). Specific pathologies associated with peripheral nerve entrapment are described in the intervention strategies section.

The pathologic reflexes (Babinski and Oppenheim), tested when an upper motor neuron lesion is suspected, are described in Chap. 2.

Morton's Test.[190] The patient is positioned in supine. The clinician grasps the foot around the metatarsal heads and squeezes the heads together. The reproduction of pain with this maneuver indicates the presence of a neuroma, or a stress fracture.

Duchenne Test.[190] The patient is positioned in supine with their legs straight. The clinician pushes through the sole on the first metatarsal head, and pushes the foot into dorsiflexion. The patient is asked to plantarflex the foot. If the medial border dorsiflexes and offers no resistance while the lateral border plantarflexes, a lesion of the superficial peroneal nerve, or a lesion of the L4, L5, or S1 nerve root is indicated.

Tinel's Sign. There are two locations around the ankle where Tinel's sign can be elicited. The anterior tibial branch of the deep peroneal nerve can be tapped on the anterior aspect of the ankle. The posterior tibial nerve may be tapped behind the medial malleolus. Tingling or paresthesia with this test is considered a positive finding.

Imaging Studies

Radiography. Bone tenderness in the posterior half of the lower 6 cm of the fibula or tibia, and an inability to bear weight immediately after injury are indications to obtain radiographs to rule out fracture of the ankle.[191–193]

If there is bone tenderness over the navicular and/or fifth metatarsal, and an inability to bear weight immediately after injury, then radiographs of the foot are indicated.[191,192]

The value of stress roentgenograms is a controversial topic, though it may be helpful in the evaluation of the sprained ankle.[22,133] The stress views include inversion to assess talar tilt and the anterior drawer stress. The accuracy of these tests increases with the use of local anesthesia, and a comparison with the uninvolved ankle.

The anterior drawer test is performed with a lateral view of the ankle in neutral position while attempting to manually translate the foot anteriorly with respect to the leg.[22,133] The sagittal plane translation of the talus with respect to the tibia is measured. When compared with the same foot unstressed, anterior subluxation of more than 3 mm is considered to indicate an ATFL injury.[194]

The talar tilt test is used more often and is felt to be more reliable. In this examination, a mortise or AP view of the ankle held in neutral position to slight plantar flexion with an inversion stress applied to the foot is obtained.[22,133] The angle to be measured is that formed by a line parallel to subchondral bone of the distal tibia and proximal talus. It is the consensus that a talar tilt test is positive when the injured ankle has a stressed tibiotalar angle of 5[195] to 15 degrees[196] greater than the uninjured side. However, the absolute number of degrees is not as important as the functional instability of the patient, as laxity does not always mean instability.[22,133]

Other imaging techniques include arthrography, peroneal tenography, and magnetic resonance imaging (MRI).

Intervention Strategies

Due to the integrated nature of the foot and ankle in functional activities, the rehabilitation can be organized around a common framework for most foot and ankle pathologies.[197]

The techniques to increase joint mobility and the techniques to increase soft tissue extensibility are described in the therapeutic techniques section.

Acute Phase

The goals during the acute phase include:

▶ Decrease pain, inflammation, and swelling.

▶ Protect the healing area from re-injury.

▶ Re-establish pain-free range of motion.

▶ Prevent muscle atrophy.

▶ Increase weight-bearing tolerance.

▶ Increase neuromuscular control.

▶ Maintain fitness levels.

▶ Attain patient independence with a home exercise program.

The control of pain, inflammation, and swelling is accomplished by applying the principles of PRICEMEM (*p*rotection, *r*est, *i*ce, *c*ompression, *e*levation, *m*anual therapy, *e*arly motion, and *m*edication). Icing for 20 to 30 minutes three to four times a day, concurrent with nonsteroidal anti-inflammatory drugs (NSAIDs) or aspirin can aid in reducing pain and swelling.

The injured ankle should be positioned and supported in the maximum amount of dorsiflexion allowed by pain and effusion as appropriate. Maximal dorsiflexion places the joint in its close-packed position or position of greatest congruency.[198] This allows for the least capsular distention and resultant joint effusion. With ankle sprains this position produces an approximation of the torn ligament ends in grade III injuries to reduce the amount of gap scarring, and reduces the tension in the grade I and II injured ligaments.[22,133]

The means by which to support or protect the joint during this phase will vary depending upon the severity of the injury, the individual patient's requirements, and the anticipated compliance of the patient to any restrictions placed on them by the physician.[22,133] For example, mild to moderate ankle sprains (grade I and II sprains) can be readily supported by the use of an elastic bandage, open Gibney strapping (with or without felt pad incorporation), taping,[199–204] or the use of some type of thermoplastic stirrup such as an Air Cast (see next section).[205,206] One of the main advantages of this type of immobilization is that pain-free protected plantar and dorsiflexion are allowed whereas inversion and eversion are minimized.

To increase range of motion, the clinician can perform gentle capsular stretches and grade I to II joint mobilizations. Exercises in this phase include towel stretches (Fig. 19-47), ankle circles and pumps, low-level biomechanical ankle platform system (BAPS) exercises (Fig. 19-48), active and active assist exercises in straight planes (plantar flexion, dorsiflexion, inversion, and eversion) and proprioceptive neuromuscular facilitation (PNF) planes. Exercises for the foot intrinsics may include toe curl exercises with a towel (Fig. 19-49), or having the patient pick up marbles from the floor with their toes and place the marbles in a small container or bowl.

Isometric exercises within the patient's pain tolerance and pain-free range of motion are initiated for all motions. These exercises are initially performed submaximally, progressing to maximal isometric contractions as tolerated. Mild manual resistive isometrics in all planes may also be started throughout the pain-free range. Active motion and exercise may also be used to effectively increase local circulation and further promote the resorption of any lingering edema.[207,208] Exercises are progressed

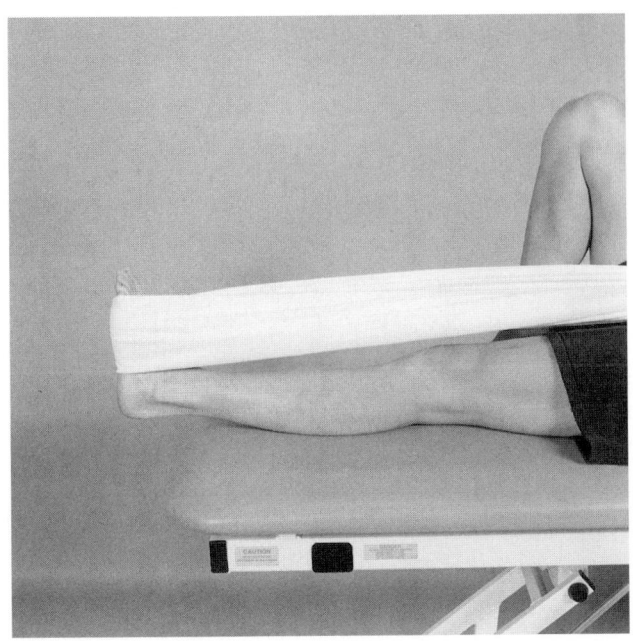

FIGURE 19-47   Towel stretch.

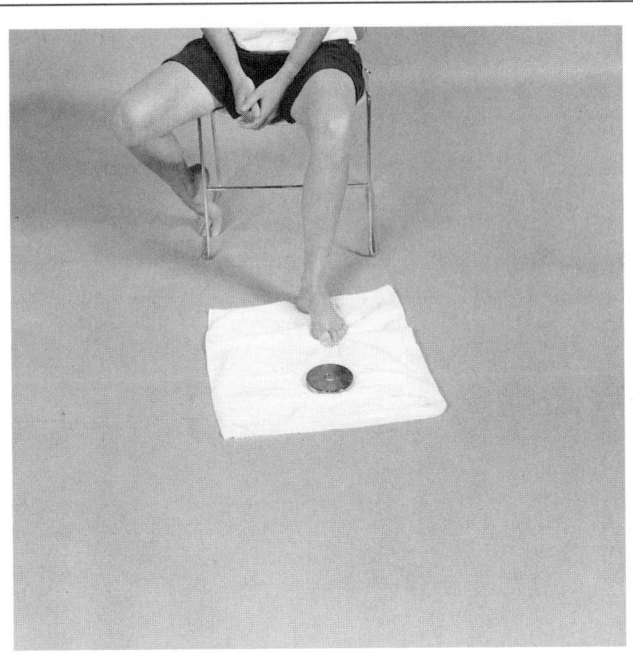

FIGURE 19-49   Towel toe curls.

to include concentric and eccentric exercises (Fig. 19-50 through 19-53) once the isometric exercises are pain-free. Seated lower extremity closed kinetic chain exercises may also be performed during this phase.

Each muscle or muscle group should be strengthened with a specific exercise which isolates the muscle or group. Resistance (rubber tubing/bands, weights, isokinetic devices, body weight exercises, etc) is increased as tolerated. Emphasis should initially

be on low resistance and endurance in all pain-free positions. As the program progresses, the joint range is increased from a stress-free position to a more stressful position. As with all exercises, the patient should become an active participant at the earliest opportunity. The exercises learned in the clinic need to be integrated appropriately into a home exercise regimen.

Pain-free weight bearing as tolerated is encouraged with the use of any appropriate assistive devices such as a cane or

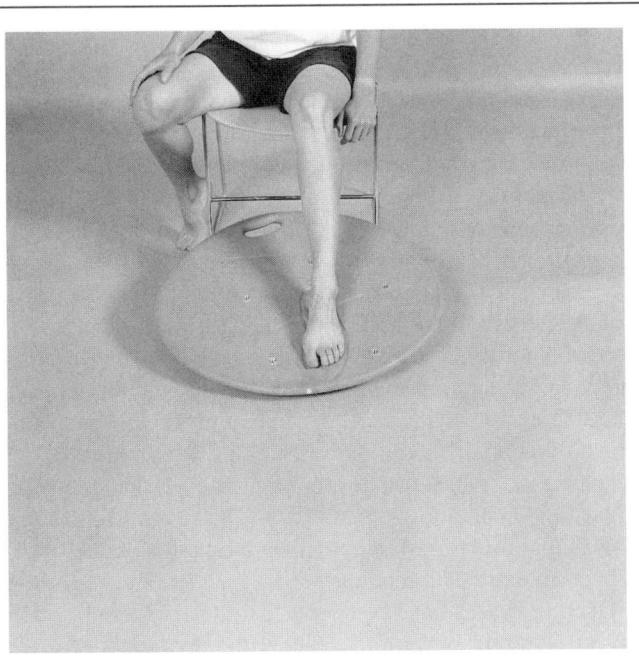

FIGURE 19-48   BAPS exercise.

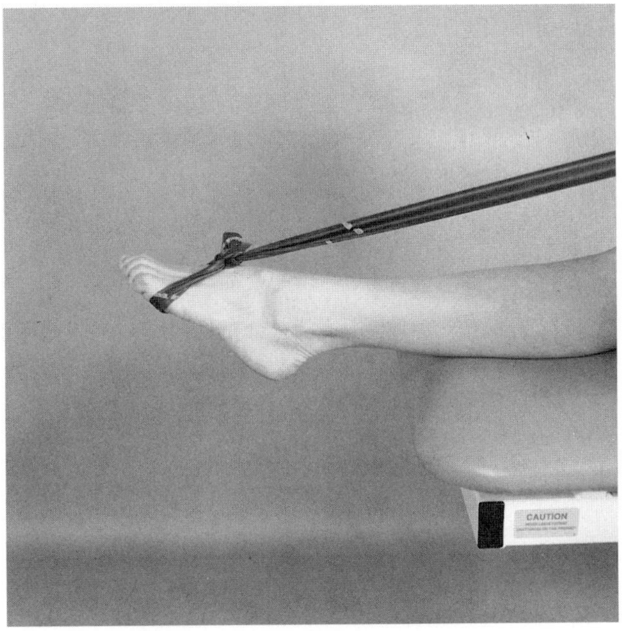

FIGURE 19-50   Resistance exercises into plantarflexion.

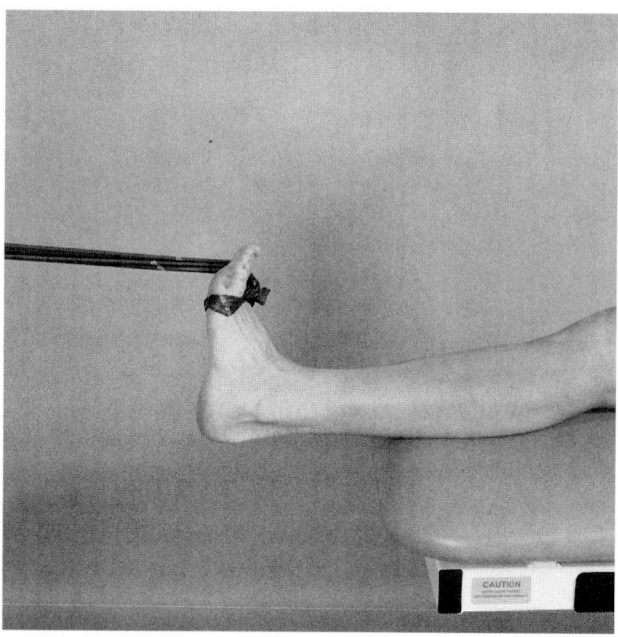

FIGURE 19-51   Resistance exercises into dorsiflexion.

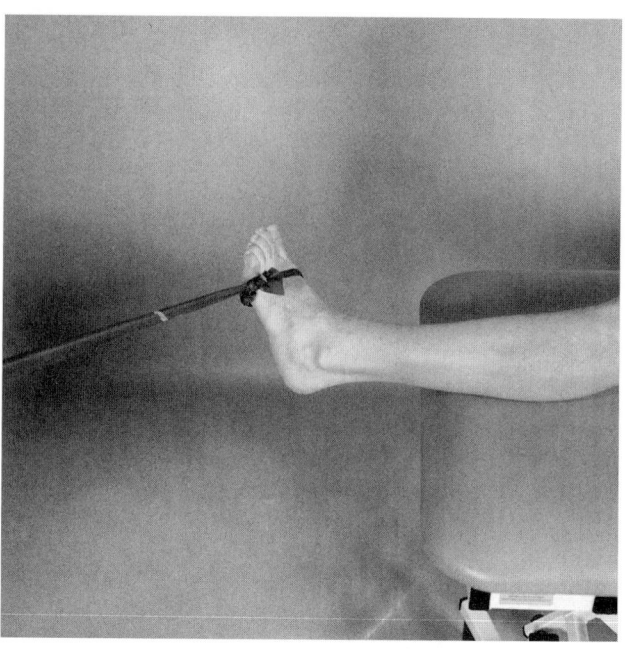

FIGURE 19-53   Resistance exercises into inversion.

crutches. During ambulation, joint protection and positioning are continued as needed using taping techniques, thermoplastic stirrups, or functional walking orthosis.[209,210] The use of crutches or other assistive devices is usually continued until the patient has a pain-free uncompensated gait. While the patient uses crutches, pain-free ankle motion during the normal gait cycle continues to be encouraged. Patients should be encouraged

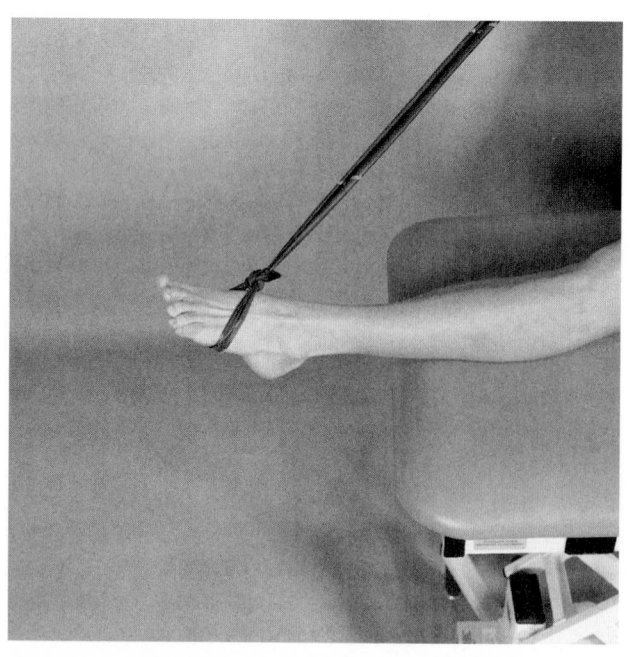

FIGURE 19-52   Resistance exercises into eversion.

to walk with as normal a gait as possible, given the limitations on ankle and knee motion.

The application of ice is continued after therapeutic activities or after prolonged weight bearing to prevent or minimize any recurrence of swelling.

For the patient to progress to the functional phase of the rehabilitation program, pain-free weight bearing and an uncompensated gait pattern must be present. At this time crutches or other assistive devices are discontinued. However, pain may still be felt with activities more vigorous than walking.

Bracing

Braces can play an important role in both the initial intervention and prevention of ankle injuries. Acutely, their role is to compress, protect, and support the ankle. They also function to limit range of motion of the injured ankle, most importantly plantar flexion, which is a precarious position for the sprained ankle.[136]

Functional braces that provide medial-lateral stabilization such as the Air Cast (Air Cast, Inc., Summit, NJ) also provide compressive force that assists in decreasing effusion.[22,133] Patients who suffer a grade III ligament injury may require more protection and support than can be afforded by a thermoplastic device. In cases such as this, consideration should be given to using a functional walking orthosis, either with a fixed ankle or a hinged ankle (which can be motion restricted) that allows only plantar flexion and dorsiflexion.[22,133] The advantage of the orthosis is that it is removable to allow the patient to continue to ice to minimize inflammation.

Overall, braces have been demonstrated to be biomechanically effective in preventing, decreasing, or slowing motions that cause injury to the lateral ankle ligaments.[103,211–214]

Although, one study[212] reported that braces were not as effective as freshly applied tape (see taping), clinically, braces appear to be as effective, if not more effective, than tape in the prevention of lateral ankle sprains.[214–218] The injury rate in one study by Sitler and colleagues[217] reported that the ankle injury rate was more than triple in the nonbraced players compared with braced players during intramural basketball at West Point.

In the presence of instability, the ankle joint is best supported by a commercial brace, with or without taping, depending on the stress of the sport.[22,133]

Night Splinting

Night splinting of the ankle in dorsiflexion has been postulated to prevent nocturnal contracture of the gastrocnemius-soleus complex, which is thought to be detrimental to plantar fascia healing.[244–246] The splint holds the ankle fixed in 5 degrees of dorsiflexion and the toes slightly dorsiflexed stretched (ie, at a functional length).[43] For most patients this orthosis reduces morning pain considerably.[246] Powell and colleagues[245] performed a crossover study using splinting with the ankle in dorsiflexion as the sole method of treatment in 47 patients. This study also showed improvement in 80 percent of involved feet.

Functional Phase

Progression to the functional phase occurs when there is minimal pain and tenderness, full PROM and strength rated at 4/5 to 5/5 with manual muscle testing as compared to the uninvolved side.[197] A recurrence of symptoms should not be provoked. The goals of this phase are:

▶ Restore normal joint kinematics.

▶ Attain full range of pain-free motion.

▶ Improve neuromuscular control of the lower extremity in a full weight-bearing posture on both level and uneven surfaces.

▶ Improve or regain lower extremity strength and endurance through integration of local and kinetic chain exercises.

▶ Return to previous level of function or recreation.

Exercises during this phase include a progression of the manually resisted exercises, and isotonic exercises with tubing or cuff weights in single planes. Closed chain exercises are progressed with a graduated increase in weight bearing. Specific joint mobilization techniques[254] and muscle stretching are initiated to begin to increase range of motion. Emphasis should also be placed on regaining any motion that was lost. Regaining dorsiflexion motion, for example, can be assisted by the use of a tilt board or heel cord stretching box.[201,210]

Proprioceptive exercises are especially important for full functional return and injury prevention.[22,133] Three factors are thought to cause functional instability of the ankle joint:[255]

▶ Anatomic or mechanical instability.

▶ Muscle weakness.

▶ Deficits in joint proprioception.

One of the all-too-common consequences of an ankle injury is an alteration of the motor conduction velocity of the peroneal nerve and the protective function of the peroneal muscles for the ankle joint.[205,256,257] A decrease in peroneal reaction time has been demonstrated to continue for up to 12 weeks after injury,[205,256] despite a nearly full return of strength (96 percent) in comparison with the contralateral side.[256] It has also been demonstrated in normal subjects that there is an increase in the latency response of the peroneal muscles with an increase in plantar flexion, indicating a loss of protective reflexes when in this position.[258] The patient must train and be rehabilitated in all potential positions of injury.[22,133]

Multidirectional, multijoint exercises should be started as early as tolerated. These include ankle proprioceptive neuromuscular facilitation (PNF) exercises, which are progressed within the patient's tolerance.[259]

Balance activities should begin in sitting until the range of motion is full and painless, at which time the exercises are gradually progressed to full weight bearing.[22,133] The greater the severity of injury, the more critical the need for multidirectional balance board activities and weight-bearing rehabilitation activities.[260–267] These activities are effective in progressing the patient toward a progressive return to function. A study by Rozzi and colleagues[164] demonstrated that a 4-week course of single leg balance training showed an improvement in balance ability in both the trained and untrained limbs. Walking or jogging progressions begin on flat surfaces, and ascending and descending stairs forward and backward, progressing to turning, changing directions, and lateral movements while running, and eccentric loading with stair running.[136]

Tests found to correlate well with good recovery are descending stairs, walking on heels and toes, and balancing on a square beam.[136,268] For some patients, the goal may be to return to sport. Progression to this level occurs when there is:[197]

▶ Full pain-free active and passive ROM.

▶ No complaints of pain or tenderness.

▶ 75 to 80 percent strength of the plantar flexors, dorsiflexors, invertors, and evertors compared to the uninvolved side.

▶ Adequate unilateral stance balance (30 seconds with eyes closed).

Before being allowed to return to full competition, the patient should be put through a functional test that simulates all requirements of his or her sport.[22,133] Observational analysis should be made of the patient's quality of movement and whether or not they are favoring the injured extremity in any way.[22,133] Activities during this phase involve cutting drills, shuttle runs, carioca crossover drills and sport-specific activities such as lay-ups and dribbling.[136]

It is important to stress to the patient that full-strength, peroneal latency response time and proprioceptive sense about the ankle may not return for many weeks following return to activity.[205,256,269]

Taping

Historically, ankle taping was the athletic trainer's method of choice to attempt to prevent ankle sprains. Ankle taping is effective in restricting the motion of the ankle and has also been proven to decrease the incidence of ankle sprains.[219–224]

However, although taping initially restricts motion, the tape loses 50 percent of its net support after as little as 10 minutes of exercise.[212,224–232] Because of this deterioration of support, and the cost of tape, removable and reusable ankle braces were designed as an alternative to taping.[22,133]

The use of tape for increased proprioception remains controversial. It is hypothesized that the tape can either provide additional cutaneous cues or may provide a general facilitation at spinal or higher levels, thereby enhancing the perception of movement signals from other proprioceptive sources,[233–236] although this has yet to be proved conclusively.[234,237,238]

The more common instabilities treated with taping include splaying of the mortise, inversion instability of the ankle, plantar instability of the talonavicular joint, and inversion or eversion instability of the talocalcaneal joint.[22,133]

▶ The mortise is taped circumferentially around the lateral and medial malleolus.

▶ Talocalcaneal instabilities are taped around the neck of the talus and the heel. With the exception of the inferior tibiofibular joint (which is a syndesmosis), the taping can effect a temporary improvement in symptoms and function.

The decision whether or not to utilize some type of protective taping or bracing upon the return to activity to prevent reinjury is a decision based upon the individual athlete and his or her case. No type of taping or bracing will prevent all injuries.[22,133]

Clinical Pearl

Often a player may argue that their performance will be adversely affected by the use of taping or bracing.[22,133] A review of the literature demonstrates that for normal athletic movement and function there does not appear to be an adverse impact on function or performance.[215,231,239–243] Indeed, one study involving soccer players demonstrated a fivefold decrease in the incidence of recurrent ankle sprains when using semi-rigid orthoses, without significantly affecting sports performance.[218]

Footwear

The type of sneaker worn during basketball, high top versus low top, has been studied and shown to have no relationship to the incidence of injury.[220] However, it does appear that increased shoe height can enhance the passive resistance to inversion when the foot is in plantar flexion, and can also increase the passive resistance afforded by tape and orthoses.[212]

One of the many contributing factors to running injuries is improper or worn out footwear. On average, running shoes wear out between 300 to 500 miles, although these figures are merely estimates and the actual distance at which a shoe breaks down may vary according to running style, training techniques and environmental conditions, including terrain and weather. Running in a shoe that no longer provides the correct protection in terms of cushioning, traction, and support may lead to heel pain, shin splints, tendonitis, and stress fractures.

Clinical Pearl

In general, a runner with a high medial longitudinal arch and a C-shaped foot, often characterized as a "supinator" tends to underpronate during midstance and should therefore be using a shoe with a softer midfoot and one that is more cushioned, especially on the lateral edge of the shoe.

Similarly, a runner with a low medial longitudinal arch, often characterized as a "pronator", tends to produce an excessive medial roll of the foot during the stance phase and should therefore be using a shoe designed for motion control of the rearfoot and with hard or rigid midsoles made from plastic or high density foam that permit only minimal pronation.[243a]

Orthotics

An orthosis can be defined as any device used to support, align, or protect joints or body segments, thus improving function.[247]

The principal purpose of a foot or ankle orthosis is to:[247]

▶ Evenly distribute the weight-bearing forces on the plantar aspect of the foot.

▶ Reduce stress on anatomic structures local or proximal to the foot and ankle by either force attenuation or control of joint motion.

▶ Prevent, correct, or compensate for the presence of foot or ankle deformities.

A wide variety of materials are available for the fabrication of custom made orthotics, which vary in elasticity, plasticity, compliance, and rigidity.

Despite the widespread use of orthoses, questions are arising as to the theoretical basis for their use for the following reasons:[247]

▶ Any definition of "normal" foot alignment assumes that anything that falls outside the criteria for "normal" must be abnormal, and associated with pathology, yet studies have shown that the criteria we use to describe "normal" apply to very few individuals, and that many asymptomatic individuals display foot abnormalities but meet those criteria.[248–250] If we are to correct a malalignment using an orthotic, we need to determine more definitively the causal relationship between the malalignment and the patient's symptoms.

▶ The determination of subtalar neutral, the measurement that is the cornerstone for the prescription of orthotics, is relatively unreliable. While the intrarater reliability in determining subtalar neutral has been found to be acceptable,[251] the interrater reliability scores have demonstrated that therapists are frequently unable to agree with other therapists in determining subtalar neutral.[248,251]

Heel Lifts

The use of heel lifts is advocated in the literature for a variety of conditions, including Achilles tendonitis and calcaneal apophysitis.[48]

The material used to make the heel lift can be modified to increase shock absorption in cases of calcaneal bruising and heel spurs.[252]

Heel Cups

Heel cups are used for similar conditions as heel lifts, with the added benefit that the heel cup is able to help redistribute the forces through the heel better, and because the medial and lateral walls contain the fat pads of the calcaneus, thus improving the natural shock absorptive ability.[44,247,253]

Wedges

Prefabricated or custom-made wedges are referred to as a "post" when used in functional foot orthoses. Wedges are typically used to slant the entire foot or part of the foot either medially or laterally, to prevent motion or change the weight-bearing aspect of the foot.

Preferred Practice Pattern 4B: Impaired Joint Mobility, Motor Function, Muscle Performance, Range of Motion Associated with Impaired Posture

Clinical findings with this pattern can include pain with sustained positions, structural deformities and deviations, limited range of motion in a noncapsular pattern of restriction, and altered kinematics.

The Pronated Foot

In the normal foot, the angle of the rearfoot and forefoot intersect at 90 degrees with a downward projection of the center of mass at 135 degrees, such that all of the forces counteract one another, resulting in zero net force and zero rotational velocity.[269a] Any changes in this anatomical relationship can affect the static equilibrium. Pronation of the foot creates an angle greater than 90 degrees between the rearfoot and forefoot. Static equilibrium can only now be maintained through a counteracting force such as the passive stretch of the passive plantar mechanism. Pronation of the foot and ankle during the stance phase of gait is essentially a temporary collapse of the ankle, rearfoot, and midfoot. This natural collapse provides a more adaptable structure that allows for shock absorption, and ground terrain changes and helps to prevent excessive strain on the joints or ligaments.[93] Some pronation of the foot is necessary during functional activities. However, excessive pronation has been linked to lower limb overuse injuries as maintenance of the equilibrium becomes the function of the muscles, specifically the peroneus brevis and the posterior tibialis.[48,270–273] Excessive pronation can occur as the result of a number of different factors. These include:[152]

▶ Congenital, including tarsal coalitions, metatarsus varus, and convex pes valgus.[4,51,274]

▶ Developmental, including talipes calcaneovalgus, talipes calcaneovarus, ligament laxity, and/or a tight Achilles tendon and forefoot varus.[4,51,274,275]

▶ Equinus at the ankle, resulting in increased dorsiflexion of the forefoot at the rearfoot around the oblique midtarsal joint axis.

▶ Subtalar varus.

▶ A plantarflexed lateral column, which results in pronation due to the fact that the fourth and fifth metatarsals are lower than the adjacent third metatarsal, which produces a pronatory force with weight bearing.

▶ Rearfoot varus associated with excessive forefoot pronation and delayed re-supination.

The patient with a symptomatic pronated foot typically complains of pain along the medial longitudinal arch. Occasionally there is pain laterally beneath the tip of the fibula secondary to impingement of the calcaneus against the fibula. The pain is usually aggravated with prolonged standing and walking, and relieved with rest.[276] Often these patients become symptomatic when they suddenly increase their level of activity.

The examination often reveals a flattening of the longitudinal arch associated with a valgus deformity of the heel, a medial bulge at the talonavicular joint, a low medial longitudinal arch, and abduction of the forefoot on the rearfoot at the transverse tarsal joint.[276,277]

Two terms can be used to describe the pronated foot: weak and hypermobile. Both the weak and hypermobile flatfoot can cause symptoms in everyday weight-bearing activities due to postural fatigue.

The Weak Foot. The weak foot produces moderate pronation. Severe pronation with flattening of the foot is associated with congenital or ligamentous laxity, and is deemed to be occurring if the foot is pronating beyond 25 percent of the stance phase.[4,120,152,278] Acquired flatfoot deformity is a symptomatic and progressive flatfoot deformity resulting from loss of function of the tibialis posterior muscle/tendon and/or the loss of integrity of the ligamentous structures supporting the joints of the arch and rearfoot. The weak foot is characterized by a general increase in the range of motion at the subtalar and midtarsal joints, with the heel positioned in valgus, and the medial arch is dropped. In addition, the forefoot is externally positioned on the rearfoot, and the foot is usually toed out.[152]

The Hypermobile Foot. Occasionally, a foot that appears normal in non–weight bearing (static examination), can excessively pronate during running (dynamic examination). Consequently, it is usual for this type of foot to only give symptoms with running, which emphasizes the importance of performing both a static and dynamic examination of the foot.

Hypermobility at the foot and ankle can lead to increased stress on the bone and soft tissues, especially the ligaments, and an overreliance on muscular support.[89]

The intervention for an abnormally and symptomatic pronated foot depends on the type, but typically involves:

▶ *Alleviation of the abnormal tissue stress.*

▶ *Stretching of the gastrocnemius-soleus complex.*

▶ *Activity and shoe modification.* Shoes that have rearfoot control, a high lacing pattern, and a straighter last may be enough to control excessive motion, particularly if it is not severe.[89,279] A straighter last is more desirable for a person with excessive pronation.

▶ *Taping.* Taping or arch strapping can be used to limit excessive pronation.[280,281]

▶ *Orthotics.*

The Flat Foot

A patient with little or no longitudinal arch with full weight bearing is said to have a flatfoot or pes planus. Flatfeet and a minimal longitudinal arch are standard in infants and common in children up to the age of 6.[282]

A flatfoot is said to be flexible if the arch can be recreated with the patient standing up on their toes. Flexible pes planus has been reported to occur in 15 percent of the general population,[283] with the majority being asymptomatic.[284] If a flatfoot is painful, other causes must be sought out, such as tarsal coalition, vertical talus, or accessory navicular.[65]

A rigid flatfoot, a relatively rare condition, positions the calcaneus in a valgus position and the midtarsal region in pronation, resulting in a displaced navicular (dorsally), and a talus that faces medially and inferiorly.

Extrinsic congenital deformities can cause abnormal pronation. These include hip dysplasia, femoral antitorsion, tibial torsions, and genu varum or valgus. These deformities produce a rotation of the lower limb, which can have the following consequences:

▶ *Excessive external rotation of the lower limb.* This may shift the center of gravity in weight bearing to the medial aspect of the foot. Ideally, the center of gravity during weight bearing should pass through the center of the foot. This increase in medial stress causes the talus to plantar flex and adduct while the calcaneus tilts laterally (into valgus).

▶ *Excessive internal rotation of the lower limb.* This produces excessive weight bearing on the lateral aspect of the foot. In an attempt to shift the center of gravity more medially, the forefoot abducts on the rearfoot, or the foot abducts on the leg. These compensations produce excessive pronation of the subtalar joint.

The Stiff Foot

Normal supination is designed to allow the foot to function as a rigid lever during push-off, torque conversion, and a lengthening mechanism of the leg.[93] An abnormally supinated foot is described as a stiff foot. The stiff foot is characterized by a high arch, increased external rotation of the tibia, increased forefoot varus, and an inability to pronate during the stance phase. Without the normal amount of pronation needed to allow the dissipation of stresses, the foot loses its ability to absorb shock.

There are three classifications of abnormal supination:[4,152]

▶ *Pes cavus.* This type is characterized by a fixed plantar flexed forefoot, or an equinus forefoot, which places the rearfoot in neutral during weight bearing.[275] The high longitudinal arch of the cavus foot results in limited weight bearing on the plantar aspect of the foot. This produces increased pressure on the heel and on the metatarsal heads.[276] The physical examination reveals a varus configuration of the heel, a marked elevation of the longitudinal arch, no medial bulge at the talonavicular joint, an adducted forefoot relative to the rearfoot, and external rotation of the leg.[276,277]

▶ *Pes cavovarus.* This type is characterized by a fixed plantar flexed medial column or first ray. This places the calcaneus in varus or inversion during weight bearing, so that the foot lands on its lateral border.[275]

▶ *Pes equinovarus.* This foot type demonstrates a fixed plantar flexed forefoot and rearfoot, with no compensation occurring with weight bearing.

The intervention for a symptomatic cavus foot is supportive, and involves having the patient wear a soft shoe with adequate padding to provide more midsole cushion for the plantar aspect of the foot.[276] Total-contact foot orthoses increase the weight-bearing surface of the foot and are recommended with this foot type.[285]

Specific Joint Deformities and Deviations
Talocrural Joint

Talipes Equinus. The lack of a minimum of 10 degrees of dorsiflexion at the talocrural joint is termed talipes equinus.[10] A common cause for a lack of dorsiflexion at the ankle is adaptive shortening of the gastrocnemius and soleus muscle groups. Other causes include trauma, spasticity structural bone deformities, and inflammatory disease. This dysfunction often results in excessive forces being transferred to the forefoot, and increased pronation at the subtalar joint.[151]

Common problems associated with this foot type include medial arch pain, posterior leg pain, plantar fasciitis, metatarsalgia, lateral ankle sprain, and talonavicular pain.[89]

Subtalar Joint

Rearfoot Varus. This is the most common structural foot deformity and is the most common abnormality of the subtalar joint. The most important component of a rearfoot varus is a calcaneal varus (subtalar varus). A calcaneus varus is characterized by an inverted position of the calcaneus when in the subtalar joint neutral position. This may result in limited eversion and pronation of the subtalar joint when the foot is in contact with the ground. The combination of calcaneal varus and any medial inclination of the tibia produces a total rearfoot varus. A 2- to 3-degree rearfoot varus is common, and generally presents no problems.[286]

The practical significance of a rearfoot varus is that at heel strike, the calcaneus is inverted more than normal and the medial condyle of the calcaneus is farther from the ground, resulting in an increase in lateral heel contact. To bring the medial side of the foot to the ground, the calcaneus must evert. Eversion of the calcaneus is produced by the subtalar joint pronation.

Thus a rearfoot varus forces the subtalar joint to go through an excessive amount of pronation. In addition, the pronation occurs too rapidly. Rapid pronation from this varus contact position can result in retrocalcaneal exostosis.[286]

Partial compensation occurs if the subtalar joint pronates abnormally, but does not have enough available pronation ROM to bring the medial condyle of the calcaneus to the ground.[127] In response to a rearfoot varus, a callus will often form under the second metatarsal head, and to a lesser degree under the third and fourth metatarsal heads.[127] The callus does not occur under the first metatarsal head because the stability of the latter depends on the peroneus longus muscle.

If no compensation occurs at the subtalar joint, the midtarsal may compensate with increased mobility and medial longitudinal arch collapse.[93]

When the rearfoot varus is large, the metatarsal joint and the forefoot may be excessively mobile when the heel rises from the ground during propulsion. In addition, the foot may not become rigid until after the heel rises, instead of just before heel rise.

Other tissue disorders that can result from rearfoot varus include plantar fasciitis, metatarsalgia, or stress factors of the second ray and hallux valgus. The proximal effects of subtalar joint compensation for a rearfoot varus are substantial. The excessive and rapid pronation that occurs during the contact phase of gait, puts a tremendous stress on the primary muscle that decelerates subtalar joint pronation, the tibialis posterior muscle, producing symptoms of overuse in this muscle.[127]

In addition to the extreme stress placed upon the tibialis posterior muscle, abnormal subtalar joint pronation may produce an excessive internal rotation of the lower leg.[127] Normally the tibia rotates an average of 19 degrees during ambulation.[27] At the beginning of the stance phase, the tibia internally rotates as the talus plantar flexes and adducts. At the end of the stance phase, the tibia must externally rotate, pushing the talus into dorsiflexion and abduction. Any extra rotation must be absorbed in the knee, hip, or sacroiliac joint, or between the vertebral segments.

The abnormal subtalar joint pronation also increases the valgus stress on the knee, and symptoms of a mild strain of the medial collateral ligament can arise.[127]

Rearfoot varus commonly occurs with tibia vara or pes cavus.[89]

Rearfoot Valgus. Rearfoot valgus involves eversion of the calcaneus when the subtalar joint is in its neutral position. This structural deformity is often associated with genu valgum, or with tibia valgus, and can lead to excessive pronation and limited supination.

Midtarsal Joint

Forefoot Varus. Forefoot varus is defined as inversion of the forefoot on the rearfoot, when the subtalar joint is held in neutral.[10] Some forefoot varus is normal, and in asymptomatic individuals, there is usually about 7 degrees of forefoot varus.[287]

This sagittal plane osseous deformity of the forefoot/first ray,[288] with increased stress applied to the medial plantar aspect of the foot, is considered to be the single most common intrinsic cause of mechanical pain and dysfunction within the foot, lower one-third of the leg, and knee (Table 19-10).[275]

Because the medial side of the foot is higher than the lateral side, the forefoot assumes an inverted or varus position. To assist the medial side of the forefoot in reaching the ground, the subtalar joint may excessively pronate as the midstance phase begins. This compensation places the midtarsal joint in its maximally mobile position, at the time when it should be in a stable supinated position (just before and during propulsion). The compensation can create:

▶ Extreme stresses on the peroneus longus and the forefoot.

▶ Dorsiflexion and subsequent hypermobility of the first ray.[127,153]

▶ Plantar fasciitis.[127]

▶ Hallux valgus, bunion deformity, and a subluxation of the first MTP joint.[275]

TABLE 19-10 Effects of a Forefoot Varus

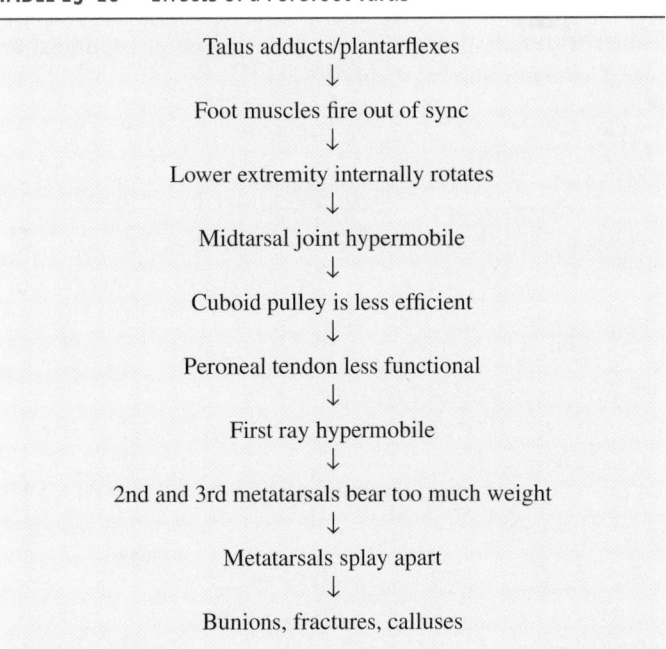

Talus adducts/plantarflexes
↓
Foot muscles fire out of sync
↓
Lower extremity internally rotates
↓
Midtarsal joint hypermobile
↓
Cuboid pulley is less efficient
↓
Peroneal tendon less functional
↓
First ray hypermobile
↓
2nd and 3rd metatarsals bear too much weight
↓
Metatarsals splay apart
↓
Bunions, fractures, calluses

From Hunter S, Prentice WE. Rehabilitation of the ankle and foot. In: Prentice WE, Voight MI, eds. *Techniques in Musculoskeletal Rehabilitation.* New York: McGraw-Hill; 2001:603–641.

Because the first ray complex cannot effectively contribute to propulsion, the second metatarsal head will experience excessive loading, with the potential for callus formation under the second metatarsal head, or metatarsalgia or stress fracture of the second metatarsal.[127,289]

In addition, the forefoot-to-rearfoot alignment in the frontal plane is abnormal, which predisposes the fifth toe to pressure from the shoe, which can result in a fifth-digit hammer toe.[152]

Terminal knee extension during the midstance phase requires the tibia to externally rotate on the femur. If the knee joint compensates by having the femur rotate medially with the tibia, the problem is transferred to a more proximal structure, mainly the hip joint, piriformis muscle, or the sacroiliac joint, increasing stress to both contractile and noncontractile tissues.[127]

Forefoot Valgus. This dysfunction occurs when the plane of the metatarsal head is in an everted, or valgus, position. Two structural types of forefoot valgus deformities exist.

▶ All of the metatarsal heads may be everted.

▶ The first metatarsal head may be plantar flexed, while the second to fifth metatarsal heads lie in the appropriate plane (pes cavovarus).

If the first ray is plantar flexed, compensation may occur at the subtalar joint in the form of rapid supination of the subtalar joint. This shifts the weight laterally to the fifth metatarsal head.[10,275] If no subtalar joint compensation occurs in response to a forefoot valgus, the body weight is borne on the medial side of the forefoot.[127] To bring the lateral side of the foot to the ground, compensatory supination at the subtalar joint is required.[127] This supination occurs at a rate that is much sooner than in a normal foot.[152] One of the distal effects of the abnormally supinated foot is that the midtarsal joint is unable to adapt to uneven surfaces, which leads to an increased susceptibility to lateral inversion sprains (Table 19-11).[127]

TABLE 19-11 Effects of a Forefoot Valgus

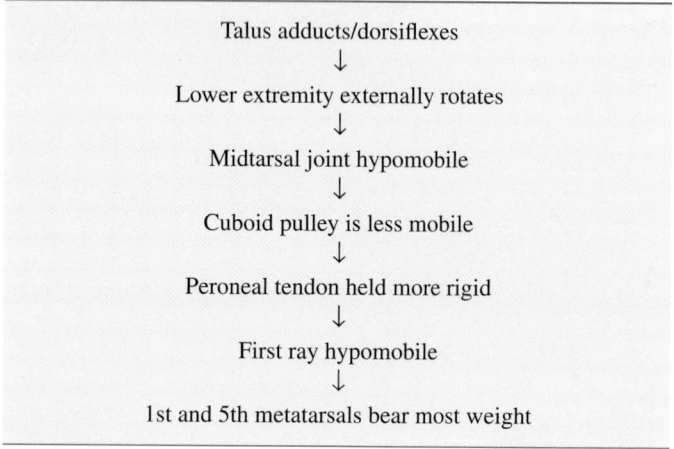

Talus adducts/dorsiflexes
↓
Lower extremity externally rotates
↓
Midtarsal joint hypomobile
↓
Cuboid pulley is less mobile
↓
Peroneal tendon held more rigid
↓
First ray hypomobile
↓
1st and 5th metatarsals bear most weight

From Hunter S, Prentice WE. Rehabilitation of the ankle and foot. In: Prentice WE, Voight MI, eds. *Techniques in Musculoskeletal Rehabilitation.* New York: McGraw-Hill; 2001:603–641.

In addition, the shock-absorbing ability of the knee is also compromised, as the necessary internal rotation of the lower leg required for flexion is delayed. This may play a role in the development of problems around the lateral aspect of the knee, or patellofemoral joint.[126,153] The increased forces may also travel up the lower extremity and contribute to the development of sacral and low back dysfunction.

Forefoot Equinus. This is also a forefoot deformity, but it occurs in the sagittal plane. The metatarsal heads, although possibly perpendicular to the calcaneal bisection, are not level with the plantar condyles of the calcaneus. This results in a relative plantar flexion of the forefoot structures when compared to the rearfoot. The functional effect of this deformity is that the ankle joint must move through a greater excursion of dorsiflexion to allow the body to move forward over the foot during the midstance phase.[127]

The subtalar joint itself is unable to compensate directly for a forefoot equinus because it has very little dorsiflexion. Thus the midtarsal joint usually becomes the source of the dorsiflexion. If the midtarsal joint is to provide the necessary dorsiflexion, the subtalar joint must be pronated. However, the time when maximum subtalar pronation is needed by the midtarsal joint (at heel rise) coincides with the time when the subtalar joint should be in a supinated position for propulsion.[127]

More proximally, if the foot and ankle are not able to provide the necessary dorsiflexion, the motion in the sagittal plane may be achieved at the knee joint. This may result in a hyperextension force at the knee as the body progresses forward over the foot and the tibia.

Combined Rearfoot and Forefoot Deformities. Combinations of deformities frequently occur together.

▶ A rearfoot varus can occur with either a forefoot varus or a forefoot valgus.[127] In a foot that exhibits a rearfoot and a forefoot varus, the compensatory subtalar joint pronation is accentuated throughout the contact, midstance, and propulsion phases of the gait cycle.[127]

▶ A rearfoot varus may be combined with a flexible forefoot valgus.[127] Clinically this foot type demonstrates a significant amount of pronation during stance. As the subtalar joint begins to pronate, the midtarsal joint mobility increases and the forefoot valgus becomes flexible.[127] The foot is abnormally pronated, but the abnormal pronation occurs at the midtarsal joint as well as at the subtalar joint.

▶ A rigid forefoot valgus can occur with a rearfoot varus.[127] This combination creates extreme bone stress in the middle of the foot, particularly the tarsal bones. Degenerative joint changes and tarsal stress fractures are potential problems, as are lateral ankle sprains and the more proximal problems that occur with a forefoot valgus.[127]

Congenital Variations of the Foot

Club Foot. The term *club foot* encompasses a wide range of deformities, most of which involve the heel to some degree. The most common clubfoot deformity is talipes equinovarus. Two categories exist: a flexible form and a resistant form. The former is amenable to conservative intervention with orthotics and footwear modification. The latter type is invariably associated with stiffness and requires surgical intervention.

Convex Pes Valgus. This deformity is also known as "rocker bottom" foot. It is characterized by a primary dorsal and lateral dislocation of the talocalcaneonavicular joint. This results in the navicular articulating with the dorsal aspect of the talus, locking it in the vertical position, and preventing normal dorsiflexion of the rearfoot.[275,290] The compensation for this loss of rearfoot dorsiflexion is dorsiflexion at the midfoot.[93]

Metatarsal Deformities. Four metatarsal deformities are commonly recognized:[288]

▶ *Metatarsus adductus.* This is a transverse plane deformity with adduction of all of the five metatarsals, which occurs at the tarsometatarsal joint.

▶ *Metatarsus varus.* This deformity is characterized by a medial subluxation of the tarsometatarsal joints with an adduction and inversion deformity of the metatarsals. This results in an inability of the forefoot to be passively abducted to the neutral position.[275]

▶ *Metatarsus adductovarus.* This is a combined transverse and frontal plane deformity of forefoot adduction and inversion that occurs at the tarsometatarsal joint.

▶ *Forefoot adductus.* This is a combined transverse and frontal plane deformity of forefoot adduction and inversion that occurs at the midtarsal joint.

Preferred Practice Pattern 4D: Impaired Joint Mobility, Motor Function, Muscle Performance, Range of Motion Associated with Connective Tissue Dysfunction

Seronegative Spondyloarthropathies

Ankylosing spondylitis (AS), psoriatic arthritis, and Reiter's syndrome are all capable of producing foot and ankle pain. Although AS predominantly affects the axial skeleton, it can also affect the MTP joints.[276]

Psoriatic arthritis usually occurs with accompanying skin lesions. However, in 10 to 15 percent of cases, no dermatologic problems exist.[276] The condition is characterized by symmetrical involvement of the hands and feet, most often at the level of the distal IP joints.[276]

Reiter's syndrome consists of a triad of conjunctivitis, urethritis, and asymmetric arthritis. This condition usually affects the knees, feet, and ankles.[276]

Traumatic Arthritis

Arthritis in the MTP joint, talocrural joint, subtalar joint, and the midfoot, is more frequently associated with repeated inversion sprain. The arthritis results in pain, swelling, and a limitation of motion in a capsular pattern. Traumatic arthritis in this region is difficult to treat conservatively, although the fitting of a heel lift in the patient's shoe allows the patient to ambulate with reduced dorsiflexion at the ankle, and can offer some short-term relief.

Hallux Rigidus

Hallux rigidus is characterized by decreased dorsiflexion of the first MTP joint, and pain and swelling in the dorsal aspect of the joint.[56] Two types of hallux rigidus have been described: adolescent and adult.

▶ *Adolescent.* The adolescent type is consistent with an osteochondritis dissecans or localized articular disorder.

▶ *Adult.* The adult type is a more generalized degenerative arthritis.[55] The cause of this degenerative process is unknown. Possible etiologies include crystal-induced arthropathy (gout, pseudogout), rheumatoid arthritis, the seronegative spondyloarthropathies, post-traumatic degeneration, an intra-articular fracture, or an osteochondrotic lesion of the first metatarsal head.[55,291] Repetitive dorsiflexion of the first MTP joint could also potentially lead to the development of hallux rigidus, although no studies have linked levels of physical activity to the development of hallux rigidus.[291]

The characteristics of both types include stiffness and pain in the MTP joint. This is associated with difficulty during the gait cycle, especially when walking or running up hills, climbing stairs, or during the toe-off phase of gait.[55] Because approximately 75 degrees of hallux dorsiflexion is needed for normal gait, limited extension of the great toe will give the feeling of vaulting over the toe. This may necessitate external rotation of the foot to allow for toe clearance. Thus patients may present with lateral stress transfer as they attempt to unload the hallux MTP joint. This may produce synovitis of the lesser MTP joints or even stress fractures of the lesser metatarsals.[55]

The dorsal metatarsal head osteophyte, or dorsal bunion, may rub against footwear, causing an abrasion or ulceration. The patient may also experience tingling and numbness on the dorsum of the toe due to compression of the cutaneous nerves.

Tenderness is usually present on palpation of the dorsal, and especially lateral, aspects of the joint. Radiographs demonstrate loss of first MTP joint space, the formation of dorsal and lateral osteophytes on the metatarsal head, and occasionally loose fragments about the joint.[169]

The initial intervention involves shoe modifications, rest, and nonsteroidal anti-inflammatory drugs. A shoe with an extra-depth toe box can be helpful to decrease dorsal pressure on the first MTP joint, while a stiff-soled shoe or a rigid custom orthotic with a Morton's extension can be helpful in limiting toe dorsiflexion. A rocker-bottom sole can also help to decrease the extension of the hallux during normal gait. An intra-articular corticosteroid injection may be considered as a temporizing measure. If symptoms increase, or when conservative measures fail, surgical intervention may provide the solution.

The most common procedure recommended is the cheilectomy, which is an excision of the dorsal 25 to 33 percent of the metatarsal head. This removes the offending osteophytes, improves toe dorsiflexion, and preserves the good articular cartilage on the middle and plantar aspects of the metatarsal head.[292] A dorsiflexion osteotomy of the proximal phalanx (Moberg procedure) may be used concurrently with a cheilectomy in selected patients to increase functional toe dorsiflexion.[293]

Tarsal Coalition

Tarsal coalition is a fibrous, cartilaginous, or bony connection of two or more bones in the midfoot or hindfoot.[65,294] It usually presents during adolescence, at an average age of 13 years,[295] when the coalition is ossifying and subtalar motion becomes more limited. Most tarsal coalitions are bilateral,[294,296] and have been reported to occur in less than 1 percent of the general population.[294] Calcaneonavicular and talocalcaneal are the most common coalitions seen.[65,294,295,297,298]

A partial or complete talocalcaneal coalition significantly alters the mechanics of the ankle joint complex, as compensatory motion occurs at the ankle joint level.[299]

The patient with a tarsal coalition typically presents with pain that is vague and has an insidious onset. They may present with a history of frequent "ankle sprains" or generalized hindfoot or midfoot pain.[295] Symptoms often begin or are exacerbated by athletic training.

The physical examination will show limited or no subtalar motion compared with the other foot and occasional tight peroneal muscles.[300] Spastic peroneals have been reported to occur in less than 1 percent of these patients.[298]

The diagnosis of such malformations is often very difficult. Plain radiographs should include AP, lateral, and oblique views of the foot.[65,294]

The goal of conservative treatment of tarsal coalition is to reduce stress in the foot, relax the peroneal muscles, and support the foot. This can usually be accomplished with orthotics and exercise, although temporary casting may be necessary.[65,294] If conservative treatment fails, however, a resection may be necessary in order to restore mobility and decrease pain.[294,295]

Hallux Valgus

Hallux valgus is the term used to describe a deformity of the first MTP joint in which the proximal phalanx is deviated laterally with respect to the first metatarsal. The term has been expanded to include varying degrees of metatarsus primus varus/valgus deviation of the proximal phalanx, medial deviation of the first metatarsal head, and bunion formation.

Hallux valgus has been observed to occur almost exclusively in populations that wear shoes, although some predisposing anatomic factors make some feet more vulnerable than others to the effects of extrinsic factors. Women have been observed to have hallux valgus at a rate of 9:1 compared with men.[301] Hallux valgus has also been reported to affect 22 to 36 percent of adolescents.[302–307]

The deformity results from a lateral subluxation of the flexor hallucis longus (FHL) muscle, which transforms the FHL

and brevis from flexors to adductors, which pull the PIP medially and the DIP laterally.[169] In addition, the abductor hallucis muscle slides underneath the metatarsal head and brings about pronation of the great toe, approaching 70 to 90 percent of pronation in severe cases.[308]

With increasing lateral deviation of the hallux, the MTP joint becomes incongruent, the sesamoids subluxate laterally, the hallux pronates, the medial aspect of the first metatarsal head becomes more prominent, and weight bearing shifts from the first metatarsal head to the second metatarsal, and possibly the third.[56,145] This weight transfer may result in the formation of a painful plantar keratosis, or a hammer toe or crossover toe deformity of the second toe.[56]

The cause of hallux valgus is unclear, but various factors are cited such as tight shoes, metatarsus primus varus, pes planus, forefoot pronation, joint hyperlaxity, and heredity.[302,303] Hallux valgus is often associated with medial deviation of the first metatarsal, known as metatarsus primus varus.[56]

A compensated bunion is a mild deformity without MTP joint subluxation and without marked lateral sesamoid subluxation.[309] A decompensated bunion is a moderate to severe deformity characterized by hallux valgus angle greater than 25 degrees, intermetatarsal angle greater than 15 degrees, lateral sesamoid subluxation, and great toe pronation.[309]

The intervention for hallux valgus should be conservative if possible. The intervention for the bunion includes wider shoes and orthotics.[302,303,305] Achilles stretching should be used in cases of Achilles contracture. A simple toe spacer can be used between the first and second toes, and a silicone bunion pad placed over the bunion may be helpful in alleviating direct pressure on the prominence.[56] In cases of pes planus associated with hallux valgus, a medial longitudinal arch support with Morton's extension under the first MTP joint may also alleviate symptoms.[56]

If pain persists, however, structural realignment of the first metatarsal varus is usually necessary, as the bunion deformity becomes more severe and decompensated.

Turf Toe

The term "turf toe" refers to a sprain of the first MTP joint.[56,64] Turf toe primarily affects football, baseball, and soccer players. Football players are at higher risk for this injury if they are tackled while landing from a jump or if another player lands on the back of their heel forcing the first MTP joint into hyperdorsiflexion.[60] Soccer players tend to develop the problem in the nonkicking foot due to the forced dorsiflexion during kicking. It was originally thought that the artificial grass surface on football fields caused athletes to stop more quickly during planting and cutting, thus slamming the toe into the front of the shoe. However, it is more likely that the lighter flexible turf shoes that are designed for the surface are more responsible. This increase in shoe flexibility causes a repetitive hyperextension injury of the great toe. The tendency of artificial turf to become hard and stiff over time may be a contributing factor.[310] The mechanism of injury can also involve hyperflexion, and varus and valgus stresses of the first MTP joint.[11,311] With forced hyperflexion of the hallux, tearing of the plantar plate and collateral ligaments can occur. In the more severe injury, the capsule can actually tear off of the metatarsal head.[64] A fracture of the sesamoids can also occur, and dorsal dislocation of the first MTP joint is possible.[56]

Clinically, patients with turf toe present with a red, swollen, stiff first MTP joint. They may have a history of a single dorsiflexion injury or multiple injuries to the great toe. The joint may be tender both plantarly and dorsally. Players may have a limp and be unable to run or jump because of pain.

Turf toe typically develops into a chronic injury, and long-term results include decreased first MTP joint motion, impaired push-off, and hallux rigidus.[311] Fifty percent of athletes will have persistent symptoms 5 years later.[311a]

Clanton and Ford[53] have classified the severity of turf toe injuries from grades I to III:

▶ A grade I sprain is a minor stretch injury to the soft tissue restraints with little pain, swelling, or disability.

▶ A grade II sprain is a partial tear of the capsuloligamentous structures with moderate pain, swelling, ecchymosis, and disability.

▶ A grade III sprain is a complete tear of the plantar plate with severe swelling, pain, ecchymosis, and inability to bear weight normally. Radiographs of the foot should be obtained to rule out fracture of the sesamoids or metatarsal head articular surface and to check joint congruity.

The initial intervention for turf toe is rest, ice, a compressive dressing, and elevation. A nonsteroidal anti-inflammatory medication is often recommended. The toe should be taped to limit dorsiflexion with multiple loops of tape placed over the dorsal aspect of the hallucal proximal phalanx and criss-crossed under the ball of the foot plantarly,[60] or a forefoot steel plate can be used.[64] Passive range-of-motion and progressive resistance exercises are begun as soon as symptoms allow.[60,169] Patients with grade I sprains are usually allowed to return to sports as soon as symptoms allow, sometimes immediately. Patients with grade II sprains usually require 3 to 14 days rest from athletic training. Grade III sprains usually require crutches for a few days and up to 6 weeks rest from sports participation. A return to sports training too early after injury could result in prolonged disability. Return to play is indicated when the toe can be dorsiflexed 90 degrees.[53]

Sprains

A sprain of a ligament is defined as an injury that stretches the fibers of the ligament. Ankle sprains are the most common injuries in sports and recreational activities,[312] and they remain a difficult diagnostic and therapeutic challenge. If left untreated, ankle sprains can lead to chronic instability and impairment.[136]

Ankle ligament injuries constitute 4.7 to 24.4 percent of all injuries incurred in an individual sport,[313] and 10 to 28 percent of all injuries that occur in running and jumping sports.[314,315] Most acute ankle injuries occur in people 21 to 30 years old, although injuries in the younger and older age groups tend to be more serious.[316] Greater than 40 percent of ankle sprains can potentially progress to chronic problems.[178,194,317-325]

Dynamic stability is provided to the lateral ankle by the strength of the peroneus longus and brevis tendons.

Stormont and colleagues[14] recently showed that ankle instability, and thus sprains, could only occur during systematic loading and unloading, but not while the ankle is fully loaded, due to the articular restraints. In the neutral position or dorsiflexion, the ankle is stable because the widest part of the talus is in the mortise. However, in plantar flexion, ankle stability is decreased as the narrow posterior portion of the talus is in the mortise.[136] Thus the most common mechanism of an ankle sprain is one of inversion and plantar flexion.[22,64] With eversion and external rotation, the deltoid and/or ligaments of the distal tibiofibular joint can be injured, producing the so-called medial and central sprains, respectively. Eversion injuries to the deltoid ligaments account for 5 percent of ankle sprains.[16,138,326]

The prognosis for ankle sprains is inversely proportional to the severity and grade of the injury (Table 19-12),[327] the age of the patient, and the recurrence rate.[22,133] The prognosis for ankle injuries is worse when the ankle has been previously sprained.[319] The prognosis is also diminished when sprains occur in younger patients,[319] presumably relating to a greater mechanistic energy of injury.[22,133]

TABLE 19-12 The West Point Ankle Sprain Grading System[327]

Criterion	Grade I	Grade II	Grade III
Location of tenderness	ATFL	ATFL, CFL	ATFL, CFL, PTFL
Edema, ecchymosis	Slight, local	Moderate, local	Significant, diffuse
Weight-bearing ability	Full or partial	Difficult without crutches	Impossible without significant pain
Ligament damage	Stretched	Partial tear	Complete tear
Instability	None	None or slight	Definite

ATFL, anterior talofibular ligament; CFL, calcaneofibular ligament; PTFL, posterior talofibular ligament.

Lateral Ankle (Inversion) Sprain. Sprains of the lateral ligamentous complex represent 85 percent of ankle ligament sprains.[202,312] In the younger population, serious ankle sprains are unusual in the skeletally immature because the ligaments are usually stronger than the bone,[296,328,329] necessitating a physeal fracture to be ruled out.[22,64]

The ATFL, which is the least elastic of the lateral ligaments,[154] is involved in 60 to 70 percent of all ankle sprains, while 20 percent involve both the ATFL and CFL.[16,138,326] The sequence of ligament tears in an inversion injury are first, the ATFL, the anterolateral capsule (which is in close proximity to the ATFL and results in hemarthrosis when torn), and the distal tibiofibular ligament. Progressive inversion strain results in a CFL tear. As the inversion force continues, the PTFL, the strongest of the lateral ligaments, ruptures.[18,202] This rupture may be associated with ankle dislocation, distal lateral malleolar avulsion or spiral fracture, medial malleolar fracture, or talar neck or medial compression fractures.[202] Most (86 percent) ankle ligament tears are midsubstance; thus only 14 percent are avulsion injuries.[138]

Lateral ligament sprains are more common than medial ligament sprains for two major reasons:[40]

▶ The lateral malleolus projects more distally than the medial malleolus, producing less bony obstruction to inversion than eversion.

▶ The deltoid ligament is much stronger than the lateral ligaments.

While a physical examination is reliable for the diagnosis of an ankle fracture,[192] the reliability for detecting lateral ankle sprains may not be as definitive, especially if the examination is performed immediately after the injury.[180] The place of a physical examination in diagnosis has been reviewed in a series of 160 patients,[180] comparing the accuracy within 48 hours of injury with that at 4 to 7 days. The specificity and sensitivity of delayed physical examination for the presence or absence of a lateral ligament injury were 84 and 96 percent, respectively, indicating that a reasonably precise clinical diagnosis is possible if the examination is delayed for about 4 days postinjury.[330]

The mechanism of injury can afford some clues. A history of a forced dorsiflexion can result in a sprain of the distal tibiofibular syndesmosis. Distal tibiofibular syndesmosis sprains are usually accompanied by complaints of pain that greatly exceed the amount of swelling and that increase with external rotation of the foot.[136] Forced plantar flexion can result in anterior capsular sprains. These are characterized by pain that worsens with passive plantar flexion and resisted dorsiflexion.[136]

No single symptom or test can provide a completely accurate diagnosis of a lateral ankle ligament rupture, but the collection of findings can be strongly indicative:[180]

▶ The absence of swelling at the time of the delayed (after 4 days) physical examination suggests that there is no ligament rupture, whereas extensive swelling at this time is indicative of ligament rupture.[331]

▶ Pain on palpation of the involved ligament suggests involvement.

▶ Presence of a hematoma suggests a rupture.

▶ Positive anterior drawer test suggests a rupture.

▶ Impairment of walking ability after injury suggests involvement.

One study[180] demonstrated that a combination of tenderness at the level of the anterior talofibular ligament, a lateral hematoma, discoloration, and a positive drawer test indicated a ligament rupture in 95 percent of cases, whereas the absence of these findings always indicated an intact ligament.

Lateral ankle sprains can be categorized as follows:

▶ Grade I sprains are characterized by minimal to no swelling and localized tenderness over the ATFL. These sprains require on the average 11.7 days before the full resumption of athletic activities.[332]

▶ Grade II sprains are characterized by localized swelling and more diffuse lateral tenderness. These sprains require approximately 2 to 6 weeks for return to full athletic function.[333,334]

▶ Grade III sprains are characterized by significant swelling, pain, and ecchymosis, and should be referred to a specialist.[335] Grade III injuries may require greater than 6 weeks to return to full function. For acute grade III ankle sprains, the average duration of disability has been reported to be anywhere from 4.5 to 26 weeks, and only 25 to 60 percent of patients are symptom free 1 to 4 years after injury.[336] Some controversy exists regarding the appropriate treatment of grade III injuries, particularly in high-level athletes.[22,133] In a summary of all prospective and controlled studies on grade III sprains, it was concluded that the long-term prognosis is good to excellent in 80 to 90 percent of patients with this injury, regardless of the type of intervention chosen.[337]

Intervention. Conservative intervention has been found to be uniformly effective in treating grade I and II ankle sprains,[338] and generally patients are completely asymptomatic and functionally stable at follow-up.

Although conservative treatment may be appropriate, the time required to return to full athletic function in any conservative program will increase as the severity of injury increases. Intervention in the acute stage centers around aggressive attempts to:

▶ Minimize effusion so as to speed healing.

▶ Promote early protected motion.

▶ Foster early supported/protected weight bearing as tolerated.

▶ Protected return to activity.

▶ Prevention of re-injury.

Early intervention incorporates cryotherapy, compression, and elevation to assist in the reduction of pain, swelling, and secondary hypoxic effects.[339] Although early motion and mobility rather than immobilization have demonstrated the stimulation of collagen bundle orientation and the promotion of healing,[340] it must be remembered that full ligamentous strength is not gained for a period of months.[341–344]

Active range-of-motion exercises, such as ankle pumping and toe curls (30 reps, 4 times/day each), are encouraged during this phase, but within pain-free limits.[141]

Protected weight bearing with an orthosis is permitted, with weight bearing to tolerance as soon as possible following injury.[23] As the healing progresses and the patient is able to bear more weight on his or her ankle, there is a corresponding increase in the use of weight-bearing (closed-chain) exercises. A useful activity during this phase is the "cross drill." The patient stands independently or with minimal external assistance on the involved limb only. The patient then moves the uninvolved limb into hip flexion, hip extension, hip abduction, and hip adduction. The exercise is performed initially on a firm surface with the eyes open. As the patient improves, the exercise is performed on a foam surface or balance board, first with the eyes open, and then with the eyes closed.

In the subacute stages of the rehabilitation process (4 to 14 days), the patient begins dynamic balance and proprioceptive exercises. The external support may still be required during this phase. Using a balance board, the patient balances on the involved limb while playing "catch" with the clinician. The intensity of this exercise can be varied by using balls of different sizes and of different weights. The clinician may also make the exercises more challenging by throwing the ball to a variety of locations. This will require a shift in the center of gravity and an instantaneous adjustment of balance from the patient.

Long-sitting gastrocnemius stretching with a strap or sheet can be introduced in this phase (6 reps of 20 seconds each) to promote ankle dorsiflexion past the neutral position, enabling a closer to normal walking pattern.[141] Open-chain (non–weight-bearing) progressive resistive exercises with elastic resistance are performed (2 sets of 30 reps each) for isolated plantar flexion, dorsiflexion, inversion, and eversion. Stationary cycling can also be performed (at a comfortable intensity for up to 30 minutes) to provide cardiovascular endurance training and controlled ankle range of motion.[144]

In the advanced healing stage (2 to 4 weeks postinjury) the goals are:

▶ The restoration of normal AROM.

▶ Normal gait without an assistive device.

▶ Pain-free performance of full weight-bearing functional activities.

▶ Enhancement of proprioception.

Activities to help achieve these goals include heel-to-toe anterior-posterior walking (10 m for 20 reps), carioca drills, and mini-trampoline balancing exercises (unilateral stance with eyes open and then closed, and catching and passing activities with a medicine ball).

Plyometric activities are introduced during the functional challenge/return to activity phase. These can include two-foot ankle hopping, single ankle hops, and then multidirection single ankle hops. If appropriate, barrier jumps or hops may be introduced.

Recurrent Ankle Sprains

The patient who suffers from recurrent sprains and functional instability poses a problem to the clinician and other members of the sports medicine team.

Recurrent ankle sprains may be due to[22,133]:

▶ Healing of the ligaments in a lengthened position.

▶ Weakness of the healed ligaments due to inherent weakness of the scar.

▶ Peroneal muscle weakness (the incompletely rehabilitated ankle sprain).

▶ Distal tibiofibular instability.

▶ Hereditary hypermobility.

▶ Loss of ankle proprioception.

▶ Impingement by the distal fascicle of the anterior tibiofibular ligament, and/or impingement of capsular scar tissue (meniscoid tissue) in the talofibular joint.

▶ Undiagnosed associated problems such as cuboid subluxation or subtalar instability.

Functional instability and loss of normal ankle kinematics as a complication of ankle sprains may lead to early degenerative changes.[175,321] Talar displacement of greater than 1 mm reduces the ankle's weight-bearing surface by 42.3 percent,[173,345,346] thus creating asymmetric load bearing of the articular surface. Thus degenerative change may be due to small amounts of articular displacement or the abnormal shearing forces of instability.

Chronic lateral instability is manifested by recurrent injuries with pain, tenderness, and sometimes bruising over the lateral ligaments.[178,319,347–350] Many, approximately 30 percent,[319] may be asymptomatic between the events. Others may manifest with chronic lateral pain, tenderness, swelling, or induration with great difficulties in sports and daily activities.[178,319,348] A history of insecurity, instability, and giving way[32,349,351] is far more important in diagnosis than the physical examination in acute and recurrent sprains.[319,352]

In general, subjective complaints include:

▶ Frequent sprains.[317,323]

▶ Difficulty running on uneven surfaces.[317]

▶ Difficulty in cutting and jumping in athletic events.[178,317,324]

▶ Feelings of "giving way."[318,320,323]

▶ Recurrent pain[178,318,320,322,323] and swelling.[317,320,322–324]

▶ Tenderness.[317,318,320]

▶ Inability to run.[194]

▶ Weakness.[178,194]

The intervention of all recurrent ankle sprains should begin with a trial of conservative management for 2 to 3 months.[194,317,325,353,354] Any or all of the following have been shown to help in some patients: a lateral heel wedge, peroneal muscle strengthening, proprioceptive/coordination exercises, taping, elastic or thermoplastic ankle supports, and/or a short leg brace.

Many patients with ankle instability can be treated satisfactorily with late repair or reconstruction of the lateral ligaments.[319,355–360]

However, in spite of surgery, some patients will be left with persistent disability including subjective or objective instability, persistent talar tilt, stretching of the ligaments, pain, stiffness, or range-of-motion limitations.[349,361]

According to Hinterman and colleagues,[21] a number of conditions can mimic ankle instability:

▶ Peroneal tendon subluxation.

▶ Instability of the Chopart joint. Inversion and plantar flexion trauma of the foot may result in avulsion by the bifurcate ligament, and sometimes, additionally by the talonavicular ligament. Injuries at the Chopart joint level are, however, frequently missed acutely and misdiagnosed as lateral ankle sprain if the clinical examination is not carefully carried out.

▶ Talocalcaneal and talonavicular coalition.

▶ Posterior tibial dysfunction.

Midfoot Sprain

A sprain of the tarsometatarsal joint usually occurs from an indirect axial load on a plantarflexed and rotated foot, with or without abduction.[362] On examination, the young patient will have tenderness to palpation directly over this area, and pain with passive midfoot pronation and supination while the rearfoot is stabilized.[362]

Radiographs of the foot should include weight-bearing AP and lateral and oblique views to rule out dislocation. The metatarsals should be lined up with their respective cuneiforms.[64]

Conservative intervention can proceed if displacement of the metatarsals on radiograph is less than 2 mm, and includes an orthotic or a fracture boot if the patient is unable to bear weight comfortably.[64] A stiff shoe, and orthotics to support the medial longitudinal arch, are recommended for return to athletics.[363]

Sinus Tarsi Syndrome

Sinus tarsi syndrome is a sprain of the subtalar joint with injury to the talocalcaneal interosseous ligament. This usually occurs after an ankle injury and is sometimes difficult to distinguish from a routine ankle sprain.[64]

Observation usually reveals swelling in the sinus tarsi. There is usually pain with palpation and pronation,[329] usually due to scarring in the soft tissue elements of the sinus tarsi.[363]

The intervention may include joint-specific mobilization and manipulation. An orthotic can be used to limit pronation and maintain the foot in a functional neutral position.

Selective cortisone injection into the subtalar joint can also be diagnostic and therapeutic.[329]

Cuboid Syndrome

Cuboid syndrome (locked cuboid, calcaneal cuboid fault syndrome, subluxed cuboid) is common but poorly recognized.[364] The calcaneocuboid joint is usually very mobile, but can be repetitively subluxed laterally and dorsally with strong forces. The subluxation is usually a temporary occurrence. The etiology has been proposed to be secondary to overuse, increasing body weight, training on uneven surfaces, or a lateral ankle or lateral foot sprain.[364,365]

Cuboid syndrome usually presents with a gradual onset of lateral midfoot pain. The pain is usually localized near the fourth and fifth metatarsals at the dorsal aspect of the cuboid or the calcaneocuboid joint.[364] Often, the patient feels as if he or she is walking with a small stone in their shoe. Maximum discomfort is elicited by pressure directed over the peroneal groove on the plantar surface of the calcaneus.[64] On occasion, the hook of the bone under the cuboid breaks or the short plantar ligament tears, producing heel pain.

Common findings in the physical examination are a subtle forefoot valgus and a pronated foot, as well as a tight peroneus longus tendon.[364,366,367] The pronated foot produces an unstable midtarsal joint.

The intervention for this condition includes a manipulation of the midfoot, stretching the peroneal tendons, and strapping/plantar padding.[364,366]

Talocrural Joint Subluxation

There are essentially two types of subluxations at this joint, anterior and posterior, which result in a loss of plantar flexion and dorsiflexion, respectively.

▶ The anterior subluxation is commonly caused by an inversion, plantar flexion force. The clinical findings include a limitation of dorsiflexion, a decreased posterior talar glide, and/or conjunct external rotation of the talus.

▶ The posterior subluxation may be from a compensatory or other type of flat foot, or from a dorsiflexion injury. The clinical findings include a loss of the plantar flexion talar swing, anterior glide, and/or medial conjunct talar rotation.

The intervention for this type of injury is usually a high velocity thrust technique applied to the joint.

Preferred Practice Pattern 4E: Impaired Joint Mobility, Motor Function, Muscle Performance, Range of Motion Associated with Localized Inflammation

The list of potential pathology for soft tissue injuries to the foot, accompanied with localized inflammation, is extensive.

Inflammation or Infection of the Nails and Skin

Subungual Hematoma. A subungual hematoma is also called "black toenails" or "runner's toe" and results from bleeding under the toenails due to chronic friction or bumping of the toe against ill-fitting shoes, or from overt trauma to the dorsal aspect of the toe.[368] Due to the extreme sensitivity of the nail bed, significant pulsating pain is often associated with this problem, with or without palpation.

In the case of poorly fitting shoes, prophylactic treatment is recommended. Athletic shoes should be one size longer than street shoes in most cases.[154]

For an existing hematoma, the treatment of choice involves decompression of the hematoma using a red-hot paper clip or 18-gauge needle, heated in an alcohol burner, which is used to burn a hole through the nail.[369]

Subungual Exostosis. A subungual exostosis is a hypertrophic bone, usually affecting the medial border of the hallux, as the result of excessive pressure, that produces pain on ambulation.[370] An accurate diagnosis of this condition requires a radiograph.[369]

Conservative intervention involves using a deep toe box and decreasing the width of hypertrophic nails.

Onychocryptosis. Onychocryptosis is more commonly referred to as ingrown toenails. It is commonly associated with a secondary pyogenic infection or paronychia.[369] Onychocryptosis without paronychia is treated conservatively by removing the offending portion of the nail, and then smoothing the nail border with a curette.[369]

Onychia. Onychia is an infection of one or both sides of the nail and nail plate, which can result from a number of factors including chronic pressure on the nail plate, allergies, nail polish, improperly cutting the nails, or certain soaps.[369]

Onychauxis. Onychauxis is an overgrowth of the nail that can be the result of microtrauma or macrotrauma, peripheral neuritis, old age, nutritional disturbances, or decreased circulation, producing future nail growth distortion.[368,369,371] The diagnosis is made by the hallmark characteristics of a hypertrophic, dystrophic, and discolored nail plate.[372]

The conservative intervention for this condition involves the mechanical or chemical debridement of the nail plate.[372]

Onychomycosis. Onychomycosis (Fig. 19-54) is a chronic fungal condition of the nails, which is often responsible for causing onychauxis.[373]

Tinea Pedis. Tinea pedis is more commonly known as athlete's foot. It usually presents with redness or itchiness, but can also appear as dry and flaky skin (Fig. 19-55).[369]

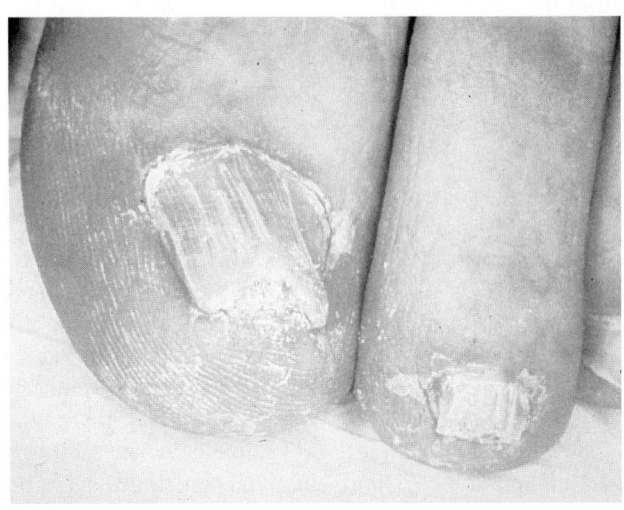

FIGURE 19-54 Onychomycosis. (Reproduced with permission from O'Connor FG, Wilder RP. *Textbook of Running Medicine.* New York: McGraw-Hill; 2001.)

Treatment is simple and involves soaking the foot in one-half cup of vinegar in a pan of water once a day and applying a topical anti-fungal agent.[369]

Blisters. Blisters occur secondary to friction and shearing and can give the clinician valuable information as to where the stresses of the foot are occurring. Besides the obvious fact that tight shoes cause blisters, other causes include excessive motion such as pronation and supination.

Tendonitis

Overuse tendonitis in the tendons spanning the ankle can be seen with training errors, sudden changes in training patterns, muscle-tendon imbalance, anatomic malalignment, improper footwear, or a sudden growth spurt.[329] Tendonitis can also be

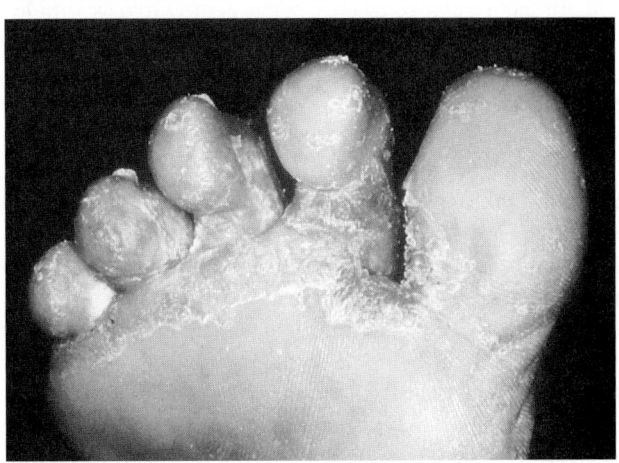

FIGURE 19-55 Tinea pedis. (Reproduced with permission from O'Connor FG, Wilder RP. *Textbook of Running Medicine.* New York: McGraw-Hill; 2001.)

seen in the adolescent that resumes play after a period of decreased training.[374]

Peroneal Tendon Tendonitis. Peroneal tendonitis is particularly common in young dancers and ice skaters, but can be seen in any running athlete. After repeated inversion strain, the sheaths of the peroneus longus and brevis tendons may be stretched and become inflamed (runner's foot). Instability between the fourth and fifth metatarsals is also associated with this disorder.

The patient usually presents with pain behind and distal to the lateral malleolus.[374] There may be associated swelling in the acute phase. There will also be pain with resisted foot eversion.

The intervention for peroneal tendonitis includes a program of stretching, strengthening, icing, and sometimes ankle bracing[374] during contact sports.

Peroneal Tendon Subluxation. Subluxation of the peroneal tendons is an uncommon but potentially disabling condition that can affect young athletes[375] and it is often difficult to distinguish from lateral ankle sprain acutely.[376]

Acute symptoms are pain at the posterior distal fibula, swelling, ecchymosis, and apprehension, or inability to evert the foot against resistance.[64] Chronic symptoms are lateral ankle pain, popping or snapping, and instability.[64] A chronic peroneal tendon subluxation can both mimic and coexist with chronic ankle instability.

In some young athletes, there may be an anatomic predisposition to peroneal tendon subluxation. These include an absent or shallow fibula groove,[85,329,377,378] possibly combined with pes planus, hindfoot valgus, or lax/absent peroneal retinaculum.[85,86,374,377,379] The retinaculum can also traumatically rupture from a violent forced dorsiflexion of the ankle with reflex contraction of the peroneal muscles and dislocation.[69,85,86,329,379–381]

Peroneal tendon subluxation can be an acute episode that turns into a chronic problem due to misdiagnosis.[64] Many of these are incorrectly diagnosed at the acute stage as simple ankle sprains.[382] The young patient may present acutely after a supposed ankle sprain with pain and swelling over the posterolateral aspect of the ankle. More commonly though, the initial presentation may be weeks to months after the injury.[69] The adolescent may complain of recurrent inversion ankle sprains and lateral ankle instability with a painful snapping across the ankle.[383] Chronic ankle instability can also contribute to chronic peroneal tendon subluxation with the development of an incompetent superficial peroneal retinaculum.[85,383] This can also be confused with the rare isolated injury to the posterior talofibular ligament.[85,86,378,379]

On physical exam, subluxation may be provoked with forceful ankle dorsiflexion and eversion. There may be pain posterior to the lateral malleolus in an acute situation, as well as a negative anterior drawer test.[64]

Many different surgical procedures have been described for chronic peroneal tendon subluxation.[85,375,379,381,382]

Tibialis Posterior Tendonitis. The tibialis posterior tendon lies just posterior to the medial malleolus and supports the medial arch of the foot. The tendon is lined with a tenosynovial sheath which can become inflamed, producing a tenosynovitis. If left untreated, the condition can progress to an eventual rupture.[384]

Posterior tibial dysfunction is a complex disorder of the hindfoot. Controversy exists as to whether persisting rotational instability after ankle sprain may cause posterior tibial dysfunction or vice versa. Posterior tibial dysfunction may cause ankle instability by overloading the ankle ligaments, especially the deltoid ligament.[47]

The pain is usually felt in one of three locations:

▶ Distal to the medial malleoli in the area of the navicular.

▶ Proximal to the medial malleoli.

▶ At the musculotendinous origin (medial shin splints), or insertion.

Posterior tibialis tendonitis is seen relatively frequently in dancers, joggers, and ice skaters, especially in those participants with a pronated foot and flattened longitudinal arch.[159] Running sports that require rapid changes in direction (basketball, tennis, soccer, and ice hockey) place increased stress across the tendon as well.[84] Contributing factors include adaptive shortening of the gastrocnemius-soleus complex, and weakness of the posterior tibialis.

On physical exam, the patient will present with pain on resisted ankle plantar flexion and inversion,[84] with tenderness to palpation along the tendon's course posterior to the medial malleolus and to its insertion into the navicular. Swelling may sometimes be seen. Sometimes pain may be secondary to an accessory navicular.[84] With a complete rupture, the navicular subluxes inferiorly, and the patient ambulates in a flat-footed position as they are unable to produce any toe-off.

Plain radiographs are rarely helpful, though magnetic resonance imaging (MRI) or bone scan[385] may also aid in the diagnosis.

The intervention for posterior tibialis dysfunction depends on the cause, but the overall approach includes tibialis posterior stretching, strengthening, orthotics, occasional casting, and icing.[84]

Patla and Abbott[160] describe a condition called tibialis posterior myofascial tightness (TPMT) as a factor in heel pain. In contrast to tibialis posterior tendonitis, TPMT is not characterized by inflammation of the tendon or tendon sheath. The patient with TPMT complains of immediate heel pain on weight bearing in the morning. The pain is increased with increased load from activities, but typically decreases during the day. There is no specific injury or activity identified as the cause. Physical findings include:[160]

▶ Depression of the medial arch with standing.

▶ Neutral or inverted calcaneus in standing.

▶ Flat foot appearance and diminished push-off with gait.

▶ Decreased full range of motion of plantar flexion and calcaneal inversion with weight bearing heel raising.

▶ Full passive range of motion of dorsiflexion and plantar flexion, but may have end-range discomfort.

▶ Posterior tibialis length test (see special tests) shows decreased extensibility and often produces pain.

The intervention for this condition is geared toward correcting the impairments of the tibialis posterior muscle. The same technique and contacts used in the test are used for treatment, except that the manual stretch is maintained for approximately 2 minutes, and is repeated approximately four times, with slightly stronger pressure used each time.

Tibialis Anterior Tendonitis. Tibialis anterior tendonitis is most commonly seen in runners. The examination will show point tenderness over the tendon as it crosses the ankle. Conservative intervention includes tibialis anterior stretching, strengthening, orthotics, and occasional casting and icing.

Flexor Hallucis Longus (FHL) Tendonitis. The FHL is lined by a tenosynovial sheath, which can become inflamed. FHL tendonitis is characterized by pain posterior to the medial malleolus, which is most often confused with posterior tibialis tendonitis.[386]

FHL tendonitis will usually present itself in the young patient as pain with resisted great toe flexion, as well as pain posterior and inferior to the medial malleolus. Dancers who assume the repeated plantar flexion posture of demipointe or pointe are particularly susceptible to FHL tendonitis, with the tendon actually locking in demipointe in the latter group.[366,387,388] It can also be seen in runners and gymnasts.

The tendon becomes inflamed due to forceful push-offs with the forefoot, where the FHL is stretched between the posterior talar tubercle and the sustentaculum tali. The tendon can also be irritated with plantar flexion, where it is compressed over the posterior talar tubercle.[386]

Conservative intervention includes icing, stretching, strengthening, decreased activity, correcting improper techniques, orthotics, a hard-soled shoe, and NSAIDs.[389]

Operative intervention typically involves releasing the tendon sheath.

Achilles Tendonitis. It is probably no accident that Homer decided that the heels of his Greek hero, Achilles, would be the one vulnerable area of the body.[390] This vulnerability of the heels continues to this day with Achilles tendonitis being the most common overuse syndrome of the lower leg,[82] accounting for 5 to 18 percent of the total number of running injuries.

The Achilles tendon is placed under extreme and rapid eccentric loading forces during such activities as running, standing up while cycling, ballet, gymnastics, soccer, and basketball.[391]

The underlying mechanism of Achilles tendonitis is not well understood, but a number of mechanisms have been proposed.

The biomechanical hypothesis is the most popular. Immediately after the foot makes contact with the ground in a supinated position, it pronates, and then supinates again as toe-off approaches.[48,123] The pronated foot imparts an internal rotation force through the tibia, whereas knee extension imparts an external rotation force through the tibia.[391] The overpronated foot places the medial aspect of the tendon under tension, generating an obligatory internal tibial rotation, which tends to draw the Achilles tendon medially.[392] The rapid and repeated transitions from pronation to supination cause the Achilles tendon to undergo a "whipping" or "bow-string" action.[393] Moreover, if the foot remains in a pronated position after knee extension has begun, the lateral tibial rotation at the knee and the medial tibial rotation at the foot results in a "wringing" or twisting action of the tendon.[48]

Another proposed mechanism involves the eccentric contraction of the triceps surae during support. Maximal triceps sural contraction is associated with adduction and supination of the foot. At heel strike the calf muscles undergo a rapid shortening, before lengthening as the tibia rotates forward over the foot. The calf muscles then shorten again during the forward propulsion phase.[394] These quick muscle action alternations may cause microtears in the tendon.

In addition to those causes already described, a number of other factors appear to contribute to the development of Achilles tendonitis:

▶ *Stretching.* In a study by McCrory and colleagues,[393] whether or not a runner incorporated stretching of the gastrocnemius into his or her training routine appeared to be a significant discriminator between the injured and uninjured cohorts. Specifically, injured runners were less likely to incorporate stretching into their regular training routines. Whether stretching habits can be related to the incidence of overuse injuries remains undetermined.[395–398]

▶ *Training variables.* The incidence of overuse injuries has been strongly associated with a faster training pace, with injured runners running at a significantly faster training pace than uninjured runners.[77,395,399] Hill training has also been suggested as an etiological factor in the onset of Achilles tendonitis.[79,394,400]

▶ *Fatigue.* Overtraining has been found to correlate to calf muscle fatigue and microtears of the tendon.[48,123]

▶ *Isokinetic variables.* Muscular insufficiency has been cited as a significant factor in the inability to eccentrically restrain dorsiflexion during the beginning of the support phase of running.[393,399–401]

▶ *Anthropometric variables.* In one study 20 percent of the injured runners with Achilles tendonitis had cavus feet.[123] Clement and coworkers,[400] after having found cavus feet to be rigid, suggested that the compensatory overpronation resulting from the inflexibility of the cavus foot is a precursor to Achilles tendonitis. Other studies have also related a high-arched foot to the incidence of various overuse syndromes.[77,272,402,403]

▶ *Age.* The role that age plays in Achilles tendonitis is inconclusive, with some studies finding a correlation,[393,404] and others[397,403,405–407] finding no associations between age and the pathogenesis of running injuries.

▶ *Shoe type.* Spike shoes lock the feet on the surface during the single support phase in running and increase the athlete's foot grip, but also transfer lateral and torque shear forces directly to the foot and ankle and through to the Achilles tendon.[392] The soles of spike shoes have minimal shock absorption, transferring the vertical force directly to the Achilles tendon.[408] This may increase the overloading of the tendon, causing microtrauma and inflammation of the Achilles tendon.

▶ *Sacroiliac joint dysfunction.* Changes in sacroiliac joint mechanics as compared with the contralateral side have also been associated with this dysfunction.[392] The primary function of the pelvis appears to be as a shock absorber, transmitting the weight of the trunk and upper extremities to the lower limbs and distributing the ground reaction forces.[9,409] The combination of ground forces, which tend to rotate the ilium posteriorly, and trunk forces provide a mechanism of stability.[9,409] Posterior dysfunction is reported to be the most common lesion of the sacroiliac articulation by several authors.[410–412] This results in a functional shortening and external rotation of the involved leg,[413–415] both of which may influence the kinematic chain of the lower extremity in the following manner:[392]

- The ankle and foot position will be in external rotation, instead of neutral, at heel strike.

- Due to the transfer of body weight over the affected leg during the rest of the stance phase, the loading of the lateral aspect of the heel will be short, the following pronation prolonged, and inversion delayed. This may decrease the amount of dorsiflexion in the ankle, thus minimizing the tension in the plantar soft tissues. This in turn decreases the leverage of the Achilles tendon,[408,416] and the truss mechanism[408] may not be activated due to insufficient hyperextension of the big toe.

- Because of the relative ineffectiveness of the foot's truss mechanism at toe-off, together with the decrease of leverage of the Achilles tendon, the triceps surae will have to activate more motor units to ensure continued performance, thus putting additional loading on the Achilles tendon.

Achilles tendonitis typically occurs as one of two types of tendonitis: insertional and noninsertional, with the former involving the tendon-bone interface, and the latter occurring just proximal to the tendon insertion on the calcaneus in or around the tendon substance.[391]

Noninsertional tendonitis can be referred to as peritendonitis, peritendonitis with tendinosis, or tendinosis.[391,417]

▶ *Peritendonitis.* The inflammation in peritendonitis is limited to the peritendon, and thickening can result.

▶ *Peritendonitis with tendinosis.* This condition describes a second stage of inflammation in which a portion of the Achilles tendon itself is involved in the disease process.

▶ *Pure tendinosis.* This condition, which typically affects the weekend warrior, is characterized by microscopic and macroscopic mucoid degeneration of the tendon.

Pain is the dominant symptom of Achilles tendonitis and is exacerbated by activity. The patient will present with insidiously increasing pain and stiffness along the Achilles tendon, sometimes with associated swelling. In the early stages of Achilles tendonitis, morning stiffness may be the only symptom, whereas pain is felt even at rest in the advanced stages.[74]

The vast majority of symptomatic patients are runners who complain of pain in the posterior aspect of the heel, about 2 cm proximal to the superior margin of the calcaneus, which increases during running activities.[75] The pain typically worsens over time, until it inhibits the individual from running, at which point they usually seek medical attention.

The differential diagnosis for posterior heel pain includes retrocalcaneal bursitis,[75] metabolic diseases, arthritis and chondropathic diseases of the ankle joint, tibia vara, os trigonum, a calcaneal contusion, plantar fasciitis, calcaneal stress fracture impingement syndrome, and stress fractures of the fibula or tibia (see Chap. 9).[392,418]

The Achilles tendon and heel may be examined with the patient in sitting or prone. Upon observation, the patient will often be found to have pronated feet and the presence of swelling is common.

Systematic palpation is performed along the tendon, over the heel, along the posterior border of the calcaneus, and down onto the heel pad. Localization of the tenderness is extremely important. Tenderness that is located 2 to 6 cm proximal to the insertion is indicative of noninsertional tendonitis, whereas pain at the bone-tendon junction is more indicative of insertional tendonitis.[391] If there is an area in the tendon itself which is discrete and painful with side-to-side pressure of the fingers, this often indicates an area of mucoid degeneration or a small partial rupture of the tendon.[75] If the tenderness is in the area of the retrocalcaneal bursa, which is noted by side-to-side pressure in that area, this is the primary area of involvement.[75]

A lack of 20 degrees of dorsiflexion in knee extension signifies gastrocnemius tightness, and inability to dorsiflex 30 degrees in knee flexion implicates the soleus as well.[75]

Analysis of gait may reveal an antalgic gait, with the involved leg held in external rotation both during stance and swing phase.

There is often pain with resisted testing of the gastrocnemius/soleus complex. The intervention for Achilles tendonitis varies, with the recommended amount of rest depending on the severity of the symptoms:[83]

▶ *Type I.*   Characterized by pain that is only experienced after activity. These patients should reduce their exercise by 25 percent.

▶ *Type II.*   Characterized by pain which occurs both during and after activity, but does not affect performance. These patients should reduce their training by 50 percent.

▶ *Type III.*   Characterized by pain during and after activity that does affect performance. These patients should temporarily discontinue running.

The conservative intervention includes Achilles stretching and strengthening, manual techniques, the correction of any lower chain asymmetries, particularly low back, pelvic, and hip flexor asymmetries, electrotherapeutic modalities as appropriate, correct shoe wear, and orthotics.[419,420]

Appropriately designed orthoses made from a mold of the foot held in subtalar neutral and non–weight bearing can be of significant benefit.[74]

Rupture of the Achilles Tendon

Rupture of the Achilles tendon was first described in 1575, and first reported in the literature in 1633.[421] The etiology of a spontaneous rupture remains incompletely understood, although a number of theories have been proposed, including microtrauma,[422] inhibitor mechanism malfunction,[423] hypoxic and mucoid tendon degeneration,[424] decreased perfusion,[425] and systemic or locally injected steroids.[426] However, the fact that the peak incidence of Achilles tendon rupture occurs in the middle age group rather than in the older population tends to lend credence to a mechanical etiology.[427] Three activities have been implicated in rupturing an Achilles tendon:[428]

▶ Pushing off with weight bearing on the forefoot while extending the knee.

▶ Sudden dorsiflexion with full weight bearing as might occur with a slip or fall.

▶ Violent dorsiflexion such as that which occurs when jumping or falling from a height and landing on a plantar-flexed foot.

The diagnosis of an Achilles tendon rupture is based almost solely on history and physical findings. The classic history is reports of sudden pain in the calf area, often associated with an audible snap, followed by difficulty in stepping off on the foot.[427] Physical examination reveals swelling of the calf as well as a palpable defect in the tendon (sometimes called a hatchet strike), as well as ecchymosis around the malleoli.[429] Perhaps the most reliable sign of a complete rupture is a positive result on the Thompson squeeze test (see Fig. 19-45).[183,430]

The conservative intervention of Achilles tendon rupture consists of short- or long-leg cast immobilization in the gravity equinus position (10 to 20 degrees of plantar flexion). However, this approach appears to result in a high incidence of re-rupture (10 to 30 percent)[431–434] and a decrease in maximal function.[423,435,436] This may be because it is impossible to restore the correct length of the Achilles tendon with nonoperative treatment.[427] The surgical intervention for Achilles tendon rupture is described in Chapter 29.

Sever's Disease (Calcaneal Apophysitis)

Sever's disease is a traction apophysitis at the insertion of the Achilles tendon, and is a common cause of heel pain in the athletically active child, with 61 percent of cases occurring bilaterally.[437]

The calcaneal apophysis serves as the attachment for the Achilles tendon superiorly and for the plantar fascia and the short muscles of the sole of the foot inferiorly.[438] This os calcis secondary center of ossification appears at age 9 and usually fuses at 16 years of age.[64] The average age of onset for this condition is 8 to 13 years.[439]

Factors involved in the etiology of Sever's disease include beginning a new sport or season, foot pronation, and a tight gastrocnemius-soleus complex.[440] There usually is a history of an increase in running activity, beginning a new sport, or the beginning of a new season.[64] Young gymnasts and dancers are particularly susceptible to this condition because of their repetitive jumping or landing from a height.[440] The tight Achilles tendon is usually associated with a recent growth spurt and is not related to a specific injury.[64]

Although radiographs are often normal, sclerosis or fragmentation of the apophysis may be seen on plain radiographs.[64]

The location of the pain differs from that of plantar fasciitis in that its focal point is more posterior than it is plantar.

The intervention for Sever's disease begins with stretching the heel cord, using heel cups or heel wedges, and avoiding barefoot walking until becoming asymptomatic.[329]

Iselin's Disease

Iselin's disease is a traction apophysitis of the tuberosity of the fifth metatarsal. It is more commonly seen in athletically active older children and adolescents. The secondary center of ossification appears as a small, shell-shaped fleck of bone oriented slightly oblique to the metatarsal shaft, and is located on the lateral plantar aspect of the tuberosity of the fifth metatarsal. This apophysis is located within the insertion site of the peroneus brevis tendon. The center appears in girls at an average of 9 years and in boys at 12 years and usually fuses to the shaft by 11 and 14 years, respectively.

The patient is usually involved in sports with running, cutting, and jumping. These activities may result in an inversion stress to this area. There is usually pain over the area but no specific history of trauma. Resisted eversion typically reproduces the pain. A bone scan will usually be positive. Iselin's disease can be differentiated from an avulsion fracture of the base of the fifth metatarsal because the apophysis is located parallel to the long axis of the shaft and an avulsion fracture is usually transverse in nature.

The intervention for Iselin's disease includes immobilization for acute pain and physical therapy for strengthening of the peroneal tendons.[441]

Plantar Fasciitis/Heel Spur Syndrome

Plantar fasciitis is an inflammatory process, secondary to repetitive stretching of the plantar fascia. Despite the fact that modern shoes are designed with every conceivable type of heel cushioning, plantar fasciitis continues to be a pervasive entity. As the plantar fascia assists in the development of the push-off power during running and jumping, it is not surprising that plantar fasciitis is particularly prevalent in joggers and tennis players, as well as in athletes participating in racquet sports, soccer, gymnastics, and basketball.[73]

Although more common in active individuals, plantar fasciitis can also affect the sedentary, though the reasons for this remain elusive. Although more common in middle-aged individuals, plantar fasciitis can occur in the younger individual, although it rarely exists alone in this age group and usually coincides with calcaneal apophysitis.[441a]

The role of the heel spur in plantar fasciitis is controversial.[73] Half of patients with plantar fasciitis have heel spurs,[442] whereas 16 to 27 percent of the population have heel spurs without symptoms.[157,443] The greater pull of the plantar fascia was thought to lead to periosteal hemorrhage and inflammatory reaction, and to laying down of new bone and heel spur formation,[444] but the heel spur is more often associated with the flexor digitorum brevis muscle than the plantar fascia.[159,389,445–449]

The etiology of plantar fasciitis is poorly understood, although a number of factors have been proposed:

▶ *Obesity.*[450]   Obesity has been shown to occur in 40% of men and 90% of women with plantar fasciitis.[442,451]

▶ *Occupational.*   There is an association between plantar fasciitis and prolonged standing or walking ("policeman's heel"),[73] or a sudden change in the stresses placed upon the feet likening this condition to other repetitive stress disorders such as carpal tunnel syndrome and tennis elbow

▶ *Acute injury.*   Although less common, plantar fasciitis may be associated with an acute injury to the heel. Some people recall stepping on a pebble, or other hard object, before pain began ("stone bruise").[73]

▶ *Anatomical.*   The heel pad is specially constructed as an efficient shock absorber to attenuate peaks in dynamic forces and to dampen vibrations.[451a] Part of the impacting energy involved in displacement of the heel pad during ambulation is dissipated, and part of the energy is recovered in the subsequent elastic recoil. Two studies that examined the mechanical properties of the heel pad[451b,451c] found that thickness and compressibility index (CI; ratio of thickness of the loaded heel pad to it unloaded) were greater in patients with plantar heel pain. This finding implies that loss of elasticity of the heel pad may be a factor in plantar heel pain syndrome.

▶ *Biomechanical causes.*   People with high arches (pes cavus) or low arches (pes planus) are at increased risk because of the increased repetitive stress being placed on the fascia.[73] Likewise, adaptive shortening of the calf muscles

and Achilles tendon, excessive rearfoot motion (especially overpronation), or a rigid varus hindfoot may also put the patient at risk by placing excess stress on the plantar fascia.[451d–g] Weakness of the intrinsic foot muscles has also been cited as a cause. These factors may increase the moment of maximum tension in the fascia, which even under normal circumstances endures tension that is approximately two times body weight during walking at the moment when the heel of the trailing leg begins to lift off the ground. Thus, an accurate history of footwear should be obtained: often patients wear shoes with poor cushioning or inadequate arch support, or they walk barefoot on hard floors.

Because chronic subcalcaneal heel pain is a common manifestation of many conditions, the following diagnoses must be excluded.

▶ *Inflammatory spondyloarthropathies.*   These disorders should be considered when multiple joints or areas are involved. Up to 16 percent of patients presenting with subcalcaneal pain will later be diagnosed with a systemic arthritic disorder.[43,73]

▶ *Calcaneal stress fracture.*[458]   The history for calcaneal stress fractures usually involves a sudden increase in a running activity, such as that seen in a military recruit at boot camp or a reservist.

▶ *Nerve entrapment.*[458–460]   Heel pain was recently reported to involve the nerve to the abductor digiti minimi, the first branch of the lateral plantar nerve.[461] In a fifth of cases of inferior heel pain, the pain may be caused by this nerve being trapped between the abductor digiti minimi muscle and the quadratus plantae muscle, or affected by inflammation of the plantar fascia.[461] Positive percussion (Tinel's sign) on the medial aspect of the heel should lead to a suspicion of entrapment of the nerve to the abductor digiti minimi or a tarsal tunnel syndrome.[43]

▶ *Tumors.*   Tumors in this area are quite rare, presenting as palpable masses or bony erosions of the calcaneus.

▶ *Infections.*[462]   As with infections in other parts of the body, there will usually be some swelling and/or erythema, and a history of malaise or fever.

▶ *Neuropathy (diabetic, alcoholic).*[458]   A history of burning pain, numbness, or paresthesias can often be elicited in patients with neuropathic pain. A thorough neurologic exam will confirm the diagnosis.

▶ *The fat pad syndrome.*[42,463]   Pain while hopping on the toes may help distinguish this entity from the fat pad syndrome.

The diagnosis of plantar fasciitis is typically made on the basis of clinical findings. Common findings include a history of pain and tenderness on the plantar medial aspect of the heel, especially during initial weight bearing in the morning. This is thought to be due to the fact that in the morning the plantar fascia is cold, contracted, or stiff.[453] The patient may also report pain that radiates up the calf and toward the toes. In severe cases, the pain may have a throbbing or burning quality. Interference with daily activities is common.[456] Plantar fasciitis is usually unilateral, although in 15 to 30 percent of people, both feet are affected.[73,457] The heel pain often decreases during the day but worsens with increased activity (such as jogging, climbing stairs, or going up on the toes) or after a period of sitting.

Upon physical examination, there will be localized pain on palpation along the medial edge of the fascia or at its origin on the anterior edge of the calcaneus, although firm finger pressure is often necessary to localize the point of maximum tenderness.[43] The main area of tenderness is typically just over and distal to the medial calcaneal tubercle, and usually there is one small exquisitely painful area. Tenderness in the center of the posterior part of the heel may be due to bruising or atrophy of the heel pad or to subcalcaneal bursitis.[442] Slight swelling in the area is common.[447] Tightness of the Achilles tendon is found in 78 percent of patients.[442,447]

To test for plantar fasciitis, the fascia needs to be put on stretch with a bowstring type test. The patient's heel is manually fixed in eversion. The clinician takes hold of the first metatarsal and places it in dorsiflexion before extending the big toe as far as possible. Pain should be elicited at the medial tubercle.

It is worth noting that almost 90 percent of patients with plantar fasciitis who undergo a conservative intervention improve significantly within 12 months, although approximately 10 percent can develop persistent and often disabling symptoms.[467] This time frame for resolution of symptoms suggests that present interventions are ineffective and that time alone heals the patient. The interventions thus far attempted include:

▶ Night splinting.

▶ Orthotics.

▶ Taping.

▶ Heel cups.

▶ Stretching and strengthening.

▶ Deep frictional massage.

▶ Corticosteroid injection.

▶ Dexamethasone iontophoresis.

▶ Shoe modifications.

▶ NSAIDs.

▶ Casting.

▶ Extracorporeal shock wave lithotripsy[465a]

▶ Radiofrequency lesioning.

▶ Open and endoscopic plantar fasciotomy and surgical neurolysis (in extremely recalcitrant cases). It has been reported that approximately 5% of patients who are diagnosed with plantar fasciitis undergo surgery for the condition.[465b,467]

A number of clinical trials have attempted to examine the efficacy of some of the interventions for plantar fasciitis. Lynch et al.[465c] performed an unblinded prospective trial of 103 subjects with plantar fasciitis randomized into one of three groups of treatment: anti-inflammatory (NSAIDS and steroid injections), accommodative (viscoelastic heel cup), or mechanical (taping for 4 weeks followed by custom orthoses). At the end of 3 months, there was no significant difference in activity level and first step pain between the groups. However, the mechanical treatment group (taping) had significantly better VAS scores than the accommodative group (heel cup) and had a significantly better rate of fair or excellent outcomes.

The University of Pittsburgh Medical Center Foot and Ankle Clinic has advocated non-surgical treatment of insertional plantar fasciitis using a standardized regimen since 1992.[465d] The regimen is as follows:

▶ Take NSAIDs as directed for 4 weeks.

▶ Go to the University of Pittsburgh Sports Medicine Clinic for a one-time instructional home exercise program of Achilles stretching (four exercises) and plantar fascia stretching (two exercises). The subject is instructed to continue the exercises for six sets, holding each for 30 sec × 3/day.

▶ Wear a night splint every night to bed.

▶ Use an orthosis or heel cup at all times when wearing shoes.

The reported outcomes in this study were not as good as the average outcome reported in other published studies with only 51 percent being asymptomatic after 4 months.[465d] The authors cited that the reasons for this were that other studies may have included subjects with causes of subcalcaneal heel pain other than true plantar fasciitis, making direct comparison difficult.

The lack of a universal intervention for plantar fasciitis, and the poor level of success, likely stems from its many causes. A poor response to an intervention may be due, in part, to inappropriate and nonspecific techniques or to inaccurate diagnosis. The etiological trauma for plantar fasciitis occurs after the peak loads of heel strike are reached as the center of mass advances beyond the ankle.[465e] This would tend to indicate that the forces associated with heel strike are not directly linked with the stresses that are applied to the plantar fascia. Indeed, the highest force loads on the foot during gait occur at the forefoot. These forces have been found to be 15 to 25 percent higher than those occurring during heel strike. Fortunately, the foot has a built in mechanism to deal with these loads—the Windlass mechanism.[465e] As the heel rises about the rotating metatarsophalangeal joints, the plantar fascia through its insertion into the bases of the digits, "winds" itself around the drumlike metatarsal heads. This creates a winchlike effect that pulls the proximal aspect of the heel closer to the ball of the foot and elevates the medial longitudinal arch, which in turn provides a stable platform upon which propulsion can occur. Critical to the efficiency of the

Windlass mechanism is the ability of the first metatarsophalangeal joint to dorsiflex during the heel raise phase of gait.[465f] An inability to dorsiflex the first MTP is called functional hallux limitus (see "Examination").[465f]

Given the number of interventions at the clinician's disposal, experimenting with several different interventions is often necessary before finding those that help. The mainstay of the intervention should include rest or at least elimination of any activity that continually provides axial loading of the heel and tensile stresses on the fascia.

Shoes that provide good shock absorption at the heel and support to the medial longitudinal arch and plantar fascia band should be recommended.[464,465] The clinician must identify any tissue overloading that is occurring, as well as any functional biomechanical deficits (plantar flexor inflexibility and weakness) and functional adaptations (running on toes, shortened stride length, foot inversion).[453]

A regimen of stretching of the gastrocnemius[455] and the medial fascial band is especially important before arising in the morning and after sedentary periods during the day, as well as before and after exercise.[465]

▶ *Gastrocnemius and soleus.* Patients are taught how to stretch the gastrocnemius and soleus components of the triceps surae independently. The stretching must be performed in such a way as to minimize stress on the plantar fascia. After a warm up, the patient stands against a wall with their hands placed against the wall. With one foot forward and one behind, the patient leans their trunk toward the wall, shifting their weight over the front foot, while straightening the knee of the back leg. The heel of the back foot should remain on the floor while the front of the foot is internally rotated and supinated, to stabilize the medial longitudinal arch, putting the foot in the close pack position, and allowing for the stretch to be isolated to the Achilles tendon.[73] The stretch is then repeated on the other leg. A similar stretch can be done by standing on a stair step with only the toes on the stairs and the back two thirds of the feet hang off the step. By leaning forward to balance, the heel, Achilles tendon, and calf will be stretched. The stretch can also be performed when standing where the heel is on the floor and the front part of the foot is on a wooden 2 × 4.

▶ *Plantar fascia stretch.* The plantar fascia stretch is performed with the patient sitting with their legs crossed, with the involved leg over the contralateral leg. Then, while using the hand on the affected side, the patient places their fingers across the base of the toes on the bottom of the foot (distal to the metatarsophalangeal joints) and pulls the toes back toward the shin until a stretch is felt in the arch of the foot. The correct stretch is confirmed by palpating the tension in the plantar fascia with the contralateral hand while performing the stretching. In a prospective randomized trial from DiGiovanni et al.[465g] One hundred and one patients who had chronic proximal plantar fasciitis for at least ten months

were randomized into one of two treatment groups. The mean age was forty-six years. All patients received prefabricated soft insoles and a three-week course of celecoxib, and they also viewed an educational video on plantar fasciitis. The patients received instructions for either a plantar fascia tissue-stretching program (Group A) or an Achilles tendon-stretching program (Group B). All patients completed the pain subscale of the Foot Function Index and a subject-relevant outcome survey that incorporated generic and condition-specific outcome measures related to pain, function, and satisfaction with treatment outcome. The patients were reevaluated after eight weeks. Eighty-two patients returned for follow-up evaluation. With the exception of the duration of symptoms ($P < .01$), covariates for baseline measures revealed no significant differences between the groups. The pain subscale scores of the Foot Function Index showed significantly better results for the patients managed with the plantar fascia-stretching program with respect to item 1 (worst pain; $P = .02$) and item 2 (first steps in the morning; $P = .006$).[465g] Analysis of the response rates to the outcome measures also revealed significant differences with respect to pain, activity limitations, and patient satisfaction, with greater improvement seen in the group managed with the plantar fascia-stretching program.

The stretches are performed twice a day, beginning with a sustained stretch for 1 minute and progressing to 3 minutes as tolerated.[461] The rest period should entail gentle dorsiflexion and plantar flexion while resting the Achilles tendon and calf on a hot pack to enhance the subsequent stretch and utilize an active rest period.[73] Massage to the foot in the area of the arch and heel or rolling the foot over a tennis ball or 15-ounce tin can may also be helpful.

Orthotics may have a role in the intervention of plantar fasciitis, but only after careful examination of the footwear to ensure a firm, well-fitting heel counter, good heel cushioning, and an adequate longitudinal arch support.[466] A wide variety of rigid, semirigid, and soft shoe inserts are available commercially, although rigid plastic orthoses rarely alleviate the symptoms and often aggravate the heel pain.[442] Orthoses made of softer materials provide cushioning by reducing the shock of walking by up to 42 percent.[43] Because the plantar fascia is stretched during flattening of the foot, orthoses should be designed to maintain the medial longitudinal arch during ambulation, and should be prescribed in full length or three-quarters length accommodative inlays of medium density plastazote.[43]

The type of orthotic prescribed depends on the findings:[73]

▶ *Normal foot.* Off-the-shelf heel cups should be used to cushion the heel. Cyriax recommended heel lifts to relieve the strain on the plantar fascia during early treatment,[132] and bilateral heel lifts of ¼ to ⅜ inch are sometimes successful, but their use should be discontinued at the earliest possible time.[75]

▶ *Pes planus (flat foot).* For this foot type, the orthotic is used to stabilize the arch and thereby decrease the strain on the plantar fascia. A University of California-Biomechanics Laboratory (UC-BL)–type of orthotic is indicated.

▶ *Pes cavus (high arch).* An excessively high arch or cavus foot can cause an inability to evert the foot to dissipate stress. In this situation, the orthotic of choice would be one that focuses on cushioning to increase the total contact area of the foot.

Taping can be considered as a means of either reinforcing the calcaneal fat pad and/or the medial longitudinal arch. The tape of choice is a low-die one-inch tape.[467a] Prior to applying tape, the patient should be relaxed, and the heel and foot placed in neutral. Excessive tension through the strips will lead to complaints during activity. Have the patient bear weight throughout the foot before applying the final closing strips. Care must be taken when applying the tape on the medial, lateral or dorsal aspect of the foot. Tension in the tape flow is critical if skin breakdown is to be avoided with repeated taping.[467a]

Recalcitrant or long-standing cases of plantar fasciitis may require casting. This can take the form of a short-leg walking cast positioned in neutral (plantigrade) for 4 to 6 weeks. Patients with severe pain and marked limitation of activity are best treated with a molded, below knee, walking cast for 3 to 4 weeks.[43] It provides relative rest, reduces pressure on the heel at heel strike, provides an arch support, and prevents tightening of the Achilles tendon.

A night splint positioned in 5 degrees of dorsiflexion is worn for an additional 6 weeks once the cast is removed, and the patient can resume the stretching and strengthening program for an additional 6 weeks once the cast is removed.[73]

A number of strengthening exercises have been devised for plantar fasciitis:

▶ *Towel curls.* A towel is placed on a smooth surface, with the foot placed on the towel. The patient is instructed to pull the towel toward the body by curling up the toes.

▶ *Marble pick-ups.* A few marbles are placed on the floor near a cup. While keeping the heel on the floor, the patient uses the toes to pick up the marbles and drop them in the cup.

▶ *Toe taps.* The patient is instructed to keep the heel on the floor and lift all of the toes off the floor. The patient is asked to tap the big toe to the floor while keeping the outside four toes in the air. Next, the patient keeps the big toe in the air while tapping the other four toes to the floor.

Bursitis

Retrocalcaneal Bursitis. Retrocalcaneal bursitis is a distinct entity denoted by pain that is anterior to the Achilles tendon, just superior to its insertion on the os calcis. This type of bursitis appears to be more common in older individuals and low-level recreational athletes.[76,468]

The bursa becomes inflamed, hypertrophied, and adherent to the underlying tendon, resulting in deep pain and visible swelling.[45,76] Characteristic findings include pain with a two-finger squeeze just superior and anterior to the Achilles insertion, and pain with passive dorsiflexion.[64]

Retrocalcaneal bursitis is treated conservatively with shoe modifications (open backed if necessary), and a heel lift.[64] In rare cases a bursectomy with associated resection of the posterior superior margin of the os calcis is necessary.

A small percentage of the population has an adventitious subcalcaneal bursa, which may become inflamed and cause heel pain.[443]

Anterior Ankle Bursitis. Anterior ankle bursitis is commonly seen in young figure skaters and ice hockey players.[64] This condition can present with swelling over the anterior ankle or over the malleoli. A doughnut pad inside the skate over the irritable area will usually decrease the pressure at this point.[64]

Haglund's Deformity. Haglund's deformity[469] refers to an abnormal prominence of the posterior superior lateral border of the calcaneus. Because of its association with various shoe types, it is often referred to as a "pump bump,"[470] high heel,[471] and winter heel.[472,473]

The prominence is frequently a bony spur or osteophyte acquired through subcutaneous pressure as the result of poorly fitting shoes in adolescent females, ice skaters, soccer players, and runners,[159] but it is also thought to be a congenital variation.

Whatever the etiology of these various prominences, they frequently aggravate the retrocalcaneal bursa on the deep surface of the Achilles tendon, producing an associated retrocalcaneal bursitis or Achilles tendonitis.[64]

On physical exam, a bump, which is 2 to 3 cm in diameter, is usually located more to the lateral side of the heel, and there is often an accompanying thickening of the overlying skin. Pain is often noted on palpation just proximal and slightly lateral to the insertion of the Achilles tendon.[465] Sometimes a varus hindfoot is found. A cavus or high-arched foot is believed to change the calcaneal position and increase the prominence of this ridge.[465]

Before intervention is initiated, the differential diagnosis must be considered, including systemic disease, Achilles tendonitis, or intrinsic conditions of the calcaneus, such as infection and tumor.[64]

Intervention involves relieving the friction imposed by the shoe counter by using a softer heel counter, increasing shoe size by one half, padding the prominence, or using a heel lift to actually raise the heel out of the shoe.[76,473,474] Achilles stretching and strengthening and the use of local modalities such as ultrasound are also recommended.[64]

Surgical excision of the deformity is reserved for persistent symptoms in the young athlete.[470,473,475]

Metatarsalgia

During the normal gait cycle, the center of pressure progresses along the plantar aspect of the foot from the heel at heel strike to the toes at toe-off. The center of pressure is initially located in the central heel, then accelerates rapidly across the midfoot to reach the forefoot, where it is located under the second and third metatarsal head, rather than under the first and fifth metatarsal head and the calcaneus, as was once thought.[56,93,98] This weight-bearing force is approximately equal to the body weight, which is more than twice the load carried by the other toes combined.

Any biomechanical intrinsic or extrinsic condition that increases stress on the metatarsal heads may result in metatarsal head pain and the development of painful plantar keratoses or calluses.[158] Plantar keratoses may be diffuse and large, or small and discrete.

▶ A Morton's foot with a short first metatarsal and a relatively long second metatarsal may result in increased loading of the second metatarsal head and the development of a painful callus.[476]

▶ Patients with abnormally lax first metatarsal-cuneiform joints resulting in a hypermobile first ray can experience increased weight bearing under the second and third metatarsals, which often results in painful diffuse calluses.[56]

▶ A prominent lateral condyle of a lesser metatarsal can result in a smaller discrete plantar keratosis, which can be exquisitely tender to palpation.

▶ A tight Achilles tendon can increase forefoot load in late stance phase and may result in metatarsalgia.[56]

▶ The use of high-heeled shoes extrinsically increases forefoot load and may lead to diffuse metatarsalgia.

The intervention for metatarsalgia involves the use of a metatarsal pad that is placed proximal to the painful metatarsal heads. Adhesive-backed metatarsal pads of different shapes and sizes are available to unload one or several metatarsal heads. Custom orthotics may also be molded specifically for the cavus foot to decrease load on the plantarflexed first and second rays in order to distribute weight evenly across the forefoot. A patient with a hypermobile first ray will benefit from a custom longitudinal arch support with medial forefoot post. A trial of Achilles stretching is helpful in the initial treatment of metatarsalgia. The wearing of high heels should be discouraged in patients with metatarsalgia.

If unresponsive to conservative intervention, surgical plantar condylectomy may be required for resolution of a discrete plantar keratosis. More generalized diffuse painful calluses such as those seen under the first and second metatarsal heads in the cavus foot may require dorsal closing wedge osteotomies of the metatarsal bases to achieve pain relief.[158]

Idiopathic Synovitis. Idiopathic synovitis of the second or third MTP joint is another cause of metatarsalgia. This condition results in painful distension of the joint, swelling of the second toe, warmth, and limited MTP joint motion.[477] Second MTP joint synovitis probably occurs as a result of attrition of the plantar plate due to a long second metatarsal.[478]

Dorsal instability of the MTP joint may develop with joint subluxation or dislocation. A hammer toe or claw toe deformity is common.

Initially the patient develops pain on palpation in the plantar and dorsal aspects of the MTP joint. Joint instability can be diagnosed with passive articular mobility testing.

Conservative intervention includes nonsteroidal anti-inflammatory medication, a metatarsal pad, taping the toe in a plantar flexed position, and an accommodative shoe. An intra-articular corticosteroid injection in combination with a rocker-sole modification has been shown to result in improvement in 93 percent of 15 cases.[479] Persistent pain in the second MTP joint despite conservative measures may necessitate operative synovectomy to avert toe dislocation or deformity.

Metatarsalgia of the Fifth Toe. This is usually due to overwork of the peroneus longus/brevis secondary to an unstable ankle. The overwork of the brevis leads to an instability of the fifth metatarsal at the intermetatarsal or cubometatarsal joints. The patient will point to the tubercle of the fifth metatarsal and complain of pain along the proximal part of the peroneus muscle. Conservative intervention involves taping a strip of tape over the dorsum of the foot and then one strip on the medial aspect, going proximal to distal. These two strips are then connected with strips of tape under the foot, across the sole.

Anterior Ankle Impingement

Anterior ankle impingement can be bony or soft tissue related. Patients with this problem usually present with anterior ankle pain exacerbated by extreme dorsiflexion.[22,64]

A bony impingement can be seen in young ballet dancers who exercise extreme ankle dorsiflexion, irritating the periosteum on the talar neck, leading to an exostosis and discomfort with pliés.[440]

A form of soft tissue impingement can be secondary to generalized synovitis or capsulitis. This can develop after acute or recurrent episodes of an inversion ankle sprain or in adolescent gymnasts who sustain repeated forced dorsiflexion in landing and dismount.

Chronic anterolateral ankle impingement due to a thickened and scarred joint capsule is a frequent sequela of recurrent ankle sprains. Wolin and associates[480] reported in 1950 that recurrent pain and swelling after injury to the lateral ligaments without instability in patients with a history of previous ankle sprains was due to hyalinized connective tissue arising from the anteroinferior portion of the talofibular joint capsule. They believed the symptoms resulted from this connective tissue becoming pinched in the talofibular joint with motion. As this mass of tissue and synovium increases in size, impingement of the tissue mass between the talus, tibia, and fibula causes further irritation and pain. This has since been confirmed arthroscopically and by MRI.[481–488]

Bassett and colleagues[489] reported a cause of chronic pain in the ankle after inversion sprain in seven patients as being due to talar impingement by a distal fascicle of the anterior inferior tibiofibular ligament.

On physical exam, there is usually pain to palpation anteriorly with no palpable swelling.[296] Plain ankle radiographs can be helpful in determining a bony problem, but a bone scan is usually necessary for a definitive diagnosis. MRI may also be diagnostic.

The intervention for the soft tissue impingement variety includes discontinuing landing temporarily, icing,[389] anti-inflammatories, and exercises to stretch the Achilles tendon and strengthen the dorsiflexors. Occasionally, a pad taped over the anterior ankle may provide temporary relief.[296] Arthroscopy may be indicated if conservative treatment fails. A partial synovectomy[490] or excision of osteophytes is successful, but must be followed by exercises to prevent recurrence.

Posterior Ankle Impingement

Posterior ankle impingement or talar compression syndrome[67] is seen most often in young female dancers, ice skaters, or gymnasts.[64] These sports require excessive plantar flexion of the ankle, compressing the posterior structures of the ankle.[67,386]

On physical exam, the patient will have pain on palpation of the posterior ankle, dramatically increased with forced plantar flexion.[64]

Plain radiographs of the ankle can be taken to rule out a bony etiology (ie, os trigonum).[67] Soft tissue etiology includes FHL irritation, thickened or invaginated posterior capsule, synovitis, and calcific debris.[386,491,492]

Sesamoiditis

This condition has been defined as inflammation and swelling of the peritendinous structures of the sesamoids. The tibial (medial) and fibular (lateral) sesamoids are situated under the first metatarsal head. These sesamoids are prone to injury in repetitive high impact and contact sports.[56] Because the tibial sesamoid bears most of the force under the first metatarsal head, it is most commonly injured.[56]

Although direct trauma or forced dorsiflexion of the great toe can acutely fracture the sesamoids, most sesamoid injuries are overuse injuries. Twelve percent of injuries to the great toe complex are sesamoid injuries.[58]

The etiologies of sesamoid injuries include stress fracture (40 percent), acute fractures (10 percent), chondromalacia, synovitis, sesamoiditis (30 percent), osteochondritis (10 percent), arthritis (5 percent), and bursitis (5 percent).[58] Bipartite or multipartite sesamoids occur in 5 to 33 percent of the population and are bilateral in 25 percent.[61,493]

The diagnosis of sesamoiditis is one of exclusion.[494] Sesamoiditis is associated with local trauma, pain on weight bearing, and plantar soft tissue swelling.[495] Passive dorsiflexion of the MTP joint while palpating the sesamoids exacerbates the pain. Sesamoidal bursitis presents with swelling, erythema, and tenderness with side-to-side pinch. A plantar fullness or fluid-filled bursal cyst may be palpated under the sesamoids.

Conservative intervention involves rest from the offending activity, nonsteroidal anti-inflammatory medication, and low heeled shoes with a soft metatarsal support proximal to the metatarsal head, to decrease the load on the involved sesamoid.[496] One or two injections of corticosteroids into the region of the sesamoids may be helpful.[56] Failure of several months of conservative care may result in the need for surgical excision of the offending sesamoid to alleviate symptoms.[496]

Medial Tibial Stress Syndrome

Exercise-induced anterior and medial leg pain has been reported to account for 60 percent of all injuries causing leg pain in athletes.[497] Over the past 30 years, a number of generic terms such as "medial tibial syndrome," "tibial stress syndrome," "shin splints," "posterior tibial syndrome," "soleus syndrome," and "periostitis" have evolved to describe exercise-related leg pain. Of all these terms, medial tibial stress syndrome (MTSS) is the most appropriate.

Neither the precise pathophysiologic mechanism nor the specific pathologic lesion in MTSS is known, although it appears to involve periosteal irritation indicated by a diffuse linear uptake on a bone scan along the length of the tibia.[498] The anatomic site of the abnormality has been fairly well localized. Initially it was thought that the tibialis posterior muscle was the source. However, recent information has identified the fascial insertion of the medial soleus as the most probable source.

The most common complaint in these patients is a dull aching pain along the middle or distal posteromedial tibia. Early in this process, the pain may occur at the beginning of a run, resolve with continued exertion, only to recur toward the end or after a workout.[499] Alternatively, the pain may only be noted toward the end of a run. At this early stage, the pain typically subsides promptly with rest.[499] With continued training the pain may become more severe, sharp, and persistent.[499] Patients may attempt trials of complete rest only to have the pain recur with resumption of training. With increasing chronicity, the pain may be present with ambulation or at rest.[499]

Overuse or weakness of the tibialis anterior, extensor digitorum longus, or extensor digitorum brevis may be causative factors in anterior shin splints, as are training errors and inadequate footwear.[89]

With the exception of pain and point tenderness at the anteromedial aspect of the tibia, which is increased with active dorsiflexion and passive stretching into plantar flexion, there are few objective findings. However, the pain is usually provoked with activity and relieved with rest.

As with most overuse injuries, the intervention for shin splints involves activity modification, followed by a gradual return to sports, making sure to identify and correct any training errors or abnormal foot biomechanics.

Preferred Practice Pattern 5F: Impaired Joint Mobility, Motor Function, Muscle Performance, Range of Motion, or Reflex Integrity Secondary to Peripheral Nerve Injury

An entrapment neuropathy is characterized by an entrapment of a peripheral nerve by fascia, a ligament, a bony groove, or a tendinous arch of a muscle origin. Sural nerve neuropraxias and peroneal nerve palsies are an infrequent complication of lateral ligamentous injuries of the ankle, but are quite problematic.[22,133] Electromyographic evaluation of patients with ankle sprains reveals that up to 80 percent of patients with severe ankle sprains have some evidence of peroneal nerve injury.[22,133]

Interdigital Neuroma

The name of the condition is a misnomer, as a true neuroma does not exist. Rather, there is a thickening of the tissues around the nerve due to perineural fibrosis, fibrinoid degeneration, demyelination, and endoneural fibrosis.[56,500] In a study of 91 patients with interdigital neuromas, the male:female ratio was 1:9.[501]

Although a common cause of this condition is chronic compression of the interdigital nerve, it can also arise due to an acute dorsiflexion injury to the toes with an associated injury to the collateral ligaments of the MTP joint.[56,155]

Symptoms are usually exacerbated with weight bearing and somewhat relieved by removing the shoe and massaging the forefoot.[56,155] Poor shoe selection, such as wearing a firm cross-training or racket shoe for long-distance running may increase the impact forces on the forefoot and contribute to neuroma symptoms.[56] Narrow shoes and high-heeled shoes have also been implicated.

Physical examination reveals tenderness in the web space plantarly between the metatarsal heads.[56] Squeezing the forefoot with one hand while carefully palpating the involved interspace with the thumb and index fingers of the other hand is usually successful in eliciting marked discomfort.[56] This compression may produce a painful audible click, known as Mulder's sign.[502] Careful palpation of the MTP joint, metatarsal head, and proximal phalanx should be performed to rule out localized joint or bone pathology such as MTP joint synovitis, stress fracture, or Freiberg's disease, which can also cause symptoms of forefoot pain.[56] A positive Tinel's sign over the tarsal tunnel or multiple symptomatic web spaces should alert the clinician to the possibility of a more proximal nerve compression or underlying peripheral neuropathy.[56] Electromyographic studies and nerve conduction velocity testing should be performed in these cases.[155]

The intervention initially entails avoiding the offending activity, cross-training in lower-impact sports and modification of footwear.[56] A switch to wider, more accommodating shoes with soft soles and better shock absorption will often improve symptoms.[56] A metatarsal pad, such as an adhesive-backed felt pad, placed proximal to the symptomatic interspace is helpful.[56] The metatarsal pad can also be incorporated into a custom-made full-length semirigid orthotic.[56] A trial of nonsteroidal anti-inflammatory drugs is indicated in an attempt to decrease inflammation around the interdigital nerve.[56] A trial of vitamin B_6 has been used successfully in the treatment of carpal tunnel syndrome and may also be useful in the treatment of interdigital neuritis.[503]

Recalcitrant cases that fail to respond to 2 to 3 months of the above conservative measures may benefit from an injection of corticosteroids into the involved interspace.[56] One to two injec-

tions can be tried, but multiple injections should be avoided as corticosteroids may cause atrophy of the plantar fat pad.[56] Surgery is the intervention of last resort.

Deep Peroneal Nerve Entrapment/Anterior Tarsal Tunnel Syndrome

Entrapment of the deep peroneal nerve was first reported in 1963,[504] and was given the name anterior tarsal tunnel syndrome in 1968.[505]

At the ankle level, both motor and sensory branches of the deep peroneal nerve are present (Fig. 19-56).

Anterior tarsal syndrome[506] occurs when there is a contusion to the terminal branch of the deep peroneal nerve, as it travels beneath the posterior tibialis and extensor hallucis brevis tendons, and above the first and second cuneiforms, where it is relatively unprotected.[507] The compression usually results from tight boots or the shoe straps of high heels, a ganglion, pes cavus, or from direct trauma.[506,508] A partial anterior tarsal tunnel syndrome[509] occurs when either the motor branch to the extensor digitorum brevis or only the sensory branch of the deep peroneal nerve is compressed beneath the inferior extensor retinaculum.[507]

Patients with anterior tarsal tunnel syndrome complain of a deep aching pain in the medial and dorsal aspect of the foot, burning around the nail of the great toe, and pins and needles at the adjacent borders of the great and second toes that are exacerbated with plantar flexion and improved with rest.[507,508,510,511]

The examination reveals weakness or atrophy of the extensor digitorum brevis muscle, and diminished movement with toe extension.[507]

Conservative intervention for these patients involves an alteration of daily and sports activities, alteration in footwear, orthotics, and if necessary NSAIDs.[507]

Surgical intervention, reserved for those who do not respond to conservative measures within 3 months, involves decompression of the nerve.[507]

Superficial Peroneal Nerve

Although injuries to the superficial nerve at the level of the ankle are relatively rare, the nerve can be stretched with lateral (inversion) ankle sprains, or become entrapped as it pierces the deep fascia to become subcutaneous about 4 to 5 inches above the lateral malleolus.[155,512–516]

Patients complain of diminished sensation on the dorsum of the foot, which is exacerbated with activity.

Tarsal Tunnel Syndrome

Tarsal tunnel syndrome (TTS) is an entrapment neuropathy of the tibial nerve as it passes through the anatomic tunnel between the flexor retinaculum and the medial malleolus (also see Chapter 9). In addition, the terminal branches of the tibial nerve, the medial, and lateral plantar nerves may be involved. These latter nerves are often called the posterior tibial nerve. The onset of TTS may be acute or insidious. Differential diagnosis includes plantar fasciitis, chronic heel pain syndrome, and

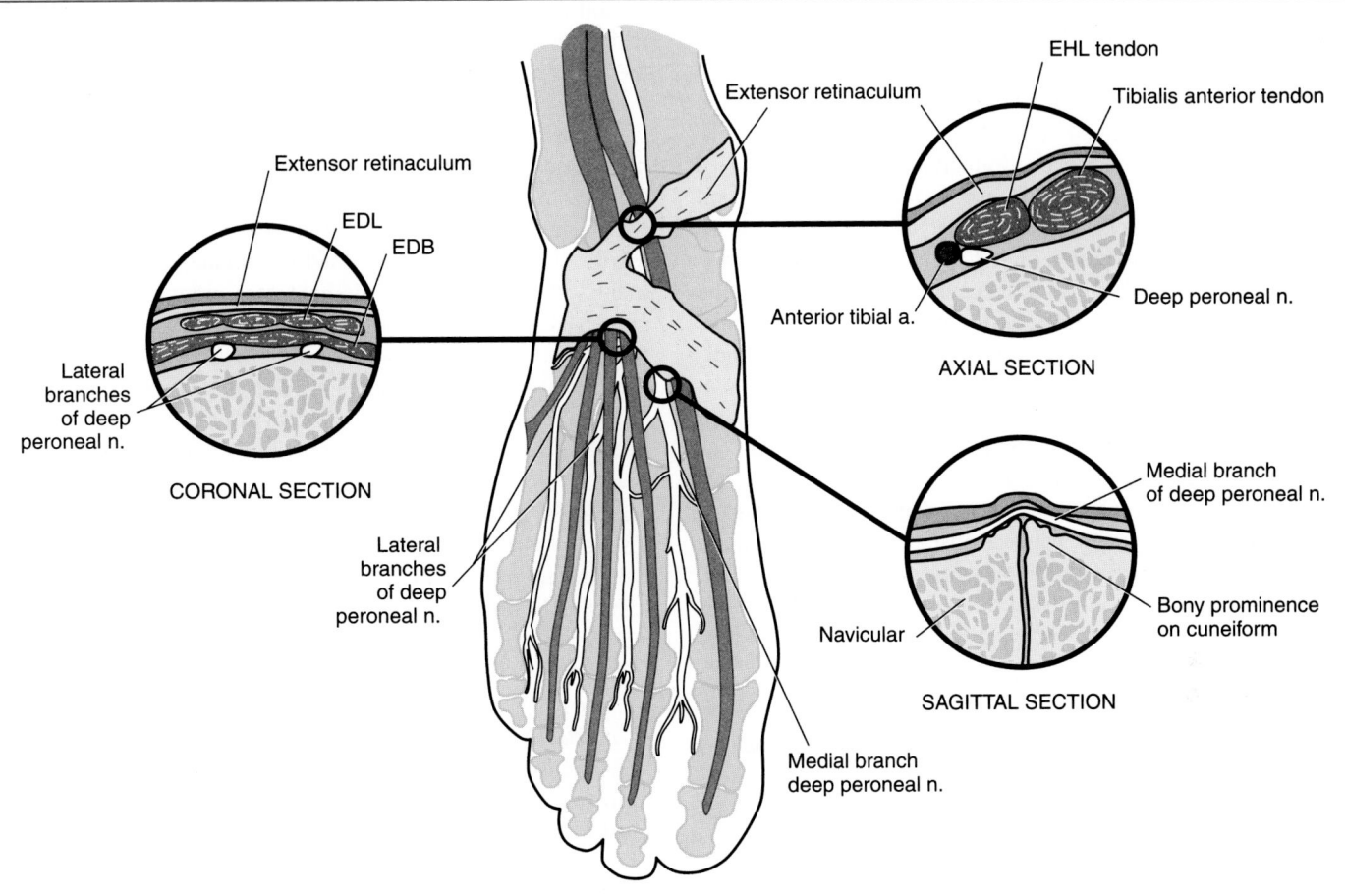

FIGURE 19-56 Sites of deep peroneal nerve entrapment. EDB, extensor digitorum brevis; EDL, extensor digitorum longus; EHL, extensor hallucis longus. (Reproduced with permission from Kelikian AS. *Operative Treatment of the Foot and Ankle.* New York: Appleton-Lange; 1999.)

flexor hallucis longus tenosynovitis. The clinical findings for TTS are outlined in Chapter 9. Etiologic factors for TTS can be classified as internal or external. Internal factors include anatomical variations such as an accessory flexor digitorum longus muscle. External factors include excessive pronation, which can tighten the flexor retinaculum and the calcaneonavicular ligament. Conservative intervention for TTS includes the use of orthotics to correct biomechanical gait abnormalities. Specifically a foot orthosis with a rearfoot varus post can limit excessive pronation. In cases of early excessive rearfoot pronation and subtalar joint pronation at heel strike, an orthosis with a deepened heel cup can help to control rearfoot motion. In cases of severe hyperpronation, a rearfoot wedge may be helpful.

Peripheral Neuropathy

Peripheral neuropathy is characterized by a progressive loss of nerve fibers that predisposes the patient to painful or insensitive extremities, vascular compromise and neuropathic ulceration.[517,518] In more severe cases, uncontrolled peripheral neuropathy can result in amputation. Affected nerve functions associated with peripheral neuropathy include reduced nerve conduction velocity, decreased temperature sensation, decreased tendon reflex response, alterations in autonomic function, and a decreased ability to detect vibration and touch. Peripheral neuropathy is a complication of both insulin dependent (type 1) and non-insulin-dependent (type 2) diabetes mellitus.[517,518]

A loss of sensation in the legs and feet prevents the patient from detecting minor cuts or trauma, which can become infected placing these patients at high risk for developing a neuropathic ulcer. Motor neuropathy may cause muscle atrophy and imbalances, which can lead to foot deformity and increased pressure on the plantar aspect of the foot. This is particularly true with the diabetic patient who participates in sports, where the forces acting on the sole of the foot can be significant. Autonomic dysfunction may lead to decreased perspiration and sebaceous oil production, which can cause dryness, cracking and, eventually, fissures in the skin. Good foot care is thus essential for these patients. It is recommended that the clinician regularly assess the general skin condition of the patient's foot and leg (dryness, cracks, and fissures) and the skin temperature.

Red and warm skin may indicate the presence of infection, cellulitis, or an undetected bone infection or fracture. Cold skin and pallor may indicate decreased blood flow. Other signs of vascular compromise can include diminished pulses and toe pressures, dry and shiny skin with no hair growth, and thickened flaky nails. Skin rashes and foul odor may be indicative of a fungal infection. Callus and corn formation, blisters, and bunions may highlight the presence of an ill-fitting shoe or a deformity (equines contracture, claw toes, and charcot arthropathy). Charcot (rocker bottom) foot occurs when the bones at the plantar aspect are prominent resulting in a diminished longitudinal arch and an increased potential for fracture. Other conditions to observe for include plantar warts and ingrown toenails.

Sensation of the foot can be tested using Semmes-Weinstein filaments, which are calibrated nylon monofilaments with increasing stiffness indicated by increasing numbers.[517,518] Protective sensation of the foot has been defined as the ability to sense a 5.07 monofilament, whereas absent sensation is defined as the inability to sense a 6.10 monofilament.[517]

The primary focus of intervention with this patient population is patient education regarding proper foot and nail inspection and care.

The following advice should be given:

▶ The feet should be washed every day in warm, not hot, water. Hot water dries the skin and can easily burn the foot. The water temperature can be tested using a thermometer. The feet should not be soaked to avoid skin maceration.

▶ The skin should be inspected at least once a day for cuts, bruises, blisters, swelling and calluses. A mirror can be used where necessary. If the skin is dry, lotion can be applied on the tops, bottoms and sides of the feet, but not between the toes, which can create a moist environment for fungal and bacterial infections.

▶ Toenails should be trimmed straight across with a nail clipper once a week. Rounding off the corners of the nails increases the potential of ingrown toenails and increases the potential for cutting the skin. If the patient has retinal neuropathy and poor eyesight, the nails are best trimmed by a family member or by a professional.

▶ The patient should avoid walking barefoot or from wearing sandals.

▶ The feet should be protected from hot or cold temperatures.

▶ The patient should exercise a little every day. Appropriate nonimpact exercises include cycling or swimming. Gait training may be appropriate to maintain mobility, and alter gait patterns to decrease abnormal plantar pressures.[517]

▶ If possible, the patient should stop smoking. Smoking causes the blood vessels to constrict.

Appropriate footwear and orthotics should be prescribed where appropriate to reduce plantar pressures, and increase the weight bearing area of the foot.[518a] The total contact cast (TCC) is considered the gold standard for ambulating patients due to its ability to reduce pressure on the midfoot and forefoot by distributing pressure over the total foot surface.[518a] Alternatively, the patient may be prescribed a prefabricated walker boot, or a bivalved ankle foot orthosis.

In the presence of a diabetic wound, frequent sharp debridement of nonviable tissue has been shown to be an effective method to speed wound healing.[518b] This can be performed with a scalpel and tweezers. Enzymatic debridement and autolytic debridement can be used as adjuncts to sharp debridement.[518b] Enzymatic debridement uses ointments that contain papain-urea or other enzymes that help break the bonds between necrotic tissue and wound bed. Autolytic debridement uses moisture retentive secondary dressings (hydrogels and hydrocolloids) to provide a moist environment, which helps to keep the wound fluids in contact with the wound bed.

Complex Regional Pain Syndrome

The more classic patient with complex regional pain syndrome will present with severe regional pain, swelling, dysesthesia to light touch (allodynia) and vasomotor instability, and the subjective report will be one of pain out of proportion to the degree of injury (see Chap. 9).[519]

Myofascial Pain Syndrome

Ankle or foot pain can arise, and trigger points in the tibialis anterior, extensor digitorum, or peroneus longus muscle are the most likely causes.[520]

Tibialis Anterior. Trigger points of this muscle can refer pain, tenderness, and stiffness deep into the anterior ankle and the great toe. These trigger points can be activated due to excessive pronation of the foot and excessive dorsiflexion.[520]

Extensor Digitorum. Trigger points of this muscle can refer pain and tenderness over the dorsum of the foot and into the middle three toes.

Peroneus Longus. Trigger points of this muscle can refer to just posterior to the lateral malleolus. This muscle is usually strained on inversion sprain injuries of the ankle and can therefore be the source of residual pain at the lateral ankle.[520]

Preferred Practice Pattern 4G: Impaired Joint Mobility, Motor Function, Muscle Performance, Range of Motion Associated with Fractures

Stress Fractures

A stress or fatigue fracture is a break that develops in bone after cyclical, submaximal loading. In the foot, the two most common locations for stress fractures are the metatarsal shaft and the calcaneus.[521]

Metatarsal Stress Fracture. Patients who abruptly increase their training, whether it be training mileage, time spent in high-impact activities, or training intensity, are susceptible to stress fractures.[56] The second and third metatarsals are the most frequently injured.[522] Military studies have found stress fractures to be more common in women, older individuals, and Caucasians.[523,524] Amenorrhea is present in up to 20 percent of vigorously exercising women, and may be as high as 50 percent in elite runners and dancers.[525] Women long-distance runners, ballet dancers, and gymnasts are notorious for dieting to achieve low body fat despite rigorous training schedules. Patients with amenorrhea for more than 6 months experience the same bone loss as postmenopausal women.[526] Whole body bone mineral density is significantly lower in amenorrheic athletes, which predisposes them to stress fracture.[526]

A recent study found the simulation of fatigue of the toe plantar flexors resulted in an increase in second metatarsal strain. Therefore muscular fatigue of the foot may play a role in the etiology of metatarsal stress fractures.[527]

Although numerous studies have attempted to correlate foot shape, footwear, and orthotics to the incidence of stress fractures, none have conclusively shown a direct relationship,[252,528–530] although one study showed a decrease in the incidence of metatarsal fractures in low-arched feet by using a semirigid orthotic.[95]

The patient with a metatarsal stress fracture usually reports mild forefoot discomfort, which may be relieved by rest, but as the stress fracture worsens, pain is experienced while walking and even at rest.[56] Occasionally, there is local point tenderness of the involved metatarsal, induration, swelling, and palpable mass.[522,531] Symptoms usually present 4 to 5 weeks after a change in training regimen.[522]

Anteroposterior, lateral, and oblique radiographs of the foot may not show a fracture for 3 to 6 weeks, although a technetium bone scan is positive as early as 48 to 72 hours after onset of symptoms.[56]

The intervention for metatarsal stress fractures includes rest from the offending activity and cross-training in a low-impact sport.[56] Weight bearing to tolerance may be allowed in comfortable shoes of choice or a wooden shoe. If weight bearing is painful, or the fracture is diagnosed late, a short leg cast or hard-soled shoe is worn for 4 to 6 weeks until healing callus is seen radiographically.[522,531]

Proximal Second Metatarsal. The proximal second metatarsal stress fracture differs from other metatarsal stress fractures because it can be difficult to heal, and may result in chronic nonunion. The anatomy in this area is such that the base of the shaft is countersunk into the bony arch of the foot and is therefore rigid (Lisfranc's joint). This tends to place an abnormal amount of stress across this area, particularly in young ballet dancers.[532–535]

Other predisposing factors can include amenorrhea, anorexia nervosa, cavus foot, and anterior ankle impingement with resulting hyperpronation.[532]

On physical exam, there will be pain in the first web space, usually accompanied by proximal second metatarsal pain.[536]

Initial foot radiographs will most often be negative; hence, a bone scan is usually necessary. The bone scan may be non-specific, with synovitis, stress reaction, and stress fracture as differential.[536]

The intervention for second metatarsal stress fracture usually consists of 6 to 8 weeks of rest in a hard shoe or cast,[532,536] with gradual return to activities when the tenderness resolves.

Navicular Stress Fracture. Although navicular stress fractures are uncommon, they are the most common midfoot fracture, and typically present with an insidious onset, or with a history of acute flexion and inversion.[11] Complaints include chronic pain that is vague in nature but tender to palpation on the dorsum of the foot and/or medial aspect of the midfoot.[522]

This condition is most commonly seen in basketball players, hurdlers, and runners, in whom repeated cyclic loading results in fatigue failure through the relatively avascular central portion of the tarsal navicular.[64,69,537] The cyclic loading across the navicular may be exacerbated due to a short first metatarsal, metatarsus adductus, or limited dorsiflexion or subtalar motion.[64]

To confirm the diagnosis, bone scan or CT scan may be necessary, as plain films are rarely diagnostic.[537]

The intervention varies according to the type of fracture. Nondisplaced fractures are treated with a short-leg non–weight-bearing cast for 6 to 8 weeks.[329,537]

If the fracture fails to heal or is displaced, operative intervention of fixation with compression screw, and additional bone grafting where necessary, is used.[329,537]

Return to sport may take as long as 16 to 20 weeks.[522]

Sesamoid Stress Fracture. The young patient with a sesamoid stress fracture will present with the insidious onset of pain and swelling over the plantar aspect of the first MTP joint.[69,538] Pain is usually aggravated by activity and relieved with rest. Differential diagnosis includes metatarsalgia, bursitis, sesamoiditis, and bipartite sesamoid.[538]

The intervention for a sesamoid fracture is initially rest from the offending high-impact activity and a wooden-soled shoe, or a short-leg cast for 6 to 8 weeks. If casted, a CT scan is performed at 8 weeks to detect signs of avascular necrosis. If avascular necrosis is present and the young patient has persistent symptoms, resection may be necessary.[59] Surgical choices include excision of the involved sesamoid or bone grafting in an attempt to achieve union and preserve the sesamoid.

An alternative treatment is the use of a "C" or "J" pad, which unloads the injured sesamoid. Pads with adhesive backing may be fixed to the insole of the shoe or may be incorporated into a custom molded orthotic to unload the sesamoid.

Fractures

Pilon Fractures. These fractures result from an axial compression force, where the tibia is driven down into the talus, splitting and shattering the distal end of the tibia and completely disrupting the ankle joint, resulting in long term morbidity in the majority of cases.[539]

Talar Dome Fractures. These are the most common chondral fractures, and are also known as osteochondritis dissecans, transchondral fractures, or flake fractures.[11]

These injuries, which present with persistent swelling, pain with walking, locking of the ankle, and crepitus, tend to present as a "sprained ankle that did not heal."[11]

Intervention varies from none, to casting, to arthroscopy for larger fragments.[11]

Talar Fractures. Major fractures of the talar head, neck, and body are associated with high-energy mechanisms, with one half of major talar injuries involving fractures of the talar neck, 15 to 20 percent involving talar body fractures, and the remainder involving talar head fractures.[11] The mechanism of injury usually involves an axial load with the foot in plantar flexion or excessive dorsiflexion, resulting in compression of the talar head against the anterior aspect of the tibia.[540]

The intervention varies according to location and severity, with non-displaced fractures treated with a short-leg non–weight-bearing cast for 6–8 weeks, and displaced fractures involving emergency reduction.[11]

Unimalleolar Fractures. Unimalleolar fractures are the most common fractures of the ankle.[11] The degree of stability of these fractures is dependent upon their location, with those located below the tibiotalar joint tending to be stable.[11] Approximately 85 percent of lateral malleolar fractures occur without damage to the medial aspect of the ankle joint, and do not cause abnormal displacement of the talus.[541,542]

Medial malleolar fractures are often seen in conjunction with other fractures.

Bimalleollar and Trimalleolar Fractures. These fractures, as their name implies, involve two or three malleoli. The bimalleolar fracture usually results from a severe pronation/abduction/external rotation force, which shears the lateral malleoli and avulses the medial malleolus. The trimalleolar fracture involves a fracture of the medial, lateral, and "posterior" malleolus, which typically results from an abduction and severe external rotation force so strong that the talus moves sufficiently posteriorly to shear off the posterior margin of the tibia.

The intervention for bimalleolar fractures remains controversial, whereas it is generally agreed that trimalleolar fractures require open reduction and internal fixation.[543]

Calcaneus. The calcaneus is the largest and most frequently fractured tarsal, accounting for over 60 percent of foot fractures,[544] and one which can be a frequent and often misdiagnosed cause of heel pain.[545] With the increasing number of middle-aged and elderly people involved in active recreational pursuits, sports medicine has had to incorporate the way these conditions are related to these different age groups.[64] Jumping activities or unaccustomed activities may precipitate crushing of the fragile architecture of an osteoporotic calcaneus, leading to fractures.[64]

Tenderness on mediolateral compression of the heel (squeeze test) should lead to a suspicion of a stress fracture of the calcaneus.[43]

Conservative intervention of calcaneal fractures has shown poor long-term clinical results with significant loss of ankle function.[546,547]

Metatarsal Fractures. All fractures of the proximal fifth metatarsal have been indiscriminately labeled a "Jones fracture." A true Jones fracture is an acute fracture of the proximal fifth metatarsal caused by forefoot adduction, that occurs at the diametaphyseal junction involving the fourth–fifth metatarsal articulation. The most common fifth metatarsal base fracture is an avulsion fracture of the tuberosity caused by traction of the peroneus brevis and lateral band of the plantar fascia during hindfoot inversion.[548]

The proximal fifth metatarsal has a poor blood supply and is at significant risk for delayed union or nonunion. These fractures should be treated with non–weight-bearing short-leg cast immobilization for 6 to 8 weeks or until healing is seen radiographically. If an established nonunion develops, screw fixation and/or bone grafting may be required.[549]

Therapeutic Techniques

Techniques to Increase Joint Mobility

Joint Mobilizations

With some slight variations, the same techniques that are used to examine the joint glides described in the test and measures sections can be used to mobilize the joints, with the clinician varying the intensity of the mobilizations based on patient response and the stage of tissue healing.

Mobilizations with Movement[550]

To Decrease Pain over the Medial Aspect of the Foot with Inversion. The pain on the medial side of the foot can be due to a positional fault of the base of the first metatarsal.[550] The patient is positioned in supine with their foot resting on the bed. The clinician stands on the involved side facing the patient's feet. Using one hand, the clinician stabilizes the shaft of the first metatarsal, while the other hand is used to grasp and stabilize the shaft of the second metatarsal. From this position, the clinician glides the base of the first metatarsal down on the second. While maintaining this glide, the patient is asked to invert the foot as the clinician applies a counterpressure up on the second metatarsal. If this maneuver is painless, the technique is repeated several times and the joint and motion is reassessed.

To Decrease Pain under the Transverse Arch (Anterior Metatarsalgia). This condition is characterized by pain under the heads of the middle metatarsals with toe flexion or extension.[550] The patient is positioned in supine with their foot resting on the bed. The clinician stands on the involved side at the foot of the bed. Using the pad of the thumb and index finger of one hand, the clinician grasps the head of one of the middle metatarsals (eg, the second). With the other thumb and index finger the clinician grasps the head of the adjacent metatarsal head (the third). The second metatarsal head is glided and held down on the third metatarsal head while the patient flexes the toes. If this is painful, the procedure is reversed so that the third metatarsal head is glided down on the second while the patient flexes their toes. The successful technique is repeated several times and the joint and range of motion is reassessed.

To Increase Ankle Plantar Flexion. The patient is positioned in supine with their knee flexed and the foot resting on the bed. The clinician stands at the foot of the bed. Using one hand, the clinician places the hypothenar eminence just proximal to the joint line and wraps the thumb and fingers around the lower leg. With the other hand, the clinician places the web space between the thumb and index finger around the talus so that the thumb and index finger slope slightly distally and lie just below the malleoli. The clinician adopts a lunge position with the legs. The tibia and fibula are glided as far posteriorly as possible using one hand. Without releasing this glide, the clinician rolls the talus ventrally with the other hand while the patient assists with the plantar flexion.

To Increase Ankle Dorsiflexion. The patient is positioned in prone with their knee extended and the ankle joint level with the end of the bed. A small towel roll is placed under the patient's ankle. The clinician stands at the foot of the bed. Using one hand, the clinician grasps the calcaneus and stabilizes it. The web space between the thumb and index finger of the other hand is wrapped around the back of the ankle. From this position, the calcaneus is pulled down towards the floor with one hand, while the other hand stabilizes the ankle (Fig. 19-57). The glide is maintained while the patient actively dorsiflexes the ankle. The maneuver is repeated several times, and the joint and range of motion are reassessed.

Techniques to Increase Soft Tissue Extensibility

Myofascial Techniques

Knee and Ankle Joint, Long-Axis Extension. The patient is positioned in supine, while the clinician stands with their back to the patient. With one hand the clinician firmly grasps the forefoot and talus. With the other hand the clinician holds the calcaneus. The clinician's elbow maintains long-axis extension, with pressure at the popliteal region. The clinician places the foot into corrective flexion-extension and abduction-adduction motions. Maintaining the above position, the clinician uses his cranial hand to create calcaneal inversion and eversion.

Muscle Energy Techniques

Gastrocnemius. Muscle imbalances of the gastrocnemius can result from chronic adaptive shortening.

The patient is positioned in supine with their knees extended, their subtalar joint in neutral, and the ankle dorsiflexed to the point of first resistance. The patient is asked to actively plantarflex their foot against the clinician's equal and opposite force (Fig. 19-58). The contraction is held for 10 seconds, and then the patient actively dorsiflexes the ankle to the new point of resistance; three to five repetitions are performed.

Soleus. The patient is positioned in prone with the knee flexed to 90 degrees, and the subtalar joint in neutral. The clinician passively dorsiflexes the patient's foot to the resistance barrier. The patient is asked to actively plantarflex against the clinician's equal and opposite force. The contraction is held for 10 seconds, after which the patient relaxes, and the ankle is passively dorsiflexed to the new barrier; three to five sets are performed before reassessing the motion.

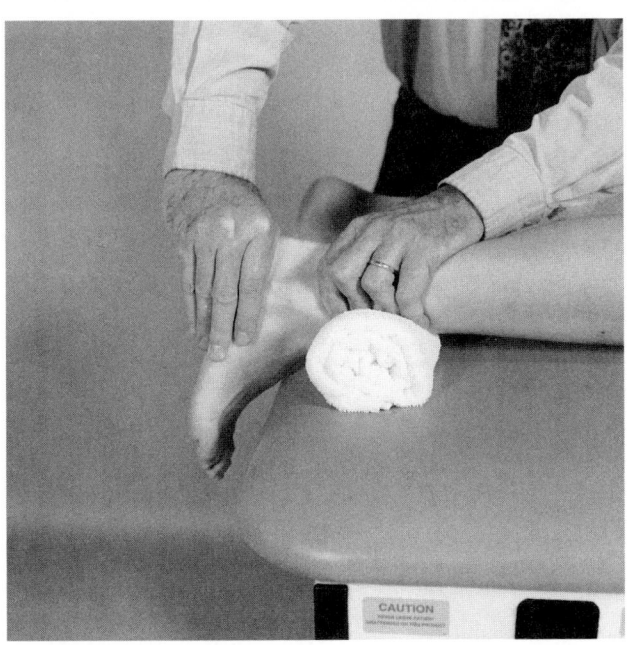

FIGURE 19-57 Technique to increase dorsiflexion.

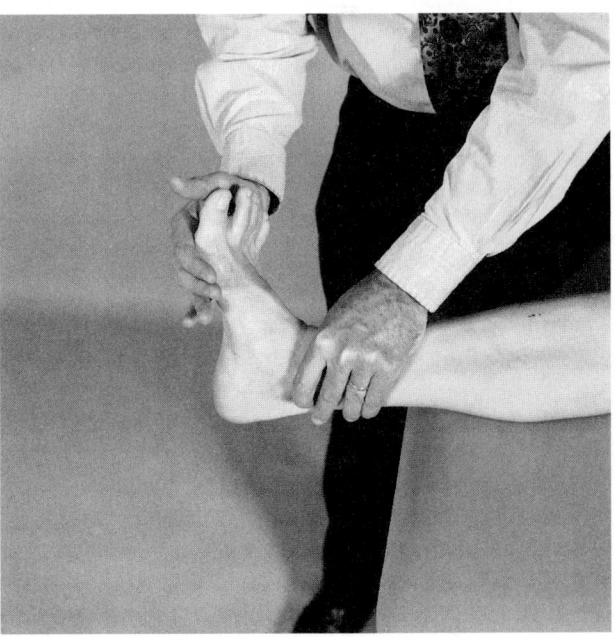

FIGURE 19-58 Gastrocnemius stretch.

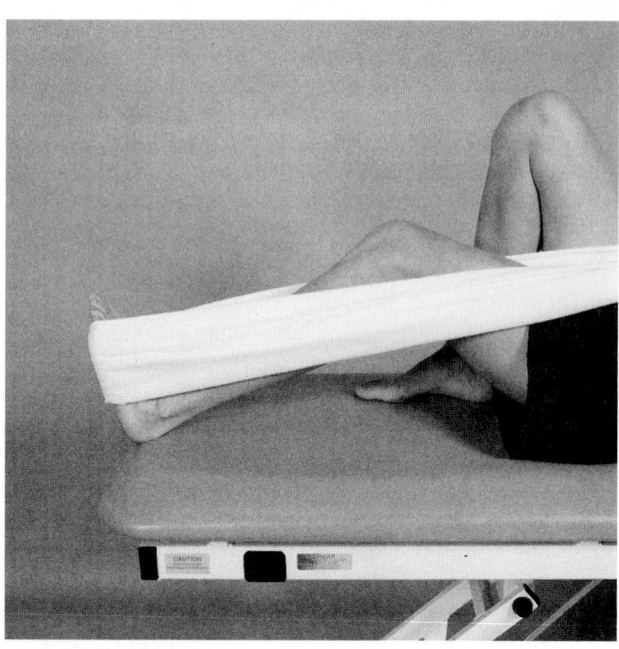

FIGURE 19-59　Soleus stretch.

Automobilization Techniques
Gastrocnemius Stretch.　See Fig. 19-47.
Soleus Stretch.　See Fig. 19-59.

CASE STUDY BILATERAL HEEL PAIN

HISTORY

History of Current Condition
54-year-old female with insidious onset of a constant dull ache in both heels, which is worse in the morning, especially when first putting her feet on the ground, and at the end of the day. The patient denies numbness or tingling in either foot or ankle area. Pain has increased this past week prompting her to see a MD, who prescribed physical therapy and an anti-inflammatory medication.

Past History of Current Condition
Bilateral heel pain of approximately 2 months duration a few years ago, which resolved spontaneously.

Past Medical/Surgical History
Unremarkable

Medications
The family of nonsteroidal anti-inflammatory drugs (NSAIDs) are prescribed for pain relief and decreasing the inflammation in the acute stage.[442]

Other Tests and Measures
Radiographs that showed presence of heel spur.

Social Habits (Past and Present)
Sedentary lifestyle.

Growth and Development
Overweight as a child.

Living Environment
Lives in a ranch-type home with carpeting throughout except for a tiled bathroom.

Occupational/Employment/School
Works in a warehouse stacking boxes of tissues. Has worked there for 6 years.

Functional Status/Activity Level
Soreness occurs first hour in morning, especially when she initially bears weight, and again at the end of the day after working. Walking on the concrete floor at work is reported to aggravate the condition.

Health Status
In general good health, but feels her pain interferes with tasks at home and at work.

QUESTIONS

1. List all of the structures that could be at fault with complaints of bilateral heel pain of an insidious onset.
2. Does the history of heel pain with initial weight bearing in the morning give the clinician any clues as to the diagnosis?
3. Why do you think the patient's symptoms are worsened with weight bearing?
4. What additional questions would you ask to help rule out referral from the hip, knee, or lumbar spine?
5. Do you have a working hypothesis at this stage? List the various tests you would use to rule out each of the possible causes.
6. Does this presentation/history warrant a scan? Why or why not?

TESTS AND MEASURES

Gait, Locomotion, and Balance
Antalgic gait bilaterally, which is more noticeable when barefoot.

Integumentary Integrity
Not tested.

Joint Integrity and Mobility
Joint glides of foot and ankle appear normal.

Motor Performance: Strength, Power, Endurance
Lower extremity strength 4+/5 bilaterally. Foot intrinsics 4/5 bilaterally.

Orthotic, Protective, Supportive Devices
Patient has not tried heel cushions, orthotics, or night splints.

Pain

Pain varies from 2 to 8/10 according to activity level and time of day. Typically the pain is worse at the beginning and at the end of the day.

Posture

Genu valgum bilaterally, and both feet pronated in weight bearing.

Range of Motion (Including Muscle Length)

Bilateral adaptive shortening of rectus femoris, hip flexors, hamstrings, and gastrocnemius. Bilateral ankle dorsiflexion at 2 degrees with knee extended, 8 degrees with knee flexed. Hallus dorsiflexion (passive) is 30 degrees on the right, 25 degrees on the left.

Reflex Integrity

Normal and symmetrical Achilles and patellar reflexes bilaterally.

EVALUATION (CLINICAL JUDGMENT)

The patient is a deconditioned moderately obese woman with soft tissue mobility restrictions and weakness in both lower extremities, which has resulted in functional limitations and pain during her duties at work and at home.

DIAGNOSIS BY PHYSICAL THERAPIST

Impaired joint mobility, motor function, muscle performance, and range of motion associated with ligament or other connective tissue disorders and localized inflammation of both heels. The provisional diagnosis is bilateral plantar fasciitis.

QUESTIONS

1. Having made the provisional diagnosis, how will you base your intervention on the phases of healing?
2. How would you describe this condition to the patient?
3. How would you describe the rationale behind your intervention to the patient?
4. How will you determine the intensity of your intervention?
5. Estimate this patient's prognosis.
6. What modalities could you use in the intervention of this patient? Why?
7. Which manual techniques would be appropriate for this patient, and what is your rationale?
8. What exercises would you prescribe? Why?

PROGNOSIS: PREDICTED OPTIMAL LEVEL OF IMPROVEMENT IN FUNCTION

The patient will demonstrate a return to normal home activities and to full work duty without pain. The duration of the intervention will be determined after assessing the patient's early response to the intervention. Goal setting is difficult with plantar fasciitis given that the condition can often last for 10–12 months. However, the clinician should address the goal setting using achievable targets and reasonable time frames.

- Pain at 2/10 or less with activity.
- Tolerance for standing increased to 30 minutes without pain.
- Normal gait pattern without assistive devices.
- Midfoot stability through exercise or orthotics.
- Ambulate in the morning without pain in 6 weeks.
- Ability to perform self-management of the condition.

PLAN OF CARE: FREQUENCY AND DURATION

2 times per week for 4 weeks. At that point, the patient will be progressed over the next 2 to 4 weeks to a home program.

INTERVENTION

The management of plantar fasciitis can involve a number of components. There is no consensus on the most effective modality or combination of modalities.

PHASE I (WEEKS 1–4)

This phase typically involves 1 to 4 physical therapy visits.

Goals

- Pain at 4/10 or less with weight-bearing activities.
- Dorsiflexion at 5 degrees with subtalar neutral and knee extended, 10 degrees with knee flexed.
- Hallux dorsiflexion at 50 degrees.
- Normal gait pattern.
- Address adaptive shortening of hip flexors, rectus femoris, hamstrings and gastrocnemius.
- Foot/ankle strength at 4+/5.

Electrotherapeutic Modalities

- Iontophoresis/phonophoresis.
- Electrical stimulation.
- Cryotherapy. Ice massage should be applied to the area 2 to 3 times daily.

Therapeutic Exercise and Home Program

- Heel cord stretching in subtalar neutral.[75]
- Specific stretching of the plantar fascia, gastrocnemius, hip flexors, hamstrings, or rectus femoris.
- Specific stretching of the toe flexors, to establish full range of motion at the MTP joint and at the great toe.
- Peroneal, gastrocnemius/soleus, and posterior tibialis strengthening.
- Foot intrinsic and other muscle strengthening.[75,554] Short and long foot flexor exercises are aggressively practiced. The patient performs towel-gripping exercises of 3 sets to fatigue, with 1-minute rests in between each. Small weights are added on the towel to increase resistance. Patients are then directed to pull with the foot into internal rotation.[73] Straight flexion and full weight-bearing arch isometrics are also prescribed.[73] The patient stands with the feet 12 inches apart and the knees

flexed over the second toe. The patient then attempts to make the medial longitudinal arch as high as possible while keeping the head of the first metatarsal on the floor. Each isometric contraction is held for a six count. The patient is progressed to 3 sets of 20.
- Cardiovascular conditioning using stationary bike, Stairmaster, and UBE (upper body ergonometer).

Patient Education

The patient should be advised against running, jumping, and athletic activities, and to avoid walking barefoot on hard surfaces. Shoes should have an arch support and cushioned heels.[555] Worn shoes may aggravate plantar fasciitis because of lack of cushioning and/or support. A laced sports shoe has been found to be more therapeutic than open sandals.[43]

Gait Training

Gait training is provided for maximal stance stability, weight-bearing as tolerated.

Manual Therapy

Manual therapy techniques for plantar fasciitis include:

- Soft issue techniques involving deep tissue massage to the plantar fascia, and techniques to stretch the gastrocnemius, and soleus.
- Myofascial release to the gastrocnemius and soleus muscles.
- Hold–relax techniques to the hip flexors, rectus femoris and hamstring muscles.

PHASE II (WEEKS 5–8)

This phase typically involves 1 to 6 physical therapy visits.

Goals
- Normal gait pattern without assistive device.
- Pain at 2/10 or less with weight-bearing activity.
- Foot and ankle strength at 5/5.
- Demonstrate compliance with home exercise program.

Therapeutic Exercise and Home Program
- Continuation of flexibility exercises, exercises for intrinsic toe flexors, plantar fascia stretches, and massage.
- Closed-chain exercises including toe and heel raises; Sport Cord for forward, backward, and sideways lunges; step up/down progression.
- Theraband strengthening exercises for foot and ankle musculature.
- Graded walking and running activities.

Neuromuscular Retraining
- BAPS.
- Forward and backward walking, progressing to hopping and jumping, if appropriate or tolerated.

Manual Therapy
- Soft tissue techniques including deep tissue massage to anterior and medial calcaneal areas.
- Manual resistive exercises in all planes of motion and in combined planes.
- Passive stretching to deficit areas.

PHASE III (WEEK 9+)

This phase typically involves compliance with the home exercise program.

Goals

The goals for this patient would differ significantly from those of an athlete. For the athlete the goals would include:

- Return to full participation of sport.
- Introduction of plyometrics if needed.

OUTCOMES

The patient's outcome depends on the level of compliance to the recommended home exercise program and intervention plan, as well as other recommended lifestyle changes. As with all musculoskeletal injuries, the return to activity must be graduated and planned. In cases where point tenderness can be elicited and all of the above measures have failed, corticosteroid injection should be considered.[73] Most physicians recommend a maximum of 2 to 3 injections. If no response is obtained after 3 injections, additional injections are not likely to be helpful.

Plantar fascia release[457] is reserved for extremely recalcitrant cases. Only those patients who fail to respond to the entire protocol for at least 6 to 12 months are considered to have failed treatment with conservative measures.[442,556]

It is anticipated that the patient will return to preinjury work level in 2–3 months, and that the recurrence of heel pain should cease within 1 year. Patient understands the strategies to self manage any minor recurrences.

CRITERIA FOR DISCHARGE

Ideally, the patient will be discharged when she reaches her established functional goals, declines further treatment, is unable to progress towards goals because of insurance authorization, or PT determines that the patient will no longer benefit from PT services.

COORDINATION, COMMUNICATION, AND DOCUMENTATION

Communicate with MD and patient regarding patient's status (directly or indirectly). Documentation will include all elements of patient management. Discharge planning will be provided.

PATIENT-RELATED INSTRUCTION

Periodic re-examination and reassessment of the home program, utilizing written instruction and illustrations. Educate patient in activities to avoid during home and work. Educate patient in the benefits of an ongoing conditioning program to prevent functional decline, and to prevent recurrence of impairments. Modeling/demonstration aids will be used for teaching.

CASE STUDY HEEL PAIN

HISTORY

History of Current Condition

A 34-year-old female complains of insidious onset of pain in the posterior aspect of the right ankle, which began about 3 months ago when she began a jogging program, but which had not worsened significantly until last week. The pain is worse in the morning and after prolonged positions. The patient denies numbness or tingling in the foot or ankle area. The increase in pain this past week had prompted the patient to visit her MD, who prescribed physical therapy, and gave her a heel lift to wear in each of her shoes.

Past History of Current Condition

Similar right posterior heel pain of approximately 1-month duration a few years ago, which resolved spontaneously.

Past Medical/Surgical History

Unremarkable.

Medications

Naproxen (daily).

Functional Status/Activity Level

Soreness occurs first hour in the morning.

Health Status

In good health, but feels the pain interferes with tasks at home and at work.

QUESTIONS

1. List the structure(s) and differential diagnoses that may be involved with complaints of unilateral heel pain related to running.
2. What does the history of no significant worsening of the pain tell the clinician?
3. Why do you think the patient's symptoms are worse after rest?
4. What additional questions would you ask?
5. What is your working hypothesis at this stage? If you have a number of hypotheses, which tests would you use to rule out each one?
6. Does this presentation/history warrant a lower quarter scanning examination? Why or why not?

TESTS AND MEASURES

Community and Work Integration/Reintegration

Patient reports spending long periods on her feet during the work day.

Gait, Locomotion and Balance

- Evidence of antalgic gait on right during stance phase.
- Premature heel-off.
- Excessive pronation during stance phase on right.
- Right lower extremity held in external rotation during gait.

Integumentary Integrity

Evidence of minimal swelling on posterior aspect of heel.

Joint Integrity and Mobility

Joint glides of foot and ankle appear normal. Crepitation felt with palpation during active dorsiflexion and plantar flexion.

Motor Performance: Strength, Power, Endurance

- Tenderness with palpation at the tenoperiosteal junction of the Achilles tendon and calcaneus.
- Pain with resisted plantar flexion, tested with repetitive heel raises.
- Lower extremity strength 4+/5 bilaterally. Foot intrinsics 4/5 bilaterally.

Pain

Pain varies from 2 to 6/10 according to activity level.

Posture

Relaxed calcaneal posture indicates excessive pronation.

Range of Motion (Including Muscle Length)

- Bilateral adaptive shortening of the hamstrings, and gastrocnemius.
- Active ankle plantar flexion at 30 degrees, dorsiflexion at 5 degrees.

EVALUATION

Impaired joint mobility, motor function, muscle performance, and range of motion associated with ligament or other connective tissue disorders and localized inflammation of the heel.

Physical therapy provisional diagnosis: Achilles tendonitis on the right.

QUESTIONS

1. Having made the provisional diagnosis, what will be your intervention?
2. How would you describe this condition to the patient?
3. How would you explain the rationale behind your intervention to the patient?
4. What activities would you advise the patient to avoid? Why?
5. How will you determine the intensity of your intervention, and which phase to initiate?
6. Estimate this patient's prognosis.
7. What modalities could you use in the intervention of this patient? Why?
8. Which manual techniques would be appropriate for this patient, and what is your rationale?
9. What exercises would you prescribe? Why?

PROGNOSIS: PREDICTED OPTIMAL LEVEL OF IMPROVEMENT IN FUNCTION

Over the course of 2 months, the patient will demonstrate the following:

- A return to normal home activities and to full work duty without pain.
- Pain at 2/10 or less with activity, and 0/10 at rest.
- AROM of involved foot and ankle to be 40 degrees of plantar flexion, and 10 degrees of dorsiflexion in subtalar neutral with the knee extended, 15 degrees with the knee flexed.
- Ratio of inversion to eversion at 2:1.
- Strength at 5/5 on manual muscle tests for gastrocnemius/soleus.

INTERVENTION

Gradual strengthening of the Achilles tendon by using active treatment regimens,[48] beginning with gentle stretching and isometric exercise in the pain-free range.

FREQUENCY AND DURATION

2 times per week for 3 weeks.

PHASE I (WEEKS 1–2)

This phase typically involves one to three physical therapy visits. The patient is advised to wear shoes that have a firm heel and a flexible forefoot.[557] Heel wedges of 12 to 15 mm are recommended in shoes as they have been shown to significantly reduce the magnitude of heel strike force during walking and running.[48,558] If the forefoot is not flexible, the lever arm of the gastrocnemius-soleus complex is increased, causing more stress across the Achilles tendon.[559]

A 0.25-inch heel lift can be placed in the shoe to lessen the amount of stress on the tendon while ambulating, as it places the ankle in slight plantar flexion.[557]

Electrotherapeutic Modalities
- Electrical stimulation.
- Cryotherapy.
- Whirlpool baths: cold or contrast.
- Iontophoresis. Ultrasound or phonophoresis could also be used depending on effectiveness. Ideally, the clinician should limit the number of electrotherapeutic modalities, unless significant benefit occurs.

Therapeutic Exercise and Home Program
- Cessation from running, jumping, and athletic activities.
- AROM for ankle, including ankle pumps and circles.
- Protection with continued use of prescribed heel lifts.
- Cardiovascular exercise using bike, swimming, or UBE, as appropriate.
- Graded gastrocnemius and soleus stretches in subtalar neutral.

Manual Therapy
Manual therapy techniques for this phase include soft tissue mobilization to the gastrocnemius and soleus, and transverse friction massage to the Achilles tendon, graded according to pain.

PHASE II (WEEK 3+)

This phase typically involves three to seven physical therapy visits.

Electrotherapeutic Modalities
Continued use of ultrasound, phonophoresis, and/or iontophoresis if effective.

Therapeutic Exercise and Home Program
- Flexibility exercises for gastrocnemius/soleus, Achilles tendon, toe flexors, plantar fascia, and hamstrings.
- Strengthening exercises using surgical tubing or cuff weights for major muscles of the lower extremity, especially the gastrocnemius/soleus group.
- Closed-chain exercises including toe raises, BAPS, ankle disks, stationary bicycle, treadmill, and Stairmaster.
- Progressive gait training for stance stability and control of excessive pronation. Consider use of orthotics to control pronation if necessary.

Neuromuscular Retraining
- Plyometrics involving step progression to hopping and jumping as tolerated, beginning with one-leg hops on the involved side, and exercises on the trampoline on both legs, before progressing to outdoor jogging uphill and downhill, and low-impact interval training.
- Lunges in forward, backward, and sideways directions.

The typical training program starts at a low impact level with low resistance and high repetitions, gradually progressing to high resistance and low repetitions, and increased speed for maximal strength and explosive strength effect.

As soon as symptoms settle, an eccentric loading program is started. This takes the following format:[557]

1. Warm-up of tendon by activity or modalities.
2. Achilles stretches (straight knee for gastrocnemius and bent knee for soleus).
3. Drop and stop exercises:

   - Stand on a block or step so the heel is unsupported.
   - Raise up on toes.
   - Allow heel to lower as far as possible.
   - Progress to dropping (lowering rapidly).
   - Perform three sets of 10 repetitions.
   - Progress as symptoms allow.

4. Repeat stretches.
5. Ice to cool down 5 to 10 minutes.

Manual Therapy
Manual therapy techniques in this phase include:

- Deep transverse friction massage to the specific lesion site in the Achilles tendon.
- Myofascial release to the hamstrings, gastrocnemius and soleus muscles as indicated for increased tissue length and elasticity.

COORDINATION, COMMUNICATION, AND DOCUMENTATION

Communicate with MD and patient regarding patient's status (directly or indirectly). Documentation will include all elements of patient management. Discharge planning will be provided.

PATIENT-RELATED INSTRUCTION

Periodic re-examination and reassessment of the home program, utilizing written instruction and illustrations. Educate patient in activities to avoid during home and work. Educate patient in the benefits of an ongoing conditioning program to prevent functional decline, and to prevent recurrence of impairments. Modeling/demonstration aids will be used for teaching.

RE-EXAMINATION

Perform selected tests and measures to evaluate patient's progress toward goals in order to modify or redirect intervention if patient fails to show progress.

CRITERIA FOR DISCHARGE

The patient will be discharged when she reaches her established functional goals, declines further treatment, is unable to progress towards goals because of complications, or PT determines that patient will no longer benefit from PT services.

OUTCOMES

The patient's outcome depends on the extent of the injury, the level of compliance to the recommended home exercise program and intervention plan, as well as other recommended lifestyle changes. It is anticipated that the patient will return to preinjury work level in 2 months, without recurrence of heel pain in the following year. Patient understands the strategies to self manage any minor recurrences.

REVIEW QUESTIONS*

1. Name the three ligaments associated with the distal tibiofibular joint.
2. Which nerve is involved with tarsal tunnel syndrome?
3. What structures maintain the longitudinal arch?
4. Supination of the foot in weight bearing is a combination of which movements of the calcaneus and talus?
5. Morton's neuroma most commonly involves which nerve?

* Additional questions to test your understanding of this chapter can be found in the Online Learning Center for *Orthopaedic Assessment, Evaluation, and Intervention* at www.duttononline.net.

REFERENCES

1. Schiowitz S. Diagnosis and treatment of the lower extremity—The knee. In: DiGiovanna EL, Schiowitz S, eds. *An Osteopathic Approach to Diagnosis and Treatment*. Philadelphia: JB Lippincott; 1991:330–346.
2. Sartoris DJ. Diagnosis of ankle injuries: the essentials. *J Foot Ankle Surg* 1994;33:101–107.
3. Sammarco GJ, Hockenbury RT. Biomechanics of the foot and ankle. In: Frankel VH, Nordin M, eds. *Basic Biomechanics of the Musculoskeletal System*. Baltimore: Williams & Wilkins; 2000.
4. Mann RA. Biomechanics of running. In: AAOS Symposium on the Foot and Leg in Running Sports. St. Louis: CV Mosby Co; 1982:30–44.
5. Cavanagh PR, Rodgers MM, Iiboshi A. Pressure distribution under symptom-free feet during barefoot standing. *Foot & Ankle International* 1987;7:262–276.
6. Gieve DW, Rashi T. Pressures under normal feet in standing and walking as measured by foil pedobarography. *Ann Rheum Dis* 1984;43:816.
7. Inman VT, Ralston HJ, Todd F. *Human Walking*. Baltimore: Williams & Wilkins; 1981.
8. Kapandji IA. *The Physiology of the Joints, Lower Limb*. New York: Churchill Livingstone; 1991.
9. Williams PL, Warwick R. *Gray's Anatomy*, 36th ed. Philadelphia: WB Saunders Co.; 1980:473–477.
10. Root M, Orien W, Weed J. *Clinical Biomechanics: Normal and Abnormal Function of the Foot*, Vol. II. Los Angeles: Clinical Biomechanics Corp.; 1977.
11. Wedmore IS, Charette J. Emergency department evaluation and treatment of ankle and foot injuries. *Emerg Med Clin North Am* 2000;18:85–113.
12. Donatelli RA. Normal anatomy and biomechanics. In: Donatelli RA, ed. *Biomechanics of the Foot and Ankle*. Philadelphia: WB Saunders; 1990:3–31.
13. Subotnick SI. Normal anatomy. In: Subotnick SI, ed. *Sports Medicine of the Lower Extremity*. Philadelphia: Churchill Livingstone; 1999:75–111.
14. Stormont DM, et al. Stability of the loaded ankle. *Am J Sports Med* 1985;13:295–300.
15. Mulfinger G, Trueta J. The blood supply to the talus. *J Bone Joint Surg* 1970;52B:160.
16. Brostrom L. Sprained ankles: I. Anatomic lesions on recent sprains. *Acta Chir Scand* 1964;128:483–495.
17. Cailliet R. *Foot and Ankle Pain*. Philadelphia: FA Davis; 1983:148–158.
18. Cox JS. Surgical and nonsurgical treatment of acute ankle sprains. *Clin Orthop* 1985;198:118–126.
19. Hamilton WG. Surgical anatomy of the foot and ankle. *Clin Symp* 1985;37:1–32.
20. Moseley HF. Traumatic disorders of the ankle and foot. *Clin Symp* 1965;17:1–30.
21. Hintermann B, et al. Biomechanics of the unstable ankle joint and clinical implications. *Med Sci Sports Exerc* 1999;31 (7 Suppl.):S459–S469.
22. Safran MR, et al. Lateral ankle sprains: a comprehensive review: part 1: etiology, pathoanatomy, histopathogenesis, and diagnosis. *Med Sci Sports Exerc* 1999;31(7 Suppl):S429–S437.
23. Hockenbury RT, Sammarco GJ. Evaluation and treatment of ankle sprains—clinical recommendations for a positive outcome. *Phys Sports Med* 2001;24:57–64.
24. Attarian DE, et al. A biomechanical study of human lateral ankle ligaments and autogenous reconstructive grafts. *Am J Sports Med* 1985;13:377–381.
25. Close JR. Some applications of the functional anatomy of the ankle joint. *J Bone Joint Surg* 1956;38-A:761–781.
26. Hintermann B, et al. Transfer of movement between calcaneus and tibia in vitro. *Clin Biomech* 1994;9:349–355.
27. Inman VT. *The Joints of the Ankle*. Baltimore: Williams & Wilkins; 1991:31–74.

28. Manter JT. Movements of the subtalar and transverse tarsal joints. *Anat Rec* 1941;80:397–400.

29. Mann RA. Functional anatomy of the ankle joint ligaments. In: Bateman JE, Trott AW, eds. *The Foot and Ankle.* New York: BC Decker Inc; 1980:161–170.

30. Burks RT, Morgan J. Anatomy of the lateral ankle ligaments. *Am J Sports Med* 1994;22:72–77.

31. Sarrafian SK. Anatomy of foot and ankle. Philadelphia: Lippincott; 1994:239–240.

32. Anderson KJ, Lecocq JF. Operative treatment of injury to the fibular collateral ligaments of the ankle. *J Bone Joint Surg* 1954;36A:825–832.

33. Colville MR, et al. Strain measurement in lateral ankle ligaments. *Am J Sports Med* 1990;18:196–200.

34. Rasmussen O. Stability of the ankle joint. *Acta Orthop Scandinavica* 1985;(Suppl. 211):56–78.

35. Renstrom PA, et al. Strain in the lateral ligaments of the ankle. *Foot Ankle* 1988;9:59–63.

36. Harper MC. Deltoid ligament: An anatomical evaluation of function. *Foot Ankle* 1987;8:19–22.

37. Siegler S, Block J, Schneck CD. The mechanical characteristics of the collateral ligaments of the human ankle joint. *Foot Ankle* 1988;8:234–242.

38. Rasmussen O, Kroman-Andersen C, Boe S. Deltoid ligament: functional analysis of the medial collateral ligamentous apparatus of the ankle joint. *Acta Orthop Scand* 1983; 54:36–44.

39. Rasmussen O, Tovberg-Jensen I. Mobility of the ankle joint: recording of rotatory movements in the talocrural joint in vitro with and without the lateral collateral ligaments of the ankle. *Acta Orthop Scand* 1982;53:155–160.

40. Attarian DE, et al. Biomechanical characteristics of human ankle ligaments. *Foot Ankle* 1985;6:54–58.

41. Isman RE, Inman VT. Anthropometric studies of the human foot and ankle. *Bull Prosthetic Res* 1969;4:97–129.

42. Jahss MH, Kummer F, Michelson JD. Investigations into the fat pads of the sole of the foot: heel pressure studies. *Foot Ankle* 1992;13:227–232.

43. Singh D, et al. Fortnightly review. Plantar fasciitis. *BMJ* 1997;315:172–175.

44. Jorgensen U, and Bojsen-Möller F. Shock absorbency factors in the shoe/heel interaction—with special focus on role of the heel pad. *Foot Ankle* 1989;9:294–299.

45. Frey CC, et al. The retrocalcaneal bursa: anatomy and bursography. *Foot Ankle* 1982;13:203–207.

46. Williams PL, et al. *Gray's Anatomy*, 37th ed. London: Churchill Livingstone; 1989.

47. Hintermann B. Tibialis posterior dysfunction: a review of the problems and personal experience. *Foot Ankle Surg* 1997;3:61–70.

48. Clement DB, Taunton JE, Smart GW. Achilles tendinitis and peritendinitis: etiology and treatment. *Am J Sports Med* 1984;12:179–183.

49. Gagey O, Hue E. Mechanics of the deltoid muscle. A new approach. *Clin Orthop Rel Res* 2000;375:250–257.

50. Bojsen-Möller F. Calcaneocuboid joint and stability of the longitudinal arch of the foot at high and low gear push off. *J Anat* 1979;129:165–176.

51. Jahss MH. *Disorders of the Foot*, Vol. 1. Philadelphia: WB Saunders; 1982.

52. Joseph J. Range of movement of the great toe in men. *J Bone Joint Surg* 1954;36B:450–457.

53. Clanton TO, Ford JJ. Turf toe injury. *Clin Sports Med* 1984;13:731–741.

54. Clanton TO, Schon LC. Athletic injuries to the soft tissues of the foot and ankle. In: Mann RA, Coughlin MJ, eds. *Surgery of the Foot and Ankle.* St. Louis: Mosby-Year Book Inc; 1993: 1095–1224.

55. Weinfeld SB, Schon LC. Hallux metatarsophalangeal arthritis. *Clin Orthop Rel Res* 1998;349:9–19.

56. Hockenbury RT. Forefoot problems in athletes. *Med Sci Sports Exerc* 1999;31(7 Suppl):S448–S458.

57. Jahss MH. The sesamoids of the hallux. *Clin Orthop* 1981; 157:88–97.

58. McBryde AM Jr, Anderson RB. Sesamoid problems in the athlete. *Clin Sports Med* 1988;7:51–60.

59. Richardson EG. Injuries to the hallucal sesamoids in the athlete. *Foot Ankle* 1987;7:229–244.

60. Sammarco GJ. Turf toe. *Instr Course Lect* 1993;42:207–212.

61. Scranton PE, Rutkowski R. Anatomic variations in the first ray. Part B. Disorders of the sesamoids. *Clin Orthop* 1980; 151:256–264.

62. Van Hal ME, et al. Stress fractures of the sesamoids. *Am J Sports Med* 1982;10:122–128.

63. Whittle AP. Fractures of the foot in athletes. *Op Tech Sports Med* 1994;2:43–57.

64. Omey ML, Micheli LJ. Foot and ankle problems in the young athlete. *Med Sci Sports Exerc* 1999;31(7 Suppl): S470–S486.

65. Sullivan JA. The child's foot. In: Morrissy RT, ed. *Lovell and Winter's Pediatric Orthopaedics.* Philadelphia: Lippincott; 1996:1077–1135.

66. Chen YJ, et al. Posterior tibial tendon tear combined with a fracture of the accessory navicular: a new subclassification? *J Trauma-Injury Infect Crit Care* 1995;39:993–996.

67. Brodsky AE, Khalil MA. Talar compression syndrome. *Am J Sports Med* 1986;14:472–476.

68. McDougall A. The os trigonum. *J Bone Joint Surg* 1955; 37B:257–265.

69. Keene JS, Lange RH. Diagnostic dilemmas in foot and ankle injuries. *JAMA* 1986;256:247–251.

70. Kelikian H, Kelikian AS. *Disorders of the Ankle.* Philadelphia: WB Saunders; 1985:1–1200.

71. Marotta JJ, Micheli LJ. Os trigonum impingement in dancers. *Am J Sports Med* 1992;20:533–536.

72. Ihle CL, Cochran RM. Fracture of the fused os trigonum. *Am J Sports Med* 1982;10:47–50.

72a. Hedrick MR, The plantar aponeurosis. Foot Ankle Int. 1996; 17:646–649.

72b. Sarrafian SK, *Anatomy of foot and ankle.* Philadelphia: Lippincott; 1994:239–240.

72c. Subotnick SI, Normal anatomy. In: Subotnick SI, ed. *Sports Medicine of the Lower Extremity.* 1999, Philadelphia: Churchill-Livingstone; 1999:75–111.

73. Charles LM. Why does my foot hurt? Plantar fasciitis. *Lippincott's Primary Care Practice* 1999;3:408–409.

74. Scioli MW. Achilles tendinitis. *Orthop Clin North Am* 1994; 25:177–182.

75. Reid DC. Heel pain and problems of the hindfoot. In: Reid DC, ed. *Sports Injury Assessment and Rehabilitation.* New York: Churchill Livingstone; 1992:437–493.

76. Myerson MS, McGarvey W. Disorders of the Achilles tendon insertion and Achilles tendonitis. *AAOS Instr Course Lect* 1999; 48:211–218.

77. Soma CA, Mandelbaum BR. Achilles tendon disorders. *Clin Sports Med* 1994;13:811–823.

78. Gerdes MH, et al. A flap augmentation technique for Achilles tendon repair. Postoperative strength and functional outcome. *Clin Orthop* 1992;280:241–246.

79. Reynolds NL, Worrell TW. Chronic Achilles peritendinitis: etiology, pathophysiology, and treatment. *J Orthop Sports Phys Ther* 1991;13:171–176.

80. Carr AJ, Norris SH. The blood supply of the calcaneal tendon. *J Bone Joint Surg* 1989;71B:100–101.

81. Lagergren C, Lindholm A. Vascular distribution in the Achilles tendon: An angiographic and microangiographic study. *Acta Chir Scand* 1958;116:491–495.

82. Nelen G, Martens M, Bursens A. Surgical treatment of chronic Achilles tendinitis. *Am J Sports Med* 1989;17:754–759.

83. Nichols AW. Achilles tendinitis in running athletes. *J Am Bd Fam Pract* 1989;2:196–203.

83a. Scioli MW. Achilles tendinitis. *Orthop Clin N Am*, 1994; 25:177–182.

83b. Reid DC. Heel pain and problems of the hindfoot. In: Reid DC, ed. *Sports Injury Assessment and Rehabilitation.* New York: Churchill-Livingstone; 1992:437–493.

83c. Myerson MS, McGarvey W. Disorders of the Achilles tendon insertion and Achilles tendonitis. *AAOS Instr Course Lect* 1999; 48:211–218.

84. Conti SF. Posterior tibial tendon problems in athletes. *Orthop Clin North Am* 1994;25:109–121.

85. Clarke HD, Kitaoka HB, Ehman RL. Peroneal tendon injuries. *Foot Ankle* 1998;19:280–288.

86. Brage ME, Hansen ST. Traumatic subluxation/dislocation of the peroneal tendons. *Foot Ankle* 1992;13:423–431.

87. Thordarson DB, et al. Dynamic support of the human longitudinal arch. *Clin Orthop* 1995;316:165–172.

88. Mann R, Inman V. Phasic activity of intrinsic muscles of the foot. *J Bone Joint Surg* 1964;46A:469–480.

89. Appling SA, Kasser RJ. Foot and Ankle. In: Wadsworth C, ed. *Current Concepts of Orthopedic Physical Therapy—Home Study Course.* La Crosse, WI: Orthopedic Section, APTA; 2001.

90. Reeser LA, Susman RL, Stern JT. Electromyographic studies of the human foot: experimental approaches to hominid evolution. *Foot Ankle* 1983;3:391–406.

91. Huang C, et al. Biomechanical evaluation of longitudinal arch stability. *Foot Ankle* 1993;14:352–357.

92. Hicks JH. Mechanics of the foot. *J Anat* 1953;87:345–357.

93. Donatelli R. Normal anatomy and pathophysiology of the foot and ankle. In: Wadsworth C, ed. *Contemporary Topics on the Foot and Ankle.* La Crosse, WI: Orthopedic Section, APTA, Inc.; 2000.

94. Hoffman PA. A statistical study of the relation between the height of the longitudinal arch and the function of the foot. *Am Med* 1907;13:467–471.

95. Simkin A, et al. Combined effect of foot structure and an orthotic device on stress fractures. *Foot Ankle* 1989;10:25–29.

96. Giladi M, et al. The low arch, a protective factor in stress fractures: a prospective study of 295 military recruits. *Orthop Review* 1985;14:709–712.

97. Cowan DN, Jones BH, Robinson JR. Foot morphological characteristics and risk of exercise-related injury. *Arch Fam Med* 1993;2:773–777.

98. Roy KJ. Force, pressure, and motion measurements in the foot. *Clin Podiatr Med Surg* 1988;5:491–508.

99. Nachbauer W, Nigg B. Effects of arch height of the foot on ground reaction forces in running. *Med Sci Sports Exerc* 1992;23:1264–1269.

100. MacConnail MA, Basmajian JV. *Muscles and Movements: A Basis for Human Kinesiology.* New York: Robert Krieger Pub. Co.; 1977.

101. Mayeaux EJ, Jr. Nail disorders. *Dermatology* 2000;27:333–351.

102. Dellon AL, Mackinnon SE. Tibial nerve branching in the tarsal tunnel. *Arch Neurol* 1984;41:645–646.

103. Vaes PH, et al. Static and dynamic roentgenographic analysis of ankle stability in braced and non-braced stable and functionally unstable ankles. *Am J Sports Med* 1998;26:692–702.

104. Edwards GS, DeLee JC. Ankle diastasis without fracture. *Foot Ankle* 1984;4:305–312.

105. Murray MP. Gait as a total pattern of movement. *Am J Phys Med* 1967;46:290.

106. Perry J. The mechanics of walking: A clinical interpretation. In: Perry J, Hislop HJ, eds. *Principles of Lower Extremity Bracing.* New York: American Physical Therapy Association; 1967:9–32.

107. Scott SH, Winter DA. Talocrural and talocalcaneal joint kinematics and kinetics during the stance phase of gait. *J Biomech* 1991;24:743–752.

108. Barnett CH, Napier JR. The axis of rotation at the ankle joint in man: Its influence upon the form of the talus and mobility of the fibula. *J Anat* 1952;86:1–9.

109. Giallonardo LM. Clinical evaluation of foot and ankle dysfunction. *Phys Ther* 1988;68:1850–1856.

110. Close JR, Inman VT. The action of the ankle joint. Prosthetic Devices Research Project. *Institute of Engineering Research* 1952;11:5.

111. Lundberg A, et al. Kinematics of the ankle/foot complex: plantar flexion and dorsiflexion. *Foot Ankle* 1989;9:194–200.

112. Levens AS, Inman VT, Blosser JA. Transverse rotations of the lower extremity in locomotion. *J Bone Joint Surg* 1948;30A:859–872.

113. Stephens MM, Sammarco GJ. The stabilizing role of the lateral ligament complex around the ankle and subtalar joints. *Foot Ankle* 1992;13:130–136.

114. O'Connor JJ, Leardini A, Catani F. The one degree of freedom nature of the human ankle/subtalar complex. *J Bone Joint Surg [Br]* 1997;79-B(Suppl III):364–365.

115. Hunt GC. Functional biomechanics of the subtalar joint. In: *Orthopaedic Physical Therapy Home Study Course 92-1: Lower Extremity.* La Crosse, WI: Orthopaedic Section, APTA, Inc.; 1992.

116. Subotnick SI. Biomechanics of the subtalar and midtarsal joints. *J Am Podiatry Assoc* 1975;65:756–764.

117. Close JR, et al. The function of the subtalar joint. *Clin Orthop* 1967;50:159–179.

118. Oatis CA. Biomechanics of the foot and ankle under static conditions. *Phys Ther* 1988;68:1815–1821.

119. Green DR, Whitney AK, Walters P. Subtalar joint motion. *J Am Podiat Med Assn* 1979;69:83–91.

120. Mann RA, Hagy J. Biomechanics of walking, running, and sprinting. *Am J Sports Med* 1980;8:345–350.

121. Carson WG. Diagnosis of extensor mechanism disorders. *Clin Sports Med* 1985;4:231–246.

122. Carson WG, et al. Patellofemoral disorders—Physical and radiographic examination. Part I. Physical examination. *Clin Orthop* 1984;185:178–186.

123. James SL, Bates BT, Osternig LR. Injuries to runners. *Am J Sports Med* 1978;6:40–49.

124. James SL. Chondromalacia patella. In: Kennedy JC, ed. *The Injured Adolescent Knee*. Baltimore: Williams & Wilkins; 1979.

125. Wright DG, Desai SM, Henderson WH. Action of the subtalar and ankle joint complex during stance phase of walking. *J Bone Joint Surg* 1964;46A:361–382.

126. McPoil TG, Jr, Brocato RS. The foot and ankle: Biomechanical evaluation and treatment. In: Gould JA, Davies GJ, eds. *Orthopaedic and Sports Physical Therapy*. St Louis: CV Mosby; 1985:313–341.

127. Tiberio D. Pathomechanics of structural foot deformities. *Phys Ther* 1988;68:1840–1849.

128. Harper MC. The lateral ligamentous support of the subtalar joint. *Foot Ankle* 1991;11:354–358.

129. Elftman H. The transverse tarsal joint and its control. *Clin Orthop Rel Res* 1960;16:41–45.

129a. Appling SA, Kasser RJ. Foot and ankle. In: Wadsworth C, ed. *Current Concepts of Orthopedic Physical Therapy—Home Study Course* La Crosse, WI: Orthopaedic Section, APTA; 2001.

129b. Bojsen-Möller F. Calcaneocuboid joint and stability of the longitudinal arch of the foot at high and low gear push off. *J Anat*, 1979; 129(1):165–176.

129c. Joseph J. Range of movement of the great toe in men. *J Bone Joint Surg* 1954; 36B:450–457.

130. Hardy RH, Clapham JCR. Observations on hallux valgus: Based on a controlled series. *J Bone Joint Surg* 1951;33B:376–391.

131. Maitland G. *Peripheral Manipulation*, 3rd ed. London: Butterworth; 1991.

132. Cyriax J. *Textbook of Orthopaedic Medicine, Diagnosis of Soft Tissue Lesions*, 8th ed. London: Bailliere Tindall; 1982.

133. Safran MR, et al. Lateral ankle sprains: a comprehensive review part 2: treatment and rehabilitation with an emphasis on the athlete. *Med Sci Sports Exerc* 1999;31(7 Suppl):S438–S447.

134. Marder RA. Current methods for the evaluation of ankle ligament injuries. *J Bone Joint Surg* 1994;76A:1103–1111.

135. Magee DJ. Lower leg, ankle, and foot. In: Magee DJ, ed. *Orthopedic Physical Assessment*. Philadelphia: WB Saunders; 2002:765–845.

136. Adamson C, Cymet T. Ankle sprains: evaluation, treatment, rehabilitation. *Maryland Med J* 1997;46:530–537.

137. Bordelon RL. Clinical assessment of the foot. In: Donatelli RA, ed. *Biomechanics of the Foot and Ankle*. Philadelphia: WB Saunders; 1990:85–98.

138. Brostrom L. Sprained ankles: III. Clinical observations in recent ligament ruptures. *Acta Chir Scand* 1965;130:560–569.

139. Cox JS. The diagnosis and management of ankle ligament injuries in the athlete. *Athl Training* 1982;18:192–196.

140. Winkel D, Matthijs O, Phelps V. Examination of the ankle and foot. In: Winkel D, Matthijs O, Phelps V, eds. *Diagnosis and Treatment of the Lower Extremities*. Gaithersburg, MD: Aspen; 1997:375–401.

141. Brosky T, et al. The ankle ligaments: consideration of syndesmotic injury and implications for rehabilitation. *J Orthop Sports Phys Ther* 1995;21:197–205.

142. Turco VJ. Injuries to the foot and ankle in athletes. *Orthop Clin North Am* 1977;8:669–682.

143. Gross MT. Lower quarter screening for skeletal malalignment—suggestions for orthotics and shoewear. *J Orthop Sports Phys Ther* 1995;21:389–405.

144. Roy S, Irvin R. *Sports Medicine—Prevention, Evaluation, Management, and Rehabilitation*. Englewood Cliffs, NJ: Prentice-Hall; 1983.

145. Mann RA. Biomechanical approach to the treatment of foot problems. *Foot Ankle* 1982;2:205–212.

146. McPoil TG, Schuit D, Knecht HG. A comparison of three positions used to evaluate tibial varum. *J Am Podiat Med Assn* 1988;78:22–28.

147. Hamill J, et al. Relationship between selected static and dynamic lower extremity measures. *Clin Biomech* 1989;4:217–225.

148. Knutzen KM, Price A. Lower extremity static and dynamic relationships with rearfoot motion in gait. *J Am Podiat Med Assn* 1994;84:171–180.

149. McPoil TG, Cornwall MW. The relationship between static lower extremity measurements and rearfoot motion during walking. *J Orthop Sports Phys Ther* 1996;24:309–314.

150. Staheli LT. Rotational problems of the lower extremity. *Orthop Clin North Am* 1987;18:503–512.

151. Hunt GC, Brocato RS. Gait and foot pathomechanics. In: Hunt GC, ed. *Physical Therapy of the Foot and Ankle*. Edinburgh: Churchill Livingstone; 1988.

152. Subotnick SI. Clinical biomechanics. In: Subotnick SI, ed. *Sports Medicine of the Lower Extremity*. Philadelphia: Churchill Livingstone; 1999:127–156.

153. Root M, Orien W, Weed J. *Clinical Biomechanics*, Vol. 2. Los Angeles: Clinical Biomechanics Corp.; 1977.

153a. Payne C, Chuter V, Miller K. Sensitivity and specificity of the functional hallux limitus test to predict foot function. *J Am Pod Med Assoc* 2002;92:269–271.

154. Reid DC. *Sports Injury Assessment and Rehabilitation*. New York: Churchill Livingstone; 1992.

155. Schon LC. Nerve entrapment, neuropathy, and nerve dysfunction in athletes. *Orthop Clin North Am* 1994;25:47–59.

156. Hertling D, Kessler RM. *Management of Common Musculoskeletal Disorders: Physical Therapy Principles and Methods*, 3rd ed. Philadelphia: Lippincott Williams & Wilkins; 1996.

157. Baxter DE. The heel in sport. *Clin Sports Med* 1994;13:683–693.

158. Baxter DE, Zingas C. The foot in running. *J Am Acad Orthop Surg* 1995;3:136–145.

159. Leach RE, Dizorio E, Harvey RA. Pathologic hindfoot conditions in the athlete. *Clin Orthop* 1983;177:116–121.

160. Patla CE, Abbott JH. Tibialis posterior myofascial tightness as a source of heel pain: diagnosis and treatment. *J Orthop Sports Phys Ther* 2000;30:624–632.

161. Rose GK, Welton GA, Marshall T. The diagnosis of flat foot in the child. *J Bone Joint Surg* 1985;67B:71–78.

162. Bojsen-Möller F, Lamoreux L. Significance of dorsiflexion of the toes in walking. *Acta Orthop Scand* 1979;50:471–479.

163. Buell T, Green DR, Risser J. Measurement of the first metatarsophalangeal joint range of motion. *J Am Podiat Med Assn* 1988;78:439–448.

164. Rozzi SL, et al. Balance training for persons with functionally unstable ankles. *J Orthop Sports Phys Ther* 1999;29:478–486.

165. Lysholm J, Gilquist J. Evaluation of knee ligament surgery results with special emphasis on the use of a scoring scale. *Am J Sports Med* 1982;10:150–154.

166. Tegner Y, et al. A performance test to monitor rehabilitation and evaluate anterior cruciate ligament injuries. *Am J Sports Med* 1986;14:156–159.

167. Noyes FR, Barber SD, Mooar LA. A rationale for assessing sports activity levels and limitations in knee disorders. *Clin Orthop* 1989;246:238–249.

168. Budiman-Mak E, Conrad KJ, Roach KE. The foot function index: a measure of foot pain and disability. *J Clin Epidemiol* 1991;44:561–570.

169. Katcherian DA. Pathology of the first ray. In: Mizel MS, Miller RA, Scioli MW, eds. *Orthopaedic Knowledge Update, Foot and Ankle.* Rosemont, IL: American Academy of Orthopaedic Surgeons; 1998:157–159.

170. Peng JR. Solving the dilemma of the high ankle sprain in the athlete. *Sports Med Arthrosc Rev* 2000;8:316–325.

171. Hopkinson WJ, et al. Syndesmosis sprains of the ankle. *Foot Ankle Int* 1990;10:325.

172. Hollis JM, Blaiser RD, Flahiff CM. Simulated lateral ankle ligamentous injury: change in ankle stability. *Am J Sports Med* 1993;23:672–677.

173. Johnson EE, Markolf K. The contribution of the anterior talofibular ligament to ankle laxity. *J Bone Joint Surg* 1983;65A:81–88.

174. Landeros O, Frost HM, Higgins CC. Anteriorly unstable ankle due to trauma: a report of 29 cases. *J Bone Joint Surg* 1966;48A:1028.

175. Landeros O, Frost HM, Higgins CC. Post traumatic anterior ankle instability. *Clin Orthop* 1968;56:169–178.

176. Frost HM, Hanson CA. Technique for testing the drawer sign in the ankle. *Clin Orthop* 1977;123:49–51.

177. Gould N, Selingson D, Gassman J. Early and late repair of lateral ligaments of the ankle. *Foot Ankle* 1980;1:84–89.

178. Staples OS. Rupture of the fibular collateral ligaments of the ankle. *J Bone Joint Surg* 1975;57A:101–107.

179. Aradi AJ, Wong J, Walsh M. The dimple sign of a ruptured lateral ligament of the ankle: brief report. *J Bone Joint Surg [Br]* 1988;70-B:327–328.

180. van Dijk CN, et al. Physical examination is sufficient for the diagnosis of sprained ankles. *J Bone Joint Surg [Br]* 1996;78-B:958–962.

181. Kleiger B. Mechanisms of ankle injury. *Orthop Clin North Am* 1974;5:127–146.

182. Katznel A, Lin M. Ruptures of the ligaments about the tibiofibular syndesmosis. *Injury* 1984;25:170–172.

183. Thompson TC, Doherty JH. Spontaneous rupture of tendon of Achilles: a new clinical diagnostic test. *J Trauma* 1962;2:126.

184. Palmer ML, Epler M. *Clinical Assessment Procedures in Physical Therapy.* Philadelphia: JB Lippincott; 1990:68–73.

185. Johnson KA. Posterior tibial tendon. In: Baxter DE, ed. *The Foot and Ankle in Sport.* St. Louis: CV Mosby; 1995.

186. Picciano AM, Rowlands MS, Worrell T. Reliability of open and closed kinetic chain subtalar joint neutral positions and navicular drop test. *J Orthop Sports Phys Ther* 1993;18:553–558.

187. Mueller MJ, Host JV, Norton BJ. Navicular drop as a composite measure of excessive pronation. *J Am Podiatr Med Assn* 1993;83:198–202.

188. Brody DM. Techniques in the evaluation and treatment of the injured runner. *Orthop Clin North Am* 1982;13:541–558.

189. Mennell JM. *Foot Pain.* Boston: Little, Brown, and Co.; 1969.

190. Evans RC. *Illustrated Essentials in Orthopedic Physical Assessment.* St. Louis: Mosby-Year Book Inc.; 1994.

191. Stiell IG, et al. Decision rules for the use of radiography in acute ankle injuries: refinement and prospective validation. *JAMA* 1994;269:1127–1132.

192. Stiell IG, et al. Implementation of the Ottawa Ankle Rules. *JAMA* 1994;271:827–832.

193. Leddy JJ, et al. Prospective evaluation of the Ottawa Ankle Rules in a University Sports Medicine Center. With a modification to increase specificity for identifying malleolar fractures. *Am J Sports Med* 1998;26:158–165.

194. Anderson KJ, Lecocq JF, Lecocq EA. Recurrent anterior subluxation of the ankle joint: A report of two cases and an experimental study. *J Bone Joint Surg* 1952;34A:853–860.

195. Cass JR, Morrey BF. Ankle instability: current concepts, diagnosis, and treatment. *Mayo Clin Proc* 1984;59:165–170.

196. Sedlin ED. A device for stress inversion or eversion roentgenograms of the ankle. *J Bone Joint Surg* 1960;42A:1184–1190.

197. Kibler BW. Rehabilitation of the ankle and foot. In: Kibler BW, Herring JA, Press JM, eds. *Functional Rehabilitation of Sports and Musculoskeletal Injuries.* Gaithersburg, MD: Aspen; 1998:273–283.

198. Kessler RM, Hertling D. Management of Common Musculoskeletal Disorders. Philadelphia: Harper and Row; 1983:379–443.

199. Hettinga DL. Inflammatory response of synovial joint structures. In: Gould JA, Davies GJ, eds. *Orthopaedic and Sports Physical Therapy.* St. Louis: CV Mosby; 1985:87–117.

200. Maadalo A, Waller JF. Rehabilitation of the foot and ankle linkage system. In: Nicholas JA, Hershman EB, eds. *The Lower Extremity and Spine in Sports Medicine.* St. Louis: CV Mosby; 1986:560–583.

201. McClusky GM, Blackburn TA, Lewis TA. A treatment for ankle sprains. *Am J Sports Med* 1976;4:158–161.

202. O'Donoghue DH. Treatment of ankle injuries. *Northwest Med* 1958;57:1277–1286.

203. Vegso JJ, Harmon LE. Non-operative management of athletic ankle injuries. *Clin Sports Med* 1982;1:85–98.

204. Wilkerson GB. Treatment of ankle sprains with external compression and early mobilization. *Phys Sports Med* 1985;13:83–90.

205. Konradsen L, Olesen S, Hansen HM. Ankle sensorimotor control and eversion strength after acute ankle inversion injuries. *Am J Sports Med* 1998;26:72–78.

206. Korkala O, et al. A prospective study of the treatment of severe tears of the lateral ligament of the ankle. *Int Orthop* 1987;11:13–17.

207. Knight KL, et al. A re-examination of Lewis' cold induced vasodilation in the finger and ankle. *Athl Training* 1980;15:248–250.

208. Knight KL, Londeree BR. Comparison of blood flow in the ankle of uninjured subjects during therapeutic applications of heat, cold, and exercise. *Med Sci Sports Exerc* 1980;12:76–80.

209. Knue J, Hitchings C. The use of a rigid stirrup for prophylactic ankle support. *Athl Training* 1982;18:121.

210. Quillen WS. An alternative management protocol for lateral ankle sprains. *J Orthop Sports Phys Ther* 1981;2:187–190.

211. Löfvenberg R, Karrholm J. The influence of an ankle orthosis on the talar calcaneal motions in chronic lateral instability of the ankle: a stereophotogrammetric analysis. *Am J Sports Med* 1993;21:224–230.

212. Shapiro MS, et al. Ankle sprain prophylaxis: an analysis of the stabilizing effects of braces and tapes. *Am J Sports Med* 1994;22:78–82.

213. Siegler S, et al. The three dimensional passive support characteristics of ankle braces. *J Orthop Sports Phys Ther* 1997;26:299–309.

214. Stover CN. Air stirrup management of ankle injuries in the athlete. *Am J Sports Med* 1980;8:360–365.

215. Gross MT, et al. Effect of ankle orthosis on functional performance for individuals with recurrent ankle sprains. *J Orthop Sports Phys Ther* 1997;25:245–252.

216. Sharpe SS, Knapik J, Jones B. Ankle braces effectively reduce recurrence of ankle sprains in female soccer players. *J Athl Training* 1997;32:21–24.

217. Sitler M, et al. The efficacy of a semirigid ankle stabilizer to reduce acute ankle injuries in basketball: a randomized clinical study at West Point. *Am J Sports Med* 1994;22:454–461.

218. Surve I, et al. A fivefold reduction in the incidence of recurrent ankle sprains in soccer players using the sport-stirrup orthosis. *Am J Sports Med* 1994;22:601–606.

219. Abdenour TE, et al. The effect of ankle taping upon torque and range of motion. *Athl Training* 1979;14:227–228.

220. Barnett JR, et al. High versus low top shoes for the prevention of ankle sprains in basketball players: a prospective randomized study. *Am J Sports Med* 1993;21:582–596.

221. Delacerde FG. Effect of underwrap conditions on the supportive effectiveness of ankle strapping with tape. *J Sports Med Phys Fitness* 1978;18:77–81.

222. Garrick JG, Requa RK. Role of external support in the prevention of ankle sprains. *Med Sci Sports Exerc* 1973;5:200–203.

223. Metcalfe RC, et al. A comparison of moleskin tape, linen tape and lace up brace on joint restriction and movement performance. *J Athl Training* 1997;32:136–140.

224. Pederson TS, et al. The effects of spatting and ankle taping on inversion before and after exercise. *J Athl Training* 1997;32:29–33.

225. Bunch RP, et al. Ankle joint support: a comparison of reusable lace on braces with taping and wrapping. *Physician Sportsmed* 1985;13:59–62.

226. Fumich RM, et al. The measured effect of taping on combined foot and ankle motion before and after exercise. *Am J Sports Med* 1981;9:165–170.

227. Glick JM, Gordon RB, Nishimoto D. The prevention and treatment of ankle injuries. *Am J Sports Med* 1976;4:136–141.

228. Laughman RK, et al. Three-dimensional kinematics of the taped ankle before and after exercise. *Am J Sports Med* 1980; 8:425–431.

229. Malina RM, Plagenz LB, Rarick GL. Effect of exercise upon measurable supporting strength of cloth and tape on ankle wraps. *Res Q* 1963;34:158–165.

230. Manfroy PP, Ashton-Miller JA, Wojtys EM. The effect of exercise, pre-wrap and athletic tape on the maximal active and passive ankle resistance to ankle inversion. *Am J Sports Med* 1997;25:156–163.

231. Paris DL, Vardaxis V, Kokkaliaris J. Ankle ranges of motion during extended activity periods while taped and braced. *J Athl Training* 1995;30:223–228.

232. Rarick GL, et al. The measurable support of the ankle joint by conventional methods of taping. *J Bone Joint Surg* 1962;44A:1183–1190.

233. Karlsson J, Andreasson GO. The effect of external ankle support in chronic lateral ankle joint instability. *Am J Sports Med* 1992;20:257–261.

234. Refshauge KM, Kilbreath SL, Raymond J. The effect of recurrent ankle inversion sprain and taping on proprioception at the ankle. *Med Sci Sports Exerc* 2000;32:10–15.

235. Gandevia SC, McCloskey DI. Joint sense, muscle sense, and their combination as position sense, measured at the distal interphalangeal joint of the middle finger. *J Physiol* 1976;260:387–407.

236. Provins KA. The effect of peripheral nerve block on the appreciation and execution of finger movements. *J Physiol* 1958;143:55–67.

237. Jerosch J, et al. The influence of orthoses on the proprioception of the ankle joint. *Knee Surg Sports Traumatol Arthrosc* 1995;3:39–46.

238. Robbins S, Waked E, Rappel R. Ankle taping improves proprioception before and after exercise in young men. *Br J Sports Med* 1995;29:242–247.

239. Lindley TR, Kernozed TW. Taping and semirigid bracing may not affect ankle functional range of motion. *J Athl Training* 1995;30:109–112.

240. MacKean LC, Bell G, Burnham RS. Prophylactic ankle bracing versus taping: effects of functional performance in female basketball players. *J Orthop Sports Phys Ther* 1995;22:77–82.

241. MacPherson K, et al. Effects of a semirigid and soft shell prophylactic ankle stabilizer on selected performance tests among high school football players. *J Orthop Sports Phys Ther* 1995;21:147–152.

242. Verbrugge JD. The effects of semirigid air stirrup bracing versus adhesive ankle taping on motor performance. *J Sports Orthop Phys Ther* 1996;23:320–325.

243. Wiley JP, Nigg BM. The effect of an ankle orthosis on ankle range of motion and performance. *J Orthop Sports Phys Ther* 1996;23:362–369.

243a. Wilk BR, Gutierrez W. Shoes and athletic injuries: analyzing shoe design, wear pattern and manufacturers' defects. *AMAA Quart,* Winter 2000:4–12.

244. Mizel MD, Marymont JV, Trapman E. Treatment of plantar fasciitis with a night splint and shoe modification consisting of a steel shank and anterior rocker bottom. *Foot Ankle Int* 1997;17:732–735.

245. Powell MW, Post WR, Keener JK. Effective treatment of chronic plantar fasciitis with dorsiflexion night splints: A cross-over prospective randomized study. *Foot Ankle Int* 1998;19:10–18.

246. Wapner KL, Sharkey PF. The use of night splints for treatment of recalcitrant plantar fasciitis. *Foot Ankle* 1991;1:135–137.

247. Cornwall MW. Foot and ankle orthosis. In: Wadsworth C, ed. *Contemporary Topics in the Foot and Ankle.* La Crosse, WI: Orthopaedic Section, APTA, Inc.; 2000.

248. Smith-Oricchio K, Harris BA. Interrater reliability of subtalar neutral, calcaneal inversion and eversion. *J Orthop Sports Phys Ther* 1990;12:10–15.

249. McPoil TG, Knecht HG, Schuit D. A survey of foot types in normal females between the ages of 18 and 30 years. *J Orthop Sports Phys Ther* 1988;9:406–409.

250. Garbalosa JC, et al. The frontal plane relationship of the forefoot to the rearfoot in an asymptomatic population. *J Orthop Sports Phys Ther* 1994;20:200–206.

251. Elveru RA, Rothstein JM, Lamb RL. Goniometric reliability in a clinical setting: subtalar and ankle measurements. *Phys Ther* 1988;68:672–677.

252. Milgrom C, et al. A prospective study of the effect of a shock-absorbing orthotic device on the incidence of stress fractures in military recruits. *Foot Ankle* 1985;6:101–104.

253. Nawoczenski DA. Orthoses for the foot. In: Nawoczenski DA, Epler ME, eds. *Orthotics in Functional Rehabilitation of the Lower Limb.* Philadelphia: WB Saunders; 1997:116–155.

254. Kaltenborn FM. *Manual Mobilization of the Extremity Joints: Basic Examination and Treatment Techniques,* 4th ed. Oslo, Norway: Olaf Norlis Bokhandel, Universitetsgaten; 1989.

255. Lentell GL, Katzman LL, Walters MR. The relationship between muscle function and ankle stability. *J Orthop Sports Phys Ther* 1990;11:605–611.

256. Kleinrensink GJ, et al. Lowered motor conduction velocity of the peroneal nerve after inversion moments. *Am J Sports Med* 1996;24:362–369.

257. Nawoczenski DA, et al. Objective evaluation of peroneal response to sudden inversion stress. *J Orthop Sports Phys Ther* 1985;7:107–109.

258. Lynch SA, et al. Electromyographic latency changes in the ankle musculature during inversion moments. *Am J Sports Med* 1996;24:362–369.

259. Voss DE, Ionta MK, Myers DJ. *Proprioceptive Neuromuscular Facilitation: Patterns and Techniques*. Philadelphia: Harper and Row; 1985:1–342.

260. Docherty CL, Moore JH, Arnold BL. Effects of strength training on strength development and joint position sense in functionally unstable ankles. *J Athl Training* 1998;33:310–314.

261. Fiore RD, Leard JS. A functional approach in the rehabilitation of the ankle and rear foot. *Athl Training* 1980;16:231–235.

262. Hoffman M, Payne VG. The effects of proprioceptive ankle disk training on healthy subjects. *J Orthop Sports Phys Ther* 1995;21:90–93.

263. Keggereis S. The construction and implementation of functional progressions as a component of athletic rehabilitation. *J Orthop Sports Phys Ther* 1985;5:14–19.

264. Mattacola CG, Lloyd JW. Effects of a 6 week strength and proprioception training program on measures of dynamic balance: a single case design. *J Athl Training* 1997;32:127–135.

265. Sheth P, et al. Ankle disk training influences reaction times of selected muscles in a simulated sprain. *Am J Sports Med* 1997;25:538–543.

266. Tropp H, Askling C, Gillquist J. Prevention of ankle sprains. *Am J Sports Med* 1985;13:259–262.

267. Wester JU, et al. Wobble board training after partial sprains of the lateral ligaments of the ankle: a prospective randomized study. *J Orthop Sports Phys Ther* 1996;23:332–336.

268. Kaikkonen A, et al. A performance test protocol and scoring scale for evaluation of ankle injuries. *Am J Sports Med* 1994;22:462–469.

269. Leanderson J, et al. Proprioception in classical ballet dancers: a prospective study on the influence of an ankle sprain proprioception in the ankle joint. *Am J Sports Med* 1996;24:370–374.

269a. Hamill J, Knutzen KM. *Biomechanical Basis of Human Movement*. Hamill J, Knutzen KM, eds. Media, Pa: Williams & Wilkins; 1995:456–488.

270. Lutter L. Injuries in the runner and jogger. *Minn Med* 1980;63:45–52.

271. Viitasalo JT, Kvist M. Some biomechanical aspects of the foot and ankle in athletes with and without shin splints. *Am J Sports Med* 1983;11:125–130.

272. Messier SP, Pittala KA. Etiologic factors associated with selected running injuries. *Med Sci Sports Exerc* 1988;20:501–505.

273. DeLacerda FG. A study of anatomical factors involved in shin splints. *J Orthop Sports Phys Ther* 1980;2:55–59.

274. Mann RA. Biomechanics of the foot. *Instruct Course Lect* 1982;31:167–180.

275. Donatelli RA. Abnormal biomechanics of the foot and ankle. *J Orthop Sports Phys Ther* 1987;9:11–16.

276. Mann RA. Pain in the foot. *Postgrad Med* 1987;82:154–162.

277. Dahle LK, et al. Visual assessment of foot type and relationship of foot type to lower extremity injury. *J Orthop Sports Phys Ther* 1991;4:70–74.

278. Buchbinder MR, Napora NJ, Biggs EW. The relationship of abnormal pronation to chondromalacia of the patella in distance runners. *J Am Podiatr Med Assoc* 1979;69:159.

279. Johanson MA, et al. Effects of three different posting methods on controlling abnormal subtalar pronation. *Phys Ther* 1994;74:149–161.

280. Hadley A, et al. Antipronation taping and temporary orthoses: effects on tibial rotation position after exercise. *J Am Podiatr Med Assn* 1999;89:118–123.

281. Keenan AM, Tanner CM. The effect of high-dye and low-dye taping on rearfoot motion. *J Am Podiatr Med Assn* 2001;91:255–261.

282. Staheli LT. Evaluation of planovalgus foot deformities with special reference to the natural history. *J Am Podiatr Med Assn* 1987;77:2–6.

283. Barry RJ, Scranton PE Jr. Flatfeet in children. *Clin Orthop* 1983;181:68–75.

284. Griffin LY. Common sports injuries of the foot and ankle seen in children and adolescents. *Orthop Clin North Am* 1994;25:83–93.

285. McPoil TG. The foot and ankle. In: Malone TR, McPoil TG, Nitz AJ, eds. *Orthopaedic and Sports Physical Therapy*. St. Louis: Mosby-Year-Book, Inc; 1997:261–293.

286. Subotnick SI. The foot and sports medicine. *J Orthop Sports Phys Ther* 1980;2:53–54.

287. Garbolosa JC, et al. Frontal plane relationship of the forefoot to the rearfoot in an asymptomatic population. *J Orthop Sports Phys Ther* 1994;20:200–206.

288. McCrea JD. *Pediatric Orthopaedics of the Lower Extremity*. Mt. Kisco, NY: Futura Publishing Co.; 1985.

289. Hutton WC, Dhanedran M. The mechanics of normal and hallux valgus feet—a quantitative study. *Clin Orthop* 1981;157:7–13.

290. Herdon CH, Heyman CH. Problems in the recognition and treatment of congenital convex pes valgus. *J Bone Joint Surg* 1963;45A:413–418.

291. Mann RA. Hallux rigidus. *Instr Course Lect* 1990;39:15–21.

292. Mann RA. Hallux rigidus: treatment by cheilectomy. *J Bone Joint Surg* 1988;70A:400–406.

293. Moberg E. A simple operation for hallux rigidus. *Clin Orthop* 1979;142:55–56.

294. Elkus RA. Tarsal coalition in the young athlete. *Am J Sports Med* 1986;14:477–480.

295. O'Neill DB, Micheli LJ. Tarsal coalition: a follow-up of adolescent athletes. *Am J Sports Med* 1989;17:544–549.

296. Hunter-Griffin LY. Injuries to the leg, ankle, and foot. In: Sullivan JA, Grana WA, eds. *The Pediatric Athlete*. Park Ridge, IL: American Academy of Orthopaedic Surgeons; 1990:187–198.

297. Mitchell GP, Gibson JMC. Excision of calcaneonavicular bar for painful spasmodic flatfoot. *J Bone Joint Surg* 1967;49B:281–287.

298. Stormont DM, Peterson HA. The relative incidence of tarsal coalition. *Clin Orthop* 1983;181:28–36.

299. Hintermann B, Nigg BM, Cole GK. Influence of selective arthrodesis on the movement transfer between calcaneus and tibia in vitro. *Clin Biomech* 1994;9:356–361.

300. Harris RI, Beath T. Etiology of peroneal spastic flatfoot. *J Bone Joint Surg* 1948;30B:624–634.

301. Frey C. Foot health and shoewear for women. *Clin Orthop Rel Res* 2000;372:32–44.

302. Geissele AE, Stanton RP. Surgical treatment of adolescent hallux valgus. *J Pediatr Orthop* 1990;10:642–648.

303. McDonald MD, Stevens DB. Modified Mitchell bunionectomy for management of adolescent hallux valgus. *Clin Orthop* 1996;332:163–169.

304. Cole S. Foot inspection of the school child. *J Am Podiatry Assoc* 1959;49:446–454.

305. Coughlin MJ. Juvenile bunions. In: Mann RA, Coughlin MJ, eds. *Surgery of the Foot and Ankle.* St. Louis: Mosby-Year Book; 1993:297–339.

306. Craigmile DA. Incidence, origin, and prevention of certain foot defects. *BMJ* 1953;2:749–752.

307. Scranton PE Jr, Zuckerman JD. Bunion surgery in adolescents: results of surgical treatment. *J Pediatr Orthop* 1984;4:39–43.

308. Mann RA. The great toe. *Orthop Clin North Am* 1989; 20:519–533.

309. Baxter DE. Treatment of the bunion deformity in athletes. *Orthop Clin North Am* 1994;25:33–39.

310. Bowers KD Jr, Martin RB. Impact absorption: new and old Astroturf at West Virginia University. *Med Sci Sports Exerc* 1974;6:217–221.

311. Rodeo SA, et al. Turf-toe: an analysis of metatarsophalangeal joint sprains in professional football players. *Am J Sports Med* 1990;18:280–285.

311a. Clanton TO, Ford JJ. Turf toe injury. *Clin Sports Med* 1984; 13:731–741.

312. Garrick JG. The frequency of injury, mechanism of injury, and epidemiology of ankle sprains. *Am J Sports Med* 1977; 5:241–242.

313. Garrick JG. Characterization of the patient population in a sports medicine facility. *Physician Sportsmed* 1985;13:73–76.

314. Barker HB, Beynnon BD, Renstrom P. Ankle injury risk factors in sports. *Sports Med* 1997;23:69–74.

315. Kaeding CC, Whitehead R. Musculoskeletal injuries in adolescents. *Primary Care Clin Office Pract* 1998;25:211–223.

316. Vargish T, et al. The ankle injury—indications for the selective use of x-rays. *Injury* 1983;14:507.

317. Brand RL, Black HM, Cox JS. The natural history of inadequately treated ankle sprains. *Am J Sports Med* 1977;5:248–249.

318. Brostrom L, Sundelin P. Sprained ankles: IV. Histologic changes in recent and "chronic" ligament ruptures. *Acta Chir Scand* 1966;132:248–253.

319. Brostrom L. Sprained ankles: V. Treatment and prognosis in recent ligament ruptures. *Acta Chir Scand* 1966;132:537–550.

320. Brostrom L. Sprained ankles: VI. Surgical treatment of "chronic" ligament ruptures. *Acta Chir Scand* 1966; 132:551–565.

321. Harrington KD. Degenerative arthritis of the ankle secondary to long standing lateral ligament instability. *J Bone Joint Surg* 1979;61A:354–361.

322. Javors JR, Violet JT. Correction of chronic lateral ligament instability of the ankle by use of the Brostrom procedure. *Clin Orthop* 1985;198:201–207.

323. Lauttamus L, Korkala O, Tanskanen P. Lateral ligament injuries of the ankle: surgical treatment of the late cases. *Ann Chir Gynaecol* 1982;71:164–167.

324. Riegler HF. Reconstruction for lateral instability of the ankle. *J Bone Joint Surg* 1984;66A:336–339.

325. Stewart MJ, Hutchings WC. Repair of the lateral ligament of the ankle. *Am J Sports Med* 1978;6:272–275.

326. Brostrom L, Liljedahl SO, Lindvall N. Sprained ankles: II. Arthrographic diagnosis of recent ligament ruptures. *Acta Chir Scand* 1965;129:485–499.

327. Gerber JP, et al. Persistent disability associated with ankle sprains: a prospective examination of an athletic population. *Foot Ankle Int* 1998;19:653–660.

328. Dias LS. Fractures of the distal tibial and fibular physes. In: Rockwood JCA, Wilkins KE, King RE, eds. *Fractures in Children.* Philadelphia: Lippincott; 1991:1314–1381.

329. McManama GB, Jr. Ankle injuries in the young athlete. *Clin Sports Med* 1988;7:547.

330. Klenerman L. The management of sprained ankle. *J Bone Joint Surg [Br]* 1998;80:11–20.

331. Prins JG. Diagnosis and treatment of injury to the lateral ligament lesion of the ankle: a comparative clinical study. *Acta Chir Scand* 1978;(Suppl)486:3–149.

332. Thorndike A. *Athletic Injuries: Prevention, Diagnosis and Treatment.* Philadelphia: Lea and Febiger; 1962.

333. Inman VT. Sprains of the ankle. In: Chapman MW, ed. *AAOS Instructional Course Lectures.* 1975:294–308.

334. O'Donoghue DH. *Treatment of Injuries to Athletes.* Philadelphia: WB Saunders; 1976:698–746.

335. Gronmark T, Johnson O, Kogstad O. Rupture of the lateral ligaments of the ankle. *Foot Ankle* 1980;1:84–89.

336. Iversen LD, Clawson DK. *Manual of Acute Orthopaedics.* Boston: Little, Brown, and Co.; 1982:231–236.

337. Kannus P, Renstrom P. Current concepts review: treatment of acute tears of the lateral ligaments of the ankle. *J Bone Joint Surg* 1991;73A:305–312.

338. Balduini FC, Tetzelaff J. Historical perspectives on injuries of the ligaments of the ankle. *Clin Sports Med* 1982;1:3–12.

339. Prentice WE. Using therapeutic modalities in rehabilitation. In: Prentice WE, Voight ML, eds. *Techniques in Musculoskeletal Rehabilitation.* New York: McGraw-Hill; 2001:289–303.

340. Eiff MP, Smith AT, Smith GE. Early mobilization versus immobilization in the treatment of lateral ankle sprains. *Am J Sports Med* 1994;22:83–88.

341. Noyes FR, et al. Biomechanics of ligament failure: II. An analysis of immobilization, exercise, and reconditioning effects in primates. *J Bone Joint Surg* 1974;56A:1406–1418.

342. Tipton CM, et al. Influence of exercise in strength of medial collateral knee ligaments of dogs. *Am J Physiol* 1970;218:894–902.

343. Tipton CM, et al. The influence of physical activity on ligaments and tendons. *Med Sci Sports Exerc* 1975;7:165–175.

344. Vailas AC, et al. Physical activity and its influence on the repair process of medial collateral ligaments. *Connect Tissue Res* 1981;9:25–31.

345. Dias LS. The lateral ankle sprain: an experimental study. *J Trauma* 1977;19:266–269.

346. Ramsey PL, Hamilton WC. Lateral talar subluxation: the effect of tibiotalar contact surfaces. *J Bone Joint Surg* 1975; 57A:567–568.

347. Brand RL, Collins MDF, Templeton T. Surgical repair of ruptured lateral ankle ligaments. *Am J Sports Med* 1981;9:40–44.

348. Freeman MAR, Dean MRE, Hanham IWF. The etiology and prevention of functional instability of the foot. *J Bone Joint Surg* 1965;47B:678–685.

349. Karlsson J, Bergstern T, Peterson L. Reconstruction of the lateral ligaments of the ankle for chronic lateral instability. *J Bone Joint Surg* 1988;70-A:581–588.

350. Ruth CJ. The surgical treatment of injuries of the fibular collateral ligaments of the ankle. *J Bone Joint Surg* 1961;43A:229–239.

351. Hintermann B. Biomechanik der Sprunggelenke: Unfallmechanismen. [Biomechanics of the ankle joint: injury mechanisms.] *Swiss Surg* 1998;4:63–69.

352. Orava S, Jaroma H, Suvela M. Radiological instability of the ankle after Evan's repair. *Acta Orthop Scand* 1983;54:734–738.

353. Nicholas JA. Ankle injuries in athletes. *Orthop Clin North Am* 1974;15:153–175.

354. Tropp H. *Functional Instability of the Ankle Joint.* Linkoping, Sweden: Linkoping University; 1985.

355. Elmslie RC. Recurrent subluxation of the ankle joint. *Ann Surg* 1934;100:364–367.

356. Hintermann B. Die anatomische Rekonstruktion des Aussenbandapparates mit der Plantarissehne. [Anatomical reconstruction of the lateral ligament complex of the ankle.] *Operat Orthop Traumatol* 1998;10:210–218.

357. Karlsson J, et al. Surgical treatment of chronic lateral instability of the ankle joint: a new procedure. *Am J Sports Med* 1989;17:268–274.

358. Karlsson J, et al. Comparison of two anatomic reconstructions for chronic lateral instability of the ankle joint. *Am J Sports Med* 1997;25:48–53.

359. Rudert M, Wülker N, Wirth CJ. Reconstruction of the lateral ligaments of the ankle using a regional periosteal flap. *J Bone Joint Surg* 1997;79-B:446–451.

360. Sammarco GJ, Diraimondo CV. Surgical treatment of lateral ankle instability syndrome. *Am J Sports Med* 1988;16:501–511.

361. Rosenbaum D, et al. Functional evaluation of the 10-year outcome after modified Evans repair for chronic ankle instability. *Foot Ankle Int* 1997;18:765–771.

362. Curtis MJ, Myerson M, Szura B. Tarsometatarsal joint injuries in the athlete. *Am J Sports Med* 1993;21:497–502.

363. Clanton TO, Porter DA. Primary care of foot and ankle injuries in the athlete. *Clin Sports Med* 1997;16:435–466.

364. Marshall P, Hamilton WG. Cuboid subluxation in ballet dancers. *Am J Sports Med* 1992;20:169–175.

365. Blakeslee TJ, Morris JL. Cuboid syndrome and the significance of midtarsal joint stability. *J Am Podiat Med Assn* 1987;77:638–642.

366. Khan K, et al. Overuse injuries in classical ballet. *Sports Med* 1995;19:341–357.

367. Newell SG, Woodie A. Cuboid syndrome. *Physician Sportsmed* 1981;9:71–76.

368. Hefland AE. Nail and hyperkeratotic problems in the elderly foot. *Am Fam Phys* 1989;39:101–110.

369. Subotnick SI. Foot injuries. In: Subotnick SI, ed. *Sports Medicine of the Lower Extremity.* Philadelphia: Churchill Livingstone; 1999:207–260.

370. Bendl BJ. Subungual exostosis. *Cutis* 1980;26:260.

371. Zook EG. The perionychium: Anatomy, physiology, and care of injuries. *Clin Plast Surg* 1981;8:27.

372. Bartolomei FJ. Onychauxis. *Clin Podiatr Med Surg* 1995;12:215–220.

373. Krausz CE. Nail survey of 12,500 patients. *Br J Chiropody* 1983;48:239.

374. Sammarco GJ. Peroneal tendon injuries. *Orthop Clin North Am* 1994;25:135–145.

375. Micheli LJ, Waters PM, Sanders DP. Sliding fibular graft repair for chronic dislocation of the peroneal tendons. *Am J Sports Med* 1989;17:68–71.

376. Clanton TO, Schon LC. Athletic injuries to the soft tissues of the foot and ankle. In: Mann RA, Coughlin MJ, eds. *Surgery of the Foot and Ankle.* St. Louis: Mosby-Year Book; 1993:1167–1177.

377. Frey CC, Shereff MJ. Tendon injuries about the ankle in athletes. *Clin Sports Med* 1988;7:103–118.

378. Niemi WJ, Savidakis J, Dejesus JM. Peroneal subluxation: a comprehensive review of the literature with case presentations. *J Foot Ankle Surg* 1997;36:141–145.

379. Stover CN, Bryan DR. Traumatic dislocation of the peroneal tendons. *Am J Surg* 1962;103:180–186.

380. Arrowsmith SR, Fleming LL, Allman FL. Traumatic dislocations of the peroneal tendons. *Am J Sports Med* 1983;11:142–146.

381. Eckert WR, Davis FA. Acute rupture of the peroneal retinaculum. *J Bone Joint Surg* 1976;58A:670–673.

382. Slatis P, Santavirta S, Sandelin J. Surgical treatment of chronic dislocation of the peroneal tendons. *Br J Sports Med* 1988;22:16–18.

383. Sobel M, Geppert MJ, Warren RF. Chronic ankle instability as a cause of peroneal tendon injury. *Clin Orthop Rel Res* 1993;296:187–191.

384. Kettlecamp D, Alexander H. Spontaneous rupture of the posterior tibialis tendon. *J Bone Joint Surg* 1969;51A:759.

385. Groshar D, et al. Scintigraphy of posterior tibial tendinitis. *J Nucl Med* 1997;38:247–249.

386. Hamilton WG, Geppert MJ, Thompson FM. Pain in the posterior aspect of the ankle in dancers. *J Bone Joint Surg* 1996;78A:1491–1500.

387. Garth WP. Flexor hallucis tendonitis in a ballet dancer. *J Bone Joint Surg* 1981;63A:1489.

388. Koleitis GJ, Micheli LJ, Klein JD. Release of the flexor hallucis longus tendon in ballet dancers. *J Bone Joint Surg* 1996;78A:1386–1390.

389. Teitz CC. Sports medicine concerns in dance and gymnastics. *Pediatr Clin North Am* 1982;29:1399–1421.

390. Morford M, Lenardon RJ. *Classical Mythology.* New York: Longman, Inc.; 1985:3329–3335.

391. Clain MR, Baxter DE. Achilles tendinitis. *Foot Ankle* 1992;13:482–487.

392. Voorn R. Case report: can sacroiliac joint dysfunction cause chronic Achilles tendinitis? *J Orthop Sports Phys Ther* 1998;27:436–443.

393. McCrory JL, et al. Etiologic factors associated with Achilles tendinitis in runners. *Med Sci Sports Exerc* 1999;31:1374–1381.

394. Smart GW, Taunton JE, Clement DB. Achilles tendon disorders in runners: a review. *Med Sci Sport Exerc* 1980;12:231–243.

395. Jacobs SJ, Berson BJ. Injuries to runners: a study of entrants to a 10,000 meter race. *Am J Sports Med* 1986;14:151–155.

396. Pinshaw R, Atlas V, Noakes TD. The nature and response to therapy of 196 consecutive injuries seen at a runners' clinic. *S Afr Med J* 1984;65:291–298.

397. Brunet ME, et al. A survey of running injuries in 1505 competitive and recreational runners. *J Sports Med Phys Fitness* 1990;30:307–315.

398. van Mechelen W, et al. Prevention of running injuries by warmup, cool-down and stretching exercises. *Am J Sports Med* 1993;21:711–719.

399. Hess GP, et al. Prevention and treatment of overuse tendon injuries. *Sports Med* 1989;8:371–384.

400. Clement DB, et al. A survey of overuse running injuries. *Physician Sportsmed* 1981;9:47–58.

401. Renstrom P, Johnson RJ. Overuse injuries in sports: a review. *Sports Med* 1985;2:316–333.

402. Lyshold J, Wiklander J. Injuries in runners. *Am J Sports Med* 1987;15:168–171.

403. Sheehan GA. An overview of overuse syndromes in distance runners. *Ann NY Acad Sci* 1977;301:877–880.

404. Barry NN, McGuire JL. Overuse syndromes in adult athletes. *Rheum Dis Clin North Am* 1996;22:515–530.

405. Gudas CJ. Patterns of lower extremity injury in 224 runners. *Exerc Sports Med* 1980;12:50–59.

406. Hogan DG, Cape RD. Marathoners over sixty years of age: results of a survey. *J Am Geriatr Soc* 1984;32:121–123.

407. Janis LR. Results of the Ohio runners sports medicine survey. *J Am Podiatr Med Assoc* 1986;10:586–589.

408. Sarrafian SK. Functional anatomy. In: *Anatomy of the Ankle and Foot*. Philadelphia: JB Lippincott; 1992:559–590.

409. Kapandji IA. *The Physiology of Joints*, Vol. 3. New York: Churchill Livingstone; 1974:54–71.

410. Grieve GP. *Common Vertebral Joint Problems*. New York: Churchill Livingstone; 1981.

411. Menell JB. *The Science and Art of Joint Manipulation, Spinal Column*, Vol. 2. London: J & A Churchill Ltd.; 1952.

412. Mennell JM. *Back Pain. Diagnosis and Treatment Using Manipulative Techniques*. Boston: Little, Brown & Co.; 1960.

413. Hartman SL. *Handbook of Osteopathic Technique*, 2nd ed. London: Unwin Hyman Ltd., Academic Division; 1990:135–143.

414. Magee DJ. Lumbar spine, pelvic joints. In: *Orthopedic Physical Assessment*. Philadelphia: WB Saunders; 1987:182–238.

415. Ombreght L, et al. Applied anatomy of the sacroiliac joint. In: *A System of Orthopaedic Medicine*. Philadelphia: WB Saunders; 1991:690–708.

416. Bojsen-Möller F. The human foot—A two-speed construction. In: Asmussen E, Jörgensen K, eds. *International Series of Biomechanics*. Baltimore: University Park Press; 1978: 261–266.

417. Puddu G, Ippolito E, Postacchini F. A classification of Achilles tendon disease. *Am J Sports Med* 1976;4:145–150.

418. Lohrer H. Seltene ursachen und differentialdiagnosen der achillodynie. *Sportverl-Sportschad* 1991;5:182–185.

419. Bates BT, et al. Foot orthotic devices to modify selected aspects of lower extremity mechanics. *Am J Sports Med* 1979; 7:338–342.

420. Leach RE, Schepsis AA. Achilles tendonitis. *Postgrad Advances in Sports Medicine—Office Study Course*. Forum Medicus, Inc.: 1986.

421. Pare A. *Les Oeuvres*, 9th ed. Lyon: Claude Rigaud et Claude Obert; 1633.

422. Fox JM, et al. Degeneration and rupture of the Achilles tendon. *Clin Orthop* 1975;107:221–224.

423. Inglis AE, et al. Surgical repair of ruptures of the tendo Achillis. *J Bone Joint Surg* 1976;58A:990–993.

424. Kager H. Zur Klinik und Diagnostik des Achillesshnenrisses. *Chirurgie* 1939;11:691–695.

425. Langergren C, Lindholm A. Vascular distribution in the Achilles tendon. *Acta Chir Scand* 1958;116:491–495.

426. Maffulli N, Dymond NP, Regine R. Surgical repair of ruptured Achilles tendon in sportsmen and sedentary patients: A longitudinal ultrasound assessment. *Int J Sports Med* 1990;11:78–84.

427. Popovic N, Lemaire R. Diagnosis and treatment of acute ruptures of the Achilles tendon: Current concepts review. *Acta Orthop Belg* 1999;65:458–471.

428. Arner O, Lindholm A, Orell SR. Histologic changes in subcutaneous rupture of the Achilles tendon. *Acta Chir Scand* 1958/1959;116:484.

429. Wills CA, et al. Achilles tendon rupture: a review of the literature comparing surgical versus nonsurgical treatment. *Clin Orthop* 1986;207:156–163.

430. Fierro NL, Sallis RE. Achilles tendon rupture: Is casting enough. *Postgrad Med* 1995;98:145–151.

431. Cetti A, et al. Operative versus non-operative treatment of Achilles tendon rupture. *Am J Sports Med* 1993;21:791–799.

432. Jacobs D, et al. Comparison of conservative and operative treatment of Achilles tendon rupture. *Am J Sports Med* 1978;6:107–111.

433. Lea RB, Smith L. Non-surgical treatment of tendo Achilles rupture. *J Bone Joint Surg* 1972;54A:1398–1407.

434. Leppilahti J, Orava S. Total Achilles tendon rupture. *Sports Med* 1998;25:79–100.

435. Soma CA, Mandelbaum BR. Repair of acute Achilles tendon ruptures. *Orthop Clin North Am* 1995;26:241–246.

436. Nistor L. Surgical and non-surgical treatment of Achilles tendon rupture. *J Bone Joint Surg* 1981;63A:394–399.

437. Micheli LJ, Ireland ML. Prevention and management of calcaneal apophysitis in children: an overuse syndrome. *J Pediatr Orthop* 1987;7:34–38.

438. Mafulli N. Intensive training in young athletes. *Sports Med* 1990;9:229–243.

439. Stanitski C. Management of sports injuries in children and adolescents. *Orthop Clin North Am* 1988;19:689–698.

440. Meeusen R, Borms J. Gymnastic injuries. *Sports Med* 1992; 13:337–356.

441. Canale ST, Williams KD. Iselin's disease. *J Pediatr Orthop* 1992;12:90–93.

441a. Omey ML, Micheli LJ. Foot and ankle problems in the young athlete. *Med Sci Sports Exer* 1999; 31(7 (Suppl)):S470–486.

442. DeMaio M, et al. Plantar fasciitis. *Orthopedics* 1993;16: 1153–1163.

443. Barrett SL, et al. Endoscopic heel anatomy: analysis of 200 fresh frozen specimens. *J Foot Ankle Surg* 1995;34:51–56.

444. DuVries HL. Heel spur (calcaneal spur). *Arch Surg* 1957; 74:536–542.

445. Tanz SS. Heel pain. *Clin Orthop* 1963;28:169–178.

446. Wolgin M, et al. Conservative treatment of plantar heel pain: long-term follow-up. *Foot Ankle* 1994;15:97–102.

447. Amis J, et al. Painful heel syndrome: radiographic and treatment assessment. *Foot Ankle* 1988;9:91–95.

448. Kier R. Magnetic resonance imaging of plantar fasciitis and other causes of heel pain. *MRI Clin North Am* 1994; 2:97–107.

449. Rubin G, Witten M. Plantar calcaneal spurs. *Am J Orthop* 1963;5:38–55.

450. Warren BL, Jones CJ. Predicting plantar fasciitis in runners. *Med Sci Sports Exerc* 1987;19:71–73.

451. Williams PL, et al. Imaging study of the painful heel syndrome. *Foot Ankle* 1987;7:345–349.

451a. Sarrafian SK. Functional anatomy of the foot and ankle. In: Sarrafian SK, ed. *Anatomy of the Foot and Ankle: Descriptive, Topographic, Functional*. Philadelphia: JB Lippincott;1993; 474–602.

451b. Prichasuk S. The heel-pad in plantar heel pain. *J Bone Joint Surg* 1994;76-B:140–142.

451c. Tsai WC, et al. The mechanical properties of the heel pad in unilateral plantar heel pain syndrome. *Foot Ankle Int* 1999; 20:663–668.

451d. Messier SP, Pittala KA. Etiologic factors associated with selected running injuries. *Med Sci Sports Exercise* 1988;20:501–505.

451e. Schepsis AA, Leach RE, Gorzyca J. Plantar fasciitis: etiology, treatment, surgical results, and review of the literature. *Clin Orthop* 1991;266:185–196.

451f. Amis J, et al. Painful heel syndrome: radiographic and treatment assessment. *Foot Ankle* 1988;9:91–95.

451g. Kibler WB, Goldberg C, Chandler TJ. Functional biomechanical deficits in running athletes with plantar fasciitis. *Am J Sports Med* 1991;19:66–71.

452. Nigg BM. Biomechanics, load analysis, and sports injuries in the lower extremities. *Sports Med* 1985;2:367–379.

453. Chandler TJ, Kibler BW. A biomechanical approach to the prevention, treatment and rehabilitation of plantar fasciitis. *Sports Med* 1993;15:344–352.

454. Schepsis AA, Leach RE, Gorzyca J. Plantar fasciitis: etiology, treatment, surgical results, and review of the literature. *Clin Orthop* 1991;266:185–196.

455. Kibler WB, Goldberg C, Chandler TJ. Functional biomechanical deficits in running athletes with plantar fasciitis. *Am J Sports Med* 1991;19:66–71.

456. Kwong PK, et al. Plantar fasciitis: mechanics and pathomechanics of treatment. *Clin Sports Med* 1988;7:119–126.

457. Furey JG. Plantar fasciitis: the painful heel syndrome. *J Bone Joint Surg* 1975;57(A):672.

458. Karr SD. Subcalcaneal heel pain. *Orthop Clin North Am* 1994;25:161–175.

459. Hendrix CL, et al. Entrapment neuropathy: the etiology of intractable chronic heel pain syndrome. *J Foot Ankle Surg* 1998;37:273–279.

460. Meyer J, Kulig K, Landel R. Differential diagnosis and treatment of subcalcaneal heel pain: a case report. *J Orthop Sports Phys Ther* 2002;32:114–124.

461. Pfeffer GB. Plantar heel pain. In: Baxter DE, ed. *The Foot and Ankle in Sport*. St. Louis: Mosby; 1995:195–206.

462. Kosinski M, Lilja E. Infectious causes of heel pain. *J Am Podiat Med Assn* 1999;89:20–23.

463. Jahss MH, et al. Investigations into the fat pads of the sole of the foot: anatomy and histology. *Foot Ankle* 1992;13:233–242.

464. Skliar JD. Heel pain syndrome. *J Foot Ankle Surg* 1998;37:548–549.

465. Van Wyngarden TM. The painful foot, part II: Common rearfoot deformities. *Am Fam Phys* 1997;55:2207–2212.

465a. Rompe JD, Schoellner C, Nafe B. Evaluation of low-energy extracorporeal shock-wave application for treatment of chronic plantar fasciitis. *J Bone Joint Surg*. 2002;84-A:335–341.

465b. Scherer PR. Heel spur syndrome. Pathomechanics and nonsurgical treatment. Biomechanics Graduate Research Group for 1988. *J Am Pod Med Assn* 1991;81:68–72.

465c. Lynch DM, et al. Conservative treatment of plantar fasciitis: a prospective study. *J Am Pod Med Assn* 1998;88:375–380.

465d. Martin RL, Irrgang JJ, Conti SF. Outcome study of subjects with insertional plantar fasciitis. *Foot Ankle Int* 1998;19:803–811.

465e. Hicks JH. Mechanics of the foot. *J Anat* 1953;87:345–357.

465f. Dananberg HJ. Functional hallux limitus and its relationship to gait efficiency. *J Am Pod Med Assn* 1986;76:648–652.

465g. DiGiovanni BF, et al. Tissue-specific plantar fascia-stretching exercise enhances outcomes in patients with chronic heel pain. A prospective, randomized study. *J Bone Joint Surg* 2003;85A:1270–1277.

466. Tanner SM, Harvey JS. How we manage plantar fasciitis. *Physician Sports Med* 1988;16:39.

467. Davis PF, Severud E, Baxter DE. Painful heel syndrome: results of nonoperative treatment. *Foot Ankle Int* 1994;15:531–535.

467a. Reid DC. Heel pain and problems of the hindfoot. In: Reid DC, ed. *Sports Injury Assessment and Rehabilitation*. New York: Churchill-Livingstone; 1992:437–493.

468. Jones D, James S. Partial calcaneal osteotomy for retrocalcaneal bursitis. *Am J Sports Med* 1984;12:72.

469. Haglund P. Beitrag zur Klinik der Achillessehne. *Z Orthop Chir* 1927;49:49–58.

470. Dickinson PH, et al. Tendo achillis bursitis: a report of twenty-one cases. *J Bone Joint Surg* 1966;48:77–81.

471. Fowler A, Philip JF. Abnormality of the calcaneus as a cause of painful heel: Its diagnosis and operative treatment. *Br J Surg* 1945;32:494–498.

472. Nisbet NW. Tendo Achilles bursitis ("winter heel"). *Br J Surg* 1954;2:1394–1395.

473. Stephens MM. Haglund's deformity and retrocalcaneal bursitis. *Orthop Clin North Am* 1994;25:41–46.

474. Taylor GJ. Prominence of the calcaneus: is operation justified? *J Bone Joint Surg* 1986;68(B):467–470.

475. Keck S, Kelley P. Bursitis of the posterior part of the heel. *J Bone Joint Surg* 1965;47(A):267–273.

476. Morton DJ. *The Human Foot: Its Evolution, Physiology, and Functional Disorders*. New York: Columbia Press; 1935:179–186.

477. Mann RA, Mizel MS. Monarticular nontraumatic synovitis of the metatarsophalangeal joint: a new diagnosis? *Foot Ankle* 1985;6:18–21.

478. Fortin PT, Myerson MS. Second metatarsophalangeal joint instability. *Foot Ankle Int* 1995;16:306–313.

479. Trepman E, Yeo SJ. Nonoperative treatment of metatarsophalangeal synovitis. *Foot Ankle Int* 1995;16:771–777.

480. Wolin I, et al. Internal derangement of the talofibular component of the ankle. *Surg Gynecol* 1950;91:193–200.

481. Ferkel RD, et al. Arthroscopic treatment of anterolateral impingement of the ankle. *Am J Sports Med* 1991;19:440–446.

482. Ferkel RD, Fischer SP. Progress in ankle arthroscopy. *Clin Orthop* 1989;240:210–220.

483. Guhl JF. Soft tissue (synovial) pathology. In: *Ankle Arthroscopy: Pathology and Surgical Technique*. Thorofare, NJ: Slack Publishing; 1993:93–135.

484. Martin DF, et al. Operative ankle arthroscopy: long-term follow-up. *Am J Sports Med* 1989;17:16–23.

485. Martin DF, Curl WW, Baker CL. Arthroscopic treatment of chronic synovitis of the ankle. *Arthroscopy* 1989;5:110–114.

486. McCarroll J, et al. Meniscoid lesions of the ankle in soccer players. *Am J Sports Med* 1987;15:255–257.

487. Reynaert P, Gelen G, Geens G. Arthroscopic treatment of anterior impingement of the ankle. *Acta Orthop Belg* 1994;60:384–388.

488. Schonholtz GJ. *Arthroscopic Surgery of the Shoulder, Elbow, and Ankle*. Springfield, IL: Charles C Thomas; 1989:69–71.

489. Bassett FH, et al. Talar impingement by the anteroinferior tibiofibular ligament. *J Bone Joint Surg* 1990;72A:55–59.

490. Thein R, Eichenblat M. Arthroscopic treatment of sports-related synovitis of the ankle. *Am J Sports Med* 1992;20:496–498.

491. Howse AJG. Posterior block of the ankle joint in dancers. *Foot Ankle* 1982;3:81–84.

492. Johnson RP, Collier BD, Carrera GF. The os trigonum syndrome, use of bone scan in the diagnosis. *J Trauma* 1984;24:761.

493. Scranton PE. Pathologic and anatomic variations of the sesamoids. *Foot Ankle* 1981;1:321–326.

494. Dobas DC, Silvers MD. The frequency of partite sesamoids of the metatarsophalangeal joint. *J Am Podiatry Assoc* 1977;67:880–882.

495. Coughlin MJ. Sesamoid pain: causes and surgical treatment. *Instr Course Lect* 1990;39:23–35.

496. Mann RA. Metatarsalgia: Common causes and conservative treatment. *Postgrad Med* 1984;75:150–167.

497. Orava S, Puranen J. Athletes' leg pain. *Br J Sports Med* 1979;13:92–97.

498. Blue JM, Mathews LS. Leg injuries. *Clin Sports Med* 1997;16:467–478.

499. Andrish JT. Leg pain. In: DeLee JC, Drez D, eds. *Orthopedic Sports Medicine*. Philadelphia: WB Saunders; 1994:1603–1607.

500. Graham CE, Graham DM. Morton's neuroma: a microscopic evaluation. *Foot Ankle* 1984;5:150.

501. Wu KK. Morton's interdigital neuroma: a clinical review of its etiology, treatment, and results. *J Foot Ankle Surg* 1996;35:112–119.

502. Mulder JD. The causative mechanism in Morton's metatarsalgia. *J Bone Joint Surg* 1951;33B:94–95.

503. Szabo RM. Carpal tunnel syndrome—general. In: Gelberman RH, ed. *Operative Nerve Repair and Reconstruction*. Philadelphia: JB Lippincott; 1991:882–883.

504. Koppell HP, Thompson WAL. *Peripheral Entrapment Neuropathies*. Baltimore: Williams & Wilkins; 1963.

505. Marinacci AA. *Applied Electromyography*. Philadelphia: Lea & Febiger; 1968.

506. Borges LF, et al. The anterior tarsal tunnel syndrome. *J Neurosurg* 1981;54:89–92.

507. Dellon AL. Deep peroneal nerve entrapment on the dorsum of the foot. *Foot Ankle* 1990;11:73–80.

508. Zengzhao L, Jiansheng Z, Li Z. Anterior tarsal syndrome. *J Bone Joint Surg* 1991;73B:470–473.

509. Krause KH, Witt T, Ross A. The anterior tarsal syndrome. *J Neurol* 1977;217:67–74.

510. Gessini L, Jandolo B, Pietrangeli A. The anterior tarsal syndrome: report of four cases. *J Bone Joint Surg* 1984;66A:786–787.

511. Ombregt L, et al. Nerve lesions and entrapment neuropathies of the lower limb. In: Ombregt L, ed. *A System of Orthopaedic Medicine*. London: WB Saunders; 1995:932–937.

512. Hyslop GH. Injuries to the deep and superficial peroneal nerves complicating ankle sprain. *Am J Surg* 1941;51:436–439.

513. Pecina M, Krmpotic-Nemanic J, Markiewitz A. *Tunnel Syndromes*. Boca Raton: CRC; 1991.

514. Acus RW, Flanagan JP. Perineural fibrosis of superficial peroneal nerve complicating ankle sprain: a case report. *Foot Ankle Int* 1991;11:233–235.

515. Meals RA. Peroneal-nerve palsy complicating ankle sprain: report of two cases and review of the literature. *J Bone Joint Surg* 1977;59-A:966–968.

516. Nitz AJ, Dobner JJ, Kersey D. Nerve injury and grades II and III ankle sprains. *Am J Sports Med* 1985;13:177–182.

517. Mueller MJ, et al. Insensitivity, limited joint mobility, and plantar ulcers in patients with diabetes mellitus. *Phys Ther* 1989;69:453–462.

518. Mueller MJ. Etiology, evaluation, and treatment of the neuropathic foot. *Crit Rev Phys Rehabil Med* 1992;3:289–309.

518a. Appling SA, Kasser RJ. Foot and ankle. In: Wadsworth C, ed. *Current Concepts of Orthopaedic Physical Therapy Home Study Course*, La Crosse, WI: Orthopaedic Section, APTA; 2001.

518b. Reddy M., et al., *Practical treatment of wound pain and trauma: a patient-centered approach. An overview.* Ostomy Wound Management, 2003. 49(4 Suppl): p. 2-15.

519. Dietz FR, Matthews KD, Montgomery WJ. Reflex sympathetic dystrophy in children. *Clin Orthop* 1990;258:225–231.

520. Smolders JJ. Myofascial pain and dysfunction syndromes. In: Hammer WI, ed. *Functional Soft Tissue Examination and Treatment by Manual Methods—The Extremities*. Gaithersburg, MD: Aspen; 1991:215–234.

521. McBryde AM Jr. Stress fractures in athletes. *J Sports Med* 1975;3:212–217.

522. Monteleone GP. Stress fractures in the athlete. *Orthop Clin North Am* 1995;26:423.

523. Brudvig TJ, Gudger TD, Obermeyer L. Stress fractures in 295 trainees: a one-year study of incidence as related to age, sex, and race. *Mil Med* 1983;148:666–667.

524. Protzman PR. Physiologic performance of women compared to men at the U.S. Military Academy. *Am J Sports Med* 1979; 7:191–196.

525. Marshall LA. Clinical evaluation of amenorrhea. In: Agostini R, Titus S, eds. *Medical and Orthopedic Issues of Active and Athletic Women*. Philadelphia: Hanley and Belfus; 1994:152–163.

526. Myburgh KH, et al. Low bone mineral density at axial and appendicular sites in amenorrheic athletes. *Med Sci Sports Exerc* 1993;25:1197–1202.

527. Sharkey NA, et al. Strain and loading of the second metatarsal during heel life. *J Bone Joint Surg* 1995;77A:1050–1057.

528. Pester S, Smith PC. Stress fractures in the lower extremities of soldiers in basic training. *Orthop Rev* 1992;21:297–303.

529. Gardner LI, et al. Prevention of lower extremity stress fractures: a controlled trial of a shock absorbent insole. *Am J Public Health* 1988;78:1563.

530. Schwellnus MP, Jordaan G, Noakes TD. Prevention of common overuse injuries by the use of shock absorbing insoles: a prospective study. *Am J Sports Med* 1990;18:636–641.

531. Gross RH. Fractures and dislocations of the foot. In: Rockwood JCA, Wilkins KE, King RE, eds. *Fractures in Children*. Philadelphia: Lippincott; 1991:1383–1453.

532. Harrington T, Crichton KJ, Anderson IF. Overuse ballet injury of the base of the second metatarsal: a diagnostic problem. *Am J Sports Med* 1993;21:591–598.

533. Hamilton WG. Foot and ankle injuries in dancers. In: Mann RA, Coughlin MJ, eds. *Surgery of the Foot and Ankle*. St. Louis: Mosby-Year Book; 1993:1241–1276.

534. Micheli LJ, Sohn RS, Solomon R. Stress fractures of the second metatarsal involving Lisfranc's joint in ballet dancers. *J Bone Joint Surg* 1985;67A:1372–1375.

535. O'Malley MJ, Hamilton WG, Munyak J. Fractures of the distal shaft of the fifth metatarsal: "dancer's fracture." *Am J Sports Med* 1996;24:240–243.

536. O'Malley MJ, et al. Stress fractures at the base of the second metatarsal in ballet dancers. *Foot Ankle* 1996;17:89–94.

537. Torg JS, et al. Stress fractures of the tarsal navicular: A retrospective review of twenty-one cases. *J Bone Joint Surg* 1982;64A:700–712.

538. Biedert R. Which investigations are required in stress fracture of the great toe sesamoids? *Arch Orthop Trauma Surg* 1993;112:94–95.

539. Bourne RB, Rorabeck CH, MacNab J. Intra-articular fractures of the distal tibia: The pilon fracture. *J Trauma* 1983;23:591–595.

540. Tomaro JE. Injuries of the leg, foot, and ankle. In: Wadsworth C, ed. *Contemporary Topics on the Foot and Ankle—Home Study Course*. La Crosse, WI: Orthopaedic Section, APTA, Inc; 2000.

541. Clarke HJ, et al. Tibio-talar stability in bimalleolar ankle fractures: a dynamic in vitro contact area study. *Foot Ankle Int* 1991;11:222–227.

542. Michelson JD, Clarke HJ, Jinnah RH. The effect of loading on tibiotalar alignment in cadaver ankles. *Foot Ankle Int* 1990;10:280–284.

543. Ho R, Abu-Laban RB. Ankle and foot. In: Rosen P, et al, eds. *Emergency Medicine: Concepts and Clinical Practice*. St. Louis: Mosby; 1998:821.

544. Starosta D, et al. Calcaneal fracture with compartment syndrome of the foot. *Ann Emerg Med* 1988;17:144.

545. Leabhart JW. Stress fractures of the calcaneus. *J Bone Joint Surg* 1959;41(A):1285–1290.

546. Kitaoka HB, et al. Displaced intra-articular fractures of the calcaneus treated non-operatively. *J Bone Joint Surg* 1994;76A:1531–1540.

547. Thoradson DB, Kreiger LE. Operative vs. non-operative treatment of intra-articular fractures of the calcaneus: a prospective randomized trial. *Foot Ankle Int* 1996;17:2–9.

548. Lawrence SJ, Botte MJ. Jones' fractures and related fractures of the proximal fifth metatarsal. *Foot Ankle* 1993;14:358–365.

549. Torg JS, et al. Fractures of the fifth metatarsal distal to the tuberosity. *J Bone Joint Surg* 1984;66A:209–214.

550. Mulligan BR. *Manual Therapy: "NAGS," "SNAGS," "PRP'S" etc.* Wellington, New Zealand: Plane View Series; 1992.

551. Forkin DM, et al. Evaluation of kinesthetic deficits indicative of balance control in gymnasts with unilateral chronic ankle sprains. *J Orthop Sports Phys Ther* 1996;23:245–250.

552. Lentell G, et al. The contributions of proprioceptive deficits, muscle function, and anatomic laxity to functional instability of the ankle. *J Orthop Sports Phys Ther* 1995;21:206–215.

553. Payne KA, Berg K, Latin RW. Ankle injuries and ankle strength, flexibility and proprioception in college basketball players. *J Athl Training* 1997;32:221–225.

554. Anderson RB, Foster MD. Operative treatment of subcalcaneal pain. *Foot Ankle* 1989;9:317–323.

555. Weiner BE, Ross AS, Bogdan RJ. Biomechanical heel pain: a case study. Treatment by use of Birkenstock sandals. *J Am Podiatry Assoc* 1979;69:723–726.

556. Gill LH. Plantar fasciitis: diagnosis and conservative management. *J Am Acad Orthop Surg* 1997;5:109–117.

557. Schunk C, Reed K. *Clinical Practice Guidelines*. Gaithersburg, MD: Aspen; 2000.

558. Lowdon A, Bader DL, Mowat AG. The effect of heel pads on the treatment of Achilles tendinitis: A double blind trial. *Am J Sports Med* 1984;12:431–435.

559. Wojtys EM. Sports injuries in the immature athlete. *Orthop Clin North Am* 1987;18:689–708.

560. Seto JL, Brewster CE. Treatment approaches following foot and ankle injury. *Clin Sports Med* 1985;13:295.

INTRODUCTION TO THE SPINE AND PELVIS

Structure

The basic building block of the spine is the vertebra. The vertebra serves as the weight-bearing unit of the vertebral column, and it is well designed for this purpose. Although a solid structure would provide the vertebral body with sufficient strength, especially for static loads, it would prove too heavy and would not have the necessary flexibility for dynamic load bearing.[1] Instead, the vertebral body is constructed with a strong outer layer of cortical bone and a hollow cavity, the latter of which is reinforced by vertical and horizontal struts called *trabeculae.*

A number of joints are associated with each vertebra. A motion segment in the vertebral column is defined as two adjacent vertebrae, the intervertebral disk (IVD), the zygapophysial or facet joints, and ligamentous structures between the vertebrae.[2] In the thoracic region, the vertebrae also form articulations with the ribs of the thoracic cage.

The IVDs of the vertebral column lie between the adjacent superior and inferior surfaces of the vertebral bodies from C2 to S1 and are similar in shape to the bodies. Each disk is composed of an inner *nucleus pulposus,* an outer *annulus fibrosus,* and limiting cartilage end plates. The annulus and end plates anchor the disk to the vertebral body. The disks contribute 20 to 25 percent of the length of the vertebral column. In cervical and lumbar regions, the IVDs are thicker anteriorly, and this contributes to the normal lordosis (see later). In the thoracic region, each of the IVDs is of uniform thickness. The IVD for each of the spinal regions is described in Chapter 20.

The paired facets or zygapophysial joints of the vertebrae are located posteriorly, and project from the neural arch of the vertebrae. The zygapophysial joints are synovial articulations.

The normal vertebral column is made up of 29 vertebrae (7 cervical, 12 thoracic, 5 lumbar, and 5 sacral) and the coccyx. The overall contour of the normal vertebral column in the coronal plane is straight. In contrast, the contour of the sagittal plane changes with development. At birth, a series of primary curves give a kyphotic posture to the whole spine. With development of the erect posture, secondary curves develop in the cervical and lumbar spines, producing a lordosis in these regions. The curves in the spinal column provide it with increased flexibility and shock-absorbing capabilities.[2] In addition, the spinal column provides support, and houses and protects vital structures, such as the spinal cord and the vertebral arteries.[3,4]

The normal coronal alignment of the spine can be altered by many conditions. *Scoliosis,* which is a descriptive term for lateral curvature, is usually accompanied by a rotational abnormality. Scoliosis can be idiopathic, a result of congenital deformity or of degeneration, or associated with numerous neuromuscular conditions. Sagittal plane alignment also can be altered by disease and injury. This alteration is manifested clinically with areas of excessive kyphosis or lordosis, or a loss of the normal curves.

The spine contains four junctions, each of which is different in posterior element orientation and spinal curvature. Transitional vertebrae can occur at any of the junctions. The transition can be "complete" but is more commonly partial. These junctions, described by Schmorl and Junghanns[5] as *ontogenically restless,* are often rich in anomalies[6]:

▶ The craniovertebral junction is located between the cervical spine and the atlas, axis, and head. This region is covered in Chapter 22.

▶ The cervicothoracic junction represents the region where the mobile cervical spine and the relatively stiffer superior segments of thoracic spine meet, and where the powerful muscles of the upper extremities and shoulder girdle insert. The cervicothoracic junction is described in Chapters 23 and 26.

▶ The thoracolumbar junction is located between the thoracic spine, with its large capacity for rotation, and the lumbar spine, with its limited rotation. This region is described in Chapter 26.

▶ The lumbosacral junction is located between the lumbar spine, with its ability to flex and extend, and the relative stiffness of the sacroiliac joints. This region is described in Chapters 25 and 27.

Spinal Motion

Movements of the spine, like those elsewhere, are produced by the coordinated action of nerves and muscles. Agonistic and synergistic muscles initiate and perform the movements, whereas the antagonistic muscles control and modify the movements. The amount of motion available at each region of the spine is a factor of a number of variables. These include:

▶ Disk–vertebral height ratio.

▶ Compliance of the fibrocartilage.

▶ Dimensions and shape of the adjacent vertebral end plates.

▶ Age.

▶ Disease.

▶ Gender.

The type of motion available is governed by:

▶ The shape and orientation of the articulations.

▶ The ligaments and muscles of the segment, and the size and location of its processes.

Including translations and rotations around three different axes, the spine is considered to possess six degrees of freedom.[7] Although the range of motion (ROM) at each vertebral segment varies, the relative amounts of motion that occur at each region, is well documented[8,9]:

▶ In the upper craniovertebral region (occiput to C2), there is comparatively little flexion-extension, whereas the mid to lower cervical spine permits increasing flexion-extension movements from approximately 10 degrees at the C2 to C3 level, to about 20 degrees at C5 to C6 and C6 to C7. Axial rotation in the upper cervical spine is 30 to 40 degrees in each direction, whereas it is 5 to 6 degrees in the lower cervical spine.

▶ Flexion-extension movements are about 4 degrees in the upper thoracic spine, 6 degrees in the midthoracic spine, and 12 degrees in the lower thoracic spine. Side bending in the upper thoracic spine is approximately 6 degrees. Axial rotation in the upper thoracic spine is 5 to 6 degrees.

▶ In the lumbar spine, there is a gradual increase of flexion-extension movements from about 12 degrees at L1 to L2, to 20 degrees at the L5 to S1 level. Side bending in the lumbar spine is greatest at L3 to L4, where it is approximately 8 to 9 degrees. Axial rotation in the lumbar spine is minimal.

▶ Although various motion patterns have been proposed for the sacroiliac joint,[10–13] the precise model for sacroiliac motion has remained fairly elusive.[14–16] Postmortem analysis has shown that until an advanced age, small movements are measurable under different load conditions.[17,18]

In general, the human zygapophysial joints of the spine are capable of only two major motions: gliding upward and gliding downward. If these movements occur in the same direction, flexion or extension occurs. If the movements occur in opposite directions, side bending occurs. Because the orientation of the articular facets does not correspond exactly to pure planes of motion, pure motions of the spine occur very infrequently.[7] In fact, most motions of the spine occur three-dimensionally because of the phenomenon of coupling. Coupling involves two or more individual motions occurring simultaneously at the segment and has been found to occur throughout the lumbar,[19] thoracic,[20] and cervical regions.[21] All normal motion in the cervical, thoracic, and lumbar regions involves both sides of the segment moving simultaneously around the same axis. That is to say, a motion of the right side of a segment produces an equal motion on the left side of that same segment. If both sides of a vertebral segment are equally impaired (equally hypomobile or hypermobile), there is no change in the axis of motion, except in the case where it ceases to exist, as in a bony ankylosis. Where a symmetric motion impairment exists, there is no noticeable deviation from the path of flexion or extension (impaired side bending and rotation), but, rather, the path is shortened with a hypomobility, or lengthened with a hypermobility.

An alteration to the structures of the motion segment can result in a loss of motion, a loss of segment integrity (instability) or a loss of function. These changes result mainly from injury, developmental changes, fusion, fracture healing, healed infection, or surgical arthrodesis.[9] The loss of motion segment integrity, which can be measured with flexion-extension roentgenograms, is defined as an anteroposterior motion of one vertebra over another that is greater than 3.5 mm in the cervical spine, greater than 2.5 mm in the thoracic spine, and greater than 4.5 mm in the lumbar spine.[22] Loss of motion segment integrity

also may be defined as a difference in the angular motion of two adjacent motion segments greater than the following:

▶ 11 degrees in the cervical spine.

▶ 15 degrees at L1 to L2, L2 to L3, and L3 to L4.

▶ 20 degrees at L4 to L5.

▶ 25 degrees between L5 and S1.

Fryette's Laws of Physiologic Spinal Motion[23]

Although listed as laws, Fryette's descriptions of spinal motion are better viewed as concepts, because they have undergone review and modifications over time. These concepts serve as useful guidelines in the evaluation and intervention of spinal dysfunction and are cited throughout many texts describing spinal biomechanics.

Fryette's First Law

"When any part of the lumbar or thoracic spine is in neutral position, side bending of a vertebra will be opposite to the side of the rotation of that vertebra."

The term *neutral*, according to Fryette, is interpreted as any position in which the zygapophysial joints are not engaged in any surface contact, and the position where the ligaments and capsules of the segment are not under tension. This law describes the coupling for the thoracic and lumbar spines. The cervical spine is not included in this law, because the zygapophysial joints of this region are always engaged. When a lumbar or thoracic vertebra is side bent from its neutral position, the vertebral body will turn toward the convexity that is being formed, with the maximum rotation occurring near the apex of the curve formed.

Dysfunctions that occur in the neutral range are termed by osteopaths *type I dysfunctions*.

Fryette's Second Law

"When any part of the spine is in a position of hyperextension or hyperflexion, the side bending of the vertebra will be to the same side as the rotation of that vertebra."

Put simply, when the segment is under load (close packed, under ligamentous tension, or in positions of flexion or extension) the coupling of side bending and rotation occur to the same side. This law describes the coupling that occurs in the C2 to T3 areas of the spine.

Dysfunctions occurring in the flexion or extension ranges are termed by osteopaths *type II dysfunctions*.

Fryette's Third Law

Fryette's third law tells us that if motion in one plane is introduced to the spine, any motion occurring in another direction is thereby restricted.

Combined Motions

It should be obvious that, irrespective of the coupling that occurs, there is a great deal of similarity between a motion involving flexion followed by left side bending, and a motion involving left side bending followed by flexion. However, although both motions have the same end result, they use different methods to arrive there. The same could be said of the following combined motions:

▶ Flexion and right side bending, followed by right side bending and flexion.

▶ Extension and right side bending, followed by right side bending and extension.

▶ Extension and left side bending, followed by left side bending and extension.

By using combined motions, the clinician can often reproduce a patient's symptom that was not reproduced using the planar motions of flexion, extension, side bending, and rotation.[24–26] However, care should be taken when utilizing combined motions, especially with the acute and subacute patient, when a reduction of symptoms through modalities and gentle exercise might be preferable to exacerbating the patient's condition through a comprehensive movement examination.

Motions that involve flexion and side bending away from the symptoms invoke a stretch to the structures on the side of the symptoms, whereas motions that involve extension and side bending toward the side of the symptoms produce a compression of the structures on the side of the symptoms.[24–26] An example of a stretching pattern would be pain on the right side of the spine that is increased with either flexion followed by a left side bending movement, or a left side bending motion followed by a flexion movement. A compression pattern would involve pain on the right side of the spine that is increased with a movement involving either extension followed by right side bending, or right side bending followed by extension.

The symptom reproduction that occurs with combined motions usually follows a logical and predictable pattern. However, there are situations in which illogical patterns are found. Because the vertebral column consists of many articulating segments, movements are complex and usually involve several segments, resulting in restrictions that may be complex and apparently illogical. An example of such a pattern would be pain on the right side of the spine that is increased with a flexion and right side bending combination, but decreased with an extension and right side bending combination. The movements just described involve a combination of stretching and compression movements. These illogical patterns typically indicate that more than one structure is involved.[24–26] Of course, they could also indicate to the clinician that the patient does not have a musculoskeletal impairment.

Spinal Locking

Spinal locking techniques employ coupling or combined movements to examine or treat the spine. The purpose of these techniques is to localize a technique to a specific segment and to protect the neighboring segments from the forces employed. Two methods of locking are commonly cited:

1. **Congruent.** Congruent or ligamentous locking involves taking the joint to its full range, using the normal coupling of side bending and rotation to tighten the ligaments and capsule, thus stabilizing the joint. The disadvantage with this type of locking is that the ligaments and capsule take the brunt of the mobilization force and, if the joint is hypermobile in that direction, further damage may ensue. This form of locking has been advocated in cases of articular instability.[27]

2. **Incongruent.** Incongruent or articular locking takes the joint to its full range while deliberately employing incongruent rotation and side bending to essentially jam the joint surfaces on each other, and so lock the joint, without tautening the capsule or ligaments. Incongruent locking tends to produce a much firmer lock, and the potential of over stretching the capsule and ligaments is minimized. It has been promoted as the locking method of choice in cases of ligamentous instability.[27] However, the presence of articular instability obviates this locking method.

Detecting the segmental level where the lock is occurring is a relatively easy process in the cervical and thoracic spine, given the accessibility of the transverse or spinous processes for palpation. Depending on the type of lock required, the patient is positioned sitting or lying supine and the clinician passively positions the cervical or thoracic spine into the desired position.

Locking of the lumbar spine, however, is a more difficult procedure, and although these techniques can be performed with the patient in the sitting position, they are easier to execute with the patient in side lying. Traditional descriptions of locking techniques for the lumbar spine include details about how to lock the spine from both above and below, with the patient positioned in side lying. Locking from above involves employing a specifically directed pull on the patients arm, whereas locking from below involves utilizing either flexion or extension of the patient's hips until motion is felt at a specific segmental level of the lumbar spine. To illustrate these concepts, a few examples follow.

Locking From Above in the Lumbar Spine

Locks from above in the lumbar spine are achieved by pulling the patient's arm that is closest to the table in a specific direction, depending on the type of lock required. Depending on the direction of the arm pull, the upper lock can be produced in either extension or flexion. More complex techniques employ an arm pull that locks the lumbar spine in a combination of extension-flexion and rotation–side bending of the lumbar spine.

Locking in Extension-Flexion

Locking in Extension. The patient is positioned side lying, facing the clinician. The patient's hips and knees are slightly flexed. To facilitate the upper lock of extension, the upper arm of the patient should be placed in a position with the elbow flexed and shoulder extended, so that the upper arm is posterior to the trunk. To ensure the upper spine is positioned in extension, the patient's lower arm is drawn vertically toward the ceiling (Fig. III-1).

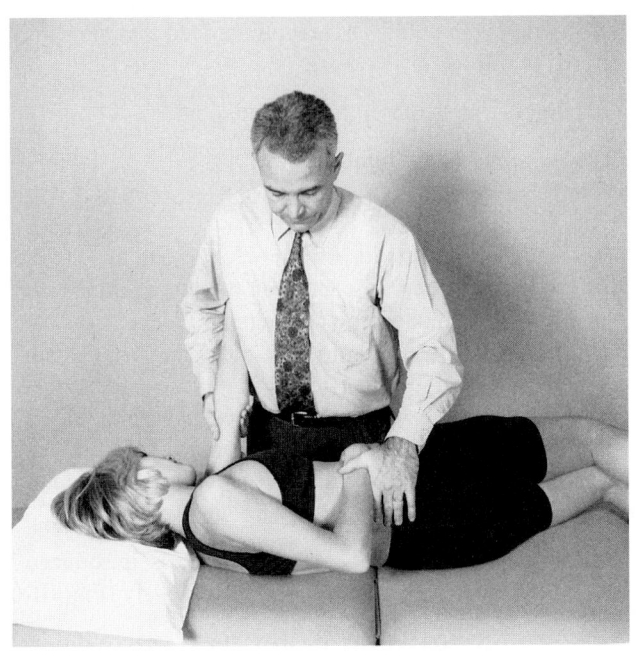

FIGURE III-1   Direction of arm pull for locking in extension from above.

Locking in Flexion.   The patient is positioned side lying, facing the clinician. The patient's hips and knees are slightly flexed. The clinician places the patient's upper arm anterior to the trunk in such a way that the palm is flat on the bed and adjacent to the patient's waist. The lower arm and shoulder girdle are then drawn forward, parallel to the table (Fig. III-2).

Locking Technique to Produce Right Side Bending.   The patient is positioned side lying, facing the clinician. The patient's hips and knees are slightly flexed. If the patient is in right side lying position, then the right arm is drawn toward the feet (i.e., caudal) (Fig. III-3).

Locking Technique to Produce Left Side Bending.   The patient is positioned side lying, facing the clinician. The patient's hips and knees are slightly flexed. If the patient is in the right side lying position, then the right arm is drawn superiorly toward the head, keeping the arm parallel to the bed.

When the preceding techniques are mastered, the clinician can progress to the more complex techniques of locking in both flexion-extension and rotation–side bending.

Locking Technique Using a Combination of Side Bending with Flexion-Extension.   The side-bending component of the lock is performed simultaneously with the flexion-extension movement by altering the direction of the arm pull.

Left Side Bending in Extension.   With the patient in the right side lying position, the right arm and shoulder girdle are drawn in a direction that is the oblique resultant of a cranial and vertical pull (Fig. III-4). This technique, with the location of the end-feel, can be used to test the ability of the joint to achieve the full ROM, or it can be used to position a patient to mobilize one side of a segment.

Right Side Bending in Flexion.   With the patient in the right side lying position, the patient's right arm and shoulder girdle are

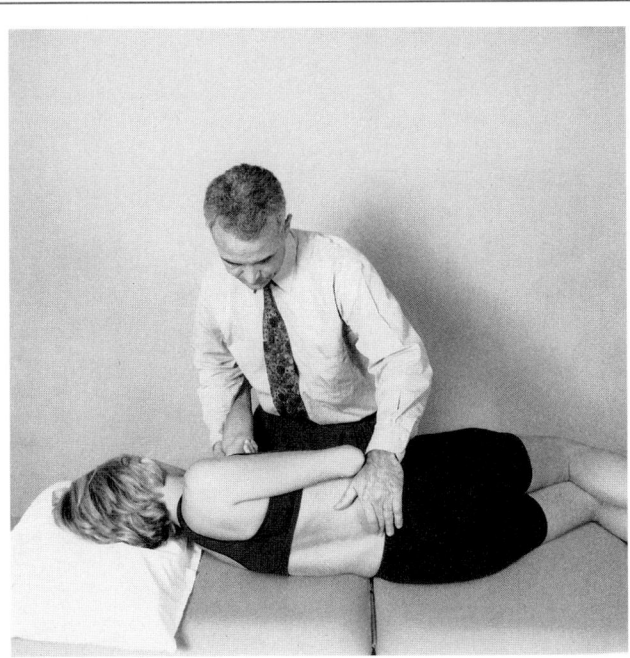

FIGURE III-2   Direction of arm pull for locking in flexion from above.

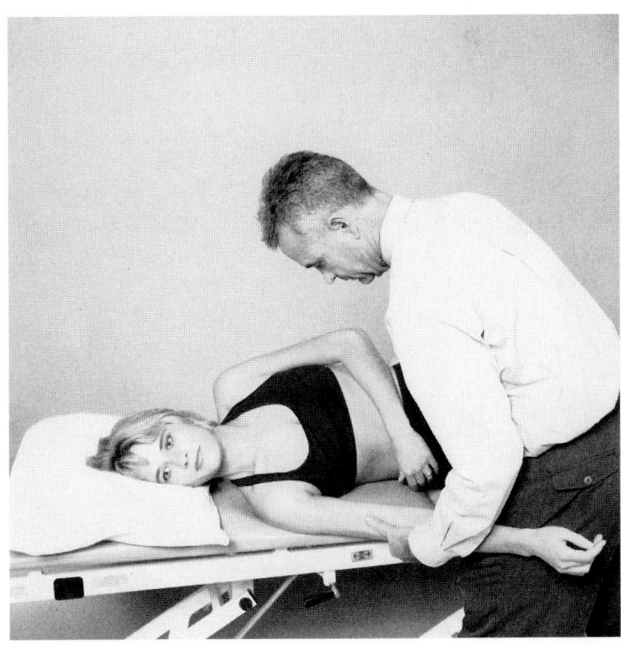

FIGURE III-3   Direction of arm pull to produce right side bending of the lumbar spine.

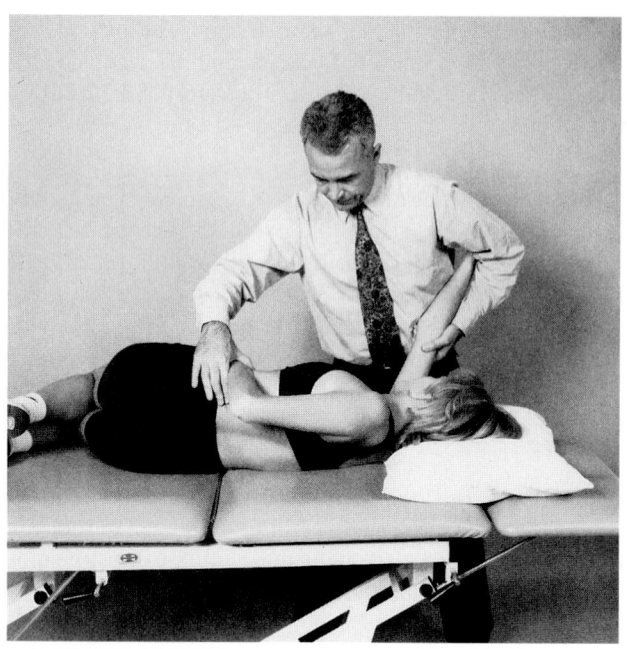

FIGURE III-4   Direction of arm pull to produce left side bending in extension.

drawn in a direction that is the oblique resultant of a caudal and horizontal pull (Fig. III-5). This technique, with the location of the end-feel, can be used to test the ability of the joint to achieve the full ROM, or it can be used to position a patient to mobilize one side of a segment.

Locking from Below in the Lumbar Spine

When locking from below, it is recommended that the spine be locked in the following sequence:

1. Flexion or extension of the lumbar spine.

2. Side bending of the lumbar spine.

3. Rotation of the lumbar spine.

The flexion-extension lock from below is achieved by positioning the patient side lying and then flexing or extending the patient's hip while monitoring the segmental level (this can be achieved using the same techniques as described for the passive physiologic intervertebral motion [PPIVM] tests described in Chapter 25). Once the segment has been flexed or extended to the correct level, the side-bending component of the lock can be introduced by using a leg pulling maneuver. For example, assuming the patient is in right side lying position:

► Right side bending of the lumbar spine is introduced by drawing the patient's upper (left) leg inferiorly (Fig. III-6).

► Left side bending of the lumbar spine is introduced by drawing the patient's lower (right) leg inferiorly (Fig. III-7).

Rotation of the lumbar spine is then used to fine tune, or localize, the lock to the specific segment.

In reality, it is difficult to be sure which type of locking is being done at any given series of spinal joints. The research into coupled movements in the lower lumbar spine has upset most of the theories on side bending–rotation coupling, and there is no reason to suppose that any other area of the spine is any more predictable (Table III-1). From the work done on the lum-

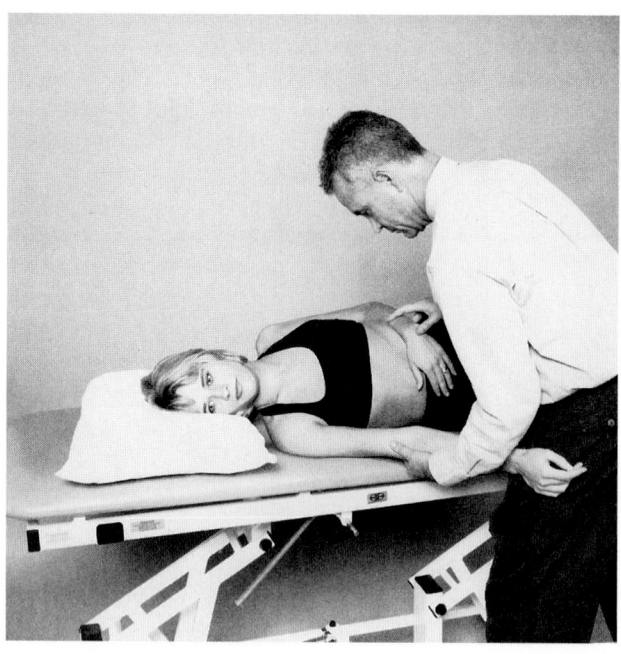

FIGURE III-5   Direction of arm pull to produce right side bending in flexion.

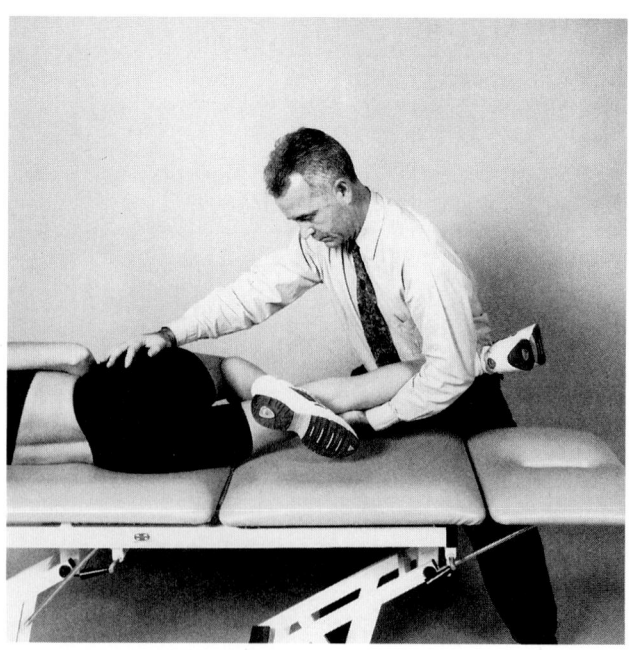

FIGURE III-6   Inferior leg pull to introduce right side bending.

The examination of the spine is complicated by the number of conditions that can cause pain in this region of the body. Borenstein and colleagues[31,32] have listed more than 50 causes of neck or back pain. In addition, there is little scientific evidence for establishment of many of the diagnostic labels attributed to spinal pain, such as instability, degenerative disk disease, and subluxation.[33]

The purpose of the examination is to correctly identify those patients who will benefit from a physical therapy intervention. To help determine the appropriateness of physical therapy, the history for the patient with spinal dysfunction should include questions on age, history of malignant disease, unexplained weight loss, intake of immunosuppressive drugs, duration of symptoms, responsiveness to previous therapy, pain that is worse at rest, history of drug use or abuse, and urinary and other infections (see Chap. 8).[33]

The correct identification of a diagnosis requires the use of evidence-based measuring tools that are valid, specific, and sensitive. There are numerous methods for examining and evaluating the spine, and each results in a conclusion that determines the course of the intervention.[34,35] Unfortunately, many of the procedures that are used today to examine the spine demonstrate methodologic shortcomings.[33–35]

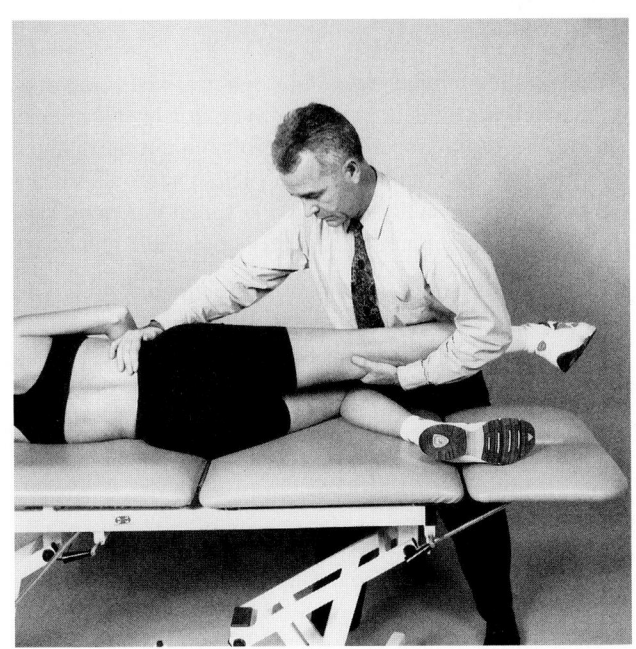

FIGURE III-7 Inferior leg pull to introduce left side bending.

TABLE III-1 Coupling in the Lumbar Spine

Author	Neutral	Flexion	Extension
Farfan[28]	—	Contralateral	Contralateral
Kaltenborn[27]	—	Ipsilateral	Ipsilateral
Grieve[7]	—	Ipsilateral	Contralateral
Fryette[23]	Contralateral	Ipsilateral	Ipsilateral
Evjenth[29]	—	Ipsilateral	Contralateral

bosacral junction, it would appear that it is perfectly possible that, when a congruent lock is applied to L4 to L5, an incongruent lock is occurring at L5 to S1. Given this, utilizing an incongruent lock to avoid ligamentous instabilities and a congruent lock to protect articular instabilities runs into difficulties because the clinician cannot be sure which is occurring at any given time, although it is probably better to avoid the direction of the instability or hypermobility.

Examination of the Spine and Pelvis

The vast majority of the diagnoses of spinal dysfunction must be considered provisional at best. Confirmation of the accuracy of the diagnosis may occur in situations in which the intervention produces improvements. However, the clinician must also take into consideration the beneficial effects of placebo. Intervention efficacy should be proven with well-executed, complete, clinical follow-up series, using validated outcome measures that demonstrate obvious, dramatic, and immediate benefits that cannot be explained by any other factors.[30]

Use of Traditional Classification Systems

In recent years, attempts have been made to use a variety of methods to classify spinal pain, particularly low back pain, into syndromes. A syndrome is a collection of signs and symptoms that, collectively, characterizes a particular condition. By classifying syndromes, it is proposed that a patient is more likely to respond to a type of intervention unique to that syndrome. The term *syndrome* implies that the specific diagnosis is unknown. In the spine, where determining a specific diagnosis has historically proven extremely difficult, syndromes have become popular. The criteria that have thus been used to categorize a syndrome include:

▶ Pathoanatomy.[36,37] This strategy involves using correlations to produce categories. The disadvantage of using pathoanatomy is the difficulty in identifying a relevant pathoanatomic cause for most patients.[38]

▶ Presence or absence of radiculopathy.[39,40]

▶ Location and type of pain.[41]

▶ Duration of the symptoms (acute, subacute, or chronic).[42]

▶ Activity and work status.[40,43]

▶ Impairments identified during the physical examination.

▶ Direction of motion that reproduces, peripheralizes, or centralizes the symptoms.[44,45]

The more common classifications are outlined next. Although the use of classification systems may have some prognostic value, their ability to direct clinicians to specific interventions that improve outcomes has not been established.[46]

Osteopathic System

Osteopaths rely on the results from the active motion tests and position tests to determine their intervention approach. *Note:* Osteopaths use the term side flexion instead of side bending.

Position Testing

Position testing involves palpation of the soft tissues over the transverse processes of the spine to determine if a rotational dysfunction is present at a segmental level when the spine is positioned in flexion or extension, compared with neutral. Theoretically, the rotational dysfunction, which is a result of the altered axis of rotation produced by the stiffer of the two sides of the segment, will be palpated as a much firmer end-feel to the palpation on that side. The direction of the rotation is named after the more posterior of the two transverse processes, and the positional name is an osteokinematic one, having no established relationship with any joint. Thus, the clinician must be very familiar with so-called layer palpation, to be sure that the palpating fingers are monitoring the positions of the transverse processes at a particular segmental level.

Position Testing in Extension. If a marked segmental rotation is evident at the limit of extension, this would indicate that one of the facets is unable to complete its inferior motion (i.e., it is being held in a relatively flexed position). The direction of the resulting rotation (denoted in terms of the anterior part of the vertebral body) informs the clinician as to which of the facets is not moving. For example, if the segment is rotated to the *left* when palpated in extension, the *right* zygapophysial joint is not moving normally. This impairment can be described in one of three ways:

1. The right zygapophysial joint cannot extend, or "close."

2. The right zygapophysial joint is flexed (F), rotated (R) and side-flexed (S) left (L) around the axis of the right zygapophysial joint.

3. The right zygapophysial joint is unable to perform any motions that require an inferior glide, such as extension, right side bending and right rotation.

FRS or extension impairments are more evident in the positional tests than ERS impairments (described next), because there is less overall motion available into extension.

Position Testing in Flexion. If a marked segmental rotation is evident in full flexion, this indicates that one of the facets cannot complete its superior motion. For example, if the segment is found to be left-rotated when palpated in flexion, the left zygapophysial joint is not moving normally.
This impairment can be described in one of three ways:

1. The left zygapophysial joint cannot flex or "open."

2. The left zygapophysial joint is extended (E), rotated (R) and side-flexed (S) left (L).

3. The left zygapophysial joint is unable to perform any motion that requires a superior glide such as flexion, right rotation, and right side bending.

Position Testing in Neutral. Positional testing is performed in the neutral spine position for three reasons:

1. If a rotational impairment of a segment exists only in neutral and is not evident in either full flexion or full extension, the cause of the impairment is probably not mechanical in origin, but rather neuromuscular. These neuromuscular impairments are usually found at the spinal junctions, particularly the thoracolumbar and cervicothoracic junctions.

2. If a marked rotation is evident at a segment, and this rotation is consistent throughout flexion, extension, and neutral, then the cause is probably an anatomic anomaly (e.g., scoliosis), rather than an articular problem.

3. If the cause of the rotational impairment is articular (zygapophysial joint), positional testing in neutral gives the clinician an idea as to the starting position of the corrective technique.

The terminology used to describe the rotational disruption of the pure spinal motions (ERS or FRS) describes the positional and kinetic impairments, only. It does not indicate what the pathology might be. Reasons for these impairments, other than movement dysfunctions, may include bony anomalies such as a deformed transverse process, compensatory adaptation, structural scoliosis, or a hemi-vertebra.

The analysis of the change in the rotational impairment between full flexion and full extension theoretically gives clues as to the pathology. Thus, in conjunction with other tests, such as active motion testing, this analysis can assist in ascertaining a biomechanical diagnosis.

Position testing has been found to be very reliable when used by experienced clinicians to identify segmental levels based on the relative position of spinous processes.[47] However, poor inter-rater reliability has been found when clinicians are asked to determine lumbar segmental abnormality using position testing,[48] or to determine the segmental level of a marked spinous process.[49]

> **Clinical Pearl**
>
> The clinician should be aware that position testing is insensitive to symmetric impairments and thus can give false negatives.

McKenzie System[44,45]

The McKenzie mechanical diagnostic and classification approach is a noninvasive and an inexpensive method of assessing patients with low back pain (LBP) that uses physical signs, symptom behavior, and their relation to end-range lumbar test movements to determine appropriate classification and intervention. The McKenzie method classifies mechanical LBP into three main syndromes: postural, dysfunction, and derangement (Fig. III-8).

The *posture syndrome* is proposed to result from sustained end-range positions and postures. The pain, which is of a gradual onset, is dull, local, midline, symmetric, and never referred.

FIGURE III-8 McKenzie classification.[35,44]

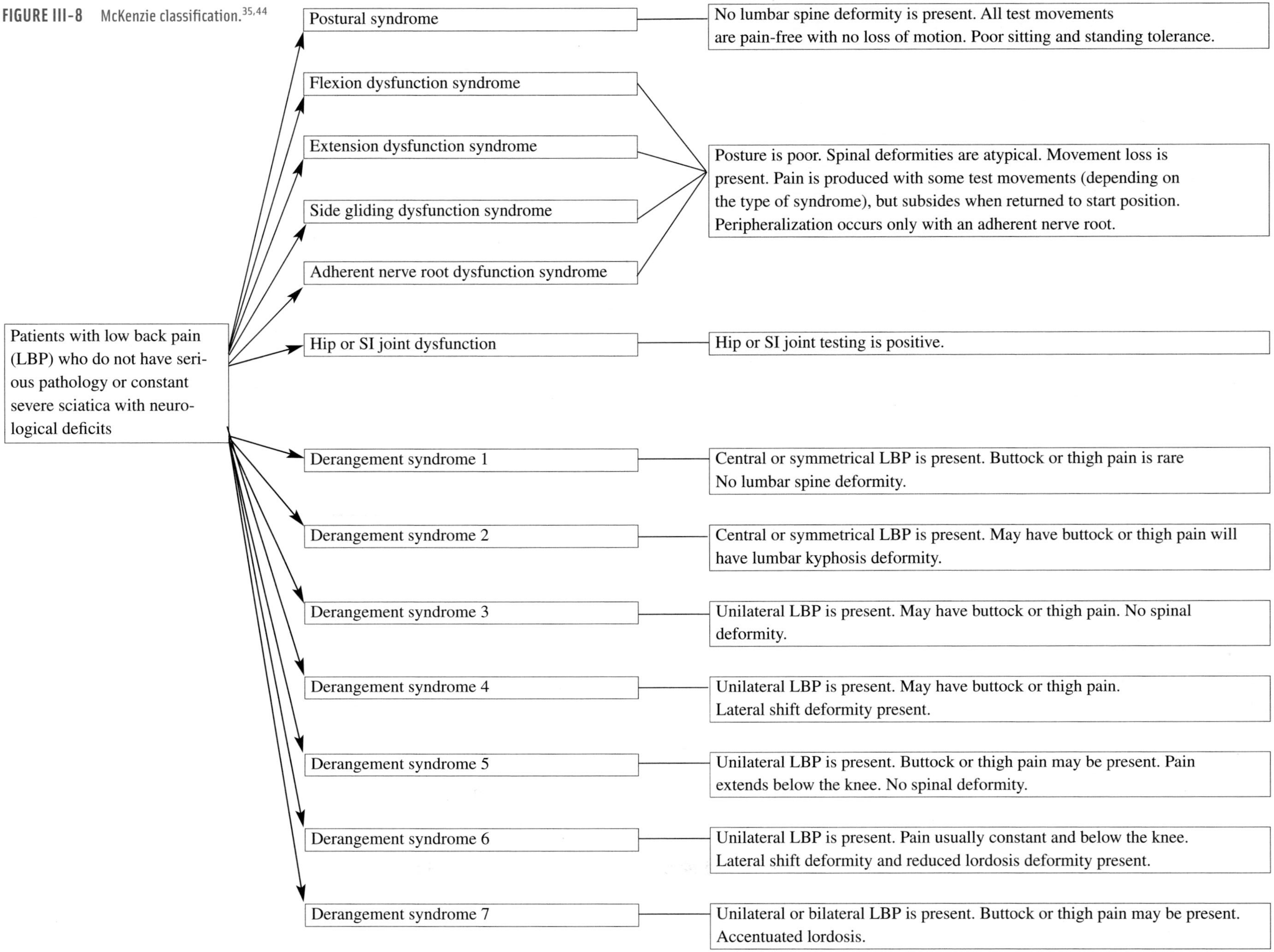

Postural syndrome	No lumbar spine deformity is present. All test movements are pain-free with no loss of motion. Poor sitting and standing tolerance.
Flexion dysfunction syndrome	Posture is poor. Spinal deformities are atypical. Movement loss is present. Pain is produced with some test movements (depending on the type of syndrome), but subsides when returned to start position. Peripheralization occurs only with an adherent nerve root.
Extension dysfunction syndrome	
Side gliding dysfunction syndrome	
Adherent nerve root dysfunction syndrome	
Hip or SI joint dysfunction	Hip or SI joint testing is positive.
Derangement syndrome 1	Central or symmetrical LBP is present. Buttock or thigh pain is rare No lumbar spine deformity.
Derangement syndrome 2	Central or symmetrical LBP is present. May have buttock or thigh pain will have lumbar kyphosis deformity.
Derangement syndrome 3	Unilateral LBP is present. May have buttock or thigh pain. No spinal deformity.
Derangement syndrome 4	Unilateral LBP is present. May have buttock or thigh pain. Lateral shift deformity present.
Derangement syndrome 5	Unilateral LBP is present. Buttock or thigh pain may be present. Pain extends below the knee. No spinal deformity.
Derangement syndrome 6	Unilateral LBP is present. Pain usually constant and below the knee. Lateral shift deformity and reduced lordosis deformity present.
Derangement syndrome 7	Unilateral or bilateral LBP is present. Buttock or thigh pain may be present. Accentuated lordosis.

Patients with low back pain (LBP) who do not have serious pathology or constant severe sciatica with neurological deficits

Prolonged postures worsen the pain, whereas movement abolishes it. On examination, the patient demonstrates no spinal deformity or loss of range, and repeated movements do not produce the symptoms. The onset of symptoms, which is time-dependent (usually occurring after more than 15 minutes), is provoked with sustained end-of-range positions.

The *dysfunction syndrome* is proposed to result from an adaptive shortening of some soft tissues and an overstretching of others. The intermittent pain associated with this syndrome is local, adjacent to the midline of the spine, and not referred. The exception occurs in the case of an adherent nerve root, where the pain may be felt in the buttock, thigh, or calf. Activities and positions at the end of range worsen the pain of this syndrome, whereas activities that avoid end ranges lessen the symptoms. On examination, the patient demonstrates a loss of motion or function, which distinguishes this syndrome from the posture syndrome. Repeated movements do not alter the symptoms, and the loss of motion, or function, may be symmetric or asymmetric.

The *derangement syndrome* is thought to result from a displacement, or an alteration in the position of joint structures. The joint structure most commonly involved is the intervertebral disk, and McKenzie divides these disturbances into posterior disk and anterior disk derangements. The posterior derangements are further subdivided into seven derangement categories. Derangements 1 through 6 describe posterior derangements, whereas derangement 7 describes the anterior derangement (see Fig. III-8).

The pain of a derangement syndrome, which is usually of a sudden onset and associated with paresthesia or numbness, is dull or sharp and can be central, unilateral, symmetric, or asymmetric. Although the pain may be referred into the buttock, thigh, leg, or foot, it varies in both intensity and distribution. Bending, sitting, or sustaining positions worsen a posterior derangement, whereas walking and standing worsen an anterior derangement. Patients with a posterior derangement often feel better when walking and lying, whereas patients with an anterior derangement usually feel better in sitting and other flexed positions. On examination, a lateral shift may be noted. There is always a loss of motion and function. Certain motions produce, increase, or cause the symptoms to peripheralize (move away from the spine), whereas other motions decrease, abolish, or centralize the symptoms.

Intervention for each of the syndromes is specific, and patients are encouraged to accept responsibility for their intervention and recovery.

The inter-rater reliability of the McKenzie method in performing clinical tests and classifying patients with LBP into syndromes has been investigated in a number of studies.[34,50–58]

Repeated movements are an integral component of the McKenzie examination and are used in an effort to reproduce the patient's symptoms. Repeated movements have been found to be a reliable part of the examination of the spine in a number of studies.[57,59]

In one study,[57] inter-tester reliability between two therapists trained in the McKenzie method seemed to be high for classifying patients with LBP into McKenzie syndromes, and excellent for judging pain status change, including the centralization phenomenon, during examination of the lumbar spine.[55,57] The results from a study by Kilpikoski also suggested that inter-tester reliability in performing clinical tests and classifying patients with LBP into the main McKenzie syndromes is high when the clinicians have been trained in the McKenzie method.[58]

Donahue and colleagues[50] suggested that the McKenzie method was unreliable for detecting the presence of a lateral shift, but that a relevant lateral component could be reliably detected using symptom response to repeated movements. In contrast, Tenhula and associates[54] noted a significant relation between positive results on a contralateral side-bending movement test and a lumbar lateral shift, indicating that the former is a useful clinical test for confirming the presence of a lateral shift in patients with LBP.

Kilby and colleagues[56] found the "McKenzie algorithm" to be reliable in the examination of pain behavior and pain response with repeated movements, but unreliable in the detection of end-range pain and lateral shift.

Riddle and Rothstein[34] found that the McKenzie approach was unreliable when physical therapists classified patients into McKenzie syndromes. They suggested that a potential source of unreliability was in determining whether the patient had a lateral shift and, if so, in which direction, and whether the patient's pain centralized or peripheralized during test movements.[34]

Treatment-based Classification (TBC) System[60,61]

This system, proposed by Delitto and colleagues,[60] uses information gathered from the physical examination and from patient self-reports of pain (pain scale and pain diagram) and disability (modified Oswestry questionnaire) to classify the patient. The classification determines whether the patient's condition is amenable to physical therapy, or whether care from another practitioner is required. The TBC system is designed for patients judged to be in the acute stage, with the determination of acuity based on the alignment of various body structures, the effect of movements on symptoms, the nature of the patient's symptoms, the degree of disability, and the goals for management, instead of strictly on the elapsed time from injury.[61]

Patients in the acute stage are those with higher levels of disability (Oswestry scores generally greater than 30), who report substantial difficulty with basic daily activities such as sitting, standing, and walking. Intervention goals are to improve the ability to perform basic daily activities, reduce disability, and permit the patient to advance in his or her rehabilitation.[61] Patients judged to be in the acute stage are assigned to a classification, which guides the initial intervention. Seven classifications are described for patients in the acute stage[60]:

1. Immobilization.
2. Lumbar mobilization.
3. Sacroiliac mobilization.
4. Extension syndrome.

5. Flexion syndrome.

6. Lateral shift.

7. Traction.

Each of the classifications has key examination findings and recommended interventions. To facilitate comparisons among classifications, these seven classifications may be collapsed further into four classifications based on similarities in the prescribed interventions.

1. Immobilization.

2. Mobilization (either sacroiliac or lumbar).

3. Specific exercise (flexion, extension, or lateral shift correction).

4. Traction.

Immobilization

The immobilization classification is purported to identify patients with lumbar segmental instability. Key examination findings are typically gleaned from the history and include a history of frequent episodes of symptoms precipitated by minimal perturbations, frequent use of manipulation with short-term relief of symptoms, trauma, or reduced symptoms with the prior use of a corset.[60]

The intervention for this category focuses on strengthening exercises for the back extensor and abdominal exercises, as well as stabilization exercises designed to improve dynamic control of the lumbar spine.[61]

Mobilization

The mobilization classification includes patients believed to have indications for either sacroiliac or lumbar region mobilization or manipulation. Mobilization of the sacroiliac region is indicated by asymmetries of the pelvic landmarks (anterior superior iliac spines, posterior superior iliac spines, and iliac crests) with the patient in the standing position, and by positive results in three of four tests as follows:

1. Asymmetry of posterior superior iliac spine heights with the patient sitting.

2. The standing flexion test.

3. The prone-knee flexion test.

4. The supine to long-sitting test.

Acute-stage intervention for this category involves a manipulation technique proposed to affect the sacroiliac joint region, muscle energy techniques, and ROM exercises for the lumbosacral spine.[61]

Lumbar mobilization is believed to be indicated by the presence of:

► Unilateral paraspinal pain in the lumbar region.

► Asymmetric amounts of lumbar side-bending ROM with the patient standing in either an "opening" pattern (limited and painful flexion and side-bending ROM to the side opposite the pain) or a "closing" pattern (limited and painful extension and side-bending ROM to the same side as the pain).

The intervention for this category consists of lumbar mobilization or manipulation techniques and ROM exercises for the lumbosacral spine.

Specific Exercise

The key examination finding that places patients into a specific exercise classification is the presence of centralization with movement of the lumbar spine based on the McKenzie method.[44] When either lumbar flexion or extension is found to produce centralization, the patient is treated with specific exercises in the direction producing the centralization. Patients also are educated to avoid positions found to peripheralize symptoms during examination.

The primary examination findings that lead to a classification of a lateral shift, in which the shoulders are offset from the pelvis in the frontal plane, are a visible frontal plane deformity and asymmetric side-bending ROM in standing. If correction of the deformity produces centralization, the patient is taught specific exercises designed to correct the lateral shift (i.e., pelvic translocation).[44]

Traction

The traction classification is reserved for patients with signs and symptoms of nerve root compression who are unable to centralize with any lumbar movements. The acute stage intervention involves the use of mechanical or autotraction[62] in an attempt to produce centralization.

Under the TBC, patients judged to be in a more chronic stage are treated with a conditioning program designed to improve strength, flexibility, and conditioning, or with a work-reconditioning program.[60]

Canadian Biomechanical Model[63]

The Canadian model is an eclectic approach founded upon an amalgam of doctrines and techniques that incorporate the biomechanical concepts of the Norwegians,[27,29,64] the selective tissue tension principles of Cyriax,[41,66] the muscle energy concepts of the American osteopaths,[67–69] the combined movement testing of Edwards,[26] the manipulative techniques of Stoddard,[70] the various approaches to stabilization therapy,[71–74] the exercise protocols of McKenzie,[44,45] the muscle balancing concepts of Janda, Jull, and Sahrmann,[75–77] and the movement re-education principles of the neurodevelopment and sensory integrationist clinicians.[78,79]

The basic tenet of the Canadian approach is that, given an understanding of the anatomy and biomechanics of a joint, segment or region, the pathologic mechanisms can be extrapolated using a series of testing procedures. These tests include the Cyriax upper and lower quarter scanning examinations for differential diagnosis (see Chap. 9), uncombined (plane) and combined movement testing, passive physiologic intervertebral motion (PPIVM) tests, passive accessory intervertebral motion (PAIVM) tests, and segmental stability tests.

Following the active motion tests, the clinician should be able to determine the planar motions (flexion, extension, and side bending and rotation to both sides) that provoke symptoms. However, the clinician cannot yet determine whether a joint or soft tissue is responsible for the pain. To help determine the presence of articular involvement, two tests are used: the PPIVM tests and the PAIVM tests.

Passive Physiologic Intervertebral Mobility Testing

The PPIVM tests are used to determine the amount of segmental mobility available in the spine. The PPIVM tests assess the ability of each segment to move through its normal range of motion. The adjacent spinous processes of the segment are palpated simultaneously, and movement between them is assessed as the segment is passively taken through its physiologic range. If both spinous processes move simultaneously, there is no movement occurring at the segment, and a hypomobility exists. If the movement between adjacent spinous processes appears excessive when compared with the level above or below, a hypermobility or instability may be suspected.

Thus, once the physiologic range has been assessed, it can be categorized as either normal, excessive, or reduced, compared with the neighboring segment. Other positive findings for a hypomobility would be a reduced range in a capsular or noncapsular pattern in the active motion tests, a reduced joint glide, and a change in the end-feel from the expected norm for that joint. The end-feel and joint glide are both tested in the PAIVM tests (discussed next).

Therefore, one of three conclusions may be drawn from the PPIVM tests:

1. The joint motion is determined to be normal. If the PPIVM test of a spinal joint has a normal range and end-feel, the joint usually can be considered normal, because in the spine, instability will invariably produce a hypermobility. However, in a peripheral joint, it is possible to have a normal range in the presence of articular instability. Thus, if a peripheral joint demonstrates a normal physiologic range, the stability of the joint needs to be tested using the segmental stability tests (see later discussion) before the clinician can deem the joint to be normal.

2. The joint motion is determined to be reduced (hypomobile). A hypomobility can be painful, suggesting an acute sprain of a structure, or painless, suggesting a contracture or an adhesion of the tested structure. If the motion is determined as being reduced (hypomobile), PAIVM testing is performed to determine, using the joint glides, whether the reduced motion is a result of an articular or extra-articular restriction.

3. The motion is determined to be excessive (hypermobile). If the motion is determined to be excessive, segmental stability tests are performed to determine whether a hypermobility or an instability is present (see later discussion).

It is worth noting that the judgments of joint stiffness made by experienced physical therapists examining patients in their own clinics have been found to have poor reliability in a number of studies. In two separate studies,[59,80] manual therapy tests that provoke patient's symptoms were found to be more reliable than judging stiffness in the spine. Smedmark and colleagues[81] investigated the inter-examiner reliability of passive intervertebral motion testing. In their study, passive intervertebral motion of the cervical spine was assessed independently by two physical therapists whose backgrounds (education and clinical experience) were equal. Sixty-one patients seeking care for cervical problems at a private clinic were included in the study, in which three segments of the cervical spine and the mobility of the first rib were graded as stiff or not stiff. Data analyzed by percentage agreement and κ coefficient indicated an inter-examiner reliability that was greater than expected by chance. Results demonstrated inter-examiner reliability of between 70 and 87 percent and κ coefficients ranging between 0.28 and 0.43, considered to be only fair to moderate.

However, in a study by Gonnella and colleagues[82] the performance of five physical therapists in evaluating passive mobility of the vertebral column of five asymptomatic endomorphic subjects was assessed for the reliability within and between therapists, the criteria for grading, and the subjects themselves. Intra-tester reliability was found to be reasonable to good; there was no inter-tester reliability. Reliability was highest at L1 to L3 and lowest at L5 to S1. Problems identified were idiosyncratic behaviors that may develop with experience, subject characteristics, and the instrument itself.

Passive Accessory Intervertebral Mobility (PAIVM) Testing

In the PAIVM tests, the clinician assesses the joint glides or accessory motions of each joint and determines the type of end-feel encountered.

Accessory motions are involuntary motions. With few exceptions, muscles cannot restrict the glides of a joint, especially if the glides are tested in the loose-pack position of a peripheral joint and at the end of available range in the spinal joints.[84] Thus, if the joint glide is restricted, the cause is an articular restriction such as the joint surface or capsule. If the glide is normal, then the restriction must be from an extra-articular source such as a peri-articular structure or muscle.

Determining the type of end-feel is very important, particularly in joints that only have very small amounts of normal range, such as those of the spine. To execute the end-feel, the point at which resistance is encountered is evaluated for quality and tenderness. Additional forces are needed as the end range of a joint is reached and the elastic limits are challenged. This space, termed the *end play zone*, requires a force of overpressure to be reached, and when that force is released, the joint springs back from its elastic limits. Because pain generally does not limit movement in specific and deliberate passive tests, the PAIVM tests are better for gauging the reliability of the limitation based on tissue resistance, rather than patient willingness, and are better at determining the pattern of restriction than the active tests. If pain is reproduced with end-feel testing, it is useful to associate the pain with the onset of tissue resistance to gain an appreciation of the acuteness of the problem (see Chap. 11).

A normal end-feel indicates normal range, whereas an abnormal end-feel suggests abnormal range, either hypomobile or hypermobile. If the articular restraints are irritable, the range will be about normal but will be accompanied by a spasmodic end-feel, because a reflex muscle contraction can prevent the motion into an abnormal, and painful, range.[84] If non-irritable, the physiologic range will be increased and the end-feel will be softer than the expected capsular one, suggesting a compromise of the structure under examination. A hard, capsular end-feel indicates a pericapsular hypomobility, whereas a jammed end-feel indicates a pathomechanical hypomobility.

The PAIVM tests can be performed symmetrically or asymmetrically. These tests are described in the relevant chapters of this text. Generally speaking, the symmetric tests are used when planar motions have produced pain in the active motion tests, whereas the asymmetric techniques are used when the combined motions have produced pain in the active motion tests.

Caution must be used when basing clinical judgments on the results of accessory motion testing alone, because few studies have examined the validity and reliability of accessory motion testing of the spine or extremities and little is known about the validity of these tests for most inferences.[85]

Hayes and Peterson[86] examined two physical therapists who used standardized positions to evaluate two knee motions and five shoulder motions. Evaluators did not interview subjects and were blinded to previous test results. Evaluators applied overpressure and noted the end-feel while subjects identified the moment their pain was reproduced. Following testing, subjects rated their pain intensity. Analyses included percentage of agreement; κ, weighted κ, and maximum κ coefficients; and confidence intervals. Analyses were repeated for subjects whose pain intensity during testing did not change between examinations. Intra-rater κ coefficients varied from 0.65 to 1.00 for end-feel, and intra-rater weighted κ coefficients varied from 0.59 to 0.87 for pain-resistance sequence. Most coefficients remained stable or improved for the unchanged subjects. Inter-rater κ coefficients for end-feel and weighted κ coefficients for pain-resistance sequence varied from −0.01 to 0.70. The authors concluded that the reliability of end-feel and pain-resistance judgments at the knee and shoulder were generally good, especially after accounting for subject change and unbalanced distributions. Inter-rater reliability, however, was generally not acceptable, even after accounting for these factors.[86]

In a separate study by the same authors,[87] the relationship between pain and normal and abnormal (pathologic) end-feels during passive physiologic motion assessment at the knee and shoulder were examined. Physical therapists examined subjects with unilateral knee or shoulder pain, and each subject was examined twice. Passive physiologic motions, two at the knee and five at the shoulder, were tested by applying an overpressure at the end of ROM, using standardized positions. Subjects reported the amount of pain (0 to 10) immediately after the evaluator recorded the end-feel. The authors concluded that abnormal (pathologic) end-feels are associated with more pain than normal end-feels during passive physiologic motion testing at the knee or shoulder. Dysfunction should be suspected when abnormal (pathologic) end-feels are present.[87]

Based on the review of the literature of the MEDLINE and CINAHL databases for the period of 1980 through 2000, using the keywords *motion palpation, accessory motion,* and *intervertebral motion,* Huijbregts[88] performed a review of 28 reliability studies. The following conclusions were made from this study:

▶ Intra-rater agreement varied from less than chance to generally moderate or substantial agreement.

▶ Inter-rater agreement only rarely exceeded poor to fair agreement.

▶ Rating scales measuring absence versus presence or magnitude of pain response yielded higher agreement values than mobility rating scales.

Segmental Stability Tests

These are tests for movements that should not exist to an appreciable degree. The tests include maneuvers that induce non-physiologic rotational, anterior, posterior, and transverse shears to the segment. The limitation in the clinical diagnosis of segmental instability lies in the difficulty of accurately detecting excessive intersegmental motion, because even conventional radiologic testing is often insensitive and unreliable.[89,90] Instability should be suspected in the presence of a positive stability test in conjunction with other clinical findings and symptoms of instability. A positive stability test in the absence of other clinical findings is probably irrelevant. Hypermobility is clinically manifested by the presence of increased physiologic range in one or more directions, or normal range with pain and spasm at the end of that range.

Research indicates that skilled clinicians can distinguish subjects with symptomatic spondylolysis from LBP based on the finding of increased intersegmental motion at the level above the pars defect.[91,92]

The various stability tests are described in the specific chapters of this text.

General Guidelines for the Intervention of Spinal Dysfunction

Numerous interventions exist for patients with spinal disorders of a neuromusculoskeletal origin, and the challenge for the clinician is to identify the most appropriate intervention. Given the exhaustive list of causes for these disorders, the choice of intervention would seem an impossible task. This is particularly true with reference to chronic low back or neck pain.

However, in most cases, the cause of spinal pain is mechanical in nature. It is likely that the direction of spinal motion that is associated with an increase in symptoms is a reflection of the movement strategies and postures that are repeated by a given individual throughout each day.[93] The most logical approach, therefore, would be to identify the primary movement or postural dysfunction, and focus the intervention on teaching the patient strategies that limit this motion, or posture. This approach should be supplemented with the following strategies:

▶ Bed rest is not recommended as an intervention for simple LBP.[94] In cases of severe pain, it may be necessary for the patient to be confined to a bed for a few days (a maximum of 2 days is recommended).[95]

▶ Joint protection techniques can reduce and control pain by minimizing repetitive movements into painful ranges of motion. In the cervical spine, this can be achieved through the use of a cervical collar with appropriate weaning. In the lumbar spine, a lumbar cushion can be used to support the spine in the position of normal lumbar lordosis.

▶ Patient education is an important component of any rehabilitative process. The patient is taught how to find the neutral position or the position of optimal function of the spine. This position is the least painful, and represents the position of minimized biomechanical stresses.[96] The patient also is advised to stay as active as possible and to continue normal daily and work activities whenever possible.[94,95]

▶ Causative factors also must be addressed. These usually include imbalances in muscle function. Once again, the patient must be taught how to correct these balances through strengthening exercises, self-stretches, or automobilization techniques.

▶ Strengthening exercises of the spine begin with single plane isometric exercises in the neutral position in the supine position, followed by the same exercises in the seated and standing positions. These exercises are progressed to isometric contractions of combined motions, and, when symptoms permit, to concentric contractions of the various local and neighboring muscle groups.

▶ Manual therapy techniques, including soft tissue techniques, mobilization, and manipulation, can be used for both the examination and intervention to determine the source and relative contribution of various structures to the pain and dysfunction of the patient, and to help decrease pain and improve mobility and function, respectively. There is moderate evidence that manipulation is more effective than a placebo for short-term pain relief of acute LBP.[95] However, the long-term effects of manipulation have not been demonstrated. Although spinal manipulation appears to increase spinal ROM and straight leg raising, it is not known to reduce an intervertebral disk herniation.[97] Complications following manipulation, although rare, can be catastrophic especially in the cervical spine.[98,99] The soft tissue techniques of stretching, deep pressure, massage, and traction can help alleviate pain, whereas myofascial techniques can be used to help stretch the noncontractile component of the soft tissue.[96]

▶ Neuromuscular control must also be reestablished. Neuromuscular control of the spine is first taught in static positions and then advanced to include control during dynamic and functional activities, through the appropriate stabilization program.[73,96]

▶ Aerobic conditioning must be maintained or improved throughout the rehabilitative process. For injuries involving the cervical and thoracic spines, this can be achieved using a stationary cycle, treadmill, or stair-stepper. For low back injuries, an upper body ergonometer can be used if the previously mentioned equipment exacerbates the symptoms.

Full restoration of spinal function can occur only when the patient is able to progress to dynamic activities involving the trunk and extremities, without the provocation of pain or the exacerbation of symptoms.

REFERENCES

1. Bogduk N, Twomey LT. Anatomy and biomechanics of the lumbar spine. In: Bogduk N, Twomey LT, eds. *Clinical Anatomy of the Lumbar Spine and Sacrum*. Edinburgh, Scotland: Churchill Livingstone; 1997:2–53,81–152,171–176.
2. White AA, Punjabi MM. *Clinical Biomechanics of the Spine*. 2nd ed. Philadelphia, Pa: JB Lippincott; 1990.
3. Alexander MJL. Biomechanical aspects of lumbar spine injuries in athletes: A review. *Can J Appl Sports Sci* 1985;10:1–20.
4. Pope MH, Lehmann TR, Frymoyer JW. Structure and function of the lumbar spine. In: Pope MH, Frymoyer JW, Andersson G, eds. *Occupational Low Back Pain*. New York, NY: Praeger; 1984:1–348.
5. Schmorl G, Junghanns H. *The Human Spine in Health and Disease*. 2nd American ed. New York, NY: Grune and Stratton; 1971.
6. Wigh R. The thoracolumbar and lumbosacral transitional junctions. *Spine* 1980;5:215–222.
7. Grieve GP. *Common Vertebral Joint Problems*. New York, NY: Churchill Livingstone; 1981.
8. White AA, Panjabi MM. *Clinical Biomechanics of the Spine*. 2nd ed. Philadelphia, Pa: JB Lippincott; 1990.
9. Cocchiarella L, Andersson GBJ, eds. *American Medical Association, Guides to the Evaluation of Permanent Impairment*. 5th ed. Chicago, Ill: AMA; 2001.
10. Aiderink GJ. The sacroiliac joint: Review of anatomy, mechanics and function. *J Orthop Sports Phys Ther* 1991;13:71.
11. Lee DG. *The Pelvic Girdle: An Approach to the Examination and Treatment of the Lumbo-Pelvic-Hip Region*. 2nd ed. Edinburgh, Scotland: Churchill Livingstone; 1999.
12. Grieve GP. The sacroiliac joint. *Physiotherapy* 1976;62:384–400.
13. Kirkaldy-Willis WH, Hill RJ. A more precise diagnosis for low back pain. *Spine* 1979;4:102–109.
14. Wang M, Bryant JT, Dumas GA. A new in vitro measurement technique for small three-dimensional joint motion and its application to the sacroiliac joint. *Med Eng Phys* 1996;18:495–501.
15. Van der Wurff P, Meyne W, Hagmeijer RHM. Clinical tests of the sacroiliac joint, a systematic methodological review. Part 2: Validity. *Man Ther* 2000;5:89–96.
16. Ross J. Is the sacroiliac joint mobile and how should it be treated? *Br J Sports Med* 2000;34:226.
17. Miller JAA, Schultz AB, Andersson GBJ. Load-displacement behaviour of sacroiliac joints. *J Orthop Res* 1987;5:92–101.
18. Vleeming A, Van Wingerden JP, Dijkstra PF. Mobility in the sacroiliac joints in the elderly: A kinematic and radiological study. *Clin Biomech* 1992;7:170–176.
19. Krag MH. *Three-dimensional Flexibility Measurements of Preload Human Vertebral Motion Segments*. New Haven, Conn: Yale University School of Medicine; 1975.

20. White AA. Analysis of the mechanics of the thoracic spine in man: An experimental study of autopsy specimens. *Acta Orthop Scand Suppl* 1969;127:1–105.

21. Farfan HF. The scientific basis of manipulative procedures. *Clin Rheum Dis* 1980;6:159–177.

22. White AA, Panjabi MM. *Clinical Biomechanics of the Spine.* Philadelphia, Pa: Lippincott-Raven; 1990:106–108.

23. Fryette HH. *Principles of Osteopathic Technique.* Carmel, Calif: Academy of Applied Osteopathy; 1980.

24. Brown L. An introduction to the treatment and examination of the spine by combined movements. *Physiotherapy* 1988;74:347–353.

25. Edwards BC. Manual of Combined Movements, 2nd ed. Edwards B, ed. St Louis, MO: Butterworth-Heinemann; 1999.

26. Edwards BC. Combined movements of the lumbar spine: Examination and treatment. In: Palastanga N, Boyling JD, eds. *Grieve's Modern Manual Therapy of the Vertebral Column.* Edinburgh, Scotland: Churchill Livingstone; 1994:561–566.

27. Kaltenborn FM. *The Spine: Basic Evaluation and Mobilization Techniques.* Wellington, New Zealand: New Zealand University Press; 1993.

28. Farfan HF. *Mechanical Disorders of the Low Back.* Philadelphia, Pa: Lea and Febiger; 1973.

29. Evjenth O, Hamberg J. *Muscle Stretching in Manual Therapy, A Clinical Manual.* Alfta, Sweden: Alfta Rehab Forlag; 1984.

30. Nachemson A. Introduction to treatment of neck and back pain. In: Nachemson AL, Jonsson E, eds. *Neck and Back Pain: The Scientific Evidence of Causes, Diagnosis, and Treatment.* Philadelphia, Pa: Lippincott Williams and Wilkins; 2000:237–239.

31. Borenstein D, Wiesel SW. *Low Back Pain: Medical Diagnosis and Comprehensive Management.* Philadelphia, Pa: Saunders; 1989:60–78.

32. Borenstein D, Wiesel SW, Boden SD. *Neck Pain: Medical Diagnosis and Comprehensive Management.* Philadelphia, Pa: Saunders; 1996.

33. Nachemson A, Vingard E. Assessment of patients with neck and back pain: A best evidence synthesis. In: Nachemson AL, Jonsson E, eds. *Neck and Back Pain: The Scientific Evidence of Causes, Diagnosis, and Treatment.* Philadelphia, Pa: Lippincott Williams and Wilkins; 2000:189–235.

34. Riddle DL, Rothstein JM. Intertester reliability of McKenzie's classifications of the syndrome types present in patients with low back pain. *Spine* 1993;18:1333–1344.

35. Riddle DL. Classification and low back pain; a review of the literature and critical analysis of selected systems. *Phys Ther* 1998;78:708–737.

36. Bernard TN, Kirkaldy-Willis WH. Recognizing specific characteristics of nonspecific low back pain. *Clin Orthop* 1987;217:266–280.

37. Mooney V. The syndromes of low back disease. *Orthop Clin North Am* 1983;14:505–515.

38. Abenhaim L, Rossingol M, Gobeille D, Bonvalot Y, Fines P, Scott S. The prognostic consequences in the making of the initial medical diagnosis of work-related back injuries. *Spine* 1995;20:791–795.

39. Bigos S, et al. *Acute Low Back Problems in Adults.* AHCPR Publication 95-0642. Rockville, Md: Agency for Health Care Policy and Research, Public Health Service, US Department of Health and Human Services; 1994.

40. Spitzer WO. Approach to the problem. Scientific approach to the assessment and management of activity-related spinal disorders: A monograph for clinicians. *Spine* 1987;12:9–11.

41. Cyriax J. *Textbook of Orthopaedic Medicine, Diagnosis of Soft Tissue Lesions.* 8th ed. London, England: Bailliere Tindall; 1982.

42. Von Korff M. Studying the natural history of back pain. *Spine* 1994;19:2041–2046.

43. Quebec Task Force on Spinal Disorders. Scientific approach to the assessment and management of activity-related spinal disorders: A monograph for clinicians. Report of the Quebec Task Force on Spinal Disorders. *Spine* 1987;12(suppl):1–59.

44. McKenzie RA. *The Lumbar Spine: Mechanical Diagnosis and Therapy.* Waikanae, New Zealand: Spinal Publications of New Zealand; 1981.

45. McKenzie RA. *The Cervical and Thoracic Spine: Mechanical Diagnosis and Therapy.* Waikanae, New Zealand: Spinal Publications of New Zealand; 1990.

46. Bouter LM, van Tulder MW, Koes BW. Methodologic issues in low back pain research in primary care. *Spine* 1998;23:2014–2020.

47. Downey BJ, Taylor NF, Niere KR. Manipulative physiotherapists can reliably palpate nominated lumbar spinal levels. *Man Ther* 1999;4:151–156.

48. Keating JC Jr, Bergmann TF, Jacobs GE, Kiner BA, Larson K. Interexaminer reliability of eight evaluative dimensions of lumbar segmental abnormality. *J Manipulative Physiol Ther* 1990;13:463–470.

49. Binkley J, Stratford PW, Gill C. Interrater reliability of lumbar accessory motion mobility testing. *Phys Ther Rev* 1995;75:786–792; discussion 793–795.

50. Donahue MS, Riddle DL, Sullivan MS. Intertester reliability of a modified version of McKenzie's lateral shift assessment obtained on patients with low back pain. *Phys Ther* 1996;76:706–726.

51. Donelson R. Reliability of the McKenzie assessment. *J Orthop Sports Phys Ther* 2000;30:770–773.

52. Donelson R, Grant W, Kamps C, Medcalf R. Pain response to sagittal end-range spinal motion. A prospective, randomized, multicentered trial. *Spine* 1991;16:S206–S212.

53. Donelson R, Silva G, Murphy K. Centralization phenomenon: Its usefulness in evaluating and treating referred pain. *Spine* 1990;15:211–213.

54. Tenhula JA, Rose SJ, Delitto A. Association between direction of lateral lumbar shift, movement tests, and side of symptoms in patients with low back pain syndromes. *Phys Ther* 1990;70:480–486.

55. Fritz JM, Delitto A, Vignovic M, Busse RG. Interrater reliability of judgements of the centralization phenomenon and status change during movement testing in patients with low back pain. *Arch Phys Med Rehabil* 2000;81:57–60.

56. Kilby J, Stigant M, Roberts A. The reliability of back pain assessment by physiotherapists using a "McKenzie algorithm." *Physiotherapy* 1990;76:579–583.

57. Razmjou H, Kramer JF, Yamada R. Intertester reliability of the McKenzie evaluation in assessing patients with mechanical low back pain. *J Orthop Sports Phys Ther* 2000;30:368–383.

58. Kilpikoski S, Airaksinen O, Kankaanpaa M, Leminen P, Videman T, Alen M. Interexaminer reliability of low back pain assessment using the McKenzie method. *Spine* 2002;27:E207–214.

59. Maher C, Adams R. Reliability of pain and stiffness assessments in clinical manual lumbar spine examination. *Phys Ther* 1994;74:801–807.

60. Delitto A, Erhard RE, Bowling RW. A treatment-based classification approach to low back syndrome: Identifying and staging patients for conservative management. *Phys Ther* 1995;75:470–489.

61. Fritz JM, George S. The use of a classification approach to identify subgroups of patients with acute low back pain. Interrater reliability and short-term treatment outcomes. *Spine* 2000;25:106–114.

62. Natchev E. *A Manual on Autotraction*. Stockholm, Sweden: Folksam Scientific Council; 1984.

63. Meadows JTS. The principles of the Canadian approach to the lumbar dysfunction patient. In: *Management of Lumbar Spine Dysfunction—Independent Home Study Course*. La Crosse, Wis: American Physical Therapy Association, Orthopaedic Section; 1999.

64. Kaltenborn FM. *Manual Mobilization of the Extremity Joints: Basic Examination and Treatment Techniques*. 4th ed. Oslo, Norway: Olaf Norlis Bokhandel, Universitetsgaten; 1989.

65. Evjenth O, Gloeck C. *Symptom Localization in the Spine and Extremity Joints*. Minneapolis, Minn: Orthopedic Physical Therapy Products; 2000.

66. Cyriax JH, Cyriax PJ. *Illustrated Manual of Orthopaedic Medicine*. London, England: Butterworth; 1983.

67. Mennell JB. *The Science and Art of Joint Manipulation*. London, England: J and A Churchill; 1949.

68. Mennell JM. *Back Pain. Diagnosis and Treatment Using Manipulative Techniques*. Boston, Mass: Little, Brown; 1960.

69. Mitchell FL, Moran PS, Pruzzo NA. *An Evaluation and Treatment Manual of Osteopathic Muscle Energy Procedures*. Manchester, Mo: Mitchell, Moran and Pruzzo; 1979.

70. Stoddard A. *Manual of Osteopathic Practice*. New York, NY: Harper and Row; 1969.

71. McGill SM, Childs A, Liebenson C. Endurance times for low back stabilization exercises: Clinical targets for testing and training from a normal database. *Arch Phys Med Rehabil* 1999; 80:941–944.

72. Richardson CA, et al. *Therapeutic Exercise for Spinal Segmental Stabilization in Low Back Pain*. London, England: Churchill Livingstone; 1999.

73. Sweeney TB, et al. Cervicothoracic muscular stabilization techniques. In: Saal JA, ed. *Physical Medicine and Rehabilitation, State of the Art Reviews: Neck and Back Pain*. Philadelphia, Pa: Hanley and Belfus; 1990:335–359.

74. Hyman J, Liebenson C. Spinal stabilization exercise program. In: Liebenson C, ed. *Rehabilitation of the Spine: A Practitioner's Manual*. Baltimore, Md: Lippincott Williams and Wilkins; 1996:293–317.

75. Jull GA, Janda V. Muscle and motor control in low back pain. In: Twomey LT, Taylor JR, eds. *Physical Therapy of the Low Back: Clinics in Physical Therapy*. New York, NY: Churchill Livingstone; 1987:258.

76. Janda V. Muscles and motor control in cervicogenic disorders: Assessment and management. In: Grant R, ed. *Physical Therapy of the Cervical and Thoracic Spine*. New York, NY: Churchill Livingstone; 1994:195–216.

77. Sahrmann SA. *Diagnosis and Treatment of Movement Impairment Syndromes*. St Louis, Mo: Mosby; 2001.

78. Knott M, Voss DE. *Proprioceptive Neuromuscular Facilitation*. 2nd ed. New York, NY: Harper and Row; 1968.

79. Feldenkrais M. *The Elusive Obvious*. Cupertino, Calif: Meta Publications; 1981.

80. Maher C, Latimer J, Adams R. An investigation of the reliability and validity of posteroanterior spinal stiffness judgments made using a reference-based protocol. *Phys Ther* 1998; 78:829–837.

81. Smedmark V, Wallin M, Arvidsson I. Inter-examiner reliability in assessing passive intervertebral motion of the cervical spine. *Man Ther* 2000;5:97–101.

82. Gonnella C, Paris SV, Kutner M. Reliability in evaluating passive intervertebral motion. *Phys Ther Rev* 1982;62:436–444.

83. Exelby L. The locked lumbar facet joint: Intervention using mobilizations with movement. *Man Ther* 2001;6:116–121.

84. Janda V. Muscles, motor regulation and back problems. In: Korr IM, ed. *The Neurological Mechanisms in Manipulative Therapy*. New York, NY: Plenum; 1978:27.

85. Riddle DL. Measurement of accessory motion: Critical issues and related concepts. *Phys Ther* 1992;72:865–874.

86. Hayes KW, Petersen CM. Reliability of assessing end-feel and pain and resistance sequence in subjects with painful shoulders and knees. *J Orthop Sports Phys Ther* 2001;31:432–445.

87. Petersen CM, Hayes KW. Construct validity of Cyriax's selective tension examination: Association of end-feels with pain at the knee and shoulder. *J Orthop Sports Phys Ther* 2000; 30:512–527.

88. Huijbregts PA. Spinal motion palpation: A review of reliability studies. *J Man Manipulative Ther* 2002;10:24–39.

89. Dvorak J, Panjabi MM, Novotny JE, Chang DG, Grob D. Clinical validation of functional flexion-extension roentgenograms of the lumbar spine. *Spine* 1991;16:943–950.

90. Pope M, Frymoyer J, Krag M. Diagnosing instability. *Clin Orthop* 1992;296:60–67.

91. Phillips DR, Twomey LT. Comparison of manual diagnosis with a diagnosis established by a uni-level spinal block procedure. In: *Proceedings of the Eighth Biennial Conference, Manipulative Therapist Association of Australia*. Perth, Australia: MTAA; 1993.

92. Avery A. *The Reliability of Manual Physiotherapy Palpation Techniques in the Diagnosis of Bilateral Pars Defects in Subjects with Chronic Low Back Pain*. Bentley, Western Australia: Curtin University of Technology; 1996.

93. Maluf KS, Sahrmann SA, Van Dillen LR. Use of a classification system to guide non-surgical management of a patient with chronic low back pain. *Phys Ther* 2000;80:1097–1111.

94. Waddell G, et al. *Low Back Pain Evidence Review*. London, England: Royal College of General Practitioners; 1996.

95. van Tulder MW, Waddell G. Conservative treatment of acute and subacute low back pain. In: Nachemson AL, Jonsson E, eds. *Neck and Back Pain: The Scientific Evidence of Causes, Diagnosis, and Treatment*. Philadelphia, Pa: Lippincott Williams and Wilkins; 2000:241–269.

96. Cole AJ, Farrell JP, Stratton SA. Functional rehabilitation of cervical spine athletic injuries. In: Kibler BW, Herring JA, Press JM, eds. *Functional Rehabilitation of Sports and Musculoskeletal Injuries*. Gaithersburg, Md: Aspen; 1998.

97. Haldeman S. Spinal manipulative therapy. A status report. *Clin Orthop Rel Res* 1983;179:62–70.

98. Kleynhans AM. Complications of and contraindications to spinal manipulative therapy. In: Haldeman S, ed. *Modern Developments in the Principles and Practice of Chiropractic*. New York, NY: Appleton-Century-Crofts; 1980.

99. Assendelft WJ, Bouter SM, Knipschild PG. Complications of spinal manipulation: A comprehensive review of the literature. *J Fam Pract* 1996;42:475–480.

CHAPTER 20

THE INTERVERTEBRAL DISK

CHAPTER OBJECTIVES

▶ *At the completion of this chapter, the reader will be able to:*

1. List the various components of the intervertebral disk.

2. Describe the chemical makeup and function of each of the intervertebral components.

3. Define the similarities and differences of the disks in each spinal area.

4. Describe the pathologic processes involved with disk degeneration and disk degradation.

5. Describe the differences between a protrusion, an extrusion, and a sequestration.

6. Identify the various forces that act on the disk and how the disk responds.

7. List the characteristics of disk impairment at each segmental level.

8. Describe the rationale for the use of the various strategies in the intervention of disk impairments.

OVERVIEW

Phylogenically, the intervertebral disk (IVD) is a relatively new structure. The IVD forms a symphysis or amphiarthrosis between two adjacent vertebrae and represents the largest avascular structure in the body.[1] In the human spinal column, the combined heights of the IVDs account for approximately 20 to 33 percent of the total length of the spinal column.[2] The presence of an IVD not only permits motion of the segment in any direction up to the point that the disk itself is stretched, but also allows for a significant increase in the weight-bearing capabilities of the spine.[3] A normally functioning disk is extremely important to permit the normal biomechanics of the spine to occur and to reduce the possibility of mechanical interference among any of the neural structures.

Although there are regional differences within the spine, all vertebral disks are composed of three parts: the annulus fibrosus; the vertebral end plate; and a central gelatinous mass, called the nucleus pulposus (Fig. 20-1).

Although the disk is incapable of independent motion, movement of the disk does occur during the clinically defined motions of flexion-extension, side bending, and axial rotation.[4] The major stresses that must be withstood by the IVD are axial compression, shearing, bending, and twisting, either singly or in combination with each other.

The role of the disk is unique because it operates as an osmotic system, holding neighboring vertebral bodies together while simultaneously pushing them apart. As such, the IVD is a dynamic structure that responds to stresses applied from vertebral movement or from static loading.

Lumbar Disks

Annulus Fibrosus

The lumbar disk is approximately cylindrical, its shape being determined by the integrity of the annulus fibrosus (AF). The AF consists of approximately 10 to 12 (often as many as 15 to 25) concentric sheets of predominantly type I collagen tissue[5] bound together by proteoglycan gel.[6] The number of annular layers decreases with age, but there is a gradual thickening of the remaining layers.[7] The fibers of the AF are oriented at about 65 degrees from vertical (Fig. 20-2). The fibers of each successive sheet or lamella maintain the same inclination of 65 degrees, but in the opposite direction to the preceding lamella, resulting in every second sheet having the same orientation. Thus, only 50 percent of the fibers are under stress with rotational forces at any given time.

Each lamella is thicker anteriorly than posteriorly, leading to the lumbar disks being thinner posteriorly than anteriorly. The wedge-shaped appearance of the disk produced by the configuration of the lamellae contributes to the normal lordosis of

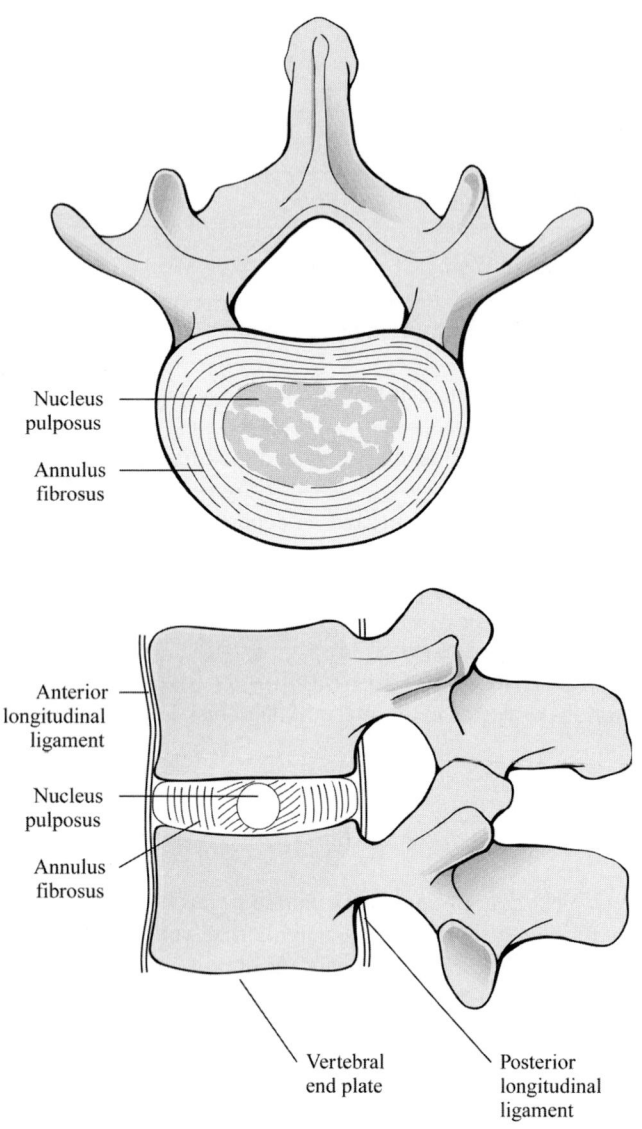

Nucleus
pulposus

Annulus
fibrosus

Anterior
longitudinal
ligament

Nucleus
pulposus

Annulus
fibrosus

Vertebral
end plate

Posterior
longitudinal
ligament

FIGURE 20-1 Intervertebral disk. (Reproduced with permission from Dutton M. *Manual Therapy of the Spine.* New York, NY: McGraw-Hill; 2002:112.)

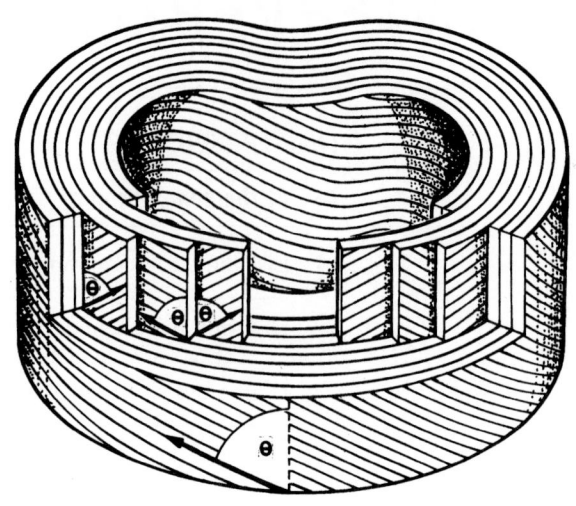

FIGURE 20-2 Annulus fibrosus. (Reproduced with permission from Bogduk N, Twomey LT. *Clinical Anatomy of the Lumbar Spine and Sacrum.* New York, NY: Churchill Livingstone; 1997:15.)

Nucleus Pulposus

The lumbar IVDs of a healthy young adult contain a nucleus pulposus (NP) that is composed of a semifluid mass of mucoid material. This material is clear, firm, and gelatinous.[9]

> ### Clinical Pearl
>
> The overall consistency of the NP changes with increased age, as the water content of the NP diminishes and subsequently becomes drier.

At birth, the water content of the NP is about 80 percent. In the elderly, the water content is about 68 percent. Most of this water content change occurs in childhood and adolescence, with only about 6 percent occurring in adulthood.[10] The portion of the NP that is not water is made up of cells that are largely chondrocytes and a matrix consisting of proteoglycans, collagen fibers, other noncollagenous proteins, and elastin.[1,11,12]

With the exception of early youth, there is no clear boundary between the NP and AF, and it resembles a transitional zone.[13] The biomechanical makeup of the NP is similar to that of the AF, except that the NP contains mostly type II collagen, as opposed to type I.[5] The collagen interacts with the ground substance to form a concentration proportional to the viscoelastic requirements of the AF.

Vertebral End Plates

Each vertebral end plate consists of a layer of hyaline and fibrocartilage about 0.6 to 1 mm thick,[14] which covers the top or bottom aspects of the disk, and separates the disk from the adjacent vertebral body. Peripherally, the end plate is surrounded by the ring apophysis.[9]

this region.[1] Although the posterior aspect of the IVD is thinner, the collagen is more tightly packed than it is anteriorly.[8] Consequently, the posterior part of the annulus will have thinner but stronger fibers, and it is capable of withstanding tension applied to this area during flexion activities and postures, which occur more frequently than with extension.[9] However, because of the predominance of flexion activities in life, fatigue damage may occur in the posterior aspect of the disk, making it a common site of injury.[1]

The outermost layer of the annulus attaches to the vertebral body by mingling with the periosteal fibers (fibers of Sharpey). The outer two thirds of the annulus fibrosus are attached firmly to the cartilaginous end plate, but the inner third is more loosely attached.[9]

At birth, the end plate is part of the vertebral body growth plate, but by approximately the 20th year, it has been separated from the body by a subchondral plate. During this time, the plate is bilaminar, with a growth zone and an articular area.[15] With aging, the growth zone becomes thinner and disappears, leaving only a thickened articular plate.

Nutrition of the disk comes via a diffusion of nutrients from the anastomosis over the AF and from the arterial plexi underlying the end plate. Although almost the entire AF is permeable to nutrients, only the center portions of the end plate are permeable. Over about 10 percent of the surface of the end plate, the subchondral bone of the centrum is deficient. At these points, the bone marrow is in direct contact with the end plate, thereby augmenting the nutrition of the disk and end plate.[16] It is possible that a mechanical pump action produced by spine motion could aid with the diffusion of the nutrients.

The two end plates of each disk, therefore, cover the NP in its entirety, but fail to cover the entire extent of the AF.

Clinical Pearl

Because of the attachment of the AF to the vertebral end plates on the periphery, the end plates are strongly bound to the IVD. In contrast, the vertebral end plates are only weakly attached to the vertebral bodies,[17] and can be completely torn from the vertebral bodies by trauma. It is for this and other morphologic reasons that the end plates are regarded as constituents of the IVD, rather than as a part of the vertebral body.[15]

Between the ages of 20 and 65 years, the end plate thins and the vascular foramina in the subchondral bone become occluded, resulting in decreased nutrition to the disk. At the same time, the underlying bone becomes weaker, and the end plate gradually bows into the vertebral body, becoming more vulnerable centrally, where it may fracture into the centrum.[9] The presence of damage to a vertebral body end plate reduces the pressure in the NP of the adjacent disk by up to 57 percent, and doubles the size of so-called stress peaks in the posterior aspect of the AF.[18]

Innervation

The outer half of the IVD, the posterior longitudinal ligament, and the dura are innervated by the sinuvertebral nerve,[19] which is considered to arise from the ventral ramus and the sympathetic trunk[20] (Fig. 20-3). The nerve endings are simple or complex, encapsulated and nonencapsulated, and exist as free nerve endings. It has been suggested that apart from a nociceptive function, these nerve endings may also have a proprioceptive function.[21,22]

Actions of the Disk During Stress

IVDs are able to distribute compressive stress evenly between adjacent vertebrae because the NP and inner AF act like a pressurized fluid, in which the pressure does not vary with location or direction.[23,24] Biomechanical studies of the IVD seem to indicate that the disk acts to provide flexibility at low loads and stability at high loads.[25,26]

Axial Compression

Axial compression or spinal loading occurs in weight bearing, whether in standing or sitting. It has been demonstrated experimentally that the AF, even without the NP, can withstand the same vertical forces that an intact disk can for short periods,[27] providing the lamellae do not buckle. However, if the compression is prolonged or if the lamellae are not held together, the sheets buckle and the system collapses on itself.

The extent and magnitude of the compression depend on the amount of applied compressive force, the disk height, and the cross-sectional area of the disk. Variations in disk height can be divided into two categories: primary disk height variations and secondary disk height changes.

1. Primary disk height variations are related to intrinsic individual factors such as body height, gender, age, disk level, and geographic region.[28,29]

2. Secondary disk height changes are associated with extrinsic factors, such as degeneration, abnormality, or clinical management. Surgical procedures, such as nucleotomy, diskectomy, and chemonucleolysis, cause a decrease in disk height, resulting from the removal of a portion of the NP or damage to the water binding capacity of the extracellular matrix.[30–32] In addition, there are diurnal changes in disk height, which are caused by fluid exchange and creep deformation.[33]

With variations in disk height, one would expect changes in mechanical behavior of the disk. An important result to

---

FIGURE 20-3 The sinuvertebral nerve. (Reproduced with permission from Dutton M. *Manual Therapy of the Spine*. New York, NY: McGraw-Hill; 2002.)

Sinuvertebral Nerve

Ascending Branch
Innervates:
• Posterior longitudinal ligament
• Posterior aspect of the superior disk
• Anterior aspect of the dura
• Spinal canal vessels

Descending Branch
Innervates:
• Posterior longitudinal ligament
• Posterior aspect of inferior disk
• Anterior aspect of the dura
• Spinal canal vessels

emerge from a recent study is that axial displacement, postero-lateral disk bulge, and tensile stress in the peripheral AF fibers are a function of axial compressive force and disk height.[34] Under the same axial force, disks with a higher height-to-area ratio generated higher values of axial displacement, disk bulge, and tensile stress on the peripheral AF fibers.

The NP is deformable but relatively incompressible. Therefore, when a load is applied to it vertically, the nuclear pressure rises, absorbing and transmitting the compression forces to the vertebral end plates and the AF.[9]

▶ The resistance of the end plate is dependent on the strength of the bone beneath and the blood capacity of the vertebral body.

▶ The AF bulges radially,[35] delaying and graduating the forces.

The peripheral pressure increases the tension on the collagen fibers, which resist it until a balance is reached, at the point when the radial pressure is matched by the collagen tension.[4]

This equilibrium achieves two things:

1. Pressure is transferred from one end plate to another, thus relieving the load on the AF.

2. The NP braces the AF and prevents it buckling under the sustained axial load.

Other structures provide resistance to axial loading of the spine:

▶ The anterior longitudinal ligament offers resistance if the spine is in its normal lordosis. The lumbar lordosis while standing is about 50 percent greater than when seated.[36]

▶ The inferior articular process can impact on the lamina below during strong lordosis.

During axial compression of the IVD:

1. Water is squeezed out of disk. The water loss is 5 to 11 percent.[37]
   a. Rapid creep occurs (1.5 mm in the first 2 to 10 minutes)[38] and then slows (to about 1 mm per hour).[27]
   b. The creep plateaus at 90 minutes.[39]
   c. Over a 16-hour day, a 10 percent loss in disk height occurs.
   d. A person's height is restored with unloading. The best unloading position is in the supine knees-up posture (better than the extended supine posture).[40]
2. The intradiskal pressure increases.

Breakdown of the System. Under normal circumstances, the NP acts like a sealed hydraulic system. Within this system the fluid pressure rises substantially when volume is increased (by fluid injection, or by imbibing[30]) and falls when volume is decreased (by surgical excision or axial compression loading).[32] By a similar mechanism, the age-related degenerative changes reduce the water content of the NP by 15 to 20 percent,[33] causing a

30 percent fall in the NP pressure.[41] In effect, the load is being transferred from the NP to the AF. The posterior AF is affected most, because it is the narrowest part of the disk and the least able to sustain large compressive strains.[34]

The end plate is also susceptible during compression, being able to withstand only about one tenth of the stress that the AF can handle.[42] Even though axial loading occurs evenly over the surface of the end plate, failure of this structure typically occurs over the NP, indicating that this central part of the end plate is weaker than the periphery.[43]

Until about 40 years of age, as much as 55 percent of the compressive load through the centrum is borne by the cancellous bone,[44] the remainder being borne by the cortical bone. After this age, horizontal trabeculae are absorbed in the center of the vertebral body, thereby weakening the part of the centrum overlying the NP. This results in only about 35 percent of the axial stress being taken by the cancellous bone, with the greater proportion now going through cortical bone.[44] Because cortical bone fails with a smaller degree of deformation than cancellous bone, compressive failure occurs much more readily in the cortical bone.[44]

Pain originating from this failure would be expected to increase during the course of a day, especially in an individual who had spent a considerable amount of time with the lumbar spine flexed (e.g., a truck driver).[45]

Distraction

Symmetric distraction of the spine is a rare force in everyday functioning and, consequently, the disk is less resistant to distraction than it is to compression.[46] Although asymmetric distraction occurs constantly with spinal movement (side bending of the spine causes ipsilateral compression and contralateral distraction), symmetric distraction, in which all points of the one vertebral body are moved an equal distance away from its adjacent body, occurs only at times such as vertical suspension or therapeutic traction.

The AF appears to bear the principal responsibility for restricting distraction, with the oblique orientation of the collagen fibers becoming more vertical as the traction force is applied. For this reason, back pain reproduced with traction may implicate the AF as the source.

Axial Rotation

About 65 percent of the resistance to IVD torsion is resisted by a combination of tension and impaction of the contralateral zygapophysial joint, and tension of the supraspinous and interspinous ligaments, with the disk contributing about 35 percent of the resistance.[47] During axial rotation, which produces torsion of the IVD, those collagen fibers of the AF that are orientated in the same direction as the twist are stretched and resist the torsional force, while the others remain relaxed, thereby sharing the stress of twisting.

During forced segmental torsion, the first structure to fail is the zygapophysial joint, which normally occurs at about 1 to 2 degrees of segmental rotation.[47] As collagen can only elongate approximately 4 percent before damage, the maximum segmental rotation at each segmental level is typically limited to about 3 degrees.[42,48] Macroscopic failure of the IVD is likely to occur only in the presence of extreme trauma, with accompanying fracture of the zygapophysial joint.[49] However, surgical incision of the zygapophysial joint, or facetectomy, which increases the amount of rotation the segment is capable of handling, also significantly increases the stress in the posterior AF fibers.[47,49]

In the absence of zygapophysial joint damage, surgical or otherwise, axial rotation must be coupled with other motions to cause disk injury.[50] For example, the combination of maximal lumbar flexion and rotation, which increases the amount of rotation before the contralateral zygapophysial joint makes contact, has been associated with trauma to the AF.[51,52]

Shear

Shear is the movement of one vertebral body across the surface of its neighbor. This movement can occur in any plane. Resistance to the shear forces is provided by a number of structures including the zygapophysial joints, the AF fibers of the IVD, and the segmental ligaments.

In forward shearing, the AF fibers on the lateral aspects of the disk predominantly resist the movement, because they lie parallel to the movement.[53] Those angled posteriorly will be relaxed during forward shearing, but tensed during backward shearing.[53] The anterior and posterior fibers will offer some contribution to anterior and posterior shearing, but this will be much less than that of the lateral fibers.[53]

The anterior and posterior fibers are primarily involved during lateral shearing, again with those orientated in the direction of the shear undergoing tension. As with torsion, only half of the fibers can contribute to the resistance and, as with torsion, shear forces are potentially very disruptive to the IVD.[53] It could be argued that the presence of free nerve endings in the outer part of the AF could indicate a nociceptive ability in the disk, and anything disturbing these endings may then be considered potentially painful, although there is no direct evidence to prove this.

Bending

Bending motions can occur in any direction, producing both a rocking motion and a translation shearing effect on the IVD. The NP tends to be compressed and the AF buckles in the direction of the rocking motion,[54] and there is a tendency for the AF to be stretched in the opposite direction, while the pressure on the posterior aspect of the NP is relieved. Although the deformation can occur in a healthy disk, displacement of the NP is prevented by the AF that encapsulates it. The AF will buckle at its compressed aspect because it is not braced by the NP, which is exerting that effect on the AF fibers at the opposite side of the disk.[42]

Alterations in Disk Structure

Although the lumbar IVD appears destined for tissue regression and destruction, it remains unclear why similar age-related changes remain asymptomatic in one individual, yet cause severe low back pain in others. The basic changes that influence the responses of the disk to aging appear to be biochemical, and may concern the collagen content levels in the NP.

There is, with age, an increase in the collagen content of both the NP and AF and a change in the type of collagen present.[55] The elastic collagen of the NP becomes more fibrous, whereas the type 1 collagen of the AF becomes more elastic.[55] Eventually, they come to resemble each other. In addition, the concentration of noncollagenous proteins increases in the NP. The change of the makeup of the collagen alters the biomechanical properties of the disk, making it less resilient, perhaps leading to changes from microtrauma.[55]

> ### Clinical Pearl
>
> In general, the IVD becomes drier, stiffer, less deformable, and less able to recover from creep with age.

It was traditionally thought that the loss of height that occurs with aging resulted from a loss in the height of the IVD. More recently, it has been demonstrated that between the ages of 20 and 70 years, the disk actually increases its height by about 10 percent, and that the loss of height with age is more likely to be caused by the erosion of the vertebral end plate.[56]

As the NP becomes more fibrous, its ability to handle compressive loading becomes compromised and more weight is taken by the AF, resulting in a separation of the lamellae and the formation of cavities within it.[55]

Degeneration

Back pain, with or without radiculopathy, is a significant clinical problem. In patients with sciatic pain (sciatica) from disk herniation, radiographic examinations such as myelograms, computed tomographic (CT) scans, and magnetic resonance imaging (MRI) scans demonstrate nerve root compression by a herniated disk. However, sciatica can have a number of causes (Table 20-1).

> ### Clinical Pearl
>
> Approximately 20% to 30% percent of individuals without any history of sciatic pain have abnormal findings in radiographic examinations.[57]

TABLE 20-1   Some Causes of Sciatica[56a]

NERVE ROOT COMPRESSION
Tumor
Abscess
Arthritis
Vertebral collapse
Inflammatory synovitis
INFLAMMATORY DISEASE OF NERVE
Toxins (alcohol, heavy metals)
Diabetes mellitus
Syphilis

Degenerative changes are the body's attempts at self-healing as the body ages. If part of this healing involves the stabilization of an unstable joint, the joint motion can be reduced by muscle spasms or by increasing the surface area of the joint.[58] The biology of IVD degeneration is not well understood, but is thought to be a normal process, as opposed to the pathologic process that occurs with degradation (see Table 20-2 and later discussion).

The diagnoses associated with degenerative disk disease include:

▶ Idiopathic low back pain.

▶ Lumbar radiculopathy.

▶ Myelopathy.

▶ Lumbar stenosis.

▶ Spondylosis.

▶ Osteoarthritis.

▶ Degenerative disk disease.

▶ Zygapophysial joint degeneration.

Disk degeneration appears to involve a structural disruption of the AF and cell-mediated changes throughout the IVD and subchondral bone.[59] Kirkaldy-Willis proposed a system to describe the spectrum of degeneration involving three stages or levels.[60] The three stages, which have essentially withstood the test of time, are defined as early dysfunction, intermediate instability, and final stabilization.

1. **Early dysfunction.** This stage is characterized by minor pathologic changes resulting in abnormal function of the posterior elements and IVD.[61] Autopsy results show that disk degeneration begins as early as 20 to 25 years of age.[62] Disk herniation most commonly occurs at the end of this stage, as splits and clefts develop in the annulus, but also may occur during the last stage. Degeneration seems to start early in the upper lumbar spine, with end plate fractures and Schmorl's nodes related to the vertical loading of those segments.[55] A Schmorl's nodule represents a dislocation of cartilage tissue through the end plate into the vertebral body. One study[63] provided evidence that a family history of operated lumbar disk herniation has a significant implication in lumbar degenerative disk disease,

indicating that there may be a genetic factor in the development of lumbar disk herniation as an expression of disk degeneration.

2. **Intermediate instability.** This stage is characterized by laxity of the posterior joint capsule and AF. Disruption of the AF is associated with back pain.[64] All skeletal tissues adapt to increased mechanical demands, but they may not always adapt quickly enough. People who suddenly change to a physically demanding occupation may subject their tissues to an increase in repetitive loading, causing fatigue damage to accumulate rapidly. The ability of spinal tissues to strengthen in response to increased muscle forces may be restricted by health and age, so that fatigue damage accumulates most rapidly in sedentary middle-aged people who suddenly become active.[65]

3. **Final stabilization.** This stage is characterized by fibrosis of the posterior joints and capsule, a loss of disk material, the formation of radial tears of the AF, and osteophyte formation.[66] Osteophyte formation around the three-joint complex increases the load-bearing surface and decreases the amount of motion, producing a stiffer and thus less painful motion segment.[59]

Clinical experience has shown that it is possible for the three-joint complex to go through all of these phases with little symptomology.

Disk Degradation

Disk degradation is a more aggressive process than the degenerative changes that occur with aging (see Table 20-2), and although the macroscopic changes are similar to those of age-related degeneration, degradation is a more accelerated process.

Under normal conditions, the NP is contained by the AF. Any disturbance of the balance of these tissue structures may lead to tissue destruction, functional impairment, and low back pain.[49] An unequal load distribution to the IVD is a major predisposing factor in radial tearing of the AF.[49] The tearing can be caused by the torsional effect of the superior vertebra rotating in a constant direction with sagittal movements. The posterolateral aspect of the AF tends to weaken first.[67] If the inner layers of the posterior AF tear in the pres-

TABLE 20-2 Comparison of Degeneration and Degradation of the Disk

Degeneration	Degradation
Changes occur to biochemistry in early adulthood and middle age	Vasculogenic degradation of nucleus
Circumferential clefting and tearing of anulus	Circumferential and radial tearing of anulus
No migration of nucleus	Nucleus migrates through radial fissures
Undisplaced	Nucleus herniates through anulus
Disk maintains or increases height	Disk is reabsorbed

ence of the NP that is still capable of bulging into the space left by the tear, the symptoms of disk disease are likely to be experienced, with the spinal canal location of disk trespass determining the type of neural compromise, clinical pain pattern, and often the outcome.[67] It must be remembered that the degree of neural compromise and potential for pain cannot be judged accurately by the size or type of disk material. Large, free fragments can often cause no neurologic deficit or pain.[68]

Three main types of lumbar disk herniation are recognized:

1. ***Contained (protrusion).*** With a contained herniation, the nuclear material bulges outward through the tear to strain, but not escape from, the outer AF or the posterior longitudinal ligament (Fig. 20-4). Contained herniations are confined to the central canal. The disk bulges against the dura and the posterior longitudinal ligament, producing a dull, poorly localized somatic-type pain in the back and sacroiliac region. Regarding the modes of lumbar disk herniation, Yasuma and colleauges[69] described the degenerative process of the matrix and concluded that most herniations are protrusions of the NP that occur before the age of 60 years, whereas after that age, prolapse of the AF predominates. Eckert and Decker[70] and Taylor and Akeson,[71] however, found cartilaginous end-plate fractures in 60 percent of herniated masses, and in approximately 50 percent of sequestrated fragments, respectively. Because the NP is usually still contained, the patient is likely to feel more pain in the morning after the NP has imbibed more fluid, because of the added volume and the subsequent increase in pressure on pain-sensitive structures. Recent attention has been given to the internal disruption of the NP in contained herniation.[72] In this condition, the NP becomes inflamed and invaginates itself between the anular layers. Compression of the disk during sitting and bending increases the pain, because the nociceptive structures within the AF are further irritated. There is usually no, or minimal, leg pain and no, or minimal, limitation in the straight leg raising (SLR) test (see Chap. 12).[72]

2. ***Extrusion (prolapse).*** With extrusion, the nuclear material remains attached to the disk, but escapes the AF or the posterior longitudinal ligament to bulge posterolaterally into the intervertebral canal (see Fig. 20-4). Once a tear to the periphery is opened for the NP, it would seem logical that further stresses can force it to migrate through the tear. However, under normal conditions, the nuclear material is intrinsically cohesive and does not herniate through the AF, even if the AF fibers are weakened by a radial incision.[73]

3. ***Sequestration.*** The migrating nuclear material escapes contact with the disk entirely and becomes a free fragment in the intervertebral canal (see Fig. 20-4).

As part of its unnatural history, the disk may or may not travel through each stage of herniation sequentially, produc-

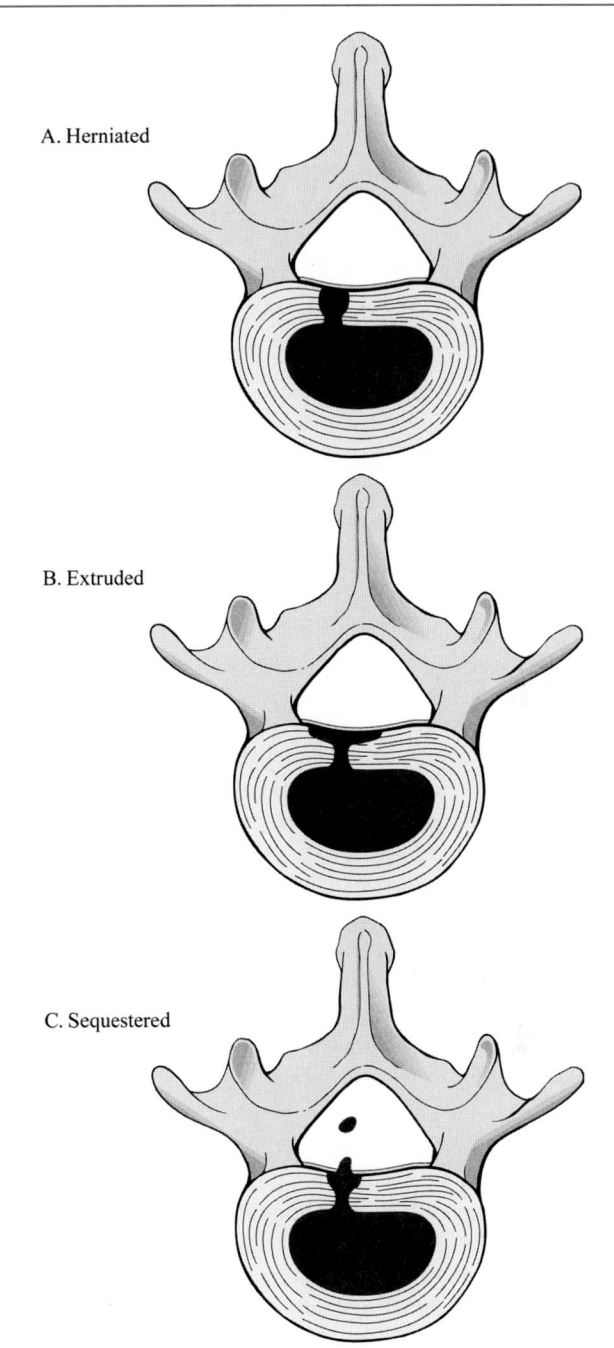

A. Herniated

B. Extruded

C. Sequestered

FIGURE 20-4 Schematic representation for herniated, extruded, and sequestered intervertebral disks. (Reproduced with permission from Dutton M. *Manual Therapy of the Spine.* McGraw-Hill; 2002:114.)

ing symptoms that range from backache to bilateral radiculopathy.

Nerve Compression

Extrusions and sequestrations impinge on nerve tissue. Central prolapses, although relatively rare, may produce upper motor neuron impairments if they occur in the cervical or thoracic spine, and bowel or bladder impairments if they occur in the lumbar spine (cauda equina syndrome).[74] A substantial compression of the root affects the nerve fibers, producing paresthesia and interference with conduction. In 1934, Mixter and Barr suggested that tissue of the IVD extrudes into the spinal canal, compressing and therefore irritating the nerve root and causing sciatic pain.[75] Although this concept was widely accepted for many years, it has now been demonstrated that mechanical compression of the nerve root alone does not explain sciatic pain and radiculopathy.[76–78] The operative finding that mechanically compressed nerve roots become tender, and results of recent histologic and biochemical studies on herniated lumbar disk tissue, led to the notion of inflammatory induced sciatic pain.[76–79] More recent models of lumbar radiculopathy suggest that the underlying mechanisms probably result, in part, from a local chemical irritant such as proteoglycans released from a disk and creating an inflammatory reaction, an autoimmune reaction from exposure to disk tissues, an increased concentration of lactic acid, or a lower pH around the nerve roots.[77,80]

Inflammation

Investigators have repeatedly demonstrated inflammatory cells, proinflammatory enzyme phospholipase A_2, immunoglobulins, and various inflammatory mediators in herniated disk tissues.[76,81] It is also thought that neovascularization in herniated disk tissue could promote the formation of granulation tissue,[78,79,82] and in association with blood vessels, deposits of immunoglobulins have been reported.[77]

The presence of inflammation in disk herniations could explain the clinical findings of improvement in radicular pain following the administration of corticosteroid or nonsteroidal anti-inflammatory drugs (NSAIDs).

Autoimmune Reaction

Several investigators have hypothesized that the adult NP is somehow concealed from the immune system, and that the exposure of nuclear disk material to the circulatory system provokes an autoimmune reaction. Some credibility is given to this idea with the identification of antibodies to NP in patients' sera and in animal models.[76,77,79]

Specific Lumbar Disk Lesions[83]

A large percentage of the mechanical causes of back pain, particularly low back pain, are attributed to pathologies of the IVD. IVD herniation in the lumbar spine may occur from adolescence into old age. Lumbar IVD herniation has a favorable prognosis in the majority of circumstances.

Several plausible diagnoses, depending on the distribution of symptoms, must be eliminated before a lumbar radiculopathy can be confirmed. These include:

▶ Hip joint pathology (degenerative joint disease, avascular necrosis, synovitis, etc.).[84]

▶ Meralgia paresthetica. This syndrome, also known as Bernhardt-Roth syndrome, is characterized by pain or dysesthesia in the anterolateral thigh caused by entrapment of the lateral femoral cutaneous nerve at the anterior superior iliac spine (see Chap. 9). Trummer and colleagues[85] reported that lumbar disk herniation could mimic meralgia paresthetica, and Kallgren and Tingle[86] noted that meralgia paresthetica could mimic lumbar radiculopathy because of the similarity of the symptoms.

▶ Irritation of the spinal nerve root by osteophytic spurs.

▶ Sacroiliac or pelvic dysfunction.

▶ Intermittent claudication of the iliac or iliofemoral arteries.

▶ Spondylolisthesis.

▶ Lateral recess stenosis.

▶ Muscle strain.

▶ Stress fracture of the lumbar/thoracic vertebra (burst and compression).

▶ Neoplasm.

▶ Isolated peripheral nerve injury or neuritis.

▶ Diabetic amyotrophy, which is relatively uncommon, can occasionally be the presenting symptom of uncontrolled diabetes mellitus.[87]

The differential diagnosis can be aided by a description of the distribution of the patient's symptoms and the results of the physical examination.

At the L1 and L2 levels, the nerves exit the intervertebral foramen above the disk. From L2 downward, the nerves leave the dura slightly more proximally than the foramen through which they pass, and at a decreasing angle of obliquity, and an increasing length within the spinal canal. The L3 nerve root travels behind the inferior aspect of the vertebral body and the L3 disk. The L4 nerve root crosses the whole vertebral body to leave the spinal canal at the upper aspect of the L4 disk at an angle of approximately 60 degrees. The L5 nerve root emerges at the inferior aspect of the fourth lumbar disk at an angle of approximately 45 degrees and crosses the fifth vertebral body to exit at the upper aspect of the L5 disk. The S1 nerve root emerges at a 30-degree angle and crosses the L5 to S1 disk.

High Lumbar Disk Lesions[88]

Although a herniated disk most commonly originates from the L4 to L5 or L5 to S1 level,[89] from 1 to 11 percent of herniated disks originate from the L1 to L2, L2 to L3, or L3 to L4 level.[90–92] Reduced motion and stress at the upper lumbar spine and the protective influence of the posterior longitudinal ligament may account for the disparity.[92]

The high lumbar radiculopathy typically does not radiate pain down the back of the leg, but instead causes an insidious onset of pain in the groin or anterior thigh that is often relieved in a flexed position and worsens with standing. The superficial cremasteric reflex is also invariably present.[93]

The differential diagnoses for upper lumbar nerve root symptoms include spondylolisthesis and an infective cause, such as diskitis or an epidural abscess.

Third Lumbar Nerve Root Compression

Compression at this level is uncommonly encountered. The clinical findings with a lesion at this level may include:

▶ Pain in the midlumbar area, upper buttock, whole anterior thigh and knee, medial knee, and just above the ankle.

▶ Dural signs of prone knee flexion and, occasionally, a positive straight leg raise (SLR).

▶ Significant motion loss of extension.

▶ Slight weakness of iliopsoas and grosser loss of quadriceps.

▶ Hypoesthesia of the medial aspect of the knee and lower leg.

▶ Absent or reduced patellar reflex.

Fourth Lumbar Nerve Root Compression

About 40 percent of IVD impairments affect this level, about an equal amount as those that affect the L5 root.[67] A disk protrusion at this level can irritate the fourth root, the fifth root, or, with a larger protrusion, both roots (Table 20-3). The clinical findings with a lesion at this level may include:

▶ Pain located in the lumbar area or iliac crest, inner buttock, outer thigh and leg, and over the foot to the great toe.

▶ Positive dural signs of SLR, bilateral and crossed SLR, and neck flexion (see Chap. 12).[94]

▶ Marked lateral deviation of the lumbar spine and gross limitation of one side flexion (both common findings).

▶ Weak dorsiflexion of the ankle.

▶ Hypoesthesia of the outer lower leg and great toe.

▶ Diminished tibialis posterior, patellar, and tibialis anterior reflexes.

Fifth Lumbar Nerve Root Compression

This level is affected as often as the fourth nerve root and frequently is compressed by the L4–5 disk as well as the L5–S1 disk (see Table 20-3). The clinical findings with a lesion at this level may include:

▶ Pain in the sacroiliac area, lower buttock, lateral thigh and leg, inner three toes, and medial sole of the foot.

▶ Positive unilateral SLR and neck flexion.[94]

▶ Lateral deviation during flexion.

▶ Weakness of peroneal, extensor hallucis, and hip abductor muscles.

▶ Hypoesthesia of outer leg and inner three toes and medial sole.

▶ Diminished peroneus longus, Achilles, and extensor hallucis reflexes.

First, Second, and Third Sacral Roots[83]

According to Cyriax, the first, second, and third sacral roots can be compressed by a fifth lumbar disk protrusion. The clinical findings with a lesion at the S1 level (see Table 20-3) may include:

▶ Pain in the low back to buttocks to sole of foot and heel.

▶ Limited SLR.

▶ Weakness of the calf muscles, peronei, and hamstrings.

▶ Atrophy of the gluteal mass (but weakness is not always detectable).

▶ Hypoesthesia in the outer two toes, outer foot, and outer leg as far as the lateral aspect of the knee.

In the second sacral root palsy, the signs are the same as for the first sacral nerve root, except that the peroneal muscles are spared and the hypoesthesia ends at the heel. With third sacral root palsy, the SLR is generally normal and no palsy is detectable. However, the patient may report pain in the groin, and pain down the inner aspect of the thigh to the knee.[74]

TABLE 20-3   Common Radicular Syndromes of the Lumbar Spine[93a]

Disk Level	Nerve Root	Motor Deficit	Sensory Deficit	Reflex Compromise
L3–4	L4	Quadriceps	Anterolateral thigh Anterior knee Medial leg and foot	Knee
L4–5	L5	Extensor hallucis longus	Lateral thigh Anterolateral leg Middorsal foot	Medial hamstrings
L5–S1	S1	Ankle plantar flexors	Posterior leg Lateral foot	Ankle

Fourth Sacral Nerve Root Compression

A lesion of this nerve root is always a concern, because a permanent palsy may lead to incontinence and impotence.[74,95] The clinical findings with a lesion at this level may include:

▶ Pain in the lower sacral, peroneal, and genital areas.

▶ Saddle area paresthesia.

▶ No positive dural signs.

▶ Possible gross limitation of all lumbar movements.

▶ Bladder, bowel, or genital dysfunction.

▶ Positive superficial anal reflex, and reduced anal wink.[93]

Vertical Prolapse (Schmorl's Node)

A Schmorl's node is the herniation of disk substance through the cartilaginous plate of the IVD into the body of the adjacent vertebra[96] (Fig. 20-5). These vertical prolapses of the disk are often asymptomatic and occur as incidental findings on radiographs. Indeed, the chronic Schmorl's node has been reported to be the most common impairment of the IVD, and of the whole spine.[97] Schmorl's nodes tend to be more common in men than women, a factor attributed to the greater spinal loads in men.[96] Theories proposed to explain the pathogenesis of Schmorl's nodes include origins that are:

▶ Developmental, in which embryonic defects such as ossification gaps, vascular channels, and notochord extrusion defects form points of weakness where Schmorl's nodes may occur.[12]

▶ Degenerative, in which the aging process produces sites of weakness in the cartilaginous endplate, resulting in formation of Schmorl's nodes.[97,98]

▶ Pathologic, where diseases weaken the IVD and/or vertebral bodies.[99,100]

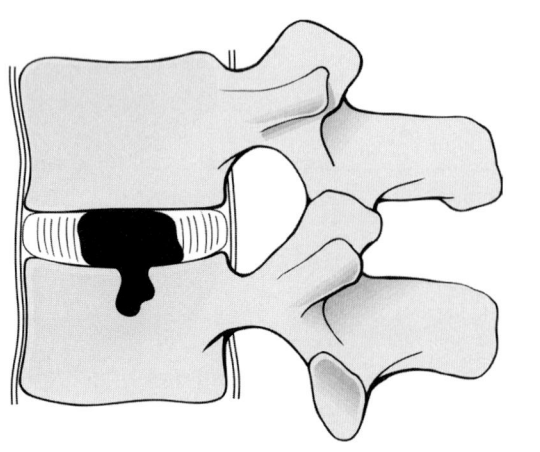

FIGURE 20-5 Lumbar degenerative disk disease and Schmorl's node. (Reproduced with permission from Dutton M. *Manual Therapy of the Spine.* New York, NY: McGraw-Hill; 2002:122.)

▶ Traumatic, in which acute and chronic trauma destroy the cartilaginous end plates, resulting in disk herniation. Although most orthopedists accept that Schmorl's nodes occur because of trauma, no studies have shown a direct causal relation between a traumatic episode and the formation of an acute Schmorl's node.

Once the Schmorl's node has occurred, subsequent proliferation of cartilage and reactive ossification may develop in the vicinity of the dislocated tissue.[101] This ossification encloses the dislocated tissue and segregates it from the spongiosa of the vertebral body. The formation of this cartilaginous cap, or calcification of the protrusion, may act to resist its expansion.[1]

Adherent Nerve Root Compression

The typical symptoms with this condition include prolonged radiculopathy with trunk or neck flexion, and protracted limitation of lower extremity motion during neurodynamic mobility testing (see Chap. 12).[102] This diagnosis should be made only after careful rejection of other more common conditions. A physical examination that reveals signs of nerve root tension (see Chap. 12) further suggests true radiculopathy.[102]

Examination

The diagnosis of a disk herniation is based largely on the history and physical examination findings and, on occasion, imaging test results. Imaging results can be misleading. Anatomic evidence of a herniated disk is found in 20 to 30 percent of imaging tests (myelography, CT, and MRI) among normal persons.[103–105] The conventional physical examination for a suspected disk herniation consists of tests for key muscle strength and lumbar range of motion, deep tendon reflex and sensory testing, and dural mobility tests such as the SLR test. It must be remembered that no single test in the physical examination has a high diagnostic accuracy alone for disk herniation.[106]

History

Various research studies have been undertaken to establish the validity of history taking for use in diagnosing a lumbar disk herniation.[103,106–108]

Clinical Pearl

Deyo and colleagues[103] reported a sensitivity for sciatic distribution of pain in the diagnosis of lumbar disk herniation of 95 percent, and calculated the likelihood of a disk herniation being present in the absence of sciatic pain as 0.1 percent. Similarly high degrees of sensitivity have been found in other studies.[106–108] Radiculopathy is such a sensitive finding (95 percent) that its absence almost rules out a clinically important disk herniation, although it is only 88 percent specific for herniation.[109] In contrast, the sensitivity of pseudoclaudication in detecting spinal stenosis is 60 percent, whereas the combination of pseudoclaudication and age greater than 50 years has a sensitivity of 90 percent (specificity, 70 percent).[109]

One study[110] showed that taking the history and MRI findings into account, elderly patients with protruded herniation were considered to be more likely to experience groin pain, with the rate of L4–5 disk involvement being higher than that of L5–S1 involvement. These results support conclusions drawn from a study by Murphey,[111] which found that groin and testicular pain are rare with L5–S1 disk disease but are fairly common with L4–5 disk disease.

In general, the presence of leg pain indicates a larger protrusion than does back pain alone.[112] Coughing, sneezing, or a Valsalva maneuver typically exacerbates the symptoms.

The patient's complaints of pain usually are related to the following factors:

▶ Whether excessive imbibition or excessive dehydration has occurred to the disk.[113] Excessive imbibition, which results from a prolonged absence from compressive forces, may place a mechanical stress on the innervated outer AF, or other posterior structures, resulting in pain and decreased mobility following recumbency. Dehydration of the disk results from the application of prolonged compressive forces, which reduces the size of the disk and allows for excessive translational segmental mobility and compression on normally unloaded segmental structures.[113] This mechanism results in increased symptoms and decreased mobility as the day progresses.

▶ Whether the nerve root is involved. An ischemic nerve root responds with an increase in symptoms if a movement increases compression to the nerve root.[113] Such movements include lumbar extension and ipsilateral side bending. This is probably why patients with nerve root involvement adopt a posture of flexion and contralateral side bending, although occasionally this posture can result in an increase in symptoms because of an increase in tension and a decrease in intraneural circulation.[113]

The ability of the disk to maintain its hydrostatic pressure is a factor of previous extrusions or sequestrations, disk surgery, and disk degeneration.[59] Theoretically, if the hydrostatic pressure is maintained following a posterolateral disk protrusion, the patient will have increased pain with flexion, flexion with contralateral rotation, or side bending.[113] These symptoms tend to be increased with repetition of those motions, but improved with motions in the opposite directions, although initially those symptoms may increase, depending on the position of the NP.[113]

Observation

Lateral Pelvic Shift. Patients with disk-related low back pain commonly present with a pelvic shift or list when acute sciatica is present. In these cases, the patient may list away from the side of the sciatica, producing a so-called sciatic scoliosis.[114] The lateral pelvic shift is perhaps the most commonly encountered. Under the McKenzie classification system (see Fig. III-8, a derangement 4 requires the presence of a relevant lateral shift deformity.[112] Determining the presence of a lateral shift deformity may help speed up the recovery from a derangement by first correcting the lateral shift deformity.[112] The direction of the list, although still controversial, is believed to result from the relative position of the disk herniation to the spinal nerve (Fig. 20-6). Theoretically, when the disk herniation is lateral to the nerve root, the patient may deviate the back away from the side of the irritated nerve, which has the effect of drawing the nerve root away from the disk fragment (Fig. 20-6). This movement is demonstrated dramatically in patients with extreme lateral disk herniations, whose efforts at side-bending to the side of the herniation markedly exaggerate the pain and paresthesia.[115] When the herniation is medial to the nerve root, the patient may list toward the side of the lesion in an effort to decompress the nerve root[116] (Fig. 20-6). It is also theorized that this is a protective position resulting from:

▶ Irritation of a zygapophysial joint.

▶ Irritation of a spinal nerve or its dural sleeve, caused by disk herniation[57] and the resulting muscle spasm.[117]

FIGURE 20-6 Nerve root compression by medial or lateral disk protrusion. (Reproduced with permission from Cipriano JJ. *Photographic Manual of Regional Orthopaedic and Neurological Tests.* 3rd ed. Baltimore, Md: Williams and Wilkins:219.)

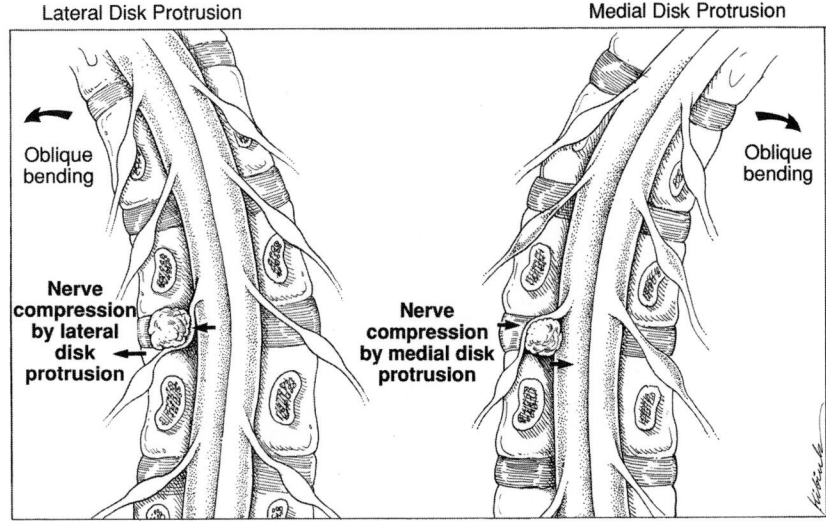

Lateral Disk Protrusion

Medial Disk Protrusion

Oblique bending

Oblique bending

Nerve compression by lateral disk protrusion

Nerve compression by medial disk protrusion

▶ Spasm of the quadratus lumborum muscle and, occasionally, the iliacus muscle.

▶ The size of the disk protrusion. In a prospective study of 45 patients with sciatic scoliotic list (Cobb's angle > 4 degrees), Suk and colleagues[115] found that the direction of sciatic scoliosis was not observed during surgery to be associated with the location of nerve root compression, but rather it was related to the side of disk herniation. Porter and Miller[118] analyzed the mechanism of sciatic scoliosis and concluded that the herniated disk was thought to be reduced in size by stretching or inward bulging at the convex side of the scoliosis, and called this phenomenon autonomic decompression.[118]

The clinician must first determine the presence of the shift, and then determine its relevance to the presenting symptoms. To determine its relevance, a side-glide test sequence can be used. The side-glide test sequence is performed by manually correcting the shift by pushing the pelvis into its correct position[112] (Fig. 20-7). If the side-glide produces either a centralization or peripheralization of the patient's symptoms, the test is considered positive for a relevant lateral shift.[119] In addition, for a lateral shift to be significant, the patient must exhibit an inability to self-correct past midline when asked to shift in the direction opposite the shift.[120]

The relevant lateral shift must be corrected, using side-glides, before the patient attempts the McKenzie extension exercises.[121] A lateral shift that is not deemed to be relevant or to be a deformity, per McKenzie's criteria, may be treated with only sagittal plane movements (e.g., extension principles).[112]

Riddle and Rothstein found that therapists agreed 60 percent of the time on the presence and direction of the lateral shift. A κ value of 0.26 was determined, indicating poor reliability.[122]

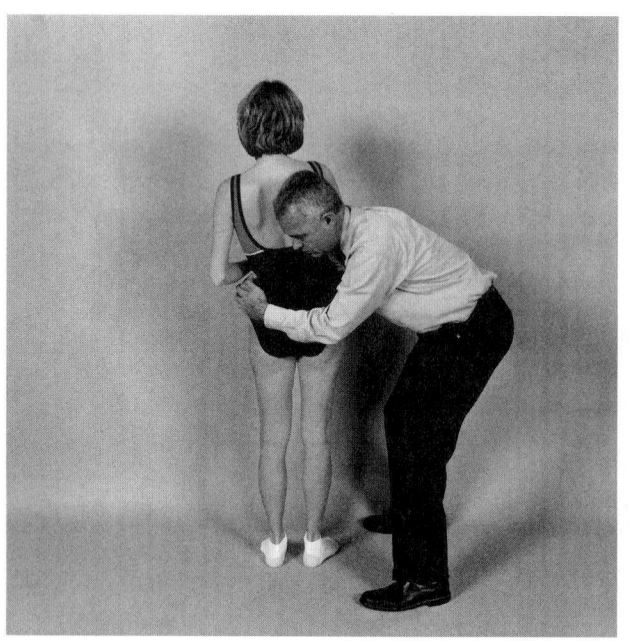

FIGURE 20-7   Manual shift correction.

A similar study by Donahue and colleagues of 49 patients with low back pain examined the amount of inter-tester agreement when assessing only the lateral shift. The amount of agreement was found to be 47 percent, statistically similar to that obtained by pure chance.[120]

Gait Analysis

Gait analysis (see Chap. 13) can provide quantitative information regarding the dynamic function of specific muscle groups. In kinetic analysis of gait, the external moments acting on the joints are calculated from force and motion measurements and body segment parameters.[123]

> **Clinical Pearl**
>
> Weakness of the gastrocnemius is a clinical sign associated with involvement of the L5–S1 disk (neurologic level S1), whereas weakness of the extensor hallucis longus is a positive sign for involvement of the L4–5 disk (neurologic L5).

Muscle weakness and reduced walking capacity are among several functional deficits associated with a lumbar herniated nucleus pulposus.[94,123]

Active Range of Motion

Trunk deviation during flexion is believed to be associated with a disk herniation, with the direction of the deviation determined by the relative position of the compression on the nerve. How the disk responds to movements depends on the activity. For example, walking appears to move the NP into a more central location, whereas prolonged sitting appears to displace the disk into a less advantageous position.[113]

Neurodynamic Mobility

The neurodynamic mobility tests to help confirm a lumbar disk herniation include SLR, bilateral SLR, crossed SLR sign, slump test, prone knee bend (femoral nerve stretch), and bowstring tests, which are described in Chapter 12.

The lower the angle of a positive SLR test, the more specific the test becomes and the larger the disk protrusion found at surgery.[103,124] A limited SLR at 60 degrees is moderately sensitive for herniated lumbar disks but nonspecific, because limitation often is observed in the absence of disk herniations.[103,125,126] Crossed SLR is less sensitive but highly specific.[125–127] Thus, the crossed SLR test suggests concordance with the diagnosis, whereas ipsilateral SLR is more effective in ruling out the diagnosis.

The femoral nerve stretch test (see Chap. 12) is probably the single best screening test to evaluate for a high lumbar radiculopathy. This test has been shown to be positive in 84 to 95 percent of patients with high lumbar disks,[31,89,128] although the test may be falsely positive in the presence of a tight iliopsoas or rectus femoris or any pathology in or about the hip joint, sacroiliac joint, and lumbar spine.

The remainder of the examination of the lumbar spine, including the key muscle tests for the myotomes and reflex testing, is described in Chapter 25. Sensation testing (light touch and pinprick) is outlined in Chapter 2.

Intervention

The natural history of radiculopathy and disk herniation is not quite as favorable as for simple low back pain, but it is still excellent, with approximately 50 percent of patients recovering in the first 2 weeks, and 70 percent recovering in 6 weeks.[129] Prognostic factors for positive outcome with conservative intervention for lumbar disk herniation are depicted in Table 20-4.

> ### Clinical Pearl
>
> Intervention focuses on a return to normal activities as soon as possible, patient education and involvement, and therapeutic exercises.

The McKenzie program (see Section III Introduction to Spine and Pelvis and Chap. 25) can be valuable to the overall intervention strategy and, if centralization of pain occurs, a good response to physical therapy can be anticipated.[130,131] The McKenzie method involves a comprehensive examination of the patient, performed in the neutral, flexed, and extended positions of the spine, for the presence of the centralization phenomenon. The same maneuvers are repeated with the trunk in the neutral position, shifted toward the side of pathology, and away from pathology. The goal is to decrease radiating symptoms into the limb and, thus, to centralize the pain. Once this centralizing position is identified, the patient is instructed to perform these maneuvers repetitively throughout the day.[78]

In addition, the patient is instructed in a spinal stabilization program in which neutral zone mechanics are practiced in various positions to decrease stress to the lumbosacral spine. The lumbar stabilization exercise progression is described in Chapter 25.

The intervention program is only as good as the concomitant home exercise program, and the clinician must continually monitor the home exercise program, evaluating the patient's knowledge of the exercises and upgrading the program when appropriate.

TABLE 20-4 Prognostic Factors of Positive Outcome with Conservative Intervention for Lumbar Disk Herniation[67]

Outcome	Factor
Favorable	Absence of crossed SLR
	Spinal motion in extension that does not reproduce leg pain
	Relief or >50% reduction in leg pain within first 6 wk of onset
	Limited psychosocial issues
	Self employed
	Educational level >12 yr
	Absence of spinal stenosis
	Progressive return of neurologic deficit within first 12 wk
Unfavorable	Positive crossed SLR
	Leg pain produced with spinal extension
	Lack of >50% reduction in leg pain within first 6 wk of onset
	Overbearing psychosocial issues
	Worker's compensation
	Educational level <12 yr
	Concommitant spinal stenosis
	Progressive neurologic deficit
	Cauda equina syndrome
Neutral	Degree of SLR
	Response to bed rest
	Response to passive care
	Gender
	Age
Questionable	Actual size of lumbar disk herniation
	Canal position of lumbar disk herniation
	Spinal level of lumbar disk herniation
	Lumbar disk herniation material

SLR, straight leg raising.

Cervical Disks

The morphology and biochemistry of the IVD have been studied extensively. However, when considering cervical IVD, it is clear that the pathology affecting the cervical IVD is different from that affecting the lumbar disk.

Differences in the Cervical Disk

In the cervical spine, there are five disks, with the first disk located between C2 and C3. The cervical disks are named after the vertebra above (the C4 disk lies between C4 and C5) (Fig. 20-8).

The IVD height-to-body height ratio (2:5) is greatest in the cervical spine, and the IVDs make up approximately 25 percent of the superior-to-inferior height of the cervical spine.[132] This increase in height ratio allows for the greatest possible range of motion.

The inferior surface of the cervical IVD is concave, and the inferior-anterior surface of the centrum projects downward to partly cover the anterior aspect.

> **Clinical Pearl**
>
> The cervical IVD, and its development, is distinctly different from that of the lumbar disk.

The cervical NP at birth constitutes no more than 25 percent of the entire disk, not 50 percent as in lumbar disks.[133] The NP sits in, or near, the center of the disk, lying slightly more posteriorly than anteriorly.

A number of features distinguish the cervical disk from the lumbar disk[134]:

▶ Anteriorly, the cervical AF consists of interwoven alar fibers, whereas posteriorly, the AF lacks any oblique fibers and consists exclusively of vertically orientated fibers.

▶ Essentially, the cervical AF has the structure of a dense anterior interosseous ligament with few fibers to contain the NP posteriorly.

▶ In no region of the cervical AF do successive lamellae exhibit alternating orientations. In fact, only in the anterior portion of the AF—where obliquely orientated fibers, upward and medially, interweave with one another—does a cruciate pattern occur.

▶ Posterolaterally, the NP is contained only by the alar fibers of the posterior longitudinal ligament, under or through which the nuclear material must pass if it is to herniate. Further protection against disk herniation is afforded by the uncovertebral joints, which reinforce the posterolateral aspect of the IVD.

▶ The absence of an AF over the uncovertebral region. In this region, collagen fibers are torn during the first 7 to 15 years of life, leaving clefts that progressively extend across the

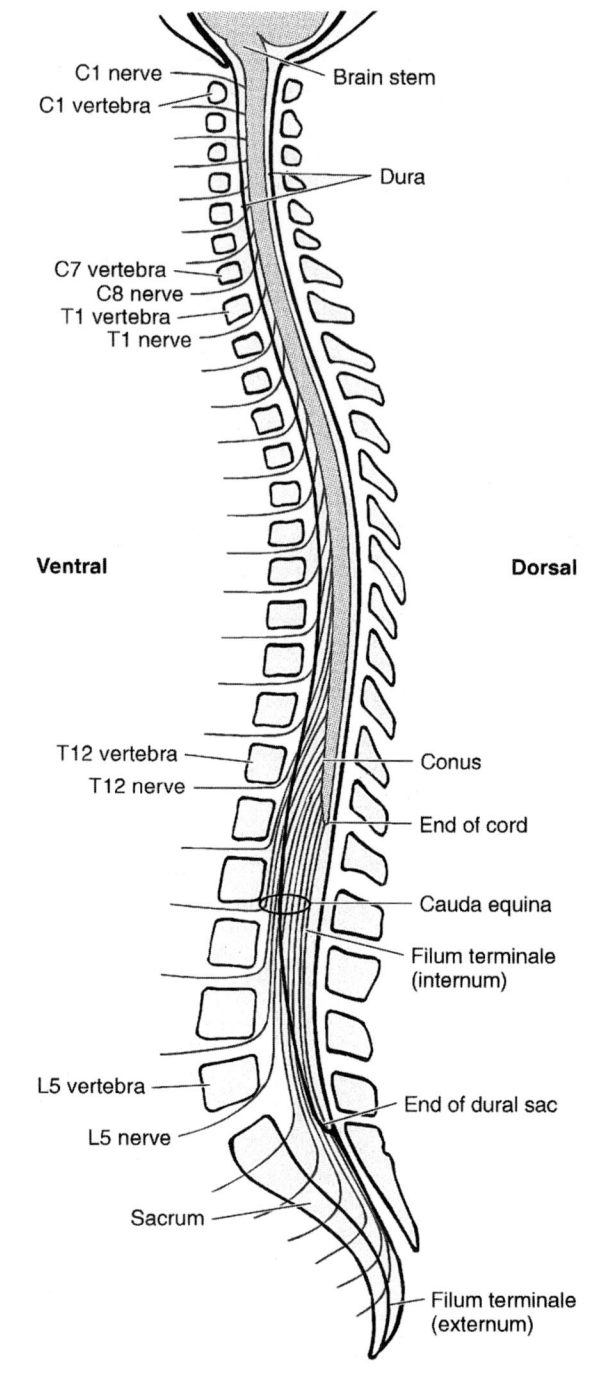

FIGURE 20-8 Schematic illustration of the relationships between the spinal nerve roots and the vertebrae. (Reproduced with permission from Dutton M. *Manual Therapy of the Spine.* New York, NY: McGraw-Hill; 2002:120.)

back of the disk. Rather than an incidental age change, this disruption has been interpreted either as enabling[135] or resulting from[136] rotatory movements of the cervical vertebrae (see next section).

▶ Axial rotation of a typical cervical vertebra occurs around an oblique axis perpendicular to the plane of its facets.[136]

As in the lumbar spine, the cervical IVD functions as a closed but dynamic system, distributing the changes in pressure equally to all components of the container (i.e., the end plates and the AF) and across the surface of the vertebral body. It has been observed that in the first and second decades of life, before complete ossification occurs, lateral tears occur in the annulus fibrosus, most probably induced by motion of the cervical spine in the bipedal posture.[137] The tears in the lateral part of the disk tend to enlarge toward the medial aspect of the IVD. The development of such tears through both sides may result in a complete transverse splitting of the disk. Such a process can be observed in the second and third decades of life in the lower cervical spine when the IVD is split in the middle into equal halves.[137] With this aging process, the NP rapidly undergoes fibrosis such that, by the third decade, there is barely any nuclear material distinguishable.[138]

These age-related changes are evident chemically and morphologically and are much more evident in the NP than in the AF. Degenerative disk disease in this region results in diminished disk height, subjecting the bony elements to increased load.[132] The splitting of the IVD in the second and third decades of life may result in segmental instability.[137] Also, such splitting of the IVD can allow the NP to move toward the spinal canal, ultimately causing disk protrusion or extrusion and resulting in spinal cord compression (myelopathy; see later discussion).[137]

Almost everyone older than 40 years of age has evidence of cervical disk degeneration.[139] According to Töndury and Theiler,[140] in the fourth and fifth decades of life, the NP usually dries out. This development can be visualized on conventional radiographs as flattening of the uncovertebral processes and narrowing of the IVD space.[141] This process may lead to a loss of elasticity and increased stresses on the vertebral end plates.

The nerve root is divided into the ventral and dorsal roots, which are responsible for motor and sensory function, respectively. Ebraheim and colleagues[141a] described the quantitative anatomy of the cervical nerve root groove and divided it into three zones: medial zone (pedicle), middle zone (vertebral artery foramen), and lateral zone. The medial zone of the cervical nerve root groove corresponds to the intervertebral foramen, and this zone is believed to play an important role in the etiology of cervical radiculopathy.[141b] The intervertebral foramen, which can be further divided into an entrance zone (medial) and exit zone (lateral), resembles a funnel in shape. The entrance zone corresponds to the narrow part of the funnel and the shape of the radicular sheath is conical, with its takeoff points from the central dural sac being the largest part.[141b] Consequently, nerve root compression occurs mostly in the entrance zone of the intervertebral foramina. Whether compression of the ventral roots, dorsal roots, or both occurs depends on various anatomic structures around the nerve roots. Anteriorly, compression of the nerve roots is likely caused by protruding disks and osteophytes of the uncovertebral region, whereas the superior articular process, the ligamentum flavum, and the periradicular fibrous tissues often affect the nerve posteriorly.[142–145] Osteophytes may develop in response to this increased stress and

from degenerative changes of the zygapophysial and uncovertebral joints. The osteophytes effectively increase the available surface area and decrease the overall force on the end plates.[146] Radicular arteries within the dural root sleeves may become compressed by osteophytes, leading to spasm and decreased vascular perfusion.[146] In addition, venous obstruction may occur, resulting in edema and additional reduction in nerve root perfusion.[146]

Cervical Disk Lesions

The cervical spine is vulnerable to the same impairments as those of the lumbar spine, and any weakness in the surrounding structures results in either a disk bulge or rupture. Considering the structure of the cervical AF, the possibilities that emerge for mechanisms of diskogenic pain are strain or tears of the anterior AF, particularly after hyperextension trauma, and strain of the alar portions of the posterior longitudinal ligament when stretched by a bulging disk.[134]

Analysis of the anatomic proportions of the cervical spine indicates that cervical diskogenic disease can have an impact on neural structures in the bony spinal canal. The available space occupied by the spinal cord and nerve roots is determined primarily by the diameter of the bony spinal canal. The anteroposterior diameter of the cervical spinal canal tends to be narrower in patients with herniation, resulting in myelopathy.[147–149] That is, patients with wide canals might be nonmyelopathic even with the same degree of herniation. Abnormalities in the osseous and the fibroelastic boundaries of the bony cervical spinal canal affect the availability of space for spinal cord and nerve roots, resulting in a stenosis. Although this stenosis often remains asymptomatic for a long time, it can become a major influence in the production of radiculomyelopathic compressive disturbances when other conditions, such as spondylosis, discal hernia, and trauma, become superimposed. One study[150] concluded that the relation between the sagittal diameter of the bony spinal canal and the sagittal diameter of the hernia determines the severity of neurologic symptoms after soft cervical disk herniation. As the resulting space for neural structures becomes smaller, the risk of developing motor or sensory disturbances increases. The "developmental sagittal diameter" of the bony cervical spinal canal is, therefore, a reliable parameter for estimating the risk of developing medullary or radicular compression by an intraspinal space-occupying process.[148,151]

In the lumbar disk, a prolapse is common. In the cervical spine, a straightforward prolapse is uncommon, and a cervical disk herniation should not be considered as a miniature version of lumbar disk herniation. It is, unlike lumbar disk herniation, extremely rare before the age of 30, with the age range of peak incidence between 45 and 54 years, and only slightly less common in the 35 to 44-year old group.[152] Acute disk herniations may result in compression of nerve roots. Cervical disks may become painful as part of the degenerative cascade, from repetitive microtrauma, or from an excessive single load. The indication that degeneration plays a greater role in cervical disk herniation may explain why cervical disk herniation is extremely rare in those younger than 30 years of age and why the mean age is around 50 years.[153,154]

The most common level of cervical nerve root involvement has been reported at the seventh (C7, 60 percent) and sixth (C6, 25 percent) disks,[145,155] followed by C4–5 disk (Table 20-5).[153,154,156] In a study of 18 cadavers by Tanaka and colleagues,[142] the C5 nerve roots were found to exit over the middle aspect of the IVD, whereas the C6 and C7 nerve roots were found to traverse the proximal part of the disk. The C8 nerve roots had little overlap with the C7–T1 disk in the intervertebral foramen. The C6 and C7 rootlets passed two disk levels in the dural sac. Also, a high incidence of the intradural connections between the dorsal rootlets of C5, C6, and C7 segments was found.[142] These intradural connections between dorsal nerve roots and the relation between the course of the nerve root and the IVD may explain the clinical variation of symptoms resulting from nerve root compression in the cervical spine.[142]

Cervical IVDs with herniation usually remain normal in height, or change only slightly without abnormality in the uncovertebral joints.[153] Sclerosis and formation of osteophytes in the uncovertebral joints accompany narrowed disks in spondylosis. These facts indicate that the uncovertebral joints bear a part of the axial load to the IVD in the cervical spine. Accordingly, disk degeneration may play a more important role than trauma in the production of herniation in the cervical spine, and it is common for a patient to awake with a cervical disk herniation, misinterpreting it as a "crick" in the neck.

Clinical Pearl

Asymptomatic cervical disk herniation is often found in MRI for other diseases.[145] Boden and colleagues[139] reported the incidence of cervical disk protrusions in the asymptomatic population to be 10 to 15 percent, depending on age.

Other factors associated with increased risk include heavy manual labor requiring lifting of more than 25 lb, smoking, and driving or operating vibrating equipment.[157]

Cervical disk degeneration occurs in a predictable fashion. The NP and AF form small cysts[69,158] and fissures as the first disruptive changes after the death of chondrocytes and the separation of fibers or fiber bundles. Subsequently, they extend and unite to form horizontal and vertical clefts.[153] Shearing stress to the disk by translational motion may lead to fibrillation of the matrix as in osteoarthritic joint cartilage. Some of the vertical clefts extend to the cartilaginous end plate, and portions of the cartilaginous end plate may be torn off.

The cervical IVD is innervated by the sinuvertebral nerve, formed by branches from the ventral nerve root and the sympathetic plexus.[158a] Once formed, the nerve turns back into the intervertebral foramen along the posterior aspect of the disk, supplying portions of the annulus, posterior longitudinal ligament, periosteum of the vertebral body and pedicle, and adjacent epidural veins. As in the lumbar spine, the pain associated with cervical disk lesions probably occurs from an inflammatory process initiated by nerve root compression, resulting in nerve root swelling.

Within the compressed nerve root, intrinsic blood vessels show increased permeability, which secondarily results in edema of the nerve root.[158b] Chronic edema and fibrosis within the nerve root can alter the response threshold and increase the sensitivity of the nerve root to pain.[158c] Neurogenic chemical mediators of pain released from the cell bodies of the sensory neurons and non-neurogenic mediators released from disk tissue may play a role in initiating and perpetuating this inflammatory response.[158d] The dorsal root ganglion has been implicated in the pathogenesis of radicular pain. Prolonged discharges originate from the cell bodies of the dorsal root ganglion as a result of brief pressure.[158b] In addition to the chemicals produced by the cell bodies of the dorsal root ganglion, the

---

TABLE 20-5   Common Radicular Syndromes of the Cervical Spine[93a]

Disk Level	Nerve Root	Motor Deficit	Sensory Deficit	Reflex Compromise
C4–5	C5	Deltoid Biceps	Anterolateral shoulder and arm	Biceps
C5–6	C6	Wrist extensors Biceps	Lateral forearm and hand Thumb	Brachoradialis Pronator Teres
C6–7	C7	Wrist flexors Triceps Finger extensors	Middle finger	Triceps
C7–T1	C8	Finger flexors Hand intrinsics	Medial forearm and hand, ring and little fingers	None
T1–T2	T1	Hand intrinsics	Medial forearm	None

membrane surrounding the dorsal root ganglion is more permeable than that around the nerve root, allowing a more florid local inflammatory response.[158b] The blood supply to the nerve root usually is not compromised by an acute herniation, unless the compression is severe.[146,159] A study involving patients under local anesthesia found that compression of the cervical nerve root produced limb pain, whereas pressure on the disk produced pain in the neck and the medial border of the scapula.[136,160] Intradiskal injection and electrical stimulation of the disk also has suggested that neck pain is referred by a damaged outer AF.[160,161] Muscle spasms of the neck also have been found after electrical stimulation of the disk.

The capacity of the disk to self-repair is limited by the fact that only the peripheral aspects of the AF receive blood, and a small amount at that.

Examination

History

It is important to obtain a detailed history to establish a diagnosis of a cervical radiculopathy and to rule out other causes, such as thoracic outlet syndrome and brachial neuritis. The clinician should first determine the main complaint (i.e., head or neck pain, numbness, weakness, decreased neck function) and location of symptoms.[135,162] Anatomic pain drawings can be helpful by supplying the clinician with a quick review of the pain pattern.

> ### Clinical Pearl
>
> Patients with a cervical disk herniation are often younger whereas patients with radicular symptoms due to cervical disk degeneration are often middle-aged.

The patient usually reports a history of neck pain before the onset of arm pain. The onset of neck and arm discomfort with cervical disk herniation is usually insidious and can range from a dull ache to severe burning pain.[135,162] The symptoms may be referred to the medial scapula initially and then along the upper or lower arm and into the hand, depending on the nerve root that is involved.[135,162] Patients with a cervical disk lesion typically have severe neck and arm pain that prevents them from getting into a comfortable position.[158b] The symptoms are usually aggravated by extension or rotation of the head to the side of the pain (the Spurling maneuver). Aggravation of the symptoms by neck extension often helps to differentiate a radicular etiology from muscular neck pain or a pathologic condition of the shoulder with secondary muscle pain in the neck.[158b] Henderson and colleagues reviewed the clinical presentations of cervical radiculopathy in 736 patients[163a]: 99.4 percent had arm pain, 85.2 percent had sensory deficits, 79.7 percent had neck pain, 71.2 percent had reflex deficits, 68 percent had motor deficits, 52.5 percent had scapular pain, 17.8 percent had anterior chest pain, 9.7 percent had headaches, 5.9 percent had anterior chest and arm pain, and 1.3 percent had left-sided chest and arm pain (cervical angina). Neurologic deficits corresponded

with the offending disk level in approximately 80 percent of patients.[158b]

C2 to C3 disk herniations are rare,[163b] in either traumatic or spontaneous etiology, and affected only 8 of 2786 patients (0.28 percent) of the surgical cervical spondylotic cases over 10 years in one study.[163c] These herniations are difficult to identify on clinical examination, because these patients usually have no specific motor weakness and reflex abnormality. Radiculopathy of the third cervical nerve root results from pathologic changes in the disk between the second and third cervical levels and is unusual. The posterior ramus of the third cervical nerve innervates the suboccipital region, and involvement of that nerve causes pain in this region, often extending to the back of the ear.

Radiculopathy of the fourth cervical nerve root may be an unexplained cause of neck and shoulder pain.[158b] Numbness extending from the caudad aspect of the neck to the superior aspect of the shoulder may be present. Difficulty with breathing during exercise may be reported in diaphragmatic involvement (C3–5).

Radiculopathy of the fifth cervical nerve root can present with numbness in an "epaulet" distribution, beginning at the superior aspect of the shoulder and extending laterally to the mid-part of the arm.[158b] The absence of pain with a range of motion of the shoulder and the absence of impingement signs at the shoulder help to differentiate radiculopathy of the fifth cervical nerve root from a pathologic shoulder condition.[158b]

Radiculopathy of the sixth cervical nerve root presents with pain radiating from the neck to the lateral aspect of the biceps, down the lateral aspect of the forearm, to the dorsal aspect of the web space between the thumb and index finger, and into the tips of those digits.[158b] Numbness occurs in the same distribution.

The seventh cervical nerve root is the most frequently involved by cervical radiculopathy. The patient has pain radiating along the back of the shoulder, often extending into the scapular region, down along the triceps, and then along the dorsum of the forearm and into the dorsum of the long finger.[158b] The patient usually pronates the forearm while trying to describe the location of the symptoms, and this is a useful observation in differentiating the hand symptoms from those of sixth cervical radiculopathy and carpal tunnel syndrome.[158b]

Radiculopathy of the eighth cervical nerve root usually presents with symptoms extending down the medial aspect of the arm and forearm and into the medial border of the hand and the ulnar two digits.[158b] Numbness usually involves the dorsal and volar aspects of the ulnar two digits and hand and may extend up the medial aspect of the forearm. The patient reports difficulty with using the hands for routine daily activities.[158b]

Patients also can present with radicular symptoms that result from other pathologies. These can include schwannomas, meningiomas, and benign or malignant vertebral body tumors.[158b] A Pancoast tumor of the apical lung can involve the caudad cervical nerve roots and, additionally, the sympathetic chain.[158b] Idiopathic brachial plexus neuritis is thought to be viral in nature and presents with severe arm pain that resolves and leaves behind polyradicular motor deficits. Polyradicular involvement also may be seen with epidural abscesses.[158b]

In middle-aged and older patients, the symptoms are often the result of degenerative changes and compression of the neural structures by osteophytes rather than disk herniation. Prior episodes of similar symptoms or localized neck pain are important for diagnosis and ultimate intervention. The older patient may have had previous episodes of neck pain, or give a history of having arthritis of the cervical spine. Leg symptoms associated with neck dysfunction, especially in the elderly, should arouse the suspicion of cervical spondylotic myelopathy.[149]

Mechanism

The position of the head and neck at the time of injury also should be noted. Acute disk herniations and sudden narrowing of the neural foramen may occur from injuries involving cervical extension, side bending, or rotation and axial loading.[164,165]

The clinician should be aware that upper trunk brachial plexus disorders can be confused with a C5 or C6 radiculopathy. This condition, often referred to as a *burner*, or *stinger*, is thought to result from either traction or compressive forces to the brachial plexus or cervical nerve roots.[166,167] At times, electrodiagnostic studies and MRI are needed to establish the diagnosis.

Peripheral nerve entrapment within the upper limb, including entrapment or compression of suprascapular, median, and ulnar nerves, also may be confused with a cervical radiculopathy[135,162]:

▶ A suprascapular neuropathy can be confused with a C5 or C6 radiculopathy, but would spare the deltoid and biceps muscles.

▶ C6 and C7 radiculopathies are most likely to be confused with median neuropathies.

▶ C8 radiculopathy must be differentiated from ulnar neuropathies and thoracic outlet syndrome.

It is important to differentiate eighth cervical radiculopathy from ulnar nerve weakness. The function of the flexor digitorum profundus in the index and long fingers and of the flexor pollicis longus in the thumb can be affected by eighth cervical radiculopathy, but they are not affected by ulnar nerve entrapment.[158b] With the exception of the adductor pollicis, the short thenar muscles are spared with ulnar nerve involvement but involved with eighth cervical or first thoracic radiculopathy.[158b] Entrapment of the anterior interosseus nerve may masquerade as eighth cervical or first thoracic radiculopathy, but it does not cause the sensory changes or have thenar muscle involvement.[158b]

Observation

The head and neck positions or motions that increase or decrease the symptoms can be used by the clinician both to help in the diagnosis and to plan the intervention. Typically, the patient with cervical radiculopathy has a head list away from the side of injury and holds the neck stiffly. These patients complain of increased posterior neck pain with neck positions that cause foraminal narrowing: extension, side bending, or rotation toward the symptomatic side.

Active Range of Motion

Active range of motion is usually reduced in the direction of pain, which is usually extension, rotation, and side bending, either toward or away from the affected nerve root. Side bending away from the affected side can cause increased displacement of a disk herniation upon a nerve root, whereas same-side bending induces pain by an impingement of a nerve root at the site of the neural foramen.[164,165]

Anterior neck pain along the sternocleidomastoid muscle belly that is aggravated by rotation to the contralateral side is most often a result of muscular strain.[158b] Pain in the posterior neck muscles that is worsened by flexion of the head suggests a myofascial etiology.[158b] Patients who present with severe pain in the suboccipital region often have pathologic changes in the upper cervical spine.[158b] The pain in these patients may radiate to the back of the ear or the lower neck. Rotation of the neck is often markedly restricted.

Palpation

On palpation, a nonspecific finding is tenderness noted along the cervical paraspinals, along the ipsilateral side of the affected nerve root, and over the upper trapezius. There may also be muscle tenderness along muscles where the symptoms are referred (e.g., medical scapula, proximal arm, and lateral epicondyle), as well as associated hypertonicity or spasm in these painful muscles.

Neurologic Testing

Manual muscle testing determines a nerve root level on physical examination and can detect subtle weakness in a myotomal, or key muscle, distribution. Weakness of shoulder abduction suggests C5 pathology, elbow flexion and wrist extension weakness suggests a C6 radiculopathy, weakness of elbow extension and wrist flexion can occur with a C7 radiculopathy, and weakness of thumb extension and ulnar deviation of the wrist is seen in C8 radiculopathies.[160] Descriptions of these muscle tests are provided in Chapter 23.

On sensory examination, a dermatomal pattern of diminished, or loss of, sensation should be present. In addition, patients with radiculitis may have hyperesthesia to light touch and pinprick examination.[160] The sensory examination can be quite subjective, however, in as much as it requires patient response.

Deep tendon reflexes are helpful (see Table 20-5). Any grade of reflex can be normal,[168] so the asymmetry of the reflexes is most helpful:

▶ The biceps brachii reflex occurs at the level of C5 to C6. The brachioradialis is another C5 to C6 reflex.

▶ The triceps reflex tests the C7 to C8 nerve roots.

▶ The pronator reflex can be helpful in differentiating C6 and C7 nerve root problems. If it is abnormal in conjunction with an abnormal triceps reflex, then the level of involvement is more likely to be C7. This reflex is performed by tapping the volar aspect of the forearm, with the forearm in a neutral position and the elbow flexed.[168,169]

Special Tests

Spurling's Test. Provocative tests for cervical radiculopathy include the foraminal compression test or Spurling's test.[170] This test is performed by asking the patient to rotate the head to the uninvolved side and then the involved side. The clinician then carefully applies a downward pressure on the head with the head in neutral. The test is considered positive if pain radiates into the limb ipsilateral to the side at which the head is rotated.[171] Neck pain with no radiation into the shoulder or arm does not constitute a positive test. Conditions such as stenosis, cervical spondylosis, osteophytes, or disk herniation are implicated with a positive test. Spurling's test has been found to be very specific (93 percent), but not sensitive (30 percent), in diagnosing acute radiculopathy.[172] Therefore, the original test is not useful as a screening test, but it is clinically useful in helping to confirm a cervical radiculopathy.

Modifications to this test have been advocated, which divide the test into three stages, each of which is more provocative.[173] If symptoms are reproduced, the clinician does not progress to the next stage. The first stage involves applying compression to the head in neutral. The second stage involves compression with the head in extension. The final stage involves compression with the head in extension and rotation to the uninvolved side, and then to the involved side.

Manual Distraction. Gentle manual cervical distraction can also be used with the patient supine as a physical examination test. A positive response is indicated by a reduction of neck or limb symptoms.

Neurodynamic Mobility Tests. Upper limb tension testing (see Chap. 12) may serve a useful role in differentiating between the involvement of neural and non-neural structures.[132]

Bakody's Sign. This test[174,175] is used to test for the presence of radicular symptoms, especially those involving the C4 or C5 nerve roots. The patient is positioned sitting or supine and is asked to elevate the arm through abduction, so that the hand or forearm rests on top of the head. If this position relieves or decreases the patient's symptoms, a cervical extradural compression problem, such as a herniated disk, or nerve root compression should be suspected. The specific segmental level can be determined by the dermatome distribution of the symptoms. If the symptoms are increased with this maneuver, the implication is that pressure is increasing in the interscalene triangle.[175]

Intervention

Little is known about the natural history of cervical radiculopathy, and there are few controlled randomized studies comparing operative with conservative intervention, although the outcome data support the concept that an extruded disk actually may have a more favorable prognosis than contained disk pathology.[176,177]

Conservative intervention consists of modified rest, a cervical collar, oral corticosteroid "dose-packs," and NSAIDs.[178,179] Oral corticosteroids have been used to reduce the associated inflammation from compression, although there is no controlled study to support their use in the intervention of cervical radiculopathy.[164,176] The beneficial effect of corticosteroids may occur as a result of the anti-inflammatory properties of these drugs. Cervical epidural corticosteroids have also been used in patients who have not responded to medications, traction, and a well-designed physical therapy program.

Exercise programs for patients with disk herniations are individualized.[162] Cervical and cervicothoracic stabilization exercises form the cornerstone of the therapeutic exercise progression (see Chap. 23). Most patients obtain analgesia using the controlled use of cervical retraction or posterior gliding of the lower cervical spine in combination with extension of the lower cervical spine and flexion of the upper cervical spine (chin tuck),[180] although repetitive use of this exercise has the potential to cause harm and should be used only as long as the patient is achieving benefit.

Surgical Intervention. Surgical intervention is reserved for patients with persistent radicular pain who do not respond to conservative measures (see later discussion).[181] In general, the decision to proceed with surgical intervention is made when a patient has significant extremity or myotomal weakness, severe pain, or pain that persists beyond an arbitrary "conservative" intervention period of 2 to 8 weeks.[182]

Thoracic Disks

Thoracic disks have been poorly researched. They are narrower and flatter than those in the cervical and lumbar spine, and contribute approximately one sixth of the length of the thoracic column.[183] Disk size in the thoracic region gradually increases from superior to inferior. The disk height-to-body height ratio is 1:5, compared with 2:5 in the cervical spine and 1:3 in the lumbar spine,[184,185] making it the smallest ratio in the spine and affording the least amount of motion.[186] Motion within the IVD is further restricted by the orientation of the lamella of the AF[53] and the relatively small NP, which is more centrally located within the AF and has a lower capacity to swell.[187] The roughly circular cross-section of the thoracic disk allows the force of torsion to be evenly distributed around its circumference, making it better able to withstand these kinds of forces.[1]

In the thoracic spine, the segmental nerve roots are situated mainly behind the inferoposterior aspect of the upper vertebral body rather than behind the disk, which reduces the possibility of root compression in impairments of the thoracic disk.[188] In a review of 280 patients, Arce and Dohrmann[189] found that thoracic disk herniation constitutes 0.25 to 0.75 percent of all disk herniations in the spine. Because the intervertebral foramina are quite large at these levels, osseous contact with the nerve roots is seldom encountered in the thoracic spine,[188] and because the dermatomes in this region have a fair amount of overlap, they cannot be relied on to determine the specific nerve root involved.

In contrast to the cervical and lumbar regions, where the spinal canal is triangular or oval in cross-section and offers a large lateral excursion to the nerve roots, the midthoracic spinal canal is small and circular, becoming triangular at the upper and lower levels. At the levels of T4 through T9, the canal is at its narrowest.[188] The spinal canal also is restricted in its size by the pedicles, remaining within the confines of the vertebrae, and not diverging as it does in the cervical spine. This would tend to predispose the spinal cord to compression more than in the cervical spine, were it not for the smaller cord size and more oval shape of the thoracic canal. Despite this, central disk protrusions are more common in the thoracic region than in other regions of the spine, and because the NP is small in the thorax, protrusions are invariably of the annular type, and nuclear protrusions are rare.[188] Complicating matters is the fact that this is an area of poor vascular supply, receiving its blood from only one radicular artery. This physiology renders the thoracic spinal cord extremely vulnerable to damage by extra-dural masses or by an overzealous manipulation.

Thoracic Disk Lesions

Herniated disks have been found at every level of the thoracic spine, although they are more common in the lower thoracic spine.[190,191]

As at the cervical and lumbar levels, the thoracic spinal nerves emerge from the cord as a large ventral and a smaller dorsal ramus, which unite to form a short spinal nerve root. There are no plexuses in this area, and the spinal nerves form the intercostal nerves.[192] The intra-spinal course of the upper thoracic nerve root is almost horizontal (as in the cervical spine). Therefore, the nerve can be compressed only by its corresponding disk. More inferiorly in the spine, however, the course of the nerve root becomes more oblique, and the lowest thoracic nerve roots can be compressed by disk impairments of two consecutive levels (T12 root by 11th or 12th disk).[192]

The major etiologic factor in most cases of thoracic disk herniation appears to be degenerative changes in the disk.[193] McKenzie[194] argues that the derangement syndrome can be divided into posterior disk derangements and anterior disk derangements because of the distinct clinical presentations. The McKenzie classification system is outlined in the introduction to Section III. Anterior derangement is rare in the thoracic spine. The following derangement patterns are seen in the thoracic spine[194]:

▶ *Derangement 1.* This type of derangement typically produces central or symmetric pain between T1 and T12. These derangements are rapidly reversible.

▶ *Derangement 2.* This type of derangement, which is rare and the result of acute trauma or serious pathology, produces an acute kyphosis.

▶ *Derangement 3.* This type of derangement typically produces unilateral or asymmetric pain across the thoracic region, with or without radiation around the chest wall. These derangements are rapidly reversible.

Clinical Pearl

The clinical manifestations of thoracic disk herniation are extremely variable and vague. This often results in long delays between presentation and diagnosis.

Midline back pain and compressive myelopathy symptoms progressing over months or years are the predominant clinical features of a thoracic disk herniation.[189] One study[195] found that 70 percent of patients had signs of spinal cord compression, but that isolated root pain occurred in only 9 percent of patients. Unusual features of thoracic disk herniation include Lhermitte's symptom precipitated by rotation of the thoracic spine,[196] neurogenic claudication with positional dependent weakness,[197] and flaccid paraplegia.[198]

The examination of the thoracic spine is detailed in Chapter 26.

Some thoracic disk herniations are asymptomatic. The incidence of asymptomatic thoracic disk protrusions is approximately 37 percent, reinforcing the view that clinicians should interpret thoracic MRI findings with caution.[190,191]

T1 and T2 Levels

Disk herniations at these levels are extremely rare.[199] This rarity may be the result of the protection afforded by the presence of the first and second ribs. Compression of the nerve at the T1 and at T2 segmental levels may result in numbness, tingling, and weakness of the hand and pain in the arm and medial forearm.[199] T1 radiculopathy also may be associated with a Horner's syndrome.[199] In addition, the patient may have reduced biceps and triceps reflexes.[199]

T2 and T3 Levels

A disk herniation at these levels is the rarest type.[200] Symptoms produced with this herniation include pain referred toward the clavicle, to the scapular spine, and down the inner side of the upper arm.[200]

T3 to T8 Levels

Compression of the nerves at these lower levels may result in symptoms that are experienced at the side or front of the trunk.[201] Compression of the dura in the thoracic spine results in unilaterally referred pain, which is extrasegmental. A T6-level compression of the dura can cause pain up to the base of the neck and down to the waist, whereas a dural compression at T12 can refer pain up to T6 and down to the sacrum.[201]

T9 to T11 Levels

Lower thoracic disk herniations have been associated with pain radiating to the buttock in some cases, confusing the diagnosis with that of a lumbosacral root compression.[202] How a herniated disk at low thoracic level could appear to be lumbosacral radiculopathy may be best explained by the anatomic arrangement of the spinal cord and vertebral bodies. In adults, the conus medullaris ends between the 12th thoracic and 3rd lumbar vertebrae, and the lumbar enlargement of the spinal cord usually locates at the lower thoracic level. Therefore, the lower thoracic disk herniation could compress the lumbosacral spinal nerves after their exit from the lumbar enlargement of the spinal cord and produce symptoms of compressive lumbosacral radiculopathy; thus, a herniation at an already tight canal may produce bilateral symptoms and sphincter disturbance, as in patients with a conus medullaris impairment.[203]

A retrospective study by Brown and colleagues[204] found that 31 of the 40 patients with symptomatic thoracic disk herniations, who were treated nonsurgically, were able to return to their previous level of activity.

Thoracic disk herniations requiring surgical management are uncommon, and account for less than 2 percent of all operations performed on herniated intervertebral disks.[205]

Electrodiagnosis

Electrodiagnostic studies are important in identifying physiologic abnormalities of the nerve root in the cervical, thoracic, and lumbar spine, and they have been shown to be a useful diagnostic test in the diagnosis of radiculopathy,[206] correlating well with findings on myelography and surgery.[207,208]

There are two parts to the electromyogram (EMG): nerve conduction studies and needle electrode examination. The nerve conduction studies are performed by placing surface electrodes over a muscle belly or sensory area and stimulating the nerve supplying either the muscle or sensory area from fixed points along the nerve. From this stimulation, the amplitude, distal latency, and conduction velocity can be measured. The amplitude reflects the number of intact axons, whereas the distal latency and conduction velocity are more of a reflection of the degree of myelination.[157,176,209]

The timing of the examination is important, because positive sharp waves and fibrillation potentials will first occur 18 to 21 days after the onset of a radiculopathy.[176,210] It is therefore best to delay this study until 3 weeks after the injury so that it can be as precise a study as possible. The primary use of electromyography is to diagnose nerve root impairment when the diagnosis is uncertain or to distinguish a radiculopathy from other impairments that are unclear on physical examination.[176] Electrodiagnostic abnormalities can persist after clinical recovery for months to years, and in some patients may persist indefinitely.[211,212]

Traction: Mechanical or Manual

Manual or mechanical traction has long been a preferred intervention throughout the spine, with the intent of improving range of motion and treating both zygapophysial joint impairments and disk herniation.[213–218] The efficacy of traction has not been scientifically proved in a randomized controlled trial, but it is commonly used and thought to be of benefit in reducing radicular pain.[180]

Traction often is applied in conjunction with the application of electrotherapeutic modalities, including moist heat and electrical stimulation over the paraspinal muscles, to aid in relaxation of the muscles and to assist in removal of the edema.[219]

For traction to be effective, the imparted force must be sufficient to overcome soft tissue resistance prior to the relaxation of the involved musculature. A cadaver study[217] demonstrated an initial average lengthening of 7.5 mm under 9 kg of lumbar traction (9 mm in younger subjects, 5.5 mm in the middle aged, and 7.5 mm in the elderly). A creep of 1.5 mm followed this lengthening during the next 30 minutes, and a set* of 2.5 mm reducing to 0.5 mm with release. Elongation of the spine was greater in the healthy spine (11 to 12 mm) and less in the spine with degenerative changes (3 to 5 mm). The creep was more rapid in the young, and there was no set in this age group. Forty percent of the lengthening was the result of straightening of lordosis, with only 0.9 mm of segmental separation, and 0.1 mm of segmental set.

A traction force of 20 to 25 lb in the cervical spine is required to completely eradicate the cervical lordosis.[220] The traction forces required to induce separation of the vertebral segments in the cervical spine have been found to be between 30 and 50 lb, with the degree of separation not significantly different at 7, 30, and 60 seconds of duration.[221]

Traction can be applied continuously or intermittently, and with the patient sitting or lying.[222] Intermittent traction produces twice as much separation as sustained traction.[220] The duration of traction recommended varies from 2 minutes to 24 hours.[223] Although separation of the vertebral segments occurs after approximately 7 seconds and requires a traction force of 20 lb in the cervical spine,[221] muscle relaxation takes as long as 20 to 25 minutes to occur.[214]

Piva and colleagues[224] recommend a trial of cervical traction if cervical flexion is the only cervical motion that is restricted.

Performed manually, traction can be very time consuming, and in the lumbar and thoracic spines, it requires a good deal of strength—approximately half a patient's body weight is needed to develop significant distraction of the vertebral bodies. However, a greater degree of specificity can be obtained using manual traction, especially if it performed using spinal locking techniques to localize the distraction to a specific level.

Vertebral axial decompression, a newer method to cause distraction, probably represents a higher-tech version of traction, although there is no evidence in the current peer-reviewed literature to support this type of intervention.

Outcome studies of traction have demonstrated varying results.[213,218] From clinical experience, it would appear that traction yields better results if at least one of the spinal motions is full and pain free. However, a one-session trial of short duration is worthwhile even if all of the motions are restricted.

Spinal traction is contraindicated in the following conditions:

▶ Acute lumbago.

▶ Instability.

▶ Respiratory or cardiac insufficiency.

▶ Respiratory irritation.

▶ Painful reactions.

▶ A large extrusion.

---

* The difference between the resting length of a structure and its length immediately after a load has been removed is called the *set*.

▶ Medial disk herniation.

▶ Altered mental state; this includes the inability of the patient to relax.

In the cervical spine, the patient position and set-up vary according to the findings. If the patient is demonstrating motor signs, the neck is positioned in 20 to 30 degrees of flexion during the traction to help "open" the anterior foramen.[223] A traction pull in 0 degrees or 20 degrees of flexion is advocated if the patient presents with a predominance of sensory symptoms and the clinician is attempting to widen the posterior foramen.[224] A traction pull of 15 degrees of extension is advocated for separation of the zygapophysial joint surfaces.[224a]

Supine cervical traction has been found to be more efficacious than seated traction in the intervention of cervical spine disorders.[225]

Electrotherapeutic and Physical Modalities

Modalities such as electrical stimulation also have been found helpful in uncontrolled studies.[164] They appear to be helpful in reducing the associated muscle pain and spasm but should be limited to the initial pain control phase of the intervention.

Once there is control of pain and inflammation, the patient's intervention should be progressed to restore full range of motion and flexibility of the spine, trunk, and extremity muscles.

Surgical Intervention

The primary rationale for surgery in any form for IVD prolapse is to relieve nerve root irritation or compression caused by herniated IVD material.

Surgery for Cervical Radiculopathy

Compressive pathologic lesions causing cervical radiculopathy (soft disk fragment herniation or spondylotic bone spurs) are most often located anterior to the nerve root.[225a] The initial surgical management for cervical radiculopathy resulting from soft disk herniation and osteophytic nerve root compression was a posterior laminectomy or a smaller keyhole foraminotomy approach that provided exposure of the nerve root.[225b] This was the only treatment for many years, and it had the advantage of preserving the spinal motion segment. Indeed, many surgeons continue to use the posterior foraminal procedure today. However, the difficulty of an indirect posterior exposure and inability to remove some ventral lesions led to the current and more common use of anterior diskectomy.[225b] These procedures were first described by Robinson and Smith in 1955[225c] and Cloward in 1958.[225d] The main disadvantage of these anterior approaches is that they required fusion of the motion segment. The interbody fusions were

used to provide inherent stability to the motion segment and to immobilize potentially painful degenerative disk and facet joints.[225b] The disadvantages of a bony fusion in a highly mobile cervical spine segment include the increased possibility of further progression of degenerative changes at other disk levels, which eventually requires further surgery.[225b] Reason suggests that preservation of motion segments by avoiding fusion where possible should be considered in patients with cervical radiculopathy.

The surgeon faces other considerations in choosing the approach, including the site of a prolapsed disk relative to the cervical spinal cord.[225e] Typically, lateral cervical disks are removed by the posterior approach, whereas the anterior approach is used with prolapsed midline disks that compromise the spinal cord, or some paramedian disks that compromise either the spinal cord or the nerve root but do not extend beyond the lateral margin of the cervical cord.[225e]

In the best-case scenario, the surgeon chooses the technique that directly eliminates the nerve-compressing pathologic lesion, while preserving the motion segment of the spine. The anterior microforaminotomy procedure has shown promising results in preserving the remaining disk in the intervertebral space as much as possible while directly eliminating the compressive pathologic lesion.[225f,225g] The advantages of this technique are many, including removal of only the offending mass, preservation of most of the disk and motion segment, a shorter operative procedure and hospital stay, avoidance of a fusion procedure and the attendant potential problems, and earlier return to full activity. The disadvantages are the long-term issues related to disk degeneration and unilateral removal of an uncovertebral joint.[225b]

Surgery for Lumbar Radiculopathy

Several characteristics of patients with sciatica appear to predict the eventual need for surgery. These include a mentally demanding job (as opposed to a mentally nondemanding job or no job); a gradual onset of pain; an increase of pain on coughing, sneezing, or straining; and difficulty putting on socks or stockings.[225h]

The aims of lumbar surgery for radiculopathy are to relieve pain and to restore neural function. Considerable literature reflects the evolution of lumbar disk surgery, the most commonly performed neurosurgical procedure. Oppenheim and Krause in 1909 were the first to remove what was thought to be a lumbar spinal tumor (enchondroma, chordoma).[225i] Other surgeries followed, leading to Mixter and Barr who systematized the diagnosis and operative treatment of lumbar disk prolapse in 1934.[225j]

Lumbar disk herniation is one of the few causes of spinal pain that can be successfully treated surgically.[225k] Several surgical options are available. The more common ones are described here.

Enzymatic Intradiskal Therapy

Enzymatic intradiskal therapy is advocated as a minimally invasive, intermediate stage between conservative management and open surgical intervention for a contained lumbar IVD prolapse.

Two enzymes are used in vivo: chymopapain and collagenase. The therapeutic concept behind intradiskal therapy is to produce a decrease in the water-binding capacity of the polysaccharide side chains. This is supposed to result in a lowering of the pressure in the IVD, with a subsequent reduction in the size of the IVD protrusion and relief of the tension on the nerve root.

The success rate of chemonucleolysis with chymopapain or collagenase has been found to be about 72 percent and 52 percent, respectively.[226,227] However, the final outcome from chemonucleolysis, followed by surgery if chemonucleolysis fails, remains poorer than the outcome from primary diskectomy.[228]

The complications associated with this procedure include allergic reactions, lumbar subarachnoid hemorrhage, and paraplegia.

Diskectomy

Diskectomy is a commonly performed surgical procedure in the general population, with high success rates reported in the literature.[229] There is now strong evidence regarding the relative effectiveness of surgical diskectomy versus chemonucleolysis versus placebo.[228]

Hemilaminectomy and Diskectomy

These diskectomies are usually approached posteriorly. Posterolateral diskectomy is used to treat herniated lumbar IVDs. The aim of a diskectomy is to decompress the involved nerve root or roots while minimizing scar tissue formation and avoiding iatrogenic nerve damage.

Percutaneous Diskectomy

Percutaneous diskectomy is a minimally invasive procedure that uses a probe for automatic aspiration of the nucleus pulposus material from the IVD. Because the probe is inserted using a cannula, the procedure causes minimal damage to the muscles, bones, and joints of the back, and no adherences in the epidural space. A short convalescence is, therefore, to be expected. This procedure is indicated for patients with radicular pain, positive SLR, and positive neurologic signs and symptoms (atrophy, weakness, sciatica) who have not responded to at least 6 weeks of conservative therapy. It also is advocated for patients with pure IVD herniation without stenosis or any other additional factors. These factors include IVD fragments in the spinal cord, severe spinal arthritis, and ligamentum flavum hypertrophy.

Microdiskectomy

A microdiskectomy is designed to decompress neural tissues by removing the IVD material that is causing the compression and irritation of the nerve root. Microdiskectomy is reported to have a high success rate, more than 90 percent in some studies.[229] Following this procedure, patients are generally able to return to their previous levels of activity, including participation in recreational sports. This surgery, however, also has been associated with a long recuperation and a protracted period of disability in some cases.[230,231]

Laser Diskectomy

As its name suggests, laser diskectomy uses a laser to remove discal tissue and thereby alleviate the pressure on the nerve root. However, because it does not address the actual pathology, its success rate is dramatically inferior to that of standard diskectomy.[232]

Laminectomy

A laminectomy is defined as the removal of a lamina. A complete laminectomy involves the removal of the entire lamina, together with the spinous process and the ligamentum flavum caudal and cranial to the lamina. The disadvantage of a complete laminectomy is that it may produce a destabilizing effect on the motion segment.[233]

Decompression

Decompression of the lumbar spine is defined as a laminectomy with partial facetectomy. Decompression also may be accompanied by partial laminectomy and canal enlargement, expansive lumbar laminoplasty, unilateral laminotomy for bilateral decompressions, or partial pediclectomy.

Fusion

There is little consensus among spine surgeons regarding the optimal indications for lumbar fusion surgery. Some surgeons believe that most patients with spinal stenosis are appropriate candidates for spinal fusion. Others believe that most of these patients should undergo only a laminectomy, because the degenerative changes that have occurred produce an inherent stability of the motion segment.

Controversy also exists regarding the use of fusion surgery versus nonsurgical approaches for degenerative disk disease with no herniation or stenosis.[234] Spinal fusion is associated with wider surgical exposure, more extensive dissection, and longer operation times than laminectomy.

As an adjunct to the excision of recurrent lumbar IVD herniations, lumbar fusion provides several theoretical advantages[235]:

▶ Reduction or elimination of segmental motion.

▶ Reduction of mechanical stresses across the degenerated disk space.

▶ Reduction of the incidence of additional herniation at the affected disk space.

Circumferential fusion has been advocated to improve fusion rates and clinical outcomes in intervention of the lumbosacral spine. Circumferential lumbar fusion can be challenging, however, requiring either thecal sac retraction and bilateral facet disruption or a posterior lumbar interbody fusion.[236]

Alternative options have included either sequential anterior and posterior fusions or a posterior lumbar interbody fusion at the time of simultaneous posterolateral fusion. In 1982, Harms and Rolinger[236] suggested the placement of bone graft and titanium mesh, via a transforaminal route, into the disk space that previously had been distracted using pedicle screw instrumentation (transforaminal lumbar interbody fusion [TLIF]).

Other options for fusing the lumbar spine include bone grafting with a posterolateral approach without instrumentation (facet fusion or intertransverse fusion), a posterolateral approach with pedicle screws, or posterior lumbar interbody fusion or anterior lumbar interbody fusion (ALIF) with bone grafts, cages, or dowels.[235]

Complications of ALIF include postoperative ileus, vascular and visceral injury, retrograde ejaculation in males, and venous thrombosis.[237] Complications of TLIF include epidural bleeding, neural injury, postsurgical instability, epidural fibrosis, and arachnoiditis.[237] Most of the complications reported for the ALIF and TLIF procedures are approach rather than device related.

Lumbar Interbody Arthrodesis

Lumbar interbody arthrodesis has become the intervention of choice for patients with disabling low back pain attributable to IVD degeneration and instability. The bone grafts available for placement include allograft and autograft.

Postsurgical Intervention

Patients who undergo spinal surgery may receive physical therapy as part of their rehabilitation. Although there is a large amount of information from evidence-based clinical practice guidelines for the management of many musculoskeletal conditions, there is relatively little information available on the physical therapy management of patients who have undergone spinal surgery.

The randomized controlled trials comparing various physical activity programs[238–241] have demonstrated the benefits of physical activity programs. These benefits have included less pain and disability, improved range of motion, and greater satisfaction with care.

Before the surgery, the patients may receive advice on spine care, postsurgical precautions, and instructions on basic exercises.

The postsurgical intervention following surgery is as varied as the number of types of surgery. The following are guidelines for postsurgical rehabilitation. The primary goals for the initial period following the surgery are:

▶ Reduction of pain and inflammation.

▶ Prevention of postsurgical complications.

▶ Protection of the surgical site.

▶ Prevention of a recurrent herniation.

▶ Maintenance of dural mobility.

▶ Improvement of function.

▶ Minimizing of the detrimental effects of immobilization.[242–247]

▶ Early return to appropriate functional activities. Patients usually are permitted to shower 1 week after the surgery.

▶ Safe return to occupational duties. Patients with a sedentary occupation may return to work within 7 to 10 days after the surgery. Prolonged positions and postures are to be avoided.

▶ Patient education on correct body mechanics and independent self-care.

The patient is given guidance on the gradual resumption of daily activities. Immobilization or prolonged rest should be avoided. Instead, the patient is encouraged to walk for short periods and distances several times a day.

Outpatient physical therapy, if appropriate, usually begins in the second or third week. The physical therapy examination includes:

▶ A thorough history.

▶ Inspection of the wound site.

▶ Anthropometric data.

▶ Postural examination.

▶ Neural examination, including neurodynamic mobility, and strength testing.

The components of the physical therapy intervention include a graded exercise program, with gentle range of motion, submaximal isometrics, and arm and leg exercises as appropriate.

Additional interventions may include electrotherapeutic modalities, physical agents, and scar massage. Patient education is very important, particularly postural education and information on body mechanics.

Progressive strengthening exercises for the spinal stabilizers usually are initiated by the fourth postoperative week.

Cardiovascular conditioning exercises are introduced at the earliest opportunity based on patient tolerance. These include riding a stationary bicycle, using an upper body ergonometer, using a stair-stepper, and swimming in a pool. The sessions for these exercises are initially brief (5 to 10 minutes) and are gradually increased up to 30 to 60 minutes.

Activities such as jogging are usually permitted at 6 to 8 weeks if there is minimal pain. When the patient does resume these activities, they should be done in the morning hours when the IVD is maximally hydrated.[248] High-impact sports such as basketball and soccer are usually permitted after the 12th week.

CASE STUDY LOW NECK PAIN

HISTORY

A 35-year-old woman presented at the clinic with what she described as a "crick" in her neck on arising from bed a few mornings ago. The patient described experiencing pain in the lower part of the neck, which radiated into the right shoulder and arm, and anteriorly and posteriorly over the upper right chest area. The patient also reported a tingling sensation over the radial aspect of the right forearm, the hand, and the fingers. The pain was reported to be aggravated by coughing, sneezing, and straining, and was disturbing her sleep. The pain was lessened by maintaining the upright position and when ambulating.

The patient's past medical and surgical history was unremarkable, and she reported being in good general health.

QUESTIONS

1. What is your working hypothesis at this time?
2. Does this presentation/history warrant a Cyriax upper quarter scanning examination? Why or why not?
3. What is the significance of pain that is aggravated by coughing, sneezing, and straining?
4. A lesion to which structure usually causes tingling sensations?

TESTS AND MEASURES

Observation of the patient revealed that the cervical lordosis was reduced and that her head was held in neutral flexion and deviation to the left. Although the history could indicate a working hypothesis of a herniated disk in the cervical region, the insidious onset, although not uncommon for the aforementioned pathology, deemed it necessary to perform an upper quarter scanning examination. In addition, the scan can be used to confirm the hypothesis while ruling out the more serious causes for these symptoms. It is always important to rule out other possible causes of neck and limb symptoms, including brachial plexus lesions, space-occupying lesions (benign or malignant tumors, cysts), thoracic outlet syndrome, nerve compression from facet or osteophyte impingement, rotator cuff tendonitis or tears, subacromial bursitis, bicipital tendonitis, and lateral epicondylitis. These disorders are distinguished by positive provocative maneuvers specific to them, in the absence of the other previously mentioned neurologic findings. The scanning examination revealed the following:

- Marked limitation of active and passive cervical motion was noted, with a spasmodic end-feel on right rotation, right side bending, and extension.
- Gentle compression through the patient's head reproduced the pain, and general distraction relieved it slightly. Performance of Spurling's test is unnecessary in this case.
- Palpable tenderness was elicited over the right aspect of the C6 to C7 segment.
- Hypoesthesia was present in the C7 dermatome.
- Triceps deep tendon reflex was hyporeflexive.
- Weakness of the C7 key muscles (elbow extensors and wrist flexors) was noted.
- Special testing revealed negative thoracic outlet testing and positive neurodynamic mobility testing in the radial and median tests.
- Negative vertebral artery involvement was found.

QUESTIONS

1. Did the scanning examination confirm the working hypothesis? How?
2. Given the findings from the scan, what is the diagnosis, or is further testing warranted?

EVALUATION

The findings from the scanning examination indicate a provisional diagnosis of compression of the seventh cervical nerve.

QUESTIONS

1. Having made the provisional diagnosis, what will be your intervention?
2. In order of priority, and based on the stages of healing, what will be the goals of your intervention?

INTERVENTION

The initial intervention is directed at the reduction of pain and inflammation, using local icing and electrotherapeutic modalities such as ultrasound and electrical stimulation, in conjunction with the nonsteroidal anti-inflammatories prescribed by the physician.[249] Manual or mechanical traction can be tried in an attempt to remove the compression from the nerve. The choice of patient position is determined by patient comfort and the ability of the clinician. Supine manual traction is easier to perform and is often more comfortable for the patient because the spine is unloaded. Once the acute phase subsides, the patient is progressed through range of motion and strengthening exercises as outlined in Chapter 23.

CASE STUDY LOW BACK AND LEG PAIN

HISTORY

A 32-year-old unemployed man presented with complaints of severe pain in the lower back that radiated into the right buttock, posterior thigh, calf, and lateral foot and two toes. The patient was a slightly obese man who had preferred to stand in the waiting room. His standing posture revealed a flexed hip and knee on the right side when weight bearing, with moderate kyphosis and a rotoscoliosis with right convexity of the lumbar spine, and shoulder girdle retraction. The pain in the back started about 2 weeks ago after sitting for a period of a few hours and initially was relieved by rest. Over the next few days, the pain gradually got worse. The patient reported the pain to be aggravated with bending at the waist and sitting, and lessened with right side lying with the hips and knees flexed. Difficulty with assuming an erect posture after lying down or sitting also was reported. The patient reported not being able to play softball or to lift and carry his 2-year-old son. Further questioning revealed that the patient had a history of minor back pain but was otherwise in good health and had no reports of bowel or bladder impairment.

QUESTIONS

1. Do you have a working hypothesis at this stage?
2. Does this presentation/history warrant a Cyriax lower quarter scanning examination? Why or why not?
3. What are the potential diagnoses for low back pain that is aggravated by bending at the waist and sitting?
4. List the conditions that could cause the distribution of symptoms described in this patient.

TESTS AND MEASURES

Prompted by the reports of a relatively insidious onset of symptoms and the report of leg pain, a lower quarter scanning examination was performed with the following findings:

- The patient demonstrated a marked restriction of gait and lumbar motion.
- Active range of lumbar motion revealed a significant restriction of trunk flexion at about 35 degrees from the kyphotic start position, which reproduced the posterior leg pain. The patient attempted to compensate during trunk flexion by bending at the hips and knees.
- The patient was unable to perform lumbar extension or right side bending because of a sharp increase in the radiation of pain into the right buttock and posterior thigh.
- Left side bending of the lumbar spine was limited by 25 percent, producing a slight ache in the right side of the low back.
- The Farfan compression test (see Chap. 25) reproduced the back, right buttock, and posterior thigh pain and posteroanterior pressure applied at the L4 and L5 segments provoked a spasmodic end-feel.
- The right straight leg raising (SLR) reproduced the radiating pain into the posterior right leg, and a hamstring spasm at 15 degrees. The application of passive ankle dorsiflexion increased the patient's symptoms. The left SLR was limited by spasm at 60 degrees, producing right low back, right buttock, and posterior thigh pain. The addition of neck flexion or dorsiflexion to the left SLR had no effect on the symptoms. The slump test was deferred as it was felt that no additional information would be achieved at the expense of aggravating the patient's condition.
- The prone knee-flexion test was negative on both sides.
- The ipsilateral and contralateral kinetic tests for the sacroiliac joint (see Chap. 27) were positive on both sides.
- Key muscle testing revealed fatigable weakness of the right ankle plantar flexors and evertors.
- Sensory testing revealed some pinprick loss over the lateral border of the right foot and toe and over the skin of the posterolateral right calf.
- Palpable tenderness of the lumbar paraspinals was noted.
- Deep tendon reflexes were decreased at the right ankle, but the spinal cord tests were unremarkable. Palpation revealed tenderness over the paravertebral area on the right side.

QUESTIONS

1. Did the lower quarter scanning examination confirm the working hypothesis? How?
2. Given the findings from the scanning examination, can a provisional diagnosis be made, or is further testing warranted? What information would further testing reveal?
3. What conditions could a positive SLR at 15 degrees with muscle spasm indicate?
4. Why do you think the prone knee-flexion test was negative?

EVALUATION

The findings in this patient indicated the presence of a prolapse, or extrusion, of the fifth lumbar disk with an isolated compression of the first sacral spinal nerve.

QUESTIONS

1. Having made the provisional diagnosis, what will be your intervention?
2. What other conditions might you suspect if your intervention does not improve the patient's condition?
3. In order of priority, and based on the stages of healing, what will be the goals of your intervention?

INTERVENTION

Caution is needed with this patient because the progression to a cauda equina syndrome is a real possibility. The intervention for this patient included:

- Manual shift correction.
- Patient education.
- Specific manual traction (see Chap. 25). The specific lumbar traction afforded the patient some relief.
- The McKenzie exercise approach.[121] The McKenzie program is initiated only after a comprehensive assessment in which the positions that centralize pain are determined.[250]
- Initiation of a walking program.

The patient was advised on a period of modified rest for 48 hours. When he returned, a series of short-duration (8 minutes), sustained mechanical traction sessions were initiated with the patient in supine 90/90 traction at 60 percent of body weight.[251] The patient was instructed on gentle active range of motion exercises of unilateral heel slides and pelvic rotations to be performed without increasing peripheral signs and symptoms. After a few sessions, the patient progressed to prone traction, posterior pelvic tilts, the McKenzie progression, and lumbar stabilization exercises.[252]

CASE STUDY SEVERE LOW BACK PAIN

HISTORY

A 49-year-old woman presented to the clinic with a 1-week history of severe low back pain. The patient experienced an acute onset of severe lumbar shooting pain that radiated immediately into the left buttock and the lateral aspect of the left leg and left foot. The pain was exacerbated by movement, sneezing, or coughing, and was lessened by resting. There was paresthesia and numbness over the lateral aspect of the left leg and foot and the dorsum of the left foot, and mild pain in the right leg. When questioned further, the patient mentioned urinary urgency. The patient's history showed that she had a history of intermittent low back pain for the past year. There was no history of back trauma. The patient had the results of a conventional computed tomographic myelogram of the lumbosacral spine with her, which were unremarkable.

QUESTIONS

1. Based on these findings, what would be your working hypothesis at this stage?
2. Does this presentation/history warrant a scanning examination? Why or why not?
3. Should the fact that there was no trauma concern the clinician?

EXAMINATION

Given the history and described symptoms, a lumbar scan was performed on this patient and elicited the following results:

- Reproduction of symptoms with end-range thoracic flexion and rotation to the left side. All other motions were normal.
- Decreased muscle strength (4/5) in foot dorsiflexors, plantar flexors, gluteus maximus, anterior tibialis, and gastrocnemius muscles on the left side.
- Reduced sensation to pinprick at the L5 and S1 dermatomes.
- Reduced ankle jerk on the left side, and plantar responses that were flexor bilaterally.
- Stretching of the sciatic nerve by an SLR test to 15 degrees reproduced the low back pain that sometimes radiated into the left leg. The crossed SLR test was negative.

EVALUATION

The patient's clinical presentation, including an acute low back pain radiating down the weak leg through the L5 and S1 dermatomes, positive SLR, and sensory and motor impairments of the corresponding roots strongly indicated acute lumbar disk disease, although there were some unusual findings. Therefore, the provisional diagnosis was a lumbar disk herniation with L5–S1 root compression.

A trial intervention of six visits was completed, but the patient failed to respond, and was referred back to her physician for further testing.

A magnetic resonance imaging study of the thoracolumbar spine showed a bulging disk and posterior osteophytes at T11 to T12, with encroachment of the underlying spinal canal and compression on the underlying cord. There was no evidence of L5 or S1 root compression at the exiting intervertebral foramina. One month later, a surgical procedure was performed to remove the bulging disk and osteophytes at T11 to T12. Following the surgery, the patient's sensory and motor deficits, and her urinary urgency, completely resolved, and the low back pain was much diminished.

REVIEW QUESTIONS*

1. What are the three components of the IVD?
2. Describe three functions of the disk.
3. Does the height of the disk increase or decrease with age?
4. Name the three stages of disk generation proposed by Kirkaldy-Willis.

5. In a large U.S. population survey, the combined prevalence of which two segmental levels accounted for 75 percent of cervical disk herniations?

---

* Additional questions to test your understanding of this chapter can be found in the Online Learning Center for *Orthopaedic Assessment, Evaluation, and Intervention* at www.duttononline.net.

REFERENCES

1. Lundon K, Bolton K. Structure and function of the lumbar intervertebral disk in health, aging, and pathological conditions. *J Orthop Sports Phys Ther* 2001;31:291–306.
2. White AA, Punjabi MM. *Clinical Biomechanics of the Spine.* 2nd ed. Philadelphia, Pa: JB Lippincott; 1990.
3. Buckwalter JA. Spine update: Aging and degeneration of the human intervertebral disc. *Spine* 1995;20:1307–1314.
4. Huijbregts PA. Lumbopelvic region: anatomy and biomechanics. In: Wadsworth C, ed. *Current Concepts of Orthopaedic Physical Therapy—Home Study Course.* La Crosse, Wis: Orthopaedic Section, American Physical Therapy Association; 2001.
5. Ghosh P, et al. Collagens, elastin and noncollagenous protein of the intervertebral disc. *Clin Orthop* 1977;129:124–132.
6. Taylor JR. The development and adult structure of lumbar intervertebral discs. *J Man Med* 1990;5:43–47.
7. Tsuji H, et al. Structural variation of the anterior and posterior annulus fibrosus in the development of the human lumbar intervertebral disc: A risk factor for intervertebral disc rupture. *Spine* 1993;18:204–210.
8. Armstrong JR. *Lumbar Disc Lesions.* 3rd ed. Edinburgh, Scotland: Churchill Livingstone; 1965.
9. Bogduk N, Twomey LT. Anatomy and biomechanics of the lumbar spine. In: Bogduk N, Twomey LT, eds. *Clinical Anatomy of the Lumbar Spine and Sacrum.* Edinburgh, Scotland: Churchill Livingstone; 1997:2–53; 81–152; 171–176.
10. Naylor A. The biophysical and biomechanical aspects of intervertebral disc herniation and degeneration. *Ann R Coll Surg Engl* 1962;31:91–114.
11. Buckwalter JA, Cooper RR, Maynard JA. Elastic fibers in human intervertebral discs. *J Bone Joint Surg* 1976;58:73–76.
12. Coventry MB, Ghormley RK, Kernohan JW. The intervertebral disc: Its microscopic anatomy and pathology. Part 1: Anatomy, development and physiology. *J Bone Joint Surg* 1945;28A:105–111.
13. Akeson WH, et al. Biomechanics and biochemistry of the intervertebral disks: The need for correlation studies. *Clin Orthop* 1977;129:133–140.
14. Eyring EJ. The biochemistry and physiology of the intervertebral disc. *Clin Orthop* 1969;67:16–28.
15. Coventry MB. Anatomy of the intervertebral disk. *Clin Orthop* 1969;67:9–17.
16. Nachemson AL. The lumbar spine: An orthopedic challenge. *Spine* 1976;1:59–71.
17. Inoue H. Three dimensional architecture of lumbar intervertebral discs. *Spine* 1981;6:138–146.
18. Adams MA, et al. Abnormal stress concentrations in lumbar intervertebral discs following damage to the vertebral body: a cause of disc failure. *Eur Spine J* 1993;1:214–221.
19. Bogduk N. The innervation of the lumbar spine. *Spine* 1983;8:286–293.
20. Edger MA, Nundy S. Innervation of the spinal dura matter. *J Neurol Neurosurg Psychiatry* 1966;29:530–534.

21. Malinsky J. The ontogenetic development of nerve terminations in the intervertebral discs of man. *Acta Anat* 1959;38:96–113.

22. Kumar S, Davis PR. Lumbar vertebral innervation and intra-abdominal pressure. *J Anat* 1973;114:47–53.

23. Adams MA, et al. Abnormal stress concentrations in lumbar intervertebral discs following damage to the vertebral body: A cause of disc failure. European Spine Society (Acromed) Award paper. *Eur Spine J* 1993;1:214–221.

24. Adams MA, et al. Posture and the compressive strength of the lumbar spine. International Society of Biomechanics Award Paper. *Clin Biomech* 1994;9:5–14.

25. Osti OL, Vernon-Roberts B, Frazer RD. Annulus tears and intervertebral disc degeneration: A study using an animal model. *Spine* 1990;15:762.

26. Panjabi M, et al. Biomechanical studies in cadaveric spines. In: Jayson MIV, ed. *The Lumbar Spine and Back Pain.* New York, NY: Churchill Livingstone; 1992:133–135.

27. Markolf KL, Morris JM. The structural components of the intervertebral disc. *J Bone Joint Surg* 1974;56A:675–687.

28. Böstman OM. Body mass index and height in patients requiring surgery for lumbar intervertebral disc herniation. *Spine* 1993;18:851–854.

29. Heliövaara M. Body height, obesity, and risk of herniated lumbar intervertebral disc. *Spine* 1987;12:469–472.

30. Andersson GBJ, Schultz AB. Effects of fluid injection on mechanical properties of intervertebral discs. *J Biomech* 1979;12:453–458.

31. Abdullah AF, et al. Surgical management of extreme lateral lumbar disc herniations. *Neurosurgery* 1988;22:648–653.

32. Brinckmann P, Grootenboer H. Change of disc height, radial disc bulge and intradiscal pressure from discectomy: An in-vitro investigation on human lumbar discs. *Spine* 1991;16:641–646.

33. Adams MA, Hutton WC. The effect of posture on the fluid content of lumbar intervertebral discs. *Spine* 1983;8:665–671.

34. Adams MA, et al. Sustained loading generates stress concentrations in lumbar intervertebral discs. *Spine* 1996;21:434–438.

35. Adams MA, Dolan P. Recent advances in lumbar spinal mechanics and their clinical significance. *Clin Biomech* 1995;10:3–19.

36. Lord MJ, et al. Lumbar lordosis: Effects of sitting and standing. *Spine* 1997;22:2571–2574.

37. Kraemer J, Kolditz D, Gowin R. Water and electrolyte content of human intervertebral discs under variable load. *Spine* 1985;10:69–71.

38. Kazarian LE. Dynamic response characteristics of the human lumbar vertebral column. *Acta Orthop Scand* 1972;146:1–86.

39. Kazarian LE. Creep characteristics of the human spinal column. *Orthop Clin North Am* 1975;6:3–18.

40. Tyrell AJ, Reilly T, Troup JDG. Circadian variation in stature and the effects of spinal loading. *Spine* 1985;10:161–164.

41. Nachemson A. Disc pressure measurements. *Spine* 1981;6:93–97.

42. Hickey DS, Hukins DWL. Relation between the structure of the annulus fibrosus and the function and failure of the intervertebral disc. *Spine* 1980;5:100–116.

43. Horst M, Brinkmann P. Measurement of the distribution of axial stress on the end plate of the vertebral body. *Spine* 1981;6:217–232.

44. Yoganandan N, et al. Functional biomechanics of the thoracolumbar vertebral cortex. *Clin Biomech* 1988;3:11–18.

45. Kelsey JL, Hardy RJ. Driving of motor vehicles as a risk factor for acute herniated lumbar intervertebral disc. *Am J Epidemiol* 1975;102:63–73.

46. Markolf KL. Deformation of the thoracolumbar intervertebral joints in response to external loads. *J Bone Joint Surg* 1972;54A:511–533.

47. Ueno K, Liu YK. A three-dimensional nonlinear finite element model of lumbar intervertebral joint in torsion. *J Biomech Eng* 1987;109:200–209.

48. White AA, Panjabi MM. *Clinical Biomechanics of the Spine.* Philadelphia: Lippincott-Raven; 1990:106–108.

49. Farfan HF, et al. The effects of torsion on the lumbar intervertebral joints: The role of torsion in the production of disc degeneration. *J Bone Joint Surg* 1970;52A:468–497.

50. Ahmed AM, Duncan MJ, Burke DL. The effect of facet geometry on the axial torque-rotation response of lumbar motion segments. *Spine* 1990;15:391–401.

51. Hindle RJ, Pearcy MJ. Rotational mobility of the human back in forward flexion. *J Biomed Eng* 1989;11:219–223.

52. Pearcy MJ. Twisting mobility of the human back in flexed postures. *Spine* 1993;18:114–119.

53. Galante JO. Tensile properties of human lumbar annulus fibrosis. *Acta Orthop Scand Suppl* 1967;100:1–91.

54. Shah JS. Structure, morphology and mechanics of the lumbar spine. In: Jayson MIV, ed. *The Lumbar Spine and Backache.* London, England: Pitman; 1980:359–405.

55. Farfan HF. *Mechanical Disorders of the Low Back.* Philadelphia, Pa: Lea and Febiger; 1973.

56. Roberts N, Gratin C, Whitehouse GH. MRI analysis of lumbar intervertebral disc height in young and older populations. *J MRI* 1997;7:880–886.

56a. Judge RD, Zuidema GD, Fitzgerald FT. Musculoskeletal system. In: Judge RD, Zuidema GD, and Fitzgerald FT, eds. *Clinical Diagnosis.* Boston, Mass: Little, Brown; 1982:365–403.

57. Bianco AJ. Low back pain and sciatica. Diagnosis and indications for treatment. *J Bone Joint Surg* 1968;50A:170.

58. Dupuis PR. The natural history of degenerative changes in the lumbar spine. In: Watkins RG, Collis JS, eds. *Principles and Techniques in Spine Surgery.* Rockville, Md: Aspen; 1987:1–4.

59. Adams MA, McNally DS, Dolan P. Stress distributions inside intervertebral discs: The effects of age and degeneration. *J Bone Joint Surg* 1996;78A:965–972.

60. Kirkaldy-Willis WH. The three phases of the spectrum of degenerative disease. In: Kirkaldy-Willis WH, ed. *Managing Low Back Pain.* New York, NY: Churchill Livingstone; 1983:75–90.

61. Miller JA, Schmatz C, Schultz AB. Lumbar disc degeneration: Correlation with age, sex, and spine level in 600 autopsy specimens. *Spine* 1988;13:173–178.

62. Kelsey JL, White AA. Epidemiology and impact of low back pain. *Spine* 1980;5:133–142.

63. Matsui H, et al. Familial predisposition for lumbar degenerative disc disease. A case-control study. *Spine* 1998;23:1029–1034.

64. Moneta GB, et al. Reported pain during lumbar discography as a function of annular ruptures and disc degeneration. *Spine* 1994;19:1968–1974.

65. Dolan P, Earley M, Adams MA. Bending and compressive stresses acting on the lumbar spine during lifting activities. *J Biomech* 1994;27:1237–1248.

66. Wedge JH. The natural history of spinal degeneration. In: Kirkaldy-Willis WH, ed. *Managing Low Back Pain.* New York, NY: Churchill Livingstone; 1983:3–8.

67. Saal JA. Natural history and nonoperative treatment of lumbar disc herniation. *Spine* 1996;21:2S–9S.

68. Rydevik B, Garfin SR. Spinal nerve root compression. In: Szabo RM, ed. *Nerve Compression Syndromes: Diagnosis and Treatment*. Thorofare, NJ: Slack; 1989:247–261.

69. Yasuma T, et al. Histological changes in aging lumbar intervertebral discs: Their role in protrusions and prolapses. *J Bone Joint Surg* 1990;72A:220–229.

70. Eckert C, Decker A. Pathological studies of intervertebral discs. *J Bone Joint Surg* 1947;29:447–454.

71. Taylor TKF, Akeson WH. Intervertebral disc prolapse: A review of morphologic and biochemical knowledge concerning the nature of prolapse. *Clin Orthop* 1971;76:54–79.

72. Jonsson B, Stromqvist B. Clinical appearance of contained and non-contained lumbar disc herniation. *J Spinal Disord* 1996;9:32.

73. Brinckmann P. Injury of the anulus fibrosus and disc protrusions. *Spine* 1986;11:149–153.

74. Kostuik JP, et al. Cauda equina syndrome and lumbar disc herniation. *J Bone Joint Surg* 1986;68A:386–391.

75. Mixter WJ, Barr JS Jr. Rupture of the intervertebral disc with involvement of the spinal canal. *N Engl J Med* 1934;211:210–215.

76. Gronblad M, et al. A controlled immuno-histochemical study of inflammatory cells in disc herniation tissue. *Spine* 1994;19:2744–2751.

77. Habtemariam A, et al. Immunocytochemical localization of immunoglobulins in disc herniations. *Spine* 1996;16:1864–1869.

78. Saal JS, et al. High levels of phospholipase A2 activity in lumbar disc herniation. *Spine* 1990;15:674–678.

79. Tolonen J, et al. Basic fibroblast growth factor immunoreactivity in blood vessels and cells of disc herniations. *Spine* 1995;20:271–276.

80. Happey T, et al. Proteoglycans and glycoproteins associated with collagen in the human intervertebral disc. *Z Klin Chem* 1971;9:79.

81. Gronblad M, et al. A controlled biochemical and immunohistochemical study of human synovial type (group II) phospholipase A2 and inflammatory cells in macroscopically normal, degenerated, and herniated human lumbar disc tissues. *Spine* 1996;22:1–8.

82. Kang JD, et al. Herniated lumbar intervertebral discs spontaneously produce matrix metalloproteinases, nitric oxide, interleukin-6, and prostaglandin E2. *Spine* 1996;21:271–277.

83. Cyriax J. *Textbook of Orthopaedic Medicine, Diagnosis of Soft Tissue Lesions*. 8th ed. London, England: Bailliere Tindall; 1982.

84. Halland AM, et al. Avascular necrosis of the hip in systemic lupus erythematosus: The role of MRI. *Br J Rheumatol* 1993;32:972–976.

85. Trummer M, et al. Lumbar disc herniation mimicking meralgia paresthetica: Case report. *Surg Neurol* 2000;54:80–81.

86. Kallgren MA, Tingle LJ. Meralgia paresthetica mimicking lumbar radiculopathy. *Anesth Analg* 1993;76:1367–1368.

87. Naftulin S, Fast A, Thomas M. Diabetic lumbar radiculopathy: Sciatica without disc herniation. *Spine* 1993;18:2419–2422.

88. Nadler SF, et al. High lumbar disc: Diagnostic and treatment dilemma. *Am J Phys Med Rehabil* 1998;77:538–544.

89. Porchet F, Frankhauser H, de Tribolet N. Extreme lateral lumbar disc herniation: A clinical presentation of 178 patients. *Acta Neurochir (Wien)* 1994;127:203–209.

90. Fontanesi G, et al. Prolapsed intervertebral disc at the upper lumbar level. *Ital J Orthop Traumatol* 1987;13:501–507.

91. Bosacco SJ, et al. High lumbar disc herniation. *Orthopedics* 1989;12:275–278.

92. Hsu K, et al. High lumbar disc degeneration: Incidence and etiology. *Spine* 1990;15:679–682.

93. Hoppenfeld S. *Physical Examination of the Spine and Extremities*. East Norwalk, Conn: Appleton-Century-Crofts; 1976.

93a. Cocchiarella L, Andersson GBJ, eds. *American Medical Association, Guides to the Evaluation of Permanent Impairment*. 5th ed. Chicago, ILL: AMA; 2001.

94. Jonsson B, Stromqvist B. The straight leg rising test and the severity of symptoms in lumbar disc herniation. *Spine* 1995;20:27–30.

95. O'Laoire SA, Crockard HA, Thomas DG. Prognosis for sphincter recovery after operation for cauda equina compression owing to lumbar disc prolapse. *BMJ* 1981;282:1852–1854.

96. Schmorl G, Junghanns H. *The Human Spine in Health and Disease*. 2nd American ed. New York, NY: Grune and Stratton; 1971.

97. Coventry MB, Ghormley RK, Kernohan JW. The intervertebral disc: Its microscopic anatomy and pathology. Part II. Changes in the intervertebral disc concomitant with age. *J Bone Joint Surg* 1945;27A:233–247.

98. Hilton RC, Ball J, Benn RT. Vertebral end plate lesions (Schmorl's nodes) in the dorsolumbar spine. *Ann Rheum Dis* 1976;35:127–132.

99. Yasuma T, Saito S, Kihara K. Schmorl's nodes: Correlation of x-ray and histological findings in postmortem specimens. *Acta Pathol Jpn* 1988;38:723–733.

100. Keyes DC, Compere EL. The normal and pathological physiology of the nucleus pulposus of the intervertebral disc. *J Bone Joint Surg* 1932;14:897–938.

101. Prescher A. Anatomy and pathology of the aging spine. *Eur J Radiol* 1998;27:181–195.

102. Butler DL, Gifford L. The concept of adverse mechanical tension in the nervous system: Part 1: Testing for "dural tension." *Physiotherapy* 1989;75:622–629.

103. Deyo RA, Rainville J, Kent DL. What can the history and physical examination tell us about low back pain? *JAMA* 1992;268:760–765.

104. Weisel SE, et al. A study of computer-assisted tomography, In: The incidence of positive CAT scans in an asymptomatic group of patients. *Spine* 1984;9:549–551.

105. Boden SD, et al. Abnormal magnetic resonance scan of the lumbar spine in asymptomatic subjects: a prospective investigation. *J Bone Joint Surg* 1990;72A:403–408.

106. Andersson GBJ, Deyo RA. History and physical examination in patients with herniated lumbar discs. *Spine* 1996;21:10S–18S.

107. Van den Hoogen HMM, et al. On the accuracy of history, physical examination, and erythrocyte sedimentation rate in diagnosing low back pain in general practice. *Spine* 1995;20:318–327.

108. Roach KE, et al. The sensitivity and specificity of pain response to activity and position in categorizing patients with low back pain. *Phys Ther* 1997;77:730–738.

109. Deyo RA. Understanding the accuracy of diagnostic tests. In: Weinstein JN, Rydevik B, Sonntag V, eds. *Essentials of the Spine*. Philadelphia, Pa: Raven; 1995:55–70.

110. Yukawa Y, et al. Groin pain associated with lower lumbar disc herniation. *Spine* 1997;22:1736–1739.

111. Murphey F. Sources and patterns of pain in disc disease. *Clin Neurosurg* 1968;15:343–351.

112. McKenzie RA. *The Lumbar Spine: Mechanical Diagnosis and Therapy*. Waikanae, New Zealand: Spinal Publications New Zealand; 1981.

113. Huijbregts PA. Lumbopelvic region: Aging, disease, examination, diagnosis, and treatment. In: Wadsworth C, ed. *Current Concepts of Orthopaedic Physical Therapy—Home Study Course.* La Crosse, Wis: Orthopaedic Section, American Physical Therapy Association; 2001.

114. Lorio MP, Bernstein AJ, Simmons EH. Sciatic spinal deformity—Lumbosacral list: An "unusual" presentation with review of the literature. *J Spinal Disord* 1995;8:201–205.

115. Suk KS, et al. Lumbosacral scoliotic list by lumbar disc herniation. *Spine* 2001;26:667–671.

116. DePalma AF, Rothman RH. *The Intervertebral Disc.* Philadelphia, Pa: Saunders; 1970.

117. Maigne R. *Diagnosis and Treatment of Pain of Vertebral Origin.* Baltimore, Md: Williams and Wilkins; 1996.

118. Porter RW, Miller CG. Back pain and trunk list. *Spine* 1986;11:596–600.

119. Battie MC, et al. Managing low back pain: Attitudes and treatment preferences of physical therapists. *Phys Ther* 1994; 74:219–226.

120. Donahue MS, Riddle DL, Sullivan MS. Intertester reliability of a modified version of McKenzie's lateral shift assessment obtained on patients with low back pain. *Phys Ther* 1996;76:706–726.

121. McKenzie RA. Manual correction of sciatic scoliosis. *N Z Med J* 1972;76:194–199.

122. Riddle DL, Rothstein JM. Intertester reliability of McKenzie's classifications of the syndrome types present in patients with low back pain. *Spine* 1993;18:1333–1344.

123. Morag E, et al. Abnormalities in muscle function during gait in relation to the level of lumbar disc herniation. *Spine* 2000;25:829–833.

124. Shiqing X, Quanzhi Z, Dehao F. Significance of straight-leg-raising test in the diagnosis and clinical evaluation of lower lumbar intervertebral disc protrusion. *J Bone Joint Surg* 1987; 69A:517–522.

125. Hakelius A, Hindmarsh J. The comparative reliability of preoperative diagnostic methods in lumbar disc surgery. *Acta Orthop Scand* 1972;43:234.

126. Hakelius A, Hindmarsh J. The significance of neurological signs and myelographic findings in the diagnosis of lumbar root compression. *Acta Orthop Scand* 1972;43:239–246.

127. Spangfort EV. The lumbar disc herniation: A computer aided analysis of 2,504 operations. *Acta Orthop Scand Suppl* 1972;142:1–95.

128. Christodoulides AN. Ipsilateral sciatica on the femoral nerve stretch test is pathognomonic of an L4/5 disc protrusion. *J Bone Joint Surg* 1989;71B:88–89.

129. Weinstein JN. A 45-year-old man with low back pain and a numb left foot. *JAMA* 1998;280:730–736.

130. Donelson R. The McKenzie approach to evaluating and treating low back pain. *Orthop Rev* 1990;19:681–686.

131. Stankovic R, Johnell O. Conservative management of acute low back pain. A prospective randomized trial: McKenzie method of treatment versus patient education in "mini back school." *Spine* 1990;15:120–123.

132. Walsh R, Nitz AJ. Cervical spine. In: Wadsworth C, ed. *Current Concepts of Orthopedic Physical Therapy—Home Study Course.* La Crosse, Wis: Orthopaedic Section, American Physical Therapy Association; 2001.

133. Taylor JR. Regional variation in the development and position of the notochordal segments of the human nucleus pulposus. *J Anat* 1971;110:131–132.

134. Mercer SB, Bogduk N. The ligaments and anulus fibrosus of human adult cervical intervertebral discs. *Spine* 1999;24:619–626.

135. Kokubun S, Sakurai M, Tanaka Y. Cartilaginous endplate in cervical disc herniation. *Spine* 1996;21:190–195.

136. Murphey F, Simmons JC. Ruptured cervical disc: experience with 250 cases. *Am J Surg* 1966;32:83.

137. Dvorak J. Epidemiology, physical examination, and neurodiagnostics. *Spine* 1998;23:2663–2673.

138. Oda J, Tanaka H, Tsuzuki N. Intervertebral disc changes with aging of human cervical vertebra: From neonate to the eighties. *Spine* 1988;13:1205–1211.

139. Boden SD, et al. Abnormal magnetic resonance scans of the cervical spine in asymptomatic subjects: A prospective investigation. *J Bone Joint Surg* 1990;72A:1178–1184.

140. Töndury G, Theiler K. *Entwicklungsgeschichte und Fehlbildung der Wirbelsäule.* Stuttgart, Germany: Hyppokrates; 1958.

141. Garvey TA, Eismont FJ. Diagnosis and treatment of cervical radiculopathy and myelopathy. *Orthop Rev* 1991;20:595–603.

141a. Ebraheim NA, et al. The quantitative anatomy of the cervical nerve root groove and the intervertebral foramen. *Spine* 1996; 21:1619–1623.

141b. Tanaka N, et al. The anatomic relation among the nerve roots, intervertebral foramina, and intervertebral discs of the cervical spine. *Spine* 2000;25:286–291.

142. Tanaka N, et al. The anatomic relation among the nerve roots, intervertebral foramina, and intervertebral discs of the cervical spine. *Spine* 2000;25:286–291.

143. Goodman BW. Neck pain. *Prim Care* 1988;15:689–707.

144. Brooker AEW, Barter RW. Cervical spondylosis: A clinical study with comparative radiology. *Brain* 1965;88:925–936.

145. Gore DR, et al. Roentgenographic findings in the cervical spine of asymptomatic people. *Spine* 1987;6:521–526.

146. Manifold SG, McCann PD. Cervical radiculitis and shoulder disorders. *Clin Orth Rel Res* 1999;368:105–113.

147. Ferguson RJ, Caplan LR. Cervical spondylitic myelopathy: History and physical findings. *Neurol Clin* 1985;3:373–382.

148. Adams CBT, Logue V. Studies in spondylotic myelopathy 2. The movement and contour of the spine in relation to the neural complications of cervical spondylosis. *Brain* 1971;94:569–586.

149. Young WF. Cervical spondylotic myelopathy: A common cause of spinal cord dysfunction in older persons. *Am Fam Phys* 2000;62:1064–1070, 1073.

150. Debois V, et al. Soft cervical disc herniation: Influence of cervical spinal canal measurements on development of neurologic symptoms. *Spine* 1996;24:1996–2002.

151. Denno JJ, Meadows GR. Early diagnosis of cervical spondylotic myelopathy: A useful clinical sign. *Spine* 1991;16:1353–1355.

152. Kondo K, et al. Protruded intervertebral cervical disc. *Minn Med* 1981;64:751–753.

153. Kokubun S. Cervical disc herniation [in Japanese]. *Rinsho Seikei Geka* 1989;24:289–297.

154. O'Laoire SA, Thomas DGT. Spinal cord compression due to prolapse of cervical intervertebral disc (herniation of nucleus pulposus): Treatment in 26 cases by discectomy without interbody bone graft. *J Neurosurg* 1983;59:847–853.

155. Ward R. Myofascial release concepts. In: Nyberg N, Basmajian JV, eds. *Rational Manual Therapies.* Baltimore, Md: Williams and Wilkins; 1993:223–241.

156. Kelsey JL. An epidemiological study of the relationship between occupations and acute herniated lumbar intervertebral discs. *Int J Epidemiol* 1975;4:197–205.

157. Leblhuber F, et al. Diagnostic value of different electrophysiologic tests in cervical disc prolapse. *Neurology* 1988;38:1879–1881.

158. Motoe T. Studies on topographic architecture of the annulus fibrosus in the developmental and degenerative process of the lumbar intervertebral disc in man [in Japanese]. *J Jpn Orthop Assoc* 1986;60:495–509.

158a. Bogduk N, Windsor M, Inglis A. The innervation of the cervical intervertebral discs. *Spine* 1988;13:2–8.

158b. Rao R. Neck pain, cervical radiculopathy, and cervical myelopathy: Pathophysiology, natural history, and clinical evaluation. *J Bone Joint Surg* 2002;84A:1872–1881.

158c. Cooper RG, et al. Herniated intervertebral disc-associated periradicular fibrosis and vascular abnormalities occur without inflammatory cell infiltration. *Spine* 1995;20:591–598.

158d. Chabot MC, Montgomery DM. The pathophysiology of axial and radicular neck pain. *Sem Spine Surg* 1995;7:2–8.

159. Farfan HF, Kirkaldy-Willis WH. The present status of spinal fusion in the treatment of lumbar intervertebral joint disorders. *Clin Orthop* 1981;158:198.

160. Chiba K. An experimental study on the pathological changes of the intervertebral disc and its surrounding tissues after intradiscal injection of various chemical substances. *J Jpn Orthop Assoc* 1993;67:1055–1069.

161. Cloward RB. The clinical significance of the sinu-vertebral nerve of the cervical spine in relation to the cervical disk syndrome. *J Neurol Neurosurg Psychiatry* 1960;23:321.

162. Saal JS, Saal JA, Yurth EF. Nonoperative management of herniated cervical intervertebral disc with radiculopathy. *Spine* 1996;21:1877–1883.

163. Bland JH. New anatomy and physiology with clinical and historical implications. In: Bland JH, ed. *Disorders of the Cervical Spine*. Philadelphia, Pa: Saunders; 1994:71–79.

163a. Henderson CM, et al. Posterior-lateral foraminotomy as an exclusive operative technique for cervical radiculopathy: A review of 846 consecutively operated cases. *Neurosurgery* 1983;13:504–512.

163b. Good DC, Couch JR, Wacaser L. Numb, clumsy hands and high cervical spondylosis. *Surg Neurol* 1984;22:285–291.

163c. Chen TY. The clinical presentation of uppermost cervical disc protrusion. *Spine* 2000;25:439–442.

164. Cole AJ, Farrell JP, Stratton SA. Cervical spine athletic injuries. *Phys Med Rehabil Clin North Am* 1994;5:37–68.

165. Marks MR. Cervical spine injuries and their neurologic implications. *Clin Sports Med* 1990;9:263–278.

166. Barnes R. Traction injuries to the brachial plexus in adults. *J Bone Joint Surg* 1949;31B:10–16.

167. Clancy WG. Brachial plexus and upper extremity peripheral nerve injuries. In: Torg JS, ed. *Athletic Injuries to the Head Neck and Face*. Philadelphia, Pa: Lea and Febiger; 1982:215–222.

168. Braddom RL. Management of common cervical pain syndromes. In: Lisa JAD, ed. *Rehabilitation Medicine: Principles and Practice*. Philadelphia, Pa: JB Lippincott; 1993:1038.

169. Malanga GA, Campagnolo DI. Clarification of the pronator reflex. *Am J Phys Med Rehabil* 1994;73:338–340.

170. Spurling RG, Scoville WB. Lateral rupture of the cervical intervertebral discs. A common cause of shoulder and arm pain. *Surg Gynecol Obstet* 1944;78:350–358.

171. Jahnke RW, Hart BL. Cervical stenosis, spondylosis, and herniated disc disease. *Radiol Clin North Am* 1991;29:777–791.

172. Tong HC, Haig AJ, Yamakawa K. The Spurling test and cervical radiculopathy. *Spine* 2002;27:156–159.

173. Bradley JP, Tibone JE, Watkins RG. History, physical examination, and diagnostic tests for neck and upper extremity problems. In: Watkins RG, ed. *The Spine in Sports*. St Louis, Mo: Mosby-Year Book; 1996:71–82.

174. Davidson RI, Dunn EJ, Metzmaker JN. The shoulder abduction test in the diagnosis of radicular pain in cervical extradural compressive monoradiculopathies. *Spine* 1981;6:441–446.

175. Evans RC. *Illustrated Essentials in Orthopedic Physical Assessment*. St Louis, Mo: Mosby-Year Book; 1994.

176. Ellenberg MR, Honet JC, Treanor WJ. Cervical radiculopathy. *Arch Phys Med Rehabil* 1994;75:342–352.

177. Reiners K, Toyka KV. Management of cervical radiculopathy. *Eur Neurol* 1995;35:313–316.

178. Grisoli F, et al. Anterior discectomy without fusion for treatment of cervical lateral soft disc extrusion: A follow-up of 120 cases. *Neurosurgery* 1989;24:853–859.

179. Gore DR, Sepic SB. Anterior cervical fusion for degenerated or protruded discs. A review of one hundred forty-six patients. *Spine* 1984;9:667–671.

180. Dreyer SJ, Boden SD. Nonoperative treatment of neck and arm pain. *Spine* 1998;23:2746–2754.

181. Dillin W, et al. Cervical radiculopathy: A review. *Spine* 1986;11:988–991.

182. Aldrich F. Posterolateral microdiscectomy for cervical monoradiculopathy caused by posterolateral soft cervical disc sequestration. *J Neurosurg* 1990;72:370–377.

183. Oliver J, Middleditch A. *Functional Anatomy of the Spine*. Oxford, England: Butterworth-Heinemann; 1991.

184. Kapandji IA. *The Physiology of the Joints, The Trunk and Vertebral Column*. New York, NY: Churchill Livingstone; 1991.

185. Reuben JD, Brown RH, Nash CL. In-vivo effects of axial loading on healthy adolescent spines. *Clin Orth Rel Res* 1979; 139:17–27.

186. DiGiovanna EL, Schiowitz S. *An Osteopathic Approach to Diagnosis and Treatment*. Philadelphia, Pa: JB Lippincott; 1991.

187. White AA. Analysis of the mechanics of the thoracic spine in man. *Acta Orthop Scand Suppl* 1969;127:1–105.

188. Lyu RK, et al. Thoracic disc herniation mimicking acute lumbar disc disease. *Spine* 1999;24:416–418.

189. Arce CA, Dohrmann GJ. Thoracic disc herniation: Improved diagnosis with computed tomographic scanning and a review of the literature. *Surg Neurol* 1985;23:356–361.

190. Wood KB, et al. The natural history of asymptomatic thoracic disc herniations. *Spine* 1997;22:525–530.

191. Wood KB, et al. Thoracic MRI evaluation of asymptomatic individuals. *J Bone Joint Surg* 1995;77A:1634–1638.

192. Gray H. *Gray's Anatomy*. Philadelphia, Pa: Lea and Febiger; 1995.

193. Martucci E, Mele C, Martella P. Thoracic intervertebral disc protrusions. *Ital J Orthop Traumatol* 1984;10:333–339.

194. McKenzie RA. *The Cervical and Thoracic Spine: Mechanical Diagnosis and Therapy*. Waikanae, New Zealand: Spinal Publications New Zealand; 1990.

195. Maiman DJ, et al. Lateral extracavitary approach to the spine for thoracic disc herniation: Report of 23 cases. *Neurosurgery* 1984;14:178–182.

196. Jamieson DRS, Ballantyne JP. Unique presentation of a prolapsed thoracic disk: Lhermitte's symptom in a golf player. *Neurology* 1995;45:1219–1221.

197. Morgenlander JC, Massey EW. Neurogenic claudication with positionally weakness from a thoracic disk herniation. *Neurology* 1989;39:1133–1134.

198. Hamilton MG, Thomas HG. Intradural herniation of a thoracic disc presenting as flaccid paraplegia: Case report. *Neurosurgery* 1990;27:482–484.

199. Kumar R, Buckley TF. First thoracic disc protrusion. *Spine* 1986;11:499–501.

200. Kumar R, Cowie RA. Second thoracic disc protrusions. *Spine* 1992;17:120–121.

201. Bland JH. Diagnosis of thoracic pain syndromes. In: Giles LGF, Singer KP, eds. *Clinical Anatomy and Management of the Thoracic Spine.* Oxford, England: Butterworth-Heinemann; 2000:145–156.

202. Albrand OW, Corkill G. Thoracic disc herniation: Treatment and prognosis. *Spine* 1979;4:41–46.

203. Byrne TN, Waxman SG. *Spinal Cord Compression: Diagnosis and Principles of Management.* Philadelphia, Pa: FA Davis; 1990.

204. Brown CW, et al. The natural history of thoracic disc herniation. *Spine* 1992;17:97–102.

205. Rothman RH, Simeone FA. *The Spine.* 3rd ed. Philadelphia, Pa: Saunders; 1992.

206. Wilbourn AJ, Aminoff MJ. The electrophysiologic examination in patients with radiculopathies. AAEE Minimonograph 32. *Muscle Nerve* 1988;11:1099–1114.

207. Herring SA, Weinstein SM. Electrodiagnosis in sports medicine. *Phys Med Rehabil State Art Rev* 1989;3:809–822.

208. Marinacci AA. A correlation between operative findings in cervical herniated disc with electromyograms and opaque myelograms. *Electromyography* 1966;6:5–20.

209. Eisen A, Aminoff MJ. Somatosensory evoked potentials. In: Aminoff MJ, ed. *Electrodiagnosis in Clinical Neurology.* New York, NY: Churchill Livingstone; 535–573.

210. Johnson EW. *Practical Electromyography.* 2nd ed. Baltimore, Md: Williams and Wilkins; 1988:229–245.

211. Speer KP, Bassett FH. The prolonged burner syndrome. *Am J Sports Med* 1990;18:591–594.

212. Bergfeld JA, Hershman E, Wilbourne A. Brachial plexus injury in sports: A five-year follow-up. *Orthop Trans* 1988;12:743–744.

213. Beurskens AJ, et al. Efficacy of traction for nonspecific low back pain: 12-week and 6-month results of a randomized clinical trial. *Spine* 1997;22:2756–2762.

214. Harris PR. Cervical traction: Review of literature and treatment guidelines. *Phys Ther* 1977;57:910–914.

215. Licht S. *Massage, Manipulation and Traction.* Huntington, NY: E Licht; 1960.

216. Natchev E. *A Manual on Autotraction.* Stockholm, Sweden: Folksam Scientific Council; 1984.

217. Twomey L. Sustained lumbar traction. An experimental study of long spine segments. *Spine* 1985;10:146–149.

218. Zylbergold RS, Piper MC. Cervical spine disorders. A comparison of three types of traction. *Spine* 1985;10:867–871.

219. Reed BV. Effect of high voltage pulsed electrical stimulation on microvascular permeability to plasma proteins: A possible mechanism of minimizing edema. *Phys Ther* 1988;68:491–495.

220. Grieve GP. Neck traction. *Physiotherapy* 1982;68:260–265.

221. Colachis SC, Strohm BR. Cervical traction: Relationship of traction time to varied tractive force with constant angle of pull. *Arch Phys Med Rehabil* 1965;46:815–819.

222. Gartland GJ. A survey of spinal traction. *Br J Phys Med* 1957;20:253–258.

223. Crue BL, Todd EM. The importance of flexion in cervical traction for radiculitis. *USAF Med* 1957;8:374–380.

224. Piva SR, Erhard R, Al-Hugail M. Cervical radiculopathy: A case problem using a decision making algorithm. *J Orthop Sports Phys Ther* 2000;30:745–754.

224a. Wong AMK, Leong CP, Chen CM. The traction angle and intervertebral separation. *Spine* 1992;17:136–138.

225. Deets D, Hands KL, Hopp SS. Cervical traction: A comparison of sitting and supine positions. *Phys Ther* 1977;57:255–261.

225a. Jho HD, Kim WK, Kim MH. Anterior microforaminotomy for treatment of cervical radiculopathy: Part 1—disc-preserving "functional cervical disc surgery." *Neurosurgery* 2002;51:46–53.

225b. Johnson JP, et al. Anterior cervical foraminotomy for unilateral radicular disease. *Spine* 2002;25:905–909.

225c. Robinson RA, Smith GW. Anterolateral cervical disc removal and interbody fusion for cervical disc syndrome. *Bull Johns Hopkins Hosp* 1955;96:223–224.

225d. Cloward RB. The anterior approach for removal of ruptured cervical discs. *J Neurosurg* 1958;15:602–614.

225e. Houser OW, et al. Cervical disk prolapse. *Mayo Clin Proc* 1995;70:939–945.

225f. Jho HD. Anterior microforaminotomy for cervical radiculopathy: Disc preservation technique. In: Rengachary SS, Wilkins RJ, eds. *Neurosurgical Operative Color Atlas,* vol 7. Baltimore, Md: Williams and Wilkins; 1998:43–52.

225g. Jho HD. Microsurgical anterior cervical foraminotomy: A new approach to cervical disc herniation. *J Neurosurg* 1996;84:155–160.

225h. Vroomen PC, de Krom MC, Knottnerus JA. When does the patient with a disc herniation undergo lumbosacral discectomy? *J Neurol Neurosurg Psych* 2000;68:75–79.

225i. Loew F, Caspar W. Surgical approach to lumbar disc herniations. *Adv Stand Neurosurg* 1978;5:153–174.

225j. Mixter WJ, Barr JS Jr. Rupture of the intervertebral disc with involvement of the spinal canal. *N Engl J Med* 1934;211:210–215.

225k. Vucetic N, et al. Diagnosis and prognosis in lumbar disc herniation. *Clin Orthop* 1999;361:116–122.

226. Nordly EJ, Wright PH. Efficacy of chymopapain in chemonucleolysis: A review. *Spine* 1994;19:2578–2583.

227. Wittenberg RH, et al. Five-year results from chemonucleolysis with chymopapain or collagenase: A prospective randomized study. *Spine* 2001;26:1835–1841.

228. Gibson JN, Grant IC, Waddell G. The Cochrane review of surgery for lumbar disc prolapse and degenerative lumbar spondylosis. *Spine* 1999;24:1820–1832.

229. Atlas SJ, et al. The Maine Lumbar Spine Study, Part II: 1-year outcomes of surgical and nonsurgical management of sciatica. *Spine* 1996;21:1777–1786.

230. Hadler NM, Carey PS, Garrett J. The influence of indemnification by workers compensation insurance on recovery from acute back ache. *Spine* 1995;20:2710–2715.

231. Junge A, Dvorak J, Ahrens S. Predictors of bad and good outcome of lumbar disc surgery: A prospective clinical study resulting in recommendations for screening to avoid bad outcomes. *Spine* 1995;20:460–468.

232. Sherk HH, et al. Laser diskectomy. *Orthopedics* 1993;16:573–576.

233. Chen WJ, et al. Surgical treatment of adjacent instability after lumbar spine fusion. *Spine* 2001;26:E519–E524.

234. Malter AD, et al. 5-year reoperation rates after different types of lumbar spine surgery. *Spine* 1998;23:814–820.

235. Vishteh AG, Dickman CA. Anterior lumbar microdiscectomy and interbody fusion for the treatment of recurrent disc herniation. *Neurosurgery* 2001;48:334–337, discussion 338.

236. Harms J, Rolinger H. A one-stage procedure in operative treatment of spondylolistheses: Dorsal traction-reposition and anterior fusion [in German]. *Z Orthop Ihre Grenzgeb* 1982; 120:343–347.

237. Phillips FM, Cunningham B. Intertransverse lumbar interbody fusion. *Spine* 2002;27:E37–E41.

238. Danielsen J, et al. Early aggressive exercise for postoperative rehabilitation after discectomy. *Spine* 2000;25:1015–1020.

239. Johannsen F, et al. Supervised endurance training compared to home training after first lumbar diskectomy: A clinical trial. *Clin Exp Rheumatol* 1994;12:609–614.

240. Kjellby-Wendt G, Styf J. Early active training after lumbar discectomy: a prospective, randomized and controlled trial. *Spine* 1998;23:2345–2351.

241. Skall F, Manniche C, Nielsen C. Intensive back exercises 5 weeks after surgery of lumbar disk prolapse: A prospective randomized multicentre trial with historical control. *Ugeskr Laeger* 1994;156:643–646.

242. Booth FW. Physiologic and biochemical effects of immobilization on muscle. *Clin Orthop Rel Res* 1987;219:15–21.

243. Eiff MP, Smith AT, Smith GE. Early mobilization versus immobilization in the treatment of lateral ankle sprains. *Am J Sports Med* 1994;22:83–88.

244. Akeson WH, et al. Collagen cross-linking alterations in the joint contractures: Changes in the reducible cross-links in periarticular connective tissue after 9 weeks immobilization. *Connect Tissue Res* 1977;5:15.

245. Akeson WH, et al. Effects of immobilization on joints. *Clin Orthop* 1987;219:28–37.

246. Akeson WH, Amiel D, Woo SLY. Immobility effects on synovial joints: The pathomechanics of joint contracture. *Biorheology* 1980;17:95–110.

247. Woo SLY, et al. Connective tissue response to immobility: A correlative study of biochemical and biomechanical measurements of normal and immobilized rabbit knee. *Arthritis Rheum* 1975;18:257–264.

248. White T, Malone T. Effects of running on intervertebral disc height. *J Orthop Sports Phys Ther* 1990;12:410.

249. Malanga GA. The diagnosis and treatment of cervical radiculopathy. *Med Sci Sports Exerc* 1997;29: S236–S245.

250. Donelson R, Silva G, Murphy K. Centralization phenomenon: Its usefulness in evaluating and treating referred pain. *Spine* 1990;15:211–213.

251. Frymoyer JW. Back pain and sciatica. *N Engl J Med* 1988; 318:291–300.

252. Vanharanta H, Videman T, Mooney V. McKenzie exercise, back track and back school in lumbar syndrome. *Orthop Trans* 1986;10:533.

VERTEBRAL ARTERY

CHAPTER OBJECTIVES

▶ *At the completion of this chapter, the reader will be able to:*

1. Describe the anatomy and distribution of the vertebral artery.

2. Describe the four commonly recognized portions of the vertebral artery.

3. Outline the causes of vertebral artery occlusion or compromise.

4. Recognize the characteristics of vertebral artery occlusion or compromise.

5. Describe the various special tests to assess the patency of the vertebrobasilar system.

OVERVIEW

The main circulation of the posterior cranial fossa originates from the vertebrobasilar artery (VBA) system. The first studies of the vertebral artery were recorded as far back as 1844.[1] In 1962, Williams and Wilson[2] provided a detailed description of vertebrobasilar artery compromise, indicating that reversible symptoms were related to an inefficiency of the basilar system.

Since that time, recognition of the importance of the vertebral artery has continued to grow, and it is now discussed in more detail than any other artery by physical therapists. For this reason the vertebral artery is afforded its own chapter. To fully comprehend its significance, a review its anatomy and function is in order.

Anatomy

The vertebral artery appears during the fifth to sixth weeks of intrauterine development, from a posterior costal anastomosis between the upper six cervical and posterolateral intersegmental arteries.[3,4]

Along its course, the artery can be viewed as having four portions: proximal, transverse, suboccipital, and intracranial[5,6] (Fig. 21-1).

The VBA system consists of three key vessels: two vertebral arteries and one basilar artery. The basilar artery is formed by the two vertebral arteries joining each other in the midline.

Proximal Portion

This portion runs from the origin of the artery to its point of entry to the cervical spine. The vertebral artery usually originates from the posterior surface of the subclavian artery, but it can also originate from the aortic arch and common carotid artery.[7]

The vertebral artery runs vertically, slightly medial and posteriorly, lateral to the longus colli and medial to the anterior scalene, to reach the transverse foramen of the lower cervical spine, although its exact direction is dependent on its exact point of origin. Its anomalous origin in this region has been suggested as a potential factor increasing the chance of blood flow compromise due to compression by the longus colli or scalene muscles.

In approximately 88 percent of individuals, the artery enters the C6 transverse foramen, but it has been shown to enter as far superior as the C4 transverse foramen.[8]

Clinical Pearl

Tortuosity and compression of this portion of the artery is common.[6] The tortuosity and compression can be congenital, muscular (resulting from compression by the longus colli and scalene),[9] or a consequence of advancing years.[10]

Transverse Portion

The second portion of the vertebral artery runs from the point of entry at the spinal column to the transverse foramen of C2 (see Fig. 21-1). As already described, the origin of this part of the artery is typically at the C6 level, but this may vary between individuals, and even from side to side in the same individual.

Throughout this section of the spinal column, the artery travels vertically in a true canal called the transverse canal. The transverse canal is formed by the bony transverse foramina at each spinal level, and the overlying anterior and posterior intertransverse muscles, the scaleni and longus coli muscles.

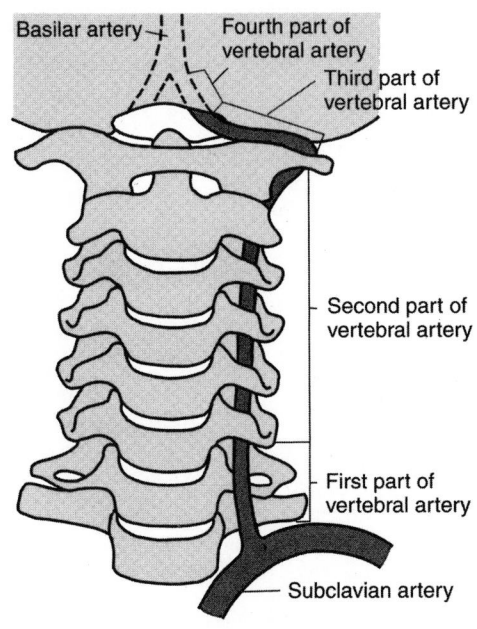

FIGURE 21-1 The four parts of the vertebral artery. (Reproduced with permission from Dutton M. *Manual Therapy of the Spine.* New York, NY: McGraw-Hill; 2002:45.)

The dimension of the transverse canal is proportionate to the diameter of the artery which is itself variable, averaging a diameter of 6 mm, about 1 to 2 mm greater than that of the artery. Within the canal, the artery is surrounded by a periosteal sheath that is adherent to the boundaries of the canal, and affords further protection for the artery. However, the artery is in close proximity to the uncinate processes of each vertebral body on its medial aspect and is prone to compression from osteophyte formation or subluxation from the zygapophysial joint.[6,11] The vertebral artery in the transverse foramen also is adjacent to the anterior spinal roots. Arterial enlargement by an intramural hematoma or a dissecting aneurysm may cause radiculopathy by compressing or stretching the spinal root.[12]

Tortuosity of this portion of the artery also can occur because of an abnormal origin of the artery from the aorta. The tortuosity is characterized by looping within the intervertebral foramina, to the extent of causing pedicle erosion and a widening of the intervertebral foramen with nerve root compression,[13] and even a fracture of the neural arch.

The proximal and suboccipital portions of the artery are more elastic and less muscular than the transverse part.[14] This variation is believed to be an adaptation to the greater mobility required in the proximal and transverse portions of the artery.

Suboccipital Portion

This portion of the artery extends from its exit at the axis to its point of penetration into the spinal canal. This portion can be further subdivided into four parts:

1. Within the transverse foramen of C2 (see Fig. 21-2). This portion lies in a complete bony canal formed by the two curves of the C2 transverse foramen. The inferior curve is almost vertical, whereas the superior curve is more horizontal and orientated laterally.

2. Between C2 and C1 (see Fig. 21-2). The second part runs vertically upward to the transverse foramen of C2. Throughout its journey, it is covered by both the levator scapulae and the inferior oblique capitis muscles. Compression of the vertebral artery may occur in conditions in which these muscles have increased tone or loss of flexibility.[15]

3. In the transverse foramen of C1 (see Fig. 21-2). In its third part, the suboccipital portion of the vertebral artery bends posteriorly and medially in the transverse foramen of C1, in which it is completely enclosed.

4. Between the posterior arch of the atlas and its entry into the foramen magnum (see Fig. 21-2). On exiting from the transverse foramen of C1, the artery and the nerve of C1 wind behind the mass of the superior articular process of the atlas to cross the posterior arch of the atlas in a groove in which the artery is held by a restraining ligament. Anomalies in this portion of the artery include ossification of the restraining ligament of the atlantal groove, turning this into a complete bony tunnel. From the medial end of this groove, the artery runs forward, inward, and upward to pierce the posterior atlanto-occipital membrane (see Fig. 21-2). The artery penetrates the dura mater on the lateral aspect of the foramen magnum about 1.5 cm lateral to the midline of the neck. This upper portion of the extracranial vertebral artery is relatively superficial and covered only by the trapezius, semispinalis, and rectus capitis muscles. Having unyielding bone beneath it, and only muscles above, the artery is vulnerable to direct blunt trauma at this part of its course, whereas in the remainder of its course, it is threatened more by penetrating trauma or disease processes, such as osteophytosis or atherosclerosis.[10,16]

Although the artery is affected by vertebral motion in the lower cervical region, it is affected even more between C2 and the occipital bone.[17]

> ### Clinical Pearl
>
> The vertebral artery is most vulnerable to compression and stretching at the level of C1 to C2, because of the amount of cervical rotation that can occur at the atlanto-axial joint.[18]

In addition, because the transverse foramen of C1 is more lateral than that of C2, the artery must incline laterally between the two vertebrae. At this point, the artery is vulnerable to impingement from:

▶ Abnormal posture.[15]

▶ Excursion of the C1 transverse mass during rotation. Approximately 50 percent of the cervical axial rotation

FIGURE 21-2 The left vertebral artery passing through a ring of bone on the arch of the atlas. (Reproduced with permission from Wilkins RH, Rengachary SS, eds. *Neurosurgery*. New York, NY: McGraw-Hill; 1996:933.)

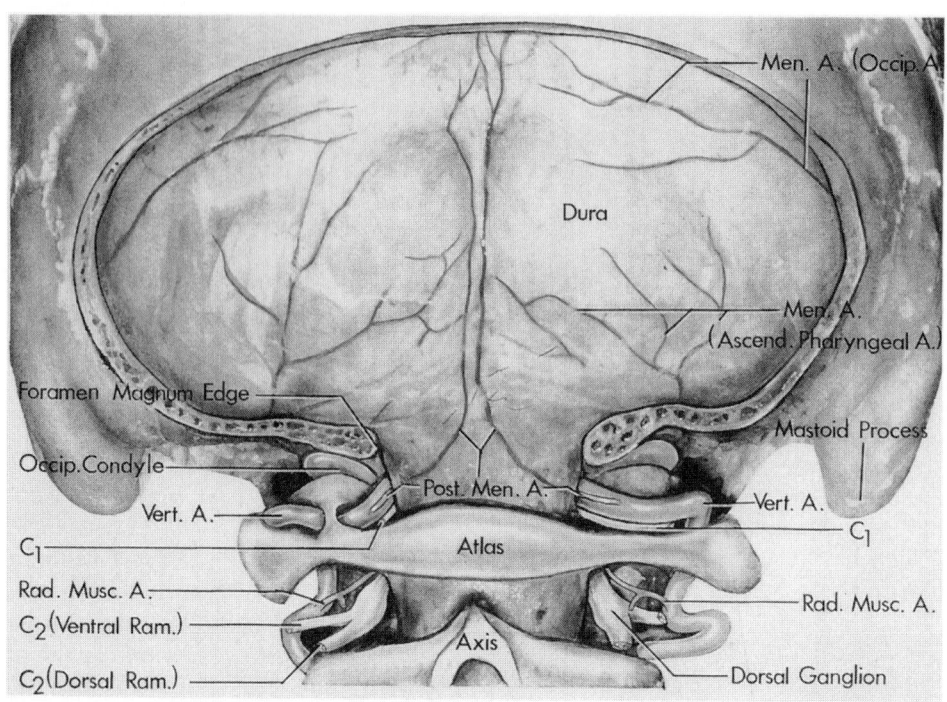

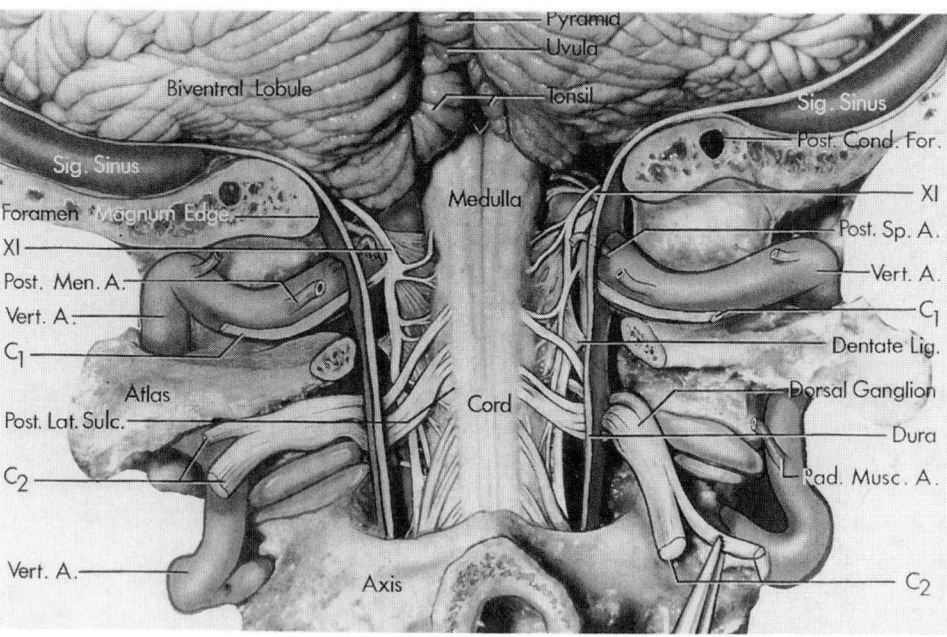

occurs between C1 and C2; hence, there is a large excursion of the transverse mass of C1 with rotation. The artery is stretched during this process, and the size of the lumen can be reduced.[17,19] Any reduction in the size of the lumina is more profound in the presence of arterial disease.

Intracranial Portion

This portion of the vertebral artery runs from its penetration of the dura mater into the arachnoid space at the level of the foramen magnum, to the formation of the basilar artery by the midline union of the two arteries at the lower border of the pons (Fig. 21-3).

FIGURE 21-3   The vertebral and basilar arteries. (Reproduced with permission from Wilkins RH, Rengachary SS, eds. *Neurosurgery.* New York, NY: McGraw-Hill; 1996:936.)

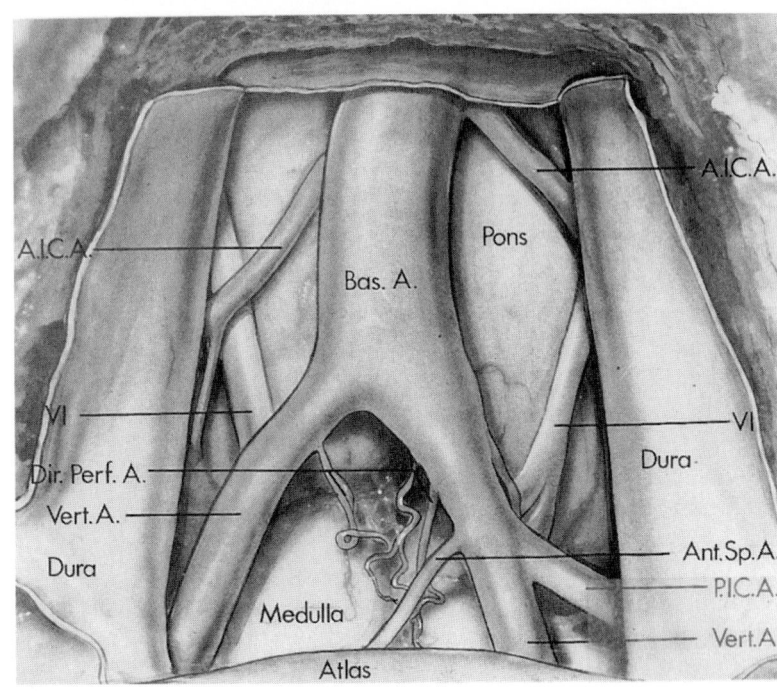

After its penetration of the cranium, the artery inclines medially toward the medulla oblongata. It courses up the front of the medulla to reach the lower border of the pons, where the artery from each side meets and unites with its partner to form the basilar artery. A major change in the structure of the artery occurs as it becomes intracranial.[6] The tunica adventitia and tunica media become thinner, and there is a gross reduction in the number of elastic fibers in these coats.[14] This decrease in elasticity can result in a distortion of the vertebral artery during head extension and rotation.[17,19,22]

Branches

In all, the vertebral arteries contribute about 11 percent of the total cerebral blood flow, the remaining 89 percent being supplied by the carotid system.[23] The vertebral artery gives off both cervical branches and cranial branches.

Cervical Branches

The cervical branches include spinal branches and muscular branches.

Spinal Branches.[12]   The vertebral arteries each give off single branches, which fuse to form the anterior spinal artery (ASA), which descends in the median anterior fissure and is additionally supplied by anterior radicular arteries (typically two to four). Whereas the ASA is bilaterally derived, the anterior radicular arteries may arise exclusively or predominately from one vertebral artery. This helps explain how a unilateral compromise of the vertebral artery may cause bilateral spinal cord infarction.

The paired posterior spinal arteries (PSAs) originate superiorly from the vertebral arteries or posterior inferior cerebellar arteries (PICAs). The PSAs also are supplied by posterior radicular arteries (usually two or three), which themselves arise exclusively or predominately from one vertebral artery, again demonstrating how a unilateral vertebral artery dissection may lead to bilateral spinal cord infarction. The PSAs supply the posterior one fifth to one quarter of the spinal cord, including the posterior columns, the posterior dorsal horns, and parts of the corticospinal and spinothalamic tracts. The ASA is the exclusive arterial supply to the gray matter of the cord. The watershed area between the PSA and ASA encompasses the anterior dorsal horns and part of the corticospinal and spinothalamic tracts.

Muscular Branches.   The muscular branches arise from the suboccipital part of the artery as it winds around the superior articular process of the atlas. They supply the deep suboccipital muscles and anastomose with the occipital and cervical arteries.

Cranial Branches

Intracranially, the vertebral artery first generates small meningeal branches, which supply the bone and dura mater of the cerebellar fossa. It is possible that ischemia of these tissues, which occurs with vertebral artery occlusion, could be responsible for the suboccipital pain that often accompanies damage to the artery.[18]

Anterior Spinal Artery.   Near the termination of the artery, the ASA arises (see Fig. 21-3). This branch unites with its opposite number in the midline and then descends along the anterior median fissure of the spinal cord, receiving reinforcement from the spinal branches of the regional arteries, either vertebral, cervical, or posterior intercostal and lumbar arteries. Together these arteries supply the spinal cord and cauda equina.

Posterior Spinal Artery.   Occasionally, the PSAs (see Fig. 21-2) arise from the vertebral arteries instead of from their more common origin, the PICA. The PSAs descend the length of the spinal cord and cauda equina on the anterior and posterior aspects of the dorsal spinal root on each side. The posterior arteries are reinforced in the same manner as the ASAs but supply less of the surface area of the cord.

Posterior Inferior Cerebellar Artery.   The PICA (see Fig. 21-3) is the largest branch of the vertebral artery, usually being formed opposite the medulla oblongata about 1 cm below the formation of the basilar artery. It supplies, either directly or indirectly, the medulla and cerebellum and, via the PSAs, the dorsal portion of the spinal cord.

Basilar Artery

The formation of the basilar artery at the lower border of the pons marks the termination of the vertebral artery. The basilar artery is formed by the union of the two vertebral arteries and runs in a fissure on the anterior surface of the pons (see Fig. 21-3). Directly, and indirectly, the basilar artery supplies the pons, the visual area of the occipital lobe, the membranous labyrinth, the medulla, the temporal lobe, the posterior thalamus, and the cerebellum.

Vertebral Artery Compromise

Damage and occlusion of the vertebral arteries is felt to occur because of the close proximity of the vertebral artery and the bony and ligamentous structures of the cervical spine.[23a] Trauma to this area may lead to thrombosis, dissection, transection, transmural hematoma, pseudoaneurysm, and spasm of the vertebral artery. Vertebral artery compromise may also occur because of atherosclerotic involvement of the artery, sickle cell disease (see Chap. 9), rheumatoid arthritis, arterial fibroplasias, an arteriovenous fistula, and a number of congenital syndromes.

Whatever the cause of vertebral artery compromise, the diagnosis requires a high index of suspicion for prompt recognition and intervention.

Occlusion

The vertebral artery is subject to occlusion from external and internal causes.

External Causes

Extracranial compression of the vertebral artery may cause neurologic symptoms, depending on the acuteness of the occlusion or the presence of underlying pathologic conditions, such as atherosclerosis, sickle cell disease, fibromuscular dysplasia, rheumatoid arthritis, or osteogenesis imperfecta.

The vertebral artery is particularly vulnerable to compression in the portion that courses through the foramina transversaria from C6 to C1. Because of its fixation to the spine in this segment, subluxations of one vertebral body on another may exert undue tension and traction on the artery. Positions of the cervical spine can cause compression of the vertebral artery.[22,29] Rotation-extension-traction appears to be the most stressful, followed by rotation-extension, rotation alone, side flexion alone, extension alone, and then flexion.[22,29,30]

Unilateral occlusion of the vertebral artery rarely results in a neurologic deficit, because of the collateral supply through the contralateral vertebral and posterior inferior cerebellar arteries.[31]

Clinical Pearl

The most common mechanism for nonpenetrating trauma injury to the vertebral artery is hyperextension of the neck, with or without rotation, or cervical side flexion.[32,33] These motions can result in stretching and tearing of the intima and media, especially at the points where the artery is tethered to a bone.[27,34]

After the primary tear of the intima, blood flows into the arterial wall between the intima and media, causing an intramural hematoma and thickening of the vessel wall. Subintimal hemorrhage can produce various degrees of stenosis; subadventitial hemorrhage can cause a pseudoaneurysm. Tearing of the artery is not always related to remarkable trauma, and so this aspect may not appear in the history unless the symptoms appear immediately following the injury. The presence of a pseudoaneurysm has been a commonly noted angiographic feature following sudden head and neck movements. In this injury, the two internal coats of the vertebral artery are torn from the tunica adventitia, which, under the influence of arterial pressure, slowly balloons out and sometimes ruptures.

There appear to be inherently weaker areas of the vertebral artery, which are subjected to great stresses during the aforementioned movements of the head. These are located[37]:

▶ At its entry point into the transverse foramen of C6.

▶ Anywhere in the bone canal secondary to fracture dislocations of the spine.

▶ Between C1 and C2. As discussed, among the possible reasons for the preponderance of lesions at this level is the large range of motion available at the atlanto-axial joint.[38] If the main restraint to atlanto-axial rotation, the alar ligament. is ruptured, the degree of this movement has been shown to increase by 30 percent.[39] Insufficiency of the alar ligament has been shown to follow rear-end collision motor vehicle accidents, and it may also exist because of a congenital defect of the dens.[40] Other contributing factors to the preponderance of lesions occurring at the second cervical joint level are the fixation of the periosteal sheath of the artery to the dura mater, the superficiality of the artery in this region, and the hard neural arch beneath the artery.

▶ During its course from the foramen of C1 to its entry point into the skull, as a result of direct trauma.

Dissection. Extracranial vertebral artery dissection is recognized with increasing frequency as a cause of stroke, and spontaneous dissections of the carotid and vertebral arteries are well-recognized causes of a stroke in young and middle-aged adults.[41–44] Traumatic dissection can also occur in the extracranial part of the internal carotid arteries, often after only moderate blunt trauma.[45]

Postmortem studies have shown that neurologic deficits, or even death, have followed posterior neck injuries by up to 8 days after the accident.[47,48] The most common clinical findings are brain stem or cerebellar ischemic symptoms preceded by severe neck pain or occipital headache, or both. Occasionally, these patients report radicular symptoms.[42]

Activities Associated with Dissection of the Vertebral Artery. A number of various, but normal, activities have been shown to produce dissection of the vertebral artery, mostly in concert with underlying predisposing factors, such as atherosclerosis and congenital anomalies, but a few apparently occurring in isolation.[36,49–54]

Cervical Manipulation and Stroke. Spinal manipulation, in particular manipulation of the upper spine, has been associated with serious adverse occurrences, including dissection of the vertebral[55] and internal carotid artery,[56] resulting in strokes[57] and at least 1 death.[58] However, the evidence implicating cervical manipulations with these serious consequences is conflicting, especially in light of the fact that even normal neck movements have been associated with spontaneous dissections. The reciprocal finding of increased blood flow through the carotid artery during vertebral artery occlusion was made by Stern,[59] who demonstrated that the flow rate in the contralateral carotid artery increased by one and half to two times with experimental occlusion of the vertebral artery. These alterations in the flow rates following an occlusion of the parallel artery serve as an apparent safety mechanism and may explain why more patients are not injured during cervical manipulation.

Despite the reports of 115 cases of cerebrovascular accidents after manipulation in English language publications during the period of 1966 to 1998 (198 articles), there is virtually no detailed information on the magnitude of forces that were exerted or the type of procedure used. It has been suggested that, in many cases, cervical manipulation may have been administered to patients who already had spontaneous dissection in progress.[62]

Internal Causes

Atherosclerosis and Thrombosis. Atherosclerosis of the extracranial part of the vertebral artery primarily affects the proximal and transverse portions, leaving the suboccipital part relatively free. Atherosclerosis in the transverse portion of the artery occurs at any level between C2 and C6 and tends to occur at levels of the artery opposite osteophytic spurs. Castaigne and colleagues[63] investigated 44 patients with vertebrobasilar artery occlusions, and found that the cause in almost 90 percent of cases was atherosclerosis, mostly affecting the proximal and intracranial portions of the artery. Approximately 40 percent of the patients in this study had concomitant carotid stenosis.

Atherosclerosis may, as with any other artery, produce signs and symptoms resulting from ischemia of the tissues supplied by the artery distal to the occlusion. However, if the contralateral artery is not occluded, and is of good caliber, the condition may be asymptomatic.

Thrombosis can occur at any level of the vertebral artery, but is more common in the suboccipital and intracranial portions than in the transverse part.[64]

Arterial Fibrodysplasia. This condition is a nonatheromatous, noninflammatory segmental angiopathy of unknown etiology. Its occurs in less than 1 percent of all patients receiving cerebral angiograms but is the third most frequent structural lesion affecting the vertebral artery following atherosclerosis and dissection.[65] Arterial fibrodysplasia is believed to be hereditary, affecting mainly young and middle-aged female patients.

Klippel-Trenaunay Syndrome. Klippel-Trenaunay syndrome consists of a constellation of anomalies, including capillary malformation, varicose veins or venous malformations, and hypertrophy of both bony and soft tissues primarily involving limbs and, to a much lesser degree, intra-abdominal, thoracic, or facial structures.[66,67] The vascular abnormalities commonly occur in the lower extremity but have been observed in other areas as well (head, neck, buttocks, abdomen, chest, and oral cavity). Klippel-Trenaunay syndrome is theorized to result from a mesodermal abnormality.[68] The syndrome is diagnosed on the basis of presence of any two of the three aforementioned features, and any intervention is based on the severity of these features.

Arteriovenous Fistulas. An arteriovenous fistula is an abnormal communication between the extracranial vertebral artery, or one its muscular or radicular branches, and an adjacent vein. It has variable causes, including traumatic dissections or dissecting aneurysms, and may occur spontaneously as a result of existing disease, such as fibromuscular dysplasia, or as a congenital condition. Most spontaneous arteriovenous fistulas occur at the level of C2 to C3 and come directly from the vertebral artery through what is believed to be a tiny rupture in the wall of the artery.[69,70] Although rare, progressive myelopathy from an intracranial arteriovenous fistula can occur.[71] In these cases, endovascular embolization, either alone or followed by surgery, is the intervention of choice.

The Clinical Manifestations of Vertebrobasilar Compromise

The clinical manifestations of vertebrobasilar compromise are difficult to distinguish from other causes of brainstem ischemia (see later), and can be subtle, intermittent, and even chronic in nature. Indeed, no single consistent pattern of neurologic signs and symptoms is pathognomonic for vertebral artery compromise. The most common presenting symptoms are vertigo, nausea, and headache.[72,73,73a,73b]

> **Clinical Pearl**
>
> Early signs of vertebral artery insufficiency include vertigo, nausea, and headache.

Vertigo. Vertigo or dizziness is a commonly reported symptom.[73,73a,73b] The examination of patients with vertigo in re-lation to vertebral artery compromise must be centered on the differentiation between central and peripheral vestibular dysfunction and cervical vertigo. Central vestibular dysfunction refers to involvement of the central processing components of the vestibular system such as the cerebellum and brainstem. Peripheral vestibular dysfunction refers to a dysfunction of the vestibular nerve and end organs. The term cervical vertigo describes the nonvestibular pathogenesis of this symptom.[73c,73d] Tatlow and Bammer[73c] proved that the cause of the vertigo in patients with vertebral artery compromise was cervical rather than vestibular. This was accomplished by placing symptomatic patients into a Stryker bed to determine whether the vertigo symptoms were being elicited by movement of the entire body, or by the movement of the head relative to the torso. Each patient that was secured within the Stryker bed had the entire body rotated up to a full 360 degrees en bloc (without movement of the head and neck relative to the torso), and the patients reported no symptoms. However, when the torso was fixed in a still position but the head and neck was moved relative to the torso, symptoms were reproduced.

Nausea. Nausea is an uneasiness of the stomach that often accompanies the urge to vomit, but doesn't always lead to the forcible voluntary or involuntary emptying of stomach contents through the mouth (vomiting). Nausea is the accompanying symptom for many different conditions, including infection, food poisoning, motion sickness, blocked intestine, illness, concussion or brain injury, appendicitis, central nervous system disorders, brain tumors, migraines, and vertebral artery compromise.

Headache. The headache associated with vertebrobasilar compromise is typically a unilateral occipital headache with associated vertigo and nausea.[73e] The pain is usually sharp and acute in its onset located on the same side as the compromise.

In addition to vertigo, nausea and headache, the following signs and symptoms have also been linked, both directly and indirectly, to vertebral artery insufficiency:[73e,26,27,73f,73g]

- ▶ Wallenberg's, Horner's, and similar syndromes.
- ▶ Bilateral or quadrilateral paresthesia.
- ▶ Hemiparesthesia.
- ▶ Ataxia.
- ▶ Scotoma (a permanent or temporary area of depressed or absent vision.)
- ▶ Nystagmus.
- ▶ Drop attack (a sudden loss of postural tone without loss of consciousness).
- ▶ Periodic loss of consciousness.
- ▶ Lip anesthesia.
- ▶ Hemifacial paralysis/anesthesia.

▶ Hyperreflexia.

▶ Positive Babinski, Hoffman, or Oppenheim signs.

▶ Clonus.

▶ Dysphasia.

▶ Dysarthria.

Clinicians need to be aware of these signs and symptoms and consider vertebral artery dissection early in the differential diagnosis because of the potential devastating neurological consequences, and in order to decrease morbidity and mortality.[73e]

Imaging Studies

Conventional angiography has long been the gold standard in the diagnosis of arterial and venous pathology in the neck. Angiography can show the arterial lumen and allows extensive characterization of dissections of the carotid and vertebral arteries.[82] Vertebral artery angiography is not, however, without risk. It is invasive and expensive. Magnetic resonance angiography (MRA) techniques are less invasive and are replacing conventional angiography as the gold standard in the diagnosis of dissections of the carotid and vertebral arteries. MRA is highly sensitive and specific in identifying stenoses and occlusions and can show the intramural hematoma itself.[83]

Ultrasonographic techniques are useful in the initial assessment of patients who are thought to have a dissection of the carotid artery.[84] Doppler sonography allows a direct visualization of the vascular tree while assessing blood flow velocity and pressure waveforms. Although the site of dissection generally is not seen, an abnormal pattern of flow is identified in more than 90 percent of patients.[84]

Vertebral Artery Examination

The testing of the vertebral artery has been a routine part of patient screening by manual therapists for many years, being first described by Maitland in 1968.[75]

A positive vertebral artery test is one in which signs or symptoms change, especially if the changes evoked include those previously mentioned. More subtle examination findings can include a significant delay in verbal responses to questions of orientation, with some inconsistency of answers; changes in pupil size; and nystagmus.[18]

It is widely recognized that passive therapeutic maneuvers applied to the cervical spine carry a small risk of iatrogenic stroke. This is especially pertinent with regard to cervical manipulations (Grade V techniques). Traditionally, clinicians have relied solely on existing manual pre-manipulative tests (see below) to determine the appropriateness of a Grade V technique, although it is not clear how sensitive these tests are.[76,77]

Ideally, before a Grade V technique is performed, more specific tests should be performed on the patient to investigate vertebral artery flow. These tests include Doppler sonography or a magnetic resonance angiography (MRA) scan (see "Imaging Studies" later).[77a] Grade V techniques should never be performed when slow blood flow of the vertebral artery is displayed on neck Doppler sonography or MRA scan.[77a]

In those cases where the clinician is to perform cervical mobilizations of Grade I–IV, rather than a Grade V thrust technique, the Australian Physiotherapy Association's Protocol for Pre-manipulative Testing of the Cervical Spine is recommended.[78] This protocol was one of the first formalized protocols designed to prevent strokes as a result of cervical manual techniques. The protocol recommends that the clinician should maintain the immediate pre-mobilization position for a minimum of 10 seconds to test the patency of the vertebrobasilar system. Others recommend assessing the patient's responses for a further 10 seconds to note any latent response.[20,31] Clinical testing of the vertebral artery should stop once positive signs or symptoms are noted. Throughout the tests, the clinician should observe the patient's eyes for possible nystagmus or changes in pupil size, and should have the patient count backward to assess their quality of speech. The patient is asked to report any changes in symptoms, however insignificant he or she may feel the changes to be.

A number of other recognized tests that may be used to assess the patency of the vertebral artery are described next.

Manual Tests

Initial Test
The initial test consists of having the patient rotate the head to each side while in sitting position. The longus colli and scalene muscles rotate the cervical spine and can squeeze the vertebral artery on the side contralateral to the rotation.[15] The presence of muscular compression of the artery can be further tested by combining cervical flexion with rotation to place the inferior oblique capitis on stretch.[15]

Barre's Test
Barre's test can be used to test for vertebral artery insufficiency, especially if the patient is unable to lie supine.

The patient is seated with the arms outstretched, forearms supinated. The patient is asked to close his or her eyes and move the head and neck into maximum extension and rotation. A positive test is one in which one of the outstretched arms sinks toward the floor and pronates, indicating the side of the compromise.

Hautard's (Hautant's, Hautart, or Hautarth) Test[79,80]
As with Barre's test, proprioceptive loss rather than dizziness is sought in Hautard's test. The test has two parts. The patient is seated. Both arms are actively flexed to 90 degrees at the shoulders. The eyes are then closed for a few seconds while the clinician observes for any loss of position of one or both arms. If the arms move, the proprioception loss has a nonvascular cause. If the first part of the test is negative, the patient is asked to extend and rotate the neck. Because the second part of the test is performed to elicit a vascular cause for the dizziness, the eyes can be open or closed. Having the eyes open allows the clinician to observe for nystagmus and changes in pupil size.

Each position is held for 10 to 30 seconds. If wavering of the arms occurs with the second part of the test, a vascular cause for the symptoms is suspected.

Cervical Quadrant Test[75]

The patient is positioned supine. The supine position is reported to result in an increase in passive motion at the cervical spine compared with sitting and may, therefore, better test the ability of the vertebral artery to sustain a stretch. The clinician passively moves the patient's head into extension and side bending. Maintaining this position, the clinician rotates the patient's head to the same side as the side bending and holds it there for 30 seconds. A positive test is one in which referring symptoms are produced if the opposite artery is involved.

DeKleyn-Nieuwenhuyse Test[81]

The patient is positioned supine. The clinician passively moves the patient's head into extension and rotation. A positive test is one in which referring symptoms are produced if the opposite artery is involved. Despite its widespread appearance in a number of texts, this test is not recommended because of the severe traction stresses it places on the vertebral artery.[80]

Progressive Testing

A series of progressive tests may be used to assess the patency of the vertebral artery. The vertebral artery is more vulnerable to compression in the region of the upper cervical spine than in the lower region.

Upper Part.   The patient is positioned supine lying, with the head supported over the edge of the table, and the clinician stands at the patient's head, facing the shoulders. With one hand, the clinician supports the mid and lower cervical spine while the other hand supports the occiput (Fig. 21-4).

1. Maintaining the lower and the midcervical spine in a neutral position, the clinician extends the craniovertebral region, holding this position for 30 seconds, and noting any symptoms or signs produced.

2. The clinician adds a compression force through the cranium and holds this force for 30 seconds, noting any symptoms or signs produced.

3. The clinician rotates the craniovertebral region to the left, holding this position for 30 seconds, and noting any symptoms or signs produced (see Fig. 21-4).

This test is repeated with the craniovertebral region rotated to the right.

Lower Part.   After a rest period of approximately 10 seconds, the patient's head is positioned so that it is resting on the table without a pillow. As before, the clinician stands at the patient's head, facing the shoulders. With one hand, the clinician palpates the cervicothoracic junction while the other hand palpates the cranium and craniovertebral joints (Fig. 21-5).

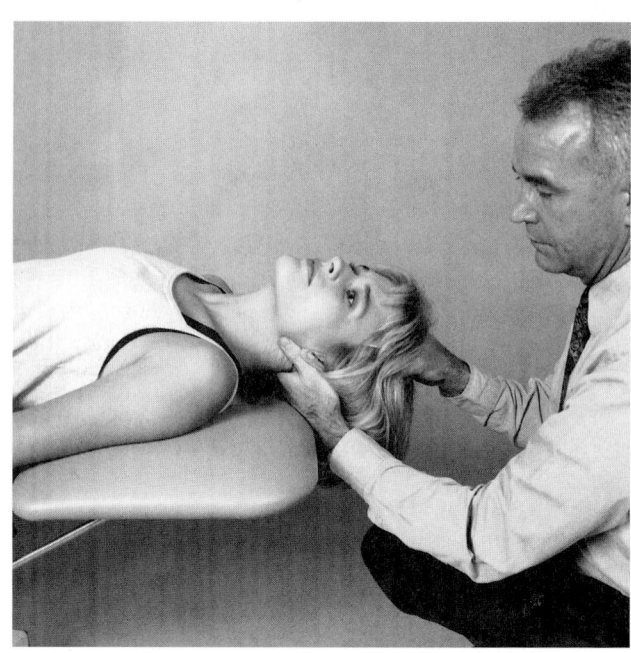

FIGURE 21-4   The upper vertebral artery test.

1. The clinician fixes the cervicothoracic junction and craniovertebral region and extends the mid and lower cervical spine. This position is held for 30 seconds, and a note is made of any symptoms or signs produced.

2. From this maximally extended position, the clinician rotates the mid-cervical spine to the left (see Fig. 21-5) and holds this position for 30 seconds, noting any symptoms or signs produced.

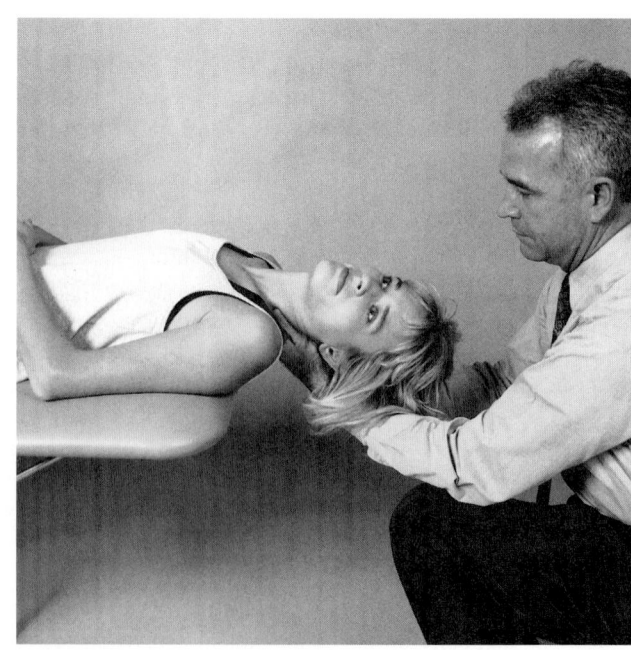

FIGURE 21-5   The lower vertebral artery test.

3. From the position of extension and left rotation, the clinician applies a traction force through the midcervical spine. This position is held for 30 seconds, and a note is made of any symptoms or signs produced.

This test is repeated with the cervical spine extended, with right rotation and traction.

Clinical Pearl

Following a positive vertebral artery test or positive responses in the history, the patient must be handled very carefully, and further intervention, particularly manipulation of the cervical spine, should not be delivered. The patient should not, under any circumstance, be allowed to leave the clinic until his or her physician has been contacted, and until the necessary arrangements have been made for the safe transport of the patient to an appropriate facility.

CASE STUDY THE DIZZY PATIENT[35]

The following case study illustrates the common history and findings for a vertebrobasilar artery insufficiency.

HISTORY

A 62-year-old woman with no history of vertigo or dizziness reported to the clinic for her scheduled physical therapy session for cervical degenerative joint disease. During the course of conversation, the patient reported experiencing dizziness after a shampoo treatment of her hair at a hairdressing salon. She had visited her hairdresser earlier that day and reported severe vertigo, occipital pain, difficulty standing, and a periodic numbness of the right arm and leg. The patient also reported hypesthesia in a glove-and-stocking type of distribution.

TESTS AND MEASURES

Most of the findings of the physical therapy examination were negative. Although deep tendon reflexes and muscle power were normal, disturbances of equilibrium were noted, and nystagmus was present.[85] Given the presence of the nystagmus, the patient was referred back to her physician for further testing.

Following magnetic resonance angiography, a diagnosis was made of vertebrobasilar artery insufficiency with cerebellar infarction caused by neck hyperextension in the hairdressing salon. The patient was treated conservatively with rest and medication, and the vertigo improved 1 week after injury, enabling the patient to walk without assistance.

DISCUSSION

Beauty parlor stroke syndrome was first described by Weintraub[86] in 1993. Since then, various authors have reported similar cases.[87,88] Because this syndrome is not recognized widely, a careful history is necessary in the presence of symptoms such as those described. Such symptoms are often thought to be nonspecific and might be attributed to neurosis, psychogenic headache, or menopause, particularly when imaging studies do not show specific findings. Routine radiography, computed tomography, and MRI studies usually do not help to identify lesions in this syndrome. Special care is therefore necessary to evaluate the clinical findings during examination of the nervous and auditory systems for back lifting or cerebellum dysfunction.

The most likely pathophysiologic mechanism of the beauty parlor stroke syndrome is stenosis of the vertebral artery caused by compression at the atlanto-occipital junction. This compression leads to damage of the intima, thrombus formation, stenosis of the artery by fibrosis, or embolism, followed by infarction of the brain stem or cerebellum.

REVIEW QUESTIONS*

1. From which artery does the vertebral artery normally arise?
2. What is the most common variation in the origin of the vertebral artery?
3. Describe the course of the third part of the artery (suboccipital).
4. List the branches generated directly by the basilar artery.
5. Which of the cranial nerves is (are) not vascularized by the vertebral artery?

---

* Additional questions to test your understanding of this chapter can be found in the Online Learning Center for *Orthopaedic Assessment, Evaluation, and Intervention* at www.duttononline.net.

REFERENCES

1. Quain R. *The Anatomy of the Arteries of the Human Body and Its Application to Pathology and Operative Surgery, with a Series of Lithographic Drawings.* London, England: Taylor and Walton; 1844.
2. Williams D, Wilson T. The diagnosis of the major and minor syndromes of basilar insufficiency. *Brain* 1962;85:741–744.
3. Padget DH. The development of cranial arteries in the human embryo. *Contrib Embryol* 1948;32:205–262.
4. Cavdar S, Arisan E. Variations in the extracranial origin of the human vertebral artery. *Acta Anat* 1989;135:236.
5. George B, Laurian C. *The Vertebral Artery: Pathology and Surgery.* New York, NY: Springer-Verlag Wien; 1987:6–22.
6. Thiel HW. Gross morphology and pathoanatomy of the vertebral arteries. *J Manipulative Physiol Ther* 1991;14:133–141.
7. Gray H. *Gray's Anatomy.* Philadelphia, Pa: Lea and Febiger; 1995.
8. Rieger P, Huber G. Fenestration and duplicate origin of the left vertebral artery in angiography. *Neuroradiology* 1983;25:45–50.
9. Powers SR, Drislane TM, Nevins S. Intermittent vertebral artery compression: A new syndrome. *Surgery* 1961;49:257–264.
10. Hadley LA. Tortuosity and deflection of the vertebral artery. *AMR* 1958;80:306–312.
11. Sheehan S, Bauer RB, Meyer JS. Vertebral artery compression in cervical spondylosis. *Neurology* 1960;10:968–986.
12. Crum B, Mokri B, Fulgham J. Spinal manifestations of vertebral artery dissection. *Neurology* 2000;55:304–306.
13. Anderson RE, Sheally CN. Cervical pedicle erosion and rootlet compression caused by a tortuous vertebral artery. *Radiology* 1970;96:537–538.

14. Wilkinson IMS. The vertebral artery: Extra and intra-cranial structure. *Arch Neurol* 1972;27:393–396.
15. Aspinall W. Clinical testing for cervical mechanical disorders which produce ischemic vertigo. *J Orthop Sports Phys Ther* 1989;11:176–182.
16. Cooper DF. Bone erosion of the cervical vertebrae secondary to tortuosity of the vertebral artery. *J Neurosurg* 1980;53:106–108.
17. DeKleyn A, Nieuwenhuyse P. Schwindelanfaalle und Nystagumus bei einer bestimmeten Lage des Kopfes. *Acta Otolaryngol* 1927;11:155–157.
18. Feudale F, Liebelt E. Recognizing vertebral artery dissection in children: A case report. *Pediatr Emerg Care* 2000;16:184–188.
19. Tatlow TWF, Bammer HG. Syndrome of vertebral artery compression. *Neurology* 1957;7:331–340.
20. Fast A, Zincola DF, Marin EL. Vertebral artery damage complicating cervical manipulation. *Spine* 1987;12:840.
21. Ouchi H, Ohara I. Extracranial abnormalities of the vertebral artery detected by selective arteriography. *J Cardiovasc Surg* 1973;18:250–261.
22. Toole J, Tucker S. Influence of head position upon cerebral circulation. *Arch Neurol* 1960;2:616–623.
23. Hardesty WH, et al. Studies on vertebral artery blood flow in man. *Surg Gyn Obstet* 1963;116:662.
23a. Giacobetti FB, et al. Vertebral artery occlusion associated with cervical spine trauma. *Spine* 1997;22:188–192.
24. Franke JP, et al. Les artéres vertébrales. Segments atlanto-axoidiens V3 et intra-cranien V4 collatérales. *Anat Clin* 1980;2:229.
25. Newton TH, Potts DG. Radiology of the skull and brain. In: *Angiography* (Books 1,3,4). St Louis: Mosby; 1974.
26. Kubernick M, Carmody R. Vertebral artery transection from blunt trauma treated by embolization. *J Trauma* 1984;24:854–856.
27. Auer RN, Krcek J, Butt JC. Delayed symptoms and death after minor head trauma with occult vertebral artery injury. *J Neurol Neurosurg Psychiatry* 1994;57:500–502.
28. Woolsey RM, Hyung CG. Fatal basilar artery occlusion following cervical spine injury. *Paraplegia* 1980;17:280–283.
29. Brown BSJ, Tissington-Tatlow WF. Radiographic studies of the vertebral arteries in cadavers. *Radiology* 1963;81:80–88.
30. Haynes MJ. Doppler studies comparing the effects of cervical rotation and lateral flexion on vertebral artery blood flow. *J Manipulative Physiol Ther* 1996;19:378–384.
31. Golueke P, Sclafani S, Phillips T. Vertebral artery injury—Diagnosis and management. *J Trauma* 1987;27:856–865.
32. Hayes P, Gerlock AJ, Cobb CA. Cervical spine trauma: A cause of vertebral artery injury. *J Trauma* 1980;20:904–905.
33. Schwarz N, et al. Injuries of the cervical spine causing vertebral artery trauma: Case reports. *J Trauma* 1991;31:127–133.
34. Bose B, Northrup BE, Osterholm JL. Delayed vertebrobasilar insufficiency following cervical spine injury. *Spine* 1985;10:108–110.
35. Endo K, et al. Cervical vertigo after hair shampoo treatment at a hairdressing salon: A case report. *Spine* 2000;25:632.
36. Nagler W. Vertebral artery obstruction by hyperextension of the neck: Report of three cases. *Arch Phys Med Rehabil* 1973;54:237–240.
37. Miyachi S, et al. Cerebellar stroke due to vertebral artery occlusion after cervical spine trauma: Two case reports. *Spine* 1994;19:83–89.
38. Panjabi M, et al. Three-dimensional movement of the upper cervical spine. *Spine* 1988;13:727.
39. Panjabi M, et al. Flexion, extension, and lateral bending of the upper cervical spine in response to alar ligament transections. *J Spinal Disord* 1991;4:157–167.
40. Jónsson H Jr, et al. Findings and outcome in whiplash-type neck distortions. *Spine* 1994;19:2733–2743.
41. Hart RG, Easton JD. Dissections. *Stroke* 1985;16:925–927.
42. Caplan LR, Zarins C, Hemmatti M. Spontaneous dissection of the extracranial vertebral artery. *Stroke* 1985;16:1030–1038.
43. Biller J, et al. Cervicocephalic arterial dissections. A ten-year experience. *Neurol Clin* 1986;1:155–182.
44. Mas JL, et al. Extracranial vertebral artery dissections: A review of 13 cases. *Stroke* 1987;18:1037–1047.
45. Mokri B. Traumatic and spontaneous extracranial internal carotid artery dissections. *J Neurol* 1990;237:356–361.
46. Biousse V, D'Anglejan J, Touboui PJ. Headache in 67 patients with extracranial internal carotid artery dissection. *Cephalalgia* 1991;11(suppl):232–233.
47. Schmitt HP, Gladisch R. Multiple Frakturen des Atlas mit zweizeitiger todlicher Vertebralisthrombose nach Schleudertrauma der Halswirbelsaule. Arch Orthop Unfall Chir 1977;87:235–244.
48. Schneider RC, Schemm GW. Vertebral artery insufficiency in acute and chronic spinal trauma. *J Neurosurg* 1961;18:348–360.
49. Sherman DG, Hart RG, Easton JD. Abrupt change in head position and cerebral infarction. *Stroke* 1981;12:2–6.
50. Hanus SH, Homer TD, Harter DH. Vertebral artery occlusion complicating yoga exercises. *Arch Neurol* 1977;34:574–575.
51. Russell WR. Yoga and vertebral artery injuries. *BMJ* 1972;1:685–690.
52. Biousse V, et al. Roller-coaster-induced vertebral artery dissection. *Lancet* 1995;346:767.
53. Goldstein SJ. Dissecting hematoma of the cervical vertebral artery. Case report. *J Neurosurg* 1982;56:451–454.
54. Wechsler B, Kim H, Hunter J. Trampolines, children, and strokes. *Am J Phys Med Rehabil* 2001;80:608–613.
55. Hillier CEM, Gross MLP. Sudden onset vomiting and vertigo following chiropractic neck manipulation. *J Postgrad Med* 1998;74:567–568.
56. Peters M, et al. Dissection of the internal carotid artery after chiropractic manipulation of the neck. *Neurology* 1995;45:2284–2286.
57. Jeret JS, Bluth MB. Stroke following chiropractic manipulation: Report of 3 cases and review of the literature. *J Neuroimaging* 2000;10:52.
58. Klougart N, Leboeuf-Yde C, Rasmussen LR. Safety in chiropractic practice, part 1: The occurrence of cerebrovascular accidents after manipulation to the neck in Denmark from 1978–1988. *J Manipulative Physiol Ther* 1996;19:371–377.
59. Stern WE. Circulatory adequacy attendant upon carotid artery occlusion. *Arch Neurol* 1969;21:455–465.
60. Assendelft WJ, Bouter SM, Knipschild PG. Complications of spinal manipulation: A comprehensive review of the literature. *J Fam Pract* 1996;42:475–480.
61. Dvorak J, Orelli F. How dangerous is manipulation to the cervical spine? Case report and results of a survey. *Man Med* 1985;2:1–4.
62. Haldeman S, Kohlbeck FJ, McGregor M. Risk factors and precipitating neck movements causing vertebrobasilar artery dissection after cervical trauma and spinal manipulation. *Spine* 1999;24:785–794.
63. Castaigne P, et al. Arterial occlusions in the vertebro-basilar system. A study of 44 patients with post-mortem data. *Brain* 1973;96:133–154.

64. Viktrup L, Knudsen GM, Hansen SH. Delayed onset of fatal basilar thrombotic embolus after whiplash injury. *Stroke* 1995; 26:2194–2196.

65. Stanley JC, et al. Extracranial internal carotid and vertebral artery fibrodysplasia. *Arch Surg* 1974;109:215–222.

66. Klippel M, Trenaunay P. Du naevus variqueux osteohypertrophique. *Arch Gen Med* 1900;185:641.

67. Capraro PA, et al. Klippel-Trenaunay syndrome. *Plast Reconstr Surg* 2002;109:2052–2060.

68. Baskerville PA, Ackroyd JS, Browse NL. The etiology of the Klippel-Trenaunay syndrome. *Ann Surg* 1985;202:624.

69. Van Dijk JM, et al. Clinical course of cranial dural arteriovenous fistulas with long-term persistent cortical venous reflux. *Stroke* 2002;33:1233–1236.

70. Nair R, et al. Spontaneous arteriovenous fistula resulting from HIV arteritis. *J Vasc Surg* 2001;33:186–187.

71. Partington MD, et al. Cranial and sacral dural arteriovenous fistulas as a cause of myelopathy. *J Neurosurg* 1992;76:615–622.

72. Ferbert A, Bruckmann H, Drummen R. Clinical features of proven basilar artery occlusion. *Stroke* 1990;21:1135–1142.

73. Aspinall W. Clinical testing for cervical mechanical disorders which produce ischemic vertigo. *J Orthop Sports Phys Ther* 1989;11:176–182.

73a. Fisher CM. Vertigo in cerebrovascular disease. *Arch Otolaryngol* 1967;85:529–534.

73b. Troost BT. Dizziness and vertigo in vertebrobasilar disease. *Stroke* 1980;11:413–415.

73c. Tatlow TWF, Bammer HG. Syndrome of vertebral artery compression. *Neurology* 1957;7:331–340.

73d. Ryan GMS, Cope S. Cervical vertigo. *Lancet* 1955;2:1355.

73e. Auer RN, Krcek J, Butt JC. Delayed symptoms and death after minor head trauma with occult vertebral artery injury. *J Neurol Neurosurg Psychiatry* 1994;57:500–502.

73f. Woolsey RM, Hyung CG. Fatal basilar artery occlusion following cervical spine injury. *Paraplegia* 1980;17:280–283.

73g. Pettman E. Stress tests of the craniovertebral joints. In: *Grieve's Modern Manual Therapy: The Vertebral Column,* Boyling JD, Palastanga N. eds. Edinburgh: Churchill Livingstone; 1994; 529–538.

74. Oas JG, Baloh RW. Vertigo and the anterior inferior cerebellar artery syndrome. *Neurology* 1992;42:2274–2279.

75. Maitland G. *Vertebral Manipulation.* Sydney, Australia: Butterworth; 1986.

76. Rivett DA, Sharples KJ, Milburn PD. Effect of pre-manipulative tests on vertebral artery and internal carotid artery blood flow. A pilot study. *J Manipulative Physiol Ther* 1999;22:368–375.

77. Grant ER. Clinical testing before cervical manipulation—can we recognise the patient at risk? In: *Proceedings of the Tenth International Congress of the World Confederation for Physical Therapy.* Sydney, Australia: WCPT 1987.

77a. Young YH, Chen CH. Acute vertigo following cervical manipulation. *Laryngoscope* 2003;113:659–662.

78. Australian Physiotherapy Association. Protocol for pre-manipulative testing of the cervical spine. *Aust J Physiother* 1988;34:97–100.

79. Evans RC. *Illustrated Essentials in Orthopaedic Physical Assessment.* St Louis, Mo: Mosby-Year Book; 1994.

80. Meadows J. *Orthopaedic Differential Diagnosis in Physical Therapy.* New York, NY: McGraw-Hill; 1999.

81. Ombregt L, et al. *A System of Orthopaedic Medicine.* London, England: Saunders; 1995.

82. Schievink WI. Spontaneous dissection of the carotid and vertebral arteries. *N Engl J Med* 2001;344:898–906.

83. Djouhri H, et al. MR angiography for the long-term follow-up of dissecting aneurysms of the extracranial internal carotid artery. *AJR Am J Roentgenol* 2000;174:1137–1140.

84. De Bray JM, et al. Ultrasonic features of extracranial carotid dissections: 47 cases studied by angiography. *J Ultrasound Med* 1994;13:659–664.

85. Sakata E, et al. Transitory, counterolling and pure/rotatory positioning nystagmus caused by cerebellar vermis lesion [in Japanese with English abstract]. *Pract Otol* 1985;78: 2729–2736.

86. Weintraub MI. Beauty parlor strokes syndrome: Report of five cases. *JAMA* 1993;269:2085–2086.

87. Nakagawa T, et al. Evaluation of vertebro-basilar hemodynamics by magnetic resonance angiography. *Equilibrium Res* 1997;56:360–365.

88. Shimura H, Yuzawa K, Nozue M. Stroke after visit to the hairdresser. *Lancet* 1997;350:1778.

CHAPTER 22

THE CRANIOVERTEBRAL JUNCTION

CHAPTER OBJECTIVES

▶ *At the completion of this chapter, the reader will be able to:*

1. Describe the anatomy of the vertebrae, ligaments, muscles, and blood and nerve supply that comprise the craniovertebral segments.

2. Describe the biomechanics of the craniovertebral joints, including coupled movements, normal and abnormal joint barriers, and kinesiology.

3. Perform a comprehensive history and systems review for the craniovertebral region.

4. Perform a detailed examination of the craniovertebral musculoskeletal system, including palpation of the articular and soft tissue structures, specific passive mobility tests, passive articular mobility tests, and stability tests.

5. Evaluate the total examination data to establish a diagnosis.

6. Apply appropriate manual techniques to the craniovertebral joints, using the correct grade, direction, and duration.

7. Describe intervention strategies based on clinical findings and established goals.

8. Evaluate intervention effectiveness in order to progress or modify intervention.

9. Plan an effective home program, and instruct the patient in this program.

10. Help the patient to develop self-reliant intervention strategies.

OVERVIEW

The craniovertebral (CV) junction is a collective term that refers to the occiput, atlas, axis, and supporting ligaments, which accounts for approximately 25 percent of the vertical height of the entire cervical spine. This junction is considered as a separate entity from the rest of the cervical spine because of its distinct embryology and anatomical structure. Kapandji[1] notes that the occiput, atlas, and axis actually form a primary kyphotic curve, and that this curve serves as a delineation between the craniovertebral region and the cervical spine proper.

Anatomy

Foramen Magnum

The general shape of the foramen magnum is oval, with the longer axis oriented in the sagittal plane (Fig. 22-1).[2] The margin of the foramen is relatively smooth and serves as the most superior attachment for a variety of the ligaments of the vertebral column. The smaller anterior region of the foramen magnum is characterized by a pair of tubercles to which the alar ligaments attach. The posterior portion of the foramen magnum houses the brain stem–spinal cord junction.

On either side of the anterolateral aspect of the foramen magnum are two ovoid projections called the occipital condyles (Fig. 22-1). The long axis of these paired occipital condyles is situated in a posterolateral to anteromedial orientation. The occipital condyles articulate with the first cervical vertebra.

Atlas

The shape of the atlas is that of a ring. The atlas is a ringlike structure that is formed by two lateral masses, which are interconnected by anterior and posterior arches (Fig. 22-2). The demarcation of the two regions is marked by a pair of tubercles to which the transverse ligament of the atlas attaches. Although the atlas has a smaller vertical dimension than any other cervical vertebrae, it is considerably wider. Because this

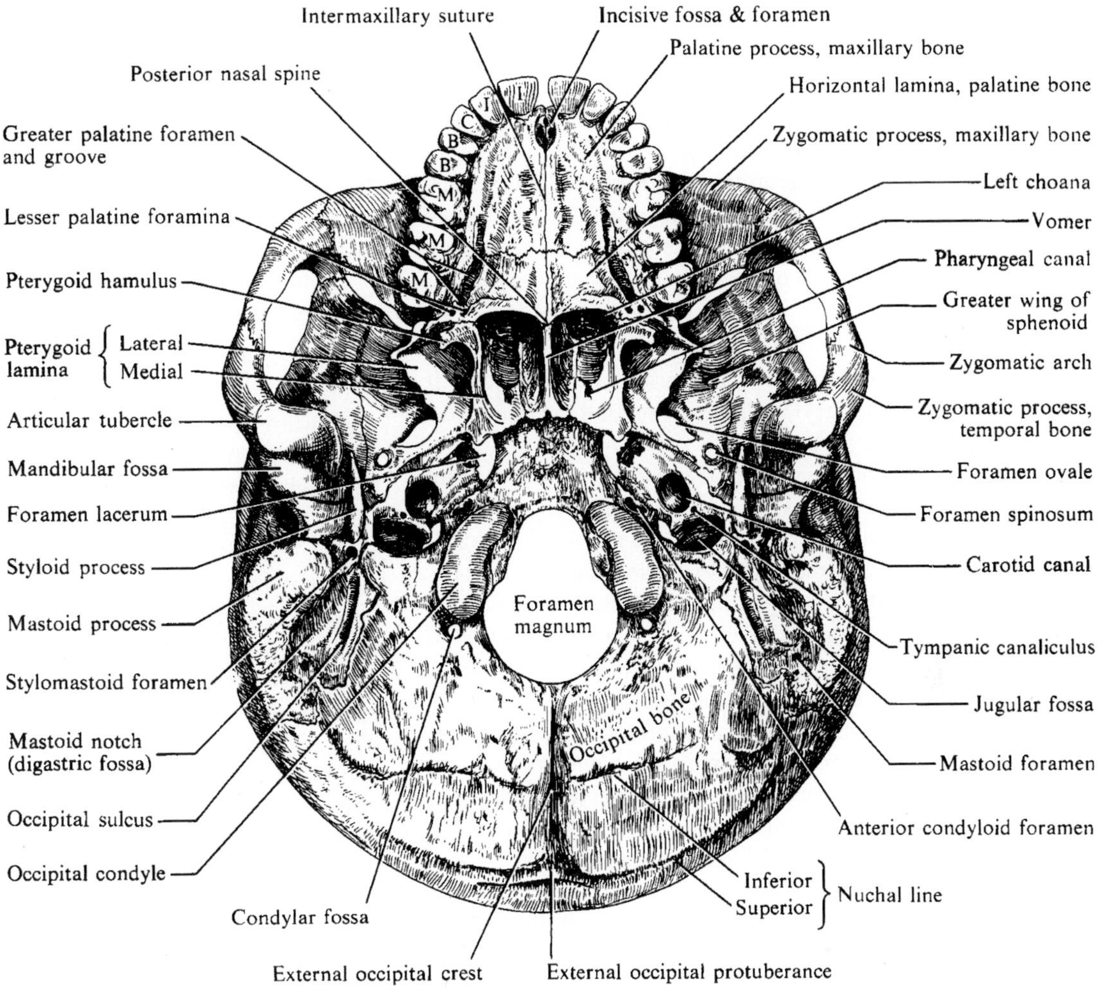

FIGURE 22-1 The foramen magnum. (Reproduced with permission from Pansky B. *Review of Gross Anatomy*. 6th ed. New York, NY: McGraw-Hill; 1996:13.)

Intermaxillary suture
Incisive fossa & foramen
Palatine process, maxillary bone
Posterior nasal spine
Horizontal lamina, palatine bone
Greater palatine foramen and groove
Zygomatic process, maxillary bone
Left choana
Vomer
Lesser palatine foramina
Pharyngeal canal
Pterygoid hamulus
Greater wing of sphenoid
Pterygoid lamina { Lateral Medial
Zygomatic arch
Articular tubercle
Zygomatic process, temporal bone
Mandibular fossa
Foramen ovale
Foramen lacerum
Foramen spinosum
Styloid process
Carotid canal
Mastoid process
Foramen magnum
Tympanic canaliculus
Stylomastoid foramen
Jugular fossa
Mastoid notch (digastric fossa)
Occipital bone
Mastoid foramen
Occipital sulcus
Anterior condyloid foramen
Occipital condyle
Inferior } Nuchal line Superior
Condylar fossa
External occipital crest
External occipital protuberance

vertebra does not have a spinous process, there is no bone posteriorly between the occipital bone and the spinous process of C2. This results in an increase in the potential for craniovertebral extension.

The superolateral aspect of each of the posterior arches has a transverse foramen to accommodate the vertebral artery

(see Chap. 21). The articular surface of the inferior facet is circular, relatively flat, and slopes inferiorly from medial to lateral. The upper articular facets of C1 are elongated from anterior to posterior, with the anterior ends closer together and more upwardly curved than their posterior counterparts.[2] This arrangement results in much more extension than flexion being

FIGURE 22-2 The atlas. (Reproduced with permission from Pansky B. *Review of Gross Anatomy*. 6th ed. New York, NY: McGraw-Hill; 1996:195.)

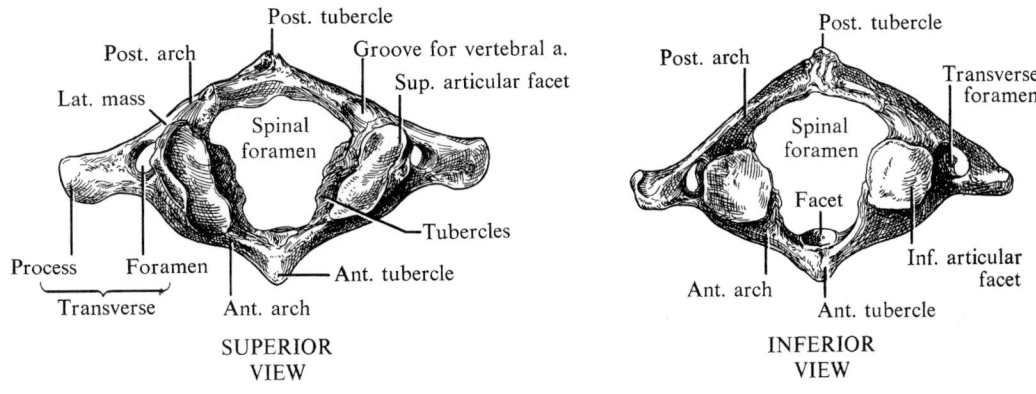

Post. tubercle
Post. arch
Groove for vertebral a.
Lat. mass
Sup. articular facet
Spinal foramen
Process
Foramen
Tubercles
Transverse
Ant. tubercle
Ant. arch
SUPERIOR VIEW

Post. tubercle
Post. arch
Transverse foramen
Spinal foramen
Facet
Ant. arch
Inf. articular facet
Ant. tubercle
INFERIOR VIEW

available at the articulation between the occipital condyles and the atlas—the occipito-atlantal joint.[3]

Occipito-atlantal Joint

The occipito-atlantal (O-A) joint represents the most superior zygapophysial joint of the vertebral column, and the only vertebral level that has an articulation characterized by a convex surface (occiput) moving on a concave joint partner (atlas).[3a] Even though these surfaces appear to be reciprocal in shape, they are not, and articular stability is only minimal.

Axis

The axis serves as a transitional vertebra (Fig. 22-3), because it is the link between the cervical spine proper and the craniovertebral region.

The dimensions of the axis are significantly different from those of the atlas. The atlas is considerably wider than the axis, but because of the long spinous process, the axis extends much farther posteriorly, and is the first palpable midline structure below the occiput.[4] Like the atlas, the transverse process of the axis has a transverse foramen to allow passage of the vertebral artery.

A unique feature of the axis is the odontoid process, or dens (Figure 22-3). The dens extends superiorly from the body to just above the C1 vertebra, before tapering to a blunt point. Very dense, thick trabecular bone is present in the center of the tip of the dens, and cortical bone at the anterior base of the body of C2 (where the anterior longitudinal ligament attaches) is uniformly thick.[4a] Hypodense bone, however, is present consistently beneath the odontoid process at the upper portion of the body of C2.[4b] This area of hypodense bone is susceptible to fracture. The anterior aspect of the dens has a hyaline cartilage-covered midline facet for articulation with the anterior tubercle of the atlas (the median A-A joint). The posterior aspect of the dens usually is marked with a groove where the transverse ligament passes. The dens functions as a pivot for the upper cervical joints, and as the center of rotation for the A-A joint. The most variable dimension of the axis is the dens angle in the sagittal plane, which can range from −2 degrees (leaning slightly anterior) to 42 degrees (leaning posterior).[4c] This extremely variable angle can make assessment of fracture reduction challenging.[4a]

Atlanto-axial Joint

This is a relatively complex articulation, which consists of:

▶ Two lateral zygapophysial joints between the articular surfaces of the inferior articular processes of the atlas and the superior processes of the axis.

▶ Two medial joints: one between the anterior surface of the dens of the axis and the anterior surface of the atlas, and the other between the posterior surface of the dens and the anterior hyalinated surface of the transverse ligament[4] (Fig. 22-3).

The relatively large superior articular facets of the axis lie lateral and anterior to the dens. These facets slope considerably downward from medial to lateral in line with the zygapophysial facets of the mid-low cervical spine.[4d] As the lateral A-A joints function to convey the entire weight of the atlas and the head to lower structures, the lamina and pedicles of the axis are quite robust.[4e] The stout, moderately long spinous process serves as the uppermost attachment for muscles that are essentially lower cervical in nature, and for muscles that act specifically on the craniovertebral joints.

One of the functions of the intervertebral disk (IVD) in the spine is to facilitate motion and provide stability (see Chap. 20). Thus, in the absence of an IVD in this region, the supporting soft tissues of the joints of the upper cervical spine must be lax to permit motion, while simultaneously being able to withstand great mechanical stresses.

Craniovertebral Ligaments

The craniovertebral region is noted for some strong ligaments, which have been the focus of a number of clinical tests to determine their efficiency in preventing unwanted and potentially dangerous movements. The controlling structures for these segments, which must be considered together, are the:

▶ ***Capsule and accessory capsular ligaments.*** The lateral capsular ligaments (anterolateral O-A ligament) of the O-A joints are typical of synovial joint capsules. These ligaments run obliquely from the basi-occiput to the transverse process of the atlas. By necessity, they are quite lax, to permit maximal motion, so they provide only moderate support to the joints during contralateral head rotation.

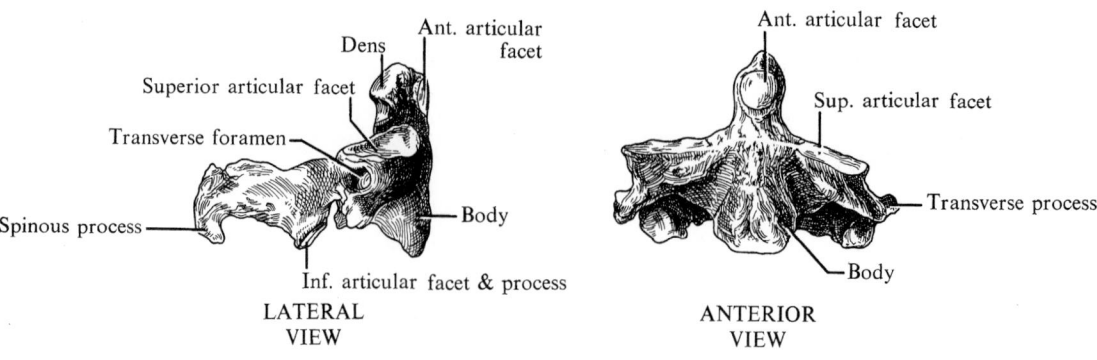

FIGURE 22-3   The axis. (Reproduced with permission from Pansky B. *Review of Gross Anatomy.* 6th ed. New York, NY: McGraw-Hill; 1996:195.)

Dens

Ant. articular facet

Superior articular facet

Transverse foramen

Spinous process

Body

Inf. articular facet & process

LATERAL VIEW

Ant. articular facet

Sup. articular facet

Transverse process

Body

ANTERIOR VIEW

▶ *Apical ligament (Fig. 22-4).* The apical ligament of the dens extends from the apex of the dens to the anterior rim of the foramen magnum. The ligament is short and thick. It runs from the top of the dens to the basi-occiput and is thought to be a remnant of the notochord. The apical ligament appears to be only a moderate stabilizer against posterior translation of the dens relative to both the atlas and the occipital bone.[4]

▶ *Vertical and transverse bands of the cruciform ligament.* (See Fig. 22-4 and later discussion.)

▶ *Alar and accessory alar ligaments.* (See Fig. 22-4 and later discussion.)

▶ *Anterior O-A membrane (see Fig. 22-4).* The anterior O-A membrane is thought to be the superior continuation of the anterior longitudinal ligament. It connects the anterior arch of vertebra C1 to the anterior aspect of the foramen magnum.

▶ *Posterior O-A membrane (see Fig. 22-4).* The posterior O-A membrane is a continuation of the ligamentum flavum. This ligament interconnects the posterior arch of the atlas and the posterior aspect of the foramen magnum, and forms part of the posterior boundary of the vertebral canal.[4]

▶ *Tectorial membrane (see Fig. 22-4).* The tectorial membrane is the most superficial of the three membranes and interconnects the occipital bone and the axis. This ligament is the superior continuation of the posterior longitudinal ligament and connects the body of vertebra C2 to the anterior rim of the foramen magnum. This bridging ligament is an important limiter of upper cervical flexion and holds the occiput off the atlas.[30]

Atlanto-axial Ligaments

The anterior atlanto-axial (anterior A-A) ligament is continuous with the anterior O-A membrane above.[31] The posterior A-A ligament interconnects the posterior arch of the atlas and the laminae of the axis.

Occipito-axial Ligaments

The O-A ligaments are very important to the stability of the upper cervical spine.

Alar Ligament[5]

The alar ligaments (see Fig. 22-4) connect the superior part of the dens to fossae on the medial aspect of the occipital condyles, although they can also attach to the lateral masses of the atlas.[32,33] A study of 44 cadavers[34] found the orientation of the ligament to be superior, posterior, and lateral. In another study,[32] 19 upper cervical spine specimens were dissected to examine the macroscopic and functional anatomy of alar ligaments. The study found that the most common orientation (10/19) was cauda-cranial, followed by transverse (5/19). In two of the specimens, a previously undescribed ligamentous connection was found between the dens and the anterior arch of the atlas, the anterior atlanto-dental ligament. In 12 specimens, the ligament also attached via caudal fibers to the lateral mass of the atlas. The posteroanterior orientation of the ligaments in 17 of the 19 subjects was directly lateral from the dens to the occipital attachment or slightly posterior.

The function of the ligament is to resist flexion, contralateral side bending, and contralateral rotation.[35] Because of the connections of the ligament, side bending of the head produces a contralateral or ipsilateral rotation of C2 depending on the source.[28]

Clinical Pearl

Insufficiency of the alar ligaments increases the potential for occipito-axial instability. The degree of instability can be determined in conjunction with other clinical findings, such as neurologic or vascular compromise, pain, and deformity.

The Cruciform Ligament

The cruciform (cross-shaped) ligament has superior, inferior, and transverse portions (Fig. 22-4). The superior and inferior portions of this ligament attach to the posterior aspect of the body of the dens and the anterior rim of the foramen magnum. The transverse portion, which stretches between tubercles on the medial aspects of the lateral masses of the atlas, connects the atlas with the dens of the axis. The transverse portion of the ligament is so distinct and important that it is often considered a separate ligament (Fig. 22-5). The major responsibility of the transverse portion is to counteract anterior translation of the atlas relative to the axis, thereby maintaining the position of the dens relative to the anterior arch of the atlas.[30]

The transverse ligament also limits the amount of flexion between the atlas and axis.[36] These limiting functions are of extreme importance because excessive movement of either type could result in the dens compressing the spinal cord, epipharynx, vertebral artery, or superior cervical ganglion. The integrity of the transverse ligament is also essential to the stability of atlas fractures; degenerative, inflammatory, and congenital disorders; and other abnormalities that affect the craniovertebral junction.

The importance of the ligament is reflected in its physical properties. Spontaneous or isolated traumatic tears of this ligament are extremely rare events. The ligament is comprised almost entirely of collagen, with a parallel orientation close to the atlas and the dens, but with an approximately 30-degree obliquity at other points in the ligament. Dvorak and colleagues[37] found the transverse ligament to be almost twice as strong as the alar ligaments, and to have a tensile strength of 330 newtons (N) (33 kg/73 lb).

Craniovertebral Muscles

Anterior Suboccipital Muscles

Rectus Capitis Anterior. The rectus capitis anterior (RCA) runs vertically. It travels deep to the longus capitis from the anterior aspect of the lateral mass of the atlas to the inferior surface of

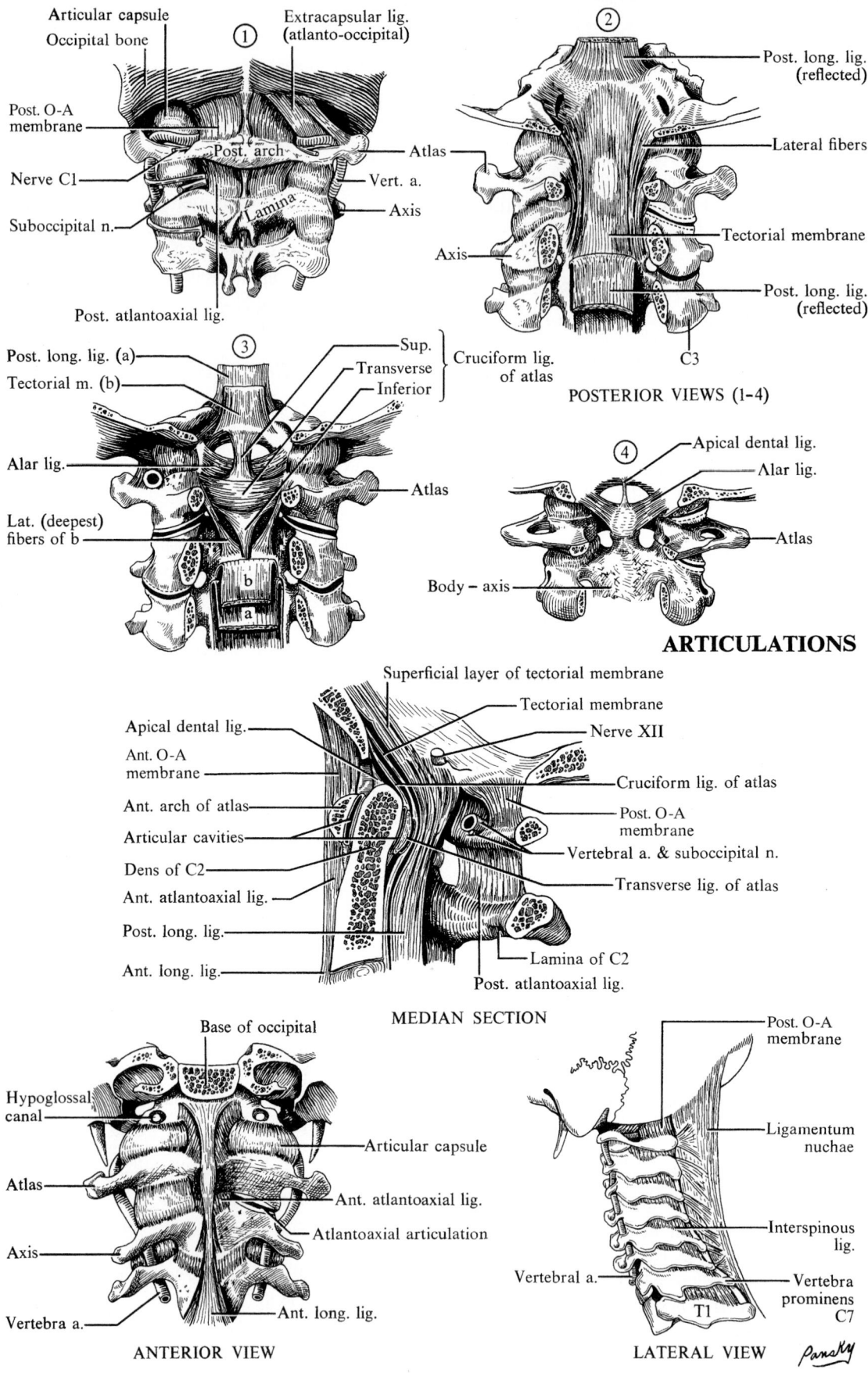

FIGURE 22-4 The ligaments of the craniovertebral region. (Reproduced with permission from Pansky B. *Review of Gross Anatomy.* 6th ed. New York, NY: McGraw-Hill; 1996:213.)

① Articular capsule
Occipital bone
Extracapsular lig. (atlanto-occipital)
Post. O-A membrane
Post. arch
Atlas
Nerve C1
Vert. a.
Lamina
Axis
Suboccipital n.
Post. atlantoaxial lig.

② Post. long. lig. (reflected)
Lateral fibers
Axis
Tectorial membrane
Post. long. lig. (reflected)
C3

POSTERIOR VIEWS (1-4)

③ Post. long. lig. (a)
Tectorial m. (b)
Sup.
Transverse
Inferior
Cruciform lig. of atlas
Alar lig.
Atlas
Lat. (deepest) fibers of b
b
a

④ Apical dental lig.
Alar lig.
Atlas
Body – axis

ARTICULATIONS

Superficial layer of tectorial membrane
Tectorial membrane
Nerve XII
Apical dental lig.
Ant. O-A membrane
Ant. arch of atlas
Articular cavities
Dens of C2
Ant. atlantoaxial lig.
Post. long. lig.
Ant. long. lig.
Cruciform lig. of atlas
Post. O-A membrane
Vertebral a. & suboccipital n.
Transverse lig. of atlas
Lamina of C2
Post. atlantoaxial lig.

MEDIAN SECTION

Base of occipital
Hypoglossal canal
Atlas
Axis
Vertebra a.
Articular capsule
Ant. atlantoaxial lig.
Atlantoaxial articulation
Ant. long. lig.

ANTERIOR VIEW

Post. O-A membrane
Ligamentum nuchae
Interspinous lig.
Vertebral a.
Vertebra prominens C7
T1

LATERAL VIEW

Pansky

994

FIGURE 22-5 The transverse ligament. (Reproduced with permission from Wilkins RH, Rengachary SS, eds. *Neurosurgery*. New York, NY: McGraw-Hill; 1996:927.)

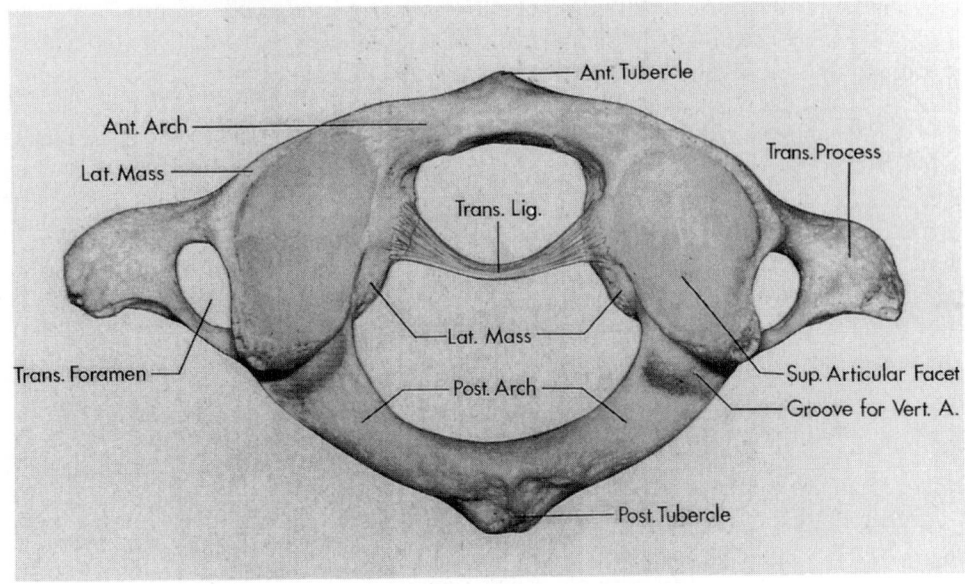

the base of the occiput, anterior to the occipital condyle (Fig. 22-6). The RCA flexes and minimally rotates the head. Thus, an adaptively shortened RCA on the right could feasibly produce a decreased left translation in extension during mobility testing of the O-A joint. The muscle is supplied by the ventral rami of C1 and C2.

Rectus Capitis Lateralis. This muscle arises from the superior surface of the C1 transverse process and inserts into the inferior surface of the jugular process of the occiput (see Fig. 22-6). It is homologous to the posterior intertransverse muscle of the spine. The rectus capitis lateralis side bends the head ipsilaterally. It is supplied by the ventral rami of C1 and C2.

Posterior Suboccipital Muscles

The posterior suboccipitals lie beneath the splenius capitis and trapezius muscles. These muscles function in the control of segmental sliding between C1 and C2[39] and may have an important

FIGURE 22-6 The anterior suboccipital muscles. (Reproduced with permission from Pansky B. *Review of Gross Anatomy*. 6th ed. New York, NY: McGraw-Hill; 1996:73.)

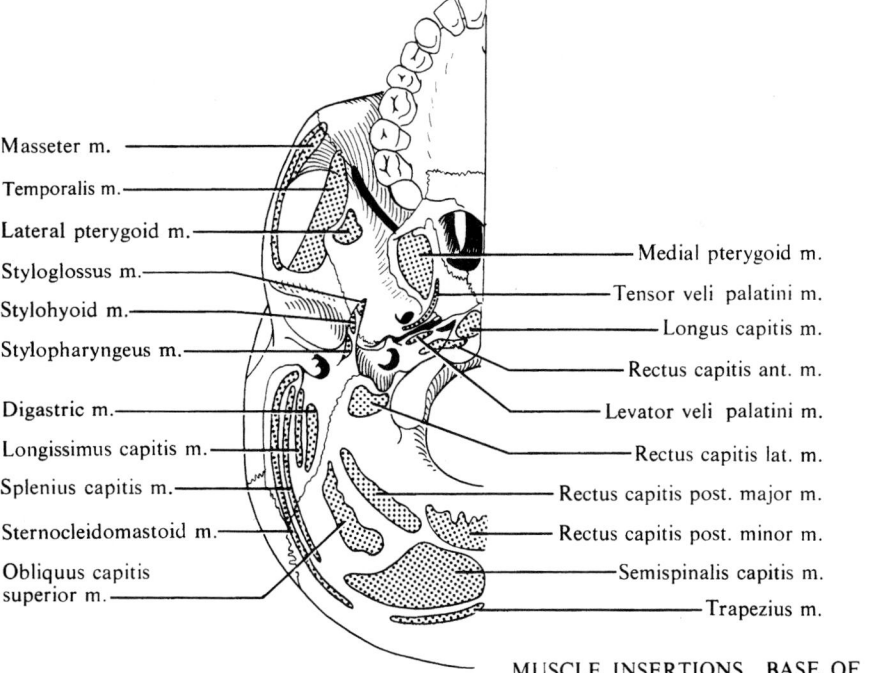

MUSCLE INSERTIONS   BASE OF SKULL

role in proprioception, having more muscle spindles than any other muscle for their size.[39] All of the posterior suboccipital muscles are innervated by the posterior ramus of C1 and also are strongly linked with the trigeminal nerve.[40,41] The suboccipitals receive their blood supply from the vertebral artery.

Rectus Capitis Posterior Major. The rectus capitis posterior major is the largest of the posterior suboccipitals. It runs from the C2 spinous process, widening as it runs cranially to attach to the lateral part of inferior nuchal line (Fig. 22-7). Located inferior and lateral to the occipital protuberances, the rectus capitis posterior major muscles, when working together, extend the head. When working individually, the muscles produce ipsilateral side bending and rotation of the head.

Rectus Capitis Posterior Minor. The rectus capitis posterior minor is a small unisegmental muscle that runs from the posterior arch tubercle of the atlas to the medial part of the inferior nuchal line (see Fig. 22-7). Because of the shortness of the atlantean tubercle, the muscle is very horizontal, running almost parallel with the occiput. The muscle functions to extend the head and provides minimal support during ipsilateral side bending of the head.

Clinical Pearl

Connective tissue attachments between the rectus capitis posterior minor and dura mater recently have been identified.[42] This finding has led to the use of cervical flexion with neurodynamic mobility tests (see Chap. 12). The differentiation between adverse neural tension and adaptive shortening of the muscle can be made by performing short neck flexion with the neural system pretensioned and then relaxed.

Inferior Oblique. This is the larger of the two oblique muscles and runs from the spinous process and lamina of the axis superolaterally to the transverse process of the atlas (see Fig. 22-7).

The inferior oblique muscle works to produce ipsilateral rotation of the atlas and skull and to control anterior translation and rotation of C1 (atlas). An adaptively shortened right inferior oblique may exert an inferior and posterior pull on the right transverse process of the atlas, producing a right rotated A-A joint.[43,44] This results in a gross limitation of left rotation of the head while in cervical flexion, but a minimal limitation of left rotation of the head in extension.

Superior Oblique. The superior oblique arises from the transverse process of the atlas and runs superoposterior and medially to the bone between the superior and inferior nuchal lines, lateral to the attachment of rectus capitis posterior major (see Fig. 22-7). Because of its posteromedial orientation, the superior oblique functions to provide contralateral rotation and ipsilateral side bending of the O-A joint when acting unilaterally. When working together, the two superior obliques can produce head extension. Dysfunction of this muscle is a common cause of chronic headaches.[45–49]

The posterior suboccipital muscles can work concentrically with the larger extensors and rotators of the cervical spine, or eccentrically, controlling the action of the flexors. Because two of these muscles parallel the occiput, their controlling influence may be more linear than angular, producing or guiding the arthrokinematic, rather than the osteokinematic, motion.[39]

Nerve Supply

The dorsal ramus of spinal nerve C1 is larger than the ventral ramus. It exits from the spinal canal by passing posteriorly between the posterior arch of the atlas and the rim of the foramen magnum, along with the vertebral artery. It then enters the

---

FIGURE 22-7 The suboccipital triangle. (Reproduced with permission from Pansky B. *Review of Gross Anatomy.* 6th ed. New York, NY: McGraw-Hill; 1996:229.)

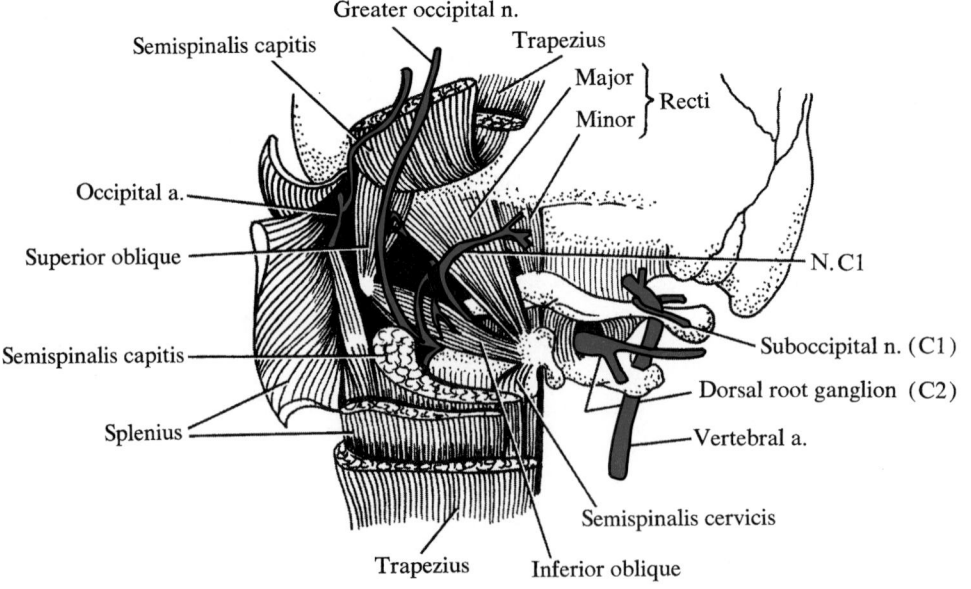

suboccipital triangle and supplies most of the muscles that form that triangle. It usually has no cutaneous distribution.

The dorsal ramus of spinal nerve C2 (see Fig. 22-7), also known as the greater occipital nerve, is larger than the ventral ramus of C2. It exits from the vertebral canal by passing through the slit between the posterior arch of the atlas and the lamina of the axis. This nerve is the largest of the cervical dorsal rami and is primarily a cutaneous nerve. It supplies most of the posterior aspect of the scalp, extending anteriorly to a line across the scalp that runs from one external auditory meatus to the other. Because this nerve has an extensive cutaneous distribution, it has a very large dorsal root ganglion. This ganglion is commonly located in a vulnerable location, almost directly between the posterior arch of C1 and the lamina of C2 (see Fig. 22-7). The interval between these two bony structures is small, and it is reduced with extension of the upper cervical spine. Given the sensitivity of the dorsal root ganglion to compression, the possible relationship between the forward head position and occipital headaches is apparent.[45–49]

Blood Supply

The intradural vertebral artery supplies the most superior segments of the cervical spinal cord (see Chap. 21). The cervical cord is supplied by two arterial systems, central and peripheral, which overlap but are discrete. The first is dependent entirely on the single anterior spinal artery (ASA). The second, without clear-cut boundaries, receives supplies from the ASA and both posterior spinal arteries.[50] Because the ASA is medial and dominant, unilateral cord infarctions are very rare. However, they may occur in the perfusion territory supplied by the ASA.[51,52] This is a result of obstruction of either a duplicated ASA[52] or obstruction of one of the sulcal arteries, which arise from the ASA and turn alternatively left or right to supply one side of the central cord.[53] Peripheral hemicord infarction may result from ischemia in the territory of the ASA[51] or posterior spinal artery.[54]

Biomechanics

The upper cervical spine is responsible for approximately 50 percent of the motion that occurs in the entire cervical spine. Motion at the A-A joint occurs relatively independently, while below C2, normal motion is a combination of motion occurring at other levels.

Articular facet asymmetry of the human upper cervical spine has been recognized for more than 30 years.[54b,54c] The implications of this anatomic observation in the human spine has been considered in relation to joint disease, specifically, facet tropism (the phenomenon observed in living tissue, of moving toward or away from a focus of stimulus), which is associated with subsequent degenerative joint disease.[54d–54f]

> ### Clinical Pearl
>
> Due to the proximity of vital structures, joint disease in this region can have severe consequences. These consequences can include:
>
> - Vertebral artery compromise.
> - Compression of the spinal cord.
> - Brainstem lesions.

Occipito-Atlantal Joint

The primary motion that occurs at this joint is flexion-extension. One cadaveric study found flexion and extension to have a combined range of 13 degrees,[11] while another cadaveric study,[12] using radiographic imaging, found the mean ranges to be:

▶ Flexion-extension: 18.6 degrees (± 0.6 degrees).

▶ Axial rotation: 3.4 degrees (± 0.4 degrees).

▶ Side bending: 3.9 degrees (± 0.6 degrees).

It is generally agreed that rotation and side bending at this joint occur to opposite sides when they are combined, and this can be demonstrated by palpating and observing the motion of the head during these movements. During occiput rotation, the atlas is felt to translate and side bend to the opposite side. Occipital rotation and, to some degree, anteroposterior translation of the occiput on C1 is limited by the alar ligaments.[13]

An early study by Werne,[14] which has since been validated with cadaveric investigations using radiographic markers[15] and computed tomographic (CT) scanning,[16] reported side bending ranges at an average of a little over 9 degrees to both sides[14–16] and rotation ranges of 2 degrees[15] to 10 to 25 degrees,[16] although the latter findings involved patients with suspected instability.

> ### Clinical Pearl
>
> Clinical studies suggest that hypermobility of this joint should only be considered as a diagnosis if the range of rotation exceeds 8 degrees, making rotational mobility and stability testing necessary at this articulation.

Atlanto-axial Joint

Ligamentous and bony structures at the atlanto-axial (A-A) joint allow for a large arc of rotation.

> ### Clinical Pearl
>
> Within the spine, only two articulations permit pure axial rotation:
>
> - The atlanto-axial joint.
> - The thoracolumbar junction.

The major motion that occurs at all three of the A-A articulations is axial rotation, totaling approximately 40 to 47 degrees to each side.[20,21] This large amount of rotation has the potential to cause compression of the vertebral artery (see Chap. 21).[22,23] As the atlas rotates, the ipsilateral facet moves posteriorly while the contralateral facet moves anteriorly, so that each facet of the atlas slides inferiorly along the convex surface of the axial facet, telescoping the head downward.

The first 25 degrees of head rotation (60 percent) occur primarily at the A-A articulations.[24] However, the axial rotation of the atlas is not a pure motion, because it is coupled with a significant degree of extension (14 degrees) and, in some cases, flexion.[25]

Flexion and extension movements of the A-A joint amount to a combined range of 10 to 15 degrees: 10 degrees of flexion, and 5 degrees of extension.[26] Flexion at the A-A joint is limited by the tectorial membrane. Extension is limited by the anterior arch of C1 as it makes contact with the odontoid process. The flexion and extension motions are associated with small anteroposterior translational movements, which can create a small space between the back of the anterior arch of the atlas and the odontoid. This space is called the atlanto-odontoid interval (ADI). Because of the arthrokinematics of the joint, flexion increases the ADI, whereas extension decreases it. Excessive gapping of the ADI can have serious consequences as it can lead to a compression of the spinal cord by the atlas.[27] An ADI of more than 3 mm in adults, and 4.5 mm in children younger than 12 years of age, detected on radiographs is indicative of gross instability secondary to a compromise of the transverse ligament (see "Transverse Ligament," later).[27] A increased ADI is associated with a history of trauma but also may be associated with severe ligamentous laxity in patients with rheumatoid arthritis, neoplastic disease, Down's syndrome, and aplasia or dysplasia of the dens.[28]

Coupling at this joint is commonly cited as contralateral side bending during rotation. However, palpation of the axis during side bending or rotation tends to argue against this.[29] If the length of the spinous process is palpated with two fingers while the subject rotates the head to the left (this holds just as well for right rotation), the superior finger is felt and seen to move to the right while the inferior finger moves to the left. This finding would imply that the vertebra of the axis has side bent to the right under the atlas, placing the A-A joint into left side bending. In this case, rotation and side bending occur to the same side.[29] However, if the spinous process is palpated while the head is side bent to the left, it will be felt to move to the right, indicating that the axis is rotating to the left. Thus, during side bending, the atlas does not rotate but, instead, appears to be translating to the contralateral side as the axis rotates under the atlas. Because the position of the joint is described by the relative motion of the superior vertebra (e.g., L4–5 flexion when L4 flexes on L5, as in forward bending, or L5 extends under L4, as in posterior pelvic tilting), the A-A joint is actually in right rotation.[29]

The direction of the conjunct rotation, therefore, appears to be dependent on the initiating movement. If the initiating movement is side bending (latexion), the conjunct rotation of the joint is to the opposite side. If the initiating movement is rotation (rotexion), the conjunct motion (side bending) is to the same side. This principle can be exploited in the assessment of the craniovertebral joints:

1. *Rotexion.* During rotation of the head to the right (rotexion):
   a. Left side bending and right rotation occur at the O-A joint, accompanied by a translation to the right.
   b. Right side bending and right rotation occur at the A-A joint and at C2 to C3.

In other words, if the head motion is initiated with rotation, ipsilateral side bending of the A-A joint and C2 to C3 occurs, whereas at the O-A joint, contralateral side bending occurs.

2. *Latexion.* Side bending of the head to the right produces:
   a. Left rotation of the O-A joint, accompanied by a translation of the occiput to the left.
   b. Left rotation of the A-A joint.
   c. Right rotation of C2 to C3.

In other words, if head motion is initiated with side bending, contralateral rotation of both the O-A and A-A joints occurs, but ipsilateral rotation occurs at C2 to C3.

Examination

The primary objective of the examination of this region is to rule out any serious injury. Once the clinician has ruled out the more insidious causes for the patient's complaints, the search can begin for a biomechanical cause for the signs and symptoms. Thus, the examination of the craniovertebral region progresses from the application of gentle stresses to the use of more assertive tests.

Because of the close relationship among the craniovertebral joints, cervical spine (see Chap. 23), and temporomandibular joint (see Chap. 24), an assessment of these areas should occur as part of a comprehensive examination of this region. The differential diagnosis for head, face, and neck pain (Table 22-1) is described in Chapter 9.

Once the neighboring areas have been cleared, a specific examination of the craniovertebral joints can begin. In general, the O-A joint is examined and treated first, otherwise the findings from a combined test of both joints would be confusing. Once the O-A joint is cleared, the examination of the A-A complex can proceed.

History

The craniovertebral region, as with the rest of the neck, is a common area for myofascial pain syndromes. These syndromes frequently are associated with complaints of headaches, local muscle soreness, and muscle spasm.[55] Pain also may be referred to this region from trigger points in the upper trapezius muscle, sternocleidomastoid muscle, digastric muscle, splenius capitis and cervicis muscles, posterior cervical muscles (semispinalis

TABLE 22-1   Pain Distribution from Cervical Structures[54a]

Structure	Pain Area
Occipital condyles	Frontal
Occipitocervical tissues	Frontal
C1 dorsal ramus	Orbit, frontal, and vertex
C1–2	Temporal, suboccipital
C3 dorsal ramus	Occiput, mastoid, frontal

capitis, semispinalis cervicis, multifidus, rotators), and suboccipital muscles (rectus capitis posterior major and minor, obliqui inferior and superior) (refer to "Intervention" section).[55]

Complaints of headaches are also common in patients with craniovertebral joint dysfunction.[56–58] Some of the more common types of headaches are described in Chapter 9. In all patients presenting with an unexplained or unusual headache, a full neurologic and general physical examination is required (Table 22-2).[59] This examination should include general appearance (including skin lesions such as rashes), vital signs (pulse, blood pressure, and temperature), mental status and speech, gait, balance and coordination, cranial nerve and long tract examination, visual fields, acuity and ophthalmoscopic fundus examination, and skull palpation.[59]

Patients who complain of headaches should be asked to describe the headache. The clinician must always be alert to the potential coincidental occurrence of secondary headache syndromes. These include headache associated with trauma, vascular disease, nonvascular intracranial disorders, substance use or withdrawal, noncephalic infections, metabolic disorders, disorders of facial or cranial structures, and cranial neuralgia.[60] Several conditions may mimic episodic or chronic tension-type headache, including muscle tension. Chronic tension-type headaches are often erroneously attributed to chronic sinusitis, but clinical and radiologic evidence must be obtained before making this diagnosis. A causal relationship between tension-type headache and oromandibular dysfunction is controversial, but the two conditions often coexist.[61] The most important structures that register pain within the skull are the blood vessels, particularly the proximal part of the cerebral arteries, as well as the large veins and venous sinuses.[62] The chronic headache of intracranial hypotension is most often distinguished by an increase of pain on standing. Descriptions such as throbbing and pounding are suggestive of a vascular origin, but can also inculpate migraine, fever, neuralgia, or hypertension. Chronic, recurrent headaches can be associated with eyestrain, excessive eating or drinking, or smoking.

Intrinsic to the understanding of the relationship of headache to the craniovertebral region are the intracranial pain pathways and their interconnections, especially the trigeminocervical pathway. The O-A joints,[56] A-A joints,[57] and C2 spinal nerve[58] all have been implicated as primary nociceptors in cervicogenic headaches. Among individuals with chronic neck pain, 58 to 88 percent describe associated headaches.[63,64] The prevalence of C2 to C3 zygapophysial joint pain has been estimated at 50 to 53 percent in those patients with a chief complaint of headaches after whiplash injury.[63,64]

The location of the headache can provide the clinician with useful information as to the source.

▶ Forehead pain may be caused by sinusitis or a muscle spasm of the occipital or suboccipital region.

▶ Occipital pain can be caused by eyestrain, herniated disk, hypertension, neuralgia, or an ear or eye disorder.

▶ Parietal pain may be indicative of meningitis or a tumor.

▶ Facial pain can be caused by sinusitis, trigeminal neuralgia, dental problems, or a tumor.

Dizziness (vertigo) and nystagmus (see "Systems Review," later) are nonspecific neurologic signs that require a careful diagnostic workup (Table 22-2). A report of vertigo, although potentially problematic, is not a contraindication to the continuation of the examination. Differential diagnosis includes primary central nervous system diseases, vestibular and ocular involvement, and, more rarely, metabolic disorders.[65] Careful questioning can help in the differentiation of central and peripheral causes of vertigo. Central vertigo is usually caused by a disturbance of the vestibular system, which can produce

TABLE 22-2 Signs and Symptoms Requiring Neurologic Assessment[64a]

Headaches that are sudden, severe, and diffuse
Headaches that awaken one from sleep
Headaches associated with projectile vomiting, but no nausea
Unilateral pulsating pain in synchrony with heartbeat
Headaches that worsen with activity or exertion
Headaches that begin or worsen with recumbency
Focal tenderness over temporal artery in someone over age 60
Sudden, intense, sharp pain of short duration that is either spontaneous or triggered by mild stimulus
Severe pain around the sinuses or teeth
Headaches associated with other symptoms
Cognitive impairment
Visual disturbances (i.e., blindness, diplopia, distortions, spots, or loss of vision on one side)
Numbness or altered sensation
Loss of strength or coordination
Loss or alteration of smell, taste, or hearing
Fever or associated systemic illness
Difficulty swallowing
Loss or impairment of voice, chronic cough

sensations of head and body rotations, to and fro movements, or up and down movements. Peripheral vertigo is manifested with general complaints such as unsteadiness and lightheadedness. Cervical vertigo may be produced by localized muscle changes and receptor irritation.[66] Some authors[67] suggest that manual therapy is indicated in patients in whom the cervical vertigo or perception of unbalance is caused by somatic dysfunction. However, this form of vertigo must always be clearly differentiated from the other causes of vertigo and the clinician must be skilled in the interpretation of such findings to reveal the source of the dizziness.

▶ Dizziness provoked by head movements or head positions could indicate an inner ear dysfunction. Dizziness provoked by certain cervical motions, particularly extension or rotation, also may indicate vertebral artery compromise (see Chap. 21). Dizziness resulting from vertebral artery compromise should be associated with other signs and symptoms, which could include neck pain and nausea. The pain associated with vertebral artery compromise develops on one side of the neck in one fourth of patients and usually is confined to the upper anterolateral cervical region.[68] Persistent isolated neck pain may mimic idiopathic carotidynia, especially if it is associated with local tenderness (see Chap. 9). Pain is also usually the initial manifestation of carotid-artery dissection, and the median time to the appearance of other symptoms is 4 days.[68]

▶ Dizziness associated with tinnitus or a hearing loss could indicate a tumor of cranial nerve VIII.

▶ Dizziness following head trauma is common and is produced if the calcareous deposits that lie on the vestibular receptors are displaced to new and sensitive regions of the ampulla of the posterior canal, evoking a hypersensitive response to stimulation with certain head positions or movements.[46,69]

Clinical Pearl

Dizziness associated with disorders of motor function, such as clumsiness, weakness, or paralysis, could suggest compromise of the vertebrobasilar system.

Systems Review

The craniovertebral region houses many vital structures. These include the spinal cord, the vertebral artery, and the brain stem. It is extremely important for the clinician to approach this area with caution and to rule out the presence of serious pathology. Craniovertebral and cranial dysfunction can be responsible for a number of signs and symptoms that may be benign or may indicate the presence of serious pathology (Table 22-3).

Due to the proximity of the cranial structures, the clinician should develop the habit of quickly screening patients with neck and head pain for their ability to orient to time, place, and name, concentrate, reason and process information, make judgments, communicate effectively, and recall information. Obtaining this information needs to be done in a sensitive

---

TABLE 22-3 Examination Findings and the Possible Conditions Causing Them[69c]

Findings	Possible Condition
Dizziness	Upper cervical impairment, vertebrobasilar ischemia, craniovertebral ligament tear; also may be relatively benign
Quadrilateral paresthesia	Cord compression, vertebrobasilar ischemia
Bilateral upper limb paresthesia	Cord compression, vertebrobasilar ischemia
Hyper-reflexia	Cord compression, vertebrobasilar ischemia
Babinski or clonus sign	Cord compression, vertebrobasilar ischemia
Consistent swallow on transverse ligament stress tests	Instability, retropharyngeal hematoma, rheumatoid arthritis
Nontraumatic capsular pattern	Rheumatoid arthritis, ankylosing spondylitis, neoplasm
Arm pain lasting > 6–9 mo	Neoplasm
Persistent root pain < 30 yr	Neoplasm
Radicular pain with coughing	Neoplasm

TABLE 22-3 *(cont.)*

Pain worsening after 1 mo	Neoplasm
> 1 level involved	Neoplasm
Paralysis	Neoplasm or neurologic disease
Trunk and limb paresthesia	Neoplasm
Bilateral root signs and symptoms	Neoplasm
Nontraumatic strong spasm	Neoplasm
Nontraumatic strong pain in elderly patient	Neoplasm
Signs worse than symptoms	Neoplasm
Radial deviator weakness	Neoplasm
Thumb flexor weakness	Neoplasm
Hand intrinsic weakness or atrophy	Neoplasm, thoracic outlet syndrome, carpal tunnel syndrome
Horner's syndrome	Superior sulcus tumor, breast cancer, cervical ganglion damage, brain stem damage
Empty end-feel	Neoplasm
Severe post-traumatic capsular pattern	Fracture
Severe post-traumatic spasm	Fracture
Loss of ROM post-trauma	Fracture
Post-traumatic painful weakness	Fracture

ROM, range of motion.

manner. Asking questions as to whether the patient knows their own name and what day it is may be considered inappropriate by some patients. Most of the concerns about the patient's mental status can be addressed through general conversation, or as part of the history. Perhaps surprisingly, the incidence of neurologic involvement in upper cervical spine injury is relatively low (18–26 percent).[69a] This may be because, when significant cord damage does occur in the upper cervical spine, the patient frequently dies because of respiratory arrest.[69b]

When compression of the spinal cord is suspected, a thorough neurologic examination should be performed. If confirmed, the appropriate medical services should be contacted. The cranial nerves should be assessed, particularly if there are complaints about vision or the patient appears to have problems with speech or swallowing. Patients with referred pain in the region of the trigeminal nerve commonly have an underlying disorder of the upper cervical spine, such as A-A instability caused by rheumatoid arthritis.[55,72] As described in Chapter 2, the various cranial nerve tests can be performed in approximately 5 minutes with practice.

The patient should be assessed for the presence of nystagmus (see Chap. 2). Nystagmus is characterized by a rhythmic movement of the eyes with an abnormal shifting away from fixation, and rapid return.[73] Failure of any one of the main control mechanisms for maintaining steady gaze-fixation (the vestibulo-ocular reflex, and a gaze-holding system [the neural integrator]) will bring about a disruption of steady fixation. Two types of abnormal fixation can result: nystagmus and saccadic intrusions or oscillations.[74,75] The essential difference between these abnormal fixations lies in the initial movement that takes the line of sight off the object of regard. In the case of nystagmus, it is a slow drift or "slow phase," often caused by a disturbance of one of the three mechanisms for gaze stability. On the other hand, with either saccadic intrusions or saccadic oscillations, it is an inappropriate fast movement that moves the eyes off target.[74,75]

The more benign types of nystagmus include the proprioceptive causes of spontaneous nystagmus, postural nystagmus, and nystagmus that is elicited with head positioning or induced by movement (vestibular nystagmus). Vestibular nystagmus occurs during self-rotation even in darkness: the inner ear contains motion detectors (vestibular labyrinth) that project to the vestibular nuclei and cerebellum (see Chap. 2). Vestibular nystagmus also can be induced by irrigating the ears with warm or cold water (caloric test). With unilateral irrigation, the conjugate nystagmus is horizontal, torsional, or oblique, depending on the position of the head. Diseases that affect the vestibular labyrinth or nerve (including the root entry zone) cause a jerk nystagmus with linear or constant velocity slow-phase drifts. Characteristically, the nystagmus increases when the eyes are turned in the direction of the quick phases (Alexander's law) and can be markedly suppressed by visual fixation.[76] The direction of the unidirectional nystagmus is related to the geometric relationship of the semicircular canals with the fast phase opposite to the side of the lesion, with a change in head position often exacerbating the nystagmus. On the other hand, a central vestibular nystagmus, which is caused by disease of the brain stem or cerebellum, is not attenuated by fixation and invariably exhibits bidirectionality to the nystagmus (i.e., left-beating on left gaze and right-beating on right gaze).[76]

The more serious causes of nystagmus include, but are not limited to, vertebrobasilar ischemia, tumors of the posterior cranial fossa, intracranial bleeding, craniocervical malformations, and autonomic dysfunction. Differentiation between the benign and serious causes of nystagmus is very important. Proprioceptive nystagmus occurs immediately upon turning the head (i.e., there is no latent period). In contrast, the ischemic type of nystagmus has a latent period and usually is only evident when the patient's neck is turned to a position and maintained there for a period of a few seconds up to 3 minutes.[66,77]

Tests and Measures

The examination is terminated if any serious signs and symptoms are produced.

Observation

The patient is observed in the sagittal, coronal, and transverse planes.

Sagittal Plane. Observing the status of the cervical curve and the relative position of the patient's chin to the chest helps to assess postural alignment in the sagittal plane. A popular view among clinicians is that habitual adoption of extreme cervical posture may account for symptoms of pain and dysfunction arising from the head and neck area.[78] The argument is that

alterations in spinal alignment may lead to changes in muscle activity and loading on the surrounding soft tissue and articular structures, which then predisposes patients to such complaints.[79,80] This argument has been supported in several studies, which have found a statistically significant correlation between the tendency to hold the head forward relative to the true vertical in the so-called *forward head posture* and symptoms of pain.[80,81] In other investigations, no such correlation has been confirmed.[82,83]

Tucking or elevation of the chin in the presence of a normal cervical curve may indicate craniovertebral dysfunction.[85]

The ears are observed for the presence of asymmetry in size, shape, or color. The top of the ear is normally in line with the eyebrow.

Coronal Plane. Alignment in the coronal plane is assessed by observing the orientation of the head relative to the trunk and shoulders, the leveling of the mastoid processes, and the symmetry of the cervical soft tissues. The face is observed for any asymmetry, or indications of bruising, puffiness, prominence, swelling, perspiration, or abnormal skin color. Any asymmetry in the relative size of the pupils of the eyes and the distance between the upper and lower lids is noted. Pupillary size differences can occur in normal individuals, but initially should arouse concern, because an abnormal unilateral change in size may be caused by an autonomic dysfunction or a central nervous system lesion.[84] The superior lid should cover a portion of the iris but not the pupil itself, unless ptosis or drooping of the eyelid is present[84] (see Chap. 2).

Missing teeth should be accounted for. Loss of teeth may be a result of trauma, avulsion, or loosening.

Transverse Plane. Alignment in the transverse plane is assessed by observing the patient from behind and noting the orientation of the head. The orientation of the head is best observed by noting any asymmetry in the position of the mastoids, which can indicate whether the head is more rotated or tilted to one side, both of which may indicate a positional fault of the craniovertebral joints. Bruising around the mastoids or around the crown of the head (Battle's sign), with a history of trauma, may indicate the presence of a cranial vault injury, such as a basilar fracture. A low hairline may indicate a condition such as Klippel-Feil syndrome,[73] defined as a short neck with decreased cervical movement and low posterior hairline. Radiologically, patients with Klippel-Feil syndrome show a failure of cervical segmentation. The etiology is unclear, but the syndrome is believed to be caused by faulty segmentation of the mesodermal somites.[86] The syndrome appears to be heterogeneous, with environmental factors possibly contributing.[87] Autosomal dominant and recessive patterns of inheritance also have been reported.[88]

Active Range of Motion, Passive Overpressure, and Resistance

Short Neck Flexion. The clinician instructs the patient to place his or her chin on the Adam's apple. This motion simulates flexion at the craniovertebral joints. If this maneuver produces tingling in the feet or electric shock sensations down the neck (Lhermitte's sign), it is highly indicative of serious pathology. Although Lhermitte's sign is not a specific symptom, it is commonly encountered in patients with meningitis and cervical spinal cord demyelination caused by multiple sclerosis.[89] The sign also has been found in many other conditions that cause a traumatic or compressive cervical myelopathy, such as cervical spondylosis, cervical instability, and epidural or subdural tumors.[90,91]

If the patient reports a pulling sensation during short neck flexion, the cervicothoracic junction may be at fault. Active neck flexion tests cranial nerve XI and the C1 and C2 myotomes, as well as muscle strength and the patient's willingness to move. Placing the neck in short neck flexion places the short neck extensors (C1), which are innervated by the spinal accessory nerve, on stretch. The clinician applies overpressure and tests the short neck extensors by asking the patient to resist (Fig. 22-8). Positive findings with this test are severe pain, nausea, muscle spasm, or cord signs, the latter of which may indicate a dens fracture or a tumor, and cause the examination to be terminated.[90] Thus, if a patient is able to flex the neck, a cervical fracture or a transverse ligament compromise can be provisionally ruled out.

Short Neck Extension. The clinician instructs the patient to look upward by only lifting the chin. The patient extends the head on the neck and the clinician attempts to lift the occiput in the direction of the ceiling (Fig. 22-9). An inability to perform this motion (in the presence of normal motion in the other planes) may indicate significant tearing of the anterior cervical

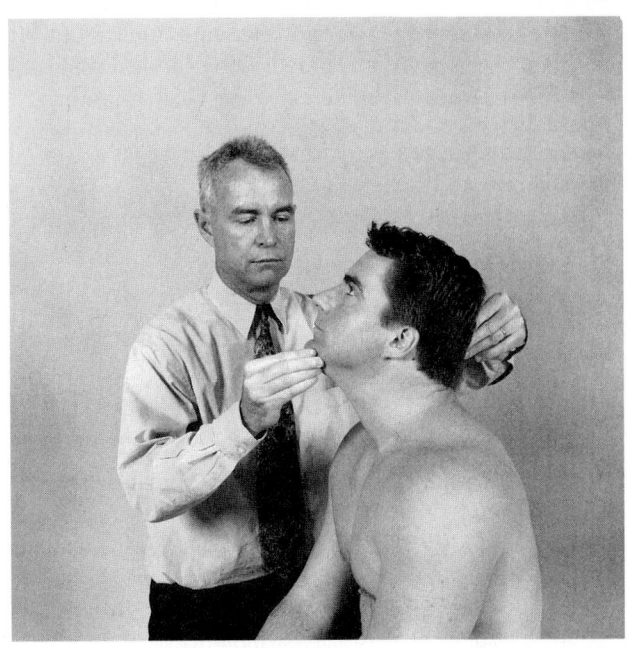

FIGURE 22-9 Short neck extension with overpressure and resistance.

structures. If this test produces tingling in the feet, it is highly suggestive of compression to the spinal cord. This compression may occur because of "buckling" of the ligamentum flavum, causing a loss of its elasticity. A loss of balance or a drop attack with this maneuver would strongly suggest a compromise of the vertebrobasilar system. A drop attack is defined as a loss of balance without a loss of consciousness. The short neck flexors (C1), which are innervated by the spinal accessory nerve, can be tested in this position by applying overpressure as though lifting the patient's chin toward the ceiling while the patient resists (see Fig. 22-9).

> **Clinical Pearl**
>
> If the neck is unstable secondary to a dens fracture or a transverse ligament tear, the patient will be unable or unwilling to flex or extend the neck in the traditional manner, often because of severe muscle spasm.

Rotation. Neck and head rotation could be considered as the functional motion of the craniovertebral joints. Thus, if the patient's symptoms and loss of motion are not reproduced with active rotation, it is doubtful that damage to tissues making up the craniovertebral joints is significant or even present. The patient is asked to perform active neck rotation. An inability to move any amount in either direction is potentially a very serious sign as it could indicate the presence of a dens fracture or a C1–C2 dislocation-fracture. Every measure must be taken to determine the cause of this inability to move. In cases of a suspected fracture or severe instability, the patient should be

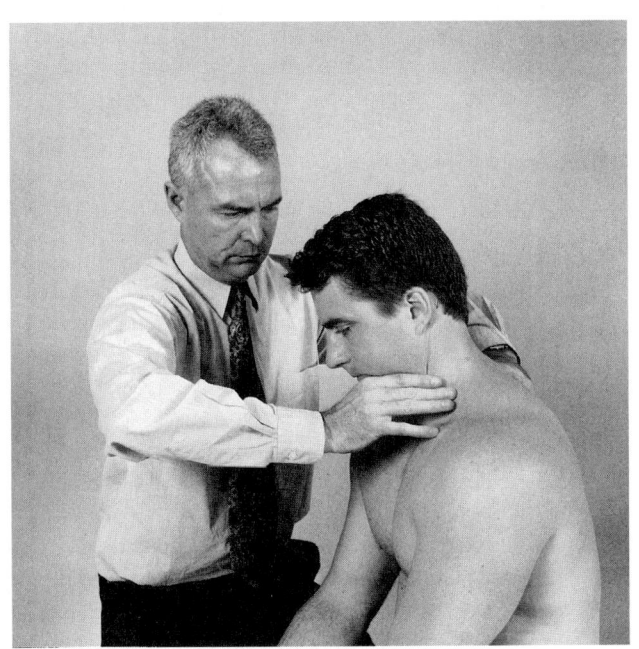

FIGURE 22-8 Short neck flexion with overpressure.

placed in a cervical collar and their physician immediately notified. In addition to the presence of a fracture, some of the other serious conditions that can be provoked by cervical rotation include vertebral artery compromise—cervical rotation is the most likely (single) motion to reproduce signs or symptoms of vertebral artery compromise (see Chap. 21).[92–94, 94a]

The findings from the cervical rotation tests may also afford the clinician some information with regard to a biomechanical lesion of the craniovertebral joints:

▶ A loss of rotation associated with pain and a history of recent trauma. This could indicate the presence of an acute/subacute, post-traumatic arthritis of the craniovertebral joints. Since it may also indicate a soft tissue injury, further testing would be required.

▶ A loss of rotation associated with pain and a history of chronic trauma. This finding could indicate a chronic painless hypomobility with an adaptive but painful ipsilateral hypermobility involving the craniovertebral joints (e.g., pain with right rotation could occur if the right O-A joint cannot flex and there is a hypermobility of the right A-A joint). It may also occur if the left O-A joint cannot extend. Again, further testing is needed to confirm this hypothesis.

▶ A loss of rotation range of motion associated with no pain, but with a history of chronic trauma. This finding, which could indicate a chronic, post-traumatic arthritis, is likely to be an incidental finding, since most patients seek help because of pain. However, depending on the extent of the loss of rotation, the patient may have become aware of a loss of function.

▶ Full rotation range of motion associated with pain and a history of chronic trauma. This could indicate a chronic fibrotic (painless) hypomobility with an adaptive but painful contralateral hypermobility (e.g., pain with right rotation could occur if the left O-A joint cannot flex and the right O-A joint develops a compensatory hypermobility).

To help the clinician differentiate between the possible biomechanical causes for this loss of rotation, the following tests can be used[94a]:

▶ *Combined motion testing (see later).*

▶ *Relevant passive joint glide.* Using the information from the combined motion tests, a joint glide is delivered at the end of range of the combined motion that reproduced the symptoms. The end-feel of the joint glide is assessed, as is pain reproduction.

▶ *Linear segmental stress tests.* These tests are used when the end feel is found to be loose compared to the other side to help determine whether the joint is hypermobile (negative stress test) or unstable (positive stress test). Linear segmental stress tests are described later.

Side Bending. The patient is asked to side bend their head around the appropriate axis. Side bending is included here for

completeness. Much more a function of the lower cervical spine, side bending of the neck is nonetheless significantly decreased in cases of craniovertebral instability or articular fixation. It could be argued that, in the presence of serious ligamentous disruption due to a subluxation of the atlas under the occiput, this motion may provoke symptoms, but it is likely that such a significant incidence of instability would be detected earlier in the examination.[94b] The side bending motions that do occur in the craniovertebral joints are essentially conjunct motions so the results from this test are unlikely to provide much in the way of additional information.

Palpation

Objective palpation of this area is guided by a sound anatomic knowledge. Palpation usually proceeds layer by layer. It should be noted that asymmetric joint geometry is common in this region.[95] For spine palpation to be a valid indicator for manual techniques, the clinician applying it must first be able to differentiate between asymmetric motion caused by vertebral dysfunction and that caused by asymmetric joint anatomy.[95] However, examination of the skin overlying the spine has been found to be very helpful, because certain skin changes in a particular location may point in the direction of a dysfunctional spinal area.[96] The skin is assessed for its thickness, moisture, and ease of displacement in all directions. Abnormal autonomic skin reactions, such as erythematous changes, increased sweat production, and pain that can be induced with minimal palpatory pressure, may indicate a segmental dysfunction.[97]

Palpation may be started at that area indicated by the patient as painful. These painful sites must be correctly localized. The bony landmarks of this region that should be routinely palpated include the occiput, mastoid, atlas, and axis.

Occiput. The clinician locates the external occipital protuberance, which is the most prominent bony structure at the occiput in the midline. By following the external occipital protuberance laterally, the clinician can locate the superior nuchal line. The semispinalis capitis muscle is located about 1½ fingerbreadths below the superior nuchal line.[97]

Mastoid. The mastoid processes are located behind each ear. Once this structure is located, the clinician moves the fingers inferiorly toward the tip of the mastoid process. Starting from the medial tip of the mastoid process, the palpating finger is moved superiorly to the upper pole of the mastoid sulcus, an important area in the examination of the irritation zones of the occiput and C1.[97]

Atlas. By placing the palpating fingers between the mastoid process and the descending ramus of the mandible, the clinician can locate the transverse process of the atlas. The inferior oblique and the superior oblique both have attachments to this site.

Axis. The spinous process of C2 is the first prominent bony landmark that is accessible to palpation below the external occipital protuberance of the occiput. The spinous process of C2 serves as the origin of the inferior oblique muscle and the rectus capitis posterior major muscle.

Positional Tests

The patient is sitting, with the clinician standing behind. With the index and middle fingers of both hands, the clinician palpates the distance between the transverse processes of the atlas and the mastoid processes of the temporal bones.

Flexion

Occipito-atlantal Joint.   With the index and middle fingers of one hand, the clinician palpates the mastoid process and the transverse process of C1 (Fig. 22-10). The patient is asked to flex the O-A joint complex. The clinician assesses the position of the occiput relative to the atlas. The other side is then tested, and a comparison is made. The side with the shortest distance between the occiput and atlas in craniovertebral flexion may be hypomobile.

Atlanto-axial Joint.   Positional testing of this joint is performed by bilaterally palpating the posterior arch of the atlas in the sub-occipital gutter and the lamina of the axis with the index and middle finger (Fig. 22-11). The joint is flexed around its axis. The clinician assesses the position of the C1 vertebra relative to C2 by noting the position of the posterior arch relative to the corresponding lamina of C2. The other side is then tested, and a comparison is made. A left posterior arch of C1 that is posterior relative to the left lamina of C2 is indicative of a left-rotated position of the C1–2 joint complex in flexion.

Extension

Occipito-atlantal Joint.   The O-A joint complex is flexed around the appropriate axis. The clinician assesses the posi-

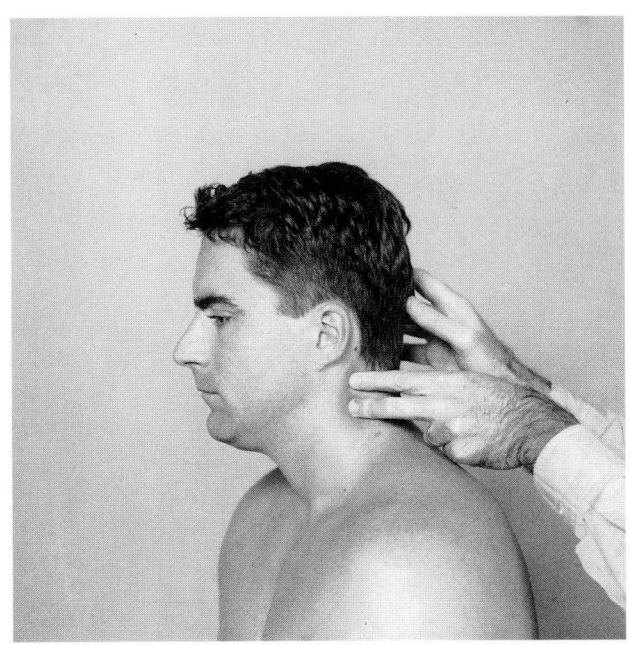

FIGURE 22-11   Position testing for atlanto-axial (A-A) joint.

tion of the occiput relative to the atlas by comparing the left with the right side. The side with the shortest distance between the occiput and atlas in craniovertebral extension may be hypomobile.

Atlanto-axial Joint.   Positional testing of this joint is performed by bilaterally palpating the posterior arch of the atlas in the sub-occipital gutter and the lamina of the axis with the index and middle fingers of both hands. The joint is extended around the appropriate axis. The clinician assesses the position of the C1 vertebra relative to C2 by noting the position of the posterior arch relative to the corresponding lamina of C2. A left posterior arch of C1 that is posterior relative to the left lamina of C2 is indicative of a left-rotated position of the C1–2 joint complex in extension.

Active Mobility of the Occiput, Atlas, and Axis

When interpreting the findings from the active mobility tests, the position of the joint at the beginning of the test should be correlated with the subsequent mobility noted, because alterations in joint mobility may merely reflect an altered starting position.[98] The patient is sitting, with the clinician standing behind. Using the thumb and index fingers of both hands, the clinician palpates each mastoid process of the temporal bones and the transverse processes of the atlas. With the middle fingers of each hand, the clinician palpates the transverse processes of the axis (Fig. 22-12).

▶ For flexion, the patient is asked to flex the head around the appropriate axis. The mastoid processes should travel posteriorly along a curved path at equal distance. The clinician notes the quantity and quality of the motions.

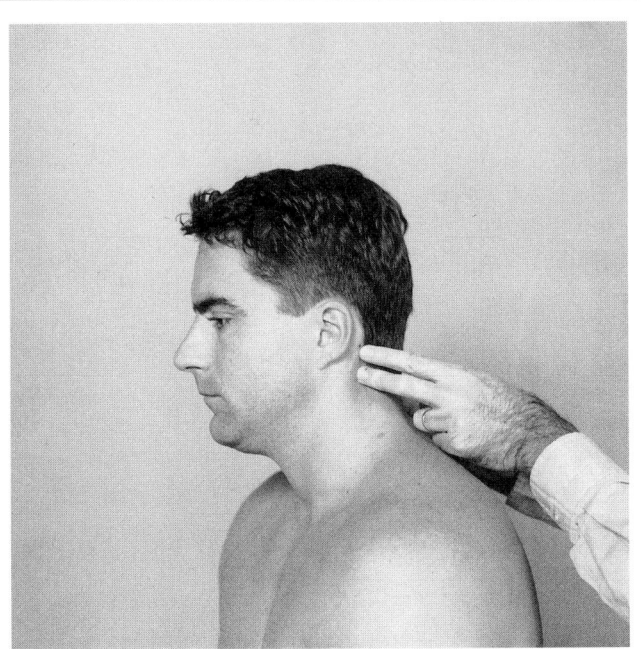

FIGURE 22-10   Position testing for occipito-atlantal (O-A) joint.

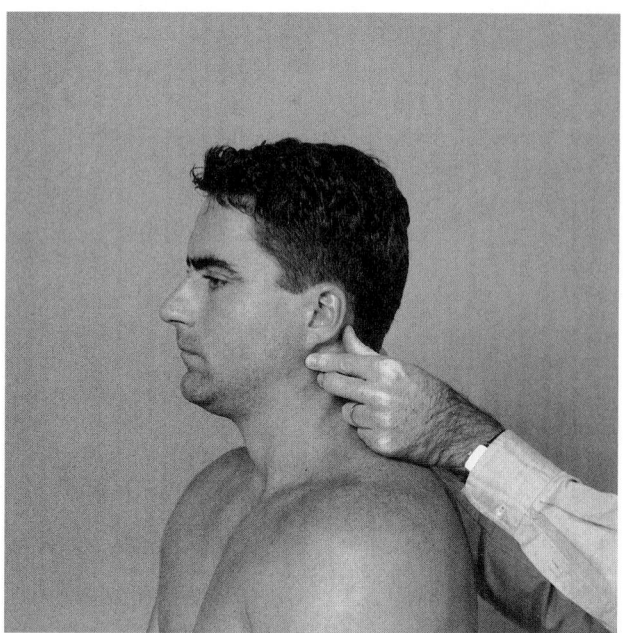

FIGURE 22-12   Active mobility testing of the O-A and A-A joints.

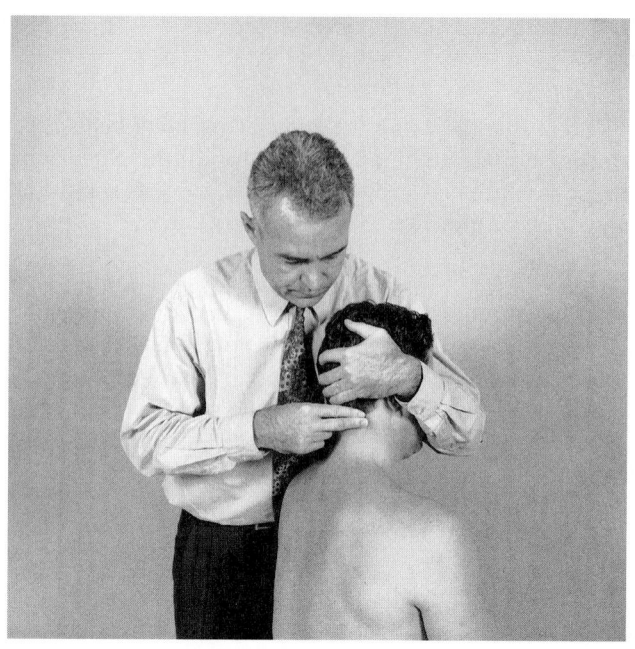

FIGURE 22-13   Mobility testing of side bending.

▶ To assess extension, the patient is asked to extend the head around the appropriate axis. The mastoid processes should travel anteriorly along a curved path at equal distance. The clinician notes the quantity and quality of the motions.

▶ To assess side bending, the patient's head is guided around the appropriate axis (Fig. 22-13). Because conjunct contralateral rotation is usually combined with side bending at this joint, the C_1 transverse process should be felt to approximate the C_2 transverse process in the coronal plane during side bending.[98]

Passive Physiologic Mobility Testing of the Occiput, Atlas, and Axis

Occipito-atlantal Joint. When mobility testing this joint, the first point to remember is that the joint is capable of flexion and extension, but that side bending and rotation also can occur, albeit slight. The second point to keep in mind is that the arthrokinematics of this joint are the reverse of those occurring in the other zygapophysial joints, and that they occur in a different plane (horizontal).

With the patient supine, the head is extended around the axis for the O-A joint (Fig. 22-14). The head is then side bent left and right. As the side bending is performed, a gradual translational force is applied in the direction opposite to the side bending. The range of movement of the side bending is assessed from side to side as is the end-feel of the translation. This procedure is then repeated for flexion.

During extension of the O-A joint (Fig. 22-14), the occipital condyles glide anteriorly to the limit of their symmetric extension range. During left side bending and right translation in extension, the coupled right rotation is produced. This rotation

causes the right occipital condyle to return toward a neutral position, while the left condyle advances toward the extension barrier. If left side bending in extension is limited, then the limiting factor is on the left joint of the segment (ipsilateral to the side bending), which is preventing the advance of the condyle into its normal position. Thus, extension and right translation

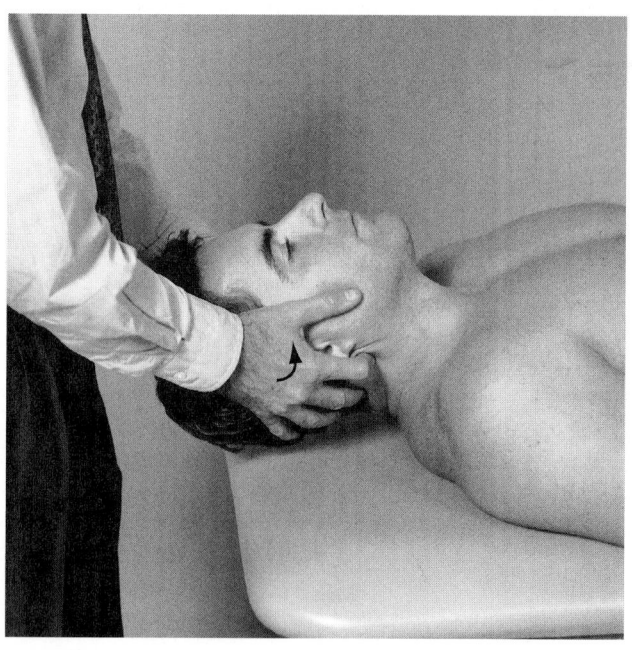

FIGURE 22-14   Passive mobility testing of O-A in extension.

TABLE 22-4   Movement Restrictions of the Craniovertebral Joints and Their Probable Causes

Movement Restriction	Probable Causes
Flexion and right side bending	Left flexion hypomobility Extensor muscle tightness Posterior capsular adhesions Left subluxation (into extension)
Extension and right side bending	Right extension hypomobility Left flexor muscle tightness Anterior capsular adhesions Right subluxation (into flexion)
Flexion and right side bending motion greater than extension and left side bending	Left capsular pattern (arthritis, arthrosis)
Flexion and right side bending equal to extension and left side bending	Left arthrofibrosis (very hard capsular end-feel)
Right side flexion in flexion and extension	Probably an anomaly

tests the anterior glide of the left O-A joint, whereas extension and left translation stresses the anterior glide of the right O-A joint (Table 22-4).

During flexion of the O-A joint, the occipital condyles glide posteriorly (Fig. 22-15). The right rotation associated with left side bending causes the left condyle to move away from the flexion barrier toward the neutral position, while the right condyle is moved posteriorly further into the flexion barrier. Thus, flexion and translation to the right tests the posterior glide of the right O-A joint, whereas flexion and left rotation tests the posterior glide of the left O-A joint (see Table 22-4).

It is apparent that the arthrokinematic and osteokinematic movements are tested simultaneously; thus, the end-feel must be used to determine the cause of the restriction. The following patterns of impairment are more or less commonly seen, and the causes of the impairments can be deduced. However, it must be remembered that deductions are only of value if the resultant intervention is successful.[29]

▶ A patient who has a subluxation into flexion (loss of anterior glide) on the right O-A joint should demonstrate decreased extension, decreased right side bending and left rotation, and a jammed end-feel with translation to left.

▶ A patient with a periarticular restriction of the left O-A joint into flexion (loss of posterior glide) should demonstrate decreased flexion, decreased right side bending and left rotation, and a capsular end-feel with translation to left.

▶ A patient with a fibrous adhesion of the right O-A joint (loss of anterior and posterior guide) should demonstrate decreased extension and right side bending, and decreased flexion and left side bending, with a hard capsular end-feel at both extremes.

▶ With motion testing, a decreased flexion and right side bending with a pathomechanic end-feel, indicates a left O-A joint subluxed into extension.

▶ With motion testing, a decreased extension and right side bending limitation indicates a capsular pattern of the right O-A joint. A decreased extension and left side bending limitation, with a spasmodic end-feel (flexion

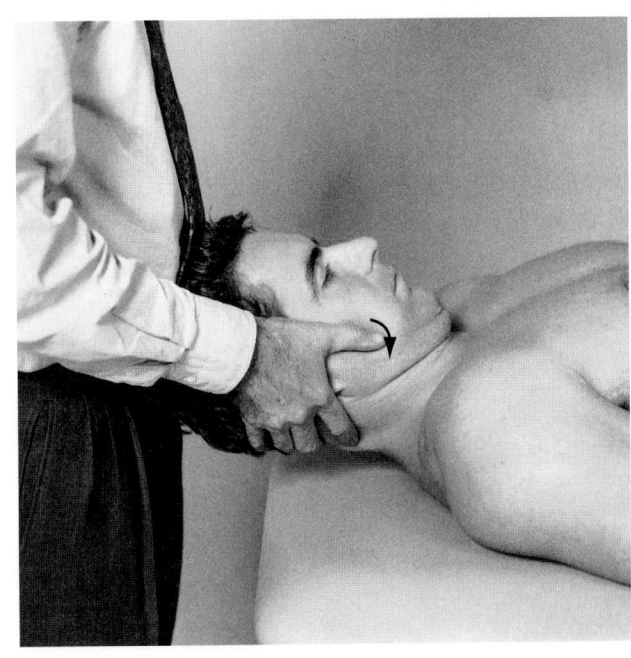

FIGURE 22-15   Passive mobility testing of O-A in flexion.

with greater range), indicates traumatic arthritis of the left O-A joint.

▶ A decreased right translation of the O-A in flexion may indicate a right posterior O-A joint dysfunction or an impaired or tight right superior oblique muscle.

Atlanto-axial Joint.   There are a number of methods to assess the passive physiologic mobility of the A-A joint. The most common method involves the patient lying supine and the clinician applying full cervical flexion, and then introducing cervical rotation. The problem with this technique is that it relies on the fact that the mid to lower cervical spine will be locked with the flexion. Because the neck often is prevented from further flexion when the chin meets the sternum, the clinician has no way of knowing whether full cervical flexion has occurred. Thus, some of the subsequent rotation may be attributed to a combination of cervical spine and A-A motion. This assumption may not be important with asymmetric lesions but can result in false negative findings with symmetric lesions.

A better method of assessment involves the use of cervical side bending. With the patient positioned in sitting, the clinician side bends the head and neck around the craniovertebral axis and then rotates the head in the direction opposite to the side bending (Fig. 22-16). The clinician assesses the amount of range available and then assesses the other side.

Combined Motion Testing

Flexion and extension at the occipito-atlantal joints involve a posterior and anterior gliding of the occipital condyles, respectively.

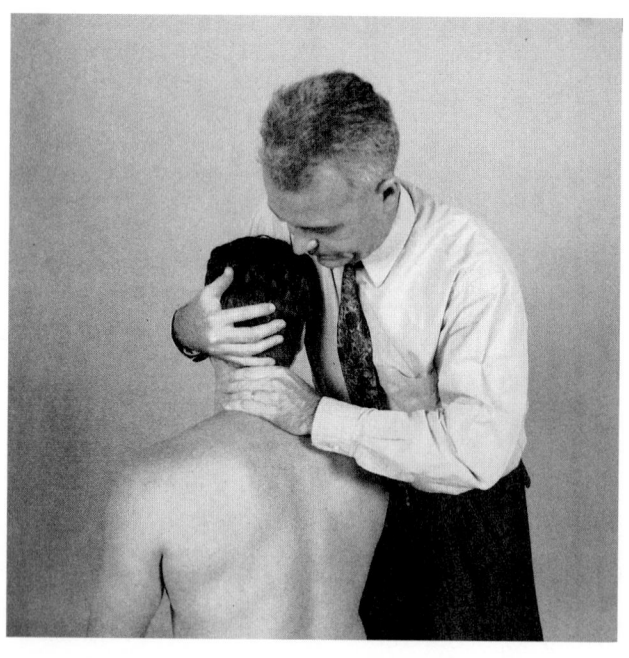

FIGURE 22-16   Passive mobility testing of A-A rotation.

The same gliding (although reciprocal in opposing facets) is utilized in rotation. At the A-A joint, flexion and extension primarily involve a "rolling" action of the condyles, with an insignificant amount of gliding. Therefore, craniovertebral flexion and extension will have a minimal effect on A-A rotation.[94a] Thus, if a symptom or range of motion is drastically altered by craniovertebral flexion or extension, an assumption could be made that the dysfunction is at the O-A joint.[94a] For example, if the right occipital condyle cannot glide posteriorly, the right joint will be unable to flex or to permit rotation to the right, as both of these motions involve a posterior glide at the right O-A joint. In the combined motion tests, the right rotation restriction will be more evident when combined with craniovertebral flexion, but will be less evident when combined with craniovertebral extension.

The findings from the combined motion tests can be used to determine which joint glide is to be assessed. For example, if it was determined in the combined motion testing that the **right** O-A joint is restricted or painful with flexion (implicating the posterior glide), the O-A joint is positioned in its extreme of flexion and right rotation (the two motions associated with a posterior glide of the right O-A joint).

Linear Segmental Stress Testing

The craniovertebral region demonstrates a high degree of mobility, but little stability, with the ligaments affording little protection during a high-velocity injury. Instability of this region can result from a number of causes:

▶ *Trauma (especially a hyperflexion injury to the neck).*

▶ *Rheumatoid arthritis, psoriatic arthritis, or ankylosing spondylitis.*   Nontraumatic hypermobility or frank instability of the O-A joint has been reported in association with rheumatoid arthritis.[99]

▶ *Corticosteroid use.*   Prolonged exposure to this class of drug can produce a softening of the dens and transverse ligament by deteriorating the Sharpey fibers, which attach the ligament to the bone. Steroid use also promotes osteoporosis, predisposing bones to fracture.

▶ *Recurrent upper respiratory tract infections or chronic sore throats in children.*   Grisel's syndrome[100] is a spontaneous A-A dislocation affecting children between the ages of 6 and 12 years. The outstanding symptom is a spontaneously arising torticollis. The most likely etiology seems to be an inflammation of the retropharyngeal space caused by upper respiratory tract infections or by adenotonsillectomy and producing pharyngeal hyperemia and bone absorption.

▶ *Congenital malformation.*   Nontraumatic hypermobility or frank instability of the O-A joint has been reported in association with congenital bony malformations.[101]

▶ *Down syndrome.*   Nontraumatic hypermobility or frank instability of the O-A joint has been reported in children and adolescents with Down syndrome.[102,103]

▶ *Immature development.* Patients younger than 12 years of age often have an immature or absent dens (see later).

▶ *Osteoporosis.*

It must be remembered that the A-A joint complex consists of three joints. The median joint, although it has no weight-bearing function, is extremely important in maintaining stability, while at the same time facilitating motion within this joint complex. Fielding and colleagues[104] found that the stability of the A-A joint depends greatly on the ligamentous structures, and on a normal and intact dens. On occasion, the integrity of the dens can be compromised because of:

1. Anomalies of the dens, including:
   a. Os odontoideum. This is a condition in which the intervertebral disk between the developing bodies of axis and atlas does not ossify.
   b. Congenital absence of the dens.
   c. An underdeveloped dens whose lack of height renders it unchecked by the transverse ligament. The body of the dens is not of sufficient size to be retained in the osseo-oligamentous ring of the atlas until a child is approximately 12 years old. Great care and justification is needed with any craniovertebral mobilization or manipulative technique with this age group.
2. Pathologies affecting the dens, including:
   a. Demineralization or resorption of the dens, such as occurs with Grisel's syndrome[100] or rheumatoid arthritis.
   b. An old, undisplaced, fracture (especially of the dens), which originally escaped diagnosis, and subsequently formed a pseudoarthrosis.

Indications for Stability Testing. The following findings are considered to be indications to perform a stability or stress tests of the craniovertebral region[90]:

▶ History of neck trauma or any of the causes of instability listed previously.

▶ Patient report of neck instability.

▶ Presence of the following signs and symptoms:

• A lump in the throat.

• Lip paresthesia.

• Nausea or vomiting.

• Severe headache and muscle spasm.

• Dizziness.

The patient is positioned supine to remove any muscular influences. If the patient is unable to lie down, the clinician may need to reconsider the appropriateness of performing these tests.

Longitudinal Stability. General traction is applied to the entire cervical region. If this maneuver does not reproduce the signs

or symptoms, C2 is stabilized so that the traction force may be directed at the craniovertebral region (Fig. 22-17).

***Anterior Shear: Transverse Ligament.*[90]** The patient is positioned supine, with his or her head cradled in the clinician's hands. The clinician locates the anterior arches of C2 by moving around the vertebra from the back to the front using the thumbs. Once the arches are located, the clinician pushes down on the anterior arches of C2 with the thumbs toward the table, while the patient's occiput and C1, cupped in the clinician's hands, is lifted, keeping the head parallel to the ceiling but in slight flexion (Fig. 22-18). The patient is instructed to keep the eyes open and to count backward aloud. The position is held for approximately 15 seconds or until an end-feel is perceived.

Coronal Stability: Alar Ligament. Rotation and side bending tighten the contralateral alar (e.g., rotation or side bending to the right tightens the left alar) whereas flexion typically tightens both alar ligaments.

The transverse process of C2 is palpated with one hand, while the patient's head is side bent or rotated (Fig. 22-19). This is a test of immediacy. If the C2 transverse process does not move as soon as the head begins to rotate, laxity of the alar ligament should be suspected.

***Transverse Shear.*[90]** Transverse shearing of the craniovertebral joints is performed with the patient supine. The clinician stabilizes the mastoid, and C1 is moved in a transverse direction, using the soft part of the metacarpophalangeal joint of the index

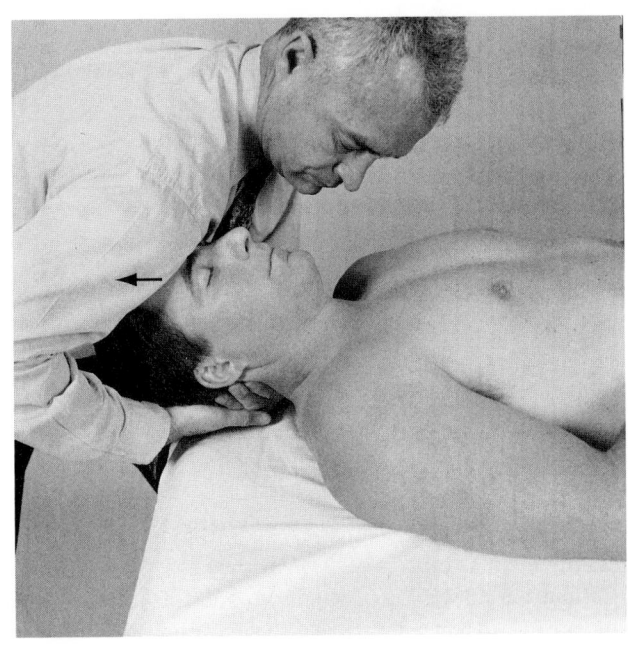

FIGURE 22-17 Longitudinal stability testing.

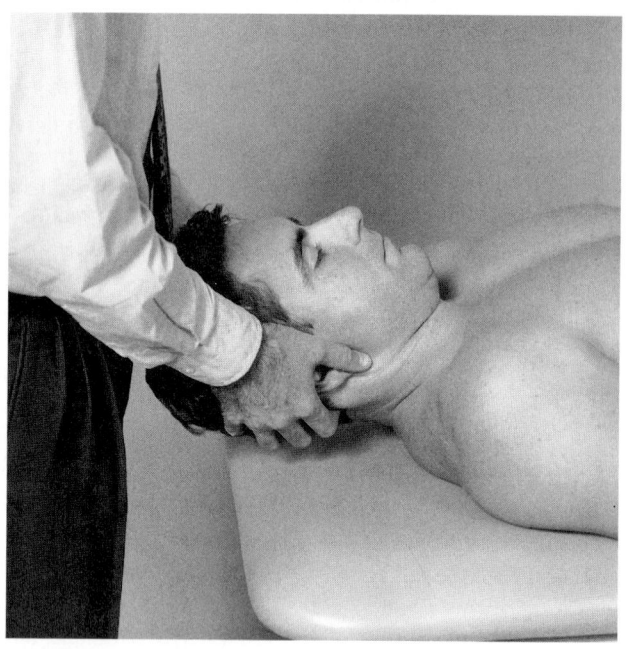

FIGURE 22-18   Transverse ligament test.

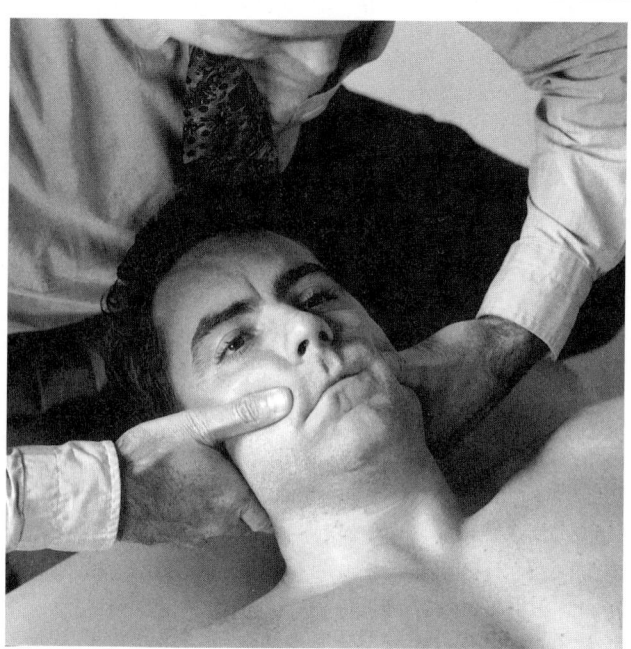

FIGURE 22-20   Translational shear of O-A joint.

move C2 transversely using the soft part of metacarpals (Fig. 22-21). No movement should be felt.

Neurologic Examination

The neurologic examination is performed to assess the normal conduction of the central and peripheral nervous systems. The presence of neurologic symptoms deserves special attention.

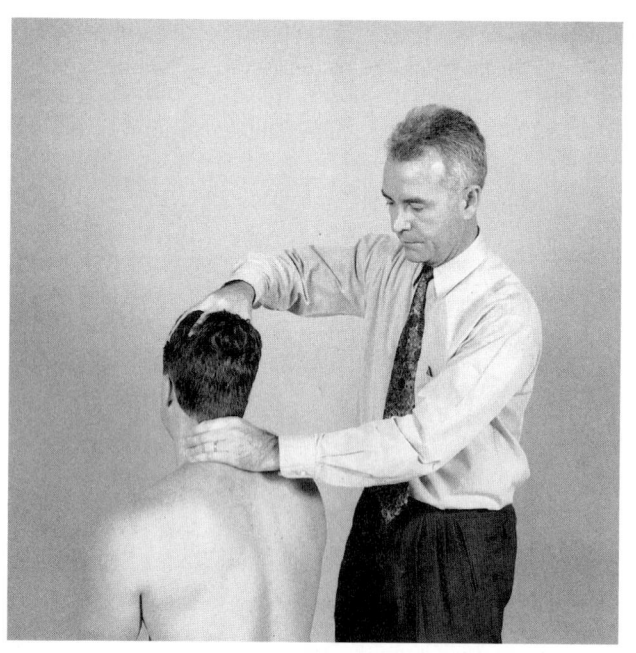

FIGURE 22-19   Alar ligament test.

finger (Fig. 22-20). The test is repeated by stabilizing C1 and translating the mastoid.

C1 and C2 can be tested similarly. The soft aspect of each second metacarpal head is placed on the opposite transverse processes and laminae of C1 and C2, with the palms facing each other. The clinician stabilizes C1 and then attempts to

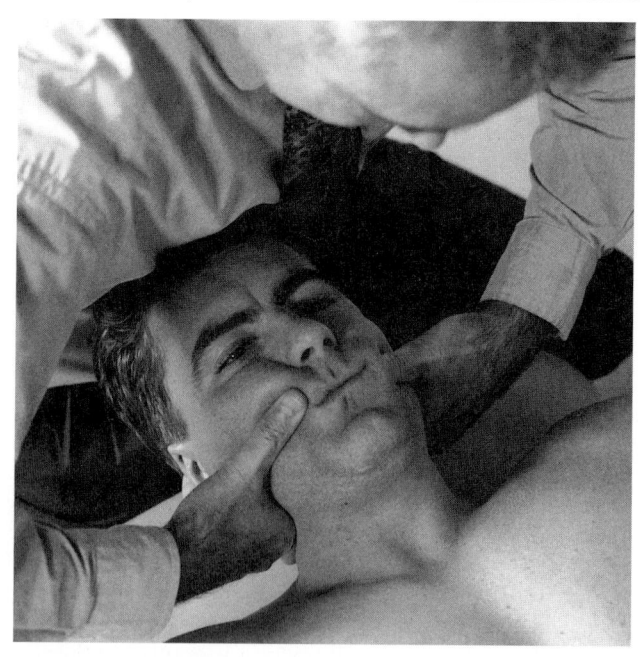

FIGURE 22-21   Translational shear of A-A joint.

Many of the symptoms that occur in an upper limb have their origins in the neck. The patient with neck trauma can report seemingly bizarre symptoms, but these need to be heeded until the clinician can rule out serious pathology. Cervical myelopathy, involving an injury to the spinal cord itself, is associated with multisegmental paresthesias, upper motor neuron (UMN) signs and symptoms such as spasticity, hyperreflexia, visual and balance disturbances, ataxia, and sudden changes in bowel and bladder function. The presence of any UMN sign or symptom requires an immediate medical referral.

In addition to the deep tendon reflexes and sensory tests outlined in Chapter 23, the clinician should perform the spinal cord reflexes of Babinski and Hoffman (see Chapter 2). Studies by Boden and colleagues[105] and Sung and Wang have demonstrated that the Hoffman test is the most sensitive reflex test in the detection of cervical myelopathy.[106]

Special Tests

Barre's Test. Barre's test can be used to assess for vertebral artery insufficiency, especially if the patient is unable to lie supine.

The patient is seated with the arms outstretched, forearms supinated. The patient is asked to close his or her eyes and move the head and neck into maximum extension and rotation (Fig. 22-22). A positive test is one in which one of the outstretched arms sinks toward the floor and pronates, indicating the side of the compromise.

For other tests for the vertebral artery, including Hautard's, and the DeKleyn-Nieuwenhuyse test, the reader is referred to Chapter 21.

Dix-Hallpike Test. This test can be used to help determine if the cause of the patient's dizziness is a vestibular impairment resulting from an accumulation of utricle debris (otoconia), which can move within the posterior semicircular canals and stimulate the vestibular sense organ (cupula). This test usually is performed only if the vertebral artery test and instability tests do not provoke symptoms.

The test involves having the patient suddenly lie down from a sitting position with the head rotated in the direction that the clinician feels is the provocative position.[69a] The end point of the test is when the patient's head overhangs the end of the table so that the cervical spine is extended (Fig. 22-23). A positive test reproduces the patient's symptoms.

Modified Sharp-Purser Test. This test was designed originally to test the sagittal stability of the A-A segment in patients with rheumatoid arthritis, because a number of pathologic conditions can affect the stability of the osseoligamentous ring of the median joints of this segment in this patient population. These changes result in degeneration and thinning of the articular cartilage between the odontoid process and the anterior arch of the atlas, or, occasionally, in softening of the dens.

The aim of the test was to determine whether the instability was significant enough to provoke central nervous system's signs or symptoms.

The patient is positioned sitting. The patient is asked to segmentally flex the head and relate any signs or symptoms that this might evoke to the clinician. In addition, a positive test may be indicated by the patient hearing or feeling a clunk. Local symptoms, such as soreness, are ignored for the purposes of evaluating the test. If no serious signs or symptoms are provoked, the clinician stabilizes C2 with one hand and applies a posteriorly oriented force to the head (Fig. 22-24).

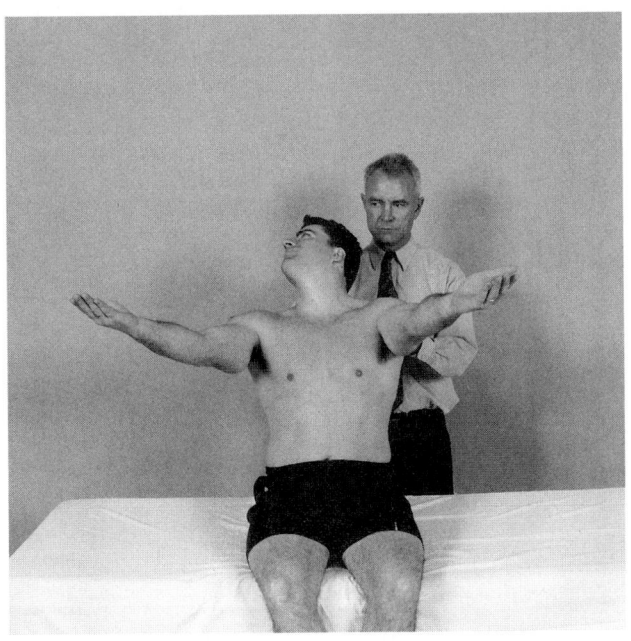

FIGURE 22-22 Barre's test.

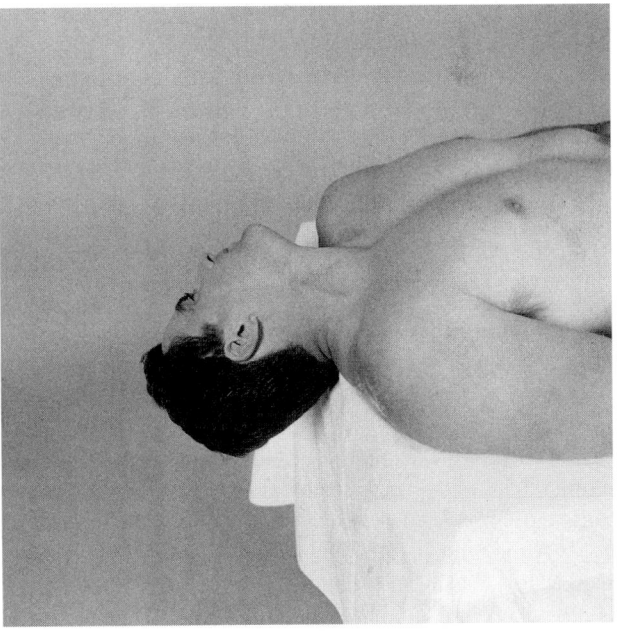

FIGURE 22-23 Dix-Hallpike test.

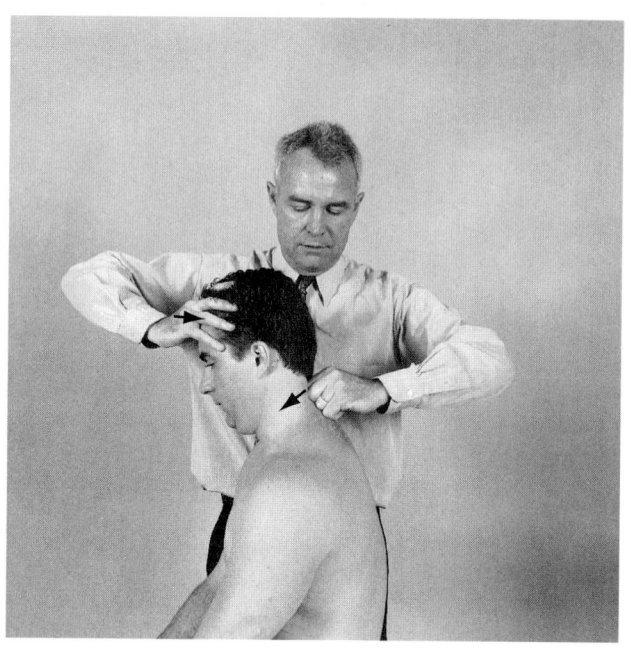

FIGURE 22-24   Modified Sharp-Purser test.

In the presence of a positive test, a provisional assumption is made that the symptoms are caused by excessive translation of the atlas, compromising one or more of the sensitive structures listed previously, and the physical examination is terminated. No intervention should be attempted other than the issuing of a cervical collar to prevent craniovertebral flexion and an immediate referral to the patient's physician.

Imaging Studies

The standard, initial cervical spine radiographic series in trauma patients includes a cross-table lateral view, an anteroposterior view, and an open-mouth view, the latter of which is used to help rule out a fracture of the dens.[106a] The usefulness of the anteroposterior view has been questioned because it provides little additional information.[106b] Although this three-view screening series can detect 65–95 percent of axis injuries,[106c,106d] the C2 vertebra often is obscured by overlying bony maxillary, mandibular, and dental structures; therefore, C2 fractures may be missed.[106a] The clinician needs to be aware of the limitations of plain radiographs, as problems exist with both specificity and sensitivity. However, radiographs can provide a gross assessment of the severity of the degenerative changes of the spine.

Thin-section CT is the best study for evaluating C2 bony fractures.[106e] Sagittal reconstruction of CT images is important because axial images may not detect a transverse odontoid fracture.[106a] Although CT is excellent in evaluating bony injuries, it can miss soft tissue and significant ligamentous injuries.[106a] Recently, therefore, dynamic flexion/extension lateral fluoroscopic evaluation has been advocated in polytrauma patients to identify occult ligamentous instabilities and confirm that the

cervical spine is uninjured.[106f] As with any diagnostic study, the findings must be correlated with the history and physical examination.

Intervention Strategies

The gamut of musculoskeletal injury to the craniovertebral region of the spine ranges from a simple strain (muscle) or sprain (ligament) to bone and neurovascular injuries. The most common injuries seen clinically are muscle strains and postural dysfunctions.

Muscle strains are common in the cervical spine because most of the cervical muscles attach via myofascial tissue inserting into the periosteum rather than by the more resilient tendon.[107] The severity of the strain is dependent on the magnitude of forces involved. If the force is sufficient, both the muscle and the associated joint become involved. In an abnormal spine, the forces needed to cause injury are reduced. Repetitive microtrauma is a common cause of craniovertebral dysfunction.

Postural dysfunctions of this region, particularly the forward head posture, usually manifest themselves at the O-A joint, resulting in fixed capital extension and a loss of O-A flexion. Patients with postural dysfunctions may develop secondary myofascial trigger points and myofascial pain syndromes. In postural dysfunctions and trauma-related injuries, other joints and regions may be involved and require further investigation.

Pain, tenderness, active range of motion restrictions, muscle imbalances, and segmental motion restrictions are common findings with craniovertebral dysfunction.

The structure at fault should determine the intervention:[98a]

▶ If ligamentous tissue damage or an intra-articular lesion are suspected, the safest initial approach would be to help in unloading the joint and controlling the extremes of motion with a soft collar for a 7 to 10 day period

▶ Within the patient's pain tolerance, contractile lesions should be treated aggressively with the emphasis on regaining maximal muscle length.[98a]

The techniques to increase joint mobility and the techniques to increase soft tissue extensibility are described later, under "Therapeutic Techniques."

A correct diagnosis can be accomplished through detailed history, and a comprehensive examination. Confirmation of the correct diagnosis can be made with an assessment of the response of the patient to the initial rehabilitation program. The intervention for the craniovertebral region may commence when the possibility of serious injury including fracture, dislocation, or injury to the spinal cord and vertebral artery have been ruled out.

Acute Phase

The goals of this phase include:

▶ Reduce pain, inflammation, and muscle spasm.

▶ Reestablish a nonpainful range of motion.

► Improve neuromuscular postural control.

► Retard muscle atrophy.

► Promote healing.

Various electrotherapeutic modalities and physical agents may be used during the acute phase to modulate pain and to decrease inflammation and muscle spasm. Therapeutic cold and electrical stimulation may be used for 48 to 72 hours. The cryotherapy is continued at home. A transcutaneous electrical nerve stimulation (TENS) unit may be prescribed to help control pain and encourage range of motion. Joint protection may be appropriate. In such cases, a soft or semirigid cervical collar may be prescribed for 7 to 10 days to reduce muscle guarding (see Chap. 23). Nonsteroidal anti-inflammatory drugs (NSAIDs) often are prescribed for 2 to 3 weeks to help decrease inflammation and to control pain, thereby increasing the potential for an early return to function. Bed rest, along with analgesics and muscle relaxants for no more than 2 to 3 days, is prescribed for patients with a severe injury. However, in less severe cases, bed rest has not been shown to improve recovery and, compared with mobilization or patient education, rest tends to prolong symptoms.[108,109]

The patient also is taught how to find the neutral position for the upper cervical spine. The neutral position is defined as the least painful position that minimizes mechanical stresses.

Range of motion exercises are initiated as early as possible, based on patient tolerance, to prevent hypomobility. Neck flexion and rotation exercises usually are performed first. Extension and side bending exercises are introduced based on the response of the patient to the flexion and rotation exercises. The rotation and side bending exercises are performed in the supine position, and then progressed to weight bearing. All of the exercises should be performed in the pain-free range.

Upper extremity range-of-motion and strengthening exercises also should be introduced to promote early integration of the entire upper kinetic chain. Important muscles to include are the rhomboids, middle and lower trapezius, latissimus dorsi, serratus anterior, and deltoid. In addition, the muscles of the rotator cuff should be strengthened.

Gentle manual techniques (see "Therapeutic Techniques," later) such as sustained or rhythmic specific traction (grade I or II) and massage also may be used. As the patient progresses, muscle stretching may be introduced. Manual techniques can have a mechanical effect on joint mobility and soft tissue extensibility. In addition, these techniques can have beneficial neurophysiologic effects, which can help alleviate pain and muscle spasm. Self-stretching and self-mobilization techniques are taught to the patient at the earliest and appropriate opportunity (see "Therapeutic Techniques," later).

Active joint protection techniques may be part of the acute phase. Joint protection exercises work by supporting the joint and reducing the applied stresses. Joint protection exercises include cervical stabilization exercises. These exercises initially are performed in single planes and in the neutral position, using submaximal isometric contractions. As with the range-of-motion exercises, it is recommended that these exercises be performed initially in the supine position, and later, sitting, as tolerance increases. As the pain-free ranges increase, the exercises are performed throughout the newly attained pain-free ranges.

Aerobic conditioning also must be included as part of the comprehensive rehabilitation program. A stationary bike, treadmill, or a stair-stepping machine can be used.

The patient is advanced to the functional phase when:

► The pain has significantly decreased so that there is minimal pain with activities of daily living.

► There is significant improvement in the pain-free ranges of motion.

Functional Phase

The duration of this phase can vary tremendously, and depends on several factors:

► Severity of the injury.

► Healing capacity of the patient.

► How the condition was managed during the acute phase.

► Level of patient involvement in the rehabilitation program.

The goals of this phase are to:

► Significantly reduce or completely resolve the patient's pain.

► Restore full and pain-free range of motion.

► Fully integrate the entire upper kinetic chain.

► Restore full cervical and upper quadrant strength and neuromuscular control.

During this phase, the range-of-motion exercises are continued until maximum range of motion is attained. The strengthening program is progressed from submaximal isometrics in single planes to maximal isometrics in single planes. Then the patient is progressed to isometrics in combined motions (flexion and side bending, extension and side bending). The strength training is then progressed to concentric and eccentric exercises in single planes using elastic tubing, pulleys, or isolation exercises. Proprioceptive neuromuscular facilitation patterns are introduced when appropriate. Elastic tubing is issued to the patient to allow training at home.

For progression to return to play, the athlete should demonstrate:

► Normal and pain-free single plane and multiplane range of motion.

► Normal cervical, cervicothoracic, glenohumeral, and scapulothoracic strength.

► Normal flexibility of cervical, cervicoscapular, and cervicothoracic musculature.

Return to sport activities should be designed to mimic the sport as closely as possible. The goal should be to improve the balance, power, and endurance of the cervical, cervicothoracic, glenohumeral, and scapulothoracic muscle groups and force couples.

Pattern 4D: Impaired Joint Mobility, Motor Function, Muscle Performance, Range of Motion Associated with Connective Tissue Dysfunction

Transverse Ligament Injuries

Injuries to the transverse ligament are classified as follows[21,27]:

▶ *Type I injuries.* Disruptions of the substance of the transverse ligament, without an osseous component.

▶ *Type II injuries.* Fractures or avulsions involving the tubercle for insertion of the transverse ligament on the C1 lateral mass, without disruption of the ligament substance.

The medical literature supports the conclusion that a type I injury is incapable of healing without surgery for internal fixation, but that most type II injuries heal when treated with an orthosis.[38]

Integration of Patterns 4B and 4D: Impaired Joint Mobility, Motor Function, Muscle Performance, Range of Motion Secondary to Impaired Posture and Connective Tissue Dysfunction

Myofascial Pain Patterns

Myofascial pain syndromes are closely associated with tender areas that have come to be known as myofascial trigger points (MTrPs; see Chap. 11). The term *myofascial trigger point* is a bit of a misnomer, because trigger points also may be cutaneous, ligamentous, periosteal, and fascial.[110] Dysfunctional joints also are associated with trigger points and tender attachment points.[111]

For a more detailed description of myofascial pain patterns, including their causes, signs and symptoms, and interventions, the reader is referred to the excellent book by Travell and Simons, *Myofascial Pain and Dysfunction: The Trigger Point Manual* (Volume 1, *The Upper Extremities*),[55] from which the following information was taken.

Trapezius. According to Travell and Simons,[55] the trapezius muscle is probably the muscle most often beset by MTrPs. In terms of the referral pain patterns that it generates, the trapezius muscle is divided into three portions: upper, middle, and lower. Activation of the MTrPs in the trapezius muscle typically is caused by sustained habitual loading, as in postural dysfunctions, tight clothing (e.g., narrow bra straps), heavy backpacks, and repetitive rotation of the head.

Upper Trapezius. Activation of the trigger points in the upper trapezius can cause a wide range of symptoms, including severe posterolateral neck pain, often constant and usually associated with temporal headache on the ipsilateral side, hypersensitivity, and pain at the angle of the jaw. Neck rotation to the opposite side usually is limited and painful.

Middle Trapezius. The most common symptoms with activation of the trigger points in this portion of the muscle are burning interscapular pain, tenderness over the acromion, and, occasionally, a referred autonomic response of pilomotor erection on the anterolateral surfaces of the ipsilateral arm.

Lower Trapezius. Activation of the trigger points in the lower trapezius can cause a variety of symptoms, which can include suprascapular, interscapular, acromial, or neck pain, or a combination of these. Neck motion usually is unaffected.

Sternocleidomastoid. Active trigger points in the sternocleidomastoid often are misdiagnosed as a typical facial neuralgia, tension headache, or cervicocephalalgia. The sternal and clavicular divisions of the sternocleidomastoid muscle have their own characteristic pain patterns. As a rule, these divisions refer pain to the face and cranium rather than the neck, although an active trigger point at the lower end of the sternal division is capable of producing referred pain over the sternum. Because trigeminal facial neuralgia is not accompanied by sternal pain, the finding of sternal pain can help in differential diagnosis.

Sternal Division. Activation of the trigger points in the sternal division can refer an aching deep pain across the mastoid, ipsilateral cheek, maxilla, supraorbital ridge, and deep within the orbit. Vertex pain, in a pattern resembling a skull cap, or sore throat and tongue pain also have been found to be associated with these trigger points.

Autonomic concomitants of these MTrPs include eye, ear, and nose symptoms. Eye symptoms include excessive lacrimation, apparent ptosis, blurring of vision, and reddening. Ear symptoms can include unilateral deafness and tinnitus. Nose symptoms can include sinus congestion on the ipsilateral side.

Clavicular Division. Activation of the trigger points in the clavicular division can refer pain to the frontal area, ipsilateral ear, and the cheek and molar areas on the ipsilateral side. Other symptoms can include postural dizziness and, in severe cases, even syncope when turning the head.

Temporalis. Activation of the trigger points in the temporalis muscle can refer pain widely throughout the temple, along the eyebrow, behind the eye, and in any or all of the upper teeth.

Masseter. Activation of the trigger points in the masseter may refer pain mainly to the lower jaw, molar teeth and related gums, and to the maxilla.

Medial Pterygoid. Activation of the trigger points in the medial pterygoid may refer pain in poorly circumscribed regions related to the mouth (tongue, pharynx, and hard palate), below and behind the temporomandibular joint, including deep in the ear, but not usually to the teeth.

Lateral Pterygoid. Activation of the trigger points in the lateral pterygoid may refer pain deep into the temporomandibular joint and to the region of the maxillary sinus.

Splenius Capitis. Activation of the trigger points in the splenius capitis can refer pain to the vertex of the head on the same side.

Splenius Cervicis. Activation of the trigger points in the splenius cervicis may refer a diffuse pain through the inside of the head, especially behind the ipsilateral eye, and sometimes to the scalp over the occiput and base of the neck. Other symptoms that may be associated with an MTrP of the splenius cervicis include blurring of near vision in the ipsilateral eye.

Semispinalis Capitis, Semispinalis Cervicis, and Multifidi. Activation of the trigger points in the semispinalis capitis, semispinalis cervicis, and multifidi may refer pain and tenderness upward to the suboccipital region and sometimes down the neck to the upper vertebral border of the scapula.

Suboccipital Muscles. Activation of the trigger points in the suboccipital muscles may refer poorly localized pain to the inside of the skull, and forward and unilaterally to the eye and forehead.

The interventions for MTrPs are outlined in Chapter 11. These include stretch and spray, muscle stripping, massage therapy, myofascial release, ischemic compression, stretching, postural correction and education to eliminate any causative or perpetuating factors, electrotherapeutic and thermal modalities, cryotherapy, injections, and joint mobilizations.

Integration of Patterns 4D and 4E: Impaired Joint Mobility, Motor Function, Muscle Performance, Range of Motion Secondary to Connective Tissue Dysfunction and Localized Inflammation

Osteoarthritis
Osteoarthrosis of the A-A joints, unrelated to trauma, is a rare cause of pain in the craniovertebral region, and an even more uncommon cause of A-A instability. It could be argued that if osteoarthrosis of the lateral mass articulations progresses, the synovitis may gradually involve the ligamentous structures, thereby weakening them and rendering them prone to rupture.[113]

Inflammatory Arthritis
The greatest risk for complications with the spondyloarthropathies in the craniovertebral region occurs at the A-A joint, where there are two different synovial articulations: the two lateral facet joints, and the articulation between the odontoid process of C2 and the anterior part of C1.[92] The transverse ligament is typically the weakest part of the complex in the presence of spondyloarthropathy.

Rheumatoid Arthritis. The most common inflammatory lesion found in the retro-odontoid space is rheumatoid arthritis, which induces abnormal proliferation of the synovial soft tissue (pannus) and frequently causes the destruction of the bony structure[114] (see Chap. 9).

Ankylosing Spondylitis. See Chapter 9.

Gout. See Chapter 9.

Craniovertebral Instability
There has been much controversy about defining and diagnosing spinal instability. Segmental spinal instability generally is defined as a greater displacement between vertebrae than under physiologic load. Therefore, maximum flexion and extension radiographs usually are used to determine hypermobility between vertebrae. Craniovertebral instability frequently is encountered in inflammatory, neoplastic, degenerative, and traumatic disorders, in addition to congenital and developmental abnormalities. Clinically, instability appears as a subluxation or spinal deformity accompanied by severe pain or neurologic deficits. Several types of craniovertebral instability are recognized; among them:

▶ ***Translational or rotary instability of C1.*** Translational anterior A-A instability is detected on lateral cervical radiographs as a widened, mobile atlantodental interval (ADI) of greater than 3 mm, caused by laxity or rupture of the transverse ligament or from an odontoid fracture.[115] Patients with congenital abnormalities of the odontoid process may develop chronic A-A subluxation. This leads to the formation of fibrous granulation tissue or a hypertrophic scar in the periodontoid or retro-odontoid epidural space, which is known as a "pseudotumor."[116] Chronic mechanical irritation associated with neck movement is speculated to be one of the causes of fibrous scar formation.[117] Posterior translation of C1 is also possible, but for this to occur, the dens or anterior arch of the atlas must be fractured or incompetent. Rotational A-A instability appears as asymmetric rotation of the C1 lateral masses on plain radiographs. Rotational subluxations that are irreducible, recurrent, or associated with transverse ligament disruption require surgery.[115] Patients with A-A subluxations exceeding 6 mm are at high risk for neurologic injury and sudden death and are, therefore, immediately considered for fusion.[118]

▶ ***Occipito-atlantal instability.*** O-A instability is demonstrated radiographically by movement between the dens and basion (the middle point on the anterior margin of the foramen magnum), by distraction or translation of the occipital condyles, or by vertical migration.[119]

Surgical stabilization is required to correct instability when conservative intervention has failed or when spontaneous healing with an orthosis, such as a halo brace, is unlikely.

Pattern 4F: Impaired Joint Mobility, Motor Function, Muscle Performance, Range of Motion, or Reflex Integrity, Secondary to Spinal Disorders

Dizziness
Dizziness is the third most common complaint among outpatients, after chest pain and fatigue.[120] There are several types of

dizziness, some benign and some serious, and it is important that the clinician be able to make the distinction. Among the cervical causes of dizziness that must be carefully considered by the clinician are the systemic, central, and peripheral causes of vertigo or dizziness.[121]

▶ Systemic causes include pharmacologic agents, hypotension, and diseases of the endocrine system.

▶ Central causes include cervical or reflex vertigo, vestibular neuritis, Ramsay Hunt syndrome, and vertebrobasilar artery dysfunction.

▶ Peripheral causes can include labyrinthitis and benign paroxysmal positional vertigo. These causes are the most frequently encountered in clinical practice.[121]

Cervical Vertigo.   Cervical vertigo is a diagnosis and a disorder that seems to be poorly understood, and yet dizziness is a common clinical symptom in patients with cervical and upper quadrant syndromes.[121] Cervical or reflex vertigo is thought to originate from a disturbance of the tonic neck reflex input from the neck to the vestibular nucleus. This disturbance can be caused by a dysfunction in the cervical joints[122] or the sternocleidomastoid.[123] As early as 1926, Barré[124] described a syndrome involving suboccipital pain and vertigo that was usually precipitated by turning the head. Ryan and Cope[125] coined the term "cervical vertigo" in 1955 for this syndrome.

Cervical vertigo symptoms appear to result from an alteration to proprioceptive spinal afferents from the mechanoreceptors of the neck, usually, but not always, resulting from trauma.[126] Macnab[127] thought that the 575 patients he studied exhibited little evidence of overt neck damage, or of neurologic damage. He thought areas other than the neck itself, such as the brain, brain stem, cranial nerves, cervical nerve roots, or inner ear, might be responsible for the symptoms. Biesinger,[128] on the other hand, proposed two possible neurologic origins:

1. A participant from the sympathetic plexus surrounding the vertebral arteries.

2. Functional disorders of proprioception in segments C1 to C2.

It would seem likely that direct damage to the vestibular apparatus, or severe damage to the vertebral artery, will produce immediate dizziness, whereas dizziness arising from the cervical joints or a less severely injured vertebral artery may not occur until the joints themselves became abnormal, or until the ischemia has had time to make itself felt.[54a] Because cervical pain also frequently is delayed, it is at least arguable that delayed dizziness commonly originates from injured cervical joints and less commonly from ischemia.[54a]

The intervention for cervical vertigo generally begins with conservative physical therapy and anti-inflammatory medications, once testing rules out an active inner ear disorder. With time and therapy, most patients with abnormal electroneurograms end up having normal results at follow-up testing.[54a]

Vestibular Neuritis.   Vestibular neuritis is thought to represent a reactivated dormant herpes infection in Scarpa's ganglion within the superior division of the vestibular nerve, which innervates the anterior and horizontal semicircular canals.[129,130]

Ramsay Hunt Syndrome.   Ramsay Hunt syndrome is caused by varicella-zoster and is a variant of vestibular neuritis, with multiple cranial nerves involved. This involvement results in facial paresis, tinnitus, hearing loss, and a vestibular defect.[131,132] It also may involve cranial nerves V, IX, and X.

Labyrinthitis.   Infection of the labyrinth can be viral or bacterial. Acute labyrinthitis usually presents with severe vertigo, sudden or progressive hearing loss, nausea, vomiting, and fever.

Benign Paroxysmal Positional Vertigo.   Benign paroxysmal positional vertigo (BPPV) is the most common cause of dizziness in the elderly, and the incidence increases with age.[131] The diagnosis usually is made solely on the basis of the history, although it is possible to confuse BPPV with orthostatic hypotension, another common cause of dizziness in the elderly. Whereas orthostatic hypotension causes dizziness when the patient sits up or stands, BPPV can occur in all positions, especially with changes in head position.

Although BPPV can be caused by head trauma, vestibular neuritis, and vestibular artery compromise, the most common cause is an accumulation of utricle debris (otoconia), which can move within the posterior semicircular canals and stimulate the vestibular sense organ (cupula), causing vertigo and nystagmus.[131]

The side of the lesion is diagnosed with a maneuver similar to the Dix-Hallpike test (see Fig. 22-23). The intervention for posterior canal BPPV involves performing a canalith-repositioning maneuver, which is designed to return the otoconia from the semicircular canals back to the macule of the utricle, from whence it can be reabsorbed.

Canalith-repositioning Procedure.[131]   The patient is seated on the end of the bed with his or her feet dangling. The clinician stands to the side of the patient, supporting the patient's head. The patient is moved into the Dix-Hallpike position, toward the side of the involved ear (see Fig. 22-23) and maintained there for 20 seconds. Then the head is slowly rotated through moderate extension of the cervical spine toward the uninvolved side (Fig. 22-25) and maintained in the new position for 20 seconds. The patient is then rolled to a side-lying position with the head turned 45 degrees down (toward the floor) (Fig. 22-26) and maintained there for 20 seconds. While keeping the head turned toward the uninvolved side and the head pitched down, the patient slowly sits up.

To maintain the otoconia in the utricle following the maneuver, the patient is fitted with a soft collar and is instructed not to bend over, lie back, move the head up or down, or tilt the head to either side for the remainder of the day.

Intervention for Dizziness.   The use of exercise in the rehabilitation of patients with unilateral peripheral vestibular hypofunction

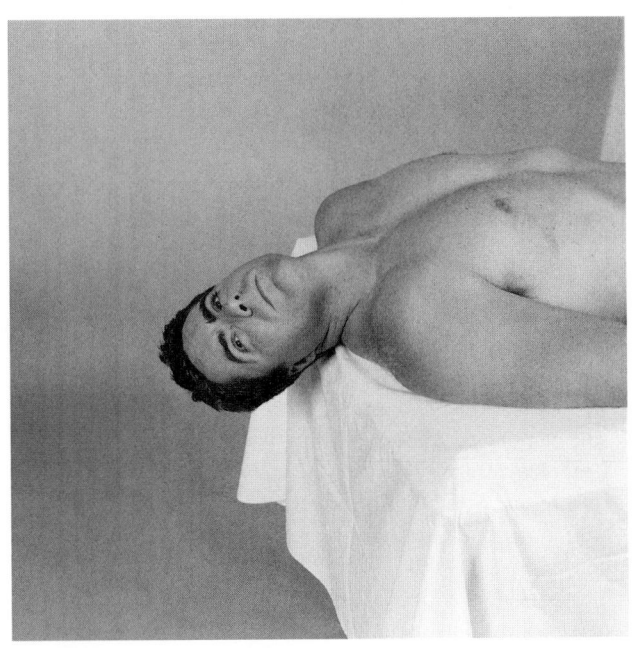

FIGURE 22-25 Benign paroxysmal positional vertigo correction: first phase.

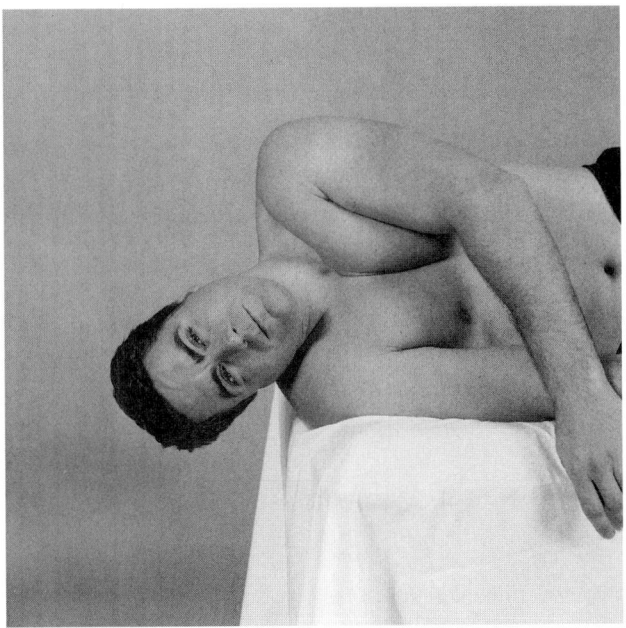

FIGURE 22-26 Benign paroxysmal positional vertigo correction: second phase.

is aimed at promoting vestibular compensation, promoting central habituation, and readjusting the vestibulo-ocular and vestibulospinal reflexes (see Chap. 2).

Animal studies[133,134] support the concepts that visuomotor experience facilitates the rate of recovery and improves the final level of recovery following vestibular dysfunction compensation.

Repetition of movements and positions that provoke dizziness and vertigo form the basic premise of habituation training, even though many of the exercises may initially increase the patient's symptoms. Several progressions have been devised (Table 22-5 and Box 22-1)

The goals of physical therapy intervention are to improve the patient's mobility, overall general physical condition and activity level, functional balance, and safety for gait and gait-related activities.

Cervical Headaches

Cervical headaches, also known as cervicogenic headaches, are difficult to define and classify because of their variable distribution and character of symptoms. The diagnosis of these headaches is usually one of exclusion in the presence of cervical abnormalities[47] (see Table 22-2). To help in the determination when examining a patient complaining of headache, the

TABLE 22-5 Cawthorne-Cooksey Exercises for Patients with Vestibular Hypofunction[135,136]

A. In bed
  1. Eye movements—at first slow, then quick
    a. Up and down
    b. From side to side
    c. Focusing on a finger moving from 3 ft to 1 ft away from face
  2. Head movements—at first slow, then quick; later with eyes closed
    a. Bending forward and backward
    b. Turning from side to side
B. Sitting
  1. Same as A1 and A2, above
  2. Shoulder shrugging and circling
  3. Bending forward and picking up objects from ground
C. Standing
  1. Same as A1 and A2 and B3, above
  2. Changing from sitting to standing position with eyes open and shut
  3. Throwing a small ball from hand to hand (above eye level).
  4. Throwing ball from hand to hand under knee
  5. Changing from sitting to standing and turning round in between
D. Moving about (in class)
  1. Circle around center person who will throw a large ball and to whom it will be returned
  2. Walk across room with eyes open and then closed
  3. Walk up and down slope with eyes open and then closed
  4. Walk up and down steps with eyes open and then closed
  5. Any game involving stooping and stretching and aiming, such as skittles, bowls, or basketball

Diligence and perseverance are required, but the earlier and more regularly the exercise regimen is carried out, the faster and more complete will be the return to normal activity.

Box 22-1 EXERCISES TO IMPROVE POSTURAL STABILITY [135]

These exercises are devised to incorporate head movement (vestibular stimulation) or to foster use of different sensory cues for balance.

1. The patient stands with his or her feet as close together as possible with both or one hand helping maintain balance by touching a wall if needed. The patient then turns his or her head to the right and to the left horizontally while looking straight ahead at the wall for 1 minute without stopping. The patient takes his or her hand or hands off the wall for longer and longer periods of the time while maintaining balance. The patient then tries moving his or her feet even closer together.

2. The patient walks, with someone for assistance if needed, as often as possible (acute disorders).

3. The patient begins to practice turning his or her head while walking. This will make the patient less stable, so the patient should stay near a wall as he or she walks.

4. The patient stands with his or her feet shoulder-width apart with eyes open, looking straight ahead at a target on the wall. He or she progressively narrows the base of support from feet apart to feet together to a semi-heel-to-toe position. The exercise is performed first with arms outstretched, then with arms close to the body, and then with arms folded across the chest. Each position is held for 15 seconds before the patient does the next-most-difficult exercise. The patient practices for a total of 5–15 minutes.

5. The patent stands with his or her feet shoulder-width apart with eyes open, looking straight ahead at a target on the wall. The patient progressively narrows his or her base of support from feet apart to feet together to a semi-heel-to-toe position. The exercise is performed with eyes closed, at first intermittently and then for longer and longer periods of time. The exercise is performed first with arms outstretched, then with arms close to the body, and then with arms folded across the chest. Each position is held for 15 seconds, and then the patient tries the next position. The patient practices for a total of 5–15 minutes.

6. A headlamp can be attached to the patient's waist or shoulders, and the patient can practice shifting weight to place the light into targets marked on the wall. This home "biofeedback" exercise can be used with the feet in different positions and with the patient standing on surfaces of different densities.

7. The patient practices standing on a cushioned surface. Progressively more difficult tasks might be hard floor (linoleum, wood), thin carpet, shag carpet, thin pillow, sofa cushion. Graded-density foam also can be purchased.

8. The patient practices walking with a more narrow base of support. The patient can do this first, touching the wall for support or for tactile cues and then gradually touching only intermittently and then not at all.

9. The patient practices turning around while walking, at first making a large circle but gradually making smaller and smaller turns. The patient must be sure to turn in both directions.

10. The patient can practice standing and then walking on ramps, either with a firm surface or with more cushioned surface.

11. The patient can practice maintaining balance while sitting and bouncing on a swiss ball or while bouncing on a trampoline. This exercise can be incorporated with attempting to maintain visual fixation of a stationary target, thus facilitating adaptation of the otolith-ocular reflexes.

12. Out in the community, the patient can practice walking in a mall before it is open and, therefore, while it is quiet; can practice walking in the mall while walking in the same direction as the flow of traffic; can walk against the flow of traffic.

---

clinician is advised to follow the simple diagnostic clinical algorithm set out below.[59]

▶ Exclude possible intracranial causes on history and physical examination. If intracranial pathology is suspected, then an urgent workup is required, which may include neuroimaging studies and laboratory investigations.

▶ Exclude headaches associated with viral or other infective illness.

▶ Exclude a drug-induced headache (see discussion that follows) or headache related to alcohol or substance abuse.

▶ Consider an exercise-related (or sex-related) headache syndrome (see Chap. 9).

▶ Differentiate between vascular, tension, cervicogenic, or other cause of headache.

Neck pain can arise from injuries of the cervical muscles, ligaments, disks, and joints. From lower cervical segments, the pain may be referred to the shoulder and upper limb (see Table 22-1). From upper segments, neck pain may be referred to the head, and manifest as headache.

According to the International Headache Society (IHS),[137] a cervicogenic headache is defined as one that meets the following criteria: (1) pain localized to the neck and occipital region that may project to the forehead, orbital region, temples, vertex, or ears; (2) pain precipitated or aggravated by specific neck movements or sustained neck posture; and (3) resistance to or limitation of active or passive physiologic and accessory neck movements or abnormal tenderness of neck muscles, or both. In addition, the IHS guidelines require radiographic examination to diagnose cervicogenic headaches. According to the IHS, radiologic examination must reveal at least one of the following: (1) movement abnormalities during flexion-extension, (2) abnormal posture, or (3) fractures, bone tumors, rheumatoid arthritis, congenital abnormalities, or other distinct pathology other than spondylosis or osteochondrosis.[137]

Clinical Pearl

Cervicogenic headaches tend to be unilateral and accompanied by tenderness of the C2 to C3 articular pillars on the affected side.[138] The patient with a cervicogenic headache usually reports a dull aching pain of moderate intensity that begins in the neck or occipital region and then spreads to include a greater part of the cranium.[139]

Cervicogenic headaches can emerge from a number of sources, including[140]:

▶ Irritation of the dorsal root ganglia and nerve root components caused by compression of the C2 dorsal root ganglia between the C1 posterior arch and the superior C2 articular process.[141]

▶ Compression of the C2 ventral ramus at the articular process of C1 to C2.[94]

▶ Entrapment of the C2 dorsal root ganglia by the C1–2 epistrophic ligament.[142]

Neck pain and headache are also the cardinal features of a whiplash mechanism,[64,143,144] but these symptoms are musculoskeletal and not neurologic in origin. According to the international classification, headache after whiplash is best classified as cervicogenic (group 11.2.1), and thus related to injured structures around the cervical spine.[137] The incidence of headache after whiplash injury is said to decrease during the first 6 months after trauma.[145] Headache after whiplash can be a result of cervical spine trauma, as listed, or from a possible coup-contrecoup injury from the rapid acceleration-deceleration of the brain in a closed calvarium. Trauma was reported in about 44 percent of 6000 headache patients in one study[146] and in about 40 percent of 96 in another,[147] with 16 percent of the 96 having been involved in a motor vehicle accident. In another study, patients who had been involved in rear-end vehicle collisions[148] were categorized in a similar fashion to the Quebec Task Force grades 1, 2, and 3. Headaches persisted at a 20-month follow-up in 70 percent of the group 3 patients and 37 percent of groups 1 and 2. Particularly relevant is the relation between a history of headache and the development of a

trauma-related headache after whiplash injury. In addition, psychological variables, which may be important in idiopathic headache,[149,150] should be evaluated in relation to the development and recovery from headache after whiplash.

Rest and minor analgesics are the best interventions for episodic tension-type headache.[60] For the prevention of episodic and chronic tension-type headaches, behavioral approaches commonly involve regular sleep and meals and avoidance of initiating or trigger factors.[60] Straightforward stress coping, meditation, or relaxation strategies best manage work-related or family stress and emotional problems. An exercise program may be helpful.[60] A systematic review of the literature for the efficacy of spinal manipulation in the intervention of chronic headache found spinal manipulative therapy to have a better effect than massage for cervicogenic headaches.[151]

Chiari Malformations

Chiari malformations are a group of disorders that manifest varying degrees of inferior displacement of the cerebellum and brainstem through the foramen magnum. Four types are recognized:[151a]

▶ *Chiari type I malformation.* This type consists of the inferior displacement of the cerebellar hemispheres (cerebellar tonsils) through the foramen magnum. This tongue-like projection of the medial inferior cerebellum envelops the medulla. The fourth ventricle is in a normal position. As the degree of descent increases, the outflow of cerebrospinal fluid (CSF) decreases, and a tubular cavitation of the upper spinal cord, called syringomyelia, then occurs. Syringomyelia is distinct from hydromyelia, which is an enlargement of the central canal of the spinal cord.

▶ *Chiari type II malformation.* Chiari type II malformation is associated with inferior displacement of the brainstem and fourth ventricle through the foramen magnum into the vertebral canal, often with hydrocephalus and meningomyelocele.

▶ *Chiari type III malformation.* This type is associated with a herniation of the cerebellum into a high cervical meningocele.

▶ *Chiari type IV malformation.* In Chiari type IV malformation, the cerebellum is generally hypoplastic.

Chiari types II through IV typically present with florid symptoms and are usually diagnosed in infancy or childhood.[151a] In contrast, in Chiari type I malformation, the signs of brainstem dysfunction evolve slowly over years, and are thus more likely than the other types to be encountered in physical therapy.

The clinical manifestations of Chiari I malformation are among the most protean in clinical medicine, which can lead to a delay in diagnosis. The most common presenting symptoms are upper extremity weakness and various pain syndromes that often include neck and arm pain.[151b] Occipital headaches, which are exacerbated by coughing, sneezing, stooping, or lifting, are also frequent.[151b] Clumsiness, upper extremity sensory changes ataxia, vertigo, hearing loss, tinnitus, dysphagia, hiccups, dysarthria, and hoarseness of voice are some of the other reported symptoms.[151b]

The diagnosis of Chiari malformation is most commonly made with MRI. If surgical intervention is necessary, it involves decompression of the Chiari malformation with or without drainage of the syringomyelia.[151a]

Pattern 4G: Impaired Joint Mobility, Motor Function, Muscle Performance, Range of Motion Associated with Fracture

Although the intervention for fractures is beyond the scope of practice for a physical therapist, being able to detect their presence, especially in this region, is critical. Clinical findings that could suggest the possibility of a craniovertebral fracture include:[151c,151d]

▶ Painful neck muscle splinting.

▶ Neck and occipital numbness.

▶ Pain and stiffness in the neck, with a reluctance to move his or her head.

▶ Presence or absence of neurological signs and symptoms.

Fractures of the Axis
There are three types of fractures of the C2 (axis) vertebra: odontoid fractures involving the dens, bilateral traumatic spondylolisthesis of the pars interarticularis ("hangman's" fracture), and nonodontoid/nonhangman's (miscellaneous) fractures.[151e]

Odontoid Fractures
Odontoid fractures are a relatively common upper cervical spine injury, comprising nearly 60 percent of all fractures of the axis and 10–18 percent of all cervical spine fractures.[151f,151g] Although odontoid fractures occur in all age groups, the mean age is approximately 47 years with a bimodal distribution.[151h] In younger patients, who comprise the first peak, these fractures are usually secondary to high-energy trauma; motor vehicle accidents are responsible for the majority of the odontoid injuries.[151f,151i] Concomitant spinal injuries are present in up to 34 percent of patients; 85 percent of these associated injuries occur in the cervical spine, with injuries of the atlas the most common.[151h,151j] The second peak in the incidence of odontoid fractures is in the elderly.[151g] In fact, odontoid fractures are the most common cervical spine fracture in patients older than age 70.[151h,151k] These fractures, unlike those in the younger patients, tend to result from low-energy injuries, such as falls from a standing height.[151h] The mechanism of injury often is hyperextension resulting in posterior displacement of the odontoid.[151h]

Described in 1974, the Anderson and D'Alonzo system divides fractures into three types based on anatomic location.[151l]

▶ *Type I.* Type I is an oblique avulsion fracture from the tip of the odontoid above the transverse ligament, attached to the alar ligament. This fracture is clinically rare, accounting

for 1–5 percent of odontoid fractures, and may be associated with occipito-atlantal dislocation.[151m]

▶ *Type II.* Type II fractures occur through the neck of the odontoid. They are the most common type of odontoid fracture (38–80 percent).

▶ *Type III.* Type III fractures extend into the body of C2. They account for 15–40 percent of all odontoid fractures.

Current management of odontoid fractures is based on three principles: timely diagnosis, reduction of the fracture, and sufficient immobilization to permit healing.[151n] Numerous treatment methods have been developed to achieve anatomic alignment and optimal stability, including cervical orthoses, Minerva jackets, halo-thoracic vests, posterior cervical fusion, and direct anterior dens screw fixation.[151o]

Jefferson Fracture. Jefferson fracture was defined as the association of a lateral mass fracture of C1 and the disruption of the C1 ring (either on the posterior or on the anterior arch).[151p] Jefferson fractures now represent a spectrum of injuries from bilateral ring fractures, to lateral mass fracture, to the pathognomonic four-point fracture (both anterior and posterior arches) of the C1 ring that the fracture was originally named for.[151q] Jefferson fracture classically results from axial loading on the atlas and is generally associated with minimal neurologic deficit and good prognosis for neurologic recovery.[151r] Presently, three general types of Jefferson fractures are described.[151s]

▶ *Type I.* Type I involves bilateral single-arch (anterior or posterior, but not both) fractures.

▶ *Type II.* Type II is the concurrent anterior and posterior arch fractures, which include the classic four-point break Jefferson fracture

▶ *Type III.* Type III is the lateral mass fracture of C1, which may extend into the anterior or the posterior osseous arch.

No prognostic significance has been attached to the different types of Jefferson fracture.[151s] Isolated Jefferson fracture can be treated effectively with external immobilization. The traditional mode of cervical immobilization is the halo vest.[151q]

Therapeutic Techniques

Techniques to Increase Soft Tissue Extensibility

Soft tissue techniques generally are applied before performing the local segmental examination and in preparation for a mobilization or manipulation intervention. Soft tissue techniques are capable of producing a strong analgesic, and relaxing, effect. With a reduction in cervical muscle tension, or spasm, it becomes much easier for the clinician to palpate and register movement.

General Kneading
General kneading techniques can be applied to the soft tissues of the craniovertebral region. These techniques are especially

useful prior to performing a specific mobilization or manipulation.

Suboccipital Massage[152]

Soft tissue techniques can be performed at several sites in the cervical region. In principle, every tender site can be treated, even though it usually involves areas of referred pain or tenderness.

The patient is positioned prone or sitting, and the head is positioned in slight flexion, without rotation. The clinician stands on the uninvolved side. While one hand supports the patient's head, the other hand palpates the suboccipital muscles. The sternocleidomastoid may need to be displaced laterally in order to palpate the muscles attaching to the transverse process of C1. The clinician locates the most tender area and places the index finger, reinforced by the middle finger, directly lateral to the tender spot (Fig. 22-27). During the massage, the index finger moves from laterally to medially and slightly cranially, while at the same time, pressure is exerted in an anteromedial and superior direction.

A similar technique is used in a combination of upper cervical traction and soft tissue mobilization of the suboccipital muscles. This technique is best performed with the patient supine, because the neck is unloaded and the patient can relax more in the supine versus seated position. While one hand grasps the patient's head, the clinician uses the fingers of the other hand to press gently into the muscles between two vertebrae. While maintaining the pressure on the muscles, a slight traction force is applied and sustained for several seconds before being released. The procedure is repeated in a rhythmic manner.

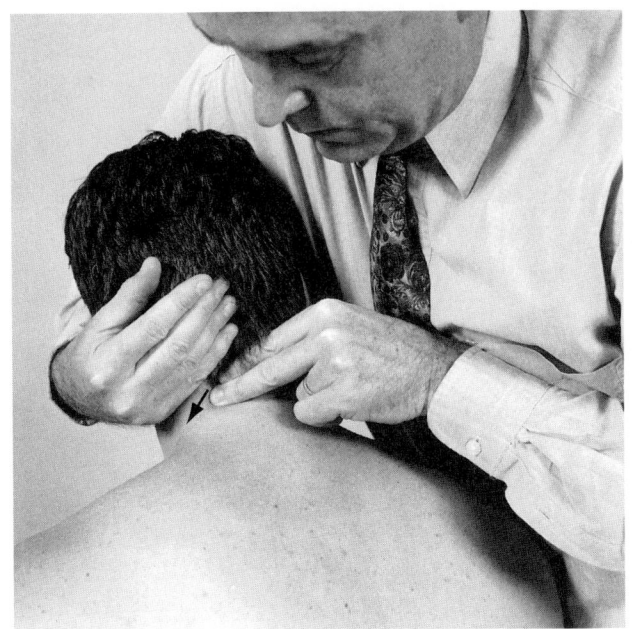

FIGURE 22-27 Suboccipital massage.

The paravertebral muscles can be treated in a similar fashion. With one hand, the clinician stabilizes the patient's head at the forehead. With the index or middle finger of the left hand, or both fingers, the clinician pulls the musculature in a lateral and anterior direction. At the same time, the hand on the patient's forehead rotates the patient's head away from the side being treated. The end position is held for 2 to 3 seconds before returning to the initial position. The clinician repeats this technique for several seconds or minutes in a rhythmic manner.

Rhythmic Flexion

The patient is positioned supine and the clinician stands at the head of the bed. The clinician cradles the patient's head in his or her hands. After first performing craniovertebral flexion, a flexion movement in the rest of the cervical spine is performed. Simultaneously, the thumb and fingers push toward each other, through the musculature, and pull in a posterior direction. The clinician begins at the level of C0 to C1, and the flexion motion is performed no further than this point. The end position is held for 2 to 3 seconds before returning to the initial position. The clinician repeats this technique several times in a rhythmic manner.

The same procedure can then be performed per segment, by shifting the hands caudally. As the successive caudal segments are localized, increasingly more flexion is performed. This technique can be used to treat all of the cervical segments.

In the same way, coupled movements in flexion can be performed. After first performing an upper cervical flexion, the clinician brings the patient's head simultaneously into flexion, ipsilateral rotation, and side bending. In this instance, pressure is emphasized on the convex side of the cervical spine.

Muscle Stretching of the Suboccipital Muscles

Rectus Capitis Posterior Major and Minor. To stretch these muscles, the patient is positioned supine. The clinician fixes C2 into craniovertebral flexion. To stretch the left muscle, a right side bending and right rotation motion is added (see Fig. 22-17) and the patient is instructed to not let the head drop back.

Inferior Oblique. To stretch the left muscle, the patient's head and neck is positioned into flexion, left side bending, and right rotation. A massage to the muscle can be applied by stroking the muscle from the C1 transverse process to the C2 spinous process, applying a force in the direction of less pain (see Fig. 22-27).

Superior Oblique. The patient is positioned sitting. The clinician places a thumb over the posterior aspect of the transverse process of C1, and the other hand wraps around the patient's head. To stretch the right superior oblique, the patient's head and neck must be placed in flexion, left side bending, and right rotation. Hold-relax or contract-relax techniques can be used.

Self-stretching

The following exercises should be performed at an intensity level that achieves an improvement without a regression of status.

Chin Retraction. The patient is seated in the correct posture. The patient is instructed to attempt to move the head, as a unit, in a posterior direction while maintaining eye level. The clinician should limit the number of chin tucks the patient performs to remove any potential for harm to the cervical structures from overuse.

C2 to C3 Side Bending and Rotation. The pattern of limitation for this area is usually one of a closing restriction. The patient is seated in the correct posture. The patient places both hands behind the neck, with the ulnar border of the little finger just below the C2 spinous process and the rest of the hand covering as much of the midcervical region as possible. The patient then simultaneously side flexes and rotates the neck and head in the direction of the restriction (Fig. 22-28), by attempting to look downward and backward (for a closing restriction).

Atlanto-axial Rotation. The patient is seated in the correct posture. The patient places both hands behind the neck, with the ulnar border of the little finger at the level of the C2 spinous process and the rest of the hand covering as much of the midcervical region as possible. The patient then gently turns the head in the direction of the restriction (Fig. 22-29). Coupled motions should be encouraged. For example, if the patient has a restriction with right rotation, right rotation and left side bending is emphasized.

Occipito-atlantal Flexion. The patient is seated in the correct posture. The patient performs a chin tuck. From the chin-tucked position, the patient is instructed to place the tips of the index and middle fingers of both hands over the anterior aspect of the

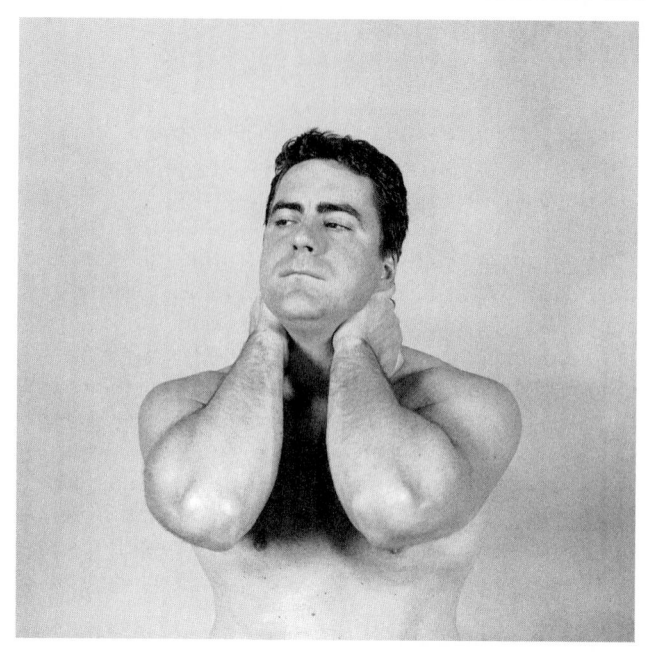

FIGURE 22-29 Technique to increase right rotation.

chin (Fig. 22-30). The fingertips provide resistance for an attempted extension movement of the head on the neck. The patient then attempts to look upward while resisting the motion with the fingertips. This is followed by relaxation and then another chin tuck.

Occipito-atlantal Extension. The patient is seated in the correct posture. The patient places both hands behind the neck, with the

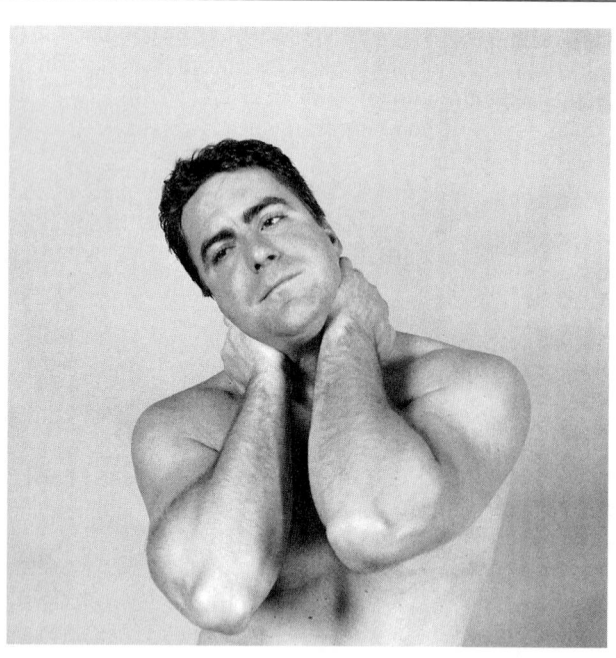

FIGURE 22-28 C2–3 side bending and rotation.

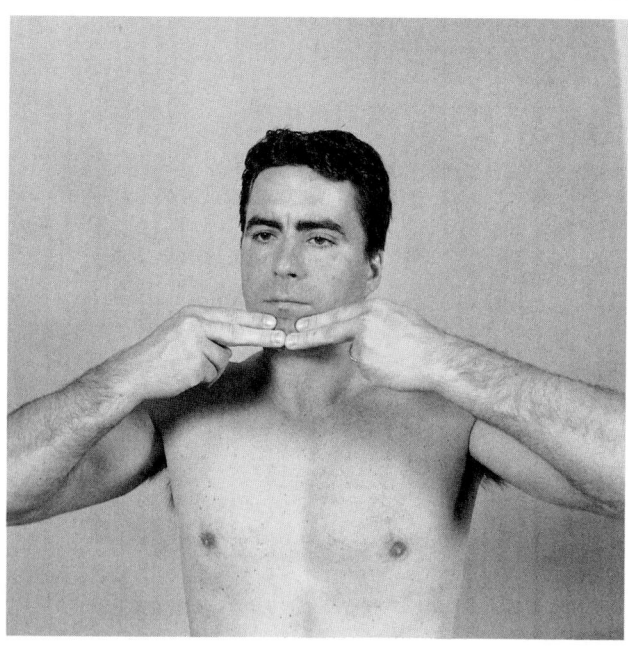

FIGURE 22-30 Home exercise for O-A flexion.

ulnar border of the little finger at the level of the C1 spinous process and the rest of the hand covering as much of the mid-cervical region as possible. The patient then gently lifts the chin around the appropriate axis (Fig. 22-31).

Techniques to Increase Joint Mobility

Joint Mobilization Techniques

Occipito-atlantal Joint

Specific Traction[152]. Specific traction is used here, as elsewhere in the spine, to apply a gentle degree of distraction and mechanical stimulation. It typically is used with acute conditions.

The patient is positioned supine. The clinician stabilizes the C1 vertebra using a wide pinch grip, and the patient's forehead is stabilized against the clinician's shoulder (see Fig. 22-17). A traction force is then applied, a graded cranial force (I to II) by the occipital hand and the chest.

Supine Technique for a Symmetrical Loss of Occipito-atlantal Extension. The patient is positioned in supine, head on a pillow, and knees flexed over a pillow. The clinician is positioned at the head of the table. The clinician cradles the patient's head in both hands with the finger pads under the occiput and places each thumb over the zygomatic arches of the patient. Using thumb pressure, the clinician tilts the patient's head into craniovertebral flexion, while the finger pads produce a posterior glide of the occipital condyles.

The joint slack is taken up. The patient is instructed to attempt to place the chin on their Adam's apple. After an isometric contraction of 3–5 seconds, the patient is instructed to relax, and the resultant joint slack is taken up by the clinician. When, following repeated muscle assisted mobilizations, no further

increased motion is apparent, it can be assumed that the inert barrier to motion has been reached. Passive soft tissue mobilization is then performed. This combination of muscle assisted and passive mobilizations is continued until no further soft tissue slack is appreciated.

Seated Technique for a Loss of Extension at the Right Occipito-atlantal Joint[152a]. The following mobilization techniques can be used for a restriction of the anterior glide of the right O-A joint. The reader is expected to extrapolate the information to produce the necessary technique for a restriction of the anterior glide of the left joint.

The patient is seated with the clinician standing on the left side. C1 is stabilized anteriorly using a wide pinch grip by the right hand and wrapping the pads of the index finger and thumbs around the front of the transverse process (Fig. 22-32). The left arm stabilizes the patient's head against the clinician's chest, and the left hand grasps the occiput. The patient's head is then extended and right side-flexed around the appropriate axes, with left translation being produced by means of the side bending until the extension barrier is reached. The mobilization is then performed by applying a graded force against the translation barrier.

Active participation from the patient can be introduced. From the motion barrier, the patient is asked to gently meet the clinician's resistance. The direction of resistance is that which facilitates further extension, right side bending, and left rotation. The isometric contraction is held for up to 5 seconds and followed by a period of complete relaxation. The joint is then passively taken to the new motion barrier. The technique is repeated three times and followed by a reexamination.

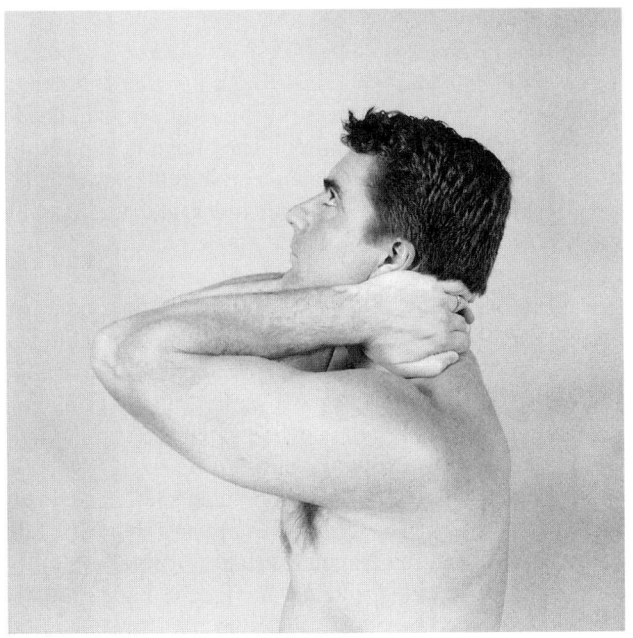

FIGURE 22-31 Home exercise for O-A extension.

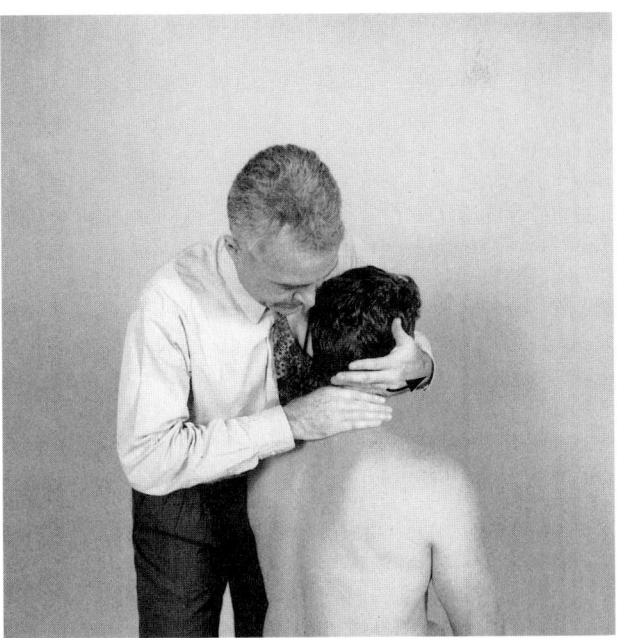

FIGURE 22-32 Mobilization of extension and right side bending of the O-A joint.

Supine Technique for an Asymmetrical Loss of Occipito-atlantal Extension (e.g., Loss of Left Occipito-atlantal Joint Extension)[94a]. The patient is positioned in supine, head on a pillow, knees flexed over a pillow. The clinician is positioned at the head of the table. The clinician cradles the patient's head in both hands. The left index and middle finger pads are placed just medial to the patient's left mastoid process, with the palm supporting the occiput. The clinician's right hand is placed over the right side of the patient's head.

Using both hands, the clinician passively moves the patient's head into cranioverbral extension and right translation, until the extension motion barrier of the left O-A joint is reached. The joint slack is taken up by the clinician using their left fingers to push upwards towards the patient's lips and the clinician's right hand, thereby inducing side-flexion of the patient's head to the left.

The patient is instructed to resist left side-flexion of the O-A joint using the command "Don't let me pull your left ear upwards." The contraction is held for 3–5 seconds and the patient is asked to relax. As the patient relaxes, the new joint slack is taken up by the clinician pushing further towards the patient's lips with the left finger pads and side-flexing the patient's head to the left with clinician's right hand. To ensure that the extension is occurring around a craniovertebral axis, the clinician looks at the patient's face. As slack is taken up, flexion of the right O-A joint should simultaneously produce chin movement towards the ceiling, while the forehead moves towards the bed. To ensure that the left side-flexion is occurring around the correct axis the clinician should note the chin movement occurring to the right while the forehead moves to the left. During the conjunct right rotation, the chin and forehead should both be seen to rotate to the right.

As with the technique to increase unilateral flexion, once the inert barrier is reached the combined passive motion into the barrier is stressed with oscillatory passive stretch and then muscle assisted mobilizations are repeated. This is continued until there is no further "give" to the motion barrier.

Supine Technique for an Asymmetrical Loss of Occipito-atlantal Flexion (e.g., Loss of Right Occipito-atlantal Joint Flexion)[94a]. The patient is positioned in supine, head on a pillow, knees flexed over a pillow. The clinician is positioned at the head of the table. The clinician cradles the patient's head in both hands so that the left hand is placed over the left side of the patient's head, and the clinician's right index and middle finger pads are placed just medial to the patient's right mastoid processes, with the palm supporting the patient's occiput.

Using both hands the clinician produces craniovertebral flexion to the barrier. At this point the patient's head is translated to the right until a firm end-feel is encountered. This maneuver induces a right translation and a right rotation at the O-A joints. The barrier to flexion of the right O-A joint is thus achieved.

Joint slack is taken up as the clinician's uses a lumbrical action to pull on the patient's right mastoid process in the direction towards the bed surface with the right index and middle fingers. Simultaneously the patient's head is side-flexed to the left

by the clinician's left hand. Using fingertip pressure through the left hand, the clinician instructs the patient: "Don't let me lift your left ear upwards." The clinician then attempts to draw the patient's left mastoid process superiorly. This produces an isometric resistance of left side-flexion of the O-A joint (and therefore, right rotation).

After a isometric contraction of 3–5 seconds, the patient is instructed to relax and as the relaxation is felt by the clinician, the resultant joint slack is taken up by the clinician by simultaneously pulling the patient's right mastoid process towards the bed (with the right hand) and side-bending the head to the left (with the left hand). When, following repeated muscle assisted mobilizations, no further increased motion is apparent, it can be assumed that the inert barrier to motion has been reached. Passive soft tissue mobilization is then achieved by pushing further into the right O-A joint flexion barrier by simultaneously pulling the right mastoid process towards the bed (right hand) and left side—bending of the head (left hand). This combination of muscle assisted and passive mobilizations is continued until no further soft tissue slack is appreciated. To ensure that the flexion is occurring around a craniovertebral axis, the clinician looks at the patient's face. As slack is taken up flexion of the right O-A joint should simultaneously produce:

▶ A downward motion of the patient's chin and an upward motion of the patient's forehead (flexion).

▶ A right-sided motion of the patient's chin with a left sided motion of the forehead (left side-flexion).

▶ A rotation of chin and forehead to the right (right rotation).

If these facial movements are not seen, then the left hand is used to ensure that these motions are occurring, thus maintaining a craniovertebral axis.

Atlanto-axial Joint

Loss of the Anterior-Inferior Glide of the Left Atlanto-axial Joint (e.g., Loss of Right Rotation in Atlanto-axial Joint—Loss of Left Anterior/Inferior Glide).[94a] The patient is positioned in supine, head on a pillow, knees flexed over a pillow. The clinician is positioned at the head of the table. The clinician cradles the patient's head in both hands. The clinician's right index and middle finger pads are placed around the *left* side of the patient's C2 neural arch, making firm contact with the left side of the C2 spinous process. The clinician's left hand supports the left side of the patient's head. The patient's head is side-flexed by clinician's left hand. Using the fingers of the right hand, the clinician feels for the C2 spinous process to move to the right. At this point, the C2 spinous process is pulled by the index and middle fingers of the right hand until the motion barrier is detected. The patient is instructed to push their head into clinician's left hand, i.e., resisted left side flexion. The C2 spinous process should be felt to move to the right and the clinician's right fingers move to fix it as the patient is instructed to relax. As patient relaxes the slack in left side flexion of the head is taken up.

This is repeated until no further motion of C2 spinous process is detected.

Thrust Techniques

Thrust techniques are similar to mobilization techniques in that the barrier or joint restriction is engaged (see Chap. 11). Although the grade V technique shares similarities with the grade IV mobilization in terms of amplitude and position in the joint's range, the grade V differs in the velocity of delivery. At the barrier or point of joint restriction, a grade V technique involves the application of a fast impulse of small amplitude to restore joint play.

The speed, force, and correct application of a manipulation are critical if serious injury is to be avoided. This is particularly true in the craniovertebral region, where an overzealous technique can result in such serious consequences as vertebral artery compromise, fracture, impingement of the spinal cord, and even death. The use of techniques that incorporate combinations of cervical rotation and extension should be avoided. In addition, clinicians should not rely exclusively on thrust techniques to achieve normal range of motion and function. It is probably advisable to use thrust techniques only in situations in which neuromuscular or grade IV mobilization techniques have failed, the patient is relaxed, and the technique is applied in a nonpainful direction. Under no circumstance should a thrust technique be repeated if the patient's symptoms are reported to worsen, or if the first technique did not succeed with little force.

Chapter 11 outlines the indications and contraindications for spinal manipulations.

Thrust Technique for the Occipito-atlantal Joint.

For the technique, the patient is positioned supine, with the clinician at the head of the table, seated to the patient's right. Contact is made by the clinician's right hand, using the web space between the thumb and the forefinger, on the inferior and right aspect of C0 (the right mastoid process). The clinician's right hand is positioned parallel to the patient's sternum and the left forearm wraps around the patient's head, so that the clinician's hand cups the patient's chin. The patient's head is then side flexed toward the clinician (to the right) around the appropriate axis (through the nose), allowing for the conjunct rotation to the left to occur (Fig. 22-33). Having taken up the slack with the right hand, the clinician applies a high-velocity, low-amplitude thrust to the mastoid in a superior direction (by the right hand), while the other hand and arm help to guide the intended movement.

Thrust Technique for the Atlanto-axial Joint.

The patient is positioned supine, with the clinician at the head of the table. The clinician supports the patient's head in his or her hands, and the posterior aspect of C1 on the right is monitored, using the index finger of the right hand. The thumbs of both hands rest on the patient's jaw and cheeks. Gripping the patient's jaw and cheeks, the clinician side flexes the patient's head to the right, either throughout the entire cervical spine (the patient's right ear is passively taken to their ipsilateral shoulder) or around the craniovertebral axis (through the nose). The head is then rotated to the left to the end of the available range (Fig. 22-34). After the

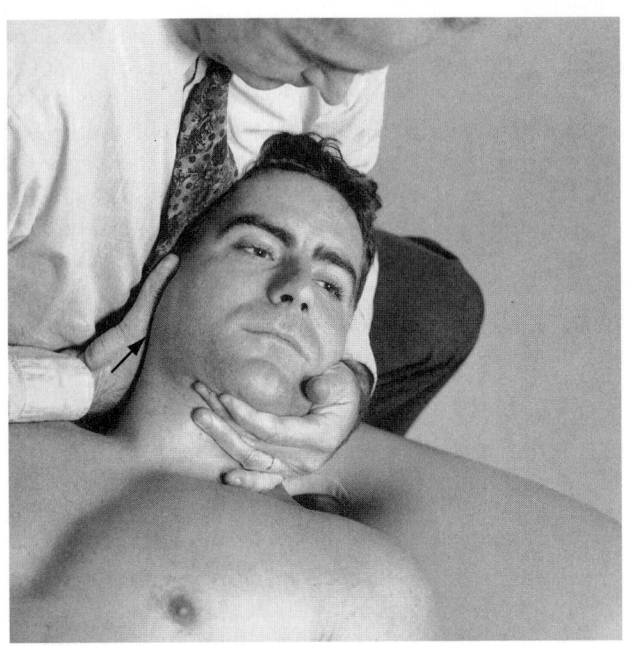

FIGURE 22-33 Thrust technique for O-A joint.

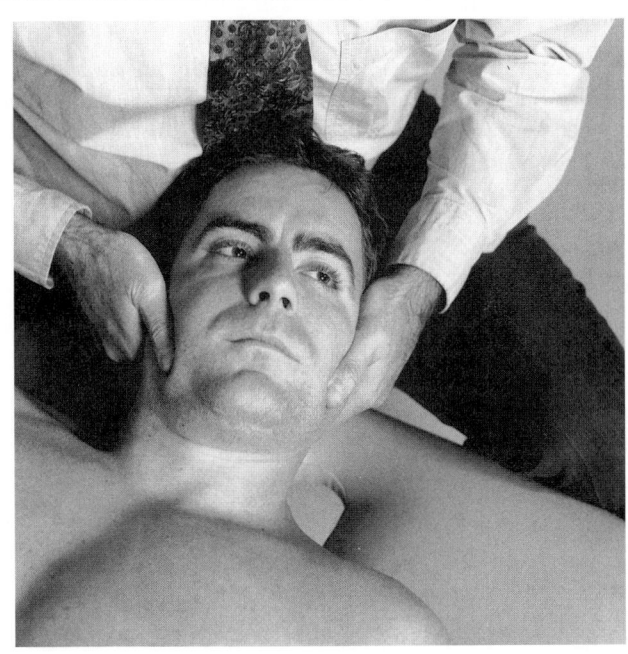

FIGURE 22-34 Thrust technique for A-A joint.

slack has been taken up into right side bending and left rotation, a high-velocity, low-amplitude thrust is then applied into left rotation by the *right* hand while the left hand guides the movement. Extra care must be taken not to be overly aggressive with this technique.

Mobilizations with Movement[153]

Upper Cervical Traction. This is an excellent technique for the intervention of upper cervical headaches. The patient is positioned sitting, with the clinician standing in front, facing the patient. The patient's head is held in neutral position against the clinician's lower chest, and the distal phalanx of the clinician's little finger is hooked around C2. The rest of the fingers wrap around the patient's head to provide firm support, and the wrist is flexed, with the forearm placed in the plane of the facets (Fig. 22-35). The lateral border of the thenar eminence of the clinician's other hand is placed directly under the little finger (see Fig. 22-35) in the gutter between the occiput and the spinous process of C2, and the palm of the hand rests on the upper back of the patient.

The clinician applies pressure on C2 using the little finger, while preventing motion of the head, so that C2 is felt to move anteriorly on C3. The end-feel is obtained and is maintained for 10 to 20 seconds.

This technique can be taught as part of the patient's home exercise program, using a towel, belt, or strap. The patient places the strap around the articular pillars of C2 and pulls gently forward while gliding the head posteriorly, without tilting it, over the strap (Fig. 22-36). The end position is maintained for 10 to 20 seconds.

To Improve Right Rotation of the Atlanto-axial Joint. The patient is positioned sitting, with the clinician sitting behind. The clinician places the thumb of one hand over the left aspect of the transverse process of C1, and the other thumb over the first thumb to help reinforce it. The remaining fingers of the hands are placed around the patient's neck and upper back, or to the side of the head (Fig. 22-37).

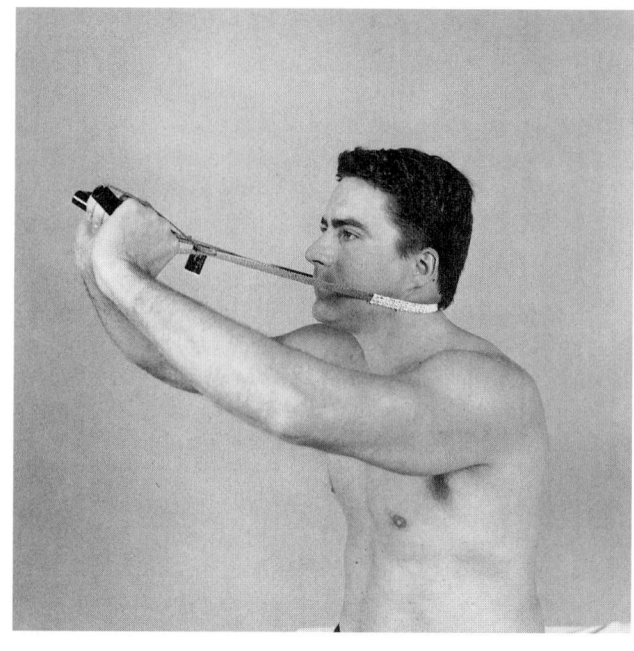

FIGURE 22-36 Home exercise for upper cervical mobilization.

The patient is asked to rotate the head and neck slowly to the right, while the clinician simultaneously assists the movement using pressure from both thumbs.

This technique can be taught as part of the patient's home exercise program, using a towel, belt, or a strap (Fig. 22-38).

The same technique can be used to improve cervical rotation to the left by altering the position of the thumbs.

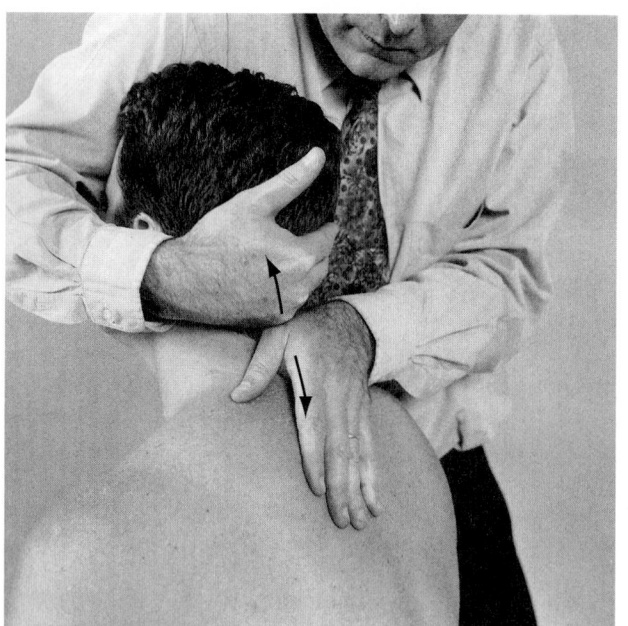

FIGURE 22-35 Upper cervical mobilization with movement.

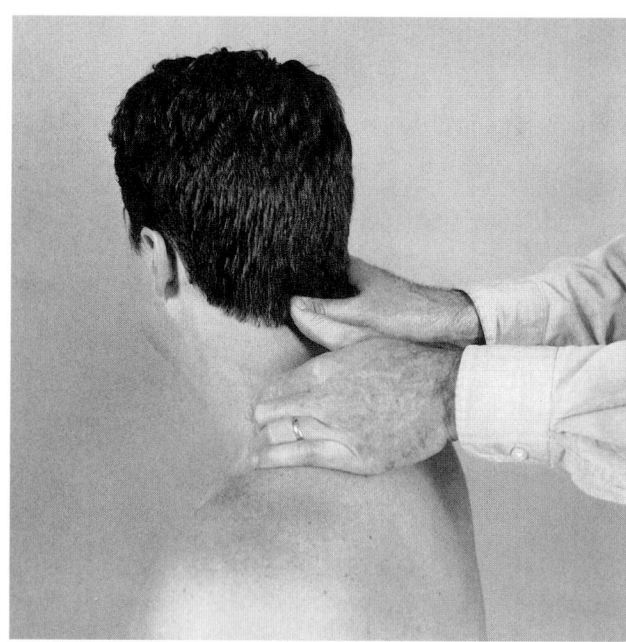

FIGURE 22-37 Home exercise to increase right rotation.

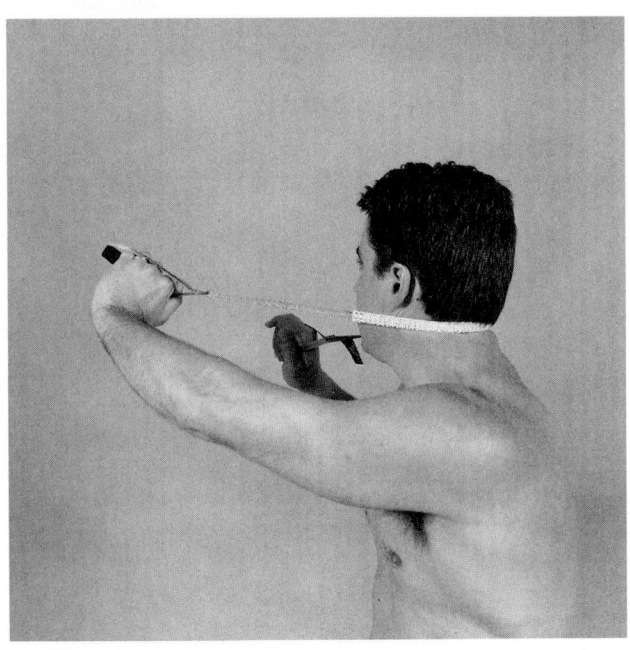

FIGURE 22-38 Home exercise for A-A rotation.

CASE STUDY HEADACHE AND NECK PAIN

HISTORY

A self-employed 42-year-old man presented to the clinic complaining of posterior upper neck pain and right suboccipital and occipital headache, which began 2 months earlier after a diving accident. He denied being knocked unconscious and could remember everything about the accident except for the period a few minutes after it. The posterior neck pain was felt immediately, but was much worse the next morning upon waking. The occipital headaches started a few days later and became worse with fatigue or exertion. The patient also reported difficulty concentrating and sleeping, and had occasional bouts of dizziness, especially when turning his head to the left, during which he would become unsteady, but denied vertigo. When the neck and occipital pain flared up, it spread from the occipital region over the head to the right eye. Previous interventions included physical therapy in the form of ultrasound, massage, spray and stretch, myofascial release, and cranial sacral therapy, which had provided no relief.

The patient had no history of back or neck pain, apart from the occasional ache, and his medical history was unremarkable.

QUESTIONS

1. List the concerns the clinician should have following this history.
2. Using a flow diagram describe how you would proceed with this patient following the history.
3. What special tests should be considered at this point?
4. Are additional questions needed with regard to the history?

TESTS AND MEASURES

Given the history, it is likely that the patient was concussive, even though he denies being unconscious. The reports of dizziness appear related to a specific movement, but because that movement is rotation of the head, further testing will be needed to rule out other causes. Some of the more insidious reasons for the headache, such as a slow intracranial hemorrhage, can be excluded, because the symptoms are not progressing and the condition is 2 months old. The type of headache associated with the patient is the typical cervicogenic headache, having a pain distribution into the occiput and occasional spreading occipitofrontally and orbitally when exacerbated, which usually is related to head and neck movements and postures. However, the neck pain and occipital headache should have responded to physical therapy. The fact that they did not suggests that inappropriate therapy may have been given.

With this type of history, it would be prudent to perform a scanning examination with the addition of cranial nerve and vertebral artery examination. The scanning examination and additional tests revealed the following findings:

• The patient had no obvious postural deficits or deformities.
• Cranial nerve testing was negative, except that during the tracking tests for the third, fourth, and sixth nerves, he experienced mild vertigo of short duration and longer-lasting nausea.
• Craniovertebral ligament stress testing was negative for both instability and symptomatology.
• Dizziness was not reproduced with the vertebral artery tests. Because the vertebral artery appeared to be normal (given the lack of cranial nerve signs and the negative tests), the Dix-Hallpike test was performed. The Dix-Hallpike test reproduced the patient's dizziness when his head was in left rotation and extension. The dizziness came on almost immediately and disappeared within 1 minute. No cranial nerve signs were discovered on testing while the patient was dizzy.
• The patient had full range cervical movements except for extension, left rotation, and right side bending.
• There were no signs of neurologic deficit. All neuromeningeal (dural and neural tension) tests were negative.
• The compression and traction tests were negative.
• Posteroanterior pressure over the spinous process of C2 and over the back of the C1 neural arch reproduced the patient's headache and local tenderness.
• The posterior suboccipital muscles were hypertonic and tender to moderate palpation.

QUESTIONS

1. Given these findings, what is your working hypothesis?
2. List some of the possible reasons for the dizziness.
3. How would you proceed?

EVALUATION

It seems probable that the occipital headache is the result of a dysfunction in the craniovertebral joints,[154,155] but exactly where this dysfunction is located cannot be ascertained as yet from the examination. Further testing is required. Passive physiologic and accessory (arthrokinematic) movement testing of the cranioverterbral area determined that there was decreased anterior glide of the right occipito-atlantal (O-A) joint with a hard end-feel and a decreased anterior glide of the right A-A joint. There also was some point tenderness over the right levator scapular and right upper trapezius.

QUESTIONS

1. Given the findings from the tests and measures, how would you explain your intervention to the patient?
2. Explain the correlation between the loss of the glides and the loss of active range of motion.
3. How would you proceed?

INTERVENTION

There is every likelihood that the patient's dizziness is caused by a musculoskeletal dysfunction within the cranioverterbral area. The goals of the intervention should be aimed at:

- Promotion and progression of healing. This is a vital component, because a considerable percentage of these patients become chronic pain sufferers.
- Control of pain and inflammation with anti-inflammatory modalities and a soft cervical collar (until capsular pattern subsides).
- Patient education.
- Preventing a dependence on health care providers.
- Restoring motion and strength, as well as neuromuscular function through:

  - Early, but gentle, mobilization exercises.[156]
  - Non–weight-bearing, progressing to weight-bearing, mid-range active exercises, and then careful full-range active movement exercises.
  - Gentle isometric exercises.
  - Intervention for specific articular impairments with stronger mobilizations, providing these do not threaten the vertebral artery.[54a]
  - Electromuscular stimulation, if no muscle tearing has occurred.

REVIEW QUESTIONS*

1. Describe the anatomy of the cranioverterbral region.
2. What structures provide stability in the cranioverterbral region?
3. Which of the following is not a suboccipital muscle: rectus capitis lateralis, rectus capitis posterior major, rectus capitis posterior minor, obliquus capitis inferior, obliquus capitis superior?
4. What is the extension of the posterior longitudinal ligament called?

5. Which muscle produces side bending of the occipito-atlantal (O-A) joint to the same side, as well as extension and contralateral rotation of the O-A?

---

* Additional questions to test your understanding of this chapter can be found in the Online Learning Center for *Orthopaedic Assessment, Evaluation, and Intervention* at www.duttononline.net.

REFERENCES

1. Kapandji IA. *The Physiology of the Joints: Annotated Diagrams of the Mechanics of the Human Joints.* 2nd ed. Edinburgh, Scotland: Churchill Livingstone; 1974.
2. Gray H. *Gray's Anatomy.* Philadelphia, Pa: Lea and Febiger; 1995.
3. Panjabi M, et al. Three-dimensional movement of the upper cervical spine. *Spine* 1988;13:727.
3a. Walsh R, Nitz AJ. Cervical spine. In: Wadsworth C, ed. *Current Concepts of Orthopaedic Physical Therapy—Home Study Course,* La Crosse, Wis: Orthopaedic Section, APTA; 2001.
4. Williams PL, et al. *Gray's Anatomy.* 37th ed. London, England: Churchill Livingstone; 1989.
4a. Sasso RC. C2 dens fractures: treatment options. *J Spinal Disorders* 2001;14:455–463.
4b. Heggeness MH, Doherty BJ. The trabecular anatomy of the axis. *Spine* 1993;18:1945–1949.
4c. Doherty BJ, Heggeness MH. Quantitative anatomy of the second cervical vertebra. *Spine* 1995;20:513–517.
4d. Ellis JH, et al. Magnetic resonance imaging of the normal cranioverterbral junction. *Spine* 1991;16:105.
4e. Pick TP, Howden R. *Gray's Anatomy,* 15th ed. New York: Barnes & Noble Books; 1995.
5. Tulsi RS. Some specific anatomical features of the atlas and axis: Dens, epitransverse process and articular facets. *Aust N Z J Surg* 1978;48:570–574.
6. Singh S. Variations of the superior articular facets of atlas vertebrae. *J Anat* 1965;99:565–571.
7. Noren R, et al. The role of facet joint tropism and facet angle in disc degeneration. *Spine* 1991;16:530–532.
8. Cassidy J, et al. Lumbar facet joint asymmetry: Intervertebral disc herniation. *Spine* 1992;17:570–574.
9. Malmavaara A, et al. Facet joint orientation, facet and costovertebral joint osteoarthritis, disc degeneration, vertebral body osteophytosis, and Schmorl's nodes in the thoracolumbar junctional region of cadaveric spines. *Spine* 1987;12:458–463.
10. Walsh R, Nitz AJ. Cervical spine. In: Wadsworth C, ed. *Current Concepts of Orthopaedic Physical Therapy—Home Study Course.* La Crosse, Wis: Orthopaedic Section, American Physical Therapy Association; 2001.
11. White AA, Panjabi MM, eds. *Clinical Biomechanics of the Spine.* Philadelphia, Pa: Lippincott-Raven; 1990:106–108.
12. Worth DR, Selvik G. Movements of the craniovertebral joints. In: Grieve G, ed. *Modern Manual Therapy of the Vertebral Column.* Edinburgh, Scotland: Churchill Livingstone; 1986:53.
13. O'Brien MF, Lenke LG. Fractures and dislocations of the spine. In: Dee R, et al, eds. *Principles of Orthopaedic Practice.* New York, NY: McGraw-Hill; 1997:1237–1293.
14. Werne S. The possibilities of movements in the cranio-vertebral joints. *Acta Orthop Scand* 1959;28:165–173.
15. Penning L, Wilmink JT. Rotation of the cervical spine. A CT study in normal subjects. *Spine* 1987;12:732–738.

16. Dvorak J, Hayek J, Zehender R. CT—functional diagnosis of the rotary instability of the upper cervical spine: 2. An evaluation on healthy adults and patients with suspected instability. *Spine* 1987;12:726–731.

17. Ellis JH, et al. Magnetic resonance imaging of the normal craniovertebral junction. *Spine* 1991;16:105.

18. Pick TP, Howden R. *Gray's Anatomy.* 15th ed. New York, NY: Barnes and Noble Books; 1995.

19. Kapandji IA. *The Physiology of the Joints, The Trunk and Vertebral Column.* New York, NY: Churchill Livingstone; 1991.

20. Braakman R, Penning L. *Injuries of the Cervical Spine.* Amsterdam, Holland: Excerpta Medica; 1971:3–30.

21. Werne S. Studies in spontaneous atlas dislocation. *Acta Orthop Scand* 1957;23(suppl) 7–12.

22. Selecki BR. The effects of rotation of the atlas on the axis: Experimental work. *Med J Aust* 1969;1:1012.

23. Fielding JW. Cineroentgenography of the normal cervical spine. *J Bone Joint Surg* 1957:39A:1280.

24. White AA, Panjabi MM. The clinical biomechanics of the occipitoatlantoaxoid complex. *Orthop Clin North Am* 1975;9:867–878.

25. Mimura M, et al. Three-dimensional motion analysis of the cervical spine with special reference to the axial rotation. *Spine* 1989;14:1135.

26. Hohl M, Baker HR. The atlanto-axial joint. *J Bone Joint Surg* 1964;46A:1739–1752.

27. Fielding JW, et al. Tears of the transverse ligament of the atlas. A clinical and biomechanical study. *J Bone Joint Surg* 1974;56A:1683–1691.

28. Vangilder JC, Menezes AH, Dolan KD. *The Craniovertebral Junction and its Abnormalities.* Mount Kisco, NY: Futura; 1987.

29. Meadows JTS. *Manual Therapy: Biomechanical Assessment and Treatment, Advanced Technique.* Lecture and video supplemental manual. Calgary, Canada: Swodeam Consulting; 1995.

30. Pal GP, Sherk HH. The vertical stability of the cervical spine. *Spine* 1988;13:447.

31. Yoganandan N, et al. Dynamic response of human cervical spine ligaments. *Spine* 1989;14:1102.

32. Dvorak J, Panjabi MM. Functional anatomy of the alar ligaments. *Spine* 1987;12:183.

33. Dvorak J, et al. CT functional diagnostics of the rotary instability of the upper cervical spine and experimental study in cadavers. *Spine* 1987;12:197–205.

34. Okazaki K. Anatomical study of the ligaments in the occipitoatlantoaxial complex [in Japanese]. *Nippon Seikeigeka Gakkai Zasshi* 1995;69:1259–1267.

35. Panjabi M. et al. Flexion, extension, and lateral bending of the upper cervical spine in response to alar ligament transections. *J Spinal Disord* 1991;4:157–167.

36. White AA, et al. Biomechanical analysis of clinical stability in the cervical spine. *Clin Orthop* 1975;109:85–96.

37. Dvorak J, et al. Biomechanics of the craniocervical region: The alar and transverse ligaments. *J Orthop Res* 1987;6:452–461.

38. Lipson SJ. Fractures of the atlas associated with fractures of the odontoid process and transverse ligament ruptures. *J Bone Joint Surg* 1977;59A:940–943.

39. Buckworth J. Anatomy of the suboccipital region. In: Vernon H, ed. *Upper Cervical Syndrome.* Baltimore, Md: Williams and Wilkins; 1988.

40. Bogduk N. Innervation and pain patterns of the cervical spine. In: Grant R, ed. *Physical Therapy of the Cervical and Thoracic Spine.* New York, NY: Churchill Livingstone; 1988.

41. Swash M, Fox K. Muscle spindle innervation in man. *J Anat* 1972;112:61–80.

42. Hack GD, et al. Anatomic relation between the rectus capitis posterior minor muscle and the dura mater. *Spine* 1995; 20:2484–2486.

43. Fryette HH. *Principles of Osteopathic Technique.* Carmel, Cal: Academy of Osteopathy; 1980.

44. DiGiovanna EL, Schiowitz S. *An Osteopathic Approach to Diagnosis and Treatment.* Philadelphia, Pa: JB Lippincott; 1991.

45. Bellavance A, et al. Cervical spine and headaches. *Neurology* 1989;39:1269–1270.

46. Bogduk N. Cervical causes of headache and dizziness. In: Grieve GP, ed. *Modern Manual Therapy of the Vertebral Column.* New York, NY: Churchill Livingstone; 1986:289–302.

47. Bogduk N. The anatomical basis for cervicogenic headache. *J Manipulative Physiol Ther* 1992;15:67–70.

48. Edmeads J. The cervical spine and headache. *Neurology* 1988;38:1874–1878.

49. Fredriksen TA, Hovdal H, Sjaastad O. Cervicogenic headache: Clinical manifestation. *Cephalalgia* 1987;7:147–160.

50. Lazorthes G. Pathology, classification and clinical aspects of vascular diseases of the spinal cord. In: Vinken PJ, Bruyn GW, ed. *Handbook of Clinical Neurology.* Oxford, England: Elsevier; 1972:494–506.

51. Baumgartner RW, Waespe W. ASA syndrome of the cervical hemicord. *Eur Arch Psychiatry Clin Neurosci* 1992; 241:205–209.

52. Wells CEC. Clinical aspects of spinovascular disease. *Proc R Soc Med* 1966;59:790–796.

53. Decroix JP, Ciaudo-Lacroix C, Lapresle J. Syndrome de Brown-Sequard du a un infarctus spinal. *Rev Neurol* 1984;140:585–586.

54. Gutowski NJ, Murphy RP, Beale DJ. Unilateral upper cervical posterior spinal artery syndrome following sneezing. *J Neurol Neurosurg Psychiatry* 1992;55:841–843.

54a. Meadows J. *A Rationale and Complete Approach to the Sub-Acute Post-MVA Cervical Patient.* Calgary, Canada: Swodeam Consulting; 1995.

54b. Tulsi RS. Some specific anatomical features of the atlas and axis: Dens, epitransverse process and articular facets. *Aust N Z J Surg* 1978;48:570–574.

54c. Singh S. Variations of the superior articular facets of atlas vertebrae. *J Anat* 1965;99:565–571.

54d. Noren R, et al. The role of facet joint tropism and facet angle in disc degeneration. *Spine* 1991;16:530–532.

54e. Cassidy J, et al. Lumbar facet joint asymmetry: Intervertebral disc herniation. *Spine* 1992;17:570–574.

54f. Malmavaara A, et al. Facet joint orientation, facet and costovertebral joint osteoarthritis, disc degeneration, vertebral body osteophytosis, and Schmorl's nodes in the thoracolumbar junctional region of cadaveric spines. *Spine* 1987;12:458–463.

55. Travell JG, Simons DG. *Myofascial Pain and Dysfunction: The Trigger Point Manual.* Baltimore, Md: Williams and Wilkins; 1983.

56. Dreyfuss P, Michaelson M, Fletcher D. Atlanto-occipital and lateral atlanto-axial joint pain patterns. *Spine* 1994;19:1125–1131.

57. Ehni GE, Benner B. Occipital neuralgia and the C1-2 arthrosis syndrome. *J Neurosurg* 1984;61:961–965.

58. Bovim G, Berg R, Dale LG. Cervicogenic headache: Anaesthetic blockade of cervical nerves (C2-5) and facet joint (C2/3). *Pain* 1992;49:315–320.

59. McCrory P. Headaches and exercise. *Sports Med* 2000; 30:221–229.

60. Welch KM. A 47-year-old woman with tension-type headaches. *JAMA* 2001;286:960–966.

61. Jensen S, Graff-Radford S. Oromandibular function and tension-type headache. In: Olesen J, Tfelt-Hansen P, Welch KMA, eds. *The Headaches*. Philadelphia, Pa: Lippincott Williams and Wilkins; 2000:593–597.

62. Wolff HG. *Headache and Other Head Pain*. New York, NY: Oxford University Press; 1987:53–76.

63. Lord SM, et al. Third occipital nerve headache: A prevalence study. *J Neurol Neurosurg Psychiatry* 1994;57:1187–1190.

64. Lord SM, et al. Chronic cervical zygapophysial joint pain after whiplash: A placebo-controlled prevalence study. *Spine* 1996;21:1737–1744.

64a. Isaacs E, Bookout M. Screening for pathological origins of head and facial pain. In: Boissonnault WG, ed. *Examination in Physical Therapy Practice: Screening for Medical Disease*. Philadelphia, Pa: Saunders; 1995:175–189.

65. Mohn A, et al. Celiac disease–associated vertigo and nystagmus. *J Pediatr Gastroenterol Nutr* 2002;34:317–318.

66. Dvorak J, Dvorak V. Differential diagnosis of vertigo. In: Gilliar WG, Greenman PE, eds. *Manual Medicine: Diagnostics*. New York, NY: Thieme; 1990:67–70.

67. Lewit K. *Manipulative Therapy in Rehabilitation of the Locomotor System*. 2nd ed. Oxford, England: Butterworth-Heinemann; 1996.

68. Silbert PL, Mokri B, Schievink WI. Headache and neck pain in spontaneous internal carotid and vertebral artery dissections. *Neurology* 1995;45:1517–1522.

69. Fast A, Zincola DF, Marin EL. Vertebral artery damage complicating cervical manipulation. *Spine* 1987;12:840.

69a. Chutkan NB, King AG, Harris MB. Odontoid fractures: Evaluation and management. *J Am Acad Ortho Surg* 1997;5:199–204.

69b. Sasso RC., C2 dens fractures: treatment options. *J Spinal Disorders* 2001;14:455–463.

69c. Meadows J. *Orthopaedic Differential Diagnosis in Physical Therapy*. New York, NY: McGraw-Hill; 1999.

70. Ono K. Myelopathic hand. New clinical signs of cervical cord damage. *J Bone Joint Surg* 1987;69:215–219.

71. Taylor JR, Twomey LT. Acute injuries to cervical joints: An autopsy study of neck sprain. *Spine* 1993;9:1115–1122.

72. Viikara-Juntura E. *Examination of the Neck. Validity of Some Clinical, Radiological and Epidemiologic Methods*. Helsinki, Finland: University of Helsinki, Institute of Occupational Health; 1988.

73. Magee DJ. Head and face. In: Magee DJ, ed. *Orthopaedic Physical Assessment*. Philadelphia, Pa: Saunders; 2002:67–120.

74. Harris C. Nystagmus and eye movement disorders. In: Taylor D, ed. *Paediatric Ophthalmology*. Oxford, England: Blackwell; 1997:869–896.

75. Dell'Osso LF, Daroff RB. Nystagmus and saccadic intrusions and oscillations. In: Glaser JS, ed. *Neuro-ophthalmology*. Baltimore, Md: Lippincott Williams and Wilkins; 1999:369–401.

76. Abadi RV. Mechanisms underlying nystagmus. *J R Soc Med* 2002;95:231–234.

77. Hulse M. *Die zervikalen Gleichgewichtsstorungen*. Berlin, Germany: Springer; 1983.

78. Johnson GM. The correlation between surface measurement of head and neck posture and the anatomic position of the upper cervical vertebrae. *Spine* 1998;23:921–927.

79. Braun BL, Amundson LR. Quantitative assessment of head and shoulder posture. *Arch Phys Med Rehabil* 1989;70:322–329.

80. Braun BL. Postural differences between asymptomatic men and women and craniofacial pain patients. *Arch Phys Med Rehabil* 1991;72:653–656.

81. Watson D, Trott P. Cervical headache: An investigation of natural head posture and upper cervical flexor muscle performance. *Cephalalgia* 1993;13:272–284.

82. Grimmer K. The relationship between cervical resting posture and neck pain. *Physiotherapy* 1996;82:45–51.

83. Griegel-Morris P, et al. Incidence of common postural abnormalities in the cervical, shoulder, and thoracic regions and their association with pain in two age groups of healthy subjects. *Phys Ther* 1992;72:426–430.

84. Kori AA, Leigh JL. The cranial nerve examination. In: Gilman S, ed. *Clinical Examination of the Nervous System*. New York, NY: McGraw-Hill; 2000:65–111.

85. Bergmann TF, Peterson DH, Lawrence DJ. *Chiropractic Technique: Principles and Procedures*. New York, NY: Churchill Livingstone; 1993.

86. McGaughran JM, Kuna P, Das V. Audiological abnormalities in the Klippel-Feil syndrome. *Arch Dis Child* 1998;79:352–355.

87. Bhandari S, Farr MJ. Case report: Klippel-Feil syndrome with coexistent hypoparathyroidism. *Am J Med Sci* 1996; 311:174–177.

88. Da-Silva EO. Autosomal recessive Klippel-Feil syndrome. *J Med Genet* 1982;19:130–134.

89. Kanchandani R, Howe JG. Lhermitte's sign in multiple sclerosis: A clinical survey and review of the literature. *J Neurol Neurosurg Psychiatry* 1982;45:308–312.

90. Pettman E. Stress tests of the craniovertebral joints. In: Boyling JD, Palastanga N, eds. *Grieve's Modern Manual Therapy: The Vertebral Column*. Edinburgh, Scotland: Churchill Livingstone; 1994:529–538.

91. Murphy DK, Gutrecht JA. Lhermitte's sign in cavernous angioma of the cervical spinal cord. *J Neurol Neurosurg Psychiatry* 1998;65:954–955.

92. Hardin J Jr. Pain and the cervical spine. *Bull Rheum Dis* 2001;50:1–4.

93. Bland JH. New anatomy and physiology with clinical and historical implications. In: Bland JH, ed. *Disorders of the Cervical Spine*. Philadelphia, Pa: Saunders; 1994:71–79.

94. Bogduk N. An anatomical basis for the neck-tongue syndrome. *J Neurol Neurosurg Psychiatry* 1981;44:202–208.

94a. Pettman E. Level III Course Notes. Berrien Springs, Michigan: North American Institute of Manual Therapy, Inc.; 2003.

94b. Fuss FK. Sagittal kinematics of the cervical spine—how constant are the motor axes? *Acta Anatomica* 1991;141:93–96.

95. Ross JK, Bereznick DE, McGill SM. Atlas-axis facet asymmetry. Implications in manual palpation. *Spine* 1999;24: 1203–1209.

96. Greenman PE. *Principles of Manual Medicine*. 2nd ed. Baltimore, Md: Williams and Wilkins; 1996.

97. Dvorak J, Dvorak V. General principles of palpation. In: Gilliar WG, Greenman PE, eds. *Manual Medicine: Diagnostics*. New York, NY: Thieme; 1990:71–75.

98. Lee DG. *A Workbook of Manual Therapy Techniques for the Upper Extremity*. 2nd ed. Delta, Canada: DOPC Delta Orthopaedic Physiotherapy Clinic. 1991:58–79.

99. Martel W. The occipito-atlanto-axial joints in rheumatoid arthritis. *Am J Roentgenol* 1961;86:223–240.

100. Parke WW, Rothman RH, Brown MJ. The pharyngovertebral veins: An anatomical rationale for Grisel's syndrome. *J Bone Joint Surg* 1984;66A:568.

101. Georgopoulos G, Pizzutillo PD, Lee MS. Occipito-atlantal instability in children. *J Bone Joint Surg* 1987;69A:429–436.

102. El-Khoury GY, et al. Posterior atlantooccipital subluxation in Down syndrome. *Radiology* 1986;159:507–509.

103. Brooke DC, Burkus JK, Benson DR. Asymptomatic occipito-atlantal instability in Down's syndrome. *J Bone Joint Surg* 1987;69A:293–295.

104. Fielding JW, Hawkins RJ, Ratzan SA. Spine fusion for atlanto-axial instability. *J Bone Joint Surg* 1976;58A:400–407.

105. Boden SD, et al. Abnormal magnetic resonance scans of the cervical spine in asymptomatic subjects: A prospective investigation. *J Bone Joint Surg* 1990;72A:1178–1184.

106. Sung RD, Wang JC. Correlation between a positive Hoffman's reflex and cervical pathology in asymptomatic individuals. *Spine* 2001;26:67–70.

106a. Sasso RC. C2 dens fractures: Treatment options. *J Spinal Disorders* 2001;14:455–463.

106b. Freemyer B, et al. Comparison of five-view and three-view cervical spine series in the evaluation of patients with cervical trauma. *Ann Emerg Med* 1989;18:818–821.

106c. Schaffer MA, Doris PE. Limitation of the cross table lateral view in detecting cervical spine injuries: A retrospective analysis. *Ann Emerg Med* 1981;10:508–513.

106d. Marchesi DG. Management of odontoid fractures. *Orthopaedics* 1997;20:911–916.

106e. Blacksin MF, Lee HJ. Frequency and significance of fractures of the upper cervical spine detected by CT in patients with severe neck trauma. *Am J Roentgenol* 1995;165:1201–1204.

106f. Harris MB, Waguespack AM, and Kronlage S. "Clearing" cervical spine injuries in polytrauma patients: Is it really safe to remove the collar? *Orthopedics* 1997;20:903–907.

107. Press JM, Herring SA, Kibler WB. *Rehabilitation of Musculoskeletal Disorders. The Textbook of Military Medicine.* Washington, DC: Borden Institute, Office of the Surgeon General; 1996.

108. McKinney LA, Dornan JO, Ryan M. The role of physiotherapy in the management of acute neck sprains following road-traffic accidents. *Arch Emerg Med* 1989;6:27–33.

109. McKinney LA. Early mobilisation and outcome in acute sprains of the neck. *BMJ* 1989;299:1006–1008.

110. Smolders JJ. Myofascial pain and dysfunction syndromes. In: Hammer WI, ed. *Functional Soft Tissue Examination and Treatment by Manual Methods—The Extremities.* Gaithersburg, Md: Aspen; 1991:215–234.

111. Liebenson C. Active muscular relaxation techniques (part 2). *J Manipulative Physiol Ther* 1990;13:2–6.

112. Harata S, Tolmo S, Kawagishi T. Osteoarthritis of the atlanto-axial joint. *Internal Orthop* 1981;5:277–282.

113. Ghanayem AJ, Leventhal M, Bohlman HH. Osteoarthrosis of the atlanto-axial joints. Long-term follow-up after treatment with arthrodesis. *J Bone Joint Surg* 1996;78A:1300–1307.

114. Semble EL, et al. Magnetic resonance imaging of the craniovertebral junction in rheumatoid arthritis. *J Rheumatol* 1988;15:1367–1375.

115. Wilson BC, Jarvis BL, Haydon RC. Nontraumatic subluxation of the atlantoaxial joint: Grisel's syndrome. *Laryngoscope* 1987;96:705–708.

116. Lansen TA, Kasoff SS, Tenner MS. Occipitocervical fusion for reduction of traumatic periodontoid hypertrophic cicatrix. Case report. *J Neurosurg* 1990;73:466–470.

117. Nishizawa S, et al. Myelopathy caused by retro-odontoid disc hernia: Case report. *Neurosurgery* 1996;39:1256–1259.

118. Papadopoulos SM, Dickman CA, Sonntag VKH. Atlantoaxial stabilization in rheumatoid arthritis. *J Neurosurg* 1991;74:1–7.

119. Dickman CA, Douglas RA, Sonntag VKH. Occipitocervical fusion: Posterior stabilization of the craniovertebral junction and upper cervical spine. *BNI Q* 1990;6:2–14.

120. Kroenke K, Mangelsdorff D. Common symptoms in ambulatory care: Incidence, evaluation, therapy and outcome. *Am J Med* 1989;86:262–266.

121. Aspinall W. Clinical testing for cervical mechanical disorders which produce ischemic vertigo. *J Orthop Sports Phys Ther* 1989;11:176–182.

122. Wyke BD. Neurology of the cervical spinal joints. *Physiotherapy* 1979;65:72–76.

123. Cohen LA. Role of eye and neck proprioceptive mechanisms in body orientation and motor coordination. *J Neurophysiol* 1961;24:1–11.

124. Barré M. Sur un syndrome sympathetique cervical posterieur et sa cause frequente: l'arthrite cervicale. *Rev Neurol* 1926;33:1246–1248.

125. Ryan GMS, Cope S. Cervical vertigo. *Lancet* 1955;2:1355.

126. Wing LW, Hargrove-Wilson W. Cervical vertigo. *Aust N Z J Surg* 1974;44:275.

127. Macnab I. Acceleration extension injuries of the cervical spine. In: Rothman RH, Simeoni FA, eds. *The Spine.* Philadelphia, Pa: Saunders; 1982:515–527.

128. Biesinger E. Vertigo caused by disorders of the cervical vertebral column. *Adv Otorhinolaryngol* 1988;39:44.

129. Furuta Y, et al. Reactivation of herpes simplex virus type 1 in patients with Bell's palsy. *J Med Virol* 1998;54:162–166.

130. Fetter M, Dichgans J. Vestibular neuritis spares the inferior division of the vestibular nerve. *Brain* 1996;119:755–763.

131. Tusa RJ. Vertigo. *Neurol Clin* 2001;19:23–55.

132. Adour KK. Otological complications of herpes zoster. *Ann Neurol* 1994;35:S62–S64.

133. Courjon JH, et al. The role of vision in compensation of vestibulo-ocular reflex after hemilabyrinthectomy in the cat. *Exp Brain Res* 1977;5:67–107.

134. Fetter M, Zee DS. Recovery from unilateral labyrinthectomy in rhesus monkeys. *J Neurophysiol* 1988;59:370–393.

135. Herdman SJ, Borello-France DF, Whitney SL. Treatment of vestibular hypofunction. In: Herdman SJ, ed. *Vestibular Rehabilitation.* Philadelphia, Pa: FA Davis; 1994:287–315.

136. Dix MR. The rationale and technique of head exercises in the treatment of vertigo. *Acta Oto-Rhino-Laryng Belg* 1979;33:370.

137. Headache Classification Committee of the International Headache Society. Classification and diagnostic criteria for headache disorders, cranial neuralgias and facial pain. *Cephalalgia* 1988;7(suppl):1–551.

138. Maigne R. La céphalée sus-orbitaire. Sa fréquente origine cervicale. Son traitement. *Ann Med Phys* 1968;39:241–246.

139. Nicholson GG, Gaston J. Cervical headache. *J Orthop Sports Phys Ther* 2001;31:184–193.

140. Sizer PS Jr, Phelps V, Brismee JM. Diagnosis and management of cervicogenic headache and local cervical syndrome with multiple pain generators. *J Man Manipulative Ther* 2002;10:136–152.

141. Lu J, Ebraheim NA. Anatomical consideration of C2 nerve root ganglion. *Spine* 1998;23:649–652.

142. Polletti CE, Sweet WH. Entrapment of the C2 root and ganglion by the atlanto-epitrophic ligament: Clinical syndrome and surgical anatomy. *Neurosurgery* 1990;27:288–290.

143. Barnsley L, et al. The prevalence of chronic cervical zygapophysial joint pain after whiplash. *Spine* 1995;20:20–26.

144. Barnsley L, Lord S, Bogduk N. The pathophysiology of whiplash. In: Malanga GA, ed. *Cervical Flexion-Extension/Whiplash Injuries. Spine: State of the Art Reviews.* Philadelphia, Pa: Hanley and Belfus; 1998:209–242.

145. Maimaris C, Barnes MR, Allen MJ. Whiplash injuries of the neck: A retrospective study. *Injury* 1988;19:393–396.

146. Braaf MM, Rosner S. Trauma of the cervical spine as a cause of chronic headache. *J Trauma* 1975;15:441–446.

147. Jull GA. Headaches associated with cervical spine: A clinical review. In: Boyling JD, Palastanga N, eds. *Grieve's Modern Manual Therapy.* Edinburgh, Scotland: Churchill Livingstone; 1994.

148. Norris SH, Watt I. The prognosis of neck injuries resulting from rear-end vehicle collisions. *J Bone Joint Surg* 1983;65:608–611.

149. Martin PR, et al. The relationship between headaches and mood. *Behav Res Ther* 1988;26:353–356.

150. Arena JG, Blanchard EB, Andrasik F. The role of affect in the etiology of chronic headache. *J Psychosom Res* 1984;28:79–86.

151. Bronfort G, et al. Efficacy of spinal manipulation for chronic headache: A systematic review. *J Manipulative Physiol Ther* 2001;24:457–466.

151a. Aferzon M, Reams CL. Radiology quiz case 2. Chiari malformation (type I). *Arch Otolaryngology–Head & Neck Surgery* 2002;128:1104,1106–1107.

151b. Piper JG, Menezes AH. Chiari malformations in the adult. In: Menezes AH, Sonntag VKH eds. *Principles of Spinal Surgery.* McGraw-Hill: New York; 1996;379–394.

151c. Lui TN, et al. C1-C2 fracture-dislocations in children and adolescents. *J Trauma-Injury Infect Crit Care* 1996;40:408–411.

151d. Wong DA, Mack RP, Craigmile TK. Traumatic atlantoaxial dislocation without fracture of the odontoid. *Spine* 1991; 16:587–589.

151e. Greene KA, et al. Acute axis fractures: Analysis of management and outcomes. *Spine* 1997;22:1843–1852.

151f. Appuzo ML, et al. Acute fractures of the odontoid process: An analysis of 45 cases. *J Neurosurg* 1978;48:85–91.

151g. Marchesi DG. Management of odontoid fractures. *Orthopaedics* 1997;20:911–916.

151h. Sasso RC. C2 dens fractures: Treatment options. *J Spinal Disorders* 2001;14:455-463.

151i. Clark CR, White AA. Fractures of the dens: a multicenter study. *J Bone Joint Surg* 1985;67A:1340–1348.

151j. Chutkan NB, King AG, Harris MB. Odontoid fractures: Evaluation and management. *J Am Acad Ortho Surg* 1997; 5:199–204.

151k. Pepin JW, Bourne RB, Hawkins RJ. Odontoid fractures, with special reference to the elderly patient. *Clin Orthop* 1985;193:178–183.

151l. Anderson LD, D'Alonzo RT. Fractures of the odontoid process of the axis. *J Bone Joint Surg* 1974;56A:1663–1674.

151m. Scott EW, Haid RW, Peace D. Type I fractures of the odontoid process: Implications for atlantoaxial instability. *J Neurosurg* 1990;72:488–492.

151n. Heller J, Levy M, Barrow D. Odontoid fracture malunion with fixed atlantoaxial subluxation. *Spine* 1993;18:311–314.

151o. Seybold EA, Bayley JC. Functional outcome of surgically and conservatively managed dens fractures. *Spine* 1998;23:1837–1846.

151p. Jefferson G. Fracture of the atlas vertebra, report of four cases and a review of those previously recorded. *Br J Surg* 1920;7:407–422.

151q. Lee TT, Green BA, Petrin DR. Treatment of stable burst fracture of the atlas (Jefferson fracture) with rigid cervical collar. *Spine* 1998;23:1963–1967.

151r. Hadley MN, et al. Acute traumatic atlas fractures: Management and long-term outcome. *Neurosurgery* 1988;23:31–35.

151s. Landells CD, Van Peteghem PK. Fractures of the atlas: Classification, treatment, and morbidity. *Spine* 1988;13:450–452.

152. Kaltenborn FM. *The Spine: Basic Evaluation and Mobilization Techniques.* Wellington: New Zealand University Press; 1993.

152a. Kaltenborn FM. *The Spine: Basic Evaluation and Mobilization Techniques.* Wellington: New Zealand University Press, 1993.

153. Mulligan BR. *Manual Therapy: "NAGS", "SNAGS", "PRP'S" etc.* Wellington, New Zealand: Plane View Series; 1992.

154. Adeboye KA, Emerton DG, Hughes T. Cervical sympathetic chain dysfunction after whiplash injury. *J R Soc Med* 2000;93:378–379.

155. Evans RW. The postconcussion syndrome and the sequelae of mild head injury. *Neurol Clin* 1992;10:815–847.

156. Nordin M. Education and return to work. In: Gunzburg R, Szpalski M, eds. *Whiplash Injuries: Current Concepts in Prevention, Diagnosis and Treatment of the Cervical Whiplash Syndrome.* Philadelphia, Pa: Lippincott-Raven; 1998:199–210.

THE CERVICAL SPINE

CHAPTER OBJECTIVES

▶ *At the completion of this chapter, the reader will be able to:*

1. Describe the anatomy of the vertebrae, ligaments, muscles, and blood and nerve supply that comprise the cervical intervertebral segment.

2. Describe the biomechanics of the cervical spine, including coupled movements, normal and abnormal joint barriers, kinesiology, and reactions to various stresses.

3. Perform a detailed objective examination of the cervical musculoskeletal system, including palpation of the articular and soft tissue structures, specific passive mobility tests, passive articular mobility tests, and stability tests.

4. Perform and interpret the results from combined motion testing.

5. Assess the static and dynamic postures of the cervical spine, and implement the appropriate intervention.

6. Apply manual therapy techniques using the correct grade, intensity, direction, and duration.

7. Evaluate intervention effectiveness in order to progress or modify the intervention.

8. Plan an effective home program, including spinal care, and instruct the patient in this program.

9. Help the patient to develop self-reliant intervention strategies.

OVERVIEW

The cervical spine consists of 37 joints, which allow for more motion than any other region of the spine. It has been estimated that the cervical spine moves about 600 times per hour with normal activity.[1] However, this degree of mobility comes with a cost. With stability being sacrificed for mobility, the cervical spine is rendered more vulnerable to both direct and indirect trauma.

Anatomically and biomechanically, the cervical spine can be divided into two areas, the upper cervical or craniovertebral region, and the mid to lower cervical region. Bogduk and Mercer[1a] further divide the cervical spine into four anatomical units: the atlas, the axis, the C2–3 junction, and the remaining cervical vertebrae. For the sake of simplicity, these units are described in separate chapters. The atlas, axis and C2–3 junction are described in Chapter 22. The remaining cervical vertebrae are described in this chapter.

The cervical spine can be the source of many pain syndromes, including neck, upper thoracic, and periscapular syndromes; cervical radiculopathy; and shoulder and elbow syndromes.[2] These syndromes may result from a vast array of causes, ranging from acute minor sprains to chronic degenerative changes that compromise the spinal cord.[3] Although most neck pain is transient and of uncertain cause, more serious causes include deceleration injuries and inflammatory diseases of the cervical articulations.[4]

It should, therefore, not be surprising that neck and upper extremity pain are common in the general population, with surveys finding the 1-year prevalence rate for neck and shoulder pain to be 16 to 18 percent.[5,6] This prevalence also is reflected in the incidence of neck pain in the outpatient physical therapy setting, which has been found to be between 15 and 34 percent.[7,8]

Anatomy

The majority of the anatomy of this region can be explained in reference to the functions that the head and neck perform on a daily basis. To carry out these various tasks, the head has to be provided with the ability to perform extensive, detailed, and, at times, very quick motions. These motions allow for precise positioning of the eyes, and the ability to respond to a host of postural changes that result from stimulation of the vestibular system.[9] In addition to providing this amount of mobility, the cervical spine has to afford some protection to several vital structures, including the spinal cord and the vertebral and carotid arteries.

Cervical Curve

The cervical spine forms a lordotic curve that develops secondary to the response of an upright posture, which initially occurs when the child begins to lift the head at 3 to 4 months. The presence of the curve allows the head and eyes to remain oriented forward, and provides a shock-absorbing mechanism to counteract the axial compressive force produced by the weight of the head.[10]

The amount of cervical lordosis is a factor of the zygapophysial joint planes, and the cervical intervertebral disks (IVDs). Under normal conditions, the C4 to C5 interspace is considered the midpoint of the curve, and the center of gravity for the skull lies anterior to the foramen magnum. The longus colli has been shown to have an important supporting role on the cervical curve.[11]

A reduction in the cervical lordotic curve because of injury or abnormal posture results in more weight being borne by the vertebral bodies and IVDs, whereas an increase in the lordosis increases the compressive load on the zygapophysial joints and posterior elements. Watson and Trout[12] have demonstrated a link between a lack of endurance capacity of the upper cervical and deep neck flexors and the forward head posture.

Cervicothoracic Junction

The cervicothoracic junction comprises the C7 to T1 segment, although functionally it includes the seventh cervical vertebra, the first two thoracic vertebrae, the first and second ribs, and the manubrium. In addition, the cervicothoracic junction forms the thoracic outlet, through which the neurovascular structures of the upper extremities pass. Lewit[13] considers the cervicothoracic junction to be the third major area of the body for musculoskeletal problems, with the cranioveretbral area and the lumbosacral junction being first and second, respectively.

Vertebrae

Compared with the rest of the spine, the vertebral bodies of the cervical spine are small and consist predominantly of trabecular (cancellous) bone.[9] The third to sixth cervical vertebrae can be considered typical, whereas the seventh is atypical. The third, fourth, and fifth vertebrae are almost identical, whereas the sixth has enough minor differences to distinguish it from the others.

The typical cervical vertebra has a larger transverse than anteroposterior dimension (Fig. 23-1). The superior aspect of the centrum is concave transversely and convex anteroposteriorly, forming a sellar surface that reciprocates with the inferior surface of the centrum, superior to it.[9] The superior surface of the vertebral body is characterized by superiorly projecting processes on their superolateral aspects. Each of these hook-shaped processes is called an uncinate process and is composed of the raised lip of the superolateral aspect of the body that articulates with a reciprocally curved surface at the synovial uncovertebral joint (see Fig. 23-2).

The anterior margin of the IVD is attached to the anterior longitudinal ligament. This surface can be palpated by the clinician and is often tender in the presence of intervertebral instability. The discal margins of the posterior surface of the vertebral body give rise to the posterior longitudinal ligament.

Variations in the lower cervical vertebrae are most commonly found in the spinous and transverse processes. The transverse processes are short and project anterolaterally and slightly inferiorly, and are typified by a foramen in each. The transverse processes of vertebrae C2 through C6 are posterior

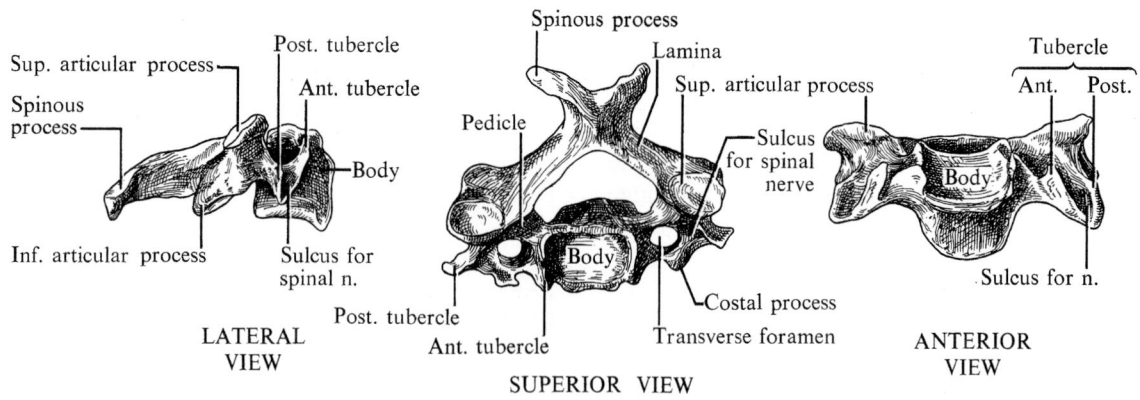

FIGURE 23-1 A cervical vertebra. (Reproduced with permission from Pansky B. *Review of Gross Anatomy.* 6th ed. New York, NY: McGraw-Hill: 1996:195.)

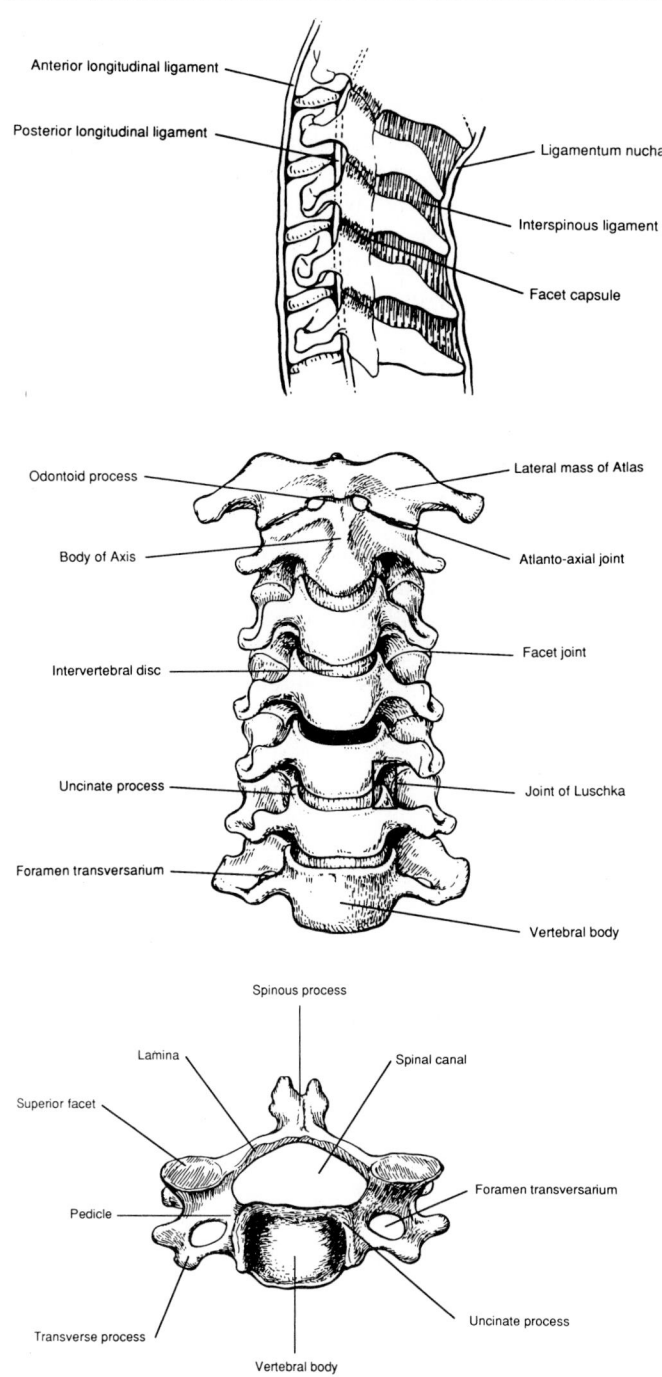

and lateral to the transverse foramina through which the vertebral artery, accessory vertebral vein, and the vertebral nerve all pass.

The transverse process consists of two parts (Fig. 23-1):

1. The anterior portion, or costal process, which ends laterally as the anterior tubercle. The longus capitis, scalenus ante-rior, and longus colli attach to this tubercle. The longus colli and scalene muscles have been implicated in the compression of the vertebral artery during rotation of the head and neck.[14] The anterior tubercle may be enlarged at the C7 vertebra, creating a cervical rib, which may be formed from either bone or fibrous tissue. If the rib is made from fibrous tissue, it will not be visible by radiograph. The anterior tubercle of the C6 vertebra, which is particularly large, is called the carotid tubercle, because it serves as the point from which the carotid pulse is taken. The anterior border of the transverse process also serves as the attachment site for the scalenus minimus.

2. The posterior portion, considered the true transverse process, ends laterally as the posterior tubercle. The posterior tubercle has attachment sites for the muscles of the splenius longissimus cervicis, iliocostalis cervicis, levator scapulae, and scalenus medius and posterior.

With the exception of the C2 vertebra, the superior aspect of the transverse process has a deep groove that mimics the orientation of the transverse process and the spinal nerve, both of which are parallel with the intervertebral foramen. The inferolateral orientation of the transverse process, and the fact that the spinal nerves are firmly anchored in the groove, makes the nerves vulnerable to a stretch injury around the distal end of the transverse process.[9]

The articular pillars and zygapophysial (facet) joints of vertebrae C2 through C7 are located approximately 1 inch lateral to the spinous processes. The articular pillar is formed by the superior and inferior articular processes of the zygapophysial joint, which bulge laterally at the pedicle-lamina junction. The articular facets on the superior articular process are concave and face superolaterally to articulate with the reciprocally curved and orientated facet on the inferior articular process of the vertebra above. The articular pillars bear a significant proportion of axial loading.[15]

As in the rest of the spine, the pedicles and laminae form the neural arch, which encloses the vertebral foramen. The pedicles project backward and laterally, whereas the long narrow laminae run posteriorly and medially, to terminate in a short bifid spinous process, which projects slightly inferiorly.[9] The seventh cervical vertebra varies from the typical cervical vertebra. In addition to possessing a much longer and monoid spinous process to which the ligamentum nuchae attaches, the seventh vertebra has wider transverse processes, no inferior uncinate facet, and no transverse foramen.

Articulations

The structure of the cervical vertebrae, combined with the orientation of the zygapophysial facets, provides very little bony stability, and the lax soft tissue restraints permit large excursions of motion.[9] A narrow space exists between the spinal cord and the vertebral canal walls in this region. There also is a very small amount of extra space in the intervertebral foramina. Thus, a relatively small change to either the vertebral canal or the dimensions of the intervertebral foramen can result in significant compression of the spinal cord or the spinal nerve, respectively.[16]

Each pair of vertebrae in this region is connected by a number of articulations: a pair of zygapophysial joints, two uncovertebral joints, and the IVD. The IVD of the cervical spine is described in Chapter 20.

Zygapophysial Joints

There are 14 zygapophysial joints from the occiput to the first thoracic vertebra. These joints are typical synovial joints and are covered with hyaline cartilage. The articular facets are teardrop-shaped, with the superior facet facing up and posteriorly, while the inferior one faces down and anteriorly. The orientation of the middle to lower zygapophysial joint planes is oblique, between the frontal and transverse planes.[17] The average horizontal angle of the joint planes is approximately 45 degrees,[18] with the upper cervical levels closer to 35 degrees, and the lower levels at approximately 65 degrees.

Clinical Pearl

Clinically, the orientation of the zygapophysial joint planes can be thought of as passing through the patient's nose.

The orientation of the zygapophysial joints permits considerable flexibility in the motions of flexion and extension, and encourages the coupling motions of rotation and side bending to the same side.

The anterior joint capsule is strong, but it is lax in neutral and extension.[19] The posterior capsule is thin and weak. This laxity allows for translation between facets. The major constraints and supports of these joints are the ligaments of the vertebral column, and the IVD.

Vascular, fat-filled, synovial intra-articular inclusions[20] have been observed in these joints. These structures have been described as fibro-adipose meniscoids, synovial folds, and capsular rims. The meniscoids consist of connective and fatty tissue that is highly vascularized and innervated.[21] In the cervical spine, the meniscoids function as space-fillers for the uneven articular surfaces, especially in regions where the elasticity of the relatively thin cartilage is not sufficient.[21] These inclusions, which are theorized to play some role in protecting the articular surfaces as they are sucked in or expelled during movements, are prone to entrapment, and can play a potential role in intra-articular fibrosis and cervical spine pain.[22] Töndury and Theiler[23] have observed that the meniscoids atrophy and virtually disappear with increasing age.

The zygapophysial joint receives its nerve supply from the medial branches of the cervical posterior rami from C2 to C8 and the recurrent meningeal (sinuvertebral) nerve. The capsular pattern of the zygapophysial joint is a limitation of extension, equal loss of rotation and side bending, with flexion unaffected.

Uncovertebral Joints

From C3 to T1, there usually are a total of ten saddle-shaped, diarthrodial articulations. These articulations, known as *joints of Luschka* or *uncovertebral joints,* are formed between the uncinate process found on the lateral aspect of the superior surface of the inferior vertebra, and the beveled inferolateral aspect of the superior vertebra[24] (see Fig. 23-2). The uncovertebral joints develop within the first 12 years of life as a result of loading from the head, and become fully developed by about 33 years of age.[25,26] Two of these uncovertebral joints are found between each pair of adjacent vertebrae in the cervical spine proper (C2–3 to C6–7). The uncovertebral joint maintains a synovial compartment and creates the posterior lateral border of the IVD.[27]

The biomechanical role of the uncovertebral joint is thought to be that of a sagitally oriented guiding rail during cervical flexion and extension that act to transfer rotation forces into side bending and posterior translation motions.[24,28,29] This function is accomplished while simultaneously ensuring that the translation between adjacent vertebral bodies is limited to the sagittal plane.[24,28,29] This stabilizing feature develops and changes with age and is based on alterations in the uncinate processes.[30]

Clinical Pearl

The uncovertebral joints serve to:

- Guide cervical flexion and extension.
- Reduce side bending of the cervical spine.
- Prevent posterior translation of neighboring vertebrae.
- Reinforce the posterolateral aspect of the IVD.[10]

Penning and Wilmink[31] highlighted a possible correlation between uncovertebral joint configuration and the coupled cervical segmental motion of side bending and axial rotation. A more recent study of the C5 to C6 segment level by Clausen and colleagues[32] found that both the zygapophysial joints and Luschka joints are the major contributors to coupled motion in the lower cervical spine, and that the uncinate processes effectively reduce motion coupling and primary cervical motion (motion in the same direction as load application), especially in response to axial rotation and side bending loads.[32]

The onset of degenerative changes in the cervical spine has been shown to occur more commonly at the midcervical level than at the lower cervical level.[33] The reasons for the different degrees of involvement are not clear. The degenerative changes result in the substitution of a hingelike motion, with the pivot point on the contralateral side, in place of the normal gliding motion at the uncovertebral joints.[9] This alteration effectively transforms the cervical segment into a sellar joint.[23,31,34]

> ### Clinical Pearl
>
> With a loss of disk height as a result of degeneration or degradation of the IVD, the potential for repeated contact between the bony surfaces of the uncovertebral joint increases. This repetitive contact may result in hypertrophic changes in the bone in the form of osteophytes.[9]

The nerve roots in the midcervical level are more predisposed to osteophytic compression because of a combination of:

▶ Higher uncinate process.

▶ Smaller anteroposterior diameter of the intervertebral foramina.

▶ Longer course of nerve roots in close proximity to the uncovertebral joints at C4 to C6 levels.

▶ Greatest segmental mobility at C5 and C6.

The vertebral artery also may be compromised in the degenerative cervical spondylotic process. When involved, the vertebral artery usually is compromised at the level of the inferior aspect of the superior vertebra, where the apical posterolateral uncovertebral osteophytes are present.

Intervertebral Foramina

The intervertebral foramina are found between all vertebrae of the spine, except in the upper cervical spine. The cervical intervertebral foramina are 4 to 5 mm long and 8 to 9 mm high. They extend obliquely anteriorly and inferiorly from the spinal canal at an angle of 45 degrees in the coronal plane.[35] The anterior boundary of the foramen is formed by the IVD and by portions of both vertebral bodies, with the zygapophysial joints serving as the posterior boundaries. The pedicles form the superior and inferior boundaries. The medial to lateral depth of the posterior wall is formed by the lateral aspect of the ligamentum flavum.

The intervertebral foramina serve as the principal routes of entry and exit for the neurovascular systems to and from the vertebral canal. Within each foramen are:

▶ A segmental mixed spinal nerve.

▶ From two to four recurrent meningeal nerves or sinuvertebral nerves.

▶ Various spinal arteries.

▶ Plexiform venous connections.

Because they contribute to the innervation of the upper limb, the lower cervical spinal nerves are quite large in diameter and nearly fill the foramina. This region is vulnerable to narrowing with certain motions, or with osteophyte growth. The dimensions of the intervertebral foramina decrease with full extension and ipsilateral side bending of the cervical spine such that uncovertebral osteophytes may compress the nerve root and cervical cord posteriorly.

The spinal nerves also are in close proximity to both the ligamentum flavum and the zygapophysial joint. Thus, zygapophysial joint arthritis or a hypertrophic ligamentum flavum can cause posterior impingement of these nerves.

Vertebral Canal

In the cervical region, the vertebral canal contains the entire cervical part of the spinal cord, as well as the upper part of the first thoracic spinal cord segment. There are eight cervical spinal cord segments, and thus eight cervical spinal nerves (see Chap. 2) on each side, but only seven cervical vertebrae.

Ligaments

Both the function and location of the ligaments in this region are similar to that of the rest of the spine. For the purposes of these descriptions, the short ligaments that interconnect adjacent vertebrae are classified as segmental, whereas those that attach to the peripheral aspects of all of the vertebrae are classified as continuous.

Continuous Ligaments

Anterior Longitudinal Ligament. The anterior longitudinal ligament (ALL) is a strong band, extending along the anterior surfaces of the vertebral bodies and IVDs, from the front of the sacrum to the anterior aspect of C2 (Fig. 23-3). The ALL is narrower in the upper cervical spine but is wider in the lower cervical spine than it is in the thoracic region. It is firmly attached to the superior and inferior end plates of the cervical vertebrae, but not to the cervical disks. In the waist of the centrum, the ligament thickens to fill in the concavity of the body. The ALL functions to restrict spinal extension and is thus vulnerable to hyperextension trauma.

Posterior Longitudinal Ligament. Lying on the anterior aspect of the vertebral canal, the posterior longitudinal ligament (PLL) extends from the sacrum to the body of the axis (C2), where it is continuous with the tectorial membrane (Fig. 23-3). The PLL travels over the posterior aspect of the centrum, attaching to the superior and inferior margins of the body, but is separated from the waist of the body by a fat pad and the basivertebral veins. In addition, this ligament attaches firmly to the posterior aspect of the IVDs, laminae of hyaline cartilage, and adjacent margins of vertebral bodies. The PLL is broader and considerably thicker in the cervical region than in the thoracic and lumbar regions.[36] The PLL functions to prevent disk protrusions and also acts as a restraint to segmental flexion of the vertebral column.

The dura mater is strongly adherent to the PLL at the level of C3 and higher, but this attachment diminishes at lower levels.

Ligamentum Nuchae. This bilaminar fibroelastic intermuscular septum spans the entire cervical spine, extending from the external occipital protuberance to the spinous process of the seventh cervical vertebra, but its connections between the occipital base and foramen magnum to the atlas and axis are considered as the most significant[37] (Fig. 23-3). From this layer, laminae are given off that attach to the posterior tubercle of the atlas and the spines of the remaining cervical vertebrae, and its importance as a posterior restraint is well accepted.[38] When the occipito-atlantal joint is flexed, the superficial fibers tighten and pull on the deep laminae, which, in turn, pull the vertebrae posteriorly, limiting the anterior translation of flexion and, therefore, flexion itself.

Segmental Ligaments

The interspinous ligaments are thin and almost membranous, interconnecting the spinous processes. The ligament is poorly developed in the upper cervical spine but well developed in the lower[36] (see Fig. 23-3).

The ligamentum flavum runs perpendicularly to the spine from C1 and C2, where it is referred to as the *posterior atlanto-axial ligament* (Fig. 23-3), to L5 and S1. This ligament connects the laminae of successive vertebrae, from the zygapophysial joint to the root of the spinous process. It is formed by collagen and yellow elastic tissue and, therefore, differs from all other ligaments of the cervical spine. The ligamentum flavum of the cervical spine is fairly long, allowing an appreciable amount of flexion to occur, while maintaining tension when the head and neck are in neutral. Scarring or fatty infiltration to the ligament in this region can compromise the degree of elasticity, making the ligament lax, particularly with cervical extension. This laxity increases the potential for the contents of the vertebral canal to be compressed by the buckling ligament.[39] Any enlargement of the ligament increases the likelihood that a spinal nerve or its posterior root will become impinged.[9] The ligament appears to function as a restrictor of flexion of the neck.

Muscles

The mass of muscle on the posterior aspect of the neck is very thick and consists of the trapezius most superficially, and the underlying levator scapulae. For the most part, the muscles of the neck function to support and move the head. In the following sections, the muscles of the cervical spine are separated into the superficial muscles, the lateral muscles, and the deep muscles.

Superficial Muscles

Trapezius. The trapezius muscle (Fig. 23-4) is the most superficial back muscle. It is a flat triangular muscle that extends over the back of the neck and well beyond the cervical region,

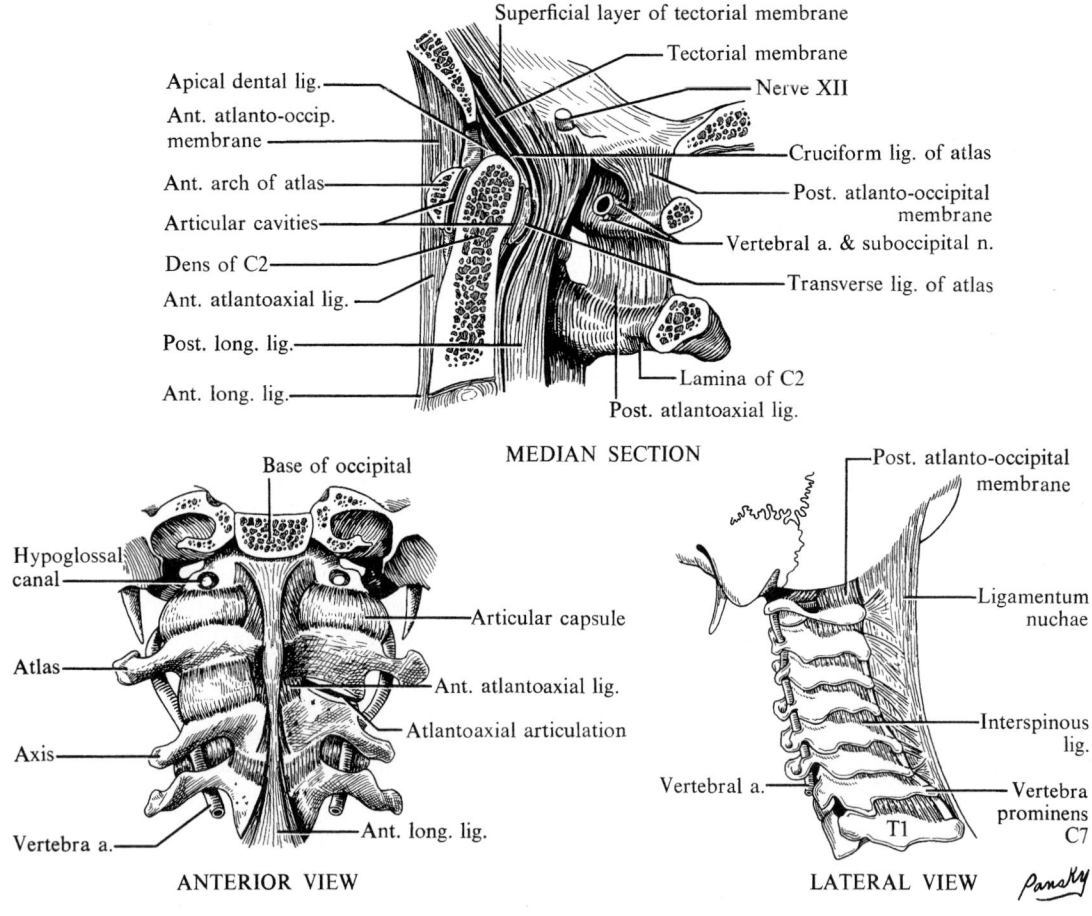

FIGURE 23-3 Anterior view, median section, and lateral view of the cervical spine. (Reproduced with permission from Pansky B. *Review of Gross Anatomy.* 6th ed. New York, NY: McGraw-Hill; 1996:213.)

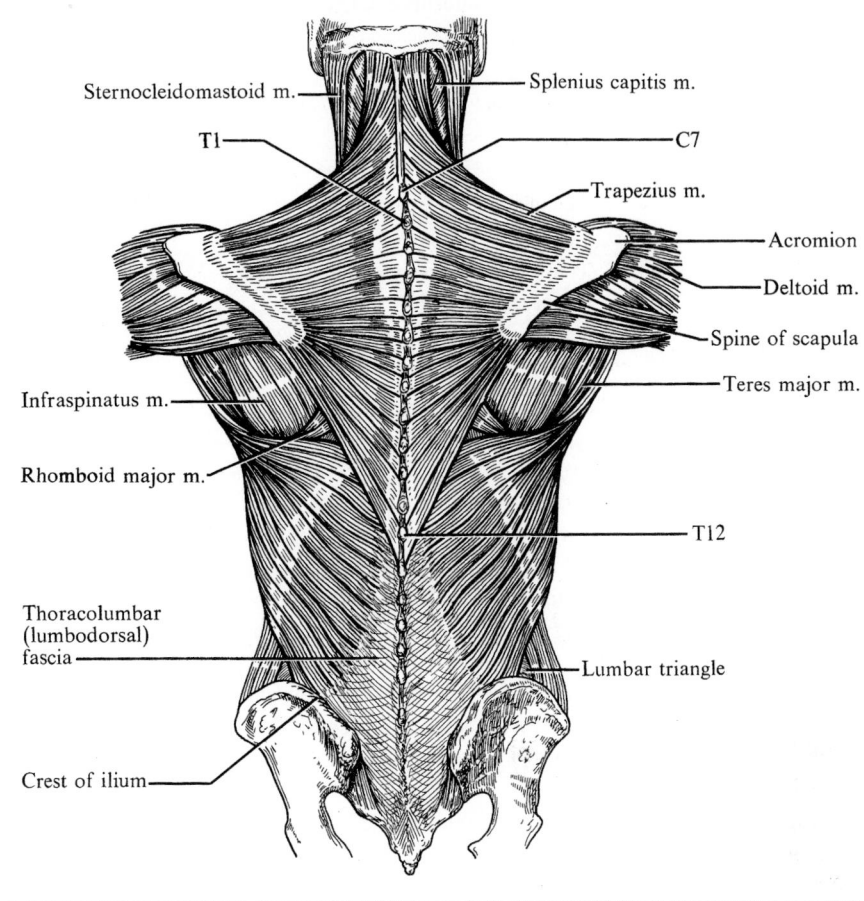

FIGURE 23-4 Superficial posterior muscles of the cervical spine. (Reproduced with permission from Pansky B. *Review of Gross Anatomy.* 6th ed. New York, NY: McGraw-Hill; 1996:201.)

arising from most of the thoracic spinous processes. Its origin, which runs from the superior nuchal line and external occipital protuberance of the occipital bone to the spinous process of T12, is the largest muscle attachment in the body. Its insertion can be traced from the entire superior aspect of the spine of the scapula, the medial aspect of the acromion, and the posterior aspect of the lateral third of the clavicle.

This muscle traditionally is divided into middle, upper, and lower parts according to anatomy and function.

▶ The middle part originates from C7 and forms the cervicothoracic part of the muscle.

▶ The lower part, attaching to the apex of the scapular spine, is relatively thin.

▶ The upper part (Table 23-1) is very thin and yet it has the most mechanical and clinical importance to the cervical spine.[40]

The innervation for the trapezius comes from the accessory nerve (CN XI) and fibers from the ventral rami of the third and fourth cervical spinal nerves, with the former speculated to provide the motor innervation, and the latter supplying the sensory information.[41] The greater occipital nerve occasionally travels through the trapezius near its superior border to reach the scalp

and can become entrapped by an adaptive shortening of the upper trapezius muscle or be traumatized by a blunt force.[42]

The different parts of this muscle provide a variety of actions on the shoulder girdle, including elevation and retraction of the scapula. When the shoulder girdle is fixed, the trapezius can produce ipsilateral side bending and contralateral rotation of the head and neck. Working together, the trapezius muscles can produce symmetric extension of the neck and head.[43] In addition, the trapezius muscle can produce scapular adduction (all three parts), and upward rotation of the scapula (primarily the superior and inferior parts). The importance of the trapezius to the shoulder joint is discussed in Chapter 14.

Sternocleidomastoid. The sternocleidomastoid (SCM; Fig. 23-5) is a fusiform muscle that descends obliquely across the side of the neck, forming a distinct landmark for palpatory purposes. It is the largest muscle in the anterior neck. It is attached inferiorly by two heads, arising from the posterior aspect of the medial third of the clavicle and the manubrium of the sternum. From here, it passes superiorly and posteriorly to attach on the mastoid process of the temporal bone. The motor supply for this muscle is from the accessory nerve (CN XI), whereas the sensory innervation is supplied from the ventral rami of C2

TABLE 23-1   Attachments of Upper Trapezius and Levator Scapulae Muscles

Muscle	Proximal	Distal	Innervation
Upper trapezius	Superior nuchal line	Lateral third of clavicle and the acromion process	Spinal accessory
	Ligamentum nuchae		
Levator scapulae	Transverse processes of upper 4 cervical vertebrae	Medial border of scapula at level of scapular superior angle	Dorsal scapular C5 (C3 and C4)

and C3.[41] This muscle can provide the clinician with information regarding the severity of symptoms, and postural impairments, because of its tendency to become prominent when hypertonic. The muscle also is involved with a condition called torticollis, a postural deformity of the neck (see Chap. 9).

In broad terms, the actions of this muscle are flexion, side bending, and contralateral rotation of the head and neck.[43] Acting together, the two muscles draw the head forward and can also raise the head when the body is supine. This head-raising action is a combination of upper cervical extension and lower cervical flexion. The muscle is also active on resisted neck flexion. With the head fixed, it is also an accessory muscle of forced inspiration.

Levator Scapulae.   The levator scapulae (Fig. 23-6) is a slender muscle attached by tendinous slips to the posterior tubercles of the transverse processes of the upper cervical vertebrae (C1–4). The levator, located deep to both the upper and middle parts of the trapezius, can be palpated just deep to the superior border of the trapezius. It descends posteriorly, inferiorly, and laterally to the superior angle and medial border of the scapula,

between the superior angle and the base of the spine (Table 23-1). The levator is the major stabilizer and elevator of the superior angle of the scapula. With the scapula stabilized, the levator produces rotation and side bending of the neck to the same side; when acting bilaterally, cervical extension is produced.[43] With a forward head posture, the potential for this extension moment increases.[9] This abnormal anterior translation is resisted by tension within the levator scapulae and the ligamentum nuchae.[44]

> ### Clinical Pearl
>
> If the levator scapulae is shorter on one side, it may provoke contralateral suboccipital muscle spasms and subsequent headaches.[9]

The levator is supplied by direct branches of the C3 and C4 cervical spinal nerves and from C5 through the dorsal scapular nerve. It is heavily innervated with muscle spindles.

Rhomboids.   The rhomboid major is a quadrilateral sheet of muscle, and the rhomboid minor muscle is small and cylindrical

FIGURE 23-5 Sternocleidomastoid muscle. (Reproduced with permission from Luttgens K, Hamilton K. *Kinesiology: Scientific Basis of Human Motion.* New York, NY: McGraw-Hill; 1997:111.)

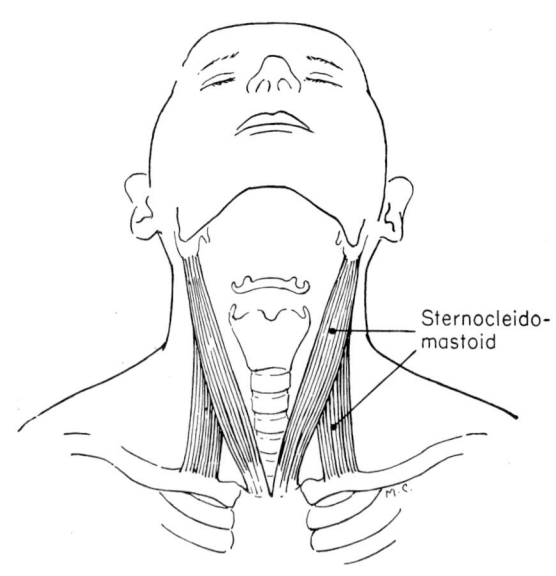

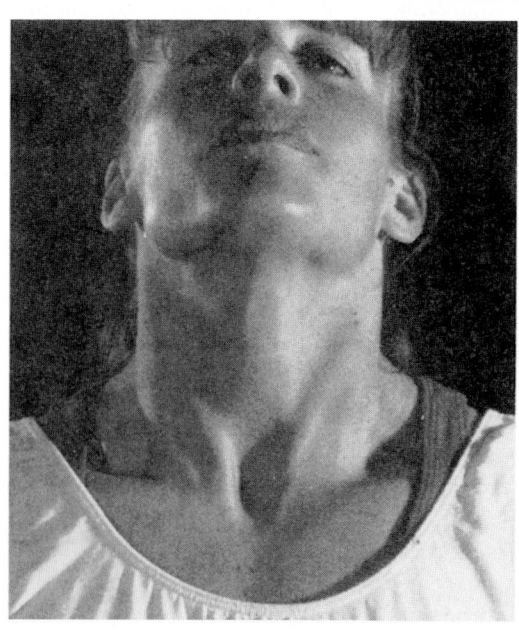

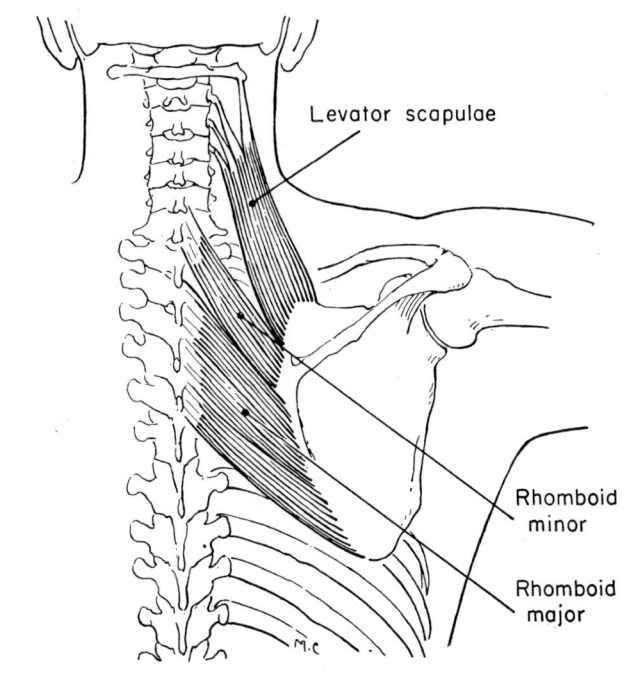

FIGURE 23-6 Levator scapulae. (Reproduced with permission from Luttgens K, Hamilton K. *Kinesiology: Scientific Basis of Human Motion.* New York, NY: McGraw-Hill; 1997:111.)

(Fig. 23-6). Together they form a thin sheet of muscle that fills much of the interval between the medial border of the scapula and the midline. Although the rhomboid minor, with its attachment to the spinous processes of C7 and T1, has a slight association with the cervical spine, the rhomboid major, arising from the spinous processes of T1 through T5, is inactive during isolated head and neck movements. The two muscles descend from their points of origin, passing laterally to the posterior aspect of the vertebral border of the scapula, from the base of the spine to the inferior angle. Both of these muscles receive their nerve supply from the dorsal scapular nerve (ventral ramus of C4–5). The principle action of these muscles is to work with the levator scapulae to control the position and movement of the scapula. Both of the muscles are involved with concentric contractions during rowing exercises or other activities involving scapular retraction.

Lateral Muscles

Scalenes. The scalenes (Fig. 23-7) extend obliquely like ladders (*scala* means ladder in Latin) and share a critical relationship with the subclavian artery. Tightness of these muscles will affect the mobility of the upper cervical spine. In addition, because of their distal attachments to the first and second ribs (Table 23-2), they can, if in spasm, elevate the ribs and be implicated in the thoracic outlet syndrome.[45,46]

Scalenus Anterior. The scalenus anterior (see Fig. 23-7) runs vertically, behind the SCM on the lateral aspect of the neck. Arising from the anterior tubercles of the C3 through C6 transverse processes, it travels to the scalene tubercle on the inner

border of the first rib. The osteal portion of the vertebral artery and the stellate ganglion are located lateral to the scalenus anterior. Acting from above, the scalenus anterior, like the rest of the scalenes, is an inspiratory muscle, even with quiet breathing.[47] Working bilaterally from below, it flexes the spine. Unilaterally, it side bends the spine ipsilaterally and rotates the spine contralaterally. It is supplied by the ventral rami of C4, C5, and C6.

Scalenus Medius. The scalenus medius (see Fig. 23-7) is the largest and longest of the group, attaching to the transverse processes of all cervical vertebrae except the atlas (although it often attaches to this) and running to the upper border of the first rib. It is separated from the anterior scalene by the carotid artery, and cervical nerve, and is pierced by the nerve to the rhomboids (dorsal scapular) and the upper two roots of the nerve to the serratus anterior (long thoracic). Working unilaterally on the cervical spine, the scalenus medius is an ipsilateral side bender of the neck. Working bilaterally, it is a cervical flexor.

Scalenus Posterior. The scalenus posterior (Fig. 23-7) is the smallest and deepest of the group, running from the posterior tubercles of the C4 through C6 transverse processes to attach to the outer aspect of the second rib. It functions to elevate or fix the second rib and side bends the neck ipsilaterally. It is innervated by the ventral rami of C5, C6, and C7.

Scalenus Minimus (Pleuralis). The scalenus minimus is a small muscle slip, running from the transverse process of C7 to the inner aspect of the first rib and the dome of the pleura. It is the suprapleural membrane that is often considered to be the expansion of the tendon of this muscle. The muscle functions to

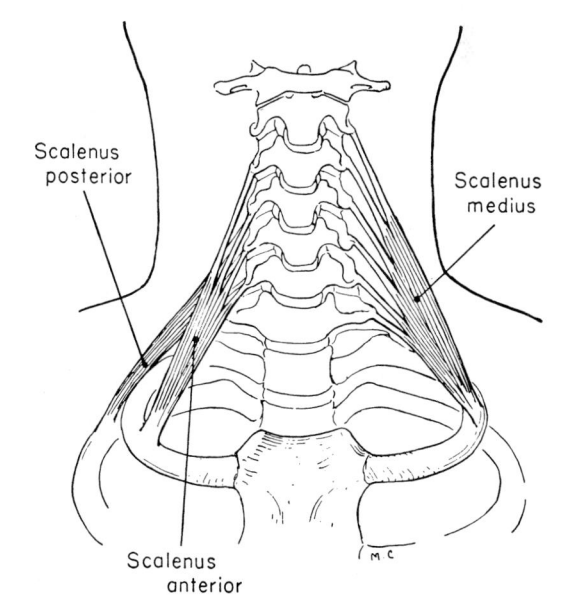

FIGURE 23-7 The scalenes. (Reproduced with permission from Luttgens K, Hamilton K. *Kinesiology: Scientific Basis of Human Motion.* New York, NY: McGraw-Hill; 1997:269.)

TABLE 23-2 Attachments of Scalene, Longus Colli, and Longus Capitis Muscles

Muscle	Proximal	Distal	Innervation
Scalenus Anterior	Anterior tubercles of C3–6	Superior crest of first rib	Ventral primary rami of cervical spinal nerves
Middle	Posterior tubercles of C2–7	Superior crest of first rib	
Posterior	Posterior tubercles of C5–7	Outer surface of second rib	
Longus colli	Anterior tubercles of C3–5 Anterior surface of C5–7, T1–3	Tubercle of the atlas, anterior tubercles of C5 and C6, anterior surface of C2–4	Ventral primary rami of cervical spinal nerves
Longus capitis	Anterior tubercles of C3–6	Inferior occipital bone, basilar portion	Ventral primary rami of cervical spine nerves

elevate the dome of the pleura during inspiration. It is innervated by the ventral ramus of C7.[48]

Platysma. The broad sheet of the platysma muscle is the most superficial muscle in the cervical region. The platsyma covers most of the anterolateral aspect of the neck, the upper parts of the pectoralis major, and deltoid, and extending superiorly to the inferior margin of the body of the mandible. As a muscle of facial expression, it cannot affect bony motion, except perhaps as a passive restraint to head extension. It is supplied by the cervical branch of CN VII (facial).

Deep Muscles of the Back

The deep or intrinsic muscles of the back are the primary movers of the vertebral column and head and are located deep to the thoracolumbar fascia. The muscles in all of these groups are segmentally innervated by the lateral branches of the dorsal rami of the spinal nerves.

Splenius Capitis. The splenius capitis (Fig. 23-8) extends upward and laterally, from the dorsal edge of the nuchal ligament and the spinous processes of the lower cervical and upper thoracic vertebrae (T4–C7), to the mastoid process of the occipital

FIGURE 23-8 Splenius capitis and cervicis. (Reproduced with permission from Luttgens K, Hamilton K. *Kinesiology: Scientific Basis of Human Motion.* New York, NY: McGraw-Hill; 1997:264.)

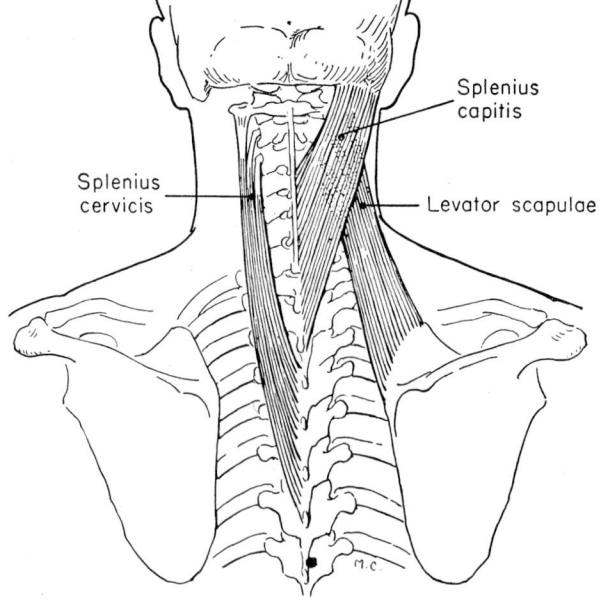
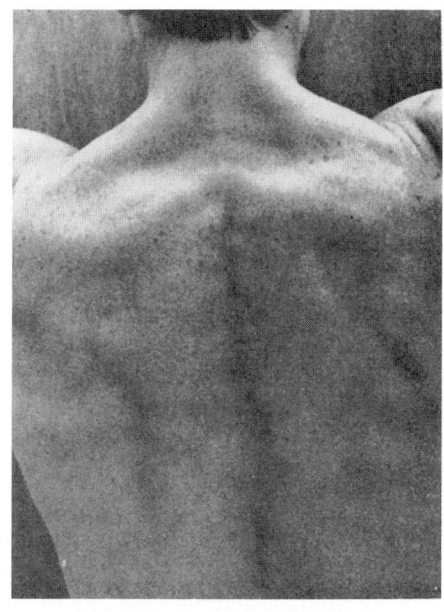

TABLE 23-3 Attachments of Splenius Capitis and Cervicis Muscles

Muscle	Proximal	Distal	Innervation
Splenius capitis	Inferior ligamentum nuchae, spinous process of C7 and T1–4 vertebrae	Mastoid process, occipital bone, and lateral third of superior nuchal line	Cervical spinal nerve and ventral primary rami of cervical spinal nerves
Splenius cervicis	Spinous processes of T3–6 vertebrae	Posterior tubercles of C1–3	

bone just inferior to the superior nuchal line, and deep to the SCM muscle.

Splenius Cervicis. The splenius cervicis (see Fig. 23-8) is just inferior and appears continuous with the capitis, extending from the spines of the third to the sixth thoracic vertebrae to the posterior tubercles of the transverse processes of the upper cervical vertebrae.

The splenius capitis and splenius cervicis muscles are two important head and neck rotators. From their attachments (Table 23-3), it is clear that these two muscles are capable of producing ipsilateral rotation, side bending, and extension at the spinal joints they cross.

Cervical Erector Spinae. The erector spinae complex spans multiple segments, forming a large musculotendonous mass consisting of the iliocostalis, longissimus, and spinalis muscles (Tables 23-4 and 23-5).

▶ The iliocostalis cervicis appears to function as a stabilizer of the cervicothoracic junction and lower cervical spine.

TABLE 23-4 Prime Movers of the Cervical Spine: Rotation and Side Bending[17]

Muscles of Rotation and Side Bending	
IPSILATERAL SIDE BENDING	IPSILATERAL ROTATION
Longissimus capitis	Splenius capitis
Intertransversarii posteriores cervices	Splenius cervices
Multifidus	Rotatores breves cervices
Rectus capitis lateralis	Rotatores longi cervices
Intertransversarii anteriores cervices	Rectus capitis posterior major
Scaleni	Obliquus capitis inferior
Iliocostalis cervicis	
CONTRALATERAL ROTATION	IPSILATERAL SIDE BENDING AND CONTRALATERAL ROTATION
Obliquus capitis superior	Sternocleidomastoid
	Scalenus anterior
	Multifidus
	Longus colli
IPSILATERAL SIDE BENDING AND IPSILATERAL ROTATION	
Longus coli	
Scalenus posterior	

▶ The semispinalis has thoracis, cervicis, and capitis divisions. The obliquus capitis superior (superior oblique) and inferior (inferior oblique), and the rectus capitis posterior major and minor (see Chap. 22) lie underneath the semispinalis capitis and splenius capitis muscles.[49] The semispinalis cervicis is a stout muscle that extends superiorly to the spinous process of vertebra C2, functioning as a strong extensor of the lower cervical spine.[9]

▶ The interspinales and intertransversarii, which interconnect the processes for which they are named, produce only minimal motion because they can influence only one motion segment, and are more likely to function as sensory organs for reflexes and proprioception.[50]

Neurology

The nerve supply to the cervical structures is rather unique because of the association some of the muscles have with the cranial nerves. The cervical spine is the only region that has more nerve roots than vertebral levels.[51] This results from the fact that the first cervical nerve root passes above the first vertebral level, between the occiput and the atlas (see Chap. 2).

In general, structures supplied by the upper three cervical nerves can cause neck and head pain (see Table 22-1), whereas the mid to lower cervical nerves can refer symptoms to the shoulder, anterior chest, upper limb, and scapular area.[3]

Cervical proprioceptive input has considerable influence on posture through the tonic neck reflex, and on eye movement and accommodation through the cervico-occular and vestibulo-ocular reflexes (see Chap. 2).[3,52,53] It is probably no accident that the two largest postural muscles of the head and neck, the trapezius and the SCM muscles, are partly innervated by the accessory nerve (CN XI).

Vascular Supply

The middle cervical segments are supplied by radicular branches off the extradural vertebral artery and are the most common segments to be affected in vertebral artery disease.[54] The vertebral artery is detailed in Chapter 21.

The common carotid artery bifurcates at the middle to upper cervical level into the internal and external carotid arteries. The carotid body, a specialized structure that senses oxygen and carbon dioxide levels in the blood, is located at this bifurcation.[51] The carotid sinus, which contains baroreceptors that monitor blood pressure, is located at a point prior to the bifurcation.[51]

TABLE 23-5 Prime Movers of the Cervical Spine: Extensors and Flexors

Extensor Muscles		Flexor Muscles
Prime Movers	Accessory Muscles	Prime Movers
Trapezius	Multifidus	Sternocleidomastoid—anterior fibers
Sternocleidomastoid—posterior fibers	Suboccipitals	Accessory muscles
Iliocostalis cervices	Rectus capitis posterior major and minor	Prevertebral muscles
Longissimus cervices	Obliquus capitis superior	Longus coli
Splenius cervices	Obliquus capitis inferior	Longus capitis
Splenius capitis		Rectus capitis anterior
Interspinales cervices		Scalene group
Spinalis cervices		Scalenus anterior
Spinalis capitis		Infrahyoid group
Semispinalis cervices		Sternohyoid
Semispinalis capitis		Omohyoid
Levator scapulae		Sternothyroid
		Thyrohyoid

Biomechanics

Although it may be clinically useful to describe the motions that occur at the cervical spine as separate motions, these motions correspond to the motion of the head alone, and do not describe what is occurring at the various segmental levels. It should be obvious that the range of head movement bears little relation to the range of neck movement, and that the total range is the sum of both the head and the neck motions.[55]

At the zygapophysial joints, there is a sagittal range of 30 to 60 degrees in each direction of flexion and extension.[56] The only significant arthrokinematic motion available to the zygapophysial joint is an inferior, medial glide of the inferior articular process of the superior facet during extension, and a superior, lateral glide during flexion. Segmental side bending is, therefore, extension of the ipsilateral joint and flexion of the contralateral joint. Rotation, coupled with ipsilateral side bending, involves extension of the ipsilateral joint and flexion of the contralateral.

Forward flexion occurs with rotation below the C5 to C6 level, and extension occurs with rotation above the C4 to C5 level. The net result is that whenever cervical spine rotation occurs, the greatest degree of weight bearing is on the anterior edge of the vertebral bodies below the C5 to C6 segments and on the posterior edge above C4 to C5 (this factor has been implicated in the cause of spondylosis in these areas).[9]

Motion within the mid to lower cervical segments involves an average of about 15 degrees of sagittal range per segment, compared with an average of about 10 degrees per segment in the lumbar spine,[57] but this can vary significantly depending on the instructions given to subjects.[58] The greatest amount of motion occurs at the C5 to C6 segment, with the C4 to C5 and C6 to C7 segments a close second.[56] A coupled translation of between 2 and 3.5 mm occurs with flexion and extension. Significant flexion occurs at C5 to C6, and ex-

tension around C6 to C7.[9] Side bending averages about 10 degrees to each side in the midcervical segments, decreasing in the caudal segments.

Flexion

Flexion is described as an anterior osteokinematic rock-tilt of the superior vertebra in the sagittal plane, a superoanterior glide of both superior facets of the zygapophysial joints, and an anterior translation-slide of the superior vertebra on the IVD. This produces a ventral compression and a dorsal distraction of the cervical disk. The uncovertebral joint lies on, or very near to, the axis of rotation for flexion and extension. Consequently, the main arthrokinematic motion that seems likely to be occurring here is an anterior spin (or very near spin).[59] This arthrokinematic spin appears especially probable as impairments of the uncovertebral joint seem to be unaffected by flexion or extension. Thus, uncovertebral restrictions may be detected in all cervical positions, although flexion partly disengages the joint because of its posterior position on the vertebra.[59]

Although all of the following anatomic movement restrictors act to some degree on most of the components of flexion, they act particularly on the associated movement component.

▶ Anterior osteokinematic motion is restrained by the extensor muscles and the posterior ligaments (posterior longitudinal, interspinous, ligamentum flavum).

▶ Superoanterior arthrokinematic is restrained by the joint capsule, whereas translation is restrained by the disk and the nuchal ligament.

Extension

Extension is described as a posterior osteokinematic sagittal rock, an inferoposterior glide and approximation of the superior facets of the zygapophysial joints, and a posterior translation of the vertebra on the disk. The uncovertebral joint undergoes a posterior arthrokinematic spin. The osteokinematic motion of extension is restricted by the anterior prevertebral muscles and the anterior longitudinal ligament. The arthrokinematic motion is restricted by the zygapophysial joint capsule.[59] The IVD restrains the posterior translation.

Side Bending

Side bending is an ipsilateral osteokinematic rock, a superoanterior glide of the contralateral superior facet, and a posteroinferior glide of the ipsilateral facet. In addition, there is a contralateral translation of the vertebra on the disk, an inferomedial glide of the ipsilateral uncovertebral joint, and a superolateral glide of the contralateral uncovertebral joint. A composite curved translation results. This curve is formed by the superoinferior linear glides of the zygapophysial joints, the oblique inferomedial and superomedial glides of the uncovertebral joints, and the linear translation across the disk.[59]

The osteokinematic rock can be limited by the contralateral scalenes and intertransverse ligaments. The uncovertebral and zygapophysial arthrokinematic motions can be limited by the joint capsule, and the translation is limited by the IVD. If the side bending is limited but the translation is okay, it is unlikely that the joint complex (the zygapophysial joint, disk, or uncovertebral joint) is impaired; instead, these findings may implicate adaptive shortening of the soft tissues.[59] However, if the translation is also limited, a problem with the joint complex also probably exists.

Rotation

Rotation is chiefly an osteokinematic motion of the vertebra about a vertical axis that is coupled with ipsilateral side bending. Presumably, the translation follows the side bending (i.e., contralateral), resulting in the same uncovertebral and zygapophysial arthrokinematic motions as does side bending.[59]

Muscle Control

The control of head and neck postures and movements is a complicated task, especially in the presence of pain or dysfunction. The muscle groups of the cervical region may be divided into those that produce movement and those that sustain postures or stabilize the segments.[60–62]

Many muscles in the neck act to provide both global and local functions, with the former having a primary role in torque production and control of the head, and latter being primarily responsible for the support and control of the spine at segmental level, and as a whole.[3,62]

The global muscles of the neck are thought to be the SCM (ventrally), and the semispinalis capitis and splenius capitis (dorsally). The local system is thought to comprise the longus capitis and colli (Table 23-2),[11] semispinalis cervicis, and multifidus.[63]

Patients with neck pain have been found to demonstrate generally less torque production in all planes, with a greater loss in the cervical flexors than extensors.[64]

Examination

The examination of the acute and recently traumatized neck is necessarily different from the routine examination of a more chronic and less irritable condition, because of the potential for the examination itself to be harmful.[65]

Where possible, the patient should be examined for central and peripheral neurologic deficit, neurovascular compromise, and serious skeletal injury, such as fractures or craniovertebral ligamentous instability. The examination must be graduated and progressive so that the testing can be discontinued at the first signs of serious pathology.[65]

Once damage to the vertebral artery (see Chap. 21) and transverse ligament (see Chap. 22) has been ruled out, the most likely pain candidates are assessed first. These include the bone, muscles, ligaments, zygapophysial joints, and IVD. In addition, because of its close proximity, a quick examination of the temporomandibular joint should be performed to rule out pain referral from this joint (see Chap. 24).

History

The cervical spine is an area with a high potential for serious injury, which makes this an area of the body that needs to be approached with caution. The history often gives the clinician clues as to the source of the patient's symptoms, the nature and location of the involved structure, the severity of the condition, and the activities or positions that appear to aggravate or improve the patient's condition (see Chap. 8).

The most common symptoms of cervical disorders are ongoing or motion-induced neck or arm pain, or both, and suboccipital headache.[21]

Winkel and colleagues[66] clinically categorize cervical disorders by the location of symptoms and the etiology of each condition:

▶ *Local cervical syndrome (LCS).* This syndrome manifests with local neck complaints, resulting from either primary or secondary disk-related conditions (see Chap. 20). A primary disk-related LCS is characterized by symptoms that may result from a protrusion, prolapse, or extrusion of the disk. A secondary disk-related LCS is characterized by symptoms resulting from gradual changes in the cervical spine that have been generated by previous degradation of the IVD. These changes include internal disk disruption and synovitis or irritation of the zygapophysial and uncovertebral joints.

▶ *Cervicobrachial syndrome.* This syndrome includes symptoms in the local cervical region, as well as in one or both upper extremities, as a result of nerve root irritation through compression or tension of the nerve root.

▶ *Cervicocephalic syndrome.* This syndrome is characterized by complaints in both the neck and head, and includes symptoms such as dizziness, tinnitus, and headache. These symptoms may result from articular, ligamentous, neurologic, organic, or vascular sources.

▶ *Cervicomedullary syndrome.* This syndrome is characterized by spinal cord symptoms associated with cord compression at the cervical spine (cervical myelopathy).

For the purposes of the examination, it is important to establish a baseline of symptoms so that the clinician is able to determine whether a particular movement aggravates or lessens the patient's symptoms. The patient should be asked to describe the symptoms (pain, paresthesia, numbness, weakness, stiffness), their location (head, neck, shoulder, arm, hand), and their nature (constant, intermittent, or variable). Radicular or referred pain may be accompanied by sensorimotor symptoms.[21] The neurologic examination attempts to differentiate between nerve root and spinal cord compression. All symptoms present should be recorded on a body diagram, even those that may initially appear unrelated. The patient's chief complaint should be determined. If pain is the major symptom, the clinician should attempt to quantify the pain using a pain rating scale. It is also appropriate at this time to establish the patient's goals.

It is important for the clinician to determine whether the patient has had successive onsets of similar symptoms in the past, because recurrent injury tends to have a detrimental affect on the potential for recovery. If the patient has had a recurrent injury, the clinician should note how often, and how easily, the injury has recurred, and the success or failure of previous interventions.

The clinician must determine whether there are musculoskeletal symptoms elsewhere. It is well established that the head, neck, upper thoracic regions, and upper extremities can be sites of referred pain. Thoracic interscapular pain, at a point level with T4 to T5, is a very common complaint, especially in women.[2] This pain is thought to be posture related.

Clinical Pearl

Referred symptoms that are cervical in origin can occur in the upper extremities, thoracic spine, scapula, and, occasionally, the upper chest. Pain may be referred to the tip of the acromion or scapular region via the cutaneous branches of the upper thoracic dorsal rami.[67] The rib articulations of cervicothoracic region may produce local pain, or refer pain to the suprascapular fossa or shoulder.[68]

Neck pain accompanied by widespread musculoskeletal pain raises the strong possibility of fibromyalgia, whereas neck pain with synovitis of peripheral joints suggests an inflammatory arthropathy, such as rheumatoid arthritis.[4] Myofascial pain syndromes are characterized by generalized aching and the presence of trigger points (see Chap. 9). The basic pathologic impairment in myofascial pain has yet to be substantiated.[69,70] In the cervical spine, myofascial pain may be a secondary tissue response to an IVD or zygapophysial joint injury.[71] The cervical zygapophysial (facet) joints can be responsible for a significant portion of chronic neck pain. Established referral zones for the cervical zygapophysial joint[72,73] overlap both myofascial and dermatomal pain patterns. Cervical zygapophysial joint

pain is typically unilateral, and is described by the patient as a dull ache. Occasionally, the pain can be referred into the cranioyertebral or interscapular regions. Pain that is constant in nature and unrelated to rest or activity may be inflammatory in origin, in which case physical therapy and, specifically, manual therapy may be inappropriate.[74]

Asking the patient to describe his or her symptoms over a 24-hour period can provide the clinician with valuable information about positions and activities that aggravate or relieve the symptoms and the duration of the symptoms. Patients who report difficulty sleeping because of pain may have an inflammatory condition.

The patient's sleeping position and habits should be investigated. Cervical symptoms often are increased when a foam or very firm pillow is used.[75] Sleeping in the prone position requires adequate cervical and upper thoracic rotation. Some degree of cervical extension also is required, depending on the number and type of pillow used.

Conditions that have a mechanical origin usually are improved with rest, although they may worsen initially on retiring.[76] Pain caused by sustained positions may awaken the patient at night but usually is relieved with a change of position.

Mechanism

The clinician must determine whether trauma occurred, and the exact mechanism. In acute sprains and strains, patients typically relate an activity that precipitated the onset of their symptoms. This may be lifting or pulling a heavy object, an awkward sleeping position, a hyperextension injury, or prolonged static postures. In whiplash-associated disorders, patients generally describe an accident in which they were unexpectedly struck from the rear, front, or side. Rotational injuries also may occur. If there were neurologic symptoms following the trauma (paresthesias, dizziness, ringing in the ears [tinnitus], visual disturbances, or loss of consciousness), more severe damage should be suspected.[77] If the patient reports electric shocklike symptoms down the spine with neck flexion (Lhermitte's sign), the clinician should consider the possibility of inflammation or irritation of the meninges.[78–80]

The onset of symptoms may provide clues as to the type of tissue involved. Muscle or ligamentous pain may either occur immediately following trauma or be delayed for several hours or days.

Clinical Pearl

An insidious onset of symptoms could suggest postural (e.g., thoracic outlet syndrome), degenerative, or myofascial origins; or a disease process, such as ankylosing spondylitis, cervical spondylosis, or facet syndrome. An insidious onset may also indicate the presence of a serious pathology such as a tumor.

Systems Review

General health questions provide information about the status of the cardiopulmonary system, the presence or absence of systemic disease, and medications the patient may be taking that might affect the examination or intervention. Warning signs in the cervical region include:

► Unexplained weight loss.

► Evidence of compromise to two or three spinal nerve roots.

► Gradual increase in pain.

► Expansion of pain in terms of the regions involved.

► Spasm with passive range of motion of the neck.

► Visual disturbances.

► Painful and weak resistive testing.

► Hoarseness.

► Limited scapular elevation.

► Horner's syndrome.

► T1 palsy (weakness and atrophy of the intrinsic muscles of the hand).

► Arm pain in a patient who is younger than 35 years old, or in a patient for more than 6 months (see Chap. 20).

► Side bending away from the painful side that cause pain (if this is the only motion that causes pain)

It also must be remembered that all cervical patients, especially the ones with a history of a hyperextension mechanism, are at potential risk for serious head and neck injuries. The following signs and symptoms demand a cautious approach or an appropriate referral:

► Recent trauma (occurring up to 6 weeks earlier).

► An acute capsular pattern.

► Severe movement loss, whether capsular or noncapsular.

► Strong spasm.

► Paresthesia.

► Segmental paresis.

► Segmental or multisegmental hyporeflexia or areflexia.

► Upper motor neuron signs and symptoms (see Chap. 2).

► Constant or continuous pain.

► Moderate to severe radiating pain.

► Moderate to severe headaches.

► Tinnitus.

► History of loss of consciousness.

► Memory loss or forgetfulness.

► Difficulties with problem solving.

► Reduced motivation.

► Irritability.

► Anxiety or depression.

► Insomnia.

Clinical Pearl

Symptoms that respond to mechanical stimuli in a predictable manner are usually considered to have a mechanical source. Symptoms that show no predictable response to mechanical stimuli are unlikely to be mechanical in origin, and their presence should alert the clinician to the possibility of a more sinister disorder or one of central initiation, autonomic, or affective nature.[74]

Neurologic Symptoms

The presence of neurologic symptoms deserves special attention. Many of the symptoms that occur in an upper limb have their origins in the neck. The patient with neck trauma can report seemingly bizarre symptoms, but these need to be heeded until the clinician can rule out serious pathology. Cervical radiculitis is most commonly associated with spinal nerve root irritation (see Chap. 20). Peripheral symptoms also can be caused by a host of other conditions, including thoracic outlet syndrome or an isolated peripheral nerve lesion.[81]

The systems review must include questions that will elicit any symptoms that might suggest a central nervous system condition or a vascular compromise to the brain. Cervical myelopathy, involving an injury to the spinal cord itself, is associated with multisegmental paresthesias, upper motor neuron (UMN) signs and symptoms such as spasticity, hyperreflexia, visual and balance disturbances, ataxia, and sudden changes in bowel and bladder function. The presence of any UMN sign or symptom requires an immediate medical referral.

Vascular Compromise

The presence of dizziness or seizures always warrants further investigation. It is not always an easy task for the clinician to determine whether the presenting dizziness is the result of a disturbed afferent input from the cervical spine, which can be extremely rewarding to treat, or has a more serious cause.[65] For example, dizziness provoked by head movements may indicate an inner ear or vertebral artery problem. A history of falling without loss of consciousness (drop attack) is strongly suggestive of vertebral artery compromise.[82] Testing of the vertebral artery (see Chap. 21) should be considered if the observation and history reveal any of the signs and symptoms that have been linked, directly or indirectly, to vertebral artery insufficiency. These include:

► Wallenberg's, Horner's, and similar syndromes.

► Bilateral or quadrilateral paresthesia.

► Hemiparesthesia.

► Ataxia.

► Nystagmus.

▶ Drop attacks.

▶ Periodic loss of consciousness.

▶ Lip anesthesia.

▶ Hemifacial paresthesia or anesthesia.

▶ Dysphasia.

▶ Dysarthria.

Headache or Facial Pain

Does the patient have headaches? If so, where? What is their frequency and intensity? Does a position alter the headache? If the patient reports relief of pain and referred symptoms with the placement of the hand or arm of the affected side on top of the head (Bakody's sign), this usually is indicative of a disk lesion of the C4 or C5 level.[83]

A history of headaches may or may not be benign, depending on the frequency and severity. Differential diagnosis is important, especially in light of the fact that there is considerable overlap in symptoms among tension headaches; cervicogenic headaches (see Chap. 22); cervical, trigeminal, and glossopharyngeal neuralgia (see Chap. 9); the headache associated with Lyme disease (see Chap. 9); migraines without aura (see Chap. 9); and temporomandibular joint dysfunction (see Chap. 24).[84] Cervicogenic headaches, which can be mild, moderate, or severe, tend to be unilateral and located in the suboccipital region, with referral to the frontal, retro-orbital, and temporal areas.[52,85] The more serious causes of headache without a history of trauma include spontaneous subarachnoid hemorrhage, vertebral artery compromise, meningitis, pituitary tumor, brain tumor, and encephalitis (see Chap. 9).

Facial pain can be the consequence of temporomandibular dysfunction, temporal arteritis, acute sinusitis, orbital disease, glaucoma, trigeminal neuralgia, referred pain, and herpes zoster (see Chap. 9).

Balance Disturbance

One of the earlier indications of a balance disturbance can be elicited during the history or systems review with correct questioning. A simple question such as "Do you have difficulty with walking or with balance?" can provide the clinician with valuable information. Positive responses may indicate a cervical myelopathy or systemic neurologic impairment.[86] Myelopathy may occur with compression of the spinal cord, and is more likely to occur at the C5 to C6 level, because in this region the spinal cord is at its widest and the spinal canal, at its narrowest.[87] Usually, narrowing of the spinal canal occurs during the end stages of degenerative disease, although structural anomalies, such as a narrowed trefoil canal or shortened pedicles, can result in congenital stenosis.[51] Depending on the cause, the onset of myelopathy can be sudden or gradual. The patient typically complains of symptoms in multiple extremities and clumsiness when performing fine motor skills.

Tests and Measures

Observation

A major contributor to cervicogenic pain is a lack of postural control resulting from poor neuromuscular function.[61,84,88,89] Sustained postures, or fatigue overloading of the deep spinal and postural muscles, can result in increased joint compressive forces and inefficient movement strategies.[69,70,90,91]

Static observation of general posture, as well as the relationship of the neck on the trunk and the head on the neck, is carried out while the patient is standing and sitting, both in the waiting area and in the examination room.

The clinician should look for gross deformities such as:

▶ Torticollis (see Chap. 9).

▶ Sprengel's deformity, a congenital elevation and medial rotation of the scapula, gives the patient the appearance of having no neck on one side, secondary to a high-riding scapula.

▶ Scars (long, transverse scars indicative of cervical surgery).

▶ Scoliosis in the thoracic spine.

▶ Muscle atrophy or hypertrophy.

▶ Swelling.

▶ Bone deformities.

▶ Autonomic skin changes (increased sweating, trophic changes, texture changes).

▶ Birthmarks.

The clinician should observe the position of the patient's head. If it is shifted to one side, a disk protrusion may be present; if deviated, acute arthritis may be the cause. Severe or constant pain usually is manifested by the patient constantly changing his or her posture, or remaining very still.

Side View

▶ The forehead should be vertical.

▶ The tip of the chin should be in line with the manubrium. If the chin is anterior to the manubrium, a forward head is present (see later discussion). The amount of forward head can be measured in two ways. The simplest method is to measure the distance between the tip of the chin and the manubrium. The more complex and expensive methods involve the use of computer-assisted digitizing systems.

▶ The clinician should observe the cervical lordosis. A flattened lordosis may be associated with stretched posterior cervical ligaments and extensor muscles, and adaptively shortened cervical flexors. An excessive lordosis is associated with a forward head, and adaptive shortening of the posterior ligaments and neck extensor muscles.

Posterior View

▶ The clinician should assess muscular asymmetry, especially in the upper trapezius and SCM (see also Chap. 14).

▶ The spinous process of the axis should be in the midline.

▶ As the patient rotates the head to each side, the tips of the transverse processes of the atlas should be felt to rotate anteriorly, and then posteriorly. Both sides are compared. The procedure is repeated for side bending. The transverse process should become less prominent, and should approximate the mastoid process, on the side of the side bending.

Anterior View

▶ The clinician should assess whether the patient's head is shifted to one side. A cervical disk protrusion (C3–4 or C4–5) can produce a horizontal side shift of the head.[59] This side shift allows the patient to maintain eye level.

▶ A slight tilt of the head is normal but may indicate an upper cervical joint dysfunction.

▶ Facial symmetry. The clinician visually splits the mass of the head into two vertical halves. Cerebral asymmetries in form and volume, associated with cranial asymmetries, are a common feature of the human race and are often associated with facial asymmetries.[92,93] This asymmetry is, in many cases, related to asymmetric cerebral growth, which is mostly accomplished in utero,[94,95] although it also may have a local origin, for instance, in the case of mandibular asymmetry.

▶ Are the shoulders level? The shoulder on the dominant side is usually lower. Is there any atrophy of the deltoid suggesting axillary nerve palsy?

Forward Head. The cervical and upper thoracic regions are highly prone to postural and degenerative dysfunctions. Poor posture and dysfunctional movement patterns may alter the normal segmental motion of the neighboring regions (Table 23-6). A forwardly inclined head (Fig. 23-9) increases the stresses at the cervicothoracic junction, and increases the craniovertebral lordosis, producing compensatory occipito-atlantal extension.

In the forward head posture, the upper trapezius can be maintained in a constant state of contraction[28] (Table 23-6). This constant state of contraction also can occur as a result of a protective mechanism for the cervical joints, ligaments, or IVD.[99]

This hypertonicity of the upper trapezius produces a paravertebral area that is broader and more prominent than normal. Tightness or adaptive shortening of the levator scapulae results in the contour of the neckline appearing as a double line (wave) where the muscle inserts into the scapula.[60] This is described as Gothic shoulders, because it is reminiscent of the form of a Gothic church tower.

Movement patterns performed on a poor postural base contribute to repetitive microtrauma of cervical structures. These structures include the zygapophysial facets, IVD, ligaments, joint capsules, and muscles, all of which are capable of propagating the cycle of pain and dysfunction.[100,101]

Active Range of Motion

The clinical examination of the mobility of the cervical spine should consist of a comparison between active and passive ranges and coupled movements of the cervical spine. Active

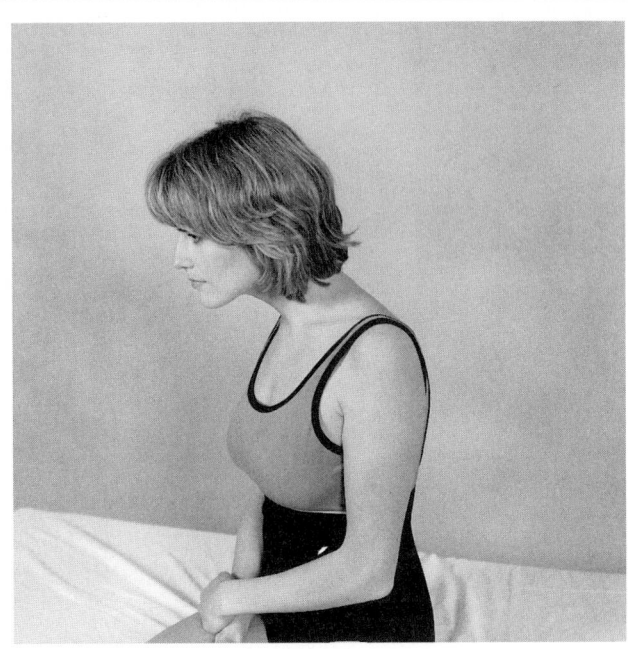

FIGURE 23-9   Extreme forward head posture.

motion induced by the contraction of the muscles determines the so-called physiologic range of motion,[102] whereas passively performed movement causes stretching of noncontractile elements, such as ligaments, and determines the anatomic range of motion. Knowledge of cervical anatomy and kinematics should assist the clinician in determining the structure responsible, based on the pattern of movement restriction noted in the physical examination (Table 23-7).

The range of motion available at the cervical spine is the result of such factors as the shape and orientation of the zygapophysial joint surfaces, the inherent flexibility of the restraining ligaments and joint capsules, and the height and pliability of the IVD.[51] As with other joints in the body, the available range of motion typically decreases with age, the only exception being the rotation available at C1 to C2, which may increase.[102]

A movement restriction is a loss of movement in a specific direction, and one in which a movement toward or away from the restriction may alter the degree and location of those symptoms. When cervical range of motion is painful or restricted, muscle pathology is suggested if the restricted motion exists in the direction opposite to the action of the involved muscles. The examiner can apply maximum resistance to the indicated muscle group(s) to verify this hypothesis.

Clinical Pearl

A motion that is restricted but painless, or normal but painful, could indicate a hypomobility. Pain that is produced by the motion that is restricted indicates an acute or subacute injury, whereas pain that is produced by the motion that is not restricted, or excessive, could indicate a hypermobility.

TABLE 23-6   Consequences of the Forward Head[96–98]

Deficit	Impairment	Effect

Cervical hyperlordosis	Overclosing of TMJ
	  Posterior compression
	  Capsular ligament injury
	  Meniscal derangement
		Trigeminal facilitation
		  Suboccipital hypertonicity
		  Scalene hypertonicity with 1st rib impairment

	Craniovertebral hyperextension
	  O-A flexion hypomobility
	  A-A rotation hypomobility
	  O-A extension hypermobility
	  Craniovertebral instability
		Trigeminal facilitation
		  Masticator hypertonicity
		  TMJ impairment

	Midcervical hyperextension
	  Flexion hypomobility
	  Extension hypermobility
	  Anterior instabilities
		C4 facilitation
		  Levator scapulae hypertonicity with adduction
		  of scapula and overuse of supraspinatus
		C5 facilitation
		  Rotator cuff hypertonicity
		  Tennis elbow

Shoulder protraction	Glenohumeral instability Acromioclavicular instability	Supraspinatus tendonitis Infraspinatus tendonitis Acromioclavicular sprain

Cervicothoracic hyperkyphosis	Extension hypomobilities	Shoulder girdle hypomobility
		  Glenohumeral instability
		  Acromioclavicular instability
		  Supraspinatus tendonitis

A-A, atlanto-axial; O-A, occipito-atlantal; TMJ, temporomandibular joint.

TABLE 23-7   Movement Restriction and Possible Causes

Movement Restriction	Possible Causes

Extension and right side bending	Right extension hypomobility
	  Left flexor muscle tightness
	  Anterior capsular adhesions
	  Right subluxation
	  Right small disc protrusion

Flexion and right side bending	Left flexion hypomobility
	  Left extensor muscle tightness
	  Left posterior capsular adhesions
	  Left subluxation

Extension and right side bending restriction greater than extension and left side bending	Left capsular pattern (arthritis, arthrosis)
Flexion and right side bending restriction equal to extension and left side flexion	Left arthrofibrosis (very hard capsular end-feel)
Side bending in neutral, flexion, and extension	Uncovertebral hypomobility or anomaly

The range of motion available in the cervical spine is a factor of the motion available at each segment, as well as the range available in the cranioverterbral joints and upper thoracic joints. Because of the close relationship of the shoulder to the cervical spine, active elevation of each upper extremity should be assessed to rule out symptom reproduction from the shoulder movements. If there is a loss of one of the cervical motions, the restricted motion should be examined more closely by separating the motion into its various components. For example, cervical rotation requires motion at the cranioverterbral joints, particularly the atlanto-axial joint, as well as segmental rotation at each of the cervical segments.

The major movements that can be assessed clinically are rotation out of neutral position, flexion-extension, and side bending (Figure 23-10 A–F). During flexion of the cervical spine, the segments below the second vertebra are blocked.[21] Therefore, rotation out of maximum flexion of the cervical spine occurs in the atlanto-axial joint. However rotation out of maximum extension occurs predominantly in the middle and lower cervical spine but includes the atlanto-axial joint, as well

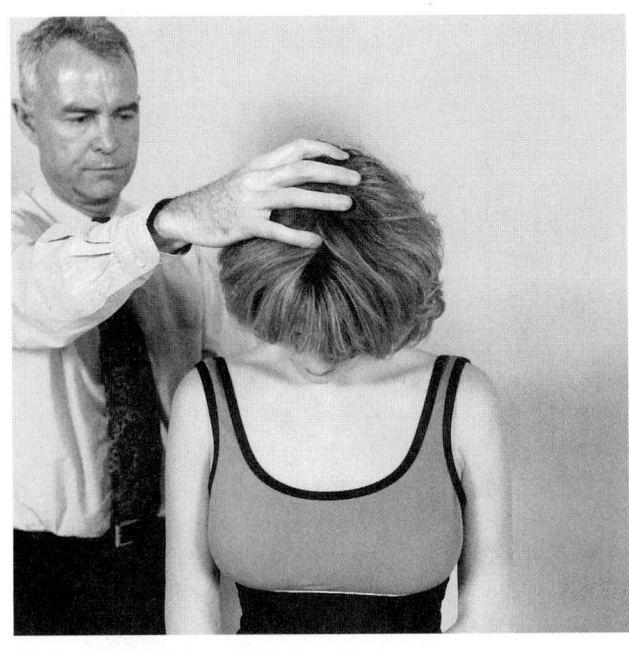

A

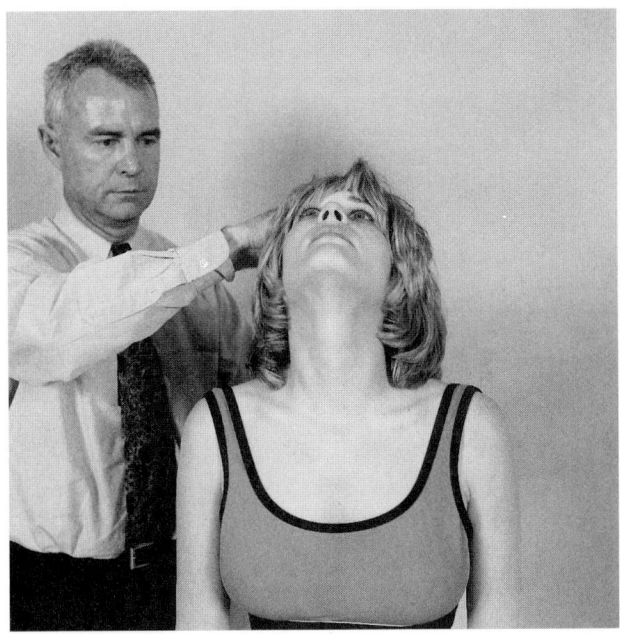

B

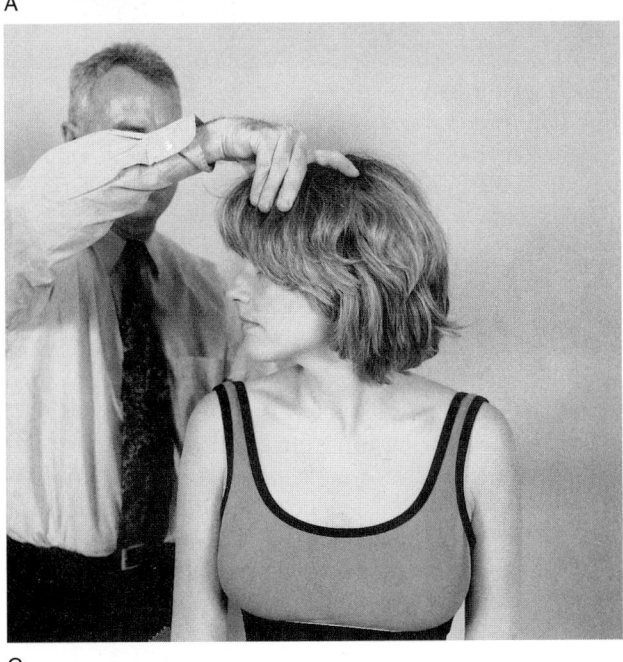

C

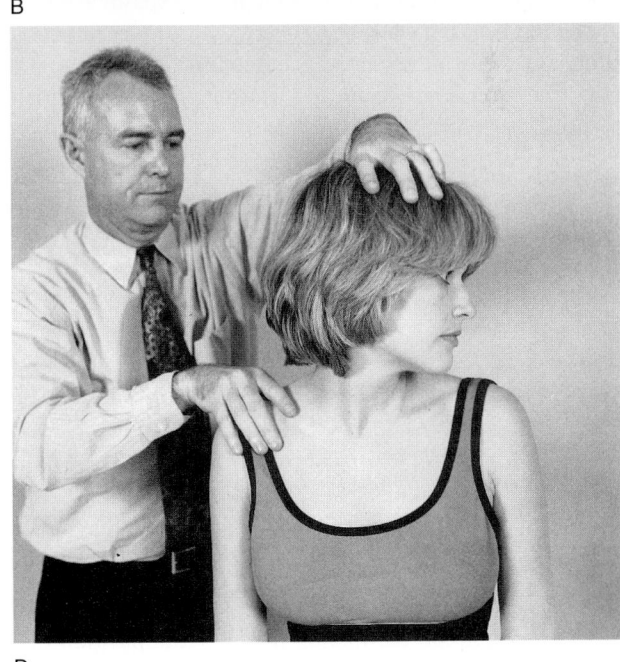

D

FIGURE 23-10 A–D Cervical active range of motion with passive overpressure and resistance. *A:* Cervical flexion *B:* Cervical extension *C:* Cervical rotation to the right *D:* Cervical rotation to the left. (*cont.*)

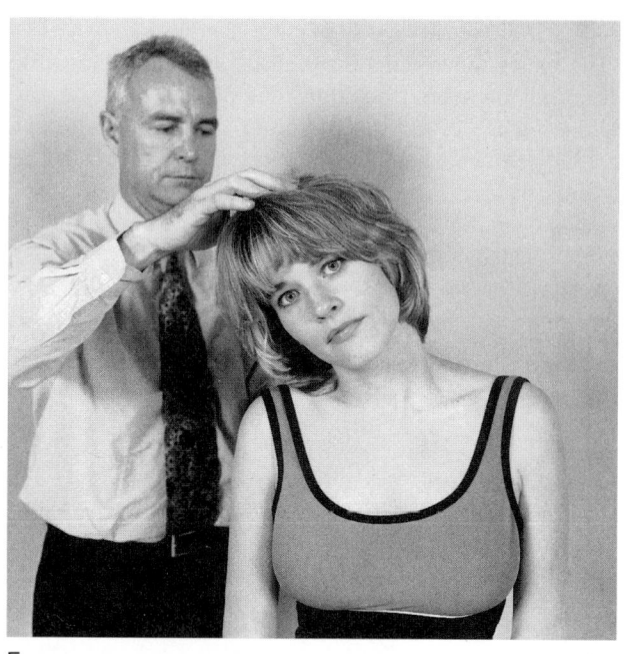

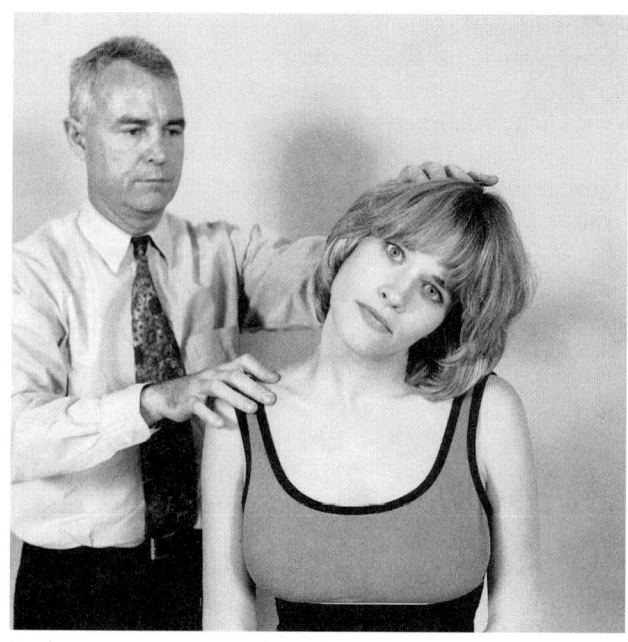

E

F

FIGURE 23-10 E–F *(cont.)* *E:* Cervical side bending to the right *F:* Cervical side bending to the left.

(see Chap. 22).[103] Each of the motions is tested with a gentle overpressure, applied at the end of range if the active range appears to be full and pain free. With the exception of rotation, the weight of the head usually provides sufficient overpressure. It is necessary to apply overpressure even in the presence of pain, in order to achieve an end-feel. If the application of overpressure produces pain, the presence of an acute muscle spasm is possible. Caution must be taken when using overpressure in the direction of rotation, especially if the rotation is combined with ipsilateral side bending and extension, because this can compromise the vertebral artery.[104] The clinician should evaluate:

▶ *Quality and quantity of the motion.* Quantity and quality of movement refers to the ability to achieve end range with curve reversal and without deviation from the intended movement plane.[105]

▶ *End-feel.*

▶ *Symptoms provoked.*

▶ *Willingness of the patient to move.*

▶ *Presence of specific patterns of restriction.* According to Cyriax,[106] the capsular pattern of the cervical spine is full flexion in the presence of limited extension, and symmetric limitation of rotation and side bending. The presence of a capsular pattern usually indicates arthritis.

When interpreting the motion findings, the position of the joint at the beginning of the test should be correlated with the subsequent mobility noted, because alterations in joint mobility may merely reflect an altered starting position.

McKenzie[76] advocates the addition of neck protrusion and neck retraction to the range of motion examination, or to specific motions, to determine if these additions affect the symptoms (see "Combined Motion Testing," later).

The inclinometer technique recommended by the American Medical Association may be used for an objective measurement of cervical motion.[107]

Flexion. An assessment of gross range of motion of cervical flexion is performed (Fig. 23-10A), and the clinician makes note of any motion that reproduces or enhances the symptoms, and the location of the symptoms. Considerable emphasis should be placed on the amount and quality of flexion available, and the symptoms it provokes, because flexion is the only motion normally tolerated well by the cervical spine.

To objectively measure cervical flexion, two inclinometers are used, which are aligned in the sagittal plane. The center of the first inclinometer is placed over the T1 spinous process. The center of the second one is placed on top of the head, parallel to a line drawn from the corner of the eye to the ear, where the temple of eyeglasses would sit. The patient is asked to flex the neck, and both inclinometer angles are recorded. The cervical flexion angle is calculated by subtracting the T1 from the calvarium inclinometer angle. The normal range of cervical flexion, measured in this manner, is 50 degrees.

If end-range flexion is immediately painful, meningitis or acute radicular pain should be ruled out. If the pain is felt after a 15- to 20-second delay, ligament pain should be suspected.

The most common restrictions to cervical flexion are an upper thoracic or cervicothoracic restriction, or an occipito-atlantal joint restriction. If, during flexion, the patient pivots the head and neck over a hypomobile and fixed cervicothoracic region, excessive motion will be noted at the levels of C4 to C6.

Flexion also may be limited by acute or severe trauma (muscle spasms straighten the lordosis), fracture dislocations, or IVD dysfunction.

Extension. Normal extension motion allows the face to be parallel with the ceiling. To objectively measure cervical extension, two inclinometers can be used, which are aligned as for measuring cervical flexion. The patient is asked to extend the neck, and both inclinometer angles are recorded. The cervical extension angle is calculated by subtracting the T1 from the calvarium inclinometer angle. The normal range of cervical extension, measured in this manner, is 60 degrees.[108]

Cervical flexion or cervical extension can provoke dizziness. This finding is thought to result from an osteophytic compression on the posterolateral aspect of the transverse foramen by the inferior articulating surface of the zygapophysial joint.[108] Cervical distraction can be applied at the point of symptom provocation. If this maneuver increases the symptoms, manual or mechanical traction should not be part of the intervention plan.

Rotation. With rotation, the chin should be in line with the acromioclavicular joint at the end of rotation (see Figure 23-10C and 23-10D). To objectively measure cervical rotation, the patient is positioned supine. One inclinometer is used, and it is aligned in the transverse plane. The base of the inclinometer is placed over the forehead. The patient is asked to rotate the neck, and the inclinometer angle is recorded. The test is repeated on the other side. The normal range of cervical rotation, measured in this manner, is 80 degrees.[107]

Limitation of or pain on cervical rotation usually suggests pathology at the C1 to C2 (atlanto-axial) segment, because most rotation occurs at this joint.[4] However, if a patient is able to achieve 40 to 50 degrees of cervical rotation while maintaining eye level, atlanto-axial involvement is unlikely. If, on the other hand, the neck has to side bend early in the active rotation range in order to achieve full motion, the atlanto-axial joint or thorax is likely to be involved. If full rotation is limited and cannot be achieved even with the substitution of neck side bending, the problem is likely with the mid to low cervical spine segments.

Two screening tests can be used to highlight the level of a rotation restriction. Both of the tests utilize rotation of the neck with the neck in various amounts of flexion.

1. Rotation with the neck in full side bending is reported to test the C1 to C2 level.

2. Rotation with the neck in a chin tuck tests the C2 to C3 level.

Side Bending. Side bending is performed to the left and right while the ipsilateral shoulder is stabilized by the clinician (see Figure 23-10E). (Stabilizing the contralateral shoulder merely tests the length of the upper trapezius, Fig. 23-10F.) To objectively measure cervical side bending, two inclinometers are used, which are aligned in the coronal plane. The center of the first inclinometer is placed over the T1 spinous process. The center of the second one is placed on top of the head, over the calvarium. The patient is asked to side bend the neck, and both inclinometer angles are recorded. The cervical side-bending angle is calculated by subtracting the T1 from the calvarium inclinometer angle. The normal range of cervical side bending, measured in this manner, is 45 degrees.[107] The range of side bending is always greater in the supine than in the sitting position.

Active side bending is typically the first motion to demonstrate problems of the cervical spine.[110] Restricted cervical side bending could be the result of joint restriction, muscle tightness, or lack of pain-free movement or extensibility of the neural tissues.[3]

Key Muscle Testing
During the resisted tests, the clinician looks for relative strength and fatigability. There are numerous smaller muscles throughout this area, so resistance needs to be applied gradually. The muscles tested are also used during the Cyriax upper quarter scanning examination. Alternates are given for each key muscle.

Resisted Cervical Rotation. Resisted cervical rotation tests the key muscle of C2.

Resisted Cervical Side Bending. Resisted side bending tests the key muscle of C3 (Fig. 23-11).

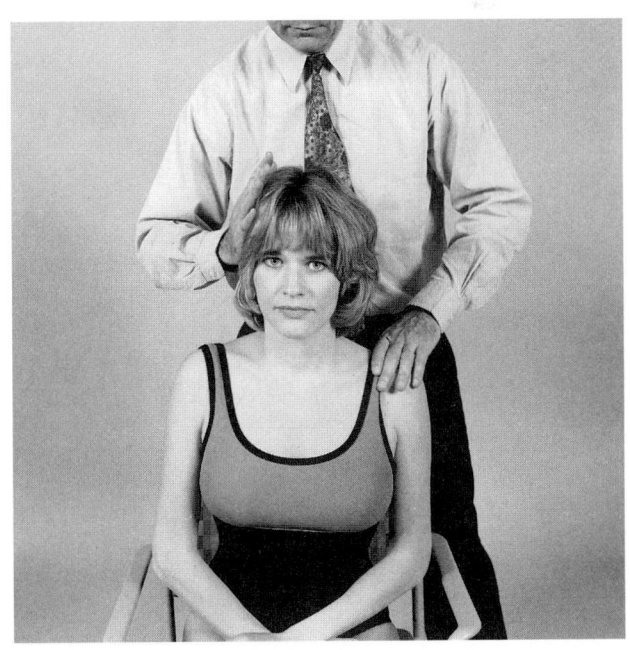

FIGURE 23-11 Resisted cervical side bending.

Scapular Elevators (C2–4). The clinician asks the patient to elevate the shoulders about one half of full elevation. The clinician applies a downward force on both shoulders while the patient resists (Fig. 23-12).

Diaphragm (C4). Using a tape measure, the clinician measures the amount of rib expansion that occurs with a deep breath (Fig. 23-13). A comparison is made to a similar measurement at rest. Four measurement positions are used:

1. Fourth lateral intercostal space.

2. Axilla.

3. Nipple line.

4. Tenth rib.

Shoulder Abduction (C5). The clinician asks the patient to abduct the arms to about 80 to 90 degrees, with the forearms in neutral. The clinician applies a downward force on the humerus while the patient resists (Fig. 23-14).

Shoulder External Rotation (C5). The clinician asks the patient to put the arms by the sides, with the elbows flexed to 90 degrees and the forearms in neutral. The clinician applies an inward force to the forearms (Fig. 23-15).

Elbow Flexion (C6). The clinician asks the patient to put the arms, with the elbows flexed to 90 degrees and the forearms supinated. The clinician applies a downward force to the forearms (Fig. 23-16).

Wrist Extension (C6). The clinician asks the patient to place the arms by the sides, with the elbows flexed to 90 degrees and the forearms, wrists, and fingers in neutral. The clinician applies a downward force to the back of the patient's hands (Fig. 23-17).

Shoulder Internal Rotation (C6). The clinician asks the patient to put the arms by the sides, with the elbows flexed to 90 degrees and the forearms in neutral. The clinician applies an outward force to the forearms (Fig. 23-18).

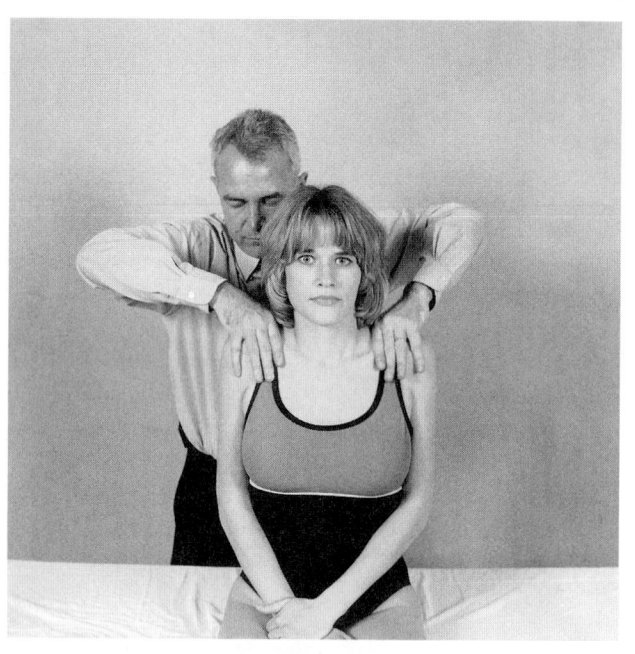

FIGURE 23-12   Resisted shoulder elevation.

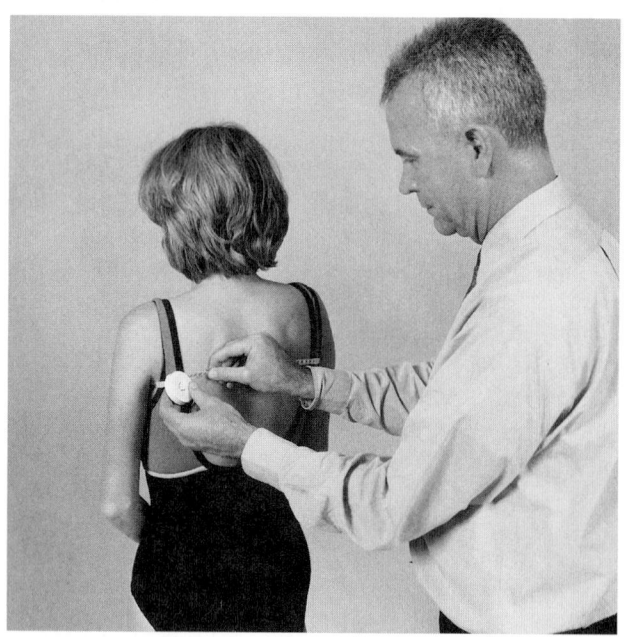

FIGURE 23-13   Chest expansion measurement.

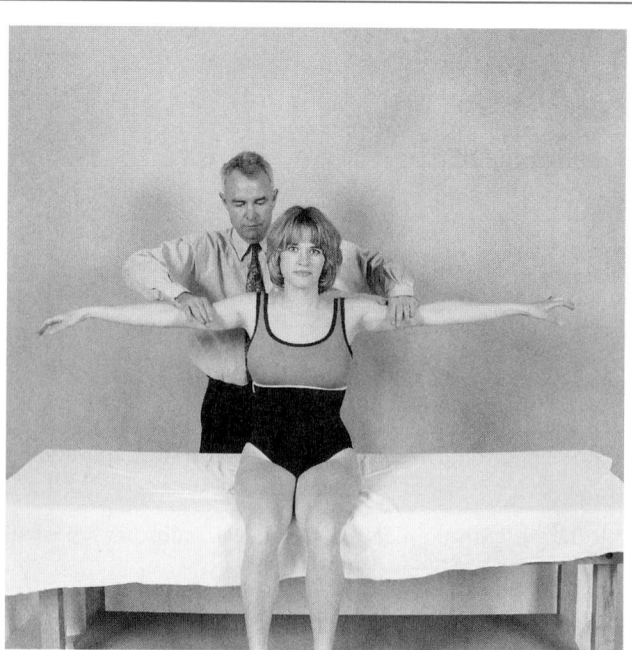

FIGURE 23-14   Resisted shoulder abduction.

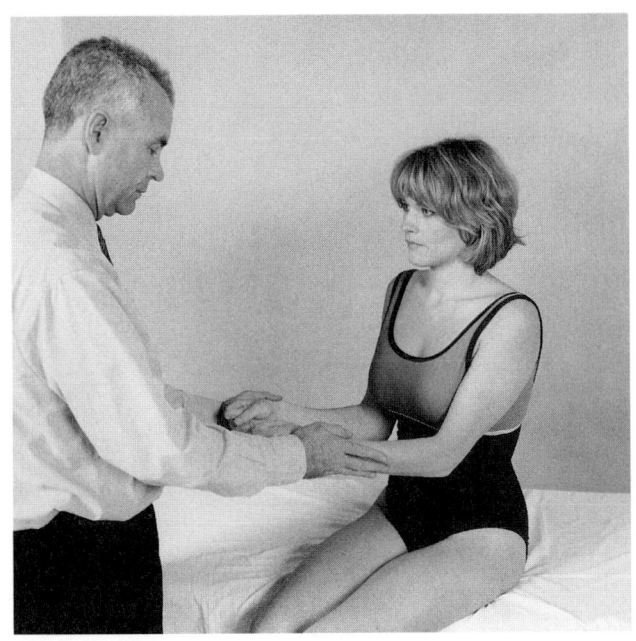

FIGURE 23-15   Resisted shoulder external rotation.

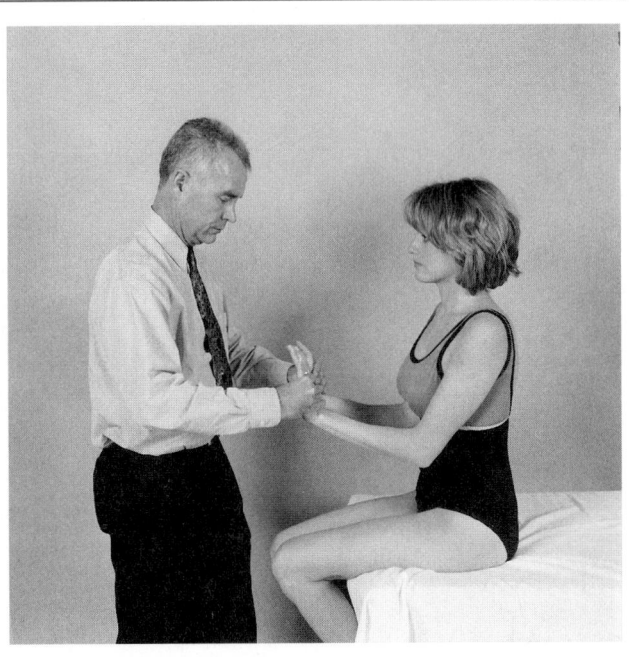

FIGURE 23-17   Resisted wrist extension.

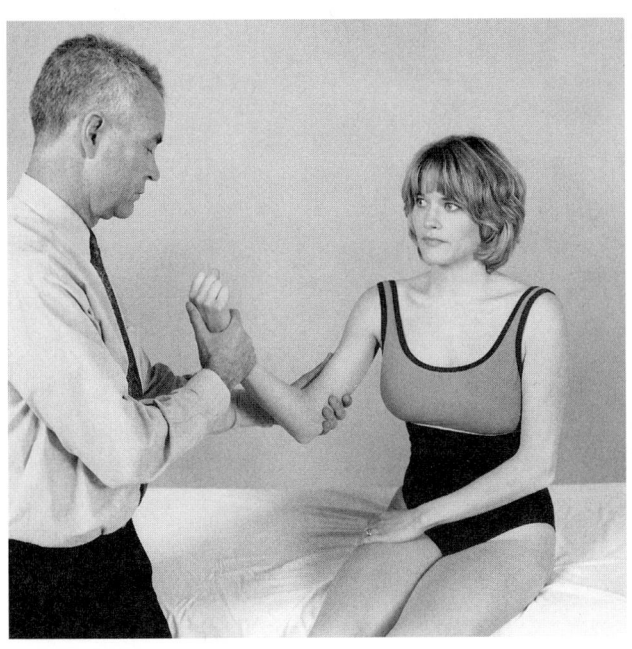

FIGURE 23-16   Resisted elbow flexion.

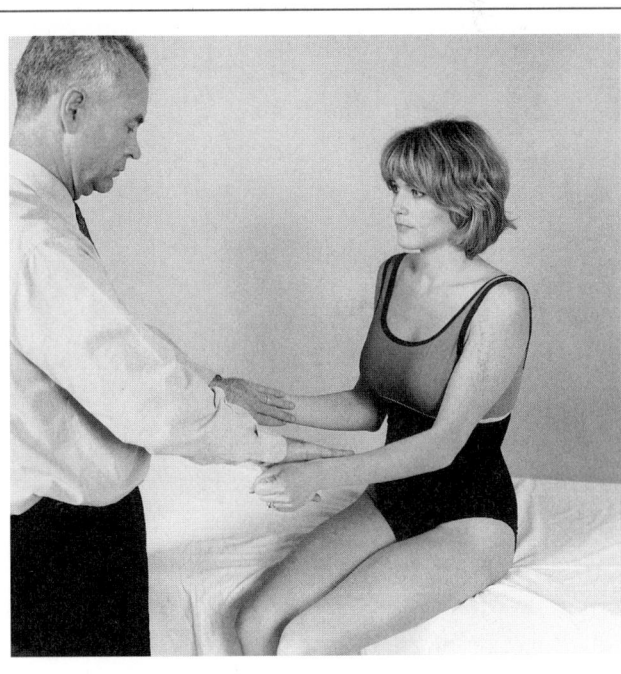

FIGURE 23-18   Resisted shoulder internal rotation.

Elbow Extension (C7).   The patient is seated with the arm out in front and elbows flexed to about 5 degrees. The clinician stands beside the patient and tests the triceps bilaterally by grasping the patient's forearms and attempting to flex the elbows (Fig. 23-19).

Wrist Flexion (C7).   The clinician asks the patient to place the arms out in front, with the elbows flexed slightly and the forearms,

wrists, and fingers in neutral. The clinician applies an upward force to the palm of the patient's hands (Fig. 23-20).

Thumb Extension (C8).   The patient extends the thumb just short of full range of motion. The clinician stabilizes the proximal interphalangeal joint of the thumb with one hand and applies an isometric force into thumb flexion with the other (Fig. 23-21).

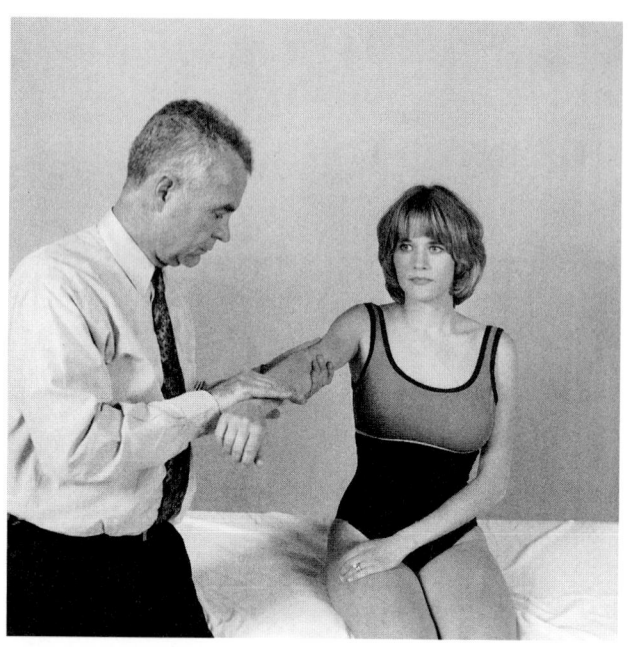

FIGURE 23-19   Resisted elbow extension.

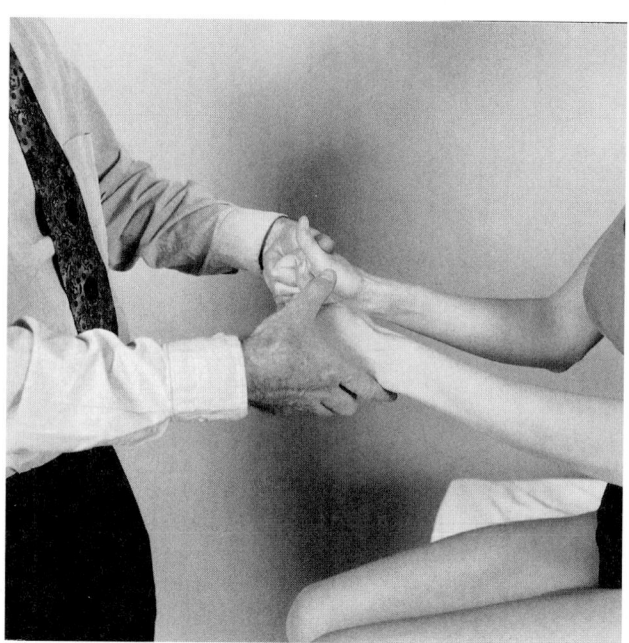

FIGURE 23-21   Resisted thumb extension.

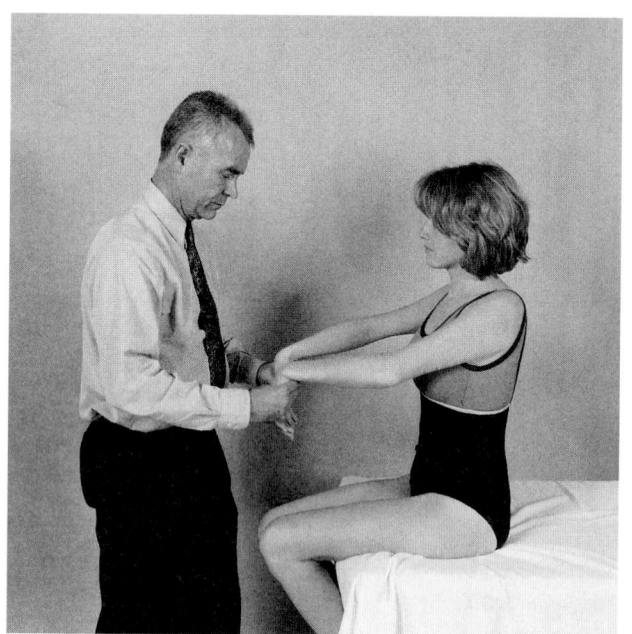

FIGURE 23-20   Resisted wrist flexion.

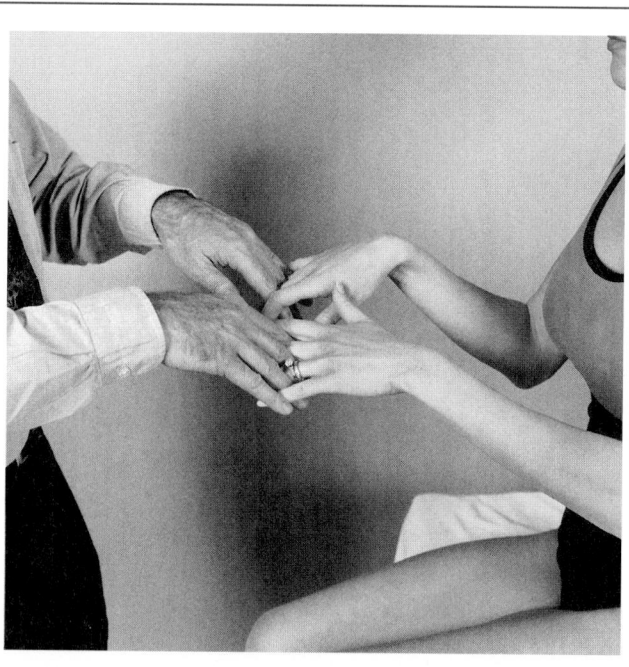

FIGURE 23-22   Strength test for finger adductors (hand intrinsics).

Hand Intrinsics (T1).   The patient is asked to squeeze the clinician's fingers between their fingers while the clinician tries to pull their fingers away (Fig. 23-22).

Combined Motion Testing

Because normal function involves complex and combined motions of the cervical spine, combined motion testing also can be used.

McKenzie[76] advocates using neck retraction and protrusion, with other motions and positions superimposed. Neck protrusion produces an extension of the upper cervical spine and flexion of the mid and lower cervical spine, whereas neck retraction produces a flexion of the upper cervical spine and an extension of the mid and lower cervical spine. Neck retraction is performed with extension (Fig. 23-23), side bending (Fig. 23-24), and rotation to both sides in sitting position and then prone,

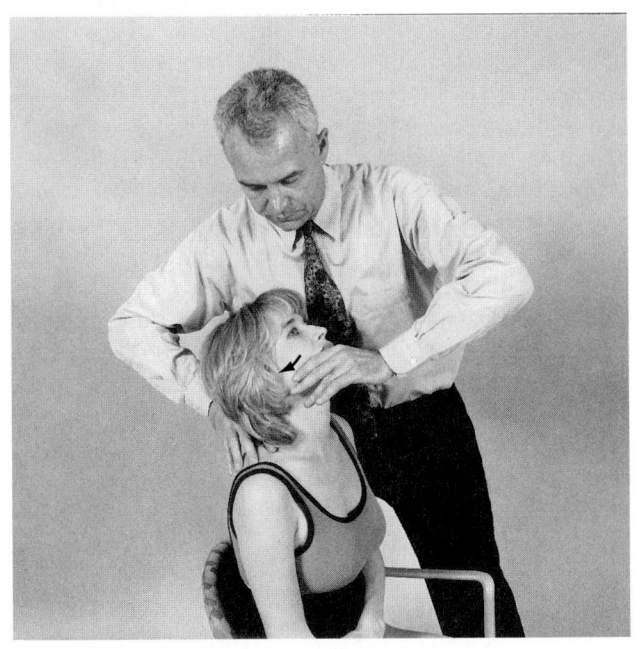

FIGURE 23-23   Neck retraction in extension.

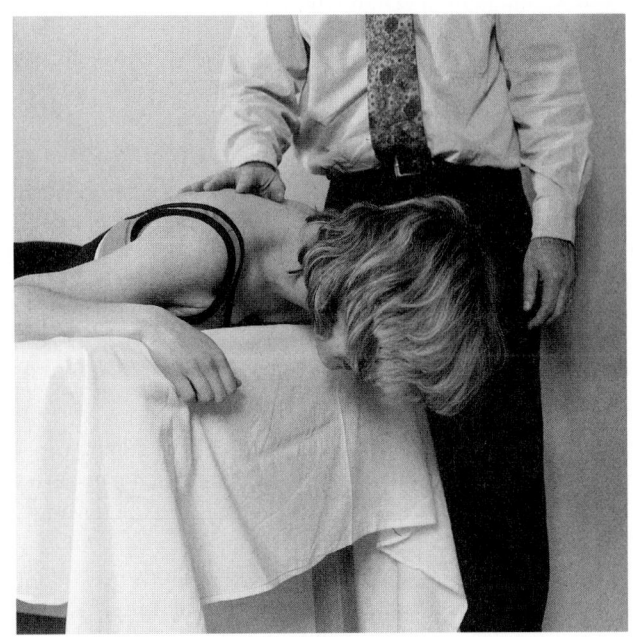

FIGURE 23-25   Neck retraction in prone: start position.

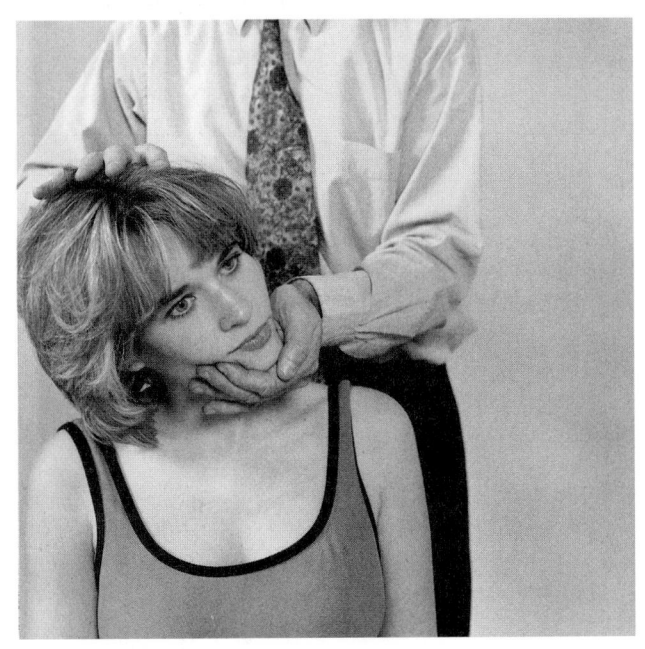

FIGURE 23-24   Neck retraction in side bending.

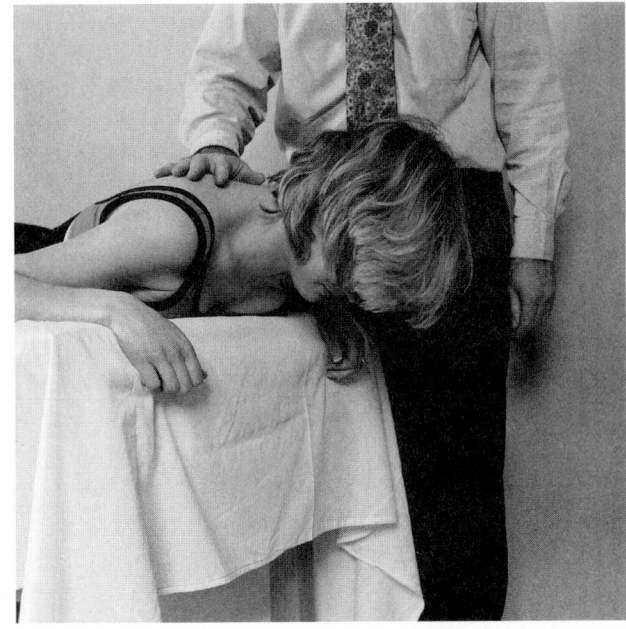

FIGURE 23-26   Neck retraction in prone: terminal position.

with the head off the end of the table (Figs. 23-25 and 23-26). The results from these motions are combined with the findings from the history and the single plane motions to categorize the symptomatic responses into one of three syndromes: postural, dysfunction, or derangement. This information can guide the clinician as to which motions to use in the intervention.

Using a biomechanical model, a restriction of cervical extension, side bending, and rotation to the same side as the pain is termed a *closing* restriction. This restriction is the most common pattern producing distal symptoms. However, a limitation in cervical flexion accompanied by the production of distal symptoms also can occur.[110] Side bending toward or away from the side of the pain also can reproduce upper extremity symptoms, depending on the cause. Pain caused by intervertebral foraminal narrowing may be increased with ipsilateral side bending. Pain caused by an IVD protrusion may be increased with contralateral side bending.

A restriction of the opposite motions (cervical flexion, side bending, and rotation to the opposite side of the pain) is termed an *opening* restriction. Opening restrictions are slightly more difficult to identify in the cervical spine because, frequently, there is no actual restriction of cervical flexion, but rather a restriction of rotation and side bending, along with reproduction of pain on the contralateral side.[110]

Muscle Length Testing

Upper Trapezius. The upper trapezius has a tendency to become adaptively shortened and overactive, which can have the effect of pulling the head laterally, as well as increasing the craniovertebral and cervical lordosis.[111]

The patient is positioned supine. The patient's head is maximally flexed, inclined to the contralateral side (Fig. 23-27), and ipsilaterally rotated. While stabilizing the head, the clinician depresses the shoulder distally. A normal finding is free movement of about 45 degrees of rotation, with a soft motion barrier. Tightness of this muscle results in a restriction in the range of motion, and a hard barrier.

Levator Scapulae. A quick test to determine the extensibility of the levator involves positioning the patient sitting erect.[110] The patient is asked to place one hand on top of the head. For example, if the length of the left levator is to be tested, the patient is asked to place the right hand on the head. The patient's neck and head are positioned in neutral, and the patient is asked to

abduct the left arm as far as possible. Normal extensibility of the levator and the rhomboids, and the absence of shoulder girdle pathology, should allow the patient to fully abduct the arm while the head is side bent away (Fig. 23-28). The test is repeated on the other side for comparison.

The more specific test involves positioning the patient supine, with the hand of the tested side behind the head. The clinician maximally flexes the patient's head, induces contralateral rotation, and inclines the head toward the contralateral side (Fig. 23-29). The clinician then depresses the patient's shoulder distally. If tightness is present, there will be tenderness at the levator insertion and a restriction of movement to less than 45 degrees.

Sternocleidomastoid. The SCM muscle has a tendency to become adaptively shortened and overactive, which can have the effect of altering the relationships between the head, neck, and shoulders, and producing restrictions at the craniovertebral and cervicothoracic junctions.[111]

The patient is positioned supine, with the head supported. From this position, the clinician induces side bending of the neck to the contralateral side, and extension of the neck (Fig. 23-30). The clinician stabilizes the scapula and rotates the patient's head and neck toward the ipsilateral side.

Scalenes. The patient is positioned supine, with the clinician at the head of the bed. The clinician side flexes and extends the head to the contralateral side, while stabilizing the shoulder (Fig. 23-31). The normal range of motion should be 45 degrees.

Neurologic Examination

The neurologic examination is performed to assess the normal conduction of the central and peripheral nervous systems, and

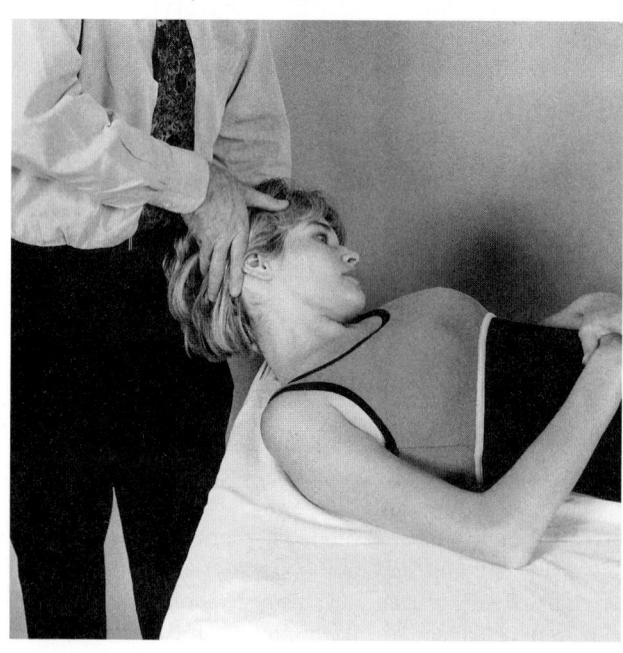

FIGURE 23-27 Muscle length test of the right upper trapezius.

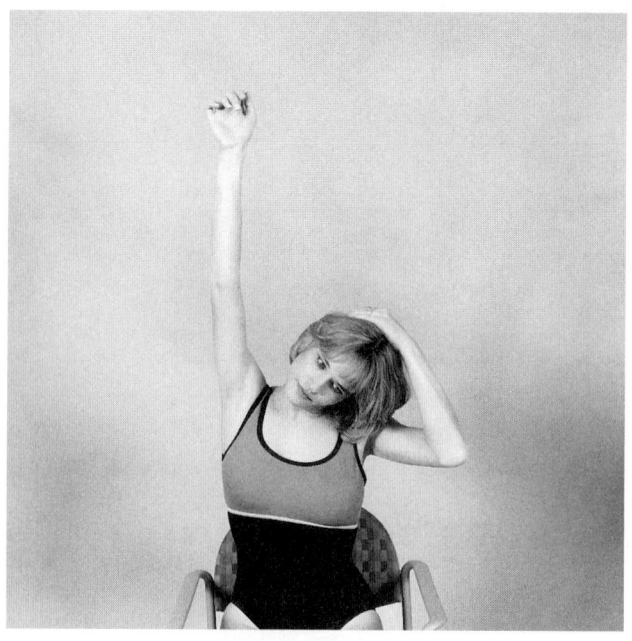

FIGURE 23-28 Muscle length test of the right levator scapulae.

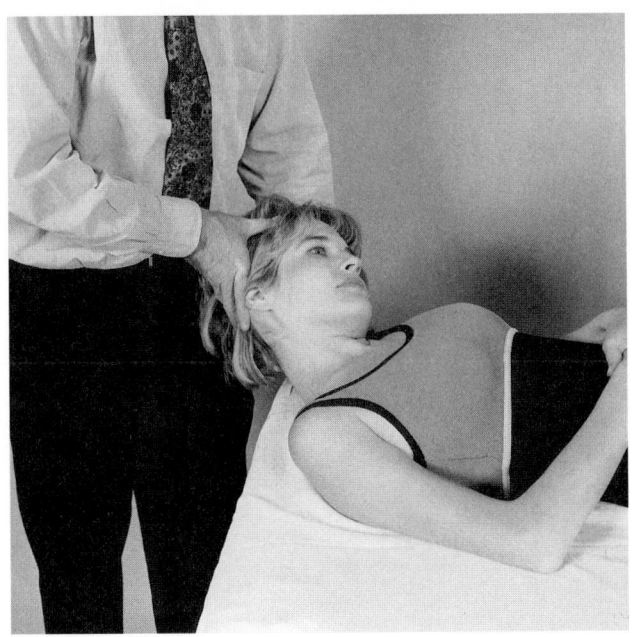

FIGURE 23-29   Muscle length test of the right levator scapulae.

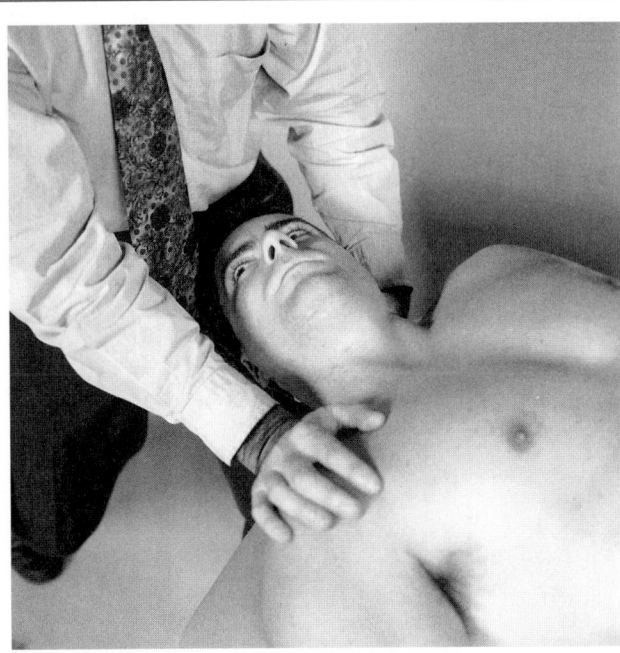

FIGURE 23-31   Muscle length test of the right scalenes.

the distributions. Light touch of hair follicles is used throughout the whole dermatome, followed by pinprick in the area of hypoesthesia. Remember that there is normally no C1 dermatome!

Deep Tendon Reflexes.   The following reflexes should be checked for differences between the two sides.

▶ C5 to C6: Brachioradialis (Fig. 23-32).

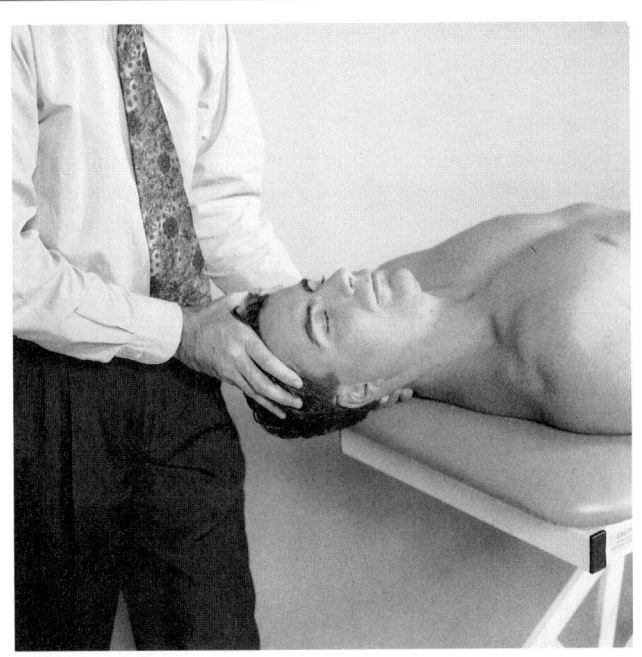

FIGURE 23-30   Muscle length test of the right sternocleidomastoid.

to help rule out such conditions as brachial neuritis and thoracic outlet syndrome. The tests for the thoracic outlet syndrome are described under "Special Tests." later.

Sensory (Afferent System).   The clinician instructs the patient to say "yes" each time he or she feels something touching the skin. The clinician notes any hypoesthesia or hyperesthesia within

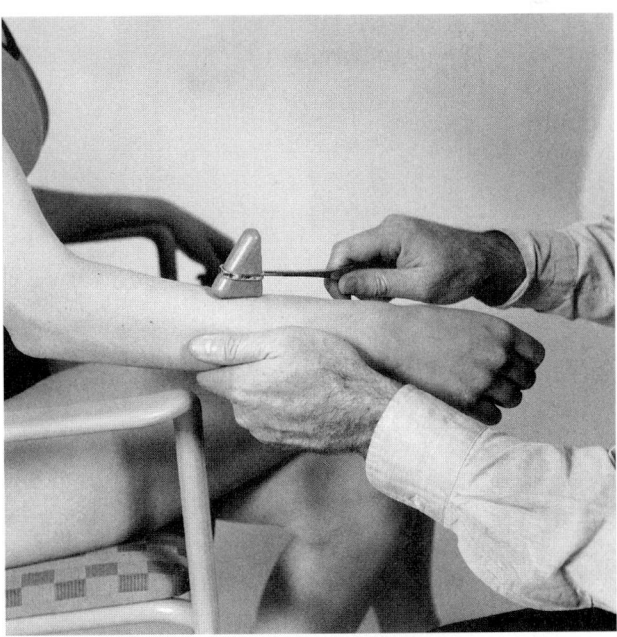

FIGURE 23-32   Brachioradialis deep tendon reflex.

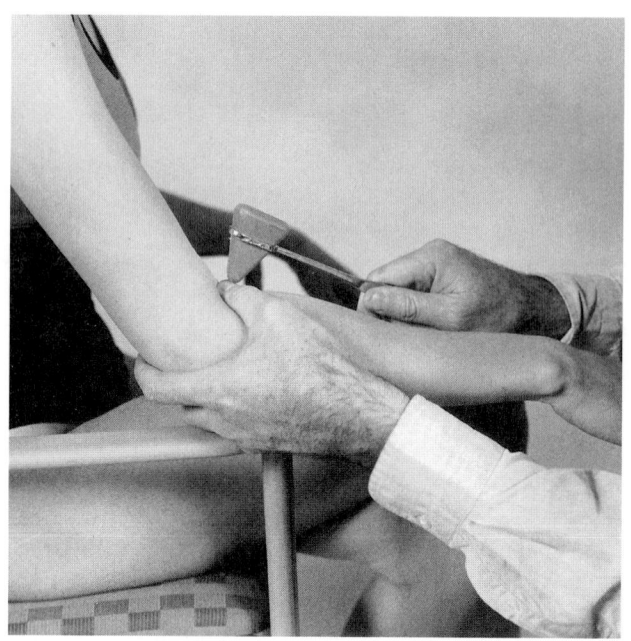

FIGURE 23-33   Biceps deep tendon reflex.

▶ C6: Biceps (Fig. 23-33).

▶ C7: Triceps (Fig. 23-34).

Pathological Reflexes.   The following reflexes are tested:
▶ Hoffmann's sign (Fig. 23-35).

▶ Babinski (Fig. 23-36).

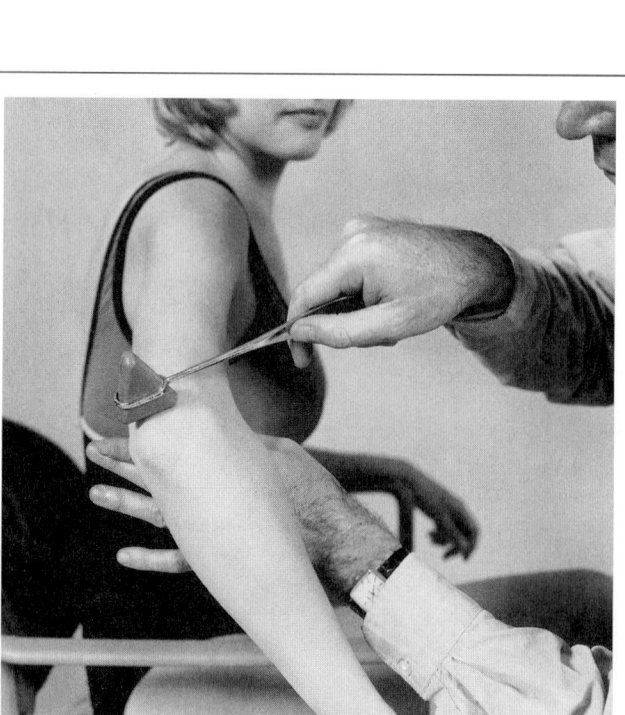

FIGURE 23-34   Triceps deep tendon reflex.

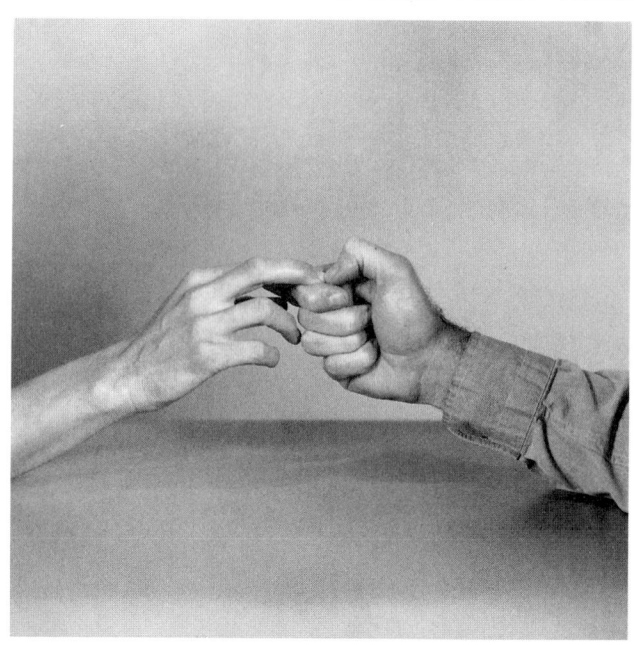

FIGURE 23-35   Hoffmann reflex.

▶ Lower limb deep tendon reflexes (Achilles, patellar) for hyperreflexia.

Segmental Palpation
The patient lies supine, and the clinician stands at the patient's head. The patient's head is rested against the clinician's thigh. Using the index fingers, the clinician slides the fingers under the

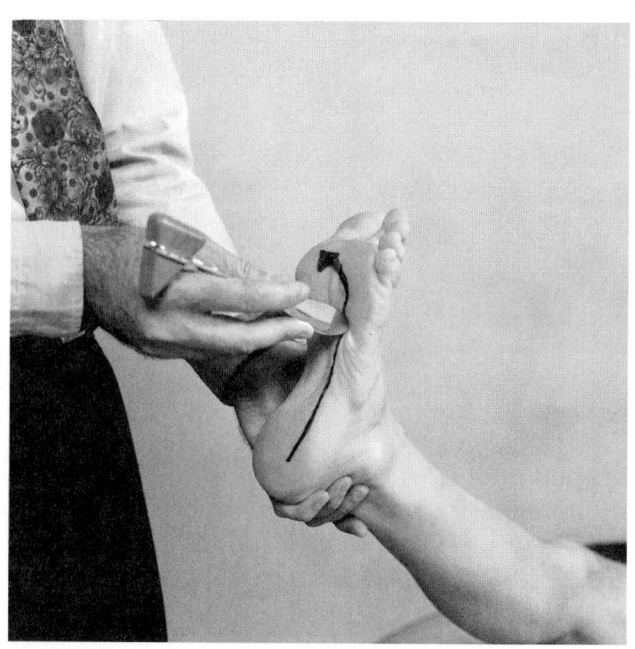

FIGURE 23-36   Babinski.

FIGURE 23-37 Palpation of the cervical structures. (Reproduced with permission from Hoppenfeld S. *Physical Examination of the Spine and Extremities.* East Norwalk, Conn: Appleton-Century-Crofts; 1976:110.)

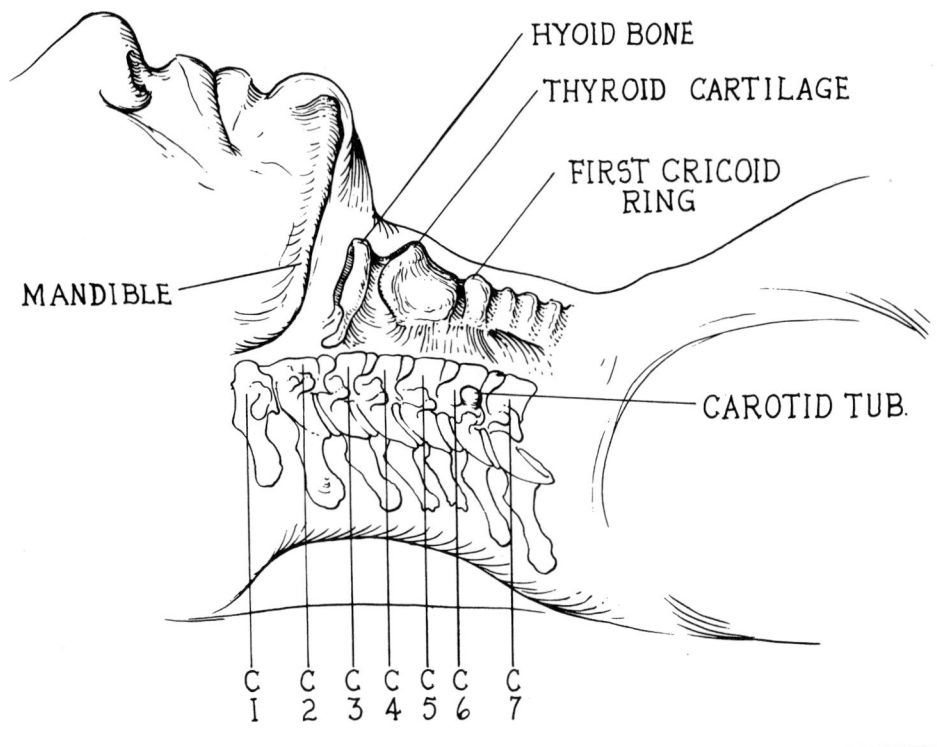

HYOID BONE

THYROID CARTILAGE

FIRST CRICOID RING

MANDIBLE

CAROTID TUB.

C C C C C C C
1 2 3 4 5 6 7

SCM and begins to palpate the anterior aspect of the cervical vertebral bodies (from C7 to C3) for tenderness. The posterior aspects can be palpated with the other hand. If palpation reveals some tenderness, the clinician can further stress the segment by gently applying a posteroanterior pressure.[112] This is accomplished using the hand under the neck and applying an anterior shear at each segmental level. This pressure should result in a slight increase in the cervical lordosis. If it results in an excessive anterior glide at the segment compared with the segment above or below, the test can be considered positive and a stability test of that segment should be performed.

According to Hoppenfeld,[113] all of the spinous processes lower than C2 are usually palpable (Fig. 23-37). The interval between the external occipital protuberance and the spine of C2 contains the posterior arch of vertebra C1, which is very deeply located and usually not palpable. The C2 spinous process can be palpated in the midline below the external occipital protuberance, the prominent midline elevation on the posteroinferior aspect of the occipital bone.[9] Occasionally, because of a bifid spine that is not symmetric, the spine may appear to be lateral to the midline, or two bony prominences may be felt at a single level between C3 and C6. C7 is usually the longest spinous process, being referred to as the *vertebra prominens,* although the spinous process of either C6 or T1 might be quite long, as well. The spinous process of C7 is located by either counting down to the correct level or by using a motion test. The motion test involves the clinician feeling for the largest spinous process located at the base of the neck and then asking the patient to extend the neck. The C6 spinous process will be felt to move anteriorly with neck extension, whereas the spinous process of C7 does not.

Muscle Function Testing: Deep Neck Flexors

The patient is positioned supine and is requested to raise the head slowly in an arclike motion. With weak deep neck flexors in the presence of a strong SCM, the jaw juts forward at the beginning of the movement, producing hyperextension of the craniovertebral junction[61] (Fig. 23-38). Confirmation is made by applying a very slight amount of resistance (2 to 4 g) against the patient's forehead.

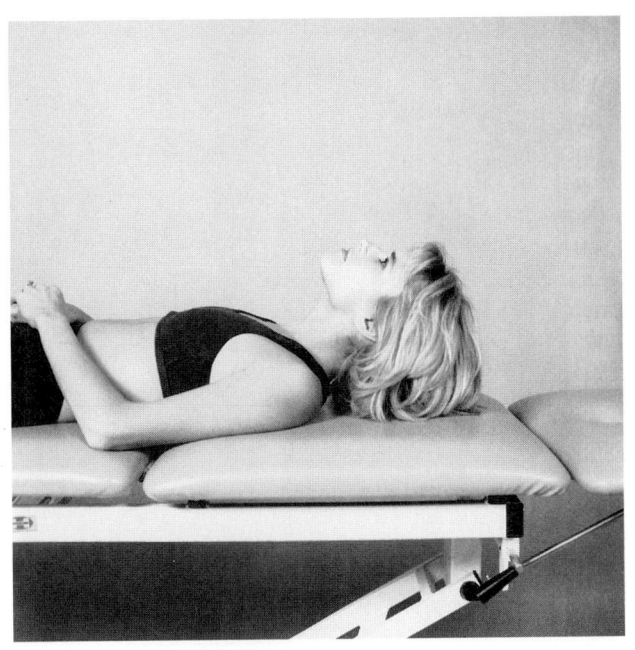

FIGURE 23-38 Muscle function testing of the deep neck flexors.

Holding Capacity of Deep Segmental and Postural Support Muscles[3]
This test is designed to assess the ability of a muscle group to sustain a low-load isometric contraction, and to replicate its function.

Deep Neck Flexors. The deep flexors of the craniovertebral and cervical regions are assessed by testing the patient's ability to sustain a precise inner range upper cervical flexion action.[3]

The patient is positioned supine, with the head supported on a folded towel, the knees flexed, and the feet flat on the bed. An inflatable pressure sensor (Stabilizer, Chattanooga, South Pacific) is positioned suboccipitally behind the neck (Fig. 23-39), and the bladder is inflated to just fill the space between the bed and the patient's neck, without exerting any pressure on the neck.

The patient is asked to bring the chin toward the sternum in a gentle and slow manner. The end-range position is sustained for 10 seconds, and the test is repeated 10 times. Ideally, the patient should increase the pressure reading by 10 mm Hg, resulting in a performance score of 100.[3]

Lower Scapular Stabilizers. The mid and lower trapezius, and serratus anterior muscles, can be assessed with the patient positioned prone, the arm slightly abducted, and the arms placed by the side of the patient. The patient is asked to sustain the scapula against the chest wall in a position of retraction and depression (Fig. 23-40), while the clinician palpates over the muscles.[3] The end-range position is sustained for 10 seconds, and the test is repeated 10 times.

Differing Philosophies

The next stage in the examination process depends on the clinician's background. Clinicians who are heavily influenced by

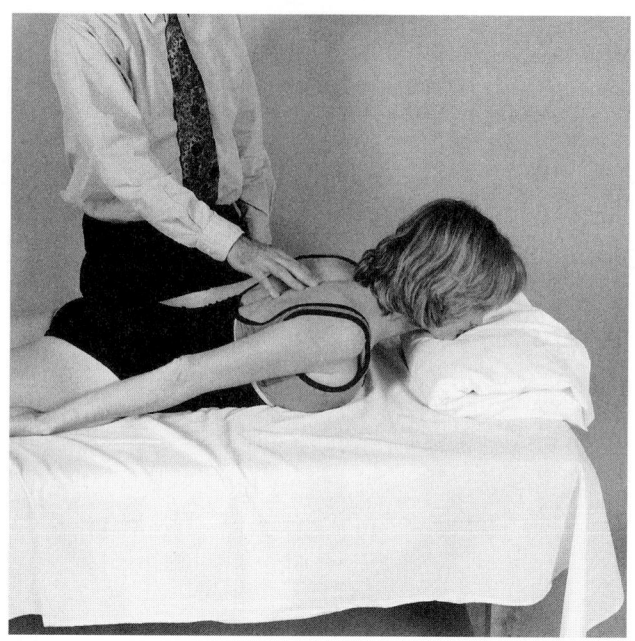

FIGURE 23-40   Testing the holding capacity of the lower scapular stabilizers.

the muscle energy techniques of the osteopaths[114] use position testing to determine the segment on which to focus. Other clinicians omit the position tests and proceed to the combined motion and passive physiologic tests.

Position Testing. The position tests are screening tests that, like all screening tests, are valuable in focusing the attention of the examiner on one segment, but not appropriate for making a definitive statement concerning the movement status of the segment. However, when combined with the results of the passive movement testing, they help to form the working hypothesis.

The patient is positioned sitting, and the clinician stands behind the patient. Using the thumbs, the clinician palpates the articular pillars of the cranial vertebra of the segment to be tested. The patient is asked to flex the neck, and the clinician assesses the position of the cranial vertebra relative to its caudal neighbor and notes which articular pillar of the cranial vertebra is the most dorsal (Fig. 23-41). A dorsal left articular pillar of the cranial vertebra relative to the caudal vertebra is indicative of a left-rotated position of the segment in flexion.[114]

In the following example, the C4 and C5 segments are used. The patient is asked to extend the joint complex, while the clinician assesses the position of the C4 vertebra relative to C5 by noting which articular pillar is the most dorsal. A dorsal left articular pillar of C4 relative to C5 is indicative of a left-rotated position of the C4–5 joint complex in extension.[114]

This test also may be performed with the patient supine. However, in the sitting position, one can better observe the effect of the weight of the head on the joint mechanics.

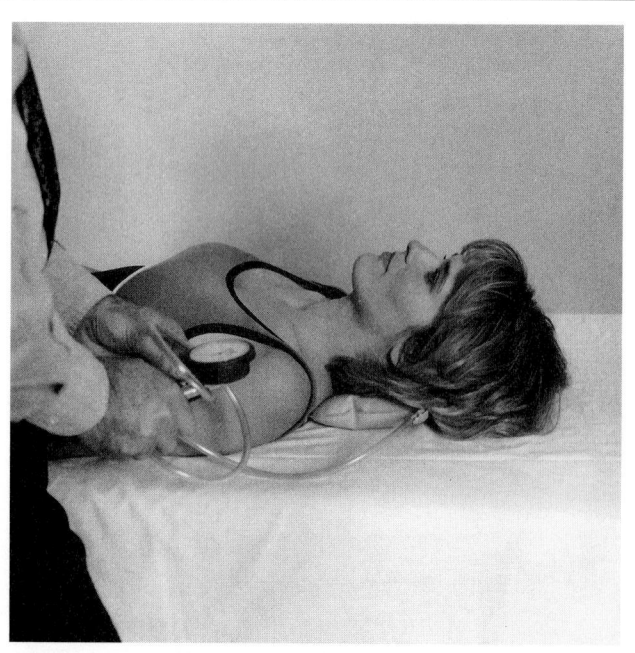

FIGURE 23-39   Testing the holding capacity of the deep neck flexors.

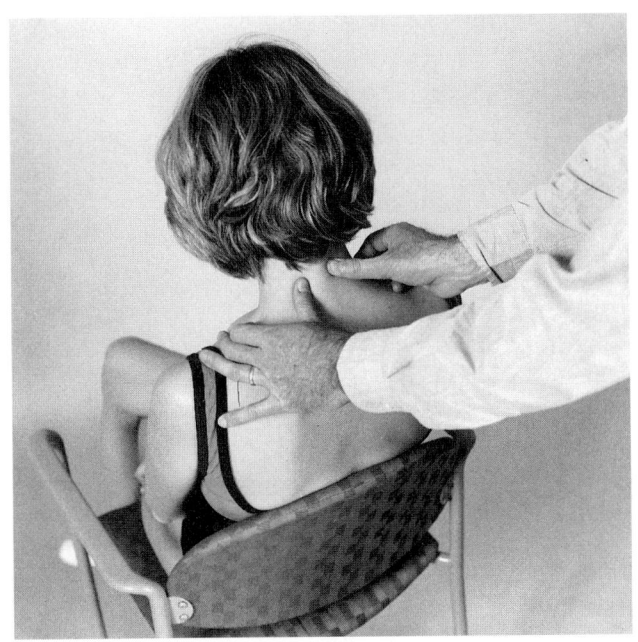

FIGURE 23-41 Position testing of the cervical spine.

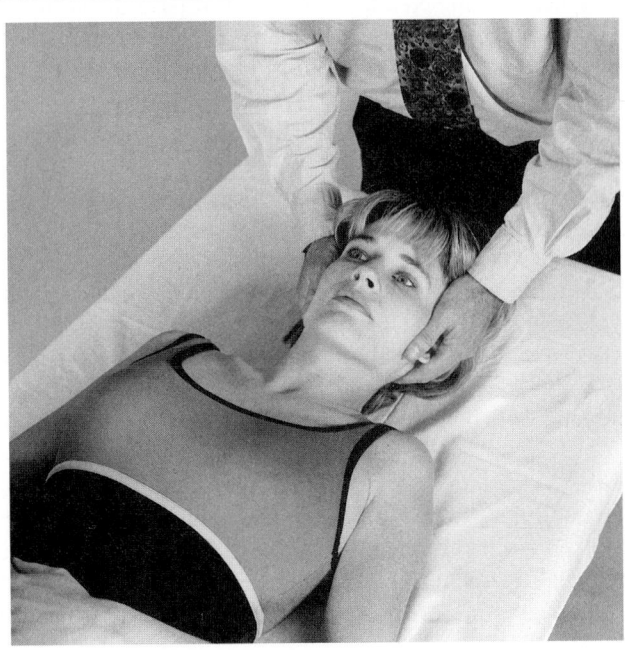

FIGURE 23-42 Translational glides of cervical spine in neutral.

Passive Physiologic Intervertebral Mobility Testing (PPIVM). These screening tests examine intersegmental mobility. As with any other screening test, these tests quickly demonstrate the need for more exhaustive testing and focus the examiner's attention on a specific level or levels and specific movement(s). Manual examination of the cervical spine by experienced clinicians has shown good sensitivity and specificity to detect the symptomatic level in spinal patients compared with other medical diagnostic tools, including radiographs.[71,115]

To test the intersegmental mobility of the midcervical region, the patient's neck is placed in the neutral position of the head on the neck, and the neck on the trunk. Once in this position, lateral glides are performed, beginning at C2 and progressing inferiorly (Fig. 23-42). The lateral glides are usually tested in one direction before repeating the process on the other side. The lateral glides result in a relative side bending of the cervical spine in the direction opposite to the glide. Light pressure from the clinician's body can be applied against the top of the patient's skull to hold the head in position. This reinforces the stabilization caused by the weight of the patient's thorax against the table. Each spinal level is glided laterally to the left and right, while the examiner palpates for muscle guarding, range of motion, end-feel, and the provocation of symptoms. Lateral glides are performed as far inferiorly as possible.

Following this procedure, the areas in which a restricted glide was found are targeted, and repetition of the lateral glides is performed in the extended and then flexed positions.

Extension. With the patient supine, and the occiput cupped, the segment is extended by lifting the superior vertebra forward (obviating the need to extend the entire spinal region) and allowing the patient's head and neck to bend over the fulcrum created by the examiner's fingers. While maintaining the extended position (by pushing the transverse processes of the segment anteriorly), the segment is side bent left and then right around its axis of motion, and translated contralaterally (Fig. 23-43). During the translation, very slight head motion should occur. Rather, a slight tilting around each segmental axis

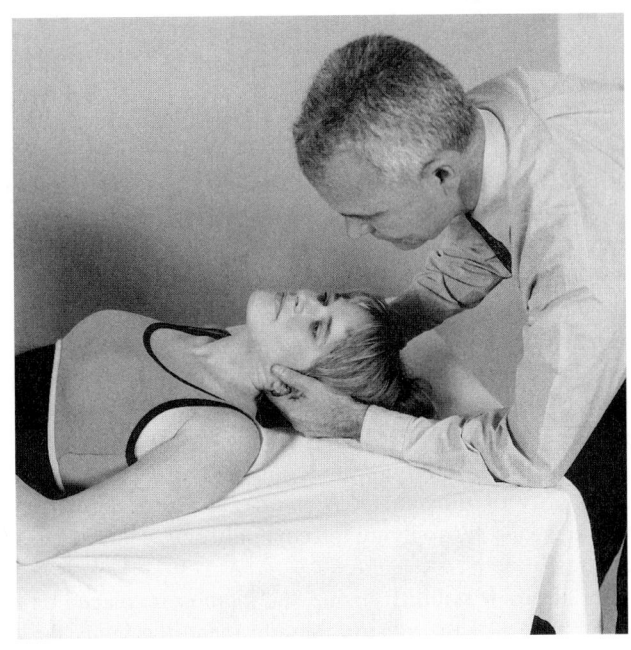

FIGURE 23-43 Translational glides of cervical spine in extension.

occurs, using gentle pressure via the fingertips or the fleshy part of the second metacarpophalangeal joint. The slight side bending before the translation is to fix the axis at that segmental level. During left side bending, the left side of the segment is maximally extended while the right side is moved toward its neutral position.

The range of motion of the side bending and the end-feel of the translation is evaluated for normal, excessive, or reduced motion states. If the end-feel of the translation is normal, but the side bending is restricted, the hypomobility is extra-articular (myofascial) (see Table 23-7).

Because of the unreliability of mobility testing in extension, the information gleaned from motion testing is more likely to be more reliable in determining the side of the closing restriction.

Flexion. The same considerations are pertinent for flexion hypomobilities. To test in flexion, the patient's head and neck are flexed without allowing a chin tuck, which would tighten the nuchal ligament. If left side bending is restricted in flexion, the right side of the segment is not flexing sufficiently (see Table 23-7).

Clinically, it would appear that the zygapophysial joints are more involved with the rotational aspect of the coupling, functioning to prevent excessive rotation, whereas the uncovertebral joints appear to be more involved with pure side bending motions. Although this concept may not hold up to scientific scrutiny, it tends to work well in the clinic. Thus, a glide restriction found in flexion, extension, and neutral would tend to implicate a problem with the uncovertebral joint.

While it is not necessary to make a diagnosis from these tests, some useful deductions can be made and these will direct the ensuing arthrokinematic tests to the appropriate joint. Remember, that if the end-feel of the glide suggests that motion is still occurring at the end of available range, the joint is *not* the cause of restriction (think *muscle*).

Cervical Stress Tests

Depending on the irritability of the segment, a variety of tests can be used to assess for instability. It is worthwhile to start gently with segmental palpation and gentle posteroanterior pressures before progressing to the other techniques. Unless indicated, the patient is positioned supine. The following tests are performed to examine segmental stability.

Posteroanterior Spring Test. The patient is positioned in prone for anterior stability testing; the clinician places his or her thumbs over the posterior aspects of the transverse processes of the inferior vertebra of the segment being tested. The vertebra is then pushed anteriorly, and the clinician feels for the quality and quantity of movement. A rotational component can be added to the test by applying force on only one of the transverse processes.

For posterior stability testing, the thumbs are placed on the anterior aspect of the superior vertebra, and the index fingers are on the posterior aspect (neural arch) of the inferior.[112] The inferior vertebra is then pushed anteriorly on the superior one,

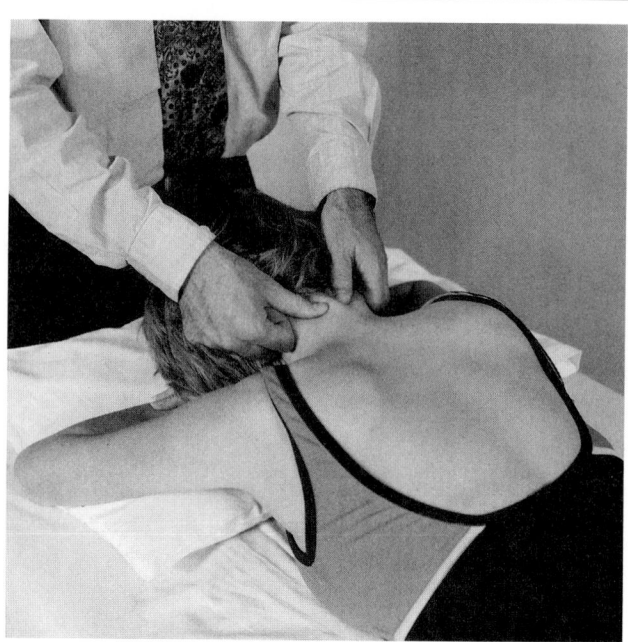

FIGURE 23-44   Posteroanterior pressures of the cervical spine.

producing a relative posterior shear of the superior segment (Fig. 23-44).

To ensure patient comfort during this test, the thumbs must be placed under (posterior to) the SCM, rather than over it, and must function merely to stabilize the maneuver, exerting no pushing force.

Transverse Shear. The transverse shear test should not be confused with the lateral glide tests previously mentioned. The lateral glide tests are used to assess joint motion, whereas the transverse shear test assesses the stability of the segment. Although motion is expected to occur in the lateral glide test, no motion should be felt to occur with the transverse shear test.[116]

The inferior segment is stabilized, and the clinician attempts to translate the superior segment transversely using the soft part of the metacarpophalangeal joint of the index finger[112] (Fig. 23-45). The end-feel should be a combination of capsular and slightly springy. The test is then reversed so that the superior segment is stabilized and the inferior segment is translated under it.

The test is repeated at each segmental level and for each side.

Craniovertebral Ligament Stress Tests. The tests for these ligaments, which include the alar and transverse ligament, are described in Chapter 22.

Distraction and Compression. The patient is supine, and the clinician stands at the patient's head. The clinician cups the patient's occiput in one hand and rests the anterior aspect of the ipsilateral shoulder on the patient's forehead. The other hand

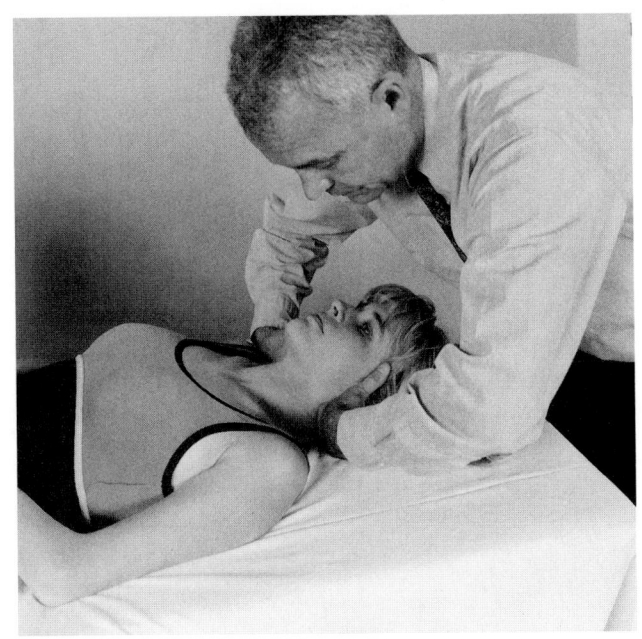

FIGURE 23-45 Transverse shear test.

stabilizes at a level close to the base of the neck[112] (Fig. 23-46). A traction-compression-traction force is applied. The clinician notes the quality and quantity of motion.

Pain reproduced with compression suggests the presence of:

▶ Disk herniation.

▶ Vertebral end plate fracture.

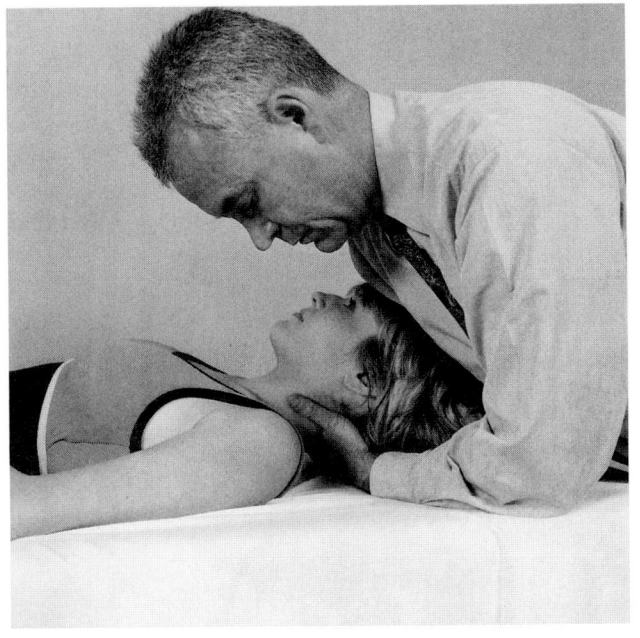

FIGURE 23-46 Cervical distraction.

▶ Vertebral body fracture.

▶ Acute arthritis or joint inflammation of a zygapophysial joint.

▶ Nerve root irritation, if radicular pain is produced.

Reproduction of pain with cervical distraction suggests the presence of:

▶ Spinal ligament tear.

▶ Tear or inflammation of the annulus fibrosis.

▶ Muscle spasm.

▶ Large disk herniation.

▶ Dural irritability (if nonradicular arm or leg pain is produced).

Functional Assessment Tests

The Neck Disability Index (NDI) is a patient survey instrument (see Table 9-7). Overall, no instrument is known to be significantly more advantageous for assessment of the neck than the NDI. The NDI is a revision of the Oswestry index and is designed to measure the level of reduction in activities of daily living in patients with neck pain. The NDI has been widely researched and validated,[117] and its test-retest reliability has been found to be 0.89.[117]

Special Tests

Temporomandibular Joint Screen. Because the temporomandibular joint (see Chap. 24) can refer pain to this region, the clinician is well advised to rule out this joint as the cause for the patient's symptoms.

The patient is asked to open and close the mouth, and to laterally deviate the jaw as the clinician observes the quality and quantity of motion and notes any reproduction of symptoms.

Lhermitte's Symptom or "Phenomenon." This is not so much a test as it is a symptom, described as an electric shocklike sensation that radiates down the spinal column into the upper or lower limbs when flexing the neck. It also may be precipitated by extending the head, coughing, sneezing, bending forward, or moving the limbs.[79] It was described in detail by Lhermitte,[118] who insisted that demyelination was the underlying pathology. Lhermitte's symptom and abnormalities in the posterior part of the cervical spinal cord on magnetic resonance imaging (MRI) are strongly associated. Smith and McDonald[119] postulated that there is an increased mechanosensitivity to traction on the cervical cord of injured axons located within the dorsal columns, causing transient activity of normally silent sensory units, as well as increasing the firing rate of spontaneously active units. Although a herniated disk is an anteriorly placed lesion, and the spinothalamic tract is usually more affected than the posterior columns, flexion of the neck will produce stretching of the posterior aspects of the cord, but not the anterior part at the site of the impairment, and this may explain this particular symptom.

Spurling's Test.   This test, designed to assess for foraminal encroachment, is described in Chapter 20.

Bakody's Sign.   This test, designed to highlight the presence of radicular symptoms in the C4 to C5 or C5 to C6 areas, is described in Chapter 20 and in the "History" section.

Brachial Plexus Tests

Stretch Test.   This test is similar to the straight leg raise for the lower extremity, because it stretches the brachial plexus. The patient is positioned sitting and is asked to side bend the head to the uninvolved side and to extend the shoulder and elbow on the involved side. Pain and paresthesia along the involved arm are indicative of a brachial plexus irritation.

Compression Test.   The patient is positioned sitting and is asked to side bend the head to the uninvolved side. The clinician applies firm pressure to the brachial plexus by squeezing the plexus between the thumb and fingers. Reproduction of shoulder or upper arm pain is positive for mechanical cervical lesions.[120]

Tinel's Sign.   The patient is positioned sitting and is asked to side bend the head to the uninvolved side. The clinician taps along the trunks of the brachial plexus using the fingertips. Local pain indicates a cervical plexus lesion. A tingling sensation in the distribution of one of the trunks may indicate a compression or neuroma of one or more trunks of the brachial plexus.[121]

Thoracic Outlet Tests.

Despite their widespread use, no studies documenting the reliability of the common thoracic outlet maneuvers of Adson's, Allen's, or the costoclavicular maneuver have been performed.[122] The specificity of these tests, determined in asymptomatic patients, has been reported to be between 18 and 87 percent,[45,123–125] whereas the sensitivity has been documented at 94 percent.[122,125]

   When performing thoracic outlet syndrome tests, either the diminution or disappearance of pulse or reproduction of neurologic symptoms indicates a positive test. However, the aim of the tests should be to reproduce the patient's symptoms rather than to obliterate the radial pulse, because more than 50 percent of normal, asymptomatic people exhibit obliteration of the radial pulse during classic provocative testing.[126]

   A baseline pulse should be established first, before performing the respective test maneuvers.

Adson's Vascular Test.   The patient extends the neck, turns the head toward the side being examined, and takes a deep breath (Fig. 23-47). This test, if positive, tends to implicate the scalenes because the test increases the tension of the anterior and middle scalenes and compromises the interscalene triangle.[127]

Allen's Pectoralis Minor Test.   The Allen test increases the tone of the pectoralis minor muscle. The shoulder of the seated patient is positioned in 90 degrees of glenohumeral abduction, 90 degrees of glenohumeral external rotation, and 90 degrees of elbow flexion on the tested side. Although the radial pulse is

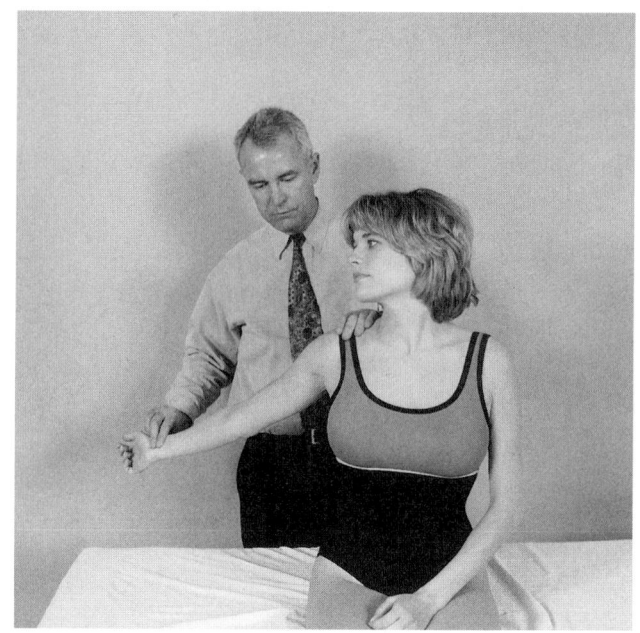

FIGURE 23-47   Adson's test.

monitored, the patient is asked to turn their head away from the tested side. This test, if positive, tends to implicate pectoralis tightness as the cause for the symptoms.

Costoclavicular Test.   During this test, the shoulders are drawn back and downward in an exaggerated military position to reduce the volume of the costoclavicular space (Fig. 23-48).

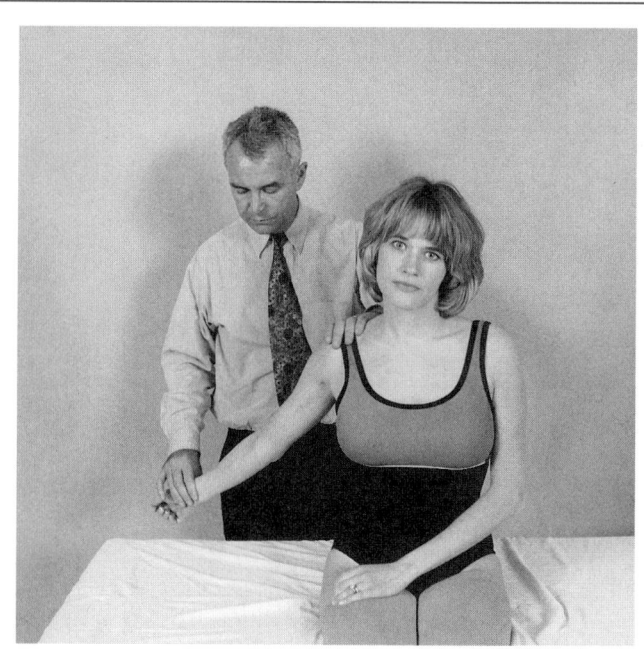

FIGURE 23-48   Costoclavicular test.

Hallstead Maneuver. The patient is positioned sitting on the edge of a table. The clinician grasps the arm on the symptomatic side, passively depresses its shoulder girdle, and then pulls the arm down towards the floor, while palpating the radial pulse (Fig. 23-49). The patient is then asked to extend the head and to turn away from the tested side. A positive test for thoracic outlet syndrome is indicated if there is an absence or diminishing of the pulse.

Roos Test.[128] The patient is positioned sitting. The arm is positioned in 90 degrees of shoulder abduction, and 90 degrees of elbow flexion. The patient is asked to perform slow finger clenching for 3 minutes (Fig. 23-50). The radial pulse may be reduced or obliterated during this maneuver, and an infraclavicular bruit may be heard. If the patient is unable to maintain the arms in the start position for 3 minutes or reports pain, heaviness, or numbness and tingling, the test is considered positive for thoracic outlet syndrome on the involved side. This test also is referred to as the hands-up test or the elevated arm stress test (EAST).

Overhead Test. The overhead exercise test is useful to detect thoracic outlet arterial compression. The patient elevates both arms overhead, and then rapidly flexes and extends the fingers (Fig. 23-51). A positive test is achieved if the patient experiences heaviness, fatigue, numbness, tingling, blanching, or discoloration of a limb within 20 seconds.[127]

Hyperabduction Maneuver (Wright Test).[123] This test is considered by many clinicians to be the best provocative test for thoracic outlet compression caused by compression in the costoclavicular space. The patient is asked to turn the head

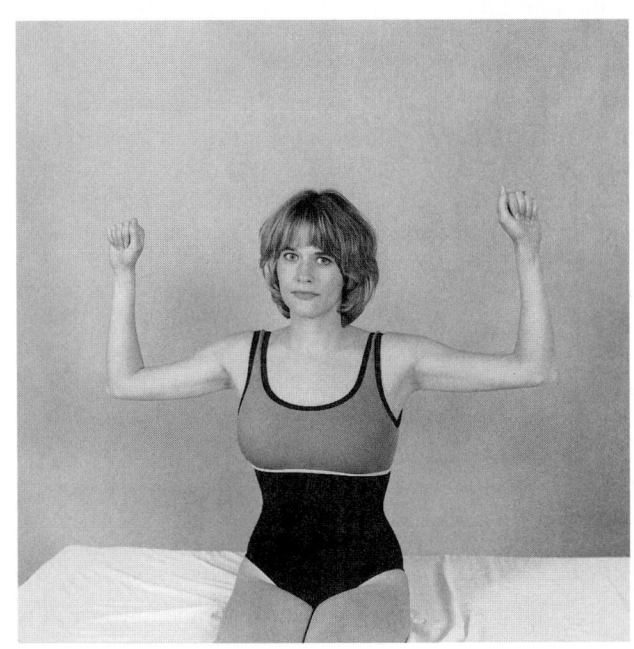

FIGURE 23-50 Roos test.

away from the side being examined, and to take a deep breath while the examiner passively abducts and externally rotates the patient's arm.

Passive Shoulder Shrug. This simple, but effective, test is used with patients who present with symptoms of thoracic outlet syndrome to help rule out this syndrome. The patient is seated

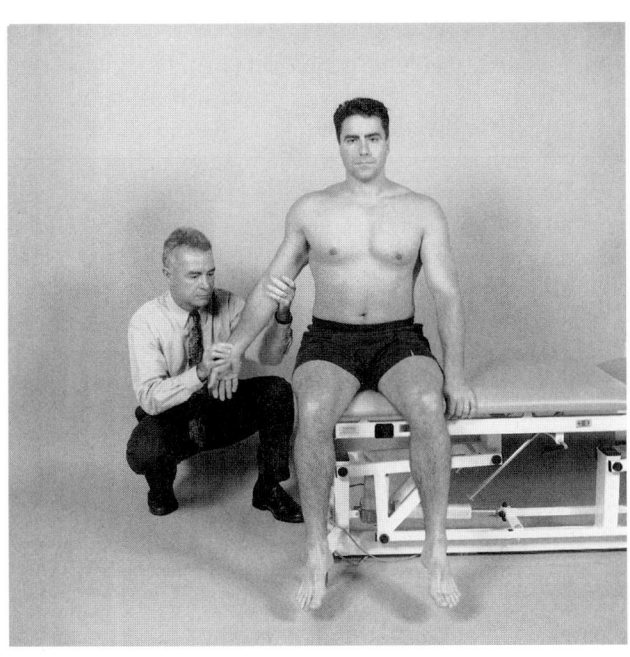

FIGURE 23-49 Hallstead maneuver.

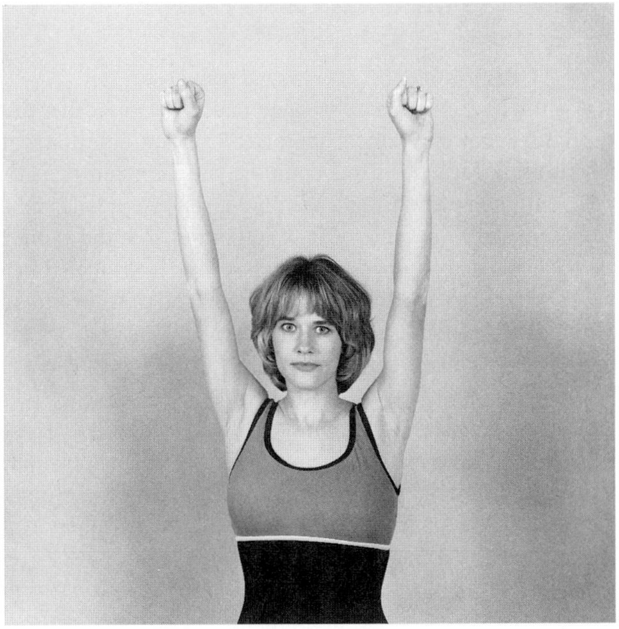

FIGURE 23-51 Overhead test.

with the arms folded, and the clinician stands behind. The clinician grasps the patient's elbows and passively elevates the shoulders up and forward. This position is maintained for 30 seconds. Any changes in the patient's symptoms are noted. The maneuver has the effect of slackening the soft tissues and the plexus.

Upper Limb Tension Tests.   The reader is encouraged to refer to Chapter 12 for the descriptions of these tests. The upper limb tension tests are equivalent to the straight leg raise test in the lumbar spine, and are designed to put stress on the neuromeningeal structures of the upper limb. Each test begins by testing the normal side first. Normal responses include:

▶ Deep stretch or ache in the cubital fossa.

▶ Deep stretch or ache into the anterior or radial aspect of forearm and radial aspect of hand.

▶ Deep stretch in the anterior shoulder area.

▶ Sensation felt down the radial aspect of the forearm.

▶ Sensation felt in the median distribution of the hand.

   Positive findings include:

▶ Production of patient's symptoms.

▶ A sensitizing test in the ipsilateral quadrant that alters the symptoms.

Cranioverebral Ligamentous Stress Tests.   These tests are described in Chapter 22

Vertebrobasilar Artery.   The examination of the vertebral artery is described in Chapter 21

Intervention Strategies

Cervical impairments have the same causes as any other areas of the body; that is, a microtraumatic or macrotraumatic impairment of the structures that compose the joint complex.

The clinician must discuss the diagnosis, prognosis, and the intervention with the patient. It is important that the clinician describe the basic anatomy and function of the cervical spine in a way that the patient will understand. Expectations of both the patient and the clinician must be clarified. Patients must realize at the outset that they are responsible for their own recovery, and must participate actively in their treatment.

Based on a working hypothesis, the physical therapy intervention needs to be precise, and guided by the impairments, functional limitations, and disability found during the examination. The intervention should aim to reverse the dysfunction and to prevent the recurrence of future episodes.

Physical therapy interventions that have included postural re-education, neck-specific strengthening and stretching exercises, and ergonomic changes at work have been shown to be beneficial in reducing neck pain and improving mobility.[129–131]

The techniques to increase joint mobility and the techniques to increase soft tissue extensibility are described later, under "Therapeutic Techniques."

Acute Phase

During the acute phase, the patient should be encouraged to perform as many activities of daily living as possible. The return to activities should be encouraged and begin within 2 to 4 days after a cervical injury, depending on severity. Rest is usually advocated in the first 24 to 72 hours, depending on the severity of the injury, to give healing a chance. Indications for rest include pain reported with all neck and head motions, however slight, and high irritability of the symptoms. Ignoring the need for rest in these situations increases the risk of delaying the recovery from the acute phase. In those situations where absolute rest is warranted, the patient is told that rest means just that. Pillows should be adjusted so that the head remains in neutral when sleeping in side lying or supine position. The patient should be cautioned about prone lying.

Patients are encouraged to take up or resume a regular activity such as walking or, later in this phase, swimming and perhaps running, or anything else that will get them back to a normal mind set about their function without reinjuring the area.

Gentle exercises are prescribed in the first part of the healing phase. The main reasons for these early exercises are:

▶ To encourage patient involvement.

▶ To provide mechanoreceptor stimulation.

▶ To control pain and inflammation.

▶ To promote healing.

▶ To maintain the newly attained ranges.

▶ To provide neuromuscular feedback.

The exercises should be performed in a non–weight-bearing position, such as supine, and are performed as gentle repetitions, well within the pain-free range. Usually, the easiest and most comfortable exercise is rotation in supine position, with the head comfortably supported. The Occipital Float (OPTP, Winnetonka, Minnesota) is a device that is extremely effective in providing support for the head and neck in the supine position (Fig. 23-52). The head is gently rolled from side to side without lifting it from the pillow. Patients perform gentle, active, small-range and amplitude rotational movements of the neck, first in one direction, then the other. The movements are repeated 10 times in each direction every waking hour. The movements are performed up to a maximum comfortable range.

To relieve muscle tension, the exercises can be done in conjunction with breathing.[65] When the patient reaches the easy end of range (at the point where the neck is about to leave its neutral zone and some tissue resistance is first being felt), the patient takes a moderate breath in, and then releases it. At the end of the release, the relaxation of the muscles allows a slight increase in range without stressing any tissues and without causing pain.

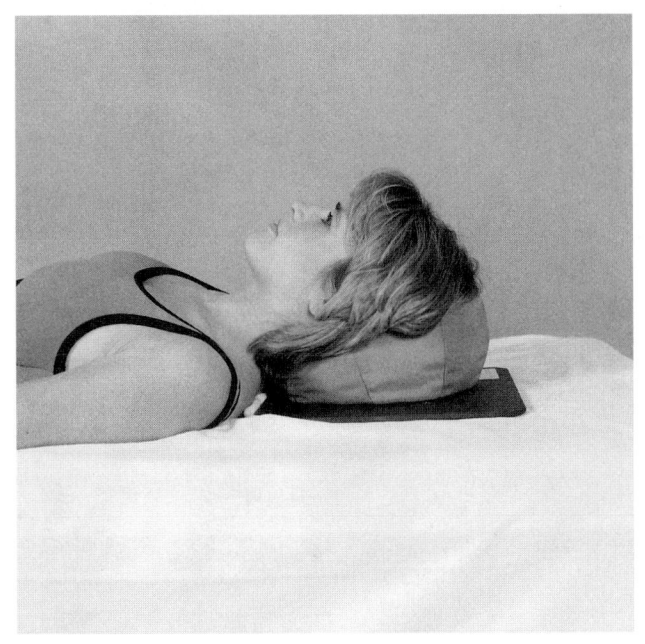

FIGURE 23-52 Occipital Float.

The other exercises prescribed early in the intervention include:

▶ Shoulder shrugging, and shoulder circumduction exercises.

▶ Hip and knee flexion–extension exercises and ankle dorsiflexion in non–weight-bearing position (to help move the dura).

▶ Isometric hip, shoulder, and abdominal exercises (using the Valsalva maneuver, not pelvic tilting or sit-ups).

As with any exercise progression, these exercises are replaced with more challenging exercises as the patient's healing progresses. Guidelines are provided for safe home exercising by teaching the patient to identify warning signs that could lead to exacerbation or recurrence of symptoms. In the event of an increase of symptoms, the techniques are adjusted by either reducing the amplitude of the movements or reducing the number of movements, or both.

Once the non–weight-bearing range of motion can be performed without an exacerbation or recurrence of symptoms, active range-of-motion exercises into cervical rotation can be initiated in the sitting and then standing positions. As range of motion and flexibility improve, cervical muscle strengthening should begin. Strengthening often begins with submaximal isometric contractions in the single planes, including flexion, extension, side bending, and rotation (Fig. 23-53A–D). These exercises usually are performed initially against manual resistance applied by the clinician and then by the patient. Isolated strengthening of weakened muscle secondary to the radiculopathy is important before advancing to the more complex exercises involving multiple muscles. Although these exercises should not cause sharp pain, they may produce mild delayed-onset muscle

soreness. Minimal resistance is used in the neutral position to aid in venous return, stimulate the mechanoreceptors in the muscle, and allay any concerns regarding weakening of the neck from disuse or a cervical collar.[65]

Other movements, such as cervical retraction, cervical protrusion, extension, flexion, rotation, side bending, or a combination of these, can be added to the program, depending on which movements are found to be beneficial during the progression.

The efficacy of electrotherapeutic modalities has not been subjected to randomized clinical trials.[132] Although passive modalities have their uses in the acute phase, the clinician should remember that they must only be used as an adjunct to the more active program, and with a specific goal in mind, such as to help in the reduction of pain and inflammation. Thus, the patient should be weaned off the use of modalities as early as possible. Cervical traction has been advocated for neck sprains, and for the pain of radiculopathy, but no clinical or statistically significant change in pain or overall range of motion has been identified.[133–136]

▶ *Ultrasound.* Pulsed ultrasound should be used precisely.[137] It can be applied to the posterior aspects of the zygapophysial joints to control pain and reduce swelling, or to a torn muscle.

▶ *Thermal agents.* Theoretically, ice is the preferred choice in the acute phase. However, ice can often increase pain that arises from trigger points. After several days, the switch can be made to the use of heat, with its ability to relax musculature, and stimulate vasodilation.[138]

▶ *Electrical muscle stimulation.*[65] Providing that none of the muscles stimulated are torn, electrical muscle stimulation can be used in the early stages as an effective pain reliever and as a venous pump. The patient is positioned supine. A small electrode is placed on each of the left and right suboccipital muscles, and a large common electrode is placed along the upper thoracic spinous process. The channels are made to stimulate asynchronously with a long "on" ramp, and a contraction length of 2 or 3 seconds (certainly no longer than 5, because this becomes uncomfortable). The session can last anywhere from a few minutes to 30 minutes, once it is established that there are no adverse effects from the intervention.

Numerous manual therapy techniques are available to the clinician, each with its own uses. These techniques, described later under "Therapeutic Techniques," can be used with hypomobilities, hypermobilities, and soft tissue injuries. The nature and location of the dysfunction, as well as the intention of its effect, guide the selection of a particular technique. Movement gained by a manual technique must be reinforced by both the mechanical and neurophysical benefits of active movement.[3]

No randomized controlled trials (RCTs) have been done on the efficacy of manipulations for patients with predominantly acute neck pain. A number of RCT studies have been done with subacute and chronic neck pain, most of which have shown that

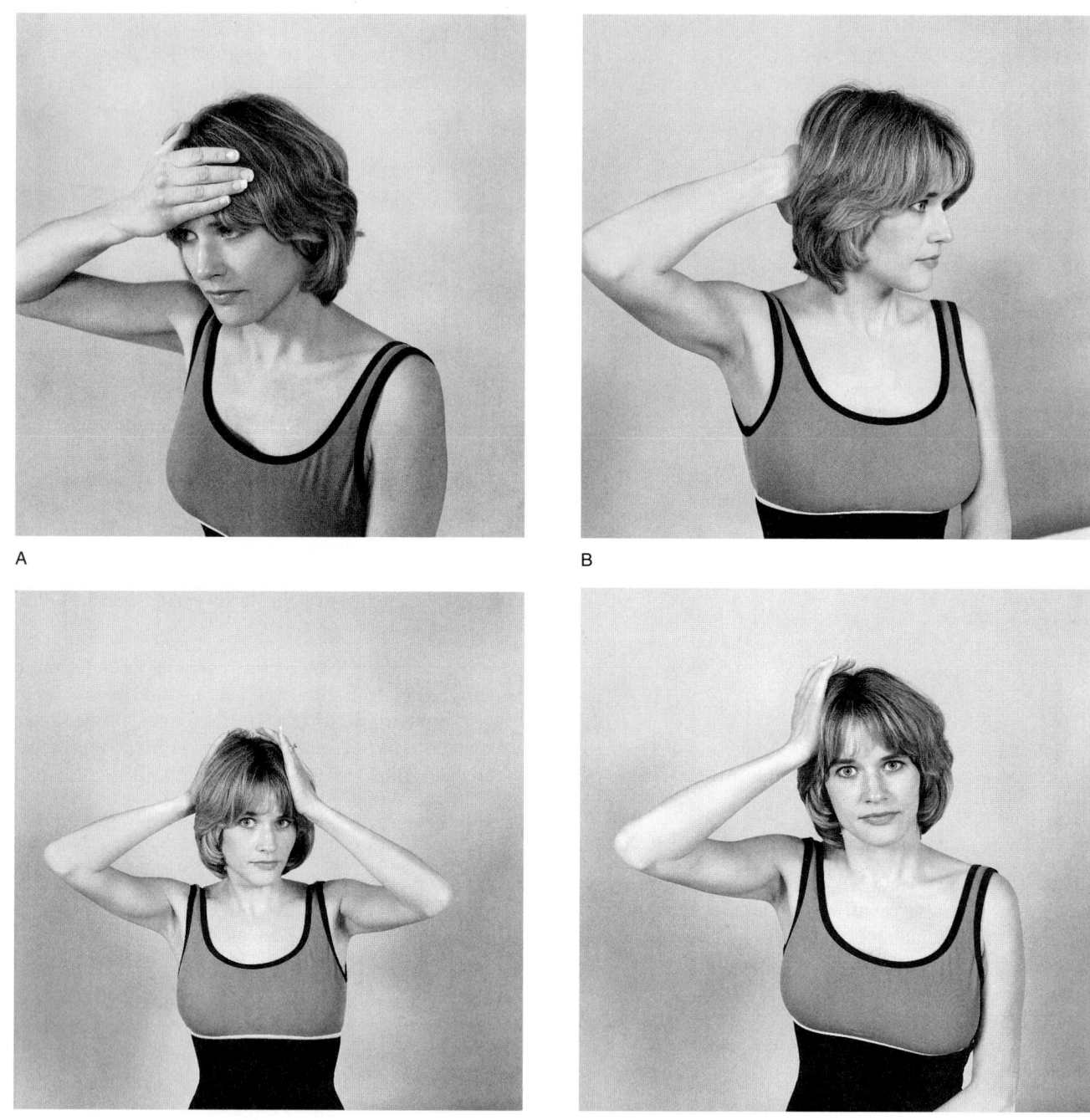

A

B

C

D

FIGURE 23-53 A–D   Cervical submaximal isometrics. *A:* Isometric cervical flexion *B:* Isometric cervical extension *C:* Isometric cervical rotation *D:* Isometric cervical side bending.

manipulation is probably slightly more effective than mobilization or other interventions.[139]

Cervical Collars

The use of cervical collars is controversial. Although several studies have concluded that the wearing of a cervical collar results in delayed recovery, these studies looked at the use of collars and other passive therapies versus other more active forms

of intervention, such as early patient activation and exercise. A study by Mealy and colleagues[140] found that early active mobilization techniques following a whiplash-associated disorder improved pain reduction and increased mobility compared with a control group receiving 2 weeks' rest with a soft cervical collar and gradual mobilization thereafter. Another study[141] found physical therapy or exact instructions in a home program of self-mobilization to be better than 2 weeks' rest with a soft collar at the 1- and 2-month follow-ups. A similar result was found at the 2-year follow-up.[142] Borchgrevink and colleagues[143] found that patients encouraged to continue with daily activities had a better outcome than patients prescribed sick leave and immobilization.

With those patients who have a severe capsular restriction of motion, a cervical collar should be issued. Soft cervical collars do not rigidly immobilize the cervical spine. They have been shown to be of benefit in the intervention of acute neck pain, if used judiciously to provide support for the head and neck in the very acute stages.[132,144]

The collar serves a number of functions, among them:

▶ Providing support in maintaining the cervical spine erect.

▶ Reminding the patient that the neck is injured and, thereby, preventing the patient from engaging in unexpected or excessive movements.

▶ Allowing the patient to rest the chin during activities, thereby offsetting the weight of the head.

▶ Allowing the patient to perform cervical rotations while the weight of the head is offset.

Prolonged reliance on the use of a collar may induce stiffness and weakness, but this can be avoided by recommending a time-limited use of the collar, which is based on specific factors such as the patient's condition and function. Certain situations warrant the use of a collar, such as long drives in a vehicle or prolonged postures of standing and sitting. However, patients should be weaned off the collar as their recovery progresses (when there is significant improvement in the range of motion and pain levels).

Functional Phase

Although strengthening exercises have been advocated for the intervention of neck pain,[145,146] only a few controlled intervention studies have been conducted to examine their benefit. However, in one randomized study, investigators found that a multimodal intervention of postural, manual, psychological, relaxation, and visual training techniques was superior to traditional approaches involving ultrasound and electric stimulation.[147] Patients returned to work earlier, and they had better results in pain intensity, emotional response, and postural disturbances.[147]

The stabilization of this region must include postural stabilization retraining of the entire spine, including the lumbar stabilization progression outlined in Chapter 25.

Cervicothoracic stabilization is a specific type of therapeutic exercise that can help the patient to (1) gain dynamic control of cervicothoracic spine forces, (2) eliminate repetitive injury to the motion segments, (3) encourage healing of the injured segment, and (4) possibly alter the degenerative process.[148]

The muscles to be strengthened include the scapular stabilizers and the deltoid. Although it is possible to isolate and strengthen these muscles individually, because they work together in functional activities, it is more prudent to strengthen them together.

Cervicothoracic Stabilization Exercises

Shoulder Shrugs. These exercises are initiated in the supine position without resistance and are progressed so that the patient performs them sitting or standing. Once they can be performed without pain, weights are added to the hands (Fig. 23-54). The shrug strengthens the upper trapezius, levator scapulae, and rhomboids.

Shoulder Circles or Squares. Shoulder circles or squares are an advanced version of shoulder shrugs. The patient is asked to elevate the shoulders, and then retract them as far as possible. While maintaining the retraction, the shoulders are depressed, and then protracted.

As with the shrugs, the circles or squares are initiated without resistance, but once they can be performed without pain, weights are added to the hands. The shoulder circles strengthen the upper trapezius, levator scapulae, and rhomboids.

Scapular Retraction. These exercises are initially performed supine, with the glenohumeral joint in internal and external rotation. The patient is asked to isometrically retract the shoulders against the bed. Once this exercise can be performed without pain, the patient performs the exercise in the side lying position and then prone or standing without resistance. Resistance is added as tolerated. Scapular retraction in internal rotation of the glenohumeral joint (Fig. 23-55) strengthens the infraspinatus, teres minor, middle and posterior deltoids, and the rhomboids. Scapular retraction in external rotation of the glenohumeral joint (Fig. 23-56) strengthens the infraspinatus, teres minor, middle and posterior deltoids, and middle trapezius.

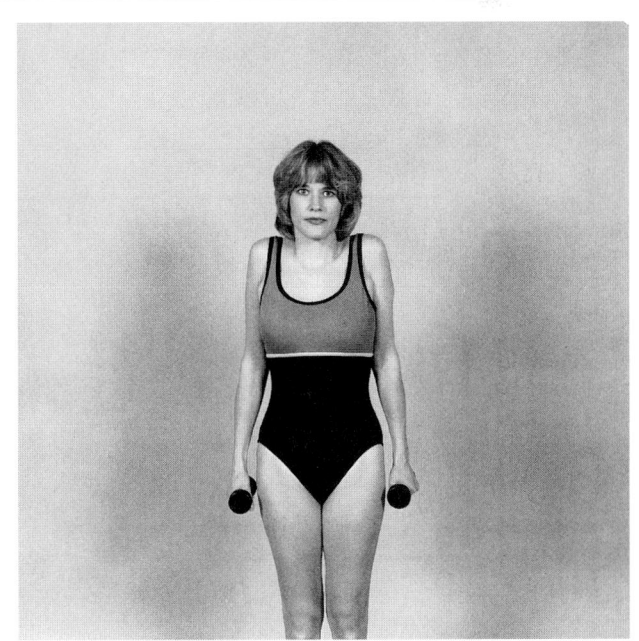

FIGURE 23-54 Shoulder shrugs.

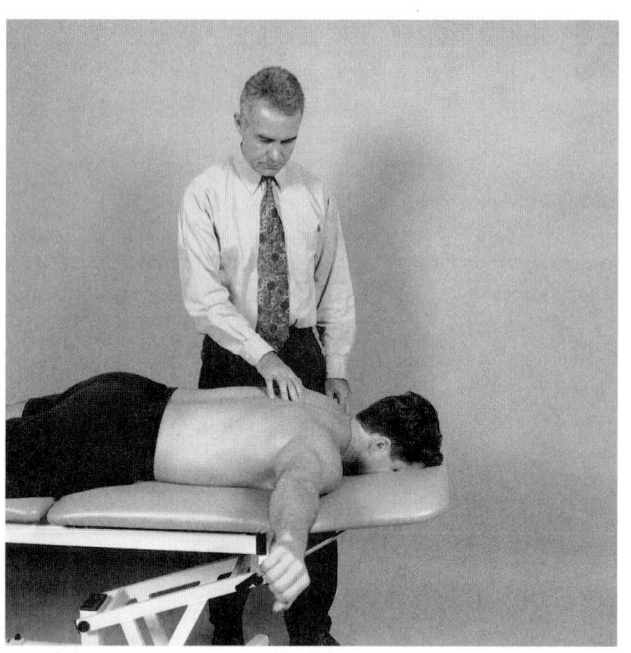

FIGURE 23-55   Scapular retraction in internal rotation of the glenohumeral joint.

Serratus Punch.   This exercise is performed initially with the patient supine, one shoulder flexed to 90 degrees, and the elbow extended. From this position, the patient raises the extended arm toward the ceiling and protracts the shoulder girdle. This exercise can be progressed by adding a weight to the hand and performing it against a wall or a chair, before progressing to a push-up on the floor.

Arm Lift.   The patient is positioned prone with his or her arms by the sides and the thumbs pointing to the ceiling. The patient is asked to raise the arms from the bed. A similar exercise can be performed on a table with the arms hanging over the edge. The patient is asked to squeeze the shoulder blades together.

Tree Hug.   The patient is asked to wrap a length of elastic tubing around the back and to hold the two ends with the thumbs pointing forward, and the arms in about 60 degrees of abduction (Fig. 23-57). From this position, the patient is asked to imagine hugging a tree and to reproduce that motion.

Upright Rows.   The muscles involved with this exercise (Fig. 23-58) include the deltoids, supraspinatus, clavicular portion of the pectoralis major, long head of the biceps, upper and lower portions of the trapezius, levator scapulae, and serratus anterior.

Elastic tubing is placed under the feet and the ends are held in each hand. Keeping the back straight, and the elbows out to the side, the patient raises their hands from about waist height to just below the chin (Fig 23-58).

Lateral Arm Raise.   This exercise (Fig. 23-59) is initiated without resistance. Once it can be performed without pain, resistance in the form of tubing or hand weights is added. Lateral arm raises involve the deltoid, supraspinatus, serratus anterior, and upper and lower trapezius.

Front Arm Raise.   Again, this exercise (Fig. 23-60) is initiated without resistance. Once it can be performed without pain, resistance in the form of tubing or hand weights is added. Front

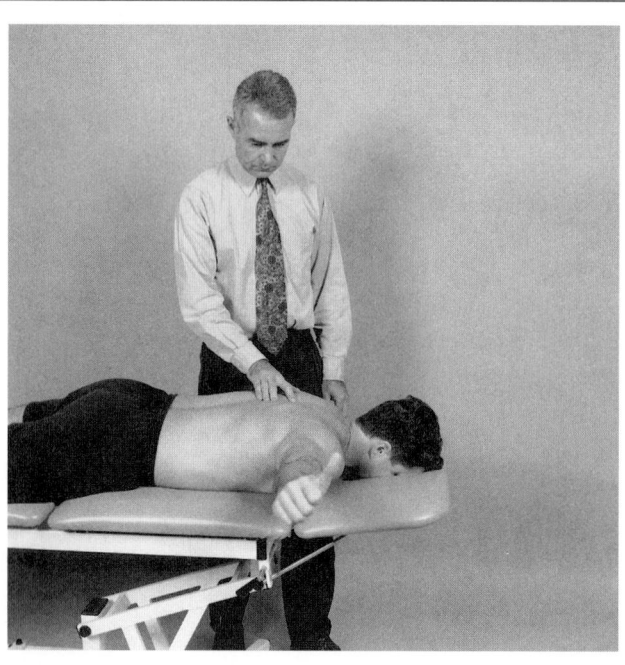

FIGURE 23-56   Scapular retraction in external rotation of the glenohumeral joint.

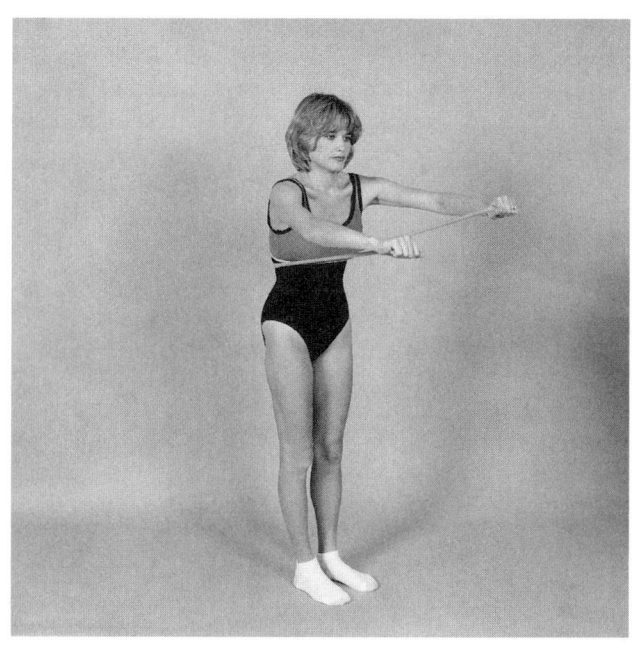

FIGURE 23-57   Tree hug.

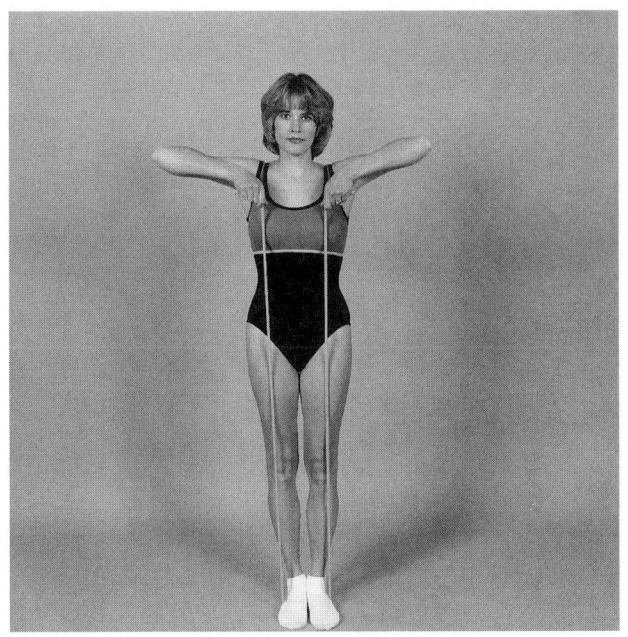

FIGURE 23-58 Upright rows.

arm raises involve the anterior deltoid, pectoralis major (upper portion), coracobrachialis, serratus anterior, and upper and lower trapezius.

Cervical Retraction.   To strengthen the cervicothoracic stabilizers, the patient is positioned prone, with the head off the end of the bed and supported in a protracted position of the neck. The patient is asked to retract the chin from this position, raising the

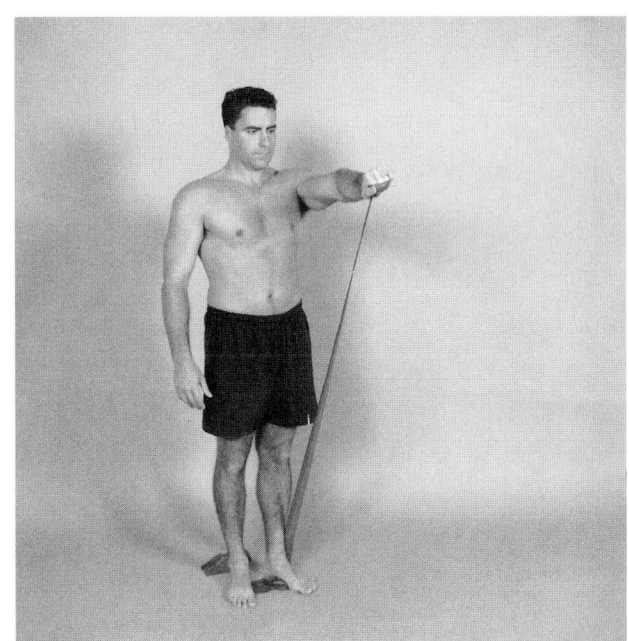

FIGURE 23-60   Front arm raise.

head toward the ceiling, while maintaining the face parallel to the floor (see Fig. 23-26).

Gravity Cervical Stabilization.   These exercises can be performed into extension (see Fig. 23-26) and side bending (Fig. 23-61) on a treatment table with the head maintaining a static position, or on a Swiss ball. Cervical side translations also can be performed against gravity.

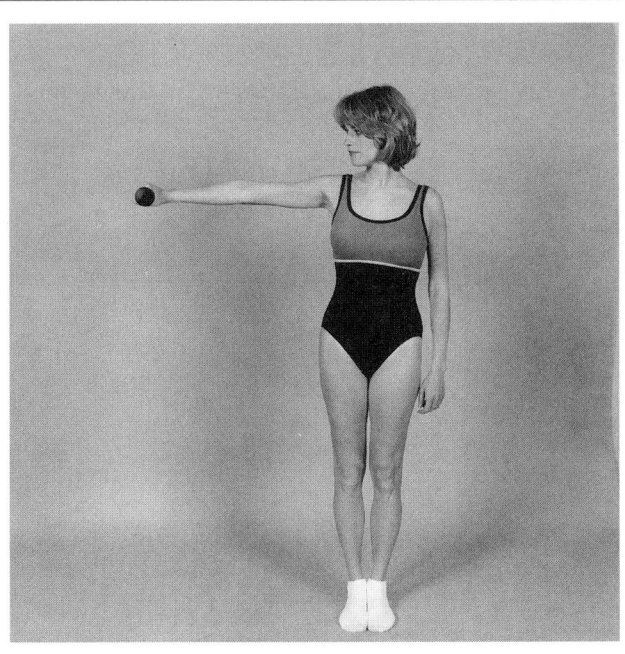

FIGURE 23-59 Lateral arm raise.

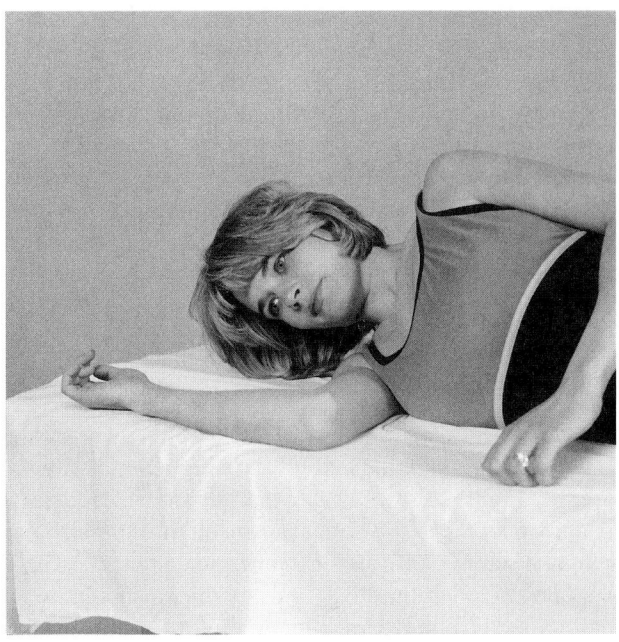

FIGURE 23-61   Cervical side bending against gravity.

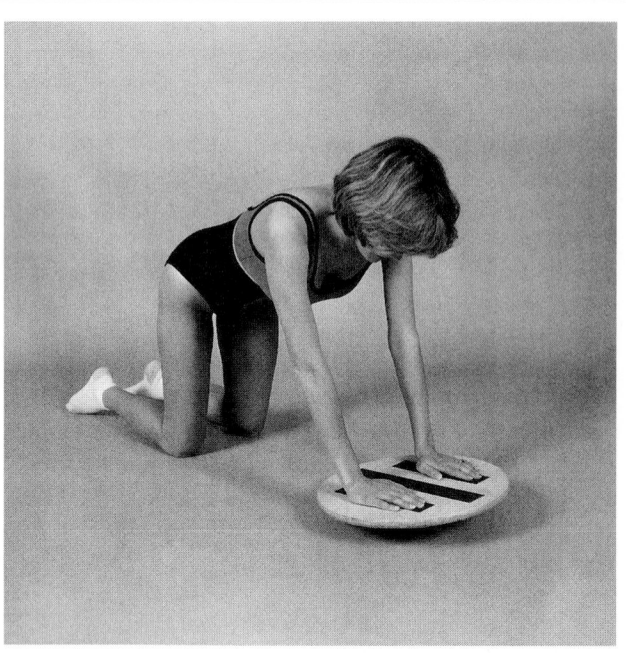

FIGURE 23-62   Close kinetic chain exercise.

Closed kinetic chain activities also can be very helpful in rehabilitating weak shoulder girdle muscles (Fig. 23-62) and the cervical stabilizers.

It should be emphasized that all exercises should be performed without pain, although some degree of postexercise soreness can be expected. Isokinetic exercises of the neck and upper extremities are not functional and are not recommended as a strengthening tool.

Strength training can progress to manually resisted cervical stabilization exercises in various planes. Cervical proprioceptive neuromuscular facilitation patterns are ideal for this purpose (Chap. 11). Muscle co-contraction of agonist and antagonist can be used for joint stabilization, by increasing joint stiffness and supporting the independent torque-producing role of the muscles that surround the joint.[149–151]

Continued efforts must be made to progressively reduce the patient's pain and advance physical function through exercise.[100] However, use of pain medication, to control pain and inflammation probably help patients to progress while experiencing considerably less pain and enabling their return to work.

Ergonomics

The patient's workstation and lifestyle ergonomics should be addressed (Table 23-8). A chair that provides adequate support and encourages the patient to maintain lumbar lordosis provides a stable platform for the cervical spine.[154] The feet should easily touch the floor, and the thighs should be horizontal to the ground. Computer monitors should be positioned to allow a slight 20-degree downward slope of the eyes.

Neuromuscular Re-education

Neuromuscular re-education exercises are designed to improve recruitment and proprioception. The coordinated activity of the upper thoracic and scapular muscles is important for the maintenance of cervicothoracic posture, and for upper limb function. Overactivity of the levator scapulae and upper trapezius is a common finding,[60,69] as is weakness of the serratus anterior, the middle and lower trapezius, and interscapular muscles.

Patients initially are positioned with front and side mirror views so that they are able to see any postural deviations of the spine, and so that they are able to see their habitual posture.[100] The clinician first helps the patient to find a neutral and balanced position of the lumbar and cervicothoracic spine by using verbal and gentle manual cues, and then helps the patient to use this position in a series of basic functional movements.[100]

Jull[3] recommends a program that emphasizes the strengthening of the deep neck flexors and scapular stabilizers, including the longus capitis muscle, longus colli muscle, serratus anterior muscle, and the lower trapezius muscle, in patients with mechanical neck pain.

Deep Neck Flexors.   The deep neck flexors are trained in the formal test position described in the section on muscle function testing, using a biofeedback pressure cuff (see Fig. 23-39), using a gradual progression.

Lower Scapular Stabilizers.   The lower scapular stabilizers are trained in the formal test position described in the section on muscle function testing (see Fig. 23-40), using a gradual progression. If the patient is unable to maintain the scapula flat against the chest wall in the prone position, the training is performed in the side lying position, adding gradual increments of arm load, and by increasing the amount of abduction until control can be maintained in 140 degrees of abduction.[3]

Proprioceptive Neuromuscular Facilitation Neck Techniques

There are two diagonals of motion for the head and neck—the upper trunk and the extremities—with each of the diagonals being composed of two antagonistic patterns.[155]

The patient is positioned sitting, and his or her head is supported by the clinician, who places one hand under the chin and the other hand under the occipital area (see Chap. 11). As the clinician applies a controlled resistance, the patient is asked to flex and rotate the neck. From this position, the patient is asked to extend the neck and rotate in the opposite direction, thereby performing the reverse diagonal.

Postural Retraining

It is important to retrain the patient to assume a correct upright and neutral spine position, and to be able to consciously activate and hold the supporting muscles in a variety of functional positions.[3] The retraining usually begins at the lumbopelvic region, ensuring that the patient does not adopt the chest-out, shoulders-back position, which results in an incorrect thoracolumbar or thoracic lordosis, rather than a correct balance between all of the spinal curves.[3]

TABLE 23-8 Workstation Setup and Keyboard Technique Checklist[152,153]

Fault	Correction
VISUAL FIELD	
Monitor positioned to side of keyboard	Monitor directly in front of chair and parallel to keyboard
Stationary monitor	Monitor mounted on adjustable support
Screen too high or too low	10–15-degree downward viewing angle to center of screen
Copy on desk surface	Copy secured along side of monitor
Glare from direct and reflected light	Clean antiglare screen (glare filter, angle screen away from window)
Overhead fluorescent lights	Task-appropriate lighting
Incorrect focal distance for visual acuity	Focal distance (eyeglasses) corrected for computer use (i.e., 20–24 in)
POSTURE	
Head forward	Ears aligned with shoulders; chin retracted
Shoulders elevated	Shoulder girdle muscle balance
Scapular winging	Scapulothoracic proximal stability
Hypertonic upper trapezii	Lower keyboard or desk height
Shoulder protraction/internal rotation	Neutral shoulder alignment
Elbow flexion > 90 degrees	Keyboard parallel to or slightly below elbow level (i.e., 80–90 degrees of elbow flexion)
Elbow flexion < 80 degrees	Keyboard moved closer to minimize reach
Wrist flexion or extension	Height of keyboard or chair adjusted to achieve wrist in position of function*
Elbows locked at sides	Arms stabilized from scapulothoracic region
Wrists against keyboard or desk edge	Hard keyboard or desk edge padded
Wrist extension	Keyboard positive incline eliminated; flat keyboard or negative incline
Wrist ulnar deviation	Re-educate neutral wrist positioning; split keyboard
Finger MCP joint hyperextension	Fingers in position of function
Flat of kyphotic back	Back supports in chair to match individual spinal contours
Stationary chair back and seat pan	Versatile chair allowing forward, upright, and reclined postures; seat pan inclined forward with "waterfall" edge
Hips lower than knees	Seat height raised; seat pan inclined to position hips slightly higher (5–10 degrees) than knees
Feet dangling	Feet flat on floor or foot rest
KEYBOARD TECHNIQUE	
Wrist extensor/flexor co-contraction	Light key-touch; relaxation-biofeedback training
Wrist ulnar deviation	Wrist aligned with forearm
Intrinsic plus keystrike	Hand postures in position of function
Intrinsic minus keystrike (zig-zag)	
Digital extensor habitus	Thumb lightly resting on spacebar; spacebar use with thumb press versus lift and strike
Thumb held in horizontal abduction and extension	
Excessive force of keystrike	Keystrike with finger press versus lift and strike; keystrike with arm bounce
Ulnar deviation at wrist and fingers with lateral key strike	Wrist aligned with forearm; use of external rotation-abduction at shoulder for lateral key reach
Excessive leaning on wrist rests	Wrist glide versus wrist rest technique
Fifth finger lateral reach and strike	Index finger use for lateral keystrike: slight supination with fifth finger keystrike
Hands play with combination keystrikes	Combination key command efficiency; macro-program development
Typing too fast	Kinesthetic awareness training
Infrequent breaks, poor work-rest cycles	Periodic rest breaks and task rotation; computer programmed to signal rest breaks

MCP, metacarpophalangeal.
*Position of function: forearm, wrist, and hand aligned, 20–30 degrees wrist extention, natural curve to digits with MCP joints at about 50 degrees of flexion, and thumb in line with radius.

Overall Strength and Fitness

It is important throughout the rehabilitation process for patients to maintain their level of cardiovascular fitness as much as possible. Aerobic exercise, which increases endurance and the general sense of well-being, should be a part of all exercise programs.[156,157] Cardiovascular conditioning should be started as soon as possible to prevent deconditioning. These exercises also serve as a great warm-up prior to a stretching program.

Practice Pattern 4B: Impaired Joint Mobility, Motor Function, Muscle Performance, Range of Motion Associated with Impaired Posture

Fiber composition studies have demonstrated that the primary dysfunction in neck muscles is a loss in the tonic supporting capacity, with the dysfunction being greater in the neck flexors, and within the neck flexors.[3,158] Several postural syndromes of the cervical have been identified over the years. A common cause of many of these syndromes is the forward head posture.

Proximal Crossed Syndrome[60,61]

This syndrome involves tightness of the levator scapulae, upper trapezius, pectoralis major and minor, SCM, and weakness of the deep neck flexors and lower scapular stabilizers. The syndrome is characterized by:

▶ Elevation and protraction of the shoulder.

▶ Rotation and abduction of the scapula.

▶ Scapular winging.

▶ Forward head (see discussion that follows).

▶ Decreased stability of the glenohumeral joint.

▶ Increased muscle activity of the levator scapula and trapezius.

The positional changes that occur with the proximal crossed syndrome may alter the structural relationships of the shoulder and the cervical spine. This alteration may result in changes in the length–tension relationships and the kinematics of the scapular and cervical muscles. The consequences of these changes may include posterior nerve root irritation, cervical radiculopathy, segmental hypermobility, and instability at C4 to C5.[76,159]

Forward Head

Abnormal posture has long been considered by many to be the cause of numerous musculoskeletal and neurovascular impairments.[40,43,53,96,160-168]

Under normal circumstances, the center of gravity (COG) for the head falls slightly anterior to the ear. The habitual placement of the head anterior to the COG of the body places undue stress on the temporomandibular joint, the cervical and upper thoracic facet joints (especially at the cervicothoracic junction), and the supporting muscles.[167,169]

For each inch that the head is anterior to the COG, the weight of the head is added to the load borne by the cervical

structures.[160] For example, the average head weighs 10 lb. If the chin is 2 inches anterior to the manubrium, 20 lb is added to the load. If normal motion is undertaken in this poor postural environment, the result may be abnormal strain placed on the joint capsule, ligaments, IVDs, levator scapulae, upper trapezius, SCM, scalene, and suboccipital muscles.

Sustained forward head postures may cause a painful fatigue in the levator scapulae, rhomboids, and lower portion of the trapezius, a condition referred to as *tired neck syndrome*.[2] The traumatized muscles may cause pain, which in turn causes the patient to restrict motion. Patients with these postural abnormalities may experience myofascial pain that can cause referral zone pain.[40] This myofascial pain is thought to be caused by waste products produced by the muscles, or from localized ischemia of those structures. An underlying cycle of abnormal relaxation in some muscles, with shortening, stretching, and a loss of tone in others, occurs during this process, with resultant joint strain and dysfunction.

Other postural adaptations associated with the forward head posture include rounded shoulders, protracted scapulae with tight anterior muscles and stretched posterior muscles, and the development of a cervicothoracic kyphosis between C4 and T4 (Table 23-6).[170-172]

These adaptations are further perpetuated by the natural cycle of aging of the spine, which involves degeneration of the disk, vertebral wedging, ligamentous calcification, and reduction in the cervical and lumbar lordoses, producing a position of spinal flexion, or stooping.

Habitual movement patterns or positions may contribute to the development of these changes and produce muscular hyperactivity, ligamentous stress, and alteration of the anatomic and biomechanical relationship of the joints. It is theorized that if a muscle lengthens as part of this compensation, muscle spindle activity increases within that muscle, producing reciprocal inhibition of the muscle's functional antagonist, and resulting in an alteration in the normal force–couple and arthrokinematic relationship, thereby effecting the efficient and ideal operation of the movement system.[89,91,170,173,174]

As the head is brought forward by flexing the cervical segments, the scalene muscles are permitted to adaptively shorten, thus lessening the support of the upper ribs. The cervical flexion is followed by an increase of the thoracic curvature, and the tension of the spinal musculature increases.[175,176] In this position, capital extension must now occur to keep the eyes horizontal and allow the individual to look ahead.[43,75,177] This occipital hyperextension of the cranium on the cervical spine has been related to head, neck, and temporomandibular joint pain. A postural-pain relationship has been described by Willford and colleagues[178] in people wearing multifocal corrective lenses.

Because the zygapophysial joints in the midcervical region incur more weight bearing, as a result of the protruding head, marginal osteophytosis may occur. The common levels for this to occur are C5 to C6 and C6 to C7. These changes also alter the scapulothoracic rhythm because of alterations in the muscle tone of the rhomboids and serratus anterior. These altered relations increase the distance between the origin and insertion of the trapezius, of the rhomboid major and minor, and of the levator scapulae, which results in further stress.

The abduction of the scapulae or protraction of the shoulders causes a lowering of the coracoid process, producing adaptive shortening of the pectoralis minor, which in turn, may flatten the anterior chest wall and alter the motion of the scapula, producing a mechanical impairment of the shoulder.

Protraction of the shoulder girdles also limits extension of the upper thoracic spine, which, in turn, limits elevation and abduction of the shoulders. This alteration can lead to a hypermobility or instability of the glenohumeral joint, and overuse syndromes of the shoulder elevators or abductors. Shoulder protraction also causes the humerus to rotate internally and so stretch the posterior glenohumeral joint capsule; in addition, it increases the anterior force at the joint as a result of gravity. The former may lead to posterior instability and rotatory hypermobility, and the latter to anterior instability and a biceps tendonitis, as this muscle becomes overused in its attempt to stabilize the glenohumeral joint.

The anteriorly displaced line of gravity induced by the forward head posture has an effect on respiration. This change in posture is postulated to have the following consequences[179]:

1. *Open-mouth breathing.*[180] Open-mouth breathing is the normal pattern of breathing for a newborn. This pattern of breathing becomes abnormal if it persists into the 5- to 7-year-old age range. A child with a long bout of sinus infections and blockages is forced to use mouth breathing as the primary method of breathing. With the development of the teeth and tongue, the oral passageway for air is gradually reduced, forcing the child to open the mouth further in order to breathe. It is postulated that this can result in[180–183]:

   a. A failure to filter inspired air of pathogens and particles. These particles go directly into the alveoli, producing an inflammatory reaction in the lungs that results in bronchospasm or asthma and stimulates a future hypersensitivity to any new particles.

   b. A failure to humidify inspired air, so that the air entering the lungs is dry.

   c. A failure to warm the inspired air. Cold or cool air entering the lungs stimulates an increased presence of white blood cells, increasing the hypersensitivity of the lungs. Early intervention with mouth breathers is essential, and it is recommended that the child be encouraged to keep the tongue against the roof of the mouth while breathing.

2. *Thoracic hyperflexion.* Although only theoretical, the thoracic compensation is necessary to counteract the backward tilting of the head and to return the eyes to a horizontal position. This compensation produces:

   a. A reduction in thoracic extension.

   b. A reduced ability of the ribs to elevate during inspiration, resulting from a reduced ability of the thoracic cavity to expand during inspiration.[181–183]

   c. An increase in the respiratory rate.[181–183]

   d. A shortening of the scalene muscles. Because of their newly acquired shortened position, the muscles have a reduced ability to contract, resulting in:

   (1) A reduced ability to elevate the first rib.

   (2) A reduced ability to increase the vertical dimension of the thoracic cavity during inspiration.[181–183]

   (3) An increase in apical breathing.[181–183]

The forces from the cervical and thoracic regions of the spine can be transmitted to the lumbar spine, increasing the lordotic curve.[184,185] The exaggeration of the lumbar curve is accompanied by a shift of the weight to the posterior part of the vertebral bodies and to the articular processes, producing maximum joint strain of the lumbosacral junction, and a forward inclination of the pelvis.

The increased forward inclination of the pelvis may produce a shortening of the erector spinae group and flexors of the hip, accompanied by a lengthening of the abdominal and hamstring muscles. These muscle imbalances serve to maintain the deformity.[97]

The intervention for postural dysfunction focuses on the correction of any strength and flexibility imbalances. Once the mechanical source is identified, the focus of the intervention is the simultaneous retraining of the muscles, by contracting the lengthened muscle when it is in a shortened position, and stretching the shortened muscle.[91]

Therapeutic exercise programs initially should focus on regaining the normal length of a muscle before strengthening the muscle, so that good movement patterns can be achieved.

Pattern 4D: Impaired Joint Mobility, Motor Function, Muscle Performance, Format Range of Motion Associated with Connective Tissue Dysfunction

Osteoarthritis

Progressive degenerative changes are expected to appear over time on radiographs as part of the natural history of the aging spine. The characteristics of degenerative joint disease and degenerative disk disease pertain to bony changes, and the two often occur concurrently.[51] Cyriax[106] reserved the term *spondylosis* for the end stage of spinal diseases, although the term is now used to describe varying levels of degenerative changes in the cervical spine.[51]

Radiographic evidence of cervical degeneration is observed in some 30-year-olds and is present in more than 90 percent of people older than 60 years of age.[186] Although aging of the cervical spine is ubiquitous, controversy remains about whether the process of spondylosis may be accelerated in patients with a history of soft tissue injuries to the neck and persistent pain. However, in the absence of pain, the finding of degenerative changes on radiographs should not be misconstrued as pathologic. One study reported evidence of cervical spondylosis in 35 percent of asymptomatic individuals.[187]

The clinical presentation of a symptomatic degenerative spine is one of a gradual onset of neck or arm symptoms, or both, that have increased frequency and severity.[51] Morning stiffness of the neck, which gradually improves throughout the day, is a common finding. However, in some cases, the patient presents with an acute stiff neck, cervical myelopathy, and vertebrobasilar insufficiency.[188]

The physical examination findings include reduced motion in the sagittal plane, with a decrease in side bending. As the degeneration progresses, a capsular pattern develops.[106]

The conservative intervention involves the use of electrotherapeutic modalities to control pain and increase the extensibility of the connective tissue. These modalities usually include moist heat, electrical stimulation, and ultrasound. Manual techniques may be used to stretch the adaptively shortened tissues. Range-of-motion exercises are performed as tolerated. These exercises initially are performed in the pain-free direction, and then in the direction of pain. As the patient regains motion, isometric exercises and cervical stabilization exercises are prescribed.

Zygapophysial Joint Dysfunction

Acute cervical joint lock, or wryneck, is a common condition of the cervical spine. The patient with this condition typically reports an onset of unilateral neck pain, or "neck locking," following sudden backward bending, side bending, or rotation of the neck, or pain that followed a sustained head position. The condition is thought to be as the result of entrapment of a small piece of synovial membrane by the facet joint.[72,189,190]

Palpation just lateral to the midline often indicates regional soft tissue changes in response to the underlying zygapophysial joint injury, and combined motion testing usually shows a closing pattern of restriction corresponding to the injured zygapophysial joint.[71]

Because traditional images (plain radiographs, computed tomography, MRI) are typically unremarkable in the presence of zygapophysial joint pain,[189] clinical suspicions of these joint injuries can be confirmed if necessary by diagnostic intra-articular zygapophysial joint injections, or a block of the joint's nerve supply.[191,192]

The conservative intervention involves the use of electrotherapeutic modalities to control pain and inflammation. Joint mobilization techniques, involving combinations of flexion or extension and rotation, with traction superimposed, are applied initially in the pain-free direction, and then in the direction of pain.

As the patient regains motion, range-of-motion exercises and isometric exercises are prescribed until full range of motion is restored, at which time the strengthening exercises are progressed.

Pattern 4E: Impaired Joint Mobility, Motor Function, Muscle Performance, Range of Motion Associated with Localized Inflammation

Whiplash-associated Disorders

Over recent years, the role of the physical therapist in the intervention of the consequences of whiplash has increased dramatically. It is thus imperative that the clinician have a strong understanding of the mechanisms that produce the myriad of symptoms associated with this disorder.

The term *whiplash injury* was introduced in 1928 by the American orthopaedist H. E. Crowe,[193] and it was defined as the effects of sudden acceleration-deceleration forces on the neck and upper trunk as a result of external forces exerting a "lash-like effect." Crowe emphasized that the term *whiplash* "describes only the manner in which a head was moved suddenly to produce a sprain in the neck."

Despite a great deal of attention, whiplash-associated disorders (WADs) remain an enigma. A lack of thorough understanding of WAD is, in part, a result of the nature of the disease itself. The subjective nature and high prevalence of the symptoms have led to controversy over their cause. These subjective complaints are most often characterized by reports of pain and suffering in the absence of focal physical findings and positive imaging studies.[194] In addition, the determination of the diagnosis has been veiled behind issues of appropriate financial compensation.[195–197]

Definition. There is little agreement as to the definition of WAD. Some authors of whiplash articles, such as Gay and Abbot,[198] do not define whiplash clearly. Neither Gotten[199] nor Macnab[200,201] offer definitions, although Macnab noted that "a significant soft tissue injury can result from the application of an extension strain to the neck by sudden acceleration."[201] Farbman[202] classified the whiplash injury as a musculoligamentous neck sprain, which did not involve nerve root damage, fractures, and other complications. Nordhoff[203] describes the whiplash injury in equally simplistic terms, as an injury that occurs because of occupant motions within a vehicle that is rapidly decelerating or accelerating, without reference to the body parts involved. Even the definition provided by the Quebec Task Force on Whiplash-associated Disorders,[204] that, for whatever reason, did not include front-end collisions, offered the following vague definition:

> *Whiplash is an acceleration-deceleration mechanism of energy transfer to the neck. It may result from rear-end or side-impact motor vehicle collisions, but can also occur through diving and other mishaps. The impact may result in bony or soft-tissue injuries (whiplash injury), which in turn may lead to a variety of clinical manifestations.*

Mechanism. A number of mechanisms have been proposed that result in a WAD. These include:

▶ Motor vehicle accidents.

▶ Sporting injuries involving a blow to the head or neck, or a heavy landing.

▶ Trauma to the neck or body.

▶ Pulls and thrusts on the arms.

▶ Falls, landing on the trunk or shoulder.

Perhaps the most common mechanism of WAD is the motor vehicle accident (MVA). According to reports, more than 1 million whiplash injuries occur each year in the United States.[196] Eighteen percent of MVAs involving passenger cars in the United States in 1994 were rear-end impacts.[205]

The extent of injury from a WAD following an MVA depends, in part, on three factors: (1) the position of the head at the point of impact (Fig. 23-63), (2) the amount of force involved, and (3) the direction of those forces (Fig. 23-64).

Head Position. Pure extension injuries seem to be uncommon in a WAD, because most injuries involve forced combinations of motion. These include a flexion or extension force applied to a rotated head and neck, resulting from a turned position on impact.[206] As many as 57 percent of persons sustaining whiplash injury, with symptoms persisting 2 years after collisions, reported having their heads rotated out of the anatomic position at

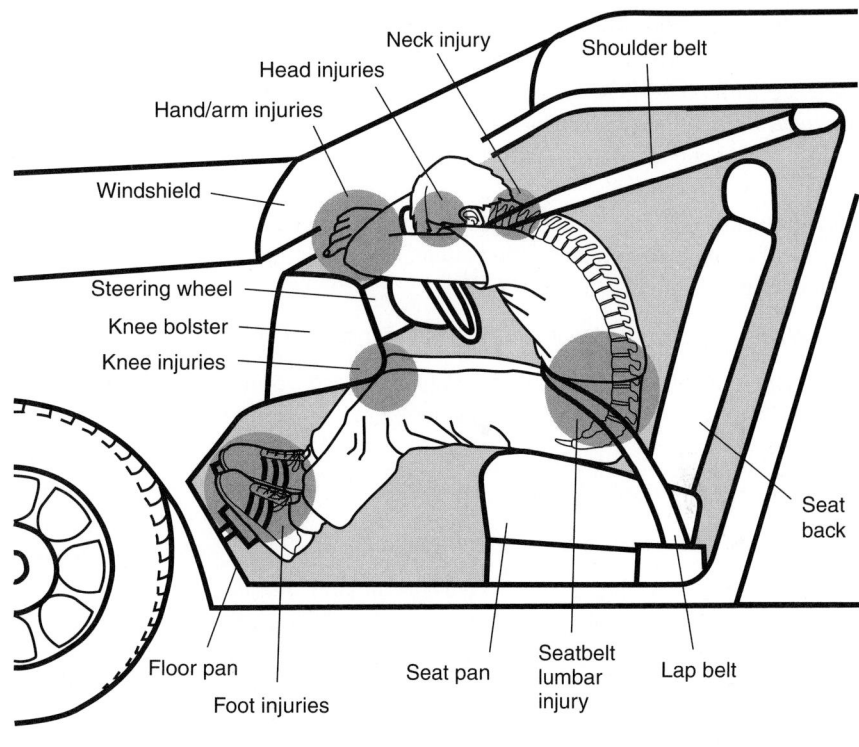

FIGURE 23-63 Human interaction with the interior of a car during a frontal crash. (Reproduced with permission from Murphy DR. *Conservative Management of Cervical Spine Syndromes.* New York, NY: McGraw-Hill; 2000:133.)

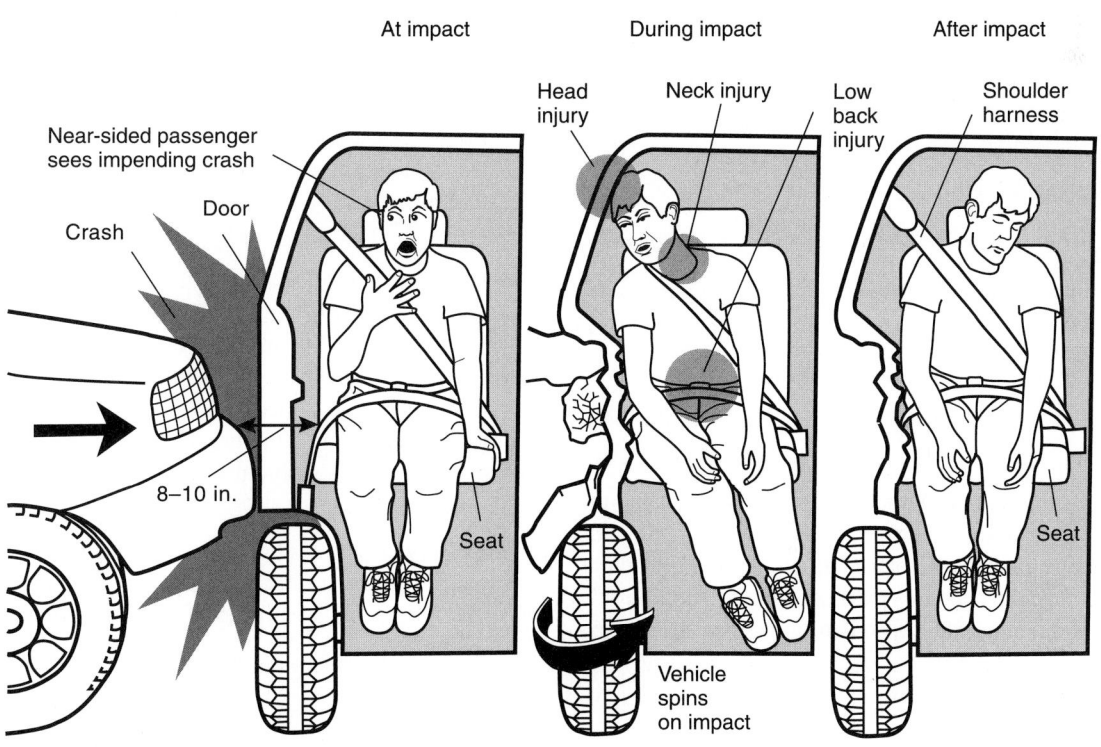

FIGURE 23-64 Occupant motion in a side crash. (Reproduced with permission from Murphy DR. *Conservative Management of Cervical Spine Syndromes.* New York, NY: McGraw-Hill; 2000:134.)

the time of impact.[207,208] In fact, head position has been reported as the only accident feature of a collision event that has a statistically significant correlation with symptom duration.[208]

Amount of Force. The amount of force applied to the neck is approximately equal to the weight of the head and the speed that the head moves. Consequently, the heavier the head or the faster it moves, the greater the stress that is put through the neck. However, it is well recognized by clinicians with any experience with post-MVA patients, that some patients who have survived high-velocity accidents do better than many who appear to have been involved in trivial impacts.

Force Direction. Force direction plays a significant role in the degree of damage sustained by the patient. The direction of the applied forces depends on[65]:

1. Where the car is hit; that is, front end, rear end, or side.

2. Symmetry of the impact; that is, directly head on or rear end, or the forward or backward side.

3. Whether the car is pushed ahead into another vehicle, the curb, or other stationary object.

4. Position of the victim in relation to the impact.

During the early phase of a rear-end collision, the occupant's trunk is forced upward toward the head, and the cervical spine undergoes a sigmoid deformation, resulting in the head being moved upward and backward.[209] During this motion, at about 100 msec after impact, the lower cervical vertebrae undergo extension, but without translation.[209] This motion causes the vertebral bodies to separate anteriorly, and the zygapophysial joints to impact posteriorly. These forces may lead to posterior dislocations.[200,210,211]

The reason for the greater severity of hyperextension injuries over the other force directions is believed to be related to several factors, including[203]:

▶ Whether the seat back breaks.

▶ Whether the occupant hits the front of the occupant space.

▶ The differential motion between the seat back and occupant.

▶ Hyperextension of the neck over the head restraint.

▶ Rebound neck flexion as the head rebounds off the head rest.

Hyperflexion injuries are typically less severe because the amount of head excursion is limited by the chin striking the chest. The damage incurred by cervical side-bending traumas depends on whether the head hits an object, or the shoulder.[65]

A number of other variables also determine the type and extent of the injury[203]:

▶ Seat position.

▶ Occupant size, height, and posture.

▶ Vehicle interior design.

▶ Size of vehicle.

▶ Sex of driver. Women generally position their seats more forward than men, which places their bodies closer to the front car structures, and therefore at higher risk of impacting the front interior.

▶ Seat belt. The subject of seatbelts is controversial, because the seatbelt appears to be responsible for more injuries than any other contact source in the car, albeit minor ones.[212] This is, in part, because of their design, which restrains only one shoulder, and because the belt acts as a fulcrum for energy concentration on the occupant.[203] As of 1997, federal law has required all passenger vehicles to have air bags. Mortality reductions in frontal collisions associated with airbags have been estimated to be no greater than 25 to 30 percent[203a] and perhaps substantially less[203b] when compared with the approximately 50 percent reduction associated with proper use of seat belts.[203c] Because airbags provide supplemental protection for occupants wearing a seat belt, it is necessary to compare the combined effect of airbags and seat belts relative to either device alone or completely unrestrained in order to adequately evaluate their effectiveness. A study by McGwin and colleagues[203d] conducted a retrospective cohort study of front seat occupants involved in police-reported, tow-away, frontal motor vehicle collisions using data from the 1995 through 2000 National Automotive Sampling System. Compared with completely unrestrained occupants, those using a seat belt alone or in combination with an airbag had a reduced overall risk of injury (relative risk, 0.42 and 0.71, respectively); no association was observed for those restrained with an airbag only (relative risk, 0.98). The study concluded that airbag deployment does not appear to significantly reduce the risk of injury either alone or in combination with seat belts.[203d] Population-based studies of airbag effectiveness against less serious injuries, which have been rare, seem to suggest that airbags may merely be altering the distribution of injuries.[203e,203f]

▶ Headrest height. Headrest height appears to play a role, with the driver often setting the head rest too low, or sitting too far forward to obtain adequate support from the head rest.[213,214] However, the fatal accidents involving hyperextension appear to occur in the absence of a head restraint, where there is no structural limitation to the head movement except anatomic structures.

Clinical Findings. It should be obvious that a meticulous examination of the traumatized patient is of paramount importance.[215] Signs and symptoms to alert the clinician include:

▶ Central nervous system signs.

▶ Periodic loss of consciousness.

▶ Patient does not move the neck, even slightly (fractured dens).

► Painful weakness of the neck muscles (fracture).

► Gentle traction and compression are painful (fracture).

► Severe muscle spasm (fracture).

► Complaints of dizziness.

The symptoms following a WAD usually begin in the neck and interscapular area within a few hours of the injury. Headaches often accompany the neck and shoulder girdle symptoms.[4]

Sources of Symptoms. The causes for symptoms following a whiplash injury are numerous. The resulting damage from a WAD can include an injury to one or more of the following types of structures:

► *Soft tissue structures.*[77] A cervical strain may be produced by an overload injury to the cervical muscle-tendon unit because of excessive forces. These forces can result in the elongation and tearing of muscles or ligaments, edema, hemorrhage, and inflammation. Many cervical muscles do not terminate in tendons, but instead attach directly to bone by myofascial tissue that blends into the periosteum.[216] Muscles respond to injury in a variety of ways, including reflex contraction, which further increases the resistance to stretch and serves as a protection to the injured muscle.

► *Joint capsule and ligaments.* Both mechanoreceptors and nociceptors have been identified in the human cervical joint capsule[217] and ligaments,[189] indicating a neural input in pain sensation and proprioception. Postmortem studies have found that after whiplash injuries, ligamentous injuries are extremely common in the cervical spine, but that herniation of the nucleus pulposus is a rare event.[218–221] The motion segment lesions found in the cervical spine included bruising and hemorrhage of the uncinate region, so-called rim lesions or transections of the anterior annulus fibrosus, rupture of the alar ligaments, and avulsions of the vertebral end plate.[218–222] As in the lumbar spine, the outer layers of the cervical annulus are innervated,[223] and are, therefore, a reasonable source of pain.[224]

► *Zygapophysial joint.* Fractures or contusions of the zygapophysial joints can occur, although postmortem studies reveal that many of these injuries are undetectable by plain radiographs.[218,225–227] Zygapophysial joint pain is the only basis for chronic neck pain after whiplash that has been subjected to scientific scrutiny.[190,228,229] However, it cannot be diagnosed clinically, or by medical imaging. The diagnosis relies on fluoroscopically guided, controlled diagnostic blocks of the painful joint. Although there is uncertainty about the exact pathway that elicits neck pain, the cervical zygapophysial joint has been identified as a source of pain in between 25 and 65 percent of people with neck pain.[189–192,230–232] Specifically, the prevalence of lower cervical facet joint pain has been reported to be 49 percent.[231] It is worth remembering that although so-called neck

sprains from motor vehicle accidents usually involve the cervical spine, one of the upper eight thoracic spinal joints is sometimes found to be affected, so these structures should be assessed in the examination of a whiplash injury.[233]

► *Central or peripheral neurologic systems.* These systems may be injured secondary to traction, impingement, hemorrhage, avulsion, or concussion. Although neck pain and headache are the two most common symptoms of a whiplash injury,[8] other symptoms such as visual disturbances, balance disorders, and altered cerebral function are reported. In 1927, Klein and Nieuwenhuyse[234] first demonstrated that simple rotation of the patient's neck, while the head was maintained fixed, caused vertigo and nystagmus. In 1976, Toglia[235] reported objective electronystagmography (ENG) abnormalities in about 57 percent of 309 patients with whiplash injuries. Wing and Hargrave-Wilson[236] reported that all of their 80 patients showed nystagmus in ENG records with the head flexed, extended, or rotated to the right and left. Abnormal peripheral vestibular function was found using platform posturography in about 90 percent of the 48 patients examined by Chester.[237] Fractures and dislocations, many causing cord damage, have been demonstrated on human victims of hyperextension injuries, who had no radiographic evidence of the severity of these lesions.[65,238]

► *Intervertebral disk.* Experimental and clinical studies have consistently demonstrated how poorly and slowly disk lesions heal after a hyperextension trauma, with very small lesions taking as long as 18 months to heal.[227,239] A follow-up study, averaging a review time of nearly eleven years,[240] found that 40 percent of patients were still having intrusive or severe symptoms (12 percent severe and 28 percent intrusive). The same study also found that in general, the symptoms did not alter after 2 years postaccident.

► *Dorsal root ganglia.*[227]

► *Vascular structures (vertebrobasilar arteries).* Postmortem studies[241] have shown that vertebral artery lesions are found in about one third of fatally injured motor vehicle accident victims with vertebral atlas injury.[242]

► *Visceral structures (secondary to ruptures, or contusions)*

The physical examination usually reveals tenderness over the transverse and spinous processes, or over the anterior vertebral body, depending on the structures involved. Depending on the severity of the strain, motion can be markedly restricted as a result of muscle guarding.

Other than perhaps to screen for possible fractures, there is no valid indication for medical imaging after whiplash, unless the patient has neurologic signs.[194] Findings on plain films are typically normal, although there may be a loss of the cervical lordosis. MRI reveals nothing but age-related changes with the same prevalence as in asymptomatic individuals.[243–245] An enticing, but small, recent study suggests that, in patients with persisting acute neck pain, single photon emission computed tomography, at 4 weeks after injury revealed occult, small fractures of the vertebral rims or the synovial joints of the neck.[246]

Intervention. Once the physician has ruled out the possibility of fracture, dislocation, IVD injury, or neurovascular compromise, a conservative approach is recommended. Initially, a cervical collar can be prescribed to reduce muscle guarding. Bed rest, along with analgesics and muscle relaxants, for no more than 2 to 3 days is prescribed for patients with a severe injury. However, in less severe cases, bed rest has not been shown to improve recovery and, when compared with mobilization or patient education, rest tends to prolong symptoms.[141,142]

Ice and electrical stimulation are applied to the neck during the first 48 to 72 hours to help control pain and inflammation. Range-of-motion exercises in the pain-free ranges of flexion and rotation are initiated as early as possible to reduce the likelihood of hypomobility. Gentle cervical isometrics also are introduced. Aggressive strengthening of the cervical musculature should not begin until full range of motion is restored. Strengthening of the trapezius muscle and other scapular stabilizers can be performed using upper extremity exercises, taking care to avoid an increase in symptoms.

Many patients improve within 8 weeks, although complete resolution is less common.[247] If pain persists for more than 3 months, more severe ligamentous, disk, associated zygapophysial joint injuries, or other factors (see later) should be suspected. If significant neck pain persists past 6 to 8 weeks, flexion and extension radiographs may be useful to exclude, or confirm, instability.

Outcomes. Studies addressing the natural history of WAD have yielded variable results. In one series, symptoms had resolved in 52 percent of patients at 8 weeks, and in 87 percent of the patients at 5 months.[248] In another series, most patients rapidly recovered following an acute injury, with some 80 percent being asymptomatic by 12 months.[207] After 12 months, between 15 and 20 percent of patients remained symptomatic, and only about 5 percent were severely affected. In addition to the distress resulting from neck and upper extremity pain, costs to society associated with absenteeism from work also are incurred.

The majority of studies reveal that, although most patients with WAD have a spontaneous resolution of symptoms, a small subgroup of patients are symptomatic beyond 1 year.[194] This group of patients constitutes the major burden to insurance companies and to health care resources, because in spite of aggressive imaging and diagnostic testing, clinicians are routinely unable to identify the specific source of these symptoms or apply interventions that are successful. It is in this small subgroup of patients with persisting chronic symptoms that the need for a better understanding of the risk factors, pathophysiology, natural history, and effectiveness of intervention options is apparent.[194]

When symptoms persist beyond 6 months, evidence for pre-existing degenerative disease is most often found.[249] Preexisting symptoms, such as headache, and radiologic degenerative changes appear to be important predictors for an unfavorable outcome.[85]

One study[207] examined a group of 117 consecutive patients, who were followed on a regular basis from shortly after the initial injury through 2 years, to determine whether preinjury status, mechanism of injury, physical examination, and somatic, radiographic, or neuropsychologic factors could be used to predict eventual outcome. At 2 years, the patients with persistent symptoms were found to have been older at the time of injury than the asymptomatic group, and had a higher incidence of pretraumatic headache. There was a higher incidence of a rotated, or inclined, head position at the time of impact, as well as a higher intensity of initial neck pain and headache, a higher incidence of initial radicular symptoms, a greater number of initial overall symptoms, and a higher average score on a multiple symptom analysis.[207]

Financial compensation, which is determined by the continued presence of pain and suffering, appears to provide a barrier to recovery and may promote persistent illness and disability. The incidence of insurance claims for whiplash is about 1 per 1000 population per year,[228] yet not all persons involved in motor vehicle crashes develop symptoms, and not all symptomatic patients experience chronic injury.

Integration of Patterns 4B, 4F, and 5F: Impaired Joint Mobility, Motor Function, Muscle Performance, Range of Motion Secondary to Impaired Posture, Systemic Dysfunction (Referred Pain Syndromes), Spinal Disorders, Myofascial Pain Dysfunction, Peripheral Nerve Entrapment

Thoracic Outlet Syndrome[127,250]

The thoracic outlet is the anatomic space bordered by the first thoracic rib, the clavicle, and the superior border of the scapula through which the great vessels and nerves of the upper extremity pass (Fig. 23-65). Thoracic outlet syndrome (TOS) is a clinical syndrome characterized by symptoms attributable to compression of the neural or vascular anatomic structures that pass through the thoracic outlet. The bony boundaries of the outlet include the clavicle, first rib, and scapula, and the outlet passage is further defined by the interscalene interval, a triangle with its apex directed superiorly. This triangle is bordered anteriorly by the anterior scalene muscle, posteriorly by the middle scalene muscle, and inferiorly by the first rib (see Fig. 23-65).

The other names used for TOS are based on descriptions of the potential sources for its compression. These names include cervical rib syndrome, scalenus anticus syndrome, hyperabduction syndrome, costoclavicular syndrome, pectoralis minor syndrome, and first thoracic rib syndrome.

TOS was first noted in 1743 when an association was made between the cervical rib and TOS, although it was not until 1818, that the medical management of thoracic outlet syndrome was discussed.[251] In the early 20th century, Adson stressed the role of the scalene muscles in neurovascular compromise, and Wright

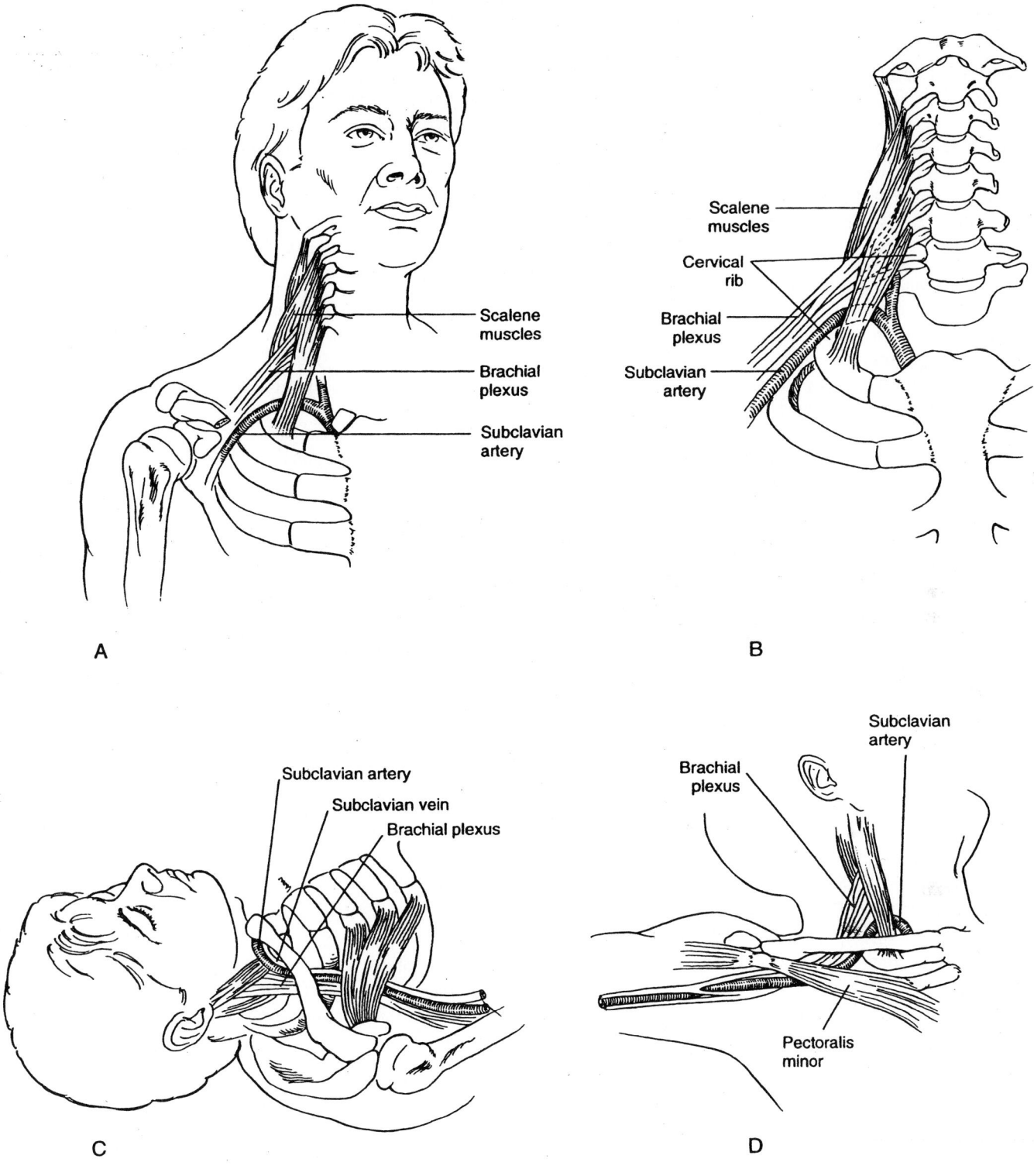

FIGURE 23-65 Sites of compression in thoracic outlet syndrome (TOS). (*A*) Scalenus anterior syndrome. (*B*) A cervical rib or a fibrous band can obstruct the neurovascular bundle. (*C*) Compression can occur between the clavicle and first rib. (*D*) Hyperabduction compresses the neurovascular bundle under the pectoralis minor tendon. (Reproduced with permission from Zachazewski JE, Magee DJ, Quillen WS. *Athletic Injuries and Rehabilitation*. Philadelphia, Pa: Saunders; 1996:447.)

showed that shoulder hyperabduction could produce thoracic outlet obstruction.[251] It was Peet[252] who coined the term "thoracic outlet syndrome" in 1956. Then, in the early 1960s, Roos[46] emphasized the importance of the first rib and its muscular and ligamentous attachments in causing thoracic outlet obstruction.

The lowest trunk of the brachial plexus, which is made up of rami from the C8 and T1 nerve roots, is the most commonly compressed neural structure in TOS. These nerve roots provide sensation to the fourth and fifth fingers of the hand and motor innervation to the hand intrinsic muscles.

The subclavian artery and the lower trunk of the plexus pass behind the clavicle, and into the costoclavicular space (see Fig. 23-65). From there they pass over the first rib, between the insertions of the anterior and middle scalene muscles, and are joined by the subclavian vein.

Thus, the course of the neurovascular bundle can be subdivided into three different sections, based on the areas of potential entrapment:

1. As the brachial plexus and subclavian artery pass through the interscalene triangle (see Fig. 23-65), interscalene triangle compression can result from injury of the scalene or scapular suspensory muscles. In some cases, fibromuscular bands can develop between the anterior and middle scalenes, or between the long transverse processes of the lower cervical vertebrae, producing entrapment. The subclavian vein is not involved, because it usually passes anterior to the anterior scalene muscle. Entrapment at this site also may result from cervical ribs, which are present in 0.2 percent of the population and occur bilaterally in 80 percent of those affected.[46] However, the presence of a cervical rib does not necessarily precipitate signs and symptoms, with fewer than 10 percent of individuals with cervical ribs ever experiencing TOS.[46]

2. As it passes the first rib, clavicle, and subclavius: the costoclavicular interval. Entrapment in this space between the rib cage and the posterior aspect of the clavicle may occur with clavicle depression, rib elevation caused by scalene hypertonicity, repetitive shoulder abduction, or a first rib-clavicular deformity. A postfracture callus formation of the first rib or clavicle can also increase the potential for entrapment.

3. As it passes the coracoid process, pectoralis minor, and clavipectoral fascia to enter the axillary fossa. At this point, the subclavian artery and vein become the axillary artery and vein. At this third site, the neurovascular bundle can be compromised with arm abduction or elevation, especially if external rotation is superimposed on the motion. Pectoralis minor tendon compression is associated with shoulder hyperabduction. During hyperabduction, the tendon insertion and the coracoid act as a fulcrum about which the neurovascular structures are forced to change direction. Hypertrophy of the pectoralis minor tendon has also been noted as a cause of outlet compression.[251]

There may be multiple points of compression of the peripheral nerves between the cervical spine and hand, in addition to the thoracic outlet. When there are multiple compression sites, less pressure is required at each site to produce symptoms. Thus, a patient may have concomitant TOS, ulnar nerve compression at the elbow, and carpal tunnel syndrome. This phenomenon has been called the *multiple crush syndrome*.[253]

Symptoms vary from mild to limb threatening, and might be ignored by many clinicians as they mimic common but difficult to treat conditions such as tension headache or fatigue syndromes. The chief complaint is usually one of diffuse arm and shoulder pain, especially when the arm is elevated beyond 90 degrees. Potential symptoms include pain localized in the neck, face, head, upper extremity, chest, shoulder, or axilla; and upper extremity paresthesias, numbness, weakness, heaviness, fatigability, swelling, discoloration, ulceration, or Raynaud phenomenon.[250] Neural compression symptoms occur more commonly than vascular symptoms.[46]

Karas[254] described five symptom patterns of thoracic outlet syndrome, characterized by the primary structures compressed.

1. The lower trunk pattern reflects lower plexus compression and manifests with pain in the supraclavicular and infraclavicular fossa, back of the neck, rhomboid area, axilla, and medial arm, and may radiate into the hand and fourth and fifth fingers. The history includes reports of feelings of coldness, or electric shock sensations in the C8 to T1, or ulnar nerve distributions.

2. The upper trunk pattern results from upper plexus compression and is distinguished by pain in the anterolateral neck, shoulder, mandible, and ear, and paresthesias that radiate into the upper chest and lateral arm in the C5 to C7 dermatomes.[126,254]

3. With venous involvement, the signs and symptoms can include swelling of the entire limb, nonpitting edema, bluish discoloration, and venous collateralization across the superior chest and shoulder.

4. Arterial involvement produces coolness, ischemic episodes, and exertional fatigue.[254]

5. The mixed pattern consists of a combination of vascular and neurologic symptoms.[254]

Mechanisms.   Proposed mechanisms for TOS include:

▶ *Traumatic.*   Twenty-one to 75 percent of TOS patients have an association with trauma.[126] This may involve macrotrauma, as in the case of a MVA, or microtrauma, as in the case of a muscle strain of the scapular stabilizers resulting from repetitive overhead activities.[255–257]

▶ *Developmental.*   During the normal growth of children and adolescents, the scapulae gradually descend upon the posterior thorax, with the descent being slightly greater in women than in men. A strain injury to the scapular suspensory muscles, which lengthen in conjunction with scapular descent during normal development, is known to be associated with TOS. These facts help to explain the rarity of symptomatic TOS until after puberty, and the increased prevalence in women.[127,258]

Diagnosis.   TOS is a clinical diagnosis, made almost entirely on the basis of the history and physical examination. To help rule out other conditions that can mimic TOS, the physical examination should include:

▶ A careful inspection of the spine, thorax, shoulder girdles, and upper extremities for postural abnormalities, shoulder asymmetry, muscle atrophy, excessively large breasts, obesity, and drooping of the shoulder girdle.

▶ Palpation of the supraclavicular fossa for fibromuscular bands, percussion for brachial plexus irritability, and auscultation for vascular bruits that appear by placing the upper extremity in the position of vascular compression.

▶ Assessment of the neck and shoulder girdle for active and passive ranges of motion, areas of tenderness, or other signs of intrinsic disease.

▶ A thorough neurologic examination of the upper extremity, including a search for sensory and motor deficits and abnormalities of deep tendon reflexes.

▶ Assessment of respiration to ensure patient is using correct abdominodiaphragmatic breathing.

▶ Assessment of the suspensory muscles: the middle and upper trapezius, levator scapulae, and SCM (thoracic outlet "openers"). These muscles typically are found to be weak.

▶ Assessment of the scapulothoracic muscles: the anterior and middle scalenes, subclavius, pectoralis minor and major (thoracic outlet "closers"). These muscles typically are found to be adaptively shortened.

▶ First rib position or presence of cervical rib.

▶ Clavicle position and history of prior fracture, producing abnormal callous formation or malalignment.

▶ Scapula position, acromioclavicular joint mobility, and sternoclavicular joint mobility.

▶ Neurophysiologic tests, which are useful to exclude coexistent pathologies such as peripheral nerve entrapment or cervical radiculopathy. An abnormal reflex F wave conduction and decreased sensory action potentials in the medial antebrachial cutaneous nerve may be diagnostic.[259]

Intervention. Conservative intervention should be attempted before surgery and should be directed toward muscle relaxation, relief of inflammation, and attention to posture. This intervention approach may require a change of occupation for the patient, because TOS is more common in those who stoop at work. Aggressive physical therapy, particularly traction, may worsen symptoms.[260]

The focus of the intervention is the correction of postural abnormalities of the neck and shoulder girdle, strengthening of the scapular suspensory muscles, stretching of the scapulothoracic muscles, and mobilization of the whole shoulder complex and the first and second ribs.

Kenny and colleagues[261] prospectively evaluated a group of 8 patients, composed mainly of middle-aged women, whose TOS was treated with a supervised physical therapy program of graduated resisted shoulder elevation exercises.[127] All patients showed major symptomatic improvement.

If symptoms progress or fail to respond within 4 months, surgical intervention should be considered.[262] Lower plexus

TOS is surgically treated by first rib and (if present) cervical rib excision.[263] Although it has been suggested that the insured patient is more likely to have an operation, results are independent of any associated litigation.[264]

Therapeutic Techniques

Techniques to Increase Joint Mobility

Joint Mobilizations

The purpose of joint mobilization techniques is to:

▶ Reduce stresses through both the fixation and leverage components of the spine.

▶ Reduce stresses through hypermobile segments by mobilizing the hypomobile joints.

▶ Reduce the overall force needed by the clinician, thus giving greater control.

The selection of a manual technique is dependent on several factors, including:

▶ The acuteness of the condition, the cause of the restriction, and the goal of the intervention. If the structure is acutely painful (pain is felt before resistance or pain is felt with resistance), pain relief, rather than a mechanical effect, is the major goal. Joint oscillations (grades I and II) that do not reach the end of range are used. The segment or joint is left in its neutral position and the mobilization is carried out from that point.

▶ Whether the restriction is symmetric, involving both sides of the segment, or asymmetric, involving only one side of the segment.

A number of specific manual techniques can be employed. Spinal locking techniques can be used to augment the comfort and safety of a manual technique. Locking is simply a method of taking up any available soft tissue tension or slack, thereby making a manual technique more specific. Two types of locking techniques are commonly advocated, craniovertebral locking and locking through segmental translation. Because of the potential for vertebral artery compromise in the craniovertebral region, the craniovertebral joints are often "locked" first before continuing motion into the middle and/or lower cervical spine joints.

Craniovertebral Locking[264a,264b]

In the following example, a left side-bending technique is used. Although this locking technique may be used with the patient positioned in sitting or supine, if it used in supine it is important to apply a small amount of compression to compensate for the loss of the spinal loading due to the weight of the head.

While palpating the C2 spinous process the clinician slowly left side-bends the patient's head. If the side bending is performed around a sagittal craniovertebral axis, the C2 spinous process should be felt to move to the right, indicating left rotation of the C2 on the C3. Maintaining the left side-bent position, the head is now rotated to the right until the C2 spinous process regains a central position. The head is again side-bent slightly to the left, and the C2 spinous process de-rotated back to midline. These motions are continued until a firm end-feel is reached. At this point, motion in the craniovertebral joints has now been exhausted, while the rest of the cervical joints remain in neutral. Being careful to maintain the position of the head, especially the right rotation, the side bending is continued left to the middle or lower cervical level required. As the cervical joints are prevented from rotating to the left, the middle cervical side bending motion is exhausted very quickly.

Segmental Translation[264a,264b]

In the following example, a left side bending of C3–4 will be described. The patient is positioned in supine, with the clinician at the head of the bed. The clinician cradles the patient's head with both hands and places the pad of the index fingers of each hand across the neural arches of C3. The clinician then applies a right translatory (shearing) force on the C3 neural arch while keeping the head and upper neck in neutral. A firm end-feel is achieved as the soft tissue slack is taken up in the joints below. Thus, at the C3–4 level there is a normal congruent set of motions occurring, e.g., left side bending/rotation with right translation. This correlates with the desired direction of the mobilization. However, at the levels below there is an incongruent set of motions occurring, e.g., right side bending/rotation with right translation, resulting in a locking of these segments.

The vast majority of biomechanical dysfunctions of the cervical spine involve the posterior quadrant (a loss of extension and a loss of side bending and rotation to one side or both). The loss of cervical flexion is usually associated with a cervical disk protrusion, a cervicothoracic dysfunction, or a craniovertebral dysfunction. However, for completeness, the techniques described here will address a loss in both the anterior and posterior quadrants.

The C4 to C5 level is used in the following examples.

Basic Techniques to Restore Motion in the Posterior Quadrant

Seated Mobilization Technique to Restore Extension and Left Side Bending-rotation. If the clinician has large hands, mobilizing into extension can be a problem, because the stabilizing hand prevents the full glide into extension from occurring. To overcome this problem, the stabilization of the inferior segment is performed by pushing the thumb up against the side of its spinous process, thereby preventing the rotation induced by the mobilization of the superior segment. For example, if the left side of C4 to C5 is being mobilized into extension, left side bending, and left rotation by the upper hand, the thumb of the inferior hand is pushed against the right side of the C5 spinous process, preventing rotation of C5 to the right (Fig. 23-66).

Supine Mobilization Technique to Restore Extension and Right Side Bending-rotation.[112] The patient is positioned supine, with the head supported on a pillow. The clinician stands at the patient's head, facing the shoulders. With the radial aspect of the right index finger, the clinician palpates the spinous process and the

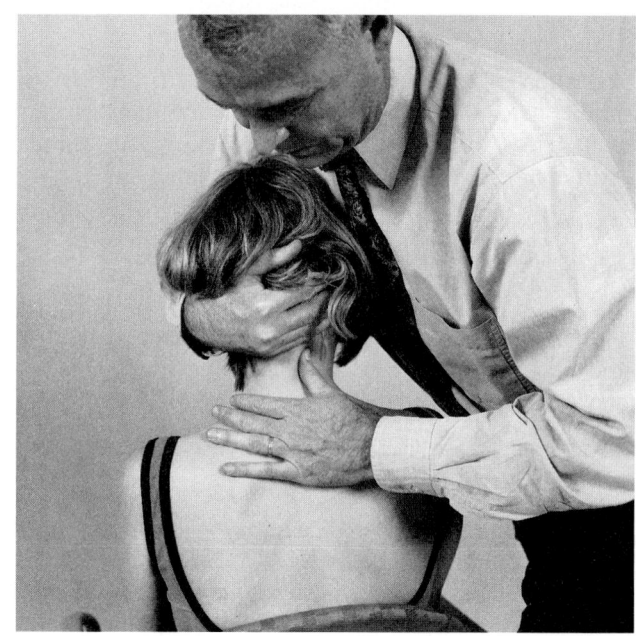

FIGURE 23-66 Seated mobilization to increase extension and left side bending rotation.

right inferior articular process of the C4 vertebra. With the other hand, the clinician supports the head and neck superior to the level being treated. A lock of the superior segment is accomplished by right side-flexing and left rotating the C3–4 joint complex, leaving the craniovertebral joints in a neutral position (Fig. 23-67). The motion barrier for extension, right side bending, and right rotation of C4 to C5 is then localized by pushing

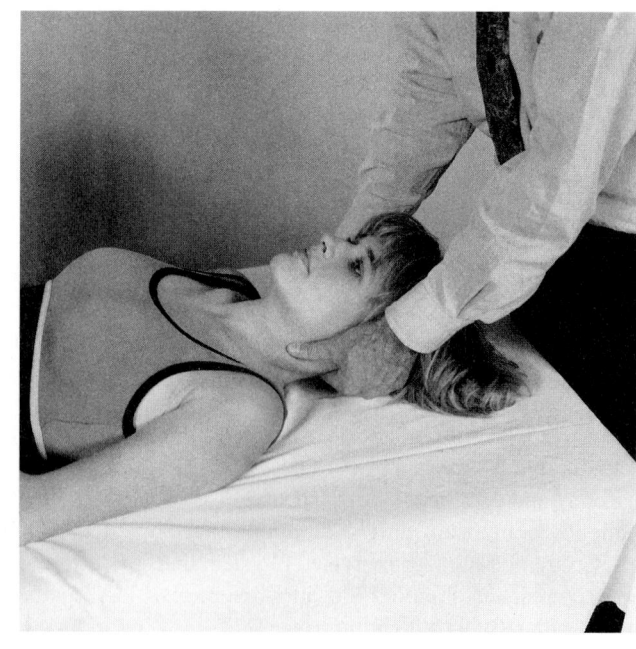

FIGURE 23-67 Supine mobilization into extension and right side bending rotation.

the right inferior articular process of C4 in a posteroinferior and medial direction on C5.

▶ *Passive.* The clinician applies a grade I to V force to the C4 vertebra to produce a posteroinferor and medial glide of the right zygapophysial joint at C4 to C5.

▶ *Active.* From the motion barrier, the patient is asked to turn the eyes in a direction that facilitates further extension, right side bending, and right rotation. The isometric contraction is held for up to 5 seconds and followed by a period of complete relaxation. The joint is then passively taken to the new motion barrier. The technique is repeated three times and followed by a reexamination of joint function.

Basic Techniques to Restore Motion in the Anterior Quadrant

Seated Mobilization Technique to Restore Flexion and Right Side Bending-rotation. The patient is positioned sitting, and the clinician stands on the right side. Using one hand, the clinician stabilizes the C5 segment using a lumbrical grip (Fig. 23-68). The other hand reaches around the head of the patient, securing it to the clinician's chest, and the ulnar border of the fifth finger is applied to the left transverse process and neural arch of C4. The C4 to C5 segment is then flexed and rotated to the right to the barrier of the left joint (see Fig. 23-68). The mobilization is carried out by the clinician applying pressure into flexion and right rotation.

▶ *Passive.* A grade I to IV mobilization force is applied to the C4 vertebra to produce a superoanterior glide at the zygapophysial joints, thus flexing the C4 to C5 joint complex and feeling the spinous processes separate.

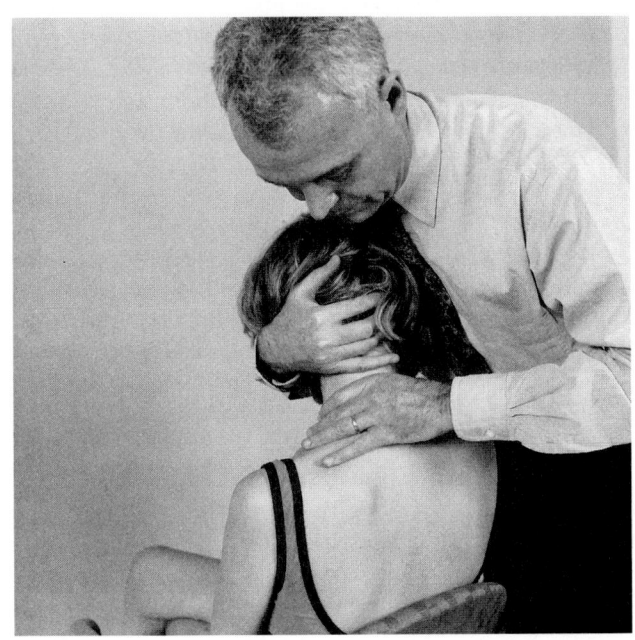

FIGURE 23-68 Seated mobilization into flexion and right side bending rotation.

▶ *Active.* At the motion barrier, the patient is instructed to turn the eyes in a direction that facilitates further flexion at C4 to C5. The isometric contraction is held for up to 5 seconds and followed by a period of complete relaxation. The joint is then passively taken to the new motion barrier. The technique is repeated three times and followed by a reexamination of joint function.

Supine Mobilization Technique to Restore Flexion and Left Side Bending-rotation. The patient is positioned supine, with the head supported. The clinician stands at the head of the table facing the patient. The C4 to C5 segment is flexed, left side bent, and right translated to bring the right joint to its flexion barrier. The clinician hooks a fingertip under the right articular process and lays a fingertip pad over the articular process on the left. The mobilization is achieved by pulling the right process cranially as steady light pressure is applied to the back of the left process to maintain a normal axis of motion.

▶ *Passive.* A grade I to V mobilization force is applied to the C4 vertebra to produce a superoanterior and medial glide of the right zygapophysial joint at C4 to C5.

▶ *Active.* At the motion barrier, the patient is instructed to turn the eyes in a direction that facilitates further flexion, left side bending, and rotation at C4 to C5. The isometric contraction is held for up to 5 seconds and followed by a period of complete relaxation. The joint is then passively taken to the new motion barrier. This technique is repeated three times and followed by a reexamination of function.

Mobilizations with Movement[265]

To Improve Flexion. The patient is positioned sitting, with the clinician standing to the side, facing the patient. The patient's head is held in neutral against the clinician's lower chest and the distal phalanx of the little finger is hooked under the spinous process of the superior vertebra of the segment being treated. The rest of the fingers wrap around the patient's neck to provide firm support, and the wrist is extended, with the forearm placed in the plane of the facets (Fig. 23-69). The lateral border of the thenar eminence of the other hand is placed below the little finger (see Fig. 23-69), and the palm of the hand rests on the upper back of the patient.

The patient is asked to flex the neck, and the glide of the superior segment is produced along the correct plane by a pull from the little finger in an anterior and superior direction, while the other hand stabilizes the lower segment.

This technique can be taught as part of the patient's home exercise program using a towel, belt, or strap.

To Improve Extension. The patient is positioned sitting, with the clinician standing to the side, facing the patient. The patient's head is held in neutral against the clinician's lower chest and the distal phalanx of the little finger is hooked under the spinous process of the superior vertebra of the segment being treated. Using a key grip between the index finger and thumb, the

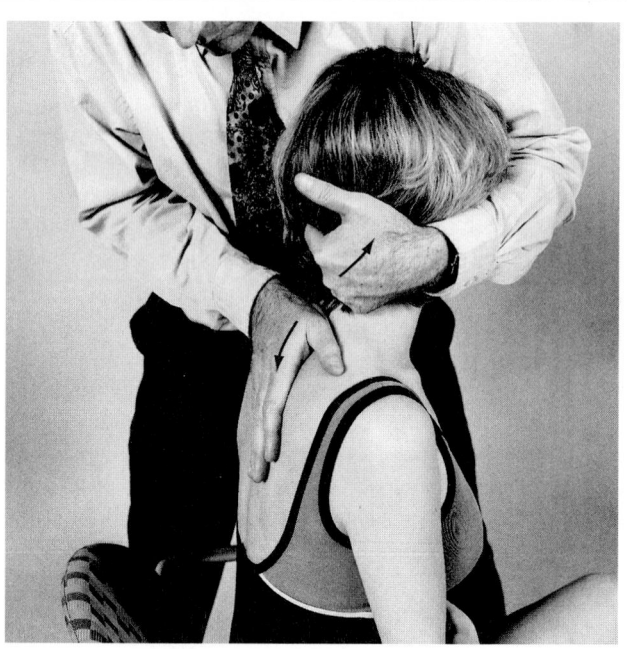

FIGURE 23-69   Mobilization with movement to improve cervical flexion.

clinician places the grip over the articular pillar on either side of the inferior spinous process of the segment (Fig. 23-70).

The patient is asked to extend the neck while the clinician simultaneously applies a glide of the inferior vertebra by pushing with the key grip hand.

This technique can be taught as part of the patient's home exercise program using a towel, belt, or a strap (Fig. 23-71).

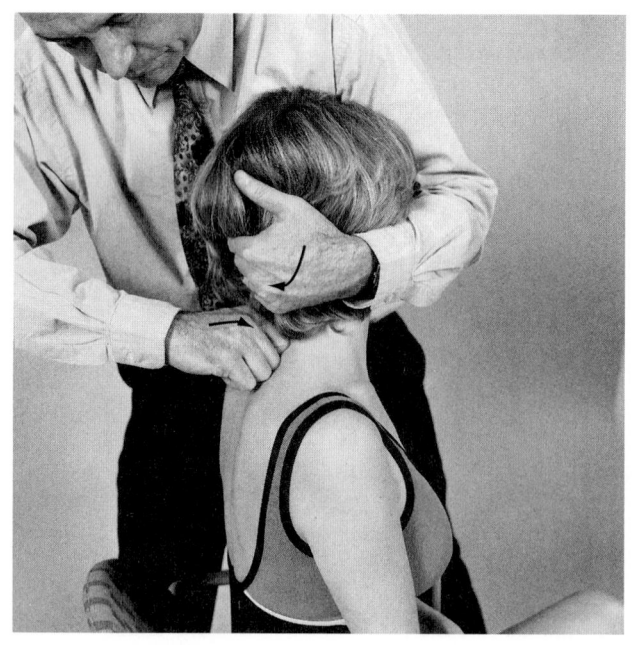

FIGURE 23-70   Mobilization with movement to improve cervical extension.

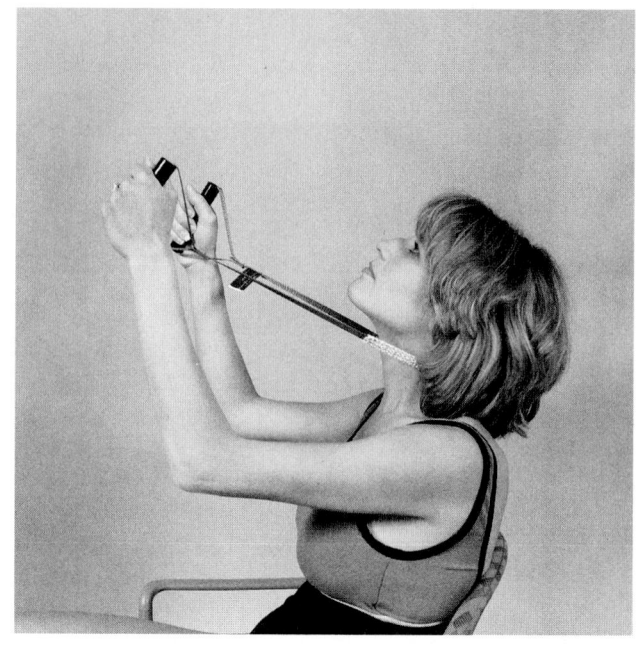

FIGURE 23-71   Home exercise to improve cervical extension.

To Improve Rotation to the Left.   The patient is positioned sitting, with the clinician sitting behind. The clinician places the thumb of one hand over the articular pillar over the left aspect of the spinous process of the superior vertebra of the segment to be treated. The other thumb is placed over the first thumb to help reinforce. The remaining fingers of the two hands are placed around the neck and upper back.

The patient is asked to rotate the head and neck slowly to the left, while the clinician simultaneously applies the glide along the correct joint plane using pressure from both thumbs.

This technique can be taught as part of the patient's home exercise program using a towel, belt, or a strap (Fig. 23-72).

The same technique can be used to improve cervical rotation to the right by altering the position of the thumbs.

Automobilizations

To Increase Side Glide.   To increase the side glide of the cervical spine, the patient is placed in the raised side-lying position, resting on the elbow, so that the body is raised at a 45-degree angle from the bed. From this position, the patient performs a side glide of the neck toward the bed, without allowing any side flexion to occur. This exercise can be progressed to the upright position, in which the patient elevates both arms and clasps the palm of the hands together. The side glide motion is performed to both sides. To add resistance to this exercise, the patient is positioned in complete side lying and the side glide is performed away from the bed. In each of these exercises, it is important that the patient incorporate a minimum amount of side-flexion of the neck.

To Increase Cervicothoracic Junction Extension.   A high-backed chair is used to stabilize the thoracic spine, with the top of the

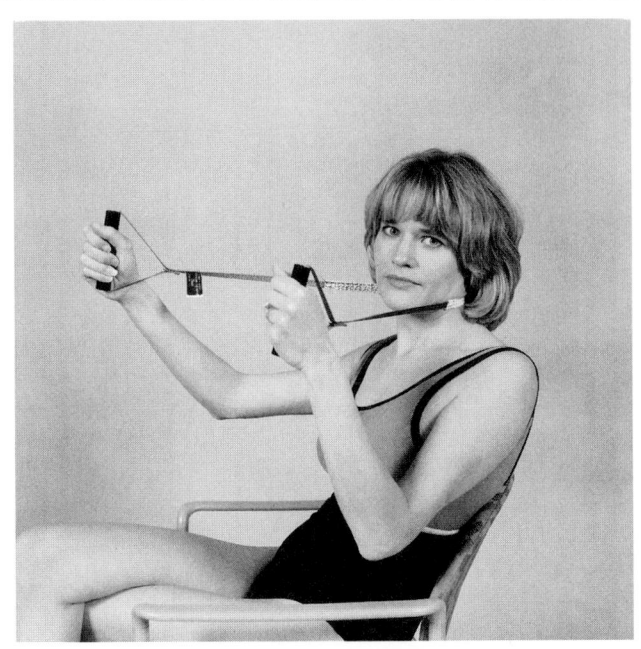

FIGURE 23-72   Home exercise to improve cervical rotation to the left.

high back positioned level with the segment just inferior to the hypomobile segment. The patient places his or her hands around the midcervical spine, with the fingers clasped together and the forearms parallel to the floor. The index fingers of the patient's clasped hands are placed over the hypermobile segment. The exercise is performed by asking the patient to raise the chin and forearms together while simultaneously maintaining the thoracic spine against the chair back (Fig. 23-73). A slight anterior force can be applied by the index fingers to prevent the hypermobile segment from extending too far. A towel or strap can be used in place of the index fingers.

Self-traction.[265]   The patient is seated. The patient places the fist of one hand with the thumb comfortably against the throat. The index finger of the other hand is placed under the occiput, and the remaining fingers are placed on the back of the head (Fig. 23-74). The patient flexes the head and neck in a forward and down direction so that the chin compresses the fist. From this position, the patient pulls the occiput superiorly and maintains the pull for 10 to 20 seconds.

Techniques to Increase Soft Tissue Extensibility

A variety of soft tissue techniques for the cervical region is available to the clinician. The choice of technique depends on the goals of the treatment and the dysfunction being treated.

Myofascial Trigger Point Therapy

Ischemic compression is advocated for myofascial trigger points and is achieved by sustaining direct pressure over a trigger point, using the thumb to apply pressure.[247] The pressure is held for 5 to 7 seconds and then quickly withdrawn.[266] The procedure is repeated on each trigger point. After each trigger point has been treated, the clinician returns to the first trigger point. The procedure is repeated three times on each trigger point.[266]

To facilitate self-treatment for inaccessible regions such as the rhomboid muscles, lying on a tennis ball or using the handle of a cane can be substituted for direct manual compression.[247]

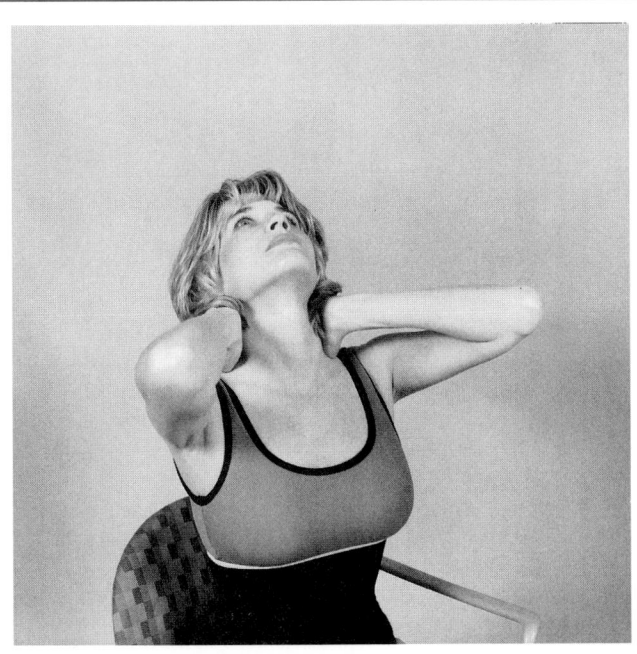

FIGURE 23-73   Cervical extension.

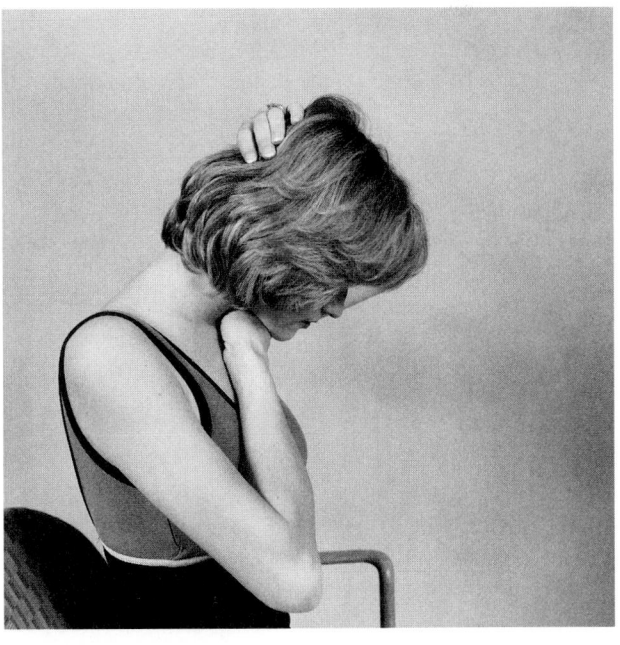

FIGURE 23-74   Self-traction technique.

General Soft Tissue Techniques

Prone. The patient is positioned prone, with the clinician standing to the side of the patient. The following areas are massaged:

▶ *Paraspinal gutter.* The clinician uses a thumb to apply a deep massage to the entire length of the paraspinal gutter.

▶ *Upper trapezius.* The clinician uses the heel of the palm and massages the upper trapezius. The clinician also can use the fingers to knead the upper trapezius muscle along the direction of its fibers.

Side Lying

Scapular Distraction. The patient is in the side lying position, and the clinician stands, facing the patient. Reaching over the back of the patient, the clinician grasps the scapula by sliding the fingers underneath and manually distracts the scapula away from the patient's back.

Scapular Rotations. The patient is in the side lying position, with the clinician standing to the side of the patient. The clinician takes the patient's arm and tucks it between his or her own arm and trunk. Reaching over the patient, the clinician grasps the whole shoulder girdle and rotates it in a full circle. This is done repeatedly, producing a rhythmic motion.

Supine. The patient is positioned supine, with the clinician at the head of the bed. The clinician wraps both hands around the back of the patient's neck, attempting to reach as low on the cervical spine as possible. The clinician then leans forward so that the front of his or her shoulder rests on the patient's forehead. By compressing the patient's head and gently grasping the back of the patient's neck, a longitudinal distraction is applied (see Fig. 23-46).

Seated. The patient is seated with the arms crossed, forearms grasped, and head resting on the hands. The clinician stands in front of the patient and threads his or her arms through the patient's arms, before resting both of his or her hands on the top, and back, of each of the patient's shoulders (Fig. 23-75). By gently leaning the patient forward, the cervical spine is extended until the stiff segment is located. Gradually, the clinician increases the amount of cervical extension by gently kneading the midscapular area. Distraction, side flexion, or rotation motions also may be introduced. Care should be taken to avoid overextending the lumbar spine during this technique by pulling the patient too far forward.

Flexibility

Various techniques can be helpful to stretch the noncontractile elements of soft tissues.[267,268] The patient may be instructed on proper stretching technique that can be done one to two times per day. Gentle, prolonged stretching is recommended. This is best done after a warm-up activity, such as using an exercise bike or brisk walking. Active or passive ranges of motion typically are more effective for the mechanical component of pain.[247]

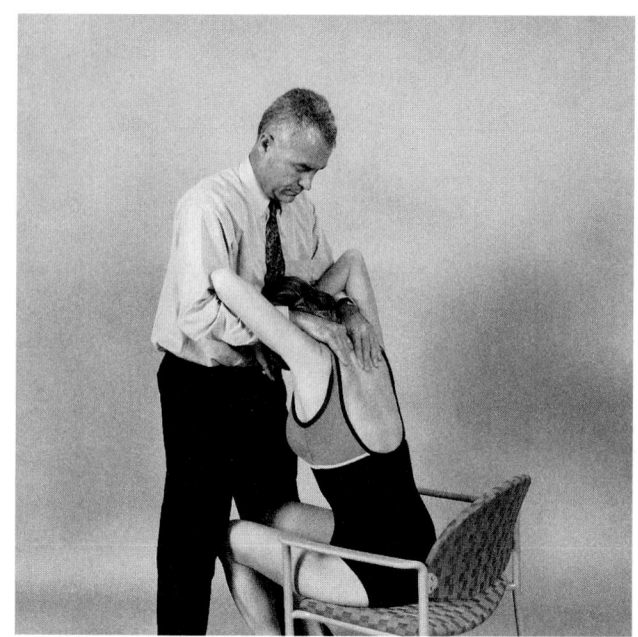

FIGURE 23-75 Seated mobilization into extension.

Muscle Stretching

Pectoralis Minor. The pectoralis minor can be stretched effectively using a corner and placing the forearms on the walls. The patient needs to avoid adopting a forward head posture during the stretch. The patient attempts to move the shoulders, against the wall, into horizontal adduction and internal rotation (Fig. 23-76). The clinician is cautioned against using this exercise with any patient with shoulder pathology, especially an anterior instability.

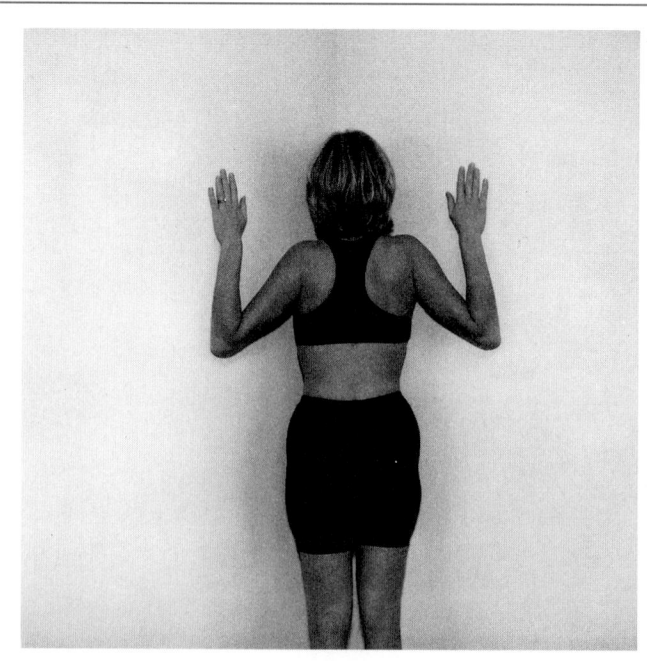

FIGURE 23-76 Pectoralis minor stretch.

Pectoralis Major. The pectoralis major can be specifically stretched if the orientation of its fibers is considered (clavicular and costosternal) by having the patient lie supine and extending the arm off the table in either approximately 140 degrees of shoulder abduction (costosternal fibers) or approximately 45 to 50 degrees of abduction (clavicular fibers).

A tight muscle is one that is hypertonic in addition to being shortened. The recommended treatment for muscle tightness is the postfacilitation stretch technique developed by Janda[89] (see Chap. 11):

1. The patient and the muscle being treated must be completely at rest.

2. The clinician is positioned so that he or she can provide sufficient resistance to the contraction by the patient.

3. The muscle to be treated is placed in its midrange.

4. The patient is asked to perform a maximal contraction of the muscle. If the clinician is unable to resist a maximal contraction, a submaximal one is used. The contraction is held for 10 seconds. After the contraction, the patient is instructed to completely let go of the muscle.

5. When the clinician is sure that the muscle is completely relaxed, a fast stretch is applied to it, and the stretch is held for 10 to 15 seconds.

6. The muscle is returned to its midrange.

7. The procedure is repeated three to five times.

Sternocleidomastoid. The SCM functions to flex and rotate the neck and extend the occipito-atlantal joint. The patient is positioned sitting or supine. The same technique that is used to assess the length of this muscle is used for the stretch (see Fig. 23-30). The patient is positioned supine, with the head supported. From this position, the clinician induces side bending of the neck to the contralateral side, and extension of the neck. The clinician stabilizes the scapula and rotates the patient's head and neck toward the ipsilateral side.

Anterior and Middle Scalenes. The patient is positioned supine. After stabilizing the first two ribs with the heel of one hand, the clinician performs passive cervical extension, contralateral side bending, and ipsilateral rotation (see Fig. 23-31).

Levator Scapulae. The same technique that is used to assess the length of this muscle is used for the stretch (see Fig. 23-29). The stretch can be passively applied by the clinician. The patient is positioned supine, with the head at the edge of the table. The elbow and hand of the side to be treated are placed above the head. The clinician stands at the head of the table and presses his or her thigh against the point of the patient's elbow, fixing it caudally. Using both hands, the clinician then flexes the neck and side flexes the patient's head to the opposite side, until resistance is felt (Fig. 23-77). The patient is then asked to look toward the treated side, a motion that is resisted by the

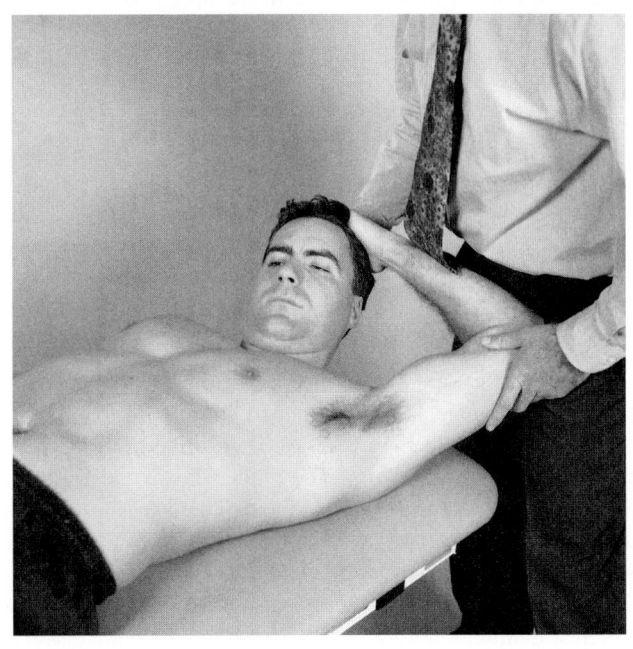

FIGURE 23-77 Levator scapulae stretch on left.

clinician. When the patient relaxes, the clinician moves the head into further side flexion and flexion.

Upper Trapezius. This procedure is similar to that of the levator scapulae except that the amount of neck flexion is reduced. The same technique that is used to assess the length of this muscle is used for the stretch (see Fig. 23-27). The patient is positioned supine, with the head at the edge of the table. The elbow and hand of the side to be treated are placed above the head. The clinician stands at the head of the table and presses his or her thigh against the point of the patient's elbow, fixing it caudally. Using both hands, the clinician then flexes the neck and side bends the patient's head to the opposite side. Rotation to the ipsilateral side is then added until resistance is felt. The patient is then asked to look toward the treated side, a motion that is resisted by the clinician. When the patient relaxes, the clinician moves the head into further flexion, side bending, and rotation.

In addition to the muscles described here, the clinician should assess the following muscles for adaptive shortening:

▶ Rectus capitis posterior major.

▶ Rectus capitis posterior minor.

▶ Obliquus capitis inferior.

▶ Obliquus capitis superior.

The stretches for these muscles are described in Chapter 22.

Self-stretching Techniques

Levator Scapulae. The patient is positioned supine, with the head on a pillow, placing the cervical spine in flexion. The patient's head is positioned in side bending and rotation in the opposite direction of the muscle to be stretched. A stretching cord with a loop at each end is given to the patient. The patient grasps one of the loops on the side of the muscle to be stretched, and places the foot on the same side as the muscle to be stretched in the loop at the opposite end of the cord. The cord is adjusted so that it is taut with the knee flexed. The patient is asked to elevate the scapula on the same side of the muscle to be stretched and to hold that position for 5 to 8 seconds before relaxing. The patient is then asked to extend the knee to exert a downward force on the scapula, via the cord, moving it into depression. The stretch is repeated three to five times.

The patient also can use the technique depicted in Figure 23-78.[269] The patient can be instructed on how to self-stretch the levator scapulae at home. The self-stretch of the left levator scapulae, depicted in Figure 23-78, is described.[269] The patient is seated with good posture. The patient flexes the neck fully. Using the fingers of the right hand, the patient grasps the left aspect of the head. Gentle pressure is applied with the fingers to side bend the head to the right while maintaining the neck flexion. The side bending continues until a gentle stretch is felt. The stretch is maintained for 8 to 10 seconds and then the patient relaxes. The stretch is repeated 10 times.

Upper Trapezius. The patient can be instructed on how to self-stretch the upper trapezius at home. The self-stretch of the left upper trapezius, depicted in Figure 23-79, is described.[269] The patient is seated with good posture. Using the fingers of the right hand, the patient grasps the left aspect of the head. Gentle pressure is applied with the fingers to side bend the head to the right. The side bending continues until a gentle stretch is felt. The stretch is maintained for 8 to 10 seconds and then the patient relaxes. The stretch is repeated 10 times.

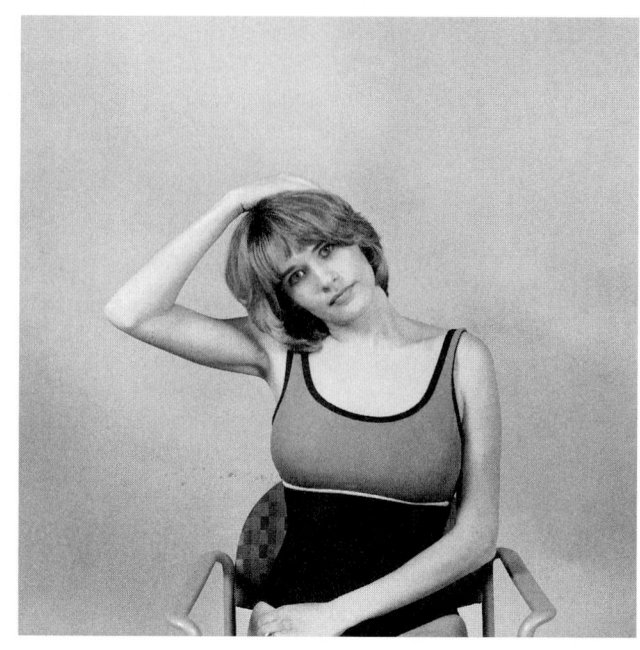

FIGURE 23-79   Self-stretch of the upper trapezius.

Three-finger Exercise. Active range of motion in the cervical spine can be increased through patient participation, using the three-finger exercise.[270] The patient's mandible rests on digits two, three, and four. The motions of flexion (Fig. 23-80), side bending (Fig. 23-81), and rotation (Fig. 23-82) can all be performed.

The patient is cautioned against reproducing sharp pain, while attempting to feel a stretch at the end of the available motion.

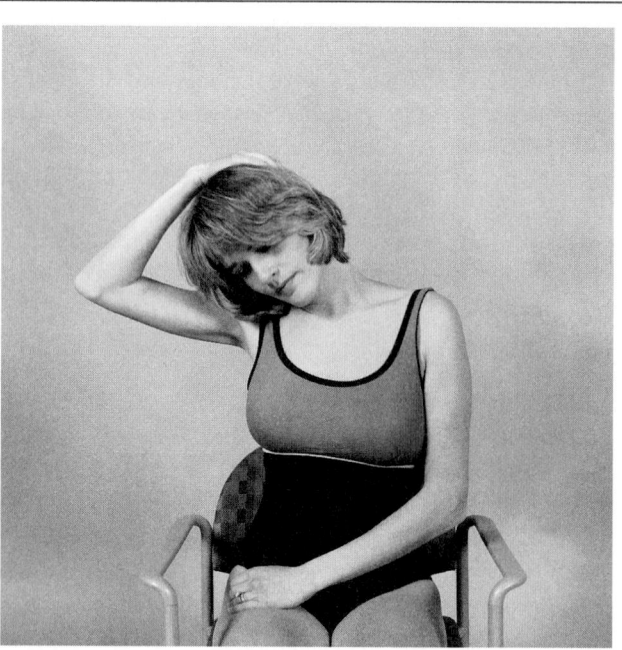

FIGURE 23-78   Self-stretch of the levator scapulae.

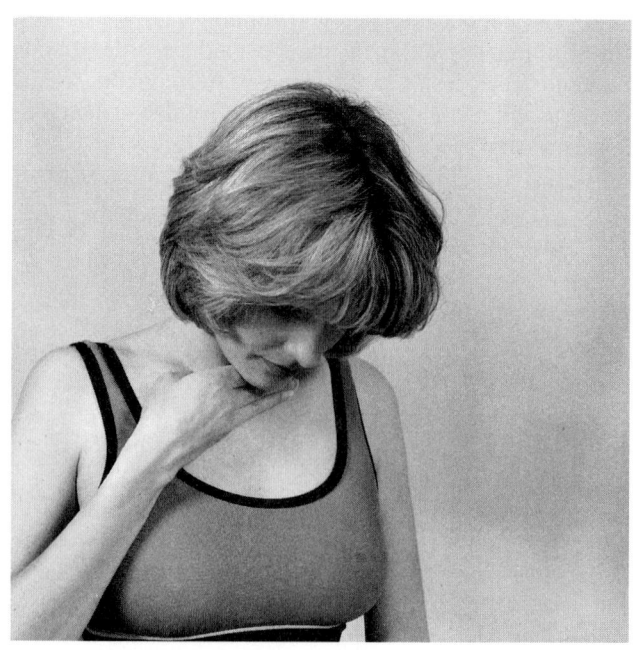

FIGURE 23-80   Three-finger exercise into cervical flexion.

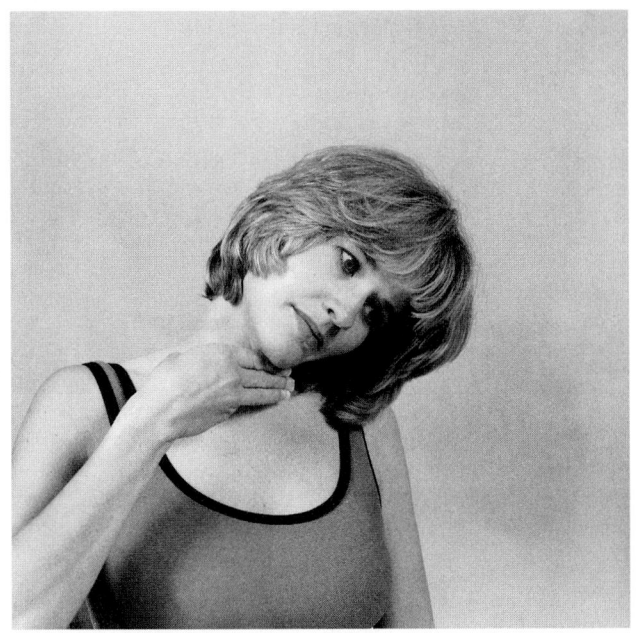

FIGURE 23-81   Three-finger exercise into cervical side bending.

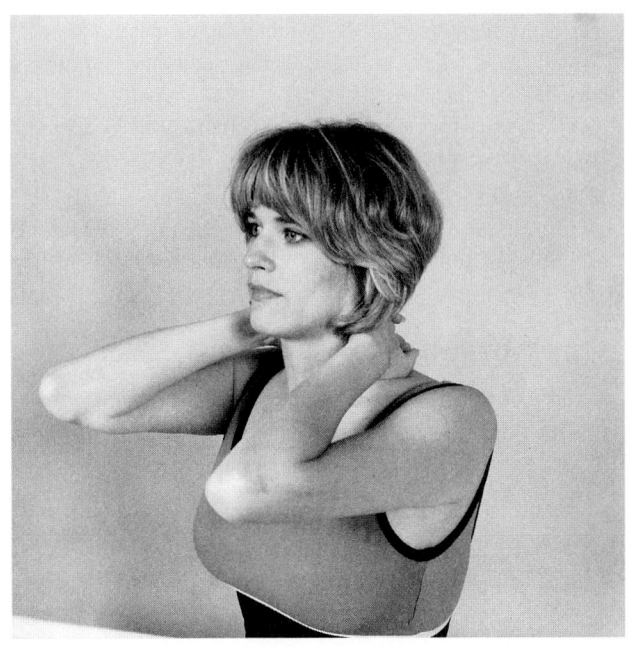

FIGURE 23-83   Three-finger exercise into cervical extension.

With a different hand position, cervical extension can be performed in a controlled and safe manner. The fingers are interlocked and placed behind the neck, with the little fingers at the segmental level below the joint restriction. Using the little finger as a fulcrum, the patient extends the cervical spine to the point just shy of pain. This position is held for a few seconds and the neck is returned to the neutral position (Fig. 83-83).

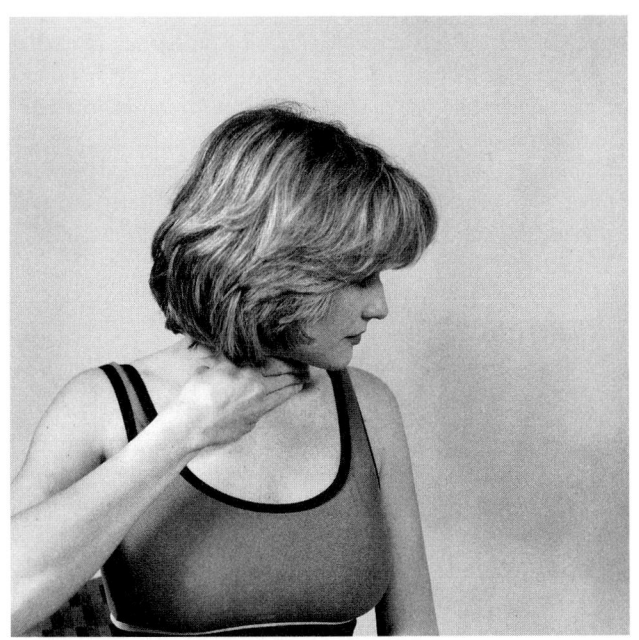

FIGURE 23-82   Three-finger exercise into cervical rotation.

CASE STUDY   NECK PAIN AND ARM PARESTHESIA

HISTORY

A 21-year-old woman presented to the clinic with complaints of right neck and shoulder pain, and paresthesias that often radiated into the medial arm, forearm, and fourth and fifth fingers of the right upper extremity. The patient also reported that her right upper extremity often felt tired and heavy, and that her right hand occasionally would appear to have a weak grip. The patient reported that her symptoms began shortly after she was involved in a motor vehicle accident about 2 months previously and have increased slightly since that time. The patient denied any history since the accident of dizziness, tinnitus, blurred vision, or headaches. No left-sided neck pain or left upper extremity symptoms were reported.

The patient described her overall health as good. Her past medical history was unremarkable, and there was no past history of any surgeries.

QUESTIONS

1. What are some of the potential causes for upper extremity paresthesias? Can you rule out any of these causes from the history given? What further questions would you ask to help rule out some of the causes?
2. Which conditions could be associated with a weak grip? Could you rule these in or out with the history?

3. Which conditions could be associated with a report of a tired and heavy upper extremity? How would you rule these in or out?
4. Would the results from any imaging studies be helpful in this case? If so, which ones and why?
5. Is an upper quarter scanning examination warranted in this case? Why or why not?
6. Is this an irritable condition? Why or why not?
7. What type of conditions were the questions about dizziness, tinnitus, blurred vision, and headaches designed to help rule out?

TESTS AND MEASURES

Because of the history of a motor vehicle accident and the presence of paresthesias, it was decided to perform an upper quarter scanning examination. The following findings were made:

- Observation—slightly obese female with rounded and depressed shoulders and a forward head posture.
- Active range of motion with passive overpressure and isometric resistance of the cervical and thoracic spine—full and pain-free.
- Neurological tests including deep tendon reflexes, sensation, and Tinel's test at the elbow and wrist—negative.
- Positive neurodynamic mobility testing of all upper limb tension tests, especially the radial and ulnar dominant tests (see Chap. 12).
- Strength testing—strong (5/5) and painful trapezius, levator scapulae, and the rhomboids on the right. Diminished grip strength (4/5) of the right hand that worsened (3+/5) when the right arm was raised overhead. Minor weakness (4+/5) of C7–T1 muscles with manual muscle testing.
- Palpation—Tenderness to palpation over the brachial plexus, no evidence of cervical rib.

QUESTIONS

1. Which conditions from your original list has the scanning examination helped to rule out? Which ones has the scanning examination not ruled out?
2. Do you have enough information to form a provisional diagnosis and begin an intervention? Why and why not?
3. Does the absence of a cervical rib with palpation necessarily rule out its presence?
4. What is your next step?

The results of the history and scanning examination are inconclusive. However, both the history and scanning examination have afforded the clinician with some useful clues that should guide the clinician to focus the examination. At this point, the most likely diagnoses are a neurological lesion (distribution of symptoms, positive neurodynamic mobility tests, weakness with muscle testing, and increased weakness with arm elevation), a vascular lesion (increased weakness with arm elevation), or both. Under further analysis it should be apparent that there are inconsistencies in the findings:

- With the exception of the hand intrinsics, the distribution of muscle weakness does not fully correlate with the symptom distribution.
- With the exception of the neurodynamic mobility tests, the neurological tests were negative.
- Active range of motion with passive overpressure and isometric resistance of the cervical and thoracic spine was full and pain-free and yet there are radicular symptoms.

It is clear that further testing is warranted. In an attempt to clarify the previously mentioned inconsistencies, the following tests were performed:

- Spurling's test to rule out foraminal encroachment—negative.
- Brachial plexus stretch test to help determine the cause of pain with palpation over the brachial plexus—positive.
- Thoracic outlet tests, including Allen's test, Adson's test, and the hyperabduction test to help rule out a vascular/neurological cause—all positive for obliteration of pulse and reproduction of symptoms.
- Muscle length tests to help determine whether posture could be a factor—decreased flexibility of the anterior and middle scalenes, pectoralis minor and major.

EVALUATION

A provisional diagnosis of thoracic outlet syndrome was made.

QUESTIONS

1. Having made a provisional diagnosis, how would you explain the cause to the patient?
2. Estimate the prognosis.
3. Which exercises would you emphasize in your intervention? Why?

The first rib was tested to see if it was elevated in relation to the other side. This was determined by palpating the first rib while passively rotating the patient's head away from the test side (rib may elevate slightly) and then extending and side bending it ipsilaterally (rib should descend). The head is then side bend contralaterally (rib should elevate). If the rib remains elevated with ipsilateral side bending of the head, a mechanical dysfunction is indicated rather than a soft tissue one.

INTERVENTION

- *Manual therapy.* Following the application of moist heat to the neck and right shoulder, the anterior and middle scalenes, and the pectoralis minor and major muscles, were manually stretched, taking care not to stress the glenohumeral joint.
- *Therapeutic exercises* to strengthen the trapezius, levator scapulae, and rhomboids on the right side were prescribed.
- *Patient-related instruction.* Explanation was given as to the cause of the patient's symptoms. The patient received instructions regarding correct posture during activities of daily living and exercises to stretch and strengthen those muscles treated in the clinic. The patient was advised to continue the exercises

at home, three to five times each day, and to expect some post-exercise soreness. The patient also received instruction on the use of heat and ice at home.

- *Goals/outcomes.* Both the patient's goals from the treatment and the expected therapeutic goals of the clinician were discussed with the patient.

CASE STUDY LOW NECK PAIN

HISTORY

A 33-year old woman presented with a diagnosis of low neck and upper back pain that, over the past few weeks, had become constant. Initially, the pain had been minimal, but it had worsened progressively. The pain was localized to the midline at the base of the neck, and there was no report of arm pain or symptoms. The patient worked as a computer operator for a local bank. Sleeping had become difficult, and all motions of the neck were reported to reproduce the symptoms. The patient denied any dizziness or nausea, or history of neck trauma.

The patient described her overall health as excellent. The past medical history was unremarkable.

QUESTIONS

1. Make a list of all of the possible causes of midline neck pain.
2. What could the gradual onset of the pain tell the clinician?
3. What is your working hypothesis at this stage? List the tests you would use to rule out the various causes of midline neck pain.
4. Should the reports of night pain concern the clinician?
5. Does this presentation/history warrant a Cyriax upper quarter scanning examination? Why or why not?

TESTS AND MEASURES

Although the onset of these symptoms had been gradual, and there was reported night pain, there were no reports of pain radiation or radiculopathy. Given the localization of the pain and the patient's occupation, an irritated postural dysfunction was suspected. With this working hypothesis, an examination was performed. The following findings were made:

- Active range of motion of the cervical spine was limited in a noncapsular pattern of decreased flexion, both rotations, both side flexions, and extension. Flexion was limited by 50 percent, rotations and side bending to both sides were limited by 30 percent, and extension by 70 percent. All of the motions reproduced the midline neck pain.
- The position tests of the cervical spine and upper thoracic spine were negative. This could indicate the joint segments were normal or that a symmetric dysfunction was present.
- The passive physiologic intervertebral mobility tests were positive for hypomobility at the C7 to T1 segment during extension.
- The posterior glides used to assess extension at C7 to T1 reproduced the pain and had a pathomechanical end-feel.

- The passive physiologic mobility and passive articular mobility tests of the first two ribs were negative.
- The passive physiologic articular intervertebral mobility testing of the upper cervical joints (see Chap. 22) revealed a bilateral loss of the posterior glide at both of the occipito-atlantal joints, with a pathomechanical end-feel.
- The Adson maneuver was positive bilaterally for a diminished pulse.
- Postural examination revealed a forward head posture.
- Point tenderness was elicited over the C7 segment, the origins of both levator scapulae, and the muscle bellies of both upper trapezius muscles.
- Flexibility testing revealed bilateral tightness of the sternocleidomastoid, scalenes, and pectoralis minor and major.
- Muscle testing revealed weakness of the rhomboids, middle and lower trapezius, and serratus anterior at a grade of 4/5.

QUESTIONS

1. Did the tests and measures confirm your working hypothesis? How?
2. Given the findings from the tests and measures, what is the diagnosis, or is further testing warranted in the form of special tests?
3. Which findings could confuse the diagnosis?

EVALUATION

A provisional diagnosis was made of an extension hypomobility at C7 to T1 and muscle imbalances of the neck and shoulder complex caused by a postural dysfunction.

QUESTIONS

1. Having made a provisional diagnosis, what will be your intervention?
2. How would you describe this condition to the patient?
3. In order of priority, and based on the stages of healing, list the various goals of your intervention.
4. How will you determine the amplitude and joint position for the intervention?
5. Is an asymmetrical or symmetrical technique more appropriate for this condition? Why?
6. Estimate this patient's prognosis.
7. What modalities could you use in the intervention of this patient?
8. What exercises would you prescribe?

INTERVENTION

A global intervention is required for this syndrome.

- The flexibility and strength deficits of the muscles are addressed.
- The hypomobile joints at C7 to T1 and the occipito-atlantal segments are mobilized
- The patient is educated on the importance of good postural habits.
- The forward head postural dysfunction is addressed.

Special attention should be applied to manually increasing extension at the cervicothoracic junction and increasing the flexion of the upper cervical joints. The following soft tissues commonly need to be addressed:

Increasing the flexibility of:
- The suboccipital extensors.
- The cervicothoracic flexors.
- The pectoralis minor.
- The sternocleidomastoid.

Correction of:
- The impaired levator scapulae and medial scapula muscles.
- The C6 to C7 hypomobility.
- The tight muscles and strengthening of the weak muscles.
- Any facilitated hypertonicity.

One of the best and most natural ways of improving posture, with little manual or other intervention by the clinician, is for the patient to initiate a walking program. Improvement should occur within 1 to 2 weeks unless there is an underlying biomechanical impairment. For more active intervention and re-educational purposes, the hypomobile joints need to be mobilized and the hypermobile ones protected. It is probably better to start the re-educational correction in the lumbar spine and thorax, addressing the cervical spine later. This tends to avoid the problem of hypermobilizing the cervical joints, which seem more vulnerable than those in the lumbar and thoracic regions.

A home exercise program is issued to reinforce the intervention.

CASE STUDY   BILATERAL ARM AND WRIST WEAKNESS

HISTORY

A 36-year-old man who sustained a left tibial plateau fracture presented at the clinic with complaints of bilateral arm and wrist weakness that had worsened progressively over the past month since his discharge from the hospital. The patient was ambulating with crutches and non–weight bearing on the left side. There was no history of cervical trauma. The patient reported no pain in his upper extremities but had noticed a mild and vague numbness in his hands. There was no report or evidence of a preceding viral infection and no proximal migration of the weakness, nor did he have any other areas of weakness. The patient did complain of pain in his axillae, and commented that his crutches had been rubbing against his axillae.[271]

QUESTIONS

1. What structure(s) could be at fault when weakness is the major complaint?
2. Why was the history of no cervical trauma pertinent?
3. Why was the statement about preceding viral infection pertinent?
4. Why was the statement about the proximal migration of the weakness pertinent?

5. What is your working hypothesis at this stage? List the various diagnoses that could present with bilateral arm numbness and the tests you would use to rule out each one.
6. Does this presentation/history warrant a scanning examination? Why or why not?

TESTS AND MEASURES

Because of the insidious nature of the patient's symptoms and the fact that the symptoms were in a distribution that could indicate a serious condition or neurologic involvement, a Cyriax upper quarter scanning examination was performed with the following findings:

- Examination of his upper extremities found that the deltoid strength at 4/5 and the biceps at 5/5.
- All radial nerve–innervated muscles from the triceps distally were 1/5 in strength.
- The wrist and finger flexors were rated at 3+/5, and the intrinsic muscles of the hand were 3−/5.
- The reflexes showed absence of triceps jerk, with preservation of the biceps jerks, which were 2+. The brachioradialis reflexes were intact up to the biceps reflex.
- There was diminished pinprick and temperature perception in the hands. These findings were present on both sides.
- The patient's axillae showed marked redness, suggestive of chronic irritation and rubbing.
- Cranial nerve function was found to be normal, as was the cervical spine.
- The lower limbs had normal strength, sensation, and reflexes.
- The patient's axillary crutches were found to be too long, with the axillary bar sitting just under the axillary fold when the patient stood erect. The patient's crutch walking technique was assessed and found to be very poor, with the patient putting all his weight on the axillary bars.

QUESTIONS

1. Did the upper quarter scanning examination confirm the working hypothesis? How?
2. List the muscles that could be used to assess the radial nerve.
3. What are the characteristics of a weakness produced by peripheral nerve palsy?
4. Given the findings from the scan, what is the diagnosis, or is further testing warranted in the form of a biomechanical examination? What information would be gained with further testing?

EVALUATION/INTERVENTION

A provisional diagnosis of crutch palsy was made based on the history and the findings from the scanning examination. The axillary crutches were initially discontinued, and a forearm-bearing walker was substituted. The patient was asked to return in 6 weeks, but to call if the symptoms did not start to improve after 2 weeks. Six weeks later, the patient's sensory function was resolved.

Examination found normal sensation in all distributions, to all assessment methods, including pinprick and temperature perception. Examination of muscle function showed full strength in all muscles innervated by the median, ulnar, musculocutaneous, and axillary nerves.

QUESTION

1. Why was the patient not treated on a regular basis in the clinic?

CASE STUDY RIGHT-SIDED NECK PAIN

HISTORY

A 45-year-old woman awoke with right-sided neck pain 10 days earlier. The pain was felt over the right neck on an intermittent basis. She related that the pain was worse with head turning to the right, and further aggravated with activities involving cervical extension. She described no neurologic pain or paresthesia. The pain sites and intensity were unchanged since the onset.

Further questioning revealed that the patient was otherwise in good health and had no reports of bowel or bladder impairment, night pain, dizziness, or radicular symptoms.

QUESTIONS

1. What structure(s) could be at fault with complaints of right-sided neck pain?
2. What should the motion pattern of restriction/pain tell you?
3. What is your working hypothesis at this stage? List the various diagnoses that could present with right-sided neck pain, and the tests you would use to rule out each one.
4. What do the questions about night pain and dizziness pertain to?
5. Does this presentation/history warrant a scanning examination? Why or why not?

TESTS AND MEASURES

Because the pain was intermittent and appeared to be related to a specific movement, the scanning examination was deferred. The tests and measures revealed the following:

- Active range of motion into flexion and left rotation and left side bending were normal.
- Extension was limited to about 50 percent of normal and reproduced the right-sided neck pain.
- Right rotation and right side bending were limited to about 50 percent of normal and reproduced the pain in the right neck and supraspinatus fossa.
- Passive physiologic intervertebral mobility tests revealed hypomobility at the right zygapophysial joints of C3 to C4.
- The pain in the right side of the neck and supraspinatus fossa was reproduced on passive articular intervertebral mobility testing with posterior glides of the right zygapophysial joints of C3 to C4.

QUESTIONS

1. Did the tests and measures confirm your working hypothesis? How?
2. Given the findings from the tests and measures, what is the diagnosis, or is further testing warranted in the form of special tests?

EVALUATION

A provisional diagnosis was made of an extension and right side bending hypomobility at C3 to C4.

QUESTIONS

1. Having made the diagnosis, what will be your intervention?
2. How would you describe this condition to the patient?
3. In order of priority, and based on the stages of healing, list the various goals of your intervention.
4. How will you determine the amplitude and joint position for the intervention?
5. What would you tell the patient about your intervention?
6. Is an asymmetric or a symmetric technique more appropriate for this condition? Why?
7. Estimate this patient's prognosis.
8. What modalities could you use in the intervention of this patient?
9. What exercises would you prescribe?

INTERVENTION

- *Manual therapy.* Following an application of moist heat, soft tissue techniques were applied to the area, followed by a specific asymmetric mobilization of the C3 to C4 segment into extension and right side bending.
- *Therapeutic exercises* of active range of motion of the cervical spine were prescribed. These were progressed to isometric resistive exercises throughout the range. Exercises for the major muscle groups of the neck and shoulder also were prescribed, in addition to aerobic exercises using a stationary bike and upper body ergometer.
- *Patient-related instruction.* Explanation was given as to the cause of the patient's symptoms. The patient was advised to avoid sudden turning of the head to the right. She was further advised to continue the exercises at home, three to five times each day, and to expect some postexercise soreness. The patient also received instruction on the use of heat and ice at home.
- *Goals/outcomes.* Both the patient's goals from the treatment and the expected therapeutic goals of the clinician were discussed with the patient. It was concluded that the clinical sessions would occur two times per week for 1 month, at which time it was hoped that the patient would be discharged to a home exercise program.

REVIEW QUESTIONS*

1. Contraction of one sternocleidomastoid muscle results in:
   A. rotation of the face to the same side
   B. sidebending of the head and neck to the opposite side

C. flexion of the head and neck

D. rotation of the face to the opposite side

2. Which of the following groups of muscles performs cervical rotation to the opposite side?

A. longus capitis, rectus capitis anterior and posterior

B. splenius cervicis, splenius capitis

C. sternocleidomastoid, scalenus anterior, obliquus capitis

D. sternocleidomastoid, scalenus medius

3. Which of the following muscles is thin and sheetlike and has fibers that extend from the chest upward over the neck?

A. levator scapula

B. buccinator

C. orbicularis oris

D. platysma

4. Which cervical structure is thought to help prevent cervical disk protrusions?

5. Which nerve trunk of the plexus is the most commonly compressed neural structure in thoracic outlet syndrome (TOS)?

---

* Additional questions to test your understanding of this chapter can be found in the Online Learning Center for *Orthopaedic Assessment, Evaluation, and Intervention* at www.duttononline.net.

REFERENCES

1. Bland JH. Diagnosis of thoracic pain syndromes. In: Giles LGF, Singer KP, Eds. *Clinical Anatomy and Management of the Thoracic Spine.* Oxford, England: Butterworth-Heinemann; 2000:145–156.

1a. Bogduk N, Mercer S. Biomechanics of the cervical spine. I. Normal kinematics. *Clin Biomech.* 2000;15:633–648.

2. Maigne JY. Cervicothoracic and thoracolumbar spinal pain syndromes. In: Giles LGF, Singer KP, eds. *Clinical Anatomy and Management of the Thoracic Spine.* Oxford, England: Butterworth-Heinemann; 2000:157–168.

3. Jull GA. Physiotherapy management of neck pain of mechanical origin. In: Giles LGF, Singer KP, eds. *Clinical Anatomy and Management of Cervical Spine Pain* London, England: Butterworth-Heinemann; 1998:168–191.

4. Hardin J Jr. Pain and the cervical spine. *Bull Rheum Dis* 2001;50:1–4.

5. Westerling D, Jonsson BG. Pain from the neck-shoulder region and sick leave. *Scand J Soc Med* 1980;8:131–136.

6. Takala J, Sievers K, Klaukka T. Rheumatic symptoms in the middle-aged population in southwestern Finland. *Scand J Rheumatol* 1982;47S:15–29.

7. Kelsey JL. An epidemiological study of the relationship between occupations and acute herniated lumbar intervertebral discs. *Int J Epidemiol* 1975;4:197–205.

8. Bovim G, Schrader H, Sand T. Neck pain in the general population. *Spine* 1994;19:1307–1309.

9. Pratt N. Anatomy of the cervical Spine. In: *Physical Therapy Home Study Course—The Cervical Spine.* La Crosse, Wis: Orthopaedic Section, American Physical Therapy Association; 1996.

10. Norkin C, Levangie P. *Joint Structure and Function: A Comprehensive Analysis.* Philadelphia, Pa: FA Davis; 1992:355–358.

11. Mayoux-Benhamou MA, et al. Longus colli has a postural function on cervical curvature. *Surg Radiol Anat* 1994;16:367–371.

12. Watson D, Trott P. Cervical headache: An investigation of natural head posture and upper cervical flexor muscle performance. *Cephalalgia* 1993;13:272–284.

13. Lewit K. *Manipulative Therapy in Rehabilitation of the Locomotor System.* 2nd ed. Oxford, England: Butterworth-Heinemann; 1996.

14. Powers SR, Drislane TM, Nevins S. Intermittent vertebral artery compression: A new syndrome. *Surgery* 1961;49:257–264.

15. Pal GP, Sherk HH. The vertical stability of the cervical spine. *Spine* 1988;13:447.

16. Yoo JU, et al. Effect of cervical motion on the neuroforaminal dimensions of the human cervical spine. *Spine* 1992;17:1131–1136.

17. Williams PL, et al. *Gray's Anatomy.* 37th ed. London, England: Churchill Livingstone; 1989.

18. White AA, Panjabi MM, eds. *Clinical Biomechanics of the Spine* Philadelphia, Pa: Lippincott-Raven; 1990:106–108.

19. Lysell E. Motion in the cervical spine: An experimental study on autopsy specimens. *Acta Orthop Scand Suppl* 1969;123:1.

20. Mercer S, Bogduk N. Intra-articular inclusions of the cervical synovial joints. *Br J Rheumatol* 1993;32:705–710.

21. Dvorak J. Epidemiology, physical examination, and neurodiagnostics. *Spine* 1998;23:2663–2673.

22. Giles LG, Taylor JR. Innervation of human lumbar zygapophysial joint synovial folds. *Acta Orthop Scand* 1987;58:43–46.

23. Töndury G, Theiler K. *Entwicklungsgeschichte und Fehlbildung der Wirbelsäule.* Stuttgart, Germany: Hyppokrates; 1958.

24. Kotani Y, et al. The role of anteromedial foraminotomy and the uncovertebral joints in the stability of the cervical spine. A biomechanical study. *Spine* 1998;23:1559–1565.

25. Tillman B, Tondury G, Ziles K. *Human Anatomy: Locomotor System.* Stuttgart, Germany: Thieme; 1987.

26. Orofino C, Sherman MS, Schechter D. Luschka's joint: A degenerative phenomenon. *J Bone Joint Surg* 1960;5A:853–858.

27. Panjabi MM, et al. Cervical human vertebrae. Quantitative three-dimensional anatomy of the middle and lower regions. *Spine* 1991;16:861–869.

28. Porterfield J, De Rosa C. *Mechanical Neck Pain: Perspectives in Functional Anatomy.* Philadelphia, Pa: Saunders; 1995:38–91.

29. Milne N. The role of zygapophysial joint orientation and uncinate processes in controlling motion in the cervical spine. *J Anat* 1991;178:189–201.

30. Yanagisawa E. Anatomy of the uncinate process. *Ear Nose Throat J* 2000;79:228.

31. Penning L, Wilmink JT. Rotation of the cervical spine. A CT study in normal subjects. *Spine* 1987;12:732–738.

32. Clausen JD, et al. Uncinate processes and Luschka joints influence the biomechanics of the cervical spine: Quantification using a finite element model of the C5-C6 segment. *J Orthop Res* 1997;15:342–347.

33. Argenson C, et al. The vertebral arteries (segment V1 and V2). *Anat Clin* 1980;2:29–41.

34. Penning L. Differences in anatomy, motion, development, and ageing of the upper and lower cervical disk segments. *Clin Biomech* 1988;3:37–47.

35. Hadley LA. Intervertebral joint subluxation, bony impingement and foramen encroachment with nerve root changes. *Am J Roentgenol* 1951;65:377–402.

36. Johnson RM, et al. Some new observations on the functional anatomy of the lower cervical spine. *Clin Orthop Rel Res* 1975;111:192–200.

37. Buckworth J. Anatomy of the suboccipital region. In: Vernon H, ed. *Upper Cervical Syndrome.* Baltimore, Md: Williams and Wilkins; 1988:28–52.

38. Fielding JW, Burstein AA, Frankel VH. The nuchal ligament. *Spine* 1976;1:3–11.

39. Penning L. Normal movements of the cervical spine. *J Roentgenol* 1978;130:317–326.

40. Travell JG, Simons DG. *Myofascial Pain and Dysfunction: The Trigger Point Manual.* Baltimore, Md: Williams and Wilkins; 1983.

41. Fitzgerald MJT, Comerford PT, Tuffery AR. Sources of innervation of the neuromuscular spindles in sternomastoid and trapezius. *J Anat* 1982;134:471–490.

42. Gray H. *Gray's Anatomy.* Philadelphia, Pa: Lea and Febiger; 1995.

43. Kendall FP, McCreary EK, Provance PG. *Muscles: Testing and Function.* Baltimore, Md: Williams and Wilkins; 1993.

44. Eliot DJ. Electromyography of levator scapulae: New findings allow tests of a head stabilization model. *J Manipulative Physiol Ther* 1996;19:19–25.

45. Rayan GM, Jensen C. Thoracic outlet syndrome: Provocative examination maneuvers in a typical population. *J Shoulder Elbow Surg* 1995;4:113–117.

46. Roos DB. The place for scalenectomy and first-rib resection in thoracic outlet syndrome. *Surgery* 1982;92:1077–1085.

47. Raper AJ, et al. Scalene and sternomastoid muscle function. *J Appl Physiol* 1966;21:497–502.

48. Pick TP, Howden R. *Gray's Anatomy.* 15th ed. New York, NY: Barnes and Noble Books; 1995.

49. Hiatt JL, Gartner LP. *Textbook of Head and Neck Anatomy.* Baltimore, Md: Williams and Wilkins; 1987.

50. Murphy DR. *Conservative Management of Cervical Spine Syndromes.* New York, NY: McGraw-Hill; 2000.

51. Walsh R, Nitz AJ. Cervical spine. In: Wadsworth C, ed. *Current Concepts of Orthopaedic Physical Therapy—Home Study Course.* La Crosse, Wis: Orthopaedic Section, American Physical Therapy Association; 2001.

52. Bogduk N. Cervical causes of headache and dizziness. In: Grieve GP, ed. *Modern Manual Therapy of the Vertebral Column.* New York, NY: Churchill Livingstone; 1986:289–302.

53. Karlberg M, Persson L, Magnusson M. Reduced postural control in patients with chronic cervicobrachial pain syndrome. *Gait Posture* 1995;3:241–249.

54. Crum B, Mokri B, Fulgham J. Spinal manifestations of vertebral artery dissection. *Neurology* 2000;55:304–306.

55. Adams CBT, Logue V. Studies in spondylotic myelopathy 2. The movement and contour of the spine in relation to the neural complications of cervical spondylosis. *Brain* 1971;94:569–586.

56. Penning L. *Functional Pathology of the Cervical Spine.* Excerpta Medica Foundation. Baltimore, Md: Williams and Wilkins; 1968.

57. Taylor JR, Twomey L. Sagittal and horizontal plane movement of the lumbar vertebral column in cadavers and in the living. *Rheum Rehabil* 1980;19:223.

58. Van Mameren H, et al. Cervical spine motions in the sagittal plane. I: Ranges of motion of actually performed movements, an x-ray cine study. *Eur J Morphol* 1990;28:47–68.

59. Meadows J, Pettman E, Fowler C. Manual therapy. In: *North American Institute of Manual Therapy Level II & III Course Notes.* Denver, Colo: NAIOMT; 1995.

60. Janda V. Muscles and motor control in cervicogenic disorders: Assessment and management. In: Grant R, ed. *Physical Therapy of the Cervical and Thoracic Spine.* New York, NY: Churchill Livingstone; 1994:195–216.

61. Jull GA, Janda V. Muscle and motor control in low back pain. In: Twomey LT, Taylor JR, eds. *Physical Therapy of the Low Back: Clinics in Physical Therapy.* New York, NY: Churchill Livingstone; 1987:258.

62. Bergmark A. Stability of the lumbar spine. *Acta Orthop Scand* 1989;60:1–54.

63. Conley MS, et al. Noninvasive analysis of human neck muscle function. *Spine* 1995;20:2505–2512.

64. Vernon HT, et al. Evaluation of neck muscle strength with a modified sphygmomanometer dynamometer: Reliabilty and validity. *J Manipulative Physiol Ther* 1992;15:343–349.

65. Meadows J. *A Rationale and Complete Approach to the Sub-Acute Post-MVA Cervical Patient.* Calgary, Canada: Swodeam Consulting; 1995.

66. Winkel D, Matthijs O, Phelps V. Cervical spine. In: Winkel D, Matthijs O, Phelps V, eds. *Diagnosis and Treatment of the Spine* Gaithersburg, Md: Aspen: 1997:542–727.

67. Maigne JY, Maigne R, Guerin-Surville H. Upper thoracic dorsal rami: Anatomic study of their medial cutaneous branches. *Surg Radiol Anat* 1991;13:109–112.

68. Bogduk N, Valencia F. Innervation and pain patterns of the thoracic spine. In: Grant R, ed. *Physical Therapy of the Cervical and Thoracic Spine.* Melbourne, Australia: Churchill Livingstone; 1994:77–88.

69. White AA, Sahrmann SA. A movement system balance approach to management of musculoskeletal pain. In: Grant R, ed. *Physical Therapy for the Cervical and Thoracic Spine.* Edinburgh, Scotland: Churchill Livingstone; 1994:347.

70. Gossman MR, Sahrmann SA, Rose SJ. Review of length-associated changes in muscle. *Phys Ther* 1982;62:1799–1808.

71. Jull G, Bogduk N, Marsland A. The accuracy of manual diagnosis for cervical zygapophysial joint pain syndromes. *Med J Aust* 1988;148:233–236.

72. Dwyer A, Aprill C, Bogduk N. Cervical zygapophysial joint pain patterns: A study from normal volunteers. *Spine* 1990; 15:453.

73. Aprill C, Dwyer A, Bogduk N. Cervical zygapophysial joint pain patterns II: A clinical evaluation. *Spine* 1990;15:458–461.

74. Magarey ME. Examination of the cervical and thoracic spine. In: Grant R, ed. *Physical Therapy of the Cervical and Thoracic Spine* New York, NY: Churchill Livingstone; 1994:109–144.

75. Grieve G. Common patterns of clinical presentation. In: Grieve GP, ed. *Common Vertebral Joint Problems.* London, England: Churchill Livingstone; 1988:283–302.

76. McKenzie RA. *The Cervical and Thoracic Spine: Mechanical Diagnosis and Therapy.* Waikanae, New Zealand: Spinal Publications New Zealand; 1990.

77. Hohl M. Soft-tissue injuries of the neck in automobile accidents. *J Bone Joint Surg* 1974;56A:1675–1682.

78. Jamieson DRS, Ballantyne JP. Unique presentation of a prolapsed thoracic disk: Lhermitte's symptom in a golf player. *Neurology* 1995;45:1219–1221.

79. Kanchandani R, Howe JG. Lhermitte's sign in multiple sclerosis: A clinical survey and review of the literature. *J Neurol Neurosurg Psychiatry* 1982;45:308–312.

80. Ventafridda V, et al. On the significance of Lhermitte's sign in oncology. *J Neurooncol* 1991;10:133–137.

81. Bush K, Hillier S. Outcome of cervical radiculopathy treated with periradicular/epidural corticosteroid injections: A prospective

study with independent clinical review. *Eur Spine J* 1996; 5:319–325.

82. Meadows J. *Orthopaedic Differential Diagnosis in Physical Therapy.* New York, NY: McGraw-Hill; 1999.

83. Foreman SM, Croft AC. *Whiplash Injuries: The Cervical Acceleration/Deceleration Syndrome.* Baltimore, Md: Williams and Wilkins; 1988.

84. Jull GA, Treleaven J, Versace G. Manual examination: Is pain a major cue to spinal dysfunction. *Aust J Physiother* 1994; 40:159–165.

85. Radanov B, et al. Factors influencing recovery from headache after common whiplash. *Br Med J* 1993;307:652–655.

86. Bradley JP, Tibone JE, Watkins RG. History, physical examination, and diagnostic tests for neck and upper extremity problems. In: Watkins RG, ed. *The Spine in Sports.* St Louis: Mosby-Year-Book; 1996.

87. Herkowitz HN. Syndromes related to spinal stenosis. In: Weinstein JN, Rydevik B, Sonntag VKH, eds. *Essentials of the Spine.* New York, NY: Raven; 1995:179–193.

88. Richardson CA, et al. *Therapeutic Exercise for Spinal Segmental Stabilization in Low Back Pain.* London, England: Churchill Livingstone; 1999.

89. Janda V. Muscle strength in relation to muscle length, pain and muscle imbalance. In: Harms-Ringdahl K, ed. *Muscle Strength.* New York, NY: Churchill Livingstone; 1993:83.

90. Janda V. Muscles, motor regulation and back problems. In: Korr IM, ed. *The Neurological Mechanisms in Manipulative Therapy.* New York, NY: Plenum; 1978:27.

91. Sahrmann SA. *Diagnosis and Treatment of Movement Impairment Syndromes.* St Louis: Mosby; 2001.

92. Geschwing N, Levitsky W. Human brain: Left-right asymmeties in temporal speech region. *Science* 1968;161:186–187.

93. Galaburda AM, le May M. Right left asymmetries in the brain. *Science* 1978;199:852–856.

94. Bledschmidt M. Principles of biodynamic differentiation in human. In: Bledschmidt M, ed. *Development of the Basicranium.* Bethesda, Md: National Institutes of Health; 1976:54–80.

95. Enlow DH. The prenatal and postnatal growth of the basicranium. In: Bedschmidt M, ed. *Development of the Basicranium.* Bethesda, Md: National Institutes of Health; 1976: 192–204.

96. Mannheimer JS. Prevention and restoration of abnormal upper quarter posture. In: Gelb H, Gelb M, eds. *Postural Considerations in the Diagnosis and Treatment of Cranio-Cervical-Mandibular and Related Chronic Pain Disorders.* St Louis, Mo: Ishiyaku EuroAmerica; 1991:93–161.

97. Troyanovich SJ, Harrison DE, Harrison DD. Structural rehabilitation of the spine and posture: Rationale for treatment beyond the resolution of symptoms. *J Manipulative Physiol Ther* 1998;21:37–50.

98. Meadows JTS. *Manual Therapy: Biomechanical Assessment and Treatment, Advanced Technique.* Lecture and video supplemental manual. 1995, Calgary, Canada: Swodeam Consulting; 1995.

99. Cloward RB. Cervical discography: A contribution to the etiology and mechanism of neck, shoulder and arm pain. *Ann Surg* 1959;150:1052–1064.

100. Sweeney TB, et al. Cervicothoracic muscular stabilization techniques. In: Saal JA, ed. *Physical Medicine and Rehabilitation, State of the Art Reviews: Neck and Back Pain.* Philadelphia, Pa: Hanley and Belfus; 1990:335–359.

101. Saal JS. Flexibility training. In: *Physical Medicine and Rehabilitation: State of the Art Reviews.* Philadelphia, Pa: Hanley and Belfus; 1987:537–554.

102. Dvorak J, et al. Age and gender related normal motion of the cervical spine. *Spine* 1992;17:S393–S398.

103. Dvorak J, et al. Motor-evoked potentials in patients with cervical spine disorders. *Spine* 1990;15:1013–1016.

104. Toole J, Tucker S. Influence of head position upon cerebral circulation. *Arch Neurol* 1960;2:616–623.

105. Jacob G, McKenzie R. Spinal therapeutics based on responses to loading. In: Liebenson C, ed. *Rehabilitation of the Spine: A Practitioner's Manual.* Baltimore, Md: Lippincott Williams and Wilkins; 1996:225–252.

106. Cyriax J. *Textbook of Orthopaedic Medicine, Diagnosis of Soft Tissue Lesions.* 8th ed. London, England: Bailliere Tindall; 1982.

107. Cocchiarella L, Andersson GBJ, eds. *American Medical Association, Guides to the Evaluation of Permanent Impairment.* 5th ed. Chicago, Ill: AMA; 2001.

108. Constantin P, Lucretia C. Relations between the cervical spine and the vertebral arteries. *ACTA Radiol* 1971;6:91–96.

109. Jirout J. The rotational component in the dynamics of the C2-3 spinal segment. *Neuroradiology* 1979;17:177–181.

110. Ehrhardt R, Bowling RW. Treatment of the cervical spine. In: *Physical Therapy Home Study Course.* La Crosse, Wis: Orthopaedic Section, American Physical Therapy Association; 1996.

111. Vasilyeva LF, Lewit K. Diagnosis of muscular dysfunction by inspection. In: Liebenson C, ed. *Rehabilitation of the Spine: A Practitioner's Manual.* Baltimore, Md: Lippincott Williams and Wilkins; 1996:113–142.

112. Lee DG. *A Workbook of Manual Therapy Techniques for the Upper Extremity.* Delta, Canada: Delta Orthopaedic Physiotherapy Clinics; 1989.

113. Hoppenfeld S. *Physical Examination of the Spine and Extremities.* East Norwalk, Conn: Appleton-Century-Crofts; 1976.

114. Mitchell FL, Moran PS, Pruzzo NA. *An Evaluation and Treatment Manual of Osteopathic Muscle Energy Procedures.* Manchester, Mo: Mitchell, Moran and Pruzzo; 1979.

115. Jensen OK, et al. Functional radiographic examination of the cervical spine in patients with post-traumatic headache. *Cephalalgia* 1990;109:275–303.

116. Pettman E. Stress tests of the craniovertebral joints. In: Boyling JD, Palastanga N, eds. *Grieve's Modern Manual Therapy: The Vertebral Column.* Edinburgh, Scotland: Churchill Livingstone; 1994:529–538.

117. Vernon H, Mior S. The neck disability index: A study of reliability and validity. *J Manipulative Physiol Ther* 1991;14:409–415.

118. Lhermitte J, Bollak NM. Les douleurs a type de decharge electrique consecutives a la flexion cephalique dans la sclerose en plaque. *Rev Neurol (Paris)* 1924;2:36–52.

119. Smith KJ, McDonald WI. Spontaneous and mechanically evoked activity due to central demyelinating lesion. *Nature* 1980;286:154–155.

120. Uchihara T, Furukawa T, Tsukagoshi H. Compression of brachial plexus as a diagnostic test of a cervical cord lesion. *Spine* 1994;19:2170–2173.

121. Landi A, Copeland S. Value of the Tinel sign in brachial plexus lesions. *Ann R Coll Surg Engl* 1979;61:470–471.

122. Marx RG, Bombardier C, Wright JG. What do we know about the reliability and validity of physical examination tests used to examine the upper extremity? *J Hand Surg* 1999;24A:185–193.

123. Wright IS. The neurovascular syndrome produced by hyperabduction of the arms. *Am Heart J* 1945;29:1–19.

124. Telford ED, Mottershead S. Pressure at the cervico-brachial junction: An operative and anatomical study. *J Bone Joint Surg* 1948;30B:249–265.

125. Winsor T, Brow R. Costoclavicular syndrome: Its diagnosis and treatment. *JAMA* 1966;196:697–699.

126. Selke FW, Kelly TR. Thoracic outlet syndrome. *Am J Surg* 1988;156:54–57.

127. Nichols AW. The thoracic outlet syndrome in athletes. *J Am Board Fam Pract* 1996;9:346–355.

128. Roos DB. Congenital anomalies associated with thoracic outlet syndrome. *J Surg* 1976;132:771–778.

129. Koes BW, et al. The effectiveness of manual therapy, physiotherapy and treatment by the general practitioner for nonspecific back and neck complaints: A randomized clinical trial. *Spine* 1992;17:28–35.

130. Foley-Nolan D, et al. Low energy high frequency pulsed electromagnetic therapy for acute whiplash disorders. A double blind randomized controlled study. *Scand J Rehabil Med* 1992; 24:51–59.

131. Giebel GD, Edelmann M, Huser R. Sprain of the cervical spine: Early functional vs. immobilization treatment [in German]. *Zentralbl Chir* 1997;122:512–521.

132. Quebec Task Force on Spinal Disorders. Scientific approach to the assessment and management of activity-related spinal disorders: A monograph for clinicians. Report of the Quebec Task Force on Spinal Disorders. *Spine* 1987; 12(suppl):1–59.

133. Zylbergold RS, Piper MC. Cervical spine disorders. A comparison of three types of traction. *Spine* 1985;10:867–871.

134. Colachis SC, Strohm BR. Cervical traction: Relationship of traction time to varied tractive force with constant angle of pull. *Arch Phys Med Rehabil* 1965;46:815–819.

135. Ellenberg MR, Honet JC, Treanor WJ. Cervical radiculopathy. *Arch Phys Med Rehabil* 1994;75:342–352.

136. Saal JS, Saal JA, Yurth EF. Nonoperative management of herniated cervical intervertebral disc with radiculopathy. *Spine* 1996;21:1877–1883.

137. Ter Haar GR, Stratford IJ. Evidence for a non-thermal effect of ultrasound. *Br J Cancer* 1982;45:172–175.

138. Michlovitz SL. The use of heat and cold in the management of rheumatic diseases. In: Michlovitz SL, ed. *Thermal Agents in Rehabilitation.* Philadelphia, Pa: FA Davis; 1990.

139. Hurwitz E, et al. Manipulation and mobilization of the cervical spine. *Spine* 1996;21:1746–1760.

140. Mealy K, Brennan H, Fenelon GC. Early mobilization of acute whiplash injuries. *BMJ* 1986;292:656–657.

141. McKinney LA, Dornan JO, Ryan M. The role of physiotherapy in the management of acute neck sprains following road-traffic accidents. *Arch Emerg Med* 1989;6:27–33.

142. McKinney LA. Early mobilisation and outcome in acute sprains of the neck. *BMJ* 1989;299:1006–1008.

143. Borchgrevink GE, et al. Acute treatment of whiplash neck sprain injuries. *Spine* 1998;23:25–31.

144. Gennis P, et al. The effect of soft cervical collars on persistent neck pain in patients with whiplash injury. *Acad Emerg Med* 1998;3:568–573.

145. Berg HE, Berggren G, Tesch PA. Dynamic neck strength training effect on pain and function. *Arch Phys Med Rehabil* 1994; 75:661–665.

146. Dyrssen T, Svedenkrans M, Paasikivi J. Muskelträning vid besvär I nacke och skuldror effektiv behandling för att minska smärtan. *Läkartidningen* 1989;86:2116–2120.

147. Provinciali L, et al. Multimodal treatment of whiplash injury. *Scand J Rehabil Med* 1996;28:105–111.

148. Cole AJ, Farrell JP, Stratton SA. Functional rehabilitation of cervical spine athletic injuries. In: Kibler BW, Herring JA, Press JM, eds. *Functional Rehabilitation of Sports and Musculoskeletal Injuries.* Gaithersburg, Md: Aspen; 1998.

149. Keshner EA, Campbell D, Katz RT. Neck muscle activiation patterns in humans during isometric head stabilization. *Exp Brain Res* 1989;75:335–344.

150. Andersson GBJ, Winters JM. Role of muscle in postural tasks: Spinal loading and postural stability. In: Winters JM, Woo SLY, eds. *Multiple Muscle Systems.* New York, NY: Springer-Verlag; 1990:375–395.

151. O'Connor JJ. Can muscle co-contraction protect knee ligaments after injury or repair? *J Bone Joint Surg* 1993;75B:41–48.

152. Rempel DM, Harrison RJ, Barnhart S. Work-related cumulative trauma disorders of the upper extremity. *JAMA* 1992; 267:838–842.

153. Armstrong TJ. Ergonomics and cumulative trauma disorders. *Hand Clin* 1986;2:553–565.

154. Black KM, McClure P, Polansky M. The influence of different sitting positions on cervical and lumbar posture. *Spine* 1996; 21:65–70.

155. Janda DH, Loubert P. A preventative program focussing on the glenohumeral joint. *Clin Sports Med* 1991;10:955–971.

156. Turk DC, Nash JM. Chronic pain: New ways to cope. In: Goleman D, Gurin J, eds. *Mind Body Medicine.* Yonkers, NY: Consumers Union of United States; 1993:111–131.

157. Jette DU, Jette AM. Physical therapy and health outcomes in patients with spinal impairments. *Phys Ther* 1996;76:930–945.

158. Uhlig Y, et al. Fiber composition and fiber transformations in the neck muscles of patients with dysfunction of the cervical spine. *J Orthop Res* 1995;13:240–249.

159. Greenfield B. Upper quarter evaluation: Structural relationships and interindependence. In: Donatelli R, Wooden M, eds. *Orthopaedic Physical Therapy.* New York, NY: Churchill Livingstone; 1989:43–58.

160. Cailliet R. *Neck and Arm Pain.* 3rd ed. Philadelphia, Pa: FA Davis; 1990.

161. Darnell MW. A proposed chronology of events for forward head posture. *J Craniomandib Prac* 1983;1:49–54.

162. Kisner C, Colby LA. *Therapeutic Exercise. Foundations and Techniques.* Philadelphia, Pa: FA Davis; 1997.

163. Kraus SL. Cervical spine influences on the craniomandibular region. In: Kraus SL, ed. *TMJ Disorders: Management of the Craniomandibular Complex.* New York, NY: Churchill Livingstone; 1988:367–396.

164. Kendall HO, Kendall FP, Boynton DA. *Posture and Pain.* Baltimore, Md: Williams and Wilkins; 1952.

165. Crawford HJ, Jull GA. The influence of thoracic posture and movement on range of arm elevation. *Physiother Theory Pract* 1993;9:143–148.

166. Adams MA, et al. Posture and the compressive strength of the lumbar spine. International Society of Biomechanics Award Paper. *Clin Biomech* 1994;9:5–14.

167. Ayub E. Posture and the upper quarter. In: Donatelli RA, ed. *Physical Therapy of the Shoulder.* New York, NY: Churchill Livingstone; 1991:81–90.

168. Janda V. On the concept of postural muscles and posture in man. *Aust J Physiother* 1983;29:83–84.

169. Turner M. Posture and pain. *Phys Ther* 1957;37:294.

170. Janda V. *Muscle Function Testing*. London, England: Butterworths; 1983:163–167.

171. Refshauge KM, Bolst L, Goodsell M. The relationship between cervicothoracic posture and the presence of pain. *J Man Manipulative Ther* 1995;3:21–24.

172. Saunders H. *Evaluation, Treatment and Prevention of Musculoskeletal Disorders*. 2nd ed. Minneapolis, MN: Viking Press; 1985.

173. Lewit K. *Manipulative Therapy in Rehabilitation of the Motor System*. 3rd ed. London, England: Butterworths; 1999.

174. Lewit K, Simons DG. Myofascial pain: Relief by post-isometric relaxation. *Arch Phys Med Rehabil* 1984;65:452–456.

175. Goldberg ME, Eggers HM, Gouras P. The ocular motor system. In: Kandel ER, Schwartz JH, Jessell TM, eds. *Principles of Neural Science*. Norwalk, Conn: Appleton & Lange; 1991:660–677.

176. Scariati P. Neurophysiology relevant to osteopathic manipulation. In: DiGiovanna EL, ed. *Osteopathic Approach to Diagnosis and Treatment*. Philadelphia, Pa: Lippincott; 1991.

177. Stratton SA, Bryan JM. Dysfunction, evaluation, and treatment of the cervical spine and thoracic inlet. In: Donatelli R, Wooden M, eds. *Orthopaedic Physical Therapy*. New York, NY: Churchill Livingstone; 1993:77–122.

178. Willford CH, et al. The interaction of wearing multifocal lenses with head posture and pain. *J Orthop Sports Phys Ther* 1996;23:194–199.

179. Lewit K. Chain reactions in disturbed function of the motor system. *J Manual Med* 1987;3:27.

180. Vig PS, et al. Quantitative evaluation of nasal airflow in relation to facial morphology. *Am J Orthod* 1981;79:263–272.

181. Lewit K. Relation of faulty respiration to posture, with clinical implications. *J Am Osteopath Assoc* 1980;79:525–529.

182. Bolton PS. The somatosensory system of the neck and its effects on the central nervous system. In: *Proceedings of the Scientific Symposium*. World Federation of Chiropractic. Ontario, Canada; 1997.

183. Chaitow L, et al. Breathing dysfunction. *J Bodywork Mov Ther* 1997;1:252–261.

184. Christie HJ, Kumar S, Warren SA. Postural aberrations in low back pain. *Arch Phys Med Rehabil* 1995;76:218–224.

185. Nachemson A, Morris JM. In vivo measurements of intradiscal pressure. *J Bone Joint Surg* 1964;46:1077.

186. Heine J. Uber die arthritis deformans. *Virchows Arch Pathol Anat* 1926;260:521–663.

187. Friedenberg ZB, Miller WT. Degenerative disc disease of the cervical spine. *J Bone Joint Surg* 1963;45:1171–1178.

188. Jeffreys E. Cervical spondylosis. In: Jeffreys E, ed. *Disorders of the Cervical Spine*. Boston, Mass: Butterworths; 1980:90–106.

189. Aprill C, Bogduk N. The prevalence of cervical zygapophysial joint pain: A first approximation. *Spine* 1992;17:744–747.

190. Bogduk N, Lord SM. Cervical zygapophysial joint pain. *Neurosurg Q* 1998;8:107–117.

191. Barnsley L, Lord S, Bogduk N. Comparative local anaesthetic blocks in the diagnosis of cervical zygapophysial joint pain. *Pain* 1993;55:99–106.

192. Barnsley L, et al. The prevalence of chronic cervical zygapophysial joint pain after whiplash. *Spine* 1995.20:20–26.

193. Crowe H. Injuries to the cervical spine. Presentation to the annual meeting of the Western Orthopaedic Association. San Francisco, Calif; 1928.

194. Spitzer WO, et al. Scientific monograph of the Quebec Task Force on Whiplash-Associated Disorders: Redefining "whiplash" and its management. *Spine* 1995;20(suppl):1S–73S. Erratum, *Spine* 1995;20:2372.

195. Reilly PA, Travers R, Littlejohn GO. Epidemiology of soft tissue rheumatism: The influence of the law. *J Rheumatol* 1991;18:1448–1449.

196. Evans RW. Some observations on whiplash injuries. *Neurol Clin* 1992;10:975–997.

197. Ferrari R, Russell AS. Epidemiology of whiplash: An international dilemma. *Ann Rheum Dis* 1999;58:1–5.

198. Gay JR, Abbott KH. Common whiplash injuries of the neck. *JAMA* 1953;152:1698–1704.

199. Gotten N. Survey of 100 cases of whiplash injury after settlement of litigation. *JAMA* 1956;162:854–857.

200. MacNab I. Acceleration injuries of the cervical spine. *J Bone Joint Surg* 1964;46A:1797–1799.

201. Macnab I. The whiplash syndrome. *Orthop Clin North Am* 1971;2:389–403.

202. Farbman AA. Neck sprain. Associated factors. *JAMA* 1973;223:1010–1015.

203. Nordhoff LS Jr. Cervical trauma following motor vehicle collisions. In: Murphy DR, ed. *Cervical Spine Syndromes*. New York, NY: McGraw-Hill; 2000:131–150.

203a. Zador PL, Ciccone MA. Automobile driver fatalities in frontal impacts: Air bags compared with manual belts. *Am J Public Health* 1993; 83:661–666.

203b. Cummings P, et al. Association of driver air bags with driver fatality: A matched cohort study. *BMJ* 2002;324:1119–1122.

203c. Evans L. The effectiveness of safety belts in preventing fatalities. *Accid Anal Prev* 1986;18:229–241.

203d. McGwin G, Jr, et al. The association between occupant restraint systems and risk of injury in frontal motor vehicle collisions. *J Trauma-Injury Infec Crit Care* 2003;54:1182–1187.

203e. Nordhoff LS, Jr. Cervical trauma following motor vehicle collisions. In: Murphy DR, ed. *Cervical Spine Syndromes*. McGraw-Hill: New York; 2000:131–150.

203f. Segui-Gomez M. Driver air bag effectiveness by severity of the crash. *Am J Public Health* 2000;90:1575–1581.

204. Scientific monograph of the Quebec Task Force on Whiplash-Associated Disorders. *Spine* 1995;20(22S):33S,38S–39S.

205. National Highway Traffic Safety Administration. *Traffic Safety Facts 1994: A Compilation of Motor Vehicle Crash Data from the Fatal Accident Reporting System and the General Estimates System*. Washington, DC: NHTSA; 1995.

206. Pennie B, Agambar L. Patterns of injury and recovery in whiplash. *Injury* 1991;22:57–60.

207. Radanov BP, Sturzenegger M, Di Stefano G. Long-term outcome after whiplash injury. A 2-year follow-up considering features of injury mechanism and somatic, radiologic, and psychosocial findings. *Med Sci Sports Exerc* 1995;74:281–297.

208. Sturzenegger M, Radanov BP, DiStefano G. The effect of accident mechanisms and initial findings on the long-term course of whiplash injury. *J Neurol* 1995;242:443–449.

209. Nikolai MD, Teasell R. Whiplash: The evidence for an organic etiology. *Arch Neurol* 2000;57:590–591.

210. Forsyth HF. Extension injury of the cervical spine. *J Bone Joint Surg* 1964;46A:1792–1797.

211. Barnes R. Paraplegia in cervical spine injuries. *J Bone Joint Surg* 1948;30B:234.

212. Carrette S. Whiplash injury and chronic neck pain. *N Engl J Med* 1994;330:1083–1084.

213. Morris F. Do headrests protect the neck from whiplash injuries? *Arch Emerg Med* 1989;6:17–21.

214. Maimaris C, Barnes MR, Allen MJ. Whiplash injuries of the neck: A retrospective study. *Injury* 1988;19:393–396.

215. Grob D. Posterior surgery. In: Gunzburg R, Szpalski M, eds. *Whiplash Injuries: Current Concepts in Prevention, Diagnosis and Treatment of the Cervical Whiplash Syndrome.* Philadelphia, Pa: Lippincott-Raven Publishers; 1998:241–246.

216. Press JM, Herring SA, Kibler WB. *Rehabilitation of Musculoskeletal Disorders. The Textbook of Military Medicine.* Washington, DC: Borden Institute, Office of the Surgeon General; 1996.

217. McLain RF. Mechanoreceptor endings in human cervical facet joints. *Spine* 1994;19:495–501.

218. Jonsson H, et al. Findings and outcomes in whiplash-type neck distortions. *Spine* 1994;19:2733–2743.

219. Jonsson H, et al. Hidden cervical spine injuries in traffic accident victims with skull fractures. *J Spinal Disord* 1991;4:251–263.

220. Rauschning W, McAfee PC, Jonsson H. Pathoanatomical and surgical findings in cervical spinal injuries. *J Spinal Disord* 1989;2:213–222.

221. Twomey LT, Taylor JR. The whiplash syndrome: Pathology and physical treatment. *J Man Manipulative Ther* 1993;1:26–29.

222. Ommaya AR. The head: Kinematics and brain injury mechanisms. In: Aldman B, Chapon A, eds. *The Biomechanics of Impact Trauma.* Amsterdam, Holland: Elsevier; 1984:117–138.

223. Mendel T, Wink CS. Neural elements in cervical intervertebral discs. *Anat Record* 1989;78A:223.

224. Cloward RB. Cervical diskography. A contribution to the etiology and mechanism of neck pain. *Ann Surg* 1959;150:1052.

225. Rauschning W, McAfee P, Jónsson H Jr. Pathoanatomical and surgical findings in cervical spine injuries. *J Spinal Disord* 1989;2:213–222.

226. Kaneoka K, et al. Motion analysis of cervical vertebrae during whiplash loading. *Spine* 1999;24:763–769.

227. Taylor JR, Twomey LT. Acute injuries to cervical joints: An autopsy study of neck sprain. *Spine* 1993;9:1115–1122.

228. Barnsley L, Lord S, Bogduk N. The pathophysiology of whiplash. In: Malanga GA, ed. *Cervical Flexion-Extension/Whiplash Injuries. Spine: State of the Art Reviews.* Philadelphia, Pa: Hanley and Belfus; 1998:209–242.

229. Winkelstein B, et al. The cervical facet capsule and its role in whiplash injury: A biomechanical investigation. *Spine* 2000;25:1238–1246.

230. Deans GT, Magalliard K, Rutherford WH. Neck sprain: A major cause of disability following car accidents. *Injury* 1987;18:10–12.

231. Lord SM, et al. Chronic cervical zygapophysial joint pain after whiplash: A placebo-controlled prevalence study. *Spine* 1996; 21:1737–1744.

232. Bogduk N. Innervation and pain patterns of the cervical spine. In: Grant R, ed. *Physical Therapy of the Cervical and Thoracic Spine.* New York, NY: Churchill Livingstone; 1988.

233. Livingston M. *Common Whiplash Injury: A Modern Epidemic.* Springfield, Ill: Charles C Thomas; 1999:65–76.

234. Klein de A, Nieuwenhuyse AC. Schwindelanfaalle und Nystagumus bei einer bestimmeten Lage des Kopfes. *Arch Otolaryngol* 1927;11:155.

235. Toglia JU. Acute flexion-extension injury of the neck. *Neurology* 1976;26:808.

236. Wing LW, Hargrove-Wilson W. Cervical vertigo. *Aust N Z J Surg* 1974;44:275.

237. Chester JB Jr. Whiplash, postural control, and the inner ear. *Spine* 1991;16:716.

238. Edeiken-Monroe B, Wagner LK, Harris JH Jr. Hyperextension dislocation of the cervical spine. *AJR Am J Roentgenol* 1986; 146:803–808.

239. Osti OL, Vernon-Roberts B, Frazer RD. Annulus tears and intervertebral disc degeneration: A study using an animal model. *Spine* 1990;15:762.

240. Gargan MF, Bannister GC. Long term prognosis of soft tissue injuries of the neck. *J Bone Joint Surg* 1990;72B:901.

241. Vanezis P. Vertebral artery injuries in road traffic accidents: A post-mortem study. *J Forensic Sci Soc* 1986;26:281–291.

242. Viktrup L, Knudsen GM, Hansen SH. Delayed onset of fatal basilar thrombotic embolus after whiplash injury. *Stroke* 1995; 26:2194–2196.

243. Borchgrevink G, et al. MR imaging and radiography of patients with cervical hyperextension-flexion injuries after car accidents. *Acta Radiol* 1995;36:425–458.

244. Ronnen HR, et al. Acute whiplash injury: Is there a role for MR imaging? A prospective study of 100 patients. *Radiology* 1996;201:93–96.

245. Ellertsson AB, Sigurjonsson K, Thorsteinsson T. Clinical and radiographic study of 100 cases of whiplash injury. *Acta Neurol Scand* 1978;57:269.

246. Seitz JP, et al. SPECT of the cervical spine in the evaluation of neck pain after trauma. *Clin Nucl Med* 1995;20:667–673.

247. Dreyer SJ, Boden SD. Nonoperative treatment of neck and arm pain. *Spine* 1998;23:2746–2754.

248. Pennie BH, Agambar LJ. Whiplash injuries. *J Bone Joint Surg* 1990;72B:277–279.

249. Helliwell PS, Evans PF, Wright V. The straight cervical spine: Does it indicate muscle spasm? *J Bone Joint Surg* 1994; 76B:103–106.

250. Thompson JF, Jannsen F. Thoracic outlet syndromes. *Br J Surg* 1996;83:435–436.

251. Strukel RJ, Garrick JG. Thoracic outlet compression in athletes: A report of four cases. *Am J Sports Med* 1978;6:35–39.

252. Peet RM, et al. Thoracic outlet syndrome: Evaluation of the therapeutic exercise program. *Proc Mayo Clin* 1956; 31:281–287.

253. MacKinnon EJ, Dellon AL. *Surgery of the Peripheral Nerve.* New York, NY: Thieme; 1988.

254. Karas SE. Thoracic outlet syndrome. *Clin Sports Med* 1990; 9:297–310.

255. Sanders RJ, et al. Scalene muscle abnormalities in traumatic thoracic outlet syndrome. *Am J Surg* 1990;159:231–236.

256. McCarthy WJ, et al. Upper extremity arterial injury in athletes. *J Vasc Surg* 1989;9:317–327.

257. Vogel CM, Jensen JE. "Effort" thrombosis of the subclavian vein in a competitive swimmer. *Am J Sports Med* 1985; 13:269–272.

258. Leffert RD. Thoracic outlet syndrome and the shoulder. *Clin Sports Med* 1983;2:439–452.

259. Nishida T, Price SJ, Minieka MM. Medial antebrachial cutaneous nerve conduction in true neurogenic thoracic outlet syndrome. *Electromyogr Clin Neurophysiol* 1993;33:285–288.

260. Cuetter AC, David MB. The thoracic outlet syndrome: Controversies, over diagnosis, over treatment, and recommendations for management. *Muscle Nerve* 1989;12:410–419.

261. Kenny RA, et al. Thoracic outlet syndrome: A useful exercise treatment option. *Am J Surg* 1993;165:282–284.

262. Silver D. Thoracic outlet syndrome. In: Sabiston DC, ed. *Textbook of Surgery: The Biological Basis of Modern Surgical Practice*. Philadelphia, Pa: Saunders; 1986:533–554.

263. Crawford FA. Thoracic outlet syndrome. *Surg Clin North Am* 1980;60:947–956.

264. Sanders RJ, Johnson RF. Medico-legal matters. In: Sanders RJ, Haug CE, eds. *Thoracic Outlet Syndrome: A Common Sequela of Neck Injuries*. Philadelphia, Pa: JB Lippincott; 1991:271–277.

264a. Pettman E. *Level III Course Notes*. Berrien Springs, Mich: North American Institute of Manual Therapy, Inc.; 2003.

264b. Evjenth O, Hamberg J. *Muscle Stretching in Manual Therapy, A Clinical Manual*. Alfta, Sweden: Alfta Rehab Forlag; 1984.

265. Mulligan BR. *Manual Therapy: "NAGS", "SNAGS", "PRP'S" etc*. Wellington, New Zealand: Plane View Series; 1992.

266. Cohen JH, Schneider MJ. Receptor-tonus technique. An overview. *Chiro Tech* 1990;2:13–16.

267. Cole AJ, Farrell JP, Stratton SA. Cervical spine athletic injuries. *Phys Med Rehabil Clin North Am* 1994;5:37–68.

268. Ward R. Myofascial release concepts. In: Nyberg N, Basmajian JV, eds. *Rational Manual Therapies*. Baltimore, Md: Williams and Wilkins; 1993:223–241.

269. Liebenson C. Manual resistance techniques and self stretches for improving flexibility and mobility. In: Liebenson C, ed. *Rehabilitation of the Spine: A Practitioner's Manual*. Baltimore, Md: Lippincott Williams and Wilkins; 1996:253–292.

270. Erhard RE. Manual therapy in the cervical spine. In: *Physical Therapy Home Study Course*. La Crosse, Wis: Orthopaedic Section, American Physical Therapy Association; 1996.

271. Raikin S, Froimson MI: Bilateral brachial plexus compressive neuropathy (crutch palsy). *J Orthop Trauma* 1997;11:136–138.

CHAPTER 24

THE TEMPOROMANDIBULAR JOINT

CHAPTER OBJECTIVES

▶ **At the completion of this chapter, the reader will be able to:**

1. Describe the anatomy of the temporomandibular joint, including the bones, ligaments, muscles, and blood and nerve supply.

2. Describe the biomechanics of the temporomandibular joint, including the movements, normal and abnormal joint barriers, kinesiology, and reactions to various stresses.

3. Summarize the various causes of temporomandibular dysfunction.

4. Describe the close association between the temporomandibular joint, the middle ear, and the cervical spine.

5. Perform a comprehensive examination of the temporomandibular musculoskeletal system, including palpation of the articular and soft tissue structures, specific passive mobility and passive articular mobility tests, and stability tests.

6. Evaluate the total examination data to establish a diagnosis.

7. Recognize the manifestations of abnormal temporomandibular joint function and develop strategies to correct these abnormalities.

8. Apply active and passive mobilization techniques to the temporomandibular joint, using the correct grade, direction, and duration.

9. Describe and demonstrate intervention strategies and techniques based on clinical findings and established goals.

10. Evaluate the intervention effectiveness in order to progress or modify an intervention.

11. Plan an effective home program and instruct the patient in this program.

OVERVIEW

Housed within the skull are the components of the stomatognathic system. The stomatognathic system comprises the temporomandibular joint (TMJ), the masticatory systems, and the related organs and tissues such as the salivary glands.[1] Due to the proximity of this system with the other structures of the head and neck, an intimate relationship exists. This relationship begins in the early stages of human embryology.

The embryologic structures from which the head, face, and neck originate are segmentally organized during development with the appearance and modification of six paired branchial or pharyngeal arches.[1] These branchial arches contain the cranial nuclei of the trigeminal nerve (ophthalmic; maxillary and mandibular), the facial, the glossopharyngeal, and the laryngeal branch of the vagus nerve as well as the hypoglossal nerve.

The first of these arches, the mandibular arch, consists of a large ventral part (mandibular process of Meckel's cartilage) and a small dorsal (maxillary) process. As development progresses, both processes disappear except for two small portions at the dorsal ends which persist. The first branchial arch forms:

▶ The mandible.

▶ The rudiments of the inner ear bones, the malleus, and incus.

► The anterior malleolar and sphenomandibular ligaments of the temporomandibular joint.

► The tensor tympani, tensor veli palatini of the inner ear.

► The mylohyoid and the anterior belly of the digastric muscle.

► The trigeminal mandibular nerve.

The second pharyngeal arch (the hyoid arch) consists of Reichert's cartilage. This arch is involved in the formation of:

► The superior component of the hyoid bone and the lesser cornu bone.

► The stapes muscle.

► The temporal styloid process.

► The stylohyoid ligament.

► The stapedius muscle.

► The stylohyoid muscle.

► The posterior belly of the digastric muscle.

► The muscles of facial expression and mastication.

► The platysma muscle.

► The glossopharyngeal nerve.

The third pharyngeal arch is involved in the formation of the greater cornu of the hyoid and its body, the stylopharyngeal muscle, and the sensory apparatus of the posterior one third of the tongue.

The fourth pharyngeal arch combines with the sixth arch to form the thyroid, cricoid, and arytenoid cartilages of the larynx. The muscles derived from this arch are the pharyngeal constrictors (the cricothyroid) and the intrinsic muscles of the larynx. The pharyngeal constrictors are innervated by the superior laryngeal branch of the vagus nerve. The intrinsic muscles of the larynx are innervated by the recurrent laryngeal branch of the vagus nerve.

In primitive creatures, and the human fetus, vibrations through the jaw are used as a basis for hearing. At around 8½ weeks, the small bones of the inner ear (the malleus, incus, and stapes) can be seen as distinct entities. The development of the malleus bone and the tensor tympani are intimately related to that of the lateral pterygoid muscle. Due to this embryological relationship, it is theorized that a spasm of the lateral pterygoid muscle can increase the tension within the tensor tympani (similar to that of a drum skin)[1a] resulting in an increased sensitivity to pitch and vibration. Theoretically this increased tension could produce sensorineural tinnitus, or ringing in the ears,[1b] a common associated symptom of a temporomandibular disorder. The term *temporomandibular disorder* (TMD) is a collective term used to describe a number of related disorders affecting the stomatognathic system and its related structures, all of which may have common symptoms. The term

TMJ as an overall descriptor of stomatognathic system dysfunction has been discontinued because it is inaccurate and misleading, and implies structural conditions when none or when many other, more important factors may be involved.[1c]

The diagnosis of TMD, like that of whiplash syndrome, remains controversial.[3] This is due in part to a paucity of studies regarding the incidence, course, management, and prognosis of claimed TMDs.[4,5] However, reports of TMD appear to be quite common. About 60 to 70 percent of the general population has at least one sign of a TMD, yet only around one in four people with signs actually is aware of or reports any symptoms,[6,7] and only about 5 percent of people with one or more signs of a TMD will actually seek an intervention.[7-9] The most common TMD by far, comprising 90 to 95 percent of all TMD cases, is a condition with multiple musculoskeletal facial pain complaints and a variety of jaw impairments, without an identified structural cause.[10]

Most of those who seek medical intervention for TMDs are female, outnumbering male patients by at least four to one.[8,9,11] The reason for the higher prevalence of TMD in women, and the overrepresentation of females at orofacial pain clinics, remains obscure. One explanation could be that women more readily seek treatment for illness than do men.[12]

TMD is best approached as a biopsychosocial dysfunction. Although TMD originally was approached as one syndrome, current research supports the view that TMD is a cluster of related disorders in the stomatognathic system that have many common symptoms.[6,13] McNeill and colleagues[14] have described three etiologic factors of TMD: (1) predisposing factors, (2) precipitating or triggering factors, and (3) perpetuating or sustaining factors[15]:

► Predisposing factors include the structural, neurologic, hormonal, and metabolic features of an individual.

► Precipitating factors generally fall into the following four categories: (1) overt, extrinsic trauma to the head, neck, or jaw; (2) repeated low-grade extrinsic trauma, such as nail biting and chewing gum; (3) repeated low-grade intrinsic trauma such as teeth clenching or bruxism (grinding teeth); and (4) stress that passes a certain threshold, which is individual for each patient.

► Perpetuating or contributing factors are those that aid in the continuation of symptoms. These can include systemic disease and cervical pathology.

Thus, the clinical course of TMD does not reflect a progressive disease but rather a complex disorder that is molded by many interacting factors, such as stress, anxiety, and depression, which serve to maintain the disease.[13] Headaches, orofacial pain, earache, and neck pain are common complaints. Persistent or recurrent pain is considered the main reason that more than 90 percent of patients with TMD seek an intervention.[8,16] A diagnosis of TMD must, therefore, include consideration of all of the following:

► Jaw muscles.

► Bone and cartilage joint structures.

► Facial structures.

► Soft tissue joint structures, including the articular disk and synovium.

► Jaw and joint function.

► Cervical and upper thoracic spine function.

► Posture and dysfunction.

► Systemic disease.

► Psychosocial issues.

Given the number of potential causes of jaw and face pain, a diagnosis of TMD can rarely be ascribed solely to the TMJ. Examples of appropriate diagnoses for TMD are more likely to include:

► Rheumatoid arthritis with synovitis, arthralgia, condylar degenerative disease, and open bite deformity.

► Chronic pain with a behavioral disorder.

► Myofascial pain and impairment.

► Internal disk derangement, with displacement and reduction.

Although dentists are the primary professionals involved in the examination and intervention of TMD, physical therapists can play an important role in assisting the dentist in restoring function to the stomatognathic system. Nonsurgical interventions such as counseling, physical therapy, pharmacotherapy, and occlusal splint therapy continue to be the most effective way of managing more than 80 percent of patients with TMD.[13]

Anatomy

The TMJ (Fig. 24-1) is a synovial, compound, modified ovoid bicondylar joint, formed between the articular eminence of the temporal bone, the intra-articular disk, and the head of the mandible.

The TMJ is unique in that, even though the joint is synovial, the articulating surfaces of the bones are covered not by hyaline cartilage, but by fibrocartilage.[17,18] Fibrocartilage has the same general properties found in hyaline cartilage, but tends to be less distensible, owing to a greater proportion of dense collagen fibers (see Chap. 1). Fibrocartilage is an avascular, alymphatic, and aneural tissue and derives its nutrition by a double-diffusion system.[19] The development of fibrocartilage over the load-bearing surface of the TMJ indicates that the joint is designed to withstand large and repeated stresses, and that this area of the joint surface has a greater capacity to repair itself than would hyaline cartilage.[20]

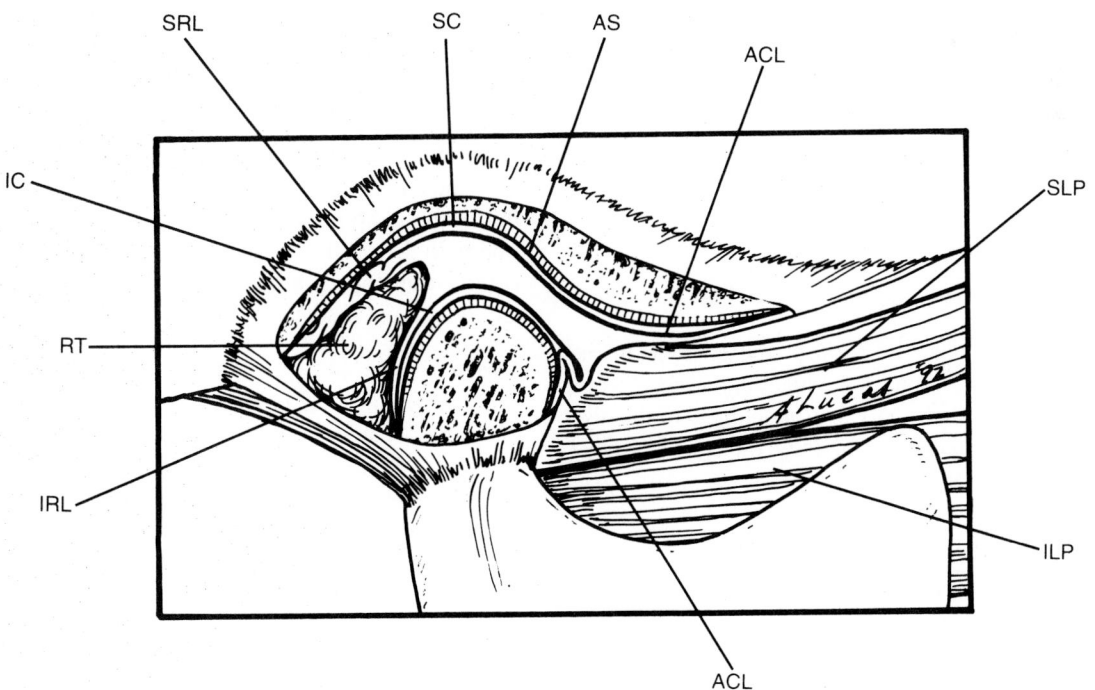

FIGURE 24-1   Lateral view of the temporomandibular joint. ACL, anterior capsular ligament; AS, articular surface; IC, inferior joint cavity; ILP, inferior lateral pterygoid muscles; IRL, inferior retrodiscal lamina; RT, retrodiscal tissues; SC, superior joint cavity; SLP, superior lateral pterygoid muscle; SRL, superior retrodiscal lamina. (Reproduced with permission from Okeson JP. *Management of Temporomandibular Disorders and Occlusion.* 4th ed. St Louis, Mo: Mosby Year Book; 1998:10.)

The area of load bearing is affected by the congruity of the contacting tooth surfaces (occlusion), head position, and the coordination of muscle function. The fibrocartilage is at its thinnest at the roof of the fossa, but load bearing here occurs only in the presence of dysfunction.[19]

The mandible works like a class-three lever, with its joint as the fulcrum. Although there is no agreement among the experts concerning force transmission through the joint, there does appear to be agreement that postural impairments of the cervical and upper thoracic spine can produce both pain and impairment of the TMJ.[6]

Fibrocartilaginous Disk

Located between the articulating surface of the temporal bone and the mandibular condyle is a fibrocartilaginous disk (sometimes inappropriately referred to as "meniscus"). The biconcave shape of the disk is determined by the shape of the condyle and the articulating fossa.[21] Rees[18] has described the fibrocartilaginous disk as having three clearly defined transverse, ellipsoidal zones that are divided into three regions—posterior band, intermediate zone, and anterior band—of which the intermediate zone makes contact with the articular surface of the condyle.

Both the disk and the lateral pterygoid muscle develop from the first branchial arch, and there is very little differentiation among the muscle, the disk, and the joint capsule.[22,23] The fibrocartilaginous disk is tethered by a number of structures:

▶ Medial and lateral collateral discal ligaments firmly attach the fibrocartilaginous disk to the medial and lateral poles of the condyle, permitting anterior and posterior rotation of the disk on the condyle during mouth opening and closing.[24,25]

▶ Posteriorly, the disk is attached by fibro-elastic tissue to the posterior mandibular fossa and the back of the mandibular condyle.[24,25]

▶ Anteriorly, the disk is attached to the upper part of the tendon of the lateral pterygoid muscle[24,25] (Fig. 24-2).

The disk usually is located on top of the condyle in the 12 o'clock to 1 o'clock position on the mandibular head when the jaw is closed.[26] Because the only firm attachment of the disk to the condyle occurs medially and laterally, the disk can move somewhat independently of the condyle.[27]

The disk effectively divides the TMJ into a lower and an upper joint cavity (see Fig. 24-2):

▶ *Lower compartment.* This compartment, bordered by the mandibular condyle and the inferior surface of the articular disk, is where, under normal conditions, the osteokinematic spin (rotation) of the condyle occurs.[6]

▶ *Upper compartment.* This compartment, bordered by the mandibular fossa and the superior surface of the

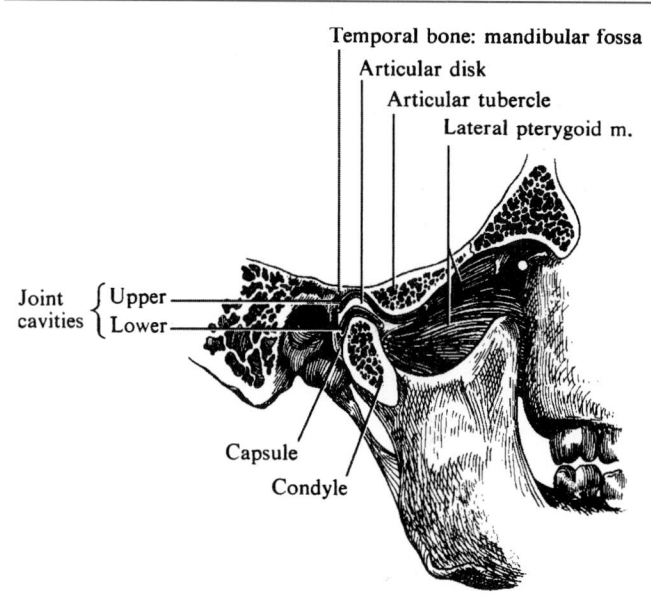

FIGURE 24-2   Sagittal section of the temporomandibular joint. (Reproduced with permission from Pansky B. *Review of Gross Anatomy.* 6th ed. New York, NY: McGraw-Hill; 1996:41.)

articular disk, primarily allows only translation of the disk and condyle along the fossa, and onto the articular eminence.[6]

Blood vessels and nerves are found only in the thickened periphery of this disk, especially its posterior attachment; its middle articular portion is avascular and aneural.[28]

Bony Anatomy

A number of bony components make up the masticatory system: the maxilla and the mandible, which support the teeth, and the temporal bone, which supports the mandible at its articulation with the skull. The sphenoid bone and the hyoid bone also could be included, because they provide important anatomic and functional links to the TMJ.

Maxilla

The borders of the maxillae extend superiorly to form the floor of the nasal cavity as well as the floor of each orbit (Fig. 24-3). Inferiorly, the maxillary bones form the palate and the alveolar ridges, which support the teeth.

Mandible

The mandible, or jaw (Fig. 24-4), which supports the lower teeth, is the largest and strongest bone in the face. It is suspended below the maxillae by muscles and ligaments that provide it with both mobility and stability. The medial surface of the mandible serves as the attachment for the medial pterygoid and the digastric muscles. The platysma, mentalis, and buccinator gain attachment on its lateral aspect.

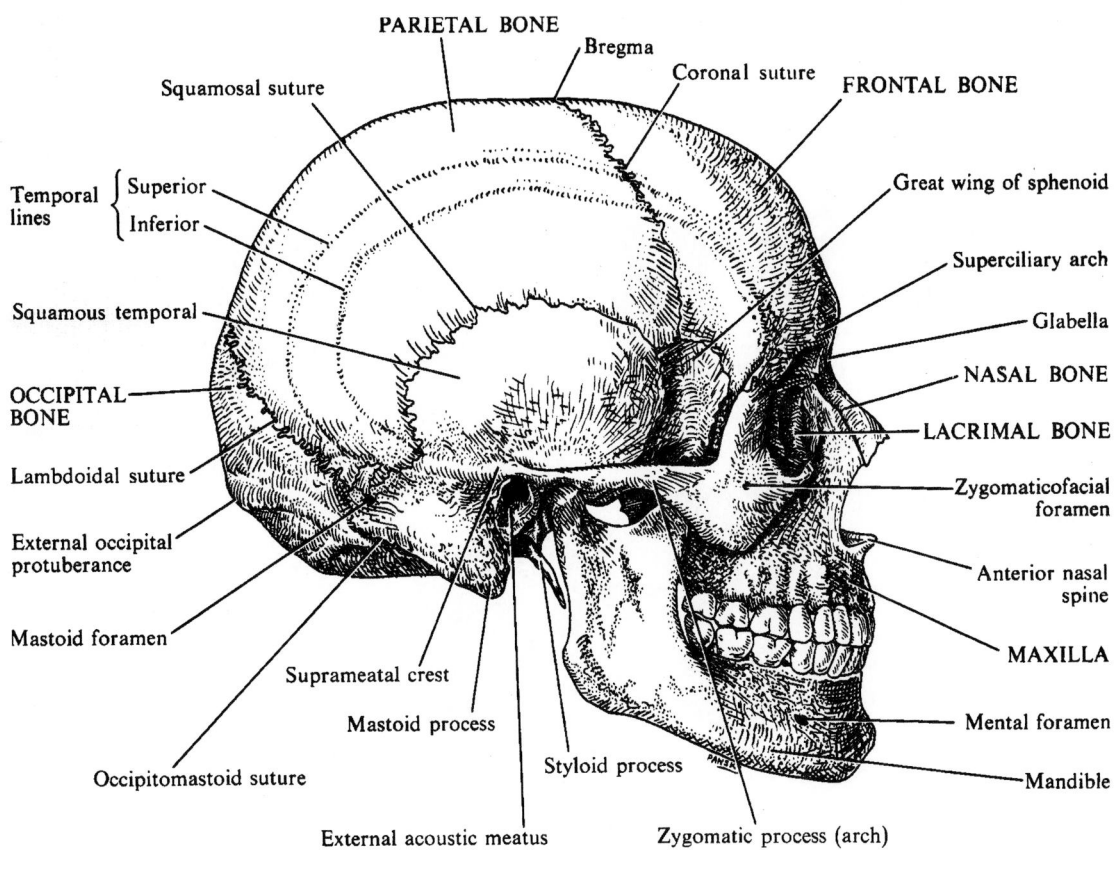

FIGURE 24-3 Lateral view of the skull showing the maxilla. (Reproduced with permission from Pansky B. *Review of Gross Anatomy*. 6th ed. New York, NY: McGraw-Hill; 1996:9.)

Two broad, vertical rami extend upward from the mandible: the condylar and the coronoid. The anterior of the two processes, the coronoid, serves as the attachment for the temporalis and masseter muscles.[29] The posterior condylar process articulates with the temporal bone.

The bony surfaces of the condyle and the articular portion of the temporal bone are made of dense cortical bone.

Temporal Bone

The articulating surface of the temporal bone is made up of a concave mandibular, or glenoid, fossa, and a convex bony prominence called the *articular eminence*.[30] The articular tubercle, situated anterior to the glenoid fossa, serves as an attachment for the temporomandibular (or lateral) ligament.[29]

Sphenoid Bone

The greater wings of the sphenoid bone form the boundaries of the anterior part of the middle cranial fossa. From these greater wings, the pterygoid laminae serve as the attachments for the medial and lateral pterygoid muscles.

Hyoid Bone

The U-shaped hyoid bone (Fig. 24-5) also is known as the skeleton of the tongue. The hyoid bone is involved with the mandible to provide reciprocal stabilization during swallowing and chewing. It also serves as the attachment for the infrahyoid muscles and for some of the extrinsic tongue muscles.

Supporting Structures

The supporting structures of the TMJ consist of periarticular connective tissue (ligament, tendon, capsule, and fascia). As its name implies, the periarticular connective tissue serves to keep the joints together and to limit the ranges of motion at the joint. For example, the ligaments of the TMJ protect and support the joint structures, and act as passive restraints to joint movement. The synovial cavities are surrounded by loose connective tissue rather than by ligaments.

The intercapsular structures are located posteriorly to the condyle. Anterior to the joint are the muscles of the medial and lateral pterygoid (see next section). There are no well-defined anterior or posterior ligaments between the mandibular condyle

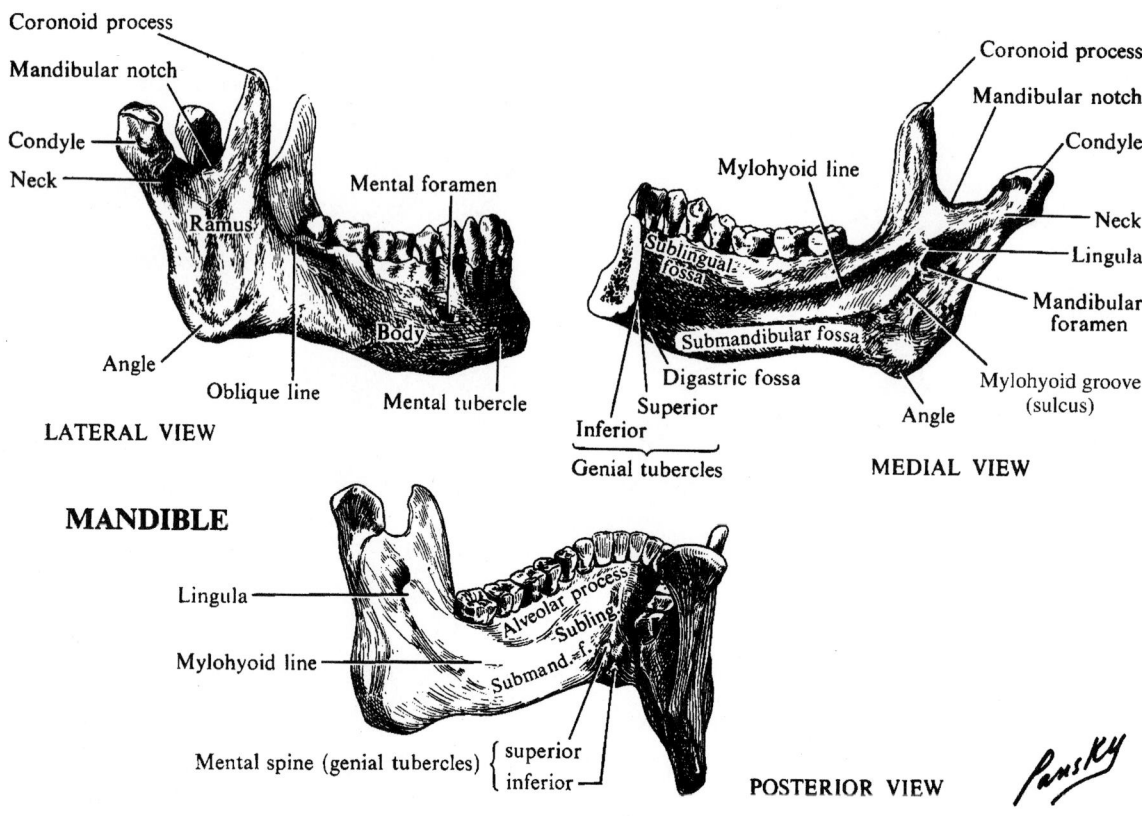

FIGURE 24-4   The mandible. (Reproduced with permission from Pansky B. *Review of Gross Anatomy*. 6th ed. New York, NY: McGraw-Hill; 1996:7.)

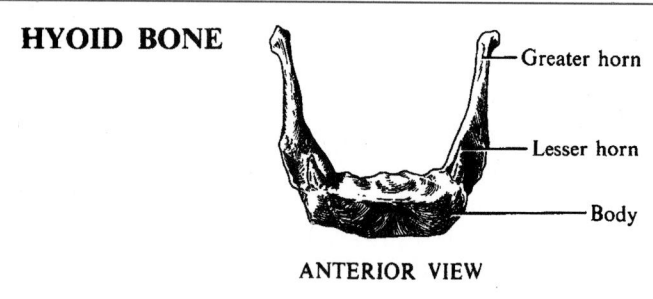

FIGURE 24-5   The hyoid bone. (Reproduced with permission from Pansky B. *Review of Gross Anatomy*. 6th ed. New York, NY: McGraw-Hill; 1996:7.)

and the temporal bone. However, two strong ligaments help to provide joint stability:

1. *Joint capsule or capsular ligament.* This structure, which surrounds the entire joint, is thought to provide proprioceptive feedback regarding joint position and movement.[31,32]

2. *Temporomandibular (or lateral) ligament.* The capsule of the TMJ is reinforced laterally by an outer oblique portion and an inner horizontal portion of the temporomandibular ligament (Fig. 24-6), which function as a suspensory mechanism for the mandible during moderate opening movements. The ligament also func-

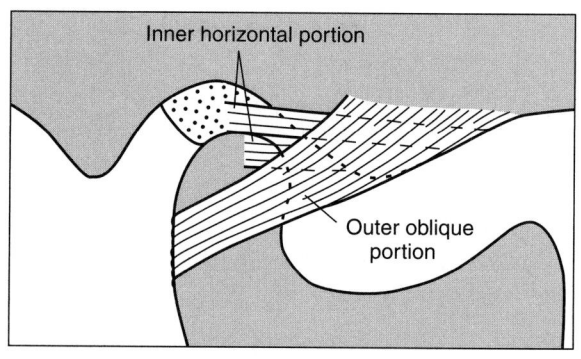

FIGURE 24-6   The temporomandibular ligament. (Reproduced with permission from Murphy DR. *Conservative Management of Cervical Spine Syndromes*. New York, NY: McGraw-Hill; 2000:581.)

tions to resist rotation, and posterior displacement of the mandible.

Two other ligaments assist with joint stability:

▶ *Stylomandibular ligament.* The stylomandibular ligament (Fig. 24-7) is a specialized band that splits away from the superficial lamina of the deep cervical fascia to run deep to both pterygoid muscles.[30] This ligament becomes taut and acts as a guiding mechanism for the mandible, keeping the condyle, disk, and temporal bone firmly opposed.

▶ *Sphenomandibular ligament.* The sphenomandibular ligament is a thin band that runs from the spine of the sphenoid bone to a small bony prominence on the medial surface of the ramus of the mandible, called the *lingula* (see Fig. 24-7). This ligament acts to check the angle of the mandible from sliding as far forward as the condyles during the translatory cycle, and serves as a suspensory ligament of the mandible during wide opening.[30] It is this ligament that hurts with any prolonged jaw opening, such as that which occurs at the dentist.

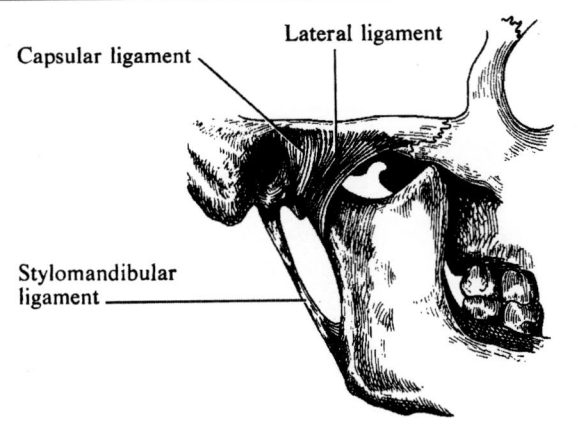

LATERAL VIEW

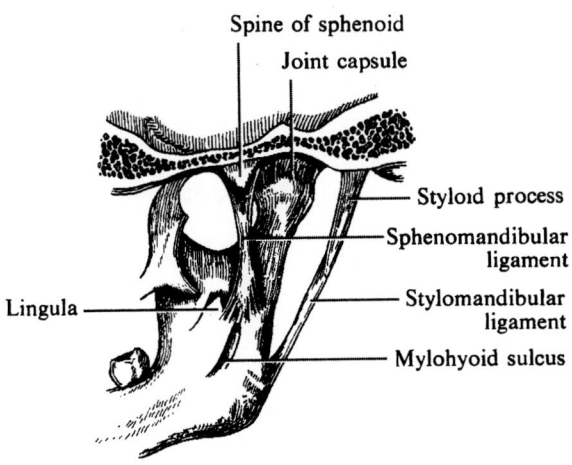

MEDIAL VIEW

FIGURE 24-7 Ligaments of the temporomandibular joint. (Reproduced with permission from Pansky B. *Review of Gross Anatomy.* 6th ed. New York, NY: McGraw-Hill; 1996:41.)

Clinical Pearl

Pinto's ligament[33] is a vestige of Meckel's cartilage, an embryologic tissue. It arises from the neck of the malleus of the inner ear and runs in a medial-superior direction to insert into the posterior aspect of the TMJ capsule and disk. Although the role of this ligament in mandibular mechanics is thought to be negligible, its relationship to the middle ear and the TMJ could be a basis for the middle ear symptoms, which are often present with TMD. Stack and Funt[34] postulated that auditory symptoms of fullness and pressure in the middle ear may be present as a result of direct transmission of TMJ capsular tension to the ossicles of the middle ear through this ligament.

Muscles

The muscles of mastication are the key muscles when discussing TMD. Three of these muscles, the masseter, medial pterygoid, and temporalis, function to raise the mandible during mouth closing. The lateral pterygoid and digastric muscles work together to depress the mandible during mouth opening.

Although these muscles work most efficiently in groups, an understanding of the specific anatomy and action(s) of the individual muscles is necessary for an appreciation of their coordinated function during masticatory activity (Tables 24-1 and 24-2).

Temporalis

The temporalis muscle (Fig. 24-8) has as its origin the floor of the temporal fossa and temporal fascia. The muscle travels inferiorly and anteriorly to insert on the anterior border of the coronoid process and anterior border of the ramus of the mandible. The temporalis muscle is innervated by a branch of the mandibular division of the trigeminal nerve. In addition to assisting with mouth closing and with side-to-side grinding of the teeth, the temporalis muscle provides a good deal of stability to the joint.

The Masseter

The masseter (Fig. 24-9) is a two-layered quadrilateral shaped muscle. The superficial portion arises from the anterior two thirds of the lower border of the zygomatic arch. The deep portion arises from the medial surface of the zygomatic arch. Both sets of fibers blend anteriorly and form a raphe with the medial pterygoid.[30] The masseter inserts on the lateral surface of the coronoid process of the mandible, upper half of the ramus and angle of the mandible. The masseter muscle is innervated by a branch of the mandibular division of the trigeminal nerve. The major function of the masseter is to elevate the mandible, thereby occluding the teeth during mastication.

The Medial Pterygoid

The medial pterygoid muscle is a thick quadrilateral muscle with a deep origin situated on the medial aspect of the mandibular

TABLE 24-1   Muscles of the Temporomandibular Joint

Muscle	Proximal	Distal	Innervation
Medial pterygoid	Medial surface of lateral pterygoid plate and tuberosity of maxilla	Medial surface of mandible close to angle	Mandibular division of trigeminal nerve
Lateral pterygoid	Greater wing of sphenoid and lateral pterygoid plate	Neck of mandible and articular cartilage	Mandibular division of trigeminal nerve
Temporalis	Temporal cranial fossa	By way of a tendon into medial surface, apex, and anterior and posterior borders of mandibular ramus	Anterior and posterior deep temporal nerves, which branch from anterior division of mandibular branch of trigeminal nerve
Masseter	Superficial portion: from anterior two thirds of lower border of zygomatic arch; deep portion from medial surface of zygomatic arch	Lateral surfaces of coronoid process of mandible, upper half of ramus, and angle of mandible	Masseteric nerve from anterior trunk of mandibular division of trigeminal nerve
Mylohyoid	Medial surface of mandible	Body of hyoid bone	Mylohyoid branch of trigeminal nerve, mandibular division
Geniohyoid	Mental spine of mandible	Body of hyoid bone	Ventral ramus of C1 via hypoglossal nerve
Stylohyoid	Styloid process of temporal bone	Body of hyoid bone	Facial nerve
Anterior and posterior digastric	Internal surface of mandible and mastoid process of temporal bone	By intermediate tendon to hyoid bone	Anterior: mandibular division of trigeminal nerve; posterior: facial nerve
Sternohyoid	Manubrium and medial end of clavicle	Body of hyoid bone	Ansa cervicalis
Omohyoid	Superior angle of scapula	Inferior body of hyoid bone	Ansa cervicalis
Sternothyroid	Posterior surface of manubrium	Thyroid cartilage	Ansa cervicalis
Thyrohyoid	Thyroid cartilage	Inferior body and greater horn of hyoid bone	C1 via hypoglossal nerve

ramus (Fig. 24-10). The muscle travels posteriorly to insert on the inferior and posterior aspects of the medial subsurface of the ramus and angle of the mandible. The medial pterygoid muscle is innervated by a branch of the mandibular division of the trigeminal nerve. Working bilaterally, and in association with the masseter and temporalis muscles, the medial pterygoids assist in mouth closing. Individually, the medial pterygoid muscle is capable of deviating the mandible toward the opposite side. The medial pterygoid muscle also acts as an assist to the lateral pterygoid and anterior fibers of the temporalis muscle to produce protrusion of the mandible.

The Lateral Pterygoid

Two divisions of the lateral pterygoid muscles are recognized, each of which is functionally and anatomically separate (Fig. 24-11). The superior head arises from the infratemporal surface of the greater wing of the sphenoid. The inferior head arises from the lateral surface of the lateral pterygoid plate. Despite several investigations,[35–37] no consensus has been reached regarding the insertion of the lateral pterygoid muscle. However, the most commonly described insertion is at the anterior aspect of the neck of the mandibular condyle and capsule of the TMJ. The lateral pterygoid muscle is

TABLE 24-2 Actions of the Temporomandibular Joint Muscles

Action	Muscles Acting
Opening of mouth	Lateral pterygoid Mylohyoid Geniohyoid Digastric
Closing of mouth	Masseter Temporalis Medial pterygoid
Protrusion of mandible	Lateral pterygoid Medial pterygoid Masseter Mylohyoid Geniohyoid Digastric Stylohyoid Temporalis (anterior fibers)
Retraction of mandible	Temporalis (posterior fibers) Masseter Digastric Stylohyoid Mylohyoid Geniohyoid
Lateral deviation of mandible	Lateral pterygoid (ipsilateral muscle) Medial pterygoid (contralateral muscle) Temporalis Masseter

innervated by a branch of the mandibular division of the trigeminal nerve.

The superior head of the lateral pterygoid is involved mainly with chewing, and functions to anteriorly rotate the disk on the condyle during the closing movement.[38,39] It has also been suggested that in normal function of the craniomandibular complex, the superior lateral pterygoid plays an important role in stabilizing and controlling the movements of the disk.[40]

The inferior head of the lateral pterygoid muscle exerts an anterior, lateral, and inferior pull on the mandible, thereby opening the jaw, protruding the mandible, and deviating the mandible to the opposite side.

Infrahyoid or "Strap" Muscles

The infrahyoid muscles comprise the sternohyoid, omohyoid, sternothyroid, and thyrohyoid muscles (Fig. 24-12).

▶ *Sternohyoid.* The sternohyoid muscle is a strap-like muscle that functions to depress the hyoid and assist in speech and mastication.

▶ *Omohyoid.* The omohyoid muscle, situated lateral to the sternohyoid, consists of two bellies and functions to depress the hyoid. In addition, the muscle has been speculated to tense the inferior aspect of the deep cervical fascia in prolonged inspiratory efforts, thereby releasing tension on the apices of the lungs and on the internal jugular vein, which are attached to this fascial layer.[30]

▶ *Sternothyroid and thyrohyoid.* The sternothyroid and thyrohyoid muscles (see Fig. 24-12) are located deep to the sternohyoid muscle. The sternothyroid muscle is involved in drawing the larynx downward, whereas the thyrohyoid depresses the hyoid and elevates the larynx.

These infrahyoid muscles are innervated by fibers from the upper cervical nerves. The nerves to the lower part of these

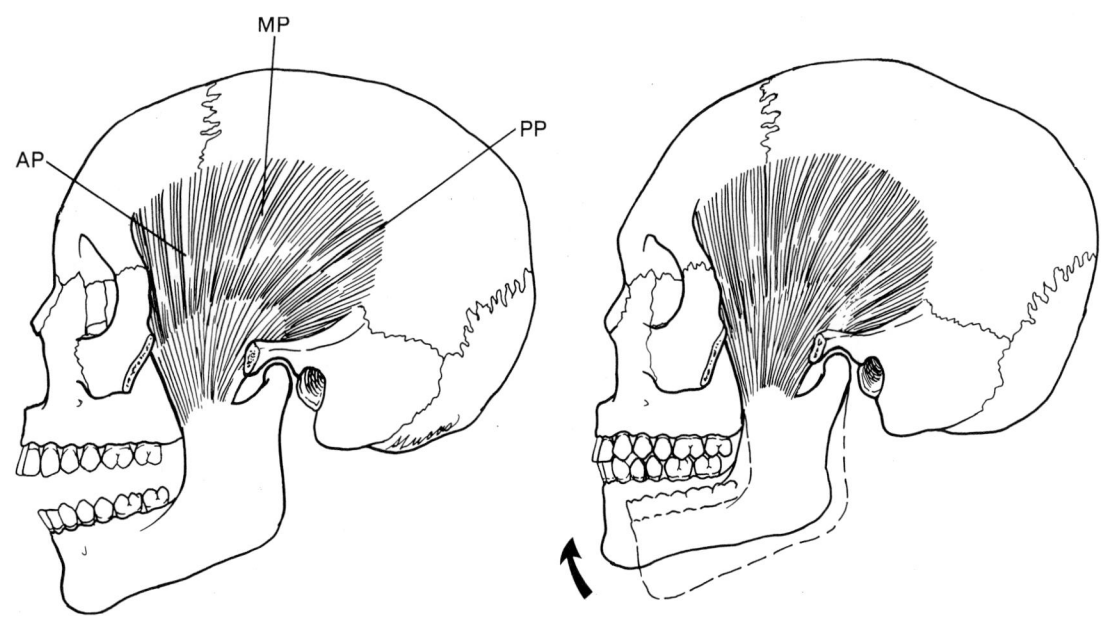

FIGURE 24-8 The temporalis muscle. AP, anterior portion; MP, middle portion; PP, posterior portion. (Reproduced with permission from Okeson JP. *Management of Temporomandibular Disorders and Occlusion.* 4th ed. St Louis, Mo: Mosby Year Book; 1998:19.)

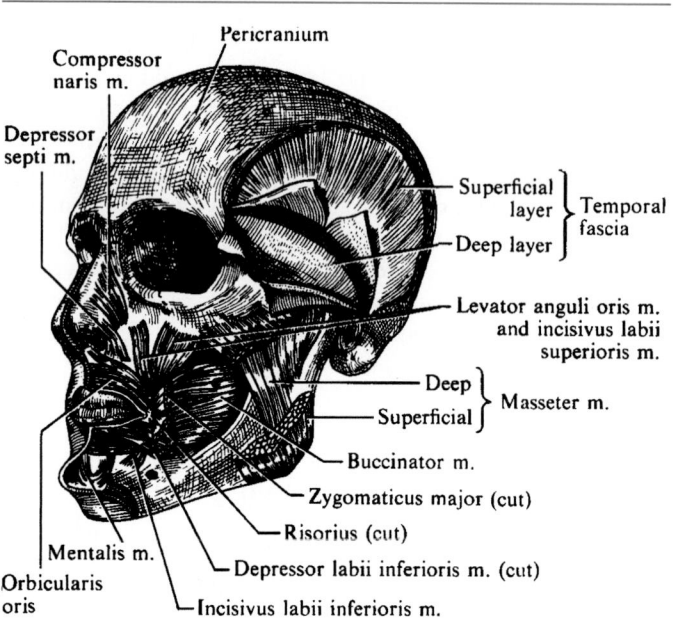

Geniohyoid. The geniohyoid muscle is a narrow muscle situated under the mylohyoid muscle (Fig. 24-13). The muscle functions to elevate the hyoid bone.

Digastric. As its name suggests, the digastric muscle consists of two bellies (Fig. 24-12). The posterior belly arises from the mastoid notch of the temporal bone, while the anterior belly arises from the digastric fossa of the mandible. The posterior belly is innervated by a branch from the facial nerve. The anterior belly is innervated by the inferior alveolar branch of the trigeminal nerve. The two bellies of the digastric muscle are joined by a rounded tendon that attaches to the body and greater cornu of the hyoid bone through a fibrous loop or sling.[30]

Bilaterally, the two bellies of the digastric muscle assist in forced mouth opening by stabilizing the hyoid. The posterior bellies are especially active during coughing and swallowing.[30]

FIGURE 24-9 The muscles of mastication (masseter muscle). (Reproduced with permission from Pansky B. *Review of Gross Anatomy.* 6th ed. New York, NY: McGraw-Hill; 1996:31.)

muscles are given off from a loop, the ansa cervicalis (cervical loop) (see Chap. 2)

Suprahyoid Muscles

The supra- and infrahyoid muscles play a major role in coordinating mandibular function, by providing a firm base on which the tongue and mandible can be moved.

> ### Clinical Pearl
>
> Working in combinations, the muscles of the TMJ are involved as follows:
>
> - Mouth opening—bilateral action of the lateral pterygoid and digastric muscles.
> - Mouth closing—bilateral action of the temporalis, masseter, and medial pterygoid muscles.
> - Lateral deviation—action of the ipsilateral masseter, and contralateral medial and lateral pterygoid muscles.
> - Protrusion—bilateral action of the lateral pterygoid, medial pterygoid, and anterior fibers of the temporalis muscles.
> - Retrusion—bilateral action of the posterior fibers of the temporalis muscle, the digastric, stylohyoid, geniohyoid, and mylohyoid muscles.

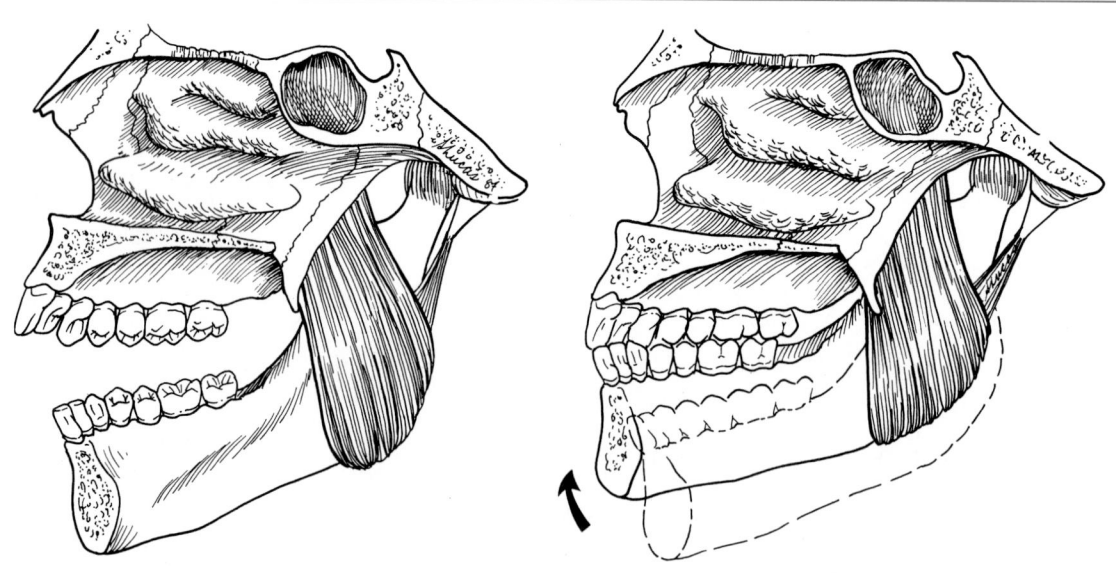

FIGURE 24-10 The medial pterygoid muscle. (Reproduced with permission from Okeson JP. *Management of Temporomandibular Disorders and Occlusion.* 4th ed. St Louis, Mo: Mosby Year Book; 1998:19.)

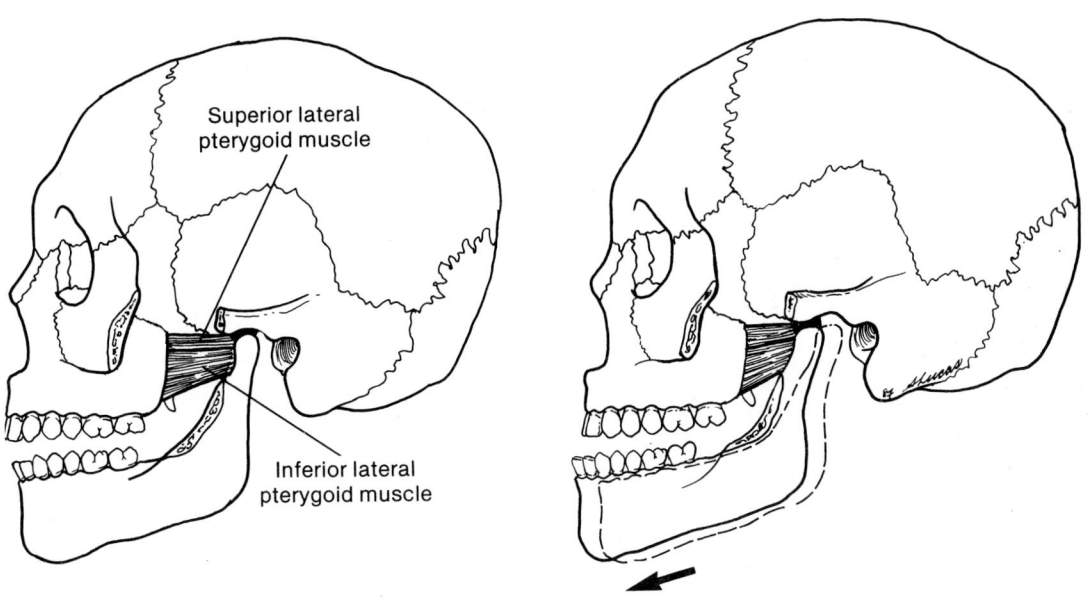

FIGURE 24-11 The inferior and superior lateral pterygoid muscles. (Reproduced with permission from Okeson JP. *Management of Temporomandibular Disorders and Occlusion.* 4th ed. St Louis, Mo: Mosby Year Book; 1998:20.)

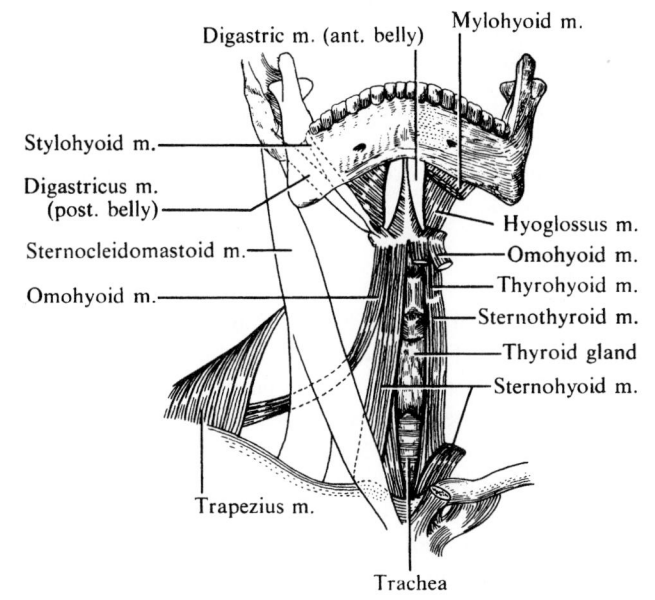

FIGURE 24-12 The hyoid muscles. (Reproduced with permission from Pansky B. *Review of Gross Anatomy.* 6th ed. New York, NY: McGraw-Hill; 1996:73.)

Mylohyoid. This flat, triangular muscle is functionally a muscle of the tongue, stabilizing or elevating the tongue during swallowing, and elevating the floor of the mouth in the first stage of deglutition.[30]

Stylohyoid. The stylohyoid muscle (Figure 24-12) elevates the hyoid and base of the tongue and has an undetermined role in speech, mastication, and swallowing.

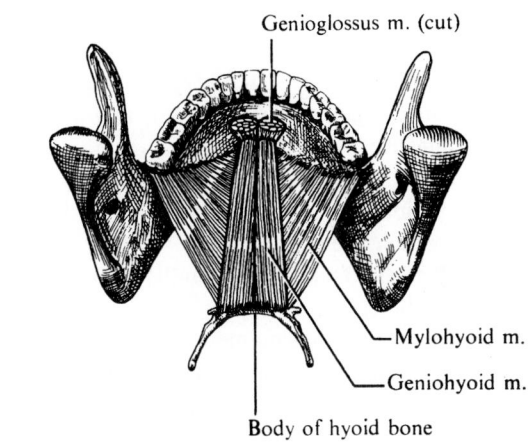

FIGURE 24-13 Muscles of the floor of the mouth. (Reproduced with permission Pansky B. *Review of Gross Anatomy.* 6th ed. New York, NY: McGraw-Hill; 1996:73.)

Nerve Supply

The TMJ is primarily supplied from three nerves that are part of the mandibular division of the fifth cranial (trigeminal) nerve (Box 24-1). Portions of the middle ear ossicles, middle ear musculature, and muscles of mastication all originate from the first branchial arch and are innervated by this nerve. Therefore, in a patient with altered bite mechanics, spasm of the muscles of mastication caused by a displaced condyle may cause neuromuscular dysfunction of all the muscles innervated by the trigeminal nerve, including the tensor palatini.[41]

Box 24-1 CHARACTERISTICS OF THE TRIGEMINAL NERVE

Motor Nucleus

The anterolateral upper pons.

Sensory Nucleus

There are two nuclei: (1) the chief sensory nucleus in the dorsal-lateral pons; and (2) the mesencephalic nucleus, which extends from the chief sensory nucleus upward through the pons to the midbrain.

Spinal Nucleus

The spinal tract consists of small and medium-sized myelinated nerve fibers and runs caudally to reach the upper cervical segments of the spinal cord. The lowest nerve fibers in the tract mix with the spinal fibers in the tract orf Lissauer.

Nerves

- Mandibular.
- Maxillary.
- Ophthalmic.

Termination

- Muscles of mastication, both pterygoids, tensor veli palatini, tensor tympani, mylohyoid, and anterior belly of digastric.
- Skin of vertex, temporal area, forehead, and face; mucosa of sinuses, nose, pharynx, anterior two thirds of tongue, and oral cavity.
- Lacrimal, parotid, and lingual glands; dura of anterior and middle cranial fossae.
- External aspect of tympanic membrane and external auditory meatus, temporomandibular joint, and teeth.
- Dilator pupillae and probably proprioceptors of extraocular muscles.
- Sensation from upper 3 or 4 cervical levels.

There is considerable clinical interest in the interactions between the cervical and craniofacial regions. This interest stems from a number of reports concerning patients who have pain in the cervical and craniofacial areas simultaneously.[27,42–45]

In the suboccipital region, a series of dense neural connections, called the *trigeminocervical complex,* exists among trigeminal, facial, glossopharyngeal, and vagus nerves, with those of the upper C1 to C4 cervical spinal nerves.[15] Postural abnormalities resulting from various acute or chronic etiologies that produce suboccipital compression may, therefore, be responsible for craniofacial pain anywhere in the head, in addition to symptoms of dizziness, or nystagmus.[5,15,46]

TMJ-related headaches usually include pain near the TMJ and ear, ear fullness, temporal headaches, and facial pain.[47] The dizziness associated with TMD tends to be of the nonvertiginous variety, with the patient complaining of unsteadiness, giddiness, or lightheadedness.[48] Although the exact mechanism is unclear, postural influences, alteration in the position of the jaw by the malocclusion, and the subsequent mismatching between the cervical muscles might be the cause.[48]

Biomechanics

The movements that occur at the TMJ are extremely complex. The TMJ has three degrees of freedom, with each of the degrees of freedom associated with a separate axis of rotation.[49] Two primary arthrokinematic movements (rotation and anterior translation) occur at this joint around three planes: sagittal, horizontal, and frontal (Fig. 24-14).

The motions of protrusion and retrusion are planar glides. In addition to the rotational motions during mouth opening and closing and lateral deviations, movements at the TMJ involve arthrokinematic rolls and slides. Thus,

▶ Mouth opening, contralateral deviation, and protrusion all involve an anterior osteokinematic rotation of the mandible and an anterior, inferior, and lateral glide of the mandibular head and disk.

▶ Mouth closing, ipsilateral deviation, and retrusion all involve a posterior osteokinematic rotation of the mandible and an anterior, inferior, and lateral glide of the mandibular head and disk.

Occlusal Position

Occlusal positions are functional positions of the TMJ. The occlusal position is defined as the point at which contact between some or all of the teeth occurs. Under normal circumstances, the upper molars rest directly on the lower molars and the upper incisors slightly override the lower incisors. The ideal position provides mutual protection of anterior and posterior teeth, comfortable and painless mandibular function, and stability.[15] The *median occlusal* position corresponds to the position in which all of the teeth are fully interdigitated[17] and is considered the start position for all mandibular motions. The median occlusal position is dependent on the presence, shape, and position of the teeth. Protrusion of the upper or lower incisors, failure of the upper incisors to overlap with the lower incisors, absent or abnormally shaped teeth, and back teeth that do not meet are all causes of malocclusion. The *centric* position is considered to be the position that implies the most retruded, unstrained position of the mandible from which lateral movements are possible and the components of the oral apparatus are the most balanced.[51] Ideally, the centric position should coincide with the median occlusal position.[51] It is worth remembering that malocclusion is probably very common in the general nonsymptomatic patient and may or may not be relevant to the presenting symptoms.[52]

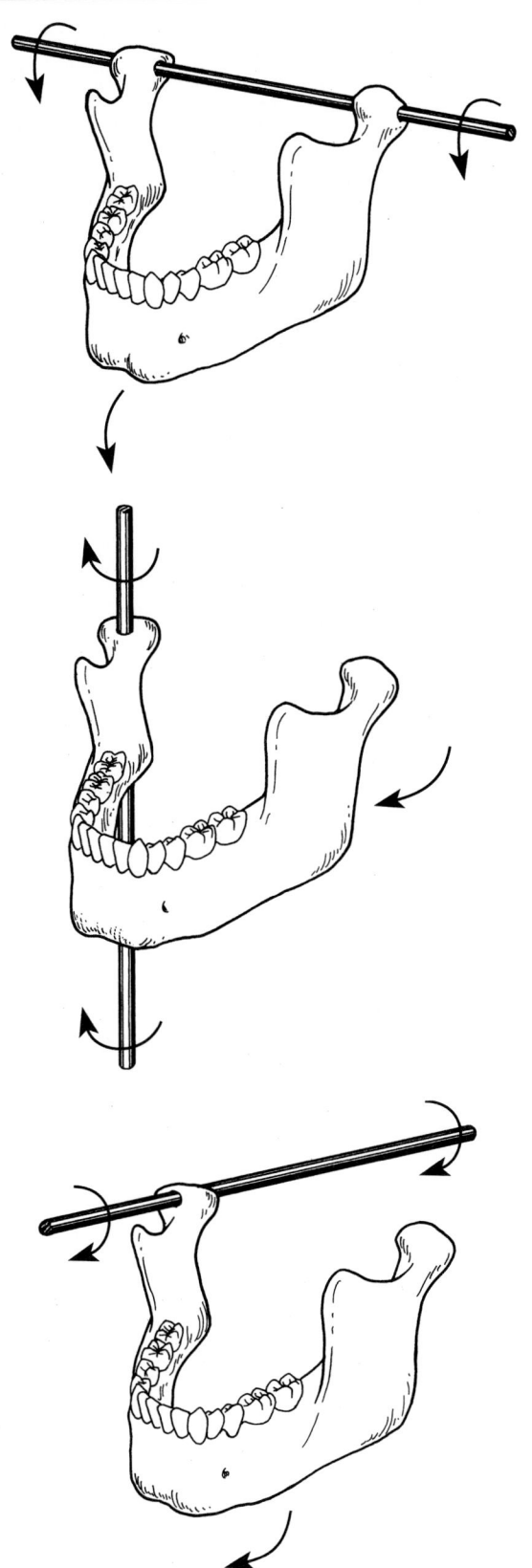

FIGURE 24-14 The axes of mandibular motion. (Reproduced with permission from Okeson JP. *Management of Temporomandibular Disorders and Occlusion.* 4th ed. St Louis, Mo: Mosby Year Book; 1998:19.)

Rather than being a primary etiologic factor in TMD, malocclusion is likely to have a secondary or contributory role.[15,53]

Mouth Opening

Mouth opening occurs in a series of steps (Table 24-3). In the erect position, the condyles begin to rotate anteriorly and translate inferiorly and laterally during the first 25° of opening as the jaw opens. This initial condylar rotation occurs as the mandibular elevators (masseter, temporalis, and medial pterygoid muscles) gradually relax and lengthen, allowing gravity to depress the mandible.[55a] The directions of the fibers of the lateral and medial temporomandibular ligaments keep the condyle from moving posteriorly. The fibrous capsule and parts of the temporomandibular ligament limit excessive lateral movement of the condyle. During the last 15° of opening, the collateral ligaments tighten and the rotation ceases, being replaced by an anterior translation of the condyles.[50] During this translation, the condyle and disk move together. The anterior translation, which is produced mainly by muscle contraction, serves to prevent mandibular encroachment of the anterior neck structures. The muscles involved with the anterior translation include the inferior head of the lateral pterygoid muscle and the anterior head of the digastric muscle.[55a] Opening is also assisted by the other suprahyoid muscles.[55a] In extremely wide opening, the functional joint contact is on the distal aspect of the condyle, and the anterior lateral aspect of the condyle contacts the posterior part of the masseter muscle. In this position, the soft tissue structures are in a position of stretch, making them more prone to dysfunction.[56]

Mouth Closing

Closing of the mouth involves a reversal of the movements described for mouth opening. The condyles translate posteriorly as a result of an interaction between the retracting portions of the masseter and temporalis muscle and the retracting portions of the mandibular depressors.[56a] As the condyles translate posteriorly and glide medially, they hinge on the disks. The disks then glide posteriorly and superiorly on the temporal bone along with the condyles (as a result of the actions of the masseter, medial pterygoid, and temporalis muscles.)[39] When the jaws are closed to maximal occlusal contact, the condyles contact the disks and the disks contact the posterior slopes of the articular tubercles and the glenoid fossae.

Protrusion

Protrusion is a forward movement of the mandible that occurs at the superior joint compartments, which consists of the disk and condyle moving downward, forward, and laterally. The muscles responsible for protrusion are the anterior fiber of the temporalis and the medial and lateral pterygoid muscles.

Retrusion

Retrusion is a backward movement of the mandible, produced by the posterior fiber of the temporalis and assisted by the suprahyoid muscles. The retrusive range is limited by the extensibility of the temporomandibular ligaments.[57]

TABLE 24-3 Arthrokinematic Steps of the Temporomandibular Joint[50]

Step	Movement
Rest position	Joint is in an open-packed position.
Rotation	There is a mid-opening. Condylar joint surfaces glide forward, inferior joint surface of disk has a relative posterior glide, upper lateral pterygoid relaxes, inferior pterygoid contracts, and posterior connective tissue is in a functional state of rest.
Functional opening	Disk and condyle experience a short anterior translatory glide, superior and inferior heads of lateral pterygoid contract to guide disk and condyle forward. Posterior connective tissue is in functional tightening.
Translation	There is full opening. Disk and condyle glide anteriorly and caudally. Superior and inferior heads of lateral pterygoid contract to guide disk and condyle fully forward. Posterior connective tissues tighten.
Closure	Surface of condyle joint glides posteriorly, and disk glides relative to anterior surface. Superior head of lateral pterygoid contracts and inferior head relaxes. Posterior connective tissue returns to its functional length.

Lateral Excursion

If a protrusion movement occurs unilaterally, it is called a *lateral excursion,* or *deviation.* For example, if only the left TMJ protrudes, the jaw deviates to the right.

Lateral movements of the mandible are the result of asymmetric muscle contractions. During lateral excursion to the right, the condyle and disk on the left side glide inferiorly, anteriorly, and laterally in the sagittal plane and medially in the horizontal plane along the articular eminence. The condyle and disk on the right side rotate laterally on a sagittal plane and translate medially in the horizontal plane while remaining in the fossa.

Clinical Pearl

The translation of the human condyle during jaw opening and during lateral jaw movements is referred to as the *Bennett shift.*

The Closed Pack and Resting Positions

The close-packed position of the TMJ is difficult to determine because the position of maximal muscle tightness is also the position of least joint surface congruity and vice versa. Rocabado[50] considers there to be two close-packed positions, named according to the end position of the mandibular head in the fossa:[50]

▶ *Anterior close-packed position.* This position is the position of maximum opening of the joint.

▶ *Posterior close-packed position.* This position is the maximum retruded position of the joint.

Under this premise, the open-packed, or "rest" position is any position away from the anterior or posterior close-packed positions of the joint.[50] The rest position, or "freeway space" corresponds to the position of the TMJ where the residual tension of the muscles is at rest and no contact occurs between maxillary and mandibular teeth. In this position, the tongue is against the palate of the mouth with its most anterior-superior tip in the area against the palate, just posterior to the rear of the upper central incisors.[58]

Capsular Pattern

The capsular pattern of the TMJ is one of motion deviation to the same side as the involved joint and a loss of functional opening.

Clinical Pearl

The significance of the rest position is that it permits the tissues of the stomatognathic system to rest and undergo repair.[59]

Examination

Given the multifactorial causes of TMD, a comprehensive examination of the entire upper quadrant, including the cervical spine and shoulders, usually is warranted. In general, the TMJ and the upper three cervical joints all refer symptoms to the head, whereas the mid to low cervical spine typically refers symptoms to the shoulder and arm.[60–62] An accurate diagnosis of TMD involves a careful evaluation of the information gleaned from the history, systems review, and tests and measures. In most chronic cases, a behavioral or psychological examination is required.[2,26,62–67] Because postural dysfunctions are closely related to TMJ symptoms, the clinician should always perform a postural examination as part of a comprehensive examination of this joint. An examination form for the TMJ examination is shown in Table 24-4.

History

During the history the clinician should observe the patient's mouth to see if the mouth is moved comfortably while speaking, or whether mouth movements appear guarded.

The clinician should determine from the patient the main reason for the visit. There are three cardinal features of TMDs, which can be local or remote:

1. ***Restricted jaw function.*** A history of limited mouth opening, which may be intermittent or progressive, is a key feature of TMD. Restricted jaw function causes considerable anxiety for the patient, who faces difficulties in everyday activities such as eating and speaking. Patients may describe a generalized tight feeling, which may indicate a muscular disorder, or the sensation that the jaw suddenly "catches" or "locks," which usually is related to mechanical interferences in the joint (internal derangement).[13] Associated signs of an internal derangement include pain and deviation of mandibular movements during opening and closing (refer to Practice Pattern 4D, under "Intervention Strategies," later).

2. ***Joint noises.*** The presence of joint noises (crepitus) of the TMJ may or may not be significant, because joint sounds occur in approximately 50 percent of healthy populations.[68] Some joint sounds, such as "soft" crepitus, are not audible to the clinician, so a stethoscope may be required. "Hard" crepitus, often described as gravelly or grating, is a diffuse sustained noise that occurs during a considerable portion of the opening or closing cycle, or both, and is evidence of a change in osseous contour.[56] Clicking is a brief noise that occurs at some point during opening, closing, or both (see the discussion of range of motion testing, later).

> **Clinical Pearl**
>
> TMJ sounds should be described and related to symptoms. Joint noise is, of itself, of little clinical importance in the absence of pain.[64,69]

---

3. ***Orofacial pain.*** Approximately half of all cases of TMD are masticatory myalgias.[70] Pain should be evaluated care-

fully in terms of its onset, nature, intensity, site, duration, aggravating and relieving factors, and, especially, how it relates to the other features such as joint noise and restricted mandibular movements.[13] The distribution of TMD symptoms can prove confusing.

> **Clinical Pearl**
>
> Pain that is centered immediately in front of the tragus of the ear and that projects to the ear, temple, cheek, and along the mandible is highly diagnostic for TMD.[71]

A gradual onset of symptoms after minor or prolonged physical activity may be indicative of a mechanical derangement.[72] Symptoms of a mechanical nature generally are eased with rest. The irritability of a disorder is determined by the degree of activity necessary to provoke a symptom response.

The severity of the symptoms, and the time before the symptoms subside, provide the clinician with valuable information regarding possible pathology.[73] Specific questions about activities and postures of a sustained nature, such as sitting, sleeping, and driving, should be asked.[74] It is important to determine:

▶ If the presenting symptoms were caused by trauma or surgery, or if the onset of pain occurred gradually. Questions should focus on any history of trauma during birth or childhood, as well as more recently.

▶ If there are any emotional factors in the patient's background that may provoke habitual protrusion or muscular tension.

▶ If the patient is aware of any parafunctional habits (cheek biting, nail biting, pencil chewing, teeth clenching, or bruxism).

▶ The behavior of symptoms over a 24-hour period. This information assists the clinician in formulating causal relationships.

▶ Whether the symptoms are improving or worsening.

▶ The relationship of eating to the symptoms. Alcohol, chocolate, and other foods can cause head pain in some individuals, suggesting a vasomotor-related pain.

▶ The patient's past dental and orthodontic history.

▶ Whether the patient has experienced any "locking" of the jaw. The patient may report the jaw suddenly "catching" or "getting stuck," which usually is related to an internal derangement.[46] Locking implies an inability to fully open or close the jaw. Locking usually is preceded by reciprocal clicking (see the discussion of range of motion testing, later). Locking of the jaw in the closed position is often caused by the condyle assuming a position that is posterior or anteromedial to the disk.

TABLE 24-4 Temporomandibular Examination Form[56]

Name: _____   General Dentist: _____
Patient's Physician: _____   Phone (home): _____
Age: _____   Phone (bus): _____
Address: _____   Chief Complaint: _____
Occupation: _____   _____
Phone: _____

Check all applicable

I. MEDICAL HISTORY

Arthritic Disease
1. Traumatic arthritis: _____
2. Osteoarthritis: _____
3. Rheumatoid arthritis: _____
4. Psoriatic arthritis: _____
5. Other: _____

ENT. Disorders
1. Salivary gland disorders: _____
2. Cysts: _____
3. Ear problems: _____
4. Polyps: _____
5. Nose/Throat problems: _____
6. Allergies: _____
7. Sinusitis: _____
8. Other: _____

Vascular Disease and Blood Dyscrasias _____

Head/Neck Trauma
Date:_____ Description:_____

Headache/Neuralgia (location, character, frequency, duration)

_____

Medication (current and past)
1. Type: _____
2. Allergy to medication: _____

Additional Medical Information (past and present)
1. Surgery: _____
2. Psychiatric: _____
3. ENT: _____
4. Orthopaedic: _____
5. Neurologic: _____
6. Internist: _____
7. Rheumatologic: _____
8. Chiropractic: _____
9. Physical therapy: _____
10. Endocrine: _____
    a. Do your nails break easily?
    b. Is your skin dry?
    c. Do you tire easily?
    d. Does the cold weather bother you?
11. Osteopathic: _____
12. Other: _____
13. Nutritional state: _____

TABLE 24-4 *(cont.)*

II. DENTAL HISTORY

A. Oral Conditions (describe general condition, presence of fixed or removable prosthesis, periodontal problems, and vertical dimension discrepancies)

_____

_____

_____

B. Last Dental Examination and Films: _____

C. Recent Dental Treatment: _____

D. Previous Orthodontic Therapy Dates: _____ **Bicuspid Extraction?** _____

E. Previous TMJ Treatment and Results (date/doctor): _____

_____

F. Pain Symptoms:
1. Date of onset: _____
2. Area of onset: _____ Right _____ Left _____
3. Type: superficial, deep, sharp, dull
4. Quality: burning, aching
5. Frequency: _____
6. Duration: constant, intermittent
7. Period of greatest intensity: _____
8. Status of pain: increased, decreased, unchanged
9. Onset: abrupt, gradual
10. Disappearance: abrupt, gradual
11. Factors alleviating pain: _____
12. Triggering devices: eating, yawning, speaking, singing, shouting
13. Pain in specific teeth: _____
14. Additional pain information: _____

G. Oral Symptoms (other than pain)
1. Jaws clenched upon awakening
2. Clenching and grinding during sleep
3. Clenching and grinding during waking hours
4. Muscle fatigue _____

H. Vertigo, Syncope, Meniere's Disease (frequency, duration, circumstances): _____

_____

I. Ear Symptoms/Joint Noises
1. Tinnitus: (R) (L)
2. Popping, clicking, or grating noises
   on opening and closing: (R) (L)
3. Stuffiness of ears: (R) (L)

J. Skeletal–Facial Deformity: _____

K. Other Complaints: _____

III. CLINICAL EXAMINATION

Reported Pain

1. Temporomandibular joint	(R) (L)		6. Shoulder	(R) (L)
2. Upper back	(R) (L)		7. Arm	(R) (L)
3. Middle back	(R) (L)		8. Fingers	(R) (L)
4. Lower back	(R) (L)		9. Chest	(R) (L)
5. Scapula area	(R) (L)		10. Occipital area	(R) (L)

Tenderness and Pain on Palpation
1. Temporalis
   a. Anterior Fibers (R) (L)
   b. Middle Fibers (R) (L)
   c. Posterior Fibers (R) (L)

TABLE 24-4 *(cont.)*

III. CLINICAL EXAMINATION

2. Masseter
   a. Zygoma   (R) (L)
   b. Body   (R) (L)
   c. Lateral surface of angle of mandible   (R) (L)
3. Digastric   (R) (L)
4. Posterior cervicals   (R) (L)
5. Trapezius   (R) (L)
6. Sternocleidomastoid   (R) (L)
7. Lateral pterygoid: insertion   (R) (L)
8. Medial pterygoid: insertion   (R) (L)
9. Mylohyoid   (R) (L)
10. Coronoid process   (R) (L)
11. TMJ lateral aspect   (R) (L)
    Lateral/Posterior aspect   (R) (L)
3a. Ear (anterior wall tenderness)   (R) (L)

TMJ Sounds

(Stethoscopic and/or digital palpation)
1. Crepitation   (R) (L)
2. Sagittal *opening* click:
   Immediate   (R) (L)
   Intermediate   (R) (L)
   Full Opening   (R) (L)
3. Sagittal *closing* click:
   Immediate   (R) (L)
   Intermediate   (R) (L)
   Terminal closure   (R) (L)
4. Nature of click (soft/loud)   (R) (L)

B. Occlusal Interferences

Left nonworking side   Right nonworking side

Protrusive   Centric Occlusion

Occlusion: Angle's class _____

Extruded labial or lingual version teeth _____

Clinical Postural Observation

1. Head posture (at rest): _____

2. Range of motion: _____

Summary of TMJ Imaging Findings: _____

Mandibular Movement

1. Widest interincisal opening _____

2. Right lateral _____ Left lateral _____

3. Pain present with movement? _____

Diagnosis: _____

Plan of Treatment: _____

Prognosis: _____

Remarks: _____

ENT, ear, nose, and throat; TMJ, temporamandibular joint.

Chronic head, neck, and back pain often are associated with psychogenic causes. Psychiatric disorders usually are manifested in patients whose afflictions seem to be excessive, or persist beyond what would be normal for that condition. The checklist outlined in Table 24-5 can be used by the clinician to identify factors that may warrant an examination by a mental health professional.

Systems Review

Clinicians often see patients with a TMD who present with nonspecific symptoms such as neck pain, headaches, earaches, and tinnitus. However, because these symptoms are not considered specific for TMDs, other possible causes should be sought and ruled out during the systems review.[76–78] Pain or dysfunction in the orofacial region often results from nonmusculoskeletal causes such as otolaryngologic, neurologic, vascular, neoplastic, psychogenic, and infectious diseases.

Unexplained weight loss, ataxia, weakness, fever with pain, nystagmus, and neurologic deficits are characteristic of intracranial disorders.[79] Neurovascular disorders are associated with migraine headache and its variants, carotidynia and cluster headaches (see Chap. 9). Neuropathic disorders include trigeminal neuralgia, glossopharyngeal neuralgia, and occipital neuralgia.

The seriousness of head, face, mouth, and neck disorders that are detectable by a careful history and physical examination run the gamut from trivial (though discomforting) viral upper respiratory tract infection to malignant tumor.[80]

Once the possibility of cervical, systemic, psychogenic, or ear or sinus problems has been ruled out, the next step is to consider the possibility of TMJ pain and impairment, particularly if the pain is accompanied by jaw clicking and limited mouth opening.[81]

Tests and Measures

Observation

The head, face, and neck are assessed for asymmetry, such as swelling or flattening of the cheek. Asymmetry is an important finding, because developmentally the facial structures evolve in

TABLE 24-5 Checklist of Psychological and Behavioral Factors[75]

Inconsistent, inappropriate, or vague reports of pain
Overdramatization of symptoms
Symptoms that vary with life events
Significant pain of > 6 months' duration
Repeated failures with conventional therapies
Inconsistent response to medications
History of other stress-related disorders
Major life events (e.g., new job, marriage, divorce, death)
Evidence of drug abuse
Clinically significant anxiety or depression
Evidence of secondary gain

Note: The significance of these factors depends on the particular patient.

a proportional relationship, some determined by genetics, others in response to the physical environment.[82] In addition, the clinician should note the presence of any abnormal cervical posture, jaw deviation, unusual dryness of the lips, changes in eye position, and signs of tissue stress such as overdeveloped masseter and mentalis muscles, or a hypertrophied lower lip.[27] The forward head posture (see Chap. 23) frequently is associated with TMD.[31,83,84] This is likely because of the direct impact a forward head posture can have on oral symmetry during occlusion. In the neutral position when tapping the teeth together, all of the teeth appear to strike simultaneously. However, if the same task is attempted while placing the head forward, it is the anterior teeth that occlude first. The consequences of this repetitive functional malocclusion during food or gum chewing should be apparent. A chronic forward head posture may result in an adaptive shortening of the deep cervical fascia and muscles, which can exaggerate the functional malocclusion.

Similarly, a lateral deviation of the jaw, evidenced by a malalignment or malocclusion of the upper and lower teeth, or hypertonus of one of the masseter muscles, may cause an adaptive shortening of the mastication muscles on the ipsilateral side of the deviation, and a lengthening of the muscles on the contralateral side. Because the role that malocclusion plays in TMD remains unclear, the relevance of the malalignment to the patient's symptoms must be determined by passively attempting to correct the deformity.[52,57] An increase in pain with the correction suggests the presence of a protective deformity.

The teeth should be examined for symmetry. Cavities, wear patterns, and restored and missing teeth should be noted. Defects in dimensions can be measured radiographically.[85] The vertical dimension of dental occlusion (i.e., depth of bite) has been implicated as a possible craniomandibular component associated with TMD.[34] It has been proposed that a deep dental overbite may have pathologic effects on cranial nerve V, the tensor veli palatini, and the soft tissue surrounding the TMJ.[34,86] Seldin[87] and Sicher[88] proposed that a deep bite results in a displaced condyle, which causes inflammation and muscle spasm in the retrodiscal tissue and muscles surrounding the TMJ. Tooth wear and fracture are often destructive signs of parafunctional habits (abrasive diet, bruxism, and teeth clenching). Loss of teeth can cause disruption in the working and nonworking interfaces of the teeth, which may cause unilateral function and subsequent overloading of the remaining teeth and the TMJ.[15]

The tongue should be examined. The tongue should appear dull red, moist, and glistening. Its anterior portion should have a smooth yet roughened appearance.[80] The posterior portion should have a smooth, slightly uneven appearance. A hairy tongue with yellow-brown to black elongated papillae on the dorsum sometimes follows antibiotic therapy.[80] A dry or white tongue may indicate a salivary gland dysfunction or an oral yeast or bacterial infection respectively.[80] The tongue is tested for frenulum length. A short frenulum may interfere with tongue function. The tongue should have no difficulty touching the hard palate behind the upper incisors.[51] A large tongue can exert excessive pressure against the teeth and may interfere with occlusion, resulting in bite marks.

The rest position of the TMJ should be noted. The clinician can locate the rest position of the TMJ by gently placing the little finger with the palmar portion facing anteriorly into the external auditory meatus. From an open-mouth position, the patient is asked to slowly close the mouth. At the point of the resting position, the patient's mandibular heads are felt to gently touch the finger. The space between the upper and lower incisors should be 2 to 4 mm. A greater distance may indicate hypermobility of both TMJs.

Range of Motion

The range of motion of the TMJ, cervical spine, craniovertebral joints, and shoulders should be assessed with active range of motion, and then with passive overpressure to assess the end-feel.

All movements of the TMJ should be smooth and without noise or pain. If pain occurs, a determination should be made as to where in the range the pain occurs, and the location of the pain. The clinician observes the opening and closing of the mouth, noting both the range and quality of movement. A Boley gauge, T-bar, or ruler, can be used to measure the range of the TMJ in millimeters.[82] The clinician can palpate over the mandible heads during opening and closing to determine whether they move together (Fig. 24-15). The clinician also notes any crepitus or clicking on opening and closing, and where they occur in the range.

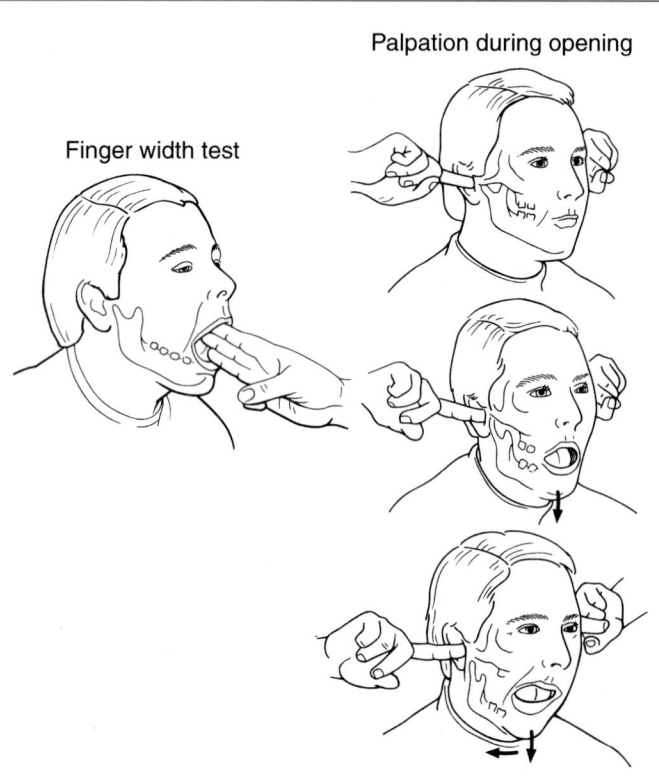

FIGURE 24-15 Mouth opening tests. (Reproduced with permission from Dutton M. *Manual Therapy of the Spine.* New York, NY: McGraw-Hill; 2002:555.)

> ### Clinical Pearl
>
> Joint clicking can be a normal occurrence or it may be caused by one of the types of internal derangement (refer to Practice Pattern 4D, later) including disk displacements, adhesive disk hypomobility, and deviation in form (articular surface damage). Clicking also may be a result of hypermobility or muscle incoordination.[89]

The type and temporal sequence of joint clicking can provide the clinician with information:

1. Reciprocal clicking is defined as clicking that occurs during opening and again during closing. The opening click occurs when the condyle moves under the posterior band of the disk until it snaps into its normal relationship on the concave surface of the disk, whereas the closing click reflects the reversal of this process.[90] Reciprocal clicks may be early, intermediate, or late depending on the degree of opening at which they occur.[50]
   a. Early clicking usually indicates a small anterior displacement.
   b. Late clicking usually indicates that the disk has been further displaced.
   Reciprocal clicking is a common finding in patients with a posterosuperior condylar positioning.[27]

2. Clicking that occurs at the end of opening often results from articular hypermobility and is accompanied by a deviation of the jaw toward the contralateral side.

3. The "soft" and "popping" opening and closing clicks associated with muscular incoordination are usually intermittent and inconsistent. They are thought to be caused by ligament movement or articular surface separation. Muscle tenderness to palpation is a frequent associated symptom.

Elevation of the Mandible (Mouth Closing). The primary muscles involved with mouth closing are the masseter, temporalis, and medial pterygoid.[51] Because the maxillary teeth are fixed, the upper midline of the incisors can be used as a landmark to assess lower jaw deviation during mouth closing. Under normal conditions, the midline relationship between the upper and lower incisors should remain constant in the closed and open positions. Overpressure can be applied to the mouth closing by placing the fingers under the chin and pushing superiorly in a controlled fashion (Fig. 24-16). The normal end-feel for mouth closing should be bone on bone (teeth contact).

Depression of the Mandible (Mouth Opening). The opening of the mouth is the most revealing and diagnostic movement for TMD.

The maximum range of motion for mouth opening is approximately 50 mm, measured between the maxillary and mandibular incisors.[71] At this extreme, the periarticular structures are stretched to 100 percent of their total length. The functional range of the motion is considered to be closer to 40 mm,

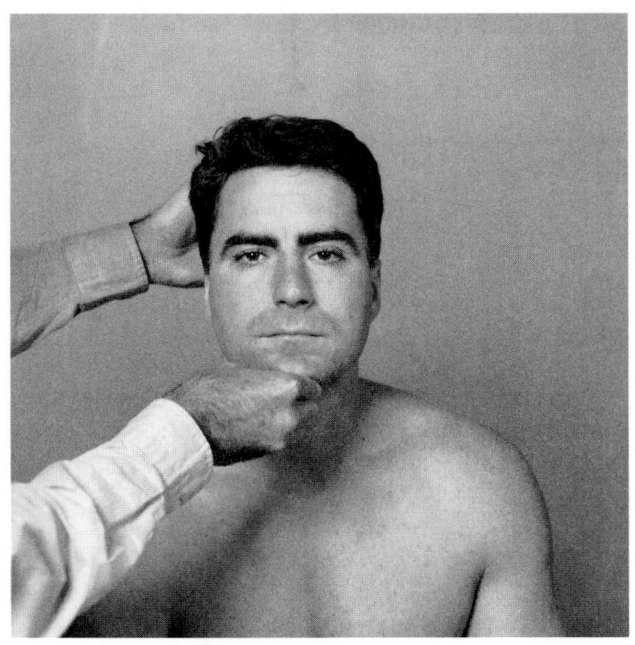

FIGURE 24-16 Mouth closing with overpressure.

or approximately a two- to three-knuckle width of the non-dominant hand[13,50,91] (see Fig. 24-15). At this point in the range, the periarticular structures are stretched to 70 to 80 percent of their total length. Excessive opening is indicated when the patient is able to insert three or more knuckles between the incisors. Excessive opening is associated with large anterior translatory movements at the beginning of mouth opening, accompanied by excessive protrusive movements of the mandible.[50]

Mouth opening may be restricted for a variety of reasons. A limited opening of the jaw may indicate joint hypomobility, muscle tightness, or the presence of trigger points within the elevator muscles: the temporalis, masseter, and medial pterygoid. Other causes of diminished mandibular opening include structural disorders of the TMJ, such as ankylosis, internal derangements, muscle contractures, and gross osteoarthritis. For example, if contracture of the masticatory muscles is present, the mandibular opening can be as limited as 10 to 20 mm between the incisors.[92]

Translation of the lateral pole of the condyle should occur after 11 mm of mouth opening. If an opening deviation occurs, it is important to note where in the opening cycle it occurs. Opening and closing deviations are observed simply by taking a small ruler or tongue depressor and laying the edge down the midline of the face.[56] While the clinician "eyes" the straight edge, the patient opens and closes the mouth slowly[89]:

▶ Limited opening with deviation to one side should alert the clinician to an internal derangement without reduction, which limits the translation on the involved side and causes the jaw to deviate toward the less-mobile side, even if that is the normally mobile side and the other side is hypermobile.

Early deviation suggests hypomobility, and late deviation indicates hypermobility.

▶ If hypomobility resulting from internal derangement with reduction of one TMJ is present, the mandible will deviate in a C pattern of motion to that side of the open mouth in the midrange of opening before returning to normal.

▶ The patient who demonstrates an S movement of the jaw while opening the mouth may have a muscle imbalance (often caused by trigeminal facilitation and masticatory hypertonicity), or it may be a momentary locking on a deranged disk. Lateral excursion of the mandible with mouth opening implicates contralateral structures such as the contralateral disk, masseter, medial and lateral pterygoid, or lateral ligaments.

Overpressure can be applied to the opening movement using a lumbrical grip placed on the patient's chin, under the bottom lip (Fig. 24-17). The overpressure is applied to ensure that the jaw is maximally depressed. The normal end-feel should be tissue stretch. Locking of the jaw can be associated with three types of abnormal end-feel[56]:

▶ *Hard.* This type of end-feel is associated with osseous abnormalities.

▶ *Springy.* This type of end-feel is associated with a displacement of the disk.

▶ *Capsular.* This type of end-feel is associated with adaptive shortening of the periarticular tissues.

Protrusive Excursion of the Mandible. The patient opens the mouth slightly and protrudes the lower jaw. The normal movement of the lower teeth is 3 to 6 mm, measured from the resting

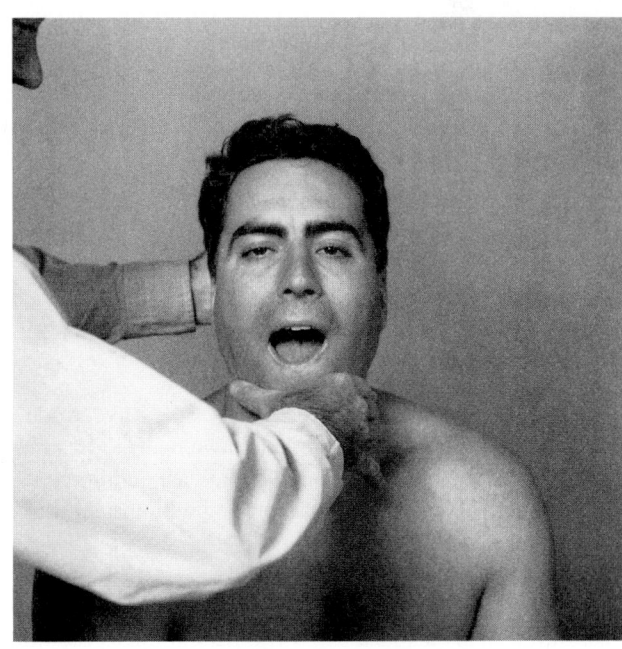

FIGURE 24-17 Mouth opening with overpressure.

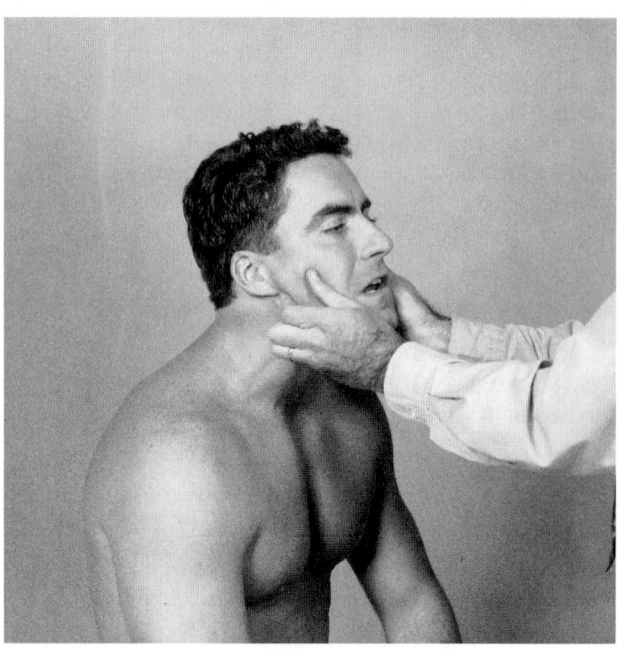

FIGURE 24-18   Passive overpressure into protrusion.

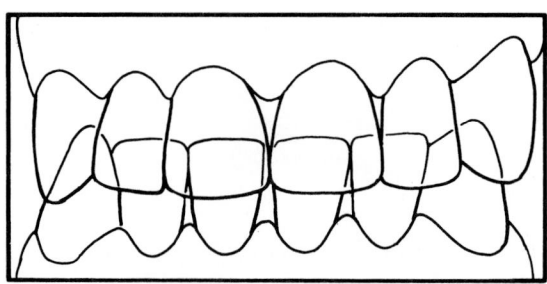

FIGURE 24-19   Maxillary and teeth alignment. (Reproduced with permission from Okeson JP. *Management of Temporomandibular Disorders and Occlusion.* 4th ed. St Louis, Mo: Mosby Year Book; 1998:84.)

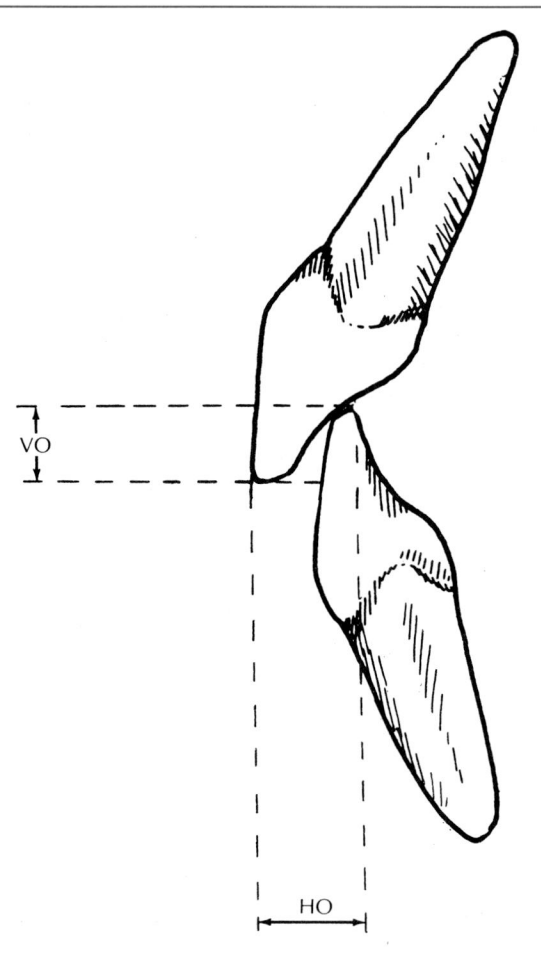

FIGURE 24-20   Normal interarch relationships. HO, horizontal; VO, vertical. (Reproduced with permission from Okeson JP. *Management of Temporomandibular Disorders and Occlusion.* 4th ed. St Louis, Mo: Mosby Year Book; 1998:85.)

position to the protruded position.[82] The amount and direction of the protrusion are noted:

▶ An abnormal protrusive position may be associated with a residual pediatric tongue thrust (deviant swallowing) or an acquired adult tongue thrust secondary to a forward head posture or habitual protrusion.

▶ Any lateral excursion of the mandible during protrusion may indicate involvement of the contralateral structures, such as the contralateral disk, masseter, medial and lateral pterygoid, or lateral ligaments.

The clinician can apply overpressure by grasping the patient's mandible with the index and middle fingers behind the mandibular angles and the thumbs on the patient's cheeks, and then gently pulling the jaw anteriorly (Fig. 24-18).

Excursion of the Mandible.   The superior and inferior incisors are assessed for any deviation of the jaw laterally (crossbite) (Fig. 24-19) or anteroposteriorly (over bite or under bite) (Fig. 24-20).

Retrusion of the Mandible.   The patient is asked to retrude the jaw as far back as possible. The normal movement is 3 to 4 mm.[57] Pain at the end range of retrusion may indicate an intracapsular injury.[6] Overpressure can be applied using a lumbrical grip positioned under the patient's bottom lip, and pushing the mandible posteriorly (Fig. 24-21).

Lateral Deviation of the Mandible.   The patient opens the mouth slightly and moves the lower jaw to the left and to the right. The right and left motions are compared. Normal range of motion

for lateral deviation is approximately one fourth of the opening range (10 to 12 mm).[32] Lateral deviation can be measured as the amount of lateral excursion between the center of the mandibular incisors and the center of the maxillary incisors. An appreciable difference between the two sides is more significant than

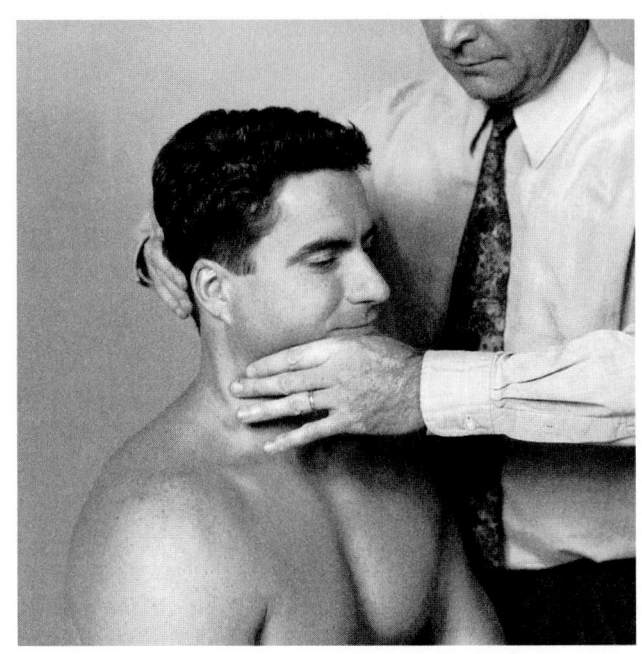

FIGURE 24-21 Passive overpressure into retrusion.

a limited range occurring bilaterally.[27] Passive overpressure can be applied in a lateral direction. Pain reported on the side away from the direction of overpressure may indicate ligamentous or joint capsule damage.[27]

Tongue Movements. Tongue movements give valuable information about the function of the hypoglossal nerve (CN XII). Any deviation or atrophy of the tongue during tongue protrusion may indicate a lesion of this nerve. Unilateral weakness of the tongue is manifested by a deviation of the protruded tongue toward the weaker side. A test for weakness of the tongue is to ask the patient to stick the tongue into the cheek while the clinician presses against the bulging cheek. A comparison is made between both sides.

Palpation

Palpation of the TMJ can be used to assess tenderness, skin temperature, muscle tone, swelling, skin moisture, and the location of trigger points. For comparison and expediency, palpation of the lateral and posterior aspects of the TMJs is performed bilaterally and simultaneously. The palpation begins with gentle touch and light pressure, because the muscles of mastication can be highly sensitive if they are in spasm. Tender areas, trigger points, and patterns of pain referral should be noted.

Anterior Aspect

Zygomatic Arch. The zygomatic arch is located anterior to the condylar process of the mandible. The temporal muscle lies above and the masseter muscle lies below the zygomatic arch.

Hyoid Bone. The hyoid bone, located anterior to the C2 and C3 vertebrae, is palpated for normal, painless movement as the patient swallows.

Digastric Muscle (Anterior Belly). The anterior belly of the digastric muscle can be palpated from its origin on the lingual side of the mandible to its tendinous insertion on the hyoid bone.

Thyroid. The thyroid cartilage, located anterior to the C4 and C5 vertebrae, is palpated and moved. Crepitation of this structure may be felt during neck extension as the cartilage becomes taut.

Lateral Aspect

Temporomandibular Joint. The clinician palpates the lateral aspect of the TMJ by placing the tip of the forefinger just anterior to the tragus of the ear (see Fig. 24-15). As the individual opens the mouth wide, the clinician's finger will identify a depression posterior to the condylar head and overlying the joint that is created by the translating condyle. Tenderness in this depression may indicate inflammation.[27] Alternatively, the lateral aspect of the joint capsule can be palpated on the lateral pole of the condyle just anterior to the tragus. To facilitate identification of the lateral pole, the patient is asked to open and lightly hold a cotton roll in the premolar region.[93]

Mandible. The mandible should be palpated along its entire length. Any asymmetry from side to side should be noted. The mandibular angle serves as an important landmark for orientation. The mandibular ramus is covered by the masseter muscle. The condylar process of the mandible is located just in front of the ear. The parotid gland is located anterior to and below the auricle, and normally extends from the sternomastoid muscle anteriorly to the masseter muscle. Enlargement of the parotid gland causes the ear lobe to move outward on the involved side. Enlargement of the parotid gland can have a number of causes, including infection, trauma, diabetes mellitus, lymphoma, or chronic alcoholism.[80] The submandibular gland is palpable in front of the mandibular angle and underneath the mandibular body, about halfway between the chin and the mandibular angle. Normally the gland has a firm, irregular consistency.

Sternocleidomastoid Muscle. The sternocleidomastoid is palpated from its dual origin on the sternum and clavicle along its course upward and posteriorly to its insertion on the mastoid process.

Trapezius Muscle. The trapezius muscle is palpated from its origin on the acromion process to its insertion along the midline of the spine to the base of the skull. The trapezius is perhaps the most common site for muscular trigger points and often refers pain to the base of the skull and the temporal region.[94]

Masseter Muscle. Both the superficial and deep portions of the masseter run from the zygomatic arch to the mandibular ramus.

The clinician should place the palpating finger against the ramus and then ask the patient to gently clench the teeth.

Temporalis Muscle.   The temporalis muscle can be palpated in front of, and above, the ear. The clinician places a finger against the temporal region and then asks the patient to gently clench the teeth.

Posterior Aspect.   Posterior TMJ palpation is performed by placing the tip of the little finger in the patient's external auditory canal and exerting anterior pressure as the patient repeatedly opens and closes the mouth.[27] Alternatively, the palpation can be performed similarly with the teeth in intercuspal position.[93] If inflammation is present, pain is felt on jaw closing as tissue is compressed between the clinician's finger and the condyle.[26] The examination also may reveal a posterosuperiorly positioned condyle and disk dysfunction. This posterosuperior position of the condyle can be a result of occlusal factors or trauma. The position results in an anteriorly displaced disk and an impingement by the condyle on the space normally occupied by the disk. This displacement may cause reciprocal clicking or locking.

The masseter, temporalis, and perihyoid muscles are palpated extraorally for hypertonicity and tenderness. In addition, the lateral aspect of the joint capsule and the lateral TMJ ligament are palpated for tenderness.

Medial Pterygoid.   The patient is asked to move the tongue to the opposite side. The clinician slides a thumb onto the medial aspect of the lower gum and toward the back of the mouth and angle of the mandible. The thumb is maintained at the bottom of the mouth to prevent the gag reflex. The insertion site for the medial pterygoid is located on the medial aspect of the mandibular angle (see Fig. 24-4).

Lateral Pterygoid.   It is questionable whether the lateral pterygoid can be palpated.[95] Nonetheless, descriptions detailing palpation of this muscle exist. The muscle is said to be palpated by sliding a thumb back to the medial aspect of the base of the upper molars. The patient is asked to open the mouth wider, and the clinician slides the thumb back and up at an angle of 45 degrees and inspects the muscle and area for tenderness.

Muscle Tests

It is important to be able to selectively stress the muscles of mastication and facial expression to determine whether they are implicated in the symptoms. All these tests cannot replace a thorough palpation of the muscles. All test positions, resisted motions, and attempted facial expressions may be used as exercises to rehabilitate any identified deficits.

Temporalis.   The patient is positioned sitting. The clinician palpates the side of the head in the temporal fossa region. The patient is asked to elevate and retract the mandible. Resistance can be applied using a tongue depressor placed between the teeth (Fig. 24-22). Both sides are tested.

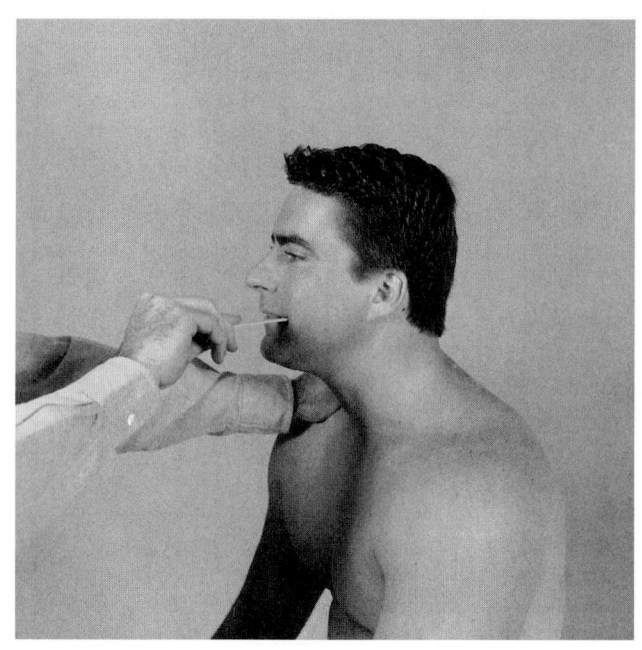

FIGURE 24-22   Resistive testing with tongue depressor.

Masseter.   The patient is positioned sitting. The clinician palpates the cheek, just above the angle of the mandible. The patient is asked to elevate the mandible, as in closing the jaw. Resistance can be applied using a tongue depressor placed between the teeth (see Fig. 24-22).

Lateral Pterygoid.   The patient is positioned sitting. The clinician palpates the pterygoid at the neck of the mandible and joint capsule. The patient is asked to protrude and depress the mandible against manual resistance.

Medial Pterygoid.   The patient is positioned sitting. The patient is asked to elevate and protrude the mandible. Resistance can be applied using a tongue depressor placed between the teeth.

Suprahyoid Muscles.   The patient is positioned sitting. The clinician palpates the floor of the mouth. The patient is asked to press the tip of the tongue against the front teeth. Resistance can be applied to the surface of the hyoid bone in an attempt to protrude the tongue.

Infrahyoid Muscles.   The patient is positioned sitting. The clinician palpates below the hyoid bone, immediately lateral to the midline. The patient is asked to swallow, while the clinician palpates for the movement of the hyoid and larynx.

Muscles of Facial Expression.   This group of muscles, most of which are innervated by the facial nerve, can be assessed by having the patient attempt to make the specific facial expression attributed to each muscle (Table 24-6). Facial strength can be evaluated with the House-Brackmann facial nerve grading

TABLE 24-6 Muscles of Facial Expression

Muscle	Action	Innervation
Occipitofrontalis	Wrinkles forehead by raising eyebrows	Facial nerve
Corrugator	Draws eyebrows together, as in frowning	Facial nerve
Procerus	Draws skin on lateral nose upward, forming transverse wrinkles over bridge of the nose	Facial nerve
Nasalis	Dilates and compresses aperture of the nostrils	Facial nerve
Orbicularis oculi	Closes eyes tightly	Facial nerve
Superior levator palpebrae	Lifts upper eyelid	Oculomotor nerve
Orbicularis oris	Closes and protrudes lips	Facial nerve
Major and minor zygomatic	Raises corners of mouth upward and laterally, as in smiling	Facial nerve
Levator anguli oris	Raises upper border of lip straight up, as in sneering	Facial nerve
Risorius	Draws corners of mouth laterally	Facial nerve
Buccinator	Presses cheeks firmly against teeth	Facial nerve
Levator labii superioris	Protrudes and elevates upper lip	Facial nerve
Depressor anguli oris and platsyma	Draws corner of mouth downward and tenses skin over neck	Facial nerve
Depressor labii inferioris	Protrudes lower lip, as in pouting	Facial nerve
Mentalis	Raises skin on chin	Facial nerve

system[96–99] (Table 24-7), which separates facial nerve paralysis into six grades, based on the severity of findings. In 1985, the American Academy of Otolaryngology, Head and Neck Surgery adopted the House-Brackmann six-point subjective grading scale as a universal standard. Parameters evaluated during the examination include:

▶ Overall macroscopic and gross appearance.

▶ Appearance at rest.

▶ Forehead movement.

▶ Eyelid closure.

▶ Mouth appearance.

▶ Synkinesis contracture or hemifacial spasm, or both.

Ligament Stress Tests.   The ligament stress tests assess the integrity of the capsule and ligaments. Positive findings include

excessive motion compared with the other side, or pain. The patient is seated.

Temporomandibular (Lateral) Ligament.   This test is only performed if there is a painful loss of active range of motion of the TMJ. The purpose of the test is to determine if the painful restriction is caused by damage to one of the ligaments or the joint capsule.

The clinician cradles and stabilizes the patient's head with one hand. The index and middle fingers of this hand can be used to palpate the joint line. The patient is asked to open their mouth to the point of restriction; mandible is positioned slightly open. The clinician places the thumb of the mobilizing hand on the ipsilateral molars of the side to be tested. The clinician then applies a downward force on the molars creating a caudal shear (Fig. 24-23). There should be slight movement with this technique and the end-feel should be capsular.

TABLE 24-7   House-Brackmann Facial Nerve Grading System[96]

Parameter	Grade I	Grade II	Grade III	Grade IV	Grade V	Grade VI
Overall appearance	Normal	Slight weakness on close inspection	Obvious but not disfiguring difference between both sides	Obvious weakness and/or disfiguring asymmetry	Only barely perceptible motion	No movement
At rest	Normal symmetry	Normal symmetry	Normal symmetry	Normal symmetry	Asymmetry	Asymmetry
Forehead movement	Normal with excellent function	Moderate-to-good function	Slight-to-moderate function	None	None	None
Eyelid closure	Normal closure	Complete with minimum effort	Complete with maximal effort	Incomplete closure with maximal effort	Incomplete closure with maximal effort	No movement
Mouth	Normal and symmetric	Slight asymmetry	Slight asymmetry with maximum effort	Asymmetry with maximum effort	Slight movement	No movement
Synkinesis contracture and/or hemifacial spasm	None	May have very slight synkinesis; no contracture or hemifacial spasm	Obvious but not disfiguring synkinesis contracture and/or hemifacial spasm	Synkinesis contracture and/or hemifacial spasm disfiguring or severe enough to interfere with function	Synkinesis contracture and/or hemifacial spasm usually absent	No movement

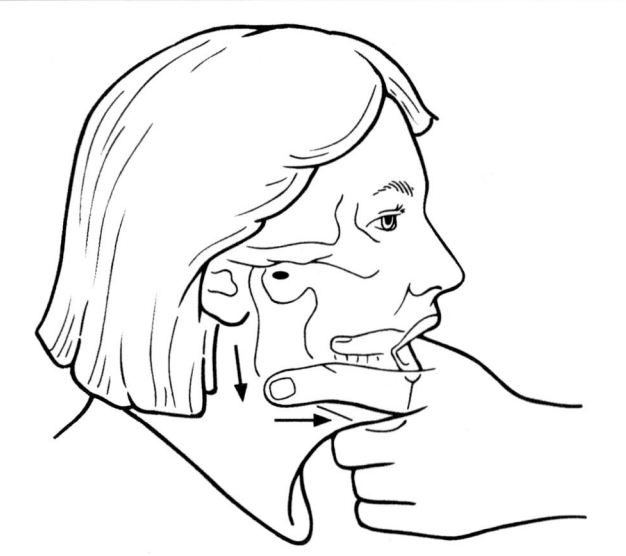

FIGURE 24-23   Caudal or inferior glide. (Reproduced with permission from Dutton M. *Manual Therapy of the Spine*. New York, NY: McGraw-Hill; 2002:556.)

Joint Capsule.   The clinician stands at the head of the patient. The patient's mandible is closed. The clinician places one hand on the top of the patient's head, and the other hand on the ramus and angle of one side. The clinician then applies a contralateral protrusion and ipsilateral deviation force (Fig. 24-24).

Joint Loading Tests

Selective loading of the TMJ may be used to help determine the presence of an intracapsular pathology. A positive finding is pain with the test. These tests include dynamic loading and joint compression.[51]

Dynamic Loading.   The patient is asked to bite forcefully on a cotton roll or tongue depressor on one side. This maneuver loads the contralateral TMJ.

Joint Compression.   The patient is positioned supine, with the clinician standing at the head of the bed. The clinician places the fingers of each hand under each side of the mandible, with the thumbs resting on the ramus. The mandible is then tipped posteriorly and inferiorly to compress the joint surfaces.

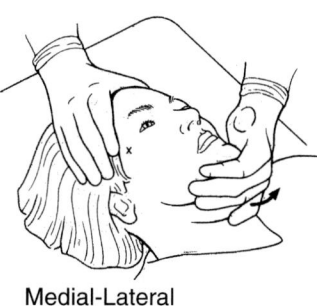

Medial-Lateral

FIGURE 24-24 Protrusion and lateral deviation. (Reproduced with permission from Dutton M, *Manual Therapy of the Spine*, McGraw-Hill, 2002.)

Passive Articular Mobility Testing

The passive articular mobility tests assess the joint glides and the end-feels. The patient and clinician setup is identical as that described above for the temporomandibular (lateral) ligament stress test.

From the end-range position (or as close as possible, given that your thumb is in the patient's mouth), the following maneuvers are performed assessing for range and end-feel. Findings are compared with each side. Pain or a restricted glide are positive findings and may indicate articular involvement or a capsular restriction. It is important to check the specific glides that are related to the loss of active motion. For example, if a patient demonstrated diminished mouth opening, the combined anterior, inferior, and lateral glide is assessed at each joint.

Limited opening can be caused by anterior disk displacement without reduction, elevator muscle spasm, or capsular restraint. By inducing a passive stretch to the joint after the patient has actively opened the mouth to the full extent, the "end-feel" can be used to differentiate between these causes. For example, if a displaced disk is responsible for limited opening, there will be a hard end-feel with little or no play. In contrast, a gummy end-feel is present when muscle spasm or capsular connective tissue is preventing full opening.[50] To help differentiate between elevator muscle spasm and a capsular restriction, passive motions can be used. With elevator muscle spasm, only vertical movement is restricted and protrusive and lateral excursions are normal. Anterior disk displacement without reduction, however, exhibits restrictions in both protrusive movements and contralateral excursions. Movement to the side of the involved joint is usually not mechanically restricted because the main movement occurring in the joint is rotation. While hypomobility may be apparent with passive articular mobility testing, hypermobility is difficult to determine with these tests.

Most of the mobility tests can also be used for mobilizations by changing the grade and the intent. The clinician should remove the thumb from the patient's mouth every 10–15 seconds to allow the patient to swallow:

▶ Inferior glide (Fig. 24-23).

▶ Anterior glide (see Fig. 24-23).

▶ Lateral glide (see Fig. 24-25).

▶ Medial glide (see Fig. 24-25).

▶ Superior glide (compression).

▶ Posterior glide with lateral excursion for the posterior ligaments (Fig. 24-26).

Neurologic Tests: Trigeminal Nerve (CN V)

Sensation. The skin near the midline (there is overlap from the ventral rami of C2 and C3 if tested too laterally) of the forehead and face can be stroked with cotton wool or tissue paper or can be tested for pinprick sensation. It is best if the testing is carried out bilaterally and simultaneously.

Reflex. The jaw jerk can be used to test trigeminal function. A lesion superior to the pons would produce hyperreflexia, and a lesion below the pons would result in hyporeflexia or areflexia. The patient's mouth is relaxed and open in the resting position. The clinician places a thumb on the mandible, then lightly taps the thumb with the pointed end of a reflex hammer (Fig. 24-27). A normal response is one in which the mouth closes.

Special Tests

At the time of writing, no routine special tests for the TMJ exist. Most, if not all, of the structures of the TMJ are isolated and tested during the standard examination described. Although cranial nerve testing is not, strictly speaking, a special test, cranial nerve testing should be performed if an injury to a cranial nerve is suspected. In addition, the special tests for thoracic outlet syndrome, brachial plexus stretching, and dural mobility should be performed to help rule out any referral of symptoms.

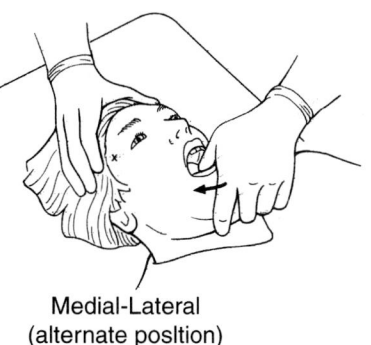

Medial-Lateral
(alternate position)

FIGURE 24-25 Caudal traction, protrusion, and medial and lateral glides. (Reproduced with permission from Dutton M. *Manual Therapy of the Spine*. New York, NY: McGraw-Hill; 2002:555.)

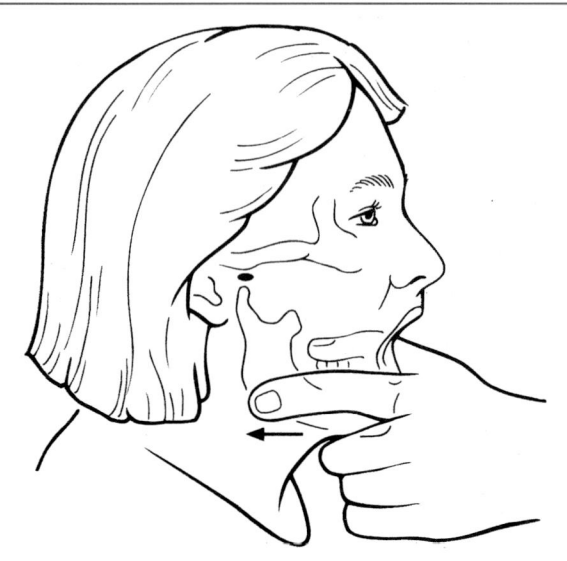

FIGURE 24-26   Posterior glide. (Reproduced with permission from Dutton M. *Manual Therapy of the Spine*. New York, NY: McGraw-Hill; 2002:556.)

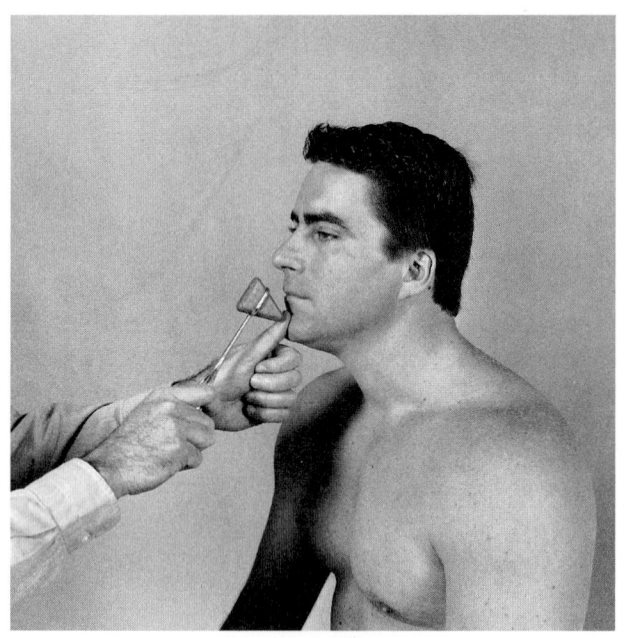

FIGURE 24-27   The jaw reflex.

Imaging Studies

With the rapid progress made in TMJ imaging techniques, many studies have focused on the importance of internal derangement and osteoarthrosis as the underlying mechanisms in the etiology of TMJ-related pain and dysfunction. Despite the limitations, plain radiographs of the TMJ, such as high-level orthopantomograms and transcranial projections, are useful ways of visualizing any gross pathologic, degenerative, or traumatic changes in the bony component of the TMJ

complex.[13,100] Magnetic resonance imaging (MRI) is currently the most accurate imaging modality for identification of disk positions of the TMJ and may be regarded as the gold standard for disk position identification purposes.[101] However, many reports question the utility of TMJ imaging studies because of the number of asymptomatic individuals who demonstrate positive signs of disk displacements and joint arthrosis (degenerative processes affecting the TMJ).[1,102] Postmortem examinations of a total of 140 persons (dental histories unknown) showed that 40 to 80 percent had joint pathology or disk displacements.[102] The relevance of bony joint arthrosis also was disputed by evidence that patients with TMJ rheumatoid arthritic pathology actually had fewer symptoms than normal individuals.[103]

Intervention Strategies

Conservative intervention for TMDs continues to be the most effective way of managing over 80 percent of patients.[104,105] A growing understanding of the natural history of TMD and some of the physical changes associated with TMD has played an important role in the intervention and management of TMD. Most instances of TMD involve masticatory muscle pains that vary in location and intensity with time. The majority of these muscle pains are self-limiting disorders that resolve without active intervention.[46]

Chronic pain associated with TMD frequently occurs because of secondary factors. These factors include a fixed head forward posture, abnormal stress levels, depression, or oral parafunctional habits (such as bruxism). This prolonged pain is frequently due to adaptive shortening of the tissues, or from a secondary hypermobility. It is likely that the longer the duration of the symptoms, the smaller the likelihood that the patient will benefit from a conservative intervention.[71] A number of authors[106,107] have recommended that the intervention for TMD should be effected at the following stages, which are, in order of importance to the patient[108]:

▶ Treatment of symptoms to reduce or eliminate pain or joint noises, or both.

▶ Treatment of the underlying cause, and to restore normal mandibular and cervical function. Selected exercises usually are performed by the patient on a regular basis to maintain muscle strength as well as joint arthrokinematic mobility in both the TMJ and cervical spine.[89]

▶ Treatment of the predisposing factor. This is best achieved with a comprehensive approach that addresses the contributing factors of poor posture, stress, depression, and oral parafunctional habits.[68,109]

Acute Phase

Acute injuries to the TMJ most frequently have a traumatic origin, such as a direct blow to the masticatory structure,[110–112] or from a sudden locking of the jaw caused by an internal derangement.[113,114]

The patient with an acute injury typically demonstrates a capsular pattern of restriction (decreased ipsilateral opening and lateral deviation to the contralateral side), with pain and tenderness on the same side. There may be ligamentous damage, which will be demonstrated on the stress tests, or muscular damage, which will become apparent on isometric testing.

Physical Therapy

The usual methods of decreasing inflammation—that is, PRICEMEM (protection, rest, ice, compression, elevation, manual therapy, early motion, and medications)—are recommended, although elevation is not applicable with the TMJ. Cold is applied to reduce edema, inflammation, and muscle spasm. The mechanism behind cryotherapy is thought to be a "counter irritation" and the production of analgesia.[116] The use of ice-filled towels soaked in warm water, applied all around the jaw, may prove beneficial in this phase. Chapman[117] concluded that local application of cold provides short-term relief of pain, possibly because of its analgesic effects and ability to reduce inflammation.

The patient should receive instruction on how to obtain the rest position of the TMJ. The rest position can be found by asking the patient to close the mouth so that the lips touch, but the teeth do not. The instruction of "lips together, teeth apart" may be used to teach the rest position for stressful situations.[118]

Motion of the TMJ should be restricted to pain-free movements. Limitation of mandibular function is encouraged to allow the rest or immobilization of the painful muscular and articular structures. Very gentle active exercises, well within the pain-free range, should be performed frequently (every hour or so) to help stimulate the mechanoreceptors and modulate pain, as well as improve vascularization.

Initial exercises during the acute stage include the so-called 6 × 6 exercise protocol of Rocabado.[119] Although the effectiveness of these exercises has not yet been subjected to formal clinical investigation, they are thought to aid in strengthening, coordination, and the reduction of muscle spasm. The goals of these exercises are to[50]:

▶ Learn a new postural position for the cervical spine, shoulder girdle, and TMJ.

▶ Restore the original muscle length.

▶ Restore normal joint mobility.

▶ Restore normal body balance.

▶ Teach the patient to use these exercises whenever the symptoms of dysfunction return.

The patient should be instructed to perform the following exercises six times each at a frequency of six times per day.

1. ***Tongue rest position, and nasal breathing.*** The patient places the tip of the tongue on the roof of the mouth, just behind the front teeth. In this position, the patient makes a "clucking" sound and gently holds the tongue against the palate with slight pressure. With the tongue in this position, the patient is asked to breathe through the nose and to use the diaphragm muscle for expiration. The use of accessory breathing muscles (pectoral, scalene, sternocleidomastoid, and intercostals) is discouraged, because they tend to promote and maintain a forward head posture.[50]

2. ***Controlled opening.*** The patient positions the tongue in the rest position and practices opening the mouth to the point where the tongue begins to leave the roof of the mouth. The patient can monitor the joint rotation by placing an index finger over the TMJ region. The patient is encouraged to chew in this nontranslatory manner.

3. ***Rhythmic stabilization.*** The patient positions the tongue in the rest position and grasps the chin with one or both hands. The patient applies a resistance sideways to the right, and then to the left. The patient then applies a resistance toward opening and closing. Throughout all of these exercises, the patient must maintain the resting jaw position at all times, and should be cautioned against the use of excessive force.

4. ***Liberation of cervical flexion.*** The patient places both hands behind the neck and interlaces the fingers to stabilize the C2 to C7 region. The neck is kept upright while the patient nods the head forward without flexing the neck. This motion produces a distraction of the occiput from the atlas and helps to counteract the craniovertebral extension produced by the forward head.

5. ***Axial neck extension.*** In one motion, the patient is asked to glide the neck backward and stretch the head upward. This exercise needs to be monitored closely to prevent a hypermobility of the cervical segments. The goal of this exercise is to improve the functional and mechanical relationship of the head to the cervical spine.

6. ***Shoulder retraction.*** In one motion, the patient is asked to pull the shoulders back and downward while squeezing the shoulder blades together. The goal of this exercise is the restoration of the shoulder girdle to an ideal postural position to establish stability of the entire head-neck-shoulder complex.

Another gentle exercise to increase joint mobility and articulation during this stage is the so-called cork exercise. The size (height) of the cork depends on the available motion. The patient holds the cork between his or her teeth while talking or reading aloud for approximately 2 minutes (Fig. 24-28). The reading or talking exercise is then repeated with the cork removed.

Neuromuscular education techniques can be used to control premature or excessive translation. Premature translation is translation that occurs before 11 mm of mouth opening. The point at which the translation occurs can be determined by palpating the lateral pole of the condyles as they move during opening. If premature translation occurs, the patient is taught to

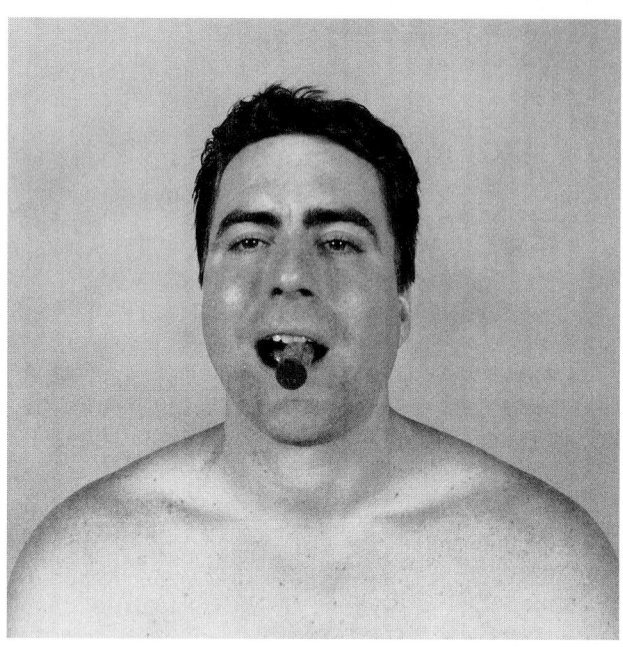

FIGURE 24-28   The cork exercise.

maintain the tongue on the posterior portion of the palate and to monitor the lateral pole of the condyles during opening to ensure that only rotation occurs during the early phase of opening.[89]

One of the most commonly overlooked problems during TMJ intervention is altered swallowing sequence and tongue position.[89] Few other forces can match the ability of the tongue to cause occlusal and skeletal deformation.[120] The presence of a residual pediatric tongue thrust or an acquired adult tongue thrust secondary to a forward head posture can affect the response to all other interventions. Presence of a tongue thrust is manifested by the hyoid moving slowly up and down during swallowing, contraction of the suboccipitals during swallowing, or head rocking and excessive lip activity during swallowing.[89] Patients with these findings should be shown the normal resting position for the tongue, and swallowing should be practiced without movement of the head and with the correct sequencing of tongue movements.[120]

Patient Education.   Perhaps the most important part of the intervention of TMD is to explain to the patient the cause and nature of the disorder, and to reassure him or her of the benign nature of the condition.[109] A successful self-care program may allow healing and prevent further injury and is often enough to control the problem.[115]

A typical self-care program includes the following: limitation of mandibular function (rest), a home exercise program, habit awareness and modification, and stress avoidance.[109]

The patient is advised to eat soft foods and avoid those that need a lot of chewing, and is discouraged from wide yawning, singing, chewing gum, and any other activities that would cause excessive jaw movement.[109] The patient's sleeping position also must be addressed. If the intrinsic ligaments are injured, the patient should be advised to sleep on the back with the mouth open and the neck supported by a cervical pillow.[68] Care must be taken to ensure that the patient does not sleep in the prone position, which stresses the cervical spine by extending and rotating it. The TMJ also receives compressive forces in this position, especially if the patient is in the habit of placing a hand under the pillow, and this can produce a sustained deviation over the course of the night.

Lastly, patients should be advised to identify source(s) of stress and to try to change their lifestyle accordingly.

Drug Intervention

The patient's physician may prescribe medications. Pharmacologic intervention in the management of chronic orofacial pain is usually considered adjunctive to a comprehensive intervention. If used properly as part of a comprehensive management program, drugs can be a valuable help in relieving symptoms.[121] However, no single drug has been proved to be effective for all cases of TMD. Thus, a wide variety of drug classes has been described for chronic orofacial pain, ranging from short-term treatment with nonsteroidal anti-inflammatory drugs (NSAIDs), corticosteroids, and muscle relaxants for pain of muscular origin to chronic administration of antidepressants for less well-characterized pain. The analgesic effect of NSAIDs is specific only in cases of TMD in which pain is the result of an inflammatory process such as synovitis or myositis. At the doses usually prescribed clinically, opiates are more effective in dampening the patient's emotional response to pain than eliminating the pain itself.[104] A need exists for well-controlled studies of drugs used for chronic orofacial pain in the relevant patient population, for periods of administration that approximate their use clinically, with appropriate indices of therapeutic efficacy and toxicity, and in comparison with a group receiving placebo medication to control for cyclic fluctuations in symptomology.[122]

Topical medications, because of their rapid onset and low side-effect profile, may offer a distinct advantage over systemic administration. To be delivered locally in the orofacial region by topical application, an agent must penetrate the natural barriers of the facial skin and oral mucosal tissues. Topical medications include lidocaine, benzocaine, and capsaicin, the latter of which is available over the counter.

Occlusal Appliance Therapy

The most common form of intervention provided by dentists for TMD is occlusal appliance therapy, alone or in combination with other interventions.[123] Occlusal appliances include bite-raising appliances, occlusal splints, or bite guards. These removable custom-made appliances are usually made of hard acrylic, which are custom made to fit over the occlusal surfaces of the teeth in one arch.[109] The function of the occlusal device is to provide a stable jaw posture by creating single contacts for all of the posterior teeth in centric relation and centric occlusion.[123]

Although occlusal appliance therapy has been shown clinically to alleviate symptoms of TMD in over 70 percent of patients, the physiologic basis of the response to treatment has never been well understood.[124,125] Malocclusion, of itself, is not established as an important factor in TMD,[53,126] because very few patients with malocclusion actually go on to develop temporomandibular pain and impairment.[127]

Functional Phase

Although the interventions for this phase are discussed separately, for optimal success they are best used in combination, and are dependent on the patient's needs.[1,71,128,129]

Postural Education

Postural education, together with patient education, should form the cornerstone of any physical therapy plan of care for patients with TMD. In a study of postural problems in 164 patients with head and neck pain, Fricton and colleagues[130] found poor sitting and standing posture in 96 percent, forward head in 84.7 percent, rounded shoulders in 82.3 percent, abnormal lordosis in 46.3 percent, and scoliosis in 15.9 percent. These findings indicate that there may be a correlation with TMJ dysfunction and poor posture, although comparisons would need to be made with a control group of normal individuals before final conclusions are drawn.

The focus of the postural intervention should be to educate the patient on correct posture of the head, neck, shoulder, and tongue in order to help minimize symptoms. Oftentimes the focus of the education is to teach the patient mental reminders to reduce the times spent in habitual positions during work and recreation. These positions, which cause an alteration in the tensile properties of the muscles and adaptive shortening of the joint capsule and ligaments, result in a variety of problems, including joint strain and improper weight bearing through the joint.[131–133] The pathologic posture then becomes associated with, or the precursor of, other deformities. A balanced and relaxed position, on the other hand, affords the best mechanical advantage for the body.[123]

Because these postural deviations do not always cause symptoms,[134] and the corrected positions require effort to maintain, patients need reassurance that the benefits in changing their posture may take time.[92,135]

Psychotherapy

Recent studies appear to suggest that TMD may be, on occasion the somatic expression of an underlying psychological or psychiatric disorder such as depression or a conversion disorder.[109,136–141] These studies have demonstrated increased psychometric scores denoting pain, chronic disability, and depression in TMD patients that far exceed the general population. Thus, in some cases referral to a psychiatrist or clinical psychologist may be a necessary part of the overall management strategy.

A study by Gardea and colleagues[142] evaluated the relative long-term efficacy of electromyographic biofeedback, cognitive-behavioral skills training (CBST), combined biofeedback and CBST, and no treatment in 108 patients suffering from chronic TMD. After an initial evaluation, patients were assigned to one of the four treatment groups. The three biobehavioral interventions consisted of 12 standardized sessions. Patients were reevaluated 1 year after completing treatment. Results demonstrated that patients who received the biobehavioral interventions reported significant improvement in subjective pain, pain-related disability, and mandibular functioning 1 year after receiving treatment. The no-treatment comparison group did not demonstrate such improvements, whereas the combined biofeedback and CBST treatment produced the most comprehensive improvements across all outcome measures.

Where persistent habits exacerbate or maintain the TMD, a more structured program of behavioral therapy may be required. Such behavioral therapy may include counseling on lifestyle, relaxation therapy, sleep interruption devices, or hypnosis.[143] Medical hypnosis has been demonstrated to be an effective treatment modality for TMD, in terms of reducing both symptoms and medical use.[144,145]

Manual Therapy

The examination sequence used to determine the appropriate manual technique to use for the TMJ is outlined in Figure 24-29. The specific manual techniques for the TMJ are described under "Therapeutic Techniques," later.

Trigger Point Therapy

Masticatory muscle pain is the one symptom for which there is the best overall evidence supporting various physical therapy interventions.[146] The most common intervention for these masticatory muscle disorders is trigger point therapy. Chapter 11 reviews the basis for the various intervention procedures for trigger points, which include deep massage, soft tissue mobilizations, postural exercises, ultrasound, acupuncture, and trigger point injections. Spray and stretch techniques also may be used. These techniques involve the application of a vapocoolant spray during the stretching of soft tissues to reduce trigger points and eliminate referred pain.[94] Vapocoolants also may be applied to rapidly cool the skin and overlying musculature during stretching. When using vapocoolants in this region, care must be taken to cover the patient's eyes and to prevent any inhalation of the vapors.

Exercise

Some evidence suggests that exercise of the specific painful area during the functional phase is effective in strengthening the muscles, improving function, and reducing pain. Tegelberg and Kopp[147] ran parallel studies of jaw exercise versus a no-treatment control in subjects with rheumatoid arthritis and ankylosing spondylitis. Significant differences were detected for both conditions in mean maximal opening, but no between-group

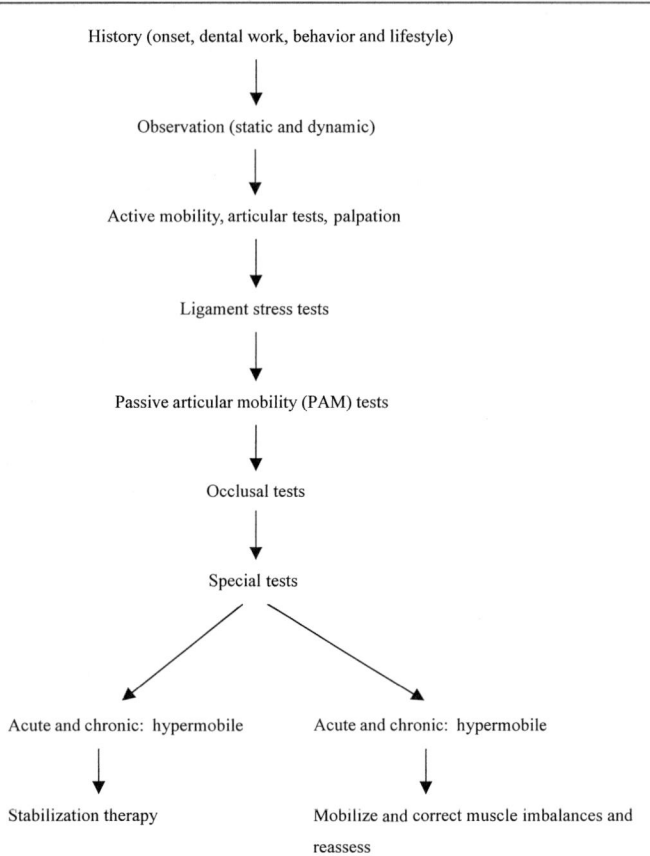

History (onset, dental work, behavior and lifestyle)

↓

Observation (static and dynamic)

↓

Active mobility, articular tests, palpation

↓

Ligament stress tests

↓

Passive articular mobility (PAM) tests

↓

Occlusal tests

↓

Special tests

Acute and chronic: hypermobile   Acute and chronic: hypermobile

↓   ↓

Stabilization therapy   Mobilize and correct muscle imbalances and
                                reassess

FIGURE 24-29   Examination sequence used to determine appropriate manual therapy technique for the TMJ. (Reproduced with permission from Dutton M. *Manual Therapy of the Spine*. New York, NY: McGraw-Hill; 2002:552.)

differences were detected for change in the subjective symptoms (pain, stiffness).

Because of the association of TMD and poor posture, the prescribed exercises for TMD include strengthening exercises for the cervicothoracic stabilizers (see Chap. 23), and the scapular stabilizers (see Chap. 14). Stretching exercises are prescribed for the scalenes, trapezius, pectoralis minor, and levator scapulae (see Chap. 23) and the suboccipital extensors (see Chap. 22).

A restriction of mouth opening is treated with range-of-motion exercises to elongate the soft tissues, and with joint mobilizations. The patient should be encouraged to begin full active range-of-motion exercises as early as tolerated (see the discussion of automobilizations under "Therapeutic Techniques," later). However, if jaw deviation is occurring, the exercises should be performed in a range in which the patient can control the deviation.

Excessive mandibular motion is treated by muscle re-education, with isometrics performed at the desired opening range.

Thermal and Electrotherapeutic Modalities

A multitude of electrotherapeutic modalities, especially ultrasound and electrical stimulation, have been applied to patients with TMDs,[13,108,148] but there appears to be little evidence that passive modalities alone can cause long-lasting reductions, and very few studies have systematically evaluated the effect of these treatments.[108,128,129,149,150] The American Academy of Craniomandibular Disorders (AACD) recommends the use of thermal and electrotherapeutic modalities and intraoral splints in conjunction with other interventions, including mobilization of the TMJ.[151]

Moist Heat Packs.   Conventional hot packs or face packs may be used in the functional stage and are applied for approximately 15 minutes. Thermotherapy is used to help the soft tissues relax and to increase circulation.

High-voltage Electric Stimulation.   High-voltage stimulators deliver a monophasic, twin-peak waveform. Because of the short duration of the twin-peak wave, high voltages with high peak current but low average current can be achieved. These characteristics provide patient comfort and safety in application. In addition, in contrast to low-voltage direct-current devices, thermal and galvanic effects are minimized.[152]

High-voltage stimulators have been applied clinically to reduce or eliminate muscle spasm and soft tissue edema, as well as for muscle re-education (non–central-nervous-system-produced muscle contraction), trigger point therapy, and increasing blood flow to tissues with decreased circulation.[62,63,152]

Ultrasound.   The effects of ultrasound are partly thermal, because of the increase in blood flow and tissue temperature produced. Thus, ultrasound may be used to help the soft tissues relax and to increase circulation. Ultrasound is an ideal modality both before and during joint and soft tissue mobilization. There is also a mechanical effect associated with ultrasound, because the sound waves produce pressure changes in the tissues, which may result in a micromassage of the tissues.[108] A 3-MHz frequency is recommended, with an intensity of between 0.75 and 1.0 W/cm^2. Tongue depressors can be inserted in the patient's mouth to apply a gentle stretch during the ultrasound treatment.[89]

Iontophoresis.   Iontophoresis may be used to introduce medications such as cortisol, dexamethasone, salicylates, and analgesics.[153,154] Kahn[155] found that following TMJ surgery, the use of iontophoresis in conjunction with ultrasound produced a decrease in pain, paresthesia, and trismus (the limitation of jaw opening caused by spasm of the masticatory muscles).

Surgical Intervention

Published reports show that about 5 percent of patients undergoing an intervention for TMD may eventually require surgery.[8,9] A range of surgical procedures is currently used to treat TMD, ranging from TMJ arthrocentesis and arthroscopy to the more complex open joint surgical procedures, referred to as *arthrotomy*.[9]

The proximity of the medial aspect of the TMJ to the structures of the infratemporal fossa raises the possibility of complications associated with TMJ surgery on the medial aspect of the joint.[156] These complications include involvement of the inferior alveolar, lingual, and auriculotemporal nerves.[157] A further study found that the location of such vital structures as the middle meningeal artery, the carotid artery, the internal jugular vein, and the trigeminal nerve, varied, increasing the likelihood of significant intra-operative or postoperative complications.[158]

In terms of intervention, the postsurgical patient is treated as though in the acute phase of healing and is progressed gradually, as outlined under "Intervention Strategies," earlier.

Practice Pattern 4D: Impaired Joint Mobility, Motor Function, Muscle Performance, Range of Motion Associated with Connective Tissue Dysfunction

Internal Derangement: Intra-articular Disk Displacement

TMJ internal derangement is one of the most common forms of TMD and is associated with characteristic clinical findings such as pain, joint sounds, and irregular or deviating jaw function.[66,159] The term *internal derangement* when related to TMD denotes an abnormal positional relationship of the articular disk to the mandibular condyle and the articular eminence.[64] This abnormal positional relationship may result in mechanical interference and restriction of the normal range of mandibular activity. Theoretically, internal derangement of the TMJ involves the anterior (and medial) displacement of the disk, resulting from the action of the upper head of the lateral pterygoid muscle, a tear or thinning of the disk, osteoarthrosis, or malocclusion.[23,40,160]

The diagnosis of internal derangement of the TMJ requires the use of a classification system. I recommend use of the following classification system devised by Pertes and Attanasio[161]:

I. Deviation in form.
   A. Frictional disk incoordination.
   B. Articular surface defects.
   C. Disk thinning and perforation.
II. Disk displacements.
   A. Partial anteromedial disk displacement.
   B. Anteromedial disk displacement with reduction.
      1. Partial.
      2. Complete.
   C. Anteromedial disk displacement with intermittent locking.
   D. Anteromedial disk displacement without reduction.
      1. Acute.
      2. Chronic.
III. Adhesive disk hypomobility.
IV. Displacement of disk-condyle complex.
   A. Subluxation.
   B. Dislocation.

Deviation in Form[161]

Frictional Disk Incoordination. Frictional disk incoordination (FDI) may occur when the intra-articular disk adheres to the eminence. FDI usually occurs after a prolonged period of TMJ inactivity, such as occurs with immobilization following surgery. Other causes of this condition include occlusion, bruxism, excessive biting force, and trauma with the teeth together. The adhesion of the disk is thought to be caused by a reduction in the lubrication, and roughness, on the articular surface of the eminence or disk. The adhesion can result in a loss of the translatory glide of the condyle, which in turn can result in excessive pressure between the disk and the eminence and a strain on the discal ligaments, predisposing the patient to a true disk displacement of the joint.

Clinical findings with this condition may include a discrete opening click with momentary discomfort, while the remainder of the translatory cycle is normally accomplished without difficulty.[162] The click associated with deviation in form caused by damage to the articular eminence or abnormal development usually occurs every time at the same point in the range of opening and closing.

The conservative intervention for this condition should focus on the elimination of any occlusal disharmony, the reduction of parafunctional habits (cheek biting, nail biting, pencil chewing, teeth clenching, or bruxism), and methods to prevent the disk-condyle complex from returning to the closed position.[6] The latter goal can be accomplished by applying a permanent stabilization splint for a few months. The splint should be fabricated without any repositioning component and should be balanced for both day and night wear. When symptoms have been reduced, the patient should be weaned off the splint during the day and eventually, night.

Articular Surface Defects. An articular surface defect located on the articulating surface of the eminence, the superior surface of the disk, or both, may cause a hindrance to the normal translatory movement of the disk.[163] The defect may be caused by trauma to the mandible when the teeth are apart, habitual abuse, and developmental and growth anomalies.[6]

Because the joint surface interference tends to occur at the same point in the translatory cycle, clinical findings for articular surface defects include a reciprocal click at the same point during both opening and closing movements. In addition, a lateral deviation frequently occurs on opening, as the patient attempts to avert the interference. Although the condition itself is painless, it can be worsened by any activities that increase intra-articular pressure.[6,164]

Conservative intervention for this condition includes habit training to develop a path of mandibular movement that avoids the interference. In addition, the patient is asked to make a conscious effort to reduce the force of chewing and eliminate parafunctional habits (cheek biting, nail biting, pencil chewing, teeth clenching, or bruxism). Chewing on the affected side, by decreasing the intra-articular pressure, also may be helpful. A stabilization splint may serve to reduce pressure on the joint structures.[6,162]

Disk Thinning and Perforation. Disk thinning can result from the application of excessive pressure on the TMJ, and can lead to a deformation of the joint structures. If overloading occurs while the teeth are together, thinning of the central part of the disk may result. Continuous pressure eventually may cause perforation of the disk.

The symptoms of disk thinning and perforation depend on the extent of damage to the disk. Theoretically, thinning of the central part of the disk should not result in pain, because that part of the disk is not innervated. However, variable joint tenderness and muscle pain often is associated with any activity that deepens the central bearing area of the disk.

If the disk should perforate, grating sounds or crepitus during the translatory cycle is likely because of damage of the articular surfaces.[165,166] Pain usually is associated with the perforation, which conversely may diminish as the extent of damage increases. The diagnosis of disk perforation usually is made by imaging, arthrography, or arthroscopy. MRI, which is ideal for visualizing disk displacement, may not be as accurate for a perforation.[54]

Conservative intervention for disk thinning usually involves the application of a stabilization splint to prevent a perforation. If perforation has occurred and the patient can no longer tolerate the symptoms, surgical intervention is indicated.

Disk Displacements.[161] Disk displacements usually are viewed as a series of progressively worsening clinical entities. A pathologic click in a disk displacement may be caused by the condyle subluxing anteriorly or medially later than normal in the opening cycle. The click also may occur as the condyle relaxes onto the disk, or it may represent the sudden snapping back of the disk by the less than adequately elastic posterior ligament of the disk.

Partial Anteromedial Disk Displacement. In a healthy joint, the center of the posterior band of the disk is in the 12-o'clock position on the condyle when the teeth are occluded. With partial anterior disk displacement, the disk is permitted to slide anteriorly on the condyle and the terminal position of the posterior band of the disk occurs anteriorly to the normal position on the condyle in the closed-joint position. The anterior displacement is thought to occur because of two factors: some thinning of the posterior band, and minimal elongation of the discal ligaments.[162]

The conservative intervention for partial displacements should focus on preventing any worsening of the disk displacement. This can be achieved using intra-oral appliances in combination with psychological stress reduction.

Anteromedial Intra-articular Disk Displacement with Reduction. Disk displacement with reduction is both an anatomic and a functional disorder that is cyclic in nature.[54] Anteromedial disk displacement with reduction is described as a unexpected alteration or interference of the disk-condyle structural relation during mandibular translation with mouth opening and closing.[68] The misalignment of the disk is thought to be the result of articular surface irregularity, disk-articular surface adherence, synovial fluid degradation, or myofascial imbalances around

the joint. In addition, this alteration or interference may be the result of increased elongation of discal ligaments and the posterior attachment, which can create an obstruction to normal condylar translation.[167]

The temporarily misaligned disk reduces or improves its structural relationship with the condyle when mandibular translation occurs with mouth opening. This change often is associated with an "opening click," and a reciprocal "closing click," which occurs just before the teeth occlude during mouth closing. Pain, if present, usually occurs at the time of the disk reduction.

Disk displacement with reduction may be characterized by five progressive stages.[82,168,169]

▶ *Stage I.* In stage I, the disk may be positioned slightly anteromedially on the mandibular head. Pain is usually mild or absent. As the disk becomes deformed from the repetitive microtrauma, it begins to interfere with the normal translation of the condyle.[68]

▶ *Stage II.* In this stage, the disk slips further anteromedially on the mandibular head. The reciprocal click described earlier may occur in the early phase of opening and late in the phase of closing (Fig. 24-30).[68] Stage II is characterized by a loss of integrity of the ligamentous and intracapsular structures. This loss of integrity may result in increased mobility and a decrease in control of the disk, which increases the potential for impingement and deformation of the disk, resulting in severe pain, and increases the potential for intermittent *open locking* or subluxation of the joint.[90] An *open lock* is characterized by two opening clicks, and two clicks on closing. During opening, the first click occurs when the condyle moves over the posterior rim of the disk, and the second click as the condyle moves over the anterior rim.[68] If, after the second click occurs on opening, the disk lies posterior to the condyle, the condyle may be prevented from sliding back.[170]

▶ *Stage III.* Stage III is often the most painful stage. This stage is characterized by a reciprocal click that occurs later in the opening cycle and earlier in the closing cycle.[68] Occasionally, the intra-articular disk becomes adherent to the mandibular condyles in both the open and closed positions. This is known as a *closed-lock* position (Fig. 24-31).[68] The sustained closed-lock condition produces a sudden limitation of opening as the disk becomes permanently lodged anteriorly, thereby interfering with the normal condylar rotation and translation.[90] This closed-lock condition results in a hard end-feel in the joint when the clinician attempts to induce a passive stretch to the joint.[50] The impingement on the posterior attachment of the disk by the condylar head may result in a prolonged stretching of the tissue. The limitation of opening usually is restricted to 25 to 30 mm. Because condylar translatory mobility commonly is hindered on the affected side only, the mandible may deviate away from the midline toward the affected side with maximal jaw opening.[68] However, if this condition is chronic, there may be no deviation or limitation of jaw opening because of

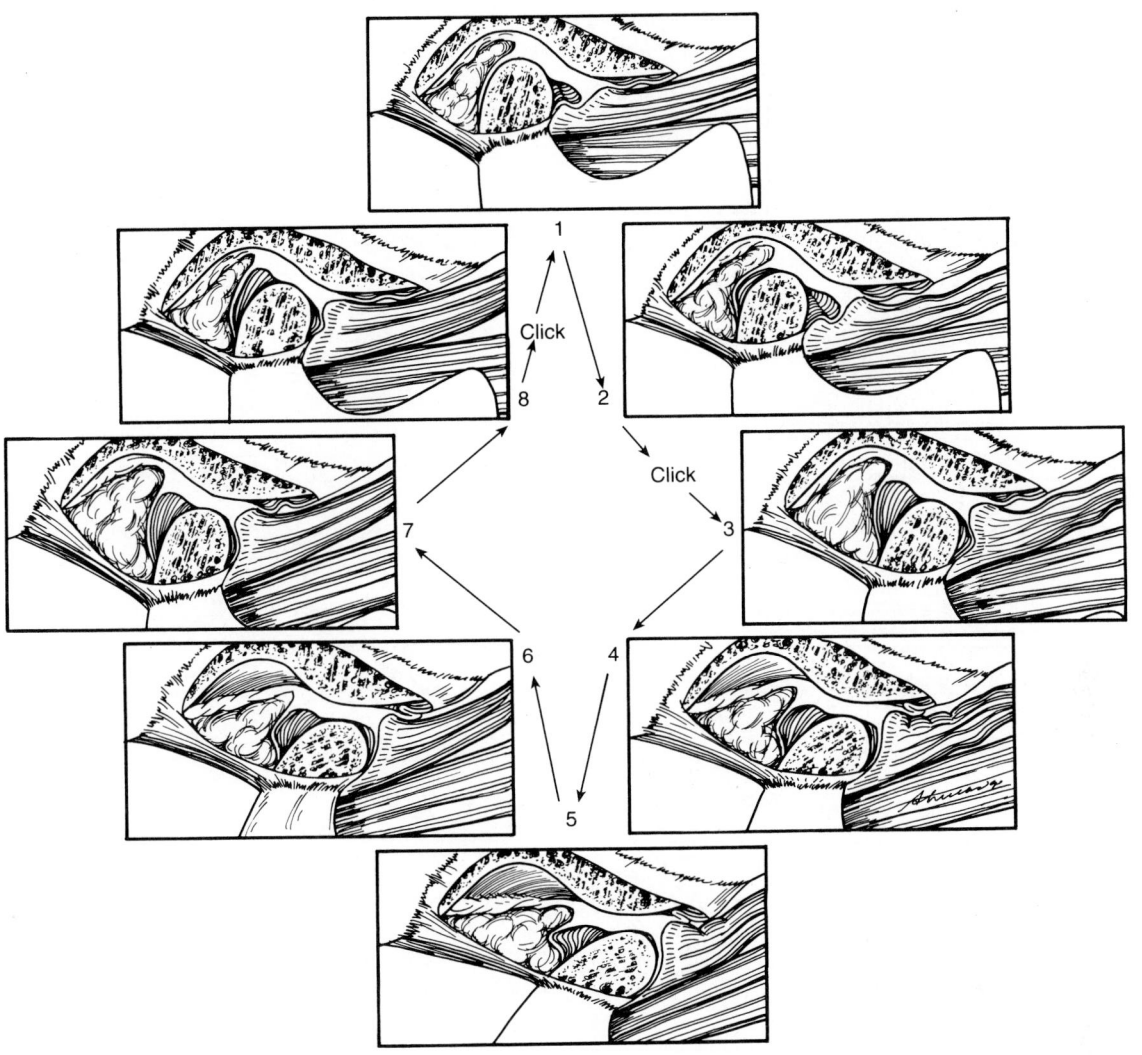

FIGURE 24-30 Reciprocal click. (Reproduced with permission from Okeson JP. *Management of Temporomandibular Disorders and Occlusion.* 4th ed. St Louis, Mo: Mosby Year Book; 1998:200.)

progressive tearing in the retrodiscal lamina. Tenderness of the masticatory muscles also may occur as a result of the protective splinting of the joint.

▶ *Stage IV.* In this stage, clicking is rare because the disk position is usually so incompatible. If clicking does occur, it is usually a single opening click because of the irregularities in translations.[68] Chronic locking with soft tissue remodeling can occur as a result of routine daily jaw function on the posteriorly or anteriorly positioned disk.[90] Known as *rotational displacement,* this condition is associated with pain and, commonly, with anterior displacement of the disk.[55]

▶ *Stage V.* This stage is characterized by radiographic degenerative changes on the condylar head and, occasionally, on the articular eminences, with evidence of remodeling and osteophytosis.[54] Marked deformity and thickening of the disk may occur, and the shape of the disk may change in con-

figuration from biconcave to biconvex. The joint space typically is narrowed to the point where bone-on-bone contact is evident, resulting in coarse crepitus with jaw motions.

Stages I and II usually are amenable to physical therapy intervention. The focus for these stages is on reducing muscle dysfunction and improving the biomechanics of the joint.[90] The intervention usually involves using mandibular-repositioning appliances that stabilize a protrusive position to keep the disk in a more optimal relationship with the condyle.[171] The primary purpose of protrusive splint therapy may be to allow repair and regeneration to occur in the retrodiscal tissue and, possibly, in the discal ligaments.[172]

The intervention for stages III through V, and those patients who are postsurgical, is directed at promoting and progressing healing, restoring joint range of motion, and reducing the inflammation associated with capsulitis.[90]

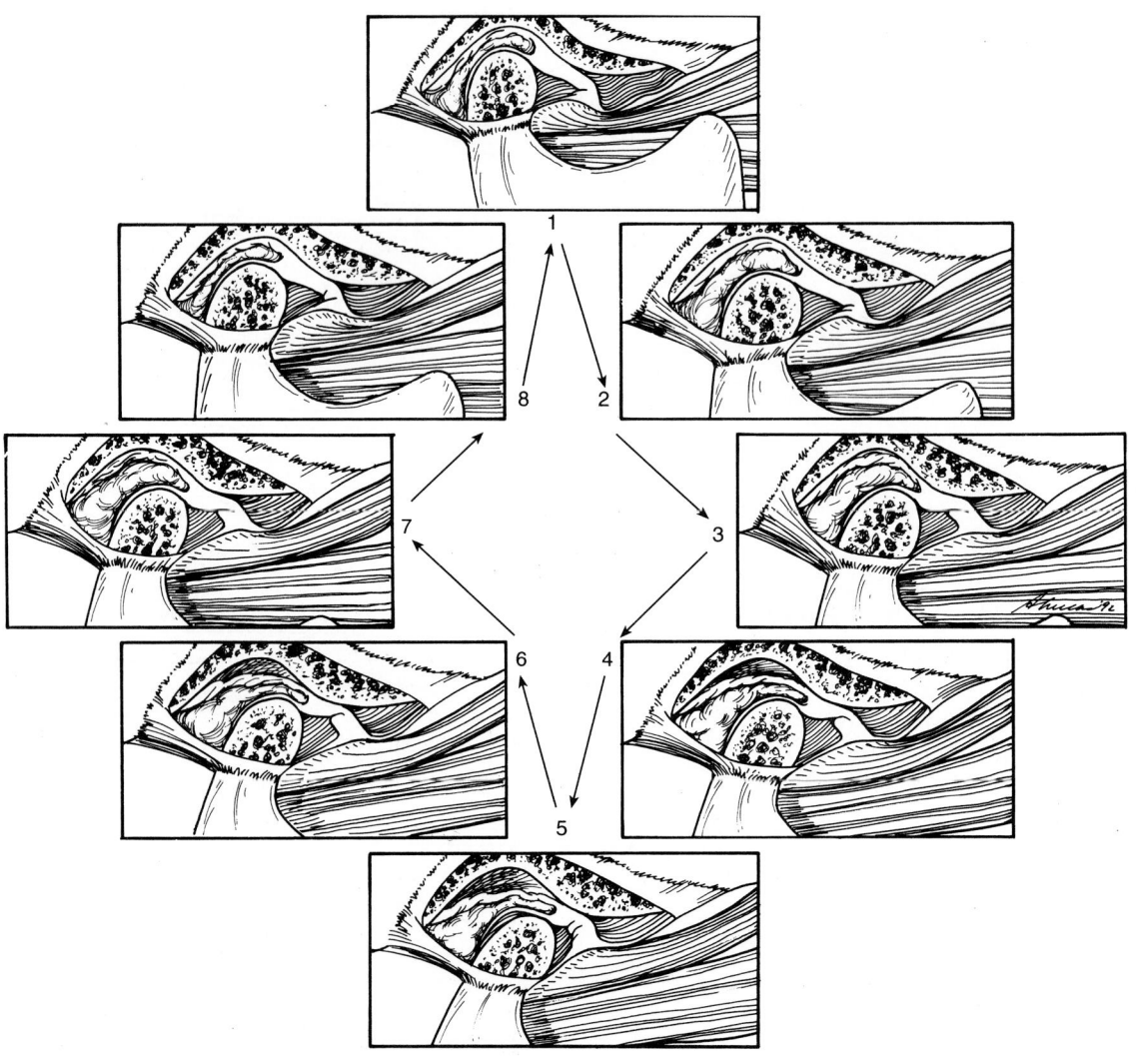

FIGURE 24-31   Closed lock. (Reproduced with permission from Okeson JP. *Management of Temporomandibular Disorders and Occlusion.* 4th ed. St Louis, Mo: Mosby Year Book; 1998:204.)

Anteromedial Disk Displacement with Intermittent Locking.   As mentioned in the previous section, if the disk remains displaced for longer periods of time, its shape becomes deformed and may slowly change from biconcave to biconvex. This change in shape makes the passage of the condyle under the disk more difficult. To return the disk, the patient must learn to move the mandible to the opposite side in order to activate the superior retrodiscal lamina.[90] Unfortunately, at this point, the retrodiscal tissue has thinned considerably and lost much of its elasticity, making disk reduction difficult to achieve.

The intermittent locking may occur at any time, but it most often occurs in the morning upon awakening, after a prolonged period of clenching, or after chewing on the involved side.[90] Conservative intervention usually involves a mandibular repositioning appliance to keep the disk in correct alignment with the condyle.

Intra-articular Disk Displacement Without Reduction.[68]   Although some patients may show progression through the various stages

of disk displacement, it is unclear why some patients remain in the category of anterior disk displacement with reduction for years, whereas others proceed to intermittent locking and anterior disk displacement without reduction within a matter of months.

Disk displacement without reduction is described as an alteration or interference of the disk-condyle structural relation that is maintained during mandibular translation. As a result of continued disk deformation along with elongation of discal ligaments and loss of tension in the posterior attachment, the disk may remain anteromedially displaced creating a "closed-lock." Contact is lost among condyle, disk, and articular eminence, and the articular disk space collapses, trapping the disk in front of the condyle and thereby preventing translation. Usually, the displacement of the disk becomes worse with jaw motions. Initially, there may be an associated locking with a sudden and marked limited jaw motion. In addition, there may be a deviation of the mandible toward the involved side during mouth opening, and a marked limitation of lateral deviation to the contralateral side.[68,90]

The limited opening resulting from anterior disk displacement without reduction may have a variety of causes. In addition to the more common causes, including muscle spasm and capsular tightness, limited mouth opening may occur when either the disk is lodged anteriorly to the condyle, or when the TMJ is dislocated or subluxed. Limited mouth opening as a result of elevator muscle spasm or capsular restraint can be differentiated by determining the end-feel. Elevator muscle spasm tends to limit only vertical movement; the protrusive and lateral excursions are usually normal. Anterior disk displacement without reduction, however, exhibits restrictions in both protrusive movements and contralateral excursions. Movement to the side of the involved joint usually is not mechanically restricted because the main movement occurring in the joint is rotation. Pain restriction may be the result of impingement on inflamed retrodiscal tissues. Secondary muscle spasm of the elevator muscles may add to the restricted opening as well as capsular involvement.

In the acute phase, joint noise is usually absent. However, crepitus may be detected as the displacement becomes chronic and changes occur in the articular surfaces. As the condition becomes chronic, the pain often is markedly reduced and the range of motion may approach normal dimensions.

The intervention for the acute phase of this type of disk displacement should focus on a reduction of the displaced disk through mobilization of the joint. Because secondary elevator muscle spasm is usually present, as well as some inflammation of joint structures, it may be of benefit for the patient to take a skeletal muscle relaxant and an NSAID prior to physical therapy session. The reduction procedure involves the patient opening the mouth as wide as is comfortable and then moving the mandible toward the opposite joint. If unsuccessful, the clinician may then attempt to reduce the disk manually through downward pressure on the last molar on the involved side.[164] Success in reducing the disk usually can be clinically determined by comparing the amount of vertical opening and contralateral movement after mobilization with the amount of movement before mobilization. This difference should be verified through imaging, because clinical criteria alone may not be accurate. Generally speaking, reductive mobilization is more successful in the more acute conditions. In cases in which changes in the connective tissue capsule may be contributing factors, manual stretching of the vertical fibers of the capsule may be indicated.

Adhesive Disk Hypomobility.[161] Although many cases of intracapsular restriction of mandibular movement or closed-lock are caused by an anterior disk displacement without reduction, another frequent abnormality of the TMJ is the formation of intra-articular adhesions. The restriction also may be caused by an adhesion occurring in the superior joint cavity between the disk and eminence, resulting in a loss of condylar translation. In addition, an adhesion may result in condylar displacement of the disk, with distortion of the disk itself on mandibular opening.[54]

Trauma frequently is implicated as a causative factor. If the trauma is slight, only mild surface damage to the disk may occur, resulting in frictional disk incoordination or an articulating surface defect. A more severe incident could cause intracapsular bleeding and effusion. Fibrosis may result, producing a reduction in the range of motion as well as degeneration. Condylar translation may be lost as a result of disk adhesion.

Clinically, adhesive disk hypomobility is indistinguishable from acute anterior disk displacement without reduction. Because translation does not occur, opening is limited. Pain is variable and may be caused by stretching of the discal ligaments, as forced opening is attempted.

The conservative intervention for adhesive disk hypomobility is specific joint mobilizations (see "Therapeutic Techniques," later).

Displacement of the Disk-Condyle Complex[161]

Subluxation. Subluxation between the disk and the articular eminence may occur as a result of excessive opening, which can force the condyle and the disk anteriorly beyond the normal limits of the translatory cycle. If the disk cannot rotate any farther posteriorly and the condyle continues to translate, a partial dislocation or subluxation can occur.

Usually, the patient has a history of jaw clicking with wide mouth opening, such as when yawning or eating or during a dental procedure. Diagnostically, for treatment purposes, this wide opening click must be differentiated from a click that signifies reduction of a displaced disk. A subluxation type of click occurs only on wide opening and not on protrusive movement or lateral excursion. The click associated with reduction of a displaced disk, however, can occur during both protrusive and contralateral excursion. Usually, pain does not accompany subluxation unless it becomes habitual.

Intervention for this condition includes habit training to voluntarily limit mouth opening within normal limits. This training should be accompanied by exercises that strengthen the elevator muscles. Occasionally, injection of a sclerosing solution to reduce the laxity of the capsule may be required.

Dislocation. Dislocation of the TMJ is caused by additional rotation of the mandibular condyle beyond its biomechanical limit, resulting in an anterior displacement of the disk beyond the articular eminence, and in direct contact between the condyle and the eminence. As opposed to subluxation, which is a partial loss of contact between the disk and the eminence, dislocation involves a collapse of the articular disk space. Because of the collapsed disk space, the superior retrodiscal lamina cannot retract the prolapsed disk. Adding to the problem is the elevator muscle spasm that frequently accompanies dislocation and preserves the decrease in articular disk space.

Some factors associated with the onset of habitual dislocation include, but are not limited to, yawning, singing, sleeping with the head resting on the forearm, manipulation of the mandible while the patient is under general anesthesia, excessive tooth abrasion, severe malocclusion, loss of dentition (leading to overclosure), and trauma.[173]

Clinical findings include an inability of the patient to close the mandible after wide mouth opening, so that the mouth becomes locked open in a prognathic position and cannot be moved vertically. An acute malocclusion is present with an anterior open bite and contact between only the most posterior teeth. Depressions may be noted in the preauricular area formerly occupied by the condyles. Pain may be variable, which increases as the patient attempts to close, thus straining the inferior retrodiscal lamina and the collateral discal ligaments.

The main objective of the intervention is to widen the articular disk space. This allows the superior retrodiscal lamina to retract the disk. Forceful closing of the mandible should be avoided. Reduction of the displaced mandible is best accomplished by having the patient yawn as widely as possible while the clinician exerts slight posterior pressure on the chin. If reduction is not achieved, placement of thumbs behind the molars and pressing down while the patient yawns may produce the reduction by increasing the additional articular space. Should these attempts at manual correction fail, the clinician may try stimulation of the gag reflex by touching a mouth mirror to the soft palate. This maneuver can result in an inhibition of elevator muscle activity, thus increasing the articular disk space.

For recurrent dislocations, the conservative approach is addressed according to the stability factors into (1) alteration of the ligaments, (2) alteration of the associated musculature, and (3) alteration of the bony anatomy[173]:

▶ Alteration to the ligaments can be achieved by the introduction of a sclerosing agent into the capsular space of the TMJ.

▶ Alteration of the associated musculature can be achieved by exercise. Strengthening the suprahyoid muscles to counterbalance the action of the lateral pterygoid muscles could, theoretically, reduce the likelihood of dislocation. The equipment to perform this type of exercise, however, is elaborate and involves considerable compliance by the patient. A more recently reported treatment modality for alteration of the musculature is the use of type A botulinum toxin (BTA). If dislocation is chronic, the patient should be taught how to self-reduce the mandible. Habit training similar to that employed for subluxation should be instituted.

▶ An alteration of bony anatomy requires a surgical eminectomy.

Arthritis

The TMJ, like other joints in the body, can become a site of osteoarthritis. Degenerative osteoarthritis may be secondary to trauma, surgery, congenital malformation, or, most commonly, long-standing disk derangement. Marginal osteophyte formation, bony erosion sclerosis, and subchondral or subcortical formation may be observed.[54] The temporomandibular disk may become distorted in shape secondary to adhesions seen in osteoarthritis.[174]

Other arthritides are known to affect the TMJ, including rheumatoid arthritis, systemic lupus erythematosus, synovial chondromatosis, ankylosing spondylitis, psoriasis, and crystalline arthritides such as calcium pyrophosphate deposition disease (CPPD) and gout.

To date, no intervention exists that can reverse the anatomic and biochemical alterations of osteoarthrosis. Thus, the intervention approach has to be aimed at restoring function and managing pain through the acute phase of the disease.

Pigmented Villonodular Synovitis

Pigmented villonodular synovitis (PVNS) is a proliferative but non-neoplastic disorder of unknown pathogenesis that affects the synovial membranes of joints.[175,176] Eighty percent of cases involve the knee, followed in order of frequency by the hip, ankle, and shoulder, with involvement of the TMJ being very rare.[177–179] The disorder is generally thought to be a benign, inflammatory process, although it may develop as an aggressive local process.

PVNS is described as expressing multiple manifestations of a histologic lesion occurring in the synovial membrane of joints. PVNS is subdivided into diffuse and localized forms, depending on the extent of synovial involvement. PVNS may extend into bone, and, in most instances, the diffuse form probably represents aggressive extra-articular extension and occasional recurrence after surgical intervention.[175]

The symptoms of PVNS of the TMJ vary but typically include swelling in the preauricular area, progressive TMJ pain during mastication, and a history of progressive difficulty in opening of the mouth.[180]

The recommended intervention for PVNS lesions involves wide synovectomy at all sites involved.[175,176]

Practice Pattern 4E: Impaired Joint Mobility, Motor Function, Muscle Performance, Range of Motion Associated with Localized Inflammation

Muscle Spasms

Muscle spasms of the mastication muscles may occur with dysfunction of the TMJ. Such dysfunctions include trauma, occlusal imbalance, changes in the vertical dimensions between the teeth, immobilization, prolonged dental procedures, chronic teeth clenching, and disease. Schwartz[181,182] hypothesized that TMD symptoms originated in mandibular muscles that went through three pathologic phases:

1. Early incoordination of muscles, producing joint clicking and recurrent subluxation.

2. A middle phase of limitation of mandibular movements by muscle spasm.

3. A final phase of muscle shortening and fibrosis, often irreversible. Psychogenic causes were the most common.

The role of cervical whiplash injuries secondary to motor vehicle accidents (MVAs) in TMD is somewhat controversial. Brooke and Stenn[183] reported that patients with post-traumatic TMD have a poor prognosis for recovery compared with non-traumatic TMD, stating as reasons the consequence of litigation and the personality of the patient. It seems plausible that an injury to the suprahyoid and infrahyoid muscles would affect the function of the mandible, thereby predisposing the joint to dysfunction. Mechanisms have been proposed to explain how an MVA trauma could cause TMDs.[184,185]

During the initial backward movement, the jaw is forced open, stretching and possibly tearing the anterior joint capsule and intra-articular disk. On the flexion phase, the jaw is snapped shut by the stretch reflex of the masticatory muscles and, in the presence of malocclusion, damages the posterior and temporal attachments of the articular cartilage and disk.

The following descriptions outline the common referral patterns of the TMJ muscles.

Temporalis. Referred pain from the temporalis muscle may extend over the temporal region, to the eyebrow and the upper teeth, and to the maxilla and TMJ.[94] Headache caused by temporalis muscle spasm is common. The patient also may feel pressure behind the eye or have increased eye fatigue.

Lateral Pterygoid. Spasm of the lateral pterygoid may cause a deep ache in the cheek area, maxilla, TMJ, or ear. Pain also is felt with chewing.

Medial Pterygoid. The medial pterygoid may refer pain behind the TMJ, deep in the ear, to the tongue, and to the back of the mouth.[94]

Masseter. Referred pain from a masseter muscle spasm may be projected to the eyebrow, maxilla, anterior mandible, and upper and lower molars.[94] The intervention for these muscle spasms includes:

▶ Application of moist heat to promote muscle relaxation.

▶ Massage of the affected muscles.

▶ Passive and active self-stretch exercises.

▶ Spray and stretch techniques.

Forced mouth opening should be avoided. In the absence of joint hypomobility, yawning exercises are recommended as a home exercise, because this activity produces a strong reflex inhibition of the mandibular elevators.[94]

The lateral pterygoid can be passively stretched with maximal retrusion, followed by rhythmic sideways oscillations. The medial pterygoid can be passively stretched with jaw opening exercises.

Travell and Simons[94] recommend the use of the mandibular self-stretch exercise for the temporalis and masseter muscles. The exercise, which consists of three steps, is performed in the sitting position facing a sink:

1. Hot packs are applied to both sides of the face.

2. The index and middle fingers are inserted below the lower incisor teeth, pads facing downward. The thumb of the same hand grasps the chin and pulls the lower jaw forward.

3. The full stretch is achieved by pulling the jaw downward while continuing to pull it forward.

Synovitis
Synovitis of the TMJ occurs when the internal lining of the joint capsule becomes inflamed, resulting in palpable tenderness of the posterior and lateral aspects of the joint. The cause of the synovitis can be[26]:

▶ Condylar impingement of the loose areolar connective tissue located immediately posterior to the condyle, which can result in significant effusion.

▶ Systemic disease, such as osteoarthritis, or rheumatoid arthritis or its variants.

▶ Infection, particularly viral.

Integration of Practice Patterns 4B and 4F: Impaired Joint Mobility, Motor Function, Muscle Performance, and Range of Motion Secondary to Impaired Posture, Systemic Dysfunction (Referred Pain Syndromes), Spinal Disorders, Myofascial Pain Dysfunction

Cervical Spine Disorders
Cervical spine disorders are common chronic conditions affecting the cervical region and related structures with or without radiation of pain toward the shoulder, arm, interscapular region, or the head.[186,187] Patients with TMD frequently report symptoms related to cervical spine disorders, and vice versa.[76,188–190] Several authors have indicated the existence of neuroanatomic and biomechanical relationships and have suggested that a dysfunction of the cervical spine may be the cause of signs and symptoms in the head.[191–202]

The masticatory and cervical muscles can affect the mandibular rest position, the mechanism of mandibular closure, and the occlusion.[203–205] Thus, a change in the mandibular rest position or habitual cervical posture can affect the occlusion and the masticatory muscles.[62,203,206–208] The most common postural abnormality in the cervical spine with direct impact on the craniofacial area and temporomandibular arthralgia is the forward head posture.[67,209–211]

Under normal circumstances, the center of gravity (COG) for the head falls slightly anterior to the ear. The forward head posture results in the habitual placement of the head anterior to the body's COG. Any increase in the sternocleidomastoid angulation, or distance from the thoracic apex to midcervical region, constitutes a forward head posture. This posture is considered to be minimal at 60 degrees, moderate at 60 to 75 degrees, and maximal at 75 to 90 degrees.[15] Associated signs include a decrease or reversal in the cervical lordosis and an increase in cranial rotation at the occipito-atlantal joint, resulting in a shortening and excessive activity of the posterior cervical muscles. The forward head posture can place undue stress on both the posterior cervical muscles and the anterior submandibular muscles by increasing their normal resting lengths. This stress also may stretch the TMJ capsule and alter the bite biomechanics of the TMJ, resulting in a posterior migration of the mandible and an altered occlusal contact pattern.

Atypical Facial Pain

Atypical facial pain is characterized by typically unilateral, dull, and relatively constant facial pain, and the presence of tender points. This condition, recently reclassified as facial pain by the International Headache Society, is not well understood and often defies all modes of intervention.[212] Many authorities believe that atypical facial pain is psychogenic.[213,214] However, it has been reported that intraoral edema and trigeminal V2 nerve distribution area tenderness were consistently found in individuals with atypical facial pain.[215] Furthermore, these individuals experienced relief of their symptoms in response to low-level helium-neon laser therapy.[215]

Bell's palsy, a common form of facial paralysis, and Ramsey Hunt syndrome, a herpetic inflammation of the geniculate or facial nerve ganglia, are described in Chapter 9.

Trigeminal Neuralgia

Trigeminal neuralgia is an intensely painful disorder of the face of brief duration (30 seconds).[216] The pain is spontaneous and can be triggered by touch, cold, shaving, brushing teeth, or make-up application.[217] The cause of trigeminal neuralgia is at present unknown, although most authors place the site of disturbance in the region of the posterior root[218,219] or in the spinal tract of the nerve.[220] Injuries to nerves and soft and hard tissues as a result of repeated traumas have been reported to produce persistent pain because of sensitization of both peripheral and central neurons.[46,221] The sensitization process has been shown to influence subsequent pain experience. Increased postoperative pain resulting from insufficient preemptive analgesia, such as incomplete use of local anesthetics or pain medication before surgery, has been well documented.[221–223] Poorly managed postoperative or posttraumatic pain also is considered to play a role in pain persistence.[221,224]

Myofascial Pain and Dysfunction

Many clinicians over the years have described numerous conditions that share features such as fatigue, pain, and other symptoms in the absence of objective findings. These include illnesses such as chronic fatigue syndrome, fibromyalgia, and TMD.

Myofascial pain and dysfunction associated with TMD generally presents with diffuse pain that is cyclic and found in several sites in the head and neck, particularly the muscles of mastication.[13] Pain is frequently at its worst in the morning, the patient often reports sore teeth from clenching, and there is often a history of stress and difficulty sleeping.[13] Masticatory muscle pain associated with TMD does not appear to progress in severity with age.[225]

The intervention for myofascial pain syndromes requires a comprehensive, and often a multidisciplinary, approach. The role of physical therapy in these syndromes is one of patient education, manual therapy techniques and electrotherapeutic modalities to reduce pain, and exercises to improve posture, reduce the adaptive shortening of tissues, and improve the strength of the postural stabilizers.

Therapeutic Techniques

Manual Therapy

The aim of manual therapy in TMD is to restore normal mandibular function using a number of techniques that serve to relieve musculoskeletal pain and promote healing of tissues.[146]

In the acute phase, manual techniques, if used at all, should be very low grade and very carefully performed, because this joint tends to be very reactive and can flare up easily. Mobilization and massage can be applied to the TMJ to reduce hypomobility and acute locking, as well as to the muscles of mastication to stretch and relax them.[90]

Muscle relaxation and soft tissue techniques often are required before mobilizations of the TMJ can be performed.

Myofascial Release

Myofascial release is a combination of direct, indirect, and reflex neural release procedures.[89] The basis of this technique is sensing palpable changes at various tissue levels and manually directing a gentle force to assist in releasing restricted tissues.

Muscle Stretching

Muscle stretching techniques can be used if the examination shows that the restriction of movement is a result of shortened muscles (or other structures). Techniques to increase the extensibility of the cervical structures are described in Chapters 22 and 23.

Joint Mobilizations

Specific joint mobilizations of the craniovertebral and cervical regions are described in Chapter 22 and Chapter 23, respectively. Specific mobilization techniques of the TMJ are indicated for decreased range of motion and pain caused by muscle contracture, disk displacement without reduction, and fibrous adhesions in the joint.[68]

During these procedures, the patient's mandible should be completely relaxed, and the patient should not attempt to open his or her mouth until instructed to do so.

Techniques to Increase Mouth Opening[50,226]

Distraction. This technique is performed to separate the joint surfaces of the TMJ to allow the disk to start repositioning on the condyle and to start realigning the fibers of the tissue caudally. The patient is positioned sitting, and the clinician stands to the patient's left side. The clinician grips the patient's head, using his or her right forearm and hand, fingers against the patient's forehead. The clinician stabilizes the patient's head between his or her hand, arm, and chest. With a medical-gloved hand, the clinician places his or her left thumb on the patient's lower molars on the right side, as far back in the mouth as possible. The clinician's index and middle fingers grip the angle of the patient's mandible of the involved side with the ring or little fingers held under the patient's mandible (depending on the size of the clinician's hand and patient's mandible). Using this grip, the clinician applies light distraction inferiorly to the patient's involved TMJ by pressing his or her thumb inferiorly against the lower molars (see Fig. 24-23).

Distraction, Anterior Glide, and Lateral Stretch.   This technique is performed to increase the anterior and inferior movement of the mandible for the patient who can only achieve slight opening of the mouth. The patient and clinician positions are the same as those described for the distraction technique. Using the same grip as described earlier, the clinician applies light distraction inferiorly to the patient's involved TMJ by pressing his or her thumb inferiorly against the lower molars. In addition to the distraction, the clinician gradually superimposes an anterior glide of the head of the mandible at the TMJ and a lateral stretch to the joint on the opposite side. Following the technique, the patient is asked to open his or her mouth as much as possible, and the newly acquired range is assessed. The procedure is repeated gradually until the patient is able to fully open his or her mouth or considerable improvement is attained.

Note: If the restriction of movement is bilateral, the technique may be performed on the opposite side.

Technique to Increase Full Mouth Closing.[226]   This technique is used to increase the posterior movement of the mandible (retraction) for the patient with an inability to fully close the mouth. The patient and clinician position is the same as described for the techniques to increase mouth opening. Using the same grip described for those techniques, the clinician gradually and maximally pushes posteriorly against the patient's involved mandible to produce a posterior glide of the head of the mandible at the TMJ (see Fig. 24-26).

Note: If the restriction of movement is bilateral, the same intervention may be performed on the patient's opposite side. The procedure is used when the patient cannot close his or her mouth.

Extraoral Lateral Glide.   This technique is used in the presence of severe pain, spasm, and marked limitation of movement caused by recent trauma.[89] The patient is positioned supine, with the head supported on a pillow. The patient is asked to rotate the head in the opposite direction of the involved TMJ. The clinician places the thumbs of both hands over the lateral pole of the condyle. Gentle oscillations are performed over the lateral pole, or more distally depending on patient tolerance.

Extraoral Depression.   This technique also is used in the presence of severe pain, spasm, and marked limitation of movement caused by recent trauma.[89] The patient is positioned supine, with the head supported on a pillow. The clinician gently grasps the angle of the mandible with the index and thumb bilaterally. Gentle oscillations are then performed in the direction of mandibular depression.

Automobilizations

Mouth-opening Exercise

In the mouth-opening exercise, the patient places the thumb on the maxillary anterior teeth and the forefinger on the mandibular anterior teeth, and creates a forceful opening. The maximal mouth opening is held for 10 seconds and repeated 10 times.

Tongue Depressor Exercise

Tongue depressors can be used to progressively increase mouth opening. The patient is asked to open the mouth as far as is comfortable. A number of tongue depressors are then placed flat in the opening so that the stack fits snugly against both the upper and lower teeth. By adding one depressor at a time to the stack, a gradual and sustained stretch can be applied to the TMJ and the structures restricting the mouth opening. Normal translation begins after 11 mm of opening, or about six tongue depressors. With the tongue depressors in position, a patient can mobilize the mandible actively into protrusion and lateral excursion.

Toothpick Exercise

This exercise can be used for patients who demonstrate lateral deviation with mouth opening or closing. The patient stands or sits facing a mirror. A thick line is drawn down the mirror using a wax crayon. The patient wedges a toothpick between the lower incisors and lines up the toothpick with the line on the mirror. As the patient opens and closes the jaw, if the line becomes visible, the patient corrects the deviation before continuing the movement. If correction is not possible, the exercise is stopped to prevent incorrect learning by the controlling muscles.

Distraction Mobilization

This technique can be taught to patients who demonstrate or report recurrent dislocations. To self-reduce a dislocation, the patient is instructed to place a gauze roll on the back inferior molars of both sides and to place his or her index fingers on the gauze. The patient opens the mouth as wide as possible and then applies a downward force on the gauze and the molars, thereby creating a joint distraction. Following a successful reduction, ice or heat (whichever produces the optimal therapeutic effect) should be applied around the TMJ.

REVIEW QUESTIONS*

1. What are the components of the stomatognathic system?
2. Which muscle develops with the fibrocartilaginous disk of the temporomandibular joint (TMJ)?
3. Which three muscles function to raise the mandible during mouth closing?
4. Which of the following alterations occurs (and may need correction via exercise) as a result of posterior capital rotation associated with the forward head posture?
    A. Adaptive shortening of the cranioverbral muscles.
    B. Forward migration of the mandible.
    C. Elongation of the submandibular muscles.
    D. Increased tension in the TMJ joint capsule.
    E. All of the above.
5. Define the rest position of the TMJ.

---

* Additional questions to test your understanding of this chapter can be found in the Online Learning Center for *Orthopaedic Assessment, Evaluation, and Intervention* at www.duttononline.net.

REFERENCES

1. Williams PL, et al. *Gray's Anatomy*, 37th ed. London: Churchill Livingstone; 1989.

1a. Ochi K, Ohashi T, Kinoshita H. Acoustic tensor tympani response and vestibular-evoked myogenic potential. *Laryngoscope.* 2002;112:2225–2229.

1b. Zipfel TE, Kaza SR, Greene JS. Middle-ear myoclonus. *J Laryngology Otology.* 2000;114:207–209.

1c. McNeill C. Temporomandibular disorders: Guidelines for diagnosis and management. *CDA J* 1991;19:15–26.

2. Okeson JP. Current terminology and diagnostic classification schemes. *Oral Surg Oral Med Oral Pathol Oral Radiol Endod* 1997;83:61–66.

3. Moses AJ. Good science, bad science, and scientific double-talk. *J Craniomandib Pract* 1996;14:170–172.

4. Ferrari R, Leonard M. Whiplash and temporomandibular disorders: A critical review. *J Am Dent Assoc* 1998;129:1739–1745.

5. Kolbinson DA, Epstein JB, Burgess JA. Temporomandibular disorders, headaches, and neck pain following motor vehicle accidents and the effects of litigation review of the literature. *J Orofacial Pain* 1996;10:101–125.

6. Bell WE. *Orofacial Pains: Classification, Diagnosis, Management.* 3rd ed. Chicago, Ill: New Year Medical Publishers; 1985.

7. Hannson T, Milner M. A study of occurrence of symptoms of diseases of the temporomandibular joint, masticatory musculature, and related structures. *J Oral Rehabil* 1975;2:313–324.

8. Dworkin SF, et al. Epidemiology of signs and symptoms in temporomandibular disorders: Clinical signs in cases and controls. *J Am Dent Assoc* 1990;120:273–281.

9. Salonen L, Hellden L. Prevalence of signs and symptoms of dysfunction in the masticatory system: An epidemiological study in an adult Swedish population. *J Craniomandib Disord Facial Oral Pain* 1990;4:241–250.

10. Stohler CS. Clinical perspectives on masticatory and related muscle disorders. In: Sessle BJ, Bryant PS, Dionne RA, eds. *Temporomandibular Disorders and Related Pain Conditions, Progress in Pain Research and Management.* Seattle, Wash: IASP Press; 1995:3–29.

11. Wänman A. Longitudinal course of symptoms of craniomandibular disorders in men and women: A 10-year follow-up study of an epidemiologic sample. *Acta Odontol Scand* 1996; 54:337–342.

12. Bush FM, et al. Analysis of gender effects on pain perception and symptom presentation in temporomandibular pain. *Pain* 1993; 53:73–80.

13. Dimitroulis G. Temporomandibular disorders: A clinical update. *BMJ* 1998;317:190–194.

14. McNeill C, et al. Craniomandibular (TMJ) disorders—the state of the art. *J Prosthet Dent* 1980;44:434–437.

15. Castaneda R. Occlusion. In: Kaplan AS, Assael LA, eds. *Temporomandibular Disorders Diagnosis and Treatment.* Philadelphia, Pa: Saunders; 1991:40–49.

16. Von Korff M, et al. Chronic pain and use of ambulatory health care. *Psychosom Med* 1991;53:61–79.

17. Sicher H, Du Brul EL. *Oral Anatomy.* 8th ed. St Louis, Mo: CV Mosby; 1988.

18. Rees LA. The structure and function of the mandibular joint. *Br Dent J* 1954;96:125.

19. Buchbinder D, Kaplan AS. Biology. In: Kaplan AS, Assael LA, eds. *Temporomandibular Disorders Diagnosis and Treatment.* Philadelphia, Pa: Saunders; 1991:11–23.

20. Mohl DN. Functional anatomy of the temporomandibular joint. In: *The President's Conference on the Examination, Diagnosis and Management of Temporomandibular Disorders.* Chicago, Ill: American Dental Association; 1983.

21. Hargreaves A. Dysfunction of the temporomandibular joints. *Physiotherapy* 1986;72:209–212.

22. Naidoo LCD. The development of the temporomandibular joint: A review with regard to the lateral pterygoid muscle. *J Dent Assoc S Africa* 1993;48:189–194.

23. Porter MR. The attachment of the lateral pterygoid muscle to the meniscus. *J Prosthet Dent* 1970;24:555–562.

24. Juniper RD. The pathogenesis and investigation of TMJ dysfunction. *Br J Oral Maxillofac Surg* 1987;25:105–112.

25. Mahan P. Temporomandibular problems: Biological diagnosis and treatment. In: Solberg WK, Clark GT, eds. *Temporomandibular Joint Problems.* Chicago, Ill: Quintessence; 1980:87–101.

26. Friedman MH, Weisberg J. Screening procedures for temporomandibular joint dysfunction. *Am Fam Physician* 1982; 25:157–160.

27. Friedman MH, Weisberg J. Application of orthopaedic principles in evaluation of the temporomandibular joint. *Phys Ther* 1982; 62:597–603.

28. Scapino RP. The posterior attachment: Its structure, function, and appearance in TMJ imaging studies. Part 2. *J Craniomandib Disord Facial Oral Pain* 1991;5:155–166.

29. Williams PL, et al. *Gray's Anatomy.* 37th ed. London, England: Churchill Livingstone; 1989.

30. Kraus SL. *TMJ Disorders: Management of the Craniomandibular Complex, Clinics in Physical Therapy.* Vol. 18. New York, NY: Churchill Livingstone; 1988.

31. Clark R, Wyke BD. Contributions of temporomandibular articular mechanoreceptors to the control of mandibular posture: An experimental study. *J Dent Assoc S Africa* 1974;2:121–129.

32. Skaggs CD. Diagnosis and treatment of temporomandibular disorders. In: Murphy ER, eds. *Cervical Spine Syndromes.* New York, NY: McGraw-Hill; 2000:579–592.

33. Pinto OF. A new structure related to the temporomandibular joint and the middle ear. *J Prosthet Dent* 1962;12:95–103.

34. Stack BC, Funt LA. Temporomandibular joint dysfunction in children. *J Pedodont* 1977;1:240–247.

35. Bittar GT, Bibb CA, Pullinger AG. Histological characteristics of the lateral pterygoid muscle insertion into the temporomandibular joint. *J Orofac Pain* 1994;8:243–249.

36. Meyenberg K, Kubick S, Palla S. Relationship of the muscles of mastication to the articular disk of the temporomandibular joint. *Helv Odont Acta* 1986;30:815–834.

37. Carpentier P, et al. Insertions of the lateral pterygoid muscle: An anatomic study of the human temporomandibular joint. *J Oral Maxillofac Surg* 1988;46:477–482.

38. McNamara JA. The independent function of the two heads of the lateral pterygoid muscle. *Am J Anat* 1973;138:197–205.

39. Luschei ES. Goodwin GM. Patterns of mandibular movement and muscle activity during mastication in the monkey. *J Neurophysiol* 1974;35:954–966.

40. Juniper RP. Temporomandibular joint dysfunction: A theory based upon electromyographic studies of the lateral pterygoid muscle. *Br J Oral Maxillofac Surg* 1984;22:1–8.

41. McDonnell JP, et al. The relationship between dental overbite and eustachian tube dysfunction. *Laryngoscope* 2001;111:310–316.

42. Franks AST. Cervical spondylosis presenting as the facial pain of temporomandibular joint disorder. *Ann Phys Med* 1968;9:193–196.

43. Trott P, Gross AN. Physiotherapy in diagnosis and treatment of the myofascial pain dysfunction syndrome. *Int J Oral Surg* 1978;7:360–365.

44. Rocabado M. Biomechanical relationship of the cranial, cervical, and hyoid regions. *J Craniomandib Pract* 1983;1:61–66.

45. Layfield SP. A whiplash injury. In: Scully RM, Barnes MR, eds. *Physical Therapy*. Philadelphia, Pa: JB Lippincott; 1989:152–168.

46. Carlsson GE, LeResche L. Epidemiology of temporomandibular disorders. In: Sessle BJ, Bryant PS, Dionne RA, eds. *Temporomandibular Disorders and Related Pain Conditions, Progress in Pain Research and Management*. Seattle, Wash: IASP Press; 1995:211–226.

47. Murphy DR. *Conservative Management of Cervical Spine Disorders*. New York, NY: McGraw-Hill; 2000.

48. Meadows J. *A Rationale and Complete Approach to the Sub-Acute Post-MVA Cervical Patient*. Calgary, Canada: Swodeam Consulting; 1995.

49. Viener AE. Oral surgery. In: Garliner D, ed. *Myofunctional Therapy*. Philadelphia, Pa: Saunders; 1976:161–182.

50. Rocabado M. Arthrokinematics of the temporomandibular joint. In: Gelb H, ed. *Clinical Management of Head, Neck and TMJ Pain and Dysfunction*. Philadelphia, Pa: Saunders; 1985:35–58.

51. Hertling D. The temporomandibular joint. In: Hertling D, Kessler RM, eds. *Management of Common Musculoskeletal Disorders*. Philadelphia, Pa: Lippincott-Raven; 1996:444–485.

52. Tsukiyama Y, Baba K, Clark GT. An evidence-based assessment of occlusal adjustment as a treatment for temporomandibular disorders. *J Prosthet Dent* 2001;86:57–66.

53. Bales JM, Epstein JB. The role of malocclusion and orthodontics in temporomandibular disorders. *J Can Dent Assoc* 1994;60:899–905.

54. Hayt MW, Abrahams JJ, Blair J. Magnetic resonance imaging of the temporomandibular joint. *Top Magn Reson Imaging* 2000;11:138–146.

55. Katzberg RW, et al. Temporomandibular joint: MR assessment of rotational and sideways disc displacements. *Radiology* 1988;169:741–748.

55a. Friedman MH, Weisberg J. Application of orthopaedic principles in evaluation of the temporomandibular joint. *Phys Ther* 1982;62:597–603.

56. Kaplan AS. Examination and diagnosis. In: Kaplan AS, Assael LA, eds. *Temporomandibular Disorders Diagnosis and Treatment*. Philadelphia, Pa: Saunders; 1991:284–311.

56a. Viener AE. Oral surgery. In: Garliner D, ed. *Myofunctional Therapy,* Philadelphia: Saunders; 1976.

57. Trott PH. Examination of the temporomandibular joint. In: Grieve G, ed. *Modern Manual Therapy of the Vertebral Column*. Edinburgh, Scotland: Churchill Livingstone; 1986:311–332.

58. Fish F. The functional anatomy of the rest position of the mandible. *Dent Prac* 1961;11:178.

59. Atwood DA. A critique of research of the rest position of the mandible. *J Prosthet Dent* 1966;16:848–854.

60. Feinstein B, et al. Experiments on pain referred from deep somatic tissues. *J Bone Joint Surg* 1954;36A:981–997.

61. Cyriax J. Rheumatic headache. *Br Med J* 1982;2:1367–1368.

62. Friedman MH, Weisberg J. *Temporomandibular Joint Disorders*. Chicago, Ill: Quintessence; 1985.

63. Okeson JP. *Orofacial Pain: Guidelines for Assessment, Diagnosis, and Management*. Chicago, Ill: Quintessence; 1996.

64. Dolwick MF. Clinical diagnosis of temporomandibular joint internal derangement and myofascial pain and dysfunction. *Oral Maxillofac Surg Clin North Am* 1989;1:1–6.

65. Hedenberg-Magnusson B, Ernberg M, Kopp S. Symptoms and signs of temporomandibular disorders in patients with fibromyalgia and local myalgia of the temporomandibular system: a comparative study. *Acta Odontol Scand* 1997; 55:344–349.

66. Isacsson G, Linde C, Isberg A. Subjective symptoms in patients with temporomandibular disk displacement versus patients with myogenic craniomandibular disorders. *J Prosthet Dent* 1989;61:70–77.

67. Kirk WS Jr, Calabrese DK. Clinical evaluation of physical therapy in the management of internal derangement of the temporomandibular joint. *J Oral Maxillofac Surg* 1989;47:113–119.

68. McNeill C. *Temporomandibular Disorders: Guidelines for Classification, Assessment and Management*. 2nd ed. Chicago, Ill: Quintessence; 1993.

69. Green CS, Laskin DM. Long term status of TMJ clicking in patients with myofascial pain dysfunction. *J Am Dent Assoc* 1988;117:461–465.

70. Marbach JJ, Lipton JA. Treatment of patients with temporomandibular joint and other facial pain by otolaryngologists. *Arch Otolaryngol* 1982;108:102–107.

71. Dimitroulis G, Dolwick MF, Gremillion HA. Temporomandibular disorders. 1. Clinical evaluation. *Aust Dent J* 1995;40:301–305.

72. Maitland G. *Vertebral Manipulation*. Sydney, Australia: Butterworth; 1986.

73. Magarey ME. Examination of the cervical and thoracic spine. In: Grant R, ed. *Physical Therapy of the Cervical and Thoracic Spine*. New York, NY: Churchill Livingstone; 1994:109–144.

74. Mannheimer JS, Dunn J. Cervical spine. In: Kaplan AS, Assael LA, eds. *Temporomandibular Disorders Diagnosis and Treatment*. Philadelphia, Pa: Saunders; 1991:50–94.

75. McNeill C, et al. Temporomandibular disorders: Diagnosis, management, education, and research. *J Am Dent Assoc* 1990; 120:253–260.

76. Clark GT, et al. Guidelines for the examination and diagnosis of temporomandibular disorders. *J Craniomandib Disord Facial Oral Pain* 1989;3:7–14.

77. Duinkerke AS, et al. Relations between TMJ pain dysfunction syndrome (PDS) and some psychological and biographical variables. *Comm Dent Oral Epidemiol* 1985;13:185–189.

78. Keith DA. Differential diagnosis of facial pain and headache. *Oral Maxillofac Surg Clin North Am* 1989;1:7–12.

79. Fricton JR, Hathaway KM. Interdisciplinary management: Address complexity with teamwork. In: Fricton JR, Kroening R, Hathaway KM, eds. *TMJ and Craniofacial Pain: Diagnosis and Management*. St Louis, Mo: IEA Inc; 1988:167–172.

80. Judge RD, Zuidema GD, Fitzgerald FT. Head. In: Judge RD, Zuidema GD, Fitzgerald FT, eds. *Clinical Diagnosis*. Boston, Mass: Little, Brown; 1982:123–151.

81. Laskin DM. Etiology of the pain-dysfunction syndrome. *J Am Dent Assoc* 1969;79:147–153.

82. Richardson JK, Iglarsh ZA. Temporomandibular joint and the cervical spine. In: Richardson JK, Iglarsh ZA, eds. *Clinical Orthopaedic Physical Therapy*. Philadelphia, Pa: Saunders; 1994:1–71.

83. Perry C. Neuromuscular control of mandibular movements. *J Prosthet Dent* 1973;30:714–720.

84. Thompson JR, Brodie AG. Factors in the position of the mandible. *J Am Dent Assoc* 1942;29:925–941.

85. Dempsey PJ, Townsend GC. Genetic and environmental contributions to variation in human tooth size. *Heredity* 2001;86:685–693.

86. Marasa FK, Ham BD. Case reports involving the treatment of children with chronic otitis media with effusion via craniomandibular methods. *J Craniomandib Pract* 1988;6:256–270.

87. Seldin HM. Traumatic temporomandibular arthritis. *N Y State Dent J* 1955;21:313–318.

88. Sicher N. Temporomandibular articulation in mandibular overclosure. *J Am Dent Assoc* 1948;36:131–139.

89. Dunn J. Physical therapy. In: Kaplan AS, Assael LA, eds. *Temporomandibular Disorders Diagnosis and Treatment.* Philadelphia, Pa: Saunders; 1991:455–500.

90. Sturdivant J, Fricton JR. Physical therapy for temporomandibular disorders and orofacial pain. *Curr Opin Dent* 1991;1:485–496.

91. Gross A, Gale EN. A prevalence study of the clinical signs associated with mandibular dysfunction. *J Am Dent Assoc* 1983; 107:932–936.

92. Fricton JR. Myofascial pain. *Baillieres Clin Rheumatol* 1994; 8:857–880.

93. Masumi S, Kim YJ, Clark GT. The value of maximum jaw motion measurements for distinguishing between common temporomandibular disorder subgroups. *Oral Surg Oral Med Oral Pathol Oral Radiol Endod* 2002;93:552–529.

94. Travell JG, Simons DG. *Myofascial Pain and Dysfunction: The Trigger Point Manual.* Baltimore, Md: Williams and Wilkins; 1983.

95. Johnstone D, Templeton M. The feasibility of palpating the lateral pterygoid. *J Prosthet Dent* 1980;44:318.

96. House JW, Brackman DE. Facial nerve grading system. *Otolaryngol Head Neck Surg* 1985;93:146–147.

97. Satoh Y, Kanzaki J, Yoshihara S. A comparison and conversion table of the House-Brackmann facial nerve grading system and the Yanagihara grading system. *Auris Nasus Larynx* 2000;27:207–212.

98. Croxson G, May M, Mester SJ. Grading facial nerve function: House-Brackmann versus Burres-Fisch methods. *Am J Otol* 1990;11:240–246.

99. Meadows A, et al. The House-Brackmann system and assessment of corneal risk in facial nerve palsy. *Eye* 2000;14:353–357.

100. Hansson LG, Hansson T, Petersson A. A comparison between clinical and radiological findings in 259 temporomandibular joint patients. *J Prosthet Dent* 1983;50:89–94.

101. Tasaki MM, Westesson PL. Temporomandibular joint: Diagnostic accuracy with sagittal and coronal MR imaging. *Radiology* 1993;186:723–729.

102. Solberg WK, Hansson TL, Nordstrom B. The temporomandibular joint in young adults at autopsy: A morphologic classification and evaluation. *J Oral Rehabil* 1985;12:303–321.

103. Ettala-Ylitalo UM, Syrjanen S, Halonen P. Functional disturbances of the masticatory system related to temporomandibular joint involvement by rheumatoid arthritis. *J Oral Rehabil* 1987; 14:415–427.

104. Goldstein BH. Temporomandibular disorders: A review of current understanding. *Oral Surg Oral Med Oral Pathol Oral Radiol Endod* 1999;88:379–385.

105. Carlsson GE. Long-term effects of treatment of craniomandibular disorders. *J Craniomand Pract* 1985;3:337–342.

106. Ogus HD, Toller PA. Common disorders of the temporomandibular joint. In: *Dental Practitioner Handbook.* Vol. 26. Bristol, England: John Wright and Son; 1986.

107. Guralnik W. The temporomandibular joint: The dentist's dilemma: Parts I and II. *Br Dent J* 1984;156:315–319,353–356.

108. Gray RJ, et al. Physiotherapy in the treatment of temporomandibular joint disorders: A comparative study of four treatment methods. *Br Dent J* 1994;176:257–261.

109. Dimitroulis G, et al. Temporomandibular disorders. 2. Nonsurgical treatment. *Aust Dent J* 1995;40:372–376.

110. Harkins SJ, Marteney JL. Extrinsic trauma: A significant precipitating factor in temporomandibular dysfunction. *J Prosthet Dent* 1985;54:271–272.

111. Pullinger AG, Seligman DA. Trauma history in diagnostic groups of temporomandibular disorders. *Oral Surg Oral Med Oral Pathol Oral Radiol Endod* 1991;71:529–534.

112. Pullinger AG, Monteiro AA. History factors associated with symptoms of temporomandibular disorders. *J Oral Rehabil* 1988;15:117–124.

113. Weinberg LA, Larger LA. Clinical report on the etiology and diagnosis of TMJ dysfunction-pain syndrome. *J Prosthet Dent* 1980;44:642–653.

114. Stenger J. Whiplash. Basal facts. *J Prosthet Dent* 1977;2:5–12.

115. Hodges JM. Managing temporomandibular joint syndrome. *Laryngoscope* 1990;100:60–66.

116. Michlovitz SL. The use of heat and cold in the management of rheumatic diseases. In: Michlovitz SL, ed. *Thermal Agents in Rehabilitation.* Philadelphia, Pa: FA Davis; 1990:67–92.

117. Chapman CE. Can the use of physical modalities for pain control be rationalized by the research evidence? *Can J Physiol Pharmacol* 1991;69:704–712.

118. Carlsson GE, Magnusson T. *Management of Temporomandibular Disorders in the General Dental Practice.* Carol Stream, Ill: Quintessence; 1999.

119. Rocabado M. Physical therapy for the post-surgical TMJ patient. *J Craniomand Disord* 1989;7:75–82.

120. Kraus SL. Cervical spine influences on the craniomandibular region. In: Kraus SL, ed. *TMJ Disorders: Management of the Craniomandibular Complex.* New York, NY: Churchill Livingstone; 1988:367–396.

121. Gangarosa LP, Mahan PE. Pharmacologic management of TMJ-MPDS. *Ear Nose Throat J* 1982;61:30–41.

122. Dionne RA. Pharmacologic treatments for temporomandibular disorders. *Oral Surg Oral Med Oral Pathol Oral Radiol Endod* 1997;83:134–142.

123. Fricton JR. Management of masticatory myofascial pain. *Semin Orthodont* 1995;1:229–243.

124. Clark GT, Adler RC. A critical evaluation of occlusal therapy. Occlusal adjustment procedures. *J Am Dent Assoc* 1985;110: 743–750.

125. Clark GT. A critical evaluation of orthopaedic interocclusal appliance therapy. Design theory and overall effectiveness. *J Am Dent Assoc* 1984;108:359–364.

126. Seligman DA, Pullinger AG. The role of intercuspal occlusal relationships in temporomandibular disorders: a review. *J Craniomandib Disord Facial Oral Pain* 1991;5:96–106.

127. Greene CS, Marbach JJ. Epidemiologic studies of mandibular dysfunction: A critical review. *J Prosthet Dent* 1982;48:184–190.

128. Feine JS, Widmer CG, Lund JP. Physical therapy: A critique. *Oral Surg Oral Med Oral Pathol Oral Radiol Endod* 1997; 83:123–127.

129. Feine JS, Lund JP. An assessment of the efficacy of physical therapy and physical modalities for the control of chronic musculoskeletal pain. *Pain* 1997;71:5–23.

130. Fricton JR, et al. Myofascial pain syndrome of the head and neck: A review of clinical characteristics of 164 patients. *Oral Surg Oral Med Oral Pathol* 1985;60:615–623.

131. Kendall FP, McCreary EK, Provance PG. *Muscles: Testing and Function.* Baltimore, Md: Williams and Wilkins; 1993.

132. Janda V. Muscle strength in relation to muscle length, pain and muscle imbalance. In: Harms-Ringdahl K, ed. *Muscle Strength.* New York, NY: Churchill Livingstone; 1993:83.

133. Sahrmann SA. *Diagnosis and Treatment of Movement Impairment Syndromes.* St Louis, Mo: Mosby; 2001.

134. Griegel-Morris P, et al. Incidence of common postural abnormalities in the cervical, shoulder, and thoracic regions and their association with pain in two age groups of healthy subjects. *Phys Ther* 1992;72:426–430.

135. Simons DG. Muscular pain syndromes. In: Fricton JR, Awad E, eds. *Advances in Pain Research and Therapy.* New York, NY: Raven Press; 1990:1–41.

136. Moss RA, Adams HE. The class of personality, anxiety and depression in mandibular pain dysfunction subjects. *J Oral Rehabil* 1984;11:233–237.

137. Rugh JD. Psychological components of pain. *Dent Clin North Am* 1987;31:579–594.

138. Cohen S, Rodriguez MS. Pathways linking affective disturbances and physical disorders. *Health Psychol* 1995;14:371–373.

139. Gatchel RJ, et al. Major psychological disorders in acute and chronic TMD: An initial examination. *J Am Dent Assoc* 1996; 127:1365–1370,1372, 1374.

140. Kight M, Gatchel RJ, Wesley L. Temporomandibular disorders: Evidence for significant overlap with psychopathology. *Health Psychol* 1999;18:177–182.

141. Korszun A, et al. The relationship between temporomandibular disorders and stress-associated syndromes. *Oral Surg Oral Med Oral Pathol Oral Radiol Endod* 1998;86:416–420.

142. Gardea MA, Gatchel RJ, Mishra KD. Long-term efficacy of biobehavioral treatment of temporomandibular disorders. *J Behav Med* 2001;24:341–359.

143. Carlsson SG, Gale EW. Biofeedback in the treatment of long-term temporomandibular joint pain: An outcome study. *Biofeedback Self Regul* 1977;2:161–165.

144. Barber J. *Hypnosis and Suggestion in the Treatment of Pain. A Clinical Guide.* New York, NY: WW Norton; 1996.

145. Simon EP, Lewis DM. Medical hypnosis for temporomandibular disorders: Treatment efficacy and medical utilization outcome. *Oral Surg Oral Med Oral Pathol Oral Radiol Endod* 2000; 90:54–63.

146. Clark GT, Adachi NY, Dornan MR. Physical medicine procedures affect temporomandibular disorders: A review. *J Am Dent Assoc* 1990;121:151–161.

147. Tegelberg A, Kopp S. Short-term effect of physical training on temporomandibular joint disorder in individuals with rheumatoid arthritis and ankylosing spondylitis. *Acta Odontol Scand* 1988;46:49–51.

148. Brazeau GA, et al. The role of pharmacy in the management of patients with temporomandibular disorders and orofacial pain. *J Am Pharm Assoc (Wash)* 1998;38:354–361; quiz 362–363.

149. Linde C, Isacsson G, Jonsson BG. Outcome of 6-week treatment with transcutaneous electric nerve stimulation compared with splint on symptomatic temporomandibular joint disk displacement without reduction. *Acta Odontol Scand* 1995;53:92–98.

150. Schiffman EL. The role of the randomized clinical trial in evaluating management strategies for temporomandibular disorders. In: Fricton JR, Dubner R, eds. *Orofacial Pain and Temporomandibular Disorders.* New York, NY: Raven Press; 1995: 415–463; Advances in Pain Research and Therapy, Vol 21.

151. Mohl ND, et al. Devices for the diagnosis and treatment of temporomandibular disorders, III: Thermography, ultrasound, electrical stimulation, and electromyographic biofeedback. *J Prosthet Dent* 1990;63:472–477.

152. Murphy GJ. Electrical physical therapy in treating TMJ patients. *J Craniomand Pract* 1983;2:67–73.

153. Gangarosa LP. *Iontophoresis in Dental Practice.* Chicago, Ill: Quintessence; 1982:13–20.

154. Gangarosa L. Iontophoresis in pain control. *Pain Digest* 1993; 3:162–174.

155. Kahn J. Iontophoresis and ultrasound for postsurgical temporomandibular trismus and paresthesias. *Phys Ther* 1980;60:307–308.

156. Weinberg S, Kryshtalskyj B. Analysis of facial and trigeminal nerve function after arthroscopic surgery of the temporomandibular joint. *J Oral Maxillofac Surg* 1996;54:40–43.

157. Loughner BA, et al. The medial capsule of the human temporomandibular joint. *J Oral Maxillofac Surg* 1997;55:363–369.

158. Talebzadeh N, Rosenstein TP, Pogrel MA. Anatomy of the structures medial to the temporomandibular joint. *Oral Surg Oral Med Oral Pathol Oral Radiol Endod* 1999;88:674–678.

159. Paesani D, et al. Prevalence of temporomandibular joint internal derangement in patients with craniomandibular disorders. *Am J Orthod Dentofacial Orthop* 1992;101:41–47.

160. Wongwatana S, et al. Anatomic basis for disk displacement in temporomandibular joint (TMJ) dysfunction. *Am J Orthod Dentofacial Orthop* 1994;105:257–264.

161. Pertes RA, Attanasio R. Internal derangements. In: Kaplan AS, Assael LA, eds. *Temporomandibular Disorders Diagnosis and Treatment.* Philadelphia, Pa: Saunders; 1991:142–164.

162. Ross JB. Diagnostic criteria and nomenclature for TMJ arthrography in sagittal section. Part I. Derangements. *J Craniomand Disord Facial Oral Pain* 1987;1:185.

163. Kondoh T, et al. Prevalence of morphological changes in the surfaces of the temporomandibular joint disc associated with internal derangement. *J Oral Maxillofac Surg* 1998;56:339–343, discussion 343–344.

164. Okeson JP. *Management of Temporomandibular Disorders and Occlusion.* 4th ed. St Louis, Mo: Mosby Year Book; 1998.

165. Stegenga B, de Bont LGM, Boering G. Osteoarthritis as the cause of craniomandibular pain and dysfunction: A unifying concept. *J Oral Maxillofac Surg* 1989;47:249.

166. Rohlin M, Westesson PL, Eriksson L. The correlation of temporomandibular joint sounds with joint morphology in fifty-five autopsy specimens. *J Oral Maxillofac Surg* 1985; 43:194.

167. Westesson PL, Brodstein SL, Liedberg J. Internal derangement of the temporomandibular joint. Morphologic description with correlation to joint function. *Oral Surg Oral Med Oral Pathol* 1985;59:323.

168. Rasmussen OC. Description of population and progress of symptoms in a longitudinal study of temporomandibular arthropathy. *Scand J Dent Res* 1981;89:196–203.

169. Wilkes CH. Internal derangement of the temporomandibular joint: Pathological variations. *Arch Otolaryngol Head Neck Surg* 1989;115:469–477.

170. Hondo T, et al. Traumatically induced posterior disc displacement without reduction of the TMJ. *J Craniomand Pract* 1994;12:128–132.

171. Lundh H, Westesson PL. Long-term follow-up after occlusal treatment to correct abnormal temporomandibular joint disk position. *Oral Surg Oral Med Oral Pathol* 1989;67:2–10.

172. Lundh H. Correction of temporomandibular joint disk displacement by occlusal therapy. *Swed Dent J Suppl* 1987;51:1–159.

173. Shorey CW, Campbell JH. Dislocation of the temporomandibular joint. *Oral Surg Oral Med Oral Pathol Oral Radiol Endod* 2000;89:662–668.

174. Scapino RP. Histopathology associated with malposition of the human temporomandibular joint disc. *Oral Surg Oral Med Oral Pathol Oral Radiol Endod* 1983;55:382.

175. Enzinger FM, Weiss SW. Benign tumors and tumor-like lesions of synovial tissue. In: Enzinger FM, Weiss SW, eds. *Soft Tissue Tumors.* St Louis, Mo: Mosby-Year Book; 1995:735–755.

176. Goldman AB, DiCarlo EF. Pigmented villonodular synovitis: Diagnosis and differential diagnosis. *Radiol Clin North Am* 1988;26:1327–1347.

177. O'Sullivan TJ, Alport EC, Whiston HG. Pigmented villonodular synovitis of the temporomandibular joint. *J Otolaryngol* 1984;13:123–126.

178. Barnard JDW. Pigmented villonodular synovitis in the temporomandibular joint: A case report. *Br J Oral Surg* 1975;13:183–187.

179. Takagi M, Ishikawa G. Simultaneous villonodular synovitis and synovial chondromatosis of the temporomandibular joint: report of case. *J Oral Surg* 1981;39:699–701.

180. Tanaka K, et al. Pigmented villonodular synovitis of the temporomandibular joint. *Arch Otolaryngol Head Neck Surg* 1997;123:536–539.

181. Schwartz LL. A temporomandibular joint pain-dysfunction syndrome. *J Chronic Dis* 1956;3:284–293.

182. Schwartz LL. Pain associated with temporomandibular joint. *J Am Dent Assoc* 1955;51:393–397.

183. Brooke RI, Stenn PG. Postinjury myofascial dysfunction syndrome: Its etiology and prognosis. *Oral Surg Oral Med Oral Pathol* 1978;45:846–850.

184. Howard RP, et al. Assessing neck extension-flexion as a basis for temporomandibular joint dysfunction. *J Oral Maxillofac Surg* 1991;49:1210–1213.

185. Howard RP, Hatsell CP, Guzman HM. Temporomandibular joint injury potential imposed by the low-velocity extension-flexion maneuver. *J Oral Maxillofac Surg* 1995;53:256–262.

186. Bland JH. Epidemiology and demographics: Phylogenesis and clinical implications. In: Bland JH, ed. *Disorders of the Cervical Spine. Diagnosis and Medical Management.* Philadelphia, Pa: Saunders; 1994:3–11.

187. Grant R. *Physical Therapy of the Cervical and Thoracic Spine.* 2nd ed. 1994, Edinburgh, Scotland: Churchill Livingstone; 1994.

188. Alanen PJ, Kirveskari PK. Occupational cervicobrachial disorder and temporomandibular joint dysfunction. *J Craniomandib Pract* 1984;3:69–72.

189. De Laat A, Meuleman H, Stevens A. Relation between functional limitations of the cervical spine and temporomandibular disorders. *J Orofacial Pain* 1993;1:109.

190. Kirveskari P, et al. Association of functional state of stomatognathic system with mobility of cervical spine and neck muscle tenderness. *Acta Odont Scand* 1988;46:281–286.

191. Bogduk N. The rationale for patterns of neck and back pain. *Patient Manage* 1984;8:13.

192. Bogduk N. Cervical causes of headache and dizziness. In: Grieve GP, ed. *Modern Manual Therapy of the Vertebral Column.* New York, NY: Churchill Livingstone; 1986:289–302.

193. Bogduk N. Innervation and pain patterns of the cervical spine. In: Grant R, ed. *Physical Therapy of the Cervical and Thoracic Spine.* New York, NY: Churchill Livingstone; 1988:72–80.

194. Bogduk N. The anatomical basis for cervicogenic headache. *J Manipulative Physiol Ther* 1992;15:67–70.

195. Bovim G, Berg R, Dale LG. Cervicogenic headache: Anaesthetic blockade of cervical nerves (C2-5) and facet joint (C2/3). *Pain* 1992;49:315–320.

196. Jull GA. Headaches associated with cervical spine: A clinical review. In: Boyling JD, Palastanga N, eds. *Grieve's Modern Manual Therapy.* Edinburgh, Scotland: Churchill Livingstone; 1994:333–348.

197. Lord SM, et al. Third occipital nerve headache: A prevalence study. *J Neurol Neurosurg Psychiatry* 1994;57:1187–1190.

198. Norris CW, Eakins K. Head and neck pain: T-M joint syndrome. *Laryngoscope* 1974;84:1466–1478.

199. de Wijer A. *Temporomandibular and Cervical Spine Disorders.* Utrecht, Netherlands: Utrecht University; 1995.

200. de Wijer A, et al. Symptoms of the cervical spine in temporomandibular and cervical spine disorders. *J Oral Rehabil* 1996;23:742–550.

201. de Wijer A, et al. Symptoms of the stomatognathic system in temporomandibular and cervical spine disorders. *J Oral Rehabil* 1996;23:733–741.

202. de Wijer A, et al. Temporomandibular and cervical spine disorders. Self-reported signs and symptoms. *Spine* 1996;21:1638–1646.

203. Mohl ND. Head posture and its role in occlusion. *N Y State Dent J* 1976;42:17–23.

204. Prieskel HW. Some observations on the postural position of the mandible. *J Prosthet Dent* 1965;15:625–633.

205. Ramfjord SP. Dysfunctional temporomandibular joint and muscle pain. *J Prosthet Dent* 1961;11:353–374.

206. Darling DW, Kraus S, Glasheen-Wray MB. Relationship of head posture and the rest position of the mandible. *J Prosthet Dent* 1984;52:111–115.

207. Goldstein DF, et al. Influence of cervical posture on mandibular movement. *J Prosthet Dent* 1984;52:421–426.

208. Robinson MJ. The influence of head position on TMJ dysfunction. *J Prosthet Dent* 1966;16:169–172.

209. Gonzalez HE, Manns A. Forward head posture: Its structural and functional influence on the stomatognathic system, a conceptual study. *Cranio* 1996;14:71–80.

210. Visscher CM, et al. Kinematics of the human mandible for different head postures. *J Oral Rehabil* 2000;27:299–305.

211. Higbie EJ, et al. Effect of head position on vertical mandibular opening. *J Orthop Sports Phys Ther* 1999;29:127–130.

212. International Headache Society. Headache classification and diagnostic criteria for headache disorders, cranial neuralgias, and facial pain. *Cephalalgia* 1988;8:19–22,71,72.

213. Feinman C, Harris ML, Cawley R. Psychogenic facial pain: Presentation and treatment. *Br Med J* 1984;288:436–438.

214. Solomon S, Lipton RB. Atypical facial pain: A review. *Semin Neurol* 1988;8:332–338.

215. Friedman MH, Weintraub MI, Forman S. Atypical facial pain: A localized maxillary nerve disorder? *Am J Pain Manage* 1995;4:149–152.

216. Appenzeller O. *Pathogenesis and Treatment of Headache.* New York, NY: Spectrum Publications; 1976.

217. Esposito CJ, Crim GA, Binkley TK. Headaches: A differential diagnosis. *J Craniomand Pract* 1986;4:318–322.

218. Wolff HG. *Headache and Other Head Pain.* New York, NY: Oxford University Press; 1987:53–76.

219. Dandy WE. An operation for the cure of tic douloureux. Partial section of the sensory root at the pons. *Arch Surg* 1929;18:687.

220. Sjoqvist O. Surgical section of pain tracts and pathways in the spinal cord and brain stem. In: *4th Congr Neurol Internat*. Paris, France: Masson; 1949.

221. Coderre TJ, et al. Contribution of central neuroplasticity to pathological pain: Review of clinical and experimental literature. *Pain* 1993;52:259–285.

222. Trowskoy M, et al. Postoperative pain after inguinal herniorraphy with different types of anesthesia. *Anesth Analg* 1990; 70:29–35.

223. McQuay J. Pre-emptive analgesia. *Br J Anesth* 1992;69:1–3.

224. Cousins M. Acute and postoperative pain. In: Wall PD, Melzack R, eds. *Textbook of Pain*. Edinburgh, Scotland: Churchill Livingstone; 1994:357–385.

225. Stohler CS. Phenomenology, epidemiology, and natural progression of the muscular temporomandibular disorders. *Oral Surg Oral Med Oral Pathol Oral Radiol Endod* 1997;83:77–81.

226. Evjenth O, Hamberg J. *Muscle Stretching in Manual Therapy, A Clinical Manual*. Alfta, Sweden: Alfta Rehab Forlag; 1984.

THE LUMBAR SPINE

CHAPTER OBJECTIVES

▶ *At the completion of this chapter, the reader will be able to:*

1. Describe the vertebrae, ligaments, muscles, and blood and nerve supply that comprise the lumbar intervertebral segment.

2. Outline the coupled movements of the lumbar spine, the normal and abnormal joint barriers, and the reactions of the various structures to loading.

3. Perform a detailed examination of the lumbar musculoskeletal system, including history, observation, palpation of the articular and soft tissue structures, specific passive mobility and passive articular mobility tests for the intervertebral joints, and stability testing.

4. Evaluate the results from the examination and establish a diagnosis.

5. Describe the common pathologies and lesions of this region.

6. Describe intervention strategies based on clinical findings and established goals.

7. Design an intervention based on patient education, manual therapy, and therapeutic exercise.

8. Apply mobilization techniques to the lumbar spine, using the correct grade, direction, and duration, and explain the mechanical and physiologic effects.

9. Evaluate intervention effectiveness in order to progress or modify the intervention.

10. Plan an effective home program, including spinal care, and instruct the patient in this program.

11. Help the patient to develop self-reliant intervention strategies.

OVERVIEW

At some time in their lives, 80 percent of the general population will experience some type of low back pain (LBP).[1] LBP is second only to the common cold as a reason for physician visits, and the most expensive source of compensated work-related injury in modern industrialized countries.[2,3] According to studies, the first episode of back pain can have differing results: 80 to 90 percent will be asymptomatic in 6 weeks, 98 percent in 24 weeks, and 99 percent in 52 weeks.[3] Thus, most cases of LBP are described as benign in nature, because the majority of patients do not appear to progress to chronic functional impairment or disability.[2,4,5] However, the small percentage of people who do become disabled with chronic LBP account for 75 to 90 percent of the cost associated with LBP.[6] This group of patients has been the focus of much research to determine factors associated with chronicity and the pathologic processes responsible.

Despite the frequency of LBP and the many studies examining it, LBP is a difficult problem to investigate and several key issues concerning its occurrence, natural history, and prognosis remain unanswered.

A broad range of risk factors is associated with the cause and course of LBP. These include, but are not limited to, occupational, psychosocial, and environmental factors.[7,8]

About 30 percent of all workers will at some time miss work because of a back ailment, and 2 to 4 percent will actually change jobs at least once because of a back problem, in addition to the ones who become disabled.[9] Physical load on the back has commonly been implicated as a risk factor for LBP and, in particular, for work-related LBP. Certain occupations and certain work tasks seem to have a higher risk of LBP.[10–13] Repeated lifting of heavy loads is considered a risk factor for LBP,[14] especially if combined with side bending and twisting.[15,16] A study of static work postures found that there was an increased risk of LBP if the work involved a predominance of sitting.[17] Exposure to whole body vibration arises in workers who operate tractors, excavators, bulldozers, forklift trucks, armored vehicles, lorries, helicopters, and many other vehicles and machines.[18] Although knowledge is incomplete, a growing body of evidence indicates that such exposure to vibration and jolting may cause an increased risk of LBP.[14,19–22] Kelsey[14] and Kelsey and Hardy[23] found that men who spend more than half their workday driving have a threefold increased risk of disk herniation.

The rate of recovery, assessed by return to work, varies only moderately by country, and is on the order of 60 to 70 percent at 6 weeks and 80 to 90 percent at 12 weeks.[24] Høgelund,[25] drawing on the literature from clinical studies of LBP and of economic, sociologic, and public policy, found evidence that return to work was related to individual as well as to work and social-environmental factors. It has also been established that people who are simultaneously subjected to demanding physical and psychosocial conditions have more LBP than people with only demanding physical or only demanding psychosocial conditions.[26]

Comorbidity may also have a deterministic effect on return to work at a variety of different levels.[27] First, specific comorbidity may slow or interfere with normal recovery from back pain. Second, comorbidity may affect an individual's general sense of health, leading to a decreased self-perception of capability. Third, health care providers or occupational health administrators may limit return to work because of comorbid conditions. This may particularly affect the physician's decision to clear an employee to return to work in positions in which the public's safety is at stake.[27]

A number of associated factors can be used to help predict the development of a complicated course of LBP. These include[28–32]:

▶ *Age older than 40 or 50 years.* The relation between chronic LBP and age over 40 or 50, with a decrease of occurrence over 60, is considered as an established fact in many reviews.[33,34] The explanation is the presence of a degenerative process and the accumulation of spinal damage associated with increasing age.

▶ *Low level of formal education and social class.* For back pain, specifically, some studies have found an inverse relation of formal education, social class, or both to the prevalence of back pain symptoms.[35–37] A tentative conclusion, although not based on an extensive literature review, indicates that lower levels of socioeconomic status and education are better predictors of adverse prognosis for occupational disability from back pain than are risk factors per se.[38]

▶ *Physical and psychosocial workload.* The relation between physical and psychosocial load at work and the occurrence of LBP has been the subject of many studies.[39,40] From these studies, it has been concluded that both work-related physical factors of flexion and rotation of the trunk and lifting at work, and low job satisfaction, are risk factors for sickness absence resulting from LBP. Four explanations for the association between psychosocial work characteristics and musculoskeletal symptoms have been suggested[41]: (1) psychosocial work characteristics can directly influence the biomechanical load through changes in posture, movement, and exerted forces; (2) these factors may trigger physiologic mechanisms, such as increased muscle tension or increased hormonal excretion, that may in the long term lead to organic changes and the development or intensification of musculoskeletal symptoms or may influence pain perception and thus increase symptoms; (3) psychosocial factors may change the ability of an individual to cope with an illness which, in turn, could influence the reporting of musculoskeletal symptoms; and (4) the association may well be confounded by the effect of physical factors at work. It seems plausible that psychosocial factors in private life also could affect musculoskeletal symptoms through the second and third mechanism.[41]

▶ *Sciatic pain.* LBP radiating to a leg (i.e., sciatic pain) seems to be a more persistent and severe type of pain than nonspecific LBP. Sciatic pain also causes more disability and longer absence from work.[34]

▶ *Low job satisfaction.* Studies have found an effect of low workplace social support and low job satisfaction. However, the effect found for low job satisfaction may be a result of insufficient adjustment for psychosocial work characteristics and physical load at work.

▶ *Smoking.* In some epidemiologic studies (mostly those of cross-sectional design), smoking has been associated with LBP.[42,43] Several possible pathophysiologic mechanisms have been proposed to explain the association. It has been suggested that smoking accelerates degeneration by impairing the blood supply to the vertebral body and nutrition of the intervertebral disk.[44] Smoking increases coughing activity, which causes an increase in intradiscal pressure.[45] Also, it has been hypothesized that the high serum proteolytic activity in the blood of cigarette smokers gains access to a previously degenerated neovascularized disk and accelerates the degenerative process. Increased proteolytic activity also may weaken the spinal ligaments, resulting in spinal instability.[46] Besides its direct harmful effects, smoking also may be an indicator of other health risk factors as well as lifestyle and behavioral patterns.[42]

▶ *Obesity.* There are several hypotheses relating to a link between obesity and LBP. Increased mechanical demands resulting from obesity have been suspected of causing LBP through excessive wear and tear,[47–50] and it has been suggested that metabolic factors associated with obesity may be detrimental.[48]

▶ *Osteoarthritis.* The link between spinal degeneration and chronic LBP often has been assumed, because the severity of the radiographic abnormalities makes it logical to infer a cause-and-effect correlation.[51–53] Conditions such as osteoarthrosis, congenital anomalies, and postural misalignments often have been assumed to relate to LBP, but the evidence to support these assumptions (with the exception of some degenerative changes) has been inconclusive.[51–53] Indeed, given the low correlation of radiographic findings and clinical signs and symptoms, some physicians feel that radiographs are not necessary initially in the workup of acute nontraumatic LBP.[52]

Given the numerous causes and types of LBP, it is imperative that any clinician examining and treating the lower back have a sound understanding and knowledge of the anatomy and biomechanics of this region. Although this knowledge is not the sole determinant of the approach to LBP, it does provide a solid framework on which to build successful management.

It is worth noting that strength, flexibility, aerobic conditioning, and postural education have all been found to have a significant preventative effect on the occurrence and recurrence of back injuries.[54–61] Thus, physical therapy, with its emphasis on the restoration of functional motion, strength, and flexibility, should be the cornerstone of both the intervention and the preventative processes in LBP. The

intervention to LBP should be dynamic and should direct the responsibility of the rehabilitative process toward the patient. The management of patients with acute LBP has two principal objectives: to relieve the acute pain and to attempt prevention of transition to chronicity.[62]

Anatomy

The lumbar spine consists of five lumbar vertebrae that, in general, increase in size from L1 to L5 in order to accommodate progressively increasing loads. Between each of the lumbar vertebrae is the intervertebral disk (IVD). The IVD of the lumbar spine is described in Chapter 20.

Vertebral Body

The anterior part of each vertebra is called the vertebral body (Fig. 25-1). The pedicles, which project from the posterior aspect of the vertebral body, represent the only connection between the posterior joints of the segment and the vertebral bodies, both of which deliver tensile and bending forces. Noticeably, the muscles that act on a lumbar vertebra pull downward, transmitting the muscular action to the vertebral body. This muscular action is borne through the pedicles, which act as levers, and thus are subjected to a certain amount of bending.[63] If the vertebral body slides forward, the inferior articular processes of that vertebra abut against the superior articular processes of the next lower vertebra and resist the slide.[63] These resistive forces are transmitted to the vertebral body along the pedicles.

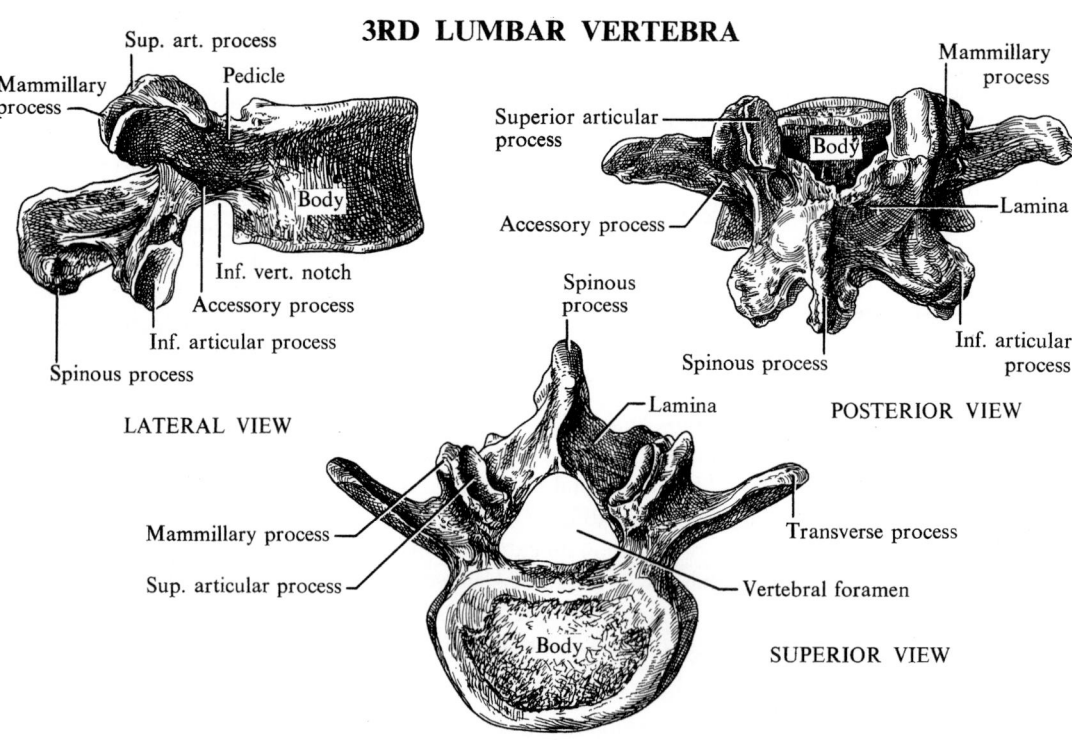

FIGURE 25-1 The lumbar vertebra. (Reproduced with permission from Pansky B. *Review of Gross Anatomy.* 6th ed. New York, NY: McGraw-Hill; 1996:199.)

3RD LUMBAR VERTEBRA

Sup. art. process
Pedicle
Mammillary process
Body
Inf. vert. notch
Accessory process
Inf. articular process
Spinous process

LATERAL VIEW

Mammillary process
Superior articular process
Body
Accessory process
Lamina
Spinous process
Spinous process
Inf. articular process

POSTERIOR VIEW

Mammillary process
Sup. articular process
Lamina
Transverse process
Vertebral foramen
Body

SUPERIOR VIEW

The lamina (see Fig. 25-1) functions to absorb the various forces that are transmitted from the spinous and articular processes. The pars interarticularis connects the vertically oriented lamina and the horizontally extending pedicle, which exposes it to appreciable bending forces.[63] The two laminae meet and fuse with one another, forming an arch of bone aptly called the vertebral, or neural, arch which serves as a bony tunnel for the spinal cord. Both the transverse and spinous processes of the vertebral body provide areas for muscle attachments.

Zygapophysial Joint

The articulations between two consecutive lumbar vertebrae form three joints. One joint is formed between the two vertebral bodies and the IVD. The other two joints are formed by the articulation of the superior articular process of one vertebra and the inferior articular processes of the vertebra above it. These latter joints are known as the zygapophysial joints.

In the intact lumbar vertebral column, the primary function of the zygapophysial joint is to protect the motion segment from anterior shear forces, excessive rotation, and flexion.[64] Additional functions include:

▶ The production of spinal motions including coupling movements.

▶ A minimal restrictor of the physiologic movements of extension and side bending.[65]

From an anteroposterior perspective, the zygapophysial joints of the lumbar spine appear straight, but when viewed from above, they are seen to be curved into a J or C shape. Their orientation varies both with the level and with the individual subject.[66] It is thought that this orientation serves to maximally restrict anterior and rotary movements, and that the C-shaped joints do better in preventing anterior displacement than the J-shaped joints, because of the curvature of the joint surfaces.[63,67] Both shapes competently prevent rotation. The area of the zygapophysial joints most involved in resisting anterior shear forces is the anteromedial part of the superior zygapophysial joint. It is this area that is most vulnerable to fibrillation.[63] The tangential splitting and vertical tearing of the cartilage that occur with aging are believed to reflect these forces, and appear to be a part of the normal degeneration of the joint.[63]

> ### Clinical Pearl
>
> At the thoracolumbar junction, the morphologic configuration of the zygapophysial joints is extremely variable. In general, there is a change from a relatively coronal orientation at T10 to T11 to a more sagittal orientation at L1 to L3, before returning to the more coronal orientation at L5 and S1. Davis[68] compared the thoracolumbar junction to a carpenter's mortise and tenon joint, which, when approximated, would have the effect of impeding all motion except flexion.[69] This appears to be particularly true with respect to axial rotation, in which there is a high degree of torsional stiffness.[70,71]

A fibrous capsule surrounds the joint on all of its aspects except the anterior aspect, which consists of the ligamentum flavum. Posteriorly, the capsule is reinforced by the deep fibers of the multifidus.[72] In lumbar extension, there is a potential for the posterior capsule to become pinched between the apex of the inferior facet and the lamina below. To prevent this, some fibers of the multifidus blend with the posterior capsular fibers and appear to keep the capsule taut.[73]

Superiorly and inferiorly, the capsule is very loose. Superiorly, it bulges toward the base of the next superior transverse process whereas, inferiorly, it does so over the back of the lamina. In both the superior and inferior poles of the joint capsule, there is a very small hole that allows the passage of fat from within the capsule to the extracapsular space.[74]

Within the zygapophysial joints, three types of intra-articular meniscoids have been noted[63]:

1. A connective tissue rim.

2. An adipose tissue pad.

3. A fibro-adipose meniscoid.

It is thought that the function of these intra-articular meniscoids is to:

▶ Fill the joint cavity.

▶ Increase the articular surface area without reducing flexibility.

▶ Protect the articular surfaces as they become exposed during extreme flexion and extension.

These menisci have been inculpated in the cause of some types of LBP, when they fail to return to their original position on recovery from a flexion or extension movement and block the joint toward the neutral position.[75]

Ligaments

Anterior Longitudinal Ligament

The anterior longitudinal ligament (ALL) covers the anterior aspects of the vertebral bodies and IVD (Fig. 25-2). The ALL extends from the sacrum along the anterior aspect of the entire spinal column, becoming thinner as it ascends.[76] The ALL is connected only indirectly with the anterior aspect of the IVD by loose areolar tissue.[63] Some of the ligament fibers insert directly into the bone or periosteum of the centrum.[77] Because of these attachments, and the pull on the bone from the ligament, it is proposed that the anterior aspect of the vertebral body becomes the site for osteophytes. The remaining ligament fibers cover two to five segments, attaching to the upper and lower ends of the vertebral body.

The ALL of the lumbar spine is under tension in a neutral position of the spine and functions to prevent overextension of the spinal segments. In addition, the ALL functions as a minor assistant in limiting anterior translation and vertical separation of the vertebral body.

The ALL receives its nerve supply from recurrent branches of the grey rami communicants.[78]

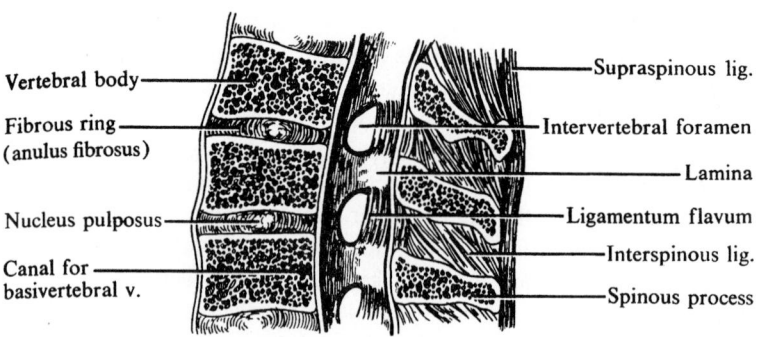

MEDIAN SECTION – LUMBAR REGION

- Vertebral body
- Fibrous ring (anulus fibrosus)
- Nucleus pulposus
- Canal for basivertebral v.
- Supraspinous lig.
- Intervertebral foramen
- Lamina
- Ligamentum flavum
- Interspinous lig.
- Spinous process

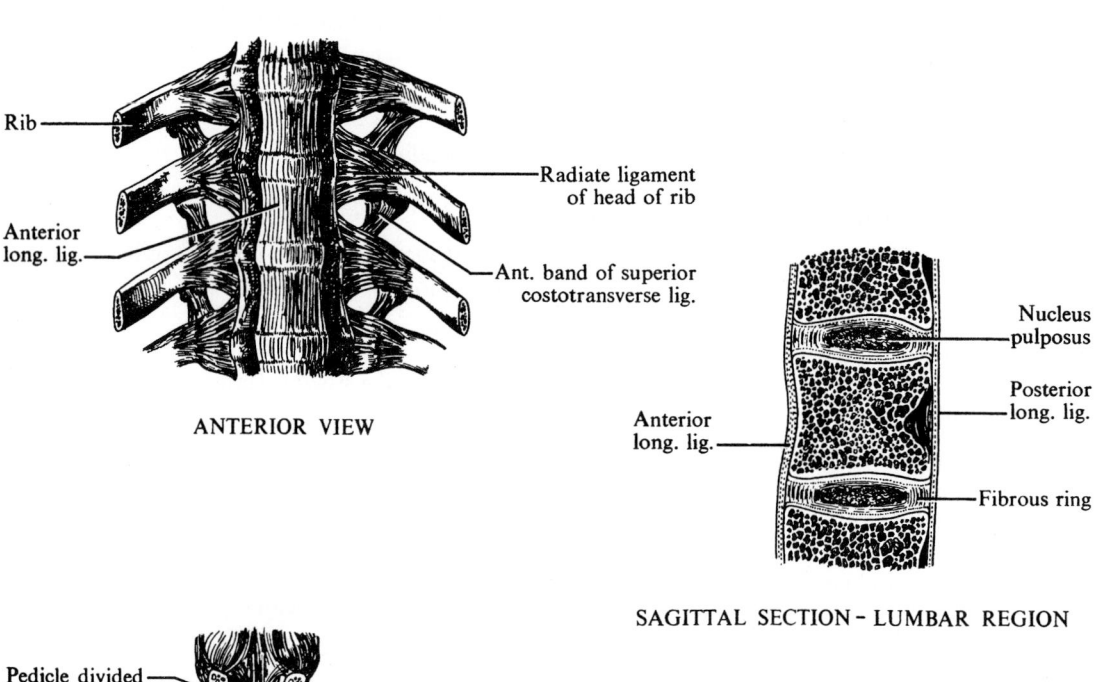

ANTERIOR VIEW

- Rib
- Anterior long. lig.
- Radiate ligament of head of rib
- Ant. band of superior costotransverse lig.

SAGITTAL SECTION – LUMBAR REGION

- Anterior long. lig.
- Nucleus pulposus
- Posterior long. lig.
- Fibrous ring

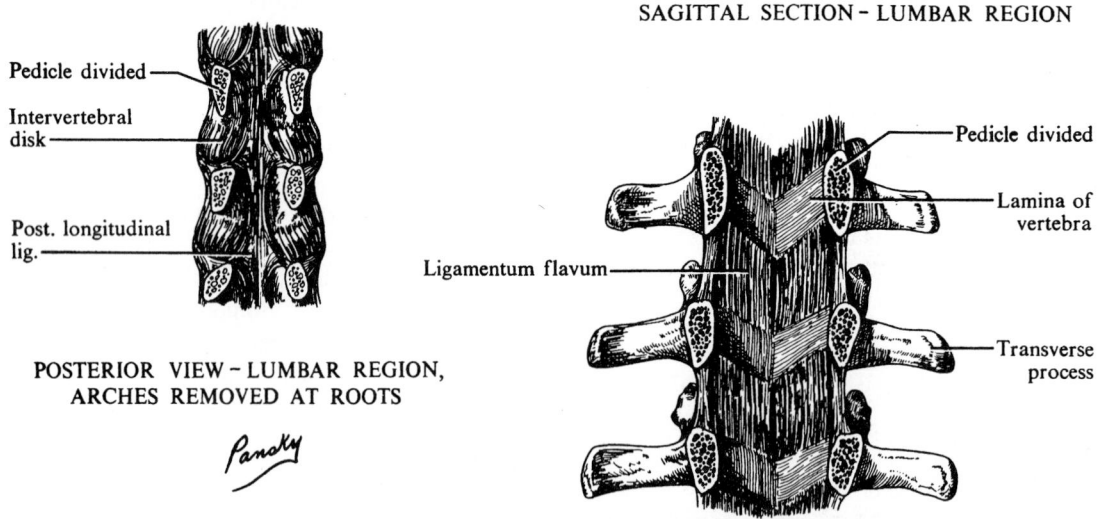

POSTERIOR VIEW – LUMBAR REGION, ARCHES REMOVED AT ROOTS

- Pedicle divided
- Intervertebral disk
- Post. longitudinal lig.

FRONT VIEW – BODIES OF VERTEBRAE REMOVED

- Pedicle divided
- Lamina of vertebra
- Ligamentum flavum
- Transverse process

FIGURE 25-2 The ligaments and articulations of the spine. (Reproduced with permission from Pansky B. *Review of Gross Anatomy*. 6th ed. New York, NY: McGraw-Hill; 1996:215.)

Posterior Longitudinal Ligament

The posterior longitudinal ligament (PLL) is found throughout the spinal column, where it covers the posterior aspect of the centrum and IVD (see Fig. 25-2). Its deep fibers span two segments, from the superior border of the inferior vertebra to the inferior margin of the superior. These fibers integrate with the superficial annular fibers to attach to the posterior margins of the vertebral bodies.[63] The more superficial fibers span up to five segments. In the lumbar spine, the ligament becomes constricted over the vertebral body and widens out over the IVD. It does not attach to the concavity of the body but is separated from it by a fat pad, which acts to block the venous drainage through the basivertebral vein during flexion, as the ligament presses it against the opening of the vein. Although the PLL is rather narrow and is not as substantial as the ALL, it is thought to be important in preventing IVD protrusion.[79] Both the ALL and the PLL have the same tensile strength per unit area.[80]

The PLL tends to tighten in traction and in posterior shearing of the vertebral body. It also acts to limit flexion over a number of segments, although because of its proximity to the center of rotation, it is less of a restraint than the ligamentum flavum.[76]

The PLL is innervated by the sinuvertebral nerve.

Ligamentum Flavum

The ligamentum flavum (LF) connects two consecutive laminae (see Fig. 25-2). This is a bilateral ligament. The medial aspect of the ligament attaches superiorly to the lower anterior surface of the lamina and the inferior surface of the pedicle.[81] The LF attaches inferiorly to the back of the lamina and the pedicle of the next inferior vertebra.[81] Its lateral portion attaches to the articular process and forms the anterior capsule of the zygapophysial joint.

The LF is formed primarily from elastin (80 percent) with the remainder (20 percent) being collagen.[82] Thus, it is an elastic ligament that is stretched during flexion and recovers its neutral length with the neutral position, or extension.

The function of the LF is to resist separation of the lamina during flexion, but there is also appreciable strain in the ligament with side bending.[63,83] Although it seems unlikely that the ligament contributes to an extension recovery from flexion, it does appear to prevent the anterior capsule from becoming nipped between the articular margins as it recoils during extension.[63] The LF is innervated by the medial branch of the dorsal ramus.[84]

Interspinous Ligament

The interspinous ligament (see Fig. 25-2) lies deeply between two consecutive spinal processes. The ligament is important for stability as it represents a major structure for the posterior column of the spine. Unlike the longitudinal ligaments, it is not a continuous fibrous band, but instead consists of loose tissue that fills the gap between the bodies of the spinous processes.[63,85] The interspinous ligament is often disrupted in traumatic cases, which results in the posterior column becoming unstable. An extensive anatomic study on the interspinous ligament showed that degenerative changes start as early as the late second

decade, with ruptures occurring in more than 20 percent of the subjects older than 20 years, particularly at L4 to L5 and L5 to S1.[86]

The ligament has three distinct parts—ventral, middle, and dorsal—of which the middle has the most clinical significance, because it is the part where ruptures tend to occur.[85]

The interspinous ligament most likely functions to resist separation of the spinous processes during flexion.[87] This ligament is supplied by the medial branch of the dorsal rami.[84]

Supraspinous Ligament

The supraspinous ligament (SSL) (see Fig. 25-2) is broad, thick, and cordlike, but it is only well developed in the upper lumbar region.[63,88] Although it joins the tips of two adjacent spinous processes, the SSL is not considered by some to be a true ligament. This is because part of it is derived from the posterior part of the interspinous ligament, although it also merges with the insertions of the lumbar dorsal muscles.[85] Because this ligament is the most superficial of the spinal ligaments and the farthest from the axis of flexion, it has a greater potential for sprains.[89] The SSL is supplied by the medial branch of the dorsal rami.[84]

Iliolumbar Ligament

The iliolumbar ligament is one of the three vertebropelvic ligaments, the others being the sacrotuberous and the sacrospinous ligaments. The ligament is variously believed to be a degenerate part of the quadratus lumborum or the iliocostalis and does not fully develop until approximately age 30.[90]

The iliolumbar ligament functions to restrain flexion, extension, axial rotation, and side bending of L5 on S1.[91] Motions at the lumbosacral joint increase by approximately 20 percent in all directions when the ligament is missing or transected.[76] The incidences of degenerative instability and isthmic lumbar spondylolisthesis also have been shown to increase in its absence.[92,93]

Pseudo Ligaments

These ligaments, the intertransverse, transforaminal, and mamillo-accessory (Fig. 25-3), resemble the membranous part of the fascial system separating paravertebral compartments and do not have any mechanical function.

Intertransverse Ligaments. These ligaments are more membranous than ligamentous. The ligament splits into dorsal and ventral portions, between which is a fat-filled recess. During flexion and extension movements, the fat can be displaced to accommodate the repositioning of the articular zygapophysial joint. The main function of the ligament appears to be to compartmentalize the anterior and posterior musculature.[63]

Transforaminal Ligaments. Occurring in about 47 percent of subjects, the transforaminal ligaments traverse the lateral end of the intervertebral foramen.[94] The most significant of these ligaments is the superior corporotransverse ligament. At L5, the fifth lumbar nerve root runs between the ligament and the ala of

FIGURE 25-3 The transforaminal ligaments. (*A*) Superior and inferior corporotransverse ligaments. (*B*) Superior transforaminal ligament. (*C*) Middle transforaminal ligament. (*D*) Inferior transforaminal ligament. (Reproduced with permission from Bogduk N, Twomey LT. *Clinical Anatomy of the Lumbar Spine and Sacrum.* New York, NY: Churchill Livingstone; 1997:52.)

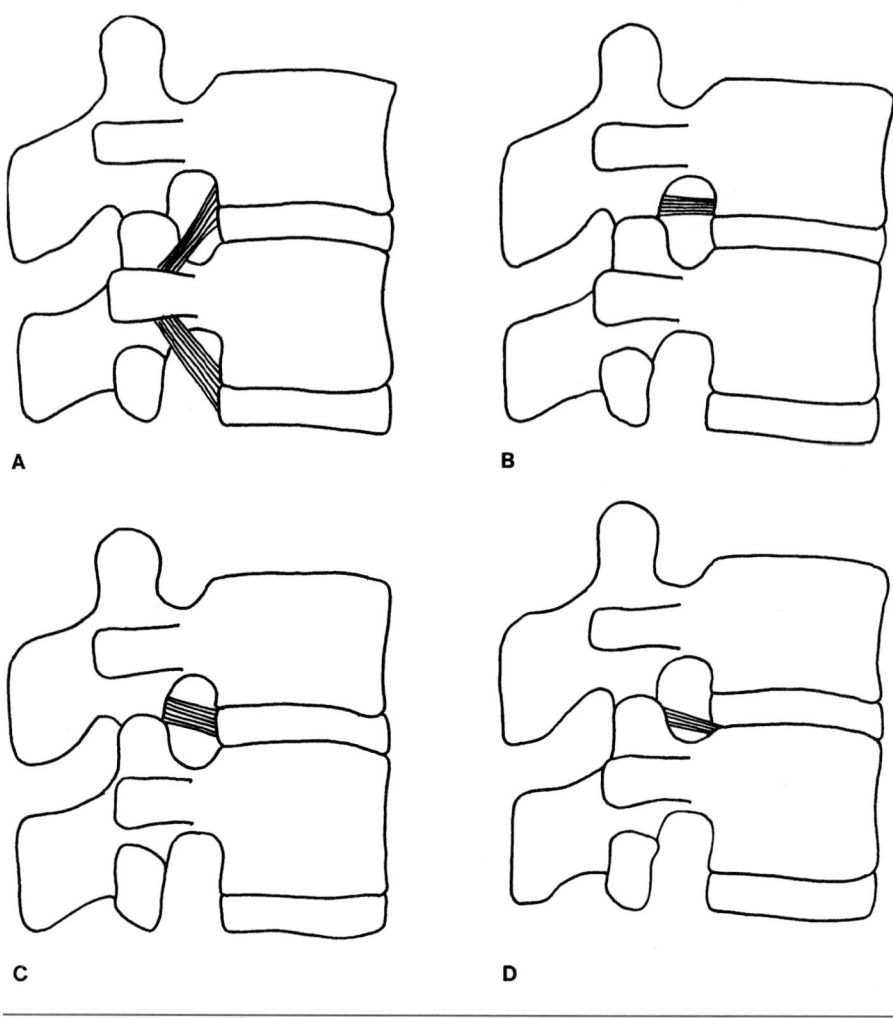

the sacrum. With marked forward slip and downward descent of L5, or with a loss of IVD height, the corporotransverse ligament can have a guillotine effect on the fifth nerve root, resulting in symptoms that can mimic an IVD herniation or a foraminal occlusion.[95]

Mamillo-accessory Ligament. This ligament runs from the accessory process of one vertebra to the mammillary process of the same vertebra.[96] The ligament forms a tunnel for the medial branch of the dorsal ramus, thereby preventing it from lifting off the neural arch. In about 10 percent of adults, the tunnel becomes ossified.[96]

Muscles

Quadratus Lumborum

The quadratus lumborum muscle is large and rectangular, with fibers that pass medially upward (Fig. 25-4). The fibers attach to:

▶ The inferior anterior surface of the 12th rib.

▶ The anterior surface of the upper four transverse processes.

▶ The anterior band of the iliolumbar ligament.

▶ The iliac crest lateral to the attachment of the iliolumbar ligament.

The muscle is active during inspiration, fixing the lowest rib to afford a stable base from which the diaphragm can act. The importance of this muscle from a rehabilitation viewpoint is its contribution as a lumbar spine stabilizer.[97] Working unilaterally, it is typically involved with side bending of the lumbar spine, especially with eccentric control of contralateral side bending. The quadratus lumborum also is very active in sustained postures and when a heavy weight is held in the opposite hand.[98,99] The quadratus lumborum is supplied by the ventral rami of T12 to L2.[100,101]

Multifidus

The lumbar multifidus is the largest of the intrinsic back muscles to cross the lumbosacral junction and lies most medially in the spinal gutter.[73] It is a fascicular muscle, with each fascicle layered on another, giving it a laminated appearance.[63] The lumbar multifidus originates in three groups, which arise from the same vertebra.

1. Laminar fibers arise from the inferoposterior edge of the lamina.

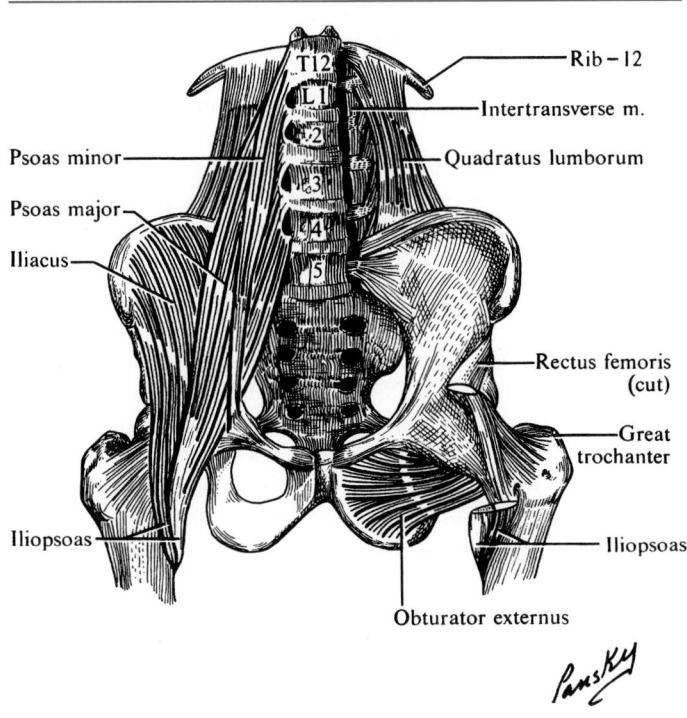

FIGURE 25-4 Psoas major and iliac muscles. (Reproduced with permission from Pansky B. *Review of Gross Anatomy*. 6th ed. New York, NY: McGraw-Hill; 1996:391.)

2. Basal fibers arise from the base of the spinous process.

3. Common tendon fibers arise from a common tendon attached to the inferior tip of the spinous process.

The lumbar multifidus has a complicated insertion (Table 25-1).

Over the past several decades, there has been much research regarding the lumbar multifidus, with particular reference to its

TABLE 25-1 Multifidus Attachments[63,101a]

Laminar	Basal	Common Tendon
L1; MP L3	MP L4	MP L5, S1, and PSIS
L2; MP L4	MP L5	MP S1 and anterolateral aspect of PSIS
L3; MP L5	MP S1	Inferior to PSIS and lateral sacrum
L4; MP S1	As common tendon	Sacrum, lateral to foramina
L5; As common tendon	As common tendon	Sacrum, medial to foramina

MP, mammillary process; PSIS, posterior superior iliac spine.

relationship to LBP, and its importance in rehabilitation. Recent in vitro biomechanical studies have shown that the lumbar multifidus is an important muscle for lumbar segmental stability through its ability to provide segmental stiffness and to control motion.[102–104] The multifidus is active in nearly all antigravity activities and appears to contribute to the stability of the lumbar spine by compressing the vertebrae together.[105]

MacIntosh and Bogduk[73] analyzed the lumbar multifidus to determine the possible actions of the muscle and its individual fibers. The study revealed that working bilaterally, the multifidus muscles can produce the rocking component of extension, but because of the muscle's vertical orientation, it cannot produce the accompanying translation.[73] Additionally, the muscle, by "bow stringing" over a number of segments, can increase the lumbar lordosis, working in a postural role.[106]

Although not considered a primary lumbar rotator,[107] the multifidus is consistently active during both ipsilateral and contralateral spinal rotation, and both multifidi are simultaneously active regardless of which way the spine is turning.[73,74] The major function of the multifidus from a biomechanical perspective is one of arthrokinematic control. It is believed that the lumbar multifidus acts as an antagonist to flexion and opposes the flexing moment of the abdominals as they rotate the trunk.[73,106,108] This synergistic function may be compromised with injury to the multifidus. Using magnetic resonance imaging, the signal intensities of the multifidus during lumbar hyperextension have been found to be markedly diminished in patients with chronic LBP compared with normal patients.[109]

Unilaterally, the multifidus muscle also should be able to produce side bending. However, its horizontal vector is very small, and it is unlikely to be an efficient side bender of the spine.[63,73]

The multifidus shares a close association with the gluteus maximus and the sacrotuberous ligament, factors that are thought to enhance sacroiliac joint and lumbar spine stability.[110–112]

The lumbar multifidus has the distinction of being innervated segmentally by the medial branch of the dorsal ramus of the same level or the level below the originating spinous process.[113,114] Because the multifidus is segmental in origin and innervation, any impairment of this muscle can produce palpable changes in the muscle, thus directing the clinician to the segment that is dysfunctional.[115]

Erector Spinae

The erector spinae is a composite muscle consisting of the iliocostalis lumborum and the thoracic longissimus. Both of these muscles are subdivided into the lumbar and thoracic longissimi and iliocostallii.[63] As a group, the muscles of the erector spinae play an important role in lumbar stabilization. The nerve supply to the erector spinae muscles is by the medial branch of the dorsal ramus of the thoracic and lumbar spinal nerves.

Longissimus Thoracis Pars Lumborum. This is a fascicular muscle that arises from the accessory processes of the lumbar vertebrae to insert into the posterior superior iliac spine and the iliac crest lateral to it (Fig. 25-5). The upper four tendons converge to form the lumbar aponeurosis that inserts lateral to the L5 fascicle.

The longissimus thoracis pars lumborum muscles have both a vertical and a horizontal vector. The vertical vector is much the larger of the two and can produce extension or side bending, depending on whether it is functioning bilaterally or unilaterally.[116] Because of its attachment to the transverse rather than the spinous process, which results in reduced leverage, the longissimus thoracis pars lumborum is much less efficient than the lumbar multifidus in producing posterior sagittal rotation.[114,117] Indeed, mathematical analysis of the lumbosacral portion of the muscle suggests that the net effect of its pull would be to produce an anterior, not a posterior, shear.[63]

Iliocostalis Lumborum Pars Lumborum.　　There are four overlying fascicles arising from the tip of the upper four transverse processes and the adjoining middle layer of the thoracolumbar fascia (see Fig. 25-5). The fibers insert onto the iliac crest, with the lower and deeper fibers attaching lateral to the posterior superior iliac spine.[117]

There is no muscular fiber from L5, but it is believed that this is represented by the iliolumbar ligament, which is completely muscular in children, becoming collagenous by approximately 30 years of age.

The vectors and actions of this muscle are similar to those of the longissimus. However, the lower and deeper fibers produce strong axial rotation and act with the multifidus as synergists to produce rotation during abdominal muscle action.[117]

Longissimus Thoracis Pars Thoracis.　　This muscle group consists of 11 to 12 pairs of muscles, which extend from the transverse processes of T2 and their ribs and run inferomedially to attach to the spinous processes of L3 to L5 and the sacral spinous processes, as well as the posterior superior iliac spine (see Fig. 25-5).

The orientation and various attachments of this muscle group allow it to act indirectly on the lumbar spine. The main action of the muscle appears to be the extension of the thoracic spine on that of the lumbar. An anatomic-mathematical study[118] suggests that 70 to 80 percent of the force required to extend the upper lumbar spine is produced from the thoracic fibers of the erector spinae, which also generate 50 percent of the force in the lower levels.

Iliocostalis Lumborum Pars Thoracis.　　The thoracic iliocostalis (Fig. 25-5) serves as the thoracic part of the iliocostalis lumborum and not the iliocostalis thoracic. It is a layered muscle consisting of inferomedially orientated fascicles attached to the following points[117]:

FIGURE 25-5　The erector spinae. (Reproduced with permission from Luttgens K, Hamilton K. *Kinesiology: Scientific Basis of Human Motion.* New York, NY: McGraw-Hill; 1997:266.)

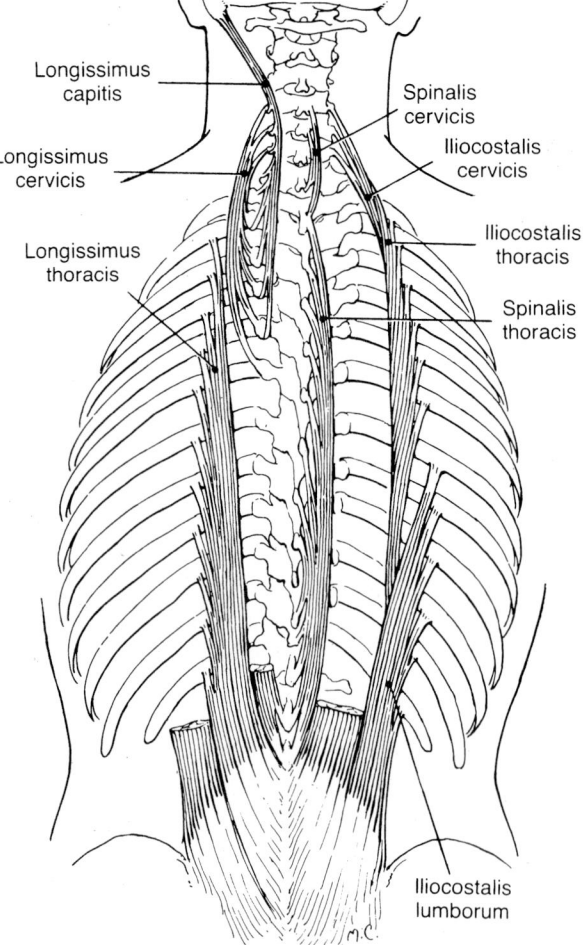
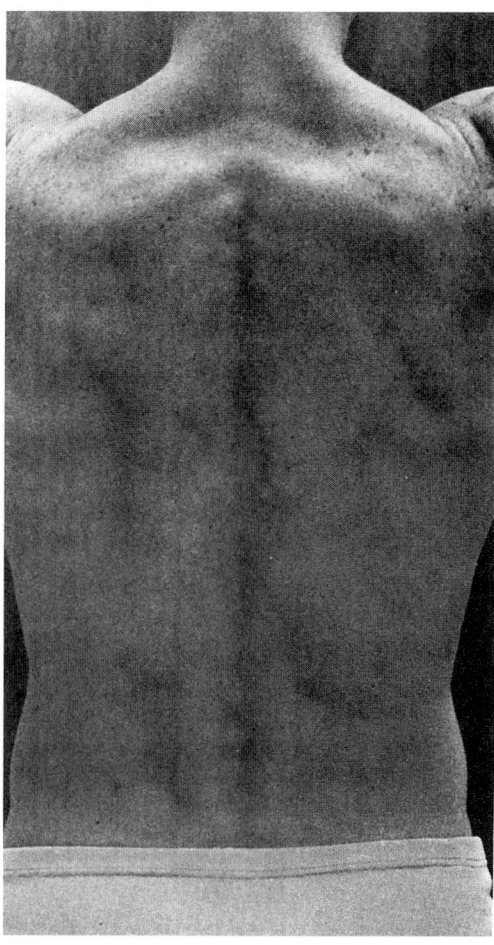

▶ Lateral part of the lower eight rib angles.

▶ Posterior superior iliac spine.

▶ Dorsal surface of the sacrum, distal to the multifidus.

This muscle completely spans the lumbar spine and is in an excellent position to extend and side bend the spine, as well as to increase the lumbar lordosis. It is a weak rotator, because the amount of rib separation on ipsilateral rotation is minor, but on contralateral rotation, it is better. It is, therefore, possible that the muscle is an effective derotator of the spine.[63]

Thoracolumbar Fascia

The thoracolumbar fascia travels from the spinous process of T12 to the posterior superior iliac spine and iliac crest (Fig. 25-6). The thoracolumbar fascia consists of three layers of connective tissue that envelop the lumbar muscles and separate them into anterior, middle, and posterior compartments or layers[119]:

1. The anterior layer covers the anterior surface of the quadratus lumborum muscle. It is attached to the anterior transverse processes, and then to the intertransverse ligaments. On the lateral side of the quadratus lumborum, it blends with the other layers of the fascia.

2. The middle layer is posterior to the quadratus lumborum, with its medial attachment to the tips of the transverse processes and the intertransverse ligaments. Laterally, it gives rise to, or is attached to, the transverse abdominal aponeurosis.

3. The posterior layer covers the lumbar musculature and arises from the spinous processes, wrapping around the muscles. It blends with the other layers of the fascia along the lateral border of the iliocostalis lumborum in a dense thickening of the fascia called the *lateral raphe*.[119] This layer consists of two laminae, a superficial one with its fibers orientated inferomedially, and a deep lamina whose fibers are inferolateral. The superficial fibers are derived from the latissimus dorsi.

The functions of the TFL are varied. The TFL:

▶ Provides muscle attachment.

▶ Stabilizes the spine against anterior shear and flexion moments.

▶ Resists segmental flexion via tension generated by the transverse abdominis on the spinous process.

▶ Assists the in transmission of extension forces during lifting activities. The posterior ligamentous system has been proposed as a model to explain some of the forces required for lifting. It is believed to transmit forces by passive resistance to flexion, from the joint capsule and extracapsular ligaments, and from the more dynamic effects of the thoracolumbar fascia.[120]

Abdominal Muscles

Rectus Abdominis. The rectus abdominis (Fig. 25-7) originates from the cartilaginous ends of the fifth through seventh ribs and xiphoid, and inserts on the superior aspect of the pubic bone.

FIGURE 25-6 The thoracolumbar fascia. (Reproduced with permission from Flynn TW. *The Thoracic Spine and Rib Cage.* Boston, Mass: Butterworth-Heinemann; 1996:21.)

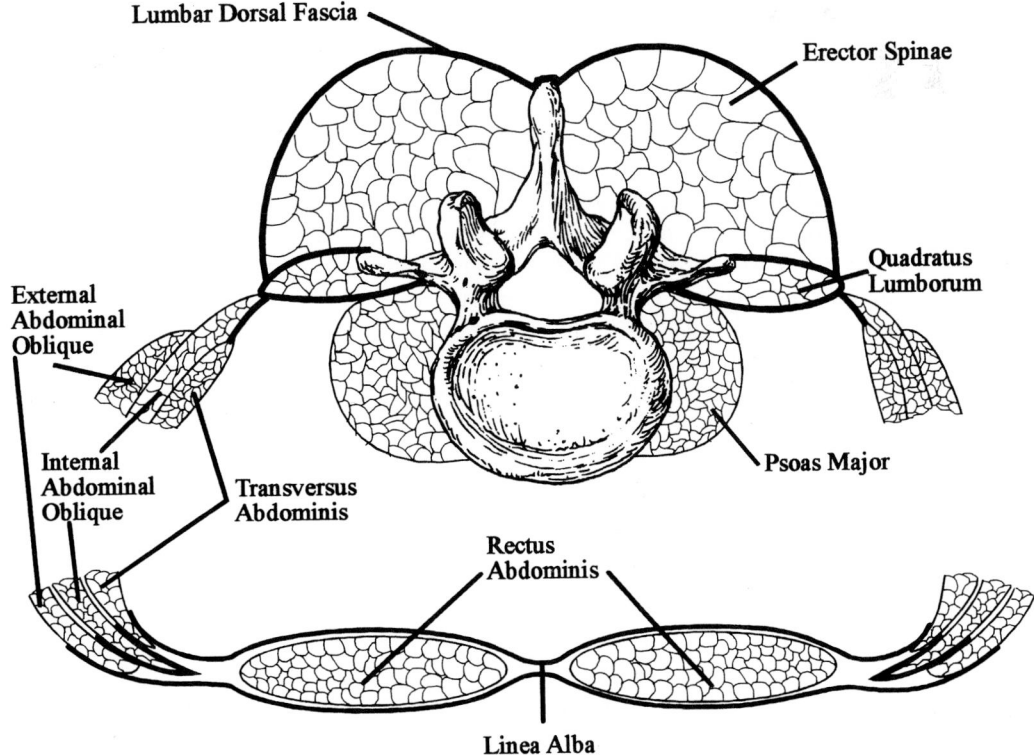

Lumbar Dorsal Fascia

Erector Spinae

External Abdominal Oblique

Internal Abdominal Oblique

Transversus Abdominis

Quadratus Lumborum

Psoas Major

Rectus Abdominis

Linea Alba

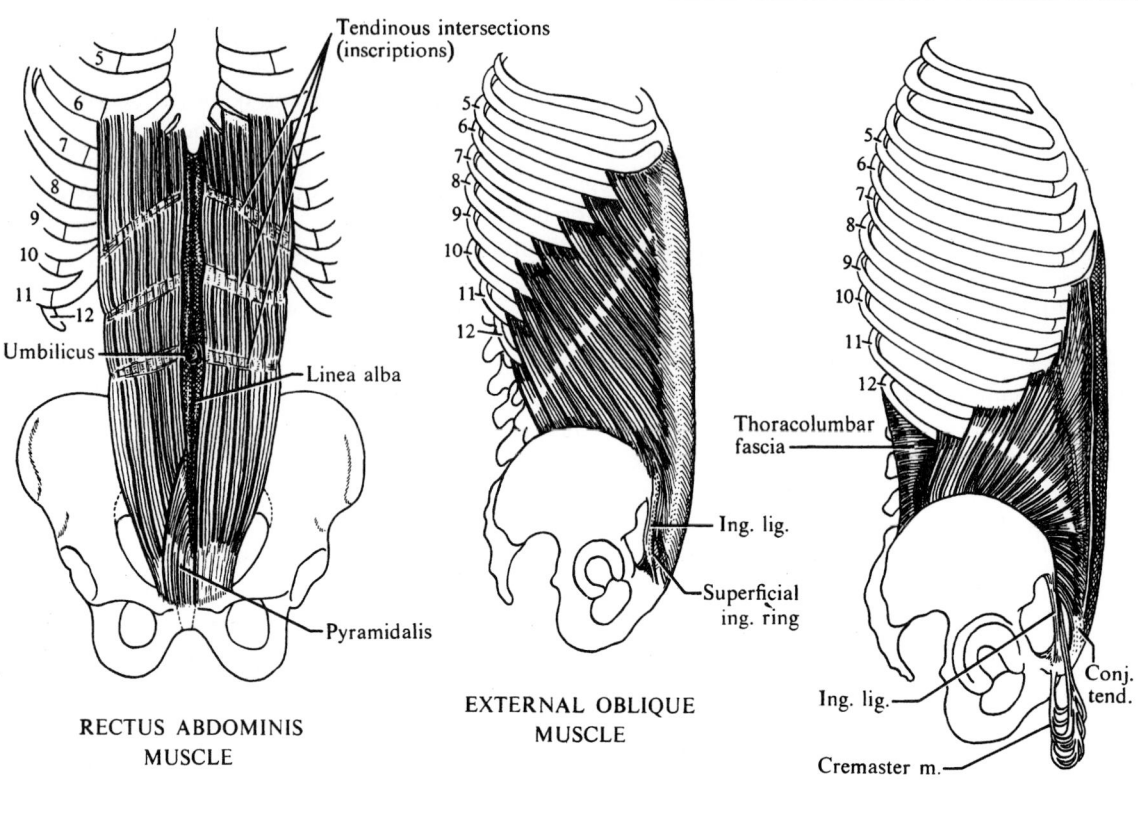

FIGURE 25-7 Abdominal muscles. (Reproduced with permission from Pansky B. *Review of Gross Anatomy.* 6th ed. New York, NY: McGraw-Hill; 1996:391.)

The muscle functions to flex the vertebral column by approximating the thorax and pelvis anteriorly.[121]

Transversus Abdominis.   The transverse abdominis muscle (Fig. 25-8) originates from the lateral one third of the inguinal ligament, the anterior two thirds of the inner lip of the iliac crest, the lateral raphe of the thoracolumbar fascia, and the internal aspects of the lower six costal cartilages, where it interdigitates with the diaphragm.[122] Its upper and middle fibers run transversely around the trunk and blend with the fascial envelope of the rectus abdominis muscle, while the lower fibers blend with the insertion of the internal oblique muscle on the pubic crest.[123]

These attachments allow the transverse abdominis muscle to exert tension on both the middle and posterior layers of the thoracolumbar fascia in the middle and lower regions of the lumbar spine.[98,122] This relationship is thought to assist in the stabilization of the lumbar motion segment.[98,99]

Internal Oblique.   The internal oblique (see Fig. 25-7), which forms the middle layer of the lateral abdominal wall, is located between the transversus abdominis and the external oblique muscles.[123] It has multiple attachments to the inguinal ligament, lateral raphe, iliac crest, pubic crest, transverse abdom-inis, and costal cartilages of the seventh through ninth costal cartilages. Because of these multiple attachment sites, the different fascicles of the muscle can have very different force vectors.

The internal oblique is active during a number of functions, including gait (most often close to initial contact[124]) and erect sitting and standing postures.[125] Acting bilaterally, the internal obliques flex the vertebral column and assist in respiration. Acting in unison, the muscle, in conjunction with the external obliques, can produce rotation of the vertebral column, bringing the thorax backward (when the pelvis is fixed), or the pelvis forward (when the thorax is fixed).[121,126]

External Oblique.   The external oblique (see Fig. 25-7) originates from the lateral aspect of the fifth through 12th ribs, and through interdigitations with the serratus anterior and latissimus dorsi. The muscle travels obliquely, medially, and inferiorly to insert into the linea alba, inguinal ligament, anterior superior iliac spine, iliac crest, and pubic tubercle.

Acting bilaterally, the external obliques flex the vertebral column and tilt the pelvis posteriorly. Acting in unison, the muscle, in conjunction with the internal obliques, can produce side bending of the vertebral column, approximating the thorax and the iliac crest laterally.[121]

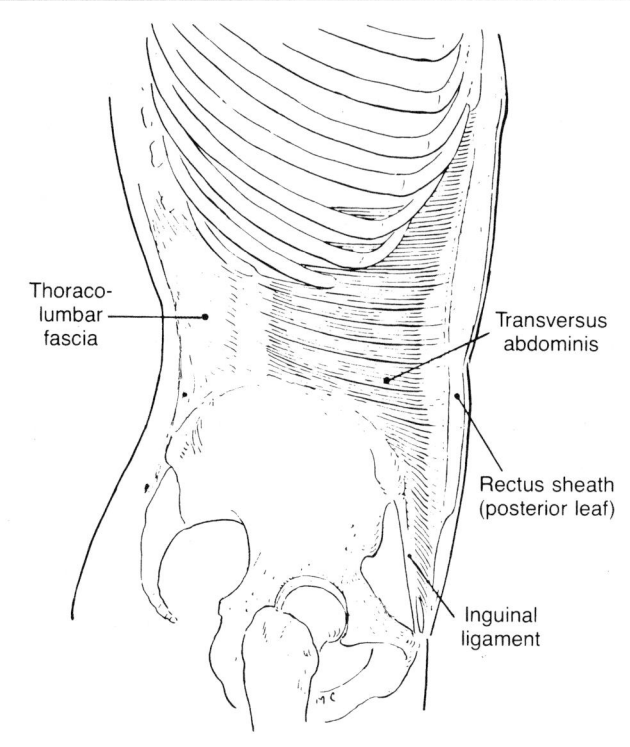

FIGURE 25-8 The transversus abdominis. (Reproduced with permission from Luttgens K, Hamilton K. *Kinesiology: Scientific Basis of Human Motion.* New York, NY: McGraw-Hill; 1997:263.)

Psoas Major

Although traditionally viewed as a muscle of the hip, the psoas major muscle combines with the iliacus muscle to directly attach the lumbar spine to the femur.[127] The psoas major originates from:

▶ Anterolateral aspects of the vertebral bodies.

▶ IVDs of T12 to L5.

▶ Transverse processes of L1 to L5.

▶ Tendinous arch spanning the concavity of the sides of the vertebral bodies.

The iliacus is attached superiorly to the iliac fossa and the inner lip of the iliac crest. Joining with the psoas major, the combined tendon passes over the superior lateral aspect of the pubic ramus and attaches to the lesser trochanter of the femur (see Fig. 25-4).

Taken individually, the iliacus and psoas major serve different functions.

▶ The psoas major is electromyographically active in many different positions and movements of the lumbar spine, and its activity can add a stabilizing effect on the lumbar spine with compressive loading.[128] With the foot fixed on the ground (closed chain), contraction of the psoas major increases the flexion of the lumbar-pelvic unit on the femur.[129]

▶ With the foot fixed on the ground, contraction of the iliacus produces an anterior torsion of the ilium, and extension of the lumbar zygapophysial joints. If there is a decrease in the length of the iliacus as a result of adaptive shortening or increased efferent neural input to the muscle, the result is an anteriorly rotated pelvis and an increase in lordosis. This may increase the anterior shear stress on the lumbosacral junction in any posture.[128]

From a clinical perspective, the iliacus and psoas major usually are considered together as the iliopsoas. Working bilaterally (insertion fixed), the iliopsoas can produce flexion of the trunk on the femur as in the sit-up from supine position, or in bending over to touch one's toes. The iliopsoas muscle also side bends the spine ipsilaterally.[128]

Working from a stable spine above (origin fixed), the iliopsoas muscle flexes the hip joint by flexing the femur on the trunk.

The iliopsoas is innervated by the ventral rami of L1 and L2.

Nerve Supply of the Lumbar Segment

The distributions of referred pain must be considered in relation to the neurologic supply of the lumbar segment. McCullogh and Waddell[130] studied the effects of electrical stimulation of spinal ligaments, muscles, the annulus fibrosus, and the nucleus pulposus and found that these structures referred pain to the buttock and upper leg, but rarely below the upper calf. The reported pain was dull and poorly localized. In contrast, stimulation of the nerve roots produced a sharper, more localized pain, often with some paresthesia. Stimulation of the L5 and S1 nerve roots nearly always radiated to or below the ankle.

The nerve supply to the lumbar spine follows a general pattern. The outer half of the IVD is innervated by the sinuvertebral nerve[131] and the grey rami communicants,[132] with the posterolateral aspect innervated by both the sinuvertebral nerve[78] and the grey rami communicants. The lateral aspect receives only sympathetic innervation.

The zygapophysial joints are innervated by the medial branches of the dorsal rami.[84,131,133] Each joint receives its nerve supply from the corresponding medial branch above and below the joint.[84,131] For instance the L4–5 joint receives its nerve supply from the medial branches of L3 and L4. The lateral branches cross the subjacent transverse process and pursue a sinuous course caudally, laterally, and dorsally through the iliocostalis lumborum.[84] They innervate that muscle, and eventually the L1 to L3 lateral branches pierce the dorsal layer of thoracolumbar fascia and become cutaneous, supplying the skin over the lateral buttock as far as the greater trochanter.[84,131] The intermediate branches run dorsally and caudally from the intertransverse spaces. They form a series of intersegmental communications within the longissimus thoracis.[84,131]

Nerve Root Canal

The nerve root canal is located at the lateral aspect of the spinal canal. The dural sac forms the medial wall of the canal, the internal aspect of the pedicle, and the lateral wall. The posterior border of the nerve root canal is formed by the ligamentum flavum, superior articular process, and lamina. The anterior border of the canal is formed by the vertebral body and IVD.

The nerve root canal can be described according to its location[134]:

▶ The entrance zone is medial and anterior to the superior articular process.

▶ The middle zone is located under the pars interarticularis of the lamina, and below the pedicle.

▶ The exit zone is the area surrounding the intervertebral foramen.

A decrease in the dimension of this canal results in a condition called lateral stenotic syndrome.[135]

Lumbar Spine Vascularization

The blood supply for the lumbar spine is provided by the lumbar arteries (Fig. 25-9), and its venous drainage occurs via the lumbar veins (Fig. 25-10).

Biomechanics

Physiologic motions at the lumbar spine joints can occur in three cardinal planes: sagittal (flexion and extension), coronal (side bending), and transverse (rotation). Including accessory motions, six degrees of freedom are available at the lumbar spine.[79]

The amount of segmental motion at each vertebral level varies. Most of the flexion and extension of the lumbar spine occurs in the lower segmental levels, whereas most of the side bending of the lumbar spine occurs in the midlumbar area.[122,136,137] Rotation, which occurs with side bending as a coupled motion, is minimal and occurs most at the lumbosacral junction.[122,136,137] The amount of range available in the lumbar spine generally decreases with age.[138]

Flexion

The lumbar spine is well designed for flexion, which is the most commonly used motion of the lumbar spine in daily activities. The flexion-extension range of the lumbar spine that occurs between vertebral segments is approximately 12 degrees in the upper lumbar spine, increasing by 1 to 2 degrees per segment to reach a maximum motion of 20 to 25 degrees between L5 and S1.[63,137]

During lumbar flexion in standing, which normally is initiated by the abdominal muscles, the entire lumbar spine leans forward, and there is a posterior sway of the pelvis as the hips flex.

Clinical Pearl

Flexion of the lumbar spine also can occur with a posterior pelvic tilt. The posterior pelvic tilt can be performed voluntarily, or it may occur as a result of weak paraspinal extensor muscles or adaptively shortened hamstring and gluteal muscles.[139]

At the vertebral level, flexion produces a combination of an anterior roll and an anterior glide of the vertebral body, and a straightening, or minimal reversal, of the lordosis.[122,137] At L4 to L5, reversal may occur, but at the L5 to S1 level, the joint will straighten but not reverse[140] unless there is pathology present. During the anterior rocking motion of the segment that occurs with flexion, the inferior facets of the superior vertebra lift upward and backward, opening a small gap between the facets. The superior vertebra translates anteriorly by approximately 5 to 7 mm, closing the gap and enhancing stability through increased tension of the joint capsule.[74] The anterior sagittal translation, or shear, is also resisted by:

▶ The superoanterior orientation of the lateral fibers of the annulus fibrosus.

▶ The iliolumbar and supraspinous ligaments at the L5 to S1 segment, with the longitudinal ligaments helping to a lesser extent.

▶ The semisagittal and sagittal orientation of the zygapophysial joints, which cause the superior facet to come against the inferior one during an anterior shear, with the highest pressure occurring on the anteromedial portion of the superior zygapophysial joint surface. The zygapophysial joints are, therefore, vital in the limitation of this anterior shear.[141]

▶ The horizontal vector of the erector spinae and the multifidus, which acts to pull the vertebrae posteriorly.

Flexion is also limited by the compressibility of the anterior structures, such as the IVD, and by the extensibility of the posterior structures of the segment (ligaments, IVD, and muscles). These structures have varying contributions to the resistance of segmental flexion, depending on the degree of flexion[142]:

▶ The joint capsule resists about 39 percent.

▶ The supraspinous and interspinous ligaments resist about 19 percent.

▶ The ligamentum flavum ligament resists about 13 percent.

▶ The IVD resists about 29 percent.

Although much emphasis has been placed on the strengthening of the rectus abdominis during lumbar spine rehabilitation, recent research has suggested that it is the contraction of the hooplike transversus abdominis that creates a rigid cylinder, resulting in enhanced stiffness of the lumbar spine.[105,143] The cross-hatch arrangement of the thoracolumbar fascia creates a pressurized visceral cavity anterior to the spine when the transversus abdominis contracts. This can result in the production of a force against the apex of the lumbar lordosis. This force is theorized to increase the stability of the lumbar spine during a variety of postures and movements.[144]

Extension

Extension movements of the lumbar spine produce a converse of those that occur in flexion. Theoretically, true extension of the lumbar spine is pathologic and depends on one's definition:

FIGURE 25-9 Arteries of the spinal cord. (Reproduced with permission from Pansky B. *Review of Gross Anatomy*. 6th ed. New York, NY: McGraw-Hill; 1996:209.)

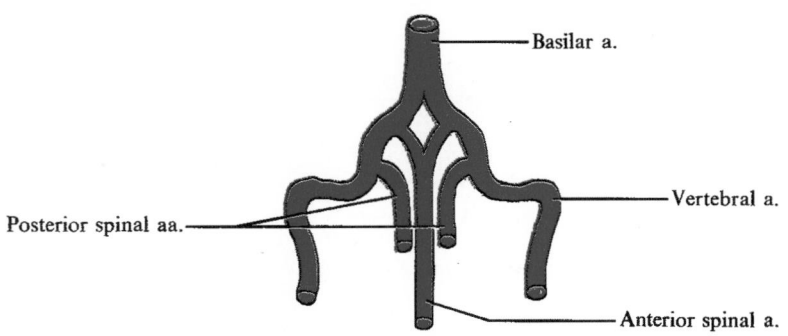

ORIGIN OF SPINAL ARTERIES (SCHEMATIC)

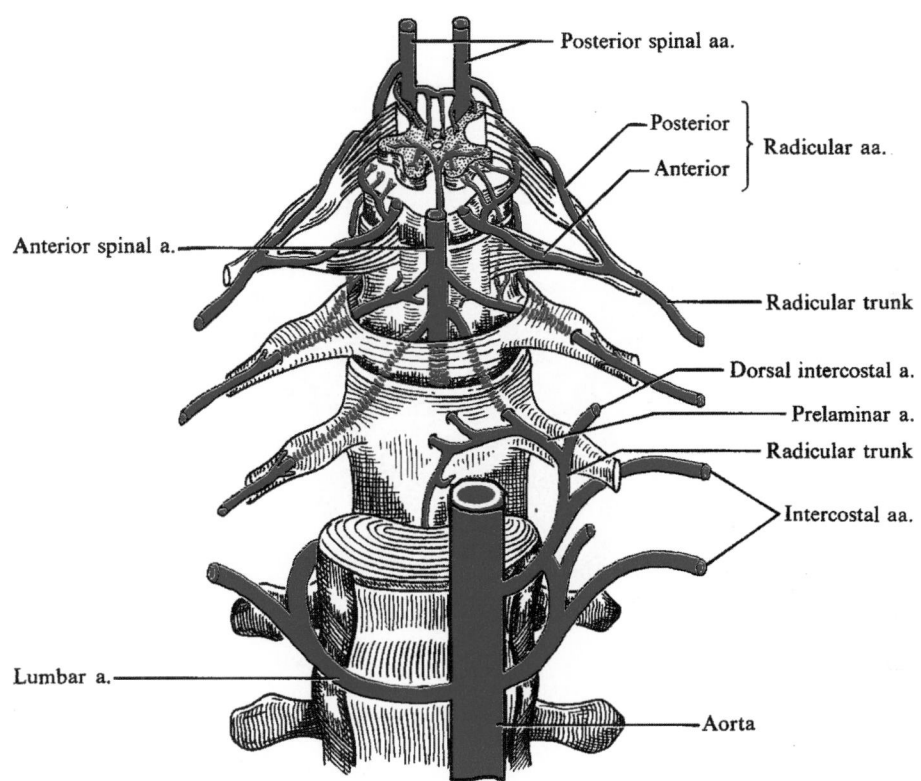

SOURCE, COURSE, AND DISTRIBUTION

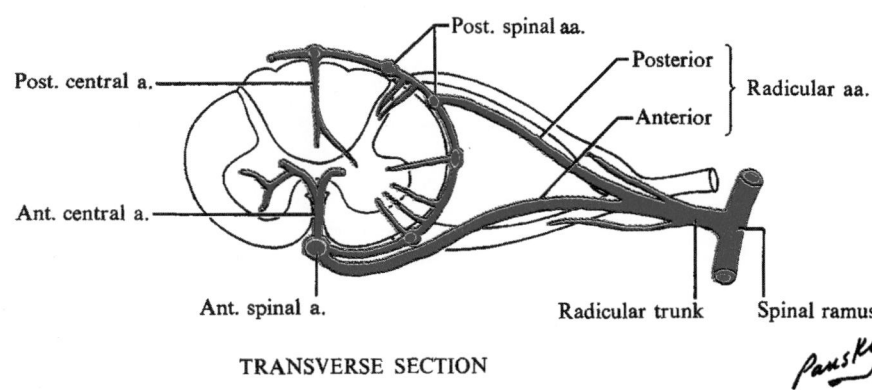

TRANSVERSE SECTION

FIGURE 25-10 Veins of the spinal cord and column. (Reproduced with permission from Pansky B. *Review of Gross Anatomy*. 6th ed. New York, NY: McGraw-Hill; 1996:211.)

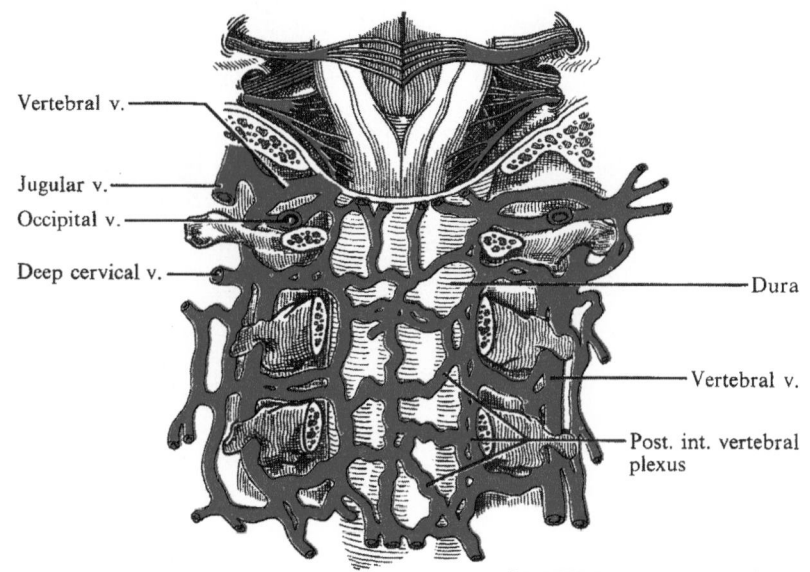

Vertebral v.
Jugular v.
Occipital v.
Deep cervical v.
Dura
Vertebral v.
Post. int. vertebral plexus

POSTERIOR VIEW – LAMINA CUT

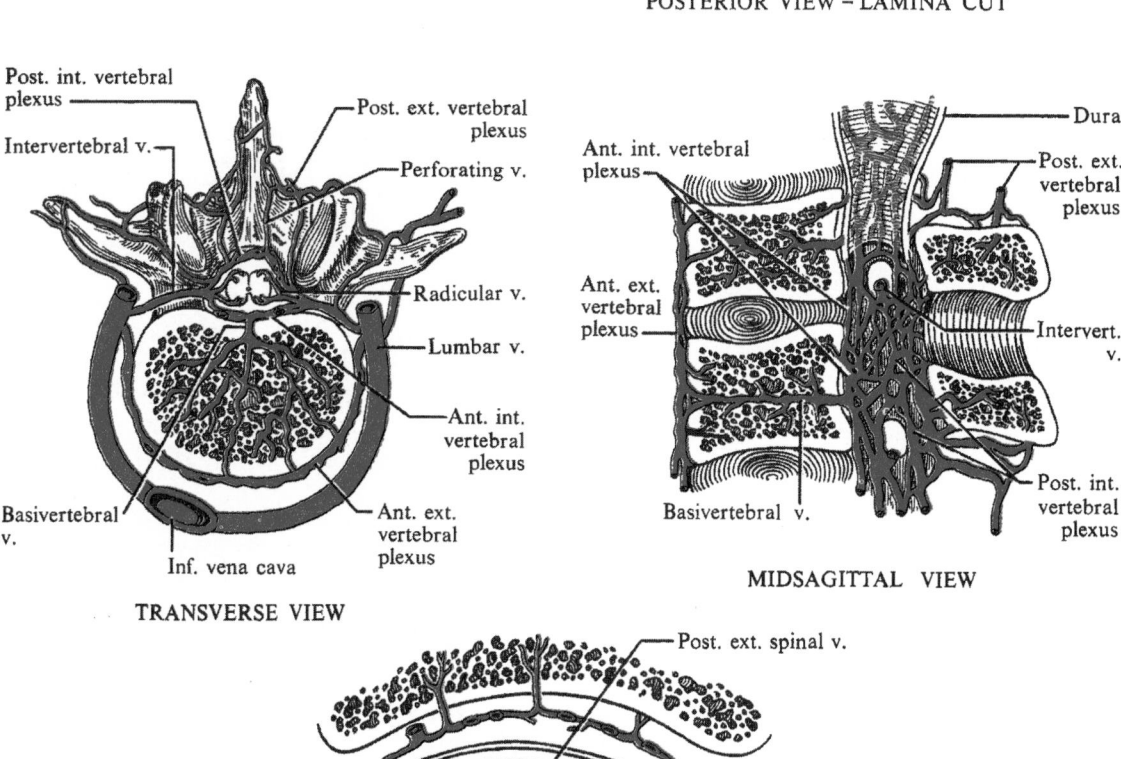

Post. int. vertebral plexus
Intervertebral v.
Post. ext. vertebral plexus
Perforating v.
Radicular v.
Lumbar v.
Ant. int. vertebral plexus
Basivertebral v.
Inf. vena cava
Ant. ext. vertebral plexus

TRANSVERSE VIEW

Ant. int. vertebral plexus
Dura
Post. ext. vertebral plexus
Ant. ext. vertebral plexus
Intervert. v.
Basivertebral v.
Post. int. vertebral plexus

MIDSAGITTAL VIEW

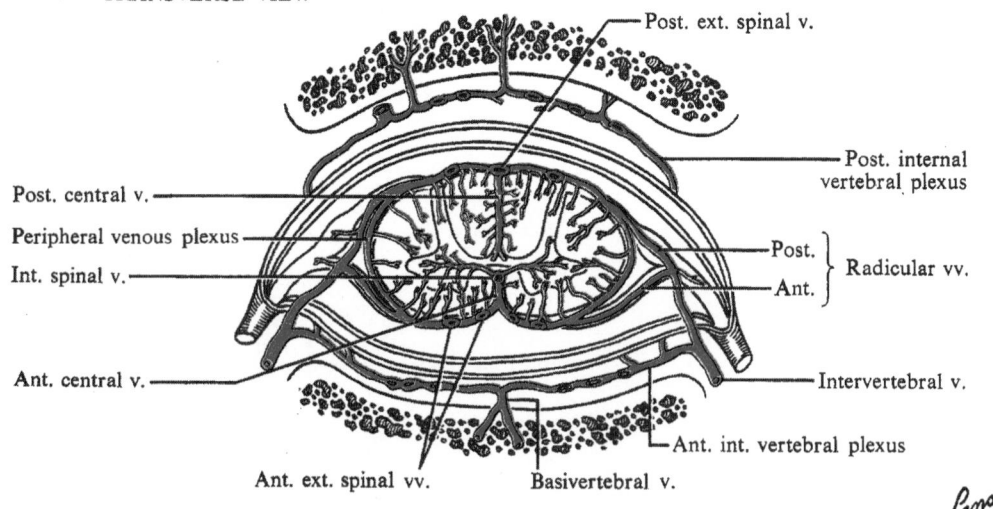

Post. ext. spinal v.
Post. central v.
Peripheral venous plexus
Int. spinal v.
Ant. central v.
Post. internal vertebral plexus
Post. } Radicular vv.
Ant. }
Intervertebral v.
Ant. int. vertebral plexus
Ant. ext. spinal vv.
Basivertebral v.

TRANSVERSE SECTION

pure extension involves a posterior roll and glide of the vertebra, and a posterior and inferior motion of the zygapophysial joints, but not necessarily a change in the degree of lordosis.[137] During lumbar extension, the inferior zygapophysial joint of the superior vertebra moves downward, impacting with the lamina below and producing a buckling of the interspinous ligament between the two spinous processes. This impaction is accentuated when the joint is subjected to the action of the back muscles.[145] If the extending force continues to be applied, especially unilaterally, the superior facets can pivot on their inferior counterparts, producing a strain on the opposite zygapophysial joint, and potentially damaging or tearing the capsule.[63]

> ### Clinical Pearl
>
> Repetitive contact of the spinous processes during the extremes of lumbar extension can lead to a periostitis called *kissing spine* or *Baastrup's disease*,[146] with resulting ligamentous laxity and hypermobility of the segment.[147]

An anterior pelvic tilt increases the lumbar lordosis and results in an anterior motion of the vertebrae and their associated structures. Although the differing terminology between true extension and the extension created by increasing the lordosis is seemingly esoteric, there are clinical implications during the examination, when the clinician is assessing the ability of the patient to assume the extended position of the lumbar spine.

Pure lumbar extension is limited by:

▶ The ability of structures anterior to the fulcrum to be elongated.

▶ The ability of the IVD to allow compression.

▶ Joint capsule tension.

▶ Passive tension of the psoas major muscle.

Axial Rotation

Rotational movements of the lumbar spine do appear to produce the appropriate motor patterns for optimal trunk muscle co-contraction and spinal stability.[148,149] The axis of rotation passes through the aspect of the IVD and vertebral body.[150] Axial rotation of the lumbar spine amounts to approximately 13 degrees to both sides. The greatest amount of segmental rotation, about 5 degrees, occurs at the L5 and S1 segment. Axial rotation of the segment involves:

▶ Twisting, or torsion, of the IVD fibers.

▶ Compression of the contralateral zygapophysial joint. For example, with left axial rotation, the right inferior zygapophysial joint will impact on the superior zygapophysial joint of the bone below.

▶ Stress on those annular fibers inclined toward the direction of rotation.

In normal segments, the zygapophysial joints protect the IVD from torsional injuries by coming into contact before microfailure of the IVD can occur. During axial rotation, tension is built in the interspinous and supraspinous ligaments, and the contralateral joint becomes impacted after 1 to 2 degrees of rotation.[151] Further movement is accommodated by compression of the articular cartilage. If this range is exceeded, any further rotation that occurs is impure. Impure rotation of the segment forces the upper vertebra to pivot backward on the impacted joint, around the newly created axis of rotation. This causes the vertebra to swing laterally and backward, increasing the potential for a lateral shear force on the annulus. At this extreme, the IVD is vulnerable to either torsional and shear forces, and the other joint capsule is placed under severe tension.[152] This combination can result in a failure of any one of these structures, resulting in any or all of the following: compression fractures of the contralateral lamina, subchondral fractures, fragmentation of the articular surface and tearing, avulsion of the ipsilateral joint capsule, or a pars interarticularis fracture.[63]

The ipsilateral joint does not normally gap during normal axial rotation, except during therapeutic manipulation.[153] Abnormal gapping has been found to occur in segments with degenerative or traumatic instability, questioning the role of therapeutic manipulation in such cases.[153]

Side Bending

Side bending of the spine is a coupled movement involving rotation. The means of how this is achieved has been the subject of debate for many years and it is difficult to ascertain how an impaired segment would behave, compared with a healthy one[154] (see the Section III introduction).

Axial Loading (Compression)

Although the IVD bears most of the compressive load of the spine in the neutral position and in the very early ranges of flexion and extension, the zygapophysial joints bear up to 25 percent of the compressive load in the middle ranges of extension.[155] The contribution of the zygapophysial joints becomes more significant during prolonged weight bearing, in the presence of IVD space narrowing, or if lumbar extension is combined with rotation.[155] In intradiscal pressure studies and electromyographic measurements of trunk muscles, in conjunction with mathematical models, investigators have estimated the compressive load on the lumbar spine to reach 1000 newtons (N) during standing and walking.[156] The compressive load on the lumbar spine is substantially higher in many lifting activities and is estimated to reach several thousand newtons.[157,158]

In the sagittal plane, when a compressive load is applied to a whole lumbar spine specimen along a vertical path, bending moments are induced because of the inherent curvature of the lumbar spine. As a result, the spine undergoes large changes in its curvature at relatively small load levels. Countless studies over the years have demonstrated that a neutral spine under compressive load results in bony failure,[159] specifically endplate fracture, and damage to the underlying trabeculae,[160] and that repeated loading reduces the ultimate strength of the end plate and can cause damage to other tissues.[161,162] A burst fracture is a vertebral fracture resulting from axial impact.[163]

> ### Clinical Pearl
>
> It is well known that during periods when the osmotic pressure within the IVD is greater than the hydrostatic pressure from axial loading (e.g., when lying in bed) the disks imbibe fluid, causing the spine to increase in length.[164–166] Patients with disk injuries should thus be advised to avoid performing full-range spinal motions (bending) shortly after rising from bed.[167,168]

Neutral Zone

From the mechanical point of view, the spinal system is highly complex and statically highly indeterminate. The *neutral zone* is a term used by Panjabi[169] to define a region of laxity around the neutral resting position of a spinal segment. The neutral zone is the position of the segment in which minimal loading is occurring in the passive structures (IVD, zygapophysial joints, and ligaments) and the active structures (the muscles and tendons that surround and control spinal motion), and within which spinal motion is produced with minimal internal resistance.[63]

Tencer and Ahmed[170] and Wilder and colleagues[171] refer to a similar concept termed a *balance point*. The balance point for a single lumbar motion segment is defined as the point of application of a compressive load that minimizes coupled flexion-extension rotations caused by the segmental bending moment.

> ### Clinical Pearl
>
> The size of the neutral zone, or balance point is determined by the integrity of the passive restraint and active control systems, which in turn are controlled by the neural system.[169]

The effectiveness of the passive support system is a factor of the ability of the ligaments, IVD, and the zygapophysial joints to resist the forces of translation, compression, and torsion. Studies have demonstrated that a larger than normal neutral zone, resulting from an accumulation of microtrauma, is related to a lack of segmental muscle control and is associated with intersegmental injury and IVD degeneration.[103,169,172–174]

Because the passive system of the spine is known to be unstable at loads far less than that of body weight,[175,176] the active and neural system must fulfill the role of maintaining postural stability, while simultaneously controlling and initiating movement.

Panjabi and colleagues[103] have studied the effect of intersegmental muscle forces on the neutral zone and range of motion of a lumbar functional spinal unit subjected to pure moments in flexion-extension, side bending, and rotation. Simulated muscle forces were applied to the spinous process of the mobile vertebra of a single motion segment using two equal and symmetric force vectors directed laterally, anteriorly, and

inferiorly. The simulated muscle force maintained or decreased the motions of the lumbar segment for intact and injured specimens with the exception of the flexion range of motion, which increased.[103]

The more recent research of Gardner-Morse and colleagues[177] and O'Sullivan and associates[178] lends support to the hypothesis of a balance point or neutral zone. They concluded that factors such as pathologic reduction in motion segment stiffness, as well as poor neuromuscular control of the spinal musculature and reduction of muscle activity, could result in a state of spinal instability.

Cholewicki and McGill[97] also reported that lumbar stability is maintained in vivo by increasing the activity (stiffness) of the lumbar segmental muscles, and they highlighted the importance of motor control to coordinate muscle recruitment between large trunk muscles and small intrinsic muscles during functional activities, to ensure stability is maintained. It is hypothesized that any change in activation may lead to increased spinal compression forces, which have been recognized as a risk factor for vertebral end-plate fracture, especially if applied repetitively.[179,180] An alternate consequence is that muscle insufficiency resulting from fatigue may shift the loading to passive tissues,[181,182] which may put the spine at increased risk of injury.

> ### Clinical Pearl
>
> Activities such as acute repetitive loading have been shown to have a significant effect on reducing the stiffness of the passive tissues of the lumbar spine, because of the viscoelastic nature of the muscles, tendons, ligaments, and IVDs.[183,184]

Intra-abdominal pressure also is thought to provide stability to the lumbar spine,[185–189] but the exact principles have yet to be specified.

The concept of different trunk muscles playing differing roles in the provision of dynamic stability to the spine was proposed by Bergmark,[190] and later refined by others.[97,98,148,191–193] The muscles of the lumbar spine can be classified functionally as either mobilizers or stabilizers.[192,193]

▶ Mobilizers function to produce movement in the sagittal plane using concentric acceleration. This particular muscle group can generate a tremendous amount of force.

▶ Stabilizers can be further divided into global and local stabilizers.[190] Global stabilizers have a role in eccentrically decelerating momentum, and controlling rotation of the spine as a whole. In contrast, the local stabilizers function to maintain a continuous low-force activity at joints in all positions and directions, and thus provide segmental joint support.

Global Muscle System

This system consists of muscles whose origins are on the pelvis and whose insertions are on the thoracic cage. These muscles include:

▶ Rectus abdominis.

▶ Internal and external obliques.

▶ Lateral fibers of the quadratus lumborum.

▶ Thoracic part of the lumbar iliocostalis.

The global muscle system acts on the trunk and spine, without being directly attached to it. These muscles appear to provide general trunk stabilization but are not capable of having a direct segmental influence on the spine. Cholewicki and McGill demonstrated that the quadratus lumborum was architecturally best suited to be the major stabilizer of the lumbar spine.[97]

Local Muscle System

The local muscle system consists of muscles that have insertions or origins at the lumbar vertebrae or pelvis and are responsible for providing segmental stability and directly controlling the lumbar segments and sacroiliac joint (see Chap. 27). These muscles include:

▶ Lumbar portions of the iliocostalis and longissimus thoracis muscles.

▶ Medial fibers of the quadratus lumborum.

▶ Diaphragm.

▶ Lumbar multifidus.

▶ Pelvic floor muscles (see Chap. 27).

▶ Transversus abdominis.

▶ Posterior fibers of the internal oblique that attach to the tensor fascia latae.

The local muscle system is important for the provision of segmental control to the spine and provides an important stiffening effect on the lumbar spine, thereby enhancing its dynamic stability.[194]

Richardson and colleagues[148] have proposed that a pressure cylinder is formed by the muscles of the local group. Under this proposal, the transversus abdominis forms the wall of the cylinder, and the muscles of the pelvic floor and diaphragm form the base and lid, respectively (Fig. 25-11). Under this system, the intra-abdominal pressure group is maintained at a level that provides spinal support (see later discussion).[112,148,187,195]

Transversus Abdominis. Recent research indicates that the transverse abdominis may have a presetting role, because it is the first trunk muscle to become active before movement initiation,[196] or perturbation.[186] Together with the internal oblique, the transversus abdominis is primarily active in providing rotational and lateral control to the spine while maintaining adequate levels of intra-abdominal pressure and imparting tension to the thoracolumbar fascia. This has the effect of increasing the stiffness of the lumbar spine.[185]

Hodges and associates[195] have made an association between the timing of the activity of the transversus abdominis and the diaphragm in motor control studies of trunk muscle activity in a

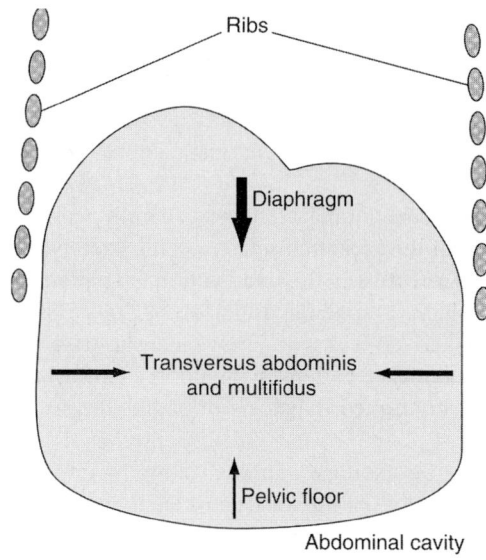

FIGURE 25-11 Local muscle system. (Reproduced with permission from Richardson CA, Jull GA, Hodges P, et al. *Therapeutic Exercise for Spinal Segmental Stabilization in Low Back Pain.* London, England: Churchill Livingstone; 1999:95.)

stabilization model. Their study found that a co-activation of the diaphragm and abdominal muscles produces a sustained increase in intra-abdominal pressure.[195]

Multifidus. The lumbar multifidus is considered to have the greatest potential to provide dynamic control to the motion segment, particularly in its neutral zone.[102,197] In a biomechanical study, Wilke and colleagues found that the lumbar multifidi are responsible for more than two thirds of the stiffness at the L4 to L5 segmental level.[174]

The lumbar multifidus, transversus abdominis, and the posterior fibers of the internal oblique are known to be tonically active during upright postures and active motions of the trunk,[198] with the transversus abdominis capable of tonic activity irrespective of trunk position, direction of movement, or loading of the spine.[185]

Breakdown of the System

As with any system, the potential for breakdown exists. In normal subjects with no history of LBP, the transverse abdominis, erector spinae, and obliques internus abdominis are recruited just prior to any limb movement.[199] Several studies indicate that the deep abdominal muscles undergo changes in their functional performance in populations with LBP.[199–201] These studies have shown that it is the local system that is particularly vulnerable to breakdown. In particular, the prevalence of LBP is being attributed to inhibition and atrophy of the multifidi and transverse abdominis, and the resultant poor neutral zone stabilization, although the reasons as to why these two muscles become inhibited and atrophied is unclear.[200,202–205]

Studies also have described subtle changes or shifts in the pattern of abdominal muscle activation in subjects with chronic LBP, in whom there is an overriding activation of the rectus abdominis during attempts to preferentially recruit the deep abdominal muscles.[206] These changes in the activation patterns result in altered patterns of synergistic control or coordination of the trunk muscles.[201,207]

Whereas conventional exercises generally work to increase the strength of the global muscles, specific exercises have been shown to be effective in the intervention for patients with LBP associated with a specific diagnosis.[54–61,178] For example, O'Sullivan and colleagues[178] have demonstrated decreased pain and disability in patients with chronic LBP who have a radiologically confirmed diagnosis of spondylolysis or spondylolisthesis.

The specific exercise approach aims to improve the dynamic stability role of the local muscles in providing stiffness to the segments of the spine and pelvis during functional postures and movements. These exercises also have proven beneficial in LBP conditions arising from the pelvic region[112,208] (see Chap. 27).

Examination

LBP can arise from a number of local structures in the lumbar spine, and from a number of sources more distal (see Chap. 9). *Idiopathic* and *nonspecific* LBP have emerged as catchall terms in the diagnosis of low back dysfunction. Indeed, up to 85 percent of patients cannot be given a definitive diagnosis because of weak associations among symptoms, pathologic changes, and imaging results.[209,210] Muscle aches, muscle sprains, tendonitis, sacroiliac and low back strain, lumbago, mechanical LBP, and lumbar strain are just some of the diagnoses currently in clinical use. This difficulty in determining a specific diagnosis stems from a variety of reasons, including the fact that multiple structures in one or more segments may be involved. These structures include the interconnecting ligaments, the outer fibers of the annulus fibrosus, zygapophysial joints, vertebral periosteum, paravertebral musculature and fascia, blood vessels, and spinal nerve roots.[209]

The physical examination of the lumbar spine must include a thorough assessment of the neuromuscular, vascular, and orthopaedic systems of the hip, lower extremities, low back, and pelvic region.[211]

History

The clinician should establish the chief complaint of the patient, in addition to the location, behavior, irritability, and severity of the symptoms. Although dysfunctions of the lumbar spine are very difficult to diagnose, the history can provide some very important clues. Applying the principles and rationale outlined in Chapter 8, the clinician uses the history to help with differential diagnosis (see Chap. 9). The clinician should explore the following factors.

Patient Age. Spondylolisthesis is more common among 10- to 20-year-olds.[212,213] Cancer, compression fractures, spinal and lateral recess stenosis, and aortic aneurysms are more common among patients older than 65 years of age.[214,215] Inflammatory spondyloarthropathy is most common in the 15- to 40-year-old age group,[209] and IVD lesions are more common in this group as well.[216] Osteoarthritis and spondylosis are more common in the 45 and older age group.[213]

Occupation. Flexion and rotation of the trunk, lifting, axial loading, sustained flexed postures, vibration, and low job satisfaction are all considered as risk factors for back pain.[217–219] The level of impairment or disability that a lesion produces is related to the type of work performed. For example, discodural back pain produces more disability in a truck driver who has to sit the whole day than in a patient who has light and varying work. For some patients, normal activities are unrestricted but their favorite sport is impossible.[213]

Mechanism of Injury. The mechanism of injury for the lumbar spine usually involves lifting, bending, or twisting, or a combination of all three.[14] However, postural ligamentous pain tends to be more frequent in patients who stand for long periods at work.[220] If an obvious cause is reported, the clinician should confirm the direction, amount, and duration of any forces involved. The forces applied to the lumbar spine and IVD vary according to the task or position of the body (Table 25-2).

Onset and History of Symptoms. When did the problem begin, how long has the patient had the problem, and have similar episodes occurred in the past? Low back disorders may be acute, chronic, or recurrent. If possible, the clinician should attempt to order the onset of symptoms chronologically, and then determine what has occurred to the symptoms since the onset. In general, a sudden onset of pain associated with an activity or movement suggests a ligament, muscle, or IVD as the source, whereas a gradual onset of symptoms suggests a degenerative process or a lesion that is increasing in size, such as a neuroma or neoplasm.[213]

The frequency of the episodes often can give the clinician an indication of severity. Stable episodes of symptoms (e.g., symptoms that only occur every few years and do not change

TABLE 25-2 Intradiskal Pressures and Forces Generated by Common Tasks[156,175,176]

Task	Total Load (kg)*
Lying supine	25
Side lying	75
Standing	150
Bending at waist in standing position	200
Sitting	175
Bending at waist in sitting position	225

*Represents total load on third lumbar disk in a 70-kg subject.

much in severity with each episode) are generally easier to treat than episodes that occur daily or weekly and appear to be worsening. If the patient has had previous similar episodes, the clinician should elicit whether the patient had interventions in the past and, if so, what was the response of the patient to these previous interventions.

Location of Pain at Present.　　Back pain may be localized centrally, unilaterally, or bilaterally. Generally speaking, the stronger the stimulus, the larger the area of pain reference. As the stimulus intensity decreases, the referred pain area becomes smaller, and localization of the pain by the patient becomes easier. The distribution of the pain should be described by the patient and outlined on a pain diagram. Central back pain is unlikely to be caused by a unilateral structure, such as a zygapophysial joint or the sacroiliac joint, and bilateral pain hardly ever has a central origin (one of the exceptions being a central IVD protrusion).[221]

▶　An inflammation of the zygapophysial joints can cause local back pain or buttock pain,[222] but it also has been associated with pain referred into the buttocks and even below the knee.[130,133,223]

▶　Groin pain, although also associated with hip pathology, is a complaint often present in patients with a high lumbar IVD herniation[224] (see Chap. 20). Upon questioning, patients with this form of groin pain often describe the pain as a dull ache lying deep beneath the skin, which they usually find difficult to localize with any degree of accuracy. Although the patient with a high lumbar IVD herniation often reports pain and numbness on physical examination, the clinician is often unable to discern any objective findings, such as tenderness, muscle weakness, or hypesthesia, except perhaps occasionally a slight hyperalgesia.[224]

▶　Leg pain reported by the patient may indicate a radiculopathy or a pseudoradiculopathy. A radiculopathy results from irritation of a spinal nerve (see Chap. 20). A pseudoradiculopathy, as its name suggests, is pain that is radicular in distribution, but is caused by something other than an irritated spinal nerve. Examples of a pseudoradiculopathy include referred pain and symptoms produced by a facilitated segment.[225] Despite the obvious differences in pathology, pseudoradiculopathy and radiculopathy have the common elements of dermatomal pain, diminished reflexes, muscle weakness, and positive nerve provocation tests.[133,225,226] Distinguishing between the two is, therefore, difficult. In general, unilateral pain with no referral below the knee may be caused by the lumbosacral structures other than the spinal nerves, whereas irritation of a spinal nerve may cause radicular symptoms below the knee.[227] On occasion, the patient may report feeling back pain more than leg pain, or vice versa. Patients who report a dominance of leg pain over back pain and whose symptoms are worsened with flexion of the lumbar spine most likely have nerve root irritation caused by an IVD herniation[227] (see Chap. 20). Patients

with bilateral root pain should be suspected of having spondylolisthesis, bilateral stenosis of the lateral spinal recesses, a narrowed spinal canal, or malignant disease.[213]

Type and Behavior of Symptoms.　　Questions related to the type and behavior of symptoms can help determine the structure involved and the stage of healing. It is important to determine whether the condition is improving or worsening. Constant pain indicates an inflammatory process. Steadily increasing pain, especially in elderly patients, may indicate malignancy.[213] Pain that is gradually expanding and increasing is associated with a lesion that is increasing in size, such as a neuroma or neoplasm.[213] Pain with movement suggests a mechanical cause of pain. If the muscles and ligaments are involved, activity will tend to decrease the pain, but the pain will worsen with repeated movements or sustained positions as the structures become fatigued or overstressed.[228,229] Dural pain tends to be diffuse, vague, and spreads upward to the chest or downward to the thighs.[221]

Symptoms of lumbosacral pathology can demonstrate a phenomenon of centralization and peripheralization.[228,230,231] Centralization of symptoms is the progressive retreat of the most distal extent of referred or radicular pain toward the lumbar spine midline. Peripheralization of symptoms indicates movement in the opposite direction. Centralization of the symptoms normally indicates improvement in the patient's condition.[232]

Diurnal or Nocturnal Variation in Symptoms.　　Complaints of morning stiffness may indicate an IVD lesion, osteoarthritis, ankylosing spondylitis, or Scheuermann's disease.

Positions or Activities That Aggravate or Relieve Symptoms (Table 25-3).　　Information about the activities or positions that aggravate or relieve the symptoms provides the clinician with an insight as to whether the patient has a mechanically related disorder or one that is nonmechanical.

In postural syndromes, the symptoms are usually increased by maintenance of a particular posture and relieved by altering the position. For example, if the patient complains of pain with standing with the feet together, the cause of the pain could be stresses on the structures caused by an increased lordosis, especially if the pain is reduced by placing one foot in front of the

TABLE 25-3　　Relieving Positions or Movements

Relieving Position or Movement	Probable Cause
Flexion	Facet joint involvement Low back strain Lateral stenosis
Extension	Disk involvement Nerve root irritation (disk herniation)
Rest	Neurogenic claudication

other, or if the pain is reduced when the lumbar lordosis is reduced with an active posterior pelvic tilt. Pain that is relieved by sitting and forward bending but aggravated by walking may indicate a zygapophysial joint problem, spondylolisthesis (in the younger patient), or lateral recess or spinal stenosis (in the elderly patient). Pain that is aggravated by sitting, stooping, or lifting, but is relieved by recumbency, and is not increased by brief periods of standing and walking may indicate an IVD lesion such as a protrusion or an annular tear.[233] If walking increases the symptoms, a lumbar extension dysfunction is probably the cause. Coughing and sneezing produce an increase in intra-abdominal pressure, which in turn causes a sudden expansion of the dura. In patients with an IVD protrusion, this expansion of the dura often causes an increase in symptoms. Pain with coughing and sneezing also occurs in patients with active sacroiliitis, because the sudden increase in intra-abdominal pressure produces a painful distraction of the sacroiliac joints.[221]

Once the motion or position that reduces the symptoms is identified, the initial focus of the intervention is teaching the patient strategies that encourage this motion or posture.

Patient's Sleeping Position. Depending on the size of the patient, prone lying tends to compress the posterior structures and aggravate a zygapophysial extension dysfunction. Persistent or progressive pain in supine lying may indicate a neurogenic or space-occupying lesion, such as an infection, swelling, or tumor. It may also indicate a zygapophysial extension dysfunction, especially if the patient has marked adaptive shortening of the hip flexors and rectus femoris.

Patient's General Health and Past Medical History. This component includes checking for a family history of rheumatoid arthritis, IVD lesions,[234] diabetes, osteoporosis, and vascular disease.

Impact of Symptoms. The effect the symptoms have on the patient's work, daily activities, and recreational pursuits can be assessed using the functional assessment tests outlined later.

Medication Use. Pain medications can mask symptoms. If the patient reports taking pain medication prior to the examination, the clinician may not obtain a true response to pain from the patient.

Clinical Pearl

In general, pain that is worse in the lower extremity than in the low back indicates a nerve root irritation, whereas pain that is worse in the low back than in the lower extremity is probably referred from a spinal structure.[235]

Systems Review

It must always be remembered that pain can be referred to the lumbar spine area from pathologic conditions in other regions. For example, reports of pain in the upper lumbar region could suggest the possibility of aortic thrombosis, neoplasm, chronic appendicitis,[236] ankylosing spondylitis, or visceral disease (see Chap. 9).

The clinician should determine whether there has been any recent and unexplained weight loss, night pain that is unrelated to movement, or changes in bowel and bladder function. Any one of these findings may indicate the presence of a serious pathology:

▶ Unexplained weight loss or night pain not associated with movement may indicate a malignancy. In many patients whose LBP is caused by infection or cancer, the pain is not relieved when the patient lies down.[237] However, this finding is not specific for the presence of these conditions.[209]

▶ Bowel or bladder dysfunction may be a symptom of severe compression of the cauda equina (cauda equina syndrome). This rare condition usually is caused by a tumor or a massive midline IVD herniation. Urinary retention with overflow incontinence is usually present, often in association with sensory loss in a saddle distribution, bilateral sciatica, and leg weakness.[209] This condition constitutes a medical emergency.

Tests and Measures

Observation

Observation involves an analysis of the entire patient in terms of how he or she moves and responds, in addition to the positions the patient adopts. Although spinal alignment provides some valuable information, a positive correlation has not been made between abnormal alignment and pain.[16,238] "Good posture" is a subjective term based on what the clinician believes to be correct, and it is highly variable.

Posterior Aspect. The shoulders and pelvis should appear fairly level, and the bony and soft tissue contours should appear symmetric. There should be no differences in the muscle bulk between both sides and regions of the erector spinae. Atrophy of the paraspinals is rare but may indicate a chronic inflammatory disease, such as ankylosing spondylitis or tuberculosis, or point to poliomyelitis or a myopathy.[221] If atrophy of the paravertebral or extremity muscles is present, the clinician must determine whether it follows a segmental or nonsegmental pattern. A predominance of the thoracolumbar portion of the erector spinae may indicate poor stabilization of this area[139] or a rotational asymmetry.[239] Asymmetric spasm of the paraspinals or gluteal muscles can make them appear more prominent compared with the normal side. The presence of spasm should alert the clinician to the presence of sciatica or a serious disease.[221]

Structural asymmetry in the lumbar region often is associated with pain. The angles of the scapulae should be level with the seventh thoracic spinous process; the iliac crests should be level.[240] The posterior superior iliac spines, medial malleoli, and lateral malleoli should all be level with their counterparts on the opposite side. Differences between the two sides may indicate a functional limb-length discrepancy. This discrepancy can be caused by altered bone length, altered mechanics, or joint dysfunction[241] (Table 25-4).

The thoracic and lumbar vertebrae should be vertically aligned. Curvature of the spine is referred to as *scoliosis*. The currently accepted definition of scoliosis is a 10-degree lateral curvature with vertebral rotation on a radiograph of the spine taken with the patient standing upright.[242] This definition is based on the fact that a graph of lateral spinal curvature of the general population is a smooth exponential function in which the sharpest change in slope occurs at 10 degrees.[243] Despite this reasonable approach to the definition of the disease state, it results in an extremely high prevalence of the disorder in the general population of 2 to 3 percent.[244] Scoliosis can be found in four forms: static, sciatic, idiopathic, and psychogenic. The latter cause is self-explanatory.

▶ *Static.* Static, or structural, scoliosis in adults may be caused by a leg-length difference (see Chap. 27), a hemivertebra, osteoporosis, osteomalacia, or compression fractures. If a platform under the heel of the shorter limb eases or even abolishes the symptoms while standing or on lumbar flexion or extension, a shoe lift is advised.[221,245]

▶ *Sciatic.* The sight of a patient with a pelvic shift or list is relatively common in patients presenting with LBP. The sciatic, or nonstructural, lumbar scoliosis results from sciatic pain caused by lumbar disk herniation a unilateral spasm of the back muscles (see Chap. 20). Sciatic scoliosis usually occurs with convexity to the symptomatic side of the herniated disk.[246] The shift is thought to result from the body finding a position of comfort and protection as a consequence of an irritation of a spinal nerve or its dural sleeve,[247] although the neuronal mechanisms of sciatic scoliosis have not been well clarified. These postural changes cannot be relieved by voluntary efforts but usually disappear after alleviation of the sciatic pain.[246] The extent of a scoliosis should be noted if it is thought to be contributing to the patient's symptoms and is occurring because of pain or dysfunction. An attempt should be made to manually correct the shift to ascertain whether this can be done

painlessly (see Chap. 20). A compensatory shift or scoliosis is often easy and painless to correct.[248,249]

▶ *Idiopathic.* The curve of an idiopathic scoliosis, present since childhood, differs from the tilt of the spine associated with recent IVD problems in that it is accompanied by a lower thoracic or lumbar rotation deformity.[221] If this deformity is not obvious in the standing posture, it should become obvious during flexion as it is manifested by the so-called *razor back eminence* of the thoracic cage.

Deformity, birthmarks, and hairy patches are all evidence of congenital deficits of the integumentary system, and can indicate underlying anomalies in the systems derived from the same embryologic segments.[250] A hairy patch or tuft that is located at the base of the lumbar spine, may indicate spina bifida occulta or diastematomyelia.[251]

Lateral Aspect. From the side, the clinician should observe the amount of lumbar lordosis and note whether it is excessive or reduced. The lumbar lordosis should appear as a smooth and gentle curve, and there should be a gradual transition at the thoracolumbar junction.

▶ An excessive lordosis may result in the pelvic crossed syndrome.[139] In this syndrome, the erector spinae and the iliopsoas are found to be adaptively shortened, and the abdominal and gluteus maximus muscles are found to be weak. As a result, this syndrome can produce adaptive shortening of the posterior longitudinal ligament, lower back extensors, and hip flexor muscles, and lengthening of the anterior longitudinal ligament and lower abdominals. An excessive lordosis also may indicate that the patient has a spondylolisthesis. With this condition, the whole spine often lies in a plane anterior to the sacrum. There may also be an associated mid- or low-lumbar shelf at the spinous processes, which if not visible, can be palpated. An anterior pelvic tilt posture also may be caused by weakness of the abdominal muscles or an adaptively shortened iliopsoas or thoracolumbar fascia, with subsequent lengthening of the hamstring and gluteal muscles.[139]

▶ A flattened back may indicate that the patient has either lumbar spinal stenosis or a lateral recessed stenosis. A flattened lordosis is caused by a posterior pelvic tilt, adaptive shortening of the hamstrings, and weakness of the hip flexor muscles.[139]

▶ A reversed lordosis, often referred to as a *sway back,* is caused by a thoracic kyphosis and a posterior pelvic tilt. This posture results in a stretching of the anterior hip ligaments, back extensors, and hip flexors; hip hyperextension; and compression of the vertebrae posteriorly.[139] Kyphosis of the lumbar spine also may indicate damage to the supraspinous ligament complex.

The type of footwear that the patient habitually wears can be a factor. For example, high-heeled footwear has a tendency to modify the pelvic angle and increase the lordosis.[252]

TABLE 25-4 Causes of Functional Limb-length Difference

Joint	Apparent Lengthening	Apparent Shortening
Sacroiliac	Anterior rotation	Posterior rotation
Hip	Lowering Extension External rotation	Hiking Flexion Internal rotation
Knee	—	Flexion Valgus Varus
Foot	Supination	Pronation

Gait. The patient's gait should be assessed. Upper lumbar or thoracolumbar instability or hypermobility often can lead to facilitation of the upper lumbar segments, with resulting psoas hypertonicity.[225,253] This may lead to reduced hip extension during gait, resulting in a shortened stride length on the involved side.[110] Body weight and ground reaction forces, generated by rapid walking, can equalize the stride length by hypermobilizing or destabilizing the lumbosacral junction or the ipsilateral sacroiliac joint.[110] The process is reinforced by the mechanical pull of the shortened psoas, and this increases the stress on the upper lumbar spine, increasing the facilitation.

Palpation

There is some disagreement as to when in the examination the palpation assessment should occur, with some authors preferring to perform this portion at the end.[254] Whenever it is performed, palpation of the lumbar spine area should be performed in a systematic manner, and in conjunction with palpation of the pelvic area, which is described in Chapter 27, and the hip area which is described in Chapter 17.

In most individuals, the midpoint of an imaginary line drawn between the iliac crests represents the L4 to L5 interspace and the level of the L4 transverse process. The transverse processes of L3, L2, and L1 each lie two fingerbreadths superior to the vertebra, respectively.[255] Alternatively, they can be found at the level of the lower pole of the spinous process of the vertebra immediately above or below. The lumbar zygapophysial joints of each motion segment are located approximately 2 to 3 cm (0.8 to 1.2 inches) lateral from the spinous processes. The reference point indicating the position of L4 is marked on the patient. The spinous process of L5 is just inferior to this point. The L5 spinous process is short, sharp, and thick compared with those of L4 and L3. The clinician should move superiorly from the L5 spinous process, carefully palpating each segmental level. Evidence of tenderness, altered temperature, muscle spasm, or abnormal alignment during palpation can highlight an underlying impairment.

Posterior Aspect. Palpation of the posterior aspect of the lumbar spine is best achieved by placing the patient in a relaxed prone position, or bent over the treatment table.

▶ The clinician moves the index and middle fingers quickly down the spine, feeling for any abnormal projections or asymmetries of the spinous processes. Any alterations in the alignment of the spinous processes in a posteroanterior direction, particularly at the L4 to L5 or L5 to S1 segmental level, may indicate the presence of a spondylolisthesis.[256] Specific pain elicited with posteroanterior pressure over the segment serves as further confirmation. Asymmetry of the spinous processes in a posteroanterior direction also may indicate wedging of a vertebral body or a complete loss of two adjacent IVD spaces.[221] Absence of a spinous process may be associated with spina bifida. Side-to-side alterations in the spinous process may indicate the presence of a rotational asymmetry of the vertebra.[239]

▶ The supraspinous ligaments should be palpated. The ligament is usually supple, springy, and nontender. Because this ligament is the most superficial of the spinal ligaments and farthest from the axis of flexion, it has a greater potential for sprains.[89]

▶ Palpation of the transverse processes of T12 and L5 presents difficulties. That of L3 is easy to feel, being usually the longest of all transverse processes; it is usually possible to feel those of L1, L2, and L4. That of L5 is covered by the posterior ilium.[257]

▶ Patients with localized tenderness over the zygapophysial joints without other root tension signs or neurologic signs may have zygapophysial joint pain.[258] This source can be confirmed if the patient responds well to intra-articular joint injections or to blocks of the medial branches of the dorsal rami.[258,259]

▶ A well-localized and tender point at the gluteal level of the iliac crest, 8 to 10 cm from the midline, may indicate the presence of Maigne's syndrome.[249] Maigne's syndrome is characterized by sacroiliac joint, low lumbar, and gluteal pain, with occasional referral to the thigh, laterally or posteriorly.

▶ Normally the skin can be rolled over the spine and gluteal region with ease. Tightness or pain produced with skin rolling may indicate some underlying pathology.[260] The source of the signs and symptoms is an irritation of the medial cutaneous branch of dorsal rami of the T12 or L1 spinal nerves as it passes through a fibro-osseous tunnel at the iliac crest.[249]

Anterior Aspect

▶ The inguinal area, located between the anterior superior iliac spine and the symphysis pubis, should be palpated carefully for evidence of tenderness, which may be indicative of a hernia, an abscess, sprain of the ligament, or an infection, if the lymph nodes are swollen and tender.

▶ In some patients, the anterior aspect of the vertebral bodies may be palpable when the patient is positioned supine with the hips flexed and feet flat on the bed. Tenderness of the anterior aspect of the vertebral bodies may indicate an irritation of the anterior longitudinal ligament, which may indicate the presence of an anterior instability.[59]

Active Movement Testing

Normal active motion, which demonstrates considerable variability between individuals, involves fully functional contractile and inert tissues and optimal neurologic function[154,261–264] (Table 25-5). However, it is the quality of motion and the symptoms provoked, rather than the quantity of motion, that are more important. The reproducibility (precision) of an individual's effort is one indicator of optimum effort. Measurements should not change significantly (more than 5 degrees) with repeated efforts.[265] The capsular pattern for the lumbar spine is normal trunk flexion, a decrease in lumbar extension with rotation, and side bending equally limited bilaterally.[266]

TABLE 25-5   Normal Active Range of Motion of the Lumbar Spine

Movement	Range
Flexion	40–60 degrees
Extension	20–35 degrees
Side bending	15–20 degrees
Axial rotation	3–18 degrees

A good view of the spine is essential during motion testing. External measurement of vertebral motion may not reflect the true intervertebral movement because of skin movement error,[267] but it is less invasive than a radiograph and more practical. Although limited spinal motion is not strongly associated with any specific diagnosis, this finding may help in the planning or monitoring of the physical therapy intervention.[209]

> ### Clinical Pearl
>
> Among the spinal motion tests, rotation, side bending, and fingertip-to-floor distance show the strongest associations with the severity of back pain.[268]

While standing, the patient performs flexion, extension, and side bending to both sides (Fig. 25-12A through D). If these motions fail to reproduce the symptoms, combined motions are introduced (see next section). The active range of motion tests should be observed in front of and behind the patient. At the end of each of the active motions, passive overpressure is applied to assess the end feel, and resistance tests are performed with the muscles in the lengthened positions.

The clinician should consider having the patient remain at the end range of each of the motion tests for 10 to 20 seconds, if sustained positions were reported to increase the symptoms. If repetitive or combined motions were reported in the history to increase the symptoms, the patient is asked to perform repeated motions. McKenzie[228] advocates the use of sustained or repeated movements of the spine in an attempt to affect nuclear position. These movements are performed to either peripheralize the symptoms lateral from the midline or distally down the extremity, or ideally to centralize the symptoms to a point more central or near midline. One study of 87 patients with leg and LBP[230] found that those patients who demonstrated excellent outcomes with the McKenzie-based interventions had reported centralization during the initial examination. Another study[231] found a significant correlation between positive diskograms and peripheralization and centralization, with the incidence of an adequate annulus being significantly greater in the centralizing patients with positive diskograms than in their peripheralizing counterparts.

During the active motions, the clinician notes the following:

▶ *Curve of the spine.*   The curve of the spine in flexion, extension, and side bending should be smooth. An angulation occurring during flexion or extension could indicate an area of instability or hypomobility. In side bending, an angulation indicates hypomobility below the level or hypermobility above the level in the lumbar spine.[260]

▶ *Presence of any deviations during or at the end of range.* Failure to recover from flexion smoothly may indicate instability.[269] This typically occurs at the end point of flexion as the patient begins to return to the erect stance and has to extend the lumbar spine by walking the hands up the thighs or by using a series of jerking motions.

▶ *Provocation of symptoms.*   The clinician should determine whether the symptoms are neurologic or non-neurologic, and how far the distribution of pain extends. Leg pain provoked by any motion other than flexion is not a good prognostic sign[266]; neither is posterior leg pain, reproduced with extension, rotation, or side bending, as this usually indicates a significant prolapse or extrusion (see Chap. 20).

▶ *Any gross limitations of motion.*   Gross limitation of both side bends may indicate ankylosing spondylitis or significant osteoarthritis.

▶ *Any compensatory motions.*

Flexion.   The first 60 degrees of forward bending, on the average, result from flexion of the lumbar motion segments, which is followed by an additional movement at the hip joints of about 25 degrees.[79] Methods to objectively measure lumbar flexion have included[262]:

▶ Measuring the distance from the fingertip to the floor after the patient bends forward. Because the contribution of hip movement in the fingertip-to-floor test has not been taken into account,[270] this test provides only a gross measurement of the lumbar flexion.

▶ The modified Schöber technique,[271] which measures the change in distance between two skin markings over the lumbar spine. A point is marked midway between the two posterior superior iliac spines, which is the level of S2. Points at 5 cm and 10 cm above that level are marked, and the distance between the three points is measured. The patient is asked to bend forward and the distance is remeasured. The distance between the two measurements is an indication of the amount of flexion occurring in the lumbar spine. This method also is prone to error, because it can measure only lower lumbar levels and may not reflect the amount of motion available in the whole lumbar spine.[272]

The more appropriate method for measuring lumbar flexion is the inclinometer technique recommended by the American Medical Association.[265] Inclinometers are small angle measuring devices that work like a plumb line, operating on the principle of gravity. An appropriate inclinometer should include a large enough dial to allow easy reading of 2-degree increments. The inclinometer technique can record regional movement of the lumbar spine rather than the combined movement of the spine and hip[273] and has been proved to correlate well with

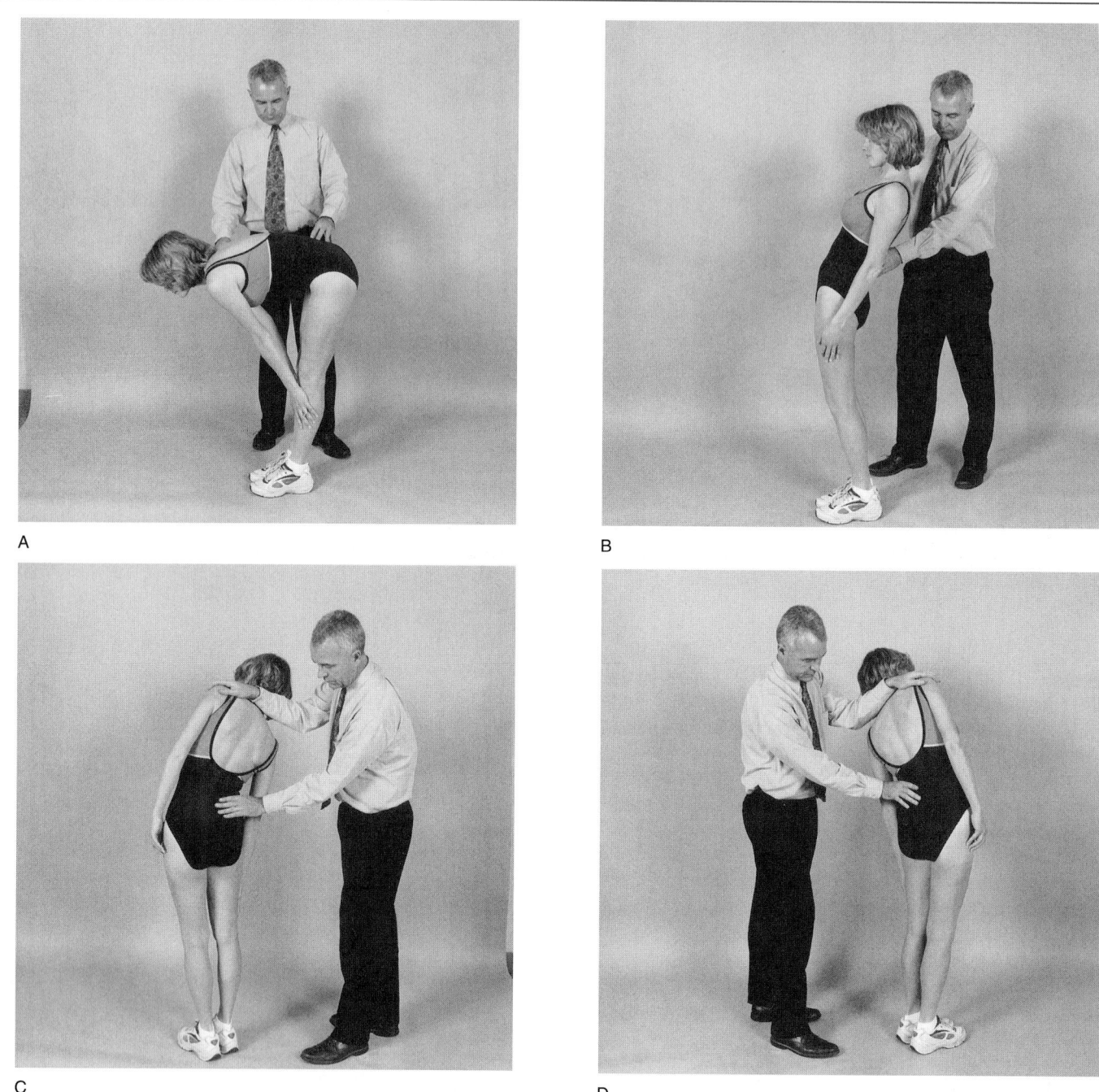

A

B

C

D

FIGURE 25-12 A–D   Active range of motion of the lumbar spine. (A) Flexion. (B) Extension. (C) Right side bending. (D) Left side bending.

measurements taken from a radiograph.[274,275] To measure lumbar flexion, two inclinometers are used, aligned in the sagittal plane. The center of the first inclinometer is placed over the T12 spinous process. The center of the second one is placed over the sacrum, midway between the posterior superior iliac spines. The patient is asked to flex the trunk as far as possible, and both inclinometer angles are recorded. The lumbar flexion angle is calculated by subtracting the sacral (hip) from the T12 inclinometer angle.

The lumbar flexion movement can be repeated with the patient sitting, as this test can help screen for the presence of rotoscoliosis.[244]

McKenzie[228] advocates the testing of lumbar flexion motion in supine as well as standing positions. In the standing position, flexion of the lumbar spine occurs from above downward, so pain at the end of the range is likely to indicate that L5 to S1 is affected. Bringing the knees to the chest in the supine position (Fig. 25-13) produces a flexion of the lumbar spine

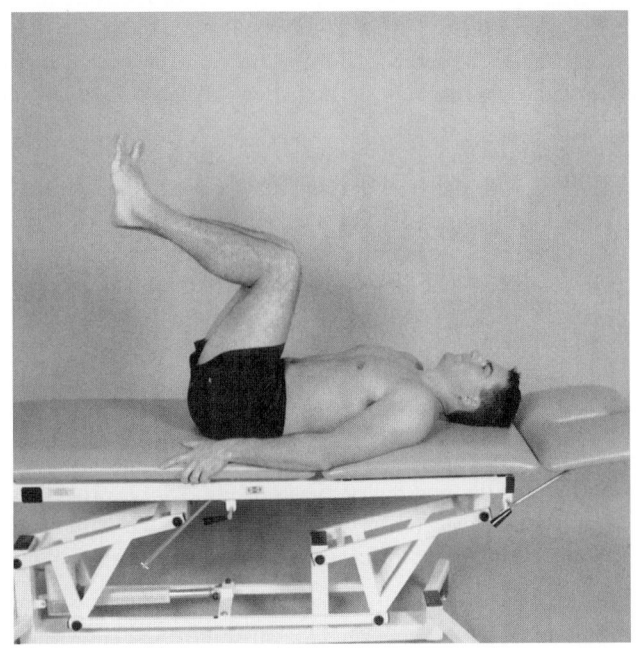

FIGURE 25-13   Lumbar flexion from below.

from below upward, so that pain at the beginning of the movement may indicate that L5 to S1 is affected.[228]

Trunk deviation during flexion is believed to be associated with an IVD herniation, with the direction of the deviation determined by the relative position of the compression on the nerve.[276] Deviations during flexion also may result from neuromeningeal adhesions, hypomobile segment(s) on the contralateral side, hypermobile segment(s) on the ipsilateral side, a structural scoliosis, and a shortened leg on the ipsilateral side.[276]

Extension.   The inclinometer technique also can be applied to the measurement of lumbar spine extension.[265] The same inclinometer positions described for flexion are used. The patient is asked to extend the trunk maximally (Fig. 25-12B). The lumbar extension angle is calculated by subtracting the sacral (hip) inclination from the T12 inclinometer angle.

Pure lumbar extension in standing involves the patient leaning back at the waist. Lumbar extension is often the stiffest and most uncomfortable movement for the patient. Thus, patients with LBP tend to utilize the protective guarding mechanism against the compression and shearing forces generated, by simply hyperextending the hips. By applying a compressive force through the patient's shoulders during the backward bending, the clinician can induce a small increase in the lumbar lordosis.

Side Bending.   Side bending range of motion has been found to be a good indicator of the degree of LBP[7] and disability.[8] In acute spinal derangements, such as a unilateral posterolateral IVD protrusion or unilateral zygapophysial joint derangement, lumbar side bending may be significantly reduced or absent on one side (usually toward the involved side). Arthritic conditions of the spine tend to demonstrate a symmetric loss of side bending to both sides.

The common method of measuring the amount of side bending is to record the distance between the fingertip and the floor at the end of the side bend, but this is merely an estimation of the flexibility of the whole spine rather than the lumbar spine.[262] Thus, it is recommended that lumbar spine movement in side bending be measured using the inclinometer technique.[265] As with the measuring of flexion-extension, two inclinometers are used, except that this time they are aligned in the frontal (coronal) plane over the T12 spinous process and sacrum (between the posterior superior iliac spines). The patient is asked to bend the trunk laterally, and both inclinometer angles are recorded. The lumbar side-bending angle is calculated by subtracting the sacral (hip) inclination from the T12 inclinometer angle.

The patient may be seen to lift one foot or bend the knees during the side-bending movements and should be reminded to maintain the feet on the floor during measurement. At the end of the side-bending motion, overpressure is applied on the shoulder opposite to the side bending to avoid any unnecessary compression (see Fig. 25-12C and 25-12D).

Axial Rotation.   Axial rotation of the spine usually is assessed in the sitting position to eliminate motion occurring from the hips. The patient, keeping the knees together, twists at the waist to each side. Axial rotation of the trunk commonly includes movement of both thoracic and lumbar segments of the spine. Overpressure may be applied at the end of range (Fig. 25-14). Normal range could indicate normalcy, hypermobility, or

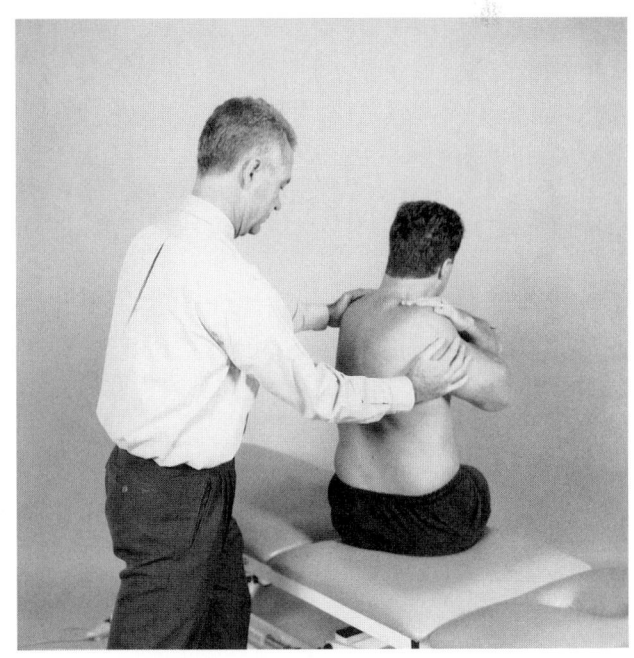

FIGURE 25-14   Lumbar rotation.

instability. Restricted range will be in either a capsular or non-capsular pattern. Pain with this maneuver can implicate a nonorganic source, an annular tear, a ligament tear, or a zygapophysial joint dysfunction.[276]

Combined Motion Testing. The combined motion tests of the lumbar spine are used to detect biomechanical impairments. Although combined motion tests do not provide information as to which segment is at fault, they may provide information as to which motion or position reproduces the pain.[277]

Combined motion tests can reproduce the pain in a structure that is either being compressed or stretched[278]:

▶ A reproduction or increase in symptoms with flexion and side bending away from the side of the symptoms may implicate pain in a structure that is being stretched.

▶ A reproduction or increase in symptoms with extension and side bending toward the side of the symptoms may implicate pain in a structure that is being compressed.

Combined motions can be performed as repetitive motions or as sustained positioning. For example, the patient can be asked to repetitively perform the combined motion of flexion and right side bending to assess for what McKenzie describes as a derangement syndrome, or the clinician can position the patient in flexion and right side bending (Fig. 25-15) to assess for what McKenzie describes as a dysfunction syndrome. Alternatively, the clinician can ask the patient to maintain the position of flexion and right side bending to assess for a postural dysfunction.[228]

Six-position Test

The six-position test is a screening tool that I have found to be particularly useful with the acute patient in helping to determine the position of comfort for the patient, and for focusing the examination and intervention. The reliability or validity of these tests has yet to be established, but they are based on applied anatomy and biomechanics. The patient is placed in the following positions:

1. Supine with the hips and knees extended (Fig. 25-16). In individuals with adaptive shortening of the rectus femoris and the iliopsoas (a common finding), this position is manifested by an inability of the posterior thighs to rest on the table. Pain in this position may indicate a lumbar extension or lumbar rotation syndrome (see "Intervention Strategies," later), especially if the next position relieves the symptoms.[279]

2. Supine in the hook-lying position, with the hips and knees flexed and the feet flat on the bed (Fig. 25-17). This is typically the most comfortable position for the patient with acute LBP, except in cases of severe stenosis or spondylolisthesis.

3. Supine with both knees held against the chest (Fig. 25-18). This position rotates the pelvis posteriorly and widens the intervertebral foramina of the lumbar segments.[229] This is normally a comfortable position for patients who have spinal stenosis, lateral recess stenosis, or a lumbar extension syndrome.

4. Supine with one knee held against the chest and the other leg lying on the bed, with the hip and knee extended (Fig. 25-19). Holding the left knee against the chest invokes a position of lumbar flexion and left side bending, which widens the intervertebral foramen on the right and narrows the intervertebral foramen on the left. Holding the

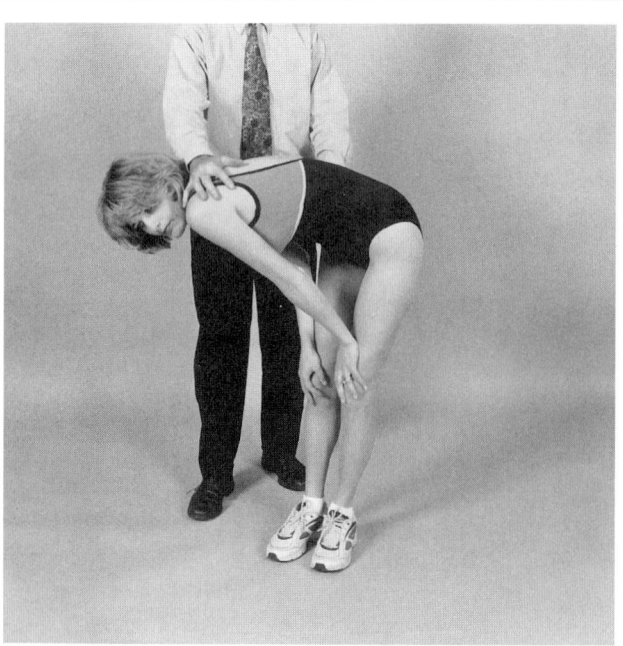

FIGURE 25-15   Lumbar flexion and right side bending.

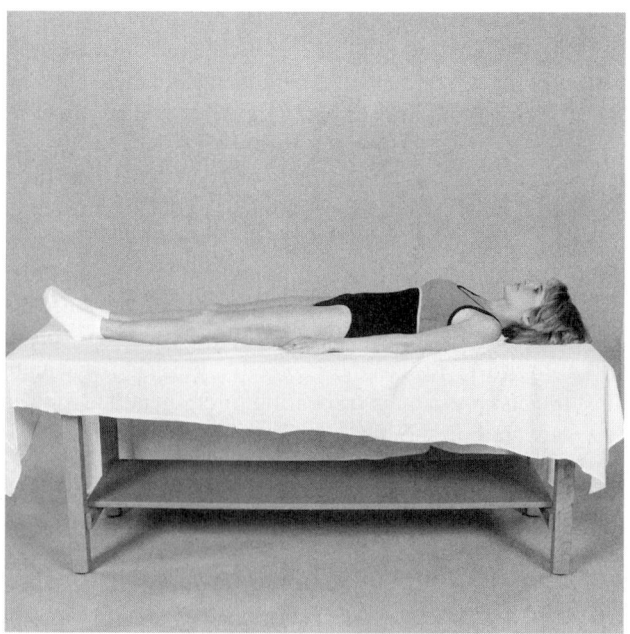

FIGURE 25-16   Supine lying.

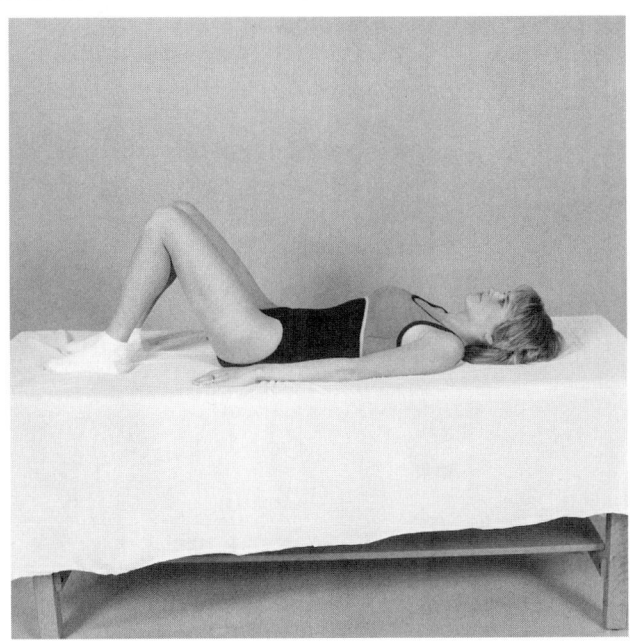

FIGURE 25-17 Hook-lying position.

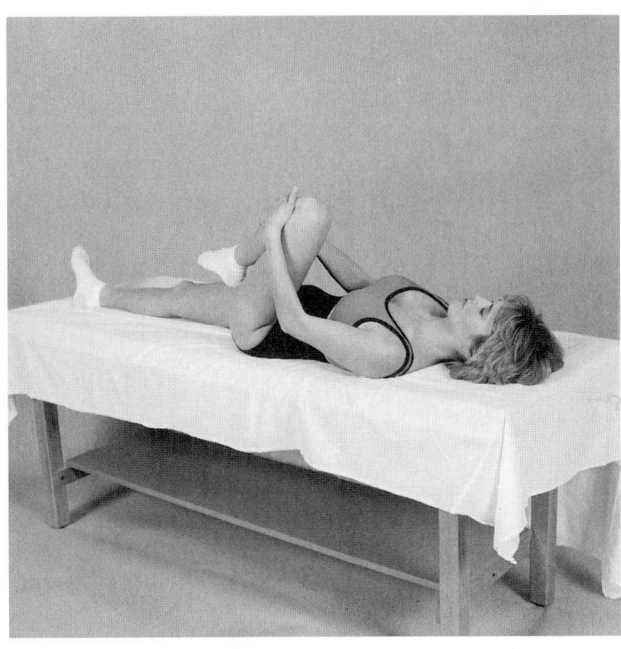

FIGURE 25-19 Single knee to chest.

right knee against the chest invokes a position of lumbar flexion and right side bending, which widens the intervertebral foramen on the left, and narrows intervertebral foramen on the right.[229] Given the amount of rotation induced with this maneuver, this test is often positive even when the position of both knees to the chest does not provoke symptoms. Occasionally though, one side may be pain free and can be used as an introductory exercise.

5. Prone lying with the legs straight (Fig. 25-20). This is typically comfortable for patients with an IVD protrusion, but uncomfortable for patients with spinal stenosis, spondylolisthesis, and an extension or a rotation syndrome[279] (see "Intervention Strategies," later).

6. Prone lying with passive knee flexion applied by the clinician (Fig. 25-21). This is a confirmatory test for the

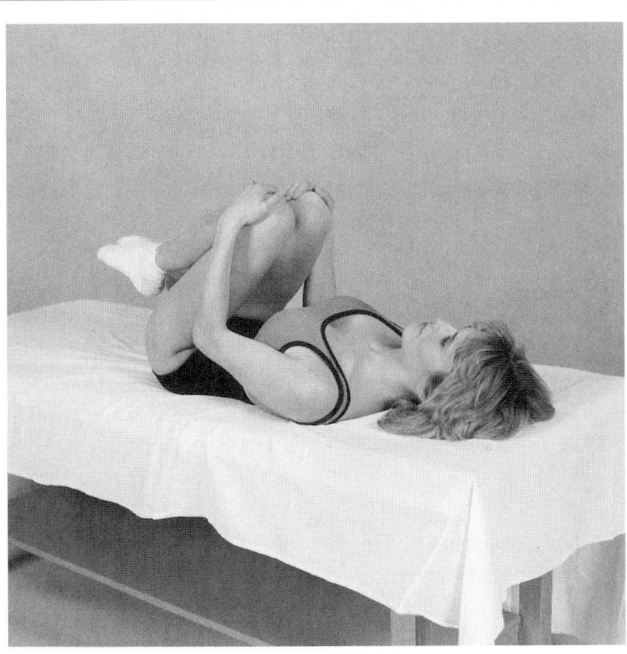

FIGURE 25-18 Double knees to chest.

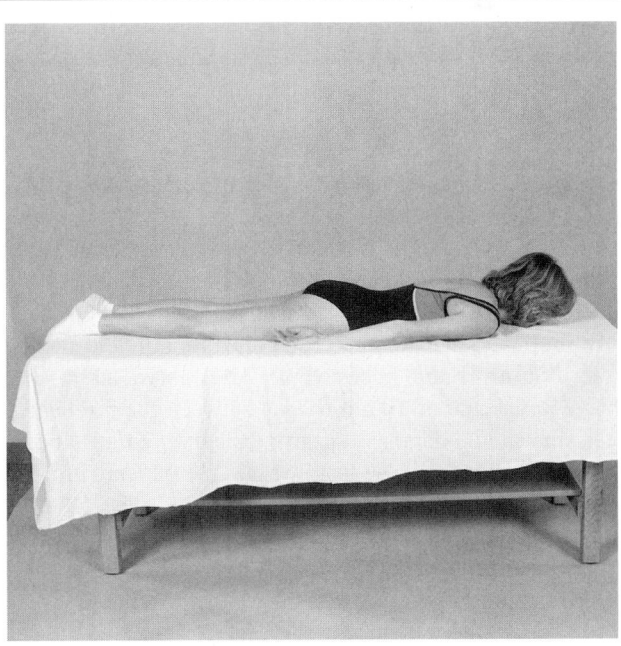

FIGURE 25-20 Prone lying.

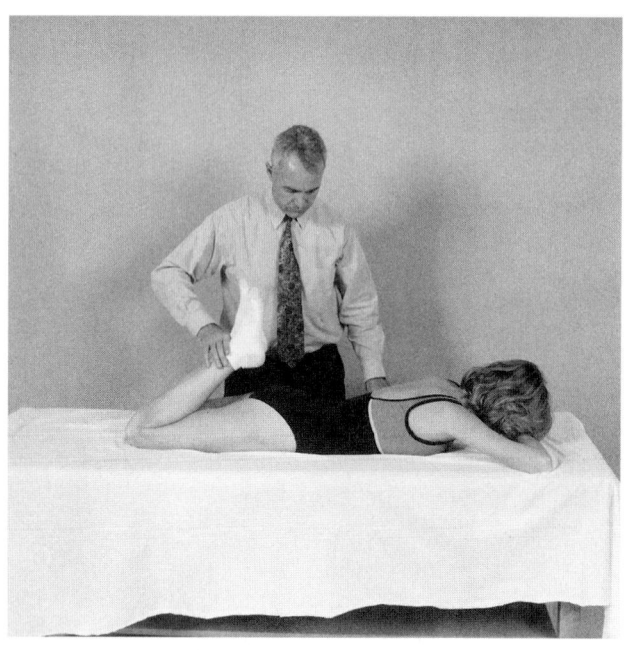

FIGURE 25-21 Prone double knee bend.

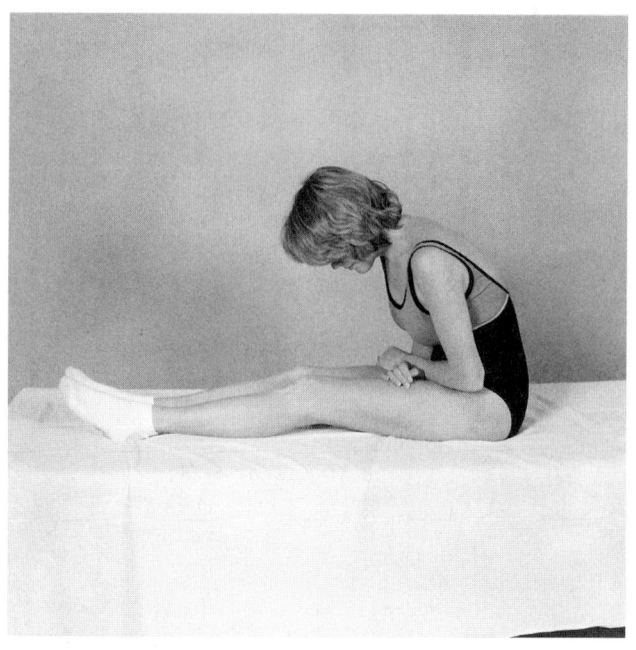

FIGURE 25-22 Erector spinae muscle length test: part 1.

previous position if it increases the symptoms in patients with spinal stenosis, spondylolisthesis, and an extension or a rotation syndrome[279] (see "Intervention Strategies," later).

The results from these tests should provide the clinician with information on the effect that pelvic tilting in a non–weight-bearing position has on the symptoms. If anterior pelvic tilting appears to aggravate the patient's symptoms, initial positions and exercises that promote posterior pelvic tilting are advocated. If posterior pelvic tilting appears to aggravate the patient's symptoms, initial positions and exercises that promote an anterior pelvic tilt are advocated.

Muscle Length

Lumbar Erector Spinae.   A simple two-part test has been described by Janda and Jull to assess the length of the erector spinae.[280] The patient is positioned on a mat table with his or her legs stretched out, keeping the pelvis as vertical as possible (if the pelvis tilts posteriorly in this position, it is a sign of adaptively shortened hamstrings). The patient is asked to move the forehead toward the knees (Fig. 25-22). An adult should achieve a distance of 10 cm or less between the forehead and knees, and should demonstrate an even curve of the spine.

The second part of the test involves the patient sitting over the end of the mat table, with the knees flexed. The patient forward bends as far as possible, attempting to move the forehead toward the knees without moving the pelvis (Fig. 25-23). If the forward bending of the trunk is greater than in the first part of the test, it is usually the result of an increased tilt of the pelvis and adaptive shortening of the hamstrings, rather than adaptive shortening of the erector spinae.

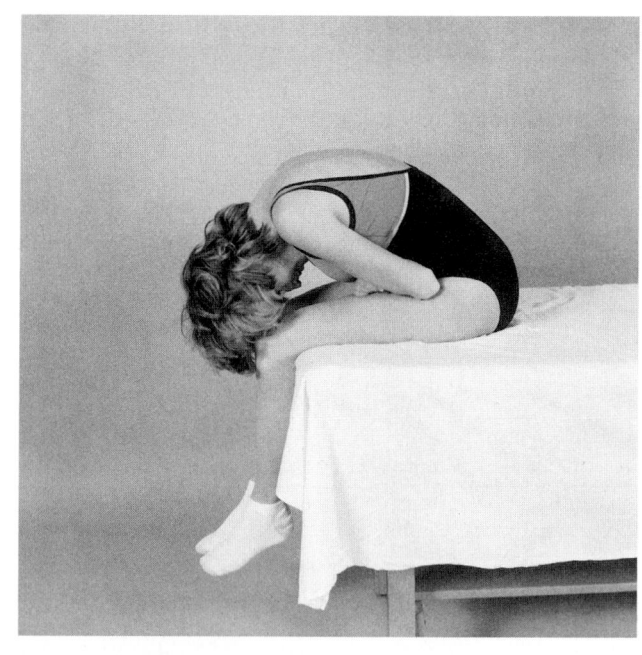

FIGURE 25-23 Erector spinae muscle length test: part 2.

Quadratus Lumborum.   The patient is in the side-lying position, with the hips and knees flexed at about 45 degrees. The patient then pushes up sideways from the table as the pelvis is monitored for movement (Fig. 25-24), while the clinician ensures that the patient's trunk does not flex or rotate during the maneuver.[280]

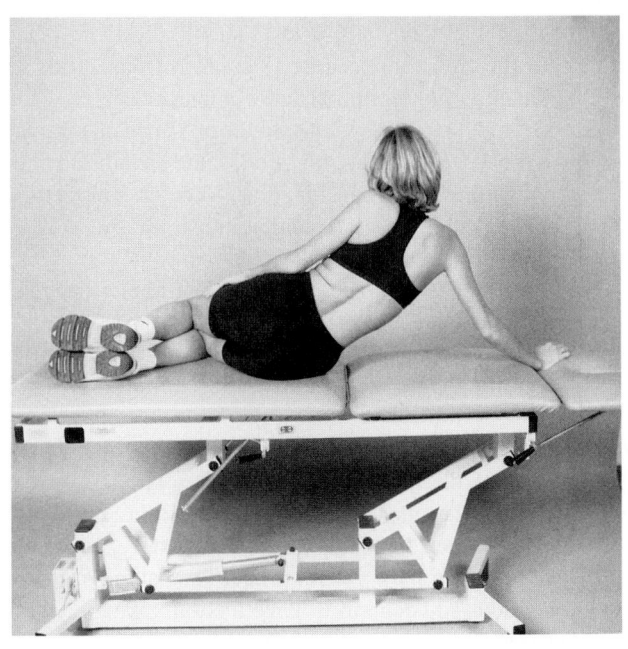

FIGURE 25-24   Quadratus lumborum muscle length.

TABLE 25-6   Key Movements of the Lumbar Quarter Scanning Examination

Segment	Movement
L1–2	Hip flexion
L3–4	Knee extension
L4	Ankle dorsiflexion
L5	Great toe extension
L5–S1	Hip extension Great toe extension
S1–2	Plantar flexion Knee flexion
S3	Foot movements produced by intrinsic muscles of foot (except abductor hallucis)

Hip Flexor and Rectus Femoris.   The tests for these muscles are described in Chapter 17.

Hamstrings.   The test for these muscles is described in Chapter 17.

Muscle Strength

Key Muscle Testing.   The key muscle tests are used as part of the lower quarter scanning examination because they examine the integrity of the neuromuscular junction and the contractile and inert components of the various muscles[266] (Table 25-6). With the isometric tests, the contraction should be held for at least 5 seconds to demonstrate any weakness. If the clinician suspects weakness, the test is repeated two to three times to assess for fatigability. The larger muscle groups, such as the quadriceps, hip extensors and calf muscles, must be tested by repetitive resistance against a load in order to sufficiently stress the muscle-nerve components.

Standing Up on the Toes (S1–2).   The patient raises both heels off the ground (Fig. 25-25). The key muscles tested during this maneuver are the plantar flexors. These are difficult muscles to fatigue, so the patient should perform 10 heel raises unilaterally, with the arms resting on the clinician's shoulders. In addition to observing for fatigability, the clinician should look for Trendelenburg's sign. A positive Trendelenburg's sign occurs when, during unilateral weight bearing, the pelvis drops toward the unsupported limb; this can indicate a number of conditions, including a hip impairment (coxa vara) or a gluteus medius weakness (see Chap. 17).

Unilateral Squat While Supported (L3–4).   The patient performs unilateral squats while supported (Fig. 25-26). The key muscles being tested during this maneuver are the quadriceps and hip extensors. Neurologic weakness of the quadriceps (L3–4) is relatively rare (see Chap. 20) and often suggests a nondiskogenic lesion, such as a neoplasm, especially if the weakness is bilateral.[276]

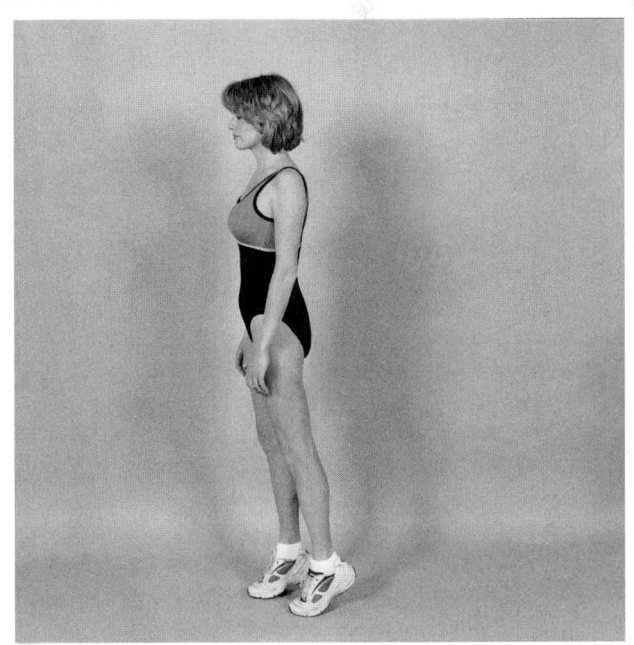

FIGURE 25-25   Standing up on toes.

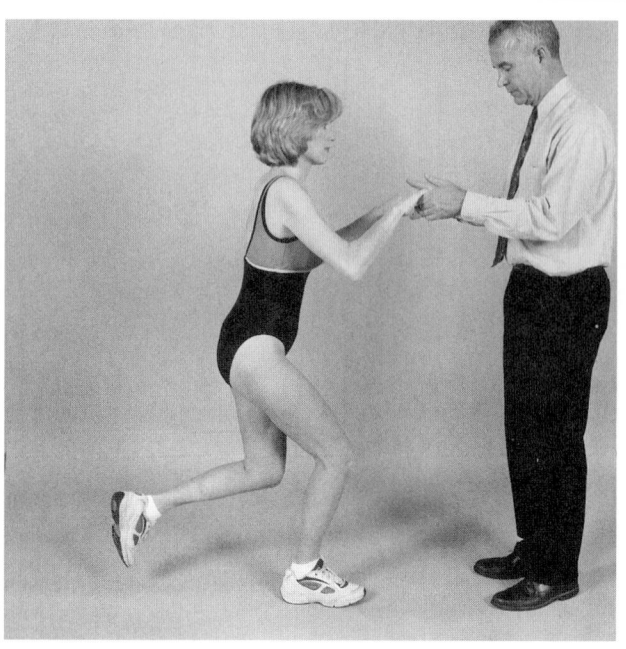

FIGURE 25-26   Unilateral squat.

Heel Walking (L4).   The patient walks toward, or away from, the clinician while weight bearing through the heels (Fig. 25-27). The key muscles being tested during this maneuver are the dorsiflexors (L4). About 40 percent of IVD lesions affect this level, about an equal amount as those that affect the L5 root.[281] An IVD protrusion of the L4–5 disk can irritate the fourth root, the fifth root, or, with a larger protrusion, both roots (see Chap. 20).

Hip Flexion (L1–2).   With palsy, the patient is unable to raise the thigh off the table. Palsy at this level should always serve as a red flag for the clinician, because IVD protrusions at this level are rare, but this is a common site for metastasis.[282] Painful weakness of hip flexion may indicate the presence of a fractured transverse process, metastatic invasion, acute spondylolisthesis, acute segmental articular dysfunction, a major contractile lesion of the hip flexors (rare), or a hip joint pathology.[276] The patient's hip is actively raised off the treatment table to about 30 to 40 degrees of flexion. The clinician then applies a resisted force proximal to the knee into hip extension (Fig. 25-28), while ensuring that the heel of the patient's foot is not contacting the examining table. Both sides are tested for comparison.

Knee Extension (L3–4).   The clinician positions the patient's knee in 25 to 35 degrees of flexion and then applies a resisted flexion force at the mid-distal shaft of the tibia (Fig. 25-29). Both sides are tested for comparison. Alternately, knee extension can be tested with the patient prone. The patient's leg is positioned in about 120 degrees of knee flexion, taking care to do this passively. The clinician rests the superior aspect of his or her shoulder against the dorsum of the patient's ankle, and grips the edges of the examining table. A force to flex the patient's knee is applied while the patient resists. Both sides are tested for comparison.

Hip Extension (L5–S1).   The patient's knee is flexed to 90 degrees, and his or her thigh is lifted slightly off the examining table by the clinician, while the other leg is stabilized. A downward force is applied to the patient's posterior thigh, while the clinician ensures that the patient's thigh is not in contact with the table. Both sides are tested for comparison.

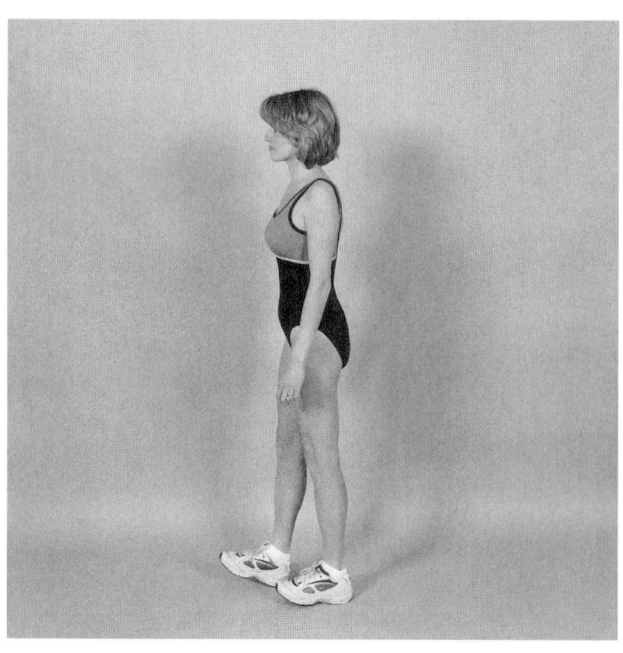

FIGURE 25-27   Heel walking.

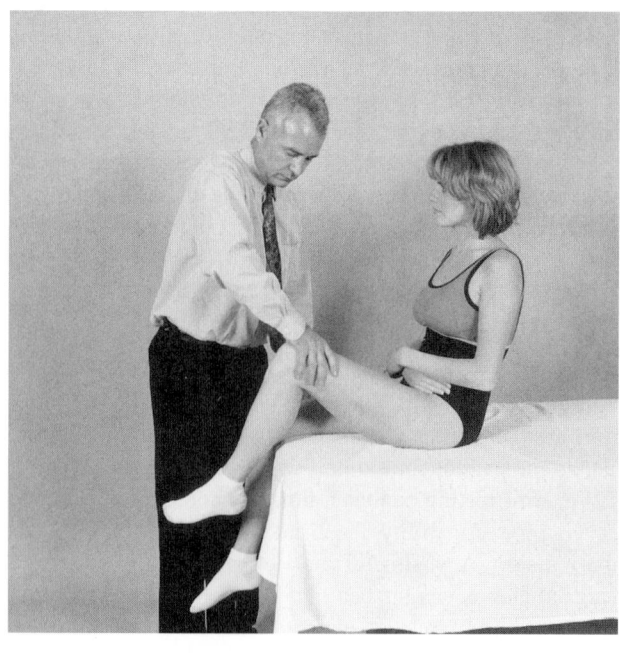

FIGURE 25-28   Resisted hip flexion.

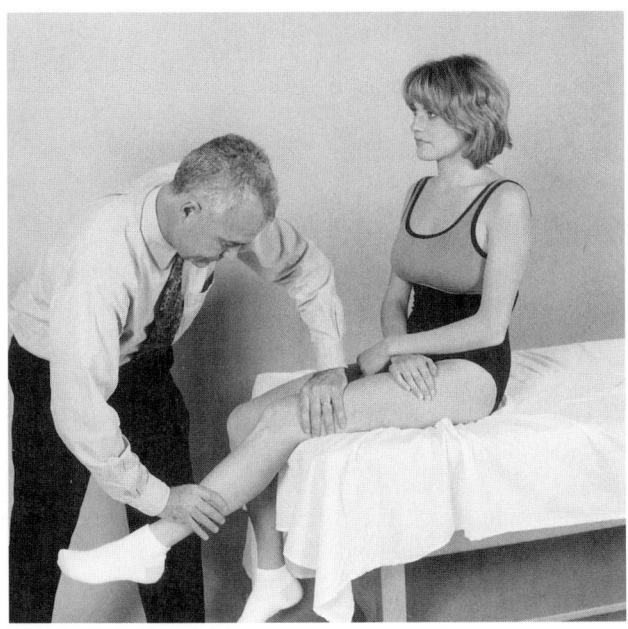

FIGURE 25-29   Resisted knee extension.

Knee Flexion (S1–2).   The patient's knee is flexed to 70 degrees, and an extension isometric force is applied just above the ankle (Fig. 25-30). Both sides are tested for comparison.

Great Toe Extension (L5).   The patient is asked to hold both big toes in a neutral position. The clinician then applies resistance to the nails of both toes (Fig. 25-31) and compares the two sides.

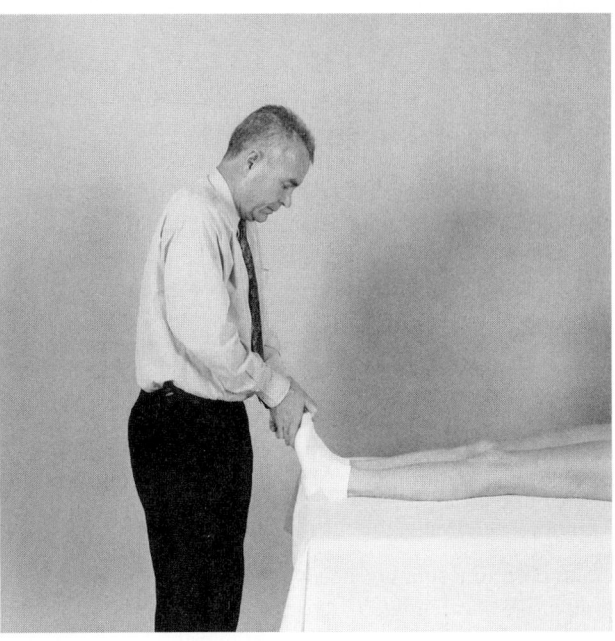

FIGURE 25-31   Resisted great toe extension.

Ankle Eversion (L5–S1).   The patient is asked to place the feet at 0 degrees of plantar and dorsiflexion relative to the leg. A resisted force is applied by the clinician to move each foot into inversion (Fig. 25-32), and a comparison is made.

Core Stability.   The term *core* is used with reference to the lumbar spine to describe a point from which the center of gravity for all movement is initiated.[103,169,283–285] The core functions to

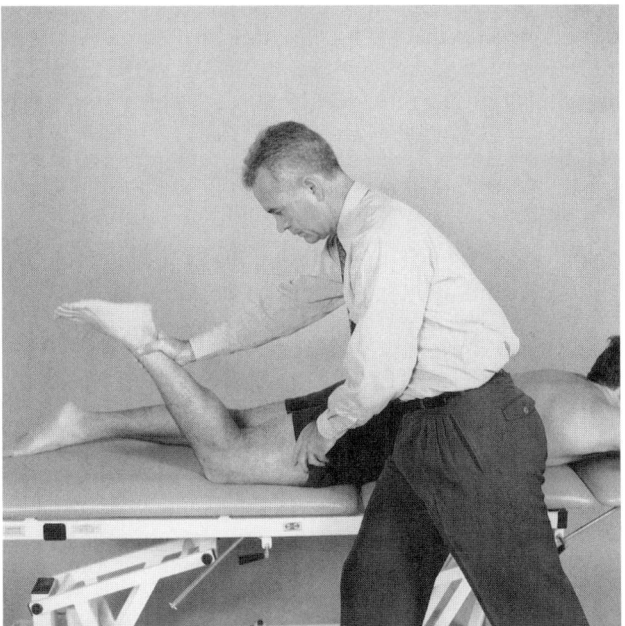

FIGURE 25-30   Resisted knee flexion.

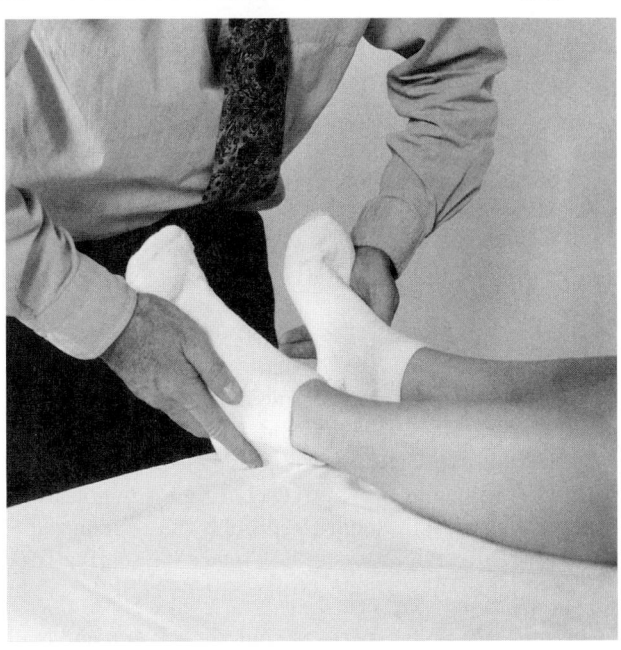

FIGURE 25-32   Resisted ankle eversion.

maintain postural alignment and dynamic postural equilibrium during functional activities.[286]

Theoretically, spinal instability occurs when there is a significant decrease in the capacity of the stabilizing systems of the spine to maintain the intervertebral neutral zone within physiologic limits, thereby preventing major deformity, neurologic deficit, or incapacitating pain.[169] The intervertebral neutral zone is the point in the range of the pelvic tilt where the pain is minimized (see the discussion under "Biomechanics," earlier).

The key muscles that influence the core include:

▶ Transversospinalis group (rotators, interspinales, intertransversarii, semispinalis, and multifidus), erector spinae, quadratus lumborum, and latissimus dorsi.

▶ Rectus abdominis, external oblique, internal oblique, and transverse abdominis.

▶ Gluteus maximus, gluteus medius, and psoas.

The core musculature needs to be examined for weakness and adaptive shortening. The rectus abdominis has a tendency to become weak, and the quadratus lumborum has a tendency to become adaptively shortened and overactive.[287]

The following tests can be used to assess the strength of the lumbar stabilizers.

Lower Abdominal Hollowing. The abdominal hollowing exercise tests the ability of the multifidus and transverse abdominis to co-contract.[148,288] These muscles are important for the provision of segmental control to the spine, because they provide an important stiffening effect on the lumbar spine, thereby enhancing dynamic stability.[194]

The patient is positioned supine. The patient is instructed to contract the deep abdominal muscles and to draw the navel up toward the chest and in toward the spine, so as to hollow the abdomen. When the muscle contracts properly, an increase in tension can be felt at a point 2 cm medial and inferior to the anterior superior iliac spine. If a bulging is felt at this point, the internal oblique is contracting rather than the transverse abdominis.[148,288] The multifidus is palpated simultaneously and should be felt to swell at a point just lateral to the spinous process.[148,288] The patient's head and upper trunk must remain stable, and he or she is not permitted to flex forward, push through the feet, or tilt the pelvis.

Spine Rotators and Multifidus Test. This test is designed to assess the ability of the spinal rotators and multifidus to stabilize the trunk during dynamic extremity movements.[289] The patient is positioned in the quadruped position, with the pelvis positioned in neutral using muscular control. The patient is then asked to perform the following maneuvers: (1) single straight arm and hold, (2) single straight leg lift and hold, and (3) contralateral straight arm and straight leg lift and hold. The scoring for this test is as follows[289]:

Normal (5) = able to perform contralateral arm and leg lift, both sides, while maintaining neutral pelvis (20- to 30-second hold).

Good (4) = able to maintain neutral pelvis while performing single leg lift, but not able to hold pelvis in neutral when doing contralateral arm and leg lift (15- to 20-second hold).

Fair (3) = Able to do single arm lift and maintain neutral pelvis (15- to 20-second hold).

Poor (2) = Unable to maintain neutral pelvis while doing single arm lift.

Trace (1) = Unable to raise arm or leg off the table to the straight position.

Abdominal Endurance Test. This test measures the endurance of the abdominals. The patient is positioned supine, with the hips flexed to approximately 45 degrees, the feet flat on the bed, and the arms by the side. A line is drawn 8 cm (for patients 40 years and older) or 12 cm (for patients younger than 40 years of age) distal to the fingers.[290] The patient is asked to tuck in the chin and to curl the trunk and touch the line with the fingers. The patient holds this position for as long as possible. The test is graded as follows[121,291]:

Normal (5) = 20- to 30-second hold.

Good (4) = 15- to 20-second hold.

Fair (3) = 10- to 15-second hold.

Poor (2) = 1- to 10-second hold.

Trace (1) = Unable to raise more than the head off the table.

Side Support or Side Bridge Test. The so-called side support or side bridge position has been identified as optimizing the challenge to the quadratus lumborum while minimizing the load on the lumbar spine.[292] The patient is in the side-lying position, with the knees flexed to 90 degrees and resting the upper body on the elbow. The test can be made more difficult by having the knees extended so that the legs are straight. The patient is asked to lift the pelvis off the table and to straighten the curve of the spine without rolling forward or backward. This position is then held. The test is graded as follows:

Normal (5) = Able to lift pelvis off the table and hold spine straight for a 20- to 30-second hold.

Good (4) = Able to lift pelvis off the table but has difficulty holding spine straight for a 15- to 20-second hold.

Fair (3) = Able to lift pelvis off the table but has difficulty holding spine straight for a 10- to 15-second hold.

Poor (2) = Able to lift pelvis off the table but cannot hold spine straight for a 1- to 10-second hold.

Trace (1) = Unable to lift pelvis off the table.

Double Straight Leg Lowering Test. The straight leg lowering test can be used to assess core strength.[178, 201,205,286,288,293–295] The patient is in the supine hook-lying position, with the hips flexed to 90 degrees, and with a pressure cuff placed under the lumbar spine at the level of L4 to L5. The cuff is inflated to 40 mm Hg. The clinician raises the patient's legs until the pelvis is seen to posteriorly rotate, and the needle on the pressure monitor begins to move. The patient is asked to perform the abdominal hollowing maneuver so as to prevent further pelvic motion, and is then asked to lower the legs toward the bed while maintaining the abdominal hollowing (Fig. 25-33). At the point when the cuff pressure is seen to increase or decrease, or when the pelvis anteriorly rotates, the test is over, and the hip angle at which this occurs is measured. This test may also be graded using the following scoring[291]:

Normal (5) = Able to reach 0 to 15 degrees from the table before pelvis tilts.

Good (4) = Able to reach 16 to 45 degrees from the table before pelvis tilts.

Fair (3) = Able to reach 46 to 75 degrees from the table before pelvis tilts.

Poor (2) = Able to reach 75 to 90 degrees from the table before pelvis tilts.

Trace (1) = Unable to hold pelvis in neutral.

A study by Youdas and colleagues[295] found that the odds of a patient having chronic LBP is increased if the score on the leg lowering test for the abdominal muscles exceeds 50 degrees for men and 60 degrees for women. Another study[296] found that there is a natural tendency for the pelvis to rotate anteriorly from very early on during this test, and that, as healthy young subjects were unable to prevent the tilting, the preceding scoring system may be questionable.

The Bent Knee Lowering Test. The lower abdominal musculature can be assessed in a similar fashion.[205,286,293] The patient is positioned supine with the knees and hips flexed to approximately 90 degrees. A pressure cuff, inflated to 40 mm Hg, is placed under the L4 to L5 segment. The patient is asked to perform the abdominal hollowing maneuver, and then to slowly lower the legs to the bed until the pressure on the monitor is seen to decrease (Fig. 25-34). The hip angle is again measured at the point where there is a change in the pressure cuff reading, or where the anterior tilt of the pelvis occurred (Fig. 23-35).

Normal (5) = Able to reach 0 to 15 degrees from the table before pelvis tilts.

Good (4) = Able to reach 16 to 45 degrees from the table before pelvis tilts.

Fair (3) = Able to reach 46 to 75 degrees from the table before pelvis tilts.

Poor (2) = Able to reach 75 to 90 degrees from the table before pelvis tilts.

Trace (1) = Unable to hold pelvis in neutral.

Trunk Raise. The trunk raise test can be used to assess the endurance of the iliocostalis lumborum (erector spinae) and the multifidus.[283,284,286,293] The patient is positioned prone, with the hands behind the back. The patient is instructed to extend at the lumbar spine by raising the chest off the bed to approximately 30 degrees (the axilla is used as the reference for the axis of the goniometer) and to hold the position for as long as possible. The clinician times the test[293]:

Normal (5) = 20- to 30-second hold.

Good (4) = 15- to 20-second hold.

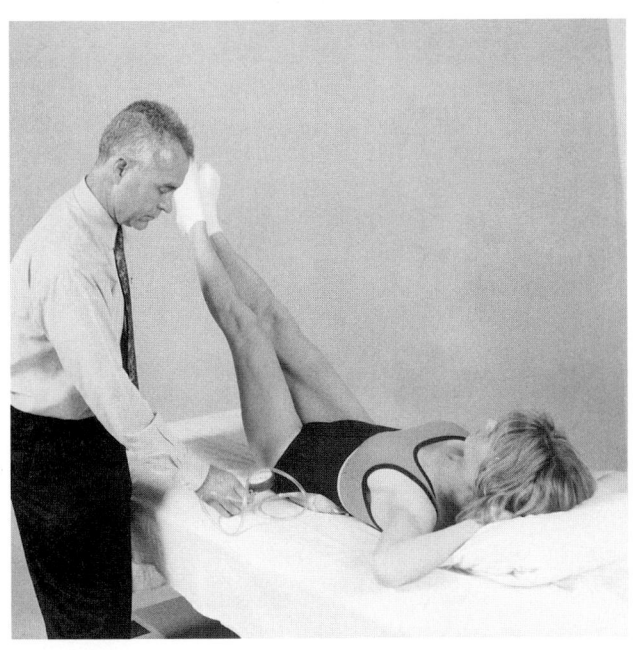

FIGURE 25-33 Straight leg lowering test.

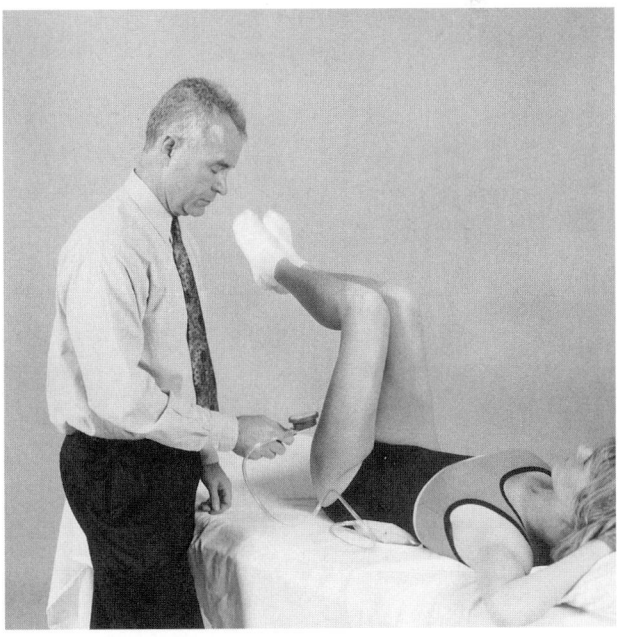

FIGURE 25-34 Bent knee lowering test: start position.

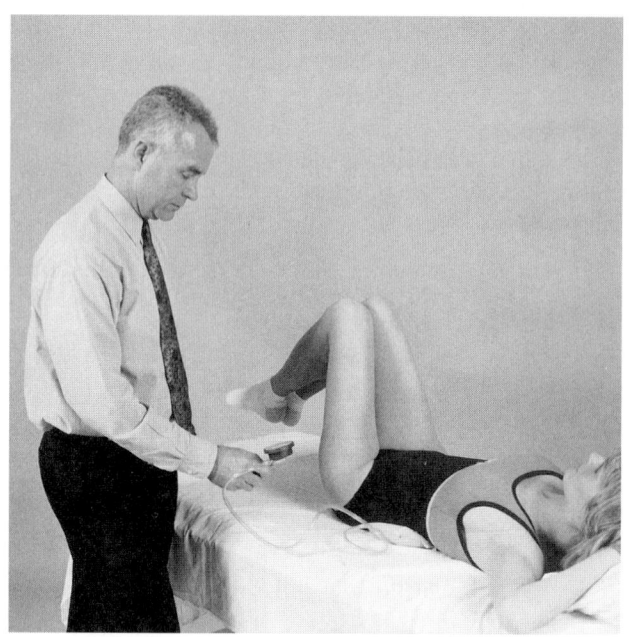

FIGURE 25-35   Bent knee lowering test: terminal position.

Fair (3) = 10- to 15-second hold.

Poor (2) = 1- to 10-second hold.

Trace (1) = Unable to raise more than the head off the table.

Lunge.   The patient is asked to perform a lunge (Fig. 25-36). The clinician notes the quality and quantity of the motion, as well as the ability of the patient to sustain the position for 30 seconds.[297] Excessive shaking of the legs with this maneuver may

indicate weakness of the lumbopelvic stabilizers or poor balance and proprioception.

Deep Tendon Reflexes

The reflexes should be assessed and graded accordingly, with any differences between the two sides noted. The tendon should be struck directly once the patient's muscles and tendons are relaxed.

Patellar Reflex (L3).   The patient is positioned sitting, with the legs hanging freely. Alternatively, both knees can be supported in flexion, with the patient positioned in supine (Fig. 25-37).

Hamstring Reflex (Semimembranosus: L5, S1; and Biceps Femoris: S1–2).   The patient is positioned prone, with the knee flexed and the foot resting on a pillow. The clinician places a thumb over the appropriate tendon and taps the thumbnail with the reflex hammer to elicit the reflex.

Achilles Reflex (S1–2).   The patient is positioned so that the ankle is slightly dorsiflexed with passive overpressure (Fig. 25-38).

Pathologic Reflexes

The following pathologic reflexes are described in Chapter 2:

▶   Babinski.

▶   Clonus.

▶   Oppenheim.

Sensory Testing

The clinician checks the dermatome patterns of the nerve roots, as well as the peripheral sensory distribution of the peripheral nerves (see Chap. 2). Dermatomes vary considerably between individuals.

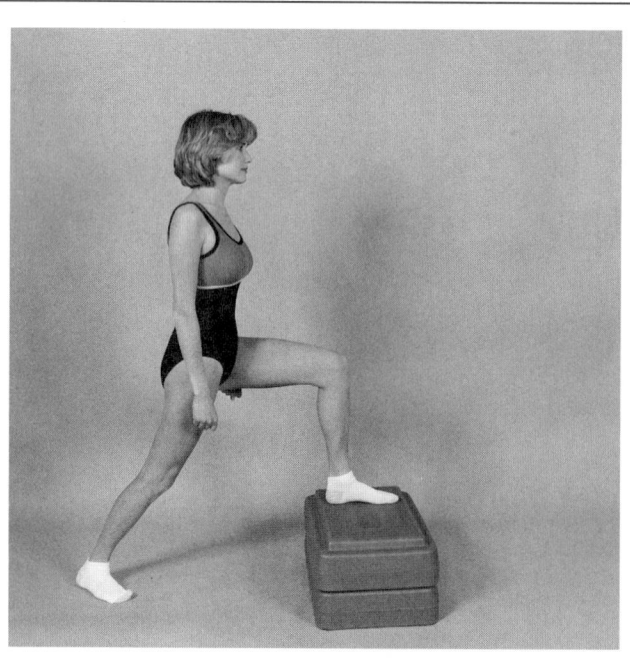

FIGURE 25-36   Lunge.

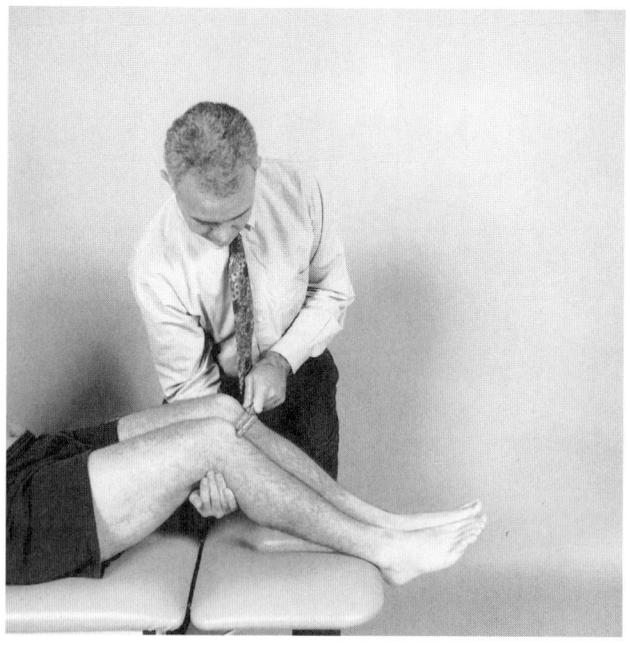

FIGURE 25-37   Patellar reflex.

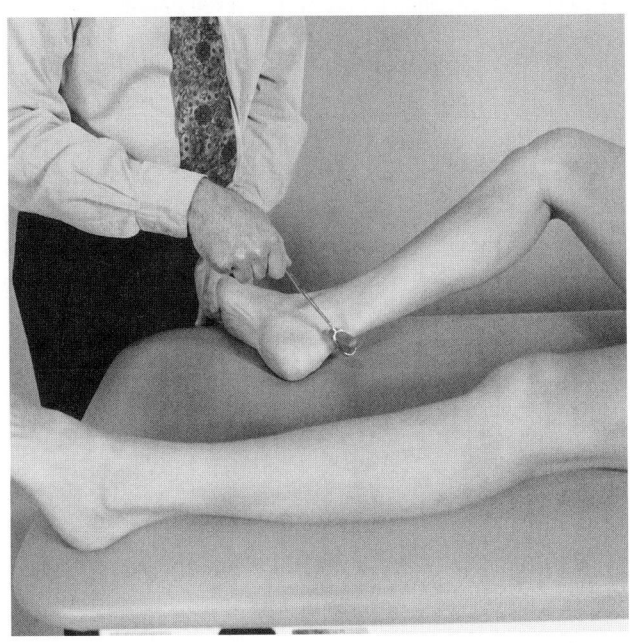

FIGURE 25-38 Achilles reflex.

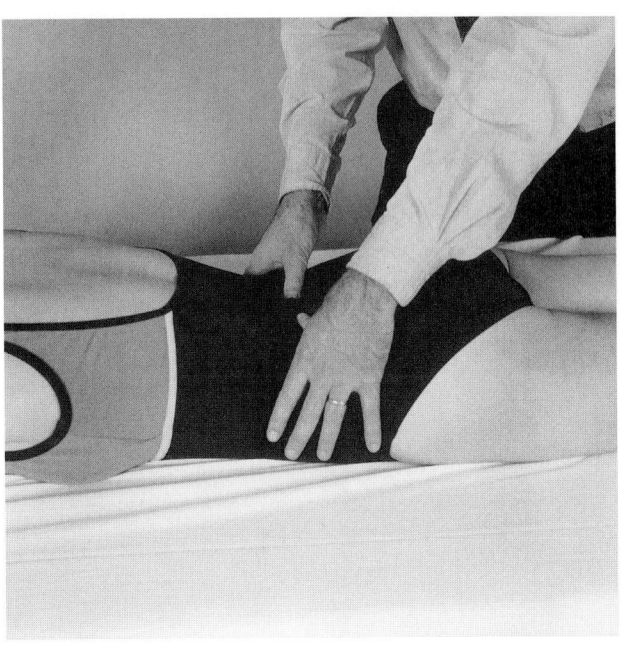

FIGURE 25-39 Position testing in neutral.

Differing Philosophies

The next stage in the examination process depends on the clinician's background. Clinicians who are heavily influenced by the muscle energy techniques of the osteopaths use position testing to determine the segment on which to focus. Other clinicians omit the position tests and proceed to the combined motion and passive physiologic tests.

Position Testing. Position testing in the lumbar spine is an osteopathic technique used to determine the level and type of zygapophysial joint dysfunction.[115,257,260,298–300] Position testing is performed with the patient in three positions: neutral (Fig. 25-39), flexion (Fig. 25-40), and extension (Fig. 25-41). The transverse processes are then layer palpated (Fig. 25-42). The findings and possible causes for the position testing are outlined in Tables 25-7 and 25-8.

Passive Physiologic Intervertebral Mobility (PPIVM) Tests.[301,302] These tests are most effectively carried out if the combined motion tests locate a hypomobility, or if the position tests are negative, rather than as the entry tests for the lumbar spine. Judgments of stiffness made by experienced physical therapists examining patients in their own clinics have been found to have poor reliability.[303]

The passive physiologic movement tests are performed into:

▶ Flexion.

▶ Extension.

▶ Rotation.

▶ Side bending.

The adjacent spinous processes of the segment are palpated simultaneously, and movement between them is assessed as the segment is passively taken through its physiologic range.

The test is used for acute and subacute patients who have pain in the cardinal motion planes. For these tests, the patient is in the side-lying position, facing the clinician. The clinician

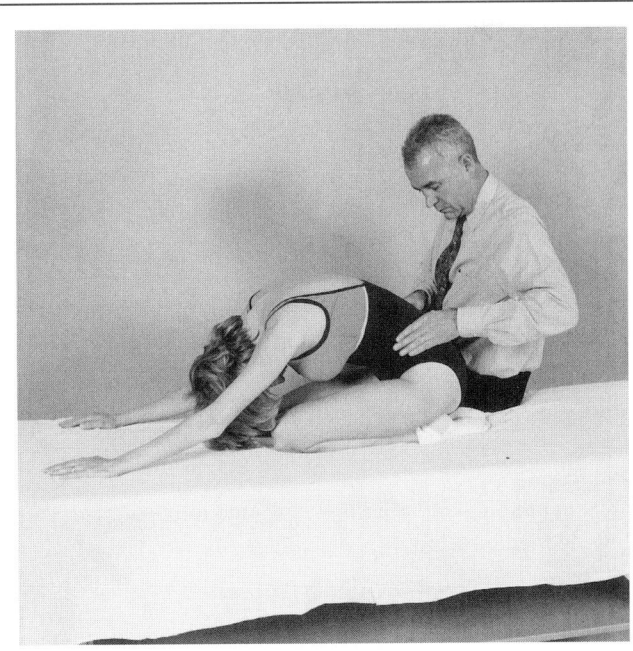

FIGURE 25-40 Position testing in flexion.

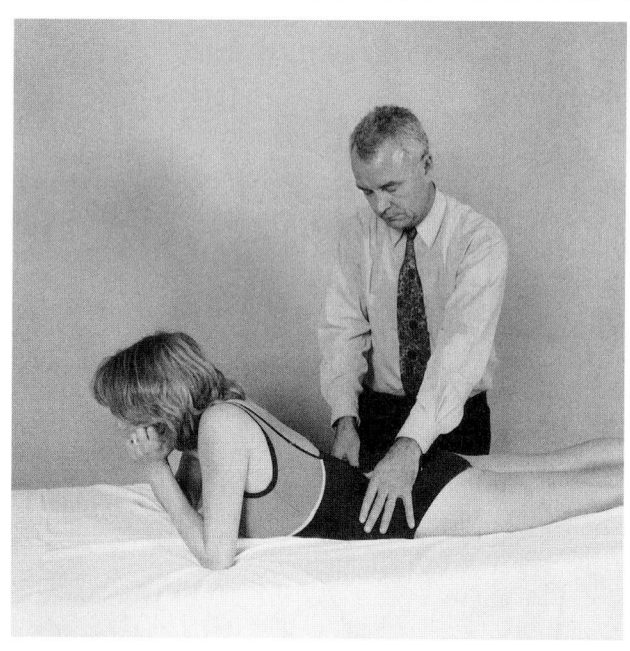

FIGURE 25-41 Position testing in extension.

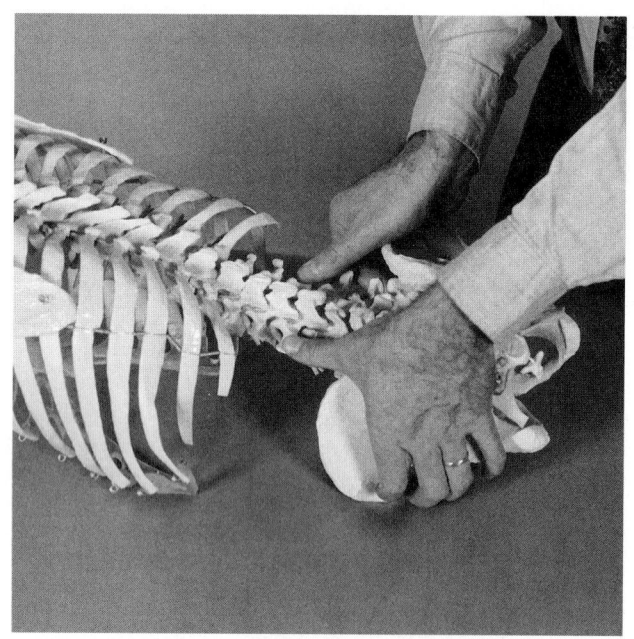

FIGURE 25-42 Layer palpation of the transverse processes. This technique also may be used for posteroanterior pressures.

may locate the patient's lumbosacral junction using one of the following methods:

▶ By locating the L5 spinous process and then moving inferiorly.

▶ By locating the posterior superior iliac spine and moving superiorly and medially.

TABLE 25-7   Causes and Findings for a Flexed Rotated Sidebent Right

Causes of an FRSR	Associated Findings
Isolated left joint extension hypomobility (FRSR)	PPIVM and PPAIVM tests in left extension quadrant are reduced
Tight left flexor muscles (FRSR)	PPIVM test in left extension quadrant is decreased PAIVM test is normal
Arthrosis or arthritis of left joint in capsular pattern (ERSL < FRSR)	PPIVM and PPAIVM tests in right flexion quadrant are more reduced than in left extension quadrant
Fibrosis of left joint (ERSL = FRSR)	PPIVM and PPAIVM tests are equally reduced in right flexion and left extension quadrants
Left posterolateral disk protrusion (ERSR < FRSR)	PPIVM tests in left extension quadrant are reduced with springy end-feel; both flexion quadrants are normal

ERSL, extended rotated sidebent left; ERSR, extended rotated sidebent right; FRSR, flexed rotated sidebent right; PPAIVM, passive physiologic accessory intervertebral movement; PPIVM, passive physiologic intervertebral mobility.

▶ By locating the spinous process of T12 and counting down to the correct level using the spinous processes.

Once located, the neutral position of the spine for flexion and extension is found by palpating the L5 spinous process and alternatively flexing and extending the hips until it is felt to rock around the flexion and extension point.

Flexion.   The patient is close to the clinician, with the underneath leg slightly flexed at the hip and knee. A small pillow or roll can be placed under the patient's waist to maintain the lumbar spine in a neutral position with respect to side bending. The test can be performed by flexing one or both of the patient's legs, but it is generally easier to use one leg. The clinician, facing the patient, palpates between two adjacent lumbar spinous processes in the interspinous space (Fig. 25-43) with the cranial hand, while the other hand grasps the patient's lower legs (Fig. 25-44). The patient's lower extremities are moved into hip and lumbar flexion and returned to neutral by the clinician, as the motion between segments is palpated. Using this general technique, the clinician works up and down the lumbar spine getting a sense of the overall motion available.

Although there is a high degree of variability in patients, segmental motion should decrease from L5 to L1.[79] A generalized

TABLE 25-8 Causes and Findings of an Extended Rotated Sidebent Left

Causes of an ERSL*	Associated Findings
Isolated left joint flexion hypomobility (ERSL)	PPIVM and PPAIVM tests in right flexion quadrant are reduced
Tight left extensor muscles (ERSL)	PPIVM test in right flexion quadrant is decreased PPAIVM is normal
Arthrosis or arthritis of left joint in capsular pattern (ERSL < FRSR)	PPIVM and PPAIVM tests are equally reduced in right flexion and left flexion quadrants
Fibrosis left joint (ERSL = FRSR)	PPIVM and PPAIVM tests are equally reduced in right and left flexion quadrants
Right posterolateral disk protrusion (ERSL < FRSL)	PPIVM tests in right extension quadrant are reduced with springy end-feel; both flexion quadrants appear normal

ERSL, extended rotated sidebent left; ERSR, extended rotated sidebent right; FRSL, flexed rotated sidebent left; FRSR, flexed rotated sidebent right; PPAIVM, passive physiologic accessory intervertebral movement; PPIVM, passive physiologic intervertebral mobility.
*An ERSR would have the same causes and findings, but on the opposite side.

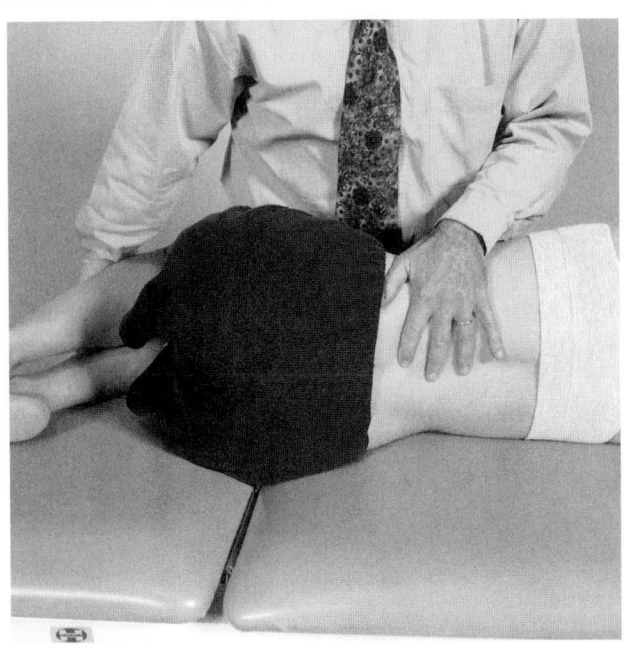

FIGURE 25-44 Passive mobility testing: flexion.

hypermobility demonstrates more motion in all of the segments, whereas an isolated hypermobile segment demonstrates more motion at only that level. Each segment is checked sequentially while moving the lumbar spine passively from neutral to full flexion.

For the mid- and upper lumbar segments, this technique can be modified for the larger patient by performing it with the patient sitting up.

Extension. Although flexion and extension can be tested together, it is more accurate to assess them separately. The patient is positioned as for flexion testing, but is oriented diagonally on the bed so that the pelvis is close to the edge, and the shoulder further from the edge. A small pillow or roll can be placed under the patient's waist to maintain the lumbar spine in a neutral position with respect to side bending. The clinician locates two adjacent spinous processes with his or her cranial hand, while the caudal arm flexes the patient's knees as much as possible before extending the patient's hips (Fig. 25-45). As the patient's knees move off the table, the clinician supports them on his or her thighs. When the patient's legs are on the table, the clinician's caudal arm is used to produce the hip and lumbar extension. The pelvis motion is felt and the spine is returned to its neutral position each time.

Side Bending. The patient is positioned side lying, with the knees and hips flexed, the thighs supported on the table, and the lower legs off the table. The lumbar spine should be in a neutral position in relation to flexion and extension. The clinician, facing the patient, places his or her cranial arm between the patient's arm and body and palpates the interspinous spaces, while

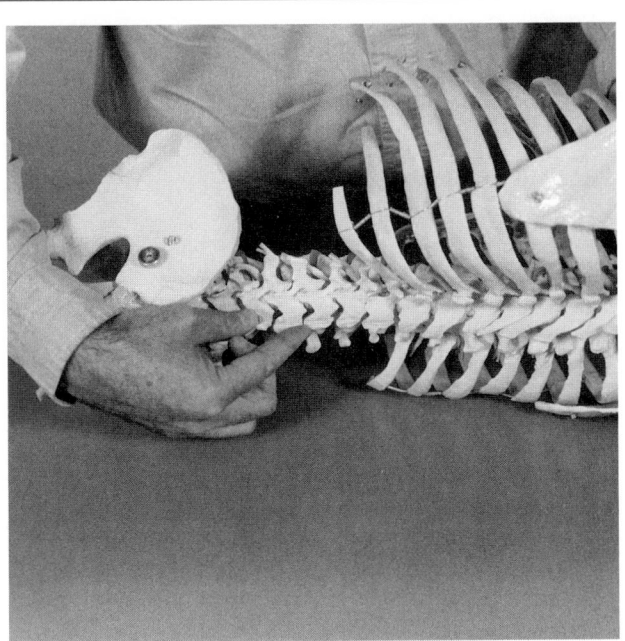

FIGURE 25-43 Intersegmental palpation.

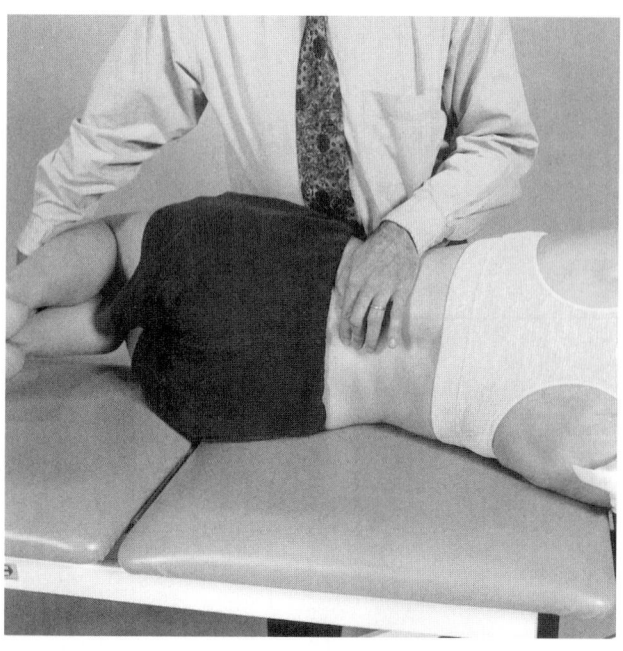

FIGURE 25-45 Passive mobility testing: extension.

the caudal hand grasps the patient's feet and ankles (Fig. 25-46). As the patient's feet and ankles are lifted toward the ceiling, the superior spinous process should be felt to move toward the table as the lumbar spine is side bent away from the table. The opposite occurs if the patient's feet are lowered off the table as the lumbar spine side bends toward the table. The direction of the leg lift represents the direction of the side bending. For example,

with the patient in the right side-lying position, right side bending (and left rotation) is introduced by lowering the feet and ankles off the table. The procedure is repeated for the other side, and the two sides are compared.

Rotation.   The patient is positioned as described for extension testing in spinal neutral, with both knees just off the table. A small pillow or roll can be placed under the patient's waist to maintain the lumbar spine in a neutral position. The interspinous spaces are palpated with the cranial hand, which is placed along the lower thoracic spine, with a reinforced finger resting against adjacent spinous processes from underneath.

The patient's pelvis is stabilized by the caudal hand, while the patient's thorax is rotated toward and away from the clinician, using the cranial hand (Fig. 25-47). As the patient's thorax is rotated away, the spinous process of the upper segment should be felt to rotate toward the table compared with the spinous process of the lower segment.

The spine is returned to neutral each time, and the clinician progresses up the spine. The process is repeated with the patient side lying on the opposite side.

Unfortunately, the PPIVM tests do not completely exclude such intersegmental impairments as minor end-range asymmetric hypomobilities or hypermobilities, because the application of side bending or rotation in neutral does not fully flex or extend the zygapophysial joints, nor is it possible to fully flex or extend both zygapophysial joints simultaneously. In order to completely flex a particular joint, the opposite joint has to move out of the fully flexed position by utilizing side bending, and allowing the increased superior glide of the superior zygapophysial joint on the opposite joint.

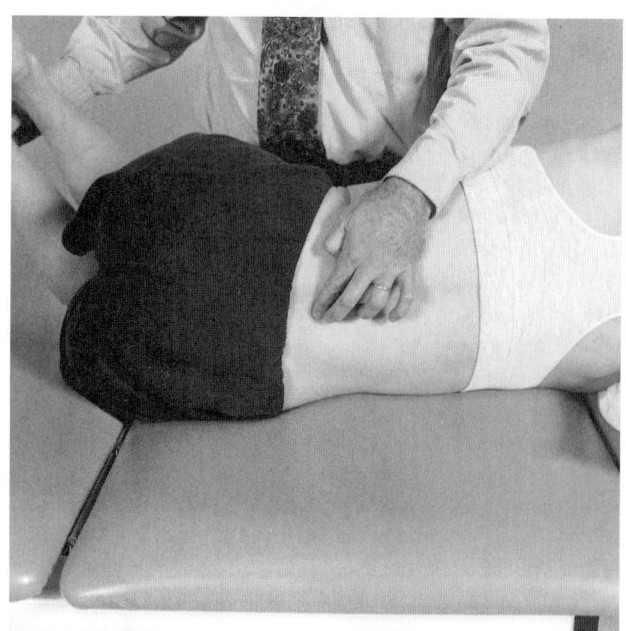

FIGURE 25-46 Passive mobility testing: Left side bending.

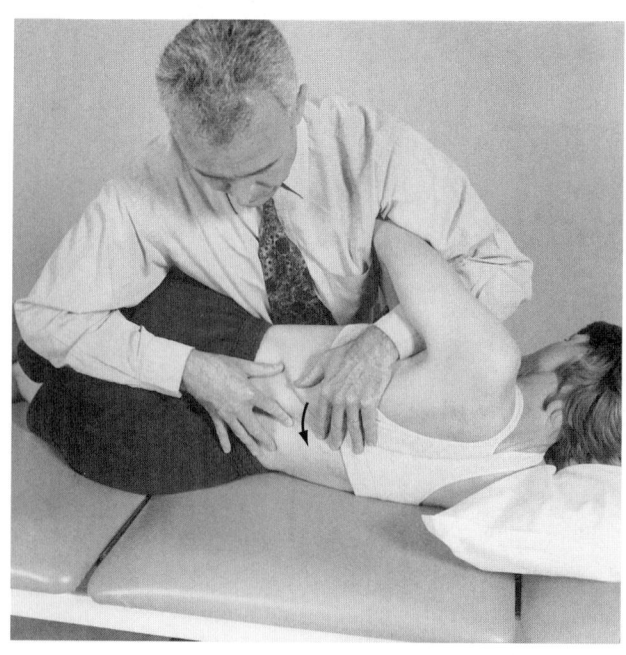

FIGURE 25-47 Passive mobility testing: Left rotation.

Passive Physiologic Accessory Intervertebral Mobility (PAIVM) Tests. These tests investigate the degree of linear or accessory glide that a joint possesses and are used on segmental levels where there is a possible hypomobility, to help determine if the motion restriction is articular, periarticular, or myofascial in origin. In other words, they assess the amount of joint motion, as well as the quality of the end-feel. The motion is assessed in relation to the patient's body type and age and the normal range for that segment, and the end-feel is assessed for:

▶ Pain.

▶ Spasm or hypertonicity.

▶ Resistance.

Several techniques have been proposed over the years to assess segmental mobility of the T10 to L5 segments, including posteroanterior pressure techniques (see later discussion). The PAIVM techniques outlined here are used to confirm the findings of the PPIVM tests by testing the joint glides of that segmental level to confirm or refute whether a hypomobility or hypermobility exists. Spinal locking techniques may be used to help localize these techniques to the specific level, or to a specific side of the segment. Descriptions of the symmetric techniques follow.

A pillow or towel roll should be placed under the lumbar spine of the patient if side bending of the lumbar spine appears to be occurring when the patient is placed in the side-lying position.

Flexion. The patient is in the side-lying position, close to the edge of the bed, with the spine supported in the neutral position, the thighs on the table, and the head resting on a pillow. The clinician faces the patient and locates the suspected segment using palpation, so that the monitoring finger is placed between the spinous processes, as in the PPIVM test (see Fig. 25-44). The clinician now flexes the patient's lumbar spine, using the patient's legs, as in the PPIVM test, until motion is felt at the superior spinous process of the monitored segment.

Stabilizing the spinous process of the superior segment with the cranial hand, the clinician straddles the transverse processes of the inferior segment with the index and middle fingers of the caudal hand and pulls the segment inferiorly, using the caudal hand and forearm (Fig. 25-48), thereby indirectly assessing the full superior linear glide of the superior segment (Fig. 25-49). The quality and quantity of the joint glide are assessed.

Extension. The patient and clinician are positioned as in the PPIVM test, with the patient positioned diagonally on the bed, hips forward, knees well flexed, and head resting on a pillow.

Having located the suspected level, the clinician extends the patient's spine to that level by pushing the patient's legs across the table until the monitoring finger detects motion at the superior spinous process (Fig. 25-50). The superior spinous process of the segment is pinched and the joint complex is passively taken into full extension by straddling the transverse processes, as for the flexion technique, and pushing the caudal vertebra

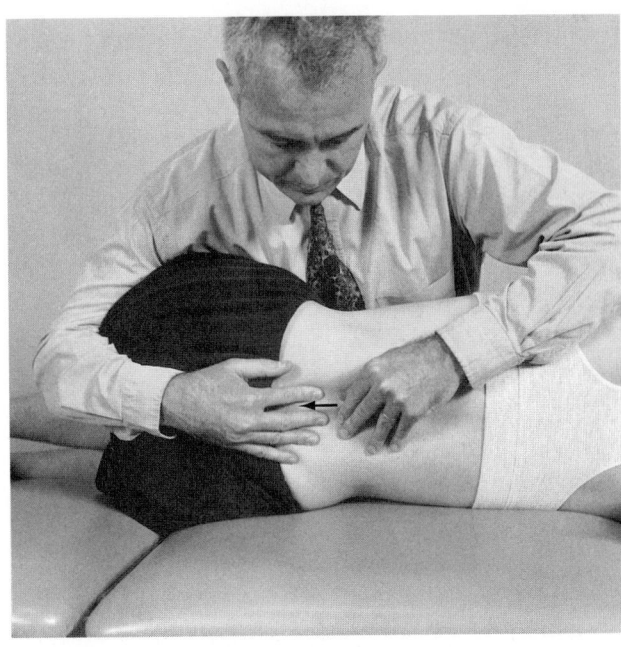

FIGURE 25-48 Passive articular mobility testing for flexion.

anteriorly (see Fig. 25-49). At the end of the available range, the transverse processes of the inferior segment are glided in a cranial direction to test the full linear glide (see Fig. 25-49). The quality and quantity of the joint glide are assessed.

Side Bending. The patient and clinician are positioned as in the PPIVM test, with the patient's hips forward, knees well flexed,

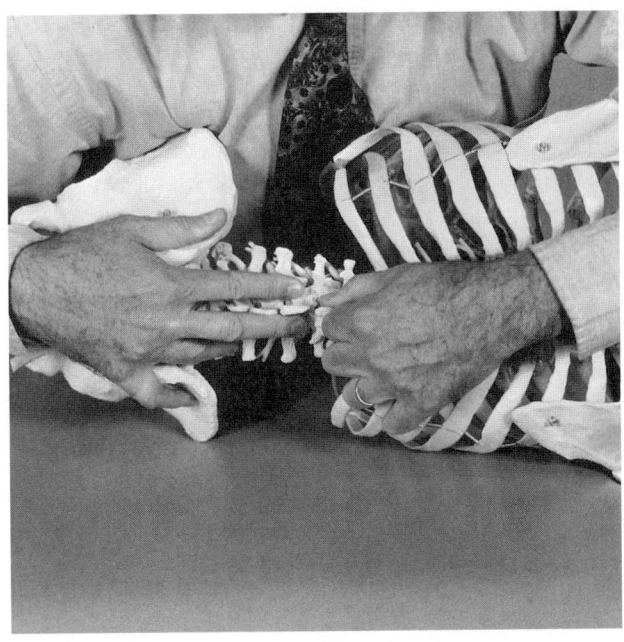

FIGURE 25-49 Passive articular mobility testing for flexion showing hand positions.

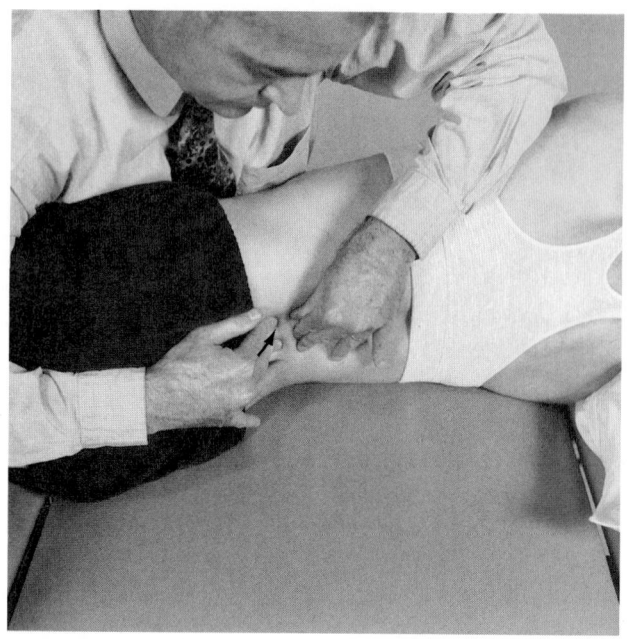

FIGURE 25-50   Passive articular mobility testing for extension.

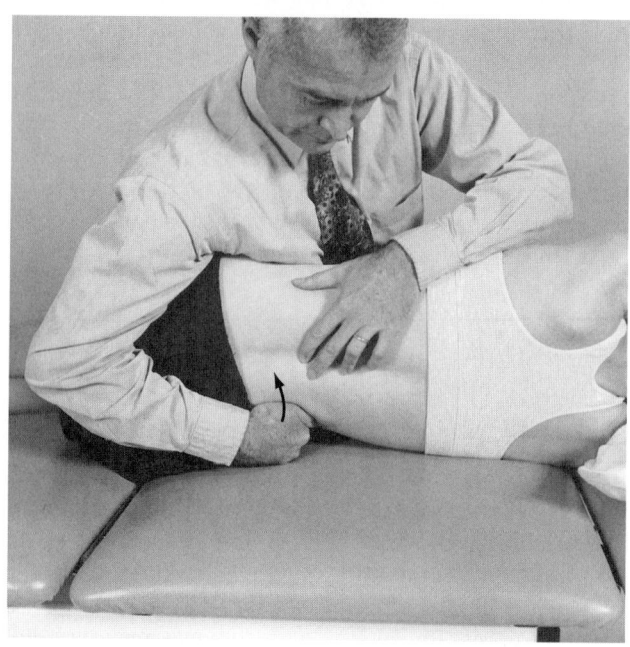

FIGURE 25-51   Passive articular mobility testing for side bending.

and head resting on a pillow. The side on which the patient lies is determined by the intent of the technique.

▶ To test the ability of the segment to side bend ipsilaterally (close), the patient lies on the side to be tested.

▶ To test the ability of the segment to side bend contralaterally (open), the patient lies with the side to be tested uppermost.

Having located the suspected level, the clinician extends or flexes the patient's spine to that level by pushing the patient's legs across the table until the monitoring finger detects motion at the superior spinous process.

The clinician places the axilla of his or her caudal arm over the iliac crest of the patient, while the index and middle fingers of the hand are placed over the spinous processes of the inferior vertebra (Fig. 25-51). The clinician firmly squeezes the patient's pelvis and upper thigh with the caudal arm and applies a force in an inferior direction toward the patient's feet, while the middle finger of the caudal hand pushes the transverse process superiorly.

The quality and quantity of the joint glide are assessed and compared with the other side.

Functional Assessment Tools

Disability and the patient's ability to function may actually be more significant to health care costs than pain alone.[304] Several instruments have been produced in the past 20 years that can provide reliable and valid methods to quantify a patient's functional status.[305]

Overall, no instrument is probably used more often for assessment of the low back than the Oswestry Low Back Disability Questionnaire (OLBDQ),[306] which has been widely researched

and validated by investigators of spinal disorders (see Table 9-6). For each section of six statements, the total score is 5; if the first statement is marked, the score is 0; if the last statement is marked, it is 5. Intervening statements are scored according to rank. If more than one box is marked in each section, the highest score is taken. If all 10 sections are completed, the score is calculated as in the following example:

16 (total scored)/50 (total possible score) × 100 = 32 percent.

If one section is missed (or not applicable), the score is calculated as follows:

16 (total scored)/45 (total possible score) × 100 = 35.5 percent.

Therefore, the final score may be summarized as:

Total score/(5 × number of questions answered) × 100 percent.

The authors suggest rounding the percentage to a whole number for convenience. The general problem with this instrument is that section 8, which deals with the impact of the pain on the patient's sex life, often is not scored by the patient, making the scoring more difficult, and less reliable.

In an attempt to devise a measurement tool in which all of the questions would be more likely to be completed, the Revised Oswestry Pain Questionnaire[307] (Table 25-9) has been recommended. Unfortunately, this questionnaire only bears a limited relationship to the original, confuses impairment with disability, uses complex wording not present in the original Oswestry, and in some sections (1, 2, and 10) does not allow for "no symptoms," which is a key feature of the original instrument.[308] A further disadvantage is that the last section carries a measurement of "changing symptoms," which is inconsistent with the theme of the original questionnaire.[308]

TABLE 25-9   Revised Oswestry Pain Questionnaire

Name: _____ Age: _____ Date of Birth: _____
Address: _____ Occupation: _____
How long have you had Low Back Pain: _____ years _____ months _____ weeks
Is this your first episode of Low Back Pain?   ❏ Yes   ❏ No

Please read: This questionnaire is designed to enable us to understand how much your Low Back Pain has affected your ability to manage your everyday activities. [Please answer each Section by marking in each Section the ONE BOX that most applies to you. We realize that you may feel that more than one statement may relate to you, but PLEASE JUST MARK THE ONE BOX WHICH MOST CLOSELY DESCRIBES YOUR PROBLEM.] Thank You.

Please complete this Questionnaire on___/ /___ and return it to us in the Pre-Paid Envelope provided.

SECTION 1—Pain Intensity
The pain comes and goes and is very mild.
The pain is mild and does not vary much.
The pain comes and goes and is moderate.
The pain is moderate and does not vary much.
The pain comes and goes and is severe.
The pain is severe and does not vary much.

SECTION 2—Personal Care
I would not have to change my way of washing or dressing in order to avoid pain.
I do not normally change my way of washing or dressing even though it causes some pain.
Washing and dressing increase the pain, but I manage *not* to change my way of doing it.
Washing and dressing increase the pain and I find it *necessary* to change my way of doing it.
Because of the pain I am unable to do *some* washing and dressing without help.
Because of the pain I am unable to do *any* washing or dressing without help.

SECTION 3—Lifting
I can lift heavy weights without extra pain.
I can lift heavy weights, but it causes extra pain.
Pain prevents me lifting heavy weights off the floor.
Pain prevents me lifting heavy weights off the floor, but I can manage if they are conveniently positioned, e.g., on a table.
Pain prevents me from lifting heavy weights, but I can manage light to medium weights if they are conveniently positioned.
I can only lift very light weights at the most.

SECTION 4—Walking
I have no pain on walking.
I have some pain on walking, but it does not increase with distance.
I cannot walk more than 1 mile without increasing pain.
I cannot walk more than ½ mile without increasing pain.
I cannot walk more than ¼ mile without increasing pain.
I cannot walk at all without increasing pain.

SECTION 5—Sitting
I can sit in any chair as long as I like.
I can sit only in my favorite chair as long as I like.
Pain prevents me sitting more than 1 hr.
Pain prevents me from sitting more than ½ hr.
Pain prevents me from sitting more than 10 min.
I avoid sitting because it increases pain straight away.

SECTION 6—Standing
I can stand as long as I want without pain.
I have some pain on standing, but it does not increase with time.
I cannot stand for longer than 1 hr without increasing pain.
I cannot stand for longer than ½ hr without increasing pain.
I cannot stand for longer than 10 min without increasing pain.
I avoid standing because it increases the pain straight away.

SECTION 7—Sleeping
I get no pain in bed.
I get pain in bed, but it does not prevent me from sleeping well.
Because of pain my normal nights sleep is reduced by less than ¼.
Because of pain my normal nights sleep is reduced by less than ½.
Because of pain my normal nights sleep is reduced by less than ¾.
Pain prevents from sleeping at all.

SECTION 8—Social Life
My social lift is normal and gives me no pain.
My social life is normal, but increases the degree of my pain.
Pain has no significant effect on my social life apart from limiting my more energetic interests, e.g., dancing, etc.
Pain has restricted my social life and I do not go out very often.
Pain has restricted my social life to my home.
I have hardly any social life because of the pain.

SECTION 9—Traveling
I get no pain while traveling.
I get some pain while traveling, but none of my usual forms of travel make it any worse.
I get extra pain while traveling, but it does not compel me to seek alternative forms of travel.
I get extra pain while traveling which compels me to seek alternative form of travel.
Pain restricts all forms of travel.
Pain prevents all forms of travel except that done lying down.

SECTION 10—Changing Degree of Pain
My pain is rapidly getting better.
My pain fluctuates, but overall is definitely getting better.
My pain seems to be getting better, but improvement is slow at present.
My pain is neither getting better nor worse.
My pain is gradually worsening.
My pain is rapidly worsening.

Anglo-European College of Chiropractic

Both the original Oswestry questionnaire and the revised version require significant time for patients to answer and for staff members to score.

The Functional Rating Index (FRI)[309] (see Table 7-8) is an instrument that is somewhat easier and quicker to use, and that emphasizes function while concurrently measuring the patient's opinion, attitude, and self-rating of disability.[310] The instrument contains 10 items that measure both pain and function of the spinal musculoskeletal system. The FRI is specifically designed to quantitatively measure the subjective perception of function and pain of the spinal musculoskeletal system in a clinical environment.[309]

Of the 10 items, 8 refer to activities of daily living that might be adversely affected by a spinal condition, and 2 refer to two different attributes of pain. Because many spinal disabilities are most likely a combination of loss of function and pain or the fear of pain, using both pain and function allows for a wider view of a patient's disability. Using a 5-point scale for each item, the patient ranks his or her perceived ability to perform a function or the quantity of pain at the present time by selecting one of the five response points (0 = no pain or full ability to function; 4 = worst possible pain and/or unable to perform this function at all).[309]

Additional research is needed to compare the sensitivity of this instrument with that of the OLBDQ to determine whether the FRI is a valuable instrument for the researcher and clinician.

The Roland-Morris Disability Questionnaire (RDQ)[311] (Table 25-10) is a health status measure designed to be completed by patients to assess physical disability due to LBP. The RDQ was derived from the Sickness Impact Profile (SIP), which is a 136-item health status measure covering all aspects of physical and mental function.[312] Twenty-four items were selected from the SIP, and each item was qualified with the phrase "because of my back pain" to distinguish back pain disability from disability resulting from other causes—a distinction that patients are, in general, able to make without difficulty.[312,313]

Patients are asked to place a check mark beside a statement if it applies to them that day, and the score is calculated by

TABLE 25-10   The Roland-Morris Disability Questionnaire

When your back hurts, you may find it difficult to do some things you normally do.

This list contains sentences that people have used to describe themselves when they have back pain. When you read them, you may find that some stand out because they describe you *today*. As you read the list, think of yourself *today*. When you read a sentence that describes you today, put a tick against it. If the sentence does not describe you, then leave the space blank and go on to the next one. Remember, only tick the sentence if you are sure it describes you today.

❑ I stay at home most of the time because of my back
❑ I change position frequently to try and get my back comfortable
❑ I walk more slowly than usual because of my back
❑ Because of my back I am not doing any of the jobs that I usually do around the house
❑ Because of my back, I use a handrail to get upstairs
❑ Because of my back, I lie down to rest more often
❑ Because of my back, I have to hold on to something to get out of an easy chair
❑ Because of my back, I try to get other people to do things for me
❑ I get dressed more slowly than usual because of my back
❑ I only stand for short periods of time because of my back
❑ Because of my back, I try not to bend or kneel down
❑ I find it difficult to get out of a chair because of my back
❑ My back is painful almost all the time
❑ I find it difficult to turn over in bed because of my back
❑ My appetite is not very good because of my back pain
❑ I have trouble putting on my socks (or stockings) because of the pain in my back
❑ I only walk short distances because of my back
❑ I sleep less well on my back
❑ Because of my back pain, I get dressed with help from someone else
❑ I sit down for most of the day because of my back
❑ I avoid heavy jobs around the house because of my back
❑ Because of my back pain, I am more irritable and bad tempered with people than usual
❑ Because of my back, I go upstairs more slowly than usual
❑ I stay in bed most of the time because of my back

adding up the number of items checked. Scores, therefore, range from 0 (no disability) to 24 (maximum disability). RDQ scores have been found to correlate well with other measures of physical function, including the physical subscales of 36-item Short Form Health Survey (SF-36), the SIP, and the OLBDQ.[312]

Special Tests

Neurodynamic Mobility Testing. The slump, bowstring, double straight leg raise, and prone knee flexion tests are described in Chapter 12.

Straight Leg Raise Test. The straight leg raise (SLR) test, which is also described in Chapter 12, should be a routine test during the examination of the lumbar spine among patients with sciatica or pseudoclaudication. However, the test is often negative in patients with spinal stenosis.[237] A leg elevation of less than 60 degrees is abnormal, suggesting compression or irritation of the nerve roots. A positive test reproduces the symptoms of sciatica, with pain that radiates below the knee, not merely back or hamstring pain.[237] Ipsilateral straight leg raising has sensitivity but not specificity for a herniated IVD, whereas crossed straight leg raising (see Chap. 12) is insensitive but highly specific. The clinician must remember that the SLR test stresses a number of structures including:

▶ Lumbosacral nerve roots.

▶ Hamstrings.

▶ Hip joint.

▶ Sacroiliac joint.

The following guidelines can be used to interpret the results from the test[314]:

▶ Symptoms reproduced in the 0- to 30-degree range may indicate hip pathology or a severely inflamed nerve root.

▶ Symptoms reproduced in the 30- to 50-degree range may indicate sciatic nerve root involvement.

▶ Symptoms reproduced in the 50- to 70-degree range may indicate hamstring involvement.

▶ Symptoms reproduced in the 70- to 90-degree range may indicate involvement of the hip and/or the sacroiliac joint.

A modification of the SLR test can be used to help detect the presence of the piriformis syndrome (see Chap. 9).

Pheasant's Test. The patient is positioned prone. While monitoring for motion at the patient's pelvis, the clinician passively flexes the patient's knees (see Fig. 25-21). Pheasant's test introduces an anterior pelvic tilt and an increase in lordosis through the pull of the rectus femoris. Once motion occurs at the pelvis, the clinician determines whether the low back symptoms have been reproduced.[315] A pulling sensation on the anterior aspect of the thighs is a normal finding. If full knee flexion is achieved before the tilting occurs, the patient is positioned in the prone-on-elbows position, and the test is repeated. Patients who test positive for this maneuver tend to have the following subjective complaints:

▶ Pain with supine lying and the legs straight, unless the rectus and hip flexors are especially flexible.

▶ Pain with prone lying on a soft mattress.

▶ Pain with sitting erect.

▶ Pain with prolonged standing.

The cause of the pain is thought to be the passive stretching or compression of pain-sensitive structures. These structures include the zygapophysial joints, the segmental ligaments, and the anterior aspect of the IVD.

Pelvic Drop Test. The patient stands with one leg on a stool. The leg on the stool is straight. The patient lowers the other leg so that the foot touches the ground and then raises the leg by hiking the hip (Fig. 25-52). Ten repetitions of this exercise without substitution should be considered normal.

Compression Test (Modified Farfan Test). The patient is positioned supine. The clinician flexes the patient's hips and knees to the point where the pelvis starts to rotate posteriorly (Fig. 25-53). The clinician then squeezes the patient's thighs against his or her chest and exerts a cranially directed pressure against the patient's feet or buttocks to flex, and apply an axial compression force to, the patient's spine.[105]

The test is positive if pain is produced. There are two scenarios for the pain production. The pain can occur before the posterior rotation of the pelvis, or during the axial loading. If it occurs before, the following may be present:

▶ Anterior spondylolisthesis.

▶ Muscle tear.

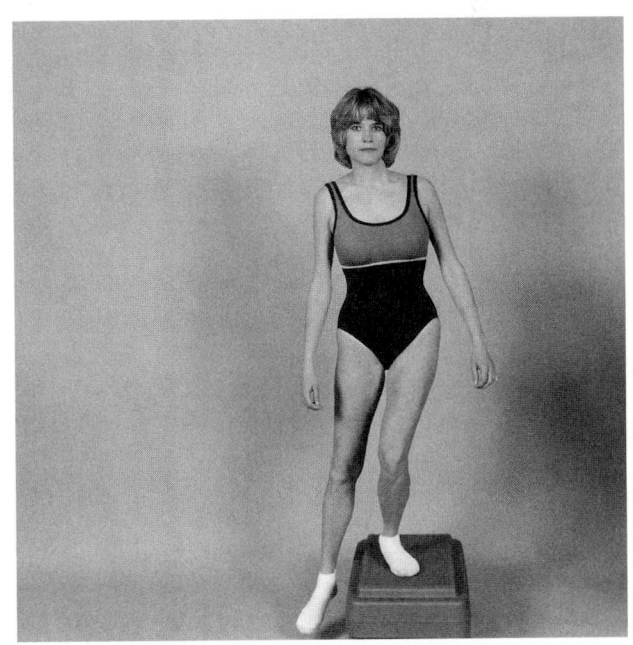

FIGURE 25-52 Pelvic drop test.

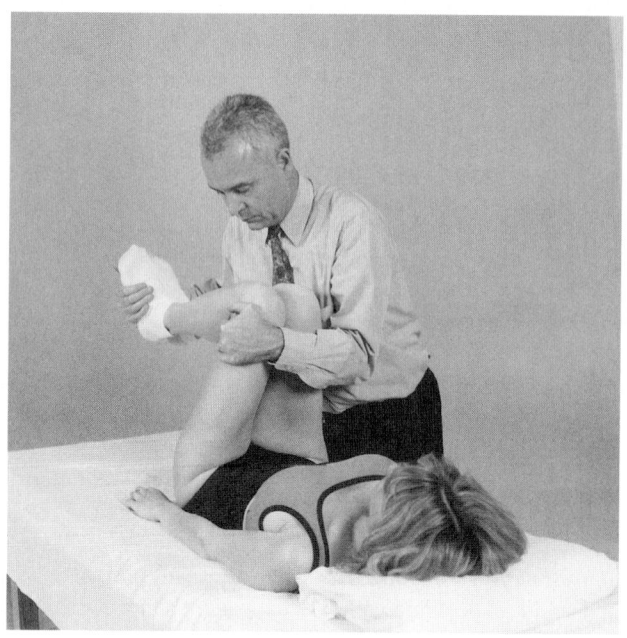

FIGURE 25-53   Farfan compression test.

▶ Acute instability.

▶ Malingering patient.

If the pain is reproduced with the axial loading, there is the possibility of an end-plate fracture or acute IVD herniation.

Anterior Sacroiliac Joint Stress Test.   The anterior stress test, also called the *gapping test,* is performed with the patient supine. The clinician stands to one side of the patient and, crossing the arms, places the palm of the hands on the patient's anterior superior iliac spines (Fig. 25-54). The crossing of the arms ensures that the applied force is in a lateral direction, thereby gapping the anterior aspect of the sacroiliac joint. The stress is maintained for 7 to 10 seconds, or until an end-feel is obtained. The procedure stresses the ventral ligament and compresses the posterior aspect of the joint. A positive test is one in which the patient's groin or sacroiliac joint pain is reproduced either anteriorly, posteriorly, unilaterally, or bilaterally.[123]

The anterior gapping test, and its posterior counterpart (see next section), are believed to be sensitive for severe arthritis or ventral ligament tears of the sacroiliac joint,[266] although they have been shown to be poorly reproducible.[316]

Posterior Sacroiliac Joint Stress Test.   The posterior stress test, also called the *compression test,* is performed with the patient in the side lying position. The clinician, standing behind the patient, applies a downward force on the side of the patient's uppermost innominate, using both hands (Fig. 25-55). The procedure creates a medial force that tends to gap the posterior aspect of the sacroiliac joint while compressing its anterior aspect. The reproduction of pain over one or both of the sacroiliac joints is considered a positive test.

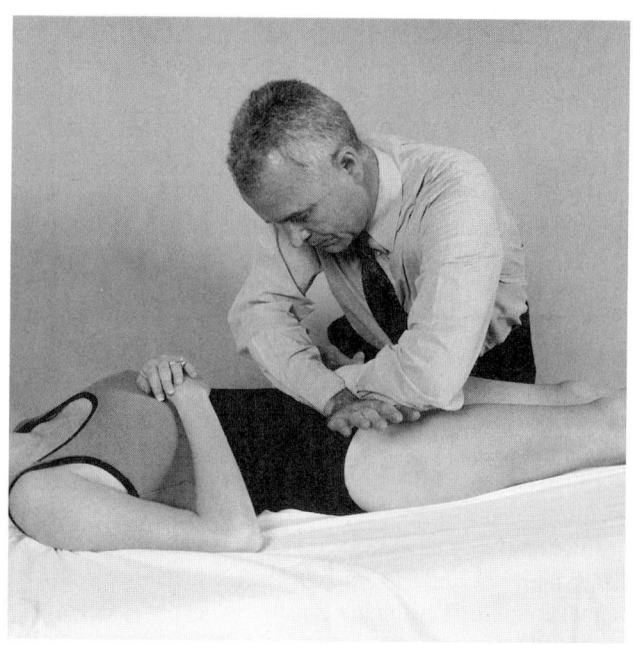

FIGURE 25-54   Anterior sacroiliac joint stress test.

The dorsal sacroiliac ligament (see Chap. 27), which is accessible just below the posterior inferior iliac spine, should be palpated for tenderness.[317]

FADE (Flexion, Adduction, Extension) Positional Test.[318]   The set-up for the FADE test is similar to that of the FABER (flexion, abduction, external rotation) test (see Chap. 17), except that the start position involves moving the patient's hip into

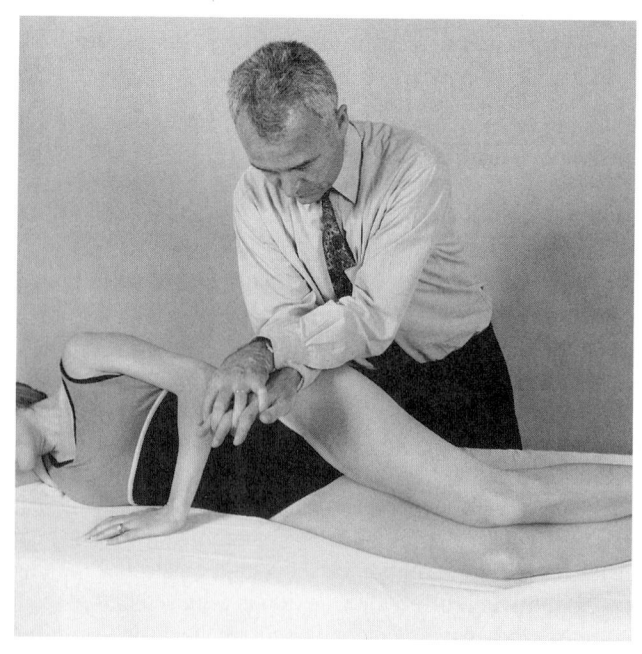

FIGURE 25-55   Posterior sacroiliac joint stress test.

McKenzie Exercises

The McKenzie exercises are a series of active and passive movements performed in the beginning, middle, and end ranges of trunk flexion, extension, and combinations of side bending and rotation called *side gliding*.[228] The end-range exercises theoretically move the nucleus pulposus (NP) away from the side of compression loading, with flexion exercises moving the NP posteriorly and extension exercises moving the NP anteriorly.[228,334–339] The midrange exercises are better suited for patients with symptoms of neural compression.[340]

Exercises typically are performed in non–weight bearing initially, and then in weight bearing, and the movement chosen is based on the ability of the exercise to centralize the patient's symptoms. Although the McKenzie maneuvers are referred to as exercises, most of the procedures are passive self-mobilizations, aimed at regaining spinal extension while concurrently maintaining flexion.

The McKenzie method has been tested for intra-observer variability, with differing results.[232,341,342] Several outcome studies have examined the effectiveness of the McKenzie method compared with that of other approaches.[343–346] Ponte and colleagues[343] compared the effectiveness of the McKenzie method with that of the Williams approach and found that the McKenzie method demonstrated greater improvements in pain intensity and lumbar range of motion than the Williams protocol.[343] However, this study had a small sample size (22 subjects), and subjects were not randomly assigned but rather assigned by the referring physician to a treatment group.

Nwuga and Nwuga[344] also compared the effectiveness of the McKenzie method with that of the Williams approach. Sixty-two female subjects, aged 20 to 40 years and all diagnosed with a prolapsed IVD in the lumbar spine, were assigned to either the McKenzie group or the Williams group. Similar conclusions were drawn from this study as from the Ponte study; namely, that the McKenzie method demonstrated greater improvements in pain intensity and lumbar range of motion than the Williams protocol.[344]

Stankovic and Johnell performed two separate outcome studies (1989 and 1994) that compared long-term patient outcomes following treatment with either the McKenzie approach or with patient education alone in a mini back school.[345,346] A mini back school involves education of the patient in the mechanics of the spine, proper posture, and safe lifting techniques. The 1989 study assessed six variables in 100 employed patients with acute LBP: return to work, sick leave during recurrences, recurrences of pain during the year of observation, pain, movement, and the patient's ability to self-help. The McKenzie method was found to be superior in four of the six variables. The two variables that showed no significant difference were sick leave during recurrences and patient's ability to self-help.[346] The 1994 study was a continuation of the 1989 study and used the same subjects. The later study showed that subjects who received McKenzie treatment had significantly fewer recurrences of pain and current episodes of sick leave compared with the subjects who received mini back school education.[345]

A randomized controlled comparative trial with an 8-month follow-up period was conducted by Petersen et al[346a] that compared the effect of the McKenzie treatment method with that of intensive dynamic strengthening training in patients with subacute or chronic low back pain. There were 260 consecutive patients with low back pain and at least 8 weeks duration of symptoms (85 percent of the patients had more than 3 months duration of symptoms). The patients were randomized into two groups: Group A was treated with the McKenzie method ($n = 132$), and Group B was treated with intensive dynamic strengthening training ($n = 128$). The treatment period for both groups was 8 weeks at an outpatient clinic, followed by 2 months of self-training at home. Treatment results were recorded at the end of the treatment period at the clinic, then 2 and 8 months after. The study concluded that the McKenzie method and intensive dynamic strengthening training seem to be equally effective in the treatment of patients with subacute or chronic low back pain.

Spinal Stabilization Exercises

The basic premise in spinal stabilization exercises is to teach the patient with LBP how to maintain functional levels by dynamically stabilizing the involved segments with increased muscular support. This increased muscular support can then be used to help maintain the neutral zone. Graded posterior pelvic tilting (Fig. 25-58) or the abdominal hollowing (Fig. 25-59)

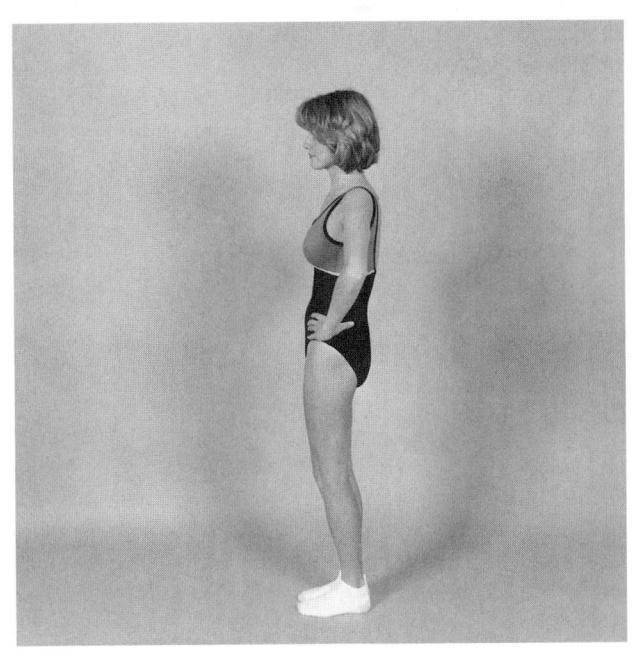

FIGURE 25-58 Posterior pelvic tilt.

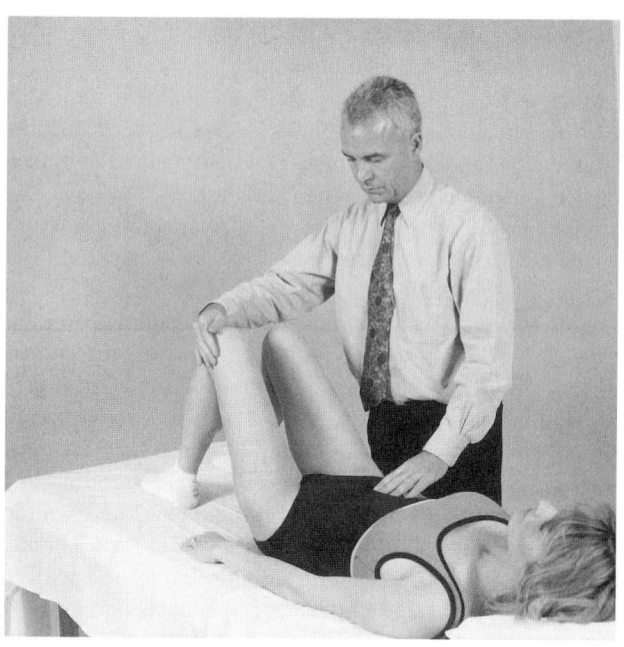

FIGURE 25-59 Abdominal hollowing.

exercises are the cornerstones of most stabilization programs.[99,148,285,297] Because the posterior pelvic tilt has the potential to preload the annulus and posterior ligaments,[168] and thus cause further injury, it should only be performed in a graded fashion to the point at which the neutral zone is located.

The four basic back support systems involved in spinal stabilization exercises include intra-abdominal pressure, the thoracolumbar fascia, the hydraulic amplifier system, and the muscular support system. Given that low back tissues may need stressing to enhance their health but too much loading can be detrimental, choosing the optimal exercise requires judgment based on clinical experience and scientific evidence.[167] Before the stabilization progression can begin, the involved structures must be permitted to heal beyond the acute stage of healing. This can be achieved with patient education and with exercises that involve extremity motion, while avoiding excessive trunk motion.

Stabilization exercises can be categorized as segmental (local) or regional (global). The global stabilization exercises are described in the "Functional Phase."

Segmental Stabilization. The segmental stabilizers, or "core" muscles, include the quadratus lumborum, transversus abdominis, internal oblique, and lumbar multifidus. These muscles surround the lumbar spine, whose primary role is considered the provision of dynamic stability and segmental control to the spine.[206] Segmental exercises are usually performed earlier in the rehabilitation process than regional exercises.

As with any other exercise progression, the lumbar stabilization exercise progression should include:

1. *Variation.* Variation to the exercises can be provided by altering[347]:
   a. Plane of motion.
   b. Range of motion.
   c. Body position.
   d. Exercise duration.
   e. Exercise frequency.
2. *A safe progression.* A safe progression is ensured if the exercises are progressed from[347]:
   a. Slow to fast.
   b. Simple to complex.
   c. Stable to unstable.
   d. Low force to high force.

The techniques to increase joint mobility and the techniques to increase soft tissue extensibility are described later, under "Therapeutic Techniques."

Acute Phase

In the acute phase of rehabilitation for the lumbar spine, the intervention goals are to:

▶ Decrease pain, inflammation, and muscle spasm.

▶ Promote healing of tissues.

▶ Increase pain-free range of segmental motion.

▶ Regain soft tissue extensibility.

▶ Regain neuromuscular control.

▶ Allow progression to the functional phase.

The recommendations concerning bed rest for common, acute LBP have changed over the years.[348] In a 1986 study by Deyo and colleagues,[349] primary care physicians in the walk-in clinic of a public hospital found that the prescription of 2 days' rest was equivalent to a prescription of 7 days in terms of pain and function. Moreover, a prescription of 2 days' rest was associated with fewer days of sick leave. In 1995, Malmivaara and colleagues[350] showed that continuation of daily activity to the extent tolerable resulted in a more rapid recovery than either bed rest or back-mobilizing exercises. The most recent guidelines (2000), based on the results of several randomized studies, advise avoiding bed rest to the extent possible.[351] A study by Rozenberg and colleagues[62] found that for patients with acute LBP, normal activity is at least equivalent to bed rest. These authors recommended that prescriptions for bed rest, and thus for sick leaves, should be limited when the physical demands of the job are similar to those for daily life activities.[62]

Pain relief may be accomplished initially by the use of modalities such as cryotherapy, and electrical stimulation, gentle exercises, and occasionally the temporary use of a spinal brace. Thermal modalities, especially ultrasound, with its ability to penetrate deeply, may be used after 48 to 72 hours. Patient education should be emphasized during this phase. Information about activities to avoid should be given, in addition to advice about positions of comfort. Once the pain and inflammation are under control, the intervention can progress toward the restoration of full strength, range of motion, and normal posture.

Manual techniques during this phase may include myofascial release, grade I and II joint mobilizations, massage, gentle stretching, and muscle energy techniques. Manual or mechanical traction may be used for patients with IVD herniations (see Chap. 20).

Range of motion for the lumbar spine is regained initially in the unloaded position of the spine, depending on patient response, in prone lying, the quadruped position, or supine lying. Initially, the exercises prescribed are those that were found to provide relief during the examination. Usually, either flexion or extension movements demonstrate benefit.

Tissue loading during walking has been found to be below levels caused by many specific rehabilitation tasks, suggesting that walking is a wise choice as an initial aerobic exercise for general back rehabilitation.[352]

O'Sullivan[59] recommends the following progression, which is based on a three-stage process of motor learning[353]:

Cognitive Stage

The cognitive stage is part of the acute phase of healing. According to Waddell,[3] 80 to 90 percent of patients with LBP will be asymptomatic in 6 weeks, 98 percent in 24 weeks, and 99 percent in 52 weeks. The purpose of this stage, which can last 3 to 6 weeks, is to increase the patient's kinesthetic awareness, and to help the patient determine a range in which he or she can function and exercise without harmful pain.[57]

The patient initially is taught to maintain controlled costal-diaphragm breathing while performing the abdominal hollowing exercise, and to maintain a neutral lordosis without the simultaneous contraction of the global muscle system. Abdominal bracing also is performed by flaring out laterally the waist region just above the iliac crest.[206]

Training may begin in a non–weight-bearing position such as supine before progressing to weight-bearing postures. Contractions initially are held for 5 seconds and gradually are increased to 60 seconds. Training is performed a minimum of once a day for 10 to 15 minutes, with emphasis on proper co-contraction of the local muscle system. Depending on the severity of the condition, this range may initially be small, permitting only upper or lower extremity motions and gentle isometrics of the spinal muscles. Specific exercises such as these have been shown to be effective for individuals with chronic LBP.[178] Research investigating different abdominal exercises has confirmed that some exercises are more specific for activating the deep abdominal muscles than others.[354] The abdominal hollowing maneuver is one exercise known to result in preferential activation of the internal oblique and transversus abdominis, with little contribution by the rectus abdominis in the pain-free population.[354] Researchers have demonstrated that an inability to perform the abdominal hollowing maneuver differentiates chronic LBP from pain-free subjects.[148,200]

Once the abdominal hollowing and abdominal bracing techniques are mastered, they are performed during lower and upper extremity open-chain activities to improve muscular endurance.[202,355] The following exercises may be superimposed on the abdominal hollowing maneuver:

▶ Supine unilateral arm elevation to a point in the range just shy of the pain.

▶ Supine bilateral arm elevation to a point in the range just shy of the pain.

▶ Supine unilateral heel slides.

▶ Supine bilateral heel slides.

Progression to dynamic functional movements with upper and lower extremity close-chain activities may be indicated after the patient is able to correctly perform the isometric and open-chain exercises without pain.[202,206] Once the patient is able to perform these exercises without significant pain, he or she can progress to more functional activities and aerobic exercises.

Associative Stage

The associative stage is the second aspect of motor learning. This phase is reserved for those patients that continue to have pain that interferes with activities of daily living or recreational activities. The focus of this stage is to refine pain-provoking movement patterns by isolating them into component parts with increased repetitions, and while maintaining the co-contraction of the local muscle group. Repetition of movement is required to increase the speed and complexity of the movements, which then become automatic. The goal for this stage is to have the patient perform activities such as sit to stand, walking, lifting, and carrying objects while maintaining a neutral lordotic curve and co-contraction of the local muscle system, and while breathing in a controlled fashion. Success at this level, which can take anywhere from 8 weeks to 4 months to achieve, depends on the level of the patient's motivation, compliance, and the severity of the pathology. During this stage, patients also are encouraged to perform regular aerobic exercise, such as walking, and to perform the co-contraction exercises in situations in which they experience or anticipate pain.

Autonomous Stage

The final stage of motor learning is the autonomous or functional phase. For many patients, the functional phase represents a personal lifetime commitment to exercise. Most, if not all, patients should be exercising independently at home or in a local gym at this stage.

Functional Phase

During this phase, the patient learns to initiate and execute functional activities without pain and while dynamically stabilizing the spine in an automatic manner.

The exercises described in the following sections have been shown to challenge muscle and enhance performance but are performed in such a way as to minimize loading of the spine to reduce the risk of injury exacerbation. Interindividual differences in injury status or training goals may allow for a continuum of required muscle stress and acceptable loading of the low back.[161]

Functional Phase Exercises

Quadratus Lumborum. The quadratus lumborum can be strengthened using the following exercise. The patient is asked to place one foot on a 20-cm (8-in) stool or step and to stand up straight. The patient then lowers the non–weight-bearing leg to the floor (see Fig. 25-52). On lowering the leg, there should be no arm abduction, anterior or pelvic motion, or trunk flexion. Nor should there be any hip adduction or internal rotation of the weight-bearing hip.

Quadruped Cat-camel Stretch.[167] The cat-camel stretch is performed by slowly moving through full spinal flexion to full extension while in the quadruped position.

Multifidus. The multifidus can be strengthened using resisted spinal extension or hyperextension exercises. Initially, these exercises can be performed in the quadruped position using single leg extension raises. These exercises can then be progressed to opposite arm and leg raises. More advanced exercises for the multifidus and the spinal extensor muscles include[129]:

▶ Back extension or hyperextension over a high bench.

▶ Modified "dead lift" (knees flexed to about 20 degrees).

▶ Seated rows.

▶ Squats.

▶ Back extension machines (with the pelvis fixated).

Functional Progression in Sitting

▶ Seated unilateral arm elevation to a point in the range just shy of the pain.

▶ Seated bilateral arm elevation to a point in the range just shy of the pain.

▶ Seated unilateral knee extension to a point in the range just shy of the pain.

▶ Seated unilateral hip flexion to a point in the range just shy of the pain.

Exercise Progressions

The following exercise progressions for the acute and functional phases have proven useful over the years in treating lumbar instabilities, and the reader is encouraged to investigate these further while individually tailoring the intervention, depending on clinical findings.[99,356–359]

The goal of the global stabilization progression is to determine the pain-free range or ranges in which the exercises are tolerated. Perhaps surprisingly, theses ranges are not always in the sagittal plane and can, in fact, involve rotary or side-bending movements.

Protection of the lumbar spine needs to be provided during these exercises to prevent an excessive amount of lordosis from occurring. For example, the exercises in the prone position should be performed with a pillow underneath the patient's abdominals to prevent excessive hyperlordosis.

Each of the progressions outlined next is listed according to an approximated degree of difficulty. The more difficult exercises incorporate dynamic stabilization exercises, which include weight shifting and extremity exercises on an unstable support such as a Swiss ball, or are performed in standing.

Supine Progression

▶ *Posterior and anterior pelvic tilting in hook-lying position.*

▶ *Posterior pelvic tilt with legs straight.*

▶ *Supine cervical flexion.* The patient is asked to lift the head from the table, attempting to touch the chin to the chest.

▶ *Unilateral shoulder flexion.* Keeping the elbows straight, the patient is asked to slowly raise one arm overhead, until he or she feels the lower back begin to arch (Fig. 25-60). The patient then slowly returns the arm to the starting position. The exercise is repeated with the other arm.

▶ *Bilateral shoulder flexion.* Keeping the elbows straight, the patient is asked to slowly raise both arms overhead, until he or she feels the lower back begin to arch. The patient then slowly returns the arms to the starting position.

▶ *Alternate knees to chest.* With arms at the sides, the patient is asked to slide one leg along the table toward the buttock. The patient is then asked to lift the knee toward the chest until the lower back starts to move toward the table. This exercise can be made more difficult by having the patient lie on a foam roll with the arms raised (Fig. 25-61).

▶ *Bilateral knees to chest.* The patient is supine lying. With arms at the sides, the patient is asked to slide both feet along the table toward the buttocks. The patient is then asked to

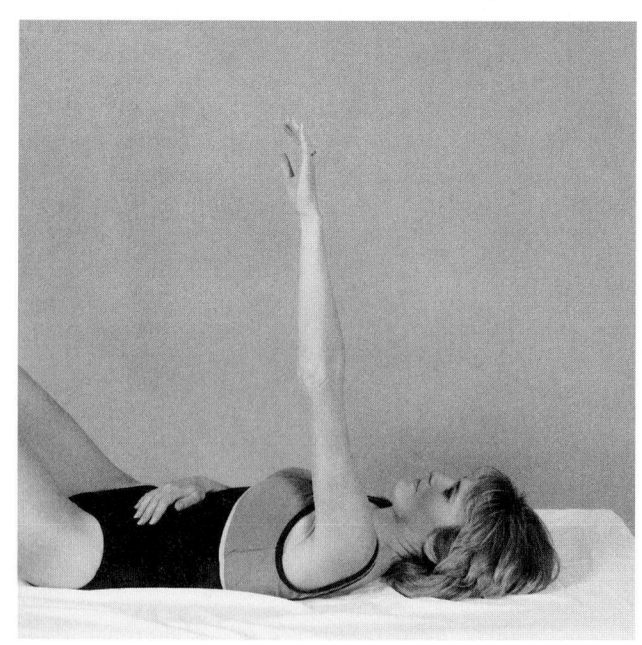

FIGURE 25-60 Unilateral shoulder flexion.

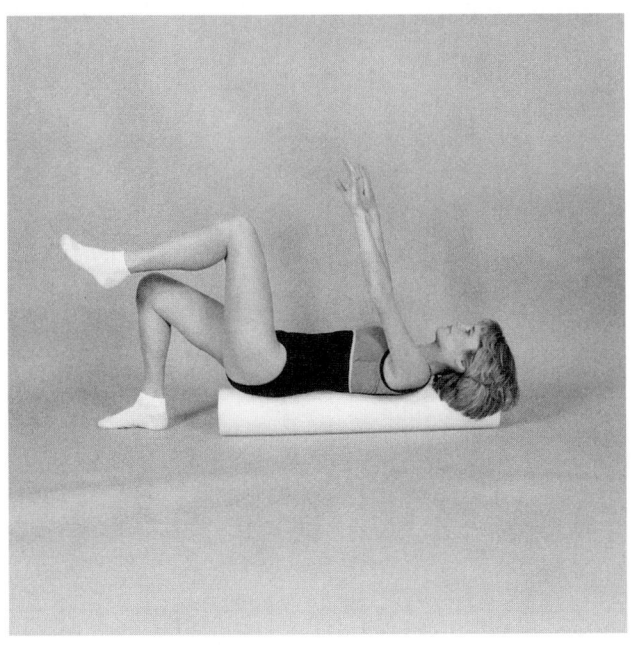

FIGURE 25-61   Alternate knees to chest.

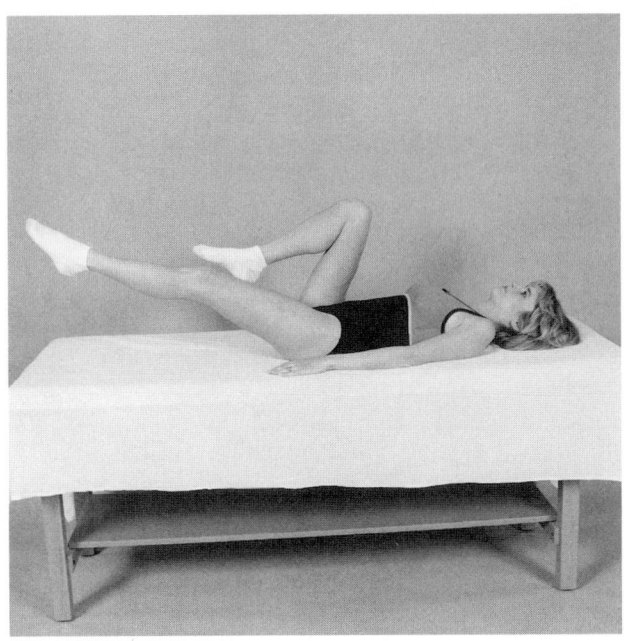

FIGURE 25-62   Alternate leg kicks.

lift both knees toward the chest until the lower back starts to move toward the table. The patient is asked to return to the starting position.

▶ *Hand to knee.* The patient starts with arms and legs straight, and arms overhead. Keeping the right elbow straight, the patient is asked to bring that arm to waist level while bringing the left knee toward the chest. The patient is then asked to touch the left knee with the right hand, before returning to the starting position.

▶ *Hands to knees.* The patient starts in the same position as for the previous exercise. Keeping the elbows straight, the patient is asked to bring both knees and arms to the waist. The patient touches the knees with the hands, before returning to the starting position.

▶ *Posterior pelvic tilt with alternating leg kicks (Fig. 25-62).*

▶ *Dead bug.* The patient maintains a posterior pelvic tilt while performing alternating leg kicks and arm raises simultaneously (Fig. 25-63).

▶ *Curl-up.* The patient is positioned supine, with the legs bent at the knees and the feet flat on the floor. The arms are folded across the chest. Concentrating on curling the upper trunk as much as possible, the patient is asked to perform an abdominal hollowing and then to raise the head and shoulders off the bed by about 30 to 45 degrees. After holding this position for 2 to 3 seconds, the patient returns to the initial position. The muscles strengthened with this exercise include the upper rectus abdominis and the internal and external obliques.

▶ *Reverse quadruped.* The patient is positioned supine, with the hips and knees flexed to approximately 90 degrees,

and the arms out in front. The position is maintained for 30 seconds.

▶ *Hip thrusts.* The patient is positioned supine, with the hips and knees flexed to approximately 90 degrees, and the arms by the sides. From this position, the patient is asked to perform a posterior pelvic tilt and lift the pelvis off the bed, while maintaining the hip and knee positions (Fig. 25-64).

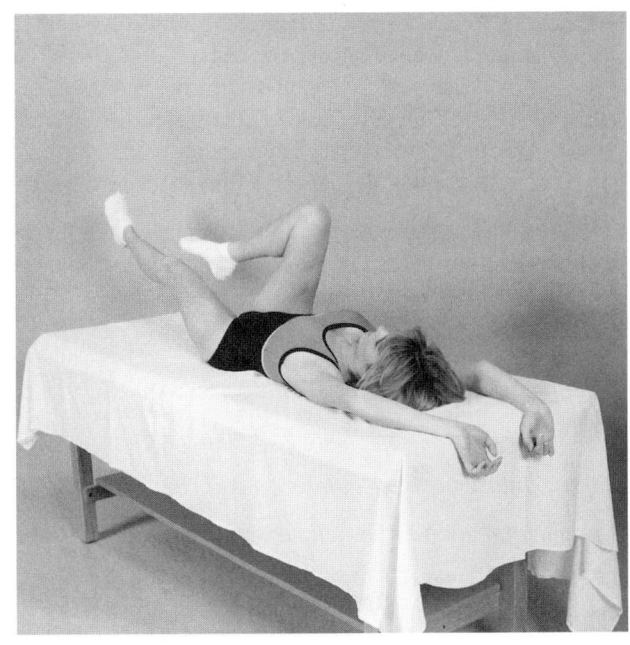

FIGURE 25-63   Dead bug exercise.

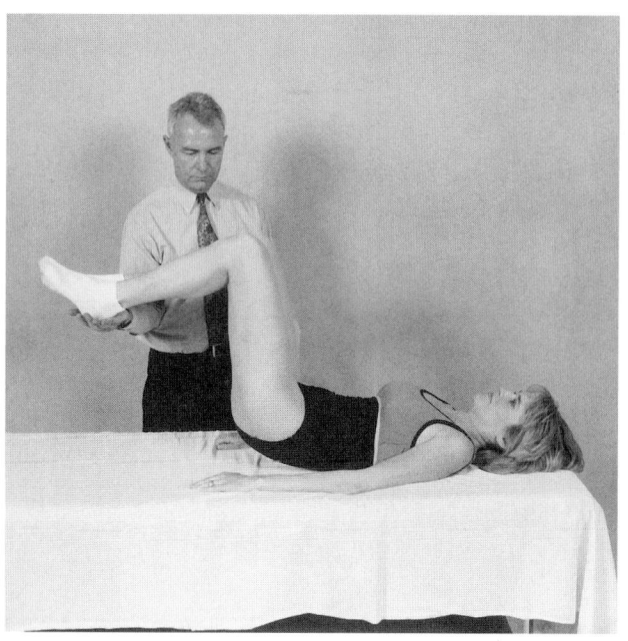

FIGURE 25-64   Hip thrusts.

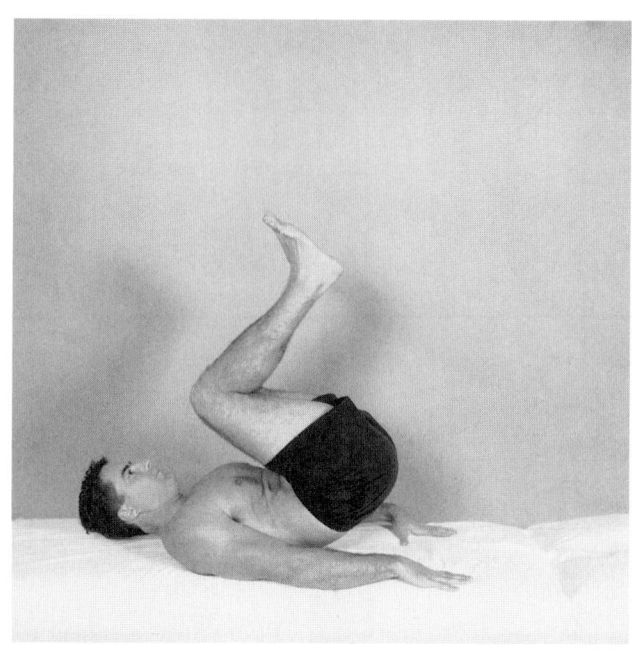

FIGURE 25-65   Reverse curl-up.

▶ *Rotational partial sit-up.* The patient is asked to cross the arms on the chest and to lift the chin toward the chest. The patient is then asked to attempt to lift the right shoulder up from the table while twisting the trunk to the left, before slowly lowering the shoulder to the table.

▶ *Reverse curl-up.* The patient is positioned supine, with the legs bent at the knees and the feet flat on the floor. The arms are by the sides. The patient is asked to perform an abdominal hollowing, and then to raise the feet off the bed until the thighs are vertical. This is the start position. From this position, the patient is asked to raise the pelvis up and toward the shoulders, keeping the knees bent tightly, until the knees are as close to the chest as possible (Fig. 25-65). The patient is allowed to push down on the bed with the hands. After holding this position for 2 to 3 seconds, the patient returns to the start position.

▶ *Bridging.* The patient is positioned supine, with the arms by the sides. The patient is asked to keep the knees bent and feet flat, and to lift the buttocks from the floor (Fig. 25-66).

▶ *Bridging with marching (Fig. 25-67).*

▶ *Bridging with feet on a Swiss ball, knees bent (Fig. 25-68).*

▶ *Bridging with feet on a Swiss ball, knees straight.*

▶ *Supine hamstring curl with Swiss ball (Fig. 25-69).*

▶ *Lying supine on a Swiss ball, knees bent (Fig. 25-70).*

▶ *Bridging on a Swiss ball and twisting torso while keeping hands together.*

▶ *Swiss ball pull-over.* The patient is positioned supine on a Swiss ball, with a medicine ball held between two hands at

waist level. The medicine ball is raised over the head and then returned to the start position.

Prone Progression

▶ *Isometric gluteal sets.* The patient is positioned prone, with a pillow under the stomach. The patient is asked to tighten the buttock muscles and to hold the contraction for 6 seconds, and then relax.

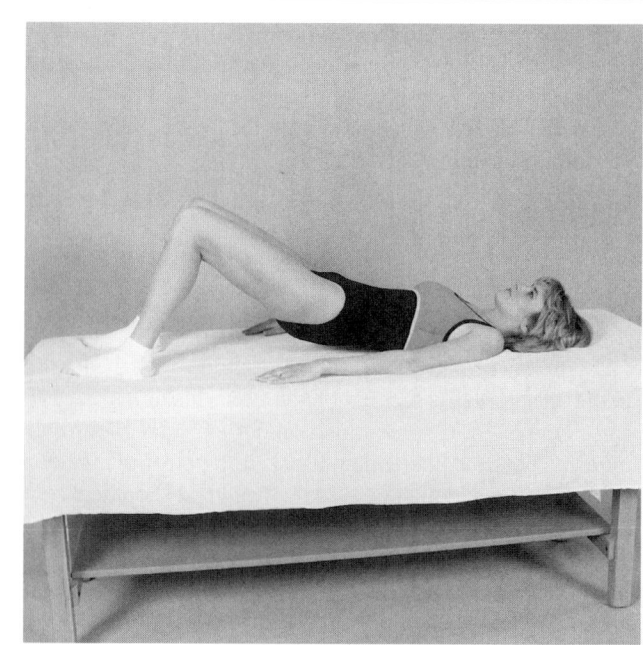

FIGURE 25-66   Bridging.

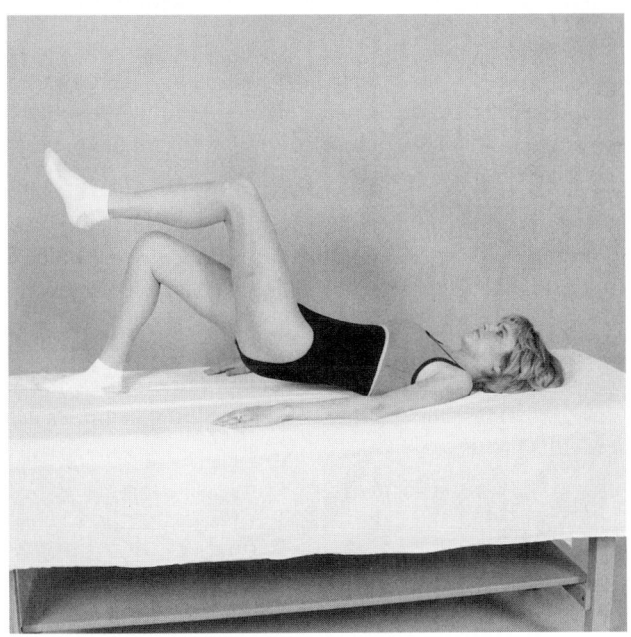

FIGURE 25-67   Bridging with marching.

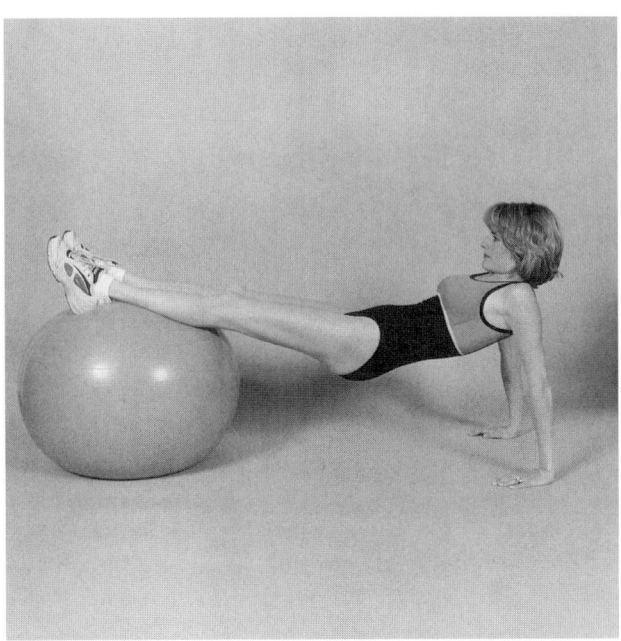

FIGURE 25-69   Hamstring curl on Swiss ball: start position.

▶ *Alternating hip extension.*   The patient is positioned prone, with a pillow under the stomach. The patient is asked to tighten the buttock and abdominal muscles, and to lift one leg 1 inch off the table. The patient then lowers the leg and performs a lift with the other leg. The knees should be kept straight, or bent, depending on the degree of difficulty desired. From the prone position, the patient is asked to flex the knee to around 90 degrees, and then to raise the thigh off

the bed, as high as is comfortable, and without introducing rotation at the lumbar spine (Fig. 25-71). The end position is held for 2 to 3 seconds, and then the thigh is returned to the bed. The exercise can be made more difficult by extending the knee and raising the straight leg from the bed.

▶ *Alternating shoulder flexion.*   The patient is positioned prone, with a pillow under the stomach. The patient is asked

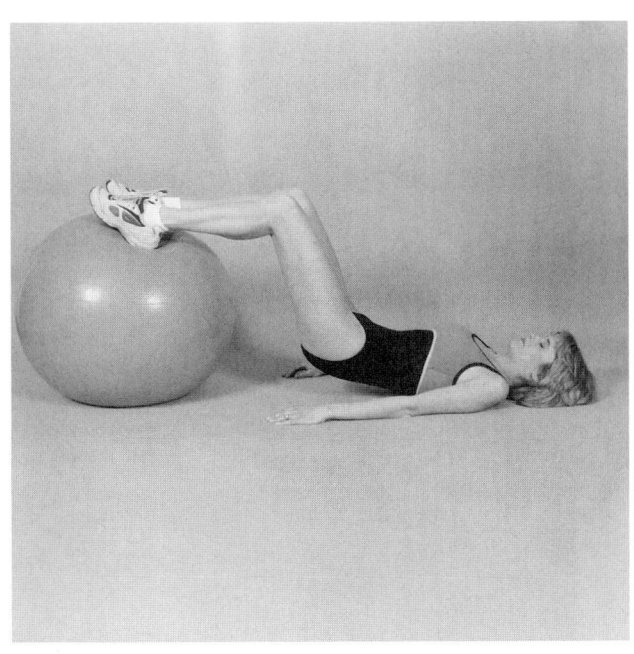

FIGURE 25-68   Bridging on Swiss ball.

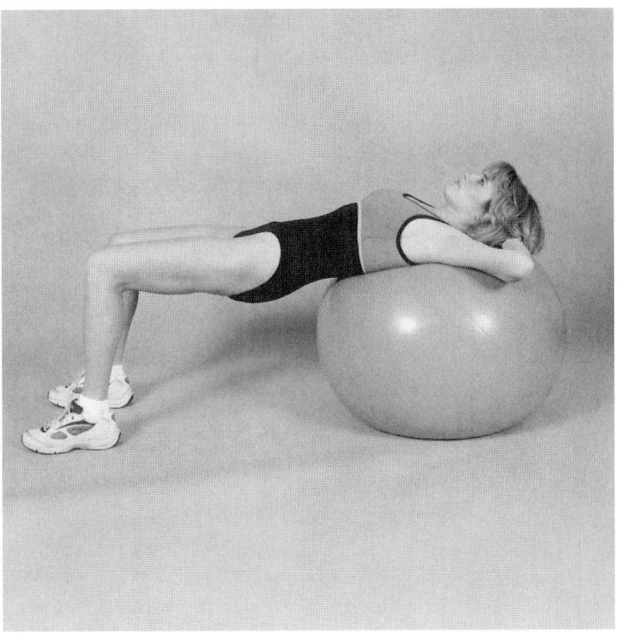

FIGURE 25-70   Supine lying on Swiss ball.

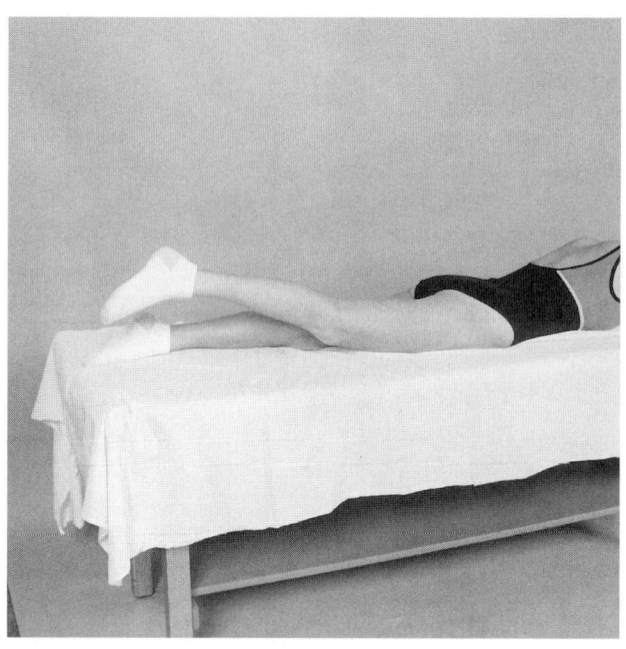

FIGURE 25-71 Alternating hip extension.

to position the arms overhead with the elbows straight, and then to tighten the abdominal muscles and lift one arm toward the ceiling, before lowering the arm to the table. This is progressed until the patient is able to raise both arms simultaneously. Then the patient is asked to raise the arms and legs alternately. Finally, the patient is asked to raise an alternate arm and leg together (Fig. 25-72).

▶ *Bilateral arm swim.*   The patient is asked to perform the arm motions of the swimmer's breast stroke.

▶ *Bilateral arm swim with hip extension.*   The patient is asked to perform the same technique as in the previous exercise, while raising one leg slightly up from the table, and keeping the knee straight.

▶ *Superman.*   With the arms overhead and knees straight, the patient is asked to raise both arms and legs toward the ceiling, while keeping the head resting on the table (Fig. 25-73).

▶ *Prone cobra (Fig. 25-74).*

▶ *Prone lying on a Swiss ball, hands touching floor (Fig. 25-75).*   This can be progressed to walking in circles using only the hands.

▶ *Prone on elbows over a Swiss ball, with unilateral hip extension.*

▶ *Push-up on a Swiss ball, feet on the floor.*

▶ *Push-up with feet on a Swiss ball.*

▶ *Push-ups between two boxes (Fig. 25-76).*

▶ *Push-up with Ab-Roller (Fig. 25-77).*

Sitting Progression

▶ Anterior and posterior pelvic tilting with soles of feet touching.

▶ Sitting balance. The patient is seated on a Swiss ball beside a chair, with the feet on the ground. Using the chair for balance, the patient lifts the feet off the floor and attempts to

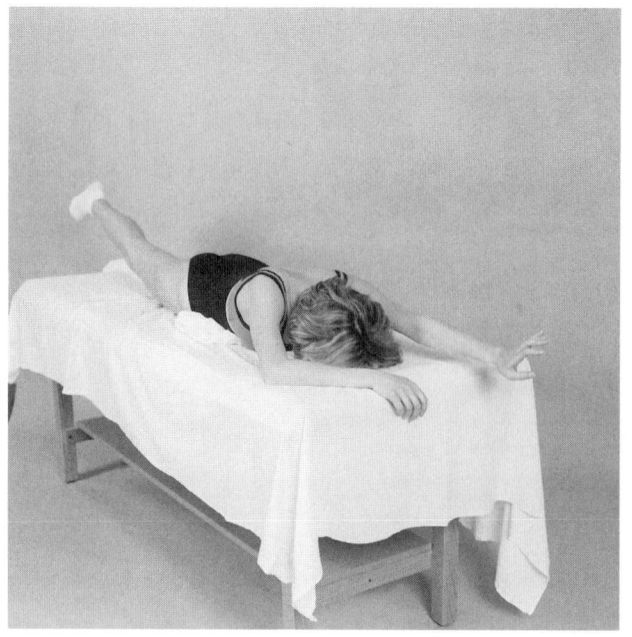

FIGURE 25-72 Alternating arm and leg raise.

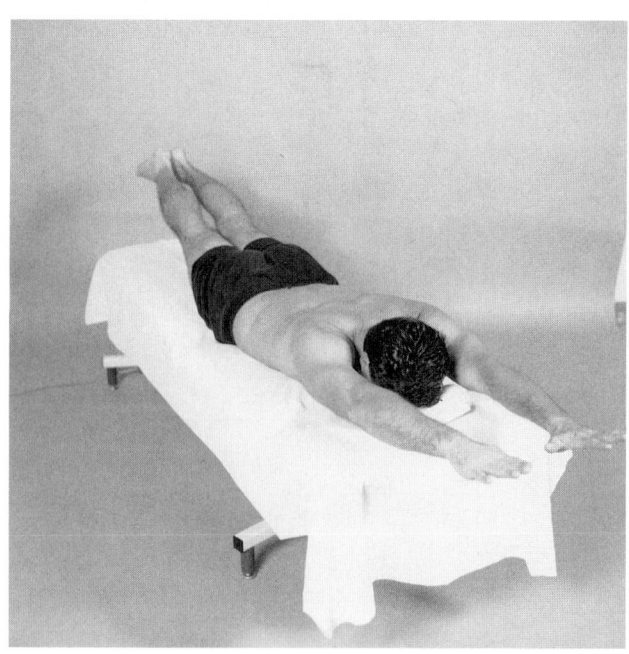

FIGURE 25-73 Superman position.

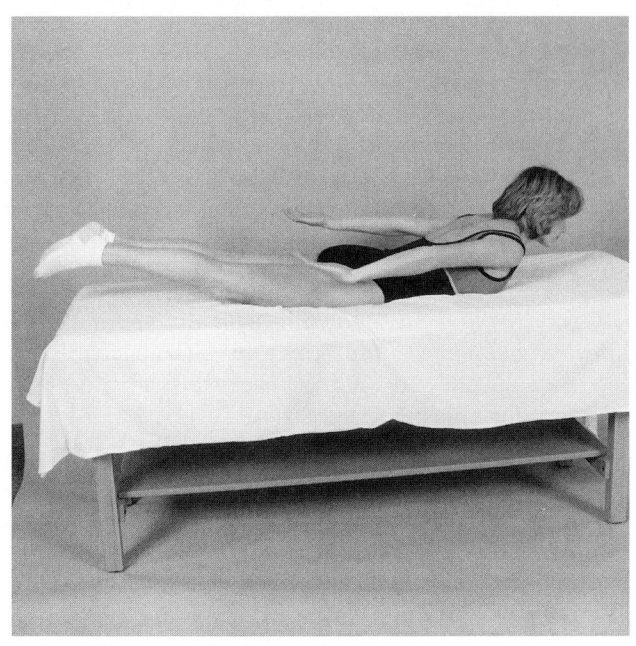

FIGURE 25-74   Prone cobra position.

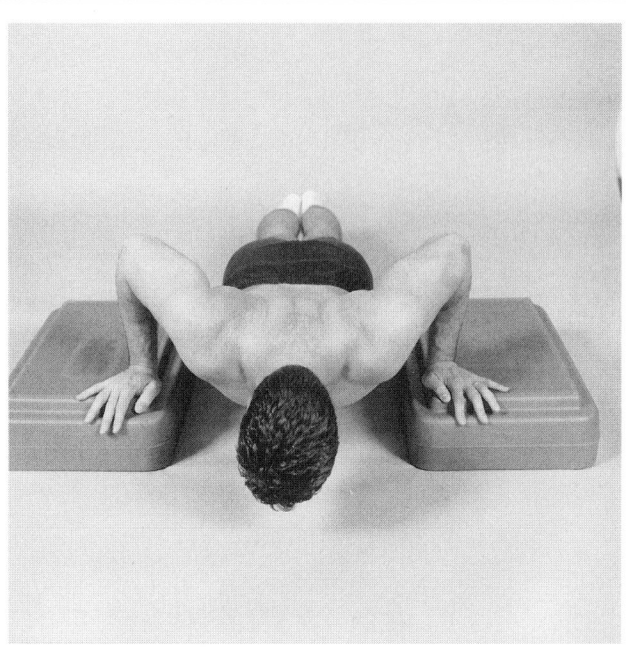

FIGURE 25-76   Push up between boxes.

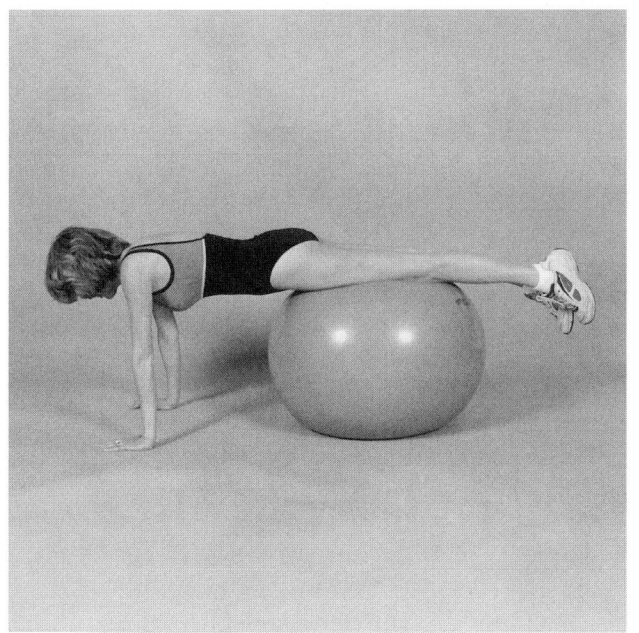

FIGURE 25-75   Prone lying on Swiss ball.

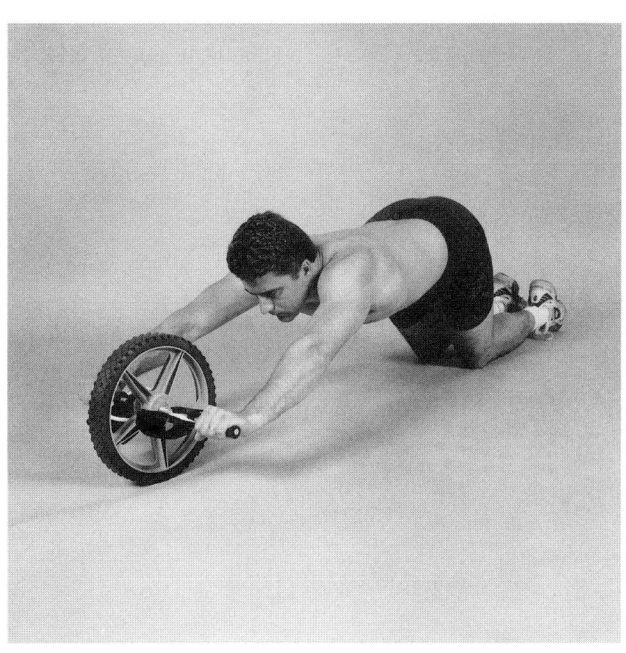

FIGURE 25-77   Push up with Ab-Roller.

sit on the Swiss ball. Gradually, the patient should decrease use of the chair for balance.

▶ Marching in place while sitting on a Swiss ball (Fig. 25-78).

▶ Sit to stand from Swiss ball.

▶ Torso twisting while holding medicine ball on a Swiss ball (Fig. 25-79).

▶ Raising medicine ball overhead while sitting on Swiss ball.

▶ Pelvic tilting on Swiss ball.

Quadruped Progression.   The patient is positioned in the quadruped position (on hands and knees) and is asked to maintain the neutral zone, or to perform an abdominal hollowing, during the following activities:

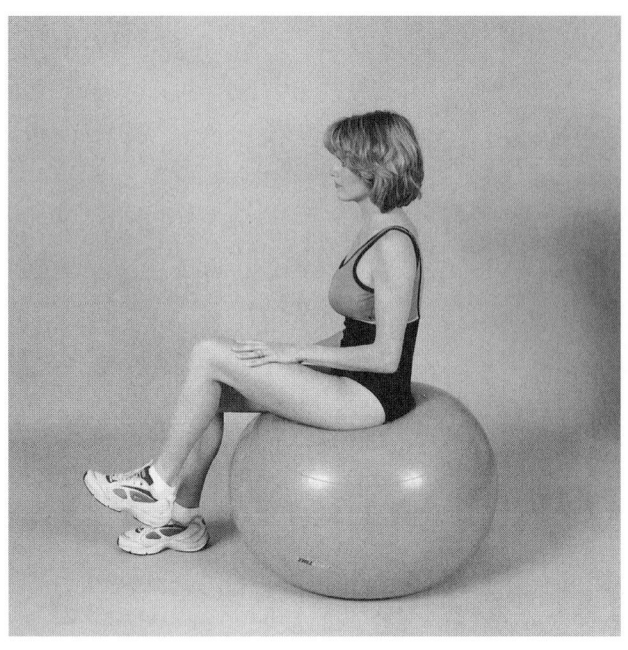

FIGURE 25-78   Marching on Swiss ball.

▶ *Unilateral shoulder flexion.*   The patient is asked to reach one arm out in front, and to prevent the hips and pelvis from rotating.

▶ *Unilateral hip extension.*   The patient is asked to reach one leg out behind, without allowing the hips and pelvis to rotate.

▶ *Weight shifting.*   The patient is asked to move the body forward and backward as far as possible while maintaining the neutral zone.

▶ *Unilateral shoulder flexion with opposite hip extension.* The patient is asked to attempt to reach one arm forward and the opposite leg backward at the same time (Fig. 25-80). The patient is asked to return to the starting position, before performing the same motion with the other arm and leg.

▶ *Weight shifting and reaching with unilateral shoulder flexion and opposite hip extension.*   The patient is asked to move the body forward and backward as far as possible while maintaining the neutral zone.

▶ *Rhythmic stabilization.*   The patient is positioned with unilateral shoulder flexion and opposite hip extension. The clinician applies perturbations to the patient while the patient attempts to resist (Fig. 25-81).

High-kneeling Progression.   The patient is in the high-kneeling position, with the hips and trunk straight. The patient is asked to maintain the neutral zone during the following activities:

▶ *Anterior and posterior pelvic tilting.*

▶ *Bilateral shoulder flexion.*   With the elbows straight, the patient is asked to raise the arms overhead as far as possible, while tightening the abdominal muscles. The patient is then asked to slowly lower the arms, while maintaining the neutral zone throughout the exercise. Resistance can be added to the arms to make the exercise more challenging.

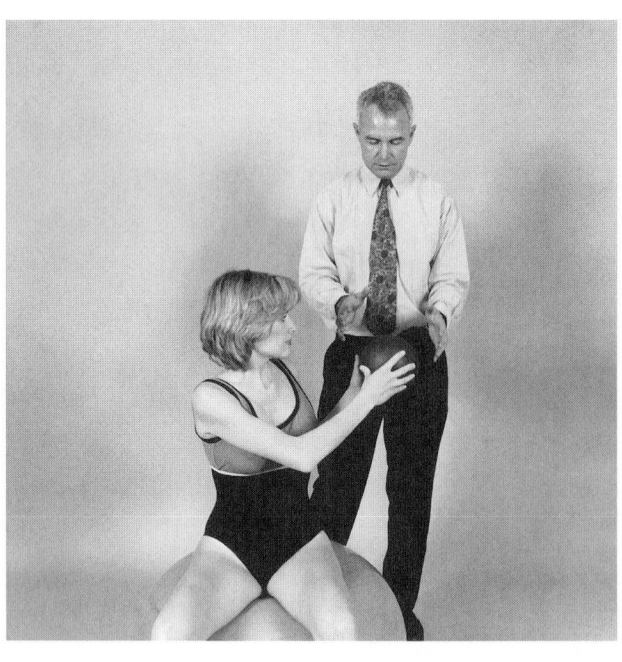

FIGURE 25-79   Torso twist on Swiss ball.

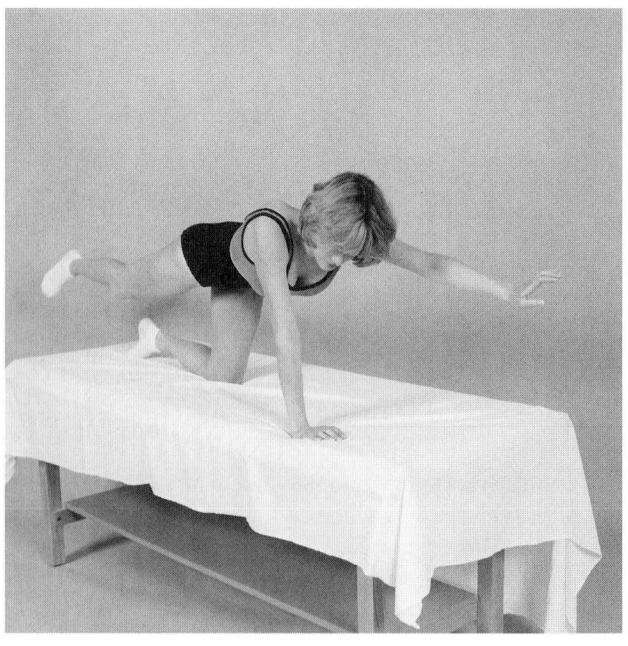

FIGURE 25-80   Leg and arm lift in quadruped.

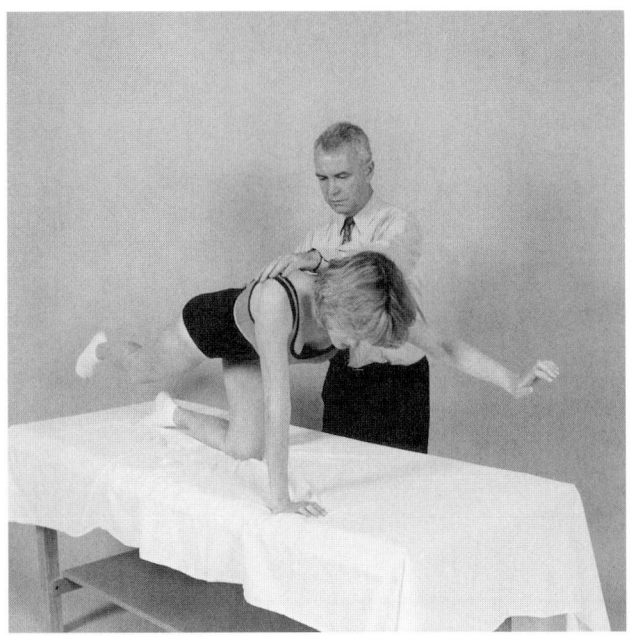

FIGURE 25-81 Rhythmic stabilization in quadruped.

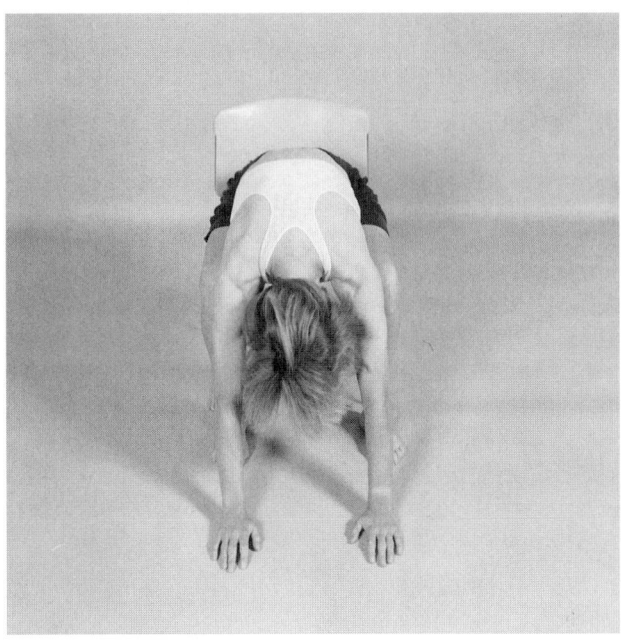

FIGURE 25-82 Seated flexion.

▶ *Alternating shoulder flexion.* With the elbows straight, the patient is asked to raise one arm overhead as far as possible while tightening the abdominals. The patient is then asked to slowly lower the arms, while maintaining the neutral zone throughout the exercise. Resistance can be added to the arms to make the exercise more challenging.

▶ *Forward bending.* The patient is asked to lower the buttocks to touch the heels of the feet, and to place the palms of the hands on the floor by the feet (Fig. 25-82). The patient is then asked to return to the starting position by reversing the motions while maintaining the neutral zone.

▶ *Full-knee to high-knee.* The patient moves from the full-kneel to the high-kneel position while maintaining a posterior pelvic tilt.

▶ *Body Blade.* The patient is asked to use a Body Blade in both hands, in various arm positions, while maintaining the neutral zone. The exercise can be performed kneeling on one knee, and then both knees (see Fig. 25-83).

Standing Progression
▶ *Bilateral shoulder flexion.* With the elbows straight, the patient is asked to raise the arms overhead as far as possible while tightening the abdominal muscles, before slowly lowering the arms, while maintaining the neutral zone throughout the exercise.

▶ *Alternating shoulder flexion.* With the elbows straight, the patient is asked to raise one arm overhead as far as pos-

sible while tightening the abdominal muscles. The patient is then asked to slowly lower the arm, while maintaining the neutral zone throughout the exercise.

▶ *Wall slides.* With the back against a wall, the patient is asked to perform a squat until the knees are bent to 60 degrees, then return to standing, while maintaining the neutral

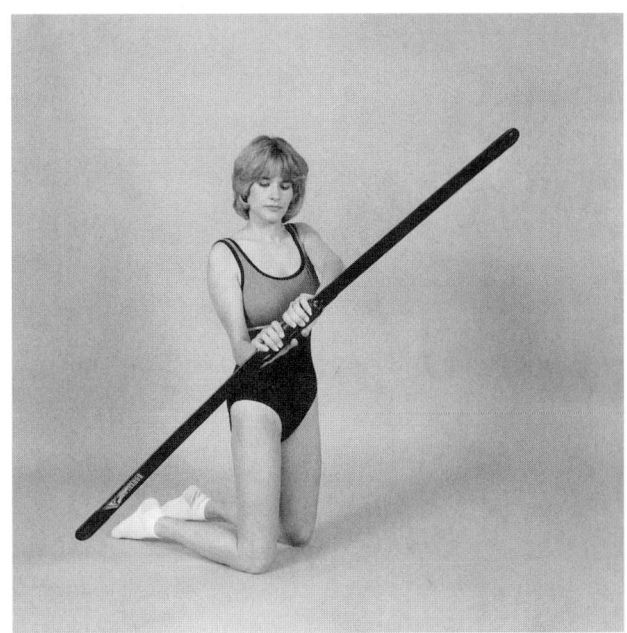

FIGURE 25-83 High-kneel position with Body Blade.

zone throughout the exercise. Modifications to this exercise include:

- A Swiss ball placed between the patient and the wall.

- A medicine ball placed between the patient's knees (Fig. 25-84).

▶ *Forward lunge.* While maintaining the neutral zone throughout the exercise, the patient is asked to step forward with one leg and lower the opposite knee to the ground. Hand weights, elastic resistance, or dumbbells can be used to make the exercise more challenging.

▶ *Backward lunge.* While maintaining the neutral zone throughout the exercise, the patient is asked to step backward with one leg, and lower the same knee to the ground, before returning to the starting position. Hand weights, elastic resistance, or dumbbells can be used to make the exercise more challenging.

▶ *Mimic sporting swing (i.e., tennis), with and without resistance, while maintaining the neutral zone.*

▶ *Medicine ball throws (chest pass, soccer throw) (Fig. 25-85).*

▶ *Medicine ball flexion and extension.* The patient stands holding a medicine ball in the hands, the ball is raised as high above the head as possible, and then in the opposite direction as the patient flexes forward, so that the ball is placed between the legs.

▶ *Medicine ball proprioceptive neuromuscular facilitation (Fig. 25-86).*

▶ *Integration of lower (Fig. 25-87) and upper kinetic chain.*

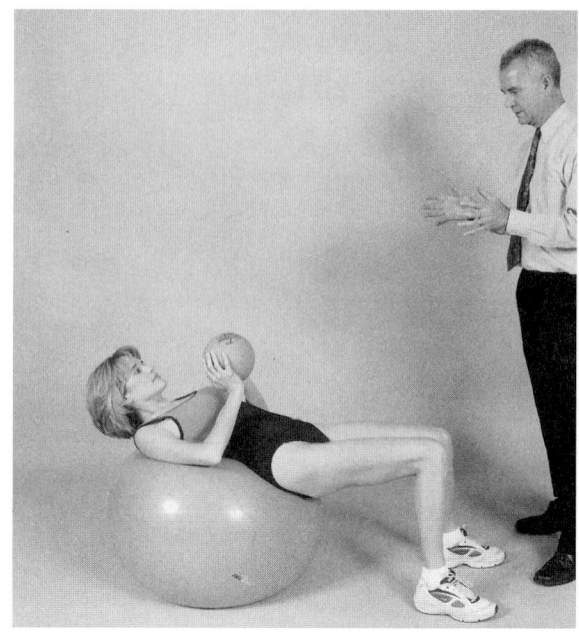

FIGURE 25-85   Medicine ball throw.

Stretching Exercises

Muscle flexibility should be addressed according to patient tolerance. Poor flexibility may cause excessive stresses to be borne by the lumbar motion segments. Adaptively shortened hip flexors and rectus femoris muscles can cause an extension and rotation hypermobility in the lumbar spine. Occasionally, stretching both the anterior and posterior thigh muscles is beneficial.

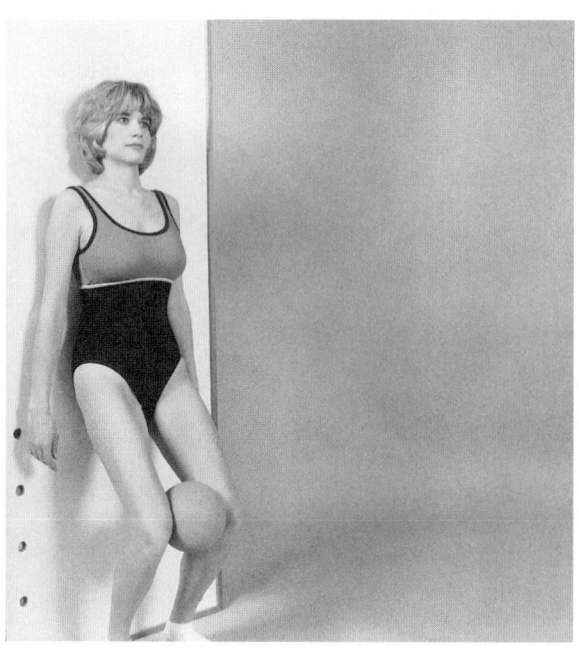

FIGURE 25-84   Wall slide with medicine ball.

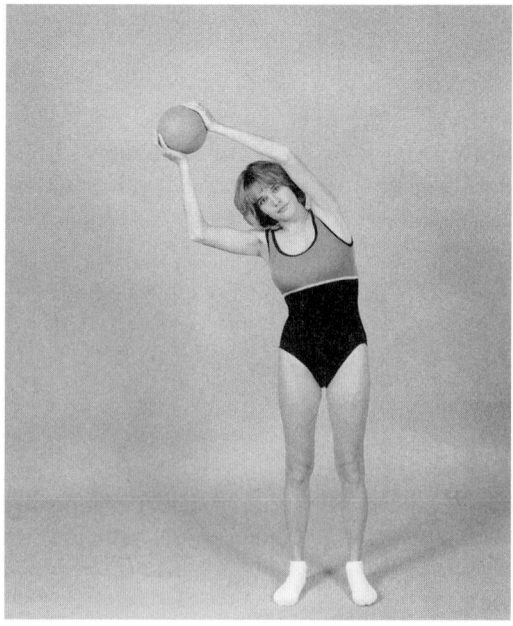

FIGURE 25-86   Medicine ball proprioceptive neuromuscular facilitation.

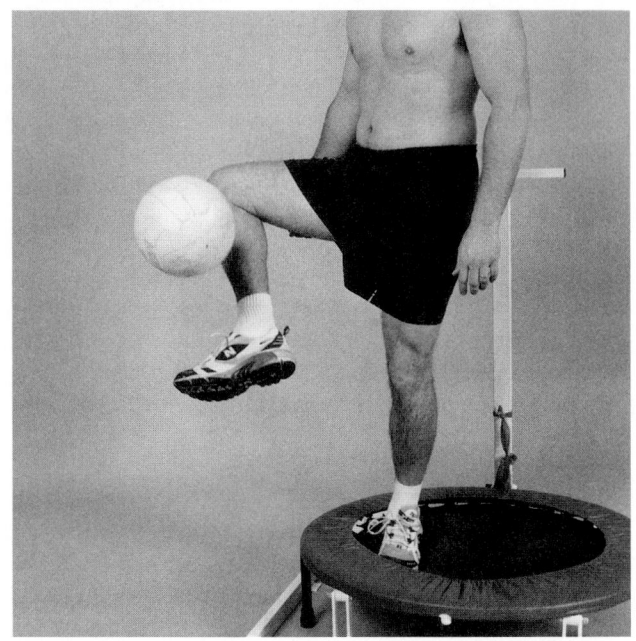

FIGURE 25-87 Integration of lower kinetic chain.

However, most of the time, only one should be stretched, and the decision is based on the diagnosis:

▶ The patient with spinal stenosis or a painful extension hypomobility, and who responds well to lumbar flexion exercises, should be taught how to stretch the hip flexors and rectus femoris while protecting the lumbar spine from excessive lordosis.

▶ The patient with a painful flexion hypomobility or IVD herniation, and who responds well to lumbar extension exercises, should be taught how to stretch the hamstrings while protecting the lumbar spine from flexing.

Stretches should be applied and then taught. The goal of stretching is to perform the technique while maintaining the pelvis in its neutral zone to avoid excessive anterior or posterior pelvic tilting.

Aerobic Exercise
The importance of aerobic exercise cannot be overemphasized, both in reducing the incidence of LBP,[360] and in the intervention for patients with LBP.[361] Aerobic fitness should be maintained. The following aerobic exercises may be used as tolerated.

▶ Walking and jogging on soft, even ground.

▶ Upper body ergonometer.

▶ Indoor cross-country skiing machines.

▶ Water aerobics.

Back School
Several back schools and back rehabilitation programs have been developed to teach people proper lifting technique and body mechanics. These programs are aimed at groups of patients. They include the provision of general information on the spine, recommended postures and activities, preventative measures, and exercises for the back.

The efficacy of back schools, however, remains controversial.[362,363] Cohen and colleagues[364] concluded that there is insufficient evidence to recommend group education for people with LBP.

Practice Pattern 4D: Impaired Joint Mobility, Motor Function, Muscle Performance, Range of Motion Associated with Capsular Restriction

Degenerative Spinal Stenosis
Degenerative spinal stenosis (DSS) is defined as narrowing of the spinal canal, nerve root canal (lateral recess), or intervertebral foramina of the lumbar spine. It is predominantly a disorder of the elderly and is the most common diagnosis associated with lumbar spine surgery in patients older than 65 years.[365]

DSS is being diagnosed more frequently. The reasons for this are the widespread use of sophisticated noninvasive imaging techniques and the increasing elderly population. Lumbar spinal stenosis may be classified as central or lateral.[366]

Central stenosis is characterized by a narrowing of the spinal canal around the thecal sac containing the cauda equina. The causes for this type of stenosis include facet joint arthrosis and hypertrophy, thickening and bulging of the ligamentum flavum, bulging of the IVD, and spondylolisthesis.

Lateral stenosis is characterized by encroachment of the spinal nerve in the lateral recess of the spinal canal or in the intervertebral foramen. Initially the depth of the canal that constituted narrowing was identified as an anteroposterior measurement,[367] but more recently the lateral width of the spinal canal has been studied.[368] The causes for this type of stenosis include facet joint hypertrophy, loss of IVD height, IVD bulging, and spondylolisthesis.

A compression of the nerve within the canal may result in a limitation of the arterial supply or claudication resulting from the compression of the venous return. Neurogenic claudication also referred to as pseudoclaudication may result in nerve root ischemia and symptomatic claudication. Neurogenic claudication is manifested as poorly localized pain, paresthesias, or cramping of one or both lower extremities, which is brought on by walking and relieved by sitting.[369] Compressive loading of the spine also can exacerbate symptoms, such as those which occur with walking. Central stenosis can result in symptoms related to cauda equina compression. Most of the compression occurs when the canal is at its narrowest diameter, with relief occurring when the diameter increases. The compression of the foraminal contents in the canal may occur more often with certain movements or changes in posture[370]:

▶ The length of the canal is shorter in lumbar lordosis than kyphosis.

▶ Extension and, to a lesser degree, side bending of the lumbar spine toward the involved side produces a narrowing of the canal.

▶ Flexion of the lumbar spine reverses the process, returning both the venous capacity, and blood flow, to the nerve.

Both the history and the examination findings are very specific.

Patients with lumbar spinal stenosis who are symptomatic often relate a long history of LBP. Unilateral or bilateral leg pain is usually a predominant symptom. Approximately 65 percent of patients with lumbar spinal stenosis present with neurogenic claudication.[369] Subjectively, the patient reports an increase in symptoms with lumbar extension activities such as walking, prolonged standing, and, to a lesser degree, side bending. On observation, the patient presents with a flattened lumbar lordosis.

The physical examination usually reveals evidence of reduced flexibility or shortening of the hip flexors (iliopsoas and rectus femoris). The hip extensor muscles (gluteus maximus and hamstrings) usually are lengthened. This lengthening places them at a mechanical disadvantage, which leads to early recruitment of the lumbar extensor muscles and may lead to excessive lumbar extension.[371]

Therapeutic exercise is one of numerous interventions that have been proposed for the conservative management of patients with lumbar spinal stenosis. Several authors advocate only the use of Williams flexion exercises because of the neuroforaminal narrowing that occurs with lumbar extension.[372,373] However, the prescribed program may need to be modified so that it does not exacerbate any coexisting orthopaedic conditions, such as osteoarthritis of the hips or knees, while still being effective.[54] The therapeutic exercise progression includes postural education; hip flexor, rectus femoris, and lumbar paraspinal stretching; lumbar (core) stabilization exercises targeting the abdominals and gluteals; aerobic conditioning; and positioning through a posterior pelvic tilt. There is some controversy as to whether the hamstrings should be stretched. Lengthening these muscles may allow the pelvis to rotate anteriorly, resulting in an increased lordosis.

Failure to respond to a conservative approach is an indication for nerve root and sinuvertebral nerve infiltration.[374] Permanent relief in lateral recess stenosis has been reported with an injection of local anesthetic around the nerve root.[375]

When nerve root infiltration fails, surgical decompression of the nerve root is indicated.

Zygapophysial Joint Dysfunction

Facet joint syndrome is a term used to describe a pain-provoking dysfunction of the zygapophysial joint.[133] This pain is the result of a lesion to the joint and its pain-sensitive structures. Zygapophysial movement dysfunctions can result from a hypomobility, or a hypermobility-instability.

Hypomobility. Hypomobility in the lumbar spine can have a variety of causes including ligament tears,[376] muscle tears or contusions,[377] lumbago,[266] intra-articular meniscoid entrapment,[378]

zygapophysial joint capsular tightness, and zygapophysial joint fixation or subluxation.[379]

Theoretically, the signs and symptoms that present with a hypomobility include unilateral LBP that is aggravated with certain movements. Given that the joint is only capable of flexion and extension movements, it is assumed that flexion or extension movements can provoke pain, particularly at the end of these ranges. These movements are tested with active range of motion and the combined motion (H and I) tests, and confirmed with the position tests of the PPIVM and PPAIVM tests.[301]

Hypomobility of the zygapophysial joint can have an extra-articular, periarticular, or pathomechanical cause, with the distinction made by the results of the end-feel obtained by the clinician during the PPIVM and PPAIVM tests.[301]

▶ *Extra-articular.* Decreased range with the PPIVM, but normal PPAIVM.

▶ *Periarticular.* Restriction of range in both PPIVM and PPAIVM tests, with a hard capsular end-feel.

▶ *Pathomechanical.* Restriction of range in both PPIVM and PPAIVM tests, with an abrupt, slightly springy end-feel.

The conservative intervention for a zygapophysial dysfunction includes specific joint mobilizations, postural education, correction of muscle imbalances and core stabilization exercises.

Instability. Lumbar instability is considered to be a significant factor in patients with chronic LBP.[380] However, there is considerable controversy as to what, exactly, constitutes spinal instability. Traditionally, the radiographic diagnosis of spondylolisthesis in patients with chronic LBP was considered to be one of the most obvious manifestations of lumbar instability.[381] However, lumbar segmental instability in the absence of radiographic findings also has been cited as a significant cause of chronic LBP.[382] The limitation in the clinical diagnosis of lumbar segmental instability lies in the difficulty of accurately detecting abnormal or excessive intersegmental motion either radiographically or through palpation.[59] Hypermobility is usually the most difficult movement impairment to diagnose in the spine, because it is not a matter of stiffness, but rather of a relative degree of looseness.[301] As with all movement impairments, instabilities or hypermobilities can be symmetric or asymmetric.

The following clinical findings (anywhere in the spinal joints) may indicate the presence of instability, and its pertinence to the presenting complaints of the patient.

History

▶ Trauma.

▶ Repeated unprovoked episode(s) of feeling unstable or giving way, following a minor provocation.

▶ Inconsistent symptomatology.

▶ Minor aching for a few days after a sensation of giving way.

► Compression symptoms (vertebrobasilar, spinal cord) that are not associated with a history of an IVD herniation or stenosis.

► Consistent clicking or clunking noises.

► Protracted pain (with full range of motion).

Observation

► Creases posteriorly or on abdomen (spondylolisthesis).

► Spinal ledging.

► Spinal angulation on full range of motion.

► Inability to recover normally from full range of motion, commonly flexion.

► Excessive active range of motion.

Physical Examination. O'Sullivan classifies instabilities according to the following patterns that each of them manifests, although he admits that these classifications have not been scientifically validated.[59]

► *Flexion pattern.* The flexion pattern is the most common. It is characterized by complaints of central back pain that is aggravated during flexion-rotational movements, and an inability to sustain semiflexed positions. On observation, there is often a loss of segmental lordosis at the level of the "unstable" motion segment, which is more noticeable in standing. This loss of lordosis is increased in flexed positions. Movements into forward flexion are associated with a tendency to flex more at the symptomatic level than at adjacent levels, and usually are associated with an arc of pain into flexion and an inability to return from flexion to neutral without use of the hands to assist in the movement. During backward bending, extension above the symptomatic segment, with an associated loss of extension at the involved segment, often is observed. Functional activities, such as squatting, sitting with knee extension or hip flexion, and sit to stand, reveal an inability to control a neutral lordosis and a preponderance to segmentally flex at the unstable motion segment. Specific muscle tests reveal an inability to perform the abdominal hollowing maneuver at the unstable motion segment. The patient also may be unable to actively produce a neutral lordotic lumbar spine posture.

► *Extension pattern.* The extension pattern is characterized by complaints of central back pain that is aggravated during extension-rotational movements, and an inability to sustain positions such as standing, overhead activities, fast walking, running, and swimming. On observation, there is often an increase in segmental lordosis at the level of the "unstable" motion segment in standing, which is often associated with an increase in segmental muscle activity at this level. Extension activities reveal segmental hinging at the involved segment, with a loss of segmental lordosis above this level and an associated postural sway. Forward bending movements

often reveal a tendency to hold the lumbar spine in lordosis, with a sudden loss of the lordosis midway through the flexion range and an arc of pain. On returning from the flexed position, there is often a tendency to hyperextend the lumbar spine segmentally before the upright posture is achieved, with pain on returning to the upright position. Specific muscle testing reveals an inability to perform the abdominal hollowing maneuver. The patient also is often unable to initiate a posterior pelvic tilt independent of hip flexion and activation of the gluteals, rectus abdominis, and external obliques.

► *Recurrent lateral shift pattern.* The lateral shift (see Chap. 20) is usually unidirectional, occurs recurrently, and is associated with unilateral LBP. The patient typically stands with a loss of lumbar segmental lordosis at the involved level and an associated lateral shift at the same level. The lateral shift is accentuated when standing on the foot ipsilateral to the shift and is observed during gait as a tendency to transfer weight through the trunk and upper body rather than through the pelvis. Sagittal spinal movements reveal a shift further laterally at midrange flexion, which is commonly associated with an arc of pain. Sit to stand and squatting are associated with a tendency toward lateral trunk shift during the movement, with increased weight bearing on the lower limb ipsilateral to the shift. Specific muscle testing reveals an inability to perform the trunk raise, with dominance of activation of the quadratus lumborum, lumbar erector spinae, and superficial multifidus on the side ipsilateral to the shift, and an inability to activate the segmental multifidus on the contralateral side to the lateral shift.

► *Multidirectional pattern.* This pattern is the most serious and debilitating of the patterns and is frequently characterized by high levels of pain and functional disability. All weight-bearing positions are normally painful, and locking of the spine occurs frequently with positions of sustained flexion, rotation, and extension. These patients exhibit great difficulty in assuming neutral lordotic spinal positions, and an inability to perform the abdominal hollowing maneuver.

Intervention. Instability of the spine is perhaps the most difficult of the motion impairments to treat. A stiff or jammed joint is a relatively simple problem that requires selecting and applying a mobilization or manipulation technique. Instability is a permanent, or at best, a semipermanent state. The intervention for a hypermobility or instability involves the removal of any abnormal stresses from the joint. If the underlying cause of the articular hypermobility is deemed to be a localized joint hypomobility, then this dysfunction must logically be dealt with first using joint mobilizations or stretching techniques.[301]

Following the diagnosis, and the correction of any articular hypomobility, the focus shifts to retraining muscles that are involved in the dynamic stabilization and segmental control of the spine. The purpose is to identify incorrect movement patterns and to isolate and retrain the movement functionally according to the patient's needs.

Movement Impairment Syndromes

Sahrmann[279] categorizes a number of movement impairment syndromes that can present in the lumbar spine as a result of an imbalance of flexibility and strength. The intervention for each of the syndromes involves a correction of these imbalances.

Flexion Syndrome. This syndrome is characterized by lumbar flexion motions that are more flexible than hip flexion motions. The syndrome is typically found in the 8- to 45-year-old age range and results in pain with positions or motions associated with lumbar flexion, because of adaptive shortening of the gluteus maximus, hamstrings, or rectus abdominis.

Extension Syndrome. This syndrome is characterized by lumbar extension motions that are more flexible than hip extension motions. Patients with this syndrome are usually older than 55 years of age, and the symptoms are increased with positions or motions associated with an increase in lumbar lordosis, because of adaptive shortening of the hip flexors and lumbar paraspinals and weakness of the external oblique muscles.

Lumbar Rotation. This syndrome is characterized by pain that is unilateral or greater on one side, and is increased with rotation to one side. No attempt is made to equate the side of rotation with the side of the symptoms. It is theorized that this syndrome is produced when one segment of the lumbar spine rotates, side bends, glides, or translates more easily than the segment above or below it. This syndrome is associated with spinal instability and can result from habitual motions or positions that involve rotation to one side, a leg-length discrepancy (see Chap. 27), or a muscle imbalance between the oblique abdominal muscles.

Lumbar Flexion with Rotation. This syndrome is characterized by pain that is unilateral or greater on one side, and is increased with the combined motion of lumbar flexion and rotation. Many of the characteristics of the lumbar flexion and lumbar rotation syndromes can be applied to this syndrome.

Lumbar Extension with Rotation. This syndrome is characterized by pain that is unilateral or greater on one side, and is increased with the combined motion of lumbar extension and rotation. Many of the characteristics of the lumbar extension and lumbar rotation syndromes can be applied to this syndrome.

Practice Pattern 4E: Impaired Joint Mobility, Motor Function, Muscle Performance, Range of Motion Associated with Localized Inflammation

Ligament Tears

As with those elsewhere in the body, ligament tears of the lumbar spine are normally traumatically induced. Knowledge of the various restraints to the various motions of the lumbar spine can aid in determining which ligament has the potential to be sprained with a given mechanism.

Iliolumbar Ligament Sprain. The iliolumbar ligament, an extremely important structure that stabilizes the lumbar spine on the sacrum and functions to anchor the L5 vertebra onto the S1 vertebral body,[90] is commonly injured.

The iliolumbar ligament sprain, also known as the iliac crest syndrome, has a classic presentation of lower lumbar pain just at or above the medial iliac crest area with radiation sometimes down the leg. On examination, the straight leg raise and Patrick (FABER) sign are both usually negative, there is no weakness or sensory impairment, and no radicular signs. The diagnosis is confirmed by deep palpation of the iliolumbar ligament in an attempt to reproduce the patient's discomfort. Njoo and colleagues[383] have provided evidence of good interobserver validity in the diagnosis of this problem in a prospective manner. A single injection of lidocaine and steroid provides effective and sustained treatment to this readily accessible area.[384]

Muscle Contusions, Strains, and Tears

Muscle injuries are associated with a history of trauma and are capable of producing a significant degree of discomfort. Two sites are commonly involved in the lumbar region, and strains and tears can occur with relatively little trauma there.[385]

1. The point where the erector spinae group of muscles joins to their common tendon just above and medial to the posterior superior iliac spines.

2. At the gluteal origin on the ala of the ilium, just lateral to the posterior iliac spines.

However, muscle pain also can be produced from excessive muscle activity or muscle guarding, which follows an injury to the spine. The intervention for muscle tears involves a gradual and controlled resumption of movements and activities.

Practice Pattern 4F: Impaired Joint Mobility, Motor Function, Muscle Performance, Range of Motion or Reflex Integrity Secondary to Spinal Disorders

Piriformis Syndrome

The sciatic nerve usually travels below the piriformis. In about 15 percent of the population, however, the tibial part of the sciatic nerve passes through either the belly of the piriformis muscle, or the piriformis has two muscle bellies, and the nerve passes between the two bellies. Consequently, contraction or tightness of the muscle can often produce radicular symptoms (see Chap. 9).

Piriformis syndrome usually is a diagnosis of exclusion once the more common causes of sciatica have been ruled out.[386] Robinson[387] listed six cardinal features of piriformis syndrome: (1) a history of trauma to the sacroiliac and gluteal regions; (2) pain in the region of the sacroiliac joint, greater sciatic notch, and piriformis muscle, extending down the lower limb and causing difficulty in walking; (3) acute exacerbation of the symptoms by lifting or stooping; (4) a palpable, sausage-shaped mass over the piriformis muscle, during an exacerbation of symptoms, that is markedly tender to pressure (this feature is pathognomonic of the syndrome); (5) a positive result on the straight leg raise test; and (6) gluteal atrophy, depending on the duration of symptoms.[386]

The intervention for piriformis syndrome depends on the suspected pathology. If muscular spasm and tightness is the suspected etiology, then an aggressive stretching and massage of the piriformis program should be instituted.[388] If this conservative approach fails, a local anesthetic block to the muscle should be considered. Surgical neurolysis is considered for recalcitrant cases.

Entrapment Neuropathy of the Medial Superior Cluneal Nerve

The cutaneous innervation of the lower lumbar and gluteal regions has been attributed to the dorsal rami of L1 to L3. Maigne and Maigne[389] observed that the cutaneous innervation of the gluteal region is derived from higher levels of the thoracolumbar region; that is, from T11 to L1. Anastomoses between these nerves also are common. Superior cluneal nerve injury is a well-known cause of chronic pain complicating bone graft harvesting from the posterior iliac crest for spinal fusion.[390,391] The medial superior cluneal (MSC) nerve is the most medial nerve of these nerves. The MSC usually crosses the posterior iliac crest at a distance of approximately 7 cm from the midline.[392] At that point, it becomes superficial by passing through an osseofibrous tunnel formed by the thoracolumbar fascia cranially and the rim of the posterior iliac crest caudally.[392] This tunnel is occasionally a site of compression for the MSC nerve.[389]

According to Maigne,[392] MSC nerve entrapment can be diagnosed and treated using the following criteria:

▶ A trigger point over the posterior iliac crest, located 7 cm from the midline (corresponding to the nerve compression zone); and

▶ Relief of symptoms by nerve block.

Integration of Practice Patterns 4H and 4I: Impaired Joint Mobility, Motor Function, Muscle Performance, Range of Motion Associated with Fractures, Joint Arthroplasty, and Soft Tissue Surgical Procedures

Spondylolisthesis

Forward slipping of one vertebral body (and the remainder of the spinal column above it) in relation to the vertebral segment immediately below it is referred to as *spondylolisthesis*. This forward slip of the vertebra is resisted by the bony block of the posterior facets, by an intact neural arch and pedicle, and, in the case of the L5 vertebra, by the iliolumbar ligament.

The most common site for spondylolysis and spondylolisthesis is L5 to S1.[393] Age appears to be an important factor in the natural history of spondylolisthesis. Children younger than age 5 rarely present with spondylolysis, and severe spondylolisthesis is equally rare. The period of most rapid slipping is between the ages of 10 and 15 years, with no more slipping occurring after the age of 20.[212] Higher-grade spondylolisthesis is twice as common in girls as in boys, and is approximately four times more common in women than men.[394]

There are two prevailing theories as to the etiology of degenerative spondylolisthesis:

1. *Dysfunction of the IVD.*[395] The IVD at the level of the spondylolisthesis is subjected to considerable anteriorly

directed shear forces, and is the main structure that opposes these shear forces, functioning to prevent against further slippage and keeping the spinal motion segment in a stable equilibrium. It is postulated that slip progression after skeletal maturity is almost always related to IVD degeneration at the slip level. As the biochemical and biomechanical integrity of the IVD is lost, the lumbosacral slip becomes unstable and progresses. Disk degeneration at the slip level, and adult slip progression, are likely to develop during the fourth and fifth decades of life. This unstable mechanical situation leads to symptoms of low back and sciatic pain, and may necessitate spinal instrumentation and fusion.

2. *Horizontalization of the lamina and the facets or sacrum morphology.*[396] A more trapezoidal shape of the vertebral body, or a dome-shaped contour of the top of the sacrum, or both, are found in individuals with slipping. There is also a greater anterior flexion of the lumbar spine than in "normal" individuals of comparable age.[397] A sagittal orientation of the facet joints also could predispose the vertebra to slip.[398]

Other factors such as the lumbosacral angle, ligamentous laxity, previous pregnancy, and hormonal factors, impose an increased stress on the L4 to L5 facet joints and, as most of the stress is placed anteriorly on the inferior facet of L4, the wear pattern is concentrated at this point, creating a more sagittally orientated joint by way of remodeling.[399]

Whatever the cause, if the syndesmosis maintains the bonds between the two halves of the neural arch, there is no mechanical instability and the patient is asymptomatic, whereas if the syndesmosis is loose, separation occurs during flexion. Repetitive flexion strains can give rise to both local and referred pain in a sciatic distribution, as a result of nerve root irritation or degenerative changes occurring in the underlying IVD.

Spondylolisthesis is graded according to the percentage of slip. Slip percentage is the distance from a line extended along the posterior cortex of the S1 body to the posteroinferior corner of the L5 vertebra,[400] divided by the anteroposterior diameter of the sacrum. Grading is then performed using the Meyerding classification,[401] as follows: grade I, 1 to 25 percent; grade II, 26 to 50 percent; grade III, 51 to 75 percent; grade IV, 76 to 100 percent; and grade V (spondyloptosis) more than 100 percent.

The spectrum of neurologic involvement runs from rare to more common in the higher-grade slips, with the majority of neurologic deficits being an L5 radiculopathy with an L5 to S1 spondylolisthesis, but cauda equina impairments can occur in grade III or IV slips. The possible pathologic changes at the adjacent instability segment include instability of the motion segment, IVD space narrowing, and stenosis caused by facet degeneration and ligament flavum hypertrophy.[402] Degeneration of the IVD above or below the fusion mass, and damage to the posterior ligament complex, also may contribute to the development of the lesions by reducing resistance to shearing forces at the intervertebral level next to the fusion.[402]

The symptoms, if they do occur, usually begin in the second decade. There is often no correlation with the degree of slip and the level of pain. This is because the forward slip of the vertebral body usually results in intervertebral foramen enlargement. It is only when the neural arch rotates on the pivot formed by its articulation with the sacrum, or there are anterior osteophytes, that encroachment occurs, resulting in nerve root irritation.

Isthmic spondylolisthesis develops as a stress fracture. In more advanced slips, there is a palpable soft tissue depression immediately above the L5 spinous process on passing the fingers down the lumbar spine, and a segmental lordosis. If an asymptomatic slip reaches 50 percent, vigorous contact sports and other activities carrying a high risk of back injury should be avoided.

Radiographic findings for these patients can be misleading. In a lateral view, taken while the patient is supine, the forward displacement often appears trivial, because it is only when the patient is standing that the true degree of slip is appreciated. Consequently, if spondylolisthesis is suspected, a lateral spot view of the lumbosacral junction must be taken while the patient stands upright, and during flexion and extension of the trunk.[403] However, a patient with LBP who demonstrates a spondylolisthesis on radiograph may have an asymptomatic spondylolisthesis, and the back pain may result from other causes.

The intervention for spondylolisthesis depends on the severity of the slip and the symptoms, and ranges from conservative to surgical. The average case is one of a limited slip and sparse clinical findings. The conservative approach includes pelvic positioning to provide symptomatic relief, lumbar stabilization exercises, and stretching of the rectus femoris and iliopsoas muscles to decrease the degree of anterior pelvic tilting. During the past decade, numerous patients with lumbar degenerative spondylolisthesis have been treated with decompression and fusion with or without instrumentation.[402] A high fusion rate and satisfactory clinical outcome have been reported. However, a few patients present with recurrent back pain and sciatica after surgery. The possible causes of postoperative pain include inadequate decompression, fibrosis, recurrent IVD herniation, adjacent stenosis, and instability.[402]

Lumbago

The term *lumbago* is used to describe local back pain of a diskogenic origin but also can be used to describe a sudden onset of persistent LBP, marked by a restriction of lumbar movements and reports of "locking." The mechanism of mechanical locking is still a contentious issue.[75,133,378] The severity of each episode varies, from incapacitating to minor discomfort. Although it can occur at any age, lumbago typically affects patients between the ages of 20 and 45 years. The mechanism of injury usually involves a sudden unguarded movement of the lumbar spine, involving either flexion or extension combined with rotation or side bending.

Hypomobilities can be classified as symmetric or asymmetric. If both sides of the joint are involved, the lesion is symmetric, whereas if only one side is involved, the lesion is asymmetric.

Lumbar Spine Surgery

Lumbar spine surgery is usually only used when conservative intervention has failed to reduce the pain or restore the normal neurologic or physiologic function (Table 25-14). The vast

TABLE 25-14   Indications for Lumbar Surgery

STRONG INDICATIONS
Cauda equina syndrome (bladder and bowel dysfunction)
Progressive neurologic symptoms and deficits
RELATIVE INDICATIONS
Severe pain, with evidence of nerve root tension
Recurrent, incapacitating episodes of sciatica
Impairment of nerve conduction
Failure to respond to conservative approach of 6–12 wk

majority of patients with IVD herniations will improve with nonsurgical intervention.

The goal of the surgery is to relieve the symptoms with as little morbidity as possible. If the quality of life or life span, reduction in pain, and improved function exceed by a sufficiently wide margin the medical risks of mortality, morbidity, and anxiety caused by the procedure, the procedure can be deemed a success.[404]

Integration of Preferred Patterns 4B and 4F: Impaired Joint Mobility, Motor Function, Muscle Performance, Range of Motion Secondary to Impaired Posture, Systemic Dysfunction (Referred Pain Syndromes), Spinal Disorders, and Myofascial Pain Dysfunction

Postural Syndromes of the Lumbar Region[103,139,169,173]

Symmetric impairments of the lumbar spine occur either as a result of acute pain, or of myofascial and articular tissue shortening from a fixed postural impairment.

A symmetric impairment will not be apparent in the flexion and extension position tests because, as both are equally impaired, there is no deviation from the path of flexion or extension, but rather the path is shortened or lengthened, depending on which type of impairment (hypomobility or hypermobility) is present. In addition, there is no apparent loss of side bending or rotation, and both sides appear equally hypomobile or hypermobile, with no change in the axis of rotation, except in the case where it ceases to exist, as in bony ankylosis.

Lower Crossed Syndrome.[139,280]   In this syndrome, the erector spinae and the iliopsoas are tight, and the abdominal and gluteus maximus are weak. This syndrome results in an anterior pelvic tilt, an increased lumbar lordosis, and a slight flexion of the hip. A number of muscles are adaptively shortened in this syndrome, including the gastrocnemius, soleus, hip adductors, and hip flexors. The hamstrings also are frequently shortened in this syndrome, and this may be a compensatory strategy to lessen the anterior tilt of the pelvis,[405] or a result of the weak glutei. Common injuries associated with this syndrome include hamstring strains, anterior knee pain, and LBP.

Therapeutic Techniques

Techniques to Increase Joint Mobility

All of the examination techniques that are used to assess joint mobility can be employed as intervention techniques. However, the intent of the technique changes from one of assessing the end-feel to one in which the application of graded mobilizations, or muscle energy techniques, is applied at the appropriate joint range. The selection of a manual technique is dependent on a number of factors, including (1) the acuteness of the condition, (2) the goal of the intervention, and (3) whether the restriction is symmetric or asymmetric.

Joint Mobilizations

Symmetric Restrictions. Symmetric restrictions are usually the result of a postural dysfunction. A number of manual techniques can be used to increase motion at a lumbar spine segment.

Symmetric Restriction of Flexion. Symmetric impairments can be treated effectively with symmetric mobilizations, at least for all but the extreme parts of the zygapophysial joint ranges. Nonacute symmetric impairments can be better treated using bilateral symmetric techniques. The L3 to L4 segment is used in the following example.[302]

The patient is in the side lying position, with the lumbar spine supported in a neutral position and the head resting on a pillow. The clinician faces the patient. Using the palpating finger of the cranial hand, the clinician palpates the interlaminar spaces of the L3 to L4 segment. Using the caudal hand, the clinician flexes the patient's hips, knees and the lower lumbar spine until L4 is felt to move. The patient's uppermost hip and knee remain flexed while the lowermost leg is extended. With the palpating finger of the caudal hand, the clinician palpates the interlaminar spaces of the L3 to L4 segment. Using the cranial hand and forearm, the clinician locks the upper lumbar spine by pulling through the patient's lowermost arm until L3 is felt to move. The direction of the arm pull determines whether the lock occurs in flexion, extension, or neutral, and whether a congruent or incongruent lock is used (see Section III Introduction). The L3 to L4 segment remains in its neutral position. The clinician fixes L4 and flexes the L3 to L4 segment to the motion barrier using the cranial hand and forearm. A grade I to IV force is applied to produce a superoanterior glide of the zygapophysial joints at L3 to L4 using the cranial hand and forearm.

Symmetric Restriction of Extension. The L3 to L4 segment is used in this example.[302] As mentioned previously, the end-feel, and the stage of healing, are used as guides to determine the intensity of the intervention.

The patient is in the side lying position, with the lumbar spine supported in a neutral position and the head resting on a pillow. The clinician faces the patient. Using the palpating finger of the cranial hand, the clinician palpates the interlaminar spaces of the L3 to L4 segment. Using the caudal hand, the clinician extends the patient's hip until L4 is felt to move. The

patient's uppermost hip and knee are flexed while the lowermost leg is extended. With the palpating finger of the caudal hand, the clinician palpates the interlaminar spaces of the L3 to L4 segment. Using the cranial hand and forearm, the clinician locks the lumbar spine by pulling through the patient's lowermost arm until L3 is felt to move. The direction of the arm pull determines whether the lock occurs in flexion, extension, or neutral, and whether a congruent or incongruent lock is used (see Section III Introduction). The L3 to L4 segment remains in its neutral position. The clinician fixes L4 by applying a posteroanterior force to the articular pillars of the L4 vertebra using the index and long fingers of the caudal hand (see Fig. 25-49). A grade I to IV force is applied to produce a posteroinferior glide of the zygapophysial joints at L3 to L4 using the cranial hand and forearm.

Asymmetric (Quadrant) Techniques. In the case of asymmetric hypomobility, the approach can be either to mobilize the stiff combined movement or to ascertain which joint and which glide is restricted and mobilize that directly, while, at the same time, safeguarding the other segments from the effect of the mobilization. For example, if right rotation–side bending and flexion are restricted, the segment can be mobilized using a flexion and right rotation mobilization technique. Alternatively, the same result would be achieved if the segment was positioned in flexion and right side bending, and a side bending mobilization was applied to increase the superior glide of the left superior zygapophysial joint (relative inferior glide of the right superior zygapophysial joint).

Asymmetric techniques may be used for any condition that allows the barrier to movement to be encroached upon. These conditions include unilateral zygapophysial joint hypomobilities, IVD protrusions, and myofascial shortening. If an appropriate bilateral hypomobility is to be treated, the clinician can utilize a bilateral asymmetric technique rather than the often-awkward symmetric technique. The only conditions that cannot be treated with asymmetric techniques are the acutely painful ones in which sub-barrier grades of mobilization must be used.

Restriction of Extension and Side Bending (Posterior Quadrant Restrictions). These impairments occur when the zygapophysial joint cannot extend and side flex. The patient typically presents with one-sided pain, which is aggravated with extension, and with side bending toward the painful side. This impairment is also known as a *closing restriction.*

The patient and clinician positioning is the same as for the side bending PPAIVM in extension (see Fig. 25-50). Once the segment has been located, the clinician pushes down on the spinous process of the superior segment using the thumb of the cranial hand while pulling up on spinous process of the lower segment with the fingers of the caudal hand. The "motion barrier" is felt, and a hold-relax technique is used to move to the new motion barrier. The process is repeated until a further increase in range is noted.

Restriction of Flexion and Side Bending (Anterior Quadrant Restrictions). These impairments occur when the zygapophysial joint cannot flex and side flex away from the side of the pain. The patient typically presents with one-sided pain, complaints of pain with flexion, and side bending away from the painful side. This impairment is also known as an *"opening" restriction.*

The patient and clinician positioning is the same as for the side bending PPAIVM in flexion (see Fig. 25-51). Once the segment has been located, the clinician pushes down on the spinous process of the superior segment using the thumb of the cranial hand while pulling up on the spinous process of the lower segment with the fingers of the caudal hand. The "motion barrier" is felt, and a hold-relax technique is used to move to the new motion barrier. The process is repeated until a further increase in range is noted.

Techniques to Increase Soft Tissue Extensibility

Muscle Energy

Erector Spinae. The patient is positioned side lying, with involved side up, or prone (Fig. 25-88). The clinician stands in front of the table, facing the patient. The involved leg is extended and adducted toward the clinician (see Fig. 25-88). The patient is instructed to attempt to rotate the spine toward the bed against equal and opposite resistance from the clinician for 10 seconds. The patient then rotates in the opposite direction and flexes the spine with assistance from the clinician. This sequence is repeated three to five times.

Quadratus Lumborum. The patient is in the side lying position, with the bottom leg flexed and the top leg extended and adducted over the edge of the table (Fig. 25-89). The patient is instructed to abduct the femur and elevate the pelvis against gravity for 10 seconds. The leg is lowered to the new barrier, and the procedure is repeated three to five times.

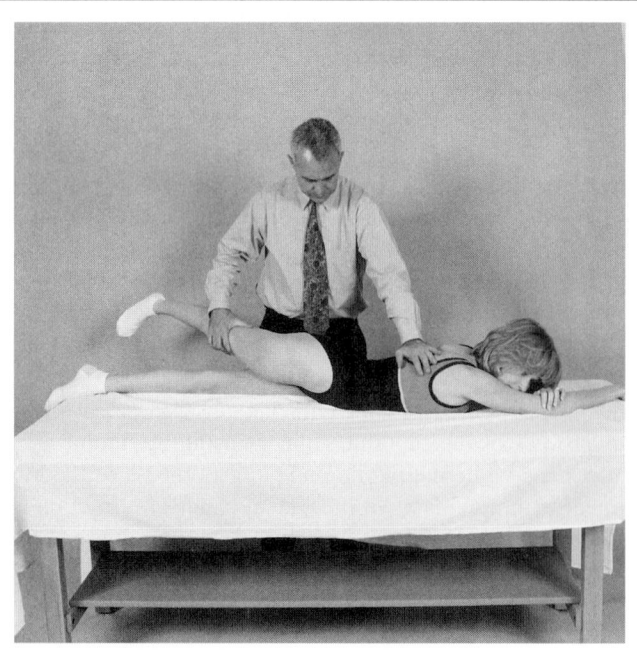

FIGURE 25-88   Erector spinae muscle energy technique.

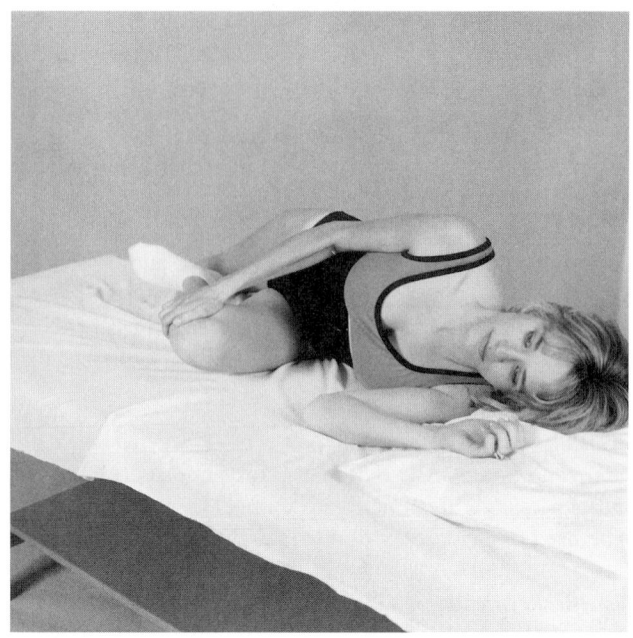

FIGURE 25-89   Quadratus lumborum muscle energy.

Myofascial Release

Lumbar Decompression.[406] Lumbar decompression is a gentle technique that may be used in the intervention for lumbar and lumbosacral dysfunction. The patient is positioned supine, with the legs straight. The clinician makes a fist with the cranial hand and places it under the patient's back in such a way as to grasp several spinous processes simultaneously between the heel of the palm and the clenched fingers. The other hand is placed over the sacrum (coming from between the patient's legs), and the elbow is rested on the table. A gentle traction force is applied to the sacrum until the fascial barrier is felt. This force is maintained until the fascial restrictions are felt to release.

Self-stretching Exercises

In addition to the manual techniques and therapeutic exercises, the following self-stretching techniques are recommended.

Hip Flexors and Rectus Femoris. These exercises are described in Chapter 17.

Hamstrings. These exercises are described in Chapter 17.

Quadratus Lumborum. This muscle can be stretched passively by side lying over a Swiss ball (Fig. 25-90), or actively in the standing position (Fig. 25-91).

Erector Spinae. This muscle group can be stretched in several ways (Figs. 25-92 through 25-95).

Piriformis. Two methods for self-stretching this muscle are shown in Figures 25-96 and 25-97.

Hip Adductor Stretch. This stretch is shown in Figure 25-98.

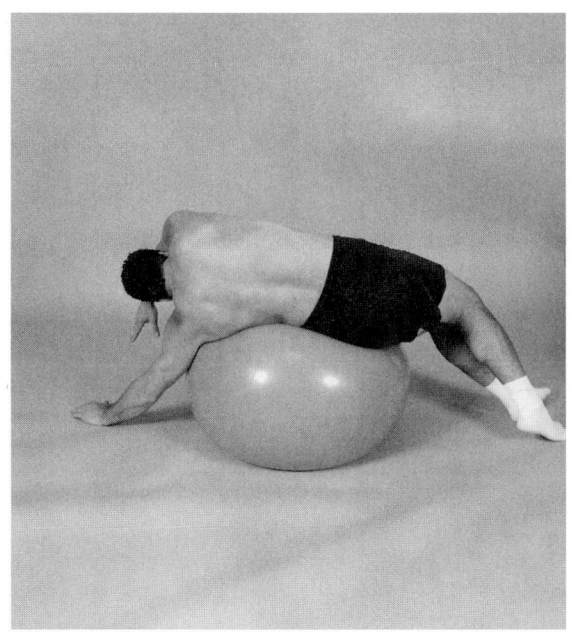

FIGURE 25-90 Quadratus lumborum stretch.

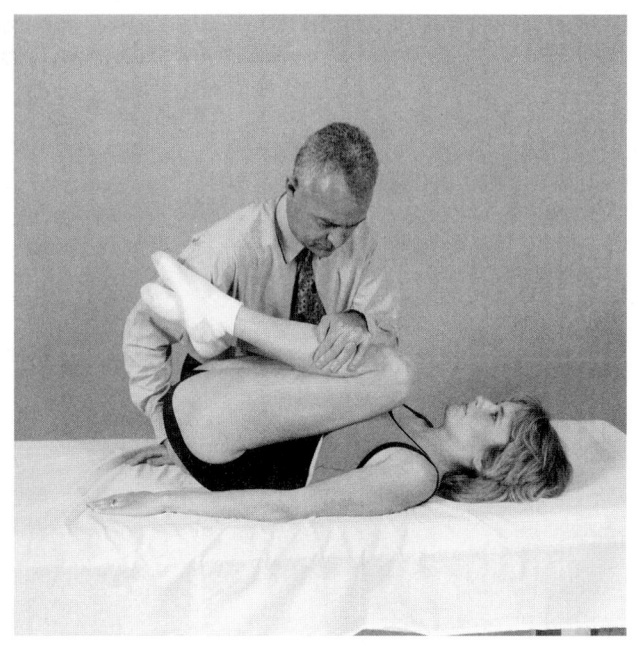

FIGURE 25-92 Erector spinae stretch, version 1.

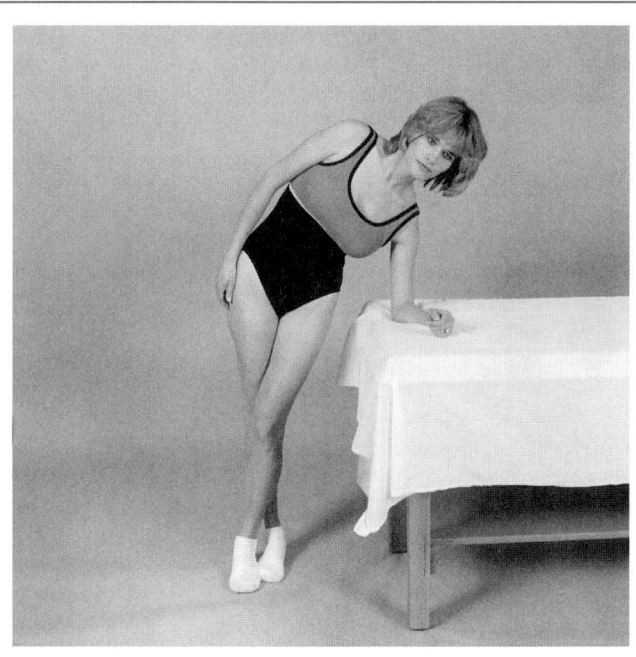

FIGURE 25-91 Quadratus lumborum stretch.

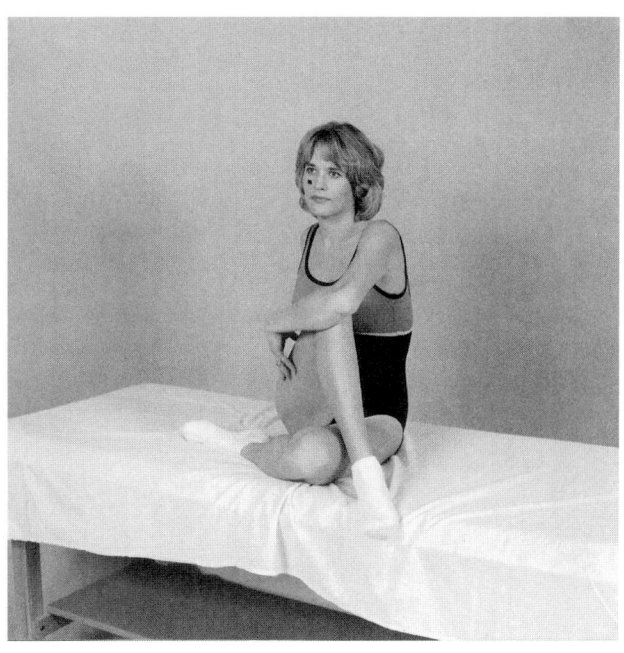

FIGURE 25-93 Erector spinae stretch, version 2.

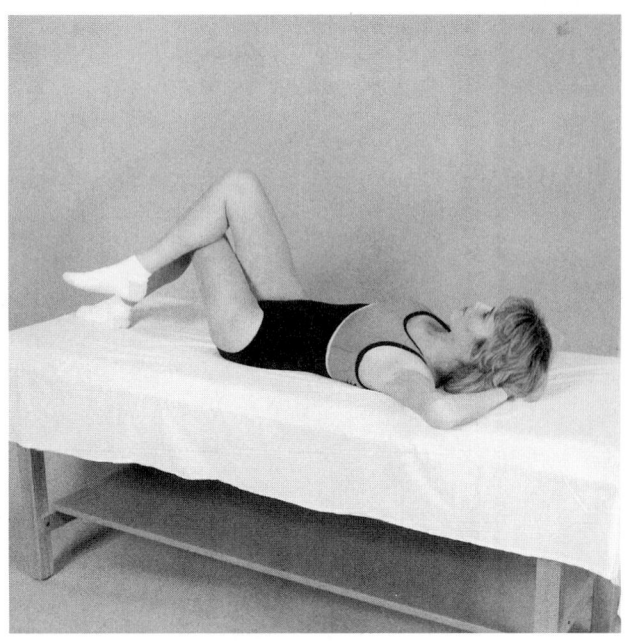

FIGURE 25-94   Erector spinae stretch, version 3.

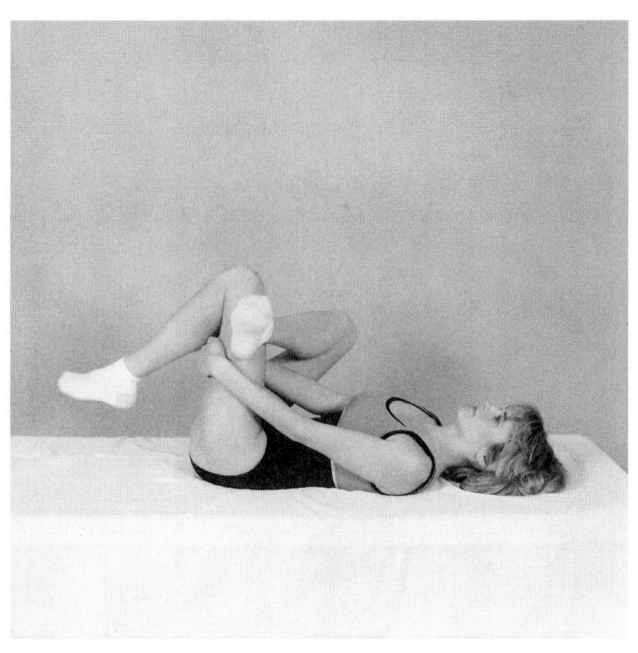

FIGURE 25-96   Piriformis stretch, version 1.

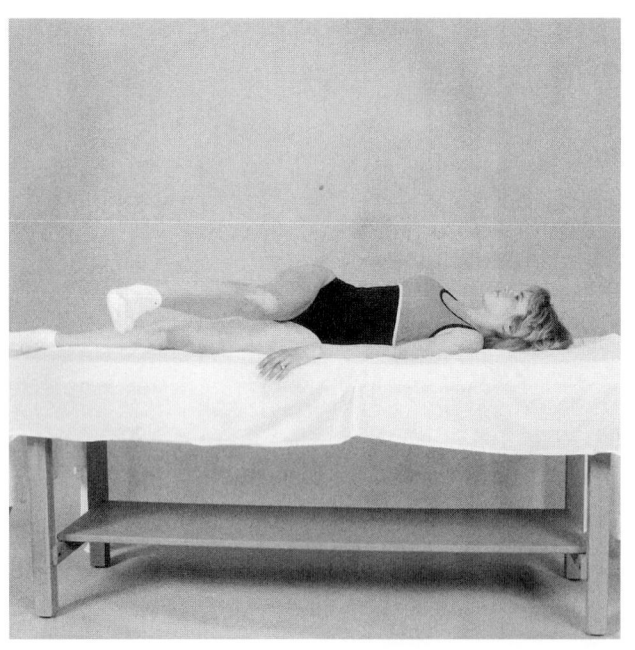

FIGURE 25-95   Erector spinae stretch, version 4.

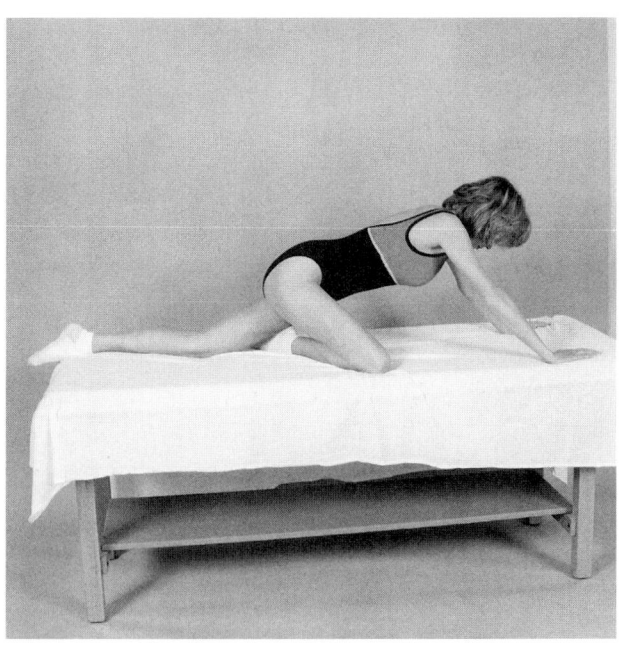

FIGURE 25-97   Piriformis stretch, version 2.

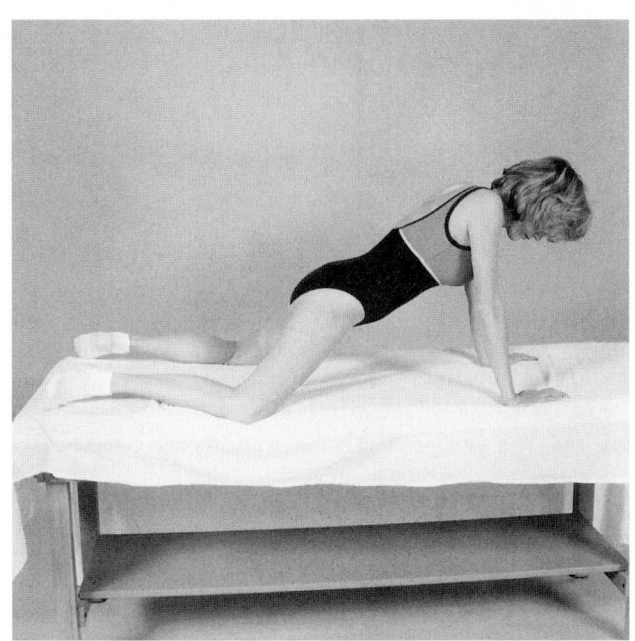

FIGURE 25-98   Hip adductor stretch.

CASE STUDY   CENTRAL LOW BACK PAIN WITH OCCASIONAL RIGHT RADIATION

HISTORY

A 58-year-old woman presented with a gradual onset of low back and sacroiliac joint pain. Her chief complaint was a "stiff" back, especially in the morning. The patient had experienced mild discomfort over several years but had noticed a recent increase in its intensity over the past few months. The pain was reported as being worse with prolonged standing, lifting, bending, and walking, and was relieved by sitting and lying down. The pain occasionally was felt in the right buttock, hip, and thigh. A recent radiograph revealed the presence of "arthritic changes" in the lumbar spine.

   The patient reported being in good general health. There were no reports of night pain, bowel and bladder changes, or pain with coughing or sneezing.

QUESTIONS

1. List the differential diagnosis for complaints of pain in the low back and sacroiliac joint.
2. What may be the significance of a history of morning stiffness?
3. List the potential reasons for the patient's symptoms being worsened with prolonged standing, lifting, bending, and walking, and improved with sitting or lying?
4. From the history, what are the indications that this may be a musculoskeletal problem?
5. Which tests could you use to rule in/rule out the potential reasons for the patient's complaints.

6. Does this presentation/history warrant a Cyriax lower quarter scanning examination? Why or why not?

EXAMINATION

Because of the insidious nature of the LBP, a lower quarter scanning examination was performed, with the following positive findings:

- Upon observation, it was noted that the patient stood with her knees slightly flexed and had a pronounced lumbar lordosis and slightly flattened buttocks.
- Active range-of-motion testing revealed a painful restriction of forward bending of 30 degrees and pain reproduced with excessive lordosis positioning.
- There was limited extensibility of the hamstrings to 45 degrees with the straight leg raise but no neurologic findings.[407]
- On palpation, the L5 spinous process was prominent and tender, and pressure against the lateral aspect of the spinous process of L5 toward the right side produced radiating pain in the L5 nerve root distribution. The pain subsided when the spinous process was pressed in the opposite direction.[408]

QUESTIONS

1. Given the findings from the scanning examination, can you determine the diagnosis, or is further testing warranted in the form of special tests? What information would you hope to gain with further testing?
2. What is the significance of the findings from the spinous process motion tests?
3. What could be the significance of the decrease in the extensibility of the hamstrings?

EVALUATION AND DIAGNOSIS

A provisional diagnosis could be made on the strength of the history—an older patient with LBP, or radicular paresthesia, or pain, that is reproduced by increasing the lordosis and that disappears on reducing the lordosis. The findings from the examination indicate the possibility of a lateral recess stenosis or a degenerative spondylolisthesis of L5.

QUESTIONS

1. Having made a provisional diagnosis, what will be your intervention?
2. How would you describe this condition to the patient?
3. How will you determine the intensity of the exercises for the intervention?
4. What would you tell the patient about your intervention?
5. Which manual techniques are appropriate for this condition? Why and why not?
6. Estimate this patient's prognosis.
7. What modalities could you use in the intervention for this patient? Why?
8. What exercises would you prescribe? Why?

INTERVENTION

A call was placed to the patient's physician to ask if a series of flexion-extension radiographs could be taken. The patient was advised to stand in the waiting room before the radiograph, to help ensure that the slippage would not be reduced during sitting. The radiographs revealed a grade II slippage. The patient returned to physical therapy for a trial period of conservative intervention. If the radiographs had not revealed any slippage, how would you have proceeded?

- *Initial symptom relief.* Electrotherapeutic modalities and thermal agents were used initially for symptomatic pain relief. The patient was educated on the use of heat and ice at home. A transcutaneous electrical nerve stimulation (TENS) unit was issued to help the patient perform activities of daily living.
- *Manual therapy.* Often the only manual intervention with this patient type is the correction of any muscle imbalances. Stretching of the hip flexors and rectus femoris while protecting the lumbar spine were performed on this patient. The stretching of the hamstrings has been a traditional adjunct to the intervention for spondylolisthesis. However, it is not clear whether this is beneficial, given the fact that adaptively shortened hamstrings may serve a protective role by decreasing the anterior tilt of the pelvis, thereby reducing the lordosis and the slip angle.
- *Therapeutic exercises.* A lumbar stabilization progression was initiated. Aerobic exercises using a stationary bike and an upper body ergometer also were prescribed.
- *Patient-related instruction.* Explanation was given as to the cause of the patient's symptoms. The patient was advised against the extremes of motion, especially activities and positions that would increase the lumbar lordosis. Prolonged standing was to be accompanied by raising one foot onto a stool. Instructions were given to sleep on the side with a pillow between the knees. The patient was advised to continue the exercises at home, three to five times each day, and to expect some postexercise soreness.
- *Goals/outcomes.* Both the patient's goals from the intervention and the expected therapeutic goals of the clinician were discussed with the patient. It was concluded that the clinical sessions would occur three times per week for 1 month, at which time a decision would be made as to the effectiveness of the lumbar stabilization exercise progression. With a strict adherence to the instructions and exercise program, it was felt that the patient would improve her functional status and ability to control the pain.

CASE STUDY LOW BACK PAIN

HISTORY

A 40-year-old man presented with a 3-month history of gradual onset of LBP with no specific mechanism of injury. The pain was felt across the lower back at the level of the belt line. The patient reported no pain in the morning upon arising. The pain began soon after reporting to work as a cashier in a grocery store, and worsened as the day wore on. The pain was also worsened with activities that involving prolonged walking or prone lying. The pain was relieved almost instantly by sitting or side lying with the knees drawn to the chest.

The patient had radiographs of the spine taken recently, which showed some evidence of arthritis but were otherwise unremarkable.

The patient reported being in good general health. There were no reports of night pain, bowel and bladder changes, or pain with coughing or sneezing.

QUESTIONS

1. List the differential diagnosis for complaints of a gradual onset of pain in the low back in this age group.
2. What may be the significance of a history of no morning pain or stiffness?
3. List the potential reasons for the patient's symptoms getting worse with prolonged standing, walking, and lying but better with sitting or the fetal position.
4. From the history, what are the indications that low back pain may be a musculoskeletal problem?
5. What is your working hypothesis at this stage? Which tests could you use to confirm or refute your hypothesis?
6. Does this presentation/history warrant a Cyriax lower quarter scanning examination? Why or why not?

EXAMINATION

Upon observation, it was noted that the patient stood with a reduced lumbar lordosis. Because of the insidious nature of the LBP, a lumbar scan was performed with the following positive findings:

- Full and pain-free range of all lumbar movements was noted, although overpressure into full extension was painful and worsened with the addition of side bending to either side.
- No dural or nerve root signs were present, but the prone knee bending test (see Chap. 8) reproduced the LBP.

The tests and measures revealed the following:

- The application of passive bilateral knee flexion (Pheasant's test) with the patient in prone, increased the symptoms.
- PPIVM testing indicated good mobility at all levels.
- PPAIVM testing indicated good mobility, with the exception of the extension glides of L3 on L4 bilaterally, which were reduced.
- Abdominal endurance was 4/5.
- Adaptive shortening of the hip flexors, hamstrings, and rectus femoris was noted.

QUESTIONS

1. Given the findings from the tests and measures, can you determine the diagnosis, or is further testing warranted in the form of special tests?
2. What might the findings from the combined motion tests indicate?
3. What is the significance of the findings from the Pheasant's test and the muscle length tests?
4. Which of the adaptive shortened muscles are likely to be more significant?
5. What other tests might you use if the intervention fails to demonstrate improvement?

EVALUATION AND DIAGNOSIS

It appeared from the examination that an otherwise healthy patient experienced pain when the tissues restraining lumbar extension were stressed. The symptoms appeared to be mechanical in nature and nonirritable. The symptom distribution was symmetric with no referral, radiation, or radiculopathy.

QUESTIONS

1. Having made a provisional diagnosis, what will be your intervention?
2. How would you describe this condition to the patient?
3. How will you determine the intensity of the exercises for the intervention?
4. What would you tell the patient about your intervention?
5. Which manual techniques are appropriate for this condition? Why and why not?
6. Estimate this patient's prognosis.
7. What modalities could you use in the intervention of this patient? Why?
8. What exercises would you prescribe? Why?

INTERVENTION

The goal of the intervention should be the removal of the aggravating stresses and the resumption of the extension motion.

- *Manual therapy.* Soft tissue techniques were applied to the area, followed by a specific mobilization of the L3 to L4 segment into symmetric extension.
- *Therapeutic exercises.* Exercises to strengthen the abdominals, gluteals, multifidus, and erector spinae were prescribed. Aerobic exercises using a stationary bike and an upper body ergonometer also were prescribed. The patient was instructed on how to stretch the hip flexors, rectus femoris, and hamstrings. The patient was progressed to a lumbar stabilization program.
- *Patient-related instruction.* Explanation was given as to the cause of the patient's symptoms. The patient was advised against sitting or standing upright. Prolonged standing was to be accompanied with the patient raising one foot onto a stool. Instructions to sleep on the side were given. The patient received instructions regarding the benefit of maintaining the neutral zone during activities of daily living, and correct lifting techniques. The patient was advised to continue the exercises at home, three to five times each day, and to expect some postexercise soreness. The patient also received instruction on the use of heat and ice at home.
- *Goals/outcomes.* Both the patient's goals from the intervention and the expected therapeutic goals of the clinician were discussed with the patient.

CASE STUDY   UNILATERAL LOW BACK PAIN

HISTORY

A 20-year-old man complained of a sudden onset of unilateral LBP. The pain was so severe as to prevent the patient from standing upright. The patient described a mechanism of bending forward quickly to catch a ball near his left foot. He immediately experienced a sharp pain in his low back and was unable to straighten up because of the pain. The patient had no past history of back pain. No spinal radiographs had been taken.[409]

QUESTIONS

1. List the differential diagnosis for complaints of a gradual onset of unilateral low back pain.
2. What may be the significance of the reported mechanism?
3. List the potential reasons for the patient being initially unable to straighten up from the flexed position.
4. From the history, what are the indications that this may be a musculoskeletal problem?
5. Would the results from imaging studies be useful in this case? Why or why not?
6. What is your working hypothesis at this stage? Which tests could you use to confirm or refute your hypothesis?
7. Does this presentation/history warrant a Cyriax lower quarter scanning examination? Why or why not?

EXAMINATION

There was no pain when the patient's back was held in flexion, but on standing upright, pain was experienced to the right of the L5 spinous process. The other lumbar ranges that were restricted included side flexion to the right and rotation to the right. All other movements were full and painless. The clinician was able to reproduce the pain with PPIVM and PPAIVM testing into flexion, but the tests into extension or right side-bending and rotation produced pain at the L4 to L5 segment, with marked spasm. Unilateral posteroanterior pressures over the right L4 to L5 zygapophysial joint also produced marked pain and spasm.

QUESTIONS

1. Given the findings from the tests and measures, can you determine the diagnosis, or is further testing warranted in the form of special tests?
2. What might the findings from the combined motion tests indicate?
3. What is the significance of the findings from the PPIVM and PPAIVM tests?
4. What other tests might you use if the intervention fails to demonstrate improvement?

EVALUATION

With this patient, the quick movement into flexion and left side-bending gapped the right lumbar zygapophysial joints, following which there was a mechanical blocking of the movements that normally appose the articular surfaces (extension, side bending, and rotation of the trunk to the right).

QUESTIONS

1. Having made a provisional diagnosis, what will be your intervention?

2. How would you describe this condition to the patient?

3. How will you determine the intensity of the exercises for the intervention?

4. Which manual techniques are appropriate for this condition? Why and why not?

5. Estimate this patient's prognosis.

6. What modalities could you use in the intervention of this patient? Why?

7. What exercises would you prescribe? Why?

INTERVENTION

- *Initial symptom relief.* Electrotherapeutic modalities and thermal agents were used initially for symptomatic pain relief. The patient was educated on the use of heat and ice at home.

- *Manual therapy.* Soft tissue techniques were applied to the area, followed by an asymmetric mobilization (grades III and IV), performed to gap the right L4 to L5 zygapophysial joint. Immediately afterward, the patient could fully extend, side flex, and rotate to the right, with some soreness experienced at the extreme of these motions. This soreness was lessened by gentle, large-amplitude posteroanterior pressures performed unilaterally over the right L4 to L5 zygapophysial joint.

- *Therapeutic exercises.* Exercises to promote spinal extension were prescribed. These consisted of a progression from prone lying, to prone on elbow, to prone push-ups. Aerobic exercises using a stationary bike and an upper body ergonometer also were prescribed.

- *Patient-related instruction.* Explanation was given as to the cause of the patient's symptoms. The patient was advised against sudden bending and twisting movements. Instructions to sleep on the side were given. The patient also received instructions regarding correct lifting techniques. The patient was advised to continue the exercises at home, three to five times each day, and to expect some postexercise soreness.

CASE STUDY CENTRAL LOW BACK PAIN

HISTORY

A 45-year-old woman was referred for LBP. She complained of pain across the center of her back at the waistline. The pain, which had started gradually many years ago, had not spread from this small area, but it had increased in intensity. The increase in intensity resulted from a bending and lifting injury a few years previously and, since that incident, the patient reported having difficulty straightening up from the bent-over position. Twisting maneuvers, whether in standing, sitting, or lying position, also produced the pain, but otherwise the woman was able to sit, stand, or walk for long periods without pain.

QUESTIONS

1. List the differential diagnosis for complaints of a gradual onset of central low back pain.

2. What may be the significance of the insidious onset?

3. List the potential reasons for the patient having difficulty straightening up from the flexed position.

4. From the history, what are the indications that this may be a mechanical problem?

5. Would the results from imaging studies be useful in this case? If so, which?

6. What is your working hypothesis at this stage? Which tests could you use to confirm or refute your hypothesis?

7. Does this presentation/history warrant a Cyriax lower quarter scanning examination? Why or why not?

EXAMINATION

Although this patient presented with an insidious onset of pain, the onset had been many years ago and the area of pain had not changed over those years. The intensity had increased, but there was no evidence of radiation, and the pain appeared to be related to movement. Thus, only a modified scan was performed with the following results:

- Flexion was full range and pain free, although the return from flexion was painful, especially the initiation. All other motions were full and pain free.

- Compression and distraction of the lumbar spine were both pain free.

- Positive Pheasant's test (see the discussion under "Special Tests," earlier in the chapter).

- No evidence of neurologic compromise was found.

The tests and measures revealed the following:

- PPIVM tests revealed good mobility at all levels of the lumbar spine.

- PPAIVM testing into extension of the L5 to S1 segment produced a spasmodic end-feel.

- The anterior shear test was positive for pain and increased motion.

- Decreased flexibility of the hip flexors, rectus femoris, and hamstrings was noted.

QUESTIONS

1. Given the findings from the tests and measures, can you determine the diagnosis, or is further testing warranted in the form of special tests?

2. What might the spasm end-feel suggest about the irritability of the condition?

3. What is the significance of the findings from the anterior shear test?

4. What is the significance of the findings from the Pheasant's test and the muscle length tests?

5. Which of the adaptive shortened muscles are likely to be more significant?

6. What other tests might you use if the intervention fails to demonstrate improvement?

EVALUATION

The history of this patient suggested instability. The possibility of an IVD herniation, degenerative changes, and zygapophysial joint impairment, need to be eliminated. In this case, the absence of neurologic symptoms and the pattern of motion restriction helped in determining the provisional diagnosis. More serious impairments also could be ruled out by the number of years that the patient had the problem.

QUESTIONS

1. Having made a provisional diagnosis, what will be your intervention?
2. How would you describe this condition to the patient?
3. How will you determine the intensity of the exercises for the intervention?
4. Which manual techniques are appropriate for this condition? Why and why not?
5. Estimate this patient's prognosis.
6. What modalities could you use in the intervention of this patient? Why?
7. What exercises would you prescribe? Why?

INTERVENTION

- *Manual therapy.* Often the only manual intervention with this patient type is the correction of any pelvic shift that is present, and the correction of any muscle imbalances. Stretching of the hip flexors and rectus femoris, while protecting the lumbar spine, were performed on this patient.
- *Therapeutic exercises.* A lumbar stabilization progression was initiated. Aerobic exercises using a stationary bike and an upper body ergometer also were prescribed.
- *Patient-related instruction.* Explanation was given as to the cause of the patient's symptoms. The patient was advised to avoid the extremes of motion, especially lumbar hyperextension. Prolonged standing was to be accompanied by raising one foot onto a stool. Instructions were given to sleep on the side with a pillow between the knees. The patient was educated about positions and activities to avoid. The patient was advised to continue the exercises at home, three to five times each day, and to expect some postexercise soreness. The patient also received instruction on the use of heat and ice at home.
- *Goals/outcomes.* Both the patient's goals from the intervention and the expected therapeutic goals of the clinician were discussed with the patient.

CASE STUDY LEG PAIN WITH WALKING

HISTORY

A 65-year-old man presented with an insidious onset of right leg symptoms, which followed a period, or distance, of walking, or occurred after a period of standing, and which disappeared when he sat down. The patient also complained of pain at night, especially when he slept on his stomach. Further questioning revealed that the patient had a history of back pain related to an occupation involving heavy lifting, but was otherwise in good health and had no reports of bowel or bladder impairment.

QUESTIONS

1. Given the age of the patient and the history, do you have a working hypothesis?
2. Why do you think the patient has pain with prone lying?
3. Is the pain at night a cause for concern in this patient? Why?
4. Does this presentation/history warrant a scanning examination? Why or why not?

EXAMINATION

A provisional diagnosis for this patient could be made on the strength of the history—an elderly patient with root pain or paresthesia that is reproduced in the erect position and immediately disappears on sitting or bending forward. This is a classic syndrome of the elderly. Despite the fact that the patient appears to fit the pattern of a syndrome, it is well worth taking the time to perform a scanning examination, particularly in view of the insidious onset of symptoms and the presence of leg symptoms. A lumbar scan revealed the following results:

- The patient was of a medium build. His standing posture revealed a flattened lumbar spine and slight flexion at the hips and knees, but was otherwise unremarkable.
- Active range-of-motion tests demonstrated a capsular pattern of restriction for the spine. During spinal extension, no symptoms were reported, but closer observation revealed very little motion occurring at the lumbar spine during this maneuver.
- When the patient was asked to perform an anterior pelvic tilt to increase the lumbar lordosis, the paresthesias into the leg were reproduced, and reversing the lordosis relieved the symptoms.
- The distribution of the paresthesia included the lateral and medial aspect of the leg and dorsum of the foot and great toe.
- The straight leg raise test was normal.
- Hip range of motion revealed a decrease in hip extension range of motion bilaterally.
- Abdominal muscle strength testing revealed weakness.
- The bicycle test of van Gelderen[410] was used to help confirm the diagnosis and to help rule out arterial claudication.

EVALUATION

The findings for this patient indicated the presence of a lateral recess spinal stenosis at the L4 to L5 level on the right side.

QUESTIONS

1. Having made the provisional diagnosis, what will be your intervention?
2. How would you describe this condition to the patient?
3. In order of priority, and based on the stages of healing, list the various goals of your intervention?
4. What would you tell the patient about your intervention?
5. Is an asymmetric or a symmetric technique more appropriate for this condition? Why?
6. Estimate this patient's prognosis.
7. What modalities could you use in the intervention for this patient?
8. What exercises would you prescribe?

INTERVENTION

- *Initial symptom relief.* Electrotherapeutic modalities and thermal agents were used initially for symptomatic pain relief. The patient was educated on the use of heat and ice at home. A TENS unit was issued to help the patient perform activities of daily living.
- *Manual therapy.* A symmetric manual traction was performed initially. Because the patient appeared to obtain good results from this, mechanical traction was introduced (see below).
- *Therapeutic exercises.* Exercises incorporating lumbar flexion were prescribed. These included posterior pelvic tilts, single and bilateral knees to chest, and seated flexion. Aerobic exercises using a stationary bike and an upper body ergometer also were prescribed.
- *Patient-related instruction.* Explanation was given as to the cause of the patient's symptoms. The patient was advised against sitting or standing upright. Prolonged standing was to be accompanied by raising one foot onto a stool. Instructions were given to sleep on the right side. Why? The patient received instructions regarding the use of posterior pelvic tilting during activities of daily living, and correct lifting techniques. The patient was advised to continue the exercises at home, three to five times each day, and to expect some postexercise soreness.
- *Goals/outcomes.* Both the patient's goals from the intervention and the expected therapeutic goals of the clinician were discussed with the patient.

CASE STUDY   RIGHT BUTTOCK PAIN

HISTORY

A 21-year-old woman presented with LBP that had occurred while playing tennis, and had been accompanied by a sharp pain in the right buttock area. The patient was able to carry on playing, and the sharp pain subsided until the following morning, when attempted to weight bear through the right leg. The pain again subsided after a hot shower and her walk to work. That evening, the patient went jogging and was forced to stop after about a mile because of the return of the sharp pain in the buttock. A hot soak eased the pain but was replaced by a dull ache that lasted several days. The patient sought medical advice and was referred to physical therapy. When asked to indicate where her pain was, she pointed to a small area, medial to the right trochanter, over the piriformis muscle. Further questioning revealed that the patient had no previous history of back pain and was otherwise in good health, with no reports of bowel or bladder impairment.

QUESTIONS

1. What structure(s) could be at fault with complaints of buttock pain?
2. What does the history of the pain tell the clinician?
3. What is your working hypothesis at this stage? List the various diagnoses that could present with buttock pain, and the tests you would use to rule out each one.
4. Does this presentation/history warrant a scan? Why or why not?

EXAMINATION

The pain was of a traumatic origin, and its intensity and behavior suggests a biomechanical cause. Observation revealed nothing remarkable. The tests and measures demonstrated the following:

- Straight plane active range of motion revealed a restriction of right side bending of 75 percent and a slight restriction of extension.
- The combined motion testing revealed a restriction of the right posterior quadrant: the combined motion of right side bending and extension at 50 percent compared with extension and left side bending, with a reproduction of the patient's pain.
- A posteroanterior pressure applied over L5 produced local tenderness.
- The PPIVM tests appeared to be positive for hypomobility at the levels of L4 to L5 and L5 to S1.
- The PPAIVM test appeared to be positive for hypomobility for extension and right side bending at the L5 to S1 level.

QUESTIONS

1. What information is gained from a positive combined motion testing?
2. Did the tests and measures confirm your working hypothesis? Why or why not?
3. If the tests and measures did not confirm your working hypothesis, what would be your course of action?
4. Given the findings from the tests and measures, what is the diagnosis, or is further testing warranted in the form of special tests? What information would be gained with further testing?
5. How can you determine whether the loss of motion is the result of an articular restriction or a myofascial restriction?

EVALUATION

The patient was provisionally diagnosed as having an articular hypomobility of extension and right side bending at the L5 to S1 level.

QUESTIONS

1. Having made the diagnosis, what will be your intervention?
2. How would you describe this condition to the patient?
3. In order of priority, and based on the stages of healing, list the various goals of your intervention.
4. How will you determine the amplitude and joint position for the intervention?
5. What would you tell the patient about your intervention?
6. Is an asymmetric or a symmetric technique more appropriate for this condition? Why?
7. What modalities could you use in the intervention for this patient?
8. What exercises would you prescribe?

INTERVENTION

- *Initial symptom relief.* Moist heat and ultrasound were applied to the area initially for symptomatic pain relief. The patient was educated on the use of heat and ice at home.
- *Manual therapy.* Following the ultrasound, soft tissue techniques were applied to the area. Given the fact that the joint glide was restricted in an asymmetric pattern, an asymmetric mobilization technique was performed to increase extension and right side bending at the L5 to S1 level. Initially, grade I and II mobilizations were used. Later, grades III and IV were introduced.
- *Therapeutic exercises.* The following exercises were prescribed:

    - Prone hip extension on the right.
    - Supine pelvic rotations in the hook-lying position.
    - Standing side bending and rotation to the right.
    - Aerobic exercises using a stationary bike and an upper body ergometer.

- *Patient-related instruction.* Explanation was given as to the cause of the patient's symptoms. Instructions were given to sleep on the side. The patient also received instructions regarding correct lifting techniques. The patient was advised to continue the exercises at home, three to five times each day, and to expect some postexercise soreness.
- *Goals/outcomes.* Both the patient's goals from the intervention and the expected therapeutic goals of the clinician were discussed with the patient.

CASE STUDY SYMMETRIC LOW BACK PAIN

HISTORY

A 30-year-old woman presented with a 3-month history of gradual onset of pain with no specific mechanism of injury. She reported no pain in the morning upon arising, but by midafternoon her low back began to ache. The pain worsened with activities that involved sustained flexion and when lifting. Sitting and lying eased the pain. The patient had radiographs taken recently, which were normal.

EXAMINATION

Upon observation, it was noted that the patient stood with a normal lumbar lordosis. Because of the insidious nature of the LBP, a lumbar scan was performed with the following findings:

- Full and pain-free range of all movements.
- No dural or nerve root signs present.

    The tests and measures revealed the following:

- Overpressure into full flexion was painful, and with the addition of side bending to either side, the pain worsened on each side.
- PPIVM testing appeared to indicate good mobility at all levels.
- PPAIVM testing appeared to indicate good mobility, with the exception of the flexion glides of L3 on L4 bilaterally, which were reduced.
- Weakness and slackness of the gluteals, erector spinae, and abdominals.

- Moderate tightness of the hamstrings, with a straight leg raise of 75 degrees bilaterally.

EVALUATION

It would appear from the examination that an otherwise healthy and mobile spine began to hurt when the tissues restraining flexion were stressed, producing a painful symmetric impairment. These structures include the posterior ligamentous and zygapophysial joint structures that were receiving poor dynamic support from the abdominals and gluteals.

INTERVENTION

This patient's condition was nonacute and the intervention was relatively straightforward.

- Explanation as to the cause of the patient's symptoms was given, as well as exercises to strengthen the lower abdominals, gluteals, and erector spinae, and exercises to stretch the hamstrings. Instructions were given on anterior pelvic tilting, and correct lifting techniques.
- The L3 to L4 segment was mobilized into symmetric flexion.
- Because the patient experienced difficulties performing the exercises correctly, a biofeedback unit was used to help teach the patient when the correct muscle was being activated, and neuromuscular (functional) electrical stimulation (NMES) was used to activate the appropriate muscles.
- The hamstring tightness was not addressed, because their tightness facilitated the posterior pelvic tilting.
- The patient received education on the maintenance of ideal body mechanics (line of gravity, use of hip, load close to body, etc.) during lifting that considered the pathology, signs, patient ability, lifting required, and potential for change. The patient was taught how to lift in the "position of power" by using a "dynamic" pelvic tilt. The dynamic pelvic tilt was taught to the patient using the following sequence:

    - The patient is positioned supine in the hook-lying position and is asked to perform a pelvic tilt and to find the "neutral zone." This exercise teaches the patient about an awareness of neutral with respect to flexion or extension. While holding the tilt, the patient is asked to straighten one leg and abduct it.
    - The patient is positioned sitting. The patient is asked to find the neutral zone using a pelvic tilt. Once the patient has achieved this, he or she is asked to stand against a wall and to find the neutral zone using a pelvic tilt. Once this is mastered, the patient is asked to maintain the neutral zone and to walk away from the wall.
    - The patient is positioned standing. The neutral zone is achieved and then maintained as the patient bends at the knees as though bending to lift an object.

REVIEW QUESTIONS*

1. Which of the spinal ligaments gives the best support against postero-lateral IVD protrusions?
2. Which lumbar ligament, consisting of five bands, prevents anterior shearing of L5 on S1?

3. Which muscles make up the erector spinae?
4. Which motions does the multifidus muscle produce?
5. Approximately what is the normal amount of lumbar range of motion with flexion and extension?

---

* Additional questions to test your understanding of this chapter can be found in the Online Learning Center for *Orthopaedic Assessment, Evaluation, and Intervention* at www.duttononline.net.

REFERENCES

1. Nathan H. Gangliform enlargement on the lateral cutaneous nerve of the thigh. *J Neurosurg* 1960;17:843.
2. Linton SJ. The socioeconomic impact of chronic back pain: Is anyone benefiting? *Pain* 1998;75:163–168.
3. Waddell G. A new clinical model for the treatment of low back pain. *Spine* 1987;12:632–643.
4. Gibson JN, Grant IC, Waddell G. The Cochrane review of surgery for lumbar disc prolapse and degenerative lumbar spondylosis. *Spine* 1999;24:1820–1832.
5. Croft PR, et al. Outcome of low back pain in general practice: A prospective study. *BMJ* 1998;316:1356–1359.
6. Indahl A, Velund L, Reikeraas O. Good prognosis for low back pain when left untampered. *Spine* 1995;20:473–477.
7. Michel A, Kohlmann T, Raspe H. The association between clinical findings on physical examination and self-reported severity in back pain: Results of a population-based study. *Spine* 1997;22:296–304.
8. Waddell G, et al. Objective clinical evaluation of physical impairment in chronic low back pain. *Spine* 1992;17:617–628.
9. Valkenberg HA, Haanen HCM. The epidemiology of low back pain. In: White AA, Gordon SL, eds. *American Academy of Orthopedic Surgeons Symposium on Idiopathic Low Back Pain.* St Louis, Mo: Mosby; 1982:9–22.
10. Riihimaki H. Epidemiology and pathogenesis of non-specific low back pain: what does the epidemiology tell us? *Bull Hosp Jt Dis* 1996;55:197–198.
11. Smedley J, et al. Prospective cohort study of predictors of incident low back pain in nurses. *BMJ* 1997;314:1225–1228.
12. Kraus JF, et al. Design factors in epidemiologic cohort studies of work-related low back injury or pain. *Am J Ind Med* 1997;32:153–163.
13. Macfarlane GJ, et al. Employment and physical work activities as predictors of future low back pain. *Spine* 1997;22:1143–1149.
14. Kelsey JL. An epidemiological study of the relationship between occupations and acute herniated lumbar intervertebral discs. *Int J Epidemiol* 1975;4:197–205.
15. Tichauer ER. *The Biomedical Basis of Ergonomics: Anatomy Applied to the Design of the Work Situation.* New York, NY: Wiley; 1978.
16. Magora A. Investigation of the relation between low back pain and occupation: 4. Physical requirements: Bending, rotation, reaching and sudden maximal effort. *Scand J Rehabil Med* 1973;5:186–190.
17. Magora A. Investigation of the relation between low back pain and occupation: 3. Physical requirements: Sitting, standing and weight lifting. *Ind Med Surg* 1972;41:5–9.
18. Palmer KT, et al. Prevalence and pattern of occupational exposure to whole body vibration in Great Britain: Findings from a national survey. *Occup Environ Med* 2000;57:229–236.
19. Backman AL. Health survey of professional drivers. *Scand J Work Environ Health* 1983;9:30–35.
20. Bongers PM, et al. Back disorders in crane operators exposed to whole-body vibration. *Int Arch Occup Environ Health* 1988;60:129–137.
21. Bongers PM, et al. Back pain and exposure to whole body vibration in helicopter pilots. *Ergonomics* 1990;33:1007–1026.
22. Pietri F, et al. Low-back pain in commercial drivers. *Scand J Work Environ Health* 1992;18:52–58.
23. Kelsey JL, Hardy RJ. Driving of motor vehicles as a risk factor for acute herniated lumbar intervertebral disc. *Am J Epidemiol* 1975;102:63–73.
24. Andersson GBJ. Epidemiological features of chronic low back pain. *Lancet* 1999;354:581–585.
25. Høgelund J. Work incapacity and reintegration: A literature review. In: Bloch FS, Prins R, eds. *Who Returns to Work and Why.* London, England: Transaction Publishing; 2001:27–54.
26. Linton S. Risk factors for neck and back pain in a working population in Sweden. *Work Stress* 1990;4:41–49.
27. Nordin M, et al. Association of comorbidity and outcome in episodes of nonspecific low back pain in occupational populations. *J Occup Environ Med* 2002;44:677–684.
28. Wipf JE, Deyo RA. Low back pain. *Med Clin North Am* 1995;79:231–246.
29. Viikari-Juntura E, et al. A lifelong prospective study on the role of psychosocial factors in neck, shoulder and low back pain. *Spine* 1991;16:1056–1061.
30. Bigos SJ, et al. A prospective study of work perceptions and psychosocial factors affecting the report of back injury. *Spine* 1991;16:1–6.
31. Dehlin O, Berg S. Back symptoms and psychological perception of work. *Scand J Rehab Med* 1977;9:61–65.
32. Leino PI, Häninen V. Psychosocial factors in relation to back and limb disorders. *Scand J Work Environ Health* 1995;21:134–142.
33. Burdorf A, Sorock G. Positive and negative evidence of risk factors for back disorders. *Scand J Work Environ Health* 1997;23:243–256.
34. Riihimaki H. Low-back pain, its origin and risk indicators. *Scand J Work Environ Health* 1991;17:81–90.
35. Croft PR, Rigby AS. Socioeconomic influences on back problems in the community in Britain. *J Epidemiol Comm Health* 1994;48:166–170.
36. Heistaro S, et al. Trends of back pain in eastern Finland, 1972–1992, in relation to socioeconomic status and behavioral risk factors. *Am J Epidemiol* 1998;148:671–682.
37. Leino-Arjas P, Hanninen K, Puska P. Socioeconomic variation in back and joint pain in Finland. *Eur J Epidemiol* 1998;14:79–87.
38. Hagen KB, et al. Socioeconomic factors and disability retirement from back pain: A 1983–1993 population-based prospective study in Norway. *Spine* 2000;25:2480–2487.
39. Hoogendoorn WE, et al. Physical load during work and leisure time as risk factors for back pain. *Scand J Work Environ Health* 1999;25:387–403.
40. Hemingway H, et al. Sickness absence from back pain, psychosocial work characteristics and employment grade among office workers. *Scand J Work Environ Health* 1997;23:121–129.
41. Hoogendoorn WE, et al. Systematic review of psychosocial factors at work and in private life as risk factors for back pain. *Spine* 2000;25:2114–2125.
42. Leboeuf-Yde C, Kyvik KO, Bruun NH. Low back pain and life style: Part I. Smoking information from a population-based sample of 29424 twins. *Spine* 1998;23:2207–2214.

43. Holmstrom EB, Lindell J, Moritz U. Low back and neck/shoulder pain in construction workers: Occupational workload and psychosocial risk factors. Part 1: Relationship to low back pain. *Spine* 1992;17:663–671.

44. Miranda H, et al. Individual factors, occupational loading, and physical exercise as predictors of sciatic pain. *Spine* 2002;27:1102–1109.

45. Kelsey JL. An epidemiological study of acute herniated lumbar intervertebral discs. *Rheumatol Rehabil* 1975;14:144–159.

46. Fogelholm RR, Alho AV. Smoking and intervertebral disc degeneration. *Med Hypotheses* 2001;56:537–539.

47. Heliövaara M. Body height, obesity, and risk of herniated lumbar intervertebral disc. *Spine* 1987;12:469–472.

48. Aro S, Leino P. Overweight and musculoskeletal morbidity: A ten-year follow-up. *Int J Obesity* 1985;9:267–275.

49. Böstman OM. Body mass index and height in patients requiring surgery for lumbar intervertebral disc herniation. *Spine* 1993;18:851–854.

50. Deyo RA, Bass JE. Lifestyle and low-back pain. The influence of smoking and obesity. *Spine* 1989;14:501–506.

51. Deyo RA, Diehl AK. Lumbar spine films in primary care: Current use and effects of selective ordering criteria. *J Gen Intern Med* 1986;1:20–25.

52. Frymoyer JW, et al. Spine radiographs in patients with low-back pain. *J Bone Joint Surg* 1984;66A:1048–1055.

53. Witt I, Vestergaard A, Rosenklint A. A comparative analysis of x-ray findings of the lumbar spine in patient with and without lumbar pain. *Spine* 1984;9:298–300.

54. Bodack MP, Monteiro M. Therapeutic exercise in the treatment of patients with lumbar spinal stenosis. *Clin Orthop Rel Res* 2001;384:144–152.

55. Caspersen CJ, Powell KE, Christenson GM. Physical activity, exercise and physical fitness. *Public Health Rep* 1985;100:125–131.

56. Danielsen J, et al. Early aggressive exercise for postoperative rehabilitation after discectomy. *Spine* 2000;25:1015–1020.

57. Janeck K, Reuven B, Romano CT. Spinal stabilization exercises for the injured worker. *Occup Med* 1998;13:199–207.

58. Kendall PH, Jenkins JM. Exercises for back ache: A double blind controlled study. *Physiotherapy* 1968;54:154–157.

59. O'Sullivan PB. Lumbar segmental "instability": Clinical presentation and specific stabilizing exercise management. *Man Ther* 2000;5:2–12.

60. Kahanovitz N, et al. Normal trunk muscle strength and endurance in women and the effect of exercises and electrical stimulation: Part 2. Comparative analysis of electrical stimulation and exercise to increase trunk muscle strength and endurance. *Spine* 1987;12:112–118.

61. Nachemson A. Work for all. For those with low back pain as well. *Clin Orthop* 1982;179:77.

62. Rozenberg S, et al. Bed rest or normal activity for patients with acute low back pain: A randomized controlled trial. *Spine* 2002;27:1487–1493.

63. Bogduk N, Twomey LT. Anatomy and biomechanics of the lumbar spine. In: Bogduk N, Twomey LT, eds. *Clinical Anatomy of the Lumbar Spine and Sacrum*. Edinburgh, Scotland: Churchill Livingstone; 1997:2–53, 81–152, 171–176.

64. Tulsi RS, Hermanis GM. A study of the angle of inclination and facet curvature of superior lumbar zygapophysial facets. *Spine* 1993;18:1311–1317.

65. Abumi K, et al. Biomechanical evaluation of lumbar stability after graded facetectomies. *Spine* 1990;15:1142–1147.

66. Haegg O, Wallner A. Facet joint asymmetry and protrusion of the intervertebral disc. *Spine* 1990;15:356–359.

67. Ahmed AM, Duncan MJ, Burke DL. The effect of facet geometry on the axial torque-rotation response of lumbar motion segments. *Spine* 1990;15:391–401.

68. Davis PR. The thoraco-lumbar mortice joint. *J Anat* 1955;89:370–377.

69. Davis PR. Engineering aspects of the spine. In: Davis PR, ed. *Mechanical Aspects of the Spine*. London, England: Mechanical Engineering Publications; 1980:33–36.

70. Singer KP, Giles LGF. Manual therapy considerations at the thoracolumbar junction: An anatomical and functional perspective. *J Manipulative Physiol Ther* 1990;13:83–88.

71. White AA. Analysis of the mechanics of the thoracic spine in man: An experimental study of autopsy specimens. *Acta Orthop Scand Suppl* 1969;127:1–105.

72. Lewin T. Osteoarthritis in lumbar synovial joints. *Acta Orthop Scand Suppl* 1964;73:1–112.

73. MacIntosh J, Bogduk N. The biomechanics of the lumbar multifidus. *Clin Biomech* 1986;1:205–213.

74. Lewin T, Moffet B, Viidik A. The morphology of the lumbar synovial intervertebral joints. *Acta Morphol Neerlando Scand* 1962;4:299–319.

75. Bogduk N, Jull G. The theoretical pathology of acute locked back: A basis for manipulative therapy. *Man Med* 1985;1:78.

76. Willard FH. The muscular, ligamentous and neural structure of the low back and its relation to low back pain. In: Vleeming A, et al, eds. *Movement, Stability and Low Back Pain*. New York, NY: Churchill Livingstone; 1997:3–36.

77. Francois RJ. Ligament insertions into the human lumbar vertebral body. *Acta Anat* 1975;91:467–480.

78. Bogduk N, Tynan W, Wilson AS. The nerve supply to the human intervertebral discs. *J Anat* 1981;132:39–56.

79. White AA, Panjabi MM, eds. *Clinical Biomechanics of the Spine*. Philadelphia, Pa: Lippincott-Raven; 1990:106–108.

80. Tkaczuk H. Tensile properties of human lumbar longitudinal ligament. *Acta Orthop Scand* 1968;115:9–69.

81. Yong-Hing K, Reilly J, Kirkaldy-Willis WH. The ligamentum flavum. *Spine* 1976;1:226–234.

82. Yahia LH, et al. Ultrastructure of the human interspinous ligament and ligamentum flavum: A preliminary study. *Spine* 1990;15:262–268.

83. Panjabi MM, Goel VK, Takata K. Physiologic strains in the lumbar ligaments: An in vitro biomechanical study. *Spine* 1983;7:192–203.

84. Bogduk N, Wilson AS, Tynan W. The human lumbar dorsal rami. *J Anat* 1982;134:383–397.

85. Heylings DJA. Supraspinous and interspinous ligaments of the human spine. *J Anat* 1978;125:127–131.

86. Newman PH. Sprung back. *J Bone Joint Surg* 1952;34B:30–37.

87. Hukins DWL, et al. Comparison of structure, mechanical properties, and function of lumbar spinal ligaments. *Spine* 1990;15:787–795.

88. Gray H. *Gray's Anatomy*. Philadelphia, Pa: Lea and Febiger; 1995.

89. Kapandji IA. *The Physiology of the Joints, The Trunk and Vertebral Column*. New York, NY: Churchill Livingstone; 1991.

90. Luk KDK, Ho HC, Leong JCY. The iliolumbar ligament. A study of its anatomy, development and clinical significance. *J Bone Joint Surg* 1986;68B:197–200.

91. Chow DHK, et al. Torsional stability of the lumbosacral junction: Significance of the iliolumbar ligament. *Spine* 1989;14:611–615.

92. Kirkaldy-Willis WH. The three phases of the spectrum of degenerative disease. In: Kirkaldy-Willis WH, ed. *Managing Low Back Pain*. New York, NY: Churchill Livingstone; 1983:75–90.

93. Seitsalo S, et al. Progression of the spondylolisthesis in children and adolescents. *Spine* 1991;16:417–421.

94. Golub BS, Silverman B. Transforaminal ligaments of the lumbar spine. *J Bone Joint Surg* 1969;51A:947–956.

95. MacNab I. *Backache*. Baltimore, Md: Williams and Wilkins; 1978:98–100.

96. Bogduk N. The lumbar mamillo-accessory ligament. Its anatomical and neurosurgical significance. *Spine* 1981;6:162–167.

97. Cholewicki J, McGill S. Mechanical stability of the in vivo lumbar spine: Implications for injury and chronic low back pain. *Clin Biomech* 1996;11:1–15.

98. Hodges PW, Richardson CA. Inefficient muscular stabilization of the lumbar spine associated with low back pain. *Spine* 1996;21:2640–2650.

99. Morgan D. Concepts in functional training and postural stabilization for the low-back-injured. *Top Acute Care Trauma Rehabil* 1988;2:8–17.

100. Williams PL, et al. *Gray's Anatomy*. 37 ed. London, England: Churchill Livingstone; 1989.

101. Hides JA, Richardson CA, Jull GA. Multifidus muscle recovery is not automatic after resolution of acute, first-episode low back pain. *Spine* 1996;21:2763–2769.

101a. Meadows J, Pettman E. *Manual Therapy: NAIOMT Level II and III Course Notes*. Denver, Colo: North American Institute of Manual Therapy; 1995.

102. Goel V, et al. A combined finite element and optimization investigation of lumbar spine mechanics with and without muscles. *Spine* 1993;18:1531–1541.

103. Panjabi M, et al. Spinal stability and intersegmental muscle forces. A biomechanical model. *Spine* 1989;14:194–199.

104. Steffen R, Nolte LP, Pingel TH. Rehabilitation of the postoperative segmental lumbar instability: A biomechanical analysis of the rank of the back muscles. *Rehabilitation* 1994;33:164–170.

105. Farfan HF. *Mechanical Disorders of the Low Back*. Philadelphia, Pa: Lea and Febiger; 1973.

106. Kalimo H, et al. Lumbar muscles: Structure and function. *Ann Med* 1989;21:353–359.

107. MacIntosh J, Pearcy M, Bogduk N. The axial torque or the lumbar back muscles: Torsion strength of the back muscles. *Aust N Z J Surg* 1993;63:205–212.

108. Donisch EW, Basmajian JV. Electromyography of deep back muscles in man. *Am J Anat* 1971;133:25–36.

109. Flicker PL, et al. Lumbar muscle usage in chronic low back pain. *Spine* 1993;18:582.

110. Lee DG. Instability of the sacroiliac joint and the consequences for gait. In: Vleeming A, ed. *Movement, Stability and Low Back Pain*. Edinburgh, Scotland: Churchill Livingstone; 1997:231.

111. Schwarzer AC, Aprill CN, Bogduk N. The sacroiliac joint in chronic low back pain. *Spine* 1995;20:31–37.

112. Snijders CJ, et al. EMG recordings of abdominal and back muscles in various standing postures: Validation of a biomechanical model on sacroiliac joint stability. *J Electromyogr Kinesiol* 1998;8:205–214.

113. Shindo H. Anatomical study of the lumbar multifidus muscle and its innervation in human adults and fetuses. *J Nippon Med School* 1995;62:439–446.

114. McIntosh JE, et al. The morphology of the lumbar multifidus muscles. *Clin Biomech* 1986;1:196–204.

115. Mitchell FL, Moran PS, Pruzzo NA. *An Evaluation and Treatment Manual of Osteopathic Muscle Energy Procedures*. Manchester, Mo: Mitchell, Moran and Pruzzo; 1979.

116. Bogduk N. A reappraisal of the anatomy of the human lumbar erector spinae. *J Anat* 1980;131:525–540.

117. McIntosh JE, Bogduk N. The morphology of the lumbar erector spinae. *Spine* 1986;12:658–668.

118. Bogduk N, Mcintosh JE, Pearcy MJ. A universal model of the lumbar back muscles in the upright position. *Spine* 1992;17:897–913.

119. Bogduk N, MacIntosh J. The applied anatomy of the thoracolumbar fascia. *Spine* 1984;9:164–170.

120. Gracovetsky S, Farfan HF, Lamy C. The mechanism of the lumbar spine. *Spine* 1981;6:249–262.

121. Kendall FP, McCreary EK, Provance PG. *Muscles: Testing and Function*. Baltimore, Md: Williams and Wilkins; 1993.

122. Huijbregts PA. Lumbopelvic region: Anatomy and biomechanics. In: Wadsworth C, ed. *Current Concepts of Orthopaedic Physical Therapy—Home Study Course*. La Crosse, Wis: Orthopaedic Section, American Physical Therapy Association; 2001.

123. Lee DG. *The Pelvic Girdle: An Approach to the Examination and Treatment of the Lumbo-pelvic-hip Region*. 2nd ed. Edinburgh, Scotland: Churchill Livingstone; 1999.

124. White SG, McNair PJ. Abdominal and erector spinae muscle activity during gait: The use of cluster analysis to identify patterns of activity. *Clin Biomech* 2002;17:177–184.

125. O'Sullivan PB, et al. The effect of different standing and sitting postures on trunk muscle activity in a pain-free population. *Spine* 2002;27:1238–1244.

126. Ng JK, et al. EMG activity of trunk muscles and torque output during isometric axial rotation exertion: A comparison between back pain patients and matched controls. *Spine* 2002;27:637–646.

127. Bogduk N, Pearcy M, Hadfield G. Anatomy and biomechanics of psoas major. *Clin Biomech* 1992;7:109–119.

128. Santaguida PL, McGill SM. The psoas major muscle: A three-dimensional geometric study. *J Biomech* 1995;28:339–345.

129. Porterfield JA, DeRosa C. *Mechanical Low Back Pain*. 2nd ed. Philadelphia, Pa: Saunders; 1998.

130. McCullough JA, Waddell G. Variation of the lumbosacral myotomes with bony segmental anomalies. *J Bone Joint Surg* 1980;62B:475–480.

131. Bogduk N. The innervation of the lumbar spine. *Spine* 1983;8:286–293.

132. Hovelacque A. *Anatomie des Nerf Craniens et Rachdiens et du Systeme Grande Sympathetique*. Paris, France: Doin; 1927.

133. Mooney V, Robertson J. The facet syndrome. *Clin Orthop* 1976;115:149–156.

134. Lee CK, Rauschning W, Glenn W. Lateral lumbar spinal canal stenosis: Classification, pathologic anatomy and surgical decompression. *Spine* 1988;13:313–320.

135. Fritz JM, Erhard R, Vignovic M. A nonsurgical treatment approach for patients with lumbar spinal stenosis. *Spine* 1997;77:962–973.

136. Kulak RF, et al. Biomechanical characteristics of vertebral motion segments and intervertebral discs. *Orthop Clin North Am* 1975;6:121–133.

137. White AA, Punjabi MM. *Clinical Biomechanics of the Spine*. 2nd ed. Philadelphia, Pa: JB Lippincott; 1990.

138. Prescher A. Anatomy and pathology of the aging spine. *Eur J Radiol* 1998;27:181–195.

139. Jull GA, Janda V. Muscle and motor control in low back pain. In: Towmey LT, Taylor JR, eds. *Physical Therapy of the Low Back: Clinics in Physical Therapy.* New York, NY: Churchill Livingstone; 1987:253–278.

140. Pearcy M, Portek I, Shepherd J. The effect of low back pain on lumbar spinal movements measured by three-dimensional X-ray analysis. *Spine* 1985;10:150–153.

141. Dunlop RB, Adams MA, Hutton WC. Disc space narrowing and the lumbar facet joints. *J Bone Joint Surg* 1984;66B:706–710.

142. Adams MA, Hutton WC. The resistance to flexion of the lumbar intervertebral joint. *Spine* 1980;5:245–253.

143. McGill SM, Norman RW. Low back biomechanics in industry: The prevention of injury through safer lifting. In: Grabiner MD, ed. *Current Issues in Biomechanics.* Champaign, Ill: Human Kinetics; 1993:69–120.

144. Aspden RM. The spine as an arch: A new mathematical model. *Spine* 1989;14:266–274.

145. El-Bohy AA, Yang KH, King AI. Experimental verification of load transmission by direct measurement of facet lamina contact pressure. *J Biomech* 1989;22:931–941.

146. Grieve G. Common patterns of clinical presentation. In: Grieve GP, ed. *Common Vertebral Joint Problems.* London, England: Churchill Livingstone; 1988:283–302.

147. Jungham H. Spondylolisthesen ohne Spalt im Zwischengelenkstuck (pseudospondylolisthesen). *Arch Orthop Unfall Chir* 1930;29:118–123.

148. Richardson CA, et al. *Therapeutic Exercise for Spinal Segmental Stabilization in Low Back Pain.* London, England: Churchill Livingstone; 1999.

149. Richardson J, Toppenberg R, Jull G. An initial evaluation of eight abdominal exercises for their ability to provide stabilisation for the lumbar spine. *Aust J Physiother* 1990;36:6–11.

150. Cossette JW, et al. The instantaneous center of rotation of the third intervertebral joint. *J Biomech* 1971;4:149–153.

151. Ueno K, Liu YK. A three-dimensional nonlinear finite element model of lumbar intervertebral joint in torsion. *J Biomech Eng* 1987;109:200–209.

152. Farfan HF, et al. The effects of torsion on the lumbar intervertebral joints: The role of torsion in the production of disc degeneration. *J Bone Joint Surg* 1970;52A:468–497.

153. McFadden KD, Taylor JR. Axial rotation in the lumbar spine and gapping of the zygapophysial joints. *Spine* 1990;15:295–299.

154. Pearcy M, Portek I, Shepherd J. Three-dimensional analysis of normal movement in the lumbar spine. *Spine* 1984;9:294–297.

155. Haher TR, et al. The role of the lumbar facets joints in spinal stability. *Spine* 1994;19:2667–2671.

156. Nachemson A. Lumbar intradiscal pressure. In: Jayson MIV, ed. *The Lumbar Spine and Back Pain.* Edinburgh, Scotland: Churchill Livingstone; 1987:191–203.

157. McGill S. Loads on the lumbar spine and associated tissues. In: Goel VK, Weinstein JN, eds. *Biomechanics of the Spine: Clinical and Surgical Perspective.* Boca Raton, Fla: CRC Press; 1990:65–95.

158. Schultz A. Loads on the lumbar spine. In: Jayson MIV, ed. *The Lumbar Spine and Back Pain.* Edinburgh, Scotland: Churchill Livingstone; 1987:204–214.

159. Brinckmann P, Biggemann M, Hilweg D. Prediction of the compressive strength of human lumbar vertebrae. *Clin Biomech* 1989;14:606–610.

160. Fyhrie DP, Schaffler MB. How human vertebral bone breaks. Paper presented at: NACOBII Congress; 1992; Chicago, Ill.

161. McGill SM. The biomechanics of low back injury: Implications on current practice in industry and the clinic. *J Biomech* 1997;30:465–475.

162. Crisco JJ, et al. Euler stability of the human ligamentous spine. Part II: Experiment. *Clin Biomech* 1992;7:27–32.

163. Holdsworth F. Fractures, dislocations, and fracture-dislocations of the spine. *J Bone Joint Surg* 1970;52A:1534–1551.

164. McGill SM, Axler CT. Changes in spine height throughout 32 hours of bedrest. *Arch Phys Med Rehab* 1996;77:1071–1073.

165. Kramer J. Pressure dependent fluid shifts in the intervertebral disc. *Orthop Clin North Am* 1977;8:211–216.

166. Adams MA, Hutton WC. The effect of posture on the fluid content of lumbar intervertebral discs. *Spine* 1983;8:665–671.

167. McGill SM. Low back exercises: Evidence for improving exercise regimes. *Phys Ther* 1998;78:754–765.

168. Adams MA, Dolan P. Recent advances in lumbar spinal mechanics and their clinical significance. *Clin Biomech* 1995;10:3–19.

169. Panjabi MM. The stabilizing system of the spine. Part 1. Function, dysfunction adaption and enhancement. *J Spinal Disord* 1992;5:383–389.

170. Tencer AF, Ahmed AM. The role of secondary variables in the measurement of the mechanical properties of the lumbar intervertebral joint. *J Biomech Eng* 1981;103:129–137.

171. Wilder DG, et al. The balance point of the intervertebral motion segment: An experimental study. *Bull Hosp Jt Dis* 1989;49:155–169.

172. Mimura M, et al. Disc degeneration affects the multidirectional flexibility of the lumbar spine. *Spine* 1994;19:1371–1380.

173. Kaigle A, Holm S, Hansson T. Experimental instability in the lumbar spine. *Spine* 1995;20:421–430.

174. Wilke H, et al. Stability of the lumbar spine with different muscle groups: A biomechanical in vitro study. *Spine* 1995;20:192–198.

175. Nachemson A, Morris JM. In vivo measurements of intradiscal pressure. *J Bone Joint Surg* 1964;46:1077.

176. Nachemson A. Disc pressure measurements. *Spine* 1981;6:93–97.

177. Gardner-Morse M, Stokes I, Laible J. Role of muscles in lumbar spine stability in maximum extension efforts. *J Orthop Res* 1995;13:802–808.

178. O'Sullivan P, Twomey L, Allison G. Evaluation of specific stabilizing exercise in the treatment of chronic low back pain with radiologic diagnosis of spondylolysis or spondylolisthesis. *Spine* 1997;22:2959–2967.

179. Bowman SM, et al. Compressive creep behavior of bovine trabecular bone. *J Biomech* 1994;27:301–310.

180. Brinckmann P, Biggemann M, Hilweg D. Fatigue fracture of human lumbar vertebrae. *Clin Biomech* 1988;3(suppl):S1–23.

181. Mannion AF, et al. The use of surface EMG power spectral analysis in the evaluation of back muscle function. *J Rehabil Res Dev* 1997;34:427–439.

182. Roy SH, De Luca CJ, Casavant DA. Lumbar muscle fatigue and chronic lower back pain. *Spine* 1989;14:992–1001.

183. Best TM, et al. Characterization of the passive responses of live skeletal muscle using the quasi-linear theory of viscoelasticity. *J Biomech* 1994;27:413–419.

184. Keller TS, Spengler DM, Hansson TH. Mechanical behavior of the human lumbar spine, I: Creep analysis during static compressive loading. *J Orthop Res* 1987;5:467–478.

185. Cresswell A, Grundstrom H, Thorstensson A. Observations on intra-abdominal pressure and patterns of abdominal intra-muscular activity in man. *Acta Physiol Scand* 1992;144:409–418.

186. Cresswell A, Oddsson L, Thorstensson A. The influence of sudden perturbations on trunk muscle activity and intra-abdominal pressure while standing. *Exp Brain Res* 1994;98:336–341.

187. Hodges PW, et al. In vivo measurement of the effect of intra-abdominal pressure on the human spine. *J Biomech* 2001;34:347–353.

188. Marras WS, Mirka GA. Intra-abdominal pressure during trunk extension motions. *Clin Biomech* 1996;11:267.

189. McGill SM, Norman RW. Reassessment of the role of intra-abdominal pressure in spinal compression. *Ergonomics* 1987;30:1565–1588.

190. Bergmark A. Stability of the lumbar spine. A study in mechanical engineering. *Acta Orthop Scand* 1989;230:20–24.

191. Stokes IAF, Gardner-Morse M. Lumbar spine maximum efforts and muscle recruitment patterns predicted by a model with multijoint muscles and joints with stiffness. *J Biomech* 1994;27:1101–1104.

192. Comerford MJ, Mottram SL. Functional stability re-training: Principles and strategies for managing mechanical dysfunction. *Man Ther* 2001;6:3–14.

193. Comerford MJ, Mottram SL. Movement and stability dysfunction-contemporary developments. *Man Ther* 2001;6:15–26.

194. Aspden RM. Review of the functional anatomy of the spinal ligaments and the lumbar erector spinae muscles. *Clin Anat* 1992;5:372–387.

195. Hodges PW, et al. Contraction of the human diaphragm during postural adjustments. *J Physiol* 1997;505:239–248.

196. Hodges P, Richardson C. Contraction of transversus abdominis invariably precedes upper limb movement. *Exp Brain Res* 1997;114:362–370.

197. McGill S. Kinetic potential of the trunk musculature about three orthogonal orthopaedic axes in extreme postures. *Spine* 1991;16:809–815.

198. Oddsson L, Thorstensson A. Task specificity in the control of intrinsic trunk muscles in man. *Acta Physiol Scand* 1990;139:123–131.

199. Hodges PW, Richardson CA. Altered trunk muscle recruitment in people with low back pain: A motor control evaluation of transversus abdominis. *Arch Phys Med Rehab* 1999;80:1005–1012.

200. Hodges P, Richardson C. Inefficient muscular stabilisation of the lumbar spine associated with low back pain: A motor control evaluation of transversus abdominis. *Spine* 1996;21:2540–2650.

201. O'Sullivan P, Twomey L, Allison G. Altered patterns of abdominal muscle activation in chronic back pain patients. *Aust J Physiother* 1997;43:91–98.

202. Stanford ME. Effectiveness of specific lumbar stabilization exercises: A single case study. *J Man Manipulative Ther* 2002;10:40–46.

203. Bierdermann HJ, et al. Power spectrum analysis of electromyographic activity. *Spine* 1991;16:1179–1184.

204. Lindgren K, et al. Exercise therapy effects on functional radiographic findings and segmental electromyographic activity in lumbar spine stability. *Arch Phys Med Rehabil* 1993;74:933–939.

205. Hodges P, Richardson C, Jull G. Evaluation of the relationship between laboratory and clinical tests of transversus abdominis function. *Physiother Res Int* 1996;1:30–40.

206. Richardson C, Jull G. Muscle control—Pain control. What exercises would you prescribe? *Man Ther* 1995;1:2–10.

207. Edgerton V, et al. Theoretical basis for patterning EMG amplitudes to assess muscle dysfunction. *Med Sci Sports Exerc* 1996;28:744–751.

208. Richardson CA, et al. The relation between the transversus abdominis muscles, sacroiliac joint mechanics, and low back pain. *Spine* 2002;27:399–405.

209. Deyo RA, Rainville J, Kent DL. What can the history and physical examination tell us about low back pain? *JAMA* 1992;268:760–765.

210. Nachemson AL. The lumbar spine: An orthopedic challenge. *Spine* 1976;1:59–71.

211. Jermyn RT. A nonsurgical approach to low back pain. *J Am Osteopath Assoc* 2001;101(suppl):S6–S11.

212. Friberg S. Studies on spondylolisthesis. *Acta Chir Orthop* 1939;60:1.

213. Ombregt L, et al, eds. *A System of Orthopaedic Medicine.* London, England: Saunders; 1995.

214. Jolles BM, Porchet F, Theumann N. Surgical treatment of lumbar spinal stenosis. Five-year follow-up. *J Bone Joint Surg* 2001;83A:949–953.

215. Bressler HB, et al. The prevalence of low back pain in the elderly. A systematic review of the literature. *Spine* 1999;24:1813–1819.

216. Frymoyer JW. Lumbar disk disease: Epidemiology. *Instr Course Lect* 1992;41:217–223.

217. Berguist-Ullman M, Larsson U. Acute low back pain in industry. A controlled prospective study with specific reference to therapy and vocational factors. *Acta Orthop Scand Suppl* 1977;170:1–117.

218. Hoogendoorn WE, et al. High physical work load and low job satisfaction increase the risk of sickness absence due to low back pain: results of a prospective cohort study. *Occup Envir Med* 2002;59:323–328.

219. Andersson GBJ. Epidemiologic aspects of low back pain in industry. *Spine* 1981;6:53–60.

220. Kelsey JL, White AA. Epidemiology and impact of low back pain. *Spine* 1980;5:133–142.

221. Ombregt L, et al. Clinical examination of the lumbar spine. In: Ombregt L, et al, eds. *A System of Orthopaedic Medicine.* London, England: Saunders; 1995:577–611.

222. Kuslich SD, Ulstrom CL, Michael CJ. The tissue origin of low back pain and sciatica. *Orthop Clin North Am* 1991;22:181–187.

223. Oesch P. Die Rolle der Zygapophysialgelenke in der Aetiologie lumbaler Rueckenschmerzen mit und ohne Ausstrahlungen. *Man Med* 1995;33:107–114.

224. Yukawa Y, et al. Groin pain associated with lower lumbar disc herniation. *Spine* 1997;22:1736–1739.

225. Korr IM. Neurochemical and neurotrophic consequences of nerve deformation. In: Glasgow EF, et al, eds. *Aspects of Manipulative Therapy.* New York, NY: Churchill Livingstone; 1985.

226. Lewit K. The contribution of clinical observation to neurobiological mechanisms in manipulative therapy. In: Korr IM, ed. *The Neurobiological Mechanisms in Manipulative Therapy.* New York, NY: Plenum Press; 1977.

227. Hall H. A simple approach to back pain management. *Patient Care* 1992;15:77–91.

228. McKenzie RA. *The Lumbar Spine: Mechanical Diagnosis and Therapy.* Waikanae, New Zealand: Spinal Publications New Zealand; 1981.

229. Jull GA. Examination of the lumbar spine. In: Grieve GP, ed. *Modern Manual Therapy of the Vertebral Column.* Edinburgh, Scotland: Churchill Livingstone; 1986:553.

230. Donelson R, Silva G, Murphy K. Centralization phenomenon: Its usefulness in evaluating and treating referred pain. *Spine* 1990;15:211–213.

231. Donelson R, et al. A prospective study of centralization in lumbar referred pain. *Spine* 1997;22:1115–1122.
232. Donelson R. The McKenzie approach to evaluating and treating low back pain. *Orthop Rev* 1990;19:681–686.
233. White AA. Injection technique for the diagnosis and treatment of low back pain. *Orthop Clin North Am* 1983;14:553–567.
234. Matsui H, et al. Familial predisposition, clustering for juvenile lumbar disc herniation. *Spine* 1992;17:1323–1328.
235. Andersson GBJ, Deyo RA. History and physical examination in patients with herniated lumbar discs. *Spine* 1996;21:10S–18S.
236. Drezner JA, Harmon KG. Chronic appendicitis presenting as low back pain in a recreational athlete. *Clin J Sports Med* 2002;12:184–186.
237. Deyo RA, Weinstein JN. Low back pain. *N Engl J Med* 2001;344:363–370.
238. Biering-Sorenson F. Low back trouble in a general population of 30-, 40-, 50- and 60-year-old men and women: Study design, representiveness and basic results. *Dan Med Bull* 1982;29:289–299.
239. Sahrmann SA. *Diagnosis and Treatment of Movement Impairment Syndromes*. St Louis, Mo: Mosby; 2001.
240. Hoppenfeld S. *Physical Examination of the Spine and Extremities*. Norwalk, Conn: Appleton-Century-Crofts; 1976.
241. Wallace L. *Lower Quarter Pain: Mechanical Evaluation and Treatment*. Cleveland, Ohio: Western Reserve Publishers; 1984.
242. Miller NH. Genetics of familial idiopathic scoliosis. *Clin Orthop Rel Res* 2002;401:60–64.
243. Kane WJ. Scoliosis prevalence: A call for a statement of terms. *Clin Orthop* 1977;126:43–46.
244. Armstrong GW, et al. Nonstandard vertebral rotation in scoliosis screening patients: Its prevalence and relation to the clinical deformity. *Spine* 1982;7:50–54.
245. Gross RH. Leg length discrepancy: How much is too much? *Orthopedics* 1978;1:307–310.
246. Finneson BE, ed. *Low Back Pain*. 2nd ed. Philadelphia, Pa: JB Lippincott; 1973:290–303.
247. Matsui H, et al. Significance of sciatic scoliotic list in operated patients with lumbar disc herniation. *Spine* 1998;23:338–342.
248. Bianco AJ. Low back pain and sciatica. Diagnosis and indications for treatment. *J Bone Joint Surg* 1968;50A:170.
249. Maigne R. *Diagnosis and Treatment of Pain of Vertebral Origin*. Baltimore, Md: Williams and Wilkins; 1996.
250. Beals RK. Anomalies associated with vertebral malformations. *Spine* 1993;18:1329.
251. Matson DD, et al. Diastematomyelia (congenital clefts of the spinal cord). *Pediatrics* 1950;6:98–112.
252. Opila KA, et al. Postural alignment in barefoot and high heeled stance. *Spine* 1988;13:542–547.
253. Korr IM. Proprioceptors and somatic dysfunction. *J Am Osteopath Assoc* 1975;74:638–650.
254. Winkel D, Matthijs O, Phelps V. *Diagnosis and Treatment of the Spine*. Gaithersburg, Md: Aspen; 1997.
255. Dvorak J, Dvorak V. Zones of irritation. In: Gilliar WG, Greenman PE, eds. *Manual Medicine: Diagnostic*. New York, NY: Thieme; 1990:219–230.
256. Nachemson A, Bigos SJ. The low back. In: Cruess RL, Rennie WRJ, eds. *Adult Orthopaedics*. New York, NY: Churchill Livingstone; 1984:843–938.
257. Bourdillon JF. *Spinal Manipulation*. 3rd ed. London, England: Heinemann; 1982.
258. Fukui S, et al. Distribution of referred pain from the lumbar zygapophysial joints and dorsal rami. *Clin J Pain* 1997;13:303–307.
259. Robert CM, Thomas H, Tery T. Facet joint injection and facet nerve block: A randomized comparison in 86 patients with chronic low back pain. *Pain* 1992;49:325–328.
260. Greenman PE. *Principles of Manual Medicine*. 2nd ed. Baltimore, Md: Williams and Wilkins; 1996.
261. Allbrook D. Movements of the lumbar spinal column. *J Bone Joint Surg* 1957;39B:339–345.
262. Ng JK, et al. Range of motion and lordosis of the lumbar spine: Reliability of measurement and normative values. *Spine* 2001;26:53–60.
263. Pearcy M, Tibrewal SB. Axial rotation and lateral bending in the normal lumbar spine measured by three-dimensional radiography. *Spine* 1984;9:582.
264. Troup JDG, Hood CA, Chapman AE. Measurements of the sagittal mobility of the lumbar spine and hips. *Ann Phys Med* 1967;9:308–321.
265. Cocchiarella L, Andersson GBJ, eds. *American Medical Association, Guides to the Evaluation of Permanent Impairment*. 5th ed. Chicago, Ill: AMA; 2001.
266. Cyriax J. *Textbook of Orthopaedic Medicine, Diagnosis of Soft Tissue Lesions*. 8th ed. London, England: Bailliere Tindall; 1982.
267. Portek I, et al. Correlation between radiographic and clinical measurement of lumbar spine movement. *Br J Rheumatol* 1983;22:197–205.
268. Michel A, Kohlmann T, Raspe H. The association between clinical findings and self-reported severity in back pain. *Spine* 1997;22:296–304.
269. Grieve GP. Lumbar instability. *Physiotherapy* 1982;68:2.
270. Helliwell P, Moll J, Wright V. Measurement of spinal movement and function. In : Jayson MIV, ed. *The Lumbar Spine and Back Pain*. Edinburgh, Scotland: Churchill Livingstone; 1992:173–205.
271. Macrae IF, Wright V. Measurement of back movement. *Ann Rheum Dis* 1969;28:584–589.
272. Miller SA, et al. Reliability problems associated with the modified Schöber technique for true lumbar flexion measurement. *Spine* 1992;17:345–348.
273. Burdett RG, Brown KE, Fall MP. Reliability and validity of four instruments for measuring lumbar spine and pelvic positions. *Phys Ther* 1986;66:677–684.
274. Adams MA, et al. An electronic inclinometer technique for measuring lumbar curvature. *Clin Biomech* 1986;1:130–134.
275. Mayer TG, et al. Use of noninvasive techniques for quantification of spinal range of motion in normal subjects and chronic low back dysfunction patients. *Spine* 1984;9:588–595.
276. Meadows J. *Orthopedic Differential Diagnosis in Physical Therapy*. New York, NY: McGraw-Hill; 1999.
277. Edwards BC. Combined movements of the lumbar spine: Examination and clinical significance. *Aust J Physiother* 1979;25:4.
278. Edwards BC. Combined movements of the lumbar spine: Examination and treatment. In: Palastanga N, Boyling JD, eds. *Grieve's Modern Manual Therapy of the Vertebral Column*. Edinburgh, Scotland: Churchill Livingstone; 1994:561–566.
279. Sahrmann SA. Movement impairment syndromes of the lumbar spine. In: Sahrmann SA, ed. *Diagnosis and Treatment of Movement Impairment Syndromes*. St Louis, Mo: Mosby; 2001:51–119.
280. Janda V. *Muscle Function Testing*. London, England: Butterworth; 1983:163–167.

281. Saal JA. Natural history and nonoperative treatment of lumbar disc herniation. *Spine* 1996;21:2S–9S.

282. Seichi A, et al. Intraoperative radiation therapy for metastatic spinal tumors. *Spine* 1999;24:470–473; discussion 474–475.

283. Gracovetsky S, Farfan HF. The optimum spine. *Spine* 1986;11:543.

284. Gracovetsky S, Farfan HF, Helleur C. The abdominal mechanism. *Spine* 1985;10:317–324.

285. Aaron G. The use of stabilization training in the rehabilitation of the athlete. In: *Sports Physical Therapy Home Study Course.* Alexandria, Va: American Physical Therapy Association, Sports Physical Therapy Section; 1996.

286. Clark MA. *Integrated Training for the New Millenium.* Thousand Oaks, Calif: National Academy of Sports Medicine; 2001.

287. Vasilyeva LF, Lewit K. Diagnosis of muscular dysfunction by inspection. In: Liebenson C, ed. *Rehabilitation of the Spine: A Practitioner's Manual.* Baltimore, Md: Lippincott Williams and Wilkins; 1996:113–142.

288. Jull G, et al. *Towards the Validation of a Clinical Test for the Deep Abdominal Muscles in Back Pain Patients.* Melbourne, Australia: Manipulative Physiotherapists Association of Australia; 1995.

289. Magee DJ. Lumbar spine. In: Magee DJ, ed. *Orthopedic Physical Assessment.* Philadelphia, Pa: Saunders; 2002:467–566.

290. Moreland J, et al. Interrater reliability of six tests of trunk muscle function and endurance. *J Orthop Sports Phys Ther* 1997;26:200–208.

291. Reese NB. *Muscle and Sensory Testing.* Philadelphia, Pa: Saunders; 1999.

292. McGill SM, Childs A, Liebenson C. Endurance times for low back stabilization exercises: Clinical targets for testing and training from a normal database. *Arch Phys Med Rehabil* 1999;80:941–944.

293. Ashmen KJ, Swanik CB, Lephart SM. Strength and flexibility characteristics of athletes with chronic low back pain. *J Sport Rehabil* 1996;5:372–387.

294. Clarkson HM. *Musculoskeletal Assessment.* 2nd ed. Philadelphia, Pa: Lippincott Williams and Wilkins; 2000.

295. Youdas JW, et al. Lumbar lordosis and pelvic inclination in adults with chronic low back pain. *Phys Ther* 2000;80:261–275.

296. Zannotti CM, et al. Kinematics of the double-leg-lowering test for abdominal muscle strength. *J Orthop Sports Phys Ther* 2002;32:432–436.

297. Hyman J, Liebenson C. Spinal stabilization exercise program. In: Liebenson C, ed. *Rehabilitation of the Spine: A Practitioner's Manual.* Baltimore, Md: Lippincott Williams and Wilkins; 1996:293–317.

298. Fryette HH. *Principles of Osteopathic Technique.* Carmel, Ca: Academy of Osteopathy; 1980.

299. Hartman SL. *Handbook of Osteopathic Technique.* 2nd ed. London, England: Unwin Hyman, Academic Division; 1990:135–143.

300. Stoddard A. *Manual of Osteopathic Practice.* New York, NY: Harper and Row; 1969.

301. Meadows JTS. The principles of the Canadian approach to the lumbar dysfunction patient. In: *Management of Lumbar Spine Dysfunction—Independent Home Study Course.* La Crosse, Wis: American Physical Therapy Association, Orthopaedic Section; 1999.

302. Lee DG, Walsh MC. *A Workbook of Manual Therapy Techniques for the Vertebral Column and Pelvic Girdle.* 2nd ed. Vancouver, Canada: Nascent; 1996.

303. Maher C, Latimer J, Adams R. An investigation of the reliability and validity of posteroanterior spinal stiffness judgments made using a reference-based protocol. *Phys Ther* 1998;78:829–837.

304. Peterson CK, Bolton JE, Wood AR. A cross-sectional study correlating lumbar spine degeneration with disability and pain. *Spine* 2000;25:218–223.

305. Millard RW, Jones RH. Construct validity of practical questionnaires for assessing disability of low-back pain. *Spine* 1991;16:835–838.

306. Fairbank J, et al. The Oswestry low back pain questionnaire. *Physiotherapy* 1980;66:271–273.

307. Hudson-Cook N, Tomes-Nicholson K, Breen A. A revised Oswestry disability questionnaire. In Roland M, Jenner J, eds. *Back Pain: New Approaches to Rehabilitation and Education.* New York, NY: Manchester University Press; 1989:187–204.

308. Fairbank J. Revised Oswestry disability questionnaire. *Spine* 2000;25:2552.

309. Feise RJ, Michael Menke J. Functional rating index: A new valid and reliable instrument to measure the magnitude of clinical change in spinal conditions. *Spine* 2001;26:78–86; discussion 87.

310. Salen BO, et al. The disability rating index: An instrument for the assessment of disability in clinical settings. *J Clin Epidemiol* 1994;47:1423–1434.

311. Roland M, Morris R. A study of the natural history of back pain, part I: The development of a reliable and sensitive measure of disability of low back pain. *Spine* 1986;8:141–144.

312. Roland M, Fairbank J. The Roland-Morris Disability Questionnaire and the Oswestry Disability Questionnaire. *Spine* 2000;25:3115–3124.

313. Ren XS. Are patients capable of attributing functional impairments to specific diseases? *Am J Public Health* 1998;88:837–838.

314. Fahrni WH. Observations on straight leg raising with special reference to nerve root adhesions. *Can J Surg* 1966;9:44–48.

315. Kirkaldy-Willis WH. *Managing Low Back Pain.* 2nd ed. New York, NY: Churchill Livingstone; 1988.

316. Potter NA, Rothstein JM. Intertester reliability for selected clinical tests of the sacroiliac joint. *Phys Ther* 1985;65:1671.

317. Vleeming A. The function of the long dorsal sacroiliac ligament: Its implication for understanding low back pain. *Spine* 1996;21:556.

318. Meadows J, Pettman E, Fowler C. Manual therapy. In: *NAIOMT Level II and III Course Notes.* Denver, Colo: North American Institute of Manual Therapy; 1995.

319. Dutton M. *Manual Therapy of the Spine: An Integrated Approach.* New York, NY: McGraw-Hill; 2002.

320. Maitland G. *Vertebral Manipulation.* Sydney, Australia: Butterworth; 1986.

321. Binkley J, Stratford PW, Gill C. Interrater reliability of lumbar accessory motion mobility testing. *Phys Ther Rev* 1995;75:786–792; discussion 793–795.

322. Bigos S, et al. *Acute Low Back Problems in Adults.* Clinical Practice Guideline No. 14. Rockville, Md: Agency for Health Care Policy and Research; 1994.

323. Boden SD, et al. Abnormal magnetic resonance scan of the lumbar spine in asymptomatic subjects: A prospective investigation. *J Bone Joint Surg* 1990;72A:403–408.

324. Weisel SE, et al. A study of computer-assisted tomography, In: The incidence of positive CAT scans in an asymptomatic group of patients. *Spine* 1984;9:549–551.

325. Deyo RA. Diagnostic evaluation of LBP: Reaching a specific diagnosis is often impossible. *Arch Intern Med* 2002;162:1444–1447; discussion 1447–1448.

326. van Tulder MW, Koes BW, Bouter LM. Conservative treatment of acute and chronic nonspecific low back pain: A systematic review of randomized controlled trials of the most common interventions. *Spine* 1997;22:2128–2156.

327. Manniche C, et al. Clinical trial of intensive muscle training for chronic low back pain. *Lancet* 1988;2:1473–1476.

328. Frost H, et al. A fitness programme for patients with chronic low back pain: 2-year follow-up of a randomised controlled trial. *Pain* 1998;75:273–279.

329. Lahad A, et al. The effectiveness of four interventions for the prevention of low back pain. *JAMA* 1994;272:1286–1291.

329a. Deyo RA, Walsh NE, Martin DC, et al. A controlled trial of transcutaneous electrical nerve stimulation (TENS) and exercise for chronic low back pain. *N Engl J Med.* 1990;322:1627–1634.

329b. Bronfort G, Goldsmith CH, Nelson CF, Boline PD, Anderson AV. Trunk exercise combined with spinal manipulative or NSAID therapy for chronic low back pain: A randomized, observer-blinded clinical trial. *J Man Physiol Ther* 1996;19:570–582.

329c. Handa N, Yamamoto H, Tani T, et al. The effect of trunk muscle exercises in patient over 40 years of age with chronic low back pain. *J Orthop Sci.* 2000;5:210–216.

330. Williams PC. *Low Back and Neck Pain-Causes and Conservative Treatment.* Springfield, Ill: Charles C Thomas; 1974.

331. Williams PC. *The Lumbosacral Spine.* New York, NY: McGraw-Hill; 1965.

332. McKenzie RA. *The Cervical and Thoracic Spine: Mechanical Diagnosis and Therapy.* Waikanae, New Zealand: Spinal Publications New Zealand; 1990.

333. Sweeney TB, et al. Cervicothoracic muscular stabilization techniques. In: Saal JA, ed. *Physical Medicine and Rehabilitation, State of the Art Reviews: Neck and Back Pain.* Philadelphia, Pa: Hanley and Belfus; 1990:335–359.

333a. Hubley-Kozey CL, McCulloch TA, McFarland DH. Chronic low back pain: A critical review of specific therapeutic exercise protocols on musculoskeletal and neuromuscular parameters. *J Man Manip Ther* 2003;11:78–87.

334. Shah JS, Hampson WGJ, Jayson MIV. The distribution of surface strain in the cadaveric lumbar spine. *J Bone Joint Surg* 1978;60B:246–251.

335. Gill K, et al. The effect of repeated extensions on the discographic dye patterns in cadaveric lumbar motion segments. *Clin Biomech* 1987;2:205–210.

336. Krag MH, et al. Internal displacement distribution from in vitro loading of human thoracic and lumbar spinal motion segments: Experimental results and theoretical predictions. *Spine* 1987;12:1001–1007.

337. Schnebel BE, et al. A digitizing technique for the study of movement of intradiscal dye in response to flexion and extension of the lumbar spine. *Spine* 1988;13:309–312.

338. Beattie P, et al. Effect of lordosis on the position of the nucleus pulposus in supine subjects. *Spine* 1994;19:2096–2102.

339. Fennell AJ, Jones AP, Hukins DWL. Migration of the nucleus pulposus within the intervertebral disc during flexion and extension of the spine. *Spine* 1996;21:2753–2757.

340. Schnebel BE, Watkins RG, Dillin W. The role of spinal flexion and extension in changing nerve root compression in disc herniations. *Spine* 1989;14:835–837.

341. Riddle DL, Rothstein JM. Intertester reliability of McKenzie's classifications of the syndrome types present in patients with low back pain. *Spine* 1993;18:1333–1344.

342. Cherkin DC, et al. A comparison of physical therapy, chiropractic manipulation and provision of an educational booklet for the treatment of patients with low back pain. *N Engl J Med* 1998;339:1021–1029.

343. Ponte DF, Jensen GJ, Kent BE. A preliminary report on the use of the McKenzie protocol versus Williams protocol in the treatment of low back pain. *J Orthop Sports Phys Ther* 1984; 6:130–139.

344. Nwuga G, Nwuga V. Relative therapeutic efficacy of the Williams and McKenzie protocols in back pain management. *Physiother Pract* 1985;2:99–105.

345. Stankovic R, Johnell O. Conservative treatment on acute low back pain: A 5 year follow-up study of two methods of treatment. *Spine* 1995;20:469–472.

346. Stankovic R, Johnell O. Conservative management of acute low back pain. A prospective randomized trial: McKenzie method of treatment versus patient education in "mini back school." *Spine* 1990;15:120–123.

346a. Petersen T, Kryger P, Ekdahl C, Olsen S, Jacobsen S. The effect of McKenzie therapy as compared with that of intensive strengthening training for the treatment of patients with subacute or chronic low back pain: A randomized controlled trial. *Spine* 2002;27:1702–1709.

347. Cook G, Voight ML. Essentials of functional exercise: A four-step clinical model for therapeutic exercise prescription. In: Prentice WE, Voight ML, eds. *Techniques in Musculoskeletal Rehabilitation.* New York, NY: McGraw-Hill; 2001:387–407.

348. Burton AK, Waddell G. Clinical guidelines in the management of low back pain. *Bailleres Clin Rheumatol* 1998;12:17–35.

349. Deyo RA, Diehl AK, Rosenthal M. How many days of bed rest for acute low back pain? A randomized clinical trial. *N Engl J Med* 1986;315:1064–1070.

350. Malmivaara A, et al. The treatment of acute low back pain: Bed rest, exercises, or ordinary activity? *N Engl J Med* 1995; 332:351–355.

351. Abenhaim L, et al. The role of activity in the therapeutic management of back pain. Report of the International Paris Task Force on back pain. *Spine* 2000;25(suppl 4S):1S–33S.

352. Callaghan JP, Patla AE, McGill SM. Low back three-dimensional joint forces, kinematics, and kinetics during walking. *Clin Biomech* 1999;14:203–216.

353. Shumway-Cook A, Woollacott M. *Motor Control—Theory and Practical Applications.* Baltimore, Md: Williams and Wilkins; 1995.

354. Strohl K, et al. Regional differences in abdominal muscle activity during various manoeuvres in humans. *J Appl Physiol* 1981;51:1471–1476.

355. Hagins M, et al. Effects of practice on the ability to perform lumbar stabilization exercises. *J Orthop Sports Phys Ther* 1999;29:546–555.

356. Edelman B. Conservative treatment considered best course for spondylolisthesis. *Orthop Today* 1989;9:6–8.

357. Saal JA. Rehabilitation of sports related lumbar spine injuries. In: Saal JA, ed. *Physical Medicine and Rehabilitation: State of the Art Reviews.* Philadelphia, Pa: Hanley and Belfus; 1987:613–638.

358. White AH. Conservative care of low back pain. In: Genant H, ed. *Spine Update 1987.* San Francisco, Calif: University of California San Francisco Press; 1987:283–285.

359. White AH. Principles for physical management of work injuries. In: Isenhagen S, ed. *Work Injury.* Gaithersburg, Md: Aspen; 1988.

360. Cady LD, et al. Strength and fitness and subsequent back injuries in firefighters. *J Occup Med* 1979;21:269–272.

361. Nutter P. Aerobic exercise in the treatment and prevention of low back pain. *Occup Med* 1988;3:137–145.

362. Daltroy LH, et al. A controlled trial of an educational program to prevent low back injuries. *N Engl J Med* 1997;337:322–328.

363. Hall H. Point of view. *Spine* 1994;21:2189.

364. Cohen JE, et al. Group education interventions for people with low back pain: An overview of the literature. *Spine* 1994; 19:1214–1222.

365. Turner JA, et al. Surgery for lumbar spinal stenosis: Attempted meta-analysis of the literature. *Spine* 1992;17:1–8.

366. Arnoldi CC, Brodsky AE, Cauchoix J. Lumbar spinal stenosis and nerve root encroachment syndromes: Definition and classification. *Clin Orthop* 1976;115:4–5.

367. Verbiest H. A radicular syndrome from developmental narrowing of the lumbar vertebral canal. *J Bone Joint Surg* 1954;26B:230.

368. Huijbregts PA. Lumbopelvic region: Aging, disease, examination, diagnosis, and treatment. In: Wadsworth C, ed. *Current Concepts of Orthopaedic Physical Therapy—Home Study Course*. La Crosse, Wis: Orthopaedic Section, American Physical Therapy Association; 2001.

369. Katz JN, et al. Degenerative lumbar spinal stenosis: Diagnostic value of the history and physical examination. *Arthritis Rheum* 1995;38:1236–1241.

370. Cailliet R. *Low Back Pain Syndrome*. Philadelphia, Pa: FA Davis; 1991:263–268.

371. Weinstein SM, Herring SA. Rehabilitation of the patient with low back pain. In: DeLisa JA, Gans BM, eds. *Rehabilitation Medicine: Principles and Practice*. Philadelphia, Pa: JB Lippincott; 1993:996–1017.

372. Fast A. Low back disorders: Conservative management. *Arch Phys Med Rehabil* 1988;69:880–891.

373. Fritz JM, Erhard RE, Vignovic M. A nonsurgical treatment approach to patients with lumbar spinal stenosis. *Phys Ther* 1997;77:962–973.

374. Dooley JF, et al. Nerve root infiltration in the diagnosis of radicular pain. *Spine* 1988;13:79–83.

375. Tajima T, Furakawa K, Kuramochi E. Selective lumbosacral radiculography and block. *Spine* 1980;5:68–77.

376. Burnell A. Injection techniques in low back pain. In: *Symposium: Low Back Pain*. Perth, Australia: Western Australian Institute of Technology; 1974.

377. Strange FG. Debunking the disc. *Proc R Soc Med* 1966;9:952–956.

378. Kraft GL, Levinthal DH. Facet synovial impingement. *Surg Gynecol Obstet* 1951;93:439–443.

379. Seimons LP. *Low Back Pain: Clinical Diagnosis and Management*. Norwalk, Conn: Appleton-Century-Crofts; 1983.

380. Friberg O. Lumbar instability: A dynamic approach by traction-compression radiography. *Spine* 1987;12:119–129.

381. Pope M, Frymoyer J, Krag M. Diagnosing instability. *Clin Orthop* 1992;296:60–67.

382. Long DM, BenDebba M, Torgenson W. Persistent back pain and sciatica in the United States: Patient characteristics. *J Spinal Disord* 1996;9:40–58.

383. Njoo KH, Vanderdoes E, Stam HJ. Inter-observer agreement on iliac crest pain syndrome in general practice. *J Rheumatol* 1995;22:1532–1535.

384. Collee G, et al. Iliac crest pain syndrome in low back pain: Frequency and features. *J Rheumatol* 1991;18:1064–1067.

385. Mennell JM. *Back Pain. Diagnosis and Treatment Using Manipulative Techniques*. Boston, Mass: Little, Brown; 1960.

386. Vandertop WP, Bosma WJ. The piriformis syndrome. A case report. *J Bone Joint Surg* 1991;73A:1095–1097.

387. Robinson DR. Pyriformis syndrome in relation to sciatic pain. *Am J Surg* 1947;73:355–358.

388. McCrory P. The "piriformis syndrome"—myth or reality? *Br J Sports Med* 2001;35:209–210.

389. Maigne JY, Maigne R. Trigger point of the posterior iliac crest: Painful iliolumbar ligament insertion or cutaneous dorsal ramus pain? An anatomic study. *Arch Phys Med Rehabil* 1991; 72:734–737.

390. Banwart JC, Asher MA, Hassanein RS. Iliac crest bone graft harvest donor site morbidity: A statistical evaluation. *Spine* 1995;20:1055–1060.

391. Fernyhough JC, et al. Chronic donor site pain complicating bone graft harvesting from the posterior iliac crest for spinal fusion. *Spine* 1992;17:1474–1480.

392. Maigne R. Low-back pain of thoraco-lumbar origin. *Arch Phys Med Rehabil* 1980;61:389–395.

393. Inoue H, Ohmori K, Miyasaka K. Radiographic classification of L5 isthmic spondylolisthesis as adolescent or adult vertebral slip. *Spine* 2002;27:831–838.

394. Dandy DJ, Shannon MJ. Lumbosacral subluxation. *J Bone Joint Surg* 1971;53B:578.

395. Rosenberg NJ. Degenerative spondylolisthesis. *J Bone Joint Surg* 1975;57A:467–474.

396. Vallois HV, Lozarthes G. Indices lombares et indice lombaire totale. *Bull Soc Anthropol* 1942;3:117.

397. Matsunaga S, et al. Natural history of degenerative spondylolisthesis: Pathogenesis and natural course of slippage. *Spine* 1990;15:1204–1210.

398. Grobler LJ, et al. Etiology of spondylolisthesis: assessment of the role played by lumbar facet joint morphology. *Spine* 1993;18:80–91.

399. Love TW, Fagan AB, Fraser RD. Degenerative spondylolisthesis: Developmental or acquired? *J Bone Joint Surg* 1999; 81B:670–674.

400. Wiltse LL, Winter RB. Terminology and measurement of spondylolisthesis. *J Bone Joint Surg* 1983;65:768–772.

401. Meyerding HW. Spondylolisthesis. *Surg Gynecol Obstet* 1932;54:371–377.

402. Chen WJ, et al. Surgical treatment of adjacent instability after lumbar spine fusion. *Spine* 2001;26:E519–E524.

403. Meschan I. Spondylolisthesis: A commentary on etiology and on improved method of roentgenographic mensuration and detection of instability. *AJR Am J Roentgenol* 1945;55:230.

404. Brook RH, et al. A method for the detailed assessment of the appropriateness of medical technologies. *Int J Technol Assess Health Care* 1986;2:53–63.

405. Lewit K. *Manipulative Therapy in Rehabilitation of the Locomotor System*. 2nd ed. Oxford, England: Butterworth-Heinemann; 1996.

406. Ramsey SM. Holistic manual therapy techniques. *Prim Care* 1997;24:759–785.

407. Barash HL. Spondylolisthesis and tight hamstrings. *J Bone Joint Surg* 1970;52:1319.

408. Spring WE. Spondylolisthesis—a new clinical test. Proceedings of the Australian Orthopedics Association. *J Bone Joint Surg* 1973;55B:229.

409. Trott PH, Grant R, Maitland GD. Manipulative therapy for the low lumbar spine: Technique selection and application to some syndromes. In: Twomey LT, Taylor JR, eds. *Clinics in Physical Therapy: Physical Therapy of the Low Back*. New York, NY: Churchill Livingstone; 1987:216–217.

410. Dyck P, Doyle JB. "Bicycle test" of van Gelderen in diagnosis of intermittent cauda equina compression syndrome. *J Neurosurg* 1977;46:667–670.

THE THORACIC SPINE AND RIB CAGE

CHAPTER OBJECTIVES

▶ *At the completion of this chapter, the reader will be able to:*

1. Describe the vertebrae, ligaments, muscles, and blood and nerve supply that comprise the thoracic intervertebral segment.

2. Outline the coupled movements of the thoracic spine, the normal and abnormal joint barriers, and the reactions of the various structures to loading.

3. Perform a detailed objective examination of the thoracic musculoskeletal system, including palpation of the articular and soft tissue structures, combined motion testing, position testing, passive articular mobility tests, and stability tests.

4. Evaluate the total examination data to establish the diagnosis and estimate the prognosis.

5. Describe the common pathologies and lesions of this region.

6. Apply manual techniques to the thoracic spine using the correct grade, direction, and duration.

7. Describe intervention strategies based on clinical findings and established goals.

8. Design an intervention plan based on patient education, manual therapy, and therapeutic exercise.

9. Evaluate intervention effectiveness in order to progress or modify an intervention.

10. Plan an effective home program, including spinal care and therapeutic exercise, and instruct the patient in this program.

OVERVIEW

The thoracic spine serves as a transitional zone between the lumbosacral region and the cervical spine. Although historically the thoracic spine has not enjoyed the same attention as other regions of the spine, it can be a significant source of local and referred pain. The thoracic spine is the most rigid region of the spine and in this area, protection of the thoracic viscera take precedence over segmental spinal mobility.

Because each thoracic vertebra is involved in at least six articulations, establishing the specific cause of thoracic dysfunction involved may not always be possible. This task is made more difficult because of the inaccessibility of most of these joints.[1]

Anatomy

The thoracic spine forms a kyphotic curve between the lordotic curves of the cervical and lumbar spines. The curve begins at T1 to T2 and extends down to T12, with the T6 to T7 disk space as the apex.[2] The thoracic kyphosis is a structural curve that is present from birth.[3] Unlike the lumbar and cervical regions, which derive their curves from the corresponding differences in intervertebral disk heights, the thoracic curve is maintained by the wedge-shaped vertebral bodies, which are about 2 mm higher posteriorly than anteriorly.

At the thoracolumbar junction, typically located between T11 and L1, the changes in curvature from one of kyphosis to one of lordosis vary quite widely according to posture, age, and previous compression fractures and resulting deformity.[4,5]

Thoracic Vertebra

The thoracic vertebrae consist of the usual elements: the vertebral body (centrum), transverse processes, and spinous process (Fig. 26-1).

Vertebral Body

The thoracic vertebral body is roughly as wide as it is long, so that its anteroposterior and mediolateral dimensions are of equal length.[6] The anterior surface of the body is convex from side to side, whereas the posterior surface is deeply concave.[6] The height, end-plate cross-sectional area, and bone mass of the vertebral bodies increases cranially to caudally, particularly in the lower levels.[7,8] Progressive wedging of the thoracic vertebral bodies occurs with increasing age in the majority of individuals, with disk space narrowing at multiple levels occurring from the third decade of life.[9] The vertebral bodies of most of the thoracic spine differ from those of the cervical and lumbar vertebrae because of the presence of a demifacet on each of their lateral aspects for articulation with the ribs (the costovertebral joint; see later discussion).

Transverse Processes

The transverse processes of the thoracic spine are oriented posteriorly (i.e., they point backward) and are located directly between the inferior articulating process and the superior articulating process of the zygapophysial joints of each level. This anatomical feature makes the transverse processes useful as palpation points when performing mobility testing in the midthorax.

The transverse processes of the first ten thoracic vertebrae differ from those of the cervical and lumbar spines because of the presence of a costal facet on the transverse process, which articulates with the corresponding rib to form the costotransverse joint (see later discussion). At the T11 and T12 levels, the costotransverse joint is absent because ribs 11 and 12 do not articulate with the transverse processes but rather with the vertebral body.

Spinous Processes

Two short and thick laminae come together to form the spinous process. The spinous processes of the thoracic region are long, slender, and triangular shaped in cross-section. Although all of the thoracic spinous processes point obliquely downward, the degree of obliquity varies. The first three spinous processes, and the last three, are almost horizontal, whereas those of the midthorax are long and steeply inclined. T7 has the greatest spinous process angulation.

As elsewhere in the spine, the thoracic vertebrae are designed to endure and distribute the compressive forces produced by weight bearing, most of which is borne by the vertebral bodies. The compressive load at T1 is approximately 9 percent of body weight, increasing to 33 percent at T8 and 47 percent at T12.[10,11]

The thoracic vertebrae are classified as typical or atypical with reference to their morphology. The typical thoracic vertebrae are found at T2 through T9, although T9 may be atypical in that its inferior costal facet is frequently absent. The atypical thoracic vertebrae are T1, T10, T11, and T12.

The first vertebra (T1) resembles C7. The centrum of T1 demonstrates a larger transverse than anteroposterior dimension of the vertebral body, being almost twice as wide as it is long, and the spinous process is usually at least as long as that of C7. There are two ovoid facets on either side of the T1 vertebral body for articulation with the head of the first rib. The inferior aspect of the vertebral body of T1 is flat and contains a small facet at each posterolateral corner for articulation with the head of the second rib.

Approximately 32 structures attach to the first rib and body of T1.[12] Because of the ringlike structure of the ribs, and their attachments both anteriorly and posteriorly, the thoracic spine and ribs can be viewed as a cagelike structure forming a series of concentric rings. Any movement occurring at the various joints of each ring (costovertebral, costotransverse, sternocostal, and zygapophysial joints) has the potential to influence motions at the other joints within the ring, or at the neighboring segments.

The third vertebra is the smallest of the thoracic vertebra. The T9 vertebra may have no demi-facets below, or it may have two demi-facets on either side (in which case, the T10 vertebra will have demi-facets only at the superior aspect). The T10

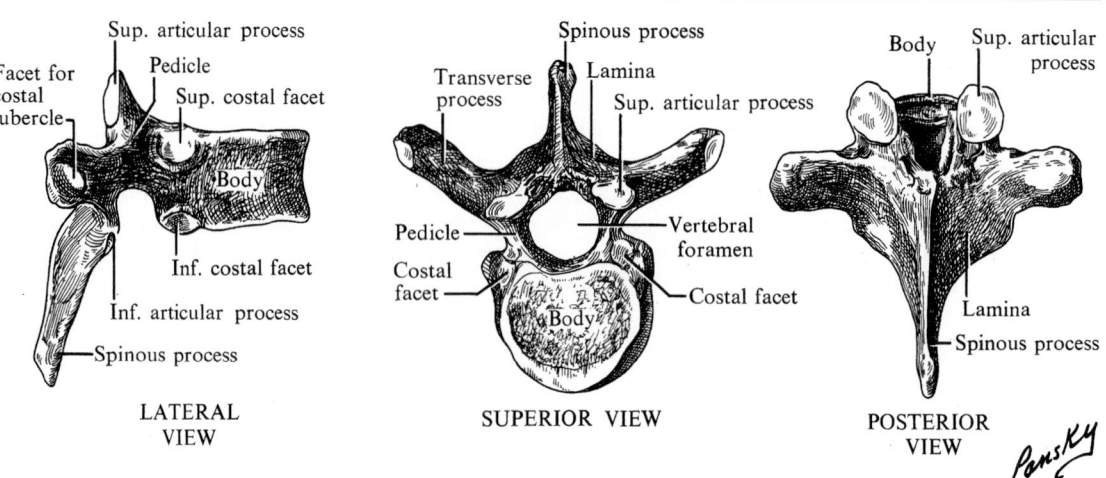

FIGURE 26-1 Thoracic vertebra. (Reproduced with permission from Pansky B. *Review of Gross Anatomy.* 6th ed. New York, NY: McGraw-Hill; 1996:195.)

LATERAL VIEW — Sup. articular process; Facet for costal tubercle; Pedicle; Sup. costal facet; Body; Inf. costal facet; Inf. articular process; Spinous process

SUPERIOR VIEW — Spinous process; Transverse process; Lamina; Sup. articular process; Pedicle; Costal facet; Body; Vertebral foramen; Costal facet

POSTERIOR VIEW — Body; Sup. articular process; Lamina; Spinous process vertebra has one full rib facet located partly on the body of the vertebra and partly on the tubercle. It does not articulate with the 11th rib, and so does not possess inferior demifacets, and occasionally there is no facet for the rib at the costotransverse joint.

The T11 and T12 segments form the thoracolumbar junction. The T11 vertebra has complete costal facets, but no facets on the transverse processes for the rib tubercle. The T12 vertebra only articulates with its own ribs and does not possess inferior demi-facets.

Ligaments

The common spinal ligaments are present at the thoracic vertebrae (Fig. 26-2), and they perform much the same function as they do elsewhere in the spine. However, the anterior longitudinal ligament in this region is narrower but thicker compared with elsewhere in the spine,[6] whereas the posterior longitudinal ligament is wider here at the level of the intervertebral disk, but narrower at the vertebral body than in the lumbar region.[13]

Intervertebral Disk

The ratio of intervertebral disk height to vertebral body height is lower in the thoracic spine (1:5) than that of the cervical (2:5) and lumbar (1:3) levels. The thoracic disks are both narrower and thinner than those of the cervical and lumbar spine, gradually increasing in size from superior to inferior (see Chap. 20). The decrease in disk height is partially responsible for the relatively low mobility demonstrated by the thoracic spine compared with the cervical and lumbar spine.

Zygapophysial Joints

The superior and inferior facets of the zygapophysial joints arise from the upper and lower parts of the pedicle of the thoracic vertebra. The superior facet lies superiorly with the articular surface on the posterior aspect, whereas the inferior facet lies inferiorly with the articular surface on the ventral aspect. The articulating facets of the thoracic zygapophysial joints are quite different from those of the cervical and lumbar spines because they are oriented in a more coronal direction, with the angle of inclination changing, depending on the segmental level:

▶ The upper segments are inclined at 45 to 60 degrees to horizontal in a similar fashion as to those of the cervical spine.

▶ The middle segments are inclined at 90 degrees to horizontal in the typical thoracic form.

▶ The lower segments are inclined as in the lumbar spine. Zygapophysial tropism (the moving toward or away from a stimulus) occurs most frequently at T11 to T12.[14] The inferior articular facets of T12 are invariably lumbar in orientation and concavity, with the orientation changing by 90 degrees at either T11 or T12, allowing pure axial rotation to occur.[15,16]

The degree of superoinferior and mediolateral orientation is slight. The superior facet arises from near the lamina-pedicle junction and faces posteriorly, superiorly, and laterally.

The inferior articulating facet arises from the laminae to face anteriorly, inferiorly, and medially, lying posterior to the superior facet of the vertebra below. The facet surfaces are concave anteriorly and convex posteriorly, bringing the axis of rotation through the centrum rather than through the spinous process, as in the lumbar vertebrae. This results in the biomechanical center of rotation coinciding with the actual center of rotation formed by body weight.[17]

The zygapophysial joints function to restrain the amount of flexion and anterior translation of the vertebral segment, and to facilitate rotation.[10] They appear to have little influence on the range of side bending.[10]

Ribs

The bony thoracic cage is formed by 12 pairs of ribs, the sternum, the clavicle, and the vertebrae of the thoracic spine. The primary function of the rib cage is to protect the heart and lungs. All of the ribs of the cage are different from each other in size, width, and curvature, although they share some common characteristics. The first rib is the shortest. The rib length increases further inferiorly until the seventh rib, after which they become progressively shorter.

The ribs are divided into two classifications: true/false and typical/atypical.

1. *True/false.* Ribs 1 through 7 are named true ribs because their cartilage attaches directly to the sternum. The remaining ribs are false ribs, so named because their distal attachment is to the costochondral cartilage of their superior neighbor.

2. *Typical/atypical.* Ribs 3 through 9 are typical ribs. The 1st, 9th, 10th, 11th and 12th ribs are considered atypical. The typical rib is characterized by a posterior end, which is composed of a head, neck, and tubercle. The head of the typical rib is characterized as two articular facets, a superior costal facet and an inferior costal facet.

   a. The superior facet attaches to the costal semilunar demifacet of the vertebra above its level.

   b. The inferior facet attaches to the costal semicircular demifacet of the vertebra of the same level.[12]

The 1st, 9th, 10th, 11th and 12th ribs are deemed atypical because they only articulate with their own vertebra via one full facet, and the lower two do not articulate with the costochondrium anteriorly.[12]

Typical Ribs

The head of the typical rib projects upward in a very similar manner to that of the uncinate process in the cervical spine and, in fact, develops in much the same way during childhood, appearing to play a similar mechanical role.[6] The head consists of a slightly enlarged posterior end, which is divided by a horizontal ridge. The ridge serves as an attachment for the intra-articular ligament. The intra-articular ligament, which travels between the head of the rib and the intervertebral disk, bisects the joint into superior and inferior portions. Each of these portions normally contains a demifacet for articulation with the synovial costovertebral joints.

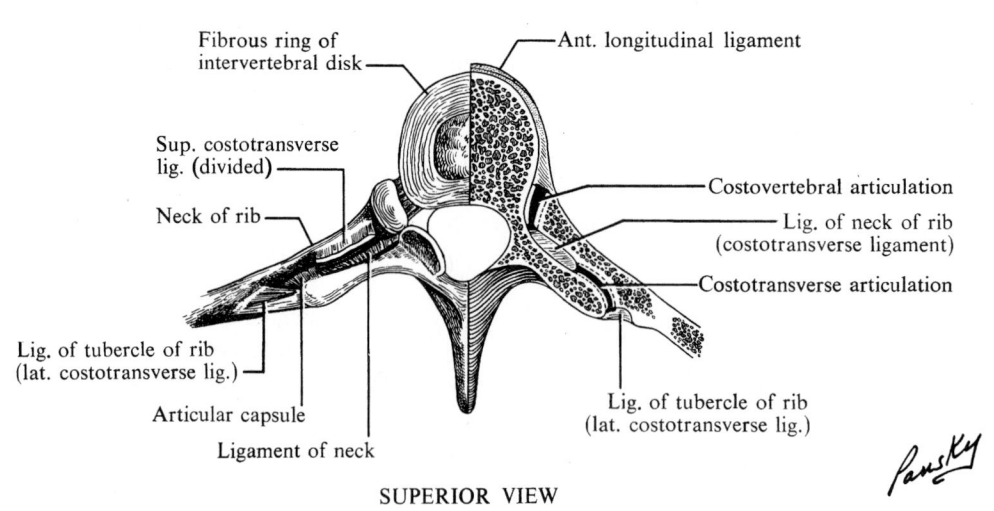

FIGURE 26-2 Costovertebral articulations. (Reproduced with permission from Pansky B. *Review of Gross Anatomy.* 6th ed. New York, NY: McGraw-Hill; 1996:217.)

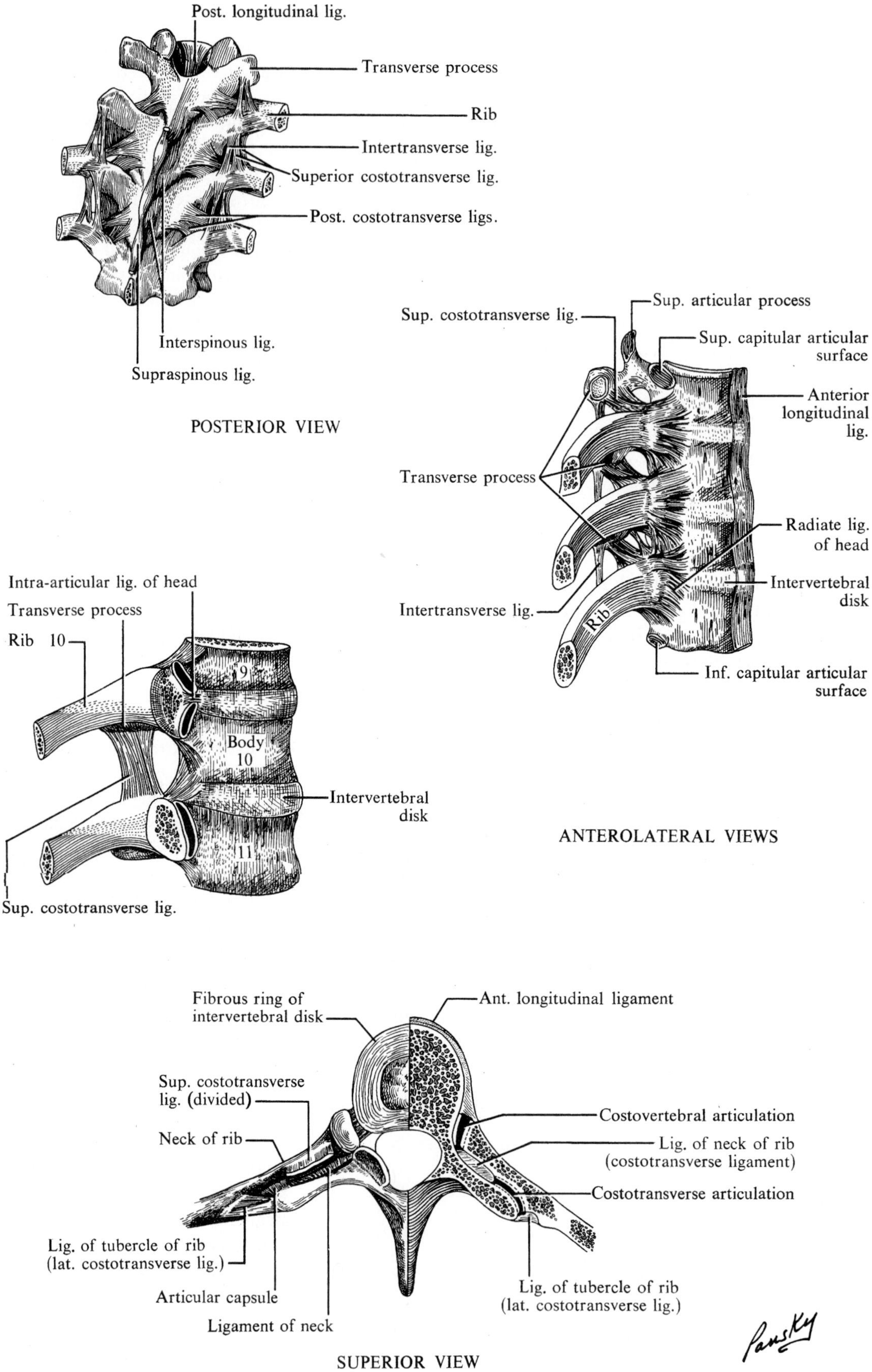

Post. longitudinal lig.

Transverse process

Rib

Intertransverse lig.

Superior costotransverse lig.

Post. costotransverse ligs.

Interspinous lig.

Supraspinous lig.

POSTERIOR VIEW

Sup. costotransverse lig.

Sup. articular process

Sup. capitular articular surface

Anterior longitudinal lig.

Transverse process

Radiate lig. of head

Intervertebral disk

Intertransverse lig.

Rib

Inf. capitular articular surface

ANTEROLATERAL VIEWS

Intra-articular lig. of head

Transverse process

Rib 10

9

Body 10

Intervertebral disk

11

Sup. costotransverse lig.

Fibrous ring of intervertebral disk

Ant. longitudinal ligament

Sup. costotransverse lig. (divided)

Neck of rib

Costovertebral articulation

Lig. of neck of rib (costotransverse ligament)

Costotransverse articulation

Lig. of tubercle of rib (lat. costotransverse lig.)

Articular capsule

Ligament of neck

Lig. of tubercle of rib (lat. costotransverse lig.)

SUPERIOR VIEW

The tubercle of the typical rib lies on the outer surface, where the neck joins the shaft, and is more prominent in the upper parts than in the lower. The articular portion of the tubercle presents an oval facet for articulation at the costotransverse joint (see Fig. 26-2).

The convex shaft of the rib is connected to the neck at the rib angle. The upper border of the shaft is round and blunt, whereas the inferior aspect is thin and sharp.[6] The anterior end of the shaft has a small depression at the tip for articulation at the costochondral joint (see Fig. 26-2).

Atypical Ribs

The atypical first rib is small but massively built. Being the most curved and the most inferiorly orientated rib, it slopes sharply downward from its vertebral articulation to the manubrium. The head is small and rounded, and articulates only with the T1 vertebra. The first costal cartilage is the shortest and this, together with the fibrous sternochondral joint, contributes to the overall stability of the first ring of the rib cage. The first rib attaches to the manubrium just under the sternoclavicular joint, and the second rib articulates with the sternum at the manubriosternal junction. The atypical second rib is longer and not as flat as the first rib. It attaches to the junction of the manubrium and the body of the sternum.

The atypical tenth rib has only a single facet on its head, because of its lack of articulation with the vertebra above. The 11th and 12th ribs do not present tubercles and have only a single articular facet on their heads. The 11th and 12th ribs remain unattached anteriorly, but end with a small piece of cartilage.

Attachment and Orientation of the Ribs

The attachment of the ribs to the sternum is variable. The upper five, six, or seven ribs have their own cartilaginous connection (see "Sternocostal Joint").[6] The cartilage of the eighth rib ends by blending with the seventh. The same situation pertains for the ninth and tenth ribs, thus giving rise to a common band of cartilage and connective tissue.

The strong ligamentous attendance, and the presence of the two joints (costovertebral and costotransverse) at each level, severely limits the amount of movement permitted here to slight gliding and spinning motions, with morphology determining the function of each rib.

The orientation of the ribs increases from being horizontal at the upper levels to being more downwardly oblique in the inferior levels of the thoracic spine (a point worth remembering when performing palpation).

> ### Clinical Pearl
>
> The cervical rib is a rare anatomic variant estimated to occur in approximately 0.5 to 1 percent of the population, and bilaterally in 66 to 80 percent of these cases.[18] Diagnosis is most often incidental, as a result of routine chest radiographs or in patients developing thoracic outlet syndrome.[18]

Costovertebral Joint

The thoracic vertebrae are connected to their adjacent vertebrae by the bilateral hyalinated, and synovial, costovertebral joints and their surrounding ligaments (see Fig. 26-2). The costovertebral articulation also forms an intimate relationship between the head of the rib and the lateral side of the vertebral body (see Fig. 26-2). The 1st, 11th, and 12th ribs articulate fully with their own vertebrae via a single costal facet, without any contact with the intervertebral disk, whereas the remaining ribs articulate with both their own vertebra, and the vertebra above, as well as with the intervertebral disk. This could potentially predispose the 1st, 11th, and 12th costovertebral joints to early arthritic changes as a result of more mechanical stress compared with the 2nd to 10th ribs.[18a]

The radiate ligament (see Fig. 26-2) connects the anterior aspect of the rib head to the bodies of two adjacent vertebrae and their intervening disk in a fanlike arrangement. Each of the three bands of the radiate ligament has different attachments.

1. The superior part runs from the head of the rib to the body of the superior vertebra.

2. The inferior part runs to the body of the inferior vertebra.

3. The intermediate part runs to the intervening disk.

Oda and colleagues[19] reported that the costovertebral joint and rib cage confer stability on the thoracic spine. They performed symmetrically applied resections of the posterior elements first, followed by resection of the bilateral costovertebral joints and then complete obliteration of the rib cage. Their conclusion was that the thoracic spine may become unstable when the posterior elements and the bilateral costovertebral joints are obliterated. In addition, there is an increase in the neutral zone and range of motion in both side bending and rotation, indicating that these joints provide a stabilizing influence during coupled motions.[19]

Feiertag and colleagues[20] reported that rib head joint resection showed significant increases in thoracic spinal motion in the sagittal and coronal planes. As the ossification of the head of the rib is not developed at the superior costovertebral joint until about age 13, younger individuals, such as gymnasts, can demonstrate a vast amount of thoracic rotation and side bending.

Costotransverse Joint

This is a synovial joint located between an articular facet on the posterior aspect of the rib tubercle and an articular facet on the anterior aspect of the transverse process, which is supported by a thin fibrous capsule (see Fig. 26-2). In the lower two thoracic vertebral segments, this articulation does not exist.

The neck of the rib lies along the entire length of the posterior aspect of the transverse process. The short and deep costotransverse ligament (see Fig. 26-2) runs posteriorly from the posterior aspect of the rib neck to the anterior aspect of its transverse process, filling the costotransverse foramen that is formed between the rib neck and its adjacent transverse process. The ligament has two divisions:

1. The superior costotransverse ligament, also known as the interosseous ligament, or ligament of the neck of the rib, is formed in two layers (see Fig. 26-2). The anterior layer, which is continuous with the internal intercostal membrane laterally, runs from the neck of the rib up and laterally to the inferior aspect of the transverse process above. The posterior layer runs up and medially from the posterior aspect of the rib neck to the transverse process above.

2. The lateral costotransverse ligament (see Fig. 26-2) runs from the tip of the transverse process laterally to the tubercle of its own rib. It is short, thick, and strong but is often damaged with direct blows to the chest (e.g., punch, kick, etc.).

Very little posteroanterior or anteromedial-posterolateral translation is available at this joint. Jiang and colleagues[21] reported that the superior costotransverse ligaments are very important in maintaining the lateral stability of the spine.

> ### Clinical Pearl
>
> Working together, the costotransverse joints and the costovertebral joints help provide stability to the thoracic spine.

Sternum

The sternum consists of three parts: the manubrium, the body, and the xiphoid process.

The manubrium (Fig. 26-3) is broad and thick superiorly and narrower and thinner inferiorly, where it articulates with the body. On either side of the suprasternal notch are articulating facets for the clavicles, and below these are the facets for the first rib. On the immediate inferolateral aspects of the manubrium are two more small facets for the cartilage of the second rib.

The articulation between the manubrium and the sternum is usually a symphysis, with the ends of the bones being lined with hyaline cartilage.

The body of the sternum is made up of the fused elements of four sternal bodies, and the vestiges of these are marked by three horizontal ridges. The upper end of the body articulates with the manubrium at the sternal angle. A facet at the superior end of the body laterally provides a joint surface common with the manubrium for the second costal cartilage. On each lateral border are four other notches that articulate with the third through sixth costal cartilages. The third rib has the deepest fossa on the sternum, indicating that it may serve as the axis for rotation and side bending during arm elevation. T7 articulates with both the sternum and the xiphoid.

The xiphisternum, or xiphoid process (see Fig. 26-3), is the smallest part of the sternum. It begins life in a cartilaginous state but, in adulthood, the upper part ossifies.

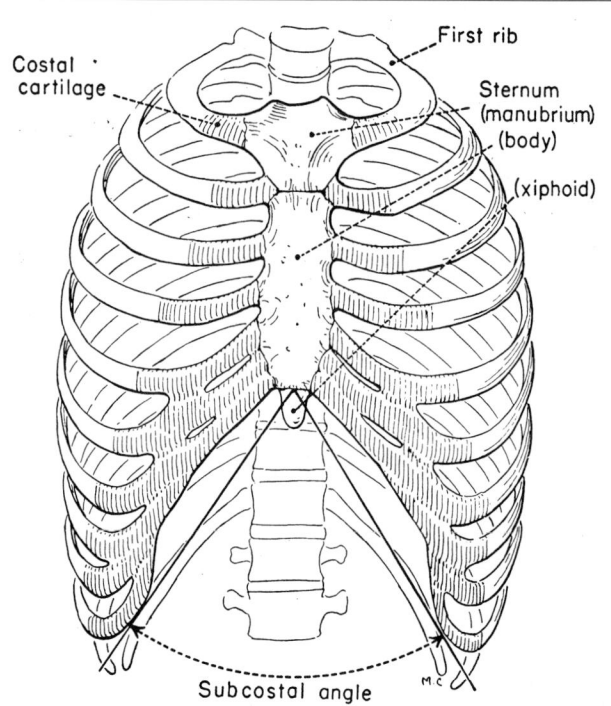

FIGURE 26-3 Manubrium and sternum. (Reproduced with permission from Luttgens K, Hamilton K. *Kinesiology: Scientific Basis of Human Motion.* New York, NY: McGraw-Hill; 1997:276.)

A study[22] examining the effect of removal of the entire sternum from the intact thorax found its removal produced an almost complete loss of the stiffening effect of the thorax.

Sternocostal Joint

The first, sixth, and seventh costal cartilages are each linked to the sternum by a synchondrosis. The second to fifth ribs are each connected to the sternum through a synovial joint, whereby the cartilage of the corresponding rib articulates with a socketlike cavity in the sternum.[23]

In all of these joints, the periosteum of the sternum and the perichondrium of the costal cartilage are continuous. A thin fibrous capsule, present in the upper seven joints, attaches to the circumference of the articular surfaces, blending with the sternocostal ligaments. The surfaces of the joints are covered with fibrocartilage and are supported by capsular, radiate sternocostal, or xiphicostal and intra-articular ligaments. The joint is capable of about 2 degrees of motion from full inspiration to full expiration and allows the full excursion of the sternum in these activities.

Muscles

A large number of muscles arise from and insert on the thoracic spine and ribs. The muscles of this region can be divided into those that are involved in spinal or extremity motion, and those that are involved in respiration (Tables 26-1 and Table 26-2).

TABLE 26-1   Muscles of Forced Expiration[24]

Primary	Accessory
Abdominal muscles	Latissimus dorsi
• Internal and external oblique	Serratus posterior inferior
• Rectus abdominis	Quadratus lumborum
• Transversus abdominis	Iliocostalis lumborum
Internal intercostals (posterior)	
Transversus thoracis	
Transverse intercostals (intima)	

TABLE 26-2   Muscles of Inspiration[24]

Primary	Accessory
Diaphragm	Scaleni
Levator costorum	Sternocleidomastoid
External intercostals	Trapezius
Internal intercostals	Serratus anterior and posterior,
(anterior)	superior and inferior
	Pectoralis major and minor
	Latissimus dorsi
	Subclavius

Spinal and Extremity Muscles

Spinal Muscles

Iliocostalis Thoracis.   The iliocostalis thoracis consists of several muscle straps that link the thoracic vertebrae and sacrum with the lower six or seven ribs. The muscle straps have a number of tendons, varying in different individuals, which insert in all angles in the lower six ribs. The function of the muscle is to extend the spine when working bilaterally, and to side bend the spine ipsilaterally when working alone. The iliocostalis consists of three subdivisions—iliocostalis lumborum, iliocostalis thoracis, and iliocostalis cervicis—which are a part of the external portion of the long erector spinae muscle group. The muscle receives its nerve supply by the dorsal rami of the thoracic nerves.

Longissimus Thoracis.   The longissimus thoracis muscles originate with the intercostalis muscles from the transverse processes of the lower thoracic vertebrae. They insert into all of the ribs and into the ends of the transverse processes of the upper lumbar vertebrae. The function of the muscle is to extend the spine when working bilaterally, and to side bend the spine ipsilaterally when working alone. The muscle is innervated by the dorsal rami of the thoracic nerves.

Spinalis Thoracis.   The spinalis thoracis muscle (spinalis dorsi) originates from the spinous processes of the upper lumbar and two lower thoracic vertebrae. It inserts in the spinous processes of the middle and upper thoracic vertebrae. The function of the

muscle is to extend the spine. The muscle is innervated by the dorsal rami of the thoracic nerves.

Semispinalis Thoracis.   The semispinalis thoracis consists of long straps of muscle that stretch along and surround the vertebrae of the spine. The muscle can have between four and eight upper ends, which originate from the transverse processes of the T6 to T10. These straps of muscle insert in the spinous processes of the first four thoracic and fifth and seventh processes of C6 to T4. The function of the muscle is to extend the spine when working bilaterally, and to rotate the spine contralaterally when working alone. The semispinalis thoracis is innervated by dorsal rami of the thoracic nerves.

Multifidus.   The multifidus is a deep back muscle that runs along the entire spine and lies deep to the erector spinae muscles. It originates from the sacrum, sacroiliac ligament, mammillary processes of the lumbar vertebrae, transverse processes of the thoracic vertebrae, and the articular processes of the last four cervical vertebrae. The multifidus consists of numerous bundles of fibers that cross over two to five vertebrae at a time and insert into the entire length of the spinous process above. The function of the muscle is to extend the spine when working bilaterally, and to minimally rotate the spine contralaterally when working alone. The thoracic multifidus is innervated by the dorsal rami of the thoracic spinal nerves.

Rotatores Thoracis (Longus and Brevis).   The rotatores muscles are deep spinal muscles that lie beneath the multifidus muscles. The rotatores brevis muscle lies just deep to the rotatores longus muscle. The rotatores muscles are the most well developed in the thoracic region. There are a total of 11 small, quadrilateral rotatores muscles on each side of the spine. Each muscle arises from the transverse process of the vertebra and extends inward to the vertebra above. The rotatores muscles help to rotate the appropriate thoracic segment. They are innervated by dorsal rami of the thoracic spinal nerves.

Intertransversarii.   The intratransversals are small muscles located between the transverse process of the vertebrae. In the thoracic region, they are single-bellied muscles and exist only from T10–11 to T12–L1. The function of the muscle is to ipsilaterally side bend the spine. The muscle is innervated by the dorsal rami of the thoracic spinal nerves.

The other spinal muscles of the thoracic region act primarily on the cervical spine. These include the trapezius, levator scapulae, and anterior, posterior, and middle scalenes (see Chap. 23).

Extremity Muscles.   The muscles of the thoracic region that act primarily on the extremities include the pectoralis major, latissimus dorsi, and serratus anterior (see Chap. 14).

Respiratory Muscles

The respiratory system is essentially a robust, multimuscle pump. Connections to the respiratory mechanism have been found to exert a strong influence on such areas as the shoulder and pelvic girdles, as well as the head and neck. The primary task of the respiratory muscles is to displace the chest wall and, therefore, move gas in and out of the lungs to maintain arterial blood gas and pH homeostasis. The importance of normal respiratory muscle function can be appreciated by considering that respiratory muscle failure caused by fatigue, injury, or disease could result in an inability to maintain blood gas and pH levels within an acceptable range, which could have lethal consequences. Restoration of the respiratory mechanism is, thus, an essential element of thoracic intervention.

The actions of various respiratory muscles, which are broadly classified as *inspiratory* or *expiratory* based on their mechanical actions, are highly redundant and provide several means by which air can be effectively displaced under a host of physiologic and pathophysiologic conditions.[25,26]

At rest, movement of air into and out of the lungs is the result of the recruitment of several muscles,[27–29] and the expiratory phase of breathing at rest also is associated with active muscle participation.[30] In the resting human, the tidal volume is primarily the result of the coordinated recruitment of a number of muscles (Table 26-1 and Table 26-2).[31,32]

Although some have argued that the performance of the respiratory muscles does not limit exercise tolerance in normal healthy adults,[33,34] heavy or prolonged exercise has been shown to impair respiratory muscle performance in humans.[35,36] Thus, an interest in the adaptability of respiratory muscles to endurance-type exercise has grown significantly during the past decade.

The primary muscles of respiration include the diaphragm, sternocostal, and intercostals. The secondary muscles of respiration are the anterior and medial scalenes, serratus anterior and posterior, trapezius pectoralis major and minor, and, with the head fixed, the sternocleidomastoid.[6]

Diaphragm

Anatomically, the diaphragm muscle may be divided into sternal, costal, and lumbar parts:

▶ The sternal fibers originate from two slips at the back of the xiphoid process.

▶ The costal fibers originate from the lower six ribs and their costal cartilages.

▶ The lumbar fibers originate from the crura of the lumbar vertebra, and the medial and lateral arcuate ligaments.

Clinical Pearl

Patients with bilateral diaphragm paralysis or severe weakness present a striking clinical picture, with orthopnea as the major symptom. Lesser degrees of diaphragm weakness, however, are hard to detect and need specific testing.

Functionally and metabolically, the diaphragm can be classified as two muscles[37,38]:

1. The crural (posterior) portion that inserts into the lumbar vertebrae.

2. The costal portion that inserts into the xiphoid process of the sternum and into the margins of the lower ribs.

Thus, the muscle is attached around the thoraco-abdominal junction circumferentially. From these attachments, the fibers arch toward each other centrally to form a large tendon. Contraction of the diaphragm pulls the large, central tendon inferiorly, producing diaphragmatic inspiration (see later discussion). The diaphragm has a phrenic C3 to C4 motor innervation and a sensory supply by the lower six intercostal nerves.

Intercostals

Between the ribs are the intercostal spaces, which are deeper both in front and between the upper ribs. Between the ribs lie the internal and external intercostal muscles, with the neurovascular bundle lying beneath each rib.

The intercostal muscles, together with the sternalis (or sternocostalis or transversalis thoracis), phylogenically form from the hypomeric muscles. These muscles correspond to their abdominal counterparts, with the sternalis being homologous to the rectus abdominis, and the intercostals homologous to the external oblique.[6]

External Intercostals. The external intercostal muscles (Fig. 26-4), of which there are 11, are laid in a direction that is superoposterior to inferoanterior (run inferiorly and medially in the front of the thorax and inferiorly and laterally in the back). Because of the oblique course of the fibers, and the fact that

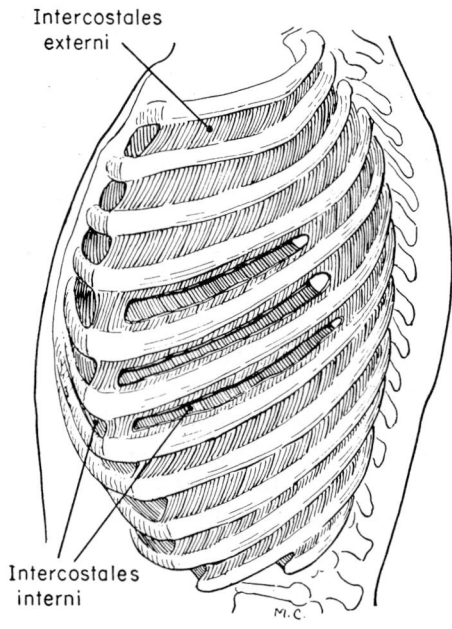

FIGURE 26-4 The intercostal muscles. (Reproduced with permission from Luttgens K, Hamilton K. *Kinesiology: Scientific Basis of Human Motion.* New York, NY: McGraw-Hill; 1997:281.)

leverage is greatest on the lower of the two ribs, the muscle pulls the lower rib toward the upper rib, which results in inspiration. The external intercostals attach to the lower border of one rib and the upper border of the rib below, extending from the tubercle to the costal cartilage. Posteriorly, the muscle is continuous with the posterior fibers of the superior costotransverse ligament. The action of the external intercostals is believed to be entirely inspiratory,[31] although the muscles also counteract the force of the diaphragm, preventing the collapse of the ribs.[28] Innervation of this muscle is supplied by the adjacent intercostal nerve.

Internal Intercostals. The internal intercostals (see Fig. 26-4), which also number 11, have their fibers in an inferoposterior to a superoanterior direction. The internal intercostals are found deep to the external intercostals and run obliquely, and perpendicular, to the externals. The posterior fibers pull the upper rib down, but only during enforced expiration.[28,31] The internal intercostals extend from the posterior rib angles to the sternum, where they end posteriorly. They are continuous with the internal membrane, which then becomes continuous with the anterior part of the superior costotransverse ligament. Innervation of this muscle group is supplied by the adjacent intercostal nerve.

Transverse Intercostals (Intima). The deepest of the intercostals, the transverse intercostals are attached to the internal aspects of two contiguous ribs. They become progressively more significant, and developed, further down the thorax. This muscle is used during forced expiration.[28,31]

Transversus Thoracis. The transversus thoracis is a triangular-shaped sheet muscle, which originates from the dorsal surface of the sternum and covers the inner surfaces of both the sternum and the second to eighth sternal costal cartilages. The apex of the muscle points cranially, with muscle slips running inferolaterally and eventually inserting on the sternal ribs quite close to the costochondral junctions. Morphologically, the transversus thoracis is similar to the ventral part of the transversus abdominis. Its function is to draw the costal cartilages down. The muscle is innervated by the adjacent intercostal nerves.

Levator Costae

These consist of 12 strong short muscles that turn obliquely (inferolaterally), parallel with the external intercostals, from the tip of the transverse process to the angle of the rib, extending from the C7 to T11 transverse processes. These muscles, which are innervated by the lateral branch of the dorsal ramus of the thoracic nerve, function to raise the rib, but their importance in respiration is argued. The levator costae also may be segmentally involved in rotation and side bending of the thoracic vertebra.

Serratus Posterior Superior

The serratus posterior superior runs from the lower part of the ligamentum nuchae, the spinous processes of C7 and T1 to T3, and their supraspinous ligaments, to the inferior border of the second through fifth ribs, lateral to the rib angle (Fig. 26-5).

The muscle receives its nerve supply from the second through fifth intercostal nerves. Its function is unclear, but it is thought to elevate the ribs.[6]

Serratus Posterior Inferior

This muscle arises from the spines and supraspinous ligaments of the two lower thoracic and the two or three upper lumbar vertebrae. It attaches to the inferior border of the lower four ribs, lateral to the rib angle (see Fig. 26-5).

The muscle receives its nerve supply from the ventral rami of the ninth through 12th thoracic nerves. Its function is unclear, but it is thought to pull the ribs downward and backward.

Vascular Supply

The blood supply to this region is provided mainly by the dorsal branches of the posterior intercostal arteries, while the venous drainage occurs through the anterior and posterior venous plexuses. The spinal cord region between T4 and T9 is poorly vascularized.[39]

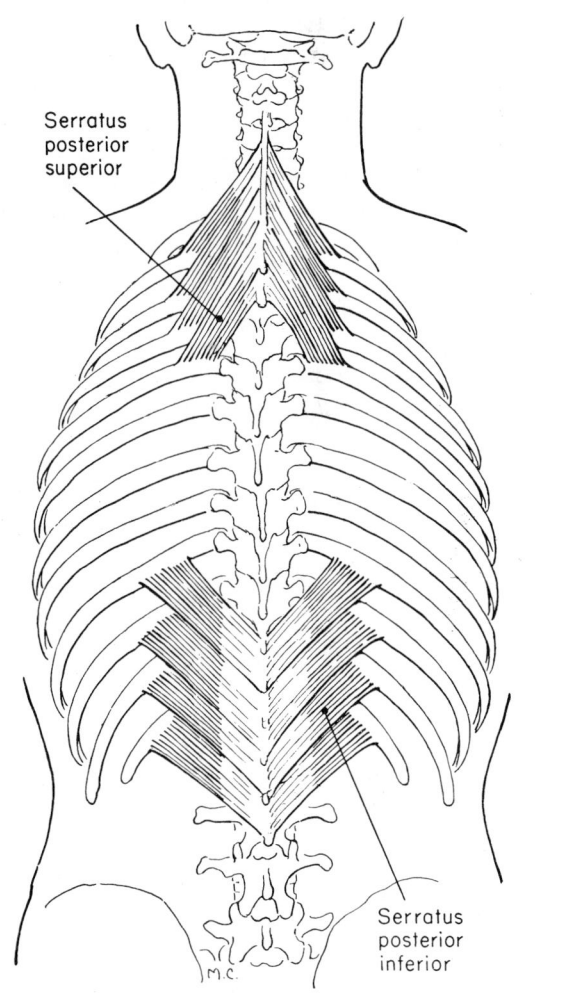

Serratus posterior superior

Serratus posterior inferior

M.C.

FIGURE 26-5 Serratus posterior. (Reproduced with permission from Luttgens K, Hamilton K. *Kinesiology: Scientific Basis of Human Motion.* New York, NY: McGraw-Hill; 1997:284.)

Neurology

The spinal canal in this region is narrow, with only a small epidural space between the cord and its osseous environment.[39] Innervation of the thoracic spinal canal is by the sinuvertebral nerve, which arises from the nerve root and reenters the epidural space.

The thoracic spinal cord is unusually susceptible to injury because it occupies a greater percentage of the total cross-sectional

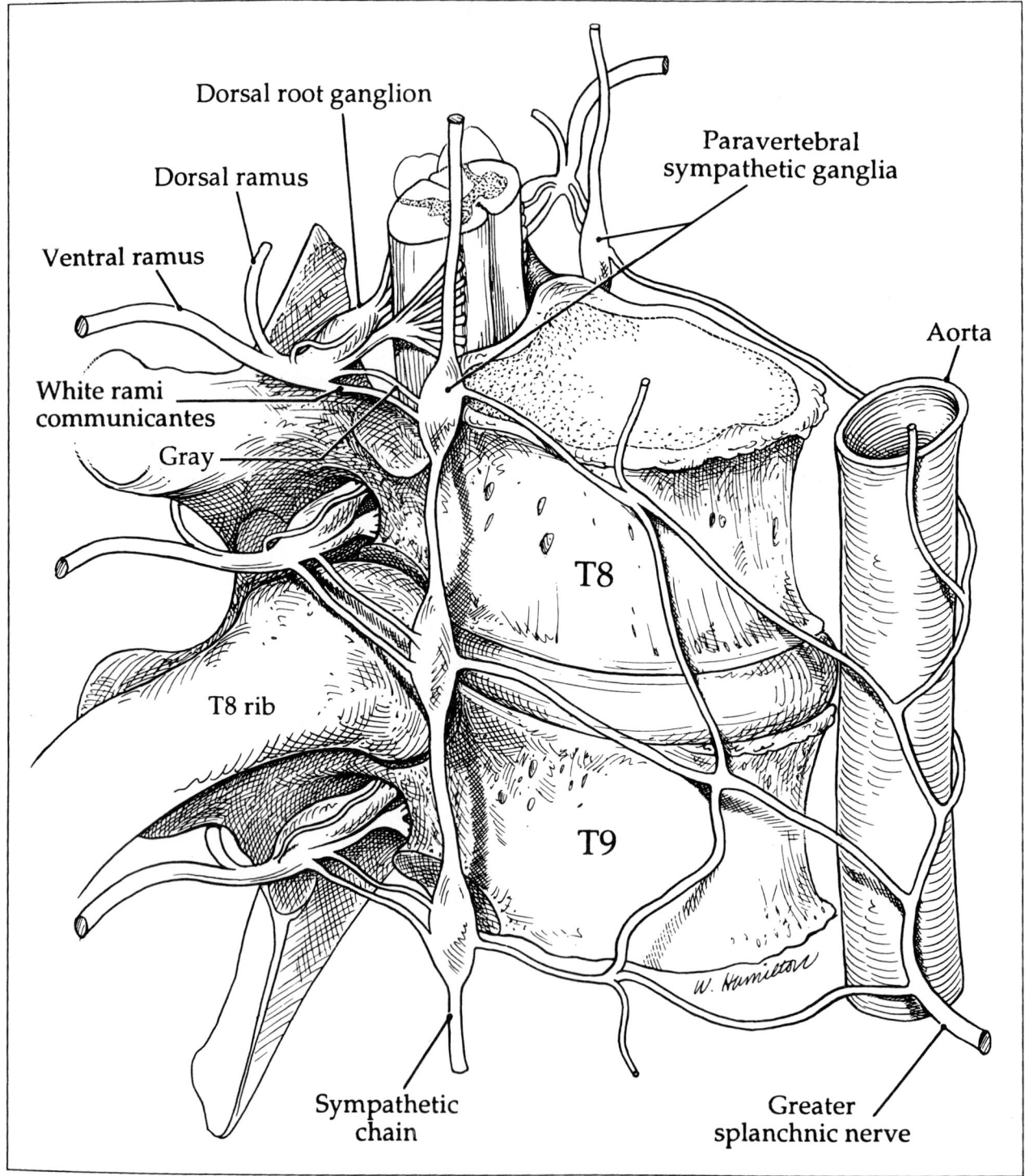

FIGURE 26-6 Nerve supply of the thoracic region. (Reproduced with permission from Harati Y. Anatomy of the spinal and peripheral autonomic nervous system. In: Low PA, ed. *Clinical Autonomic Disorders: Evaluation and Management.* Boston, Mass: Little, Brown; 1997:21.)

area of its surrounding spinal canal than do the cervical or lumbar sections of the spinal cord, and the thoracic cord is tightly packed in the canal and easily injured by displaced fragments of bone or disk material.[39a] Furthermore, the blood supply of the midthoracic spinal cord is tenuous. Thus, seemingly trivial injuries can disrupt the blood supply to a substantial portion of the thoracic cord, resulting in devastating neurologic deficits.[39b]

In the thoracic region, there is great variability in the topography of the nerves and the structures that they serve (Fig. 26-6).[40] Typically, the spinal root arises from the lateral end of the spinal nerve but, in 25 percent of cases, the spinal root is made up of two parts that arise from the superior border of the spinal nerve.[41] The thoracic spinal nerves are segmented into dorsal primary and ventral primary divisions (see Chap. 2). As elsewhere, the dermatomes of this region are considered to represent the cutaneous region innervated by one spinal nerve through both of its rami.[42]

The ventral rami (anterior branches) from T2 through T11 become intercostal nerves. The intercostal nerves supply the intercostal muscles, the costotransverse joints, the parietal pleura, and the body wall of the thorax and part of the abdomen. The ventral rami above T2 and below T11 form the somatic plexuses that innervate the extremities (Fig. 26-6). (The anterior primary ramus innervates the skin [dermatome], muscles [myotome], and bone [sclerotome] of the extremities, the anterolateral trunk, and the neck via its lateral and anterior branches).

The distribution of all dorsal rami is similar. The branches of these rami supply the skin of the medial two thirds of the back and neck, the deep muscles of the back and neck (lateral branches), the zygapophysial joints (medial branches),[43] and the ligamentum flavum.

The peripheral nerves, which travel through the thoracic spine and chest wall, include the dorsal scapular, thoracodorsal, and long thoracic nerves (see Chap. 2).

Biomechanics

The thoracic spinal segments possess the potential for a unique array of movements. However, there is very little agreement in the literature with regard to the biomechanics of the thoracic spine, and most of the current understanding is based largely on the ex vivo studies of White[10] and Panjabi and colleagues[44,45] as well as a variety of so-called clinical models.[15,46]

It can be assumed that, because of the modifying influence of the cagelike structure of the ribs and the kyphotic shape of the curve, the biomechanics of the thoracic spine are considerably different from those of the lumbar and cervical regions. The rib cage and its articulations provide a significant degree of stability. Andriacchi[22] performed a computer simulation analysis to determine the effect of the rib cage on the stiffness properties of the normal spine during flexion, extension, side bending, and axial rotation, and found them to be greatly enhanced by the presence of the rib cage for all four motions, especially extension. This increased stability and reduced mobility of the thoracic segments has been reported to produce three primary effects[11,47]:

1. It influences the motions available in other regions of the spine and in the shoulder girdle.

2. It increases the potential for postural impairments in this region.[48]

3. It provides an important weight-bearing mechanism for the vertebral column.[49] The load-bearing capacity of the spine has been found to be up to three times greater with an intact rib cage.[22,50]

Other biomechanical studies have investigated the effects of anterior and posterior sequential destabilization conditions on functional unit mechanics.[50a,50b] Using dog cadavers, the earlier studies concluded that the costovertebral joints play an important role in providing stability to the thoracic spine, especially under side bending and axial rotation loading.[50a,50b] However, because of the anatomic differences between human and dog spines, these studies were of limited value. A more recent in vitro study by Oda and colleagues[50c] investigated the biomechanical properties of the human thoracic spine, The purpose of this study was to indicate the mechanical significance of the anterior and posterior stabilizers, and to compare the effects of sequential destabilization conditions on functional unit mechanics. Sixteen functional spinal units with intact costovertebral joints were obtained from six human cadavers and randomized into two groups based on destabilization procedures: group 1, anterior-to-posterior sequential resection; and group 2, posterior-to-anterior sequential destabilization. The following destabilization procedure was performed in group 1: (1) total diskectomy and transection of the anteroposterior longitudinal ligaments, preserving the bilateral rib head joints (disk); (2) resection of the right rib head joint, including radiate and intra-articular ligaments; (3) removal of the right costotransverse joint, including costotransverse and superior costotransverse ligaments; and (4) resection of the left rib head joint. For group 2, the following destabilization procedure was performed: (1) laminectomy combined with bilateral medial facetectomy at the medial margin of the pedicles, (2) bilateral total facetectomy, (3) resection of the right costovertebral joint, and (4) removal of the left costovertebral joint. The costovertebral joint was defined as the costotransverse joint and rib head joint.

Biomechanical testing was performed after each destabilization procedure, and the range of motion under maximum load was calculated. The following conclusions were made from this study:

▶ The intervertebral disk can be regarded as the most important stabilizer in the thoracic functional unit mechanics.

▶ The rib head joints serve as stabilizing structures to the human thoracic spine under flexion–extension, side bending, and axial rotation loading, and resection after diskectomy increases range of motion by approximately 80 percent under all loading modes.

▶ The lateral portion of the facet joints plays an important role in providing spinal stability.

▶ In the thoracic spine, total resection of the posterior ligamentous complex leads to an approximately 40 percent increase in range of motion under flexion–extension, side bending, and axial rotation loading.

Flexion

Flexion of the thoracic spine in weight bearing is initiated by the abdominal muscles and, in the absence of resistance, is continued by gravity, with the spinal erector muscles eccentrically controlling the descent. Flexion also may occur during bilateral scapular protraction.

There are about 4 to 5 degrees of flexion available at the upper thoracic levels, 6 to 8 degrees in the middle layers, and 9 to 15 degrees in the lower levels,[10] giving an overall total range for thoracic flexion of 20 to 45 degrees.[51] End-range flexion is resisted by the posterior half of annulus, and by the impaction of the zygapophysial joints.

According to Lee,[16] flexion of the cervicothoracic region consists of an anterior rotation of the head of the rib and a superoanterior glide of the zygapophysial joints, whereas extension and arm elevation in this region consists of a posterior sagittal rotation and posterior translation of the superior vertebra. This latter action pushes the superior aspect of the head of the rib posteriorly at the costovertebral joint, producing a posterior rotation of the rib (the anterior aspect travels superiorly, while the posterior aspect travels inferiorly).[16]

In the remainder of the thorax, flexion results from the superior facets (i.e., the inferior articular processes of the superior vertebra of the segment) gliding superiorly and anteriorly[15] (Table 26-3). This motion at the zygapophysial joint is accompanied by an anterior translation of the superior vertebra, and a slight distraction of the centrum. It seems likely that the anterior vertebral translation produces a similar motion in the ribs, with a superior glide occurring at the costotransverse joint (Fig. 26-7). During this motion, the anterior aspects of the ribs approximate each other, while the posterior aspects separate.

Studies have shown that the thoracic zygapophysial facets play an important role in stabilization of the thoracic spine during flexion loading.[44,52]

Extension

Extension of the thoracic spine is produced principally by the lumbar extensors and results in an inferior glide of the superior facet of the zygapophysial joint (see Table 26-3). One to 2 degrees of extension is available at each thoracic segment, giving an overall average of 15 to 20 degrees of thoracic extension for the entire thoracic spine.

Extension of the thoracic spine is restrained by the relative stiffness of the anterior intervertebral disk; the anterior longitudinal ligament; bony contact of the posterior elements, including the inferior facet onto the lamina below; and the spinous processes.[11,44] Given the location of the axis of rotation for extension, which is close to the moving segment, more translation than rotation occurs during extension.[53]

The joint motions occurring with extension are essentially the opposite of those of flexion. The translation of the vertebra occurs in a posterior direction, with an accompanying slight compression of the centra. The posterior translation that occurs with extension is controlled by the posteriorly directed lamellae of the annulus, and by the capsule of the zygapophysial joint.

FIGURE 26-7 The osteokinematic and arthrokinematic motion proposed to occur during forward bending. (Reproduced with permission from Lee DG. *Manual Therapy for the Thorax—A Biomechanical Approach.* Delta, Canada: Delta Orthopedic Physiotherapy Clinic; 1994:27.)

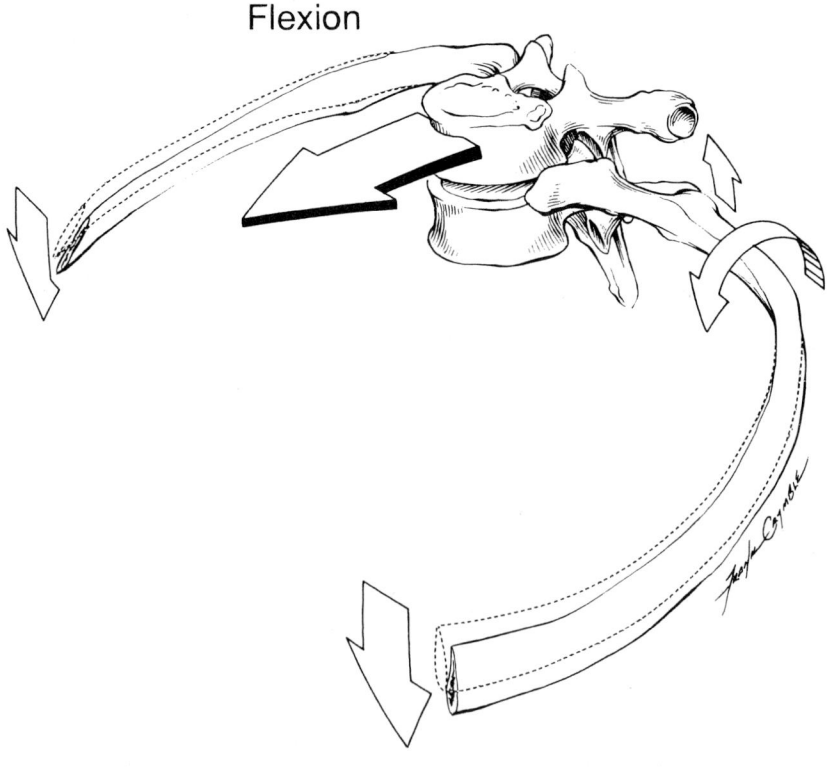

Flexion

TABLE 26-3 Biomechanics of the Thorax

Vertebromanubrial (T1–2)			
Motions	Z Joint	Rib Motion	Costotransverse Joint
Flexion	Superoanterior glide	Anterior rotation	NA
Extension	Inferoposterior glide	Posterior rotation	NA
Latexion	Ipsilateral coupling	NA	NA
Rotexion	Ipsilateral coupling	NA	NA
Inspiration	NA	Elevation	NA
Expiration	NA	Depression	NA

Vertebrosternal (T3–7)			
Motions	Z Joint	Rib Motion	Costotransverse Joint
Flexion	Superoanterior glide	Varies (very mobile) antero-posterior rotation	Superior-inferior glide (varies)
Extension	Posteroinferior glide	Varies (very mobile) antero-posterior rotation	Superior-inferior glide (varies)
Latexion	Ipsilateral sidebend and contralateral rotation	Ipsilateral—anterior rotation, Contralateral—posterior rotation	Ipsilateral—superior glide Contralateral—inferior glide
Rotexion	Ipsilateral sidebend and ipsilateral rotation	Ipsilateral—posterior rotation Contralateral—anterior rotation	Ipsilateral—inferior glide Contralateral—superior glide
Inspiration	NA	Posterior rotation bilaterally	Inferior glide
Expiration	NA	Anterior rotation bilaterally	Superior glide

Vertebrochonral (T8–10)			
Motions	Z Joint	Rib Rotation	Costotransverse Joint
Flexion	Superoanterior glide	Anterior rotation	Superior medial posterior (SMP) glide
Extension	Inferoposterior glide	Posterior rotation	Inferior lateral anterior (ILA) glide
Latexion	Varies	NA	Apex in line with trochanter Ipsilateral—SMP Contralateral—ILA If not, the reverse occurs
Rotexion	Ipsilateral—inferior glide Contralateral—superior glide	NA	Ipsilateral—ILA then anteromedial Contralateral—SMP then posterolateral glide
Inspiration	NA	NA	Inferior lateral anterior (ILA) glide
Expiration	NA	NA	Superior medial posterior (SMP) glide

NA, not applicable.

The transitional region between the thoracic and lumbar spine can produce an inflexion point that may serve to reduce the bending forces in the sagittal plane.[3] However, stiffness in this area also may result in the thoracic spine pivoting over the thoracolumbar region, thereby increasing the risk of compression fracture.[54]

In addition to those motions occurring at the zygapophysial joints and the vertebral body during thoracic extension, motion also occurs at the rib articulations. The ribs rotate posteriorly, with the posterior aspects approximating and the anterior aspects separating, and an inferior glide occurs at the costotransverse joint.[16]

Side Bending

Side bending of the thoracic spine is initiated by the ipsilateral abdominals and erector muscles, and then continued by gravity. A total of 25 to 45 degrees of side bending is available in the thoracic spine, at an average of about 3 to 4 degrees to each side per segment, with the lower segments averaging slightly more, at 7 to 9 degrees, each.[10,55]

At the zygapophysial joints, the primary motion involves the ipsilateral superior facet gliding inferiorly, and the contralateral gliding superiorly (see Table 26-3). In effect, the ipsilateral zygapophysial joint extends while the contralateral flexes. Side bending is restrained by the compression of the intervertebral disk and approximation of the ribs.

Side bending in the upper thoracic spine is associated with ipsilateral rotation and ipsilateral translation.[56] According to Lee,[16] the coupling that occurs in the rest of the thoracic spine depends on which of the two coupling motions initiates the movement. If side bending initiates the movement, it is called *latexion,* and the biomechanics consist of side bending, contralateral rotation, and ipsilateral translation. The mechanism of this coupling, or actually tripling, is not certain, and one must guard against strong conclusions. The postulated mechanism is as follows: With side bending, a contralateral convex curve is produced. This causes the ribs on the convex side of the curve to separate and those on the concave side to approximate.[16] Trunk side bending is essentially halted, by soft tissue tension or rib approximation, or both, and the ribs become fixed. Further side bending is modified by the fixed ribs.[16] The ipsilateral articular facet of the transverse process glides inferiorly on its rib, resulting in a relative anterior rotation of the neck of the rib, while the contralateral transverse process glides superiorly, producing a posterior rotation of the rib neck[16] (Fig. 26-8). The effect of these bilateral rib rotations is to force the superior vertebra into rotation away from the direction of side bending.

Rotation

Axial rotation (rotexion) is produced either by the abdominal muscles and other trunk rotators, or by unilateral elevation of the arm. Pure axial rotation (twisting) can only occur at two points in the spine: at the thoracolumbar and cervicothoracic junctions. The axis of rotation lies within the vertebral body in the midthoracic joints, but anterior to the vertebral body in the upper and lower joints.[57] Almost pure rotation can occur in the midthoracic region, whereas, in the upper and lower segments, rotation can be associated with side bending to either side (see Table 26-3).

A total of 35 to 50 degrees of rotation is available in the thoracic spine.[10,55] Segmental axial rotation in the thoracic spine averages 7 degrees in the upper thoracic area, about 5 degrees in the middle thoracic spine, and 2 to 3 degrees in the last two or three segments.[10,51,58] Torsional stiffness is enhanced in the thoracolumbar region by the mortise-type morphology of the

zygapophysial joints and the near sagittal alignment of the upper lumbar articulations.[11,14,49,54,59]

According to MacConaill and Basmajian,[17] thoracic segmental rotation is coupled with contralateral side bending and contralateral translation. However, this finding deviates from what is generally observed clinically, where the coupling of rotation and side bending that occurs seems to depend on the segmental level and the integrity of the joint.

Respiration

The ribs function as levers, with the fulcrum represented by the rib angle, the effort arm represented by the neck, and the load arm represented by the shaft. Because of the relatively small size of the rib neck, a small movement at the rib neck will produce a large degree of movement in the shaft.

The shapes of the articular facets of the upper six ribs would suggest that the upward and downward gliding movements that occur would produce spinning of the neck of the rib. In fact, the main movement in the upper six ribs during respiration and other movements is one of rotation of the neck of the rib, with only small amounts of superior and inferior motion. In the seventh through tenth ribs, the principal movement is upward, backward, and medially during inspiration, with the reverse occurring during expiration.[15]

Because the anterior end of the ribs is lower than the posterior, when the ribs elevate, they rise upward while the rib neck drops down. In the upper ribs, this results in an anterior elevation (pump handle) and in the middle and lower ribs (excluding the free ribs), a lateral elevation (bucket handle), with the former movement increasing the anteroposterior diameter of the thoracic cavity, and the latter increasing the transverse diameter.

Both kinds of rib motion are produced by the action of the diaphragm. The seventh through tenth ribs act to increase the abdominal cavity free space to afford space for the descending diaphragm. As the ends of these ribs are elevated, they push up on each other, lifting each successive rib upward and finally lifting the sternum. The two lower ribs are depressed by the quadratus lumborum to provide a stable base of action for the diaphragm.

Quiet respiration involves very little zygapophysial joint motion.

Inspiration

During inspiration, the diaphragm descends and pulls the central tendon inferiorly through the fixed 12th ribs and L1 to L3. When the maximum extensibility (distention) of the abdominal wall is reached, the central tendon becomes stationary. Further contraction of the diaphragm produces an elevation and posterior rotation of the lower six ribs, with torsion of the anterior costal cartilage, and an anterosuperior thrust of the sternum (and eventually the inferior aspect of the manubrium).

During inspiration in the normal population, because the second rib is longer than the first, the superior aspect of the manubrium is forced to tilt posteriorly as its inferior edge is moved anteriorly. As the top of the manubrium tilts back, the clavicle rolls anteriorly. Because the lower ribs are longer, the inferior sternum moves further anteriorly than the superior section during

FIGURE 26-8 The osteokinematic and arthrokinematic motion proposed to occur during side bending. (Reproduced with permission from Lee DG. *Manual Therapy for the Thorax—A Biomechanical Approach*. Delta, Canada: Delta Orthopedic Physiotherapy Clinic; 1994:37.)

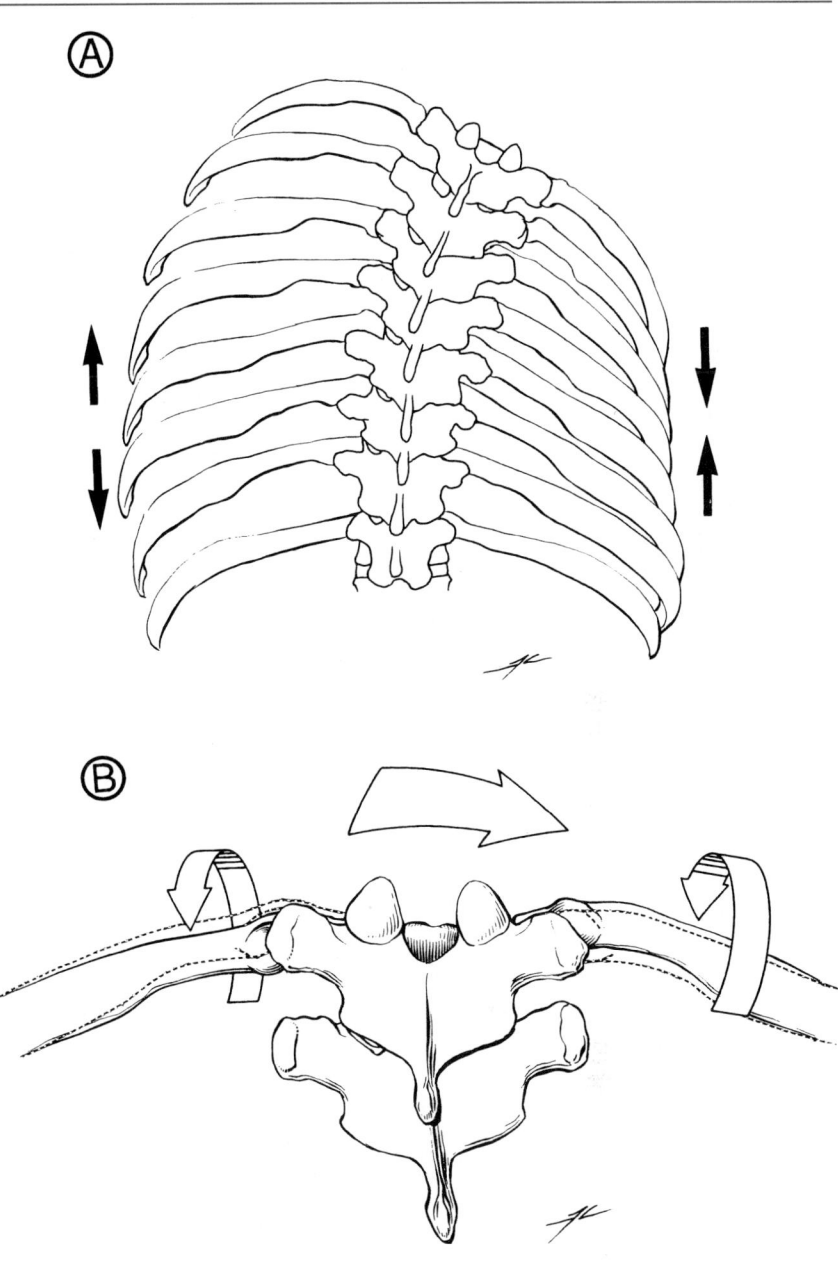

inspiration. The manubriosternal junction acts as the hinge for this motion. If this joint stiffens or ossifies, respiratory function will suffer. In addition, if the central tendon stiffens, inspiration will have to be accomplished with the ribs moving laterally.

Forced inspiration produces an increase in the activity level of the diaphragm, intercostals, scaleni, and quadratus lumborum. In addition, new activity occurs in the sternocleidomastoid, trapezius, both pectorals, and serratus anterior.

During inspiration, the ribs move with the sternum in an upward and forward direction, increasing the anteroposterior diameter of the chest while posteriorly rotating. The tubercles and costotransverse joints of[16]:

▶ T1 through T7 glide inferiorly.

▶ T8 through T10 glide in an anterolateral and inferior direction.

▶ T11 and T12 remain stationary, except for slight caliper motion increasing the lateral dimension.

Expiration

Quiet expiration occurs passively. During forced expiration, there is activity in a number of muscles (Table 26-1). During expiration, the ribs rotate anteriorly and the tubercles and costotransverse joints of[16]:

▶ T1 through T7 glide superiorly.

▶ T8 through T10 glide in a posteromedial and superior direction.

▶ T11 and T12 remain stationary, except for slight caliper motion decreasing the lateral dimension.

TABLE 26-4 Rib Dysfunctions[60]

Dysfunction	Rib Angle	Intercostal Space	Anterior Rib	Thoracic Findings
Anterior subluxation	Less prominent	Tender	More prominent	NA
Posterior subluxation	More prominent	Tender	Less prominent	NA
External rib torsion	Prominent and tender superior border	Wide above, narrow below	NA	ERS, ipsilateral at the level above
Internal rib torsion	Prominent and tender inferior border	Narrow above, wide below	NA	FRS contralateral at the level above

ERS, extended, rotated, and side flexed; FRS, flexed, rotated, and side flexed; NA, not applicable.

It may be possible to detect a subluxation of the costotransverse joints by palpating the ipsilateral transverse process and rib during inspiration and thoracic side bending.[16] For example, a superior subluxation of the right rib may produce:

▶ Decreased inferior glide of the rib.

▶ Decreased thoracic motion in the directions of left side bending and right rotation.

The findings for other rib dysfunctions are outlined in Table 26-4.

Examination

Differential diagnosis of thoracic pain can be difficult, because of the complicated biomechanics and function of the region, the proximity to vital organs, and the many articulations. Bogduk and Valencia[60a] have cited the following anatomical structures as possible causes of thoracic spine pain: posterior thoracic muscles, spinous processes, anterior and posterior longitudinal ligaments, vertebral bodies, zygapophysial and costotransverse joints, inferior articular process, pars interarticularis, intervertebral disk, nerve root, joint meniscus, and dura mater. Pain arising from inflammation of the axial spine can mimic a variety of serious conditions, including cardiac and pulmonary pathology, renal colic, fracture, tumor, or numerous visceral and retroperitoneal abnormalities, including abdominal aortic aneurysm.[60b]

The thoracic spine is less commonly implicated in musculoskeletal pain syndromes than the lumbar and cervical spines, and when it is implicated, there is some disagreement as to whether the ribs or the intervertebral joints are the major source of the biomechanical dysfunction. Complicating matters is the fact that pain arising from the thoracic spinal joints has considerable overlap and can refer symptoms to distal regions (groin, pubis, and lower abdominal wall; see Chap. 9). The pathology and manifestations of thoracic disk herniations are described in Chapter 20. Apart from musculoskeletal lesions, the thoracic spine is also a common source of systemic pain, and the phenomenon of referred pain poses more diagnostic difficulties in the thoracic spine than in any other region of the vertebral column.[60a]

History

The history should include the chief complaints and a pain drawing.

The clinician must determine whether the pain is provoked or alleviated with movement or posture (musculoskeletal pain), respiration (rib dysfunction or pleuritic pain), eating or drinking (gastric pain), or exertion (rib dysfunction or cardiac pain).

Visceral pain tends to be vague and dull, and may be accompanied by nausea and sweating (see Chap. 9). To help differentiate between visceral pain and musculoskeletal pain, the clinician should focus on the relationship of specific movements or activities. Any information regarding the onset, as well as aggravating factors, is important, especially if the pain appears only during certain positions or movements, which would suggest a musculoskeletal lesion. Pulling and pushing activities typically worsen thoracic symptoms. Deep breathing or arm elevation tends to aggravate a rib dysfunction. Aggravation of pain by coughing, sneezing, or deep inspiration tends to implicate the costovertebral joint.[61] Chronic problems in this area tend to result from postural dysfunctions. Pain of a mechanical origin tends to worsen throughout the day but is relieved with rest.

The patient is asked to describe the quality of the pain. Thoracic nerve root pain is often sharp, stabbing, and severe, although it also can have a burning quality. Nerve pain usually is referred in a sloping band along an intercostal space.[62] Vascular pain and visceral pain often are described as being poorly localized and achy. A sudden onset of pain related to trauma could indicate a fracture, muscle strain, or ligament sprain.

> ### Clinical Pearl
>
> Pain from a musculoskeletal lesion in this area can vary from a dull ache to a feeling of local fatigue and cramping. Musculoskeletal pain is usually sharp and well localized, whereas muscle or tendon pain is typically dull and aching. Bone pain usually feels very deep and boring.

The patient should be asked to point to the area of pain. If the patient has difficulty localizing the pain, the clinician should suspect referred pain as the source.

The administration of the Oswestry Low Back Disability Questionnaire, Functional Rating Scale, and McGill Pain Questionnaire may be helpful in determining the quality of pain and its effect on function.[63–65]

Systems Review

Thoracic pain may originate from just about all of the viscera (Table 26-5; see also Chap. 9). Both visceral and somatic afferent nerves transmit pain messages from a peripheral stimulus and converge on the same projection neurons in the dorsal horn.

The thoracolumbar outflow of the autonomic nervous system (see Chap. 2) has its location here. Stimulation of this outflow can lead to the presence of facilitated segments, and trophic changes in the skin of the periphery.[66]

Systemic illnesses, such as rheumatoid arthritis and malignancy, and conditions causing referred pain must be included in the differential diagnosis. Nonmusculoskeletal causes of thoracic pain can include[67]:

▶ Dissecting aortic aneurysm.

▶ Myocardial infarction.

▶ Intercostal neuralgia.

▶ Pleural irritation. When the tissues of an irritated pleura are stretched, chest pain can result. This pain can be increased by breathing, as well as by trunk movements, a situation that could lead the clinician to believe that the problem is musculoskeletal.

▶ Tumor.

▶ Acute thoracic disk herniation (see Chap. 20).

Questions should be asked with regard to bowel and bladder function; upper and lower extremity numbness, tingling, or weakness; and visual or balance disorders. These symptoms may indicate compromise to the spinal cord, cauda equina, or central nervous system.

Questions also must be asked about unexplained weight loss, fever, chills, and night pain. These symptoms often are associated with cancer or systemic disease, although night pain may just be because the patient has an increased, and fixed, kyphosis, and needs a softer bed to accommodate the deformity.[68]

Tests and Measures

Observation

The patient should be suitably disrobed to expose as much of this region as is necessary. As a quick orientation to the relationship of the bony structures (Fig. 26-9), the clinician should confirm the following findings:

▶ The spine of the scapula is level with the spinous process of T3.

▶ The inferior angle of the scapula is in line with the spinous processes of T7 through T9.

▶ The medial border of the scapula is parallel with the spinal column and about 5 cm lateral to the spinous processes.

▶ The iliac crests are level and symmetric. One crest higher than the other could suggest a leg-length discrepancy, an iliac rotation, or both.

▶ The shoulder heights are level. A normal variant is that individuals carry their dominant shoulder slightly lower than the nondominant side.

The clinician also should evaluate the following:

▶ Smoothness of the thoracic curve. By running the palm of the hand down the midline of the patient's thoracic spine, the clinician can determine the smoothness of the

TABLE 26-5 Symptoms and Possible Causes of Thoracic Pain

Indication	Possible Condition
Severe bilateral root pain in elderly	Neoplasm (most common areas for metastasis are lung, breast, prostate, and kidney)
Wedging/compression fracture	Osteoporotic (estrogen deficiency) or neoplastic fracture
Onset-offset of pain unrelated to trunk movements	Ankylosing spondylitis, visceral
Decreased active motion: contralateral side flexion painful, with both rotations full	Neoplasm
Severe chest wall pain without articular pain	Visceral
Spinal cord signs and symptoms	Spinal cord pressure or ischemia
Pain onset related to eating or diet	Visceral

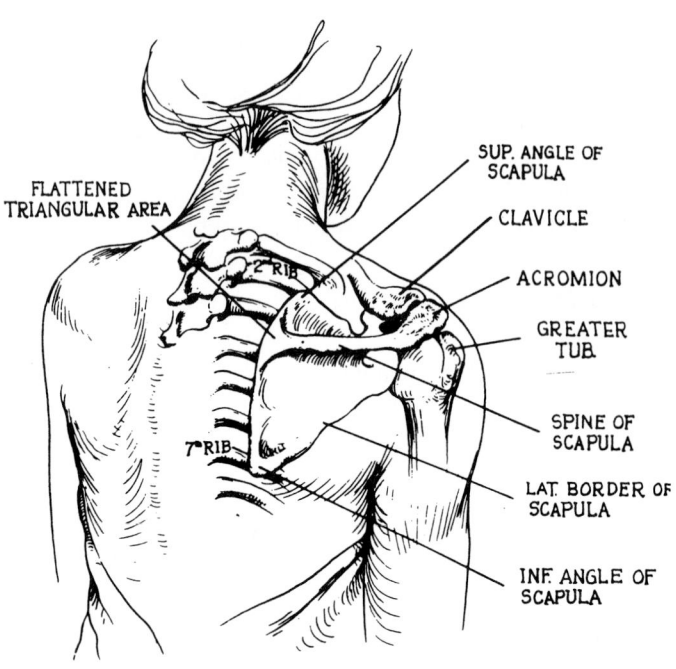

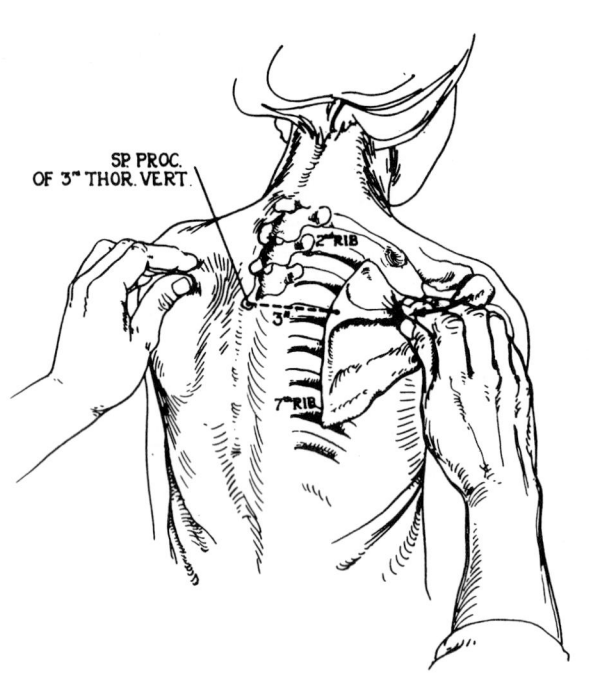

FIGURE 26-9 Palpation landmarks in the thoracic region.

curvature. Any areas of flatness could suggest a vertebral dysfunction such as an opening restriction (ERS lesion), whereas areas of relative increased curvature suggest a closing restriction (FRS lesion); refer to the introduction to Section III.

▶ Degree of thoracic kyphosis. As elsewhere in the spine, posture has an important influence on the available range of motion of the neighboring joints. Conversely, changes in the lumbar posture, such as excessive lordosis, and changes in the cervical spine, such as those rendered by a forward head position, can affect the thoracic spine. The increased lumbar lordosis increases the stresses applied to the thoracolumbar junction, whereas the forward head increases the stresses at the cervicothoracic junction.

The thoracic spine adopts a natural kyphotic curve, which is an increased convexity of the thoracic vertebrae. Varying degrees of kyphosis can occur in the thoracic spine. It is known that the thoracic kyphosis increases with age,[69] and in women more than men.[70] The appearance of increased kyphosis in the young is typically postural, but could be the result of Scheuermann's disease, or ankylosing spondylitis.[11,71] The degree of curvature of the spine also has been found to be diurnal, with a slight flattening of the thoracic kyphosis occurring overnight.[72] Attempts to define the "normal" thoracic kyphosis have demonstrated considerable variation in the asymptomatic population,[48,73] suggesting that any individual differences reflect normal variations rather than deviations.

It has been theorized by a number of authors[74–79] that postural dysfunctions in this region create an imbalance between agonists and antagonists, producing adaptive shortening and weakness. It is likely that these changes are degenerative in nature, resulting from a change in intervertebral disk height. Disk height changes commonly are seen in the upper and midthoracic segments[80] and may result in an alteration of the kyphotic curve, with subsequent compensatory changes in load bearing and movement. These altered load-bearing patterns may result in a compression of the anterior aspect of the thoracic intervertebral disks, and a stretching of the thoracic extensors and the middle and lower trapezius. The posterior ligaments also are lengthened. In addition, the kyphotic posture is associated with adaptive shortening of the anterior longitudinal ligament, the upper abdominals, and the anterior chest muscles. The common kyphotic deformities include[81]:

- *Dowager's hump.* This deformity is characterized by a severely kyphotic upper dorsal region, which results from multiple anterior wedge compression fractures in several vertebrae of the middle to upper thoracic spine, usually caused by postmenopausal osteoporosis or long-term corticosteroid therapy (specificity, 0.99).[82]

- *Hump back.* This deformity is a localized, sharp, posterior angulation, called *gibbus,* produced by an anterior wedging of one of two thoracic vertebra as a result of infection (tuberculosis), fracture, or congenital bony anomaly of the spine.[71]

- *Round back.* This deformity is characterized by decreased pelvic inclination and excessive kyphosis.

- *Flat back.* This deformity is characterized by decreased pelvic inclination, increased kyphosis, and a mobile thoracic spine

▶ *Pelvic heights.* A significant leg-length discrepancy (greater than $1/2$ inch) can alter the lateral curvature of the spine, resulting in compensation.

▶ *Amount of lateral curvature of the thoracic spine.* When observing the thoracic spine, it is important to note the morphologic latitude of the spinal curvature.[83] Two terms, *scoliosis* and *rotoscoliosis,* are used to describe the lateral curvature of the spine. Scoliosis is the older term and refers to an abnormal side bending of the spine, but gives no reference to the coupled rotation that also occurs. Rotoscoliosis is a more detailed definition, used to describe the curve of the spine by detailing how each vertebra is rotated and side flexed in relation to the vertebra below. For example, with a left lumbar convexity, the L5 vertebra would be found to be side flexed to the right and rotated to the left in relation to the sacrum. The same would be true with regard to the relation between L4 and L5. This rotation, toward the convexity, continues in small increments until the apex at L3. L2, which is above the apex, is right rotated and right side-flexed in relation to L3. The small increments of right rotation continue up until the thoracic spine, where the side bending and rotation return to the neutral position.

Scoliosis is never normal, although most cases are idiopathic, manifesting in the preadolescent years.[1,84] An abnormal lateral thoracic curve is described as being structural or functional, and can produce a fixed deformity or a changeable adaptation, respectively, with the rib hump occurring on the convex side of the curve. Persistent scoliosis during forward bending (Adam's sign) is indicative of a structural curve. Structural curves may be genetic, congenital, or idiopathic, producing a structural change to the bone and a loss of spinal flexibility. With a structural scoliosis, the vertebral bodies rotate toward the convexity of the curve, producing a distortion.[85] The distortion in the thoracic spine is called a *rib hump*. The rotation of the vertebral bodies causes the spinous processes to deviate toward the concave side. The curvature results in an adaptive shortening of the intrinsic trunk muscles on the concave side, and lengthening of the intrinsic muscles on the convex side.

The curve patterns are named according to the level of the apex of the curve. For example, a right thoracic curve has a convexity toward the right, and the apex of the curve is in the thoracic spine. There may be a number of curves spanning the thoracic and lumbar region, and the clinician should determine if the curvature is:

- *Contributing to the patient's pain.* Frequently, these curves can be asymptomatic. A slight lateral curve in the coronal plane is thought to result from right-hand dominance, or the presence of the aorta.[86]

- Nonstructural, in which case the patient is able to correct the curves relatively easily.

- Adaptive, resulting from poor posture, nerve root irritation, leg-length discrepancy, atrophy, or hip contracture.

▶ *Chest wall shape.* On the anterior aspect of the thoracic region, the clinician should look for evidence of deformity.

- *Barrel chest.* In this deformity, a forward and upward projecting sternum increases the anteroposterior diameter. The barrel chest results in respiratory difficulty, stretching of the intercostal and anterior chest muscles, and adaptive shortening of the scapular adductor muscles.

- *Pigeon chest.* In this deformity, a forward and downward projecting sternum increases the anteroposterior diameter. The pigeon chest results in a lengthening of the upper abdominal muscles and an adaptive shortening of the upper intercostal muscles.

- *Funnel chest.* In this deformity, a posterior-projecting sternum occurs secondary to an outgrowth of the ribs.[87] The funnel chest results in adaptive shortening of the upper abdominals, shoulder adductors, pectoralis minor, and intercostal muscles, and in lengthening of the thoracic extensors and middle and upper trapezius.

▶ *Motion of the ribs during quiet breathing.*

▶ *Asymmetry in muscle bulk, prominence, or length.* According to Sahrmann,[88] shortness of the rectus abdominis results in anterior rib cage depression, shortness of the internal oblique results in an increase in the infrasternal angle, and shortness of the external oblique results in a decreased angle. Rotatores atrophy could suggest nerve palsy, whereas rotatores hypertonicity could suggest a segmental facilitation.[78,89]

▶ *Any lesions, swellings, or scars on the back and chest.* This is a common area for the characteristic lesion pattern of herpes zoster (shingles), which follows the course of the affected nerve (see Chap. 9).

Gait

The analysis of the patient's gait pattern can provide valuable information as to whether the condition originates in the spine or lower extremities, and discloses gross weakness of the muscles that affect gait[71] (see Chap. 13). For example, a decreased arm swing during gait can indicate stiffness of the thoracic segments.

Palpation

The spinous processes of the thoracic vertebrae are readily palpated (see Fig. 26-9), because they are not covered by muscle or thick connective tissue.[71] The landmarks outlined in Table 26-6 may be helpful to determine the segmental level involved.

The spinous processes have varying degrees of obliquity, and if they are used as landmarks, this obliquity must be understood and exploited.

TABLE 26-6   Anterior and Posterior Palpation Points of the Thoracic Region

Anterior Aspect	Posterior Aspect
Suprasternal notch	Spinous and associated transverse processes
Manubriosternal angle	T2—level with base of spine of scapula
Xiphoid process	Spinal gutter (rotatores)
Infrasternal angle	Erector spinae
Sternochondral junctions	Rib angles
Costal cartilage	Rib shafts Rib shafts and rib joint line of costotransverse joint C6—locate largest spinous process at base of neck, and have patient extend neck; first spinous process to move anteriorly under your finger is C6

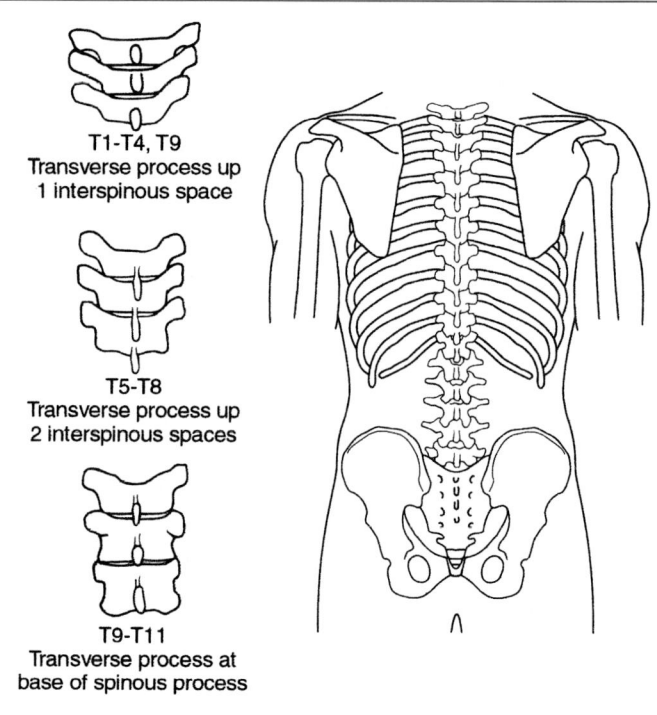

FIGURE 26-10   The rule of three. (Reproduced with permission from Dutton M. *Manual Therapy of the Spine.* New York, NY: McGraw-Hill; 2002:420.)

Clinical Pearl

The areas of spinous process obliquity may be divided into four regions by the so-called rule of three[90] (Fig. 26-10).

- First group of three spinous processes (T1–3). These spinous processes are level with vertebral body of the same level.
- Second group of three spinous processes (T4–6). These spinous processes are level with the disk of the inferior level. This can be estimated at about 3 fingerbreadths.
- Third group of three spinous processes (T7–9). These spinous processes are level with the vertebral body of the level below.
- The fourth group of three spinous processes reverses the obliquity:
  - T10 is level with the vertebral body of the vertebra below (same as T7–9).
  - T11 is level with the disk of the inferior vertebra (same as T6).
  - T12 is level with its own vertebral body (same as T3).

The first rib is located 45 degrees medially to the junction of the posterior scalene and trapezius (see Fig. 26-9). Palpation of the first rib during respiration can detect the presence of asymmetry. Palpation of the first rib also can be performed during testing of the active motions of cervical rotation and side bending in patients with suspected brachialgia. The clinician

passively rotates the patient's cervical spine away from the involved side. From this position, the neck is side bent as far as is comfortable, moving the ear to the chest (Fig. 26-11). A restriction occurring in the second part of the test indicates a positive test for brachialgia. This test has been found to have excellent

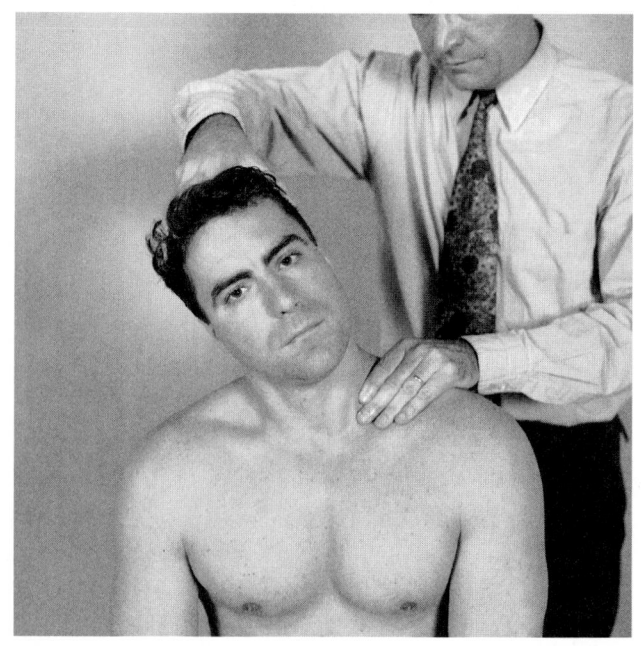

FIGURE 26-11   First rib test.

interrater reliability (κ = 1.0) and good agreement, with cineradiographic findings (κ = 0.84).

The transverse processes are roughly level with their own body. The costal cartilages of the second rib articulate with the junction between the sternum and manubrium (Fig. 26-12).

Palpation of the soft tissues of the region is important. The clinician should note the presence of any tenderness, temperature changes, and muscle spasm. A comparison should be made between the firmness and tenderness of the paravertebral muscles, and their relationship from side to side.

Screening Tests

A few simple screening tests can help differentiate between a rib dysfunction and a thoracic joint dysfunction.

Rib Spring Test. The patient is positioned prone, and the clinician stands on one side of the patient. Reaching over the patient, the clinician spreads the length of the thumb over the right rib in question and applies a posteroanterior force (Fig. 26-13). This is the equivalent of a left rotation of the thoracic spine. The clinician then repeats the posteroanterior force on the rib, except this time, the rotation of the thoracic spine is blocked by the clinician placing the ulnar border of the other hand over a group of left transverse processes (Fig. 22-14). Pain produced with this maneuver implicates the rib, because the thoracic spine is stabilized.

Thoracic Spring Test. The patient is positioned as previously. Spring testing in a posteroanterior direction is applied using the palm of the hand, with the elbows locked over the spinous processes of the thoracic spine (Fig. 26-14). These spring tests

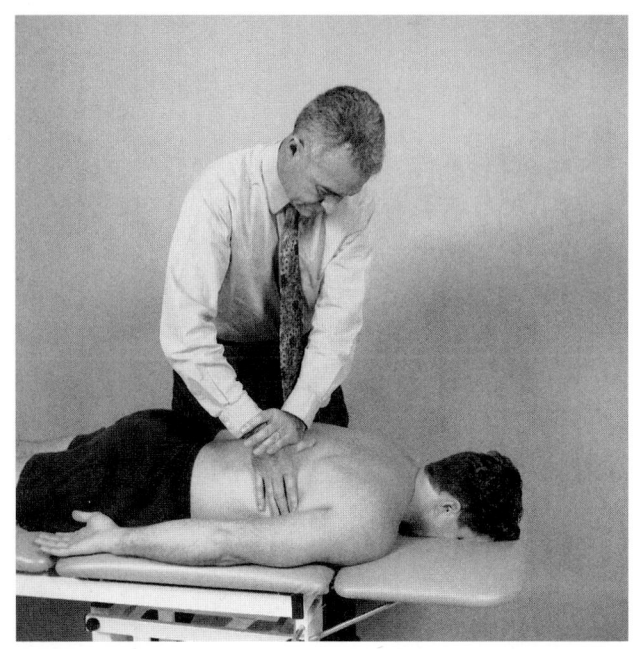

FIGURE 26-13 Rib springing.

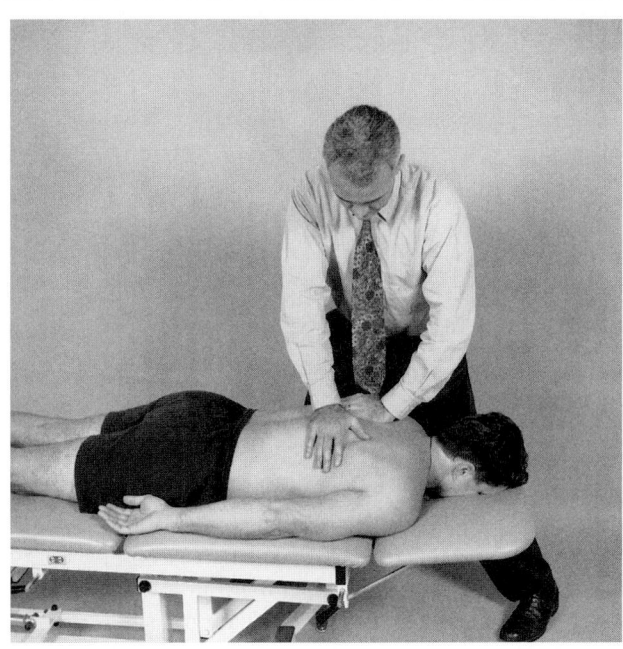

FIGURE 26-14 Rib springing with thoracic motion blocked.

are provocative for pain but also may be used for a gross assessment of mobility.

Reflex Hammer Test. The patient is sitting, and the clinician uses a reflex hammer to tap over each spinous process (Fig. 26-15). If tenderness is encountered, especially in a patient with a history of trauma to the area, a fracture must be ruled out.

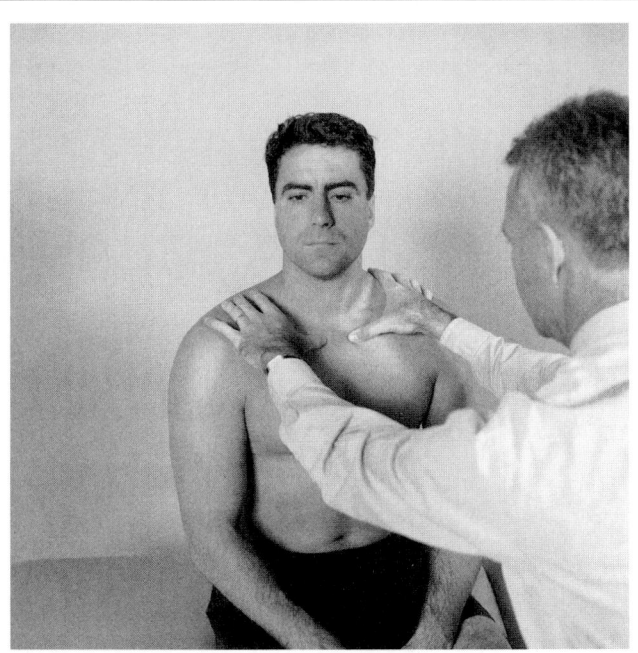

FIGURE 26-12 Palpation of the manubriosternal junction.

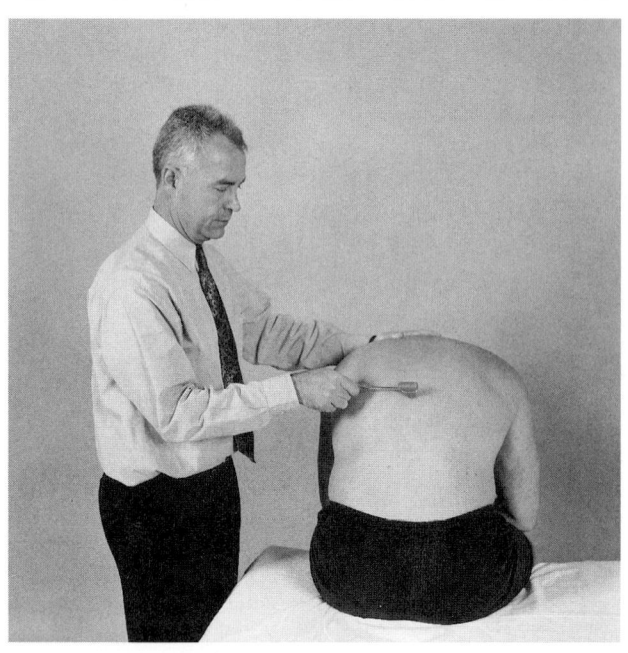

FIGURE 26-15   Reflex hammer test.

Neck Flexion.   The patient is seated and is asked to fully flex the neck. Neck flexion in this position stretches the dura of the cervical and thoracic regions. Pain with neck flexion may suggest a diagnosis such as dural irritation or meningitis.

Chest Expansion Measurement.   Ankylosing spondylitis is a disease that can produce an ossification of the anterior longitudinal ligament, the thoracic disk, and the thoracic zygapophysial joints. Findings of ankylosing spondylitis are common in the thoracic region, making chest expansion measurements a requirement in this region. Decreased expansion can highlight the presence of ankylosing spondylitis, but also may be the result of diaphragm palsy (C4), intercostal weakness, pulmonary (pleura) problems, old age, a rib fracture, or a chronic lung condition. Respiratory excursion is measured at three levels using a tape measure placed circumferentially around the chest at the level of the axilla, the xiphoid level, and the tenth rib level. Comparisons are made between the measurements taken at the position of maximum expiration and the measurement taken at full inspiration. The normal difference between inspiration and expiration is 3 to 7.5 cm (1 to 3 in).[91]

T1 to T2 Dural Stretch.   The patient is seated and is asked to protract and retract the shoulders. Scapular approximation pulls on the thoracic extent of the dura mater via the first and second thoracic nerves.[71] A positive response of symptom reproduction should lead the clinician to suspect an upper thoracic disk protrusion, or a space-occupying lesion, such as a tumor.[23]

Deep Breathing and Flexion.   This test can be used for patients who complain of pain with thoracic flexion. The patient is

seated with the thoracic spine positioned in neutral. The patient is asked to inhale fully and then to flex the thoracic spine until the pain is felt. At this point, the patient maintains the position of flexion and slowly exhales. If further flexion can be achieved after exhalation, the source of the pain is likely to be the ribs rather than the thoracic spine.[92]

Active Motion Testing

Active range-of-motion tests are used to determine the osteokinematic function of two adjacent thoracic vertebrae during active motions, to identify which joints are dysfunctional, as well as the specific direction of motion loss.[93] Active range of motion initially is performed globally, looking for abnormalities, such as asymmetric limitations of motion. A specific examination is then performed on any region that appears to have either excessive or reduced motion. If the history indicated that the patient's symptoms were altered with repetitive motions or sustained positions, these movements and postures should be included. Various techniques are used to correctly assess each area of the thoracic spine.

Movement restriction of the upper thoracic spine may be secondary to pain or a result of adaptive shortening of connective tissue or muscle.[1] Because of the relationship that the first two ribs share with the zygapophysial joints as part of the manubrial ring, associated movement dysfunction of these ribs is common. Physiologic movement in the thoracic spine decreases with age. Midthoracic hypomobilities are the most common thoracic presentation,[94] with the movement restrictions being more common in the sagittal and frontal planes, particularly extension and side bending.[1] Most of the trunk rotation below the level of C2 occurs in the thoracic spine.

The clinician should look for capsular or noncapsular patterns of restriction, pain, or painful weakness (possible fracture or neoplasm). The capsular pattern of the thoracic spine appears to be symmetric limitation of rotation and side bending, extension loss, and least loss of flexion. Joint capsular lesions demonstrate a capsular pattern as equal and grossly severe limitation of movement in every direction.[71] With an asymmetric impairment, such as trauma, the capsular pattern appears to be an asymmetric limitation of rotation and side bending, extension loss, and a lesser loss of flexion.

Overpressure applied at the end of the available range of motion is used to take the joint from its physiologic barrier to its anatomic barrier. During overpressure, an increase in resistance to motion should be felt. The end-feels should be noted.

▶ If the normal elastic end-feel of thoracic rotation is replaced by a stiffer one, it may indicate the presence of osteoporosis or ankylosing spondylitis.

▶ During forward flexion, the nonstructural scoliosis disappears, whereas the structural scoliosis does not.

▶ If side bending is more seriously affected than rotation, neoplastic disease of the viscera or chest wall may be present.[68]

▶ If, during side bending, the ipsilateral paraspinal muscles demonstrate a contracture (Forestier's bowstring sign), ankylosing spondylitis may be present.[95]

▶ Side bending away from the painful side, which is the only painful and limited movement, almost always indicates a severe extra-articular impairment, such as a pulmonary or abdominal tumor or a spinal neurofibroma. The functional examination normally confirms the patient history.

▶ A marked restriction of motion in a noncapsular pattern with one or more spasmodic end-feels could indicate a thoracic disk herniation.

▶ Anterior or lateral pain with resisted thoracic rotation could indicate a muscle tear. Localized pain with resisted testing could indicate a rib fracture.

Because of the length of the spine in this region, it is important to ensure that all parts of the thoracic spine are involved in the range-of-motion testing. Motion in the thoracic spine requires a synchronous movement between the intervertebral and zygapophysial joints, and the rib articulations. Thus, the presence of joint dysfunction or degeneration, or structural changes in the spinal curvature, will influence the amount of available range of motion, and the pattern of these coupled motions.[11]

Clinical Pearl

It is important to remember that maximum arm elevation requires motion in the upper thoracic segments.

The inclinometer techniques recommended by the American Medical Association are used to objectively measure thoracic motion.[96]

Flexion (Fig. 26-16). To measure thoracic flexion, two inclinometers are used and are aligned in the sagittal plane. The center of the first inclinometer is placed over the T1 spinous process. The center of the second one is placed over the T12 spinous process. The patient is asked to slump forward as though trying to place the forehead on the knees, and both inclinometer angles are recorded. The thoracic flexion angle is calculated by subtracting the T12 from the T1 inclinometer angle. The patient should be able to flex approximately 20 to 45 degrees.[51,93] The clinician observes for any paravertebral fullness during flexion, which might indicate hypertonus from a facilitated segment. The thoracic spine during flexion should curve forward in a smooth and even manner. There should be no evidence of segmental rotation or side bending. To decrease pelvic and hip movements, McKenzie advocates examining thoracic flexion with the patient seated.[97]

Extension. The clinician places one hand and arm across the upper chest region of the patient, and the other hand over the spinous processes of the lower thoracic spine. The patient is guided into a backward slump (Fig. 26-17). Overpressure is applied by the arm across the front of the patient, while avoiding any anterior translation occurring at the lumbar spine.

Thoracic extension may be measured using the same technique and inclinometer positions as described for flexion. The

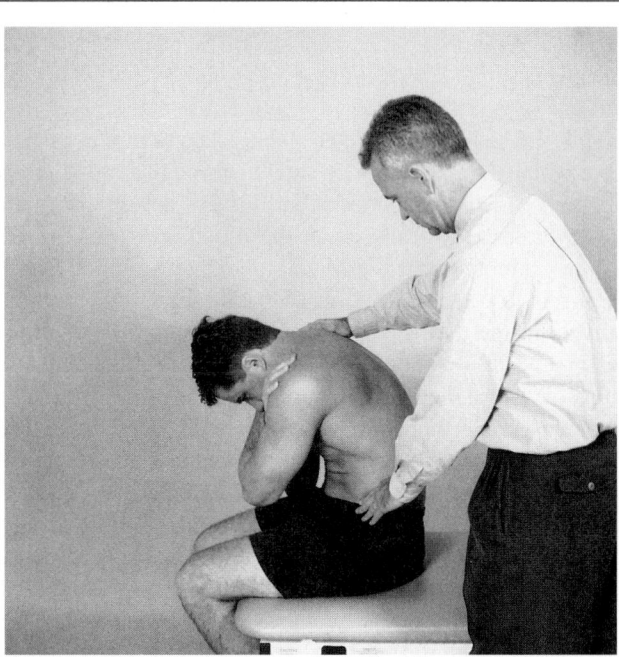

FIGURE 26-16 Active thoracic flexion.

thoracic extension angle is calculated by subtracting the T12 from the T1 inclinometer angle. The patient should be able to extend approximately 15 to 20 degrees.[93] Alternatively, thoracic extension can be measured using a tape measure. The distance between two points (the C7 and T12 spinous processes) is measured. A 2.5-cm difference between neutral and extension measurements is considered normal.[95,98] During

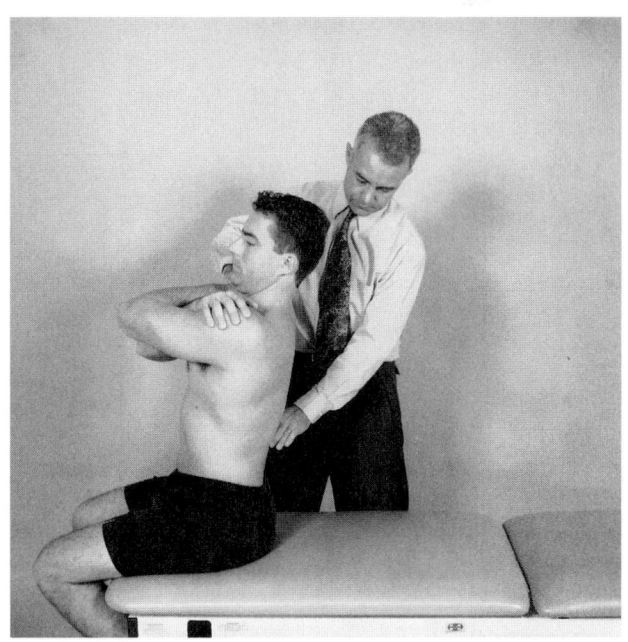

FIGURE 26-17 Active thoracic extension.

thoracic extension, the thoracic curve should curve backward or straighten. As with flexion, there should be no evidence of segmental rotation or side bending.

Rotation.   The patient is seated and is asked to turn to each side at the waist. Overpressure is applied through both shoulders (Fig. 26-18). This motion tests the ability of the ribs and the superior vertebrae to translate in the direction opposite to the rotation—a motion that is essential if complete rotation and side bending is to occur. A total of 35 to 50 degrees of rotation is available in the thoracic spine.[10,55] Active thoracic rotation of 20 degrees or less results in an impairment of function during activities of daily living involving the thoracic spine.[95] Pavelka[99] devised a simple objective clinical method to measure thoracolumbar rotation using a tape measure that can be used to detect asymmetries in rotation. The tape is placed over the L5 spinous process and over the jugular notch on the superior aspect of the manubrium. A measurement is taken before and after full trunk rotation. The measurements from each side are then compared.

Side Bending.   A total of 25 to 45 degrees of side bending is available in the thoracic spine.[10,55] Using a hand placed against the patient's side, the patient is asked to side bend over the clinician's hand. Overpressure is applied through the contralateral shoulder to avoid compression (Fig. 26-19). Side bending can be measured objectively using a tape measure.[91] Two ink marks are placed on the skin of the lateral trunk. The upper mark is made at a point where a horizontal line through the xiphisternum crosses the coronal line. The lower mark is made at the highest point on the iliac crest. The distance between the two marks is measured in centimeters with the patient standing erect, and again after full ipsilateral side bending. The second

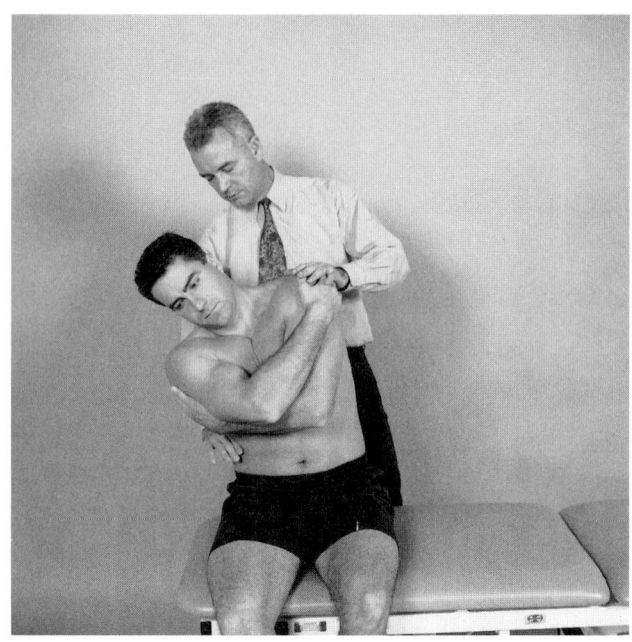

FIGURE 26-19   Active thoracic side bending.

measurement is subtracted from the first and the remainder is taken as an index of lateral spinal mobility.

> ### Clinical Pearl
>
> A finding of painful and limited side bending away from the painful side, with both rotations free from pain, should always create a suspicion of serious lesions.[71]

Inspiration and Expiration.   The motions of the ribs are palpated during breathing. If a rib stops moving in relation to the other ribs during inspiration, it is classified as a *depressed rib*.[90,100] If a rib stops moving in relation to the other ribs during expiration, it is classified as an *elevated rib*.[90,100] Because of the interrelationship of all of the ribs, if a depressed rib is implicated, it is usually the most superior depressed rib that causes the most significant dysfunction. In contrast, if an elevated rib is implicated, it is usually the most inferior restricted rib that causes the most significant dysfunction.[90,100]

Resisted Testing

Resistance applied at the point of overpressure can give the clinician an indication of the integrity of the musculotendinous units of this area. Resistance is applied at the end range of flexion, extension, rotation, and side bending while the clinician looks for pain, weakness, or painful weakness. Pain that is exacerbated with motion, but not with resisted isometric contraction, suggests a ligamentous lesion.[93]

Static Postural Testing

Thoracic pain of a postural origin is difficult to provoke with active motion and resistive testing. McKenzie[97] recommends

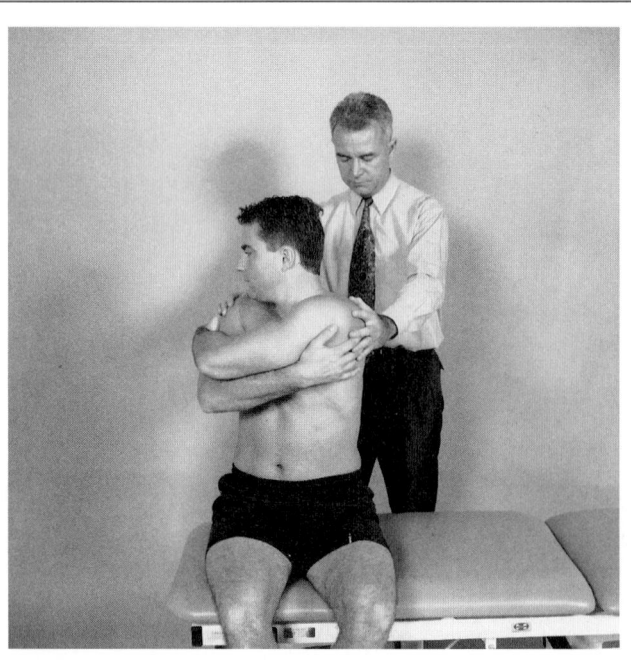

FIGURE 26-18   Active thoracic rotation.

placing the patient in a position for approximately 3 minutes to load the structures sufficiently to provoke postural pain. The following positions are used.

Flexion in Sitting. The patient is positioned so that the thoracic spine is slouched and the back is fully rounded.

Prone Lying. The patient lies in the prone position with the thoracic spine fully extended and the weight supported by the hands. The lower thoracic spine and lumbar spine (T4–5 to L1) are allowed to sag into the treatment table.

Supine Lying in Extension. The patient is positioned supine over the end of the treatment table so that the head, neck, and shoulders are unsupported down to the level of T4. Care must be taken with this maneuver, and it should not be attempted with patients who have a history of cervical pathology, or a history that may indicate the potential for vertebrobasilar artery compromise. This test also can be performed with the patient in the prone on elbows position.

Differing Philosophies

The next stage in the examination process depends on the clinician's background. For clinicians who are heavily influenced by the muscle energy techniques of the osteopaths, position testing is used to determine the segment on which to focus. Other clinicians omit the position tests and proceed to the combined motion and passive physiologic tests.

Position Testing: Spinal. The vertebrae may be tested for positional symmetry. If an ERS or FRS is present, passive mobility testing will definitively diagnose the movement impairment. The upper thoracic joints (C7–T4) can be assessed using the cervical techniques described in Chapter 23. The following techniques can be used for the T4 to T12 levels.

Example: T7 to T8. The patient is positioned sitting, with the clinician standing behind. Using the thumbs, the clinician palpates the transverse processes of the T7 vertebra. The joint is tested in the following manner:

▶ The joint complex is flexed, and an evaluation is made as to the position of the T7 vertebra relative to T8 by noting which transverse process is the most posterior. A posterior left transverse process of T7 relative to T8 is indicative of a left-rotated position of the T7 to T8 complex in flexion.

▶ The joint complex is extended, and an evaluation is made as to the position of the T7 vertebra in relation to T8 by noting which transverse process is the most posterior. A posterior left transverse process of T7 relative to T8 is indicative of a left-rotated position of the T7 to T8 joint complex in extension.

Once a segment has been localized by one of the preceding techniques, the arthrokinematics of the segment can be tested using the following passive mobility tests, which incorporate

specific symmetric or asymmetric motions. Care in the interpretation of the passive mobility tests is important, because local tenderness in the thoracic region is common, especially over the spinous processes as a result of the proximity of the dorsal rami over the apex of these bony prominences.[11,101]

Combined Motion Testing. Normal function involves complex and combined motions of the thoracic spine, combined motion testing can also be used. The motions tested include forward flexion with side bending, extension with side bending, side bending with flexion, and side bending with extension. The results from these motions are combined with the findings from the history and the single plane motions to categorize the symptomatic responses. This information can guide the clinician when determining which motions to use in the intervention.

Passive Mobility Testing. The upper thoracic joints (C7–T4) can be assessed using the cervical techniques described in Chapter 23. The following techniques can be used for the T4 to T12 levels.

Flexion of the Zygapophysial Joints. The patient is seated at the end of the table, with arms folded and hands resting on the shoulders. The clinician stands by the side of the patient and reaches around the front of the patient with one arm and hand. The clinician then applies a slight pressure with the sternum against the patient's shoulder so that the patient is gently squeezed. Using the other hand to monitor intersegmental motion between the spinous processes (Fig. 26-20), the clinician flexes the thoracic spine (Fig. 26-21). The quantity and quality of motion is noted and is compared with the levels above and below.

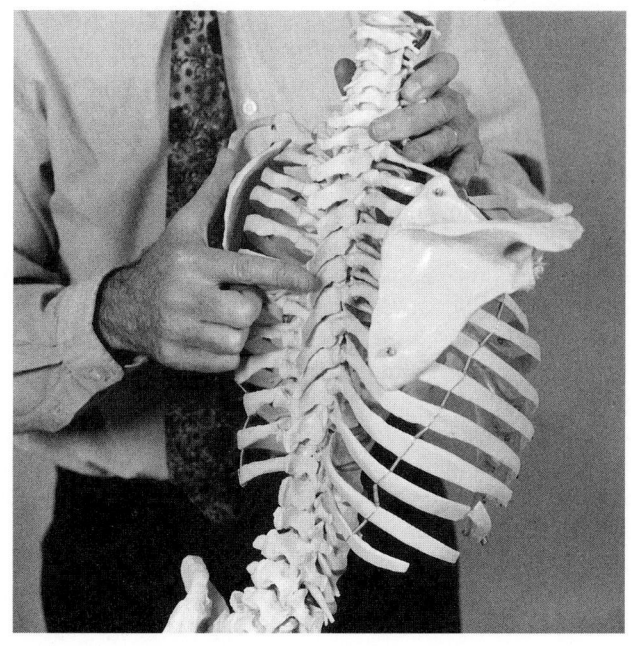

FIGURE 26-20 Intersegmental palpation.

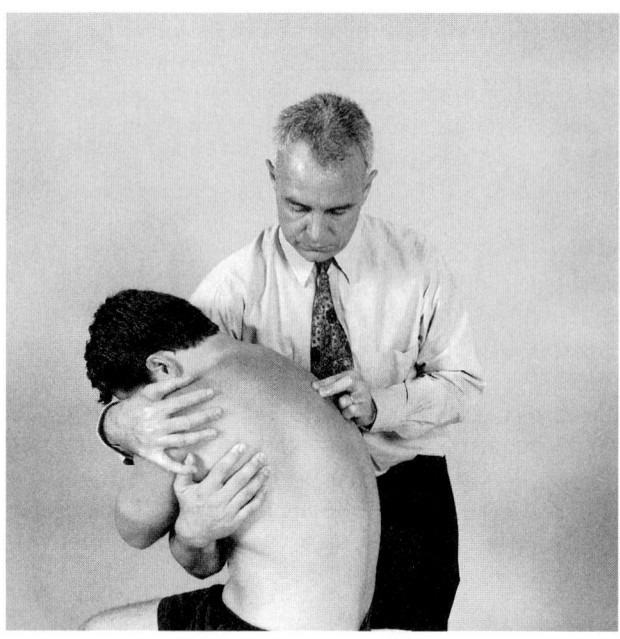

FIGURE 26-21   Passive mobility testing: flexion.

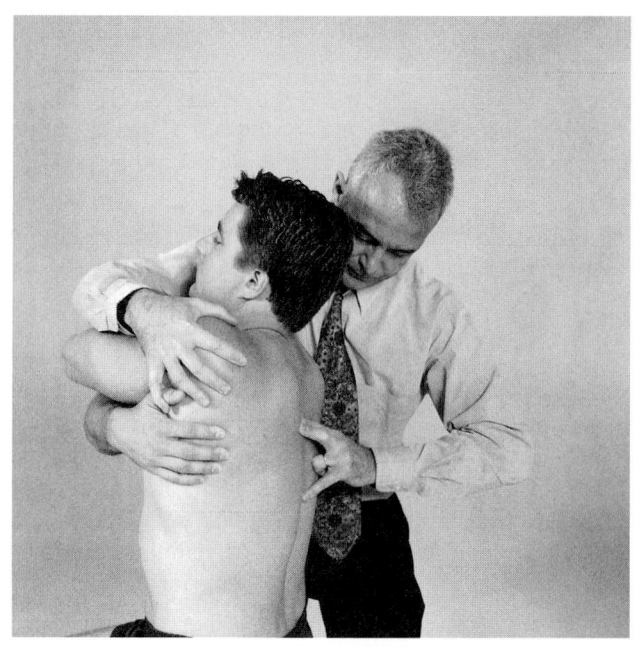

FIGURE 26-22   Passive mobility testing: extension.

Extension of the Zygapophysial Joints.   The patient is seated with the arms folded, one hand on top of the shoulder and the other hand under the opposite axilla. The clinician stands to the side of the patient. While palpating the interspinous spaces or the transverse processes of the level to be tested with one hand, the clinician wraps the other arm around the front of the patient and rests that hand on the patient's contralateral shoulder (Fig. 26-22). Crouching slightly, the clinician then places his or her anterior shoulder region against the lateral aspect of the patient's shoulder. Using the other hand to monitor intersegmental motion between the spinous processes, the clinician extends the thoracic spine (Fig. 26-22). The quantity and quality of motion is noted and compared with the levels above and below.

Combined Motions of the Zygapophysial Joints.   The patient is seated with one hand on top of one of the shoulders and the other hand under the opposite axilla. The clinician stands to the side of the patient. While palpating the interspinous spaces or the transverse processes of each level with one hand, the clinician wraps the other arm around the front of the patient, under the patient's crossed arms, resting his or her hand on the patient's contralateral shoulder. Crouching slightly, the clinician then places the anterior shoulder region against the lateral aspect of the patient's shoulder. Side bending and rotation of the patient's thoracic spine is then performed away from the clinician (Fig. 26-23) as the clinician lifts with his or her body. The palpating hand palpates the concave side of the curve.

Costal Examination.   It is well worth postponing the costal, or rib, examination until after the thoracic spinal joints have been examined and treated, or the testing of these joints has proved negative.

All of the ribs move with complex combinations of what is often described as "pump handle," "bucket handle," or caliper motion. Pump handle (anterior) motion is analogous to flexion-extension, bucket handle (lateral rib) motion is analogous to adduction-abduction, and caliper motion is analogous to internal and external rotation.

The first rib has an equal proportion of pump and bucket handle motion, whereas the sternal ribs have a greater proportion

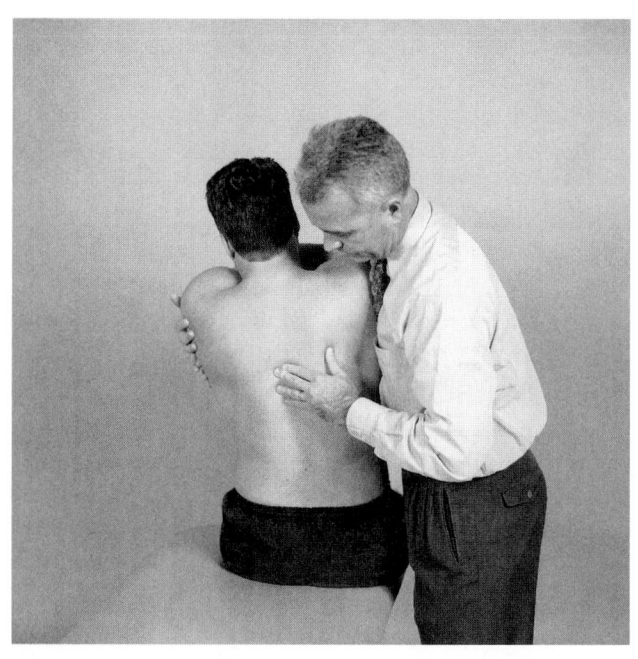

FIGURE 26-23   Passive mobility testing: side bending and rotation.

of pump handle motion. Ribs 8 through 10 have a greater proportion of bucket handle motion.

Manubrium Motion Testing. Cervicothoracic flexion and extension require motion to occur at a number of joints, including the manubriosternal junction, sternoclavicular joints, and manubriocostal junction anteriorly, and the vertebral segments of T1 to T4 and their attachments posteriorly. Theoretically, because of the ringlike structure of the thoracic cage, movements of the manubrium during cervical motion should mimic those of the spine. Thus, palpation of the manubrium (Fig. 26-12) during cervical motions can give the clinician a method of screening for biomechanical dysfunction of the joints that comprise this ring. For example, during cervical extension, the ring complex of T1 should be felt to rotate posteriorly while the manubrium tilts posteriorly. During flexion the converse occurs, with the ring rotating anteriorly and the manubrium tilting anteriorly. During side bending of the cervical spine, the manubrium should be felt to tilt in the same direction as the side bend. Manubrial motion restrictions can be described using the ERS and FRS terminology.

For example, an FRSR (closing) restriction on the left at T1 will produce the following findings at the manubrium when the patient attempts to extend the cervical spine: The ring will rotate to the right, making the left side of the manubrium tilt anteriorly. However, during cervical flexion, no significant deficits should be noted.

In contrast, an ERSL (opening) restriction demonstrates the following findings when the patient attempts to flex the cervical spine: The ring will rotate to the left causing the right side of the manubrium to move anteriorly. However, during cervical extension, no significant deficits should be noted.

The second and third "rings" of the thoracic spine can be assessed in a similar manner.

Manubrial motion also can be assessed during respiration. Under normal circumstances, the manubrium should elevate with inspiration and depress with expiration. In addition, during inspiration, the superior aspect of the manubrium tilts posteriorly, while the inferior aspect moves anteriorly. The process reverses during expiration.

Palpation. Surface landmarks can be used to locate the ribs. The fifth rib passes directly under, or slightly inferior to, the male mammary nipples (see Fig. 26-9). To palpate the rib angles of the interscapular ribs, the shoulders are positioned in horizontal adduction. The rib angles of 3 through 10 can then be felt about 2 to 5 cm lateral to the spinous processes (Fig. 26-24).

When palpating anteriorly, on the sternum, a rib dysfunction will be highlighted by the presence of asymmetry and should be compared with the posterior findings. A prominent rib angle on the back and a depression of that rib at the sternum indicates a posterior subluxation, the reverse occurring in an anterior subluxation, whereas a rib that is prominent both anteriorly and posteriorly indicates a single rib torsion.

Passive Mobility Examination of Ribs 2 Through 10: Bucket and Pump Handle Motion. For rib elevation, the overpressure is

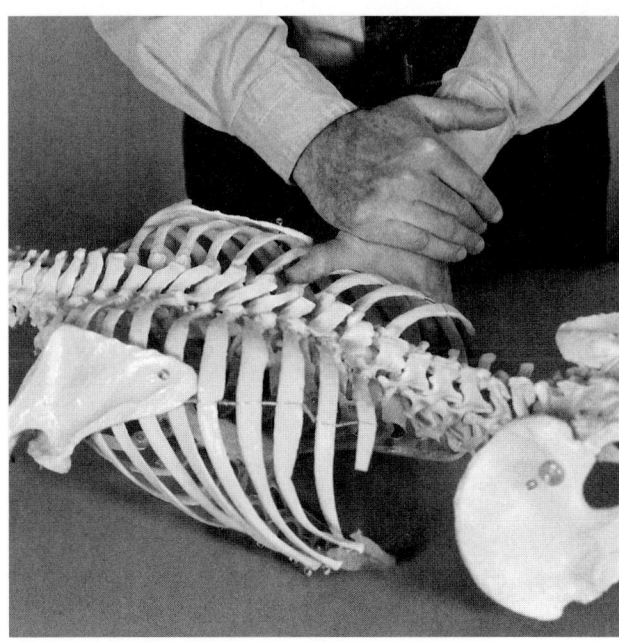

FIGURE 26-24 Palpation of rib angles.

applied by grasping the patient's arm above the elbow and rocking the arm into hyperabduction for the lower ribs (so-called bucket; Fig. 26-25), and flexion for the upper seven ribs (so-called pump; Fig. 26-26).

Neurologic Tests

A neurologic deficit is very difficult to detect in the thoracic spine. In this region, one dermatome may be absent with no loss of sensation.[102]

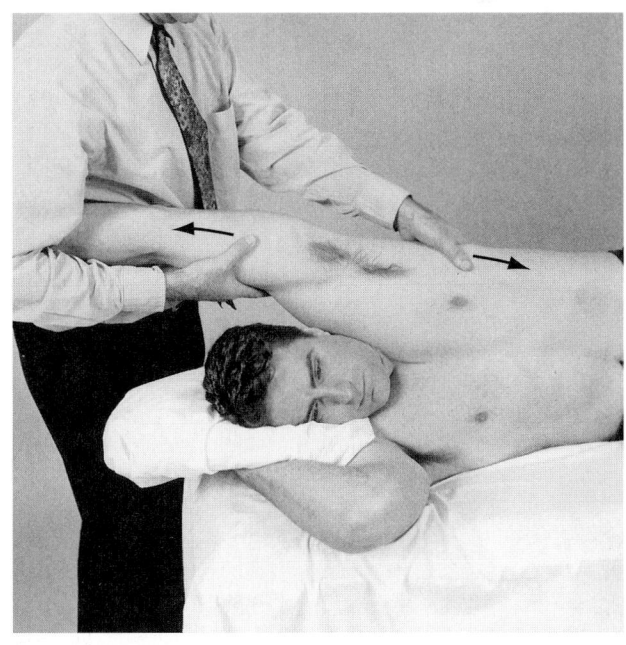

FIGURE 26-25 Bucket handle motion.

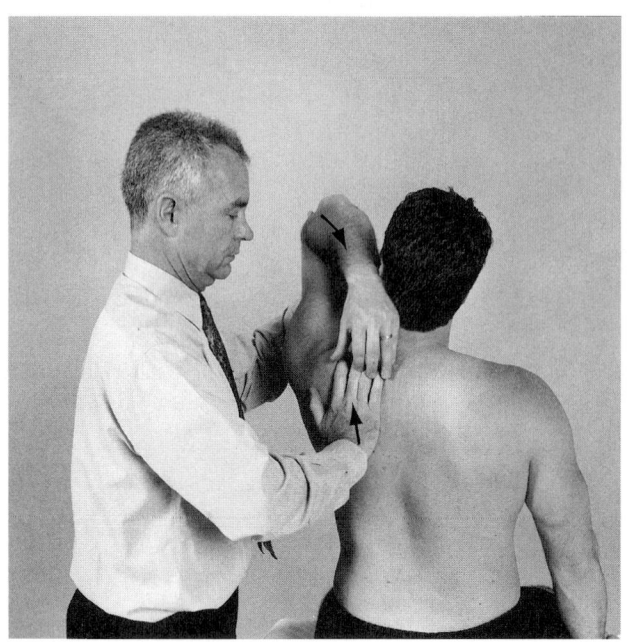

FIGURE 26-26   Pump handle motion.

Sensation should be tested over the abdomen. The area just below the xiphoid process is innervated by T8, the umbilicus by T10, and the lower abdominal region, level with the anterior superior iliac spines, by T12.[68] Too much overlap exists above T8 to make sensation testing reliable.

Because of the proximity and vulnerability of the spinal cord in this region, long tract signs (Babinski, Oppenheim, clonus, deep tendon reflexes) should be routinely assessed. Several tests have been devised to help assess the integrity of the neurologic system in this area.

Beevor's Sign (T7–12).   The patient is positioned supine, with the knees flexed and both feet flat on the bed. The patient is asked to raise the head against resistance, cough, or attempt to sit up with the hands resting behind their head[103] (Fig. 26-27). The clinician observes for motion at the umbilicus, which should remain in a straight line. If the umbilicus deviates diagonally, a weakness in the diagonally opposite set of three abdominal muscles is suggested. If it moves distally, weak upper abdominals are suggested; if proximally, weak lower abdominals are suggested. For example, if the umbilicus moves upward and to the right, the muscles in the lower left quadrant must be weak. The weakness may be a result of spinal nerve root palsy, in this case the 10th, 11th, and 12th thoracic nerves on the left.[104]

Clinical Pearl

Beevor's sign is a common finding in patients with facioscapulohumeral dystrophy, even before functional weakness of abdominal wall muscles is apparent, but is absent in patients with other facioscapulohumeral disorders.[105]

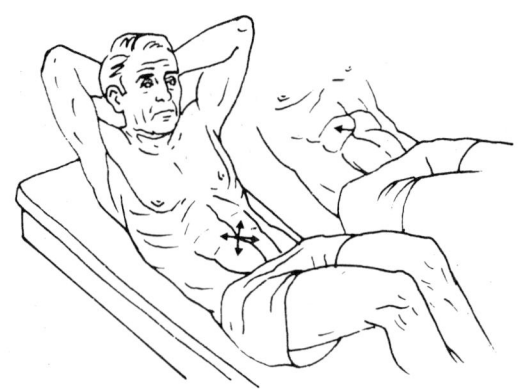

FIGURE 26-27   Beevor's sign. (Reproduced with permission from Haldeman S, ed. *Principles and Practice of Chiropractic.* Norwalk, Conn: Appleton and Lange; 1992:286.)

Slump Test.   This neurodynamic mobility test is described in Chapter 12.

Abdominal Cutaneous Reflex.   To test the abdominal cutaneous reflex, deep stroking over the abdominal muscles is performed using the handle of a reflex hammer (Fig. 26-28). Each quadrant is tested by etching diagonal lines around the patient's umbilicus. The clinician observes for symmetry of skin rippling or displacement of the umbilicus.

Lhermitte's Symptom.   This impairment usually is considered to be a lesion to the cervical spinal cord (see Chap. 23), and it is associated with demyelination, prolapsed cervical disk, neck trauma, or subacute combined degeneration of the cord. Because the thoracic cord is immobilized by the denticulate ligaments, flexion will produce only limited stretching of the cord, and thus less excursion. Lhermitte's symptom, characterized by an electric shocklike sensation into the spinal cord and limbs during neck

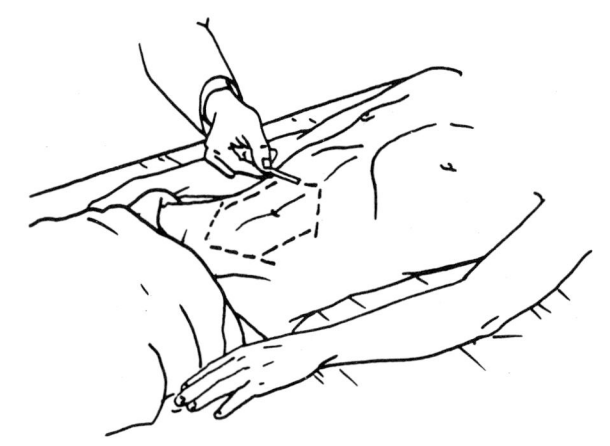

FIGURE 26-28   Superficial abdominal reflexes. (Reproduced with permission from Haldeman S, ed. *Principles and Practice of Chiropractic.* Norwalk, Conn: Appleton and Lange; 1992:286.)

flexion, may be present in the thoracic spine with compression of the thoracic cord by metastatic malignant deposits,[106] impairments of the thoracic vertebrae,[107] and thoracic spinal tumors.[108]

Brown-Séquard Syndrome. This syndrome is characterized by ipsilateral flaccid segmental palsy, ipsilateral spastic palsy below the impairment, and ipsilateral anesthesia, loss of proprioception, loss of appreciation of the vibration of a tuning fork (dysesthesia). Contralateral discrimination of pain sensation and thermoanesthesia may be present and are both noted below the impairment. If a neurologic impairment is suspected, the clinician must first exclude a neoplastic process, infectious process, or fracture, and then consider a disk protrusion. A nondiscal disorder of the thoracic spine could include a neurofibroma; some of the signs to help confirm its presence are:

▶ The patient reports preferring to sleep sitting up.

▶ The pain, which slowly increases over a period of months, is felt mainly at night and is uninfluenced by activities.

▶ The patient reports a band-shaped area of numbness that is related to one dermatome.

▶ The patient reports the presence of pins and needles sensations in one or both feet, or reports any other sign of cord compression.

Brown-Séquard syndrome symptoms also may occur with an idiopathic spinal cord herniation.[108a] This syndrome is caused by damage to the lateral funiculus of the spinal cord.[108a] The spinal cord frequently is shifted ventrolaterally, and sometimes rotated toward the side of tethering,[108a] which might cause unilateral damage of the lateral funiculus. For the diagnosis of spinal cord herniation, magnetic resonance imaging (MRI) and computed tomography (CT) myelography are essential. An MRI myelogram can show acute, angular, ventral deviation of the spinal cord in the sagittal plane.[108b] CT myelograms can detect ventral or ventrolateral shifts of the spinal cord and, sometimes, an extradural cyst in the ventral epidural space.[108b]

Functional Outcomes

As yet, there are no specific measures for functional loss and disability in patients with a thoracic dysfunction. Until such time, the reader is recommended to use the Neck Disability Index (NDI) (see Table 9-7) for dysfunctions that originate above the level of the T4 disk, and the Roland-Morris Disability Questionnaire,[109,110] (see Table 25-1) for pain originating below the T4 disk level.[46] In addition, the Oswestry Low Back Disability Questionnaire and the Functional Rating Scale can be used.

| Intervention Strategies

Because of the complexity of this area, interventions for thoracic and rib dysfunctions require a multifaceted and eclectic approach. It is essential that the impairments, functional limitations, and disability found during the examination guide the intervention.

Once the causes for referral of symptoms have been ruled out, dysfunctions of the thoracic spine and rib cage may be categorized as somatic or biomechanical.

The intervention approach for the upper thoracic spine is similar to that of the cervical spine (see Chap. 23), whereas the approach for the lower thoracic spine is similar to that of the lumbar spine (see Chap. 25). The approach to the midthoracic region is variable and depends on the cause. This region is prone to both postural and biomechanical dysfunctions. Fortunately, there are a number of very effective techniques for the thoracic spine. The techniques to increase joint mobility and the techniques to increase soft tissue extensibility are described later, under "Therapeutic Techniques."

Acute Phase

In the acute phase of rehabilitation for the thoracic spine, the intervention goals are to:

▶ Decrease pain, inflammation, and muscle spasm.

▶ Promote healing of tissues.

▶ Increase pain-free range of vertebral and costal motion.

▶ Regain soft tissue extensibility.

▶ Regain neuromuscular control.

▶ Initiate postural education.

▶ Promote correct breathing.

▶ Educate the patient about activities to avoid and positions of comfort.

▶ Allow progression to the functional phase.

Pain relief may be accomplished initially by the use of modalities such as cryotherapy and electrical stimulation, gentle exercises, and occasionally the temporary use of a spinal brace. Thermal modalities—especially ultrasound, with its ability to penetrate deeply—may be used after 48 to 72 hours. Ultrasound is the most common clinically used deep-heating modality to promote tissue healing.[111–113]

Electrical stimulation can be used in the thoracic region to:

▶ Create a muscle contraction through nerve or muscle stimulation. The purpose of this muscle contraction and stimulation is to create a muscle pump to aid in the healing process. Electrical stimulation of muscles for the correction of scoliosis has not been found to be effective in preventing scoliosis progression.[114]

▶ Decrease pain through the stimulation of sensory nerves (TENS).

▶ Provide muscle re-education and facilitation through both motor and sensory stimulation.

Once the pain and inflammation are controlled, the intervention can progress toward the restoration of full strength, range of motion, and normal posture. Range-of-motion exercises are initiated at the earliest opportunity. These are performed during the early stages in the pain-free ranges. Submaximal isometric exercises are then performed throughout the pain-free ranges. These exercises are progressed as the range of motion and strength increase.

Manual techniques during this phase may include myofascial release, grade I and II joint mobilizations, massage, gentle stretching, and muscle energy techniques.

Functional Phase

The duration of this phase can vary tremendously and depends on several factors:

▶ Severity of the injury.

▶ Healing capacity of the patient.

▶ How the condition was managed during the acute phase.

▶ Level of patient involvement in the rehabilitation program.

The goals of this phase are:

▶ To achieve significant reduction or to complete resolution of the patient's pain.

▶ Restoration of full and pain-free vertebral and costal range of motion.

▶ Full integration of the entire upper and lower kinetic chains.

▶ Complete restoration of respiratory function.

▶ Restoration of thoracic and upper quadrant strength and neuromuscular control.

During this phase, the patient learns to initiate and execute functional activities without pain and while dynamically stabilizing the spine in an automatic manner.

The exercises prescribed must challenge and enhance muscle performance while minimizing loading of the thoracic spine and ribs to reduce the risk of injury exacerbation. Interindividual differences in injury status or training goals may allow for a continuum of required muscle stress and acceptable loading of the spine.[115]

The stabilization of this region must include postural stabilization retraining of the entire spine, including the stabilization progressions outlined in Chapters 23 and 25. Cervicothoracic stabilization (see Chap. 23) and lumbar stabilization (see Chap. 25) are specific types of therapeutic exercise that can help the patient to (1) gain dynamic control of spine forces, (2) eliminate repetitive injury to the motion segments, (3) encourage healing of the injured segment, and (4) possibly alter the degenerative process.[115a]

Practice Pattern 4B: Impaired Joint Mobility, Motor Function, Muscle Performance, Range of Motion Associated with Impaired Posture

Postural Dysfunction

Postural dysfunctions of the thoracic spine are relatively common. Postural pain is not typically reproducible with the typical physical examination, and the diagnosis is based solely on the history of pain following sustained positions or postures. Occasionally, patients with this type of pain may report that their pain is aggravated by stress, fatigue, or changes in the weather.[116]

Maigne's Thoracic Pain of Lower Cervical Origin. Although the pain from this condition may originate in the thoracic spine, Maigne[94] believes that the vast majority of these cases originate from the lower three cervical segments. The typical patient is female, with complaints of stiffness and tenderness of the shoulder girdle and thoracic muscle groups, particularly the interscapular muscles. The chief complaint is often described as a unilateral and intense pain, which is increased with sustained positions of sitting, and the lifting and carrying of heavy weights. The pain generally is decreased with rest, although it can sometimes be worse in the morning upon awakening. There may also be accompanying cervical and low back pain associated with postural habits or standing or sitting positions.

The physical examination usually reveals tenderness at the level of T5 to T6 (interscapular point), 1 to 2 cm lateral of the midline. Mild pressure at this point is sufficient to reproduce the patient's pain.

The intervention for this condition involves a therapeutic trial of cervical mobilization.

Abnormal Pelvic Tilting. Good mobility of the pelvis in all directions is important for the thoracic spine. Two postural deviations are associated with pelvic tilting:

1. Posterior pelvic tilting in the sitting position produces an increase in the flexion of the lumbar and thoracic spine, and a forward head posture. This posture is thought to result in a dorsal shifting of the thoracic disk, which places a stress on the posterior longitudinal ligament and the dura mater, producing both local and nonsegmental referrals of pain. This condition can be treated by having the patient sit on a wedge that tilts the pelvis anteriorly.

2. Anterior pelvic tilting in the standing position (usually caused by adaptive shortening of the rectus femoris and iliopsoas muscles) causes the trunk to lean backward and results in overstretching of the rectus abdominis and a pulling forward of the shoulders, shortening of the posterior neck muscles, and increased extension of the atlanto-occipital joint.[60] This condition can be treated by having the patient perform posterior pelvic tilts while standing, or stand with one foot in front of the other.

Postural Syndromes. The combination of adaptive shortening and weakness of muscles in one region affects posture and can contribute to thoracic spine problems. Jull and Janda[75] describe the *pelvic crossed syndrome*. In this syndrome, the erector spinae and iliopsoas are tight, and the abdominals and gluteus maximus are weak. This syndrome promotes an anterior pelvic tilt, an increased lumbar lordosis, and a slight flexion of the hip. The hamstrings frequently are shortened in this syndrome, and this may be a compensatory strategy to lessen the anterior tilt of the pelvis,[117] or because the glutei are weak. The syndrome promotes an increased lumbar lordosis, an increased thoracic kyphosis, and a compensatory increase in cervical lordosis to keep the head and eyes level.

Jull and Janda also described the *upper crossed syndrome*.[118] This syndrome involves adaptive shortening of the levator scapulae, upper trapezius, pectoralis major and minor, and sternocleidomastoid, and weakness of the deep neck flexors and lower scapular stabilizers. The syndrome produces elevation and protraction of the shoulder and rotation and abduction of the scapula, together with scapular winging. It also produces a forward head and hypermobility of the C4 to C5 and T4 segments.

The intervention for these postural dysfunctions includes simple measures such as reassurance, postural education, and the correction of muscle imbalances with strengthening and stretching exercises.

Precordial Catch Syndrome. This is a benign self-limiting condition occurring mainly in adolescents and young adults.[119,120] It is characterized by sharp, stabbing pain in the precordial and left parasternal region that does not radiate. This pain usually lasts a few seconds and may occur at rest or with mild to moderate exercise.[119] When occurring at rest, it is often associated with being seated in a slouched position and may be relieved by stretching into a more upright position.[121] It affects males and females equally but is uncommon after the age of 35 years.[120] The etiology of this condition is unknown, but it may originate from the pleura.[120] After excluding other causes, management consists of explanation, reassurance, postural education, and exercises to correct any muscle imbalances.

Clinical Pearl

Patients with any form of postural dysfunction often benefit from the movement therapies of the Alexander technique, Feldenkrais method, Trager psychophysical integration, Pilates, and tai chi chuan[122–128] (see Chap. 10).

Practice Pattern 4D: Impaired Joint Mobility, Motor Function, Muscle Performance, Range of Motion Associated with Ligament or Other Connective Tissue Disorders

Zygapophysial Joint Dysfunction

Apart from the upper and lower segments of this region, little is known about the extent or patterns of thoracic zygapophysial joint degeneration. However, these joints have been found to be potential sources of local and referred pain.[129]

The pathomechanics describing mechanical dysfunction in this region are largely based on expert opinion and the principles of anatomy and biomechanics. Given the controversy surrounding the nature of coupled motions in the thoracic spine, and the number of structures involved in executing motion at

these levels, the clinician is advised to diagnose dysfunction in this region based on restrictions of motion, rather than on specific structures.

Restriction of motion can have many causes in this region, including zygapophysial joint hypomobility, soft tissue contracture, and costovertebral-costotransverse joint hypomobility. Differentiation among these structures, to find the specific cause of dysfunction, requires a great deal of expertise.

For the sake of simplicity, and because the spinous and transverse processes are more easily palpated in this region, the osteopathic approach of diagnosing a positional dysfunction using position testing is recommended.

As elsewhere in the spine, dysfunctions can be either symmetric or asymmetric. Symmetric impairments are more common in the thoracic region than in the lumbar, particularly in the upper and cervicothoracic spine as a result of fixed postural impairments. These, of course, will not be apparent on position testing and must be sought after when the position tests are negative. If no asymmetry is found on position testing, then the segment of interest should be separately passively flexed, extended, and rotated in all directions.

To determine which lesion is present, layer palpation is used. The position of the superior vertebra and the posteroanterior relationship of the transverse processes to the coronal body plane is noted and compared with the level above and below, in thoracic flexion and then extension (see "Position Testing: Spinal," earlier).

Rib Dysfunction

The costovertebral joint may be involved in inflammatory or degenerative joint disease. Complaints of symptoms in these joints are common in conditions such as ankylosing spondylitis as a result of synovitis. The clinical features of severe arthropathy of the costovertebral joint include pain with deep breathing, trunk rotation, sneezing, or coughing. CT scans are helpful in confirming the diagnosis. Inflammation of the costovertebral joint commonly causes localized pain about 3 to 4 cm from the midline, where the rib articulates with the transverse process and the vertebral body.[61]

According to the osteopaths, rib dysfunctions are described as structural, torsional, or respiratory.[90,130,131]

▶ *Structural.* Structural rib dysfunctions are true joint subluxations that occur secondary to trauma. These dysfunctions are extremely painful and significantly reduce motion of the ribs during inspiration and expiration. The most important landmarks for structural rib dysfunctions are the rib angle and the anterior rib. Ribs can sublux anteriorly or posteriorly (see Table 26-4). The first rib can sublux superiorly.

▶ *Torsional.* As their name suggests, these rib dysfunctions are twisting injuries, in which the rib is held in a position of internal or external rotation. These dysfunctions affect the thoracic spine motions as well as the motions of respiration (see Table 26-4).

▶ *Respiratory.* Respiratory rib dysfunctions usually are related to poor posture and result in a restriction of either inspiration or expiration.

The intervention for costovertebral dysfunctions involves mobilization and manipulation techniques or local anesthetic injections, or both.

Practice Pattern 4E: Impaired Joint Mobility, Motor Function, Muscle Performance, Range of Motion Associated with Localized Inflammation

Tietze Syndrome

Tietze syndrome is a local inflammation of the costosternal cartilage, which most commonly affects the second and third costochondral junctions.[23,132] Tietze syndrome also may affect any of the cartilaginous articulations of the chest wall, including the sternoclavicular joints.[133]

The clinical findings for this condition include a history of a gradual or sudden onset of pain in the involved region, which is increased with deep inspiration, coughing, or sneezing. Upon physical examination, there is often a localized swelling of the costosternal cartilage.

This is a self-limiting condition, which can last from weeks to years. The intervention can involve local injections of corticosteroid and specific joint mobilizations to the costovertebral articulations.

Muscle Strains

Muscle strains are common in the thoracic region and are characterized by localized pain and tenderness, which is exacerbated with isometric testing or passive stretching of the muscle. Although it is difficult to isolate muscles in this region, the clinician can determine the directions that alleviate the symptoms and those that do not. A gradual strengthening and gentle passive stretching program into the painless directions is initially performed, before progressing as tolerated into the painful directions.

Intercostal Muscles. Injuries to intercostal muscles are mainly caused by trauma after unaccustomed or excessive muscular activity.[134] There may be a specific incident before the onset of pain, such as lifting a heavy object, or symptoms may be of gradual onset with no obvious inciting event.[135] In athletes, a premature return to heavy training after a period of rest or deconditioning may predispose to muscular injuries. Intercostal muscle injuries are more likely in sports in which upper body activity is extreme, such as rowing.[135] However, intercostal pain can occur in the presence of persistent coughing as a result of such conditions as an upper respiratory tract infection.

Diagnosis is based on pain between the ribs that is worse on movement, deep inspiration, or coughing. This pain is associated with tenderness in the same area on palpation. Plain radiographs are normal unless there is underlying lung disease or infection, and diagnosis may be dependent on exclusion of more serious pathology, such as cardiac chest pain, in the absence of a clear history of injury.[135]

The intervention for intercostals muscle strains includes anti-inflammatory medications, the avoidance of exacerbating activities, and the treatment of any underlying pathology where appropriate.

Contusions

The severity of soft tissue injury to the chest wall is dependent on the mechanism of injury and the degree of protection between the traumatic force and the chest wall.[39b] Chest injury is commonly produced by the restraining influence of the diagonal component of a seat belt. Seat belt injuries occur predominantly on the side of the belt and, hence, occur on different sides in drivers and passengers.[39b] These injuries take the form of abrasions, ecchymoses, and friction burns, producing an imprint of the belt.[39b]

Trauma to the female breast can be produced by a combination of compression and shearing stress produced by a seat belt, and subcutaneous rupture of breast tissue can occur.[135a] The presence of a persistent breast mass after trauma must always be taken seriously, because trauma may draw attention to an unsuspected carcinoma.[39b]

Chest trauma can result in disruption of subcutaneously placed pacemaker generators or leads, long-term indwelling central venous catheters, or subcutaneous portions of arterial bypass grafts.[39b] Severe skeletal trauma to the chest wall can be associated with large chest wall hematomas or collections of air within the chest wall, which can communicate with the intrathoracic space.[39b]

The conservative intervention for thoracic cage contusions depends on the severity of the injury and the tissues involved. Typically, the initial intervention for soft tissue injury is cryotherapy with rest. Gentle, pain-free, active range-of-motion exercises are introduced as tolerated. Once the acute phase is over, thermal modalities are used and the range-of-motion exercises progressed to strengthening exercises in all planes.

Practice Pattern 4G: Impaired Joint Mobility, Motor Function, Muscle Performance, Range of Motion Associated with Fractures

Thoracic Vertebral Fractures

Fractures of the thoracic spine account for 25 to 30 percent of all spinal fractures.[135b] These fractures are most often a result of hyperflexion or axial loading injuries[135c] and less commonly attributable to rotational stresses, side bending, horizontal shear, and hyperextension. The most common fractures seen in the thoracic spine are anterior wedge compression fractures and burst fractures[135d] (see Chap. 9). Most thoracic spine fractures occur between the 9th and 11th vertebral bodies. Multiple fractures are found in 10 percent of all patients with a spine fracture; therefore, evaluation of the entire spine is necessary, because up to 80 percent of these additional fractures are noncontiguous.[135e] Only 12 percent of patients with fracture– dislocations of the thoracic spine are neurologically intact, and 62 percent of patients with thoracic spine fracture–dislocations have complete neurologic deficits.[39b]

Rib Fractures

Fractured ribs can lacerate the pleura, lung, or abdominal organs. Fractures to the upper ribs, clavicle, and upper sternum can signal brachial plexus or vascular injury. Isolated fractures of the ribs, clavicle, or scapula seldom represent significant injuries in and of themselves, but they do reflect the magnitude of force imparted, particularly in older patients with noncompliant chest walls.[135f] Fractured rib ends can lacerate the pleura or lung, resulting in hemothorax or pneumothorax.[39b] There is a much greater incidence of rib fractures in older patients, whose ribs are relatively inelastic, compared with the incidence of rib fractures in children, whose ribs are more pliable and resilient.[39b] For this reason, a posttraumatic pneumothorax in older patients is almost always associated with one or more rib fractures, whereas children can sustain a pneumothorax or major internal thoracic injury after trauma without an associated rib fracture.

Fractures of the first three ribs in particular indicate significant energy transfer because they are well protected by the shoulder girdles and associated musculature.[39b] Fractures to the upper ribs, clavicle, and upper sternum are accompanied by brachial plexus or vascular injury in 3 to 15 percent of patients.[135g] Fractures of the 10th, 11th, or 12th ribs are associated with injury to the liver, kidneys, or spleen and should prompt confirmation of organ injury with CT.[39b] Double fractures of three or more adjacent ribs or contiguous combined rib and sternal or costochondral fractures, or single fracture of four or more contiguous ribs, can produce a focal area of chest wall instability. Paradoxical movement of a "flail" segment during the respiratory cycle can impair respiratory mechanics, promote atelectasis, and impair pulmonary drainage.

The common findings for a rib fracture are described in Chapter 9. A key factor in the intervention of rib fractures is believed to be adequate pain control to allow early aggressive respiratory care and, hence, prevent the development of pulmonary complications.

Early intervention includes assistance with coughing, intracostal nerve blocks, and muscle relaxants. Adhesive strapping or taping should be avoided because it can inhibit deep inspiration and may contribute to atelectasis.[136] Simple rib fractures become stable in 1 to 2 weeks, with firm healing by callus in approximately 6 weeks.[136]

Scheuermann's Disease

Scheuermann's disease, which is found in approximately 10 percent of the population and in males and females equally, typically is seen in pubescent athletes.[137]

The disease involves a defect to the ring apophysis of the vertebral body and anterior wedging of the affected vertebrae, as a result of a flexion overload of the anterior vertebral body.[138] The end plate can crack, thus making it possible for disk material to bulge into the vertebral body (Schmorl's node). According to McKenzie,[97] the extension dysfunction develops in patients with Scheuermann's disease as a result of adaptive shortening from poor postural habits, or from derangement or trauma and the healing process.

Clinical findings include evidence of a thoracic kyphosis and pain with thoracic extension and rotation.

The intervention depends on the severity but typically involves postural education, a modification of the aggravating

activity, exercise (seated rotation, and extension in lying exercises), or bracing. The exercise program involves the stretching of the pectoralis major and minor muscles, and muscle strengthening exercises for the thoracic spine extensors and the scapular adductors.[23]

Scapular Fractures

Fractures of the scapula are relatively rare, because of the thick muscles lying both superficial and deep to the scapula, and the energy-absorbing ability of the scapula to move on the chest wall.[138a] As a result of the large amount of force required to fracture a scapula, these fractures are often associated with other major injuries. For example, the incidence of pneumothorax in patients with fracture of a scapula is over 50 percent.[138b] Associated injuries that are directly related to the fractured scapula include injuries of the suprascapular nerve, axillary nerve, axillary artery, and subclavian artery.[39b] The body of the scapula is the most frequent site of fracture, followed by the neck and glenoid.[138c] The spine, coracoid, and acromion are less frequently fractured.[138c] Scapular fractures may not be recognized on the initial chest radiograph because frequently they are radiographically obscure, and because they are commonly associated with multiple other regional injuries, such as clavicular and rib fractures, subcutaneous air, pneumothorax, and pulmonary contusion.[39b]

Sternal Fractures. The tremendous force necessary to cause a fracture of the sternum has led to the belief that the presence of a sternal fracture is a harbinger of severe associated injuries. The association of seat belt wearing with sternal fractures is well known.[138d] A proportional increase in incidence of 100 percent in drivers and 150 percent in front seat passengers has been noted since the enactment of seat belt legislation.[138e] Sternal fractures as such do not generally cause problems either in healing or by direct damage to adjacent structures. Dislocation of the sternoclavicular joint with posterior displacement of the inner end of the clavicle may cause compression of the trachea and the adjacent great vessels, with significant clinical consequences.[138f]

Integration of Practice Patterns 4B and 4F: Impaired Joint Mobility, Motor Function, Muscle Performance, Range of Motion Secondary to Impaired Posture, Systemic Dysfunction (Referred Pain Syndromes), Spinal Disorders, and Myofascial Pain Dysfunction

Referred Pain

Referred pain to this area is extremely common. Referred pain is characterized by a poorly localized pain that is nontender to palpation and does not change with movements or alterations of posture (see Table 26-5).

T4 Syndrome

The name of this syndrome is a bit of a misnomer, because the syndrome can additionally affect the T2 to T7 levels, although it always includes the T4 segment. The T4 syndrome has an unknown etiology, although it is believed to result from a sympathetic reaction to a hypomobile segment, because the symptoms appear to resolve in response to manual therapy techniques to the thoracic segments.[139–141] In the thorax, the sympathetic trunks lie on or just lateral to the costovertebral joints. These trunks may undergo mechanical deformation with abnormal posture (forward head, accentuated thoracic kyphosis, and protracted shoulder girdle), trauma, or pulling and reaching activities, producing pain and sympathetic epiphenomena.[142]

Neurovascular symptoms are not a feature of this syndrome, though a differential diagnosis should consider such conditions.[139] The upper extremity symptoms are glovelike in distribution and are not segmentally related.[140] Nocturnal symptoms are common, usually occurring in side lying or supine position.[140] More women are affected by this condition than men, in a ratio of more than 3:1.[143]

Clinical findings include local tenderness of bony points, positive slump test, positive upper limb tension tests, depression or prominence of one or more spinous processes, and local thickening and stiffness of one segment,[143] although gross cervical and thoracic motions are usually normal.[139]

The differential diagnosis includes carpal tunnel syndrome, thoracic outlet syndrome, cervical disk disease, vascular disease, and neurologic disease.[139]

The intervention for this condition involves mobilization and manipulation of the involved segment, of which T4 is the most frequently involved, followed by an exercise progression emphasizing upper thoracic flexibility and muscle strength. Butler[144] recommends using both upper limb tension tests and also the slump test, with combinations of thoracic rotation and side bending.

Notalgia Paresthetica[145]

The name of this condition comes from the Greek root meaning "pain in the back." Clinically, this condition consists of pruritus and localized dysesthesia and hyperesthesia in the distribution of one of the cutaneous dorsal rami of the upper thoracic area.

The recommended intervention for this condition is an injection of corticosteroid.

Therapeutic Techniques

Techniques to Increase Joint Mobility

Joint Mobilizations

Mobilization and manipulation techniques in this region are highly effective for restoring thoracic spinal or rib joint mobility.[16,67,146,147] The purpose of these techniques is to be able to isolate a mobilization to a specific level, and in so doing:

▶ Reduce stresses through both the fixation and leverage components of the spine.

▶ Reduce stresses through the hypermobile segments.

▶ Reduce the overall force needed by the clinician, thus giving greater control.

The selection of a manual technique is dependent on a number of factors, including the acuteness of the condition and the restriction to the movement that is encountered. Oftentimes, the same techniques that were used to examine the segment can be used for the intervention, the difference being the intent of the clinician and the goal of the intervention. For example, if stretching of the mechanical barrier rather than pain relief is the immediate objective of the intervention, a mobilization technique is carried out at the end of the available range.

To achieve this, the antagonist muscle must be relaxed, and this is most easily accomplished by the hold-relax technique. After this has been gained (and sometimes before and after), there is some minor pain to be dealt with, using grade IV oscillations, after which the joint capsule can be stretched, using either grade IV++ or prolonged stretch techniques. The prolonged stretch or the strong oscillations are continued for as long as the clinician can maintain good control. At the point where control is about to be lost, several isometric contractions to the agonists and the antagonists are demanded of the patient's muscles in the new range, to give the central nervous system information about the newly acquired range. To complete the re-education, concentric and eccentric retraining is carried out through the whole range of the joint. Active exercises are continued at home and at work on a regular and frequent basis to reinforce the re-education.

Long Sit Superior Distraction. The patient is positioned on the treatment table in the long sit, with the buttocks on the edge of the back of the table and the hands on the back of the neck, fingers interlocked. The clinician stands behind the patient, and places a small towel roll at the T6 level. The towel roll is held in place by the clinician's chest (made easier if the clinician turns slightly so that the side of the chest is used). The clinician threads his or her arms under the patient's armpits and places the heel of the palms under the patient's forearms. The patient is asked to flex the neck. A stride stance (one foot in front of the other) is adopted by the clinician (Fig. 26-29) and, while keeping the elbows close together, the clinician gently rocks the patient backward and forward. After two or three rocks, the traction force is applied as the clinician shifts his or her body weight from the forward leg to the back, while lifting the patient and pushing the patient's forearms toward the ceiling.

Long Sit Inferior Distraction. The patient is positioned on the mat table in the long sit, with the buttocks on the edge of the table and the hands on the back of the neck, fingers interlocked. The clinician stands behind the patient and places a small towel roll at the T5 level. The towel roll is held in place by the clinician's chest (made easier if the clinician turns slightly so that the side of the chest is used). The patient is asked to cross the arms over the chest and to lean back against the clinician's shoulder. The clinician reaches around the patient and grasps the patient's lower elbow in both hands, wedging his or her forearms under the infraglenoid tubercle area of the patient's scapula (Fig. 26-30). The segment is extended as much as is comfortable, and the patient's upper body is lifted by a graded

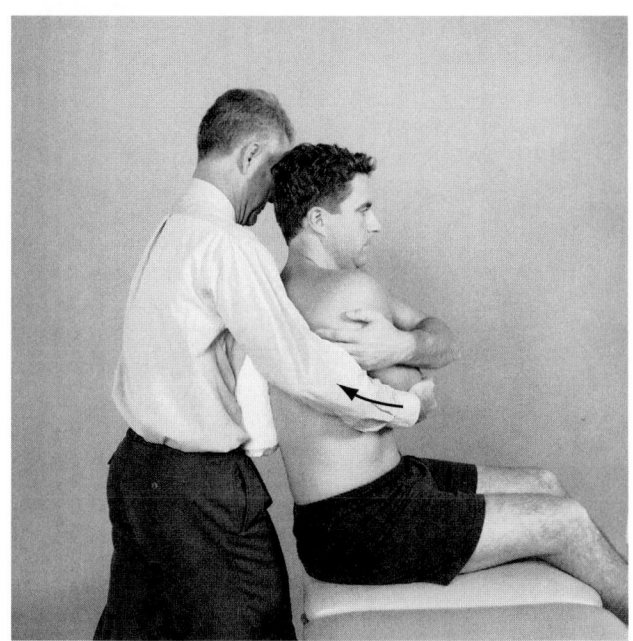

FIGURE 26-29 Long sit superior distraction.

squeezing of the clinician's arms together underneath the scapula. The patient's buttocks should not be lifted off the bed.

Longitudinal Distraction. The patient is in the side lying position, with the head supported on a pillow and the arms crossed to the opposite shoulders. The method of arm crossing depends on the size and flexibility of the patient. The larger, heavier, and less flexible patient crosses the arms as in Figure 26-31A. The

smaller, lighter, and more flexible patient crosses the arms as in Figure 26-31B. If the patient crosses his or her arms as in Figure 26-31A, the clinician stands on the side of the patient so that the patient's arm resting on the chest is nearest to the clinician.

With the tubercle of the scaphoid bone placed against the lateral aspect of the spinous process, and the flexed proximal interphalangeal joint of the middle finger placed on the other side of the spinous process, the transverse processes of the inferior vertebra are palpated and fixed, blocking the inferior ring complex (Fig. 26-32). Thus, the spinous process of T5 nestles in the

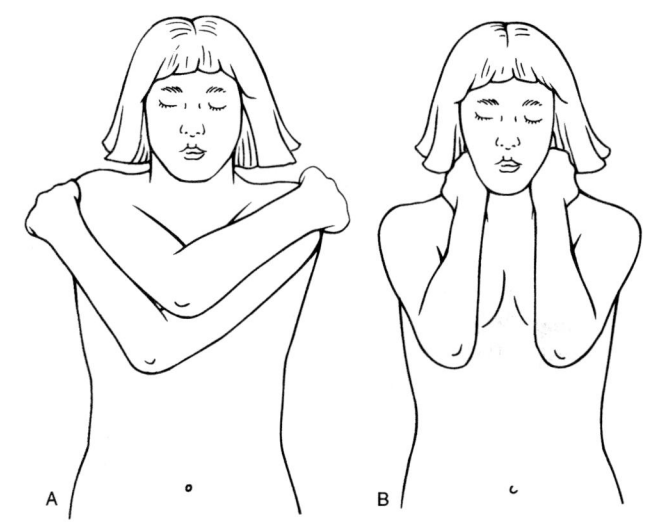

FIGURE 26-31 Arm positions for patients. **A.** Arm position for the larger, heavier patient. **B.** Arm position for the smaller, lighter patient (Reproduced with permission from Dutton M. *Manual Therapy of the Spine.* New York, NY: McGraw-Hill; 2002:435.)

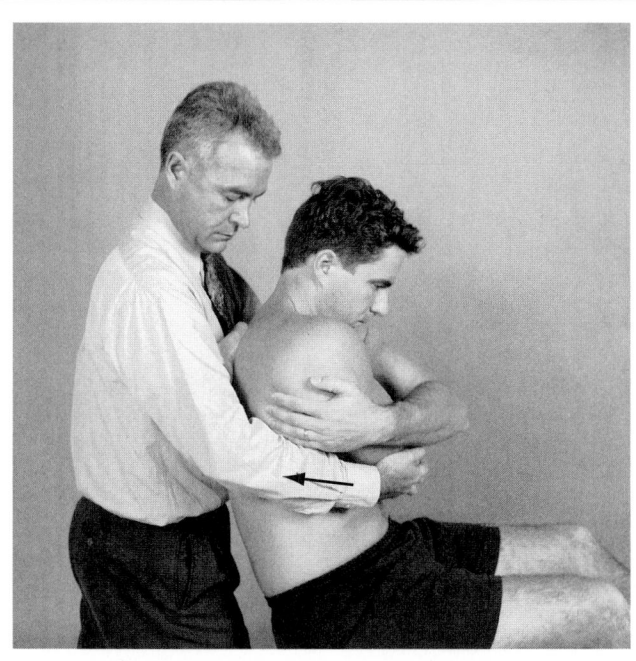

FIGURE 26-30 Long sit inferior distraction.

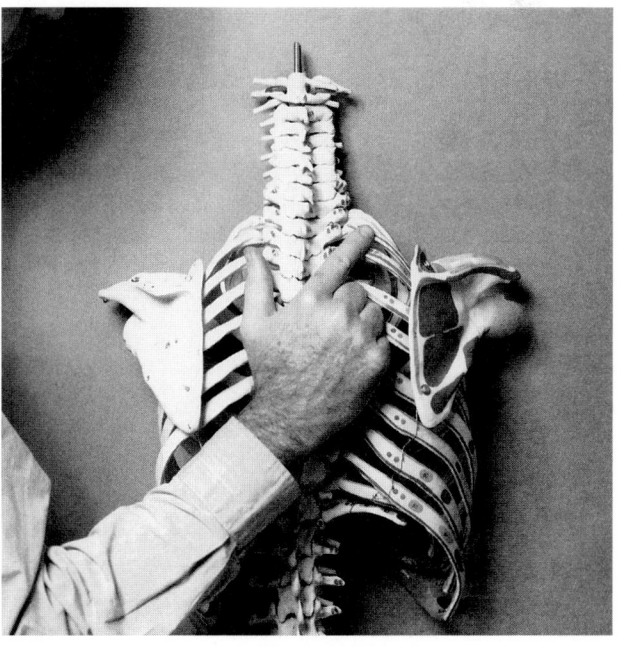

FIGURE 26-32 Hand position on skeleton.

space created by the extended index finger (Fig. 26-33). The other hand and arm lie across and on top of the patient's crossed arms to control the thorax. Segmental localization is achieved by flexing or extending the joint to the motion barrier using the hand and arm controlling the thorax. This localization is maintained by having the clinician's body lean on the patient's elbows as the clinician reaches around the neck and back of the patient and supports the thorax, while rolling the patient supine or semisupine (only until contact is made between the table and the dorsal hand) (Fig. 26-34). The thoracic curve above the treated segment is maintained either by the clinician or by raising the table end. A minimum amount of the patient's body weight should be resting on the clinician's right hand to prevent a painful compression against the contact hand. From this position, a mobilizing force applied in a superior direction (up the bed), will tend to produce a distraction of the segment, whereas a mobilizing force applied in a posterior direction (down into the bed), will tend to produce a gapping of the segment. The amplitude of the technique can be graded from I to V.

Mobilizations with Movement

The sustained neutral apophyseal glide (SNAG) techniques described by Mulligan[148] are particularly useful in the spine because they are performed with the spine under normal physiologic weight bearing, and they combine active and passive physiologic motions with accessory glides along the zygapophysial joint plane.[11]

Technique to Improve Extension. In this example, the clinician is attempting to restore extension at the midthoracic region. The patient is positioning astride on one end of the table, with the thighs supported in order to stabilize the pelvis, and the hands

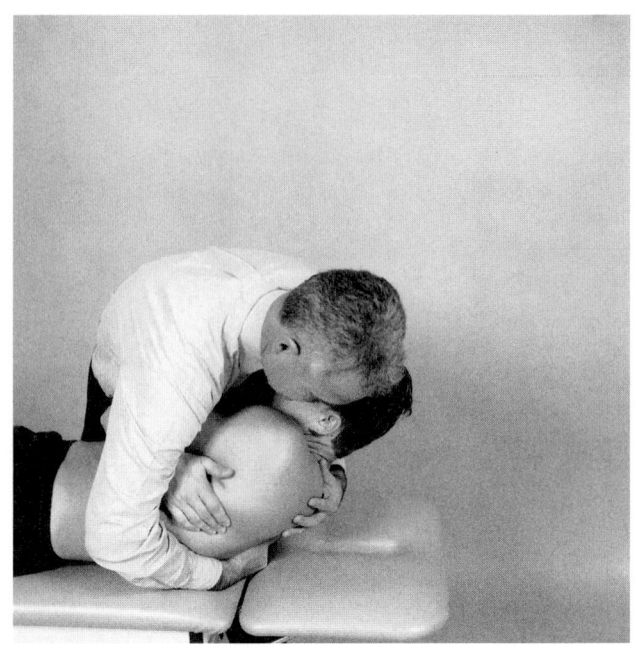

FIGURE 26-34 Prethrust position.

positioned behind the head (Fig. 26-35). The clinician stands slightly behind and to the side of the patient. One arm is wrapped around the front of the patient at the level of the suspected lesion (see Fig. 26-35). The ulnar border of the other hand is placed over the inferior spinous process, or articular pillar of the involved segment, and acts as the fulcrum for the extension movement. The patient is asked to extend the spine

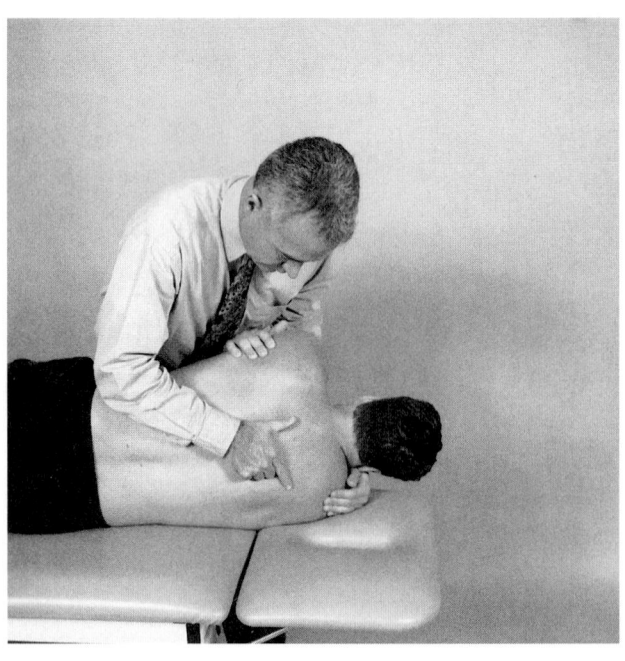

FIGURE 26-33 Hand position on patient.

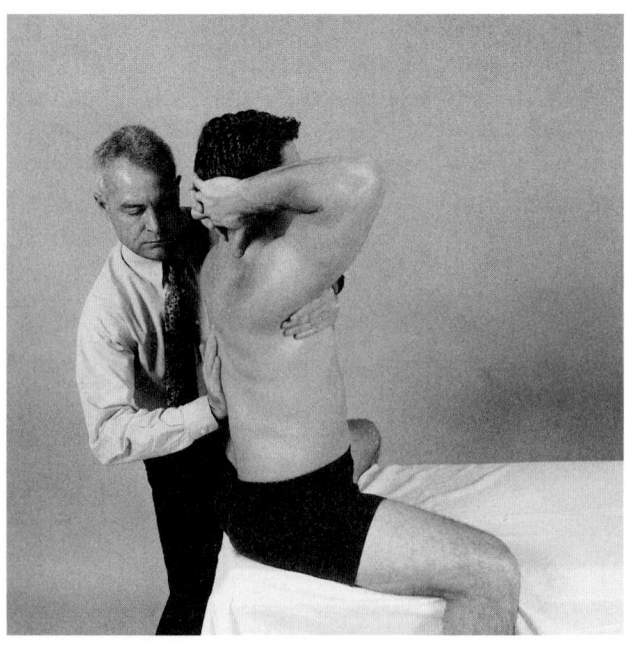

FIGURE 26-35 Mobilization with movement to increase extension.

over the clinician's hand while the clinician simultaneously performs a gliding force to the inferior aspect of the segment, along the plane of the joint (see Fig. 26-35).

Technique to Improve Flexion.   A similar technique to the preceding one can be used to increase flexion at the midthoracic region. As for the extension mobilization with movement, the patient is positioned astride on one end of the table, with the thighs supported in order to stabilize the pelvis, and the clinician stands slightly behind and to the side of the patient. One arm is wrapped around the front of the patient at the level of the suspected lesion. This arm serves as the fulcrum for the flexion movement. The ulnar border of the other hand is placed over the superior spinous process or articular pillar of the involved segment. The patient is asked to flex forward while the clinician simultaneously performs a gliding force along the plane of the joint.

Techniques to Increase Soft Tissue Extensibility

Muscle Energy

When the myofascial structures are thought to be the main cause of the motion restriction, the muscle energy techniques can be used. The motion barrier is localized and, from this position, the patient is instructed to hold still while the clinician applies resistance to the trunk. The direction of the applied resistance is determined by the neurophysiologic effect desired from the technique. For example, to increase thoracic spine extension, the patient is positioned sitting, with the clinician standing to one side. The patient places each hand behind the neck (Fig. 26-36), and the clinician uses one hand to squeeze the patient's elbow together. With the other hand, the clinician monitors thoracic spine motion as the patient's thoracic spine is passively moved to the limit of extension. The patient is asked to gently contract the shoulder extensors for 5 seconds (see Fig. 26-36). This contraction is resisted isometrically by the clinician, after which the patient is instructed to completely relax. The new barrier to thoracic extension is localized, and the mobilization repeated three times.

Automobilization Techniques

Barrel Hug Stretch.   This exercise can be used in the clinic or at home to maintain or increase the motions gained with manual techniques in midthoracic flexion or side bending.[46]

The patient is positioned sitting, with a Swiss ball in the lap. If a Swiss ball is not available, the patient is asked to imagine that he or she has a 55-gallon drum in the lap and to attempt to get both arms around it (Fig. 26-37). The patient should bend forward so that the apex of the curve is at the point of greatest flexion restriction.

While squeezing the Swiss ball, the patient moves into the desired direction. For example, if the restriction of motion is flexion and right rotation, the patient moves into this direction. This position is held for 30 to 90 seconds and is then repeated 3 to 5 times. The patient also can use deep breathing to increase the stretch, breathing out at the end of available range.

To focus on the left side of the midthoracic spine, the patient is asked to turn the trunk slightly to the right and place more weight on the left hip.

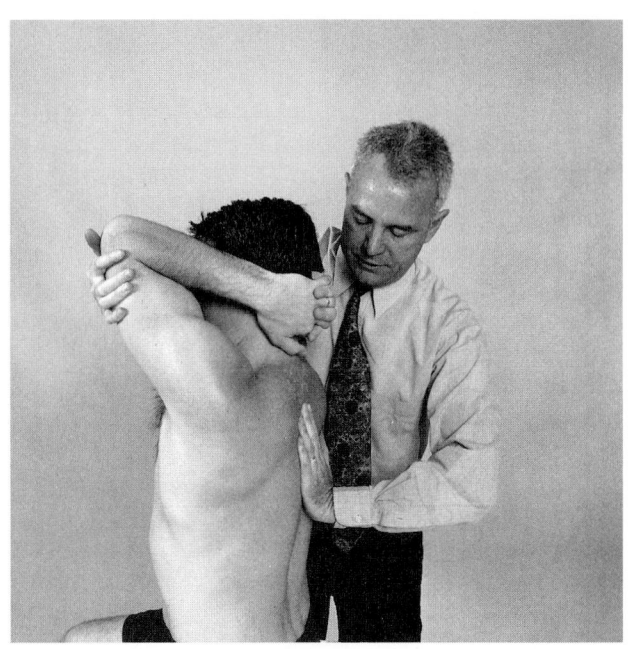

FIGURE 26-36   Muscle energy technique to increase thoracic extension.

Lower Trapezius.   This exercise is used to promote or maintain extension in the T6 through T10 region.[46] The patient is kneeling, with both arms outstretched in front and resting on a chair, traction stool, or Swiss ball (Fig. 26-38). The clinician ensures that the patient's head is in line with the upper back. The patient is asked to allow the upper back to slump toward the floor while maintaining the buttocks in a tucked position to prevent an increase in lumbar lordosis. From this position, the patient is

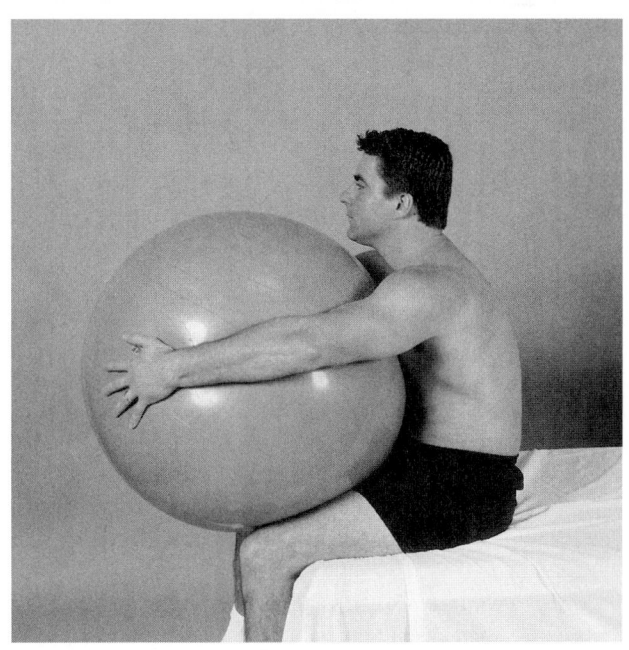

FIGURE 26-37   Barrel hug stretch.

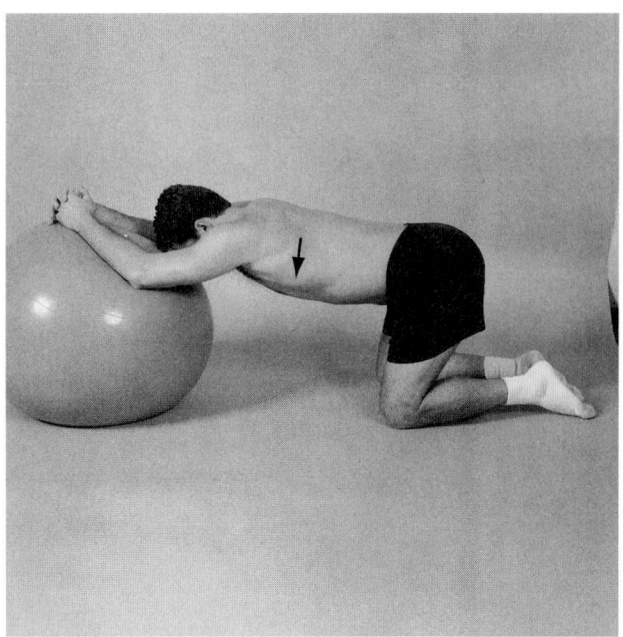

FIGURE 26-38   Lower trapezius exercise and stretch.

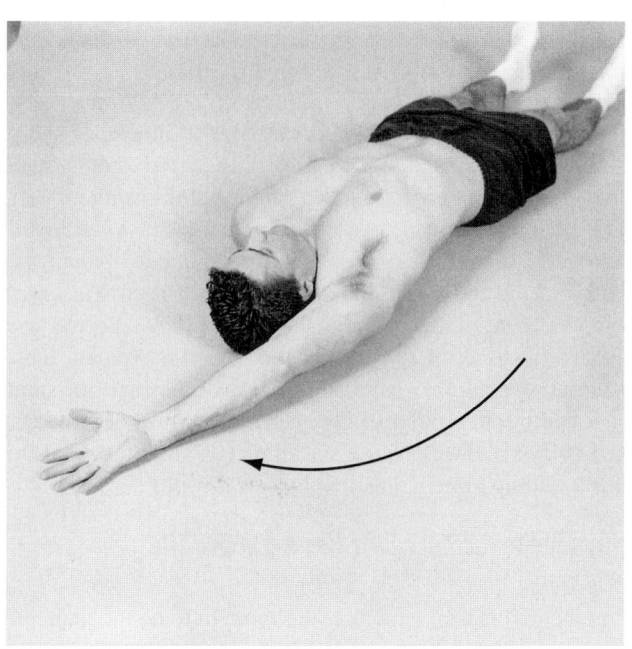

FIGURE 26-39   Shoulder sweep.

asked to raise the hand of the involved side off the stool by about 2 to 3 inches and to maintain the position for 5 to 10 seconds.

This technique can be prescribed to a patient following a manual technique to increase extension in the midthoracic spine.

Shoulder Sweep. This exercise is used to mobilize the chest wall and to integrate upper extremity function with thoracic spine and rib cage motion.[46]

The patient is positioned supine on the floor or on a mat table, with the hips and knees flexed to about 90 degrees (Fig. 26-39). A small pillow may be placed under the patient's head for comfort. The patient is asked to reach forward and place the palm of the hand as far in front as is comfortable. While maintaining contact with the floor, the patient moves the hand above the head and to the other side of the body, making a large circle around their body (see Fig. 26-39). Manual assistance applied to the scapula or rib cage can be used as can deep breathing, in order to move into the restricted ranges.

Thoracic Spine Flexion. The patient kneels in front of a Swiss ball. After clasping the hands together, the patient places his or her forearms on the Swiss ball and leans into the ball, rolling the ball away slightly (Fig. 26-40). While applying some body weight through the forearms, the patient arches the thoracic spine as far as is comfortable. This position is held for 8 to 10 seconds, after which the patient relaxes. The exercise is repeated 8 to 10 times.

Thoracic Spine Extension. It is advised that the clinician monitor this exercise in case the patient loses his or her balance. The patient sits on a Swiss ball, with the feet on the ground. Once the patient has good sitting balance, he or she attempts to lie

supine on the ball, and then places the hands behind the head (Fig. 26-41). The patient is then instructed to move the top of the head toward the floor in an attempt to fully extend the thoracic spine. This position is held for 8 to 10 seconds, after which the patient relaxes. The exercise is repeated 8 to 10 times. This exercise can be made more challenging by moving the hands from behind the head, out to the sides and back again while maintaining the balance (Fig. 26-42).

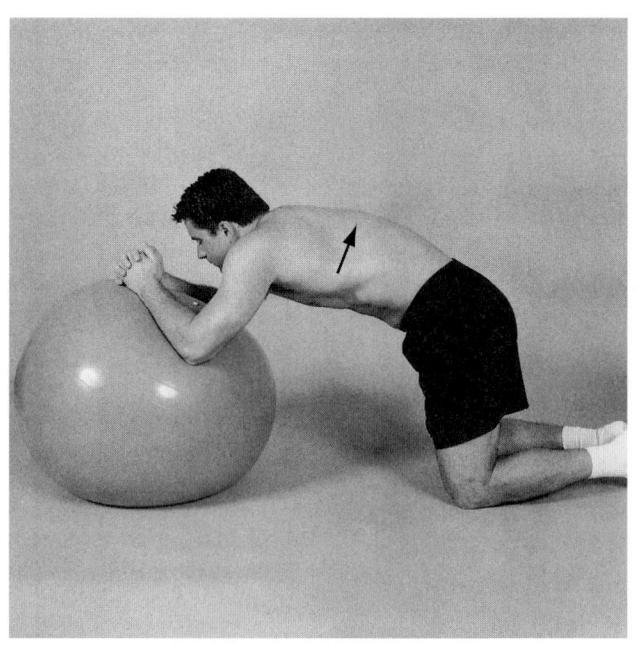

FIGURE 26-40   Thoracic spine flexion.

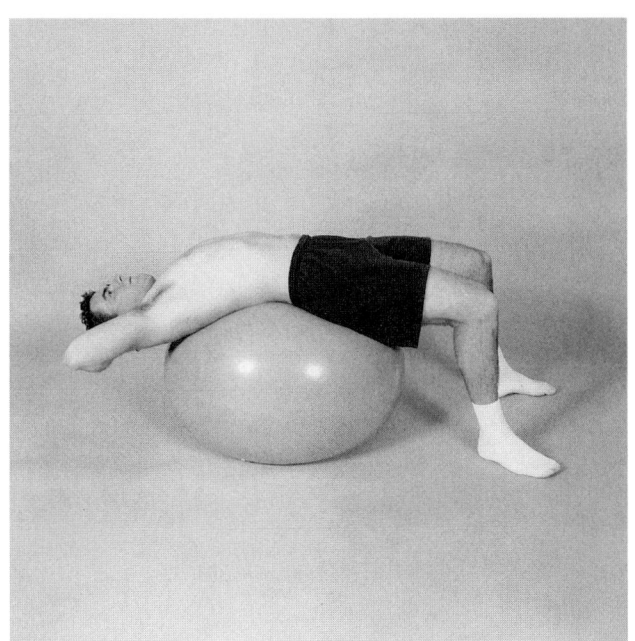

FIGURE 26-41 Thoracic spine extension with Swiss ball.

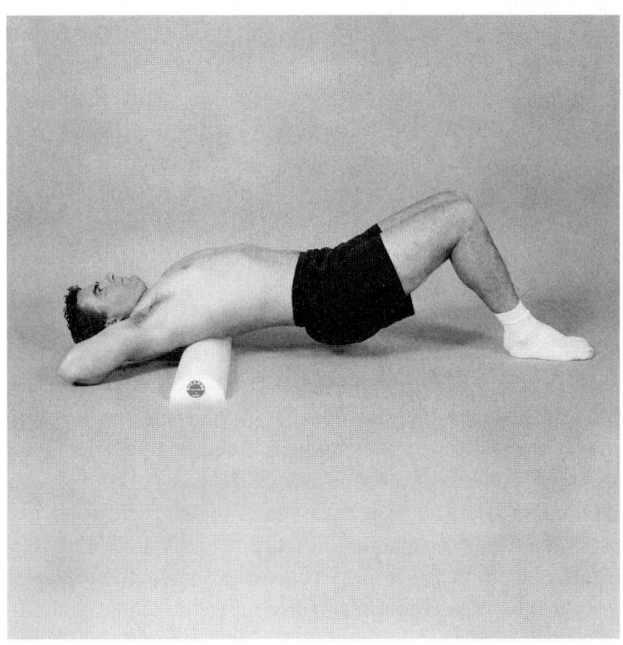

FIGURE 26-43 Thoracic spine extension using foam roll.

recommended for the athletic population, only. The patient kneels with his or her back facing the Swiss ball. Using one leg at a time, the patient reaches back with the foot and places it on top of the Swiss ball. Once both feet are on the ball, the legs are straightened and the weight of the body is primarily borne through the arms. Using the dorsum of the feet and the anterior legs, the patient induces a rotation to the thoracic region by twisting at the waist (Fig. 26-44) while maintaining

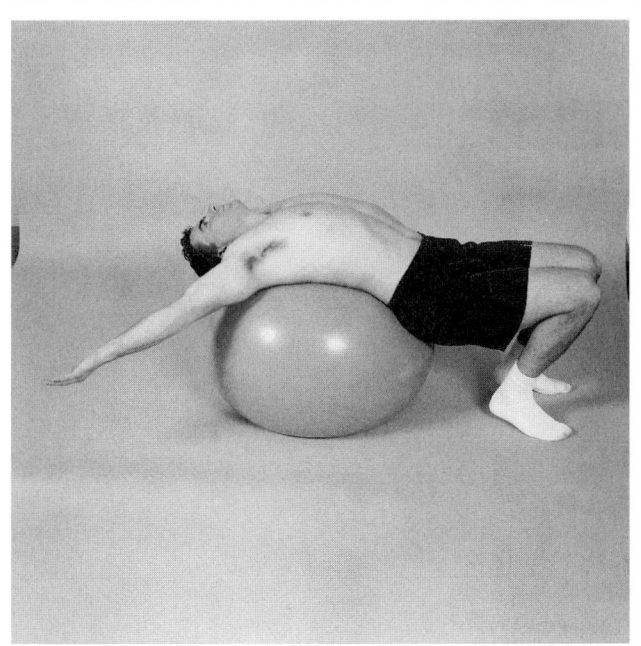

FIGURE 26-42 Thoracic spine extension on Swiss ball with arms spread.

If the patient is unable to maintain his or her balance on the Swiss ball, a foam roll may be used (Fig. 26-43). The foam roll also allows the clinician to focus the extension exercise on a specific segment.

Thoracic Spine Rotation. The following Swiss ball exercises to improve thoracic rotation range of motion and strength are

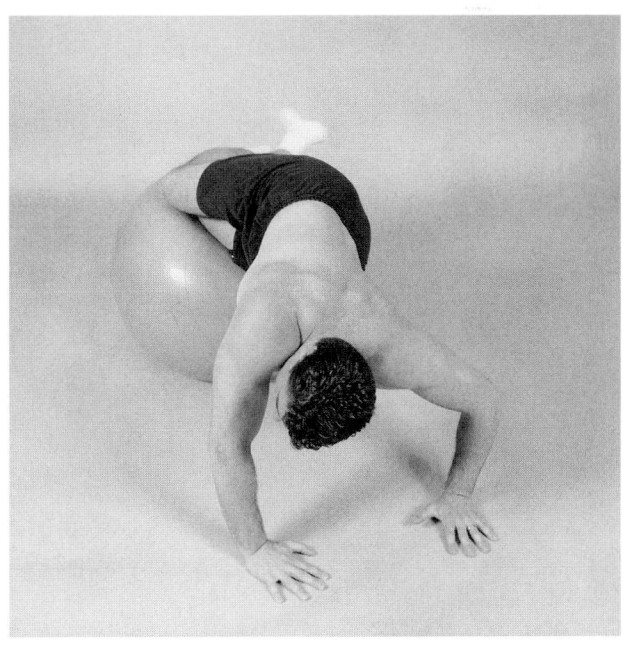

FIGURE 26-44 Thoracic spine rotation with lower trunk and extremity rotation.

balance through the arms. This position is held for 8 to 10 seconds, after which the patient relaxes. The exercise is repeated 8 to 10 times. This exercise can be made more challenging by placing the pelvis on the ball so that the legs are suspended in the air (Fig. 26-45). By alternatively moving the legs into hip flexion and extension, rotation of the thoracic spine can be achieved while maintaining balance with the arms (see Fig. 26-45).

For the nonathletic population, thoracic rotation exercises can be performed using a firmer base of support. The patient kneels in front of a wobble board and places both hands on the board. Once good balance is achieved, the patient is asked to raise one arm out to the side as high as is comfortable while keeping both knees on the floor (Fig. 26-46). This position is held for 8 to 10 seconds, after which the patient relaxes. The exercise is repeated 8 to 10 times.

Thoracic rotation exercises can also be performed in the supine position. The patient lies supine with both knees bent and feet placed on the floor. The arms are abducted to approximately 90 degrees (Fig. 26-47). Keeping the trunk against the floor the patient lowers their thighs to one side and then the other (see Fig. 26-47) as far as is comfortable. This position is held for 8 to 10 seconds, after which the patient relaxes. The exercise is repeated 8 to 10 times.

Thoracic Spine Side Bending. The patient kneels to the side of a Swiss ball. The patient is asked to lean sideways over the ball and, with the arm closest to the ball, to attempt to touch the floor on the other side of the ball (Fig. 26-48) without losing balance. This position is held for 8 to 10 seconds, after which the patient relaxes. The exercise is repeated 8 to 10 times.

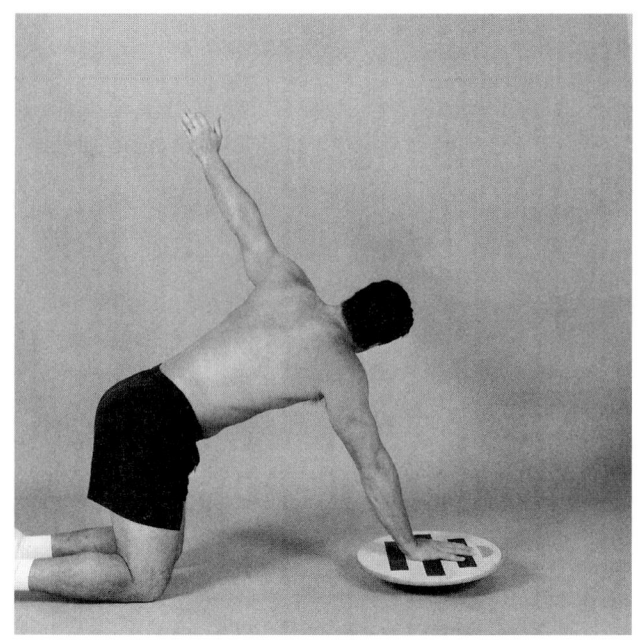

FIGURE 26-46   Thoracic spine rotation in kneeling position using wobble board.

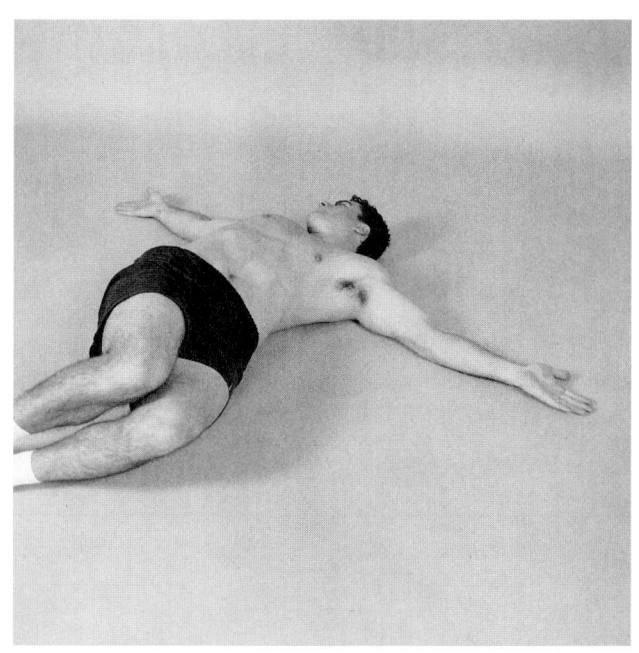

FIGURE 26-47   Thoracic spine rotation using pelvic rotations.

Rib Techniques

Myofascial Stretch into Extension. The patient is positioned supine, and the clinician stands at the head of the bed. The patient elevates both arms over the head and reaches around the back of the clinician's thighs. By having the patient hold a towel in this position, the clinician can place both of his or her hands under the patient's rib cage and pull the rib cage in an anterior

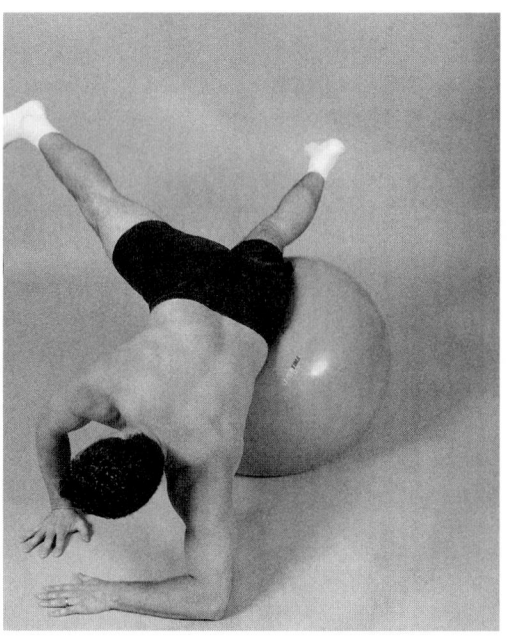

FIGURE 26-45   Thoracic spine rotation with upper trunk rotation.

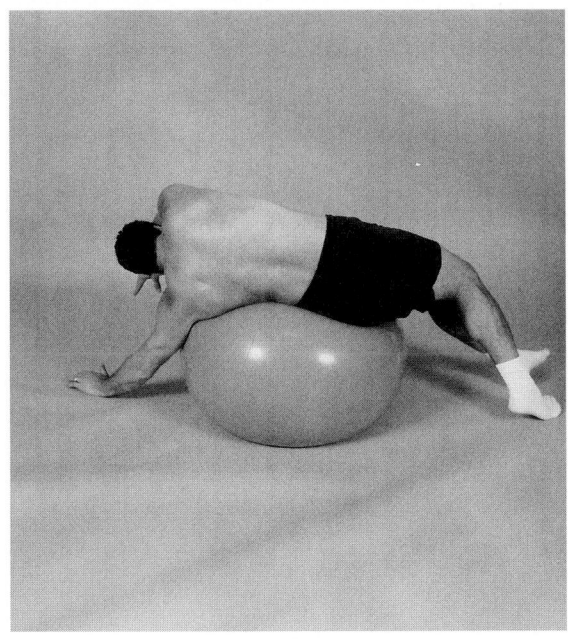

FIGURE 26-48 Thoracic spine side bending over Swiss ball.

and cranial direction, thereby encouraging thoracic extension (Fig. 26-49). A belt wrapped around the patient at the correct level can make this technique more specific.

Bucket Handle Stretch. The patient is positioned side lying. The clinician fully abducts the patient's uppermost arm, grasping it above the elbow. The arm is taken into hyperabduction, thereby fully expanding the rib cage on the uppermost

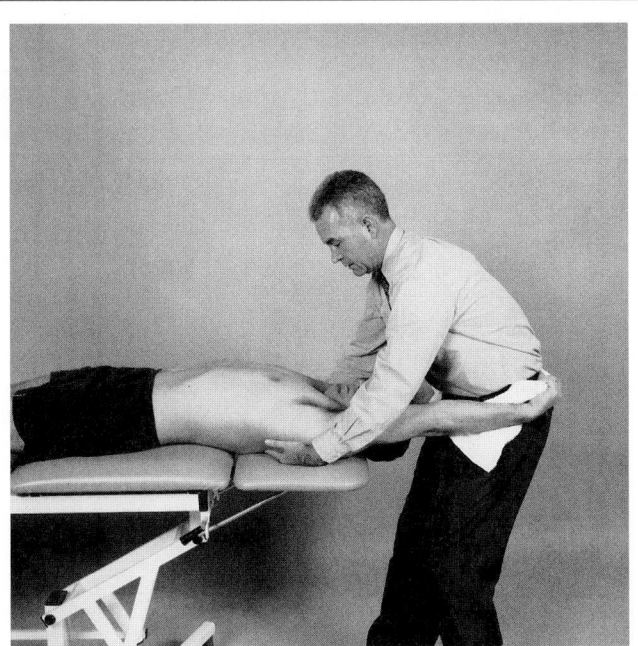

FIGURE 26-49 Rib stretch.

side (Fig. 26-25). Muscle energy techniques also can be incorporated. By adjusting the point of stabilization, this technique can be used to treat inspiration and expiration restricted impairments, for example, a rib dysfunction at ribs 4 and 5, as follows:

▶ *Inspiration restriction.* The clinician stabilizes the fifth rib with the heel of one hand while moving the uppermost arm into sufficient flexion with the other arm.

▶ *Expiration restriction.* While holding the arm in sufficient flexion with one hand, the clinician uses the heel of the other hand to mobilize the fourth rib inferiorly and distally.

Pump Handle Stretch. A similar technique to the one previously described can be used to treat ribs demonstrating a restriction of the pump handle action. The clinician stabilizes the inferior rib with the heel of one hand while moving the uppermost arm into sufficient flexion with the other arm (Fig. 26-26).

CASE STUDY RIGHT ANTERIOR CHEST PAIN

HISTORY

A 25-year-old man presented at the clinic complaining of pain in his right anterior chest. About 1 month previously, the patient had experienced a sudden and sharp pain in his right posterior chest at the midscapular level during a tug of war game at his company's picnic. The posterior chest pain subsided very quickly and did not bother him for the rest of the game. However, the next morning, pain was felt in the anterior aspect of the chest. This anterior chest pain eased off over the next few days with rest, but recurred as soon as the patient returned to weight lifting.[68]

QUESTIONS

1. Given the mechanism of injury, what structure(s) could be at fault?
2. Should the report of anterior chest pain concern the clinician in this case?
3. What is your working hypothesis at this stage? List the various diagnoses that could present with anterior chest pain, and the tests you would use to rule out each one.
4. Why did the pain shift from posterior thoracic to anterior thoracic?
5. Does this presentation/history warrant a scan? Why or why not?

EXAMINATION

On observation, the patient was a healthy looking male with no obvious postural deficits. The patient had presented with pain following a specific mechanism of injury, but because the pain had shifted, a scan was considered necessary. A modification of a thoracic and cervical scan revealed the following:

• The patient demonstrated full range of cervical motion.
• The patient demonstrated full range of thoracic motion, although overpressure with rotation to the right produced the anterior chest pain.

- The slump, neck flexion, and scapular retraction tests were all negative.
- The neurologic tests were negative.
- The compression, traction, and posteroanterior pressures were all pain free.
- Anteroposterior pressure over the right fifth costochondral joint reproduced the patient's pain.
- All other tests were negative.

QUESTIONS

1. Did the scanning examinations confirm the working hypothesis? How?
2. Given the findings from the scanning examination, what is your provisional diagnosis, or is further testing warranted in the form of special tests? What information would be gained with further testing?
3. Has it been determined why the pain shifted from a posterior thoracic to an anterior thoracic location?

The results of the Cyriax scanning examination seemed to indicate costochondritis of the fifth rib. However, the original mechanism had produced posterior thoracic pain. Further examination is needed. The subsequent examination revealed the following:

- The position tests for the thoracic spine were negative.
- The screening test was positive for a rib impairment (positioning the thoracic spine in extreme flexion and having the patient take in a deep breath reproduced the pain, as did positioning the thoracic spine in extreme extension and having the patient take a deep breath out).
- The passive mobility tests for the thoracic spine were negative.

Once the thoracic spine has been ruled out, a rib examination must be performed to confirm a musculoskeletal cause for the patient's symptoms. The rib examination revealed that the posterior rib joint glides were all full and pain free, except for the fifth rib, which appeared to have lost all of its glides.

EVALUATION

The patient was diagnosed with a fifth costotransverse or costovertebral joint subluxation, or both, with a loss of anterior rotation of the rib. The costochondritis probably resulted from abnormal stresses being imparted to this area as a result of the subluxation and provides a good example of the silent hypomobile joint producing pain in a nearby joint.

QUESTIONS

1. Having made the provisional diagnosis, what will be your intervention?
2. How would you describe your findings to the patient?
3. In order of priority, and based on the stages of healing, list the various goals of your intervention.

4. How will you determine the amplitude and joint position for the intervention?
5. Estimate this patient's prognosis.
6. What modalities could you use in the intervention of this patient?

INTERVENTION

- *Electrotherapeutic modalities and thermal agents.* At the initial session, a moist heat pack was applied to the thoracic spine when the patient arrived. Electrical stimulation with a medium frequency of 50 to 120 pulses per second was applied with the moist heat to aid in pain relief. Ultrasound at 1 MHz also could be administered to the articulation in question in lieu of the moist heat. An ice pack was applied to the area at the end of the treatment session.
- *Manual therapy.* Following the application of heat, general stretch techniques were applied to the area followed by a mobilization and manipulation of the fifth rib.
- *Therapeutic exercises.* To maintain the mobility gained, the patient was instructed to perform specific mid-thoracic right side bending and left rotation. The exercises are performed in the pain-free range and should not aggravate any symptoms. Aerobic exercises using a stationary bike and the treadmill also could be prescribed.
- *Patient-related instruction.* Explanation was given as to the cause of the patient's symptoms. The patient was advised to continue the exercises at home, performing ten repetitions, ten times per day and to expect some postexercise soreness. The patient also received instruction on the use of heat and ice at home.
- *Goals/outcomes.* Both the patient's goals from the intervention and the expected therapeutic goals of the clinician were discussed with the patient. It was concluded that the clinical sessions would occur for three more visits spread over a month, at which time it was hoped that the patient would be discharged to a home exercise program.

CASE STUDY BILATERAL AND CENTRAL UPPER THORACIC PAIN

HISTORY

A 30-year-old housewife presents at the clinic with a 3-day history of constant central and bilateral upper thoracic pain that is deep, dull, and can be felt in the front of the chest when the pain is aggravated. The pain is reported to be worse with flexion motions but is improved with lying on a hard surface. Further questioning revealed that the patient had a history of minor back pain but was otherwise in good health and had no report of bowel or bladder impairment.

QUESTIONS

1. What structure(s) could be at fault with central and bilateral upper thoracic pain as the major complaint?
2. Should the report of anterior chest pain concern the clinician in this case?

3. Why was the statement about "no reports of bowel or bladder impairment" pertinent?
4. What is your working hypothesis at this stage? List the various diagnoses that could manifest with central and bilateral upper thoracic pain and the tests you would use to rule out each one.
5. Does this presentation/history warrant a scanning examination? Why or why not?

EXAMINATION

The pain appears to be related to specific motions and positions, is of short duration, and is nonradicular in nature. Therefore, a scanning examination may not be warranted at this time. Active motion testing of the thoracic spine revealed the following:

- Flexion was limited and painful, with a minimal loss of rotation and side bending bilaterally. Extension appeared normal.
- Combined motion testing revealed an increase in pain with flexion and side bending to both sides, and side bending to both sides and flexion.
- Position testing was normal.
- Symmetric passive mobility tests revealed decreased flexion at T5 to T6.
- Confirmatory posteroanterior pressures revealed pain over T5 and T6.

QUESTIONS

1. Did the active motion testing confirm the working hypothesis? How?
2. What information was gathered from the combined motion tests?
3. Using the results of the combined motion tests, is it possible to determine the specific segment at fault?
4. Given the findings from the examination, what is the diagnosis, or is further testing warranted in the form of special tests? What information would be gained with further testing?

EVALUATION

The patient is presenting with the signs of a symmetric flexion hypomobility at T5 to T6. A hypomobility may present as a bilateral or unilateral capsular, or noncapsular hypomobility, or as a unilateral or bilateral hypermobility. If a bilateral arthritis is present, then extension and both side flexions and rotations will be decreased, with flexion being less affected. If it is unilateral, then there will be greater loss of extension than flexion, and one rotation and side bending will be decreased more than the other. A unilateral capsular pattern of the right zygapophysial joint will demonstrate, on position testing, as a large FRSL and a smaller ERSR.

QUESTIONS

1. Having made the provisional diagnosis, what will be your intervention?
2. In order of priority, and based on the stages of healing, list the various goals of your intervention.

3. How will you determine the amplitude and joint position for the intervention?
4. Is an asymmetric or symmetric technique more appropriate for this condition? Why?
5. Estimate this patient's prognosis.
6. What modalities could you use in the intervention of this patient?

INTERVENTION

Following thermotherapy to the area (moist heat or ultrasound), general stretch techniques were applied to the area, followed by a specific mobilization to increase flexion at T5 to T6. To maintain the mobility gained, the patient was instructed to perform specific midthoracic flexion exercises in the pain-free range. Aerobic exercises using a stationary bike and the treadmill also were prescribed. An ice pack was applied to the area at the end of the treatment session. An explanation was given as to the cause of the patient's symptoms. The patient was advised to continue the exercises at home, performing ten repetitions, ten times per day and to expect some postexercise soreness. The patient also received instruction on the use of heat and ice at home.

Both the patient's goals from the treatment and the expected therapeutic goals of the clinician were discussed with the patient. It was concluded that the clinical sessions would occur two times per week for 3 weeks, at which time the plan was to discharge the patient to a home exercise program. With adherence to the instructions and exercise program, it was felt that the patient would make a full return to function.

CASE STUDY INTERSCAPULAR PAIN

HISTORY

A 21-year-old woman presented with a 1-week history of left-sided interscapular pain that started at work. The patient worked as a computer operator. The pain was reported to be aggravated by lying prone, deep breathing in, and standing or sitting erect. Further questioning revealed that the patient had a history of this pain over the past few months, but that it had not been as intense as currently. The patient was otherwise in good health and had no reports of bowel or bladder impairment.

QUESTIONS

1. List the structures that can produce interscapular pain.
2. Given the fact that this patient works at a computer, what could be the cause of her pain?
3. What is your working hypothesis at this stage? List the various diagnoses that could manifest with interscapular pain, and the tests you would use to rule out each one.
4. Does this presentation/history warrant a scan? Why or why not?

TESTS AND MEASURES

The examination revealed the following results:

- With plane motions, the pain was reproduced with extension, and with left side bending.

- The combined movement of extension, left rotation, and left side bending reproduced the pain.
- The passive mobility tests revealed decreased motion at the T5 to T6 level into extension, and decreased motion into left side bending.
- Posteroanterior pressure over T6 revealed extreme tenderness.
- With the joint glide tests, the inferior joint glide at the T5 to T6 zygapophysial joint was reduced on the left side.

QUESTIONS

1. Did the active motion testing confirm the working hypothesis? How?
2. What was the purpose of the combined motion test, if two aggravating motions had already been found?
3. Given the findings from the examination, what is the diagnosis, or is further testing warranted in the form of special tests? What information would be gained with further testing? How would you rule out Maigne's thoracic pain of lower cervical origin?

EVALUATION

A preliminary diagnosis of a unilateral restriction of extension at the T5 to T6 level or an FRSR of T5 was made.

QUESTIONS

1. Having made the provisional diagnosis, what will be your intervention?
2. In order of priority, and based on the stages of healing, list the various goals of your intervention.
3. How will you determine the amplitude and joint position for the intervention?
4. Is an asymmetric or symmetric technique more appropriate for this condition? Why?
5. Estimate this patient's prognosis.
6. What modalities could you use in the intervention of this patient?

INTERVENTION

Following thermotherapy to the area (moist heat or ultrasound), general stretch techniques were applied to the area, followed by a specific mobilization to restore the extension glide on the left at the T5 to T6 level. To maintain the mobility gained, the patient was instructed to perform specific midthoracic left side bending in slight extension frequently (up to ten repetitions, several times per day) in the pain-free range. Explanation was given as to the cause of the patient's symptoms. The patient was advised to expect some postexercise soreness. The patient also received instruction on the use of heat and ice at home. Both the patient's goals from the treatment and the expected therapeutic goals of the clinician were discussed with the patient. It was concluded that the clinical sessions would occur once per week for a month, at which time the patient would be discharged to a home exercise program.

REVIEW QUESTIONS*

1. In the thoracic region, in which plane are the facet joints oriented?
2. Which are the atypical ribs, and why are they atypical?
3. What is the joint where the rib and the vertebra meet called?
4. Which structures modify and restrict rotation in the thoracic region?
5. Which ribs demonstrate bucket handle movement and which display pump handle motions?

---

* Additional questions to test your understanding of this chapter can be found in the Online Learning Center for *Orthopaedic Assessment, Evaluation, and Intervention* at www.duttononline.net.

REFERENCES

1. Singer KP, Edmondston SJ. Introduction: the enigma of the thoracic spine. In: Giles LGF, Singer KP, eds. *Clinical Anatomy and Management of Thoracic Spine Pain*. Oxford, England: Butterworth-Heinemann; 2000.
2. Bradford S. Juvenile kyphosis. In: Bradford DS, et al, eds. *Moe's Textbook of Scoliosis and Other Spinal Deformities*. Philadelphia, Pa: Saunders; 1987:347.
3. Frazer JE. *Frazer's Anatomy of the Human Skeleton*. London, England: Churchill Livingstone; 1965.
4. Singer KP, Jones T, Breidahl PD. A comparison of radiographic and computer-assisted measurements of thoracic and thoracolumbar sagittal curvature. *Skel Radiol* 1990;19:21–26.
5. Willen J, et al. The natural history of burst fractures in the thoracolumbar spine T12 and L1. *J Spinal Disord* 1990;3:39–46.
6. Gray H. *Gray's Anatomy*. Philadelphia, Pa: Lea and Febiger; 1995.
7. Panjabi MM, Takata K, Goel V. Thoracic human vertebrae. Quantitative three-dimensional anatomy. *Spine* 1991;16:888–901.
8. Edmondston SJ, et al. In-vitro relationships between vertebral body density, size and compressive strength in the elderly thoracolumbar spine. *Clin Biomech* 1994;9:180–186.
9. Wood KB, et al. Thoracic MRI evaluation of asymptomatic individuals. *J Bone Joint Surg* 1995;77A:1634–1638.
10. White AA. An analysis of the mechanics of the thoracic spine in man. *Acta Orthop Scand Suppl* 1969;12:78–92.
11. Edmondston SJ, Singer KP. Thoracic spine: Anatomical and biomechanical considerations for manual therapy. *Man Ther* 1997;2:132–143.
12. Williams PL, ed. *Gray's Anatomy*. 38th ed. New York, NY: Churchill Livingstone; 1995.
13. Rouviere H. *Anatomie Humaine. Descriptive et Topographique*. Paris, France: Masson; 1927.
14. Singer KP, Breidahl PD, Day RE. Posterior element variation at the thoracolumbar transition: A morphometric study using computed tomography. *Clin Biomech* 1989;4:80–86.
15. Lee DG. Biomechanics of the thorax. In: Grant R, ed. *Physical Therapy of the Cervical and Thoracic Spine*. New York, NY: Churchill Livingstone; 1988:47–76.
16. Lee DG. *Manual Therapy for the Thorax—A Biomechanical Approach*. Delta, Canada: Delta Orthopedic Physiotherapy Clinic; 1994.
17. MacConnail MA, Basmajian JV. *Muscles and Movements: A Basis for Human Kinesiology*. New York, NY: Robert Krieger; 1977.

18. King TC, Smith CR. Chest wall, pleura, lung, and mediastinum. In: Schwartz SI, Shires GT, Spencer FC, eds. *Principles of Surgery*. New York, NY: McGraw-Hill; 1989:627.

18a. Nathan H, et al. The costovertebral joints: Anatomical-clinical observations in arthritis. *Arthritis Rheum* 1964;7:228–240.

19. Oda I, et al. Biomechanical role of the posterior elements, costovertebral joints, and rib cage in the stability of the thoracic spine. *Spine* 1996;21:1423–1429.

20. Feiertag MA, et al. The effect of different surgical releases on thoracic spinal motion. *Spine* 1995;20:1604–1611.

21. Jiang H, Raso JV, Moreau MJ. Quantitative morphology of the lateral ligaments of the spine. Assessment of their importance in maintaining lateral stability. *Spine* 1994;19:2676–2682.

22. Andriacchi T, et al. A model for studies of mechanical interactions between the human spine and rib cage. *J Biomech* 1974;7:497–505.

23. Winkel D, Matthijs O, Phelps V. Thoracic spine. In: Winkel D, Matthijs O, Phelps V, eds. *Diagnosis and Treatment of the Spine*. Gaithersburg, Md: Aspen; 1997:389–541.

24. Kendall HO, Kendall FP, Boynton DA. *Posture and Pain*. Baltimore, Md: Williams and Wilkins; 1952.

25. Whitelaw WA. Recruitment patterns of respiratory muscles. In: *Breathlessness: The Campbell Symposium*. Hamilton, Canada: Boehringer Ingelheim; 1992.

26. De Troyer A. Actions and load sharing between respiratory muscles. In: *Breathlessness: The Campbell Symposium*. Hamilton, Canada: Boehringer Ingelheim; 1992.

27. Grassino AE. Limits of maximal inspiratory muscle function. In: *Breathlessness: The Campbell Symposium*. Hamilton, Canada: Boehringer Ingelheim; 1992.

28. De Troyer A, Sampson MG. Activation of the parasternal intercostals during breathing efforts in human subjects. *J Appl Physiol* 1982;52:524–529.

29. Estenne M, Ninane V, Troyer AD. Triangularis sterni muscle use during eupnea in humans: Effect of posture. *Respir Physiol* 1988;74:151–162.

30. De Troyer A, et al. Triangularis sterni muscle use in supine humans. *J Appl Physiol* 1987;62:919–925.

31. Taylor A. The contribution of the intercostal muscles to the effort of respiration in man. *J Physiol* 1960;151:390–402.

32. Whitelaw WA, Feroah T. Patterns of intercostal muscle activity in humans. *J Appl Physiol* 1989;67:2087–2094.

33. Nava S, et al. Respiratory muscle fatigue does not limit exercise performance during moderate endurance run. *J Sports Med Phys Fitness* 1992;32:39–44.

34. Brooks G, Fahey T. *Fundamentals of Human Performance*. New York, NY: Macmillan; 1987.

35. Johnson B, Babcock M, Dempsey J. Exercise-induced diaphragmatic fatigue in healthy humans. *J Physiol* 1993; 460:385–405.

36. Mador M, et al. Diaphragmatic fatigue after exercise in healthy subjects. *Am Rev Resp Dis* 1993;148:1571–1575.

37. De Troyer A, et al. The diaphragm: Two muscles. *Science* 1981;213:237–238.

38. De Troyer A, et al. Action of the costal and crural parts of the diaphragm during breathing. *J Appl Physiol* 1982;53:30–39.

39. Dommisse GF. The blood supply of the spinal cord. *J Bone Joint Surg* 1974;56B:225.

39a. Groskin SA. Selected topics in chest trauma. *Radiology* 1992;183:605–617.

39b. Collins J. Chest wall trauma. *J Thorac Imag* 2000;15:112–119.

40. Groen GJ, Stolker RJ. Thoracic neural anatomy. In: Giles LGF, Singer KP, eds. *Clinical Anatomy and Management of the Thoracic Spine*. Oxford, England: Butterworth-Heinemann; 2000:114–141.

41. Hovelacque A. *Anatoime des neufs craniens et radichiens et du sisteme grand sympathetique chez l'homme*. Paris, France: Gaston Doin et Cie; 1927.

42. Haymaker W, Woodhall B. *Peripheral Nerve Injuries. Principles of Diagnosis*. London, England: Saunders; 1953.

43. Bogduk N, Marsland A. The cervical zygapophysial joint as a source of neck pain. *Spine* 1988;13:610.

44. Panjabi MM, Hausfeld JN, White AA. A biomechanical study of the ligamentous stability of the thoracic spine in man. *Acta Orthop Scand* 1981;52:315–326.

45. Panjabi MM, Brand RA, White AA. Mechanical properties of the human thoracic spine. *J Bone Joint Surg* 1976;58A:642–652.

46. Flynn TW. Thoracic spine and chest wall. In: Wadsworth C, ed. *Current Concepts of Orthopedic Physical Therapy—Home Study Course*. La Crosse, Wis: Orthopaedic Section, American Physical Therapy Association; 2001.

47. Refshauge KM, Bolst L, Goodsell M. The relationship between cervicothoracic posture and the presence of pain. *J Man Manipulative Ther* 1995;3:21–24.

48. Raine S, Twomey LT. Attributes and qualities of human posture and their relationship to dysfunction or musculoskeletal pain. *Crit Rev Phys Rehabil Med* 1994;6:409–437.

49. Singer KP, Malmivaara A. Pathoanatomical characteristics of the thoracolumbar junctional region. In: Giles LGF, Singer KP, eds. *Clinical Anatomy and Management of the Thoracic Spine*. Oxford, England: Butterworth-Heinemann; 2000:100–113.

50. Shea KG, et al. *The Contribution of the Rib Cage to Thoracic Spine Stability*. Burlington, Vt: International Society for the Study of the Lumbar Spine; 1996.

50a. Takeuchi T, et al. Biomechanical role of the intervertebral disc and costovertebral joint in stability of the thoracic spine: A canine model. *Spine* 1999;24:1414–1420.

50b. Oda I, et al. Biomechanical role of the posterior elements, costovertebral joints, and rib cage in the stability of the thoracic spine. *Spine* 1996;21:1423–1429.

50c. Oda I, et al. An in vitro human cadaveric study investigating the biomechanical properties of the thoracic spine. *Spine* 2002;27:E64–E70.

51. Raou RJP. *Recherches sur la mobilité vertebrale en fonction des types rachidiens*. Paris, France: Thèse; 1952.

52. White AA, Hirsch C. The significance of the vertebral posterior elements in the mechanics of the thoracic spine. *Clin Orthop* 1971;81:2–14.

53. Panjabi MM, et al. Thoracic spine centers of rotation in the sagittal plane. *J Orthop Res* 1984;1:387–394.

54. Levine A, Edwards C. Lumbar spine trauma. In: Camins E, O'Leary P, eds. *The Lumbar Spine*. New York, NY: Raven; 1987:183–212.

55. Gonon JP, et al. Utilité de l'analyse cinématique de radiographies dynamiques dans le diagnostic de certaines affections de la colonne lombaire. In: Simon L, Rabourdin JP, eds. *Lombalgies et médecine de rééducation*. Paris, France: Masson; 1983:27–38.

56. Panjabi MM, Brand RA, White AA. Three-dimensional flexibility and stiffness properties of the human thoracic spine. *J Biomech* 1976;9:185.

57. Davis PR. The medial inclination of the human thoracic intervertebral articular facets. *J Anat* 1959;93:68–74.

58. Singer KP, Day RE, Breidahl PD. In vivo axial rotation at the thoracolumbar junction: An investigation using low dose CT in healthy male volunteers. *Clin Biomech* 1989;4:80–86.

59. Singer KP. The thoracolumbar mortice joint: Radiological and histological comparisons. *Clin Biomech* 1989;4:137–143.

60. Ellis JJ, Johnson GS. Myofascial considerations in somatic dysfunction of the thorax. In: Flynn TW, ed. *The Thoracic Spine and Rib Cage: Musculoskeletal Evaluation and Treatment.* Boston, Mass: Butterworth-Heinemann; 1996:211–262.

60a. Bogduk N, Valencia F. Innervation and pain patterns of the thoracic spine. In: Grant R, ed. *Physical Therapy of the Cervical and Thoracic Spine.* Melbourne, Australia: Churchill Livingstone; 1994:77–88.

60b. Le T, et al. Costovertebral joint erosion in ankylosing spondylitis. *Am J Phys Med Rehabil* 2001;80:62–64.

61. Murtagh JE, Kenna CJ. *Back Pain and Spinal Manipulation.* 2nd ed. Oxford, England: Butterworth-Heinemann; 1997.

62. Lyu RK, et al. Thoracic disc herniation mimicking acute lumbar disc disease. *Spine* 1999;24:416–418.

63. Melzack R. The McGill Pain Questionnaire: Major properties and scoring methods. *Pain* 1975;1:277.

64. Feise RJ, Michael Menke J. Functional rating index: A new valid and reliable instrument to measure the magnitude of clinical change in spinal conditions. *Spine* 2001;26:78–86; discussion 87.

65. Fairbank J. Revised Oswestry Disability questionnaire. *Spine* 2000;25:2552.

66. Lewit K. Chain reactions in disturbed function of the motor system. *J Manual Med* 1987;3:27.

67. Grieve GP. *Common Vertebral Joint Problems.* New York, NY: Churchill Livingstone; 1981.

68. Meadows J. *Orthopedic Differential Diagnosis in Physical Therapy.* New York, NY: McGraw-Hill; 1999.

69. Singer KP, Giles LGF. Manual therapy considerations at the thoracolumbar junction: an anatomical and functional perspective. *J Manipulative Physiol Ther* 1990;13:83–88.

70. Gelb DE, et al. An analysis of sagittal spinal alignment in 100 asymptomatic middle and older aged volunteers. *Spine* 1995;20:1351–1358.

71. Bland JH. Diagnosis of thoracic pain syndromes. In: Giles LGF, Singer KP, eds. *Clinical Anatomy and Management of the Thoracic Spine.* Oxford, England: Butterworth-Heinemann; 2000:145–156.

72. Wing P, Tsang I, Gagnon F. Diurnal changes in the profile shape and range of motion of the back. *Spine* 1992;17:761–766.

73. Beck A, Killus J. Normal posture of the spine determined by mathematical and statistical methods. *Aerospace Med* 1973;44:1277–1281.

74. White AA, Sahrmann SA. A movement system balance approach to management of musculoskeletal pain. In: Grant R, ed. *Physical Therapy for the Cervical and Thoracic Spine.* Edinburgh, Scotland: Churchill Livingstone; 1994:347.

75. Jull GA, Janda V. Muscle and Motor control in low back pain. In: Twomey LT, Taylor JR, eds. *Physical Therapy of the Low Back: Clinics in Physical Therapy.* New York, NY: Churchill Livingstone; 1987:258.

76. Jull GA. Physiotherapy management of neck pain of mechanical origin. In: Giles LGF, Singer KP, eds. *Clinical Anatomy and Management of Cervical Spine Pain.* London, England: Butterworth-Heinemann; 1998:168–191.

77. Crawford HJ, Jull GA. The influence of thoracic posture and movement on range of arm elevation. *Physiother Theory Pract* 1993;9:143–148.

78. Vasilyeva LF, Lewit K. Diagnosis of muscular dysfunction by inspection. In: Liebenson C, ed. *Rehabilitation of the Spine: A Practitioner's Manual.* Baltimore, Md: Lippincott Williams and Wilkins; 1996:113–142.

79. Lewit K. Relation of faulty respiration to posture, with clinical implications. *J Am Osteopath Assoc* 1980;79:525–529.

80. Crawford R, Singer KP. Normal and degenerative anatomy of the thoracic intervertebral discs. In: *Proceedings of Manipulative Physiotherapists Association of Australia: 9th Biennial Conference.* Melbourne, Australia: Gold Coast; 1995.

81. Wiles P, Sweetnam R. *Essentials of Orthopedics.* London, England: JA Churchill; 1965.

82. Deyo RA, Rainville J, Kent DL. What can the history and physical examination tell us about low back pain? *JAMA* 1992;268:760–765.

83. Stagnara P, et al. Reciprocal angulation of vertebral bodies in a sagittal plane: Approach to references for the evaluation of kyphosis and lordosis. *Spine* 1982;7:335–342.

84. McKenzie RA. Manual correction of sciatic scoliosis. *N Z Med J* 1972;76:194–199.

85. Keim HA. *The Adolescent Spine.* New York, NY: Springer-Verlag; 1982.

86. Ombregt L, et al, eds. *A System of Orthopedic Medicine.* London, England: Saunders; 1995.

87. Sutherland ID. Funnel chest. *J Bone Joint Surg* 1958;40B:244–251.

88. Sahrmann SA. *Diagnosis and Treatment of Muscle Imbalances Associated with Regional Pain Syndromes* [lecture outline]. New Brunswick, NJ; 1991.

89. Lewit K. The contribution of clinical observation to neurobiological mechanisms in manipulative therapy. In: Korr IM, ed. *The Neurobiological Mechanisms in Manipulative Therapy.* New York, NY: Plenum Press; 1977:65–78.

90. Mitchell FL, Moran PS, Pruzzo NA. *An Evaluation and Treatment Manual of Osteopathic Muscle Energy Procedures.* Manchester, Mo: Mitchell, Moran and Pruzzo; 1979.

91. Moll JMH, Wright V. Measurement of spinal movement. In: Jayson MIV, ed. *The Lumbar Spine and Back Pain.* New York, NY: Grune and Stratton; 1981:93–112.

92. Evjenth O, Gloeck C. *Symptom Localization in the Spine and Extremity Joints.* Minneapolis, Minn: Orthopedic Physical Therapy Products; 2000.

93. Lawrence DJ, Bakkum B. Chiropractic management of thoracic spine pain of mechanical origin. In: Giles LGF, Singer KP, eds. *Clinical Anatomy and Management of Thoracic Pain.* Oxford, England: Butterworth-Heinemann; 2000:244–256.

94. Maigne R. *Diagnosis and Treatment of pain of Vertebral Origin.* Baltimore, Md: Williams and Wilkins;1996.

95. Evans RC. *Illustrated Essentials in Orthopedic Physical Assessment.* St Louis, Mo: Mosby-Year Book; 1994.

96. Cocchiarella L, Andersson GBJ, eds. *American Medical Association, Guides to the Evaluation of Permanent Impairment.* 5th ed. Chicago, Ill: AMA; 2001.

97. McKenzie RA. *The Cervical and Thoracic Spine: Mechanical Diagnosis and Therapy.* Waikanae, New Zealand: Spinal Publications New Zealand; 1990.

98. Magee DJ. *Orthopedic Physical Assessment.* Philadelphia, Pa: Saunders; 1997.

99. Pavelka K. Rotationsmessung der Wirbelsaule. *Z Rheumaforsch* 1970;29:366.

100. Stoddard A. *Manual of Osteopathic Practice*. New York, NY: Harper and Row; 1969.

101. Maigne JY, Maigne R, Guerin-Surville H. Upper thoracic dorsal rami: Anatomic study of their medial cutaneous branches. *Surg Radiol Anat* 1991;13:109–112.

102. Magee DJ. Cervical spine. In Magee DJ, ed. *Orthopedic Physical Assessment*. Philadelphia, Pa: Saunders; 1992:34–70.

103. Post M. *Physical Examination of the Musculoskeletal System*. Chicago, Ill: Year Book; 1987.

104. Hoppenfeld S. *Orthopedic Neurology—A Diagnostic Guide to Neurological Levels*. Philadelphia, Pa: JB Lippincott; 1977:97–98.

105. Awerbuch GI, Nigro MA, Wishnow R. Beevor's sign and facioscapulohumeral dystrophy. *Arch Neurol* 1990;47:1208–1209.

106. Ventafridda V, et al. On the significance of Lhermitte's sign in oncology. *J Neurooncol* 1991;10:133–137.

107. Ongerboer de Visser BW. Het teken van Lhermitte bij thoracale wervelaandoeningen. *Ned Tijdschr Geneeskd* 1980;124:390–392.

108. Broager B. Lhermitte's sign in thoracic spinal tumour. Personal observation. *Acta Neurochir (Wien)* 1978;106:127–135.

108a. Borges LF, Zervas NT, Lehrich JR. Idiopathic spinal cord herniation: A treatable cause of the Brown-Sequard syndrome: Case report. *Neurosurgery* 1995;36:1028–1031.

108b. Aizawa T, et al. Idiopathic herniation of the thoracic spinal cord: Report of three cases. *Spine* 2001;26:E488–E491.

109. Hudson-Cook N, Tomes-Nicholson K, Breen A. A revised Oswestry disability questionnaire. In: Roland M, Jenner J, eds. *Back Pain: New Approaches to Rehabilitation and Education*. New York, NY: Manchester University Press; 1989:187–204.

110. Roland M, Morris R. A study of the natural history of back pain, part I: The development of a reliable and sensitive measure of disability of low back pain. *Spine* 1986;8:141–144.

111. Klaffs CE, Arnheim DD. *Modern Principles of Athletic Training*. St Louis, Mo: CV Mosby; 1989.

112. Lehmann JF, Silverman DR, et al. Temperature distributions in the human thigh produced by infrared, hot pack and microwave applications. *Arch Phys Med Rehabil* 1966;47:291.

113. Prentice WE. Using therapeutic modalities in rehabilitation. In: Prentice WE, Voight ML, eds. *Techniques in Musculoskeletal Rehabilitation*. New York, NY: McGraw-Hill, 2001:289–303.

114. Durham JW, Moskowitz K, Whitney J. Surface electrical stimulation versus brace in treatment of idiopathic scoliosis. *Spine* 1990;15:888–892.

115. McGill SM. The biomechanics of low back injury: Implications on current practice in industry and the clinic. *J Biomech* 1997;30:465–475.

115a. Cole AJ, Farrell JP, Stratton SA. Functional rehabilitation of cervical spine athletic injuries. In: Kibler BW, Herring JA, Press JM, eds. *Functional Rehabilitation of Sports and Musculoskeletal Injuries*. Gaithersburg, Md: Aspen; 1998:127–148.

116. Corrigan B, Maitland GD. *Practical Orthopaedic Medicine*. Boston, Mass: Butterworth; 1985.

117. Lewit K. *Manipulative Therapy in Rehabilitation of the Motor System*. 3rd ed. London, England: Butterworth; 1999.

118. Janda V. Muscles and motor control in cervicogenic disorders: Assessment and management. In: Grant R, ed. *Physical Therapy of the Cervical and Thoracic Spine*. New York, NY: Churchill Livingstone; 1994:195–216.

119. Pickering D. Precordial catch syndrome. *Arch Dis Child* 1981;56:401–403.

120. Sparrow M, Bird E. "Precordial catch": A benign syndrome of chest pain in young persons. *N Z Med J* 1978;88:325–326.

121. Fam AG, Smythe HA. Musculoskeletal chest wall pain. *Can Med Assoc J* 1985;133:379–389.

122. Brennan R. *The Alexander Technique: Natural Poise for Health*. New York, NY: Barnes and Noble Books; 1991.

123. Buchanan PA, Ulrich BD. The Feldenkrais method: A dynamic approach to changing motor behavior. *Res Q Exerc Sport* 2001;72:315–323.

124. Lake B. Acute back pain: Treatment by the application of Feldenkrais principles. *Aust Fam Physician* 1985;14:1175–1178.

125. Watrous I. The Trager approach: An effective tool for physical therapy. *Phys Ther For* 1992; April 10.

126. Witt P. Trager psychophysical integration: An additional tool in the treatment of chronic spinal pain and dysfunction. *Trager J* 1987;2:4–5.

127. Witt P, Parr C. Effectiveness of Trager psychophysical integration in promoting trunk mobility in a child with cerebral palsy, a case report. *Phys Occup Ther Pediatr* 1988;8:75–94.

128. Blum CL. Chiropractic and Pilates therapy for the treatment of adult scoliosis. *J Manipulative Physiol Ther* 2002;25:E3.

129. Dreyfuss P, Tibiletti C, Dreyer SJ. Thoracic zygapophysial joint pain patterns. A study in normal volunteers. *Spine* 1994;15:453–457.

130. Greenman PE. *Principles of Manual Medicine*. 2nd ed. Baltimore, Md: Williams and Wilkins; 1996.

131. Bourdillon JF. *Spinal Manipulation*. 3rd ed. London, England: Heinemann; 1982.

132. Dunlop R. Tietze revisited. *Clin Orthop* 1969;62:223–225.

133. Gill G. Epidemic of Tietze's syndrome. *BMJ* 1977;2:499.

134. Morgan-Hughes J. Painful disorders of muscle. *Br J Hosp Med* 1979;360:362–365.

135. Gregory PL, Biswas AC, Batt ME. Musculoskeletal problems of the chest wall in athletes. *Sports Med* 2002;32:235–250.

135a. Eastwood DS. Subcutaneous rupture of the breast: A seat-belt injury. *Br J Surg* 1972;59:491–492.

135b. Pal J, Mulder D, Brown RA, Fleiszer D. Assessing multiple trauma: Is the cervical spine enough? *J Trauma* 1988;28:1282–1284.

135c. Daffner R. *Imaging of Vertebral Trauma*. Rockville, Ill: Aspen; 1988.

135d. El-Khoury GY, Whitten CG. Trauma to the upper thoracic spine: Anatomy, biomechanics, and unique imaging features. *AJR* 1993;160:95–102.

135e. Gupta A, El Masri W. Multilevel spinal injuries. *J Bone Joint Surg* 1989;71B:692–695.

135f. Mirvis SE, Templeton P. Imaging in acute thoracic trauma. *Sem Roentgenol* 1992;27:184–210.

135g. Greene R. Lung alterations in thoracic trauma. *J Thorac Imag* 1987;2:1–11.

136. Reid ME. Bone trauma and disease of the thoracic spine and ribs. In: Flynn TW, ed. *The Thoracic Spine and Rib Cage*. Boston, Mass: Butterworth-Heinemann; 1996:87–105.

137. Bradford DS, et al. *Moe's Textbook of Scoliosis and other Spinal Deformities*. 2nd ed. Philadelphia, Pa: Saunders; 1987.

138. Benson MK, Byrnes DP. The clinical syndromes and surgical treatment of thoracic intervertebral disc prolapse. *J Bone Joint Surg* 1975;57B:471–477.

138a. Rowe CR. Fractures of the scapula. *Surg Clin North Am* 1963;43:1565–1571.

138b. McLennan JG, Ungersma J. Pneumothorax complicating fracture of the scapula. *J Bone Joint Surg* 1982;64A:598–599.

138c. McGinnis M, Denton JR. Fractures of the scapula: A retrospective study of 40 fractured scapulae. *J Trauma* 1989;29:1488–1493.

138d. Fletcher BD, Brogdon BG. Seat-belt fractures of the spine and sternum. *JAMA* 1967;200:177–178.

138e. Rutherford WH, et al. The medical effects of seat belt legislation in the United Kingdom. DHSS (Office of the Chief Scientist) HMSO Research Report No. 13; 1985.

138f. Gazak S, Davidson SJ. Posterior sternoclavicular dislocations: Two case reports. *J Trauma* 1984;24:80–82.

139. DeFranca GG, Levine LJ. The T4 syndrome. *J Manipulative Physiol Ther* 1995;18:34–37.

140. McGuckin N. The T4 syndrome. In: Grieve GP, ed. *Modern Manual Therapy of the Vertebral Column*. New York, NY: Churchill Livingstone; 1986:370–376.

141. Maitland G. *Vertebral Manipulation*. Sydney, Australia: Butterworth; 1986.

142. Butler DL, Slater H. Neural injury in the thoracic spine: A conceptual basis for manual therapy. In: Grant R, ed. *Physical Therapy of the Cervical and Thoracic Spine*. New York, NY: Churchill Livingstone; 1994:313–338.

143. Grieve GP. Thoracic musculoskeletal problems. In: Boyling JD, Palastanga N, eds. *Grieve's Modern Manual Therapy of the Vertebral Column*. Edinburgh, Scotland: Churchill Livingstone; 1994:401–428.

144. Butler, DS. Mobilization of the Nervous System. 1992, New York, NY: Churchill Livingstone.

145. Maigne JY. Cervicothoracic and thoracolumbar spinal pain syndromes. In: Giles LGF, Singer KP, eds. *Clinical Anatomy and Management of the Thoracic Spine*. Oxford, England: Butterworth-Heinemann; 2000:157–168.

146. Haldeman S. Spinal manipulative therapy in sports medicine. *Clin Sports Med* 1986;5:277–293.

147. Hartman SL. *Handbook of Osteopathic Technique*. 2nd ed. London, England: Unwin Hyman; 1990:135–143.

148. Mulligan BR. *Manual Therapy: "NAGS," "SNAGS," "PRPS"* etc. Wellington, New Zealand: Plane View Series; 1992.

CHAPTER 27

THE SACROILIAC JOINT

CHAPTER OBJECTIVES

▶ *At the completion of this chapter, the reader will be able to:*

1. Describe the anatomy of the bones, ligaments, muscles, and blood and nerve supply that comprise the sacroiliac region.

2. Describe the biomechanics of the sacroiliac joint, including coupled movements, normal and abnormal joint barriers, kinesiology, and reactions to various stresses.

3. Perform a detailed objective examination of the sacroiliac musculoskeletal system, including palpation of the articular and soft tissue structures, specific passive mobility tests, passive articular mobility tests, and stability tests.

4. Evaluate the total examination data to establish the diagnosis.

5. Describe intervention strategies based on clinical findings and established goals.

6. Design an intervention based on patient education, manual therapy, and therapeutic exercise.

7. Apply active and passive mobilization techniques, and combined movements to the sacroiliac joint, in any position using the correct grade, direction, and duration.

8. Describe the common pathologies and lesions of this region.

9. Evaluate intervention effectiveness in order to progress or modify an intervention.

10. Plan an effective home program and instruct the patient in this program.

OVERVIEW

The sacroiliac joint, which serves as the point of intersection between the spinal and the lower extremity joints, is the least understood and, therefore, one of the most controversial and interesting areas of the spine.

Grieve[1] has proposed that the sacroiliac joint, together with the other areas of the spine that serve as transitional areas, is of prime importance in understanding vertebral joint problems. This level of importance is perhaps surprising, because isolated pelvic impairments are rare. However, findings for sacroiliac joint dysfunction appear to be common, and the literature is replete with intervention techniques aimed at correcting pelvic dysfunctions.[2-12] This may be explained by the fact that, in addition to producing pain on its own, the pelvic joints often can refer pain.[13]

The level of interest surrounding this joint dates back to the Middle Ages, a time when the burning of witches was commonplace.[14] It was noticed after these burnings that three of the bones were not destroyed: a large triangular bone, and two very small bones. It can only be assumed that some degree of significance was given to the large triangular bone as it was deemed a sacred bone, and was thus called the sacrum. It is unclear what significance was given to the two smaller bones, the sesamoid bones of the great toe.

Despite these illustrious beginnings for the sacrum, it was not until about 100 years ago that significant attention was applied to the study of pelvic anatomy and function, and its relationship to low back and pelvic pain. At the start of the 20th century, sacroiliac joint strain was thought to be the most common cause of sciatica.[15] Then, in 1934, Mixter and Barr[16] reported that sciatica could be caused by a prolapsed intervertebral disk, and the interest in the sacroiliac joint as a source of sciatica dwindled.

Since then, there have been periods when the joint has been blamed for almost all low back and leg pain, and times when it has only been considered a problem during pregnancy.

Anatomy

Anatomically, the sacroiliac joint is a large diarthrodial joint that connects the spine with the pelvis. Three bones comprise the sacroiliac joint, two innominates, and the sacrum.

Innominates

The ilium, ischium, and pubic bone fuse at the acetabulum to form each innominate. The ilium of each of the two innominates articulate with the sacrum, forming the sacroiliac joint, and the pubic bone of each of the innominates articulate with each other at the symphysis pubis.[17]

Sacrum

The sacrum (Fig. 27-1), a strong and triangular bone located between the two innominates, provides stability to this area and transmits the weight of the body from the mobile vertebral column to the pelvic region. The sacrum base is above and anterior, and its apex below and posterior (Fig. 27-1). Five centra fuse to form the central part of the sacrum, which contains remnants of the intervertebral disks enclosed by bone. The sacrum has four pairs of pelvic sacral foramina for transmission of the ventral primary rami of the sacral nerves, and four pairs of dorsal sacral foramina for transmission of the dorsal primary rami.

The transverse processes of the first sacral vertebra fuse with the costal elements, to form the ala and lateral crests (see Fig. 27-1). The ala of the sacrum forms the superolateral portions of the base.

The superior articular processes of the sacrum (Fig. 27-1), which are concave and oriented posteromedially, extend upward from the base, to articulate with the inferior articular processes of the fifth lumbar vertebra.

On the dorsal surface of the sacrum is a midline ridge of bone called the median sacral crest (see Fig. 27-1), which represents the fusion of the sacral spinous processes of S1 to S4. Projecting posteriorly from this crest are four spinous tubercles. The fused laminae of S1 to S5, which are located lateral to the median sacral crest, form the intermediate sacral crest (Fig. 27-1).

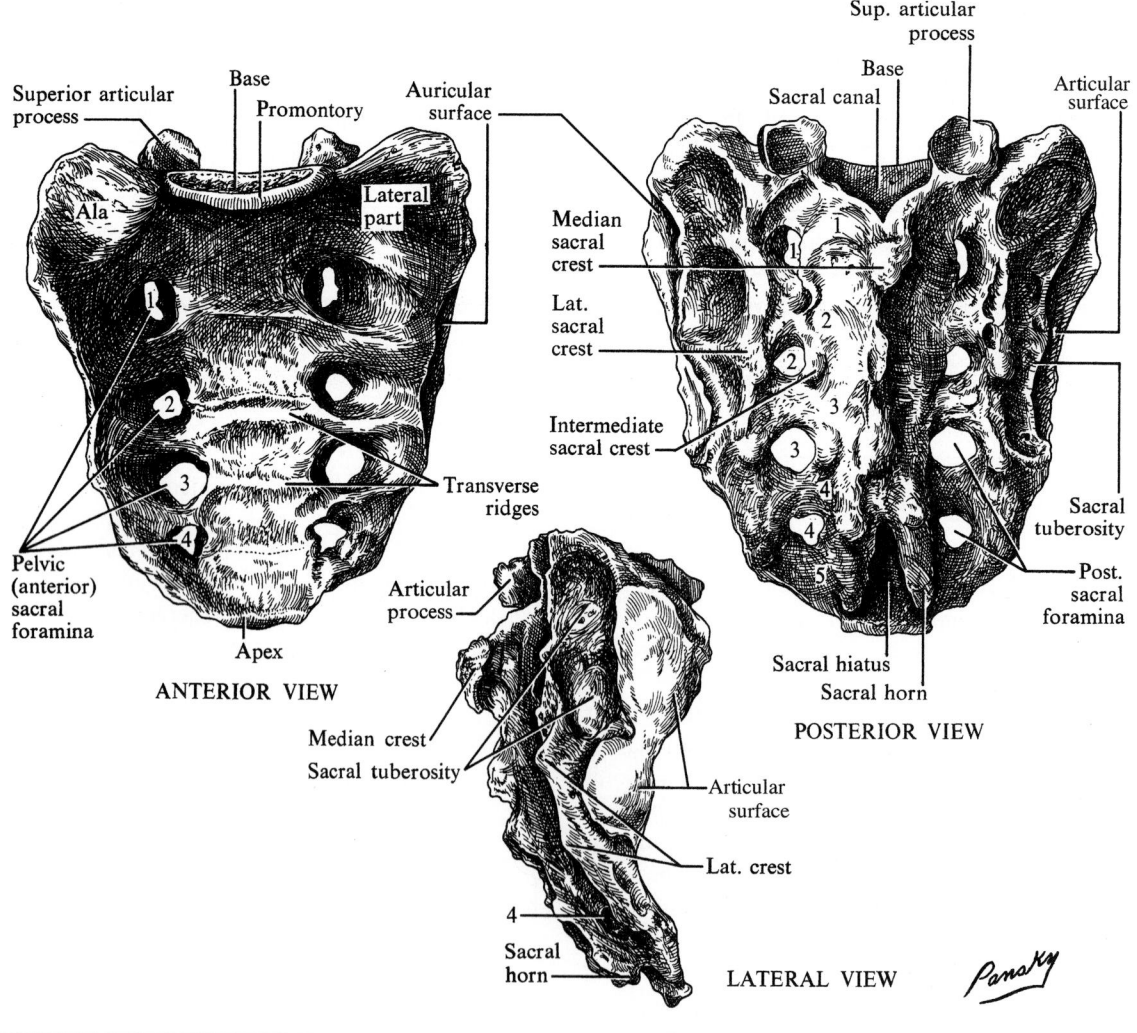

FIGURE 27-1   The sacrum. (Reproduced with permission from Pansky B. *Review of Gross Anatomy*. 6th ed. New York, NY: McGraw-Hill; 1996:199.)

The sacral hiatus (see Fig. 27-1) exhibits bilateral downward projections that are called the *sacral cornua*. These projections represent the inferior articular processes of the fifth sacral vertebra, and are connected to the coccyx via the intercornual ligaments. On the inferolateral borders of the sacrum, about 2 cm to either side of the sacral hiatus, are the inferior lateral angles. The triangular sacral canal (see Fig. 27-1) houses the cauda equina.

In addition to the more commonly considered bones and joints are those of the coccygeal spine (Fig. 27-2).

Sacroiliac Joint

The articulating surfaces of this joint differ, with the iliac joint surfaces formed from fibrocartilage, and the sacral surfaces formed from hyaline cartilage.[18] The hyaline cartilage is three to five times thicker than the fibrocartilage,[19] so that between the sacral and iliac auricular surfaces, the sacroiliac joint is deemed a synovial articulation or diarthrosis.[20]

The inverted, L-shaped, auricular articular surface of the sacrum (Fig. 27-1) is contained entirely by the costal elements of the first three sacral segments. The short (superior) arm of this L-shape lies in a craniocaudal plane, within the first sacral segment, and corresponds to the depth of the sacrum (see Fig. 27-1). It is widest superiorly and anteriorly. The long (inferior) arm of the L-shape lies in an anteroposterior plane, within the second and third sacral segments, and represents the length of the sacrum from top to bottom. It is widest inferiorly and posteriorly. There are large irregularities on each articular surface[21] that are roughly, though not exactly, reciprocal, with the sacral contours being generally deeper.[22,23] In addition to the larger irregularities, there are smaller horizontal crests and hollows that run anteroposteriorly.

Variations in the sacroiliac joint morphology are so common that they have been classified as type A, being less vertical than type B, and type C as an asymmetric mixture of types A and B.[5] Each of these variants can alter the function of the pelvis and its influence on the lumbar lordosis.[24]

> ### Clinical Pearl
>
> The configuration of the sacroiliac joints is extremely variable from person to person, and between genders in terms of morphology and mobility.[23,25,26] However, it has been determined that many of these differences are not pathologic, but rather are normal adaptations.[25]

The articulating surfaces of the joint respond differently to the aging process, with early degenerative changes occurring on the iliac surface rather than on both surfaces of the joint simultaneously.[27] Other changes associated with aging include the development of intra-articular fibrous connections.[28] However, even with severe degenerative changes, the sacroiliac joint rarely fuses.[20]

The sacroiliac joint can be the site of manifestation for several disease processes, including sacroiliac tuberculosis,

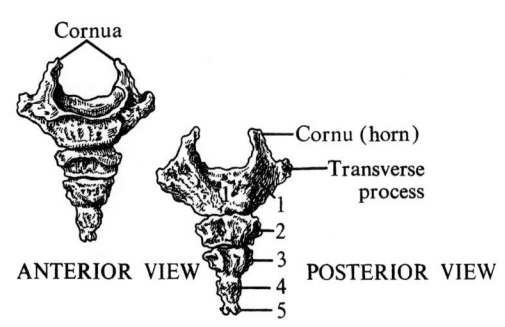

FIGURE 27-2 The coccyx. (Reproduced with permission from Pansky B. *Review of Gross Anatomy.* 6th ed. New York, NY: McGraw-Hill; 1996:199.)

spondyloarthropathy (ankylosing spondylitis), and crystal and pyogenic arthropathies.

Joint Capsule

The sacroiliac joint capsule, consisting of two layers, is extensive and very strong. It attaches to both articular margins of the joint and is thickened inferiorly.

Ligaments

Like other synovial joints, the sacroiliac joint is reinforced by ligaments, but the ligaments of the sacroiliac joint are some of the strongest and toughest ligaments of the body (Fig. 27-3).

Anterior Sacroiliac (Articular)

The anterior sacral ligament (Fig. 27-3) is an anteroinferior thickening of the fibrous capsule, which is relatively weak and thin compared with the rest of the sacroiliac ligaments. The ligament extends between the anterior and inferior borders of the iliac auricular surface and the anterior border of the sacral auricular surface.[20] The anterior sacral ligament is better developed near the arcuate line and the posterior inferior iliac spine (PSIS), where it connects the third sacral segment to the lateral side of the preauricular sulcus.

Because of its thinness, this ligament is often injured and can be a source of pain. It can be palpated at Baer's sacroiliac (SI) point*[29] and can be stressed using the anterior distraction and posterior compression pain provocation tests (see later discussion).

Interosseus Sacroiliac (Articular)

This is a strong, short ligament located deep to the dorsal sacroiliac ligament, and forms the major connection between the sacrum and the innominate, filling the irregular space posterosuperior to the joint between the lateral sacral crest and the iliac tuberosity.[30] The deep portion sends fibers cranially and caudally from behind the auricular depressions. The superficial portion is

---

* Baer's SI point has been described as being on a line from the umbilicus to the anterior superior iliac spine, 5 cm from the umbilicus.

FIGURE 27-3 Anterior and posterior views of the sacrum. (Reproduced with permission from Pansky B. *Review of Gross Anatomy.* 6th ed. New York, NY: McGraw-Hill; 1996:511.)

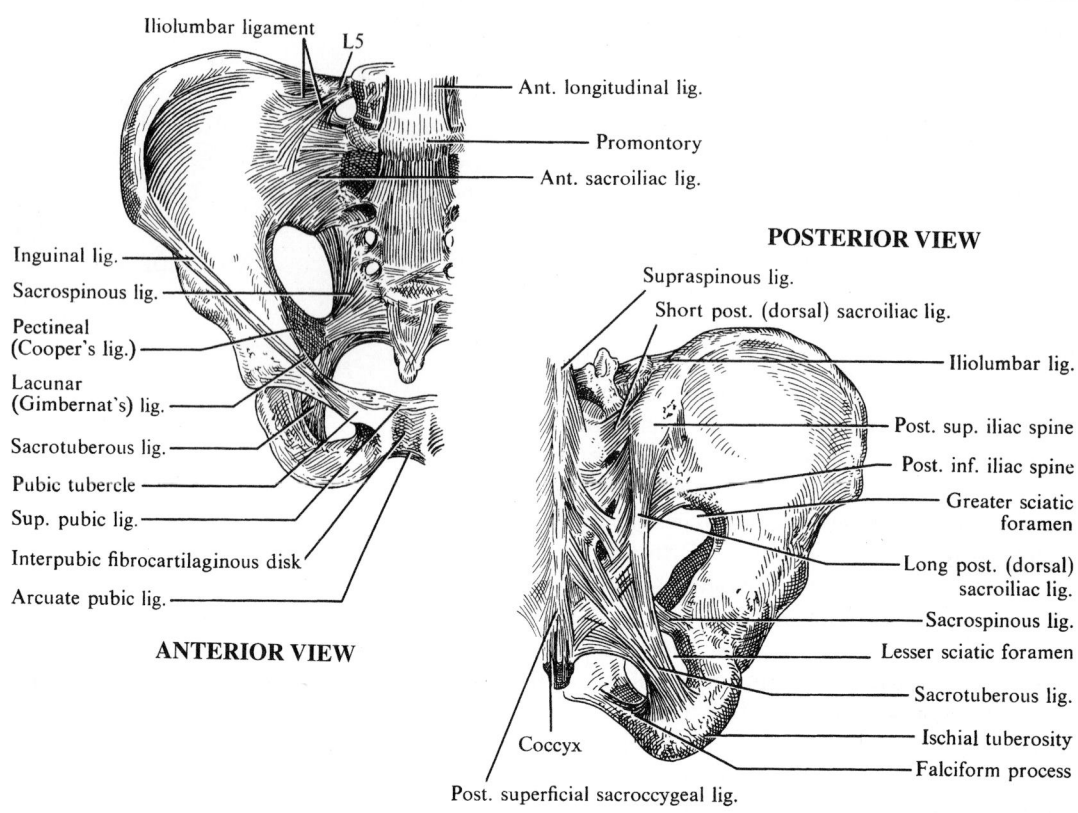

a fibrous sheet connecting the cranial and dorsal margins of the sacrum to the ilium, forming a layer that limits direct palpation of the sacroiliac joint. The interosseous sacroiliac ligament functions to resist anterior and inferior movement of the sacrum.

Dorsal Sacroiliac (Articular)

The dorsal sacroiliac ligament, or long ligament (see Fig. 27-3), which is easily palpable in the area directly caudal to the PSIS, connects the PSIS (and a small part of the iliac crest) with the lateral crest of the third and fourth segments of the sacrum.[17] This is a very tough and strong ligament. The fibers from this ligament are multidirectional and blend laterally with the sacrotuberous ligament. It also has attachments medially to the erector spinae[31] and multifidus muscles,[32] and the thoracodorsal fascia. Thus, contractions of the various muscles that attach to this ligament can result in a tightening of the ligament.

Directly caudal to the PSIS, the ligament is so solid and stout that one can easily think a bony structure is being palpated. Complicating matters is the fact that the skin overlying the ligament is a frequent source of pain.[33] The lateral expansion of the long ligament in the region directly caudal to the PSIS varies between 15 and 30 mm. The length, measured between the PSIS and the third and fourth sacral segments, varies between 42 and 75 mm. The lateral part of the dorsal ligament is continuous with fibers passing between ischial tuberosity and iliac bone.

At the cranial side, the dorsal ligament is attached to the PSIS and the adjacent part of the ilium, at the caudal side to the

lateral crest of the third and fourth, and occasionally to the fifth, sacral segments.[31]

Nutation (anterior motion) of the sacrum appears to slacken the dorsal ligament, whereas counternutation (posterior motion) tautens the ligament.[31]

Sacrotuberous (Extra-articular)

This ligament (see Fig. 27-3) is composed of three large fibrous bands, broadly attached by its base to the PSIS, the lateral sacrum, and partly blended with the dorsal sacroiliac ligament. Its oblique, lateral fibers descend and attach to the medial margin of the ischial tuberosity, spanning the piriformis muscle from which it receives some fibers. The medial fibers, running anteroinferior and laterally, have an attachment to the transverse tubercles of S-3, S-4, and S-5, and the lateral margin of the coccyx. To the posterior surface of the sacrotuberous ligament are attached the lowest fibers of the gluteus maximus and the piriformis, the contraction of which produces increased tension in the ligament.[36] Superficial fibers on the inferior aspect of the ligament can continue into the tendon of the biceps femoris.

In addition to stabilizing against nutation of the sacrum, the sacrotuberous ligament also counteracts against the dorsal and cranial migration of the sacral apex during weight bearing.[34,35]

Sacrospinous (Extra-articular)

Thinner than the sacrotuberous ligament, this triangular-shaped ligament extends from the ischial spine to the lateral margins of the sacrum and coccyx, and laterally to the spine of the ischium

FIGURE 27-4 Two views of the symphysis pubis. (Reproduced with permission from Pansky B. *Review of Gross Anatomy.* 6th ed. New York, NY: McGraw-Hill; 1996:511.)

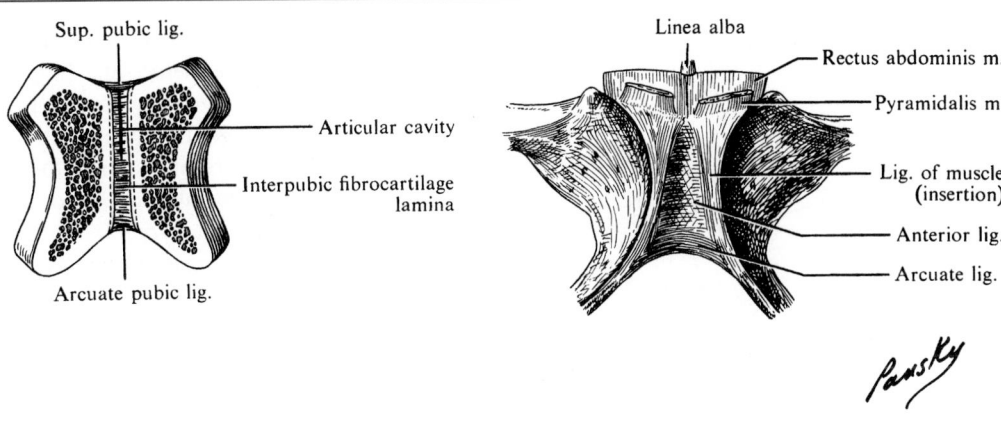

(see Fig. 27-3). The ligament runs anterior (deep) to the sacrotuberous ligament to which it blends, and attaches to the capsule of the sacroiliac joint.[32]

The sacrotuberous and sacrospinous ligaments, which convert the greater and lesser sciatic notches into the greater and lesser foramen respectively, oppose forward tilting of the sacrum on the innominates during weight bearing of the vertebral column.

Iliolumbar (Indirect)

A description of the anatomy of the iliolumbar ligament, is provided in Chapter 25.

Pubic Symphysis

The pubic symphysis is classified as a symphysis because it has no synovial tissue or fluid, and it contains a fibrocartilaginous lamina or disk (Fig. 27-4). The bone surfaces of the joint are covered with hyaline cartilage, but are kept apart by the presence of the disk.

The supporting ligaments of this joint are[22]:

▶ Superior pubic ligament, a thick fibrous band (Fig. 27-4).

▶ Inferior arcuate pubic ligament, which attaches to the inferior pubic rami bilaterally and blends with the articular disk (Fig. 27-4).

▶ Posterior pubic ligament, a membranous structure that blends with the adjacent periosteum.

▶ Anterior ligament, a very thick band that contains both transverse and oblique fibers (Fig. 27-4).

The pubic symphysis is a common source of groin pain, particularly in athletes.

Muscles

Lee[12] lists 35 muscles that attach directly to the sacrum or innominate, or both (Table 27-1). A muscle attaching to a bone has the potential for moving that bone, although the degree of potential varies. Rather than producing movement at the sacroiliac joint, the muscles around the pelvis are more likely involved directly or indirectly in providing stability to the joint.

Piriformis

This muscle (Fig. 27-5) arises from the anterior aspect of the S2, S3, and S4 segments of the sacrum, as well as the capsule of the sacroiliac joint, and the sacrotuberous ligament. It exits from the pelvis via the greater sciatic foramen, before attaching to the upper border of the greater trochanter of the femur.

The piriformis primarily functions to produces external rotation and abduction of the femur, but is also thought to function as an internal rotator and abductor of the hip if the hip joint is flexed beyond 90 degrees. It also helps to stabilize the sacroiliac joint, although too much tension from it can restrict motion of this joint.[37] The piriformis has been implicated as the source for a number of conditions in this area, including:

▶ *Entrapment neuropathies of the sciatic nerve (piriformis syndrome*[38–44]*).* Piriformis syndrome is described in Chapter 9.

▶ *Trigger and tender points.*[45]

TABLE 27-1 Muscles That Attach to the Sacrum, Ilium, or Both

Latissimus dorsi	Gluteus madius
Erector spinae	Gluteus maximus
Semimembranosus	Quadratus femoris
Semitendonosus	Superior gemellus
Biceps femoris	Gracilis
Sartorius	Iliacus
Inferior gamellus	Adductor magnus
Multifidus	Rectus femoris
Obturator internus	Quadratus lumborum
Obturator externus	Pectineus
Piriformis	Psoas minor
Tensor fascia lata	Adductor brevis
External oblique	Adductor longus
Internal oblique	Levator ani
Transversus abdominis	Sphincter urethrae
Rectus abdominis	Superficial transverse
Pyramidalis	perineal ischiocavernous
Gluteus minimus	Coccygeus

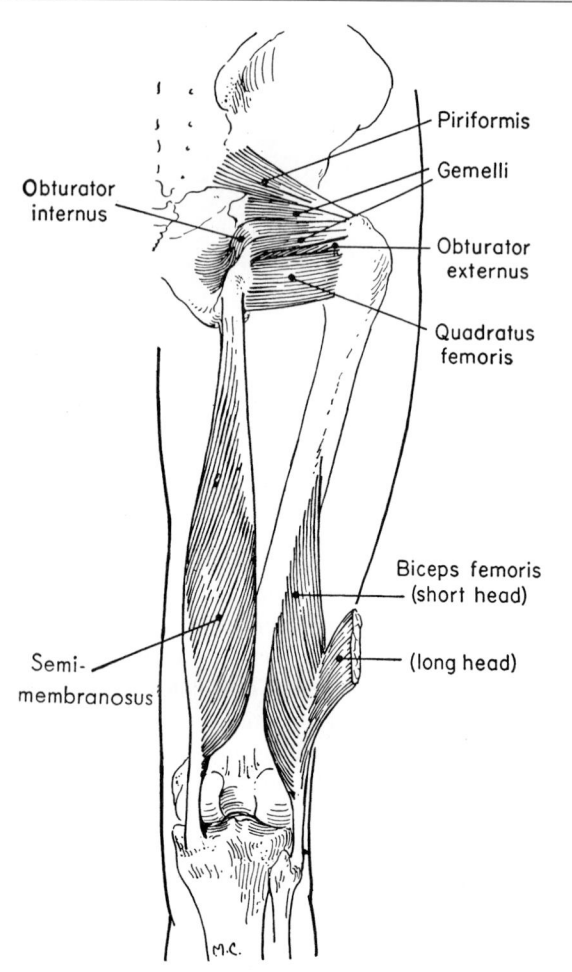

FIGURE 27-5   Deep posterior muscles of the thigh. (Reproduced with permission from Luttgens K, Hamilton K. *Kinesiology: Scientific Basis of Human Motion*. New York, NY: McGraw-Hill; 1997:194.)

Multifidus

The anatomy of the multifidus muscle is described in Chapter 25. Some of the deepest fibers of the multifidus attach to the capsules of the zygapophysial joints[46] and are located close to the centers of rotation for spinal motion. They connect adjacent vertebrae at appropriate angles, and their geometry remains relatively constant through a range of postures, thereby enhancing spinal stability.[47]

Erector Spinae

For a detailed description of the anatomy of the erector spinae, refer to Chapter 25. Through its extending effect on the spine and its substantial sacral attachments, the erector spinae might be thought to promote sacral nutation, although this has not been proven.

Gluteus Maximus

This is one of the strongest muscles in the body (see Chap. 17). It arises from the posterior gluteal line of the innominate, the dorsum of the lower lateral sacrum and coccyx, the aponeurosis

of erector spinae muscle, the superficial laminae of the posterior thoracodorsal fascia, and the fascia covering the gluteus medius muscle, before attaching to the gluteal tuberosity. In the pelvis, the gluteus maximus blends with the ipsilateral multifidus, through the raphe of the thoracodorsal fascia,[32] and the contralateral latissimus dorsi, through the superficial laminae of the thoracodorsal fascia.[48] Some of its fibers attach to the sacrotuberous ligament. When these fibers contract, tension in the sacrotuberous ligament is increased.[49]

Iliacus

This muscle arises from the iliac fossa, the iliac crest, the anterior sacroiliac ligament, the inferior fibers of the iliolumbar ligament,[50] and the lateral aspect of the sacrum. As it travels distally, its fibers merge with the lateral aspect of the psoas major tendon to form the iliopsoas, which continues onto the lesser trochanter of the femur, sending some fibers to the hip joint capsule as it passes.

Long Head of the Biceps Femoris

The long head of the biceps femoris originates from the ischial tuberosity and sacrotuberous ligament. In addition to functioning as a hip extensor and knee flexor, the long head of the biceps femoris, due to its connections to the sacrotuberous ligament, may also have a proprioceptive role during activities such as gait.

Pelvic Floor Musculature

The term "pelvic floor muscles" primarily refers to the levator ani, a muscle group composed of the pubococcygeus, puborectalis, and iliococcygeus. The levator ani muscles join the coccygeus muscles to complete the pelvic floor. The pelvic floor muscles work in a coordinated manner to increase intra-abdominal pressure, provide rectal support during defecation, inhibit bladder activity, help to support the pelvic organs, and assist in lumbopelvic stability.[51]

Levator Ani.   The levator ani (Fig. 27-6) originates anteriorly from the pelvic surface of the pubis, posteriorly from the inner surface of the ischial spine, and from the obturator fascia. It inserts on the front and sides of the coccyx, to the sides of the rectum, and into the perineal body. The levator ani forms the floor of the pelvic cavity, functions to constrict the lower end of the rectum and vagina, and can also be activated during forced expiration.

The muscle, which consists of anterior, intermediate, and posterior fibers, is innervated by the muscular branches of the pudendal plexus.

Anterior Fibers.   The anterior fibers insert into the perineal body, comprise the levator prostatae or sphincter vaginae, and form a sling around the prostate or vagina.

Intermediate Fibers
▶ ***Puborectalis.***   The puborectalis (see Fig. 27-6) originates at the pubis and forms a sling around the junction of the rectum and anal canal. The muscle pulls the anorectal junction anteriorly, assisting the external sphincter in anal closure.

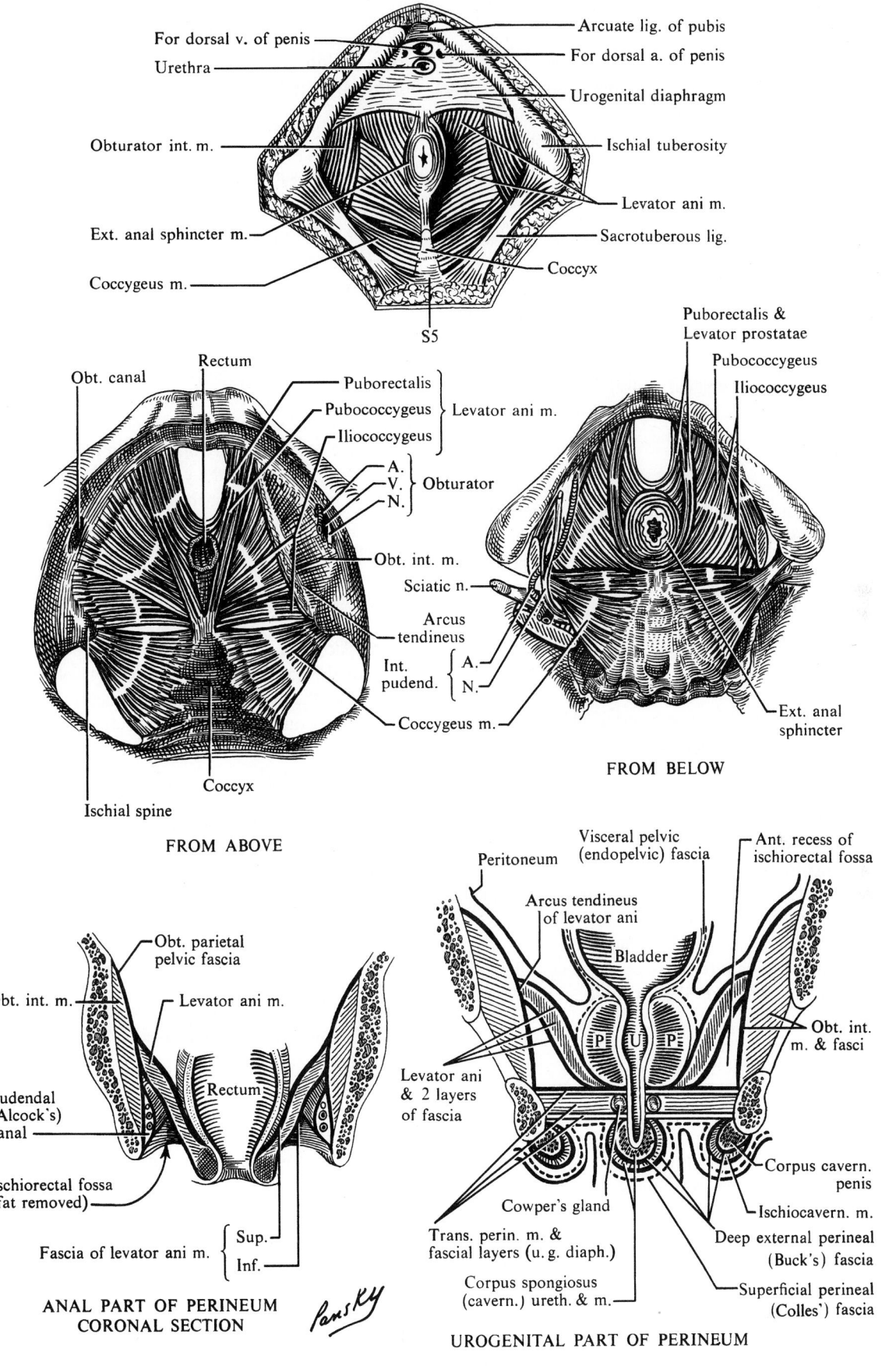

FIGURE 27-6   Pelvic floor musculature: male pelvis. (Reproduced with permission from Pansky B. *Review of Gross Anatomy.* 6th ed. New York, NY: McGraw-Hill; 1996:461.)

▶ *Pubococcygeus.* The pubococcygeal muscle (see Fig. 27-6) arises from the pubis and its superior ramus, and passes posteriorly to insert into the anococcygeal body between the coccyx and anal canal. The muscle functions to pull the coccyx forward. It also serves to elevate the pelvic organs, and to compress the rectum and vagina.

Posterior Fibers. The iliococcygeal muscle (see Fig. 27-6) arises from the arcus tendineus and ischial spine and inserts onto the last segment of the coccyx and anococcygeal body. The muscle functions to pull the coccyx from side to side, and to elevate the rectum.

Levator Plate. The pubococcygeal muscle and the iliococcygeal muscle unite posterior to the anorectal junction to form the levator plate, which inserts into the coccyx.

Coccygeus. This muscle (Fig. 27-6) arises from the pelvic surface of the ischial spine and sacrospinous ligament and inserts on the coccyx margin, and side of the lowest segment of the sacrum. Supplied by the muscular branches of the pudendal plexus, the coccygeus functions to pull forward and support the coccyx. In addition, the coccygeus muscle provides support for the pelvic contents and the sacroiliac joint.

Neurology

It remains unclear precisely how the anterior and posterior aspects of the sacroiliac joint are innervated, although the anterior portion of the joint likely receives innervation from the posterior rami of the L2 to S2 roots.[54] Contribution from these root levels is highly variable and may differ among the joints of given individuals.[55] Additional innervation to the anterior joint may arise directly from the obturator nerve, superior gluteal nerve, or lumbosacral trunk.[23,56] The posterior portion of the joint is likely innervated by the posterior rami of L4 to S3, with a particular contribution from S1 and S2.[57] An additional autonomic component of the joint's innervation further increases the complexity of its neural supply and likely adds to the variability of pain referral patterns from this area.[56,58]

Biomechanics

The motions at the lumbar spine predominantly occur around the sagittal plane and comprise flexion and extension, whereas the motions occurring at the hip occur in three planes, and include the one motion that the lumbar spine does not tolerate well, rotation. Thus, the pelvic area must function to absorb the majority of the lower extremity rotation, while still permitting motion to occur,[59] particularly during bipedal gait.[60]

Although sacroiliac joint mobility under normal circumstances is very limited, movement has been demonstrated.[61–64] It is likely that the movement of the pelvis is in the nature of deformations and slight gliding motions around a number of undefined axes, with the joints of the pelvic ring deforming in response to body weight and ground reaction forces. Motion at the sacroiliac joint is facilitated by several features, including:

▶ The fibrocartilaginous surfaces of the innominate facets, which are deformable, especially during weight bearing, when the surfaces are forced together.

▶ The pubic symphysis. If the innominates are moving at the sacroiliac joint, then they must also be moving at their anterior junction, which would allow for an immediate, and almost perfect, reciprocal motion.

Models of Sacroiliac Motion

There is very little agreement, either among or even within disciplines, about the biomechanics of the pelvic complex. The results from the numerous studies on mobility of the sacroiliac joint have led to a variety of different hypotheses and models of pelvic mechanics over the years. The various models of sacroiliac joint motion are described to give the reader an appreciation of the complexity of this region. It is felt that a deeper understanding of these models will help the clinician in the examination and subsequent intervention. In addition, these models are mentioned in many orthopaedic and manual therapy texts.

Osteopathic Model

Most of the earlier osteopathic models of sacral motion only considered the primary motions of sacral flexion (nutation) and extension (counternutation), which were deemed to occur around four axes:

1. A posterior extra-articular axis.

2. An anterior extra-articular axis.

3. An intra-articular axis at the convergence of the limbs.

4. An axis with a slide along the inferior limb.

In addition, three other axes at S1, S2, and S3 were theorized to accommodate respiratory, sacroiliac, and iliosacral motions, respectively.

Later theories also included two oblique axes about which the sacrum rotated in an oblique fashion. These axes were named after the upper corner of the sacrum from which they emerge. Thus, the axis running from the superior right corner to the inferior left was termed the *right oblique axis,* and, that axis running from the superior and left corner to the inferior right, the *left oblique axis.*

It was proposed that the innominate rotated anteriorly and posteriorly, depending on the motion occurring. A clear distinction was made between sacroiliac impairment and iliosacral impairment. Despite the obvious fact that the two lesions were describing a dysfunction of the same joint, the distinction has survived.

Chiropractic Model

A model of pelvic mechanics developed by Illi[65] is still regarded by many chiropractors as the most complete.[66] Illi proposed that the sacroiliac joint is most active during locomotion, with movement occurring mainly in the oblique sagittal plane. In this proposal, each sacroiliac joint goes through two full cycles of alternating flexion and extension during gait, with the motion at one joint mirrored by the motion at the opposing joint. Illi suggests that as one innominate flexes (anteriorly rotates), the ipsilateral sacral base moves anterior and inferior, and as the other innominate extends (posteriorly rotates), the sacral base on that side moves posterior and superior. If the described actions of the sacrum are visualized as one continuous motion, it can be viewed as an oblique and horizontal figure eight. He further postulates that alternating movements of flexion act through the iliolumbar ligament to dampen motion at L5 and, hence, the whole spine. As the innominate moves posteriorly, L5 is pulled posteriorly and inferiorly through tension in the iliolumbar ligament, and the rest of the lumbar spine undergoes coupled motion in slight rotation and side bending.

Functional Biomechanical Model

The functional biomechanical model of sacroiliac joint motion is based on the work of Vleeming[67] and Snijders.[68] This model proposes that small amounts of motion occur at the sacroiliac joint and that sacroiliac dysfunction is the result of impaired load transfer through the sacroiliac joints.

Sacral Motion. Vleeming and colleagues[67] have proposed that when the sacrum nutates, or flexes, relative to the innominate, a small linear glide occurs between the two L-shaped articular surfaces of the sacroiliac joint. The shorter of the two lengths, level with S1, lies in a vertical plane, whereas the longer length, spanning S2 to S4, lies in an anteroposterior plane.

1. During sacral nutation (Fig. 27-7), the sacrum glides inferiorly down the short length, and posteriorly along the long length. This motion is resisted by a number of factors that include:
   a. The wedge shape of the sacrum.
   b. The ridges and depressions of the articular surfaces.
   c. The friction coefficient of the joint surface.

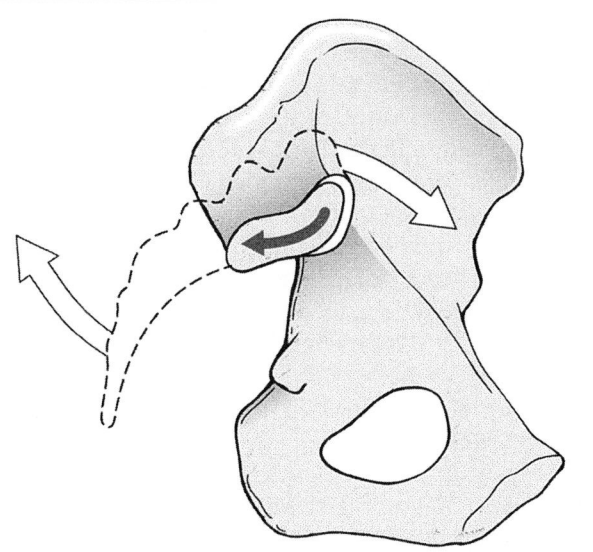

FIGURE 27-7 Sacral nutation. (Reproduced with permission from Dutton M. *Manual Therapy of the Spine.* New York, NY: McGraw-Hill; 2002:452.)

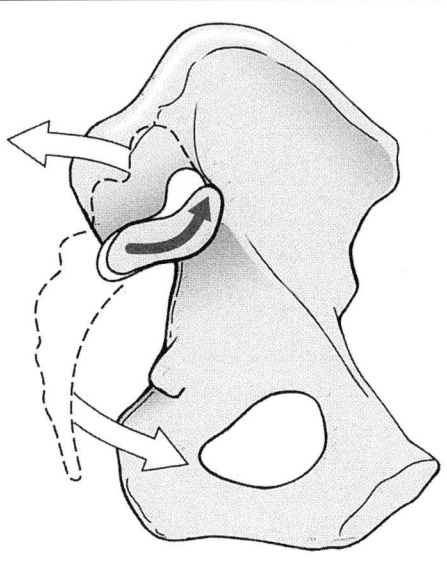

FIGURE 27-8 Sacral counternutation. (Reproduced with permission from Dutton M. *Manual Therapy of the Spine.* New York, NY: McGraw-Hill; 2002:452.)

   d. The integrity of the dorsal, interosseous and sacrotuberous ligaments, supported by the muscles that insert into the ligaments.
2. During sacral counternutation, or extension (Fig. 27-8), the sacrum glides anteriorly along the longer length and superiorly up the shorter length. This motion is resisted by the dorsal sacroiliac ligament,[31] which is supported by the contraction of the multifidus.

Innominate Motion. Innominate motion is induced by hip motion, as in extension of the lower extremity, or during trunk motion when bending forward at the waist. When the innominate rotates anteriorly (Fig. 27-9), it glides in the direction of the short length of the "L" and posteriorly along the longer length of the "L" of the sacroiliac joint, in exactly the same way as the motion that occurs during counternutation of the sacrum. When the innominate rotates posteriorly (Fig. 27-10), it glides in the direction along the longer length of the "L" and superiorly up the short length of the "L" of the sacroiliac joint, in exactly the same way as the motion that occurs during nutation of the sacrum.

Innominate Rotation. The direction of the innominate rotation depends on the initiating movement.

▶ During hip flexion, the ipsilateral innominate posteriorly rotates while the sacrum rotates to the same side as the flexed femur. The posterior rotation of the innominate positions the anterior superior iliac spine (ASIS) in an upward position. If the femur is extended, the ipsilateral innominate anteriorly rotates, and the sacrum rotates to the contralateral side to the extended femur (Table 27-2).

▶ During an anterior pelvic tilt on a relatively fixed femur, an anterior rotation of the innominate occurs. The converse holds true for posterior rotation. Thus, during a posterior pelvic tilt, the innominate posteriorly rotates.

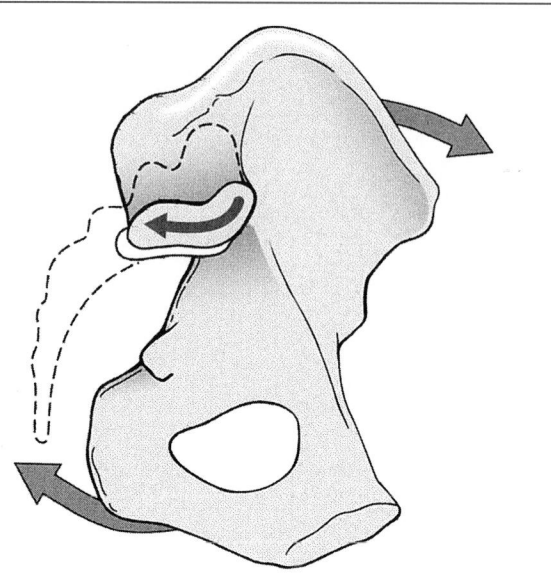

FIGURE 27-9 Anterior rotation of the innominate. (Reproduced with permission from Dutton M. *Manual Therapy of the Spine.* New York, NY: McGraw-Hill; 2002:453.)

Functional Movements. The functional biomechanical model can be used to help explain the integration of lumbar–pelvic–hip movements that occurs during the planar motions of the lumbar spine.

Forward Bending. Sacral flexion, or nutation, involves an anterior rotation in the sagittal plane, so that the anterior aspect of the sacrum inclines downward. If this sacral flexion occurs from top to bottom (as part of lumbar flexion), it results in flexion of the sacrum. However if the sacral flexion occurs from bottom to top (as part of a posterior pelvic tilt or hip flexion), the sacrum extends.

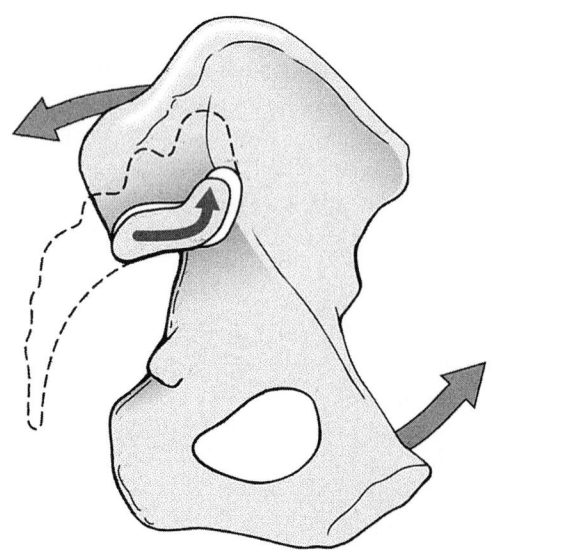

FIGURE 27-10 Posterior rotation of the innominate. (Reproduced with permission from Dutton M. *Manual Therapy of the Spine.* New York, NY: McGraw-Hill; 2002:453.)

TABLE 27-2   Hip Motion and Innominate Motions

Hip Motion	Motion of Ipsilateral Innominate
Flexion	Posterior rotation
Extension	Anterior rotation
Internal rotation	Internal rotation (inflare)
External rotation	External rotation (outflare)
Abduction	Superior glide
Adduction	Inferior glide

During forward bending at the waist, a combination of anterior and outward rotation of both innominates results in the approximation and superior motion of both PSISs, while the sacrum nutates (Table 27-3). After about 60 degrees of forward bending, the innominates continue to rotate anteriorly, but the sacrum no longer nutates.[12] If the sacrum remains nutated throughout forward bending, the sacroiliac joint remains compressed and stable. However, if the sacrum is forced to counternutate earlier in the range, as in individuals with tight hamstrings, less compression occurs, thereby increasing the reliance on dynamic stabilization provided by muscles and thus making the sacroiliac joint more vulnerable to injury.[12]

Backward Bending. Backward bending at the waist, or extension of the spine, involves a combination of an anterior displacement of the pelvic girdle and an inferior motion of both posterior superior iliac spines. A slight posterior innominate rotation occurs and the sacrum remains nutated (Table 27-3).

Side Bending. During right side bending, the right innominate rotates anteriorly and the sacrum right side bends. Motion of the innominate during side bending likely results from ground reaction forces.[69] As side bending to the right occurs, the right leg takes more weight, and so is compressed. This downward body weight force, together with the upward ground reaction force, results in anterior rotation (extension) of the innominate, causing a slight flexion of the hip. This hip flexion, together with the flattening of the foot and hyperextension of the knee, effectively allows the leg to shorten in response to these compressive forces. It is interesting that in non–weight bearing, anterior innominate rotation results in a leg-length increase, whereas in weight bearing, an anterior rotation produces a leg-length decrease. In fact, it is the same mechanism in both cases.[69] In non–weight bearing, the anterior rotation of the innominate pushes the femur downward. Because there is no resistance under the foot, and no force to flex the hip, the leg can lengthen. In weight bearing, ground reaction forces push the innominate superiorly because of the inability of the leg to lengthen during the side bending.

Trunk Rotation. During axial rotation of the trunk to the left, the right innominate rotates anteriorly, while the left innominate rotates posteriorly. Simultaneously, counternutation of the sacrum occurs at the right sacroiliac joint, and nutation occurs at the left

TABLE 27-3 Lumbar Motions and Sacroiliac Motions

Lumbar Motion	Innominate Motion	Sacrum Motion
Flexion	Anterior rotation	Nutation, then counternutation
Extension	Slight posterior rotation	Nutation
Rotation	*Ipsilateral:* Posterior rotation *Contralateral:* Anterior rotation	Nutates ipsilaterally
Side bending	*Ipsilateral:* Anterior rotation *Contralateral:* Posterior rotation	*Ipsilateral:* Side bends ipsilaterally *Contralateral:* Side bends contralaterally

sacroiliac joint. The motion of the innominates during trunk rotation allows the sacrum to rotate osteokinematically while maintaining a more or less vertical orientation.

Gait Biomechanics. The following description of gait biomechanics is based on the functional biomechanical model of sacroiliac joint motion and is, at this time, hypothetical. As described in Chapter 13, an efficient gait requires, amongst other things, a fully functioning lumbar–pelvic–hip complex. As the right leg approaches initial contact, the pelvic girdle is rotated counterclockwise in the transverse plane, translated anteriorly, and adducted on the femoral head. The right innominate is posteriorly rotated, and the left innominate is anteriorly rotated. The anterior rotation of the left innominate pulls the sacrum into right rotation.

At this point in the gait cycle, the lower lumbar vertebrae flex, and side bend contralaterally, adopting the same direction of rotation as the sacrum,[70] with the iliolumbar ligament modifying the motion at the L5 to S1 segment.[71] The lumbar rotation and side bending appear to occur in an isolated manner, and are out of phase with each other; when the spine is side bent maximally, it is rotated the least, and vice versa. This unusual coupling is thought to allow:

▶ The facet column on the non–weight-bearing leg to function as a mobile adaptor, so that the spine is in a loose-pack position at initial contact.

▶ The opposite facet column to function as a rigid lever, so that the spine is in a close-pack position during the weight bearing phases of gait.

Just before the right foot makes initial contact and the left foot begins the swing phase, tension within the interosseous ligament, biceps femoris, and sacrotuberous ligament increases on the right side.[72] This increase in tension contributes to the stabilization of the sacroiliac joint on the side of initial contact.[12]

From initial contact to midstance, the ipsilateral gluteus medius and contralateral adductors are active to stabilize the pelvic girdle on the femoral head. During this period of double support, the lumbar spine is initially in a position of neutral

with reference to side bending. However, as the left foot comes off the ground, the pelvis lists to the left. This list is controlled by the right hip abductors and right lumbar side flexors. To compensate for this list, the lumbar spine side bends to the right.

During the right single leg stance phase:

▶ The pelvic girdle translates anteriorly, and adducts on the right femoral head.

▶ The right innominate begins to rotate anteriorly, relative to the sacrum, and the left innominate rotates posteriorly.

▶ The biceps femoris relaxes and the gluteus maximus becomes more active.[72] Simultaneously, the contralateral latissimus dorsi fires.[73] Together, these two muscles tense the thoracodorsal fascia, which helps to stabilize the sacroiliac joint.[12]

In the early stance phase on the right, with the shoulders in opposite position to the pelvis, the lumbar spine is positioned in right side bending and left rotation, rotating in the same direction as the sacrum. At midstance on the right, the pelvis has reached a position of neutral rotation in the transverse plane, a motion that is controlled by the hip external rotators on the right.

During the late stance on the right leg, the pelvis continues to rotate in a clockwise direction, and the lumbar spine is now in a position of full left rotation and slight side bending to the right.

The displacement of the center of gravity is exaggerated when the sacroiliac joint is unstable, and compensation results through a transfer of weight laterally over the involved limb, thus reducing the vertical shear forces through the joint.[74] In a noncompensated gait pattern, the patient often demonstrates a Trendelenburg gait which serves to reduce the vertical shear force.

Form Closure and Force Closure. Snijders[75] and Vleeming[25,76] defined kinetics within the lumbar–pelvic–hip region by introducing the concepts of "extrinsic" and "intrinsic" stability of the pelvic girdle and the self-locking mechanism (see later discussion). Their work instituted the terms *form closure* and *force closure* to describe the passive and active forces that help to stabilize the pelvis and the sacroiliac joint.

Form Closure.   Form closure refers to a state of stability within the pelvic mechanism, with the degree of stability dependent on its anatomy, with no need for extra forces to maintain the stable state of the system.[68] The following anatomic structures are proposed to assist with form closure:

▶ The congruity of the articular surfaces and the friction coefficient of the articular cartilage. Both the coarseness of the cartilage and the complementary grooves and ridges increase the friction coefficient, and thus contribute to form closure, by resisting against horizontal and vertical translations.[23] In infants, the joint surfaces are very planar, but between the ages of 11 and 15 years, the characteristic ridges and humps that make up the mature sacrum begin to form. By the third decade, the superficial layers of the fibrocartilage are fibrillated, and crevice formation and erosion has begun. By the fourth and fifth decades, the articular surfaces increase irregularity and coarseness, and the wedging is incomplete.[20]

▶ The integrity of the ligaments.

▶ The shape of the closely fitting joint surfaces.

The integrity of form closure is clinically evaluated with the long-arm and short-arm shear tests, discussed later.

Force Closure.   Force closure requires intrinsic and extrinsic forces to keep the sacroiliac joint stable.[68] These dynamic forces involve the neurological and myofascial systems, and gravity. Together, these components produce a self-locking mechanism for the sacroiliac joint.

Critical to the functioning of the self-locking mechanism is the ability of the sacrum to nutate, because nutation of the sacrum winds up most of the sacroiliac joint ligaments, particularly the sacrospinous, sacrotuberous, and the interosseous ligaments.[67,68,76a] In addition, the ligaments posterior to the joint approximate the posterior iliac bones when placed under tension during sacral nutation.[67]

Just as nutation of the sacrum enhances the self-locking mechanism, counternutation of the sacrum, which occurs during activities such as the end range of forward-bending, sacral sitting, long sitting, and hip hyperextension, reduces the self-locking mechanism.[67]

In addition to the ligamentous contribution to the force closure system, kinetic analysis of the pelvic girdle by Vleeming et al. have identified a number of muscles that resist translational forces and which are specifically important to the force-closure mechanism: the erector spinae, gluteus maximus, latissimus dorsi, and biceps femoris (see Chap. 25).[67,76b] Two other muscle groups, an "inner muscle unit" and an "outer muscle unit" also play an important role.[52,53,12] The inner muscle unit consists of:

▶ *The muscles of the pelvic floor.*   Hemborg et al.[78] have demonstrated that the pelvic floor muscles co-activate with the transversus abdominis during lifting tasks.

▶ *Transverse abdominis.*

▶ *Multifidus.*

▶ *The diaphragm.*

The outer muscle unit consists of four systems: the posterior oblique system (latissimus dorsi, gluteus maximus, and thoracolumbar fascia), the deep longitudinal system (erector spinae, deep lamina of the thoracolumbar fascia, sacrotuberous ligament, and biceps femoris), the anterior oblique system (external and internal oblique, contralateral adductors of the thigh, and the intervening anterior abdominal fascia), and the lateral system (gluteus medius–minimus and contralateral adductors of the thigh). The outer muscle unit is proposed to contribute to the force closure mechanism in the following manner:[12]

▶ *Posterior oblique system.*   The gluteus maximus, which blends with the thoracodorsal fascia, and the contralateral latissimus dorsi contribute to force closure of the sacroiliac joint posteriorly by approximating the posterior aspects of the innominates. This oblique system is a significant contributor to load transference through the pelvic girdle during the rotational activities of gait.

▶ *Deep longitudinal system.*   This system, serves to counteract any anterior shear or sacral nutation forces as well as to facilitate compression through the sacroiliac joints. As mentioned in the anatomy section, the long head of the biceps femoris muscle controls the degree of nutation via its connections to the sacrotuberous ligaments.[76c]

▶ *Anterior oblique system.*   The oblique abdominals, acting as phasic muscles, initiate movements[53] and are involved in all movements of the trunk and upper and lower extremities, except when the legs are crossed.[79]

▶ *Lateral system.*   The lateral system functions to stabilize the pelvic girdle on the femoral head during gait through a coordinated action.

It is important that the length and strength of the muscle units are assessed, as is the ability of the sacrum to nutate.

Weakness or insufficient recruitment and/or unbalanced muscle function within the lumbar–pelvic–hip region can reduce the force closure mechanism, which can result in compensatory movement strategies.[74] These compensatory movement strategies and/or patterns of muscle imbalance may produce a sustained counternutation of the sacrum, thereby "unlocking" the mechanism and rendering the sacroiliac joint vulnerable to injury. This "unlocked" position of the pelvis may also increase shear forces at the lumbar spine and abnormal loading of the lumbar disks.

Examination

Most investigators agree that no single test can be used confirm the diagnosis of sacroiliac joint dysfunction. Diagnostic physical examination tests that are commonly used to determine a diagnosis include[55]:

► Direct tenderness.

► Soft tissue examination for zones of hyperirritability and tissue texture changes.

► Evaluation of referral zones.

► Associated fascial or musculotendonous restrictions.

► Regional abnormal length-strength muscle relationships.

► Postural analysis.

► True leg-length and functional leg-length determination.

► Static and dynamic osseous landmark examinations.

► Provocative testing, including traditional orthopaedic tests, motion demand tests, and ligament tension tests.

Although traditionally assumed to be reliable and diagnostically useful, none of these tests has ever been validated against an independent criterion standard.[55] As a consequence, controversy exists about which group of tests is the best.

Under the premise that a relationship exists between pelvic asymmetry and low back pain, orthopaedic, osteopathic, and physical therapy texts promote the use of pain provocation (symptom-based) tests and static (positional) or dynamic (motion or functional) tests.[1,10,12,37,80–83]

The use of static tests has been questioned,[84–88] although Cibulka and colleagues[89] found the results from these tests reliable, Levangie[88] found a weak association between standing PSIS asymmetry and low back pain, at least in selected groups. The problems with static testing are:

► Determining whether the asymmetry noted is normal or abnormal.

► Determining which side is abnormal.

► Determining whether the asymmetry is too asymmetric or not asymmetric enough. If the right innominate is anteriorly rotated, compared with the left, is it rotated too much, too little, or just the right amount compared with its starting position? Because the starting position is not known, the degree of rotation cannot be assessed.

The dynamic tests do not fair much better. Dreyfuss and colleagues[55] reported 20 percent positive findings in one or more of the dynamic (motion or functional) tests in a group of asymptomatic people. An example of a dynamic test is the standing flexion test. The standing flexion test has been used frequently to analyze sacroiliac joint mobility and has been used by most health professions to determine the side of the impairment. The test is performed as follows. Each PSIS is palpated with the thumb placed under it caudally. The patient then bends forward at the waist. Providing there is no impairment in the sacroiliac joint or the lower lumbar spine, as the patient bends forward, both thumbs should move cranially. If the joint is "blocked," it moves upward further in relation to the other side.[87] Thus far, reliability studies of the standing flexion test show it to lack sufficient diagnostic power.[87,90,91] This shortfall may be because the compression of

the joints caused by the sacral nutation in the early to midranges of forward flexion likely limits movement of the sacroiliac joint.[92]

Some studies have reported that pain provocation tests have a good interexaminer reliability,[87,93] but they have not been found reliable by others.[90,94]

This is likely because the pain provocation tests have only been found reliable in identifying sacroiliac joint dysfunction in certain populations, such as patients with posterior pelvic pain during or following pregnancy.[94a]

Given the questionable reliability and validity of the tests for the sacroiliac joint, the clinician should guard against forming a diagnosis based on the results of a few tests. Ideally, the diagnosis needs to be based on the results from a thorough biomechanical examination that includes pain provocation and static and dynamic tests. As several recent studies have found improved inter-rater reliability in the diagnosis of low back pain when using a combination of physical examination procedures as opposed to a single model approach,[94b–94f] it might be logical to assume that a similar approach would work with the sacroiliac joint.

In most cases, an examination of the pelvic joints is of little use if the lumbar spine and hip joints have not been previously cleared by examination or intervention, because both of these joints can refer pain to this area and may also profoundly affect the function of the sacroiliac joint.

History

A history of low back pain or leg pain, or both, warrants an examination of the lumbo–pelvic–hip complex.

Mechanical pain resulting from sacroiliac joint dysfunction may manifest as sacral pain but may also refer pain distally. Sacroiliac joint problems can refer pain to the PSIS, iliac fossa, medial buttock, and superior lateral and posterior thigh.[95] Pain also may be referred to the sacrum from a distant structure, including the contralateral sacrospinalis muscle,[96] the ipsilateral interspinous ligaments of L3 to S2,[97] and the L4 to L5 facet joints.[98] In addition, it is well established that dysfunctional pelvic floor muscles can contribute to the symptoms of interstitial cystitis and the so-called urethral syndrome, which is urgency-frequency with or without chronic pelvic pain.[99–101] In general, unilateral pain with no referral below the knee may be caused by the sacroiliac joint, whereas irritation of a spinal nerve may cause radicular symptoms below the knee.[102] Pubic symphysis dysfunction typically results in localized pain, or groin pain, which is aggravated by activities involving the hip adductor or rectus abdominis muscles.[103]

The following findings are likely to be present with a sacroiliac joint dysfunction[13,55,104,105]:

► A history of sharp pain that awakens the patient from sleep upon turning in bed.

► Pain with walking, ascending or descending stairs, rising to stand from a sitting position, or hopping or standing on the involved leg.

► A positive straight leg raise at, or near, the end of range (occasionally early in the range when hyperacute), pain, and sometimes limitation on extension and ipsilateral side bending of the trunk.

Systems Review

Given the number of visceral organs in the vicinity of the sacroiliac joint, the clinician must complete a thorough systems review to rule out a visceral source for the symptoms. A Cyriax scanning examination (see Chap. 9) should be performed on any patient who presents with an insidious onset of pelvic pain. The scanning examination, which includes the primary stress tests (anterior and posterior distraction) can be used to detect sacroiliitis resulting from microtraumatic arthritis, macrotraumatic arthritis, or systemic arthritis (e.g., ankylosing spondylitis, Reiter's syndrome), or the more serious pathologies grouped under the sign of the buttock (see Chap. 17). Primary breast, lung, and prostate cancers are among the most common cancers to metastasize to the axial skeleton, including the pelvic ring.[106] A further source of sacral pain can be a stress fracture of the sacrum, which can be associated with a wide range of extrinsic and intrinsic risk factors (see "Intervention Strategies," later), and an equally wide range of symptoms and signs.[107]

Tests and Measures

Observation

The observation should begin with an overall assessment of posture to check for the presence of asymmetry. The clinician should observe the degree of tilt at the pelvis. The question of cause and effect should be raised. An anterior pelvic tilt causes an increase in the lumbar lordosis and thoracic kyphosis. The anterior pelvic tilt results in a stretching of the abdominals and the sacrotuberous, sacroiliac, and sacrospinous ligaments, and an adaptive shortening of the hip flexors, hamstrings, and erector spinae. A posterior pelvic tilt results in a lengthening of the hip flexors, hamstrings, and erector spinae, and adaptive shortening of the abdominals and gluteals.

A lateral pelvic tilt, in which one iliac crest is higher than the other, may be caused by scoliosis with ipsilateral lumbar convexity, a leg-length discrepancy, or shortening of the contralateral quadratus lumborum. This position results in adaptive shortening of the ipsilateral hip abductors and contralateral hip adductors, and weakness of the contralateral hip abductors.

There appears to be a strong correlation between the position of the pelvis and the forward head.[108] If the pelvic landmarks are asymmetric and the patient has a forward head, the clinician should attempt to correct the forward head. If the attempted correction of the forward head worsens the pelvic asymmetry and increases the symptoms, the intervention should be aimed at correcting the asymmetry. If the attempted correction of the forward head improves the pelvic symmetry and the symptoms, the subsequent intervention should be aimed at correcting the forward head.[109]

> ### Clinical Pearl
>
> The pelvic crossed syndrome (see Chap. 25) produces an increase in anterior tilt accompanied by an increase in lumbar lordosis.

Hip Range of Motion

Range of motion of the hip, including internal and external rotation, is performed to help rule out pain referred from the hip joint. A unilateral limitation of hip motion, in which one of the motions is unequal between the left and right sides, has been observed in patients with disorders of the sacroiliac joint.[64,110–112]

However, the evidence to demonstrate whether hip motion is limited in patients with signs of sacroiliac joint dysfunction is inconclusive. LaBan and colleagues[103] noted asymmetry in hip abduction and external rotation in patients with inflammation of the sacroiliac joints. Dunn and colleagues[113] reported limited hip mobility in patients with infection of the sacroiliac joint; however, no mention was made as to which movements were limited.

Others have described cases in which patients with low back pain had unilateral, limited internal hip rotation and excessive external hip rotation, and also exhibited signs of sacroiliac joint dysfunction. A recent study by Cibulka and colleagues[110] attempted to determine whether a characteristic pattern of hip range of motion existed in patients with low back pain, and whether those classified as having sacroiliac joint dysfunction have a different pattern of hip range of motion compared with those with unspecified low back pain. The study found that patients with low back pain, who had signs suggesting sacroiliac joint regional pain, had significantly more hip external than internal rotation range of motion on one side. The authors concluded that identifying unilateral hip range of motion asymmetry in patients with low back pain may help in diagnosing sacroiliac joint regional pain.[110]

Lumbosacral Screen

This screening test assesses the overall function of the lumbo–pelvic–hip complex, and if negative, would indicate that these regions are not the source of pain. However, as with any screening test, the results from this test should be combined with other test results before a definitive conclusion is drawn.

The patient is asked to stand with the feet shoulder-width apart. The patient is asked to forward bend and then to rotate to the left while in full flexion. The patient is then asked to backward bend and then to rotate to the left while backward bent.

The test is then repeated using forward flexion and right rotation, and backward bending and right rotation. The clinician notes the quality and quantity of motion and whether any of the motions reproduce the patient's pain. Whether or not motions occur at the sacroiliac joint during these maneuvers, it cannot be argued that the lumbar spine, and hip joints are all moved through substantial ranges during these tests. Thus, full and pain-free motion with the tests tends to rule out a mechanical source of pain at these joints.

Landmark Palpation

The palpation of landmarks can be used to locate areas of tenderness rather than for detecting pelvic asymmetry, because as pelvic landmark asymmetry is probably the norm, "positive" findings are likely to be misleading.[88] The various landmarks of the pelvis are palpated with the patient positioned standing, sitting, and prone lying.

The following landmarks and structures are palpated:

► *Iliac crest.* The iliac crests on both sides are located using the medial aspects of the index fingers. The crest heights should be level (Fig. 27-11).

► *Anterior superior iliac spine (ASIS) (see Fig. 27-11).* These structures are located anteriorly to the iliac crests. An inferior ASIS relative to the other side may indicate a rotated innominate.[8] In the supine position, if the innominate is anteriorly rotated, the leg will be longer on that side, but if posteriorly rotated, the leg will be shorter.[8] Tenderness of the ASIS may indicate a so-called hip pointer injury or injury to the inguinal ligament.

► *Posterior superior iliac spine (PSIS).* These structures are located posteriorly to the iliac crests and approximately 2–3 cm beneath the dimples of the lumbar spine, and level with the S2 spinous process (Fig. 27-12). To assess the levels of the PSIS relative to the opposite side, the clinician hooks the thumbs under both PSIS. A superior PSIS relative to the other side may indicate a rotated innominate.[8] Slightly medially and distal to the PSIS are the sacroiliac joints.

► *Pubic symphysis and pubic tubercles.* The pubic tubercles are lateral to the pubic symphysis (Fig. 27-11).

► *Thoracodorsal fascial attachments.*

► *Dorsal ligament (see Fig. 27-3).*

► *Greater trochanter (Fig. 27-12).*

► *Ischial tuberosity and the sacrotuberous ligament (medial to the tuberosity).* The ischial tuberosity serves as the attachment for the hamstrings and the sacrotuberous ligament. The ischial bursa also is located here. According to osteopathic doctrine, the sacrotuberous ligament is firm on the side of an anteriorly rotated innominate, and taut on the side of a posteriorly rotated innominate.[8] The patient is positioned prone, and the clinician stands at the patient's side. With the heel of the hands, the clinician locates the ischial tuberosities through the soft tissue at the gluteal folds (see Fig. 27-12). Then, with the thumbs, the clinician palpates the inferomedial aspect of the ischial tuberosities. From this point, the clinician slides the thumbs superolaterally and palpates the sacrotuberous ligament (see Fig. 27-3). The clinician then compares the relative tension between the left and right sides.

► *Sacral sulcus and sacral base.* From the PSIS, the clinician moves in a thumb width, and then up a thumb width (see Fig. 27-1).

► *Inferior lateral angle.* These structures are level with the prominent part of the tail bone.

► *L5 segment.* The clinician palpates medially along the iliac crest. L5 is usually level with the point at which the palpating finger begins to descend on the crest. The L5–S1 zygapophysial joints are located half way between the L5 spinous process and the ipsilateral PSIS (see Fig. 27-12).

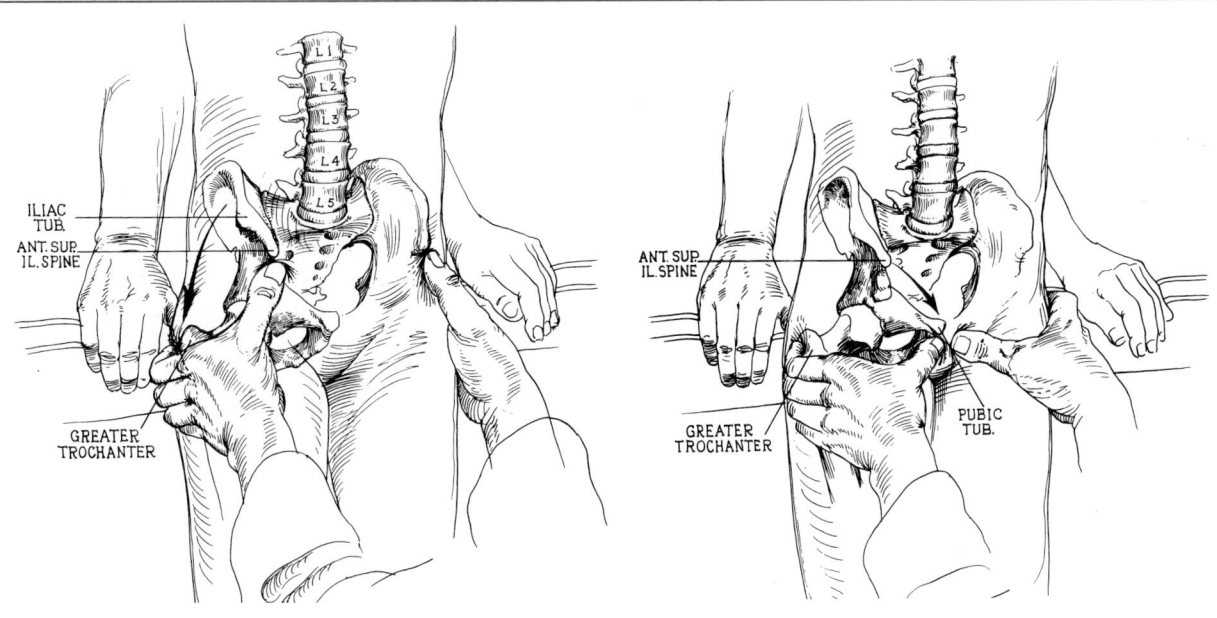

FIGURE 27-11 Palpation landmarks of the hip and pelvis.

FIGURE 27-12 Bony landmarks. (Reproduced with permission from Hoppenfeld S. *Physical Examination of the Spine and Extremities.* Norwalk, Conn: Appleton-Century-Crofts; 1976:146.)

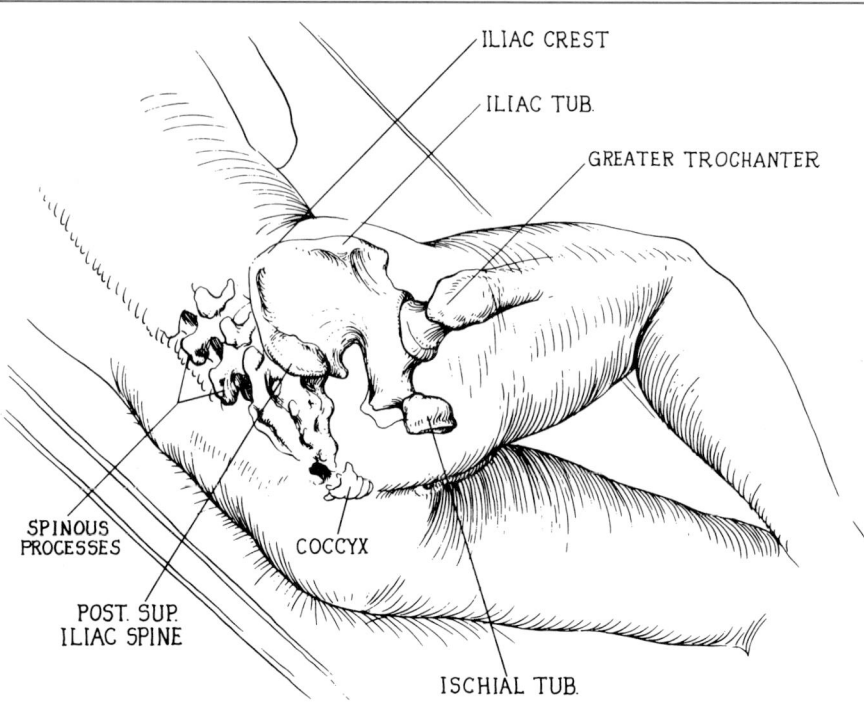

ILIAC CREST

ILIAC TUB.

GREATER TROCHANTER

SPINOUS PROCESSES

COCCYX

POST. SUP. ILIAC SPINE

ISCHIAL TUB.

▶ *Lumbosacral angle.* An increased or decreased lumbosacral angle on one side may indicate a rotated innominate. Although very difficult to measure without radiographs, the normal lumbosacral angle (the angle the sacrum makes with the lumbar spine) is approximately 140 degrees from the vertical.

▶ *S2 segment.* S2 is normally level with the PSIS.

Weight-bearing Kinetic Tests

The kinetic tests, as a group, include both weight-bearing and non–weight-bearing tests. These tests are designed to assess the osteokinematics occurring at the sacroiliac joint during patient-generated movements. The tests assess the mobility of the innominate, and the ability of the sacrum to nutate (ipsilateral test) and to side bend (contralateral test). Because these movements are difficult to observe, bony landmarks are palpated during the movements. The tests for the right side are described.

Ipsilateral Flexion Kinetic Test (Gillet Test). The ipsilateral flexion kinetic test[114] assesses the mobility of the short arm of the auricular surface, and the ability of the ipsilateral innominate to rotate posteriorly. With the patient standing, the clinician palpates the inferior aspect of the right PSIS with one thumb, while the left thumb palpates the median sacral crest (S2) directly parallel. The clinician then asks the patient to flex the right hip as far as is comfortable (Fig. 27-13). The patient may steady himself or herself using a hand against a wall or similar stable object.

During this maneuver, the lumbar spine side bends to the left and rotates to the right. The clinician should feel the right

innominate rotate posteriorly, and the sacrum to rotate to the left (nutate on the right).

A positive ipsilateral flexion kinetic test is observed when the thumb on the inferior aspect of the PSIS moves cranially instead of caudally, and the patient hikes the right side of the pelvis or leans excessively away from the tested side, indicating a dysfunction of the ipsilateral sacroiliac joint or the lumbar spine.

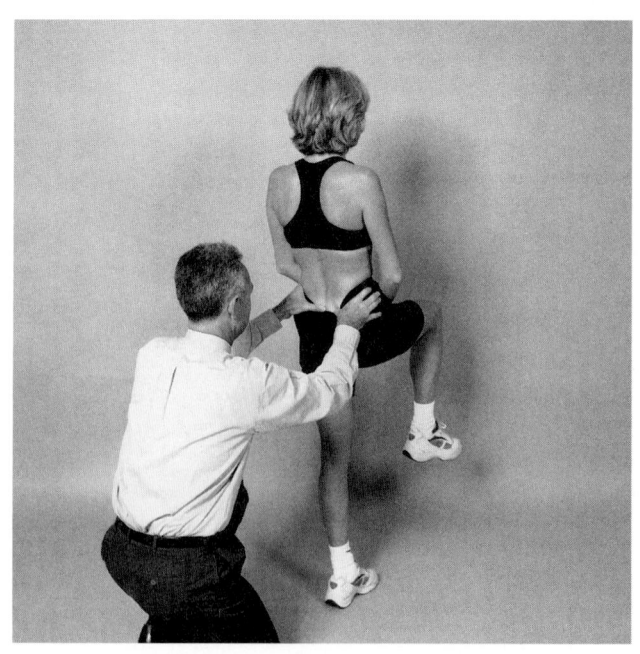

FIGURE 27-13 Ipsilateral kinetic flexion test.

The test is repeated on the other side, and the results are compared.

Ipsilateral Extension Kinetic Test. This test serves as a functional mobility test of the sacroiliac joint. The clinician palpates under the right PSIS with one thumb, and at the median sacral crest (S2) directly parallel with the opposite thumb (Fig. 27-14). The patient extends the right hip, with the knee extended, into varying degrees of hip extension, while the clinician notes the superolateral displacement of the PSIS relative to the sacrum.

Both sides are tested. The right extension test examines the ability of the right innominate to rotate anteriorly, and the sacrum to right rotate (counternutate). The left extension test examines the ability of the left innominate to rotate anteriorly, and the sacrum to left rotate (counternutate.)

Summary of Findings. The potential impairments within the pelvic girdle, which render the ipsilateral kinetic tests positive, include[10]:

▶ Anteriorly or posteriorly rotated innominate of the ipsilateral side (intra-articular or extra-articular in origin).

▶ Pubic symphysis impairment on the ipsilateral side.

▶ Innominate flare on the ipsilateral side.

▶ Subluxed innominate on the ipsilateral side (intra-articular in origin).

Contralateral Flexion Kinetic Test.[10] This test evaluates the mobility of the long arm of the auricular surface, and the ability of the sacrum to side bend to the opposite side of the hip flexion.

With the patient standing, the clinician places the left thumb on the medial sacral crest of the sacrum (S2), and the right thumb on the right PSIS. The patient is asked to flex the left hip to 90 degrees (Fig. 27-15). During this movement, the clinician's left thumb, on the sacral crest, travels caudally initially because of the posterior rotation of the left innominate, which produces a right side bending and left rotation of the sacrum (conjunct rotation).

In addition, the lumbar vertebral bodies will rotate to the left because of the influence of the iliolumbar ligament on L5.

When the contralateral kinetic test is positive, the left thumb travels caudally or it does not move, indicating that the sacrum is unable to side bend.

The potential sacroiliac impairments that render the contralateral kinetic test positive include[10]:

▶ Sacral torsion.

▶ Sacral nutation or counternutation.

The ipsilateral and contralateral kinetic tests are evaluated on both sides for comparison.

Non–Weight-bearing Kinetic Tests[115]

The patient is positioned prone. The clinician palpates the PSIS on one side, and the median sacral crest (S2), and asks the patient to flex the ipsilateral knee. During this maneuver, the clinician should feel an anterior rotation of the ipsilateral innominate (Fig. 27-16).

Using the same palpation points, the patient then flexes the other knee. The clinician should feel a relative posterior rotation of the innominate during this maneuver. The two tests are repeated on the other side.

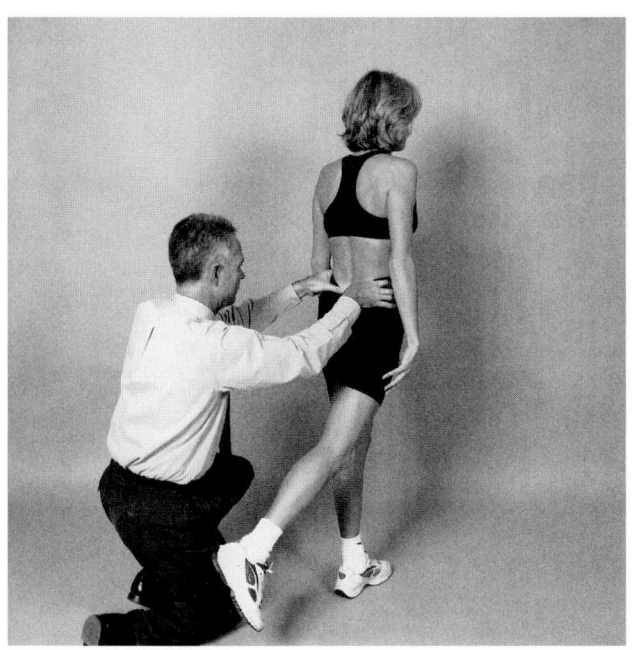

FIGURE 27-14 Ipsilateral extension kinetic test.

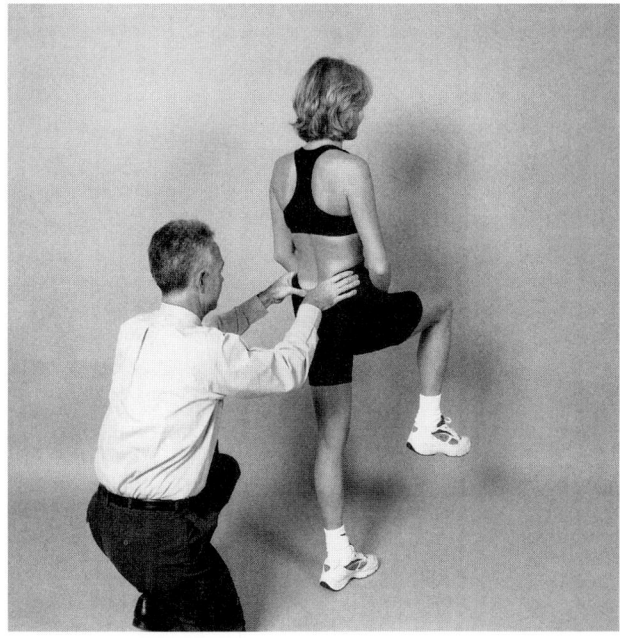

FIGURE 27-15 Contralateral kinetic flexion test.

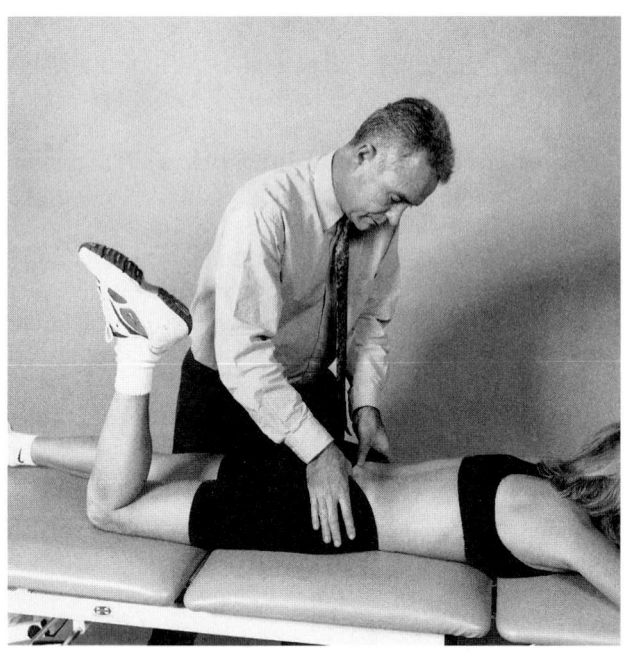

FIGURE 27-16　Non–weight-bearing kinetic test.

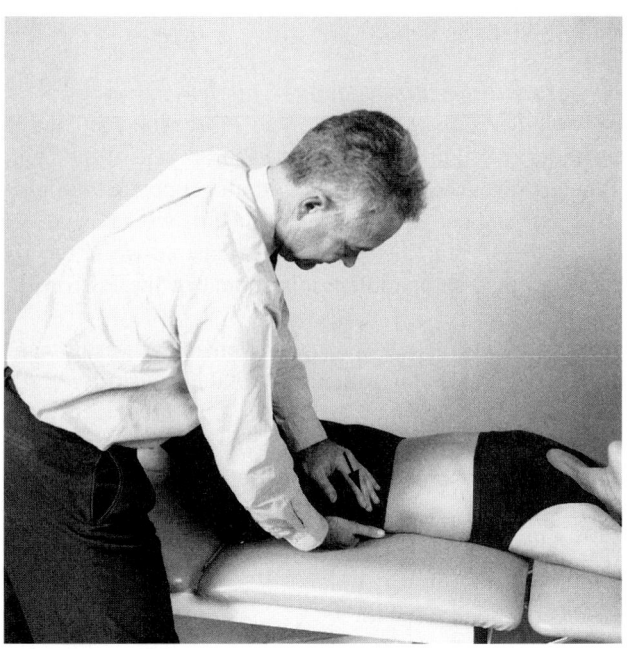

FIGURE 27-17　Short-arm test.

If an unstable subluxation exists (i.e., where the subluxation reduces spontaneously) it is likely to be discernible as a hypomobility on the weight-bearing tests when body weight subluxes it, but appear normal with the non–weight-bearing tests when it is reduced (Table 27-4).

Short- and Long-arm Tests[116]

To confirm or refute the findings from the kinetic tests, the short- and long-arm tests are performed. These tests can also be used to assess the efficiency of the form closure mechanism of the sacroiliac joint.

Short-arm Test.　The short-arm test is designed to confirm or refute the findings of the ipsilateral kinetic tests. The following description is for a test of the left side of the sacrum. The patient lies supine with the legs straight, while the clinician stands on the left side of the patient. The clinician slides his or her right hand under the left side of the patient's lumbar spine, and palpates the left sacral base with the index and long finger. With the left hand, the

clinician grasps the anterior aspect of the patient's left innominate and ASIS (Fig. 27-17). From this position, the clinician stabilizes the left sacral base and sulcus with the right hand, and pushes the left innominate down toward the bed, using the left hand. Slight motion should be felt before a ligamentous end-feel is reached. A loss of motion or pain reproduction compared with the contralateral side indicates dysfunction and confirms the findings of the ipsilateral kinetic test.

Long-arm Test.　The long-arm test is designed to confirm or refute the findings of the contralateral kinetic tests. The following description is for a test of the right side of the sacrum. The palpation and stabilization points are the same as for the short-arm test. The patient's right hip is flexed to about 45 degrees with one hand. Using the heel of the right hand, the clinician pushes down the length of the flexed femur, while stabilizing the sacral base with the left hand (Fig. 27-18). Again, slight motion should be felt (although a little more than with the short-arm test) before a solid ligamentous end-feel is reached. There

TABLE 27-4　Comparison of Weight-bearing and Non–weight-bearing Tests

Weight-bearing Tests	Non–weight-bearing Tests	Indication
+	+	Stable subluxation or severe pericapsular hypomobility
+	−	Unstable subluxation
−	+	Myofascial or mild to moderate pericapsular hypomobility
−	−	Normal or hypermobile or unstable, but no subluxing

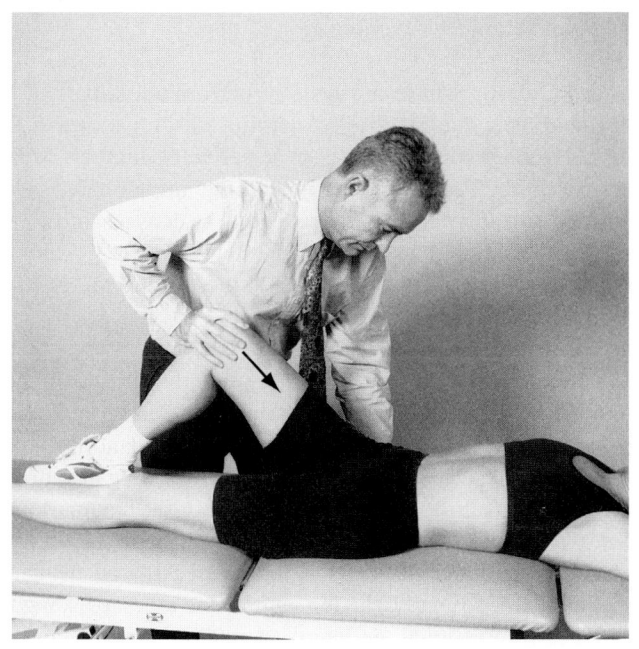

FIGURE 27-18 Long-arm test.

should be no pain. A loss of motion or pain reproduction compared with the contralateral side indicates dysfunction and confirms the findings of the contralateral kinetic test.

Summary of Findings from the Biomechanical Examination.

Following the weight-bearing and non–weight-bearing tests and the confirmatory long- and short-arm tests, the clinician should be able to determine the side of the lesion and the type of biomechanical dysfunction. (See "Sacral Torsion" discussion later.)

However, if the tests just described proved negative, the source of the lesion lies elsewhere, and further investigation is required.

Pelvic Floor Palpation

Manual palpation of the pelvic floor is performed on the advice of a physician, or if there is strong evidence of pelvic floor dysfunction. These techniques should only be performed by clinicians with formal training.

The patient is positioned in the lithotomy position: supine with the thighs supported in a position of 90 degrees of hip flexion and 90 degrees of knee flexion. The initial physical examination is performed via the rectum or vagina using a gloved index finger. The clinician palpates the whole pelvic floor, including the urinary and anal sphincter, iliococcygeus, obturator internus, and piriformis, looking for evidence of tightness, tenderness, taut bands, and pain radiation that reproduces the patient's symptoms.[99]

In women, the tenderness is usually evident lateral to the urethra (urinary sphincter and pubourethralis muscle [muscle fiber of the pubococcygeus]), whereas in men, the pain is typically lateral to the prostate, in the puborectalis muscle (muscle fiber of the pubococcygeus).[99]

Once the sources of the pain have been located, the clinician treats these structures with digital compression, stretching, and strumming perpendicular to the affected muscle bundles (see "Intervention Strategies," later).

Special Tests

Sacroiliac Joint Stress Tests. A positive stress test is one that reproduces unilateral or bilateral sacroiliac pain, either anteriorly or posteriorly.[117] A positive stress test indicates the presence of inflammation, but does not give any information as to the cause. If either test is positive in the patient who has recently fallen, there is a possibility that a fracture of the pelvis exists.[118]

Anterior Gapping Test. The anterior gapping stress test, also called the anterior sacroiliac joint stress test, is described in Chapter 25. This test and its posterior counterpart, described here, are believed to be sensitive for severe arthritis or ventral ligament tears,[117] although they have been shown to be poorly reproducible.[87]

Posterior Distraction Test. The patient is in the side-lying position, and the clinician applies pressure to the lateral side of the ilium, thereby compressing the anterior aspect of the joint and gapping its posterior aspect. The dorsal and interosseus ligaments are among the strongest in the body and are not usually torn by trauma, but may be attenuated by prolonged or repeated stress. This test is less sensitive for arthritis because of the reduced leverage available to the clinician and, when positive, indicates severe arthritis. The test also indirectly assesses the ability of the sacrum to counternutate.

Pubic Stress Tests.[115] The patient is positioned supine, and the clinician stands at the patient's side. With the heel of one hand, the clinician palpates the superior aspect of the superior ramus of one pubic bone, and with the heel of the other hand, palpates the inferior aspect of the superior ramus of the opposite pubic bone (Fig. 27-19). Fixing one pubic bone, the clinician applies a slow, steady, inferosuperior force to the other bone and, noting the quantity and end-feel of motion, as well as the reproduction of any symptoms, the clinician then switches hands and repeats the test so that both sides are stressed superiorly and inferiorly.

> ### Clinical Pearl
>
> In some cases of trauma, or occasionally with child bearing, the pubis can become destabilized. This is a very severe and painful impairment, and one that is not easily missed. The pain is local to the pubic area, the patient is quite disabled with all movements, and weight-bearing postures are very painful. The impairment generally shows up on one-legged weight-bearing radiographs and often requires surgical intervention to stabilize the symphysis.

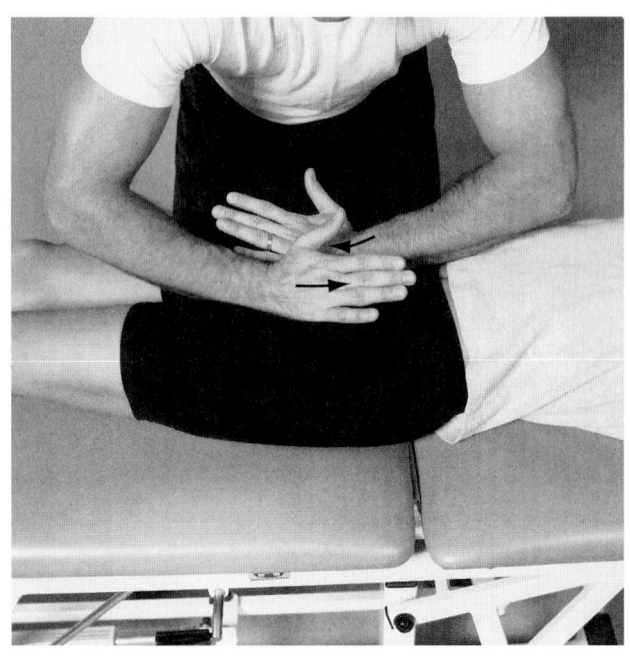

FIGURE 27-19   Pubic stress test.

Sacrotuberous Ligament Stress Test.   The performance and interpretation of this test rely on the patient having no hip joint pathology and full hip range of motion. The patient is positioned supine. The clinician flexes and adducts the patient's hip by moving the patient's knee toward the opposite shoulder. This maneuver is reported, in an otherwise normal hip joint, to stretch the sacrotuberous ligament and to cause the sacrum to nutate.[12,119] This force is maintained for about 20 seconds, and any reproduction of symptoms is noted. Pain in the sacroiliac joints is considered a positive test, but this finding must be incorporated with other clinical findings such as palpation of the sacrotuberous ligament for tenderness, before drawing any conclusions.

Sacral Compression Test.   The patient is positioned prone on a firm surface, and the clinician stands at the patient's side. With one hand, the clinician palpates the inferior aspect of the sacrum in the midline and reinforces this hand with the other. The clinician then applies an anterior force to the apex of the sacrum, thus forcing the sacrum to counternutate. This force is maintained for about 20 seconds, and the reproduction of symptoms is noted. The test is considered positive if pain is reproduced over the sacroiliac joints or the dorsal sacroiliac ligament, or both.[120]

Rotational Stress Test.[120]   The patient is positioned prone, and the clinician stands at the patient's side. The clinician places a thumb over the transverse process of L5 on one side to stabilize the segment against rotation. The clinician uses the other hand to pull up the contralateral iliac crest from the bed, thereby inducing a rotational stress at the lumbosacral junction. Pain produced with this maneuver may indicate an iliolumbar ligament

or anterior sacroiliac ligament tear, or a dysfunction of the lumbosacral junction, or a combination of these.

Leg-length Tests.   These are usually performed as part of the bony landmark examination. Anatomic discrepancies in leg length can predispose patients to a pelvic or lumbar impairment, or both. Posterior rotation of the innominate on the sacrum results in a decrease in leg length, as does an anterior rotation of the innominate on the contralateral side.[66] Although not exact measurements of leg length, these tests can highlight any significant asymmetries.

Prone Test.   Chiropractors assess leg length with the patient prone. The comparative lengths of the legs are compared by observing the heels or medial malleoli. If a discrepancy is noted, the knees are flexed to 90 degrees while maintaining a neutral of hip rotation (neutral upright position), and the landmarks are reassessed to screen for a shortened tibia. The patient is then positioned supine, and the leg lengths are reassessed using the same landmarks. Finally, the leg lengths are assessed using the long sit test. Functional leg length inequality that is secondary to sacroiliac subluxation or dysfunction may reverse from the supine to sitting position, whereas anatomic leg-length inequality or functional inequality secondary to dysfunction at other sites likely will not.[66]

Standing Leg-length Test.   The iliac crest palpation and book correction (ICPBC) method for assessing leg length is used in many clinics. The patient stands with the feet shoulder width apart. The clinician palpates the iliac crests and compares the relative heights for asymmetry. The asymmetry identified is corrected using a book opened to the required number of pages. The iliac crest heights are reassessed. If the iliac crests are level, the thickness of the book correction is measured. One study with 34 healthy subjects found the ICPBC technique for measuring leg-length discrepancy to be highly reliable and moderately valid when there is no history of pelvic deformity and the iliac crests can be readily palpated.[121]

Functional Leg Length.   The patient stands with the feet shoulder width apart. The clinician palpates the iliac crests, ASISs, and the PSISs and compares the relative heights for asymmetry. The patient is then positioned with the subtalar joints in neutral, the toes pointing forward, and the knees fully extended. The same landmarks are reassessed. If the second position corrects any asymmetry found in the first position, the test is positive for a functional leg-length discrepancy and indicates that the leg is structurally normal but has abnormal joint mechanics.

Seated Flexion Test (Piedallu's Sign).   The patient sits with the legs over the end of the table and feet supported.[8] In this position, innominate motion is severely abbreviated, because sitting places the innominates near the end of their extension range. The test is performed as follows. Each PSIS is palpated with the thumb placed under it caudally. The patient then bends forward at the waist. Providing there is no impairment in the sacroiliac joint or the lower lumbar spine, as the patient bends forward, both thumbs should move cranially. If the joint is "blocked," it moves upward further in relation to the other side.[87] The test is purported by osteopaths to help distinguish between a sacroiliac lesion and an iliosacral lesion when compared with the results of the standing flexion test.[5–7]

Long Sit Test. The long sit test is used to indicate the direction of the rotation that the innominate has adopted, and is used in conjunction with the standing flexion test. After noting the side of the impairment obtained from the standing flexion test, the clinician observes whether the medial malleolus on that side moves distally or proximally during the long sit test. Rotation about a coronal axis, whose resultant movement leads to an increase in the length of a limb, is defined as extension. If it shortens the length of the limb, it is defined as flexion. Thus, if the apparent shorter leg becomes longer during the test, the innominate on that side is purportedly held in a posteriorly rotated malposition, whereas if the apparent longer leg becomes shorter during the test, the innominate on that side is allegedly held in an anteriorly rotated malposition.

The problems with this test involve the maneuver itself. To ask patients who are experiencing some degree of discomfort to raise themselves off the bed from a supine position into a long sit position without any twisting or use of the arms is unnecessarily painful. In addition, for the successful completion of the maneuver, the patient needs 90 degrees of hip flexion and hamstring length.

Sign of the Buttock. The test for this syndrome is described here because its underlying pathologies occur in the lower quadrant. The sign of the buttock is not a single sign, as the name would suggest, but rather a collection of signs indicating that a serious pathology is present posterior to the axis of flexion and extension in the hip. Among the causes of the syndrome are osteomyelitis, infectious sacroiliitis, fracture of the sacrum or pelvis, septic bursitis, ischiorectal abscess, gluteal hematoma, gluteal tumor, and rheumatic bursitis.

The patient lies supine, and the clinician performs a passive unilateral straight leg raise. If a unilateral restriction is noted, the clinician flexes the knee and notes whether the hip flexion increases. If the restriction was caused by the lumbar spine or hamstrings, the hip flexion should increase. The sign of the buttock test is positive if the hip flexion does not increase when the knee is flexed. If the sign of the buttock is encountered, the patient must be immediately returned to his or her physician for further investigation.

Gaenslen's Test. The patient is positioned supine at the edge of the bed. The leg furthest from the edge of the bed (nontested leg) is flexed at the hip and knee and held by the patient with both arms. The clinician stabilizes the pelvis and passively positions the upper leg (test leg) into hyperextension at the hip, so that it hangs over the edge of the table.[122] The clinician applies

a further stretch to the test leg into hip extension and adduction. Pain with this maneuver is considered a positive test for a sacroiliac joint lesion, pubic symphysis instability, hip pathology, or an L4 nerve root lesion. The test also stresses the femoral nerve.

Yeoman's Test. This test[123] is performed with the patient positioned prone. The clinician stabilizes the patient's sacrum with the palm of one hand. With the other hand, the clinician grasps the patient's distal thigh and extends the patient's hip. At the end of the available motion, the hip is hyperextended so that the innominate is forced into anterior rotation. A positive test produces pain over the sacroiliac joint. Other structures that are stressed with this maneuver include the lumbar spine, hip joint, and iliopsoas muscle.

Patrick's (FABER or Figure-Four) Test. The patient is positioned supine. The test leg is positioned so that the sole of the foot rests against the side of the other knee (or on top of the knee of the opposite leg; see Fig. 17-22). This position flexes, abducts, and externally rotates the femur at the hip joint. The clinician slowly lowers the knee of the test leg toward the bed. At the end of available motion, the pelvis is stabilized, and overpressure is applied. Pain with this maneuver indicates hip joint pathology, pubic symphysis instability, sacroiliac joint dysfunction, or an iliopsoas muscle spasm.[124]

Active Straight Leg Raise (ASLR) Test. When performed passively, the straight leg raise test is usually associated with assessment of neurodynamic mobility or hamstring length. When performed actively, the straight leg raise test has been recommended as a disease severity scale for patients with posterior pelvic pain after pregnancy.[125–127] It seems that the integrity of the function to transfer loads between the lumbosacral spine and legs is tested by the ASLR test.

Intervention Strategies

Thus far, the success of interventions at this joint has been mixed, due in part to the poor reliability with many of the examinations used. The success of any intervention depends on the quality and accuracy of the examination and the subsequent evaluation. It follows that if the examination gives an inaccurate diagnosis, the intervention may have a mixed result. Given that the chosen intervention for the sacroiliac joint, like the spine, depends largely on the philosophy or background the clinician uses to establish the diagnosis, a variety of diagnoses for the same biomechanical dysfunction can arise. However, although the philosophies may differ, the principles behind the interventions for sacroiliac joint impairments should remain constant:

▶ A joint that has reduced motion (hypomobility) requires mobilizing techniques and exercises that are designed to restore normal optimal alignment and mobility.

▶ A joint that demonstrates excessive motion (hypermobility and/or instability) requires techniques and exercises that are designed to stabilize or balance forces around the hypermobile or unstable joint.[127a]

The techniques and exercises used for the sacroiliac joint should always be based on the stage of healing and patient tolerance, and must take into account the influences that the lumbar spine and hip can have on this area.

A great number of structures can produce low back, pelvic, or groin pain of a serious nature (see Chap. 9). Some conditions predispose these joints to isolated impairments, as a result of either gross trauma or a lack of integrity of the joint surfaces and ligamentous support:

▶ Until about the age of 11 years, the sacroiliac joint is quite planar, with very few ridges to provide support to the joint.

▶ The release of the hormone relaxin during pregnancy causes a decrease in the tensile strength of all of the ligaments in the body. This ligamentous laxity continues to occur for up to 3 months after the pregnancy.[128] Because the pelvic area relies heavily on its ligaments for stability, the area becomes vulnerable to injury with even minor trauma.

▶ Significant high-velocity trauma to the pelvic complex, such as that occurring during a motor vehicle accident, can produce a subluxation of the sacroiliac joint.

In normal healthy adults, the pelvic complex is a structure that is not prone to injury. Lesions that occur at the sacroiliac joint typically occur as sprains, a result of a combination of an innominate and sacral motions due to the ligamentous relationship that the joints share.

Acute Phase
In the acute phase of rehabilitation for the sacroiliac joint the intervention goals are:

▶ Decrease pain, inflammation, and muscle spasm.

▶ Increase weight bearing tolerance, where appropriate.

▶ Promote healing of tissues through sufficient stabilization (may require belt).

▶ Increase pain-free range of sacroiliac joint motion.

▶ Regain soft tissue extensibility around the pelvic region.

▶ Regain neuromuscular control.

▶ Allow progression to the functional stage.

Pain relief may be accomplished initially by the use of cryotherapy, and electrical stimulation (TENS), gentle muscle setting exercises, and occasionally the temporary use of a sacroiliac belt (see below). These measures are particularly indicated when the joint has been demonstrated to be inflamed by the stress tests. Thermal modalities, especially ultrasound with its ability to penetrate deeply, may be used after 48 to 72 hours. Ultrasound is the most common clinically used deep heating modality to promote tissue healing.[128a–128c]

Various investigators have advocated the use of orthoses in the intervention of this region,[128d–128f] but no prospective studies have been done to evaluate the effectiveness of bracing. Clinicians often correct leg length discrepancies of greater than 0.5 in, as such inequalities have been described as altering normal sacroiliac joint function.[128d]

Sacroiliac joint and pelvic stabilization orthoses have been employed in an attempt to limit sacroiliac joint motion and improve proprioception.[128g] Not much force from these belts (20–50 Newtons) to afford relief to the patient.[128g] The elastic ones tend to be better than the firm ones, but I have not had much success with the sacrum-shaped patches. The position of the belt in terms of its height on the ilium should be experimented with to find the optimal position for pain relief. The recommended position is just above the greater trochanter.[128h] A bicycle inner tube can be used as an sacroiliac belt, as this is the right width and has the correct degree of elasticity. The following conditions appear to respond well to bracing:

1. Sacroiliitis.

2. Sacroiliac hypermobility/instability: (pre and postpartum and micro-traumatic).

3. Pubic instability (may afford some relief).

Once the pain and inflammation is under control, the intervention can progress towards the restoration of full strength, range of motion, and normal posture. Range of motion exercises are initiated at the earliest opportunity. These are performed during the early stages in the pain-free ranges. Submaximal isometric exercises are then performed throughout the pain-free ranges. These exercises are progressed as the range of motion and strength increases.

Aggressive manual therapy has a very limited place in the intervention of the acutely inflamed joint. In almost every case, the presence of a positive stress test contraindicates the use of passive mobilization or manipulation for that joint. However, mobilization, or manipulation of the contralateral joint may reduce the stress on the painful and inflamed articulation. Gentle manual techniques such as myofascial release, grade I-II joint mobilizations, massage, gentle stretching, and muscle energy techniques should be attempted and continued if effective.

Functional Phase
The duration of this phase can vary tremendously, and depends upon several factors:

▶ The severity of the injury.

▶ The healing capacity of the patient.

▶ How the condition was managed during the acute phase.

▶ The level of patient involvement in their rehabilitation program.

The goals of this phase are:

▶ To significantly reduce or to completely resolve the patient's pain.

▶ To restore full and pain-free sacroiliac joint range of motion.

▶ To integrate the lower kinetic chains into the rehabilitation.

▶ Complete restoration of gait, where appropriate.

▶ The restoration of pelvic and lower quadrant strength and neuromuscular control.

During this stage, the patient learns to initiate and execute functional activities without pain and while dynamically stabilizing the sacroiliac joint in an automatic manner.

Muscle imbalances around this joint complex also are common. A biomechanical model has been proposed[68,129–131] that can explain how specific exercise may help in the conservative management of problems associated with the mechanical control of the sacroiliac joints. A recent study by Richardson and colleagues[132] found that contraction of the transversus abdominis significantly decreases the laxity of the sacroiliac joint, and that this decrease in laxity is larger than that caused by a bracing action using all the lateral abdominal muscles. The abdominal drawing-in maneuver is one exercise known to result in preferential activation of the internal oblique and transversus abdominis. The exercises used in the lumbopelvic stabilization exercise progression are described in detail in Chapter 25. Exercises more specific to the sacroiliac joints are described under "Therapeutic Techniques" later.

The exercises prescribed must challenge and enhance muscle performance while minimizing loading of the sacroiliac joint to reduce the risk of injury exacerbation. Inter-individual differences in injury status and/or training goals may allow for a continuum of required muscle stress and acceptable loading of the spine and sacroiliac joint.[132a]

Stabilization exercises and joint positioning can help the patient to (1) gain dynamic control of spine forces, (2) eliminate repetitive injury to the motion segments, (3) encourage healing of the injured segment, and (4) possibly alter the degenerative process.[132b]

The techniques to increase joint mobility and the techniques to increase soft tissue extensibility are described under "Therapeutic Techniques," later.

In addition to the exercise program, the patient should be educated on the trunk and lower extremity positions to avoid (those that produce an excessive or sustained sacral counternutation) and those to adopt (the positions that enhance sacral nutation).

Integration of Practice Patterns 4D and 4E: Impaired Joint Mobility, Motor Function, Muscle Performance, Range of Motion Associated with Connective Tissue Dysfunction and Localized Inflammation

Urinary Incontinence

Urinary incontinence includes the various types of incontinence: stress incontinence (loss of bladder control associated with increased abdominal pressure that occurs during coughing or exercise), urge incontinence (a sudden urge to urinate), or mixed incontinence (a combination of stress and urge incontinence).[132c] One of the contributing factors to urinary incontinence can be a weakness of the pelvic floor musculature. Although often associated with aging, incontinence due to pelvic floor muscle weakness is not an automatic response to aging and many patients have achieved significant improvement through behavior modification, muscle re-education and pelvic floor muscle strengthening (see "Pelvic Floor Exercises").[132d,132e] Behavior modification techniques include timed voiding schedules, proper toileting techniques, dietary modification, and patient education. Muscle re-education is primarily used for those patients who do not demonstrate improvement with the pelvic floor muscle strengthening program after approximately 4 weeks. Muscle re-education can be achieved in a number of ways:

▶ *Biofeedback.* A study by Cardozo et al.[132f] reported improvements in 81 per cent of patients with urge incontinence who were treated with biofeedback.

▶ *Acupuncture.* A study by Philp et al.[132j] reported improvements in 77 percent of patients with urge incontinence who were treated with acupuncture.

▶ *Electrical stimulation (ES).* Various forms of electrical stimulation have been used in the treatment of female urinary incontinence. ES is an option for patients who demonstrate difficulty with identifying the pelvic floor muscles or with producing a contraction of these muscles. Transvaginal stimulation with a removable electrode has been in clinical use in Europe and North America for three decades. The typical neuromuscular stimulation system is a portable electrical pulse generator powered by a 9 volt alkaline battery. A fully insertable vaginal electrode, which is composed of silicone rubber is commonly used. Two randomized studies have reported the usefulness of transvaginal electrical stimulation.[132g,132h] In the Sand et al.[5] study comparisons of changes from baseline between active-device and control patients showed that active-device patients had significantly greater improvement in weekly ($p = .009$) and daily ($p = .04$) leakage episodes, pad testing ($p = .005$), and vaginal muscle strength ($p = .02$) when compared with control subjects. Significantly greater improvement was also found for both visual analog scores of urinary incontinence ($p = .007$) and stress incontinence ($p = .02$), as well as for subjective reporting of frequency of urine loss ($p = .002$), and urine loss with sneezing, coughing, or laughing ($p = .02$), when compared with controls. In the Smith et al.[5] study, of the patients using electrical stimulation in the stress urinary incontinence group, 66 percent improved and 72 percent of the patients with detrusor instability treated with electrical stimulation improved. These rates were not considered statistically significant when compared to traditional therapy, but the authors concluded that electrical stimulation was as safe and at least as effective as properly performed Kegel and drug therapy in the treatment of stress urinary incontinence and detrusor instability. A typical protocol is outlined below:[132i]

▶ For patients with urge incontinence: 12.5 Hz for 15 minutes, twice a day

▶ For patients with stress incontinence: 50 Hz for 15 minutes, twice a day

▶ For patients with mixed incontinence: 12.5 Hz for 15 minutes a day and 50 Hz for 15 minutes a day

Spondyloarthropathies

The spondyloarthropathies are a group of inflammatory arthritic conditions that share certain clinical and laboratory features (see Chap. 9).[133]

▶ An inflammatory arthritis, which manifests with pain associated with stiffness.

▶ The absence of a rheumatoid factor; hence the distinction of the group as "seronegative" spondyloarthropathies.

▶ The tendency for the arthritis to be asymmetric and involve the lower extremities.

▶ Often, inflammation at the insertion of tendons into bone (enthesitis), accompanied by certain extra-articular features, including skin and mucous membrane impairments, bowel complaints, eye involvement, and aortic root dilation.

▶ The familial aggregation, which occurs within each condition and among the entities within the group.

▶ An association with HLA-B27, documented in the diseases included in this group.

Ankylosing Spondylitis

Ankylosing spondylitis (Bekhterev's or Marie-Strümpell disease) is a chronic rheumatoid disorder that is usually progressive, resulting in a full ankylosing of the sacroiliac joints.[133] Men generally have the more severe form affecting the spine, whereas in women, the peripheral joints are more often affected.

The typical radiographic changes are seen primarily in the axial skeleton, especially in the sacroiliac, intervertebral, zygapophysial, costovertebral, and costotransverse joints.[134] In addition, ankylosing spondylitis is one of the most common rheumatic disorders associated with radiologic abnormalities of the pubic symphysis, with pubic synchondrosis present in 20 to 25 percent of patients.[135] In fact, changes of the symphysis can sometimes precede spine involvement.[135]

Tests to discriminate sacroiliac joint tenderness caused by ankylosing spondylitis from that caused by mechanical spine conditions have traditionally included passive hip extension, anteroposterior pressure applied to the sacrum, and the primary stress tests. However, these tests have been found to be poorly reproducible and inaccurate in making any distinction.[87]

Although radiologic evidence of sacroiliitis is accepted as being obligatory for the diagnosis of ankylosing spondylitis, the clinical signs (see Chap. 9) may predate radiologic abnormalities by months or even years.[133]

Groin Pain

Chronic pain in the groin region (see Chap. 17) is a difficult clinical problem to evaluate, and in many cases, the cause of the pain is poorly understood. The differential diagnosis of groin pain and tenderness includes adductor muscle strain, prostatitis, orchitis, inguinal hernia, urolithiasis, ankylosing spondylitis, Reiter's syndrome, hyperparathyroidism, metastasis, osteitis pubis, stress fracture, rheumatoid arthritis tendonitis, degenerative joint disease of the hip, bursitis, stress fracture, conjoint tendon strains, inguinal ligament enthesopathy, and entrapment of the lateral cutaneous nerve of the thigh.[136–138]

In addition, nerve entrapment syndromes have been described as a possible cause of adductor region pain, with the anterior division of the obturator nerve in the thigh,[139] the ilioinguinal nerve, and the genitofemoral nerve having all been inculpated.[140]

Osteitis Pubis

Many theories have been put forward concerning the etiology and progression of this disease, but the cause of osteitis pubis remains unclear.

Osteitis pubis is seen in athletes who participate in activities that create continual shearing forces at the pubic symphysis, as with unilateral leg support or acceleration-deceleration forces required during multidirectional activities. These include such activities as running, race walking, gymnastics, soccer, basketball, rugby, and tennis. Pain with walking can be in one or several of many distributions: perineal, testicular, suprapubic, inguinal, and in the scrotum and perineum.[141] Overuse is the most likely etiology of the inflammation, and the process is usually self limiting.[141]

Osteitis pubis has been likened to gracilis syndrome, an avulsion fatigue fracture involving the bony origin of the gracilis muscle at the pubic symphysis and occurring in relation to the directional pull of the gracilis.[142] However, osteitis pubis does not necessarily involve a fracture. The process could be the result of stress reaction, which might be associated with several biomechanical abnormalities.

Osteitis pubis usually appears during the third and fourth decades of life, occurring more commonly in men.[143] The pain or discomfort can be located in the pubic area, one or both groins, and the lower rectus abdominis muscle. Symptoms of osteitis pubis have been described as "groin burning," with discomfort while climbing stairs, coughing, or sneezing.

During the physical examination, pain can be elicited by having the patient squeeze a fist between the knees with resisted long and flexed adductor contraction. Range of motion in one or both hips may be decreased. An adductor muscle spasm might occur with limited abduction and a positive cross-leg test[144,145] (Fig. 27-20). A soft tissue mass with calcification, and an audible or palpable click over the symphysis might be detected during daily activities.[141]

Correct examination of this region involves examining the position of the pelvic girdle. The normal position for the pelvic bowl is 45 degrees in the sagittal plane and 45 degrees in the coronal plane. Pubic motion is assessed by locating the pubic crest and then gently testing the mobility of each available direction.

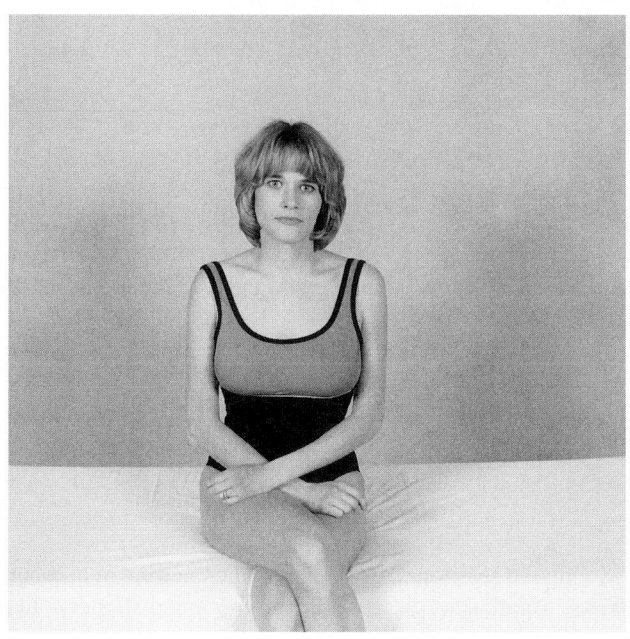

FIGURE 27-20 Cross-leg test.

Dysfunction of this articulation may be primary or secondary and, when present, is always treated first, because a loss of function or integrity of this joint disrupts the mechanics of the entire pelvic complex. The impairment pattern is determined by palpating the position of the pubic tubercles and correlating the findings with the side of the positive kinetic test, with the restricted side indicating the side of the impairment.

An altered positional relationship within the pelvic girdle is significant only if a mobility restriction of the sacroiliac joint or pubic symphysis, or both, is found. The inguinal ligament is usually very tender to palpation on the side of the impairment. It is common to find the pubic symphysis held in one of the four following positions:

1. Anteroinferior.

2. Posterosuperior.

3. Anterosuperior.

4. Posteroinferior.

These articular dysfunctions are treated using manual techniques (see "Therapeutic Techniques" section).

Intervention for the inflammatory type of osteitis pubis is conservative and most athletes return to their respective sports within a few days to weeks.[146] The intervention includes plenty of rest from weight-bearing activities, a course of nonsteroidal anti-inflammatory medicine, and physical therapy to gently mobilize, stretch, and strengthen the muscles about the groin.[147] Patients should be able to swim for exercise.

An intervention protocol for osteitis pubis is outlined in Box 27-1.

Box 27-1 INTERVENTION PROTOCOL FOR OSTEITIS PUBIS [148]

Phase I

1. Static adduction against a soccer ball placed between feet when lying supine. Each adduction is held for 30 sec and is repeated ten times.
2. Abdominal sit-ups performed both in straight direction and in oblique direction. Patient performs five sets to fatigue.
3. Combined abdominal sit-up and hip flexion (crunch). Patient starts from supine position and with a soccer/basketball placed between knees. Patient performs five sets to fatigue.
4. Balance training on wobble board for 5 min.
5. One-foot exercises on sliding board, with parallel feet as well as with a 90-degree angle between feet.

Five sets of 1-min continuous work are performed with each leg, and in both positions.

Phase II (from third week)

1. Leg abduction and adduction exercises in side lying position on side. Patient performs five series of ten repetitions of each exercise.
2. Low-back extension exercises while in prone position over end of treatment table. Patient performs five series of ten repetitions.
3. One-leg weight-pulling abduction-adduction, standing. Patient performs five series of ten repetitions for each leg.
4. Abdominal sit-ups both in straightforward direction and in oblique direction. Patient performs five sets to fatigue.
5. One-leg coordination exercise flexing and extending knee and swinging arms in same rhythm (cross-country skiing on one leg). Patient performs five sets of ten repetitions for each leg.
6. Skating movements on sliding board. This is performed five times for 1-min continuous work.

Symphysis Pubic Dysfunction

Symphysis pubic dysfunction (SPD) describes the situation where the ligaments between the pubic symphysis become stretched and allow the bones to move with respect to each other. In severe cases rupture of the symphysis may occur. This more severe form is called diastasis symphysis pubis (DSP). SPD commonly occurs during pregnancy, and should always be considered when examining patients in the postpartum period who are experiencing suprapubic, sacroiliac, or thigh pain. The associated ligamentous laxity during pregnancy is in response to the hormones progesterone and relaxin. Causes unrelated to pregnancy include the possibility of a structural misalignment of the pelvis. This pelvic misalignment results in increased pressure on the pubic symphysis cartilage, with subsequent pain.

The symptoms of SPD and DSP vary from person to person. On examination, the patient typically demonstrates an antalgic, waddling gait. Subjectively the patient reports pain with any activity that involves lifting one leg at a time or parting the legs. Lifting the leg to put on clothes, getting out of a car, bending over, turning over in bed, sitting down or getting up, walking up stairs, standing on one leg, lifting heavy objects, and walking in general are all painful. Patients may also report that the hip joint seems stuck in place or they describe having to wait for it to 'pop into place' before being able to walk. Radiological evaluation may occasionally be useful in confirming the diagnosis.[147a] The amount of symphyseal separation does not always correlate with severity of symptoms or the degree of disability. Therefore, the intervention is based on the severity of symptoms rather than the degree of separation as measured by imaging studies.[147a] Palpation reveals anterior pubic symphyseal tenderness. Occasional clicking can be felt or heard. The findings on the physical examination include positive sacroiliac joint stress tests (compression, distraction, and FABER tests). The range of hip movements will be limited by pain, and there is an inability to stand on one leg. Characteristic pain can often be evoked by bilateral pressure on the trochanters or by hip flexion with the legs in extension. However, such maneuvers may result in severe pain or muscle spasm and are not necessary for diagnosis.

In cases of DSP, there is likely an associated anterior-posterior (A-P) compression (common) or a vertical shear (rare) fracture. Three types of DSP are described, indicating the severity of the injury.[147b]

► Type 1 involves minor anterior damage, mild (less than 2.5 cm) pubic symphysis diastasis, and/or (vertical) pubic rami fractures.

► Type II has wide diastasis of the symphysis pubis, disruption of the anterior sacroiliac ligament complex, and (hinging) of the iliac bone on the sacrum at the intact posterior sacroiliac joint

► Type III designates total disruption of the sacroiliac joint, a diastasis of greater than 2.5 cm has been shown to indicate disruption of the anterior sacroiliac joint at least, but it is frequently associated with total sacroiliac joint disruption.

Although the symptoms can be dramatically severe in presentation for SPD and DSP, a conservative management approach is often effective in cases of SPD. In more severe cases, the interventions can include bed rest in the lateral decubitus position, pelvic support with a brace or girdle, ambulation with assistance or devices such as walkers and graded exercise protocols.[147a] In all cases, patient education is extremely important in terms of providing advice on how to avoid stress to the area. Many of the suggestions to give include:

► Use a pillow between the legs when sleeping.

► Keep the legs and hips parallel and as symmetrical as possible when moving or turning in bed.

► A waterbed mattress may be helpful.

► Silk/satin sheets and night garments may make it easier to turn over in bed.

► Swimming may help relieve pressure on the joint (the breaststroke may prove aggravating).

► Deep water aerobics or deep water running using floatation devices may be helpful as well.

► Keep the legs close together and move symmetrically when turning.

► When standing, stand symmetrically, with the weight evenly distributed through both legs.

► Sit down to get dressed, especially when putting on underwear or pants.

► Avoid "straddle" movements.

► Swing the legs together as a unit when getting in and out of cars; use plastics or something smooth and slippery (like a garbage bag) on the car seat.

► An ice pack may feel soothing and help reduce inflammation in the pubic area; painkillers may also help.

► Move slowly and without sudden movements.

► If sex is uncomfortable, use pillows under the knees, or try other positions.

► If bending over to pick up objects is difficult, use specific devices.

Resolution of symptoms in approximately 6 to 8 weeks with no lasting sequela is the most common outcome in SDP and DSP.[147a] Occasionally, patients report residual pain requiring several months of physical therapy but long-term impairment is unusual. Surgical intervention is rarely required but may be utilized in cases of inadequate reduction, recurrent diastasis, or persistent symptoms.

Coccydynia

Coccygeal pain is relatively common. The coccyx can move anteriorly or posteriorly. There are a number of ligaments around this area, which can be injured:

► *Ventral.*

  • Lateral sacrococcygeal.

  • Ventral ligament of the coccyx (caudal extension of the anterior longitudinal ligament).

► *Dorsal.*

  • Superficial dorsal sacrococcygeal (caudal extension of the ligamentum flavum).

  • Deep dorsal sacrococcygeal (caudal extension of the posterior longitudinal ligament).

  • Intercornual ligament.

The dominant muscle in this area is the levator ani, which has connections with:

▶ Iliococcygeal ligament.

▶ Pubococcygeal ligament.

Coccydynia tends to occur when the coccyx becomes stuck into flexion with an accompanying deviation. The causes can be muscle scarring or trauma.

Correction of this impairment involves grasping the coccyx after inserting the index finger in the anal canal. The coccyx is distracted and pulled posteriorly, while pulling laterally on the medial surface of the ischial tuberosity.

Sacral Torsions

It would appear from the anatomy and biomechanics of this region that the pelvic complex is anatomically and functionally a contiguous circle, or ring, and that isolated impairments to this region probably only occur when a high degree of trauma is involved. With less severe trauma, impairments seem to occur in combination with an injury to one part of the ring, having repercussions at other parts within the ring.

Based on osteopathic doctrine, the sacroiliac, lumbosacral, and pubic symphysis joints can adopt one of four pathologic positions:

1. One side of the sacrum is nutated while the ipsilateral innominate is posteriorly rotated. The pubic tubercle is superior on the side of the posteriorly rotated innominate.

2. One side of the sacrum is counternutated while the ipsilateral innominate is anteriorly rotated. The pubic tubercle is inferior on the side of the anteriorly rotated innominate.

3. One side of the sacrum is nutated while the ipsilateral innominate is anteriorly rotated. The pubic tubercle is inferior on the side of the anteriorly rotated innominate.

4. One side of the sacrum is counternutated while the ipsilateral innominate is posteriorly rotated. The pubic tubercle is superior on the side of the posteriorly rotated innominate.

The biomechanical examination should determine which of the four scenarios is occurring. Two sacral torsion syndromes are recognized, referred to as type I and type II.[10]

Type I Sacral Torsion. The left sacral torsion syndrome exists when the anterior sacrum is held in a left-rotated position and the lumbar vertebrae adapt by following the first law of physiologic spinal motion, side flexing to the right and rotating to the left.[10] A left torsion of the sacrum is defined as an unphysiologic occurrence. Arthrokinematically, the sacrum glides anteroinferiorly along the short length on the right joint and posteroinferiorly along the long arm on the left joint.[120] A review of Fryette's laws of physiologic spinal motion[5] helps explain the effect on the lumbar spine when the sacrum is held in this unphysiologic position:

Law I. Whenever the spine moves from neutral, side bending occurs before rotation except during pure flexion or extension. The side bending produces a bending movement about which the rotation occurs. This combined motion is referred to as *latexion,* and the side bending and rotation occur to opposite sides; the vertebral body rotates into the convexity of the curve. Spinal impairments presenting as latexion are referred to as type I impairments.[10] Anterior sacral torsions are thus classified as type I impairments.[10]

Law II. From a position of full flexion or full extension, rotation precedes side bending when movement other than a return to neutral occurs. This combined motion is referred to as *rotexion,* and the rotation and side bending occur to the same side; the vertebral body rotates into the concavity of the curve. Spinal impairments presenting as rotexion are referred to as type II impairments.[10] Posterior sacral torsions are thus classified as type II impairments.[10]

With left sacral torsion, the sacrum will have moved inferiorly and posteriorly on the left articular surface, and inferiorly and anteriorly on the right. Relative to the sacrum, the left innominate will have moved superiorly, and anteriorly, and the right innominate will have moved posteriorly.[10] If the lumbosacral angle is increased, and the iliolumbar ligaments have, therefore, become taut, the right iliolumbar ligament pulls on the posterior aspect of the right transverse processes of the fifth and sometimes the fourth lumbar vertebrae, and they will move with the innominates—superiorly and anteriorly on the left and posteriorly on the right.[10] Applying the second law of Fryette, the vertebrae are now in a right-rotated and right side-flexed position. The lumbar vertebrae above L5 and L4 gradually counter-rotate, producing the appearance of a left convexity.[10]

If the lumbosacral angle is in neutral, with no tension on the iliolumbar ligaments, the fifth lumbar vertebra will be free to follow Fryette's first law of physiologic spinal motion, side bending to the right and rotating to the left.[10] The remainder of the lumbar spine will follow L5, side bending to the right and producing a convexity to the left.

Type II Sacral Torsion. The type II sacral torsion syndrome exists when the anterior surface of the sacrum is held in a left-rotated position and the lower lumbar vertebrae follow the second law of physiologic motion; L5 and L4 rotate and side bend to the right.[10] The clinical appearance of the type II sacral torsion is very similar to that of acute lumbar disk prolapse, and the history is often helpful in differentiating the two (i.e., type II sacral torsion are not aggravated by sitting, whereas the patient with an acute lumbar disk prolapse finds this position intolerable). This impairment occurs more frequently on the right side.

The intervention for these scenarios can then be approached in one of two ways:

1. Addressing all of the deficits simultaneously.

2. Addressing all of the deficits individually.

Practice Pattern 4G: Impaired Joint Mobility, Motor Function, Muscle Performance, Range of Motion Associated with Fracture

Sacral Stress Fracture

Repetitive loading on the body can lead to the development of stress fractures. Stress fractures have been described as a cause of back pain, especially fractures of the pelvis and pars interarticularis of the sacrum.[149] Back and buttock pain caused by sacral stress fractures are less common but may occur in athletes and in the elderly.[150] Fractures in the latter group have been reported both with and without trauma.

The cause of sacral stress fractures is controversial. These fractures are believed to result from stress concentration of the vertical body forces, which are dissipated from the spine to the sacrum and sacral alae and then onto the iliac wings.[151] In addition to abnormal stresses on normal bone, normal stress on abnormal bone can produce these fractures, especially in the elderly. Patients who sustain such insufficiency fractures may have predisposing factors, including idiopathic osteoporosis, irradiation-induced osteoporosis, steroid-induced osteoporosis, or osteoporosis associated with malignancy.[149] Another cause cited for sacral fractures is progressive *insufficiency* of the supporting muscles.[152] These fatigue fractures may result from the transfer of loading forces directly to the bone, without absorption of some energy by the muscles. Other reported causes of sacral stress fractures are differences in physical demands, environmental and genetic influences, training methods, footwear, and intensity of training.[152] Atwell and Jackson[153] suggested that leg-length inequality may increase the stress on one side of the sacrum, but this has not been proven by biomechanical analysis.[149]

Patients with sacral stress fractures typically present with low back pain and sacral pain that may radiate into the buttocks. However, pain may be referred to the groin and, occasionally, down the leg.[153] In the case of an athlete, the history may reveal a recent history of stress fracture in the same area, or a rapid increase in training intensity prior to the onset of symptoms.[107] Insufficiency fractures of the sacrum in nonathletes have been reported to mimic disk disease, spinal stenosis, and tumors.[154] Irritation of the cauda equina or sacral nerve roots may explain the wide variety of symptoms seen in patients with sacral stress fractures.[149,155]

Physical examination may not provide reliable signs initially, because many of these patients have diffuse low back, sacral, and buttock pain. However, most patients will have localized tenderness over the sacrum and sacroiliac joint.[149–151,153–155] Tenderness in the upper gluteal areas tends to be coexistent with sacral stress fractures, and tenderness in this region may contribute to the impression that the origin of the pain is centered in the more proximal lumbar spine.[149] Most patients are neurologically intact, with no signs of nerve root irritation. The Patrick's, or the FABER (flexion, abduction, external rotation), test may or may not be positive, and it cannot be depended on in making a diagnosis.[149]

The most sensitive method of evaluating the sacrum for occult stress fractures and other bone lesions is three-phase scintigraphy.[156] This bone imaging technique can help detect stress fractures as early as several days after the fracture occurs. In contrast, plain radiographs of the lumbosacral spine and the pelvis, although useful to rule out other causes of back pain, are not helpful in diagnosing sacral stress fractures.[150]

Patients with sacral stress fractures recover quickly with rest. Most patients are able to return to their normal activity levels in 4 to 6 weeks with no long-term sequelae.[149] Anti-inflammatory agents and analgesics may be used as adjunctive treatment for patient comfort. Cycling or running in a pool may be used until weight-bearing activities are tolerated.

Therapeutic Techniques

Normally, pelvic impairments are presented as isolated entities when, in fact, clinically, they tend to occur in combination. Therefore, an intervention progression is necessary. It is recommended that pelvic impairments are treated in the following order:

1. Segmental restrictive faults of the lumbar spine.

2. Normalization of muscle imbalances in hip adductors, hip flexors, hamstrings, and rectus femoris.

3. Pubic symphysis impairment.

4. Sacral torsion syndrome.

5. Innominate subluxation.

6. Innominate rotation.

7. Innominate flare.

8. Correction of any imbalance of the lower limb and foot.

Several interventions for the sacroiliac joint have been adopted by the various disciplines. These interventions consist of manual therapy, therapeutic exercises, orthoses, modalities, and education.

It is essential that the impairments, functional limitations, and disability found during the examination guide the intervention.

Manual Therapy

This technique has a very limited place as an intervention for the acutely inflamed joint. In almost every case, the presence of a positive stress test contraindicates the use of passive mobilization or manipulation for that joint. However, it is theorized that mobilization or manipulation of the contralateral joint can reduce the stress on the painful and inflamed articulation. One theoretical explanation for the clinical effect achieved by manipulation-mobilization of the sacroiliac joint is that manipulation results in a reduction of subluxation of the joint.

The majority of sacroiliac joint impairments comprise a number of structural changes, which occur simultaneously. These structural changes can be treated individually or as part of a combined intervention strategy.

Muscle energy techniques are most effective in cases of myofascial or mild pericapsular hypomobility, and less useful in cases of very stiff joints or subluxations. Among the individual conditions that are more amenable to this type of technique are[8]:

▶ Inferior or superior pubic symphysis.

▶ Innominate flexion hypomobility (anterior rotation).

▶ Innominate extension hypomobility (posterior rotation).

▶ Forward sacral torsion (left on left or right on right).

▶ Backward sacral torsion (left on right or right on left).

Probably the least used technique in the sacroiliac joint is passive mobilization, but it can be more specific than muscle energy. The principles of mobilization that pertain to other joints also apply here.

Muscle Energy Techniques to Restore Pubic Symphyseal Joint Dysfunction

Superior Pubic Symphyseal Joint (Left Side). The patient is positioned supine, lying near the left side of the bed and with the lower extremity hanging off the edge of the bed. The clinician stands on the patient's left side and supports the patient's left leg with one hand, while stabilizing the patient's right ASIS with the other hand. The clinician slowly guides the patient's left leg toward the floor, while also slightly abducting it, until the motion barrier is reached. From this position, the patient is asked to lift the left knee "up and in," against the clinician's unyielding counterforce. The contraction is held for 3 to 5 seconds, and the maneuver is repeated three to five times. Improvement of position and decreased pain on palpating the inguinal ligament should be found if the technique has been successful. By restoring the inferior component of the impairment complex, the anterior positional displacement also is corrected.

Inferior Pubic Symphyseal Joint (Right Side). The patient is positioned supine, lying near the right side of the bed. The clinician standing to the patient's right, flexes the patient's hip and knee, and places the closed fist of the right hand under the patient's right ischial tuberosity (Fig. 27-21). From this position, the patient is asked to attempt to straighten the right leg against the unyielding counterforce of the clinician. The contraction is held for 3 to 5 seconds, and the maneuver is repeated three to five times, following which the positional findings and kinetic test are retested.

Inferior or Superior Pubic Symphyseal Joint (Modified Shotgun). The patient is positioned supine, with the knees and hips flexed so the soles of the feet rest on the bed (Fig. 27-22). The clinician is at the patient's feet and holds the patient's knees together. The patient is asked to try to abduct, or open, the legs against the clinician's unyielding counterforce. The contraction is held for 3 to 5 seconds, and the maneuver is repeated three to five times, following which the positional findings and kinetic test are retested.

Next, the clinician abducts the patient's legs, while keeping the feet together (Fig. 27-23). The patient is then asked to

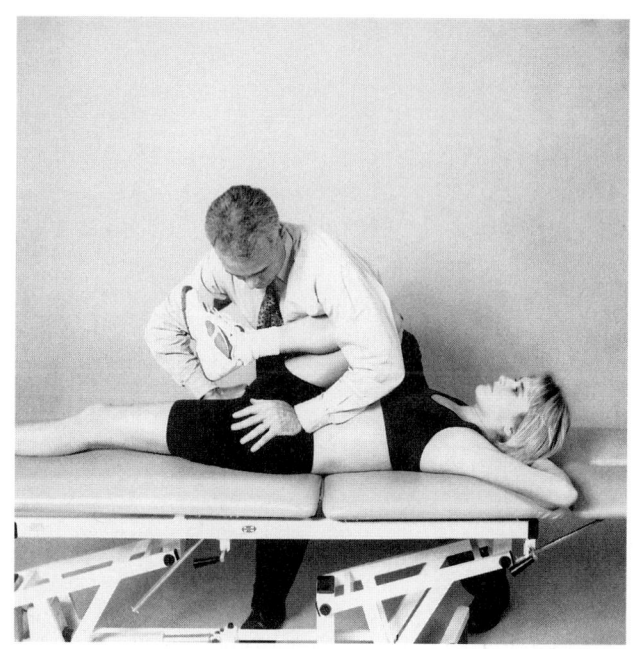

FIGURE 27-21   Patient and clinician positions for pubic symphysis mobilization.

adduct, or close, the legs against the clinician's unyielding counterforce. The contraction is held for 3 to 5 seconds, and the maneuver is repeated three to five times, following which the positional findings and kinetic test are retested.

Home Exercise. This technique can be performed at home, using a strap or belt for the abduction component (Fig. 27-24) and a rolled towel for the adduction part (Fig. 27-25).

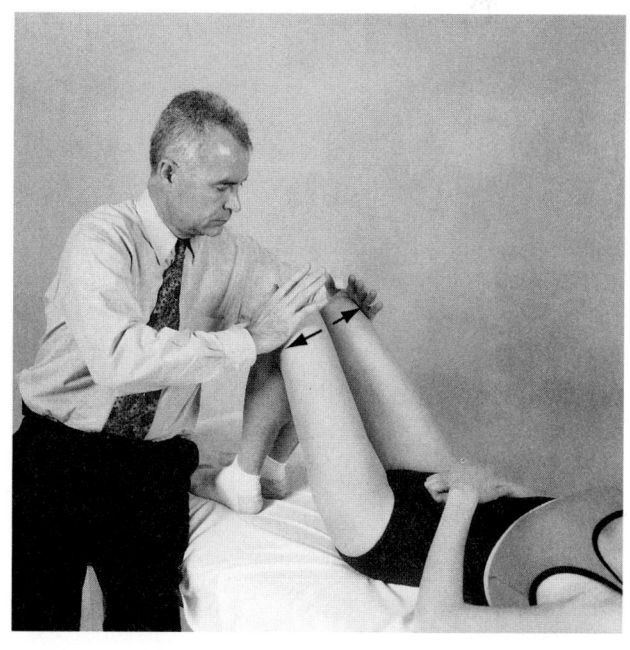

FIGURE 27-22   Modified shotgun, initial maneuver.

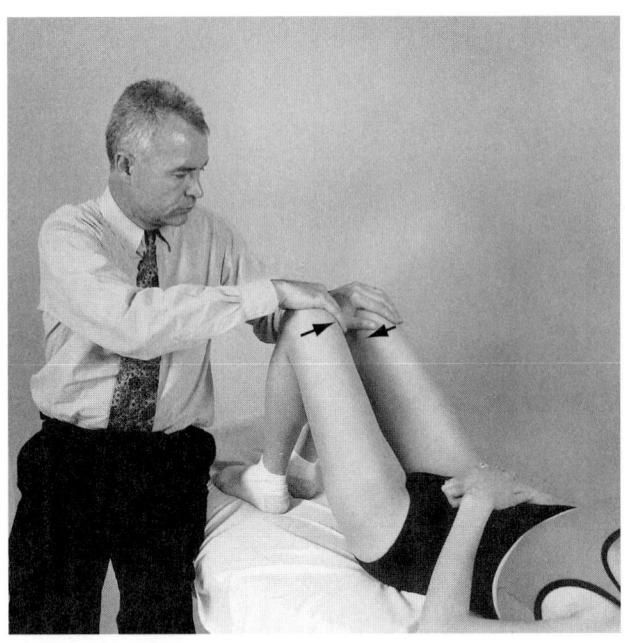

FIGURE 27-23   Modified shotgun, second maneuver.

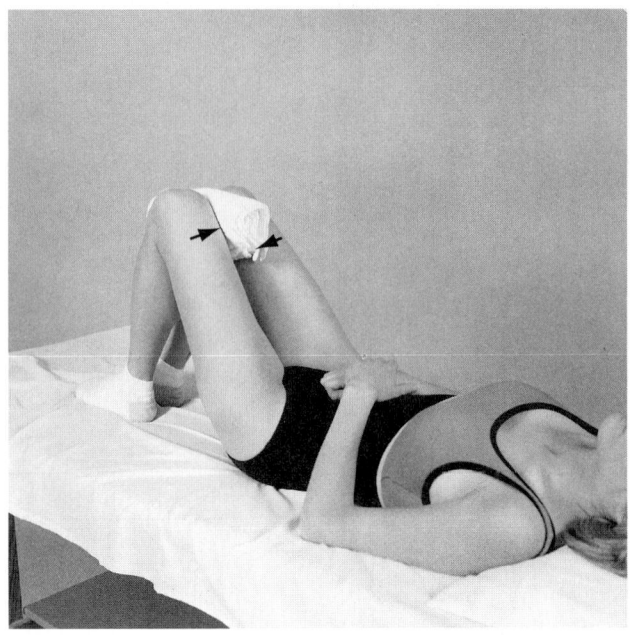

FIGURE 27-25   Home exercise for pubic dysfunction, version 2.

Mobilization Techniques to Restore Anterior Rotation of the Right Innominate

Passive Mobilization.   The patient is in the supine lying position, and the clinician stands on the right side of the patient. Sliding the left hand under the patient's buttock, the clinician stabilizes the apex of the sacrum and places the heel of the right hand on the patient's right iliac crest. Using a series of small

oscillations, the clinician rotates the right innominate anteriorly (Fig. 27-26). By altering the angle of the anterior rotation, the clinician can find the direction that is the most comfortable and efficient.

After a number of these oscillations, the patient is positioned in prone lying with the right ASIS off the edge of the

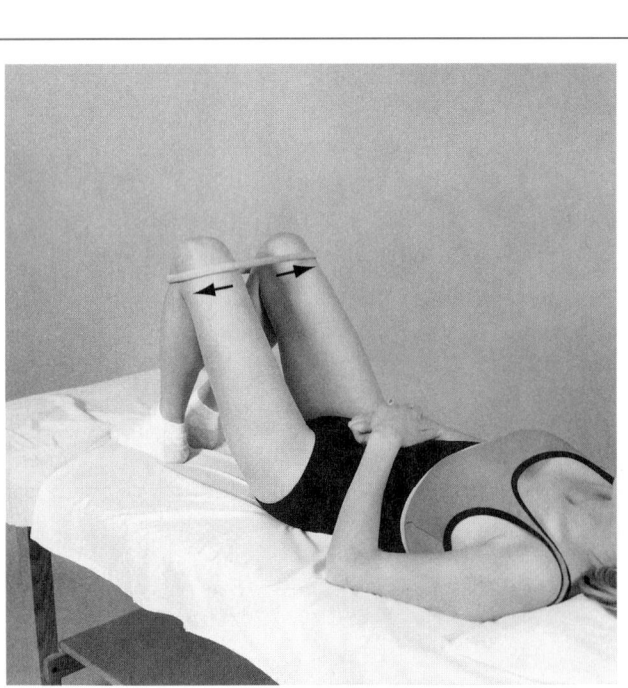

FIGURE 27-24   Home exercise for pubic dysfunction, version 1.

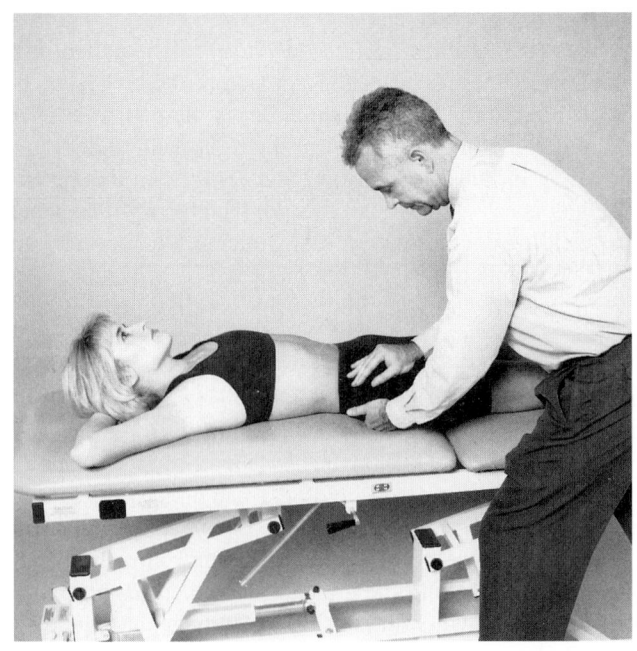

FIGURE 27-26   Patient and clinician positions for passive mobilization into anterior rotation of the right innominate.

table. Ensuring that the motion of the patient's right ASIS into anterior rotation is not blocked by the table, the clinician passively rotates the right innominate anteriorly with a series of small oscillations. As more motion is gained, the clinician places a pillow under the right thigh of the patient, or elevates the end of the table, and the patient's left leg is lowered off the side of the bed. In this position, the clinician continues to mobilize the right innominate into anterior rotation.

Muscle energy can be incorporated into the technique. As the clinician stabilizes the apex of the sacrum, the patient is instructed to push the right hip into the pillow or table while keeping the right leg straight, thereby using the rectus femoris, sartorius, and iliopsoas muscles. By inserting a hand between the patient's thigh and the table, the clinician can monitor the force of the hip flexion.

Active Mobilization: Method One. The patient is in the left side-lying position, facing away from the clinician and with the left hip fully flexed. Grasping the anterior aspect of the patient's right thigh, the clinician passively extends the patient's right hip, while monitoring the right posterior inferior iliac spine, S2, and the ischial tuberosity with the other hand, until motion occurs. At the motion barrier, the patient performs an isometric contraction of right hip flexion against the clinician's resistance (Fig. 27-27). The patient relaxes, and the right hip is extended to the new barrier.

Active Mobilization: Method Two. The patient is in the left side-lying position, facing the clinician and with the left hip flexed to about 90 degrees. The clinician stabilizes the patient's left leg using his or her thigh. The patient's right hip is passively extended to the motion barrier and is both supported in this position, and prevented from moving into adduction. The clinician leans onto the patient and places the heel of his or her right hand over the apex of the sacrum. The left arm and hand of the clinician are placed between the patient's legs (Fig. 27-28). The patient is then instructed to push the right hip into flexion against the clinician's body. The patient then relaxes, the right hip is moved to the new barrier to hip extension, and the process is repeated.

Active Mobilization: Method Three. The patient is in the prone lying position, with the clinician standing on the patient's left side. With the right hand, the clinician supports the anterior aspect of the patient's right thigh, at a point just above the knee. The clinician places the heel of his or her left hand over the patient's right posterior inferior iliac spine. Extending the right hip until motion at the lumbosacral junction is perceived (Fig. 27-29), the clinician localizes the motion barrier. The patient is instructed to flex the right hip against the clinician's resistance. This isometric contraction is held up to 5 seconds, following which the patient is instructed to completely relax. The new barrier to anterior rotation is achieved by further extension of the hip. The mobilization is repeated three times and followed by a reexamination of function.

Home Exercise to Produce Anterior Rotation of the Innominate. The patient is positioned supine, with the uninvolved extremity flexed to the chest and the involved leg close to the edge of the bed. The patient lowers the involved leg toward the floor,

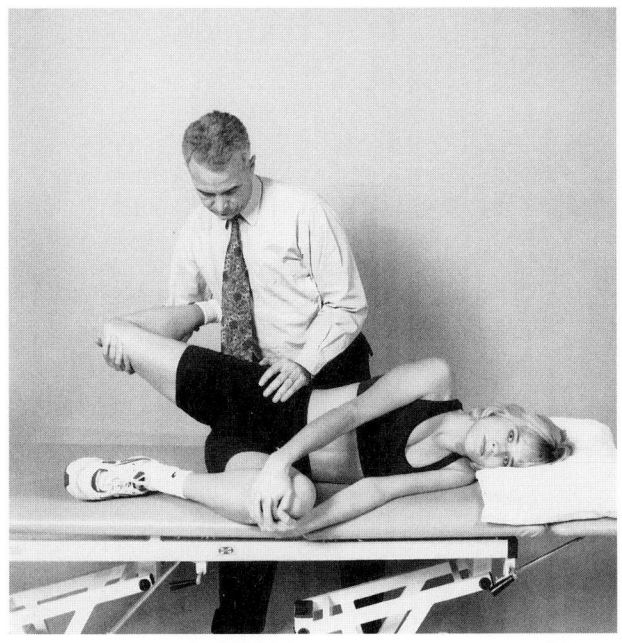

FIGURE 27-27 Patient and clinician positions for active mobilization into anterior rotation of the right innominate: method 1.

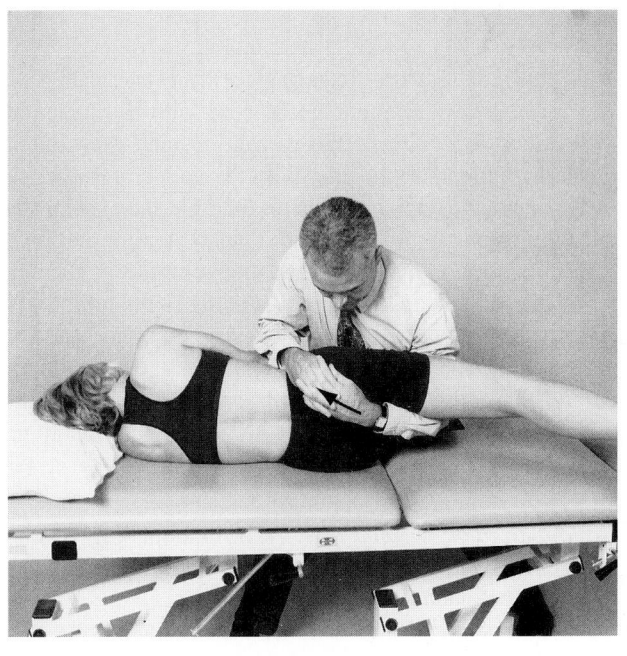

FIGURE 27-28 Patient and clinician positions for active mobilization into anterior rotation of the right innominate: method 2.

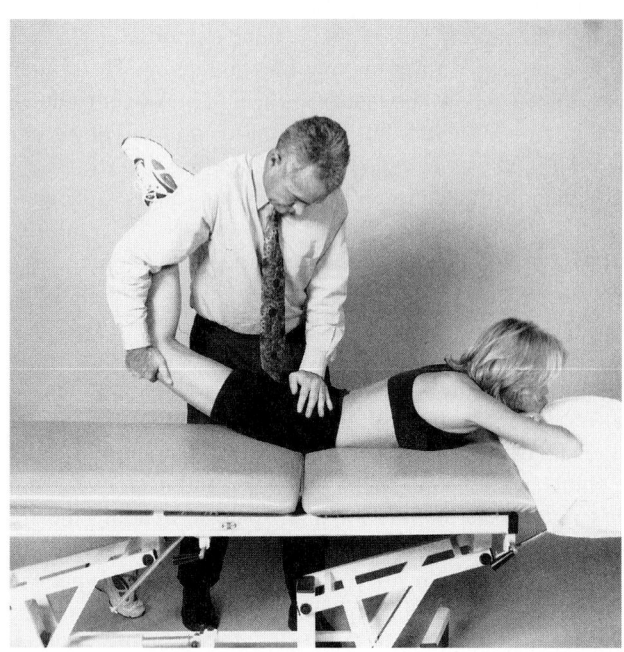

FIGURE 27-29 Patient and clinician positions for active mobilization into anterior rotation of the right innominate: method 3.

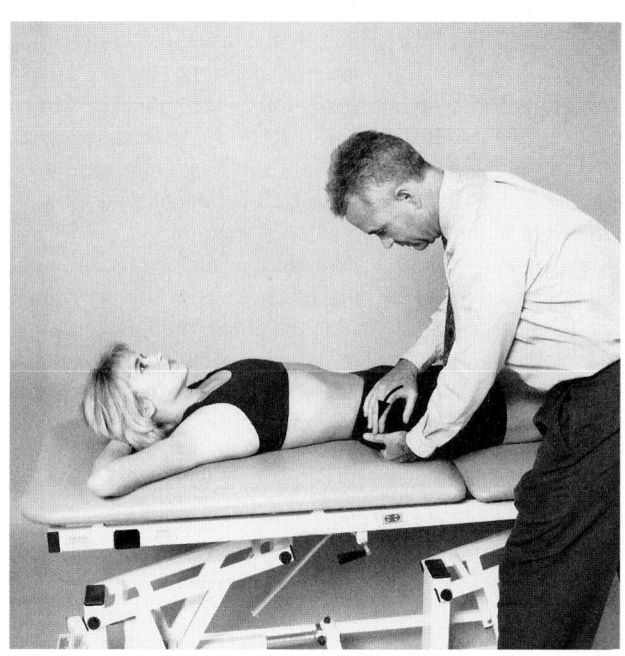

FIGURE 27-30 Patient and clinician positions for passive mobilization into posterior rotation of the right innominate.

producing a combined motion of hip extension and slight abduction, until the motion barrier is reached. From this position, the patient performs an isometric contraction of the hip adductor muscles for 3 to 5 seconds. The patient then initiates slight hip flexion and holds this position for 3 to 5 seconds. Following each contraction, the patient moves the leg into further hip extension to localize the new barrier. The exercise is repeated three to five times.

Techniques to Restore Posterior Rotation of the Right Innominate

Passive Mobilization. Patient lies supine with the knees and hips flexed to the point of the restriction, and the clinician stands at the patient's right side. With the long and ring fingers of the left hand, the clinician palpates the right sacral sulcus just medial to the posterior inferior iliac spine to monitor motion between the right innominate bone and the sacrum. With the index finger of the same hand, the clinician palpates the lumbosacral junction to note any movement between the pelvic girdle and the L5 vertebra. The heel of the right hand is placed on the right ASIS and iliac crest (Fig. 27-30). A grade II to IV posterior rotation force is applied to the right ASIS and iliac crest to produce an anterosuperior glide at the sacroiliac joint.

Active Mobilization: Method One. The patient is positioned supine near the end of the bed, with the clinician standing on the right side. If necessary, a towel roll is placed under the patient's lumbar spine. With the index and middle fingers of the left hand, the clinician palpates the lumbosacral junction and the sacral sulcus. With the right hand, the clinician cups the right ischial tuberosity and, by leaning onto the patient's right

leg, passively flexes the patient's right hip to the point of restriction (Fig. 27-31). Further hip flexion rotates the innominate posteriorly, and this is applied until the motion at the lumbosacral junction is perceived. The sacroiliac joint motion barrier has then been reached. The patient is asked to

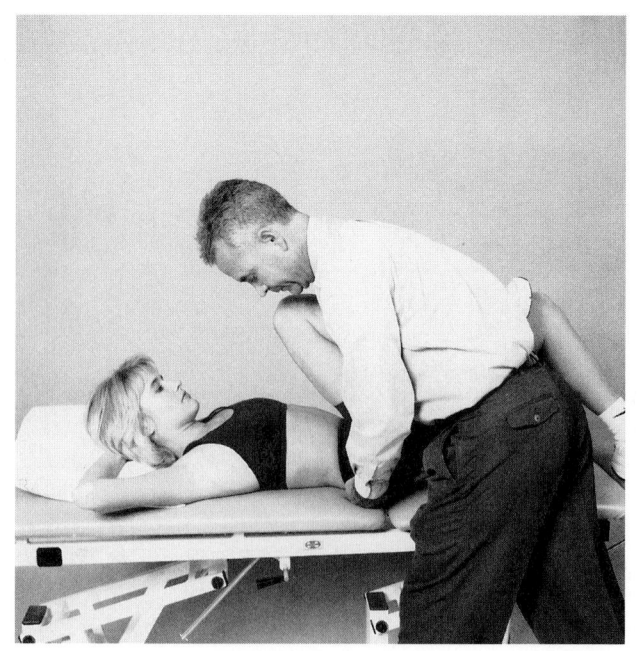

FIGURE 27-31 Patient and clinician positions for passive mobilization into posterior rotation of the right innominate: method 1.

extend the right hip against the clinician's chest. This isometric contraction is held up to 5 seconds, following which the patient is instructed to completely relax. The new barrier to posterior rotation is localized by further flexion of the hip joint. This mobilization is repeated three times and followed by a reexamination.

Active Mobilization: Method Two. The patient is in the left side-lying position, facing the clinician. The patient's left leg is stabilized by the clinician, or by a belt. The patient's right leg is placed around the trunk of the clinician and the right hip is flexed to the barrier. The right leg must not be allowed to adduct. The right innominate is grasped by both hands (Fig. 27-32). The patient is then instructed to extend the right hip against the clinician's trunk. If the patient keeps the right knee flexed (see Fig. 27-32), only the gluteus maximus is used for the contraction. By keeping the right leg straight, the patient utilizes the hamstrings, as well as the gluteus maximus (Fig. 27-33). This isometric contraction is held up to 5 seconds, following which the patient is instructed to completely relax. The new barrier to posterior rotation is localized by further flexion of the hip joint. This mobilization is repeated three times and followed by a reexamination.

Active Mobilization: Method Three. The patient is in the prone lying position, with the right hip and leg over the edge of the table. The clinician stands at the patient's right side. The patient's right foot is placed between the clinician's legs and held there. While monitoring the sacral sulcus with the index finger of the left hand, the clinician moves the patient's right leg to the

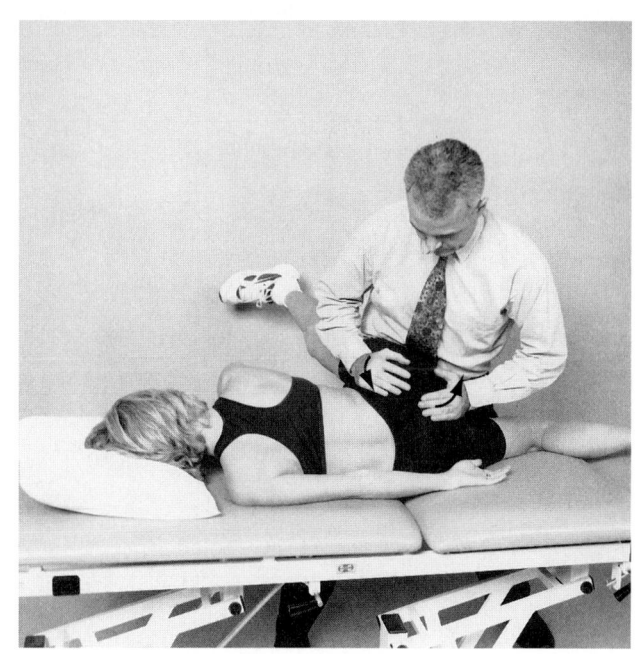

FIGURE 27-33 Patient and clinician positions for active mobilization into posterior rotation of the right innominate using gluteus maximus and hamstrings: method 2.

barrier (Fig. 27-34). The patient is asked to gently push the right foot toward the foot of the table. This movement is resisted by the clinician's left leg, and after 3 to 5 seconds, the patient is told to relax. Once again, when full relaxation has occurred, the slack is taken up, and the patient's right leg is moved in the

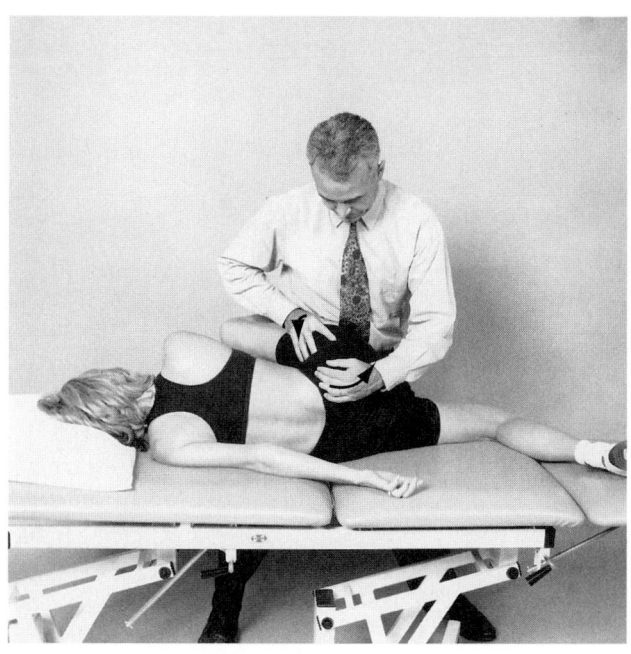

FIGURE 27-32 Patient and clinician positions for active mobilization into posterior rotation of the right innominate using gluteus maximus: method 2.

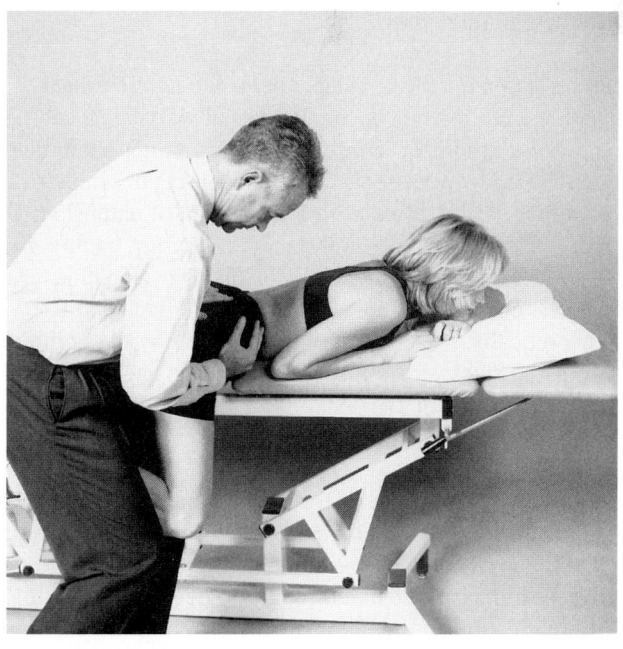

FIGURE 27-34 Patient and clinician positions for active mobilization into posterior rotation of the right innominate: method 3.

TABLE 27-5 Clinical Characteristics of an Osteopathic Sacral Torsion

	Anterior Torsion (L on L)	Posterior Torsion (R on L)
Sacral sulcus position	Deep on right	Prominent on right
Inferior lateral angle position	Prominent on left	Deep on left
Lumbar extension	Increased or normal	Decreased
Amount of lordosis	Increased or normal	Flat
Application of PA pressure to sacrum	Possible	No or limited motion
L5	Side bent right, rotated left	Side bent left, rotated left

L, left; PA, posteroanterior; R, right.

direction of hip flexion until the monitoring finger indicates the new barrier has been reached. This mobilization is repeated three times and followed by a reexamination.

Home Exercise to Produce a Posterior Rotation of the Innominate. The patient is positioned prone, with the uninvolved extremity hanging over the edge of the bed and the involved leg flexed to the chest. Once the motion barrier is engaged, the patient attempts to gently extend the hip of the involved side against an unyielding counterforce for about 3 to 5 seconds. Upon relaxation, the patient further flexes and posteriorly rotates the involved hip to localize the new motion barrier. The exercise is repeated three to five times.

Techniques to Correct a Counternutation of the Sacrum on the Right

This is not a motion that occurs in normal walking. It can only occur when the lumbar spine is operating in non-neutral mechanics and is always associated with a non-neutral impairment of the lumbar spine, often with a restriction of extension. The clinical findings for a counternutated sacrum on the right (a right-on-left posterior sacral torsion, using osteopathic terminology) are outlined in Table 27-5.

Theoretically, the correction is produced by the combined action of the right piriformis, pulling on the sacrum, and the gluteus medius, with the tendon of the tensor fascia latae, pulling on the innominate.

Active Mobilization: Method One. The patient is in the left side-lying position, facing the clinician. The L5–S1 junction is palpated with the right hand. The clinician positions the patient by placing the lumbar spine in left rotation (see the introduction to Part III). The clinician then grasps the patient's left ankle and moves the left hip into extension until motion is felt at the sacral base (Fig. 27-35). The patient is asked to resist the clinician's attempt to move the hip into further extension. This resistance is achieved by activation of the erector spinae and the left iliopsoas muscles. The patient relaxes, and the clinician locates the new motion barrier.

Active Mobilization: Method Two. The patient is in the left side-lying position, facing the clinician. The L5–S1 junction is palpated with the right hand. The clinician locks down from above, using an extension and right rotation lock of the lumbar spine. The clinician extends the patient's left leg until the sacral base is felt to move. The patient's right hip is passively flexed to

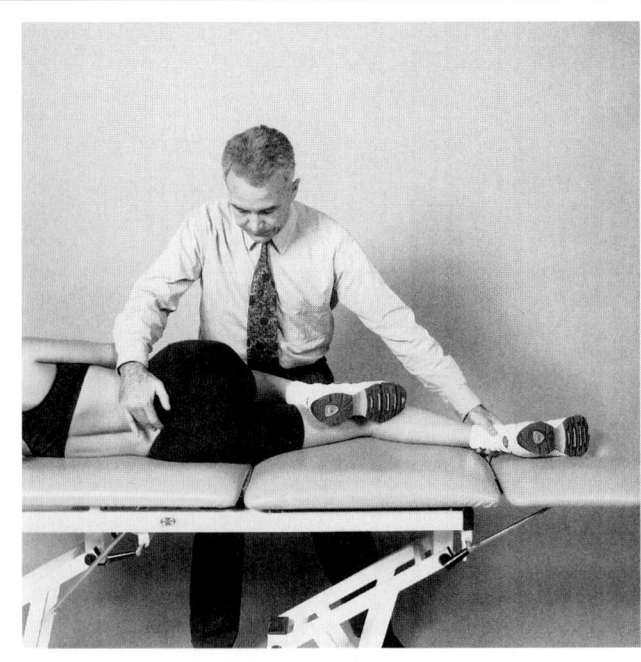

FIGURE 27-35 Patient and clinician positions for active mobilization to correct a counternutation of the sacrum on the right.

about 90 degrees, producing a posterior rotation of the right innominate, and the leg is positioned so that the knee is off the edge of the bed (Fig. 27-36). The patient is asked to abduct the right leg toward the ceiling against the resistance of the clinician. The piriformis is an abductor of the hip when the hip is flexed to 90 degrees, and its contraction produces a right nutation of the sacrum. The contraction and relaxation is repeated, and the patient is re-assessed

Thrust Technique for a Right-on-Left Correction. A thrust technique also may be used to correct a posterior sacral torsion. The patient lies supine, with the fingers laced together behind the neck and the elbows forward. The patient's pelvis should be close to the clinician (at the side of the table). The patient's feet and upper trunk are moved to the opposite side of the table, producing a right side bend of the trunk. Leaning over the patient, the clinician threads his or her right forearm, from the lateral side, through the gap between the patient's left arm and chest, and grasps the edge of the table, thereby rotating the patient's thorax away, without losing the patient's right side bending, until the patient's left innominate just begins to lift off the table. The clinician holds the left innominate down and takes up any slack by slightly increasing the rotation, without losing the side bend. The correction is made by a high-velocity, low-amplitude thrust using the left hand in a posterior direction (Fig. 27-37). The patient is then re-examined.

Home Exercise. The patient is in the left side-lying position, with the right leg off the edge of the table and the left knee flexed. The patient rotates the trunk so that his or her right hand

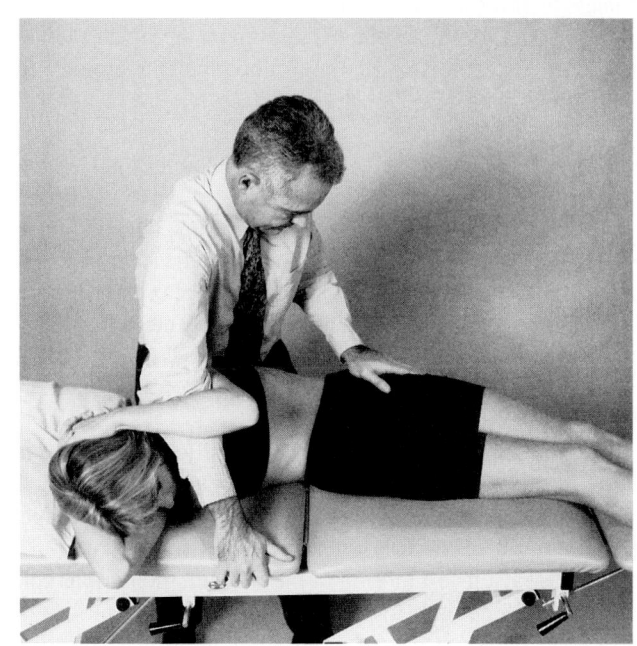

FIGURE 27-37 Patient and clinician positions for thrust technique, right-on-left correction.

is able to grasp the left knee or the edge of the table, and orients the face toward the ceiling (Fig. 27-38). From this position, the patient inhales slightly and attempts to lift the right leg toward the ceiling, using only slight movement. The isometric contraction is held for 3 to 5 seconds, and the exercise is repeated three to five times.

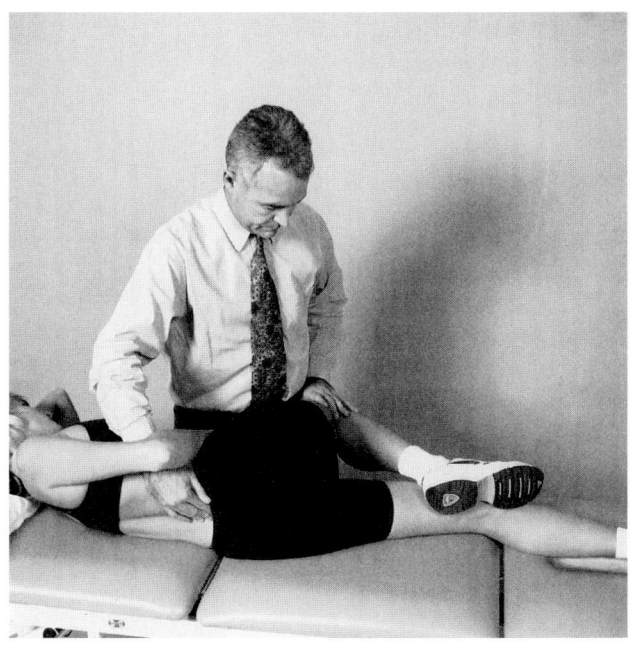

FIGURE 27-36 Active mobilization technique for a right-on-left correction.

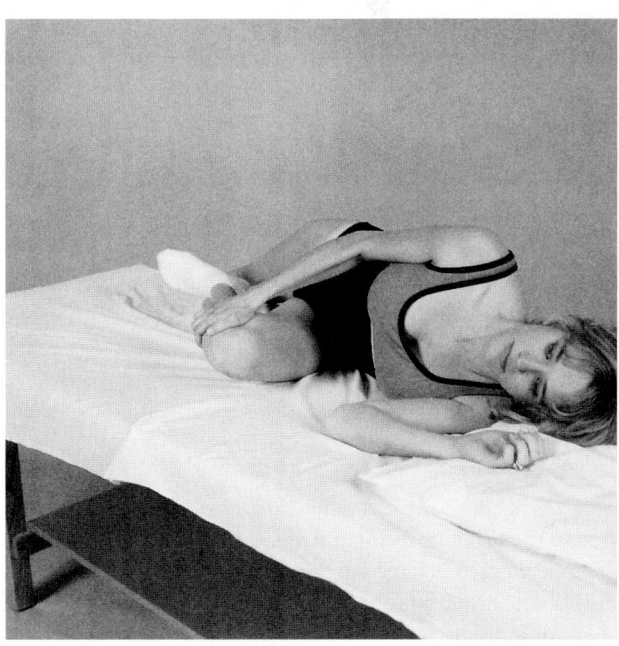

FIGURE 27-38 Home exercise for sacral counternutation.

Techniques to Treat a Nutated Sacrum on the Right

The clinical findings for a nutated sacrum on the right (a left-on-left anterior sacral torsion, using osteopathic terminology) are outlined in Table 27-5.

Active Mobilization. Because the inferior lateral angle is both posterior and caudal on the left side, a number of muscles around the hip are utilized to pull the sacrum into the correct position. With a nutated sacrum on the right, the right piriformis is often tight, so this technique attempts to relax the right piriformis and its antagonists, the right hip internal rotators, through a reciprocal inhibition of the right piriformis. At the same time, a pull from the left piriformis is encouraged to help pull the sacrum into its correct position.

The patient is in the left side-lying position, facing the clinician. Because the dysfunction is a nutated sacrum on the right (left on left), the patient is positioned to encourage a counternutation of the sacrum on the right (right on left). To produce a right-on-left motion of the sacrum, the lumbar spine is positioned in flexion (which extends the sacrum, pulling the right sacral base posteriorly) and right rotation (which will also pull the right sacral base posteriorly), by flexing the lumbar spine from below, using the legs. The patient's trunk is placed into rotation into the table by placing the patient's right arm over the edge of the table and his or her left arm behind the torso, so that the chest is resting on the table. This position is accentuated by asking the patient to reach toward the floor with the right hand. The clinician flexes the patient's hips by grasping the patient's feet and ankles with their left hand, while palpating for motion at the patient's sacral base with the right hand. The patient's thighs are supported on the clinician's thighs.

With the patient's lower legs off the edge of the table (Fig. 27-39), the patient's left piriformis is placed on stretch, producing a passive right rotation of the sacrum. The patient is asked to perform lateral rotation of the left hip and medial rotation of the right hip simultaneously. After each 3- to 5-second contraction, the slack is taken up and the new motion barrier is located while the L5–S1 junction is palpated. It is important that the L5–S1 junction remain in neutral throughout the procedure. At the new motion barrier, the clinician grasps the patient's ankles and raises them to the ceiling, until the sacral base begins to move. At this point, the patient is asked to either push the feet toward the ceiling against the clinician's resistance, or to push the feet down toward the floor against the clinician's resistance. After a 3- to 5-second contraction, the patient relaxes, and the clinician raises the patient's feet toward the ceiling.

Home Exercise to Treat a Left-on-Left Sacral Torsion. The patient is in the left side-lying position, with both feet and knees positioned near the edge of the bed. The patient may reach toward the floor with the right hand to increase rotation of the lumbar spine to the left. From this position, both feet are lowered off the bed toward the floor, creating left side bending of the lumbar spine, to the motion barrier (Fig. 27-40). The

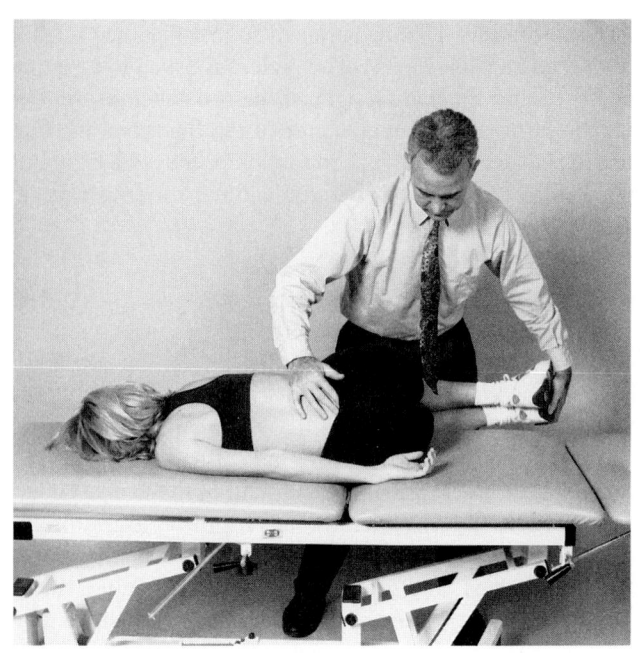

FIGURE 27-39 Patient and clinician positions for active mobilization technique, left-on-left correction.

patient then attempts to lift the feet towards the ceiling, using only slight movement, while taking and holding a deep breath. The isometric contraction is held for 3 to 5 seconds, at which point the patient exhales and lowers the feet toward the new motion barrier. The exercise is repeated three to five times.

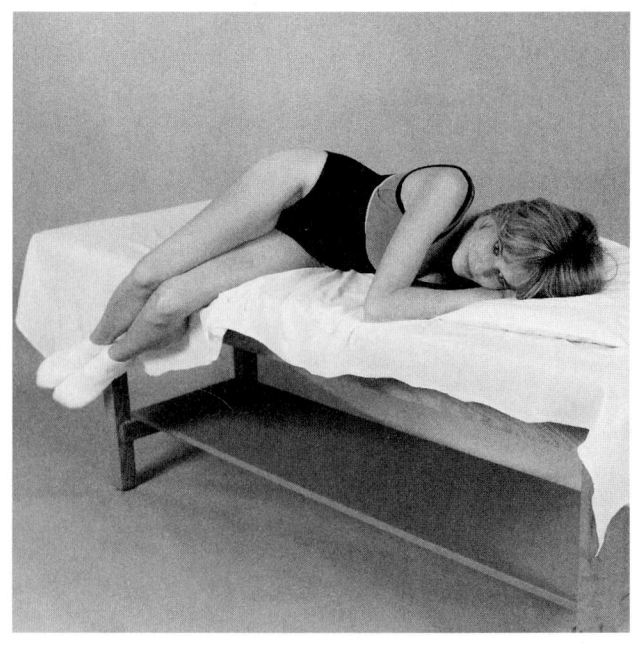

FIGURE 27-40 Home exercise for a left-on-left sacral torsion.

Myofascial Release of Pelvic Floor Trigger Points

As with the examination techniques for the pelvic floor muscles, it is very important that these techniques be performed only on the advice of a physician, or if there is strong evidence of pelvic floor dysfunction. The techniques should be performed only by clinicians with formal training.

For all of these techniques, the patient is positioned in the lithotomy position: supine with the thighs supported in a position of 90 degrees of hip flexion and 90 degrees of knee flexion. The clinician inserts a gloved index finger via the rectum or vagina.

Lateral Stretching.[99] The clinician locates the tender area identified in the pelvic floor examination. In women, the tender areas in the urinary sphincter and periurethral tissues are compressed against the symphysis pubis, combined with a lateral traction force (Fig. 27-41). The initial light pressure is increased according to tolerance.

Following several of these lateral stretches, the clinician applies posterior traction via the vagina or rectum (Fig. 27-42). The patient is asked to contract isometrically against the finger, to inhibit muscle tension and result in an increased lengthening of the anterior contracted muscles, with a reduction of trigger points in the levator muscles. The isometric contractions are repeated several times.

A similar technique is used in men, except that the focus is directed to the endopelvic fascia and pubococcygeus muscle lateral to the prostatic edge (Fig. 27-43).

Obturator Internus.[99] In addition to the urogenital diaphragm, the obturator internus is a common source of myofascial trigger points associated with the urgency-frequency syndrome. The patient is positioned as shown in Figure 27-44 and is asked to abduct the thigh against resistance by pushing the knee laterally. This has the affect of causing the obturator internus to contract, shorten, and widen under the levator muscle, making it easier to first identify, and then to apply the compression and stretching techniques.

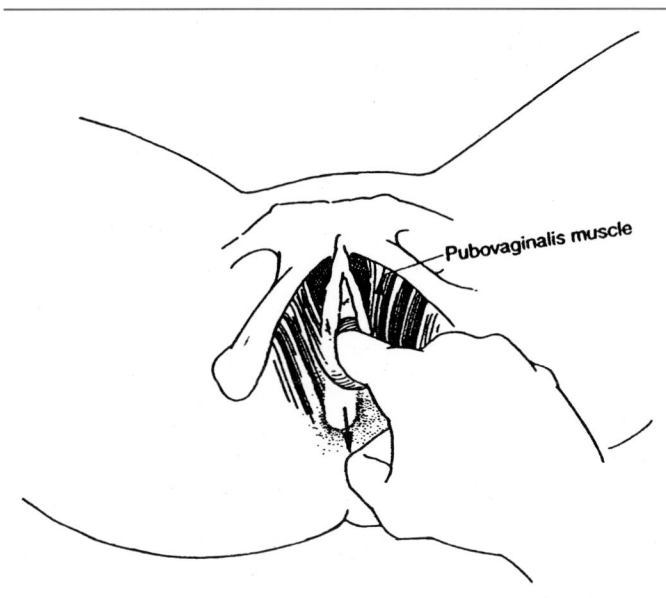

FIGURE 27-42 Posterior stretching of the pubovaginalis muscle. (Reproduced with permission from Weiss JM. Pelvic floor myofascial trigger points: Manual therapy for interstitial cystitis and the urgency-frequency syndrome. *J Urol* 2001;166:2228.)

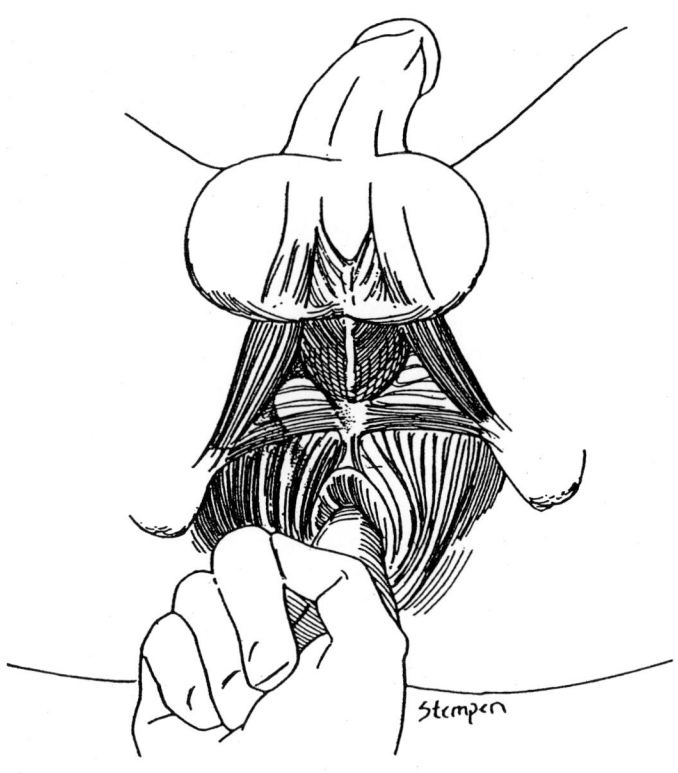

FIGURE 27-43 Lateral and inferior stretching of the puboprostate, urogenital diaphragm, and urinary sphincter. (Reproduced with permission from Weiss JM. Pelvic floor myofascial trigger points: Manual therapy for interstitial cystitis and the urgency-frequency syndrome. *J Urol* 2001;166:2228.)

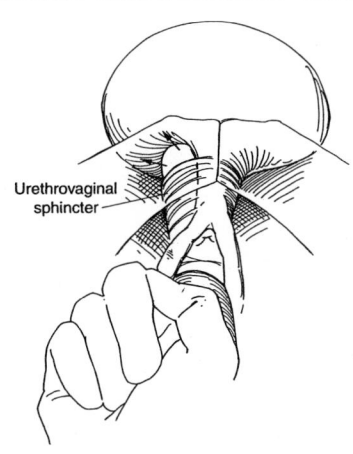

FIGURE 27-41 Lateral stretching and compression of the urinary sphincter. (Reproduced with permission from Weiss JM. Pelvic floor myofascial trigger points: Manual therapy for interstitial cystitis and the urgency-frequency syndrome. *J Urol* 2001;166:2227.)

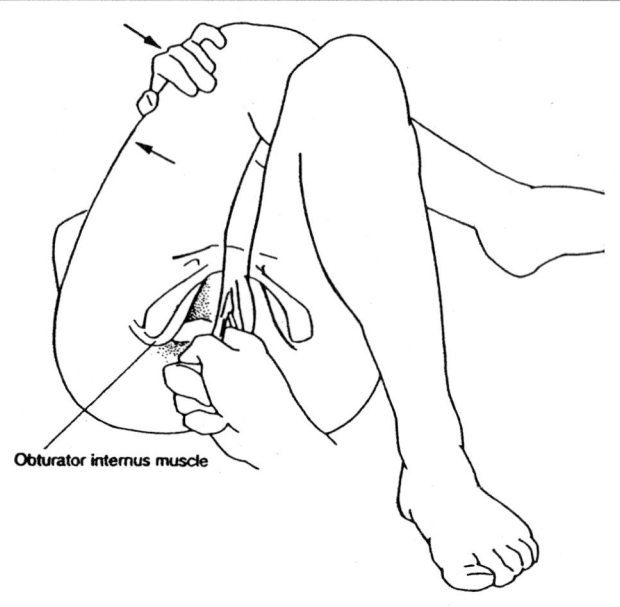

FIGURE 27-44 Compression and stretching of the obturator internus muscle assisted by external stretching. (Reproduced with permission from Weiss JM. Pelvic floor myofascial trigger points: Manual therapy for interstitial cystitis and the urgency-frequency syndrome. *J Urol* 2001;166:2228.)

Therapeutic Exercise

For the most part, exercises are avoided in the acute phase, because they tend to increase the symptoms. The same principles apply here as elsewhere: stretch those muscles that are tight or shortened, and strengthen those muscles that are found to be weak. Intervention strategies should emphasize pelvic stabilization,[157] the elimination of trunk and lower extremity muscle imbalances, and the correction of gait abnormalities.[158] Corrective exercises also may be used to position the innominate bone in proper relation to the sacrum. Postural correction and the correction of compensatory movements need to be addressed. As symptoms are controlled, therapy should be advanced to activity-specific stabilization exercises to facilitate return to function at the patient's occupation, sport, or avocational activities.

Flexibility

The muscles to be stretched around this joint complex are usually the erector spinae, quadratus lumborum, rectus femoris, iliopsoas, tensor fascia lata, hip adductors, and the deep external rotators of the hip, especially the piriformis, and gluteus maximus.[35,36]

In addition, the clinician must address any flexibility deficits found in the following muscles, or muscle groups:

▶ *Hamstrings.* The hamstrings are stretched as a group, although it is the biceps femoris that is attached to the sacrotuberous ligament and that can have potential influences on the sacroiliac joint.[35,36]

▶ *Lumbosacral fascia.*

▶ *Abdominals.*

Stabilization Exercises

Exercise is an important aspect of intervention for musculoskeletal impairments. No group of exercises is exclusive for the sacroiliac joint, so it is necessary to approach the rehabilitation of this region by including the lumbar spine and hip joints. The focus of the therapeutic exercises for this region is to augment the force-closure mechanism and to reduce any stress that could prove detrimental to the sacroiliac complex.

The strengthening component of the exercises is aimed at improving the function of the muscles of the inner and outer groups. The appropriate muscles must be isolated and then retrained to increase their strength and endurance, and to automatically recruit to support and protect the region.

A four-stage program has been designed to isolate and retrain the inner and outer muscle groups.[12,52,53]

Stage 1

▶ *Levator ani.* The patient is first taught the location of the levator ani. To strengthen the muscle, the patient is asked to shorten the distance between the coccyx and the pubic symphysis and to hold the contraction for 10 seconds (Fig. 27-45). When the muscle contracts properly, the transverse abdominis muscle can be felt to contract at a point 2 cm medial and inferior to the ASIS, there is no contraction of the buttocks, and by carefully palpating the sacral apex, the sacrum is felt to counternutate as the levator ani contracts. The exercise is repeated ten times.

▶ *Transversus abdominis/multifidus.* To test for isolation of the transversus abdominis, the patient is positioned prone, and a pressure biofeedback unit is placed underneath the abdomen[52,53] (Fig. 27-46). The cuff is inflated to a base

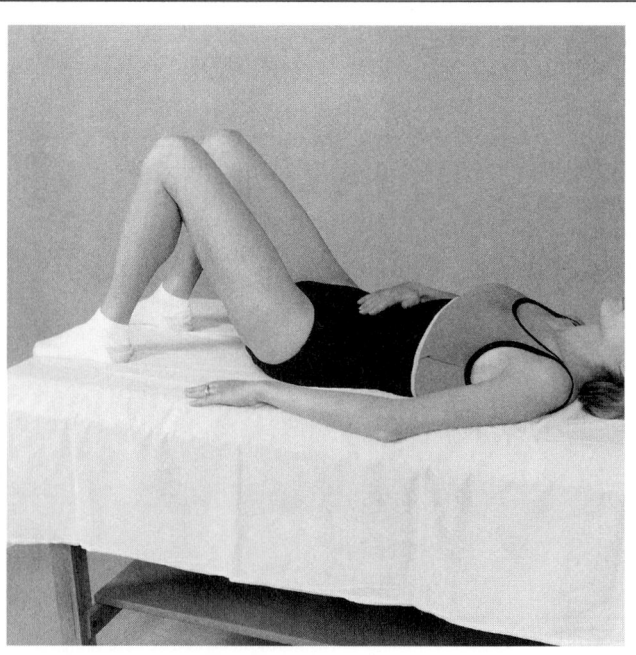

FIGURE 27-45 Levator ani exercise.

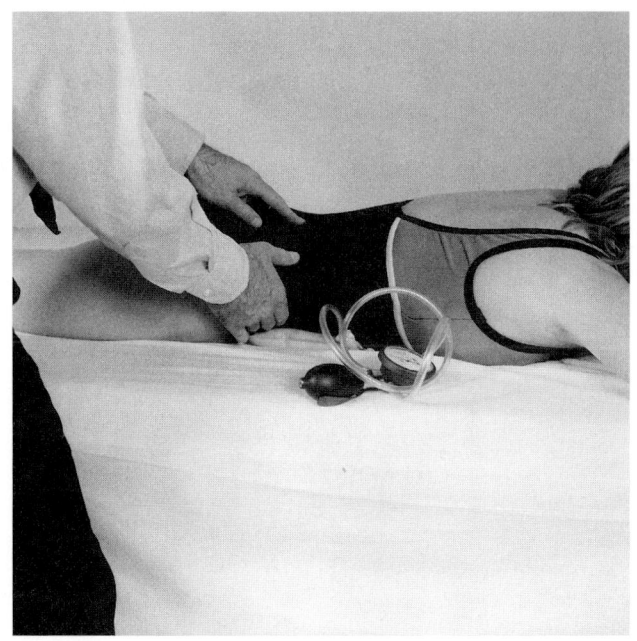

FIGURE 27-46 Isolation of the transversus abdominis.

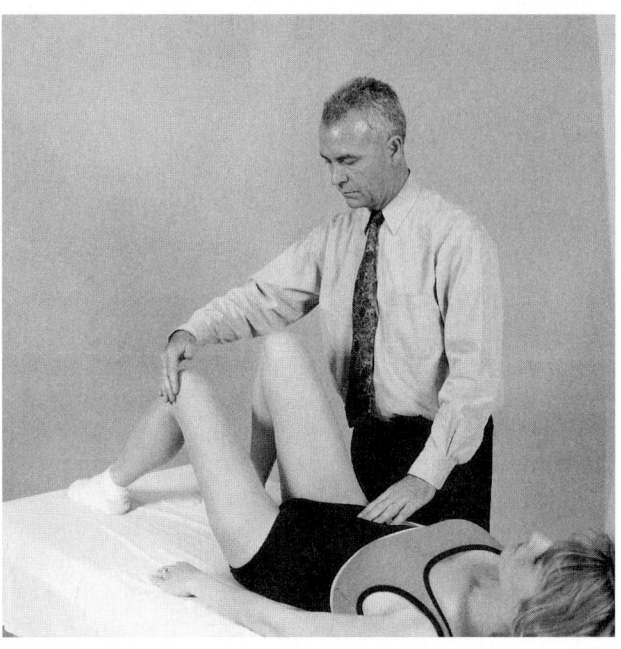

FIGURE 27-47 Exercise for the inner muscle group.

level of 70 mm Hg. The patient is asked to draw the navel up and in toward the chest (abdominal hollowing). When the muscle contracts properly, an increase in tension can be felt at a point 2 cm medial and inferior to the ASIS. If a bulging is felt at this point, the internal oblique is contracting. The multifidus is palpated simultaneously and should be felt to swell at a point just lateral to the spinous process.

If a pressure biofeedback unit is not available, an alternative technique can be used to test these muscles, in which the patient assumes the quadruped position on the hands and knees. The patient's shoulders and hips are centered over the hands and knees, and the lumbar spine is in a neutral position. The patient is asked to take a deep breath in, breathe out, and then draw the navel up toward the spine (abdominal hollowing).[53] If performed correctly, the lower abdomen should elevate before the upper abdomen. There should be no expansion or contraction of the lower rib cage, and the oblique muscles should not contract. The multifidus can be tested in this position by having the patient make the muscle harden under the clinician's fingers.

Stage 2. The stabilization program is progressed to the next stage with the introduction of lower or upper extremity motion, which changes the focus of the program from the inner muscle group to the outer muscle group.

In the supine position with the hips and knees flexed, the patient is asked to isolate the inner muscle group, while maintaining the lumbar spine in a neutral position. From this position, the patient is asked to slowly let the knee fall to one side (Fig. 27-47). Alternatively, the patient may extend the leg with the foot supported on the table.

The next step in the progression involves asking the patient to slowly extend this leg while maintaining the hip and knee flexed (with the foot lifted) to 45 degrees above the table (Fig. 27-48). This exercise initially is performed unilaterally and then is progressed to alternate leg extensions. The same exercises may be performed sitting on a gym ball or lying supine on a long roll. By making the base unstable, the exercise becomes more difficult without having to progress to the next stage.

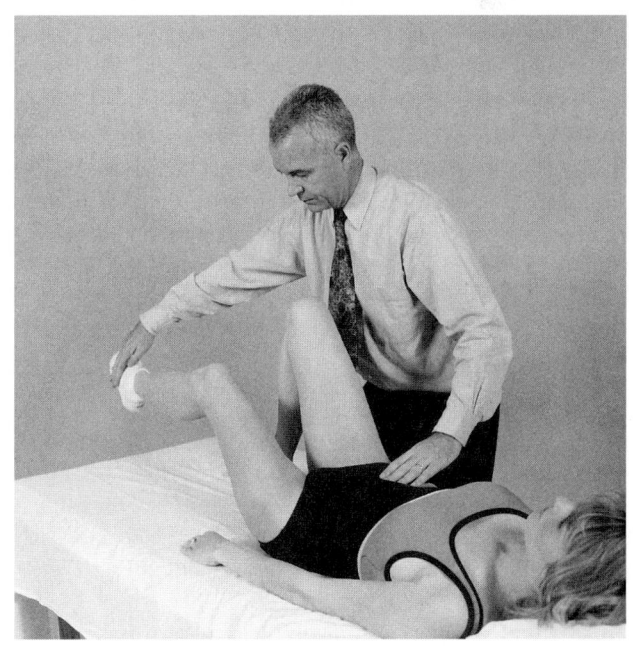

FIGURE 27-48 Exercise progression for the inner muscle group.

Exercising on a gym ball requires core stability (inner muscle group control), coordination, and appropriate postural reflexes. While sitting on the ball, the patient is asked to contract the muscles of the inner muscle group. This contraction is maintained while the patient moves forward and back, and up and down on the ball. The patient is instructed to incorporate the co-contraction of the inner muscle group into their activities of daily living.

If the individual muscles of the outer muscle group are weak or poorly recruited, the exercise program should include isolation and training at this time.

▶ *Posterior oblique system.* In the posterior oblique system, it is common to find the gluteus maximus both lengthened and weak.[12] Having the patient squeeze the buttocks together and sustain the contraction for 10 seconds isolates the gluteus maximus. A surface electromyography unit can provide a useful biofeedback system for this muscle. The exercise is progressed by having the patient lie prone over a gym ball and asking him or her initially to recruit the inner muscle group and then to extend the hip while the knee is flexed. Lifting the extended thigh increases the degree of difficulty. Leg extension machines can help to strengthen the gluteus maximus. Initially, the patient exercises in the supine position with one or both feet on the foot plate. Functional training is introduced by having the patient practice going from sitting to standing with a stabilized trunk, using primarily the gluteus maximus muscle.

▶ *Lateral system.* In the lateral system, the posterior fibers of the gluteus medius are often weak, which can have a marked effect on walking and load transference through the hip joint.[74] Isolation of the gluteus medius is taught in the side-lying position with a pillow placed between the knees. The exercise is progressed by asking the patient to lift the knee off the pillow and then to extend the knee while maintaining the correct position of the trunk and hip. Resistance can be added using elastic tubing or a cuff weight.

▶ *Anterior oblique system.* Isolation of the anterior oblique system involves training the specific contraction of the external and internal oblique abdominals. When the external obliques contract bilaterally, the infrasternal angle narrows, whereas when the internal obliques contract bilaterally, the infrasternal angle widens. The patient is taught to palpate the lateral costal margin and to specifically widen and narrow the infrasternal angle through specific contraction of the oblique abdominals.

The progression includes activation of the anterior and posterior oblique systems and differentiation of trunk from thigh motion. To begin, the patient is supine with the hips and knees flexed. The patient is instructed to bridge and then to rotate the trunk and pelvic girdle at the hip joints in the unsupported position, while maintaining the lumbar joints in a neutral position (Fig. 27-49).

Stage 3. Stage 3 exercises involve controlled motion of the "unstable region."[52] Because this stage is much more advanced, it is only used when required by an individual's work or sport.

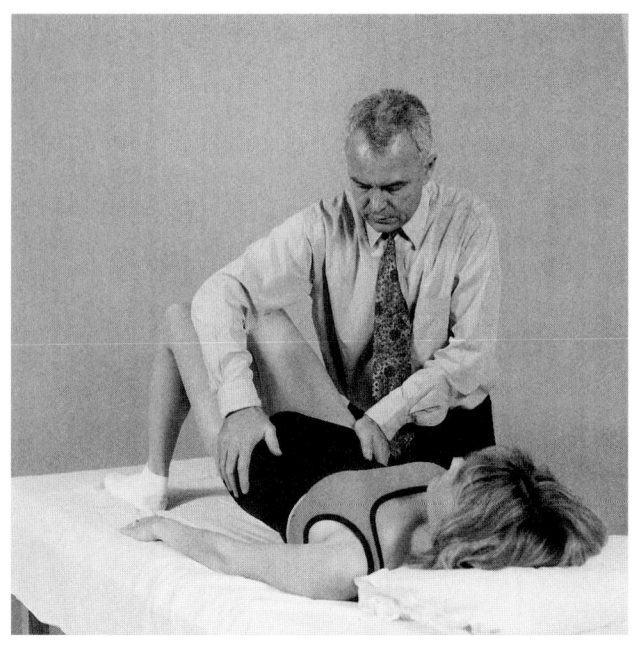

FIGURE 27-49 Bridge and trunk rotation exercise.

The protocol includes concentric and eccentric work with variable resistance in all three planes.

Stage 4.[52] Stage 4 of the protocol involves stabilization during high-speed motions. Very few people require stage 4 stabilization, particularly in view of the fact that high-speed exercise tends to reduce the stabilizing capability of the trunk muscles.[53]

Pelvic Floor Exercises[51]

In 1948 Kegel first advocated pelvic floor muscle (PFM) exercise to enhance urethral resistance and promote urinary control.[157a] The application of Kegel exercises has been broadened to various applications but the concentration continues to be considered a useful adjunct in the management of functional urinary incontinence. Many studies have shown that the success of PFM exercise for female stress urinary incontinence depends on the degree and duration of treatment, and close supervision by a physical therapist.[157b] The patients are initially educated in pelvic floor muscle awareness. Several teaching methods can be used, including verbal cues, visualization with an anatomical model, palpation, objective pelvic floor muscle contraction at the anus or base of the penis, or biofeedback with electromyography recordings via a rectal probe.[157c] The method chosen depends on the patient's baseline awareness, coordination and comfort level. The palpation method is performed as follows:

The patient is asked to sit forward on a chair with their legs apart, their spine extended, and their feet flat on the floor. The clinician and patient each place a hand anterior to the anterior superior iliac spine (ASIS) and along the inguinal region to feel the contraction of the transverse abdominis and the internal obliques. The fingers are also spread superiorly to feel the weight of the belly and the rectus abdominis. The patient is asked to "move the urethra and vagina gently upward" and to maintain the contraction for endurance.

Bracing. The patient is asked to sit forward on a chair with their legs apart, their spine extended, and their feet flat on the floor. The patient is asked to "push their abdomen out" without using an inspiratory effort, to isometrically contract the upper and lower rectus abdominis in its outer range. The patient is taught to initiate, and hold, this action during a defecatory urge.

Abdominal Drawing-in. The patient is positioned in supine with the spine in neutral and the abdominal wall relaxed. The patient is asked to draw the lower part of the abdomen up and in towards the spine without moving the trunk or pelvis, or using an inspiratory effort, thereby contracting the transverse abdominis and the internal obliques. This exercise is taught in a variety of patient positions, with the appropriate muscles being palpated by the patient and clinician, and the use of normal breathing.

Other exercises are added as tolerated. For the following four exercises the patient is positioned in the supine, hook-lying position:[157c]

▶ *Exercise 1.* The patient performs a PFM contraction with a posterior pelvic tilt.

▶ *Exercise 2.* The patient performs a PFM contraction with a bridging motion.

▶ *Exercise 3.* The patient performs a PFM contraction with hip adduction against a pillow between the knees.

▶ *Exercise 4.* The patient performs a PFM contraction with hip external rotation against an elastic exercise band.

Swissball exercises may then be added.[157c,157d] The patient is positioned sitting on a Swissball:

▶ *Exercise 1.* The patient performs a PFM contraction with a posterior pelvic tilt in the sagittal plane while rolling on the ball.

▶ *Exercise 2.* The patient performs a PFM contraction with a posterior pelvic tilt in the oblique plane while rolling on the ball.

▶ *Exercise 3.* The patient bounces vertically on the Swissball while performing a PFM contraction during each ascending movement.

▶ *Exercise 4.* The patient performs a PFM contraction while rolling on the ball from sitting to standing for functional training with transfers.

CASE STUDY LEFT-SIDED LOW BACK AND BUTTOCK PAIN

HISTORY

A 47-year-old man presented at the clinic who had developed left-sided low back and buttock pain while at work 2 weeks previously. When describing the mechanism of injury, the patient reported feeling something "pop" in his low back during a lifting maneuver that involved bending forward and twisting to the right. The pain was now localized to an area slightly inferior to the left posterior superior iliac spine, which he reported as being very tender to the touch. The pain was aggravated with forward bending and turning at the waist to the left in the sitting position. The patient reported sleeping well, if he remained prone, and there were no complaints of paresthesias or anesthesias. The patient denied any neurologic symptoms related to cauda equina or spinal cord involvement. He was in otherwise good health.

QUESTIONS

1. Given a distinct mechanism of injury, what type of structure(s) could be at fault with complaints of left-sided low back and buttock pain?

2. What does the region of *localized* tenderness tell the clinician?

3. Why do you think the patient is sleeping well in the prone position?

4. What is your working hypothesis at this stage? List the various diagnoses that could manifest with low back and buttock pain, and the tests you would use to rule out each one.

5. Does this presentation/history warrant a scan? Why or why not?

EXAMINATION

The patient had a specific mechanism of injury, and although the pain distribution initially was more widespread, the presence of a very localized area of pain suggested a musculoskeletal impairment and so a scanning examination was deferred. If this hypothesis proved incorrect, a lumbosacral scan may be necessary.

The patient's standing posture was unremarkable. Active range-of-motion testing for the lumbar spine revealed pain and restriction with forward flexion, right side bending, and left rotation. There was palpable tenderness along the S3 to S4 level on the sacrum. However, a number of structures in this specific area are capable of producing pain. The iliolumbar ligament was examined, but the tests were negative. The anterior and posterior stress tests for the sacroiliac joint also were assessed to help rule out sacroiliac joint inflammation. The anterior test was negative and although the posterior test caused a slight increase in symptoms, it was not considered a positive test. The resisted tests of the major hip muscles were negative.

The dorsal sacroiliac ligament was assessed. The patient was positioned prone, and the clinician, while palpating the tender area with one hand, pushed the sacral base anteriorly with the palm of the other hand, thereby producing a sacral nutation. The tenderness lessened according to the patient. To produce a counternutation, and therefore stress the dorsal sacroiliac ligament, both inferior lateral angles were pushed anteriorly. This maneuver immediately caused a significant increase in the patient's pain. It was decided to use a functional test for the dorsal sacroiliac ligament.

The patient was positioned supine, with both legs straight. The patient was asked to perform a straight leg raise with the left leg and to hold the leg about 5 degrees off the bed. Because the initial 5 degrees of a straight leg raise produces an anterior rotation of the innominate and a counternutation force of the sacrum on the ipsilateral side, a positive finding for this test is the reproduction of pain, or weakness. Slight modifications to the test were used to help in the confirmation.

- The right knee was flexed, and the patient was asked to perform a straight leg raise with the right leg. Flexing the contralateral knee to the straight leg raise has the effect of relaxing the lumbar spine while maintaining the counternutation on the ipsilateral side. If this maneuver decreases the pain, a muscle imbalance is probably present (quadratus lumborum, multifidus, etc.).
- The patient was asked to lift the right shoulder off the bed against manual resistance from the clinician, while performing the straight leg raise on the right. This maneuver tests the ability of the anterior oblique system of force closure.
- The sacroiliac joint was manually compressed via the innominates as in the posterior stress test of the sacroiliac joint, while the patient performed a straight leg raise on the right. Compressing the innominates produces a slight counternutation of the sacrum.

All of the modifications produced an increase in the patient's symptoms, confirming a provisional diagnosis of a sprained left dorsal sacroiliac ligament.

QUESTIONS

1. Based on the provisional diagnosis, what will be your intervention?
2. How would you describe this condition to the patient?
3. In order of priority, and based on the stages of healing, list the various goals of your intervention.
4. How will you determine the amplitude and joint position for the intervention?
5. What would you tell the patient about your intervention?
6. Estimate this patient's prognosis.
7. What modalities could you use in the intervention of this patient?
8. What exercises would you prescribe?

INTERVENTION

- *Electrotherapeutic modalities and thermal agents.* Moist heat may be applied over the dorsal sacroiliac ligament. Electrical stimulation with a medium frequency of 50 to 120 pulses per second may be applied with the moist heat to aid in pain relief. Ultrasound at 1 MHz may be administered prior to any manual techniques to increase the extensibility of the tissues. An ice pack may be applied to the area at the end of the treatment session if the patient reports an increase in symptoms.
- *Manual therapy.* Transverse frictional massage was applied to the tender aspect of the ligament.
- *Therapeutic exercises.* To strengthen the opposite gluteus maximus, exercises involving the ipsilateral latissimus dorsi,

and the erector spinae of both sides, were prescribed. These exercises could include:

- Lunges. The patient grasps a weight in the right hand and is asked to perform a lunge, leading with the left leg, while swinging the right arm into shoulder extension.
- To strengthen the erector spinae, the patient wears a rucksack containing cuff-weights on the front of the trunk throughout the therapeutic exercise session.
- Lateral pull-downs and seated rows strengthen the latissimus dorsi.

Aerobic exercises using a stationary bike and upper body ergonometer to maintain aerobic fitness also were prescribed.

- *Patient-related instruction.* Explanation was given as to the cause of the patient's symptoms. The patient was advised against bending forward and twisting to the right when standing, and forward bending and turning at the waist to the left when sitting. The patient was instructed to continue sleeping in the prone position. The patient received instructions regarding correct lifting techniques. The patient was advised to continue the exercises at home, three to five times each day, and to expect some postexercise soreness. The patient also received instruction on the use of heat and ice at home.
- *Goals/outcomes.* Both the patient's goals from the treatment and the expected therapeutic goals of the clinician were discussed with the patient.

CASE STUDY TAIL BONE PAIN

HISTORY

A 26-year-old woman presented to the clinic two weeks after a fall down stairs with her 3-month-old infant in her arms. The infant was unhurt, and the patient had landed in a sitting position. Immediately after the accident, the patient was able to walk, but pain persisted in the anal region.

EXAMINATION

On examination, the only positive findings were pain with sitting, and palpable tenderness at the level of the sacrococcygeal joint. On rectal examination, a painful anterior displacement of the joint was confirmed.

INTERVENTION

Correction for this impairment involves grasping the coccyx, after inserting the index finger in the anal canal. The coccyx is distracted and pulled posteriorly, while the clinician pulls laterally on the medial surface of the ischial tuberosity.

CASE STUDY RIGHT-SIDED LOW BACK AND BUTTOCK PAIN

HISTORY

A 22-year-old male soccer player presented at the clinic with complaints of right-sided low back and buttock pain, which occurred after an overzealous right-legged kick against a missed target about

2 weeks previously. Initially the pain had been intense, but it had now subsided to a dull ache, which was aggravated with weight bearing on one limb, bending backward, walking, and supine lying with the extremity in extension. The patient reported sleeping well, and there were no complaints of paresthesia or anesthesia. The patient denied any neurologic symptoms related to cauda equina or spinal cord involvement. He appeared to be in good health.

QUESTIONS

1. What structure(s) could be at fault with complaints of right-sided low back and buttock pain?
2. What does the history of the pain tell the clinician?
3. Why do you think the patient is sleeping well?
4. What information does the history of no paresthesia or anesthesia give the clinician?
5. What questions would you ask to help rule out cauda equina impairment?
6. What questions would you ask to help rule out spinal cord impairment?
7. What is your working hypothesis at this stage? List the various diagnoses that could present with low back and buttock pain, and the tests you would use to rule out each one.
8. Does this presentation/history warrant a scan? Why or why not?

EXAMINATION

Based on the history and the specific mechanism of injury that suggests a musculoskeletal impairment, the Cyriax scanning examination was deferred. An observation of the patient's gait revealed a shortened stance phase and a marked vertical limp. His standing posture was unremarkable. The combined motion tests of lumbosacral motion were positive in the posterior right quadrant, but the test was negative if sacral motion was prevented. Because of this finding, a sacroiliac examination was initiated, which revealed the following:

- The left iliac crest was inferior relative to the right in the standing and sitting positions, but superior relative to the right in lying. This reversal in position of the crests from sitting and standing to lying is thought to occur because of the release of tension from the iliopsoas and quadratus lumborum muscles which, in the standing position, counteract the effects of gravity. Relaxation of these muscles in the supine position allows the true position of the left iliac crest relative to the sacrum to be seen.
- The left anterior superior iliac spine (ASIS) was slightly anterior relative to the right in the standing and sitting positions.
- The lumbar spine had a left convexity.
- Point tenderness was elicited on the crest of the left ilium at the origin of the lateral margin of the iliocostalis lumborum muscle, and the left iliotibial band.
- A trigger point was found deep in the buttock within the piriformis muscle.

- The weight-bearing ipsilateral kinetic test was positive on the right, but negative in the non–weight-bearing position.
- The corresponding short-arm test was restricted.
- The contralateral kinetic test was positive on the left, but negative in the non–weight-bearing position.
- The corresponding long-arm test was restricted.
- In the prone position, fullness was found posterior to the left transverse process of the fifth lumbar vertebra, the lumbar lordosis was accentuated, the sacral sulcus was deeper on the right than on the left, and the sacral lateral angle (ILA) was posterior and inferior on the left.
- With sacral stabilization through the left innominate, which was prevented from rotating anteriorly by the application of a caudal counter force against the inferior aspect of the ASIS, extension and medial rotation of the right innominate was passively induced, and a hard capsular end-feel was gained.
- With passive physiologic mobility testing, innominate motion was restricted on the right.

QUESTIONS

1. Give some reasons as to why the combined motion tests could be positive?
2. Did the sacral examination confirm your working hypothesis? How?
3. What was the reason for the left convexity in the lumbar spine?
4. What information was gathered from the modified combined motion test?
5. Given the findings from the tests and measures, what is the diagnosis, or is further testing warranted in the form of special tests?
6. What information would be gained with further testing?

EVALUATION

It was deduced from the clinical findings that the patient had a loss of the anterior rotation of the right innominate, and a loss of the counternutation of the sacrum on the right (a type I left sacral torsion syndrome.)[10]

QUESTIONS

1. Based on the provisional diagnosis, what will be your intervention?
2. How would you describe this condition to the patient?
3. In order of priority, and based on the stages of healing, list the various goals of your intervention.
4. How will you determine the amplitude and joint position for the intervention?
5. What would you tell the patient about your intervention?
6. Estimate this patient's prognosis.
7. What modalities could you use in the intervention of this patient?
8. What exercises would you prescribe?

INTERVENTION

- *Manual therapy.* After the application of heat to the area (heating pad, or ultrasound), soft tissue techniques were applied, followed by a specific mobilization. The manual intervention for this condition involves the correction of the loss of the anterior rotation of the right innominate and a loss of the counternutation of the sacrum on the right. These asymmetries are treated separately, using any one of the previously outlined techniques.
- *Therapeutic exercises.* Exercises to strengthen the abdominals, the gluteals, the multifidus, and the erector spinae were prescribed. Aerobic exercises using a stationary bike and upper body ergometer to maintain aerobic fitness also were prescribed.
- *Patient-related instruction.* Explanation was given as to the cause of the patient's symptoms. Instructions to sleep on the side were given. The patient received instructions regarding correct lifting techniques. The patient was advised to continue the exercises at home, three to five times each day, and to expect some postexercise soreness. The patient also received instruction on the use of heat and ice at home.
- *Goals/outcomes.* Both the patient's goals from the treatment and the expected therapeutic goals of the clinician were discussed with the patient.

CASE STUDY RIGHT-SIDED LOW BACK BUTTOCK AND POSTERIOR THIGH PAIN

HISTORY

A 35-year-old woman who was 7 months' pregnant presented at the clinic with an insidious onset of right-sided low back, buttock, and right posterior thigh pain. She described the onset as occurring during the previous month, and could not remember any particular event that precipitated the pain. The pain was aggravated by bending forward or to her left side, and was alleviated with sitting or supine lying. The patient reported sleeping well, and there were no complaints of paresthesias or anesthesias. The patient denied any neurologic symptoms related to cauda equina or spinal cord involvement. She appeared to be in good health.

QUESTIONS

1. What structure(s) could be at fault with complaints of right-sided low back and posterior thigh pain?
2. What does the history of the onset tell the clinician?
3. What effect does pregnancy have on ligamentous structures?
4. What information does the history of no paresthesia or anesthesia give the clinician?
5. What is your working hypothesis at this stage? List the various diagnoses that could manifest with low back and buttock pain, and the tests you would use to rule out each one.
6. Does this presentation/history warrant a scan? Why or why not?

EXAMINATION

The patient appeared to be a healthy, pregnant woman. However, because of the insidious onset of her symptoms and the fact that she was experiencing a potential radiculopathy, a lumbar and sacroiliac scan was performed, which revealed the following positive findings:

- Restriction of forward bending.
- Restriction of left side bending.

Both motions reproduced the posterior thigh pain and a "pulling sensation" over the right lower lumbar area. Because the neurologic tests were negative, an assumption was made that the posterior thigh pain was referred, and a further investigation was initiated. The H and I test (Chap. 25) was positive in the anterior right quadrant, indicating a flexion and right side-bending restriction, but the test was negative if sacral motion was prevented. Because of this finding, a sacroiliac examination was initiated, which revealed the following:

- The left iliac crest was inferior relative to the right in the standing position, but superior relative to the right in sitting.[10,120]
- The left anterior superior iliac (ASIS) was considerably more ventral relative to the right in standing and sitting.[10,120]
- The lumbar spine demonstrated a left convexity.
- Point tenderness was elicited at the origin of the left iliocostalis on the left iliac crest, and the left iliotibial band.
- The ipsilateral and contralateral kinetic tests were positive on the left as were their corresponding short- and long-arm tests.[10,120]
- In the supine position, the right iliac crest was superior relative to the left.[10,120]
- In the prone position, fullness was felt posterior to the right transverse process of the fifth lumbar vertebra, the lumbar lordosis was decreased, the sacral sulcus was deeper on the right than on the left, the sacral inferior lateral angle (ILA) was posterior on the left, and the sacral ILA was inferior on the left.[10,120]
- With passive physiologic mobility testing, the sacrum was stabilized through the left innominate, which was prevented from rotating posteriorly by the application of a caudal counter force against the superior aspect of the ASIS, the right innominate was then rotated passively into flexion and lateral rotation, and a hard capsular end-feel was gained.[10,120]

QUESTIONS

1. Did the sacral examination confirm your working hypothesis? How?
2. Why were the lumbar motions of forward bending and left side bending restricted?
3. Given the findings from the tests and measures, what is the diagnosis, or is further testing warranted in the form of special tests? What information would be gained with further testing?

EVALUATION

Based on the clinical findings of a loss of the posterior rotation of the right innominate and a loss of the nutation of the sacrum on the right, the diagnosis of a type II left sacral torsion was made.[10]

QUESTIONS

1. Based on the provisional diagnosis, what will be your intervention?
2. How would you describe this condition to the patient?
3. In order of priority, and based on the stages of healing, list the various goals of your intervention.
4. How will you determine the amplitude and joint position for the intervention?
5. What would you tell the patient about your intervention?
6. Estimate this patient's prognosis.
7. What modalities could you use in the intervention of this patient?
8. What exercises would you prescribe?

INTERVENTION

- *Electrotherapeutic modalities and thermal agents.* A moist heat pack was applied to the sacroiliac joint. Because the patient was pregnant, it was felt that the use of electrical stimulation and ultrasound was contraindicated. An ice pack may be applied to the area at the end of the treatment session, if the patient reports an increase in symptoms.
- *Manual therapy.* After the application of moist heat to the area, soft tissue techniques were applied, followed by a specific mobilization. The manual intervention for this condition involves the correction of the loss of the posterior rotation of the right innominate and loss of the nutation of the sacrum on the right. These asymmetries are treated separately, using any one of the previously outlined techniques.
- *Therapeutic exercises.* Exercises to strengthen the abdominals, the gluteals, the multifidus, and the erector spinae were prescribed.
- *Patient-related instruction.* Explanation was given as to the cause of the patient's symptoms. Instructions to sleep on the side were given. The patient received instructions regarding correct lifting techniques. The patient was advised to continue the exercises at home, three to five times each day, and to expect some postexercise soreness. The patient also received instruction on the use of heat and ice at home.
- *Goals/outcomes.* Both the patient's goals from the treatment and the expected therapeutic goals of the clinician were discussed with the patient.

CASE STUDY PUBIC PAIN

HISTORY

A 44-year-old man came to the clinic complaining of worsening abdominal and midline pelvic pain. The pain had developed gradually, and there was no report of recent direct trauma or acute injury. The pain was aggravated with forced flexion at the waist, and the Valsalva maneuver, but the patient reported no pain at rest. The pain, described as a sharp, "stabbing" sensation, remained fairly localized to his upper pelvis and lower abdominal area.

The patient had no history of abdominal or genitourinary diseases or surgeries, and he had not experienced similar symptoms in the past. A review of systems was unremarkable. He denied dysuria, hematuria, diarrhea, constipation, fever, chills, or weight change.[146]

The patient frequently participated in physical activity and played soccer, averaging four games per week, an increase from his usual level of commitment. An inguinal hernia had been ruled out by his physician.

QUESTIONS

1. What structure(s) could be at fault when abdominal and midline pelvic pain is the major complaint?
2. What is the significance of the Valsalva maneuver?
3. Why are the questions with regard to dysuria, hematuria, diarrhea, constipation, fever, chills, or weight change pertinent?
4. What does no pain at rest suggest?
5. What is your working hypothesis at this stage? List the various diagnoses that could manifest with this pain and the tests you would use to rule out each one.
6. Does this presentation/history warrant a scan? Why or why not?

EXAMINATION

Given the location of the patient's symptoms, and the relatively insidious onset, a lower quarter scanning examination was performed with the following findings:

- The patient demonstrated full range of motion of his lumbar spine without spasm.
- Straight leg raise testing was negative.
- His gait was moderately wide based, and he had full range of motion of knees and hips, although hip flexion, abduction, and external rotation (the FABER test) produced some pubic discomfort.
- Femoral pulses were 2+ bilaterally.
- Special tests revealed palpable tenderness of the pubic symphysis and inguinal ligament bilaterally. The sacroiliac kinetic tests and pubic stress tests were positive.

QUESTIONS

1. Did the scanning examination confirm the working hypothesis? How?
2. Why were the femoral pulses assessed?
3. Why were the kinetic tests performed?
4. Given the findings from the scanning examination, what is the diagnosis, or is further testing warranted in the form of special tests? What information would be gained with further testing?

EVALUATION

The findings for this patient's symphysis tenderness were consistent with osteitis pubis.

QUESTIONS

1. Having confirmed the diagnosis, what will be your intervention?
2. In order of priority, and based on the stages of healing, list the various goals of your intervention.
3. Estimate this patient's prognosis.
4. What modalities could you use in the intervention of this patient?
5. What exercises would you initiate?

INTERVENTION

This condition is traditionally slow to heal. If mobilizations are used, only one direction needs to be chosen for correction, because the other direction occurs as a result of the osteokinematic motion. Improvement of position and decreased pain on palpating the inguinal ligament should be found if the technique has been successful. By restoring the posterior component of the impairment complex, the superior positional displacement also is corrected.

Alternatively, the modified shotgun technique can be applied to the adductors for impairments that do not respond to the preceding techniques. The short adductors cross the inferior aspect of the pubic articulation in a cruciate manner, and, when recruited, bring the joint into a level position. Because a slight "popping" noise often is elicited as the clinician overcomes the muscle resistance by a short high-velocity movement in the opposite direction, which can be of concern and surprise to the patient, a preliminary word of warning is necessary.

Following the intervention, the kinetic test and positional findings are reevaluated. If no improvement is seen, a sacroiliac impairment is the probable cause.

REVIEW QUESTIONS*

1. Which sacroiliac joint ligament forms the major connection between the sacrum and the innominate, filling the irregular space posterior-superior to the joint between the lateral sacral crest, and the iliac tuberosity?
2. Which sacral motion places tension on the dorsal sacroiliac ligament of the sacroiliac joint?
3. What are the muscle actions of the piriformis muscle?
4. Which muscle group comprises the pelvic floor muscle group?
5. During right side bending, which sacral and right innominate motions are purported to occur?

* Additional questions to test your understanding of this chapter can be found in the Online Learning Center for *Orthopaedic Assessment, Evaluation, and Intervention* at www.duttononline.net.

REFERENCES

1. Grieve GP. *Common Vertebral Joint Problems*. New York, NY: Churchill Livingstone; 1981.
2. Cibulka MT. The treatment of the sacroiliac joint component to low back pain: A case report. *Phys Ther* 1992;72:917–922.
3. Grieve GP. The sacroiliac joint. *Physiotherapy* 1976;62:384–400.
4. Huston C. The sacroiliac joint. In: Gonzalez EG, ed. *The Nonsurgical Management of Acute Low Back Pain*. New York, NY: Demos Vermande; 1997:137–150.
5. Fryette HH. *Principles of Osteopathic Technique*. Carmel, Calif: Academy of Osteopathy; 1980.
6. DiGiovanna EL, Schiowitz S. *An Osteopathic Approach to Diagnosis and Treatment*. Philadelphia, Pa: JB Lippincott; 1991.
7. Hartman SL. *Handbook of Osteopathic Technique*. 2nd ed. London, England: Unwin Hyman, Academic Division; 1990: 135–143.
8. Mitchell FL, Moran PS, Pruzzo NA. *An Evaluation and Treatment Manual of Osteopathic Muscle Energy Procedures*. Manchester, Mo: Mitchell, Moran and Pruzzo; 1979.
9. Stoddard A. *Manual of Osteopathic Practice*. New York, NY: Harper and Row; 1969.
10. Fowler C. Muscle energy techniques for pelvic dysfunction. In: Palastanga N, Boyling JD, eds. *Grieve's Modern Manual Therapy: The Vertebral Column*. Edinburgh, Scotland: Churchill Livingstone; 1986:781–792.
11. Lee DG, Walsh MC. *A Workbook of Manual Therapy Techniques for the Vertebral Column and Pelvic Girdle*. 2nd ed. Vancouver, Canada: Nascent; 1996.
12. Lee DG. *The Pelvic Girdle: An Approach to the Examination and Treatment of the Lumbo-pelvic-hip Region*. 2nd ed. Edinburgh, Scotland: Churchill Livingstone; 1999.
13. Schwarzer AC, Aprill CN, Bogduk N. The sacroiliac joint in chronic low back pain. *Spine* 1995;20:31–37.
14. Pettman E. *Level One Course Notes*. Portland, Oregon: North American Institute of Orthopedic Manual Therapy; 1990.
15. Goldthwaite JE, Osgood RB. A consideration of the pelvic articulations from an anatomical, pathological, and clinical consideration. *Boston Med Surg J* 1905;152:593–634.
16. Mixter WJ, Barr JS Jr. Rupture of the intervertebral disc with involvement of the spinal canal. *N Engl J Med* 1934;211:210–215.
17. Williams PL, et al. *Gray's Anatomy*. 37th ed. London, England: Churchill Livingstone; 1989.
18. Schunke GB. The anatomy and development of the sacro-iliac joint in man. *Anat Rec* 1938;72:313.
19. MacDonald GR, Hunt TE. Sacro-iliac joint observations on the gross and histological changes in the various age groups. *Can Med Assoc J* 1951;66:157.
20. Bowen V, Cassidy JD. Macroscopic and microscopic anatomy of the sacroiliac joint from embryonic life until the eighth decade. *Spine* 1980;6:620.
21. Weisl H. The articular surfaces of the sacro-iliac joint and their relation to the movements of the sacrum. *Acta Anat* 1954;22:1.
22. Kapandji IA. *The Physiology of the Joints, The Trunk and Vertebral Column*. New York, NY: Churchill Livingstone; 1991.
23. Solonen KA. The sacroiliac joint in the light of anatomical roentgenographical and clinical studies. *Acta Orthop Scand* 1957;26:9.
24. Erdmann H. Die Verspannung des Wirbelsockels im Beckenring. In: Junghanns H, ed. *Wirbelsäule in Forschung und Praxis*. Stuttgart, Germany: Hippokrates; 1956:51.
25. Vleeming A, et al. Relation between form and function in the sacroiliac joint. 1: Clinical anatomical aspects. *Spine* 1990; 15:130–132.

26. Kissling RO, Jacob HAC. The mobility of the sacroiliac joints in healthy subjects. *Bull Hosp Joint Dis* 1996;54:158–164.

27. Resnick D, Niwayama G, Goergen TG. Degenerative disease of the sacroiliac joint. *Invest Radiol* 1975;10:608–621.

28. Vleeming A, et al. Mobility in the SI-joints in old people: A kinematic and radiological study. *Clin Biomech* 1992;7:170–176.

29. Mennell JB. *The Science and Art of Joint Manipulation.* London, England: J and A Churchill; 1949.

30. Meadows J, Pettman E. *Manual Therapy: NAIOMT Level II & III Course Notes.* Denver, Colo: North American Institute of Manual Therapy; 1995.

31. Vleeming A. The function of the long dorsal sacroiliac ligament: Its implication for understanding low back pain. *Spine* 1996;21:556.

32. Willard FH. The muscular, ligamentous and neural structure of the low back and its relation to low back pain. In: Vleeming A, et al, eds. *Movement, Stability and Low Back Pain.* Edinburgh, Scotland: Churchill Livingstone; 1997:3–36.

33. Fortin JD, Pier J, Falco F. Sacroiliac joint injection: Pain referral mapping and arthrographic findings. In: Vleeming A, et al, eds. Movement, Stability and Low Back Pain. Edinburgh, Scotland: Churchill Livingstone; 1997:271.

34. Vleeming A, Stoeckart R, Snijders CJ. The sacrotuberous ligament: A conceptual approach to its dynamic role in stabilizing the sacroiliac joint. *Clin Biomech* 1989;4:201–203.

35. Vleeming A, et al. Load application to the sacrotuberous ligament. *Clin Biomech* 1989;4:204–209.

36. Van Wingerden JP, et al. A functional-anatomical approach to the spine-pelvis mechanism: Interaction between the biceps femoris muscle and the sacrotuberous ligament. *Eur Spine J* 1993;2:140–142.

37. Bourdillon JF. *Spinal Manipulation.* 3rd ed. London, England: Heinemann; 1982.

38. Beaton LE, Anson BJ. The sciatic nerve and the piriformis muscle: Their interrelation a possible cause of coccygodynia. *J Bone Joint Surg* 1938;20:686–688.

39. Durrani Z, Winnie AP. Piriformis muscle syndrome: An underdiagnosed cause of sciatica. *J Pain Symptom Manage* 1991;6: 374–379.

40. Julsrud ME. Piriformis syndrome. *J Am Podiatr Med Assoc* 1989;79:128–131.

41. Pace JB, Nagle D. Piriformis syndrome. *West J Med* 1976; 124:435–439.

42. Pfeifer T, Fitz WFK. Das Piriformis-Syndrom. *Zeitschr Orthop* 1989;127:691–694.

43. Solheim LF, Siewers S, Paus B. The piriformis syndrome. Sciatic nerve entrapment treated with section of the piriformis muscle. *Acta Orthop Scand* 1981;52:73–75.

44. Steiner C, et al. Piriformis syndrome: Pathogenesis, diagnosis, and treatment. *J Am Osteopath Assoc* 1987;87:318–323.

45. Travell JG, Simons DG. *Myofascial Pain and Dysfunction—The Trigger Point Manual.* Baltimore, Md: Williams and Wilkins; 1983.

46. McIntosh JE, et al. The morphology of the lumbar multifidus muscles. *Clin Biomech* 1986;1:196–204.

47. McGill SM. Kinetic potential of the lumbar trunk musculature about three orthogonal orthopaedic axes in extreme postures. *Spine* 1991;16:809–815.

48. Vleeming A, et al. The posterior layer of the thoracolumbar fascia: Its function in load transfer from spine to legs. *Spine* 1995;20:753–758.

49. Dorman T. Pelvic mechanics and prolotherapy. In: Vleeming A, et al, eds. *Movement, Stability and Low Back Pain.* Edinburgh, Scotland: Churchill Livingstone; 1997:507.

50. Bogduk N, Pearcy M, Hadfield G. Anatomy and biomechanics of psoas major. *Clin Biomech* 1992;7:109–119.

51. Markwell SJ. Physical therapy management of pelvic/perineal and perianal pain syndromes. *World J Urol* 2001;19:194–199.

52. Richardson CA, Jull GA, Hodges P, Hides J. *Therapeutic Exercise for Spinal Segmental Stabilization in Low Back Pain.* London, England: Churchill Livingstone; 1999.

53. Richardson C, Jull G. Muscle control—Pain control. What exercises would you prescribe? *Manual Ther* 1995;1:2–10.

54. Bogduk N. The sacroiliac joint. In: Bogduk N, ed. *Clinical Anatomy of the Lumbar Spine and Sacrum.* New York, NY: Churchill Livingstone; 1997:177–186.

55. Dreyfuss P, et al. The value of medical history and physical examination in diagnosing sacroiliac joint pain. *Spine* 1996; 21:2594–2602.

56. Pitkin HC, Pheasant HC. Sacrarthrogenic telalgia I: A study of referred pain. *J Bone Joint Surg* 1936;18:111–133.

57. Grob KR, Neuhuber WL, Kissling RO. Innervation of the sacroiliac joint of the human. *Z Rheumatol* 1995;54:117–122.

58. Inman VT, Saunders JB. Referred pain from skeletal structures. *J Nerv Ment Dis* 1944;99:660–667.

59. Duckworth JWA. The anatomy and movements of the sacroiliac joints. In: Wolff HD, ed. *Manuelle Medizin und ihre wissenschaftlichen Grundlagen.* Heidelberg, Germany: Physikalische Medizin; 1970:56.

60. Basmajian JV, Deluca CJ. *Muscles Alive: Their Functions Revealed by Electromyography.* Baltimore, Md: Williams and Wilkins; 1985.

61. Miller JAA, Schultz AB, Andersson GBJ. Load displacement behavior of sacroiliac joints. *J Orthop Res* 1987;5:92–101.

62. Sturesson B, Uden A, Vleeming A. A radiostereometric analysis of the movements of the sacroiliac joints in the reciprocal straddle position. *Spine* 2000;25:214–217.

63. Egund N, et al. Movements in the sacroiliac joints demonstrated with roentgen stereophotogrammetry. *Acta Radiol Diagn* 1978; 19:833–846.

64. Smidt GL, et al. Sacroiliac kinematics for reciprocal straddle positions. *Spine* 1995;20:1047–1054.

65. Illi F. *The Vertebral Column: Lifeline of the Body.* Chicago, Ill: National College of Chiropractic; 1951.

66. Bergmann TF, Peterson DH, Lawrence DJ. *Chiropractic Technique: Principles and Procedures.* New York, NY: Churchill Livingstone; 1993.

67. Vleeming A, Snijders CJ, Stoeckart R, Mens JMA: The role of the sacroiliac joints in coupling between spine, pelvis, legs and arms. In: Vleeming A, Mooney V, Dorman T, et al., eds. Movement, stability and low back pain. Edinburgh: Churchill Livingstone, 1997;53.

68. Snijders CJ, Vleeming A, Stoeckart R, et al. Biomechanics of the interface between spine and pelvis in different postures. In: Vleeming A, Mooney V, Dorman T, et al, eds. *Movement, Stability and Low Back Pain.* Edinburgh, Scotland: Churchill Livingstone; 1997:103.

69. Meadows JTS. *Manual Therapy: Biomechanical Assessment and Treatment, Advanced Technique.* Lecture and video supplemental manual. Calgary, Canada: Swodeam Consulting; 1995.

70. Gracovetsky S, Farfan HF. The optimum spine. *Spine* 1986; 11:543.

71. Pearcy M, Tibrewal SB. Axial rotation and lateral bending in the normal lumbar spine measured by three-dimensional radiography. *Spine* 1984;9:582.

72. Inman VT, Ralston HJ, Todd F. *Human Walking*. Baltimore, Md: Williams and Wilkins; 1981.

73. Gracovetsky S. Linking the spinal engine with the legs: a theory of human gait. In: Vleeming A, et al, eds. *Movement, Stability and Low Back Pain*. Edinburgh, Scotland: Churchill Livingstone; 1997:243.

74. Lee DG. Instability of the sacroiliac joint and the consequences for gait. In: Vleeming A, et al, eds. *Movement, Stability and Low Back Pain*. Edinburgh, Scotland: Churchill Livingstone; 1997:231.

75. Snijders CJ, Vleeming A, Stoeckart R. Transfer of lumbo-sacral load to iliac bones and legs. 2: Loading of the sacroiliac joints when lifting in a stooped posture. *Clin Biomech* 1993; 8:295–301.

76. Vleeming A, et al. Relation between form and function in the sacroiliac joint. I: Biomechanical aspects. *Spine* 1990;15: 130–132.

76a. Franke BA. Formative dynamics: The pelvic girdle. *J Man Manip Ther* 2003;11:12–40.

76b. Vleeming A, Pool-Goudzwaard AL, Stoeckart R, Snijders CJ. The posterior layer of the thoracolumbar fascia: Its function in load transfer from spine to legs. *Spine* 1995;20:753–758.

76c. Van Wingerden JP, Vleeming A, Snijders CJ, Stoeckart R. A functional-anatomical approach to the spine-pelvis mechanism: interaction between the biceps femoris muscle and the sacro-tuberous ligament. *Eur Spine J* 1993;2:140–142.

77. Vleeming A, et al. The role of the sacroiliac joints in coupling between spine, pelvis, legs and arms. In: Vleeming A, et al, eds. *Movement, Stability and Low Back Pain*. Edinburgh, Scotland: Churchill Livingstone; 1997:53.

78. Hemborg B, Moritz U, Lowing H. Intra-abdominal pressure and trunk muscle activity during lifting. IV. The causal factors of the intra-abdominal pressure rise. *Scand J Rehab Med* 1985;17:25–38.

79. Snijders CJ, Slugter AHE, Van Strik R, et al. Why leg-crossing? The influence of common postures on abdominal muscle activity. *Spine* 1995;20:1989–1993.

80. Borenstein D, Wiesel SW. *Low Back Pain: Medical Diagnosis and Comprehensive Management*. Philadelphia, Pa: Saunders; 1989:60–78.

81. Greenman PE. *Principles of Manual Medicine*. 2nd ed. Baltimore, Md: Williams and Wilkins; 1996.

82. Kirkaldy-Willis WH. *Managing Low Back Pain*. 2nd ed. New York, NY: Churchill Livingstone; 1988.

83. Palmer ML, Epler M. *Clinical Assessment Procedures in Physical Therapy*. Philadelphia, Pa: JB Lippincott; 1990:68–73.

84. Beal MC. The sacroiliaca problem: Review of anatomy, mechanics, and diagnosis. *J Am Osteopath Assoc* 1981;81:667–679.

85. Carmichael JP. Inter- and intra-examiner reliability of palpation for sacroiliac joint dysfunction. *J Manipulative Physiol Ther* 1987;10:164–171.

86. Herzog W, et al. Reliability of motion palpation procedures to detect sacro-iliac joint fixations. *J Manipulative Physiol Ther* 1988;11:151–157.

87. Potter NA, Rothstein JM. Intertester reliability for selected clinical tests of the sacroiliac joint. *Phys Ther* 1985;65:1671.

88. Levangie PK. The association between static pelvic asymmetry and low back pain. *Spine* 1999;24:1234–1242.

89. Cibulka MT, Delitto A, Koldehoff RM. Changes in innominate tilt after manipulation of sacro-iliac joint in patients with low back pain. An experimental study. *Phys Ther* 1988;68:1359–1363.

90. McCombe PF, et al. Reproducibility of physical signs in low back pain. *Spine* 1989;14:908–918.

91. Kirkaldy-Willis WH, Hill RJ. A more precise diagnosis for low back pain. *Spine* 1979;4:102–109.

92. Sturesson B, Uden A, Vleeming A. A radiostereometric analysis of the movements of the sacroiliac joints during the standing flexion test. *Spine* 2000;25:364–368.

93. Laslett M, Williams M. The reliability of selected pain provocation tests for sacroiliac joint pathology. *Spine* 1994;19:1243–1249.

94. Maigne JY, Aivaliklis A, Pfefer F. Results of sacroiliac joint double block and value of sacroiliac pain provocation tests in 54 patients with low back pain. *Spine* 1996;21:1889–1892.

94a. Ostgaard HC. Lumbar back and posterior pelvic pain in pregnancy. In: Vleeming A, Mooney V, Dorman T, et al, eds. *Movement, Stability, and Low Back Pain*. Edinburgh: Churchill Livingstone 1997;411–420.

94b. Dreyfuss P, Michaelson M, Pauza K, et al. The value of medical history and physical examination in diagnosing sacroiliac joint pain. *Spine* 1996;21:2594–2602.

94c. Maigne JY, Aivaliklis A, Pfefer F. Results of sacroiliac joint double block and value of sacroiliac pian provocation tests in 54 patients with low back pain. *Spine* 1996;21:1889–1892.

94d. Potter NA, Rothstein JM. Intertester reliability for selected clinical tests of the sacroiliac joint. *Phys Ther* 1985;65:1671.

94e. Van der Wurff P, Meyne W, Hagmeijer RHM. Clinical tests of the sacroiliac joint, a systematic methodological review. Part 2: Validity. *Man Ther* 2000;5:89–96.

94f. Hesch J. Evaluation and treatment of most common patterns of sacroiliac joint dysfunction. In: Vleeming A, Mooney V, Dorman T, et al, eds. *Movement, Stability, and Low Back Pain*. Edinburgh: Churchill Livingstone, 1997;535–545.

95. Fortin JD, et al. Sacroiliac joint pain referral maps upon applying a new injection/arthrography technique. Part I: Asymptomatic volunteers. *Spine* 1994;19:1475–1482.

96. Kellgren JH. Observations on referred pain arising from muscle. *Clin Sci* 1938;3:175–190.

97. Kellgren JH. On the distribution of pain arising from deep somatic structures with charts of segmental pain areas. *Clin Sci* 1939;4:35–46.

98. McCall IW, Park WM, O'Brien JP. Induced pain referral from posterior lumbar elements in normal subjects. *Spine* 1979; 4:441–446.

99. Weiss JM. Pelvic floor myofascial trigger points: Manual therapy for interstitial cystitis and the urgency-frequency syndrome. *J Urol* 2001;166:2226–2231.

100. Raz S, Smith RB. External sphincter spasticity syndrome in female patients. *J Urol* 1976;115:443.

101. Lilius HG, Oravisto KJ, Valtonen EJ. Origin of pain in interstitial cystitis. *Scand J Urol Nephrol* 1973;7:150.

102. Hall H. A simple approach to back pain management. *Patient Care* 1992;15:77–91.

103. LaBan MM, et al. Symphyseal and sacroiliac joint pain associated with pubic symphysis instability. *Arch Phys Med Rehabil* 1978;59:470–472.

104. Alderink GJ. The sacroiliac joint: Review of anatomy, mechanics, and function. *J Orthop Sports Phys Ther* 1991;13:71–84.

105. DonTigny RL. Function and pathomechanics of the sacroiliac joint. A review. *Phys Ther* 1985;65:35–44.

106. Fornasier VL, Horne JG. Metastases to the vertebral column. *Cancer* 1975;36:590–594.

107. Boissonnault WG, Thein-Nissenbaum JM. Differential diagnosis of a sacral stress fracture. *J Orthop Sports Phys Ther* 2002;32:613–621.

108. Brugger A. Die Funktionskrankheiten des Bewegungsapparates. *Funktionskrankheiton des Bewegungsapparates* 1986;1:69–129.

109. Silverstolpe L. A pathological erector spinae reflex—a new sign of mechanical pelvic dysfunction. *J Manual Med* 1989;4:28.

110. Cibulka MT, et al. Unilateral hip rotation range of motion asymmetry in patients with sacroiliac joint regional pain. *Spine* 1998;23:1009–1015.

111. Papadopoulos SM, McGillicuddy JE, Albers JW. Unusual cause of piriformis muscle syndrome. *Arch Neurol* 1990;47:1144–1146.

112. Vandertop WP, Bosma WJ. The piriformis syndrome. A case report. *J Bone Joint Surg* 1991;73A:1095–1097.

113. Dunn EJ, et al. Pyogenic infections of the sacro-iliac joint. *Clin Orthop* 1976;118:113–117.

114. Gillet H, Liekens M. *Belgian Chiropractic Research Notes.* 12th ed. Huntington Beach, Calif: 1985.

115. Lee DG. *A Workbook of Manual Therapy Techniques for the Upper Extremity.* 2nd ed. Delta, Canada: DOPC (Delta Orthopaedic Physiotherapy Clinic); 1991:58–79.

116. Lee DG. *A Workbook of Manual Therapy Techniques for the Upper Extremity.* Delta, Canada: Delta Orthopedic Physiotherapy Clinics; 1989.

117. Cyriax J. *Textbook of Orthopaedic Medicine, Diagnosis of Soft Tissue Lesions.* 8th ed. London, England: Bailliere Tindall; 1982.

118. Van Deursen LL, et al. The value of some clinical tests of the sacroiliac joint. *J Manual Med* 1990;5:96–99.

119. Porterfield JA, DeRosa C. *Mechanical Low Back Pain.* 2nd ed. Philadelphia, Pa: Saunders; 1998.

120. Lee DG. Clinical manifestations of pelvic girdle dysfunction, In: Palastanga N, Boyling JD, eds. *Grieve's Modern Manual Therapy: The Vertebral Column.* Edinburgh, Scotland: Churchill Livingstone; 1994:453–462.

121. Hanada E, et al. Measuring leg-length discrepancy by the "iliac crest palpation and book correction" method: Reliability and validity. *Arch Phys Med Rehabil* 2001;82:938–942.

122. Hoppenfeld S. Physical examination of the hip and pelvis. In: *Physical Examination of the Spine and Extremities.* Norwalk, Conn: Appleton-Century-Crofts; 1976:143.

123. Yeoman W. The relation of arthritis of the sacro-iliac joint to sciatica, with an analysis of 100 cases. *Lancet* 1928;2:1119–1122.

124. Evans RC. *Illustrated Essentials in Orthopedic Physical Assessment.* St Louis, Mo: Mosby-Year Book; 1994.

125. Mens JM, et al. Validity of the active straight leg raise test for measuring disease severity in patients with posterior pelvic pain after pregnancy. *Spine* 2002;27:196–200.

126. Mens JMA, et al. Validity and reliability of the active straight leg raise test as diagnostic instrument in posterior pelvic pain since pregnancy. *Spine* 2001;26:1167–1171.

127. Mens JMA, et al. The active straight-leg-raising test and mobility of the pelvic joints. *Eur Spine J* 1999;8:468–473.

127a. Franke BA. Formative dynamics: The pelvic girdle. *J Man Manip Ther* 2003;11:12–40.

128. Lynch FW. The pelvic articulation during pregnancy, labor and the puerperium. An X-ray study. *Surg Gynecol Obstet* 1920; 30:575–580.

128a. Klaffs CE, Arnheim DD. *Modern Principles of Athletic Training.* St Louis: CV Mosby, 1989.

128b. Lehmann JF, Silverman DR, et al. Temperature distributions in the human thigh produced by infrared, hot pack and microwave applications. *Arch Phys Med Rehabil* 1966;47:291.

128c. Prentice WE. Using therapeutic modalities in rehabilitation. In: Prentice WE, Voight ML, eds. *Techniques in Musculoskeletal Rehabilitation,* New York: McGraw-Hill; 2001:289–303.

128d. Cibulka MT, Koldehoff RM. Leg length disparity and its effect on sacroiliac joint dysfunction. *Clin Manage* 1986;6:10–11.

128e. Fitch RR. Mechanical lesions of the sacroiliac joints. *Am J Orthop Surg* 1908;6:693–698.

128f. Fortin JD. Sacroiliac joint dysfunction. A new perspective. *J Back Musculoskel Rehab* 1993;3:31–43.

128g. Vleeming A, et al. An integrated therapy from peripartum pelvic instability: A study of the biomechanical effects of pelvic belts. *Am J Obstet Gynecol* 1992;166:1243–1247.

128h. Huston C. The sacroiliac joint. In: Gonzalez EG, ed. *The Nonsurgical Management of Acute Low Back Pain.* New York: Demos Vermande; 1997;137–150.

129. Hoek van Dijke GA, et al. A biomechanical model on muscle forces in the transfer of spinal load to the pelvis and legs. *J Biomech* 1999;32:927–933.

130. Snijders CJ, et al. Oblique abdominal muscle activity in standing and in sitting on hard and soft seats. *Clin Biomech* 1995;10:73–78.

131. Snijders CJ, et al. EMG recordings of abdominal and back muscles in various standing postures: Validation of a biomechanical model on sacroiliac joint stability. *J Electromyogr Kinesiol* 1998;8:205–214.

132. Richardson CA, et al. The relation between the transversus abdominis muscles, sacroiliac joint mechanics, and low back pain. *Spine* 2002;27:399–405.

132a. McGill SM. The biomechanics of low back injury: Implications on current practice in industry and the clinic. *J Biomech* 1997;30:465–475.

132b. Cole AJ, Farrell JP, Stratton SA. Functional rehabilitation of cervical spine athletic injuries. In: Kibler BW, Herring JA, Press JM, eds. *Functional Rehabilitation of Sports and Musculoskeletal Injuries.* Gaithersburg Md: Aspen; 1998;127–148.

132c. Markwell SJ. Physical therapy management of pelvi/perineal and perianal pain syndromes. *World J Urol* 2001;19:194–199.

132d. Cammu H, Van Nylen M. Pelvic floor muscle exercises: Five years later. *Urology* 1995;45:113–117.

132e. Bo K, Talseth T. Five-year follow-up of pelvic floor exercises for treatment of stress incontinence. *Neurol Urodyn* 1994;13:374–375.

132f. Cardozo LD, Abrams PD, Stanton SL, Feneley RC. Idiopathic bladder instability treated by biofeedback. *British J Urology* 1978;50:521–523.

132g. Sand PK, Richardson DA, Staskin DR, et al. Pelvic floor electrical stimulation in the treatment of genuine stress incontinence: A multicenter, placebo-controlled trial. *Am J Obstet Gynecol* 1995;173:72–79.

132h. Smith JJ III. Intravaginal stimulation randomized trial. *J Urology* 1996;155:127–130.

132i. Wilson F. In Control: Incontinence treatment goes beyond Kegel exercises. *ADVANCE Directors Rehabil* 2003;12(5):73–75.

132j. Philp T, Shah PJ, Worth PH. Acupuncture in the treatment of bladder instability. *Br J Urol* 1988;61(6):490–493.

133. Gladman DD. Clinical aspects of the spondyloarthropathies. *Am J Med Sci* 1998;316:234–238.

134. Jajic Z, Jajic I, Grazio S. Radiological changes of the symphysis in ankylosing spondylitis. *Acta Radiol* 2000;41:307–30^.

135. Jajic I. *Ankylosing Spondylitis*. Zagreb, Yugoslavia: Školska knjiga; 1978.

136. Ashby EC. Chronic obscure groin pain is commonly caused by enthesopathy: "Tennis elbow" of the groin. *Br J Surg* 1994; 81:1632–1634.

137. Martens MA, Hansen L, Mulier JC. Adductor tendinitis and musculus rectus abdominis tendonopathy. *Am J Sports Med* 1987;15:353–356.

138. Zimmerman G. Groin pain in athletes. *Aust Fam Physician* 1988;17:1046–1052.

139. Bradshaw C, et al. Obturator neuropathy a cause of chronic groin pain in athletes. *Am J Sports Med* 1997;25:402–408.

140. Thompson WAL, Kopell HP. Peripheral entrapment neuropathies of the upper extremity. *N Engl J Med* 1959;260:1261–1265.

141. Middleton R, Carlisle R. The spectrum of osteitis pubis. *Compr Ther* 1993;19:99–105.

142. Wiley JJ. Traumatic osteitis pubis: the gracilis syndrome. *Am J Sports Med* 1983;11:360–363.

143. Fricker PA, Tauton JE, Ammann W. Osteitis pubis in athletes. Infection, inflammation, or injury? *Sports Med* 1991;12:266–279.

144. Barry NN, McGuire JL. Overuse syndromes in adult athletes. *Rheum Dis Clin North Am* 1996;22:515–530.

145. Grace JN, et al. Wedge resection of the symphysis pubis for the treatment of osteitis pubis. *J Bone Joint Surg* 1989; 71A:358–364.

146. Andrews SK, Carek PJ. Osteitis pubis: A diagnosis for the family physician. *J Am Board Fam Pract* 1998;11:291–295.

147. Holt MA, et al. Treatment of osteitis pubis in athletes. *Am J Sports Med* 1995;23:601–606.

147a. Snow RE, Neubert AG. Peripartum pubic symphysis separation: A case series and review of the literature. *Obstet Gyn Sur* 1997;52:438–443.

147b. Bellabarba C, et al. Midline sagittal sacral fractures in anterior-posterior compression pelvic ring injuries. *J Orthop Trauma* 2003;17:32–37.

148. Holmich P, et al. Effectiveness of active physical training as treatment for long-standing adductor-related groin pain in athletes: Randomised trial. *Lancet* 1999;353:439–443.

149. McFarland EG, Giangarra C. Sacral stress fractures in athletes. *Clin Orthop* 1996;329:240–243.

150. Shah MK, Stewart GW. Sacral stress fractures: An unusual cause of low back pain in an athlete. *Spine* 2002;27:E104–E108.

151. Holtzhausen LM, Noakes TD. Stress fracture of the sacrum in two distance runners. *Clin J Sports Med* 1992;2:139–142.

152. Volpin G, et al. Stress fractures of the sacrum following strenuous activity. *Clin Orthop* 1989;243:184–188.

153. Atwell EA, Jackson DW. Stress fractures of the sacrum in runners. *Am J Sports Med* 1991;19:531–533.

154. Cooper KL, Beabout JAW, Swee RG. Insufficiency fractures of the sacrum. *Radiology* 1985;156:15–20.

155. Byrnes DP, et al. Sacral fractures and neurological damage. *J Neurosurg* 1977;47:459–462.

156. Keats TE. *Radiology of Musculoskeletal Stress Injury*. Chicago, Ill: Year Book; 1990.

157. DonTigney RL. Function and pathomechanics of the sacroiliac joint. A review. *Phys Ther* 1985;65:35–44.

157a. Kegel AH. Physiologic therapy for urinary stress incontinence. *JAMA* 1951;146:915.

157b. Kari B, Hagen RH, Kvarstein B, Jorgensen J, Larsen S. Pelvic floor muscle exercise for the treatment of female stress urinary incontinence. *Neurol Urodyn* 1990;47:489–495.

157c. Parekh AR, Feng MI, Kirages D, et al. The role of pelvic floor exercises on post-prostatectomy incontinence. *J Urol* 2003;170:130–133.

157d. Carriere B. *The Swiss Ball: Theory, Basic Exercises and Clinical Applications*. New York: Springer-Verlag: 1997.

158. Greenman PE. Clinical aspects of the sacroiliac joint in walking. In: Vleeming A, et al, eds. *Movement, Stability and Low Back Pain*. Edinburgh, Scotland: Churchill Livingstone; 1997:235–241.

159. Cibulka MT, Koldehoff RM. Leg length disparity and its effect on sacroiliac joint dysfunction. *Clin Man* 1986;6:10–11.

160. Fitch RR. Mechanical lesions of the sacroiliac joints. *Am J Orthop Surg* 1908;6:693–698.

161. Fortin JD. Sacroiliac joint dysfunction. A new perspective. *J Back Musculoskel Rehab* 1993;3:31–43.

162. Vleeming A, et al. An integrated therapy from peripartum pelvic instability: A study of the biomechanical effects of pelvic belts. *Am J Obstet Gynecol* 1992;166:1243–1247.

POSTSURGICAL REHABILITATION

Overview

Although many musculoskeletal conditions can be treated conservatively, surgical intervention is often indicated for cases in which a sufficient traumatic or degenerative injury has occurred. The typical criteria for surgical intervention includes:[1,2]:

▶ Failure to respond to a 4- to 6-month course of conservative measures.

▶ Severe levels of pain that significantly limit the performance of daily activities and personal care.

▶ Gross joint instability fracture, and abnormal joint alignment, with accompanying loss of function.

Over the years, the number of surgical procedures for orthopaedic conditions has increased considerably. However, although surgery can often correct the presenting problem, for the postsurgical patient to return to an appropriate level of function, some form of postsurgical rehabilitation usually is required. Indeed, a number of studies have reported that skilled intervention following most surgical procedures of the musculoskeletal system allows patients to achieve greater independence and control over their lives in a shorter timeframe, than do patients who do not receive these interventions.[3,4]

Postsurgical Complications

Although surgical procedures can offer many benefits, they are not without their complications. Some of the more serious of these complications include:

▶ *Postsurgical infection.* Postsurgical infections are perhaps the greatest challenge facing the modern-day surgeon. At any one time, 9 percent of hospitalized patients are being treated for an infection they acquired there.[5] *Staphylococcus aureus*, coagulase-negative staphylococci, *Enterococcus* spp., and *Escherichia coli* remain the most frequently isolated pathogens. An increasing proportion of infections are caused by antimicrobial-resistant pathogens, such as methicillin-resistant *S. aureus* (MRSA), or by *Candida albicans*.[6] Microorganisms may contain or produce toxins and other substances that increase their ability to invade a host, produce damage within the host, or survive on or in host tissue. For example, many gram-negative bacteria produce endotoxin, which stimulates cytokine production. In turn, cytokines can trigger the systemic inflammatory response syndrome that sometimes leads to multiple system organ failure.[6] In certain kinds of surgical procedures, some patient characteristics have been found to be possibly associated with an increased risk of an infection. These include co-incident remote site infections or colonization, diabetes, cigarette smoking, systemic steroid use, obesity (> 20 percent of ideal body weight), extremes of age, poor nutritional

status, and perioperative transfusion of certain blood products.[6–8] Although physical therapists are not directly involved in surgical procedures, they are a potential mode of transmission for infections. Hand washing has been found to be an important infection control measure, although improving compliance with hand washing has been a challenge for most hospital infection control programs.[9]

▶ *Deep vein thrombosis.* A thrombus, or blood clot, is an obstruction of the venous or arterial system. If a thrombus is located in one of the superficial veins, it is usually self-limiting, whereas a deep vein thrombosis (DVT) can result in a pulmonary embolus (see later), which is life threatening. DVT is caused by an alteration in the normal coagulation system. This alteration in the fibrinolytic system, which acts as a system of checks and balances, results in a failure to dissolve the clot. If the clot becomes dislodged, it enters into the circulatory system, through which it can travel to become lodged in the lungs (pulmonary embolism), obstructing the pulmonary artery or branches, which supply the lungs with blood. If the clot is large and completely blocks a vessel, it can cause sudden death. Certain patients are at increased risk for DVT. Those undergoing orthopaedic surgery, such as joint replacements, are particularly susceptible, as are patients with paralysis. Other risk factors include advancing age, family history of DVT, estrogen use, pregnancy, obesity, and prolonged air flights.[10] Any form of prolonged immobility causes blood circulation to become sluggish, resulting in venous stasis and increasing the risk for DVT. The association of DVT with venous stasis was first proposed by Virchow in 1859.[11] A recent study indicated that up to 60 percent of patients undergoing total hip replacement surgery may develop a DVT without preventative treatment.[12,13] Clinical signs of a DVT include swelling of the extremity, tenderness or a feeling of cramping of the calf muscles that increases when the ankle is dorsiflexed (positive Homan's sign) or with weight bearing, and inflammation and discoloration or redness of the extremity.

• *Prevention is the key with DVT.* Surgical patients are usually prescribed anti-coagulant drugs such as warfarin (Coumadin). These drugs work by altering the body's normal blood-clotting process. Counteracting the effects of immobility can also prevent DVT. A recent study has shown that substantial hyperemia (a mean 22 percent increase in venous outflow) occurs after the performance of active ankle pumps for 1 minute, and venous outflow remains greater than the baseline level for 30 minutes, reaching a maximum 12 minutes after these exercises.[13] Although this does not provide sufficient evidence that exercise alone prevents DVT, it suggests that the active ankle pump does influence venous hemodynamics.

• *Pulmonary embolus.* This is a potentially fatal, but rare, complication following major surgery, which requires the immediate notification of the nursing staff and physician. Clinical signs range from tachypnea or dyspnea, wheezing, tachycardia, and hypotension to severe cardiopulmonary shock.

▶ *Poor wound healing.* Wound-healing abnormalities cause great physical and psychological stress to affected patients and are extremely expensive to treat. The rate of healing in acute surgical wounds is affected by both extrinsic factors (surgical technique, tension of wound suturing, maintenance of adequate oxygenation, cigarette smoking, prevention or eradication of infection, and types of wound dressing) and intrinsic factors (presence of shock or sepsis, control of diabetes mellitus, and the age, nutritional, and immune status of the patient).[14] Although many studies have documented relationships between malnutrition and poor wound healing, the optimal nutrient intake to promote wound healing is unknown. It is known, however, that vitamins A, C, and E, protein, arginine, zinc, and water play a role in the healing process.[15]

▶ *Scars and adhesions.* Surgery is a form of controlled macrotrauma to the musculoskeletal system. The tissues respond to this trauma in much the same way that they do to any other form of trauma or injury. As part of the postsurgical rehabilitation process, the involved structure usually is immobilized, to protect the surgical site from injury. However, prolonged immobilization of a connective tissue can produce significant changes in its histochemical and biomechanical structure. These changes include a fibrofatty infiltration, which can progress into fibrosis, creating adhesions around the healing site, and an increase in the microscopic cross-linking of collagen fibers, resulting in an overall loss of extensibility of the connective tissues.[16–20] Unlike connective tissue, which is mature and stable with limited pliability, scar tissue is more vulnerable to breakdown.[21–25] Fortunately, controlled and skilled therapeutic interventions can reverse the detrimental effects of short-term immobilization. These include mobilization of the connective tissue with passive mobility techniques or active range of motion, which help to restore the extensibility of the tissue. To assist with the overall healing of the incision, scar mobilization techniques may be performed to the patient's tolerance with lotion and Roylan 50/50, Otoform K, and Elastomer.

Postsurgical Examination

Detailed descriptions of actual surgical procedures are not presented in Chapters 28 and 29. Although it is important for the clinician to be familiar with surgical techniques, such a wide variety of procedures are used for each surgical technique, that it would be futile to attempt to describe all of them here. These details can be found in numerous texts and journal articles. Ideally, the clinician should establish a rapport with local surgeons, and arrange times to view the surgical procedures frequently performed on patients encountered in the clinic.

Although each patient is approached as an individual with differing needs and responses to surgery, the postsurgical examination should follow a systematic plan, which includes the following components.

History and Systems Review

Details about the type of procedure performed are noted, as well as the location, nature, and behavior of symptoms. The clinician asks about the patient's current and previous functional status, and discusses with the patient, his or her functional goals and predicted outcomes. Questions regarding the patient's past medical and surgical history provide the clinician with information that may influence the choice of intervention.

Tests and Measures

Pain
The patient's subjective complaints of pain are measured and reported on a visual analog scale.

Cardiovascular Status
The clinician should determine whether circulatory and pulmonary complications exist, such as thrombophlebitis, deep vein thrombosis, or pneumonia.

Integumentary Integrity
The clinician should observe and palpate around the incision, check the integrity and mobility of the scar, and determine the degree of edema, crepitus, and tenderness. Abnormal redness, swelling, or increased heat could indicate an infection, especially if accompanied by fever.

Range of Motion
The range of motion of the involved area can be assessed. Where possible and appropriate, the range of motion is assessed actively. Otherwise, the clinician assesses the available passive range of motion, taking care to not over-stress the healing structures, and to observe any range limitations related to the procedure.

Joint Integrity and Mobility
A general examination of the healing area is performed, checking the musculature, tendons, and ligaments, where appropriate.

Muscle Performance
Resisted testing can be performed on the muscles that are not directly related to the surgery site. The clinician examines the patient's ability to perform isometric exercises pertinent to the postsurgical protocol.

Posture
The clinician ensures that the patient is positioned appropriately and is avoiding positions that are contraindicated as a result of the surgery.

Function
The clinician should determine the patient's level of functional independence, noting which functional tasks (transfers, bed

mobility, and ambulation) the patient is able to perform independently. The patient should be provided with a safe and efficient means of ambulation, if appropriate.

Post-surgical Rehabilitation

Traditional interventions for postsurgical patients have involved adhering to exercise protocols designed by the surgeon performing the operation in order to limit post-surgical stress. This has led to an emphasis on interventions based solely on exercises linked to time frames, a sort of "cookbook" approach, rather than a comprehensive approach designed in conjunction with the physical therapist, based on clinical findings and individual consideration.

Among the key factors that must be considered in the postsurgical rehabilitation are[26]:

▶ Type of surgery.

▶ Patient's age.

▶ Patient's physical status, including weight, and other medical conditions, such as any history of cardiovascular or peripheral vascular disease, or diabetes.

▶ Social lifestyle of the patient.

▶ Preoperative joint contracture or muscle atrophy.

▶ Method of fixation.

▶ Surrounding soft tissues involved.

▶ Degree of correction of biomechanical alignment.

▶ Functional and recreational goals of the patient.

These factors may influence the rate at which the patient progresses through the rehabilitation process, as well as determine the extent of functional return that can be expected in the long term.

The purpose of including Chapters 28 and 29 is not to provide the reader with a series of rigid protocols for each of the postsurgical conditions presented. Given the wide variety of protocols available, that would be an impossible task. Instead, the goal is to provide the reader with guidelines for goal setting and interventions based on the stages of healing of the various tissues. Through the use of these guidelines, the reader should be able to establish efficient intervention plans that include the establishment of appropriate goals, the use of pertinent modalities, therapeutic exercise, manual techniques, and the prescription of a comprehensive home program. The stages of healing described in Chapter 5 should not be viewed as distinct entities or as rigid templates, but as a continuum that must be modified based on clinical findings and subjective responses. For example, responses to an intervention that indicate an overly aggressive approach include:

▶ Increased area of pain.

▶ Pain at rest that lasts longer than 2 hours after exercising.[27]

▶ Pain that alters the performance of an activity or exercise in a detrimental manner.[27]

Obviously, each surgical procedure is different, as is the healing capacity of each individual. In addition, each surgeon has his or her opinion as to the intensity of the postsurgical intervention. These opinions must always be respected. The descriptions of the postsurgical interventions outlined in Chapters 28 and 29 are based on personal experience. Most of the exercises listed are described in more detail in the respective joint chapters earlier in this text, as are the rationales behind the therapeutic progressions. The point at which the tools of intervention are used following surgery may vary, and although estimated timetables are provided with each of the protocols, the intention is to provide the clinician with intervention ideas rather than a regimented time scale.

Realistic goalsetting is important following surgery. Postsurgical rehabilitation goals should be based on the status of the uninvolved extremity, as long as the uninvolved extremity has no deficits. For cases in which the uninvolved extremity does have deficits, the clinician should use the guidelines from expected norms. The patient should be involved in the goal setting process when possible.

REFERENCES

1. Daigneault J, Cooney, LM Jr. Shoulder pain in older people. *J Am Geriatr Soc* 1998;46:1144–1151.
2. Burkhart SS. A 26-year-old woman with shoulder pain. *JAMA* 2000;284:1559–1567.
3. Jennings JJ, Gerard F. Total hip replacement in patients with rheumatoid arthritis. *South Med J* 1978;71:1112.
4. Opitz JL. Total joint arthroplasty: Principles and guidelines for postoperative physiatric management. *Mayo Clin Proc* 1979;54–602.
5. Kmietowicz Z. Hospital infection rates in England out of control. *BMJ* 2000;320:534.
6. Mangram AJ, et al. Guideline for prevention of surgical site infection, 1999. Centers for Disease Control and Prevention (CDC) Hospital Infection Control Practices Advisory Committee. *Am J Infect Control* 1999;27:97–132.
7. Nagachinta T, et al. Risk factors for surgical-wound infection following cardiac surgery. *J Infect Dis* 1987;156:967–973.
8. Lilienfeld DE, et al. Obesity and diabetes as risk factors for postoperative wound infections after cardiac surgery. *Am J Infect Control* 1988;16:3–6.
9. Boyce J. Is it time for action: Improving hand washing hygiene in hospitals. *Ann Intern Med* 1999;130:153–155.
10. Gorman WP, Davis KR, Donnelly R. ABC of arterial and venous disease. Swollen lower limb-1: General assessment and deep vein thrombosis. *BMJ* 2000;320:1453–1456.
11. Virchow R. Die cellular pathologie. In: *Ihrer Begrundung auf physiologische und pathologische Gewebelehre.* Berlin, Germany: Hirschwald, 1859.
12. McNally MA, Mollan RAB. Total hip replacement, lower limb blood flow and venous thrombogenesis. *J Bone Joint Surg* 1993; 75B:640–644.
13. McNally MA, Mollan RAB. The effect of active movement of the foot on venous blood flow after total hip replacement. *J Bone Joint Surg* 1997;79A:1198–1201.
14. Thomas DR. Age-related changes in wound healing. *Drugs Aging* 2001;18:607–620.

15. Scholl D, Langkamp-Henken B. Nutrient recommendations for wound healing. *J Intravenous Nurs* 2001;24:124–132.

16. Akeson, WH, et al. The connective tissue response to immobility: Biochemical changes in periarticular connective tissue of the immobilized rabbit knee. *Clin Orthop* 1973;93:356–362.

17. Akeson WH, Amiel D, Woo SLY. Immobility effects on synovial joints: The pathomechanics of joint contracture. *Biorheology* 1980;17:95–110.

18. Woo SLY, et al. Connective tissue response to immobility: A correlative study of biochemical and biomechanical measurements of normal and immobilized rabbit knee. *Arthritis Rheum* 1975; 18:257–264.

19. Woo SLY, et al. Mechanical properties of tendons and ligaments. II. The relationships of immobilization and exercise on tissue remodeling. *Biorheology* 1982;19:397–408.

20. Akeson WH, et al. Collagen cross-linking alterations in the joint contractures: Changes in the reducible cross-links in periarticular connective tissue after 9 weeks immobilization. *Connect. Tissue Res* 1977;5:15.

21. Light KE, Nuzik S. Low-load prolonged stretch vs high-load brief stretch in treating knee contractures. *Phys Ther* 1984;64:330–333.

22. Arem A, Madden J. Effects of stress on healing wounds: Intermittent non-cyclical tension. *J Surg Res* 1971;42:528–543.

23. Clayton ML Wier, GJ. Experimental investigations of ligamentous healing. *Am J Surg* 1959;98:373–378.

24. Forrester JC, et al. Wolff's law in relation to the healing skin wound. *J Trauma* 1970;10:770–779.

25. Salter RB, et al. The biological effect of continuous passive motion on the healing of full-thickness defects in articular cartilage. *J Bone Joint Surg* 1980;62A:1232–1251.

26. Auberger SS, Mangine RE. *Innovative Approaches to Surgery and Rehabilitation, in Physical Therapy of the Knee.* New York, NY: Churchill Livingstone; 1988:233–262.

27. O'Connor FG, Sobel JR, Nirschl, RP. Five step treatment for overuse injuries. *Phys Sports Med* 1992;20:128.

CHAPTER 28

POSTSURGICAL REHABILITATION OF THE UPPER EXTREMITY

Procedures Involving the Shoulder

Anterior Capsular Reconstruction of the Shoulder

When the glenohumeral joint subluxes or dislocates, either traumatically or atraumatically, significant capsular stretching can occur. Capsular stretching, in turn, can result in glenohumeral joint laxity or instability, depending on the severity. If the stretching occurs to such an extent that it results in the stripping of the anterior capsule from the glenoid labrum, it is referred to as a *Bankart* lesion.[1] To regain shoulder stability, lesions such as the Bankart may require surgical repair, with the aim of alleviating pain while permitting the range of motion (ROM) and strength to return to premorbid levels.[2–6]

Indications

The extent and direction of the joint instability, and the physical requirements of the patient, determine whether the initial approach is conservative or surgical. The conservative approach includes a program of deltoid, rotator cuff, and scapular stabilizer muscle strengthening (see Chap. 14).[7–10] Surgical intervention is reserved for patients who remain symptomatic or disabled following the conservative intervention, or those whose instability is so gross that conservative intervention is not deemed appropriate.[11]

Procedure

A number of surgical procedures exist for instability of the shoulder; they include the open anterior capsulolabral reconstruction, arthroscopic reconstruction, and the thermal capsulorrhaphy.[11]

The proposed advantages of arthroscopic stabilization over the traditional open repairs include smaller skin incisions, more complete inspection of the glenohumeral joint, the ability to treat intra-articular lesions, access to all areas of the glenohumeral joint for repair, less soft-tissue dissection, and maximum preservation of external rotation.[12] One study, with a 2- to 5-year follow-up, showed good or excellent results in 49 of 53 patients treated with arthroscopic repair for anteroinferior glenohumeral instability.[13] These results are equivalent to those for the open repair.

Thermal capsular modification to treat shoulder instability is a relatively recent procedure. The thermal capsulorrhaphy technique applies thermal energy, laser, or radiofrequency to the capsular tissues. Ultimately, this shrinks (denatures) the collagen, which tightens the entire anterior and inferior capsule. To resolve posterior instability, the surgeon introduces the thermal capsulorrhaphy probe posteriorly, directly heating the tissue of the posterior capsule. One of the advantages of this procedure is that the patient is often permitted to perform active range of motion (AROM) within 3 days of the surgery.[14,15] Whether this translates into better outcomes has yet to be determined. Currently, only one clinical study showing the long-term outcome of patients treated with this technology has been published in a peer reviewed journal.[16] Twenty-eight of the 30 patients had a satisfactory result, and two had recurrent instability. These results were comparable to those of another group of patients treated by the same authors with arthroscopic capsular shift.[16]

Several complications have been mentioned with the thermal capsulorrhaphy procedure.[14,15] These include:

▶ The potential effect of thermal necrosis of capsular nerve endings on proprioception.

▶ The strength of the capsular tissue after thermal shrinkage, and the effect this could have on subsequent open or arthroscopic capsulorrhaphy.

Postsurgical Rehabilitation

The following protocol is based on the open anterior capsulolabral reconstruction procedure. Following the surgical repair, the surgeon moves the patient's arm through the ranges of motion and notes any areas of tension on the repair, so that postsurgical ROM limits can be set. Following the closing of the skin, the arm typically is splinted or immobilized.

The surgeon sees the patient during the first 24 hours after surgery and the bandages are changed. The bandages are usually replaced with sterile adhesive bandage strips or gauze and tape after another 72 hours. The patient is instructed not to submerge the incision in water during the first postoperative week. The period of immobilization is dependent on the surgical procedure, and may also be dependent on how loose the shoulder was preoperatively and what additional procedures were performed. In general, patients with anterior instability following an anterior capsular reconstruction are immobilized for 2 weeks in 90 degrees of abduction, 45 degrees of external rotation, and 30 degrees of forward flexion,[4] whereas patients with posterior instability are immobilized for 3 to 4 weeks in neutral to external rotation. During this period of immobilization, only ROM exercises for the hand, wrist, and elbow are permitted, with the exception of pendulum exercises, although this can vary, with a few protocols allowing AROM of the shoulder earlier.[17]

The patient is instructed to apply an ice pack to the surgical shoulder for 15 minutes, three times per day, for 48 hours. The patient is advised that he or she may experience some normal bruising and swelling at the surgical site, and to watch for and report any signs and symptoms of infection (e.g., a persistent fever higher than 38°C [101°F] and lasting more than a few days, large areas of redness around the incisions sites). The patient is instructed to return for a postoperative office visit, usually 1 week after surgery. He or she may return to work at approximately 7 days postoperatively, depending on surgeon preference and patient occupation. The surgeon also may order light duties with limited shoulder involvement for a specified period of time, if appropriate, depending on the patient's occupation. Return to unrestricted activity usually occurs by 3 to 6 months after surgery.[16]

The goals of the rehabilitation process are to restore functional flexibility and to strengthen the rotator cuff muscles and scapular stabilizers, while protecting the healing capsule.

Phase 1 (Day 3 to 3 Weeks Post-surgery). This phase typically involves 6 to 9 physical therapy sessions.

Goals

▶ Reports of pain to be 2 to 3/10 or less.

▶ Allow healing progression of sutured capsule.

▶ Retard muscle atrophy and enhance dynamic stability.

▶ Minimize detrimental effects of immobilization.[18–23]

▶ Ensure patient compliance with postsurgical restrictions.

▶ Restore ROM. Passive range of motion (PROM) to be within 60 percent compared with the uninvolved extremity, with the exception of external rotation.

▶ Patient to be able to don and doff splint independently.

Electrotherapeutic and Physical Modalities

▶ Cryotherapy can be used to help decrease pain and inflammation during the first 2 to 3 days, before progressing to the thermal modalities. Thermal modalities during the first weeks also are used to decrease muscle co-contraction and promote tissue healing by increasing local blood flow.[24,25] Moist heat can be applied before exercise to encourage relaxation of the shoulder muscles after the first 2 to 3 days. Thermal modalities typically are discontinued by the fourth week.[26]

▶ The patient usually is prescribed medications by his or her physician, which also can help control pain and inflammation.[27]

▶ With the physician's permission, electrical stimulation can be used for edema reduction, muscle re-education, and pain control.[28–31]

Therapeutic Exercise and Home Program. The splint is removed for these exercises.

▶ Passive shoulder ROM should include wand or cane exercises into flexion and abduction, using tolerance or surgical restrictions as a guide. Depending on the procedure, active shoulder abduction and external rotation exercises in the scapular plane are initiated, with the aim of discontinuing the splint once the patient is able to abduct beyond 90 degrees.

▶ Codman's pendulum exercises are performed with the elbow supported. Depending on the procedure, and physician orders about ROM restrictions, gentle pulley exercises of flexion to 90 degrees and elevation in the scapular plane to 60 degrees can be performed.

▶ Gentle shoulder isometrics are initiated for internal and external rotation, flexion, extension, and abduction to retard muscle atrophy, with the arm below 90 degrees of abduction and 90 degrees of flexion.[32]

▶ Shoulder shrugs and shoulder retraction exercises are initiated.

▶ AROM is performed to elbow, wrist, and hand, including elbow flexion and extension, forearm pronation and supination, wrist flexion and extension, and hand opening and closing.

▶ Grip exercises for the wrist and hand can be initiated using ball squeezes, therapeutic putty, or a hand exerciser.

A progressive cardiovascular program is initiated, using a walking program or a stationary bike.

Manual Therapy

▶ The soft tissue techniques of soft tissue mobilization, myofascial release, and trigger point therapy are appropriate.

▶ Joint mobilizations of grades I and II can be used for pain relief, with grades III and IV being applied to specific areas of hypomobility in the cervical and thoracic spines, as appropriate.

▶ Passive, pain-free ROM is performed into all planes, making sure not to stress external rotation.

Phase 2 (3 Weeks to 2 Months Postsurgery). This phase involves three to eight physical therapy sessions.

Goals

▶ Shoulder AROM to be within 90 percent compared with the uninvolved extremity, with the exception of external rotation.

▶ Muscle strength to be at 4/5, or better, compared with the other side by the eighth week.

▶ Patient to have the ability to reach and lift 5 to 7 lb in front of the trunk and overhead by the eighth week.

▶ Achieve normal glenohumeral rhythm as compared to the uninvolved side.

Therapeutic Exercise and Home Program. Once the patient has regained active elevation to within 20 to 30 degrees compared with the uninvolved side, and rotation is about 50 to 60 percent of the uninvolved side, gentle muscle strengthening of the shoulder can begin.[11] The following resistive exercises can generally be initiated by the third week postsurgery, with an emphasis on internal and external rotation.

▶ The supraspinatus is exercised actively in isolation using the so-called empty can position (internal rotation of the shoulder, thumb pointing to the floor, and abduction of the shoulder to 90 degrees while maintaining a position of 30 degrees anterior to the midfrontal plane).

▶ Horizontal abduction is initiated by week 4 and typically is performed actively in the prone position, whereas horizontal adduction begins 1 week later and is performed supine.

▶ Deltoid strengthening and shoulder proprioceptive neuromuscular facilitation patterns are introduced based on patient tolerance, and within the postsurgical range limitations.

▶ Internal and external rotation strengthening exercises are performed within permitted ranges with the arm at the side. Using an axillary roll emphasizes the teres minor muscle; omission of the roll emphasizes the infraspinatus muscle.

▶ Active shoulder extension is performed in the prone position.

▶ Resisted exercises are added to the elbow and wrist.

▶ Gentle hands-and-knees rocking is initiated and progresses to gentle three-point rocking.

▶ The stretching phase of the program is initiated after about 6 weeks, taking care to observe the restrictions imposed by the surgery. For anterior instability repairs, external rotation typically is limited to minus 15 degrees compared with the uninvolved side, and internal rotation is limited similarly for posterior instability repairs. In fact, it is a good idea to allow the patient to achieve the last 15 degrees of each motion at his or her own speed, rather than risk overstretching the capsule too early, and possibly compromising the repair.

▶ The cardiovascular program is progressed to include the use of an upper body ergometer, beginning with a 3- to 5-minute session with low resistance, alternating the direction every other minute.

Manual Therapy
▶ The clinician continues with those soft tissue techniques that remain effective.

▶ Joint mobilization is progressed into all planes of glenohumeral motion using progressive grades, while still maintaining caution when stressing the anterior capsule.

▶ Manual resisted exercises are performed in diagonal or functional patterns, taking special care with external rotation.

▶ Rhythmic stabilization exercises are performed with the arm elevated to a comfortable level.

▶ Assisted stretching is performed by the clinician to the shoulder complex, with emphasis on the subscapularis and latissimus dorsi.

Phase 3 (2 Months +). This phase involves two to three further physical therapy sessions.

Goals
▶ Achieve all rehabilitation goals of strength, ROM, and function.

▶ Patient to be compliant and independent with home exercise program and its progression for the next 3 to 6 months.

Therapeutic Exercise and Home Program
▶ Eccentric cuff exercises are initiated and progressed.

▶ Scapular stabilization exercises are progressed, beginning with wall push-ups, then hands-and-knees rocking, then hands-and-knees push-up, and finally the full push-up (where appropriate), emphasizing the push-up plus phase of the exercise. Chest presses and scapular retractions can be initiated.

▶ The Body Blade can be used to address neuromuscular and proprioception retraining.

▶ Plyometrics are progressed. Medicine ball throwing progresses from the single-arm underhand pass to the two-handed toss, followed by the overhead toss. Progressions of these exercises include increasing the number of throws, the speed of the throw, and the distances thrown.

▶ Isokinetic training is usually reserved for athletic populations. This form of training is initiated when the patient can lift at least 5 lb in side-lying external rotation, and 10 to 15 lb in side-lying internal rotation without pain.[33] Isokinetic testing typically is performed at 6 months.[4] Activity- and sport-specific drills are initiated once the involved side has achieved 70 to 80 percent of the strength of the uninvolved side, tested isokinetically (120 degrees/sec for internal rotation and 240 degrees/sec for external rotation.)[33]

Acromioplasty

Repetitive impingement of the rotator cuff and the subacromial structures in the subacromial space between the humeral head and the coracoacromial arch is a common cause of shoulder pain and results in a condition called *subacromial impingement syndrome* (see Chap. 14). Continued impingement of the rotator cuff against the overlying acromion is the principal cause of rotator cuff tears.[34–36]

Indications

An acromioplasty typically is performed on patients with a clinical diagnosis of subacromial impingement syndrome who have persistent pain and loss of function, and who have failed a conservative intervention, including rehabilitation, activity modification, anti-inflammatory medications, and subacromial cortisone injections.[37] An acromioplasty also is a routine procedure for virtually all patients undergoing a rotator cuff repair.

Procedures

Acromioplasty can be performed as an open procedure or arthroscopically. Acromioplasty procedures can be complicated by deltoid detachment, compromise of the deltoid lever arm, anterosuperior instability, and adhesions of the rotator cuff tendons under the bleeding cancellous bone of the osteotomized acromion.

Open decompression was described by Neer for stage II and III lesions in 1972.[34] Neer identified the acromial contact area for the rotator cuff as anterior rather than lateral and believed that the development of a traction spur within the coracoacromial ligament or an osteophyte in the distal clavicle played a role in patients' symptoms. The Neer procedure includes debridement of the subacromial bursa and resection of the coracoacromial ligament and the anteroinferior acromion, as well as any underhanging osteophytes from the acromioclavicular joint. As part of this procedure, the deltoid muscle is split in line with its fibers approximately 5 mm anterior to the acromioclavicular joint for a distance of 3 to 4 cm distally. This approach leaves a strong, healthy cuff of tissue that allows for a secure repair of the deltoid split, but can cause postoperative weakening of the deltoid.[34,38,39] Neer's initial results, as well as other follow-up studies with regard to this and similar procedures, have shown excellent outcomes, with success rates based on functional outcome from 80 to 95 percent.[34,40]

In 1982, Ellman described an arthroscopic technique to decompress the subacromial space while also sparing the origin of the deltoid.[41] This subacromial decompression procedure involves a release of the coracoacromial ligament, resection of the undersurface of the anterior acromion, and debridement of any hypertrophic bursa. Ellman reported satisfactory results in 88 percent of patients at 2 to 5 years of follow-up.[42] Many variations of this technique have since been reported.

Advocates of the open approach point to its technical simplicity and shorter operating time, whereas arthroscopists claim better cosmesis and deltoid preservation, and faster recovery.[43,44]

In a prospective, randomized, controlled, blinded clinical trial, Spangehl and colleagues[45] examined the outcomes of 71 patients with a clinical diagnosis of impingement syndrome who were randomized to arthroscopic or open acromioplasty. Their study found that both techniques resulted in significant improvement for pain and function, with the open technique being slightly superior.[45]

The postsurgical rehabilitation program following both procedures is similar.

Postsurgical Rehabilitation

The aim of postsurgical rehabilitation is to increase the size of the subacromial space through therapeutic exercises that enhance the surgical decompression, without overloading the healing tissues. Depending on the surgeon's protocol and the surgical findings, the patient may be prescribed a sling or shoulder immobilizer to be used for 1 to 5 days following the surgery. The purpose of the sling is to decrease the forces on the supraspinatus tendon by centralizing the humeral head in the glenoid fossa.

Phase 1 (Day 1 to 6 Weeks Postsurgery). This phase typically involves one to six physical therapy sessions.

Goals
▶ Improve patient comfort through a decrease in pain and inflammation to 5/10 or less.

▶ Minimize cervical spine stiffness and loss of range.

▶ Retard muscle atrophy.

▶ Minimize detrimental effects of immobilization and activity restriction.[18–23]

▶ Protect the surgical site.

▶ Involved shoulder passive range of motion (PROM) to be at 75 to 90 percent of the uninvolved side by the third week. The goal is to achieve full and supple PROM by 6 weeks.

▶ Maintain range of motion (ROM) and fitness of other components of the kinetic chain (neck, elbow, wrist, and hand).

▶ Manual muscle strength in the uninvolved areas to be at 4+/5.

▶ Manual muscle testing of rotators to be at 3 to 4/5.

▶ Restore or maintain scapular and scapulothoracic mobility.

▶ Patient to be independent with home exercise program.

Electrotherapeutic and Physical Modalities
▶ Cryotherapy is used in the first few days during the acute phase. The thermal and deep thermal modalities can be used once the acute phase of healing has subsided.

▶ The patient usually is prescribed medications by the physician, which can help control pain and inflammation but also may mask the patient's symptoms.[27]

▶ The clinician should determine whether a scalene block was performed, because this can delay the onset of postsurgical pain.

Therapeutic Exercise and Home Program
▶ Codman's pendulum, passive elevation using a table, and external rotation using a cane are started the afternoon of surgery. Passive extension is avoided initially to prevent stress on the deltoid repair, if applicable. PROM exercises have been shown to prevent the degenerating effects of immobilization, provide nourishment to the articular cartilage, and assist in collagen synthesis and organization.[46–48] The

degree of movement is guided by the stability of the operative repair.[32]

▶ The patient also can begin exercises to help regain scapular control by the second week. These exercises include isometric scapular pinches and scapular elevation; gentle closed-chain weight shifts with hands on table, shoulder flexed less than 60 degrees, and abducted less than 45 degrees; and the use of a tilt board or circular board to perform weight shifts with the same range limitations.[32]

▶ The patient also performs active range of motion (AROM) of the cervical spine, elbow, wrist, and hand.

Fitness of the rest of the kinetic chain is maintained with[32]:

▶ Lower extremity anaerobic agility drills, where appropriate.

▶ Lower extremity strengthening by machines.

▶ Flexibility exercises, especially to those areas shown to be adaptively shortened during the examination.

▶ A walking or running program, initiated at the earliest opportunity, for cardiovascular conditioning. Alternatively, a lower extremity ergometer, such as a stair stepper stationary bike, can be used. An upper body ergometer (UBE) may be used by the end of the third week, making sure that the patient avoids internal rotation at the glenohumeral joint to avoid provoking an impingement. The UBE sessions begin with 3- to 5-minute bouts with low resistance, alternating the direction every other minute.

At approximately 3 to 7 days postsurgery, the patient may begin submaximal, pain-free isometrics into internal and external rotation, and progressive resisted exercises (PREs) are initiated at 3 weeks for elbow flexion and extension. At approximately 1 to 2 weeks, depending on patient tolerance, the patient progresses from active assistive range of motion (AAROM) exercises to AROM against gravity. This can include active elevation, side-lying internal and external rotation exercises, and scapular retraction. According to patient tolerance, these exercises are progressed to include resistance. The initiation of the strengthening program is dictated by pain and tissue response, and the exercises are performed in a range below 90 degrees of elevation to avoid the potential for impingement. The resistance should be light, initially, but progressed as strength improves. Emphasis is placed on proper mechanics, proper technique, and joint stabilization.[32]

Manual Therapy
▶ The soft tissue techniques of soft tissue mobilization, myofascial release, and trigger point therapy are appropriate.

▶ Joint mobilizations of grades I and II can be used for pain relief, with grades III and IV being applied to specific areas of hypomobility in the cervical and thoracic spine.

▶ Passive, pain-free ROM is performed, taking care not to overstress the healing tissues.

Phase 2 (6 Weeks to 9 Weeks Postsurgery). This phase typically involves three to six physical therapy sessions.

Goals
▶ AROM to be at 90 degrees of abduction without substitution from the scapulothoracic region by the beginning of this phase.

▶ Reports of pain to be 2/10 or less.

▶ Achieve normal shoulder arthrokinetics in single, then multiple, planes of motion.[32]

▶ Patient to be able to perform functional activities, including pain-free driving and dressing, and report an increase in sleep duration, compared with initial examination.

▶ Achieve normal kinetic chain and force generation patterns, and restoration of normal strength ratios of the involved and uninvolved arms, by the eighth week.

Therapeutic Exercise and Home Program
▶ Scapular proprioceptive neuromuscular facilitation patterns are performed in diagonals, initially without resistance.

▶ Internal and external rotation PREs are performed in varying angles of elevation with the elbow flexed to 90 degrees. Strengthening of the deltoid, infraspinatus, scapular rotators, and biceps is progressed.

▶ The supraspinatus is exercised in isolation using the so-called empty can position (internal rotation of the shoulder, thumb pointing to the floor, and abduction of the shoulder to 90 degrees while maintaining a position of 30 degrees anterior to the midfrontal plane).[49]

▶ Horizontal adduction in the supine position is performed, and progressed to horizontal abduction in the prone position.

▶ Aerobic exercises. The UBE sessions are progressed from low-intensity and short-duration sessions to sessions that are longer in duration and higher in intensity, alternating the direction every 5 minutes.

Neuromuscular Retraining. Neuromuscular and proprioceptive retraining can be initiated in this phase and can include:

▶ Gentle multidirectional hand-heel rocking in the quadruped position, progressing to three-point rocking, and the push-up progression of wall push-ups and hand-knee push-ups. Care must be taken during these exercises to avoid hand positions that place the glenohumeral joint in internal rotation.

▶ Medicine ball catch and push activities, and other plyometric activities, can be initiated by about the seventh week.[32]

▶ A Body Blade also can be introduced during this phase, working in all planes of motion, especially the transverse plane.

Manual Therapy

▶ The clinician continues with those soft tissue techniques that remain effective.

▶ Joint mobilization is progressed into all planes of glenohumeral motion using progressive grades to stretch the glenohumeral capsule and inhibit muscle guarding and inhibition through receptor facilitation.[50,51] Joint mobilizations also may be necessary in the other joints of the shoulder complex, including the sternoclavicular, acromioclavicular, and scapulothoracic joints.

▶ Manual resisted exercises are performed in diagonal or functional patterns.[52,53]

▶ Assisted stretching is performed by the clinician to the shoulder complex, with particular emphasis on stretching the posterior capsule.

Phase 3 (Week 10+). This phase typically involves one to three physical therapy sessions.

Goals

▶ Pain-free AROM to be at 100 percent compared with the uninvolved side.

▶ Reports of pain to be 0/10 at rest, and 2/10 or less with functional activity or exercise.

▶ Strength of shoulder muscles to be at 4/5 or equal to the uninvolved shoulder.

▶ Functional performance to include reaching and lifting 5 to 8 lb in front of trunk, and lifting 5 to 10 lb overhead

Therapeutic Exercise and Home Program. The exercise program is progressed during this phase to include isotonic exercises, emphasizing eccentric contractions. The resisted exercises are performed in straight planes, the scaption plane, and functional diagonal planes (proprioceptive neuromuscular facilitation). It is important that the patient continue to perform the exercises correctly. Surgical tubing can be used to exercise the muscles under a constant load during the exercise.[54] The muscles should be worked at varying speeds and angles, simulating sports-specific or functional activities.

▶ Rowing is a good overall exercise for the shoulder muscles and strengthens all portions of the trapezius, levator scapula, and rhomboids.

▶ The military press is also a good exercise, particularly for the upper trapezius and deltoid, but it is recommended that dumbbells be used for this exercise so that the internal-rotated position of the glenohumeral joint can be avoided.

▶ The Body Blade can be used, with the patient performing contractions throughout the range. Other proprioceptive exercises include weight-bearing exercises in prone over a swiss ball, push-offs from the swiss ball, and seated shoulder depressions using a swiss ball.

▶ Kinetic chain exercises also are performed, including exercises that incorporate lower extremity and trunk exercises to promote co-contractions and enhance dynamic joint stability (see Chap. 10).[27,32,55–57]

▶ Plyometrics are progressed from performing the underhand pass, to the two-handed toss, and, finally, the overhead pass. Progressions are made in the number of throws, speed of the throw, and distances thrown. Other plyometric exercises for this phase include[32]:

• *Wall push-ups.* The push-up-plus exercise can be added to help strengthen the serratus anterior.

• *Corner push-ups.*

• *Tubing.* Tubing exercises may be used to mimic any of the needed motions in throwing or serving.

• *Medicine balls.* These are very effective plyometric devices, because the weight of the ball creates a pre-stretch and an eccentric load when it is caught, and then creates a resistance and a powerful agonist contraction to propel it forward again.[32]

The criteria for return to play should include a normal clinical examination, normal shoulder arthrokinetics, and normal kinetic chain integration.[32]

Patients are advised to continue the ROM and strengthening exercises for 1 year.[58]

Rotator Cuff Repair

The patient with a symptomatic, rotator cuff-deficient glenohumeral joint poses a complex problem for the orthopaedic team, and several surgical options are available, depending on the presentation.[59,60]

Indications

The indications for a rotator cuff repair are persistent pain that interferes with activities of daily living, work, or sports; patients who are unresponsive to a 4- to 6-month period of conservative care; or active young patients (younger than 50 years of age) with an acute full-thickness tear.[58]

Procedure

The surgical intervention for a rotator cuff repair is based on the size of the tear, the patient's age and activity level, and the level of function and pain.[61] Two of the more common techniques are the open rotator cuff repair and the arthroscopic repair.

The role of arthroscopy in the treatment of rotator cuff lesions is evolving. The procedure has advanced remarkably over the past two decades,[62] from its original use as a diagnostic tool to an effective treatment option for patients with stage II impingement and acromioclavicular joint arthritis.[41,43,44] In the past, arthroscopic techniques were reserved for small or moderately-sized partial- or full-thickness tears of the supraspinatus or infraspinatus.[63–65] Recently, repair of full-thickness rotator cuff tears using an arthroscopic technique has been described.[66-69]

The advantages of arthroscopic repair appear to include smaller skin incisions, glenohumeral joint inspection, treatment of intra-articular lesions, avoidance of deltoid detachment, less soft tissue dissection, and less pain.[58,66,69]

The open technique involves a vertical incision over the anterior shoulder. The deltoid is divided to allow access to the rotator cuff and subacromial space. An anterior and inferior acromioplasty is performed, and the rotator cuff is inspected, because the method of repair is dependent on the extent of the tear.

The coracoacromial ligament, an important structure in restraining upward migration of the humerus, is not resected unless major tightness is present or exposure is needed.[70]

Regardless of the technique chosen, open or arthroscopic, the speed of the postsurgical rehabilitation remains unchanged, because the limiting factor—tendon-to-bone healing—remains a constant. In addition, the speed of the progression is a factor of the status of the deltoid muscle, the size of the tear, and the ability to move the shoulder without injuring the tissues.[71,72]

Postsurgical Rehabilitation

For the first 6 weeks postoperatively, the arm is typically protected in a sling or on a small abduction pillow. Depending on the surgeon, a continuous passive motion machine may be prescribed to prevent the degenerating effects of immobilization, provide nourishment to the articular cartilage, and assist in collagen synthesis and organization.[46-48,72] However, manual passive range of motion (PROM) exercises have been found to be more cost-effective and to yield results similar to those of a continuous passive motion machine.[72] The degree of movement permitted during the first 6 weeks is guided by the stability of the operative repair.[32] External rotation motion beyond neutral is usually restricted for the first 4 weeks.[70]

The following rehabilitation protocol is designed for the active recreational athlete.

Phase 1 (Day 1 to 6 Weeks Postsurgery). This phase typically involves one to six physical therapy sessions.

Goals

▶ Improve patient comfort through a decrease in pain and inflammation to 5/10 or less.

▶ Minimize cervical spine stiffness and loss of range.

▶ Retard muscle atrophy.

▶ Minimize detrimental effects of immobilization.[18-23]

▶ Protect the surgical site.

▶ Involved shoulder PROM to be at 50 to 60 percent of the uninvolved side by 3 to 4 weeks postsurgery. Therefore, the patient should achieve at least 45 degrees of passive external rotation and 120 degrees of passive forward flexion.

▶ Maintain range of motion (ROM) and strength of other components of the kinetic chain (cervical elbow, wrist, and hand).

▶ Manual muscle strength in the uninvolved areas to be at 4+/5.

▶ Initiate scapular control; involved side and uninvolved side scapular asymmetry to be less than 1.5 cm with the lateral scapular slide test (see Chap. 14).[32]

▶ Patient to be independent with home exercise program.

Electrotherapeutic and Physical Modalities. Cryotherapy can be used, as well as the athermal modalities such as ultrasound. The patient usually is prescribed medications by the physician, which can also help control the pain and inflammation.[27]

Therapeutic Exercise and Home Program. The splint or abduction pillow is removed for the exercises.

▶ Codman's pendulum, passive elevation using a table, and external rotation exercises using a cane are started the afternoon of surgery. These exercises are continued at home for 6 weeks. Passive extension is avoided initially to prevent stress on the deltoid repair.

▶ The patient also can begin exercises to help regain scapular control. These exercises include isometric scapular pinches and scapular elevation; gentle closed-chain weight shifts, with hands on table, shoulder flexed less than 60 degrees and abducted less than 45 degrees; and the use of a tilt board or circular board to perform weight shifts with the same range limitations.[32]

▶ The patient also performs active range of motion (AROM) of the cervical spine and elbow, and strengthening of the wrist and hand.

Fitness of the rest of the kinetic chain is maintained with[32]:

▶ Aerobic exercises, such as running, bicycling, or stepping.

▶ Lower extremity anaerobic agility drills, where appropriate.

▶ Lower extremity strengthening by machines.

▶ Flexibility exercises to those areas found to be adaptively shortened during the examination.

At approximately 3 to 4 weeks, the patient may begin submaximal, pain-free isometrics of the shoulder girdle muscles.

At approximately 5 to 6 weeks, the patient progresses from PROM exercises to active assistive range of motion (AAROM) to AROM against gravity.

Manual Therapy

▶ The soft tissue techniques of soft tissue mobilization, myofascial release, and trigger point therapy are appropriate.

▶ Joint mobilizations of grades I and II can be used for pain relief, with grades III and IV being applied to specific areas of hypomobility in the cervical and thoracic spine.

▶ Passive, pain-free ROM is performed into elevation and external rotation, taking care not to overstress the healing tissues.

Phase 2 (6 Weeks to 11 Weeks Postsurgery).   The sling or immobilizer is discarded. During this phase, which typically involves four to six physical therapy sessions, the emphasis is on regaining ROM rather than strength.

Goals

▶ Active assisted motion with cane to be above 90 degrees of abduction.

▶ Reports of pain to be at 2/10 or less.

▶ Cervical AROM to be within normal limits.

▶ Achieve normal shoulder arthrokinetics in single, then multiple, planes of motion.[32]

▶ Patient to be able to perform functional activities, including pain-free driving, dressing, and increase in sleep duration, compared with initial evaluation.

▶ Achieve appropriate kinetic chain and force generation patterns.

Therapeutic Exercise and Home Program.   At 6 weeks, patients should be performing AAROM. Once pain is controlled, AROM is performed in straight planes, the scaption plane, and functional planes (proprioceptive neuromuscular facilitation),[73] initially moving in the 0- to 70-degree range and progressing according to tolerance, and the patient's ability to perform the movements correctly.

▶ Internal and external rotation exercises are performed with the arm at the side, and the elbow flexed to 90 degrees. Using an axillary roll emphasizes the teres minor muscle; omission of the roll emphasizes the infraspinatus muscle.

▶ The supraspinatus is exercised in isolation using the so-called empty can position (internal rotation of the shoulder, thumb pointing to the floor, abduction of the shoulder to 90 degrees while maintaining a position of 30 degrees anterior to the midfrontal plane).[49]

▶ Horizontal adduction in the supine position is performed, and is progressed to horizontal abduction in the prone position.

▶ Shoulder shrugs are performed, as well as scapular retraction and depression.

▶ The muscles of the elbow, wrist, and hand are strengthened using grip exercises and the hand exerciser.

▶ An upper body ergonometer (UBE) can be used for cardiovascular conditioning, making sure that the patient avoids internal rotation at the glenohumeral joint to avoid provoking an impingement. The UBE sessions begin with 3- to 5-minute bouts with low resistance, alternating the direction every other minute.

Neuromuscular Retraining.   Neuromuscular and proprioceptive retraining can be initiated in this phase and can include:

▶ Gentle multidirectional rocking in quadruped position, progressing to three-point rocking, and the push-up progression of wall push-ups and hand-knee push-ups. Care must be taken during these exercises to avoid hand positions that place the glenohumeral joint in internal rotation.

▶ Medicine ball catch and push activities can be initiated.[32]

▶ A Body Blade also can be introduced during this phase, working in all planes of motion, especially the transverse plane.

Manual Therapy

▶ The clinician continues with those soft tissue techniques that remain effective.

▶ Joint mobilization is progressed into all planes of glenohumeral motion using progressive grades to stretch the glenohumeral capsule and inhibit muscle guarding and inhibition through receptor facilitation.[50,51] Joint mobilizations also may be necessary in the other joints of the shoulder complex, including the sternoclavicular, acromioclavicular, and scapulothoracic joints.

▶ Manual resisted exercises are performed in diagonal or functional patterns.[52,53]

▶ Assisted stretching is performed by the clinician to the shoulder complex, with particular emphasis on stretching the posterior capsule.

Phase 3 (Week 12+).   At 12 weeks after surgery, isotonic resisted exercises are commenced and stretching is continued. This phase typically involves one to three physical therapy sessions.

Goals

▶ Pain-free AROM to be at 90–100 percent compared with the uninvolved side.

▶ Reports of pain to be 0/10 at rest, and 2/10 or less with functional activity or exercise.

▶ Strength of shoulder muscles to be at 4/5 or equal to the uninvolved shoulder.

▶ Functional performance should include reaching and lifting 5 lb in front of trunk, and lifting 5 to 10 lb overhead.

Therapeutic Exercise and Home Program.   The exercise program is progressed during this phase to include isotonic exercises, emphasizing eccentric contractions. Scapulothoracic (scapular stabilizing) exercises also are begun at this stage. The initiation of the strengthening program is dictated by pain and tissue response, and is performed in a range below 90 degrees of elevation to avoid the potential for impingement. The resistance should be light, initially, and progressed as strength and ROM improves. Emphasis is placed on proper mechanics, proper technique, and joint stabilization.[32]

The resisted exercises are performed in straight planes, the scaption plane, and functional planes (proprioceptive neuromuscular facilitation). It is important that the patient continue to perform the exercises correctly. Surgical tubing can be used to exercise the muscles under a constant load during the exercise.[54] The muscles should be worked at varying speeds and angles, simulating sports-specific or functional activities.

▶ Kinetic chain exercises. These include exercises that incorporate lower extremity and trunk exercises to promote co-contractions and enhance dynamic joint stability (see Chap. 10).[27,32,55–57]

▶ Plyometrics are progressed from the underhand pass, to the two-handed toss, and, finally, the overhead pass. Progressions are made in the number of throws, speed of the throw, and distances thrown. Other plyometric exercises for this phase include[32]:

  • *Wall push-ups.*

  • *Corner push-ups.*

  • *Tubing.* Tubing exercises may be used to mimic any of the needed motions in throwing or serving.

▶ The UBE sessions are progressed from low-intensity and short-duration sessions to sessions that are longer in duration and higher in intensity, alternating the direction every 5 minutes. The use of the UBE can be complimented with a walking or running program, or the use of a lower extremity ergometer, such as a stair-stepper or cross-country ski machine.

▶ Isokinetic training if appropriate, is initiated when the patient can lift at least 5 lb in side-lying external rotation, and 10 to 15 lb in side-lying internal rotation without pain.[4,33] The recommended speed for starting is 200 degrees/sec.[74]

Patients are advised to continue the ROM and strengthening exercises for 6 months to 1 year.[58]

Total Shoulder Arthroplasty

A total shoulder arthroplasty (TSA) is a surgical option for elderly patients with cuff-deficient arthritic shoulders.[59] Other patients who may require a TSA include those with bone tumors, rheumatoid arthritis, Paget's disease, avascular necrosis of the humeral head, fracture dislocations, and recurrent dislocations.[75,76]

Indications

The main indication for surgical intervention is unremitting pain, rather than decreased motion, and a failure of conservative measures. Additional considerations include patient age, activity level, job requirements, and general health.[59]

A course of preoperative intervention is recommended. This should include an assessment of range of motion, scapular mobility, muscle imbalances, and pain. The key muscles to examine preoperatively for strength include the rotator cuff, deltoid, trapezius, rhomboids, serratus anterior, latissimus dorsi, teres major, and pectoralis major and minor.[26] The patient should be provided with exercise instruction and patient education on postsurgical precautions. A course of shoulder stretching before a prosthetic arthroplasty may improve postsurgical function.[77]

Procedure

The TSA is a very difficult procedure, and the outcome depends on the skill of the reconstruction, the soft tissue repair, the orientation of the implants, and the success of the rehabilitation.[75,78–80] The total shoulder replacement provides significantly greater pain relief than hemiarthroplasty, with approximately 80 percent of patients reporting pain relief after hemiarthroplasty versus more than 90 percent after shoulder replacement.[80]

Three types of replacement components are used:

1. *Unconstrained.* This is the most widely used component and consists of a humeral component that exists with a scapular component.

2. *Constrained.* This type is designed for patients who have severe deterioration of the rotator cuff, but with a functioning deltoid. The glenoid and humeral components are coupled and fixed to bone.

3. *Semiconstrained.* This type involves the use of a smaller and spherical humeral head with a head neck angle of 60 degrees, which reportedly permits increased range of motion (ROM).

The unconstrained technique and the postsurgical rehabilitation that follows this procedure are described in this section.

Although surgical techniques vary, most involve the dissection of the subscapularis or a rotator cuff repair, or a combination of both. The patient usually is placed in a sling or an elastic shoulder immobilizer following the operation, which positions the humerus in adduction, internal rotation, and slight forward flexion. An abduction splint may be issued if a rotator cuff repair is performed, and is worn for 4 to 6 weeks, according to the surgeon's instructions.

Postsurgical Rehabilitation

The final outcome following shoulder arthroplasty will depend on many factors, including the quality of the soft tissue (especially the status of the rotator cuff), the quality of the bone, the type of implant and fixation used, the patient's expectations, and the quality of the rehabilitation program.[26] Only the surgeon knows the extent of soft tissue damage and repair, and the guidelines communicated to the clinician must be strongly adhered to. Typically, the only motions not allowed in the early weeks are active internal rotation, and active and passive external rotation beyond 35 to 40 degrees.

Phase 1 (0 to 3 Weeks). This phase typically involves one to four physical therapy sessions. Sometimes, a continuous passive motion machine (CPMM) is prescribed by the physician. The shoulder immobilizer is worn between exercise sessions, and at night.

Goals
- ▶ Reports of pain to be 5/10 or less with motion, and 2/10 or less at rest.

- ▶ Increase shoulder passive range of motion (PROM) to 70 percent of the uninvolved side. Emphasis throughout the rehabilitation phase should be on the restoration of external rotation, which can be a challenge. A loss of external rotation will affect function more significantly than any other reduction in range.[81] Patients can tolerate a 90-degree loss of glenohumeral elevation, but will have difficulty tolerating more than a 45-degree loss of external rotation without marked functional impairment in activities such as dressing, reaching, and combing hair.[26]

- ▶ Minimize detrimental effects of immobilization.[18–23]

- ▶ Maintain elbow, wrist, and hand motion of the involved extremity.

- ▶ Educate the patient on correct positioning of the involved upper extremity.

Electrotherapeutic and Physical Modalities
- ▶ Cryotherapy using ice packs should be applied frequently throughout the first 1 to 2 days postsurgery to help with pain and inflammation.

- ▶ Pain management also may consist of high-rate, conventional transcutaneous electrical nerve stimulation. With the physician's permission, electrical stimulation also can be used for edema reduction and muscle re-education.[28–31]

- ▶ Moist heat can be applied prior to exercise to encourage relaxation of the shoulder muscles after the first few days. Electrotherapeutic and physical modalities typically are discontinued by the fourth week.[26]

Therapeutic Exercise and Home Program. For a patient with an intact rotator cuff, therapeutic exercise is typically initiated 24 to 48 hours after the surgery and is usually performed twice daily until the PROM is at 140 degrees of passive forward flexion and scapular plane elevation, and 30 to 40 degrees of external rotation (humerus positioned in neutral to 30 degrees of abduction). These exercises may be delayed for approximately 3 weeks if subscapularis reattachment or lengthening was performed.[59] The patient is advised to place a pillow under the humerus, to position it in slight forward flexion, whenever he or she is lying supine.

The exercises during the first 1 to 3 days postsurgery include:

- ▶ *Codman's pendulum exercises.* The patient bends forward at the waist until the thoracic spine is parallel to the floor and the arm hangs freely. By using positions of forearm pronation and supination, the patient induces internal and external rotation at the shoulder. The patient also performs circumduction in a clockwise and counter-clockwise direction by rocking the trunk while allowing the arm to hang freely. Each exercise is performed for 30 to 60 seconds and is repeated every 2 to 3 hours.

- ▶ *Active assistive range of motion (AAROM) of arm elevation in the scapular plane with the patient supine.* The patient grasps the involved wrist with the uninvolved hand, then slowly elevates the arm as high as can be tolerated. At the maximum point in the available range, the position is held for about 5 seconds before the arm is gradually returned to the start position. This exercise is repeated 10 times.

- ▶ *PROM/AAROM external rotation with a cane.* The patient is positioned supine, with a towel roll placed under the elbow (to prevent glenohumeral extension), and the arm positioned in slight abduction. The patient holds a cane in both hands, then gently rotates the involved arm into glenohumeral external rotation. If the subscapularis is divided and repaired, the patient is cautioned against active internal rotation and passive external rotation beyond 35 to 40 degrees. Care must be taken to produce the rotation at the glenohumeral joint and not to merely extend the elbow. The cane should remain in line with the motion, perpendicular to the humerus.[26] At the maximum point in the allowed range, the position is held for about 30 to 60 seconds, before the arms are gradually returned to the start position. This is repeated 10 times. This exercise is progressed, at about the seventh to tenth day, to having the patient standing facing a doorway, with the elbow at 90 degrees and the humerus beside the body. With the palm flat on the doorway, the patient slowly turns the body away, creating an external rotation motion at the glenohumeral joint. At the maximum point in the allowed range, the position is held for about 5 seconds before the arm is gradually returned to the start position. This is repeated 10 times.

- ▶ *Assisted elevation with a pulley (day 5).* The pulley is positioned over a door approximately 1 foot higher than the reach of the uninvolved shoulder, and slightly behind the patient. The patient is in the sitting position, with the back to the door. The patient uses the uninvolved extremity to pull the involved extremity into maximum, but tolerable, elevation. The patient is cautioned against using muscles (supraspinatus and deltoid) to control the descent of the arm. This exercise is performed for 60 to 90 seconds. Pulley exercises are postponed for the first 3 weeks if a rotator cuff repair was part of the procedure.[59]

- ▶ *AAROM into abduction with the patient supine.* The patient is instructed on how to use the uninvolved arm to assist in the elevation of the other arm by intertwining the hand and fingers. The hands are brought over the head and then clasped behind the neck. From this position, the elbows are brought gently down to the table with the patient actively horizontally abducting, followed by horizontally adducting, the shoulder to bring the elbows together. The exercise is performed for 30 to 60 seconds.

▶ *AAROM internal rotation (day 10).* The patient is positioned supine, with both arms as close to 90 degrees of abduction as can be tolerated, with towel rolls under each elbow. Holding a cane with both hands, the patient slowly lowers the cane toward the abdomen, taking care to keep the elbow bent and the cane parallel to the humerus. At the maximum point in the available range, the position is held for about 5 seconds before the arms are gradually returned to the start position. This is repeated 10 times.

▶ *AAROM into horizontal adduction (weeks 3 to 4).* The patient, positioned standing, uses the uninvolved extremity to lift the involved extremity to shoulder height. The patient then pushes the involved extremity across the front of the body, keeping the arm parallel to the floor. At the maximum point in the available range, the position is held for about 5 seconds before the extremity is gradually returned to the start position. This is repeated 10 times

▶ *Gentle isometrics.* Gentle isometrics for internal rotation, external rotation, and abduction in neutral (week 3).

▶ *Exercises to help regain scapular control (week 3).* These exercises include isometric scapular pinches and scapular elevation; gentle closed-chain weight shifts, with hands on table, shoulder flexed less than 60 degrees and abducted less than 45 degrees; scaption exercises; and the use of a tilt board or circular board to perform weight shifts with the same range limitations.[32]

▶ Grip-and-release exercises for the hand, wrist circles, and active pronation and supination of the forearm.

▶ Active flexion and extension of the elbow.

▶ Shoulder circles and gentle shoulder retraction and protraction.

▶ A cardiovascular program of walking or lower extremity cycling.

Manual Therapy. PROM of the involved shoulder is performed in the pain-free ranges.

▶ *Elevation in the scapular plane.* The patient is positioned supine, with the clinician standing on the involved side. The clinician applies a gentle distraction force on the humerus while elevating the patient's arm in the plane of the scapula. At the maximum point in the available range, the position is held for about 5 seconds, before the arm is gradually returned to the start position. This is repeated 10 times.

▶ *External rotation.* The patient is positioned supine, with the arm abducted slightly and supported under the elbow with a towel roll. The clinician stands on the involved side. Keeping the patient's elbow flexed, the clinician passively externally rotates the patient's arm by taking the hand away from the body, while ensuring that the motion occurring is external rotation at the glenohumeral joint. At the maximum point in the available range, the position is held for about 5 seconds, before the arm is gradually returned to the start position. This is repeated 10 times.

Phase 2 (Weeks 4 to 6). This phase typically involves two to four physical therapy sessions.

Goals

▶ ROM at 80 percent compared with the uninvolved side.

▶ Pain to be at 2/10 or less for activities of daily living.

▶ Muscle strength to be at 3+/5 on manual muscle test for shoulder girdle musculature.

▶ Patient to be able to perform functional activities, including combing hair, reaching into a cupboard, or lifting light items above shoulder height.

Therapeutic Exercise and Home Program. Therapeutic exercises include a continuation of PROM until range is at 160 degrees of elevation and 60 degrees of external rotation. Progression to AAROM is also advocated. AROM exercises typically begin by the 6th week postsurgery although this varies. Exercises for this phase typically include:

▶ Strengthening of biceps, triceps, and forearm.

▶ Scapular stabilizer strengthening.

At 6 weeks postsurgery, a stretching program to achieve the remaining 20 degrees of motion in all directions can also be initiated. These exercises include:

▶ *Door frame stretch.* The patient stands in a doorway, with both arms elevated to shoulder height and both hands braced against the door frame with the elbows flexed to 90 degrees so that the humerus is parallel to the floor. The patient then leans forward, which forces the shoulder into external rotation and slight extension. At the maximum point in the available range, the position is held for about 5 seconds, before the patient gradually returns to the start position. This exercise is repeated 10 times.

▶ *AAROM of internal rotation utilizing a door frame, or by positioning the involved arm behind the back.* The patient moves the other arm into extension while keeping the humerus in a sagittal plane, and moves the wrist further up the back. This is progressed to assisted internal rotation using a towel, or a countertop.

▶ *Assisted adduction and posterior capsule stretch.* The patient pulls the involved arm across the torso, under the chin.

There is a considerable difference in opinion as to when strengthening of the rotator cuff should occur, ranging from week 1 to week 12. These discrepancies are a result of the surgical procedure performed. Patients with shoulder replacement for primary osteoarthritis may start strengthening 10 to 14 days after surgery, and stretching may be unnecessary. If the greater tuberosity is salvaged and reattached to the prosthesis, the physician should be consulted prior to initiating eccentric loading. Strengthening exercises, at 4 weeks, include:

▶ Active flexion in the supine position. This is progressed to active assisted elevation to 90 degrees, followed by eccentric anterior deltoid, and supraspinatus, through lowering of the involved arm from 90 to 0 degrees in supine. When the patient is able to perform this exercise supine using 5 lb, the exercise is progressed to being performed in the sitting and standing positions.

▶ *Isometric scapular plane elevation.* The patient faces a wall with the fist against the wall. The patient attempts to flex the arm against the wall, without any movement occurring.

▶ Isometric exercises into abduction, extension, and internal rotation, against a firm surface.

▶ Deltoid strengthening with active abduction in sitting (6 weeks).

▶ Resisted internal rotation with surgical tubing (8 weeks).

▶ Resisted external rotation with surgical tubing (8 weeks).

▶ Rhythmic stabilization.

▶ Introduction of an upper body ergonometer.

Neuromuscular Retraining. At the 4- to 6-week period after the surgery, neuromuscular and proprioceptive retraining are further progressed. Scapular stabilization exercises are initiated, beginning with wall push-ups, then hands-and-knees rocking, then a hands-and-knees push-up.

Manual Therapy
▶ The soft tissue techniques of soft tissue mobilization, myofascial release, and trigger point therapy are applied, as necessary.

Phase 3 (Week 9+)
Goals
▶ Improve shoulder strength and endurance to equal that of the uninvolved side.

▶ Improve functional capacity.

Therapeutic Exercise and Home Program. This phase typically involves a continued progression of previous ROM exercises to restore functional ROM, and strengthening of the deltoid, rotator cuff, and scapular muscles. Elbow flexion and extension strengthening exercises also are progressed. Closed chain exercises are progressed to include therapeutic ball exercises against a wall, wall push-ups, chest presses, and scapular retraction.

Manual Therapy. Joint mobilizations are continued, if necessary, to restore functional ROM.

Procedures Involving the Elbow

Ulnar Collateral Ligament Reconstruction
The anterior oblique band of the ulnar collateral ligament is particularly vulnerable to microtearing, attenuation, weakening, and eventual rupture in throwing sports such as baseball or javelin. Reconstruction of this ligament is one of the most common surgeries performed on the throwing athlete, and centers on the restoration of the anterior oblique band of the ulnar collateral ligament, with the use of an autologous free tendon graft.

Indications
The main indication for surgical intervention is a failure of conservative measures in a well-motivated athlete. Additional considerations include patient age, activity level, job requirements, general health, and general integrity of the uninvolved elbow.[59,82,83]

Procedure
The detached ulnar collateral ligament is reattached to its point of origin or insertion. Posterior olecranon osteophytes, if present, are removed, and bone holes are drilled in the humerus and ulna, resulting in trauma to the bone. Depending on the type of surgery, the iliotibial band, palmaris longus tendon, or plantaris tendon can be used as the graft.[84] The ulnar nerve typically is mobilized and transposed during the procedure, which can result in neurologic symptoms after the surgery. Following surgery, the elbow typically is immobilized in a posterior splint for 7 to 10 days at 90 degrees of flexion, in neutral rotation,[84] or in a bulky dressing.

Postsurgical Rehabilitation
Only the surgeon knows the extent of soft tissue damage and repair, and the guidelines communicated to the clinician must be strongly adhered to.

Phase 1 (0 to 3 Weeks). This phase typically involves one to four physical therapy sessions.

Goals
▶ Protect healing tissue.

▶ Promote scar mobilization.

▶ Reports of pain to be at 5/10 or less with motion, 2/10 or less at rest.

▶ Increase elbow active range of motion (AROM) to 70 percent of the uninvolved side. Emphasis throughout the rehabilitation phase should be on the restoration of elbow extension, although the elbow should not extend beyond 20 degrees in the first 2 weeks.

▶ Minimize detrimental effects of immobilization.[18–23]

▶ Maintain shoulder, wrist, and hand motion of the involved extremity.

Electrotherapeutic and Physical Modalities
▶ Cryotherapy, using ice packs, should be applied frequently throughout the day to help with pain and inflammation.

▶ Moist heat can be applied 2 to 3 days after the surgery and prior to exercise to encourage relaxation of the muscles, and to increase the extensibility of the joint capsule. Thermal modalities typically are discontinued by the fourth week.[26]

▶ With the physician's permission, electrical stimulation can be used for edema reduction, muscle re-education, and pain control.[28–31]

Therapeutic Exercise and Home Program

▶ Codman's exercises for the shoulder. The patient bends forward at the waist until the thoracic spine is parallel to the floor and the arm hangs freely. The patient performs circumduction in a clockwise and counter-clockwise direction by rocking the trunk and allowing the arm to hang freely. Each exercise is performed for 30 to 60 seconds.

▶ Gentle grip-and-release exercises for the hand, wrist circles, and AROM of wrist and hand during the first week. These are repeated 10 times.

▶ AROM exercises of the elbow, within the guidelines, are started at 10 days postsurgery.[83]

▶ Wrist isometrics, typically initiated by week 2.

▶ Shoulder submaximal isometrics, except internal and external rotation; shoulder shrugs; and gentle shoulder retraction.

▶ Very gentle elbow flexion-extension isometrics initiated by week 2.

▶ Application of functional brace (week 2) with a range-of-motion (ROM) limitation from 30 to 100 degrees of elbow motion. The brace is advanced to 15 to 110 degrees by week 3, and increased thereafter at 5 degrees of extension and 10 degrees of flexion per week, so that at week 6, full ROM (0 to 145 degrees) should be achieved.[85]

▶ A cardiovascular program of walking or lower extremity cycling.

Manual Therapy. Passive range of motion (PROM) is performed in the pain-free ranges.

Phase 2 (Weeks 4 to 8). This phase typically involves 4 to 12 physical therapy sessions.

Goals

▶ Gradual increase in AROM to 100 percent, compared with the uninvolved side by week 6.

▶ Reports of pain to be at 2/10 or less for activities of daily living.

▶ Muscle strength to be at 3+/5 on manual muscle test for elbow musculature.

▶ Patient to be able to perform functional activities, combing hair, reaching into a cupboard, or lifting light items to shoulder height.

Therapeutic Exercise and Home Program

▶ The elbow AROM exercises are progressed until the elbow ROM is normal.

▶ At 6 weeks, unrestricted PROM exercises for the elbow are initiated.

▶ Light resistance progressive resisted exercises (PREs) of wrist curls, wrist extension, pronation, and supination. Elbow flexion and extension PREs are initiated at 6 to 8 weeks postsurgery, depending on tissue response and the stage of healing. These exercises are progressed as tolerated.

▶ Progression of shoulder strengthening, emphasizing strength of rotator cuff and scapular stabilizers.[84] Moderate strengthening of the internal or external rotators should be avoided until the 6th to 12th week, because of the valgus stresses placed on the elbow during these exercises.

▶ At week 6, the functional brace is set at 0 to 130 degrees. At this point, the patient's AROM should be 0 to 145 degrees.[85] The functional brace is usually discontinued by week 8.[84]

Manual Therapy

▶ The soft tissue techniques of soft tissue mobilization, myofascial release, and trigger point therapy are applied, as necessary.

▶ Joint mobilizations of grades I and II can be used for relief of any residual pain, with grades III and IV being applied to specific areas of hypomobility to restore normal arthrokinematics.

Phase 3 (Weeks 9 to 13)
Goals

▶ Improve upper extremity strength, endurance, and power to equal that of the uninvolved side.

▶ Maintain full AROM of elbow.

▶ Improve functional capacity.

▶ Achieve gradual initiation of sports-specific activities as appropriate.

Therapeutic Exercise and Home Program. This phase typically involves a continued progression of previous ROM and strengthening exercises to restore functional ROM, and strength of the shoulder, elbow, and wrist musculature.

▶ Eccentric exercises for elbow flexors and extensors.

▶ Isotonic exercises for forearm and wrist.

▶ Thrower's Ten program[85] for shoulder (see Chap. 14) for pitchers.

▶ Closed-chain exercises, to include therapeutic ball exercises against a wall, wall push-ups, biomechanical ankle platform system (BAPS) board exercises, Fitter board exercises (see Chap. 10), and chest presses and pulls.

▶ Plyometric exercises with a medicine ball.

▶ Light sporting activities by week 11.[85]

Manual Therapy

▶ Joint mobilizations are continued, if necessary, to restore functional ROM.

▶ Manual resistance of proprioceptive neuromuscular facilitation patterns at the shoulder and elbow are incorporated to increase strength in the functional planes.[86]

▶ Stretching and flexibility techniques are used to restore, or maintain, full elbow, shoulder, and wrist ROM.[84]

Phase 4: Return to Sport. Refer to Chapter 15.

Procedures Involving the Forearm, Wrist, and Hand

Flexor Tendon Repair

One of the main purposes of the hand is to grasp; therefore, the loss of flexor tendons imposes a catastrophic functional loss.[87] The purpose of a flexor tendon repair is to restore maximum active flexor tendon gliding to ensure effective finger joint motion.

Most flexor tendon ruptures occur silently after prolonged inflammatory tenosynovitis, although the causes also can be traumatic. When all nine flexor tendons to the digits have ruptured, little can be done. Single tendon ruptures are more common, and the flexor pollicis longus tendon is the most vulnerable to attrition rupture where it crosses the scaphotrapezial joint, and where local synovitis can create a sharp spike of bone that abrades against this spur and ruptures during use. The flexor digitorum profundus (FDP) tendon to the index finger also is at risk from this bony spur.[88]

Tendon injuries are classified into five zones, according to the level of injury. The zone within which the tendon is repaired dictates to some extent the intervention.

▶ *Zone 1.* This zone extends from the insertion of the FDP in the middle phalanx to that of the flexor digitorum superficialis (FDS) in the base of the distal phalanx. Injuries at this level involve isolated lacerations of the FDS.

▶ *Zone 2.* This is the region in which both flexor tendons travel within the fibro-osseous tunnel from the A1 pulley (see Fig. 28-1) to the FDP insertion. Usually, both flexor tendons are injured at this level.

▶ *Zone 3.* The area in the palm between the distal border of the carpal tunnel and the proximal border of the A1 pulley comprises zone 3. Common digital nerves and vessels, lumbrical muscles, and one or both flexor tendons may be injured in this region.

▶ *Zone 4.* This zone consists of that segment of the flexor tendons covered by the transverse carpal ligament. Injuries at this level involve median or ulnar nerves and tendons.

▶ *Zone 5.* The forearm from the musculotendonous junction of the extrinsic flexors to the proximal border of the transverse

carpal ligament comprises zone 5. Interference with tendon gliding is less of a problem in this region.

Indications

The indications for a tendon surgical repair are normally based on the level of functional loss.

Procedure

There are a number of different procedures and rehabilitation protocols for flexor tendon repairs. In brief, the retracted ends of the tendon are retrieved either by hand and wrist positioning or with a surgical instrument. Although it is not within the scope of this text to discuss suturing techniques, it is important to mention that several suturing methods have been found to withstand an early active mobilization protocol such as the one presented here. They include the Savage, Silfverskiold (modified Kirchmayer or modified Kessler),[89,90] Tang,[91] Robertson,[92] and cruciate[93] methods. In all of these methods, the anatomic relationship between the FDS and the FDP is maintained.

Postsurgical Rehabilitation

The rate of tendon healing depends on adequate nutrition (through vascular and synovial fluid perfusion), the part of the tendon affected, and the presence of the vinculum.

Early postoperative protected mobilization of repaired tendons was popularly adopted as the postoperative treatment protocol after tendon repair.[94–100]

However, in recent years, based on an improved understanding of connective tissue physiology and the success achieved with other types of surgical repairs, various active mobilization protocols have been attempted to obtain better function of repaired tendons.[97,98,101] It has been demonstrated that active mobilizations of the tendons are a more effective way to increase excursion and decrease adhesions of repaired tendons.[101–106] In addition, the tension added to the repaired tendon by active mobilization seems to help initiate proliferation of the tenocytes, and increase the rate of collagen synthesis of the repaired tendon, thereby enhancing the tendon healing process.[107,108]

However, care must be taken when prescribing active mobilization exercises, because active finger motion generates far more tension in the flexor tendons (1 to 29 newtons [N]) than passive motion of the tendons (1 to 9 N), and 15 to 50 N against moderate or maximum resistance.[109,110] Considering the resistance of the sheath during tendon gliding and a decrease in suture strength during the initial weeks after repair, most investigators believe that sufficient suture strength is vital to the performance of gentle or moderate active finger motion.[89,92,93]

Researchers have shown that early mobilization can prevent the formation of scar tissue without jeopardizing tendon healing, and they have developed many different forms of early mobilization programs.[111] Kleinert and colleagues introduced a program of early controlled motion after flexor tendon repair using a dorsal splint with a rubber-band traction device and early active extension of the digit against the tension of the passive rubber-band flexion.[112] In the original Kleinert protocol,

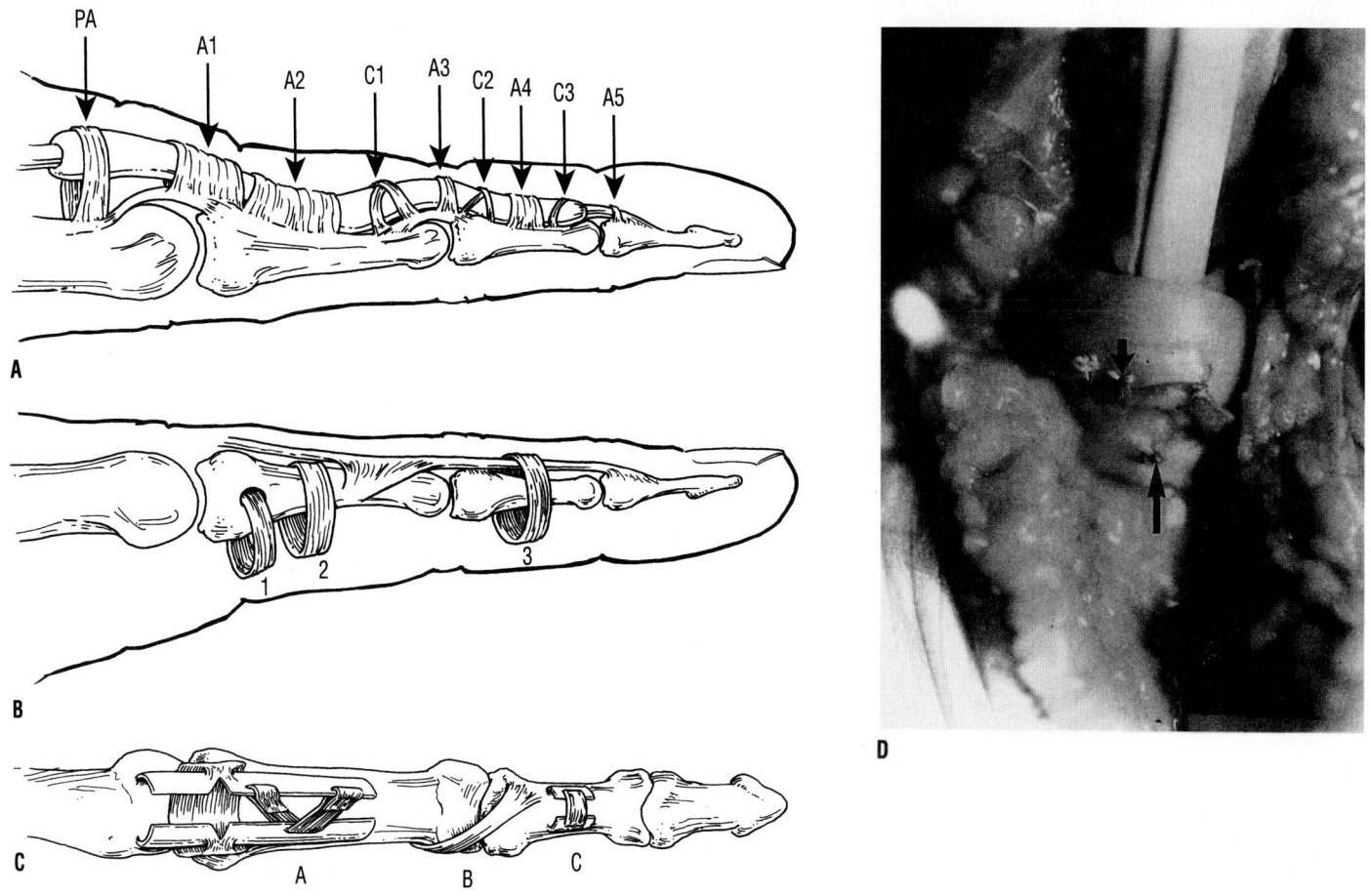

FIGURE 28-1 *A.* The positions of the annular (A) and cruciate (C) pulleys are marked. In addition to the classic pulleys of the fibro-osseous sheath, the palmar aponeurotic pulley (PA) must be taken into consideration *B.* Methods of A2 and A4 pulley reconstruction. *C.* Reconstruction of the pulleys using the residual rim of the flexor sheath is Illustrated. *D.* An A2 pulley reconstruction using a tendon graft wrapped around the proximal phalanx. (Reproduced with permission from Herndon JH. *Surgical Reconstruction of the Upper Extremity.* Stamford Conn: Appleton and Lange; 1999.)

the dorsal protective splint blocked the wrist at 45 degrees of flexion and the metacarpophalangeal (MCP) joints at 10 to 20 degrees. More recent adaptations to the protocol splint the wrist in 10 to 30 degrees of wrist flexion, 40 to 60 degrees of MCP flexion, and full extension at the interphalangeal (IP) joint. Dynamic traction, provided by rubber bands connected between fingertips and volar aspects of the wrist, maintains the involved digits in flexion to further relax the tendon and prevent inadvertent active flexion.[113] The patient actively extends the fingers to the limits of the splint and then relaxes, so that the tension in the rubber bands returns the fingers to their previous flexed position.

Until recently, this technique was well accepted and was subjected to several modifications.[111,114–116] The most important change was the introduction of a palmar pulley by Slattery and McGrouther.[115] This application redirects the line of the pull into the palm to increase distal interphalangeal (DIP) joint motion, minimizing adhesions, and allowing differential gliding of FDS and FDP tendons.[113] However, one of the complications of the Kleinert traction splint can be the development of

permanent flexion contracture of the IP joints, because the traction places the proximal interphalangeal (PIP) joint in 60 to 90 degrees of flexion.[117] Even the addition to the Kleinert protocol of passive motion to the IP joints only slightly reduces the incidence of this complication, from 29 to 40 percent to 24 percent.[104,118]

Thus, the more recent protocols have advocated the removal of the traction from the intervention. Several postsurgical protocols and modifications exist, based on individual characteristics, the zone involved, the suture strength, and physician preferences. The modified Duran program, which emphasizes early passive mobilization, and the early activation-tenodesis protocols are presented here; both approaches commonly are used after a surgical repair to zones I to III. Whichever protocol is used, a dorsal blocking splint is fitted for continual wear, which positions the wrist and hand in 20 degrees of wrist flexion, 70 degrees of MCP flexion, and full extension of the PIPs and DIPs. If a nerve repair is involved, the IP joints may be flexed to 10 degrees, depending on the tension on the nerve repair. The splint is worn with the IP joints free during the day at all times except for hand hygiene and physical therapy sessions.[119] At night, the IP joints are held in neutral with Velcro straps. The passive range of motion (PROM) exercises are initiated within the restraints of the dorsal blocking splint every 2 hours throughout the day.

In the active mobilization protocol, a tenodesis splint is fitted, using a dynamic hinge to serve as the wrist component. The tenodesis splint allows full wrist flexion, while limiting wrist extension to a maximum of 30 degrees, MCP flexion to 70 degrees, and IP joints to neutral. The PROM exercises are performed within the dorsal blocking splint and the tenodesis exercises are continued within the confines of the tenodesis splint. At approximately 3 weeks postsurgery, the parameters of the splint are changed to place the wrist in neutral, and the MCPs in 40 to 50 degrees of flexion.

Both splints typically are discontinued at 4 to 5 weeks postsurgery.

Phase 1 (Day 5 to 3 Weeks). This phase typically involves four to six physical therapy sessions. The sutures typically are removed 10 to 14 days after the surgery.

Goals

▶ Stabilize and protect the surgical site with proper use of splints.

▶ Decrease edema to within 50 percent of the uninvolved side.

▶ Encourage tendon gliding.

▶ Increase PROM of all digits to 80 percent of normal, compared with the uninvolved side, while preventing tendon rupture.

▶ Decrease scar density.

▶ Minimize detrimental effects of immobilization, including flexion contractures.[18–23]

▶ Maintain full range of motion of all uninvolved joints of the involved upper extremity.

▶ Promote independent self-care within the limits of postsurgical restrictions.

Therapeutic Exercise. Based on the observation that 3 to 5 mm of tendon excursion is necessary to prevent adhesion formation, and that active extension of IP joints has been shown to successfully reduce the development of flexion contracture,[113,120,121] the following exercise protocol is recommended.

None of the exercises should result in an increase in pain, edema, or stiffness.

▶ Early controlled and protected passive extension exercises of the PIP and DIP joints.[113]

▶ Passive flexion exercises, performed by the patients themselves on involved and uninvolved digits, are performed for isolated MCP, PIP, and DIP flexion followed by full passive flexion of these three joints.

▶ Passive IP extension is followed by active extension of the IP joints within the splint at about 3 to 4 weeks postsurgery, if permitted by the physician, with the MCP joint held at 90 degrees of flexion to avoid excessive tension on the repair site.[113] Neuromuscular electrical stimulation may be added after the patient has been performing active flexion exercises for 3 to 5 days.

▶ Passive closing of the fist is initiated, followed by active extension, if permitted by the physician.

All passive exercises are repeated 10 times, and each position is held for 5 seconds. Patients are instructed to keep the hand and limb elevated for edema control, and not to actively flex the involved digit or digits.

If the patient is placed on the early activation-tenodesis protocol, the following exercises can be performed, in the absence of swelling, within 72 hours after the surgery:

▶ Place and hold fisting exercises, if permitted by the physician. Place and hold exercises involve having the patient press the finger or fingers passively into full flexion with the uninvolved hand. Then, on releasing the pressure of the uninvolved hand, the patient attempts to hold the flexed position of the fingers. Place and hold fisting is the least stressful active motion for the tendon.

▶ Short arc active flexion and extension exercises. The patient is asked to actively bring the digits to the tips of the opposed thumb, then actively extend the digits (with the wrist positioned in neutral or out of the splint).

At the beginning of the third week, the patient begins active fist making with the wrist in neutral (the FDP has the greatest excursion in this position). In addition, the patient begins active hook fist exercises with the wrist positioned in 40 to 45 degrees of flexion to produce differential gliding between the FDS and FDP.

Manual Therapy. Manual therapy techniques are not initiated until 2 weeks postsurgery, following suture removal. They include soft tissue techniques of:

▶ Retrograde massage for edema reduction.

▶ Soft tissue mobilization.

▶ Scar massage.

Phase 2 (Weeks 4 to 6). This phase typically involves four to six physical therapy sessions. Between the fourth and fifth weeks, the dorsal splint is removed. The splint application for patients with median or ulnar nerve injuries, or both, typically is continued for 6 weeks.[113]

Goals

▶ Wrist and hand PROM to be within normal limits compared with the uninvolved side.

▶ Edema to be within 25 percent or less of uninvolved side.

▶ Decreased scar density.

▶ Reports of pain to be at 3/10 or less with activity, and 0/10 at rest.

Therapeutic Exercise. Patients are instructed to avoid simultaneous wrist and finger extension during this phase.

Passive exercises are continued after removal of the splint, as in phase 1, with the wrist positioned in approximately 10 degrees of extension. The tendon glide is assessed. If less than 50 degrees of difference exists between total active motion and total passive motion, the preceding intervention continues until 6 weeks postsurgery. If more than 50 degrees of difference between total active motion and total passive motion exists, the following exercises are added:

▶ Active straight fisting with the wrist in neutral.

▶ Gentle passive PIP extension, with MCPs and wrist slightly flexed. This is progressed to PIP extension, with the wrist in neutral, and with only the MCPs flexed. This "shelf" position allows increased tendon excursion into the palm.

By the fourth week, depending on where the tendon was lacerated and repaired, the following exercises should be added:

▶ Isolated tendon excursion exercises. For these exercises, the patient is instructed to flex the IPs while actively extending the MCPs, and then to extend the digits.

▶ Active wrist flexion.

▶ Gradual increase of wrist extension with the digits held in flexion (blocking exercises).

▶ Light passive IP stretching exercises.

Manual Therapy
▶ The soft tissue techniques of soft tissue mobilization and transverse friction massage may be applied to the scars.

▶ Joint mobilization with grades III to V can be used for hypomobility in the carpal and MCP joints (see Chap. 16).

Phase 3 (Weeks 6 to 12)
Goals
▶ Active range of motion (AROM) of digit and thumb to be within 80 percent of normal compared with the uninvolved side.

▶ Demonstrate independence with activities of daily living (ADLs) and vocational function.

▶ Return to presurgical unrestricted activity level.

Therapeutic Exercise. At 6 weeks postsurgery, the tendon glide is assessed. If the tendon glide is improving, the preceding program is maintained. If there is no increase in active motion, the following exercises are added:

▶ Sustained gripping.

▶ Hand helper with one rubber band.

▶ Putty scraping using fingers.

▶ Use of heavier putty (progressing from very light to light or medium).

At the seventh week, the patient should begin light resistance for prehensile activities with a gradual progression. These activities can include foam gripping, and therapeutic putty, with the patient using stroking motions, and gradually increasing the intensity.[119]

At the eighth week, the patient's PROM should be within normal limits, compared with the uninvolved side. However, the patient must avoid heavy resistance activities until the 12th week, at which time heavy resistance exercise, and use of the hand in all ADLs, is usually permitted.

At about 10 to 12 weeks, the patient is permitted to resume use of the hand for light ADLs, such as using a spoon, tying laces, and brushing teeth. Heavy and sustained lifting and tight gripping should be avoided for approximately 14 to 16 weeks. Additional exercises are introduced:

▶ Active prehensile tasks with light resistance, such as the nine-hole pegboard.

▶ Active IP and MCP flexion exercises of increasing intensity, with MCP blocking occurring with IP flexion, except to the small finger FDP because of the diameter and poor blood supply to this tendon.

Manual Therapy
▶ The soft tissue techniques of soft tissue mobilization and transverse friction massage are continued, as appropriate.

▶ Joint mobilizations are used for any joints in which hypomobility persists.

Carpal Tunnel Release

Carpal tunnel syndrome (CTS) is by far the most common type of peripheral nerve entrapment and is a significant cause of morbidity. CTS prevalence in general population has been estimated at 3.8 percent.[122] Conservative intervention for CTS typically involves activity modification, wrist splints, anti-inflammatory or analgesic medications (or both), and, occasionally, injections of corticosteroids into the carpal canal (see Chap. 16).

Indications

Patients with CTS who do not improve with conservative measures often are referred for surgical decompression of the carpal tunnel. Approximately 250,000 to 300,000 carpal tunnel releases are performed annually in the United States.[123] The surgery is reported to relieve symptoms in 70 to 90 percent of patients.[124–126]

Procedure

Various surgical techniques are available for the carpal tunnel release. However, there has been considerable discussion about which method is the most effective. The technique can be endoscopic or open, with the former being used more commonly recently. The advantages of the endoscopic technique is that it offers decreased scar formation, and the ability to avoid an incision directly over the carpal tunnel between the thenar and hypothenar muscles, which is a sensitive region of the hand.[127]

Whichever technique is used, a carpal tunnel release generally involves a division of the transverse carpal ligament, thereby increasing the tunnel volume[128] and reducing the compression of the median nerve.[129] In the presence of thenar muscle atrophy, constant loss of sensibility along the median nerve distribution, and severe pain, an internal neurolysis may be performed in addition to the carpal tunnel release.

Following carpal tunnel release procedures, a bulky dressing is applied immediately after surgery, which is changed to a smaller dressing after several days.[127] The patient may be fitted with a splint to keep the wrist in slight extension, but leaving the metacarpophalangeal (MCP) and interphalangeal (IP) joints free. If used, the splint remains in place for approximately 10 days. It has been proposed that the positioning of the splint may be associated with differential outcomes,[130] although studies have demonstrated no significant difference in outcome between patients treated with and without immobilization after surgery.[131]

Postsurgical Rehabilitation

The postsurgical rehabilitation for carpal tunnel release is highly variable. In addition to the typical examination described for the postsurgical examination (see Section IV introduction), the clinician must also assess:

▶ *Finger dexterity.* Finger dexterity typically is examined using a nine-hole pegboard, and a score is recorded for the amount of time in seconds it takes the patient to put the nine pegs into the board, one at a time, compared with the uninvolved hand or with the established norms.[132]

▶ *Grip strength.* Grip strength may be measured anywhere from 3 to 6 weeks postsurgery, using a dynamometer with the handle positioned at the second setting.[133,134] The patient is seated with the shoulder adducted, in neutral rotation, the elbow flexed to 90 degrees, and the forearm in neutral position and unsupported.[135] Three grip measurements are taken and documented and compared with the established norms.[136]

▶ *Pinch strength.* A pinch meter is used about 3 weeks after surgery to measure two types of pinch, the three-point pinch and the lateral pinch, and the measurements are recorded and compared with the established norms.[136]

▶ *Sensibility.* Sensibility is assessed using the Semmes-Weinstein Pressure Esthesiometer Kit (see Chap. 16).

▶ *Neural tension.* Upper limb tension testing of the median nerve is appropriate to assess for neural adhesions (see Chap. 12).

Phase 1 (Weeks 0 to 3). This phase typically involves three to six physical therapy sessions.

Goals

▶ Reports of pain to be 3/10 or less with activity, and 0/10 at rest.

▶ Protect incision and prevent infection or postsurgical complications.

▶ Manage edema.

▶ Minimize detrimental effects of immobilization.[18–23]

▶ Wrist range of motion (ROM) to be within 80 percent of normal compared with the uninvolved side.

▶ Maintain elbow and shoulder ROM of the involved side.

Electrotherapeutic and Physical Modalities

▶ Cryotherapy can be used to help with pain and inflammation, as can the athermal and deep thermal modalities. These modalities also are used to increase elasticity of tissues, decrease co-contraction, and promote tissue healing.[24,25]

▶ Phonophoresis, iontophoresis, and high-voltage galvanic stimulation can all be used to reduce local swelling and pain.[24,25]

▶ Transcutaneous electrical nerve stimulation (TENS) is not recommended for pain management in these cases because it may irritate the median nerve and heighten pain.

Therapeutic Exercise

▶ The patient performs active range of motion (AROM) of shoulder, elbow, and forearm in all planes.

▶ The patient is instructed in tendon gliding exercises to prevent adhesions of the tendons and nerves,[137–140] as follows:

• IP flexion or "hook fist."

• Straight fingers, wrist in neutral.

• Table top wrist extension.

• MCP flexion, followed by proximal interphalangeal (PIP) flexion, "straight fist."

• Full fisting, active assisted and gentle.

▶ The patient performs thumb flexion, extension, and opposition.

▶ The patient performs digit abduction and adduction.

Once the sutures are removed after 10 to 14 days, the patient can progress to AROM exercises of the wrist, including extension, radial deviation, and ulnar deviation. One study[141] looked at the effects of splinting versus ROM exercises following carpal tunnel release and reported significantly fewer days away from work, fewer days to resume activities of daily living, and significantly less pain in patients who received unrestricted ROM hand exercises compared with those who received splints.

Wrist flexion usually is avoided until at least 3 weeks after the surgery to prevent bowstringing of the flexor tendons through the healing carpal ligament. Strengthening of the forearm, elbow, and shoulder girdle is initiated on the 28th day after surgery.

By the third to sixth week, the patient should be performing gentle strengthening with a foam ball or therapeutic putty, and isometrics in the neutral wrist position, for wrist extension and flexion.[142] Strengthening exercises are not initiated if significant pain or moderate amounts of edema persist.

Sensory Retraining. The patient performs sensory retraining through scar desensitization once the surgical incision is closed. This can include manual self-massage of the scar or the use of a mini-vibrator, gripping of different textured materials, and rubbing the scar with different textured materials.[143] Fluidotherapy and rice gripping also can be used.

Manual Therapy. The following soft tissue techniques are advocated:

▶ Soft tissue mobilization of the thenar eminence.

▶ Gentle friction massage to reduce scar adhesion to tendons, skin, and nerves following suture removal, usually after 2 weeks.

▶ Manual lymphatic drainage using a light retrograde massage.

Therapeutic Devices and Equipment

▶ A scar conformer can be fabricated, which will be worn by the patient at night for about 3 months. The patient also must be educated to inspect the scar daily for signs of irritation, skin maceration, or heat rash, and to inform the clinician if they occur.

▶ A customized or prefabricated wrist splint is worn at night and during strenuous activity to maintain the wrist in the neutral position.

Functional Activities. The patient should be encouraged to use the involved hand for self-care, while avoiding wrist flexion, forceful or repetitive gripping, and lifting more than 4 lb.

Phase 2 (Weeks 4 to 6). This phase typically involves four to six physical therapy sessions and focuses on strengthening and education.

Goals

▶ Achieve 100 percent of ROM for wrist and thumb compared with the uninvolved side.

▶ Reports of pain to be at 3/10 or less.

▶ Decrease sensitivity of scar, and increase scar mobility.

▶ Resolve edema in fingers.

▶ Grip strength to be at approximately 15 lb by the sixth week after surgery.

▶ Prehensile motor performance (grip and pinch) to be at 90 percent of uninvolved hand using nine-hole peg test.

▶ Absence of any scar adhesion.

▶ Patient to be able to make a full fist to distal IP crease.

▶ Patient to be able to lift and carry 3 to 5 lb with involved hand.

Electrotherapeutic and Physical Modalities. Moist heat is applied before the exercises, and ice is applied after the intervention sessions.

Therapeutic Exercise. Exercises during this phase include a continuation of the exercises in phase 1, as follows:

▶ The isometric exercises initiated in phase 1 are progressed to isotonic strengthening, avoiding specific strengthening in radial deviation to prevent tenosynovitis of the abductor pollicis longus and brevis.

▶ Specific median nerve-gliding exercises are initiated. Each of the following exercises is maintained for 7 seconds and repeated five times each session:

  • The wrist are in neutral, with the fingers and thumb in flexion.

  • The wrist is in neutral, with the fingers and thumb extended.

  • The wrist and fingers are extended, with the thumb in neutral.

  • The wrist, fingers, and thumb are extended.

  • The wrist, fingers, and thumb are extended, with the forearm supinated.

  • The wrist, fingers, and thumb are extended, with the forearm supinated, and the other hand gently stretches the thumb.

▶ Resisted gripping with light resistive therapeutic putty can begin 3 to 6 weeks after the surgery, limited to two 3-minute sessions every day.[127] The progression of the putty grade is determined by motor performance and pinch assessment results.

▶ Progressive resisted exercises of the wrist flexors and extensors are added when pain is controlled.[142] Resistance begins with ½ lb, and is progressed to 5 lb, as tolerated.

Manual Therapy

▶ Joint mobilizations include anteroposterior glides of the distal radius and proximal carpal row, mobilizations of the distal radioulnar joint, and scaphoid distractions.

▶ Soft tissue techniques include scar massage to reduce adhesions.

▶ Passive stretching is performed into thumb abduction and wrist extension.

▶ The previously described median nerve glides are performed with the patient supine, the shoulder abducted to

110 degrees, the forearm supinated, and the elbow, wrist, and fingers extended.

▶ Upper extremity proprioceptive neuromuscular facilitation patterns are performed gently, focusing on the hand component.

Functional Activities. Work simulation activities are initiated using minimal torque and progressing as tolerated. The patient is educated about workstation setup as appropriate (see Table 23-8). Patients who are involved in repetitive activities at work should be advised to perform their activities with the wrist positioned in neutral.

Phase 3 (Weeks 6 to 12). This phase typically involves two to three physical therapy sessions.

Goals
▶ Prehensile (grip and pinch) motor performance to be at 100 percent compared with the other side.

▶ Patient to have adequate strength to return to work activities full time.

▶ Patient to be independent with self-management of symptoms.

Therapeutic Exercise. The exercises of phase are continued and progressed as tolerated. Large muscle group exercises using the full kinetic chains are recommended in this phase.

REVIEW QUESTIONS*

1. What are some of the surgical procedures that can be used to treat instability of the shoulder?
2. What are some of the purported advantages for arthroscopic surgical techniques over the open repair techniques?
3. The period of immobilization following shoulder surgery depends on the procedure. The position of immobilization also varies according to the procedure. Which position is the shoulder immobilized in following an anterior stabilization procedure?
4. True or false: A progressive cardiovascular program can be initiated in the very early stages following upper extremity surgery.
5. An acromioplasty is typically performed on which group of patients?

---

* Additional questions to test your understanding of this chapter can be found in the Online Learning Center for *Orthopaedic Assessment, Evaluation, and Intervention* at www.duttononline.net.

REFERENCES

1. Duthie R, Bentley G, eds. *Mercer's Orthopedic Surgery.* 8th ed. Baltimore, Md: University Park Press; 1983:886–890.
2. Jobe FW, Moynes DR, Brewster CE. Rehabilitation of shoulder joint instabilities. *Orthop Clin North Am* 1987;18:473–482.
3. Jobe CM, et al. Anterior shoulder instability, impingement and rotator cuff tear. In: Jobe FW, ed. *Operative Techniques in Upper Extremity Sports Injuries.* St Louis, Mo: Mosby-Year Book; 1996:164–272.
4. Jobe FW, Glousman RE. Anterior capsulolabral reconstruction. In: Paulos LE, Tibone JE, eds. *Operative Technique in Shoulder Surgery.* Gaithersburg, Md: Aspen; 1992:65–90.
5. DePalma AF. *Surgery of the Shoulder.* 2nd ed. Philadelphia, Pa: Lippincott: 1973.
6. Jackson D, Einhorn A. Rehabilitation of the shoulder. In: Jackson DW, ed. *Shoulder Surgery in the Athlete.* Rockville, Md: Aspen; 1985:69–87.
7. Burkhead WZ Jr, Rockwood CA Jr. Treatment of instability of the shoulder with an exercise program. *J Bone Joint Surg* 1992; 74A:890–896.
8. Hawkins RJ, Koppert G, Johnston G. Recurrent posterior instability (subluxation) of the shoulder. *J Bone Joint Surg* 1984; 66A:169–174.
9. Jobe FW, et al. The shoulder in sports. In: Rockwood CA Jr, Matsen FA III, eds. *The Shoulder.* Philadelphia, Pa: Saunders; 1990:963–967.
10. Matsen FA, Harryman DT, Sidles JA. Mechanics of glenohumeral instability. *Clin Sports Med* 1991;10:783–788.
11. Wirth MA, Groh GI, Rockwood CA Jr. Capsulorrhaphy through an anterior approach for the treatment of atraumatic posterior glenohumeral instability with multidirectional laxity of the shoulder. *J Bone Joint Surg* 1998;80A:1570–1578.
12. McIntyre LF, Caspari RB, Savoie FH III. The arthroscopic treatment of multidirectional shoulder instability: Two-year results of a multiple suture technique. *Arthroscopy* 1997;13: 418–425.
13. Gartsman GM, Roddey TS, Hammerman SM. Arthroscopic treatment of anterior-inferior glenohumeral instability. Two to five-year follow-up. *J Bone Joint Surg* 2000;82A:991–1003.
14. Wong KL, Williams GR. Complications of thermal capsulorrhaphy of the shoulder. *J Bone Joint Surg* 2001;83A:151–155.
15. Anderson K, et al. Risk factors for early failure after thermal capsulorrhaphy. *Am J Sports Med* 2002;30:103–107.
16. Savoie FH, Field LD. Thermal versus suture treatment of symptomatic capsular laxity. *Clin Sports Med* 2000;19:63–75.
17. Montgomery WH III, Jobe FW. Functional outcomes in athletes after modified anterior capsulolabral reconstruction. *Am J Sports Med* 1994;22:352–358.
18. Booth FW. Physiologic and biochemical effects of immobilization on muscle. *Clin Orthop Rel Res* 1987;219:15–21.
19. Eiff MP, Smith AT, Smith GE. Early mobilization versus immobilization in the treatment of lateral ankle sprains. *Am J Sports Med* 1994;22:83–88.
20. Akeson WH, et al. Collagen cross-linking alterations in the joint contractures: Changes in the reducible cross-links in periarticular connective tissue after 9 weeks immobilization. *Connect Tissue Res* 1977;5:15.
21. Akeson WH, et al. Effects of immobilization on joints. *Clin Orthop* 1987;219:28–37.
22. Akeson WH, Amiel D, Woo SLY. Immobility effects on synovial joints: The pathomechanics of joint contracture. *Biorheology* 1980;17:95–110.
23. Woo SLY, et al. Connective tissue response to immobility: A correlative study of biochemical and biomechanical measurements of normal and immobilized rabbit knee. *Arthritis Rheum* 1975; 18:257–264.

24. Haralson K. Physical modalities. In: Banwell BF, Gall V, eds. *Physical Therapy Management of Arthritis.* New York, NY: Churchill Livingstone; 1987:98–108.

25. Marino M. Principles of therapeutic modalities: Implications for sports medicine. In: Nicholas JA, Hershman EB, eds. *The Lower Extremity and Spine in Sports Medicine.* St Louis, Mo: CV Mosby; 1986:195–244.

26. Brown DD, Friedman RJ. Postoperative rehabilitation following total shoulder arthroplasty. *Orthop Clin North Am* 1998; 29:535–547.

27. Kibler WB, Livingston B, Bruce R. Current concepts in shoulder rehabilitation. *Adv Op Orthop* 1996;3:249–301.

28. Goth RS, et al. Electrical stimulation effect on extensor lag and length of hospital stay after total knee arthroplasty. *Arch Phys Med Rehabil* 1994;75:957.

29. Lamboni P, Harris B. The use of ice, air splints, and high voltage galvanic stimulation in effusion reduction. *Athl Training* 1983;18:23–25.

30. McMiken DF, Todd-Smith M, Thompson C. Strengthening of human quadriceps muscles by cutaneous electrical stimulation. *Scand J Rehabil Med* 1983;15:25–28.

31. Walker RH, et al. Postoperative use of continuous passive motion, transcutaneous electrical nerve stimulation, and continuous cooling pad following total knee arthroplasty. *J Arthroplasty* 1991;6:151–156.

32. Kibler WB. Shoulder rehabilitation: principles and practice. *Med Sci Sports Exerc* 1998;30:40–50.

33. Jobe FW, Bradley JP. The diagnosis and nonoperative treatment of shoulder injuries in athletes. *Clin Sports Med* 1989; 8:419–439.

34. Neer CS II. Anterior acromioplasty for the chronic impingement syndrome in the shoulder: A preliminary report. *J Bone Joint Surg* 1972;54A:41–50.

35. Gohlke F, Essigkrug B, Schmitz F. The pattern of the collagen fiber bundles of the capsule of the glenohumeral joint. *J Shoulder Elbow Surg* 1994;3:111–128.

36. Nakajima T, et al. Histologic and biomechanical characteristics of the supraspinatus tendon: Reference to rotator cuff tearing. *J Shoulder Elbow Surg* 1994;3:79–87.

37. Levy O, Copeland SA. Regeneration of the coracoacromial ligament after acromioplasty and arthroscopic subacromial decompression. *J Shoulder Elbow Surg* 2001;10:317–320.

38. Kumar VP, et al. The anatomy of the anterior origin of the deltoid. *J Bone Joint Surg* 1997;79B:680–683.

39. Torpey BM, et al. The deltoid muscle origin: Histologic characteristics and effects of subacromial decompression. *Am J Sports Med* 1998;26:379–383.

40. Neer CS, Poppen NK. Supraspinatus outlet. *Orthop Trans* 1987; 11:234.

41. Ellman H. Arthroscopic subacromial decompression: Analysis of one- to three-year results. *Arthroscopy* 1987;3:173–181.

42. Ellman H, Kay SP. Arthroscopic subacromial decompression for chronic impingement: 2- to 5-year results. *J Bone Joint Surg* 1991;73B:395–401.

43. Gartsman GM. Arthroscopic acromioplasty for lesions of the rotator cuff. *J Bone Joint Surg* 1990;72A:169–180.

44. Altchek DW, et al. Arthroscopic acromioplasty: Technique and results. *J Bone Joint Surg* 1990;72A:1198–1207.

45. Spangehl MJ, et al. Arthroscopic versus open acromioplasty: A prospective, randomized, blinded study. *J Shoulder Elbow Surg* 2002;11:101–107.

46. Grieve GP. Manual mobilizing techniques in degenerative arthrosis of the hip. *Bull Orthop Section APTA* 1977;2:7.

47. Frank C, et al. Physiology and therapeutic value of passive joint motion. *Clin Orthop* 1984;185:113.

48. Salter RB, et al. The biological effect of continuous passive motion on the healing of full-thickness defects in articular cartilage. *J Bone Joint Surg* 1980;62A:1232–1251.

49. Townsend J, et al. Electromyographic analysis of the glenohumeral muscles during a baseball rehabilitation program. *Am J Sports Med* 1991;3:264–272.

50. Wyke BD. The neurology of joints. *Ann R Coll Surg Engl* 1967; 41:25–50.

51. Freeman MAR, Wyke BD. An experimental study of articular neurology. *J Bone Joint Surg* 1967;49B:185.

52. Wilk KE, Arrigo C. Current concepts in the rehabilitation of the athletic shoulder. *J Orthop Sports Phys Ther* 1993;18:365.

53. Wilk KE, Arrigo C, Andrews JR. Current concepts in rehabilitation of the athlete's shoulder. *J South Orthop Assoc* 1994; 3:216–231.

54. Anderson L, et al. The effects of a Theraband exercise program on shoulder internal rotation strength. *Phys Ther* 1992;72:540.

55. Gray GW. Closed chain sense. *Fitness Management* 1992;8: 31–33.

56. Kibler BW. Closed kinetic chain rehabilitation for sports injuries. *Phys Med Rehabil North Am* 2000;11:369–384.

57. Kibler WB. Kinetic chain concept. In: Ellenbecker TS, ed. *Knee Ligament Rehabilitation.* Philadelphia, Pa: Churchill Livingstone; 2000:301–306.

58. Gartsman GM. Arthroscopic rotator cuff repair. *Clin Orthop Rel Res* 2001;390:95–106.

59. Zeman CA, et al. The rotator cuff-deficient arthritic shoulder: Diagnosis and surgical management. *J Am Acad Orthop Surg* 1998;6:337–348.

60. Neer CSI, Watson KC, Stanton FC. Recent experience in total shoulder replacement. *J Bone Joint Surg* 1982;64:319–337.

61. Daigneault J, Cooney LM Jr. Shoulder pain in older people. *J Am Geriatr Soc* 1998;46:1144–1151.

62. Norberg FB, Field LD. Repair of the rotator cuff: Mini-open and arthroscopic repairs. *Clin Sports Med* 2000;19:77–99.

63. Ellman H. Diagnosis and treatment of incomplete rotator cuff tears. *Clin Orthop* 1990;254:64–74.

64. Esch JC. Arthroscopic subacromial decompression: Results according to the degree of rotator cuff tear. *Arthroscopy* 1988; 4:241–249.

65. Gartsman GM, Milne J. Partial articular surface tears of the rotator cuff. *J Shoulder Elbow Surg* 1995;4:409–416.

66. Gartsman GM, Brinker MR, Khan M. Early effectiveness of arthroscopic repair for full-thickness tears of the rotator cuff: An outcome analysis. *J Bone Joint Surg* 1998;80A:33–40.

67. Gartsman GM, Hammerman SM. Full-thickness tear: Arthroscopic repair. *Orthop Clin North Am* 1997;28:83–98.

68. Gleyze P, et al. Arthroscopic rotator cuff repair: A multicentric retrospective study of 87 cases with anatomical assessment. *Rev Chir Orthop Reparatrice Appar Mot* 2000;86:566–574.

69. Gartsman GM, Hammerman SM. Arthroscopic rotator cuff repair: Operative technique. *Oper Tech Shoulder Elbow Surg* 2000;1:2–8.

70. Nirschl RP. Prevention and treatment of elbow and shoulder injuries in the tennis player. *Clin Sports Med* 1988;7:289–308.

71. Marks PH, Warner JJP, Irrgang JJ. Rotator cuff disorders of the shoulder. *J Hand Ther* 1994;7:90–98.

72. LaStayo PC, et al. Continuous passive motion after repair of the rotator cuff: A prospective outcome study. *J Bone Joint Surg* 1998;80A:1002–1011.

73. Osternig LR, et al. Differential responses to proprioceptive neuromuscular facilitation stretch techniques. *Med Sci Sports Exerc* 1990;22:106.

74. Brewster C, Moynes-Schwab DR. Rehabilitation of the shoulder following rotator cuff injury or surgery. *J Orthop Sports Phys Ther* 1993;18:422–426.

75. Sisk TD, Wright PE. Arthroplasty of the shoulder and elbow. In: Crenshaw AH, ed. *Campbell's Operative Orthopedics*. St Louis, Mo: Mosby; 1992:287–309.

76. Bergmann G. Biomechanics and pathomechanics of the shoulder joint with reference to prosthetic joint replacement. In: Koelbel R, et al, eds. *Shoulder Replacement*. Berlin, Germany: Springer-Verlag; 1987:33.

77. Williams GR Jr, Rockwood CA Jr. Massive rotator cuff defects and glenohumeral arthritis. In: Friedman RJ, ed. *Arthroplasty of the Shoulder*. New York, NY: Thieme; 1994:204–214.

78. Neer CS II, Craig EV, Fukuda H. Cuff-tear arthropathy. *J Bone Joint Surg* 1983;65A:1232–1244.

79. Cofield RH. Degenerative and arthritic problems of the glenohumeral joint. In: Rockwood CA, Master R, eds. *The Shoulder*. Philadelphia, Pa: Saunders; 1990:678–745.

80. Gartsman GM, Roddey TS, Hammerman SM. Shoulder arthroplasty with or without resurfacing of the glenoid in patients who have osteoarthritis. *J Bone Joint Surg* 2000;82A:26–34.

81. Brems JJ. Rehabilitation following shoulder arthroplasty. In: Friedman RJ, ed. *Arthroplasty of the Shoulder*. New York, NY: Thieme; 1994:99–112.

82. Thompson WH, et al. Ulnar collateral ligament reconstruction in athletes: Muscle-splitting approach without transposition of the ulnar nerve. *J Shoulder Elbow Surg* 2001;10:152–157.

83. Conway JE, et al. Medial instability of the elbow in throwing athletes: Treatment by repair or reconstruction of the ulnar collateral ligament. *J Bone Joint Surg* 1992;74A:67–83.

84. Azar FM, et al. Operative treatment of ulnar collateral ligament injuries of the elbow in athletes. *Am J Sports Med* 2000;28:16–23.

85. Wilk KE, Arrigo C, Andrews JR. Rehabilitation of the elbow in the throwing athlete. *J Orthop Sports Phys Ther* 1993;17:305–317.

86. Wilk KE, et al. Rehabilitation following elbow surgery in the throwing athlete. *Oper Tech Sports Med* 1996;4:114–132.

87. Ertel AN, Millender LH, Nalebuff E. Flexor tendon ruptures in patients with rheumatoid arthritis. *J Hand Surg Am* 1988;13A:860–866.

88. Mannerfelt L, Norman O. Attrition rupture of flexor tendons in rheumatoid arthritis caused by bony spurs in the carpal tunnel. A clinical and radiological study. *J Bone Joint Surg* 1969;51B:270–277.

89. Silfverskiold KL, May EJ, Tornvall AH. Gap formation during controlled motion after flexor tendon repair in zone II: A prospective clinical study. *J Hand Surg Am* 1992;17:539.

90. Silfverskiold KL, May EJ. Flexor tendon repair in zone II with a new suture technique and early program combining passive and active flexion. *J Hand Surg* 1994;19:53.

91. Tang JB, et al. Double and multiple looped suture tendon repair. *J Hand Surg Br* 1994;19:699.

92. Robertson GA, Al-Qattan MM. A biomechanical analysis of a new interlock suture technique for flexor tendon repair. *J Hand Surg Br* 1992;17:92.

93. McLarney E, Hoffman H, Wolfe SW. Biomechanical analysis of the cruciate four-strand flexor tendon repair. *J Hand Surg Am* 1999;24:295.

94. Ejeskar A. Flexor tendon repair in no-man's-land: Results of primary repair with controlled mobilization. *J Hand Surg Am* 1984;9:171.

95. Strickland JW, Glogovac SV. Digital function following flexor tendon repair in zone II: A comparison of immobilization and controlled passive motion techniques. *J Hand Surg Am* 1980;5:537.

96. Chow JA, et al. A combined regimen of controlled motion following flexor tendon repair in "no man's land." *Plast Reconstr Surg* 1987;9:447–455.

97. Cullen KW, et al. Flexor tendon repair in zone 2 followed by controlled active mobilisation. *J Hand Surg* 1989;14B:392–395.

98. Elliot D, et al. The rupture rate of acute flexor tendon repairs mobilized by the controlled active motion regimen. *J Hand Surg* 1994;19B:607–612.

99. Lister GD, et al. Primary flexor tendon repair followed by immediate controlled mobilization. *J Hand Surg* 1977;2:441–451.

100. Tang JB, Shi D. Subdivision of flexor tendon "no man's land" and different treatment methods in each subzone. *Clin Med J* 1992;105:60–69.

101. Taras JS, et al. The double-grasping and cross-stitch for acute flexor tendon repair: Applications with active motion. *Atlas Hand Clin* 1996;1:13–28.

102. Aoki M, et al. Biomechancial and histological characteristics of canine flexor tendon repair using early postoperative mobilization. *J Hand Surg* 1997;22A:107–114.

103. Panchal J, Mehdi S, Donoghue JO. The range of excursion of flexor tendons in zone V: A comparison of active vs passive flexor mobilization regimes. *Br J Plast Surg* 1997;50:517–522.

104. Small JO, Bernnen MD, Colville J. Early active mobilisation following flexor tendon repair in zone 2. *J Hand Surg Br* 1989; 14:383–391.

105. Ingari JV, Pederson WC. Update on tendon repair. *Clin Plast Surg* 1997;24:161.

106. Gelberman RH, Siedel DB, Woo SLY. Healing of digital flexor tendons: Importance of the interval from injury to repair. A biomechanical, biochemical, and morphological study in dogs. *J Bone Joint Surg* 1991;73A:66–75.

107. Hitchcock TF, et al. The effect of immediate constrained digital motion on the strength of flexor tendon repairs in chickens. *J Hand Surg* 1987;12A:590–595.

108. Kubota H, et al. Effect of motion and tension on injured flexor tendons in chickens. *J Hand Surg* 1996;21A:456–463.

109. Schuind F, et al. Flexor tendon forces: In vivo measurements. *J Hand Surg* 1992;17A:291–298.

110. Urbaniak JR, Cahill JD, Mortenson R. Tendon suturing methods: Analysis of tensile strengths. In: Hunter JM, Schnieder LH, eds. *AAOS Symposium on Tendon Surgery in the Hand*. St Louis, Mo: CV Mosby; 1975:70–80.

111. Stewart KM. Review and comparison of current trends in the postoperative management of tendon repair. *Hand Clin* 1991;7:447–460.

112. Kleinert HE, et al. Primary repair of flexor tendons. *Orthop Clin North Am* 1973;4:865–876.

113. Cetin A, et al. Rehabilitation of flexor tendon injuries by use of a combined regimen of modified Kleinert and modified Duran techniques. *Am J Phys Med Rehabil* 2001;80:721–728.

114. Strien G. Postoperative management of flexor tendon injuries. In: Hunter JM, Schneider LH, Mackin EJ, eds. *Rehabilitation of*

the Hand: Surgery and Therapy. St Louis, Mo: CV Mosby; 1990:390–409.

115. Slattery PG, McGrouther DA. A modified Kleinert controlled mobilization splint following flexor tendon repair. *J Hand Surg* 1984;9B:217–218.

116. Dovelle S, Heeter PK. The Washington regimen: Rehabilitation of the hand following flexor tendon injuries. *Phys Ther* 1989;69:1034–1040.

117. Taras JS, Gray RM, Culp RW. Complications of flexor tendon injuries. *Hand Clin* 1994;10:93–109.

118. May EJ, Silverskiold KL, Sollerman CJ. Controlled mobilization after flexor tendon repair in zone II: A prospective comparison of three methods. *J Hand Surg* 1992;17:942–952.

119. Kitsis CK, et al. Controlled active motion following primary flexor tendon repair: A prospective study over 9 years. *J Hand Surg Br* 1998;23:344–349.

120. Cannon NM, Strickland JW. Therapy following flexor tendon surgery. *Hand Clin* 1985;1:147.

121. Duran RJ, Houser RG. Controlled passive motion following flexor tendon repair in zones 2 and 3. In: *American Academy of Orthopedic Surgeons: Symposium on Flexor Tendon Surgery in the Hand.* St Louis, Mo: CV Mosby; 1975.

122. Atroshi I, et al. Prevalence of carpal tunnel syndrome in a general population. *JAMA* 1999;282:153–158.

123. Keller RB, et al. Maine Carpal Tunnel Study: Small area variations. *J Hand Surg Am* 1998;23:697–710.

124. Brown RA, et al. Carpal tunnel release: A prospective, randomized, blind assessment trial of open and endoscopic methods of transverse carpal ligament release. *J Bone Joint Surg* 1993;75A:1585–1592.

125. Hybbinette CH, Mannerfelt M. The carpal tunnel syndrome: A retrospective study of 400 operated patients. *Acta Orthop Scand* 1975;46:610–620.

126. Kulick MI, et al. Long-term analysis of patients having surgical treatment for carpal tunnel syndrome. *J Hand Surg Am* 1986;11:59–66.

127. Trumble TE, Gilbert M, McCallister MV. Endoscopic versus open surgical treatment of carpal tunnel syndrome. *Neurosurg Clin North Am* 2001;12:255–266.

128. Richman JA, et al. Carpal tunnel syndrome: Morphologic changes after release of the transverse carpal ligament. *J Hand Surg* 1989;14A:852–857.

129. Okutsu I, et al. Measurement of pressure in the carpal canal before and after endoscopic management of carpal tunnel syndrome. *J Bone Joint Surg* 1989;71A:679–683.

130. Feuerstein M, et al. Clinical management of carpal tunnel syndrome: A 12 year review of outcomes. *Am J Ind Med* 1999; 35:232–245.

131. Bury TF, Akelman E, Weiss AP. Prospective, randomized trial of splinting after carpal tunnel release. *Ann Plast Surg* 1995; 35:19–22.

132. Mathiowetz V, et al. Adult norms for the nine-hole peg test of finger dexterity. *Occup Ther J Res* 1985;5:24.

133. American Society for Surgery of the Hand. *The Hand: Examination and Diagnosis.* Aurora, Colo: ASSH; 1978.

134. American Society for Surgery of the Hand. *The Hand: Examination and Diagnosis.* 2nd ed. New York, NY: Churchill Livingstone; 1983.

135. Fess EE. Grip strength. In: American Society of Hand Therapists, ed. *Clinical Assessment Recommendations.* Chicago, Ill: ASHT; 1992.

136. Mathiowetz V, et al. Grip and pinch strength: normative data for adults. *Arch Phys Med Rehabil* 1985;66:69.

137. Totten PA, Hunter JM. Therapeutic techniques to enhance nerve gliding in thoracic outlet syndrome and carpal tunnel syndrome. *Hand Clin* 1991;7:505–520.

138. Wilgis EF, Murphy R. The significance of longitudinal excursion in peripheral nerves. *Hand Clin* 1986;2:761–766.

139. McLellan DL, Swash M. Longitudinal sliding of the median nerve during movements of the upper limb. *J Neurol Neurosurg Psychiatry* 1976;39:566–570.

140. Rozmaryn LM, et al. Nerve and tendon gliding exercises and the conservative management of carpal tunnel syndrome. *J Hand Ther* 1998;11:171–179.

141. Cook AC, et al. Early mobilization following carpal tunnel release: A prospective randomized study. *J Hand Surg* 1995;20:228–230.

142. Kasch M. Therapists evaluation and treatment of upper extremity cumulative trauma disorders. In: Hunter JM, Mackin EJ, Callahan AD, eds. *Rehabilitation of the Hand: Surgery and Therapy.* St Louis, Mo: Mosby; 1995:101–139.

143. Waylett-Rendall J. Use of therapeutic modalities in upper extremity rehabilitation. In: Hunter JM, Mackin EJ, Callahan AD, eds. *Rehabilitation of the Hand: Surgery and Therapy.* St Louis, Mo: Mosby; 1995:156–172.

CHAPTER 29

POSTSURGICAL REHABILITATION OF THE LOWER EXTREMITY

Procedures Involving the Hip

Total Hip Arthroplasty

The total hip arthroplasty (THA), a common procedure performed in many acute care hospitals, is used in cases of severe joint damage resulting from osteoarthritis, rheumatoid arthritis, and avascular necrosis.[1] It is one of the most successful and cost-effective interventions in medicine.[2,3] After THA surgery, many patients typically are able to return to participation in activities that were too painful before surgery.[4,5]

Indications

The most common indications for a THA are[6]:

▶ *Pain.* Pain is the principal indication for hip replacement. This includes pain with movement and pain at rest. A significant amount of pain may be reliably relieved as early as 1 week after surgery.[7]

▶ *Functional limitations.* Capsular contractions and joint deformity cause a decreased range of motion in the hip, with subsequent functional restrictions.

▶ *Loss of mobility.* There are certain patient subgroups in which joint stiffness, without hip pain, is an indication for surgery. These groups include patients with ankylosing spondylitis.

▶ *Radiographic indications of intra-articular disease.* Although radiographic changes are considered in the decision to operate, the more significant determinant is the severity of symptoms.

Contraindications for THA, both absolute and relative, include but are not limited to the following:

▶ Active infection.

▶ Younger age. Although most THAs are performed in patients between 60 and 80 years of age, hip replacement occasionally is performed in younger patients, including those in their teens and early 20s.[8,9]

▶ Obesity.

▶ Planned return to high-impact sports or occupations.

▶ Arterial insufficiency.

▶ Neuromuscular disease.

▶ Mental illness.

Procedure

A number of factors determine the procedure used by the surgeon, including surgeon familiarity and comfort, patient size, and scars from previous surgery or trauma.

The first successful THA was developed by John Charnley in the 1960s. This procedure used a transtrochanteric lateral approach. Three other approaches have evolved since: the anterolateral approach, the direct lateral approach, and the posterolateral approach.[2] Controversy remains as to which approach results in the lowest complication rate.[3–8]

▶ *Anterolateral approach.* There are numerous variations of the anterolateral approach. All variations approach the hip through the interval between the tensor fascia lata and the gluteus medius muscle. Some portion of the hip abductor is released from the greater trochanter, and the hip is dislocated anteriorly.[9]

▶ *Direct lateral approach.* The direct lateral approach leaves the posterior portion of the gluteus medius attached to the greater trochanter. Because the posterior soft tissues and capsule are left intact, this approach is preferred in the more noncompliant patients to prevent postsurgical dislocation.[9]

▶ *Posterolateral approach.* The posterolateral approach gains access to the hip joint by splitting the gluteus maximus muscle. The short external rotators are then released, and the hip abductors are retracted anteriorly. The femur is then dislocated posteriorly. Although the posterior approach may allow for maintenance of abductor strength,[10] it generally results in a higher postsurgical dislocation rate.[7,8]

Both the anterolateral and the posterolateral approaches appear to result in decreased blood loss[5] and fewer hematomas,[5] compared with the transtrochanteric approach. The advantages of the anterolateral approach are the lower dislocation rates[4,6] and the excellent acetabular exposure. The disadvantage of the anterolateral approach is an increase in antalgic gait (at least temporarily).[3,4] Although several studies[3,4,10] imply weakening of the abductor muscles as a result of the anterolateral approach, only one study[10] has found a statistically significant increase in weakness of the abductors with this approach.

Although the posterolateral approach has remained essentially unchanged, the anterolateral approach has been modified by several surgeons to decrease gluteus medius disruption and, it is hoped, to decrease postoperative abductor muscle dysfunction and resultant limp.[3,4,6,8] However, no studies from the past decade have yet compared abductor muscle dysfunction in the posterolateral approach versus a modified anterolateral approach.

A number of criteria must be met for the long-term success of the implant. These include adequate fixation, adequate strength and wear resistance, biological and biomechanical compatibility.[11–13]

▶ *Fixation.* Two types of fixation are recognized: cemented and cementless.[14,15] There are a number of disadvantages to the traditional method of cementing. These include poor tensile and compressive strengths of the acrylic cement.[16] Cementless technology was introduced as a strategy to improve the results of cemented hip replacement in the 1970s. Excellent bone ingrowth has been demonstrated in porous-coated implants inserted without cement.[17] There is no universal agreement on indications for cementless versus cemented hip replacement. However, it is generally agreed that the primary indication for a cementless THA is the young, active individual, usually younger than age 65 physiologically.[9]

▶ *Adequate strength and wear resistance.* In the early years of hip replacement, fracture of the femoral stem was a problem. This problem has been largely resolved by the use of improved metal processing. Polyethylene wear undoubtedly has been the major long-term problem of THA. The use of a ceramic femoral head has been advocated, especially in young, active patients, because it produces less polyethylene wear compared with a conventional metal femoral head.

▶ *Biological compatibility.* The primary fixation mode of cementless acetabular components is mechanical and is dependent on a physical interlock between the cup and the reamed acetabulum.[18] Secondary fixation is biological and is achieved by means of bone growth onto or into the substrate at the implant-bone interface. The fixation surface of cementless metal-backed sockets typically consists of a porous coating of beads or fiber metal, a titanium plasma-sprayed surface, various sintered surface textures, or a bioactive ceramic coating such as hydroxyapatite or tricalcium phosphate.[18] For long-term stability, it is essential that this direct bond between the implant and the bone be maintained. The production of particulate wear debris from implant materials and subsequent osteolysis has been recognized as the major cause of long-term failure in THA. Using cell cultures, Vermes and colleagues[19] demonstrated that metallic particulate debris affected osteoblast function through two distinct mechanisms: a direct negative effect on cellular function by the phagocytosis itself, and an effect mediated through cytokines, which cause a downregulation of procollagen α_1 gene expression along with decreased cell proliferation. Moreover, this study demonstrated that osteoblasts stimulated by particulate debris produced interleukin-6 and prostaglandin E_2, leading to the activation of osteoclast function.

▶ *Biomechanical compatibility.* Prosthetic impingement resulting from poor positioning, the head-neck ratio, and the presence of a modular head with an extended sleeve has been implicated in decreasing the postsurgical range of motion (ROM) at the hip after THA. Additional factors, such as osseous impingement and soft-tissue tension, can further decrease the range.

Several complications are associated with THA. These include, but are not limited to:

▶ *Deep vein thrombosis (DVT).* DVT is the most common complication following THA (see Section IV introduction).[9] Peak incidence occurs at 5 to 10 days postsurgery.[20] However, the period of increased risk can be up to 3 months after surgery.[21]

▶ *Heterotopic ossification.* Heterotopic ossification is a well-known complication of surgical approaches to the hip that involve dissection of the gluteal muscles.[22,23] The exact mechanism for heterotopic bone formation has not been thoroughly elucidated; however, it appears to involve pluripotent mesenchymal cell differentiation into osteoprogenitor cells after tissue injury or dissection.[24,25] This process begins as soon as 16 hours after injury and is maximal at 36 to 48 hours.[25] The surgical approach to the acetabulum appears to be a major risk factor for heterotopic ossification. Posterior and extensile approaches to the acetabulum may result in a prevalence of ossification of up to 50 percent.[26] Additional reported risk factors for heterotopic ossification include thoracic and abdominal trauma, male gender, T-type fracture, delay in fracture fixation, and closed head injury.[27]

▶ *Femoral fractures.* Fracture of the femur in association with THA is a challenging complication that has been well described.[28–32] The prevalence of these fractures has ranged from 0.1 percent (7 of 5400)[30] to 20 percent (16 of 79).[31] Risk factors include female gender, rheumatoid arthritis, cortical perforation, osteopenia, osteoporosis, preoperative femoral deformity, a revision operation, osteolysis, and loosening of the stem.[30,32]

▶ *Dislocation.* Dislocation of the total hip replacement remains a common and potentially extremely problematic complication. As many as 85 percent of dislocations are reported to occur within 2 months after THA.[33] Dislocation is more common in elderly people, particularly those with impaired cognition and balance and vibration sensitivity.[34] It occurs more commonly in women.[35] There is also a correlation with history of trauma or developmental dysplasia of the hip.[8] Patients with cerebral dysfunction or excessive alcohol use also are at higher risk.[36] Dislocation rate is a factor of many other requirements, including component position, technical errors, imbalance of tissues, surgical approach, and patient compliance.[37]

▶ *Neurovascular injury.* A review of the literature reveals that the prevalence of nerve palsy following THA varies from 0.08 to 7.5 percent, depending on the study, with an overall prevalence of 1 percent.[38] The peroneal division of the sciatic nerve is involved in almost 80 percent of cases, with the femoral nerve and the obturator nerve involved less frequently.[38] There are many proposed causes for neuropathy associated with THA, including direct trauma; excessive tension because of an increase in limb length, or offset, or both; bleeding, or compression, or both, by a hematoma; and unknown.[38–40]

Presurgery Evaluation and Education

At many institutions, patients attend a presurgery class 7 to 10 days before surgery. These preoperative training sessions have been shown to improve motivation, understanding, and compliance during rehabilitation of the postsurgical patient.[41,42] The class instructors usually include a case nurse, dietitian, and physical therapist.

► The case nurse reviews how to make the home safe; what to expect before, during, and after surgery; how to prevent dislocations; what medications will be used; and what type of transport is needed to bring the patient home. He or she also brings in pictures of the operating room and samples of equipment. A case nurse reviews the patient's history before admissions, and a home assessment is performed 6 weeks preoperatively.

► The dietitian discusses which foods help healing, and how to cope with decreased appetite and depression, which are both common after surgery.

► The physical therapist discusses the postsurgical physical therapy program and shows each patient how to use an appropriate assistive device for gait. An assessment is made of general strength, ROM, neurologic status, endurance, and safety awareness. The patient receives instruction on the early postoperative exercises, pertinent hip precautions, and safe transfer techniques. Upper body exercises are taught to help the patient walk with crutches. Function can be assessed using the Harris Hip Scale (see Table 17-10) or a similar standard outcome measurement for the hip.

Patients and their caregivers are encouraged to ask questions and complete forms used to calculate their current function. The patients receive booklets on diet, exercise, home safety, and discharge planning.

Postsurgical Rehabilitation

Following the surgery, thromboembolic disease (TED) hose are placed on the patient. For patients who have undergone either a posterolateral approach or a transtrochanteric approach, a triangular foam cushion is strapped between the legs to keep the hip in an abducted position. Patients at high risk of dislocation, such as those who have undergone a postrevision arthroplasty or those with cognitive impairments, may need to wear a hip abduction orthosis that maintains the hip in abduction for 6 to 12 weeks. These orthoses may make ambulation difficult if the abduction is more than 5 to 10 degrees.

The staples usually are removed after 12 to 14 days. Hip precautions must be maintained at all times, as follows:

► For the posterolateral approach, this involves avoidance of flexion of the hip beyond 90 degrees, and minimal adduction or internal rotation of the hip.

► Following a lateral or anterolateral approach, the patient should avoid extension, external rotation, and adduction across midline.

These precautions must be maintained for at least 6 weeks, or until the surgeon decides otherwise.

A review of the literature reveals inconsistent practice patterns in the physical therapy management of THA patients.[43] The postsurgical rehabilitation program that follows is based on the consensus found.[44–46] The program is divided into two components: the inpatient stay, and the outpatient course of intervention.

Phase 1: Inpatient Phase (24 Hours to Discharge). This phase typically involves four to ten physical therapy sessions. Ideally, the patient will have attended a preoperative training session. Patients should be evaluated routinely for peripheral nerve function on a daily basis.[38] If a palsy is detected, a knee immobilizer (for femoral nerve palsy) should be used with ambulation, additional exercises focusing on strengthening the affected muscles and stretching the antagonists to prevent joint contractures should be prescribed, and the patient should be fitted with the appropriate orthotic (ankle foot orthoses [AFOs] with sciatic palsy) to allow physical therapy to proceed.[38]

Goals

► Prevent postsurgical complications, including:

• DVT.

• Postoperative infection.

• Detrimental effects of immobilization.[47–52]

• Pulmonary embolus.

• Reports of pain to be 7/10 or less. Increasing or severe buttock pain may indicate a hematoma.

• Patient to achieve an independent or minimally supervised functional level for:

• Transfers in and out of bed.

• Transfers on and off a commode.

• Transfers up and down from a chair of varying heights.

► Gait training at a household level with the appropriate assistive device for 100 feet.

► Independence with stair negotiation (one or more steps), consistent with the patient's home environment, with appropriate assistive device and with and without a handrail.

► Independence with the home exercise program, which will be performed two to three times a day.

- Independence with THA precautions, and correct application of them into any permitted functional activity.

The patient should be repositioned every 2 hours by the nursing staff. The skin, especially on the heels, is checked regularly for breakdown. The patient is provided with information on assistive devices, such as an elevated seat and the reacher.

Electrotherapeutic and Physical Modalities.   Modalities that reduce pain and swelling (ice and elevation) are initiated as early as possible. With the physician's permission, electrical stimulation can be used for edema reduction, muscle re-education, and pain control.[53–56]

Therapeutic Exercise and Home Program.   The therapeutic exercise program typically begins within 24 hours after the surgery.[43,57] Exercises may include:

▶ Resistive exercises to the uninvolved extremities.

▶ Ankle pumps (not circles, so as to prevent any inadvertent rotation at the hip) for both lower extremities.

▶ Quadriceps sets, gluteal sets, and hamstring sets of the involved leg.

▶ Deep-breathing exercises.

▶ Active and isometric hip abduction of the involved leg (day 2).[43] These exercises are deferred initially if a trochanteric osteotomy has been performed.

▶ Active assistive hip and knee flexion (heel slides) to the involved limb. These are performed while maintaining the hip ROM within the guidelines specified by the surgeon (day 2).[43] The patient can use a sheet to help with this exercise (Fig. 29-1).

▶ Short arc quads of the involved leg (day 2).[43]

Functional Training.   On the first day after the surgery, the clinician begins transfer training and instructs the patient with regard to bed mobility. Training includes transfers from supine to sitting in the bed, and then from sit to stand, while observing all of the necessary hip precautions.[43] If permitted by the surgeon, the patient can be shown how to transfer to an appropriate bedside chair. The patient is encouraged to sit in the chair for about 30 to 60 minutes, depending on tolerance, which can be measured using the vital signs of pulse and blood pressure, as well as subjective complaints such as light headedness or dizziness.

Gait training with crutches or walker usually is begun on the second day following surgery.[43] The patient's assistive device is adjusted to the correct height. Close attention must be paid to these patients during gait training, because of their balance deficiencies and the potential for temporary postural hypotension.

▶ The weight-bearing status of the patient with a noncemented THA is decided by the surgeon. It can vary from non–weight bearing to toe-touch weight bearing, to partial

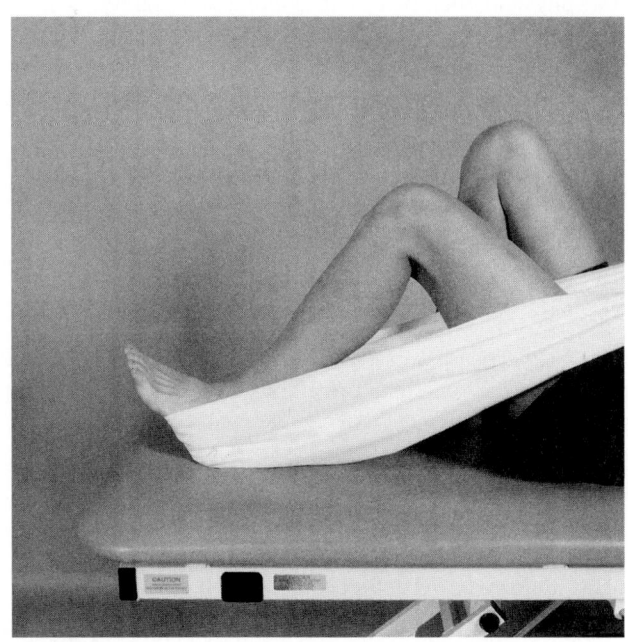

FIGURE 29-1   Heel slide with sheet.

weight bearing. Toe-touch weight bearing involves applying no more than 10 percent of body weight. It has been described as analogous to walking on eggshells. Partial weight bearing is a difficult concept for most patients to grasp. Using a description such as "half of body weight" usually helps. Force platforms are available to measure these forces directly and can provide beneficial feedback for the patient.

▶ The weight-bearing status for the patient with a cemented THA is usually partial weight bearing for 6 weeks prior to full weight bearing, although some surgeons permit weight bearing as tolerated with a walker immediately.

Normalization of the gait pattern should be taught early. Stand-to-pivot transfers also should be taught to prevent the patient from rotating at the involved hip.

Stair negotiation, based on the patient's home situation, is typically taught on day 3.[43]

Home Care Phase (1 to 7 Days).   If functional independence is required before a patient returns home, the patient typically is transferred to an acute or subacute care setting. If adequate home care and safe transport are available, the patient is allowed to return home.

Munin and colleagues[58] in one study determined certain markers that were predictive of patients who would require an inpatient rehabilitation program versus direct discharge to home. Those patients determined to be at high risk were 70 years of age or older, 51 percent lived alone, and many had a number of comorbid conditions.

A physical home care assessment usually occurs within 24 hours after hospital discharge. During this phase, the role of the physical therapist is to address any safety concerns, including moving or adjusting the height of furniture, the removal of any throw rugs, review of sitting and sleeping positions and hip precautions, and progression of home exercise program.

Weight-bearing exercises, such as seated heel raises (Fig. 29-2), and mini-squats against a wall usually are introduced at this time.

The patient's gait training should be advanced to independence with crutches or walker.

Phase 2: Outpatient Phase (Week 2 to 8).   This phase typically lasts 2 to 6 weeks and may involve six to nine physical therapy sessions.

Goals

▶ Reports of pain to be 5/10 or less.

▶ Hip ROM to be 70 to 90 degrees of hip flexion.

▶ Balance and proprioception to be at 50 percent of the uninvolved leg, as measured by single-leg stance time, if weight-bearing status permits.

▶ Strength to be 3/5 to 4/5 on the involved lower extremity.

▶ Patient to achieve independence with all transfers.

▶ Patient to have a normal gait pattern with an assistive device on level surfaces.

Electrotherapeutic and Physical Modalities.   Superficial thermal modalities may be used in this phase.

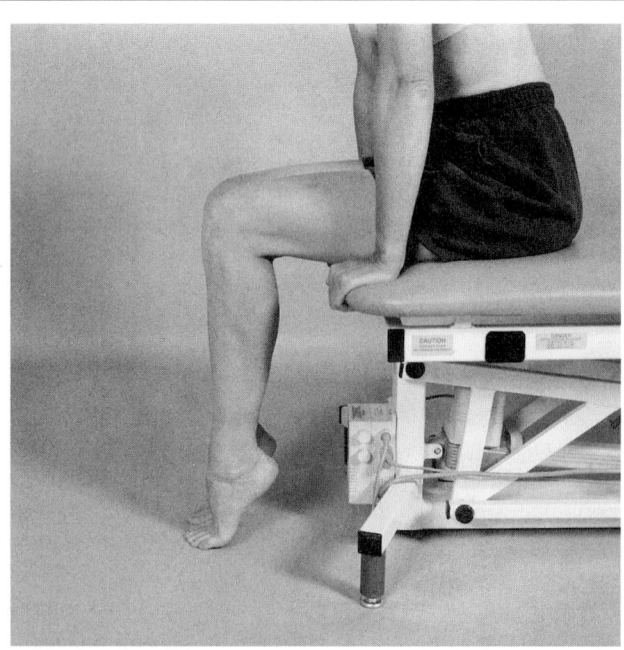

FIGURE 29-2   Seated heel raises.

Therapeutic Exercise.   Weakness following a THA is common and can lead to diminished protection of the implant fixation surfaces during activities.[59]

▶ Flexibility exercises are performed within the limitations of hip precautions to the following muscle groups:

  • Iliopsoas.

  • Quadriceps and rectus femoris.

  • Gastrocnemius and soleus.

  • Hamstrings.

▶ Lower extremity strengthening exercises include:

  • Non–weight-bearing exercises of heel slides, hip abduction in the supine position, straight leg raises, and short arc quads.

  • Weight-bearing exercises of weight shifting, modified wall slide squats to approximately 45 degrees of hip flexion, modified lunges (anterior and lateral), and step-ups and step-downs.

▶ Upper extremity strengthening exercises are initiated as needed.

▶ Cardiovascular conditioning is begun through use of an upper body ergonometer.

Neuromuscular Retraining

▶ BAPS (biomechanical ankle platform system) board exercises in sitting or standing position, with weight-bearing restrictions observed.

▶ Biased stance balance-and-reach activities involving reaching arms forward at shoulder height and waist height.

Functional Training

▶ Gait training is performed on level and stairs with appropriate assistive device. The patient can be advanced to a single-point cane as and if appropriate. A four-point cane may be used as an interim device.

▶ Transfers are progressed to all surfaces, when permitted.

▶ Patients usually are permitted to drive 3 to 4 weeks after surgery.

Manual Therapy.   Manual therapy techniques include:

▶ Soft tissue techniques and mobilization of the posterolateral or anterolateral hip.

▶ Scar mobilization.

▶ Contract-relax techniques within the limits of the hip precautions.

▶ Passive stretching of lateral hip, knee, and lumbar spine within the limits of the precautions.

Phase 3 (Week 9+)

Goals

▶ Reports of pain to be 2/10 or less with activity of the involved leg, and 0/10 at rest.

▶ Hip ROM to be at 90 degrees of flexion.

▶ Involved lower extremity muscle strength to be at 4/5 with manual muscle testing.

▶ Patient to be independent with ambulation, and with no gait dysfunction.

▶ Balance and proprioception to be at 80 percent, compared with the uninvolved leg, as measured by single-leg stance time.

▶ Patient to be independent with stair negotiation without an assistive device.

▶ Patient to demonstrate functional independence in activities of daily living.

▶ Patient to achieve return to employment or previous hobbies, as indicated.

Therapeutic Exercise

▶ Phase 1 exercises are progressed, with the addition of increased resistance as appropriate. Weakness of hip muscles has been shown to exist up to 2 years postsurgery. Therefore, the therapeutic exercise program should be continued for at least 1 year, and preferably longer, until the involved limb strength is equal to that of the uninvolved.[60]

▶ Treadmill exercises are initiated, as well as other low-impact forms of conditioning, as appropriate.

Neuromuscular Retraining. Single-leg balance-and-reach exercises are performed, including reaching arms forward, reaching opposite leg forward, and reaching opposite leg laterally.

Outcomes

Various clinical rating systems may be used for the outcome measurement of osteoarthritis interventions for the hip, most of which are designed for evaluating postoperative outcome after arthroplasty.[61]

Lavernia and colleagues[62] have analyzed quality of life following THA, and their findings indicate that THA is extremely cost-effective compared with medical interventions in other disciplines.

In the past decade, much discussion has focused on the use of patient-directed outcome measurement instruments such as the Medical Outcomes Study 26-Item Short-Form Health Survey (SF-36), the Harris Hip Scale, and the Western Ontario and McMaster University Osteoarthritis Index (WOMAC) in the evaluation of patients who have had a THA. In a study by Soderman and Malchau,[63] in which a Harris hip score was assigned to 350 patients who had had a THA and already had been assigned SF-36 and WOMAC scores, all three instruments were found to be valid, reproducible, and reliable. There was also good interobserver reliability among the investigators who assigned the Harris hip scores, and the correlation was especially good with regard to pain and function.[63] Soderman and Malchau concluded that the Harris scale was as valid for outcome measurement as the SF-36 and the WOMAC.[63]

Procedures Involving the Knee

Total Knee Arthroplasty

Total knee arthroplasty (TKA) has been shown to be an effective long-term intervention for the elderly population to relieve knee pain, improve function, increase social mobility and interaction, and contribute to psychological well-being.[64–66]

Indications

Although pain and loss of function are the primary reasons for a TKA, the procedure can also be used to correct knee instability and lower extremity alignment and for the treatment of isolated but severe patellofemoral disease.[67,68] Because TKA generally is contraindicated in younger and more active patients, those with unicompartmental osteoarthritis of the knee may be considered candidates for a high tibial osteotomy or a distal femoral osteotomy. The high tibial osteotomy is used with isolated medial compartment arthritis. The distal femoral osteotomy is used in lateral compartment arthritis. The short-term results for these procedures have been very successful,[69,70] even to the point where the need for TKA is eliminated.[71] However, permanent pain relief with high tibial osteotomy is as yet unlikely.

Absolute and relative contraindications for a TKA include, but are not limited to:

▶ Active infection of the knee.

▶ Significant genu recurvatum.

▶ Severe obesity.

▶ Return to high-impact sports or occupations.

▶ Arterial insufficiency.

▶ Neuropathic joint.

▶ Mental illness.

Procedure

Several techniques are at the surgeon's disposal. The choice of approach is determined by surgeon familiarity and comfort. Three approaches are commonly described: anterior, subvastus, and lateral.[72]

1. ***Anterior approach.*** The anterior approach is generally through an anterior midline longitudinal skin incision and median parapatellar arthrotomy. The advantages of this approach include its extensile potential and its wide exposure medially and laterally. The disadvantages include its violation

of the quadriceps mechanism, and the potential for patellar devascularization.[72]

2. **Subvastus approach.** The subvastus approach uses the same midline anterior skin incision as the anterior approach. The advantages of this approach include maintenance of the quadriceps mechanism with decreased postoperative pain and earlier functional recovery.[72] The disadvantages include its somewhat limited exposure.

3. **Lateral approach.** The lateral approach occurs lateral to the patella and through the medial edge of Gerdy's tubercle. Proponents of this technique feel that it is a superior method in the correction of valgus deformity.[72]

Most primary arthroplasties rely upon the patient's anatomy to confer stability to the articulation. Anatomic structures that can confer stability include the posterior cruciate ligament (PCL) and a balancing of the soft tissues around the knee. The fate of the PCL in primary TKA is controversial. If the PCL is sacrificed, a posterior stabilizer (see below) is used. However, the long-term results of PCL-retaining and posterior-stabilized TKAs are similar.[73,74] PCL substitution may be indicated in patients requiring TKA who present with end-stage degenerative joint disease with varus or valgus malalignment and associated flexion contracture, with a combined deformity greater than 15 degrees.[75,76]

Many early designs of TKA replaced only the tibiofemoral joint and did not address the patellofemoral articulation. The posterior stabilizer was developed to increase the arc of motion of these earlier models and thereby improve the functional results of TKA. Although the range of motion (ROM) improved substantially with these components, patellofemoral complications emerged as a major problem after knee replacement. Errors in sizing, alignment, and rotation of the tibial and femoral component eventually were appreciated as contributing factors to many of these patellofemoral problems. In addition, many of these complications appear to be secondary to patellar resurfacing, which may be part of the procedure. Whether to resurface the patella remains among the most controversial topics in TKA.

Surprisingly high loads are transmitted across the patellofemoral articulation (see Chap. 18). Following a knee replacement, there is a decrease in the contact area and consequent increase in the contract stress.[77] A study by Matsuda and colleagues[77] showed that resurfacing the patella decreased the contact area to a greater degree compared with not resurfacing the patella. In addition, kinematic studies of motion of the patellofemoral joint after knee replacement have consistently shown some degree of altered kinematics.[78]

Postsurgical Rehabilitation

Preoperative instruction is believed to be invaluable in the early postoperative setting. Preoperative instruction should include education regarding the ice-compression-elevation program, ROM exercises, isometric quadriceps strengthening, patellofemoral mobilization, and gait training with the appropriate postoperative assistive devices.[79]

Complications associated with TKA include[80]:

► Thromboembolic disease.

► Fat embolism.

► Poor wound healing.

► Infection.

► Periprosthetic fractures.

► Neurologic problems. Peroneal nerve palsy is the most common neurologic complication of TKA.

► Vascular problems. Injuries to the superficial femoral, popliteal, and genicular vessels have all been reported following TKA.

► Arthrofibrosis.

► Disruption of the extensor mechanism.

Postoperative rehabilitation for primary TKA continues to be studied in an effort to decrease the cost while still providing the quality of clinical results expected by the surgeon and the patient.[81]

A review of the literature reveals inconsistent practice patterns in the physical therapy management of TKA patients.[43] The postsurgical rehabilitation program that follows is based on the consensus found.[46,82,83] The program is divided into two components: the inpatient stay, and the outpatient course.

The success of the rehabilitation program for this patient population is dependent on knowledge of the surgical procedure, communication with the surgeon and the patient, and, above all, the ability of the rehabilitation team to educate the patient to participate actively in the treatment program.[79]

Phase 1: Inpatient Phase (1 Day until Discharge).[43] This phase typically involves four to ten physical therapy sessions.

The subject of continuous passive motion device use following a TKA has been debated for years, with some surgeons advocating and others opposing its use. The modality of continuous passive motion was introduced to the orthopaedic community in 1980,[84] although Coutts and colleagues[85] should be given credit for introducing it for the postoperative rehabilitation of patients who underwent TKA.

The use of a continuous passive motion device for postoperative TKA rehabilitation has been promoted as a means to facilitate a more rapid recovery by improving flexion range, decreasing length of hospital stay, and lowering the amount of narcotic use.[56,86–95] However, other studies have shown that the effect of continuous passive motion machines on analgesia consumption, ROM, hospital stay, and complications has been variable.[96–98]

Thus, the use of continuous passive motion after primary TKA remains controversial[99]:

► Data support its use to decrease the rate of manipulation for poor ROM after TKA.

► The ultimate ROM probably is not increased by the use of continuous passive motion after TKA.

▶ Because of standardized inpatient hospital clinical pathways, the length of hospital stay is not decreased by the use of continuous passive motion and, depending on the hospital involved, the overall cost is not increased.

▶ Wound complications probably are not increased with the use of continuous passive motion, provided good technique is used in wound closure and gradual increase in ROM occurs during the first 4 days postoperatively.

It is still not clear whether ROM is achieved faster and whether the prevalence of deep vein thrombosis (DVT) and analgesics use are decreased with continuous passive motion. Although it appears that the use of a continuous passive motion device does help regain knee flexion quicker, it is not as effective in the enhancement of knee extension.[93,100,101]

If ligament instability is present in the days immediately following the surgery, a postoperative knee brace is used, which initially is adjusted to a 0- to 90-degree position. The brace functions to allow free movement in the 0- to 90-degree range, while preventing varus and valgus forces to the knee, and thus assists in maintaining the corrective alignment obtained in surgery.[79]

Goals

▶ Prevent postoperative complications, including DVT, infection, and pulmonary embolus.

▶ Reports of pain to be 5/10 or less.

▶ Minimize detrimental effects of immobilization.[47–52]

▶ Patient to achieve an independent or supervised functional level for:

• Transfers in and out of bed, on and off a commode, up and down from an appropriate chair (high or elevated).

• Ambulation at a household level with an appropriate assistive device.

• Stair negotiation of one or more steps, as dictated by home environment, with appropriate assistive device and with or without handrail.

• Adherence to weight-bearing status.

▶ Active assistive ROM to be at 5 to 90 degrees of involved knee motion or better.

▶ Patient to achieve functional straight leg raise without extensor lag.

▶ Motor performance to be at 3/5 on manual muscle test.

Electrotherapeutic and Physical Modalities. Modalities to reduce pain and swelling (ice and elevation) are initiated as early as possible. With the physician's permission, electrical stimulation can be used for edema reduction, muscle re-education, and pain control.[53–56] The use of neuromuscular electrical stimulation (NMES) has been shown to reduce extensor lag and the length

of stay in the acute care setting when used in conjunction with a continuous passive motion machine.[53]

Hecht and colleagues[102] compared the effectiveness of local applications of cold and heat in conjunction with exercise versus exercise alone on postsurgical pain of the knee. The application of cold with exercise was rated as providing significantly greater relief than the application of heat plus exercise or exercise alone, and swelling also was significantly decreased in the group that received the cold therapy. No other significant differences between groups were found.

Therapeutic Exercise and Home Program. Exercise encourages early enforcement of quadriceps activity and passive ROM, as well as reduction of joint effusion.[79] The patient is instructed to perform sets of 10 repetitions of isometric contractions during every waking hour, focusing on breathing normally during these exercises.[79] These exercises usually are initiated on the first or second postoperative day[43] and include:

▶ Resistive exercises to the uninvolved extremities.

▶ Deep breathing exercises.

▶ Proper elevation and positioning of the involved lower extremity.

▶ Active assistive knee flexion and extension to the involved knee. If continuous passive motion is ordered, it typically is applied immediately after surgery in the recovery room to patient tolerance, so as not to irritate the soft tissue response to the surgery. The patient is encouraged to remain on the unit for 10 to 12 hours each day, with gradual increases in both extension and flexion ranges as tolerated.

▶ Ankle pumps, quadriceps sets, gluteal sets, hamstring sets, heel slides.

▶ Straight leg raising.[43] During the early days postoperatively, leg raises are limited to the supine and prone positions to prevent the varus and valgus forces associated with hip abduction and adduction in the initial healing phase.[79] Cemented fixation allows for these movements at 2 weeks postsurgery. However, in uncemented knee replacements, hip abduction and adduction are not permitted until 4 to 6 weeks, pending sufficient bony ingrowth on radiographic examination.[79]

▶ Seated knee extension.[43]

▶ Standing knee flexion of the involved leg.

Functional Training. Functional training includes:

▶ Transfer training in and out of bed, from bed to and from chair, and to and from commode or elevated toilet seat.

▶ Gait training, including instruction on weight-bearing status, use of an assistive device, and stair negotiation. Ambulation on different levels can occur by the second or third day, if appropriate.[43] The correct progression of weight bearing is crucial to the overall success of the joint replacement, and depends on the type of fixation and alignment.[79] In patients with porous-coated prostheses, limited weight bearing is essential to allow for sufficient bony in-growth into the prosthesis, and to prevent loosening of the appliance and premature failure of the surgical alignment.[79] Full weight bearing generally is allowed at 6 weeks, based on a radiographic examination and the patient's body weight.[79]

Manual Therapy. Manual therapy techniques include patellar mobilization and soft tissue techniques. Because unrestricted patellofemoral mobility is essential for normal knee motion, mediolateral and superior patellofemoral mobilizations are initiated as early as the second postoperative day.[79]

The patient is discharged from the hospital to home or an extended care facility when medically stable. To be discharged to home, the patient should be able to demonstrate 80 to 90 degrees of active or active assisted knee motion,[43] transfer supine to sit and sit to stand, ambulate 100 feet, and ascend and descend three steps,[103] or more, as the home environment dictates.[43]

If functional independence is required before a patient returns home, the patient typically is transferred to an acute or subacute care setting. If adequate home care and safe transport are available, the patient is allowed to return home.

Home Care Phase (1 to 2 Weeks). This phase typically involves a visit from a physical therapist for 3 days a week. A physical home care assessment usually occurs within 24 hours after hospital discharge.

During this phase, the role of the physical therapist is to address any safety concerns, including moving or adjusting the height of furniture, removal of any throw rugs, review of sitting and sleeping positions, and progression of the home exercise program. Weight-bearing exercises typically are introduced at this time. These include seated heel raises (see Fig. 29-2), sit-to-stand exercises, mini-lunges (weight shifting), and mini-squats.

Specific transfers in the home and car are practiced. Gait training is advanced to crutches or cane, depending on the patient's balance. Once patients are no longer homebound, they begin outpatient physical therapy.

Phase 2: Outpatient (Weeks 3 to 6). This phase typically involves three to eight physical therapy sessions.

Goals

▶ Patient to demonstrate functional independence with gait and an assistive device on level surfaces and stairs.

▶ Patient to normalize gait pattern as necessary.

▶ Patient to achieve independence with basic activities of daily living (ADLs). ADLs may cause pain at this time. The patient should be advised against overactivity.

▶ Active range of motion (AROM) of involved knee flexion to be at 110 to 125 degrees. This degree of knee flexion is necessary for successful stair negotiation, and for sitting on a regular toilet seat.[104]

▶ AROM of knee extension to be at 0 degrees, to normalize gait.[105–108]

▶ Motor performance to be at 4/5 for the involved extremity, demonstrated by single-leg half squat at 65 percent of body weight.

▶ Reports of pain to be 3/10 or less.

Electrotherapeutic and Physical Modalities. Electrical muscle stimulation (NMES) is used in this phase of rehabilitation, with particular attention to the vastus medialis obliquus. Once full extension is achieved, NMES is applied throughout ROM and during multiple-angle isometrics, including those angles at which the quadriceps appears to function less efficiently.[79] In the more advanced stages of weight bearing, NMES is applied in the standing position to enforce strengthening of the quadriceps in the end range of extension, while incorporating proprioceptive training through the closed kinetic chain.[79]

Therapeutic Exercise and Home Program. The exercise program during this phase can include:

▶ Aerobic conditioning (stationary cycling, upper body ergonometer). Through seat adjustment on the stationary bicycle, emphasis can be placed on either flexion or extension, maintaining a comfortable, slow cadence so as not to traumatize the joint at its end range, while gaining the benefit of prolonged stretch and high repetition.[79] The reciprocal pattern of bicycling incorporates multiple joint motions and strengthening through a functional pattern of movement.[79] Because most of this patient population has had a limited activity level since prior to surgery, it is not long before this cycling program becomes an aerobic activity, and therefore affects cardiovascular endurance as well.[79]

▶ Aquatic therapy (deep-water jog, squats, straight leg raises, step-up exercises), if available.

▶ Isotonic exercises with ankle weights or surgical tubing. These exercises include knee extension, knee flexion, straight leg raising in all four planes (flexion, extension, adduction, abduction), and bridging.

▶ Side-lying hip external rotation (Fig. 29-3). The patient lies on the uninvolved side, with the shoulders and hips perpendicular to the table and the knees flexed to about 45 degrees. The patient lifts the top knee toward the ceiling, maintaining the pelvic position and contact of the feet.

▶ Flexibility exercises. A basic flexibility program is introduced, which includes stretches of those two-joint muscle groups that cross the knee joint, in particular, the hamstrings, gastrocnemius, and quadriceps.[79]

▶ Weight-bearing exercises, including partial lunges, leg press, bilateral heel raises, wall slides, and partial squats.

Neuromuscular Training. The following exercises may be performed, based on the goals of the intervention:

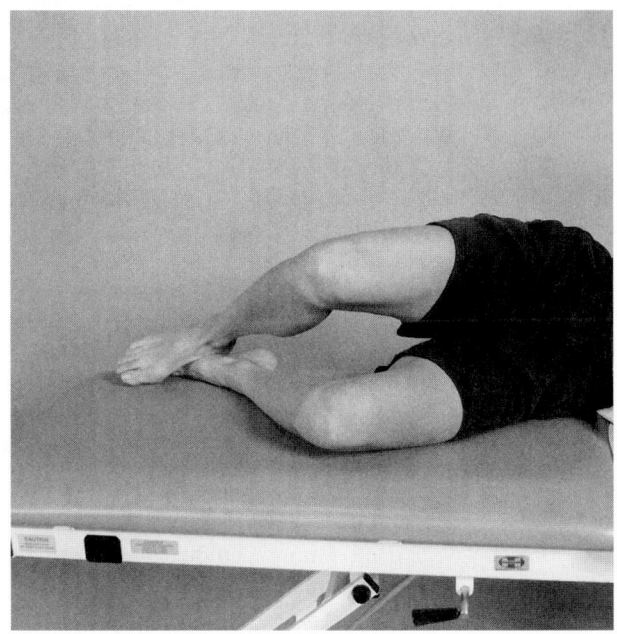

FIGURE 29-3 Side-lying hip external rotation.

- Balance-and-reach exercises (Fig. 29-4).
- Backward walking.
- BAPS (biomechanical ankles platform system).
- Toe-heel walking (Fig. 29-5).
- Side-stepping.

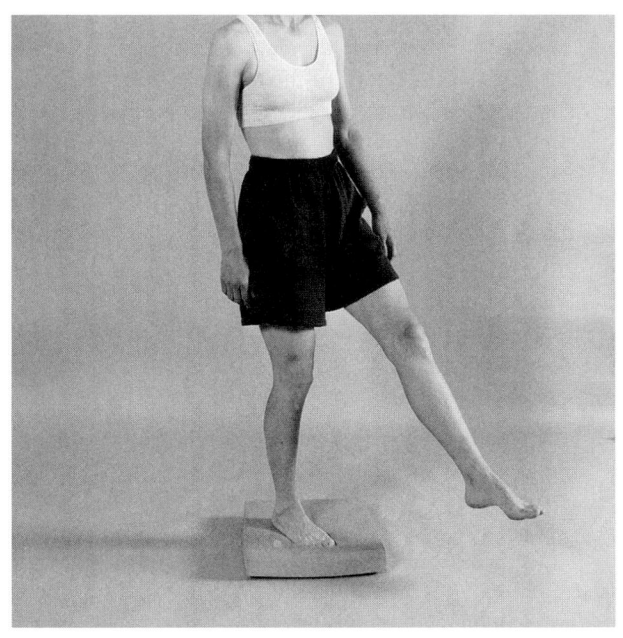

FIGURE 29-4 Balance-and-reach exercise.

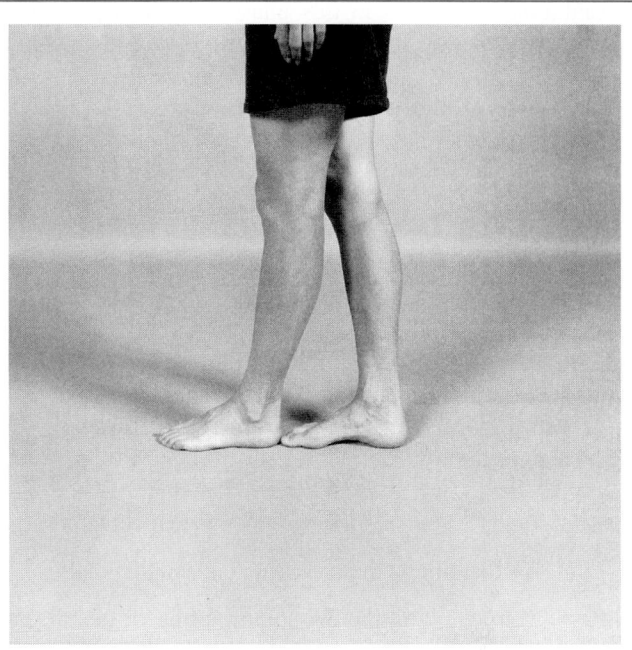

FIGURE 29-5 Toe-heel walking.

- Mini-trampoline exercises.
- Single limb balancing on the involved leg.

Manual Therapy. Manual therapy during this phase includes joint mobilizations to the patella, as appropriate, and soft tissue techniques to stretch the surrounding musculature.

Phase 3 (Weeks 7 to 12). This phase typically involves 3 to 12 physical therapy sessions.

Goals

- Patient to achieve independence and pain-free motion with all ADLs.
- Patient to have independent, normal gait pattern with single-point cane over all surfaces.
- Patient to achieve return to employment or previous hobbies as indicated.
- AROM to be at 0 to 115 degrees.
- Motor performance to be at 5–/5 on manual muscle testing, or equal to the uninvolved leg.
- Reports of pain to be at 2/10 or less.

Therapeutic Exercise

- Emphasis is placed on remaining muscle performance and ROM deficits.
- Self-stretching exercises are performed.
- Gait training is advanced to use of a single-point cane on stairs and all surfaces.

► Endurance activities in this phase shift to a progressive walking program. The program begins with 8- to 10-minute walking sessions, progressing to 60-minute walks, as tolerated.[79] The level of activity achieved after a TKA is dependent on a number of factors. The most significant consideration for patients and orthopaedic surgeons in considering athletic activity after knee replacement is wear at the weight-bearing surface.

Neuromuscular Retraining.   Various techniques and changes in direction can be applied to lateral step-ups to make the exercise more difficult and challenging to the proprioceptive system.[79] Higher levels of balance board activities are introduced. Walking activities may be progressed to include side-stepping and quick changes in direction.[79]

Manual Therapy.   Manual therapy techniques include:

► Joint mobilization to the patella as indicated.

► Passive stretching of the two joint muscles of the knee and hip (gastrocnemius, hamstrings, rectus femoris).

Outcomes

Traditionally, clinical rating scores have been used to assess results following TKA. These rating systems typically aggregate weighted scores for pain, ROM, stability, alignment, and functional ability.

The use of patient-reported outcome measures for assessing the outcomes of TKA has been emphasized in the orthopaedic literature over the past 10 years.[109] Patient self-reported measures of outcome, such as the Western Ontario and McMaster University Osteoarthritis Index (WOMAC)[110] and the Medical Outcomes Study 36-Item Short-Form Health Survey (SF-36),[111,112] have now been accepted by the orthopaedic community.[109]

Both the condition-specific WOMAC and the generic SF-36 capture the improvement in pain in patients undergoing comprehensive inpatient rehabilitation intervention sufficiently well.[113]

Anterior Cruciate Ligament Reconstruction

Despite recent improvements in efficiency, reconstruction of the anterior cruciate ligament (ACL) remains costly in terms of patient disability and medical care. Postsurgical rehabilitation, which plays a major factor in the functional outcome of these patients, has been a topic of much discussion regarding costs and effects. In addition, guidelines for postsurgical ACL rehabilitation vary considerably in the literature.[114] However, it is generally acknowledged that the quality of the rehabilitation, rather than the quantity is critical to the success of the intervention.[115,116]

Indications

Treatment options or indications are based on[117,118]:

► *Amount of knee instability.*   Surgical treatment usually is recommended for young adult athletes because they have

more years to develop degenerative joint conditions from chronic rotary knee instabilities caused by ACL deficiencies.

► *Presence of meniscal tears.*   It is becoming clear that a torn ACL that is associated with a meniscal injury needs particular attention, because the menisci contribute to stability of the knee.[119,120] The loss of the stabilizing effect of the meniscus appears to predispose patients who have a torn ACL to osteoarthrosis.[121–126]

► *Skeletal maturity of patients.*   The decision to perform surgery on children with open growth plates who are diagnosed with complete ACL disruption remains questionable. This is because of the potential damage to the growth plates, which may result in growth arrest.[127,128] The risk of growth disturbance appears to be low if young athletes are within 1 year of skeletal maturity at the time of surgery.[129]

► *Expected levels of patients' participation in future sports activities.*   The expected future activity levels and participation in sports activities for the younger patient often are more vigorous than those for middle-aged adult athletes.[130]

Procedure

Surgical treatment for patients undergoing ACL reconstruction procedures involves the use of grafts to replace their damaged cruciate ligament. The graft is placed through drilled femoral and tibial tunnels, and anchored in place at the proximal and distal attachment sites with a fixation device. Graft options include the use of autologous, allogenous, or synthetic grafts.

Autologous grafts are harvested from patients. They consist of tendons, or tendons with attached bone blocks. These grafts usually are taken from the involved extremity. The two most common autologous grafts harvested for ACL reconstruction procedures are the hamstring and patellar tendons. These grafts are used frequently because they are easy to harvest. Autologous grafts also allow return of the patient's proprioceptive response, a proven stabilizing mechanism for ACL-deficient knee joints.[131] When the semitendonosus and gracilis tendons are used together, the strength of the hamstring graft far exceeds that of the ACL. Patellar tendons also are reliable autologous grafts for ACL-deficient knee joints[132] and are used frequently because they maintain their inherent strength, and they consist of bone-tendon-bone contacts. Postoperative complications to patients' remaining patellar tendons are rare and may be minimized by careful attention to surgical technique.

Ideally, the biomechanical properties of a replacement graft should be similar to the patient's original ACL. Graft elongation behavior at the time of reconstruction has been shown to have a significant influence on the long-term anteroposterior laxity of the knee after healing. However, measurement of the length of the graft immediately following reconstruction is inadequate for determining the anteroposterior laxity and biomechanical behavior of the graft after full healing.[133,134] Instead, measurement of the elongation behavior of the graft throughout flexion-extension of the knee immediately following its fixation may provide important information for predicting the long-term laxity behavior of the knee.[133,134]

Another critical consideration for choosing a graft is the type of fixation device it requires. One recent advance for ACL reconstruction procedures has been the development of a new titanium-alloy graft fixation device, which is used to secure the proximal graft site and may be used with autologous or allogenous grafts. Avoidance of a second incision is another positive aspect of this fixation device.[135]

Postsurgical Rehabilitation

Typically, the patient is discharged on the first postoperative day following an ACL reconstruction. Just as delayed repair of an ACL-deficient knee enhances the patient's postoperative recovery, early rehabilitation after an ACL reconstruction is vital for optimal surgical results. The patient is usually permitted to shower after the second postoperative day, with bathing permitted after the sutures are removed, usually in 10 to 14 days. Following the surgery, the most common brace used is the knee immobilizer or locked drop-lock knee extension brace, weight bearing as tolerated, with crutches. The brace is worn 24 hours a day, and is only unlocked or removed for bathing and appropriate exercises. The patient is instructed on the use of crutches prior to discharge. The crutches are discontinued when the patient can stand on the involved leg with the brace unlocked, or once the patient can ambulate without limping.[136]

A patient may drive an automobile when he or she has full control of the surgical limb and is pain free.

No single postsurgical rehabilitation protocol has been universally successful for all patients. Until such time, rehabilitation protocols will continue to evolve as our knowledge of the structure and function of the ACL grows. Factors such as age, sex, chronicity of injury, associated pathology, range of motion (ROM), patient activity level, attitude, and motivation must all be considered in the rehabilitation program.[117]

Phase 1 (Weeks 0 to 4). This phase typically involves 10 to 12 physical therapy sessions.

Goals

▶ Promote wound healing and protect the surgical site.

▶ Minimize edema and pain.

▶ Minimize detrimental effects of immobilization.[47–52]

▶ Passive range of motion (PROM) to be 0 to 120 degrees of knee flexion.

▶ Patient to achieve independence with transfers of sit to stand and supine to sit, without assisting the involved leg.

▶ Patient to achieve full weight bearing with ambulation. Crutches are used with weight bearing as tolerated. The restoration of normal functional walking, stair climbing, running, and sports-specific activities in a specified time is an important component of the rehabilitation process. The

period of protected weight bearing after ACL reconstruction varies. Shelbourne and Nitz[137] have advocated an advanced and accelerated protocol. This protocol is based on observations that patients who did not comply with the traditional postoperative restrictions had more rapid improvement, without adverse results.[138] The theorized advantages of immediate weight bearing include facilitation of isometric activity to the muscles surrounding the joint, thereby reducing effusion and counteracting the reflex inhibition of the quadriceps mechanism.[139,140] The benefits of isometric activity are:

• Increased earlier articular cartilage compression and nutrition.[138]

• Maintenance of subchondral bone strength.[138]

• Decreased peripatellar fibrosis.[138]

• A lower incidence of anterior knee pain.[141] The presence of anterior knee pain may be attributed to decreased vastus medialis oblique activity and the inability to control the patella early during rehabilitation.[138] In a study by Tyler and colleagues,[138] patients who were allowed to bear weight early had a pronounced and significant increase in early quadriceps vastus medialis oblique electromyography activity at 2 weeks and less anterior knee pain. The beneficial effects of early capture of the quadriceps include early patellar mobility and earlier compressive loads on the patella.[138] The disadvantages are early loss of graft fixation and subsequent instability, although more rigid graft fixation techniques have decreased this possibility.[138]

▶ Patient to have controlled-balance double limb support.

▶ Patient to have controlled dynamic stability of the uninvolved leg.

▶ Patient able to ambulate without an assistive device for household and limited community distances.

▶ Patient to have improved quadriceps control, demonstrated by straight leg raise without extensor lag.

Electrotherapeutic and Physical Modalities. Ice, passive motion, and elevation may be used to help control muscle inhibition, and control pain.[142–145]

With the physician's permission, electrical stimulation can be used for edema reduction, muscle re-education, and pain control.[53–56] Electrical stimulation also can be used to assist in obtaining a quadriceps contraction. This often is performed in conjunction with electrical stimulation to the hamstrings to facilitate a co-contraction.[146] Neuromuscular electrical stimulation (NMES) has been shown to be either as effective as[55,147] or more effective[148] than isometric exercises in increasing muscle strength. However, NMES is recommended only in patients in whom an early aggressive rehabilitation regimen of exercises is contraindicated or not available.

Therapeutic Exercise

▶ *Continuous passive motion (CPM) machine.* In the immediate postoperative period, ice and the CPM machine have traditionally been used as part of a program intended to decrease pain and swelling and to restore full motion. Several recent studies have failed to demonstrate any clinically important or long-lasting benefits of either the CPM machine[149–152] or cold therapy,[143,153] although it has been documented that patients placed in immediate postoperative CPM require less pain medication, and that patient comfort is increased, allowing for enhancement of the rehabilitation process.[154]

▶ *ROM exercises.* The clinician should ensure immediate active extension to 0 degrees after surgery, while avoiding hyperextension. Achieving early quadriceps control in the terminal inner range, while maintaining graft integrity, is essential to prevent a flexion contracture, and for avoiding a flexed knee gait pattern.[155] Increased attention is now being paid to regaining the strength, timing, and control of the quadriceps muscle, and the restoration of early full extension, without compromising the integrity of the graft. A loss of 5 to 10 degrees of extension can result in significant disability, not only in athletes, but also in activities of daily living. Many factors can cause a loss of ROM, but delaying an ACL reconstruction procedure in an acutely injured knee, in addition to early postoperative rehabilitation, appears to help to prevent flexion contractures.[156,157]

▶ *Strengthening.* A major area of controversy revolves around the relative value of strengthening quadriceps versus hamstrings.[158] Quadriceps rehabilitation after surgery was de-emphasized in the 1970s and 1980s because of the potential for anterior tibial translation resulting from quadriceps contraction, and subsequent loosening or stretching of the graft.[155,159–161] Instead, rehabilitation of the hamstring muscles was emphasized because of their ability to generate posterior tibial translation and thus protect the graft. This emphasis on retraining, together with traditional blocking of extension, proved unsatisfactory, resulting in development of a flexion contracture, patellofemoral pain, and marked quadriceps weakness.[162] Although there have been changes in rehabilitation trends,[163,164] persistent, substantial deficits in quadriceps strength continue to be reported.[155,165–168] There have also been several reports of minor deficits in hamstring strength after ACL reconstructions. Quadriceps strength deficits of between 20 percent[165,167] and 41 percent[169] compared with deficits in the leg that was not treated have been recorded, and in some cases these deficits have been identified for as long as 4 years after surgery.[165] A 4 to 1 emphasis on quadriceps to hamstring exercise is now recommended in an effort to equalize the quadriceps/hamstring ratio from its normal 3:2 to a 1:1 ratio.[101]

- Isometrics, including so-called spider killers, are initiated along with ankle pumps. Spider killer exercises require that the patient perform the isometric contraction of the hamstrings and quadriceps while applying pressure to the ground via the heel (pretending that a spider is under the heel), to mimic a weight-bearing environment.

- Isometric quadriceps contractions are performed in complete, supported extension. Biofeedback or electrical stimulation may be used to facilitate the contraction.[170]

- Isometric quadriceps contractions are performed at 0 and at 90 degrees, with and without electrical stimulation.[170]

- Passive stretch sessions of 10 minutes are initiated to regain terminal knee extension. These include sessions of prone knee hangs (Fig. 29-6) and supine passive knee extension with a towel roll under the heel (Fig. 29-7).

- Supine wall slides (heel-unsupported hangs) are used to help regain knee flexion.

- Hip active range of motion (AROM) exercises. Straight leg raises in all four planes are used. Initially the brace is kept locked for these exercises until sufficient muscle control has been achieved.

- Supine heel slides and standing hamstring curls with and without resistance as tolerated (Fig. 29-8).

- Supine bridges.

- The supine leg press exercise, and the incline sled, can be initiated with the brace locked from 0 to 90 degrees, as indicated, to help strengthen plantar flexion and initial bilateral squatting activity in the 20- to 70-degree range, progressing to 0 to 90 degrees.

- Standing heel raises.

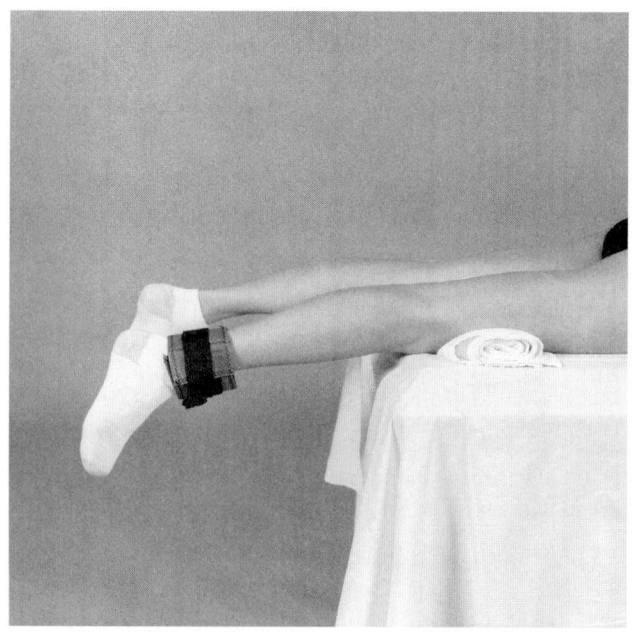

FIGURE 29-6 Prone knee hangs.

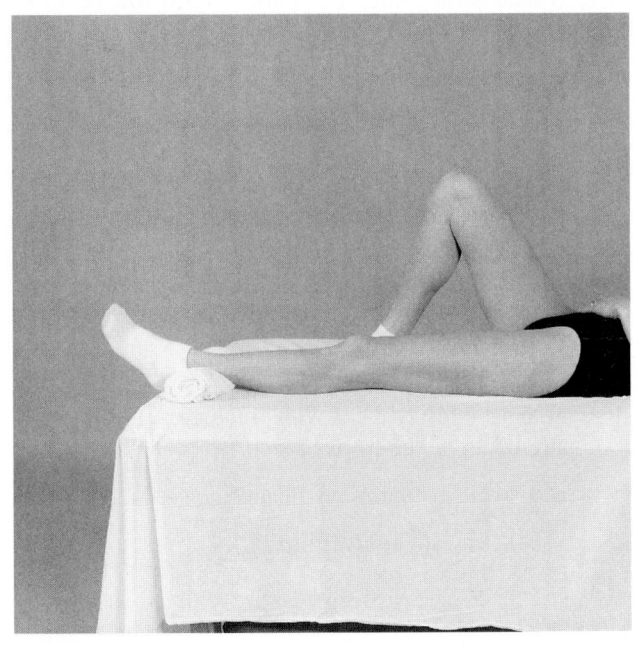

FIGURE 29-7   Supine passive knee extension.

- Seated hamstrings (carpet drags), prone hamstring curls, sports cord knee flexion.[170]

- Seated leg extension from 90 to 45 degrees is performed with no resistance other than gravity.

- Flexibility exercises for hamstrings, quadriceps, gastrocnemius and soleus, iliotibial band, and iliopsoas.[170]

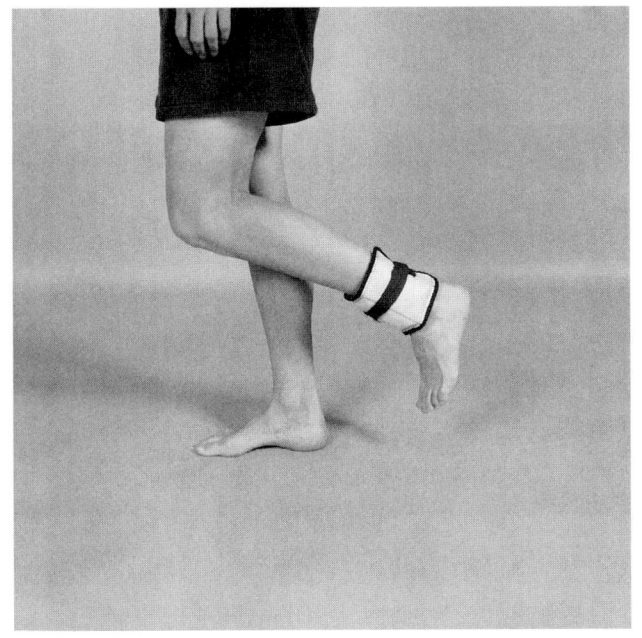

FIGURE 29-8   Standing hamstring curls with resistance.

- Cardiovascular exercises using an upper body ergonometer.

- Upper and midbody strengthening program.[170]

By the second week of the program, the patient should be progressed to:

▶ Bilateral mini-squats (0 to 40 degrees).[170]

▶ Bilateral leg press.

▶ Toe and heel raises.[170]

By the third week, the patient should be progressed to[170]:

▶ Walking on heels.

▶ Standing balance and proprioceptive exercises.

In the early stages, as the ROM increases, hamstring muscle strengthening is progressed from isometric contractions of the hamstring muscle at various joint angles within the available range, to concentric contractions of the hamstrings.

Exercises that safely strain the ACL following reconstruction include[171]:

▶ Isometric hamstring contractions at all knee flexion angles.

▶ Contraction of the dominant quadriceps muscle with the knee flexed at 60 degrees or greater (isometric quadriceps, simultaneous quadriceps and hamstring contractions, and active flexion-extension between 40 and 90 degrees of flexion).

▶ Concentric exercises of the hamstrings can be achieved by positioning the patient supine with a Swiss ball at the feet. The heel of the involved leg is placed on the ball and the patient is asked to perform a heel slide from the bridge position. This elevation of the leg also serves to reduce joint effusion.

Gait Training.   The clinician should advise the patient that acquiring dynamic stability of the knee typically takes 4 to 6 weeks. The brace is kept locked at 0 degrees with ambulation until the patient is able to perform a straight leg raise with no extensor lag.

Walking exercises are initiated once the crutches have been discontinued and may include the use of a treadmill.

Neuromuscular Retraining.   The complex kinematics of the knee depend on both mechanical stability and dynamic interaction between the central nervous system and the joint.[172,173] Between 1 and 2 percent of the volume of the ACL consists of mechanoreceptors, most of which are subsynovial, close to the femoral and tibial insertion of the ligament.[172]

Lorentzon and colleagues[174] found a significantly lower mechanical output in the ACL-deficient leg, and suggested that the observed decreases in isokinetic performance of the quadriceps muscles can best be explained by diminished activation of normally functioning muscle fibers resulting from the deficient sensory feedback from the mechanoreceptors of the torn ACL. This loss of proprioception and muscle activation may disturb the dynamic stabilization of the knee joint and endanger a graft after ACL reconstruction. A voluntary-activation deficit in patients with subacute ACL rupture also has been described by Snyder-Mackler and colleagues,[139] although the neurophysiologic mechanisms of voluntary muscle activation deficits are not yet fully understood.

There is evidence that knee joint receptors contribute to the regulation of muscle tone in posture and movement via influence on the γ muscle loop to regulate joint stiffness and joint stability.[175] It has been shown that unilateral acute inflammation increases the effectiveness of tonic descending inhibition, resulting in less hyperexcitability for the afferent input from the inflamed knee as well as for the input from regions of the contralateral leg.[176,177] Although these experiments do not explain entirely the neurophysiology of voluntary-activation deficits, they do point toward central mechanisms adjusting the bilateral fusimotor-muscle-spindle system in cases of joint pathology.[178]

This would call into question whether it is useful to attempt to overcome a voluntary-activation deficit of the quadriceps and, therefore, interfere with its regulatory effect.[178] The results of previous studies[179] showing that joint pathology without instability causes a voluntary-activation deficit clearly support a nonspecific reaction functioning as a "protection reflex" to avoid further joint or soft tissue damage.[178]

A longitudinal study concluded that most of the proprioceptive recovery from an ACL reconstruction occurred between 3 and 6 months after the reconstruction, with further improvement after that period in the midrange position.[172] These results are clinically important because they support the concept that the patient can be allowed to return gradually to his or her previous level of activity after 3 to 4 months, and that an earlier return to full activity could be dangerous because of the proprioceptive deficit still present at this time.[172]

Exercises to enhance neuromuscular activity include:

► Lower extremity proprioceptive neuromuscular facilitation (PNF) patterns with the brace locked at 0 degrees.[180]

► Step-up activities initiated with the brace unlocked, but limited.

► Stationary cycling. Because at least 100 degrees of flexion is required for a complete crank cycle, the bike should only be used once that range is established. The clinician should ensure that the seat is at the correct height to avoid the potential for developing patellofemoral symptoms.[181]

► Single-leg stance, beginning with the uninvolved leg, and progressing to the involved leg.

► Balance-and-reach leg (see Fig. 29-4) and arm exercises.[136]

► Lunge exercises in anterolateral, lateral, posterolateral, and posterior directions on the uninvolved leg.[136]

Manual Therapy. Manual therapy techniques include:

► Patellofemoral and tibiofemoral mobilizations. These are performed if there is any residual loss of motion caused by

a restricted joint glide. The patient is instructed in self-mobilization of the patella.

► Gastrocnemius stretching.

Phase 2 (Weeks 5 to 8). This phase typically involves six to nine physical therapy sessions.

Goals

► Patient to achieve normal heel-toe gait pattern without assistive device on level surfaces.

► Discontinue use of immobilizer, if still used.

► Patient to have full AROM, with emphasis on full extension compared with the uninvolved side.

► Patient to achieve controlled balance single limb support.

► Patient able to walk up to 1 mile.

► Patient able to tolerate standing for 1 hour.

► Strength to be at 70 percent of the uninvolved leg, as measured by one-repetition maximum leg press test.

► Patient able to perform a unilateral squat with full body weight from 0 to 90 degrees.

► Patient to have normal patellar ROM.

Therapeutic Exercise. The brace initially is worn for the exercises as well as for gait activities.

► The exercise intensity for the quadriceps femoris is increased from AROM to progressive resistive exercises.

► Full arc quads are introduced by week 6, together with bilateral semi-squats, and cariocas.[170]

► Step-ups, mini-squats, and other closed-chain exercises are introduced by week 6. The mini-squats should be performed with the trunk flexed, because this has been shown to increase hamstring activity and the posterior drawer force on the tibia.[182] Resistance can be added by using elastic tubing, or by adding cuff weights or shoulder weights.

► Single-leg hops begin in week 8, together with unilateral eccentric leg press and unilateral mini-squats (0 to 40 degrees).[170]

► For the athletic population, isokinetic exercises are performed in the 90- to 30-degree range of knee flexion at high speeds (360 degrees or more per second) and 70 percent or less of maximal effort, once pain and swelling are controlled. The exercises are limited to the range outside of the crepitus. More emphasis is placed on regaining quadriceps control, as this group is likely to be weak following the surgery.[183] At around 6 to 8 weeks, once there is good quadriceps control, isokinetic hip flexion and extension exercises are performed.

► Stair-stepper and cross-country ski machine exercises, and pool walking, can be initiated gradually to improve aerobic conditioning, with the goal for the duration being 20 to 30 minutes at or above the target heart rate.[184,185]

▶ By 6 weeks after surgery, the hamstrings may be exercised throughout the ROM,[186] with the patient performing 3 sets to fatigue at 40 to 60 percent of the one-repetition maximum.[187]

Manual Therapy.   Joint mobilizations are continued as needed to maintain extension and improve flexion.

Lower extremity (hip and knee) PNF patterns are initiated at 6 to 8 weeks after surgery.[180] The patterns to emphasize with these patients, are the D1 hip extension pattern (extension, abduction, internal rotation), D2 hip extension pattern (extension, adduction, external rotation), and the knee flexion patterns, all of which facilitate hamstring activity.[180]

Delsman and Losee[188] studied the leg press movement and found it closely correlated to both D1 and D2 extension patterns (hip extension, knee extension, tibial rotation). The study also demonstrated that the leg press greatly decreased ACL stress compared with isolated knee extension exercises.[180]

Gait Training.   Gait training focuses on normalizing the gait pattern. By the end of this phase, patients should be able to walk through figure-of-eight and box patterns.

Neuromuscular Retraining.   Balance exercises during this phase include BAPS (biomechanical ankle platform system) and balance board,[183] and balance-and-reach exercises involving balancing on the involved leg and reaching in various directions, heights, and distances. Other balance activities include:

▶ Single-leg stance with eyes closed.

▶ Double-leg stance on a wobble board, progressing to wobble board on one leg.

▶ Single-leg stance on a trampoline, throwing a ball ahead, and progressing to throwing the ball in different directions.[136]

Neuromuscular stimulation exercises during this phase include:

▶ Jumping rope gently.

▶ Stepping activities, which are advanced from stepping to jump-ups on a height basis (2 to 6 inches), and in different directions.

▶ Lateral shuffle (no cross-over steps).

Phase 3 (Week 9+).   This phase typically includes 14 to 21 physical therapy sessions.

Goals.   The goal of the early phase of rehabilitation following ACL reconstruction is to return the patient to "daily life" functions within the first 3 months.[189] The next step in the rehabilitation process is for the patient to return to full recreational and sports activities, as previously indicated by the patient. For this to be achieved, the patient must build up tolerance to stressful weight-bearing activities to equal that of the uninvolved leg.

Therapeutic Exercise

▶ Stool walking is initiated, in which the patient sits on a wheeled stool and propels around using the legs only (Fig. 29-9).

▶ Stair-stepper exercises, both forward and backward facing.

▶ Jumping rope normally (12th week).

▶ Jogging (12th week).

▶ Stationary bike.

Neuromuscular Retraining.   Agility training is performed in conjunction with perturbation training to allow for carryover of improvements in postural and dynamic knee stability into more sport-specific movement.[190]

▶ Balance beam walking.

▶ Two-legged hops.

▶ Two-legged jumps on a trampoline.[136]

▶ Slide board exercises.

▶ Wobble board exercises, on a single leg with eyes closed.[136]

▶ Balance-and-reach exercises (see Fig. 29-4).[136]

▶ Lunges in multiple directions.[136]

▶ Jump-ups and jump-downs with a 6- to 18-inch box.

Gait Training.   Resistance in the form of surgical tubing is added to gait activities, which include backward, sideways, and diagonal walking.

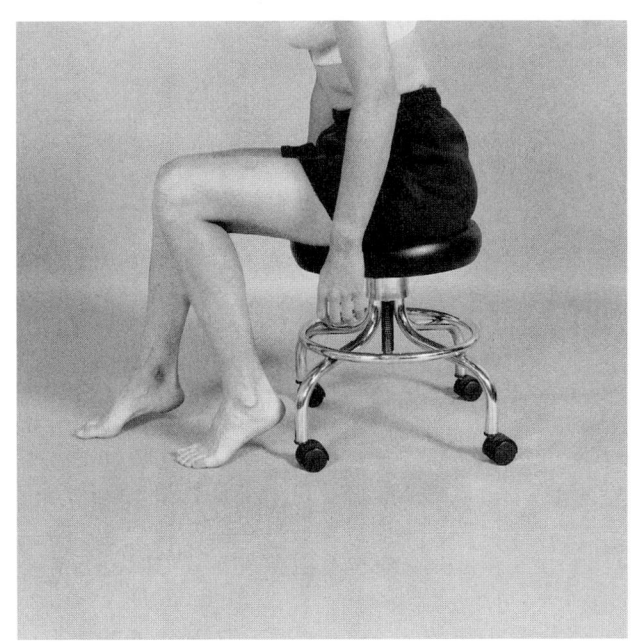

FIGURE 29-9   Stool walking.

Return to Sport. The time at which the patient returns to sport depends on the demands of that sport and the individual recovery speed. Ideally, this should not occur until the patient has regained more than 80 percent of functional strength, endurance, and agility of the uninvolved extremity.[117,191,192]

A number of objective tests can be used to assess a patient's readiness to return to sport, the most useful being functional testing (see Chap. 18):

► *Hop and stop.*[193,194]

► *Vertical jump.*[194–197]

► *Figure-of-eight running.* Patients run in figure-of-eight circles of varying diameters (4 to 8 m), three times in one direction and three times in the other direction, and their time is recorded.

► *Single-leg hop.*[194–196,198,199] The patient stands on the involved leg and performs a long jump–type movement. The distance from take-off toe to landing heel and is measured and compared with that for the uninvolved leg.

► *Six-meter single-leg hop.*[194–196,198] The clinician marks off a distance of 6 m, and the patient performs single-leg hops over the distance. The time taken is measured and compared with that for the uninvolved leg.

► *Triple jump.*[189,195]

The two-legged tests and figure-of-eight tests have been correlated to daily life function, and the one-legged tests are highly correlated to knee instability.[189]

The patient must be progressed gradually toward the performance of these tests. The plyometric and agility drills that follow can help in that progression.[136,200]

► Single-leg jumps on a trampoline.

► Bounding for distance.

► Running in a figure-of-eight.

► Vertical jumps.

► Scissor jumps.

► Forward and sideways lunges.

► Hopping onto a BAPS board.

► Step-offs from a BAPS board.

► Cutting and agility drills.

DeMaio and colleauges[183] advocate the use of the functional progression in Table 29-1. The patient can progress though each step in the progression only if asymptomatic.

Bracing. A derotational brace may be used for activities of daily living to keep the patient's knee from internally or externally rotating. The use of a knee orthosis is recommended for patients whose KT-1000 test result increases 2 to 3 mm over the previous test (if used), for those who complain of the knee

TABLE 29-1 Functional Progression Following Anterior Cruciate Ligament Reconstruction

1. 15 heel raises.
2. Walking at a fast pace.
3. Jumping on both legs.
4. Hopping on the involved leg.
5. Jogging straight.
6. Jogging straight and on curves.
7. Running straight at ½ speed, ¾ speed, and then full speed.
8. Running large figure-8s (20 yards) at ½ speed, ¾ speed, and then full speed.
9. Running small figure-8s (10 yards) at ½ speed, ¾ speed, and then full speed.
10. Cariocas (grape-vine or cross-over drill) performed in both directions.
11. Running on uneven terrain; running up, down, and sideways on hills.
12. Cutting (wearing athletic shoes on asphalt) at ½ speed, ¾ speed, and then full speed.
13. Cutting (wearing spikes on grass) at ½ speed, ¾ speed, and then full speed.

giving way, or those in whom the bracing appears to change muscle firing patterns.[201,202]

Bracing is continued for 1 to 2 years after surgery during any sports activity. It can take up to 12 months for the graft to resemble the normal ACL and possibly 24 months for it to progress to the preinjury strength level.[203]

Sleeves. Several studies have shown that patients after ACL rupture display decreased proprioception,[204–206] and to some extent this remains, even after reconstruction.[173,207] It also has been shown that patient satisfaction does not correlate well with knee joint stability following ACL reconstruction, but rather correlates with the residual level of proprioception.[173,207] This finding suggests that the ability to provide functional knee joint stability through neuromuscular control is an important factor after ACL reconstruction.[208]

An elastic bandage has been found to improve joint position sense in patients with disturbed proprioception.[209,210] In addition, a recent study revealed that an elastic compression sleeve reduced the sway in the anteroposterior direction during balance by as much as 20 percent, and the force requirements for the postural adjustments were reduced by 5 percent, indicating that the integration of afferent and efferent pathways (e.g., inter-joint and muscle coordination) was significantly refined.[208]

Meniscal Repair

The intervention options for meniscal tears include no intervention, partial meniscectomy, or meniscal repair. Determinations as to the course of treatment are based on several variables. These include the patient's age, the chronicity of the injury, the patient's activity requirements, and arthroscopic findings as to the location and length of the tear.

Traditional thinking viewed the menisci as essentially functionless.[211] Thus, meniscal lesions were treated by total meniscectomy.[212–216] This attitude changed as studies were published noting the harmful long-term effects of a total meniscectomy, including an increase in peak stresses on the tibial plateaus by up to 70 percent after meniscectomy,[217,218] ligamentous laxity, persistent pain and effusion, gait abnormalities, and varus angulation, all of which worsened with increased time from meniscectomy.[219–223]

These findings and the development of arthroscopic techniques led to increased emphasis on partial meniscectomy. Although initial reports were positive,[224–226] later studies indicated that the severity of post-partial meniscectomy changes correlated with the amount of meniscal tissue removed.[227]

The outer 25 to 30 percent of the menisci is known to be vascular.[228] Tears in the vascular region are repairable, as well as tears extending into the avascular midsubstance, if vascularity is stimulated through abrasion of the perimeniscal synovium or implantation of a fibrin clot, or both.[124,229–231] Success rates for meniscal repairs have been reported to be about 90 percent at follow-up, from 3 to 5 years after surgery.[232–234]

Next to an adequate blood supply, the most important factor influencing the prognosis of the meniscus repair is stability of the anterior cruciate ligament.

Indications

The principal indications for meniscal repair are a peripheral, longitudinal, full-thickness meniscal tear, with no secondary disruptions, that lies within the peripheral vascular zone. The tear should be at least 10 cm in length.[235]

Postsurgical Rehabilitation

There is no consistent agreement as to the best postsurgical protocol following meniscal repair. Most protocols cover three basic issues: motion, weight bearing, and return to pivoting sports.[235]

► *Motion.* Some surgeons advocate an initial immobilization in extension. Others advocate immobilization in various positions of flexion. Still others advocate limited early motion.

► *Weight bearing.* Some surgeons permit no weight bearing (the duration of this restriction varies). Others permit partial weight bearing. Still others place no restriction on immediate weight bearing.

► *Pivoting sports.* Some surgeons permit the athlete to return to sports after 4 months, others wait 6 months, and still others recommend an even longer wait.

The postsurgical rehabilitation program that follows is based on the consensus found.[235]

Phase 1 (Weeks 0 to 4). This phase typically involves two to eight physical therapy sessions. If the number of patient visits must be managed, fewer treatments are necessary in the initial phases of rehabilitation if pain and swelling are under control, and range of motion (ROM) is progressing without complications.

Goals

► Control inflammation, pain, and edema.

► Observe for possible complications (peroneal and saphenous nerve palsies, deep infections, deep vein thrombosis, cellulitis, complex regional pain syndrome, and thrombophlebitis).

► Minimize detrimental effects of immobilization.[47–52]

► Patient to increase weight-bearing activities. The weight-bearing status of the patient varies from non-weight bearing to weight bearing as tolerated. Recent studies have shown similar success rates between conservative rehabilitation programs and those with early, full weight bearing and unrestricted ROM, known as *accelerated programs.*[232,235,236]

► Knee ROM to be at 0 to 130 degrees.

► Strength of hamstrings and quadriceps to be at 4/5 with manual muscle test.

► Patient to have no extensor lag with the straight leg raise.

► Reports of pain to be 1/10 or less at rest, and 2/10 or less after light activity.

► Ensure correct gait pattern and weight bearing, with or without assistive device.

► Patient to be able to negotiate stairs with an assistive device.

► Patient to achieve independent transfers.

► Begin progression into neuromuscular training.

Electrotherapeutic and Physical Modalities

► Cryotherapy.[142]

► Electrical stimulation for edema reduction, muscle reeducation, and pain control.[53–56]

Therapeutic Exercise

► Active range of motion (AROM)/Active assistive range of motion (AAROM) of knee within the constraints of the bracing. Meniscal repairs of the outer third and large meniscal tears are typically braced at 0 to 90 degrees for up to 14 days. Meniscal repairs to the avascular zone may be braced at 20 to 70 degrees, with a gradual increase to 0 degrees of extension and 90 degrees of flexion occurring over 7 to 10 days. The ROM should not be forced and should be performed within tolerance, because knee flexion pulls the medial and lateral meniscus posteriorly, which can place increased stress on the repaired and healing tissues.[228,237]

► Submaximal isometrics of the quadriceps, hip abductors, hip adductors, hamstrings, and hip extensors. Co-contractions of the hamstrings and quadriceps are encouraged.

▶ Hamstring stretches.

▶ Gastrocnemius (Fig. 29-10) and soleus (Fig. 29-11) stretching with a towel or sheet in the long sit position.

▶ Ankle progressive resistive exercises using surgical tubing.

▶ Wall slides or passive heel slides (see Fig. 29-1), depending on weight-bearing status.

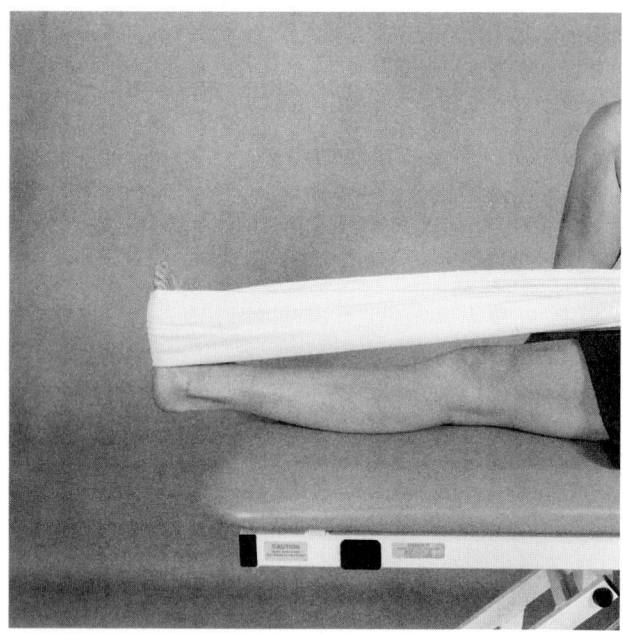

FIGURE 29-10   Gastrocnemius stretch.

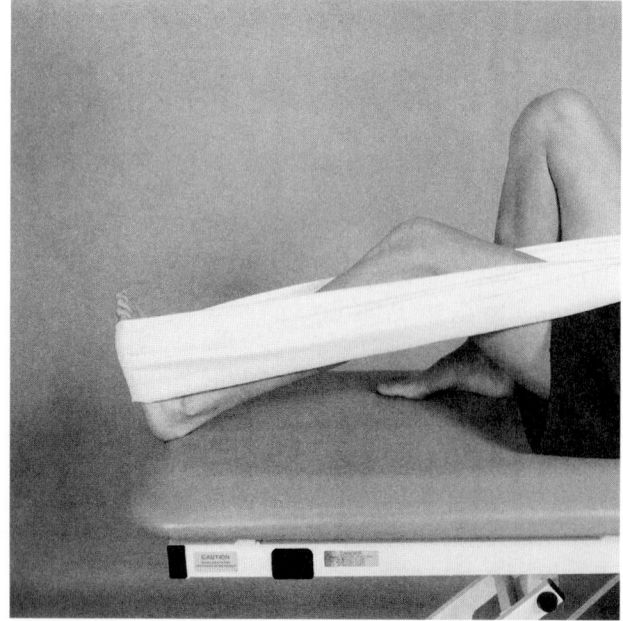

FIGURE 29-11   Soleus stretch.

▶ Heel raises while standing or using an incline squat machine, depending on weight-bearing status.

▶ Straight leg raising in all four planes (flexion, abduction, adduction, and extension), with the addition of cuff weights or tubing, as tolerated.

▶ Low-resistance, moderate-speed stationary cycling once knee flexion is 110 degrees.

▶ Standing terminal knee extension with surgical tubing (Fig. 29-12).

▶ Aquatic therapy or swimming, if available.

▶ Leg press machine within appropriate ranges (less than 90 degrees of knee flexion).

Manual Therapy.   Manual therapy techniques include:

▶ Passive range of motion (PROM) of knee flexion-extension within tolerated or restricted range.

▶ Passive stretching of the gastrocnemius, soleus, and hamstrings.

▶ Patellar mobilizations. Patellar taping may be necessary to correct patellar tracking.[238,239]

▶ Gentle scar massage of incisions after 10 days.

▶ Tibiofemoral mobilizations (third to fourth week), as needed.

Gait Training.   Crutches should be used until adequate strength, ROM, and normal gait biomechanics are achieved. Adherence to the weight-bearing instructions is critical.

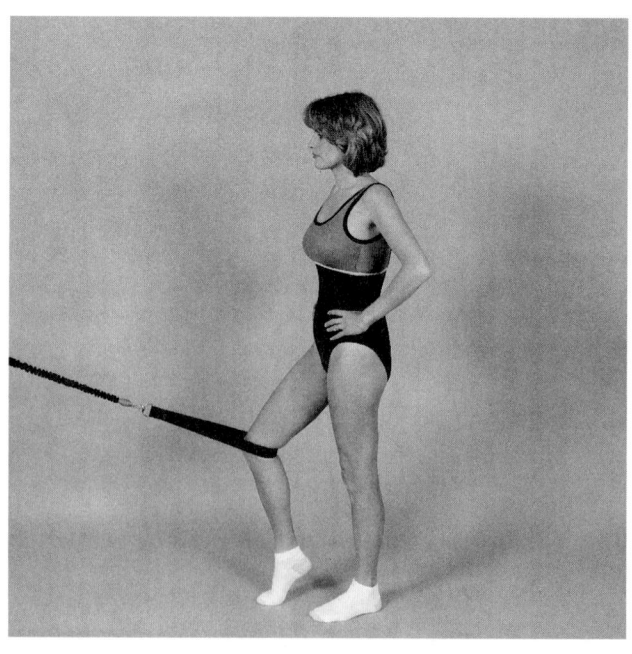

FIGURE 29-12   Terminal knee extension.

Phase 2 (Weeks 5 to 12). This phase typically involves 6 to 14 physical therapy sessions.

Goals

▶ Strength to be at 70 percent of the uninvolved leg, as measured in a weight-bearing exercise, such as a leg press.

▶ Proprioception to be at 70 percent of the uninvolved leg, as measured by the single-leg stance time.

▶ Patient to have full AROM.

▶ Patient to achieve normal gait and standing tolerance.

▶ Continue progression to functional activities.

Therapeutic Exercise

▶ Isotonic progression for hamstrings.

▶ Stationary cycling at various speeds, resistance, and duration.

▶ Stair-stepper, treadmill, and cross-country ski machine exercises.

▶ Progression to a walking-running program.

▶ Stretching of quadriceps and iliopsoas.

Manual Therapy. Joint mobilization of the tibiofemoral joint at end ranges is performed, if needed.

Neuromuscular Retraining

▶ Weight-bearing exercises, including heel raises, lateral step-up, forward step-ups and step-downs, wall squats (knee flexion at 45 to 60 degrees), and partial lunges, with constant re-assessment of response in terms of pain and swelling.

▶ Balance activities, including BAPS (biomechanical ankle platform system), balance board, and trampoline, with reach-and-balance activities.

▶ Steamboats with elastic tubing (Fig. 29-13).

Phase 3 (Weeks 13 to 24). This phase typically involves two to five physical therapy sessions.

Goals

▶ Patient to have full, pain-free AROM compared with the uninvolved side.

▶ Reports of pain to be 0/10 for activities of daily living, and 2/10 or less with activity.

▶ Strength to be at 90 to 100 percent of the uninvolved leg, as measured by a single closed-kinetic chain exercise, such as the leg press.

▶ Patient to have a normal gait pattern without an assistive device.

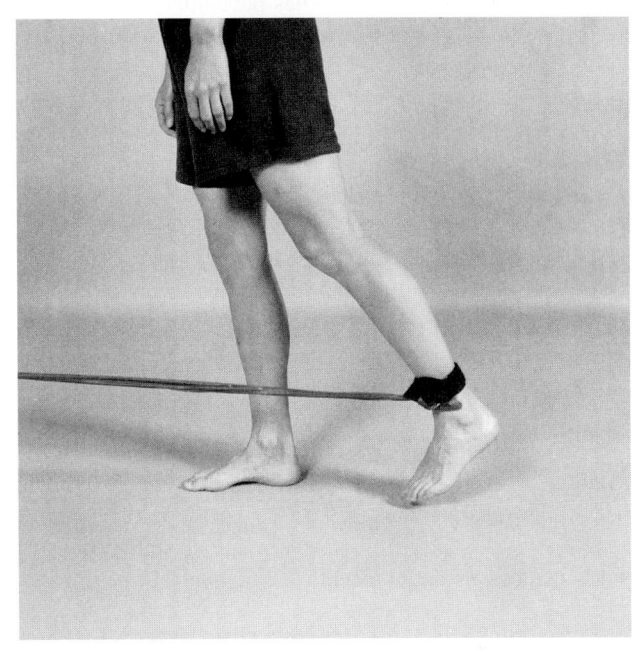

FIGURE 29-13 Steamboats.

▶ Patient to achieve appropriate isokinetic test results for progression to running and agility program (70 percent of the uninvolved extremity).

▶ Patient to achieve appropriate isokinetic test results for return to sport (10 percent of the uninvolved extremity).[236]

▶ Patient able to return to sport or previous functional status.

Therapeutic Exercise

▶ Progression of exercises outlined in phase 2 is continued.

▶ Jog-walk program is increased to 1½ miles over 3 weeks.

▶ Once sprinting is tolerated, cutting and twisting movements can be added in the form of carioca, figure-of-eight, circle running, and cutting.

Neuromuscular Retraining. Progression of the exercises in phase 2 is continued.

Note: The intervention of meniscal injuries has undergone a substantial evolution in the past decade, resulting in an increased understanding of meniscal function and the long-term effects of meniscectomy. Current research has begun to focus on techniques for preservation of meniscal tissue.

Allograft Meniscal Transplantation.[240] Studies demonstrating the ability of meniscal tissue to heal if attached to a well-vascularized periphery led to the hypothesis that transplanted allographic meniscal tissue would have the potential to revascularize and function within the recipient's knee.[241–245]

Meniscal transplantation was first performed in humans in 1984 by Milachowski and colleagues.[246] Since that time, preliminary reports and case studies have appeared in the literature. These reports have shown good or satisfactory results in 85 to 95 percent of patients.[242,246–249]

The topic of postoperative rehabilitation for the meniscal transplant is not fully developed within the current literature. Most reports advocate the use of a brace on the involved knee, 5 to 6 weeks of partial or non–weight-bearing status on the involved extremity, and immediate ROM of the knee joint.[242,247,249,250]

Restoring full extension immediately after surgery is emphasized, particularly in medial transplants, because this often involves removal and reattachment of the posterior oblique ligament and deep portion of the medial collateral ligament. Loss of motion after anterior cruciate ligament reconstruction has been correlated with repairs of these structures.[251]

As rehabilitation progresses, closed kinetic chain activities are limited from 0 to 60 degrees of flexion, because the load borne by the menisci increases as the knee approaches 90 degrees.[217] Proprioceptive training is emphasized, because the menisci contain mechanoreceptors and likely have a proprioceptive role.[252]

Based on the findings from a variety of studies,[242–246,248] the initiation of functional activities can occur at approximately 9 months, with a full return to functional activities at about 1 year after surgery.

The functional progression initially includes jogging, and progresses to running straight ahead. Cutting activities, which are added slowly, are monitored carefully. Returning to hard cutting and pivoting activities following meniscal transplant surgery is not recommended because of the high stresses these activities place on the menisci and the increased risk of reinjury they present.

Procedures Involving the Foot and Ankle

Achilles Tendon Repair

Indications
Because re-ruptures are known to occur in as many as 30 percent of patients undergoing conservative treatment for Achilles tendon rupture, surgical repair often is advocated for these injuries.[253–255] Other indications for surgical intervention appear to be the better prognosis afforded, restoration of the continuity of the tendon, facilitation of healing, and restoration of maximum muscle function.

Procedure
The literature is replete with descriptions of various techniques with which to repair the ruptured Achilles tendon. The surgical procedure, which ideally is performed within 1 week of rupture, can be performed under local, spinal, epidural, or general anesthesia. Surgical exposure of the tear typically involves a transverse, medial, or longitudinal incision, which varies in length from 6 to 10 cm, with the patient positioned prone. The severed ends of the tendon are brought together and then sutured, with the ankle in a neutral position. The ankle is then taken through

a range of motion to evaluate the integrity of the repair, and, often, a cast is applied.

The length of time that the cast remains on the patient varies according to the surgical technique. A study[256] that involved early active motion of the ankle and weight bearing, without casting, demonstrated remarkable functional recovery without serious complications. If casting is used, it incorporates varying degrees of plantar flexion (typically 10 to 20°) to protect the repair from stress. Because long-term immobilization impairs the recovery of the injured tendon and delays remodeling of newly formed collagen fibrils,[257] casting has become less popular.

After the cast is removed, the patient can be fitted with a short walking cast for about 4 weeks, and permitted partial weight bearing. If early weight bearing is the aim, the patient is issued a specially designed shoe that has a 3-cm heel lift, or a removable ankle-foot-orthosis with a rocking sole.[258]

Postsurgical Rehabilitation
Early controlled mobilization and passive motion are advocated for all tendon injuries.[259–262]

Phase 1 (Day 1 to Week 3).   This phase typically involves three to six physical therapy sessions.

Goals

▶ Control edema.

▶ Protect the repair site.

▶ Minimize scar adhesion.

▶ Minimize detrimental effects of immobilization.[47–52]

▶ Begin progression to full weight bearing with normal gait pattern with an assistive device, as necessary.

▶ Ankle range of motion (ROM) to be at 5 degrees of dorsiflexion with the subtalar joint in neutral and knee extended, and 10 degrees with the knee flexed.

▶ Reports of pain to be at 5/10 or less.

▶ Strength to be at a minimum of 4/5 in all of the major muscle groups of the involved lower extremity, with the exception of the plantar flexors.

▶ Minimize aerobic deconditioning.

Electrotherapeutic and Physical Modalities

▶ Cryotherapy for edema.

▶ Pulsed ultrasound, progressing to continuous ultrasound.

▶ With the physician's permission, electrical stimulation can be used for edema reduction, muscle re-education, and pain control.[53–56]

Therapeutic Exercise

▶ General lower extremity stretches are performed, as indicated (hamstrings, hip flexors, and rectus femoris).

Gastrocnemius and soleus stretching gradually is introduced by the third week.

▶ Active range of motion (AROM) of the ankle out of the splint is begun on the second day postsurgery. Plantar flexion-dorsiflexion exercises are performed three times daily, with two sets of five repetitions. By the second week, a progression is made to two sets of 20, three times a day. Active ROM exercises of inversion-eversion and circumduction are initiated during week 2.

▶ Foot and ankle isometric exercises into eversion-inversion and plantar flexion-dorsiflexion are initiated in week 2. By the third week, the exercises are progressed to using bands or tubing.

▶ Toe curls with a towel and weight are initiated in week 2.

▶ Proprioceptive neuromuscular retraining of the lower extremity is initiated.

▶ Gait training in a walker splint (partial weight bearing or full weight bearing) begins 2 weeks after the surgery on the day the sutures are removed, or after 3 weeks.[263] A heel lift or cam walker (Fig. 29-14) can be used to maximize comfortable propulsion in the terminal stance phase, if appropriate.

▶ Cardiovascular exercise using an upper body ergonometer and stationary bicycle is initiated. A stationary bicycle is excellent for gradually increasing the length and intensity of exercise.[264] Although a stair-stepper machine can be used, care must be taken with the intensity to prevent an overuse injury.

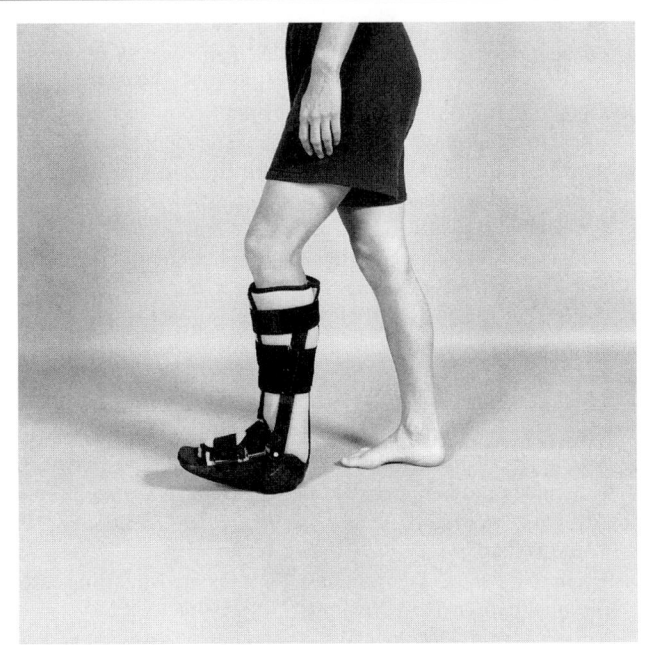

FIGURE 29-14 A cam walker.

Manual Therapy. Manual therapy techniques include:

▶ Manual resistive exercises to foot and ankle.

▶ Soft tissue techniques, including gentle transverse frictional massage to the surgical scar and tendon repair, and myofascial techniques to the gastrocnemius and soleus muscles.

▶ Joint mobilization for talocrural dorsiflexion-plantar flexion, and rearfoot and midfoot inversion-eversion.

Phase 2 (Weeks 4 to 6). This phase typically involves three to six physical therapy sessions.

Goals

▶ Patient to achieve an unassisted, normal gait pattern with maximized propulsive phase on all surfaces and stairs and without protective boot.

▶ Restore full AROM in all four planes (plantar flexion, dorsiflexion, eversion, and inversion).

▶ Restore normal foot and ankle arthrokinematics.

▶ Strength to be at 5/5 for all major muscle groups with manual muscle testing, with the exception of plantar flexion.

▶ Begin return to full activities of daily living and vocational function.

▶ Reports of pain to be 2/10 or less.

▶ Proprioceptive and neuromuscular reactions to be equal to the uninvolved side.

▶ Maintain cardiovascular conditioning.

Therapeutic Exercise

▶ Continuation of ankle flexibility exercises with progressively greater efforts, positioning the knee at full extension and flexed to 35 to 40 degrees.

▶ Progressive close chain calf strengthening and ankle stabilizer strengthening.

▶ Progression of cardiovascular training from stationary bike (pedal under midfoot until 10 to 12 weeks postsurgery) to treadmill to stair-stepper or cross-country ski machine.

▶ Proprioceptive neuromuscular retraining progression.

▶ Progressive walking and running activities on all surfaces.

Manual Therapy. Manual therapy techniques include:

▶ Manual resistance exercises.

▶ Mobilizations to ankle, rearfoot, and midfoot, as indicated.

Gait Training. As indicated, gait is progressed from partial weight bearing to full load by weeks 5 to 6.[263]

Phase 3 (Weeks 6 to 15). This phase typically involves four to six physical therapy sessions.

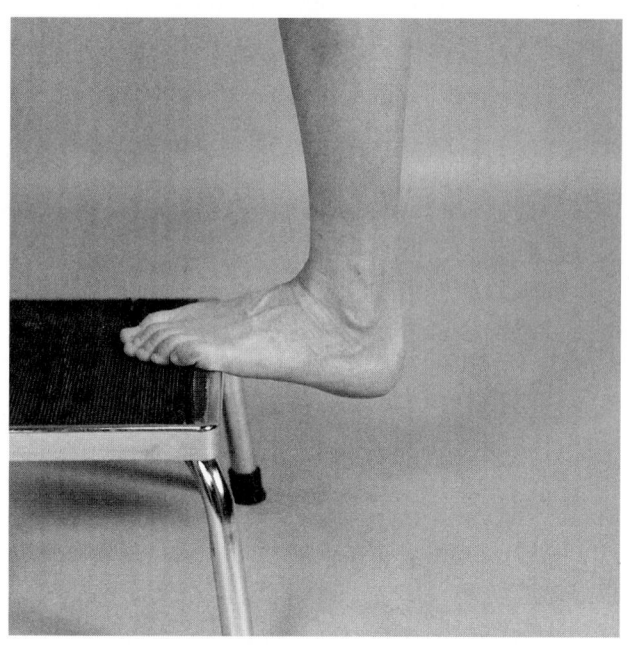

FIGURE 29-15   Single-leg heel raising and lowering.

Goals

▶ Initiate running program.

▶ Improve balance and coordination.

▶ Increase velocity of activities.

▶ Return to pre-operative level of activity or sport.

Therapeutic Exercise

▶ Strengthening can be progressed to proprioceptive neuromuscular facilitation patterns and isokinetics, as tolerated. One study noted that 6 months of rehabilitation after surgical intervention was not sufficient to recover concentric, and especially eccentric, plantar flexion muscle strength compared with the noninvolved side.[265]

▶ Double heel raise and lowering exercises are initiated on a level surface. These exercises are progressed to single heel raises. When tolerated, the exercise is progressed to single-leg heel raising and lowering over the edge of a step (Fig. 29-15). Varying speeds of single heel raising are then introduced

Once a normal gait pattern is established, the patient can begin a running progression, sport-specific skill development, and functional activities.

REVIEW QUESTIONS

1. What are the four most common approaches employed with a total hip arthroplasty?

2. What is a common, but preventable life-threatening condition that can follow any type of surgery?

3. What are some of the risk factors associated with a DVT?

4. What are some of the signs and symptoms associated with heterotopic ossificans?

5. What are the common post-surgical motion precautions following a posterolateral approach at the hip?

* Additional questions to test your understanding of this chapter can be found in the Online Learning Center for *Orthopaedic Assessment, Evaluation, and Intervention* at www.duttononline.net.

REFERENCES

1. Harris WH. Traumatic arthritis of the hip after dislocation and acetabular fractures. Treatment by mold arthroplasty: An end-result study using a new method of result evaluation. *J Bone Joint Surg* 1969;51:737–755.

2. Ritter MA, et al. A clinical comparison of the anterolateral and posterolateral approaches to the hip. *Clin Orthop* 2001;385:95–99.

3. Baker AS, Bitounis VC. Abductor function after total hip arthroplasty: An electromyographical and clinical review. *J Bone Joint Surg* 1989;71B:47–50.

4. Frndak PA, Mallory TH, Lombardi AV. Translateral surgical approach to the hip: The abductor muscle "split". *Clin Orthop* 1993;295:135–141.

5. Roberts JM, et al. A comparison of the posterolateral and anterolateral approaches to total hip arthroplasty. *Clin Orthop* 1984; 187:205–210.

6. Mulliken BD, et al. A modified direct lateral approach in total hip arthroplasty: A comprehensive review. *J Arthroplasty* 1998;13:737–747.

7. Hedlundh U, et al. Surgical experience related to dislocation after total hip arthroplasty. *J Bone Joint Surg* 1996;78B:206–209.

8. Mallory TH, et al. Dislocation after total hip arthroplasty using the anterolateral abductor split approach. *Clin Orthop* 1999; 358:166–172.

9. Dee R, DiMaio F, Pae R. Inflammatory and degenerative disorders of the hip joint. In: Dee R, et al, eds. *Principles of Orthopaedic Practice*. New York, NY: McGraw-Hill; 1997:839–893.

10. Gore DR, et al. Anterolateral compared to posterior approach in total hip arthroplasty: Differences in component positioning, hip strength, and hip motion. *Clin Orthop* 1982;165:180–187.

11. Turek SL, ed. *Orthopaedics: Principles and Their Application*. Philadelphia, Pa: JB Lippincott; 1984:1141.

12. Walker PS. Innovation in total hip replacement—when is new better? *Clin Orthop* 2000;381:9–25.

13. American Academy of Orthopaedic Surgeons. *Orthopaedic Knowledge Update 4: Home Study Syllabus*. Rosemont, Ill: AAOS; 1992.

14. Engh CA, Glassman AH, Suthers KE. The case for porous-coated hip implants: The femoral side. *Clin Orthop* 1990;261:63.

15. Mulroy RD Jr, Harris WH. The effect of improved cementing techniques on component loosening in total hip replacement: An 11 year radiographic review. *J Bone Joint Surg* 1990; 72B:757.

16. Evans BG, et al. The rationale for cemented total hip arthroplasty. *Orthop Clin North Am* 1993;24:599–610.

17. Engh CA, et al. Histological and radiographic assessment of well functioning porous coated acetabular components. *J Bone Joint Surg* 1993;75A:814–824.

18. Tonino A, et al. Hydroxyapatite-coated acetabular components. Histological and histomorphometric analysis of six cups retrieved at autopsy between three and seven years after successful implantation. *J Bone Joint Surg* 2001;83A:817–825.

19. Vermes C, et al. The effects of particulate wear debris, cytokines, and growth factors on the functions of MG-63 osteoblasts. *J Bone Joint Surg* 2001;83A:201–211.

20. Anderson FA, Wheeler HB. Natural history and epidemiology of venous thromboembolism. *Orthop Rev* 1994;23:5–9.

21. Lotke P, Steinberg ME, Ecker ML. Significance of deep venous thrombosis in the lower extremity after total joint arthroplasty. *Clin Orthop* 1994;299:25–30.

22. Brooker AF, et al. Ectopic ossification following total hip replacement. Incidence and a method of classification. *J Bone Joint Surg* 1973;55A:1629–1632.

23. Morrey BF, Adams RA, Cabanela ME. Comparison of heterotopic bone after anterolateral, transtrochanteric, and posterior approaches for total hip arthroplasty. *Clin Orthop* 1984;188:160–167.

24. Sawyer JR, et al. Heterotopic ossification: Clinical and cellular aspects. *Calcif Tissue Int* 1991;49:208–215.

25. Ayers DC, Pellegrini VD Jr, Evarts CM. Prevention of heterotopic ossification in high-risk patients by radiation therapy. *Clin Orthop* 1991;263:87–93.

26. Bosse MJ, et al. Heterotopic ossification as a complication of acetabular fracture. Prophylaxis with low-dose irradiation. *J Bone Joint Surg* 1988;70A:1231–1237.

27. Burd TA, Lowry KJ, Anglen JO. Indomethacin compared with localized irradiation for the prevention of heterotopic ossification following surgical treatment of acetabular fractures. *J Bone Joint Surg* 2001;83A:1783–1788.

28. Bethea JS III, et al. Proximal femoral fractures following total hip arthroplasty. *Clin Orthop* 1982;170:95–106.

29. Johansson JE, et al. Fracture of the ipsilateral femur in patients with total hip replacement. *J Bone Joint Surg* 1981;63A:1435–1442.

30. McElfresh EC, Coventry MB. Femoral and pelvic fractures after total hip arthroplasty. *J Bone Joint Surg* 1974;56A:483–492.

31. Stuchin SA. Femoral shaft fracture in porous and press-fit total hip arthroplasty. *Orthop Rev* 1990;19:153–159.

32. Crockarell JR Jr, Berry DJ, Lewallen DG. Nonunion after periprosthetic femoral fracture associated with total hip arthroplasty. *J Bone Joint Surg* 1999;81:1073–1079.

33. Li E, et al. The natural history of a posteriorly dislocated total hip replacement. *J Arthroplasty* 1999;14:964–968.

34. Hedlundh U, et al. Muscular and neurologic function in patients with recurrent dislocation after total hip arthroplasty: A matched controlled study of 65 patients using dual-energy X-ray absorptiometry and postural stability tests. *J Arthroplasty* 1999;14:319–325.

35. Woo RY, Morrey BF. Dislocations after total hip arthroplasty. *J Bone Joint Surg* 1982;64A:1295–1306.

36. Paterno SA, Lachiewicz PF, Kelley SS. The influence of patient-related factors and the position of the acetabular component on the rate of dislocation after total hip replacement. *J Bone Joint Surg* 1997;79A:1202–1210.

37. Demos HA, et al. Instability in primary total hip arthroplasty with the direct lateral approach. *Clin Orthop* 2001;393:168–180.

38. Schmalzried TP, Noordin S, Amstutz HC. Update on nerve palsy associated with total hip replacement. *Clin Orthop* 1997;344:188–206.

39. Edwards BN, Tullos HS, Noble PC. Contributory factors and etiology of sciatic nerve palsy in total hip replacement. *Clin Orthop* 1987;218:136–141.

40. Cohen B, Bhamra M, Ferris BD. Delayed sciatic nerve palsy following total hip replacement. *Br J Clin Pract* 1991;45:292–293.

41. Petty W. *Total Joint Replacement.* Philadelphia, Pa: Saunders; 1991.

42. Brady LP. A multi-faceted approach to prevention of thromboembolism: A report of 529 cases. *South Med J* 1977;70:546.

43. Enloe LJ, et al. Total hip and knee replacement treatment programs: A report using consensus. *J Orthop Sports Phys Ther* 1996;23:3.

44. Burton DS, Inmrie SH. Total hip arthroplasty and postoperative rehabilitation. *Phys Ther* 1973;53:132–140.

45. Kaye G. The cementless total hip arthroplasty. *Physiotherapy* 1982;68:394–398.

46. Schunk C, Reed K. *Clinical Practice Guidelines.* Gaithersburg, Md: Aspen; 2000.

47. Booth FW. Physiologic and biochemical effects of immobilization on muscle. *Clin Orthop* 1987;219:15–21.

48. Eiff MP, Smith AT, Smith GE. Early mobilization versus immobilization in the treatment of lateral ankle sprains. *Am J Sports Med* 1994;22:83–88.

49. Akeson WH, et al. Collagen cross-linking alterations in the joint contractures: Changes in the reducible cross-links in periarticular connective tissue after 9 weeks immobilization. *Connect Tissue Res* 1977;5:15.

50. Akeson WH, et al. Effects of immobilization on joints. *Clin Orthop* 1987;219:28–37.

51. Akeson WH, Amiel D, Woo SLY. Immobility effects on synovial joints: The pathomechanics of joint contracture. *Biorheology* 1980;17:95–110.

52. Woo SLY, et al. Connective tissue response to immobility: A correlative study of biochemical and biomechanical measurements of normal and immobilized rabbit knee. *Arthritis Rheum* 1975;18:257–264.

53. Goth RS, et al. Electrical stimulation effect on extensor lag and length of hospital stay after total knee arthroplasty. *Arch Phys Med Rehabil* 1994;75:957.

54. Lamboni P, Harris B. The use of ice, air splints, and high voltage galvanic stimulation in effusion reduction. *Athl Training* 1983;18:23–25.

55. McMiken DF, Todd-Smith M, Thompson C. Strengthening of human quadriceps muscles by cutaneous electrical stimulation. *Scand J Rehabil Med* 1983;15:25–28.

56. Walker RH, et al. Postoperative use of continuous passive motion, transcutaneous electrical nerve stimulation, and continuous cooling pad following total knee arthroplasty. *J Arthroplasty* 1991;6:151–156.

57. Powell M. *Orthopaedic Nursing and Rehabilitation.* 9th ed. Edinburgh, Scotland: Churchill Livingstone; 1986.

58. Munin MC, et al. Predicting discharge outcome after elective hip and knee arthroplasty. *Am J Phys Med Rehabil* 1995;74:294.

59. Sheh C, et al. Muscle recovery and the hip joint after total hip replacement. *Clin Orthop* 1994;302:115.

60. Shih CH, et al. Muscular recovery around the hip joint after total hip arthroplasty. *Clin Orthop* 1993;303:115–120.

61. Bellamy N, et al. Recommendations for a core set of outcome measures for future phase III clinical trials in knee, hip, and hand osteoarthritis: Consensus development at OMERACT III. *J Rheumatol* 1997;24:799–802.

62. Lavernia CJ, et al. Revision and primary hip and knee arthroplasty. A cost analysis. *Clin Orthop* 1995;311:136–141.

63. Soderman P, Malchau H. Is the Harris hip score system useful to study the outcome of total hip replacement? *Clin Orthop* 2001;384:189–197.

64. Rorabeck CH, Murray P. The benefit of total knee arthroplasty. *Orthopaedics* 1996;19:777–779.

65. Diduch DR, et al. Total knee replacement in young, active patients. Long-term follow-up and functional outcome. *J Bone Joint Surg* 1997;79A:575–582.

66. Ritter MA, et al. Long-term survival analysis of a posterior cruciate-retaining total condylar total knee arthroplasty. *Clin Orthop* 1994;309:136–145.

67. Greenfield B, Tovin BJ, Bennett JG. Knee. In: Wadsworth C, ed. *Current Concepts of Orthopaedic Physical Therapy*. La Crosse, Wis: Orthopaedic Section, American Physical Therapy Association; 2001.

68. Kolettis GT, Stern SH. Patellar resurfacing for patellofemoral arthritis. *Orthop Clin North Am* 1992;23:665–673.

69. Aglietti P, et al. Tibial osteotomy for the varus osteoarthritic knee. *Clin Orthop* 1983;176:239–251.

70. Insall JN, Shoji H, Mayer V. High tibial osteotomy: A five year evaluation. *J Bone Joint Surg* 1974;56A:1397–1405.

71. Windsor RE, Insall JN, Vince KG. Technical considerations of total knee arthroplasty after proximal tibial osteotomy. *J Bone Joint Surg* 1988;70A:547–555.

72. Larcom P, Lotke PA. Treatment of inflammatory and degenerative conditions of the knee. In: Dee R, et al, eds. *Principles of Orthopaedic Practice*. New York, NY: McGraw-Hill; 1997:945–983.

73. Aglietti P, et al. The Insall-Burstein total knee replacement in osteoarthritis: A 10-year minimum follow-up. *J Arthroplasty* 1999;14:560–565.

74. Banks SA, Markovich GD, Hodge WA. In vivo kinematics of cruciate-retaining and substituting knee arthroplasties. *J Arthroplasty* 1997;12:297–304.

75. Laskin RS. Total knee replacement with posterior cruciate ligament retention in patients with a fixed varus deformity. *Clin Orthop* 1996;331:29–34.

76. Laskin RS, et al. The posterior-stabilized total knee prosthesis in the knee with a severe fixed deformity. *Am J Knee Surg* 1988;1:199–203.

77. Matsuda S, et al. Patellofemoral joint after total knee arthroplasty: Effect on contact area and contact stress. *J Arthroplasty* 1997;12:790–797.

78. Chew JTH, et al. Differences in patellar tracking and knee kinematics among three different total knee designs. *Clin Orthop* 1997;345:87–98.

79. Auberger SS, Mangine RE. Innovative approaches to surgery and rehabilitation. In: Margine, RE ed. *Physical Therapy of the Knee*. New York, NY: Churchill Livingstone; 1988:233–262.

80. Ecker ML, Lotke PA. Postoperative care of the total knee patient. *Orthop Clin North Am* 1989;20:55–62.

81. Kumar PJ, et al. Rehabilitation after total knee arthroplasty: A comparison of 2 rehabilitation techniques. *Clin Orthop* 1996;331:93–101.

82. Manske PR, Gleeson P. Rehabilitation program following polycentric total knee arthroplasty. *Phys Ther* 1987;57:915–918.

83. Waters EA. Physical therapy management of patients with total knee replacement. *Phys Ther* 1974;54:936–942.

84. Salter RB, et al. The biological effect of continuous passive motion on the healing of full-thickness defects in articular cartilage. *J Bone Joint Surg* 1980;62A:1232–1251.

85. Coutts RD, et al. The role of continuous passive motion in the postoperative rehabilitation of the total knee patient. *Orthop Trans* 1982;6:277–278.

86. Johnson DP. The effect of continuous passive motion on wound-healing and joint mobility after knee arthroplasty. *J Bone Joint Surg* 1990;72A:421–426.

87. Basso M, Knapp L. Comparison of two continuous passive motion protocols for patients with total knee implants. *Phys Ther* 1987;67:360–363.

88. Colwell CW Jr, Morris BA. The influence of continuous passive motion on the results of total knee arthroplasty. *Clin Orthop* 1992;276:225–228.

89. Coutts RD. Continuous passive motion in the rehabilitation of the total knee patient. It's role and effect. *Orthop Rev* 1986;15:27.

90. Coutts RD, Toth C, Kaita JH. The role of continuous passive motion in the postoperative rehabilitation of the total knee patient. In: Hungerford DS, ed. *Total Knee Arthroplasty: A Comprehensive Approach*. Baltimore, Md: Williams and Wilkins; 1984:126–132.

91. Jordan LR, Siegel JL, Olivo JL. Early flexion routine, an alternative method of continuous passive motion. *Clin Orthop* 1995;315:231–233.

92. Maloney WJ, et al. The influence of continuous passive motion on outcome in total knee arthroplasty. *Clin Orthop* 1990;256:162–168.

93. Vince KG, et al. Continuous passive motion after total knee arthroplasty. *J Arthroplasty* 1987;2:281–284.

94. Wasilewski SA, et al. Value of continuous passive motion in total knee arthroplasty. *Orthopaedics* 1990;13:291–295.

95. McInnes J, et al. A controlled evaluation of continuous passive motion in patients undergoing total knee arthroplasty. *JAMA* 1992;268:1423–1428.

96. Nadler SF, Malanga GA, Zimmerman JR. Continuous passive motion in the rehabilitation setting. *Am J Phys Med Rehabil* 1993;72:162–165.

97. Ritter MA, Gandolf VS, Holston KS. Continuous passive motion versus physical therapy in total knee arthroplasty. *Clin Orthop* 1989;244:239–243.

98. Romness DW, Rand JA. The role of continuous passive motion following total knee arthroplasty. *Clin Orthop* 1988;226:34–37.

99. Lachiewicz PF. The role of continuous passive motion after total knee arthroplasty. *Clin Orthop* 2000;380:144–150.

100. Chiarello CM, Gunderson L, O'Halloran T. The effect of continuous passive motion duration and increment on range of motion in total knee arthroplasty patients. *J Orthop Sports Phys Ther* 1997;25:119.

101. Irrgang JJ. Rehabilitation for nonoperative and operative management of knee injuries. In: Fu FH, Harner CD, Vince KG, eds. *Knee Surgery*. Baltimore, Md: Williams and Wilkins; 1994:485–507.

102. Hecht PJ, et al. Effects of thermal therapy on rehabilitation after total knee arthroplasty: A prospective randomized study. *Clin Orthop* 1983;178:198–201.

103. Shields RK, et al. Reliability, validity, and responsiveness of functional tests in patients with total joint replacement. *Phys Ther* 1995;75:169.

104. Aliga NA. New venues for joint replacement rehab. *Adv Dir Rehabil* 1998;17:43.

105. Murray MP. Gait as a total pattern of movement. *Am J Phys Med* 1967;46:290.

106. Giannini S, et al. Terminology, parameterization and normalization in gait analysis. In: *Gait Analysis: Methodologies and Clinical Applications*. Washington, DC: IOS Press; 1994:65–88.

107. Kerrigan DC, et al. A tool to assess biomechanical gait efficiency; a preliminary clinical study. *Am J Phys Med Rehabil* 1996;75:3–8.

108. Saunders JBD, Inman VT, Eberhart HD. The major determinants in normal and pathological gait. *J Bone Joint Surg* 1953; 35A:543–558.

109. Lingard EA, et al. Validity and responsiveness of the Knee Society Clinical Rating System in comparison with the SF-36 and WOMAC. *J Bone Joint Surg* 2001.83A:1856–1864.

110. Bellamy N, et al. Validation study of WOMAC: A health status instrument for measuring clinically important patient relevant outcomes to antirheumatic drug therapy in patients with osteoarthritis of the hip or knee. *J Rheumatol* 1988;15:1833–1840.

111. McHorney CA, et al. The MOS 36-item Short-Form Health Survey (SF-36): III. Tests of data quality, scaling assumptions, and reliability across diverse patient groups. *Med Care* 1994;32:40–66.

112. Ware JE Jr, et al. *SF-36 Health Survey: Manual and Interpretation Guide*. Boston, Mass: Health Institute; 1993.

113. Angst F, et al. Responsiveness of the WOMAC osteoarthritis index as compared with the SF-36 in patients with osteoarthritis of the legs undergoing a comprehensive rehabilitation intervention. *Ann Rheum Dis* 2001;60:834–840.

114. Fischer DA, et al. Home based rehabilitation for anterior cruciate ligament reconstruction. *Clin Orthop* 1998;347:194–199.

115. Baratta R, et al. Muscular coactivation: The role of the antagonist musculature in maintaining knee stability. *Am J Sports Med* 1988;16:113–122.

116. Bryant JT, Cooke TD. Standardized biomechanical measurement for varus-valgus stiffness and rotation in normal knees. *J Orthop Res* 1988;6:863–870.

117. Williams JS, Bernard RB. Operative and nonoperative rehabilitation of the ACL-injured knee. *Sports Med Arthritis Rev* 1996;4:69–82.

118. Keays SL, Bullock-Saxton J, Keays AC. Strength and function before and after anterior cruciate ligament reconstruction. *Clin Orthop* 2000;373:174–183.

119. Hefzy MS, Grood ES. Ligament restraints in anterior cruciate ligament-deficient knees. In: Jackson DW, et al, eds. *The Anterior Cruciate Ligament. Current and Future Concepts*. New York, NY: Raven; 1993:141–151.

120. Levy IM, Torzilli PA, Warren RF. The effect of medial meniscectomy on anterior-posterior motion of the knee. *J Bone Joint Surg* 1982;64A:883–888.

121. Frank CB, Jackson DW. The science of reconstruction of the anterior cruciate ligament. *J Bone Joint Surg* 1997;79:1556–1576.

122. Daniel DM, et al. Fate of the ACL-injured patient. A prospective outcome study. *Am J Sports Med* 1994;22:632–644.

123. Ferretti A, et al. Osteoarthritis of the knee after ACL reconstruction. *Int Orthop* 1991;15:367–371.

124. Henning CE. Current status of meniscal salvage. *Clin Sports Med* 1990;9:567–576.

125. Shirakura K, et al. The natural history of untreated anterior cruciate tears in recreational athletes. *Clin Orthop* 1995;317:227–236.

126. Sommerlath K, Lysholm J, Gillquist J. The long-term course after treatment of acute anterior cruciate ligament ruptures. A 9 to 16 year followup. *Am J Sports Med* 1991;19:156–162.

127. Janarv PM, et al. Anterior cruciate ligament injuries in skeletally immature patients. *J Pediatr Orthop* 1996;16:673.

128. Parker AW, Drez D, Cooper JL. Anterior cruciate injuries in patients with open physes. *Am J Sports Med* 1994;22:47.

129. Busch MT. Sports medicine. In: Morrissey RT, Weinstein SL, eds. *Lovell and Winter's Pediatric Orthopaedics*. Philadelphia, Pa: JB Lippincott; 1996:886–889.

130. Micheli LJ, Jenkins M. Knee injuries. In: Micheli LF, ed: *The Sports Medicine Bible*. Scranton, Pa: Harper and Row; 1995:130.

131. Koenig VS, Barrett GR. Endoscopic anterior cruciate ligament reconstruction. *Today's OR Nurse* 1995;18:6.

132. Moyen B, Lerat JL. Artificial ligaments for anterior cruciate replacement. *J Bone Joint Surg* 1994;76:173.

133. Beynnon BD, et al. The elongation behavior of the anterior cruciate ligament graft in vivo: A long-term follow-up study. *Am J Sports Med* 2001;29:161–166.

134. Tohyama H, et al. The effect of anterior cruciate ligament graft elongation at the time of implantation on the biomechanical behavior of the graft and knee. *Am J Sports Med* 1996;24:608–614.

135. Barrett GR, Papendick L, Miller C. Endobutton endoscopic fixation technique in anterior cruciate ligament reconstruction. *Arthroscopy* 1995;11:340.

136. Risberg MA, et al. Design and implementation of a neuromuscular training program following anterior cruciate ligament reconstruction. *J Orthop Sports Phys Ther* 2001;31:620–631.

137. Shelbourne KD, Nitz P. Accelerated rehabilitation after anterior cruciate ligament reconstruction. *Am J Sports Med* 1990;18:292–299.

138. Tyler TF, et al. The effect of immediate weightbearing after anterior cruciate ligament reconstruction. *Clin Orthop* 1998; 357:141–148.

139. Snyder-Mackler L, et al. Reflex inhibition of the quadriceps femoris muscle after injury or reconstruction of the anterior cruciate ligament. *J Bone Joint Surg* 1994;76A:555–560.

140. Stockmeyer SA. An interpretation of the approach of Rood to the treatment of neuromuscular dysfunction. *Am J Phys Med Rehabil* 1967;46:901–956.

141. O'Neill DB. Arthroscopically assisted reconstruction of the anterior cruciate ligament. *J Bone Joint Surg* 1996;78A:803–813.

142. Knight KL. *Cryotherapy: Theory, Technique, and Physiology*. Chattanooga, Tenn: Chattanooga Corp; 1985.

143. Daniel DM, Stone ML, Arendt DL. The effect of cold therapy on pain, swelling, and range of motion after anterior cruciate ligament reconstructive surgery. *Arthroscopy* 1994;10:530–533.

144. Michlovitz SL. The use of heat and cold in the management of rheumatic diseases. In: Michlovitz SL, ed. *Thermal Agents in Rehabilitation*. Philadelphia, Pa: FA Davis; 1990.

145. Jensen K, Graf BK. The effects of knee effusion on quadriceps strength and knee intraarticular pressure. *Arthroscopy* 1993; 9:52–56.

146. O'Connor JJ. Can muscle co-contraction protect knee ligaments after injury or repair? *J Bone Joint Surg* 1993;75B:41–48.

147. Laughman RK, et al. Strength changes in the normal quadriceps femoris muscle as a result of electrical stimulation. *Phys Ther* 1983;63:494–499.

148. Delitto A, et al. Electrical stimulation versus voluntary exercise in strengthening thigh musculature after anterior cruciate ligament surgery. *Phys Ther* 1988;68:660–663.

149. Engstrom B, Wredmark T. Continuous passive motion in rehabilitation after anterior cruciate ligament reconstruction. *Knee Surg Sports Traumatol Arthrosc* 1995;3:18–20.

150. Noyes FR, Mangine RE, Barber S. Early knee motion after open and arthroscopic anterior cruciate ligament reconstruction. *Am J Sports Med* 1987;15:149–160.

151. Richmond JC, Gladstone J, MacGillivray J. Continuous passive motion after arthroscopically assisted anterior cruciate ligament reconstruction: Comparison of short-versus long-term use. *Arthroscopy* 1991;7:39–44; erratum, 1991;7:256.

152. Rosen MA, Jackson DW, Atwell EA. The efficacy of continuous passive motion in the rehabilitation o anterior cruciate ligament reconstructions. *Am J Sports Med* 1992;20:122–127.

153. Konrath GA, et al. The use of cold therapy after anterior cruciate ligament reconstruction. A prospective randomized study and literature review. *Am J Sports Med* 1996;24:629–633.

154. McCarthy MR, et al. The effects of immediate continuous passive motion on pain during the inflammatory phase of soft tissue healing following anterior cruciate ligament reconstruction. *J Orthop Sports Phys Ther* 1993;17:100.

155. Hungerford DS, Barry M. Biomechanics of the patellofemoral joint. *Clin Orthop* 1979;144:9–15.

156. Shelbourne KD, et al. Arthrofibrosis in acute anterior cruciate ligament reconstruction. The effect of timing of reconstruction and rehabilitation. *Am J Sports Med* 1991;19:332–336.

157. Graf BK, et al. Risk factors for restricted motion after anterior cruciate reconstruction. *Orthopaedics* 1994;17:909–912.

158. Ferretti A, et al. Knee ligament injuries in volleyball players. *Am J Sports Med* 1992;20:203–207.

159. Draganich LF, Vahey JW. An in vitro study of anterior cruciate ligament strain induced by quadriceps and hamstrings forces. *J Orthop Res* 1990;8:57–63.

160. Dufek JS, Bates BT. The evaluation and prediction of impact forces during landings. *Med Sci Sports Exerc* 1990;22:370–377.

161. Griffin JW, et al. Eccentric muscle performance of elbow and knee muscle groups in untrained men and women. *Med Sci Sports Exerc* 1993;25:936–944.

162. Hahn T, Foldspang A. The Q angle and sport. *Scand J Med Sci Sports* 1997;7:43–48.

163. Hewett TE, Riccobene JV, Lindenfeld TN. The effect of neuromuscular training on the incidence of knee injury in female athletes: A prospective study. *Am J Sports Med* 1999;27:699–706.

164. Hewett TE, et al. Plyometric training in female athletes. *Am J Sports Med* 1996;24:765–773.

165. Grana WA, Moretz JA. Ligamentous laxity in secondary school athletes. *JAMA* 1978;240:1975–1976.

166. Hagood S, et al. The effect of joint velocity on the contribution of the antagonist musculature to knee stiffness and laxity. *Am J Sports Med* 1990;18:182–187.

167. Houseworth, SW, et al. The intercondylar notch in acute tears of the anterior cruciate ligament: A computer graphics study. *Am J Sports Med* 1987;15:221–224.

168. Ireland ML, Wall C. Epidemiology and comparison of knee injuries in elite male and female United States basketball athletes. *Med Sci Sports Exerc* 1990;22(suppl):S82.

169. Harner CD, et al. Detailed analysis of patients with bilateral anterior cruciate ligament injuries. *Am J Sports Med* 1994; 22:37–43.

170. Tyler TF, McHugh MP. Neuromuscular rehabilitation of a female Olympic ice hockey player following anterior cruciate ligament reconstruction. *J Orthop Sports Phys Ther* 2001;31:577–587.

171. Beynnon BD, Johnson RJ. Anterior cruciate ligament injury rehabilitation in athletes. *Sports Med* 1996;22:54–64.

172. Fremerey RW, et al. Proprioception after rehabilitation and reconstruction in knees with deficiency of the anterior cruciate ligament: a prospective, longitudinal study. *J Bone Joint Surg* 2000;82B:801–806.

173. Barrett DS. Proprioception and function after anterior cruciate ligament reconstruction. *J Bone Joint Surg* 1991;73B:833–837.

174. Lorentzon R, et al. Thigh musculature in relation to chronic anterior cruciate ligament tear: Muscle size, morphology, and mechanical output before reconstruction. *Am J Sports Med* 1989;17:423–429.

175. Johansson H, Sjolander P, Sojka P. Actions on gamma-motoneurons elicited by electrical stimulation of joint afferent fibres in the hind limb of the cat. *J Physiol (Lond)* 1986; 375:137–152.

176. Schaible HG, et al. Changes in tonic descending inhibition of spinal neurons with articular input during the development of acute arthritis in the cat. *J Neurophysiol* 1991;66:1021–1032.

177. Neugebauer V, Schaible HG. Evidence for a central component in the sensitization of spinal neurons with joint input during development of acute arthritis in cat's knee. *J Neurophysiol* 1990;64:299–311.

178. Urbach D, et al. Bilateral deficit of voluntary quadriceps muscle activation after unilateral ACL tear. *Med Sci Sports Exerc* 1999;31:1691–1696.

179. Shakespeare DT, et al. Reflex inhibition of the quadriceps after meniscectomy: Lack of association with pain. *Clin Physiol* 1985;5:137–144.

180. Engle RP, Canner GC. Proprioceptive neuromuscular facilitation (PNF) and modified procedures for anterior cruciate ligament (ACL) instability. *J Orthop Sports Phys Ther* 1989;11:230.

181. Ericson MO, Nisell R. Tibiofemoral joint forces during ergometer cycling. *Am J Sports Med* 1986;14:285–290.

182. Ohkoshi Y, et al. Biomechanical analysis of rehabilitation in the standing position. *Am J Sports Med* 1991;19:605–611.

183. DeMaio M, et al. Advanced muscle training after ACL reconstruction: Weeks 6–52. *Orthopaedics* 1992;15:757–767.

184. Klaffs CE, Arnheim DD. *Modern Principles of Athletic Training*. St Louis, Mo: CV Mosby; 1989.

185. Onieal ME. *Athletic Training and Sports Medicine*. 2nd ed. Park Ridge, Ill: American Academy of Orthopaedic Surgeons; 1991.

186. Yasuda K, Sadaki T. Exercise after anterior cruciate ligament reconstruction: The force exerted on the tibia by the separate isometric contractions of the quadriceps of the hamstrings. *Clin Orthop* 1987;220:275–283.

187. DeLorme T, Watkins A. *Techniques of Progressive Resistance Exercise*. New York, NY: Appleton-Century; 1951.

188. Delsman PA, Losee GM. Isokinetic shear forces and their effect on the quadriceps active drawer. *Med Sci Sports Exerc* 1984;16:151.

189. Risberg MA, Ekeland A. Assessment of functional tests after anterior cruciate ligament surgery. *J Orthop Sports Phys Ther* 1994;19:212.

190. Williams GR, et al. Dynamic knee stability: Current theory and implications for clinicians and scientists. *J Orthop Sports Phys Ther* 2001;31:546–566.

191. Malone T, et al. Neuromuscular concepts. In: Ellenbecker TS, ed. *Knee Ligament Rehabilitation*. Philadelphia, Pa: Churchill Livingstone; 2000:399–411.

192. Malone TR, Garrett WE Jr. Commentary and historical perspective of anterior cruciate ligament rehabilitation. *J Orthop Sports Phys Ther* 1992;15:265.

193. Juris PM, et al. A dynamic test of lower extremity function following anterior cruciate ligament reconstruction and rehabilitation. *J Orthop Sports Phys Ther* 1997;26:184.

194. Fitzgerald GK, et al. Hop tests as predictors of dynamic knee stability. *J Orthop Sports Phys Ther* 2001;31:588–597.

195. Bolga LA, Keskula DR. Reliability of lower extremity functional performance tests. *J Orthop Sports Phys Ther* 1997;26:138.

196. Barber SD, et al. Quantitative assessment of functional limitations in normal and anterior cruciate ligament-deficient knees. *Clin Orthop* 1990;255:204–214.

197. Blackburn JR, Morrissey MC. The relationship between open and closed kinetic chain strength of the lower limb and jumping performance. *J Orthop Sports Phys Ther* 1998;27:430–435.

198. Daniel D, et al. Quantification of knee instability and function. *Contemp Orthop* 1982;5:83–91.

199. Ageberg E, Zatterstrom R, Moritz U. Stabilometry and one-leg hop test have high test-retest reliability. *Scand J Med Sci Sports* 1998;8:198–202.

200. Cerulli G, et al. Proprioceptive training and prevention of anterior cruciate ligament injuries in soccer. *J Orthop Sports Phys Ther* 2001;31:655–660.

201. Branch TP, Hunter R, Donath M. Dynamic EMG analysis of anterior cruciate deficient legs with and without bracing during cutting. *Am J Sports Med* 1989;17:35–41.

202. Branch TP, Hunter RE. Functional analysis of anterior cruciate ligament braces. *Clin Sports Med* 1990;9:771–797.

203. Campbell J, Cambell Jr TE. Anterior cruciate ligament reconstruction: Using patellar tendon grafts. *AORN J* 1990; 51:944–946.

204. Barrack RL, Skinner HB, Buckley SL. Proprioception in the anterior cruciate deficient knee. *Am J Sports Med* 1989;17:1–6.

205. Beard DJ, et al. Proprioception after rupture of the anterior cruciate ligament. An objective indication of the need for surgery? *J Bone Joint Surg* 1993;75B:311–315.

206. Corrigan JP, Cashman WF, Brady MP. Proprioception in the cruciate deficient knee. *J Bone Joint Surg* 1992;74B:247–250.

207. Shirashi M, et al. Stabilometric assessment in the anterior cruciate ligament reconstructed knee. *Clin J Sports Med* 1996;6:32–39.

208. Kuster MS, et al. The benefits of wearing a compression sleeve after ACL reconstruction. *Med Sci Sports Exerc* 1999;31:368–371.

209. Barrett DS, Cobb AG, Bentley G. Joint proprioception in normal, osteoarthritic and replaced knees. *J Bone Joint Surg* 1991;73B:53–56.

210. Sell S, Zacher J, Lack S. Disorders of proprioception of arthrotic knee joint. *Z Rheumatol* 1993;52:150–155.

211. Fairbank TJ. Knee joint changes after meniscectomy. *J Bone Joint Surg* 1948;30B:664–670.

212. Ghormley RK. Late changes as a result of internal derangements of the knee. *Am J Surg* 1948;76:496–501.

213. Helfet AJ. Mechanism of derangements of the medial semilunar cartilage and their management. *J Bone Joint Surg* 1959; 41B:319–336.

214. Lipscomb PR, Henderson MS. Internal derangements of the knee. *JAMA* 1947;135:827–831.

215. Smillie IS. *Injuries of the Knee Joint*. London, England: Churchill Livingstone; 1971.

216. Smillie IS. Observations of the regeneration of the semilunar cartilages in man. *Br J Surg* 1944;31:398–401.

217. Ahmed AM, Burke DL. In-vitro measurement of static pressure distribution in synovial joints: I. Tibial surface of the knee. *J Biomech Eng* 1983;105:216–225.

218. Kurosawa H, Fukubayashi T, Nakajima H. Lode-bearing mode of the knee joint: Physical behaviour of the knee joint with or without menisci. *Clin Orthop* 1980;149:283–290.

219. Appel H. Late results after meniscectomy in the knee joint. A clinical and roentgenographic follow-up investigation. *Acta Orthop Scand Suppl* 1970;133:1–111.

220. Jackson JP. Degenerative changes in the knee after meniscectomy. *Br Med J* 1968;2:525–527.

221. Johnson RJ, et al. Factors affecting late results after meniscectomy. *J Bone Joint Surg* 1974;56A:719–729.

222. Jones RE, Smith EC, Reisch JS. Effects of medial meniscectomy in patients older than forty years. *J Bone Joint Surg* 1978; 60A:783–786.

223. Tapper EM, Hoover NW. Late results after meniscectomy. *J Bone Joint Surg* 1969;51A:517–526.

224. McGinty JB, Geuss LF, Marvin RA. Partial or total meniscectomy: A comparative analysis. *J Bone Joint Surg* 1977;59A:763–766.

225. Northmore-Ball MD, Dandy DJ. Long-term results of arthroscopic partial meniscectomy. *Clin Orthop* 1982;167:34–42.

226. Whipple TL, Caspari RB, Meyers JF. Arthroscopic meniscectomy: An interim report at 3 to 4 years after operation. *Clin Orthop* 1984;183:105–114.

227. Cox JS, et al. The degenerative effects of partial and total resection of the medial meniscus in dogs' knees. *Clin Orthop* 1975;109:178–183.

228. Arnoczky SP, Warren RF. Microvasculature of the human meniscus. *Am J Sports Med* 1982;10:90–95.

229. Arnoczky SP, et al. The effect of cryopreservation on canine menisci: A biochemical, morphologic, biomechanical evaluation. *J Orthop Res* 1988;6:1–12.

230. Henning CE, Lynch MA, Yearout KM. Arthroscopic meniscal repair using an exogenous fibrin clot. *Clin Orthop* 1990;252:64–72.

231. Henning CE, Lynch MA, Glick C. An in vivo strain gauge study of elongation of the anterior cruciate ligament. *Am J Sports Med* 1985;13:22–26.

232. DeHaven KE, Black KP, Griffiths HJ. Open meniscus repair-technique and two to nine year results. *Am J Sports Med* 1989;17:788–795.

233. Jensen NC, et al. Arthroscopic repair of the ruptured meniscus: One to 6.3 years follow-up. *Arthroscopy* 1994;10:211–214.

234. Miller DB. Arthroscopic meniscal repair. *Am J Sports Med* 1988;16:315–320.

235. Barber FA, Click SD. Meniscus repair rehabilitation with concurrent anterior cruciate reconstruction. *Arthroscopy* 1997;13:433.

236. Shelbourne KD, et al. Rehabilitation after meniscal repair. *Clin Sports Med* 1996;15:595.

237. Bullough PG, Vosburgh F, Arnoczky SP. The menisci of the knee. In: Insall, JN, ed. *Surgery of the Knee*. New York, NY: Churchill Livingstone; 1983:135–146.

238. McConnell J. Conservative management of patellofemoral problems. In: Grelsamer RP, McConnell J, eds. *The Patella. A Team Approach*. Gaithersburg, Md: Aspen; 1998:119–136.

239. Grelsamer RP, McConnell J. Conservative management of patellofemoral problems. In: Grelsamer RP, McConnell J, eds. *The Patella: A Team Approach*. Gaithersburg, Md: Aspen; 1998:109–118.

240. Fritz JM, Irrgang JJ, Harner CD. Rehabilitation following allograft meniscal transplantation: A review of the literature and case study. *J Orthop Sports Phys Ther* 1996;24:98–106.

241. De Boer HH, Koudstaal J. Failed meniscus transplantation. A report of three cases. *Clin Orthop* 1994;306:155–162.

242. Veltri DM, et al. Current status of allographic meniscal transplantation. *Clin Orthop* 1994;306:155–162.

243. Arnoczky SP, Warren RF, McDevitt CA. Meniscal replacement using a cryopreserved allograft. An experimental study in dogs. *Clin Orthop* 1990;252:121–128.

244. Jackson DW, et al. Meniscal transplantation using fresh and cryopreserved allografts. *Am J Sports Med* 1992;20:644–656.

245. Mikic ZD, Tubic MV, Lazetic AB. Allograft meniscus transplantation in the dog. *Acta Orthop Scand* 1993;64:329–332.

246. Milachowski KA, Weismeier K, Wirth CJ. Homologous meniscal transplantation: Experimental and clinical results. *Int Orthop* 1989;13:1–11.

247. Garrett JC, Stevenson RN. Meniscal transplantation in the human knee: A preliminary report. *Arthroscopy* 1991;7:57–62.

248. De Boer HH, Koudstaal J. The fate of meniscus cartilage after transplantation of cryopreserved nontissue-antigen-matched allograft. *Clin Orthop* 1991;266:145–151.

249. Van Arkel ERA, De Boer HH. Human meniscal transplantation. *Agents Action Suppl* 1993;39:243–246.

250. Stone KR, Rosenberg TD. Surgical technique of meniscal replacement. *Arthroscopy* 1993;9:234–237.

251. Harner CD, et al. Loss of motion after anterior cruciate ligament reconstruction. *Am J Sports Med* 1992;20:499–506.

252. Assimakopoulos AP, et al. The innervation of the human meniscus. *Clin Orthop* 1992;275:232–236.

253. Edna TH. Non-operative treatment of Achilles tendon ruptures. *Acta Orthop Scand* 1980;51:991–993.

254. Haggmark T, et al. Calf muscle atrophy and muscle function after non-operative vs operative treatment of Achilles tendon ruptures. *Orthopaedics* 1986;9:160–164.

255. Hart TJ, et al. Diagnosis and treatment of the ruptured Achilles tendon. *J Foot Surg* 1988;27:30–39.

256. Aoki M, et al. Early active motion and weightbearing after cross-stitch Achilles tendon repair. *Am J Sports Med* 1998;26:794–800.

257. Gelberman RH, et al. Effects of early intermittent passive mobilization on healing canine flexor tendons. *J Hand Surg* 1982; 7A:170–175.

258. Speck M, Klaue K. Early full weightbearing and functional treatment after surgical repair of acute Achilles tendon rupture. *Am J Sports Med* 1998;26:789–793.

259. Akeson WH, et al. Biochemical changes in periarticular connective tissue of the immobilized rabbit knee. *Clin Orthop* 1973; 93:356–362.

260. Amiel D, Woo SLY, Harwood FL. The effect of immobilization on collagen turnover in connective tissue: A biochemical-biomechanical correlation. *Acta Orthop Scand* 1982;53:325–332.

261. Frank C, et al. Normal ligament properties and ligament healing. *Clin Orthop* 1985;196:15–25.

262. Gelberman RH, Siedel DB, Woo SLY. Healing of digital flexor tendons: Importance of the interval from injury to repair. A biomechanical, biochemical, and morphological study in dogs. *J Bone Joint Surg* 1991;73A:66–75.

263. Soma CA, Mandelbaum BR. Achilles tendon disorders. *Clin Sports Med* 1994;13:811–823.

264. Fierro NL, Sallis RE. Achilles tendon rupture: Is casting enough? *Postgrad Med* 1995;98:145–151.

265. Alfredson H, Pietila T, Lorentzon R. Chronic Achilles tendinitis and calf muscle strength. *Am J Sports Med* 1996;24:829–833.

SOLUTIONS FOR REVIEW QUESTIONS

CHAPTER 1

1. Macrophages, mast cells, and fibroblasts.
2. Hyaline cartilage, fibrocartilage, and elastic cartilage.
3. Fascia.
4. Type 1.
5. The epitenon.

CHAPTER 2

1. E.
2. A.
3. A.
4. A.
5. C.

CHAPTER 3

1. The anatomical reference position for the human body is described as the erect standing position with the feet just slightly separated and the arms hanging by the side, the elbows straight, and with the palms of the hand facing forward.
2. Frontal, lateral, or coronal plane.
3. Transverse or horizontal.
4. Sagittal.
5. Flexion, extension, hyperextension, dorsiflexion, and plantar flexion.

CHAPTER 4

1. Body weight, friction, and air or water resistance.
2. Macrotrauma.
3. Crimp.
4. False. It is better designed to resist tensile loading.
5. Osteoarthritis.

CHAPTER 5

1. Primary injuries can be self-inflicted, caused by another individual or entity, or caused by the environment. Secondary injuries are essentially the inflammatory response that occurs with the primary injury.
2. Microtraumatic injuries occur as the result of a cumulative repetitive overload, incorrect mechanics, and/or frictional resistance. Macrotraumatic injuries occur with a sudden overloading of the musculoskeletal tissues.
3. (1) Coagulation and inflammation stage. (2) Migratory and proliferative stage. (3) Remodeling stage.
4. Neutrophils are white blood cells of the polymorphonuclear (PMN) leukocyte subgroup that appear during the inflammation stage. Neutrophils are filled with granules of toxic chemicals (phagocytes) that enable them to bind to microorganisms, internalize them, and kill them.
5. Monocytes are white blood cells of the mononuclear leukocyte subgroup. The monocytes migrate into tissues and develop into macrophages, and provide immunological defenses against many infectious organisms.

CHAPTER 6

1. Extensibility, elasticity, irritability, and the ability to develop tension.
2. The erector spinae, the biceps brachii, the long head of the triceps brachii, the hamstrings, and the rectus femoris.
3. Isometric, concentric, and eccentric.
4. An isotonic contraction is a contraction in which the tension within the muscle remains constant as the muscle shortens or lengthens.
5. True.

CHAPTER 7

1. An impairment represents the consequences of disease, pathological processes, or lesions.
2. Disability.
3. Contextual variables.
4. A physical therapy diagnosis is a diagnostic label that identifies the impact of a condition on function. A medical diagnosis is based on a pathology.
5. Range of motion testing, strength testing, and gait assessment.

CHAPTER 8

1. Empathy is the ability to see another person's viewpoint, so that a deep and true understanding of what the person is experiencing can be made.
2. An *examination* refers to the gathering of data and information concerning a topic. An *evaluation* refers to the making of a value judgment based on the collected data and information.

3. The history, systems review, and tests and measures.
4. Congestive heart failure, hypothyroidism, or cancer.
5. *Cauda equina* syndrome is associated with compression of the spinal nerve roots that supply neurologic function to the bladder and bowel.

CHAPTER 9

1. Viscerogenic, vasculogenic, neurogenic, psychogenic, and spondylogenic.
2. The intentional production of false symptoms or the exaggeration of symptoms that truly exist.
3. False.
4. L4–L5.
5. Migraine.

CHAPTER 10

1. Coordination, communication, and documentation; patient/client-related instruction; and direct interventions.
2. PRICEMEM (Protection, Rest, Ice, Compression, Elevation, Manual therapy, Early motion, and Medications).
3. Stimulation of the large fiber joint afferents of the joint capsule, soft tissue, and joint cartilage, which aids in pain reduction; stimulation of endorphins, which aids in pain reduction; a decrease of intra-articular pressure, which aids in pain reduction; the mechanical effect which increases joint mobility; the remodeling of local connective tissue; the increase of the gliding of tendons within their sheaths; and an increase in joint lubrication.
4. The inflammatory stage of healing.
5. The clinical aims during the inflammatory phase are to avoid painful positions, improve range of motion, reduce muscle atrophy through gentle isometric muscle setting, and to maintain aerobic fitness.

CHAPTER 11

1. When there is mild pain; a nonirritable condition demonstrated by pain that is provoked by motion but which disappears very quickly; intermittent musculoskeletal pain; the pain reported by the patient is either relieved by rest or by particular motions or positions; and the pain is altered by postural changes or movement.
2. Any five from the following: Bacterial infection, malignancy, systemic localized infection, sutures, recent fracture, cellulitis, febrile state, hematoma, an acute circulatory condition, an open wound, osteomyelitis, advanced diabetes, hypersensitivity of the skin, constant severe pain.
3. Traumatic hyperemia, pain relief, and decreasing scar tissue.
4. Strain–counterstrain, or functional techniques.
5. Joint mobilizations.

CHAPTER 12

1. Posture, direct trauma, extremes of motion, electrical injury, and compression.
2. Double-crush syndrome.
3. Visible atrophy, pain with palpation, diminished active and passive range of motion in the same direction, and weakness in the muscle distribution of a peripheral nerve.
4. L4–S2.
5. 30–70 degrees.

CHAPTER 13

1. The swing period begins as the foot is lifted from the ground and ends with initial contact with the ipsilateral foot.
2. The four intervals of the swing period include *pre-swing, initial swing, midswing,* and *terminal swing.*
3. Normal cadence is considered to be between 90 and 120 steps per minute.
4. False.
5. Stability of the weight-bearing foot throughout the stance period, foot clearance of the non–weight-bearing foot in swing, appropriate prepositioning of the foot for initial contact, and adequate step length.

CHAPTER 14

1. External rotation > abduction > internal rotation in a 3:2:1 ratio.
2. D.
3. Subscapularis, teres major, pectoralis major, and latissimus dorsi.
4. Infraspinatus, teres minor, and posterior deltoid.
5. Supraspinatus, infraspinatus, teres minor, and pectoralis major.

CHAPTER 15

1. False. It is the anterior band of the ulnar collateral ligament.
2. Full elbow extension and maximum forearm supination.
3. Pronator quadratus, pronator teres, flexor carpi radialis.
4. Posteriorly (especially posterior-lateral).
5. A.

CHAPTER 16

1. The scaphoid and the lunate.
2. Hamate, capitate, trapezoid, trapezium.
3. Ulnar nerve and artery.
4. D.
5. B.

CHAPTER 17

1. Extension, internal rotation, and abduction–adduction.
2. Laterally, inferiorly, and anteriorly.
3. Ligamentum teres.
4. External rotation, abduction, and extension.
5. Gluteus medius.

CHAPTER 18

1. Lateral collateral ligament.
2. Improve the weight-bearing capacity of the knee; decrease friction; and act to restrict anterior tibial translation.
3. Femoral.
4. Genu valgum.
5. Inferior facet.

CHAPTER 19

1. Anterior tibiofibular, posterior tibiofibular, and interosseous.
2. Tibial.
3. A combination of ligaments, tendons, and muscle.
4. Calcaneal inversion, talar abduction, and talar dorsiflexion external rotation of the tibia.
5. The interdigital nerve.

CHAPTER 20

1. Nucleus pulposus, vertebral end plate, and anulus fibrosis.
2. It permits range of motion between vertebrae, maintains contiguity between the vertebral bodies, attenuates, and transfers vertebral loading.
3. Usually increases between the ages of 20 and 70 years.
4. The three stages are defined as dysfunction, instability, and stabilization.
5. C5–6 and C6–7.

CHAPTER 21

1. The usual site of origin is from the proximal part of the subclavian artery.
2. Four percent of the left arteries arise from the aorta. In this variation, the artery runs vertically and slightly medial and posterior to reach the transverse foramen of the lower cervical spine, although its exact direction is dependent on its exact point of origin (any anomalies result in tortuosity). The typical point of entry is at the C6 transverse foramen, but 10 percent of the population has entry points from C5 to C7. Also, the postsubclavian artery could have a kink in it.

3. Divided into four parts: (1) Within the transverse foramen of C2. The C2 vertebral foramen has two curves: the inferior curve is almost vertical, whereas the superior curve is more horizontal and orientated laterally. (2) Between C2 and C1. The second part runs vertically upward in the transverse foramen of C2 and is covered by the levator scapulae and the inferior capitis muscles. (3) In the transverse foramen of C1. In the third part, the suboccipital portion of the vertebral artery bends backward and medially in the transverse foramen of C1. (4) Between the posterior arch of the atlas and its entry into the foramen magnum. On exiting the transverse foramen of C1, the artery behind the mass of the superior articular process of the atlas to cross the posterior arch of the atlas in a groove in which it is held by a restraining ligament. From the medial end of this groove, the artery runs forwards, inwards, and upwards to pierce the posterior atlanto-occipital membrane with the nerve of C1 which separates it from the posterior arch of the atlas. It penetrates the dural matter on the lateral aspect of the foramen magnum, about 1.5 cm lateral to the midline of the neck. The artery is vulnerable to direct blunt trauma in this portion.
4. (1) Pontine branches—pons. (2) Anterior inferior cerebellar artery—pons and cerebellum. (3) Superior cerebellar artery—pons midbrain and cerebellum. (4) Internal auditory (labyrinthine)—membranous labyrinth and 8th cranial nerve (vestibulocochlear). (5) Superior cerebral—thalamus (central), temporal lobe (temporal branch of the cortical), and the occipital lobe (calcarine branch of the cortical).
5. Olfactory (CN1).

CHAPTER 22

1. Occipito-atlantal (O-A) joint: Occipital condyles are bi-convex and articulate with the superior facets of the atlas, which are biconcave. The atlanto-axial (A-A) joint has two lateral and two median articulations. The lateral articulations are biconvex, with lax capsular ligaments allowing for good mobility. The median articulations are formed between the posterior surface of the dens and the anterior aspect of the transverse ligament.
2. Dens, alar ligament, transverse ligament, and tectorial membrane.
3. Rectus capitis lateralis.
4. Tectorial membrane.
5. Obliquus capitis superior.

CHAPTER 23

1. D.
2. C.
3. D.
4. Uncinate process.
5. Lowest (C8–T1).

CHAPTER 24

1. The temporomandibular joint (TMJ), the masticatory systems, and the related organs and tissues such as the salivary glands. It also includes the muscles of facial expression.
2. The lateral pterygoid muscle.
3. Masseter, temporalis, and medial pterygoid.
4. E.
5. The position when the tongue is against the palate of the mouth and the teeth are not in contact.

CHAPTER 25

1. Posterior longitudinal ligament.
2. Iliolumbar ligament.
3. E.
4. Lumbar extension, ipsilateral side bending, and contralateral rotation of the lumbar spine.
5. Approximately 60 degrees of flexion and 25 degrees of extension.

CHAPTER 26

1. Coronally (to facilitate rotation).
2. Ribs 1, 10, 11, and 12 are atypical, because they only articulate with their own vertebra and do not possess inferior demifacets.
3. Costovertebral.
4. Ribs.
5. T1 to T6 = pump handle; T7 to T12 = bucket handle.

CHAPTER 27

1. The interosseous ligament.
2. Counternutation (posterior motion).
3. The piriformis primarily functions to produce external rotation and abduction of the femur, but is also thought to function as an internal rotator and abductor of the hip if the hip joint is flexed beyond 90 degrees.

4. The levator ani, a muscle group composed of the pubococcygeus, puborectalis, and iliococygeus.
5. The right innominate rotates anteriorly, and the sacrum right side flexes and left rotates.

CHAPTER 28

1. The open anterior capsulolabral reconstruction, arthroscopic reconstruction and the thermal capsulorrhaphy.
2. The proposed advantages of arthroscopic repairs include smaller skin incisions, more complete inspection of the glenohumeral joint, the ability to treat intra-articular lesions, access to all areas of the glenohumeral joint for repair, less soft-tissue dissection, and maximum preservation of external rotation.
3. In general, following an anterior capsular reconstruction the shoulder is immobilized in 90 degrees of abduction, 45 degrees of external rotation, and 30 degrees of forward flexion.
4. True.
5. Those with a clinical diagnosis of impingement syndrome who have persistent pain, and loss of function, and who have failed a conservative intervention including rehabilitation, activity modification, anti-inflammatory medications, and subacromial cortisone injections.

CHAPTER 29

1. The transtrochanteric lateral approach, the anterior–lateral approach, the direct lateral approach and the posterior–lateral approach.
2. Deep vein thrombosis with subsequent pulmonary embolism.
3. Advancing age, family history of DVT, estrogen use, pregnancy, obesity, and prolonged flights.
4. Decreased range of motion, pain, swelling, and erythema.
5. Avoidance of flexion of the hip beyond 90 degrees, and minimal adduction or internal rotation of the hip.

INDEX